SKIN
Pathology

SECOND EDITION

Commissioning Editor: Michael J. Houston
Project Development Manager: Sheila Black
Project Manager: Nora Naughton, Samantha Gear
Design Manager: Sarah Russell

SKIN
Pathology

SECOND EDITION

David Weedon AO MD FRCPA

Clinical Professor of Pathology
University of Queensland
Senior Visiting Pathologist
Royal Brisbane Hospital,
Brisbane
Sullivan Nicolaides Pathology (a division of Sonic Healthcare)
Australia

Contributor
Geoffrey Strutton MB BS FRCPA

Senior Anatomical Pathologist
Princess Alexandra Hospital
Brisbane
Australia

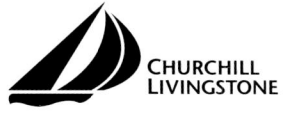
CHURCHILL
LIVINGSTONE

EDINBURGH LONDON NEW YORK OXFORD PHILADELPHIA ST LOUIS SYDNEY TORONTO 2002

CHURCHILL LIVINGSTONE
An imprint of Elsevier Science Limited

First edition 1997
Second edition 2002
   Reprinted 2002 (twice), 2003

ISBN 0-443-07069-5

British Library Cataloguing in Publication Data
A catalogue record for this book is available from the British Library

Library of Congress Cataloging in Publication Data
A catalog record for this book is available from the Library of Congress

Note
Medical knowledge is constantly changing. As new information becomes available, changes in treatment, procedures, equipment and the use of drugs become necessary. The author, contributor and the publishers have taken care to ensure that the information given in this text is accurate and up to date. However, readers are strongly advised to confirm that the information, especially with regard to drug usage, complies with the latest legislation and standards of practice.

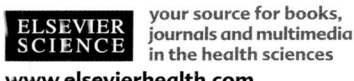
your source for books, journals and multimedia in the health sciences
www.elsevierhealth.com

The publisher's policy is to use paper manufactured from sustainable forests

Printed in China
C/04

Contents

5 The skin in systemic and miscellaneous diseases

6 Infections and infestations

7 Tumors

Preface

The response to the last edition of the book was most gratifying, encouraging me to expend the many hours of personal effort that are necessary to update a book of this size and complexity. Although I am mindful of the perceived shortcomings of a basically solo-authored book, I have declined offers of assistance with the writing, preferring to keep an element of continuity and to avoid entities 'slipping through the cracks', as inevitably occurs with multi-authored books. Nevertheless, I have been most fortunate in once again having the assistance of Geoffrey Strutton, who has extensively revised Chapter 41.

It is fashionable these days to have Mission Statements (and new logos) despite the lack of any evidence that they improve quality or morale. Nevertheless, it is relevant to the reader and potential purchasers to outline the mission of this book. It is my desire to produce a textbook of dermato-pathology that is comprehensive, applicable to the daily practice of the subject, and which contains recent references from accessible journals that are relevant to dermatopathology. It is my strongly held view that many clinical aspects are relevant. So often, an absurd or irrelevant diagnosis can be made on a slide if it is interpreted in the absence of clinical history.

Because I am frequently asked at meetings whether I could possibly have read all the references included (the enquirers are obviously unaware of my obsessive personality, and my one a.m. starts, six days a week), a brief outline of the reference acquisition follows. It is my practice to scan every issue of 34 titles, marking them off on a list as this is completed. I try to scan additional journals on display at the Medical Library. Every relevant article is then photocopied (one or more pages) and filed by Chapter and entity grouping. Each reference is allocated a number and eventually read or scanned prior to its incorporation into the text.

As I stated in the Preface to the previous edition, we are indeed 'coming nearer and nearer to the very essence of phenomena', to use the words of Louis Pasteur. However, despite further advances in our knowledge of molecular pathology, there are still many gaps in the jig-saw puzzle of life. This edition hopefully adds a few more pieces.

On a personal level, I was pleased when the last edition of this book won the Advanced Author Book Category of the Medical Society of London Medical Book Awards in 1998.

A successful and satisfying life in Dermatopathology requires many things — interesting material, an appropriate work environment, time to think and reflect, and colleagues. In this latter category I must acknowledge Professor W. St C. Symmers, who was instrumental in my acceptance of the task of writing the first edition, my former senior partner John Sullivan, John Kerr of 'apoptosis fame', and A. Bernard Ackerman, who despite expressing opposition to the concept of apoptosis still remains a friend and my original mentor in dermatopathology. I hasten to add that responsibility for any errors, omissions or departures from orthodox/accepted wisdom is mine alone.

Finally, my thanks are due to my secretary, Pam Kent, who spent hours at the photocopy machine, ever longer hours at the keyboard and who typed the entire manuscript, now in excess of one million words. Once again, Graeme Dean assisted with the technical aspects of reference sorting and computer typesetting. Cleo Wilkinson assisted with many library-related matters. The staff at Elsevier Science have given helpful advice throughout this project. In particular, Michael Houston assisted with the pre-production stages of the project.

Brisbane, Queensland, Australia
May 2002

David Weedon

Introduction

An approach to the interpretation of skin biopsies

INTRODUCTION

Unfortunately, dermatopathology requires years of training and practice to achieve an acceptable level of diagnostic skill. Many have found this process an exciting and challenging one, well worth the expenditure of time and intellectual effort. To the trainee, there seems to be an endless number of potential diagnoses in dermatopathology, with many bewildering names. However, if a logical approach is adopted, the great majority of skin biopsies can be diagnosed specifically and the remainder can be partly categorized into a particular group of diseases. It should not be forgotten that the histopathological features of some dermatoses are not diagnostically specific and it may only be possible in these circumstances to state that the histopathological features are 'consistent with' the clinical diagnosis.

The interpretation of many skin biopsies requires the identification and integration of two different, morphological features – the *tissue reaction pattern* and the *pattern of inflammation*. This is a crude algorithmic approach; more sophisticated ones usually hinder rather than enhance the ability to make a specific diagnosis.

Tissue reaction patterns are distinctive morphological patterns which categorize a group of cutaneous diseases. Within each of these histopathological categories there are diseases which may have similar or diverse clinical appearances and etiologies. Some diseases may show histopathological features of more than one reaction pattern at a particular time or during the course of their evolution.

The *pattern of inflammation* refers to the distribution of the inflammatory cell infiltrate within the dermis and/or the subcutaneous tissue. There are several distinctive patterns of inflammation (see below): their recognition assists in making a specific diagnosis.

Some dermatopathologists base their diagnostic approach on the inflammatory pattern, while others look first to see if the biopsy can be categorized into one of the 'tissue reactions' and use the pattern of inflammation to further categorize the biopsy within each of these reaction patterns. In practice, the experienced dermatopathologist sees these two aspects (tissue reaction pattern and inflammatory pattern) simultaneously, integrating and interpreting the findings in a matter of seconds.

The categorization of inflammatory dermatoses by their tissue reactions will be considered first.

Tissue reaction patterns

There are many different reaction patterns in the skin, but the majority of inflammatory dermatoses can be categorized into six different patterns. For convenience, these will be called the *major tissue reaction patterns*. There are a number of other diagnostic reaction patterns which occur much less commonly than the major group of six, but which are nevertheless specific for other groups of dermatoses. These patterns will be referred to as *minor tissue reaction patterns*. They will be considered after the major reaction patterns.

Patterns of inflammation

There are four patterns of cutaneous inflammation characterized on the basis of distribution of inflammatory cells within the skin:

1. superficial perivascular inflammation
2. superficial and deep dermal inflammation
3. folliculitis and perifolliculitis
4. panniculitis.

There are numerous dermatoses showing a superficial perivascular inflammatory infiltrate in the dermis and a limited number in the other categories. Sometimes panniculitis and folliculitis are regarded as major tissue reaction patterns, because of their easily recognizable pattern.

MAJOR TISSUE REACTION PATTERNS

A significant number of inflammatory dermatoses can be categorized into one of the following six major reaction patterns, the key morphological feature of which is included in parentheses:

1. *lichenoid* (basal cell damage; interface dermatitis)
2. *psoriasiform* (regular epidermal hyperplasia)
3. *spongiotic* (intraepidermal intercellular edema)
4. *vesiculobullous* (blistering within or beneath the epidermis)
5. *granulomatous* (chronic granulomatous inflammation)
6. *vasculopathic* (pathological changes in cutaneous blood vessels).

Each of these reaction patterns will be discussed in turn, together with a list of the dermatoses found in each category.

THE LICHENOID REACTION PATTERN ('INTERFACE DERMATITIS')

The lichenoid reaction pattern ('interface dermatitis') (see Ch. 3, pp. 31–74) is characterized by *epidermal basal cell damage*, which may be manifested by cell death and/or basal vacuolar change (known in the past as 'liquefaction degeneration'). The basal cell death usually presents in the form of shrunken eosinophilic cells, with pyknotic nuclear remnants, scattered along the basal layer of the epidermis (Fig. 1.1). These cells are known as Civatte bodies. They are undergoing death by apoptosis, a morphologically distinct type of cell death seen in both physiological and pathological circumstances (see p. 32). Sometimes the basal cell damage is quite subtle with only an occasional Civatte body and very focal vacuolar change. This is a feature of some drug reactions.

The term 'interface dermatitis' is sometimes used synonymously with the lichenoid reaction pattern, although it is not usually applied to the subtle variants. At other times, it is used for the morphological subset (see below) in which inflammatory cells extend into the basal layer or above. The term is widely used despite its lack of precision. It is a pattern, not a diagnosis.

A distinctive subgroup of the lichenoid reaction pattern is the *poikilodermatous pattern*, characterized by mild basal damage, usually of vacuolar type, associated with epidermal atrophy, pigment incontinence and dilatation of vessels in the papillary dermis (Fig. 1.2). It is a feature of the various types of poikiloderma (see p. 54).

The specific diagnosis of a disease within the lichenoid tissue reaction requires an assessment of several other morphological features. These include:

1. the *type of basal damage* (vacuolar change is sometimes more prominent than cell death in lupus erythematosus, dermatomyositis, the poikilodermas and drug reactions);

2. the *distribution of the accompanying inflammatory cell infiltrate* (the infiltrate touches the undersurface of the basal layer in lichen planus and its variants, early lichen sclerosus et atrophicus, and in disseminated superficial actinic porokeratosis; it obscures the dermoepidermal interface (so-called 'interface dermatitis') in erythema multiforme, paraneoplastic pemphigus, fixed drug eruptions and acute pityriasis lichenoides (PLEVA) and it involves

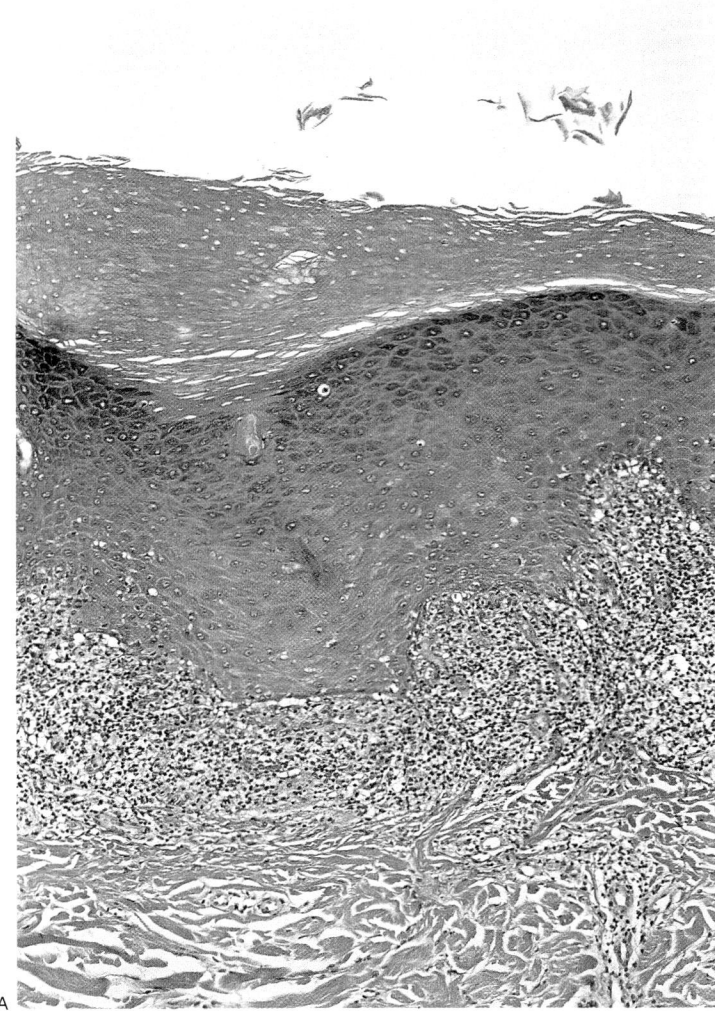

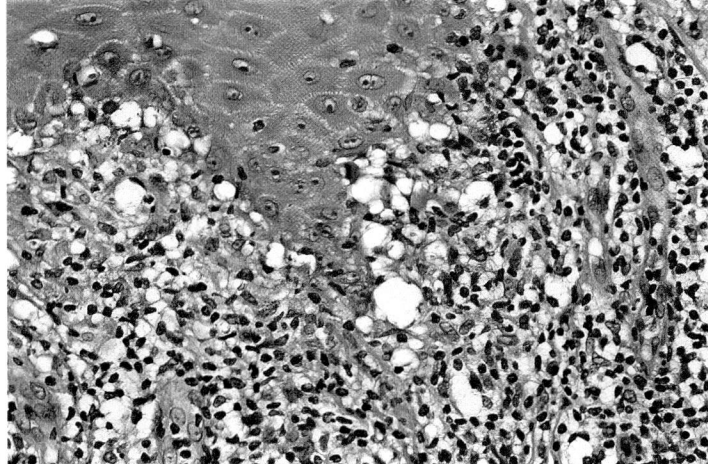

Fig. 1.1 **The lichenoid reaction pattern.** There are shrunken keratinocytes with pyknotic nuclear remnants (Civatte bodies) in the basal layer. These cells are undergoing death by apoptosis. There is also focal vacuolar change. (H & E)

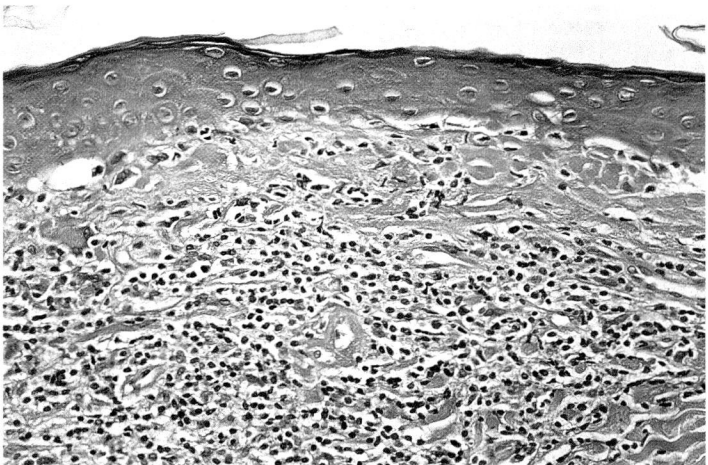

Fig. 1.2 **The poikilodermatous variant of the lichenoid reaction pattern.** It is characterized by mild vacuolar change of the basal layer of the epidermis, mild epidermal atrophy, and dilatation of vessels in the papillary dermis. (H & E)

some of the sun exacerbated lichen planus variants, e.g. lichen planus actinicus); and

4. the presence of *satellite cell necrosis* (lymphocyte-associated apoptosis) – defined here as two or more lymphocytes in close proximity to a Civatte body (a feature of graft-versus-host reaction, regressing plane warts, erythema multiforme and some drug reactions).

The diseases showing the lichenoid reaction pattern are listed in Table 1.1.

Table 1.1 **Diseases showing the lichenoid reaction pattern ('interface dermatitis')**

Lichen planus
Lichen planus variants
Lichen nitidus
Lichen striatus
Lichen planus-like keratosis
Lichenoid drug eruptions
Fixed drug eruptions
Erythema multiforme
Graft-versus-host disease
Eruption of lymphocyte recovery
AIDS interface dermatitis
Lupus erythematosus
Dermatomyositis
Poikiloderma congenitale
Congenital telangiectatic erythema
Lichen sclerosus et atrophicus
Dyskeratosis congenita
Pityriasis lichenoides
Persistent viral reactions
Perniosis
Paraneoplastic pemphigus
Lichenoid purpura
Lichenoid contact dermatitis
Late secondary syphilis
Porokeratosis
Drug eruptions
Phototoxic dermatitis
Prurigo pigmentosa
Erythroderma
Mycosis fungoides
Regressing warts and tumors
Lichen amyloidosus
Vitiligo
Lichenoid tattoo reaction

the deep as well as the superficial part of the dermis in lupus erythematosus, syphilis, photolichenoid eruptions and some drug reactions);

3. the presence of *prominent pigment incontinence* (as seen in drug reactions, the poikilodermas, lichenoid reactions in dark-skinned people and

THE PSORIASIFORM REACTION PATTERN

The psoriasiform reaction pattern was originally defined as the cyclic formation of a suprapapillary exudate with focal parakeratosis related to it (see Ch. 4, pp. 75–96). The concept of the 'squirting dermal papilla' was also put forward with the suggestion that serum and inflammatory cells escaped from the blood vessels in the papillary dermis and passed through the epidermis to form the suprapapillary exudate referred to above. The epidermal hyperplasia which also occurred was regarded as a phenomenon secondary to these other processes. From a morphological viewpoint, the psoriasiform tissue reaction is defined as *epidermal hyperplasia in which there is elongation of the rete ridges, usually in a regular manner* (Fig. 1.3).

It is acknowledged that this latter approach has some shortcomings, as many of the diseases in this category, including psoriasis, show no significant epidermal hyperplasia in their early stages. Rather, dilated vessels in the papillary dermis and an overlying suprapapillary scale (indicative of the 'squirting papilla') may be the dominant features in early lesions of psoriasis. Mitoses are increased in basal keratinocytes in this pattern, particularly in active lesions of psoriasis.

Diseases showing the psoriasiform reaction pattern are listed in Table 1.2.

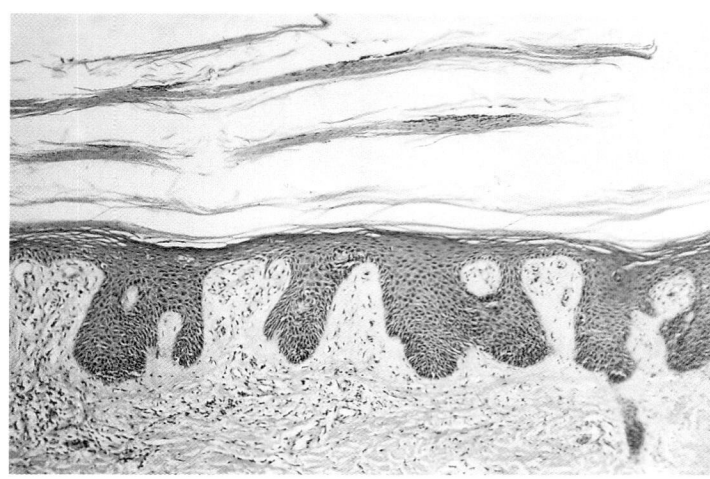

Fig. 1.3 **The psoriasiform reaction pattern** showing epidermal hyperplasia with regular elongation of the rete processes. There are several layers of scale resulting from intermittent 'activity' of the process. (H & E)

Table 1.2 **Diseases showing the psoriasiform reaction pattern**

Psoriasis
AIDS-associated psoriasiform dermatitis
Pustular psoriasis
Reiter's syndrome
Pityriasis rubra pilaris
Parapsoriasis
Lichen simplex chronicus
Subacute and chronic spongiotic dermatitides
Erythroderma
Mycosis fungoides
Chronic candidosis and dermatophytoses
Inflammatory linear verrucous epidermal nevus (ILVEN)
Norwegian scabies
Bowen's disease (psoriasiform variant)
Clear cell acanthoma
Lamellar ichthyosis
Pityriasis rosea ('herald patch')
Pellagra
Acrodermatitis enteropathica
Glucagonoma syndrome
Secondary syphilis

THE SPONGIOTIC REACTION PATTERN

The spongiotic reaction pattern (see Ch. 5, pp. 97–128) is characterized by *intraepidermal intercellular edema (spongiosis)*. It is recognized by the presence of widened intercellular spaces between keratinocytes, with elongation of the intercellular bridges (Fig. 1.4). The spongiosis may vary from microscopic foci to grossly visible vesicles. This reaction pattern has been known in the past as the 'eczematous tissue reaction'. Inflammatory cells are present within the dermis, and their distribution and type may aid in making a specific diagnosis within this group. This is the most difficult reaction pattern in which to make a specific clinicopathological diagnosis; often a diagnosis of 'spongiotic reaction consistent with …' is all that can be made.

The major diseases within this tissue reaction pattern (atopic dermatitis, allergic and irritant contact dermatitis, nummular dermatitis and seborrheic dermatitis) all show progressive psoriasiform hyperplasia of the epidermis with chronicity (Fig. 1.5). This change is usually accompanied by diminishing spongiosis, but this will depend on the activity of the disease. Both patterns may be present in the same biopsy. The psoriasiform hyperplasia is, in part, a response to chronic rubbing and scratching.

Five patterns of spongiosis can be recognized:

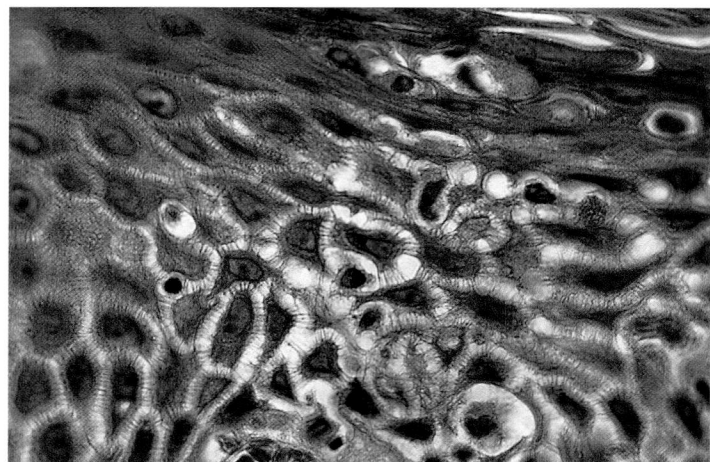

Fig. 1.4 **The spongiotic reaction pattern.** There is mild intercellular edema with elongation of the intercellular bridges. (H & E)

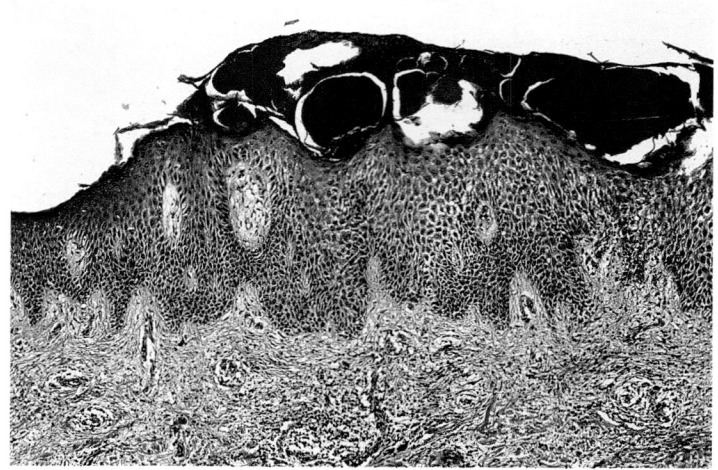

Fig. 1.5 **The spongiotic reaction pattern in a lesion of some duration.** Psoriasiform hyperplasia coexists with the spongiosis. (H & E)

1. *neutrophilic spongiosis* (where there are neutrophils within foci of spongiosis);
2. *eosinophilic spongiosis* (where there are numerous eosinophils within foci of spongiosis);
3. *miliarial (acrosyringial) spongiosis* (where the edema is related to the acrosyringium);
4. *follicular spongiosis* (where the spongiosis is centered on the follicular infundibulum); and
5. *haphazard spongiosis* (the other spongiotic disorders in which there is no particular pattern of spongiosis).

The diseases showing the spongiotic reaction pattern are listed in Table 1.3.

THE VESICULOBULLOUS REACTION PATTERN

In the vesiculobullous reaction pattern, there are *vesicles or bullae at any level within the epidermis or at the dermoepidermal junction* (see Ch. 6, pp. 129–191). A specific diagnosis can usually be made in a particular case by assessing three features – the anatomical level of the split, the underlying mechanism responsible for the split and, in the case of subepidermal lesions, the nature of the inflammatory infiltrate in the dermis.

The *anatomical level of the split* may be subcorneal, within the stratum malpighii, suprabasal or subepidermal. The *mechanism responsible* for vesiculation may be exaggerated spongiosis, intracellular edema and ballooning (as occurs in viral infections such as herpes simplex), or acantholysis. Acantholysis is the loss of coherence between epidermal cells. It may be a primary phenomenon or secondary to inflammation, ballooning degeneration (as in viral infections of the skin), or epithelial dysplasia. In the case of subepidermal blisters, electron microscopy and immunoelectron microscopy could be used to make a specific diagnosis in most cases. In practice, the subepidermal blisters are subdivided on the basis of the *inflammatory cell infiltrate within the dermis*. Knowledge of the immunofluorescence findings is often helpful in categorizing the subepidermal blistering diseases.

Table 1.4 lists the various vesiculobullous diseases, based on the anatomical level of the split and, in the case of subepidermal lesions, the predominant inflammatory cell within the dermis.

THE GRANULOMATOUS REACTION PATTERN

This group of diseases (see Ch. 7, pp. 193–220) is characterized by the presence of *chronic granulomatous inflammation*; that is, localized collections of epithelioid cells usually admixed with giant cells, lymphocytes, plasma cells, fibroblasts and non-epithelioid macrophages (Fig. 1.6). Five histological types of granuloma can be identified on the basis of the constituent cells and other changes within the granulomas – sarcoidal, tuberculoid, necrobiotic, suppurative and foreign body. A miscellaneous category is usually added to any classification.

Sarcoidal granulomas are composed of epithelioid cells and giant cells, some containing asteroid bodies or other inclusions. The granulomas are often referred to as 'naked granulomas', in that they have only a sparse 'clothing' of peripheral lymphocytes and plasma cells, in contrast to tuberculoid granulomas that usually have more abundant lymphocytes. Some overlap occurs between sarcoidal and tuberculoid granulomas.

Tuberculoid granulomas resemble those seen in tuberculosis, although caseation necrosis is not always present. The giant cells that are present within the granuloma are usually of Langhans type.

Necrobiotic granulomas are composed of epithelioid cells, lymphocytes and occasional giant cells associated with areas of 'necrobiosis' of collagen.

Table 1.3 **Diseases showing the spongiotic reaction pattern**

Neutrophilic spongiosis

Pustular psoriasis
IgA pemphigus
Infantile acropustulosis
Acute generalized exanthematous pustulosis
Palmoplantar pustulosis
Dermatophytosis/candidosis
Beetle (*Paederus*) dermatitis
Pustular contact dermatitis

Eosinophilic spongiosis

Pemphigus (precursor lesions)
Herpetiform pemphigus
Pemphigus vegetans
Bullous pemphigoid
Idiopathic eosinophilic spongiosis
Eosinophilic, polymorphic, and pruritic eruption
Allergic contact dermatitis
Protein contact dermatitis
Arthropod bites
Eosinophilic folliculitis
Incontinentia pigmenti (first stage)

Miliarial spongiosis

Miliaria

Follicular spongiosis

Infundibulofolliculitis
Atopic dermatitis (follicular lesions)
Apocrine miliaria
Eosinophilic folliculitis

Other spongiotic disorders

Irritant contact dermatitis
Allergic contact dermatitis
Nummular dermatitis
Sulzberger–Garbe syndrome
Seborrheic dermatitis
Atopic dermatitis
Papular dermatitis
Pompholyx
Hyperkeratotic dermatitis of the hands
Juvenile plantar dermatosis
Vein graft donor-site dermatitis
Stasis dermatitis
Autoeczematization
Pityriasis rosea
Papular acrodermatitis of childhood
Spongiotic drug reactions
Chronic superficial dermatitis
Blaschko dermatitis
Psoriasis (spongiotic and site variants)
Light reactions
Dermatophytoses
Arthropod bites
Grover's disease (spongiotic variant)
Toxic shock syndrome
PUPPP
Erythema annulare centrifugum
Pigmented purpuric dermatoses
Pityriasis alba
Eruption of lymphocyte recovery
Lichen striatus
Erythroderma
Mycosis fungoides

Table 1.4 **Vesiculobullous diseases**

Intracorneal and subcorneal blisters	Paraneoplastic pemphigus
	Bullous fixed drug eruption
Skin peeling syndrome	Lichen sclerosus et atrophicus
Impetigo	Lichen planus pemphigoides
Staphylococcal 'scalded skin' syndrome	Polymorphous light eruption
Dermatophytosis	Fungal infections
Pemphigus foliaceus and erythematosus	Dermal allergic contact dermatitis
Herpetiform pemphigus	Bullous leprosy
Subcorneal pustular dermatosis	Bullous mycosis fungoides
IgA pemphigus	
Infantile pustular dermatoses	**Subepidermal blisters with eosinophils***
Acute generalized exanthematous pustulosis	
Miliaria crystallina	Wells' syndrome
	Bullous pemphigoid
Intraepidermal (stratum malpighii) blisters	Pemphigoid gestationis
	Arthropod bites (in sensitized individuals)
Spongiotic blistering diseases	Drug reactions
Palmoplantar pustulosis	Epidermolysis bullosa
Amicrobial pustulosis of autoimmune diseases	
Viral blistering diseases	**Subepidermal blisters with neutrophils***
Epidermolysis bullosa (Weber–Cockayne type)	
Friction blister	Dermatitis herpetiformis
	Linear IgA bullous dermatosis
Suprabasilar blisters	Cicatricial pemphigoid
	Ocular cicatricial pemphigoid
Pemphigus vulgaris and vegetans	Localized cicatricial pemphigoid
Paraneoplastic pemphigus	Deep lamina lucida (anti-p105) pemphigoid
Hailey–Hailey disease	Anti-p200 pemphigoid
Darier's disease	Bullous urticaria
Grover's disease	Bullous acute vasculitis
Acantholytic solar keratosis	Bullous lupus erythematosus
	Erysipelas
Subepidermal blisters with little inflammation	Sweet's syndrome
	Epidermolysis bullosa acquisita
Epidermolysis bullosa	
Porphyria cutanea tarda and pseudoporphyria	**Subepidermal blisters with mast cells**
Bullous pemphigoid (cell-poor variant)	
Burns and cryotherapy	Bullous urticaria pigmentosa
Toxic epidermal necrolysis	
Suction blisters	**Miscellaneous blistering diseases**
Blisters overlying scars	
Bullous solar elastosis	Drug overdose-related bullae
Bullous amyloidosis	Methyl bromide-induced bullae
Waldenström's macroglobulinemia	Etretinate-induced bullae
Drug reactions	PUVA-induced bullae
Kindler's syndrome	Cancer-related bullae
	Lymphatic bullae
Subepidermal blisters with lymphocytes	Bullous eruption of diabetes mellitus
Erythema multiforme	

*Varying admixtures of eosinophils and neutrophils may be seen in cicatricial pemphigoid and late lesions of dermatitis herpetiformis.

Sometimes the inflammatory cells are arranged in a palisade around the areas of necrobiosis. The term 'necrobiosis' has been criticized because it implies that the collagen (which is not a vital structure) is 'necrotic'. The process of necrobiosis is characterized by an accumulation of acid mucopolysaccharides between the collagen bundles and degeneration of some interstitial fibroblasts and histiocytes.

Suppurative granulomas have neutrophils within and sometimes surrounding the granuloma. The granulomatous component is not always well formed.

Foreign body granulomas have multinucleate, foreign body giant cells as a constituent of the granuloma. Foreign material can usually be visualized in sections stained with hematoxylin and eosin, although at other times it requires the use of polarized light for its detection.

The identification of organisms by the use of special stains (the periodic acid Schiff and other stains for fungi and stains for acid-fast bacilli) or by culture may be necessary to make a specific diagnosis. Organisms are usually scanty in granulomas associated with infectious diseases. The distribution of the granulomas (they may be arranged along nerve fibers in tuberculoid leprosy) may assist in making a specific diagnosis.

It should also be noted that many of the infectious diseases listed in Table 1.5 as causing the granulomatous tissue reaction can also produce inflammatory reactions that do not include granulomas, depending on the stage of the disease and the immune status of the individual.

THE VASCULOPATHIC REACTION PATTERN

The vasculopathic reaction pattern (see Ch. 8, pp. 221–278) includes a clinically heterogeneous group of diseases which have in common *pathological changes in blood vessels*. The most important category within this tissue reaction pattern is *vasculitis*, which can be defined as an inflammatory process involving the walls of blood vessels of any size (Fig. 1.7). Some dermato-pathologists insist on the presence of fibrin within the vessel wall before they will accept a diagnosis of vasculitis. This criterion is far too restrictive and it

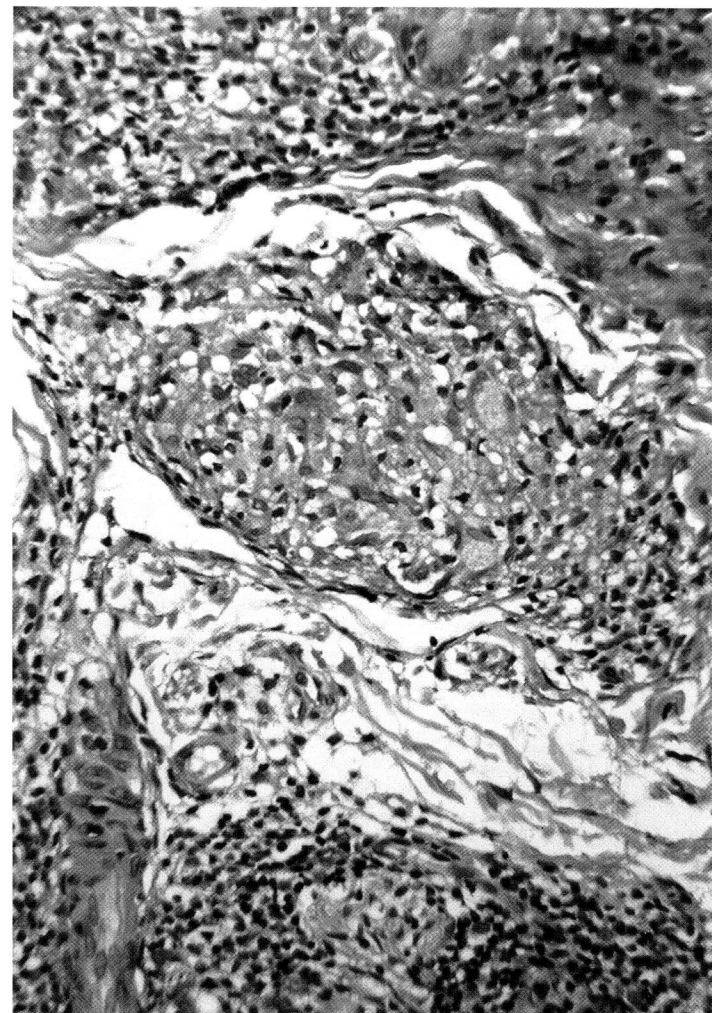

Fig. 1.6 **The granulomatous reaction pattern.** A small tuberculoid granuloma is present in the dermis. (H & E)

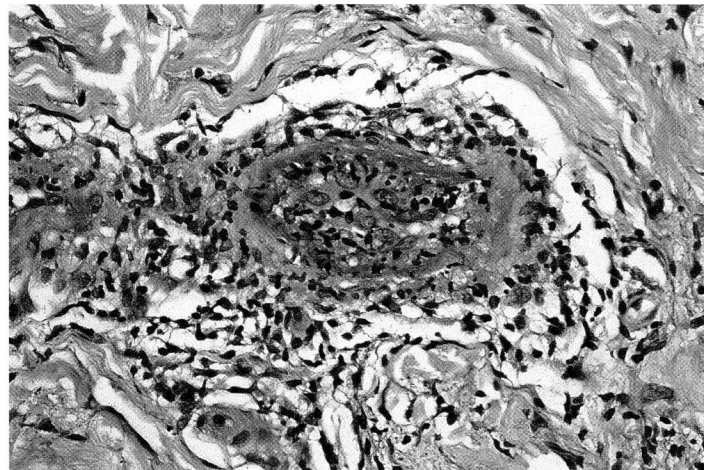

Fig. 1.7 **Acute vasculitis.** Neutrophils are present in the wall of a vessel which also shows extravasation of fibrin. (H & E)

Table 1.5 **Diseases causing the granulomatous reaction pattern**

Sarcoidal granulomas

Sarcoidosis
Blau's syndrome
Reactions to foreign materials
Secondary syphilis
Sézary syndrome
Herpes zoster scars
Systemic lymphomas
Common variable immunodeficiency

Tuberculoid granulomas

Tuberculosis
Tuberculids
Leprosy
Late syphilis
Leishmaniasis
Protothecosis
Rosacea
Perioral dermatitis
Lupus miliaris disseminatus faciei
Crohn's disease

Necrobiotic granulomas

Granuloma annulare
Necrobiosis lipoidica
Necrobiotic xanthogranuloma
Rheumatoid nodules
Rheumatic fever nodules
Reactions to foreign materials and vaccines

Suppurative granulomas

Chromomycosis and phaeohyphomycosis
Sporotrichosis
Non-tuberculous mycobacterial infection
Blastomycosis
Paracoccidioidomycosis
Coccidioidomycosis
Blastomycosis-like pyoderma
Mycetoma, nocardiosis and actinomycosis
Cat-scratch disease
Lymphogranuloma venereum
Pyoderma gangrenosum
Ruptured cysts and follicles

Foreign body granulomas

Exogenous material
Endogenous material

Miscellaneous granulomas

Melkersson–Rosenthal syndrome
Cutaneous histiocytic lymphangitis
Elastolytic granulomas
Annular granulomas in ochronosis
Granulomas in immunodeficiency disorders
Interstitial granulomatous dermatitis
Interstitial granulomatous drug reaction
Granulomatous T-cell lymphomas

ignores the fact that exudative features, such as fibrin extravasation, are not prominent in chronic inflammation in any tissue of the body. On the other hand, a diagnosis of vasculitis should not be made simply because there is a perivascular infiltrate of inflammatory cells. Notwithstanding these comments,

in resolving and late lesions of vasculitis there may only be a tight perivascular inflammatory cell infiltrate, making it difficult to make a diagnosis of vasculitis. The presence of endothelial swelling in small vessels and an increase in fibro-histiocytic cells (a 'busy dermis') and sometimes acid mucopolysaccharides in the dermis are further clues which assist in confirming that a resolving vasculitis is present. Although it is useful to categorize vasculitis into acute, chronic lymphocytic and granulomatous forms, it should be remembered that

Table 1.6 **Diseases showing the vasculopathic reaction pattern**

Non-inflammatory purpuras	**Neutrophilic dermatoses**
Traumatic purpura	Sweet's syndrome
Psychogenic purpura	Bowel-associated dermatosis-arthritis syndrome
Drug purpura	Rheumatoid neutrophilic dermatosis
Bleeding diatheses	Acute generalized pustulosis
Senile purpura	Behçet's disease
	Abscess-forming neutrophilic dermatosis
Vascular occlusive diseases	
Warfarin necrosis	**Chronic lymphocytic vasculitis**
Atrophie blanche (livedoid vasculopathy)	Toxic erythema
Disseminated intravascular coagulation	Connective tissue disease
Purpura fulminans	PUPPP
Thrombotic thrombocytopenic purpura	Prurigo of pregnancy
Thrombocythemia	Gyrate and annular erythemas
Cryoglobulinemia	Pityriasis lichenoides
Cholesterol embolism	Pigmented purpuric dermatoses
Antiphospholipid syndrome	Malignant atrophic papulosis (Degos)
Factor V Leiden mutation	Perniosis
Sneddon's syndrome	Rickettsial and viral infections
CADASIL	Pyoderma gangrenosum
Miscellaneous conditions	Polymorphous light eruption (variant)
	TRAPS
Urticarias	Sclerosing lymphangitis of the penis
	Leukemic vasculitis
Acute vasculitis	
Leukocytoclastic (hypersensitivity) vasculitis	**Vasculitis with granulomatosis**
Henoch–Schönlein purpura	Crohn's disease
Eosinophilic vasculitis	Drug reactions
Rheumatoid vasculitis	Herpes zoster
Urticarial vasculitis	Infectious granulomatous diseases
Mixed cryoglobulinemia	Wegener's granulomatosis
Hypergammaglobulinemic purpura	Lymphomatoid granulomatosis
Hypergammaglobulinemia D syndrome	Allergic granulomatosis
Septic vasculitis	Lethal midline granuloma
Erythema elevatum diutinum	Giant cell (temporal) arteritis
Granuloma faciale	Takayasu's arteritis
Localized chronic fibrosing vasculitis	
Microscopic polyangiitis (polyarteritis)	**Miscellaneous vascular disorders**
Polyarteritis nodosa	Vascular calcification
Kawasaki disease	Pericapillary fibrin cuffs
Superficial thrombophlebitis	Vascular aneurysms
Miscellaneous associations	Erythermalgia
	Cutaneous necrosis and ulceration

an acute vasculitis may progress with time to a chronic stage. Fibrin is rarely present in these late lesions.

Other categories of vascular disease include non-inflammatory purpuras, vascular occlusive diseases and urticarias. The purpuras are characterized by extravasation of erythrocytes and the vascular occlusive diseases by fibrin and/or platelet thrombi or, rarely, other material in the lumen of small blood vessels. The urticarias are characterized by increased vascular permeability, with escape of edema fluid and some cells into the dermis. The neutrophilic dermatoses are included also because they share some morphological features with the acute vasculitides.

The diseases showing the vasculopathic reaction pattern are listed in Table 1.6.

MINOR TISSUE REACTION PATTERNS

'Minor tissue reaction patterns' is a term of convenience for a group of reaction patterns in the skin that are seen much less frequently than the six major patterns already discussed. Like the major reaction patterns, each of the patterns to be considered below is diagnostic of a certain group of diseases of the skin. Sometimes, a knowledge of the clinical distribution of the lesions (e.g. whether they are localized, linear, zosteriform or generalized) is required before a specific clinicopathological diagnosis can be made. The minor tissue reaction patterns to be discussed, with their key morphological feature in parentheses, are:

1. *epidermolytic hyperkeratosis* (hyperkeratosis with granular and vacuolar degeneration)
2. *acantholytic dyskeratosis* (suprabasilar clefts with acantholytic and dyskeratotic cells)
3. *cornoid lamellation* (a column of parakeratotic cells with absence of an underlying granular layer)
4. *papillomatosis* – 'church-spiring' (undulations and protrusions of the epidermis)
5. *angiofibromas* (increased dermal vessels with surrounding fibrosis)
6. *eosinophilic cellulitis with 'flame figures'* (dermal eosinophils and eosinophilic material adherent to collagen bundles)

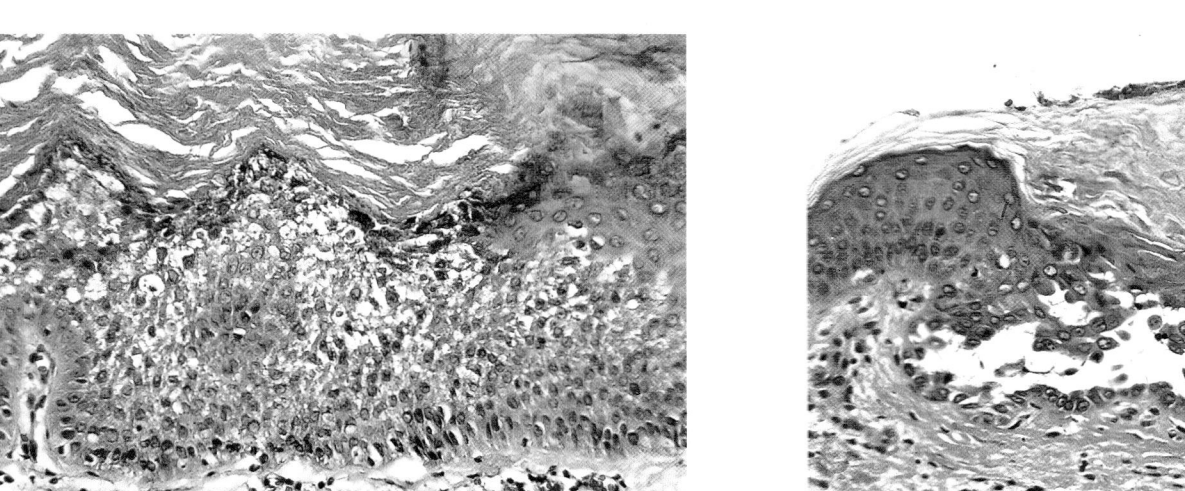

Fig. 1.8 **Epidermolytic hyperkeratosis** characterized by granular and vacuolar degeneration of the upper layers of the epidermis and overlying hyperkeratosis. (H & E)

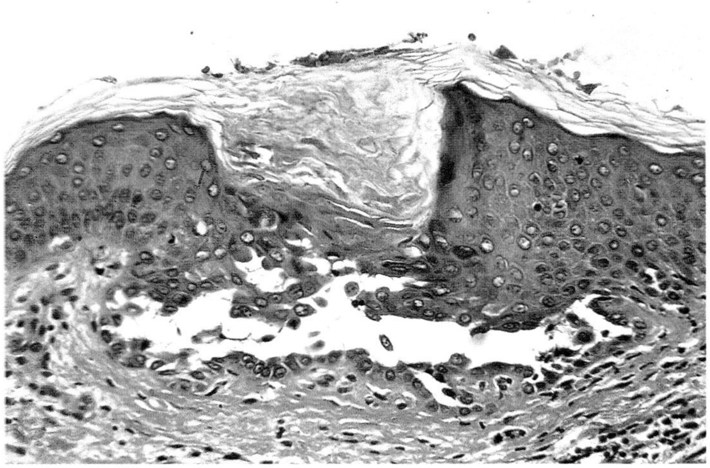

Fig. 1.9 **Acantholytic dyskeratosis** with suprabasal clefting and dyskeratotic cells in the overlying epidermis. (H & E)

7. *transepithelial elimination* (elimination of material via the epidermis or hair follicles).

The first four patterns listed are all disorders of epidermal maturation and keratinization. They will be discussed briefly below and in further detail in Chapter 9, pages 281–320. Angiofibromas are included with tumors of fibrous tissue in Chapter 34, pages 918–920, while eosinophilic cellulitis is discussed with the cutaneous infiltrates in Chapter 40, pages 1059–1061. Transepithelial elimination is a process that may occur as a secondary event in a wide range of skin diseases. It is discussed below.

EPIDERMOLYTIC HYPERKERATOSIS

The features of the epidermolytic hyperkeratotic reaction pattern are *compact hyperkeratosis accompanied by granular and vacuolar degeneration of the cells of the spinous and granular layers* (Fig. 1.8). This pattern may occur in diseases or lesions which are generalized (bullous ichthyosiform erythroderma), systematized (epidermal nevus variant), palmar-plantar (a variant of palmoplantar keratoderma), solitary (epidermolytic acanthoma), multiple and discrete (disseminated epidermolytic acanthoma) or follicular (nevoid follicular hyperkeratosis). Rarely, this pattern may be seen in solar keratoses. Not uncommonly, epidermolytic hyperkeratosis is an incidental finding in a biopsy taken because of the presence of some other lesion.

ACANTHOLYTIC DYSKERATOSIS

Acantholytic dyskeratosis is characterized by *suprabasilar clefting with acantholytic and dyskeratotic cells at all levels of the epidermis* (see p. 294) (Fig. 1.9). It may be a generalized process (Darier's disease), a systematized process (a variant of epidermal nevus), transient (Grover's disease), palmar-plantar (a very rare form of keratoderma), solitary (warty dyskeratoma), an incidental finding or a feature of a solar keratosis (acantholytic solar keratosis).

CORNOID LAMELLATION

Cornoid lamellation (Fig. 1.10) is localized faulty keratinization characterized by a thin column of parakeratotic cells with an absent or decreased underlying granular zone and vacuolated or dyskeratotic cells in the spinous layer (see p. 292). Although cornoid lamellation is a characteristic feature of

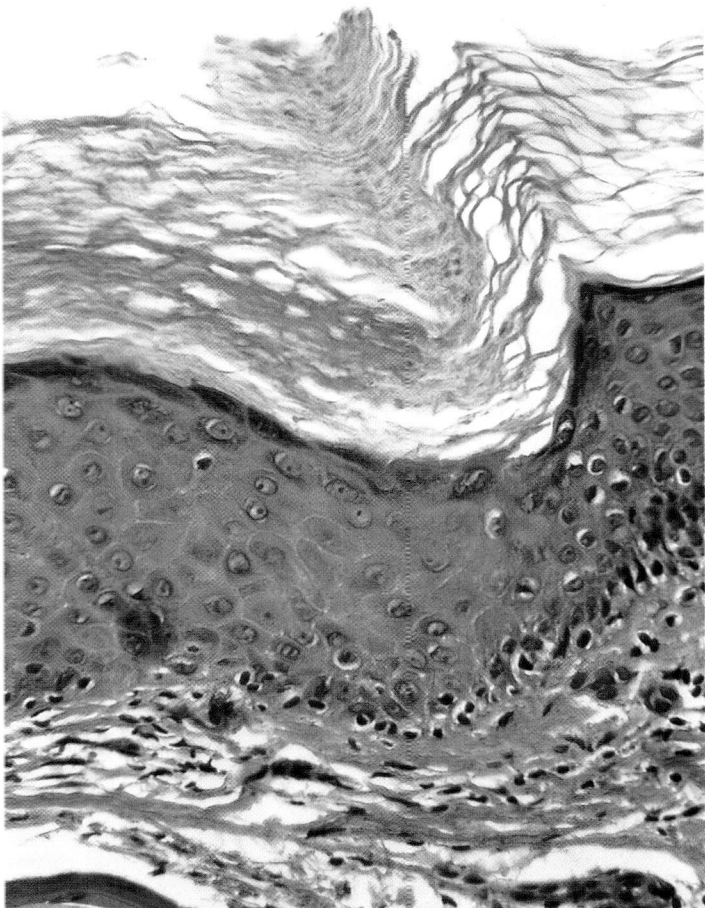

Fig. 1.10 **A cornoid lamella in porokeratosis.** A thin column of parakeratotic cells overlies a narrow zone in which the granular layer is absent. (H & E)

porokeratosis and its clinical variants, it can be found as an incidental phenomenon in a range of inflammatory, hyperplastic and neoplastic conditions of the skin.

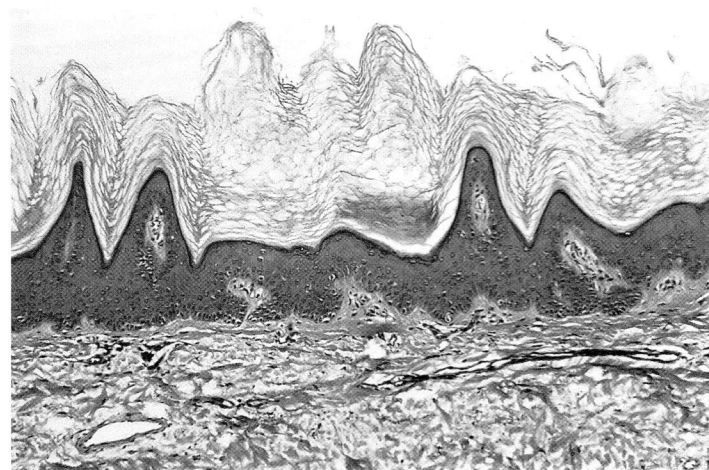

Fig. 1.11 **Papillomatosis ('church-spiring').** This is acrokeratosis verruciform s. (H & E)

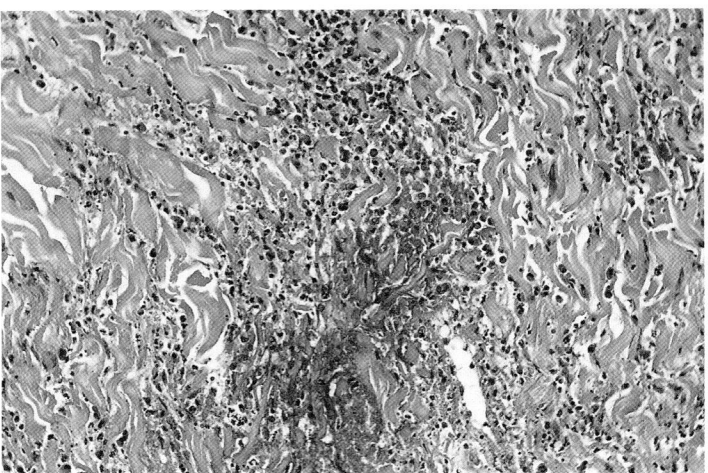

Fig. 1.12 **Eosinophilic cellulitis with flame figures.** (H & E)

Table 1.7 **Lesions showing papillomatosis**

Seborrheic keratosis
Acrokeratosis verruciformis
Verruca vulgaris
Epidermodysplasia verruciformis
Verruca plana
Stucco keratosis
Tar keratosis
Arsenical keratosis
Solar keratosis
Acanthosis nigricans
Reticulated papillomatosis
Epidermal nevus
Verrucous carcinoma
Keratosis follicularis spinulosa
Multiple minute digitate keratoses
Hyperkeratosis lenticularis
Rubbed and scratched skin

PAPILLOMATOSIS ('CHURCH-SPIRING')

Papillomatosis refers to the presence of undulations or projections of the epidermal surface (Fig. 1.11). This may vary from tall 'steeple-like' projections to quite small, somewhat broader elevations of the epidermal surface. The term 'church-spiring' is sometimes used to refer to these changes. The various lesions showing papillomatosis are listed in Table 1.7.

ACRAL ANGIOFIBROMAS

The acral angiofibroma reaction pattern is characterized by an *increase in the number of small vessels, which is associated with perivascular and, sometimes, perifollicular fibrosis* (see p. 918). The fibrous tissue usually contains stellate cells. The conditions showing this reaction pattern are listed in Table 1.8.

Table 1.8 **Conditions showing an angiofibromatous pattern**

Adenoma sebaceum (tuberous sclerosis)
Angiofibromas in syndromes – MEN I, neurofibromatosis
Subungual and periungual fibroma
Acquired acral fibrokeratoma
Fibrous papule of the nose
Pearly penile papules
Familial myxovascular fibromas

EOSINOPHILIC CELLULITIS WITH 'FLAME FIGURES'

In eosinophilic cellulitis with 'flame figures' there is *dermal edema with an infiltration of eosinophils and some histiocytes and scattered 'flame figures'* (Fig. 1.12). 'Flame figures' result from the adherence of amorphous or granular eosinophilic material to collagen bundles in the dermis. They are small, poorly circumscribed foci of apparent 'necrobiosis' of collagen, although they are eosinophilic rather than basophilic as seen in the usual 'necrobiotic' disorders.

Eosinophilic cellulitis with 'flame figures' can occur as part of a generalized cutaneous process known as Wells' syndrome (see p. 1060). This reaction pattern, which may represent a severe urticarial hypersensitivity reaction to various stimuli, can also be seen, rarely, in biopsies from arthropod reactions, other parasitic infestations, internal cancers, bullous pemphigoid, dermatitis herpetiformis, diffuse erythemas and *Trichophyton rubrum* infections. The 'flame figures' of eosinophilic cellulitis resemble the Splendore–Hoeppli deposits which are sometimes found around parasites in tissues.

TRANSEPITHELIAL ELIMINATION

The term 'transepithelial elimination' was coined by Mehregan for a biological phenomenon whereby materials foreign to the skin are eliminated through pores between cells of the epidermis or hair follicle or are carried up between cells as a passive phenomenon, during maturation of the epidermal cells.[1] The validity of this hypothesis has been confirmed using an animal model.[2] The process of transepithelial elimination can be recognized in tissue sections by the presence of pseudoepitheliomatous hyperplasia or expansion of hair follicles (Fig. 1.13). These downgrowths of the epidermis or follicle usually surround the material to be eliminated, and the term 'epidermal vacuum cleaner' can be applied to them. Various tissues, substances or organisms can be eliminated from the dermis in this way, including elastic fibers, collagen, erythrocytes, amyloid, calcium salts, bone, foreign material, inflammatory cells and debris, fungi and mucin.[3–16] The various disorders (also known as 'perforating disorders') which may show transepithelial elimination are listed in Table 1.9.

The apparent transepithelial elimination of a sebaceous gland has been reported.[17] This process was probably an artifact of tissue sectioning.

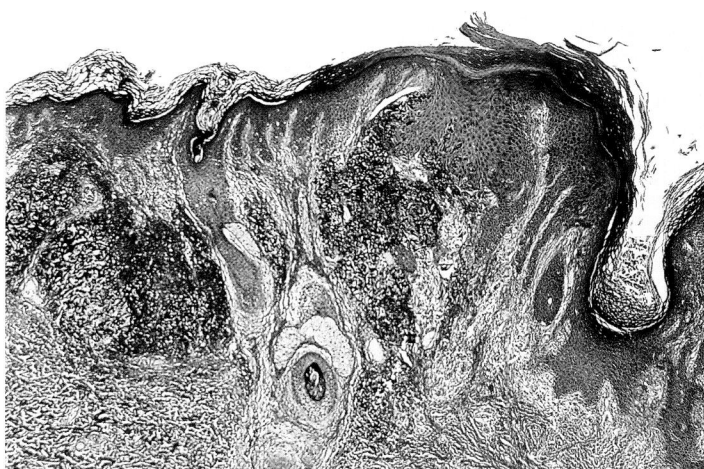

Fig. 1.13 Transepithelial elimination of solar elastotic material is occurring through an enlarged follicular infundibulum. (Verhoeff van Gieson)

Table 1.9 **Diseases in which transepithelial elimination may occur**

Necrobiosis lipoidica
Necrobiotic xanthogranuloma
Perforating folliculitis
Pseudoxanthoma elasticum
Elastosis perforans serpiginosa
Reactive perforating collagenosis
Calcaneal petechiae ('black heel')
Amyloidosis
Chondrodermatitis nodularis helicis
Urate crystals
Calcinosis cutis
Osteoma cutis
Deep mycoses
Cutaneous tuberculosis
Blastomycosis-like pyoderma
Granuloma inguinale
Sarcoidosis
Foreign body granulomas
Suture material
Lichen nitidus
Papular mucinosis
Acne keloidalis nuchae
Solar elastosis
Post-cryotherapy injury
Cutaneous tumors

PATTERNS OF INFLAMMATION

Four patterns of inflammation can be discerned in biopsies taken from the various inflammatory diseases of the skin – superficial perivascular inflammation, superficial and deep dermal inflammation, folliculitis and perifolliculitis, and panniculitis. Superficial band-like infiltrates are not included as a separate category as they are usually associated with the lichenoid reaction pattern (interface dermatitis) or the infiltrate is merely an extension of a superficial perivascular infiltrate.

SUPERFICIAL PERIVASCULAR INFLAMMATION

Superficial perivascular inflammation is usually associated with the spongiotic, psoriasiform or lichenoid reaction patterns. On some occasions, diseases

which are usually regarded as showing the spongiotic reaction pattern have only very mild spongiosis which may not always be evident on casual inspection of one level of a biopsy. This should be kept in mind when a superficial perivascular inflammatory reaction is present.

Causes of a superficial perivascular infiltrate, in the absence of spongiosis or another reaction pattern, include the following:

- drug reactions
- dermatophytoses
- viral exanthems
- chronic urticaria
- erythrasma
- superficial annular erythemas
- pigmented purpuric dermatoses
- resolving dermatoses.

SUPERFICIAL AND DEEP DERMAL INFLAMMATION

Superficial and deep dermal inflammation may accompany a major reaction pattern, as occurs in discoid lupus erythematosus in which there is a concomitant lichenoid reaction pattern, and in photocontact allergic dermatitis in which there is a spongiotic reaction pattern in addition to the dermal inflammation. This pattern of inflammation may also occur in the absence of any of the six major reaction patterns already discussed. The predominant cell type is usually the lymphocyte but there may be a variable admixture of other cell types (Fig. 1.14). The often quoted mnemonic of diseases causing this pattern of inflammation is the eight 'L' diseases – *l*ight reactions, *l*ymphoma (including pseudolymphomas), *l*eprosy, *l*ues (syphilis), *l*ichen striatus, *l*upus erythematosus, *l*ipoidica (includes necrobiosis lipoidica and incomplete forms of granuloma annulare) and *l*epidoptera (used incorrectly in the mnemonic to refer to arthropod bites and other parasitic infestations). To the eight 'L diseases' should be added 'DRUGS' – *d*rug reactions, as well as *d*ermatophyte infections, *r*eticular erythematous mucinosis, *u*rticaria (chronic urticaria and the urticarial stages of bullous pemphigoid and herpes gestationis), *g*yrate erythemas (deep type) and *s*cleroderma (particularly the localized variants).

This list is obviously incomplete but it covers most of the important diseases having this pattern of inflammation. For example, the vasculitides and

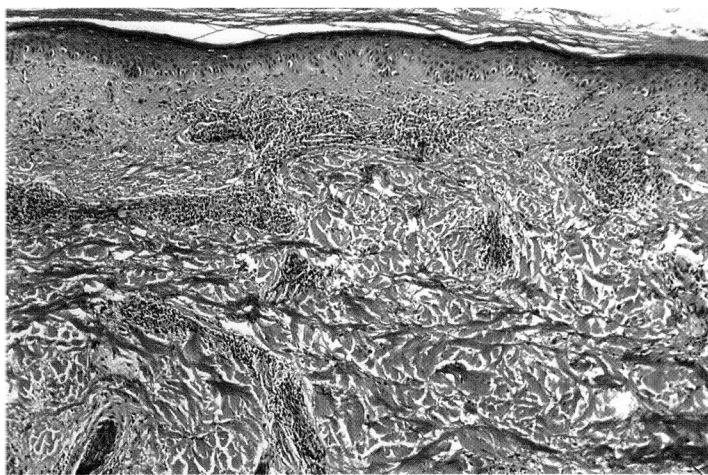

Fig. 1.14 There is a superficial and deep perivascular infiltrate of lymphocytes. The presence of mild lichenoid changes suggests a diagnosis of lupus erythematosus. (H & E)

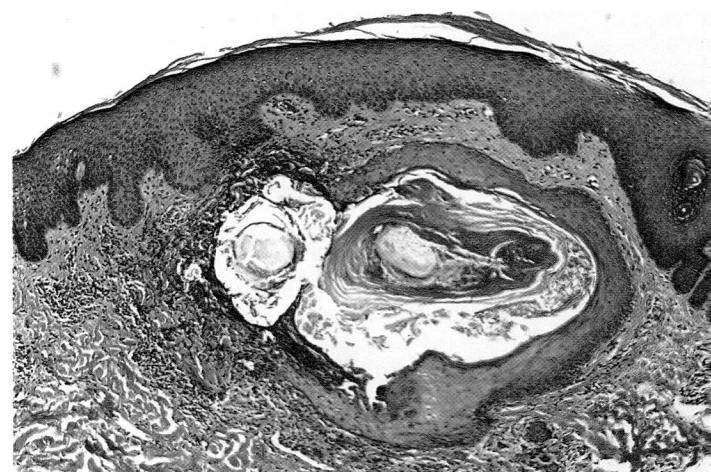

Fig. 1.15 **The acute folliculitis has ruptured with extension of the inflammatory infiltrate into the adjacent dermis.** (H & E)

various granulomatous diseases have superficial and deep inflammation in the dermis but they have been excluded from the mnemonics because they constitute major reaction patterns. It is always worth keeping in mind these mnemonics when a superficial and deep infiltrate is present in tissue sections.

FOLLICULITIS AND PERIFOLLICULITIS

Inflammation of the hair follicle (folliculitis) usually extends into the adjacent dermis, producing a perifolliculitis (Fig. 1.15). For this reason, these two patterns of inflammation are considered together. There are several ways of classifying the various folliculitides, the most common being based on the anatomical level of the follicle (superficial or deep) that is involved. This distinction is not always clearcut and, in some cases of folliculitis due to an infectious agent, the follicle may be inflamed throughout its entire length. The folliculitides are discussed in further detail in Chapter 15, pages 457–466.

Infectious agents are an important cause of folliculitis and perifolliculitis, and diseases showing this pattern of inflammation are sometimes subclassified into 'infective' and 'non-infective' groups. If this etiological classification is used in conjunction with the anatomical level of the follicle most affected by the inflammation, four groups of folliculitides are produced. The important diseases in each of these groups are listed in parentheses:

1. *superficial infective folliculitis* (impetigo, some fungal infections, herpes simplex folliculitis, folliculitis of secondary syphilis)
2. *superficial non-infective folliculitis* (infundibulofolliculitis, actinic folliculitis, acne vulgaris(?), acne necrotica, eosinophilic pustular folliculitis)
3. *deep infective folliculitis* (kerion, favus, pityrosporum folliculitis, Majocchi's granuloma, folliculitis decalvans, furuncle, herpes simplex folliculitis)
4. *deep non-infective folliculitis* (hidradenitis suppurativa, dissecting cellulitis of the scalp, acne conglobata, perforating folliculitis).

In sections stained with hematoxylin and eosin, the division into superficial or deep folliculitis can usually be made, except in cases with overlap features. Further subdivision into infective and non-infective types may require the use of special stains for organisms. It should be remembered that the involved hair follicle may not be present in a particular histological section, and serial sections may need to be studied. An apparent 'uneven vasculitis' (involving a localized part of the biopsy) is a clue to the presence of a folliculitis in a deeper plane of section.

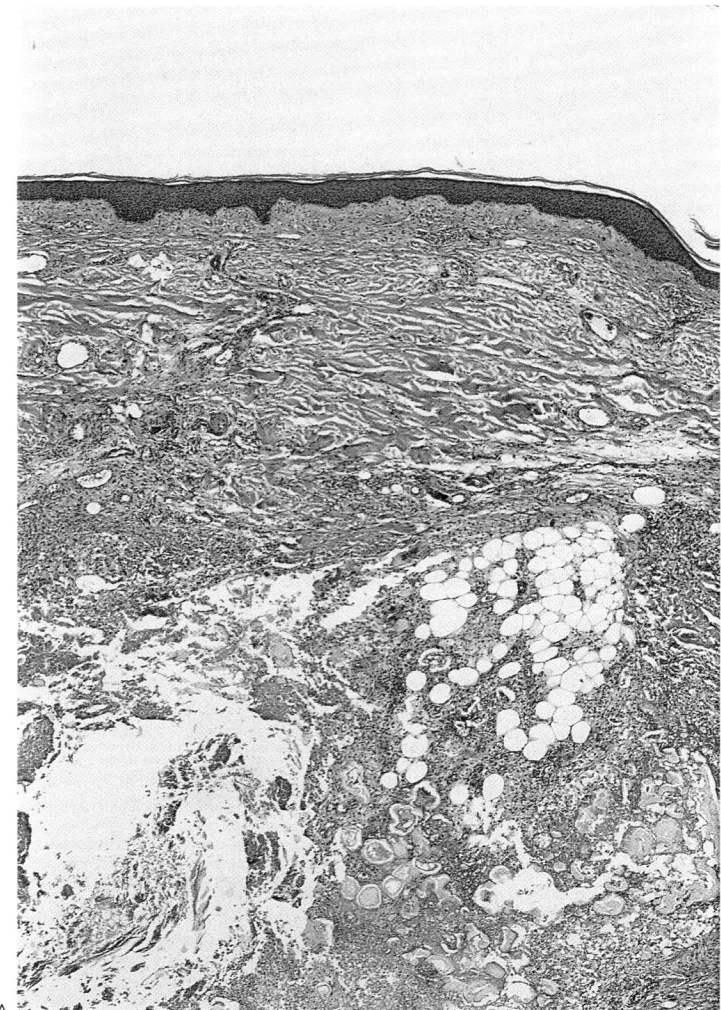

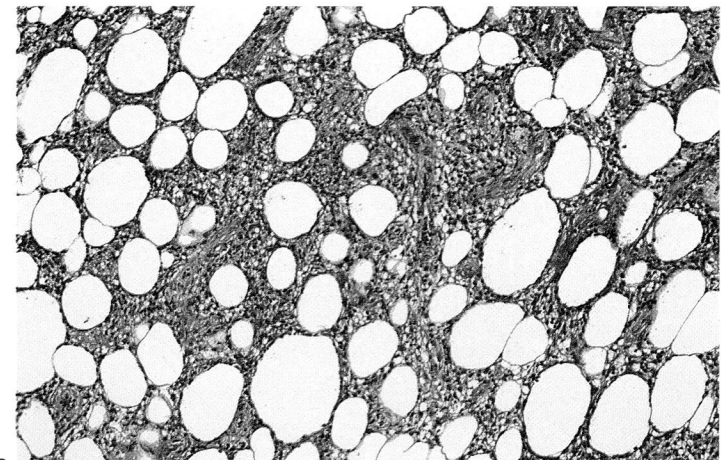

Fig. 1.16 **(A) A panniculitis of lobular type** is present in a case of pancreatic panniculitis. **(B) Another example of a lobular panniculitis** in a patient with erythema induratum–nodular vasculitis. (H & E)

PANNICULITIS

Inflammatory lesions of the subcutaneous fat can be divided into three distinct categories: *septal panniculitis*, in which the inflammation is confined to the interlobular septa of the subcutis; *lobular panniculitis*, in which the

Table 1.10 **Diseases causing a panniculitis**

Septal panniculitis

Erythema nodosum
Necrobiosis lipoidica
Scleroderma

Lobular panniculitis

Erythema induratum – nodular vasculitis
Subcutaneous fat necrosis of the newborn
Sclerema neonatorum
Cold panniculitis
Weber–Christian disease
α_1-antitrypsin deficiency
Cytophagic histiocytic panniculitis
Panniculitis-like T-cell lymphoma
Pancreatic panniculitis
Lupus panniculitis
Connective tissue panniculitis
Poststeroid panniculitis
Lipodystrophy syndromes
Membranous lipodystrophy
Lipodermatosclerosis
Factitial panniculitis
Traumatic fat necrosis
Infective panniculitis
Non-infective neutrophilic panniculitis
Eosinophilic panniculitis

Panniculitis secondary to large vessel vasculitis

Cutaneous polyarteritis nodosa
Superficial migratory thrombophlebitis

REFERENCES

1 Mehregan AH. Elastosis perforans serpiginosa. A review of the literature and report of 11 cases. Arch Dermatol 1968; 97: 381–393.
2 Bayoum A-HM, Gaskell S, Marks R. Development of a model for transepidermal elimination. Br J Dermatol 1978; 99: 611–620.
3 Woo TY, Rasmussen JE. Disorders of transepidermal elimination. Part 1. Int J Dermatol 1985; 24: 267–279.
4 Woo TY, Rasmussen JE. Disorders of transepidermal elimination. Part 2. Int J Dermatol 1985; 24: 337–348.
5 Patterson JW. The perforating disorders. J Am Acad Dermatol 1984; 10: 561–581.
6 Jones RE Jr. Questions to the Editorial Board and other authorities. Am J Dermatopathol 1984; 6: 89–94.
7 Goette DK. Transepithelial elimination of altered collagen after intralesional adrenal steroid injections. Arch Dermatol 1984; 120: 539–540.
8 Goette DK, Berger TG. Acne keloidalis nuchae. A transepidermal elimination disorder. Int J Dermatol 1987; 26: 442–444.
9 Goette DK. Transepidermal elimination of actinically damaged connective tissue. Int J Dermatol 1984; 23: 669–672.
10 Goette DK, Odom RB. Transepithelial elimination of granulomas in cutaneous tuberculosis and sarcoidosis. J Am Acad Dermatol 1986; 14: 126–128.
11 Goette DK. Transepithelial elimination of Monsel's solution-induced granuloma. J Cutan Pathol 1984; 11: 158–161.
12 Goette DK, Robertson D. Transepithelial elimination in chromomycosis. Arch Dermatol 1984; 120: 400–401.
13 Batres E, Klima M, Tschen J. Transepithelial elimination in cutaneous sarcoidosis. J Cutan Pathol 1982; 9: 50–54.
14 Goette DK. Transepithelial elimination of suture material. Arch Dermatol 1984; 120: 1137–1138.
15 Goette DK. Transepithelial elimination of benign and malignant tumors. J Dermatol Surg Oncol 1987; 13: 68–73.
16 Chang P, Fernandez V. What are the perforating diseases? Int J Dermatol 1993; 32: 407–408.
17 Weigand DA. Transfollicular extrusion of sebaceous glands: natural phenomenon or artifact? A case report. J Cutan Pathol 1976; 3: 239–244.

inflammation involves the entire fat lobule and often the septa as well; and *panniculitis secondary to vasculitis involving large vessels in the subcutis*, in which the inflammation is usually restricted to the immediate vicinity of the involved vessel (Fig. 1.16). The various panniculitides are listed in Table 1.10. They are discussed further in Chapter 17, pages 521–536.

Diagnostic clues

In the previous chapter, an orderly approach to the diagnosis of inflammatory skin lesions was discussed. This chapter records in table form some useful points that may assist in reaching a correct diagnosis. Many of the clues that follow produce diagnostic lists that are not necessarily related to tissue reaction, etiology or pathogenesis.

Some of the clues that follow are original observations; many have been around for decades. An acknowledgement should be made here of the work of Bernard Ackerman, who has contributed more 'clues' to diagnostic dermatopathology than anyone else.

Like all 'short cuts', the following 'clues' must be used with caution. They are not absolute criteria for diagnosis and they are not invariably present at all stages of a disease. An attempt has been made to group the clues into several sections.

FEATURES OF PARTICULAR PROCESSES

SIGNS OF PHOTOSENSITIVITY (Fig. 2.1)

- Dilated vessels in the upper dermis
- Stellate fibroblasts/dendrocytes
- Deep elastotic fibers
- Deep extension of the infiltrate
- Epidermal 'sunburn' cells.

Note: The duration of the process and the underlying nature of the light reaction will influence the response. Only one or two features may be present, e.g. sunburn cells (apoptotic keratinocytes) are confined to phototoxic and photosensitive drug eruptions.

SIGNS OF RUBBING/SCRATCHING (Fig. 2.2)

Acute, severe: Pale pink epidermis, sometimes with loss of cell borders; pin-point erosions or larger ulcers; fibrin below the epidermis.

Chronic, persistent: Psoriasiform epidermal hyperplasia; vertical streaks of collagen in the papillary dermis; stellate fibroblasts/dendrocytes; fibroplasia of varying amounts; enlarged follicular infundibula (as prurigo nodularis commences); compact orthokeratosis.

SUBTLE CLUES TO DRUG REACTIONS

- Superficial dermal edema
- Activated lymphocytes
- Eosinophils and/or plasma cells
- Red cell extravasation
- Endothelial swelling of vessels
- Exocytosis of lymphocytes
- Apoptotic keratinocytes.

The changes present will mirror the clinical types of reaction. In morbilliform reactions, lymphocytes extend into the lower epidermis and the apoptotic keratinocytes are in the basal layer.

CLUES TO ELASTIC TISSUE ALTERATIONS

- Small blue coiled/clumped fibers (PXE)
- Wavy epidermis (particularly in children)

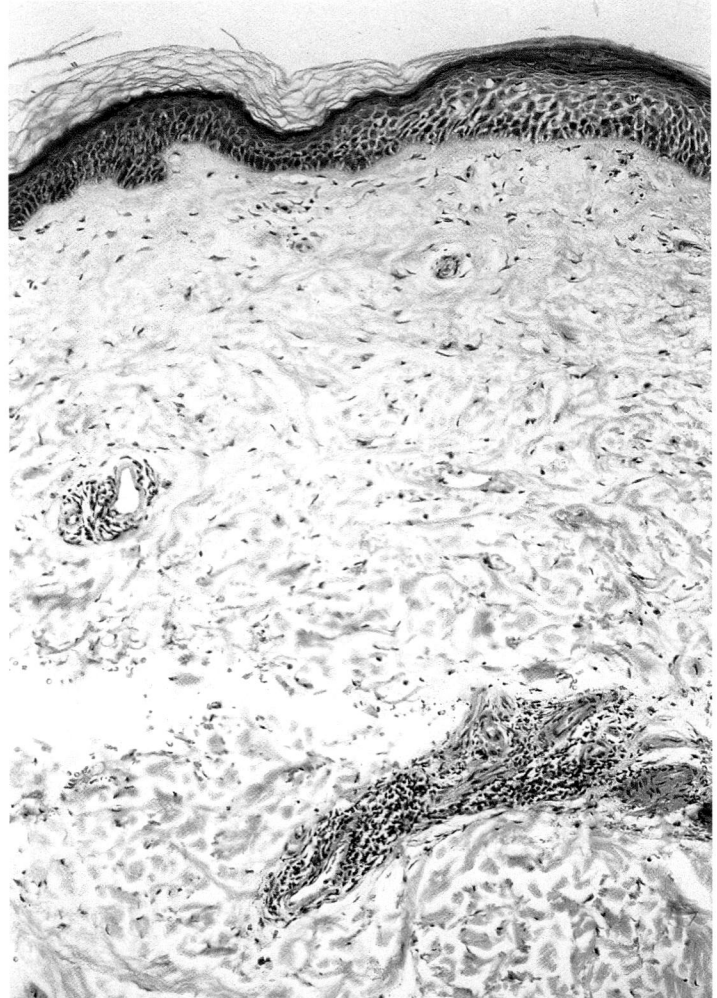

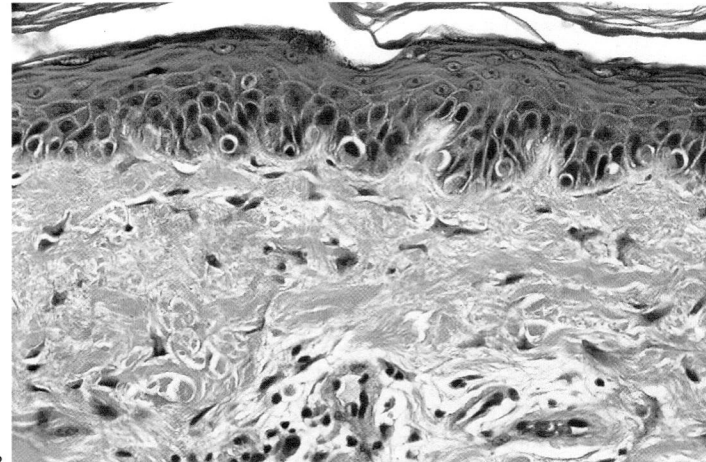

Fig. 2.1 **Photosensitivity reaction. (A)** Note the mild telangiectasia, scattered stellate cells, deep extension of the infiltrate and mild deep solar elastosis. **(B)** Note the stellate cells. (H & E)

- Elastophagocytosis
- Dispersed neutrophils (early cutis laxa)
- Unusually thickened collagen (connective tissue nevus).

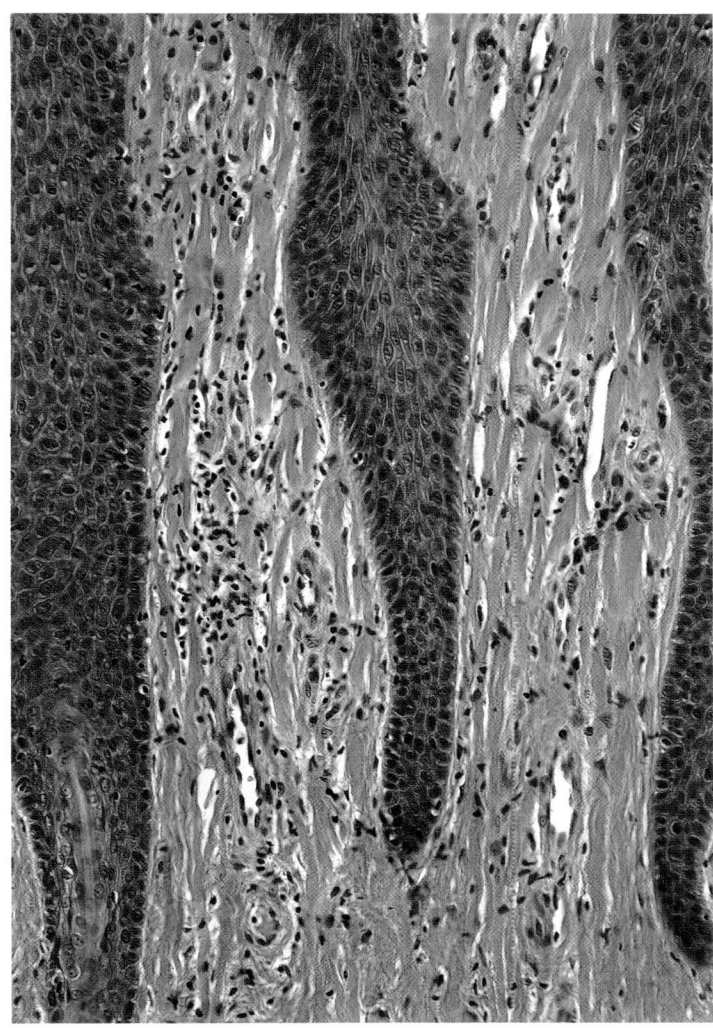

Fig. 2.2 **Chronic rubbing leading to vertical collagen in the papillary dermis and psoriasiform hyperplasia of the epidermis.** (H & E)

CLUES TO DEFICIENCY STATES

- Confluent parakeratosis
- Superficial epidermal necrosis and/or pallor
- Mild psoriasiform hyperplasia
- Hemorrhage (in pellagra and mixed deficiencies).

CLUES TO FUNGAL INFECTIONS (Fig. 2.3)

Basically, these features should prompt the performance of a PAS stain. Many simulants exist.

- Compact orthokeratosis with no other explanation
- Layering of epidermal cornification ('sandwich sign')
- Neutrophils in the epidermis/stratum corneum
- Spongiosis, particularly palmoplantar
- Suppurative folliculitis.

SUBTLE CLUES TO A FOLLICULITIS (Fig. 2.4)

These signs refer to a likely folliculitis at deeper levels of the biopsy.

- Neutrophils on top of the stratum corneum

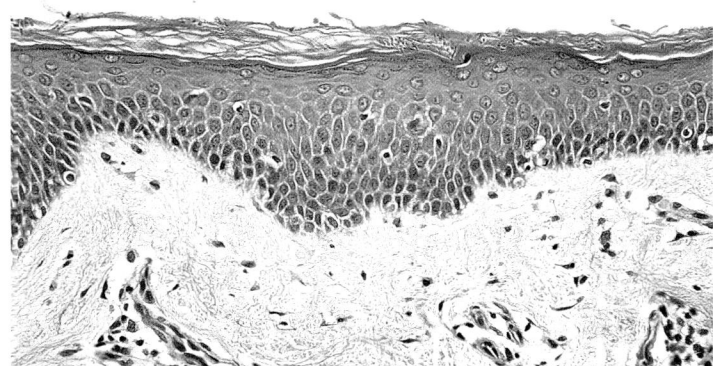

Fig. 2.3 **Dermatophyte.** The fungal elements are present in the region with compact orthokeratosis. Note the adjacent normal 'basket-weave' pattern. (H & E)

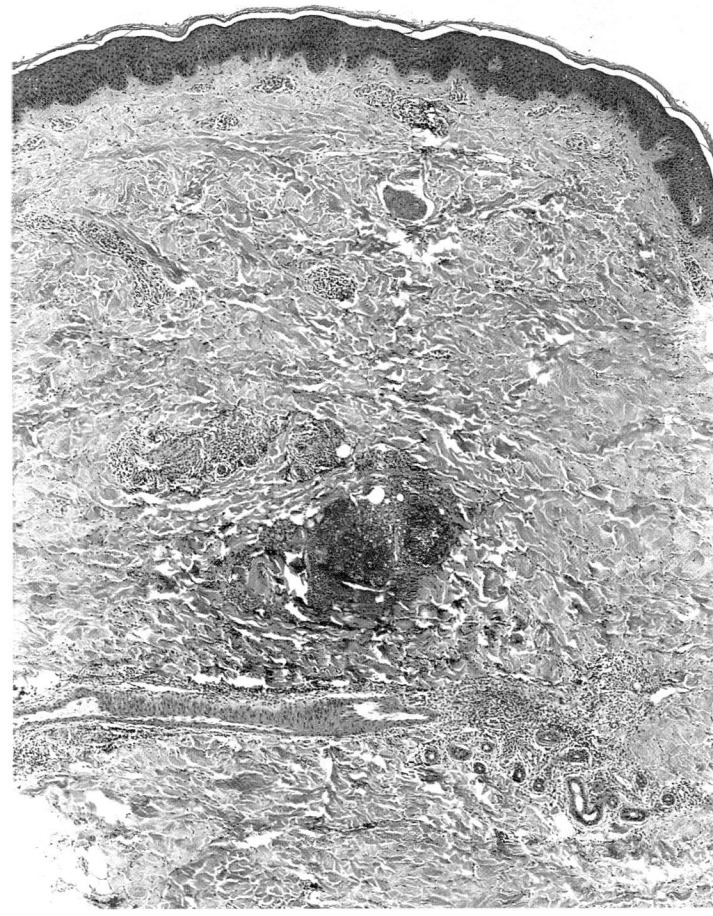

Fig 2.4 **Folliculitis.** There is deep dermal inflammation and an 'uneven vasculitis' more superficially. A ruptured and inflamed follicle was present on deeper levels. (H & E)

- Neutrophils at the edge of the tissue section
- Uneven vasculitis (centered in one small area) – miliaria may do the same
- Focal splaying of neutrophils and dust in mid dermis.

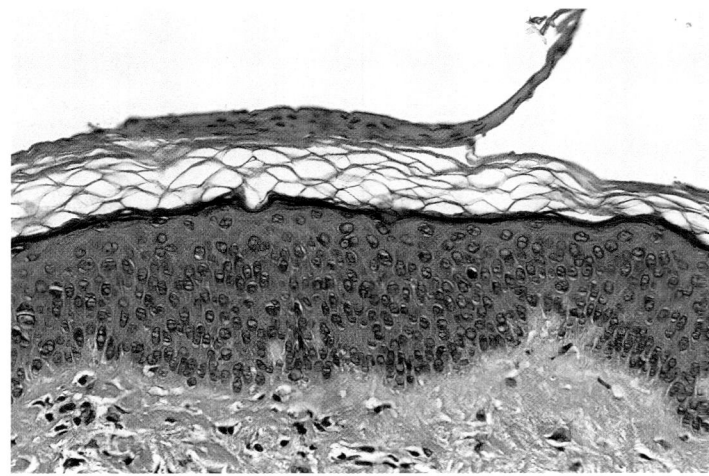

Fig. 2.5 **'Last week's sign'.** The return to the production of normal basket-weave keratin beneath a layer of parakeratosis suggests there is little on-going activity in this region. (H & E)

'LAST WEEK'S SIGN' (Fig. 2.5)

This refers to a dermatosis, no longer active, which is 'playing itself out'. It was presumably more active some days earlier.

- Parakeratosis overlying basket-weave orthokeratin (the key feature)
- Mild hyperplasia of the epidermis
- Mild dermal inflammation.

HISTOLOGICAL FEATURES – WHAT DO THEY SUGGEST?

SUPERFICIAL AND DEEP INFLAMMATION (Fig. 2.6)

The presence of a superficial and deep inflammatory cell infiltrate within the dermis should trigger the mnemonic '8Ls + DRUGS'.

8Ls

- Light reactions
- Lymphoma
- Leprosy
- Lues
- Lichen striatus
- Lupus erythematosus
- Lipoidica (necrobiosis)
- Lepidoptera (and other arthropods)

DRUGS

- Dermatophyte
- Reticular erythematous mucinosis
- Urticarial stages (BP)
- Gyrate erythemas
- Scleroderma (localized)
- And, of course, drug reactions

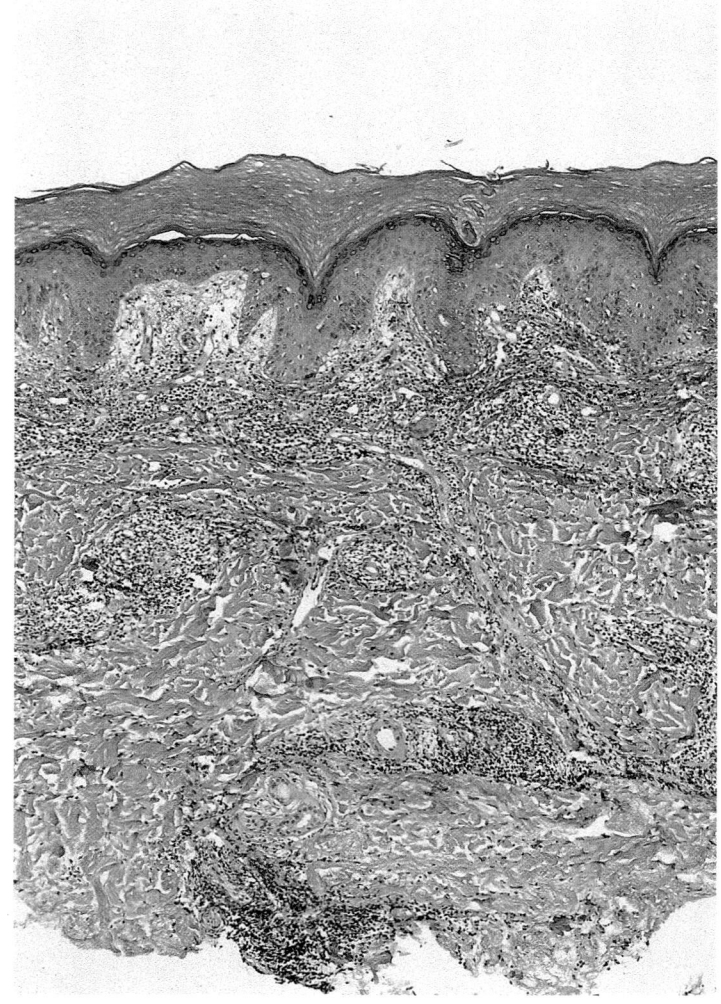

Fig. 2.6 **A superficial and deep dermal infiltrate.** This is one of the 'L' diseases – polymorphous *light* eruption. (H & E)

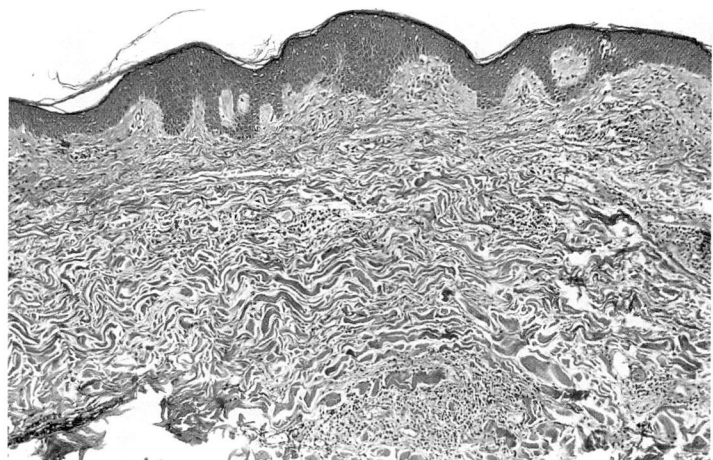

Fig. 2.7 **A 'busy' dermis.** There is hypercellularity in this case of interstitial granulomatous drug reaction. (H & E)

A 'BUSY' DERMIS (Fig. 2.7)

'Busy' refers to a dermis that appears focally hypercellular on scanning magnification and is not usually due to the usual inflammatory infiltrates.

- Incomplete form of granuloma annulare
- Interstitial granulomatous dermatitis
- Interstitial granulomatous drug reaction
- Resolving vasculitis (increased mucin also)
- Chronic photodermatoses
- Folliculitis – at deeper levels (cells are neutrophils and dust)
- Subtle breast carcinoma recurrence
- Desmoplastic melanoma (also perivascular lymphocytes)
- Kaposi's sarcoma (early stage).

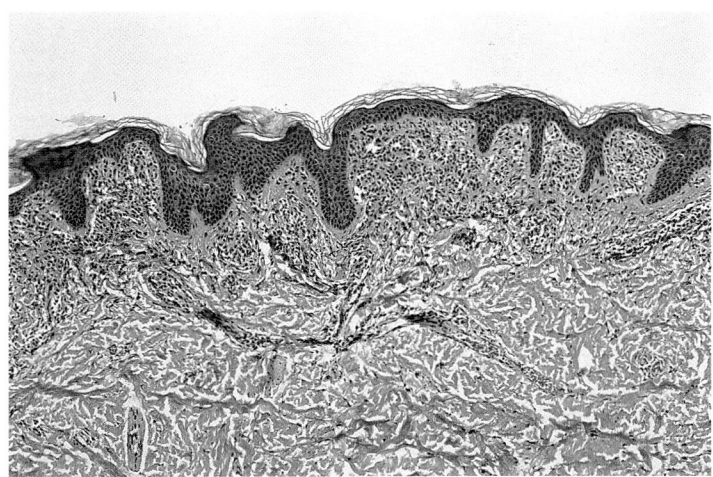

Fig. 2.8 **The papillary dermis is filled.** This is mastocytosis. (H & E)

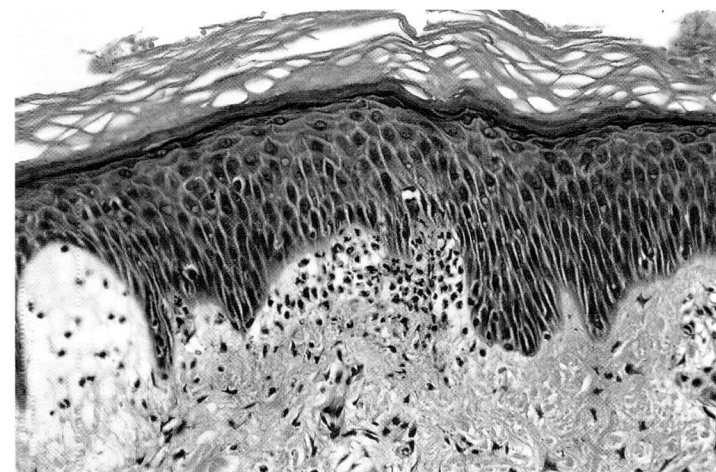

Fig. 2.9 **Dermal papillary microabscess.** This is dermatitis herpetiformis. (H & E)

ABSENT STRATUM CORNEUM

- Staphylococcal scalded skin syndrome
- Pemphigus foliaceus
- Peeling skin syndrome
- Psoriatic erythroderma (psoriasiform hyperplasia present)
- Artifacts.

FILLED PAPILLARY DERMIS (Fig. 2.8)

The low power impression is that of a variably hypercellular papillary dermis. Excluded from consideration are nodular and diffuse infiltrates also involving the reticular dermis.

- Most of the lichenoid tissue reactions
- Pigmented purpuric dermatoses
- Cutaneous T-cell lymphoma
- Parapsoriasis (if not included above)
- Some mastocytomas
- Early lichen sclerosus et atrophicus.

PAPILLARY MICROABSCESSES (Fig. 2.9)

- Dermatitis herpetiformis
- Linear IgA disease
- Cicatricial pemphigoid
- Localized cicatricial pemphigoid
- Bullous lupus erythematosus
- Epidermolysis bullosa acquisita
- Drugs
- Hypersensitivity vasculitis (rare)
- Rheumatoid neutrophilic dermatosis
- Pemphigoid gestationis (eosinophils)
- Deep lamina lucida pemphigoid
- Generalized exanthematous pustulosis (rare).

THICKENED BASEMENT MEMBRANE (Fig. 2.10)

- Lupus erythematosus
- Dermatomyositis (less so)
- Lichen sclerosus et atrophicus.

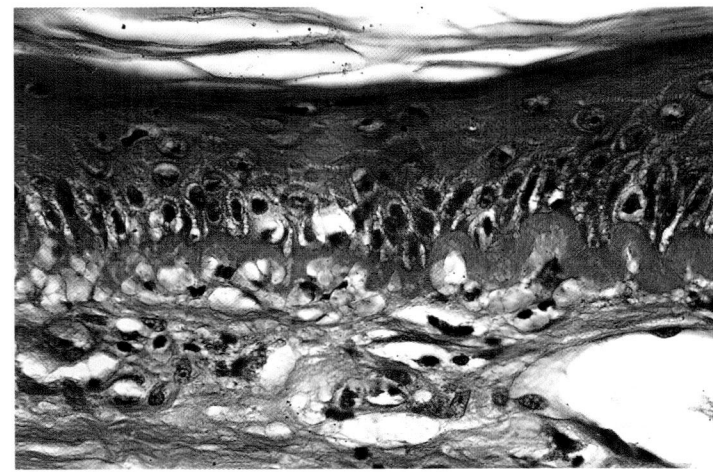

Fig. 2.10 **Thickened basement membrane and mild basal vacuolar change.** This is an example of systemic lupus erythematosus. (H & E)

MID-DERMAL INFILTRATE AND MUCIN (Fig. 2.11)

- Cutaneous lupus erythematosus
- Reticular erythematous mucinosis (REM).

Other signs will usually allow these diagnoses, but sometimes REM will present with very little deep infiltrate. Biopsies appear to have a 'mid-dermal plexus'. Dermatomyositis can have mucin, but the infiltrate is only superficial. Perifollicular mucin can be seen in Carney's complex.

EPIDERMOTROPISM AND EXOCYTOSIS (Fig. 2.12)

The terms 'epidermotropism' and 'exocytosis' are often used interchangeably. It is best to restrict them as follows:

Exocytosis: Random emigration of inflammatory cells through the epidermis; some cells will reach the surface. It is common in inflammatory dermatoses. In the spongiotic tissue reaction, it may be a striking feature in nummular dermatitis and spongiotic drug reactions.

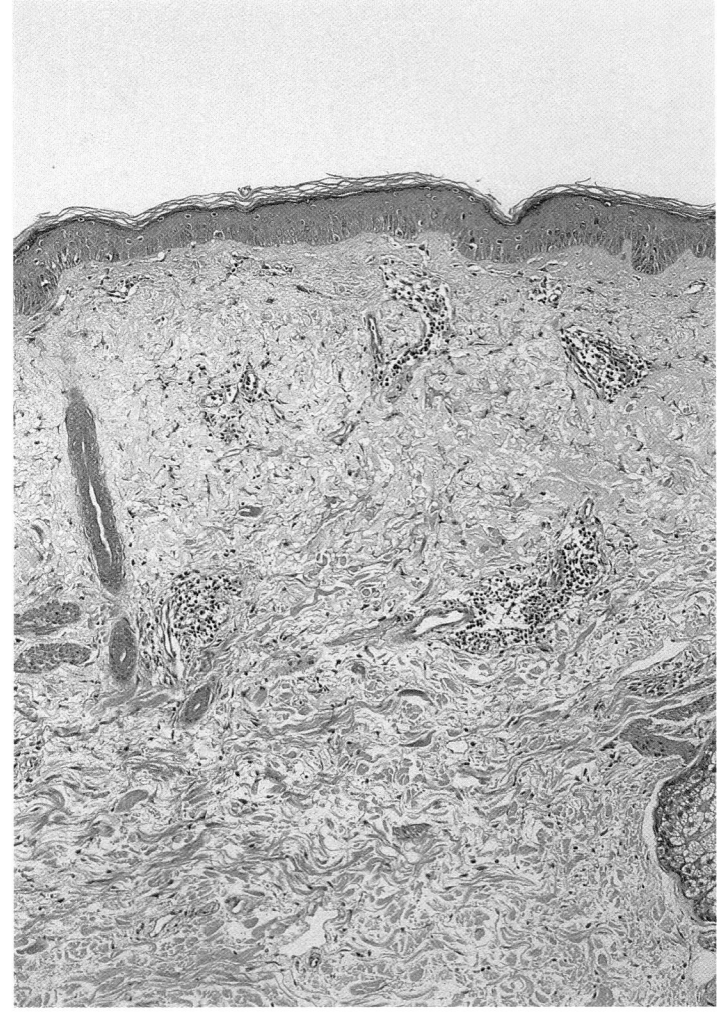

Fig. 2.11 **A 'mid-dermal plexus' with perivascular inflammation is present.** Lupus and reticular erythematous mucinosis (REM) can do this (they may be the one condition). The mucin is difficult to appreciate. (H & E)

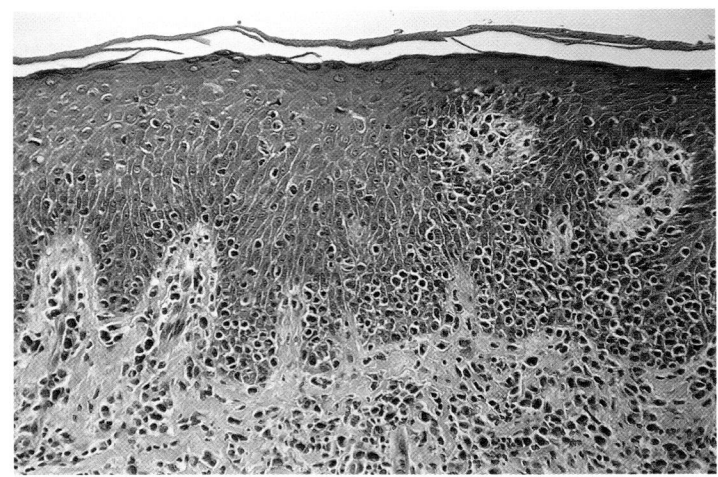

Fig. 2.12 **Epidermotropism.** The cells are confined to the lower one-third to one-half of the epidermis. (H & E)

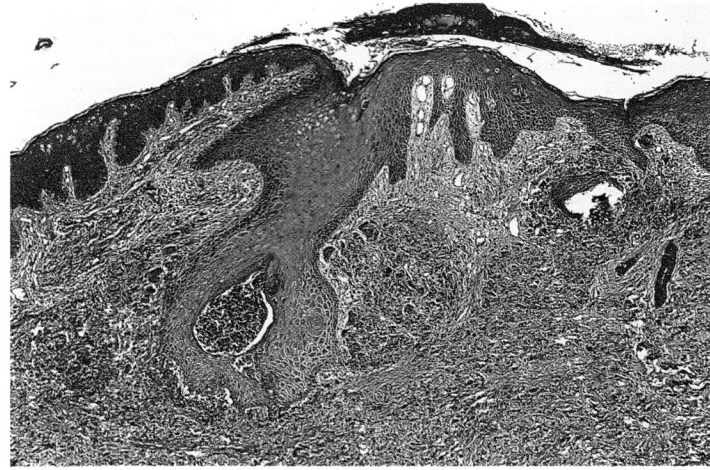

Fig. 2.13 **Epidermal 'vacuum cleaner'.** The acanthotic downgrowth serves as a site for transepidermal elimination of elastotic material in this case of perforating pseudoxanthoma elasticum. (H & E)

Epidermotropism: Refers to directed emigration of lymphocytes; it usually involves only the lower one-third to half of the epidermis. The cells have a tendency to aggregate. There is little, if any, accompanying spongiosis. It is a feature of mycosis fungoides.

THE EPIDERMAL/FOLLICULAR 'VACUUM CLEANER' (Fig. 2.13)

The epidermal/follicular 'vacuum cleaner' is the author's term for the irregular epidermal hyperplasia ± enlarged follicular infundibula, associated with the transepidermal elimination of material from the dermis. It can be subtle following cryotherapy to sun damaged skin; it may be the cause of a persistent lesion at the site, often mistaken as a clinical recurrence.

PARAKERATOSIS AS A HELPFUL SIGN

Lipping: See below.
Mounds: Pityriasis rosea, erythema annulare centrifugum.

Neutrophils: Psoriasis (neutrophils in 'summits' of mounds). Dermatophyte infection. Secondary bacterial infection.
Overlying orthokeratosis: Healing lesion or intermittent activity, particularly a spongiotic process.
Alternating: Alternating orthokeratosis and parakeratosis in a horizontal direction is seen in ILVEN and in a horizontal and vertical direction in pityriasis rubra pilaris.
Broad thick zones: Psoriasis, glucagonoma and deficiency states (epidermal pallor is not invariable), pityriasis lichenoides, granular parakeratosis.

PARAKERATOTIC FOLLICULAR LIPPING

- Seborrheic dermatitis
- Pityriasis rubra pilaris (follicular lesions)
- Spongiotic processes, or psoriasis, on the face. The large number of follicles on the face means that they are more likely to be involved incidentally in any condition with parakeratosis.

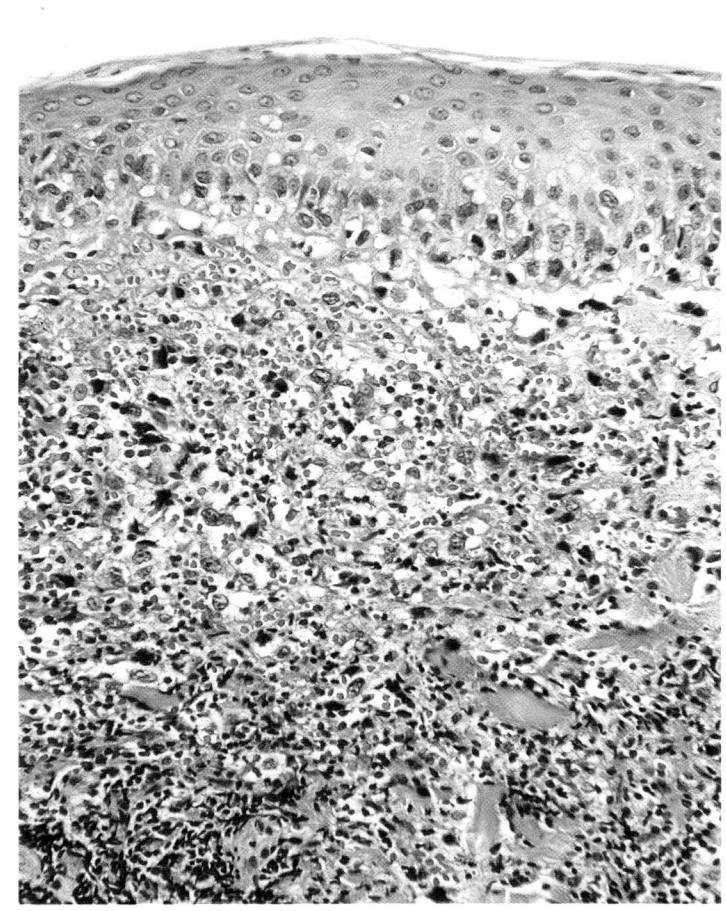

Fig. 2.14 **'Chunks of coal'.** Cells with large, dark, hyperchromatic nuclei are present in the dermis in this case of lymphomatoid papulosis. (H & E)

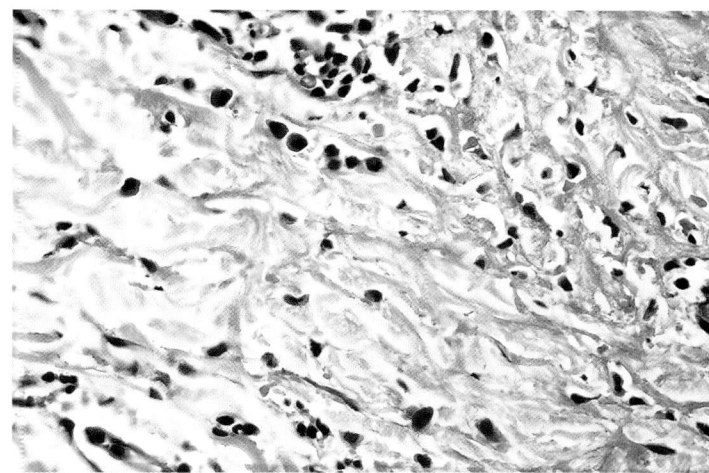

Fig. 2.15 **Interstitial eosinophils in an insect bite reaction.** (H & E)

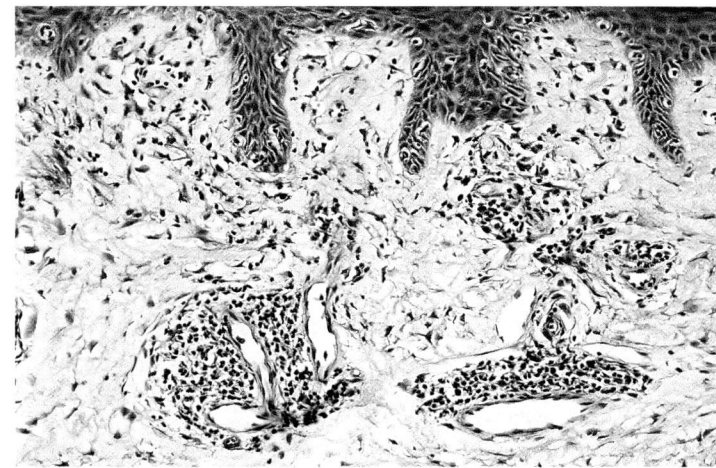

Fig. 2 16 **The 'bare underbelly' sign.** Note the paucity of lymphocytes on the undersurface of the superficial vascular plexus. (H & E)

'CHUNKS OF COAL' (Fig. 2.14)

Large atypical lymphoid cells within a heavy mixed infiltrate occur in lymphomatoid papulosis. The cells have been likened to 'chunks of coal'.

INTERSTITIAL EOSINOPHILS (Fig. 2.15)

'Interstitial eosinophils' refers to the presence of eosinophils between collagen bundles and away from vessels. Perivascular eosinophils are also present.

- Arthropod bites
- Cnidarian contact
- Other parasite infestations
- Drug reactions
- Toxic erythema of pregnancy
- Annular erythemas of infancy
- Wells' syndrome
- Dermal hypersensitivity
- Hypereosinophilic syndrome
- Urticaria
- Urticarial stages of bullous pemphigoid, pemphigoid gestationis
- Internal malignancy (rare).

Large numbers of eosinophils in suspected bite reactions suggest scabies or a hypersensitive state to the arthropod. Prebullous pemphigoid also has numerous eosinophils.

'BOTTOM-HEAVY' INFILTRATES

Dense lymphoid infiltrates may be found in the lower dermis in the following circumstances:

- Cutaneous lymphoma
- Herpes folliculitis
- Hidradenitis suppurativa (mixed infiltrate + scarring).

THE 'BARE UNDERBELLY' SIGN (Fig. 2.16)

In some cases of mycosis fungoides, the lymphocytes are present on the upper (epidermal) side of the superficial vascular plexus with few, if any, on the undersurface. This is possibly a reflection of their directed migration to the epidermis. It is an unreliable sign, but a striking one in some cases.

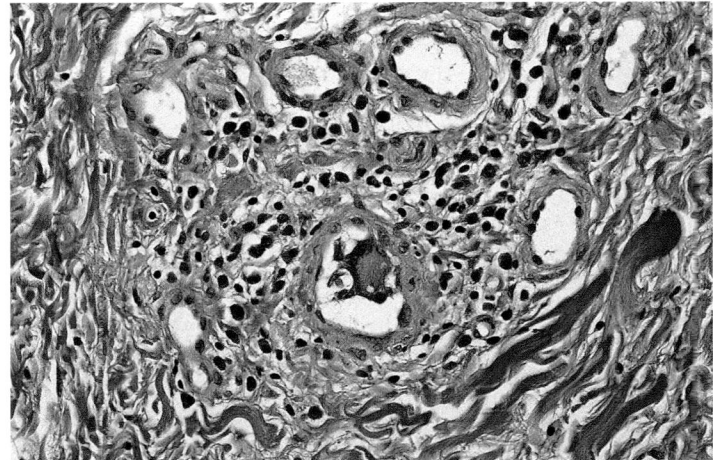

Fig. 2.17 **An intraluminal giant cell.** The patient had chronic infections of the genital and inguinal region. (H & E)

INTRALUMINAL GIANT CELLS/HISTIOCYTES
(Fig. 2.17)

- Melkersson–Rosenthal syndrome
- Recurrent genitocrural infections
- Cutaneous histiocytic lymphangitis (angioendotheliomatosis)
- Rosai – Dorfman disease.

INTRAVASCULAR LEUKOCYTES

Leukocytes (eosinophils and/or neutrophils) are often present in the lumen of small vessels in the upper dermis in urticaria, even in the absence of accompanying vasculitis, and in lymphomatoid papulosis.

HIGH APOPTOTIC (DYSKERATOTIC) KERATINOCYTES (Fig. 2.18)

Presumptive apoptotic keratinocytes (the author has not stained them or examined them ultrastructurally in most entities listed) may occur in the spinous layer in:

- Lichenoid tissue reaction – true 'interface-obscuring' subtype
- Drug reactions

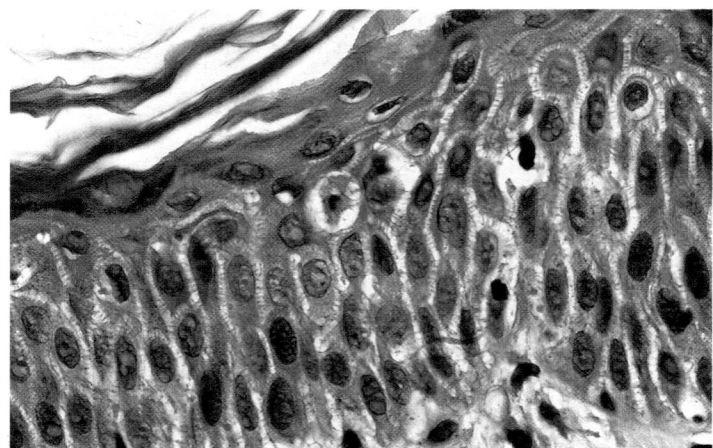

Fig. 2.18 **High apoptotic keratinocytes in a drug reaction.** (H & E)

- Light reactions
- Resolving viral and putative viral lesions
- AIDS-related sebopsoriasis
- Incontinentia pigmenti (second stage)
- Tumors (e.g. Bowen's disease)
- Rarely in normal skin and other inexplicable circumstances
- Near an excoriation
- Glucagonoma syndrome
- Acrodermatitis enteropathica
- Bazex's syndrome.

VERTICAL COLLAGEN BUNDLES

Vertically oriented collagen bundles in the reticular dermis (usually combined with other bundles in random array) are seen in:

- Collagenous and elastotic plaques of the hand
- Digital fibromatosis of childhood
- Acral fibrokeratomas.

LOOSE PINK FIBRILLARY COLLAGEN (Fig. 2.19)

If such tissue is surrounded by a granulomatous rim with foreign body giant cells, this is probably tophaceous gout in which the crystals have dissolved out in aqueous solutions.

EXTRAVASATED ERYTHROCYTES

- Vasculitides of all types
- Pigmented purpuric eruptions (included above)
- Certain drug eruptions
- Some viral, rickettsial infections, septicemia and erysipelas
- Some arthropod reactions
- Pityriasis rosea (often into basal epidermis)
- Bleeding diatheses – purpura, DIC
- Scurvy
- Kaposi's sarcoma
- Lichen sclerosus et atrophicus
- Biopsy trauma.

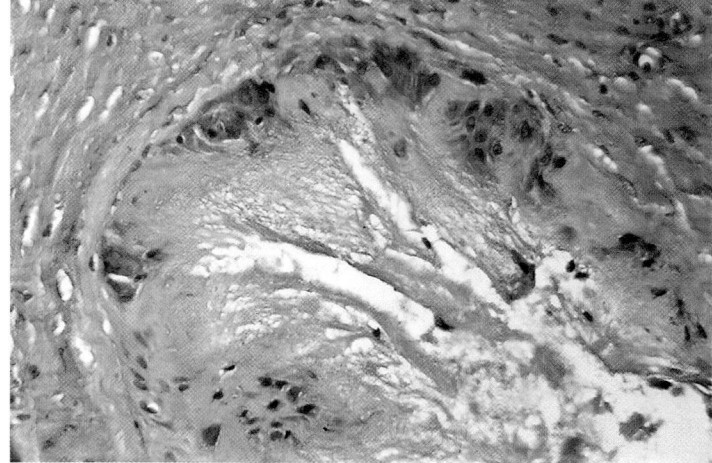

Fig. 2.19 **Giant cells surround eosinophilic material in this tophaceous gout that was fixed in formalin, dissolving out the urate crystals.** (H & E)

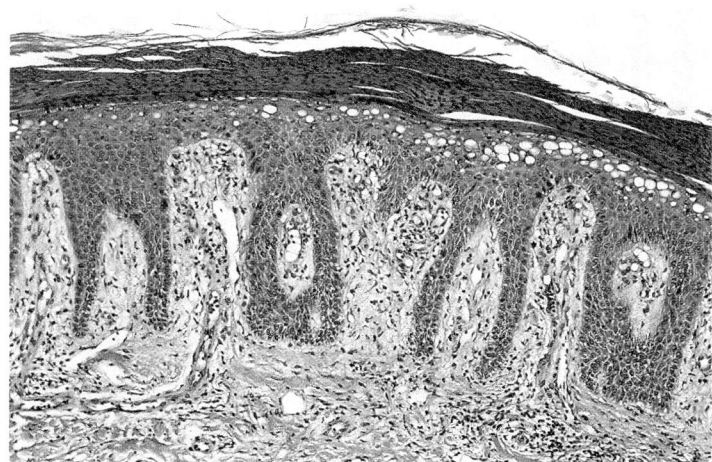

Fig. 2.20 **Pale cells are present in the upper epidermis in this case of glucagonoma syndrome.** (H & E)

- Trichotillomania
- Stasis dermatitis
- Porphyria cutanea tarda (in blister)
- Discoid lupus erythematosus.

PALLOR OF EPIDERMAL CELLS (Fig. 2.20)

- Pellagra
- Acrodermatitis enteropathica
- Glucagonoma syndrome
- Hartnup disease
- Deficiency of M-subunit, LDH
- Acroerythema
- Spongiotic diseases (variable)
- Clear cell acanthoma
- Clear (pale) cell acanthosis
- Clear cell papulosis
- Pagetoid dyskeratosis
- Colloid keratosis.

Note: This list could include other conditions but they are usually diagnosed by other clues (e.g. lichen planus, pityriasis lichenoides chronica and orf).

CLEAR CELL TUMORS

Epidermal-derived
- Clear cell acanthoma
- Bowen's disease
- Basal cell carcinoma
- Squamous cell carcinoma.

Adnexal tumors
- Paget's disease
- Clear cell syringoma
- Clear cell hidradenoma (apocrine hidradenoma)
- Clear cell hidradenocarcinoma (apocrine hidradenocarcinoma)
- Clear cell eccrine carcinoma
- Clear cell myoepithelioma
- Tricholemmoma

- Tricholemmal carcinoma
- Sebaceous adenoma
- Sebaceous carcinoma.

Nevomelanocytic
- Balloon cell nevus
- Balloon cell melanoma
- Clear cell melanoma
- Clear cell sarcoma.

Mesenchymal
- Clear cell dermatofibroma
- Clear cell atypical fibroxanthoma
- Clear cell fibrous papule.

Salivary gland
- Acinic cell carcinoma
- Hyalinizing clear cell carcinoma
- Clear cell mucoepidermoid carcinoma.

Metastases
- Renal cell carcinoma
- Breast carcinoma
- Hepatocellular carcinoma
- Pulmonary adenocarcinoma and mesothelioma.

CLUES TO A PARTICULAR DISEASE

CLUES TO HERPES FOLLICULITIS (Fig. 2.21)

- Bottom-heavy infiltrate
- Sebaceitis
- Lichenoid changes around follicle ± epidermis
- Necrotic lower follicle
- Multinucleate epithelial cells, on searching.

CLUES TO GROVER'S DISEASE

- Focal acantholytic dyskeratosis with spongiosis
- Late lesions have elongated rete ridges and may resemble an early solar keratosis

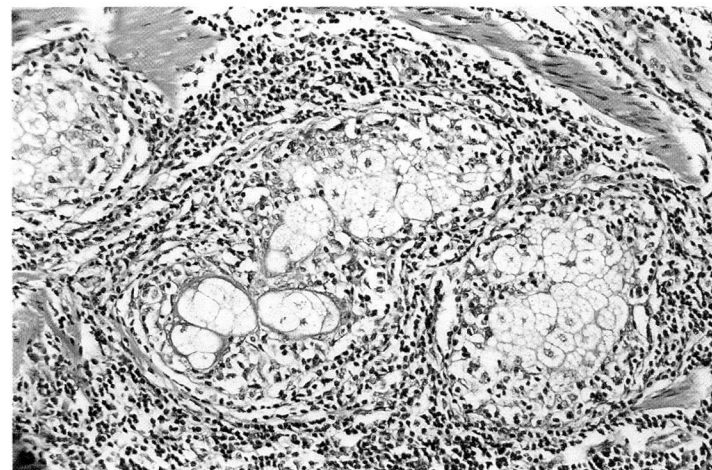

Fig. 2.21 **'Sebaceitis' in a case of herpes folliculitis.** (H & E)

- Eosinophils and less thick parakeratotic plugs may distinguish it from Darier's disease.

CLUES TO CICATRICIAL PEMPHIGOID

- Subcutaneous blister with neutrophils
- Split may extend down follicles
- Dermal fibrosis (detected early by the presence of parallel collagen, on polarization)
- Extruded sebaceous gland within the blister.

Remember that even early lesions may show dermal fibrosis because blisters tend to recur at the site of a previous one.

CLUES TO MYCOSIS FUNGOIDES (Fig. 2.22)

- Pautrier's microabscesses (only present in one-third)
- Haloed lymphocytes
- Epidermotropism without spongiosis
- Lymphocytes aligned within the basal layer
- Hyperconvoluted intraepidermal lymphocytes
- Epidermal lymphocytes larger than dermal ones

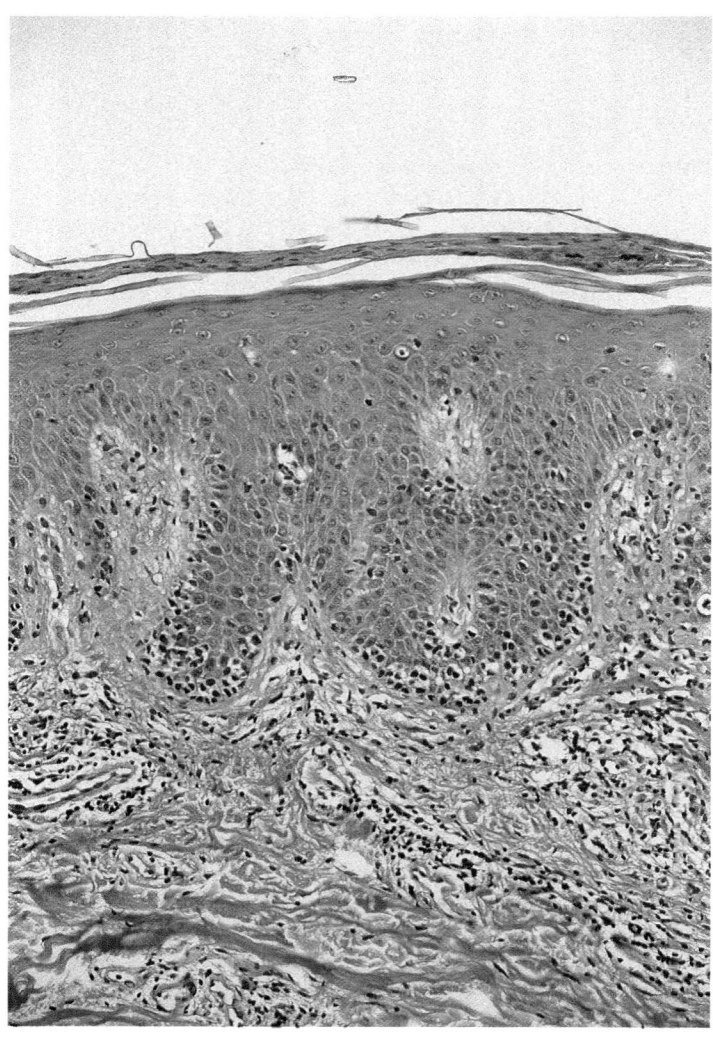

Fig. 2.22 **Mycosis fungoides.** Note the epidermotropism and haloed lymphocytes within the epidermis. (H & E)

- Filling of the papillary dermis
- The 'bare underbelly' sign (unreliable)
- Fibrotic, thickened papillary dermis.

CLUES TO ALOPECIA AREATA

- Virtually all terminal follicles in the same stage
- 'Swarm of bees' (lymphocytes) in the hair bulb.

CLUES TO ANDROGENIC ALOPECIA

- Progressive decrease in follicular size
- Follicles do not extend into subcutis.

LATE BULLOUS LESIONS

Dermatitis herpetiformis: Intracorneal nuclear dust aggregates.
Pemphigus foliaceus: Dyskeratotic cells with hyperchromatic nuclei in granular layer.

GRANULOMA ANNULARE VERSUS NECROBIOSIS LIPOIDICA

Necrobiosis lipoidica: Likened to 'stacks of plates' with multilayered necrobiosis and 'open ends'; thickened collagen bundles may be seen within palisaded granulomas. Numerous plasma cells favor this diagnosis.
Granuloma annulare: Usually not multilayered and open ended, but palisading continues around the edges of the palisading granulomas; central acid mucopolysaccharides; plasma cells uncommon.

GRANULOMA ANNULARE VERSUS LICHEN NITIDUS

In disseminated granuloma annulare small, poorly formed granulomas may develop in the upper dermis, sometimes mimicking lichen nitidus. Granuloma annulare does not usually have claw-like acanthotic downgrowths at the edge; it often has focal 'necrobiosis'.

CLUES TO TRICHOEPITHELIOMA (OVER BCC)

- Papillary mesenchymal bodies ('stromal induction')
- CD34$^+$ stromal cells around the island
- No clefts around the nests
- Ruptured keratinous cysts
- Only basal layer *bcl*-2 expression
- A central dell/depression in the skin surface.

CLUES TO KAPOSI'S SARCOMA

- Abnormal tissue spaces in the dermis
- Promontory sign (small vessel protruding into an abnormal space)
- Hemosiderin and plasma cells
- Stuffing of all dilated neoplastic vessels with erythrocytes in the absence of plasma
- Established lesions have the usually documented features.

CLUES TO BACILLARY ANGIOMATOSIS

Pyogenic granuloma-like lesion with nuclear dust and clumps of purplish material.

GENERAL HELPFUL HINTS AND CAUTIONS

BEWARE OF KERATOACANTHOMA SIMULANTS

- Clinically, squamous cell carcinomas may grow quickly in the very elderly, simulating a keratoacanthoma.
- Squamous cell carcinomas overlying rigid structures (e.g. cartilage of ear, base of nose or bone of the tibia) may have infolding of margins simulating the architecture of a keratoacanthoma.
- Keratoacanthomas have a unique pattern of cell differentiation (pink cytoplasm and large central cells).

BE CAUTIOUS WITH AMYLOID STAINS

- In solar elastotic skin, false-positive staining may occur with Congo red, as differentiation may not remove all the stain from elastotic collagen.
- A progressive stain (alkaline Congo red) may be better in these circumstances.
- False-negative reactions may occur with the Congo red stain in macular amyloidosis.
- The crystal violet stain is the most useful stain for amyloid keratin (AK).

'DO SERIALS, NOT DEEPERS'

If suppurative granulomas are present, a fungal element (e.g. asteroid body in sporotrichosis) is usually present in each granuloma. Serial sections will ensure that the entire focus is sampled. Random deeper levels may miss the organism.

FUNGI MAY BE MISSED ON PAS STAIN (Fig. 2.23)

- 'Dead' fungi do not always stain with the PAS method.
- The equine fungus *Phythium* does not stain.

The silver methenamine method will stain the fungi in both cases, but it is not always reliable with the zygomycoses.

DERMAL NEUTROPHILS – OFTEN FORGOTTEN

Dermal and/or subcutaneous neutrophils may be seen in numerous conditions. They are discussed in Chapter 40 (p. 1058). The author has temporarily 'missed' some of the following conditions through failure to think of them.

- Infections
- Acute cutis laxa
- α_1-antitrypsin deficiency
- Eruptive xanthoma (extracellular lipid may assist)
- Folliculitis on deeper levels
- Excoriation on deeper levels
- Neutrophilic urticaria
- Erythema nodosum leprosum
- Dermatomyositis
- Polymorphous light eruption.

See Chapter 40 (Table 40.1) for a complete list.

THE DEMONSTRATION OF CRYPTOCOCCI
(Fig 2.24)

- Cryptococci are doubly refractile.
- They are mucicarmine positive.
- On alcian blue-PAS, a beautiful contrast is seen between cell wall and capsule.

THE EDGE OF BOWEN'S DISEASE

Pagetoid cells are often present at the edge of Bowen's disease. They may simulate melanoma or Paget's disease in small (2 or 3 mm) punch biopsies.

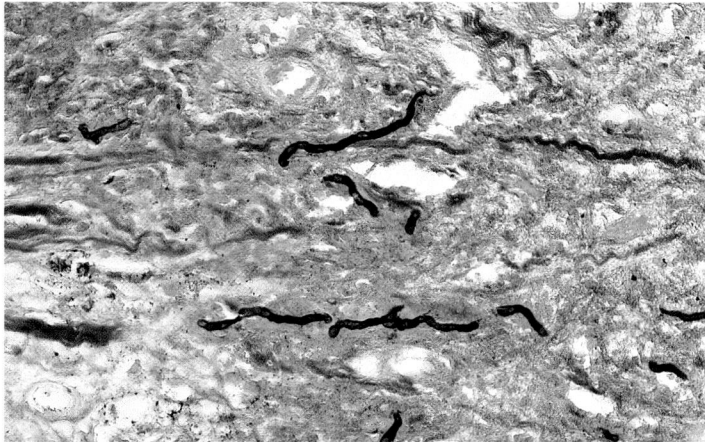

Fig. 2.23 **Equine fungus which is demonstrable only with silver stains.** (Silver methenamine)

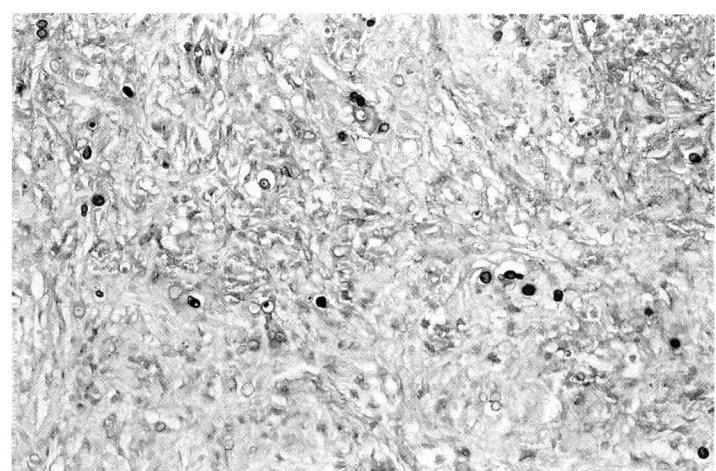

Fig. 2.24 **Cryptococcus.** The capsule stains light blue and the cell wall a reddish color. (Alcian blue-PAS)

FALSE-NEGATIVE IMMUNOPEROXIDASE

The use of microwaves for fixation may release excess antigens leading to the prozone phenomenon. A false negative results, although some staining may occur at the periphery of the tumor. The dilution of the antisera used must be changed in these circumstances.

MISCELLANEOUS HINTS

- Psoriasis is a 'mitotic disease'. Look for mitoses in basal keratinocytes.
- In hypertrophic lichen planus the lichenoid activity may be confined to the tips of the rete pegs.
- Early lichen sclerosus et atrophicus may have licheroid histological features.

Tissue reaction patterns

The lichenoid reaction pattern ('interface dermatitis')

INTRODUCTION

The lichenoid reaction pattern (lichenoid tissue reaction, interface dermatitis) is characterized histologically by epidermal basal cell damage.[1-3] This takes the form of cell death and/or vacuolar change (liquefaction degeneration). The cell death usually involves only scattered cells in the basal layer which become shrunken with eosinophilic cytoplasm. These cells, which have been called Civatte bodies, often contain pyknotic nuclear remnants. Sometimes, fine focusing up and down will reveal smaller cell fragments, often without nuclear remnants, adjacent to the more obvious Civatte bodies.[4] These smaller fragments have separated from the larger bodies during the process of cell death. Ultrastructural studies have shown that the basal cells in the lichenoid reaction pattern usually die by apoptosis, a comparatively recently described form of cell death, which is quite distinct morphologically from necrosis.[5,6]

Before discussing the features of apoptosis, mention will be made of the term '**interface dermatitis**', which is widely used. It has been defined as a dermatosis in which the infiltrate (usually composed mostly of lymphocytes) appears 'to obscure the junction when sections are observed at scanning magnification'.[7] The term is not used uniformly or consistently. Some apply it to most dermatoses with the lichenoid tissue reaction. Others use it for the subgroup in which the infiltrate truly obscures the interface (erythema multiforme, fixed drug eruption, paraneoplastic pemphigus, some cases of subacute lupus erythematosus and pityriasis lichenoides). The infiltrate may obscure the interface in lymphomatoid papulosis, but basal cell damage is not invariable. Many apply the term, also, to lichen planus and variants, in which the infiltrate characteristically 'hugs' the basal layer without much extension into the epidermis beyond the basal layer. The author prefers the traditional term 'lichenoid' for this group of dermatoses because it is applicable more consistently than interface dermatitis and it is less likely to be applied as a 'final sign-out diagnosis', which is often the case with the term interface dermatitis. The term is so entrenched that it is unlikely to disappear from the lexicon of dermatopathology.

In *apoptosis*, single cells become condensed and then fragment into small bodies by an active budding process (Fig. 3.1). In the skin, these condensed apoptotic bodies are known as Civatte bodies (see above). The smaller apoptotic bodies, some of which are beyond the resolution of the light microscope, are usually phagocytosed quickly by adjacent parenchymal cells or by tissue macrophages.[5] Cell membranes and organelles remain intact for some time in apoptosis, in contradistinction to necrosis where breakdown of these structures is an integral and prominent part of the process. Keratinocytes contain tonofilaments which act as a 'straitjacket' within the cell, and therefore budding and fragmentation are less complete in the skin than they are in other cells in the body undergoing death by apoptosis. This is particularly so if the keratinocyte has accumulated filaments in its cytoplasm, as occurs with its progressive maturation in the epidermis. The term 'dyskeratotic cell' is usually used for these degenerate keratinocytes. The apoptotic bodies that are rich in tonofilaments are usually larger than the others; they tend to 'resist' phagocytosis by parenchymal cells, although some are phagocytosed by macrophages. Others are extruded into the papillary dermis, where they are known as *colloid bodies*. These bodies appear to trap immunoglobulins non-specifically, particularly the IgM molecule, which is larger than the others.

Some of the diseases included within the lichenoid reaction pattern show necrosis of the epidermis rather than apoptosis; in others, the cells have accumulated so many cytoplasmic filaments prior to death that the actual mechanism – apoptosis or necrosis – cannot be discerned by light or electron

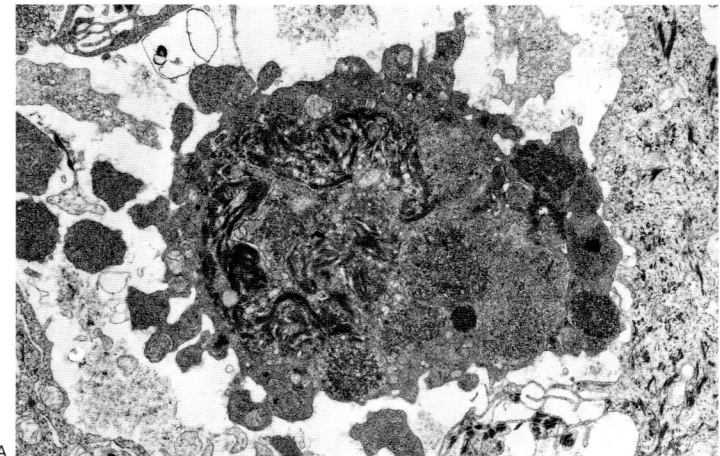

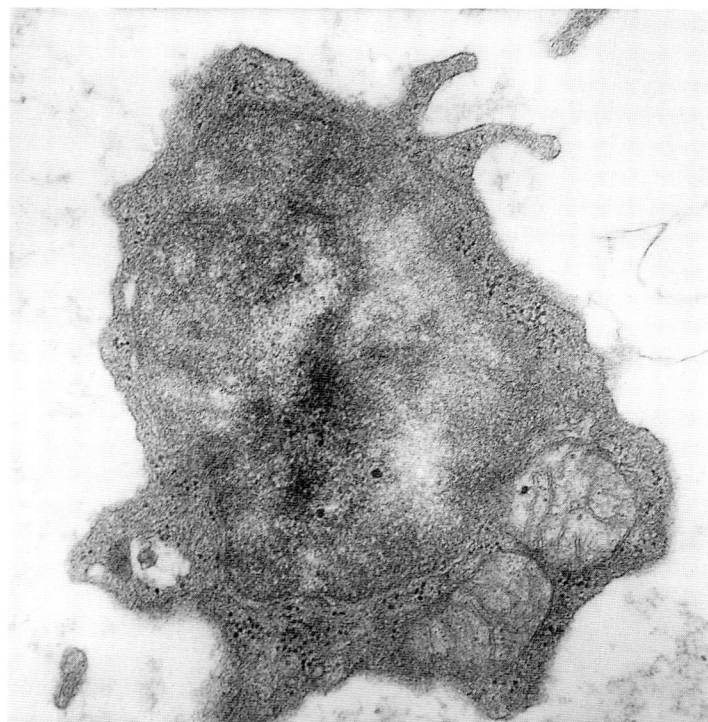

Fig. 3.1 **(A) Apoptosis of a basal keratinocyte in lichen planus.** There is surface budding and some redistribution of organelles within the cytoplasm. Electron micrograph × 12000. **(B) A tiny budding fragment in which the mitochondria have intact cristae.** (× 25000)

microscopy. The term 'filamentous degeneration' has been suggested for these cells;[8] on light microscopy, they are referred to as 'dyskeratotic cells' (see above). It should be noted that apoptotic keratinocytes have been seen in normal skin, indicating that cell deletion also occurs as a normal physiological phenomenon.[9-11] As Afford and Randhawa have so eloquently stated 'Apoptosis is the genetically regulated form of cell death that permits the safe disposal of cells at the point in time when they have fulfilled their intended biological function.'[12] It also plays a role in the elimination of the inflammatory infiltrate at the end stages of wound healing.[13]

Although it is beyond the scope of this book, readers interested in apoptosis and the intricate mechanisms of its control should read the excellent studies published on this topic.[14-22] Ackerman has continued to present a minority view that apoptosis is a type of necrosis.[23] In reality, each is a distinctive form of cell death.

Vacuolar change (liquefaction degeneration) is often an integral part of the basal damage in the lichenoid reaction. Sometimes it is more prominent than the cell death. It results from intracellular vacuole formation and edema, as well as from separation of the lamina densa from the plasma membrane of the basal cells. Vacuolar change is usually prominent in lupus erythematosus, particularly the acute systemic form, and in dermatomyositis and some drug reactions.

As a consequence of the basal cell damage, there is variable *melanin incontinence* resulting from interference with melanin transfer from melanocytes to keratinocytes, as well as from the death of cells in the basal layer.[1] Melanin incontinence is particularly prominent in some drug-induced and solar-related lichenoid lesions, as well as in patients with marked racial pigmentation.

Another feature of the lichenoid reaction pattern is a variable *inflammatory cell infiltrate*. This varies in composition, density and distribution according to the disease. An assessment of these characteristics is important in distinguishing the various lichenoid dermatoses. As apoptosis, unlike necrosis, does not itself evoke an inflammatory response, it can be surmised that the infiltrate in those diseases with prominent apoptosis is of pathogenetic significance and not a secondary event.[5] Furthermore, apoptosis is the usual method of cell death resulting from cell-mediated mechanisms, whereas necrosis and possibly vacuolar change result from humoral factors, including the deposition of immune complexes.

One study has given some insight into the possible mechanisms involved in the variability of expression of the lichenoid tissue reaction in several of the diseases within this group. The study examined the patterns of expression of the intercellular adhesion molecule-1 (ICAM-1).[24] Keratinocytes in normal epidermis have a low constitutive expression of ICAM-1, rendering the normal epidermis resistant to interaction with leukocytes. Therefore, induction of ICAM-1 expression may be an important factor in the induction of leukocyte-dependent damage to keratinocytes.[24] In lichen planus, ICAM-1 expression is limited to basal keratinocytes, while in subacute cutaneous lupus erythematosus there is diffuse epidermal ICAM-1 expression, sometimes with basal accentuation. This pattern is induced by ultraviolet radiation and possibly mediated by tumor necrosis factor-α. In erythema multiforme, there is strong basal expression of ICAM-1, with cell surface accentuation and similar pockets of suprabasal expression, probably induced by herpes simplex virus infection.[24]

In summary, the lichenoid reaction pattern includes a heterogeneous group of diseases which have in common basal cell damage.[25] The histogenesis is also diverse and includes cell-mediated and humoral immune reactions and possibly ischemia in one condition. Scattered apoptotic keratinocytes can also be seen in the sunburn reaction in response to ultraviolet radiation;[26,27] these cells are known as 'sunburn cells'.[28] A specific histological diagnosis can usually be made by attention to such factors as:

- the nature and extent of the basal damage
- the nature, composition and distribution of the inflammatory reaction
- the amount of melanin incontinence which results from the basal damage
- the coexistence of another tissue reaction[29]
- other individual characteristics.[2]

These points are considered further in Tables 3.1, 3.2 and 3.3.

A discussion of the various lichenoid (interface) dermatoses follows. The conditions listed as 'other lichenoid (interface) diseases' are discussed only briefly as they are considered in detail in other chapters.

Table 3.1 **Key histopathological features of various lichenoid diseases**

Disease	Histopathological features
Lichen planus	Prominent Civatte bodies, band-like inflammatory infiltrate, wedge-shaped hypergranulosis. Hypertrophic form has changes limited to the tips of the acanthotic downgrowths and often superadded lichen simplex chronicus. The infiltrate extends around hair follicles in lichen planopilaris. Pigment incontinence is conspicuous in erythema dyschromicum perstans.
Lichen nitidus	Focal (papular) lichenoid lesions; some giant cells; dermal infiltrate often 'clasped' by acanthotic downgrowths.
Lichen striatus	Clinically linear; irregular and discontinuous lichenoid reaction; infiltrate sometimes around follicles and sweat glands.
Lichen planus-like keratosis	Solitary; prominent Civatte body formation; solar lentigo often at margins.
Lichenoid drug eruptions	Focal parakeratosis; eosinophils, plasma cells and melanin incontinence may be features. Deep extension of the infiltrate occurs in photolichenoid lesions.
Fixed drug eruptions	Interface-obscuring infiltrate, often extends deeper than erythema multiforme; cell death often above basal layer; neutrophils often present.
Erythema multiforme	Interface-obscuring infiltrate; sometimes subepidermal vesiculation and variable epidermal cell death.
Graft-versus-host disease	Basal vacuolation; scattered apoptotic keratinocytes, sometimes with attached lymphocytes ('satellite cell necrosis'); variable lymphocytic infiltrate.
Lupus erythematosus	Mixed vacuolar change and Civatte bodies. SLE has prominent vacuolar change and minimal cell death. Discoid lupus away from the face has more cell death and superficial and deep infiltrate; mucin; follicular plugging; basement membrane thickening. Some cases resemble erythema multiforme with cell death at all layers.
Dermatomyositis	May resemble acute lupus with vacuolar change, epidermal atrophy, some dermal mucin; infiltrate usually superficial and often sparse.
Poikiloderma	Vacuolar change; telangiectasia; pigment incontinence; late dermal sclerosis.
Pityriasis lichenoides	Acute form combines lymphocytic vasculitis with epidermal cell death; interface-obscuring infiltrate; focal hemorrhage; focal parakeratosis.
Paraneoplastic pemphigus	Erythema multiforme-like changes with suprabasal acantholysis and clefting; subepidermal clefting sometimes present.

LICHENOID (INTERFACE) DERMATOSES

LICHEN PLANUS

Lichen planus, a relatively common eruption of unknown etiology, displays violaceous, flat-topped papules, which are usually pruritic.[30,31] A network of fine white lines (Wickham's striae) may be seen on the surface of the papules. There is a predilection for the flexor surface of the wrists, the trunk, the thighs and the genitalia. Palmoplantar lesions appear to be more common than once thought.[32] Oral lesions are common; rarely the esophagus is also involved.[33,34] Lesions localized to the lip,[35] vulva[36,37] and to an eyelid[38] have been reported. Nail changes occur[39,40] and, as with oral lesions, these may be the only manifestations of the disease.[41] Clinical variants include atrophic,

Table 3.2 **Diagnoses associated with various pathological changes in the lichenoid reaction pattern**

Pathological change	Possible diagnoses
Vacuolar change	Lupus erythematosus, dermatomyositis, drugs and poikiloderma
Interface-obscuring infiltrate	Erythema multiforme, fixed drug eruption, pityriasis lichenoides (acute), paraneoplastic pemphigus, lupus erythematosus (some)
Purpura	Lichenoid purpura
Cornoid lamella	Porokeratosis
Deep dermal infiltrate	Lupus erythematosus, syphilis, drugs, photolichenoid eruption
'Satellite cell necrosis'	Graft-versus-host disease, eruption of lymphocyte recovery, erythema multiforme, paraneoplastic pemphigus, regressing plane warts, drug reactions
Prominent pigment incontinence	Poikiloderma, drugs, 'racial pigmentation' and an associated lichenoid reaction, erythema dyschromicum perstans and related entities
Eccrine duct involvement	Erythema multiforme (drug induced), lichen striatus, keratosis lichenoides chronica, periflexural exanthem of childhood

Table 3.3 **Diseases with the lichenoid and one or more coexisting tissue reaction patterns**

Additional pattern	Possible diagnosis
Spongiotic	Drug reactions (see spongiotic drug reactions), lichenoid contact dermatitis, lichen striatus
Granulomatous	Lichen nitidus, lichen striatus (rare), secondary syphilis, herpes zoster infection, tinea capitis, *Mycobacterium marinum*, *M. haemophilum*, drug reactions (often in setting of Crohn's disease or rheumatoid arthritis – atenolol, allopurinol, captopril, enalapril, simvastatin, diclofenac)
Vasculitic	Pityriasis lichenoides, perniosis (some cases), pigmented purpuric dermatosis (lichenoid variant), persistent viral reactions, including herpes simplex
Vasculitic/spongiotic	Gianotti–Crosti syndrome, some other viral/putative viral diseases, rare drug reactions

annular, hypertrophic, linear, zosteriform,[42] erosive, actinic, follicular, erythematous and bullous variants. They are discussed further below. Spontaneous resolution of lichen planus is usual within 12 months, although post-inflammatory pigmentation may persist for some time afterwards.[43]

Familial cases are uncommon, and rarely these are associated with HLA-D7.[44–46] An association with HLA-DR1 has been found in non-familial cases.[47] There is an increased frequency of HLA-DR6 in Italian patients with hepatitis C virus-associated oral lichen planus.[48] Lichen planus is rare in children.[49–54] Lichen planus has been reported in association with immunodeficiency states,[55] internal malignancy,[56,57] primary biliary cirrhosis,[58,59] peptic ulcer (but not *Helicobacter pylori* infection),[60] chronic hepatitis C infection,[61–69] hepatitis B vaccination,[70–75] pemphigus,[76] porphyria cutanea tarda,[77] ulcerative colitis,[78] a Becker's nevus,[79] and lichen sclerosus et atrophicus with coexisting morphea.[80] Reports linking lichen planus to infection with human papillomavirus may be a false-positive result.[81,82] Squamous cell carcinoma is a rare complication of the oral and vulval cases of lichen planus and of the hypertrophic and ulcerative

variants (see below).[83–86] A contact allergy to metals, flavorings and plastics may be important in the etiology of oral lichen planus.[87]

Cell-mediated immune reactions appear to be important in the pathogenesis of lichen planus.[88] It has been suggested that these reactions are precipitated by an alteration in the antigenicity of epidermal keratinocytes, possibly caused by a virus or a drug or by an allogeneic cell.[89] Keratinocytes in lichen planus express HLA-DR on their surface and this may be one of the antigens which has an inductive or perpetuating role in the process.[90–92] Keratinocytes also express fetal cytokeratins (K13 and K8/18) but whether they are responsible for triggering the T-cell response is speculative.[93] The cellular response, initially, consists of CD4$^+$ lymphocytes;[94] they are also increased in the peripheral blood.[95] In recent years attention has focused on the role of cytotoxic CD8$^+$ lymphocytes in a number of cell-mediated immune reactions in the skin. They appear to play a significant role as the effector cell, whereas the CD4$^+$ lymphocyte, usually present in greater numbers, plays its traditional 'helper' role. In lichen planus, CD8$^+$ cells appear to recognize an antigen associated with MHC class I on lesional keratinocytes, resulting in their death by apoptosis.[96] The recruitment of lymphocytes to the interface region may be the result of the chemokine MIG (monokine induced by interferon-γ).[97] Lymphokines produced by these T lymphocytes, including interferon-γ, interleukins-1β, -4 and -6 and tumor necrosis factor, may have an effector role in producing the apoptosis of keratinocytes.[93,99] A unique subclass of cytotoxic T lymphocyte (γδ) is also found in established lesions.[100] Langerhans cells are increased and it has been suggested that these cells initially process the foreign antigen.[91] Factor XIIIa-positive cells and macrophages expressing lysozyme are found in the dermis.[94] Matrix metalloproteinases may play a concurrent role by destroying the basement membrane. Evidence from an animal model suggests that keratinocytes require cell survival signals, derived from the basement membrane, to prevent the onset of apoptosis.[101]

Most studies have found no autoantibodies and no alteration in serum immunoglobulins in lichen planus.[102] However, a lichen planus-specific antigen has been detected in the epidermis and a circulating antibody to it has been found in the serum of individuals with lichen planus.[103] Its pathogenetic significance remains uncertain.

Replacement of the damaged basal cells is achieved by an increase in actively dividing keratinocytes in both the epidermis and the skin appendages. This is reflected in the pattern of keratin expression, which resembles that seen in wound healing; keratin 17 (K17) is found in suprabasal keratinocytes.[104]

Histopathology[105]

The basal cell damage in lichen planus takes the form of multiple, scattered Civatte bodies (Fig. 3.2). Eosinophilic colloid bodies, which are PAS positive and diastase resistant, are found in the papillary dermis (Fig. 3.3). They measure approximately 20 μm in diameter. The basal damage is associated with a band-like infiltrate of lymphocytes and some macrophages which press against the undersurface of the epidermis (Fig. 3.4). Occasional lymphocytes extend into the basal layer, where they may be found in close contact with basal cells and sometimes with Civatte bodies. The infiltrate does not obscure the interface or extend into the mid-epidermis, as in erythema multiforme and fixed drug eruptions. Karyorrhexis is sometimes seen in the dermal infiltrate.[106] Rarely, plasma cells are prominent in the cutaneous lesions;[107–109] they are invariably present in lesions adjacent to or on mucous membranes. There is variable melanin incontinence but this is most conspicuous in lesions of long duration and in dark-skinned people.

Other characteristic epidermal changes include hyperkeratosis, wedge-shaped areas of hypergranulosis related to the acrosyringia and acrotrichia,

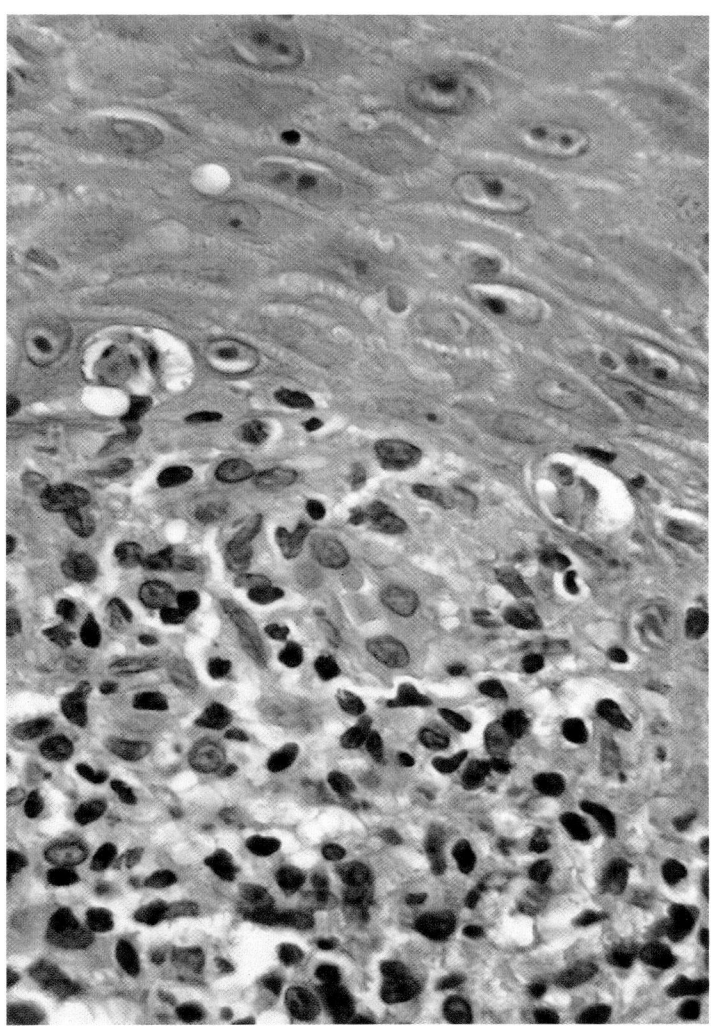

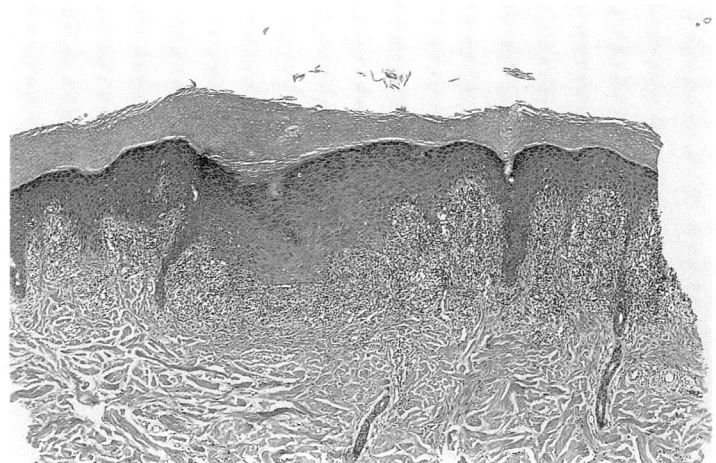

Fig. 3.4 **Lichen planus.** A band-like infiltrate of lymphocytes fills the papillary dermis and touches the undersurface of the epidermis. (H & E)

(Caspary–Joseph spaces)[110] may form at the dermoepidermal junction secondary to the basal damage. The eccrine duct adjacent to the acrosyringium is sometimes involved.[111] A variant in which the lichenoid changes were localized entirely to the acrosyringium has been reported.[112] Transepidermal elimination with perforation is another rare finding.[113] The formation of milia may be a late complication.[114]

Ragaz and Ackerman have studied the evolution of lesions in lichen planus.[105] They found an increased number of Langerhans cells in the epidermis in the very earliest lesions, before there was any significant infiltrate of inflammatory cells in the dermis. In resolving lesions, the infiltrate is less dense and there may be minimal extension of the inflammatory infiltrate into the reticular dermis.

As already mentioned, some diseases exhibiting the lichenoid tissue reaction may also show features of another tissue reaction pattern as a major or minor feature. These conditions are listed in Table 3.3.

Direct immunofluorescence of involved skin shows colloid bodies in the papillary dermis, staining for complement and immunoglobulins, particularly IgM. An irregular band of fibrin is present along the basal layer in most cases. Often there is irregular extension of the fibrin into the underlying papillary dermis (Fig. 3.5). Immunofluorescent analysis of the basement membrane zone, using a range of antibodies, suggests that disruption occurs in the lamina lucida region.[115] Other studies have shown a disturbance in the epithelial anchoring system.[116]

Electron microscopy

Ultrastructural studies have confirmed that lymphocytes attach to basal keratinocytes, resulting in their death by apoptosis.[4,5,117] Many cell fragments, beyond the limit of resolution of the light microscope, are formed during the budding of the dying cells. The cell fragments are phagocytosed by adjacent keratinocytes and macrophages.[118] The large tonofilament-rich bodies that result from redistribution of tonofilaments during cell fragmentation appear to resist phagocytosis and are extruded into the upper dermis, where they are recognized on light microscopy as colloid bodies.[119] Various studies have confirmed the epidermal origin of these colloid bodies.[120,121] There is a suggestion from some experimental work that sublethal injury to keratinocytes may lead to the accumulation of tonofilaments in their cytoplasm. Some apoptotic bodies contain more filaments than would be accounted for by a simple redistribution of the usual tonofilament content of the cell.

Fig. 3.2 **Lichen planus.** Two apoptotic keratinocytes (Civatte bodies) are present in the basal layer of the epidermis. An infiltrate of lymphocytes touches the undersurface of the epidermis. (H & E)

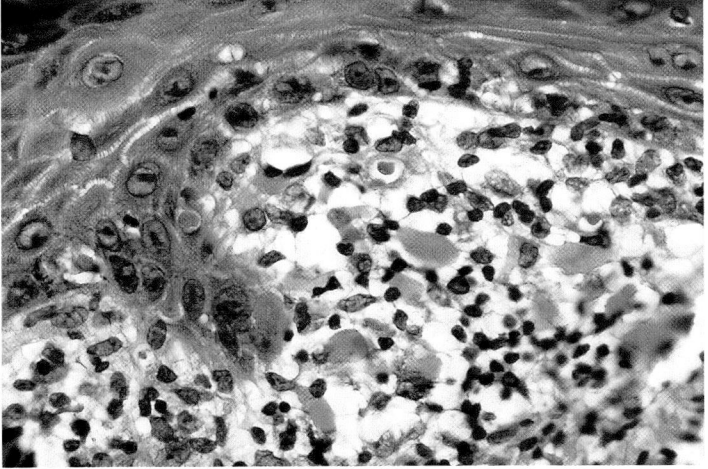

Fig. 3.3 **Lichen planus.** There are numerous colloid bodies in the papillary dermis. (H & E)

and variable acanthosis. At times the rete ridges become pointed, imparting a 'saw tooth' appearance to the lower epidermis. There is sometimes mild hypereosinophilia of keratinocytes in the malpighian layer. Small clefts

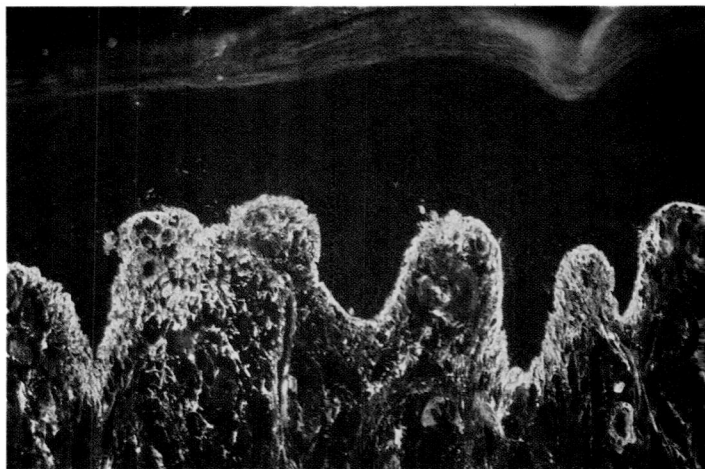

Fig. 3.5 **Lichen planus.** A band of fibrin involves the basement membrane zone and extends into the papillary dermis. (Direct immunofluorescence)

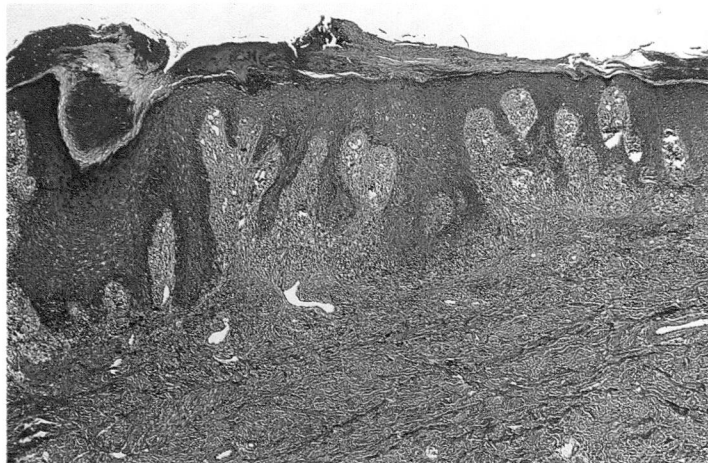

Fig. 3.6 **Hypertrophic lichen planus.** The epidermis shows irregular hyperplasia. The dermal infiltrate is concentrated near the tips of the rete ridges. (H & E)

LICHEN PLANUS VARIANTS

A number of clinical variants of lichen planus occur. In some, typical lesions of lichen planus are also present. These variants are discussed in further detail below.

Atrophic lichen planus

Atrophic lesions may resemble porokeratosis clinically. Typical papules of lichen planus are usually present at the margins. A rare form of atrophic lichen planus is composed of annular lesions.[122–124] Experimentally, there is an impaired capacity of the atrophic epithelium to maintain a regenerative steady state.

Histopathology

The epidermis is thin and there is loss of the normal rete ridge pattern. The infiltrate is usually less dense than in typical lichen planus.

Hypertrophic lichen planus

Hypertrophic lesions are usually confined to the shins, although sometimes they are more generalized. They appear as single or multiple pruritic plaques, which may have a verrucous appearance;[125] they usually persist for many years. Rarely, squamous cell carcinoma develops in lesions of long standing.[126] Cutaneous horns, keratoacanthoma and verrucous carcinoma may also develop in hypertrophic lichen planus.[127–129]

Hypertrophic lichen planus has been reported in several patients infected with the human immunodeficiency virus.[130]

Histopathology

The epidermis shows prominent hyperplasia and overlying orthokeratosis (Fig. 3.6). At the margins there is usually psoriasiform hyperplasia representing concomitant changes of lichen simplex chronicus secondary to the rubbing and scratching. If the epidermal hyperplasia is severe it may mimic a squamous cell carcinoma on a shave biopsy.[131] Vertically oriented collagen ('vertical-streaked collagen') is present in the papillary dermis in association with the changes of lichen simplex chronicus.

The basal cell damage is usually confined to the tips of the rete ridges and may be missed on casual observation (Fig. 3.7). The infiltrate is not as dense or as band-like as in the usual lesions of lichen planus. A few eosinophils and plasma cells may be seen in some cases in which the ingestion of beta blockers can sometimes be incriminated.

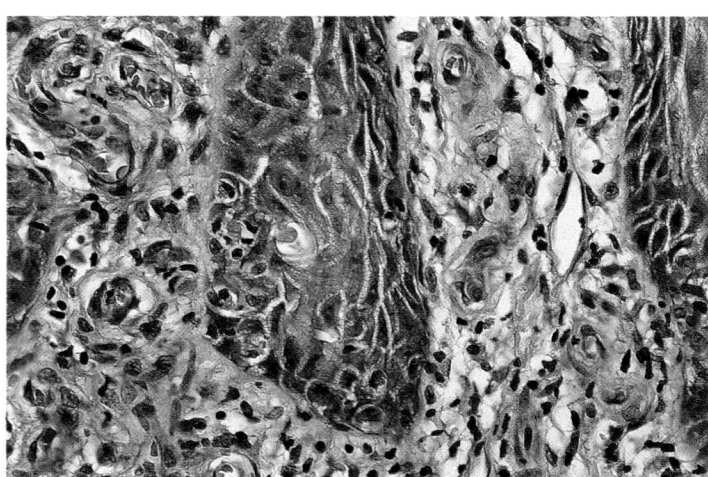

Fig. 3.7 **Hypertrophic lichen planus.** There are a number of civalte bodies near the tips of the rete ridges.

Xanthoma cells have been found in the dermis, localized to a plaque of hypertrophic lichen planus, in a patient with secondary hyperlipidemia.[132] This is an example of dystrophic xanthomatization.

Linear lichen planus

Linear lichen planus is a rare variant which must be distinguished from linear nevi and other dermatoses with linear variants.[133,134] Linear lichen planus usually involves the limbs. It may follow the lines of Blaschko.[135]

Ulcerative (erosive) lichen planus

Ulcerative lichen planus (erosive lichen planus) is characterized by ulcerated and bullous lesions on the feet.[136] Mucosal lesions, alopecia and more typical lesions of lichen planus are sometimes present. Squamous cell carcinoma may develop in lesions of long standing. Variants of ulcerative lichen planus involving the perineal region,[137] penis,[138] the mouth[139] or the vulva, vagina and mouth – the vulvovaginal-gingival syndrome[140–142] – have been reported. A patient with erosive lesions of the flexures has been reported.[143]

Castleman's tumor (giant lymph node hyperplasia) and malignant lymphoma are rare associations of erosive lichen planus;[144,145] long-term therapy with hydroxyurea and infection with hepatitis C are others.[146]

Antibodies directed against a nuclear antigen of epithelial cells have been reported in patients with erosive lichen planus of the oral mucosa.[147]

Histopathology

There is epidermal ulceration with more typical changes of lichen planus at the margins of the ulcer. Plasma cells are invariably present in cases involving mucosal surfaces. Eosinophils were prominent in the oral lesions of a case associated with methyldopa therapy.

Lichen planus erythematosus

Lichen planus erythematosus has been challenged as an entity. Non-pruritic, red papules, with a predilection for the forearms, have been described.[125]

Histopathology

A proliferation of blood vessels may be seen in the upper dermis in addition to the usual features of lichen planus.

Erythema dyschromicum perstans

Erythema dyschromicum perstans (ashy dermatosis, lichen planus pigmentosus)[148] is a slowly progressive, asymptomatic, ash-colored or brown macular hyperpigmentation[149-151] which has been reported from most parts of the world; it is most prevalent in Latin America. Lesions are often quite widespread, although there is a predilection for the trunk. Unilateral[152] and linear lesions[153] have been described. Activity of the disease may cease after several years.

Erythema dyschromicum perstans has been regarded as a macular variant of lichen planus[154] on the basis of the simultaneous occurrence of both conditions in several patients[151,155,156] and similar immunopathological findings.[157,158] Paraphenylenediamine has been incriminated in its etiology,[154] although this has not been confirmed. This condition has also been reported in patients with HIV infection.[159]

Lichen planus pigmentosus, originally reported from India, is thought by some to be the same condition,[150,154] although this has been disputed.[160,161] It has been reported in association with a head and neck cancer and with concurrent acrokeratosis paraneoplastica (see p. 575). Both conditions cleared after treatment of the cancer.[162]

Histopathology[149]

In the active phase, there is a lichenoid tissue reaction with basal vacuolar change and occasional Civatte bodies (Fig. 3.8). The infiltrate is usually quite mild in comparison to lichen planus. Furthermore, there may be deeper extension of the infiltrate. There is prominent melanin incontinence and this is the only significant feature in older lesions. The pigment usually extends deeper in the dermis than in postinflammatory pigmentation of other causes.[160] Cases reported as lichen planus pigmentosus (see above) have similar histological features.[161]

Immunofluorescence has shown IgM, IgG and complement-containing colloid bodies in the dermis, as in lichen planus. Apoptosis and residual filamentous bodies are present on electron microscopy.[149]

Lichen planus actinicus

Lichen planus actinicus is a distinct clinical variant of lichen planus in which lesions are limited to sun-exposed areas of the body.[163,164] It has a predilection for certain races,[165] particularly young individuals of Oriental origin. There is some variability in the clinical expression of the disease in different countries and this has contributed to the proliferation of terms used – lichen planus tropicus,[166] lichen planus subtropicus,[167] lichenoid melanodermatitis[168] and summertime actinic lichenoid eruption (SALE).[164,169] More recently it has

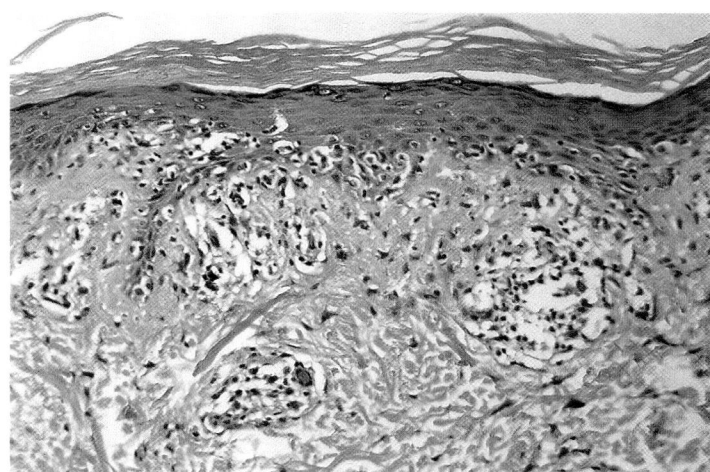

Fig. 3.8 **Erythema dyschromicum perstans.** There is patchy basal cell damage and some pigment incontinence. (H & E)

been suggested that SALE is an actinic variant of lichen nitidus. The development of pigmentation in some cases[170] has also led to the suggestion that there is overlap with erythema dyschromicum perstans (see above).[155] The pigmentation may take the form of melasma-like lesions.[171,172] Lesions have been induced by repeated exposure to ultraviolet radiation.[173]

Histopathology[167]

The appearances resemble lichen planus quite closely,[174] although there is usually more marked melanin incontinence[164,173] and there may be focal parakeratosis.[163] The inflammatory cell infiltrate in lichen planus actinicus is not always as heavy as it is in typical lesions of lichen planus.

Numerous immunoglobulin-coated cytoid bodies are usually present on direct immunofluorescence.[175]

Lichen planopilaris

Lichen planopilaris (follicular lichen planus) is a clinically heterogeneous variant of lichen planus in which keratotic follicular lesions are present, often in association with other manifestations of lichen planus.[176-178] The most common and important clinical group is characterized by scarring alopecia of the scalp, which is generalized in about half of these cases. The keratotic follicular lesions and associated erythema are best seen at the margins of the scarring alopecia.[179] In this group, changes of lichen planus are present or develop subsequently in approximately 50% of cases.[179] The Graham Little–Piccardi–Lassueur syndrome is a rare but closely related entity in which there is cicatricial alopecia of the scalp, follicular keratotic lesions of glabrous skin, and variable alopecia of the axillae and groins.[178,180,181] Two other clinical groups occur but they have not received as much attention.[177] In one, there are follicular papules, without scarring, usually on the trunk and extremities. In the other, which is quite rare, there are plaques with follicular papules, usually in the retroauricular region, although other sites can be involved.[177] This variant has been called lichen planus follicularis tumidus.[182]

Rare variants of lichen planopilaris include a linear form[183-185] and the presence of lesions confined to the vulva.[186]

Histopathology[176,177,179]

In lichen planopilaris, there is a lichenoid reaction pattern involving the basal layer of the follicular epithelium, with an associated dense perifollicular infiltrate of lymphocytes and a few macrophages (Fig. 3.9). The changes involve the infundibulum and the isthmus of the follicle. Unlike lupus erythe-

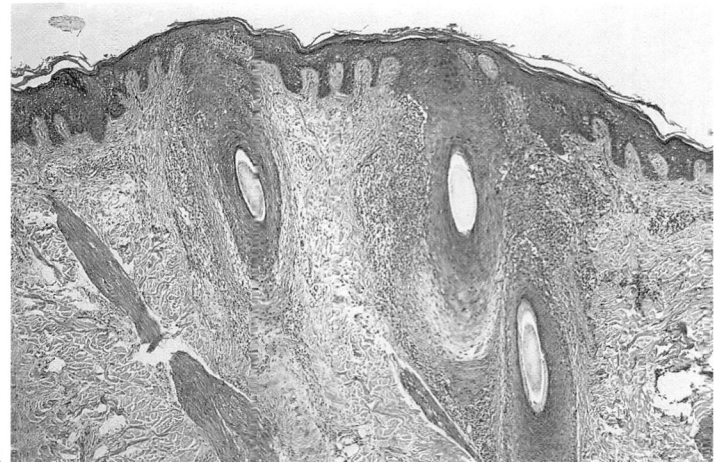

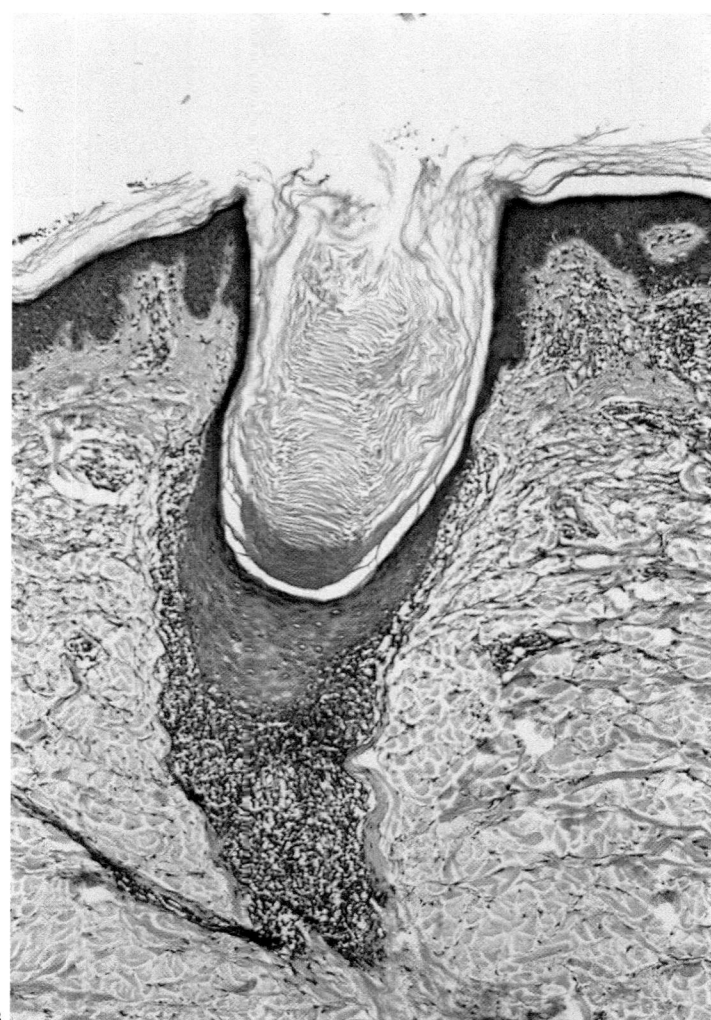

Fig. 3.9 **Lichen planopilaris.** The lichenoid infiltrate is confined to a perifollicular location. Two different cases – **(A)** and **(B)**. (H & E)

matosus, the infiltrate does not extend around blood vessels of the mid and deep plexus. The interfollicular epidermis is involved in up to one-third of cases with scalp involvement[177,179,187] and in the rare plaque type (see above). It is not usually involved in the variant with follicular papules on the trunk and extremities.[177] If scarring alopecia develops there is variable perifollicular

fibrosis and loss of hair follicles which are replaced by linear tracts of fibrosis.[187] The papillary dermis may also be fibrosed. In advanced cases of scarring alopecia, the diagnostic features may no longer be present. The term 'pseudopelade' has been used by some for cases of end-stage scarring alopecia.

Direct immunofluorescence shows colloid bodies containing IgG and IgM in the dermis adjacent to the upper portion of the involved follicles.[178,188] In one report, linear deposits of immunoglobulins were found along the basement membrane of the hair follicles (of the scalp) in all cases. Fibrin was present in one case; cytoid bodies were not demonstrated.[189] It should be noted that the lesions were of long standing (3–7 years).[189]

Lichen planus pemphigoides

This rare disease is characterized by the coexistence of lichen planus and a heterogenous group of subepidermal blistering diseases resembling bullous pemphigoid.[190–192] There are tense bullae, often on the extremities, which may develop in normal or erythematous skin or in the lesions of lichen planus.[193–196] They do not necessarily recur with subsequent exacerbations of the lichen planus.[197,198] Oral lesions are exceedingly rare.[199] Lichen planus pemphigoides has been reported in children.[197,198] Rare clinical presentations include a unilateral distribution and onset following PUVA therapy.[200,201] Similar lesions have been induced by the anti-motion sickness drug cinnarizine and by the ACE inhibitor ramipril.[202,203]

Lichen planus pemphigoides is different from **bullous lichen planus**[204] in which vesicles or bullae develop only in the lichenoid papules, probably as a result of unusually severe basal damage and accompanying dermal edema.[205,206]

The pathogenesis of lichen planus pemphigoides appears to be due to epitope spreading. It has been suggested that damage to the basal layer in lichen planus may expose or release a basement membrane zone antigen, which leads to the formation of circulating antibodies and consequent blister formation.[207–209] The target antigen is a novel epitope (MCW-4) within the C-terminal NC16A domain of the 180 kd bullous pemphigoid antigen (BP180, type XVII collagen).[210–212]

Lichenoid erythrodermic bullous pemphigoid is a rare disease reported in African patients. It differs from lichen planus pemphigoides by the presence of a desquamative erythroderma and frequent mucosal lesions.[213]

Histopathology

A typical lesion of lichen planus pemphigoides consists of a subepidermal bulla which is cell poor, with only a mild, perivascular infiltrate of lymphocytes, neutrophils and eosinophils.[214] The presence of neutrophils and eosinophils has not been mentioned in all reports. Sometimes a lichenoid infiltrate is present at the margins of the blister[205] and there are occasional degenerate keratinocytes in the epidermis overlying the blister.[193] Lesions which arise in papules of lichen planus show predominantly the features of lichen planus; a few eosinophils and neutrophils are usually present, in contrast to bullous lichen planus in which they are absent.[193] In one report, a pemphigus vulgaris-like pattern was present in the bullous areas.[215]

Direct immunofluorescence of the bullae will usually show IgG, C3 and C9 neoantigen in the basement membrane zone and there is often a circulating antibody to the basement membrane zone.[216,217] Indirect split-skin immunofluorescence has shown binding to the roof of the split.[208]

Electron microscopy

In lichen planus pemphigoides the split occurs in the lamina lucida, as it does in bullous pemphigoid.[208,218] Immunoelectron microscopy has shown that the localization of the immune deposits may resemble that seen in bullous pemphigoid, cicatricial pemphigoid or epidermolysis bullosa acquisita, evidence of a heterogeneous disorder.[219]

Keratosis lichenoides chronica

Keratosis lichenoides chronica is characterized by violaceous, papular and nodular lesions in a linear and reticulate pattern on the extremities and a seborrheic dermatitis-like facial eruption.[220-226] Oral ulceration and nail involvement may occur.[227,228] It is a rare condition, particularly in children.[229,230] The condition is possibly an unusual chronic variant of lichen planus, although this concept has been challenged.[231,232]

Keratosis lichenoides chronica may be associated with internal diseases such as glomerulonephritis and lymphoproliferative disorders.[231,233]

Histopathology

There is a lichenoid reaction pattern with prominent basal cell death and focal basal vacuolar change.[234] The inflammatory infiltrate usually includes a few plasma cells and sometimes there is deeper perivascular and periappendageal cuffing.[235] Telangiectasia of superficial dermal vessels is sometimes noted.[236] Epidermal changes are variable, with alternating areas of atrophy and acanthosis sometimes present, as well as focal parakeratosis. Cornoid lamellae and amyloid deposits in the papillary dermis have been recorded.[232] Numerous IgM-containing colloid bodies are usually found on direct immunofluorescence.[227]

The term '**lichen planoporitis**' was used for a case with the clinical features of keratosis lichenoides chronica and histologic changes that included a lichenoid reaction centered on the acrosyringium and upper eccrine duct with focal squamous metaplasia of the upper duct and overlying hypergranulosis and keratin plugs.[237] Ruben and LeBoit have also reported eccrine duct involvement in a case of keratosis lichenoides chronica.[238]

Lupus erythematosus–lichen planus overlap syndrome

Lupus erythematosus–lichen planus overlap syndrome is a heterogeneous entity in which one or more of the clinical, histological and immunopathological features of both diseases are present.[239,240] Some cases may represent the co-existence of lichen planus and lupus erythematosus, while in others the ultimate diagnosis may depend on the course of the disease.[241,242] In most cases, the lupus erythematosus is of the chronic discoid or systemic type; rarely, it is of the subacute type.[243] Before the diagnosis of an overlap syndrome is entertained, it should be remembered that some lesions of cutaneous lupus erythematosus may have numerous Civatte bodies and a rather superficial inflammatory cell infiltrate which at first glance may be mistaken for lichen planus. The use of an immunofluorescent technique using patient's serum and autologous lesional skin as a substrate may assist in the future in elucidating the correct diagnosis in some of these cases.[244]

LICHEN NITIDUS

Lichen nitidus is a rare, usually asymptomatic chronic eruption characterized by the presence of multiple, small flesh-colored papules, 1–2 mm in diameter.[245,246] The lesions have a predilection for the upper extremities, chest, abdomen and genitalia of children and young adult males.[245,247] Familial cases are rare.[248] Nail changes[249,250] and involvement of the palms and soles[251-253] have been reported. It has been suggested that cases reported in the past as summertime actinic lichenoid eruption (SALE) should be re-classified as actinic lichen nitidus.[254,255]

Although regarded originally as a variant of lichen planus, lichen nitidus is now considered a distinct entity of unknown etiology. The lymphocytes in the dermal infiltrate in lichen nitidus express different markers from those in lichen planus.[256]

Histopathology

A papule of lichen nitidus shows a dense, well-circumscribed, subepidermal infiltrate, sharply limited to one or two adjacent dermal papillae.[245] Claw-like, acanthotic rete ridges, which appear to grasp the infiltrate, are present at the periphery of the papule (Fig. 3.10). The inflammatory cells push against the undersurface of the epidermis, which may be thinned and show overlying parakeratosis. Occasional Civatte bodies are present in the basal layer.

In addition to lymphocytes, histiocytes and melanophages, there are also epithelioid cells and occasional multinucleate giant cells in the inflammatory infiltrate.[257] Rarely, plasma cells are conspicuous.[258] The appearances are sometimes frankly granulomatous and these lesions must be distinguished from disseminated granuloma annulare in which the infiltrate may be superficial and the necrobiosis sometimes quite subtle. Lichen nitidus also needs to be distinguished from an early lesion of lichen scrofulosorum. While the infiltrate in lichen nitidus 'hugs' the epidermis and expands the dermal papilla, the granulomas in lichen scrofulosorum do not cause widening of the papillae. Furthermore, in lichen scrofulosorum there may be mild spongiosis and exocytosis of neutrophils into the epidermis.[259]

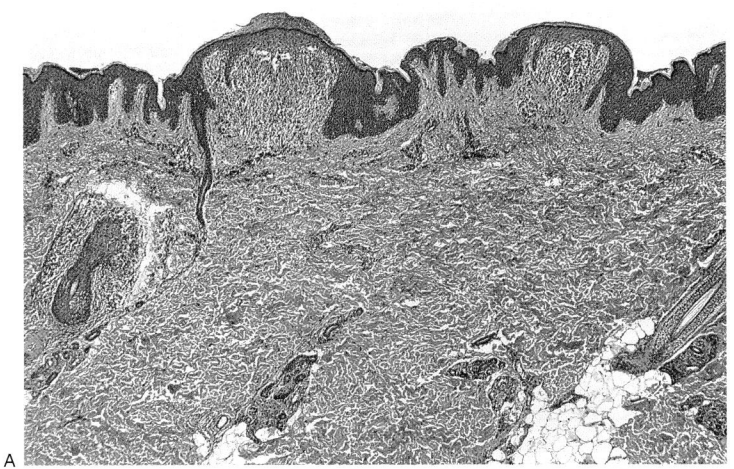

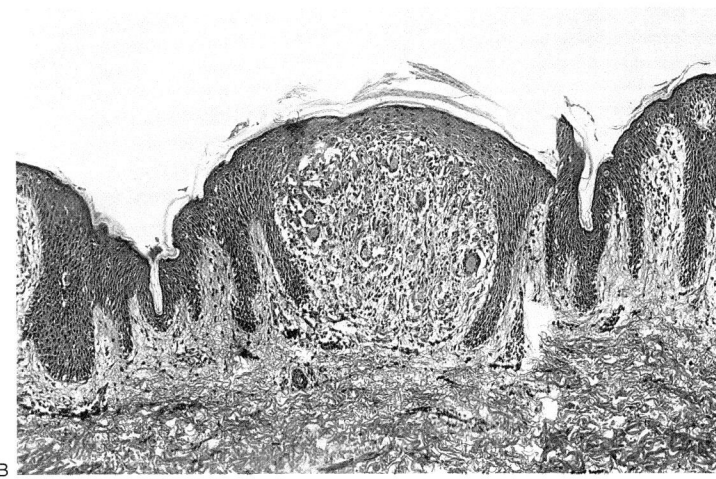

Fig. 3.10 **Lichen nitidus. (A)** There are two discrete foci of inflammation involving the superficial dermis. **(B)** Claw-like downgrowths of the rete ridges are present at the margins of these foci. (H & E)

Rare changes that have been reported include subepidermal vesiculation,[260] transepidermal elimination of the inflammatory infiltrate[257,261,262] and the presence of perifollicular granulomas.[263]

Direct immunofluorescence is usually negative, a distinguishing feature from lichen planus.

Electron microscopy

The ultrastructural changes in lichen nitidus are similar to those of lichen planus.[264]

LICHEN STRIATUS

Lichen striatus is a linear, papular eruption of unknown etiology which may extend in a continuous or interrupted fashion along one side of the body, usually the length of an extremity.[255] Annular[266] and bilateral forms[267] have been reported. The lesions often follow Blaschko's lines.[268–271] Nail changes are not uncommon.[272] Lichen striatus has a predilection for female children and adolescents. An unusual presentation in children is the presence of linear lesions on the nose with some overlap features with lupus erythematosus.[273] Spontaneous resolution usually occurs after 1 or 2 years. A history of atopy is sometimes present in affected individuals.[274]

Lichen striatus has been reported following BCG vaccination[271] and following a flu-like illness.[275]

Histopathology[265, 276–278]

There is a lichenoid reaction pattern with an infiltrate of lymphocytes, histiocytes and melanophages occupying three or four adjacent dermal papillae.[278] The overlying epidermis is acanthotic with mild spongiosis associated with exocytosis of inflammatory cells. Small intraepidermal vesicles containing Langerhans cells are present in half of the cases.[279] Dyskeratotic cells are often present at all levels of the epidermis; such cells are uncommon in linear lichen planus.[280] There is usually mild hyperkeratosis and focal parakeratosis.[265] The dermal papillae are mildly edematous. The infiltrate is usually less dense than in lichen planus and it may extend around hair follicles or vessels in the mid-plexus. Eccrine extension of the infiltrate is often present (Fig. 3.11).[276,277] A monoclonal population of T cells has been reported in one case but excluded in others.[281]

Electron microscopy

Dyskeratotic cells similar to the corps ronds of Darier's disease have been described in the upper epidermis.[277] The Civatte bodies in the basal layer show the usual changes of apoptosis on electron microscopy.

LICHEN PLANUS-LIKE KERATOSIS

Lichen planus-like keratosis is a commonly encountered entity in routine histopathology.[282–287] Synonyms used for this entity include solitary lichen planus, benign lichenoid keratosis,[283] lichenoid benign keratosis[284,285] and involuting lichenoid plaque.[286] It should not be confused with lichenoid actinic (solar) keratosis[288] in which epithelial atypia is a prerequisite for diagnosis.[289] Lichen planus-like keratoses are usually solitary, discrete, slightly raised lesions of short duration, measuring 3–10 mm in diameter. The sudden appearance of the lesion is often a striking feature. Lesions are violaceous or pink, often with a rusty tinge.[282] There may be a thin, overlying scale. There is a predilection for the arms and presternal area of middle-aged and elderly women. Lesions are sometimes mildly pruritic or 'burning'.[283] Clinically, lichen planus-like keratosis is usually misdiagnosed as a basal cell carcinoma or Bowen's disease.

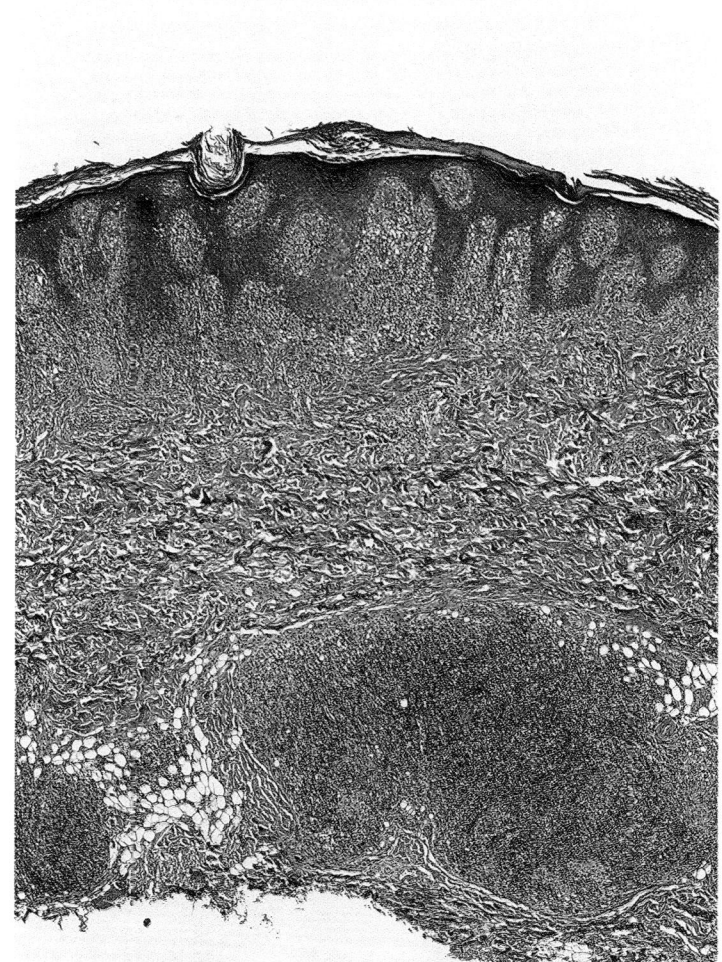

Fig. 3.11 **Lichen striatus.** This case has a florid perieccrine infiltrate of lymphocytes. (H & E)

Lichen planus-like keratosis is a heterogeneous condition which usually represents the attempted cell-mediated immune rejection of any of several different types of epidermal lesion. In most instances this is a solar lentigo,[282,290,291] but in some lesions there is a suggestion of an underlying seborrheic keratosis, large cell acanthoma or even a viral wart.[292] Constant pressure was incriminated in one case.[293] In one study, a contiguous solar lentigo was present in only 7% of cases and a seborrheic keratosis in 8.4%.[287] These findings do not accord with the author's own experiences.

Histopathology[284,285,291]

There is a florid lichenoid reaction pattern with numerous Civatte bodies in the basal layer and accompanying mild vacuolar change (Fig. 3.12). The infiltrate is usually quite dense and often includes a few plasma cells and eosinophils, in addition to the lymphocytes and macrophages. The infiltrate may obscure the dermoepidermal interface. Pigment incontinence may be prominent. There may be mild atypia but this is never as marked as it is in a lichenoid solar keratosis.[27]

There is often mild hyperkeratosis and focal parakeratosis.[287] Hypergranulosis is not as pronounced as in lichen planus. A contiguous solar lentigo or large cell acanthoma is sometimes seen.[294]

Usually cell death is scattered and of apoptotic type. At times confluent necrosis occurs and in these cases subepidermal clefting may result. There is

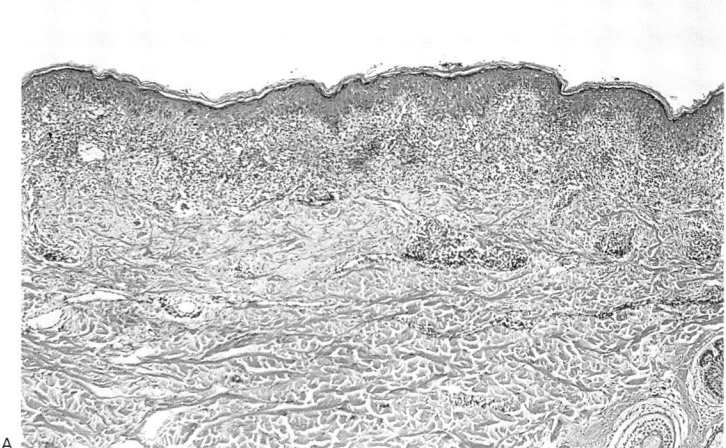

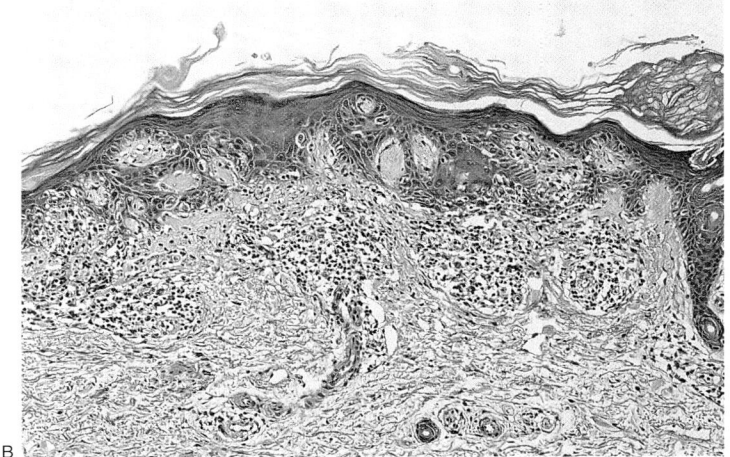

Fig. 3.12 **(A) Lichen planus-like keratosis. (B)** There is a lichenoid reaction pattern with some deeper extension of the infiltrate than is usual in lichen planus. (H & E)

Table 3.4 **Drugs producing a lichenoid (interface) pattern (but excluding cases with only rare apoptotic keratinocytes)**

Lichen planus pemphigoides: cinnarizire, ramipril

Lichenoid drug eruption: amlodipine, antimalarials, arsenicals, beta blockers, captopril, carbamazepine, chlorpropamide, cyanamide, dapsone, docetaxel, enalapril, ethambutol, gold, granulocyte colony-stimulating factor (local), hepatitis B vaccination, indapamide, indoramin, interferon alfa-2b, intravenous immunoglobulins, iodides, lansoprazole, metformin, methyldopa, naproxen, omeprazole, pantoprazole, penicillamine, phenothiazine, quinidine, quinine, simvastatin, spironolactone, streptomycin, suramin, tiopronin

Photolichenoid drug eruption: pyrazinamide, sparfloxacin, tetracycline, thiazides, torsemide

Fixed drug eruption: acetaminophen, amoxicillin, carbamazepine, ciprofloxacin, clarithromycin, clioquinol, colchicine, dimenhydrinate, diphenhydramine, eperisone hydrochloride, erythromycin, feprazone, fluconazole, griseofulvin, ibuprofen, iomeprol, lactose, lamotrigine, mefenamic acid, metramizole, metronidazole, minocycline, naproxen, nimesulide, nystatin, paclitaxel, paracetamol, penicillin, phenolphthalein, phenylbutazone, phenylpropanolamine hydrochloride, phenytoin, pseudoephedrine, quinine, sulfamethoxazole, sulfonamides, tartrazene, temazepam, terbinafine, tetracyclines, theophylline, ticlopidine, tinidazole, tranexamic acid, tranquilizers, trimethoprim, tropisetron

Erythema multiforme/TEN: acarbose, allopurinol, amifostine, aminopenicillins, bezafibrate, bupropion, carbamazepine, ceftazidime, chloroquine, cimetidine, ciprofloxacin, clindamycin, clobazam, clonazepam, cocaine, cyclophosphamide, cytosine arabinoside, diacerein, doxycycline, ethambutol, etretinate, famotidine, gemeprost, griseofulvin, indapamide, indomethacin, isoxicam, lamotrigine, latanoprost eye drops, mefloquine, methotrexate, mifepristone, nevirapine, nitrogen mustard, nystatin, oxaprozin, phenylbutazone, phenytoin, piroxicam, ranitidine, ritodrine, sertraline, sulfamethoxazole, suramin, terbinafine, theophylline, ticlopidine, trichloroethylene, trimethoprim, valproic acid, vancomycin

Subacute lupus erythematosus: antihistamines, calcium channel blockers, captopril, cilazapril, cinnarizine, diltiazem, griseofulvin, naproxen, nifedipine, oxyprenolol, piroxicam, ranitidine, terbinafine, thiazides, verapamil

Systemic lupus erythematosus: allopurinol, atenolol, captopril, carbamazepine, chlorpromazine, clonidine, danazol, ethosuximide, griseofulvin, hydralazine, hydrochlorothiazide, isoniazid, lithium, lovastatin, mesalazine, methimazole, methyldopa, minocycline, penicillin, penicillamine, phenobarbitone, phenylbutazone, phenytoin, piroxicam, practolol, primidone, procainamide, propylthiouracil, quinidine, streptomycin, sulfonamides, terbinafine, tetracycline derivatives, thiamazole, trimethadione, valproate.

also a rare 'creeping' form in which there is focal acute activity and other areas with few lymphocytes, little if any apoptotic cell death, and some melanin incontinence. A careful search for a cornoid lamella of porokeratosis should always be made when these changes are present.

The recent attempt to classify 'lichenoid keratoses' into three groups – lichen planus-like keratosis, seborrheic keratosis-like lichenoid keratosis, and lupus erythematosus-like lichenoid keratosis – deserves some comment.[295] The seborrheic keratosis-like variant is best called an irritated (lichenoid) seborrheic keratosis and the lupus erythematosus-like variant is simply a lesion with some basal clefting (see above).

Direct immunofluorescence shows colloid bodies containing IgM and some basement membrane fibrin.[284] Immunohistochemistry shows fewer Langerhans cells in the epidermis than in lichen planus.[295]

LICHENOID DRUG ERUPTIONS

A lichenoid eruption has been reported following the ingestion of a wide range of chemical substances and drugs.[297,298] The eruption may closely mimic lichen planus clinically, although at other times there is eczematization and more pronounced, residual hyperpigmentation. Some of the β-adrenergic blocking agents produce a psoriasiform pattern clinically but lichenoid features histologically.[299,300] Discontinuation of the drug usually leads to clearing of the rash over a period of several weeks.[301]

Lichenoid eruptions have been produced by gold,[302] gold-containing liquor,[303,304] methyldopa,[305] β-adrenergic blocking agents,[306] penicillamine,[307] quinine,[308] quinidine,[309] synthetic antimalarials[310] and ethambutol.[311] Less common causes of a lichenoid reaction are captopril,[312] enalapril,[313] amlodipine,[314] naproxen,[315,316] dapsone, simvastatin,[317] indapamide, arsenicals, iodides, carbamazepine,[318] phenothiazine derivatives, chlorpropamide,[319] suramin,[320] tiopronin,[321] docetaxel,[322] cyanamide,[323] omeprazole, lansoprazole, pantoprazole,[324] spironolactone,[325] metformin,[326] indoramin,[327] interferon alfa-2b intravenous immunoglobulin[328] and streptomycin.[329] Thiazides, some tetracyclines, sparfloxacin,[330] torsemide (a loop diuretic)[331] and pyrazinamide[332] may produce lesions in a photodistribution.[333] A lichenoid stomatitis, which may take time to clear after cessation of the drug, can be produced by methyldopa and rarely by lithium carbonate[334] or propranolol. Contact with color film developer may produce a lichenoid photodermatitis.[301] A topical mixture of the local anesthetic agents lidocaine and prilocaine produced basal clefting similar to epidermolysis bullosa simplex with basophilic granules in the cleft.[335] A lichen planus-like eruption has been reported at sites repeatedly exposed to methacrylic acid esters used in the car industry[336] and also at injection sites of granulocyte colony-stimulating factor.[337] A list of the drugs that produce lichenoid eruptions is included in Table 3.4.

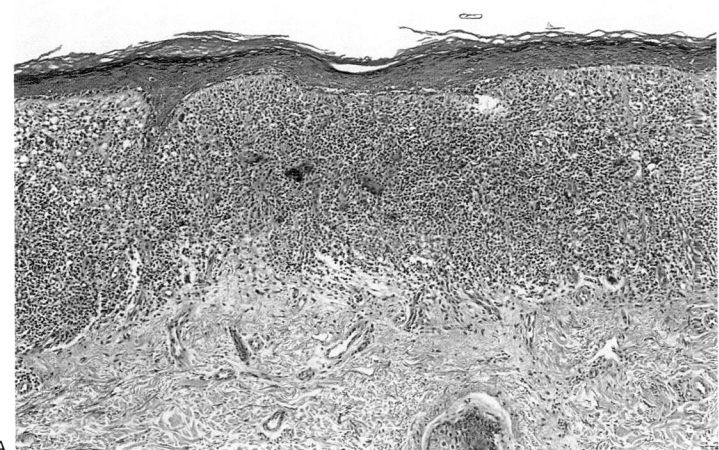

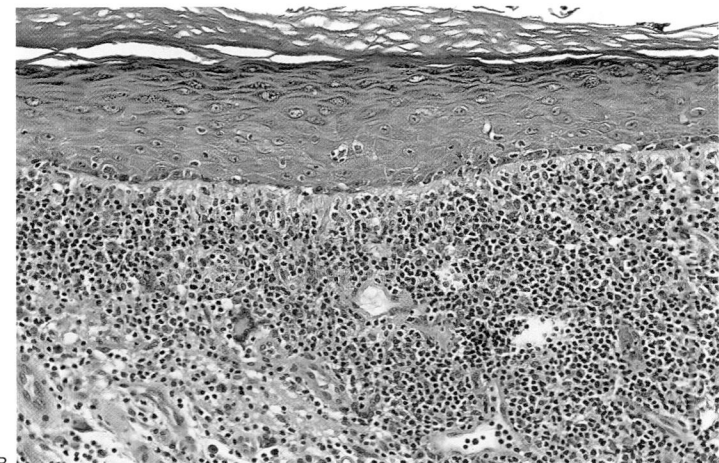

Fig. 3.13 **(A) Giant cell lichenoid dermatitis. (B)** There are several multinucleate giant cells in the lichenoid infiltrate. (H & E)

Histopathology[301,338]

Lichenoid drug eruptions usually differ from lichen planus by the presence of focal parakeratosis and mild basal vacuolar change, as well as a few eosinophils and sometimes plasma cells in the infiltrate. These features are said to be more common in non-photodistributed lesions, whereas photodistributed lesions may mimic lichen planus.[339] There is often more melanin incontinence than in lichen planus. The infiltrate is often less dense and less band-like than in lichen planus itself. A few inflammatory cells may extend around vessels in the mid and lower dermis. Sometimes the histological features closely simulate those of lichen planus.[339] A few eosinophils in the infiltrate may be the only clue to the diagnosis. An unusual lichenoid reaction with epidermotropic multinucleate giant cells in the inflammatory infiltrate has been reported in patients taking a variety of drugs.[340] The term '**giant cell lichenoid dermatitis**' has been used for this pattern (Fig. 3.13).[341] One patient subsequently developed sarcoidosis.[341] It has recently been reported in herpes zoster scars, particularly in bone marrow recipients.[342]

FIXED DRUG ERUPTIONS

A fixed drug eruption is a round or oval erythematous lesion which develops within hours of taking the offending drug and which recurs at the same site with subsequent exposure to the drug.[343] Lesions may be solitary or multiple.

A bullous variant with widespread lesions also occurs.[344,345] Fixed eruptions subside on withdrawal of the drug, leaving a hyperpigmented macule.[346] Non-pigmenting lesions have been described[347–349] and depigmented areas may be the result in patients whose skin is naturally heavily pigmented. Sometimes there is a burning sensation in the erythematous lesions, but systemic manifestations such as malaise and fever are uncommon.[343] Rare clinical variants include eczematous, urticarial, linear,[350,351] 'wandering'[352] and erythema dyschromicum perstans-like[353] types. An interesting presentation concerns the fixed drug eruption that developed in a male after coitus, which was thought to have resulted from the trimethoprim-sulfamethoxazole that his wife was taking.[354] Common sites of involvement include the face, lips,[355] buttocks and genitals.[356] Paronychia is a rare presentation.[357]

In one series of 446 cases of drug eruption, 92 (21%) were instances of fixed drug eruptions and, of these, 16 were bullous and generalized.[358] Over 100 drugs have been incriminated, but the major offenders are sulfonamides,[359] particularly the combination of trimethoprim-sulfamethoxazole,[354,360,361] tetracyclines,[361–363] tranquilizers, quinine, phenolphthalein (in laxatives) and some analgesics.[364] Specific drugs incriminated in some recent reports in the literature include minocycline,[363] nystatin,[365] colchicine,[366] clioquinol,[367] penicillin,[368] amoxicillin,[369] erythromycin,[370] clarithromycin,[371] ciprofloxacin,[372] tranexamic acid,[373] griseofulvin,[374] terbinafine,[375] dimenhydrinate (Gravol),[376–378] diphenhydramine,[379] paclitaxel,[380] temazepam,[381] mefenamic acid,[345,382] carbamazepine,[383,384] acetaminophen (paracetamol),[385–392] fluconazole,[393] feprazone,[394] tartrazine,[395] ticlopidine,[396] phenytoin,[384] lamotrigine,[397] pseudoephedrine,[398,399] iomeprol,[400] phenylpropanolamine hydrochloride,[401] tropisetron,[402] metramizole,[361] phenylbutazone,[361] naproxen,[403] ibuprofen,[404] eperisone hydrochloride,[405] lactose,[406] metronidazole,[407] tinidazole,[407] nimesulide[408] and theophylline.[353] More complete lists are included in several reviews of the subject.[343,364] The drugs responsible are also listed in Table 3.4. Two different drugs were involved in one patient.[409] In yet another report, three different drugs each produced a fixed drug eruption at a different site.[410] It has been suggested that the distribution of lesions is influenced by the drug in question; tetracyclines tend to involve the glans penis, while pyrazolones affect mainly the lips and mucosae.[360] There are rare reports of fixed food eruptions. Lentils[411] and strawberries[412] have been implicated. Foods may sometimes produce a flare in a fixed drug eruption.[413]

Numerous studies have attempted to elucidate the pathogenesis of fixed eruptions. It appears that the offending drug acts as a hapten and binds to a protein in basal keratinocytes and sometimes melanocytes.[343] As a consequence, an immunological reaction is stimulated, which probably takes the form of an antibody-dependent, cellular cytotoxic response.[414] Lymphocytes attack the drug-altered epidermal cells. Suppressor/cytotoxic lymphocytes play a major role in this process and in preserving the cutaneous memory function which characterizes a fixed eruption.[415] Keratinocytes at the site of a fixed drug eruption express one of the cell adhesion molecules (ICAM-1) that is involved in the adherence reaction between lymphocytes and epidermal keratinocytes.[416] It has been suggested that localized expression of this adhesion antigen may be one factor that explains the site specificity of fixed drug eruptions.[416] These findings have been incorporated into the following hypothesis: that the causative drug activates mast cells or keratinocytes to release cytokines or induces keratinocytes to express adhesion molecules on their surfaces, leading to the activation of epidermal T cells.[417] This theory has been put forward in an attempt to explain the early onset of symptoms, which occur much earlier than traditional cell-mediated responses could produce.

There appears to be a genetic susceptibility to fixed drug eruptions, with an increased incidence of HLA-B22.[418]

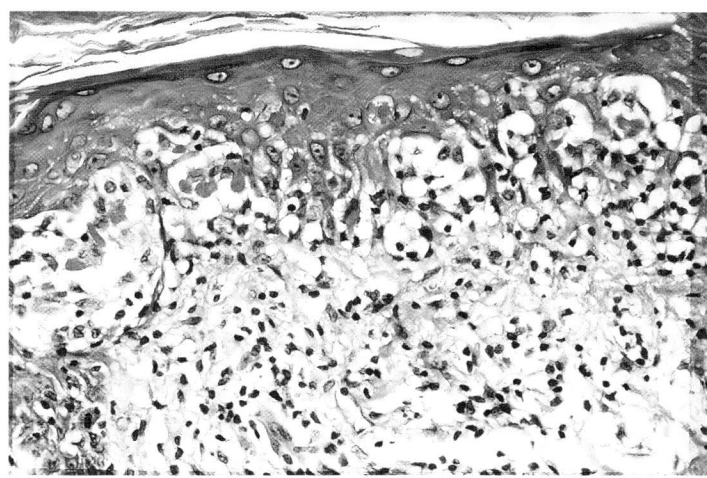

Fig. 3.14 **Fixed drug eruption.** Dead keratinocytes are present in the basal layer and at higher levels of the epidermis. Lymphocytes extend into the epidermis. (H & E)

Histopathology[343,419]

Established lesions show a lichenoid reaction pattern with prominent vacuolar change and Civatte body formation (Fig. 3.14). The degenerate keratinocytes usually show less shrinkage than in lichen planus. The inflammatory infiltrate tends to obscure the dermoepidermal interface, as in erythema multiforme and some cases of pityriasis lichenoides et varioliformis acuta (PLEVA). The infiltrate often extends into the mid and upper epidermis producing death of keratinocytes above the basal layer (Fig. 3.15). Fixed drug eruptions can usually be distinguished from erythema multiforme by the deeper extension of the infiltrate, the presence of a few neutrophils, and the more prominent melanin incontinence in fixed eruptions.

Based on one study,[419] it appears that very early lesions may show epidermal spongiosis, dermal edema and neutrophil microabscesses and numerous eosinophils in the dermis. These features have usually disappeared after several days, although some eosinophils persist.

The clinical variants of fixed drug eruption have not been documented very well, except for the bullous form which results when subepidermal clefting occurs. This may be misdiagnosed as erythema multiforme. Spongiotic vesiculation is present in the eczematous variant and a picture resembling an urticarial reaction is seen in others. Vasculitis is another pattern seen, rarely, in fixed drug eruptions.[388] In the non-pigmenting variant there is a mild perivascular and interstitial mixed inflammatory infiltrate in the dermis.[348]

Electron microscopy

There is prominent clumping of tonofilaments in the cytoplasm of basal keratinocytes, which provides an explanation for the bright eosinophilic cytoplasm and the comparatively small amount of shrinkage that these cells undergo during cell death.[346] There is also condensation of nuclear chromatin. Intracytoplasmic desmosomes are sometimes seen. Filamentous bodies, composed of filaments which are less electron dense than in the intact cells, are quite numerous.[420] These contain some melanosomes and sometimes nuclear remnants.[346] They are sometimes phagocytosed by adjacent keratinocytes or macrophages.[346] The accumulation of tonofilaments may represent a response by keratinocytes to sublethal injury or some other stimulus. It has the effect of masking the exact mode of death – apoptosis or necrosis. The term 'filamentous degeneration' has some merit in these circumstances.

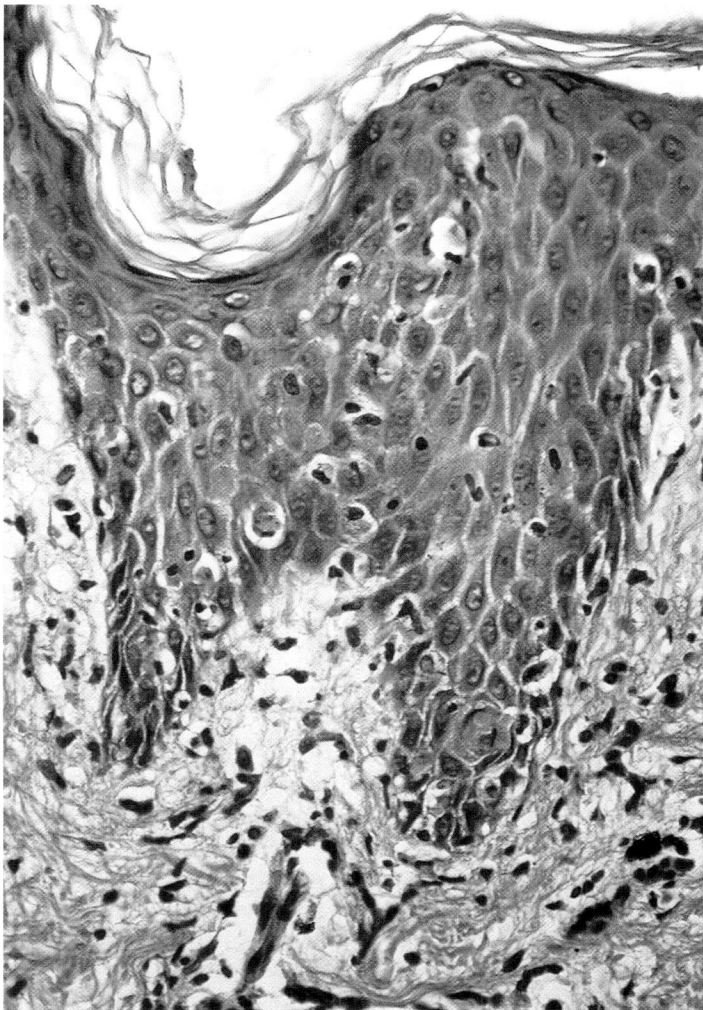

Fig. 3.15 **Fixed drug eruption.** The infiltrate of lymphocytes extends some distance into the epidermis resulting in cell death in the basal layer and above. (H & E)

ERYTHEMA MULTIFORME

Erythema multiforme is a self-limited, sometimes episodic disease of the skin, which may also involve the mucous membranes. It is characterized by a pleomorphic eruption consisting of erythematous macules, papules, urticarial plaques, vesicles and bullae.[421,422] Individual lesions may evolve through a papular, vesicular and target (iris) stage in which bullae surmount an erythematous maculopapule.[423] Lesions tend to be distributed symmetrically with a predilection for the extremities, particularly the hands.

Clinical variants

In the past, erythema multiforme was classified into *erythema multiforme minor* and *erythema multiforme major*, the latter being characterized by a severe and sometimes fatal illness in which fever, systemic symptoms and severe oral lesions were usually present.[423–426] The term *Stevens–Johnson syndrome* was also applied to these severe cases with oral involvement. Recently, an attempt has been made to distinguish Stevens–Johnson syndrome from erythema multiforme major with mucosal lesions on the basis of their different *cutaneous* lesions and their etiology;[427] their *mucosal* lesions are similar. Stevens–Johnson syndrome is said to be characterized by flat atypical target lesions or purpuric macules, that are widespread or limited to the trunk.

Erythema multiforme major with mucosal lesions has typical or raised atypical target lesions, located on the extremities and/or the face.[427] Using these definitions, Stevens–Johnson syndrome is usually related to drugs and erythema multiforme to herpes or other infections.[427,428]

These criteria have been criticized on the basis that they ignore the fundamental clinical differences between these two related conditions.[429] Namely, Stevens–Johnson syndrome is associated with systemic symptoms and involvement of internal organs, whereas erythema multiforme is not.[429] **Toxic epidermal necrolysis** (see below) has variously been regarded as a separate entity or as representing the severe end of the spectrum of erythema multiforme major or Stevens–Johnson syndrome.[430,431] Some clinicians have arbitrarily diagnosed toxic epidermal necrolysis when blisters and peeling involved more than 30% of the total body surface area and Stevens–Johnson syndrome when mucosal lesions were present and blistering involved less than 30% of the body surface.[432] An international group has attempted to standardize the terminology by defining five clinical categories – bullous erythema multiforme, Stevens–Johnson syndrome, overlap Stevens–Johnson syndrome/toxic epidermal necrolysis, toxic epidermal necrolysis with 'spots' (widespread purpuric macules or target lesions), and toxic epidermal necrolysis without 'spots'.[432,433] The strategy behind this approach is summed up by two of the experts in this area: 'Our current concept is to separate an EM spectrum (EM minor combined with EM major), from an SJS/TEN spectrum.'[434] Many clinicians use only three categories – erythema multiforme, Stevens–Johnson syndrome and toxic epidermal necrolysis – making comparative studies of this clinical spectrum difficult.

Two further clinical subgroups have been delineated: *recurrent erythema multiforme* and a rare *persistent* form. The persistent form has been associated with an underlying malignancy and with Epstein–Barr virus infection.[435,436] The recurrent form is frequently associated with recurring infections with the herpes simplex virus.[437] Rarely it is associated with hepatitis C infection.[438] Sometimes the recurrent lesions mimic polymorphous light eruption by having a photodistribution.[439] Patients with certain HLA types – B35, B62 (B15) and DR53 – are more susceptible to this recurrent form.[440]

Unusual clinical presentations include the limitation of lesions to areas of lymphatic obstruction,[441] to nevi[442,443] or to Blaschko's lines,[444] a photosensitive eruption[445] and the development of eruptive nevocellular nevi following severe erythema multiforme.[446] Leukoderma is a rare complication.[447]

Etiology and pathogenesis

Over 100 different causal factors have been implicated, including viral and bacterial infections, drugs and several associated neoplastic conditions.[448,449] Infection with herpes simplex type 1 is a common precipitating factor for minor forms,[450] while *Mycoplasma pneumoniae* infection[451] and drugs are often incriminated in the more severe cases.[424,452] A recent study of erythema multiforme in children found that the minor forms were due to herpes simplex and the cases with Stevens–Johnson syndrome to *Mycoplasma pneumoniae* infection. Drugs were rarely implicated in this age group.[453] Infection with Epstein–Barr virus has been associated with both minor and persistent erythema multiforme.[435,454] Other infections to be associated with erythema multiforme include cytomegalovirus,[455] Lyme disease (in its early stages)[456,457] and hepatitis B.[458] It has also followed hepatitis B immunization.[459]

Numerous drugs have been involved, most commonly the sulfonamides and non-steroidal anti-inflammatory drugs.[449,460,461] They often produce a severe reaction. Specific drugs incriminated include ciprofloxacin,[462] nystatin,[463] the aminopenicillins,[464] doxycycline,[465,466] cimetidine, suramin,[467] theophylline,[468] allopurinol, etretinate,[469] terbinafine,[470–474] griseofulvin,[475] clonazepam,[476] acarbose,[477] ticlopidine,[396] sertraline,[478] amifostine,[479]

cyclophosphamide,[480] lamotrigine,[481,482] bezafibrate,[483] cocaine,[484] bupropion,[485] topical nitrogen mustard,[486] mefloquine,[487] trichloroethylene,[488] and nevirapine.[489]

Erythema multiforme has been reported in association with an allergic contact dermatitis; plants, woods,[490] epoxy sealants and diphencyprone (used in the treatment of warts) have been incriminated.[491–493] An erythema multiforme-like reaction has been reported following the intravenous injection of vinblastine in the vicinity,[494] and at sites of radiation therapy in patients taking antiepileptic drugs.[495]

Erythema multiforme appears to result from a cell-mediated immune reaction to one of the many agents listed above. In the case of herpes simplex, lymphocytes home to viral antigen-positive cells containing the herpes DNA polymerase gene (*Pol*).[496,497] The term HAEM (herpes-associated erythema multiforme) is used for these cases. The virus often remains in affected cutaneous sites for up to 3 months or more following resolution of the erythema multiforme, suggesting that the skin may function as a site of viral persistence.[498,499] Herpes simplex virus can be detected in up to three-quarters of patients with erythema multiforme, on paraffin embedded biopsy material.[500–502] Two classes of lymphocytes appear to be involved in this cell-mediated reaction. They are T lymphocytes carrying the Vβ2 phenotype[503] and CD8+ cells with natural killer-cell activity.[504] The effector cytokine may well be interferon-γ in cases of HAEM, while in drug-induced erythema multiforme major/Stevens–Johnson syndrome/toxic epidermal necrolysis, tumor necrosis factor (TNF-α) produces the epidermal destruction.[461,505,506] The finding of autoantibodies against desmoplakin I and II is probably an epiphenomenon.[507–509]

Histopathology[424,510,511]

In established lesions, there is a lichenoid (interface) reaction pattern with a mild to moderate infiltrate of lymphocytes, some of which move into the basal layer, thereby obscuring the dermoepidermal interface (Fig. 3.16). Some of the intraepidermal lymphocytes are of the large granular subtype.[512] This is associated with prominent epidermal cell death, which is not confined to the basal layer. Apoptosis is the mechanism of cell death.[513] There is also basal vacuolar change and some epidermal spongiosis.[510] One study has found that an acrosyringeal concentration of apoptotic keratinocytes in erythema multiforme is a clue to a drug etiology. These changes are likely to be accompanied by an inflammatory infiltrate containing eosinophils.[514]

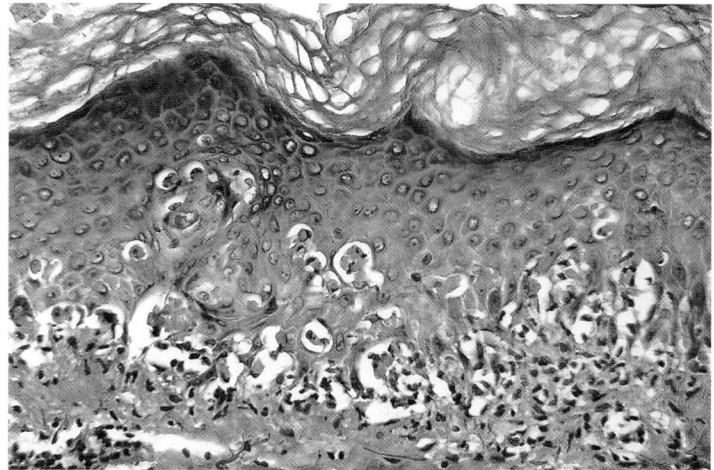

Fig. 3.16 **Erythema multiforme.** Cell death involves keratinocytes within and above the basal layer. The infiltrate of lymphocytes tends to obscure the dermoepidermal interface. (H & E)

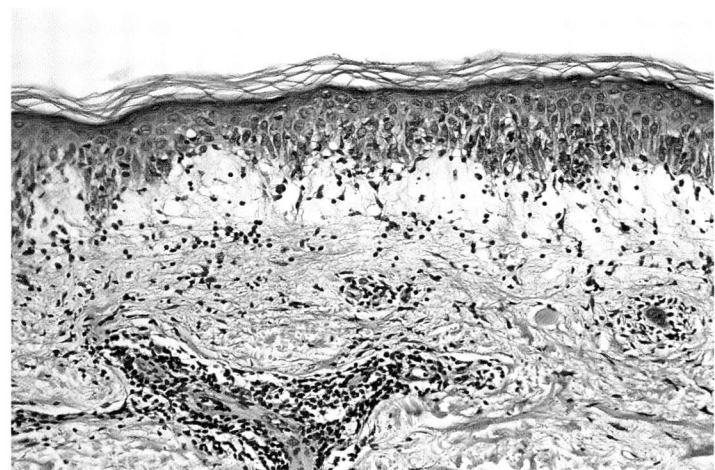

Fig. 3.17 **Erythema multiforme with early subepidermal vesiculation.** (H & E)

Vesicular lesions are characterized by clefting at the dermoepidermal junction and prominent epidermal cell death in the overlying roof (Fig. 3.17). This may involve single cells or groups of cells, or take the form of confluent necrosis.

The dermal infiltrate in erythema multiforme is composed of lymphocytes and a few macrophages involving the superficial and mid-dermal vessels and a more dispersed infiltrate along and within the basal layer. In severe cases of erythema multiforme showing overlap features with toxic epidermal necrolysis (see below), the infiltrate may be quite sparse with confluent necrosis of the detached overlying epidermis. Eosinophils are not usually prominent in erythema multiforme, although they have been specifically mentioned as an important feature in some reports.[510,515–517] We have seen a case with numerous dermal eosinophils with eosinophilic microabscesses in the epidermis.[518] Likewise, a vasculitis has been noted by some,[519] but specifically excluded by most.[510,511,520] Nuclear dusting, not related to blood vessels, is sometimes present.[521]

Erythema multiforme has been divided in the past into epidermal, dermal and mixed types based on the corresponding predominant histological features.[521] In the epidermal type there was prominent epidermal damage. In the dermal type there was pronounced dermal papillary edema leading to subepidermal vesiculation; some basal epidermal damage was to be seen in some areas of the biopsy. It seems likely that diseases other than erythema multiforme – severe urticarias and urticarial vasculitis – have been included in this category of dermal erythema multiforme. There is little merit in the continued separation of these three histological subtypes.[522] The rare cases with subcorneal pustules are probably not variants of erythema multiforme as reported.[523]

Erythema multiforme-like changes can be seen in some biopsies of paraneoplastic pemphigus (see p. 152). Usually, foci of suprabasal acantholysis will be seen in some areas of the biopsy. Distinctive immunofluorescence changes are also present in paraneoplastic pemphigus.

Erythema multiforme-like changes can be seen in biopsies taken from the hypersensitivity reactions to phenytoin, carbamazepine and related drugs. Interestingly, the clinical picture does not resemble erythema multiforme.

Direct immunofluorescence shows intraepidermal cytoid bodies, representing degenerate keratinocytes, which stain in a homogeneous pattern usually with IgM and sometimes C3.[524] Frequently, there is granular staining for C3 along the dermoepidermal junction and, in early lesions, also in papillary dermal vessels.[525,526] The presence of properdin suggests activation of the alternate complement pathway.[526]

Toxic epidermal necrolysis

Toxic epidermal necrolysis, regarded as the most severe form of an erythema multiforme spectrum, presents with generalized tender erythema which rapidly progresses into a blistering phase with extensive shedding of skin.[526–534] Erosive mucosal lesions are usually present. The mortality approaches 35%.[534,535] The risk of death can be predicted from the quantitative 'severity of illness' score.[536] The extent of the necrolysis (skin shedding) is one of the principal prognostic factors, and a classification system based on the extent of epidermal detachment has therefore been proposed:[434,537]

1. Stevens–Johnson syndrome – mucosal erosions and epidermal detachment below 10% of total body area;
2. Stevens–Johnson syndrome/toxic epidermal necrolysis overlap – epidermal detachment between 10 and 30%;
3. Toxic epidermal necrolysis – epidermal detachment more than 30%.

Drugs are incriminated in the etiology in the majority of cases,[538] particularly sulfonamides,[539] anticonvulsants[540–543] and non-steroidal anti-inflammatory drugs, such as phenylbutazone, isoxicam and piroxicam.[544,545] Specific drugs implicated include allopurinol,[546,547] ranitidine,[548,549] clindamycin,[550] chloroquine,[551] famotidine,[552] indapamide,[553] clobazam,[554] oxaprozin,[555] diacerein,[556] methotrexate,[557,558] cytosine arabinoside,[559] lamotrigine,[560,561] carbamazepine,[562,563] latanoprost eye drops, trimethoprim-sulfamethoxazole,[564] ceftazidime,[565] vancomycin,[565] ciprofloxacin,[566] nevirapine,[567,568] mefloquine,[487] mifepristone/gemeprost,[569] ritodrine/indomethacin/betamethasone therapy for preterm labor,[570] phenytoin[543] and ethambutol.[543]

The pathogenesis is uncertain but it appears that most patients with toxic epidermal necrolysis have an abnormal metabolism of the offending drug, which leads to an increased production of reactive metabolites.[434,541] Some genetic susceptibility is suggested by the increased incidence of HLA-B12 in affected individuals.[571] Epidermal necrosis is probably mediated by cytotoxic lymphokines, such as tumor necrosis factor-α.[461,505,572] Apoptosis of keratinocytes also occurs.[573] The action of cytokines would explain the apparent discrepancy between the extent of the damage and the paucity of the dermal infiltrate. The final pathway leading to epidermal death is not known but disturbances in intracellular Ca^{2+} homeostasis have been postulated.[574] The majority of non-keratinocytic cells in the epidermis are $CD8^+$ lymphocytes and macrophages, while the lymphocytes in the papillary dermis are $CD4^+$.[575–577] Factor XIIIa-positive dendrocytes in the dermis may also play a role.[461] The reactive metabolites of the offending drug possibly behave as haptens, adhere to epidermal cells and provoke an immune response.[434] Prompt withdrawal of the offending drug should be a priority. This reduces the risk of death by about 30% per day.[578] Patients on corticosteroid therapy may still develop toxic epidermal necrolysis; corticosteroids may delay the onset of the disease, but not halt its progression.[579] Patients infected with the human immunodeficiency virus may develop toxic epidermal necrolysis similar to immunocompetent patients.[580]

Histopathology[529,581]

There is a subepidermal bulla with overlying confluent necrosis of the epidermis and a sparse perivascular infiltrate of lymphocytes (Fig. 3.18). In early lesions there is some individual cell necrosis which may take the form of satellite cell necrosis with an adjacent lymphocyte or macrophage. This has been likened to the changes of graft-versus-host disease (see below).[528,582] In established lesions of toxic epidermal necrolysis there is full thickness epidermal necrosis which is not seen in GVHD.[582] A more prominent dermal infiltrate is seen in those cases which overlap with erythema multiforme. Sweat ducts show a variety of changes ranging from basal cell apoptosis to necrosis of the duct.[583]

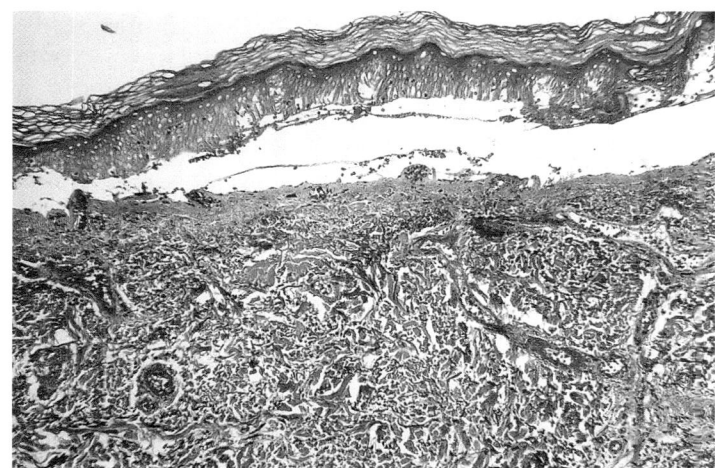

Fig. 3.18 **Toxic epidermal necrolysis.** There is a subepidermal cell-poor blister with epidermal necrosis in the roof. (H & E)

A diffuse deposition of immunoreactants has been found in the mid-epidermis on immunofluorescence.[584]

GRAFT-VERSUS-HOST DISEASE

Graft-versus-host disease (GVHD) is a systemic syndrome with important cutaneous manifestations. It is usually seen in patients receiving allogeneic immunocompetent lymphocytes in the course of bone marrow transplants used in the treatment of aplastic anemia,[585] leukemia or in immunodeficiency states.[456,586–590] Acute GVHD develops in approximately half of HLA-matched recipients of allogeneic bone marrow.[591] It may also occur following maternofetal blood transfusions in utero,[592] intrauterine exchange transfusions and the administration of non-irradiated blood products to patients with disseminated malignancy and a depressed immune system.[593–598] It is seen only rarely after solid organ transplantation.[599] It is also less common with cord-blood than with bone marrow transplants in children receiving either product from HLA-identical siblings.[600] Rarely, immunocompetent patients are at risk, particularly those subject to cardiac surgery.[601–603] The acute stage can be precipitated in some individuals by autologous and syngeneic bone marrow transplantation;[604–606] chronic lesions (see below), particularly lichenoid ones, are rare.[607] GVHD has been reported in patients with a thymoma or lymphoma.[608–610]

There is an early acute phase with vomiting, diarrhea, hepatic manifestations and an erythematous macular rash.[588,611,612] Uncommonly, there are follicular papules[613] or blisters;[614] rarely, toxic epidermal necrolysis ensues.[588,615] Ichthyosiform features may occur in both the acute and chronic forms.[616,617] Localization to an area of skin affected by piebaldism has been reported.[618] The chronic stage develops some months or more after the transplant. A preceding acute stage is present in 80% of these patients.[588,619] Chronic GVHD has an early lichenoid phase which resembles lichen planus and includes oral lesions.[620,621] Linear lichenoid lesions have been reported both in a dermatomal distribution and following Blaschko's lines.[622–626] Rarely, dermatomal lesions occur at sites of varicella-zoster infection.[626,627] A poikilodermatous phase may precede the eventual sclerodermoid phase. The lesions of the latter may be localized[628] or generalized.[588] Other late manifestations include alopecia, a lupus erythematosus-like eruption, cicatrizing conjunctivitis,[629] pyogenic granuloma and angiomatous lesions,[630] wasting, diffuse melanoderma,[631] esophagitis, liver disease and the sicca syndrome. Acute GVHD may be a late manifestation, following the suspension or tapering of immunosuppressive drugs.

The pathogenesis appears to be complex,[632] but the essential factor is the interaction of donor cytotoxic T lymphocytes with recipient minor histocompatibility antigens.[633–635] Several effector cell populations appear to be involved.[636,637] Young rete ridge keratinocytes[638] and Langerhans cells[635,639] are preferred targets. The acute stage is associated with HLA-DR expression of keratinocytes.[640–642] Factor XIIIa-positive dermal dendrocytes appear to play some role,[643,644] possibly in the regulation of the connective tissue remodeling that follows epidermal destruction.

Histopathology[588,645]

In early *acute lesions* there is a sparse superficial perivascular lymphocytic infiltrate with exocytosis of some inflammatory cells into the epidermis. The number of these cells correlates positively with the probability of developing more severe, acute GVHD.[646,647] This is accompanied by basal vacuolation. Established lesions are characterized by more extensive vacuolation and lymphocytic infiltration of the dermis and scattered, shrunken, eosinophilic keratinocytes with pyknotic nuclei, at all levels of the epidermis.[588] These damaged cells are often accompanied by two or more lymphocytes, producing the picture known as 'satellite cell necrosis' (lymphocyte-associated apoptosis) (Fig. 3.19).[648] A similar picture is sometimes seen in subacute radiation dermatitis (see p. 596)[649] and in the cutaneous eruption of lymphocyte recovery (see below). Distinction from a drug eruption can sometimes be difficult.[650,651] The presence of eosinophils is generally taken to favor a drug reaction, but this is not a correct assumption as eosinophils are occasionally seen in GVHD.[652] Fulminant lesions in the acute stage resemble those seen in toxic epidermal necrolysis with subepidermal clefting and full thickness epidermal necrosis. These various changes are often graded as to severity.[653] However, the biopsy findings after bone marrow transplantation correlate poorly with the clinical severity of the skin rash and in predicting progression of the disease to a more severe clinical state.[654,655] The following scheme has been proposed by Horn:[656]

Grade 0: normal skin
Grade 1: basal vacuolar change
Grade 2: dyskeratotic cells in the epidermis and/or follicle, dermal lymphocytic infiltrate
Grade 3: fusion of basilar vacuoles to form clefts and microvesicles
Grade 4: separation of epidermis from dermis.

In the early *chronic phase*, the lichenoid lesions closely resemble those of lichen planus, although the infiltrate is not usually as dense.[657] Sometimes the pattern may even resemble that seen in acute GVHD.[658] Pigment incontinence may be prominent. Biopsies taken from follicular papules resemble lichen planopilaris.[613,620] A rare manifestation is so-called 'columnar epidermal necrosis' characterized by small foci of total epidermal necrosis accompanied by a lichenoid tissue reaction.[659] Immunofluorescence shows a small amount of IgM and C3 in colloid bodies in the papillary dermis and some immunoglobulins on necrotic keratinocytes.[620,621]

In the late *sclerodermoid phase*, there are mild epidermal changes such as atrophy and basal vacuolation. There is thickening of dermal collagen bundles which assume a parallel arrangement. The dermal fibrosis, which may result in atrophy of skin appendages, usually extends into the subcutis, resulting in septal hyalinization.[645] Subepidermal bullae were present in one reported case.[660]

The recently introduced immunomodulatory agent roquinimex has produced eccrine sweat gland necrosis in a number of instances.[661]

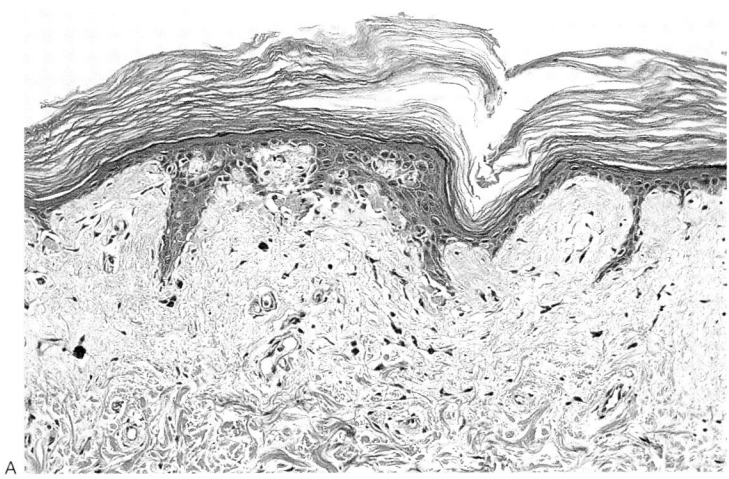

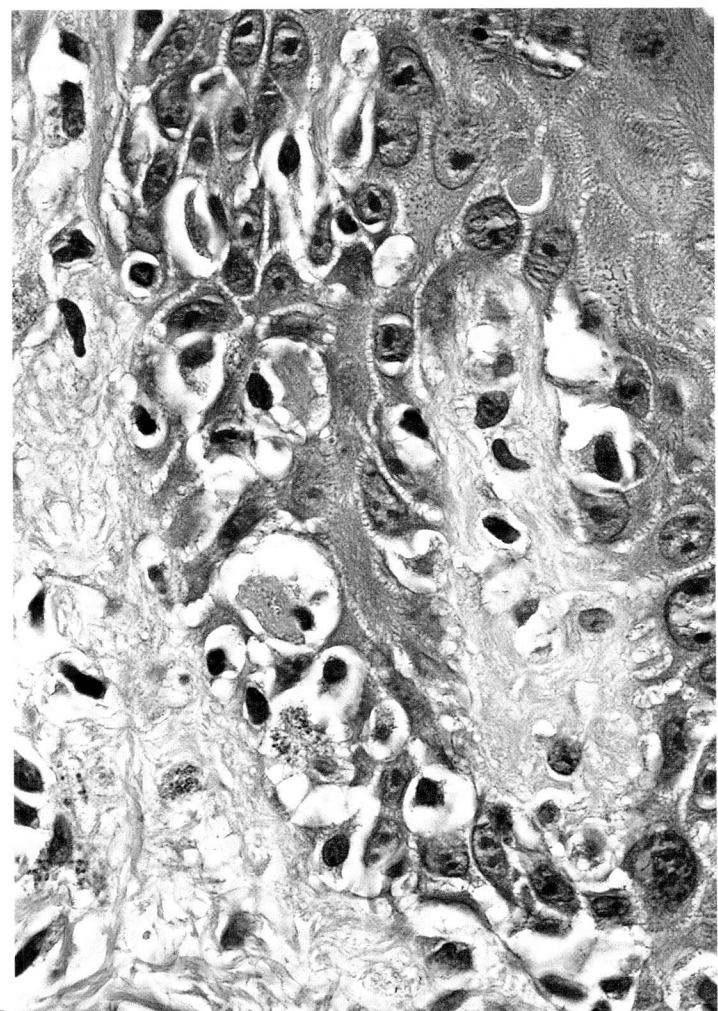

Fig. 3.19 **(A) Graft-versus-host disease. (B)** Lymphocytes are in close apposition to apoptotic keratinocytes. (H & E)

Electron microscopy

Ultrastructural examination shows 'satellite cell necrosis' in both stages with lymphocytes in close contact with occasional keratinocytes,[662] some of which show the changes of apoptosis. The term 'lymphocyte-associated apoptosis' is therefore more appropriate than 'satellite cell necrosis'.[663] Lymphocytes are also in contact with melanocytes[664] and Langerhans cells, the latter being reduced in number. Melanosomes may be increased in the melanocytes. The late sclerotic phase is distinct from scleroderma, with some apoptotic cells in the epidermis and numerous active fibroblasts in the upper dermis.[665]

ERUPTION OF LYMPHOCYTE RECOVERY

The original description of this 'entity' involved patients who developed a maculopapular eruption after receiving cytoreductive therapy (without bone marrow transplant) for acute myelogenous leukemia.[666] The lesions usually developed 14–21 days later, coincident with the return of lymphocytes to the circulation.[656] The histological similarities between this eruption and those seen in mild GVHD and the eruption associated with the administration of cyclosporin A, led to the suggestion that all three conditions represent variations on the theme of lymphocyte recovery.[656]

Histopathology

The eruption is characterized by an upper dermal perivascular infiltrate of small T lymphocytes with accompanying vascular dilatation. There is mild exocytosis of lymphocytes with occasional apoptotic keratinocytes. Lymphocytes are sometimes seen in apposition with these degenerate cells ('satellite cell necrosis'). The appearances resemble mild GVHD.[667] In one report, Pautrier-like microabscesses containing CD4+ cells were present in the epidermis, mimicking mycosis fungoides.[668]

The systemic administration of recombinant cytokines prior to marrow recovery leads to a relatively heavy lymphocytic infiltrate with nuclear pleomorphism and hyperchromasia.[669]

AIDS INTERFACE DERMATITIS

A lichenoid reaction pattern with interface changes resembling those seen in erythema multiforme or fixed drug eruptions has been reported in some patients with the acquired immunodeficiency syndrome and in whom the clinical presentation suggested a drug reaction.[670] The patients had numerous opportunistic infections and all had received at least one medication prior to the onset of the rash. It has been suggested that systemic and cutaneous immune abnormalities may be relevant in the pathogenesis.[670]

There is little justification for the continuation of this diagnosis as a discrete entity.

LUPUS ERYTHEMATOSUS

Lupus erythematosus is a chronic inflammatory disease of unknown etiology which principally affects middle-aged women. It has traditionally been regarded as an immune disorder of connective tissue, along with scleroderma and dermatomyositis. However, a striking feature of cutaneous biopsies is the presence in most cases of the lichenoid reaction pattern (interface dermatitis). It may not be present in tumid forms, in lupus profundus (panniculitis) and in lymphocytic infiltration of the skin, if indeed this is truly a variant of lupus erythematosus.

Three major clinical variants are recognized – chronic discoid lupus erythematosus which involves only the skin, systemic lupus erythematosus which is a multisystem disease, and subacute lupus erythematosus in which distinct cutaneous lesions are sometimes associated with mild systemic illness.[671,672] Some overlap exists between the histological changes seen in these various clinical subsets.[673] There are several less common clinical variants which will be considered after a discussion of the major types.

Discoid lupus erythematosus

The typical lesions of discoid lupus erythematosus are sharply demarcated, erythematous, scaly patches with follicular plugging. They usually involve the skin of the face, often in a butterfly distribution on the cheeks and bridge of the nose. The neck, scalp, lips,[674] oral mucosa[675] and hands are sometimes involved. Periorbital localization has been reported.[676] The lesions may undergo atrophy and scarring. Cicatricial alopecia may result from scalp involvement.[677] Squamous cell carcinoma is a rare complication in any site.[678,679] Discoid lupus erythematosus is rare in children.[680–682]

A *hypertrophic variant* of discoid lupus erythematosus in which verrucous lesions develop, usually on the arms, has been reported.[683,684] Lupus erythematosus hypertrophicus et profundus is a very rare destructive variant of hypertrophic discoid lupus erythematosus with a verrucous surface and eventual subcutaneous necrosis.[685]

Annular lesions, resembling erythema multiforme, may rarely develop acutely in patients with all forms of lupus erythematosus.[686] This syndrome, known as **Rowell's syndrome**, is also characterized by a positive test for rheumatoid factor and speckled antinuclear antibodies.[686–692] The antiphospholipid syndrome may also be present.[693]

Papulonodular lesions associated with diffuse dermal mucin are uncommon manifestations of chronic cutaneous lupus erythematosus.[694,695] This mucinosis has presented as periorbital edema.[696] This variant is part of the spectrum of tumid lupus erythematosus (see below).

Tumid lupus erythematosus (lupus erythematosus tumidus)[697] consists of erythematous plaques and sometimes papules on the face, neck and upper trunk. Lesions may have a fine scale and be pruritic.[698] It usually occurs in a setting of discoid lupus erythematosus but sometimes systemic lupus erythematosus has been present.[699] This variant is part of a spectrum that includes the papulonodular type (see above).

Lymphocytic infiltration of the skin (of Jessner and Kanof) is now regarded as a variant of discoid lupus erythematosus.[700,701] Although various studies in the 1980s concluded that they were separate entities on the basis of the direct immunofluorescence, the usual absence of epidermal damage and the phenotype of the infiltrating lymphocytes, recent studies have suggested that it may be part of the tumid spectrum of discoid lupus erythematosus. Provocative phototesting gives similar results.[701]

Linear lesions, often following the lines of Blaschko, have been reported.[702–706]

Discoid lesions may be seen in up to 20% of individuals with systemic lupus erythematosus,[707] often as a presenting manifestation. It is therefore difficult to estimate accurately the incidence of the progression of the discoid to the systemic form. This is in the order of 5–10%[708–710] and is most likely in those who present abnormal laboratory findings, such as a high titer of antinuclear antibody (ANA) and antibodies to DNA, from the beginning of their illness.[711] Approximately 70% of patients possess low titers of anti-Ro/SSA antibodies and it remains to be seen whether such patients are at greater risk of progression to the systemic form.[710,712] Some patients with localized lesions may progress to more widespread disease.[713] Visceral manifestations are absent in uncomplicated discoid lupus erythematosus. An increased incidence of various haplotypes has been found.[714,715] It has been suggested that genes encoding immunoregulatory molecules may determine individual susceptibility to lupus erythematosus.[716] Lesions resembling discoid or subacute lupus erythematosus can be found in the female carriers of X-linked chronic granulomatous disease[717–722] and rarely in an autosomal form of that disease.[723,724] Discoid lupus erythematosus has also been reported in association with a deficiency of C5[725] and other immunodeficiency syndromes.[726]

Histopathology[673,727]

Discoid lupus erythematosus is characterized by a lichenoid reaction pattern and a superficial and deep dermal infiltrate of inflammatory cells which have a tendency to accumulate around the pilosebaceous follicles (Fig. 3.20). In scalp lesions with scarring alopecia, there is considerable reduction in the size of sebaceous glands and the lymphocytic infiltrate is maximal around the mid-follicle at the level of the sebaceous gland.[677] The lichenoid reaction (interface dermatitis) takes the form of vacuolar change ('liquefaction degeneration'), although there are always scattered Civatte bodies (apoptotic keratinocytes). In lesions away from the face the number of Civatte bodies is always much greater and a few colloid bodies may be found in the papillary dermis (Fig. 3.21). In older lesions, there is progressive thickening of the basement membrane, which is best seen with a PAS stain. Other epidermal changes include hyperkeratosis, keratotic follicular plugging and some atrophy of the malpighian layer.[728]

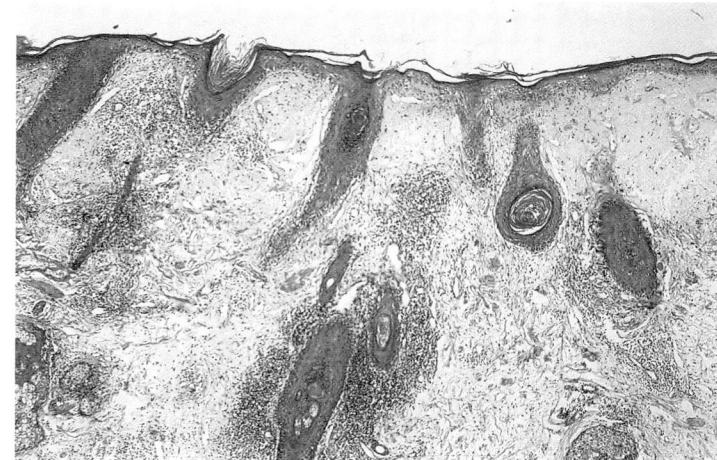

Fig. 3.20 **Discoid lupus erythematosus.** The dermal infiltrate is both superficial and deep with perifollicular accentuation. (H & E)

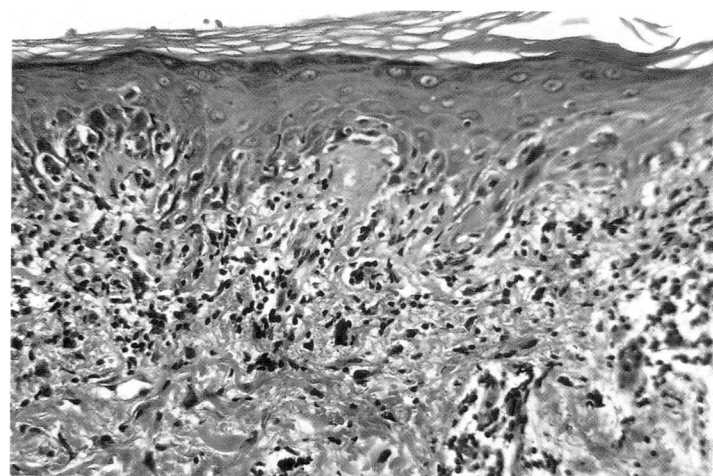

Fig. 3.21 **Discoid lupus erythematosus.** There is more cell death and less vacuolar change in the basal layer than usual. Distinction from the subacute form is difficult in these cases. (H & E)

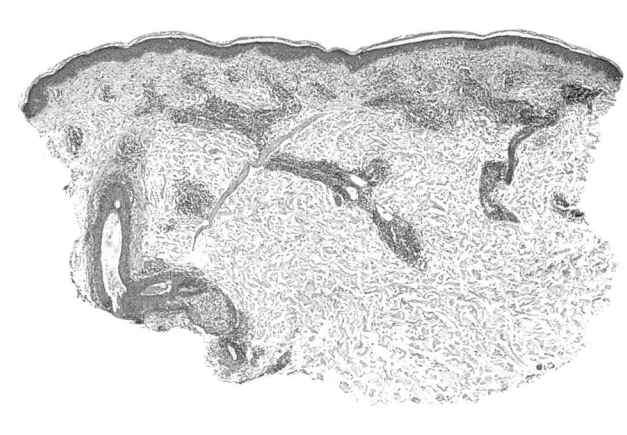

A

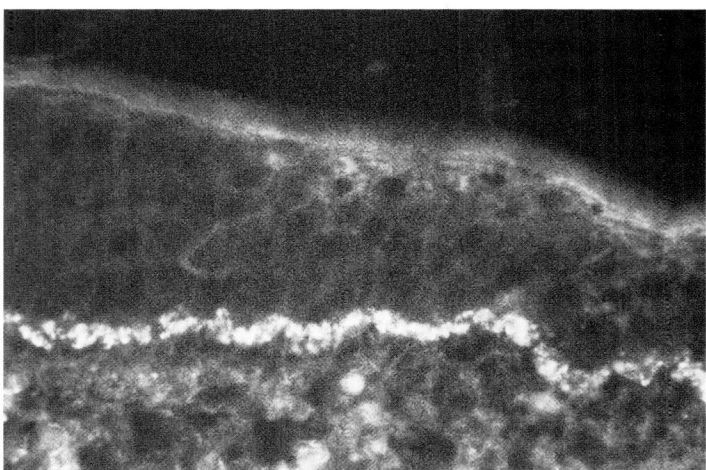

Fig. 3.23 **Discoid lupus erythematosus.** A broad band of C3 is present along the basement membrane zone. (Direct immunofluorescence)

superficial edema are also seen in the papillary dermis in some early lesions. Mucin is sometimes increased, but only rarely are there massive amounts.[730] Calcification has been reported on a few occasions.[731,732]

In *tumid lesions* there is increased dermal mucin often accompanied by subepidermal edema (Fig. 3.22). Some cases have only a sparse inflammatory cell infiltrate, while others have a heavy infiltrate of lymphocytes and less mucin.[733] Epidermal involvement is uncommon.[698,734]

In *hypertrophic lesions* there is prominent hyperkeratosis and epidermal hyperplasia. There may be a vague resemblance to a superficial squamous cell carcinoma.[735,736] Elastic fibers are often present between epidermal cells at the tips of the epidermal downgrowths.

Direct immunofluorescence of involved skin in discoid lupus will show the deposition of immunoglobulins, particularly IgG and IgM, along the basement membrane zone in 50–90% of cases (Fig. 3.23).[737–743] The incidence is less than 50% in the author's experience; perhaps this is a reflection of subtropical cases in Caucasians. Complement components are present less frequently. This so-called 'lupus band test' is positive much less often in lesions from the trunk.[744] A positive lupus band test should always be interpreted in conjunction with the clinical and histological findings,[745] as it may be obtained in chronic light-exposed skin[746] and some other conditions.[747]

Electron microscopy

There is some disorganization of the basal layer, scattered apoptotic keratinocytes and reduplication of the basement membrane.[684] Indeterminate cells, dendritic macrophages and unusual dendritic cells with short and blunt dendrites have been reported in the dermis.[748]

Subacute lupus erythematosus

Subacute lupus erythematosus is characterized by recurring, photosensitive, non-scarring lesions which may be annular or papulosquamous in type.[749–751] They are widely distributed on the face, neck, upper trunk and extensor surfaces of the arms.[752] A case with only acral lesions has been reported.[753] The patients frequently have a mild systemic illness with musculoskeletal complaints and serological abnormalities, but no renal or central nervous system disease.[754,755] Severe visceral involvement is most uncommon.[756] Cases with overlap features between the systemic and subacute forms have been reported.[757–759] Rare clinical presentations have included erythroderma,[760] a poikilodermatous pattern,[761] pityriasiform lesions,[762] the simultaneous occurrence of Sweet's syndrome[763] and an association with the ingestion of

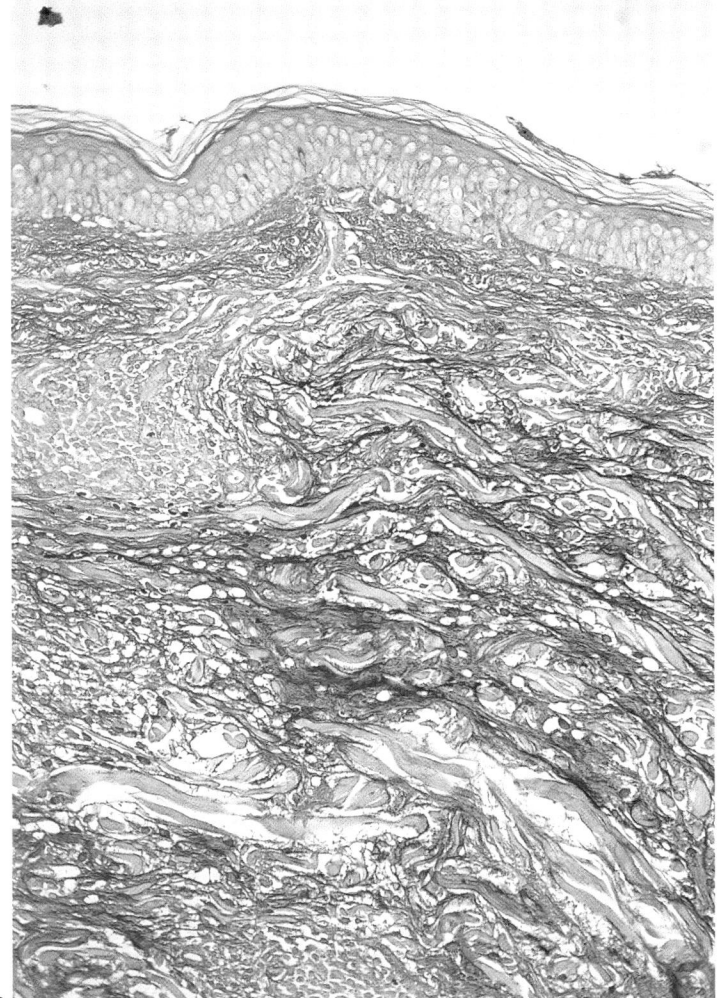

B

Fig. 3.22 **Discoid lupus of tumid type. (A)** There is a superficial and deep dermal infiltrate (H & E). **(B)** Dermal mucin is greatly increased. (Alcian blue)

The dermal infiltrate is composed predominantly of lymphocytes with a few macrophages. Atypical lymphocytes, mimicking mycosis fungoides, have been reported in one case.[729] Occasionally there are a few plasma cells and rarely there are neutrophils and nuclear dust in the superficial dermis in active lesions. Plasma cells are prominent in oral lesions.[675] Fibrin extravasation and

thiazide,[764] terbinafine,[765,766] antihistamines,[767] calcium channel blockers[768] and griseofulvin.[769] It has also been induced by radiation therapy.[770] It has been reported in a patient with hepatocellular carcinoma.[771] An interesting finding is that smokers with cutaneous lupus erythematosus are less responsive to antimalarial treatment than non-smokers.[772]

The test for ANA is often negative if mouse liver is used as the test substrate, but positive if human Hep-2 cells are used.[773] There is a high incidence of the anticytoplasmic antibody Ro/SSA;[774–779] it is found in a higher incidence in those with annular rather than papulosquamous lesions.[780] This antibody is also found in systemic lupus erythematosus, neonatal lupus erythematosus, in the lupus-like syndrome that may accompany homozygous C2 deficiency[781–784] and in Sjögren's syndrome.[785,786] The Ro/SSA antigen is now known to be localized in the epidermis and it is thought that antibodies to this antigen are important in the initiation of tissue damage.[787] Antigen expression is higher in photosensitive forms of lupus erythematosus.[788] However, the antibody titer does not correlate with the activity of the skin disease.[789]

Histopathology[790]

The histopathological features differ only in degree from those seen in discoid lupus.[754,791] Usually there is more basal vacuolar change, epidermal atrophy and dermal edema and superficial mucin than in discoid lupus, but less hyperkeratosis, pilosebaceous atrophy, follicular plugging, basement membrane thickening and cellular infiltrate (Fig. 3.24).[790–793] The pattern can be characterized as a pauci-inflammatory, vacuolar, lymphocytic interface dermatitis.[733] Apoptotic keratinocytes (Civatte bodies) are sometimes quite prominent in subacute lupus erythematosus; they may be found at various levels within the epidermis, resembling erythema multiforme[794] (Fig. 3.25).[795] Furthermore, the infiltrate is usually confined more to the upper dermis than in discoid lupus.[790,796] The above features relate to the more common annular form which may resemble erythema multiforme to varying degrees.[692] The papulosquamous form of subacute lupus erythematosus has no distinguishing features to permit differentiation from the discoid form.[792]

The lupus band test (see above) shows immunoglobulins at the dermo-epidermal junction in approximately 60% of cases. The band is usually not as thick or as intensely staining as in discoid lupus erythematosus. Very fine, dust-like particles of IgG (a speckled pattern) have been described predominantly, but not exclusively, in the cytoplasm of basal cells[796–799] and also in the cellular infiltrate in the dermis.[800] This pattern is not specific for subacute cutaneous

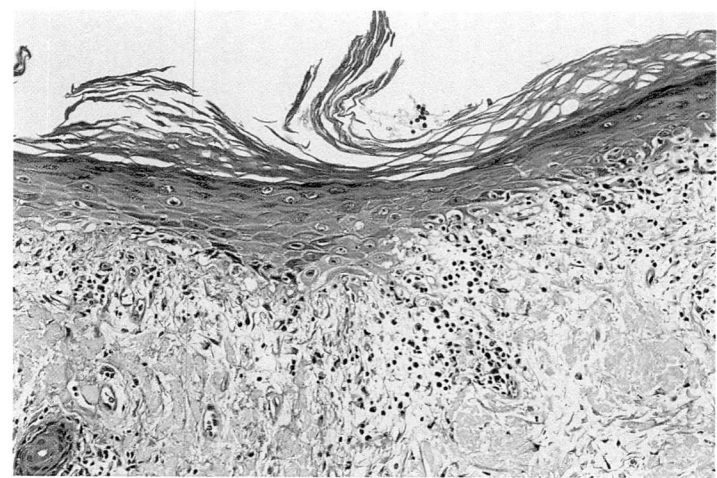

Fig. 3.24 **Subacute lupus erythematosus** with patchy basal vacuolar change and occasional Civatte bodies. (H & E)

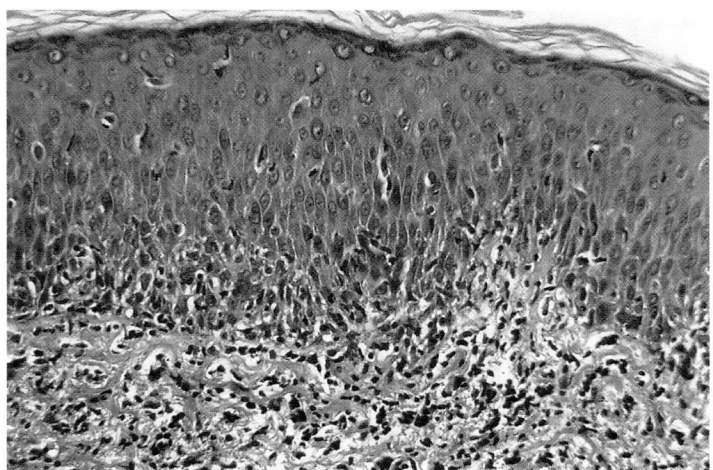

Fig. 3.25 **Subacute lupus erythematosus.** The infiltrate extends into the lower epidermis and cell death occurs at a slightly higher level than usual. This variant can be mistaken for erythema multiforme. (H & E)

lupus erythematosus or the presence of Ro/SSA antibodies. Dust-like particles were found in only 3% of cases in one recent study.[801]

Systemic lupus erythematosus

In systemic lupus erythematosus (SLE) the changes in the skin are part of a much more widespread disorder. Four clinical manifestations are particularly important as criteria for the diagnosis of SLE: skin lesions, renal involvement, joint involvement and serositis.[671] The coexistence of the first two of these manifestations is sufficient to justify a strong presumption of the diagnosis.

Cutaneous lesions take the form of erythematous, slightly indurated patches with only a little scale. They are most common on the face, particularly the malar areas. The lesions are usually more extensive and less well defined than those of discoid lupus erythematosus and devoid of atrophy. Scarring is an important complication of all forms of lupus erythematosus.[802] The lesions may spread to the chest and other parts of the body. In some instances, they may be urticarial,[803] bullous,[804–806] mucinous,[807] purpuric or, rarely, ulcerated. It is important to remember that skin lesions do not develop at all in about 20% of patients with SLE; approximately the same proportion have discoid lesions of the type seen in chronic discoid lupus erythematosus, but usually without scarring.[808] This latter group often has less severe disease.[707] The digits, calves and heels are involved in the rare chilblain (pernictic) lupus which results from microvascular injury in the course of SLE.[809–811] Red lunulae have been reported in association with chilblain lupus and also as an isolated phenomenon in SLE.[812–814] Subclinical inflammatory alopecia has also been reported.[815] A spectrum of elastic tissue changes can occur in patients with lupus erythematosus. They range from mid-dermal elastolysis to anetoderma (see p. 394).

SLE may coexist with other diseases such as rheumatoid arthritis, scleroderma,[816] dermatomyositis, Sjögren's syndrome (sometimes with associated annular erythema),[817] eosinophilic fasciitis,[818] autoimmune thyroiditis,[819] ulcerative colitis,[820] myasthenia gravis,[821] pemphigus,[821] gout,[822] alopecia areata,[823] sarcoidosis,[824] porphyria cutanea tarda,[825] Sweet's syndrome,[826] psoriasis,[827] pyodermatitis vegetans,[828] cutaneous T-cell lymphoma,[829] dermatitis herpetiformis,[830] acanthosis nigricans[671] and various complement deficiencies.[831–835] It has been suggested that some patients with photosensitive lupus erythematosus represent the coexistence of a photodermatosis such as polymorphous light eruption.[836] Many of these associated conditions represent the chance coexistence of the two diseases, although the occurrence of SLE with diseases such as scleroderma, dermatomyositis and rheumatoid arthritis has been included in the concept of mixed connective disease, an ill-defined condition with various overlap features and the presence of ribonucleoprotein antibody (see p. 351).[837,838]

Joint symptoms, serositis and renal disease are frequent.[671] Rare manifestations include vegetations on the valve leaflets in the heart, vasculitis,[839] diffuse pulmonary interstitial fibrosis, peripheral neuropathy and ocular involvement.[671] Neurological manifestations are not uncommon and occasionally these are thromboembolic in nature, related to the presence of circulating anticardiolipin antibodies (the 'lupus anticoagulant') (see p. 226).[840–842] Cutaneous infarction[843–845] and ulceration[846] are other rare manifestations of this circulating antibody. However, digital necrosis can occur in patients with SLE in the absence of this antiphospholipid syndrome.[847]

SLE usually runs a chronic course with a series of remissions and exacerbations. The commonest causes of death are renal failure and vascular lesions of the central nervous system.[848] The 10-year survival rate currently exceeds 90%.[671] In a recent review of 57 children with SLE, eight had died, six from severe infection and two from renal failure.[849]

Investigations

Various laboratory investigations are undertaken in the diagnostic study of patients with suspected lupus erythematosus.[850–852] The LE cell preparation is now of historical interest only and it has been replaced as a screening test by the immunofluorescent detection of circulating antinuclear antibodies (ANA).[853] Various patterns of immunofluorescence, corresponding to different circulating antibodies, can be seen; the incidence of positivity depends on the substrate used.[854] A homogeneous staining pattern is usually obtained. This test is positive in more than 90% of untreated patients, many of the negative cases belonging to the subset with anti-Ro/SSA antibodies (see p. 50).

Much more specific for the diagnosis is the detection of antibodies to double-stranded DNA. They are found in over 50% of cases and the titer may be used to monitor the progress of treatment.[671] The presence of these antibodies is often associated with renal disease. They are usually detected by a radioimmunoassay method.

Other antibodies may also be detected, including rheumatoid factor and antibodies to extractable nuclear antigen (ENA). Anti-α-fodrin antibodies, commonly found in patients with Sjögren's syndrome, are seen in a small number of patients with SLE.[855] Antineutrophil cytoplasmic antibodies (ANCA) have been present in many patients with minocycline-induced lupus-like syndrome.[856] False-positive serological tests for syphilis are sometimes present.[671] Antibodies to cytoplasmic keratin proteins in the epidermis have been detected in patients with SLE. Their presence appears to correlate with the finding of cytoplasmic deposits of immunoglobulin in epidermal keratinocytes.[857,858] Antibodies to basement membrane antigens are sometimes found in the sera of patients with no evidence of bullous lesions.[859]

Etiology

Altered immunity, drugs, viruses, genetic predisposition, hormones and ultraviolet light may all contribute to the etiology and pathogenesis of lupus erythematosus.[671] Immunological abnormalities are a key feature. Various autoantibodies are often present and high levels of antibodies against double-stranded DNA have been considered specific for SLE. Immune complexes are found in about 50% of affected individuals[708] and those containing DNA appear to be responsible for renal injury. Vascular injury may result from the deposition of these complexes.[860] There have been conflicting reports on the role of the various T-cell subsets.[861–863] However, CD4+ αβ T cells infiltrate the papillary dermis and appear to play some role in the basal damage.[864]

Increased cytokine production, particularly IFN-γ, has been noted.[865] A similar mechanism appears to be responsible in discoid lupus erythematosus.[866] It appears that dysregulation of T lymphocytes causes the activation of B cells, producing various autoantibodies of pathogenetic significance.[867] Interestingly, a chimeric CD4-monoclonal antibody has been used successfully in the treatment of severe cutaneous lupus erythematosus.[868] Other immunological findings include a reduction in epidermal Langerhans cells, loss of HLA-DR surface antigens on dermal capillaries and a small percentage of Leu 8-positive cells in the dermal infiltrate.[862,869,870] HLA-DR is expressed on epidermal keratinocytes, while ICAM-1 is expressed on keratinocytes, dermal inflammatory cells and endothelial cells.[870]

In a small but important proportion of cases the onset of systemic lupus is quite clearly related to the ingestion of drugs.[671] Those incriminated include procainamide,[871] isoniazid, hydralazine,[872] quinidine,[873] minocycline,[874–877] penicillamine,[878] sulfonamides,[879] terbinafine,[880,881] chlorpromazine,[882] phenylbutazone, hydrochlorothiazide,[883] methimazole,[884] carbamazepine,[885] atenolol,[886] practolol, phenobarbitone and phenytoin. A recent review also lists allopurinol, captopril, clonidine, danazol, ethosuximide, griseofulvin, lithium, lovastatin, mesalazine, methyldopa, penicillin, piroxicam, primidone, propylthiouracil, streptomycin, thiamazole, trimethadione and valproate.[852] A new anti-angiogenesis drug (COL-3) used in the treatment of cancer can also induce SLE.[887] Oral contraceptives may sometimes result in a flare-up of the disease. Withdrawal of the drug is usually followed by slow resolution of the process. Exposure to insecticides has also been incriminated.[888,889] Procainamide-induced SLE, which is the best studied of the drug-related cases, has a low incidence of renal involvement.[671] High titers of leukocyte-specific ANA are present in those with clinical disease.[890]

The role of viruses is still controversial. Structures resembling paramyxovirus have been demonstrated on electron microscopy, particularly in endothelial cells, in SLE and also in discoid lupus erythematosus.[891] There is doubt about the nature of these inclusions. Rare cases associated with parvovirus B19 have been reported.[733]

Familial cases have been recorded, usually in siblings, but also in successive generations. The disease has been observed in numerous pairs of identical twins. Several HLA types have been incriminated.[892]

The role of sunlight in inducing and exacerbating cutaneous lupus of all types is well documented.[893–896] Ultraviolet (UV)-B irradiation is the most frequent inducer of skin lesions in photosensitive lupus, although very high doses of UVA may trigger lesions in some patients.[897] The mechanism of action appears to be the stimulation of keratinocytes to translocate cytoplasmic and nuclear antigens, such as SSA and SSB. Ultraviolet irradiation also stimulates keratinocytes and fibroblasts to release cytokines, such as tumor necrosis factor-α and interleukin-1α. A rare allele (-308A, TNF2) of the TNF-α promotor gene is strongly linked to subacute lupus erythematosus.[897] Sunlight-induced damage of cellular DNA contributes ultimately to the formation of immune complexes which may be of pathogenetic significance.

Finally, the occurrence of both systemic and subacute lupus erythematosus in association with cancer, albeit rarely, raises the possibility of a paraneoplastic association.[457,898]

Histopathology[673]

The cutaneous lesions of systemic lupus erythematosus show prominent vacuolar change involving the basal layer. Civatte body formation is not usually a feature. Edema, small hemorrhages and a mild infiltrate of inflammatory cells, principally lymphocytes, are present in the upper dermis. Eosinophils may be present in drug-induced cases. Fibrinoid material is deposited in the dermis around capillary blood vessels, on collagen and in the interstitium. It sometimes contributes to thickening of the basement

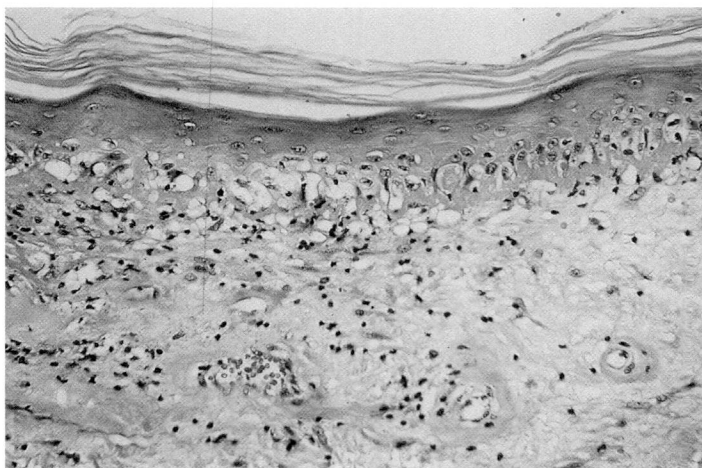

Fig. 3.26 **Acute lupus erythematosus.** There is thickening of the basement membrane zone as well as vacuolar change and Civatte bodies. (H & E)

membrane zone (Fig. 3.26). The main constituents of this thickened zone are type IV and type VII collagen.[899] Mucin can be demonstrated by special stains[900] and its presence may be helpful in distinguishing the lesions of SLE from polymorphous light eruption.[901] The term 'cutaneous lupus mucinosis' has been used for cases with abundant dermal mucin.[807] A vasculitis, usually of leukocytoclastic type is sometimes present. It may be complicated by thrombosis.

The subset of patients who have antibodies to Ro/SSA show additional vascular changes not usually seen in those without these antibodies. They include telangiectasia, endothelial cell necrosis and luminal deposits of fibrin.[733]

In chilblain lupus, a lichenoid (vacuolar interface) reaction overlies a lymphocytic vasculitis involving both the superficial and deep plexuses.

Hematoxyphile bodies – altered nuclei that are the tissue equivalent of the LE cells in the blood – are found rarely in the skin, in contrast to visceral lesions in which they are not infrequent.

The incidence of a positive lupus band test will depend on the site biopsied.[902] Involved skin is positive in almost 100% of cases, while uninvolved skin from sun-exposed areas is positive in about 90% of cases.[903] Biopsies of uninvolved skin from sun-protected areas are positive in only one-third of cases. Positive tests are obtained from sun-exposed skin in one-third or more of normal controls,[904–906] although the staining pattern is usually weak.[904] The lupus band test may be negative in remissions, very early lesions and some cases of drug-induced lupus erythematosus.[907] The test is useful in excluding diseases that are clinically similar to SLE.[908] Membrane attack complex (MAC) is deposited in a granular pattern along the basement membrane zone in approximately 75% of patients with cutaneous lupus erythematosus.[909] It is also found in subacute lupus erythematosus.[910] It may be a useful adjunct to the lupus band test.[909] Another finding on direct immunofluorescence is epidermal nuclear staining, usually for IgG. It is found in only a small percentage of cases but it may correlate with oral involvement.[911] Immunoelectron microscopy has shown that the immunoglobulin deposits are predominantly in the papillary dermis, just beneath the basal lamina.[912] The deposition appears to damage both type IV and type VII collagen.[913] DNA is a major component of the complexes.

LUPUS ERYTHEMATOSUS VARIANTS

The traditional variants of lupus erythematosus (discoid, subacute and systemic) have already been discussed. This section covers uncommon, but distinct, clinico-pathological variants.

Neonatal lupus erythematosus

Neonatal lupus erythematosus is a rare syndrome[914–918] characterized by a transient lupus dermatitis developing in the neonatal period, accompanied by a variety of hematological and systemic abnormalities,[919,920] including congenital heart block.[921,922] Cutaneous lesions resemble those seen in subacute cutaneous lupus erythematosus;[923] telangiectatic macules may be a feature.[924,925] Periorbital, scalp and extremity lesions are common.[926] Depigmented lesions are rare,[927] so too are cutaneous erosions[928] and lupus panniculitis.[929] Approximately 20% of the mothers have SLE at the time of the birth and a similar percentage will subsequently develop it.[921] Others may have Sjögren's syndrome or, uncommonly, a vasculitis.[930] The Ro/SSA antibody is present in infants and mothers in nearly all cases[923,926,931–934] and it has been suggested that this is of maternal origin and crosses the placenta, where it is subsequently destroyed by the infant.[935,936] Antibodies to α-fodrin,[937] La/SSB and U₁RNP have been detected in some cases.[938–942] The anticardiolipin antibody has been reported in a baby with neonatal lupus erythematosus.[943] Successive siblings may be affected with this condition.[944]

The histological features resemble those seen in subacute lupus erythematosus.[945]

Bullous lupus erythematosus

A rare form of SLE, bullous lupus erythematosus, is a skin eruption which clinically and histologically closely resembles dermatitis herpetiformis.[946–949] Rare clinical variants include a localized linear form[950] and one in which milia develop.[951] The blisters are subepidermal with neutrophils in the papillary dermis and some lymphocytes around vessels in the superficial plexus.[952] Bullae have been reported in a case of discoid lupus erythematosus[953] and also following steroid withdrawal in SLE.[806] Linear or mixed linear and granular deposits of IgG are found along the basement membrane zone.[954] IgA and/or IgM may also be present.[955,956] The immunoreactants are deposited beneath the lamina densa.[952]

There appear to be at least two immunologically distinct subtypes characterized by the presence or absence of circulating and/or tissue-bound autoantibodies to type VII collagen.[956–959] Patients with autoantibodies to type VII collagen are similar but not identical to patients with epidermolysis bullosa acquisita[960] (see p. 148). The autoantibodies appear to recognize the same non-collagenous (NC1) domain.[961] In other cases, various components of the basement membrane zone may be targeted. In one case there were autoantibodies to the bullous pemphigoid antigen (BP230), laminin-5, laminin-6 and type VII collagen.[962]

Lupus panniculitis

Lupus panniculitis (lupus profundus) presents clinically as firm subcutaneous inflammatory nodules, from 1–4 cm or more in diameter, situated on the head, neck, arms, abdominal wall, thighs or buttocks.[963,964] There are isolated reports of breast involvement (lupus mastitis)[965] and also of linear lesions.[966] Lupus panniculitis is a rare complication which may precede the development of overt systemic or discoid lupus erythematosus.[967] A patient with widespread lesions in the setting of a partial deficiency of C4 has been reported.[968] In some cases the lesions subside without any other sign of the disease.[969] The clinical diagnosis may be difficult if there are no other manifestations of lupus erythematosus. The lesions may be misdiagnosed as deep morphea.[970] Lupus panniculitis is discussed in more detail with the panniculitides (Ch. 17, p. 529).

DERMATOMYOSITIS

Dermatomyositis is characterized by the coexistence of a non-suppurative myositis (polymyositis) and inflammatory changes in the skin.[971–974] Cutaneous lesions may precede the development of muscle involvement by up to two years or more.[975–977] Cases without muscle involvement (amyopathic dermatomyositis, dermatomyositis sine myositis) exist.[978–981] Amyopathic dermatomyositis is defined as the finding of dermatomyositis in the absence of any clinical or laboratory signs of muscle disease for at least two years after the onset of skin pathology.[982] Dermatomyositis may occur in either sex and at any age. Those cases commencing in childhood are sometimes considered as a separate clinical group, because of the greater incidence in them of multiorgan disease.[983–987] Rarely this includes a necrotizing vasculitis that may involve the gut and other organs with a fatal outcome.[983]

The skin lesions are violaceous or erythematous, slightly scaly lesions with a predisposition for the face, shoulders, the extensor surfaces of the forearms and the thighs.[988] Poikilodermatous features (telangiectasia, hyperpigmentation and hypopigmentation) may be present.[989] Photosensitivity is sometimes present.[990] Other characteristic findings are nail fold changes, gingival telangiectases,[991] purplish discoloration and edema of the periorbital tissues (heliotrope rash) and atrophic papules or plaques over the knuckles (Gottron's papules).[989] Plaques of calcification sometimes develop.[992,993] Unusual presentations include as an isolated flagellate eruption on the back,[994,995] as a plaque-like mucinosis,[996,997] the presence of follicular keratotic papules with some features of pityriasis rubra pilaris,[998–1000] lesions resembling malignant atrophic papulosis[1001] and as a panniculitis,[1002,1003] erythroderma[1004] or vesiculobullous eruption.[1005]

Other clinical features include the presence of proximal muscle weakness and elevation of certain serum enzymes such as creatine phosphokinase.[988,1006] Muscle ultrasound is sometimes abnormal in patients with dermatomyositis and normal muscle enzyme levels.[1007] Raynaud's phenomenon, dysphagia, Sjögren's syndrome, retinopathy and overlap features with scleroderma[1008,1009] and with lupus erythematosus sometimes occur.[989,1010] Interstitial lung disease is an uncommon but debilitating complication which is usually associated with the presence of the anti-Jo-1 antibody.[1011,1012] Other autoantibodies, such as to histone, are sometimes present.[1013]

An underlying malignancy is present in 10% or more of cases.[1014–1024] Predictive factors for malignancy include male gender and older age of onset.[1025] The cutaneous manifestations may precede the diagnosis of the malignancy by up to a year or more. Amyopathic cases of paraneoplastic dermatomyositis have been reported.[1026] Subepidermal vesiculation is an uncommon finding in dermatomyositis; its presence may be related to the occurrence of an internal malignancy.[1005,1027] Bullous pemphigoid has also been recorded as a coexisting disease.[1028]

The etiology and pathogenesis are unknown but immunological mechanisms are probably involved. In addition to the various autoantibodies that are often present, activated T cells and natural killer cells have been demonstrated in biopsied muscle.[988] In the skin, the infiltrate consists predominantly of macrophages expressing HLA-DR and of T cells, especially of the CD4 subset.[1029] The deposition of membrane attack complex of complement (MAC) has been demonstrated along the dermoepidermal junction and in some dermal blood vessels.[1030] There are elevated levels of soluble vascular cell adhesion molecule-1 (sVCAM-1).[1031] A dermatomyositis-like syndrome has been associated with certain viral illnesses, including parvovirus B19,[1032] with toxoplasmosis[1033] and leishmaniasis.[1034] It has followed administration of hydroxyurea[1035–1041] and of penicillamine.[988] Dermatomyositis has developed in pregnancy with rapid improvement following delivery[1042] and in the postpartum period.[1043] It has been reported in a patient with hereditary complement (C9) deficiency.[1044] Cytoplasmic inclusions resembling the paramyxovirus-like structures seen in lupus erythematosus (see p. 51) have also been found in blood vessels in cases of dermatomyositis.[1045]

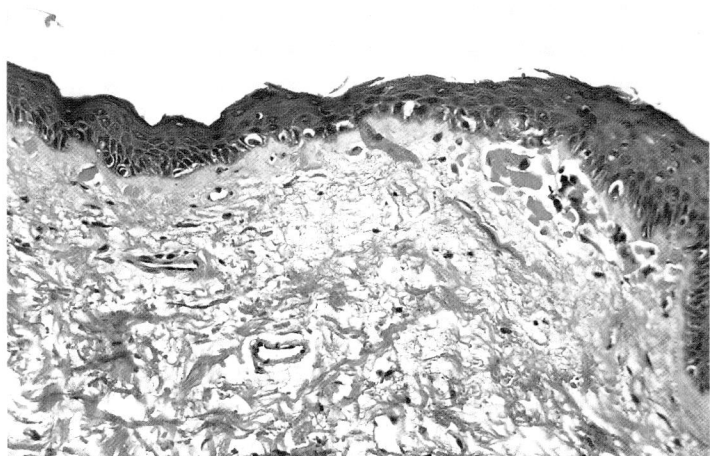

Fig. 3.27 **Dermatomyositis.** The changes are quite subtle with mild basal vacuolar change and several colloid bodies in the papillary dermis. The appearances may be indistinguishable from acute lupus erythematosus although in the latter disease basement membrane thickening may be more pronounced and colloid bodies less frequent than in dermatomyositis. (H & E)

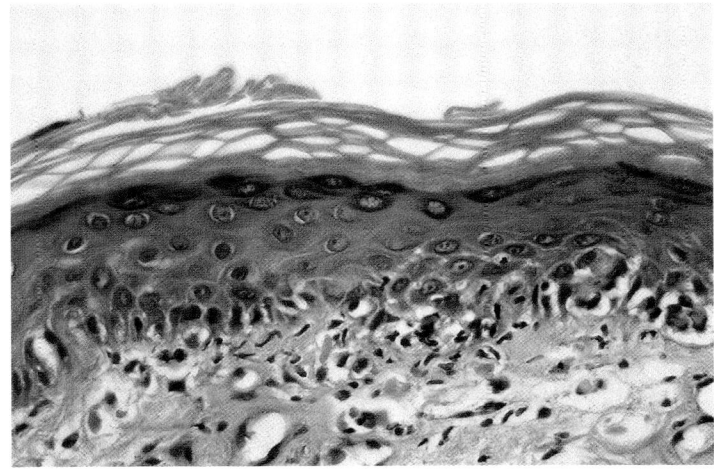

Fig. 3.28 **Dermatomyositis.** The lichenoid reaction pattern is more obvious in this case. The appearances are indistinguishable from cutaneous lupus erythematosus. (H & E)

Histopathology[1046]

The histological changes are quite variable. At times the changes are subtle (Fig. 3.27) with only a sparse superficial perivascular infiltrate of lymphocytes, associated with variable edema and mucinous change in the upper dermis.[1046] More often, there are the features of a lichenoid tissue reaction consisting of vacuolar change in the basal layer. Only occasional Civatte bodies are present, if any (Fig. 3.28). A few neutrophils are sometimes present in the infiltrate, particularly in those cases with fibrinoid material in the papillary dermis and around superficial vessels. Diffuse dermal neutrophilia and leukocytoclastic vasculitis are rare findings.[1047] The basement membrane is often thickened. These appearances are indistinguishable from those of acute lupus erythematosus.

At other times, there are additional features of epidermal atrophy, melanin incontinence and dilatation of superficial vessels (poikilodermatous changes).[1046] A biopsy from a Gottron's papule will show mild hyperkeratosis and some acanthosis, in addition to the basal vacuolar change.[1048]

Unusual findings include subepidermal vesiculation, a lobular panniculitis and dystrophic calcification.[1002,1003,1049–1051] The vesicular lesions are cell poor with abundant edema fluid. Necrosis of the roof sometimes occurs. An osteogenic sarcoma developed in an area of heterotopic ossification in one case of dermatomyositis.[1052]

In the Wong type of dermatomyositis, in which pityriasis rubra pilaris-like lesions are present, there is follicular hyperkeratosis with destruction of hair follicles. Cornoid lamellation has been seen in one of these cases.[1000]

Intercellular deposits of immunoglobulins have been reported in the epidermis of nail fold biopsies.[1053] Colloid bodies containing IgM are sometimes quite prominent in the papillary dermis. The lupus band test is usually negative although it was positive in a significant number of cases in one series.[1054] Vascular deposits of C_{5b-9} are found in dermatomyositis but not in lupus erythematosus.[1055] Immunoglobulins, including IgA, have been reported in muscle biopsies in dermatomyositis.[1056]

POIKILODERMAS

The poikilodermas are a heterogeneous group of dermatoses characterized clinically by erythema, mottled pigmentation and, later, epidermal atrophy. These changes result from basal vacuolar change with consequent melanin incontinence and variable telangiectasia of blood vessels in the superficial dermis (Fig. 3.29). For this reason, Pinkus included the poikilodermatous pattern as a subgroup of the lichenoid tissue reaction.[1]

Four distinct groups of poikilodermatous dermatoses are found:

1. the genodermatoses poikiloderma congenitale (Rothmund–Thomson syndrome), congenital telangiectatic erythema (Bloom's syndrome) and dyskeratosis congenita;
2. a stage in the evolution of early mycosis fungoides;
3. a variant of dermatomyositis and less frequently of SLE;
4. a miscellaneous group which may follow radiation, cold and heat injury, prolonged exposure to sunlight (poikiloderma of Civatte) and ingestion of drugs (arsenicals and busulfan) or which may occur in the evolution of chronic graft-versus-host reaction.[1057]

The three genodermatoses mentioned above are distinct clinical entities, but the poikiloderma which may precede mycosis fungoides (poikiloderma atrophicans vasculare) is now regarded as an early stage in the evolution of mycosis fungoides. Likewise, poikilodermatomyositis represents a clinico-pathological variant of dermatomyositis rather than a disease sui generis.

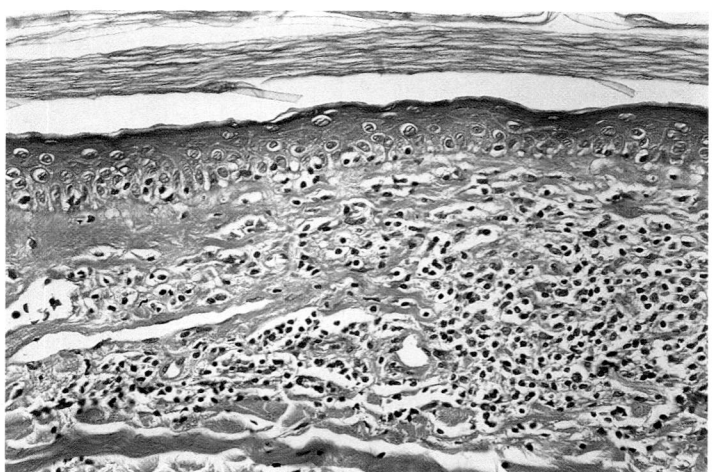

Fig. 3.29 **The poikilodermatous reaction pattern in a case of mycosis fungoides.** (H & E)

Poikiloderma of Civatte is probably not a distinct entity.[1058,1059] It has been suggested that some poikilodermas are possibly related in some way to a graft-versus-host reaction.[1057]

POIKILODERMA CONGENITALE

Over 200 cases of poikiloderma congenitale (Rothmund–Thomson syndrome) have now been reported in the English literature.[1060,1061] It is an autosomal recessive, multisystem disorder which affects principally the skin, eyes and skeletal system.[1062–1068] A reticular erythematous eruption commences in the first year of life and this is followed by the development of areas of hyperpigmentation. Warty keratoses may appear on the hands, elbows, knees and feet. Other clinical features include a short stature, cataracts, hypogonadism, mental retardation, photosensitivity to ultraviolet A radiation[1060,1069] and, rarely, the development of skin cancers,[1070] hematologic malignancies[1071,1072] and osteogenic sarcoma.[1073,1074] Sometimes only a few of these features are present in an individual case, illustrating the variable presentation of this syndrome.[1075] Reduced DNA repair capacity might be related to the photosensitivity in early childhood.[1076] There appears to be instability in chromosome 8, sometimes leading to trisomy 8 or other abnormalities.[1075] The condition appears to be genetically heterogeneous. Some cases are due to mutations in the *RECQ4* helicase gene which maps to chromosome 8q24.3.[1077]

Hereditary sclerosing poikiloderma

Hereditary sclerosing poikiloderma (of Weary) is an autosomal dominant disorder with many similar clinical features.[1078] However, there are linear hyperkeratotic and sclerotic bands in the flexural areas, sclerosis of the palms and soles, and clubbing of the nails.[1079]

Kindler's syndrome

Kindler's syndrome, initially thought to represent the association of poikiloderma congenitale with dystrophic epidermolysis bullosa,[1080] is now regarded as a distinct but related entity.[1081–1083] Similar cases have been reported under the title *hereditary acrokeratotic poikiloderma*.[1084,1085] Both groups of cases are characterized by acral bullae and keratoses with poikilodermatous changes.[1081] Photosensitivity is often present in Kindler's syndrome.[1086] Abnormalities in keratin 5 or 14 have been postulated.[1087]

Another variant with poikiloderma, traumatic bulla formation and pitted palmoplantar keratoderma has been reported.[1088]

Histopathology

There are the usual poikilodermatous features of hyperkeratosis, epidermal atrophy, basal vacuolar change, numerous telangiectatic vessels, scattered dermal melanophages and a variable upper dermal inflammatory cell infiltrate.

The keratotic (warty) lesions show hyperkeratosis, a normal or thickened epidermis and some loss of cell polarity, with dyskeratotic cells also present.[1062]

The bullae in *Kindler's syndrome* are subepidermal and cell poor, although ultrastructural studies have shown that the split can occur at several levels within the dermoepidermal junction zone, including within the basal cells.[1086,1087,1089,1090]

CONGENITAL TELANGIECTATIC ERYTHEMA

Congenital telangiectatic erythema is a rare autosomal recessive disorder usually known by the eponymous designation Bloom's syndrome. In addition to the telangiectatic, sun-sensitive facial rash, there is stunted growth, proneness to respiratory and gastrointestinal infections, chromosomal abnormalities and a variety of congenital malformations.[1091–1093] The facial rash has lupus-like qualities.[1094] Various chromosomal breakages are found in cultured lymphocytes, the most characteristic being a high rate of sister chromatid exchanges during metaphase.[1095] As a consequence, there is a significant tendency to develop various malignancies,[1096] particularly acute leukemia and lymphoma.[1091,1097] The gene responsible has been mapped to chromosome 15q26.1.[1093]

Histopathology
The facial rash consistently shows dilatation of dermal capillaries. There is usually only a mild perivascular infiltrate of lymphocytes. Basal vacuolar change may occur but does not usually result in pigment incontinence.

DYSKERATOSIS CONGENITA

Dyskeratosis congenita is a rare, sometimes fatal genodermatosis characterized primarily by the triad of reticulate hyperpigmentation, nail dystrophy and leukokeratosis of mucous membranes.[1098,1099] Other less constant features include a Fanconi-type pancytopenia,[1100–1102] eye and dental changes, mental deficiency, deafness,[1103] intracranial calcification,[1104] palmoplantar hyperkeratosis, scarring alopecia[1105] and an increased incidence of malignancy, particularly related to the mucous membranes.[1103,1106] Bone marrow failure is the major cause of premature death.

Although found predominantly in Caucasian males, it has been reported in several races and occasionally in females.[1107] Most cases are inherited as a sex-linked recessive trait,[1103] but several kindreds with autosomal dominant inheritance have been reported.[1108] The gene, *DKC1*, which encodes a 514 amino acid protein, dyskerin, is located at Xp28.[1109] The disease is predominantly caused by missense mutations in this gene.[1110] It is thought that dyskerin is a nucleolar protein that is responsible for some early steps in ribosomal-RNA processing.[1109]

The skin changes, which may resemble poikiloderma, usually develop on the face, neck and upper trunk in childhood. It has been suggested that there may be pathogenetic features in common with graft-versus-host disease.[1098]

Histopathology
Usually there are mild hyperkeratosis, epidermal atrophy, prominent telangiectasia of superficial vessels and numerous melanophages in the papillary dermis. Less constant features include mild basal vacuolar change, fibrosis of the upper dermis and a mild lymphocytic infiltrate beneath the epidermis.[1098] Civatte bodies have not been recorded.

OTHER LICHENOID (INTERFACE) DISEASES

In addition to the dermatoses discussed above, a number of other important diseases may show features of the lichenoid reaction pattern. They have been discussed more fully in other chapters, but they are also included here for completeness. Only the salient histological features are mentioned.

LICHEN SCLEROSUS ET ATROPHICUS

In early lesions, the inflammatory infiltrate is quite heavy with band-like qualities mimicking lichen planus. Both vacuolar change and apoptotic basal keratinocytes are present. The infiltrate is eventually pushed downwards by an expanding zone of edema and sclerosis (see p. 354).

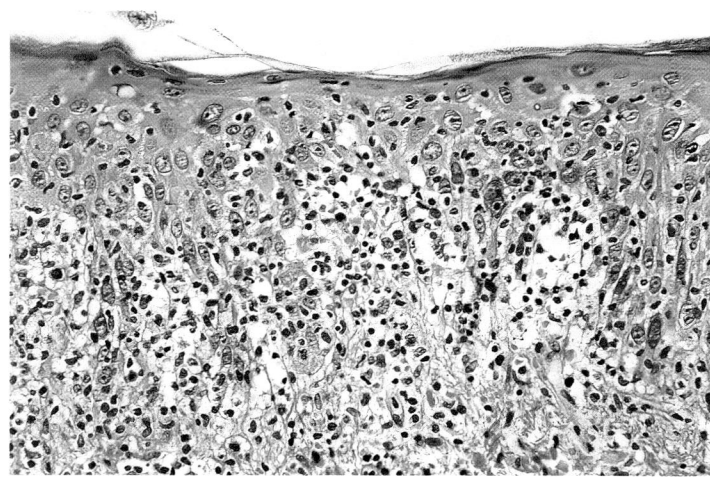

Fig. 3.30 **Pityriasis lichenoides** (acute form). The dermoepidermal interface is obscured by the inflammatory cell infiltrate. (H & E)

PITYRIASIS LICHENOIDES

In the acute form of pityriasis lichenoides, pityriasis lichenoides et varioliformis acuta (PLEVA), there is a heavy lymphocytic infiltrate which obscures the dermoepidermal interface in much the same way as it does in erythema multiforme and fixed drug eruption (Fig. 3.30). This may be associated with focal epidermal cell death and overlying parakeratosis or confluent epidermal necrosis.[1111] The dermal infiltrate varies from a mild lymphocytic vasculitis to a heavy infiltrate which also extends between the vessels and is accompanied by variable hemorrhage. The dermal infiltrate is often wedge-shaped in distribution with the apex towards the deep dermis. PLEVA is considered further with the lymphocytic vasculitides in Chapter 8 (p. 246).

PERSISTENT VIRAL REACTIONS

There is increasing recognition that viral and putative viral infections may be followed by a spectrum of cutaneous reactions that often includes the lichenoid tissue reaction. Examples include lichenoid lymphocytic vasculitis (see p. 243) which occurs with persistent herpes simplex infection, the Gianotti–Crosti syndrome (see p. 706)[1112] and reactions resembling mild pityriasis lichenoides. A chronic lichenoid dermatosis has been reported in several patients as an unusual manifestation of both herpes simplex and varicella-zoster infection. There was a lichenoid reaction but no cytolytic host response.[1113] Late stages of pityriasis rosea (included here as a putative viral infection) often show prominent epidermal cell death. Basal vacuolar change is usually present in these various reactions.

Asymmetric periflexural exanthem of childhood, also known as unilateral laterothoracic exanthem, is a putative viral disease with pruritic, unilateral macules and papules. It has a distinctive perisudoral CD8+ infiltrate at the interface. Lymphocytes have also been found around the eccrine coils. Apoptotic basal keratinocytes are also present.[1114,1115]

PERNIOSIS

In some cases of perniosis, a mild lichenoid reaction is present. It is mostly focal. The changes are more prominent in cases of chilblain lupus (lupus pernio). There is usually no parakeratosis, unlike pityriasis lichenoides which also combines a lichenoid and vasculitic tissue reaction. In perniosis there is usually a thick layer of orthokeratin reflecting the acral site.

PARANEOPLASTIC PEMPHIGUS

Paraneoplastic pemphigus (see p 152) resembles erythema multiforme, with a lichenoid tissue reaction and dyskeratotic cells at different levels of the epidermis. Usually, foci of suprabasal acantholysis and clefting are also present. Subepidermal clefting has also been reported.

LICHENOID PURPURA

Some lesions of pigmented purpuric dermatosis may show lichenoid as well as purpuric and chronic vasculitic features (see p. 247). The presence of purpura and hemosiderin are important clues to the diagnosis.

LICHENOID CONTACT DERMATITIS

A lichenoid contact dermatitis has been seen after contact with rubber and certain clothing dyes, and following contact with chemicals used in the wine industry. In two personally studied cases, there was a patchy, band-like dermal infiltrate of lymphocytes with a few eosinophils and very mild basal spongiosis.

LATE SECONDARY SYPHILIS

Some lesions of late secondary syphilis show a lichenoid reaction pattern (see p. 651). There is usually extension of the inflammatory infiltrate into the mid and deep dermis. Plasma cells are usually present in the infiltrate.

POROKERATOSIS

In lesions of porokeratosis, particularly the disseminated superficial actinic form, a lichenoid tissue reaction associated with a heavy superficial lymphocytic infiltrate can occur. A careful search will reveal the diagnostic cornoid lamella at the periphery of the infiltrate. The lichenoid infiltrate may be directed against the abnormal epidermal clones which emerge in this condition. Porokeratosis is considered in detail in Chapter 9 (p. 292).

DRUG ERUPTIONS

The lichenoid reaction pattern is a prominent feature in lichenoid and fixed drug eruptions. In many other drug-induced cutaneous reactions, a very occasional Civatte body (apoptotic keratinocyte) may be seen in the basal layer or at a higher level within the epidermis. There may be an associated exocytosis of a few lymphocytes. Apoptotic cells are a valuable clue to the drug etiology of an otherwise non-specific spongiotic tissue reaction (see p. 114). These cells are usually easier to find in morbilliform drug eruptions.

PHOTOTOXIC DERMATITIS

In a phototoxic dermatitis there are scattered apoptotic keratinocytes (dyskeratotic cells, sunburn cells) at all levels of the epidermis. In severe cases confluent necrosis may be present. There is some telangiectasia of superficial dermal vessels, but very little dermal inflammation.

PRURIGO PIGMENTOSA

A patchy lichenoid reaction with associated melanin incontinence is seen in this uncommon condition (see p. 332).

ERYTHRODERMA

A lichenoid reaction is present in some patients with erythroderma (see p. 576). Many of these cases may be drug induced.

MYCOSIS FUNGOIDES

A subset of patients with mycosis fungoides has lichenoid changes on biopsy. One study has found that lichenoid changes tend to be associated with intense pruritus and may connote a poor prognosis.[1116] The presence of basal epidermotropism, nuclear atypia in the lymphocytes, and the presence of eosinophils and sometimes plasma cells in the dermal infiltrate are helpful in identifying the underlying mycosis fungoides.[1116]

REGRESSING WARTS AND TUMORS

The regression of viral warts, particularly plane warts, is associated with a lichenoid reaction pattern and exocytosis of cells into the epidermis. Keratinocytes in the stratum malpighii, presumably expressing viral antigen, are attacked by lymphocytes, resulting in death of the keratinocytes by apoptosis. Sometimes two or more lymphocytes 'surround' a keratinocyte, similar to the 'satellite cell necrosis' (lymphocyte-associated apoptosis) of graft-versus-host disease.

A lichenoid reaction pattern can be associated with a variety of epidermal tumors, where it appears to represent the attempted immunological regression of those lesions. This may be seen in seborrheic keratoses (the so-called 'irritated' seborrheic keratosis), solar keratoses (lichenoid solar keratoses) and intraepidermal carcinomas. The lichen planus-like keratosis represents a similar reaction in a solar lentigo and probably some other epithelial lesions.

A similar mechanism is involved in the partial regression of basal and squamous cell carcinomas and other cutaneous tumors. However, these circumstances do not conform to the definition of the lichenoid reaction pattern, namely basal epidermal cell damage. Accordingly they will not be considered further in this section.

LICHEN AMYLOIDOSUS

In lichen amyloidosus there is an accumulation of filamentous material in basal cells, with their eventual death. The filamentous material is extruded into the dermis in a manner similar to the formation of colloid bodies. The basal cells possibly die by apoptosis but the accumulation of the filamentous material obscures this basic process (see p. 432).

VITILIGO

In active lesions of vitiligo, careful search will often reveal an occasional lymphocyte in contact with a melanocyte. The destruction of melanocytes by lymphocyte-mediated apoptosis would explain the features of vitiligo (see p. 323).

LICHENOID TATTOO REACTION

A lichenoid reaction, localized to the red areas, is a rare complication in a tattoo.

REFERENCES

Introduction

1 Pinkus H. Lichenoid tissue reactions. Arch Dermatol 1973; 107: 840–846.
2 Weedon D. The lichenoid tissue reaction. Int J Dermatol 1982; 21: 203–206.
3 Patterson JW. The spectrum of lichenoid dermatitis. J Cutan Pathol 1991; 18: 67–74.
4 Weedon D. Apoptosis in lichen planus. Clin Exp Dermatol 1980; 5: 425–430.
5 Weedon D, Searle J, Kerr JFR. Apoptosis. Its nature and implications for dermatopathology. Am J Dermatopathol 1979; 1: 133–144.
6 Weedon D. Apoptosis. Adv Dermatol 1990; 5: 243–256.
7 LeBoit PE. Interface dermatitis. How specific are its histopathologic features? Arch Dermatol 1993; 129: 1324–1328.
8 Hashimoto K. Apoptosis in lichen planus and several other dermatoses. Acta Derm Venereol 1976; 56: 187–210.
9 Grubauer G, Romani N, Kofler H et al. Apoptotic keratin bodies as autoantigen causing the production of IgM-anti-keratin intermediate filament autoantibodies. J Invest Dermatol 1986; 87: 466–471.
10 Campisi J. The role of cellular senescence in skin aging. J Invest Dermatol (Symposium Proceedings) 1998; 3: 1–5.
11 Haake AR, Roublevskaia I, Cooklis M. Apoptosis: a role in skin aging? J Invest Dermatol (Symposium Proceedings) 1998; 3: 28–35.
12 Afford S, Randhawa S. Apoptosis. J Clin Pathol: Mol Pathol 2000; 53: 55–63.
13 Edwards MJ, Jones DW. Programmed cell death in human acute cutaneous wounds. J Cutan Pathol 2001; 28: 151–155.
14 Norris DA. Differential control of cell death in the skin. Arch Dermatol 1995; 131: 945–948.
15 Pileri S, Poggi S, Sabattini E et al. Apoptosis as programmed cell death (PCD): *Cupio dissolvi* in cell life. Curr Diagn Pathol 1994; 1: 48–55.
16 Kerr JFR, Winterford CM, Harmon BV. Apoptosis. Its significance in cancer and cancer therapy. Cancer 1994; 73: 2013–2026.
17 Raskin CA. Apoptosis and cutaneous biology. J Am Acad Dermatol 1997; 36: 885–896.
18 Cummings MC, Winterford CM, Walker NI. Apoptosis. Am J Surg Pathol 1997; 21: 88–101.
19 Chiodino C, Cesinaro AM, Ottani D et al. Expression of the novel inhibitor of apoptosis survivin in normal and neoplastic skin. J Invest Dermatol 1999; 113: 415–418.
20 Godar DE. Light and death: photons and apoptosis. J Invest Dermatol (Symposium Proceedings) 1999; 4: 17–23.
21 Leonard JV, Schapira AHV. Mitochondrial respiratory chain disorders II: neurodegenerative disorders and nuclear gene defects. Lancet 2000; 355: 389–394.
22 Sellheyer K, Krahl D, Ratech H. Distribution of Bcl-2 and Bax in embryonic and fetal human skin. Antiapoptotic and proapoptotic proteins are differentially expressed in developing skin. Am J Dermatopathol 2001; 23: 1–7.
23 Malmusi M, Ackerman AB. Apoptosis is a type of necrosis. Part 1 – The importance of historical perspective and of definition. Dermatopathology: Practical & Conceptual 1998; 4: 15–27.
24 Bennion SD, Middleton MH, David-Bajar KM et al. In three types of interface dermatitis, different patterns of expression of intercellular adhesion molecule-1 (ICAM-1) indicate different triggers of disease. J Invest Dermatol 1995; 105: 71S–79S.
25 Oliver GF, Winkelmann RK, Muller SA. Lichenoid dermatitis: A clinicopathologic and immunopathologic review of sixty-two cases. J Am Acad Dermatol 1989; 21: 284–292.
26 Godar DE. UVA1 radiation triggers two different final apoptotic pathways. J Invest Dermatol 1999; 112: 3–12.
27 Okamoto H, Mizuno K, Itoh T et al. Evaluation of apoptotic cells induced by ultraviolet light B radiation in epidermal sheets stained by the TUNEL technique. J Invest Dermatol 1999; 113: 802–807.
28 Gilchrest BA, Soter NA, Stoff JS, Mihm MC Jr. The human sunburn reaction: histologic and biochemical studies. J Am Acad Dermatol 1981; 5: 411–422.
29 Magro CM, Crowson AN. Lichenoid and granulomatous dermatitis. Int J Dermatol 2000; 39: 126–133.

Lichenoid (interface) dermatoses

30 Boyd AS, Neldner KH. Lichen planus. J Am Acad Dermatol 1991; 25: 593–619.
31 Marshman G. Lichen planus. Australas J Dermatol 1998; 39: 1–13.
32 Sánchez-Pérez J, Rios Buceta L, Fraga J, García-Díez A. Lichen planus with lesions on the palms and/or soles: prevalence and clinicopathological study of 36 patients. Br J Dermatol 2000; 142: 310–314.
33 Jobard-Drobacheff C, Blanc D, Quencez E et al. Lichen planus of the oesophagus. Clin Exp Dermatol 1988; 13: 38–41.
34 Evans AV, Fletcher CL, Owen WJ, Hay RJ. Oesophageal lichen planus. Clin Exp Dermatol 2000; 25: 36–37.

35 Itin PH, Schiller P, Gilli L, Buechner SA. Isolated lichen planus of the lip. Br J Dermatol 1995; 132: 1000–1002.
36 Lewis FM, Shah M, Harrington CI. Vulval involvement in lichen planus: a study of 37 women. Br J Dermatol 1996; 135: 89–91.
37 Lewis FM. Vulval lichen planus. Br J Dermatol 1998; 138: 569–575.
38 Vogel PS, James WD. Lichen planus of the eyelid: An unusual clinical presentation. J Am Acad Dermatol 1992; 27: 638–639.
39 Peluso AM, Tosti A, Piraccini BM, Cameli N. Lichen planus limited to the nails in childhood: case report and literature review. Pediatr Dermatol 1993; 10: 36–39.
40 Tosti A, Peluso AM, Fanti PA, Piraccini BM. Nail lichen planus: clinical and pathologic study of twenty-four patients. J Am Acad Dermatol 1993; 28: 724–730.
41 Colver GB, Dawber RPR. Is childhood idiopathic atrophy of the nails due to lichen planus? Br J Dermatol 1987; 116: 709–712.
42 Lutz M, Perniciaro C, Lim K. Zosteriform lichen planus without evidence of herpes simplex or varicella-zoster by polymerase chain reaction: report of two cases. J Cutan Pathol 1997; 24: 109 (abstract).
43 Irvine C, Irvine F, Champion RH. Long-term follow-up of lichen planus. Acta Derm Venereol 1991; 71: 242–244.
44 Mahood JM. Familial lichen planus. A report of nine cases from four families with a brief review of the literature. Arch Dermatol 1983; 119: 292–294.
45 Kofoed ML, Wantzin GL. Familial lichen planus. J Am Acad Dermatol 1985; 13: 50–54.
46 Graells J, Notario J, Badia F. Lichen planus in monozygotic twins. Clin Exp Dermatol 1998; 23: 299.
47 Powell FC, Rogers RS, Dickson ER, Moore SB. An association between HLA DR1 and lichen planus. Br J Dermatol 1986; 114: 473–478.
48 Carrozzo M, Francia di Celle P, Gandolfo S et al. Increased frequency of HLA-DR6 allele in Italian patients with hepatitis C virus-associated oral lichen planus. Br J Dermatol 2001; 144: 803–808.
49 Cottoni F, Ena P, Tedde G, Montesu MA. Lichen planus in children: a case report. Pediatr Dermatol 1993; 10: 132–135.
50 Milligan A, Graham-Brown RAC. Lichen planus in children – a review of six cases. Clin Exp Dermatol 1990; 15: 340–342.
51 Kanwar AJ, Handa S, Ghosh S, Kaur S. Lichen planus in childhood: a report of 17 patients. Pediatr Dermatol 1991; 8: 288–291.
52 Sharma R, Maheshwari V. Childhood lichen planus: a report of fifty cases. Pediatr Dermatol 1999; 16: 345–348.
53 Aste N, Pau M, Ferreli C, Biggio P. Lichen planus in a child requiring circumcision. Pediatr Dermatol 1997; 14: 129–130.
54 Nanda A, Al-Ajmi HS, Al-Sabah H et al. Childhood lichen planus: a report of 23 cases. Pediatr Dermatol 2001; 18: 1–4.
55 Flamenbaum HS, Safai B, Siegal FP, Pahwa S. Lichen planus in two immunodeficient hosts. J Am Acad Dermatol 1982; 6: 918–920.
56 Helm TN, Camisa C, Liu AY et al. Lichen planus associated with neoplasia: a cell-mediated immune response to tumor antigens? J Am Acad Dermatol 1994; 30: 219–224.
57 Gibson GE, Murphy GM. Lichen planus and carcinoid tumour. Clin Exp Dermatol 1997; 22: 180–182.
58 Epstein O. Lichen planus and liver disease. Br J Dermatol 1984; 111: 473–475.
59 Rebora A. Lichen planus and the liver. Int J Dermatol 1992; 31: 392–395.
60 Vainio E, Huovinen S, Liutu M et al. Peptic ulcer and *Helicobacter pylori* in patients with lichen planus. Acta Derm Venereol 2000; 80: 427–429.
61 Jubert C, Pawlotsky J-M, Pouget F et al. Lichen planus and hepatitis C virus-related chronic active hepatitis. Arch Dermatol 1994; 130: 73–76.
62 Cribier B, Garnier C, Laustriat D, Heid E. Lichen planus and hepatitis C virus infection: an epidemiologic study. J Am Acad Dermatol 1994; 31: 1070–1072.
63 Sanchez-Perez J, De Castro M, Buezo GF et al. Lichen planus and hepatitis C virus: prevalence and clinical presentation of patients with lichen planus and hepatitis C virus infection. Br J Dermatol 1996; 134: 715–719.
64 Chuang T-Y, Stitle L, Brashear R, Lewis C. Hepatitis C virus and lichen planus: a case-control study of 340 patients. J Am Acad Dermatol 1999; 41: 787–789.
65 Mignogna MD, Muzio LL, Favia G et al. Oral lichen planus and HCV infection: a clinical evaluation of 263 cases. Int J Dermatol 1998; 37: 575–578.
66 Bellman B, Reddy R, Falanga V. Generalized lichen planus associated with hepatitis C virus immunoreactivity. J Am Acad Dermatol 1996; 35: 770–772.
67 Mignogna MD, Muzio LL, Russo LL et al. Oral lichen planus: different clinical features in HCV-positive and HCV-negative patients. Int J Dermatol 2000; 39: 134–139.
68 Tucker SC, Coulson IH. Lichen planus is not associated with hepatitis C virus infection in patients from North West England. Acta Derm Venereol 1999; 79: 378–379.
69 Jury CS, Munro CS. Linear lichen planus related to hepatitis C infection? Br J Dermatol 2000; 142: 836–837.

70 Aubin F, Angonin R, Humbert P, Agache P. Lichen planus following hepatitis B vaccination. Arch Dermatol 1994; 130: 1329–1330.

71 Saywell CA, Wittal RA, Kossard S. Lichenoid reaction to hepatitis B vaccination. Australas J Dermatol 1997; 38: 152–154.

72 Ferrando MF, Doutre MS, Beylot-Barry M et al. Lichen planus following hepatitis B vaccination. Br J Dermatol 1998; 139: 350.

73 Schupp P, Vente C. Lichen planus following hepatitis B vaccination. Int J Dermatol 1998; 38: 799–800.

74 Rebora A, Rongioletti F, Drago F, Parodi A. Lichen planus as a side effect of HBV vaccination. Dermatology 1999; 198: 1–2.

75 Usman A, Kimyai-Asadi A, Stiller MJ, Alam M. Lichenoid eruption following hepatitis B vaccination: first North American case report. Pediatr Dermatol 2001; 18: 123–126.

76 Neumann-Jensen B, Worsaae N, Dabelsteen E, Ullman S. Pemphigus vulgaris and pemphigus foliaceus coexisting with oral lichen planus. Br J Dermatol 1980; 102: 585–590.

77 Creamer D, McGregor JM, McFadden J, Hawk JLM. Lichenoid tissue reaction in porphyria cutanea tarda. Br J Dermatol 1999; 141: 123–126.

78 Gruppo Italiano Studi Epidemiologici in Dermatologia. Epidemiological evidence of the association between lichen planus and two immune-related diseases. Alopecia areata and ulcerative colitis. Arch Dermatol 1991; 127: 688–691.

79 Terheyden P, Hornschuh B, Karl S et al. Lichen planus associated with Becker's nevus. J Am Acad Dermatol 1998; 38: 770–772.

80 Connelly MG, Winkelmann RK. Coexistence of lichen sclerosus, morphea, and lichen planus. Report of four cases and review of the literature. J Am Acad Dermatol 1985; 12: 844–851.

81 Boyd AS, Leonardi CL. Absence of human papillomavirus infection in cutaneous lichen planus. J Am Acad Dermatol 1997; 36: 267–268.

82 Boyd AS, Annarella M, Rapini RP et al. False-positive polymerase chain reaction results for human papillomavirus in lichen planus. Potential laboratory pitfalls of this procedure. J Am Acad Dermatol 1996; 35: 42–46.

83 Yesudian P, Rao R. Malignant transformation of hypertrophic lichen planus. Int J Dermatol 1985; 24: 177–178.

84 Odukoya O, Gallagher G, Shklar G. A histologic study of epithelial dysplasia in oral lichen planus. Arch Dermatol 1985; 121: 1132–1136.

85 Dwyer CM, Kerr REI, Millan DWM. Squamous carcinoma following lichen planus of the vulva. Clin Exp Dermatol 1995; 20: 171–172.

86 Lewis FM, Harrington CI. Squamous cell carcinoma arising in vulval lichen planus. Br J Dermatol 1994; 131: 703–705.

87 Yiannias JA, el-Azhary RA, Hand JH et al. Relevant contact sensitivities in patients with the diagnosis of oral lichen planus. J Am Acad Dermatol 2000; 42: 177–182.

88 Shai A, Halevy S. Lichen planus and lichen planus-like eruptions: pathogenesis and associated diseases. Int J Dermatol 1992; 31: 379–384.

89 Morhenn VB. The etiology of lichen planus. A hypothesis. Am J Dermatopathol 1986; 8: 154–156.

90 Shiohara T, Moriya N, Tanake Y et al. Immunopathologic study of lichenoid skin diseases: correlation between HLA-DR-positive keratinocytes or Langerhans cells and epidermotropic T cells. J Am Acad Dermatol 1988; 18: 67–74.

91 Shiohara T, Moriya N, Tsuchiya K et al. Lichenoid tissue reaction induced by local transfer of Ia-reactive T-cell clones. J Invest Dermatol 1986; 87: 33–38.

92 Shiohara T, Moriya N, Mochizuki T, Nagashima M. Lichenoid tissue reaction (LTR) induced by local transfer of Ia-reactive T-cell clones. II. LTR by epidermal invasion of cytotoxic lymphokine-producing autoreactive T cells. J Invest Dermatol 1987; 89: 8–14.

93 Biermann H, Rauterberg EW. Expression of fetal cytokeratins in epidermal cells and colloid bodies in lichen planus. J Cutan Pathol 1998; 25: 35–43.

94 Akasu R, From L, Kahn HJ. Lymphocyte and macrophage subsets in active and inactive lesions of lichen planus. Am J Dermatopathol 1993; 15: 217–223.

95 Mauduit G, Fernandez-Bussy R, Thivolet J. Sequential enumeration of peripheral blood T cell subsets in lichen planus. Clin Exp Dermatol 1984; 9: 256–262.

96 Sugerman PB, Satterwhite K, Bigby M. Autocytotoxic T-cell clones in lichen planus. Br J Dermatol 2000; 142: 449–456.

97 Spandau U, Toksoy A, Goebeler M et al. MIG is a dominant lymphocyte-attractant chemokine in lichen planus lesions. J Invest Dermatol 1998; 111: 1003–1009.

98 Shiohara T, Moriya N, Nagashima M. The lichenoid tissue reaction. A new concept of pathogenesis. Int J Dermatol 1988; 27: 365–374.

99 Shiohara T. The lichenoid tissue reaction. An immunological perspective. Am J Dermatopathol 1988; 10: 252–256.

100 Gadenne A-S, Strucke R, Dunn D et al. T-cell lines derived from lesional skin of lichen planus patients contain a distinctive population of T-cell receptor γδ-bearing cells. J Invest Dermatol 1994; 103: 347–351.

101 Zhou XJ, Sugerman PB, Savage NW, Walsh LJ. Matrix metalloproteinases and their inhibitors in oral lichen planus. J Cutan Pathol 2001; 28: 72–82.

102 Shuttleworth D, Graham-Brown RAC, Campbell AC. The autoimmune background in lichen planus. Br J Dermatol 1986; 115: 199–203.

103 Olsen RG, du Plessis DP, Schultz EJ, Camisa C. Indirect immunofluorescence microscopy of lichen planus. Br J Dermatol 1984; 110: 9–15.

104 Schofield JK, De Berker D, Milligan A et al. Keratin expression in cutaneous lichen planus. Histopathology 1995; 26: 153–158.

105 Ragaz A, Ackerman AB. Evolution, maturation, and regression of lesions of lichen planus. New observations and correlations of clinical and histologic findings. Am J Dermatopathol 1981; 3: 5–25.

106 Patel GK, Inalöz HS, Marks R. The significance of karyorrhexis in lichen planus. J Eur Acad Dermatol Venereol 2000; 14: 515–516.

107 Lupton GP, Goette DK. Lichen planus with plasma cell infiltrate. Arch Dermatol 1981; 117: 124–125.

108 Roustan G, Hospital M, Villegas C et al. Lichen planus with predominant plasma cell infiltrate. Am J Dermatopathol 1994; 16: 311–314.

109 Van Praag MCG, Boom BW, van Hees CLM et al. Classical and ulcerative lichen planus with plasma cell infiltrate. Arch Dermatol 1991; 127: 264–265.

110 Ross TH. Caspary–Joseph spaces: a comment on priority. Int J Dermatol 1977; 16: 842–843.

111 Akosa AB, Lampert IA. Sweat gland abnormalities in lichenoid dermatosis. Histopathology 1991; 19: 345–349.

112 Enhamre A, Lagerholm B. Acrosyringeal lichen planus. Acta Derm Venereol 1987; 67: 346–350.

113 Hanau D, Sengel D. Perforating lichen planus. J Cutan Pathol 1984; 11: 176–178.

114 Lucke T, Fallowfield M, Burden D. Lichen planus associated with milia. Clin Exp Dermatol 1999; 24: 266–269.

115 Smoller BR, Glusac EJ. Immunofluorescent analysis of the basement membrane zone in lichen planus suggests destruction of the lamina lucida in bullous lesions. J Cutan Pathol 1994; 21: 123–128.

116 Haapalainen T, Oksala O, Kallioinen M et al. Destruction of the epithelial anchoring system in lichen planus. J Invest Dermatol 1995; 105: 100–103.

117 Burkhart CG. Ultrastructural study of lichen planus: an evaluation of the colloid bodies. Int J Dermatol 1981; 20: 188–192.

118 Metze D. Explaining clinical features and histopathologic findings by electron microscopy: lichen planus. Dermatopathology: Practical & Conceptual 1998; 4: 28–29.

119 Ebner H, Gebhart W. Epidermal changes in lichen planus. J Cutan Pathol 1976; 3: 167–174.

120 Danno K, Horio T. Sulphydryl crosslinking in cutaneous apoptosis: a review. J Cutan Pathol 1982; 9: 123–132.

121 Gomes MA, Staquet MJ, Thivolet J. Staining of colloid bodies by keratin antisera in lichen planus. Am J Dermatopathol 1981; 3: 341–347.

122 Friedman DB, Hashimoto K. Annular atrophic lichen planus. J Am Acad Dermatol 1991; 25: 392–394.

123 Requena L, Olivares M, Piqué E et al. Annular atrophic lichen planus. Dermatology 1994; 189: 95–98.

124 Matsuura C, Tsukifuji R, Shinkai H. Annular lichen planus showing a change in metallothionein expression on immunohistochemistry. Br J Dermatol 1998; 138: 1043–1045.

125 Fox BJ, Odom RB. Papulosquamous diseases: a review. J Am Acad Dermatol 1985; 12: 597–624.

126 Jayaraman M, Janaki VR, Yesudian P. Squamous cell carcinoma arising from hypertrophic lichen planus. Int J Dermatol 1995; 34: 70–71.

127 Castaño E, López-Ríos F, Alvarez-Fernández JG et al. Verrucous carcinoma in association with hypertrophic lichen planus. Clin Exp Dermatol 1997; 22: 23–25.

128 Badell A, Marcoval J, Gallego I et al. Keratoacanthoma arising in hypertrophic lichen planus. Br J Dermatol 2000; 142: 380–382.

129 Sharma VK, Achar A, Ramam M, Singh MK. Multiple cutaneous horns overlying lichen planus hypertrophicus. Br J Dermatol 2001; 144: 424–425.

130 Rippis GE, Becker B, Scott G. Hypertrophic lichen planus in three HIV-positive patients: a histologic and immunological study. J Cutan Pathol 1994; 21: 52–58.

131 Tan E, Malik R, Quirk CJ. Hypertrophic lichen planus mimicking squamous cell carcinoma. Australas J Dermatol 1998; 39: 45–47.

132 Weedon D, Robertson I. Lichen planus and xanthoma. Arch Dermatol 1977; 113: 519.

133 Hartl C, Steen KH, Wegner H et al. Unilateral linear lichen planus with mucous membrane involvement. Acta Derm Venereol 1999; 79: 145–146.

134 Mizoguchi S, Setoyama M, Kanzaki T. Linear lichen planus in the region of the mandibular nerve caused by an allergy to palladium in dental metals. Dermatology 1998; 196: 268–270.

135 Long CC, Finlay AY. Multiple linear lichen planus in the lines of Blaschko. Br J Dermatol 1996; 135: 275–276.

136 Crotty CP, Su WPD, Winkelmann RK. Ulcerative lichen planus. Follow-up of surgical excision and grafting. Arch Dermatol 1980; 116: 1252–1256.

137 Rowland Payne CME, McPartlin JF, Hawley PR. Ulcerative perianal lichen planus. Br J Dermatol 1997; 136: 479.

138 Alinovi A, Barella PA, Benoldi D. Erosive lichen planus involving the glans penis alone. Int J Dermatol 1983; 22: 37–38.

139 Schlesinger TE, Camisa C, Gay JD, Bergfeld WF. Oral erosive lichen planus with epidermolytic hyperkeratosis during interferon alfa-2b therapy for chronic hepatitis C virus infection. J Am Acad Dermatol 1997; 36: 1023–1025.

140 Eisen D. The vulvovaginal-gingival syndrome of lichen planus. The clinical characteristics of 22 patients. Arch Dermatol 1994; 130: 1379–1382.

141 Lewis FM, Shah M, Harrington CI. Vulval involvement in lichen planus: a study of 37 women. Br J Dermatol 1996; 135: 89–91.

142 Vente C, Reich K, Rupprecht R, Neumann C. Erosive mucosal lichen planus: response to topical treatment with tacrolimus. Br J Dermatol 1999; 140: 338–342.

143 Higgins CR, Handfield-Jones S, Black MM. Erosive, flexural lichen planus – an uncommon variant. Clin Exp Dermatol 1993; 18: 169–170.

144 Ashinoff R, Cohen R, Lipkin G. Castleman's tumor and erosive lichen planus: coincidence or association? J Am Acad Dermatol 1989; 21: 1076–1080.

145 Lee Y-S, Fong P-H. Extensive ulcerative and erosive lichenoid dermatosis in a patient with malignant lymphoma. Am J Dermatopathol 1993; 15: 576–580.

146 Renfro L, Kamino H, Raphael B et al. Ulcerative lichen planus-like dermatitis associated with hydroxyurea. J Am Acad Dermatol 1991; 24: 143–145.

147 Parodi A, Cardo PP. Patients with erosive lichen planus may have antibodies directed to a nuclear antigen of epithelial cells: a study of the antigen nature. J Invest Dermatol 1990; 94: 689–693.

148 Bhutani LK, Bedi TR, Pandhi RK, Nayak NC. Lichen planus pigmentosus. Dermatologica 1974; 149: 43–50.

149 Person JR, Rogers RS III. Ashy dermatosis. An apoptotic disease? Arch Dermatol 1981; 117: 701–704.

150 Tschen JA, Tschen EA, McGavran MH. Erythema dyschromicum perstans. J Am Acad Dermatol 1980; 2: 295–302.

151 Novick NL, Phelps R. Erythema dyschromicum perstans. Int J Dermatol 1985; 24: 630–633.

152 Urano-Suehisa S, Tagami H, Iwatsuki K. Unilateral ashy dermatosis occurring in a child. Arch Dermatol 1984; 120: 1491–1493.

153 Palatsi R. Erythema dyschromicum perstans. A follow-up study from Northern Finland. Dermatologica 1977; 155: 40–44.

154 Bhutani LK. Ashy dermatosis or lichen planus pigmentosus: what is in a name? Arch Dermatol 1986; 122: 133.

155 Naidorf KF, Cohen SR. Erythema dyschromicum perstans and lichen planus. Arch Dermatol 1982; 118: 683–685.

156 Berger RS, Hayes TJ, Dixon SL. Erythema dyschromicum perstans and lichen planus: are they related? J Am Acad Dermatol 1989; 21: 438–442.

157 Miyagawa S, Komatsu M, Okuchi T et al. Erythema dyschromicum perstans. Immunopathologic studies. J Am Acad Dermatol 1989; 20: 882–886.

158 Baranda L, Torres-Alvarez B, Cortes-Franco R et al. Involvement of cell adhesion and activation molecules in the pathogenesis of erythema dyschromicum perstans (Ashy dermatitis). Arch Dermatol 1997; 133: 325–329.

159 Molinero J, Vilata JJ, Nagore E et al. Ashy dermatosis in an HIV antibody-positive patient. Acta Derm Venereol 2000; 80: 78–79.

160 Sanchez NP, Pathak MA, Sato SS et al. Circumscribed dermal melaninoses: classification, light, histochemical, and electron microscopic studies on three patients with the erythema dyschromicum perstans type. Int J Dermatol 1982; 21: 25–31.

161 Vega ME, Waxtein L, Arenas R et al. Ashy dermatosis and lichen planus pigmentosus: a clinicopathologic study of 31 cases. Int J Dermatol 1992; 31: 90–94.

162 Sassolas B, Zagnoli A, Leroy J-P, Guillet G. Lichen planus pigmentosus associated with acrokeratosis of Bazex. Clin Exp Dermatol 1994; 19: 70–73.

163 Salman SM, Kibbi A-G, Zaynoun S. Actinic lichen planus. A clinicopathologic study of 16 patients. J Am Acad Dermatol 1989; 20: 226–231.

164 Isaacson D, Turner ML, Elgart ML. Summertime actinic lichenoid eruption (lichen planus actinicus). J Am Acad Dermatol 1981; 4: 404–411.

165 Singh OP, Kanwar AJ. Lichen planus in India: an appraisal of 441 cases. Int J Dermatol 1976; 15: 752–756.

166 El Zawahry M. Lichen planus tropicus. Dermatol Int 1965; 4: 92–95.

167 Dilaimy M. Lichen planus subtropicus. Arch Dermatol 1976; 112: 1251–1253.

168 Verhagen ARHB, Koten JW. Lichenoid melanodermatitis. A clinicopathological study of fifty-one Kenyan patients with so-called tropical lichen planus. Br J Dermatol 1979; 101: 651–658.

169 Bedi TR. Summertime actinic lichenoid eruption. Dermatologica 1978; 157: 115–125.

170 Salman SM, Khallouf R, Zaynoun S. Actinic lichen planus mimicking melasma. A clinical and histopathologic study of three cases. J Am Acad Dermatol 1988; 18: 275–278.

171 Al-Fouzan AS, Hassab-el-Naby HMM. Melasma-like (pigmented) actinic lichen planus. Int J Dermatol 1992; 31: 413–415.

172 Aloi F, Solaroli C, Giovannini E. Actinic lichen planus simulating melasma. Dermatology 1997; 195: 69–70.

173 Van der Schroeff JG, Schothorst AA, Kanaar P. Induction of actinic lichen planus with artificial UV sources. Arch Dermatol 1983; 119: 498–500.

174 Macfarlane AW. A case of actinic lichen planus. Clin Exp Dermatol 1989; 14: 65–68.

175 Albers SE, Glass LF, Fenske NA. Lichen planus subtropicus: direct immunofluorescence findings and therapeutic response to hydroxychloroquine. Int J Dermatol 1994; 33: 645–647.

176 Waldorf DS. Lichen planopilaris. Arch Dermatol 1966; 93: 684–691.

177 Matta M, Kibbi A-G, Khattar J et al. Lichen planopilaris: a clinicopathologic study. J Am Acad Dermatol 1990; 22: 594–598.

178 Horn RT Jr, Goette DK, Odom RB et al. Immunofluorescent findings and clinical overlap in two cases of follicular lichen planus. J Am Acad Dermatol 1982; 7: 203–207.

179 Mehregan DA, Van Hale HM, Muller SA. Lichen planopilaris: clinical and pathologic study of forty-five patients. J Am Acad Dermatol 1992; 27: 935–942.

180 Bardazzi F, Landi C, Orlandi C et al. Graham Little–Piccardi–Lasseur syndrome following HBV vaccination. Acta Derm Venereol 1999; 79: 93.

181 Samtsov AV, Bozhchenko AA. Histopathological features of Lassueur–Graham–Little syndrome. Am J Dermatopathol 2000; 22: 352 (abstract).

182 Vázquez García J, Pérez Oliva N, Peireio Ferreirós MM, Toribio J. Lichen planus follicularis tumidus with cysts and comedones. Clin Exp Dermatol 1992; 17: 346–348.

183 Kuster W, Kind P, Holzle E, Plewig G. Linear lichen planopilaris of the face. J Am Acad Dermatol 1989; 21: 131–132.

184 Gerritsen MJP, de Jong EMGJ, van de Kerkhof PCM. Linear lichen planopilaris of the face. J Am Acad Dermatol 1998; 38: 633–635.

185 Yanaru E, Ueda M, Ichihashi M. Linear lichen planopilaris of the face treated with low-dose cyclosporin A. Acta Derm Venereol 2000; 80: 212.

186 Grunwald MH, Zvulunov A, Halevy S. Lichen planopilaris of the vulva. Br J Dermatol 1997; 136: 477–478.

187 Annessi G, Lombardo G, Gobello T, Puddu P. A clinicopathologic study of scarring alopecia due to lichen planus. Comparison with scarring alopecia in discoid lupus erythematosus and pseudopelade. Am J Dermatopathol 1999; 21: 324–331.

188 Smith WB, Grabski WJ, McCollough ML, Davis TL. Immunofluorescence findings in lichen planopilaris: a contrasting experience. Arch Dermatol 1992; 128: 1405–1406.

189 Ioannides D, Bystryn J-C. Immunofluorescence abnormalities in lichen planopilaris. Arch Dermatol 1992; 128: 214–216.

190 Tamada Y, Yokochi K, Nitta Y et al. Lichen planus pemphigoides: identification of 180 kd hemidesmosome antigen. J Am Acad Dermatol 1995; 32: 883–887.

191 Joshi RK, Atukorala DN, Abanmi A, Al Awadi T. Lichen planus pemphigoides. Is it a separate entity? Br J Dermatol 1994; 130: 537–538.

192 Willstead E, Bhogal BS, Das AK et al. Lichen planus pemphigoides: a clinicopathological study of nine cases. Histopathology 1991; 19: 147–154.

193 Lang PG Jr, Maize JC. Coexisting lichen planus and bullous pemphigoid or lichen planus pemphigoides? J Am Acad Dermatol 1983; 9: 133–140.

194 Archer CB, Cronin E, Smith NP. Diagnosis of lichen planus pemphigoides in the absence of bullae on normal-appearing skin. Clin Exp Dermatol 1992; 17: 433–436.

195 Fivenson DP, Kimbrough TL. Lichen planus pemphigoides: Combination therapy with tetracycline and nicotinamide. J Am Acad Dermatol 1997; 36: 638–640.

196 Nousari HC, Goyal S, Anhalt GJ. Successful treatment of resistant hypertrophic and bullous lichen planus with mycophenolate mofetil. Arch Dermatol 1999; 135: 1420–1421.

197 Hernando LB, Sabastián FV, Sánchez JH et al. Lichen planus pemphigoides in a 10-year-old girl. J Am Acad Dermatol 1992; 26: 124–125.

198 Paige DG, Bhogal BS, Black MM, Harper JI. Lichen planus pemphigoides in a child – immunopathological findings. Clin Exp Dermatol 1993; 18: 552–554.

199 Maceyko RF, Camisa C, Bergfeld WF, Valenzuela R. Oral and cutaneous lichen planus pemphigoides. J Am Acad Dermatol 1992; 27: 889–892.

200 Sapadin AN, Phelps RG, Fellner MJ, Kantor I. Lichen planus pemphigoides presenting with a strikingly unilateral distribution. Int J Dermatol 1998; 37: 942–946.

201 Kuramoto N, Kishimoto S, Shibagaki R, Yasuno H. PUVA-induced lichen planus pemphigoides. Br J Dermatol 2000; 142: 509–512.

202 Miyagawa S, Ohi H, Muramatsu T et al. Lichen planus pemphigoides-like lesions induced by cinnarizine. Br J Dermatol 1985; 112: 607–613.

203 Ogg GS, Bhogal BS, Hashimoto T et al. Ramipril-associated lichen planus pemphigoides. Br J Dermatol 1997; 136: 412–414.

204 Camisa C, Neff JC, Rossana C, Barrett JL. Bullous lichen planus: diagnosis by indirect immunofluorescence and treatment with dapsone. J Am Acad Dermatol 1986; 14: 464–469.

205 Oomen C, Temmerman L, Kint A. Lichen planus pemphigoides. Clin Exp Dermatol 1986; 11: 92–96.

59

206 Gawkrodger DJ, Stavropoulos PG, McLaren KM, Buxton PK. Bullous lichen planus and lichen planus pemphigoides – clinico-pathological comparisons. Clin Exp Dermatol 1989; 14: 150–153.

207 Prost C, Tesserand F, Laroche L et al. Lichen planus pemphigoides: an immuno-electron microscopic study. Br J Dermatol 1985; 113: 31–36.

208 Bhogal BS, McKee PH, Wonjnarowska F et al. Lichen planus pemphigoides: an immunopathological study. J Cutan Pathol 1989; 16: 297 (abstract).

209 Okochi H, Nashiro K, Tsuchida T et al. Lichen planus pemphigoides: case report and results of immunofluorescence and immunoelectron microscopic study. J Am Acad Dermatol 1990; 22: 626–631.

210 Zillikens D, Caux F, Mascaro JM Jr et al. Autoantibodies in lichen planus pemphigoides react with a novel epitope within the C-terminal NC16A domain of BP180. J Invest Dermatol 1999; 113: 117–121.

211 Hsu S, Ghchestani RF, Uitto J. Lichen planus pemphigoides with IgG autoantibodies to the 180 kd bullous pemphigoid antigen (type XVII collagen). J Am Acad Dermatol 2000; 42: 136–141.

212 Skaria M, Salomon D, Jaunin F et al. IgG autoantibodies from a lichen planus pemphigoides patient recognize the NC16A domain of the bullous pemphigoid antigen 180. Dermatology 1999; 199: 253–255.

213 Joly P, Tanasescu S, Wolkenstein P et al. Lichenoid erythrodermic bullous pemphigoid of the African patient. J Am Acad Dermatol 1998; 39: 691–697.

214 Mora RG, Nesbitt LT Jr, Brantley JB. Lichen planus pemphigoides: clinical and immunofluorescent findings in four cases. J Am Acad Dermatol 1983; 8: 331–336.

215 Feuerman EJ, Sandbank M. Lichen planus pemphigoides with extensive melanosis. Arch Dermatol 1971; 104: 61–67.

216 Hintner H, Sepp N, Dahlback K et al. Deposition of C3, C9 neoantigen and vitronectin (S-protein of complement) in lichen planus pemphigoides. Br J Dermatol 1990; 123: 39–47.

217 Swale VJ, Black MM, Bhogal BS. Lichen planus pemphigoides: two case reports. Clin Exp Dermatol 1998; 23: 132–135.

218 Murphy GM, Cronin E. Lichen planus pemphigoides. Clin Exp Dermatol 1989; 14: 322–324.

219 Bouloc A, Vignon-Pennamen M-D, Caux F et al. Lichen planus pemphigoides is a heterogeneous disease: a report of five cases studied by immunoelectron microscopy. Br J Dermatol 1998; 138: 972–980.

220 Nabai H, Mehregan AH. Keratosis lichenoides chronica. Report of a case. J Am Acad Dermatol 1980; 2: 217–220.

221 Ryatt KS, Greenwood R, Cotterill JA. Keratosis lichenoides chronica. Br J Dermatol 1982; 106: 223–225.

222 Mehregan AH, Heath LE, Pinkus H. *Lichen ruber moniliformis* and *lichen ruber verrucosus et reticularis* of Kaposi. J Cutan Pathol 1984; 11: 2–11.

223 Grunwald MH, Hallel-Halevy D, Amichai B. Keratosis lichenoides chronica: response to topical calcipotriol. J Am Acad Dermatol 1997; 37: 263–264.

224 Konstantinov KN, Søndergaard J, Izuno G, Obreshkova E. Keratosis lichenoides chronica. J Am Acad Dermatol 1998; 38: 306–309.

225 Criado PR, Valente NYS, de Souza Sittart JA et al. Keratosis lichenoides chronica: report of a case developing after erythroderma. Australas J Dermatol 2000; 41: 247–249.

226 Avermaete A, Kreuter JA, Stücker M et al. Keratosis lichenoides chronica: characteristics and response to acitretin. Br J Dermatol 2001; 144: 422–424.

227 Kersey P, Ive FA. Keratosis lichenoides chronica is synonymous with lichen planus. Clin Exp Dermatol 1982; 7: 49–54.

228 Lang PG Jr. Keratosis lichenoides chronica. Successful treatment with psoralen-ultraviolet-A therapy. Arch Dermatol 1981; 117: 105–108.

229 Torrelo A, Mediero IG, Zambrano A. Keratosis lichenoides chronica in a child. Pediatr Dermatol 1994; 11: 46–48.

230 Arata J, Seno A, Tada J et al. Peculiar facial erythematosquamous lesions in two siblings with cyclical summer improvement and winter relapse: a variant of keratosis lichenoides chronica? J Am Acad Dermatol 1993; 28: 870–873.

231 Masouyé I, Saurat J-H. Keratosis lichenoides chronica: the centenary of another Kaposi's disease. Dermatology 1995; 191: 188–192.

232 Stefanato CM, Youssef EAH, Cerio R et al. Atypical Nekam's disease – keratosis lichenoides chronica associated with porokeratotic histology and amyloidosis. Clin Exp Dermatol 1993; 18: 274–276.

233 Lombardo GA, Annessi G, Baliva G et al. Keratosis lichenoides chronica. Report of a case associated with B-cell lymphoma and leg panniculitis. Dermatology 2000; 201: 261–264.

234 Petrozzi JW. Keratosis lichenoides chronica. Possible variant of lichen planus. Arch Dermatol 1976; 112: 709–711.

235 Ruben BS, Barr RJ, Bukaty LM et al. Lichen ruber acuminatus verrucosus et reticularis and lichen ruber moniliformis: modern examples of antique diseases. J Cutan Pathol 1997; 24: 120 (abstract).

236 David M, Filhaber A, Rotem A et al. Keratosis lichenoides chronica with prominent telangiectasia: response to etretinate. J Am Acad Dermatol 1989; 21: 1112–1114.

237 Kossard S, Lee S. Lichen planoporitis: keratosis lichenoides chronica revisited. J Cutan Pathol 1998; 25: 222–227.

238 Ruben BS, LeBoit PE. Keratosis lichenoides chronica is authentic! Dermatopathology: Practical & Conceptual 1997; 3: 310–312.

239 Van der Horst JC, Cirkel PKS, Nieboer C. Mixed lichen planus-lupus erythematosus disease: a distinct entity? Clinical, histopathological and immunopathological studies in six patients. Clin Exp Dermatol 1983; 8: 631–640.

240 Inalöz HS, Chowdhury MMU, Motley RJ. Lupus erythematosus/lichen planus overlap syndrome with scarring alopecia. J Eur Acad Dermatol Venereol 2001; 15: 171–174.

241 Ahmed AR, Schreiber P, Abramovits W et al. Coexistence of lichen planus and systemic lupus erythematosus. J Am Acad Dermatol 1982; 7: 478–483.

242 Plotnick H, Burnham TK. Lichen planus and coexisting lupus erythematosus versus lichen planus-like lupus erythematosus. J Am Acad Dermatol 1986; 14: 931–938.

243 Grabbe S, Kolde G. Coexisting lichen planus and subacute cutaneous lupus erythematosus. Clin Exp Dermatol 1995; 20: 249–254.

244 Camisa C, Neff JC, Olsen RG. Use of direct immunofluorescence in the lupus erythematosus/lichen planus overlap syndrome: an additional diagnostic clue. J Am Acad Dermatol 1984; 11: 1050–1059.

245 Lapins NA, Willoughby C, Helwig EB. Lichen nitidus. A study of forty-three cases. Cutis 1978; 21: 634–637.

246 Chen W, Schramm M, Zouboulis ChC. Generalized lichen niticus. J Am Acad Dermatol 1997; 36: 630–631.

247 Lestringant GG, Piletta P, Feldman R et al. Coexistence of atopic dermatitis and lichen nitidus in three patients. Dermatology 1996; 192: 171–173.

248 Kato N. Familial lichen nitidus. Clin Exp Dermatol 1995; 20: 336–338.

249 Kellett JK, Beck MH. Lichen nitidus associated with distinctive nail changes. Clin Exp Dermatol 1984; 9: 201–204.

250 Bettoli V, De Padova MP, Corazza M, Virgili A. Generalized lichen nitidus with oral and nail involvement in a child. Dermatology 1997; 194: 367–369.

251 Coulson IH, Marsden RA, Cook MG. Purpuric palmar lichen nitidus – an unusual though distinctive eruption. Clin Exp Dermatol 1988; 13: 347–349.

252 Munro CS, Cox NH, Marks JM, Natarajan S. Lichen nitidus presenting as palmoplantar hyperkeratosis and nail dystrophy. Clin Exp Dermatol 1993; 18: 381–383.

253 De Eusebio Murillo E, Sánchez Yus E, Novo Lens R. Lichen nitidus of the palms: a case with peculiar histopathologic features. Am J Dermatopathol 1999; 21: 161–164.

254 Hussain K. Summertime actinic lichenoid eruption, a distinct entity, should be termed *actinic lichen nitidus*. Arch Dermatol 1998; 134: 1302–1303.

255 Kanwar AJ, Kaur S. Lichen nitidus actinicus. Arch Dermatol 1999; 135: 714.

256 Smoller BR, Flynn TC. Immunohistochemical examination of lichen nitidus suggests that it is not a localized papular variant of lichen planus. J Am Acad Dermatol 1992; 27: 232–236.

257 Bardach H. Perforating lichen nitidus. J Cutan Pathol 1981; 8: 111–116.

258 Eisen RF, Stenn J, Kahn SM, Bhawan J. Lichen nitidus with plasma cell infiltrate. Arch Dermatol 1985; 121: 1193–1194.

259 Khopkar U, Joshi R. Distinguishing lichen scrofulosorum from lichen nitidus. Dermatopathology: Practical & Conceptual 1999; 5: 44–45.

260 Jetton RL, Eby CS, Freeman RG. Vesicular and hemorrhagic lichen nitidus. Arch Dermatol 1972; 105: 430–431.

261 Banse-Kupin L, Morales A, Kleinsmith D. Perforating lichen nitidus. J Am Acad Dermatol 1983; 9: 452–456.

262 Itami A, Ando I, Kukita A. Perforating lichen nitidus. Int J Dermatol 1994; 33: 382–384.

263 Madhok R, Winkelmann RK. Spinous, follicular lichen nitidus associated with perifollicular granulomas. J Cutan Pathol 1988; 15: 245–248.

264 Clausen J, Jacobsen FK, Brandrup F. Lichen nitidus: electron microscopic and immunofluorescent studies. Acta Derm Venereol 1982; 62: 15–19.

265 Zhang Y, McNutt NS. Lichen striatus. Histological, immunohistochemical, and ultrastructural study of 37 cases. J Cutan Pathol 2001; 28: 65–71.

266 Nutter AF, Champion RH. Lichen striatus occurring as an annular eruption: an acquired 'locus minoris resistentiae'. Br J Dermatol 1979; 101: 351–352.

267 Aloi F, Solaroli C, Pippione M. Diffuse and bilateral lichen striatus. Pediatr Dermatol 1997; 14: 36–38.

268 Jordá E, Zayas AI, Revert A et al. A lichen striatuslike eruption adopting the morphology of Blaschko lines. Pediatr Dermatol 1991; 8: 120–121.

269 Taieb A, El Youbi A, Grosshans E, Maleville J. Lichen striatus: a Blaschko linear acquired inflammatory skin eruption. J Am Acad Dermatol 1991; 25: 637–642.

270 Kennedy D, Rogers M. Lichen striatus. Pediatr Dermatol 1996; 13: 95–99.

271 Hwang SM, Ahn SK, Lee SH, Choi EH. Lichen striatus following BCG vaccination. Clin Exp Dermatol 1996; 21: 393–394.

272 Tosti A, Peluso AM, Misciali C, Cameli N. Nail lichen striatus: Clinical features and long-term follow-up of five patients. J Am Acad Dermatol 1997; 36: 908–913.

273 Lee M-W, Choi J-H, Sung K-J et al. Linear eruptions of the nose in childhood: a form of lichen striatus? Br J Dermatol 2000; 142: 1208–1212.

274 Toda K-I, Okamoto H, Horio T. Lichen striatus. Int J Dermatol 1986; 25: 584–585.

275 Patrizi A, Neri I, Fiorentini C et al. Simultaneous occurrence of lichen striatus in siblings. Pediatr Dermatol 1997; 14: 293–295.

276 Reed RJ, Meek T, Ichinose H. Lichen striatus: a model for the histologic spectrum of lichenoid reactions. J Cutan Pathol 1975; 2: 1–18.

277 Charles CR, Johnson BL, Robinson TA. Lichen striatus. A clinical, histologic and electron microscopic study of an unusual case. J Cutan Pathol 1974; 1: 265–274.

278 Stewart WM. Pathology of lichen striatus. Br J Dermatol (Suppl) 1976; 14: 18–19.

279 Gianotti R, Restano L, Grimalt R et al. Lichen striatus – a chameleon: an histopathological and immunohistological study of forty-one cases. J Cutan Pathol 1995; 22: 18–22.

280 Herd RM, McLaren KM, Aldridge RD. Linear lichen planus and lichen striatus – opposite ends of a spectrum. Clin Exp Dermatol 1993; 18: 335–337.

281 Rose C, Hauber K, Starostik P et al. Lichen striatus: a clinicopathologic study with follow-up in 13 patients. Am J Dermatopathol 2000; 22: 354 (abstract).

282 Laur WE, Posey RE, Waller JD. Lichen planus-like keratosis. A clinicohistopathologic correlation. J Am Acad Dermatol 1981; 4: 329–336.

283 Goette DK. Benign lichenoid keratosis. Arch Dermatol 1980; 116: 780–782.

284 Berger TG, Graham JH, Goette DK. Lichenoid benign keratosis. J Am Acad Dermatol 1984; 11: 635–638.

285 Scott MA, Johnson WC. Lichenoid benign keratosis. J Cutan Pathol 1976; 3: 217–221.

286 Berman A, Herszenson S, Winkelmann RK. The involuting lichenoid plaque. Arch Dermatol 1982; 118: 93–96.

287 Prieto VG, Casal M, McNutt NS. Lichen planus-like keratosis. A clinical and histological reexamination. Am J Surg Pathol 1993; 17: 259–263.

288 Tan CY, Marks R. Lichenoid solar keratosis – prevalence and immunologic findings. J Invest Dermatol 1982; 79: 365–367.

289 King TW, Ackerman AB. What is the clue and what is the diagnosis? Lichen planus-like keratosis or lichenoid solar keratosis? Dermatopathology: Practical & Conceptual 1999; 5: 37–40.

290 Goldenhersh MA, Barnhill RL, Rosenbaum HM, Stenn KS. Documented evolution of a solar lentigo into a solitary lichen planus-like keratosis. J Cutan Pathol 1986; 13: 308–311.

291 Barranco VP. Multiple benign lichenoid keratoses simulating photodermatoses: evolution from senile lentigines and their spontaneous regression. J Am Acad Dermatol 1985; 13: 201–206.

292 Glaun RS, Dutta B, Helm KF. A proposed new classification system for lichenoid keratosis. J Am Acad Dermatol 1996; 35: 772–774.

293 Ramesh V, Kulkarni SB, Misra RS. Benign lichenoid keratosis due to constant pressure. Australas J Dermatol 1998; 39: 177–178.

294 Frigy AF, Cooper PH. Benign lichenoid keratosis. Am J Clin Pathol 1985; 83: 439–443.

295 Jang K-A, Kim S-H, Choi J-H et al. Lichenoid keratosis: a clinicopathologic study of 17 patients. J Am Acad Dermatol 2000; 43: 511–516.

296 Prieto VG, Casal M, McNutt NS. Immunohistochemistry detects differences between lichen planus-like keratosis, lichen planus, and lichenoid actinic keratosis. J Cutan Pathol 1993; 20: 143–147.

297 Halevy S, Sandbank M, Livni E. Macrophage migration inhibition factor release in lichenoid drug eruptions. J Am Acad Dermatol 1993; 29: 263–265.

298 Halevy S, Shai A. Lichenoid drug eruptions. J Am Acad Dermatol 1993; 29: 249–255.

299 Gange RW, Levene GM. A distinctive eruption in patients receiving oxprenolol. Clin Exp Dermatol 1979; 4: 87–97.

300 Cochran REI, Thomson J, Fleming K, McQueen A. The psoriasiform eruption induced by practolol. J Cutan Pathol 1975; 2: 314–319.

301 Almeyda J, Levantine A. Lichenoid drug eruptions. Br J Dermatol 1971; 85: 604–607.

302 Penneys NS. Gold therapy: dermatologic uses and toxicities. J Am Acad Dermatol 1979; 1: 315–320.

303 Russell MA, Langley M, Truett AP III et al. Lichenoid dermatitis after consumption of gold-containing liquor. J Am Acad Dermatol 1997; 36: 841–844.

304 Smith KE, Fenske NA. Cutaneous manifestations of alcohol abuse. J Am Acad Dermatol 2000; 43: 1–16.

305 Burry JN. Ulcerative lichenoid eruption from methyldopa. Arch Dermatol 1976; 112: 880.

306 O'Brien TJ, Lyall IG, Reid SS. Lichenoid eruption induced by sotalol. Australas J Dermatol 1994; 35: 93–94.

307 Van Hecke E, Kint A, Temmerman L. A lichenoid eruption induced by penicillamine. Arch Dermatol 1981; 117: 676–677.

308 Meyrick Thomas RH, Munro DD. Lichen planus in a photosensitive distribution due to quinine. Clin Exp Dermatol 1986; 11: 97–101.

309 Maltz BL, Becker LE. Quinidine-induced lichen planus. Int J Dermatol 1980; 19: 96–97.

310 Bauer F. Quinacrine hydrochloride drug eruption (tropical lichenoid dermatitis). J Am Acad Dermatol 1981; 4: 239–248.

311 Grossman ME, Warren K, Mady A, Satra KH. Lichenoid eruption associated with ethambutol. J Am Acad Dermatol 1995; 33: 675–676.

312 Phillips WG, Vaughan-Jones S, Jenkins R, Breathnach SM. Captopril-induced lichenoid eruption. Clin Exp Dermatol 1994; 19: 317–320.

313 Roten SV, Mainetti C, Donath R, Saurat J-H. Enalapril-induced lichen planus-like eruption. J Am Acad Dermatol 1995; 32: 293–295.

314 Swale VJ, McGregor JM. Amlodipine-associated lichen planus. Br J Dermatol 2001; 144: 920–921.

315 Heymann WR, Lerman JS, Luftschein S. Naproxen-induced lichen planus. J Am Acad Dermatol 1984; 10: 299–301.

316 Özkan Ş, Izler F, Fetil E et al. Naproxen-induced lichen planus bullosus. Acta Derm Venereol 1999; 79: 329–330.

317 Roger D, Rolle F, Labrousse F et al. Simvastatin-induced lichenoid drug eruption. Clin Exp Dermatol 1994; 19: 88–89.

318 Atkin SL, McKenzie TMM, Stevenson CJ. Carbamazepine-induced lichenoid eruption. Clin Exp Dermatol 1990; 15: 382–383.

319 Franz CB, Massullo RE, Welton WA. Lichenoid drug eruption from chlorpropamide and tolazamide. J Am Acad Dermatol 1990; 22: 128–129.

320 Lowitt MH, Eisenberger M, Sina B, Kao GF. Cutaneous eruptions from suramin. Arch Dermatol 1995; 131: 1147–1153.

321 Fiérard E, Delaporte E, Flipo R-M et al. Tiopronin-induced lichenoid eruption. J Am Acad Dermatol 1994; 31: 665–667.

322 Chu C-Y, Yang C-H, Yang C-Y et al. Fixed erythrodysaesthesia plaque due to intravenous injection of docetaxel. Br J Dermatol 2000; 142: 808–811.

323 Aguilar A, Gallego MA, Pigué E. Lichenoid drug eruption due to cyanamide. Int J Dermatol 1999; 38: 950–951.

324 Bong JL, Lucke TW, Douglas WS. Lichenoid drug eruption with proton pump inhibitors. BMJ 2000; 320: 283.

325 Clark C, Douglas WS. Lichenoid drug eruption induced by spironolactone. Clin Exp Dermatol 1998; 23: 43–44.

326 Azzam H, Bergman R, Friedman-Birnbaum R. Lichen planus associated with metformin therapy. Dermatology 1997; 194: 376.

327 Farrell AM, Bunker CB. Cutaneous eruption due to indoramin. Clin Exp Dermatol 1998; 23: 233.

328 Yockey SMD, Ahmed I. Intravenous immunoglobulin-induced lichenoid dermatitis: a unique adverse reaction. Mayo Clin Proc 1997; 72: 1151–1152.

329 Fellner MJ. Lichen planus. Int J Dermatol 1980; 19: 71–75.

330 Hamanaka H, Mizutani H, Shimizu M. Sparfloxacin-induced photosensitivity and the occurrence of a lichenoid tissue reaction after prolonged exposure. J Am Acad Dermatol 1998; 38: 945–949.

331 Byrd DR, Ahmed I. Photosensitive lichenoid reaction to torsemide – a loop diuretic. Mayo Clin Proc 1997; 72: 930–931.

332 Choonhakarn C, Janma J. Pyrazinamide-induced lichenoid photodermatitis. J Am Acad Dermatol 1999; 40: 645–646.

333 Jones HE, Lewis CW, Reisner JE. Photosensitive lichenoid eruption associated with demeclocycline. Arch Dermatol 1971; 106: 58–63.

334 Hogan DJ, Murphy F, Burgess WR et al. Lichenoid stomatitis associated with lithium carbonate. J Am Acad Dermatol 1985; 13: 243–246.

335 Hoss DM, Gross EG, Grant-Kels JM. Histopathology of an adverse reaction to a eutectic mixture of the local anesthetics lidocaine and prilocaine. J Cutan Pathol 1999; 26: 100–104.

336 Kawamura T, Fukuda S, Ohtake N et al. Lichen planus-like contact dermatitis due to methacrylic acid esters. Br J Dermatol 1996; 134: 358–360.

337 Villiard AM, Lavenue A, Balme B et al. Lichenoid cutaneous drug reaction at injection sites of granulocyte colony-stimulating factor (filgrastim). Dermatology 1999; 198: 301–303.

338 Hawk JLM. Lichenoid drug eruption induced by propranolol. Clin Exp Dermatol 1980; 5: 93–96.

339 West AJ, Berger TG, LeBoit PE. A comparative histopathologic study of photodistributed and nonphotodistributed lichenoid drug eruptions. J Am Acad Dermatol 1990; 23: 689–693.

340 Gonzalez JG, Marcus MD, Santa Cruz DJ. Giant cell lichenoid dermatitis. J Am Acad Dermatol 1986; 15: 87–92.

341 Goldberg LJ, Goldberg N, Abrahams I et al. Giant cell lichenoid dermatitis: a possible manifestation of sarcoidosis. J Cutan Pathol 1994; 21: 47–51.

342 Córdoba S, Fraga J, Bartolomé B et al. Giant cell lichenoid dermatitis within herpes zoster scars in a bone marrow recipient. J Cutan Pathol 2000; 27: 255–257.

343 Korkij W, Soltani K. Fixed drug eruption. A brief review. Arch Dermatol 1984; 120: 520–524.

344 Baird BJ, De V Ilez RL. Widespread bullous fixed drug eruption mimicking toxic epidermal necrolysis. Int J Dermatol 1988; 27: 170–174.

345 Sowden JM, Smith AG. Multifocal fixed drug eruption mimicking erythema multiforme. Clin Exp Dermatol 1990; 15: 387–388.

346 Masu S, Seiji M. Pigmentary incontinence in fixed drug eruptions. Histologic and electron microscopic findings. J Am Acad Dermatol 1983; 8: 525–532.

347 Shelley WB, Shelley ED. Non pigmenting fixed drug eruption as a distinctive reaction pattern: examples caused by sensitivity to pseudoephedrine hydrochloride and tetrahydrozoline. J Am Acad Dermatol 1987; 17: 403–407.

348 Krivda SJ, Benson PM. Nonpigmenting fixed drug eruption. J Am Acad Dermatol 1994; 31: 291–292.

349 Roetzheim RG, Herold AH, Van Durme DJ. Nonpigmenting fixed drug eruption caused by diflunisal. J Am Acad Dermatol 1991; 24: 1021–1022.

350 Sigal-Nahum M, Konqui A, Gaulier A, Sigal S. Linear fixed drug eruption. Br J Dermatol 1988; 118: 849–851.

351 Özkaya-Bayazit E, Baykal C. Trimethoprim-induced linear fixed drug eruption. Br J Dermatol 1997; 137: 1028–1030.

352 Guin JD, Haynie LS, Jackson D, Baker GF. Wandering fixed drug eruption: a mucocutaneous reaction to acetaminophen. J Am Acad Dermatol 1987; 17: 399–402.

353 Mizukawa Y, Shiohara T. Fixed drug eruption presenting as erythema dyschromicum perstans: a flare without taking any medications. Dermatology 1998; 197: 383–385.

354 Gruber F, Stasić A, Lenković M, Brajac I. Postcoital fixed drug eruption in a man sensitive to trimethoprim-sulphamethoxazole. Clin Exp Dermatol 1997; 22: 144–145.

355 Chan HL. Fixed drug eruptions. A study of 20 occurrences in Singapore. Int J Dermatol 1984; 23: 607–609.

356 Kuokkanen K. Erythema fixum of the genitals and the mucous membranes. Int J Dermatol 1974; 13: 4–8.

357 Baran R, Perrin C. Fixed-drug eruption presenting as an acute paronychia. Br J Dermatol 1991; 125: 592–595.

358 Kauppinen K, Stubb S. Drug eruptions: causative agents and clinical types. Acta Derm Venereol 1984; 64: 320–324.

359 Shukla SR. Drugs causing fixed drug eruptions. Dermatologica 1981; 163: 160–163.

360 Thankappan TP, Zachariah J. Drug-specific clinical pattern in fixed drug eruptions. Int J Dermatol 1991; 30: 867–870.

361 Mahboob A, Haroon TS. Drugs causing fixed eruptions: a study of 450 cases. Int J Dermatol 1998; 37: 833–838.

362 Tham SN, Kwok YK, Chan HL. Cross-reactivity in fixed drug eruptions to tetracyclines. Arch Dermatol 1996; 132: 1134–1135.

363 Correia O, Delgado L, Polónia J, Genital fixed drug eruption: cross-reactivity between doxycycline and minocycline. Clin Exp Dermatol 1999; 24: 137.

364 Kauppinen K, Stubb S. Fixed eruptions: causative drugs and challenge tests. Br J Dermatol 1985; 112: 575–578.

365 Pareek SS. Nystatin-induced fixed eruption. Br J Dermatol 1980; 103: 679–680.

366 Mochida K, Teramae H, Hamada T. Fixed drug eruption due to colchicine. Dermatology 1996; 192: 61.

367 Janier M, Vignon MD. Recurrent fixed drug eruption due to clioquinol. Br J Dermatol 1995; 133: 1013–1014.

368 Coskey RJ, Bryan HG. Fixed drug eruption due to penicillin. Arch Dermatol 1975; 111: 791–792.

369 Arias J, Férnandez-Rivas M, Panadero P. Selective fixed drug eruption to amoxycillin. Clin Exp Dermatol 1995; 20: 339–340.

370 Pigatto PD, Riboldi A, Riva F, Altomare GF. Fixed drug eruption to erythromycin. Acta Derm Venereol 1984; 64: 272–273.

371 Hamamoto Y, Ohmura A, Kinoshita E, Muto M. Fixed drug eruption due to clarithromycin. Clin Exp Dermatol 2001; 26: 48–49.

372 Dhar S, Sharma VK. Fixed drug eruption due to ciprofloxacin. Br J Dermatol 1996; 134: 156–158.

373 Kavanagh GM, Sansom JE, Harrison P et al. Tranexamic acid (Cyklokapron®)-induced fixed-drug eruption. Br J Dermatol 1993; 128: 229–230.

374 Savage J. Fixed drug eruption to griseofulvin. Br J Dermatol 1977; 97: 107–108.

375 Munn SE, Russell Jones R. Terbinafine and fixed drug eruption. Br J Dermatol 1995; 133: 815–816.

376 Hogan DJ, Rooney ME. Fixed drug eruption due to dimenhydrinate. J Am Acad Dermatol 1989; 20: 503–504.

377 Gonzalo-Garijo MÁ, Revenga Arranz F. Fixed drug eruption due to dimenhydrinate. Br J Dermatol 1996; 135: 661–662.

378 Smola H, Kruppa A, Hunzelmann N et al. Identification of dimenhydrinate as the causative agent in fixed drug eruption using patch-testing in previously affected skin. Br J Dermatol 1998; 138: 920–921.

379 Dwyer CM, Dick D. Fixed drug eruption caused by diphenhydramine. J Am Acad Dermatol 1993; 29: 496–497.

380 Young PC, Montemarano AD, Lee N et al. Hypersensitivity to paclitaxel manifested as a bullous fixed drug eruption. J Am Acad Dermatol 1996; 34: 313–314.

381 Archer CB, English JSC. Extensive fixed drug eruption induced by temazepam. Clin Exp Dermatol 1988; 13: 336–338.

382 Long CC, Finlay AY, Marks R. Fixed drug eruption to mefenamic acid: a report of three cases. Br J Dermatol 1992; 126: 409–411.

383 Shuttleworth D, Graham-Brown RAC. Fixed drug eruption due to carbamazepine. Clin Exp Dermatol 1974; 9: 424–426.

384 Chan HL, Tan KC. Fixed drug eruption to three anticonvulsant drugs: An unusual case of polysensitivity. J Am Acad Dermatol 1997; 36: 259.

385 Duhra P, Porter DI. Paracetamol-induced fixed drug eruption with positive immunofluorescence findings. Clin Exp Dermatol 1990; 15: 296–297.

386 Meyrick Thomas RH, Munro DD. Fixed drug eruption due to paracetamol. Br J Dermatol 1986; 115: 357–359.

387 Kawada A, Hiruma M, Noguchi H, Ishibashi A. Fixed drug eruption induced by acetaminophen in a 12-year-old girl. Int J Dermatol 1996; 35: 148–149.

388 Harris A, Burge SM. Vasculitis in a fixed drug eruption due to paracetamol. Br J Dermatol 1995; 133: 790–791.

389 Ko R, Tanaka M, Murata T, Nishikawa T. Papular fixed drug eruption mimicking folliculitis due to acetaminophen. Clin Exp Dermatol 2000; 25: 96–97.

390 Hern S, Harman K, Clement M, Black MM. Bullous fixed drug eruption due to paracetamol with an unusual immunofluorescence pattern. Br J Dermatol 1998; 139: 1129–1131.

391 Sehgal VN. Paracetamol-induced bilateral symmetric, multiple fixed drug eruption (MFDE) in a child. Pediatr Dermatol 1999; 16: 165–166.

392 Silva A, Proença E, Carvalho C et al. Fixed drug eruption induced by paracetamol. Pediatr Dermatol 2001; 18: 163–164.

393 Heikkilä H, Timonen K, Stubb S. Fixed drug eruption due to fluconazole. J Am Acad Dermatol 2000; 42: 883–884.

394 Pellicano R, Lomuto M, Ciavarella G et al. Fixed drug eruptions with feprazone are linked to HLA-B22. J Am Acad Dermatol 1997; 36: 782–784.

395 Orchard DC, Varigos GA. Fixed drug eruption to tartrazine. Australas J Dermatol 1997; 38: 212–214.

396 Yosipovitch G, Rechavia E, Feinmesser M, David M. Adverse cutaneous reactions to ticlopidine in patients with coronary stents. J Am Acad Dermatol 1999; 41: 473–476.

397 Hsiao C-J, Lee JY-Y, Wong T-W, Sheu H-M. Extensive fixed drug eruption due to lamotrigine. Br J Dermatol 2001; 144: 1289–1291.

398 Alanko K, Kanerva L, Mohell-Talolahti B et al. Nonpigmented fixed drug eruption from pseudoephedrine. J Am Acad Dermatol 1996; 35: 647–648.

399 Hindioğlu U, Şahin S. Nonpigmenting solitary fixed drug eruption caused by pseudoephedrine hydrochloride. J Am Acad Dermatol 1998; 38: 499–500.

400 Watanabe H, Sueki H, Nakada T et al. Multiple fixed drug eruptions caused by iomeprol (Iomeron®), a nonionic contrast medium. Dermatology 1999; 198: 291–294.

401 Heikkilä H, Kariniemi A-L, Stubb S. Fixed drug eruption due to phenylpropanolamine hydrochloride. Br J Dermatol 2000; 142: 845–847.

402 Bernand S, Scheidegger EP, Dummer R, Burg G. Multifocal fixed drug eruption to paracetamol, tropisetron and ondansetron induced by interleukin 2. Dermatology 2000; 201: 148–150.

403 Gonzalo MA, Alvarado MI, Fernández L et al. Fixed drug eruption due to naproxen: lack of cross-reactivity with other propionic acid derivatives. Br J Dermatol 2001; 144: 1291–1292.

404 Jara MD, Montero AP, Gracia Bara MT et al. Allergic reactions due to ibuprofen in children. Pediatr Dermatol 2001; 18: 66–67.

405 Choonhakarn C. Non-pigmenting fixed drug eruption: a new case due to eperisone hydrochloride. Br J Dermatol 2001; 144: 1288–1289.

406 Cox NH, Duffey P, Royle J. Fixed drug eruption caused by lactose in an injected botulinum toxin preparation. J Am Acad Dermatol 1999; 40: 263–264.

407 Thami GP, Kanwar AJ. Fixed drug eruption due to metronidazole and tinidazole without cross-sensitivity to secnidazole. Dermatology 1998; 196: 368.

408 Robalo Cordeiro M, Gonçalo M, Fernandes B et al. Positive lesional patch tests in fixed drug eruptions from nimesulide. Contact Dermatitis 2000; 43: 307.

409 Kanwar AJ, Majid A, Singh M, Malhotra YK. An unusual presentation of fixed drug eruption. Dermatologica 1982; 164: 115–116.

410 Bhargava P, Kuldeep CM, Mathur NK. Polysensitivity and familiar occurrence in fixed drug eruption. Int J Dermatol 1997; 36: 236.

411 Yanguas I, Oleaga JM, González-Güemes M et al. Fixed food eruption caused by lentils. J Am Acad Dermatol 1998; 38: 640–641.

412 Kelso JM. Fixed food eruption. J Am Acad Dermatol 1996; 35: 638–639.

413 Shiohara T, Kokaji T. Polysensitivity in fixed drug eruption. J Am Acad Dermatol 1997; 37: 1017.

414 Smoller BR, Luster AD, Krane JF et al. Fixed drug eruptions: evidence for a cytokine-mediated process. J Cutan Pathol 1991; 18: 13–19.

415 Hindsen M, Christensen OB, Gruic V, Lofberg H. Fixed drug eruption: an immunohistochemical investigation of the acute and healing phase. Br J Dermatol 1987; 116: 351–360.

416 Shiohara T, Nickoloff BJ, Sagawa Y et al. Fixed drug eruption. Expression of epidermal keratinocyte intercellular adhesion molecule-1 (ICAM-1). Arch Dermatol 1989; 125: 1371–1376.

417 Shiohara T. What is new in fixed drug eruption? Dermatology 1995; 191: 185–187.

418 Pellicano R, Ciavarella G, Lomuto M, Di Giorgio G. Genetic susceptibility to fixed drug eruption: evidence for a link with HLA-B22. J Am Acad Dermatol 1994; 30: 52–54.

419 Van Voorhees A, Stenn KS. Histological phases of bactrim-induced fixed drug eruption. The report of one case. Am J Dermatopathol 1987; 9: 528–532.

420 Komura J, Yamada M, Ofuji S. Ultrastructure of eosinophilic staining epidermal cells in toxic epidermal necrolysis and fixed drug eruption. Dermatologica 1969; 139: 41–48.

421 Tonnesen MG, Soter NA. Erythema multiforme. J Am Acad Dermatol 1979; 1: 357–364.

422 Ledesma GN, McCormack PC. Erythema multiforme. Clin Dermatol 1986; 4: 70–80.

423 Huff JC, Weston WL, Tonnesen MG. Erythema multiforme: a critical review of characteristics, diagnostic criteria, and causes. J Am Acad Dermatol 1983; 8: 763–775.

424 Howland WW, Golitz LE, Weston WL, Huff JC. Erythema multiforme: clinical, histopathologic, and immunologic study. J Am Acad Dermatol 1984; 10: 438–446.

425 Ting HC, Adam BA. Stevens–Johnson syndrome. A review of 34 cases. Int J Dermatol 1985; 24: 587–591.

426 Leenutaphong V, Sivayathorn A, Suthipinittharm P, Sunthonpalin P. Stevens–Johnson syndrome and toxic epidermal necrolysis in Thailand. Int J Dermatol 1993; 32: 428–431.

427 Assier H, Bastuji-Garin S, Revuz J, Roujeau J-C. Erythema multiforme with mucous membrane involvement and Stevens–Johnson syndrome are clinically different disorders with distinct causes. Arch Dermatol 1995; 131: 539–543.

428 Côté B, Wechsler J, Bastuji-Garin S et al. Clinicopathologic correlation in erythema multiforme and Stevens–Johnson syndrome. Arch Dermatol 1995; 131: 1268–1272.

429 Bystryn J-C. Erythema multiforme with mucous membrane involvement and Stevens–Johnson syndrome are clinically different disorders. Arch Dermatol 1996; 132: 711.

430 Ruiz-Maldonado R. Acute disseminated epidermal necrosis types 1, 2, and 3: Study of sixty cases. J Am Acad Dermatol 1985; 13: 623-635.

431 Lever WF. My concept of erythema multiforme. Am J Dermatopathol 1985; 7: 141–142.

432 Rasmussen JE. Erythema multiforme. Should anyone care about the standards of care? Arch Dermatol 1995; 131: 726–729.

433 Bastuji-Garin S, Rzany B, Stern RS et al. Clinical classification of cases of toxic epidermal necrolysis, Stevens–Johnson syndrome, and erythema multiforme. Arch Dermatol 1993; 129: 92–96.

434 Roujeau J-C, Revuz J. Toxic epidermal necrolysis: an expanding field of knowledge. J Am Acad Dermatol 1994; 31: 301–302.

435 Drago F, Parodi A, Rebora A. Persistent erythema multiforme: report of two new cases and review of literature. J Am Acad Dermatol 1995; 33: 366–369.

436 Drago F, Romagnoli M, Loi A, Rebora A. Epstein–Barr virus-related persistent erythema multiforme in chronic fatigue syndrome. Arch Dermatol 1992; 128: 217–222.

437 Schofield JK, Tatnall FM, Leigh IM. Recurrent erythema multiforme: clinical features and treatment in a large series of patients. Br J Dermatol 1993; 128: 542–545.

438 Dumas V, Thieulent N, Souillet AL et al. Recurrent erythema multiforme and chronic hepatitis C: efficacy of interferon alpha. Br J Dermatol 2000; 142: 1248–1249.

439 Wolf P, Soyer HP, Fink-Puches R et al. Recurrent post-herpetic erythema multiforme mimicking polymorphic light and juvenile spring eruption: report of two cases in young boys. Br J Dermatol 1994; 131: 364–367.

440 Schofield JK, Tatnall FM, Brown J et al. Recurrent erythema multiforme: tissue typing in a large series of patients. Br J Dermatol 1994; 131: 532–535.

441 Heng MCY, Feinberg M. Localized erythema multiforme due to lymphatic obstruction. Br J Dermatol 1982; 106: 95–97.

442 Pariser RJ. 'Nevocentric' erythema multiforme. J Am Acad Dermatol 1994; 31: 491–492.

443 Cox NH. 'Nevocentric' erythema multiforme: not unique. J Am Acad Dermatol 1995; 33: 319.

444 Micalizzi C, Farris A. Erythema multiforme along Blaschko's lines. J Eur Acad Dermatol Venereol 2000; 14: 203–204.

445 Shiohara T, Chiba M, Tanaka Y, Nagashima M. Drug-induced, photosensitive, erythema-multiforme-like eruption: possible role for cell adhesion molecules in a flare induced by Rhus dermatitis. J Am Acad Dermatol 1990; 22: 647–650.

446 Soltani K, Bernstein JE, Lorincz AL. Eruptive nevocytic nevi following erythema multiforme. J Am Acad Dermatol 1979; 1: 503–505.

447 Fustes-Morales AJ, Soto-Romero I, Estrada Z et al. Unusual leukoderma after erythema multiforme: a case report. Pediatr Dermato 2001; 18: 120–122.

448 Margolis RJ, Bhan A, Mihm MC Jr, Bernhardt M. Erythema multiforme in a patient with T cell chronic lymphocytic leukemia. J Am Acad Dermatol 1986; 14: 618–627.

449 Ledesma GN, McCormack PC. Erythema multiforme. Clin Dermatol 1986; 4: 70–80.

450 Weston WL, Brice SL. Atypical forms of herpes simplex-associated erythema multiforme. J Am Acad Dermatol 1998; 39: 124–126.

451 Tay Y-K, Huff JC, Weston WL. Mycoplasma pneumoniae infection is associated with Stevens–Johnson syndrome, not erythema multiforme (von Hebra). J Am Acad Dermatol 1996; 35: 757–760.

452 Dikland WJ, Orange AP, Stolz E, Van Joost T. Erythema multiforme in childhood and early infancy. Pediatr Dermatol 1986; 3: 135–139.

453 Léauté-Labrèze C, Lamireau T, Chawki D et al. Diagnosis, classification, and management of erythema multiforme and Stevens–Johnson syndrome. Arch Dis Child 2000; 83: 347–352.

454 Hughes J, Burrows NP. Infectious mononucleosis presenting as erythema multiforme. Clin Exp Dermatol 1993; 18: 373–374.

455 Koga T, Kubota Y, Nakayama J. Erythema multiforme-like eruptions induced by cytomegalovirus infection in an immunocompetent adult. Acta Derm Venereol 1999; 79: 166.

456 Lesire V, Machet L, Toledano C et al. Atypical erythema multiforme occurring at the early phase of Lyme disease? Acta Derm Venereol 2000; 80: 222.

457 Schuttelaar M-LA, Laeijendecker R, Heinhus RJ, Van Joost Th. Erythema multiforme and persistent erythema as early cutaneous manifestations of Lyme disease. J Am Acad Dermatol 1997; 37: 873–875.

458 Tabata N, Kato T, Noguchi K et al. Erythema multiforme following the exacerbation of hepatitis B virus infection. Int J Dermatol 1999; 38: 52–53.

450 Loche F, Schwarze HP, Thedenat B et al. Erythema multiforme associated with hepatitis B immunization. Clin Exp Dermatol 2000; 25 167–169.

460 Chan H-L, Stern RS, Arndt KA et al. The incidence of erythema multiforme, Stevens–Johnson syndrome, and toxic epidermal necrolysis. Arch Dermatol 1990; 126: 43–47.

461 Paquet P, Paquet F, Al Saleh W et al. Immunoregulatory effector cells in drug-induced toxic epidermal necrolysis. Am J Dermatopathol 2000; 22: 413–417.

462 Win A, Evers ML, Chmel H. Stevens–Johnson syndrome presumably induced by ciprofloxacin. Int J Dermatol 1994; 33: 512–514.

463 Garty B-Z. Stevens–Johnson syndrome associated with nystatin treatment. Arch Dermatol 1991; 127: 741–742.

464 Strom BL, Carson JL, Halpern AC et al. A population-based study of Stevens–Johnson syndrome. Incidence and antecedent drug exposures. Arch Dermatol 1991; 127: 831–838.

465 Curley RK, Verbov JL. Stevens–Johnson syndrome due to tetracyclines – a case report (doxycycline) and review of the literature. Clin Exp Dermatol 1987; 12: 124–125.

466 Lewis-Jones MS, Evans S, Thompson CM. Erythema multiforme occurring in association with lupus erythematosus during therapy with doxycycline. Clin Exp Dermatol 1988; 13: 245–247.

467 Katz SK, Medenica MM, Kobayashi K et al. Erythema multiforme induced by suramin. J Am Acad Dermatol 1995; 32: 292–293.

468 Brook U, Singer L, Fried D. Development of severe Stevens–Johnson syndrome after administration of slow-release theophylline. Pediatr Dermatol 1989; 6: 126–129.

469 David M, Sandbank M, Lowe NJ. Erythema multiforme-like eruptions associated with etretinate therapy. Clin Exp Dermatol 1989; 14: 230–232.

470 Todd P, Halpern S, Munro DD. Oral terbinafine and erythema multiforme. Clin Exp Dermatol 1995; 20: 247–248.

471 McGregor JM, Rustin MHA. Terbinafine and erythema multiforme. Br J Dermatol 1994; 131: 587–588.

472 Rzany B, Mockenhaupt M, Gehring W, Schöpf E. Stevens–Johnson syndrome after terbinafine therapy. J Am Acad Dermatol 1994; 30: 509.

473 Goeteyn V, Naeyaert JM, Lambert J et al. Is systemic autoimmune disease a risk factor for terbinafine-induced erythema multiforme? Br J Dermatol 2000; 142: 578–579.

474 Gupta AK, Lynde CW, Lauzon GJ et al. Cutaneous adverse effects associated with terbinafine therapy: 10 case reports and a review of the literature. Br J Dermatol 1998; 138: 529–532.

475 Rustin MHA, Bunker CB, Dowd PM, Robinson TWE. Erythema multiforme due to griseofulvin. Br J Dermatol 1989; 120: 455–458.

476 Amichai B, Grunwald MH. Erythema multiforme due to clonazepam – supportive

evidence from the macrophage migration inhibition factor test. Clin Exp Dermatol 1998; 23: 206–207.

477 Kono T, Hayami M, Kobayashi H et al. Acarbose-induced generalised erythema multiforme. Lancet 1999; 354: 396–397.

478 Jan V, Toledano C, Machet L et al. Stevens–Johnson syndrome after sertraline. Acta Derm Venereol 1999; 79: 401.

479 Lale Atahan İ, Özyar E, Sahin Ş et al. Two cases of Stevens–Johnson syndrome: toxic epidermal necrolysis possibly induced by amifostine during radiotherapy. Br J Dermatol 2000; 143: 1072–1073.

480 Assier-Bonnet H, Araczingi S, Cadranel J et al. Stevens–Johnson syndrome induced by cyclophosphamide: report of two cases. Br J Dermatol 1996; 135: 864–866.

481 Sachs B, Rönnau AC, von Schmiedeberg S et al. Lamotrigine-induced Stevens–Johnson syndrome: demonstration of specific lymphocyte reactivity in vitro. Dermatology 1997; 195: 60–64

482 Yalçin B, Karaduman A. Stevens–Johnson syndrome associated with concomitant use of lamotrigine and valproic acid. J Am Acad Dermatol 2000; 43: 898–899.

483 Sawamura D, Umeki K. Stevens–Johnson syndrome associated with bezafibrate. Acta Derm Venereol 2000; 80: 457.

484 Hofbauer GFL, Burg G, Nestle FC. Cocaine-related Stevens–Johnson syndrome. Dermatology 2000; 201: 258–260.

485 Lineberry TW, Peters GE Jr, Bostwick JM. Bupropion-induced erythema multiforme. Mayo Clin Proc 2001; 76: 664–666.

486 Newman JM, Rindler JM, Bergfeld WF, Brydon JK. Stevens–Johnson syndrome associated with topical nitrogen mustard therapy. J Am Acad Dermatol 1997; 36: 112–114.

487 Smith HR, Croft AM, Black MM. Dermatological adverse effects with the antimalarial drug mefloquine: a review of 74 published case reports. Clin Exp Dermatol 1999; 24: 249–254.

488 Goon AT, Lee L-T, Tay Y-K et al. A case of trichloroethylene hypersensitivity syndrome. Arch Dermatol 2001; 137: 274–276.

489 Metry DW, Lahart CJ, Farmer KL, Hebert AA. Stevens–Johnson syndrome caused by the antiretroviral drug nevirapine. J Am Acad Dermatol 2001; 44: 354–357.

490 Shimizu S, Chen K-R, Pratchyaprui: W-O, Shimizu H. Tropical-wood-induced bullous erythema multiforme. Dermatology 2000; 200: 59–62.

491 Puig L, Fernández-Figueras M-T, Montero M-A et al. Erythema-multiforme-like eruption due to topical contactants: expression of adhesion molecules and their ligands and characterization of the infiltrate. Contact Dermatitis 1995; 33: 329–332.

492 Whitfield MJ, Rivers JK. Erythema multiforme after contact dermatitis in response to an epoxy sealant. J Am Acad Dermatol 1991; 25: 386–388.

493 Puig L, Alegre M, Cuatrecasas M, De Moragas JM. Erythema multiforme-like reaction following diphencyprone treatment of plane warts. Int J Dermatol 1994; 33: 201–203.

494 Arias D, Requena L, Hasson A et al. Localized epidermal necrolysis (erythema multiforme-like reaction) following intravenous injection of vinblastine. J Cutan Pathol 1991; 18: 344–346.

495 Duncan KO, Tigelaar RE, Bolognia JL. Stevens–Johnson syndrome limited to multiple sites of radiation therapy in a patient receiving phenobarbital. J Am Acad Dermatol 1999; 40: 493–496.

496 Kokuba H, Imafuku S, Huang S et al. Erythema multiforme lesions are associated with expression of a herpes simplex virus (HSV) gene and qualitative alterations in the HSV-specific T-cell response. Br J Dermatol 1998; 138: 952–964.

497 Aurelian L, Kokuba H, Burnett JW. Understanding the pathogenesis of HSV-associated erythema multiforme. Dermatology 1998; 197: 219–222.

498 Brice SL, Leahy MA, Ong L et al. Examination of non-involved skin, previously involved skin, and peripheral blood for herpes simplex virus DNA in patients with recurrent herpes-associated erythema multiforme. J Cutan Pathol 1994; 21: 408–412.

499 Imafuku S, Kokuba H, Aurelian L, Burnett J. Expression of herpes simplex virus DNA fragments located in epidermal keratinocytes and germinative cells is associated with the development of erythema multiforme lesions. J Invest Dermatol 1997; 109: 550–556.

500 Aslanzadeh J, Helm KF, Espy MJ et al. Detection of HSV-specific DNA in biopsy tissue of patients with erythema multiforme by polymerase chain reaction. Br J Dermatol 1992; 126: 19–23.

501 Miura S, Smith CC, Burnett JW, Aurelian L. Detection of viral DNA within skin of healed recurrent herpes simplex infection and erythema multiforme lesions. J Invest Dermatol 1992; 98: 68–72.

502 Darragh TM, Egbert BM, Berger TG, Yen TSB. Identification of herpes simplex virus DNA in lesions of erythema multiforme by the polymerase chain reaction. J Am Acad Dermatol 1991; 24: 23–26.

503 Kokuba H, Imafuku S, Burnett JW, Aurelian L. Longitudinal study of a patient with herpes-simplex-virus-associated erythema multiforme: viral gene expression and T cell repertoire usage. Dermatology 1999; 198: 233–242.

504 Pham N, Phelps RG. The role of natural killer cells and natural killer like T cells in erythema multiforme type reactions. J Cutan Pathol 2000; 27: 568–569 (abstract).

505 Paquet P, Piérard GE. Erythema multiforme and toxic epidermal necrolysis: a comparative study. Am J Dermatopathol 1997; 19: 127–132.

506 Kokuba H, Aurelian L, Burnett J. Herpes simplex virus associated erythema multiforme (HAEM) is mechanistically distinct from drug-induced erythema multiforme: interferon-γ is expressed in HAEM lesions and tumor necrosis factor-α in drug-induced erythema multiforme lesions. J Invest Dermatol 1999; 113: 808–815.

507 Foedinger D, Sterniczky B, Elbe A et al. Autoantibodies against desmoplakin I and II define a subset of patients with erythema multiforme. J Invest Dermatol 1996; 106: 1012–1016.

508 Johnson SM, Smoller BR, Horn TD. Erythema multiforme associated human autoantibodies against desmoplakin I and II. J Invest Dermatol 1999; 112: 395.

509 Foedinger D, Elbe-Bürger A, Sterniczky B et al. Erythema multiforme associated human autoantibodies against desmoplakin I and II: biochemical characterization and passive transfer studies into newborn mice. J Invest Dermatol 1998; 111: 503–510.

510 Bedi TR, Pinkus H. Histopathological spectrum of erythema multiforme. Br J Dermatol 1976; 95: 243–250.

511 Ackerman AB, Penneys NS, Clark WH. Erythema multiforme exudativum: distinctive pathological process. Br J Dermatol 1971; 84: 554–566.

512 Ford MJ, Smith KL, Croker BP et al. Large granular lymphocytes within the epidermis of erythema multiforme lesions. J Am Acad Dermatol 1992; 27: 460–462.

513 Inachi S, Mizutani H, Shimizu M. Epidermal apoptotic cell death in erythema multiforme and Stevens–Johnson syndrome. Contribution of perforin-positive cell infiltration. Arch Dermatol 1997; 133: 845–849.

514 Zohdi-Mofid M, Horn TD. Acrosyringeal concentration of necrotic keratinocytes in erythema multiforme: a clue to drug etiology. J Cutan Pathol 1997; 24: 235–240.

515 Patterson JW, Parsons JM, Blaylock WK, Mills AS. Eosinophils in skin lesions of erythema multiforme. Arch Pathol Lab Med 1989; 113: 36–39.

516 Rzany B, Hering O, Mockenhaupt M et al. Histopathological and epidemiological characteristics of patients with erythema exudativum multiforme major, Stevens–Johnson syndrome and toxic epidermal necrolysis. Br J Dermatol 1996; 135: 6–11.

517 Solomon AR. The histological spectrum of the reactive inflammatory vesicular dermatoses. Dermatol Clin 1985; 3: 171–183.

518 Wells JM, Weedon D, Muir JB. Erythema multiforme: a case with unusual histopathological features. Australas J Dermatol 2000; 41: 257–259.

519 Reed RJ. Erythema multiforme. A clinical syndrome and a histologic complex. Am J Dermatopathol 1985; 7: 143–152.

520 Ackerman AB. Erythema multiforme. Am J Dermatopathol 1985; 7: 133–139 (Editor's note).

521 Orfanos CE, Schaumburg-Lever G, Lever WF. Dermal and epidermal types of erythema multiforme. A histopathologic study of 24 cases. Arch Dermatol 1974; 109: 682–688.

522 Ackerman AB. Dermal and epidermal types of erythema multiforme. Arch Dermatol 1975; 111: 795.

523 Reichert-Penetrat S, Barbaud A, Antunes A et al. An unusual form of Stevens–Johnson syndrome with subcorneal pustules associated with *Mycoplasma pneumonice* infection. Pediatr Dermatol 2000; 17: 202–204.

524 Finan MC, Schroeter AL. Cutaneous immunofluorescence study of erythema multiforme: correlation with light microscopic patterns and etiologic agents. J Am Acad Dermatol 1984; 10: 497–506.

525 Imamura S, Yanase K, Taniguchi S et al. Erythema multiforme: demonstration of immune complexes in the sera and skin lesions. Br J Dermatol 1980; 102: 161–166.

526 Grimwood R, Huff JC, Weston WL. Complement deposition in the skin of patients with herpes-associated erythema multiforme. J Am Acad Dermatol 1983; 9: 199–203.

527 Matsuoka LY, Wortsman J, Stanley JR. Epidermal autoantibodies in erythema multiforme. J Am Acad Dermatol 1989; 21: 677–680.

528 Merot Y, Saurat JH. Clues to pathogenesis of toxic epidermal necrolysis. Int J Dermatol 1985; 24: 165–168.

529 Goldstein SM, Wintroub BW, Elias PM. Toxic epidermal necrolysis. Unmuddying the waters. Arch Dermatol 1987; 123: 1153–1156.

530 Lyell A. Toxic epidermal necrolysis (the scalded skin syndrome): a reappraisal. Br J Dermatol 1979; 100: 69–86.

531 Lyell A. Requiem for toxic epidermal necrolysis. Br J Dermatol 1990; 122: 837–838.

532 Roujeau J-C, Chosidow O, Saiag P, Guillaume J-C. Toxic epidermal necrolysis (Lyell syndrome). J Am Acad Dermatol 1990; 23: 1039–1058.

533 Avakian R, Flowers FP, Araujo OE, Ramos-Caro FA. Toxic epidermal necrolysis: a review. J Am Acad Dermatol 1991; 25: 69–79.

534 Parsons JM. Toxic epidermal necrolysis. Int J Dermatol 1992; 31: 749–768.

535 Revuz J, Penso D, Roujeau J-C et al. Toxic epidermal necrolysis. Clinical findings and prognosis factors in 87 patients. Arch Dermatol 1987; 123: 1160–1165.

536 Bastuji-Garin S, Fouchard N, Bertocchi M et al. SCORTEN: a severity-of-illness score for toxic epidermal necrolysis. J Invest Dermatol 2000; 115: 149–153.

537 Roujeau J-C. The spectrum of Stevens–Johnson syndrome and toxic epidermal necrolysis: a clinical classification. J Invest Dermatol 1994; 102: 28S–30S.

538 Kaufman DW. Epidemiologic approaches to the study of toxic epidermal necrolysis. J Invest Dermatol 1994; 102: 31S–33S.

539 Roujeau J-C, Guillaume J-C, Fabre J-P et al. Toxic epidermal necrolysis (Lyell syndrome). Incidence and drug etiology in France, 1981–1985. Arch Dermatol 1990; 126: 37–42.

540 Sherertz EF, Jegasothy BV, Lazarus GS. Phenytoin hypersensitivity reaction presenting with toxic epidermal necrolysis and severe hepatitis. Report of a patient treated with corticosteroid 'pulse therapy'. J Am Acad Dermatol 1985; 12: 178–181.

541 Wolkenstein P, Charue D, Laurent P et al. Metabolic predisposition to cutaneous adverse drug reactions. Arch Dermatol 1995; 131: 544–551.

542 Creamer JD, Whittaker SJ, Kerr-Muir M, Smith NP. Phenytoin-induced toxic epidermal necrolysis: a case report. Clin Exp Dermatol 1996; 21: 116–120.

543 Pasricha JS, Khaitan BK, Shantharaman R et al. Toxic epidermal necrolysis. Int J Dermatol 1996; 35: 523–527.

544 Guillaume J-C, Roujeau J-C, Revuz J et al. The culprit drugs in 87 cases of toxic epidermal necrolysis (Lyell's syndrome). Arch Dermatol 1987; 123: 1166–1170.

545 Stotts JS, Fang ML, Dannaker CJ, Steinman HK. Fenoprofen-induced toxic epidermal necrolysis. J Am Acad Dermatol 1988; 18: 755–757.

546 Dan M, Jedwab M, Peled M, Shibolet S. Allopurinol-induced toxic epidermal necrolysis. Int J Dermatol 1984; 23: 142–144.

547 Brand R, Rohr JB. Toxic epidermal necrolysis in Western Australia. Australas J Dermatol 2000; 41: 31–33.

548 Miralles ES, Núñez M, del Olmo N, Ledo A. Ranitidine-induced toxic epidermal necrolysis in a patient with idiopathic thrombocytopenic purpura. J Am Acad Dermatol 1995; 32: 133–134.

549 Vélez A, Moreno J-C. Second case of ranitidine-related toxic epidermal necrolysis in a patient with idiopathic thrombocytopenic purpura. J Am Acad Dermatol 2000; 42: 305.

550 Paquet P, Schaaf-Lafontaine N, Piérard GE. Toxic epidermal necrolysis following clindamycin treatment. Br J Dermatol 1995; 132: 665–666.

551 Boffa MJ, Chalmers RJG. Toxic epidermal necrolysis due to chloroquine phosphate. Br J Dermatol 1994; 131: 444–445.

552 Brunner M, Vardarman E, Goldermann R et al. Toxic epidermal necrolysis (Lyell syndrome) following famotidine administration. Br J Dermatol 1995; 133: 814–815.

553 Partanen J, Pohjola-Sintonen S, Mäkijärvi M. Toxic epidermal necrolysis due to indapamide. Arch Dermatol 1993; 129: 793.

554 Redondo P, Vicente J, España A et al. Photo-induced toxic epidermal necrolysis caused by clobazam. Br J Dermatol 1996; 135: 999–1002.

555 Carucci JA, Cohen DE. Toxic epidermal necrolysis following treatment with oxaprozin. Int J Dermatol 1999; 38: 233–234.

556 Dereure O, Hillaire-Buys D, Augias D et al. Fatal toxic epidermal necrosis: responsibility of diacerein? a controversy. Dermatology 1998; 196: 431.

557 Wong KC, Kennedy PJ, Lee S. Clinical manifestations and outcomes in 17 cases of Stevens–Johnson syndrome and toxic epidermal necrolysis. Australas J Dermatol 1999; 40: 131–134.

558 Primka EJ III, Camisa C. Methotrexate-induced toxic epidermal necrolysis in a patient with psoriasis. J Am Acad Dermatol 1997; 36: 815–818.

559 Özkan A, Apak H, Celkan T et al. Toxic epidermal necrolysis after the use of high-dose cytosine arabinoside. Pediatr Dermatol 2001; 18: 38–40.

560 Vukelić D, Božinović D, Tešović G et al. Lamotrigine and toxic epidermal necrolysis. Dermatology 1997; 195: 307.

561 Bhushan M, Brooke R, Hewitt-Symonds M et al. Prolonged toxic epidermal necrolysis due to Lamotrigine. Clin Exp Dermatol 2000; 25: 349–351.

562 Jarrett P, Rademaker M, Havill J, Pullon H. Toxic epidermal necrolysis treated with cyclosporin and granulocyte colony stimulating factor. Clin Exp Dermatol 1997; 22: 146–147.

563 Dhar S, Todi SK. Are carbamazepine-induced Stevens–Johnson syndrome and toxic epidermal necrolysis more common in nonepileptic patients? Dermatology 1999; 199: 194.

564 Yang C-h, Yang L-J, Jaing T-H, Chan H-L. Toxic epidermal necrolysis following combination of methotrexate and trimethoprim-sulfamethoxazole. Int J Dermatol 2000; 39: 621–623.

565 Thestrup-Pedersen K, Hainau B, Al'Eisa A et al. Fatal toxic epidermal necrolysis associated with ceftazidine and vancomycin therapy: a report of two cases. Acta Derm Venereol 2000; 80: 316–317.

566 Livasy CA, Kaplan AM. Ciprofloxacin-induced toxic epidermal necrolysis: a case report. Dermatology 1997; 195: 173–175.

567 Wetterwald E, Le Cleach L, Michel C et al. Nevirapine-induced overlap Stevens–Johnson syndrome/toxic epidermal necrolysis. Br J Dermatol 1999; 140: 980–982.

568 Phan TG, Wong RCW, Crotty K, Adelstein S. Toxic epidermal necrolysis in acquired immunodeficiency syndrome treated with intravenous gammaglobulin. Australas J Dermatol 1999; 40: 153–157.

569 Lecorvaisier-Pieto C, Joly P, Thomine E et al. Toxic epidermal necrolysis after mifepristone/gemeprost-induced abortion. J Am Acad Dermatol 1996; 35: 112.

570 Claessens N, Delbeke L, Lambert J et al. Toxic epidermal necrolysis associated with treatment for preterm labor. Dermatology 1998; 196: 461–462.

571 Roujeau J-C, Huynh TN, Bracq C et al. Genetic susceptibility to toxic epidermal necrolysis. Arch Dermatol 1987; 123: 1171–1173.

572 Paquet P, Nikkels A, Arrese JE et al. Macrophages and tumour necrosis factor α in toxic epidermal necrolysis. Arch Dermatol 1994; 130: 605–608.

573 Paul C, Wolkenstein P, Adle H et al. Apoptosis as a mechanism of keratinocyte death in toxic epidermal necrolysis. Br J Dermatol 1996; 134: 710–714.

574 Paquet P, Piérard GE. Epidermal calprotectin in drug-induced toxic epidermal necrolysis. J Cutan Pathol 1999; 26: 301–305.

575 Correia O, Delgado L, Ramos JP et al. Cutaneous T-cell recruitment in toxic epidermal necrolysis. Further evidence of CD8+ lymphocyte involvement. Arch Dermatol 1993; 129: 466–468.

576 Friedman PS, Strickland I, Pirmohamed M, Park BK. Investigation of mechanisms in toxic epidermal necrolysis induced by carbamazepine. Arch Dermatol 1994; 130: 598–604.

577 Villada G, Roujeau J-C, Clérici T et al. Immunopathology of toxic epidermal necrolysis. Arch Dermatol 1992; 128: 50–53.

578 Garcia-Doval I, LeCleach L, Bocquet H et al. Toxic epidermal necrolysis and Stevens–Johnson syndrome. Does early withdrawal of causative drugs decrease the risk of death? Arch Dermatol 2000; 136: 323–327.

579 Guibal F, Bastuji-Garin S, Chosidow O et al. Characteristics of toxic epidermal necrolysis in patients undergoing long-term glucocorticoid therapy. Arch Dermatol 1995; 131: 669–672.

580 Saiag P, Caumes E, Chosidow O et al. Drug-induced toxic epidermal necrolysis (Lyell syndrome) in patients infected with the human immunodeficiency virus. J Am Acad Dermatol 1992; 26: 567–574.

581 Westly ED, Wechsler HL. Toxic epidermal necrolysis. Granulocytic leukopenia as a prognostic indicator. Arch Dermatol 1984; 120: 721–726.

582 Stone N, Sheerin S, Burge S. Toxic epidermal necrolysis and graft vs. host disease: a clinical spectrum but a diagnostic dilemma. Clin Exp Dermatol 1999; 24: 260–262.

583 Akosa AB, Elhag AM. Toxic epidermal necrolysis. A study of the sweat glands. J Cutan Pathol 1995; 22: 359–364.

584 King T, Helm TN, Valenzuela R, Bergfeld WF. Diffuse intraepidermal deposition of immunoreactants on direct immunofluorescence: a clue to the early diagnosis of epidermal necrolysis. Int J Dermatol 1994; 33: 634–636.

585 Hood AF, Soter NA, Rappeport J, Gigli I. Graft-versus-host reaction. Cutaneous manifestations following bone marrow transplantation. Arch Dermatol 1977; 113: 1087–1091.

586 Breathnach SM, Katz SI. Immunopathology of cutaneous graft-versus-host disease. Am J Dermatopathol 1987; 9: 343–348.

587 Tawfik N, Jimbow K. Acute graft-vs-host disease in an immunodeficient newborn possibly due to cytomegalovirus infection. Arch Dermatol 1989; 125: 1685–1688.

588 Harper JI. Graft versus host reaction: etiological and clinical aspects in connective tissue diseases. Semin Dermatol 1985; 4: 144–151.

589 Richter HI, Stege H, Ruzicka T et al. Extracorporeal photopheresis in the treatment of acute graft-versus-host disease. J Am Acad Dermatol 1997; 36: 787–789.

590 Johnson ML, Farmer ER. Graft-versus-host reactions in dermatology. J Am Acad Dermatol 1998; 38: 369–392.

591 Darmstadt GL, Donnenberg AD, Vogelsang GB et al. Clinical, laboratory, and histopathologic indicators of the development of progressive acute graft-versus-host disease. J Invest Dermatol 1992; 99: 397–402.

592 Alain G, Carrier C, Beaumier L et al. In utero acute graft-versus-host disease in a neonate with severe combined immunodeficiency. J Am Acad Dermatol 1993; 29: 862–865.

593 Held JL, Druker BJ, Kohn SR et al. Atypical, nonfatal, transfusion-associated, acute graft-versus-host disease in a patient with Hodgkin's disease. J Am Acad Dermatol 1992; 26: 261–262.

594 Hull RJ, Bray RA, Hillyer C, Swerlick RA. Transfusion-associated chronic cutaneous graft-versus-host disease. J Am Acad Dermatol 1995; 33: 327–332.

595 Aricò M, Noto G, Pravatà G et al. Transfusion-associated graft-versus-host disease – report of two further cases with an immunohistochemical analysis. Clin Exp Dermatol 1994; 19: 36–42.

596 Fernández-Herrera J, Valks R, Feal C et al. Induction of hyperacute graft-vs-host disease after donor leukocyte infusions. Arch Dermatol 1999; 135: 304–308.

597 Tanei R, Ohta Y, Ishihara S et al. Transfusion-associated graft-versus-host disease: an in situ hybridization analysis of the infiltrating donor-derived cells in the cutaneous lesion. Dermatology 1999; 199: 20–24.

598 Jones-Caballero M, Fernández-Herrera J, Córdoba-Guijarro S et al. Sclerodermatous graft-versus-host disease after donor leucocyte infusion. Br J Dermatol 1998; 139: 889–892.

599 Schmuth M, Vogel W, Weinlich G et al. Cutaneous lesions as the presenting sign of acute graft-versus-host disease following liver transplantation. Br J Dermatol 1999; 141: 901–904.

600 Rocha V, Wagner JE Jr, Sobocinski KA et al. Graft-versus-host disease in children who have received a cord-blood or bone marrow transplant from an HLA-identical sibling. N Engl J Med 2000; 342: 1846–1854.

601 Tanaka K, Aki T, Shulman HM et al. Two cases of transfusion-associated graft-vs-host disease after open heart surgery. Arch Dermatol 1992; 128: 1503–1506.

602 Sola MA, España A, Redondo P et al. Transfusion-associated acute graft-versus-host disease in a heart transplant recipient. Br J Dermatol 1995; 132: 626–630.

603 Rubeiz N, Taher A, Salem Z et al. Post-transfusion graft-versus-host disease in two immunocompetent patients. J Am Acad Dermatol 1993; 28: 862–865.

604 Hood AF, Vogelsang GB. Black LP et al. Acute graft-vs-host disease. Development following autologous and syngeneic bone marrow transplantation. Arch Dermatol 1987; 123: 745–750.

605 Ferrara JLM. Syngeneic graft-vs-host disease. Arch Dermatol 1987; 123: 741–742.

606 Gaspari AA, Cheng SF, DiPersio JF, Rowe JM. Roquinimex-induced graft-versus-host reaction after autologous bone marrow transplantation. J Am Acad Dermatol 1995; 33: 711–717.

607 Martin RW III, Farmer ER, Altomonte VL et al. Lichenoid graft-vs-host disease in an autologous bone marrow transplant recipient. Arch Dermatol 1995; 131: 333–335.

608 Holder J, North J, Bourke J et al. Thymoma-associated cutaneous graft-versus-host-like reaction. Clin Exp Dermatol 1997; 22: 287–290.

609 Scarisbrick JJ, Wakelin SH, Russell-Jones R. Cutaneous graft-versus-host-like reaction in systemic T-cell lymphoma. Clin Exp Dermatol 1999; 24: 382–384.

610 Parkes IR, Zaki I, Stevens A et al. Graft-versus-host disease-like eruption in a patient with non-Hodgkin's lymphoma. Br J Dermatol 1997; 137: 137–139.

611 Mascaro JM, Rozman C, Palou J et al. Acute and chronic graft-vs-host reaction in skin: report of two cases. Br J Dermatol 1980; 102: 461–466.

612 Mauduit G, Claudy A. Cutaneous expression of graft-v-host disease in man. Semin Dermatol 1988; 7: 149–155.

613 Friedman KJ. LeBoit PE. Farmer ER Acute follicular graft-vs-host reaction. Arch Dermatol 1988; 124: 688–691.

614 Schauder CS, Hymes SR, Rapini RP, Zipf TF. Vesicular graft-versus-host disease. Int J Dermatol 1992; 31: 509–510.

615 Villada G, Roujeau J-C, Cordonnier C et al. Toxic epidermal necrolysis after bone marrow transplantation: study of nine cases. J Am Acad Dermatol 1990; 23: 870–875.

616 Sale GE, Shulman HM, Schubert MM et al. Oral and ophthalmic pathology of graft versus host disease in man: predictive value of the lip biopsy. Hum Pathol 1981; 12: 1022–1030.

617 Chao S-C, Tsao C-J, Liu C-L, Lee JY-Y. Acute cutaneous graft-versus-host disease with ichthyosiform features. Br J Dermatol 1998; 139: 553–555.

618 Chow RKP, Stewart WD, Ho VC. Graft-versus-host reaction affecting lesional skin but not normal skin in a patient with piebaldism. Br J Dermatol 1996; 134: 134–137.

619 Matsuoka LY. Graft versus host disease. J Am Acad Dermatol 1981; 5: 595–599.

620 Saurat JH, Gluckman E. Lichen-planus-like eruption following bone marrow transplantation: a manifestation of the graft-versus-host disease. Clin Exp Dermatol 1977; 2: 335–344.

621 Saurat JH. Cutaneous manifestations of graft-versus-host disease. Int J Dermatol 1981; 20: 249–256.

622 Freemer CS, Farmer ER, Corio RL et al. Lichenoid chronic graft-vs-host disease occurring in a dermatomal distribution. Arch Dermatol 1994; 130: 70–72.

623 Wilson BB, Lockman DW. Linear lichenoid graft-vs-host disease. Arch Dermatol 1994; 130: 1206–1207.

624 Beers B, Kalish RS, Kaye VN, Dahl MV. Unilateral linear lichenoid eruption after bone marrow transplantation: an unmasking of tolerance to an abnormal keratinocyte clone? J Am Acad Dermatol 1993; 28: 888–892.

625 Kikuchi A, Okamoto S-i, Takahashi S et al. Linear chronic cutaneous graft-versus-host disease. J Am Acad Dermatol 1997; 37: 1004–1006.

626 Baselga E, Drolet BA, Segura AD et al. Dermatomal lichenoid chronic graft-vs-host disease following varicella-zoster infection despite absence of viral genome. J Cutan Pathol 1996; 23: 576–581.

627 Lacour J-P, Sirvent N, Monpoux F et al. Dermatomal chronic cutaneous graft-versus-host disease at the site of prior herpes zoster. Br J Dermatol 1999; 141: 587–589.

628 Van Vloten WA, Scheffer E, Dooren LJ. Localized scleroderma-like lesions after bone marrow transplantation in man. A chronic graft versus host reaction. Br J Dermatol 1977; 96: 337–341.

629 Marzano AV, Facchetti M, Berti E, Caputo R. Chronic graft-vs-host disease with severe

630 Barnadas MA, Brunet S, Sureda A et al. Exuberant granulation tissue associated with chronic graft-versus-host disease after transplantation of peripheral blood progenitor cells. J Am Acad Dermatol 1999; 41: 876–879.

631 Aractingi S, Janin A, Devergie A et al. Histochemical and ultrastructural study of diffuse melanoderma after bone marrow transplantation. Br J Dermatol 1996; 134: 325–331.

632 Snover DC. Acute and chronic graft versus host disease: histopathological evidence for two distinct pathogenetic mechanisms. Hum Pathol 1984; 15: 202–205.

633 Breathnach SM. Current understanding of the aetiology and clinical implications of cutaneous graft-versus-host disease. Br J Dermatol 1986; 114: 139–143.

634 Gomes MA, Schmitt DS, Souteyrand P et al. Lichen planus and chronic graft-versus-host reaction. In situ identification of immunocompetent cell phenotypes. J Cutan Pathol 1982; 9: 249–257.

635 Breathnach SM, Katz SI. Cell-mediated immunity in cutaneous disease. Hum Pathol 1986; 17: 162–167.

636 Horn TD, Haskell J. The lymphocytic infiltrate in acute cutaneous allogeneic graft-versus-host reactions lacks evidence for phenotypic restriction in donor-derived cells. J Cutan Pathol 1998; 25: 210–214.

637 Horn TD. Effector cells in cutaneous graft-versus-host disease. Who? what? when? where? how? Br J Dermatol 1999; 141: 779–780.

638 Sale GE, Shulman HM, Gallucci BB, Thomas ED. Young rete ridge keratinocytes are preferred targets in cutaneous graft-versus-host disease. Am J Pathol 1985; 118: 278–287.

639 Sloane JP, Thomas JA, Imrie SF et al. Morphological and immunohistological changes in the skin in allogeneic bone marrow recipients. J Clin Pathol 1984; 37: 919–930.

640 Dreno B, Milpied N, Harousseau JL et al. Cutaneous immunological studies in diagnosis of acute graft-versus-host disease. Br J Dermatol 1986; 114: 7–15.

641 Lever R, Turbitt M, MacKie R et al. A perspective study of the histological changes in the skin in patients receiving bone marrow transplants. Br J Dermatol 1986; 114: 161–170.

642 Favre A, Cerri A, Bacigalupo A et al. Immunohistochemical study of skin lesions in acute and chronic graft versus host disease following bone marrow transplantation. Am J Surg Pathol 1997; 21: 23–34.

643 Yoo YH, Park BS, Whitaker-Menezes D et al. Dermal dendrocytes participate in the cellular pathology of experimental acute graft-versus-host disease. J Cutan Pathol 1998; 25: 426–434.

644 Hermanns-Lê T, Paquet P, Piérard-Franchimont C et al. Regulatory function of factor-XIIIa-positive dendrocytes in incipient toxic epidermal necrolysis and graft-versus-host reaction. A hypothesis. Dermatology 1999; 198: 184–186.

645 Wick MR, Moore SB, Gastineau DA, Hoagland HC. Immunologic, clinical, and pathologic aspects of human graft-versus-host disease. Mayo Clin Proc 1983; 58: 603–612.

646 Hymes SR, Farmer ER, Lewis PG et al. Cutaneous graft-versus-host reaction: prognostic features seen by light microscopy. J Am Acad Dermatol 1985; 12: 468–474.

647 Norton J, Sloane JP. Epidermal damage in skin of allogeneic marrow recipients: relative importance of chemotherapy, conditioning and graft v. host disease. Histopathology 1992; 21: 529–534.

648 Langley RGB, Walsh N, Nevill T et al. Apoptosis is the mode of keratinocyte death in cutaneous graft-versus-host disease. J Am Acad Dermatol 1996; 35: 187–190.

649 LeBoit PE. Subacute radiation dermatitis: a histologic imitator of acute cutaneous graft-versus-host disease. J Am Acad Dermatol 1989; 20: 236–241.

650 Kohler S, Chao NJ, Smoller BR. Reassessment of histologic parameters in the diagnosis of acute graft versus host disease. J Cutan Pathol 1996; 23: 54 (abstract).

651 Connors J, Drolet B, Walsh J et al. Morbilliform eruption in a liver transplantation patient. Arch Dermatol 1996; 132: 1161–1163.

652 Nghiem P. The "drug vs graft-vs-host disease" conundrum gets tougher, but there is an answer. The challenge to dermatologists. Arch Dermatol 2001; 137: 75–76.

653 Massi D, Franchi A, Pimpinelli N et al. A reappraisal of the histopathologic criteria for the diagnosis of cutaneous allogeneic acute graft-vs-host disease. Am J Clin Pathol 1999; 112: 791–800.

654 Kohler S, Hendrickson MR, Chao NJ, Smoller BR. Value of skin biopsies in assessing prognosis and progression of acute graft-versus-host disease. Am J Surg Pathol 1997; 21: 988–996.

655 Zhou Y, Barnett MJ, Rivers JK. Clinical significance of skin biopsies in the diagnosis and management of graft-vs-host disease in early postallogeneic bone marrow transplantation. Arch Dermatol 2000; 136: 717–721.

656 Horn TD. Acute cutaneous eruptions after marrow ablation: roses by other names? J Cutan Pathol 1994; 21: 385–392.

657 Saurat JH, Gluckman E, Bussel A et al. The lichen planus-like eruption after bone marrow transplantation. Br J Dermatol 1975; 92: 675–681.

658 Horn TD, Zahurak ML, Atkins D et al. Lichen planus-like histopathologic characteristics in the cutaneous graft-vs-host reaction. Arch Dermatol 1997; 133: 961–965.

cicatrizing conjunctivitis mimicking cicatricial pemphigoid. Br J Dermatol 2000; 143: 209–210.

659 Saijo S, Honda M, Sasahara Y et al. Columnar epidermal necrosis. A unique manifestation of transfusion-associated cutaneous graft-vs-host disease. Arch Dermatol 2000; 136: 743–746.

660 Hymes SR, Farmer ER, Burns WH et al. Bullous sclerodermalike changes in chronic graft-vs-host disease. Arch Dermatol 1985; 121: 1189–1192.

661 Ohsuga Y, Rowe JM, Liesveld J et al. Dermatologic changes associated with roquinimex immunotherapy after autologous bone marrow transplant. J Am Acad Dermatol 2000; 43: 437–441.

662 Rozman C, Mascaro JM, Granena A et al. Ultrastructural findings in acute and chronic graft-vs-host reaction of the skin. J Cutan Pathol 1980; 7: 354–363.

663 Slavin RE. Lymphocyte-associated apoptosis in AIDS, in bone-marrow transplantation, and other conditions. Am J Surg Pathol 1987; 11: 235–238.

664 Claudy AL, Schmitt D, Freycon F, Boucheron S. Melanocyte-lymphocyte interaction in human graft-versus-host disease. J Cutan Pathol 1983; 10: 305–311.

665 Janin-Mercier A, Saurat JH, Bourges M et al. The lichen planus like and sclerotic phases of the graft versus host disease in man: an ultrastructural study of six cases. Acta Derm Venereol 1981; 61: 187–193.

666 Horn TD, Redd JV, Karp JE et al. Cutaneous eruptions of lymphocyte recovery. Arch Dermatol 1989; 125: 1512–1517.

667 Bauer DJ, Hood AF, Horn TD. Histologic comparison of autologous graft-vs-host reaction and cutaneous eruption of lymphocyte recovery. Arch Dermatol 1993; 129: 855–858.

668 Gibney MD, Penneys NS, Nelson-Adesokan P. Cutaneous eruption of lymphocyte recovery mimicking mycosis fungoides in a patient with acute myelocytic leukemia. J Cutan Pathol 1995; 22: 472–475.

669 Horn T, Lehmkuhle MA, Gore A et al. Systemic cytokine administration alters the histology of the eruption of lymphocyte recovery. J Cutan Pathol 1996; 23: 242–246.

670 Rico MJ, Kory WP, Gould EW, Penneys NS. Interface dermatitis in patients with the acquired immunodeficiency syndrome. J Am Acad Dermatol 1987; 16: 1209–1218.

671 Tuffanelli DL. Lupus erythematosus. J Am Acad Dermatol 1981; 4: 127–142.

672 Gilliam JN, Sontheimer RD. Distinctive cutaneous subsets in the spectrum of lupus erythematosus. J Am Acad Dermatol 1981; 4: 471–475.

673 Clark WH, Reed RJ, Mihm MC. Lupus erythematosus. Histopathology of cutaneous lesions. Hum Pathol 1973; 4: 157–163.

674 Coulson IH, Marsden RA. Lupus erythematosus cheilitis. Clin Exp Dermatol 1986; 11: 309–313.

675 Shklar G, McCarthy PL. Histopathology of oral lesions of discoid lupus erythematosus. A review of 25 cases. Arch Dermatol 1978; 114: 1031–1035.

676 Cyran S, Douglas MC, Silverstein JL. Chronic cutaneous lupus erythematosus presenting as periorbital edema and erythema. J Am Acad Dermatol 1992; 26: 334–338.

677 Wilson CL, Burge SM, Dean D, Dawber RPR. Scarring alopecia in discoid lupus erythematosus. Br J Dermatol 1992; 126: 307–314.

678 Sulica VI, Kao GF. Squamous-cell carcinoma of the scalp arising in lesions of discoid lupus erythematosus. Am J Dermatopathol 1988; 10: 137–141.

679 Sherman RN, Lee CW, Flynn KJ. Cutaneous squamous cell carcinoma in black patients with chronic discoid lupus erythematosus. Int J Dermatol 1993; 32: 677–679.

680 George PM, Tunnessen WW Jr. Childhood discoid lupus erythematosus. Arch Dermatol 1993; 129: 613–617.

681 Magaña M, Vazquez R. Discoid lupus erythematosus in childhood. Pediatr Dermatol 2000; 17: 241–242.

682 McMullen EA, Armstrong KDB, Bingham EA, Walsh MY. Childhood discoid lupus erythematosus: a report of two cases. Pediatr Dermatol 1998; 15: 439–442.

683 Rubenstein DJ, Huntley AC. Keratotic lupus erythematosus: treatment with isotretinoin. J Am Acad Dermatol 1986; 14: 910–914.

684 Santa Cruz DJ, Uitto J, Eisen AZ, Prioleau PG. Verrucous lupus erythematosus: ultrastructural studies on a distinct variant of chronic discoid lupus erythematosus. J Am Acad Dermatol 1983; 9: 82–90.

685 Otani A. Lupus erythematosus hypertrophicus et profundus. Br J Dermatol 1977; 96: 75–78.

686 Parodi A, Drago EF, Varaldo G, Rebora A. Rowell's syndrome. Report of a case. J Am Acad Dermatol 1989; 21: 374–377.

687 Fiallo P, Tagliapietra A-G, Santoro G, Venturino E. Rowell's syndrome. Int J Dermatol 1995; 34: 635–636.

688 Zeitouni NC, Funaro D, Cloutier RA et al. Redefining Rowell's syndrome. Br J Dermatol 2000; 142: 343–346.

689 Fitzgerald EA, Purcell SM, Kantor GR, Goldman HM. Rowell's syndrome: report of a case. J Am Acad Dermatol 1996; 35: 801–803.

690 Shteyngarts AR, Warner MR, Camisa C. Lupus erythematosus associated with erythema multiforme: Does Rowell's syndrome exist? J Am Acad Dermatol 1999; 40: 773–777.

691 Child FJ, Kapur N, Creamer D, Kobza Black A. Rowell's syndrome. Clin Exp Dermatol 1999; 24: 74–77.

692 Massone C, Parodi A, Rebora A. Erythema multiforme-like subacute cutaneous lupus erythematosus: a new variety? Acta Derm Venereol 2000; 80: 308–309.

693 Marzano AV, Berti E, Gasparini G, Caputo R. Lupus erythematosus with antiphospholipid syndrome and erythema multiforme-like lesions. Br J Dermatol 1999; 141: 720–724.

694 Lowe L, Rapini RP, Golitz LE, Johnson TM. Papulonodular dermal mucinosis in lupus erythematosus. J Am Acad Dermatol 1992; 27: 312–315.

695 Lee WS, Chung J, Ahn SK. Mucinous lupus alopecia associated with papulonodular mucinosis as a new manifestation of lupus erythematosus. Int J Dermatol 1996; 35: 72–73.

696 Williams WL, Ramos-Caro FA. Acute periorbital mucinosis in discoid lupus erythematosus. J Am Acad Dermatol 1999; 41: 871–873.

697 Sontheimer RD. Questions answered and a $1 million question raised concerning lupus erythematosus tumidus. Is routine laboratory surveillance testing during treatment with hydroxychloroquine for skin disease really necessary? Arch Dermatol 2000; 136: 1044–1049.

698 Dekle CL, Mannes KD, Davis LS, Sangueza OP. Lupus tumidus. J Am Acad Dermatol 1999; 41: 250–253.

699 Ruiz H, Sánchez JL. Tumid lupus erythematosus. Am J Dermatopathol 1999; 21: 356–360.

700 Weyers W, Bonczkowitz M, Weyers I. LE or not LE – that is the question. An unsuccessful attempt to separate lymphocytic infiltration from the spectrum of discoid lupus erythematosus. Am J Dermatopathol 1993; 20: 225–232.

701 Weber F, Schmuth M, Fritsch P, Sepp N. Lymphocytic infiltration of the skin is a photosensitive variant of lupus erythematosus: evidence by phototesting. Br J Dermatol 2001; 144: 292–296.

702 Abe M, Ishikawa O, Miyachi Y. Linear cutaneous lupus erythematosus following the lines of Blaschko. Br J Dermatol 1998; 139: 307–310.

703 Bouzit N, Grézard P, Wolf F et al. Linear cutaneous lupus erythematosus in an adult. Dermatology 1999; 199: 60–62.

704 Lipsker D, Heid E. Cutaneous lupus erythematosus following the lines of Blaschko. Dermatology 1999; 199: 373.

705 Green JJ, Baker DJ. Linear childhood discoid lupus erythematosus following the lines of Blaschko: a case report with review of the linear manifestations of lupus erythematosus. Pediatr Dermatol 1999; 16: 128–133.

706 Davies MG, Newman P. Linear cutaneous lupus erythematosus in association with ipsilateral submandibular myoepithelial sialadenitis. Clin Exp Dermatol 2001; 26: 56–58.

707 Callen JP. Systemic lupus erythematosus in patients with chronic cutaneous (discoid) lupus erythematosus. Clinical and laboratory findings in seventeen patients. J Am Acad Dermatol 1985; 12: 278–288.

708 Rowell NR. The natural history of lupus erythematosus. Clin Exp Dermatol 1984; 9: 217–231.

709 Millard LG, Rowell NR. Abnormal laboratory test results and their relationship to prognosis in discoid lupus erythematosus. A long-term follow-up of 92 patients. Arch Dermatol 1979; 115: 1055–1058.

710 Provost TT. The relationship between discoid and systemic lupus erythematosus. Arch Dermatol 1994; 130: 1308–1310.

711 Callen JP, Fowler JF, Kulick KB. Serologic and clinical features of patients with discoid lupus erythematosus: relationship of antibodies to single-stranded deoxyribonucleic acid and of other antinuclear antibody subsets to clinical manifestations. J Am Acad Dermatol 1985; 13: 748–755.

712 Lee LA, Roberts CM, Frank MB et al. The autoantibody response to Ro/SSA in cutaneous lupus erythematosus. Arch Dermatol 1994; 130: 1262–1268.

713 Paroci A, Massone C, Cacciapuoti M et al. Measuring the activity of the disease in patients with cutaneous lupus erythematosus. Br J Dermatol 2000; 142: 457–460.

714 Fowler JF, Callen JP, Stelzer GT, Cotter PK. Human histocompatibility antigen associations in patients with chronic cutaneous lupus erythematosus. J Am Acad Dermatol 1985; 12: 73–77.

715 Donnelly AM, Halbert AR, Rohr JB. Discoid lupus erythematosus. Australas J Dermatol 1995; 36: 3–12.

716 Millard TP, McGregor JM. Molecular genetics of cutaneous lupus erythematosus. Clin Exp Dermatol 2001; 26: 184–191.

717 Garioch JJ, Sampson JR, Seywright M, Thomson J. Dermatoses in five related female carriers of X-linked chronic granulomatous disease. Br J Dermatol 1989; 121: 391–396.

718 Barton LL, Johnson CR. Discoid lupus erythematosus and X-linked chronic granulomatous disease. Pediatr Dermatol 1986; 3: 376–379.

719 Sillevis Smitt JH, Weening RS, Krieg SR, Bos JD. Discoid lupus erythematosus-like lesions in carriers of X-linked chronic granulomatous disease. Br J Dermatol 1990; 122: 643–650.

720 Llorente CP, Amorós JI, Ortiz de Frutos FJ et al. Cutaneous lesions in severe combined immunodeficiency: two case reports and a review of the literature. Pediatr Dermatol 1991; 8: 314–321.

721 Hudson-Peacock MJ, Joseph SA, Cox J et al. Systemic lupus erythematosus complicating

complement type 2 deficiency: successful treatment with fresh frozen plasma. Br J Dermatol 1997; 136: 388–392.

722 Córdoba-Guijarro S, Feal C, Daucén E et al. Lupus erythematosus-like lesions in a carrier of X-linked chronic granulomatous disease. J Eur Acad Dermatol Venereol 2000; 14: 409–411.

723 Stalder JF, Dreno B, Bureau B, Hakim J. Discoid lupus erythematosus-like lesions in an autosomal form of chronic granulomatous disease. Br J Dermatol 1986; 114: 251–254.

724 Ortiz-Romero PL, Corell-Almuzara A, Lopez-Estebaranz JL et al. Lupus like lesions in a patient with X-linked chronic granulomatous disease and recombinant X chromosome. Dermatology 1997; 195: 280–283.

725 Ashgar SS, Venneker GT, van Meegen M et al. Hereditary deficiency of C5 in association with discoid lupus erythematosus J Am Acad Dermatol 1991; 24: 376–378.

726 Wolpert KA, Webster ADB, Whittaker SJ. Discoid lupus erythematosus associated with a primary immunodeficiency syndrome showing features of non-X-linked hyper-IgM syndrome. Br J Dermatol 1998; 138: 1053–1057.

727 Winkelmann RK. Spectrum of lupus erythematosus. J Cutan Pathol 1979; 6: 457–462

728 Di Leonardo M, Ackerman AB. Atrophic lichen planus vs. chronic discoid lupus erythematosus vs. disseminated superficial actinic porokeratosis. Dermatopathology: Practical & Conceptual 1997; 3: 14.

729 Friss AB, Cohen PR, Bruce S, Duvic M. Chronic cutaneous lupus erythematosus mimicking mycosis fungoides. J Am Acad Dermatol 1995; 33: 891–895.

730 Weigand DA, Burgdorf WHC, Gregg LJ. Dermal mucinosis in discoid lupus erythematosus. Report of two cases. Arch Dermatol 1981; 117: 735–738.

731 Ueki H, Takei Y, Nakagawa S. Cutaneous calcinosis in localized discoid lupus erythematosus. Arch Dermatol 1980; 116: 196–197.

732 Kabir DI, Malkinson FD. Lupus erythematosus and calcinosis cutis. Arch Dermatol 1969; 100: 17–22.

733 Crowson AN, Magro C. The cutaneous pathology of lupus erythematosus: a review. J Cutan Pathol 2001; 28: 1–23.

734 Kuhn A, Richter-Hintz D, Oslislo C et al. Lupus erythematosus tumidus. A neglected subset of cutaneous lupus erythematosus: Report of 40 cases. Arch Dermatol 2000; 36: 1033–1041.

735 Uitto J, Santa-Cruz DJ, Eisen AZ, Leone P. Verrucous lesions in patients with discoid lupus erythematosus. Clinical, histopathological and immunofluorescence studies. Br J Dermatol 1978; 98: 507–520.

736 Perniciaro C, Randle HW, Perry HO. Hypertrophic discoid lupus erythematosus resembling squamous cell carcinoma. Dermatol Surg 1995; 21: 255–257.

737 Weigand DA. The lupus band test: a re-evaluation. J Am Acad Dermatol 1984; 11: 230–234.

738 Williams REA, MacKie RM, O'Keefe R, Thomson W. The contribution of direct immunofluorescence to the diagnosis of lupus erythematosus. J Cutan Pathol 1989; 16: 122–125.

739 De Jong EMGJ, van Erp PEJ, Ruiter DJ, van de Kerkhof PCM. Immunohistochemical detection of proliferation and differentiation in discoid lupus erythematosus. J Am Acad Dermatol 1991; 25: 1032–1038.

740 Sugai SA, Gerbase AB, Cernea SS et al. Cutaneous lupus erythematosus: direct immunofluorescence and epidermal basal membrane study. Int J Dermatol 1992; 31: 260–264.

741 Kulthanan K, Pinkaew S, Suthipinittharm P. Diagnostic value of IgM deposition at the dermo-epidermal junction. Int J Dermatol 1998; 37: 201–205.

742 Kulthanan K, Roongphiboolsopit P, Chanjanakijskul S, Kullavanijaya P. Chronic discoid lupus erythematosus in Thailand: direct immunofluorescence study. Int J Dermatol 1996; 35: 711–714.

743 Ng PPL, Tan SH, Koh ET, Tan T. Epidemiology of cutaneous lupus erythematosus in a tertiary referral centre in Singapore. Australas J Dermatol 2000; 41: 229–233.

744 Weigand DA. Lupus band test: anatomical regional variations in discoid lupus erythematosus. J Am Acad Dermatol 1986; 14: 426–428.

745 Al-Suwaid AR, Venkataram MN, Bhushnurmath SR. Cutaneous lupus erythematosus: comparison of direct immunofluorescence findings with histopathology. Int J Dermatol 1995; 34: 480–482.

746 Gruschwitz M, Keller J, Hornstein OP. Deposits of immunoglobulins at the dermo-epidermal junction in chronic light-exposed skin: what is the value of the lupus band test? Clin Exp Dermatol 1988; 13: 303–308.

747 Wojnarowska F, Bhogal B, Black MM. The significance of an IgM band at the dermo-epidermal junction. J Cutan Pathol 1986; 13: 359–362.

748 Mori M, Pimpinelli N, Romagnoli P et al. Dendritic cells in cutaneous lupus erythematosus: a clue to the pathogenesis of lesions. Histopathology 1994; 24: 311–321.

749 Callen JP, Kulick KB, Stelzer G, Fowler JF. Subacute cutaneous lupus erythematosus. Clinical, serologic, and immunogenetic studies of forty-nine patients seen in a nonreferral setting. J Am Acad Dermatol 1986; 5: 1227–1237.

750 Norris DA. Pathomechanisms of photosensitive lupus erythematosus. J Invest Dermatol 1993; 100: 58S–68S.

751 Watanabe T, Tsuchida T, Ito Y et al. Annular erythema associated with lupus erythematosus/Sjögren's syndrome. J Am Acad Dermatol 1997; 36: 214–218.

752 Harper JI. Subacute cutaneous lupus erythematosus (SCLE): a distinct subset of LE. Clin Exp Dermatol 1982; 7: 209–212.

753 Scheinman PL. Acral subacute cutaneous lupus erythematosus: an unusual variant. J Am Acad Dermatol 1994; 30: 800–801.

754 Sontheimer RD, Thomas JR, Gilliam JN. Subacute cutaneous lupus erythematosus. A cutaneous marker for a distinct lupus erythematosus subset. Arch Dermatol 1979; 115: 1409–1415.

755 De Silva BD, Plant W, Kemmett D. Subacute cutaneous lupus erythematosus and life-threatening hypokalaemic tetraparesis: a rare complication. Br J Dermatol 2001; 144: 622–624.

756 Weinstein CL, Littlejohn GO, Thomson NM, Hall S. Severe visceral disease in subacute cutaneous lupus erythematosus. Arch Dermatol 1987; 123: 638–648.

757 Chlebus E, Wolska H, Blaszczyk M, Jablonska S. Subacute cutaneous lupus erythematosus versus systemic lupus erythematosus: Diagnostic criteria and therapeutic implications. J Am Acad Dermatol 1998; 38: 405–412.

758 Callen JP. Subacute cutaneous lupus erythematosus versus systemic lupus erythematosus. J Am Acad Dermatol 1999; 39: 129.

759 Callen JP. Is subacute cutaneous lupus erythematosus a subset of systemic lupus erythematosus or a distinct entity? Br J Dermatol 2001; 144: 450–451.

760 DeSpain J, Clark DP. Subacute cutaneous lupus erythematosus presenting as erythroderma. J Am Acad Dermatol 1988; 19: 388–392.

761 generalized poikiloderma. J Am Acad Dermatol 2000; 42: 286–288.

762 Caproni M, Cardinali C, Salvatore E, Fabbri P. Subacute cutaneous lupus erythematosus with pityriasis-like cutaneous manifestations. Int J Dermatol 2001; 40: 59–62.

763 Levenstein MM, Fisher BK, Fisher LL, Pruzanski W. Simultaneous occurrence of subacute lupus erythematosus and Sweet syndrome. A marker of Sjögren syndrome? Int J Dermatol 1991; 30: 640–643.

764 Fine RM. Subacute cutaneous lupus erythematosus associated with hydrochlorothiazide therapy. Int J Dermatol 1989; 28: 375–376.

765 Brooke R, Coulson IH, Al-Dawoud A. Terbinafine-induced subacute cutaneous lupus erythematosus. Br J Dermatol 1998; 139: 1132–1133.

766 Bonsmann G, Schiller M, Luger TA, Ständer S. Terbinafine-induced subacute cutaneous lupus erythematosus. J Am Acad Dermatol 2001; 44: 925–931.

767 Crowson AN, Magro CM. Lichenoid and subacute cutaneous lupus erythematosus-like dermatitis associated with antihistamine therapy. J Cutan Pathol 1999; 26: 95–100.

768 Crowson AN, Magro CM. Subacute cutaneous lupus erythematosus arising in the setting of calcium channel blocker therapy. Hum Pathol 1997; 28: 67–73.

769 Miyagawa S, Okuchi T, Shiomi Y, Sakamoto K. Subacute cutaneous lupus erythematosus lesions precipitated by griseofulvin. J Am Acad Dermatol 1989; 21: 343–346.

770 Balabanova MB, Botev IN, Michailova JI. Subacute cutaneous lupus erythematosus induced by radiation therapy. Br J Dermatol 1997; 137: 648–649.

771 Ho C, Shumack SP, Morris D. Subacute cutaneous lupus erythematosus associated with hepatocellular carcinoma. Australas J Dermatol 2001; 42: 110–113.

772 Jewell ML, McCauliffe DP. Patients with cutaneous lupus erythematosus who smoke are less responsive to antimalarial treatment. J Am Acad Dermatol 2000; 42: 983–987.

773 Deng J-S, Sontheimer RD, Gilliam JN. Relationship between antinuclear and anti-Ro/SS-A antibodies in subacute cutaneous lupus erythematosus. J Am Acad Dermatol 1984; 11: 494–499.

774 Wechsler HL, Stavrides A. Systemic lupus erythematosus with anti-Ro antibodies: clinical, histologic, and immunologic findings. Report of three cases. J Am Acad Dermatol 1982; 6: 73–83.

775 Wermuth DJ, Geoghegan WD, Jordon RE. Anti-Ro/SS antibodies. Association with a particulate (large speckledlike thread) immunofluorescent nuclear staining pattern. Arch Dermatol 1985; 121: 335–338.

776 Dore N, Synkowski D, Provost TT. Antinuclear antibody determinations in Ro(SSA)-positive, antinuclear antibody-negative lupus and Sjögren's syndrome patients. J Am Acad Dermatol 1983; 8: 611–615.

777 Sontheimer RD. Questions pertaining to the true frequencies with which anti-Ro/SS-A autoantibody and the HLA-DR3 phenotype occur in subacute cutaneous lupus erythematosus patients. J Am Acad Dermatol 1987; 16: 130–134.

778 Provost TT, Watson R, Simmons-O'Brien E. Significance of the anti-Ro (SS-A) antibody in evaluation of patients with cutaneous manifestations of a connective tissue disease. J Am Acad Dermatol 1996; 35: 147–169.

779 Parodi A, Drosera M, Barbieri L, Rebora A. Counterimmunoelectrophoresis, ELISA and immunoblotting detection of anti-RO/SSA antibodies in subacute cutaneous lupus erythematosus. A comparative study. Br J Dermatol 1998; 138: 114–117.

780 Bielsa I, Herrero C, Ercilla G et al. Immunogenetic findings in cutaneous lupus erythematosus. J Am Acad Dermatol 1991; 25: 251–257.

781 Sontheimer RD. Immunological significance of the Ro/SSA antigen-antibody system. Arch Dermatol 1985; 121: 327–330.

782 Callen JP, Hodge SJ, Kulick KB et al. Subacute cutaneous lupus erythematosus in multiple members of a family with C2 deficiency. Arch Dermatol 1987; 123: 66–70.

783 Tsutsui K, Imai T, Hatta N et al. Widespread pruritic plaques in a patient with subacute cutaneous lupus erythematosus and hypocomplementemia: Response to dapsone therapy. J Am Acad Dermatol 1996; 35: 313–315.

784 Magro CM, Crowson AN. The cutaneous pathology associated with seropositivity for antibodies to SSA (RO). A clinicopathologic study of 23 adult patients without subacute cutaneous lupus erythematosus. Am J Dermatopathol 1999; 21: 129–137.

785 Provost TT, Talal N, Harley JB et al. The relationship between anti-Ro (SS-A) antibody-positive Sjögren's syndrome and anti-Ro (SS-A) antibody-positive lupus erythematosus. Arch Dermatol 1988; 124: 63–71.

786 Lee LA. Anti-Ro (SSA) and anti-La (SSB) antibodies in lupus erythematosus and in Sjögren's syndrome. Arch Dermatol 1988; 124: 61–62.

787 Jones SK, Coulter S, Harmon C et al. Ro/SSA antigen in human epidermis. Br J Dermatol 1988; 118: 363–367.

788 Ioannides D, Golden BD, Buyon JP, Bystryn J-C. Expression of SS-A/RO and SS-B/La antigens in skin biopsy specimens of patients with photosensitive forms of lupus erythematosus. Arch Dermatol 2000; 136: 340–346.

789 Purcell SM, Lieu TS, Davis BM, Sontheimer RD. Relationship between circulating anti-Ro/SS-A antibody levels and skin disease activity in subacute cutaneous lupus erythematosus. Br J Dermatol 1987; 117: 277–287.

790 Bangert JL, Freeman RG, Sontheimer RD, Gilliam JN. Subacute cutaneous lupus erythematosus and discoid lupus erythematosus. Comparative histopathologic findings. Arch Dermatol 1984; 120: 332–337.

791 Jerdan JS, Hood AF, Moore GW, Callen JP. Histopathologic comparison of the subsets of lupus erythematosus. Arch Dermatol 1990; 126: 52–55.

792 Bielsa I, Herrero C, Collado A et al. Histopathologic findings in cutaneous lupus erythematosus. Arch Dermatol 1994; 130: 54–58.

793 Murphy JK, Stephens C, Hartley T et al. Subacute cutaneous lupus erythematosus – the annular variant. A histological and ultrastructural study of five cases. Histopathology 1991; 19: 329–336.

794 Baima B, Sticherling M. Apoptosis in different cutaneous manifestations of lupus erythematosus. Br J Dermatol 2001; 144: 958–966.

795 Herrero C, Bielsa I, Font J et al. Subacute cutaneous lupus erythematosus: clinicopathologic findings in thirteen cases. J Am Acad Dermatol 1988; 19: 1057–1062.

796 David-Bajar KM, Bennion SD, DeSpain JD et al. Clinical, histologic, and immunofluorescent distinctions between subacute cutaneous lupus erythematosus and discoid lupus erythematosus. J Invest Dermatol 1992; 99: 251–257.

797 Nieboer C, Tak-Diamand Z, van Leeuwen-Wallau HE. Dust-like particles: a specific direct immunofluorescence pattern in sub-acute cutaneous lupus erythematosus. Br J Dermatol 1988; 118: 725–729.

798 Valeski JE, Kumar V, Forman AB et al. A characteristic cutaneous direct immunofluorescent pattern associated with Ro(SS-A) antibodies in subacute cutaneous lupus erythematosus. J Am Acad Dermatol 1992; 27: 194–198.

799 David-Bajar KM. Subacute cutaneous lupus erythematosus. J Invest Dermatol 1993; 100: 2S–8S.

800 Lipsker D, Di Cesare M-P, Cribier B et al. The significance of the 'dust-like particles' pattern of immunofluorescence. A study of 66 cases. Br J Dermatol 1998; 138: 1039–1042.

801 Parodi A, Caproni M, Cardinali C et al. Clinical, histological and immunopathological features of 58 patients with subacute cutaneous lupus erythematosus. Dermatology 2000; 200: 6–10.

802 Goodfield M. Measuring the activity of disease in cutaneous lupus erythematosus. Br J Dermatol 2000; 142: 399–400.

803 Matthews CNA, Saihan EM, Warin RP. Urticaria-like lesions associated with systemic lupus erythematosus: response to dapsone. Br J Dermatol 1978; 99: 455–457.

804 Barton DD, Fine J-D, Gammon WR, Sams WM Jr. Bullous systemic lupus erythematosus: an unusual clinical course and detectable circulating autoantibodies to the epidermolysis bullosa acquisita antigen. J Am Acad Dermatol 1986; 15: 369–373.

805 Camisa C, Sharma HM. Vesiculobullous systemic lupus erythematosus. Report of two cases and a review of the literature. J Am Acad Dermatol 1983; 9: 924–933.

806 Callen JP. Cutaneous bullae following acute steroid withdrawal in systemic lupus erythematosus. Br J Dermatol 1981; 105: 603–606.

807 Kanda N, Tsuchida T, Watanabe T, Tamaki K. Cutaneous lupus mucinosis: a review of our cases and the possible pathogenesis. J Cutan Pathol 1997; 24: 553–558.

808 Watanabe T, Tsuchida T. Classification of lupus erythematosus based upon cutaneous manifestations. Dermatology 1995; 190: 277–283.

809 Millard LG, Rowell NR. Chilblain lupus erythematosus (Hutchinson). A clinical and laboratory study of 17 patients. Br J Dermatol 1978; 98: 497–506.

810 Aoki T, Ishizawa T, Hozumi Y et al. Chilblain lupus erythematosus of Hutchinson responding to surgical treatment: a report of two patients with anti-Ro/SS-A antibodies. Br J Dermatol 1996; 134: 533–537.

811 Stainforth J, Goodfield MJD, Taylor PV. Pregnancy-induced chilblain lupus erythematosus. Clin Exp Dermatol 1993; 18: 449–451.

812 Yell JA, Mbuagbaw J, Burge SM. Cutaneous manifestations of systemic lupus erythematosus. Br J Dermatol 1996; 135: 355–362.

813 García-Patos V, Bartralot R, Ordi J et al. Systemic lupus erythematosus present with red lunulae. J Am Acad Dermatol 1997; 36: 834–836.

814 Wollina U, Barta U, Uhlemann C, Oelzner P. Lupus erythematosus-associated red lunula. J Am Acad Dermatol 1999; 41: 419–421.

815 Vendrell P, Sánchez JL. Subclinical inflammatory alopecia in systemic lupus erythematosus. Dermatopathology: Practical & Conceptual 2000; 6: 46–48.

816 Nitta Y, Muramatsu M. A juvenile case of overlap syndrome of systemic lupus erythematosus and polymyositis, later accompanied by systemic sclerosis with the development of anti-Scl 70 and anti-Ku antibodies. Pediatr Dermatol 2000; 17: 381–383.

817 Ruzicka T, Faes J, Bergner T et al. Annular erythema associated with Sjögren's syndrome: a variant of systemic lupus erythematosus. J Am Acad Dermatol 1991; 25: 557–560

818 Gallardo F, Vadillo M, Mitjavila F, Servitje O. Systemic lupus erythematosus after eosinophilic fasciitis: A case report. J Am Acad Dermatol 1998; 38: 283–285.

819 Van der Meer-Roosen CH, Maes EPJ, Faber WR. Cutaneous lupus erythematosus and autoimmune thyroiditis. Br J Dermatol 1979; 101: 91–92.

820 Stevens HP, Ostlere LS, Rustin MHA. Systemic lupus erythematosus in association with ulcerative colitis: related autoimmune diseases. Br J Dermatol 1994; 130: 385–389.

821 Cruz PD Jr, Coldiron BM, Sontheimer RD. Concurrent features of cutaneous lupus erythematosus and pemphigus erythematosus following myasthenia gravis and thymoma. J Am Acad Dermatol 1987; 16: 472–480.

822 DeCastro P, Jorizzo JL, Solomon AR et al. Coexistent systemic lupus erythematosus and tophaceous gout. J Am Acad Dermatol 1985; 13: 650–654.

823 Werth VP, White WL, Sanchez MR, Franks AG. Incidence of alopecia areata in lupus erythematosus. Arch Dermatol 1992; 128: 368–371.

824 Aronson PJ, Fretzin DF, Morgan NE. A unique case of sarcoidosis with coexistent collagen vascular disease. J Am Acad Dermatol 1985; 13: 886–89.

825 Gibson GE, McEvoy MT. Coexistence of lupus erythematosus and porphyria cutanea tarda in fifteen patients. J Am Acad Dermatol 1998; 38: 569–573.

826 Goette DK. Sweet's syndrome in subacute cutaneous lupus erythematosus. Arch Dermatol 1985; 121: 789–791.

827 Hays SB, Camisa C, Luzar MJ. The coexistence of systemic lupus erythematosus and psoriasis. J Am Acad Dermatol 1984; 10: 619–622.

828 Khorshid SM, Beynon HLC, Rustin MHA. Lupus erythematosus vegetans. Br J Dermatol 1999; 141: 893–896.

829 McBurney EI, Hickham PR, Garry RF, Reed RJ. Lupus erythematosus-like features in patients with cutaneous T-cell lymphoma. Int J Dermatol 1998; 37: 579–585.

830 Thomas JR III, Su WPD. Concurrence of lupus erythematosus and dermatitis herpetiformis. A report of nine cases. Arch Dermatol 1983; 119: 740–745.

831 Taieb A, Hehunstre J-P, Goetz J et al. Lupus erythematosus panniculitis with partial genetic deficiency of C2 and C4 in a child. Arch Dermatol 1986; 122: 576–582.

832 Massa MC, Connolly SM. An association between C1 esterase inhibitor deficiency and lupus erythematosus: report of two cases and review of the literature. J Am Acad Dermatol 1982; 7: 255–264.

833 Komine M, Matsuyama T, Nojima Y et al. Systemic lupus erythematosus with hereditary deficiency of the fourth component of complement. Int J Dermatol 1992; 31: 653–656.

834 Stone NM, Williams A, Wilkinson JD, Bird G. Systemic lupus erythematosus with C1q deficiency. Br J Dermatol 2000; 142: 521–524.

835 Lipsker DM, Schreckenberg-Gilliot C, Uring-Lambert B et al. Lupus erythematosus associated with genetically determined deficiency of the second component of the complement. Arch Dermatol 2000; 136: 1508–1514.

836 Hasan T, Nyberg F, Stephansson E et al. Photosensitivity in lupus erythematosus, UV photoprovocation results compared with history of photosensitivity and clinical findings. Br J Dermatol 1997; 136: 699–705.

837 Rasmussen EK, Ullman S, Hoier-Madsen M et al. Clinical implications of ribonucleoprotein antibody. Arch Dermatol 1987; 123: 601–605.

838 Sharp GC, Anderson PC. Current concepts in the classification of connective tissue diseases. Overlap syndromes and mixed connective tissue disease (MCTD). J Am Acad Dermatol 1980; 2: 269–279.

839 Callen JP, Kingman J. Cutaneous vasculitis in systemic lupus erythematosus. A poor prognostic indicator. Cutis 1983; 32: 433–436.

840 Yasue T. Livedoid vasculitis and central nervous system involvement in systemic lupus erythematosus. Arch Dermatol 1986; 122: 66–70.

841 Weinstein C, Miller MH, Axtens R et al. Livedo reticularis associated with increased titers

of anticardiolipin antibodies in systemic lupus erythematosus. Arch Dermatol 1987; 123: 596–600.

842 Alarcón-Segovia D, Pérez-Ruiz A, Villa AR. Long-term prognosis of antiphospholipid syndrome in patients with systemic lupus erythematosus. JAI 2000; 15: 157–161.

843 Dodd HJ, Sarkany I, O'Shaughnessy D. Widespread cutaneous necrosis associated with the lupus anticoagulant. Clin Exp Dermatol 1985; 10: 581–586.

844 Amster MS, Conway J, Zeid M, Pincus S. Cutaneous necrosis resulting from protein S deficiency and increased antiphospholipid antibody in a patient with systemic lupus erythematosus. J Am Acad Dermatol 1993; 29: 853–857.

845 Chtourou M, Aubin F, Savariault I et al. Digital necrosis and lupus-like syndrome preceding ovarian carcinoma. Dermatology 1998; 196: 348–349.

846 Grob J-J, Bonerandi J-J. Cutaneous manifestations associated with the presence of the lupus anticoagulant. J Am Acad Dermatol 1986; 15: 211–219.

847 Vocks E, Welcker M, Ring J. Digital gangrene: a rare skin symptom in systemic lupus erythematosus. J Eur Acad Dermatol Venereol 2000; 14: 419–421.

848 Rasaratnam I, Ryan P. Lupus: advances and remaining challenges. Med J Aust 1995; 163: 398–399.

849 Wananukul S, Watana D, Pongprasit P. Cutaneous manifestations of childhood systemic lupus erythematosus. Pediatr Dermatol 1998; 15: 342–346.

850 Deegan MJ. Systemic lupus erythematosus. Some contemporary laboratory aspects. Arch Pathol Lab Med 1980; 104: 399–404.

851 Hochberg MC, Boyd RE, Ahearn JM et al. Systemic lupus erythematosus: a review of clinico-laboratory features and immunogenetic markers in 150 patients with emphasis on demographic subsets. Medicine (Baltimore) 1985; 64: 285–295.

852 Mutasim DF, Adams BB. A practical guide for serologic evaluation of autoimmune connective tissue diseases. J Am Acad Dermatol 2000; 42: 159–174.

853 Lerner EA, Lerner MR. Whither the ANA? Arch Dermatol 1987; 123: 358–362.

854 Sontheimer RD, Deng J-S, Gilliam JN. Antinuclear and anticytoplasmic antibodies. Concepts and misconceptions. J Am Acad Dermatol 1983; 9: 335–343.

855 Watanabe T, Tsuchida T, Kanca N et al. Anti-α-fodrin antibodies in Sjögren syndrome and lupus erythematosus. Arch Dermatol 1999; 135: 535–539.

856 Dunphy J, Oliver M, Rands A_ et al. Antineutrophil cytoplasmic antibodies and HLA class II alleles in minocycline-induced lupus-like syndrome. Br J Dermatol 2000; 142: 461–467.

857 Sontheimer RD. Antibodies inside our keratinocytes? Arch Dermatol 1993; 129: 1184–1186.

858 Ioannides D, Bystryn J-C. Association of tissue-fixed cytoplasmic deposits of immunoglobulin in epidermal keratinocytes with lupus erythematosus. Arch Dermatol 1993; 129: 1130–1135.

859 Ishikawa O, Zaw KK, Miyachi Y et al. The presence of anti-basement membrane zone antibodies in the sera of patients with non-bullous lupus erythematosus. Br J Dermatol 1997; 136: 222–226.

860 Belmont HM, Abramson SB, Lie JT. Pathology and pathogenesis of vascular injury in systemic lupus erythematosus. Arthritis Rheum 1996; 39: 9–22.

861 Kohchiyama A, Oka D, Ueki H. T-cell subsets in lesions of systemic and discoid lupus erythematosus. J Cutan Pathol 1985; 12: 493–499.

862 Andrews BS, Schenk A, Barr R et al. Immunopathology of cutaneous human lupus erythematosus defined by murine monoclonal antibodies. J Am Acad Dermatol 1986; 15: 474–481.

863 Hasan T, Stephansson E, Ranki A. Distribution of naive and memory T-cells in photoprovoked and spontaneous skin lesions of discoid lupus erythematosus and polymorphous light eruption. Acta Derm Venereol 1999; 79: 437–442.

864 Kita Y, Kuroda K, Mimori T et al. T cell receptor clonotypes in skin lesions from patients with systemic lupus erythematosus. J Invest Dermatol 1998; 110: 41–46.

865 Stein LF, Saed GM, Fivenson DP. T-cell cytokine network in cutaneous lupus erythematosus. J Am Acad Dermatol 1997; 37: 191–196.

866 Toro JR, Finlay D, Dou X et al. Detection of type 1 cytokines in discoid lupus erythematosus. Arch Dermatol 2000; 136: 1497–1501.

867 Musette P. T cells in systemic lupus erythematosus. Dermatology 1998; 196: 281–282.

868 Prinz JC, Meurer M, Reiter C et al. Treatment of severe cutaneous lupus erythematosus with a chimeric CD4 monoclonal antibody, cM-T412. J Am Acad Dermatol 1996; 34: 244–252.

869 Ashworth J, Turbitt M, MacKie R. A comparison of the dermal lymphoid infiltrates in discoid lupus erythematosus and Jessner's lymphocytic infiltrate of the skin using the monoclonal antibody Leu 8. J Cutan Pathol 1987; 14: 198–201.

870 Tebbe B, Mazur L, Stadler R, Orfanos CE. Immunohistochemical analysis of chronic discoid and subacute cutaneous lupus erythematosus – relation to immunopathological mechanisms. Br J Dermatol 1995; 132: 25–31.

871 Ullman S, Wiik A, Kobayasi T, Halberg P. Drug-induced lupus erythematosus syndrome. Acta Derm Venereol 1974; 54: 387–390.

872 Peterson LL. Hydralazine-induced systemic lupus erythematosus presenting as pyoderma gangrenosum-like ulcers. J Am Acad Dermatol 1984; 10: 379–384.

873 Lavie CJ, Biundo J, Quinet RJ et al. Systemic lupus erythematosus (SLE) induced by quinidine. Arch Intern Med 1985; 145: 446–448.

874 Gordon PM, White MI, Herriot R et al. Minocycline-associated lupus erythematosus. Br J Dermatol 1995; 132: 120–121.

875 Crosson J, Stillman MT. Minocycline-related lupus erythematosus with associated liver disease. J Am Acad Dermatol 1997; 36: 867–868.

876 Corona R. Minocycline in acne is still an issue. Arch Dermatol 2000; 136: 1143–1145.

877 Schlienger RG, Bircher AJ, Meier CR. Minocycline-induced lupus. A systematic review. Dermatology 2000; 200: 223–231.

878 Burns DA, Sarkany I. Penicillamine induced discoid lupus erythematosus. Clin Exp Dermatol 1979; 4: 389–392.

879 Adams JD. Drug induced lupus erythematosus – a case report. Australas J Dermatol 1978; 19: 31–32.

880 Holmes S, Kemmett D. Exacerbation of systemic lupus erythematosus induced by terbinafine. Br J Dermatol 1998; 139: 1133.

881 Murphy M, Barnes L. Terbinafine-induced lupus erythematosus. Br J Dermatol 1998; 138: 708–709.

882 Pavlidakey GP, Hashimoto K, Heller GL, Daneshvar S. Chlorpromazine-induced lupuslike disease. Case report and review of the literature. J Am Acad Dermatol 1985; 13: 109–115.

883 Goodrich AL, Kohn SR. Hydrochlorothiazide-induced lupus erythematosus: a new variant? J Am Acad Dermatol 1993; 28: 1001–1002.

884 Kawachi Y, Nukaga H, Hoshino M et al. ANCA-associated vasculitis and lupus-like syndrome caused by methimazole. Clin Exp Dermatol 1995; 20: 345–347.

885 Reiffers-Mettelock J, Hentges F, Humbel R-L. Syndrome resembling systemic lupus erythematosus induced by carbamazepine. Dermatology 1997; 195: 306–307.

886 McGuiness M, Frye RA, Deng J-S. Atenolol-induced lupus erythematosus. J Am Acad Dermatol 1997; 37: 298–299.

887 Ghate JV, Turner ML, Rudek MA et al. Drug-induced lupus associated with COL-3. Report of 3 cases. Arch Dermatol 2001; 137: 471–474.

888 Beer KR, Lorincz AL, Medenica MM et al. Insecticide-induced lupus erythematosus. Int J Dermatol 1994; 33: 860–862.

889 Curtis CF. Insecticide-induced lupus erythematosus. Int J Dermatol 1996; 35: 74–75.

890 Gorsulowsky DC, Bank PW, Goldberg AD et al. Antinuclear antibodies as indicators for the procainamide-induced systemic lupus erythematosus-like syndrome and its clinical presentations. J Am Acad Dermatol 1985; 12: 245–253.

891 Haustein U-F. Tubular structures in affected and normal skin in chronic discoid and systemic lupus erythematosus: electron microscopic studies. Br J Dermatol 1973; 89: 1–13.

892 Arnett FC. HLA and genetic predisposition to lupus erythematosus and other dermatologic disorders. J Am Acad Dermatol 1985; 13: 472–481.

893 Lehmann P, Holzle E, Kind P et al. Experimental reproduction of skin lesions in lupus erythematosus by UVA and UVB radiation. J Am Acad Dermatol 1990; 22: 181–187.

894 Zamansky GB. Sunlight-induced pathogenesis in systemic lupus erythematosus. J Invest Dermatol 1985; 85: 179–180.

895 McGrath H Jr. Ultraviolet A1 (340–400 nm) irradiation and systemic lupus erythematosus. J Invest Dermatol (Symposium Proceedings) 1999; 4: 79–84.

896 Lee LA, Farris AD. Photosensitivity diseases: cutaneous lupus erythematosus. J Invest Dermatol (Symposium Proceedings) 1999; 4: 73–78.

897 Werth VP, Zhang W, Dortzbach K, Sullivan K. Association of a promoter polymorphism of tumor necrosis factor-α with subacute cutaneous lupus erythematosus and distinct photoregulation of transcription. J Invest Dermatol 2000; 115: 726–730.

898 Brenner S, Golan H, Gat A, Bialy-Golan A. Paraneoplastic subacute cutaneous lupus erythematosus: report of a case associated with cancer of the lung. Dermatology 1997; 194: 172–174.

899 Sellheyer K. What makes up the basement membrane in cutaneous lupus erythematosus? Dermatopathology: Practical & Conceptual 2000; 6: 174–176.

900 Rongioletti F, Rebora A. Papular and nodular mucinosis associated with systemic lupus erythematosus. Br J Dermatol 1986; 115: 631–636.

901 Panet-Raymond G, Johnson WC. Lupus erythematosus and polymorphous light eruption. Differentiation by histochemical procedures. Arch Dermatol 1973; 108: 785–787.

902 Jacobs MI, Schned ES, Bystryn J-C. Variability of the lupus band test. Results in 18 patients with systemic lupus erythematosus. Arch Dermatol 1983; 119: 883–889.

903 Monroe EW. Lupus band test. Arch Dermatol 1977; 113: 830–834.

904 Leibold AM, Bennion S, David-Bajar K, Schleve MJ. Occurrence of positive immunofluorescence in the dermo-epidermal junction of sun-exposed skin of normal adults. J Cutan Pathol 1994; 21: 200–206.

905 Al-Fouzan AS, Hassab-El-Naby HMM, Dvorak R. How reliable is the basement membrane

phenomenon in the diagnosis of systemic lupus erythematosus? Int J Dermatol 1995; 34: 330–332.

906 Fabré VC, Lear S, Reichlin M et al. Twenty percent of biopsy specimens from sun-exposed skin of normal young adults demonstrate positive immunofluorescence. Arch Dermatol 1991; 127: 1006–1011.

907 Dahl MV. Usefulness of direct immunofluorescence in patients with lupus erythematosus. Arch Dermatol 1983; 119: 1010–1017.

908 George R, Kurian S, Jacob M, Thomas K. Diagnostic evaluation of the lupus band test in discoid and systemic lupus erythematosus. Int J Dermatol 1995; 34: 170–173.

909 Helm KF, Peters MS. Deposition of membrane attack complex in cutaneous lesions of lupus erythematosus. J Am Acad Dermatol 1993; 28: 687–691.

910 Magro CM, Crowson AN, Harrist TJ. The use of antibody to C5b–9 in the subclassification of lupus erythematosus. Br J Dermatol 1996; 134: 855–862.

911 Burrows NP, Bhogal BS, Russell Jones R, Black MM. Clinicopathological significance of cutaneous epidermal nuclear staining by direct immunofluorescence. J Cutan Pathol 1993; 20: 159–162.

912 Pehamberger H, Konrad K, Holubar K. Immunoelectron microscopy of skin in lupus erythematosus. J Cutan Pathol 1978; 5: 319–328.

913 Mooney E, Gammon WR, Jennette JC. Characterization of the changes in matrix molecules at the dermoepidermal junction in lupus erythematosus. J Cutan Pathol 1991; 18: 417–422.

914 Lee LA, Weston WL. Neonatal lupus erythematosus. Semin Dermatol 1988; 7: 66–72.

915 Esterly NB. Neonatal lupus erythematosus. Pediatr Dermatol 1986; 3: 417–424.

916 Hetem MB, Takada MH, Velludo MASL, Foss NT. Neonatal lupus erythematosus. Int J Dermatol 1996; 35: 42–44.

917 Kaneko F, Tanji O, Hasegawa T et al. Neonatal lupus erythematosus in Japan. J Am Acad Dermatol 1992; 26: 397–403.

918 Hogan PA. Neonatal lupus erythematosus. Australas J Dermatol 1995; 36: 39–40.

919 Watson RM, Lane AT, Barnett NK et al. Neonatal lupus erythematosus. A clinical, serological and immunofluorescence study with review of the literature. Medicine (Baltimore) 1984; 63: 362–378.

920 Watson R, Kang JE, May M et al. Thrombocytopenia in the neonatal lupus syndrome. Arch Dermatol 1988; 124: 560–563.

921 Draznin TH, Esterly NB, Furey NL, De Bofsky H. Neonatal lupus erythematosus. J Am Acad Dermatol 1979; 1: 437–442.

922 Watson RM, Scheel JN, Petri M et al. Neonatal lupus erythematosus. Report of serological and immunogenetic studies in twins discordant for congenital heart block. Br J Dermatol 1994; 130: 342–348.

923 Lee LA. Neonatal lupus erythematosus. J Invest Dermatol 1993; 100: 9S–13S.

924 Thornton CM, Eichenfield LF, Shinall EA et al. Cutaneous telangiectases in neonatal lupus erythematosus. J Am Acad Dermatol 1995; 33: 19–25.

925 Paton S, Wiss K, Lyon N et al. Neonatal lupus erythematosus and maternal lupus erythematosus mimicking HELLP syndrome. Pediatr Dermatol 1993; 10: 177–181.

926 Weston WL, Morelli JG, Lee LA. The clinical spectrum of anti-Ro-positive cutaneous neonatal lupus erythematosus. J Am Acad Dermatol 1999; 40: 675–681.

927 Jenkins RE, Kurwa AR, Atherton DJ, Black MM. Neonatal lupus erythematosus. Clin Exp Dermatol 1994; 19: 409–411.

928 Crowley E, Frieden IJ. Neonatal lupus erythematosus: an unusual congenital presentation with cutaneous atrophy, erosions, alopecia, and pancytopenia. Pediatr Dermatol 1998; 15: 38–42.

929 Nitta Y. Lupus erythematosus profundus associated with neonatal lupus erythematosus. Br J Dermatol 1997; 136: 112–114.

930 Borrego L, Rodríguez J, Soler E et al. Neonatal lupus erythematosus related to maternal leukocytoclastic vasculitis. Pediatr Dermatol 1997; 14: 221–225.

931 Lumpkin LR III, Hall J, Hogan JD et al. Neonatal lupus erythematosus. A report of three cases associated with anti-Ro/SSA antibodies. Arch Dermatol 1985; 121: 377–381.

932 Lin RY, Cohen-Addad N, Krey PR et al. Neonatal lupus erythematosus, multiple thromboses, and monoarthritis in a family with Ro antibody. J Am Acad Dermatol 1985; 12: 1022–1025.

933 Miyagawa S, Shinohara K, Fujita T et al. Neonatal lupus erythematosus: Analysis of HLA class II alleles in mothers and siblings from seven Japanese families. J Am Acad Dermatol 1997; 36: 186–190.

934 Yukiko N. Immune responses to SS-A 52-kDa and 60-kDa proteins and to SS-B 50-kDa protein in mothers of infants with neonatal lupus erythematosus. Br J Dermatol 2000; 142: 908–912.

935 Provost TT. Commentary: neonatal lupus erythematosus. Arch Dermatol 1983; 119: 619–622.

936 Nitta Y, Ohashi M, Morikawa M, Ueki H. Significance of tubuloreticular structures forming in Daudi cells cultured with sera from mothers bearing infants with neonatal lupus erythematosus. Br J Dermatol 1994; 131: 525–531.

937 Miyagawa S, Yanagi K, Yoshioka A et al. Neonatal lupus erythematosus: maternal IgG antibodies bind to a recombinant NH$_2$-terminal fusion protein encoded by human α-fodrin cDNA. J Invest Dermatol 1998; 111: 1189–1192.

938 Lee LA, Frank MB, McCubbin VR, Reichlin M. Autoantibodies of neonatal lupus erythematosus. J Invest Dermatol 1994; 102: 963–966.

939 Neidenbach PJ, Sahn EE. La (SS-B)-positive neonatal lupus erythematosus: report of a case with unusual features. J Am Acad Dermatol 1993; 29: 848–852.

940 Dugan EM, Tunnessen WW, Honig PJ, Watson RM. U$_1$RNP antibody-positive neonatal lupus. Arch Dermatol 1992; 128: 1490–1494.

941 Solomon BA, Laude TA, Shalita AR. Neonatal lupus erythematosus: discordant disease expression of U$_1$RNP-positive antibodies in fraternal twins – is this a subset of neonatal lupus erythematosus or a new distinct syndrome? J Am Acad Dermatol 1995; 32: 858–862.

942 Sheth AP, Esterly NB, Ratoosh SL et al. U$_1$RNP positive neonatal lupus erythematosus: association with anti-La antibodies? Br J Dermatol 1995; 132: 520–526.

943 Katayama I, Kondo S, Kawana S et al. Neonatal lupus erythematosus with a high anticardiolipin antibody titer. J Am Acad Dermatol 1989; 21: 490–492.

944 Gawkrodger DJ, Beveridge GW. Neonatal lupus erythematosus in four successive siblings born to a mother with discoid lupus erythematosus. Br J Dermatol 1984; 111: 683–687.

945 Maynard B, Leiferman KM, Peters MS. Neonatal lupus erythematosus. J Cutan Pathol 1991; 18: 333–338.

946 Olansky AJ, Briggaman RA, Gammon WR et al. Bullous systemic lupus erythematosus. J Am Acad Dermatol 1982; 7: 511–520.

947 Camisa C. Vesiculobullous systemic lupus erythematosus. J Am Acad Dermatol 1988; 18: 93–100.

948 Lalova A, Pramatarov K, Vassileva S. Facial bullous systemic lupus erythematosus. Int J Dermatol 1997; 36: 369–371.

949 Yung A, Oakley A. Bullous systemic lupus erythematosus. Australas J Dermatol 2000; 41: 234–237.

950 Roholt NS, Lapiere JC, Wang JI et al. Localized linear bullous eruption of systemic lupus erythematosus in a child. Pediatr Dermatol 1995; 12: 138–144.

951 Don PC. Vesiculobullous lupus erythematosus with milial formation. Int J Dermatol 1992; 31: 793–795.

952 Rappersberger K, Tschachler E, Tani M, Wolff K. Bullous disease in systemic lupus erythematosus. J Am Acad Dermatol 1989; 21: 745–752.

953 Quirk CJ, Heenan PJ. Bullous discoid lupus erythematosus: a case report. Australas J Dermatol 1979; 20: 85–87.

954 Burge S, Schomberg K, Wonjnarowska F. Bullous eruption of SLE – a case report and investigation of the relationship of anti-basement-membrane-zone antibodies to blistering. Clin Exp Dermatol 1991; 16: 133–138.

955 Tani M, Shimizu R, Ban M et al. Systemic lupus erythematosus with vesiculobullous lesions. Immunoelectron microscopic studies. Arch Dermatol 1984; 120: 1497–1501.

956 Gammon WR, Briggaman RA. Bullous SLE: a phenotypically distinctive but immunologically heterogeneous bullous disorder. J Invest Dermatol 1993; 100: 28S–34S.

957 Burrows NP, Bhogal BS, Black MM et al. Bullous eruption of systemic lupus erythematosus: a clinicopathological study of four cases. Br J Dermatol 1993; 128: 332–338.

958 Tsuchida T, Furue M, Kashiwado T, Ishibashi Y. Bullous systemic lupus erythematosus with cutaneous mucinosis and leukocytoclastic vasculitis. J Am Acad Dermatol 1994; 31: 387–390.

959 Fujii K, Fujimoto W, Ueda M et al. Detection of anti-type VII collagen antibody in Sjögren's syndrome/lupus erythematosus overlap syndrome with transient bullous systemic lupus erythematosus. Br J Dermatol 1998; 139: 302–306.

960 Janniger CK, Kowalewski C, Mahmood T et al. Detection of anti-basement membrane zone antibodies in bullous systemic lupus erythematosus. J Am Acad Dermatol 1991; 24: 643–647.

961 Shirahama S, Furukawa F, Yagi H et al. Bullous systemic lupus erythematosus: Detection of antibodies against noncollagenous domain of type VII collagen. J Am Acad Dermatol 1998; 38: 844–848.

962 Chan LS, Lapiere J-C, Chen M et al. Bullous systemic lupus erythematosus with autoantibodies recognizing multiple skin basement membrane components, bullous pemphigoid antigen 1, laminin-5, laminin-6, and type VII collagen. Arch Dermatol 1999; 135: 569–573.

963 Burrows NP, Walport MJ, Hammond AH et al. Lupus erythematosus profundus with partial C4 deficiency responding to thalidomide. Br J Dermatol 1991; 125: 62–67.

964 Ahmed I, Ahmed D. Lupus erythematosus panniculitis: a unique subset of lupus erythematosus. J Cutan Pathol 2000; 27: 547 (abstract).

965 Cernea SS, Kihara SM, Sotto MN, Vilela MAC. Lupus mastitis. J Am Acad Dermatol 1993; 29: 343–346.

966 Tada J, Arata J, Katayama H. Linear lupus erythematosus profundus in a child. J Am Acad Dermatol 1991; 24: 871–874.

967 Caproni M, Palleschi GM, Papi C, Fabbri P. Discoid lupus erythematosus lesions developed on lupus erythematosus profundus nodules. Int J Dermatol 1995; 34: 357–359.

968 Nousari HC, Kimyai-Asadi A, Provost TT. Generalized lupus erythematosus profundus in a patient with genetic partial deficiency of C4. J Am Acad Dermatol 1999; 41: 362–364.

969 Watanabe T, Tsuchida T. Lupus erythematosus profundus: a cutaneous marker for a distinct clinical subset? Br J Dermatol 1996; 134: 123–125.

970 Stork J, Vosmik F. Lupus erythematosus panniculitis with morphea-like lesions. Clin Exp Dermatol 1994; 19: 79–82.

971 Callen JP. Dermatomyositis and polymyositis update on current controversies. Australas J Dermatol 1987; 28: 62–67.

972 Dawkins MA, Jorizzo JL, Walker FO et al. Dermatomyositis: A dermatology-based case series. J Am Acad Dermatol 1998; 38: 397–404.

973 Kovacs SO, Kovacs SC. Dermatomyositis. J Am Acad Dermatol 1998; 39: 899–920.

974 Callen JP. Dermatomyositis. Lancet 2000; 355: 53–57.

975 Rockerbie NR, Woo TY, Callen JP, Giustina T. Cutaneous changes of dermatomyositis precede muscle weakness. J Am Acad Dermatol 1989; 20: 629–632.

976 Euwer RL, Sontheimer RD. Amyopathic dermatomyositis (dermatomyositis sin, myositis). Presentation of six new cases and review of the literature. J Am Acad Dermatol 1991; 24: 959–966.

977 Kagen LJ. Amyopathic dermatomyositis. Arch Dermatol 1995; 131: 1458–1459.

978 Stonecipher MR, Jorizzo JL, White WL et al. Cutaneous changes of dermatomyositis in patients with normal muscle enzymes: dermatomyositis sine myositis? J Am Acad Dermatol 1993; 28: 951–956.

979 Caproni M, Salvatore E, Bernacchi E, Fabbri P. Amyopathic dermatomyositis: report of three cases. Br J Dermatol 1998; 139: 1116–1118.

980 Olhoffer IH, Carroll C, Watsky K. Dermatomyositis sine myositis presenting with calcinosis universalis. Br J Dermatol 1999; 141: 365–366.

981 Erel A, Toros P, Tokçaer AB, Gürer MA. Amyopathic dermatomyositis. Int J Dermatol 2000; 39: 771–773.

982 Hess Schmid M, Trüeb RM. Juvenile amyopathic dermatomyositis. Br J Dermatol 1997; 136: 431–433.

983 Winkelmann RK. Dermatomyositis in childhood. Clin Rheumat Dis 1982; 8: 353–381.

984 Woo TR, Rasmussen J, Callen JP. Recurrent photosensitive dermatitis preceding juvenile dermatomyositis. Pediatr Dermatol 1985; 2: 207–212.

985 Pope DN, Strimling RB, Mallory SB. Hypertrichosis in juvenile dermatomyositis. J Am Acad Dermatol 1994; 31: 383–387.

986 Kavanagh GM, Colaco CB, Kennedy CTC. Juvenile dermatomyositis associated with partial lipoatrophy. J Am Acad Dermatol 1993; 28: 348–351.

987 Olson JC. Juvenile dermatomyositis. Semin Dermatol 1992; 11: 57–64.

988 Callen JP. Dermatomyositis. Dis Mon 1987; 33: 237–305.

989 Callen JP. Dermatomyositis – an update 1985. Semin Dermatol 1985; 4: 114–125.

990 Cheong W-K, Hughes GRV, Norris PG, Hawk JLM. Cutaneous photosensitivity in dermatomyositis. Br J Dermatol 1994; 131: 205–208.

991 Ghali FE, Stein LD, Fine J-D et al. Gingival telangiectases. An underappreciated physical sign of juvenile dermatomyositis. Arch Dermatol 1999; 135: 1370–1374.

992 Kawakami T, Nakamura C, Hasegawa H et al. Ultrastructural study of calcinosis universalis with dermatomyositis. J Cutan Pathol 1986; 13: 135–143.

993 Ichiki Y, Akiyama T, Shimozawa N et al. An extremely severe case of cutaneous calcinosis with juvenile dermatomyositis, and successful treatment with diltiazem. Br J Dermatol 2001; 144: 894–897.

994 Jara M, Amérigo J, Duce S, Borbujo J. Dermatomyositis and flagellate erythema. Clin Exp Dermatol 1997; 21: 440–441.

995 Bachmeyer C, Blum L, Danne O, Aractingi S. Isolated flagellate eruption in dermatomyositis. Dermatology 1998; 197: 92–93.

996 Kaufmann R, Greiner D, Schmidt P, Wolter M. Dermatomyositis presenting as plaque-like mucinosis. Br J Dermatol 1998; 138: 889–892.

997 del Pozo J, Almagro M, Martínez W et al. Dermatomyositis and mucinosis. Int J Dermatol 2001; 40: 120–124.

998 Requena L, Grilli R, Soriano L et al. Dermatomyositis with a pityriasis rubra pilaris-like eruption: a little-known distinctive cutaneous manifestation of dermatomyositis. Br J Dermatol 1997; 136: 768–771.

999 Lister RK, Cooper ES, Paige DG. Papules and pustules of the elbows and knees: an uncommon clinical sign of dermatomyositis in Oriental children. Pediatr Dermatol 2000; 17: 37–40.

1000 Lupton JR, Figueroa P, Berberian BJ, Sulica VI. An unusual presentation of dermatomyositis: The type Wong variant revisited. J Am Acad Dermatol 2000; 43: 908–912.

1001 Tsao H, Busam K, Barnhill RL, Haynes HA. Lesions resembling malignant atrophic papulosis in a patient with dermatomyositis. J Am Acad Dermatol 1997; 36: 317–319.

1002 Chao Y-Y, Yang L-J. Dermatomyositis presenting as panniculitis. Int J Dermatol 2000; 39: 141–144.

1003 Molnár K, Kemény L, Korom I, Dobozy A. Panniculitis in dermatomyositis: report of two cases. Br J Dermatol 1998; 139: 161–163.

1004 Nousari HC, Kimyai-Asadi A, Spegman DJ. Paraneoplastic dermatomyositis presenting as erythroderma. J Am Acad Dermatol 1998; 39: 653–654.

1005 McCollough ML, Cockerell CJ. Vesiculo-bullous dermatomyositis. Am J Dermatopathol 1998; 20: 170–174.

1006 Bohan A, Peter JB, Bowman RL, Pearson CM. A computer-assisted analysis of 153 patients with polymyositis and dermatomyositis. Medicine (Baltimore) 1977; 56: 255–286.

1007 Stonecipher MR, Jorizzo JL, Monu J et al. Dermatomyositis with normal muscle enzyme concentrations. Arch Dermatol 1994; 130: 1294–1299.

1008 Mimori T. Scleroderma-polymyositis overlap syndrome. Clinical and serologic aspects. Int J Dermatol 1987; 26: 419–425.

1009 Orihara T, Yanase S, Furuya T. A case of sclerodermatomyositis with cutaneous amyloidosis. Br J Dermatol 1985; 112: 213–219.

1010 Rowell NR. Overlap in connective tissue diseases. Semin Dermatol 1985; 4: 136–143.

1011 Phillips TJ, Leigh IM, Wright J. Dermatomyositis and pulmonary fibrosis associated with anti-Jo-1 antibody. J Am Acad Dermatol 1987; 17: 381–382.

1012 Knoell KA, Hook M, Grice DP, Hendrix JD Jr. Dermatomyositis associated with bronchiolitis obliterans organizing pneumonia (BOOP). J Am Acad Dermatol 1999; 40: 328–330.

1013 Kubo M, Ihn H, Yazawa N et al. Prevalence and antigen specificity of anti-histone antibodies in patients with polymyositis/dermatomyositis. J Invest Dermatol 1999; 112: 711–715.

1014 Basset-Seguin N, Roujeau J-C, Gherardi R et al. Prognostic factors and predictive signs of malignancy in adult dermatomyositis. A study of 32 cases. Arch Dermatol 1990; 126: 633–637.

1015 Lakhanpal S, Bunch TW, Ilstrup DM, Melton LJ III. Polymyositis-dermatomyositis and malignant lesions: does an association exist? Mayo Clin Proc 1986; 61: 645–653.

1016 Cox NH, Lawrence CM, Langtry JAA, Ive FA. Dermatomyositis. Disease associations and an evaluation of screening investigations for malignancy. Arch Dermatol 1990; 126: 61–65.

1017 Manchul LA, Jin A, Pritchard KI et al. The frequency of malignant neoplasms in patients with polymyositis-dermatomyositis. A controlled study. Arch Intern Med 1985; 145: 1835–1839.

1018 Bernard P, Bonnetblanc J-M. Dermatomyositis and malignancy. J Invest Dermatol 1993; 100: 128S–132S.

1019 Roselino AMF, Souza CS, Andrade JM et al. Dermatomyositis and acquired ichthyosis as paraneoplastic manifestations of ovarian tumor. Int J Dermatol 1997; 36: 611–614.

1020 Davis MDP, Ahmed I. Ovarian malignancy in patients with dermatomyositis and polymyositis: A retrospective analysis of fourteen cases. J Am Acad Dermatol 1997; 37: 730–733.

1021 Leow Y-H, Goh CL. Malignancy in adult dermatomyositis. Int J Dermatol 1997; 36: 904–907.

1022 Mallon E, Osborne G, Dinneen M et al. Dermatomyositis in association with transitional cell carcinoma of the bladder. Clin Exp Dermatol 1999; 24: 94–96.

1023 Hill CL, Zhang Y, Sigurgeirsson B et al. Frequency of specific cancer types in dermatomyositis and polymyositis: a population-based study. Lancet 2001; 357: 96–100.

1024 Borgia F, Vaccaró M, Guarneri F et al. Dermatomyositis associated with IgG myeloma. Br J Dermatol 2001; 144: 200–201.

1025 Chen Y-J, Wu C-Y, Shen J-L. Predicting factors of malignancy in dermatomyositis and polymyositis: a case-control study. Br J Dermatol 2001; 144: 825–831.

1026 Goyal S, Nousari HC. Paraneoplastic amyopathic dermatomyositis associated with breast cancer recurrence. J Am Acad Dermatol 1999; 41: 874–875.

1027 Kubo M, Sato S, Kitahara H et al. Vesicle formation in dermatomyositis associated with gynecologic malignancies. J Am Acad Dermatol 1996; 34: 391–394.

1028 Glover M, Leigh I. Dermatomyositis pemphigoides: a case with coexistent dermatomyositis and bullous pemphigoid. J Am Acad Dermatol 1992; 27: 849–852.

1029 Hausmann G, Herrero C, Cid MC et al. Immunopathologic study of skin lesions in dermatomyositis. J Am Acad Dermatol 1991; 25: 225–230.

1030 Mascaró JM Jr, Hausmann G, Herrero C et al. Membrane attack complex deposits in cutaneous lesions of dermatomyositis. Arch Dermatol 1995; 131: 1386–1392.

1031 Kubo M, Ihn H, Yamane K et al. Increased serum levels of soluble vascular cell adhesion molecule-1 and soluble E-selectin in patients with polymyositis/dermatomyositis. Br J Dermatol 2000; 143: 392–398.

1032 Crowson AN, Magro CM, Dawood MR. A causal role for parvovirus B19 infection in adult dermatomyositis and other autoimmune syndromes. J Cutan Pathol 2000; 27: 505–515.

1033 Harland CC, Marsden JR, Vernon SA, Allen BR. Dermatomyositis responding to treatment of associated toxoplasmosis. Br J Dermatol 1991; 125: 76–78.

1034 Daudén E, Peñas PF, Rios L et al. Leishmaniasis presenting as a dermatomyositis-like eruption in AIDS. J Am Acad Dermatol 1996; 35: 316–319.

1035 Senet P, Aractingi S, Porneuf M et al. Hydroxyurea-induced dermatomyositis-like eruption. Br J Dermatol 1995; 133: 455–459.

1036 Varma S, Lanigan SW. Dermatomyositis-like eruption and leg ulceration caused by hydroxyurea in a patient with psoriasis. Clin Exp Dermatol 1999; 24: 164–166.

1037 Suehiro M, Kishimoto S, Wakabayashi T et al. Hydroxyurea dermopathy with a dermatomyositis-like eruption and a large leg ulcer. Br J Dermatol 1998; 139: 748–749.

1038 Daoud MS, Gibson LE, Pittelkow MR. Hydroxyurea dermopathy: A unique lichenoid eruption complicating long-term therapy with hydroxyurea. J Am Acad Dermatol 1997; 36: 178–182.

1039 Rocamora V, Puig L, Alomar A. Dermatomyositis-like eruption following hydroxyurea therapy. J Eur Acad Dermatol Venereol 2000; 14: 227–228.

1040 Kirby B, Gibson LE, Rogers S, Pittelkow M. Dermatomyositis-like eruption and leg ulceration caused by hydroxyurea in a patient with psoriasis. Clin Exp Dermatol 2000; 25: 256.

1041 Vassallo C, Passamonti F, Merante S et al. Muco-cutaneous changes during long-term therapy with hydroxyurea in chronic myeloid leukaemia. Clin Exp Dermatol 2001; 26: 141–148.

1042 Harris A, Webley M. Usherwood M, Burge S. Dermatomyositis presenting in pregnancy. Br J Dermatol 1995; 133: 783–785.

1043 Kanoh H, Izumi T, Seishima M et al. A case of dermatomyositis that developed after delivery: the involvement of pregnancy in the induction of dermatomyositis. Br J Dermatol 1999; 141: 897–900.

1044 Ichikawa E, Furuta J, Kawachi Y et al. Hereditary complement (C9) deficiency associated with dermatomyositis. Br J Dermatol 2001; 144: 1080–1083.

1045 Hashimoto K, Robinson L, Velayos E, Niizuma K. Dermatomyositis. Electron microscopic, immunologic, and tissue culture studies of paramyxovirus-like inclusions. Arch Dermatol 1971; 103: 120–135.

1046 Janis JF, Winkelmann RK. Histopathology of the skin in dermatomyositis. Arch Dermatol 1968; 97: 640–650.

1047 Ito A, Funasaka Y, Shimoura A et al. Dermatomyositis associated with diffuse dermal neutrophilia. Int J Dermatol 1995; 34: 797–798.

1048 Hanno R, Callen JP. Histopathology of Gottron's papules. J Cutan Pathol 1985; 12: 389–394.

1049 Sabroe RA, Wallington TB, Kennedy CTC. Dermatomyositis treated with high-dose intravenous immunoglobulins and associated with panniculitis. Clin Exp Dermatol 1995; 20: 164–167.

1050 Fusade T, Belanyi P, Joly P et al. Subcutaneous changes in dermatomyositis. Br J Dermatol 1993; 128: 451–453.

1051 Neidenbach PJ, Sahn EE, Helton J. Panniculitis in juvenile dermatomyositis. J Am Acad Dermatol 1995; 33: 305–307.

1052 Eckardt JJ, Ivins JC, Perry HO, Unni KK. Osteosarcoma arising in heterotopic ossification of dermatomyositis: case report and review of the literature. Cancer 1981; 48: 1256–1261.

1053 Chen Z, Maize JC, Silver RM et al. Direct and indirect immunofluorescent findings in dermatomyositis. J Cutan Pathol 1985; 12: 18–27.

1054 Vaughan Jones SA, Black MM. The value of direct immunofluorescence as a diagnostic aid in dermatomyositis – a study of 35 cases. Clin Exp Dermatol 1997; 22: 77–81.

1055 Magro CM, Crowson AN. The immunofluorescent profile of dermatomyositis: a comparative study with lupus erythematosus. J Cutan Pathol 1997; 24: 543–552.

1056 Alexander CB, Croker BP, Bossen EH. Dermatomyositis associated with IgA deposition. Arch Pathol Lab Med 1982; 106: 449–451.

Poikilodermas

1057 Person JR, Bishop GF. Is poikiloderma a graft-versus-host-like reaction? Am J Dermatopathol 1984; 6: 71–72.

1058 Canizares O. Poikiloderma of Civatte. Arch Dermatol 1968; 98: 429–431.

1059 Katoulis AC, Stavrianeas NG, Georgala S et al. Familial cases of poikiloderma of Civatte: genetic implications in its pathogenesis? Clin Exp Dermatol 1999; 24: 385–387.

1060 Berg E, Chuang T-Y, Cripps D. Rothmund-Thomson syndrome. A case report, phototesting, and literature review. J Am Acad Dermatol 1987; 17: 332–338.

1061 Moss C. Rothmund–Thomson syndrome: a report of two patients and a review of the literature. Br J Dermatol 1990; 122: 821–829.

1062 Shuttleworth D, Marks R. Epidermal dysplasia and skeletal deformity in congenital poikiloderma (Rothmund–Thomson syndrome). Br J Dermatol 1987; 117: 377–384.

1063 Roth DE, Campisano LC, Callen JP et al. Rothmund–Thomson syndrome: a case report. Pediatr Dermatol 1989; 6: 321–324.

1064 Tong M. Rothmund–Thomson syndrome in fraternal twins. Pediatr Dermatol 1995; 12: 134–137.

1065 Collins P, Barnes L, McCabe M. Poikiloderma congenitale: case report and review of the literature. Pediatr Dermatol 1991; 8: 58–60.

1066 Vennos EM, Collins M, James WD. Rothmund–Thomson syndrome: review of the world literature. J Am Acad Dermatol 1992; 27: 750–762.

1067 Blaustein HS, Stevens AW, Stevens PD, Grossman ME. Rothmund–Thomson syndrome associated with annular pancreas and duodenal stenosis: a case report. Pediatr Dermatol 1993; 10: 159–163.

1068 Snels DGCTM, Bouwes Bavinck JN, Muller H, Vermeer BJ. A female patient with the Rothmund–Thomson syndrome associated with anhidrosis and severe infections of the respiratory tract. Dermatology 1998; 196: 260–263.

1069 Nanda A, Kanwar AJ, Kapoor MM et al. Rothmund–Thomson syndrome in two siblings. Pediatr Dermatol 1989; 6: 325–328.

1070 Simmons IJ. Rothmund–Thomson syndrome: a case report. Australas J Dermatol 1980; 21: 96–99.

1071 Porter WM, Hardman CM, Abdalla SH, Powles AV. Haematological disease in siblings with Rothmund–Thomson syndrome. Clin Exp Dermatol 1999; 24: 452–454.

1072 Narayan S, Fleming C, Trainer AH, Craig JA. Rothmund–Thomson syndrome with myelodysplasia. Pediatr Dermatol 2001; 8: 210–212.

1073 Dick DC, Morley WN, Watson JT. Rothmund–Thomson syndrome and osteogenic sarcoma. Clin Exp Dermatol 1982; 7: 119–123.

1074 Judge MR, Kilby A, Harper JI. Rothmund–Thomson syndrome and osteosarcoma. Br J Dermatol 1993; 129: 723–725.

1075 Pujol LA, Erickson RP, Heidenreich RA, Cunniff C. Variable presentation of Rothmund–Thomson syndrome. Am J Med Genet 2000; 95: 204–207.

1076 Shinya A, Nishigori C, Moriwaki S-I et al. A case of Rothmund–Thomson syndrome with reduced DNA repair capacity. Arch Dermatol 1993; 129: 332–336.

1077 Lindor NM, Furuichi Y, Kitao S et al. Rothmund–Thomson syndrome due to RECQ4 helicase mutations: report and clinical and molecular comparisons with Bloom syndrome and Werner syndrome. Am J Med Genet 2000; 90: 223–228.

1078 Grau Salvat C, Pont V, Cors JR, Aliaga A. Hereditary sclerosing poikiloderma of Weary: report of a new case. Br J Dermatol 1999; 140: 366–368.

1079 Greer KE, Weary PE, Nagy R, Robinow M. Hereditary sclerosing poikiloderma. Int J Dermatol 1978; 17: 316–322.

1080 Bordas X, Palou J, Capdevila JM, Mascaro JM. Kindler's syndrome. Report of a case. J Am Acad Dermatol 1982; 6: 263–265.

1081 Forman AB, Prendiville JS, Esterly NB et al. Kindler syndrome: report of two cases and review of the literature. Pediatr Dermatol 1989; 6: 91–101.

1082 Ban M, Hosoe H, Yamada T et al. Kindler's syndrome with recurrence of bullae in the fifth decade. Br J Dermatol 1996; 135: 503–504.

1083 Krunic ALJ, Ljiljana M, Novak A et al. Hereditary bullous acrokeratotic poikiloderma of Weary–Kindler associated with pseudoainhum and sclerotic bands. Int J Dermatol 1997; 36: 529–533.

1084 Weary PE, Manley WF Jr, Graham GF. Hereditary acrokeratotic poikiloderma. Arch Dermatol 1971; 103: 409–422.

1085 Draznin MB, Esterly NB, Fretzin DF. Congenital poikiloderma with features of hereditary acrokeratotic poikiloderma. Arch Dermatol 1978; 114: 1207–1210.

1086 Hovnanian A, Blanchet-Bardon C, de Prost Y. Poikiloderma of Theresa Kindler: report of a case with ultrastructural study, and review of the literature. Pediatr Dermatol 1989; 6: 82–90.

1087 Haber RM, Hanna WM. Kindler syndrome. Clinical and ultrastructural findings. Arch Dermatol 1996; 132: 1487–1490.

1088 Person JR, Perry HO. Congenital poikiloderma with traumatic bulla formation, anhidrosis, and keratoderma. Acta Derm Venereol 1979; 59: 347–351.

1089 Şentürk N, Usubütün A, Şahin S et al. Kindler syndrome: Absence of definite ultrastructural feature. J Am Acad Dermatol 1999; 40: 335–337.

1090 Suga Y, Tsuboi R, Hashimoto Y et al. A Japanese case of Kindler Syndrome. Int J Dermatol 2000; 39: 284–286.

1091 Gretzula JC, Hevia O, Weber PJ. Bloom's syndrome. J Am Acad Dermatol 1987; 17: 479–488.

1092 Landau JW, Sasaki MS, Newcomer VD, Norman A. Bloom's syndrome. The syndrome of telangiectatic erythema and growth retardation. Arch Dermatol 1966; 94: 687–694.

1093 Reddy BSN, Kochhar AM, Anitha M, Bamezai R. Bloom's syndrome – a first report from India. Int J Dermatol 2000; 39: 760–763.

1094 Grob M, Wyss M, Spycher MA et al. Histopathologic and ultrastructural study of lupus-like skin lesions in a patient with Bloom syndrome. J Cutan Pathol 1998; 25: 275–279.

1095 Dicken CH, Dewald G, Gordon H. Sister chromatid exchanges in Bloom's syndrome. Arch Dermatol 1978; 114: 755–760.

1096 Brothman AR, Cram LS, Bartholdi MF, Kraemer PM. Preneoplastic phenotype and chromosome changes of cultured human Bloom syndrome fibroblasts (strain GM 492). Cancer Res 1986; 46: 791–797.

1097 German J, Bloom D, Passarge E. Blooms syndrome XI. Progress report for 1983. Clin Genet 1984; 25: 166–174.

1098 Ling NS, Fenske NA, Julius RL et al. Dyskeratosis congenita in a girl simulating chronic graft-vs-host disease. Arch Dermatol 1985; 121: 1424–1428.

1099 Reichel M, Grix AC, Isseroff RR. Dyskeratosis congenita associated with elevated fetal hemoglobin, X-linked ocular albinism, and juvenile-onset diabetes mellitus. Pediatr Dermatol 1992; 9: 103–106.

1100 Gutman A, Frumkin A, Adam A et al. X-linked dyskeratosis congenita with pancytopenia. Arch Dermatol 1978; 114: 1667–1671.

1101 Phillips RJ, Judge M, Webb D, Harper JI. Dyskeratosis congenita: delay in diagnosis and successful treatment of pancytopenia by bone marrow transplantation. Br J Dermatol 1992; 127: 278–280.

1102 Ivker RA, Woosley J, Resnick SD. Dyskeratosis congenita or chronic graft-versus-host disease? A diagnostic dilemma in a child eight years after bone marrow transplantation for aplastic anemia. Pediatr Dermatol 1993; 10: 362–365.

1103 Connor JM. Teague RH. Dyskeratosis congenita. Report of a large kindred. Br J Dermatol 1981; 105: 321–325.

1104 Mills SE, Cooper PH, Beacham BE, Greer KE. Intracranial calcifications and dyskeratosis congenita. Arch Dermatol 1979; 115: 1437–1439.

1105 Milgrom H, Stoll HL, Crissey JT. Dyskeratosis congenita. A case with new features. Arch Dermatol 1964; 89: 345–349.

1106 Moretti S, Spallanzani A, Chiarugi A et al. Oral carcinoma in a young man: a case of dyskeratosis congenita. J Eur Acad Dermatol Venereol 2000; 14: 123–125.

1107 Joshi RK, Atukorala DN, Abanmi A, Kudwah A. Dyskeratosis congenita in a female. Br J Dermatol 1994; 130: 520–522.

1108 Tchou P-K, Kohn T. Dyskeratosis congenita: an autosomal dominant disorder. J Am Acad Dermatol 1982; 6: 1034–1039.

1109 McGrath JA. Dyskeratosis congenita: new clinical and molecular insights into ribosome function. Lancet 1999; 353: 1204–1205.

1110 Knight SW, Heiss NS, Vulliamy TJ et al. X-linked dyskeratosis congenita is predominantly caused by missense mutations in the DKC1 gene. Am J Hum Genet 1999; 65: 50–58.

Other lichenoid (interface) diseases

1111 Suárez J, López B, Villaba R, Perera A. Febrile ulceronecrotic Mucha–Habermann disease: a case report and review of the literature. Dermatology 1996; 192: 277–279.

1112 Stefanato CM, Goldberg LJ, Andersen WK, Bhawan J. Gianotti–Crosti syndrome presenting as lichenoid dermatitis. Am J Dermatopathol 2000; 22: 162–165.

1113 Nikkels AF, Sadzot-Delvaux C, Rentier B et al. Low-productive alpha-herpesviridae infection in chronic lichenoid dermatoses. Dermatology 1998; 196: 442–446.

1114 Gutzmer R, Herbst RA, Kiehl P et al. Unilateral laterothoracic exanthem (asymmetrical periflexural exanthem of childhood): Report of an adult patient. J Am Acad Dermatol 1997; 37: 484–485.

1115 Coustou D, Léauté-Labrèze C, Bioulac-Sage P et al. Asymmetric periflexural exanthem of childhood. A clinical, pathologic, and epidemiologic prospective study. Arch Dermatol 1999; 135: 799–803.

1116 Guitart J, Peduto M, Caro WA, Roenigk HH. Lichenoid changes in mycosis fungoides. J Am Acad Dermatol 1997; 36: 417–422.

The psoriasiform reaction pattern

4

INTRODUCTION

The psoriasiform reaction pattern is defined morphologically as the presence of epidermal hyperplasia with elongation of the rete ridges in a regular manner. This definition encompasses a heterogeneous group of dermatological conditions. This morphological concept is much broader than the pathogenetic one, outlined by Pinkus and Mehregan.[1] They considered the principal features of the psoriasiform tissue reaction to be the formation of a suprapapillary exudate with parakeratosis, secondary to the intermittent release of serum and leukocytes from dilated blood vessels in the papillary dermis (the so-called 'squirting papilla').

The increased mitotic activity of the epidermis which results in the elongated rete ridges and the psoriasiform epidermal hyperplasia is presumed to be secondary to the release of various mediators from the dilated vessels in the papillary dermis in psoriasis. These aspects are discussed in further detail below. The epidermal hyperplasia in lichen simplex chronicus may be related to chronic rubbing and irritation, while in Bowen's disease there is increased mitotic activity of the component cells. In many of the conditions listed the exact pathogenesis of the psoriasiform hyperplasia remains to be elucidated.

Psoriasis is the prototype of the psoriasiform reaction pattern, but it should be noted that early lesions of psoriasis and pustular psoriasis show no epidermal hyperplasia, although there is evidence of a 'squirting papilla' in the form of dilated vessels and exocytosis of inflammatory cells with neutrophils collecting in the overlying parakeratotic scale.

The major psoriasiform dermatoses – psoriasis, pustular psoriasis, Reiter's syndrome, pityriasis rubra pilaris, parapsoriasis and its variants and lichen simplex chronicus – will be considered first.[2] The other dermatoses listed as causes of the psoriasiform reaction pattern have been discussed in detail in other chapters. They are included again here for completeness, with a brief outline of the features which distinguish them from the other psoriasiform dermatoses.

MAJOR PSORIASIFORM DERMATOSES

This group of dermatoses is characterized, as a rule, by regular epidermal hyperplasia, although in the early stages such features are usually absent. Psoriasis, which is the prototype for this tissue reaction, will be considered first.

PSORIASIS

Psoriasis (psoriasis vulgaris) is a chronic, relapsing, papulosquamous dermatitis characterized by abnormal hyperproliferation of the epidermis.[2] It affects approximately 2% of the population and involves all racial groups, although it is rare in South American Indians.[3–5] There is a genetic proclivity to psoriasis, but no precise mode of inheritance is clear.[6–9] A recessive mode of inheritance has been suggested in Swedish patients.[10] Concordance in monozygotic twins varies from 35% to 70% or more.[6,11]

Since 1994, four main genetic loci (on chromosomes 17q, 4q, 1q and 6p) have been under investigation.[12–14] More recent studies suggest that there is a major susceptibility region for psoriasis on chromosome 6p21.3, near to HLA-C.[15–19] It has been estimated that the proportion of genetic susceptibility attributable to this gene (Psors1) is about 30%.[20] Attempts to link this gene to the S gene (corneodesmosin), also near to HLA-C, have been unsuccessful.[10] However, the gene Psors 1 shows epistasis with genes at other locations, such

as on 1p.[21] Another study of psoriasis in Chinese has suggested that the MICA gene, another HLA-related gene on chromosome 6p21.3, may be a candidate gene.[22]

Psoriasis is associated with HLA-Cw6, B13 and B17 on serology,[6,23,24] and more specifically with HLA-Cw*0602 by PCR.[18,25,26] A recent study has shown that all patients with guttate psoriasis carried this allele compared with 20% of the control population.[27]

Psoriasis typically consists of well-circumscribed erythematous patches with a silvery white scale (plaque form). Characteristic bleeding points develop when the scale is removed (Auspitz's sign).[28] Pruritus is sometimes present.[29] There is a predilection for the extensor surfaces of the extremities, including the elbows and knees, and also the sacral region, scalp and nails.[30,31] A scarring alopecia is rare.[32,33] The lips are not commonly involved[34] and oral lesions in the form of whitish areas on the mucosa are quite rare.[35] Penile lesions are more common in uncircumcised men.[36] Lesions may develop at sites of trauma.

In 5% or more of psoriatics, a seronegative polyarthritis develops.[3] Bilateral upper limb lymphedema has been reported in a patient with arthritis.[37] Psoriasis has also been reported in association with vitiligo,[38] gout,[39] diabetes,[40] ankylosing spondylitis, ILVEN,[41] benign migratory glossitis (geographic tongue),[42] minor hair shaft abnormalities,[43] gliadin antibodies[44,45] and inflammatory bowel disease.[46] Its association with bullous pemphigoid and other bullous diseases,[47–49] perforating folliculitis,[50] lupus erythematosus,[51] Kawasaki disease,[52] prolactinoma,[53] CD4[+] lymphocytopenia,[54] epidermal nevi, multiple exostoses and surgical scars[55] is probably a chance occurrence. There is a slight increase in the incidence of lymphoma and carcinoma of the larynx in patients with psoriasis, which is unrelated to mode of treatment.[56,57]

The mean age of onset of psoriasis is approximately 25 years, although it also develops sporadically in older persons, in whom it tends to have a milder course.[6,58,59] Childhood cases are not uncommon,[60,61] particularly in Scandinavia, where the disease commences in childhood in a high proportion of cases.[62] Congenital onset is a rare occurrence.[63] A family history of psoriasis and an association with HLA-Cw6 are often present in those with early onset.[64,65] Psoriasis usually runs a chronic course, although spontaneous or treatment-induced remissions may occur. It can have a significant effect on the quality of life in those persons with the disease.[66]

Clinical variants

Several clinical variants of psoriasis have been recognized. *Guttate psoriasis* consists of 1–5 mm erythematous papules, which eventually develop a fine scale. It may be preceded by a streptococcal pharyngitis.[67–70] T lymphocytes specific for group A streptococcal antigens have been isolated from lesions of guttate psoriasis.[71] There is a predilection for the trunk and it is more common in children.[72] Clearing may occur spontaneously in weeks or months. Psoriasis begins as the guttate form in 15% or more of cases.[65] *Erythrodermic psoriasis* develops in approximately 2% of psoriatics and it accounts for 20% or more of erythrodermas.[73–75] It is a severe form with a high morbidity and an unpredictable course. Erythrodermic psoriasis may be precipitated by administration of systemic steroids, by the excess use of topical steroids or by a preceding illness; it may develop as a complication of phototherapy.[73] *Sebopsoriasis* consists of yellowish-red, less well-marginated lesions, often distributed in seborrheic regions of the body.[76] Rare clinical variants include a nevoid form,[77] photosensitive psoriasis,[78] follicular psoriasis,[75,80] psoriasis spinulosa,[72,81] congenital erythrodermic psoriasis,[82] rupioid psoriasis,[83] annular verrucous psoriasis,[84] erythema gyratum repens-like psoriasis,[85] and linear psoriasis,[51,86] although the occurrence of a linear form of psoriasis is not accepted by some authorities. Psoriasiform napkin dermatitis may also be a variant of psoriasis.[87] Pustular psoriasis is regarded as a discrete entity.

Cases reported as *psoriasiform acral dermatitis* are now thought to represent a variant of psoriasis in children and not a discrete entity. This variant is characterized by cutaneous involvement of the digits without nail dystrophy.[88]

Trigger factors

Specific factors may trigger the onset or exacerbation of psoriasis. Trauma, infections[89] and drugs are accepted triggers, while the roles of climate, hormonal factors, cigarette smoking,[90,91] alcohol,[91] internal malignancy[92,93] and stress[94] are sometimes disputed.[6] Psoriasis may actually improve during pregnancy.[95] The development of lesions in response to trauma (Koebner reaction) is present in approximately one-third of cases.[96] The role of infections has already been mentioned as a trigger factor in guttate psoriasis.[67] Various drugs may precipitate or exacerbate psoriasis,[97] particularly lithium;[98,99] other drugs include quinidine,[100] clonidine, iodine, carbamazepine,[101,102] olanzapine,[103] terbinafine,[104,105] indomethacin,[100] various beta-blocker drugs,[106,107] terfenadine,[108] isotretinoin, interferon-α,[90,109] interleukin-2,[110] antimalarials and, rarely, the non-steroidal anti-inflammatory drugs and the angiotensin-converting enzyme (ACE) inhibitors.[111] A psoriasiform eruption has been reported as a complication of several beta-blocker drugs,[112] with fluorescein sodium used in angiography,[113] with the oral hypoglycemic agent glibenclamide,[114] with icodextrin[115] and with terbinafine (see above).[116] The reactions caused by some of the beta-blocker drugs have a lichenoid histology despite their clinical appearance.

Pathogenesis of psoriasis

Psoriasis is a complex disease in which numerous abnormal findings have been reported.[117] Despite this, the primary (initiating) alteration is unknown. It appears that the molecular phenotype necessary for the clinical expression of psoriasis is present in all keratinocytes and includes a capacity for hyper-proliferation and altered differentiation. Control of the expression of this phenotype involves the keratinocytes themselves, as well as cells of the immune system and various cytokines.[118–120] Many of the changes in these elements may be epiphenomena or secondary and tertiary events in the pathogenetic cascade. As mentioned already, the primary alteration is not known, although it may involve the signal-transducing system of epidermal keratinocytes or the transcription regulatory elements associated with one or more cytokines.[121,122] Stimulation of the immune system by superantigens has also been put forward as a primary event (see below). It is possible that different etiologies may initiate psoriasis in the genetically susceptible individual.

As the earliest detectable morphological change in psoriasis involves blood vessels in the papillary dermis, some research has focused on their role in the pathogenetic cascade.[123,124] Vascular changes in psoriasis include dilatation and tortuosity of vessels in the papillary dermis, as well as angiogenesis (neovascularization) and the formation of high endothelial venules, which are specialized postcapillary venules lined by tall columnar or cuboidal endothelial cells. These factors are important in expanding the size of the microcirculation which may, in turn, facilitate the trafficking of T lymphocytes, of the Th1 subclass, into the skin.[125] The high endothelial venules play an important role in the cutaneous recruitment of circulating lymphocytes.[126] Angiogenesis is stimulated by factors such as interleukin-8 and transforming growth factor-α (TGF-α).[123,127] The presence of angiogenesis in psoriasis has been challenged. Using three-dimensional reconstructions, it has been suggested that downgrowths of the rete ridges include the vessels of the horizontal plexus giving the appearance of intrapapillary capillaries.[128] This study has not been confirmed.

Recruitment of lymphocytes to the papillary dermis is an important factor.[129] This is aided by various chemoattractants such as platelet-activating factor and leukotriene B$_4$.[130] Some of these lymphocytes are already activated before entering the skin, while still circulating in the blood stream.[131] The lymphocytes bind to endothelial cells in venules in the papillary dermis as a consequence of the enhanced expression of various adhesion molecules by endothelial cells.[132] They then diapedese transendothelially and pass through the vessel wall into the papillary dermis. Neutrophils will subsequently leave the vessels in a similar way and migrate into the stratum corneum. Chemotactic factors such as C5a anaphylatoxin are important in their recruitment.[133]

While the importance of T lymphocytes in the pathogenesis of psoriasis is accepted,[134,135] there has been some dispute over the relative importance of CD4+ and CD8+ lymphocytes.[136] The T cells in lesional dermis are predominantly CD4+. Cells migrating into the epidermis are mostly CD8+. Which type produces keratinocyte proliferation by the release of mediators (cytokines) is still disputed.[137] Both now appear to be involved.[138–140] CD8+ cells in the epidermis express the Vβ T-cell receptor subgroups Vβ3 and Vβ13.1.[141] Another study has shown an increase in the Vβ2 receptor in skin-homing lymphocytes in psoriasis.[142]

As mentioned above, leukocytes bind to endothelial cells in the papillary dermis, prior to their passage from the vessels. This process is under the control of adhesion molecules, which can be classified into three distinct groups:

1. the immunoglobulin gene superfamily which includes ICAM-1 (CD54) and ICAM-2 and VCAM-1 (vascular cell adhesion molecule-1)
2. integrins[143]
3. selectins (the most important of which is E-selectin).

One or more of these adhesion molecules leads to the selective adhesion of CD4, CD45RO helper T cells.[130] Various cytokines appear to induce the enhanced expression of these adhesion molecules in psoriasis; they include interleukin-1 (IL-1), interleukin 2 (IL-2), TNF-α, interferon-γ (IFN-γ) and interleukin-4 (IL-4).[129,144] On the other hand, ultraviolet-B radiation reduces the adhesive interactions and expression of adhesion molecules, possibly explaining its mode of action in the treatment of psoriasis.[145] Serum levels of soluble E-selectin correlate with the extent of psoriatic lesions.[146]

There is a complex interplay between the various cytokines found in the skin in psoriasis; some cytokines have more than one action. They are produced mostly by lymphocytes, although keratinocytes release at least two.[119,147,148] Their many functions include stimulation of keratinocytes,[149] vascular changes (see above), control of lymphocyte trafficking (see above) and stimulation of neutrophil chemotaxis. Exacerbations of psoriasis are preceded by a rapid increase in neutrophil chemotaxis. Interleukin-8 (IL-8) is a cytokine with possibly more chemotactic activity than the various complement factors.[150,151] Another is psoriasin, a protein belonging to the S100 family. It is a potent inflammatory mediator.[152] The importance of the cytokines in the pathogenesis is shown by the downregulatory effects of cyclosporine on cytokines and cytokine receptors in the treatment of psoriasis.[153,154] The role of the various cytokines in psoriasis has recently been reviewed.[155] They are summarized in Table 4.1.

The final pathway in the pathogenesis of psoriasis involves the stimulation of keratinocytes by factors such as IL-8, TGF-α, IFN-γ and the phospholipase C/protein kinase C signal transduction system (see below). IFN-γ, which plays an important role in the growth stimulation of keratinocyte stem cells in psoriasis, can be produced by mast cells as well as lymphocytes.[156] There is also an overexpression of the CXC chemokines, interleukin-8 (IL-8) and GRO/melanoma growth-stimulatory activity (GRO-α).[157] They are potent activators of neutrophils and lymphocytes but also stimulate proliferation of

Table 4.1 **Cytokines in the pathogenetic cascade***

Pathogenetic cascade		Cytokines involved
Endothelial activation and vascular changes ↓	→	IL-1, IL-6, IL-8, TNF-α, TGF-α/β, IFN-γ, endothelin-1
Lymphocyte recruitment ↓	→	IL-1, IL-8, MCP-1, TNF-α, psoriasin, CD11a/CD18
Keratinocyte–lymphocyte interactions ↓	→	IL-1, IL-7, IL-8, TNF-α, IFN-γ, CD11a/CD18
Amplification of inflammatory mechanisms ↓	→	IL-1, IL-2, IL-6, IL-3, TNF-α, IFN-γ, amphiregulin, MCP-1
Keratinocyte proliferation	→	IL-1, IL-3, IL-6, IL-3, GM-CSF, IFN-γ, TGF-α, EGF, amphiregulin, endothelin-1, insulin growth factor, TGF-β receptors, GRO-α, phospholipase C/protein kinase C system

* After Bonifati and Ameglio[155]

keratinocytes.[157] These factors produce an alteration in the turnover time for the epidermis: 3–4 days in psoriasis compared with the usual 13 days in normal skin.[158] It has been estimated that there is a 12-fold increase in the number of basal and suprabasal keratinocytes in cell cycling.[159] TGF-α, which is elevated in psoriasis, is predominantly synthesized in subcorneal keratinocytes.[160] It is a potent mitogen that can also stimulate angiogenesis. In contrast, TGF-β has an inhibitory effect on epithelial cell proliferation. Downregulation of its receptor in psoriatic epidermis has the effect of diminishing this inhibitory influence.[161] Amphiregulin, a cytokine which acts as an epidermal growth factor, is also increased in psoriatic keratinocytes.[162] Transgenic mice, engineered to overproduce amphiregulin, develop a psoriasis-like phenotype suggesting that a genetically transmitted alteration of amphiregulin synthesis may be a possible cause of the cascade of events in psoriasis.[155] The existence of an increased number of epidermal growth factor receptors (EGF-R), resulting from their persistence at all levels of the epidermis instead of just the basal layer, may be just as important.[159,163] Associated with this hyperproliferation of keratinocytes is an increase in apoptosis and a reduction in the number of bcl-2-positive cells in the basal layer.[164] A senescence switch involving p16 may prevent malignant transformation of this upregulated epidermis.[165]

As a consequence of the hyperproliferation of keratinocytes, there is enhanced expression of keratins K6, K16 and K17[166] and reduced amounts of the keratins indicative of differentiation (K1, K2 and K10). There is a unique subpopulation of cells in psoriatic epidermis that coexpress K6 and K10.[167] There are also alterations in cell-surface glycoconjugates.[168]

The role of microbiological superantigens in the pathogenesis of psoriasis is gaining acceptance, although formal proof of a pathogenic role is still lacking.[169–174] Superantigens are toxins of microbial origin that not only stimulate certain classes of T cells[175] but also have the capability to interact directly (without prior processing) with MHC class II molecules: this leads to considerable T-cell activation and cytokine release.[176] Streptococcal antigens can function as superantigens and it is suggested that they may act as the initiating factor in some cases of guttate psoriasis.[177] A recent study has confirmed that prior pharyngeal infection is a risk factor for guttate psoriasis.[178] Peripheral blood lymphocytes from patients with psoriasis are generally hyporesponsive to streptococcal superantigens,[179] but there is a subpopulation of CD4+ cells that produces interferon-γ (IFN-γ) in response to this antigen.[180] Superantigens produced by *Staphylococcus aureus* may also be triggering factors.[181] Patients with psoriasis harbor human papillomavirus type 5 (HPV-5) in a significant number of cases.[182] Antibodies to HPV-5, one of the types associated with epidermodysplasia verruciformis, appear to be generated in the epidermal repair process, but whether they contribute to a proliferation of keratinocytes in psoriasis is not known.[182] The high prevalence of cytomegalovirus antigenemia in psoriasis is possibly related to reactivation

of the virus by elevated levels of tumor necrosis factor-α (TNF-α).[183,184] These disparate findings remain to be integrated into a unitarian theory of pathogenesis.

Other findings in psoriasis that may play some role in the pathogenetic cascade include the increased expression of heat shock proteins by keratinocytes,[185] excessive activation of a phospholipase C/protein kinase C signal transduction system which stimulates keratinocyte proliferation[122,186] and increased lysophosphatidyl choline activity in lesional skin. This substance is a lysophospholipid which is chemotactic for monocytes and stimulates the expression of certain adhesion molecules – VCAM-1 and ICAM-1.[187] The finding of immunoreactants in the stratum corneum and the dermis is not thought to be of major pathogenetic significance.[188] There is an upregulation of the gap junction protein connexin 26 between keratinocytes of psoriasis.[189] There is also an overexpression of matrix metalloproteinases 2 (MMP-2) and 9 (MMP-9).[190,191] The significance of these findings is uncertain. Increased levels of elafin, also termed skin-derived anti-leukoproteinase (SKALP), are found in subcorneal keratinocytes of psoriatic lesions.[192] It is a potent elastase inhibitor which may protect the epidermis from the proteolytic activity of neutrophils.[192] The exact role of neuropeptides (including substance P) remains to be clarified. They provide a possible explanation for the triggering action of stress in the exacerbation of psoriasis.[193] Increased serum cortisol levels are another possible mechanism by which stress influences psoriasis.[194]

In concluding this section, it should not be forgotten that psoriasis is characterized by erythematosquamous lesions. The erythematous nature of the lesions results from the dilatation and increase in vessels in the dermal papillae, which have a thin, overlying layer of epidermal keratinocytes. The clinical thickening of the lesions results from the psoriasiform epidermal hyperplasia brought about by increased mitotic activity in basal keratinocytes through the action of various cytokines with growth factor activity. The scale is composed of parakeratotic cells, resulting from increased transit time, and a focal admixture of neutrophils.[195] All of these features are possibly the consequence of an autoreactive inflammatory process mediated by T lymphocytes of the Th1 subclass.[154] This cytokine profile may be the result of local factors and not determined by a specific genotype.[196]

Therapy

Specific treatments are beyond the scope of this book. However, in psoriasis, the effects of various therapies targeted at different components of the pathogenetic cascade give further insight into this complex process. Some therapies target keratinocyte differentiation and hyperproliferation, or the dilatation of vessels in the papillary dermis, while others exert their effect on T lymphocytes or various cytokines.[197]

Induction of apoptosis in epidermal keratinocytes appears to be the mechanism responsible for the involution of the psoriatic hyperplasia that follows PUVA, narrowband UVB, and topical zinc pyrithione therapy.[198–201] Subepidermal blisters may result from massive basal apoptosis after UVB therapy with the TL-01 lamp.[200] Clinical clearance of psoriasis using 6-thioguanine involves cutaneous T-cell depletion by apoptosis.[202,203] A monoclonal antibody against CD4 is another potential treatment method for psoriasis.[204]

Topical calcitriol appears to target several different pathways in the pathogenetic cascade, producing decreased keratinocyte proliferation, normalized differentiation of keratinocytes and decreased immune activation. It also normalizes the expression of adhesion molecules.[205–207] Etretinate[208] and other retinoids such as acitretin[209] have a similar action on keratinocytes as well as an inhibitory effect on tissue inflammation.

Cyclosporine, which is an effective treatment for severe psoriasis, appears to interfere with the expression of keratinocyte adhesion molecules.[210] It also normalizes the basal lamina and the overexpression of cyclins.[211–213]

Daclizumab, a humanized antibody to the α-subunit (CD25) of the interleukin-2 (IL-2) receptor has been used with limited success in the treatment of psoriasis.[214] IL-2 is a major stimulus for T-cell growth.

The administration of a single dose of an antibody to CD11a (a subunit of leukocyte-function associated antigen (LFA-1) important in T-cell activation, cytotoxic function and emigration into the skin), appears to improve psoriasis.[215]

The pulsed dye laser has been used in some cases of psoriasis. It targets the dilated vessels in the papillary dermis. It has met with some success, although lesions with tortuous blood vessels in the papillary dermis responded poorly to this therapy.[216]

Histopathology[2, 70, 217–220]

Psoriasis is a dynamic process and consequently the histopathological changes vary during the evolution and subsequent resolution of individual lesions. The earliest changes, seen in lesions of less than 24 hours' duration, consist of dilatation and congestion of vessels in the papillary dermis and a mild, perivascular, lymphocytic infiltrate, with some adjacent edema. There is also some exocytosis of lymphocytes into the epidermis overlying the vessels and this is usually associated with mild spongiosis (Fig. 4.1). The epidermis is otherwise normal. This is soon followed by the formation of mounds of parakeratosis, with exocytosis of neutrophils through the epidermis to reach the summits of these parakeratotic foci.[221] There is often overlying orthokeratosis of normal basket-weave type and loss of the underlying granular layer. At this papular stage, increased mitotic activity can be seen in the basal layer of the epidermis associated with a modest amount of psoriasiform acanthosis (Fig. 4.2). Keratinocytes in the upper epidermis show some cytoplasmic pallor. Vessels in the papillary dermis are still dilated and somewhat tortuous, and their lumen may contain neutrophils. Very few neutrophils are ever present in the perivascular infiltrate: this consists mainly of lymphocytes, Langerhans cells and indeterminate cells.[222] A few extravasated erythrocytes may also be present. These changes can also be seen in guttate psoriasis although the epidermal hyperplasia is usually mild in this variant of psoriasis.[2]

In early plaques of psoriasis and in 'hot spots' of more established plaques,[223] there are mounds of parakeratosis containing neutrophils, which usually migrate to the upper layers (summits) of these mounds (Fig. 4.3). With time, confluent parakeratosis develops (Fig. 4.4). Several layers of parakeratosis containing neutrophils, with intervening layers of orthokeratosis, are sometimes present. While intracorneal collections of neutrophils (Munro microabscesses) are common, similar collections in the spinous layer (spongiform pustules of Kogoj) are less so. They are also much smaller than in pustular psoriasis. These pustules contain lymphocytes in addition to

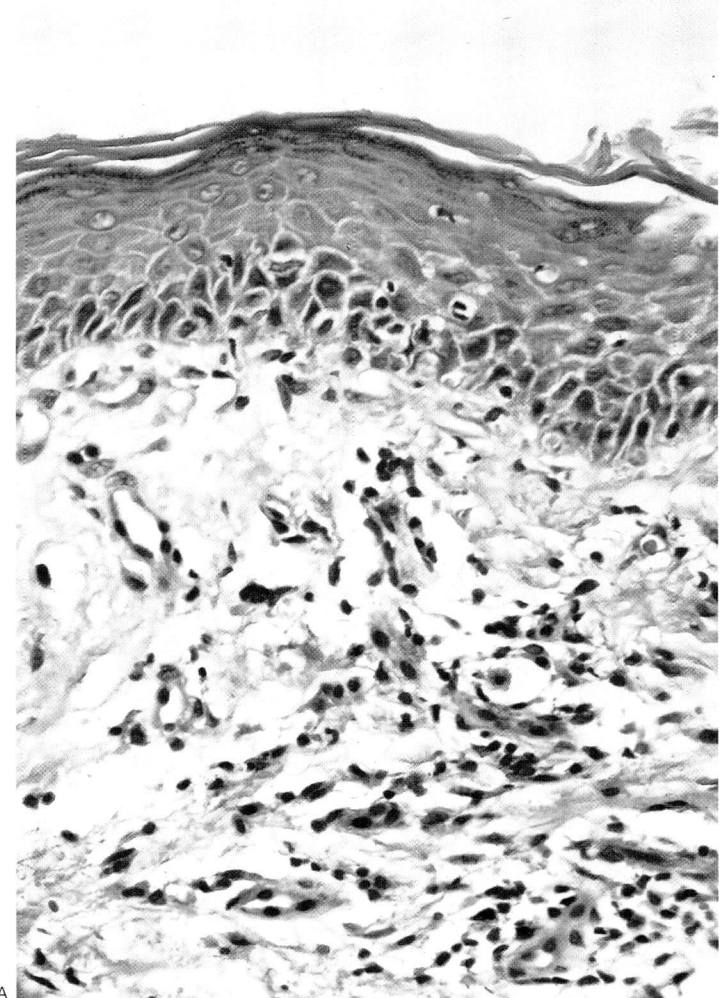

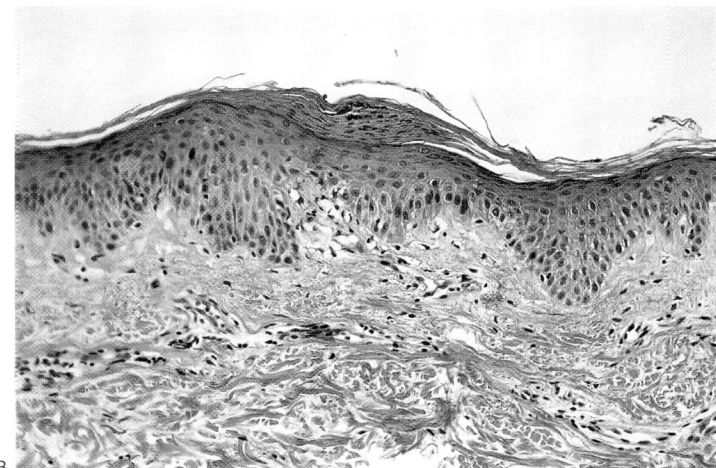

Fig. 4.1 **Psoriasis. (A)** A very early lesion with dilated vessels in a dermal papilla, perivascular cuffing with lymphocytes, and exocytosis of lymphocytes and a neutrophil or two. **(B)** A slightly later stage with neutrophils migrating to the summits of the parakeratotic mounds. (H & E)

neutrophils. The epidermis now shows psoriasiform (regular) hyperplasia, with relatively thin suprapapillary plates overlying the dilated vessels of the papillary dermis (Fig. 4.5). A few mononuclear cells are usually present in the lower layers of the suprapapillary epidermis. The dermal inflammatory cell infiltrate is usually a little heavier than in earlier lesions. It includes activated T

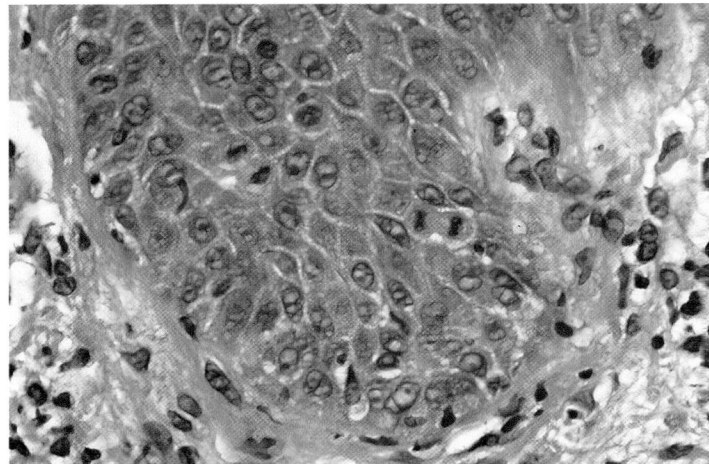

Fig. 4.2 **Psoriasis.** Mitoses are evident in keratinocytes within the epidermis. (H & E)

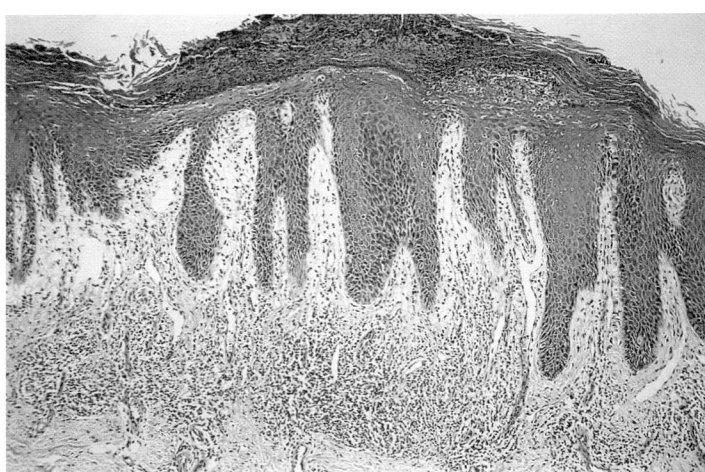

Fig. 4.4 **Psoriasis.** Confluent parakeratosis overlies an epidermis showing psoriasiform hyperplasia. (H & E)

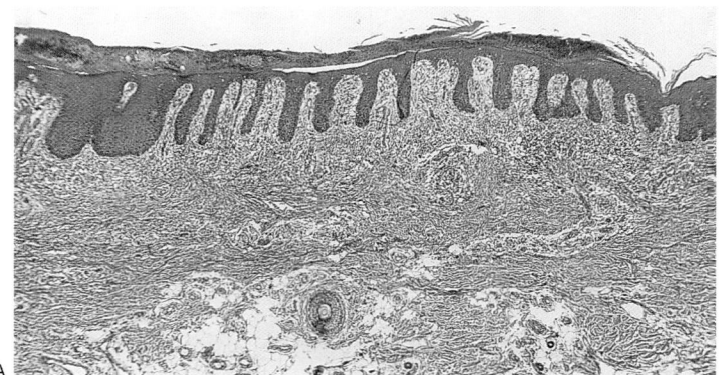

A

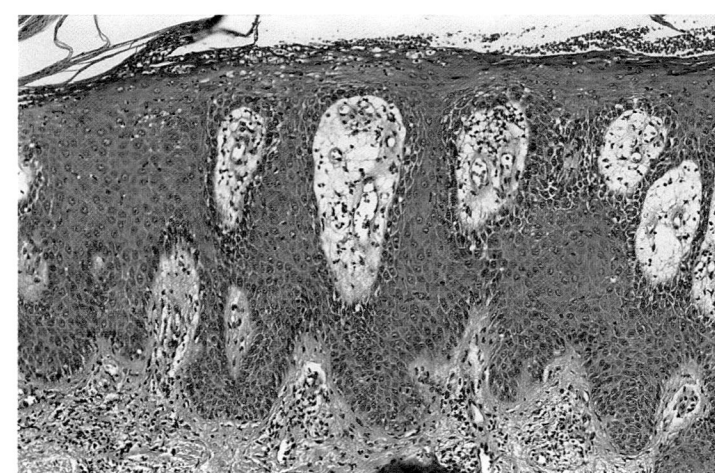

Fig. 4.5 **Psoriasis.** The dilated vessels in the papillary dermis are well shown. The suprapapillary epidermis ('plate') is relatively thin. (H & E)

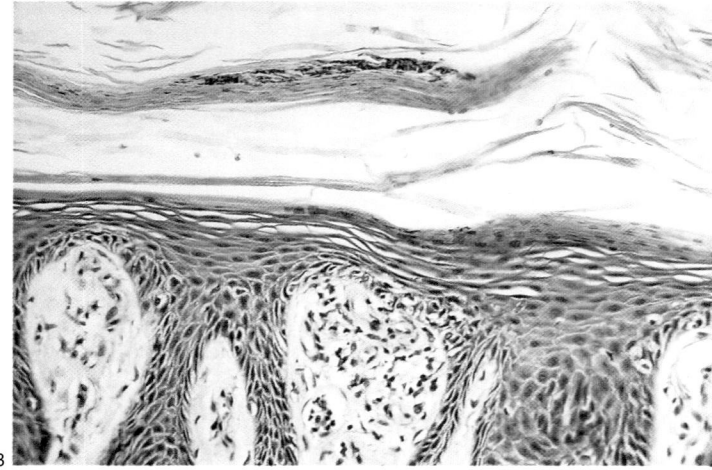

B

Fig. 4.3 **Psoriasis. (A)** There is psoriasiform hyperplasia of the epidermis. **(B)** Neutrophils are present in the upper layers of the overlying parakeratotic scale – neutrophils migrating to the 'summits' of the parakeratotic mounds. (H & E)

With time, there may be club-shaped thickening of the lower rete pegs with coalescence of these in some areas (Fig. 4.6).[218,219] Later lesions show orthokeratosis, an intact granular layer and some thickening of the suprapapillary plates. Exocytosis of inflammatory cells is usually mild. The finding in one patient of numerous fatty vacuoles in the papillary dermis – pseudolipomatosis cutis (see p. 957) – is of doubtful significance.[227] Differentiation of late lesions of psoriasis from lichen simplex chronicus may be difficult, although in the latter condition the suprapapillary plates and granular layer are usually more prominent and there may be vertically oriented collagen bundles in the papillary dermis.[2] If psoriatic plaques are rubbed or scratched, the histopathological features of the underlying psoriasis may be obscured by these superimposed changes.

In resolving or treated plaques of psoriasis there is a progressive diminution in the inflammatory infiltrate, a reduction in the amount of epidermal hyperplasia, and restoration of the granular layer.[217] Vessels in the papillary dermis are still dilated, although by now there is an increase in fibroblasts in this region with mild fibrosis.[217] Only after 10–14 weeks of treatment do the histological appearances return to normal.[228]

Minor changes which have been reported in psoriasis of the scalp include mild sebaceous gland atrophy, a decrease in hair follicle size, and thinner hair

lymphocytes,[224] fewer Langerhans cells than in earlier lesions and very occasional neutrophils.[222] A subset of spindle-shaped macrophages, situated along the basement membrane, has been described as a characteristic feature. These so-called 'lining cells' are positive for CD11c. Plasma cells and eosinophils are usually absent,[219] but eosinophil cationic protein has been identified, particularly in the upper third of the epidermis in psoriasis.[225] Plasma cells may be present in patients with HIV infection.[226]

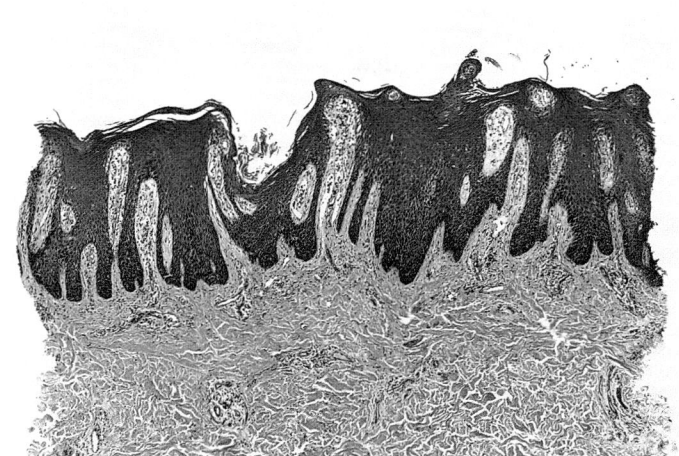

Fig. 4.6 **Psoriasis.** There is some coalescence of the tips of the rete pegs. (H & E)

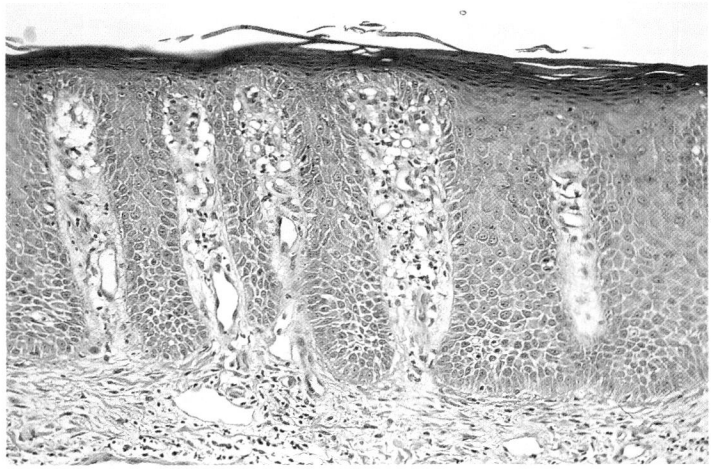

Fig. 4.7 **Psoriasis.** There is mild spongiosis at the tips of the rete pegs. (H & E)

shafts.[229] Munro microabscesses are said to be uncommon in this region.[219] Another regional variation is the lessened epidermal hyperplasia in psoriasis of the penis and vulva;[219] spongiosis may be present.

Spongiosis has already been mentioned as a feature of the early lesions of psoriasis, and of psoriasis occurring in various regions such as the hands and feet and genital regions. It may also occur in erythrodermic psoriasis (see below). Ackerman has also drawn attention to its presence in other situations. The author has now seen several cases that caused diagnostic confusion, initially because of significant spongiosis, but which, over time, have evolved into classic psoriasis. Their initial biopsies showed spongiosis, mounds of parakeratosis containing neutrophils, dilated vessels in the papillary dermis and a mild, superficial perivascular infiltrate of lymphocytes. The term *spongiotic psoriasis* is an appropriate designation for these cases (Fig. 4.7).

In *erythrodermic psoriasis*, the appearances may resemble those described in early lesions of psoriasis, possibly a reflection of the early medical intervention that usually occurs in this condition.[230] Dilatation of superficial vessels is usually quite prominent. A cornified layer is usually absent. Sometimes the histological changes do not resemble those of psoriasis at all.

In *follicular psoriasis*, there is follicular plugging with marked parakeratosis in the mid-zone of the ostium.[79] The dermal inflammatory infiltrate is both perivascular and perifollicular.

In *annular verrucous psoriasis*, there is exaggerated papillomatosis resulting in finger-like projections of the epidermis.[84]

Skin tumors have developed at sites treated with PUVA therapy,[231,232] particularly after prolonged exposure.[56,233,234] Prolonged UVB therapy results in the accumulation of DNA photoproducts in the cells, although adaptive responses occur.[235] The use of coal tar does not produce any appreciable increase in skin cancers.[236] Variants of seborrheic keratosis have also been reported in psoriatic patients receiving treatment with ultraviolet radiation.[237] Of relevance is the controversy over whether patients with psoriasis have an inherently low risk of developing skin cancer,[238] although recent studies suggest that this is not so.[239–241] Another rare complication of treatment is cutaneous ulceration, which has been reported following methotrexate therapy.[242]

Differential diagnosis

The histopathological differentiation of psoriasis from *chronic eczematous dermatitis*, particularly seborrheic dermatitis, is sometimes difficult. The presence of prominent spongiosis involving the rete ridges generally rules out psoriasis, while the presence of a leukocytic exudate, other than in a folliculocentric distribution, is quite uncommon in seborrheic dermatitis.[1] In seborrheic dermatitis there is often less epidermal hyperplasia than in psoriasis. Spongiotic psoriasis (see above) can be very difficult to distinguish from other spongiotic processes. The presence of mounds of parakeratosis containing neutrophils and a dermal infiltrate that is usually mild are clues to the diagnosis of psoriasis.

The features that distinguish psoriasis from *lichen simplex chronicus* have been discussed above. Spongiosis is sometimes present in the rete ridges in this latter condition if it is superimposed on an eczematous process.

In *pityriasis rubra pilaris*, there is mild to moderate psoriasiform hyperplasia, parakeratotic lipping of follicles and, in some lesions, alternating zones of orthokeratosis and parakeratosis in both horizontal and vertical directions.

Pustular psoriasis has more prominent spongiform pustulation than psoriasis vulgaris, particularly at the shoulders of the lesions.

Electron microscopy[243]

There are numerous cytoplasmic organelles in the keratinocytes, reflecting their hyperactivity. These are decreased with treatment.[244] Tonofilaments and desmosomes are reduced in number and size and there is also a reduction in the number of keratohyaline granules.[243] Vessels in the papillary dermis are dilated with abundant fenestrations.[243] Neutrophils are said to be polar in shape with ruffled cell membranes.[245]

AIDS-ASSOCIATED PSORIASIFORM DERMATITIS

Psoriasis, seborrheic dermatitis and cases with overlap features may occur in patients infected with the human immunodeficiency virus (HIV).[246–249] The term 'AIDS-associated psoriasiform dermatitis' has been used, particularly for those cases with features of both conditions. Interestingly, there is often more uniformity in the histopathological expression than in the clinical presentations. In some circumstances, onset of the disease, or its exacerbation, has been associated with the initial seroconversion. In others, exacerbations are associated with cutaneous or systemic infections. The severity of the disease is variable.

Histopathology

The epidermis shows psoriasiform hyperplasia, but unlike psoriasis, there is no thinning of the suprapapillary plate. There are scattered apoptotic keratinocytes within the epidermis, usually associated with some lymphocyte exocytosis. Perivascular lymphocytes in the dermis may show karyorrhexis, giving rise to small amounts of nuclear dust. Plasma cells are often present in small numbers.[226]

PUSTULAR PSORIASIS

Pustular psoriasis is a rare, acute form of psoriasiform dermatosis characterized by the widespread eruption of numerous sterile pustules on an erythematous base and associated with constitutional symptoms.[74,250–252] Skin tenderness, a neutrophil leukocytosis and an absolute lymphopenia[253] may precede the onset of the pustules. These may continue to develop in waves for several weeks or longer before remitting. Arthritis,[254] generalized erythroderma,[254] hypocalcemia[255] and lesions of the mucous membranes, including fissured tongue and benign migratory glossitis (geographical tongue), may develop in the course of the disease.[256] Amyloidosis,[257] acute respiratory distress syndrome[258] and a bullous disorder[259] are extremely rare complications.

Several clinical variants of pustular psoriasis are recognized.[250,254] The *Von Zumbusch type* is the most common variant. It has an explosive onset and a mortality as high as 30% in some of the earlier series. *Impetigo herpetiformis* is a controversial entity defined by some on the basis of flexural involvement with centripetal spread of the pustules and by others as a variant of pustular psoriasis occurring in pregnancy.[260–264] Onset in pregnancy is usually in the third trimester, although it develops earlier in subsequent pregnancies.[265–267] It usually remits post partum, but may flare with the use of oral contraceptives.[268] Fetal mortality is high as a consequence of placental insufficiency.[268] A subset related to hypoparathyroidism with hypocalcemia is sometimes included in impetigo herpetiformis.[269-271] The *acral variant* of pustular psoriasis arises in a setting of acrodermatitis continua which is a localized pustular eruption of one or more digits with displacement and dystrophy of the nails.[250,272–274] The development of generalized pustular psoriasis in acrodermatitis continua has a bad prognosis.[250,272] Other variants include an *exanthematic form*,[250,272,275] an *annular variant*[276,277] with some resemblance to subcorneal pustular dermatosis, a *linear variant*[278,279] and a *localized form* which consists of pustular psoriasis developing in pre-existing plaques of psoriasis.[250,254] Some of the cases reported in the past as exanthematous variants may represent examples of acute generalized exanthematous pustulosis (see p. 136).[280] A case of pustular psoriasis limited to the penis has been reported.[281] There was no pre-existing condition.

Generalized pustular psoriasis may develop in three main clinical settings.[250] In the first group there is a long history of psoriasis of early onset. In these cases the pustular psoriasis is often precipitated by some external provocative agent (see below). In the second group, there is preceding psoriasis of atypical form, in which the onset was relatively late in life. Precipitating factors are not usually present. In the third group, pustular psoriasis arises without pre-existing psoriasis. Pustular psoriasis may rarely develop as a consequence of persistent pustulosis of the palms and soles. Familial cases of pustular psoriasis[282,283] and onset in childhood have also been reported.[282–286] In children, pustular psoriasis can be complicated by sterile, lytic lesions of bones.[285,287] The development of renal failure and cholestatic jaundice in one patient may have been a coincidence.[288]

Numerous factors have been implicated in precipitating pustular psoriasis.[289] These include infections, sunlight, burns,[290] ultraviolet radiation from tanning salon use,[277] alcohol, malignancy, metabolic and endocrine factors, pregnancy,[291] emotional stress and drugs. The drugs include lithium,[292] iodides, non-steroidal anti-inflammatory agents including phenylbutazone,[293] beta-blockers,[294] penicillin and related drugs,[289] procaine, cyclosporine,[295,296] oral terbinafine,[297,298] sulfonamides, morphine, hydroxychloroquine,

progesterone,[299] nystatin and topical calcipotriol.[300] The withdrawal of steroids is a common precipitating factor which may be included in this category.

One of the most striking features of pustular psoriasis is the enhanced chemotaxis of neutrophils, which is even more marked than in psoriasis.[301,302] The chemotactic factors in the affected areas of skin include leukotrienes, complement products and cathepsin 1.[303]

Histopathology[304, 305]

The diagnostic feature is the presence of intraepidermal pustules at various stages of development (Fig. 4.8). In early lesions, the epidermis is usually only slightly acanthotic, while psoriasiform hyperplasia is seen only in older and persistent lesions (Fig. 4.9). Mitoses are usually present within the epidermis. Neutrophils migrate from dilated vessels in the papillary dermis into the epidermis. They aggregate beneath the stratum corneum and in the upper malpighian layer between degenerate and thinned keratinocytes to form the so-called 'spongiform pustules of Kogoj' (Fig. 4.10).[306] The subcorneal pustules have a thin roof of stratum corneum. In later lesions these are replaced by scale crusts with collections of neutrophils trapped between parakeratotic layers. A few eosinophils may be present in the infiltrate.

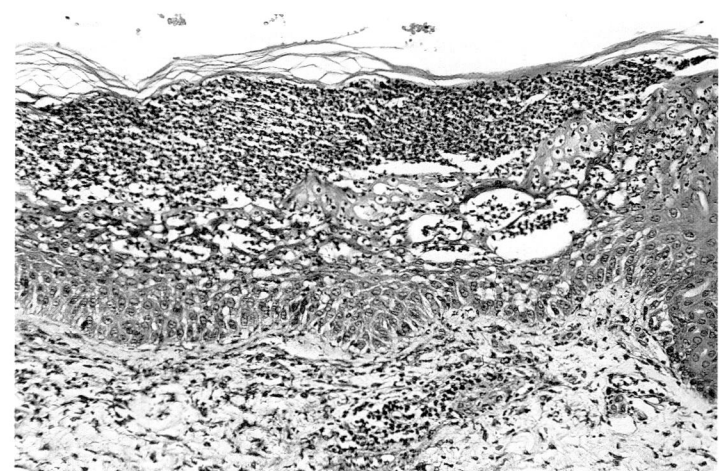

Fig. 4.8 **Early pustular psoriasis.** There is a heavy infiltrate of neutrophils in the upper layers of the epidermis and beneath the stratum corneum. (H & E)

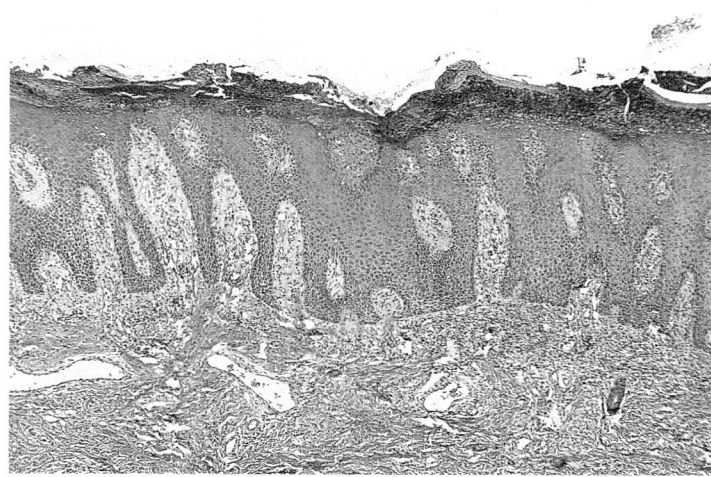

Fig. 4.9 **Pustular psoriasis (old lesion).** There is pronounced psoriasiform hyperplasia of the epidermis and spongiform pustulation in the upper layers. (H & E)

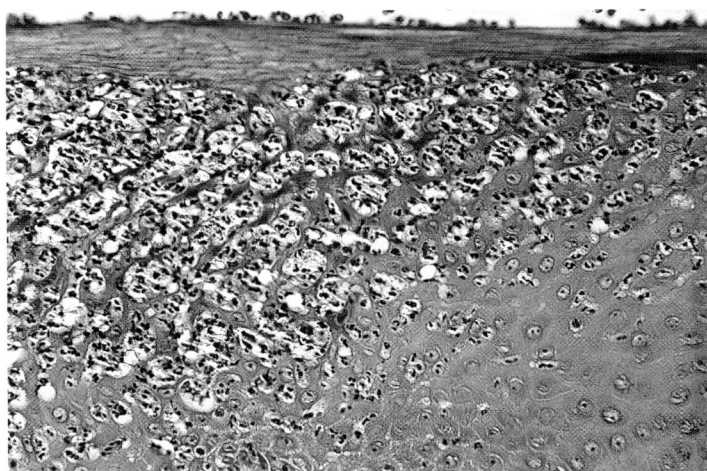

Fig. 4.10 **Pustular psoriasis.** A spongiform pustule of Kogoj is shown. (H & E)

The blood vessels in the papillary dermis are usually dilated and there is a perivascular infiltrate of lymphocytes and a few neutrophils. Large mono-nuclear cells were noted in the pustules and in the dermis in one report of impetigo herpetiformis.[307] They were thought to be specific for this variant of pustular psoriasis, although they were specifically excluded in a subsequent report of this condition.[307]

Electron microscopy[303]

Multipolypoid herniations of basal keratinocytes have been described protruding into the dermis through large gaps in the basal lamina. Neutrophil proteases are probably responsible for this change. In another study there were gaps between the endothelial cells of dermal blood vessels.[308]

REITER'S SYNDROME

Reiter's syndrome is usually defined as the triad of non-gonococcal urethritis, ocular inflammation and arthritis.[309] The presence of mucocutaneous lesions is sometimes included as a fourth feature.[310] Reiter's syndrome occurs in approximately 30% of patients with reactive arthritis, which in turn develops in 1–3% of patients with sexually acquired, non-gonococcal infections of the genital tract.[309,311] Reiter's syndrome has also been associated with certain bacterial gut infections, including those due to *Shigella flexneri*, *Yersinia enterocolitica*[312] and, rarely, *Campylobacter jejuni*.[313] The genital infectious agent which is usually incriminated is *Chlamydia trachomatis*, but *Ureaplasma urealyticum* and species of *Mycoplasma* have also been isolated.[309,313] Chlamydial elementary bodies have been detected by immunofluorescence and monoclonal antibodies in the synovium of patients with reactive arthritis, which to date has always been sterile by conventional cultures.[314] *Chlamydia*-specific antigens have been detected in a biopsy of the cutaneous lesions of Reiter's syndrome.[315] Reiter's syndrome has also been induced by systemic interferon-α treatment.[316]

There is genetic susceptibility to the development of reactive arthritis and Reiter's syndrome and this is manifest by the presence of the histocompatibility antigen HLA-B27.[312,317] Other clinical features of Reiter's syndrome include a marked preponderance in males, a mean age of onset in the third decade of life and a variable, often relapsing course.[317–319] Some cases begin in childhood.[320] An association with the acquired immunodeficiency syndrome has been reported.[321,322]

The mucocutaneous lesions, already alluded to, include a circinate balanitis with perimeatal erosions and mucosal ulcers.[323] Involvement of the vulva is

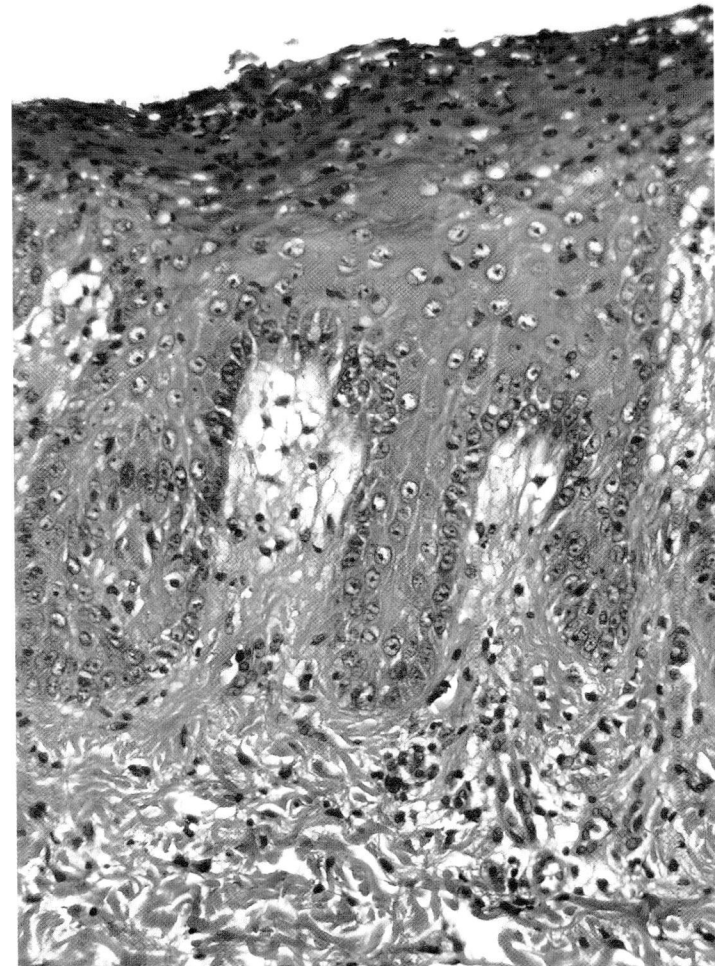

Fig. 4.11 **Reiter's syndrome.** The appearances may be indistinguishable from pustular psoriasis. (H & E)

rare.[324] In 10–30% of cases there are crusted erythematous papules and plaques with a predilection for the soles of the feet, genitalia, perineum, buttocks, scalp and extensor surfaces of the extremities.[319] Some lesions may be frankly pustular, resembling pustular psoriasis. These cutaneous lesions are known by the name 'keratoderma blennorrhagica'. They usually heal after several weeks, without scarring. Ackerman believes that Reiter's syndrome is a variant of psoriasis.[325]

Histopathology

In most biopsies, the cutaneous lesions of Reiter's syndrome are indistinguish-able from pustular psoriasis. Accordingly, there is psoriasiform epidermal hyperplasia with a thick horny layer (Fig. 4.11). This is most prominent in lesions on the palms and soles and least prominent in penile and buccal lesions. Spongiform pustulation with exocytosis of neutrophils is another conspicuous feature.[326] A variable inflammatory cell infiltrate, usually including a few neutrophils, is present in the upper dermis.[327] A mild, leukocytoclastic vasculitis has been observed in the papillary dermis of several cases.[315]

Various histological features have been claimed to be more suggestive of Reiter's syndrome than pustular psoriasis. These include a thicker horny layer, larger spongiform pustules, eczematous changes, a thicker suprapapillary plate of epidermis, the presence of neutrophils in the dermis and the absence of clubbing of the rete ridges. The horny layer is sometimes more loosely attached than in pustular psoriasis, leading to its partial detachment during processing of the specimen. These various features are usually not sufficiently different from the findings in pustular psoriasis to allow a confident distinction to be made between the two conditions on biopsy material.

PITYRIASIS RUBRA PILARIS

Pityriasis rubra pilaris is a rare, erythematosquamous dermatosis of unknown etiology characterized by small follicular papules with a central keratin plug, perifollicular erythema with a tendency to become confluent but with islands of sparing, palmoplantar keratoderma, often with edema, and pityriasis capitis.[328–332] The condition often begins with a seborrheic dermatitis-like rash on the face or scalp which rapidly spreads downwards.[333–335] In other patients, particularly juveniles, the disease starts on the lower half of the body.[336,337] Some patients may become erythrodermic.[338–340] A variable degree of pruritus is often present.[341] Cases with localized lesions, restricted often to the elbows and knees, occur. Severe forms of pityriasis rubra pilaris have been reported in patients infected with the human immunodeficiency virus (HIV).[342–346] Cystic acne may coexist.[343]

Pityriasis rubra pilaris has been reported as the initial manifestation of internal neoplasia.[347] A rare familial form with autosomal dominant inheritance occurs.[348]

Nail changes,[328,349] alopecia[329,330] and, rarely, multiple seborrheic keratoses or cutaneous malignancies may occur in patients with pityriasis rubra pilaris.[350,351] The age of onset and clinical course are quite variable.[352,353] For this reason, the clinical classification into five types, as proposed by Griffiths, has not been used here.[354] Complete remission occurs within 6 months to 2 years in about 50% of cases.[355,356]

Although there is some resemblance to vitamin A deficiency (phrynoderma), serum vitamin A levels are normal.[338] Reduced levels of retinol-binding protein (the specific carrier of vitamin A) have been reported,[357] but the results of this work have not been confirmed.[358,359] Epidermal cell kinetics show an increased rate of cell proliferation.[360,361]

Histopathology[2,338,362]

The changes are most marked when erythema is greatest, and least impressive in biopsies of follicular papules.[331] There is diffuse orthokeratosis with spotted parakeratosis which also forms a collarette around the follicular ostia (Fig. 4.12). Some follicular plugging is often present (Fig. 4.13).[363] Parakeratosis is not prominent in early lesions. These changes may be stated in another way – alternating orthokeratosis and parakeratosis in both vertical and horizontal directions (Fig. 4.14).[362] However, many cases will be missed if this criterion is too rigidly applied. There is also acanthosis: this is never as regular as that seen in psoriasis. There are broad rete ridges and thick suprapapillary plates. Hypergranulosis is often prominent and this may be focal or confluent.[362] An unusual perinuclear vacuolization is sometimes seen in cells in the malpighian layer and there may be some vacuolar change involving the pilary outer root sheath. Spongiosis, usually mild, is present in about 10% of cases.[364] There is a superficial perivascular and perifollicular lymphocytic infiltrate in the dermis. While the infiltrate is usually mild, a heavy infiltrate, which is rarely lichenoid in distribution, is sometimes present.[365] Eosinophils and plasma cells are occasionally present in the infiltrate.[366] Folliculitis is a rare complication.[353] Another rare histological finding is the presence of focal acantholytic dyskeratosis in the lesions of pityriasis rubra pilaris.[351,367–370] Epidermolytic hyperkeratosis has been reported in one case.[366]

In contrast to pityriasis rubra pilaris, vitamin A deficiency shows no focal parakeratosis, irregular acanthosis or dermal inflammatory infiltrate.[329]

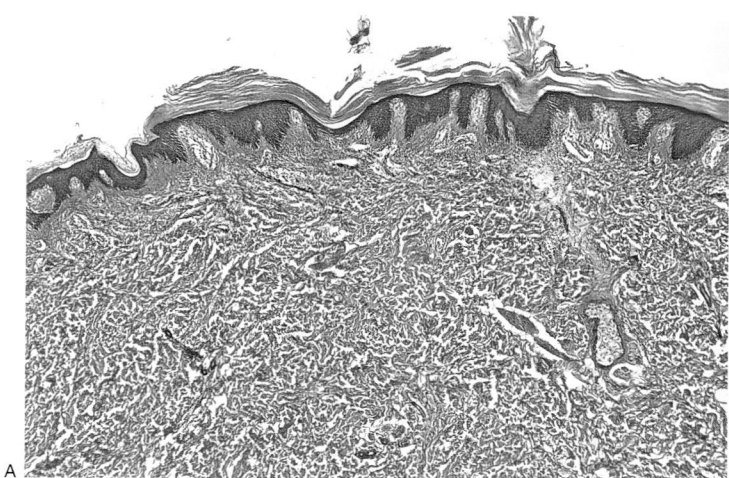

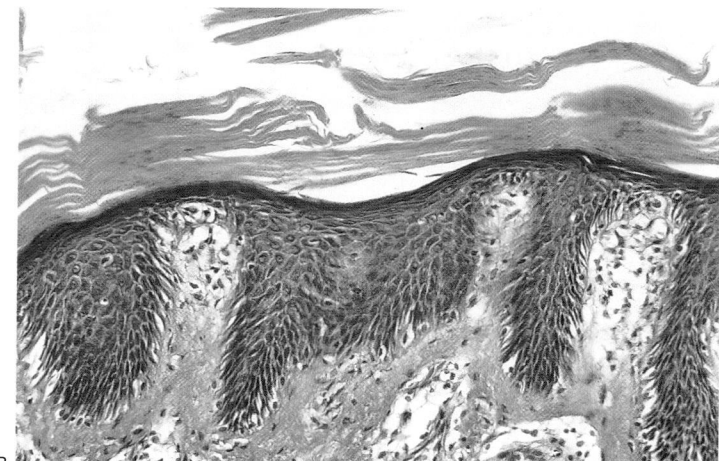

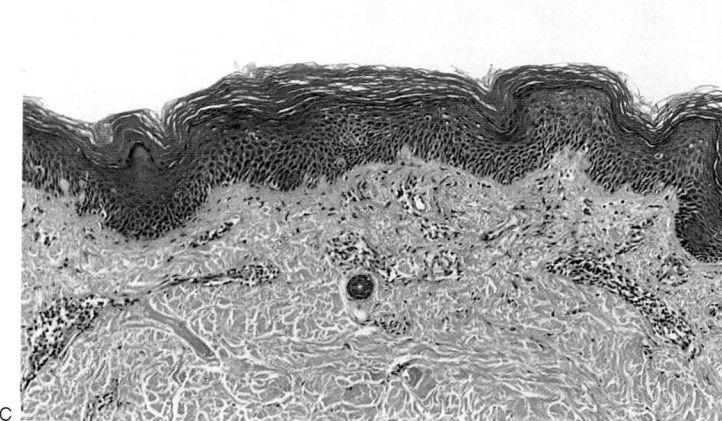

Fig. 4.12 **Pityriasis rubra pilaris. (A)** As it should be, with psoriasiform hyperplasia and overlying 'geometric' parakeratosis. **(B)** High power view of the case shown in (A). **(C)** As it sometimes is, with atypical features. The author has missed more cases of this disease (on the initial biopsy) than any other. (H & E)

Electron microscopy

Tonofilaments and desmosomes are decreased, but there are large numbers of keratinosomes and lipid-like vacuoles in the parakeratotic areas.[371] The basal lamina is focally split, containing gaps.[371]

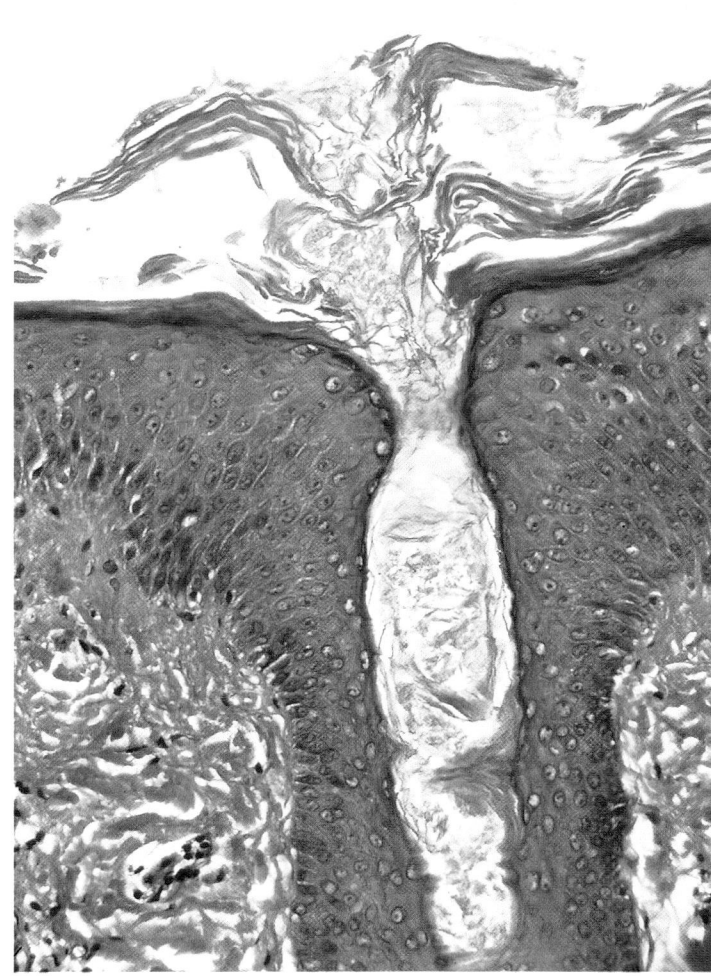

Fig. 4.13 **Pityriasis rubra pilaris.** There is mild keratotic follicular plugging and lipping. (H & E)

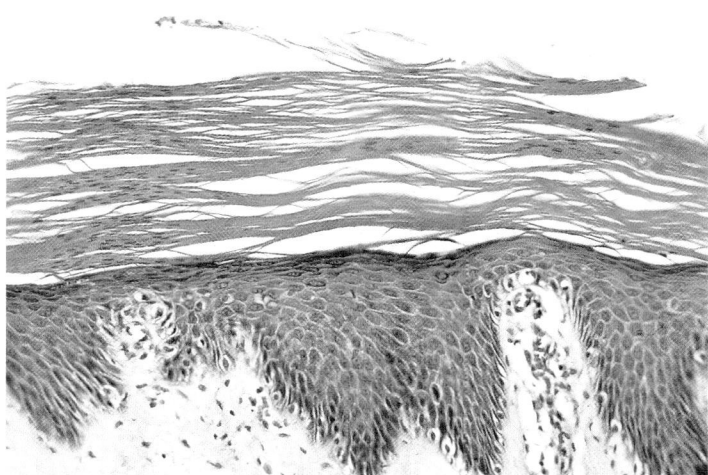

Fig. 4.14 **Pityriasis rubra pilaris.** There is alternating orthokeratosis and parakeratosis in both a horizontal and a vertical direction. (H & E)

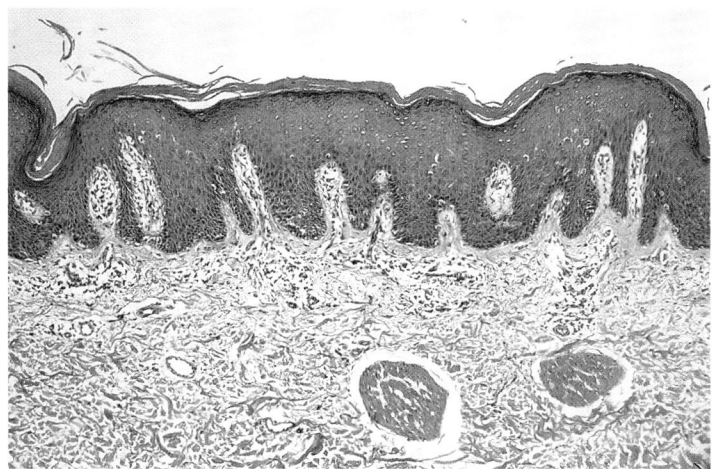

Fig. 4.15 **Chronic superficial dermatitis** with psoriasiform hyperplasia, thick suprapapillary 'plates' of epidermis and a mild, superficial lymphocytic infiltrate with some upward spread. (H & E)

PARAPSORIASIS

The term 'parapsoriasis', as originally introduced, referred to a heterogeneous group of asymptomatic, scaly dermatoses with some clinical resemblance to psoriasis.[372–374] These conditions were further characterized by chronicity and resistance to therapy. Three distinct entities are now recognized as having been included in the original concept of 'parapsoriasis' – pityriasis lichenoides, chronic superficial dermatitis (small plaque parapsoriasis, digitate dermatosis) and large plaque parapsoriasis (atrophic parapsoriasis, retiform parapsoriasis, patch-stage mycosis fungoides).[373]

Confusion has arisen because of the retention of the term 'parapsoriasis' for two distinct conditions. In the United States, the term 'parapsoriasis en plaque' is usually used to refer to the entity that in the United Kingdom is called chronic superficial dermatitis.[375] The term 'parapsoriasis' is also used for a condition with large plaques, which in 10–30% of cases progresses to a frank T-cell lymphoma of the skin.[376] Studies have indicated monoclonal populations of T cells in 20% or more of cases of large plaque parapsoriasis.[377]

Brief mention will be made of the three entities included in the original concept of parapsoriasis.

Pityriasis lichenoides shows features of both a chronic lymphocytic vasculitis and the lichenoid tissue reaction (see p. 246). It should no longer be considered as a variant of parapsoriasis.

Chronic superficial dermatitis (small plaque parapsoriasis) resembles a 'mild eczema' and it is therefore discussed in detail on page 115, as part of the spongiotic tissue reaction. The spongiosis is often quite mild and in chronic lesions may be absent. In these circumstances, the epidermal acanthosis may assume psoriasiform proportions, hence its mention here also. It differs from psoriasis by the absence of dilated vessels in the papillary dermis and the absence of neutrophil exocytosis. Furthermore, chronic superficial dermatitis lacks a thin suprapapillary plate and there is a paucity of mitoses in the keratinocytes (Fig. 4.15). Lymphocytes with a normal mature morphology are often found in the papillary dermis in chronic superficial dermatitis. This feature, combined with the regular acanthosis and focal parakeratosis, allows a diagnosis to be made in many cases with the scanning power of the light microscope. A dominant clonal pattern of T cells has been identified in some cases.[378,379] Accordingly, it is often regarded as an early stage of cutaneous T-cell lymphoma.

Large plaque parapsoriasis, the third entity included originally as 'parapsoriasis', may also show features of psoriasiform epidermal hyperplasia, although in atrophic and poikilodermatous lesions the epidermis is thin with loss of the rete ridge pattern. Basal vacuolar change and epidermotropism of lymphocytes are usually present. Large plaque parapsoriasis, a stage in the evolution of mycosis fungoides, is considered with other cutaneous lymphoid infiltrates on page 1105.

Finally, brief mention will be made of the term 'guttate parapsoriasis'. This term has been used in the past synonymously with both pityriasis lichenoides and chronic superficial dermatitis. It is best avoided.[374]

LICHEN SIMPLEX CHRONICUS

Lichen simplex chronicus ('circumscribed neurodermatitis') is an idiopathic disorder in which scaly, thickened plaques develop in response to persistent rubbing of pruritic sites.[380,381] There is a predilection for the nape of the neck, the ulnar border of the forearms, the wrists, the pretibial region, the dorsa of the feet and the perianal and genital region.[381–383] Atopic individuals are more prone than others to develop lichen simplex chronicus.[384]

Kinetic studies have shown epidermal cell proliferation similar to that seen in psoriasis although the transit time of the cells is not as fast.[382] There is also an increase in mitochondrial enzymes in keratinocytes and in the number of melanocytes in the basal layer.[385] Although these kinetic aspects are known, there is still no explanation for the pathogenesis of these plaques and the underlying pruritus; it is apparent, however, that self-induced trauma plays an important localizing role.[382]

Histopathology[381,386]

A thick layer of compact orthokeratosis (resembling that seen on normal palms and soles) is present, overlying hypergranulosis. Focal zones of parakeratosis are sometimes interspersed with the orthokeratosis, but there is not the confluent parakeratosis of psoriasis.[382] The epidermis shows psoriasiform hyperplasia with thicker rete ridges of less even length than in psoriasis. Epidermal thickness and volume are greater than in psoriasis.[382] Minimal papillomatosis is sometimes present in a few areas. Focal excoriation is another change that may be seen in lichen simplex chronicus.

There is marked thickening of the papillary dermis with bundles of collagen arranged in vertical streaks (Fig. 4.16).[386] Scattered inflammatory cells and some fibroblasts are usually present in this region of the dermis.

Regional variations occur in lichen simplex chronicus. Epidermal hyperplasia is usually quite mild in lesions on the lip, while vertical-streaked collagen is unusual in lesions on the scalp or in mucocutaneous regions such as the vulva and perianal area.[386]

Changes like those of lichen simplex chronicus may be superimposed on other dermatoses such as lichen planus (hypertrophic lichen planus), mycosis fungoides, actinic reticuloid and eczematous dermatitides including atopic dermatitis.[381,384] These changes are particularly prominent in some solar keratoses of the hands or forearms.

The term 'prurigo nodularis' (see p. 756) is used for lesions with a nodular clinical appearance and prominent epidermal hyperplasia of pseudo-epitheliomatous rather than psoriasiform type. At times, lesions with overlapping clinical and histopathological features of both lichen simplex chronicus and prurigo nodularis are found.

OTHER PSORIASIFORM DERMATOSES

This group of other psoriasiform dermatoses has been arbitrarily separated from the so-called 'major psoriasiform dermatoses' because of their inclusion in various other chapters, on the basis of their etiology or of other histopathological features.

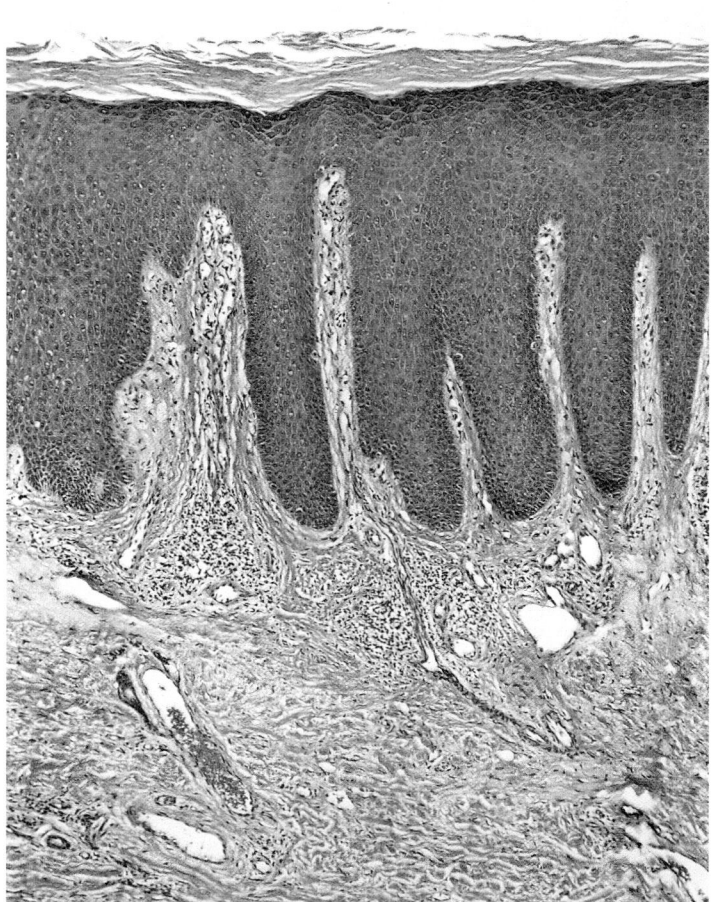

Fig. 4.16 **Lichen simplex chronicus.** The rete pegs are thinner than usual but the vertical 'streaking' of collagen in the papillary dermis is well developed. (H & E)

SUBACUTE AND CHRONIC SPONGIOTIC DERMATITIDES

The various 'eczematous' dermatitides (allergic contact dermatitis, seborrheic dermatitis, nummular dermatitis and atopic dermatitis) may show prominent psoriasiform epidermal hyperplasia in their subacute and chronic stages.

Histopathology

In subacute lesions, spongiosis is usually sufficiently obvious to allow a correct diagnosis. In some chronic lesions, particularly if activity has been dampened by treatment prior to the taking of a biopsy, the spongiosis may be quite mild or even absent. The features which distinguish chronic seborrheic dermatitis from psoriasis have been discussed on page 81. In some cases of chronic atopic and nummular dermatitis the epidermal hyperplasia is not as regular and as even as that seen in psoriasis, although this is by no means invariable. The presence of eosinophils and plasma cells in the superficial dermis would tend to exclude psoriasis. They may be found in any of the chronic spongiotic dermatitides that may simulate psoriasis histopathologically. The changes of lichen simplex chronicus may be superimposed on these chronic spongiotic dermatitides (Fig. 4.17).

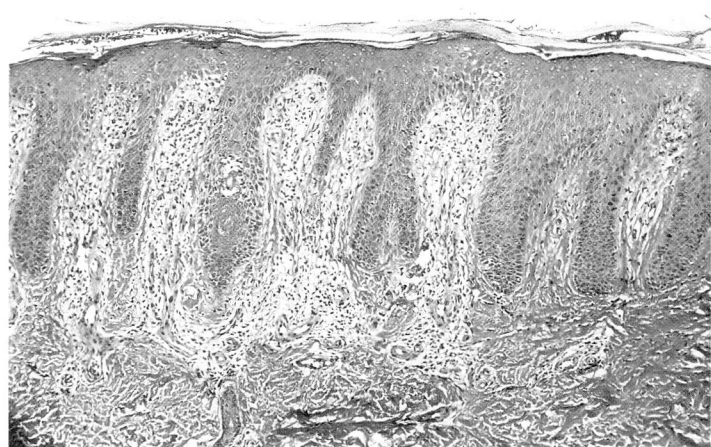

Fig. 4.17 **Chronic allergic contact dermatitis** with psoriasiform hyperplasia of the epidermis and small foci of spongiosis. (H & E)

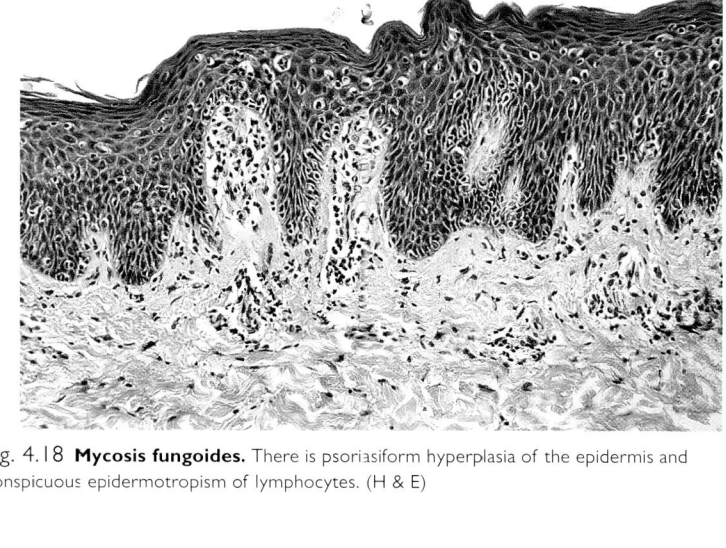

Fig. 4.18 **Mycosis fungoides.** There is psoriasiform hyperplasia of the epidermis and conspicuous epidermotropism of lymphocytes. (H & E)

ERYTHRODERMA

Erythroderma (exfoliative dermatitis) is a cutaneous reaction pattern characterized by erythema, edema and scaling of all or most of the skin surface, often accompanied by pruritus (see p. 576). It may complicate a pre-existing dermatosis, follow the ingestion of a drug or be associated with an internal cancer or with cutaneous T-cell lymphoma.

Histopathology

The findings are variable and often non-specific. Psoriasiform hyperplasia, sometimes accompanied by mild spongiosis, may be present in cases of erythroderma not thought to be of psoriatic origin, while presumptive cases of erythrodermic psoriasis may show only non-specific changes in the epidermis. The difficulties encountered in an attempted histopathological diagnosis of erythroderma are mentioned on page 577.

MYCOSIS FUNGOIDES

Mycosis fungoides is a cutaneous T-cell lymphoma with three clinical stages – patch, plaque and tumor. Its varied clinical features are discussed on page 1104.

Histopathology

Psoriasiform hyperplasia of the epidermis is not uncommon in mycosis fungoides. It is usually of mild to moderate proportions. The presence of epidermotropism and variable cytological atypia of the lymphocytic infiltrate are features which distinguish this condition from other psoriasiform dermatoses (Fig. 4.18).

CHRONIC CANDIDOSIS AND DERMATOPHYTOSES

Psoriasiform epidermal hyperplasia may be present in lesions of chronic candidosis (see p. 665) and, rarely, in chronic dermatophyte infections, most notably in tinea imbricata.

Histopathology

The rete ridges are not unusually long in the psoriasiform hyperplasia of chronic candidosis. There are usually a few neutrophils and some serum in the overlying parakeratotic scale. Fungal elements, in the form of yeasts and pseudohyphae, may be sparse and difficult to find with the PAS stain. They are often more readily seen in methenamine silver preparations.

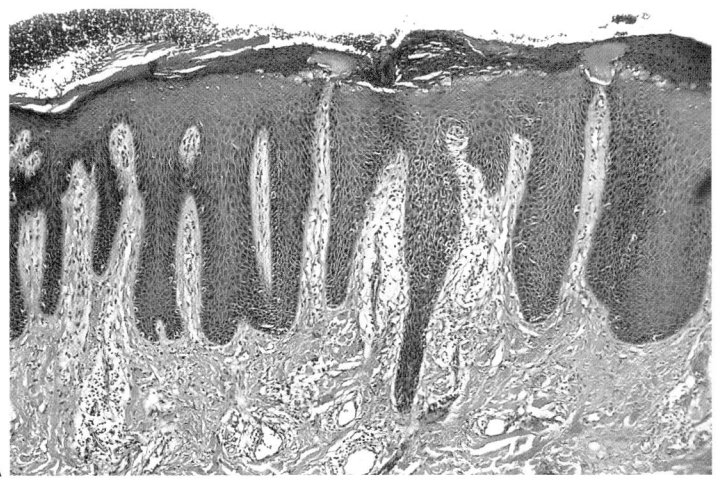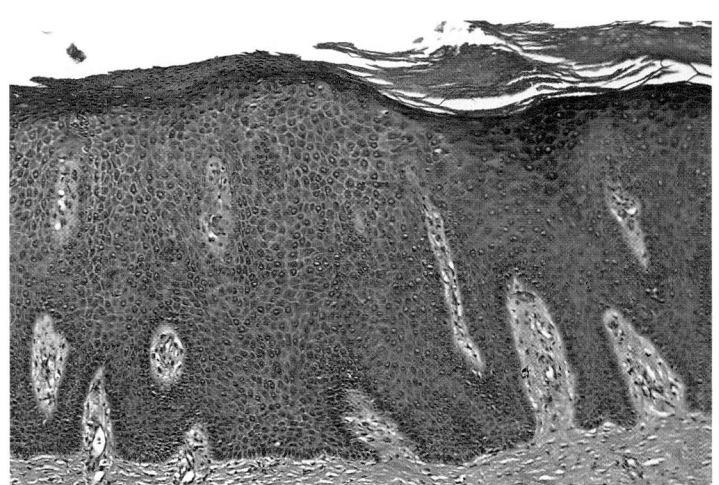

Fig. 4.19 **Inflammatory linear verrucous epidermal nevus (ILVEN). (A)** Note the psoriasiform epidermal hyperplasia. **(B)** There are broad zones of parakeratosis alternating with orthokeratosis. The granular layer is absent beneath the parakeratotic zones. (H & E)

Hyphae and spores are usually abundant in the thick stratum corneum in tinea imbricata.

INFLAMMATORY LINEAR VERRUCOUS EPIDERMAL NEVUS

The acronym ILVEN is often used in place of the more cumbersome inflammatory linear verrucous epidermal nevus. This condition is a variant of epidermal nevus which usually presents as a pruritic, linear eruption on the lower extremities (see p. 755). It must be distinguished from linear psoriasis.

Histopathology
The characteristic feature is the presence of alternating zones of orthokeratosis and parakeratosis in a horizontal direction, overlying a psoriasiform epidermis (Fig. 4.19). The zones of parakeratosis overlie areas of agranulosis. Focal mild spongiosis is often present as well.

NORWEGIAN SCABIES

Norwegian (crusted) scabies is a rare form of scabies which is usually found in the mentally and physically debilitated; it also occurs in immunosuppressed individuals (see p. 741). There are widespread crusted and secondarily infected hyperkeratotic lesions.

Histopathology
Overlying the psoriasiform epidermis there is a very thick layer of orthokeratosis and parakeratosis containing numerous scabies mites at all stages of development. The appearances are characteristic (Fig. 4.20).

BOWEN'S DISEASE

There is a variant of Bowen's disease in which the epidermis shows psoriasiform hyperplasia (see p. 763). It has no distinguishing clinical features.

Histopathology
There is psoriasiform hyperplasia with a thick suprapapillary plate. Atypical keratinocytes usually involve the full thickness of the epidermis; sometimes

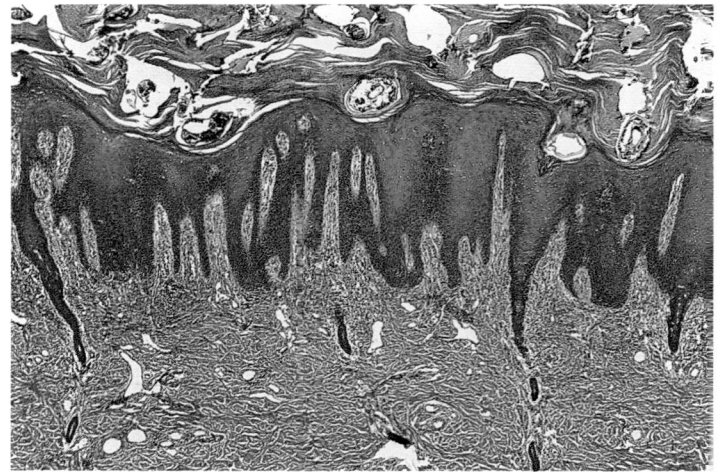

Fig. 4.20 **Norwegian scabies.** The thick stratum corneum which overlies the psoriasiform epidermis contains a number of scabies mites. (H & E)

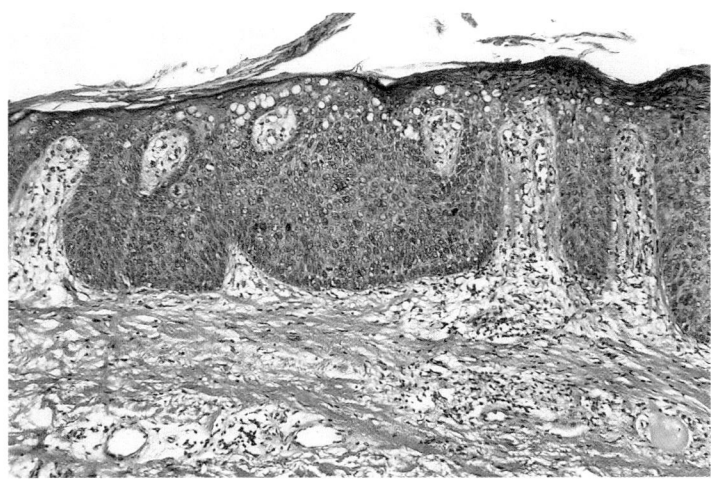

Fig. 4.21 **Bowen's disease.** There is psoriasiform epidermal hyperplasia and full thickness atypia. (H & E)

there is sparing of the basal layer and the acrosyringium (Fig. 4.21). Mitoses and dyskeratotic cells are usually present. Uncommonly, the psoriasiform variant of Bowen's disease is composed of pale pagetoid cells.

CLEAR CELL ACANTHOMA

The clear (pale) cell acanthoma presents as a papulonodular lesion, usually on the lower parts of the legs (see p. 759).

Histopathology
The characteristic feature is the presence of a well-demarcated area of psoriasiform epidermal hyperplasia in which the cells have palely staining cytoplasm. Exocytosis of inflammatory cells may also be present. The pale keratinocytes contain abundant glycogen.

LAMELLAR ICHTHYOSIS

This is a rare, severe, autosomal recessive form of ichthyosis (see p. 284). It is usually manifest at birth.

Histopathology
There is prominent orthokeratosis and focal parakeratosis overlying a normal or thickened granular layer. Psoriasiform epidermal hyperplasia is sometimes present, although usually the epidermis shows only moderate acanthosis. Psoriasiform hyperplasia is also found in some cases of ichthyosis congenita (see p. 284) and Netherton's syndrome (see p. 286). Biopsies of the ichthyosis linearis circumflexa that is a component of Netherton's syndrome may be misdiagnosed as congenital psoriasis (Fig. 4.22).

PITYRIASIS ROSEA

The 'herald patch' of pityriasis rosea may show the psoriasiform tissue reaction (see p. 112).

Histopathology
There is usually acanthosis and only mild psoriasiform hyperplasia. Small 'Pautrier simulants', composed of inflammatory cells in a spongiotic focus, are often seen. There is usually focal parakeratosis overlying the epidermis.

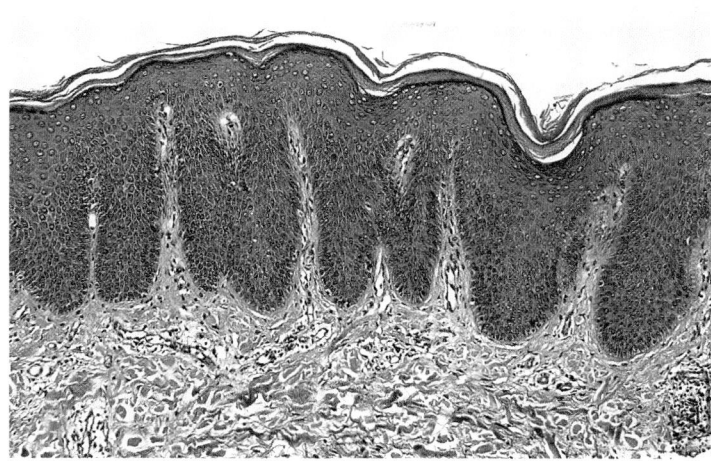

Fig. 4.22 **Ichthyosis linearis circumflexa.** Distinguishing this lesion from psoriasis is sometimes difficult. (H & E)

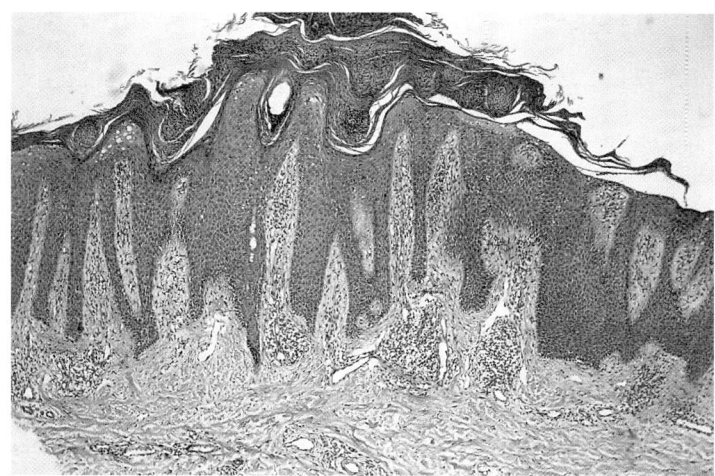

Fig. 4.23 **Glucagonoma syndrome.** There is very little vacuolation of keratinocytes, although it was present in another biopsy from this patient. (H & E)

PELLAGRA

Pellagra is caused by an inadequate amount of niacin (nicotinic acid) in the tissues. Skin lesions include a scaly erythematous rash in sun-exposed areas, sometimes with blistering, followed by hyperpigmentation and epithelial desquamation (see p. 547).

Histopathology

The findings are not usually diagnostic. Sometimes there is psoriasiform acanthosis with pallor of the upper epidermis and overlying orthokeratosis and focal parakeratosis. The psoriasiform acanthosis is more common in mixed nutritional deficiency states.

ACRODERMATITIS ENTEROPATHICA

Acrodermatitis enteropathica, a rare disorder resulting from zinc deficiency, presents with periorificial and acral lesions which may be eczematous, vesiculobullous, pustular or an admixture of these patterns (see p. 551).

Histopathology

In established lesions there is confluent parakeratosis overlying psoriasiform epidermal hyperplasia. The upper layers of the epidermis show a characteristic pallor and sometimes there is focal necrosis or subcorneal clefting. The epidermal pallor disappears in late lesions.

GLUCAGONOMA SYNDROME

Necrolytic migratory erythema is the term used for the cutaneous lesions of the glucagonoma syndrome. This syndrome in most cases is a manifestation of a glucagon-secreting islet cell tumor of the pancreas (see p. 552).

Histopathology

The changes may resemble those seen in acrodermatitis enteropathica with psoriasiform hyperplasia, upper epidermal pallor and overlying confluent parakeratosis. At other times there is focal or confluent necrosis of the upper epidermis with a preceding phase of pale, vacuolated keratinocytes. Subcorneal or intraepidermal clefting and pustulation may develop. Psoriasiform epidermal hyperplasia of any significant degree is present in only a minority of cases (Fig. 4.23).

SECONDARY SYPHILIS

The great imitator, syphilis, can sometimes present lesions, in the secondary phase, with a psoriasiform pattern (see p. 651).

Histopathology

It should be stressed that there is considerable variation in the histopathological appearances of secondary syphilis. Psoriasiform hyperplasia is more often seen in late lesions of secondary syphilis. A lichenoid tissue reaction may also be present and this combination of tissue reactions is very suggestive of syphilis, particularly if the infiltrate in the dermis forms in both the superficial and deep parts (Fig. 4.24). Plasma cells are commonly present, but they are not invariable.

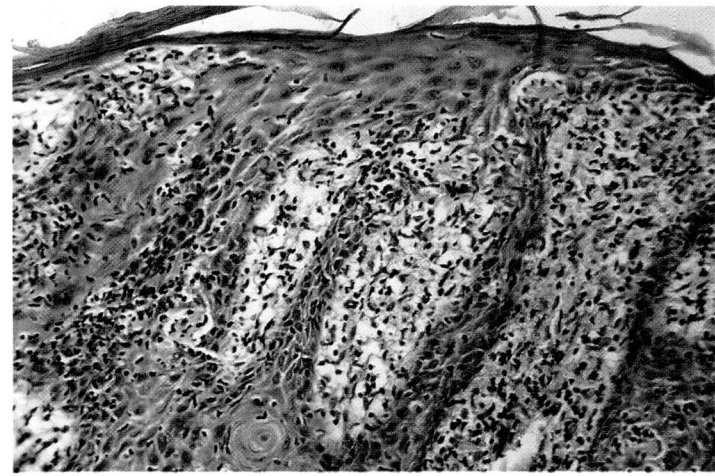

Fig. 4.24 **Late secondary syphilis.** The epidermal hyperplasia is less regular than is usual in psoriasiform hyperplasia. There are focal lichenoid changes. (H & E)

Table 4.2 **Histopathological features of the various psoriasiform diseases**

Disease	Histopathological features
Psoriasis	Progressive psoriasiform epidermal hyperplasia, initially mild; mitoses in basal keratinocytes; dilated vessels in dermal papillae; parakeratosis, initially focal and containing neutrophils, later confluent with few neutrophils; thinning of the suprapapillary epidermis
Pustular psoriasis	Spongiform pustulation overshadows epidermal hyperplasia, except in lesions of some duration when both are present
Reiter's syndrome	Closely resembles pustular psoriasis; the overlying, thick scale crust often detaches during processing
Pityriasis rubra pilaris	Alternating orthokeratosis and parakeratosis, vertically and horizontally; follicular plugging with parafollicular (lipping) parakeratosis; mild to moderate epidermal hyperplasia; no neutrophil exocytosis
Parapsoriasis	Variable epidermal hyperplasia; the superficial perivascular or band-like infiltrate involves the papillary dermis ('spills upwards'); some exocytosis/epidermotropism; probably represents early cutaneous lymphoma
Lichen simplex chronicus	Conspicuous psoriasiform hyperplasia, sometimes irregular; prominent granular layer with patchy parakeratosis; thick suprapapillary epidermal plates; thick collagen in vertical streaks in papillary dermis; variable inflammatory infiltrate and plump fibroblasts
Chronic spongiotic dermatitides	Progressive psoriasiform hyperplasia, usually with diminishing spongiosis eventually merging with picture of lichen simplex chronicus; chronic nummular lesions 'untidy' with mild exocytosis; eosinophils may be present in nummular and allergic contact lesions; chronic seborrheic dermatitis may mimic psoriasis but no neutrophils, less hyperplasia and sometimes perifollicular parakeratosis
Erythroderma	Variable psoriasiform hyperplasia; usually focal spongiosis; no distinguishing features
Mycosis fungoides	Epidermotropism; papillary dermal infiltrate of lymphocytes with variable cytological atypia
Chronic candidosis and dermatophytoses	Psoriasiform hyperplasia not as regular or as marked as in psoriasis; spongiform pustules or neutrophils in parakeratotic scale; fungal elements may be sparse in candidosis.
ILVEN	Papillated psoriasiform hyperplasia with foci of parakeratosis overlying hypogranulosis; often focal mild spongiosis; may have alternating orthokeratosis and parakeratosis in a horizontal direction
Norwegian scabies	Marked orthokeratosis and scale crust; numerous mites, larvae and ova in the keratinous layer
Bowen's disease (psoriasiform type)	Full thickness atypia of keratinocytes but basal layer sometimes spared; cells sometimes pale staining
Clear cell acanthoma	Pallor of keratinocytes but no atypia; abundant glycogen; some exocytosis of inflammatory cells
Lamellar ichthyosis	Mild psoriasiform hyperplasia with a thick compact or laminated orthokeratin layer overlying a prominent granular layer
Pityriasis rosea (herald patch)	Mild psoriasiform hyperplasia; spongiosis and exocytosis of lymphocytes leading to 'mini-Pautrier simulants'; focal parakeratosis
Pellagra, acrodermatitis enteropathica and glucagonoma syndrome	Mild to moderate psoriasiform hyperplasia; the upper epidermis shows pallor and ballooning progressing sometimes to necrosis, vesiculation or pustulation (not in pellagra); confluent parakeratosis overlying these changes; many cases of pellagra show mild, even non-specific changes
Secondary syphilis	Superficial and deep dermal infiltrate which often includes plasma cells; may have lichenoid changes or granuloma formation in late stages

REFERENCES

Introduction

1 Pinkus H, Mehregan AH. The primary histologic lesions of seborrheic dermatitis and psoriasis. J Invest Dermatol 1966; 46: 109–116.
2 Barr RJ, Young EM Jr. Psoriasiform and related papulosquamous disorders. J Cutan Pathol 1985; 12: 412–425.

Major psoriasiform dermatoses

3 Watson W. Psoriasis: epidemiology and genetics. Dermatol Clin 1984; 2: 363–371.
4 Bell LM, Sedlack R, Beard CM et al. Incidence of psoriasis in Rochester, Minn, 1980–1933. Arch Dermatol 1991; 127: 1184–1137.
5 Christophers E. Psoriasis – epidemiology and clinical spectrum. Clin Exp Dermatol 2001; 26: 314–320.
6 Krueger GG, Eyre RW. Trigger factors in psoriasis. Dermatol Clin 1984; 2: 373–381.
7 Swanbeck G, Inerot A, Martinsson T, Wahlstrom J. A population genetic study of psoriasis. Br J Dermatol 1994; 131: 32–39.
8 Elder JT, Nair RP, Guo S-W et al. The genetics of psoriasis. Arch Dermatol 1994; 130: 216–224.
9 Krueger GG, Duvic M. Epidemiology of psoriasis: clinical issues. J Invest Dermatol 1994; 102: 14S–18S.
10 Enerbäck C, Enlund F, Inerot A et al. S gene (corneodesmosin) diversity and its relationship to psoriasis: high content of cSNP in the HLA-linked S gene. J Invest Dermatol 2000; 114: 1158–1163.

11 Duffy DL, Spelman LS, Martin NG. Psoriasis in Australian twins. J Am Acad Dermatol 1993; 29: 428–434.
12 Stern RS. Epidemiology of psoriasis. Dermatol Clin 1995; 13: 717–722.
13 Burden AD, Javed S, Bailey M et al. Genetics of psoriasis: paternal inheritance and a locus on chromosome 6p. J Invest Dermatol 1998; 110: 958–960.
14 Capon F, Novelli G, Semprini S et al. Searching for psoriasis susceptibility genes in Italy: genome scan and evidence for a new locus of chromosome 1. J Invest Dermatol 1999; 112: 32–35.
15 Balendran N, Clough RL, Arguello JR et al. Characterization of the major susceptibility region for psoriasis at chromosome 6p21.3. Int J Dermatol 1999; 113: 322–328.
16 Barker JNWN. The genes that cause psoriasis. Clin Exp Dermatol 2000; 25: 165–166.
17 Nair RP, Stuart P, Henseler T et al. Localization of psoriasis-susceptibility locus PSORS1 to a 60-kb interval telomeric to HLA-C. Am J Hum Genet 2000; 66: 1833–1844.
18 Gonzalez S, Martinez-Borra J, Sanchez del Río J et al. The OTF3 gene polymorphism confers susceptibility to psoriasis independent of the association of HLA-Cw*0602. J Invest Dermatol 2000; 115: 824–828.
19 Barker JNWN. Genetic aspects of psoriasis. Clin Exp Dermatol 2001; 26: 321–325.
20 Burden AD. Identifying a gene for psoriasis on chromosome 6 (Psors 1). Br J Dermatol 2000; 143: 238–241.
21 Veal CD, Clough RL, Barber RC et al. Identification of a novel psoriasis susceptibility locus at 1p and evidence of epistasis between PSORS1 and candidate loci. J Med Genet 2001; 38: 7–13.
22 Cheng L, Zhang SZ, Xiao CY et al. The A5.1 allele of the major histocompatibility complex class I chain-related gene A is associated with psoriasis vulgaris in Chinese. Br J Dermatol 2000; 143: 324–329.

23 Tiilikainen A, Lassus A, Karvonen J et al. Psoriasis and HLA-CW6. Br J Dermatol 1980; 102: 179–184.

24 Elder JT, Nair RP, Voorhees JJ. Epidemiology and the genetics of psoriasis. J Invest Dermatol 1994; 102: 24S–27S.

25 Mallon E, Young D, Bunce M et al. HLA-Cw*0602 and HIV-associated psoriasis. Br J Dermatol 1998; 139: 527–533.

26 Mallon E, Bunce M, Wojnarowska F, Welsh K. HLA-CW*0602 is a susceptibility factor in type 1 psoriasis, and evidence A1a-73 is increased in male type 1 psoriatics. J Invest Dermatol 1997; 109: 183–186.

27 Mallon E, Bunce M, Savoie H et al. HLA-C and guttate psoriasis. Br J Dermatol 2000; 143: 1177–1182.

28 Fry L. Psoriasis. Br J Dermatol 1988; 119: 445–461.

29 Gupta MA, Gupta AK, Kirkby S et al. Pruritus in psoriasis. Arch Dermatol 1988; 124: 1052–1057.

30 Van der Kerkhof PCM. Clinical features. In: Mier PD, van der Kerkhof PCM, eds. Textbook of psoriasis. Edinburgh: Churchill Livingstone, 1986; 13–39.

31 Boisseau-Garsaud A-M, Beylot-Barry M, Doutre M-S et al. Psoriatic onycho-pachydermo-periostitis. Arch Dermatol 1996; 132: 176–180.

32 Bardazzi F, Fanti PA, Orlandi C et al. Psoriatic scarring alopecia: observations in four patients. Int J Dermatol 1999; 38: 765–768.

33 Cockayne SE, Messenger AG. Familial scarring alopecia associated with scalp psoriasis. Br J Dermatol 2001; 144: 425–427.

34 Baumal A, Kantor I, Sachs P. Psoriasis of the lips. Report of a case. Arch Dermatol 1961; 84: 185–187.

35 Rudolph RI, Rudolph LP. Intraoral psoriasis vulgaris. Int J Dermatol 1975; 14: 101–104

36 Mallon E, Hawkins D, Dinneen M et al. Circumcision and genital dermatoses. Arch Dermatol 2000; 136: 350–354.

37 Böhm M, Riemann B, Luger TA, Bonsmann G. Bilateral upper limb lymphoedema associated with psoriatic arthritis: a case report and review of the literature. Br J Dermatol 2000; 143: 1297–1301.

38 Koransky JS, Roenigk HH Jr. Vitiligo and psoriasis. J Am Acad Dermatol 1982; 7: 183–189.

39 Fordham JN, Storey GO. Psoriasis and gout. Postgrad Med J 1982; 58: 477–480.

40 Henseler T, Christophers E. Disease concomitance in psoriasis. J Am Acad Dermatol 1995; 32: 982–986.

41 Menni S, Restano L, Gianotti R, Boccardi D. Inflammatory linear verrucous epidermal nevus (ILVEN) and psoriasis in a child? Int J Dermatol 2000; 39: 30–32.

42 Gonzaga HFS, Torres EA, Alchorne MMA, Gerbase-Delima M. Both psoriasis and benign migratory glossitis are associated with HLA-Cw6. Br J Dermatol 1996; 135: 368–370.

43 Plozzer C, Coletti C, Kokelj F, Trevisan G. Scanning electron microscopy study of hair shaft disorders in psoriasis. Acta Derm Venereol 2000; suppl 211: 9–11.

44 Michaëlsson G, Gerdén B, Hagforsen E et al. Psoriasis patients with antibodies to gliadin can be improved by a gluten-free diet. Br J Dermatol 2000; 142: 44–51.

45 Chalmers RJG, Kirby B. Gluten and psoriasis. Br J Dermatol 2000; 142: 5–7.

46 Yates VM, Watkinson G, Kelman A. Further evidence for an association between psoriasis, Crohn's disease and ulcerative colitis. Br J Dermatol 1982; 106: 323–330.

47 Grunwald MH, David M, Feuerman EJ. Coexistence of psoriasis vulgaris and bullous diseases. J Am Acad Dermatol 1985; 13: 224–228.

48 Chen K-R, Shimizu S, Miyakawa S et al. Coexistence of psoriasis and an unusual IgG-mediated subepidermal bullous dermatosis: identification of a novel 200-kDa lower lamina lucida target antigen. Br J Dermatol 1996; 134: 340–346.

49 Endo Y, Tamura A, Ishikawa O et al. Psoriasis vulgaris coexistent with epidermolysis bullosa acquisita. Br J Dermatol 1997; 137: 783–786.

50 Patterson JW, Graff GE, Eubanks SW. Perforating folliculitis and psoriasis. J Am Acad Dermatol 1982; 7: 369–376.

51 Baselga E, Puig L, Llobet J et al. Linear psoriasis associated with systemic lupus erythematosus. J Am Acad Dermatol 1994; 30: 130–133.

52 Han M-H, Jang K-A, Sung K-J et al. A case of guttate psoriasis following Kawasaki disease. Br J Dermatol 2000; 142: 548–550.

53 Sánchez Regaña M, Umbert Millet P. Psoriasis in association with prolactinoma: three cases. Br J Dermatol 2000; 143: 864–867.

54 Hardman CM, Baker BS, Lortan J et al. Active psoriasis and profound CD4+ lymphocytopenia. Br J Dermatol 1997; 136: 930–932.

55 Paslin DA. Psoriasis on scars. Arch Dermatol 1973; 108: 665–666.

56 Hannuksela-Svahn A, Pukkala E, Läärä E et al. Psoriasis, its treatment, and cancer in a cohort of Finnish patients. J Invest Dermatol 2000; 114: 587–590.

57 Margolis D, Bilker W, Hennessy S et al. The risk of malignancy associated with psoriasis. Arch Dermatol 2001; 137: 778–783.

58 Christophers E, Henseler T. Characterization of disease patterns in nonpustular psoriasis. Semin Dermatol 1985; 4: 271–275.

59 Swanbeck G, Inerot A, Martinsson T et al. Age at onset and different types of psoriasis. Br J Dermatol 1995; 133: 768–773.

60 Choi YJ, Hann SK, Chang S-N, Park W-H. Infantile psoriasis: successful treatment with topical calcipotriol. Pediatr Dermatol 2000; 17: 242–244.

61 Raychaudhuri SP, Gross J. A comparative study of pediatric onset psoriasis with adult onset psoriasis. Pediatr Dermatol 2000; 17: 174–178.

62 Nyfors A, Lemholt K. Psoriasis in children. A short review and a survey of 245 cases. Br J Dermatol 1975; 92: 437–442.

63 Lerner MR, Lerner AB. Congenital psoriasis. Report of three cases. Arch Dermatol 1972; 105: 598–601.

64 Farber EM, Mullen RH, Jacobs AH, Nall L. Infantile psoriasis: a follow-up study. Pediatr Dermatol 1986; 3: 237–243.

65 Lowe NJ. Psoriasis. Semin Dermatol 1988; 7: 43–47.

66 Wahl A, Loge JH, Wiklund I, Hanestad BR. The burden of psoriasis: a study concerning health-related quality of life among Norwegian adult patients with psoriasis compared with general population norms. J Am Acad Dermatol 2000; 43: 803–808.

67 Whyte HJ, Baughman RD. Acute guttate psoriasis and streptococcal infection. Arch Dermatol 1964; 89: 350–356.

68 Wilson AGMcT, Clark I, Heard SR et al. Immunoblotting of streptococcal antigens in guttate psoriasis. Br J Dermatol 1993; 128: 151–158.

69 Telfer NR, Chalmers RJG, Whale K, Colmar G. The role of streptococcal infection in the initiation of guttate psoriasis. Arch Dermatol 1992; 128: 39–42.

70 Christophers E, Kiene P. Guttate and plaque psoriasis. Dermatol Clin 1995; 13: 751–756.

71 Baker BS, Bokth S, Powles A et al. Group A streptococcal antigen-specific T lymphocytes in guttate psoriatic lesions. Br J Dermatol 1993; 128: 493–499.

72 Beylot C, Puissant A, Bioulac P et al. Particular clinical features of psoriasis in infants and children. Acta Derm Venereol (Suppl) 1979; 87: 95–97.

73 Boyd AS, Menter A. Erythrodermic psoriasis. Precipitating factors, course and prognosis in 50 patients. J Am Acad Dermatol 1989; 21: 985–991.

74 Prystowsky JH, Cohen PR. Pustular and erythrodermic psoriasis. Dermatol Clin 1995; 13: 757–770.

75 Salleras M, Sanchez-Regaña M, Umbert P. Congenital erythrodermic psoriasis: case report and literature review. Pediatr Dermatol 1995; 12: 231–234.

76 Kerl H, Pachinger W. Psoriasis: odd varieties in the adult. Acta Derm Venereol (Suppl) 1979; 87: 90–94.

77 Atherton DJ, Kahana M, Russell-Jones R. Naevoid psoriasis. Br J Dermatol 1989; 120: 837–841.

78 Ros A-M. Photosensitive psoriasis. Semin Dermatol 1992; 11: 267–268.

79 Stankler L, Ewen SWB. Follicular psoriasis. Br J Dermatol 1981; 104: 153–156.

80 Ploysangam T, Mutasim DF. Follicular psoriasis: an under-reported entity. A report of five cases. Br J Dermatol 1997; 137: 988–991.

81 Lucky PA, Carter DM. Psoriasis presenting as cutaneous horns. J Am Acad Dermatol 1981; 5: 681–683.

82 Chang SE, Choi JH, Koh JK. Congenital erythrodermic psoriasis. Br J Dermatol 1999; 140: 538–539.

83 Murakami T, Ohtsuki M, Nakagawa H. Rupioid psoriasis with arthropathy. Clin Exp Dermatol 2000; 25: 409–412.

84 Erkek E, Bozdoğan Ö. Annular verrucous psoriasis with exaggerated papillomatosis. Am J Dermatopathol 2001; 23: 133–135.

85 Jablonska S, Blaszczyk M, Kozlowska A. Erythema gyratum repens-like psoriasis. Int J Dermatol 2000; 39: 695–697.

86 Al-Fouzan AS, Hassab-El-Naby HMM, Nanda A. Congenital linear psoriasis: a case report. Pediatr Dermatol 1990; 7: 303–306.

87 Neville EA, Finn OA. Psoriasiform napkin dermatitis – a follow-up study. Br J Dermatol 1975; 92: 279–285.

88 Patrizi A, Bardazzi F, Neri I, Fanti PA. Psoriasiform acral dermatitis: a peculiar clinical presentation of psoriasis in children. Pediatr Dermatol 1999; 16: 439–443.

89 Henderson CA, Highet AS. Acute psoriasis associated with Lancefield Group C and Group G cutaneous streptococcal infections. Br J Dermatol 1988; 118: 559–562.

90 Funk J, Langeland T, Schrumpf E, Hanssen LE. Psoriasis induced by interferon-α. Br J Dermatol 1991; 125: 463–465.

91 Higgins E. Alcohol, smoking and psoriasis. Clin Exp Dermatol 2000; 25: 107–110.

92 Bhate SM, Sharpe GR, Marks JM et al. Prevalence of skin and other cancers in patients with psoriasis. Clin Exp Dermatol 1993; 18: 401–404.

93 Hughes BR, Cotterill JA. The relationship of psoriasis to malignancy: a clinical report. Clin Exp Dermatol 1993; 18: 41–44.

94 Farber EM, Rein G, Lanigan SW. Stress and psoriasis. Psychoimmunologic mechanisms. Int J Dermatol 1991; 30: 8–10.

95 Boyd AS, Morris LF, Phillips CM, Menter MA. Psoriasis and pregnancy: hormone and immune system interaction. Int J Dermatol 1996; 35: 169–172.

96 Melski JW, Bernhard JD, Stern RS. The Koebner (isomorphic) response in psoriasis. Arch Dermatol 1983; 119: 655–659.

97 Abel EA. Diagnosis of drug-induced psoriasis. Semin Dermatol 1992; 11: 269–274.

98 Skott A, Mobacken H, Starmark JE. Exacerbation of psoriasis during lithium treatment. Br J Dermatol 1977; 96: 445–448.

99 Sarantidis D, Waters B. A review and controlled study of cutaneous conditions associated with lithium carbonate. Br J Psychiatry 1983; 143: 42–50.

100 Harwell WB. Quinidine-induced psoriasis. J Am Acad Dermatol 1983; 9: 278.

101 Redondo P, Vázquez-Doval J. Carbamazepine and psoriasis. J Am Acad Dermatol 1998; 39: 808–809.

102 Brenner S, Golan H, Lerman Y. Psoriasiform eruption and anticonvulsant drugs. Acta Derm Venereol 2000; 80: 382.

103 Ascari-Raccagni A, Baldari U, Rossi E, Alessandrini F. Exacerbation of chronic large plaque psoriasis associated with olanzapine therapy. J Eur Acad Dermatol Venereol 2000; 14: 315–316.

104 Gupta AK, Sibbald RG, Knowles SR et al. Terbinafine therapy may be associated with the development of psoriasis de novo or its exacerbation: Four case reports and a review of drug-induced psoriasis. J Am Acad Dermatol 1997; 36: 858–862.

105 Pauluzzi P, Boccucci N. Inverse psoriasis induced by terbinafine. Acta Derm Venereo 1999; 79: 389.

106 Gold MH, Holy AK, Roenigk HH Jr. Beta-blocking drugs and psoriasis. J Am Acad Dermatol 1988; 19: 837–841.

107 Gawkrodger DJ, Beveridge GW. Psoriasiform reaction to atenolol. Clin Exp Dermatol 1984; 9: 92–94.

108 Harrison PV, Stones RN. Severe exacerbation of psoriasis due to terfenadine. Clin Exp Dermatol 1988; 13: 275.

109 Wolfe JT, Singh A, Lessin SR et al. De novo development of psoriatic plaques in patients receiving interferon alfa for treatment of erythrodermic cutaneous T-cell lymphoma. J Am Acad Dermatol 1995; 32: 887–893.

110 Lee RE, Gaspari AA, Lotze MT et al. Interleukin 2 and psoriasis. Arch Dermatol 1988; 124: 1811–1815.

111 Gilleaudeau P, Vallat VP, Carter DM, Gottlieb AB. Angiotensin-converting enzyme inhibitors as possible exacerbating drugs in psoriasis. J Am Acad Dermatol 1993; 28: 490–492.

112 Steinkraus V, Steinfath M, Mensing H. β-adrenergic blocking drugs and psoriasis. J Am Acad Dermatol 1992; 27: 266–267.

113 Mayama M, Hirayama K, Nakano H et al. Psoriasiform drug eruption induced by fluorescein sodium used for fluorescein angiography. Br J Dermatol 1999; 140: 982–984.

114 Goh CL. Psoriasiform drug eruption due to glibenclamide. Australas J Dermatol 1987; 28: 30–32.

115 Valance A, Lebrun-Vignes B, Descamps V et al. Icodextrin cutaneous hypersensitivity. Report of 3 psoriasiform cases. Arch Dermatol 2001; 137: 309–310.

116 Wach F, Stolz W, Hein R, Landthaler M. Severe erythema annulare centrifugum-like psoriatic drug eruption induced by terbinafine. Arch Dermatol 1995; 131: 960–961.

117 Kirby B, Griffiths CEM. Psoriasis: the future. Br J Dermatol 2001; 144 (Suppl 58): 37–43.

118 Griffiths TW, Griffiths CEM, Voorhees JJ. Immunopathogenesis and immunotherapy of psoriasis. Dermatol Clin 1995; 13: 739–749.

119 Kaduce DP, Krueger GG. Pathogenesis of psoriasis. Current concepts. Dermatol Clin 1995; 13: 723–737.

120 Nickoloff BJ. The cytokine network in psoriasis. Arch Dermatol 1991; 127: 871–884.

121 Iizuka H, Takahashi H. Psoriasis, involucrin, and protein kinase C. Int J Dermatol 1993 32: 333–338.

122 Venneker GT, Das PK, Meinardi MMHM et al. Glycosylphosphatidylinositol (GPI)-anchored membrane proteins are constitutively down-regulated in psoriatic skin. J Pathol 1994 172: 189–197.

123 Creamer JD, Barker JNWN. Vascular proliferation and angiogenic factors in psoriasis. Clin Exp Dermatol 1995; 20: 6–9.

124 Goodfield M, Macdonald Hull S, Holland D et al. Investigations of the 'active' edge of plaque psoriasis: vascular proliferation precedes changes in epidermal keratin. Br J Dermatol 1994; 131: 808–813.

125 Van de Kerkhof PCM, Gerritsen MJP, De Jong EMGJ. Transition from symptomless to lesional psoriatic skin. Clin Exp Dermatol 1996; 21: 325–329.

126 Lowe PM, Lee M-L, Jackson CJ et al. The endothelium in psoriasis. Br J Dermatol 1995; 132: 497–505.

127 Sweet WL, Smoller BR. Differential proliferation of endothelial cells and keratinocytes in psoriasis and spongiotic dermatitis. J Cutan Pathol 1997; 24: 356–363.

128 Bacharach-Buhles M, El Gammal S, Panz B, Altmeyer P. In psoriasis the epidermis, including the subepidermal vascular plexus, grows downwards into the dermis. Br J Dermatol 1997; 136: 97–101.

129 Griffiths CEM. Cutaneous leukocyte trafficking and psoriasis. Arch Dermatol 1994; 130: 494–499.

130 Wakita H, Takigawa M. E-selectin and vascular cell adhesion molecule-1 are critical for initial trafficking of helper-inducer/memory T cells in psoriatic plaques. Arch Dermatol 1994; 130: 457–463.

131 Jeffes EWB III, Lee GC, Said S et al. Elevated numbers of proliferating mononuclear cells in the peripheral blood of psoriatic patients correlate with disease severity. J Invest Dermatol 1995; 105: 733–738.

132 Chin Y-H, Falanga V, Taylor JR et al. Adherence of human helper/memory T-cell subsets to psoriatic dermal endothelium. J Invest Dermatol 1990; 94: 413–417.

133 Takematsu H, Tagami H. Quantification of chemotactic peptides (C5a anaphylatoxin and IL-8) in psoriatic lesional skin. Arch Dermatol 1993; 129: 74–80.

134 Horrocks C, Holder JE, Berth-Jones J, Camp RDR. Antigen-independent expansion of T cells from psoriatic skin lesions: phenotypic characterization and antigen reactivity. Br J Dermatol 1997; 137: 331–338.

135 Sánchez-Regaña M, Catasús M, Creus L, Umbert P. Serum neopterin as an objective marker of psoriatic disease activity. Acta Derm Venereol 2000; 80: 185–187.

136 Chang JCC, Smith LR, Froning KJ et al. Persistence of T-cell clones in psoriatic lesions. Arch Dermatol 1997; 133: 703–708.

137 Prinz JC. Which T cells cause psoriasis? Clin Exp Dermatol 1999; 24: 291–295.

138 Austin LM, Ozawa M, Kikuchi T et al. The majority of epidermal T cells in psoriasis vulgaris lesions can produce type 1 cytokines, interferon-γ, interleukin-2, and tumor necrosis factor-α, defining TC1 (cytotoxic T lymphocyte) and TH1 effector populations: a type 1 differentiation bias is also measured in circulating blood T cells in psoriatic patients. J Invest Dermatol 1999; 113: 752–759.

139 Nickoloff BJ. The immunologic and genetic basis of psoriasis. Arch Dermatol 1999; 135: 1104–1110.

140 Austin LM, Coven TR, Bhardwaj N et al. Intraepidermal lymphocytes in psoriatic lesions are activated GMP-17(TIA-1)+ CD8+ CD3+ CTLs as determined by phenotypic analysis. J Cutan Pathol 1998; 25: 79–88.

141 Gottlieb AB. Immunopathogenesis of psoriasis. The road from bench to bedside is a 2-way street. Arch Dermatol 1997; 133: 781–782.

142 Davison S, Allen M, Harmer A et al. Increased T-cell receptor Vβ2 chain expression in skin homing lymphocytes in psoriasis. Br J Dermatol 1999; 140: 845–848.

143 Peñas PF, Gómez M, Buezo GF et al. Differential expression of activation epitopes of β1 integrins in psoriasis and normal skin. J Invest Dermatol 1998; 111: 19–24.

144 Petzelbauer P, Pober JS, Keh A, Braverman IM. Inducibility and expression of microvascular endothelial adhesion molecules in lesional, perilesional, and uninvolved skin of psoriatic patients. J Invest Dermatol 1994; 103: 300–305.

145 Cai J-P, Harris K, Falanga V et al. UVB therapy decreases the adhesive interaction between peripheral blood mononuclear cells and dermal microvascular endothelium, and regulates the differential expression of CD54, VCAM-1, and E-selectin in psoriatic plaques. Br J Dermatol 1996; 134: 7–16.

146 Szepietowski J, Wasik F, Bielicka E et al. Soluble E-selectin serum levels correlate with disease activity in psoriatic patients. Clin Exp Dermatol 1999; 24: 33–36.

147 Chang EY, Hammerberg C, Fisher G et al. T-cell activation is potentiated by cytokines released by lesional psoriatic, but not normal, epidermis. Arch Dermatol 1992; 128: 1479–1485.

148 Veale D, Rogers S, Fitzgerald O. Immunolocalization of adhesion molecules in psoriatic arthritis, psoriatic and normal skin. Br J Dermatol 1995; 132: 32–38.

149 Strange P, Cooper KD, Hansen ER et al. T-lymphocyte clones initiated from lesional psoriatic skin release growth factors that induce keratinocyte proliferation. J Invest Dermatol 1993; 101: 695–700.

150 Schröder J-M, Gregory H, Young J, Christophers E. Neutrophil-activating proteins in psoriasis. J Invest Dermatol 1992; 98: 241–247.

151 Kulke R, Todt-Pingel I, Rademacher D et al. Co-localized overexpression of GRO-α and Il-8 mRNA is restricted to the suprapapillary layers of psoriatic lesions. J Invest Dermatol 1996; 106: 526–530.

152 McMenamin ME, Sweeney EC. Psoriasis and eczema. Curr Diagn Pathol 1997; 4: 20–27.

153 Prens EP, Van Joost Th, Hegmans JPJJ et al. Effects of cyclosporine on cytokines and cytokine receptors in psoriasis. J Am Acad Dermatol 1995; 33: 947–953.

154 Rappersberger K, Meingasner JG, Fialla R et al. Clearing of psoriasis by a novel immunosuppressive macrolide. J Invest Dermatol 1996; 106: 701–710.

155 Bonifati C, Ameglio F. Cytokines in psoriasis. Int J Dermatol 1999; 38: 241–251.

156 Ackermann L, Harvima IT, Pelkonen J et al. Mast cells in psoriatic skin are strongly positive for interferon-gamma. Br J Dermatol 1999; 140: 624–633.

157 Kulke R, Bornscheuer E, Schlüter C et al. The CXC receptor 2 is overexpressed in psoriatic epidermis. J Invest Dermatol 1998; 110: 90–94.

158 Champion RH. Psoriasis. Br Med J 1986; 292: 1693–1696.

159 Bos JD. The pathomechanisms of psoriasis; the skin immune system and cyclosporin. Br J Dermatol 1988; 118: 141–155.

160 Watts P, Stables GS, Akhurst RJ, MacKie RM. Localization of transforming growth factor-alpha RNA and protein in the skin of psoriatic patients receiving therapy. Br J Dermatol 1994; 131: 64–71.

161 Leivo T, Leivo I, Kariniemi A-L et al. Down-regulation of transforming growth factor-β receptors I and II is seen in lesional but not non-lesional psoriatic epidermis. Br J Dermatol 1998; 138: 57–62.

162 Piepkorn M. Overexpression of amphiregulin, a major autocrine growth factor for cultured human keratinocytes, in hyperproliferative skin diseases. Am J Dermatopathol 1996; 18: 165–171.

163 Nanney LB, Yates RA, King LE Jr. Modulation of epidermal growth factor receptors in psoriatic lesions during treatment with topical EGF. J Invest Dermatol 1992; 98: 296–301.

164 Bianchi L, Farrace MG, Nini G, Piacentini M. Abnormal bcl-2 and 'tissue' transglutaminase expression in psoriatic skin. J Invest Dermatol 1994; 103: 829–833.

165 Nickoloff BJ. Creation of psoriatic plaques: the ultimate tumor suppressor pathway. A new model for an ancient T-cell-mediated skin disease. Viewpoint. J Cutan Pathol 2001; 28: 57–64.

166 Leigh IM, Navsaria H, Purkis PE et al. Keratins (K16 and K17) as markers of keratinocyte hyperproliferation in psoriasis in vivo and in vitro. Br J Dermatol 1995; 133: 501–511.

167 Mommers JM, van Rossum MM, van Erp PEJ, van de Kerkhof PCM. Changes in keratin 6 and keratin 10 (co-)expression in lesional and symptomless skin of spreading psoriasis. Dermatology 2000; 201: 15–20.

168 Ishida-Yamamoto A, Senshu T, Takahashi H et al. Decreased deiminated keratin K1 in psoriatic hyperproliferative epidermis. J Invest Dermatol 2000; 114: 701–705.

169 Pérez-Lorenzo R, Zambrano-Zaragoza JF, Saul A et al. Autoantibodies to autologous skin in guttate and plaque forms of psoriasis and cross-reaction of skin antigens with streptococcal antigens. Int J Dermatol 1998; 37: 524–531.

170 Nickoloff BJ, Wrone-Smith T. Superantigens, autoantigens, and pathogenic T cells in psoriasis. J Invest Dermatol 1998; 110: 459–460.

171 Boehncke W-H, Zollner TM, Dressel D, Kaufmann R. Induction of psoriasiform inflammation by a bacterial superantigen in the SCID-hu xenogeneic transplantation model. J Cutan Pathol 1997; 24: 1–7.

172 Fry L. Role of microbes in psoriasis. Clin Exp Dermatol 2000; 25: 164.

173 Jappe U. Superantigens and their association with dermatological inflammatory diseases: facts and hypotheses. Acta Derm Venereol 2000; 80: 321–328.

174 Prinz JC. Psoriasis vulgaris – a sterile antibacterial skin reaction mediated by cross-reactive T cells? An immunological view of the pathophysiology of psoriasis. Clin Exp Dermatol 2001; 26: 326–332.

175 Leung DYM, Walsh P, Giorno R, Norris DA. A potential role for superantigens in the pathogenesis of psoriasis. J Invest Dermatol 1993; 100: 225–228.

176 Skov L, Baadsgaard O. Bacterial superantigens and inflammatory skin diseases. Clin Exp Dermatol 2000; 25: 57–61.

177 Herbst RA, Hoch O, Kapp A, Weiss J. Guttate psoriasis triggered by perianal streptococcal dermatitis in a four-year-old boy. J Am Acad Dermatol 2000; 42: 885–887.

178 Naldi L, Peli L, Parazzini F et al. Family history of psoriasis, stressful life events, and recent infectious disease are risk factors for a first episode of acute guttate psoriasis: Results of a case-control study. J Am Acad Dermatol 2001; 44: 433–438.

179 Horiuchi N, Aiba S, Ozawa H et al. Peripheral blood lymphocytes from psoriatic patients are hyporesponsive to β-streptococcal superantigens. Br J Dermatol 1998; 138: 229–235.

180 Brown DW, Baker BS, Ovigne J-M et al. Skin CD4+ T cells produce interferon-γ in vitro in response to streptococcal antigens in chronic plaque psoriasis. J Invest Dermatol 2000; 114: 576–580.

181 Sayama K, Midorikawa K, Hanakawa Y et al. Superantigen production by Staphylococcus aureus in psoriasis. Dermatology 1998; 196: 194–198.

182 Favre M, Majewski S, Noszczyk B et al. Antibodies to human papillomavirus type 5 are generated in epidermal repair processes. J Invest Dermatol 2000; 114: 403–407.

183 Asadullah K, Prösch S, Audring H et al. A high prevalence of cytomegalovirus antigenaemia in patients with moderate to severe chronic plaque psoriasis: an association with systemic tumour necrosis factor α overexpression. Br J Dermatol 1999; 141: 94–102.

184 Kirby B, Al-Jiffri O, Cooper RJ et al. Investigation of cytomegalovirus and human herpes viruses 6 and 7 as possible causative antigens in psoriasis. Acta Derm Venereol 2000; 80: 404–406.

185 Puig L, Fernández-Figueras MT, Ferrándiz C et al. Epidermal expression of 65 and 72 kd heat shock proteins in psoriasis and AIDS-associated psoriasiform dermatitis. J Am Acad Dermatol 1995; 33: 985–989.

186 Pike MC, Lee CS, Elder JT et al. Increased phosphatidylinositol kinase activity in psoriatic epidermis. J Invest Dermatol 1989; 92: 791–797.

187 Ryborg AK, Gron B, Kragballe K. Increased lysophosphatidylcholine content in lesional psoriatic skin. Br J Dermatol 1995; 134: 398–402.

188 Gottlieb AB. Immunologic mechanisms in psoriasis. J Am Acad Dermatol 1988; 18: 1376–1380.

189 Labarthe M-P, Bosco D, Saurat J-H et al. Upregulation of connexin 26 between keratinocytes of psoriatic lesions. J Invest Dermatol 1998; 111: 72–76.

190 Fleischmajer R, Kuroda K, Hazan R et al. Basement membrane alterations in psoriasis are accompanied by epidermal overexpression of MMP-2 and its inhibitor TIMP-2. J Invest Dermatol 2000; 115: 771–777.

191 Buisson-Legendre N, Emonard H, Bernard P, Hornebeck W. Relationship between cell-associated matrix metalloproteinase 9 and psoriatic keratinocyte growth. J Invest Dermatol 2000; 115: 213–218.

192 Tanaka N, Fujioka A, Tajima S et al. Levels of proelafin peptides in the sera of the patients with generalized pustular psoriasis and pustulosis palmoplantaris. Acta Derm Venereol 2000; 80: 102–105.

193 Raychaudhuri SP, Rein G, Farber EM. Neuropathogenesis and neuropharmacology of psoriasis. Int J Dermatol 1995; 34: 685–693.

194 Weigl BA. Immunoregulatory mechanisms and stress hormones in psoriasis (part 1). Int J Dermatol 1998; 37: 350–357.

195 van de Kerkhof PCM. Neutrophils in psoriasis: cause or effect? Clin Exp Dermatol 2000; 25: 165.

196 Craven NM, Jackson CW, Kirby B et al. Cytokine gene polymorphisms in psoriasis. Br J Dermatol 2001; 144: 849–853.

197 Duvic M, Asano AT, Hager C, Mays S. The pathogenesis of psoriasis and the mechanism of action of tazarotene. J Am Acad Dermatol 1998; 39: S129–S133.

198 Coven TR, Burack LH, Gilleaudeau P et al. Narrowband UV-B produces superior clinical and histopathological resolution of moderate-to-severe psoriasis in patients compared with broadband UV-B. Arch Dermatol 1997; 133: 1514–1522.

199 Laporte M, Galand P, Fokan D et al. Apoptosis in established and healing psoriasis. Dermatology 2000; 200: 314–316.

200 Calzavara-Pinton PG, Zane C, Candiago E, Facchetti F. Blisters on psoriatic lesions treated with TL-01 lamps. Dermatology 2000; 200: 115–119.

201 Rowlands CG, Danby FW. Histopathology of psoriasis treated with zinc pyrithione. Am J Dermatopathol 2000; 22: 272–276.

202 Murphy FP, Coven TR, Burack LH et al. Clinical clearing of psoriasis by 6-thioguanine correlates with cutaneous T-cell depletion via apoptosis. Arch Dermatol 1999; 135: 1495–1502.

203 Mason C, Krueger GG. Thioguanine for refractory psoriasis: a 4-year experience. J Am Acad Dermatol 2001; 44: 67–72.

204 Gottlieb AB, Lebwohl M, Shirin S et al. Anti-CD4 monoclonal antibody treatment of moderate to severe psoriasis vulgaris: Results of a pilot, multicenter, multiple-dose, placebo-controlled study. J Am Acad Dermatol 2000; 43: 595–604.

205 Reichrath J, Horf R, Chen TC et al. Expression of integrin subunits and CD44 isoforms in psoriatic skin and effects of topical calcitriol application. J Cutan Pathol 1997; 24: 499–506.

206 Savoia P, Novelli M, De Matteis A et al. Effects of topical calcipotriol on the expression of adhesion molecules in psoriasis. J Cutan Pathol 1998; 25: 89–94.

207 Rizova E, Corroller M. Topical calcitriol – studies on local tolerance and systemic safety. Br J Dermatol 2001; 144 (Suppl 58): 3–10.

208 Gottlieb SL, Hayes E, Gilleaudeau P et al. Cellular actions of etretinate in psoriasis: enhanced epidermal differentiation and reduced cell-mediated inflammation are unexpected outcomes. J Cutan Pathol 1996; 23: 404–418.

209 Katz HI, Waalen J, Leach EE. Acitretin in psoriasis: An overview of adverse effects. J Am Acad Dermatol 1999; 41: S7–S12.

210 Servitje O, Bordas X, Serón D et al. Changes in T-cell phenotype and adhesion molecules expression in psoriatic lesions after low-dose cyclosporin therapy. J Cutan Pathol 1996; 23: 431–436.

211 Toti P, Pellegrino M, Villanova M et al. Altered expression of the α2 laminin chain in psoriatic skin: the effect of treatment with cyclosporin. Br J Dermatol 1998; 139: 375–379.

212 Miracco C, Pellegrino M, Flori ML et al. Cyclin D1, B and A expression and cell turnover in psoriatic skin lesions before and after cyclosporin treatment. Br J Dermatol 2000; 143: 950–956.

213 Ho VCY, Griffiths CEM, Berth-Jones J et al. Intermittent short courses of cyclosporine microemulsion for the long-term management of psoriasis: A 2-year cohort study. J Am Acad Dermatol 2001; 44: 643–651.

214 Krueger JG, Walters IB, Miyazawa M et al. Successful in vivo blockade of CD25 (high-affinity interleukin 2 receptor) on T cells by administration of humanized anti-Tac antibody to patients with psoriasis. J Am Acad Dermatol 2000; 43: 448–458.

215 Gottlieb A, Krueger JG, Bright R et al. Effects of administration of a single dose of a humanized monoclonal antibody to CD11a on the immunobiology and clinical activity of psoriasis. J Am Acad Dermatol 2000; 42: 428–435.

216 Zelickson BD, Mehregan DA, Wendelschfer-Crabb G et al. Clinical and histologic evaluation of psoriatic plaques treated with a flashlamp pulsed dye laser. J Am Acad Dermatol 1996; 35: 64–68.

217 Ragaz A, Ackerman AB. Evolution, maturation, and regression of lesions of psoriasis. Am J Dermatopathol 1979; 1: 199–214.

218 Gordon M, Johnson WC. Histopathology and histochemistry of psoriasis. I. The active lesion and clinically normal skin. Arch Dermatol 1967; 95: 402–407.

219 Stadler R, Schaumberg-Lever G, Orfanos CE. Histology. In: Mier PD, van de Kerkhof PCM, eds. Textbook of psoriasis. Edinburgh: Churchill Livingstone, 1986; 40–54.

220 Cox AJ, Watson W. Histological variations in lesions of psoriasis. Arch Dermatol 1972; 106: 503–506.

221 Jablonska S, Chowaniec O, Beutner EH et al. Stripping of the stratum corneum in patients with psoriasis. Production of prepinpoint papules and psoriatic lesions. Arch Dermatol 1982; 118: 652–657.

222 Bieber T, Braun-Falco O. Distribution of CD1a-positive cells in psoriatic skin during the evolution of the lesions. Acta Derm Venereol 1989; 69: 175–178.

223 Griffin TD, Lattanand A, Van Scott EJ. Clinical and histologic heterogeneity of psoriatic plaques. Therapeutic relevance. Arch Dermatol 1988; 124: 216–220.

224 De Panfilis G, Manara GC, Ferrari C et al. Further characterization of the 'incipient lesion of chronic stationary type psoriasis vulgaris in exacerbation'. Acta Derm Venereol (Suppl) 1989; 146: 26–30.

225 Lundin A, Fredens K, Michaelsson G, Venge P. The eosinophil granulocyte in psoriasis. Br J Dermatol 1990; 122: 181–193.

226 Horn TD, Herzberg GZ, Hood AF. Characterization of the dermal infiltrate in human immunodeficiency virus-infected patients with psoriasis. Arch Dermatol 1990; 126: 1462–1465.

227 Lee J, Bhawan J, Rothman K. Massive papillary dermal fatty infiltration in a patient with psoriasis. J Cutan Pathol 1995; 22: 182–184.

228 Gottlieb SL, Heftler NS, Gilleaudeau P et al. Short-contact anthralin treatment augments therapeutic efficacy of cyclosporine in psoriasis: a clinical and pathologic study. J Am Acad Dermatol 1995; 33: 637–645.

229 Headington JT, Gupta AK, Goldfarb MT et al. A morphometric and histologic study of the scalp in psoriasis. Arch Dermatol 1989; 125: 639–642.

230 Tomasini C, Aloi F, Solaroli C, Pippione M. Psoriatic erythroderma: a histopathologic study of forty-five patients. Dermatology 1997; 194: 102–106.

231 Maddin WS, Wood WS. Multiple keratoacanthomas and squamous cell carcinoma occurring at psoriatic treatment sites. J Cutan Pathol 1979; 6: 96–100.

232 Kahn JR, Chalet MD, Lowe NJ. Eruptive squamous cell carcinomata following psoralen-UVA phototoxicity. Clin Exp Dermatol 1986; 11: 398–402.

233 Stern RS, Laird N. The carcinogenic risk of treatments for severe psoriasis. Cancer 1994; 73: 2759–2764.

234 Studniberg HM, Weller P. PUVA, UVB, psoriasis and nonmelanoma skin cancer. J Am Acad Dermatol 1993; 29: 1013–1022.

235 Bataille V, Bykov VJ, Sasieni P et al. Photoadaptation to ultraviolet (UV) radiation in vivo: photoproducts in epidermal cells following UVB therapy for psoriasis. Br J Dermatol 2000; 143: 477–483.

236 Pittelkow MR, Perry HO, Muller SA et al. Skin cancer in patients with psoriasis treated with coal tar. Arch Dermatol 1981; 117: 465–468.

237 Gupta AK, Siegel MT, Noble SC et al. Keratoses in patients with psoriasis: a prospective study in fifty-two inpatients. J Am Acad Dermatol 1990; 23: 52–55.

238 Kocsard E. The rarity of solar keratoses in psoriatic patients: preliminary report. Australas J Dermatol 1976; 17: 65–66.

239 Halprin KM, Comerford M, Taylor JR. Cancer in patients with psoriasis. J Am Acad Dermatol 1982; 7: 633–638.

240 Frentz G, Olsen JH. Malignant tumours and psoriasis: a follow-up study. Br J Dermatol 1999; 140: 237–242.

241 Murphy GM. Skin cancer in patients with psoriasis – many intertwined risk factors. Br J Dermatol 1999; 141: 1001–1003.

242 Pearce HP, Braunstein Wilson B. Erosion of psoriatic plaques: An early sign of methotrexate toxicity. J Am Acad Dermatol 1996; 35: 835–838.

243 Kanerva L, Lauharanta J, Niemi K-M, Lassus A. Light and electron microscopy of psoriatic skin before and during retinoid (Ro 10-9359) and retinoid-PUVA treatment. J Cutan Pathol 1982; 9: 175–188.

244 Kanerva L. Electron microscopy of the effects of dithranol on healthy and on psoriatic skin. Am J Dermatopathol 1990; 12: 51–62.

245 Cox NH. Morphological assessment of neutrophil leucocytes in psoriasis. Clin Exp Dermatol 1986; 11: 340–344.

246 Kaplan MH, Sadick NS, Wieder J et al. Antipsoriatic effects of zidovudine in human immunodeficiency virus-associated psoriasis. J Am Acad Dermatol 1989; 20: 76–82.

247 Obuch ML, Maurer TA, Becker B, Berger TG. Psoriasis and human immunodeficiency virus infection. J Am Acad Dermatol 1992; 27: 667–673.

248 Jaffe D, May LP, Sanchez M, Moy J. Staphylococcal sepsis in HIV antibody seropositive psoriasis patients. J Am Acad Dermatol 1991; 24: 970–972.

249 Montazeri A, Kanitakis J, Bazex J. Psoriasis and HIV infection. Int J Dermatol 1996; 35: 475–479.

250 Lyons JH III. Generalized pustular psoriasis. Int J Dermatol 1987; 26: 409–418.

251 Zelickson BD, Muller SA. Generalized pustular psoriasis. A review of 63 cases. Arch Dermatol 1991; 127: 1339–1345.

252 Tay Y-K, Tham S-N. The profile and outcome of pustular psoriasis in Singapore: a report of 28 cases. Int J Dermatol 1997; 36: 266–271.

253 Sauder DN, Steck WD, Bailin PB, Krakauer RS. Lymphocyte kinetics in pustular psoriasis. J Am Acad Dermatol 1981; 4: 458–460.

254 Baker H, Ryan TJ. Generalized pustular psoriasis. A clinical and epidemiological study of 104 cases. Br J Dermatol 1968; 80: 771–793.

255 Stewart AF, Battaglini-Sabetta J, Millstone L. Hypocalcemia-induced pustular psoriasis of von Zumbusch. Ann Intern Med 1984; 100: 677–680.

256 Hubler WR Jr. Lingual lesions of generalized pustular psoriasis. Report of five cases and a review of the literature. J Am Acad Dermatol 1984; 11: 1069–1076.

257 Mackie RM, Burton J. Pustular psoriasis in association with renal amyloidosis. Br J Dermatol 1974; 90: 567–571.

258 Sadeh JS, Rudikoff D, Gordon ML et al. Pustular and erythrodermic psoriasis complicated by acute respiratory distress syndrome. Arch Dermatol 1997; 133: 747–750.

259 Saeki H, Hayashi N, Komine M et al. A case of generalized pustular psoriasis followed by bullous disease: an atypical case of bullous pemphigoid or a novel bullous disease? Br J Dermatol 1996; 134: 152–155.

260 Lotem M, Katzenelson V, Rotem A et al. Impetigo herpetiformis: a variant of pustular psoriasis or a separate entity? J Am Acad Dermatol 1989; 20: 338–341.

261 Lee SH, Hunt MJ, Barnetson R StC. Pustular psoriasis of pregnancy. Australas J Dermatol 1995; 36: 199–200.

262 Rackett SC, Baughman RD. Impetigo herpetiformis and Staphylococcus aureus lymphadenitis in a pregnant adolescent. Pediatr Dermatol 1997; 14: 387–390.

263 Katsambas A, Stavropoulos PG, Katsiboulas V et al. Impetigo herpetiformis during the puerperium. Dermatology 1999; 198: 400–402.

264 Breier-Maly J, Ortel B, Breier F et al. Generalized pustular psoriasis of pregnancy (impetigo herpetiformis). Dermatology 1999; 198: 61–64.

265 Ott F, Krakowski A, Tur E et al. Impetigo herpetiformis with lowered serum level of vitamin D and its diminished intestinal absorption. Dermatologica 1982; 164: 360–365.

266 Beveridge GW, Harkness RA, Livingstone JRB. Impetigo herpetiformis in two successive pregnancies. Br J Dermatol 1966; 78: 106–112.

267 Bajaj AK, Swarup V, Gupta OP, Gupta SC. Impetigo herpetiformis. Dermatologica 1977; 155: 292–295.

268 Oumeish OY, Farraj SE, Bataineh AS. Some aspects of impetigo herpetiformis. Arch Dermatol 1982; 118: 103–105.

269 Moynihan GD, Ruppe JP Jr. Impetigo herpetiformis and hypoparathyroidism. Arch Dermatol 1985; 121: 1330–1331.

270 Thio HB, Vermeer BJ. Hypocalcemia in impetigo herpetiformis: a secondary transient phenomenon? Arch Dermatol 1991; 127: 1587–1588.

271 Holm AL, Goldsmith LA. Impetigo herpetiformis associated with hypocalcemia of congenital rickets. Arch Dermatol 1991; 127: 91–95.

272 Ryan TJ, Baker H. The prognosis of generalized pustular psoriasis. Br J Dermatol 1971; 85: 407–411.

273 Van der Kerkhof PCM, Steijlen PM, Raymarkers RAP. Acrodermatitis continua of Hallopeau in a patient with myelodysplastic syndrome. Br J Dermatol 1996; 134: 754–757.

274 Piraccini BM, Tosti A, Iorizzo M, Misciali C. Pustular psoriasis of the nails: treatment and long-term follow-up of 46 patients. Br J Dermatol 2001; 144: 1000–1005.

275 Matsumura N, Takematsu H, Saijo S et al. Exanthematic type of pustular psoriasis consisting of two types of pustular lesion. Acta Derm Venereol 1991; 71: 442–444.

276 Judge MR, McDonald A, Black MM. Pustular psoriasis in childhood. Clin Exp Dermatol 1993; 18: 97–99.

277 Rosen RM. Annular pustular psoriasis induced by UV radiation from tanning salon use. J Am Acad Dermatol 1991; 25: 336–337.

278 Kanoh H, Ichihashi N, Kamiya H et al. Linear pustular psoriasis that developed in a patient with generalized pustular psoriasis. J Am Acad Dermatol 1998; 39: 635–637.

279 Özkaya-Bayazit E, Akasya E, Büyükbabani N, Baykal C. Pustular psoriasis with a striking linear pattern. J Am Acad Dermatol 2000; 42: 329–331.

280 Whittam LR, Wakelin SH, Barker JNWN. Generalized pustular psoriasis or drug-induced toxic pustuloderma? The use of patch testing. Clin Exp Dermatol 2000; 25: 122–124.

281 Quan MB, Ruben BS. Pustular psoriasis limited to the penis. Int J Dermatol 1996; 35: 202–204.

282 Hubler WR Jr. Familial juvenile generalized pustular psoriasis. Arch Dermatol 1984; 120: 1174–1178.

283 Khan SA, Peterkin GAG, Mitchell PC. Juvenile generalized pustular psoriasis. A report of five cases and a review of the literature. Arch Dermatol 1972; 105: 67–72.

284 McGibbon DH. Infantile pustular psoriasis. Clin Exp Dermatol 1979; 4: 115–118.

285 Ivker RA, Grin-Jorgensen CM, Vega VK et al. Infantile generalized pustular psoriasis associated with lytic lesions of the bone. Pediatr Dermatol 1993; 10: 277–282.

286 Zelickson BD, Muller SA. Generalized pustular psoriasis in childhood. Report of thirteen cases. J Am Acad Dermatol 1991; 24: 186–194.

287 Prose NS, Fahrner LJ, Miller CR, Layfield L. Pustular psoriasis with chronic recurrent multifocal osteomyelitis and spontaneous fractures. J Am Acad Dermatol 1994; 31: 376–379.

288 Li SP-S, Tang WY-M, Lam W-Y, Wong S-N. Renal failure and cholestatic jaundice as unusual complications of childhood pustular psoriasis. Br J Dermatol 2000; 143: 1292–1296.

289 Katz M, Seidenbaum M, Weinrauch L. Penicillin-induced generalized pustular psoriasis. J Am Acad Dermatol 1987; 17: 918–920.

290 Gniadecki R, Petersen CS, Rossen K. Localized pustular psoriasis with onycholysis representing a Köbner phenomenon. Acta Derm Venereol 2000; 80: 208.

291 Finch TM, Tan CY. Pustular psoriasis exacerbated by pregnancy and controlled by cyclosporin A. Br J Dermatol 2000; 142: 582–584.

292 Lowe NJ, Ridgway HB. Generalized pustular psoriasis precipitated by lithium carbonate. Arch Dermatol 1978; 114: 1788–1789.

293 Reshad H, Hargreaves GK, Vickers CFH. Generalized pustular psoriasis precipitated by phenylbutazone and oxyphenbutazone. Br J Dermatol 1983; 108: 111–113.

294 Hu C-H, Miller AC, Peppercorn R, Farber EM. Generalized pustular psoriasis provoked by propanolol. Arch Dermatol 1985; 121: 1326–1327.

295 Mahendran R, Grech C. Generalized pustular psoriasis following a short course of cyclosporin (Neoral). Br J Dermatol 1998; 139: 934.

296 De Silva BD, Benton EC, Tidman MJ. Generalized pustular psoriasis following withdrawal of oral cyclosporin treatment for palmo-plantar pustulosis. Clin Exp Dermatol 1999; 24: 10–13.

297 Papa CA, Miller OF. Pustular psoriasiform eruption with leukocytosis associated with terbinafine. J Am Acad Dermatol 1998; 39: 115–117.

298 Wilson NJE, Evans S. Severe pustular psoriasis provoked by oral terbinafine. Br J Dermatol 1998; 139: 168.

299 Murphy FR, Stolman LP. Generalized pustular psoriasis. Arch Dermatol 1979; 115: 1215–1216.

300 Georgala S, Rigopoulos D, Aroni K, Stratigos JT. Generalized pustular psoriasis precipitated by topical calcipotriol cream. Int J Dermatol 1994; 33: 515–516.

301 Kaminski M, Szmurlo A, Pawinska M, Jablonska S. Decreased natural killer cell activity in generalized pustular psoriasis (von Zumbusch type). Br J Dermatol 1984; 110: 565–568.

302 Ternowitz T, Thestrup-Pedersen K. Neutrophil and monocyte chemotaxis in pustulosis palmo-plantaris and pustular psoriasis. Br J Dermatol 1985; 113: 507–513.

303 Heng MCY, Heng JA, Allen SG. Electron microscopic features in generalized pustular psoriasis. J Invest Dermatol 1987; 89: 187–191.

304 Shelley WB, Kirschbaum JO. Generalized pustular psoriasis. Arch Dermatol 1961; 84: 123–128.

305 Kingery FAJ, Chinn HD, Saunders TS. Generalized pustular psoriasis. Arch Dermatol 1961; 84: 912–919.

306 Neumann E, Hard S. The significance of the epidermal sweat duct unit in the genesis of pustular psoriasis (Zumbusch) and the microabscess of Munro-Sabouraud. Acta Derm Venereol 1974; 54: 141–146.

307 Piérard GE, Piérard-Franchimont C, de la Brassinne M. Impetigo herpetiformis and pustular psoriasis during pregnancy. Am J Dermatopathol 1983; 5: 215–220.

308 Braverman IM, Cohen I, O'Keefe E. Metabolic and ultrastructural studies in a patient with pustular psoriasis (von Zumbusch). Arch Dermatol 1972; 105: 189–196.

309 Keat A. Reiter's syndrome and reactive arthritis in perspective. N Engl J Med 1983; 309: 1606–1615.

310 Calin A. Reiter's syndrome. Med Clin North Am 1977; 61: 365–376.

311 Editorial. Treating Reiter's syndrome. Lancet 1987; 2: 1125–1126.

312 Leirisalo M, Skylv G, Kousa M et al. Followup study on patients with Reiter's disease and reactive arthritis, with special reference to HLA-B27. Arthritis Rheum 1982; 25: 249–259.

313 Bengtsson A, Ahlstrand C, Lindstrom FD, Kihrstrom E. Bacteriological findings in 25 patients with Reiter's syndrome (reactive arthritis). Scand J Rheumatol 1983; 12: 157–160.

314 Keat A, Dixey J, Sonnex C et al. Chlamydia trachomatosis and reactive arthritis: the missing link. Lancet 1987; 1: 72–74.

315 Magro CM, Crowson AN, Peeling R. Vasculitis as the basis of cutaneous lesions in Reiter's disease. Hum Pathol 1995; 26: 633–638.

316 Cleveland MG, Mallory SB. Incomplete Reiter's syndrome induced by systemic interferon α treatment. J Am Acad Dermatol 1993; 29: 788–789.

317 Hart HH, McGuigan LE, Gow PJ, Grigor RR. Reiter's syndrome: chronicity of symptoms and employment. Aust NZ J Med 1986; 16: 452–456.

318 Butler MJ, Russell AS, Percy JS, Lentle BC. A follow-up study of 48 patients with Reiter's syndrome. Am J Med 1979; 67: 808–810.

319 Marks JS, Holt PJL. The natural history of Reiter's disease – 21 years of observations. Q J Med 1986; 60: 685–697.

320 Zivony D, Nocton J, Wortmann D, Esterly N. Juvenile Reiter's syndrome: A report of four cases. J Am Acad Dermatol 1998; 38: 32–37.

321 Williams HC, Du Vivier AWP. Etretinate and AIDS-related Reiter's disease. Br J Dermatol 1991; 124: 389–392.

322 Romaní J, Puig L, Baselga E, De Moragas JM. Reiter's syndrome-like pattern in AIDS-associated psoriasiform dermatitis. Int J Dermatol 1996; 35: 484–488.

323 Callen JP. The spectrum of Reiter's disease. J Am Acad Dermatol 1979; 1: 75–77.

324 Edwards L, Hansen RC. Reiter's syndrome of the vulva. Arch Dermatol 1992; 128: 811–814.

325 Mahmood A, Ackerman AB. Reiter's syndrome is psoriasis! Dermatopathology: Practical & Conceptual 2000; 6: 337–339.

326 Jaramillo D, Leon W, Cardenas V, Cortes A. Reiter's syndrome, immunodepression and strongyloidiasis. J Cutan Pathol 1978; 5: 200–208.

327 Shatin H, Canizares O, Ladany E. Reiter's syndrome and keratosis blennorrhagica. Arch Dermatol 1960; 81: 551–555.

328 Gelmetti C, Schiuma AA, Cerri D, Gianotti F. Pityriasis rubra pilaris in childhood: a long term study of 29 cases. Pediatr Dermatol 1986; 3: 446–451.

329 Lamar LM, Gaethe G. Pityriasis rubra pilaris. Arch Dermatol 1964; 89: 515–522.

330 Griffiths WAD. Pityriasis rubra pilaris – an historical approach. 2. Clinical features. Clin Exp Dermatol 1976; 1: 37–50.

331 Griffiths WAD. Pityriasis rubra pilaris. Clin Exp Dermatol 1980; 5: 105–112.

332 Albert MR, Mackool BT. Pityriasis rubra pilaris. Int J Dermatol 1999; 38: 1–11.

333 Shvili D, David M, Mimouni M. Childhood-onset pityriasis rubra pilaris with immunologic abnormalities. Pediatr Dermatol 1987; 4: 21–23.

334 Jacyk WK. Pityriasis rubra pilaris in black South Africans. Clin Exp Dermatol 1999; 24: 160–163.

335 Varma S, Logan RA. Exanthematic pityriasis rubra pilaris. Br J Dermatol 1999; 141: 769–771.

336 Griffiths A. Pityriasis rubra pilaris. Etiologic considerations. J Am Acad Dermatol 1984; 10: 1086–1088.

337 Shahidullah H, Aldridge RD. Changing forms of juvenile pityriasis rubra pilaris – a case report. Clin Exp Dermatol 1994; 19: 254–256.

338 Niemi K-M, Kousa M, Storgards K, Karvonen J. Pityriasis rubra pilaris. A clinico-pathological study with a special reference to autoradiography and histocompatibility antigens. Dermatologica 1976; 152: 109–118.

339 Dicken CH. Treatment of classic pityriasis rubra pilaris. J Am Acad Dermatol 1994; 31: 997–999.

340 Duncan KO, Imaeda S, Milstone LM. Pneumocystis carinii pneumonia complicating methotrexate treatment of pityriasis rubra pilaris. J Am Acad Dermatol 1998; 39: 276–278.

341 Neess CM, Hinrichs R, Dissemond J et al. Treatment of pruritus by capsaicin in a patient with pityriasis rubra pilaris receiving RE-PUVA therapy. Clin Exp Dermatol 2000; 25: 209–211.

342 Miralles ES, Núñez M, De Las Heras ME et al. Pityriasis rubra pilaris and human immunodeficiency virus infection. Br J Dermatol 1995; 133: 990–993.

343 Martin AG, Weaver CC, Cockerell CJ, Berger TG. Pityriasis rubra pilaris in the setting of HIV infection: clinical behaviour and association with explosive cystic acne. Br J Dermatol 1992; 126: 617–620.

344 Auffret N, Quint L, Domart P et al. Pityriasis rubra pilaris in a patient with human immunodeficiency virus infection. J Am Acad Dermatol 1992; 27: 260–261.

345 Menni S, Brancaleone W, Grimalt R. Pityriasis rubra pilaris in a child seropositive for the human immunodeficiency virus. J Am Acad Dermatol 1992; 27: 1009.

346 Blauvelt A, Nahass GT, Pardo RJ, Kerdel FA. Pityriasis rubra pilaris and HIV infection. J Am Acad Dermatol 1991; 24: 703–705.

347 Sánchez-Regaña M, López-Gil F, Salleras M, Umbert P. Pityriasis rubra pilaris as the initial manifestation of internal neoplasia. Clin Exp Dermatol 1995; 20: 436–438.

348 Vanderhooft SL, Francis JS, Holbrook KA et al. Familial pityriasis rubra pilaris. Arch Dermatol 1995; 131: 448–453.

349 Sonnex TS, Dawber RPR, Zachary CB et al. The nails in adult type 1 pityriasis rubra pilaris. J Am Acad Dermatol 1986; 15: 956–960.

350 Cohen PR, Prystowsky JH. Pityriasis rubra pilaris: a review of diagnosis and treatment. J Am Acad Dermatol 1989; 20: 801–807.

351 Tannenbaum CB, Billick RC, Srolovitz H. Multiple cutaneous malignancies in a patient with pityriasis rubra pilaris and focal acantholytic dyskeratosis. J Am Acad Dermatol 1996; 35: 781–782.

352 Davidson CL Jr, Winkelmann RK, Kierland RR. Pityriasis rubra pilaris. A follow-up study of 57 patients. Arch Dermatol 1969; 100: 175–178.

353 Castanet J, Lacour JPh, Perrin C et al. Juvenile pityriasis rubra pilaris associated with hypogammaglobulinaemia and furunculosis. Br J Dermatol 1994; 131: 717–719.

354 Piamphongsant T, Akaraphant R. Pityriasis rubra pilaris: a new proposed classification. Clin Exp Dermatol 1994; 19: 134–138.

355 Sørensen KB, Thestrup-Pedersen K. Pityriasis rubra pilaris: a retrospective analysis of 43 patients. Acta Derm Venereol 1999; 79: 405–406.

356 Selvaag E, Hædersdal M, Thomsen K. Pityriasis rubra pilaris: a retrospective study of 12 patients. J Eur Acad Dermatol Venereol 2000; 14: 514–515.

357 Finzi AF, Altomare G, Bergamaschini L, Tucci A. Pityriasis rubra pilaris and retinol-binding protein. Br J Dermatol 1981; 104: 253–256.

358 Van Voorst Vader PC, van Oostveen F, Houthoff HJ, Marrink J. Pityriasis rubra pilaris vitamin A and retinol-binding protein: a case study. Acta Derm Venereol 1984; 64: 430–432.

359 Stoll DM, King LE, Chytil F. Serum levels of retinol binding protein in patients with pityriasis rubra pilaris. Br J Dermatol 1983; 108: 375.

360 Ralfs IG, Dawber RPR, Ryan TJ, Wright NA. Pityriasis rubra pilaris: epidermal cell kinetics. Br J Dermatol 1981; 104: 249–252.

361 Marks R, Griffiths A. The epidermis in pityriasis rubra pilaris: a comparison with psoriasis. Br J Dermatol (Suppl) 1973; 9: 19–20.

362 Soeprono FF. Histologic criteria for the diagnosis of pityriasis rubra pilaris. Am J Dermatopathol 1986; 8: 277–283.

363 Koehn GG. Dramatic follicular plugging in pityriasis rubra pilaris. J Am Acad Dermatol 1990; 23: 526–527.

364 Clayton BD, Jorizzo JL, Hitchcock MG et al. Adult pityriasis rubra pilaris: A ten-year case series. J Am Acad Dermatol 1997; 36: 959–964.

365 Hashimoto K, Fedoronko L. Pityriasis rubra pilaris with acantholysis and lichenoid histology. Am J Dermatopathol 1999; 21: 491–493.

366 Magro CM, Crowson AN. The clinical and histomorphological features of pityriasis rubra pilaris. A comparative analysis with psoriasis. J Cutan Pathol 1997; 24: 416–424.

367 Kao GF, Sulica VI. Focal acantholytic dyskeratosis occurring in pityriasis rubra pilaris Am J Dermatopathol 1989; 11: 172–176.

368 Shulman KJ, Magro CM, Crowson AN. Acantholytic pityriasis rubra pilaris: a unique variant. J Cutan Pathol 1996; 23: 61 (abstract).

369 Howe K, Foresman P, Griffin T, Johnson W. Pityriasis rubra pilaris with acantholysis. J Cutan Pathol 1996; 23: 270–274.

370 Cowen P, O'Keefe R. Pityriasis rubra pilaris and focal acantholytic dyskeratosis. Australas J Dermatol 1997; 38: 40–41.

371 Kanerva L, Lauharanta J, Niemi K-M, Lassus A. Ultrastructure of pityriasis rubra pilaris with observations during retinoid (etretinate) treatment. Br J Dermatol 1983; 108: 653–663.

372 Everett MA, Headington JT. Parapsoriasis. JCE Dermatology 1978; 17 (12): 12–24.

373 Bennaman O, Sanchez JL. Comparative clinicopathological study on pityriasis lichenoides chronica and small plaque parapsoriasis. Am J Dermatopathol 1988; 10: 189–196.

374 Lambert WC, Everett MA. The nosology of parapsoriasis. J Am Acad Dermatol 1981; 5: 373–395.

375 Altman J. Parapsoriasis: a histopathologic review and classification. Semin Dermatol 1984; 3: 14–21.

376 Lazar AP, Caro WA, Roenigk HH Jr, Pinski KS. Parapsoriasis and mycosis fungoides: the Northwestern University experience, 1970 to 1985. J Am Acad Dermatol 1989; 21: 919–923.

377 Kikuchi A, Naka W, Harada T et al. Parapsoriasis en plaques: its potential for progression to malignant lymphoma. J Am Acad Dermatol 1993; 29: 419–422.

378 Haeffner AC, Smoller BR, Zepter K, Wood GS. Differentiation and clonality of lesional lymphocytes in small plaque parapsoriasis. Arch Dermatol 1995; 131: 321–324.

379 Burg G, Dummer R. Small plaque (digitate) parapsoriasis is an 'abortive cutaneous T-cell lymphoma' and is not mycosis fungoides. Arch Dermatol 1995; 131: 336–338.

380 Shaffer B, Beerman H. Lichen simplex chronicus and its variants. Arch Dermatol 1951; 64: 340–351.

381 Kouskoukis CE, Scher RK, Ackerman AB. The problem of features of lichen simplex chronicus complicating the histology of diseases of the nail. Am J Dermatopathol 1984; 6: 45–49.

382 Marks R, Wells GC. Lichen simplex: morphodynamic correlates. Br J Dermatol 1973; 88: 249–256.

383 Porter WM, Bewley A, Dinneen M et al. Nodular lichen simplex of the scrotum treated by surgical excision. Br J Dermatol 2001; 144: 915–916.

384 Singh G. Atopy in lichen simplex (neurodermatitis circumscripta). Br J Dermatol 1973; 89: 625–627.

385 Marks R, Wells GC. A histochemical profile of lichen simplex. Br J Dermatol 1973; 88: 557–562.

386 Ackerman AB. Subtle clues to diagnosis by conventional microscopy. Marked compact hyperkeratosis as a sign of persistent rubbing. Am J Dermatopathol 1980; 2: 149–152.

The spongiotic reaction pattern

INTRODUCTION

The spongiotic tissue reaction is characterized by the presence of intra-epidermal and intercellular edema (spongiosis) (Fig. 5.1). It is recognized by the widened intercellular spaces between keratinocytes, with elongation of the intercellular bridges (Fig. 5.2).[1] The foci of spongiosis may vary from microscopic in size to grossly identifiable vesicles and even bullae. Mild spongiosis is well seen in semithin sections.[2] Inflammatory cells, usually lymphocytes but sometimes eosinophils or even neutrophils, are also present.[1]

The spongiotic tissue reaction is a histopathological concept and not a clinical one, although several of the many diseases with this tissue reaction have been included, in the past, in the category of 'eczemas'. This term (derived from Greek elements which mean 'boiling over') has fallen into some disrepute in recent years because it lacks precision.[3–5] The 'eczemas' all show epidermal spongiosis at some stage of their evolution, even though this has been disputed for atopic eczema. Clinically, the various spongiotic disorders may present with weeping crusted patches and plaques, as in the so-called 'eczemas', or as erythematous papules, papulovesicles and even vesiculobullous lesions. Resolving lesions and those of some duration may show a characteristic collarette of scale.

The mechanism involved in the collection of the intercellular fluid is controversial. It is generally accepted that the fluid comes from the dermis and, in turn, from blood vessels in the upper dermis. Various immunological reactions are involved in some of the diseases discussed in this chapter, but in others the etiology of this fluid extravasation from vessels remains to be elucidated. The controversy also involves the mechanism by which the dermal edema fluid enters the epidermis.[6,7] One concept is that an osmotic gradient develops towards the epidermis, drawing fluid into it.[6] The opposing view suggests that hydrostatic pressure leads to the epidermal elimination of dermal edema.[8] The latter explanation does not satisfactorily explain the absence of spongiosis in pronounced urticarial reactions. Perhaps both mechanisms are involved to a varying degree. The spongiotic tissue reaction is a dynamic process.[9] Vesicles come and go and they can be situated at different levels in the epidermis.[9] Parakeratosis forms above areas of spongiosis, probably as a result of an acceleration in the movement of keratinocytes towards the surface, although disordered maturation may contribute.[10] Small droplets of plasma may accumulate in the mounds of parakeratosis, contributing to the appearance of the collarettes of scale mentioned above.[10]

Simulants of the spongiotic tissue reaction

There are several categories of disease in which casual histological examination may show a simulation of the spongiotic reaction pattern: they are excluded from consideration here.[1] Diseases that present a lichenoid reaction pattern with obscurement of the dermoepidermal interface (such as pityriasis lichenoides, erythema multiforme and fixed drug eruption) or prominent vacuolar change (variants of lupus erythematosus) may show some spongiosis above the basal layer. They are not included among the diseases considered in this chapter.

Certain viral exanthems and morbilliform drug eruptions show mild epidermal spongiosis, but it is usually limited to the basal layer of the epidermis. Other viral diseases, such as herpes simplex and herpes zoster, show ballooning degeneration of keratinocytes with secondary acantholysis. Some spongiosis is invariably present but it is overshadowed by the other changes. Primary acantholytic disorders leading to vesiculation are also excluded. Mild spongiosis is seen overlying the dermal papillae in early lesions of psoriasis, but again this disease is not usually regarded as a spongiotic disorder.

The accumulation of acid mucopolysaccharides in the follicular infundibulum in follicular mucinosis may simulate spongiosis. Stains for mucin, such as the colloidal iron stain, will confirm the diagnosis, if any doubt exists.

Finally, the Pautrier microabscesses of mycosis fungoides may be simulated by the collections of mononuclear cells that sometimes accumulate in spongiotic dermatitis. In spongiotic dermatitis, the cellular collections often assume a vase-like shape, with the lips of the vase situated at the interface between the granular and cornified layers.[11] The intraepidermal collections of mononuclear cells express CD1a, S100 protein, CD36 and CD68. They lack CD14 which is found on mature Langerhans cells. Their phenotype suggests derivation from circulating monocytes and differentiation into mature Langerhans cells.[12]

Patterns of spongiosis

There are four special patterns of spongiosis which can be distinguished morphologically from the more usual type. These special patterns are *neutrophilic spongiosis*, in which there are numerous neutrophils associated with epidermal spongiosis, *eosinophilic spongiosis*, characterized by the presence of numerous eosinophils within the spongiotic foci, *miliarial spongiosis*, in

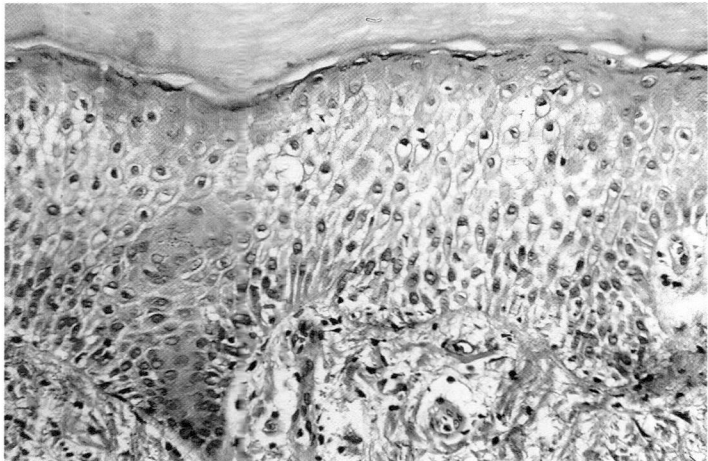

Fig. 5.1 **The spongiotic reaction pattern.** There is mild intracellular edema leading to pallor of the keratinocytes, in addition to the intercellular edema. (H & E)

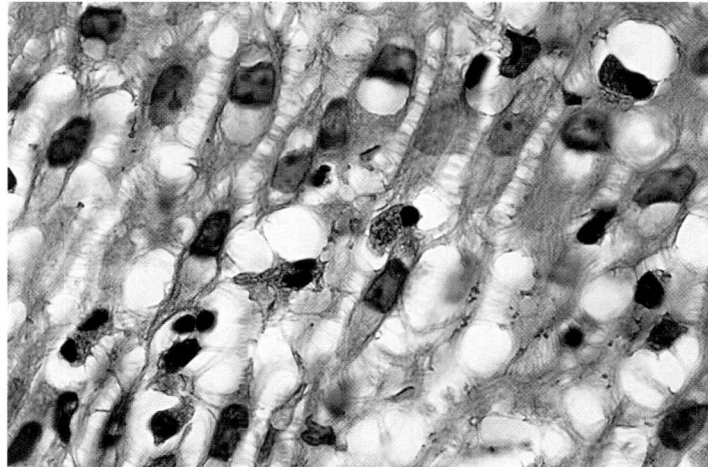

Fig. 5.2 **The spongiotic reaction pattern.** Note the elongation of the intercellular bridges resulting from the intercellular edema. Occasional eosinophils are present within the epidermis. (H & E)

which the edema is centered on the acrosyringium, and *follicular spongiosis*, in which there is involvement of the follicular infundibulum. Sometimes serial sections are required before it is appreciated that the spongiosis is related to the acrosyringium or acrotrichium. Diseases in these special categories will be discussed first, followed by a description of the more usual type of spongiotic disorders.

NEUTROPHILIC SPONGIOSIS

Neutrophilic spongiosis is characterized by the presence of neutrophils within spongiotic foci in the epidermis (Fig. 5.3). The term spongiform pustular dermatitis can be used for a severe form of neutrophilic spongiosis in which pustules can be seen clinically and histologically. Subcorneal pustules are excluded from this category. Ackerman states that neutrophils are absent in 'authentic' spongiotic dermatitides,[13] but a case can be made for including the following conditions in this histological pattern:

- pustular psoriasis
- Reiter's syndrome
- IgA pemphigus
- herpetiform pemphigus
- infantile acropustulosis
- acute generalized exanthematous pustulosis
- palmoplantar pustulosis
- staphylococcal toxic shock syndrome
- neisserial infections
- dermatophytoses
- candidosis
- beetle *(Paederus)* dermatitis
- pustular contact dermatitis
- amicrobial pustulosis associated with autoimmune diseases.

Reiter's syndrome (see p. 83) shares histological features with pustular psoriasis. It will not be considered further. In infantile acropustulosis (see p. 136) there are variable numbers of eosinophils admixed with the neutrophils. In palmoplantar pustulosis (see p. 137) large vesicles are the dominant feature with only some neutrophilic spongiosis at the edges. This tissue reaction can also be seen in the staphylococcal toxic shock syndrome (see p. 619) and in infections with *Neisseria* sp. (see p. 624). Pustular contact dermatitis is

considered later in this chapter (see p. 106). Amicrobial pustulosis associated with autoimmune diseases and herpetiform pemphigus are discussed in Chapter 6 (see pp 138 and 134 respectively).

PUSTULAR PSORIASIS

In both pustular psoriasis (see p. 82) and Reiter's syndrome (see p. 83) there is characteristic spongiform pustulation.

IgA PEMPHIGUS

IgA pemphigus is a vesiculobullous disease (see p. 135) with a variable expression, accounting for the many titles applied to this condition in the past. There are subcorneal and/or intraepidermal pustules with usually only mild acantholysis. IgA is deposited in the epidermis in an intercellular position.

ACUTE GENERALIZED EXANTHEMATOUS PUSTULOSIS

Acute generalized exanthematous pustulosis is a rapidly evolving pustular eruption (see p. 136), usually associated with the ingestion of drugs, particularly antibiotics. There are subcorneal and superficial intraepidermal pustules. Subepidermal pustules are sometimes present with prominent neutrophil exocytosis and neutrophilic spongiosis.

DERMATOPHYTOSES AND CANDIDOSIS

Neutrophilic spongiosis can be found with dermatophyte infection and also with the yeast *Candida*. The presence of neutrophils in the epidermis and/or overlying stratum corneum should always lead to the performance of a PAS stain.

BEETLE *(PAEDERUS)* DERMATITIS

Vesicular dermatitis, characterized by areas of neutrophilic spongiosis, results from contact with various beetles (order Coleoptera).[14,15] Bullae and small pustules may even result. The term Paederus dermatitis is used for the reaction produced by the genus *Paederus*, of which there are several hundred species capable of producing a form of acute irritant contact dermatitis.[15] The irritant substance is pederin, a highly toxic alkaloid produced by members of this genus. Localized erythema occurs first, followed by blisters after 2–4 days, associated with increasing pain.[14] Lesions are commonly linear due to crushing of the beetle on the skin, followed by its wiping off the skin. The delay in the appearance of the lesions may lead to lack of recognition of the causal event.

Histopathology
Early lesions show neutrophilic spongiosis leading to vesiculation and eventual reticular necrosis of the epidermis. This is followed by confluent epidermal necrosis, usually with a surviving layer of suprabasal cells. Scattered acantholytic cells may be present. The large number of intraepidermal neutrophils, combined with areas of confluent necrosis and reticular degeneration, are characteristic. Older lesions show irregular acanthosis and pallor of superficial keratinocytes, with overlying parakeratotic scale containing a neutrophil exudate.[14]

A similar spongiotic and vesicular dermatitis, with the addition of vasculitis, has been produced by the hide beetle, *Dermestes peruvianus*.[16]

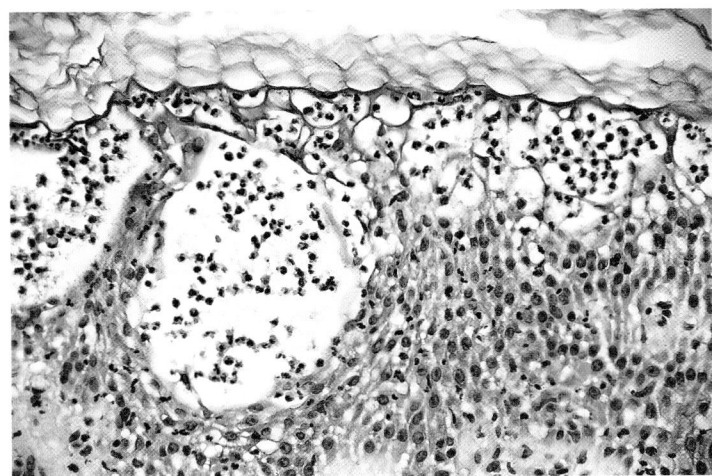

Fig. 5.3 **Neutrophilic spongiosis** characterized by the presence of neutrophils within spongiotic vesicles. (H & E)

EOSINOPHILIC SPONGIOSIS

Eosinophilic spongiosis is a histological reaction pattern characterized by the presence of epidermal spongiosis associated with the exocytosis of eosinophils into the spongiotic foci.[17] Microabscesses, containing predominantly eosinophils, are formed.

Eosinophilic spongiosis is found in a heterogeneous group of dermatoses,[18] most of which are considered elsewhere. It can be seen in the following conditions:

- pemphigus (precursor lesions)
- pemphigus vegetans
- bullous pemphigoid
- cicatricial pemphigoid
- herpes gestationis
- idiopathic eosinophilic spongiosis
- eosinophilic, polymorphic, and pruritic eruption
- allergic contact dermatitis
- atopic dermatitis
- arthropod bites
- eosinophilic folliculitis (Ofuji's disease)
- incontinentia pigmenti (first stage)
- drug reactions
- 'id' reactions.

PEMPHIGUS (PRECURSOR LESIONS)

Eosinophilic spongiosis may occur in the preacantholytic stage of both pemphigus foliaceus and pemphigus vulgaris.[17,19–21] In these early stages, direct immunofluorescence demonstrates the presence of IgG in the intercellular areas of the epidermis.[19] In those patients whose disease evolves into pemphigus foliaceus, the initial clinical presentation may resemble dermatitis herpetiformis.[20,22] Some of these cases have been reported in the literature as herpetiform pemphigus.[23,24]

Histopathology
The pattern is that described for eosinophilic spongiosis (Fig. 5.4). Acantholysis and transitional forms between eosinophilic spongiosis and the usual histological findings in pemphigus may be present.

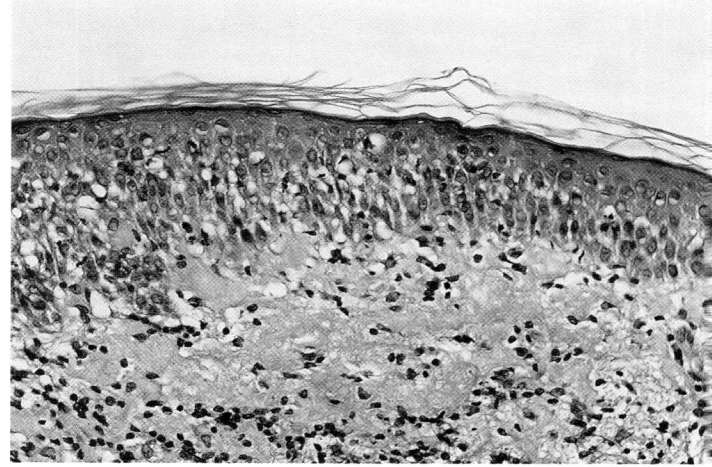

Fig. 5.4 **Eosinophilic spongiosis** as a precursor of pemphigus foliaceus. (H & E)

PEMPHIGUS VEGETANS

Eosinophils are often prominent within the vesicles of pemphigus vegetans. Acantholysis, epidermal hyperplasia and the absence of spongiosis adjacent to the suprabasal vesicles usually allow the diagnosis of pemphigus vegetans to be made.

BULLOUS PEMPHIGOID

Eosinophilic spongiosis is an uncommon finding in the urticarial stage of bullous pemphigoid and in erythematous patches adjacent to characteristic bullae in later stages of the disease.[25] In one case, the eosinophilic spongiosis preceded the diagnosis of bullous pemphigoid by 13 years.[26] There is usually a prominent dermal infiltrate of eosinophils, and IgG is demonstrable along the basement membrane zone.

IDIOPATHIC EOSINOPHILIC SPONGIOSIS

Several cases have been recorded in which a localized, recurrent bullous eruption has been associated with the histological appearance of eosinophilic spongiosis.[27] Polycythemia rubra vera was present in one case.[28]

EOSINOPHILIC, POLYMORPHIC, AND PRURITIC ERUPTION

Eosinophilic, polymorphic, and pruritic eruption, associated with the use of radiotherapy, particularly for carcinoma of the breast, has not been well characterized.[29] Similar cases have been reported in the past, often without histological confirmation, under several different designations, including erythema multiforme and bullous pemphigoid after radiation therapy.[29] The rash is widespread, polymorphic and intensely pruritic, commencing during radiotherapy and lasting several weeks or months. The lesions are usually erythematous papules, measuring 3–10 mm in diameter. Wheals, vesicles and tense subepidermal blisters are less common.

Histopathology
The variable histological appearances reflect the polymorphic nature of the rash. There is usually spongiosis with focal spongiotic vesiculation. There may be some acanthosis in lesions of longer duration and secondary changes of rubbing and scratching. The dermal infiltrate is usually superficial and deep and of moderate severity. Extension into the subcutis sometimes occurs. Eosinophils are always present. There is usually some eosinophilic spongiosis; an eosinophilic panniculitis is much less common. If bullae are present, they usually resemble bullous pemphigoid. There are no features of erythema multiforme, despite the earlier publications attributing this condition to erythema multiforme.

ALLERGIC CONTACT DERMATITIS

Eosinophilic spongiosis may be seen in allergic contact dermatitis (see p. 104).

ARTHROPOD BITES

Eosinophilic spongiosis is occasionally seen in the reaction to the bite of certain arthropods, particularly the scabies mite (see p. 737).

EOSINOPHILIC FOLLICULITIS

In eosinophilic folliculitis (Ofuji's disease – see p. 460) the eosinophilic spongiosis involves the follicular infundibulum; sometimes the immediately adjacent epidermis is also involved.

INCONTINENTIA PIGMENTI

In the first stage of incontinentia pigmenti (see p. 333) there is prominent exocytosis of eosinophils into the epidermis and foci of eosinophilic spongiosis (Fig. 5.5). Occasional dyskeratotic keratinocytes may also be present.

MILIARIAL SPONGIOSIS

Miliarial spongiosis is characterized by intraepidermal edema centered on the acrosyringium. It is characteristic of the various clinical forms of miliaria.

MILIARIA

The miliarias are a clinically heterogeneous group of diseases which occur when the free flow of eccrine sweat to the skin surface is impeded. Three

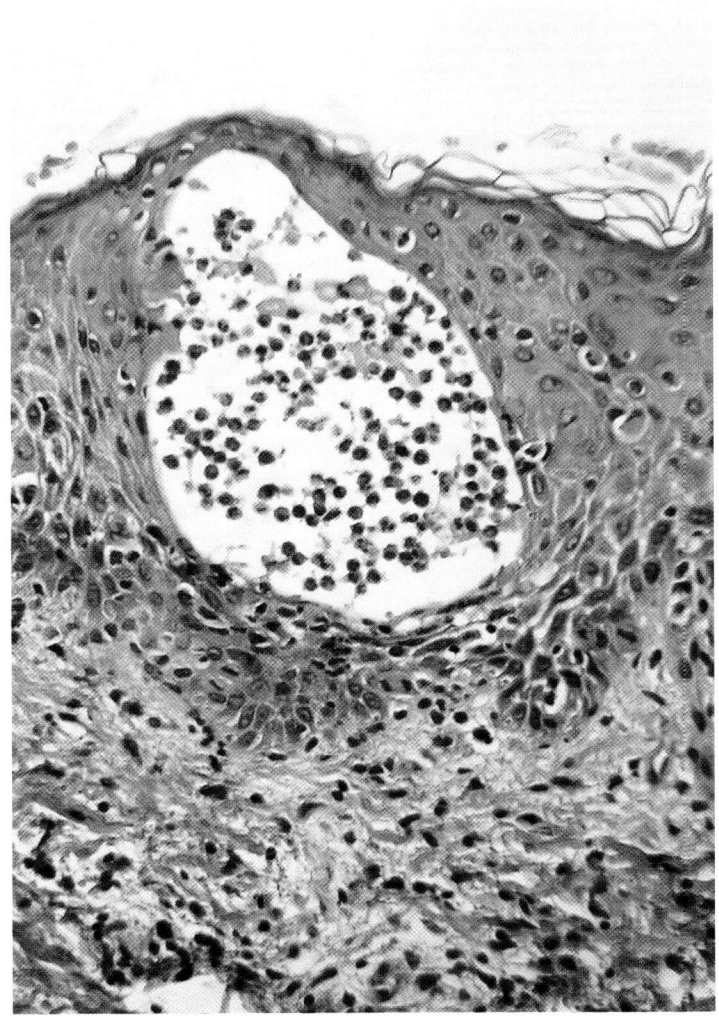

Fig. 5.5 **Eosinophilic spongiosis** in the first stage of incontinentia pigmenti. (H & E)

variants of miliaria have been defined according to the depth at which this sweat duct obstruction occurs.

Miliaria crystallina (miliaria alba), which results from superficial obstruction in the stratum corneum, is characterized by asymptomatic, clear, 1–2 mm vesicles which rupture easily with gentle pressure.[30] Congenital onset is exceedingly rare.[31]

Miliaria rubra (prickly heat) consists of small, discrete, erythematous papulovesicles with a predilection for the clothed areas of the body.[32] The lesions are often pruritic. In severe cases, with recurrent crops of lesions, anhidrosis may result.[33] Occasionally, pustular lesions (miliaria pustulosa) may coexist.

Miliaria profunda refers to the development of flesh-colored papules resembling gooseflesh, associated with obstruction of the sweat duct near the dermoepidermal junction.[34,35] It usually follows severe miliaria rubra and is associated with anhidrosis. A case has been reported in which large white plaques with an erythematous border were present.[36] The lesions expanded centrifugally until they were several centimeters or more in diameter. They were localized to sites at which occlusive tape had been applied.[36]

Although it has been presumed since the last century that obstruction of the eccrine duct is involved in the pathogenesis of the miliarias, the nature of this obstruction and its etiology have been the subject of much debate.[34] The first demonstrable histological change is the accumulation of PAS-positive, diastase-resistant material in the distal pore,[34] although this has not always been found.[37] This material has been designated 'extracellular polysaccharide substance (EPS)'.[38] It is likely that there is an earlier stage of obstruction, which cannot be demonstrated in tissue sections. After several days, a keratin plug forms as part of the repair process, leading to further obstruction of the duct, often at a deeper level. Various factors may contribute to the initial duct obstruction.[39,40] These include changes in the horny layer related to excess sweating, the presence of sodium chloride in more than isotonic concentration[37] and lipoid depletion. In many cases there is an increase in the number of resident aerobic bacteria, particularly cocci.[34,41–43] Certain strains of *Staphylococcus epidermidis* produce the PAS-positive material known as EPS (see above) and these organisms may play a central role in the pathogenesis of miliaria.[38] Miliaria have also developed at the site of previous radiotherapy; there was associated keratotic plugging of the eccrine orifices.[44]

Histopathology

In *miliaria crystallina* there is a vesicle within or directly beneath the stratum corneum. There is often a thin, orthokeratotic layer forming the roof of the vesicle and a basket-weave layer of keratin in the base. A PAS-positive plug may be seen in the distal sweat pore.

Miliaria rubra is characterized by variable spongiosis and spongiotic vesiculation related to the epidermal sweat duct unit and the adjacent epidermis (Fig. 5.6). There is a small number of lymphocytes in the areas of spongiosis. An orthokeratotic or parakeratotic plug may overlie the spongiosis.[32] Sometimes there is edema in the papillary dermis adjacent to the point of entry of the eccrine duct into the epidermis (Fig. 5.7). A mild lymphocytic infiltrate is usually present in this region. If the edema is pronounced, leading to subepidermal vesiculation, then *miliaria profunda* is said to be present.

Less commonly, there is only slight spongiosis in the region of the acrosyringium in miliaria rubra associated with dilatation of the terminal eccrine duct.[32] It should be remembered that not all eccrine ducts are involved.

The secretory acini show few changes in the miliarias.[32] They may be mildly dilated. Often there is slight edema of the connective tissue between the secretory units. Lymphocytes are not usually present, unless there is a prominent inflammatory cell infiltrate elsewhere in the dermis.

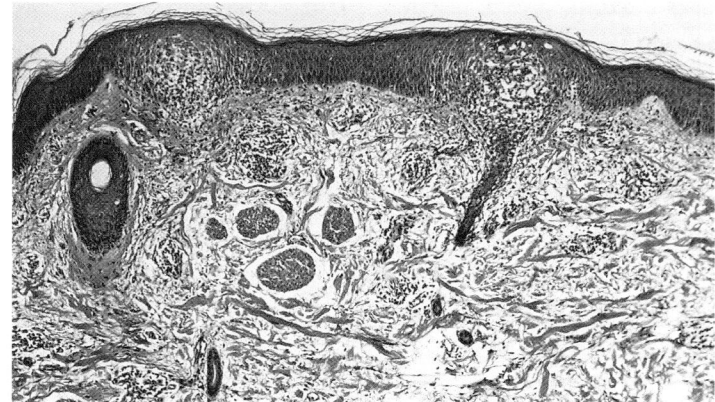

Fig. 5.6 **Miliaria rubra.** The spongiosis is related to the acrosyringium. (H & E)

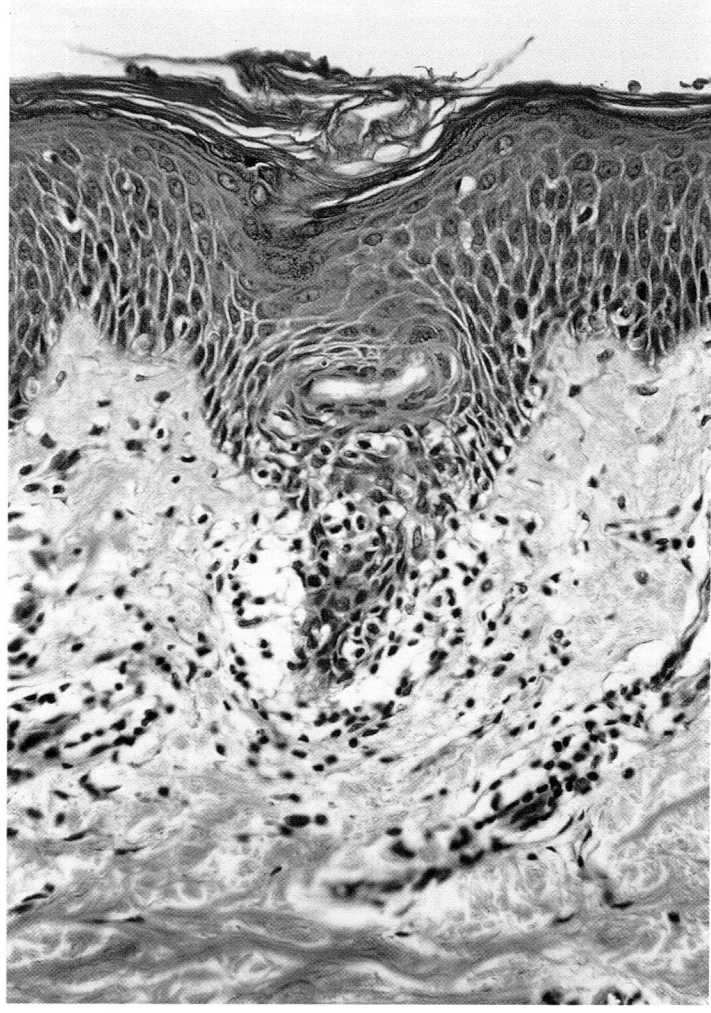

Fig. 5.7 **Miliaria rubra.** There is edema in the wall of the eccrine duct as it enters the epidermis and also in the adjacent papillary dermis. (H & E)

FOLLICULAR SPONGIOSIS

Follicular spongiosis refers to the presence of intercellular edema in the follicular infundibulum (Fig. 5.8). It occurs in a limited number of circumstances:

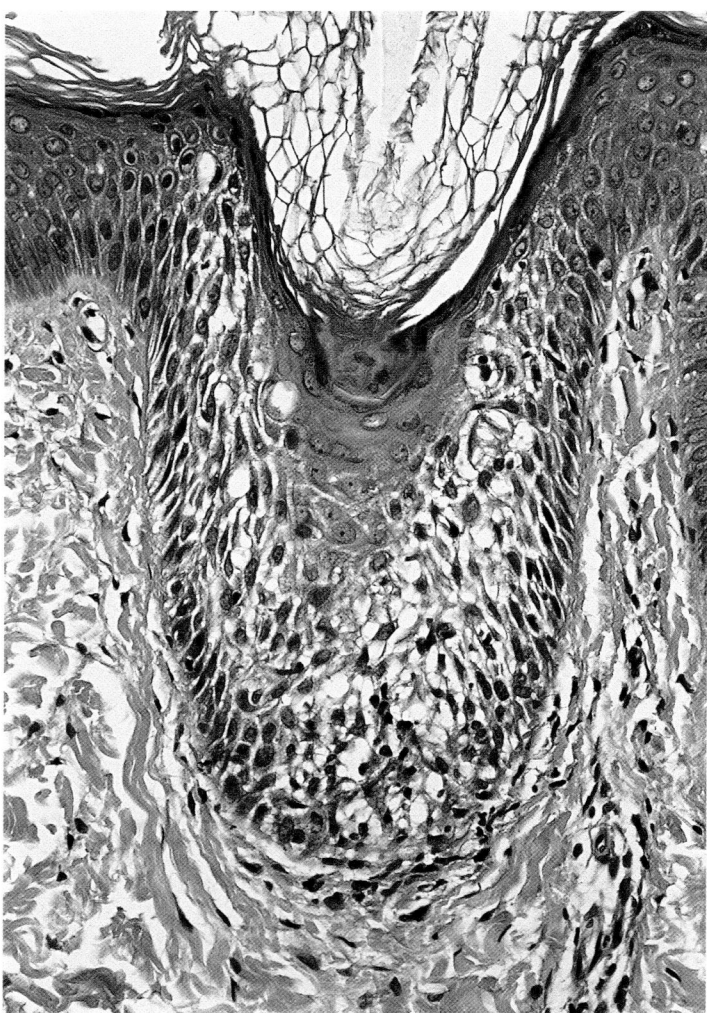

Fig. 5.8 **Follicular spongiosis.** The patient had follicular lesions on the trunk as a manifestation of atopic dermatitis. (H & E)

- infundibulofolliculitis
- atopic dermatitis (follicular lesions)
- apocrine miliaria
- eosinophilic folliculitis.

INFUNDIBULOFOLLICULITIS

Infundibulofolliculitis, also known as disseminate and recurrent infundibulofolliculitis, presents as a follicular, often pruritic, papular eruption with a predilection for the trunk and proximal parts of the extremities of young adult males.[45–48] It occurs almost exclusively in black patients. Although the lesions resemble those seen in some cases of atopic dermatitis, the individuals studied so far have not been atopic.[49]

Histopathology[45,47,49]

There is spongiosis of the follicular infundibulum with exocytosis of lymphocytes (Fig. 5.9). A few neutrophils are sometimes present. There is widening of the follicular ostium and focal parakeratosis of the adjacent epidermis. Occasional follicles contain a keratin plug.[49] The follicular infundibulum is often hyperplastic. There is usually a slight infiltrate of lymphocytes around the follicles and around the blood vessels in the superficial part of the dermis. Mast cells may be increased.

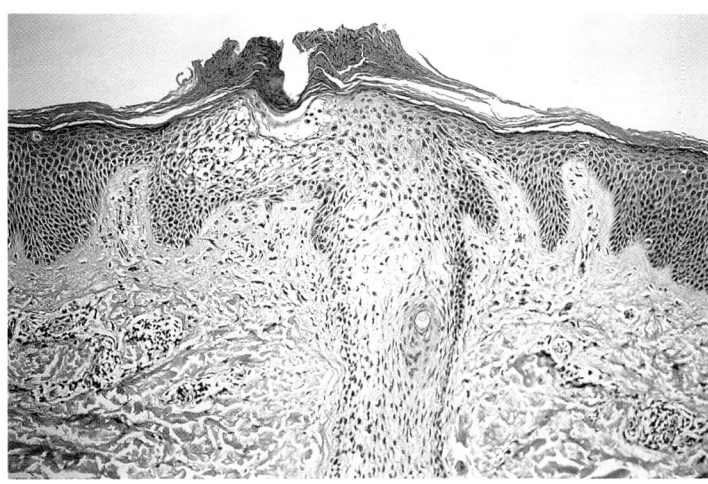

Fig. 5.9 **Infundibulofolliculitis.** There is follicular spongiosis, focal parakeratosis and a mild inflammatory cell infiltrate in the dermis. (H & E)

ATOPIC DERMATITIS

Some patients with atopic dermatitis develop small follicular papules, often on the trunk.

Histopathology

There is spongiosis of the follicular infundibulum with exocytosis into this region of the epidermis. Usually no neutrophils are present. The adjacent epidermis may show mild acanthosis and sometimes focal parakeratosis. The histopathology resembles that seen in infundibulofolliculitis.

APOCRINE MILIARIA

Apocrine miliaria (Fox–Fordyce disease) presents as a chronic papular eruption, usually limited to the axilla (see p. 486). It results from rupture of the intrainfundibular portion of the apocrine duct.

Histopathology

Serial sections may be required to demonstrate the spongiosis of the follicular infundibulum adjacent to the point of entry of the apocrine duct. There may be a few neutrophils in the associated inflammatory response.

EOSINOPHILIC FOLLICULITIS

Eosinophilic folliculitis (Ofuji's disease) is characterized by eosinophilic spongiosis centered on the follicular infundibulum. It is discussed in detail on page 460.

OTHER SPONGIOTIC DISORDERS

Most of the other diseases in which the spongiotic reaction pattern occurs show spongiosis distributed randomly through the epidermis with no specific localization to the acrosyringium or follicular infundibulum, which indeed are often spared.

It is sometimes quite difficult to make a specific histopathological diagnosis of some of the diseases in this category. Often a diagnosis of 'spongiotic dermatitis consistent with …' is as specific as one can be.

IRRITANT CONTACT DERMATITIS

Irritant contact dermatitis is an inflammatory condition of the skin produced in response to the direct toxic effect of an irritant substance.[50] The most commonly encountered of these irritants include detergents, solvents, acids and alkalis.[50-52] Other agents include wool fibers,[53] fiberglass,[53,54] sunscreen preparations,[55] propylene glycol[56] and plants,[57] particularly the milky sap of members of the family Euphorbiaceae.[58,59] Even airborne substances in droplet, particulate or volatile form can cause this type of dermatitis.[60] Chemically induced irritant contact dermatitis is a leading cause of occupational disease with important economic consequences,[61] accordingly protective creams are being developed and evaluated to assist in the control of this important problem.[62,63]

Our knowledge of irritant contact dermatitis is limited in spite of the fact that it is more common than allergic contact dermatitis, from which it may be difficult to distinguish.[64] Irritant reactions vary from simple erythema to purpura, eczematous reactions, vesiculobullous lesions and even epidermal necrosis with ulceration. Lesions are often more glazed than allergic reactions and subject to cracking, fissuring and frictional changes.[51] Irritant reactions occur at the site of contact with the irritant; in the case of airborne spread, the eyelids are a common site of involvement.[60,65] Pustular reactions have been reported with heavy metals, halogens and other substances.[66,67] These responses are assumed to be irritant in type. Acute ulceration is a severe reaction that may follow contact with alkalis, including cement.[68,69]

A special variant of irritant contact dermatitis is seen in association with urostomies. Eventually pseudoverrucous papules and nodules may develop in the perianal region.[70] Other stomas may also be associated with irritant reactions.[71] Granuloma gluteale infantum (a misnomer because there are no granulomas) is probably a diaper-related irritant dermatitis in which *Candida albicans* may also play a role (see p. 666).[72]

Susceptibility to irritant dermatitis is variable, although approximately 15% of the population have heightened sensitivity of their skin which appears to result from a thin, permeable stratum corneum.[64] There are differences in skin sensitivity in different regions of the body.[73,74] Atopic individuals are more susceptible,[75] and both irritants and an atopic diathesis have been incriminated in the etiology of occupational dermatitis of the hands.[64,76,77] Cumulative irritancy, in which multiple subthreshold damage to the skin occurs, may also be seen with agents in cosmetics, for example.[51,61,78] Delayed irritancy is another variant of irritant contact dermatitis in which the clinical changes are not manifest until 8–24 hours after the exposure.[79] Susceptibility to irritants is also more common in the winter months, apparently as a result of changes in the barrier functions of the stratum corneum.[80]

Irritants may act in several different ways. They may remove surface lipids and water-holding substances (as with surfactants contained in household cleaning products),[81,82] damage cell membranes or denature epidermal keratins.[83] They may have a direct cytotoxic effect. Some irritants are also chemotactic for neutrophils in vitro, while others may lead to the liberation of cytokines and other inflammatory mediators; tumor necrosis factor has been implicated as an important cytokine in irritant reactions.[78] The pathogenesis of irritant contact dermatitis continues to be poorly understood, although evidence is emerging that a very complex reaction pattern occurs, involving immunoregulatory processes.[84,85]

Cytokine expression in allergic and irritant contact reactions differs surprisingly little.[86] They are similar at 72 hours after the application of the respective experimental contactant although, at 6 hours, the irritant reaction expresses higher levels.[87] Cytokines that are increased include IL-1α, IL-1β, IL-2, IL-6, IFN-γ and TNF-α.[86,87] Apoptosis of epidermal Langerhans cells is produced by some irritants but not others.[88]

Histopathology

The changes observed in irritant contact dermatitis vary with the nature of the irritant, including its mode of action and its concentration.[83,89] A knowledge of these factors helps to explain the conflicting descriptions in the literature.[90] Furthermore, many of the histopathological studies have been performed on animals, which are particularly liable to develop epidermal necrosis and dermoepidermal separation with neutrophil infiltration when exposed to high concentrations of irritants.[39,91] In humans, high concentrations of an irritant will produce marked ballooning of keratinocytes in the upper epidermis with variable necrosis ranging from a few cells to confluent areas of the epidermis (Fig. 5.10).[92–94] Neutrophils are found in the areas of ballooning and necrosis, and mild spongiosis is also present in the adjacent epidermis (Fig. 5.11).[94]

If low and medium concentrations of an irritant are applied, the histopathological spectrum of the reactions produced often mimics that seen in allergic contact dermatitis, with epidermal spongiosis, mild superficial dermal edema and a superficial, predominantly perivascular infiltrate of lymphocytes (Fig. 5.12).[89,90,95] The lymphocytes are of helper/inducer type.[50] Langerhans cells are found diffusely through the upper dermis from day 1 to day 4 following contact with the irritant; this is in contrast to allergic contact dermatitis in which these cells are more perivascular in location and persist in the dermis for a longer period.[50] Occasional apoptotic keratinocytes may be seen in the epidermis in irritant reactions.[96,97] In the recovery phase of irritant dermatitis mild epidermal hyperplasia is often present. Psoriasiform hyperplasia may develop in chronic irritant reactions.

Pustular reactions show subcorneal vesicles with neutrophils, cellular debris and a fibrinous exudate. There are also some neutrophils in the upper dermal infiltrate.

A recent detailed study using various irritants and human volunteers has confirmed the marked variability in histopathological responses, depending on the chemical used.[83] For example, propylene glycol produced hydration of corneal cells and a prominent basket-weave pattern.[83] Nonanoic acid resulted in tongues of eosinophilic keratinocytes with shrunken nuclei in the upper epidermis; croton oil caused a spongiotic tissue reaction resembling allergic contact dermatitis.[83] Sodium lauryl sulfate produced a thick zone of parakeratosis; dithranol caused some basal spongiosis and pallor of superficial keratinocytes; benzalkonium resulted in mild spongiosis, sometimes accompanied by foci of necrosis in the upper spinous layers.[83] The ultrastructural changes also varied widely with the different irritants.[83] It is obvious that further studies using other potential human irritants are needed to increase our understanding of the diversity of irritant reactions.

ALLERGIC CONTACT DERMATITIS

Allergic contact dermatitis is an inflammatory disorder which is initiated by contact with an allergen to which the person has previously been sensitized.[50,79] The prevalence of contact dermatitis (both irritant and allergic) in the general population in the USA has been variably estimated to be between 1.5% and 5.4%.[64] It is uncommon in children.[98] Allergic contact dermatitis is less frequent than irritant dermatitis, but both are a significant occupational problem.[99]

Clinically, there may be erythematous papules, small vesicles or weeping plaques, which are usually pruritic. The lesions develop 12–48 hours after exposure to the allergen. In the case of cosmetic reactions, the face, eyelids and neck are commonly involved, but the lesions may extend beyond the zone of contact, in contrast to irritant reactions.[100,101] With occupational exposures, the hands are frequently involved.[102,103] Stasis dermatitis of the lower parts of the legs is particularly susceptible to allergic contact reactions. Rarely reported allergic reactions include follicular or pustular lesions,[104]

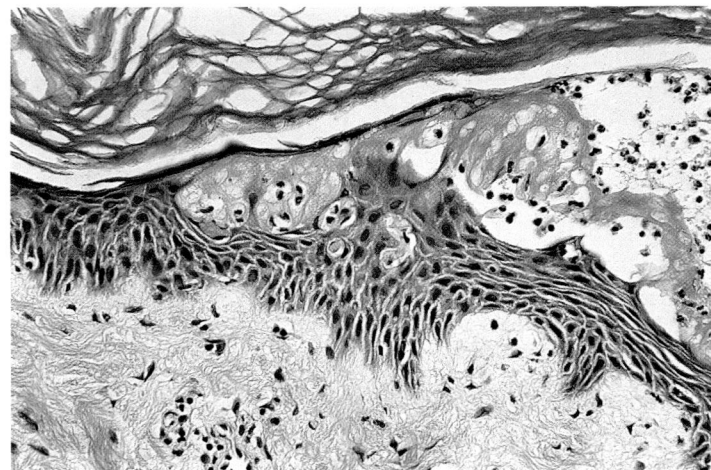

Fig. 5.10 **Irritant contact dermatitis** with superficial epidermal necrosis, edema and some neutrophils. (H & E)

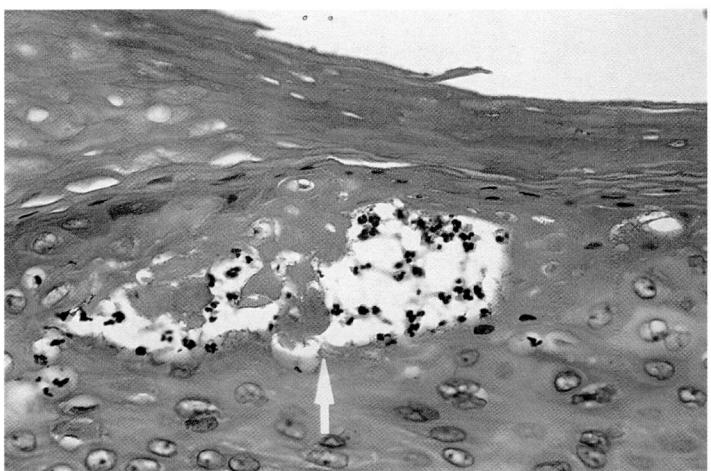

Fig. 5.11 **Irritant contact dermatitis.** There is focal ballooning and necrosis of keratinocytes in the upper epidermis together with spongiosis and a mild infiltrate of neutrophils. (H & E) (Photograph kindly supplied by Dr JJ Sullivan)

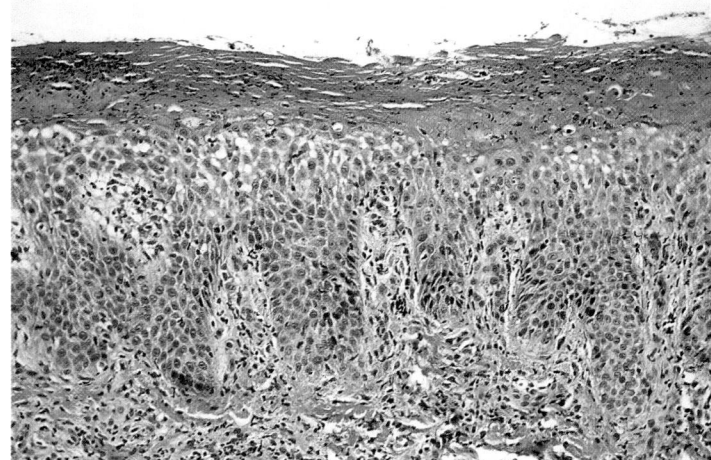

Fig. 5.12 **Mixed irritant and allergic contact dermatitis.** (H & E)

systemic contact reactions and urticarial,[105] granulomatous,[106] leukodermic[107] or erythema multiforme-like lesions.[108–110] Purpuric lesions, which may go on to resemble pigmented purpuric dermatosis, are a rare manifestation of contact allergy. They usually result from contact with resins or textile dyes, particularly Disperse Blue.[111] Resolution of allergic contact dermatitis usually occurs 2–3 weeks after the withdrawal of the relevant allergen or cross-sensitizing agent.

Etiology

Numerous agents have been incriminated in the etiology of allergic contact dermatitis.[112] They include cosmetics, foodstuffs, plants,[113,114] topical medicaments and industrial chemicals.[115] Reactions to cosmetics may result from the fragrances, preservatives[116–118] or lanolin base.[100,119–130] Foodstuffs that have been implicated include flavorings, spices,[131] animal and fish proteins, olive oil,[132] flour additives,[133] citrus fruits,[134] macadamia nuts,[135] mangos,[136] cinnamon,[137] onions, spinach,[138] asparagus,[139] garlic and chives.[140–143] Preservatives used in animal feed and in other industries may produce an occupational dermatitis.[144,145] The plants include poison ivy,[146–149] various members of the Compositae family,[146,150–152] melaleuca (tea tree) oil,[153,154] the latex of mangrove trees,[155] *Agave americana*,[156] tulips,[157] sunflower[158] and *Alstroemeria* (Peruvian lily).[159,160] Plant particles and some chemicals may give rise to contact reactions by airborne spread.[65,161–163] In the past, topical medicaments such as penicillin, sulfonamides, mercurials and antihistamines were the most common sensitizers.[164] Currently neomycin, benzocaine, ethylenediamine (a stabilizer), parabens preservatives and propylene glycol are common causes of such reactions.[56,164,165] Other sensitizers include potassium dichromate, gold,[166] mercury,[167] nickel salts (see below), formaldehyde,[168] chemicals in rubber,[169–174] color film developers,[175] acrylic and epoxy resins,[176–180] immersion oil,[161] coloring agents, henna,[181] 'paint-on' tattoos,[182–184] textile dyes,[185–188] disposable gloves,[189,190] cinnamic aldehyde, quarternium-15 and phenylenediamine.[191,192] Less common causes include doxepin cream,[193] ciclopirox olamine (topical antifungal),[194] vitamin E preparations,[164] topical corticosteroids,[195–210] non-steroidal anti-inflammatory drugs (NSAIDs),[211] bacitracin,[212] mupirocin,[213] enoxolone,[214] lanoconazole,[215] propacetamol,[216] surgical adhesive materials,[217,218] topical amide anesthetics,[219–222] idoxuridine,[223] unna boots,[224] benzalkonium chloride,[225] plastic banknotes,[226] oils used in aromatherapy,[227] tear gas (2-chloroacetophenone),[228] fluorouracil[229] and psoralens.[230] Allergic contact dermatitis can be provoked or intensified by chemically related substances. These cross-sensitization reactions are an important clinical problem.[164]

Nickel allergy is an important cause of morbidity, especially from hand dermatitis.[231–239] The prevalence of nickel allergy is much lower in men: there is evidence to suggest that ear piercing followed by the use of nickel-containing earrings accounts for this difference.[232] Avoidance of skin contact with and dietary intake of nickel is difficult to achieve.[235]

The specific allergen responsible for allergic contact dermatitis can be identified using a patch test.[240–245] However, these reactions are not always reproducible at sequential or concomitant testing. Confocal reflectance microscopy has been used to study allergic contact dermatitis.[246] Initial studies are promising.

Pathogenesis

Allergic contact dermatitis is a special type of delayed hypersensitivity reaction.[247,248] In cases produced by chemicals, an associated irritant reaction is often present.[249] The compound responsible for the allergic reaction is usually of low molecular weight (a hapten) and lipid soluble.[250] After penetrating the skin, the hapten becomes bound to a structural or cell surface protein, usually by a covalent bond, thus forming a complete antigen.[64,251,252] This antigen is processed by Langerhans cells, and possibly macrophages,[253] and then presented to T lymphocytes.[254,255] The actual way in which the Langerhans cells interact with the antigen and lymphocytes is not known,

although the dendritic nature of Langerhans cells obviously assists in their antigen-presenting role.[64,256,257] Keratinocyte-derived cytokines influence this initial phase of the response.[258] Keratinocytes can mature functionally and become potent antigen-presenting cells in the same way that Langerhans cells do.[259] This induction phase is followed by migration of T lymphocytes to the regional lymph nodes where there is clonal expansion of specifically sensitized lymphocytes.[231] On second and subsequent exposures to the allergen, the elicitant response occurs with proliferation of T lymphocytes both in the skin and regional lymph nodes.[212,250,260] The homing of lymphocytes to the antigen-exposed skin involves various cell adhesion molecules, such as lymphocyte function-associated antigen-1 (LFA-1).[255,261,262] Lymphocytes liberate various cytokines in the affected area of skin,[247] including IL-1α, IL-1β, IL-2, IL-4, IL-6, IFN-γ and TNF-α,[86,87,235] leading to a further influx of inflammatory cells, particularly non-sensitized lymphocytes and some eosinophils. The role of IL-12, produced by keratinocytes subject to stimulation with allergens, needs clarification in further studies.[263] Basophils may play a role in a very limited group of circumstances.[251,264] Epidermal proliferation is also stimulated.[265] The actual pathogenesis of the spongiosis still requires elucidation. Hypersensitivity to an allergen may persist for prolonged periods, although in a proportion of cases it subsides or disappears with time.[266]

Histopathology [93,94]

Allergic contact dermatitis is characterized in the very early stages by spongiosis, which is most marked in the lower epidermis. This is followed by the formation of spongiotic vesicles at different horizontal and vertical levels of the epidermis. This often has a very ordered pattern (Figs 5.13 and 5.14). When present, it allows a distinction to be made from nummular dermatitis, which may, at times, closely mimic allergic contact dermatitis histopathologically (see below).

The upper dermis contains a mild to moderately heavy infiltrate of lymphocytes, macrophages and Langerhans cells, with accentuation around the superficial plexus. Eosinophils are usually present, but in some cases only in small numbers.[267] There is exocytosis of lymphocytes and sometimes eosinophils. Eosinophilic spongiosis is a rare pattern. In contrast, exocytosis of eosinophils is uncommon in nummular dermatitis, although exocytosis of lymphocytes and occasional neutrophils is characteristic.

In lesions that persist, scale crust and epidermal hyperplasia develop and the dermal inflammatory cell infiltrate becomes denser. Chronic lesions may show little spongiosis but prominent epidermal hyperplasia of psoriasiform type.[267] Mild fibrosis may develop in the papillary dermis.

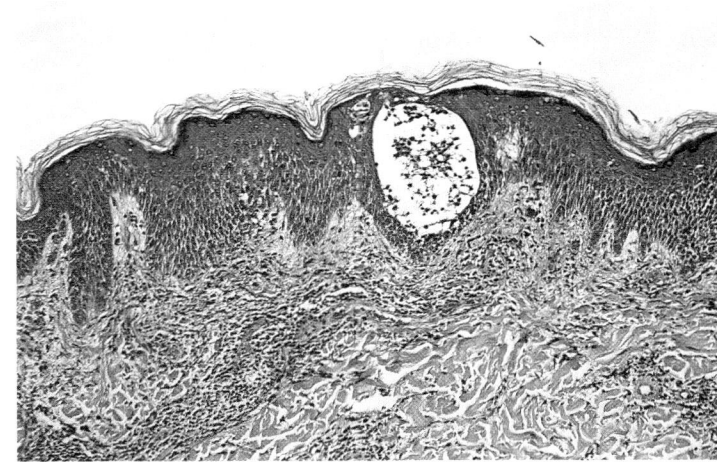

Fig. 5.13 **Allergic contact dermatitis.** There is spongiotic vesiculation. (H & E)

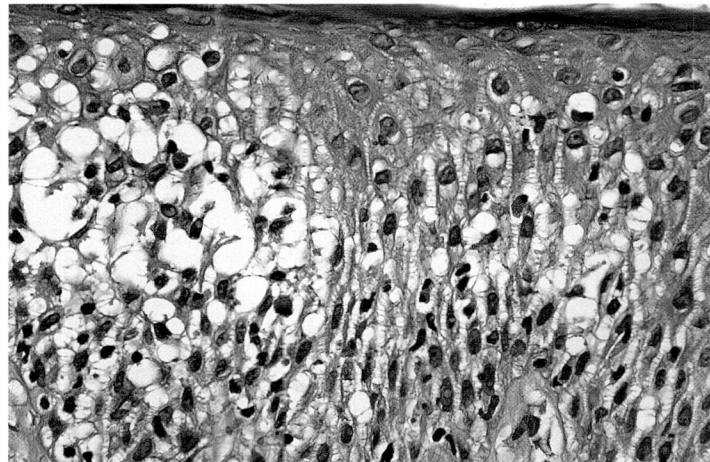

Fig. 5.14 **Allergic contact dermatitis** with exocytosis of eosinophils and lymphocytes into the spongiotic epidermis. (H & E)

Marker studies have shown that the lymphocytes are predominantly helper T cells with CD4 (Leu 3) positivity.[268] The cells are often positive for Leu 8 and 9, markers which are uncommon in the lymphocytes in mycosis fungoides.[268]

Special variants of allergic contact dermatitis

There are several histologically distinct variants of contact dermatitis, some of which may involve an irritant rather than an allergic mechanism. Urticarial (see p. 228) and systemic contact (see p. 114) variants are discussed elsewhere. The status of the erythema multiforme-like pattern,[108,109] and a personally studied lichenoid reaction resulting from contact with chemicals in the wine industry is uncertain. The various types of contact dermatitis are shown in Table 5.1.

Pustular contact dermatitis shows exocytosis of neutrophils and the formation of subcorneal pustules.[104] Neutrophilic spongiosis is sometimes present. Contact with cement may produce this pattern.

Purpuric contact dermatitis, from contact with textile dyes and resins (see above), usually shows a mild lymphocytic vasculitis with red cell extravasation.[111] With time, many cases go on to resemble one of the pigmented purpuric dermatoses (see p. 247) with the accumulation of

Table 5.1 **Clinicopathologic variants of contact dermatitis**

Allergic
Dermal
Erythema multiforme-like
Follicular
Granulomatous
Ichthyosiform
Irritant
Leukodermic
Lichenoid
Lymphomatoid
Photoallergic
Phototoxic
Protein
Purpuric
Pustular
Systemic
Urostomy-associated
Urticarial

hemosiderin in the upper dermis. In one case of acute purpuric dermatitis from contact with *Agave americana*, a leukocytoclastic vasculitis was present.[269]

Dermal contact dermatitis, another special variant of allergic contact reaction, has been poorly documented. Mild edema of the papillary dermis can be seen in many cases of the usual type of allergic contact dermatitis, but more pronounced edema may result from exposure to topical neomycin and to zinc and nickel salts. Such cases are called dermal contact dermatitis (Fig. 5.15). Autoeczematization (see p. 112) produces a similar pattern.

Photoallergic contact dermatitis is considered with the photosensitivity disorders (see Ch. 21, p. 601). The histopathological changes may resemble those seen in allergic contact dermatitis. In cases of some months' duration there is often telangiectasia of superficial vessels, increased and more deeply extending elastotic fibers, deep perivascular extension of the infiltrate, and stellate cells in the upper one-third of the dermis.

Granulomatous contact dermatitis refers to the presence of granulomas in the dermis resulting from a contactant. Sarcoidal granulomas have been found at the sites of ear piercing with gold earrings.[106] Dermal granulomas have resulted from the use of propolis, a resinous beehive product used in folk medicine.[270] In the papular lesions that result from penetration of the allergen into the dermis in 'bindii' (*Soliva pterosperma*) dermatitis, there is a mixed dermal infiltrate with some foreign body giant cells.[271,272] Marked edema of the papillary dermis is usually present and draining sinuses may form.[271]

Lymphomatoid contact dermatitis is a poorly understood variant of allergic contact dermatitis in which the histological appearances may simulate cutaneous T-cell lymphoma.[273–275] There is a heavy infiltrate of lymphocytes in the upper dermis in a so-called 'T-cell pattern' of distribution. Most of the reported cases have resulted from contact with chemicals or metals, such as nickel or gold.[276–278] The author has seen a recurrent case (Fig. 5.16), with a heavy superficial dermal infiltrate, that resulted from contact with Noogoora Burr (*Xanthium occidentale*). Drugs have rarely been implicated.[279]

Leukodermic contact dermatitis is characterized by hypopigmentation occurring at sites of allergic contact dermatitis, as a consequence of post-inflammatory melanin incontinence. It results, uncommonly, from the destruction of melanocytes or from a reduction in melanin synthesis. Betel chewing and contact with lubricants can rarely produce a vitiligo-like leukoderma as a consequence of melanocyte destruction.[107,217] This is strictly an irritant rather than an allergic contact mechanism.

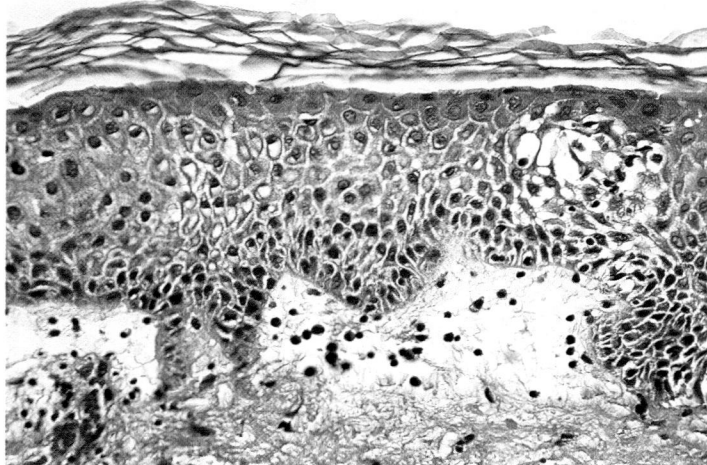

Fig. 5.15 **Allergic contact dermatitis** with prominent edema of the papillary dermis. Certain specific contactants are usually associated with this pattern (see text). It also resembles the reaction seen in autosensitization. (H & E)

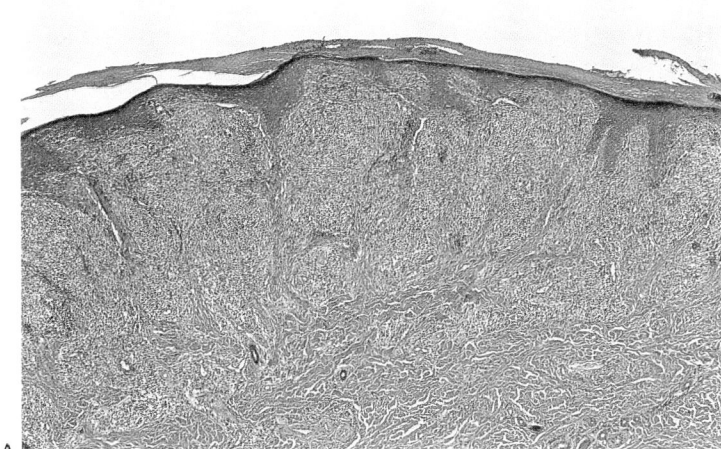

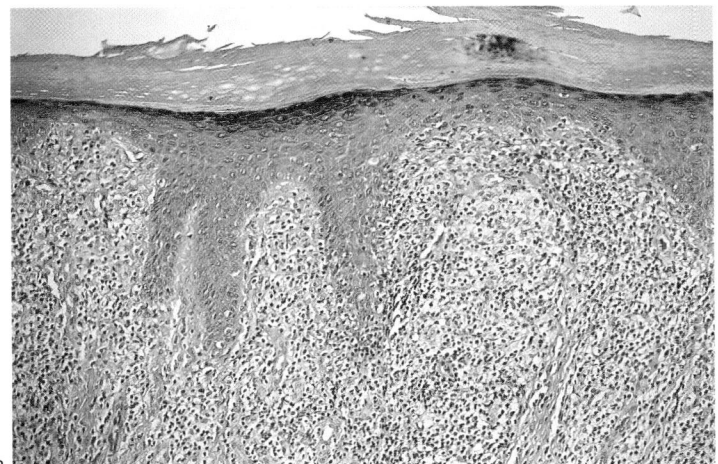

Fig. 5.16 (A) Lymphomatoid contact dermatitis. (B) A dense infiltrate of lymphocytes, some mildly atypical, fill the upper dermis. The eruption developed on several occasions after contact with Noogoora Burr. (H & E)

Follicular contact dermatitis has been reported following contact with formaldehyde and polyoxyethylene laurylether (used in cosmetics).[280] The papules show follicular spongiosis.

Ichthyosiform contact dermatitis has been reported following the use of cetrimide. It is regarded as an acquired form of ichthyosis.

PROTEIN CONTACT DERMATITIS

Protein contact dermatitis usually presents as a chronic eczema with episodic acute exacerbations a few minutes after contact with the offending agent.[281] The lesions are usually confined to the hands and forearms because occupational allergens are usually involved. Patch testing is usually negative when read at 48 hours. Approximately 50% of those involved are atopic.

It appears that a combined type I and IV immunological reaction is present. The causative 'protein' is either a fruit, vegetable, plant, animal protein, grain or enzyme.[281–286]

Histopathology

No distinguishing histological features have been recorded for this variant of contact dermatitis. There may be more edema of the papillary dermis than in allergic contact dermatitis.

NUMMULAR DERMATITIS

Nummular dermatitis (nummular eczema) commences with tiny papules and papulovesicles that become confluent and group themselves into coin-shaped patches which may be single or multiple.[287,288] The surface is usually weeping or crusted and the margins are flat. Central clearing may occur. Sites of predilection include the dorsum of the hands, the extensor surface of the forearms, the lower part of the legs, the outer aspect of the thighs and the posterior aspect of the trunk.[288] The course is usually chronic with remissions and exacerbations.[287,289]

The etiology is unknown but numerous factors have been implicated over the years, often with very little basis. External irritants, cold, dry weather and a source of infection are factors which may aggravate nummular dermatitis.[289,290] In one series, all the cases were said to be related to varicose veins and/or edema of the legs, suggesting stasis with autoeczematization as an etiological factor.[291] Several drugs, such as methyldopa, latanoprost eye drops,[292] gold and antimycobacterial drugs in combination, appear to provoke nummular eczema.[293] Mercury in dental fillings has also been implicated.[294] There is no evidence for an atopic basis, as once thought.[287,288,295]

Histopathology[288,291,296]

The appearances vary with the chronicity and activity of the lesion. In early lesions there is epidermal spongiosis and sometimes spongiotic vesiculation associated with some acanthosis and exocytosis of inflammatory cells, including lymphocytes and occasional neutrophils. The spongiotic vesicles sometimes contain inflammatory cells,[291] simulating Pautrier microabscesses. There is progressive psoriasiform epidermal hyperplasia but this is not always as uniform as in allergic contact dermatitis (see above), which otherwise closely mimics nummular dermatitis. Scale crust often forms above this thickened epidermis. There is a superficial perivascular infiltrate in the dermis composed of lymphocytes, some eosinophils and occasional neutrophils and plasma cells. Nummular dermatitis often has an 'untidy appearance' microscopically (Fig. 5.17).

Progressive rubbing and scratching of individual lesions lead to ulceration or the superimposed changes of lichen simplex chronicus.

SULZBERGER–GARBE SYNDROME

A rare entity, of doubtful status, Sulzberger–Garbe syndrome is also known as 'the distinctive exudative discoid and lichenoid chronic dermatosis of Sulzberger and Garbe'.[297,298] It is regarded by some as a variant of nummular dermatitis,[296] although there are clinical differences. These include larger lesions, intense pruritus, a high prevalence of penile and facial lesions, and a predilection for Jewish males.[299]

Histopathology[296,299]

The histological changes are usually indistinguishable from those of nummular dermatitis. Dilatation of superficial vessels with endothelial swelling and perivascular edema have been regarded as characteristic features,[297] although not universally accepted.[296]

SEBORRHEIC DERMATITIS

Seborrheic dermatitis is a chronic dermatosis of disputed histogenesis. It has a prevalence of 1–3% in the general population.[300,301] It consists of erythematous, scaling papules and plaques, sometimes with a greasy yellow appearance, with a characteristic distribution on the scalp, ears, eyebrows, eyelid margins and nasolabial area – the so-called 'seborrheic areas'.[300,302]

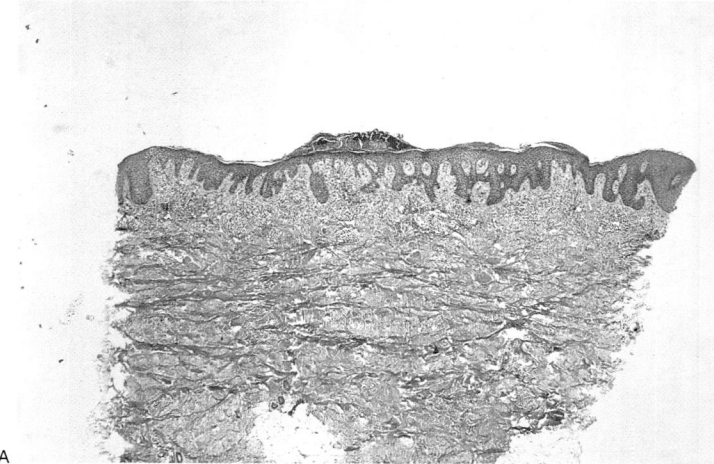

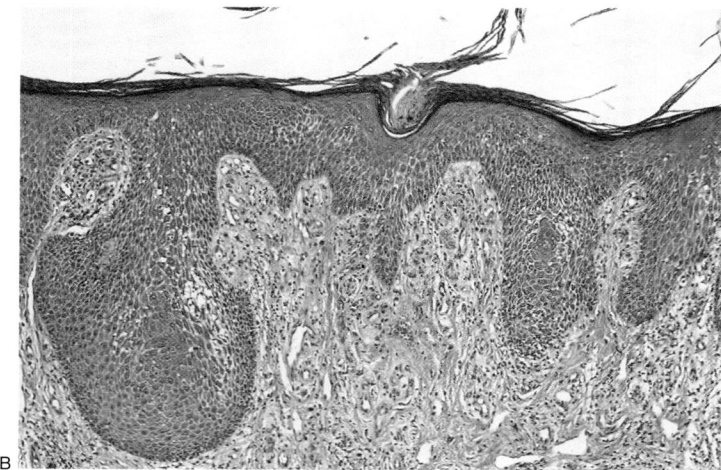

Fig. 5.17 **(A) Nummular dermatitis. (B)** There is spongiosis, irregular acanthosis and exocytosis of inflammatory cells. (H & E)

Less commonly, it may involve other hair-bearing areas of the body, particularly the flexures and pectoral region. Males are more commonly affected.[300] Seborrheic dermatitis is not usually seen until after puberty; the exact nosological position of cases reported in infancy (infantile seborrheic eczema) is uncertain[303] and their occurrence may represent another variant of the atopic tendency.[304–308]

Seborrheic dermatitis is one of the most common cutaneous manifestations of the acquired immunodeficiency syndrome (AIDS), affecting 20–80% of patients.[309–311] In these circumstances, it is often quite severe and atypical in distribution. Seborrheic dermatitis is also seen with increased frequency in association with a number of medical disorders which include Parkinson's disease,[312] epilepsy, congestive heart failure, obesity, chronic alcoholism, Leiner's disease (exfoliative dermatitis of infancy) and zinc deficiency.[302,309] The high prevalence of seborrheic dermatitis in mountain guides (16%) may be the result of UV-induced immunosuppression from the occupational sun exposure.[313] Seborrheic dermatitis may occur as a reaction to arsenic, gold, chlorpromazine, methyldopa[302] and cimetidine.[314]

Pityriasis amiantacea

Pityriasis amiantacea consists of asbestos-like sticky scales, which bind down tufts of hair, involving localized areas of the scalp.[315–317] Scarring alopecia is a rare complication.[318] Seborrheic dermatitis is often present, although it is uncertain whether the two conditions are related.[316]

Dandruff

Dandruff is an extremely common affliction of the scalp. It has been regarded as a mild expression of seborrheic dermatitis by some and as a completely separate disorder by others.[300,319,320] It is best regarded as a reactive response of the epidermis to various stimuli, particularly species of *Malassezia*.[88,321]

Pathogenesis of seborrheic dermatitis

Traditionally, seborrheic dermatitis has been regarded as a dysfunction of sebaceous gland activity, often associated with an oily complexion. This view was supported by its localization to the 'seborrheic areas' of the body. A more recent study has shown, however, that the sebum excretion rate is not increased in patients with seborrheic dermatitis.[322] The role of *Malassezia sp.* (*Pityrosporum*) in the etiology is also controversial.[323–325] This organism is usually quantitatively increased in both seborrheic dermatitis and dandruff but there is dispute about whether this is causal or a secondary event related to the increased keratin scale.[326–329] The organism's role in HIV-related cases is doubted;[330] no quantitative differences are usually observed in the number of yeasts in HIV-related and non-HIV-related seborrheic dermatitis.[329] There is some evidence favoring an abnormal immune response to *Malassezia furfur* and possibly other organisms as well, although this has been refuted in recent studies.[331–335] Other possible explanations include the production of an inflammatory mediator or alterations in lipase activity by *Malassezia*.[334] *Malassezia furfur* seems to play no role in the pathogenesis of the infantile form, further evidence that it may be a different disease.[336] A reclassification of the various species of *Malassezia* took place a few years ago (see p. 666). To date, few papers have appeared linking specific species in the new classification to this disease.

Histopathology[337,338]

The changes are those of an acute, subacute or chronic spongiotic dermatitis depending on the age of the lesion biopsied (Figs 5.18 and 5.19). In *acute lesions* there is focal, usually mild, spongiosis with overlying scale crust containing a few neutrophils; the crust is often centered on a follicle. The papillary dermis is mildly edematous; the blood vessels in the superficial vascular plexus are dilated and there is a mild superficial perivascular infiltrate of lymphocytes, histiocytes and occasional neutrophils.[339] There is some exocytosis of inflammatory cells but this is not as prominent as it is in nummular dermatitis.

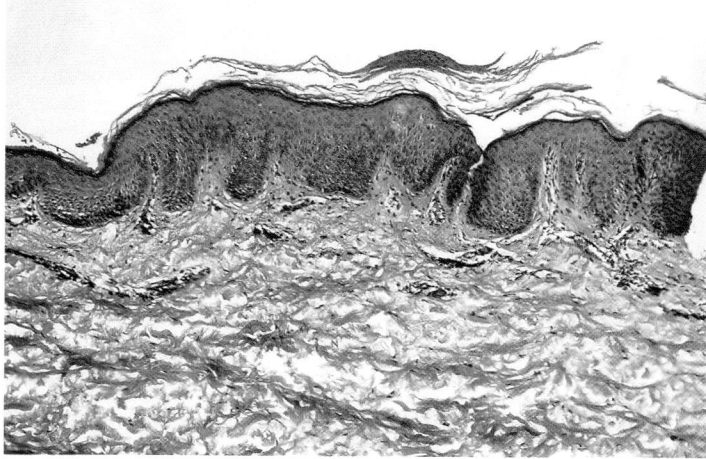

Fig. 5.18 **Seborrheic dermatitis.** Spongiosis is not a feature in this biopsy. There is psoriasiform hyperplasia of the epidermis and focal parakeratosis. (H & E)

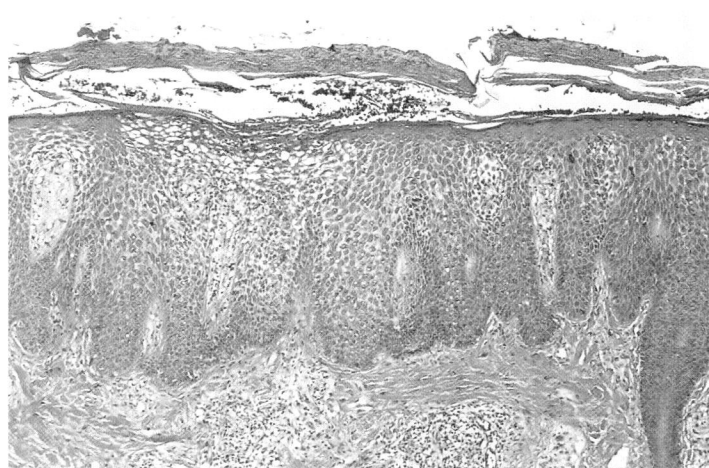

Fig. 5.19 **Subacute seborrheic dermatitis** with spongiosis and parakeratosis in a folliculocentric distribution. (H & E)

In *subacute lesions* there is also psoriasiform hyperplasia, initially slight, with mild spongiosis and the other changes already mentioned. Numerous yeast-like organisms can usually be found in the surface keratin.

Chronic lesions show more pronounced psoriasiform hyperplasia and only minimal spongiosis. Sometimes the differentiation from psoriasis can be difficult but the presence of scale crusts in a folliculocentric distribution favors seborrheic dermatitis.

The seborrheic dermatitis related to AIDS shows spotty cell death of keratinocytes, increased exocytosis of leukocytes, and some plasma cells and neutrophils in the superficial dermal infiltrate.[310]

Pityriasis amiantacea
There is spongiosis of both the follicular and surface epithelium with parakeratotic scale at the follicular ostia.[315] Parakeratotic scale is layered around the outer hair shafts in an 'onion skin' arrangement.[315] Sebaceous glands are sometimes shrunken.

Dandruff
There are no spongiotic or inflammatory changes in dandruff, but only minute foci of parakeratosis scattered within the thickened orthokeratotic scale.[339]

ATOPIC DERMATITIS

Atopic dermatitis (atopic eczema) is a chronic, pruritic, inflammatory disease of the skin which usually occurs in individuals with a personal and/or family history of atopy (asthma, allergic rhinitis and atopic dermatitis).[340–347] It is a common disorder with an incidence of approximately 1–2%;[341] its prevalence appears to be increasing in children, particularly in the Western world, where incidences as high as 15–20% have been recorded.[348–359] Onset is usually in infancy or childhood.[343,360]

The diagnosis of atopic dermatitis is made on the basis of a constellation of major and minor clinical features.[340,342,361–364] Its distinction from infantile seborrheic dermatitis is sometimes difficult.[304,345] Major criteria for the diagnosis of atopic dermatitis include the presence of pruritus, chronicity and a history of atopy, as well as lesions of typical morphology and flexural distribution.[342,361] In infants and young children there is an erythematous, papulovesicular rash with erosions involving the face and extensor surfaces of the arms and legs.[365] This progresses with time to a scaly, lichenified derma-

titis with a predilection for the flexures of the arms and legs.[366] Involvement of the hands and feet may occur at a later stage. The vulva is sometimes involved.[367,368] Itchy follicular papules on the trunk are quite common in oriental and black patients.[369,370] A patient with linear distribution of the lesions has been reported.[371]

Minor clinical features[340,342,372] include xerosis, which may be focal or generalized, elevated IgE, interleukin-2 receptor (IL-2R),[373] eosinophil cationic protein (ECP),[374,375] E-selectin[376–379] and IgG$_4$ in the serum,[366,380,381] increased colonization of the skin with *Staphylococcus aureus*,[382,383] a greater risk of viral and fungal infections of the skin,[384] pityriasis alba,[365] rippled hyper-pigmentation,[385] reduced numbers of melanocytic nevi,[386] keratosis pilaris, cheilitis, nipple eczema, food intolerance, orbital darkening, white dermatographism and an increased incidence of dermatitis of the hands, including pompholyx and irritant dermatitis.[387,388] The ethnic background of the patient appears to influence the phenotype and the relative incidence of the various minor clinical features in atopic dermatitis.[389]

Atopic dermatitis-like skin lesions can be seen in a number of genodermatoses, the most important of which is ichthyosis vulgaris.[365] They also occur in the Wiskott–Aldrich syndrome,[390,391] in ataxia-telangiectasia and in some patients with phenylketonuria.[365] The incidence is probably not increased in Down syndrome.[392]

The course of atopic dermatitis is one of remissions and exacerbations; the symptom-free periods tend to increase with age.[342] There is also a tendency towards spontaneous remission in adult life, although some recent studies have shown lower remission rates than previously thought.[393] Outcome studies, including the response to various treatments,[394–402] rely on consistency in the measurement of disease activity/severity. Unfortunately, there is less consistency than is desirable between the various severity scales.[403] Some children with atopic dermatitis will develop allergic respiratory diseases later in childhood. Positive skin-prick tests to food allergens, severe skin disease and a high serum IgE level are risk factors for the later development of allergic respiratory disease.[404]

Pathogenesis of atopic dermatitis
Although the etiology and pathogenesis of atopic dermatitis are still unclear, evidence suggests that IgE-mediated late phase responses, as well as cytokine imbalances and cell-mediated reactions (T-lymphocyte activation), contribute in some way.[405–418] Expressed more specifically, there is an expansion of the skin-homing type 2 cytokine-secreting T cells, leading to increased levels of interleukin-4, -10 and -13 and of IgE.[419–425] There is a corresponding decrease in interferon-γ (IFN-γ).[394,419,420] The IgE-mediated reactions may be to ingested food[366,426–429] or to inhaled or contactant aeroallergens[430–432] such as human dander,[433] grass pollens[434] and house dust mites.[435–443] Dust mite elimination has a beneficial effect on the control of atopic dermatitis.[442,444] Recently, antigens of *Staphylococcus aureus* and other bacteria have been considered as possible stimulants of the IgE response.[419,445,446] About 10% of patients have normal serum IgE levels (non-allergic atopic dermatitis). Studies of this group have shown a lack of interleukin-13-induced B-cell activation, resulting in decreased IgE production.[447]

Cellular changes in atopic dermatitis, in addition to the increase in skin-homing type 2 T lymphocytes, include an increase in inflammatory dendritic cells in the epidermis (either altered Langerhans cells or cells derived from the CD34 subset of dendritic cells)[347] and an increased life span of eosinophils.[347] Langerhans cells appear to be hyperstimulatory.[411,448–450]

Changes in mediators and receptors occur,[451] but there have been conflicting results depending on the model used and the method of measurement. No single cytokine can be said to have a pivotal role. Increased expression of

Fc receptors for IgG[452] and of integrins is present.[378] Prostaglandins may not be as important as previously thought.[453]

Patients with atopic dermatitis have a reduced itch threshold[454] and greater skin 'irritancy'.[455] It appears that mast cell mediators other than histamine are involved in the pruritus.[456,457]

Genetic factors also appear to be involved in the pathogenesis of atopic dermatitis in some way.[453] This is confirmed by the frequent presence of a family history of atopy and the high concordance in twins.[458–460] There is some allelic association with chromosomes 11q13,13q12–14 and 5q31–33.[461,462] Interestingly, the gene for the beta subunit of FcγRI, the high affinity receptor for IgE, has been localized to chromosome 11q12–13.[416] Another candidate gene on chromosome 16p11–p12 is associated with the IL 4R gene.[463] Finally, the reduced barrier function in atopic dermatitis results from ceramide deficiency in the stratum corneum, as a consequence of the abnormal expression of the enzyme sphingomyelin deacylase.[464]

Histopathology[341,465–468]

Atopic dermatitis presents the typical spectrum of acute, subacute and chronic phases as seen in some other spongiotic (eczematous) processes.[467] As such, the biopsy appearances may be indistinguishable from those seen in nummular dermatitis and allergic contact dermatitis. Subtle features, to be listed below, may sometimes allow the diagnosis to be made on biopsy, although most often the dermatopathologist is restricted to describing the findings as 'consistent with atopic dermatitis'.

Acute lesions show spongiosis and some spongiotic vesiculation,[468] even though some authorities deny the presence of spongiosis in atopic dermatitis. There is usually some intracellular edema as well, leading to pallor of the cells in the lower epidermis.[466] Exocytosis of lymphocytes is usually present, although it is never a prominent feature. There is a perivascular infiltrate of lymphocytes and macrophages around vessels of the superficial plexus, but there is no significant increase in mast cells or basophils in acute lesions.[466] The mast cells present are in different stages of degranulation, indicating activation of these cells.[413] Occasional eosinophils may be present.

Subacute lesions show irregular acanthosis of the epidermis with eventual psoriasiform hyperplasia. With increasing chronicity of the lesion, the changes of rubbing and scratching become more obvious and the spongiosis less so.

Chronic lesions show hyperkeratosis, moderate to marked psoriasiform hyperplasia and variable, but usually only mild spongiosis. Mast cells are now significantly increased in the superficial perivascular infiltrate.[465,466] Small vessels appear prominent due to an increase in their number and a thickening of their walls which involves both endothelial cells and the basement membrane.[466] Demyelination, focal vacuolation and fibrosis of cutaneous nerves are also observed.[465,466] Epidermal keratinocytes produce increased amounts of neurotrophin-4 in the chronic pruriginous lesions of atopic dermatitis. It may be responsible for the nerve hypertrophy that is sometimes seen.[469] Langerhans cells are increased in both the epidermis and the dermis.[470–472] With further lichenification of the lesions, there is prominent hyperkeratosis and some vertical streaking of collagen in the papillary dermis, the changes recognized as lichen simplex chronicus. Collagen types I and III increase in the dermis following PUVA therapy.[473] Lichenified lesions have an increased number of mast cells in the dermis.[474]

If dry skin is biopsied in patients with atopic dermatitis there is usually focal parakeratosis, mild spongiosis and a mild perivascular infiltrate involving the superficial plexus.[475] There is focal hypergranulosis in those with dry skin alone,[476] but a reduced granular layer in those who have concurrent ichthyosis vulgaris.[475]

The rippled hyperpigmentation ('dirty neck') seen in approximately 2% of atopics results from melanin incontinence (see p. 334). Amyloid-like material has been seen on electron microscopy, but not on light microscopy, using the Congo red stain.[477]

Infective dermatitis, a recently delineated entity in children and young adults, has similar clinical and histopathological features (see p. 1116). It appears to be caused by infection with human T-lymphotropic virus type I (HTLV-1).

As already mentioned, there are several morphological features which, if present, favor the diagnosis of atopic dermatitis over the other spongiotic dermatitides which it closely resembles. The assessment of these features is somewhat subjective and, in some, it involves the use of techniques that are not routine. Features favoring the diagnosis of atopic dermatitis include prominence of small blood vessels in the papillary dermis, atrophy of sebaceous glands (this change is usually present only in those who have concomitant ichthyosis vulgaris)[475] and an increase in epidermal volume without psoriasiform folding of the dermoepidermal interface (Fig. 5.20).[478] This latter change is a useful clue to the diagnosis of atopic dermatitis. Eosinophils and basophils are usually more prominent in the infiltrate of allergic contact dermatitis than in atopic dermatitis. Despite this relative paucity of eosinophils in atopic dermatitis, eosinophil major basic protein has been reported in the upper dermis in a fibrillar pattern.[479] The diagnostic value of this feature requires further study, as do the findings of perivascular IgE[480] and intercellular epidermal staining for IgE, HLA-DR and CD1a in atopic dermatitis.[481] This also applies to the finding of a predominantly T helper-cell infiltrate in atopic dermatitis[471,472] and a T suppressor-cell infiltrate in allergic contact dermatitis;[480] the latter finding does not accord with the results of other studies.[268]

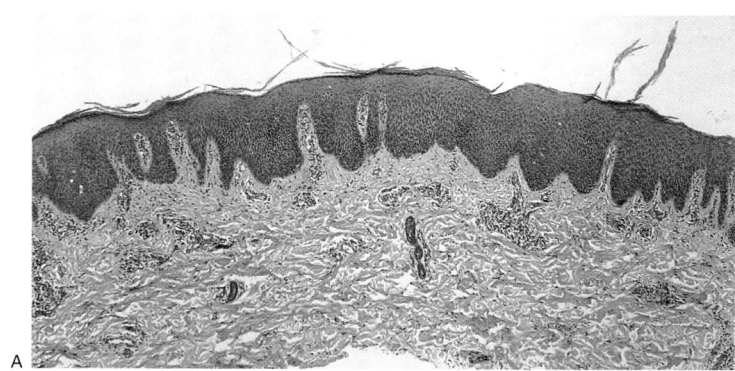

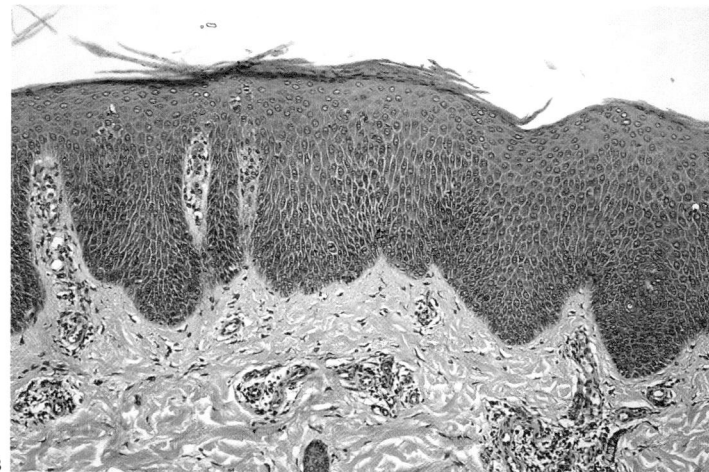

Fig. 5.20 **(A) Atopic dermatitis. (B)** There is an increase in epidermal volume which is associated with only partial psoriasiform folding. Focal parakeratosis is also present. (H & E)

PAPULAR DERMATITIS

Papular dermatitis (subacute prurigo, 'itchy red bump' disease) presents as a pruritic papular eruption with superimposed secondary changes due to excoriation.[482] The lesions tend to be symmetrically distributed on the trunk, the extensor surfaces of the extremities, face, neck and buttocks.

The etiology is unknown, although some patients have an atopic background. The earlier view that this may be a form of *Cheyletiella* dermatitis is no longer tenable (see p. 742).

Histopathology

There is variable epidermal spongiosis and focal parakeratosis. Excoriation and changes of rubbing and scratching are usually present. There is a mild superficial perivascular infiltrate of lymphocytes with a few eosinophils. These changes are not diagnostically specific, being present in other endogenous dermatitides.

POMPHOLYX

Pompholyx (acral vesicular dermatitis, dyshidrotic eczema) is a common, recurrent, vesicular eruption of the palms and soles which is one of several clinical expressions of so-called 'chronic hand dermatitis'.[483,484] It consists of deep-seated vesicles, often with a burning or itching sensation, most commonly involving the palms, volar aspects of the fingers and sometimes the sides of the fingers.[484] Lesions usually resolve after several weeks, leading to localized areas of desquamation.

The term 'dyshidrotic eczema' was introduced because of a mistaken belief that the pathogenesis of this condition involved hypersecretion of sweat and its retention in the acrosyringia.[485] The term should be avoided. Pompholyx is a spongiotic dermatitis, the expression of which is modified by the thickened stratum corneum of palmar and plantar skin which reduces the possibility of rupture of the vesicles. Episodes may be precipitated by infections, including dermatophyte infections at other sites ('id reaction' – p. 112),[486] contact sensitivity to various allergens such as medicaments, mercury in amalgam fillings,[294] nickel[486] and emotional stress.[487] An atopic diathesis is sometimes present;[488] many cases are idiopathic.[489]

Histopathology[485]

Pompholyx is characterized by spongiosis of the lower malpighian layer with subsequent confluence of the spongiotic foci to form an intraepidermal vesicle (Fig. 5.21). The expanding vesicles displace acrosyringia at the outer margin of the vesicles. There is a thick, overlying stratum corneum, characteristic of palms and soles. Other changes include a sparse, superficial perivascular infiltrate of lymphocytes with some exocytosis of these cells. Some persons develop pompholyx-like vesicles that soon evolve into pustules with histopathological features of pustulosis palmaris (see p. 137). A PAS stain should always be performed on vesicular lesions of the palms and soles, particularly if there are any neutrophils within the vesicles or stratum corneum, as dermatophyte infections may mimic the lesions of pompholyx (Fig. 5.22).

Allergic contact dermatitis of the palms and soles may also be difficult to distinguish from pompholyx. In the former condition, mild spongiosis may be present adjacent to the vesicles, and there are sometimes eosinophils in the inflammatory infiltrate.

HYPERKERATOTIC DERMATITIS OF THE PALMS

A somewhat neglected entity, hyperkeratotic dermatitis of the palms is a clinical variant of chronic hand dermatitis.[483,490] It presents as a sharply marginated, fissure-prone, hyperkeratotic dermatitis which is limited usually to the palms and occurs chiefly in adults. Involvement of the volar surfaces of the fingers is quite common. Plantar lesions are rare. The cause of the condition is unknown.

Histopathology

The appearances are those of a chronic spongiotic dermatitis with spongiosis and psoriasiform hyperplasia of the epidermis, although the elongation of the rete ridges is usually not as regular as in psoriasis. There is overlying compact orthokeratosis with small foci of parakeratosis. There is a moderately heavy chronic inflammatory cell infiltrate in the papillary dermis, predominantly in a perivascular location. Lymphocyte exocytosis is quite prominent in the epidermis, but there are usually no neutrophils. The amount of spongiosis allows a distinction to be made from psoriasis.

JUVENILE PLANTAR DERMATOSIS

Juvenile plantar dermatosis is a condition which affects children between the ages of 3 and 14.[491] It presents as a shiny, scaly, erythematous disorder of

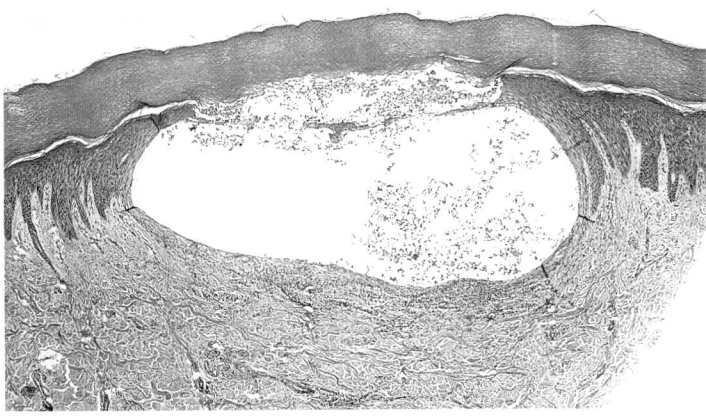

Fig. 5.21 **Pompholyx.** A unilocular vesicle is present within the epidermis. There is no spongiosis in the adjacent epidermis. (H & E)

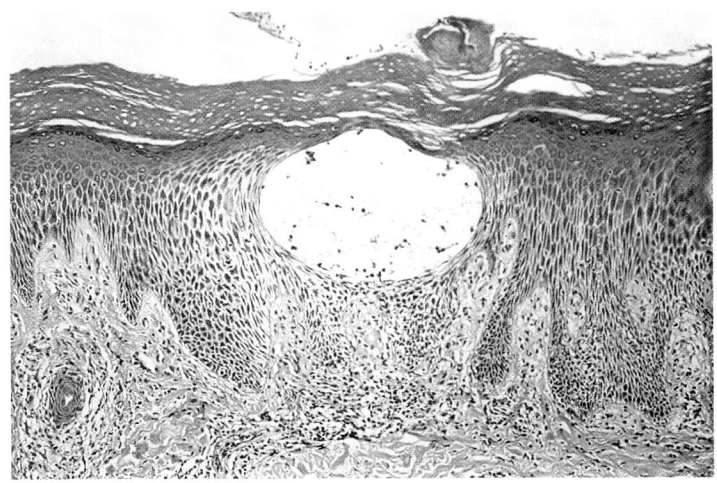

Fig. 5.22 **Dermatophyte infection of the hands.** There are only scattered neutrophils in the spongiotic vesicle, testimony to the necessity to keep a fungal infection in mind when the spongiotic reaction pattern is present on the hands or feet. (H & E)

weight-bearing areas of the feet.[492] Fissuring subsequently develops. Sometimes the hands, particularly the fingertips, are also affected. Most cases improve over the years.

The etiology is uncertain, with conflicting evidence on the role of atopy and of footwear.[493,494] **Dermatitis palmaris sicca** is a related lesion of the palms.[495]

Histopathology[492,496,497]

Juvenile plantar dermatosis shows variable parakeratosis and hypogranulosis overlying psoriasiform acanthosis. A distinctive feature is the presence of spongiosis, mild spongiotic vesiculation, vacuolization of keratinocytes and exocytosis of lymphocytes, localized to the epidermis surrounding the acrosyringium.[492] Lymphocytes are present in the upper dermis around the sweat ducts at their point of entry into the acrosyringium.[492] Ducts and acrosyringia are not dilated.[496]

VEIN GRAFT DONOR-SITE DERMATITIS

A subacute spongiotic dermatitis has been recorded in several patients at the site from which a saphenous vein graft was removed.[498] There was a sensory peripheral neuropathy in the distribution of the dermatitis. Other changes reported at donor sites include the presence of localized myxedema in Graves' disease, and the formation of an indurated linear plaque resulting from cutaneous sclerosis (see p. 355). Cellulitis of the lower leg is another complication.

STASIS DERMATITIS

Stasis dermatitis (hypostatic dermatitis) is a common disorder of middle-aged and older individuals. It is a consequence of impaired venous drainage of the legs.[499] In the early stages, there is edema of the lower one-third of the legs, which have a shiny and erythematous appearance. Subsequently, dry and scaly or crusted and weeping areas may develop.[499] Sometimes the changes are most prominent above the medial malleoli. Affected areas become discolored, due in part to the deposition of hemosiderin in the dermis. Ulceration is a frequent complication of stasis dermatitis of long standing.[499] Stasis dermatitis of the abdominal wall has been reported in the Budd–Chiari syndrome.[500]

Affected skin is unusually sensitive to contactants and, not infrequently, topical medications applied to these areas result in an eczematous reaction which can be quite widespread. This process of 'autoeczematization' is poorly understood (see below).

Histopathology[499,501]

Stasis dermatitis is unlikely to be biopsied unless complications such as ulceration, allergic contact dermatitis or basal cell carcinoma arise. In stasis dermatitis, the spongiosis is usually mild, although spongiotic vesiculation may develop if there is a superimposed contact dermatitis. Focal parakeratosis and scale crusts may also be present.

The dermal changes are usually prominent and include a proliferation of small blood vessels in the papillary dermis. This neovascularization may lead occasionally to the formation of a discrete papule. There is variable fibrosis of the dermis which can be quite prominent in cases of long standing. Abundant hemosiderin is present throughout the dermis. It is not localized to the upper third of the dermis, as occurs in the pigmented purpuric dermatoses (see p. 247). The veins in the deep dermis and subcutis are often thick walled.

AUTOECZEMATIZATION

Autoeczematization (autosensitization) is characterized by the dissemination, often widespread and quick, of a previously localized 'eczematous' process.[502] The term is often used with less precision to apply to other autosensitization reactions, whereby an inflammatory dermatitis develops at a site distant to the original inflammatory process or insult. The term 'id reaction' has also been applied to this latter group, which now seems less common than previously.

Included in the broad concept of autosensitization/autoeczematization are the distant reactions to localized dermatophyte infections (for example, pompholyx of the hands in response to dermatophyte infection elsewhere), to localized bacterial infections, scabies, burns and ionizing radiation,[502] and also to stasis dermatitis (see above). Generalization of a localized cutaneous eruption has been reported following the use of systemic prednisolone.[503] The development of recalcitrant eczema in patients with lymphoma or leukemia may result from a similar mechanism.[504]

The mechanism responsible for these reactions involves an abnormal immune response to autologous skin antigens.[505] Activated T lymphocytes appear to mediate this response.[506,507]

Histopathology

The histopathological reactions have not been widely studied. In cases of dissemination of an originally localized process, the changes will usually mimic those seen in the initial lesions. In other instances, the generalized reaction is that of a spongiotic process of variable intensity. In the author's experience, there has often been some edema of the superficial papillary dermis with some large (presumably activated) lymphocytes in the upper dermis. These two features may also be seen in spongiotic drug reactions (see p. 114) and dermal, systemic and protein contact dermatitis (see p. 107). Dermal edema may also be seen in the pompholyx associated with this process of autoeczematization (see p. 111). However, when epidermal spongiosis is associated with subepidermal edema and a history of rapid generalization of an initially localized lesion, autoeczematization will usually be present (Fig. 5.23).

PITYRIASIS ROSEA

Pityriasis rosea is a common, acute, self-limited dermatosis in which oval, salmon-pink, papulosquamous lesions develop on the trunk, neck and proximal extremities.[508] Lesions often follow the lines of skin cleavage. A scaly

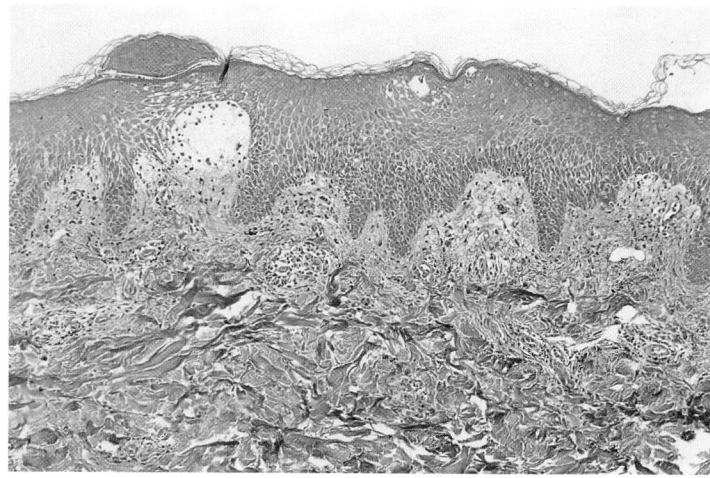

Fig. 5.23 **Autoeczematization.** This case shows spongiosis and characteristic subepidermal edema. (H & E)

plaque 2–10 cm in diameter, the 'herald patch', may develop on the trunk 1–2 weeks before the other lesions. Pityriasis rosea has been reported at all ages,[509] but the majority of patients are between 10 and 35 years.[510] Clinical variants include those with acral or facial involvement,[509] oral lesions,[511] a unilateral or local distribution,[512,513] or the presence of pustular, purpuric or vesicular lesions.[508,514,515]

The etiology is unknown, but an infectious etiology, particularly a virus, has long been suspected. This is supported by a history of a preceding upper respiratory tract infection in some patients,[516] occasional involvement of close-contact pairs,[510] case clustering,[517] modification of the disease by the use of convalescent serum or erythromycin,[518] and the development of a pityriasis rosea-like eruption in some cases of infection by ECHO 6 virus and by *Mycoplasma*.[508] There has been recent interest in the role of human herpesvirus-6 (HHV-6) and -7 (HHV-7) in the etiology of pityriasis rosea. While HHV-6 and HHV-7 may play a role in some patients,[519–521] the low detection rate of HHV-7 DNA sequences argues against a causative role for this virus.[522] In the case of HHV-6, reactivation of the virus during the early stages of the disease might explain its detection in some cases.[523] Particles resembling togavirus or arenavirus have been found on electron microscopy of a herald patch,[524] suggesting that this might be the inoculation site. No virus has ever been cultured.[525] Immunological reactions,[526] particularly cell-mediated, have also been regarded as important.[527]

A pityriasis rosea-like eruption has been reported in association with the administration of many drugs,[508] including gold, bismuth, arsenicals, ketotifen, clonidine, barbiturates, methoxypromazine, omeprazole,[528] terbinafine, benfluorex,[529] pyribenzamine, penicillamine, isotretinoin, metronidazole[530] and captopril.[531] A pityriasis rosea-like eruption has also been recorded as a complication of graft-versus-host reaction, following bone marrow transplantation.[532]

Histopathology[527,533,534]

Although the lesions are clinically papulosquamous, microscopy shows a spongiotic tissue reaction. The histopathological features are not pathognomonic, although in most cases they are sufficiently characteristic to allow the diagnosis to be made, even without a clinical history (Fig. 5.24). The epidermis often has a vaguely undulating appearance. There is usually focal parakeratosis, sometimes with the formation of parakeratotic mounds. There is a diminution of the granular layer and focal spongiosis with lymphocyte exocytosis (Fig. 5.25). Small spongiotic vesicles, sometimes simulating Pautrier microabscesses because of the aggregation of lymphocytes within them, are a characteristic feature; they are present in most cases if several levels are examined. Dyskeratotic cells may be seen at all levels of the epidermis; they are more common in the herald patch. Apoptotic keratinocytes are present in the lower epidermis in lesions undergoing involution. Multinucleate epidermal cells are uncommon. Focal acantholytic dyskeratosis has been reported once.[535]

The papillary dermis shows some edema and sometimes homogenization of collagen. There may be some melanin incontinence. Red cell extravasation is common in the upper dermis and may extend into the lower layers of the epidermis. There is a mild to moderate lymphohistiocytic infiltrate in the upper dermis, with some eosinophils in the infiltrate in older lesions.

Electron microscopy

Ultrastructural examination has confirmed the presence of dyskeratotic cells in some patients.[536] These cells show aggregation of tonofilaments, some cytoplasmic vacuoles and intracytoplasmic desmosomes.[537] Cytolytic degeneration of keratinocytes adjacent to Langerhans cells has been reported in a herald patch.[538] Virus-like particles were seen in one study.[536]

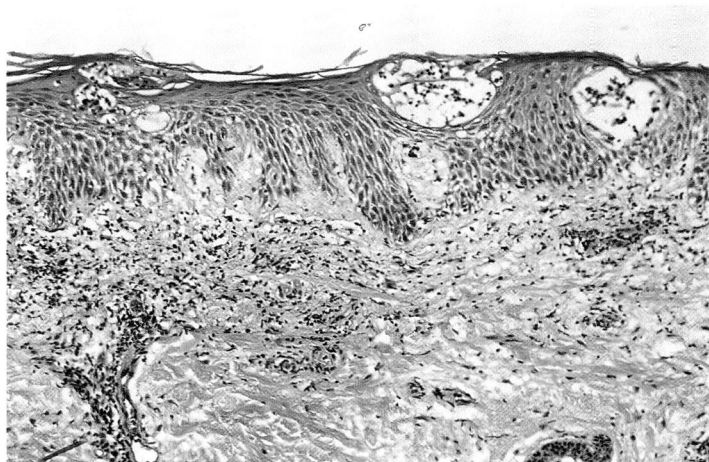
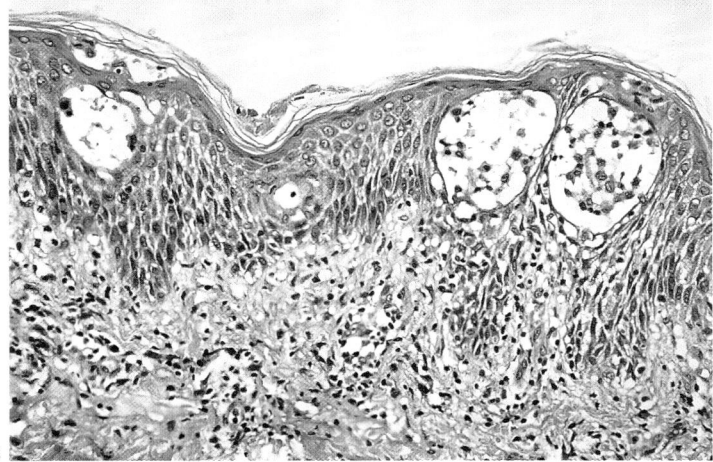

Fig. 5.24 **Pityriasis rosea. (A)** The spongiotic vesicles may contain more lymphocytes than one usually sees in spongiotic foci. **(B)** These 'Pautrier-like' foci are a characteristic feature. This case is more spongiotic than usual. (H & E)

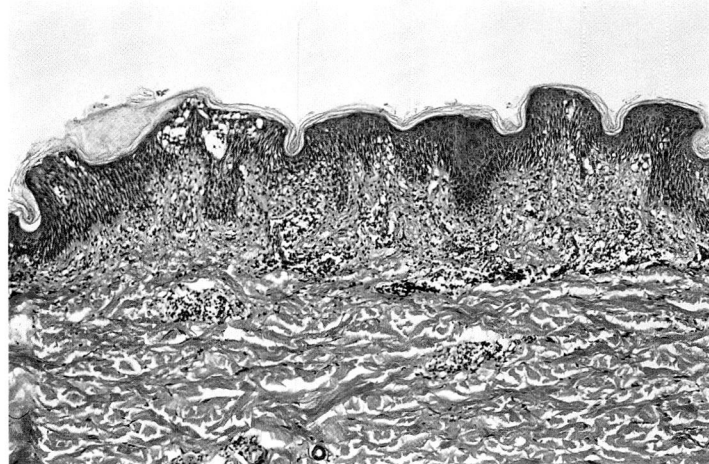

Fig. 5.25 **Pityriasis rosea.** Note the undulating epidermis and the small Pautrier-like foci. (H & E)

PAPULAR ACRODERMATITIS OF CHILDHOOD

Papular acrodermatitis of childhood (Gianotti–Crosti syndrome) is an uncommon, self-limited disease of low infectivity characterized by the triad of an erythematous papular erupt on of several weeks' duration, localized to the face and limbs, mild lymphadenopathy, and acute hepatitis which is usually anicteric.[539–541] The skin lesions are flat-topped papules 1–2 mm in diameter, which sometimes coalesce. An isomorphic response (Koebner phenomenon) is often present.[542] The lesions may be mildly pruritic. Hepatitis B surface antigen is often present in the serum.[543–545]

It is now apparent that other viral infections, in particular infection with the Epstein–Barr virus,[546,547] coxsackie virus A16,[548] parainfluenza virus, hepatitis A virus,[549] hepatitis C virus,[550] human immunodeficiency virus[551] and cytomegalovirus,[552] are rarely associated with a similar acral dermatitis;[553,554] hepatitis and lymphadenopathy are not commonly present in these circumstances.[553,554] Gianotti used the term 'papulovesicular acrorelated syndrome' for these cases.[541,555] Although infections associated with these other viruses often pursue a longer course and may have tiny vesicular lesions, individual cases occur which closely resemble those associated with the hepatitis B virus. Accordingly, it seems best to group all these virus-related disorders under the term Gianotti–Crosti syndrome.

In the author's experience, there is an increasing incidence of cutaneous reactions to viral and presumptive viral infections, ranging from those resembling Gianotti–Crosti syndrome at one end of the spectrum to others with histological features of mild pityriasis lichenoides. The clinical expression and distribution of these changes is somewhat variable, making the delineation of a specific clinicopathological entity a difficult task.

Histopathology[556]

Although the changes are not diagnostically specific, they are often sufficiently characteristic at least to suggest the diagnosis. The appearances at low magnification often suggest that three tissue reactions – lichenoid, spongiotic and vasculitic – are simultaneously present.[553] On closer inspection there is prominent exocytosis of mononuclear cells into the lower epidermis. This is usually associated with some basal vacuolar change, but cell death is not a conspicuous feature.[557] The spongiosis is usually mild, but small spongiotic vesicles, containing a few inflammatory cells and resembling those of pityriasis rosea, may be present (see above). Although most observers specifically deny the presence of a vasculitis, because of the absence of fibrin,[539] there is always a tight perivascular infiltrate of lymphocytes associated with variable endothelial swelling. In many instances the changes merit a diagnosis of lymphocytic vasculitis.[553] The inflammatory infiltrate not only fills the papillary dermis and extends into the epidermis, but it usually involves the mid and even the lower dermis to a lesser extent. There is often some edema of the papillary dermis. Epidermal spongiosis is less prominent in cases related to the hepatitis B virus.

SPONGIOTIC DRUG REACTIONS

Spongiotic reactions to drugs occur in several different clinical and pathogenetic settings, although in some instances the precise mechanism that results in the spongiosis is unknown (see Table 5.2). A delayed hypersensitivity response is usually suspected.[558] The three major categories of spongiotic drug reactions are provocation of an endogenous dermatitis, systemic contact reactions, and a miscellaneous group. Excluded from this discussion are the spongiotic reactions resembling pityriasis rosea produced by gold,[559] captopril[531] and other drugs, the phototoxic and photoallergic reactions produced by a variety of drugs,[560,561] and allergic contact dermatitis resulting from the topical application of various substances. Although there is mild spongiosis in the exanthematous (morbilliform) eruptions, these are histopathologically distinct from the other spongiotic reactions.

Table 5.2 **Drugs causing spongiosis***

Allergic contact dermatitis: Amide anesthetics, antihistamines (topical), bacitracin, benzocaine, corticosteroids, cosmetics, doxepin, ethylenediamine, fluorouracil, formaldehyde, idoxuridine, lanoconazole, melaleuca (tea-tree) oil, mupirocin, neomycin, nickel, NSAIDs, parabens, phenylenediamine, propacetamol, propylene glycol, psoralens, vitamin E preparations

Nummular dermatitis: Antimycobacterial drugs (in combination), gold, latanoprost eye drops, mercury (in dental fillings), methyldopa

Seborrheic dermatitis: Arsenic, chlorpromazine, cimetidine, gold, methyldopa

Pityriasis-rosea like: Barbiturates, benfluorex, bismuth, captopril, clonidine, enalapril, gold, isotretinoin, ketotifen, methoxypromazine, metronidazole omeprazole, penicillamine, pyribenzamine, terbinafine

Systemic contact dermatitis: Aminophylline, amoxicillin, ampicillin, chloral hydrate, cimetidine, cinnamon oil, clonidine, codeine, disulfiram, diuretics, erythromycin, gentamicin, hydroxyurea, hypoglycemic agents, immunoglobulins, isoniazid, minoxidil, neomycin, procaine, quinine, sweetening agents (artificial), synergistins, thiamine

Non-specific spongiosis: The most common causes (leading to biopsy) are ACE inhibitors, allopurinol, atenolol, calcium channel blockers, NSAIDs (some) and thiazide diuretics (particularly compound ones such as Moduretic). Specific drugs include calcitonin, estrogen, fluoxetine (Prozac), gold, indomethacin, immunoglobulin infusion, interleukins, nifedipine, paroxetine (Aropax), phenytoin sodium, piroxicam, progesterone, sulfasalazine, tamoxifen and subcutaneous injection of danaparoid, GMCSF, heparin, vitamin K

Photoallergic dermatitis: Alprazolam, amlodipine, ampiroxicam, chlordiazepoxide, chlorpromazine, clofibrate, cyclamates, diphenhydramine, droxicam, fenofibrate, flutamide, griseofulvin, ibuprofen, ketoprofen, lomefloxacin, piketoprofen, piroxicam, pyridoxine, quinidine, quinine, ranitidine, sertraline, sulfonamides, tegafur, tetracyclines, thiazides, tolbutamide, triflusal

Phototoxic dermatitis (spongiosis variable; apoptosis ballooning and/or necrosis may be present): Amiodarone, carbamazepine, doxycycline, dyes (some clothing), fleroxacin, non-steroidal anti-inflammatory drugs, oflaxacin, phenothiazines, retinoids, sulfonamides, tetrazepam, thiazides, thioxanthenes

* Excluded from consideration are the drugs causing neutrophilic and eosinophilic spongiosis as precursors of vesiculobullous diseases, and the chemicals (largely industry-related) producing irritant contact dermatitis.

Reactions resembling seborrheic or nummular dermatitis have been reported following the use of latanoprost eye drops for lowering intraocular pressure,[292] and the ingestion of various drugs including cimetidine, methyldopa[293] and antituberculous therapy.[293] This is assumed to be a *provocation reaction* in an individual with a predisposition to the development of an endogenous dermatitis.[293]

Systemic contact dermatitis results from the administration of an allergen to an individual who has been sensitized to that agent by previous contact with it or with a related substance.[558] Systemic contact dermatitis may present as an exacerbation of vesicular hand dermatitis, as an eczematous flare at sites of previously positive patch tests, or as a systemic eczematous eruption with a predisposition for the buttocks, genital areas, elbow flexures, axillae, eyelids and side of the neck.[562] The term 'baboon syndrome' was coined for this eruption.[562] This is an important category of spongiotic drug reaction in which numerous drugs have been incriminated. They include antibiotics used topically as well as systemically, such as neomycin, erythromycin,[363] ampicillin, amoxicillin,[564] synergistins[565] and gentamicin, as well as procaine, quinine, chloral hydrate, cimetidine,[566] clonidine, minoxidil, codeine, disulfiram, thiamine, isoniazid, cinnamon oil, hydroxyurea,[567] mercury vapor,[568] papaya juice,[569] aminophylline (crossreacting with ethylenediamine, a stabilizer in creams)[570] and certain oral hypoglycemic agents, diuretics and sweetening agents which crossreact with sulfonamides.[562,571,572] Ingestion of derivatives of the lacquer tree (*Rhus*), used in traditional (folk) medicine,[573] and the intravenous infusion of immunoglobulins[574] are two additional causes of systemic contact dermatitis.

The *miscellaneous category* of drugs producing the spongiotic tissue reaction undoubtedly includes agents that should be more appropriately included in other categories. For example, thiazide diuretics are usually included among the agents that produce photosensitive eruptions but it appears that, on occasions, an eruption is produced which is not confined to sun-exposed areas.[575,576] Other drugs in this miscellaneous category include calcium channel blockers (such as nifedipine), calcitonin, sulfasalazine,[576] indomethacin,[576] fluoxetine (Prozac),[577] paroxetine (Aropax), allopurinol,[576] piroxicam,[578] tamoxifen and phenytoin sodium (sensitivity reaction).[579] The subcutaneous injection of heparin, semisynthetic heparinoids (such as danaparoid) or vitamin K_1 may produce an eczematous plaque.[580–583] The infusion of IL-2 or human immune globulin[584] and the subcutaneous injection of either IL-6 or granulocyte-monocyte colony-stimulating factor (GMCSF) have been associated with a spongiotic tissue reaction.[585–588] Gold, in addition to causing a pityriasis rosea-like reaction, also produces an eczematous eruption which may last for up to 12 months after the cessation of gold therapy.[589,590] Estrogen and progesterone (usually endogenous) have been associated with a spongiotic reaction.[591–593] They produce recurrent skin eruptions premenstrually. Other patterns (urticaria and erythema multiforme) have been attributed to these hormones.[594]

The incidence of spongiotic drug reactions is difficult to assess. Some reports make no mention of this type of reaction. One study reported that approximately 10% of cutaneous drug reactions were of 'eczematous' type.[595] In addition to generalized papules and eczematous plaques, a fixed eczematous eruption can also occur, the agents responsible usually being antibiotics.

Histopathology

By definition, there is epidermal spongiosis: this may occur at all levels of the epidermis. Spongiotic vesiculation is sometimes present. A characteristic feature is the presence of exocytosis of lymphocytes and occasionally of eosinophils. Often there is more exocytosis than would be expected for the amount of spongiosis in the region (Fig. 5.26). Rare Civatte bodies (apoptotic cells) are almost invariably present, but a careful search is usually necessary to find these (Fig. 5.27). Small spongiotic vesicles containing lymphocytes are a characteristic feature of pityriasis rosea-like eruptions (Fig. 5.28). In exanthematous eruptions the spongiosis and exocytosis are confined to the basal layers of the epidermis in a rather characteristic pattern.[596] Other epidermal changes in spongiotic drug reactions include variable parakeratosis and, in chronic lesions, some acanthosis.

The papillary dermis shows mild to moderate edema and there is a predominantly perivascular infiltrate of lymphocytes. Occasional eosinophils are often present, but this is not invariable. Some of the lymphoid cells appear to be larger than the usual mature lymphocyte. In a study of gold-induced reactions the lymphocytes were characterized as T-helper cells.[590] Another feature of the infiltrate is its tendency to extend into the mid dermis, somewhat deeper than is usual with other spongiotic disorders. Red cell extravasation is sometimes present in the upper dermis.[590] Pigment incontinence is uncommon.

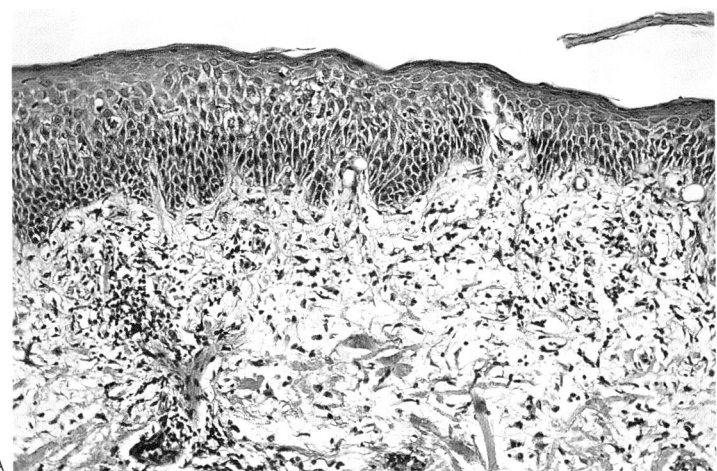

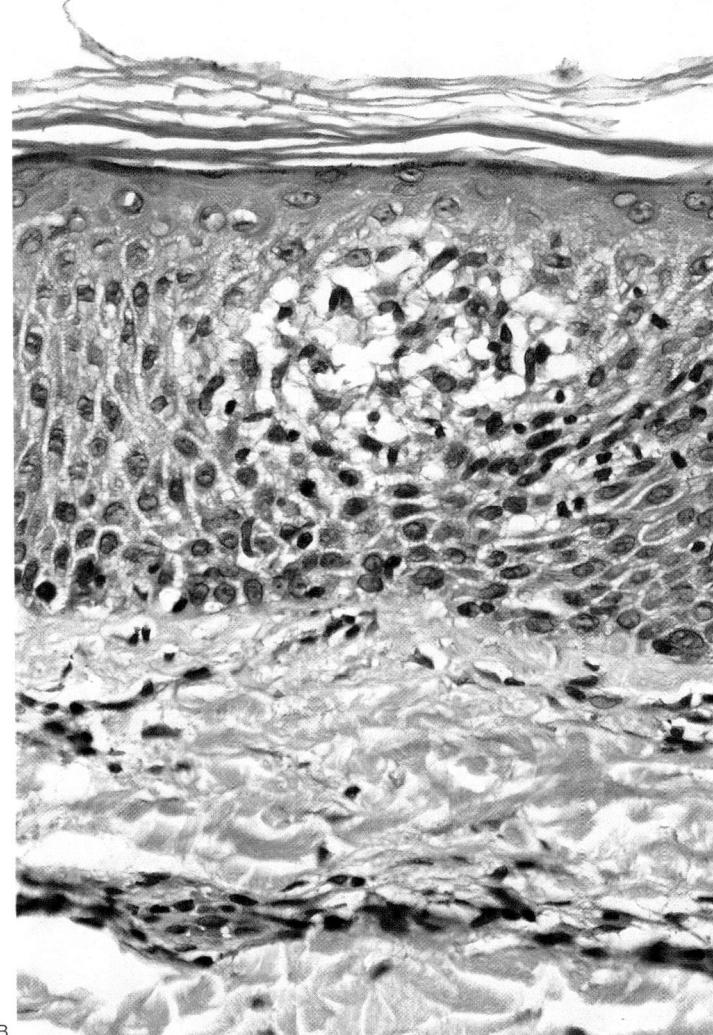

Fig. 5.26 **(A) Spongiotic drug reaction. (B)** There is more exocytosis of inflammatory cells in spongiotic drug reactions than in most other spongiotic diseases. (H & E)

CHRONIC SUPERFICIAL DERMATITIS

Chronic superficial dermatitis (persistent superficial dermatitis, small plaque parapsoriasis,[597] digitate dermatosis[598]) is characterized by well-defined, round to oval patches with a fine 'cigarette-paper' scale, usually situated on the trunk and proximal parts of the extremities.[597,599] Individual lesions measure 2–5 cm in diameter, although larger patches, sometimes with a digitate pattern, may be found on the lower limbs, particularly the thighs.[600] The lesions usually have a reddish-brown color, although the hue is yellowish in a small number

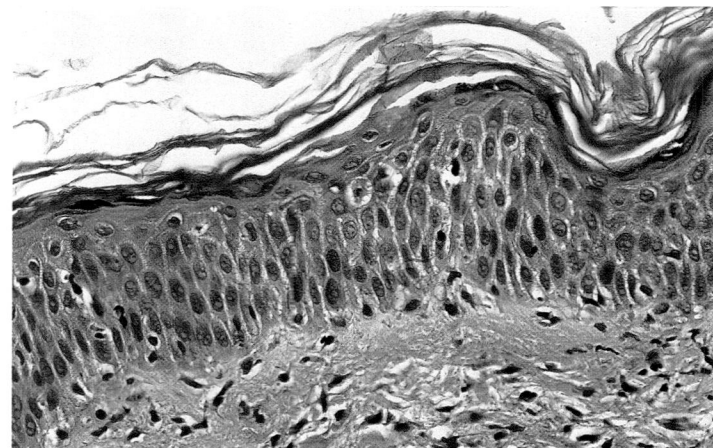

Fig. 5.27 **Spongiotic drug reaction**. The spongiosis is minimal in this area of the biopsy. Note the exocytosis of lymphocytes and an apoptotic keratinocyte. (H & E)

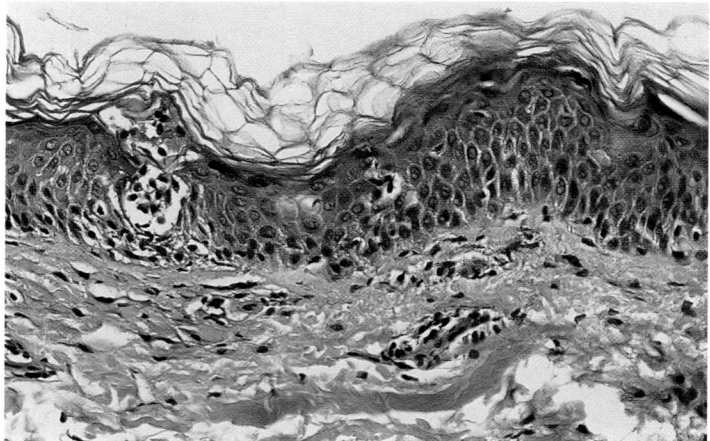

Fig. 5.28 **Spongiotic drug reaction** with pityriasis rosea-like features. An ACE inhibitor was implicated. (H & E)

of cases.[601] The term 'xanthoerythrodermia perstans' was applied in the past to these latter cases.[598,602]

Onset of the disease is usually in middle life and there is a male predominance. The lesions are mostly asymptomatic and persistent, although a minority clear spontaneously.[603] Chronic superficial dermatitis, unlike large plaque parapsoriasis, with which it has been confused in the past, does not appear to progress to lymphoma,[550] despite the recent findings of a dominant T-cell clone in some cases.[604] For various reasons, Ackerman and colleagues regard it as an early stage of mycosis fungoides.[605,606] Others have called it an 'abortive' lymphoma[607,608] or a distinct disorder 'only weakly associated with mycosis fungoides'.[609] Until the clinical significance of clonality and the chain of events leading to tumor progression are better understood, the true nature of this process will remain speculative.

Histopathology[597,600]

Although chronic superficial dermatitis is classified with the spongiotic tissue reaction, it must be emphasized that in this condition the spongiosis is usually only focal and mild. There is usually focal parakeratosis or focal scale crust formation, implying preceding spongiosis. The epidermis is usually acanthotic and, in older lesions, there may be psoriasiform hyperplasia.

A mild infiltrate of lymphocytes and occasional histiocytes is present around blood vessels in the superficial plexus. Cells often extend high in the papillary dermis, a characteristic feature. Exocytosis of these cells is common, but mild (Fig. 5.29). There are no interface changes as in pityriasis lichenoides chronica and no atypical lymphoid cells as may occur in mycosis fungoides.

BLASCHKO DERMATITIS

In 1990, Grosshans and Marot described an adult male with acquired, unilateral, relapsing inflammatory lesions, in a linear arrangement along Blaschko's lines.[610] The designations 'acquired relapsing self-healing Blaschko dermatitis' and 'Blaschkitis'[611] have since been applied.[612] The etiology is unknown, but genomic mosaicism has been suggested as the explanation for the distribution. The histopathology is characterized by an acute or subacute spongiotic dermatitis with spongiotic vesiculation.[612]

PSORIASIS

Spongiosis can occur in the early stages of psoriasis associated with lymphocyte exocytosis. It can be seen in established lesions of psoriasis on the palms and soles, leading to difficulties in distinguishing these cases from allergic contact dermatitis. The presence of mounds of scale crust, regularly distributed within the cornified layer (akin to the mounds of parakeratosis containing neutrophils at their summits seen in psoriasis elsewhere on the body), is characteristic of psoriasis on volar surfaces.[13] Spongiosis is often present in erythrodermic psoriasis.

Rarely, an established case of psoriasis will show mild spongiosis, sometimes associated with features seen in the glucagonoma syndrome (see p. 552), such as mild epidermal vacuolation and intracorneal neutrophils.

LIGHT REACTIONS

Epidermal spongiosis may be seen in photoallergic dermatitis (see p. 601), phototoxic dermatitis (see p. 599), the so-called 'eczematous' form of polymorphous light eruption, and certain persistent light reactions such as actinic reticuloid (see p. 604).

Histopathology
Photoallergic and phototoxic reactions are akin to allergic contact and irritant contact reactions respectively. They may be morphologically indistinguish-

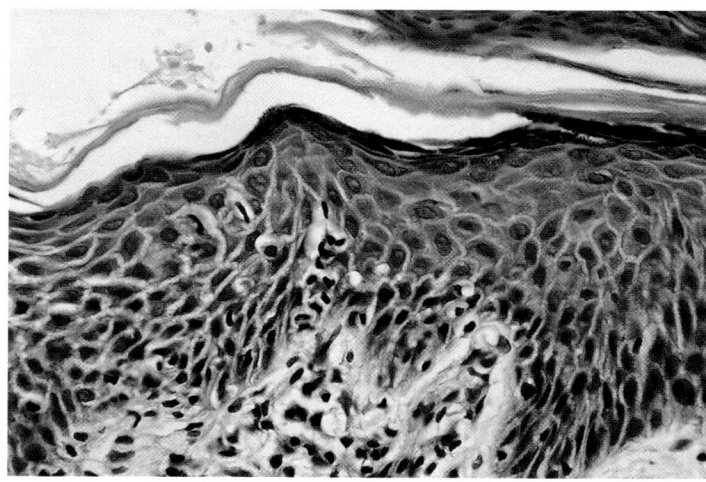

Fig. 5.29 **Chronic superficial dermatitis.** The epidermis is only mildly spongiotic and there is focal exocytosis of mature lymphocytes into the epidermis. (H & E)

able, although in some photoallergic reactions the inflammatory cell infiltrate extends deeper in the dermis. There is usually a superficial and deep perivascular infiltrate of lymphocytes in the papulovesicular form (so-called 'eczematous' type) of polymorphous light eruption. The epidermis shows variable spongiosis leading to spongiotic vesiculation.

Actinic reticuloid may have a mildly spongiotic epidermis. However, the diagnosis is usually made on the basis of the dense, polymorphous infiltrate in the upper dermis which includes some large lymphoid cells with hyperchromatic nuclei and stellate fibroblasts.

DERMATOPHYTOSES

Dermatophyte infections can present with a spongiotic dermatitis, and clinically they can mimic a range of 'eczematous' dermatitides.

Histopathology
In addition to the spongiosis, the stratum corneum is usually abnormal, with compact orthokeratosis or parakeratosis sandwiched between orthokeratotic layers or the presence of neutrophils in the stratum corneum. Sometimes spongiotic pustules are present. The presence of neutrophils within the epidermis or stratum corneum warrants a careful search for hyphae, including the use of the PAS stain.

ARTHROPOD BITES

Epidermal spongiosis is a common finding in certain arthropod bite reactions, particularly scabies. Vesicles and rarely bullous lesions may develop in response to some arthropods. The spongiosis is usually of eosinophilic type (see p. 100), but certain beetles can produce neutrophilic spongiosis. Contact with moths of the genus *Hylesia* is said to cause vesicular lesions. Although not arthropod related, mention should be made here of cercarial dermatitis (see p. 732), which can mimic a bite reaction.

Histopathology
There is variable spongiosis, sometimes leading to spongiotic vesiculation. Exocytosis of eosinophils through the epidermis may be present, but eosinophilic spongiosis is quite uncommon. The dermis contains a superficial and deep perivascular infiltrate of lymphocytes and eosinophils; characteristically, there are interstitial eosinophils.

GROVER'S DISEASE

There is a rare variant of Grover's disease, clinically indistinguishable from the other histopathological variants, in which spongiosis is present (see p. 297).

Histopathology
Suprabasal clefting with some overlying dyskeratotic cells and grains will be found in addition to the spongiosis.

TOXIC SHOCK SYNDROME

Small foci of spongiosis containing a few neutrophils and scattered degenerate keratinocytes are a feature of this rare staphylococcal toxin syndrome (see p. 619).

PUPPP

PUPPP (pruritic urticarial papules and plaques of pregnancy), also known as toxic erythema of pregnancy (see p. 244), presents as an intensely pruritic eruption of papules and urticarial plaques towards the end of pregnancy.

Histopathology
The tissue reaction is a subtle lymphocytic vasculitis with variable edema of the papillary dermis. Epidermal spongiosis is present in one-third of cases. There may be focal parakeratosis as well.

ERYTHEMA ANNULARE CENTRIFUGUM

There are one or more annular, erythematous lesions which may spread outwards or remain stationary. A fine scale is sometimes present inside the advancing edge (see p. 245). The annular erythema of Sjögren's syndrome is sometimes spongiotic.[613]

Histopathology
A biopsy through the advancing edge will show focal spongiosis and parakeratosis with an underlying superficial perivascular infiltrate of lymphocytes, often with a 'coat-sleeve' appearance. There are some similarities to pityriasis rosea, although a biopsy taken at right angles to the edge of erythema annulare centrifugum will show a much more localized process. A variant without spongiosis and with a deep as well as superficial inflammatory infiltrate also occurs.

PIGMENTED PURPURIC DERMATOSES

Epidermal spongiosis, usually mild, may be present in several clinical variants of the pigmented purpuric dermatoses (see p. 247). The presence of a superficial, band-like infiltrate of inflammatory cells, often associated with a lymphocytic vasculitis, and the deposition of hemosiderin in the upper dermis usually overshadow the spongiosis. Lesions of purpuric contact dermatitis (see p. 106) may closely resemble those of the pigmented purpuric dermatoses.

PITYRIASIS ALBA

Pityriasis alba consists of variably hypopigmented, slightly scaly patches, usually on the head and neck of atopic individuals (see p. 327).

Histopathology
Pityriasis alba should be considered if there is mild epidermal spongiosis with minimal exocytosis and focal parakeratosis in the clinical setting of hypopigmented lesions. There is a reduction in melanin in the basal layer of the epidermis.

ERUPTION OF LYMPHOCYTE RECOVERY

Mild epidermal spongiosis is usually present (see p. 47).

LICHEN STRIATUS

Lichen striatus is a linear, papular eruption with a predilection for children and adolescents (see p. 40). There is a lichenoid tissue reaction involving a number of adjacent dermal papillae. The overlying epidermis is acanthotic with mild spongiosis and exocytosis of inflammatory cells. In summary, it is a lichenoid/spongiotic dermatosis.

ERYTHRODERMA

Erythroderma (exfoliative dermatitis) may complicate various spongiotic dermatitides, including atopic dermatitis, seborrheic dermatitis, photosensitive eczematous processes (for example, actinic reticuloid), nummular dermatitis, stasis dermatitis and contact dermatitis (see p. 576).

Histopathology

The underlying, pre-existing dermatosis is not always diagnosable when erythroderma supervenes. Often the amount of spongiosis is mild, even in cases with a pre-existing spongiotic dermatitis; there may even be psoriasiform hyperplasia of the epidermis without spongiosis in these circumstances. Spongiosis is usually present in the congenital erythroderma accompanying Omenn's syndrome.[614]

MYCOSIS FUNGOIDES

Mycosis fungoides is a cutaneous T-cell lymphoma which evolves through several clinical stages (see p. 1104). An unequivocal diagnosis is sometimes difficult to make in the early stages of the disease.

Histopathology

There has been controversy in the past regarding the presence or absence of spongiosis in lesions of mycosis fungoides.[615,616] In one study, slight spongiosis was found in 38% of lesions in the patch/plaque stage and moderate spongiosis in a further 17%.[616] There was no microvesiculation.[616] The epidermis appears to contain increased amounts of acid mucopolysaccharides. Other features which allow mycosis fungoides to be distinguished from other spongiotic disorders include the presence of a band-like infiltrate of lymphocytes (some atypical) and often eosinophils and plasma cells in the upper dermis associated with papillary dermal fibrosis. There is usually prominent epidermotropism of the lymphoid cells.

Spongiosis may also be found in the Sézary syndrome (see p. 1110).

ACROKERATOSIS PARANEOPLASTICA

Acrokeratosis paraneoplastica (Bazex's syndrome) is characterized by mild spongiosis (see p. 575). Other changes include hyperkeratosis, focal parakeratosis, exocytosis of lymphocytes and scattered apoptotic keratinocytes.

Table 5.3 **Histopathological features of the spongiotic diseases (excluding eosinophilic, miliarial and follicular variants)**

Disease	Histopathological features
Irritant contact dermatitis	Superficial ballooning, necrosis and neutrophils; mild irritants produce spongiotic dermatitis mimicking allergic contact dermatitis, although superficial apoptotic keratinocytes may also be present
Allergic contact dermatitis	Variable spongiosis and vesiculation at different horizontal and vertical levels, with an 'ordered' pattern; mild exocytosis; progressive psoriasiform hyperplasia with chronicity; usually eosinophils in superficial dermal infiltrate; superficial dermal edema
Protein contact dermatitis	No distinguishing features recorded; an urticarial component may be present
Nummular dermatitis	May mimic allergic contact dermatitis but usually more 'untidy'. Neutrophils may be in dermal infiltrate and even the epidermis; the psoriasiform hyperplasia in chronic cases may show variable thickening of adjacent rete pegs
Seborrheic dermatitis	Variable spongiosis and psoriasiform hyperplasia depending on activity and chronicity. Scale crust and spongiosis may localize to follicular ostia
Atopic dermatitis	Mimics other spongiotic diseases with variable spongiosis (usually quite mild) and psoriasiform hyperplasia; subtle features include prominence of vessels in the papillary dermis, increased epidermal volume without necessarily producing psoriasiform folding; eosinophil major basic protein present, sometimes disproportionate to eosinophils
Pompholyx	Vesiculation with peripheral displacement of acrosyringia; process usually more sharply defined than allergic contact dermatitis of palms and soles; some evolve into picture of pustulosis palmaris with neutrophils (important to exclude fungi in these cases with PAS stain)
Stasis dermatitis	Mild spongiosis only; proliferation of superficial dermal vessels; extravasation of erythrocytes; abundant hemosiderin
Autoeczematization	Variable spongiosis; edema of papillary dermis and activated lymphocytes often present
Pityriasis rosea	Undulating epidermis with focal parakeratosis and spongiotic vesicles, sometimes resembling small Pautrier microabscesses; lymphocyte exocytosis; sometimes erythrocyte extravasation in papillary dermis; 'herald patch' is more psoriasiform
Papular acrodermatitis of childhood	Three tissue reaction patterns (lichenoid, spongiotic and lymphocytic vasculitis) often present; small spongiotic vesicles resembling pityriasis rosea may be present
Spongiotic drug reactions	Spongiosis with conspicuous exocytosis of lymphocytes relative to the amount of spongiosis; rare apoptotic keratinocytes; eosinophils, plasma cells and activated lymphocytes may be in superficial dermal infiltrate; may show mid-dermal spillover; sometimes superficial dermal edema
Chronic superficial dermatitis	Only mild spongiosis and focal parakeratosis with variable psoriasiform hyperplasia; superficial perivascular infiltrate with characteristic upward extension and mild exocytosis
Light reactions	Variable, usually mild spongiosis; superficial and deep perivascular dermal inflammation; a deep infiltrate is not invariable in lesions of short duration; subepidermal edema in some cases of polymorphous light eruption; stellate fibroblasts, vertical collagen streaking, variable psoriasiform hyperplasia and some atypical lymphocytes with exocytosis in actinic reticuloid; scattered 'sunburn cells' in phototoxic lesions (sometimes with only mild other changes); deeply extending, straight, basophilic (elastotic) fibers in lesions of long duration
Dermatophytoses	Neutrophils in stratum corneum, or compact orthokeratosis or 'sandwich sign' should alert observer to perform a PAS stain. Spongiotic vesicles may form on palms and soles
Arthropod bites	Spongiotic vesicles containing variable numbers of eosinophils; superficial and deep dermal inflammation with interstitial eosinophils
Grover's disease	Spongiosis with focal acantholysis in the spongiotic variant; untidy superficial dermal inflammation

Table 5.3 **Histopathological features of the spongiotic diseases (excluding eosinophilic, miliarial and follicular variants) (Continued)**

Disease	Histopathological features
Toxic erythema of pregnancy	Spongiosis mild and inconstant; variable papillary dermal edema; tight superficial perivascular infiltrate sometimes extending to mid dermis; interstitial eosinophils in some cases
Erythema annulare centrifugum	Mild spongiosis and focal parakeratosis at periphery of lesion; mild perivascular cuffing with lymphocytes
Pigmented purpuric dermatoses	Spongiosis mild and inconstant; lymphocytic vasculitis with variably dense infiltrate in the papillary dermis; hemosiderin in the upper dermis
Pityriasis alba	Clinical diagnosis; mild focal spongiosis with minimal parakeratosis
Erythroderma	Mild spongiosis; variable psoriasiform hyperplasia; appearances depend on underlying disease; a difficult diagnosis without clinical history
Mycosis fungoides	Mild spongiosis, variable epidermal hyperplasia and epidermal mucinosis; epidermotropism, often with Pautrier microabscesses; variable cytological atypia of lymphocytes which extend upwards into the papillary dermis

REFERENCES

Introduction

1 Ackerman AB. More about spongiosis. Am J Dermatopathol 1984; 6: 419–420.
2 Russell Jones R. The histogenesis of eczema. Clin Exp Dermatol 1983; 8: 213–225.
3 Ackerman AB, Ragaz A. A plea to expunge the word 'eczema' from the lexicon of dermatology and dermatopathology. Am J Dermatopathol 1982; 4: 315–326.
4 Sulzberger MB. Eczema viewed from the perspective of 60 years' experience. Am J Dermatopathol 1982; 4: 337–338.
5 Altekrueger I, Ackerman AB. 'Eczema revisited'. A status report based upon current textbooks of dermatology. Am J Dermatopathol 1994; 16: 517–522.
6 Stenn KS, Balin AK, Higgins T, Stenn JO. Spongiosis. J Am Acad Dermatol 1981; 5: 213–214.
7 Russell Jones R. Spongiosis – a passive phenomenon? J Am Acad Dermatol 1982; 6: 547–549.
8 Russell Jones R. PEEPO: papular eruption with elimination of papillary oedema. Br J Dermatol 1982; 106: 393–400.
9 Russell Jones R, McDonald DM. Eczema. Immunopathogenesis and histogenesis. Am J Dermatopathol 1982; 4: 335–336.
10 Ackerman AB. Subtle clues to histopathologic findings from gross pathology (clinical lesions). Collarettes of scales as signs of spongiosis. Am J Dermatopathol 1979; 1: 267–272.
11 LeBoit PE, Epstein BA. A vase-like shape characterizes the epidermal-mononuclear cell collections seen in spongiotic dermatitis. Am J Dermatopathol 1990; 12: 612–616.
12 Candiago E, Marocolo D, Manganoni MA et al. Nonlymphoid intraepidermal mononuclear cell collections (pseudo-Pautrier abscesses). Am J Dermatopathol 2000; 22: 1–6.

Neutrophilic spongiosis

13 Ackerman AB. Histologic diagnosis of inflammatory skin diseases. An algorithmic method based on pattern analysis, 2nd edn. Baltimore: Williams & Wilkins, 1997.
14 Banney LA, Wood DJ, Francis GD. Whiplash rove beetle dermatitis in central Queensland. Australas J Dermatol 2000; 41: 162–167.
15 Şendur N, Şavk E, Karaman G. Paederus dermatitis: a report of 46 cases in Aydın, Turkey. Dermatology 1999; 199: 353–355.
16 Ramachandran S, Hern J, Almeyda J et al. Contact dermatitis with cervical lymphadenopathy following exposure to the hide beetle, Dermestes peruvianus. Br J Dermatol 1997; 136: 943–945.

Eosinophilic spongiosis

17 Emmerson RW, Wilson-Jones E. Eosinophilic spongiosis in pemphigus. Arch Dermatol 1968; 97: 252–257.
18 Ruiz E, Deng J-S, Abell EA. Eosinophilic spongiosis: a clinical, histologic, and immunopathological study. J Am Acad Dermatol 1994; 30: 973–976.
19 Knight AG, Black MM, Delaney TJ. Eosinophilic spongiosis. A clinical histological and immunofluorescent correlation. Clin Exp Dermatol 1976; 1: 141–153.
20 Brodersen I, Frentz G, Thomsen K. Eosinophilic spongiosis in early pemphigus foliaceus. Acta Derm Venereol 1978; 58: 368–369.
21 Cooper A, Le Guay J, Wells JV. Childhood pemphigus initially seen as eosinophilic spongiosis. Arch Dermatol 1981; 117: 662–663.
22 Osteen FB, Wheeler CE Jr, Briggaman RA, Puritz EM. Pemphigus foliaceus. Early clinical appearance as dermatitis herpetiformis with eosinophilic spongiosis. Arch Dermatol 1976; 112: 1148–1152.
23 Jablonska S, Chorzelski TP, Beutner EH, Chorzelska J. Herpetiform pemphigus, a variable pattern of pemphigus. Int J Dermatol 1975; 14: 353–359.

24 Marsden RA, Dawber RPR, Millard PR, Mowat AG. Herpetiform pemphigus induced by penicillamine. Br J Dermatol 1977; 97: 451–452.
25 Nishioka K, Hashimoto K, Katayama I et al. Eosinophilic spongiosis in bullous pemphigoid. Arch Dermatol 1984; 120: 1166–1168.
26 Ameen M, Pembroke AC, Black MM, Russell-Jones R. Eosinophilic spongiosis in association with bullous pemphigoid and chronic lymphocytic leukaemia. Br J Dermatol 2000; 143: 421–424.
27 Kennedy C, Hodge L, Sanderson KV. Eosinophilic spongiosis: a localized bullous dermatosis unassociated with pemphigus. Clin Exp Dermatol 1978; 3: 117–122.
28 Black MM. Eosinophilic spongiosis with polycythaemia rubra vera. Proc R Soc Med 1977; 70: 139–140.
29 Rueda RA, Valencia IC, Covelli C et al. Eosinophilic, polymorphic, and pruritic eruption associated with radiotherapy. Arch Dermatol 1999; 135: 804–810.

Miliarial spongiosis

30 Gupta AK, Ellis CN, Madison KC, Voorhees JJ. Miliaria crystallina occurring in a patient treated with isotretinoin. Cutis 1986; 38: 275–276.
31 Arpey CJ, Nagashima-Whelan LS, Chren M-M, Zaim MT. Congenital miliaria crystallina: case report and literature review. Pediatr Dermatol 1992; 9: 283–287.
32 O'Brien JP. A study of miliaria rubra, tropical anhidrosis and anhidrotic asthenia. Br J Dermatol 1947; 59: 124–158.
33 O'Brien JP. Tropical anhidrotic asthenia. Its definition and relationship to other heat disorders. Arch Intern Med 1948; 81: 799–831.
34 Holzle E, Kligman AM. The pathogenesis of miliaria rubra. Role of the resident microflora. Br J Dermatol 1978; 99: 117–137.
35 Kirk JF, Wilson BB, Chun W, Cooper PH. Miliaria profunda. J Am Acad Dermatol 1996; 35: 854–856.
36 Rogers M, Kan A, Stapleton K, Kemp A. Giant centrifugal miliaria profunda. Pediatr Dermatol 1990; 7: 140–146.
37 Loewenthal LJA. The pathogenesis of miliaria. The role of sodium chloride. Arch Dermatol 1961; 84: 2–17.
38 Mowad CM, McGinley KJ, Foglia A, Leyden JJ. The role of extracellular polysaccharide substance produced by Staphylococcus epidermidis in miliaria. J Am Acad Dermatol 1995; 33: 729–733.
39 O'Brien JP. The aetiology of poral closure. II. The role of staphylococcal infection in miliaria rubra and bullous impetigo. J Invest Dermatol 1950; 15: 102–133.
40 Sulzberger MB, Griffin TB. Induced miliaria, postmiliarial hypohidrosis, and some potential sequelae. Arch Dermatol 1969; 99: 145–149.
41 Henning DR, Griffin TB, Maibach HI. Studies on changes in skin surface bacteria in induced miliaria and associated hypohidrosis. Acta Derm Venereol 1972; 52: 371–375.
42 Lyons RE, Levine R, Auld D. Miliaria rubra. A manifestation of staphylococcal disease. Arch Dermatol 1962; 86: 282–286.
43 Singh E. The role of bacteria in anhidrosis. Dermatologica 1973; 146: 256–261.
44 Kossard S, Commens CA. Keratotic miliaria precipitated by radiotherapy. Arch Dermatol 1988; 124: 855–856.

Follicular spongiosis

45 Hitch JM, Lund HZ. Disseminate and recurrent infundibulo-folliculitis. Report of a case. Arch Dermatol 1968; 97: 432–435.
46 Hitch JM, Lund HZ. Disseminate and recurrent infundibulo-folliculitis. Arch Dermatol 1972; 105: 580–583.
47 Thew MA, Wood MG. Disseminate and recurrent infundibulo-folliculitis. Report of a second case. Arch Dermatol 1969; 100: 728–733.

48 Soyinka F. Recurrent disseminated infundibulofolliculitis. Int J Dermatol 1973; 12: 314–317.

49 Owen WR, Wood C. Disseminate and recurrent infundibulofolliculitis. Arch Dermato 1979; 115: 174–175.

Other spongiotic disorders

50 Marks JG Jr, Zaino RJ, Bressler MF, Williams JV. Changes in lymphocyte and Langerhans cell populations in allergic and irritant contact dermatitis. Int J Dermatol 1987; 26: 354–357.

51 Rietschel RL. Irritant contact dermatitis. Dermatol Clin 1984; 2: 545–551.

52 Willis CM, Stephens CJM, Wilkinson JD. Experimentally-induced irritant contact dermatitis. Determination of optimum irritant concentrations. Contact Dermatitis 1988; 18: 20–24.

53 Hatch KL, Maibach HI. Textile fiber dermatitis. Contact Dermatitis 1985; 12: 1–11.

54 Chen JY, Phillips R, Lewis AT et al. Irritant contact dermatitis secondary to fiberglass: an unusual presentation. Int J Dermatol 2000; 39: 372–374.

55 Foley P, Nixon R, Marks R et al. The frequency of reactions to sunscreens: results of a longitudinal population-based study on the regular use of sunscreens in Australia. Br J Dermatol 1993; 128: 512–518.

56 Catanzaro JM, Smith JG Jr. Propylene glycol dermatitis. J Am Acad Dermatol 1991; 24: 90–95.

57 Lear JT, Tan BB, Lovell CR, English JSC. Irritant contact dermatitis from *Cerastium tomentosum* (snow-in-summer). Contact Dermatitis 1996; 35: 182.

58 Webster GL. Irritant plants in the spurge family (Euphorbiaceae). Clin Dermatol 1986; 4: 36–45.

59 Worobec SM, Hickey TA, Kinghorn AD et al. Irritant contact dermatitis from an ornamental Euphorbia. Contact Dermatitis 1981; 7: 19–22.

60 Dooms-Goossens AE, Debusschere KM, Gevers DM et al. Contact dermatitis caused by airborne agents. A review and case reports. J Am Acad Dermatol 1986; 15: 1–10.

61 Wigger-Alberti W, Krebs A, Elsner P. Experimental irritant contact dermatitis due to cumulative epicutaneous exposure to sodium lauryl sulphate and toluene: single and concurrent application. Br J Dermatol 2000; 143: 551–556.

62 Patterson SE, Williams JV, Marks JG Jr. Prevention of sodium lauryl sulfate irritant contact dermatitis by Pro-Q aerosol foam skin protectant. J Am Acad Dermatol 1999; 40: 783–785.

63 Wigger-Alberti W, Caduff L, Burg G, Elsner P. Experimentally induced chronic irritant contact dermatitis to evaluate the efficacy of protective creams in vivo. J Am Acad Dermatol 1999; 40: 590–596.

64 Andersen KE, Benezra C, Burrows D et al. Contact dermatitis. A review. Contact Dermatitis 1987; 16: 55–78.

65 Björkner BE. Industrial airborne dermatoses. Dermatol Clin 1994; 12: 501–509.

66 Wahlberg JE, Maibach HI. Sterile cutaneous pustules: a manifestation of primary irritancy? Identification of contact pustulogens. J Invest Dermatol 1981; 76: 381–383.

67 Dooms-Goossens A, Loncke J, Michiels JL et al. Pustular reactions to hexafluorosilicate in foam rubber. Contact Dermatitis 1985; 12: 42–47.

68 Rycroft RJG. Acute ulcerative contact dermatitis from Portland cement. Br J Dermato 1980; 102: 487–489.

69 Fischer G, Commens C. Cement burns: rare or rarely reported? Australas J Dermatol 1986; 27: 8–10.

70 Goldberg NS, Esterly NB, Rothman KF et al. Perianal pseudoverrucous papules and nodules in children. Arch Dermatol 1992; 128: 240–242.

71 Lyon CC, Smith AJ, Griffiths CEM, Beck MH. The spectrum of skin disorders in abdominal stoma patients. Br J Dermatol 2000; 143: 1248–1260.

72 de Zeeuw R, van Praag MCG, Oranje AP. Granuloma gluteale infantum: a case report. Pediatr Dermatol 2000; 17: 141–143.

73 Van der Valk PGM, Maibach HI. Potential for irritation increases from the wrist to the cubital fossa. Br J Dermatol 1989; 121: 709–712.

74 Elsner P, Wilhelm D, Maibach HI. Sodium lauryl sulfate-induced irritant contact dermatitis in vulvar and forearm skin of premenopausal and postmenopausal women. J Am Acad Dermatol 1990; 23: 648–652.

75 Shmunes E. Contact dermatitis in atopic individuals. Dermatol Clin 1984; 2: 561–566.

76 Rystedt I. Atopy, hand eczema, and contact dermatitis: summary of recent large scale studies. Semin Dermatol 1986; 5: 290–300.

77 Goh CL. An epidemiological comparison between hand eczema and non-hand eczema. Br J Dermatol 1988; 118: 797–801.

78 Elsner P. Irritant dermatitis in the workplace. Dermatol Clin 1994; 12: 461–467.

79 Krasteva M. Contact dermatitis. Int J Dermatol 1993; 32: 547–560.

80 Agner T, Serup J. Seasonal variation of skin resistance to irritants. Br J Dermatol 1989; 121: 323–328.

81 Effendy I, Maibach HI. Surfactants and experimental irritant contact dermatitis. Contact Dermatitis 1995; 33: 217–225.

82 Piérard GE, Goffin V, Hermanns-Lê T et al. Surfactant-induced dermatitis: comparison of corneosurfametry with predictive testing on human and reconstructed skin. J Am Acad Dermatol 1995; 33: 462–469.

83 Willis CM, Stephens CJM, Wilkinson JD. Epidermal damage induced by irritants in man: a light and electron microscopic study. J Invest Dermatol 1989; 93: 695–699.

84 Brand ChU, Hunziker Th, Schaffner Th et al. Activated immunocompetent cells in human skin lymph derived from irritant contact dermatitis: an immunomorphological study. Br J Dermatol 1995; 132: 39–45.

85 Brasch J, Burgard J, Sterry W. Common pathogenetic pathways in allergic and irritant contact dermatitis. J Invest Dermatol 1992; 98: 166–170.

86 Brand ChU, Hunziker Th, Yawalkar N, Braathen LR. IL-1β protein in human skin lymph does not discriminate allergic from irritant contact dermatitis. Contact Dermatitis 1996; 35: 152–156.

87 Ulfgren A-K, Klareskog L, Lindberg M. An immunohistochemical analysis of cytokine expression in allergic and irritant contact dermatitis. Acta Derm Venereol 2000; 80: 167–170.

88 Forsey RJ, Shahidullah H, Sands C et al. Epidermal Langerhans cell apoptosis is induced in vivo by nonanoic acid but not by sodium lauryl sulphate. Br J Dermatol 1998; 139: 453–461.

89 Willis CM, Young E, Brandon DR, Wilkinson JD. Immunopathological and ultrastructural findings in human allergic and irritant contact dermatitis. Br J Dermatol 1986; 115: 305–316.

90 Nater JP, Hoedemaeker PJ. Histological differences between irritant and allergic patch test reactions in man. Contact Dermatitis 1976; 2: 247–253.

91 Mahmoud G, Lachapelle JM, van Neste D. Histological assessment of skin damage by irritants: its possible use in the evaluation of a 'barrier cream'. Contact Dermatitis 1984; 11: 179–185.

92 Nater JP, Baar AJM, Hoedemaeker PJ. Histological aspects of skin reactions to propylene glycol. Contact Dermatitis 1977; 3: 181–185.

93 Taylor RM. Histopathology of contact dermatitis. Clin Dermatol 1986; 4: 18–22.

94 Ackerman AB, Niven J, Grant-Kels JM. Differential diagnosis in dermatopathology. Philadelphia: Lea & Febiger, 1982; 14–17.

95 Reitamo S, Tolvanen E, Konttinen YT et al. Allergic and toxic contact dermatitis: inflammatory cell subtypes in epicutaneous test reactions. Br J Dermatol 1981; 105: 521–527.

96 Lindberg M. Studies on the cellular and subcellular reactions in epidermis at irritant and allergic dermatitis. Acta Derm Venereol (Suppl) 1982; 105: 1–45.

97 Kanerva L. Electron microscopic observations of dyskeratosis, apoptosis, colloid bodies and fibrillar degeneration after skin irritation with dithranol. J Cutan Pathol 1990; 17: 37–44.

98 Manzini BM, Ferdani G, Simonetti V et al. Contact sensitization in children. Pediatr Dermatol 1998; 15: 12–17.

99 De Groot AC, Beverdam EGA, Ayong CT et al. The role of contact allergy in the spectrum of adverse effects caused by cosmetics and toiletries. Contact Dermatitis 1988; 19: 195–201.

100 Eiermann HJ, Larsen W, Maibach HI, Taylor JS. Prospective study of cosmetic reactions: 1977–1980. J Am Acad Dermatol 1982; 6: 909–917.

101 Rotstein E, Rotstein H. The ear-lobe sign: A helpful sign in facial contact dermatitis. Australas J Dermatol 1997; 38: 215–216.

102 Smith HR, Armstrong DKB, Wakelin SH et al. Descriptive epidemiology of hand dermatitis at the St. John's contact dermatitis clinic 1983–97. Br J Dermatol 2000; 142: 284–287.

103 Schwanitz HJ, Uter W. Interdigital dermatitis: sentinel skin damage in hairdressers. Br J Dermatol 2000; 142: 1011–1012.

104 Burkhart CG. Pustular allergic contact dermatitis: a distinct clinical and pathological entity. Cutis 1981; 27: 630–638.

105 Goh CL. Urticarial papular and plaque eruptions. A noneczematous manifestation of allergic contact dermatitis. Int J Dermatol 1989; 28: 172–176.

106 Armstrong DKB, Walsh MY, Dawson JF. Granulomatous contact dermatitis due to gold earrings. Br J Dermatol 1997; 136: 776–778.

107 Iliev D, Elsner P. An unusual hypopigmentation in occupational dermatology: presentation of a case and review of the literature. Dermatology 1998; 196: 248–250.

108 Meneghini CL, Angelini G. Secondary polymorphic eruptions in allergic contact dermatitis. Dermatologica 1981; 163: 63–70.

109 Koch P, Bahmer FA. Erythema-multiforme-like, urticarial papular and plaque eruptions from bufexamac: report of 4 cases. Contact Dermatitis 1994; 31: 97–101.

110 Kurumaji Y. Photo Koebner phenomenon in erythema-multiforme-like eruption induced by contact dermatitis due to bufexamac. Dermatology 1998; 197: 183–186.

111 Lazarov A, Cordoba M. Purpuric contact dermatitis in patients with allergic reaction to textile dyes and resins. J Eur Acad Dermatol Venereol 2000; 14: 101–105.

112 Kuiters GRR, Sillevis Smitt JH, Cohen EB, Bos JD. Allergic contact dermatitis in children and young adults. Arch Dermatol 1989; 125: 1531–1533.

113 Cook DK, Freeman S. Allergic contact dermatitis to plants: An analysis of 68 patients tested at the Skin and Cancer Foundation. Australas J Dermatol 1997; 38: 129–131.

114 Mark KA, Brancaccio RR, Soter NA, Cohen DE. Allergic contact and photoallergic contact dermatitis to plant and pesticide allergens. Arch Dermatol 1999; 135: 67–70.

115 Lee PA, Freeman S. Allergic contact dermatitis due to para-tertiary-butylcatechol in a resin operator. Australas J Dermatol 1999; 40: 49–50.

116 Van Ginkel CJW, Rundervoort GJ. Increasing incidence of contact allergy to the new preservative 1,2-dibromo-2,4-dicyanobutane (methyldibromoglutaronitrile). Br J Dermatol 1995; 132: 918–920.

117 De Groot AC, van Ginkel CJW, Weijland JW. Methyldibromoglutaronitrile (Euxyl K 400): An important "new" allergen in cosmetics. J Am Acad Dermatol 1996; 35: 743–747.

118 Jackson JM, Fowler JF. Methyldibromoglutaronitrile (Euxyl K400): A new and important sensitizer in the United States? J Am Acad Dermatol 1998; 38: 934–937.

119 Larsen WG, Maibach HI. Fragrance contact allergy. Semin Dermatol 1982; 1: 85–90.

120 Larsen WG. Perfume dermatitis. J Am Acad Dermatol 1985, 12: 1–9.

121 Cronin E. 'New' allergens of clinical importance. Semin Dermatol 1982; 1: 33–41.

122 Rademaker M. Allergy to lichen acids in a fragrance. Australas J Dermatol 2000; 41: 50–51.

123 Frosch PJ, Johansen JD, Menné T et al. Lyral® is an important sensitizer in patients sensitive to fragrances. Br J Dermatol 1999; 141: 1076–1083.

124 Buckley DA, Wakelin SH, Seed PT et al. The frequency of fragrance allergy in a patch-test population over a 17-year period. Br J Dermatol 2000; 142: 279–283.

125 Beck MH. Fragrance allergy. Br J Dermatol 2000; 142: 203–204.

126 Thomson KF, Wilkinson SM. Allergic contact dermatitis to plant extracts in patients with cosmetic dermatitis. Br J Dermatol 2000; 142: 84–88.

127 Johansen JD, Rastogi SC, Menné T. Contact allergy to popular perfumes; assessed by patch test, use test and chemical analysis. Br J Dermatol 1996; 135: 419–422.

128 Mackenzie-Wood AR, Freeman S. Severe allergy to sorbolene cream. Australas J Dermatol 1997; 38: 33–34.

129 Brand R, Delaney TA. Allergic contact dermatitis to cocamidopropylbetaine in hair shampoo. Australas J Dermatol 1998; 39: 121–122.

130 Johansen JD, Skov L, Volund A et al. Allergens in combination have a synergistic effect on the elicitation response: a study of fragrance-sensitized individuals. Br J Dermatol 1998; 139: 264–270.

131 Kanerva L, Estlander T, Jolanki R. Occupational allergic contact dermatitis from spices. Contact Dermatitis 1996; 35: 157–162.

132 Isaksson M, Bruze M. Occupational allergic contact dermatitis from olive oil in a masseur. J Am Acad Dermatol 1999; 40: 312–315.

133 Morren M-A, Janssens V, Dooms-Goossens A et al. α-Amylase, a flour additive: an important cause of protein contact dermatitis in bakers. J Am Acad Dermatol 1993; 29: 723–728.

134 Cardullo AC, Ruszkowski AM, DeLeo VA. Allergic contact dermatitis resulting from sensitivity to citrus peel, geraniol, and citral. J Am Acad Dermatol 1989; 21: 395–397.

135 Knight TE, Hausen BM. Dermatitis in a nutshell: Occupational exposure to *Macadamia integrifolia*. J Am Acad Dermatol 1996; 35: 482–484.

136 Calvert ML, Robertson I, Samaratung H. Mango dermatitis: allergic contact dermatitis to *Mangifera indica*. Australas J Dermatol 1996; 37: 59–60.

137 Nixon R. Cinnamon allergy in a baker. Australas J Dermatol 1995; 36: 41.

138 Maillard H, Machet L, Meurisse Y et al. Cross-allergy to latex and spinach. Acta Derm Venereol 2000; 80: 51.

139 Rademaker M, Yung A. Contact dermatitis to *Asparagus officinalis*. Australas J Dermatol 2000; 41: 262–263.

140 Hausen BM, Hjorth N. Skin reactions to topical food exposure. Dermatol Clin 1984; 2: 567–578.

141 Nethercott JR, Holness DL. Occupational dermatitis in food handlers and bakers. J Am Acad Dermatol 1989; 21: 485–490.

142 Eming SA, Piontek J-O, Hunzelmann N et al. Severe toxic contact dermatitis caused by garlic. Br J Dermatol 1999; 141: 391–392.

143 Rafaat M, Leung AKC. Garlic burns. Pediatr Dermatol 2000; 17: 475–476.

144 Taran JM, Delaney TA. Allergic contact dermatitis to 1,2-benzisothiazolin-3-one in the carpet industry. Australas J Dermatol 1997; 38: 42–43.

145 Rubel DM, Freeman S. Allergic contact dermatitis to ethoxyquin in a farmer handling chicken feeds. Australas J Dermatol 1998; 39: 89–91.

146 Mitchell JC, Rook AJ. Diagnosis of contact dermatitis from plants. Semin Dermatol 1982; 1: 25–32.

147 Hurwitz RM, Rivera HP, Guin JD. Black-spot poison ivy dermatitis. An acute irritant contact dermatitis superimposed upon an allergic contact dermatitis. Am J Dermatopathol 1984; 6: 319–322.

148 Williams JV, Light J, Marks JG Jr. Individual variations in allergic contact dermatitis from urushiol. Arch Dermatol 1999; 135: 1002–1003.

149 Brook I, Frazier EH, Yeager JK. Microbiology of infected poison ivy dermatitis. Br J Dermatol 2000; 142: 943–946.

150 Gordon LA, Compositae dermatitis. Australas J Dermatol 1999; 40: 123–130.

151 Stingeni L, Agea E, Lisi P, Spinozzi F. T-lymphocyte cytokine profiles in Compositae airborne dermatitis. Br J Dermatol 1999; 141: 689–693.

152 Goulden V, Wilkinson SM. Patch testing for Compositae allergy. Br J Dermatol 1998; 138: 1018–1021.

153 Knight TE, Hausen BM. Melaleuca oil (tea tree oil) dermatitis. J Am Acad Dermatol 1994; 30: 423–427.

154 Rubel DM, Freeman S, Southwell IA. Tea tree oil allergy: what is the offending agent? Report of three cases of tea tree oil allergy and review of the literature. Australas J Dermatol 1998; 39: 244–247.

155 Kumarasinghe SPW, Seneviratne R. Skin and eye injury due to latex of *Excoecaria agallocha*. Australas J Dermatol 1998; 39: 275–276.

156 Brenner S, Landau M, Goldberg I. Contact dermatitis with systemic symptoms from *Agave americana*. Dermatology 1998; 196: 408–411.

157 Gette MT, Marks JE Jr. Tulip fingers. Arch Dermatol 1990; 126: 203–205.

158 Gómez E, Garcia R, Galindo PA et al. Occupational allergic contact dermatitis from sunflower. Contact Dermatitis 1996; 35: 139–190.

159 Marks JG Jr. Allergic contact dermatitis to *Alstroemeria*. Arch Dermatol 1988; 124: 914–916.

160 Thiboutot DM, Hamory BH, Marks JG Jr. Dermatoses among floral shop workers. J Am Acad Dermatol 1990; 22: 54–58.

161 Géraut C, Tripodi D. 'Airborne' contact dermatitis due to Leica immersion oil. Int J Dermatol 1999; 38: 676–679.

162 Spiewak R, Skorska C, Dutkiewicz J. Occupational airborne contact dermatitis caused by thyme dust. Contact Dermatitis 2001; 44: 235–239.

163 Estlander T, Jolanki R, Alanko K, Kanerva L. Occupational allergic contact dermatitis caused by wood dusts. Contact Dermatitis 2001; 44: 213–217.

164 Fisher AA. Contact dermatitis from topical medicaments. Semin Dermatol 1982; 1: 49–57.

165 Hogan DJ. Allergic contact dermatitis to ethylenediamine. A continuing problem. Dermatol Clin 1990; 8: 133–136.

166 Möller H. Clinical response to gold as a circulating contact allergen. Acta Derm Venereol 2000; 80: 111–113.

167 Koch P, Bahmer FA. Oral lesions and symptoms related to metals used in dental restorations: A clinical, allergological, and histologic study. J Am Acad Dermatol 1999; 41: 422–430.

168 Fowler JF Jr, Skinner SM, Belsito DV. Allergic contact dermatitis from formaldehyde resins in permanent press clothing: an underdiagnosed cause of generalized dermatitis. J Am Acad Dermatol 1992; 27: 962–968.

169 Conde-Salazar L, del-Río E, Guimaraens D, Domingo AG. Type IV allergy to rubber additives: a 10-year study of 686 cases. J Am Acad Dermatol 1993; 29: 76–180.

170 Warshaw EM. Latex allergy. J Am Acad Dermatol 1998; 39: 1–24.

171 Wilkinson SM, Burd R. Latex: A cause of allergic contact eczema in users of natural rubber gloves. J Am Acad Dermatol 1998 38: 36–42.

172 Wakelin SH, White IR. Natural rubber latex allergy. Clin Exp Dermatol 1999; 24: 245–248.

173 Holme SA, Lever RS. Latex allergy in atopic children. Br J Dermatol 1999; 140: 919–921.

174 Gibbon KL, McFadden JP, Rycroft RJG et al. Changing frequency of thiuram allergy in healthcare workers with hand dermatitis. Br J Dermatol 2001; 144: 347–350.

175 Brancaccio RR, Cockerell CJ, Belsito D, Ostreicher R. Allergic contact dermatitis from color film developers: clinical and histologic features. J Am Acad Dermatol 1993; 28: 827–830.

176 Hemmer W, Focke M, Wantke F et al. Allergic contact dermatitis to artificial fingernails prepared from UV light-cured acrylates. J Am Acad Dermatol 1996; 35: 377–380.

177 Guin JD, Baas K, Nelson-Adesokan P. Contact sensitization to cyanoacrylate adhesive as a cause of severe onychodystrophy. Int J Dermatol 1998; 37: 31–36.

178 Woollons A, Voyce ME, Darley CR, Price ML. Allergic contact dermatitis to acrylates in diathermy plates. Br J Dermatol 1998; 138: 1094–1095.

179 Morgan VA, Fewings JM. 1,6-hexanediol diacrylate: a rapid and potent sensitizer in the printing industry. Australas J Dermatol 2000; 41: 190–192.

180 Rademaker M. Occupational epoxy resin allergic contact dermatitis. Australas J Dermatol 2000; 41: 222–224.

181 Lestringant GG, Bener A, Frossard PM. Cutaneous reactions to henna and associated additives. Br J Dermatol 1999; 141: 598–600.

182 Tosti A, Pazzaglia M, Bertazzoni M. Contact allergy from temporary tattoos. Arch Dermatol 2000; 136: 1061–1062.

183 Mohamed M, Nixon R. Severe allergic contact dermatitis induced by paraphenylenediamine in paint-on temporary 'tattoos'. Australas J Dermatol 2000; 41: 168–171.

184 Le Coz CJ, Lefebvre C, Keller F, Grosshans E. Allergic contact dermatitis caused by skin painting (pseudotattooing) with black henna, a mixture of henna and p-phenylenediamine and its derivatives. Arch Dermatol 2000; 136: 1515–1517.

185 Hatch KL, Maibach HI. Textile dye dermatitis. J Am Acad Dermatol 1985; 12: 1079–1092.

186 Hatch KL, Maibach HI. Textile dermatitis: an update. (I). Resins, additives and fibers. Contact Dermatitis 1995; 32: 319–326.

187 Hatch KL, Maibach HI. Textile dye dermatitis. J Am Acad Dermatol 1995; 32: 631–639.

188 Su JC, Horton JJ. Allergic contact dermatitis from azo dyes. Australas J Dermatol 1997; 38: 48–49.

189 Maso MJ, Goldberg DJ. Contact dermatoses from disposable glove use: a review. J Am Acad Dermatol 1990; 23: 733–737.

190 Kanerva L. Occupational protein contact dermatitis and paronychia from natural rubber latex. J Eur Acad Dermatol Venereol 2000; 14: 504–506.

191 Storrs FJ, Rosenthal LE, Adams RM et al. Prevalence and relevance of allergic reactions in patients patch tested in North America – 1984 to 1985. J Am Acad Dermatol 1989; 20: 1038–1045.

192 Westphal GA, Reich K, Schulz TG et al. N-acetyltransferase 1 and 2 polymorphisms in *para*-substituted arylamine-induced contact allergy. Br J Dermatol 2000; 142: 1121–1127.

193 Shelley WB, Shelley ED, Talanin NY. Self-potentiating allergic contact dermatitis caused by doxepin hydrochloride cream. J Am Acad Dermatol 1996; 34: 143–144.

194 Foti C, Diaferio A, Bonamonte D. Allergic contact dermatitis from ciclopirox olamine. Australas J Dermatol 2001; 42: 145.

195 Guin JD. Contact sensitivity to topical corticosteroids. J Am Acad Dermatol 1984; 10: 773–782.

196 Dooms-Goossens AE, Degreef HJ, Marien KJC, Coopman SA. Contact allergy to corticosteroids: a frequently missed diagnosis? J Am Acad Dermatol 1989; 21: 538–543.

197 Lauerma A, Reitamo S. Contact allergy to corticosteroids. J Am Acad Dermatol 1993; 28: 618–622.

198 Burden AD, Beck MH. Contact hypersensitivity to topical corticosteroids. Br J Dermatol 1992; 127: 497–500.

199 Räsänen L, Hasan T. Allergy to systemic and intralesional corticosteroids. Br J Dermatol 1993; 128: 407–411.

200 Lepoittevin J-P, Drieghe J, Dooms-Goossens A. Studies in patients with corticosteroid contact allergy. Arch Dermatol 1995; 131: 31–37.

201 Lauerma AI, Kanerva L. Contact allergy to corticosteroids. Int J Dermatol 1996; 35: 92–93.

202 Okano M. Contact dermatitis due to Budesonide: report of five cases and review of the Japanese literature. Int J Dermatol 1994; 3: 709–715.

203 Dooms-Goossens A, Meinardi MMHM, Bos JD, Degreef H. Contact allergy to corticosteroids: the results of a two-centre study. Br J Dermatol 1994; 130: 42–47.

204 Wilkinson SM. Hypersensitivity to topical corticosteroids. Clin Exp Dermatol 1994; 19: 1–11.

205 Thomson KF, Wilkinson SM, Powell S, Beck MH. The prevalence of corticosteroid allergy in two U.K. centres: prescribing implications. Br J Dermatol 1999; 141: 863–866.

206 Wilkinson SM, Jones MF. Corticosteroid usage and binding to arginine: determinants of corticosteroid hypersensitivity. Br J Dermatol 1996; 135: 225–230.

207 Lutz ME, el-Azhary RA. Allergic contact dermatitis due to topical application of corticosteroids: review and clinical implications. Mayo Clin Proc 1997; 72: 1141–1144.

208 Lutz ME, el-Azhary RA, Gibson LE, Fransway AF. Contact hypersensitivity to tixocortol pivalate. J Am Acad Dermatol 1998; 38: 691–695.

209 English JSC. Corticosteroid-induced contact dermatitis: a pragmatic approach. Clin Exp Dermatol 2000; 25: 261–264.

210 Poon E, Fewings JM. Generalized eczematous reaction to budesonide in a nasal spray with cross-reactivity to triamcinolone. Australas J Dermatol 2001; 42: 36–37.

211 Ophaswongse S, Maibach H. Topical nonsteroidal antiinflammatory drugs: allergic and photoallergic contact dermatitis and phototoxicity. Contact Dermatitis 1993; 29: 57–64.

212 Held JL, Kalb RE, Ruszkowski AM, DeLeo V. Allergic contact dermatitis from bacitracin. J Am Acad Dermatol 1987; 17: 592–594.

213 Zappi EG, Brancaccio RR. Allergic contact dermatitis from mupirocin ointment. J Am Acad Dermatol 1997; 36: 266.

214 Tanaka S, Otsuki T, Matsumoto Y et al. Allergic contact dermatitis from enoxolone. Contact Dermatitis 2001; 44: 192.

215 Taniguchi S, Kono T. Allergic contact dermatitis due to lanoconazole with no cross-reactivity to other imidazoles. Dermatology 1998; 196: 366.

216 Barbaud A, Reichert-Penetrat S, Trechot P et al. Occupational contact dermatitis to propacetamol. Dermatology 1997; 195: 329–331.

217 Dwyer P, Freeman S. Allergic contact dermatitis to adhesive tape and contrived disease. Australas J Dermatol 1997; 38: 141–144.

218 Scalf LA, Fowler JF Jr. Peristomal allergic contact dermatitis due to Gantrez in Stomahesive paste. J Am Acad Dermatol 2000; 42: 355–356.

219 Curley RK, Macfarlane AW, King CM. Contact sensitivity to the amide anesthetics lidocaine, prilocaine, and mepivacaine. Case report and review of the literature. Arch Dermatol 1986; 122: 924–926.

220 Handfield-Jones SE, Cronin E. Contact sensitivity to lignocaine. Clin Exp Dermatol 1993; 18: 342–343.

221 Kearney CR, Fewings J. Allergic contact dermatitis to cinchocaine. Australas J Dermatol 2001; 42: 118–119.

222 Erdmann SM, Sachs B, Merk HF. Systemic contact dermatitis from cinchocaine. Contact Dermatitis 2001; 44: 260–261.

223 Amon RB, Lis AW, Hanifin JM. Allergic contact dermatitis caused by idoxuridine. Arch Dermatol 1975; 111: 1581–1584.

224 Praditsuwan P, Taylor JS, Roenigk HH Jr. Allergy to Unna boots in four patients. J Am Acad Dermatol 1995; 33: 906–908.

225 Wong DA, Watson AB. Allergic contact dermatitis due to benzalkonium chloride in plaster of Paris. Australas J Dermatol 2001; 42: 33–35.

226 Mohamed M, Delaney TA, Horton JJ. Allergic contact dermatitis to plastic banknotes. Australas J Dermatol 1999; 40: 164–166.

227 Schaller M, Korting HC. Allergic airborne contact dermatitis from essential oils used in aromatherapy. Clin Exp Dermatol 1995; 20: 143–145.

228 Treudler R, Tebbe B, Blume-Peytavi U et al. Occupational contact dermatitis due to 2-chloroacetophenone tear gas. Br J Dermatol 1999; 140: 531–534.

229 Goette DK, Odom RB. Allergic contact dermatitis to topical fluorouracil. Arch Dermatol 1977; 113: 1058–1061.

230 Takashima A, Yamamoto K, Kimura S et al. Allergic contact and photocontact dermatitis due to psoralens in patients with psoriasis treated with topical PUVA. Br J Dermatol 1991; 124: 37–42.

231 Benezra C, Foussereau J. Allergic contact dermatitis – a chemical-clinical approach. Semin Dermatol 1982; 1: 73–83.

232 McDonagh AJG, Wright AL, Cork MJ, Gawkrodger DJ. Nickel sensitivity: the influence of ear piercing and atopy. Br J Dermatol 1992; 126: 16–18.

233 Burrows D. Is systemic nickel important? J Am Acad Dermatol 1992; 26: 632–635.

234 Lidén C, Menné T, Burrows D. Nickel-containing alloys and platings and their ability to cause dermatitis. Br J Dermatol 1996; 134: 193–198.

235 Troost RJJ, Kozel MMA, van Helden-Meeuwsen CG et al. Hyposensitization in nickel allergic contact dermatitis: clinical and immunologic monitoring. J Am Acad Dermatol 1995; 32: 576–583.

236 Shah M, Lewis FM, Gawkrodger DJ. Nickel as an occupational allergen. A survey of 368 nickel-sensitive subjects. Arch Dermatol 1998; 134: 1231–1236.

237 Cavani A, Mei D, Guerra E et al. Patients with allergic contact dermatitis to nickel and nonallergic individuals display different nickel-specific T cell responses. Evidence for the presence of effector CD8+ and regulatory CD4+ T cells. J Invest Dermatol 1998; 111: 621–628.

238 Nielsen NH, Menné T, Kristiansen J et al. Effects of repeated skin exposure to low nickel concentrations: a model for allergic contact dermatitis to nickel on the hands. Br J Dermatol 1999; 141: 676–682.

239 Gawkrodger DJ, Lewis FM, Shah M. Contact sensitivity to nickel and other metals in jewelry reactors. J Am Acad Dermatol 2000; 43: 31–36.

240 Fisher AA. New advances in contact dermatitis. Int J Dermatol 1977; 16: 552–568.

241 Memon AA, Friedmann PS. Studies on the reproducibility of allergic contact dermatitis. Br J Dermatol 1996; 134: 208–214.

242 Cohen DE, Brancaccio R, Andersen D, Belsito DV. Utility of a standard allergen series alone in the evaluation of allergic contact dermatitis: A retrospective study of 732 patients. J Am Acad Dermatol 1997; 36: 914–918.

243 Shah M, Lewis FM, Gawkrodger DJ. Patch testing in children and adolescents: Five years' experience and follow-up. J Am Acad Dermatol 1997; 37: 964–968.

244 Marks JG Jr, Belsito DV, DeLeo VA et al. North American Contact Dermatitis Group patch test results for the detection of delayed-type hypersensitivity to topical allergens. J Am Acad Dermatol 1998; 38: 911–918.

245 Schnuch A, Geier J, Uter W, Frosch PJ. Patch testing with preservatives, antimicrobials and industrial biocides. Results from a multicentre study. Br J Dermatol 1998; 138: 467–476.

246 González S, González E, White WM et al. Allergic contact dermatitis: Correlation of in vivo confocal imaging to routine histology. J Am Acad Dermatol 1999; 40: 708–713.

247 Nishioka K. Allergic contact dermatitis. Int J Dermatol 1985; 24: 1–8.

248 Bergstresser PR. Immune mechanisms in contact allergic dermatitis. Dermatol Clin 1990; 8: 3–11.

249 Zhang L, Tinkle SS. Chemical activation of innate and specific immunity in contact dermatitis. J Invest Dermatol 2000; 115: 168–176.

250 Bergstresser PR. Immunologic mechanisms of contact hypersensitivity. Dermatol Clin 1984; 2: 523–532.

251 Bergstresser PR. Contact allergic dermatitis. Old problems and new techniques. Arch Dermatol 1989; 125: 276–279.

252 Basketter D, Dooms-Goossens A, Karlberg A-T, Lepoittevin J-P. The chemistry of contact allergy: why is a molecule allergenic? Contact Dermatitis 1995; 32: 65–73.

253 De Panfilis G, Giannotti B, Manara GC et al. Macrophage-T lymphocyte relationships in man's contact allergic reactions. Br J Dermatol 1983; 109: 183–189.

254 Breathnach SM. Immunologic aspects of contact dermatitis. Clin Dermatol 1986; 4: 5–17.

255 Kalish RS. Recent developments in the pathogenesis of allergic contact dermatitis. Arch Dermatol 1991; 127: 1558–1563.

256 Giannotti B, De Panfilis G, Manara GC et al. Langerhans cells are not damaged in contact allergic reactions in humans. Am J Dermatopathol 1986; 8: 220–226.

257 Katz SI. The role of Langerhans cells in allergic contact dermatitis. Am J Dermatopathol 1986; 8: 232–233.

258 Kondo S, Sauder DN. Epidermal cytokines in allergic contact dermatitis. J Am Acad Dermatol 1995; 33: 786–800.

259 Nakano Y. Antigen-presenting cell function of epidermal cells activated by hapten application. Br J Dermatol 1998; 138: 786–794.

260 Friedman P. The systemic nature of contact hypersensitivity. Acta Derm Venereol 2000; 80: 81.

261 Kondo S, Kono T, Brown WR et al. Lymphocyte function-associated antigen-1 is required for maximum elicitation of allergic contact dermatitis. Br J Dermatol 1994; 131: 354–359.

262 Garioch JJ, MacKie RM, Campbell I, Forsyth A. Keratinocyte expression of intercellular adhesion molecule 1 (ICAM-1) correlated with infiltration of lymphocyte function associated antigen 1 (LFA-1) positive cells in evolving allergic contact dermatitis reactions. Histopathology 1991; 19: 351–354.

263 Yawalkar N, Brand CU, Braathen LR. Interleukin-12 expression in human afferent lymph derived from the induction phase of allergic contact dermatitis. Br J Dermatol 1998; 138: 297–300.

264 Mahapatro D, Mahapatro RC. Cutaneous basophil hypersensitivity. Am J Dermatopathol 1984; 6: 483–489.

265 Le TKM, Van der Valk PGM, Schalkwijk J, van de Kerkhof PCM. Changes in epidermal proliferation and differentiation in allergic and irritant contact dermatitis reactions. Br J Dermatol 1995; 133: 236–240.

266 Keczkes K, Basheer AM, Wyatt EH. The persistence of allergic contact sensitivity: a 10-year follow-up in 100 patients. Br J Dermatol 1982; 107: 461–465.

267 White CR Jr. Histopathology of exogenous and systemic contact eczema. Semin Dermatol 1990; 9: 226–229.

268 Wood GS, Volterra AS, Abel EA et al. Allergic contact dermatitis: novel immunohistologic features. J Invest Dermatol 1986; 87: 688–693.

269 Ricks MR, Vogel PS, Elston DM, Hivnor C. Purpuric agave dermatitis. J Am Acad Dermatol 1999; 40: 356–358.

270 Teraki Y, Shiohara T. Propolis-induced granulomatous contact dermatitis accompanied by marked lymphadenopathy. Br J Dermatol 2001; 144: 1277–1278.

271 Commens C, McGeogh A, Bartlett B, Kossard S. Bindii (Jo Jo) dermatitis (*Soliva pterosperma* [Compositae]). J Am Acad Dermatol 1984; 10: 768–773.

272 Hogan PA. Bindii dermatitis. Australas J Dermatol 1997; 38: 224–225.

273 Orbaneja JG, Diez LI, Lozano JLS, Salazar LC. Lymphomatoid contact dermatitis. Contact Dermatitis 1976; 2: 139–143.

274 Ecker RI, Winkelmann RK. Lymphomatoid contact dermatitis. Contact Dermatitis 1981; 7: 84–93.

275 Wall LM. Lymphomatoid contact dermatitis due to ethylenediamine dihydrochloride. Contact Dermatitis 1982; 8: 51–54.

276 Marliere V, Beylot-Barry M, Doutre MS et al. Lymphomatoid contact dermatitis caused by isopropyl-diphenylenediamine: two cases. J Allergy Clin Immunol 1998; 102: 152–153.

277 Houck HE, Wirth FA, Kauffman CL. Lymphomatoid contact dermatitis caused by nickel. Am J Contact Dermat 1997; 8: 175–176.

278 Fleming C, Burden D, Fallowfield M, Lever R. Lymphomatoid contact reaction to gold earrings. Contact Dermatitis 1997; 37: 298–299.

279 Braun RP, French LE, Feldmann R et al. Cutaneous pseudolymphoma, lymphomatoid contact dermatitis type, as an unusual cause of symmetrical upper eyelid nodules. Br J Dermatol 2000; 143: 411–414.

280 Kimura M, Kawada A. Follicular contact dermatitis due to polyoxyethylene laurylether. J Am Acad Dermatol 2000; 42: 879–880.

281 Janssens V, Morren M, Dooms-Goossens A, Degreef H. Protein contact dermatitis: myth or reality? Br J Dermatol 1995; 132: 1–6.

282 Boehncke W-H, Pillekamp H, Gass S, Gall H. Occupational protein contact dermatitis caused by meat and fish. Int J Dermatol 1998; 37: 358–360.

283 Kumar A, Freeman S. Protein contact dermatitis in food workers. Case report of a meat sorter and summary of seven other cases. Australas J Dermatol 1999; 40: 138–140.

284 Guin JD, Styles A. Protein-contact eczematous reaction to cornstarch in clothing. J Am Acad Dermatol 1999; 40: 991–994.

285 Weinberg JM, Haimowitz JE, Spiers EM, Mowad CM. Fish skin-induced dermatitis. J Eur Acad Dermatol Venereol 2000; 14: 222–223.

286 Guin JD, France G. Protein contact dermatitis from pecan. Contact Dermatitis 2000; 43: 309–310.

287 Hellgren L, Mobacken H. Nummular eczema – clinical and statistical data. Acta Derm Venereol 1969; 49: 189–196.

288 Sirot G. Nummular eczema. Semin Dermatol 1983; 2: 68–74.

289 Rietschel RL, Ray MC. Nonatopic eczemas. J Am Acad Dermatol 1988; 18: 569–573.

290 Aoyama H, Tanaka M, Hara M et al. Nummular eczema: an addition of senile xerosis and unique cutaneous reactivities to environmental aeroallergens. Dermatology 1999; 199: 135–139.

291 Bendl BJ. Nummular eczema of stasis origin. Int J Dermatol 1979; 18: 129–135.

292 Rowe JA, Hattenhauer MG, Herman DC. Adverse side effects associated with latanoprost. Am J Ophthalmol 1997; 124: 683–685.

293 Church R. Eczema provoked by methyl dopa. Br J Dermatol 1974; 91: 373–378.

294 Adachi A, Horikawa T, Takashima T, Ichihashi M. Mercury-induced nummular dermatitis. J Am Acad Dermatol 2000; 43: 383–385.

295 Krueger GG, Kahn G, Weston WL, Mandel MJ. IgE levels in nummular eczema and ichthyosis. Arch Dermatol 1973; 107: 56–58.

296 Stevens DM, Ackerman AB. On the concept of distinctive exudative discoid and lichenoid chronic dermatosis (Sulzberger–Garbe). Is it nummular dermatitis? Am J Dermatopathol 1984; 6: 387–395.

297 Sulzberger MB. Distinctive exudative discoid and lichenoid chronic dermatosis (Sulzberger and Garbe) re-examined – 1978. Br J Dermatol 1979; 100: 13–20.

298 Rongioletti F, Corbella L, Rebora A. Exudative discoid and lichenoid chronic dermatosis (Sulzberger–Garbe). A fictional disease? Int J Dermatol 1989; 28: 40–243.

299 Freeman K, Hewitt M, Warin AP. Two cases of distinctive exudative discoid and lichenoid chronic dermatosis of Sulzberger and Garbe responding to azathioprine. Br J Dermatol 1984; 111: 215–220.

300 Kligman AM, Leyden JJ. Seborrheic dermatitis. Semin Dermatol 1983; 2: 57–59.

301 Webster G. Seborrheic dermatitis. Int J Dermatol 1991; 30: 843–844.

302 Fox BJ, Odom RB. Papulosquamous diseases: a review. J Am Acad Dermatol 1985; 12: 597–624.

303 Thomsen K. Seborrhoeic dermatitis and napkin dermatitis. Acta Derm Venereol (Suppl) 1981; 95: 40–42.

304 Podmore P, Burrows D, Eedy DJ, Standord CF. Seborrhoeic eczema – a disease entity or a clinical variant of atopic eczema? Br J Dermatol 1986; 115: 341–350.

305 Podmore P, Burrows D, Eedy D. T-cell subset assay. A useful differentiating marker of atopic and seborrheic eczema in infancy? Arch Dermatol 1988; 124: 1235–1238.

306 Yates VM, Kerr REI, Mackie R. Early diagnosis of infantile seborrhoeic dermatitis and atopic dermatitis – clinical features. Br J Dermatol 1983; 108: 633–638.

307 Yates VM, Kerr REI, Frier K et al. Early diagnosis of infantile seborrhoeic dermatitis and atopic dermatitis – total and specific IgE levels. Br J Dermatol 1983; 108: 639–645.

308 Tollesson A, Frithz A, Berg A, Karlman G. Essential fatty acids in infantile seborrheic dermatitis. J Am Acad Dermatol 1993; 28: 957–961.

309 Mathes BM, Douglass MC. Seborrheic dermatitis in patients with acquired immunodeficiency syndrome. J Am Acad Dermatol 1985; 13: 947–951.

310 Soeprono FF, Schinella RA, Cockerell CJ, Comite SL. Seborrheic-like dermatitis of acquired immunodeficiency syndrome. A clinicopathologic study. J Am Acad Dermatol 1986; 14: 242–248.

311 Froschl M, Land HG, Landthaler M. Seborrheic dermatitis and atopic eczema in human immunodeficiency virus infection. Semin Dermatol 1990; 9: 230–232.

312 Binder RL, Jonelis FJ. Seborrheic dermatitis in neuroleptic-induced Parkinsonism. Arch Dermatol 1983; 119: 473–475.

313 Moehrle M, Dennenmoser B, Schlagenhauff B et al. High prevalence of seborrhoeic dermatitis on the face and scalp in mountain guides. Dermatology 2000; 201: 146–147.

314 Kanwar AJ, Majid A, Garg MP, Singh G. Seborrheic dermatitis-like eruption caused by cimetidine. Arch Dermatol 1981; 117: 65–66.

315 Knight AG. Pityriasis amiantacea: a clinical and histopathological investigation. Clin Exp Dermatol 1977; 2: 137–143.

316 Hersle K, Lindholm A, Mobacken H, Sandberg L. Relationship of pityriasis amiantacea to psoriasis. A follow-up study. Dermatologica 1979; 159: 245–250.

317 Ring DS, Kaplan DL. Pityriasis amiantacea: a report of 10 cases. Arch Dermatol 1993; 129: 913–914.

318 Langtry JAA, Ive FA. Pityriasis amiantacea, an unrecognized cause of scarring alopecia, described in four patients. Acta Derm Venereol 1991; 71: 352–353.

319 Leyden JJ, McGinley KJ, Kligman AM. Role of microorganisms in dandruff. Arch Dermatol 1976; 112: 333–338.

320 Shuster S. The aetiology of dandruff and the mode of action of therapeutic agents. Br J Dermatol 1984; 111: 235–242.

321 Baroni A, De Rosa R, De Rosa A et al. New strategies in dandruff treatment: growth control of Malassezia ovalis. Dermatology 2000; 201: 332–336.

322 Burton JL, Pye RJ. Seborrhoea is not a feature of seborrhoeic dermatitis. Br Med J 1983; 286: 1169–1170.

323 Ashbee HR, Ingham E, Holland KT, Cunliffe WJ. The carriage of Malassezia furfur serovars A, B and C in patients with pityriasis versicolor, seborrhoeic dermatitis and controls. Br J Dermatol 1993; 129: 533–540.

324 Hay RJ, Graham-Brown RAC. Dandruff and seborrhoeic dermatitis: causes and management. Clin Exp Dermatol 997; 22: 3–6.

325 Faergemann J, Bergbrant I-M, Dohsé M et al. Seborrhoeic dermatitis and Pityrosporum (Malassezia) folliculitis: characterization of inflammatory cells and mediators in the skin by immunohistochemistry. Br J Dermatol 2001; 144: 549–556.

326 Ford GP, Farr PM, Ive FA, Shuster S. The response of seborrhoeic dermatitis to ketoconazole. Br J Dermatol 1984; 111: 603–607.

327 Faergemann J, Fredriksson T. Tinea versicolor with regard to seborrheic dermatitis. An epidemiological investigation. Arch Dermatol 1979; 115: 966–968.

328 Skinner RB Jr, Noah PW, Taylor RM et al. Double-blind treatment of seborrheic dermatitis with 2% ketoconazole cream. J Am Acad Dermatol 1985; 12: 852–856.

329 Schechtman RC, Midgley G, Hay RJ. HIV disease and Malassezia yeasts: a quantitative study of patients presenting with seborrhoeic dermatitis. Br J Dermatol 1995; 133: 694–698.

330 Wikler JR, Nieboer C, Willemze R. Quantitative skin cultures of Pityrosporum yeasts in patients seropositive for the human immunodeficiency virus with and without seborrheic dermatitis. J Am Acad Dermatol 1992; 27: 37–39.

331 Bergbrant I-M, Faergemann J. Seborrhoeic dermatitis and Pityrosporum ovale: a cultural and immunological study. Acta Derm Venereol 1989; 69: 332–335.

332 Broberg A, Faergemann J. Infantile seborrhoeic dermatitis and Pityrosporum ovale. Br J Dermatol 1989; 120: 359–362.

333 Heng MCY, Henderson CL, Barker DC, Haberfelde G. Correlation of Pityrosporum ovale density with clinical severity of seborrheic dermatitis as assessed by a simplified technique. J Am Acad Dermatol 1990; 23: 82–86.

334 Parry ME, Sharpe GR. Seborrhoeic dermatitis is not caused by an altered immune response to Malassezia yeast. Br J Dermatol 1998; 139: 254–263.

335 Bergbrant I-M, Andersson B, Faergemann J. Cell-mediated immunity to Malassezia furfur in patients with seborrhoeic dermatitis and pityriasis versicolor. Clin Exp Dermatol 1999; 24: 402–406.

336 Tollesson A, Frithz A, Stenlund K. Malassezia furfur in infantile seborrheic dermatitis. Pediatr Dermatol 1997; 14: 423–425.

337 Pinkus H, Mehregan AH. The primary histologic lesion of seborrheic dermatitis and psoriasis. J Invest Dermatol 1966; 46: 109–116.

338 Barr RJ, Young EM Jr. Psoriasiform and related papulosquamous disorders. J Cutan Pathol 1985; 12: 412–425.

339 Ackerman AB. Histologic diagnosis of inflammatory skin diseases. Philadelphia: Lea & Febiger, 1978; 239–240.

340 Hanifin JM, Rajka G. Diagnostic features of atopic dermatitis. Acta Derm Venereol (Suppl) 1980; 92: 44–47.

341 Hanifin JM. Atopic dermatitis. J Am Acad Dermatol 1982; 6: 1–13.

342 Hanifin JM. Clinical and basic aspects of atopic dermatitis. Semin Dermatol 1983; 2: 5–19.

343 Kang K, Tian R. Atopic dermatitis. An evaluation of clinical and laboratory findings. Int J Dermatol 1987; 26: 27–32.

344 Roth HL. Atopic dermatitis revisited. Int J Dermatol 1987; 26: 139–149.

345 Graham-Brown RAC. Atopic dermatitis. Semin Dermatol 1988; 7: 37–42.

346 Rothe MJ, Grant-Kels JM. Atopic dermatitis: An update. J Am Acad Dermatol 1996; 35: 1–13.

347 Thestrup-Pedersen K, Ring J. Atopic dermatitis: summary of the 1st Georg Rajka Symposium 1998 and a literature review. Acta Derm Venereol 1999; 79: 257–264.

348 Kay J, Gawkrodger DJ, Mortimer MJ, Jaron AG. The prevalence of childhood atopic eczema in a general population. J Am Acad Dermatol 1994; 30: 35–39.

349 Williams HC. Is the prevalence of atopic dermatitis increasing? Clin Exp Dermatol 1992; 17: 385–39 .

350 Larsen FS, Diepgen T, Svensson A. The occurrence of atopic dermatitis in North Europe: an international questionnaire study. J Am Acad Dermatol 1996; 34: 760–764.

351 Mar A, Tam M, Jolley D, Marks R. The cumulative incidence of atopic dermatitis in the first 12 months among Chinese, Vietnamese, and Caucasian infants born in Melbourne, Australia. J Am Acad Dermatol 1999; 40: 597–602.

352 Marks R, Kilkenny M, Plunkett A, Merlin K. The prevalence of common skin conditions in Australian school students: 2. Atopic dermatitis. Br J Dermatol 1999; 140: 468–473.

353 Dotterud LK, Odland JØ, Falk ES. Atopic diseases among adults in the two geographically related arctic areas Nikel, Russia and Sør-Varanger, Norway: possible effects of indoor and outdoor air pollution. J Eur Acad Dermatol Venereol 2000; 14: 107–111.

354 McNally NJ, Williams HC, Phillips DR, Strachan DP. Is there a geographical variation in eczema prevalence in the U.K.? Evidence from the 1958 British birth cohort study. Br J Dermatol 2000; 142: 712–720.

355 Schäfer T, Krämer U, Vieluf D et al. The excess of atopic eczema in East Germany is related to the intrinsic type. Br J Dermatol 2000; 143: 992–998.

356 Laughter D, Istvan JA, Tofte SJ, Hanifin JM. The prevalence of atopic dermatitis in Oregon schoolchildren. J Am Acad Dermatol 2000; 43: 649–655.

357 Foley P, Zuo Y, Plunkett A, Marks R. The frequency of common skin conditions in preschool-age children in Australia. Atopic dermatitis. Arch Dermatol 200 ; 137: 293–300.

358 Williams HC. Epidemiology of atopic dermatitis. Clin Exp Dermatol 2000; 25: 522–529.

359 Thestrup-Pedersen K. Clinical aspects of atopic dermatitis. Clin Exp Dermatol 2000; 25: 535–543.

360 Bannister MJ, Freeman S. Adult-onset atopic dermatitis. Australas J Dermatol 2000; 41: 225–228.

361 Williams HC, Burney PGJ, Hay RJ et al. I. Derivation of a minimum set of discriminators for atopic dermatitis. Br J Dermatol 1994; 131: 383–396.

362 Sehgal VN, Jain S. Atopic dermatitis: clinical criteria. Int J Dermatol 1993; 32: 628–637.

363 Williams HC. Diagnostic criteria for atopic dermatitis. Where do we go from here? Arch Dermatol 1999; 135: 583–586.

364 Firooz A, Davoudi SM, Farahmand AN et al. Validation of the diagnostic criteria for atopic dermatitis. Arch Dermatol 1999; 135: 514–516.

365 Heskel N, Lobitz WC Jr. Atopic dermatitis in children: clinical features and management. Semin Dermatol 1983; 2: 39–44.

366 Sampson HA. The role of food allergy and mediator release in atopic dermatitis. J Allergy Clin Immunol 1988; 81: 635–645.

367 Fischer G, Rogers M. Vulvar disease in children: a clinical audit of 130 cases. Pediatr Dermatol 2000; 17: 1–6.

368 Crone AM, Stewart EJC, Wojnarowska F, Powell SM. Aetiological factors in vulvar dermatitis. J Eur Acad Dermatol Venereol 2000; 14: 181–186.

369 Ofuji S, Uehara M. Follicular eruptions of atopic dermatitis. Arch Dermatol 1973; 107: 54–55.

370 Rencic A, Cohen BA. Prominent pruritic periumbilical papules: a diagnostic sign in pediatric atopic dermatitis. Pediatr Dermatol 1999; 16: 436–438.

371 Taieb A. Linear atopic dermatitis ('naevus atopicus'): a pathogenetic clue? Br J Dermatol 1994; 131: 134–135.

372 Böhme M, Svensson Å, Kull I, Wahlgren C-F. Hanifin's and Rajka's minor criteria for atopic dermatitis: Which do 2-year-olds exhibit? J Am Acad Dermatol 2000; 43: 785–792.

373 Piletta PA, Wirth S, Hommel L et al. Circulating skin-homing T cells in atopic dermatitis. Arch Dermatol 1996; 132: 1171–1176.

374 Czech W, Krutmann J, Schöpf E, Kapp A. Serum eosinophil cationic protein (ECP) is a sensitive measure for disease activity in atopic dermatitis. Br J Dermatol 1992; 126: 351–355.

375 Kapp A, Czech W, Krutmann J, Schöpf E. Eosinophil cationic protein in sera of patients with atopic dermatitis. J Am Acad Dermatol 1991; 24: 555–558.

376 Czech W, Schöpf E, Kapp A. Soluble E-selectin in sera of patients with atopic dermatitis and psoriasis – correlation with disease activity. Br J Dermatol 1996; 134: 17–21.

377 Wakita H, Sakamoto T, Tokura Y, Takigawa M. E-selectin and vascular cell adhesion molecule-1 as critical adhesion molecules for infiltration of T lymphocytes and eosinophils in atopic dermatitis. J Cutan Pathol 1994; 21: 33–39.

378 Furue M, Koga T, Yamashita N. Soluble E-selectin and eosinophil cationic protein are distinct serum markers that differentially represent clinical features of atopic dermatitis. Br J Dermatol 1999; 140: 67–72.

379 Wolkerstorfer A, Laan MP, Savelkoul HFJ et al. Soluble E-selectin, other markers of inflammation and disease severity in children with atopic dermatitis. Br J Dermatol 1998; 138: 431–435.

380 Gondo A, Saeki N, Tokuda Y. IgG4 antibodies in patients with atopic dermatitis. Br J Dermatol 1987; 117: 301–310.

381 Shehade SA, Layton GT, Stanworth DR. IgG4 and IgE antibodies in atopic dermatitis and urticaria. Clin Exp Dermatol 1988; 13: 393–396.

382 Lever R, Hadley K, Downey D, Mackie R. Staphylococcal colonization in atopic dermatitis and the effect of topical mupirocin therapy. Br J Dermatol 1988; 119: 189–198.

383 Higaki Y, Hauser C, Rilliet A, Saurat J-H. Increased in vitro cell-mediated immune response to staphylococcal antigens in atopic dermatitis. J Am Acad Dermatol 1986; 15: 1204–1209.

384 Bork K, Brauninger W. Increasing incidence of eczema herpeticum: analysis of seventy-five cases. J Am Acad Dermatol 1988; 19: 1024–1029.

385 Hughes BR, Cunliffe WJ. Rippled hyperpigmentation resembling macular amyloidos s – a feature of atopic eczema. Clin Exp Dermatol 1990; 15: 380–381.

386 Broberg A, Augustsson A. Atopic dermatitis and melanocytic naevi. Br J Dermatol 2000; 142: 306–309.

387 Svensson A. Hand eczema: an evaluation of the frequency of atopic background and the difference in clinical pattern between patients with and without atopic dermatitis. Acta Derm Venereol 1988; 68: 509–513.

388 Lee H-J, Ha S-J, Ahn W-K et al. Clinical evaluation of atopic hand-foot dermatitis. Pediatr Dermatol 2001; 18: 102–106.

389 Lee H-J, Cho S-H, Ha S-J et al. Minor cutaneous features of atopic dermatitis in South Korea. Int J Dermatol 2000; 39: 337–342.

390 Peacocke M, Siminovitch KA. Wiskott–Aldrich syndrome: new molecular and biochemical insights. J Am Acad Dermatol 1992; 27: 507–519.

391 Feliciani C, Castellaneta M, Amatetti M et al. Non-lethal Wiskott–Aldrich syndrome: atopic dermatitis-like lesions persist after splenectomy. Int J Dermatol 2000; 39: 398–400.

392 Schepis C, Barone C, Siragusa M, Romano C. Prevalence of atopic dermatitis in patients with Down syndrome: A clinical survey. J Am Acad Dermatol 1997; 36: 1019–1021.

393 Williams HC, Strachan DP. The natural history of childhood eczema: observations from the British 1958 birth cohort study. Br J Dermatol 1998; 139: 834–839.

394 Boguniewicz M, Leung DYM. Atopic dermatitis. A question of balance. Arch Dermatol 1998; 134: 870–871.

395 Hanifin JM, Chan S. Biochemical and immunologic mechanisms in atopic dermatitis: New targets for emerging therapies. J Am Acad Dermatol 1999; 41: 72–77.

396 Abeck D, Schmidt T, Fesq H et al. Long-term efficacy of medium-dose UVA1 phototherapy in atopic dermatitis. J Am Acad Dermatol 2000; 42: 254–257.

397 Reitamo S, Wollenberg A, Schöpf E et al. Safety and efficacy of 1 year of tacrolimus ointment monotherapy in adults with atopic dermatitis. Arch Dermatol 2000; 136: 999–1006.

398 Mills LB, Mordan LJ, Roth HL et al. Treatment of severe atopic dermatitis by topical immune modulation using dinitrochlorobenzene. J Am Acad Dermatol 2000; 42: 687–689.

399 Uehara M, Sugiura H, Sakurai K. A trial of Oolong tea in the management of recalcitrant atopic dermatitis. Arch Dermatol 2001; 137: 42–43.

400 Harper J, Green A, Scott G et al. First experience of topical SDZ ASM 981 in children with atopic dermatitis. Br J Dermatol 2001; 144: 781–787.

401 Luger T, van Leent EJM, Graeber M et al. SDZ ASM 981: an emerging safe and effective treatment for atopic dermatitis. Br J Dermatol 2001; 144: 788–794.

402 Griffiths CEM. Ascomycin: an advance in the management of atopic dermatitis. Br J Dermatol 2001; 144: 679–681.

403 Charman C, Williams H. Outcome measures of disease severity in atopic eczema. Arch Dermatol 2000; 136: 763–769.

404 Patrizi A, Guerrini V, Ricci G et al. The natural history of sensitizations to food and aeroallergens in atopic dermatitis: a 4-year follow-up. Pediatr Dermatol 2000; 17: 261–265.

405 Zachary CB, MacDonald DM. Quantitative analysis of T-lymphocyte subsets in atopic eczema, using monoclonal antibodies and flow cytofluorimetry. Br J Dermatol 1983; 108: 411–422.

406 Hall TJ, Rycroft R, Brostoff J. Decreased natural killer cell activity in atopic eczema. Immunology 1985; 56: 337–344.

407 Uehara M, Sawai T. A longitudinal study of contact sensitivity in patients with atopic dermatitis. Arch Dermatol 1989; 125: 366–368.

408 Nicolas JF, Thivolet J. Immunologic features of atopic dermatitis. Semin Dermatol 1988; 7: 156–162.

409 Clark RAF. Cell-mediated and IgE-mediated immune responses in atopic dermatitis. Arch Dermatol 1989; 125: 413–416.

410 Holden CA. Atopic dermatitis – messengers, second messengers and cytokines. Clin Exp Dermatol 1993; 18: 201–207.

411 Cooper KD. Atopic dermatitis: recent trends in pathogenesis and therapy. J Invest Dermatol 1994; 102: 128–137.

412 Bos JD, Wierenga EA, Smitt JHS et al. Immune dysregulation in atopic eczema. Arch Dermatol 1992; 128: 1509–1512.

413 Horsmanheimo L, Harvima IT, Järvikallio A et al. Mast cells are one major source of interleukin-4 in atopic dermatitis. Br J Dermatol 1994; 131: 348–353.

414 Halbert AR, Weston WL, Morelli JG. Atopic dermatitis: is it an allergic disease? J Am Acad Dermatol 1995; 33: 1008–1018.

415 Hanifin JM. Assembling the puzzle pieces in atopic inflammation. Arch Dermatol 996; 132: 1230–1232.

416 Cox HE, Moffatt MF, Faux JA et al. Association of atopic dermatitis to the beta subunit of the high affinity immunoglobulin E receptor. Br J Dermatol 1998; 138: 182–187.

417 Bang K, Lund M, Wu K et al. CD4+ CD8+ (thymocyte-like) T lymphocytes present in blood and skin from patients with atopic dermatitis suggest immune dysregulation. Br J Dermatol 2001; 144: 1140–1147.

418 Wollenberg A, Kraft S, Oppel T, Bieber T. Atopic dermatitis: pathogenetic mechanisms. Clin Exp Dermatol 2000; 25: 530–534.

419 Sperhake K, Neuber K, Enssle K, Ring J. Effects of recombinant human soluble interleukin-4 receptor on interleukin-4/staphylococcal enterotoxin B-stimulated peripheral mononuclear cells from patients with atopic eczema. Br J Dermatol 1998; 139: 784–790.

420 Vestergaard C, Bang K, Gesser B et al. A Th2 chemokine, TARC, produced by keratinocytes may recruit CLA+CCR4+ lymphocytes into lesional atopic dermatitis skin. J Invest Dermatol 2000; 115: 640–646.

421 Teraki Y, Hotta T, Shiohara T. Increased circulating skin-homing cutaneous lymphocyte-associated antigen (CLA)+ type 2 cytokine-producing cells, and decreased CLA+ type 1 cytokine-producing cells in atopic dermatitis. Br J Dermatol 2000; 143: 373–378.

422 Ishii N, Takahashi K, Sugita Y, Nakajima H. Atopic dermatitis apparently caused by type 2 CD8+ T cells in an AIDS patient. Clin Exp Dermatol 1998; 23: 121–122.

423 Kallmann B-A, Kolb H, Hüther M et al. Interleukin-10 is a predominant cytokine in atopic dermatitis. Arch Dermatol 1996; 132: 1133–1134.

424 Banfield CC, Callard RE, Harper JI. The role of cutaneous dendritic cells in the immunopathogenesis of atopic dermatitis. Br J Dermatol 2001; 144: 940–946.

425 Leung DYM, Soter NA. Cellular and immunologic mehanisms in atopic dermatitis. J Am Acad Dermatol 2001; 44: S1–S12.

426 Esterly NB. Significance of food hypersensitivity in children with atopic dermatitis. Pediatr Dermatol 1986; 3: 161–174.

427 Guillet G, Guillet M-H. Natural history of sensitizations in atopic dermatitis. Arch Dermatol 1992; 128: 187–192.

428 Binkley KE. Role of food allergy in atopic dermatitis. Int J Dermatol 1992; 31: 611–614.

429 Tanaka M, Aiba S, Matsumura N et al. IgE-mediated hypersensitivity and contact sensitivity to multiple environmental allergens in atopic dermatitis. Arch Dermatol 1994; 130: 1393–1401.

430 Wananukul S, Huiprasert P, Pongprasit P. Eczematous skin reactions from patch testing with aeroallergens in atopic children with and without atopic dermatitis. Pediatr Dermatol 1993; 10: 209–213.

431 Darsow U, Vieluf D, Ring J. Evaluating the relevance of aeroallergen sensitization in atopic eczema with the atopy patch test: A randomized. double-blind multicenter study. J Am Acad Dermatol 1999; 40: 187–193.

432 Darsow U, Ring J. Airborne and dietary allergens in atopic eczema: a comprehensive review of diagnostic tests. Clin Exp Dermatol 2000; 25: 544–551.

433 Yu B, Sawai T, Uehara M et al. Immediate hypersensitivity skin reactions to human dander in atopic dermatitis. Arch Dermatol 1988; 124: 1530–1533.

434 Darsow U, Behrendt H, Ring J. Gramineae pollen as trigger factors of atopic eczema: evaluation of diagnostic measures using the atopy patch test. Br J Dermatol 1997; 137: 201–207.

435 Elliston WL, Heise EA, Huntley CC. Cell-mediated hypersensitivity to mite antigens in atopic dermatitis. Arch Dermatol 1982; 18: 26–29.

436 Beck H-I, Korsgaard J. Atopic dermatitis and house dust mites. Br J Dermatol 1989; 120: 245–251.

437 Norris PG, Schofield O, Camp RDR. A study of the role of house dust mite in atopic dermatitis. Br J Dermatol 1988; 118: 435–440.

438 Imayama S, Hashizume T, Miyahara H et al. Combination of patch test and IgE for dust mite antigens differentiates 130 patients with atopic dermatitis into four groups. J Am Acad Dermatol 1992; 27: 531–538.

439 Colloff MJ. Exposure to house dust mites in homes of people with atopic dermatitis. Br J Dermatol 1992; 127: 322–327.

440 Ricci G, Patrizi A, Specchia F et al. Mite allergen (Der p 1) levels in houses of children with atopic dermatitis: the relationship with allergometric tests. Br J Dermatol 1999; 140: 651–655.

441 Fitzharris P, Riley G. House dust mites in atopic dermatitis. Int J Dermatol 1999; 38: 173–175.

442 Friedmann PS. Dust mite avoidance in atopic dermatitis. J Am Acad Dermatol 1999; 24: 433–437.

443 Varela P, Selores M, Gomes E et al. Immediate and delayed hypersensitivity to mite antigens in atopic dermatitis. Pediatr Dermatol 1999; 16: 1–5.

444 Ricci G, Patrizi A, Specchia F et al. Effect of house dust mite avoidance measures in children with atopic dermatitis. Br J Dermatol 2000; 143: 379–384.

445 Yoshino T, Asada H, Sano S et al. Impaired responses of peripheral blood mononuclear cells to staphylococcal superantigen in patients with severe atopic dermatitis: a role of T cell apoptosis. J Invest Dermatol 2000; 114: 281–288.

446 Jahreis A, Beckheinrich P, Haustein U-F. Effects of two novel cationic staphylococcal proteins (NP-tase and p70) and enterotoxin B on IgE synthesis and interleukin-4 and interferon-γ production in patients with atopic dermatitis. Br J Dermatol 2000; 142: 680–687.

447 Akdis CA, Akdis M, Simon D et al. T cells and T cell-derived cytokines as pathogenic factors in the nonallergic form of atopic dermatitis. J Invest Dermatol 1999; 113: 628–634.

448 Najem N, Hull D. Langerhans cells in delayed skin reactions to inhalant allergens in atopic dermatitis – an electron microscopic study. Clin Exp Dermatol 1989; 14: 218–222.

449 Wollenberg A, Kraft S, Hanau D, Bieber T. Immunomorphological and ultrastructural characterization of Langerhans cells and a novel, inflammatory dendritic epidermal cell (IDEC) population in lesional skin of atopic eczema. J Invest Dermatol 1996; 106: 446–453.

450 Oppel T, Schuller E, Günther S et al. Phenotyping of epidermal dendritic cells allows the differentiation between extrinsic and intrinsic forms of atopic dermatitis. Br J Dermatol 2000; 143: 1193–1198.

451 Boone M, Lespagnard L, Renard N et al. Adhesion molecule profiles in atopic dermatitis vs. allergic contact dermatitis: pharmacological modulation by cetirizine. J Eur Acad Dermatol Venereol 2000; 14: 263–266.

452 Kiekens RCM, Thepen T, Bihari IC et al. Expression of Fc receptors for IgG during acute and chronic cutaneous inflammation in atopic dermatitis. Br J Dermatol 2000; 142: 1106–1113.

453 Leonhardt A, Krauss M, Gieler U et al. In vivo formation of prostaglandin E1 and prostaglandin E2 in atopic dermatitis. Br J Dermatol 1997; 136: 337–340.

454 Morren M-A, Przybilla B, Bamelis M et al. Atopic dermatitis: triggering factors. J Am Acad Dermatol 1994; 31: 467–473.

455 Nassif A, Chan SC, Storrs FJ, Hanifin JM. Abnormal skin irritancy in atopic dermatitis and in atopy without dermatitis. Arch Dermatol 1994; 130: 1402–1407.

456 Rukwied R, Lischetzki G, McGlone F et al. Mast cell mediators other than histamine induce pruritus in atopic dermatitis patients: a dermal microdialysis study. Br J Dermatol 2000; 142: 1114–1120.

457 Greaves M. Mast cell mediators other than histamine induced pruritus in atopic dermatitis patients – a dermal microdialysis study. Br J Dermatol 2000; 142: 1079–1080.

458 Larsen FS, Holm NV, Henningsen K. Atopic dermatitis. A genetic-epidemiologic study in a population-based twin sample. J Am Acad Dermatol 1986; 15: 487–494.

459 Bradley M, Kockum I, Söderhäll C et al. Characterization by phenotype of families with atopic dermatitis. Acta Derm Venereol 2000; 80: 106–110.

460 Harris JM, Cullinan P, Williams HC et al. Environmental associations with eczema in early life. Br J Dermatol 2001; 144: 795–802.

461 Coleman R, Trembath RC, Harper JI. Genetic studies of atopy and atopic dermatitis. Br J Dermatol 1997; 136: 1–5.

462 Beyer K, Nickel R, Freidhoff L et al. Association and linkage of atopic dermatitis with chromosome 13q12–14 and 5q31–33 markers. J Invest Dermatol 2000; 115: 906–908.

463 Oiso N, Fukai K, Ishii M. Interleukin 4 receptor α chain polymorphism Gln551Arg is associated with adult atopic dermatitis in Japan. Br J Dermatol 2000; 142: 1003–1006.

464 Hara J, Higuchi K, Okamoto R et al. High-expression of sphingomyelin deacylase is an important determinant of ceramide deficiency leading to barrier disruption in atopic dermatitis. J Invest Dermatol 2000; 115: 406–413.

465 Mihm MC Jr, Soter NA, Dvorak HF, Austen KF. The structure of normal skin and the morphology of atopic eczema. J Invest Dermatol 1976; 67: 305–312.

466 Soter NA, Mihm MC JR. Morphology of atopic eczema. Acta Derm Venereol (Suppl) 1980; 92: 11–15.

467 White CR Jr. Histopathology of atopic dermatitis. Semin Dermatol 1983; 2: 34–38.

468 Hurwitz RM, DeTrana C. The cutaneous pathology of atopic dermatitis. Am J Dermatopathol 1990; 12: 544–551.

469 Grewe M, Vogelsang K, Ruzicka T et al. Neurotrophin-4 production by human epidermal keratinocytes: increased expression in atopic dermatitis. J Invest Dermatol 2000; 114: 1108–1112.

470 Uno H, Hanifin JM. Langerhans cells in acute and chronic epidermal lesions of atopic dermatitis, observed by L-dopa histofluorescence, glycol methacrylate thin section, and electron microscopy. J Invest Dermatol 1980; 75: 52–60.

471 Uehara M. Clinical and histological features of dry skin in atopic dermatitis. Acta Derm Venereol (Suppl) 1985; 114: 82–86.

472 Beran D, Kossard S, Freeman S et al. Immune mechanisms in atopic dermatitis: studies and hypothesis. Australas J Dermatol 1986; 27: 112–117.

473 Mempel M, Schmidt T, Boeck K et al. Changes in collagen I and collagen III metabolism in patients with generalized atopic eczema undergoing medium-dose ultraviolet A1 phototherapy. Br J Dermatol 2000; 142: 473–480.

474 Sugiura H, Hirota Y, Uehara M. Heterogeneous distribution of mast cells in lichenified lesions of atopic dermatitis. Acta Derm Venereol (Suppl) 1989; 144: 115–118.

475 Uehara M, Miyauchi H. The morphologic characteristics of dry skin in atopic dermatitis. Arch Dermatol 1984; 120: 1186–1190.

476 Finlay AY, Nicholls S, King CS, Marks R. The 'dry' non-eczematous skin associated with atopic eczema. Br J Dermatol 1980; 103: 249–256.

477 Humphreys F, Spencer J, McLaren K, Tidman MJ. An histological and ultrastructural study of the 'dirty neck' appearance in atopic eczema. Clin Exp Dermatol 1996; 21: 17–19.

478 Van Neste D, Douka M, Rahier J, Staquet MJ. Epidermal changes in atopic dermatitis. Acta Derm Venereol (Suppl) 1985; 114: 67–71.

479 Leiferman KM, Ackerman SJ, Sampson HA et al. Dermal deposition of eosinophil-granule major basic protein in atopic dermatitis. N Engl J Med 1985; 313: 282–285.

480 Lever R, Turbitt M, Sanderson A, Mackie R. Immunophenotyping of the cutaneous infiltrate and of the mononuclear cells in the peripheral blood in patients with atopic dermatitis. J Invest Dermatol 1987; 89: 4–7.

481 Bieber T, Dannenberg B, Ring J, Braun-Falco O. Keratinocytes in lesional skin of atopic eczema bear HLA-DR, CD1a and IgE molecules. Clin Exp Dermatol 1989; 14: 35–39.

482 Clark AR, Jorizzo JL, Fleischer AB. Papular dermatitis (subacute prurigo, "itchy red bump" disease): Pilot study of phototherapy. J Am Acad Dermatol 1998; 38: 929–933.

483 Epstein E. Hand dermatitis: practical management and current concepts. J Am Acad Dermatol 1984; 10: 395–424.

484 Menne T, Hjorth N. Pompholyx – dyshidrotic eczema. Semin Dermatol 1983; 2: 75–80.

485 Kutzner H, Wurzel RM, Wolff HH. Are acrosyringia involved in the pathogenesis of 'dyshidrosis'? Am J Dermatopathol 1986; 8: 109–116.

486 Meneghini CL, Angelini G. Contact and microbial allergy in pompholyx. Contact Dermatitis 1979; 5: 46–50.

487 Miller RM, Coger RW. Skin conductance conditioning with dyshidrotic eczema patients. Br J Dermatol 1979; 101: 435–440.

488 Norris PG, Levene GM. Pompholyx occurring during hospital admission for treatment of atopic dermatitis. Clin Exp Dermatol 1987; 12: 189–190.

489 Vocks E, Plötz SG, Ring J. The dyshidrotic eczema area and severity index – a score developed for the assessment of dyshidrotic eczema. Dermatology 1999; 198: 265–269.

490 Hersle K, Mobacken H. Hyperkeratotic dermatitis of the palms. Br J Dermatol 1982; 107: 195–202.

491 Mackie RM, Hussain SL. Juvenile plantar dermatosis: a new entity? Clin Exp Dermatol 1976; 1: 253–260.

492 Ashton RE, Russell Jones R, Griffiths A. Juvenile plantar dermatosis. A clinicopathologic study. Arch Dermatol 1985; 121: 225–228.

493 Young E. Forefoot eczema – further studies and a review. Clin Exp Dermatol 1986; 11: 523–528.

494 Verbov J. Juvenile plantar dermatosis. Acta Derm Venereol (Suppl) 1989; 144: 153–154.

495 Lim KB, Tan T, Rajan VS. Dermatitis palmaris sicca – a distinctive pattern of hand dermatitis. Clin Exp Dermatol 1986; 11: 553–559.

496 Van Diggelen MW, van Dijk E, Hausman R. The enigma of juvenile plantar dermatosis. Am J Dermatopathol 1986; 8: 336–340.

497 Shrank AB. The aetiology of juvenile plantar dermatosis. Br J Dermatol 1979; 100: 641–648.

498 Hruza LL, Hruza GJ. Saphenous vein graft donor site dermatitis. Arch Dermatol 1993; 129: 609–612.

499 Beninson J, Livingood CS. Stasis dermatitis. In: Demis DJ, ed. Clinical dermatology. Philadelphia: Harper & Row, 1986: unit 7.44; 1–6.

500 Sivaram M, Chawla Y, Kumar B. Stasis dermatitis – a new cutaneous manifestation of Budd–Chiari syndrome. Int J Dermatol 1998; 37: 397–398.

501 Weedon D. Unpublished observations.

502 Roa WHY, Gardiner DB, Krause BE, Chan LS. Generalized autosensitization to a localized eczematoid dermatitis induced by ionizing radiation. J Am Acad Dermatol 1994; 30: 489–490.

503 Harris A, McFadden JP. Dermatitis following systemic prednisolone: patch testing with prednisolone eye drops. Australas J Dermatol 2000; 41: 124–125.

504 Callen JP, Bernardi DM, Clark RAF, Weber DA. Adult-onset recalcitrant eczema: A marker of noncutaneous lymphoma or leukemia. J Am Acad Dermatol 2000; 43: 207–210.

505 González-Amaro R, Baranda L, Abud-Mendoza C et al. Autoeczematization s associated with abnormal immune recognition of autologous skin antigens. J Am Acad Dermatol 1993; 28: 56–60.

506 Cunningham MJ, Zone JJ, Petersen MJ, Green JA. Circulating activated (DR-positive) T lymphocytes in a patient with autoeczematization. J Am Acad Dermatol 1986; 14: 1039–1041.

507 Kasteler JS, Petersen MJ, Vance JE, Zone JJ. Circulating activated T lymphocytes in autoeczematisation. Arch Dermatol 1992; 128: 795–798.

508 Parsons JM. Pityriasis rosea update: 1986. J Am Acad Dermatol 1986; 15: 159–167.

509 Hendricks AA, Lohr JA. Pityriasis rosea in infancy. Arch Dermatol 1979; 115: 896–897.

510 Chuang T-Y, Ilstrup DM, Perry HO, Kurland LT. Pityriasis rosea in Rochester, Minnesota, 1969 to 1978. A 10-year epidemiologic study. J Am Acad Dermatol 1982; 7: 80–89.

511 Kay MH, Rapini RP, Fritz KA. Oral lesions in pityriasis rosea. Arch Dermatol 1985; 121: 1449–1451.

512 Del Campo DV, Barsky S, Tisocco L, Gruszka RJ. Pityriasis rosea unilateralis. Int J Dermatol 1983; 22: 312–313.

513 Ahmed I, Charles-Holmes R. Localized pityriasis rosea. Clin Exp Dermatol 2000; 25: 624–626.

514 Garcia RL. Vesicular pityriasis rosea. Arch Dermatol 1976; 112: 410.

515 Pierson JC, Dijkstra JWE, Elston DM. Purpuric pityriasis rosea. J Am Acad Dermatol 1993; 28: 1021.

516 Chuang T-Y, Perry HO, Ilstrup DM, Kurland LT. Recent upper respiratory tract infection and pityriasis rosea: a case-control study of 249 matched pairs. Br J Dermatol 1983; 108: 587–591.

517 Messenger AG, Knox EG, Summerly R et al. Case clustering in pityriasis rosea: support for role of an infective agent. Br Med J 1982; 284: 371–373.

518 Sharma PK, Yadav TP, Gautam RK et al. Erythromycin in pityriasis rosea: A double-blind, placebo-controlled clinical trial. J Am Acad Dermatol 2000; 42: 241–244.

519 Kosuge H, Tanaka-Taya K, Miyoshi H et al. Epidemiological study of human herpesvirus-6 and human herpesvirus-7 in pityriasis rosea. Br J Dermatol 2000; 143: 795–798.

520 Drago F, Ranieri E, Brusati C et al. Pityriasis rosea, HHV-7 and multiple sclerosis. A coincidence? Br J Dermatol 2000; 142: 1250–1251.

521 Offidani A, Pritelli E, Simonetti O et al. Pityriasis rosea associated with herpesvirus 7 DNA. J Eur Acad Dermatol Venereol 2000; 14: 313–314.

522 Kempf W, Adams V, Kleinhans M et al. Pityriasis rosea is not associated with human herpesvirus 7. Arch Dermatol 1999; 135: 1070–1072.

523 Yasukawa M, Sada E, Machino H, Fujita S. Reactivation of human herpesvirus 6 in pityriasis rosea. Br J Dermatol 1999; 140: 169–170.

524 Aoshima T, Komura K, Ofuji S. Virus-like particles in the herald patch of pityriasis rosea. Dermatologica 1981; 162: 64–65.

525 Hudson LD, Adelman S, Lewis CW. Pityriasis rosea. Viral complement fixation studies. J Am Acad Dermatol 1981; 4: 544–546.

526 Burch PRJ, Rowell NR. Pityriasis rosea – an autoaggressive disease? Br J Dermatol 1970; 82: 549–560.

527 Aiba S, Tagami H. Immunohistologic studies in pityriasis rosea. Evidence for cellular immune reaction in the lesional epidermis. Arch Dermatol 1985; 121: 761–765.

528 Buckley C. Pityriasis rosea-like eruption in a patient receiving omeprazole. Br J Dermatol 1996; 135: 660–661.

529 Loche F, Thouvenin MD, Bazex J. Pityriasis-rosea-like eruption due to benfluorex. Dermatology 2000; 201: 75.

530 Maize JC, Tomecki KJ. Pityriasis rosea-like drug eruption secondary to metronidazole. Arch Dermatol 1977; 113: 1457–1458.

531 Wilkin JK, Kirkendall WM. Pityriasis rosea-like rash from captopril. Arch Dermatol 1982; 118: 186–187.

532 Spelman LJ, Robertson IM, Strutton GM, Weedon D. Pityriasis rosea-like eruption after bone marrow transplantation. J Am Acad Dermatol 1994; 31: 348–351.

533 Panizzon R, Bloch PH. Histopathology of pityriasis rosea Gibert. Qualitative and quantitative light-microscopic study of 62 biopsies of 40 patients. Dermatologica 1982; 165: 551–558.

534 Bunch LW, Tilley JC. Pityriasis rosea. A histologic and serologic study. Arch Dermatol 1961; 84: 79–86.

535 Stern JK, Wolf JE Jr, Rosen T. Focal acantholytic dyskeratosis in pityriasis rosea. Arch Dermatol 1979; 115: 497.

536 El-Shiemy S, Nassar A, Mokhtar M, Mabrouk D. Light and electron microscopic studies of pityriasis rosea. Int J Dermatol 1987; 26: 237–239.

537 Okamoto H, Imamura S, Aoshima T et al. Dyskeratotic degeneration of epidermal cells in pityriasis rosea: light and electron microscopic studies. Br J Dermatol 1982; 107: 189–194.

538 Takaki Y, Miyazaki H. Cytologic degeneration of keratinocytes adjacent to Langerhans cells in pityriasis rosea (Gibert). Acta Derm Venereol 1976; 56: 99–103.

539 Gianotti F. The Gianotti–Crosti syndrome. JCE Dermatol 1979; 18(2): 15–25.

540 Eiloart M. The Gianotti–Crosti syndrome. Report of forty-four cases. Br J Dermatol 1966; 78: 488–492.

541 Caputo R, Gelmetti C, Ermacora E et al. Gianotti–Crosti syndrome: a retrospective analysis of 308 cases. J Am Acad Dermatol 1992; 26: 207–210.

542 Strate EG, Esterly NB. Human immunodeficiency virus and the Gianotti–Crosti syndrome. Arch Dermatol 1995; 131: 108–109.

543 Schneider JA, Poley JR, Millunchick EW et al. Papular acrodermatitis (Gianotti–Crosti syndrome) in a child with anicteric hepatitis B, virus subtype adw. J Pediatr 1982; 101: 219–222.

544 Lee S, Kim KY, Hahn CS et al. Gianotti–Crosti syndrome associated with hepatitis B surface antigen (subtype adr). J Am Acad Dermatol 1985; 12: 629–633.

545 Ishimaru Y, Ishimaru H, Toda G et al. An epidemic of infantile papular acrodermatitis (Gianotti's disease) in Japan associated with hepatitis-B surface antigen subtype ayw. Lancet 1976; 1: 707–709.

546 Konno M, Kikuta H, Ishikawa N et al. A possible association between hepatitis-B antigen-negative infantile papular acrodermatitis and Epstein–Barr virus infection. J Pediatr 1982; 101: 222–224.

547 Iosub S, Santos C, Gromisch DS. Papular acrodermatitis with Epstein–Barr virus infection. Clin Pediatr 1984; 23: 33–34.

548 James WD, Odom RB, Hatch MH. Gianotti–Crosti-like eruption associated with coxsackievirus A-16 infection. J Am Acad Dermatol 1982; 6: 862–866.

549 Sagi EF, Linder N, Shouval D. Papular acrodermatitis of childhood associated with hepatitis A virus infection. Pediatr Dermatol 1985; 3: 31–33.

550 Liehr H, Seelig R, Seelig HP. Cutaneous papulo-vesicular eruptions in non-A, non-B hepatitis. Hepatogastroenterology 1985; 32: 11–14.

551 Blauvelt A, Turner ML. Gianotti–Crosti syndrome and human immunodeficiency virus infection. Arch Dermatol 1994; 130: 481–483.

552 Berant M, Naveh Y, Weissman I. Papular acrodermatitis with cytomegalovirus hepatitis. Arch Dis Child 1984; 58: 1024–1025.

553 Spear KL, Winkelmann RK. Gianotti–Crosti syndrome. A review of ten cases not associated with hepatitis B. Arch Dermatol 1984; 120: 891–896.

554 Taïeb A, Plantin P, Du Pasquier P et al. Gianotti–Crosti syndrome: a study of 26 cases. Br J Dermatol 1986; 115: 49–59.

555 Gianotti F. Papular acrodermatitis of childhood and other papulo-vesicular acro-located syndromes. Br J Dermatol 1979; 100: 49–59.

556 Winkelmann RK, Bourlond A. Infantile lichenoid acrodermatitis. Report of a case of Gianotti–Crosti syndrome. Arch Dermatol 1965; 92: 398–401.

557 Rubenstein D, Esterly NB, Fretzin D. The Gianotti–Crosti syndrome. Pediatrics 1978; 61: 433–437.

558 Fisher AA. Systemic contact-type dermatitis due to drugs. Clin Dermatol 1986; 4: 58–69.

559 Räsänen L, Kaipiainen-Seppänen O, Myllykangas-Luosujärvi R et al. Hypersensitivity to gold in gold sodium thiomalate-induced dermatosis. Br J Dermatol 1999; 141: 683–688.

560 Rosen C. Photo-induced drug eruptions. Semin Dermatol 1989; 8: 149–157.

561 Youn JI, Lee HG, Yeo UC, Lee YS. Piroxicam photosensitivity associated with vesicular hand dermatitis. Clin Exp Dermatol 1993; 18: 52–54.

562 Menne T, Veien NK, Maibach HI. Systemic contact-type dermatitis due to drugs. Semin Dermatol 1989; 8: 144–148.

563 Goossens C, Sass U, Song M. Baboon syndrome. Dermatology 1997; 194: 421–422.

564 Köhler LD, Schönlein K, Kautzky F, Vogt HJ. Diagnosis at first glance: the Baboon syndrome. Int J Dermatol 1996; 35: 502–503.

565 Michel M, Dompmartin A, Szczurko C et al. Eczematous-like drug eruption induced by synergistins. Contact Dermatitis 1996; 34: 86–87.

566 Helmbold P, Hegemann B, Dickert C, Marsch WCh. Symmetric psychotropic and nonpigmenting fixed drug eruption due to cimetidine (so-called baboon syndrome). Dermatology 1998; 197: 402–403.

567 Chowdhury MMU, Patel GK, Inaloz HS, Holt PJA. Hydroxyurea-induced skin disease mimicking the baboon syndrome. Clin Exp Dermatol 1999; 24: 336–337.

568 Bartolome B, Cordoba S, Sanchez-Perez J et al. Baboon syndrome of unusual origin. Contact Dermatitis 2000; 43: 113.

569 Iliev D, Elsner P. Generalized drug reaction due to papaya juice in throat lozenges. Dermatology 1997; 194: 364–366.

570 VanArsdel PP Jr. Allergy and adverse drug reactions. J Am Acad Dermatol 1982; 6: 833–845.

571 Swinyer LJ. Determining the cause of drug eruptions. Dermatol Clin 1983; 1: 417–431.

572 Bruynzeel DP, van Ketel WG. Patch testing in drug eruptions. Semin Dermatol 1989; 8: 196–203.

573 Park SD, Lee S-W, Chun J-H, Cha S-H. Clinical features of 31 patients with systemic contact dermatitis due to the ingestion of *Rhus* (lacquer). Br J Dermatol 2000; 142: 937–942.

574 Barbaud A, Tréchot P, Granel F et al. A baboon syndrome induced by intravenous human immunoglobulins: report of a case and immunological analysis. Dermatology 1999; 199: 258–260.

575 Addo HA, Ferguson J, Frain-Bell W. Thiazide-induced photosensitivity: a study of 33 subjects. Br J Dermatol 1987; 116: 749–760.

576 Weedon D. Unpublished observations.

577 Beer K, Albertini J, Medinica M, Busbey S. Fluoxetine-induced hypersensitivity. Arch Dermatol 1994; 130: 803–804.

578 Bigby M, Stern R. Cutaneous reactions to nonsteroidal anti-inflammatory drugs. A review. J Am Acad Dermatol 1985; 12: 866–876.

579 Stanley J, Fallon-Pellicci V. Phenytoin hypersensitivity reaction. Arch Dermatol 1978; 114: 1350–1353.

580 Tuneu A, Moreno A, de Moragas JM. Cutaneous reactions secondary to heparin injections. J Am Acad Dermatol 1985; 12: 1072–1077.

581 Klein GF, Kofler H, Wolf H, Fritsch PO. Eczema-like, erythematous, infiltrated plaques: a common side effect of subcutaneous heparin therapy. J Am Acad Dermatol 1989; 21: 703–707.

582 Tuppal R, Tremaine R. Cutaneous eruption from vitamin K₁ injection. J Am Acad Dermatol 1992; 27: 105–106.

583 Bircher AJ, Flückiger R, Buchner SA. Eczematous infiltrated plaques to subcutaneous heparin: a type IV allergic reaction. Br J Dermatol 1990; 123: 507–514.

584 Whittam LR, Hay RJ, Hughes RAC. Eczematous reactions to human immune globulin. Br J Dermatol 1997; 137: 481–482.

585 Wolkenstein P, Chosidow O, Wechsler J et al. Cutaneous side effects associated with interleukin 2 administration for metastatic melanoma. J Am Acad Dermatol 1993; 28: 66–70.

586 Blessing K, Park KGM, Heys SD et al. Immunopathological changes in the skin following recombinant interleukin-2 treatment. J Pathol 1992; 167: 313–319.

587 Fleming TE, Mirando WS, Soohoo LF et al. An inflammatory eruption associated with recombinant human IL-6. Br J Dermatol 1994; 130: 534–536.

588 Mehregan DR, Fransway AF, Edmonson JH, Leiferman KM. Cutaneous reactions to granulocyte-monocyte colony-stimulating factor. Arch Dermatol 1992; 128: 1055–1059.

589 Penneys NS. Gold therapy: dermatologic uses and toxicities. J Am Acad Dermatol 1979; 1: 315–320.

590 Ranki A, Niemi K-M, Kanerva L. Clinical, immunohistochemical, and electron-microscopic findings in gold dermatitis. Am J Dermatopathol 1989; 11: 22–28.

591 Shelley WB, Shelley ED, Talanin NY, Santoso-Pham J. Estrogen dermatitis. J Am Acad Dermatol 1995; 32: 25–31.

592 Herzberg AJ, Strohmeyer CR, Cirillo-Hyland VA. Autoimmune progesterone dermatitis. J Am Acad Dermatol 1995; 32: 335–338.

593 Kumar A, Georgouras KE. Oestrogen dermatitis. Australas J Dermatol 1999; 40: 96–98.

594 Ródenas JM, Herranz MT, Tercedor J. Autoimmune progesterone dermatitis: treatment with oophorectomy. Br J Dermatol 1998; 139: 508–511.

595 Kauppinen K, Stubb S. Drug eruptions: causative agents and clinical types. A series of in-patients during a 10-year period. Acta Derm Venereol 1984; 64: 320–324.

596 Fellner MJ, Frutkin L. Morbilliform eruptions caused by penicillin. A study by electron microscopy and immunologic tests. J Invest Dermatol 1970; 55: 390–395.

597 Bennaman O, Sanchez JL. Comparative clinicopathological study on pityriasis lichenoides chronica and small plaque parapsoriasis. Am J Dermatopathol 1988; 10: 189–196.

598 Hu C-H, Winkelmann RK. Digitate dermatosis. A new look at symmetrical, small plaque parapsoriasis. Arch Dermatol 1973; 107: 65–69.

599 Calnan CD, Meara RH. Parapsoriasis en plaque and chronic superficial dermatitis. Trans St John's Hosp Dermatol Soc 1956; 37: 12–13.

600 Lambert WC, Everett MA. The nosology of parapsoriasis. J Am Acad Dermatol 1981; 5: 373–395.

601 Bluefarb SM. The clinical implications of parapsoriasis. Int J Dermatol 1980; 19: 556–557.

602 Goldberg LC. Xantho-erythrodermia perstans (Crocker). Arch Dermatol 1963; 88: 901–907.

603 Samman PD. The natural history of parapsoriasis en plaques (chronic superficial dermatitis) and prereticulotic poikiloderma. Br J Dermatol 1972; 87: 405–411.

604 Haeffner AC, Smoller BR, Zepter K, Wood GS. Differentiation and clonality of lesional lymphocytes in small plaque parapsoriasis. Arch Dermatol 1995; 131: 321–324.

605 Ackerman AB, Schiff TA. If small plaque (digitate) parapsoriasis is a cutaneous T-cell lymphoma, even an 'abortive' one, it must be mycosis fungoides! Arch Dermatol 1996; 132: 562–566.

606 King-Ismael D, Ackerman AB. Guttate parapsoriasis/digitate dermatosis (small plaque parapsoriasis) is mycosis fungoides. Am J Dermatopathol 1992; 14: 518–530.

607 Burg G, Dummer R. Small plaque (digitate) parapsoriasis is an 'abortive cutaneous T-cell lymphoma' and is not mycosis fungoides. Arch Dermatol 1995; 131: 336–338.

608 Burg G, Dummer R, Nestle FO et al. Cutaneous lymphomas consist of a spectrum of nosologically different entities including mycosis fungoides and small plaque parapsoriasis. Arch Dermatol 1996; 132: 567–572.

609 Sterry W. Thoughts about parapsoriasis. Dermatopathology: Practical & Conceptual 2000; 6: 52–54.

610 Grosshans E, Marot L. Blaschkite de l'adulte. Ann Dermatol Venereol 1990; 117: 9–15.

611 Betti R, Vergani R, Gualandri L, Crosti C. Acquired self-healing Blaschko dermatitis in an adult. Australas J Dermatol 1998; 39: 271–272.

612 Megahed M, Reinauer S, Scharffetter-Kochanek K et al. Acquired relapsing self-healing Blaschko dermatitis. J Am Acad Dermatol 1994; 31: 849–852.

613 Haimowitz JE, McCauliffe DP, Seykora J, Werth VP. Annular erythema of Sjögren's syndrome in a white woman. J Am Acad Dermatol 2000; 42: 1069–1073.

614 Rybojad M, Cambiaghi S, Moraillon I et al. Omenn's reticulosis associated with the nephrotic syndrome. Br J Dermatol 1996; 135: 124–127.

615 Sanchez JL, Ackerman AB. The patch stage of mycosis fungoides. Criteria for histologic diagnosis. Am J Dermatopathol 1979; 1: 5–26.

616 Nickoloff BJ. Light-microscopic assessment of 100 patients with patch/plaque-stage mycosis fungoides. Am J Dermatopathol 1988; 10: 469–477.

The vesiculobullous reaction pattern

INTRODUCTION

The vesiculobullous reaction pattern is characterized by the presence of vesicles or bullae at any level within the epidermis or at the dermoepidermal junction. Pustules, which are vesicles or bullae containing numerous neutrophils or eosinophils, are included in this reaction pattern. Vesiculobullous lesions result from a defect, congenital or acquired, in the adhesion of keratinocytes. Accordingly, it is important to have an understanding of the mechanisms involved in normal epidermal cohesion.

Epidermal cohesion

The epidermis is a dynamic structure held together by adhesion molecules which have an important role in cell–cell and cell–matrix adhesion, as well as in the transmission of signals, in both directions, across the cell membrane.[1,2] Signal transmission is also a function of gap junctions, composed of various polypeptides, the most important of which are connexins.[3] Their role in cell–cell adhesion appears to be a minor one. Adhesion molecules are transmembrane proteins, the extracellular domains of which are homophilic and the intracellular portions linked to the cytoskeleton of the cell.

There are four major families of adhesion molecules – cadherins, integrins, selectins and the immunoglobulin superfamily – which are localized to two specialized intercellular junctions known as *desmosomes* (including hemidesmosomes) and the *adherens junction*. Focal adhesions (labile structures seen in cultured keratinocytes and postulated to exist in the skin) are included with the latter group. Desmosomes are well-defined, plaque-like areas of point contact that are easily seen in the spinous layer. The adherens junction is less well defined. Some work suggests that it may be situated near desmosomes.[4] Desmosomes and adherens junctions further differ from one another in three respects:

1. the subclass of adhesion molecule present;
2. the composition of the cytoplasmic plaque (see below); and
3. the nature of the associated cytoskeletal element.

These aspects will be considered further in the sections discussing adhesion molecules and cytoplasmic plaques.

Adhesion molecules

As indicated above, there are four families of adhesion molecules. They are sometimes divided into two groups – those which mediate cell–cell adhesion, such as the cadherins and immunoglobulin superfamily, and those which mediate cellular adhesion to matrix molecules such as the selectins. The integrins are capable of mediating both types of adhesion. The cadherins are the most important group in keratinocyte cohesion, although the integrins have a role in basal cells, particularly in the hemidesmosomes. Only brief mention will be made of the other families in the discussion that follows.

Cadherins

The cadherins are calcium-dependent adhesion molecules which extracellularly can attach to other cadherins; that is, they are homophilic.[2] There are two major subfamilies of cadherins: the first, known as *classic cadherins* (E-cadherin), are found in the adherens junctions where their cytoplasmic domains link with cytoplasmic anchoring molecules (including β catenin, type XIII collagen[5] and vinculin) in the cytoplasmic plaques and which, in turn, connect with actin filaments of the cytoskeleton; the second group of cadherins, which are localized to desmosomes (*desmosomal cadherins*), are linked eventually to keratin intermediate filaments via plakoglobin and the desmoplakins of the cytoplasmic plaques.[6] There are two major groups of desmosomal cadherins – the *desmogleins* and the *desmocollins*. Both have

been mapped to chromosome 18.[6] To date, three desmoglein and three desmocollin genes have been identified.

The *desmogleins*, which have large cytoplasmic domains, exhibit a tissue- and differentiation-specific pattern of expression.[7] Of the three desmogleins, desmoglein 1 is expressed primarily in the upper layers of the epidermis. It is the target antigen in pemphigus foliaceus. Desmoglein 2 is found in simple epithelia and basal epidermis, while desmoglein 3 is found primarily in the spinous layer. It is the target antigen in pemphigus vulgaris.[7]

Less is known about the *desmocollins*. They have shorter intracytoplasmic domains than the desmogleins. They may play a key role in initiating desmosome assembly.[6] Both IgA pemphigus and pemphigus foliaceus (particularly the endemic form) may sometimes be associated with autoantibodies to desmocollin.

Integrins

The integrin family of adhesion molecules is involved in cell–cell and cell–matrix adhesions, particularly in the hemidesmosomes of basal keratinocytes and the 'focal adhesions' of cultured keratinocytes. Integrins are heterodimers with an α and a β chain. Fourteen α and eight β chains have been described, but only a limited number of permutations have so far been described in the skin – α2β1, α3β1, α6β4.[8] The first two subtypes are found in the lateral and basal aspects of basal cells, while α6β4 is located in the hemidesmosomes. Epiligrin is an adhesive ligand for α3β1 and α6β4 integrins. Other extracellular matrix ligands include laminin and fibronectin.[8] The laminins are of great importance in maintaining epidermal adhesion to the dermis.[9]

Immunoglobulin superfamily

The immunoglobulin superfamily has one or more immunoglobulin-like domains. Included in this group are molecules concerned with adhesion to lymphocytes and the intercellular adhesion molecule (ICAM). They have no significant role in keratinocyte cohesion.[2]

Selectins

The selectins are mainly involved in endothelial cell adhesion. They have no significant role in the epidermis.[2]

Cytoplasmic plaques

Cytoplasmic plaques are dense, submembranous regions of the intercellular junctions, measuring 14–20 nm in thickness. They are composed of filament-binding proteins which connect with the cytoplasmic domain of the cadherins and the filaments of the cytoskeleton. In desmosomes, the plaques connect with keratin intermediate filaments, while in the adherens junctions, they connect with actin filaments.

The composition of the cytoplasmic plaques is different in the two junctions; only *plakoglobin* is common to both. In the adherens junctions, the cytoplasmic plaques contain α and β *catenins*. In desmosomes, the cytoplasmic plaques consist primarily of *desmoplakins 1 and 2*, antibodies to which are found in paraneoplastic pemphigus. The desmoplakins play a pivotal role in anchoring the network of intermediate filaments to desmosomes.[10] Other proteins (such as IFAP-300) may enhance this association.[11] The desmoplakins, along with the bullous pemphigoid (230 kd) antigen and plectin, belong to the so-called 'intermediate filament-associated proteins.'[6] An absence of plectin from the hemidesmosomes has been found in a variant of epidermolysis bullosa simplex with associated muscular dystrophy. Autoantibodies to plectin (450 kd) have been reported in a patient with a bullous pemphigoid-like eruption.[12] Other constituents of the desmosomal cytoplasmic plaque include desmocalmin,[1] pinin, envoplakin and plakophilin 1, 2 and 3.[13] Absence of plakophilin 1 has been associated with skin fragility and hypohidrotic ectodermal dysplasia.[14]

In summary, epidermal cohesion is a complex process involving the adhesion molecule families – cadherins and integrins – concentrated in areas known as desmosomes and adherens junctions. They have extracellular domains (homophilic in the case of cadherins), and intracellular ones which connect with filament-binding proteins (plakoglobin and catenins or desmoplakins) in cytoplasmic plaques. These proteins connect with filaments of the cytoskeleton, such as actin and keratin intermediate filaments.

Classification of vesiculobullous diseases

Early lesions should always be biopsied to ensure that a histopathological diagnosis can be made. Once regeneration of the epidermis commences or secondary changes such as infection or ulceration occur, accurate diagnosis of a vesiculobullous lesion may not always be possible. Furthermore, in some blistering diseases, special techniques such as direct immunofluorescence, split-skin immunofluorescence[15-18] or electron microscopy may assist in making the diagnosis. Identification of the target antigen may be of diagnostic importance in some of the autoimmune blistering diseases (Table 6.1). Interestingly, some of the same structural proteins targeted by autoantibodies in patients with acquired autoimmune bullous disorders are mutated in some patients with inherited bullous diseases.[19]

There are three morphological features that may need to be assessed in the diagnosis of vesiculobullous lesions. They are:

1. the anatomical level of the split
2. the mechanism responsible for the split
3. the inflammatory cell component (in the case of subepidermal blisters).

These various aspects will be considered in greater detail.

Anatomical level of the split

The blister may form at any one of four different anatomical levels. The split may be subcorneal (intracorneal splitting is included in this category), within the spinous or malpighian layers, suprabasilar, or beneath the epidermis (subepidermal). In the case of subepidermal blisters there are several different anatomical levels that may be involved but these are 'submicroscopic' and require the use of electron microscopy or other special techniques (see below) for their elucidation.

The mechanism responsible for the split

There are several mechanisms by which blistering can result – spongiosis, acantholysis and ballooning degeneration of keratinocytes. *Spongiosis* refers to the presence of intercellular edema. In some of the disorders showing the spongiotic reaction pattern (see Ch. 5, pp. 97–128) the edema may be so pronounced that there is breakdown of the intercellular connections, leading to vesicle formation. Clinically visible vesicles occur in a small proportion of cases with the spongiotic reaction pattern. *Acantholysis* refers to the loss of attachments between keratinocytes, resulting in the formation of rounded, detached cells within the blister. Acantholysis may result from damage to the intercellular connections due to the deposition of immune complexes, as in pemphigus, or from abnormalities of the tonofilament–desmosome complexes, which may be an acquired abnormality or have a heredofamilial basis. Acantholysis may also occur secondary to other processes such as ballooning degeneration. *Ballooning degeneration* of keratinocytes refers to the swelling of these cells which follows their infection with certain viruses. The ballooning results in rupture of desmosomal attachments and vesicle formation. Sometimes a few acantholytic cells are present in vesicles as an

Table 6.1 **Autoimmune bullous diseases – target antigens**

Disease	Target antigen (molecular wt – kd)	Site of antigen	Other minor antigens reported and comments
Pemphigus foliaceus	Desmoglein 1 (160)	Desmosomes of upper epidermis	Desmocollin – antibodies to this alone in some endemic cases
Herpetiform pemphigus	Desmoglein 1	Desmosomes of upper epidermis	Desmoglein 3
IgA pemphigus (SPD type)	Desmocollin 1	Desmosomes (transmembrane)	
IgA pemphigus (IEN type)	Desmoglein 1 or 3	Desmosomes	
Pemphigus vulgaris	Desmoglein 3 (130)	Desmosomes of lower epidermis	Desmocollin, 85 kd antigen (in pemphigus vulgaris–Neumann), desmoglein 1
Epidermolysis bullosa acquisita	Type VII collagen (290)	Anchoring fibrils	Similar antigen in bullous SLE
Paraneoplastic pemphigus	Desmoplakin 1 (250) Multiple plakins and desmogleins	Cytoplasmic plaques	Envoplakin, BP230, periplakin, γ-catenin, HD1/plectin, desmoglein 1 and 3, 170 kd
Bullous pemphigoid	BPAg1 (230) BPAg2 (180)	Hemidesmosome Transmembrane protein (NC16A domain)	80% have antibodies to 230, 30% to 180, and 20% only to 180 kd antigen Others reported – 240, 190, 138, 120, 125, 105 kd, plectin
Pemphigoid gestationis	BPAg2 (180)	See above	Others reported – 200 kd, BP230
Dermatitis herpetiformis	?Tissue transglutaminase	Gut, ?site in skin	IgA deposits haphazard in papilla
Linear IgA bullous dermatosis	LAD-1 – ladinin (97) 285 kd (10–15% of cases)	Anchoring filament Sublamina densa	97 kd and 120 kd antigens are degradation products of BP180 NC-1 domain of type VII collagen and others
Ocular cicatricial pemphigoid	Not named (45)	Conjunctiva	IgA antibody
Cicatricial pemphigoid	BPAg2 (180) Epiligrin	Against extracellular (C-terminal) domain α3 subunit of laminin 5	? other epitopes exist on antigen Epiligrin cases uncommon (10% or more)
Deep lamina lucida pemphigoid	105 kd	Lower lamina lucida	Clinically resembles TEN, pemphigus vulgaris
Anti-p200 pemphigoid	200 kd	Lower lamina lucida	Clinically resembles BP, DH or LABD

incidental phenomenon, resulting from the action of enzymes released by neutrophils in the accompanying inflammatory infiltrate. The presence of a few acantholytic cells in these circumstances should not be misinterpreted as indicating that acantholysis is the pathogenetic mechanism responsible for the blister in such a case. *Junctional separation* is sometimes included as a mechanism of blister formation but it is a heterogeneous process involving different mechanisms and different anatomical levels within the basement membrane zone.

Inflammatory cell component

In the case of subepidermal blisters, it is usual to subclassify them further on the basis of the predominant cell in the inflammatory infiltrate in the underlying dermis. In some subepidermal blisters, the proportion of eosinophils and neutrophils may vary from case to case and with the age of the lesion. These caveats must always be kept in mind when a subepidermal blister with neutrophils or eosinophils is biopsied. The presence of neutrophils within intraepidermal blisters may also have relevance to the diagnosis, even though this aspect is not used in the subclassification of intraepidermal blisters.

Other morphological features

Although the key features in the assessment of any vesiculobullous lesion are the anatomical level of the split, the mechanism responsible for the split and the nature of the inflammatory cell infiltrate, as discussed above, the presence of changes in keratinocytes may assist in making a diagnosis in several diseases. Examples include the presence of dyskeratotic cells in Darier's disease, the presence of multinucleate giant cells in certain virus-induced blisters, and confluent epidermal necrosis in toxic epidermal necrolysis and in severe erythema multiforme. Shrunken keratinocytes (Civatte bodies) may be seen in bullous lichen planus, bullous fixed drug eruptions, erythema multiforme and paraneoplastic pemphigus.

INTRACORNEAL AND SUBCORNEAL BLISTERS

In this group of vesiculobullous diseases the split occurs within the stratum corneum or directly beneath it. In addition to the conditions discussed below, subcorneal blisters or pustules have been reported uncommonly as a manifestation of epidermolysis bullosa simplex, acute generalized pustulosis and other pustular vasculitides, and pyoderma gangrenosum (see p. 251).[20] There has been one report of a patient with vegetative plaques resembling pemphigus vegetans and a subcorneal spongiform pustule with marked acanthosis of the epidermis on histological examination.[21] Subcorneal splitting is usually present in the **peeling skin syndrome**. It may be congenital (see p. 304) or acquired. Azathioprine has been implicated in acquired cases.[22]

Other causes of intracorneal or subcorneal blisters are discussed below.

IMPETIGO

Impetigo is an acute superficial pyoderma which occurs predominantly in childhood (see p. 132). *Staphylococcus aureus* is the usual organism isolated from this condition. There are two clinical forms of impetigo – a common vesiculopustular type and a rare bullous type.

Histopathology

In impetigo there are subcorneal collections of neutrophils. A few acantholytic cells are sometimes present, particularly in bullous impetigo, as a result of the action of enzymes released from neutrophils. Acantholysis is never as prominent in impetigo as it is in pemphigus foliaceus. Gram-positive cocci can usually be demonstrated in impetigo, another distinguishing feature of this condition.

Subcorneal pustules, sometimes resembling impetigo, can be seen in some cases of listeriosis.

STAPHYLOCOCCAL 'SCALDED SKIN' SYNDROME

The staphylococcal 'scalded skin' syndrome (SSSS) is discussed in detail with the bacterial infections on page 618. It results from the production of an epidermolytic toxin by certain strains of *Staphylococcus aureus*.[23]

Histopathology

It is usually difficult to obtain an intact blister in the staphylococcal 'scalded skin' syndrome, as the stratum corneum may be cast off during the biopsy procedure or the subsequent processing of the specimen. A few acantholytic cells and neutrophils are usually present in intact blisters or on the surface of the epidermis if its roof has been shed (Fig. 6.1). Organisms are not usually present in the affected skin, in contrast to bullous impetigo. There is usually only a sparse inflammatory cell infiltrate in the upper dermis, in contrast to bullous impetigo and pemphigus foliaceus in which the infiltrate is usually heavier.

DERMATOPHYTOSIS

Subcorneal and intraepidermal blisters are sometimes seen in the dermatophytoses, particularly on the hands and feet. The presence of neutrophils in the stratum corneum or within the epidermis should always prompt consideration of an infectious etiology, including fungi. Candidosis is another uncommon cause of subcorneal blistering.

PEMPHIGUS FOLIACEUS

Pemphigus foliaceus, which accounts for approximately 10% of all cases of pemphigus, is one of the less severe forms of the disease.[24,25] There are recurrent crops of flaccid bullae that readily rupture, resulting in shallow

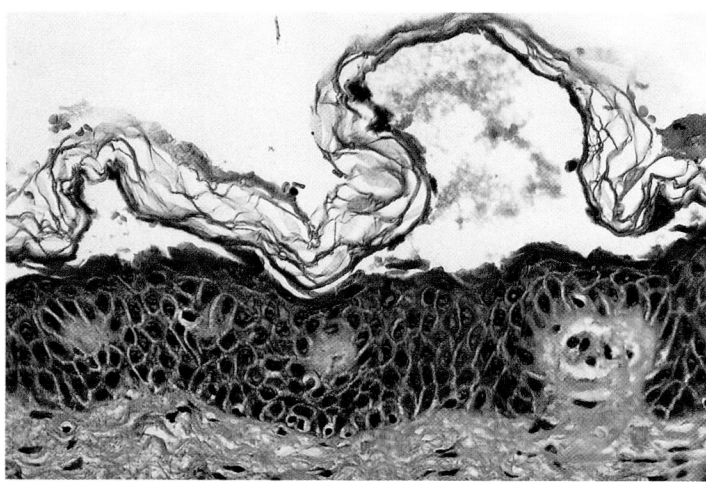

Fig. 6.1 **Staphylococcal 'scalded skin' syndrome.** A thin layer of normal stratum corneum forms the roof of the blister. There is no inflammation. (H & E)

erosions and crusted erythematous plaques.[26,27] A stinging or burning sensation is sometimes present. Lesions may be localized to the face and trunk initially, but the condition usually spreads to involve large areas of the body. However, mucous membrane involvement is rare.[28,29] No age, including childhood,[30–35] is exempt, although the majority of cases present in late middle life. Postpartum onset[36] and neonatal involvement, following passive transfer of antibodies across the placenta, have been reported.[37,38]

Rare clinical presentations have included lesions resembling eruptive seborrheic keratoses[39–41] and in other instances erythematous and vesicular lesions suggestive of dermatitis herpetiformis.[42–47] This latter group, also known as *pemphigus herpetiformis* and *herpetiform pemphigus*, has auto-antibodies directed against desmoglein 1, indicating its close relationship to pemphigus foliaceus (see below).[48,49] Rarely, the clinical and histological features of pemphigus foliaceus may change to those of pemphigus vulgaris; the antibody profile also changes.[50] A case with features of both pemphigus vulgaris and pemphigus foliaceus has been reported.[51]

Pemphigus foliaceus has been reported in association with bullous pemphigoid,[52,53] lupus erythematosus,[54] rheumatoid arthritis, IgA nephropathy,[55] myasthenia gravis,[28,56] thymoma,[57,58] lymphoma,[59] prostate cancer,[60] herpes simplex infection,[61] HIV infection,[62] silicosis,[63] lichen planus,[64] Graves' disease[54] and mycosis fungoides.[65] Pemphigus foliaceus may be induced by sunlight.[66] It has also been associated with the use of penicillamine,[67] bucillamine,[68] gold, pyritinol, rifampin (rifampicin),[69] captopril,[70,71] enalapril,[72] ramipril,[73] fosinopril,[74] cephalosporins, levodopa, aspirin,[75] methimazole (thiamazole) and α-mercaptopropionylglycine (tiopronin).[76–78] Some drugs that contain thiol groups can produce acantholysis, *in vitro*, in human skin explants.[79]

Pemphigus foliaceus is the most common form of pemphigus complicating the use of penicillamine.[67,80,81] Pemphigus develops in nearly 10% of those taking penicillamine for prolonged periods and it may persist for many months after the drug is discontinued.[82] Sometimes the eruption that ensues is not typical of a specific type of pemphigus but shares clinical or immunohistological features of different types of the disease.[83–85]

Pathogenesis

Pemphigus foliaceus results from the formation of autoantibodies, mainly of the IgG_4 subclass, which react with several different antigenic epitopes on the amino-terminal region of desmoglein 1, a 160 kd transmembrane glycoprotein, which is present in desmosomes.[7,86–90] In certain cases, the antibodies appear to react with desmocollins, the other subtype of desmosomal cadherins, or other antigens.[91–94] The expression of desmoglein 1 is highest in specimens from the upper torso, but excluding the scalp.[95,96] It is expressed primarily in the upper layers of the epidermis.[7] Desmoglein 1 is expressed at a much lower level than desmoglein 3 in oral mucosa.[97] This suggests that desmoglein 3 may be sufficient for cell–cell adhesion in oral mucosa, with consequently no oral involvement in patients with pemphigus foliaceus.[97] Neonates are protected from the effect of the passive transfer of maternal autoantibodies across the placenta by possessing desmoglein 3 in the upper levels of the epidermis.[98,99] The antibodies found in patients with drug-induced pemphigus[100,101] and in some patients with pemphigus vulgaris also react with desmoglein 1.[102] The antibodies themselves are pathogenic,[90] but complement, including the terminal complement sequence (membrane attack complex),[103] is also an important mediator in the detachment of the epidermal cells. The use of plasminogen activator knockout mice suggests that there is no requirement for proteases in blister formation.[66,104] Antibody levels fluctuate during the course of the disease and have some correlation with disease activity. The availability of recombinant desmoglein 1 has

facilitated the development of antigen-specific plasmapheresis as a therapeutic strategy.[90]

Endemic pemphigus foliaceus

The variant endemic pemphigus foliaceus is also known by the Portuguese expression *fogo selvagem* ('wild fire') and as Brazilian pemphigus foliaceus.[105–107] It affects mostly children and young adults and is endemic in certain rural areas of South America, particularly parts of Brazil.[108,109] An endemic form of pemphigus has recently been reported in Tunisia.[110] The epidemiology strongly suggests an environmental factor,[111] possibly a virus, and this is supported by the finding of elevated levels of thymosin α 1 in many affected individuals.[112,113] The endemic variant has an abrupt onset and a variable course.[114] Sunlight can exacerbate the condition.[115] Improvement has been recorded in a patient who developed HIV infection.[116] Familial cases occur in 10%, in contrast to their rarity in the more usual form of pemphigus foliaceus.[17,118] In many cases, the circulating intercellular antibodies have similar antigenic specificity to those found in the non-endemic form of the disease[119–121] although, in some, antibodies to the desmocollins, rather than to desmoglein 1, have been present. Furthermore, their localization may be at a different site on the cell surface (see below).[122] The prevalence of anti-bodies against desmoglein 1 is high among normal subjects living in endemic areas, and the onset of the disease is preceded by a sustained antibody response.[123] Circulating antibodies, using indirect immunofluorescence and human skin as substrate, can be demonstrated in 70% of cases.[124] Of interest is the finding that the intraperitoneal injection into mice of IgG from patients with endemic pemphigus foliaceus causes acantholysis in the animals.[125] In addition to the humoral–immune response, cell-mediated mechanisms involving $CD4^+$ lymphocytes are also involved.[126]

Histopathology

Established lesions of pemphigus foliaceus of both the endemic and non-endemic forms show a superficial bulla with the split high in the granular layer or directly beneath the stratum corneum.[127] The bulla contains fibrin, some neutrophils and scattered acantholytic keratinocytes. No bacteria are present, unlike bullous impetigo.[127]

The earliest change appears to be the formation of vacuoles in the intercellular spaces in the upper layers of the epidermis.[128] These expand, leading to cleft formation. Uncommonly, eosinophilic spongiosis is seen as a precursor lesion, and transitions between this picture and that of pemphigus foliaceus may be seen. Eosinophilic spongiosis appears to be more common in pemphigus foliaceus in some African races.[41] Neutrophilic spongiosis is a rare occurrence in pemphigus foliaceus;[129] its occurrence is usually related to the deposition of IgA, or the herpetiform type (herpetiform pemphigus).[46]

In late lesions of pemphigus foliaceus the epidermis may be hyperplastic, with overlying focal parakeratosis and some orthokeratosis.[130] Dyskeratotic cells with hyperchromatic nuclei and somewhat resembling the 'grains' found in Darier's disease are a distinctive feature of the granular layer (Fig. 6.2).

The superficial dermis is edematous with a mixed inflammatory cell infiltrate which usually includes both eosinophils and neutrophils. In drug-induced lesions, eosinophils may predominate in the dermal infiltrate.

With direct immunofluorescence, there is intercellular staining for IgG and C3 in both affected and normal skin.[131,132] Sometimes the staining is localized to the upper levels of the epidermis (Fig. 6.3).[133,134] Rarely, these immuno-reactants may be present along the basement membrane, even in cases that clinically resemble pemphigus foliaceus rather than pemphigus erythematosus (see below).[135] In a few instances, IgA rather than IgG has been present in the intercellular regions.[136,137] The term 'IgA pemphigus' has been used for these

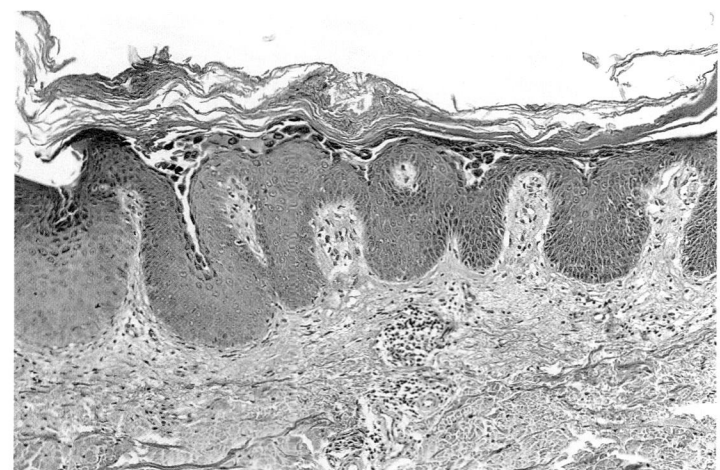

Fig. 6.2 **Pemphigus foliaceus.** Dyskeratotic cells with hyperchromatic nuclei are a distinctive feature in the granular layer in this older lesion.

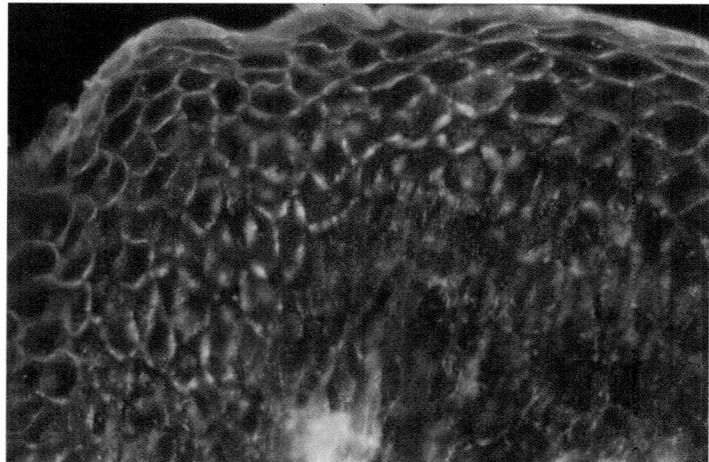

Fig. 6.3 **Pemphigus foliaceus.** The intercellular IgG is deposited throughout much of the epidermis but spares the basal layer. (Direct immunofluorescence)

cases. Indirect immunofluorescence demonstrates circulating antibodies in nearly 90% of cases of non-endemic pemphigus foliaceus.[138]

Electron microscopy
Acantholysis in pemphigus foliaceus appears to result from separation of the non-specific junctions and subsequent rupture of desmosomal junctions.[130] The tonofilament–desmosomal complexes remain intact, although irregular bundles of tonofilaments are found within the acantholytic cells.[139] Internalization of intact desmosomes also occurs.[140] Immunoelectron microscopy shows immunoglobulins deposited over the plasma membrane of the keratinocytes and permeating the desmosomal junctions in the endemic form,[122,139] while in the usual form there is affinity for desmosomes and separated attachment plaques in the upper layers of the epidermis.[141–143]

PEMPHIGUS ERYTHEMATOSUS

Pemphigus erythematosus (Senear–Usher syndrome), which accounts for approximately 10% of all cases of pemphigus,[25,144] is a variant of pemphigus foliaceus which combines some of the immunological features of both pemphigus and lupus erythematosus.[26] It usually develops insidiously with erythematous, scaly and crusted plaques in a butterfly distribution over the nose and malar areas.[145] It may also involve other 'seborrheic areas' such as the scalp, pectoral and interscapular regions, as well as intertriginous areas. Usually, there is no visceral involvement. Pemphigus erythematosus may persist almost indefinitely as a localized disease.[44] Sunlight sometimes adversely affects its course.[24] This condition is extremely rare in children.[146]

Pemphigus erythematosus is occasionally found in association with other autoimmune diseases, especially myasthenia gravis with an accompanying thymoma.[147] Rare cases of concurrent pemphigus erythematosus and systemic lupus erythematosus have been documented.[148] There are reports of its association with parathyroid adenoma,[149] internal cancers,[150] burns[151] and X-radiation. Drugs which may induce pemphigus erythematosus[145] include ceftazidime,[152] penicillamine,[153–155] propranolol,[145] captopril,[156] pyritinol,[145] thiopronine[157] and heroin.[158]

Antinuclear antibodies and circulating antibodies to the intercellular regions are often present. Antibodies to DNA are usually absent.[155]

Histopathology
The appearances are identical to those of pemphigus foliaceus, with a subcorneal blister containing occasional acantholytic cells (see above).[159] Eroded and crusted lesions may develop.

Direct immunofluorescence usually demonstrates IgG and/or complement, both in the intercellular spaces and at the dermoepidermal junction.[160,161] The intercellular staining may be more pronounced in the upper layers of the epidermis. The lupus band test is sometimes positive in uninvolved skin.[155]

HERPETIFORM PEMPHIGUS

Brief mention has already been made of the occurrence of cases with the clinical features of dermatitis herpetiformis and the immunopathology of pemphigus, usually the foliaceus type (see above).[42–49] Such cases account for approximately 7% of all cases of pemphigus.[162] Clinically, there are erythematous, urticarial plaques and vesicles in herpetiform arrangement. Severe pruritus is often present.[162] Mucous membranes are uncommonly involved. It has been reported in association with psoriasis[163] and with endemic pemphigus foliaceus.[164] Cases may evolve into pemphigus foliaceus.

Most cases have circulating autoantibodies to desmoglein 1, the pemphigus foliaceus antigen. A few cases with antibodies to the pemphigus vulgaris antigen, desmoglein 3, have been reported.[165,166]

Histopathology
The characteristic features of herpetiform pemphigus are eosinophilic spongiosis with the formation of intraepidermal vesicles. Variable numbers of neutrophils may be present, leading to the formation of neutrophilic spongiosis or subcorneal pustules with both eosinophils and neutrophils. Acantholysis is minimal or absent.

Direct immunofluorescence shows the deposition of IgG, with or without C3, on the cell surfaces of keratinocytes, as seen in pemphigus. There is usually superficial accentuation,[163] but in cases with antibodies to desmoglein 3, the deposition may be more prominent on the lower layers of the epidermis.[166]

SUBCORNEAL PUSTULAR DERMATOSIS

Subcorneal pustular dermatosis is a chronic, relapsing, vesiculopustular dermatosis with a predilection for the trunk, particularly intertriginous areas, and the flexor aspect of the limbs.[167–170] It usually spares the face and mucous membranes, and there are usually no constitutional symptoms.[171,172] The condition is more common in women, particularly occurring in the fourth and fifth decades of life. Cases purporting to be subcorneal pustular dermatosis in children[173] have been disputed.[174]

The pustules are flaccid. They are initially sterile but secondary infection sometimes develops. A transient erythematous flare surrounds the pustules in the early stages.[168]

The etiology and pathogenesis remain unknown. A small number of patients have had an associated monoclonal gammopathy, most commonly of IgA type.[171,175–178] Some of these cases have been associated with intercellular deposits of IgA and would now be reclassified as IgA pemphigus (see below). Whether subcorneal pustular dermatosis survives as an entity must await further reports. Pyoderma gangrenosum has been described in patients with subcorneal pustular dermatosis, usually in association with an IgA monoclonal gammopathy.[179,180] In two cases, the lesions of subcorneal pustular dermatosis developed several hours after the performance of echography.[181] Other rare associations include aplastic anemia,[182] multiple sclerosis[183] and systemic lupus erythematosus. Subcorneal pustular dermatosis is regarded by some authorities as a variant of pustular psoriasis.[184,185] This confusion has arisen, in part, because cases not conforming to the original 1956 description of Sneddon and Wilkinson have been reported misleadingly as cases of subcorneal pustular dermatosis. Some of these cases have been examples of the annular variant of pustular psoriasis.[169,186] It should be noted that seven of the 23 purported cases of subcorneal pustular dermatosis seen at the Mayo Clinic subsequently developed generalized pustular psoriasis.[187]

Pustular eruptions with some histological or clinical resemblance to subcorneal pustular dermatosis have been reported following the ingestion of isoniazid,[188] diltiazem,[189] paclitaxel,[190] the cephalosporins[191] and amoxicillin.[192] New lesions have been precipitated in a patient with subcorneal pustular dermatosis following the ingestion of dapsone and of quinidine sulfate.[193] Sterile, subcorneal pustules sometimes form in pustular vasculitis.

Tumor necrosis factor-α is increased in subcorneal pustular dermatosis; it may be responsible, in part, for the activation of neutrophils that is a feature of this condition.[194]

Histopathology

The subcorneal pustule is filled with neutrophils, with an occasional eosinophil. Neutrophils also migrate through the epidermis, but they do not form spongiform pustules.[169] The pustule appears to 'sit' on the epidermis (Fig. 6.4)

and usually it causes no depression of the latter. An occasional acantholytic cell may be present in older lesions, a result of the activity of the proteolytic enzymes released from neutrophils.[169] Mitotic figures are usually absent within the epidermis, unlike pustular psoriasis.[195]

A mixed superficial perivascular inflammatory cell infiltrate is present in the underlying dermis. In early lesions the infiltrate includes quite a few neutrophils.

Direct immunofluorescence is usually negative, although immunoreactants have been described in the epidermis in rare cases.[175] Several cases have been reported of a condition resembling subcorneal pustular dermatosis clinically but in which a biopsy of the lesions showed intercellular IgA. Such cases have recently been classified as IgA pemphigus, although a case could be made for the retention of some of them as variants of subcorneal pustular dermatosis.[196] This subject is discussed further in the section on IgA pemphigus (see below).

IgA PEMPHIGUS

IgA pemphigus is characterized by the presence of a vesiculobullous eruption, with variable acantholysis and the presence of intercellular deposits of IgA within the epidermis.[136,137,162,197–201] Circulating IgA antibodies are present in approximately half of the cases, while an IgA monoclonal gammopathy is present in nearly 20% of cases.[199,202] Other terms used for this entity include intraepidermal IgA pustulosis,[202] intraepidermal neutrophilic IgA dermatosis (IEN type),[198,203,204] IgA herpetiform pemphigus, intercellular IgA vesiculo-pustular dermatosis,[205] subcorneal pustular dermatosis with IgA deposition[206] and intercellular IgA dermatosis.[207]

IgA pemphigus is a clinically heterogeneous condition reflecting differences in the autoantigens involved.[208] Two distinct groups are now recognized: the first with a subcorneal pustule, resembling subcorneal pustular dermatosis (SPD type), and IgA deposition confined to the upper epidermis;[206,209] and a second group, which sometimes presents with clinical herpetiform lesions[210,211] and intraepidermal pustules, associated with a more widespread distribution of IgA throughout the epidermis (IEN type).[198] The presence of cases with overlap features supports the notion that this is one disease with variable expression.[199,210] In a review of the 49 cases published up to the year 2000, 25 were of the SPD type, 19 were of the IEN type and the other 5 cases were unclassified.[212] In 6 of the SPD type, a monoclonal IgA gammopathy was present. Some of these cases have been previously diagnosed as subcorneal pustular dermatosis (see above). In studies of the subcorneal group, the antibodies have recognized bovine desmocollins

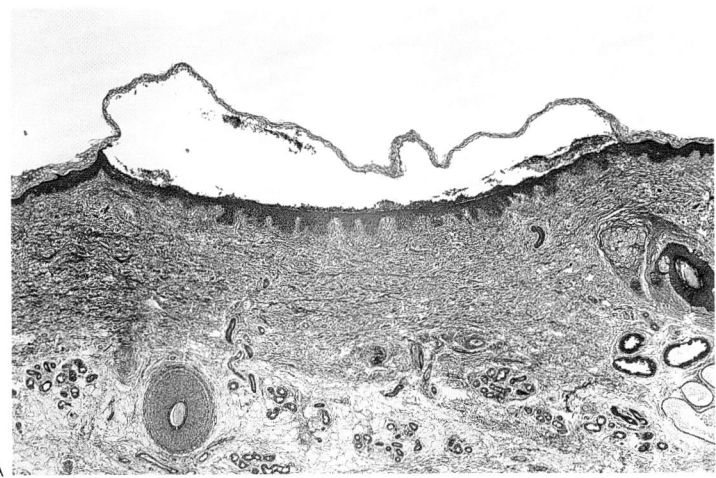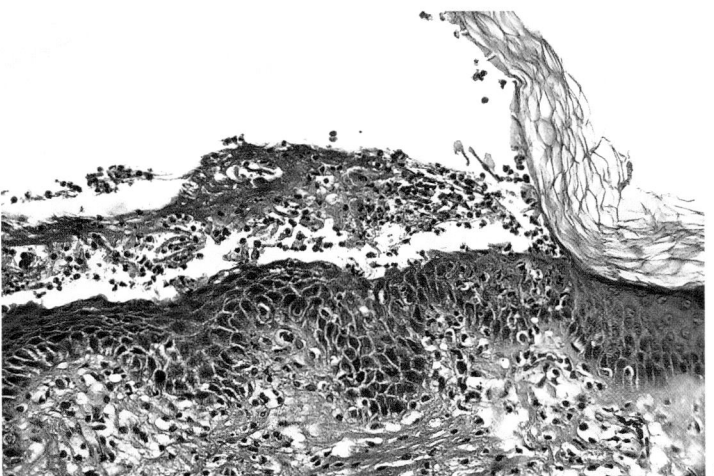

Fig. 6.4 **(A) Subcorneal pustular dermatosis. (B)** The subcorneal pustule contains fibrin and a modest number of neutrophils. (H & E)

and/or human desmocollin 1, or neither,[201,205,212–214] while in the intra-epidermal group the antibodies have been variously characterized as reacting to desmoglein 1 or desmoglein 3.[199,205,208,215]

Cases have been reported in children[207,216] and in adult males with HIV infection.[204,217]

Histopathology

In the SPD type there are subcorneal pustules with variable, but usually mild acantholysis, while in the IEN type there are intraepidermal pustules. There is usually a mixed inflammatory cell infiltrate in the underlying dermis. A case of IgA pemphigus (foliaceus) has been reported which resembled the more usual cases of pemphigus foliaceus without any neutrophilic infiltration.[137] Neutrophilic spongiosis, suggestive of IgA pemphigus, has been reported in a case of pemphigus foliaceus devoid of IgA. A rare variant of the IEN type, which occurred in a child on immunosuppressive drugs, had features of pemphigus vegetans with epidermal hyperplasia and intraepidermal pustules.[218]

Electron microscopy

On immunoelectron microscopy the deposits have been found along the keratinocyte cell membrane and not confined to the region of the desmosomes.[219]

INFANTILE ACROPUSTULOSIS

Infantile acropustulosis is an uncommon pustular dermatosis characterized by recurrent crops of intensely pruritic vesiculopustules on the distal parts of the extremities of infants.[220–228] The lesions measure 1–2 mm in diameter. Its onset is at birth or in the first few months of life, and resolution occurs at 2–3 years of age. There is a predilection for black males. The etiology is unknown, although some cases are said to have followed scabies.[225,229–231] Peripheral eosinophilia and atopy[223] have been present in several patients.

Infantile acropustulosis, erythema neonatorum toxicum and transient neonatal pustular melanosis can be grouped together as the 'pustular dermatoses of infancy' (see below) because of their overlapping clinical and histological features. Three other neonatal pustular eruptions will be mentioned for completeness. **Transient cephalic neonatal pustulosis** is thought to be related to infection with *Malassezia* sp. (see p. 666),[232] while **congenital erosive and vesicular dermatosis**, which heals with a characteristic reticulated supple scarring, is of unknown etiology.[233] In the only case of this latter condition in which histology was performed on an early lesion, there were erosions (precluding epidermal assessment) and a neutrophilic dermatosis.[233] An unusual vesiculopustular eruption has been reported in infants with **Down syndrome and myeloproliferative disorders**.[234,235] There were immature myeloid cells in subcorneal spongiotic vesicles.

The condition originally reported in infants as 'eosinophilic pustular folliculitis' has a predilection for the scalp.[236] It has been renamed 'eosinophilic pustulosis of the scalp' on the basis of an interfollicular, rather than a follicular infiltrate. It has been claimed that 'this disorder has more clinicopathological similarities with acropustulosis of infancy than with Ofuji's disease' – see page 460.[236,237]

Histopathology[224]

In early lesions there is an intraepidermal pustule containing neutrophils and sometimes varying numbers of eosinophils.[225] This progresses to form a subcorneal pustule. There is a sparse perivascular mixed inflammatory cell infiltrate in the upper dermis.

ERYTHEMA TOXICUM NEONATORUM

Erythema toxicum neonatorum is a common entity which appears within the first few days of life as erythematous macules, papules and pustules, mostly located on the trunk.[238–242] There is no racial predilection. The lesions resolve within a few days leaving no sequelae. The etiology remains elusive.[243]

Histopathology[238, 244]

There are subcorneal or intraepidermal pustules, filled with eosinophils and related to the orifices of the pilosebaceous follicles.[238] An inflammatory infiltrate composed predominantly of eosinophils is present in the upper dermis in the vicinity of the follicles, and there is some exocytosis of these cells into the epithelium of the involved follicles.[238]

The histological appearances resemble those of eosinophilic pustular folliculitis but the clinical features of the two conditions differ.[245]

TRANSIENT NEONATAL PUSTULAR MELANOSIS

Transient neonatal pustular melanosis is an uncommon condition that presents at birth with pigmented macules, often with a distinct collarette of scale, and vesiculopustules which are clustered beneath the chin, on the forehead, the neck and the back, and sometimes on the extremities.[246–248] The vesiculopustules usually resolve after several days, often transforming into pigmented macules. The pigmented lesions persist for several weeks or more and then slowly fade.[246] The etiology of the condition is unknown, but there appears to be a predilection for black races.[246] Furthermore, there is an increased incidence of squamous metaplasia in the placentas of affected neonates.[228]

Histopathology[246]

The vesiculopustules are intracorneal or subcorneal collections of neutrophils, admixed with fibrin and a few eosinophils. There may be a mild infiltrate of inflammatory cells around vessels in the upper dermis.

The pigmented macules show increased melanin in the basal and suprabasal keratinocytes but, surprisingly, there is no melanin in the dermis.

ACUTE GENERALIZED EXANTHEMATOUS PUSTULOSIS

Acute generalized exanthematous pustulosis, also known as toxic pustuloderma, is an uncommon, rapidly evolving pustular eruption characterized by the development of sterile, miliary pustules on an erythematous background. The lesions may have a targetoid appearance.[41] Fever and a peripheral blood leukocytosis are usually present. The eruption occurs within hours or days of the ingestion of certain drugs and resolves rapidly after cessation of the offending agent.[249] In a small number of cases a viral infection, including enterovirus or cytomegalovirus, has been implicated.[250,251] The lesions are non-follicular, in contrast to the follicular pustules that may occur in the anticonvulsant hypersensitivity syndrome.[252] Some patients have a history of underlying psoriasis, ulcerative colitis or thyroiditis. The lesions of acute generalized exanthematous pustulosis can usually be distinguished from pustular psoriasis.[253,254]

Numerous drugs have been implicated in the etiology, particularly antibiotics of the β lactam, cephalosporin and macrolide type.[255] Specific drugs implicated include carbamazepine, furosemide (frusemide), acetaminophen (paracetamol), allopurinol,[41,256] itraconazole,[257,258] quinidine,[255] diltiazem,[259–262] pholcodine,[263] trimethoprim–sulfamethoxazole,[264,265] cephalexin,[265] chloramphenicol,[266] gentamicin,[267] teicoplanin,[268] roxithromycin,[269] vancomycin, doxycycline, nystatin,[270] erythromycin, penicillin, ciprofloxacin, amoxicillin,[271,272] terbinafine,[273–276] ceftriaxone,[277] icodextrin,[278] mercury, thalidomide,[279] intracavernous prostaglandin E_1,[280] ticlopidine,[281] phenytoin, metronidazole,[282] nifedipine, olanzapine,[283] clemastine,[284] paracetamol with bromhexine,[285] chromium picolinate,[286] chemotherapy drugs,[287] enalapril,[288] imipenem,[265] cimetidine,[289] antimalarials such as chloroquine, proguanil and hydroxychloroquine,[290,291] and traditional remedies including the ingestion of lacquer chicken.[289,292] A full list of implicated drugs was published in a recent review.[249] Cutaneous patch testing, using the suspected drug, may be used to confirm the diagnosis.

It has been suggested that patients who develop this eruption have an underlying tendency to develop a pattern of immune dysregulation characterized by a T-helper 1 (Th1) cytokine pattern.[254]

Histopathology

The usual picture is a subcorneal or superficial intraepidermal pustule with mild spongiform pustulation at the margins (Fig. 6.5). This latter change is never as prominent as the spongiform pustules seen in pustular psoriasis. There is usually some exocytosis of neutrophils adjacent to the pustules. Scattered apoptotic keratinocytes are often present.[269]

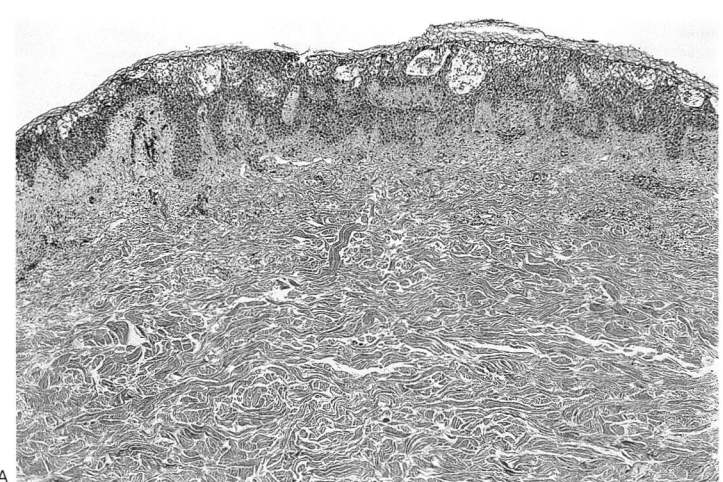

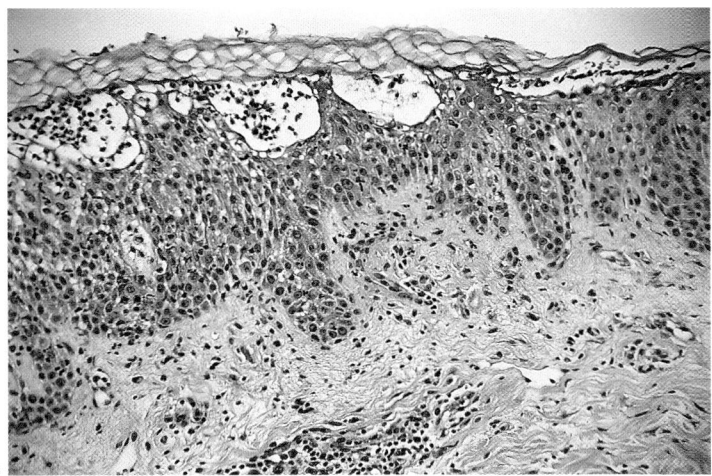

Fig. 6.5 **(A) Acute generalized exanthematous pustulosis. (B)** There is superficial epidermal pustulation and neutrophilic spongiosis. (H & E)

The papillary dermis is usually edematous and there is a heavy mixed inflammatory cell infiltrate in the upper dermis. Eosinophils are often present, a distinguishing feature from pustular psoriasis. In a small number of cases a leukocytoclastic vasculitis is present. Less commonly, this is associated with subepidermal pustulation which may be in continuity with the intraepidermal pustules.[289] Similar cases have been reported in the past as acute generalized pustulosis or included with the pustular vasculitides.

MILIARIA CRYSTALLINA

The condition known as miliaria crystallina is associated with small 1–2 mm vesicles which rupture easily (see p. 101).

Histopathology

The vesicle forms within or directly beneath the stratum corneum. It is centered on the acrosyringium.

INTRAEPIDERMAL BLISTERS

The term 'intraepidermal blister' refers to the formation of lesions within the malpighian layers; it does not include those vesiculobullous diseases in which the split occurs beneath the stratum corneum or in a suprabasilar position. It should be noted, however, that biopsies from some of the diseases listed as forming subcorneal or suprabasilar blisters may sometimes show splitting within the malpighian layers. This is particularly likely in lesions of some days' duration in which regeneration of the epidermis may alter the level of the split.

Intraepidermal blisters usually form as the outcome of spongiosis or ballooning degeneration. The primary acantholytic diseases usually form blisters that are subcorneal or suprabasilar in position, before regeneration occurs. Most of the intraepidermal blistering diseases have been discussed elsewhere but, with the exception of hydroa vacciniforme (see p. 601), they are mentioned below.

SPONGIOTIC BLISTERING DISEASES

Although most of the diseases that produce the spongiotic reaction pattern (see Ch. 5, pp. 97–128) can sometimes be associated with clinically visible vesicles and even bullae, the ones most often associated with blisters are allergic contact dermatitis, nummular dermatitis, pompholyx, polymorphous light eruption (vesicular type), insect bite reactions, incontinentia pigmenti (first stage) and miliaria rubra. The presence of spongiosis adjacent to the vesicle or elsewhere in the biopsy is the clue to this group of blistering diseases. Eosinophils are prominent in the infiltrate in insect bite reactions and incontinentia pigmenti.

The bullae that sometimes form in acrodermatitis enteropathica (see p. 551) are intraepidermal in location. Intraepidermal or subcorneal clefting can also occur in the glucagonoma syndrome (see p. 552).

Palmoplantar pustulosis commences as a spongiotic vesicle but pustulation rapidly ensues (see below).

PALMOPLANTAR PUSTULOSIS

In palmoplantar pustulosis there are erythematous scaly plaques with recurrent sterile pustules symmetrically distributed on the palms and soles.[293–295] Initially, only a palm or a sole may be involved.[296] Onset of the disease is usually between the ages of 40 and 60 years. Women are predominantly affected.[296] Palmoplantar pustulosis is sometimes associated with a focus of infection somewhere in the body,[297] although elimination of the infectious process has no influence on the course of the disease,[293,298] which is usually protracted and somewhat unpredictable. Low-dose cyclosporin appears to be effective in the treatment of this condition.[299]

Psoriasis is present in at least 6% of cases; some studies have shown a much greater incidence.[300] However, unlike psoriasis, there are no clear associations with any particular HLA type.[301] There is also a difference in the surface receptors on neutrophils in the two conditions.[302] Both psoriasis and palmoplantar pustulosis may be precipitated by lithium.[303] Furthermore, a seronegative spondyloarthropathy is sometimes present.[304] There is also an increased incidence of osteoarthritis.[305] An association with Sweet's syndrome has been reported.[295]

Other clinical findings in palmoplantar pustulosis include the presence of sternocostoclavicular ossification in 10% of cases,[304] lytic, but sterile, bone lesions[306] and an increased incidence of autoantibodies to thyroid antigens.[307,308]

Palmoplantar pustulosis has been regarded as a form of psoriasis, a bacterid (an inflammatory reaction at a site remote from that of a bacterial infection presumed to be of pathogenetic significance) and a distinct clinicopathological entity, probably with an immunological pathogenesis.[309,310] The last of these theories is supported by the finding of increased numbers of Langerhans cells in active lesions.[307] There is some evidence that the very rare acute form of palmoplantar pustulosis, which may progress into the chronic form, is a bacterid with an associated vasculitis.[311] It has also been linked to smoking[308,312] and metal allergy.[313] It has been suggested that the acrosyringium is the target for the inflammation.[308]

Histopathology[310]

The earliest lesion is a spongiotic vesicle in the lower malpighian layer which contains mononuclear cells and some neutrophils.[293] This progresses to a unilocular well-delimited pustule within the epidermis and extending upwards to the undersurface of the stratum corneum (Fig. 6.6).[293] There may be overlying, focal parakeratosis. In the dermis, a mixed perivascular and diffuse infiltrate of inflammatory cells is present.

Controversy exists as to whether it is possible to differentiate pustular psoriasis and palmoplantar pustulosis on histopathological grounds.[314]

Spongiform pustulation is often present at the upper margins of the pustule in palmoplantar pustulosis but the focus is usually much smaller than that seen in pustular psoriasis.[314] Sometimes there is spongiosis without associated pustulation; this feature is not present in pustular psoriasis.[314] Eosinophils may be present in palmoplantar pustulosis, a finding not usually seen in pustular psoriasis.[308]

Immunoreactants are present in the stratum corneum in some cases of palmoplantar pustulosis.[315]

AMICROBIAL PUSTULOSIS ASSOCIATED WITH AUTOIMMUNE DISEASES

The rare disease amicrobial pustulosis associated with autoimmune diseases, known by the acronym APAD, is a chronic relapsing eruption involving predominantly the main cutaneous flexures, external auditory canal and scalp. It has been reported in association with various autoimmune diseases.[316,317] Some improvement has occurred after oral zinc supplementation.[316]

Histopathology

There are high intraepidermal spongiform pustules in an acanthotic epidermis. There is usually overlying parakeratosis containing neutrophil debris. A mixed perivascular infiltrate of neutrophils and lymphocytes is present in the upper dermis.

VIRAL BLISTERING DISEASES

Intraepidermal vesicles are seen in herpes simplex, herpes zoster, varicella, hand, foot and mouth disease, and some cases of milker's nodule and orf. In the case of herpes simplex, herpes zoster and varicella there is ballooning degeneration of keratinocytes with secondary acantholysis of cells. Multinucleate keratinocytes, some with intranuclear inclusion bodies, may also be seen. In hand, foot and mouth disease there is both spongiosis and intracellular edema, while in milker's nodule and orf there may be pronounced intracellular edema with pallor and degeneration of keratinocytes in the upper layers of the epidermis. These conditions are discussed in Chapter 26, pages 696–700.

EPIDERMOLYSIS BULLOSA (WEBER–COCKAYNE TYPE)

In the Weber–Cockayne type of epidermolysis bullosa simplex (see p. 144), the split is usually in the mid or upper layers of the epidermis, although in induced blisters the split develops in the basal layer. An occasional dyskeratotic cell may be present in the epidermis.

FRICTION BLISTER

Friction blisters are produced at sites where the epidermis is thick and firmly attached to the underlying dermis, as on the palms, soles, heels and the back of the fingers.

Histopathology

The blister usually forms just beneath the stratum granulosum. The keratinocytes in the base of the blister show variable edema and pallor and even degenerative changes.

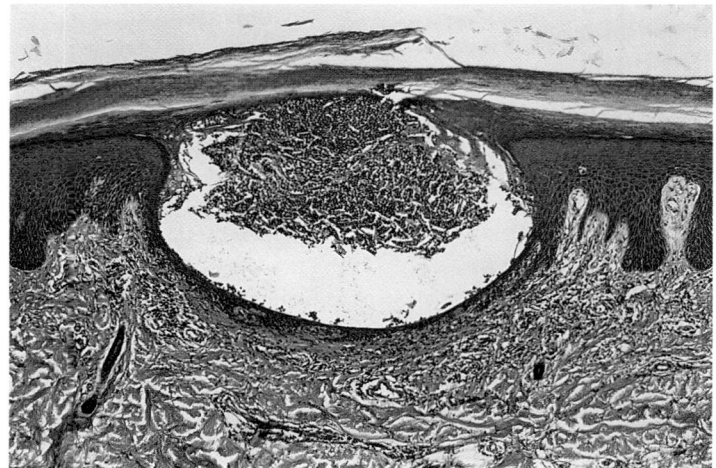

Fig. 6.6 **Palmoplantar pustulosis.** There is a well-delimited, unilocular pustule extending to the undersurface of the stratum corneum. (H & E)

SUPRABASILAR BLISTERS

The suprabasilar blistering diseases – pemphigus vulgaris, pemphigus vegetans, Hailey–Hailey disease (familial benign chronic pemphigus), Darier's disease, Grover's disease (transient acantholytic dermatosis) and acantholytic solar keratosis – all result from acantholysis. Suprabasal acantholysis has been reported in one case of necrolytic migratory erythema. It may sometimes be seen in paraneoplastic pemphigus. In blisters of some days' duration, the split may be present at a higher level within the epidermis as a result of epidermal growth.

PEMPHIGUS VULGARIS

Pemphigus vulgaris is a rare vesiculobullous condition which accounts for approximately 80% of all cases of pemphigus.[318-321] The initial presentation is often with oral blisters,[322,323] ulcers and erosions, which are followed within weeks to months by the development of cutaneous lesions.[26] Nail involvement is relatively rare.[324] Skin lesions take the form of flaccid blisters on a normal or erythematous base; there is a predilection for the trunk, groins, axillae, scalp, face and pressure points.[26] Penile involvement is rare.[325] The blisters break easily, giving eroded and crusted areas. Application of pressure to a blister leads to its extension (Nikolsky's sign).[318] Burning and itching may be present.[322] The lesions generally heal without scarring.[26]

In addition to oral lesions, which eventually develop in 80–90% of cases,[326,327] other mucosal surfaces may be involved. These include the conjunctiva[328] and larynx[144,329] and, rarely, the esophagus,[330,331] urethra, anorectum, vulva, vagina and cervix.[332-334]

Rare clinical presentations include localized lesions, bilateral foot ulcers,[335] lesions limited to the surgical area after mastectomy,[336] the development of lesions in childhood,[337-339] in siblings[340] or in a familial setting,[341] the development of transient blisters in a neonate whose mother has pemphigus,[342-348] the development of nodular,[349] vegetative[350] or acanthosis nigricans-like lesions,[351] and the coexistence of pemphigus vulgaris with bullous pemphigoid.[352,353] Rarely, the clinical and histological features of pemphigus vulgaris may change to those of pemphigus foliaceus;[354,355] the antibody profile also changes.[356,357] Cases with overlap features also occur.[51] Internal cancer,[358,359] Castleman's disease,[360,361] thymoma,[57,358,362] myasthenia gravis,[363] localized scleroderma,[364] Graves' disease,[365] silicosis,[366] systemic lupus erythematosus,[367] oral submucosal fibrosis[368] and oral herpes simplex or HIV infection[369,370] are rare clinical associations. There is an increased susceptibility to the development of autoimmune diseases in the family members of patients with pemphigus vulgaris.[371,372] Several HLA types are prevalent in patients with pemphigus vulgaris.[373,374]

The prognosis has improved considerably in recent years, although the mortality is still 5–15%; deaths result from infections complicating corticosteroid therapy[375,376] and biochemical abnormalities associated with extensive disease.[377] In one recent study, complete and long-lasting remissions were induced in 25%, 50%, and 75% of patients 2, 5, and 10 years, respectively, after diagnosis.[378] The use of cyclosporin as an adjuvant to corticosteroids offers no therapeutic advantages and increases complications.[379] Plasmapheresis, which reduces the levels of circulating pemphigus antibodies more rapidly than conventional therapy, has been used in the treatment of pemphigus vulgaris.[380-382] The titer of circulating antibodies to the pemphigus vulgaris antigen (desmoglein 3) tends to parallel disease activity; they can be measured by ELISA methods.[383-387]

Etiology and pathogenesis
The antibodies in pemphigus vulgaris are directed against the so-called 'pemphigus vulgaris antigen', also termed desmoglein 3, a 130 kd polypeptide which, like the pemphigus foliaceus antigen, is a member of the desmoglein subfamily of the cadherin supergene family.[388,389] The antigen is localized to the desmosomes of keratinocytes, particularly the extracellular domain.[142,390,391] Epitope mapping suggests that a segment containing amino-terminal residues 1–161 of desmoglein 3 contains the critical antigens recognized by the autoantibodies in pemphigus vulgaris sera.[392] This segment is considered to include structures essential for cell–cell adhesion.[392] The cytoplasmic 'tail' of the pemphigus vulgaris antigen, like other desmogleins, binds to the plakoglobin inside keratinocytes.[388,393,394] More than 50% of sera from patients with pemphigus vulgaris also contain autoantibodies against desmoglein 1. These antibodies also appear to be pathogenic.[395] The antibodies against both desmoglein 1 and desmoglein 3 have predominant IgG₄ subclass specificity.[395,396] Antibodies in the IgA and IgE class have also been detected.[397] Patients with mucosa-dominant disease have antibodies only against desmoglein 3.[398] The development of antibodies to desmoglein 1 in these patients is sometimes accompanied by changes in the clinical expression of the disease, such as the development of generalized cutaneous lesions.[399-403] In pemphigus vulgaris, the antibodies produced by circulating B cells tend to bind preferentially to desmosomes in the lower epidermis, reflecting differences in the relative expression of the different cadherins in different levels of the epidermis.[142,404] This antibody binding may be followed by internalization of some desmosomes.[405] Antibodies will only cause cell separation (acantholysis) where the antigen is the principal adhesion molecule and others are unable to compensate.[406] Cholinergic receptors on keratinocytes also play a role in cell adhesion. Autoantibodies to these receptors can induce clinical features resembling pemphigus in desmoglein 3-deficient knockout mice.[407,408] There is also upregulation of P-cadherin expression in lesional skin.[409] Another protein involved in cellular adhesion is focal adhesion kinase (p125ᶠᵃᵏ). Its upregulation in lesional skin may be a reactive or reparative response to acantholysis.[410] The desmosomal damage and consequent acantholysis may follow the activation of complement[86,103,411,412] or local stimulation of the plasminogen–plasmin system, independent of complement.[413-415] However, studies using plasminogen activator knockout mice suggest that this system is not necessary for blister formation.[104] Experimental evidence suggests that antibodies may eventually generate desmosomes lacking desmoglein 3, resulting in acantholysis.[416] Other mechanisms involved in acantholysis include the release of keratinocyte-derived cytokines such as interleukin-1 (IL-1) and tumor necrosis factor-α.[417] Activated mononuclear cells are present in lesional skin and may contribute to the pathogenesis.[418] Autoreactive T lymphocytes that respond to epitopes located on desmoglein 3 have been identified, confirming a role for cell-mediated as well as humoral responses in pemphigus vulgaris.[419-421] T cells that react against desmoglein 1 are sometimes present.[422] Various inflammatory mediators have been isolated from blister fluid and these presumably have a role in eliciting the accompanying inflammatory response.[423] What stimulates the formation of antibodies is unknown, although minor trauma,[25,424,425] surgery,[426] ionizing radiation,[427] thermal burns,[428] PUVA therapy,[429] viral infection[430] and exposure to chemicals[431] have occasionally been documented prior to the onset of the disease. Antidesmoglein autoantibodies are sometimes found in patients with no bullous disease. For example, they have been found in some patients with silicosis,[432] and in relatives of patients with pemphigus vulgaris.[433] The term 'contact pemphigus' has been used for cases which have followed contact with chemicals, usually pesticides.[434-436] There are also cases in which rifampin (rifampicin),[437] norfloxacin,[438] ampicillin,[439] interleukin-2,[440] penicillin,[441] captopril,[442,443] enalapril,[444] quinapril,[74] cilazapril,[445] typhoid and influenza vaccination,[446,447] diclofenac,[448] penicillamine,[449] dipyrone,[450] nifedipine,[451] and possibly other

drugs[78,452] have precipitated pemphigus vulgaris. Drugs with thiol groups have a particular capacity to precipitate or exacerbate pemphigus.[453] Incidental acantholysis has been found in two biopsies from a patient on enalapril who had no clinical features of pemphigus vulgaris.[454]

The role of various foods in the precipitation of pemphigus has been studied.[455,456] Possible candidates include thiol-containing foods (garlic, onion, leek, shallots), thiocyanates (mustards), phenols (artificial sweeteners, preservatives, colorings) and tannins (certain fruits).[456,457]

The finding of HHV-8 DNA sequences in lesional skin may indicate trophism for pemphigus lesions rather than an etiologic role.[458]

Histopathology

Established lesions of pemphigus vulgaris are suprabasal bullae with acantholysis (Fig. 6.7). The clefting may extend down adnexal structures. The basal cells lose their intercellular bridges but they remain attached to the dermis, giving a 'tombstone appearance'.[459] The blister cavity usually contains a few acantholytic cells which often show degenerative changes. Occasionally, a few eosinophils or neutrophils are present in the cavity.[26]

The earliest changes in pemphigus vulgaris consist of edema and disappearance of the intercellular bridges of keratinocytes in the lower epidermis (Fig. 6.8). This leads to acantholysis and subsequent suprabasal blisters. Eosinophilic spongiosis and subepidermal splitting are two rare presentations of pemphigus vulgaris.[460] Vegetative lesions show epidermal hyperplasia but a paucity of eosinophils, in contrast to pemphigus vegetans. Acanthomas resembling seborrheic keratosis may form at the sites of previous blisters.[461]

Dermal changes are of little significance. There is usually a mild, superficial, mixed inflammatory cell infiltrate which usually includes scattered eosinophils. There are no histological features that differentiate drug-associated pemphigus vulgaris from idiopathic cases.[462] Direct immunofluorescence usually demonstrates IgG in the intercellular regions of the epidermis in and around the affected parts of the skin or mucous membrane (Fig. 6.9);[463,464] IgG_1 and IgG_4 are the subclasses of IgG found most commonly in patients with active lesions;[465] C3, IgM and IgA are present less frequently.[463,466] Patients in clinical remission, who have positive direct immunofluorescence on a skin biopsy, are more likely to relapse than those with negative immunofluorescence findings.[467,468] Circulating intercellular antibodies are present in 80–90% of patients with pemphigus vulgaris, although they may be absent in early cases.[138,469,470] Their demonstration depends to some extent on the substrate used; monkey esophagus gives a higher yield of positive results than guinea-pig esophagus or human skin.[471] Pemphigus-like antibodies have also been reported in a wide range of inflammatory dermatoses, as well as following burns.[469,472]

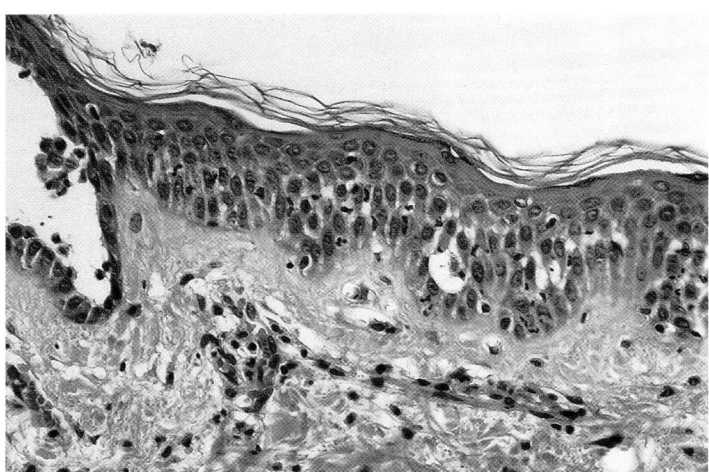

Fig. 6.8 **Pemphigus vulgaris.** The earliest changes are intercellular edema and disappearance of the intercellular bridges in the lower epidermis. (H & E)

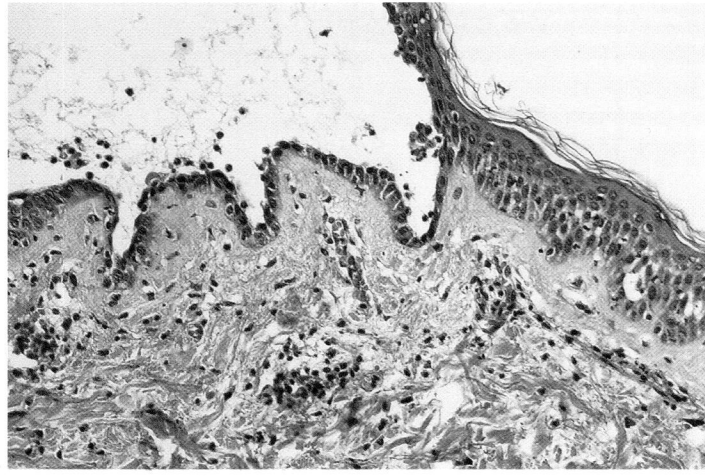

Fig. 6.7 **(A) Pemphigus vulgaris. (B)** The suprabasal blister contains a few acantholytic cells. (H & E)

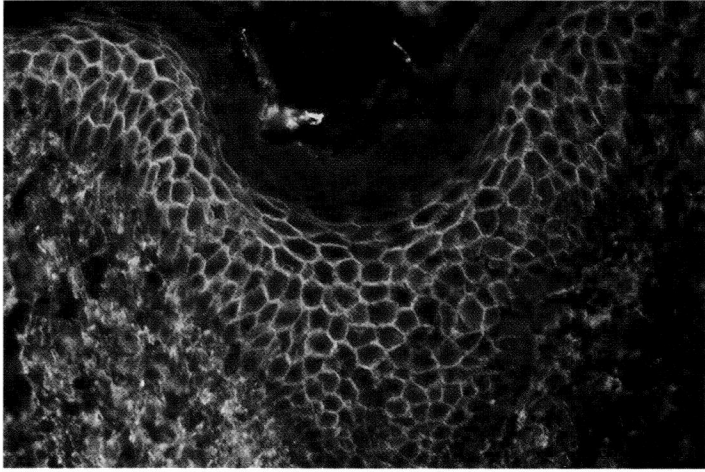

Fig. 6.9 **Pemphigus vulgaris.** IgG is deposited in the intercellular regions of the epidermis. The upper layers are spared. (Direct immunofluorescence)

Electron microscopy[26]

There is dissolution of the intercellular attachments, leading to a widening of the intercellular spaces and eventual separation of the desmosomal attachment plaques.[473] As acantholysis progresses, the desmosomes gradually disappear, followed by retraction of the tonofilaments to the perinuclear area. The keratinocytes often develop numerous, interdigitating processes. Immunoelectron microscopy shows that the immunoglobulins are deposited on the surface of the epidermal cells in a discontinuous globular pattern in the region of the intercellular domains of desmosomes.[474]

PEMPHIGUS VEGETANS

Pemphigus vegetans is a rare variant of pemphigus vulgaris[24] which differs from it by the presence of vegetating erosions, primarily affecting flexural areas.[319,475–477] Two variants of pemphigus vegetans have been recognized.[475] In the *Neumann type* the initial lesions are vesicular and erosive, resembling pemphigus vulgaris, but the lesions progressively evolve into vegetating plaques. The less common *Hallopeau type* commences with pustular lesions and has a relatively benign course with few, if any, relapses.[478–480]

Oral lesions are almost invariably present in pemphigus vegetans and these may be the presenting or dominant feature.[481,482] Some of these cases may represent **pyodermatitis–pyostomatitis vegetans (pyoderma vegetans)**, a condition which has often been confused with pemphigus vegetans.[483] In pyodermatitis–pyostomatitis vegetans annular pustular lesions on the skin may precede, accompany or follow the usually extensive vegetating oral lesions.[483–485] Most cases are associated with inflammatory bowel disease, particularly ulcerative colitis.[486]

Sometimes the surface of the tongue in pemphigus vegetans assumes a cerebriform pattern.[487] Similar thickening of the epidermis of the scalp may rarely lead to the clinical picture of cutis verticis gyrata.[487] Localization to the vulva has been reported.[488] Another clinical feature is the frequent presence of eosinophilia in the peripheral blood.[475] Cases induced by the ingestion of the drugs captopril and enalapril and by the intranasal use of heroin have been reported.[489–491]

Immunological studies[492] provide further evidence for the close relationship between pemphigus vegetans and pemphigus vulgaris.[493,494] Circulating antibodies have been found in patients with pemphigus vegetans of the Neumann type that precipitate with the 130 and 85 kd polypeptides of the pemphigus vulgaris antigen, but there appear to be additional antibodies directed against as yet uncharacterized antigens.[492] In the Hallopeau type, antibodies to a 130 kd polypeptide have been detected.[495] The antibodies appear to belong to the IgG_2 and IgG_4 subclass, with strong complement fixation.[495]

Histopathology[475,487,492]

In the early pustular lesions of the *Hallopeau type*, the appearances resemble those of eosinophilic spongiosis with transmigration of eosinophils into the epidermis and the formation of spongiotic microvesicles and eosinophilic microabscesses.[479] Charcot–Leyden crystals have been seen within these microabscesses.[496] Sporadic acantholytic cells may be present, although they are not usually seen in Tzanck smears prepared from the pustules.[487]

In early lesions of the *Neumann type* there are intraepidermal vesicles with suprabasal acantholysis but no eosinophilic microabscesses.

The vegetative lesions of both types of pemphigus vegetans are similar, with hyperkeratosis, some papillomatosis and prominent acanthosis with downward proliferation of the rete ridges (Fig. 6.10). There are suprabasal lacunae containing some eosinophils. A few acantholytic cells may be present, particularly in the Neumann type.

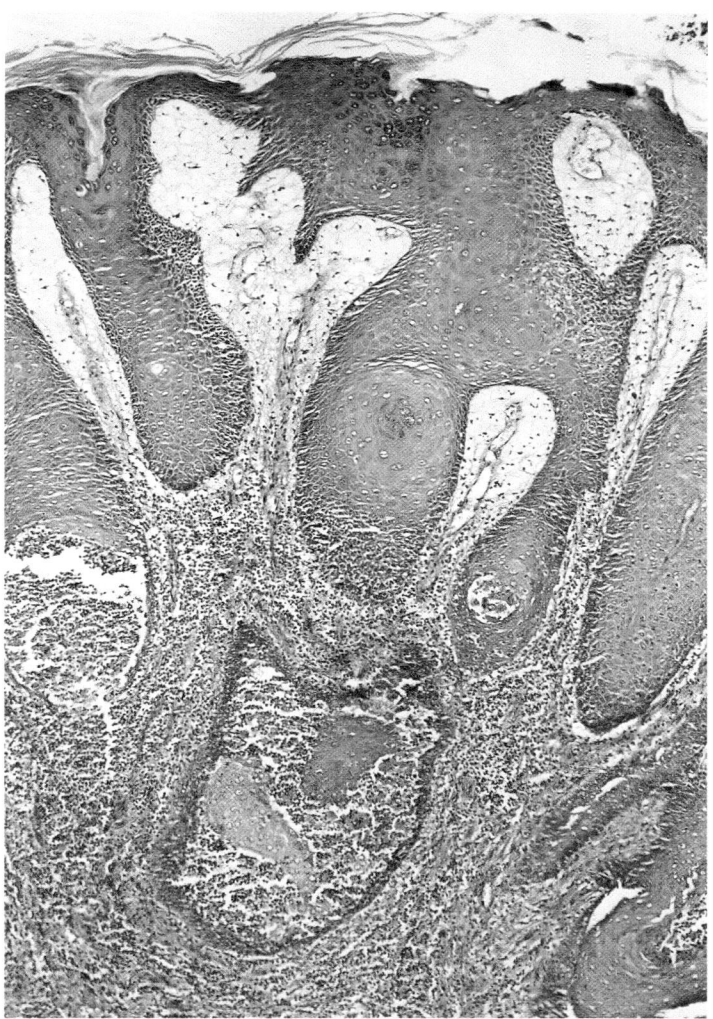

Fig. 6.10 **Pemphigus vegetans.** Suprabasal clefts containing eosinophils are present in the markedly acanthotic epidermis. (H & E)

In both types of pemphigus vegetans the upper dermis contains a heavy infiltrate of lymphocytes and eosinophils, together with some neutrophils. There may be edema of the papillary dermis.

The histological features of **pyodermatitis–pyostomatitis vegetans (pyoderma vegetans)** show some similarities to pemphigus vegetans. There are intraepithelial and subepithelial microabscesses with an admixture of neutrophils and eosinophils (Fig. 6.11).[483] There is a moderately heavy, mixed inflammatory cell infiltrate in the underlying dermis. The lesions are usually more inflammatory than the lesions of pemphigus vegetans. Epithelial hyperplasia is variable and usually more marked in oral lesions. Acantholysis is focal and never severe.[483] Direct immunofluorescence is negative, if misdiagnosed cases of pemphigus vegetans are excluded.

The direct immunofluorescence findings in pemphigus vegetans are similar to those in pemphigus vulgaris with the intercellular deposition of IgG and C3.[497] Circulating antibodies to the intercellular region are usually detectable by indirect immunofluorescence.

Electron microscopy[497,498]

There is a reduction in tonofilaments and desmosomes in keratinocytes in skin adjoining the lesion; only rare desmosomes are found in affected skin.[498] Migration of eosinophils into the epidermis through a damaged basement membrane is frequently observed.

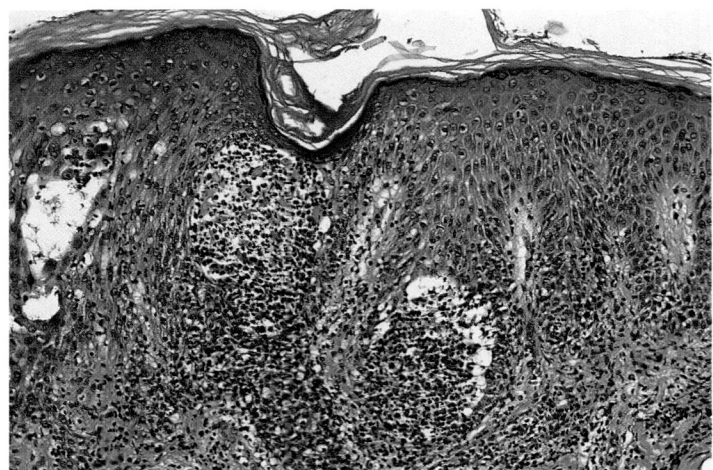

Fig. 6.11 **Pyoderma vegetans in a patient with inflammatory bowel disease.** There are intraepidermal pustules with many eosinophils and epidermal hyperplasia. (H & E)

PARANEOPLASTIC PEMPHIGUS

Paraneoplastic pemphigus (see p. 152) has polymorphous skin lesions with features of both erythema multiforme and pemphigus vulgaris clinically and histologically. Rarely, lesions may resemble bullous pemphigoid. A lichenoid tissue reaction is usually present.

HAILEY–HAILEY DISEASE

Hailey–Hailey disease (familial benign chronic pemphigus) is an uncommon genodermatosis with recurrent, erythematous, vesicular plaques which progress to small flaccid bullae with subsequent rupture and crusting. This condition is discussed on page 298.

Histopathology
Early lesions show suprabasilar clefting with acantholytic cells lining and within the clefts. Widespread partial acantholysis at different levels of the epidermis gives rise to the 'dilapidated brick wall' appearance that is so characteristic of the disease. In contrast to Darier's disease, corps ronds are infrequent and grains are rare. Pemphigus vulgaris usually has less acantholysis and more cells showing pronounced dyskeratosis than Hailey–Hailey disease. Direct immunofluorescence is negative.

DARIER'S DISEASE

Darier's disease is an autosomal dominant genodermatosis with greasy, crusted papules and papulovesicles, mainly in the seborrheic areas of the head, neck and trunk. It is characterized by the minor tissue reaction pattern known as acantholytic dyskeratosis; it is discussed in Chapter 9 (p. 296).

Histopathology
The papulovesicles of Darier's disease show suprabasilar clefting with acantholysis and dyskeratotic cells in the form of corps ronds and grains. There is an overlying keratin plug composed of orthokeratotic and parakeratotic material.

Darier's disease shows more dyskeratosis than pemphigus vulgaris and less acantholysis than Hailey–Hailey disease.

GROVER'S DISEASE

Grover's disease, also referred to as transient acantholytic dermatosis, is characterized by the sudden onset of small, sometimes crusted, erythematous papules and papulovesicles, particularly on the upper part of the trunk. Like Darier's disease it shows acantholytic dyskeratosis; it is discussed in Chapter 9 (p. 297).

Histopathology
Four histological patterns may be seen in Grover's disease – the Darier-like pattern, the Hailey–Hailey-like pattern, the pemphigus vulgaris-like pattern and the spongiotic pattern. Subtle histopathological features may allow a lesion of Grover's disease to be distinguished from the three diseases which Grover's disease may resemble microscopically. Lesions of Grover's disease usually have a much thinner keratin plug than those in Darier's disease. The size of an individual lesion and the extent of the acantholysis are usually less in Grover's disease than in either Hailey–Hailey disease or pemphigus vulgaris. Furthermore, the pemphigus vulgaris-like lesions of Grover's disease sometimes involve the epidermis adjacent to a hair follicle, in contrast to the random distribution and the more extensive lesions of pemphigus vulgaris itself.

ACANTHOLYTIC SOLAR KERATOSIS

Acantholytic solar keratoses are not always clinically distinct from other types of solar keratosis; they may sometimes resemble a superficial basal cell carcinoma.

Histopathology
Acantholytic solar keratoses are characterized by suprabasilar clefting with acantholytic cells both in the cleft and in its margins. Atypical (dysplastic) keratinocytes are also present. The underlying dermis shows variable solar elastosis. The presence of dysplastic epithelial cells distinguishes acantholytic solar keratosis from the other suprabasilar diseases.

SUBEPIDERMAL BLISTERS – A CLASSIFICATION

As stated in the Introduction to this chapter, the classification of the subepidermal blistering diseases is usually based on the pattern of inflammation in the underlying dermis.[499] Some overlap occurs between the various categories, particularly with subepidermal vesiculobullous diseases in which neutrophils or eosinophils are the predominant cell in the dermal infiltrate.

The use of special techniques – such as electron microscopy, immunoelectron microscopy, direct immunofluorescence using salt-split skin, and immunoperoxidase techniques using monoclonal antibodies directed against various components of the basement membrane zone – has allowed many of the subepidermal blistering diseases to be characterized, in recent times, on the basis of the anatomical level of the split within the basement membrane zone. These techniques have little practical application in most laboratories at present; in routine practice, the nature of the dermal infiltrate is used to distinguish the various subepidermal blistering diseases.

Some knowledge of the basement membrane zone and the various antigens associated with it is required for a proper understanding of the subepidermal blistering diseases.

The epidermal basement membrane

Basement membranes are thin, extracellular matrices which separate epithelia and endothelium from their underlying connective tissue.[500–503] In the skin, basement membranes are found at the dermoepidermal junction, in the walls of blood vessels and surrounding the various adnexal structures.[500] The discussion that follows relates to the epidermal basement membrane, which has four major structural components: proceeding from the epidermis to the dermis, they are the basal cell plasma membrane, the lamina lucida, the lamina densa and the sublamina densa zone including the anchoring fibrils (Fig. 6.12).[501,502] In addition to these structural components there are numerous antigenic epitopes within this region.[504–506] Much of our knowledge about the basement membrane has been gained in recent times; it now appears that the PAS-positive basement membrane, visualized by light microscopists for decades, encompasses more than the true basement membrane.[501]

It should also be noted that there are structural and functional changes in the various components of this region with aging, probably giving a less effective epidermal anchoring system.[507]

Plasma membrane

The plasma membrane incorporates the hemidesmosomes, which are studded along the basal surface of the keratinocytes.[501] Tonofilaments, composed of the intermediate keratin filaments K5 and K14, insert into the hemidesmosomes. Small anchoring filaments extend between the plasma membrane and the underlying lamina densa,[502] bridging the lamina lucida. The hemidesmosomes contain the major 230 kd bullous pemphigoid antigen (BPAg1), α6β4 integrin and the minor (180 kd) bullous pemphigoid antigen (BPAg2). The extracellular domains of α6β4 integrin (a receptor for extracellular matrix molecules) and BPAg2 extend into the lamina lucida at the site where anchoring filaments are located.[508] Their interaction is necessary for the stabilization of the hemidesmosome structure.[509] α6β4 integrin is able to transduce signals from the extracellular matrix to the interior of the cell.[510] The 97 kd antigen, autoantibodies to which are found in some patients with linear IgA bullous dermatosis, is a degradation product of BP180, one of the bullous pemphigoid antigens.

Lamina lucida

The lamina lucida is a relatively electron-lucent zone, 20–40 nm in thickness, which is contiguous with the plasma membrane of the overlying basal keratinocytes.[511] The lamina lucida is the weakest link in the dermoepidermal junction and it represents a plane which is easily severed.[502] The anchoring filaments bridge the lamina lucida and insert into the lamina densa. It is possible that some filaments pass through the lamina densa and bind directly to anchoring fibrils in the sublamina densa region.[508] There are multiple antigens associated with the lamina lucida, particularly the anchoring filaments. They include laminin 5, laminin 6, uncein (also called 19-DEJ-1 antigen), laminin 1, nidogen (which connects laminin to type IV collagen in the lamina densa) and epiligrin.[504,508,512–514] Laminin 5 is a heterotrimeric protein consisting of three polypeptide chains, α3, β3 and γ2, each encoded by a distinct gene, *LAMA3*, *LAMB3* and *LAMC2*, respectively.[515] When antibodies to laminin 5 are injected into adult mice, subepidermal blisters result.[9] Epiligrin, the antigen recognized in one form of cicatricial pemphigoid, is the α3 subunit of laminin 5.[516,517] Epiligrin was once thought to be in the lower lamina lucida, possibly at a lower level than the antigenic activity of other forms of laminin 5. Uncein (19-DEJ-1) is absent from nearly all cases of junctional epidermolysis bullosa regardless of disease subtype,[514] whereas laminin 5 (as detected by the monoclonal antibody to GB3) is feebly expressed in all cases of the Herlitz subtype of junctional epidermolysis bullosa and 50% of the other subtypes. Autoantibodies to uncein appear to characterize an

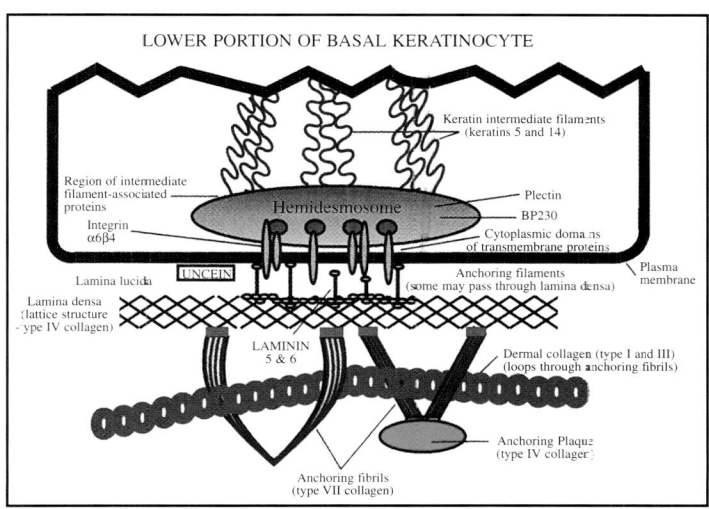

Fig. 6.12 **Schematic representation of the basement membrane zone** (not to scale).

exceedingly rare subepidermal blistering disease.[518] Fibronectin, which is not confined to a single ultrastructural region, binds to collagen and other components of this zone.[519]

Lamina densa

The lamina densa, which is of epidermal origin, is approximately 30–60 nm in width.[502] It is present just beneath the lamina lucida and it rests on the underlying dermal connective tissue.[511] The lamina densa has been referred to in the past as the basal lamina, but this term has also been applied to the lamina lucida and the lamina densa together.[502,504,520] The lamina densa consists of a lattice network of structural proteins. The main component is type IV collagen, which is thought to provide the basement membrane with much of its strength.[500,521] It consists of six genetically different chains (α1–α6); it is produced by both keratinocytes and fibrocytes.[522] Type IV collagen is resistant to human skin collagenase but is a substrate for various neutral proteases derived from mast cells, macrophages and granulocytes.[500] Other antigenic components are laminin 1, nidogen, percelan (formerly termed heparan sulfate proteoglycan) and chondroitin sulfate proteoglycan.[504,508,522–524]

Sublamina densa

The sublamina densa zone has a variety of components but the major ones are the anchoring fibrils which are the strongest mechanism in securing the epidermis to the dermis.[501] The anchoring fibrils are curved structures with irregularly spaced crossbanding of their central portion.[501] They fan out at either end, inserting into the lamina densa above and 'anchoring plaques' in the papillary dermis. These 'anchoring plaques' are composed of type IV collagen and probably laminin and other components.[525] Many fibrils form a sling around islands of type I and III collagen, and possibly oxytalan fibers, both ends of the sling inserting into the lamina densa.[501,525] The anchoring fibrils are composed of type VII collagen.[525,526] Anchoring fibrils vary in their density in different regions of the body.[524] The antigens AF-1 and AF-2 are associated with the sublamina densa zone. They may represent components of the anchoring fibrils additional to type VII collagen.[504] The antibody LH 7:2 reacts with the central region of the N-terminal non-collagenous domain of type VII collagen.[527] Antigens located in this region include the EBA (epidermolysis bullosa acquisita) antigen which is localized in part of the type VII collagen structure and the 285 kd protein recognized in some cases of linear IgA bullous dermatosis.

Further reference to the basement membrane zone and the antigens within it will be made in the descriptions of the subepidermal blistering diseases that follow.

SUBEPIDERMAL BLISTERS WITH LITTLE INFLAMMATION

This heterogeneous group of vesiculobullous diseases includes variants of epidermolysis bullosa, porphyria cutanea tarda, the cell-poor type of bullous pemphigoid, burns, toxic epidermal necrolysis, suction blisters, the blisters that sometimes form over dermal scar or solar elastotic tissue, and some bullous drug reactions.

EPIDERMOLYSIS BULLOSA

The term 'epidermolysis bullosa' is applied to a heterogeneous group of non-inflammatory disorders characterized by the development of blisters or erosions following minor trauma of the skin.[523,528–532] Spontaneous blister formation may occur in some individuals. The clinical presentation may range from minimal involvement of the hands and feet to severe, life-threatening, generalized blistering with dystrophic changes and extracutaneous involvement.[533]

Epidermolysis bullosa is usually inherited as an autosomal dominant or recessive disorder, although an acquired form (see below) has also been recognized.[529] The incidence of the hereditary forms is 1:50 000 births; the more severe recessive forms have an incidence of 1:200 000 to 1:500 000 births.[533] In a study from Northern Ireland, 48 new cases of epidermolysis bullosa were recorded during a 23-year period (1962–1984). Of these 48 cases, 31 (65%) were of simplex type, one (2%) was of junctional type, 12 (25%) were of dystrophic type and the remaining 4 (8%) were of the acquisita type.[534] In another study from Scotland (population 5 million), 259 individuals with epidermolysis bullosa were identified. Of these, 149 had the simplex form, 108 the dystrophic form and 2 the junctional form.[535]

These mechanobullous diseases are best classified into three subgroups on the basis of the level at which the skin separates.[536,537] The three subgroups are:

1. *epidermolytic* (epidermolysis bullosa simplex)
2. *junctional* (junctional epidermolysis bullosa)
3. *dermolytic* (dystrophic epidermolysis bullosa).

For convenience, all forms of epidermolysis bullosa will be considered together because in the majority of cases the appearances on light microscopy are those of a cell-poor subepidermal blister. Routine histology is usually insufficient to allow classification of the various subtypes.[538] However, the use of immunohistochemical markers for type IV collagen and keratin may assist considerably in the subclassification of an individual case. In epidermolytic (simplex) forms, keratin is usually seen in the floor of the blister. The molecular defects, as currently known,[539] are listed in Table 6.2. A proposal to add a fourth subgroup of hemidesmosomal cases, to include the plectin-deficient variant of epidermolysis bullosa simplex with muscular dystrophy, has not been incorporated into the most recent classification.[540,541] The epidermolytic (simplex) group, which involves lysis of basal cells, will be considered first.

Epidermolysis bullosa simplex

Epidermolysis bullosa simplex, one of the three major subgroups of epidermolysis bullosa, is a mechanobullous disorder characterized by intraepidermal

Table 6.2 **Revised classification of inherited epidermolysis bullosa (EB)**

Major EB type	Subtype	Molecular defect
Simplex (epidermolytic)	Köbner	K5, K14
	Weber–Cockayne	K5, K14
	Dowling–Meara	K5, K14
	Muscular dystrophy	Plectin
Junctional	Herlitz	Laminin 5*
	Non Herlitz	Laminin 5; type XVII collagen (BP180)
	Pyloric atresia	α6β4 integrin
Dystrophic (dermolytic)	Dominant dystrophic	Type VII collagen
	Recessive dystrophic (Hallopeau–Siemens)	Type VII collagen
	Recessive dystrophic (non HS)	Type VII collagen

* Laminin 5 is composed of three distinct laminin chains (α3, β3, γ2); mutations in any of the encoding genes may be responsible for this phenotype.

cleavage, usually through the basal layer of cells.[528,542] There are several distinct clinical variants.[543] Most cases have a mild clinical expression with blisters which heal without scarring, and an autosomal dominant inheritance.[544,545] Rare cases with an autosomal recessive inheritance and a more severe clinical course, sometimes with associated neuromuscular disease (particularly muscular dystrophy), have been reported.[546–548] Not all recessive forms have severe disease.[549] A prenatal diagnosis can be made using fetal skin biopsy samples.[514,550,551] Analysis of fetal DNA using chorionic villi or amniotic fluid cells is now the preferred technique.[514,552,553]

The molecular basis of the simplex subgroup appears to reside in defects that disrupt the assembly, structure and/or function of the keratin inter-mediate filament skeleton of the basal keratinocyte – the coexpressed peptides keratin 5 and 14.[554–557] It appears that mutations in certain locations of the keratins (usually the ends of conserved α-helical rod domains) are more likely to produce the severe forms, such as the Dowling–Meara type (see below).[558] Four major subtypes of epidermolysis bullosa simplex are recognized in the latest classification (see Table 6.2).

Generalized (Köbner) type
The generalized (Köbner) clinical variant is characterized by the development of serous blisters at birth or in early infancy.[559,560] Blisters may involve the whole body, but they are preferentially distributed on the hands and feet.[528] Cases with oral involvement or with keratoderma of the palms and soles have been reported.[561] The lesions tend to be worse in warmer weather, a feature present in several other variants. This variant results from a mutation in either the keratin 5 or keratin 14 gene.[562]

Localized (Weber–Cockayne) type
The localized (Weber–Cockayne) form appears to be a localized variant of the Köbner type in which lesions are confined to the hands and feet.[528,543] Onset is usually within the first 2 years of life, although it may be delayed into adolescence or beyond.[563] A kindred with autosomal recessive inheritance has been reported.[564] The disorder results from a mutation in either the keratin 5 or keratin 14 gene, or both.[554,565]

Epidermolysis bullosa herpetiformis (Dowling–Meara)
Epidermolysis bullosa herpetiformis (the Dowling–Meara subtype) is characterized by the development in the first few months of life of serous or hemorrhagic blisters on the trunk, face and extremities.[566,567] The blisters may have a herpetiform arrangement.[568] Inflammatory lesions may be present and these sometimes heal with transitory milia or pigmentation. Mucosal lesions

and nail involvement may occur, as may keratoderma of the palms and soles.[569–571] Some improvement occurs with age. This variant has distinct ultrastructural features with clumping of tonofilaments.[566,572–575] Although mutations may occur in either keratin 5 or keratin 14 in this variant,[576–579] reports suggest that codon 125 of keratin 14 is frequently involved.[570,580,581]

Epidermolysis bullosa simplex with muscular dystrophy (EBS-MD)

EBS-MD is a rare variant in which a defect in plectin (which is probably identical to HD-1) has been found.[582] Plectin is a 500 kd cytoskeleton-associated protein which links the keratin intermediate filaments to the transmembrane proteins of the hemidesmosomes.[583–585] Decayed teeth, urethral strictures, mild palmoplantar hyperkeratosis, respiratory complications[586] and alopecia may also occur.[587] The muscular dystrophy may be of late onset.[588,539] The majority of patients are products of consanguineous marriage and have homozygous plectin gene mutations.[587] The gene for plectin, *PLEC1*, is located on chromosome 8q24.

Other variants

Exceedingly rare variants include the *Ogna type* in which there are acral sanguineous blebs and a generalized bruising tendency,[533] the *Fischer* and *Gedde–Dahl type*[528] in which the blistering tendency is accompanied by mottled pigmentation of the skin[528,590,591] and the *superficial type* in which there is subcorneal cleavage mimicking the 'scalded skin' or peeling skin syndromes.[592] They are not included in the most recent classification. The variant with mottled pigmentation described by Fischer and Gedde–Dahl (see above) is now known as EB-MP.[593] The genetic basis of this type, in five unrelated families, has been ascribed to a heterozygous point mutation in the non-helical V1 domain of K5.[593] Acral blistering begins in early childhood. Isolated reports claiming new clinical variants appear from time to time.[548,594–596] The *Bart type*, in which there is congenital localized absence of the skin associated with trauma-induced blisters, is not a specific form of epidermolysis bullosa as sometimes claimed; it has been reported in association with the various subtypes of epidermolysis bullosa, including the simplex type.[597–600] However, a study of descendants from the original case of Bart's syndrome has revealed it to be a subtype of dominantly inherited dystrophic (dermolytic) epidermolysis bullosa with the gene on chromosome 3p, at or near the site of the gene encoding type VII collagen.[601] The absence of skin may follow the lines of Blaschko.[602]

Histopathology

In epidermolysis bullosa simplex the cleavage is so low in the epidermis that in routine paraffin sections the blister may appear to be a cell-poor subepidermal blister (Fig. 6.13).[544] With thin plastic-embedded sections, fragments of basal keratinocytes may be observed in the blister base;[544] the PAS-positive basement membrane is also found in that position. Immunofluorescence or immunoperoxidase techniques can also be used to confirm the level of the split. These methods will show that the bullous pemphigoid antigen, laminin, type IV collagen and the LDA-1 antigen (a component of the lamina densa) are all present in the base of the bulla.[603,604] Fragments of keratinocyte containing keratin can be detected in the base by the use of the monoclonal antibody MNF116.[605] It also strongly stains the basal keratinocytes.

In the Weber–Cockayne subtype, the level of the split is usually in the mid or upper epidermis (Fig. 6.14), although induced blisters develop in the basal layer.[606,607] In one case which clinically resembled this subtype, suprabasal acantholysis resembling Hailey–Hailey disease was present.[608] In epidermolysis bullosa herpetiformis (Dowling–Meara) a number of eosinophils may be found in the underlying papillary dermis.[609,610] They are not specific for this

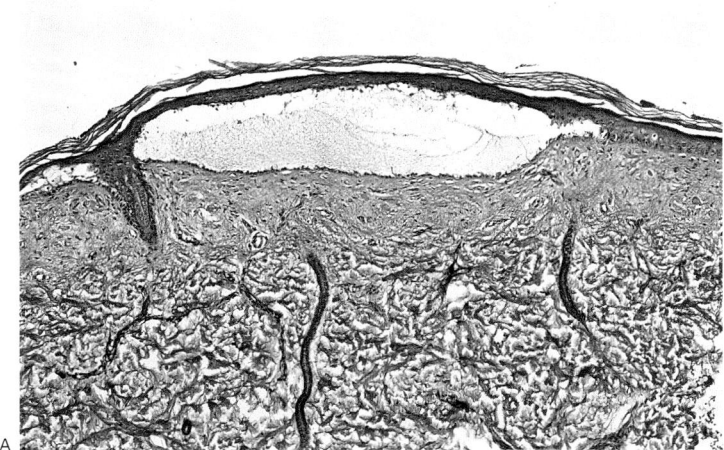

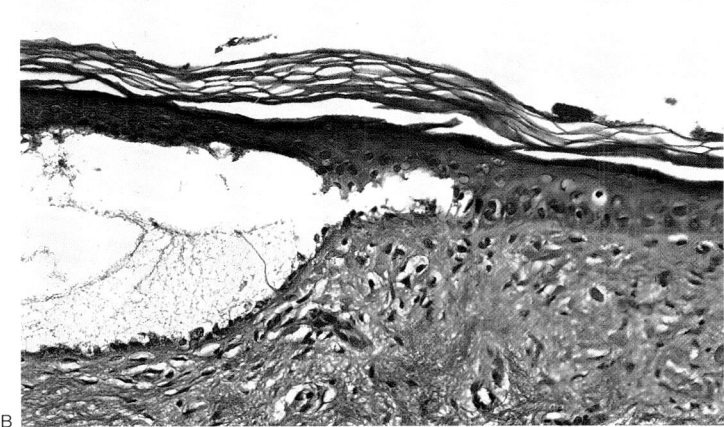

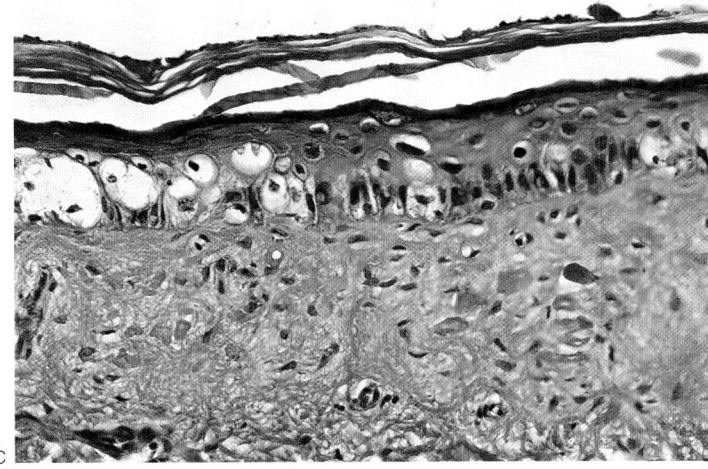

Fig. 6.13 **Epidermolysis bullosa simplex. (A)** Cleavage in the base of the epidermis. **(B)** Fragments of the basal keratinocytes are present in the floor of the blister. There is no dermal inflammation. **(C)** There is vacuolar change within keratinocytes, prior to cleavage. (H & E)

variant and may be found in other subtypes. In EBS-MD, the blister formation always occurs just above the hemidesmosome. The expression of plectin is absent or markedly reduced.[587] A rare variant with subcorneal splitting has been reported (see above);[592] a variant with enlarged dyskeratotic basal cells which have eosinophilic clumps in the cytoplasm and show some atypical mitoses is also rare.[611]

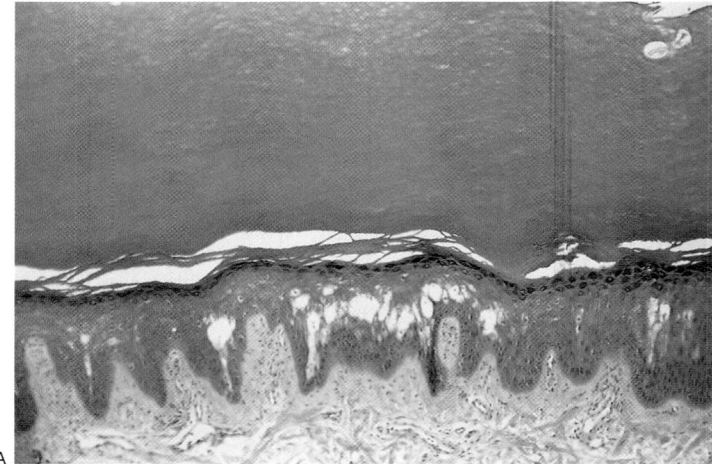

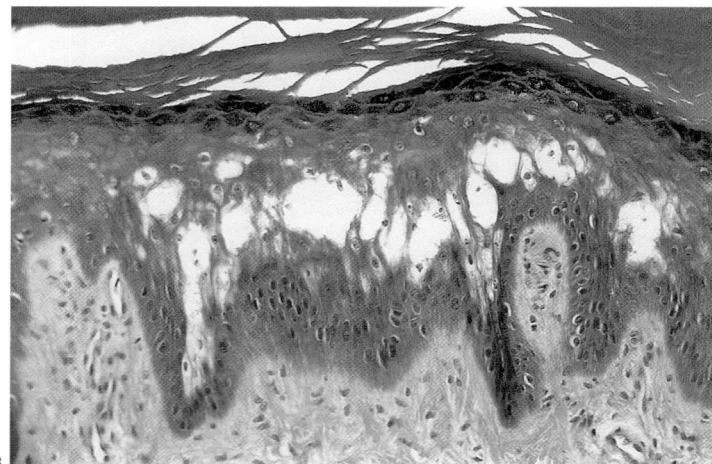

Fig. 6.14 **(A) Epidermolysis bullosa** (Weber–Cockayne type). **(B)** The split is in the mid-epidermis. (H & E)

Transient intraepidermal blisters with the appearances of epidermolysis bullosa simplex can be seen at the donor sites of skin grafts taken for use in patients who have had toxic epidermal necrolysis.[612]

Electron microscopy
There is some perinuclear edema and subnuclear cytolysis of the basal cells[561] but organelles are usually intact. In epidermolysis bullosa herpetiformis the cytolysis is preceded by aggregation and clumping of the tonofilaments which are attached to the hemidesmosomes at the dermoepidermal junction.[566,569,613] The tonofilament clumps may be round or 'whisk type'.[568] The basement membrane zone is intact in all variants of epidermolysis bullosa simplex.

Junctional epidermolysis bullosa

Junctional ('lamina lucidolytic') epidermolysis bullosa (JEB) is an extremely rare group of mechanobullous diseases characterized by autosomal recessive inheritance, lesions that heal without scarring (although in time atrophy may develop) and separation between the basal cells and the lamina lucida due to reduced numbers/function of the hemidesmosomes.[536,614,615] Three subtypes of junctional epidermolysis bullosa are recognized in the latest classification of epidermolysis bullosa.[541]

- Herlitz type (JEB-H)
- non-Herlitz type (JEB-nH)
- pyloric atresia type (JEB-PA).

The non-Herltz group includes cases previously reported as generalized atrophic benign epidermolysis bullosa – GABEB, a designation that will be difficult to dislodge from the literature.

Six antigenic defects have been detected in the basement membrane zone in cases of JEB.[616–620] Originally they were detected by the absence of reactivity using immunofluorescent techniques and either a GB3 monoclonal antibody or a murine monoclonal antibody 19-DEJ-1.[621,622] More specific monoclonal antibodies may now be used. The six genes and the associated protein encoded by them are as follows:

- *LAMA3* – α3 subunit of laminin 5
- *LAMB3* – β3 subunit of laminin 5
- *LAMC2* – γ2 subunit of laminin 5
- *COL17A1/BPAg2* – type XVII collagen (BP180)
- *ITGA6* – α6 integrin
- *ITGB4* – β4 integrin.

Mutations in laminin 5 have been demonstrated in cases of Herlitz (JEB-H) and non-Herltz (JEB-nH) type.[623] Other patients with JEB-rH may have mutations in the *COL17A1/BPAg2* gene. Mutations in either of the genes encoding α6β4 integrin underlie JEB-PA. Uncein, a poorly understood protein on the anchoring filaments and recognized by the monoclonal antibody 19-DEJ-1, is absent in nearly all patients with junctional epidermolysis bullosa and 25% of those with the recessive dystrophic (dermolytic) form.[513,624,625] Interestingly, two acquired subepidermal blistering diseases (cell poor), one with autoantibodies to uncein and the other with antibodies to the β subunit of laminin 5, have recently been reported.[626] The term 'acquired junctional epidermolysis bullosa' is appropriate for these cases.[518] The various molecular abnormalities in JEB appear to affect certain critical intracellular functions of hemidesmosomes, such as the normal connections with keratin intermediate filaments.[627]

Reduced adhesion of keratinocytes in culture has also been reported;[628] this appears to result from defective hemidesmosome synthesis.[629]

Three variants are included in the latest classification.[541]

Junctional epidermolysis bullosa – Herlitz type (JEB-H)
JEB-H, known in the past as epidermolysis bullosa atrophicans gravis (epidermolysis bullosa letalis), has severe generalized involvement with acral accentuation.[630–632] Erosions and bullae are present at birth. Large non-healing areas of granulation tissue develop on the nape of the neck and in the perioral region. Most affected individuals die in early infancy but a few have survived for longer periods.[528] Clinical associations have included anemia, oral lesions, blepharitis, anonychia and epithelial separation in various internal organs.[633,634] Defects in all three polypeptide chains (α3, β3 and γ2) of laminin 5 have been recorded in different families.[515,635–637] Mutations in the *LAMB3* gene on chromosome 1q32, particularly the mutation R635X, are found more often than mutations in the other two genes for laminin 5.[638–641]

Junctional epidermolysis bullosa – non-Herlitz (JEB-nH)
JEB-nH, known in the past as epidermolysis bullosa atrophicans mitis (generalized atrophic benign epidermolysis bullosa – GABEB), is a generalized form in which lesions heal with atrophy and mild scarring, but there are no milia or contractures.[642–648] There may be some improvement with age. Alopecia and absence of pubic and axillary hair are other clinical features.[533] Multiple squamous cell carcinomas of the skin may develop in adult life.[649] At least two different molecular defects have been reported in this subtype. Most of the mutations involve the *COL17A1/BPAg2* gene, responsible for the formation of the 180 kd bullous pemphigoid antigen (BP180, type XVII collagen).[650–654] A minority of the mutations involve the *LAMB3* gene,

encoding the β3 polypeptide of laminin 5.[655,656] A patient with defects in both genes (digenic) has been reported.[657] In a few cases a deficiency of LAD-1, a portion of the extracellular domain of BP180, has been present.[658–660] A mosaic expression of BP180, LAD-1 and uncein has been reported in one patient.[661]

Junctional epidermolysis bullosa with pyloric atresia (JEB-PA)

The variant of junctional epidermolysis bullosa with pyloric atresia may also present with aplasia cutis congenita and/or ureterovesical junction obstruction.[614,662–671] The molecular defect involves α6β4 integrin, a heterodimeric protein which has been isolated from most epithelial linings. Mutations in either the α6 or β4 gene have been associated with JEB-PA.[619,672] Mutations in β4 are more common. Rarely, pyloric atresia occurs in the setting of epidermolysis bullosa simplex.[673,674]

Other variants of junctional epidermolysis bullosa

Several other variants of JEB have long been recognized, but they are not included as major subtypes in the recent classification. *Epidermolysis bullosa atrophicans inversa* has truncal blistering with acral sparing.[536] Improvement occurs with age. Chymotrypsin, a proteolytic enzyme thought to digest laminin, was increased in the serum in one reported case.[675] *Epidermolysis bullosa atrophicans localisata* has its onset in early childhood. Lesions are restricted to the soles and pretibial area.[533,676] *Epidermolysis bullosa junctionalis progressiva* is a rare form which presents with nail dystrophy followed some years later by acral blisters.[625,677,678] Partial deafness is sometimes present. *Cicatricial junctional epidermolysis bullosa* clinically resembles the dystrophic forms, with lesions present at birth which heal with scarring.[388,679] Contractures and scarring of the anterior nares may develop, as may oral and laryngeal lesions.[679]

Histopathology

The junctional forms appear as subepidermal, cell-poor blisters with the PAS-positive basement membrane in the floor. Laminin and type IV collagen can also be demonstrated in the base of the blister; the bullous pemphigoid antigen can be detected in the roof.[604,642] If atrophy develops, there is thinning of the epidermis and flattening of the rete ridges. Dermal fibrosis is present in the cicatricial variant.

Electron microscopy

The various junctional forms cannot be distinguished ultrastructurally. They all show separation through the lamina lucida with variable hypoplasia of the hemidesmosomes.[680,681] Disruption of the basement membrane and an increase in dermal fibroblasts are present in the cicatricial variant.[679] Amorphous deposits have been reported in the lamina lucida in epidermolysis bullosa progressiva but this finding has not been confirmed subsequently.[677]

Dermolytic (dystrophic) epidermolysis bullosa

The dermolytic (dystrophic) forms of epidermolysis bullosa present with trauma-induced blistering which is followed by the formation of scars and milia.[682–684] The new classification recognizes three major subtypes although traditionally six have been reported, three of which are inherited in an autosomal dominant fashion. The remainder are recessive in type, and in these cases the lesions tend to be more severe. A transient neonatal variant (transient bullous dermolysis of the newborn), which does not fit into any of these six subtypes, has also been reported (see below). Antenatal diagnosis of dermolytic (dystrophic) epidermolysis bullosa can be made by fetal skin biopsy,[685] although analysis of fetal DNA obtained from chorionic sampling or amniotic fluid cells allows the diagnosis to be made more accurately and in the first trimester.[686,687] The challenges of gene therapy are now being addressed.[688,689]

Other clinical features which may be present include nail dystrophy[690] and oral[662] and gastrointestinal lesions,[691] particularly esophageal webs and strictures;[692] congenital localized absence of the skin,[598,693,694] anemia, growth retardation and poor nutrition may also be present.[695,696] Squamous cell carcinomas of the skin are an uncommon complication,[688,697,698] which may be linked to the persistent growth-activated immunophenotype of epidermal keratinocytes that has been found in this disease.[699] Mutant p53 protein is found in only one-quarter of the tumors, possibly a reflection of their well-differentiated nature.[700] Atypical melanocytic lesions have been reported in one case.[701] Systemic amyloidosis is a rare complication.[702,703]

The dermolytic (dystrophic) variants are all characterized by the development of a split below the lamina densa in the region of the anchoring fibrils. These fibrils are usually absent or severely diminished in the severe recessive form and reduced in number in many of the other types.[704,705] In cases with normal numbers of anchoring fibrils it is assumed that they may be qualitatively changed.[706] Abnormal collagenase activity has been demonstrated in some of the recessive forms but it appears to play a minor pathogenetic role.[707–709] Nevertheless, it is interesting that drugs which inhibit collagenase and proteases have a favorable therapeutic effect on the course of the disease.[533,710,711]

Type VII collagen, the major if not the exclusive component of the anchoring fibrils, is markedly reduced or absent in all but rare cases of the recessive form; it is also reduced or 'defective' in many of the dominant forms of dermolytic (dystrophic) epidermolysis bullosa.[706,712–717] Rare cases of the recessive variants with normal type VII collagen (such as the inversa form) may represent mutations affecting interactions of the anchoring fibrils with other components of the basement membrane zone or in the structural assembly of the fibrils.[718,719] Elastic microfibrils might contribute to dermal–epidermal adherence in areas with intact skin but an absence of anchoring fibrils.[720]

The synthesis of type VII collagen is under the control of the gene *COL7A1*, on chromosomal locus 3p21.[721] There is a strong genetic linkage between this gene and both the dominant and recessive forms of dermolytic (dystrophic) epidermolysis bullosa.[721,722] A glycine-to-arginine substitution in the triple helical domain of type VII collagen, a mutation designated as G2043R, is the classic mutation in the dominant forms.[723–725] Numerous different mutations have been reported.[726–728] Most *COL7A1* mutations are unique to individual families, and therefore it is usually necessary to screen all 118 exons of the gene to determine the molecular pathology in a patient with dystrophic epidermolysis bullosa.[729–734] Several recurrent mutations have been reported.[735,736] The less severe forms of recessive dermolytic (dystrophic) epidermolysis bullosa have been found to be heterozygous for the usual defect in *COL7A1*, but with a further different mutation in the other allele.[737,738]

Studies with cultured keratinocytes have produced conflicting results with reports of reduced production of type VII collagen,[739] but sometimes with normal amounts of collagen VII mRNA,[740] normal production[717] and even intracellular accumulation.[741]

Five other basement membrane components – 19-DEJ-1, KF1, AF1/AF2, the 105 kd antigen and chondroitin-6-sulfate proteoglycan – have been reported to be defective, in varying degrees, in some patients with the dermolytic (dystrophic) form.[742] These abnormalities are probably secondary phenomena resulting from the altered structural integrity of the basement membrane zone.

The various clinical types of dermolytic epidermolysis bullosa are discussed below, commencing with the three dominant forms. The transient form will be considered last.

Dermolytic epidermolysis bullosa, hyperplastic variant (Cockayne–Touraine)

In this dominant form, blisters commence at birth or in early childhood, but they are usually not debilitating.[743] There is a predilection for acral regions, particularly the extensor surfaces.[536] The scars that develop may be hypertrophic.[533] This variant and the Pasini variant (see below) are allelic and differences in their clinical presentation may reflect the precise position of the glycine substitution along the type VII collagen molecule.[723] These two forms have been combined as dominant dystrophic epidermolysis bullosa in the new classification.[541] Their clinical differences warrant their continued separation.

Dermolytic epidermolysis bullosa, albopapuloid variant (Pasini)

Generalized blistering and erosions commence at birth or in infancy.[536] Pale papules (albopapuloid lesions) develop on the trunk at puberty.[744] Cultured fibroblasts from the skin of affected individuals accumulate excess amounts of glycosaminoglycans; the significance of this is uncertain.[743] Several different mutations in COL7A1 have been reported.[745]

Pretibial epidermolysis bullosa

Pretibial epidermolysis bullosa is a rare dominant dystrophic form associated with pretibial blisters which usually develop between the ages of 11 and 24 years.[746–748] Albopapuloid lesions are occasionally present.[528,749] The inflammatory nature of some lesions may mask the diagnosis for some time.[750] The anchoring fibrils are sparse and rudimentary in both lesional and non-predilected normal skin.[749] A linkage to the collagen type VII gene COL7A1 has been found.[751,752]

Dermolytic epidermolysis bullosa (Hallopeau–Siemens)

Dermolytic epidermolysis bullosa, an autosomal recessive variant, is highly debilitating and characterized by large flaccid bullae on any part of the skin from birth.[744] There is a range of severity, with a shortened lifespan in the severe (gravis) forms.[533,536,753] The scarring often leads to digital fusion and so-called 'mitten' deformities.[744,754] The oral, esophageal, anal and vaginal mucosae are frequently involved with the development of fibrous strictures.[755] Sparse hair, dystrophic teeth, keratitis[756] and growth retardation are common features.[536] A variant with progressive, symmetrical, centripetal involvement exists.[536, 757] Sclerodermoid lesions have been reported in one patient with this disorder.[758] Heterozygotes appear to have diminished numbers of anchoring fibrils.[759]

Localized dermolytic epidermolysis bullosa

Blisters develop on the extremities in early childhood.[528] There is some improvement with age. A variant with prurigo nodularis-like lesions has been reported as *epidermolysis bullosa pruriginosa*.[760,761] The molecular pathology in this pruriginous variant suggests that other factors in addition to the inherent COL7A1 mutation(s) may be responsible for this distinctive phenotype.[762]

Dermolytic epidermolysis bullosa inversa (recessive dystrophic epidermolysis bullosa inversa)

In dermolytic epidermolysis bullosa inversa, blisters develop in the skin of the axillae, neck and lower part of the trunk with sparing of the extremities.[763,764] Milia are often absent. Mucosal involvement is common and the tongue may be bound to the floor of the mouth.[763] Ultrastructural analysis reveals absent or rudimentary anchoring fibrils, although type VII collagen is present on immunofluorescence.[765] This implies a defect in the supramolecular aggregation of collagen VII into anchoring fibrils.[764–766]

Transient bullous dermolysis of the newborn

Transient bullous dermolysis of the newborn is a rare variant, probably a dominant form, which is characterized by a self-limited course and the presence of abundant type VII collagen within the cytoplasm of basilar and, to a lesser extent, suprabasilar keratinocytes.[767–771] There is only patchy basement membrane zone staining for type VII collagen, but this reverts to normal with clinical improvement. This condition may result from delay in the transport and integration of type VII collagen or excessive phagocytosis by basal keratinocytes.[772] In addition, there are mutations in the COL7A1 gene.[773,774] Small amounts of similar cytoplasmic type VII collagen can be seen, from time to time, in other types of dermolytic (dystrophic) epidermolysis bullosa, particularly during wound healing in severe forms of the disease.[775]

Histopathology

Routine light microscopy is of little value in the diagnosis of the dermolytic forms of epidermolysis bullosa.[618] There is a cell-poor, subepidermal blister. Uncommonly, there are sparse eosinophils in the dermis;[610] they were numerous in one case.[776] Superficial dermal scarring and milia are often present. The PAS-positive basement membrane, the bullous pemphigoid antigen, laminin and types IV and V collagen are all found in the roof of the blister.[603,777] Staining is weak or absent with antibodies to KF-1, AF-1 and AF-2, which are all components of the anchoring fibrils.[533,604,618] If a monoclonal antibody to type VII collagen is used (LH 7:2 or commercial preparations), staining will occur in the genetically dominant dermolytic forms but only weakly or not at all in the recessive forms.[682,714,778] Studies have shown that LH 7:2 reacts with the central region of the N-terminal non-collagenous domain of type VII collagen.[527]

Electron microscopy

The anchoring fibrils are usually totally absent in the generalized recessive form and diminished in number in both the localized recessive and the dominant variants.[536,705] The split occurs beneath the lamina densa.[613] Perinuclear stellate inclusions are seen in basilar keratinocytes in transient bullous dermolysis of the newborn.[772] They represent cytoplasmic type VII collagen.

Epidermolysis bullosa acquisita

Epidermolysis bullosa acquisita (dermolytic pemphigoid, EBA) is a rare, non-hereditary, subepidermal bullous disorder with heterogeneous clinical features.[779–781] Typically, there are non-inflammatory bullae which develop in areas subjected to minor trauma such as the extensor surface of the limbs.[782] Rare cases have been precipitated by prolonged sun exposure.[783] The lesions eventually heal leaving atrophic scars and milia. In up to 50% of cases the initial presentation is with widespread inflammatory bullae, which are not precipitated by trauma and which heal without scarring.[779,784,785] Some such cases, if not all, eventually evolve into the non-inflammatory (mechanobullous), scarring type.[779] At times the clinical presentation may mimic bullous pemphigoid,[786,787] localized cicatricial pemphigoid,[788,789] cicatricial pemphigoid[790] or linear IgA bullous dermatosis.[791] The confocal laser scanning microscope has been used with some success in distinguishing bullous pemphigoid from epidermolysis bullosa acquisita.[792]

Involvement of the mucous membranes occurs in 30–50% of cases.[793] This usually takes the form of oral erosions and blisters, but ocular involvement can also occur.[794] A variant with ocular involvement, sometimes severe, and IgA autoantibodies has been reported.[791,795] Vesicular cystitis,[796] esophageal webs[797] and scarring alopecia[798] are rarely present.[799]

Onset of the disease is usually in mid-adult life, although some cases have been reported in children.[800–811] Its course is usually chronic and there is great variability in severity and evolution.[779,812,813]

Epidermolysis bullosa acquisita has been associated with various systemic diseases, particularly those with a presumed immune pathogenesis.[779,782] They include systemic lupus erythematosus,[814,815] rheumatoid arthritis, inflammatory bowel disease[798,816] (particularly Crohn's disease),[817] chronic thyroiditis, HIV infection,[818] amyloidosis,[819] mixed cryoglobulinemia[820] and the multiple endocrinopathy syndrome.[821] Its association with a benign schwannoma was probably coincidental.[822] Its onset has also been triggered by pregnancy[823] and by penicillamine.

Earlier views[824] that this condition was not a distinct entity but a variant of cicatricial pemphigoid were put to rest by the discovery of the epidermolysis bullosa acquisita (EBA) antigen.[825–828] This antigen, with a molecular weight of 290 kd, has been identified as type VII collagen,[829–831] a major component of the anchoring fibrils.[830] It appears to be synthesized by both fibroblasts and keratinocytes.[827] The initiating event in this dermatosis is probably the formation and binding of antibody to the carboxyl terminal region of type VII collagen.[829,832] Multiple epitopes exist on the N-terminal non-collagenous domain of type VII collagen, capable of binding the autoantibodies in this disease.[833] Passive transfer of these autoantibodies from a patient with severe EBA produced comparable changes when injected subcutaneously into neonatal mice.[834] An infant with multiple tense blisters and autoantibodies to both the EBA antigen and BP180, has been reported.[835]

Antibodies to type VII collagen are also found in many cases of bullous systemic lupus erythematosus.[781,836] Patients who develop apparent EBA in association with systemic lupus erythematosus (SLE) have been regarded as a subset of the bullous eruption of SLE.[837,838]

Intravenous immunoglobulins have been used successfully in the treatment of EBA.[839,840]

Histopathology[779]

There is a subepidermal bulla with fibrin and only a few inflammatory cells in the lumen.[841] The roof of the blister is usually intact and there may be a few dermal fragments attached to the epidermis.[842] In non-inflammatory lesions (Fig. 6.15) there is a sparse lymphocytic infiltrate around the vessels of the superficial vascular plexus, while in inflammatory lesions there is a heavy upper dermal inflammatory infiltrate in which neutrophils predominate.[784] The neutrophils often form papillary microabscesses. Some eosinophils may also be present. The histological heterogeneity presumably results from the heterogeneity of the immune complexes that are deposited, some having greater ability than others to generate complement-derived chemotaxis. In older lesions there will be some dermal scarring and also milia.

With the PAS stain, the basement membrane is split, and most of the PAS-positive material is attached to the blister roof.[841] Laminin and type IV collagen can be identified by immunoperoxidase techniques in the roof of the blister.[843,844] This technique is helpful if facilities are not available for immuno-electron microscopy or split-skin immunofluorescence (see below).

Direct immunofluorescence shows linear deposition of immunoglobulins, particularly IgG, and of complement (including the complement components C3b and C5)[845] along the basement membrane zone in nearly all lesions;[798,819] cases reported without immunoreactants may form a distinct subgroup.[842,846,847] Circulating IgG class antibodies to the basement membrane zone are present in up to 50% of cases.[848,849] IgA autoantibodies have been detected in a significant number of cases.[850] When salt-split skin is used as a substrate, these antibodies bind to the dermal floor, in contrast to bullous pemphigoid antibodies which bind to the epidermal roof. Some doubts have been expressed on the reliability of this technique in the diagnosis of EBA.[851,852] The presence of epidermal-binding antibodies, which are sometimes found in EBA, may be a consequence of epitope spreading, a phenomenon observed in other immunobullous diseases.[853,854] In one case, antibodies

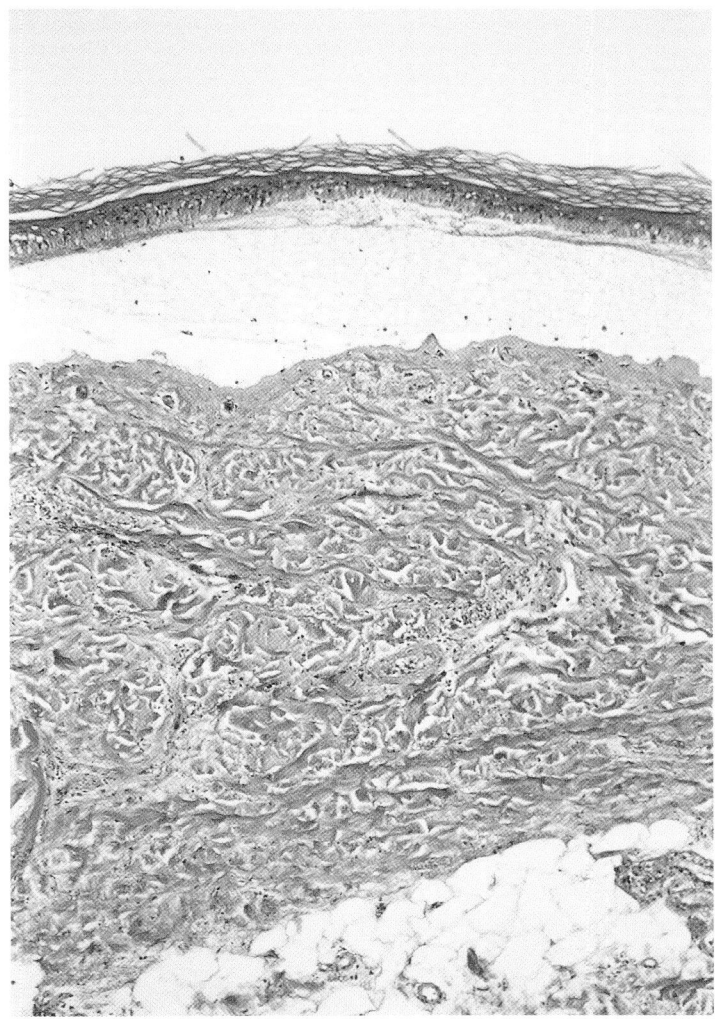

Fig. 6.15 **Epidermolysis bullosa acquisita (EBA).** This is a non-inflammatory lesion. (H & E)

to laminin α3 were detected in addition to the usual antibodies to type VII collagen.[854] The site of the deposits can be determined by the fluorescence overlay antigen mapping (FOAM) technique, although this is a more complex technique than the salt-split skin method.[855]

Electron microscopy

The split usually occurs in the superficial dermis below the lamina lucida.[856] In some of the inflammatory variants, however, splitting may occur within the lamina lucida, possibly as a result of leukocyte-derived proteolytic enzymes acting on the lamina lucida, which appears to be a *locus minoris resistentiae*.[857,858] Electron-dense amorphous deposits are present beneath the lamina densa. On immunoelectron microscopy, the immunoreactants which correspond with the electron-dense deposits noted on routine electron microscopy are found within and/or below the lamina densa, sometimes covering the anchoring fibrils.[812,858–860] In one report, the site of the deposits varied depending on whether pre-embedding or postembedding immunogold techniques were used.[861]

PORPHYRIA CUTANEA TARDA

Blisters can develop in light-exposed areas, particularly the dorsum of the hands, in porphyria cutanea tarda.

Histopathology

The blisters are subepidermal, with preservation of the dermal papillae in the floor of the lesion ('festooning'; Fig. 6.16). Hyaline material, which is PAS positive and diastase resistant, is present in the walls of the small vessels in the upper dermis and sometimes in the basement membrane of the epidermis. There is usually no inflammatory infiltrate, although patchy hemorrhage is sometimes present in the blister and the underlying dermis.

BULLOUS PEMPHIGOID (CELL-POOR TYPE)

If a biopsy is taken from a bullous lesion in bullous pemphigoid which does not have an erythematous base, the lesion will often have few inflammatory cells in the dermis. This is in contrast to lesions with an erythematous base which usually have a heavier dermal infiltrate, including many eosinophils.

BURNS AND CRYOTHERAPY

Subepidermal blisters may develop in second-degree thermal burns and following electrodesiccation therapy. Rarely, thermal burns are produced by a high-intensity fiberoptic light source used in transillumination for the diagnosis of pneumothorax.[862] Delayed postburn blisters may develop months after the initial burn.[863] They are subepidermal in type. A bullous pemphigoid-like eruption has also been reported after a chemical burn.[864] Hemorrhagic blisters may develop after cryotherapy (see p. 150). They are usually cell poor initially; neutrophils may be present in older lesions, particularly if the lesion becomes infected. Bullous dermatitis artefacta, probably produced by an aerosol spray resulting in cryoinjury, has been reported.[865]

The epidermis is usually necrotic; vertical elongation of keratinocytes is a conspicuous feature after electrodesiccation. The basket-weave pattern of the stratum corneum is usually preserved. A distinctive feature of burns and electrodesiccation is the fusion of collagen bundles in the upper dermis; they have a refractile eosinophilic appearance.

TOXIC EPIDERMAL NECROLYSIS

Toxic epidermal necrolysis, which is now regarded as the most severe form of an erythema multiforme spectrum, presents with generalized tender erythema which rapidly progresses to a blistering phase with extensive shedding of the skin. There is a subepidermal bulla with confluent necrosis of the overlying epidermis (Fig. 6.17). The perivascular infiltrate of lymphocytes, if present at all, is usually sparse, justifying categorization of the condition as a cell-poor blistering disease. Cases with features overlapping those of erythema multiforme are sometimes seen.

Mustard gas, used in chemical warfare, can result in bullae with full-thickness epidermal necrosis resembling toxic epidermal necrolysis.[866] In the early stages, the epidermal keratinocytes are swollen and hydropic; many have pyknotic nuclei.[867,868]

Sometimes, chemotherapy-induced acral erythema can progress to a subepidermal bullous lesion with epidermal necrosis.[869]

SUCTION BLISTERS

Blisters induced by suction are subepidermal in type, in contrast to friction blisters which develop within the epidermis. The dermal papillae are usually preserved in suction blisters ('festooning'). Suction blisters may be a manifestation of dermatitis artefacta.

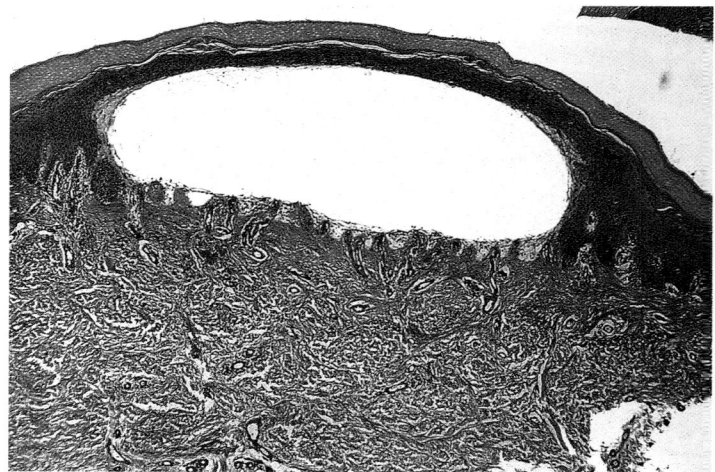

Fig. 6.16 **Porphyria cutanea tarda.** There is a cell-poor, subepidermal bulla with preservation of the dermal papillae in the floor ('festooning'). (Periodic acid–Schiff)

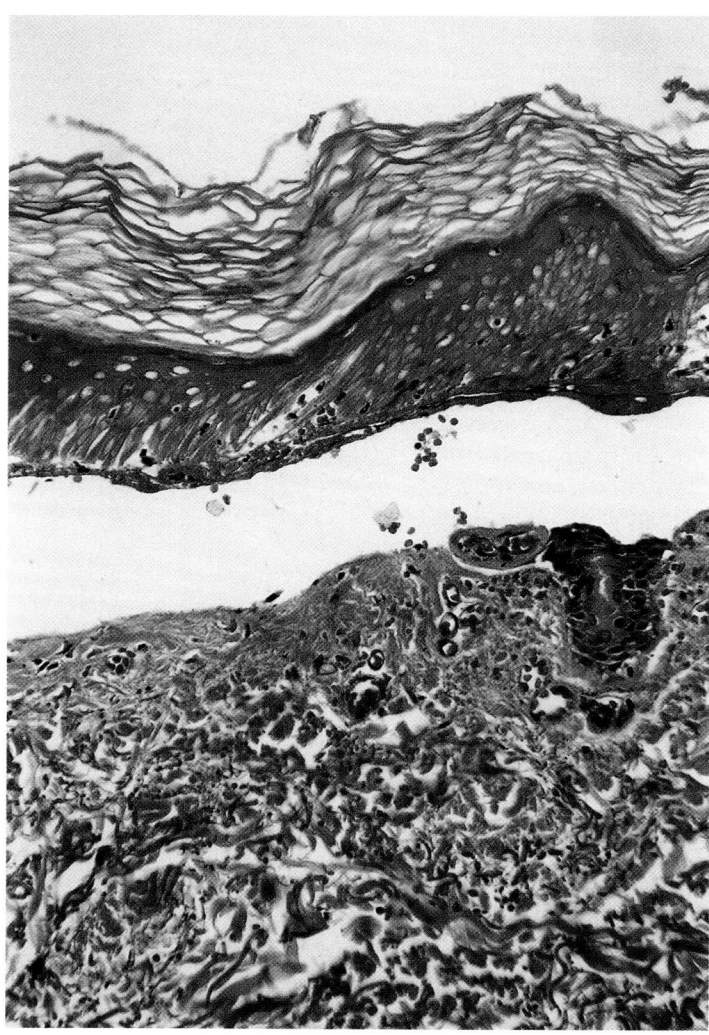

Fig. 6.17 **Toxic epidermal necrolysis.** This lesion is characterized by a cell-poor, subepidermal blister with necrosis of the overlying epidermis. There is a surviving sweat duct in the base of the blister. (H & E)

BLISTERS OVERLYING SCARS

Subepidermal clefting sometimes occurs overlying a dermal scar, particularly if this involves the papillary as well as the reticular dermis. The clefting is usually an incidental histological finding without obvious clinical manifestations. The finding of scar tissue in the base of the blister in association with a clinical history of surgery or some other trauma at the affected site characterizes this entity (Fig. 6.18).

Subepidermal bullae, with a slight lymphocytic infiltrate, have been reported in grafted leg ulcers 4–8 weeks after the operation.[870] The pathogenetic mechanism is not currently known.

BULLOUS SOLAR ELASTOSIS

The blisters that occur rarely in areas of severe solar elastosis are intradermal rather than subepidermal. A thin grenz zone of papillary dermis overlies them.

BULLOUS AMYLOIDOSIS

Rarely, bullae may form above the amyloid deposits in the skin in primary systemic amyloidosis (see p. 430). The split is usually in the upper dermis. There are characteristic hyaline deposits of amyloid in the base of the blister. Hemorrhage is often present.

A poikilodermatous, bullous form of amyloidosis, with the split at the level of the lamina lucida, has been reported.[871] A few cases of a subepidermal bullous dermatosis have been reported in **Waldenström's macroglobulinemia**.[872] Separation occurs at the site of the IgM deposits.[872,873]

BULLOUS DRUG REACTION

Subepidermal bullae are an uncommon manifestation of a drug reaction. The inflammatory cell infiltrate in the dermis may be variable in intensity and composition. One category is cell poor and resembles porphyria cutanea tarda (pseudoporphyria).

In contrast to porphyria cutanea tarda, drug-induced pseudoporphyria has less PAS-positive material in vessel walls and less obvious 'festooning'

(persistence of dermal papillae in the base of the blister). A rare eosinophil may be present in the dermis in the drug-induced cases; this is not a feature of porphyria cutanea tarda.

Cell-poor subepidermal bullae have been reported following the infusion of ε-aminocaproic acid.[874] Fibrin thrombi were present in vessels in the papillary dermis.

This is a convenient place to tabulate all drugs producing a vesiculobullous pattern (see Table 6.3). Specific references are included in the text in the appropriate section of this chapter.

Table 6.3 **Drugs causing vesiculobullous and pustular reactions**

Subcorneal pustular dermatosis-like: amoxicillin, cephalosporins. dapsone, diltiazem, isoniazid, paclitaxel, quinidine

Acute generalized exanthematous pustulosis: acetaminophen (paracetamol), allopurinol, amoxicillin, antimalarials, ceftriaxone, cephalexin, chemotherapy drugs, chloramphenicol, chloroquine, chromium picolinate, cimetidine, ciprofloxacin, clemastine, diltiazem, doxycycline, enalapril, erythromycin, gentamicin, hydroxychloroquine, icodextrin, imipenem, itraconazole, mercury, metronidazole, nifedipine, nystatin, olanzapine, penicillin, phenytoin, pholcodine, proguanil, prostaglandin E_1, quinidine, roxithromycin, teicoplanin, terbinafine, thalidomide, ticlopidine, trimethoprim–sulfamethoxazole, vancomycin

Pemphigus foliaceus and erythematosus: aspirin, bucillamine, captopril, ceftazidine, cephalosporins, enalapril, fosinopril, gold, heroin, levodopa, methimazole, penicillamine, propanolol, pyritinol, ramipril, rifampin (rifampicin), thiol-containing drugs, thiopronine

Pemphigus vulgaris and vegetans: ampicillin, captopril, cilazapril, diclofenac, dipyrone, enalapril, heroin, influenza immunization, interleukin-2, nifedipine, norfloxacin, penicillamine, penicillin, phenols, quinapril, rifampin (rifampicin), tannins, thiol-containing foods, typhoid immunization

Subepidermal (cell poor) – pseudoporphyria: chlorthalidone, etretinate, flutamide, furosemide (frusemide), isotretinoin, mefenamic acid, nabumetone, nalidixic acid, naproxen, oxaprozin, pravastatin, pyridoxine, sulfonamides, tetracyclines

Subepidermal (lymphocytes ± eosinophils – erythema multiforme/TEN): acarbose, allopurinol, amifostine, aminopenicillins, bezafibrate, carbamazepine, ceftazidime, chloroquine, cimetidine, ciprofloxacin, clindamycin, clobazam, clonazepam, cocaine, cyclophosphamide, cytosine arabinoside, diacerein, doxycycline, ethambutol, etretinate, famotidine, gemeprost, griseofulvin, indapamide, indomethacin, isoxicam, lamotrigine, latanoprost eye drops, mefloquine, methotrexate, mifepristone, nevirapine, nitrogen mustard, nystatin, oxaprozin, phenylbutazone, phenytoin, piroxicam, ranitidine, ritodrine, sertraline, sulfamethoxazole, suramin, terbinafine, theophylline, ticlopidine, trichloroethylene, trimethoprim, valproic acid, vancomycin

Subepidermal (eosinophils) – bullous pemphigoid: ampicillin, antipsychotic drugs, bumetanide, captopril, cephalexin, chloroquine, ciprofloxacin, doxazosin, enalapril, fluorouracil (topical), fluoxetine, furosemide (frusemide), ibuprofen, influenza immunization, levobunolol (ophthalmic), neuroleptics, nifedipine, novoscabin, penicillamine, penicillin and derivates, serratiopeptidase, sulfasalazine, tetanus immunization

Subepidermal (neutrophils) – linear IgA bullous dermatosis: amiodarone, atorvastatin, captopril, cefamandole, ceftriaxone, diclofenac, furosemide (frusemide), glibenclamide, interleukin-2, lithium carbonate, metronidazole, naproxen, penicillin, phenytoin, piroxicam, sodium hypochlorite (contact), somatostatin, trimethoprim–sulfamethoxazole, vancomycin

Subepidermal (scarring) – cicatricial pemphigoid: azathioprine, clonidine, practolol

Subepidermal (vasculitis): some of the drugs producing a leukocytoclastic vasculitis (see Ch. 8) may result in blister formation, but this is not a consistent feature of any particular drug

Subepidermal (necrosis) – drug overdose-related bullae: amitryptyline, barbiturates, carbamazepine, clobazam, diazepam, heroin, imipramine, methadone, morphine

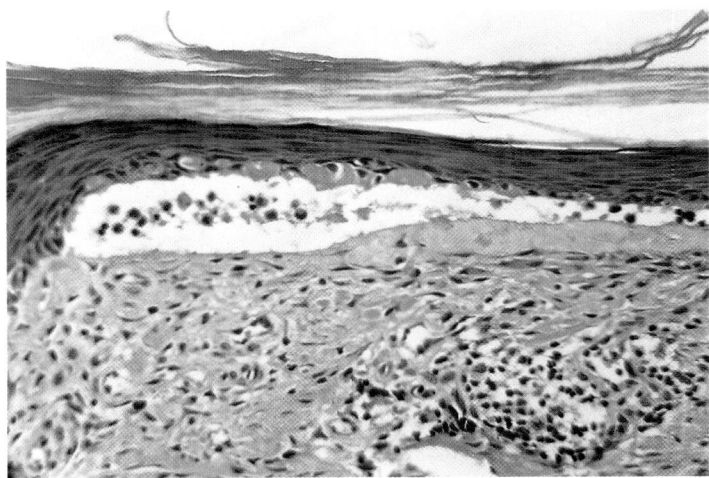

Fig. 6.18 **Subepidermal clefting overlying scar tissue.** (H & E)

KINDLER'S SYNDROME

Kindler's syndrome, a poikilodermatous genodermatosis, is characterized by bullae that are subepidermal and cell poor (see p. 54). Ultrastructural studies have shown that the split can occur at several levels within the dermo-epidermal junction zone, including within the basal cells.

SUBEPIDERMAL BLISTERS WITH LYMPHOCYTES

All of the conditions in this group, with the exception of paraneoplastic pemphigus, have been discussed in other chapters. Accordingly, these other conditions will be given only brief mention here.

ERYTHEMA MULTIFORME

The vesiculobullous lesions in erythema multiforme result from damage to the basal cells of the epidermis. Accordingly, this condition is considered among the lichenoid reaction patterns (see Ch. 3, p. 43). Erythema multiforme is characterized by a subepidermal blister with a mild to moderately heavy infiltrate of lymphocytes in the underlying dermis. The infiltrate, which may include a few eosinophils, extends to the level of the mid dermis. The epidermis overlying the blister may show necrosis which may be confluent or involve only small groups of cells. Apoptotic keratinocytes are usually present in the epidermis adjacent to the blister.

PARANEOPLASTIC PEMPHIGUS

Paraneoplastic pemphigus is an entity characterized by polymorphous skin lesions with features of both erythema multiforme and pemphigus vulgaris in association with internal neoplasms, especially non-Hodgkin's lymphoma.[875–879] Several patients with chronic lymphocytic leukemia treated with fludarabine have developed paraneoplastic pemphigus.[880] Other associations have included Hodgkin's disease,[881] thymoma[882,883] and Castleman's disease.[884–890] Since its original description, the clinical and immunopathological spectrum of paraneoplastic pemphigus has expanded. At least six clinical variants are now recognized:

- erythema multiforme-like
- pemphigoid-like[891–894]
- pemphigus-like (foliaceus, vulgaris and vegetans)[895,896]
- GVHD-like[897]
- lichen planus pemphigoides- or erosive lichen planus-like[898–901]
- cicatricial pemphigoid-like.[902,903]

Unusual presentations have included onset following systemic interferon[904] or radiotherapy,[905] localization to a radiation field,[875] elevated levels of IL-6,[906] onset in childhood or adolescence,[907,908] the presence of annular lesions,[909] and the absence of a detectable neoplasm.[910,911] Other features of this condition include the presence of mucosal erosions, pseudomembranous conjunctivitis, corneal melting or severe pulmonary involvement that may lead to respiratory failure.[885,912,913] Patients with paraneoplastic pemphigus usually have a poor prognosis, although several cases of prolonged survival have been reported.[914,915]

Antibodies have been detected to multiple antigens, including members of the plakin family as well as the desmogleins. Specifically they include:

- desmoplakin I (250 kd)
- envoplakin (210 kd), originally thought to be desmoplakin II[916]
- bullous pemphigoid antigen (230 kd)
- periplakin (190 kd)[917–919]
- γ-catenin (plakoglobin – 82 kd)[920]
- HD1/plectin (500 kd)[921,922]
- an unidentified 170 kd antigen
- desmoglein I and II.[923–925]

Antibodies to one or both of the desmogleins are usually, but not always, present.[926] Epitope spreading is probably responsible for the diversity of the antibodies and the clinicopathological changes.[927,928] The initial lichenoid reaction may promote the exposure of self-antigens and the development of subsequent and progressive humoral autoimmunity.[928] The diversity of auto-antibodies that may deposit in the skin, lungs and other organs has led to the suggestion of the encompassing term 'paraneoplastic autoimmune multiorgan syndrome' or PAMS.[900]

In addition to this humoral component, there appears to be a major contribution of cytotoxic T lymphocytes to the pathogenesis.[897]

Histopathology

The histological features are variable, reflecting the polymorphous clinical features (Fig. 6.19). There is usually a lichenoid tissue reaction (interface dermatitis) with exocytosis of lymphocytes, apoptotic (dyskeratotic) keratinocytes and basal vacuolar change. These features are usually combined with suprabasal acantholysis and clefting, but this change is not invariably found even when multiple sections are examined.[929–931] In one study, 27% of cases had suprabasal acantholysis alone.[932] Focal epidermal spongiosis is often present. Subepidermal clefting is uncommonly a major feature. Rarely, verrucous lesions with acanthosis and papillomatosis have been seen. Suprabasal acantholysis has been seen in a malignant melanoma. The authors suggested that this was a localized variant of paraneoplastic pemphigus.[933]

The dermal infiltrate is often heavy and band-like, although there is usually some extension of the infiltrate into the reticular dermis. Most of the cells are lymphocytes but occasional eosinophils and neutrophils may also be present.[934]

Direct immunofluorescence shows intercellular and basement membrane staining with C3 and/or IgG, reminiscent of pemphigus erythematosus.[934,935] Indirect immunofluorescence using murine bladder epithelium shows

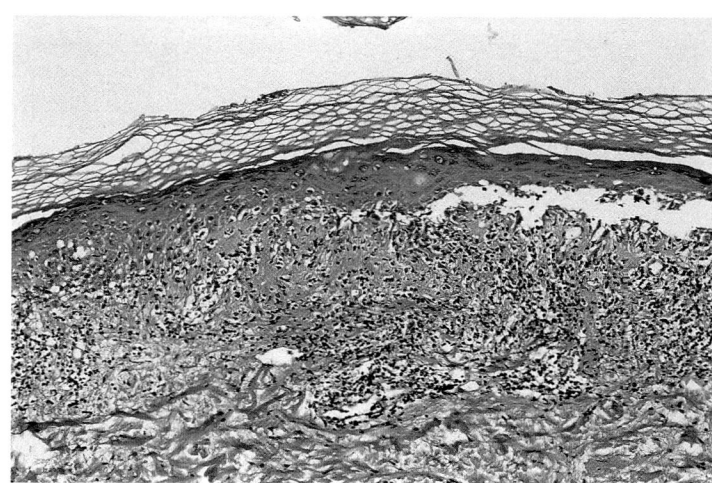

Fig. 6.19 **Paraneoplastic pemphigus.** There are erythema multiforme-like changes in one area and pemphigus vulgaris-like changes in others. (H & E)

intercellular staining of the epithelium.[936] This test was originally regarded as highly specific and sensitive, although one study has reported negative findings in nearly 25% of cases.[937]

FIXED DRUG ERUPTIONS

A bullous variant of fixed drug eruption has been described. The lesions resemble those seen in erythema multiforme; in fixed drug eruptions there is usually deeper extension of the inflammatory cell infiltrate in the dermis, with more eosinophils and sometimes neutrophils in the infiltrate, and melanin in macrophages and lying free in the upper dermis. The inflammatory cell infiltrate tends to obscure the dermoepidermal interface (interface dermatitis) adjacent to the blister in both erythema multiforme and fixed drug eruptions.

LICHEN SCLEROSUS ET ATROPHICUS

Lichen sclerosus et atrophicus is a chronic dermatosis affecting predominantly the anogenital region of middle-aged and elderly women. Infrequently, hemorrhagic bullae develop. There is a broad zone of edema or partly sclerotic collagen in the base of the blister with telangiectatic vessels and some hemorrhage. Beneath this edematous/sclerotic zone there is an infiltrate of lymphocytes which is predominantly perivascular in position.

LICHEN PLANUS PEMPHIGOIDES

Lichen planus pemphigoides is characterized by the development of tense blisters, often located on the extremities, in a patient with lichen planus. There is a mild perivascular infiltrate of lymphocytes and sometimes there are a few eosinophils and neutrophils beneath the blister. Occasional Civatte bodies are usually present in the basal layer at the margins of the blister. Direct immunofluorescence will usually demonstrate IgG and C3 in the basement membrane zone.

If the bullae develop in papules of lichen planus, as opposed to otherwise uninvolved skin, there is usually a much heavier dermal infiltrate which is superficial and band-like in distribution. There are numerous Civatte bodies in the overlying and adjacent basal keratinocytes. The term 'bullous lichen planus' is used in these circumstances.

POLYMORPHOUS LIGHT ERUPTION

Papulovesicular lesions and, rarely, bullae may occur as a clinical subset of polymorphous light eruption. The lesions develop several hours after exposure to the sun. There is pronounced subepidermal edema leading to blister formation. In early lesions the collagen fibers are separated by the edema fluid, giving a cobweb-like appearance. Extravasation of red blood cells may be present in this region. A characteristic feature is the presence of a perivascular infiltrate of lymphocytes which involves not only the superficial dermis but also the deep dermis.

FUNGAL INFECTIONS

Pronounced subepidermal edema leading to vesiculation is a rare manifestation of a fungal infection. It may also be seen in the autoeczematous reaction ('id reaction') to a fungus (see p. 112).

DERMAL ALLERGIC CONTACT DERMATITIS

This poorly understood variant of allergic contact dermatitis may result from contact with various agents, in particular neomycin and zinc and nickel salts. There is pronounced subepidermal edema leading to vesiculation. The lymphocytes in the infiltrate do not extend as deeply in the dermis as they do in polymorphous light eruption. Epidermal spongiosis is often present and it distinguishes this condition from the other subepidermal blistering diseases.

BULLOUS LEPROSY

Subepidermal bullae are an exceedingly rare manifestation of borderline lepromatous leprosy. Lymphocytes and small collections of macrophages, some with foamy cytoplasm, are present in the dermis; they also surround small cutaneous nerves. Acid-fast bacilli are present within the macrophages.

BULLOUS MYCOSIS FUNGOIDES

Bullae are a very rare manifestation of mycosis fungoides. They are usually subepidermal in location but intraepidermal splitting has been recorded. The presence of atypical lymphocytes in the underlying dermis and of Pautrier microabscesses in the epidermis characterizes this condition.

SUBEPIDERMAL BLISTERS WITH EOSINOPHILS

Eosinophils are a conspicuous and major component of the inflammatory cell infiltrate in the bullae and in the dermis in bullous pemphigoid and pemphigoid gestationis. They are also found in certain arthropod reactions, particularly in sensitized individuals, and in some bullous drug reactions. Vesiculobullous lesions, resembling insect bites, have been reported in patients with chronic lymphocytic leukemia.[938] Eosinophils may be the predominant cell type in some cases of dermatitis herpetiformis (particularly lesions that are more than 48 hours old) and of cicatricial pemphigoid. They are also present in the subepidermal blisters that sometimes develop in Wells' syndrome (see p. 1060).

BULLOUS PEMPHIGOID

Bullous pemphigoid is a chronic subepidermal blistering disease that occurs primarily in the elderly.[939–941] Multiple, tense bullae of varying size develop on normal or erythematous skin. Individual lesions may measure several centimeters in diameter. In addition, there may be erythematous macules, urticarial plaques and crusted erosions.[942] Annular lesions have been reported.[943] Eczematous or urticarial lesions, usually pruritic, may precede by weeks or months the occurrence of bullous lesions.[944–946] Rarely, this prodromal phase of bullous pemphigoid does not progress to a blistering stage.[947,948] Uncommon presentations of bullous pemphigoid include as an erythroderma,[949–951] or figurate erythema,[952,953] the development of lesions localized to one area of the body,[954] such as the vulva,[955–957] the legs (particularly the pretibial skin),[958–961] the paralyzed side in hemiplegia,[962] a stoma site[963] or the palms and soles,[964] and the development of a hemorrhagic pompholyx.[965–968] The localized variants of bullous pemphigoid must be distinguished from localized cicatricial pemphigoid in which scarring occurs (see p. 163) and from acute edema blisters which may form on the legs in association with rapidly developing edema.[969] In established cases of bullous pemphigoid, bullae are found on the lower part of the abdomen, in the groins and on the flexor surface of the arms and legs. Oral lesions are present in 10–40% of cases, but involvement of other mucosal surfaces is quite rare.[973–972] Eosinophilia in the blood and elevated serum IgE and eosinophil cationic protein levels are often present.[942,973–975] The disease tends to involve older people,[942,976] but its occurrence in young adults[977] and children has been reported.[978–984] An association with HLA-DQ7 has been reported in men.[985] Bullous pemphigoid is the most common subepidermal bullous disease with an annual incidence, in a recent French series, of seven cases per 1 000 000 people.[986] It accounts for approximately 80% of all subepidermal autoimmune bullous diseases.[987]

Several rare clinical variants of bullous pemphigoid have been reported (see below). Immunoelectron microscopy of these variants has shown that the immunoreactants deposit in the same position in the basement zone as they do in bullous pemphigoid; this justifies their inclusion as variants of bullous pemphigoid.[961,988,989]

Vesicular pemphigoid

There is a chronic eruption of small vesicles which are often pruritic and occasionally grouped, resembling dermatitis herpetiformis.[990,991] Progression to typical bullous pemphigoid sometimes occurs.[990] Autoantibodies in this variant can be heterogeneous.[992,993] In one case they were to plectin[994] and, in another, to desmoplakin.[995]

Pemphigoid vegetans

Pemphigoid vegetans is a rare variant that resembles pemphigus vegetans clinically with purulent and verrucous vegetating lesions in intertriginous areas, particularly the groins.[996–1000] Inflammatory bowel disease is usually present in patients with this form of bullous pemphigoid.[996] The autoantibodies, which are primarily in the IgG$_4$ subclass, react with the 230 kd major bullous pemphigoid antigen.[999]

Polymorphic pemphigoid

This term 'polymorphic pemphigoid' has been used for cases with features of both dermatitis herpetiformis and bullous pemphigoid.[1001,1002] Some of these cases would now be regarded as examples of linear IgA disease.[1003] The probable coexistence of bullous pemphigoid and dermatitis herpetiformis has also been reported.[1004]

Pemphigoid excoriée

The term 'pemphigoid excoriée' was given to a case in which the bullae were localized to areas of chronic excoriation.[1005]

Pemphigoid nodularis

Pemphigoid nodularis is a rare variant combining features of prurigo nodularis with those of bullous pemphigoid, often in the same lesion.[959,1006–1009] The verrucous papules or nodules may persist or resolve with scarring. Sometimes the nodules precede the onset of blisters by several months.[1010] A case with hyperkeratotic islands within areas of denuded blisters, reported as 'pemphigoid en cocarde', is best regarded as a variant of pemphigoid nodularis.[1011]

A wide range of diseases, many of presumed autoimmune origin, is reported in association with bullous pemphigoid.[1012] They include rheumatoid arthritis,[1013] systemic lupus erythematosus,[1014–1016] primary biliary cirrhosis,[1017] ulcerative colitis,[1018] alopecia areata,[1019] diabetes mellitus,[1020] thyroid disease,[1021,1022] multiple sclerosis,[1023] amyotrophic lateral sclerosis,[1024] leukocytoclastic vasculitis,[1025] a myelodysplastic syndrome,[1026] silicosis,[1027] neurofibromatosis,[1028] C4 deficiency,[1029] autoimmune thrombocytopenia,[1030] acanthosis palmaris,[1031] immune complex nephritis,[1032–1034] pemphigus,[1035]

psoriasis[1036–1038] and internal or cutaneous cancer.[1039–1044] It now appears, however, that the association of bullous pemphigoid with autoimmune diseases and with internal cancer is not statistically significant.[1045,1046]

Bullous pemphigoid runs a chronic course of months to years, with periods of remission and exacerbation.[377] Death is now uncommon in this disease because of improved management.[377] Death is more likely in elderly patients with extensive disease, and in those with antibodies to BP180 (see below).[1047]

Pathogenesis

The initial event in the pathogenesis of bullous pemphigoid appears to be the binding of autoantibodies to a transmembrane antigen associated with the lamina lucida and the hemidesmosomes of basal keratinocytes (the bullous pemphigoid antigen).[1048–1052] The bullous pemphigoid antigen shows molecular heterogeneity:[940,1053–1056] one antigen (BP230, BPAg1) is a 230 kd polypeptide which is assembled in macromolecular aggregates within the hemidesmosomes;[1057,1058] the other (BP180, BPAg2) is a 180 kd transmembrane glycoprotein with both intracellular and extracellular relationships with the hemidesmosomes.[1059–1061]

BP180 consists of an intracellular N-terminal portion, a transmembrane region and a long collagenous extracellular domain (type XVII collagen) that spans the lamina lucida and extends to the lamina densa.[1062] A non-collagenous stretch of this ectodomain, designated NC16A, harbors four major epitopes recognized by serum samples from patients with bullous pemphigoid.[1063–1065] A portion of the extracellular domain of BP180 is identical to an antigen found in linear IgA bullous dermatosis, LABD97. Antibodies may occur to this segment in bullous pemphigoid.[1066] Male patients are more likely to have antibodies to BP180, whereas antibodies to BP230 occur with equal frequency.[1067] A defect in the BP180 gene is the defect in the so-called 'GABEB variant' of junctional epidermolysis bullosa, also known as junctional epidermolysis bullosa, non-Herlitz type (see p. 146).

BP230, a member of the plakin family of proteins and regulated by homeoprotein transcription factors,[1068] is restricted to the intracellular hemidesmosomal plaque. Autoantibodies to this antigen were originally thought not to be involved in the initiation of the disease.[1065,1069] However, their role may have been underestimated as it appears that they may precipitate and perpetuate the disease.[1070] Molecular genetic studies have revealed distinct chromosomal localizations for the two bullous pemphigoid antigens.[1056] The major antigenic epitopes of the 230 kd protein map within the C-terminal end.[1071] Autoantibodies to this antigen or a complex of this with the 180 kd antigen are present in up to 80% of patients with bullous pemphigoid, and to the 180 kd antigen (BP180) in approximately 30% of patients.[1072,1073] Approximately 20% of patients have antibodies directed solely to BP180.[1072] The clinical expression of the disease has been thought to be the same, no matter which antigen is present.[1074] However, recent studies have found evidence that antibodies to the 180 kd antigen (BP180, BPAg2) are more often associated with oral lesions, a disease less responsive to steroids, and poor prognosis.[1075,1076] Serum levels of autoantibodies to BP180 correlate with disease activity.[1065,1077] IgG$_4$, IgG$_1$ and IgE are the major immunoglobulins targeting the NC16A domain of BP180 in bullous pemphigoid.[1078,1079] IgA autoantibodies to various antigens have also been found.[1080,1081] Their presence is not associated with any clinical differences; nor is the presence of antibodies to the C-terminal region of BP180, as found in cicatricial pemphigoid.[1082] In rare cases, antibodies have been described to other antigens – 190 kd,[1083] 105 kd, 120 kd,[1084] 240 and 138 kd,[1085] 125 kd[1086] – and to plectin[1087] and desmoplakin.[1088] It is worth noting that the bullous pemphigoid antigens are distinct from α6/β4 integrin, another major antigen localized on the hemidesmosomes.[1089] This antigen is usually destroyed in areas of blistering.[8] Following the fixation of antibody to the bullous pemphigoid antigens, complement is activated leading to the chemotaxis of neutrophils and eosinophils.[411] Mast cells, eotaxin and IL-5 may also be important in the recruitment of eosinophils.[1090–1092] The neutrophils and eosinophils release proteolytic enzymes which appear to be responsible for the initial stages of blister formation.[86,975,1093] Antibodies binding antigenic sites on the intracellular domains of BP180 may also play a role in the blister formation. Whether this results from internalization of immune complexes or epitope spreading remains to be determined.[1094–1096] Vascular permeability factor is strongly expressed in bullous pemphigoid, leading to increased microvascular permeability, followed by papillary edema which, in turn, contributes to the formation of the blister.[1097]

Experimentally, autoantibodies to BP180 trigger a signal transducing event that leads to the release of interleukin-6 (IL-6) and interleukin-8 (IL-8) from cultured human keratinocytes.[1098] In another experiment, T-cell lines from patients with bullous pemphigoid reacted with the same epitopes on the BP180 ectodomain as did the autoantibodies,[1099] supporting a role for cellular mechanisms in the pathogenesis of bullous pemphigoid.[1099–1101]

Etiologic triggers

Although the pathogenetic mechanisms involved in blister formation are reasonably well understood, what triggers the formation of the antibodies to the hemidesmosome antigens is unknown. Drugs have been incriminated in a few cases, although there is some evidence that the antibodies involved in drug-related cases are, in part, different from those found in usual cases of bullous pemphigoid. The implicated drugs include penicillin derivatives,[1102–1104] sulfasalazine, ibuprofen,[1105] phenacetin,[1106] enalapril,[1107] captopril, novoscabin, levobunolol ophthalmic solution,[1108] tetracoq, influenza, tetanus and other vaccinations,[1109–1113] nifedipine,[1114,1115] doxazosin,[1114] serratiopeptidase,[1116] cephalexin,[1117] bumetanide,[1118] fluoxetine,[1119] chloroquine,[1120] antipsychotic drugs,[1121] ciprofloxacin,[1122] furosemide (frusemide),[1123,1124] neuroleptics,[1125] penicillamine[1126] and topical fluorouracil.[1106] Trauma,[1124,1127] burns,[864,1128–1130] phototherapy[1131] and radiation[1132–1134] have been implicated in a very small number of cases.

Histopathology[499,1135]

In bullous pemphigoid there is a unilocular subepidermal blister, eosinophils being the predominant cell in the dermis and blister cavity (Fig. 6.20). If the biopsy is taken from a bulla on otherwise normal-appearing skin, there is only a sparse dermal infiltrate; bullae with an erythematous base have a much heavier infiltrate of inflammatory cells in the upper dermis. Eosinophilic 'flame figures' are a rare finding.[1136] In addition to eosinophils there are some neutrophils and lymphocytes. Eosinophilic spongiosis may be seen in the clinically erythematous skin bordering the blister.[1137]

In lesions of several days' duration, the blister may appear intraepidermal in location at its periphery as a result of regeneration. Sometimes epidermal necrosis occurs in the roof of the blister.[1138] There are no isolated, necrotic, basal keratinocytes in the roof of early blisters, as sometimes are seen in pemphigoid gestationis.

The variants of bullous pemphigoid (see above) show some distinguishing histological features reflecting their different clinical appearances. In *vesicular pemphigoid* the lesions are quite small (Fig. 6.21), while in *pemphigoid vegetans* there is usually prominent acanthosis of the epidermis. Acanthosis is also present in *pemphigoid nodularis*; in addition there is overlying hyperkeratosis and mild papillomatosis.

Prodromal lesions of bullous pemphigoid show edema of the papillary dermis and a superficial and mid-dermal perivascular infiltrate with numerous eosinophils, occasional lymphocytes and rare neutrophils. Interstitial

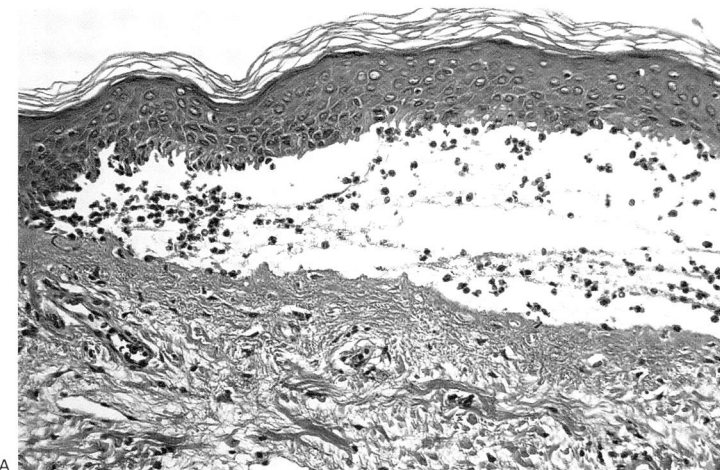

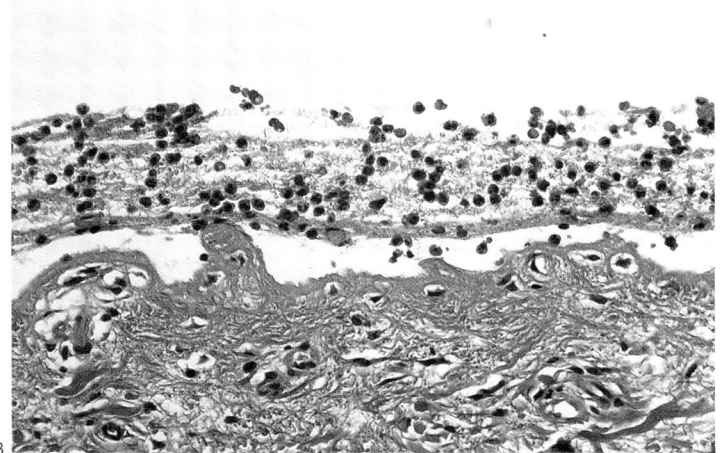

Fig. 6.20 **Bullous pemphigoid. (A)** There is a subepidermal blister, the lumen of which contains eosinophils. **(B)** There are relatively few eosinophils ('cell poor') in the dermis. (H & E)

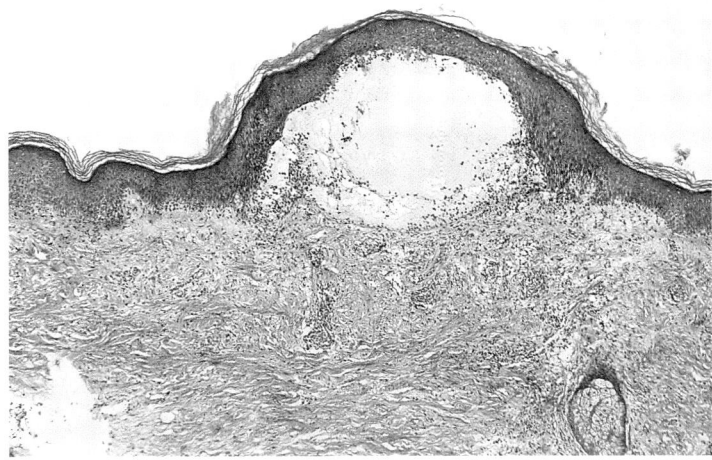

Fig. 6.21 **Vesicular pemphigoid.** There is a small subepidermal blister. (H & E)

eosinophils may also be present. There are usually more eosinophils than in an arthropod bite reaction. A few eosinophils are found within the epidermis (Fig. 6.22).

A case that commenced with the histological features of erythema multiforme and progressed to bullous pemphigoid has been reported.[1139]

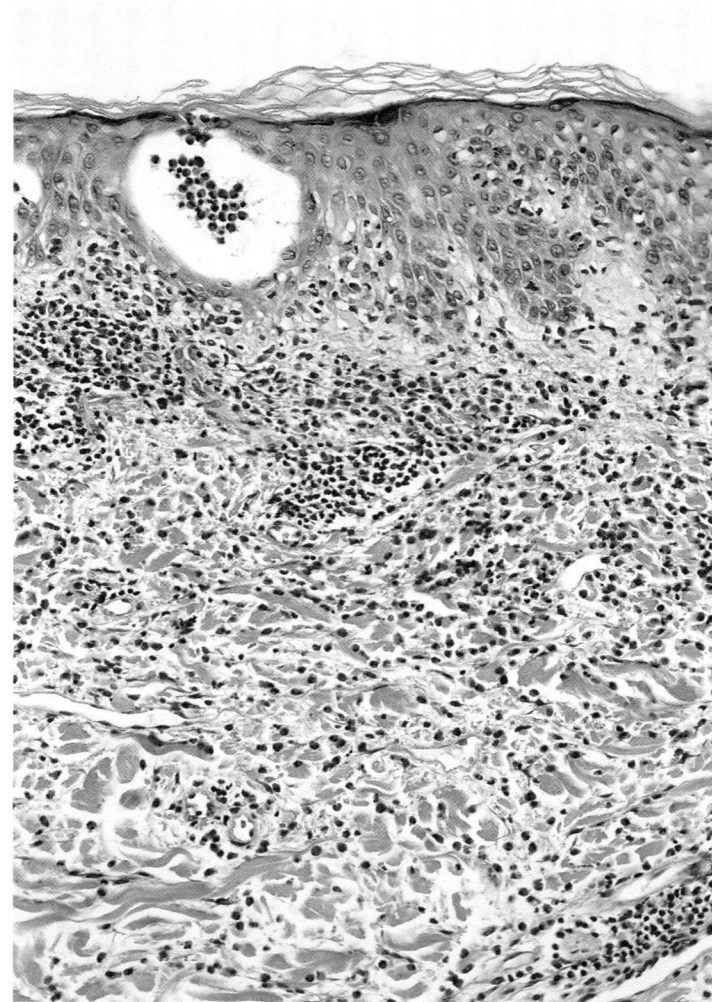

Fig. 6.22 **Bullous pemphigoid, prodromal stage.** There is focal eosinophilic spongiosis, and numerous dermal eosinophils are present. (H & E)

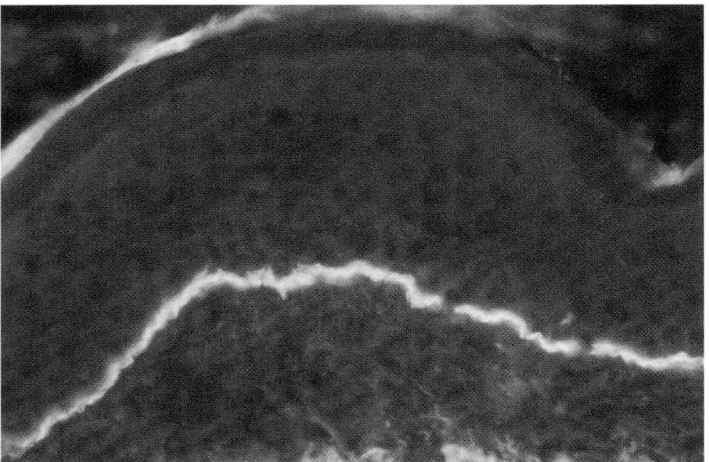

Fig. 6.23 **Bullous pemphigoid.** The basement membrane zone shows a linear pattern of staining for C3. (Direct immunofluorescence)

non-bullous dermatoses. Localization of the target antigen is possible if the substrate is salt-split skin.[1157,1158] A further method to help localize the anatomical level of the split is staining for type IV collagen; it is present in the base of the blister. Basement membrane zone antibodies have also been detected by indirect immunofluorescence in the urine of patients with bullous pemphigoid.[1159]

Electron microscopy[939,1090,1160,1161]

In the cell-poor blisters there is focal thinning and disruption of anchoring filaments with formation of the split in the lamina lucida. In the cell-rich lesions there is more extensive damage in the basement membrane zone following the migration of eosinophils into this region. There is disintegration of the lamina lucida and fragmentation of anchoring fibrils and hemidesmosomes. The basal cells may show some vacuolization.

Immunoelectron microscopy shows that the immunoreactants are in the lamina lucida and in the vicinity of the cytoplasmic plaque of the basal cell hemidesmosomes.[981,1050] Some deposits are located on the intracellular portion of the hemidesmosomes.[1162] There are no deposits beneath melanocytes.

PEMPHIGOID GESTATIONIS

Pemphigoid gestationis (also known as herpes gestationis) is a rare, pruritic, vesiculobullous dermatosis of pregnancy and the puerperium.[1163–1170] It occurs in approximately 1 in 50 000 pregnancies and rarely in association with hydatidiform mole[1168,1171] and choriocarcinoma.[1172] The onset of the disease is usually in the second or third trimester of pregnancy with the development of papules and urticarial plaques, initially localized to the periumbilical region. Subsequently, the lesions spread to involve the trunk and extremities, becoming vesiculobullous in form.[1163] Untreated, the lesions persist through the pregnancy, but they subside within several days or weeks of delivery;[1173] persistence for many months or years has been reported.[1174–1176] Oral contraceptives sometimes cause exacerbations.[1177] Cases with overlap features with bullous pemphigoid have been reported, as has the conversion of pemphigoid gestationis to bullous pemphigoid.[1178,1179]

Pemphigoid gestationis usually recurs in subsequent pregnancies and at an earlier stage.[1180] 'Skipped' pregnancies are more likely to occur following a change in paternity or when the mother and fetus are fully compatible at the HLA-D locus.[1170,1172]

There were no features to suggest paraneoplastic pemphigus. In another case, suprabasal acantholysis preceded the development of bullous pemphigoid.[1140]

Direct immunofluorescence almost invariably shows a linear, homogeneous deposition of IgG and/or C3 along the basement membrane zone of the skin around the lesion (Fig. 6.23).[1141–1143] In early stages of the disease only C3 may be present. IgM and IgA are present in approximately 20% of cases.[1144] Using salt-split skin, the immunoreactants are found on the epidermal side of the preparation, in contrast to epidermolysis bullosa acquisita where they are found on the dermal side.[1145] Uncommonly, deposits are found on the dermal side in bullous pemphigoid, but the reasons for this are unclear;[1146–1148] it has been suggested that extracellular epitopes of the 180 kd antigen are separated from the epidermis during the salt-splitting process.[1149] A new technique, fluorescence overlay antigen mapping (FOAM), can be used to increase the sensitivity and resolution capability of conventional immunofluorescence microscopy.[1150] Microwave irradiation in urea may be used to retrieve the bullous pemphigoid antigen from paraffin-embedded material.[1151]

Circulating anti-basement membrane zone antibodies, usually of IgG class, are present in 60–80% of patients, depending on the substrate used.[1152–1155] Their titer does not correlate with disease activity or severity. Antibodies may be absent when circulating immune complexes are formed.[1156] Similar antibodies are present in some cases of cicatricial pemphigoid and, rarely, in

Most reports have shown an increased fetal morbidity and mortality related to premature delivery, but in one large study there was no increase in spontaneous abortions or stillbirths.[1181,1182] Only rarely does the infant develop transient vesicular lesions resembling those of the mother.[1180,1183,1184]

Pemphigoid gestationis has been reported in association with other autoimmune diseases, particularly Graves' disease.[1170,1185,1186] It also occurs more frequently in patients with the HLA antigens DR3-DR4.[1172,1187-1189] This HLA phenotype is thought to confer a state of heightened immune responsiveness.[1172] A major initiating event in pemphigoid gestationis is the aberrant expression of the class II molecules of the major histocompatibility complex in the placenta.[1190,1191] Using sensitive techniques it has been found that all patients with pemphigoid gestationis possess a circulating autoantibody of IgG_1 class (the pemphigoid gestationis factor) which has complement-binding activity.[1192-1194] This antibody is directed against a placental matrix antigen which crossreacts with an antigen in the basement membrane of skin.[1172] The antigen has been further characterized as a basement zone glycoprotein of 180 kd which is similar to the bullous pemphigoid antigen (BP180). Epitope mapping analyses have revealed that both bullous pemphigoid and pemphigoid gestationis sera react with one of four (possibly five) epitopes within the non-collagenous domain (NC16A) of BP180.[1195] The major epitopes targeted have been called MCW-1 and MCW-2. There is no reaction to MCW-4, the site targeted in lichen planus pemphigoides.[1195] Some binding of antibody to BP230 may occur.[1196] Antibodies in both the IgG_3 and IgG_1 subclasses have been found.[1195] A cytotoxic anti-HLA antibody has also been demonstrated.[1197,1198] They may develop coincidentally with the anti-basement membrane zone antibodies, reflecting a common immunological event.[1199] Activation of complement and the release of toxic cationic proteins from eosinophils have an effector role in the formation of the cutaneous lesions.[1200]

Histopathology [1177,1180,1201]

In early urticarial lesions there is marked edema of the papillary dermis and a superficial and mid-dermal infiltrate of lymphocytes, histiocytes and eosinophils. The infiltrate is predominantly perivascular in location. Overlying the tips of the dermal papillae there is often focal spongiosis and, sometimes, necrosis of basal keratinocytes. The vesiculobullous lesions that form are subepidermal. They contain eosinophils, lymphocytes and histiocytes; a similar infiltrate is present in the superficial dermis (Fig. 6.24). The eosinophils usually form microabscesses in the dermal papillae. A small number of neutrophils may also be present.

Direct immunofluorescence shows C3 and, sometimes, IgG in a linear pattern along the basement membrane zone.[1180,1202,1203] These immunoreactants are found in the lamina lucida, as in bullous pemphigoid.[1204,1205] That is, using salt-split skin, the immunoreactants are on the epidermal side. One case with coexisting intercellular IgG deposits has been reported.[1206] Eosinophil major basic protein can also be detected in the upper dermis by immunofluorescent techniques.[1200] It is more abundant than in PUPPP (see p. 244).[1207] Circulating anti-basement membrane zone antibodies are uncommon.[1208] As mentioned above, a circulating factor (the pemphigoid gestationis factor), which fixes complement at the dermoepidermal junction of normal human skin, is found in 80% of cases;[1209,1210] this figure increases to 100% if sensitive techniques are used.[1172]

Electron microscopy [1201,1202,1211]

The cleavage occurs at the level of the sub-basal dense plate.[1181] Cleavage through upper hemidesmosomal structures can occur in parallel. Degenerative changes are present in some of the basal cells.[1202]

ARTHROPOD BITES

The bite of certain arthropods will result in a bullous lesion in susceptible individuals.[1212] There may be a subepidermal blister or a mixed intraepidermal and subepidermal lesion with thin strands of keratinocytes bridging the bulla (Fig. 6.25). Eosinophils are usually present in the blister. The dermal infiltrate consists of lymphocytes and eosinophils around vessels in the superficial and deep dermis; interstitial eosinophils are also present.

DRUG REACTIONS

Certain drugs may produce a vesiculobullous eruption which resembles bullous pemphigoid both clinically and histologically. At other times the resemblance is less complete. The second generation quinolones (such as ciprofloxacin and lomefloxacin) may produce subepidermal blisters with a mixed cellular infiltrate, including eosinophils.[1213] The reaction is often photo-exacerbated.

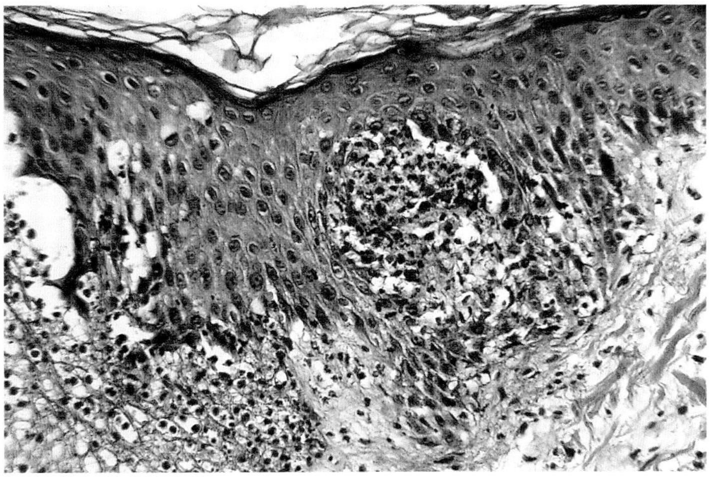

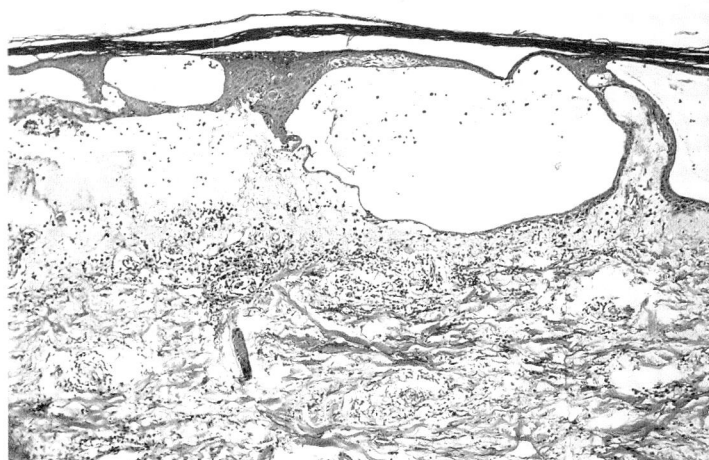

Fig. 6.24 Pemphigoid gestationis. There is subepidermal clefting with both neutrophils and eosinophils in the dermal infiltrate. (H & E)

Fig. 6.25 Arthropod bite reaction in a sensitized person. Thin columns of surviving keratinocytes produce a characteristic multilocular blister which is both intraepidermal and subepidermal. There are many eosinophils in the inflammatory infiltrate. (H & E)

EPIDERMOLYSIS BULLOSA

Eosinophils have been found in the bullae of all three major subtypes of epidermolysis bullosa, particularly in blisters biopsied in the neonatal period. The presence of eosinophils does not appear to characterize any particular subtype.[610]

SUBEPIDERMAL BLISTERS WITH NEUTROPHILS

Neutrophils are a major component of the inflammatory cell infiltrate in the dermis in early lesions of dermatitis herpetiformis and in linear IgA bullous dermatosis, cicatricial pemphigoid, ocular cicatricial pemphigoid and localized cicatricial pemphigoid. Bullae are an uncommon manifestation of urticaria, acute vasculitis, lupus erythematosus, erysipelas and Sweet's syndrome. Neutrophils are abundant in some inflammatory forms of epidermolysis bullosa acquisita and in the recently described entities of deep lamina lucida (anti-p105) pemphigoid and anti-p200 pemphigoid. A 'superficial neutrophilic dermolysis with subepidermal bulla formation' has been reported in a patient with hepatobiliary disease.[1214]

DERMATITIS HERPETIFORMIS

Dermatitis herpetiformis is a rare, chronic, subepidermal blistering disorder characterized by the presence of intensely pruritic papules and vesicles, granular deposition of IgA in the dermal papillae, and a high incidence of gluten-sensitive enteropathy.[1215–1219] It is of uncertain pathogenesis.

The cutaneous papulovesicles have a characteristic herpetiform grouping and a predilection for extensor surfaces, usually in symmetrical distribution.[1216] Sites of involvement include the elbows, the knees, the shoulders, the nape of the neck, the sacral area and the scalp; mucous membranes are infrequently involved.[1220–1222] In addition to papulovesicles, excoriations are almost invariably present. Bullae are quite uncommon.[1216] Onset of the disease is most frequent in early adult life, but it may occur at any age, including childhood.[1223,1224] There is a male preponderance; in women with the disease, perimenstrual exacerbations sometimes occur.[1225] The HLA antigens B8, DR3, DQ2, and DQ8 on chromosome 6, are increased in frequency in those with the disease.[1226–1229] The concordance of dermatitis herpetiformis and celiac disease occurs in monozygous twins.[1229]

A gluten-sensitive enteropathy is present in approximately 90% of cases, although clinical symptoms of this are quite uncommon. A gluten-free diet usually leads to a reversal of the intestinal villous atrophy and improved control of the skin lesions.[1230] This diet also has a protective effect against the development of lymphoma.[1231] There is also a high incidence of gluten-sensitive enteropathy in relatives, although very few of the relatives with an enteropathy have dermatitis herpetiformis.[1232]

Circulating antibodies to reticulin,[1233] gliadin,[1234] nuclear components, human jejunum,[1235] gastric parietal cells[1236] and thyroid antigens[1237] have been reported in variable percentages. Only the presence of IgA-class endomysial antibodies is of diagnostic importance.[1233,1238–1241] They are present in 70% of patients with dermatitis herpetiformis on a normal diet and in 100% of those with villous atrophy.[1242] The autoantigen of endomysial antibodies in celiac disease is tissue transglutaminase (tTG), an enzyme involved in crosslinking certain intracellular and extracellular molecules.[1243] Gluten challenge usually converts seronegative cases to seropositive, while a gluten-free diet results in a rapid decrease in the titer of various antibodies.[1242,1244,1245] Demonstration of this antibody to tTG may assist in making a diagnosis of dermatitis herpetiformis when clinical and histological features are equivocal.[1246,1247]

Dermatitis herpetiformis has been associated sporadically with auto-immune thyroid disease,[1248] ulcerative colitis,[1249–1251] systemic lupus erythematosus,[1252] rheumatoid arthritis,[1248] Sjögren's syndrome,[1250,1253] Addison's disease,[1254] primary biliary cirrhosis,[1255] lichen planopilaris,[1256] atopic disorders,[1257] vitiligo, alopecia areata[1250] and immune complex nephritis.[1258] Although there are reports of its association with internal cancers, only the development of intestinal lymphomas appears to be of statistical significance.[1040,1259]

If untreated, dermatitis herpetiformis has a protracted course although there may be long periods of remission.[1260,1261] Individual lesions persist for days to weeks. Iodine and non-steroidal anti-inflammatory drugs may provoke or exacerbate the disease in susceptible individuals.[1262,1263] Two cases of dermatitis herpetiformis precipitated by the use of a commercial cleaning solution have been reported.[1264]

Pathogenesis

The pathogenesis of dermatitis herpetiformis is still unknown, but it has been suggested that IgA antibodies formed in the gut somehow fix to the skin.[1260,1265,1266] The role of the IgA autoantibodies to tissue transglutaminase remains to be clarified. They are not present in other immunobullous diseases. The deposits are partly localized to the microfibrillar bundles in the dermal papillae, possibly to fibrillin-reactive fibrils.[1267] Other studies have shown a haphazard distribution of the deposits.[1268,1269] The IgA deposited in the skin was originally thought to be of A_1 class only,[1270] but IgA_2 has also been detected in these deposits.[1271] Whatever the mechanism involved in the formation and deposition of IgA deposits, it appears that the final common pathway involves activation of the complement system followed by chemotaxis of neutrophils into the papillary dermis.[1266] Cytokines such as endothelial leukocyte adhesion molecule (ELAM), IL-8 and granulocyte-macrophage colony-stimulating factor (GM-CSF) also contribute to the infiltration and activation of neutrophils.[1272,1273] Enzymes released from these neutrophils alter or destroy at least two basement membrane components (laminin and type IV collagen), contributing to the formation of blisters.[1274]

Although most studies have focused on the role of immune complexes in the pathogenesis of dermatitis herpetiformis, it appears that activated T cells may also be involved.[1275] Most of the T cells are CD45RO-positive memory cells;[1275] they do not bear the γ/δ receptor.[1276] Recent work suggests that cytokines from CD4$^+$ lymphocytes of the Th2 subtype play an important role in the pathogenesis of dermatitis herpetiformis.[1273,1277]

Histopathology[1216]

Early lesions are characterized by collections of neutrophils and a varying number of eosinophils at the tips of edematous dermal papillae, resulting in the so-called 'papillary microabscesses' (Fig. 6.26). Fibrin is also present near the tips of the dermal papillae, imparting a 'necrotic' appearance. An occasional acantholytic basal cell may also be found above the tips of the papillae.

In lesions of 36–48 hours' duration, the number of eosinophils in the infiltrate is proportionately increased. Some fragmentation of neutrophils is also present. Very occasionally, intraepidermal collections of neutrophils appear to be present, such cases requiring distinction from the very rare condition known as IgA pemphigus.

In older lesions, subepidermal vesiculation occurs, although initially the interpapillary ridges remain attached, leading to multilocularity of the vesicle;[1278] after a few days the attachments break down with the formation of a unilocular blister. The vesicles contain fibrin, neutrophils, eosinophils and

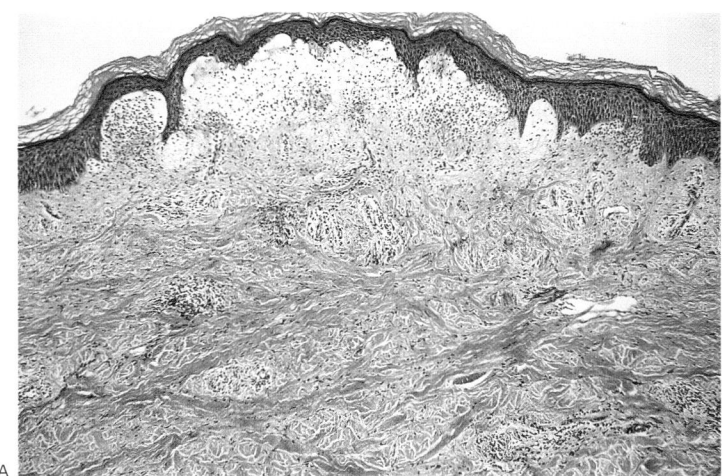

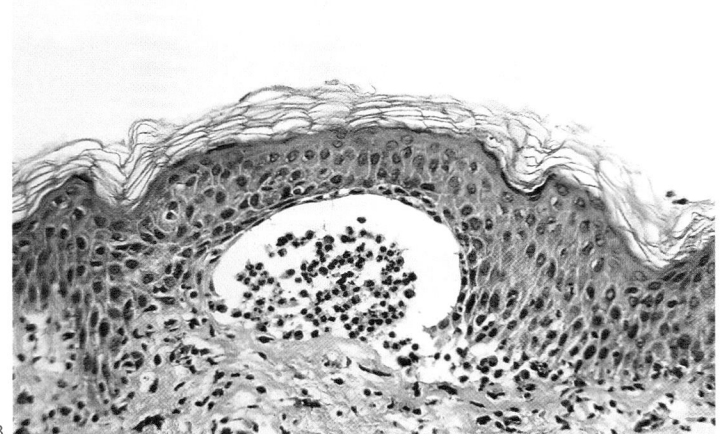

Fig. 6.26 **Dermatitis herpetiformis. (A)** There is a subepidermal blister. **(B)** A microabscess is present in a dermal papilla. (H & E)

very occasional 'shadow' epidermal cells.[1236] Aggregates of nuclear dust are sometimes present in the stratum corneum in the old (resolving) lesions.[1279]

Blood vessels in the upper and mid dermis are surrounded by an infiltrate of lymphocytes and histiocytes with a variable admixture of neutrophils and eosinophils. A vasculitis is rarely present. In urticarial lesions there is also marked edema of the upper dermis. Neutrophils may not be prominent in such lesions.

The histological distinction between dermatitis herpetiformis and linear IgA disease is almost impossible,[1280] although subtle distinguishing features have been reported[1278,1281] (see p. 160). Older lesions of dermatitis herpetiformis may resemble bullous pemphigoid, although eosinophils are usually more prominent in the latter condition.[1278] Rare cases with overlap features between dermatitis herpetiformis and other bullous diseases, including bullous pemphigoid, have been reported.[1282–1285] This is thought to be due to epitope spreading.[1286] It should be remembered that dermal papillary microabscesses can be seen not only in dermatitis herpetiformis but also in cicatricial pemphigoid, localized cicatricial pemphigoid, bullous lupus erythematosus, linear IgA bullous dermatosis and deep lamina lucida pemphigoid. Papillary microabscesses also form in pemphigoid gestationis but they are composed of eosinophils in most cases. Neutrophils are also found in some cases of epidermolysis bullosa acquisita.

Direct immunofluorescence shows granular deposits of IgA in the dermal papillae of perilesional and uninvolved skin, although the deposition is not uniform (Fig. 6.27).[1287,1288] The deposition is greatest in normal skin adjacent to an active lesion.[1289] A fibrillar pattern is sometimes recognized.[1290] Interestingly, IgA is not found in the skin in celiac disease without skin lesions.[1291] Experience has shown that if IgA is not detected, the disorder usually turns out to be a dermatosis other than dermatitis herpetiformis,[1292] although rarely IgA is found on a second biopsy when it was not demonstrated on the initial examination.[1293] In a small number of cases with negative immunofluorescent findings, antibodies to tTG will be present; such cases respond to a gluten-free diet.[1294] An immunohistochemical technique using the avidin–biotin–peroxidase complex and paraffin-embedded material has been found to be as effective as direct immunofluorescence in detecting IgA.[1295] Other immunoglobulins, particularly IgM, are present in almost 30% of all cases, while C3 is found in approximately 50%.[466,1293] Most studies have recorded a diminution in the quantity of IgA and in the incidence of C3 deposition in patients on a gluten-free diet.[1296]

The exact nosological position of cases with a granular linear pattern of IgA is uncertain,[1216] but they are best regarded as a subgroup of dermatitis herpetiformis.[1217]

Electron microscopy

Many early studies suggested that the blister formation occurred below the lamina lucida, corresponding to the site of the neutrophilic infiltrate. A more recent study has demonstrated the split within the lamina lucida.[1297]

Immunoelectron microscopy confirms that the IgA is present in clumps in the dermal papillae. Initially, the IgA was thought to be associated with microfibrillar bundles,[1298] but more recent studies have shown a somewhat haphazard deposition which only sometimes involves the microfibrillar bundles.[1268,1269]

LINEAR IgA BULLOUS DERMATOSIS

Linear IgA bullous dermatosis (linear IgA disease) is a rare, sulfone-responsive, subepidermal blistering disorder of unknown etiology in which smooth linear deposits of IgA are found in the basement membrane zone.[1217,1299–1303] There are two clinical variants – chronic bullous dermatosis of childhood and adult linear IgA bullous dermatosis. They are now regarded as different expressions of the same disease[1304] as both variants share the same target antigen (a 97 kd or 285 kd antigen in the upper lamina lucida).

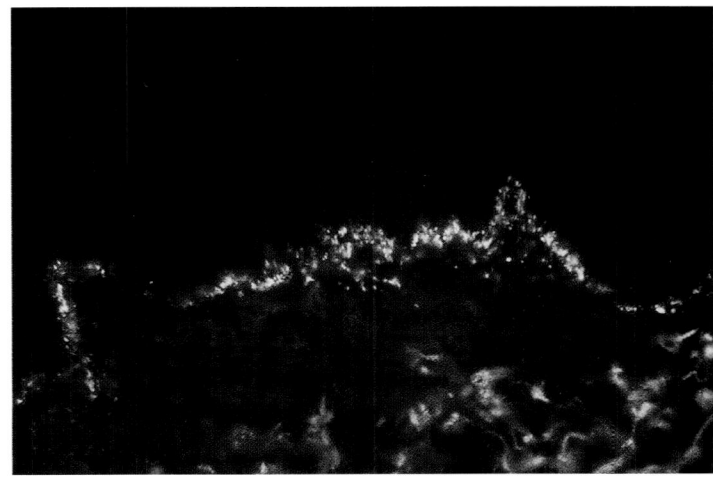

Fig. 6.27 **Dermatitis herpetiformis.** There are granular deposits of IgA in the dermal papillae. (Direct immunofluorescence)

Chronic bullous dermatosis of childhood

Chronic bullous dermatosis of childhood, known in the past as juvenile dermatitis herpetiformis,[1305] juvenile pemphigoid[1306] and linear IgA disease of childhood, is characterized by the abrupt onset, in the first decade of life, of large, tense bullae on a normal or erythematous base.[1300,1307–1310] They have a predilection for the perioral and genital regions, as well as the lower part of the abdomen and the thighs.[1311] Often there is a polycyclic grouping, the so-called 'cluster of jewels' sign.[1300] The disease usually runs a benign course with remission after several months or years.[1312,1313] In one series, 12% of the cases persisted beyond puberty.[1300] The entity known as childhood cicatricial pemphigoid appears to be a variant of chronic bullous dermatosis of childhood and is characterized by severe scarring lesions of mucosae, particularly the conjunctiva.[1300,1314]

Adult linear IgA bullous dermatosis

Adult linear IgA bullous dermatosis was originally regarded as a subgroup of dermatitis herpetiformis, but it is now known to differ from dermatitis herpetiformis by the absence of gluten-sensitive enteropathy[1315,1316] and IgA antiendomysial antibodies,[1239,1240] although antigliadin antibodies are sometimes present.[1234] Adult linear IgA bullous dermatosis has a heterogeneous clinical presentation which may clinically resemble dermatitis herpetiformis, bullous pemphigoid or other bullous disorders.[1001,1317–1321] Sometimes the lesions have an annular configuration.[1322] Bullae usually involve the trunk and limbs; facial and perineal lesions are not as frequent as in the childhood form.[1299] Rarely, the lesions are limited to seborrheic areas.[1323] An association with sarcoidosis,[1324] psoriasis,[1325] ulcerative colitis,[1326,1327] lymphocytic colitis,[1328] rheumatoid arthritis,[1329] lymphoma,[1330,1331] other malignant tumors,[1332–1336] immune complex glomerulonephritis[1337,1338] and chronic renal failure[1339] has been reported. The disease has also followed the therapeutic use of captopril,[1340] somatostatin,[1341] atorvastatin,[1342] furosemide (frusemide),[1343] glibenclamide,[1344] penicillin, cefamandole, interleukin-2,[1345] ceftriaxone and metronidazole,[1346] trimethoprim–sulfamethoxazole,[1341] lithium carbonate,[1347] amiodarone,[1348,1349] phenytoin,[1341,1350,1351] vancomycin[1352–1357] and non-steroidal anti-inflammatory drugs[1299,1358] such as piroxicam, naproxen and diclofenac.[1359] Contact with sodium hypochlorite and a burn from boiling methyl alcohol have also been incriminated.[1360,1361] The onset of the drug-related cases is usually within 4–14 days of the administration of the implicated drug.[1341] The eruption is self-limited and heals within several weeks of the cessation of the drug. In contrast, the usual adult case runs a chronic course and lesions may persist indefinitely.[1299,1362,1363] An improvement often occurs during pregnancy, although a relapse is frequent at approximately 3 months post partum.[1364] The childhood form often has remissions, and complete clearing sometimes occurs.

In both the adult and the childhood forms the lesions may be pruritic or burning.[1299] Hemorrhagic bullae may form.[1308] Mucosal involvement occurs in 80% or more of adults but less frequently in children.[1365–1367] Scarring conjunctival lesions sometimes develop.[1366,1368] Such cases may represent IgA variants of cicatricial pemphigoid.[1369,1370] Other findings have included severe arthralgia[1304] and the presence of organ-specific antibodies and of various histocompatibility antigens (Cw7, DR3), some of which differ from those found in dermatitis herpetiformis.[1227,1371] However, the incidence of HLA-B8 is increased in both dermatitis herpetiformis and chronic bullous dermatosis of childhood and marginally so in the adult form of the latter.[1299]

Pathogenesis

Linear IgA bullous dermatosis is a heterogeneous disease with regard to the localization of target antigens and antibody deposition.[1372–1377] The antigen for the major type (the lamina lucida type) was originally reported to be a 97 kd protein (ladinin) or a 120 kd protein (LAD-1).[1378,1379] It is now known that these proteins are a degradation product of the 180 kd bullous pemphigoid antigen (BP180). It has been suggested that the target antigen involves epitopes in the NC16A domain of BP180, although it has been claimed recently that the target is in the adjacent 15th collagenous domain.[1380–1385] In 10–15% of cases, the IgA autoantibodies are to antigens in the lamina densa; the antigen in many instances is not known.[1386] In some cases the antigen is type VII collagen, specifically the NC-1 domain, the immunodominant epitope for epidermolysis bullosa acquisita.[1387] It has been suggested that these cases be called IgA epidermolysis bullosa acquisita.[1388] Other target antigens have included 100 and 145 kd proteins,[1389] and 200 and 280 kd hemidesmosomal proteins distinct from any known target antigen in this region.[1390] Childhood cases with IgA antibodies against BP180 or BP230 have been reported.[1084,1391] The target antigen in drug-induced forms is also heterogeneous.[1344,1392] Studies using indirect immunofluorescence on salt-split skin have usually localized the target antigen to the upper lamina lucida, while studies using immunoelectron microscopy have shown a number of cases with deposits in the sublamina densa region of the dermis.[1374] In one series of 46 cases, only 4 had sublamina densa deposits.[1373] Circulating IgA antibodies are found in approximately 70% of childhood cases, but in only 20% of adult cases.[1299] A higher yield is obtained using split skin as the substrate.[1393] These antibodies are thought to have some pathogenetic significance despite their low incidence in the adult forms of the disease. In a small number of cases, circulating IgG antibodies are present as well.[1394,1395] Such cases have been called linear IgA/IgG bullous dermatosis (LAGBD). The antibodies appear to target the ectodomain of BP180.[1396] The clinical appearance and the histology of these cases resemble linear IgA bullous dermatosis.[1397–1399]

It appears that in both idiopathic and drug-induced cases, cytokines produced by CD4+ lymphocytes, enzymes released by neutrophils and eosinophils, and IgA deposits in the basement membrane zone all contribute to the specific tissue lesions.[1346,1400]

Histopathology

Linear IgA bullous dermatosis is a subepidermal blistering disease in which neutrophils are usually the predominant cell in the infiltrate. Accordingly, many cases are indistinguishable on light microscopy from dermatitis herpetiformis, with the presence of dermal papillary microabscesses.[1319] Some adult cases may mimic bullous pemphigoid by having a predominance of eosinophils in the infiltrate.[1299] No attempt has yet been made to ascertain whether the type of the predominant cell in the infiltrate is merely a reflection of the age of the lesion. Eosinophils are sometimes the predominant cell in the drug-precipitated cases.[1341,1353] A scanty infiltrate of lymphocytes usually surrounds the small vessels in the superficial plexus.

Attempts have been made to establish criteria for the distinction of linear IgA bullous dermatosis from dermatitis herpetiformis.[1278,1281] Fibrin is present at the tips of the dermal papillae with underlying leukocytoclasis in nearly all cases of dermatitis herpetiformis.[1278] However, these changes are also present in three-quarters of the cases of linear IgA disease.[1278] Furthermore, the neutrophil infiltration in this latter condition tends to be more widespread than that in dermatitis herpetiformis in which there is relative sparing of the rete tips between each dermal papilla (Fig. 6.28).[1281] In most cases it is impossible to distinguish between the two conditions.

Direct immunofluorescence reveals a homogeneous linear pattern of IgA deposition along the basement membrane zone of non-lesional skin.[1240] This is the only immunoreactant in nearly 80% of cases.[1299] In the remainder, IgG, IgM and/or C3 may be present (see above).[1299,1401,1402] It was initially thought that the IgA was exclusively IgA1, but IgA2 may be involved in some

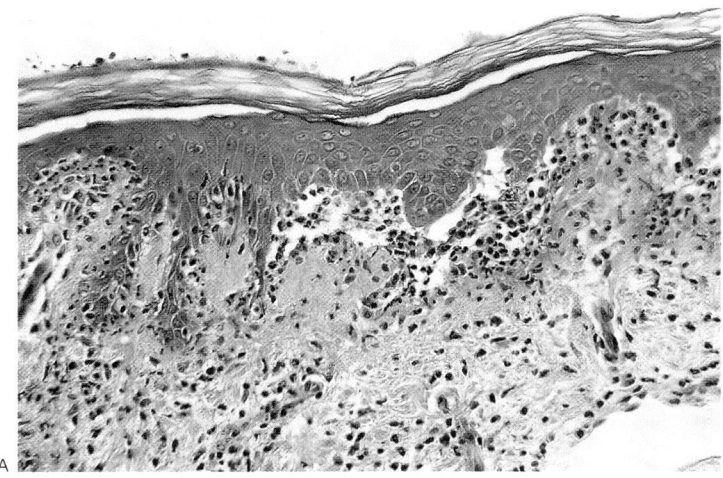

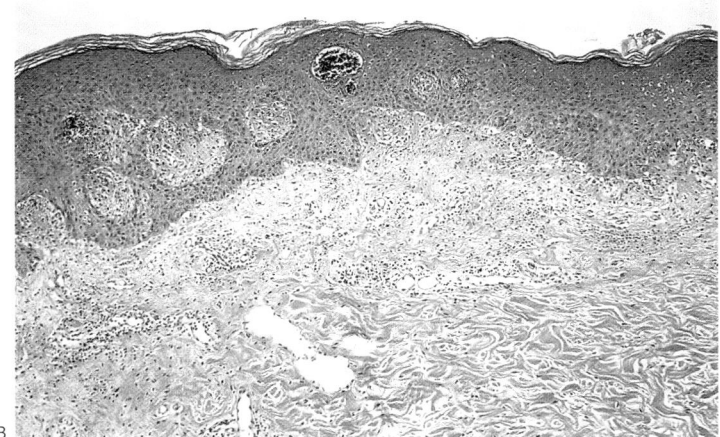

Fig. 6.28 **Linear IgA bullous dermatosis. (A)** There is a subepidermal blister with neutrophils in the lumen and in the base. **(B)** They are dispersed in the papillary dermis of the adjacent skin. (H & E)

cases.[1403–1405] It has been suggested, on the basis of two cases, that lesions on the volar surface of the forearm may not contain immunoreactants even though they are present in lesions from other body sites.[1406] Until this is clarified, this site should probably be avoided at biopsy. As already mentioned, circulating IgA antibodies are found more often in childhood than in adult cases. The deposition of IgA in a linear fashion along the basement membrane is not specific for linear IgA bullous dermatosis, as it may also be found in several bullous dermatoses and cutaneous diseases.[1407] Incidentally, IgA is deposited along the basement membrane of the eccrine secretory coils in patients with alcoholic liver disease.[1408]

Electron microscopy
Most of the ultrastructural studies have been directed at ascertaining the site of deposition of the IgA, rather than the anatomical level of the split within the basement membrane zone.[1409] In some studies the split has been within the lamina lucida,[1409,1410] while in others it has been below the basal lamina, as in dermatitis herpetiformis.[1411] Most immunoelectron microscopical studies have shown that the deposits are below the lamina densa, as in epidermolysis bullosa acquisita,[1412,1413] or on either side of the lamina densa in a mirror image pattern.[1414] A few studies, involving small numbers of cases, have demonstrated deposits within the lamina lucida.[1347,1415] In contrast, split-skin studies have shown that the IgA is deposited at a higher level in the basement

membrane zone. These conflicting results have already been discussed (see above). They are a reflection of the heterogeneous nature of the condition.

CICATRICIAL PEMPHIGOID

Cicatricial pemphigoid (benign mucous membrane pemphigoid) is an uncommon, chronic, vesiculobullous disease that is distinguished clinically by its predilection for oral and ocular mucous membranes and a tendency for the lesions to scar.[1416–1420] It occurs predominantly in older age groups, but there are several reports of the disease in children and adolescents.[1421,1422] There is a female predominance.[1417]

The mouth is the most frequent site of onset and is eventually involved in 85% of cases.[1423] There are erosions, irregular ulcers and vesiculobullous lesions. Ocular involvement is also common and corneal and conjunctival scarring may lead to blindness.[1368,1417] Some of these cases may represent ocular cicatricial pemphigoid, a unique disease in which there is an IgA antibody that binds to a 45 kd basement membrane antigen. In cicatricial pemphigoid, skin lesions occur in about 25% of cases, but in only 10% is the skin the initial site of involvement.[1416,1424] There may be scattered tense bullae which heal without scarring or several areas of erythema with blisters which often heal with scarring.[44] There is a tendency for blisters to recur in the same area. Generalized cutaneous lesions resembling bullous pemphigoid are uncommon.[1425] Some of these cases may represent so-called 'disseminated cicatricial pemphigoid' (see p. 162). The face, neck, upper trunk, scalp and, to a lesser extent, the axillae and distal parts of the limbs are the usual sites of cutaneous lesions.[1416,1426,1427] The external genitalia,[1428] larynx,[1429–1431] pharynx, anus, esophagus,[1432] middle ear[1433] and nail plates[1434] may also be involved.[1417] Coexistence with thymoma,[1435] carcinoma of the pancreas,[1436] stomach,[1437] and lung,[903,1438] and with rheumatoid arthritis,[1439] systemic lupus erythematosus[1440] and other autoimmune diseases,[1441] as well as an association with the ingestion of practolol[1442] and clonidine,[1443] have also been reported. Generalization of the disease has followed the use of azathioprine therapy.[1444] The antiepiligrin variant (see below) appears to be associated with an increased relative risk for cancer.[1445]

The relationship of cicatricial pemphigoid to several other subepidermal bullous diseases has been a matter for discussion and some controversy.[1446–1450]

Pathogenesis
Cicatricial pemphigoid is a heterogeneous group of diseases that share the same clinical phenotype. One group has autoantibodies that target multiple sites on the extracellular (C-terminal) domain of BP180, whereas in bullous pemphigoid and pemphigoid gestationis (herpes gestationis) sera target the NC16A domain.[1082,1451] The second group, which accounts for 10% or more of cases, has IgG autoantibodies directed against epiligrin.[516,517,1452–1458] Epiligrin is now known to be laminin 5, a heterotrimeric ($\alpha3\beta3\gamma2$) adhesion molecule that is a component of the anchoring filaments. Virtually all patients have pathogenic antibodies that bind the $\alpha3$ subunit, but there have been occasional cases where the antibodies have been directed against the $\beta3$ and $\gamma2$ subunits of laminin 5.[1431,1459–1462] Interestingly, a deficiency of laminin 5 is present in the lethal (Herlitz) junctional form of epidermolysis bullosa (see p. 146). In one case of antiepiligrin cicatricial pemphigoid, there was an underlying gastric carcinoma producing laminin 5.[1463] Antibodies to laminin 6 are sometimes found.[1464,1465] In another case, there were antibodies against both laminin 5 and the 180 kd bullous pemphigoid antigen (BP 80).[1466] IgG4 autoantibodies were found to predominate in one study of antiepiligrin cicatricial pemphigoid.[1467] Several cases of cicatricial pemphigoid have had autoantibodies directed against a 230–240 kd antigen, a 45 kd antigen or a 168 kd mucosal antigen or antigens that could not be characterized.[1463–1471]

Finally, the existence of a rare, scarring, bullous eruption with linear IgA at the dermoepidermal junction raises the question of the relationship of these cases to cicatricial pemphigoid and linear IgA bullous dermatosis.[1314,1472–1476] In one case,[1475] the IgA antibody bound a distinct set of antigens (180 and 130 kd), quite different from those in any other bullous disease.

Histopathology

In cicatricial pemphigoid there is a subepidermal blister which shows a variable infiltrate of cells in its base, depending on the age of the lesion. In lesions of less than 48 hours' duration there are neutrophil microabscesses in the dermal papillae resembling those seen in dermatitis herpetiformis.[1477] With increasing age of the lesion there are increasing numbers of eosinophils and later of lymphocytes and a reducing number of neutrophils. There are always fewer eosinophils than in bullous pemphigoid.[1417]

Scarring may be present even in early lesions if the biopsy site corresponds to an area of previous blister formation and subsequent scarring (Fig. 6.29). The earliest stages of scarring may be detected by examination under polarized light. New collagen bundles are arranged parallel to the surface rather than in the usual haphazard distribution.

The presence of a sebaceous gland within the blister is said to be a clue to the diagnosis of cicatricial pemphigoid.[1478] It presumably results from extension of the blister along the edge of the pilosebaceous unit.

Direct immunofluorescence shows linear deposits of IgG and often of C3 along the basement membrane zone in approximately 80% of cases.[1479,1480] The yield is higher in buccal mucosa than in skin.[1446,1481] A similar band often extends along the basement membrane of the appendages; it has also been reported in a similar position in the mucous glands of the oropharynx.[482] IgA and other immunoglobulins may also be present in approximately 20% of cases,[1477] but only rarely (see above) is IgA the only immunoglobulin present.[1314,1479] Using salt-split skin, two different patterns can be seen.[1469] In the antiepiligrin group (see above) the deposits are found on the dermal side, while in the other group they are on the epidermal side.

Circulating antibodies to basement membrane zone were initially found in only 20% of cases, but the use of multiple substrates, including salt-split skin, and/or the use of concentrated serum samples will increase considerably the number of positives obtained.[1483–1485] IgA antibodies are frequently present.[486,1487] Their presence may signify a more severe and persistent disease.[1488] Serial titers of these circulating IgG and IgA antibodies correlate with disease activity.[1485] Circulating pemphigus-like antibodies have been demonstrated in several cases; they are of doubtful significance and probably the result of epitope spreading.[1489]

Electron microscopy

Most studies have shown that the split occurs in the lower lamina lucida, although it has been suggested that a lower level (the lamina densa) would be more in keeping with the presence of scarring.[1490,1491] Ultrastructural studies that were carried out prior to the recognition of the two distinct immuno-pathological groups need to be interpreted with this in mind.[1491] In the antiepiligrin group, the deposits are found in the lower lamina lucida and in the adjacent lamina densa, while in the other group they are at a higher level in the lamina lucida, spilling on to the hemidesmosomes.[1447,1448] Further studies are needed to confirm these findings.

OCULAR CICATRICIAL PEMPHIGOID

Ocular cicatricial pemphigoid is a rare disease characterized by the linear deposition of IgG and/or IgA along the basement membrane zone of conjunctival biopsies. The disease appears to be unique on the basis of a 45 kd antigen that binds IgA antibodies.[1479,1492] It is possible that this is an antigenically heterogeneous entity.[1449]

A case of ocular cicatricial pemphigoid in which oral pemphigus vulgaris also occurred has been reported.[1493]

LOCALIZED CICATRICIAL PEMPHIGOID

Localized cicatricial pemphigoid (Brunsting–Perry type) is characterized by the occurrence of one or more scarring, plaque-like lesions, usually on the head and neck, but without involvement of mucous membranes, even during prolonged follow-up.[1494–1498] The temple is the most frequent site,[1499,1500] but lesions have been reported elsewhere[1501] and also in tissue transplanted to the site of a pre-existing lesion.[1496] The exact relationship of this condition to cicatricial pemphigoid is speculative, although they are thought to be closely related diseases.[1497] Rare cases may progress to a generalized bullous eruption that heals with scarring, but in contrast to cicatricial pemphigoid, there is no mucous membrane involvement. The term 'disseminated cicatricial pemphigoid' has been used for these cases.[1502] Other cases have been claimed to represent localized acquired epidermolysis bullosa.[1503] The exact nosological position of this 'entity' must await further studies. In one case, antibodies to a 180 kd antigen were present.[1504]

Localized cicatricial pemphigoid should also be distinguished from 'localized pemphigoid' which is a variant of bullous pemphigoid in which lesions are localized to one area, such as the vulva,[955,956] pretibial region, a stoma site or the palms and soles.[954,963] In contrast to localized cicatricial pemphigoid, the lesions in 'localized pemphigoid' do not scar. It is uncertain whether all cases of 'localized pemphigoid' are variants of bullous pemphigoid: underlying vascular disease and lymphatic obstruction have been present in some cases in the pretibial region.[958] Furthermore, direct immunofluorescence is sometimes negative in these cases.[958] The author has seen several such cases; it appears to be a 'neglected' entity. Pretibial epidermolysis bullosa also needs to be considered in these circumstances; it usually presents in the first three decades of life.

Histopathology[1496]

There is a subepidermal blister with a mixture of neutrophils, eosinophils and lymphocytes, similar to that seen in cicatricial pemphigoid. The proportion of

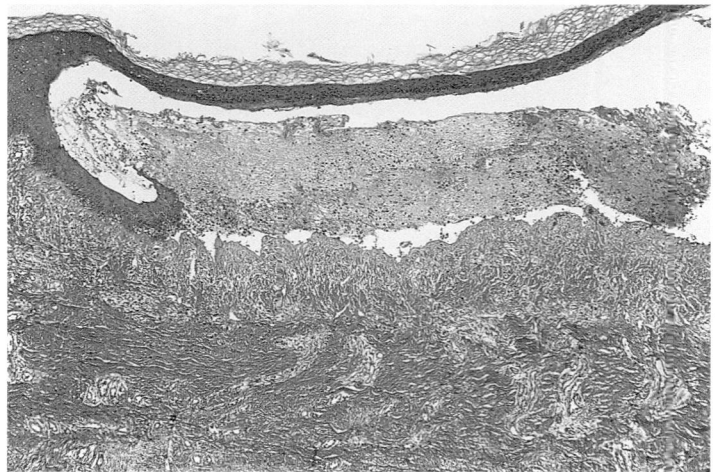

Fig. 6.29 **Cicatricial pemphigoid.** Scar tissue is present in the dermis beneath the subepidermal blister. Because blisters have a tendency to recur at the site of a previous lesion, scarring may be present in the dermis beneath a 'new' blister. (H & E)

the various cell types in the infiltrate depends on the age of the lesion biopsied. Small papillary microabscesses are present in lesions less than 48 hours old (Fig. 6.30).[1499] There is variable fibrosis in the dermis, depending on the presence of a previous blister at the site of biopsy.

In the pretibial form of 'localized pemphigoid' there is only a sparse dermal inflammatory cell infiltrate associated with neovascularization of the papillary dermis.[958] There may be some fibrosis of the dermis, but this is rarely a prominent feature.

Immunofluorescence of localized cicatricial pemphigoid usually shows basement membrane zone IgG and/or C3.[1496] Indirect immunofluorescence for circulating antibodies is usually negative.[1496]

Electron microscopy
Ultrastructural studies have shown that the blister forms below the basal lamina.[1497] The basal lamina and anchoring fibrils are well preserved and attached to the intact epidermis which forms the roof of the blister.[1497]

DEEP LAMINA LUCIDA (ANTI-P105) PEMPHIGOID

Deep lamina lucida (anti-p105) pemphigoid appears to be a unique non-scarring, subepidermal bullous dermatosis with extensive bullae and erosions on mucous membrane and skin resembling toxic epidermal necrolysis or pemphigus vulgaris.[1505–1507] The target antigen has a molecular weight of 105 kd.

Histopathology
There is a subepidermal blister with neutrophils in the papillary dermis, resembling dermatitis herpetiformis. Direct immunofluorescence shows linear IgA and C3 along the basement membrane zone. The deposits are in the lower lamina lucida, reacting with a 105 kd antigen.[1505,1506]

ANTI-P200 PEMPHIGOID

Anti-p200 pemphigoid, a unique subepidermal blistering disease, has the clinical appearance of bullous pemphigoid, dermatitis herpetiformis or linear IgA bullous dermatosis combined with linear deposits of IgG and C3 along the basement membrane.[1508] The antibodies are directed against a 200 kd protein

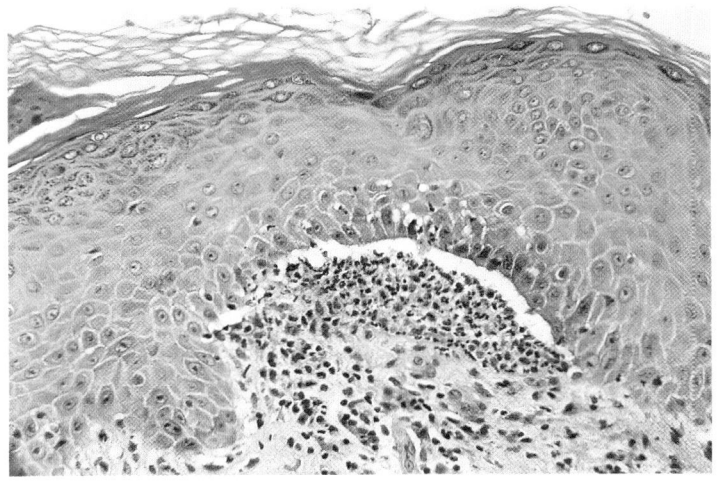

Fig. 6.30 **Localized cicatricial pemphigoid.** A neutrophil microabscess is present in a dermal papilla, similar to the picture in dermatitis herpetiformis. (H & E)

in the lower lamina lucida which is distinct from either laminin 5 or type VII collagen.[1509–1511]

Histopathology
There is a subepidermal blister with dermal papillary microabscesses and some admixed eosinophils. Too few cases have been studied to know whether the presence of eosinophils is influenced by the age of the blister that is biopsied.

BULLOUS URTICARIA

Bullae are an uncommon manifestation of urticaria and result from severe edema of the papillary dermis. Neutrophils and eosinophils are present in the upper dermis; sometimes a mixed infiltrate of lymphocytes and eosinophils is present.

BULLOUS ACUTE VASCULITIS

If bullae form in acute vasculitis they are sometimes hemorrhagic. The vessels in the underlying dermis show the typical features of an acute vasculitis. Leukocytoclasis may be a conspicuous feature. A vasculitis is usually present in the bullous lesions associated with septicemia caused by *Vibrio vulnificus*[1512] and, rarely, by *Escherichia coli*,[1513] *Yersinia enterocolitica* and *Morganella morganii*.[1514] Subepidermal bullae have also been reported in the toxic shock syndrome.[1515]

BULLOUS LUPUS ERYTHEMATOSUS

A vesiculobullous eruption is an uncommon manifestation of systemic lupus erythematosus. The lesions vary in appearance from herpetiform vesicles to large hemorrhagic bullae. Sometimes the lesions are limited to sun-exposed areas of the body.

Bullous lupus erythematosus shares with epidermolysis bullosa acquisita the presence of autoantibodies to type VII collagen, although not all patients have these autoantibodies.

Bullae are exceedingly rare in dermatomyositis.

Histopathology[1516]
The appearances closely resemble dermatitis herpetiformis with subepidermal splitting and papillary microabscesses (Fig. 6.31). Nuclear dust is prominent in the papillae and sometimes around superficial blood vessels. The neutrophils tend to extend more deeply in the papillary dermis and around vessels than they do in dermatitis herpetiformis. Vacuolar change is not usually present although occasional Civatte bodies are sometimes seen.

Immunoelectron microscopy shows the deposits (IgG, C3 and often IgA) deep to the anchoring fibrils in the upper dermis.

ERYSIPELAS

In erysipelas, subepidermal blisters may form as a result of massive edema in the upper dermis. Elongated rete ridges may bridge the blister and connect with the underlying dermis. The neutrophilic infiltrate is usually only mild, although there are numerous extravasated erythrocytes.

SWEET'S SYNDROME

Bullae are quite uncommon in Sweet's syndrome. Sometimes there is severe edema of the upper dermis mimicking early blister formation, but the clinical

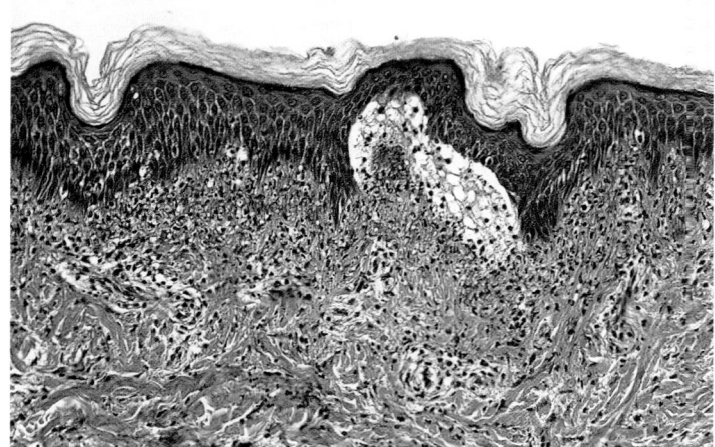

Fig. 6.31 **Bullous lupus erythematosus.** Neutrophils are present in the superficial dermis in a more dispersed arrangement than in dermatitis herpetiformis. There is a small subepidermal blister. (H & E)

appearances suggest an urticarial plaque, not a blister. There is a heavy infiltrate of neutrophils in the upper and mid dermis, often with leukocytoclasis. There is no fibrinoid change in vessel walls.

EPIDERMOLYSIS BULLOSA ACQUISITA

Neutrophils are present in the dermis in the inflammatory variant of this disease (see p. 149).

SUBEPIDERMAL BLISTERS WITH MAST CELLS

BULLOUS MASTOCYTOSIS

Bullous lesions are an uncommon manifestation of mastocytosis in neonates and infants (see p. 1065). There are usually numerous mast cells in the dermis beneath the blister.

MISCELLANEOUS BLISTERING DISEASES

The *miscellaneous category* of blistering diseases includes several very rare entities in which the anatomical level of the split is variable or the disease does not fit appropriately into one of the categories of subepidermal blistering diseases already mentioned. Penicillamine may produce blisters at different anatomical levels in the epidermis, resembling either pemphigus foliaceus or pemphigus vulgaris. An unusual bullous eruption has been reported in a patient receiving intravenous trimethoprim–sulfamethoxazole.[1517] The blisters occurred below the lamina densa yet produced no scarring. On light microscopy they were subepidermal with a light, mixed inflammatory cell infiltrate.[1517]

Blisters have been reported on the knees from repeated kneeling in church ('prayer' or 'pew' blisters).[1518] No histology was performed.

Unusual blisters resembling bubble wrap developed after occupational skin injury with 35% hydrogen peroxide.[1519] Numerous vacuolar structures were observed in the epidermis, dermis and subcutis. The vacuoles were considered to be 'oxygen bubbles'.[1519]

The bullous lesions that develop rarely in diabetes mellitus (see p. 556) may be subepidermal or intraepidermal; so too may the blisters associated with non-01 *Vibrio cholerae* infection (see p. 621). Infection may have been the precipitating cause of two cases reported as IgE bullous disease.[1520] There were subepidermal bullae resembling bullous pemphigoid but no immunoreactants, other than deposits of IgE on inflammatory cells within the dermis.[1520]

Bullae may be a manifestation of the rare genodermatoses pachyonychia congenita (see p. 292) and Kindler's syndrome (see p. 54). Small, hemorrhagic blisters have been reported in one case of Wilson's disease.[1521] A subepidermal bullous eruption has been reported in patients with reflex sympathetic dystrophy.[1522]

The following entities are discussed further below:

- drug overdose-related bullae
- methyl bromide-induced bullae
- etretinate-induced bullae
- PUVA-induced bullae
- cancer-related bullae
- lymphatic bullae.

DRUG OVERDOSE-RELATED BULLAE

Bullae, tense vesicles, erosions and dusky erythematous plaques may develop at sites of pressure in patients with drug-induced or carbon monoxide-induced coma, particularly if the coma is deep.[1523] Drugs involved have included morphine, heroin, methadone, barbiturates,[1524] imipramine, carbamazepine,[1525] amitryptyline,[1526] clobazam[1527] and diazepam.[1528] Rarely, this entity has developed in association with other neurological disorders;[1528] it followed treatment with the β-adrenergic antagonist atenolol in a patient with pheochromocytoma.[1529] Similar blisters have developed in a patient with a coma due to diabetic ketoacidosis.[1530]

The lesions are believed to result from tissue ischemia, which in turn is related to local pressure and to systemic hypoxia.[1531]

Histopathology[1531–1534]

The blisters that form are predominantly subepidermal, but there is also spongiosis in the overlying epidermis which may lead to the formation of intraepidermal vesicles as well. There is focal necrosis of keratinocytes in and adjacent to the acrosyringium; sometimes the epithelium in the pilosebaceous follicles also shows focal necrosis. The secretory cells of the sweat glands beneath the bullae are necrotic. The basement membrane of the sweat glands may also be destroyed but the myoepithelial cells usually survive. In the dermis there is only a sparse inflammatory cell infiltrate which includes some neutrophils. Some arterioles show necrosis of their walls with a mild perivascular infiltrate of neutrophils. Thrombi are not usually seen, but are more common in non-drug-induced coma.[1535]

METHYL BROMIDE-INDUCED BULLAE

A vesiculobullous eruption has been reported following occupational exposure to high concentrations of methyl bromide used in fumigation.[1536]

Histopathology[1536]

The bullae induced by methyl bromide are subepidermal in location and associated with marked edema of the upper dermis. The dermal infiltrate is composed of neutrophils, eosinophils and a few lymphocytes. The infiltrate is distributed around blood vessels in the upper dermis.

Another feature of this entity is the presence of spongiosis of the epidermis and necrosis of epidermal keratinocytes. Neutrophils infiltrate the epidermis.

Similar changes have been reported following skin exposure to nitrogen and sulfur mustard.[1537]

ETRETINATE-INDUCED BULLAE

Increased skin fragility and subepidermal blistering are rare complications of therapy with etretinate.[1538] The blisters rapidly ulcerate; they are followed by some scarring.

Histopathology[1538]

Intact blisters are difficult to obtain. Clefting appears to occur at the dermo-epidermal junction. The overlying epidermis may show spongiosis. The dermal infiltrate includes plasma cells, eosinophils and neutrophils.

PUVA-INDUCED BULLAE

Blisters may develop on the limbs in 10% of patients receiving therapy with psoralens plus long-wave ultraviolet light (PUVA).[1539] The lesions appear to result from friction and minor trauma. The mechanism remains to be determined although the blisters apparently develop as a result of damage to the basal and suprabasal layers of the epidermis.[1539] Blisters have also been reported following ruby laser treatment for incontinentia pigmenti.[1540]

Histopathology[1539]

The blistering appears to form in the basal layer of the epidermis as damaged basal cells are sometimes seen in the base of the blisters. There is swelling and destruction of keratinocytes in the overlying epidermis. Apoptotic cells ('sunburn cells') are sometimes present. The dermis contains a very sparse, mixed inflammatory cell infiltrate.

CANCER-RELATED BULLAE

Several patients with cancer have developed bullae in association with gyrate lesions.[1541,1542] Uncommonly, the bullae are related to trauma.[1542] Bullae have been reported in a patient with multiple myeloma, but there were no gyrate lesions.[1543,1544] An unusual pustular eruption, with epidermal spongiosis containing immature myeloid cells, has been reported in infants with Down syndrome and a congenital leukemoid reaction.[234,235]

Not included in this category are the bullous eruptions, resembling bullous pemphigoid and epidermolysis bullosa acquisita, that sometimes develop in patients with cancer.

Histopathology[1542]

The cancer-related bullae with gyrate lesions are usually subepidermal in location, and the inflammatory cell infiltrate in the dermis is mild and of mixed type. Direct immunofluorescence may show IgG and C3 in the basement membrane zone.[1542]

LYMPHATIC BULLAE

Subepidermal bullae are a very rare complication of lymphedema or of a lymphatic fistula.[1545,1546] Uncommonly, vesicular lesions are due to markedly dilated lymphatics in the papillary dermis.[1547] Interference with lymphatic drainage has been postulated as a possible mechanism for the bullae that have been described over laser-resurfaced skin.[1548]

The blisters that develop near fractures, adjacent to joints or areas of limited skin mobility, result from massive subepidermal edema leading to separation of the epidermis which becomes necrotic.[1549] They are mentioned here for completeness.

REFERENCES

Introduction

1 Burge S. Cohesion in the epidermis. Br J Dermatol 1994; 131: 153–159.
2 Freemont T. The significance of adhesion molecules in diagnostic histopathology. Curr Diagn Pathol 1995; 2: 101–110.
3 Macari F, Landau M, Cousin P et al. Mutation in the gene for connexin 30.3 in a family with erythrokeratodermia variabilis. Am J Hum Genet 2000; 67: 1296–1301.
4 Haftek M, Hansen MU, Kaiser HW et al. Interkeratinocyte adherens junctions: immunocytochemical visualization of cell-cell junctional structures, distinct from desmosomes, in human epidermis. J Invest Dermatol 1996; 106: 498–504.
5 Peltonen S, Hentula M, Hägg P et al. A novel component of epidermal cell-matrix and cell-cell contacts: transmembrane protein type XIII collagen. J Invest Dermatol 1999; 113: 635–642.
6 Amagai M. Adhesion molecules. I: Keratinocyte-keratinocyte interactions; cadherins and pemphigus. J Invest Dermatol 1995; 104: 146–152.
7 Kowalczyk AP, Anderson JE, Borgwardt JE et al. Pemphigus sera recognize conformationally sensitive epitopes in the amino-terminal region of desmoglein-1. J Invest Dermatol 1995; 105: 147–152.
8 Venning VA, Allen J, Aplin JD et al. The distribution of α6β4 integrins in lesional and non-lesional skin in bullous pemphigoid. Br J Dermatol 1992; 127: 103–111.
9 Lazarova Z, Yee C, Cheng P, Yancey K. Anti-laminin 5 IgG induces subepidermal blisters in adult murine skin as well as human skin grafted onto SCID mice. J Invest Dermatol 1996; 106: 812 (abstract).
10 Borrslaeger EA, Corcoran CM, Stappenbeck TS, Green KJ. Displacement of desmoplakin from cell-cell interfaces disrupts anchorage of intermediate filament bundles and alters junction assembly. J Invest Dermatol 1996; 106: 832 (abstract).
11 Skalli O, Goldman RD, Steinert PM. IFAP-300 is associated with the anchorage of keratin intermediate filaments to desmoplakin at desmosomal junctions in epidermal cells. J Invest Dermatol 1996; 96: 835.
12 Fujiwara S, Kohno K, Iwamatsu A et al. Identification of a 450-kDa human epidermal autoantigen as a new member of the plectin family. J Invest Dermatol 1996; 106: 1125–1130.
13 Diaz LA, Giudice GJ. End of the century overview of skin blisters. Arch Dermatol 2000; 136: 106–112.
14 McGrath JA, Hoeger PH, Christiano AM et al. Skin fragility and hypohidrotic ectodermal dysplasia resulting from ablation of plakophilin 1. Br J Dermatol 1999; 140: 297–307.
15 Gammon WR, Fine J-D, Forbes M, Briggaman RA. Immunofluorescence on split skin for the detection and differentiation of basement membrane zone autoantibodies. J Am Acad Dermatol 1992; 27: 79–87.
16 Kirtschig G, Wojnarowska F. Autoimmune blistering diseases: an up-date of diagnostic methods and investigations. Clin Exp Dermatol 1994; 19: 97–112.
17 Willsteed EM, Bhogal BS, Das A et al. An ultrastructural comparison of dermo-epidermal separation techniques. J Cutan Pathol 1991; 18: 8–12.
18 Peters MS. Ultrastructural evidence for the use of NaCl-split skin in the evaluation of subepidermal bullous diseases. J Cutan Pathol 1991; 18: 1–2.
19 Yarcey KB. From bedside to bench and back. The diagnosis and biology of bullous diseases. Arch Dermatol 1994; 130: 983–987.

Intracorneal and subcorneal blisters

20 Wilkinson DS. Pustular dermatoses. Br J Dermatol (Suppl) 1969; 3: 38–45.
21 Tagami H, Iwatsuki K, Shirahama S, Yamada M. Pustulosis vegetans. Arch Dermatol 1984; 120: 1355–1359.
22 Hermanns-Lê T, Piérard GE. Azathioprine-induced skin peeling syndrome. Dermatology 1997; 194: 175–176.
23 Feldman SR. Bullous dermatoses associated with systemic disease. Dermatol Clin 1993; 11: 597–609.
24 Ryan JG. Pemphigus. A 20-year survey of experience with 70 cases. Arch Dermatol 1971; 104: 14–20.
25 Beutner EH, Chorzelski TP. Studies on etiologic factors in pemphigus. J Cutan Pathol 1976; 3: 67–74.
26 Korman N. Pemphigus. J Am Acad Dermatol 1988; 18: 1219–1238.

27 Koulu L, Stanley JR. Clinical, histologic, and immunopathologic comparison of pemphigus vulgaris and pemphigus foliaceus. Semin Dermatol 1988; 7: 82–90.

28 Imamura S, Takigawa M, Ikai K et al. Pemphigus foliaceus, myasthenia gravis, thymoma and red cell aplasia. Clin Exp Dermatol 1978; 3: 285–291.

29 Perry HO, Brunsting LA. Pemphigus foliaceus. Further observations. Arch Dermatol 1965; 91: 10–23.

30 Jones SK, Schwab HP, Norris DA. Childhood pemphigus foliaceus: case report and review of the literature. Pediatr Dermatol 1986; 3: 459–463.

31 Sotiriou L, Herszenson S, Jordon RE. Childhood pemphigus foliaceus. Report of a case. Arch Dermatol 1980; 116: 679–680.

32 Yorav S, Trau H, Schewack-Millet M. Pemphigus foliaceus in an 8-year-old girl. Int J Dermatol 1989; 28: 125–126.

33 Goodyear HM, Abrahamson EL, Harper JI. Childhood pemphigus foliaceus. Clin Exp Dermatol 1991; 16: 229–230.

34 Mehravaran M, Morvay M, Molnár K et al. Juvenile pemphigus foliaceus. Br J Dermatol 1998; 139: 496–499.

35 Aboobaker J, Morar N, Ramdial PK, Hammond MG. Pemphigus in South Africa. Int J Dermatol 2001; 40: 115–119.

36 Nousari HC, Kimyai-Asadi A, Ketabchi N et al. Severe nonendemic pemphigus foliaceus presenting in the postpartum period. J Am Acad Dermatol 1999; 40: 845–846.

37 Walker DC, Kolar KA, Hebert AA, Jordon RE. Neonatal pemphigus foliaceus. Arch Dermatol 1995; 131: 1308–1311.

38 Avalos-Diaz E, Olague-Marchan M, López-Swiderski A et al. Transplacental passage of maternal pemphigus foliaceus autoantibodies induces neonatal pemphigus. J Am Acad Dermatol 2000; 43: 1130–1134.

39 Bruckner N, Katz RA, Hood AF. Pemphigus foliaceus resembling eruptive seborrheic keratoses. Arch Dermatol 1980; 116: 815–816.

40 Kahana M, Trau H, Schewack-Millet M, Sofer E. Pemphigus foliaceus presenting as multiple giant seborrheic keratoses. J Am Acad Dermatol 1984; 11: 299–300.

41 Mahé A, Flageul B, Ciss I et al. Pemphigus in Mali: a study of 30 cases. Br J Dermatol 1996; 134: 114–119.

42 Emmerson RW, Wilson Jones E. Eosinophilic spongiosis in pemphigus. Arch Dermatol 1968; 97: 252–257.

43 Knight AG, Black MM, Delaney TJ. Eosinophilic spongiosis. A clinical histological and immunofluorescent correlation. Clin Exp Dermatol 1976; 1: 141–153.

44 Lever WF. Pemphigus and pemphigoid. A review of the advances made since 1964. J Am Acad Dermatol 1979; 1: 2–31.

45 Morini JP, Jomaa B, Gorgi Y et al. Pemphigus foliaceus in young women. An endemic focus in the Sousse area of Tunisia. Arch Dermatol 1993; 129: 69–73.

46 Huhn KM, Tron VA, Nguyen N, Trotter MJ. Neutrophilic spongiosis in pemphigus herpetiformis. J Cutan Pathol 1996; 23: 264–269.

47 Shimizu K, Hashimoto T, Wang N et al. A case of herpetiform pemphigus associated with autoimmune hemolytic anemia: detection of autoantibodies against multiple epidermal antigens. Dermatology 1996; 192: 179–182.

48 Santi CG, Maruta CW, Aoki V et al. Pemphigus herpetiformis is a rare clinical expression of nonendemic pemphigus foliaceus, fogo selvagem, and pemphigus vulgaris. J Am Acad Dermatol 1996; 34: 40–46.

49 Verdier-Sevrain S, Joly P, Thomine E et al. Theopronine-induced herpetiform pemphigus: report of a case studied by immunoelectron microscopy and immunoblot analysis. Br J Dermatol 1994; 130: 238–240.

50 Ishii K, Amagai M, Ohata Y et al. Development of pemphigus vulgaris in a patient with pemphigus foliaceus: Antidesmoglein antibody profile shift confirmed by enzyme-linked immunosorbent assay. J Am Acad Dermatol 2000; 42: 859–861.

51 Izumi T, Seishima M, Satoh S et al. Pemphigus with features of both vulgaris and foliaceus variants, associated with antibodies to 160 and 130 kDa antigens. Br J Dermatol 1998; 139: 688–692.

52 Korman NJ, Stanley JR, Woodley DT. Coexistence of pemphigus foliaceus and bullous pemphigoid. Arch Dermatol 1991; 127: 387–390.

53 Ishiko A, Hashimoto T, Shimizu H et al. Combined features of pemphigus foliaceus and bullous pemphigoid: immunoblot and immunoelectron microscopic studies. Arch Dermatol 1995; 131: 732–734.

54 Levine L, Bernstein JE, Soltani K et al. Coexisting childhood pemphigus foliaceus and Graves' disease. Arch Dermatol 1982; 118: 602–604.

55 Perez GL, Agger WA, Abellera RM, Dahlberg P. Pemphigus foliaceus coexisting with IgA nephropathy in a patient with psoriasis vulgaris. Int J Dermatol 1995; 34: 794–795.

56 Kaufman AJ, Ahmed AR, Kaplan RP. Pemphigus, myasthenia gravis, and pregnancy. J Am Acad Dermatol 1988; 19: 414–418.

57 Patten SF, Dijkstra JWE. Associations of pemphigus and autoimmune disease with malignancy or thymoma. Int J Dermatol 1994; 33: 836–842.

58 Ng PPL, Ng SK, Chng HH. Pemphigus foliaceus and oral lichen planus in a patient with systemic lupus erythematosus and thymoma. Clin Exp Dermatol 1998; 23: 181–184.

59 Cowley NC, Neill SM, Staughton RCD. Pemphigus foliaceus and non-Hodgkin's lymphoma. Int J Dermatol 1994; 33: 510–511.

60 Ota M, Sato-Matsumura KC, Matsumura T et al. Pemphigus foliaceus and figurate erythema in a patient with prostate cancer. Br J Dermatol 2000; 142: 816–818.

61 Palleschi GM, Falcos D, Giacomelli A, Caproni M. Kaposi's varicelliform eruption in pemphigus foliaceus. Int J Dermatol 1996; 35: 809–810.

62 Lateef A, Packles MR, White SM et al. Pemphigus vegetans in association with human immunodeficiency virus. Int J Dermatol 1999; 38: 778–781.

63 Ueki H, Takao J, Yamasaki F et al. Pemphigus foliaceus associated with silicosis. Br J Dermatol 2000; 143: 456–457.

64 Neumann-Jensen B, Worsaae N, Dabelsteen E, Ullman S. Pemphigus vulgaris and pemphigus foliaceus coexisting with oral lichen planus. Br J Dermatol 1980; 102: 585–590.

65 Sarnoff DS, DeFeo CP. Coexistence of pemphigus foliaceus and mycosis fungoides. Arch Dermatol 1985; 121: 669–672.

66 Kano Y, Shimosegawa M, Mizukawa Y, Shiohara T. Pemphigus foliaceus induced by exposure to sunlight. Dermatology 2000; 201: 132–138.

67 Santa Cruz DJ, Prioleau PJ, Marcus MD, Uitto J. Pemphigus-like lesions induced by D-penicillamine. Analysis of clinical, histopathological, and immunofluorescence features in 34 cases. Am J Dermatopathol 1981; 3: 85–92.

68 Ogata K, Nakajima H, Ikeda M et al. Drug-induced pemphigus foliaceus with features of pemphigus vulgaris. Br J Dermatol 2001; 144: 421–422.

69 Lee CW, Lim JH, Kang HJ. Pemphigus foliaceus induced by rifampicin. Br J Dermatol 1984; 111: 619–622.

70 Blanken R, Doeglas HMG, De Jong MCJM et al. Pemphigus-like eruption induced by d-penicillamine and captopril in the same patient. Acta Derm Venereol 1983; 68: 456–457.

71 Kaplan RP, Potter TS, Fox JN. Drug-induced pemphigus related to angiotensin-converting enzyme inhibitors. J Am Acad Dermatol 1992; 26: 364–366.

72 Shelton RM. Pemphigus foliaceus associated with enalapril. J Am Acad Dermatol 1991; 24: 503–504.

73 Vignes S, Paul C, Flageul B, Dubertret L. Ramipril-induced superficial pemphigus. Br J Dermatol 1996; 135: 657–658.

74 Ong CS, Cook N, Lee S. Drug-related pemphigus and angiotensin converting enzyme inhibitors. Australas J Dermatol 2000; 41: 242–246.

75 Goldberg I, Kashman Y, Brenner S. The induction of pemphigus by phenol drugs. Int J Dermatol 1999; 38: 888–892.

76 Lucky PA, Skovby F, Thier SO. Pemphigus foliaceus and proteinuria induced by α-mercaptopropionylglycine. J Am Acad Dermatol 1983; 8: 667–672.

77 Pisani M, Ruocco V. Drug-induced pemphigus. Clin Dermatol 1986; 4: 118–132.

78 Anhalt GJ. Drug-induced pemphigus. Semin Dermatol 1989; 8: 166–172.

79 De Dobbeleer G, Godfrine S, Gourdain J-M et al. In vitro acantholysis induced by D-penicillamine, captopril, and piroxicam on dead de-epidermized dermis. J Cutan Pathol 1992; 19: 181–186.

80 Bialy-Golan A, Brenner S. Penicillamine-induced bullous dermatoses. J Am Acad Dermatol 1996; 35: 732–742.

81 Peñas PF, Buezo GF, Carvajal I et al. D-Penicillamine-induced pemphigus foliaceus with autoantibodies to desmoglein-1 in a patient with mixed connective tissue disease. J Am Acad Dermatol 1997; 37: 121–123.

82 Walton S, Keczkes K, Robinson EA. A case of penicillamine-induced pemphigus, successfully treated by plasma exchange. Clin Exp Dermatol 1987; 12: 275–276.

83 Troy JL, Silvers DN, Grossman ME, Jaffe IA. Penicillamine-associated pemphigus: is it really pemphigus? J Am Acad Dermatol 1981; 4: 547–555.

84 Bahmer FA, Bambauer R, Stenger D. Penicillamine-induced pemphigus foliaceus-like dermatosis. Arch Dermatol 1985; 121: 665–668.

85 Velthuis PJ, Hendrikse JC, Nefkens JJ. Combined features of pemphigus and pemphigoid induced by penicillamine. Br J Dermatol 1985; 112: 615–619.

86 Jordon RE, Kawana S, Fritz KA. Immunopathologic mechanisms in pemphigus and bullous pemphigoid. J Invest Dermatol 1985; 85: 72s–78s.

87 Rubinstein N, Stanley JR. Pemphigus foliaceus antibodies and a monoclonal antibody to desmoglein I demonstrate stratified squamous epithelial-specific epitopes of desmosomes. Am J Dermatopathol 1987; 9: 510–514.

88 Labib RS, Camargo S, Futamura S et al. Pemphigus foliaceus antigen: characterization of a keratinocyte envelope associated pool and preparation of a soluble immunoreactive fragment. J Invest Dermatol 1989; 93: 272–279.

89 Allen EM, Giudice GJ, Diaz LA. Subclass reactivity of pemphigus foliaceus autoantibodies with recombinant human desmoglein. J Invest Dermatol 1993; 100: 685–691.

90 Amagai M, Hashimoto T, Green KJ et al. Antigen-specific immunoadsorption of pathogenic autoantibodies in pemphigus foliaceus. J Invest Dermatol 1995; 104: 895–901.

91 Dmochowski M, Hashimoto T, Chidgey MAJ et al. Demonstration of antibodies to bovine desmocollin isoforms in certain pemphigus sera. Br J Dermatol 1995; 133: 519–525.

92 Chorzelski TP, Hashimoto T, Nishikawa T et al. Unusual acantholytic bullous dermatosis associated with neoplasia and IgG and IgA antibodies against bovine desmocollins I and II. J Am Acad Dermatol 1994; 31: 351–355.

93 Ghohestani R, Joly P, Gilbert D et al. Autoantibody formation against a 190-kDa antigen of the desmosomal plaque in pemphigus foliaceus. Br J Dermatol 1997; 137: 774–779.

94 Kazerounian S, Mahoney MG, Uitto J, Aho S. Envoplakin and periplakin, the paraneoplastic pemphigus antigens, are also recognized by pemphigus foliaceus autoantibodies. J Invest Dermatol 2000; 115: 505–507.

95 Ioannides D, Hytiroglou P, Phelps RG, Bystryn J-C. Regional variation in the expression of pemphigus foliaceus, pemphigus erythematosus, and pemphigus vulgaris antigens in human skin. J Invest Dermatol 1991; 96: 159–161.

96 Ruocco V, Brenner S, Ruocco E et al. Different patterns of *in vitro* acantholysis in normal human skin samples explanted from different sites of the body. Int J Dermatol 1998; 37: 18–22.

97 Shirakata Y, Amagai M, Hanakawa Y et al. Lack of mucosal involvement in pemphigus foliaceus may be due to low expression of desmoglein 1. J Invest Dermatol 1998; 110: 76–78.

98 Wu H, Wang ZH, Yan A et al. Protection against pemphigus foliaceus by desmoglein 3 in neonates. N Engl J Med 2000; 343: 31–35.

99 Edelson RL. Pemphigus – decoding the cellular language of cutaneous autoimmunity. N Engl J Med 2000; 343: 60–61.

100 Korman NJ, Eyre RW, Zone J, Stanley JR. Drug-induced pemphigus: autoantibodies directed against the pemphigus antigen complexes are present in penicillamine and captopril-induced pemphigus. J Invest Dermatol 1991; 96: 273–276.

101 Brenner S, Bialy-Golan A, Anhalt GJ. Recognition of pemphigus antigens in drug-induced pemphigus vulgaris and pemphigus foliaceus. J Am Acad Dermatol 1997; 36: 919–923.

102 Emery DJ, Diaz LA, Fairley JA et al. Pemphigus foliaceus and pemphigus vulgaris autoantibodies react with the extracellular domain of desmoglein-1. J Invest Dermatol 1995; 104: 323–328.

103 Kawana S, Geoghegan WD, Jordon RE, Nishiyama S. Deposition of the membrane attack complex of complement in pemphigus vulgaris and pemphigus foliaceus skin. J Invest Dermatol 1989; 92: 588–592.

104 Mahoney MG, Wang ZH, Stanley JR. Pemphigus vulgaris and pemphigus foliaceus antibodies are pathogenic in plasminogen activator knockout mice. J Invest Dermatol 1999; 113: 22–25.

105 Diaz LA, Sampaio SA, Rivitti EA. Endemic pemphigus foliaceus (fogo selvagem). I. Clinical features and immunopathology. J Am Acad Dermatol 1989; 20: 657–669.

106 Crosby DL, Diaz LA. Endemic pemphigus foliaceus. Fogo selvagem. Dermatol Clin 1993; 11: 453–462.

107 Zaitz C, Campbell I, Alves GF. Endemic pemphigus foliaceus (fogo selvagem). Int J Dermatol 2000; 39: 812–814.

108 Diaz LA, Sampaio SAP, Rivitti EA et al. Endemic pemphigus foliaceus (fogo selvagem): II. Current and historic epidemiologic studies. J Invest Dermatol 1989; 92: 4–12.

109 Friedman H, Campbell I, Rocha-Alvarez R et al. Endemic pemphigus foliaceus (fogo selvagem) in Native Americans from Brazil. J Am Acad Dermatol 1995; 32: 949–956.

110 Joly P, Mokhtar I, Gilbert D et al. Immunoblot and immunoelectronmicroscopic analysis of endemic Tunisian pemphigus. Br J Dermatol 1999; 140: 44–49.

111 Tur E, Brenner S. The role of the water system as an exogenous factor in pemphigus. Int J Dermatol 1997; 36: 810–816.

112 Roscoe JT, Naylor PH, Diaz LA et al. Elevated thymosin alpha 1 levels in Brazilian pemphigus foliaceus. Br J Dermatol 1986; 115: 147–150.

113 Ahmed AR, Rosen GB. Viruses in pemphigus. Int J Dermatol 1989; 28: 209–217.

114 Robledo MA, de Prada C S, Jaramillo D, Leon W. South American pemphigus foliaceus: study of an epidemic in El Bagre and Nechi, Colombia 1982 to 1986. Br J Dermatol 1988; 118: 737–744.

115 Reis VMS, Toledo RP, Lopez A et al. UVB-induced acantholysis in endemic pemphigus foliaceus (fogo selvagem) and pemphigus vulgaris. J Am Acad Dermatol 2000; 42: 571–576.

116 Cunha PR, Focaccia RR, Diaz LA. Evolution of endemic pemphigus foliaceus (fogo selvagem) after HIV-1 infection. J Am Acad Dermatol 1995; 32: 809–811.

117 Voelter WW, Newell GB, Schwartz SL et al. Familial occurrence of pemphigus foliaceus. Arch Dermatol 1973; 108: 93–94.

118 Feinstein A, Yorav S, Movshovitz M, Schewach-Millet M. Pemphigus in families. Int J Dermatol 1991; 30: 347–351.

119 Roscoe JT, Diaz L, Sampaio SAP et al. Brazilian pemphigus foliaceus autoantibodies are pathogenic to BALB/c mice by passive transfer. J Invest Dermatol 1985; 85: 538–541.

120 Stanley JR, Klaus-Kovtun V, Sampaio SAP. Antigenic specificity of fogo selvagem autoantibodies is similar to North American pemphigus foliaceus and distinct from pemphigus vulgaris autoantibodies. J Invest Dermatol 1986; 87: 197–201.

121 Rivitti EA, Sanches JA, Miyauchi LM et al. Pemphigus foliaceus autoantibodies bind both epidermis and squamous mucosal epithelium, but tissue injury is detected only in the epidermis. J Am Acad Dermatol 1994; 31: 954–958.

122 Akiyama M, Hashimoto T, Sugiura M, Nishikawa T. Ultrastructural localization of Brazilian pemphigus foliaceus (fogo selvagem) antigens in cultured human squamous cell carcinoma cells. Br J Dermatol 1993; 128: 378–383.

123 Warren SJP, Lin M-S, Giudice GJ et al. The prevalence of antibodies against desmoglein 1 in endemic pemphigus foliaceus in Brazil. N Engl J Med 2000; 343: 23–30.

124 Rowilson-Cunha P, Bystryn J-C. Sensitivity of indirect immunofluorescence and immunoblotting for the detection of intercellular antibodies in endemic pemphigus foliaceus (fogo selvagem). Int J Dermatol 1999; 38: 41–45.

125 Futamura S, Martins C, Rivitti EA. Ultrastructural studies of acantholysis induced in vivo by passive transfer of IgG from endemic pemphigus foliaceus (fogo selvagem). J Invest Dermatol 1989; 93: 480–485.

126 Santi CG, Sotto MN. Immunopathologic characterization of the tissue response in endemic pemphigus foliaceus (fogo selvagem). J Am Acad Dermatol 2001; 44: 446–450.

127 Kouskoukis CE, Ackerman AB. What histologic finding distinguishes superficial pemphigus and bullous impetigo? Am J Dermatopathol 1984; 6: 179–181.

128 Kouskoukis CE, Ackerman AB. Vacuoles in the upper part of the epidermis as a clue to eventuation of superficial pemphigus and bullous impetigo. Am J Dermatopathol 1984; 6: 183–186.

129 Hoss DM, Shea CR, Grant-Kels JM. Neutrophilic spongiosis in pemphigus. Arch Dermatol 1996; 132: 315–318.

130 Castro RM, Roscoe JT, Sampaio SAP. Brazilian pemphigus foliaceus. Clin Dermatol 1983; 1: 22–41.

131 Bhogal B, Wojnarowska F, Black MM et al. The distribution of immunoglobulins and the C3 component of complement in multiple biopsies from the uninvolved and perilesional skin in pemphigus. Clin Exp Dermatol 1986; 11: 49–53.

132 De Messias IT, von Kuster LC, Santamaria J, Kajdacsy-Balla A. Complement and antibody deposition in Brazilian pemphigus foliaceus and correlation of disease activity with circulating antibodies. Arch Dermatol 1988; 124: 1664–1668.

133 Rodriguez J, Bystryn J-C. Pemphigus foliaceus associated with absence of intercellular antigens in lower layers of epidermis. Arch Dermatol 1977; 113: 1696–1699.

134 Hernandez C, Amagai M, Chan LS. Pemphigus foliaceus: preferential binding of IgG1 and C3 at the upper epidermis. Br J Dermatol 1997; 136: 249–252.

135 Maize JC, Green D, Provost TT. Pemphigus foliaceus: a case with serologic features of Senear-Usher syndrome and other autoimmune abnormalities. J Am Acad Dermatol 1982; 7: 736–741.

136 Beutner EH, Chorzelski TP, McDonough Wilson R et al. IgA pemphigus foliaceus. Report of two cases and a review of the literature. J Am Acad Dermatol 1989; 20: 89–97.

137 Neumann E, Dmochowski M, Bowszyc J et al. The occurrence of IgA pemphigus foliaceus without neutrophilic infiltration. Clin Exp Dermatol 1994; 19: 56–58.

138 Jiao D, Bystryn J-C. Sensitivity of indirect immunofluorescence, substrate specificity, and immunoblotting in the diagnosis of pemphigus. J Am Acad Dermatol 1997; 37: 211–216.

139 Sotto MN, Shimizu SH, Costa JM, De Brito T. South American pemphigus foliaceus: electron microscopy and immunoelectron localization of bound immunoglobulin in the skin and oral mucosa. Br J Dermatol 1980; 102: 521–527.

140 Tada J, Hashimoto K. Curvicircular intracytoplasmic membranous structures in keratinocytes of pemphigus foliaceus. J Cutan Pathol 1996; 23: 511–517.

141 Iwatsuki K, Takigawa M, Jin F, Yamada M. Ultrastructural binding site of pemphigus foliaceus autoantibodies: comparison with pemphigus vulgaris. J Cutan Pathol 1991; 18: 160–163.

142 Shimizu H, Masunaga T, Ishiko A et al. Pemphigus vulgaris and pemphigus foliaceus sera show an inversely graded binding pattern to extracellular regions of desmosomes in different layers of human epidermis. J Invest Dermatol 1995; 105: 153–159.

143 Shimizu H, Masunaga T, Ishiko A et al. Demonstration of desmosomal antigens by electron microscopy using cryofixed and cryosubstituted skin with silver-enhanced gold probe. J Histochem Cytochem 1994; 42: 687–692.

144 Rosenberg FR, Sanders S, Nelson CT. Pemphigus. A 20-year review of 107 patients treated with corticosteroids. Arch Dermatol 1976; 112: 962–970.

145 Amerian ML, Ahmed AR. Pemphigus erythematosus. Senear-Usher syndrome. Int J Dermatol 1985; 24: 16–25.

146 Lyde CB, Cox SE, Cruz PD Jr. Pemphigus erythematosus in a five-year-old child. J Am Acad Dermatol 1994; 31: 906–909.

147 Van Joost T, Stolz E, Blog FB et al. Pemphigus erythematosus: clinical and histo-immunological studies in two unusual cases. Acta Derm Venereol 1984; 64: 257–260.

148 Ngo AW, Straka C, Fretzin D. Pemphigus erythematosus: a unique association with systemic lupus erythematosus. Cutis 1986; 38: 160–163.

149 Basler RSW. Senear-Usher syndrome with parathyroid adenoma. Br J Dermatol 1974; 91: 465–467.

150 Saikia NK, MacConnell LES. Senear-Usher syndrome and internal malignancy. Br J Dermatol 1972; 87: 1–5.

151 Chorzelski T, Jablonska S, Beutner EH, Kowalska M. Can pemphigus be provoked by a burn? Br J Dermatol 1971; 85: 320–325.

152 Pellicano R, Iannantuono M, Lomuto M. Pemphigus erythematosus induced by ceftazidime. Int J Dermatol 1993; 32: 675–676.

153 Kennedy C, Hodge L, Sanderson KV. Skin changes caused by D-penicillamine treatment of arthritis. Clin Exp Dermatol 1978; 3: 107–116.

154 De Jong MCJM, Doeglas HMG, Dijkstra JWE. Immunohistochemical findings in a patient with penicillamine pemphigus. Br J Dermatol 1980; 102: 333–337.

155 Amerian ML, Ahmed AR. Pemphigus erythematosus. Presentation of four cases and review of literature. J Am Acad Dermatol 1984; 10: 215–222.

156 Parfrey PS, Clement M, Vandenburg MJ, Wright P. Captopril-induced pemphigus. Br Med J 1980; 281: 194.

157 Alinovi A, Benoldi D, Manganelli P. Pemphigus erythematosus induced by thiopronine. Acta Derm Venereol 1982; 62: 452–454.

158 Fellner MJ, Wininger J. Pemphigus erythematosus and heroin addiction. Int J Dermatol 1978; 17: 308–311.

159 Ahmed AR. Pemphigus: current concepts. Ann Intern Med 1980; 92: 396–405.

160 Chorzelski T, Jablonska S, Blaszczyk M. Immunopathological investigations in the Senear-Usher syndrome (coexistence of pemphigus and lupus erythematosus). Br J Dermatol 1968; 80: 211–217.

161 Bean SF, Lynch FW. Senear-Usher syndrome (pemphigus erythematosus). Immunofluorescent studies in a patient. Arch Dermatol 1970; 101: 642–645.

162 Robinson ND, Hashimoto T, Amagai M, Chan LS. The new pemphigus variants. J Am Acad Dermatol 1999; 40: 649–671.

163 Morita E, Amagai M, Tanaka T et al. A case of herpetiform pemphigus coexisting with psoriasis vulgaris. Br J Dermatol 1999; 141: 754–755.

164 Cunha PR, Jiao D, Bystryn J-C. Simultaneous occurrence of herpetiform pemphigus and endemic pemphigus foliaceus (fogo selvagem). Int J Dermatol 1997; 36: 850–854.

165 Ishii K, Amagai M, Komai A et al. Desmoglein 1 and desmoglein 3 are the target autoantigens in herpetiform pemphigus. Arch Dermatol 1999; 135: 943–947.

166 Kubo A, Amagai M, Hashimoto T et al. Herpetiform pemphigus showing reactivity with pemphigus vulgaris antigen (desmoglein 3). Br J Dermatol 1997; 137: 109–113.

167 Sneddon IB, Wilkinson DS. Subcorneal pustular dermatosis. Br J Dermatol 1956; 68: 385–394.

168 Sneddon IB. Subcorneal pustular dermatosis. Int J Dermatol 1977; 16: 640–644.

169 Sneddon IB, Wilkinson DS. Subcorneal pustular dermatosis. Br J Dermatol 1979; 100: 61–68.

170 Kono T, Terashima T, Oura H et al. Recalcitrant subcorneal pustular dermatosis and bullous pemphigoid treated with mizoribine, an immunosuppressive, purine biosynthesis inhibitor. Br J Dermatol 2000; 143: 1328–1329.

171 Dallot A, Decazes JM, Drouault Y et al. Subcorneal pustular dermatosis (Sneddon-Wilkinson disease) with amicrobial lymph node suppuration and aseptic spleen abscesses. Br J Dermatol 1988; 119: 803–807.

172 Zachariae COC, Rossen K, Weismann K. An unusual severe case of subcorneal pustular dermatosis treated with cyclosporine and prednisolone. Acta Derm Venereol 2000; 80: 386–387.

173 Johnson SAM, Cripps DJ. Subcorneal pustular dermatosis in children. Arch Dermatol 1974; 109: 73–77.

174 Limmer BL. Subcorneal pustular dermatosis vs pustular psoriasis. Arch Dermatol 1974; 110: 131.

175 Kasha EE Jr, Epinette WW. Subcorneal pustular dermatosis (Sneddon-Wilkinson disease) in association with a monoclonal IgA gammopathy: a report and review of the literature. J Am Acad Dermatol 1988; 19: 854–858.

176 Marsden JR, Millard LG. Pyoderma gangrenosum, subcorneal pustular dermatosis and IgA paraproteinaemia. Br J Dermatol 1986; 114: 125–129.

177 Lautenschlager S, Itin PH, Hirsbrunner P, Buchner SA. Subcorneal pustular dermatosis at the injection site of recombinant human granulocyte-macrophage colony-stimulating factor in a patient with IgA myeloma. J Am Acad Dermatol 1994; 30: 787–789.

178 Bauwens M, De Coninck A, Roseeuw D. Subcorneal pustular dermatosis treated with PUVA therapy. A case report and review of the literature. Dermatology 1999; 198: 203–205.

179 Scerri L, Zaki I, Allen BR. Pyoderma gangrenosum and subcorneal pustular dermatosis, without monoclonal gammopathy. Br J Dermatol 1994; 130: 398–399.

180 Powell FC, Su WPD, Perry HO. Pyoderma gangrenosum: Classification and management. J Am Acad Dermatol 1996; 34: 395–409.

181 Ingber A, Ideses C, Halevy S, Feuerman EJ. Subcorneal pustular dermatosis (Sneddon-Wilkinson disease) after a diagnostic echogram. Report of two cases. J Am Acad Dermatol 1983; 9: 393–396.

182 Park B-S, Cho K-H, Eun H-C, Youn J-I. Subcorneal pustular dermatosis in a patient with aplastic anemia. J Am Acad Dermatol 1998; 39: 287–289.

183 Köhler LD, Möhrenschlager M, Worret WI, Ring J. Subcorneal pustular dermatosis (Sneddon-Wilkinson disease) in a patient with multiple sclerosis. Dermatology 1999; 199: 69–70.

184 Sanchez N, Ackerman AB. Subcorneal pustular dermatosis: a variant of pustular psoriasis. Acta Derm Venereol (Suppl) 1979; 85: 147–151.

185 Chimenti S, Ackerman AB. Is subcorneal pustular dermatosis of Sneddon and Wilkinson an entity sui generis? Am J Dermatopathol 1981; 3: 363–376.

186 Wolff K. Subcorneal pustular dermatosis is not pustular psoriasis. Am J Dermatopathol 1981; 3: 381–382.

187 Sanchez NP, Perry HO, Muller SA, Winkelmann RK. Subcorneal pustular dermatosis and pustular psoriasis. A clinicopathologic correlation. Arch Dermatol 1983; 119: 715–721.

188 Yamasaki R, Yamasaki M, Kawasaki Y, Nagasako R. Generalized pustular dermatosis caused by isoniazid. Br J Dermatol 1985; 112: 504–506.

189 Lambert DG, Dalac S, Beer F et al. Acute generalized exanthematous pustular dermatitis induced by diltiazem. Br J Dermatol 1988; 118: 308–309.

190 Weinberg JM, Egan CL, Tangoren IA et al. Generalized pustular dermatosis following paclitaxel therapy. Int J Dermatol 1997; 36: 559–560.

191 Stough D, Guin JD, Baker GF, Haynie L. Pustular eruptions following administration of cefazolin: a possible interaction with methyldopa. J Am Acad Dermatol 1987; 16: 1051–1052.

192 Shuttleworth D. A localized recurrent pustular eruption following amoxycillin administration. Clin Exp Dermatol 1989; 14: 367–368.

193 Halevy S, Ingber A, Feuerman J. Subcorneal pustular dermatosis – an unusual course. Acta Derm Venereol 1983; 63: 441–444.

194 Grob JJ, Mege JL, Capo C et al. Role of tumor necrosis factor-α in Sneddon-Wilkinson subcorneal pustular dermatosis. J Am Acad Dermatol 1991; 25: 944–947.

195 Ryan TJ. Sneddon and Wilkinson's pustular dermatosis does exist. Am J Dermatopathol 1981; 3: 383–384.

196 Wallach D, Janssen F, Vignon-Pennamen M-D et al. Atypical neutrophilic dermatosis with subcorneal IgA deposits. Arch Dermatol 1987; 123: 790–795.

197 Hashimoto T, Inamoto N, Nakamura K, Nishikawa T. Intercellular IgA dermatosis with clinical features of subcorneal pustular dermatosis. Arch Dermatol 1987; 123: 1062–1065.

198 Prost C, Intrator L, Wechsler J et al. IgA autoantibodies bind to pemphigus vulgaris antigen in a case of intraepidermal neutrophilic IgA dermatosis. J Am Acad Dermatol 1991; 25: 846–848.

199 Miyagawa S, Hashimoto T, Ohno H et al. Atypical pemphigus associated with monoclonal IgA gammopathy. J Am Acad Dermatol 1995; 32: 352–357.

200 Gruss C, Zillikens D, Hashimoto T et al. Rapid response of IgA pemphigus of subcorneal pustular dermatosis type to treatment with isotretinoin. J Am Acad Dermatol 2000; 43: 923–926.

201 Niimi Y, Kawana S, Kusunoki T. IgA pemphigus: A case report and its characteristic clinical features compared with subcorneal pustular dermatosis. J Am Acad Dermatol 2000; 43: 546–549.

202 Wallach D. Intraepidermal IgA pustulosis. J Am Acad Dermatol 1992; 27: 993–1000.

203 Kuan Y-Z, Chiou H-T, Chang H-C et al. Intraepidermal neutrophilic IgA dermatosis. J Am Acad Dermatol 1990; 22: 917–919.

204 Muldrow ME, Orr LK, Huff JC. Intraepidermal neutrophilic IgA dermatosis in a patient with advanced human immunodeficiency virus infection. Arch Dermatol 1997; 133: 667–668.

205 Ebihara T, Hashimoto T, Iwatsuki K et al. Autoantigens for IgA anti-intercellular antibodies of intercellular IgA vesiculopustular dermatosis. J Invest Dermatol 1991; 97: 742–745.

206 Todd DJ, Bingham EA, Walsh M, Burrows D. Subcorneal pustular dermatosis and IgA paraproteinaemia: response to both etretinate and PUVA. Br J Dermatol 1991; 125: 387–389.

207 Teraki Y, Amagai N, Hashimoto T et al. Intercellular IgA dermatosis of childhood. Arch Dermatol 1991; 127: 221–224.

208 Harman KE, Holmes G, Bhogal BS et al. Intercellular IgA dermatosis (IgA pemphigus) – two cases illustrating the clinical heterogeneity of this disorder. Clin Exp Dermatol 1999; 24: 464–466.

209 Supapannachart N, Mutasim DF. The distribution of IgA pemphigus antigen in human skin and the role of IgA anti-cell surface antibodies in the induction of intraepidermal acantholysis. Arch Dermatol 1993; 129: 605–608.

210 Chorzelski TP, Beutner EH, Kowalewski C et al. IgA pemphigus foliaceus with a clinical presentation of pemphigus herpetiformis. J Am Acad Dermatol 1991; 24: 839–844.

211 Hodak E, David M, Ingber A et al. The clinical and histopathological spectrum of IgA-pemphigus – report of two cases. Clin Exp Dermatol 1990; 15: 433–437.

212 Yasuda H, Kobayashi H, Hashimoto T et al. Subcorneal pustular dermatosis type of IgA pemphigus: demonstration of autoantibodies to desmocollin-1 and clinical review. Br J Dermatol 2000; 143: 144–148.

213 Hashimoto T, Amagai M, Garrod DR, Nishikawa T. Human desmocollin 1 (Dsc1) is an autoantigen for subcorneal pustular dermatosis type of intercellular IgA vesiculopustular dermatosis (IgA pemphigus). J Invest Dermatol 1996; 106: 832 (abstract).

214 Hashimoto T, Kiyokawa C, Mori O et al. Human desmocollin 1 (Dsc 1) is an autoantigen for the subcorneal pustular dermatosis type of IgA pemphigus. J Invest Dermatol 1997; 109: 127–131.

215 Hashimoto T, Komai A, Futei Y et al. Detection of IgA autoantibodies to desmogleins by an enzyme-linked immunosorbent assay. The presence of new minor subtypes of IgA pemphigus. Arch Dermatol 2001; 137: 735–738.

216 Caputo R, Pistritto G, Gianni E et al. IgA pemphigus in a child. J Am Acad Dermatol 1991; 25: 383–386.

217 Myers SA, Rico MJ. Intraepidermal neutrophilic IgA dermatosis in an HIV-infected patient. J Am Acad Dermatol 1994; 31: 502–504.

218 Weston WL, Friednash M, Hashimoto T et al. A novel childhood pemphigus vegetans variant of intraepidermal neutrophilic IgA dermatosis. J Am Acad Dermatol 1998; 38: 635–638.

219 Kim S-C, Won JH, Chung J, Bang DS. IgA pemphigus: report of a case with immunoelectron localization of bound IgA in the skin. J Am Acad Dermatol 1996; 34: 852–854.

220 Kahana M, Schewach-Millet M, Feinstein A. Infantile acropustulosis – report of a case. Clin Exp Dermatol 1987; 12: 291–292.

221 Newton JA, Salisbury J, Marsden A, McGibbon DH. Acropustulosis of infancy. Br J Dermatol 1986; 115: 735–739.

222 Jennings JL, Burrows WM. Infantile acropustulosis. J Am Acad Dermatol 1983; 9: 733–738.

223 McFadden N, Falk ES. Infantile acropustulosis. Cutis 1985; 36: 49–51.

224 Vignon-Pennamen M-D, Wallach D. Infantile acropustulosis. A clinicopathologic study of six cases. Arch Dermatol 1986; 122: 1155–1160.

225 Bundino S, Zina AM, Ubertalli S. Infantile acropustulosis. Dermatologica 1982; 165: 615–619.

226 Dromy R, Raz A, Metzker A. Infantile acropustulosis. Pediatr Dermatol 1991; 8: 284–287.

227 Truong AL, Esterly NB. Atypical acropustulosis in infancy. Int J Dermatol 1997; 36: 688–691.

228 van Praag MCG, van Rooij RWG, Folkers E et al. Diagnosis and treatment of pustular disorders in the neonate. Pediatr Dermatol 1997; 14: 131–143.

229 Prendiville JS. Infantile acropustulosis – how often is it a sequela of scabies? Pediatr Dermatol 1995; 12: 275–276.

230 Humeau S, Bureau B, Litoux P, Stalder J-F. Infantile acropustulosis in six immigrant children. Pediatr Dermatol 1995; 12: 211–214.

231 Mancini AJ, Frieden IJ, Paller AS. Infantile acropustulosis revisited: history of scabies and response to topical corticosteroids. Pediatr Dermatol 1998; 15: 337–341.

232 Bardazzi F, Patrizi A, Neri I. Transient cephalic neonatal pustulosis. Arch Dermatol 1997; 133: 528–529.

233 Sidhu-Malik NK, Resnick SD, Wilson BB. Congenital erosive and vesicular dermatosis healing with reticulated supple scarring: report of three new cases and review of the literature. Pediatr Dermatol 1998; 15: 214–218.

234 Lerner LH, Wiss K, Gellis S, Barnhill R. An unusual pustular eruption in an infant with Down syndrome and a congenital leukemoid reaction. J Am Acad Dermatol 1996; 35: 330–333.

235 Nijhawan A, Baselga E, Gonzalez-Ensenat MA et al. Vesiculopustular eruptions in Down syndrome neonates with myeloproliferative disorders. Arch Dermatol 2001; 137: 760–763.

236 Taïeb A, Bassan-Andrieu L, Maleville J. Eosinophilic pustulosis of the scalp in childhood. J Am Acad Dermatol 1992; 27: 55–60.

237 Vicente J, España A, Idoate M et al. Are eosinophilic pustular folliculitis of infancy and infantile acropustulosis the same entity? Br J Dermatol 1996; 135: 807–809.

238 Freeman RG, Spiller R, Knox JM. Histopathology of erythema toxicum neonatorum. Arch Dermatol 1960; 82: 586–589.

239 Marino LJ. Toxic erythema present at birth. Arch Dermatol 1965; 92: 402–403.

240 Schachner L, Press S. Vesicular, bullous and pustular disorders in infancy and childhood. Pediatr Clin North Am 1983; 30: 609–629.

241 Esterly NB. Vesiculopustular eruptions in the neonate. Australas J Dermatol 1991; 32: 1–12.

242 Marchini G, Ulfgren A-K, Loré K et al. Erythema toxicum neonatorum: an immunohistochemical analysis. Pediatr Dermatol 2001; 18: 177–187.

243 Chang MW, Jiang SB, Orlow SJ. Atypical erythema toxicum neonatorum of delayed onset in a term infant. Pediatr Dermatol 1999; 16: 137–141.

244 Luders D. Histologic observations in erythema toxicum neonatorum. Pediatrics 1960; 26: 219–224.

245 Lucky AW, Esterly NB, Heskel N et al. Eosinophilic pustular folliculitis in infancy. Pediatr Dermatol 1984; 1: 202–206.

246 Ramamurthy RS, Reveri M, Esterly NB et al. Transient neonatal pustular melanosis. J Pediatr 1976; 88: 831–835.

247 Auster B. Transient neonatal pustular melanosis. Cutis 1978; 22: 327–328.

248 Barr RJ, Globerman LM, Werber FA. Transient neonatal pustular melanosis. Int J Dermatol 1979; 18: 636–638.

249 Sidoroff A, Halevy S, Bavinck JNB et al. Acute generalized exanthematous pustulosis (AGEP) – a clinical reaction pattern. J Cutan Pathol 2001; 28: 113–119.

250 Haro-Gabaldón V, Sánchez-Sánchez-Vizcaino J, Ruiz-Avila P et al. Acute generalized exanthematous pustulosis with cytomegalovirus infection. Int J Dermatol 1996; 35: 735–737.

251 Eeckhout I, Noens L, Ongenae K et al. Acute generalized exanthematous pustulosis: a case with a lymphoma-like presentation. Dermatology 1997; 194: 408–410.

252 Kleier RS, Breneman DL, Boiko S. Generalized pustulation as a manifestation of the anticonvulsant hypersensitivity syndrome. Arch Dermatol 1991; 127: 1361–1364.

253 Roujeau J-C, Bioulac-Sage P, Bourseau C et al. Acute generalized exanthematous pustulosis. Analysis of 63 cases. Arch Dermatol 1991; 127: 1333–1338.

254 Smith KJ, Norwood C, Pehoushek P, Skelton H. Is acute generalized exanthematous pustulosis an eruption associated with a T helper 1 pattern of cytokine dysregulation? J Cutan Pathol 2000; 27: 572 (abstract).

255 Moreau A, Dompmartin A, Castel B et al. Drug-induced acute generalized exanthematous pustulosis with positive patch tests. Int J Dermatol 1995; 34: 263–266.

256 Boffa MJ, Chalmers RJG. Allopurinol-induced toxic pustuloderma. Br J Dermatol 1994; 131: 447.

257 Heymann WR, Manders SM. Itraconazole-induced acute generalized exanthemic pustulosis. J Am Acad Dermatol 1995; 32: 130–131.

258 Park YM, Kim JW, Kim CW. Acute generalized exanthematous pustulosis induced by itraconazole. J Am Acad Dermatol 1997; 36: 794–796.

259 Wakelin SH, James MP. Diltiazem-induced acute generalised exanthematous pustulosis. Clin Exp Dermatol 1995; 20: 341–344.

260 Knowles S, Gupta AK, Shear NH. The spectrum of cutaneous reactions associated with diltiazem: Three cases and a review of the literature. J Am Acad Dermatol 1998; 38: 201–206.

261 Vicente-Calleja JM, Aguirre A, Landa N et al. Acute generalized exanthematous pustulosis due to diltiazem: confirmation by patch testing. Br J Dermatol 1997; 137: 837–839.

262 Jan V, Machet L, Gironet N et al. Acute generalized exanthematous pustulosis induced by diltiazem: value of patch testing. Dermatology 1998; 197: 274–275.

263 Lee S, Artemi P, Holt D. Acute generalized exanthematous pustulosis. Australas J Dermatol 1995; 36: 25–27.

264 Bissonnette R, Tousignant J, Allaire G. Drug-induced toxic pustuloderma. Int J Dermatol 1992; 31: 172–174.

265 Spencer JM, Silvers DN, Grossman ME. Pustular eruption after drug exposure: is it pustular psoriasis or a pustular drug eruption? Br J Dermatol 1994; 130: 514–519.

266 Lee A-Y, Yoo S-H. Chloramphenicol induced acute generalized exanthematous pustulosis proved by patch test and systemic provocation. Acta Derm Venereol 1999; 79: 412–413.

267 Sawhney RA, Dubin DB, Otley CC et al. Generalized exanthematous pustulosis induced by medications. Int J Dermatol 1996; 35: 826–827.

268 Chu C-Y, Wu J, Jean S-S, Sun C-C. Acute generalized exanthematous pustulosis due to teicoplanin. Dermatology 2001; 202: 141–142.

269 Ohtsuka T, Yamakage A, Yamazaki S. Acute generalized exanthematous pustulosis – an apoptotic process as suggested by immunohistochemical analysis? Dermatology 1998; 197: 188–189.

270 Küchler A, Hamm H, Weidenthaler-Barth B et al. Acute generalized exanthematous pustulosis following oral nystatin therapy: a report of three cases. Br J Dermatol 1997; 137: 808–811.

271 Corbalán-Vélez R, Peón G, Ara M, Carapeto F-J. Localized toxic follicular pustuloderma. Int J Dermatol 2000; 39: 209–211.

272 Meadows KP, Egan CA, Vanderhooft S. Acute generalized exanthematous pustulosis (AGEP), an uncommon condition in children: case report and review of the literature. Pediatr Dermatol 2000; 17: 399–402.

273 Bennett ML, Jorizzo JL, White WL. Generalized pustular eruptions associated with oral terbinafine. Int J Dermatol 1999; 38: 596–600.

274 Condon CA, Downs AMR, Archer CB. Terbinafine-induced acute generalized exanthematous pustulosis. Br J Dermatol 1998; 138: 709–710.

275 Kempinaire A, De Raeve L, Merckx M et al. Terbinafine-induced acute generalized exanthematous pustulosis confirmed by a positive patch-test result. J Am Acad Dermatol 1997; 37: 653–655.

276 Dupin N, Gorin I, Djien V et al. Acute generalized exanthematous pustulosis induced by terbinafine. Arch Dermatol 1996; 132: 1253–1254.

277 Belgodère X, Olivier V, Basteri M et al. Acute generalized exanthematous pustulosis following administration of ceftriaxone. Int J Dermatol 2000; 39: 558–559.

278 Valance A, Lebrum-Vignes B, Descamps V et al. Icodextrin cutaneous hypersensitivity. Report of 3 psoriasiform cases. Arch Dermatol 2001; 137: 309–310.

279 Darvay A, Basarab T, Russell-Jones R. Thalidomide-induced toxic pustuloderma. Clin Exp Dermatol 1997; 22: 297–299.

280 Gallego I, Badell A, Notario J et al. Toxic pustuloderma induced by intracavernous prostaglandin E_1. Br J Dermatol 1997; 136: 975–976.

281 Cannavò SP, Borgia F, Guarneri F, Vaccaro M. Acute generalized exanthematous pustulosis following use of ticlopidine. Br J Dermatol 2000; 142: 577–578.

282 Watsky KL. Acute generalized exanthematous pustulosis induced by metronidazole: the role of patch testing. Arch Dermatol 1999; 135: 93–94.

283 Adams BB, Mutasim DF. Pustular eruption induced by olanzapine, a novel antipsychotic agent. J Am Acad Dermatol 1999; 41: 851–853.

284 Feind-Koopmans A, van der Valk PGM, Steijlen PM, van de Kerkhof PCM. Toxic pustuloderma associated with clemastine therapy. Clin Exp Dermatol 1996; 21: 293–295.

285 Halevy S, Cohen AD, Livni E. Acute generalized exanthematous pustulosis associated with polysensitivity to paracetamol and bromhexine: the diagnostic role of *in vitro* interferon-γ release test. Clin Exp Dermatol 2000; 25: 652–654.

286 Young PC, Turiansky GW, Bonner MW, Benson PM. Acute generalized exanthematous pustulosis induced by chromium picolinate. J Am Acad Dermatol 1999; 41: 820–823.

287 Valks R, Fraga J, Muñoz E et al. Acute generalized exanthematous pustulosis in patients receiving high-dose chemotherapy. Arch Dermatol 1999; 135: 1418–1420.

288 Ferguson JE, Chalmers RJG. Enalapril-induced toxic pustuloderma. Clin Exp Dermatol 1996; 21: 54–55.

289 Burrows NP, Russell Jones R. Pustular drug eruptions: a histopathological spectrum. Histopathology 1993; 22: 569–573.

290 Wilairatana P, Looareesuwan S, Riganti M et al. Pustular eruption in a malaria patient treated with chloroquine. Int J Dermatol 1997; 36: 634–635.

291 Janier M, Froidevaux D, Lons-Danic D, Daniel F. Acute generalized exanthematous pustulosis due to the combination of chloroquine and proguanil. Dermatology 1998; 196: 271.

292 Park YM, Park JG, Kang H et al. Acute generalized exanthematous pustulosis induced by ingestion of lacquer chicken. Br J Dermatol 2000; 143: 230–232.

Intraepidermal blisters

293 Uehara M. Pustulosis palmaris et plantaris: evolutionary sequence from vesicular to pustular lesions. Semin Dermatol 1983; 2: 51–56.

294 Rosen K. Pustulosis palmoplantaris and chronic eczematous hand dermatitis. Acta Derm Venereol (Suppl) 1988; 137: 7–52.

295 van de Kerkhof PCM. Pustulosis palmaris et plantaris. J Eur Acad Dermatol Venereol 2000; 14: 248.

296 Hellgren L, Mobacken H. Pustulosis palmaris et plantaris. Prevalence, clinical observations and prognosis. Acta Derm Venereol 1971; 51: 284–288.

297 Jansen CT, Hollmen A, Pajarre R, Terho P. Antichlamydial antibodies in chronic palmoplantar pustulosis. Acta Derm Venereol 1980; 60: 263–266.

298 Paller AS, Packman L, Rich K et al. Pustulosis palmaris et plantaris: its association with chronic recurrent multifocal osteomyelitis. J Am Acad Dermatol 1985; 12: 927–930.

299 Erkko P, Granlund H, Remitz A et al. Double-blind placebo-controlled study of long-term low-dose cyclosporin in the treatment of palmoplantar pustulosis. Br J Dermatol 1998; 139: 997–1004.

300 Thomsen K, Osterbye P. Pustulosis palmaris et plantaris. Br J Dermatol 1973; 89: 293–296.

301 Ward JM, Barnes RMR. HLA antigens in persistent palmoplantar pustulosis and its relationship to psoriasis. Br J Dermatol 1978; 99: 477–483.

302 Iwatsuki K, Imaizumi S, Tsugiki M et al. Alterations of surface receptors on intralesional neutrophils in pustular psoriasis and palmo-plantar pustulosis. Br J Dermatol 1985; 112: 53–56.

303 White SW. Palmoplantar pustular psoriasis provoked by lithium therapy. J Am Acad Dermatol 1982; 7: 660–662.

304 Jurik AG, Ternowitz T. Frequency of skeletal disease, arthro-osteitis, in patients with pustulosis palmoplantaris. J Am Acad Dermatol 1988; 18: 666–671.

305 Torii H, Nakagawa H, Ishibashi Y. Osteoarthritis in 84 Japanese patients with palmoplantar pustulosis. J Am Acad Dermatol 1994; 31: 732–735.

306 Sofman MS, Prose NS. Dermatoses associated with sterile lytic bone lesions. J Am Acad Dermatol 1990; 23: 494–498.

307 Rosen K, Jontell M, Mobacken H, Rosdahl I. Epidermal Langerhans' cells in patients with pustulosis palmoplantaris treated with etretinate or etretinate + methoxsalen photochemotherapy. Acta Derm Venereol 1988; 68: 218–223.

308 Eriksson M-O, Hagforsen E, Lundin IP, Michaélsson G. Palmoplantar pustulosis: a clinical and immunohistological study. Br J Dermatol 1998; 138: 390–398.

309 Goette DK, Morgan AM, Fox BJ, Horn RT. Treatment of palmoplantar pustulosis with intralesional triamcinolone injections. Arch Dermatol 1984; 120: 319–323.

310 Stevens DM, Ackerman AB. On the concept of bacterids (pustular bacterid, Andrews). Am J Dermatopathol 1984; 6: 281–286.

311 Burge SM, Ryan TJ. Acute palmoplantar pustulosis. Br J Dermatol 1985; 113: 77–83.

312 Hagforsen E, Einarsson A, Aronsson F et al. The distribution of choline acetyltransferase- and acetylcholinesterase-like immunoreactivity in the palmar skin of patients with palmoplantar pustulosis. Br J Dermatol 2000; 142: 234–242.

313 Nakamura K, Imakado S, Takizawa M et al. Exacerbation of pustulosis palmaris et plantaris after topical application of metals accompanied by elevated levels of leukotriene B_4 in pustules. J Am Acad Dermatol 2000; 42: 1021–1025.

314 Thormann J, Heilesen B. Recalcitrant pustular eruptions of the extremities. J Cutan Pathol 1975; 2: 19–24.

315 Takematsu H, Ohkohchi K, Tagami H. Demonstration of anaphylatoxins C3a, C4a and C5a in the scales of psoriasis and inflammatory pustular dermatoses. Br J Dermatol 1986; 114: 1–6.

316 Bénéton N, Wolkenstein P, Bagot M et al. Amicrobial pustulosis associated with autoimmune diseases: healing with zinc supplementation. Br J Dermatol 2000; 143: 1306–1310.

317 Stefanidou MP, Kanavaros PE, Stefanaki KS, Tosca AD. Amicrobial pustulosis of the folds. A cutaneous manifestation associated with connective tissue disease. Dermatology 1998; 197: 394–396.

Suprabasilar blisters

318 Ahmed AR. Clinical features of pemphigus. Clin Dermatol 1983; 1: 13–21.

319 Becker BA, Gaspari AA. Pemphigus vulgaris and vegetans. Dermatol Clin 1993; 11: 429–452.

320 Micali G, Musumeci ML, Nasca MR. Epidemiologic analysis and clinical course of 84 consecutive cases of pemphigus in eastern Sicily. Int J Dermatol 1998; 37: 197–200.

321 Tsankov N, Vassileva S, Kamarashev J et al. Epidemiology of pemphigus in Sofia, Bulgaria. A 16-year retrospective study (1980–1995). Int J Dermatol 2000; 39: 104–108.

322 Meurer M, Millns JL, Rogers RS III, Jordon RE. Oral pemphigus vulgaris. A report of ten cases. Arch Dermatol 1977; 113: 1520–1524.

323 Sirois DA, Fatahzadeh M, Roth R, Ettlin D. Diagnostic patterns and delays in pemphigus vulgaris: experience with 99 patients. Arch Dermatol 2000; 136: 1569–1570.

324 Engineer L, Norton LA, Ahmed AR. Nail involvement in pemphigus vulgaris. J Am Acad Dermatol 2000; 43: 529–535.

325 Sami N, Ahmed AR. Penile pemphigus. Arch Dermatol 2001; 137: 756–758.

326 Shklar G, Cataldo E. Histopathology and cytology of oral lesions of pemphigus. Arch Dermatol 1970; 101: 635–641.

327 Scully C, Paes De Almeida O, Porter SR, Gilkes JJH. Pemphigus vulgaris: the manifestations and long-term management of 55 patients with oral lesions. Br J Dermatol 1999; 140: 84–89.

328 Bean SF, Holubar K, Gillett RB. Pemphigus involving the eyes. Arch Dermatol 1975; 111: 1484–1486.

329 Hale EK, Bystryn J-C. Laryngeal and nasal involvement in pemphigus vulgaris. J Am Acad Dermatol 2001; 44: 609–611.

330 Kaneko F, Mori M, Tsukinaga I, Miura Y. Pemphigus vulgaris of esophageal mucosa. Arch Dermatol 1985; 121: 272–273.

331 Goldberg NS, Weiss SS. Pemphigus vulgaris of the esophagus in women. J Am Acad Dermatol 1989; 21: 1115–1118.

332 Sagher F, Bercovici B, Romem R. Nikolsky sign on cervix uteri in pemphigus. Br J Dermatol 1974; 90: 407–411.

333 Lonsdale RN, Gibbs S. Pemphigus vulgaris with involvement of the cervix. Br J Dermatol 1998; 138: 363–365.

334 Batta K, Munday PE, Tatnall FM. Pemphigus vulgaris localized to the vagina presenting as chronic vaginal discharge. Br J Dermatol 1999; 140: 945–947.

335 Tan HH, Tay YK. An unusual case of pemphigus vulgaris presenting as bilateral foot ulcers. Clin Exp Dermatol 2000; 25: 224–226.

336 Shirahama S, Furukawa F, Takigawa M. Recurrent pemphigus vulgaris limited to the surgical area after mastectomy. J Am Acad Dermatol 1998; 39: 352–355.

337 Ahmed AR, Salm M. Juvenile pemphigus. J Am Acad Dermatol 1983; 8: 799–807.

338 Bjarnason B, Flosadóttir E. Childhood, neonatal, and stillborn pemphigus vulgaris. Int J Dermatol 1999; 38: 680–688.

339 Harangi F, Várszegi D, Schneider I, Zombai E. Complete recovery from juvenile pemphigus vulgaris. Pediatr Dermatol 2001; 18: 51–53.

340 Reohr PB, Mangklabruks A, Janiga AM et al. Pemphigus vulgaris in siblings: HLA-DR4 and HLA-DQw3 and susceptibility to pemphigus. J Am Acad Dermatol 1992; 27: 189–193.

341 Starzycki Z, Chorzelski TP, Jablonska S. Familial pemphigus vulgaris in mother and daughter. Int J Dermatol 1998; 37: 211–214.

342 Hup JM, Bruinsma RA, Boersma ER, de Jong MCJM. Neonatal pemphigus vulgaris: transplacental transmission of antibodies. Pediatr Dermatol 1986; 3: 468–472.

343 Moncado B, Sandoval-Cruz JM, Baranda L, Garcia-Reyes J. Neonatal pemphigus. Int J Dermatol 1989; 28: 123–124.

344 Grunwald MH, Zamora E, Avinoach I et al. Pemphigus neonatorum. Pediatr Dermatol 1993; 10: 169–170.

345 Goldberg NS, DeFeo C, Kirshenbaum N. Pemphigus vulgaris and pregnancy: risk factors and recommendations. J Am Acad Dermatol 1993; 28: 877–879.

346 Tope WD, Kamino H, Briggaman RA et al. Neonatal pemphigus vulgaris in a child born to a woman in remission. J Am Acad Dermatol 1993; 29: 480–485.

347 Hern S, Vaughan Jones SA, Setterfield J et al. Pemphigus vulgaris in pregnancy with favourable foetal prognosis. Clin Exp Dermatol 1998; 23: 260–263.

348 Chowdhury MMU, Natarajan S. Neonatal pemphigus vulgaris associated with mild oral pemphigus vulgaris in the mother during pregnancy. Br J Dermatol 1998; 139: 500–503.

349 Ohta M, Yamamoto M, Utani A et al. Pemphigus vulgaris presenting as a nodular lesion. J Am Acad Dermatol 1990; 23: 522–523.

350 Faber WR, Neumann HAM, Flinterman J. Persistent vegetating and keratotic lesions in patients with pemphigus vulgaris during immunosuppressive therapy. Br J Dermatol 1983; 109: 459–463.

351 Coverton RW, Armstrong RB. Acanthosis nigricans developing in resolving lesions of pemphigus vulgaris. Arch Dermatol 1982; 118: 115–116.

352 Leibovici V, Ron N, Goldenhersh M, Holubar K. Coexistence of pemphigus and bullous pemphigoid. Int J Dermatol 1989; 28: 259–260.

353 Kore-eda S, Horiguchi Y, Ohtoshi E et al. A case of autoimmune bullous dermatosis with features of pemphigus vulgaris and bullous pemphigoid. Am J Dermatopathol 1995; 17: 511–516.

354 Iwatsuki K, Takigawa M, Hashimoto T et al. Can pemphigus vulgaris become pemphigus foliaceus? J Am Acad Dermatol 1991; 25: 797–800.

355 Chang SN, Kim S-C, Lee I-J et al. Transition from pemphigus vulgaris to pemphigus foliaceus. Br J Dermatol 1997; 137: 303–305.

356 Kawana S, Hashimoto T, Nishikawa T, Nishiyama S. Changes in clinical features, histologic findings, and antigen profiles with development of pemphigus foliaceus from pemphigus vulgaris. Arch Dermatol 1994; 130: 1534–1538.

357 Komai A, Amagai M, Ishii K et al. The clinical transition between pemphigus foliaceus and pemphigus vulgaris correlates well with the changes in autoantibody profile assessed by an enzyme-linked immunosorbent assay. Br J Dermatol 2001; 144: 1177–1182.

358 Younus J, Ahmed AR. The relationship of pemphigus to neoplasia. J Am Acad Dermatol 1990; 23: 498–502.

359 Kanwar AJ, Dawn G, Dhar S, Gangopadhyay M. Pemphigus vulgaris and renal cell carcinoma. Int J Dermatol 1996; 35: 723–724.

360 Gili A, Ngan B-Y, Lester R. Castleman's disease associated with pemphigus vulgaris. J Am Acad Dermatol 1991; 25: 955–959.

361 Saito K, Morita M, Enomoto K. Bronchiolitis obliterans with pemphigus vulgaris and Castleman's disease of hyaline-vascular type: an autopsy case analyzed by computer-aided 3-D reconstruction of the airway lesions. Hum Pathol 1997; 28: 1310–1312.

362 Norris DL, Saywell MS, Strutton GM, Stephenson GJ. Pemphigus vulgaris associated with spindle cell thymoma. Australas J Dermatol 1993; 34: 97–102.

363 Vetters JM, Saikia NK, Wood J, Simpson JA. Pemphigus vulgaris and myasthenia gravis. Br J Dermatol 1973; 88: 437–441.

364 Chan LS, Cooper KD. Coexistence of pemphigus vulgaris and progressive localized scleroderma. Arch Dermatol 1989; 125: 1555–1557.

365 Hamlet KR, Stevens SR, Gushurst C et al. Juvenile pemphigus vulgaris associated with Graves' disease. J Am Acad Dermatol 1995; 33: 132–134.

366 Yamagami Y, Kohda M, Mimura S, Ueki H. Pemphigus vulgaris associated with silicosis. Dermatology 1998; 197: 55–57.

367 Kuchabal DS, Kuchabal SD, Pandit AM, Nashi HK. Pemphigus vulgaris associated with systemic lupus erythematosus. Int J Dermatol 1998; 37: 636–638.

368 Hay RJ, Calnan CD. Oral submucosal fibrosis in a patient with pemphigus vulgaris. Clin Exp Dermatol 1979; 4: 381–383.

369 Brown P, Taylor B. Herpes simplex infection associated with pemphigus vulgaris. Case report and literature review. J Am Acad Dermatol 1989; 21: 1126–1128.

370 Capizzi R, Marasca G, De Luca A et al. Pemphigus vulgaris in a human-immunodeficiency-virus-infected patient. Dermatology 1998; 197: 97–98.

371 Firooz A, Mazhar A, Ahmed AR. Prevalence of autoimmune diseases in the family members of patients with pemphigus vulgaris. J Am Acad Dermatol 1994; 31: 434–437.

372 Kirtschig G, Mittag H, Wolf M et al. Three different autoimmune bullous diseases in one family: is there a common genetic base? Br J Dermatol 1999; 140: 322–327.

373 Lombardi ML, Mercuro O, Ruocco V et al. Common human leukocyte antigen alleles in pemphigus vulgaris and pemphigus foliaceus Italian patients. J Invest Dermatol 1999; 113: 107–110.

374 Hertl M, Karr RW, Amagai M, Katz SI. Heterogeneous MHC II restriction pattern of autoreactive desmoglein 3 specific T cell responses in pemphigus vulgaris patients and normals. J Invest Dermatol 1998; 110: 388–392.

375 Seidenbaum M, David M, Sandbank M. The course and prognosis of pemphigus. A review of 115 patients. Int J Dermatol 1988; 27: 580–584.

376 Martin FJ, Pérez-Bernal AM, Camacho F. Pemphigus vulgaris and disseminated nocardiosis. J Eur Acad Dermatol Venereol 2000; 14: 416–418.

377 Savin JA. The events leading to the death of patients with pemphigus and pemphigoid. Br J Dermatol 1979; 101: 521–534.

378 Herbst A, Bystryn J-C. Patterns of remission in pemphigus vulgaris. J Am Acad Dermatol 2000; 42: 422–427.

379 Ioannides D, Chrysomallis F, Bystryn J-C. Ineffectiveness of cyclosporine as an adjuvant to corticosteroids in the treatment of pemphigus. Arch Dermatol 2000; 136: 868–872.

380 Stanley JR. Therapy of pemphigus vulgaris. Arch Dermatol 1999; 135: 76–78.

381 Turner MS, Sutton D, Sauder DN. The use of plasmapheresis and immunosuppression in the treatment of pemphigus vulgaris. J Am Acad Dermatol 2000; 43: 1058–1064.

382 Piontek J-O, Borberg H, Sollberg S et al. Severe exacerbation of pemphigus vulgaris in pregnancy: successful treatment with plasma exchange. Br J Dermatol 2000; 143: 455–456.

383 Lenz P, Amagai M, Volc-Platzer B et al. Desmoglein 3-ELISA. A pemphigus vulgaris-specific diagnostic tool. Arch Dermatol 1999; 135: 143–148.

384 Amagai M, Komai A, Hashimoto T et al. Usefulness of enzyme-linked immunosorbent assay using recombinant desmogleins 1 and 3 for serodiagnosis of pemphigus. Br J Dermatol 1999; 140: 351–357.

385 Nishikawa T. Desmoglein ELISAs. A novel diagnostic tool for pemphigus. Arch Dermatol 1999; 135: 195–196.

386 Harman KE, Gratian MJ, Seed PT et al. Diagnosis of pemphigus by ELISA: a critical evaluation of two ELISAs for the detection of antibodies to the major pemphigus antigens, desmoglein 1 and 3. Clin Exp Dermatol 2000; 25: 236–240.

387 Gaspari AA. Advances in laboratory evaluation of pemphigus vulgaris. Arch Dermatol 1999; 135: 1418.

388 Plott RT, Amagai M, Udey MC, Stanley JR. Pemphigus vulgaris antigen lacks biochemical properties characteristic of classical cadherins. J Invest Dermatol 1994; 103: 168–172.

389 Stanley JR. The unexpected pathophysiologic link between pemphigus and chronic urticaria. Clin Exp Dermatol 2000; 25: 158.

390 Iwatsuki K, Takigawa M, Imaizumi S, Yamada M. In vivo binding site of pemphigus vulgaris antibodies and their fate during acantholysis. J Am Acad Dermatol 1989; 20: 578–582.

391 Wilson CL, Dean D, Wojnarowska F. Pemphigus and the terminal hair follicle. J Cutan Pathol 1991; 18: 428–431.

392 Futei Y, Amagai M, Sekiguchi M et al. Use of domain-swapped molecules for conformational epitope mapping of desmoglein 3 in pemphigus vulgaris. J Invest Dermatol 2000; 115: 829–834.

393 Amagai M, Kárpáti S, Klaus-Kovtun V et al. Extracellular domain of pemphigus vulgaris antigen (desmoglein 3) mediates weak homophilic adhesion. J Invest Dermatol 1994; 102: 402–408.

394 Müller E, Caldelari R, de Bruin A et al. Pathogenesis in pemphigus vulgaris: a central role for the armadillo protein plakoglobin. J Invest Dermatol 2000; 115: 332 (abstract).

395 Ding X, Diaz LA, Fairley JA et al. The anti-desmoglein 1 autoantibodies in pemphigus vulgaris sera are pathogenic. J Invest Dermatol 1999; 112: 739–743.

396 Kricheli D, David M, Frusic-Zlotkin M et al. The distribution of pemphigus vulgaris-IgG subclasses and their reactivity with desmoglein 3 and 1 in pemphigus patients and their first-degree relatives. Br J Dermatol 2000; 143: 337–342.

397 Spaeth S, Riechers R, Borradori L et al. IgG, IgA and IgE autoantibodies against the ectodomain of desmoglein 3 in active pemphigus vulgaris. Br J Dermatol 2001; 144: 1183–1188.

398 Amagai M, Tsunoda K, Zillikens D et al. The clinical phenotype of pemphigus is defined by the anti-desmoglein autoantibody profile. J Am Acad Dermatol 1999; 40: 167–170.

399 Miyagawa S, Amagai M, Iida T et al. Late development of antidesmoglein 1 antibodies in pemphigus vulgaris: correlation with disease progression. Br J Dermatol 1999; 141: 1084–1087.

400 Amagai M. Towards a better understanding of pemphigus autoimmunity. Br J Dermatol 2000; 143: 237–238.

401 Harman KE, Gratian MJ, Bhogal BS et al. A study of desmoglein 1 autoantibodies in pemphigus vulgaris: racial differences in frequency and the association with a more severe phenotype. Br J Dermatol 2000; 143: 343–348.

402 Ding X, Aoki V, Mascaro JM Jr et al. Mucosal and mucocutaneous (generalized) pemphigus vulgaris show distinct autoantibody profiles. J Invest Dermatol 1997; 109: 592–596.

403 Harman KE, Seed PT, Gratian MJ et al. The severity of cutaneous and oral pemphigus is related to desmoglein 1 and 3 antibody levels. Br J Dermatol 2001; 144: 775–780.

404 Nishifuji K, Amagai M, Kuwana M et al. Detection of antigen-specific B cells in patients with pemphigus vulgaris by enzyme-linked immunospot assay: requirement of T cell collaboration for autoantibody production. J Invest Dermatol 2000; 114: 88–94.

405 Iwatsuki K, Han G-W, Fukuti R et al. Internalization of constitutive desmogleins with the subsequent induction of desmoglein 2 in pemphigus lesions. Br J Dermatol 1999; 140: 35–43.

406 Burge SM, Wilson CL, Dean D, Wojnarowska F. An immunohistological study of desmosomal components in pemphigus. Br J Dermatol 1993; 128: 363–370.

407 Nguyen VT, Lee TX, Ndoye A et al. The pathophysiological significance of nondesmoglein targets of pemphigus autoimmunity. Arch Dermatol 1998; 134: 971–980.

408 Grando SA. Autoimmunity to keratinocyte acetylcholine receptors in pemphigus. Dermatology 2000; 201: 290–295.

409 Hakuno M, Akiyama M, Shimizu H et al. Upregulation of P-cadherin expression in the lesional skin of pemphigus, Hailey-Hailey disease and Darier's disease. J Cutan Pathol 2001; 28: 277–281.

410 Penneys NS. Focal adhesion kinase is expressed in acantholytic keratinocytes associated with pemphigus vulgaris and pemphigus foliaceus. Br J Dermatol 1996; 135: 592–594.

411 Anhalt GJ, Patel H, Diaz LA. Mechanisms of immunologic injury. Pemphigus and bullous pemphigoid. Arch Dermatol 1983; 119: 711–714.

412 Lapiere J-C, Guitart J, Ettlin DA et al. Preferential activation of the complement system in the lower epidermis of patients with pemphigus vulgaris. Br J Dermatol 1998; 139: 851–854.

413 Fabbri P, Lotti T, Panconesi E. Pathogenesis of pemphigus. Int J Dermatol 1985; 24: 422–425.

414 Xue W, Hashimoto K, Toi Y. Functional involvement of urokinase-type plasminogen activator receptor in pemphigus acantholysis. J Cutan Pathol 1998; 25: 469–474.

415 Schaefer BM, Jaeger C, Kramer MD. Plasminogen activator system in pemphigus vulgaris. Br J Dermatol 1996; 135: 726–732.

416 Aoyama Y, Kitajima Y. Pemphigus vulgaris-IgG causes a rapid depletion of desmoglein 3 (Dsg3) from the Triton X-100 soluble pools, leading to the formation of Dsg3-depleted desmosomes in a human squamous carcinoma cell line, DJM-1 cells. J Invest Dermatol 1999; 112: 67–71.

417 Feliciano C, Toto P, Amerio P et al. In vitro and in vivo expression of interleukin-1α and tumor necrosis factor-α mRNA in pemphigus vulgaris: interleukin-1α and tumor necrosis factor-α are involved in acantholysis. J Invest Dermatol 2000; 114: 71–77.

418 Zillikens D, Ambach A, Zentner A et al. Evidence for cell-mediated immune mechanisms in the pathology of pemphigus. Br J Dermatol 1993; 128: 636–643.

419 Lin M-S, Swartz SJ, Lopez A et al. Development and characterization of T cell lines responding to desmoglein-3. J Invest Dermatol 1996; 106: 832 (abstract).

420 Hertl M, Amagai M, Sundaram H et al. Recognition of desmoglein 3 by autoreactive T cells in pemphigus vulgaris patients and normals. J Invest Dermatol 1998; 110: 62–66.

421 Eming R, Büdinger L, Riechers R et al. Frequency analysis of autoreactive T-helper 1 and 2 cells in bullous pemphigoid and pemphigus vulgaris by enzyme-linked immunospot assay. Br J Dermatol 2000; 143: 1279–1282.

422 Lin M-S, Swartz SJ, Lopez A et al. Lymphocytes from a subset of patients with pemphigus vulgaris respond to both desmoglein-3 and desmoglein-1. J Invest Dermatol 1997; 109: 734–737.

423 Grando SA, Glukhenky BT, Drannik GN et al. Mediators of inflammation in blister fluids from patients with pemphigus vulgaris and bullous pemphigoid. Arch Dermatol 1989; 125: 925–930.

424 Kaplan RP, Detwiler SP, Saperstein HW. Physically induced pemphigus after cosmetic procedures. Int J Dermatol 1993; 32: 100–103.

425 Mehregan DR, Roenigk RK, Gibson LE. Postsurgical pemphigus. Arch Dermatol 1992; 128: 414–415.

426 Micali G, Nasca MR, Musumeci ML, Innocenzi D. Postsurgical pemphigus. Dermatology 1998; 197: 192–193.

427 Low GJ, Keeling JH. Ionizing radiation-induced pemphigus. Arch Dermatol 1990; 126: 1319–1323.

428 Hogan P. Pemphigus vulgaris following a cutaneous thermal burn. Int J Dermatol 1992; 31: 46–49.

429 Fryer EJ, Lebwohl M. Pemphigus vulgaris after initiation of psoralen and UVA therapy for psoriasis. J Am Acad Dermatol 1994; 30: 651–653.

430 Tufano MA, Baroni A, Buommino E et al. Detection of herpesvirus DNA in peripheral blood mononuclear cells and skin lesions of patients with pemphigus by polymerase chain reaction. Br J Dermatol 1999; 141: 1033–1039.

431 Krain LS. Pemphigus. Epidemiologic and survival characteristics of 59 patients, 1955–1973. Arch Dermatol 1974; 110: 862–865.

432 Ueki H, Kohda M, Nobutoh T et al. Antidesmoglein autoantibodies in silicosis patients with no bullous diseases. Dermatology 2001; 202: 16–21.

433 Brandsen R, Frusic-Zlotkin M, Lyubimov H et al. Circulating pemphigus IgG in families of patients with pemphigus: Comparison of indirect immunofluorescence, direct immunofluorescence, and immunoblotting. J Am Acad Dermatol 1997; 36: 44–52.

434 Vozza A, Ruocco V, Brenner S, Wolf R. Contact pemphigus. Int J Dermatol 1996; 35: 199–201.

435 Brenner S, Wolf R, Ruocco V. Contact pemphigus: a subgroup of induced pemphigus. Int J Dermatol 1994; 33: 843–845.

436 Orion E, Barzilay D, Brenner S. Pemphigus vulgaris induced by diazinon and sun exposure. Dermatology 2000; 201: 378–379.

437 Gange RW, Rhodes EL, Edwards CO, Powell MEA. Pemphigus induced by rifampicin. Br J Dermatol 1976; 95: 445.

438 Ramsay B, Woodrow D, Cream JJ. An acantholytic bullous eruption after norfloxacin. Br J Dermatol 1993; 129: 500.

439 Brenner S, Livni E. Macrophage migration inhibition factor in pemphigus vulgaris. Arch Dermatol 1986; 14: 453–455.

440 Prussick R, Plott RT, Stanley JR. Recurrence of pemphigus vulgaris associated with interleukin 2 therapy. Arch Dermatol 1994; 130: 890–893.

441 Fellner MJ, Mark AS. Penicillin- and ampicillin-induced pemphigus vulgaris. Int J Dermatol 1980; 19: 392–393.

442 Butt A, Burge SM. Pemphigus vulgaris induced by captopril. Br J Dermatol 1995; 132: 315–316.

443 Ruocco V, Satriano RA, Guerrera V. "Two-step" pemphigus induction by ACE-inhibitors. Int J Dermatol 1992; 31: 33–36.

444 De Angelis E, Lombardi ML, Grassi M, Ruocco V. Enalapril: a powerful in vitro non-thiol acantholytic agent. Int J Dermatol 1992; 31: 722–724.

445 Orion E, Gazit E, Brenner S. Pemphigus vulgaris possibly triggered by cilazapril. Acta Derm Venereol 2000; 80: 220.

446 Bellaney GJ, Rycroft RJG. Pemphigus vulgaris following a hyperimmune response to typhoid booster. Clin Exp Dermatol 1996; 21: 434–436.

447 Mignogna MD, Lo Muzio L, Ruocco E. Pemphigus induction by influenza vaccination. Int J Dermatol 2000; 39: 800.

448 Matz H, Bialy-Golan A, Brenner S. Diclofenac: a new trigger of pemphigus vulgaris? Dermatology 1997; 195: 48–49.

449 Shapiro M, Jimenez S, Werth VP. Pemphigus vulgaris induced by D-penicillamine therapy in a patient with systemic sclerosis. J Am Acad Dermatol 2000; 42: 297–299.

450 Brenner S, Bialy-Golan A, Crost N. Dipyrone in the induction of pemphigus. J Am Acad Dermatol 1997; 36: 488–490.

451 Brenner S, Ruocco V, Bialy-Golan A et al. Pemphigus and pemphigoid-like effects of nifedipine on in vitro cultured normal human skin explants. Int J Dermatol 1999; 38: 36–40.

452 Mutasim DF, Pelc NJ, Anhalt GJ. Drug-induced pemphigus. Dermatol Clin 1993; 11: 463–471.

453 Ruocco V, Sacerdoti G. Pemphigus and bullous pemphigoid due to drugs. Int J Dermatol 1991; 30: 307–312.

454 Lo Schiavo A, Guerrera V, Cozzani E et al. In vivo enalapril-induced acantholysis. Dermatology 1999; 198: 391–393.

455 Tur E, Brenner S. Contributing exogenous factors in pemphigus. Int J Dermatol 1997; 36: 888–893.

456 Tur E, Brenner S. Diet and pemphigus. In pursuit of exogenous factors in pemphigus and fogo selvagem. Arch Dermatol 1998; 134: 1406–1410.

457 Brenner S, Ruocco V, Ruocco E et al. In vitro tannin acantholysis. Int J Dermatol 2000; 39: 738–742.

458 Memar OM, Rady PL, Goldblum RM et al. Human herpesvirus 8 DNA sequences in blistering skin from patients with pemphigus. Arch Dermatol 1997; 133: 1247–1251.

459 Moy R, Jordon RE. Immunopathology in pemphigus. Clin Dermatol 1983; 1: 72–81.

460 Smolle J, Kerl H. Pitfalls in the diagnosis of pemphigus vulgaris (early pemphigus vulgaris with features of bullous pemphigoid). Am J Dermatopathol 1984; 6: 429–435.

461 Yesudian PD, Krishnan SGS, Jayaraman M et al. Postpemphigus acanthomata: a sign of clinical activity? Int J Dermatol 1997; 36: 194–196.

462 Landau M, Brenner S. Histopathologic findings in drug-induced pemphigus. Am J Dermatopathol 1997; 19: 411–414.

463 Judd KP, Lever WF. Correlation of antibodies in skin and serum with disease severity in pemphigus. Arch Dermatol 1979; 115: 428–432.

464 Helander SD, Rogers RS III. The sensitivity and specificity of direct immunofluorescence testing in disorders of mucous membranes. J Am Acad Dermatol 1994; 30: 65–75.

465 David M, Katzenelson V, Hazaz B et al. Determination of IgG subclasses in patients with pemphigus with active disease and in remission. Arch Dermatol 1989; 125: 787–790.

466 Maurice PDL, Allen BR, Marriott DW et al. Skin immunofluorescence in the diagnosis of primary bullous diseases – a review of 279 cases. Clin Exp Dermatol 1986; 11: 352–364.

467 David M, Weissman-Katzenelson V, Ben-Chetrit A et al. The usefulness of immunofluorescent tests in pemphigus patients in clinical remission. Br J Dermatol 1989; 120: 391–395.

468 Ratnam KV, Pang BK. Pemphigus in remission: value of negative direct immunofluorescence in management. J Am Acad Dermatol 1994; 30: 547–550.

469 Fellner MJ, Fukuyama K, Moshell A, Klaus MV. Intercellular antibodies in blood and epidermis. Br J Dermatol 1973; 89: 115–126.

470 Harman KE, Gratian MJ, Bhogal BS et al. The use of two substrates to improve the sensitivity of indirect immunofluorescence in the diagnosis of pemphigus. Br J Dermatol 2000; 142: 1135–1139.

471 Feibelman C, Stolzner G, Provost TT. Pemphigus vulgaris. Superior sensitivity of monkey esophagus in the determination of pemphigus antibody. Arch Dermatol 1981; 117: 561–562.

472 Ahmed AR, Workman S. Anti-intercellular substance antibodies. Presence in serum samples of 14 patients without pemphigus. Arch Dermatol 1983; 119: 17–21.

473 Grando SA, Terman AK, Stupina AS et al. Ultrastructural study of clinically uninvolved skin of patients with pemphigus vulgaris. Clin Exp Dermatol 1991; 16: 359–363.

474 Zhou S, Ferguson DJP, Allen J, Wojnarowska F. The location of binding sites of pemphigus vulgaris and pemphigus foliaceus autoantibodies: a post-embedding immunoelectron microscopic study. Br J Dermatol 1997; 136: 878–883.

475 Ahmed AR, Blose DA. Pemphigus vegetans. Neumann type and Hallopeau type. Int J Dermatol 1984; 23: 135–141.

476 Rackett SC, Rothe MJ, Hoss DM et al. Treatment-resistant pemphigus vegetans of the scalp. Int J Dermatol 1995; 34: 865–866.

477 Sillevis Smitt JH, Mulder TJ, Albeda FW, Van Nierop JC. Pemphigus vegetans in a child. Br J Dermatol 1992; 127: 289–291.

478 Nelson CG, Apisarnthanarax P, Bean SF, Mullins JF. Pemphigus vegetans of Hallopeau. Immunofluorescent studies. Arch Dermatol 1977; 113: 942–945.

479 Pearson RW, O'Donoghue M, Kaplan SJ. Pemphigus vegetans. Its relationship to eosinophilic spongiosis and favorable response to dapsone. Arch Dermatol 1980; 116: 65–68.

480 Neumann HAM, Faber WR. Pyodermite végétante of Hallopeau. Immunofluorescence studies performed in an early disease stage. Arch Dermatol 1980; 116: 1169–1171.

481 Woo TY, Solomon AR, Fairley JA. Pemphigus vegetans limited to the lips and oral mucosa. Arch Dermatol 1985; 121: 271–272.

482 Sawai T, Kitazawa K, Danno K et al. Pemphigus vegetans with oesophageal involvement: successful treatment with minocycline and nicotinamide. Br J Dermatol 1995; 132: 668–670.

483 Storwick GS, Prihoda MB, Fulton RJ, Wood WS. Pyodermatitis-pyostomatitis vegetans: a specific marker for inflammatory bowel disease. J Am Acad Dermatol 1994; 31: 336–341.

484 Mehravaran M, Kemény L, Husz S et al. Pyodermatitis-pyostomatitis vegetans. Br J Dermatol 1997; 137: 266–269.

485 O'Hagan AH, Irvine AD, Allen GE, Walsh M. Pyodermatitis-pyostomatitis vegetans: evidence for an entirely mucocutaneous variant. Br J Dermatol 1998; 139: 552–553.

486 Bianchi L, Carrozzo AM, Orlandi A et al. Pyoderma vegetans and ulcerative colitis. Br J Dermatol 2001; 144: 1224–1227.

487 Premalatha S, Jayakumar S, Yesudian P, Thambiah AS. Cerebriform tongue – a clinical sign in pemphigus vegetans. Br J Dermatol 1981; 104: 587–591.

488 Wong KT, Wong KK. A case of acantholytic dermatosis of the vulva with features of pemphigus vegetans. J Cutan Pathol 1994; 21: 453–456.

489 Pinto GM, Lamarão P, Vale T. Captopril-induced pemphigus vegetans with Charcot-Leyden crystals. J Am Acad Dermatol 1992; 27: 281–284.

490 Bastiaens MT, Zwan NV-V, Verschueren GLA et al. Three cases of pemphigus vegetans: induction by enalapril – association with internal malignancy. Int J Dermatol 1994; 33: 168–171.

491 Downie JB, Dicostanzo DP, Cohen SR. Pemphigus vegetans – Neumann variant associated with intranasal heroin abuse. J Am Acad Dermatol 1998; 39: 872–875.

492 Parodi A, Stanley JR, Ciaccio M, Rebora A. Epidermal antigens in pemphigus vegetans. Report of a case. Br J Dermatol 1988; 119: 799–802.

493 Roerigk HH Jr, Fowler-Bergfeld W. Pemphigus vulgaris-vegetans. Arch Dermatol 1969; 99: 123–124.

494 Matsubara M, Tamaki T, Sato M et al. An unusual form of pemphigus vegetans. Acta Derm Venereol 1981; 61: 259–261.

495 Hashizume H, Iwatsuki K, Takigawa M. Epidermal antigens and complement-binding anti-intercellular antibodies in pemphigus vegetans, Hallopeau type. Br J Dermatol 1993; 129: 739–743.

496 Kuo T-T, Wang CN. Charcot-Leyden crystals in pemphigus vegetans. J Cutan Pathol 1986; 13: 242–245.

497 Guerra-Rodrigo F, Morias Cardoso JP. Pemphigus vegetans. Immunofluorescent and ultrastructural studies in a patient. Arch Dermatol 1971; 104: 412–419.

498 Higashida T, Hino H, Kobayasi T. Desmosomes in pemphigus vegetans. Acta Derm Venereol 1981; 61: 107–113.

Subepidermal blisters – a classification

499 Farmer ER. Subepidermal bullous diseases. J Cutan Pathol 1985; 12: 316–321.

500 Sage H. Collagens of basement membranes. J Invest Dermatol 1982; 79: 51s–59s.

501 Eady RAJ. The basement membrane. Interface between the epithelium and the dermis: structural features. Arch Dermatol 1988; 124: 709–712.

502 Katz SI. The epidermal basement membrane zone – structure, ontogeny, and role in disease. J Am Acad Dermatol 1984; 11: 1025–1037.

503 Fine J-D. Structure and antigenicity of the skin basement membrane zone. J Cutan Pathol 1991; 18: 401–409.

504 Fine J-D. Antigenic features and structural correlates of basement membranes. Relationship to epidermolysis bullosa. Arch Dermatol 1988; 124: 713–717.

505 Mellerio JE. Molecular pathology of the cutaneous basement membrane zone. Clin Exp Dermatol 1999; 24: 25–32.

506 Allen J, Schomberg K, Wojnarowska F. Physicochemical characterization and differentiation of the components of the cutaneous basement membrane zone. Br J Dermatol 1997; 137: 907–915.

507 Le Varlet B, Chaudagne C, Saunois A et al. Age-related functional and structural changes in human dermo-epidermal junction components. J Invest Dermatol (Symposium Proceedings) 1998; 3: 172–179.

508 Yancey KB. Adhesion molecules. II. Interactions of keratinocytes with epidermal basement membrane. J Invest Dermatol 1995; 104: 1008–1014.

509 Hopkinson SB, Findlay K, deHart GW, Jones JCR. Interaction of BP180 (type XVII collagen) and α6 integrin is necessary for stabilization of hemidesmosome structure. J Invest Dermatol 1998; 111: 1015–1022.

510 Borradori L, Sonnenberg A. Structure and function of hemidesmosomes: more than simple adhesion complexes. J Invest Dermatol 1999; 112: 411–418.

511 Tidman MJ, Eady RAJ. Ultrastructural morphometry of normal human dermal-epidermal junction. The influence of age, sex, and body region on laminar and nonlaminar components. J Invest Dermatol 1984; 83: 448–453.

512 Fine J-D, Horiguchi Y, Couchman JR. 19-DEJ-1, a hemidesmosome-anchoring filament complex-associated monoclonal antibody. Arch Dermatol 1989; 125: 520–523.

513 Jonkman MF, De Jong MCJM, Heeres K et al. Generalized atrophic benign epidermolysis bullosa. Arch Dermatol 1996; 132: 145–150.

514 Fine J-D. International Symposium on Epidermolysis Bullosa. J Invest Dermatol 1994; 103: 839–843.

515 McGrath JA, Kivirikko S, Ciatti S et al. A recurrent homozygous nonsense mutation within the LAMA3 gene as a cause of Herlitz junctional epidermolysis bullosa in patients of Pakistani ancestry: evidence for a founder effect. J Invest Dermatol 1996; 106: 781–784.

516 Kirtschg G, Marinkovich MP, Burgeson RE, Yancey KB. Anti-basement membrane autoantibodies in patients with anti-epiligrin cicatricial pemphigoid bind the α subunit of laminin 5. J Invest Dermatol 1995; 105: 543–548.

517 Domloge-Hultsch N, Anhalt GJ, Gammon WR et al. Antiepiligrin cicatricial pemphigoid. Arch Dermatol 1994; 130: 1521–1529.

518 Horiguchi Y, Ueda M, Shimizu H et al. An acquired bullous dermatosis due to an autoimmune reaction against uncein. Br J Dermatol 1996; 134: 934–938.

519 Kaminska R, Helisalmi P, Harvima RJ et al. Focal dermal-epidermal separation and fibronectin cleavage in basement membrane by human mast cell tryptase. J Invest Dermatol 1999; 113: 567–573.

520 Fleischmajer R, Kühn K, Sato Y et al. There is temporal and spatial expression of α1 (IV), α2 (IV), α5 (IV), α6 (IV) collagen chains and β1 integrins during the development of the basal lamina in an "in vitro" skin model. J Invest Dermatol 1997; 109: 527–533.

521 Stanley JR, Woodley DT, Katz SI, Martin GR. Structure and function of basement membrane. J Invest Dermatol 1982; 79: 69s–72s.

522 Sellheyer K. Which cells produce the basement membrane? Dermatopathology: Practical & Conceptual 2000; 6: 63–64.

523 Uitto J, Christiano AM. Inherited epidermolysis bullosa. Clinical features, molecular genetics, and pathoetiologic mechanisms. Dermatol Clin 1993; 11: 549–563.

524 Eady RAJ, McGrath JA, McMillan JR. Ultrastructural clues to genetic disorders of skin: the dermal-epidermal junction. J Invest Dermatol 1994; 103: 13S–18S.

525 Burgeson RE. Type VII collagen, anchoring fibrils, and epidermolysis bullosa. J Invest Dermatol 1993; 101: 252–255.

526 Smith LT, Sakai LY, Burgeson RE, Holbrook KA. Ontogeny of structural components at the dermal-epidermal junction in human embryonic and fetal skin: the appearance of anchoring fibrils and type VII collagen. J Invest Dermatol 1988; 90: 480–485.

527 Tanaka T, Takahashi K, Furukawa F, Imamura S. The epitope for anti-type VII collagen monoclonal antibody (LH7:2) locates at the central region of the N-terminal non-collagenous domain of type VII collagen. Br J Dermatol 1994; 131: 472–476.

Subepidermal blisters with little inflammation

528 Haber RM, Hanna W, Ramsay CA, Boxall LBH. Hereditary epidermolysis bullosa. J Am Acad Dermatol 1985; 13: 252–278.

529 Gedde-Dahl T Jr. Sixteen types of epidermolysis bullosa. Acta Derm Venereol (Suppl) 1981; 95: 74–87.

530 Abahussein AA, Al Zayir AA, Mostafa WZ, Okoro AN. Inherited epidermolysis bullosa. Int J Dermatol 1993; 32: 561–568.

531 Eady RAJ. Epidermolysis bullosa: to split and to clump. Pediatr Dermatol 1992; 9: 36 –364.

532 Uitto J, Pulkkinen L. Epidermolysis bullosa in Mexico. Int J Dermatol 2000; 39: 433–435.

533 Tabas M, Gibbons S, Bauer EA. The mechanobullous diseases. Dermatol Clin 1987; 5: 123–136.

534 McKenna KE, Walsh MY, Bingham EA. Epidermolysis bullosa in Northern Ireland. Br J Dermatol 1992; 127: 318–321.

535 Horn HM, Priestley GC, Eady RAJ, Tidman MJ. The prevalence of epidermolysis bullosa in Scotland. Br J Dermatol 1997; 136: 560–564.

536 Pearson RW. Clinicopathologic types of epidermolysis bullosa and their nondermatological complications. Arch Dermatol 1988; 124: 718–725.

537 Fine J-D, Bauer EA, Briggaman RA et al. Revised clinical and laboratory criteria for subtypes of inherited epidermolysis bullosa. J Am Acad Dermatol 1991; 24: 119–135.

538 Bergman R. Immunohistopathologic diagnosis of epidermolysis bullosa. Am J Dermatopathol 1999; 21: 185–192.

539 Hsu TM, Kwok P-Y. Advances in molecular medicine. J Am Acad Dermatol 2001; 44: 847–855.

540 Fine J-D, McGrath J, Eady RAJ. Inherited epidermolysis bullosa comes into the new millenium: A revised classification system based on current knowledge of pathogenetic mechanisms and the clinical, laboratory, and epidemiologic findings of large, well-defined patient cohorts. J Am Acad Dermatol 2000; 43: 135–137.

541 Fine J-D, Eady RAJ, Bauer EA et al. Revised classification system for inherited epidermolysis bullosa: Report of the Second International Consensus Meeting on diagnosis and classification of epidermolysis bullosa. J Am Acad Dermatol 2000; 42: 1051–1066.

542 Sanchez G, Seltzer JL, Eisen AZ et al. Generalized dominant epidermolysis bullosa simplex: decreased activity of a gelatinolytic protease in cultured fibroblasts as a phenotypic marker. J Invest Dermatol 1983; 81: 576–579.

543 Horn HM, Tidman MJ. The clinical spectrum of epidermolysis bullosa simplex. Br J Dermatol 2000; 142: 468–472.

544 Eady RAJ, Tidman MJ. Diagnosing epidermolysis bullosa. Br J Dermatol 1983; 108 621–626.

545 Hu Z, Smith L, Martins S et al. Partial dominance of a keratin 14 mutation in epidermolysis bullosa simplex – increased severity of disease in a homozygote. Invest Dermatol 1997; 109: 360–364.

546 Salih MAM, Lake BD, El Hag MA, Atherton DJ. Lethal epidermolytic epidermolysis bullosa: a new autosomal recessive type of epidermolysis bullosa. Br J Dermatol 1985; 113: 135–143.

547 Fine J-D, Stenn J, Johnson L et al. Autosomal recessive epidermolysis bullosa simplex. Arch Dermatol 1989; 125: 931–938.

548 Abanmi A, Joshi RK, Atukorala DN et al. Autosomal recessive epidermolysis bullosa simplex. A case report. Br J Dermatol 1994; 130: 115–117.

549 Batta K, Rugg EL, Wilson NJ et al. A keratin 14 'knockout' mutation in recessive epidermolysis bullosa simplex resulting in less severe disease. Br J Dermatol 2000; 143: 621–627.

550 Holbrook KA, Smith LT, Elias S. Prenatal diagnosis of genetic skin disease using fetal skin biopsy samples. Arch Dermatol 1993; 129: 1437–1454.

551 Shimizu H, Horiguchi Y, Suzumori K et al. Successful prenatal exclusion of an unspecified subtype of severe epidermolysis bullosa. Int J Dermatol 1998; 37: 364–359.

552 Christiano AM, Uitto J. DNA-based prenatal diagnosis of heritable skin diseases. Arch Dermatol 1993; 129: 1455–1459.

553 Akiyama M, Holbrook KA. Analysis of skin-derived amniotic fluid cells in the second trimester; detection of severe genodermatoses expressed in the fetal period. J Invest Dermatol 1994; 103: 674–677.

554 Ehrlich P, Sybert VP, Spencer A, Stephens K. A common keratin 5 gene mutation in epidermolysis bullosa simplex – Weber-Cockayne. J Invest Dermatol 1995; 104: 877–879.

555 Chen H, Bonifas JM, Matsumura K et al. Keratin 14 gene mutations in patients with epidermolysis bullosa simplex. J Invest Dermatol 1995; 105: 629–632.

556 Fuchs E, Coulombe P, Cheng J et al. Genetic bases of epidermolysis bullosa simplex and epidermolytic hyperkeratosis. J Invest Dermatol 1994; 103: 25S–30S.

557 Leigh IM, Lane EB. Mutations in the genes for epidermal keratins in epidermolysis bullosa and epidermolytic hyperkeratosis. Arch Dermatol 1993; 129: 1571–1577.

558 Goldsmith LA. Mutations in epidermolysis bullosa simplex. J Invest Dermatol 1995; 105: 529–531.

559 Ito M, Okuda C, Shimizu N et al. Epidermolysis bullosa simplex (Koebner) is a keratin disorder. Arch Dermatol 1991; 127: 367–372.

560 Kawana S, Hashimoto I, Nishiyama S. Epidermolysis bullosa simplex with transient erythema circinatum. Br J Dermatol 1994; 131: 571–576.

561 Haber RM, Ramsay CA, Boxall LBH. Epidermolysis bullosa simplex with keratoderma of the palms and soles. J Am Acad Dermatol 1985; 12: 1040–1044.

562 Galligan P, Listwan P, Siller GM, Rothnagel JA. A novel mutation in the L12 domain of keratin 5 in the Köbner variant of epidermolysis bullosa simplex. J Invest Dermatol 1998; 111: 524–527.

563 DesGroseilliers J-P, Brisson P. Localized epidermolysis bullosa. Report of two cases and evaluation of therapy with glutaraldehyde. Arch Dermatol 1974; 109: 70–72.

564 Fine J-D, Johnson L, Wright T, Horiguchi Y. Epidermolysis bullosa simplex: identification of a kindred with autosomal recessive transmission of the Weber-Cockayne variety. Pediatr Dermatol 1989; 6: 1–5.

565 Müller FB, Küster W, Bruckner-Tuderman L, Korge BP. Novel K5 and K14 mutations in German patients with the Weber-Cockayne variant of epidermolysis bullosa simplex. J Invest Dermatol 1998; 111: 900–902.

566 Hacham-Zadeh S, Rappersberger K, Livshin R, Konrad K. Epidermolysis bullosa herpetiformis Dowling-Meara in a large family. J Am Acad Dermatol 1988; 18: 702–706.

567 Fine J-D, Eady RAJ. Tetracycline and epidermolysis bullosa simplex. A new indication for one of the oldest and most widely used drugs in dermatology? Arch Dermatol 1999; 135: 981–982.

568 Kitajima Y, Jokura Y, Yaoita H. Epidermolysis bullosa simplex, Dowling-Meara type. A report of two cases with different types of tonofilament clumping. Br J Dermatol 1993; 128: 79–85.

569 Buchbinder LH, Lucky AW, Ballard E et al. Severe infantile epidermolysis bullosa simplex: Dowling-Meara type. Arch Dermatol 1986; 122: 190–198.

570 Shemanko CS, Horn HM, Keohane SG et al. Laryngeal involvement in the Dowling-Meara variant of epidermolysis bullosa simplex with keratin mutations of severely disruptive potential. Br J Dermatol 2000; 142: 315–320.

571 Shemanko CS, Mellerio JE, Tidman MJ et al. Severe palmo-plantar hyperkeratosis in Dowling-Meara epidermolysis bullosa simplex caused by a mutation in the keratin 14 gene (KRT14). J Invest Dermatol 1998; 111: 893–895.

572 Tidman MJ, Eady RAJ, Leigh IM, MacDonald DM. Keratin expression in epidermolysis bullosa simplex (Dowling-Meara). Acta Derm Venereol 1988; 68: 15–20.

573 Kates SG, Sueki H, Honig PJ, Murphy GF. Immunohistochemical and ultrastructural characterization of tonofilament and hemidesmosome abnormalities in a case of epidermolysis bullosa herpetiformis (Dowling-Meara). J Am Acad Dermatol 1992; 27: 929–934.

574 McGrath JA, Ishida-Yamamoto A, Tidman MJ et al. Epidermolysis bullosa simplex (Dowling-Meara). A clinicopathological review. Br J Dermatol 1992; 126: 421–430.

575 Furumura M, Imayama S, Hori Y. Three neonatal cases of epidermolysis bullosa herpetiformis (Dowling-Meara type) with severe erosive skin lesions. J Am Acad Dermatol 1993; 28: 859–861.

576 Ishida-Yamamoto A, McGrath JA, Chapman SJ et al. Epidermolysis bullosa simplex (Dowling-Meara type) is a genetic disease characterized by an abnormal keratin-filament network involving keratins K5 and K14. J Invest Dermatol 1991; 97: 959–968.

577 Müller FB, Anton-Lamprecht I, Küster W, Korge BP. A premature stop codon mutation in the 2B helix termination peptide of keratin 5 in a German epidermolysis bullosa simplex Dowling-Meara case. J Invest Dermatol 1999; 112: 988–990.

578 Sørensen CB, Ladekjær-Mikkelsen A-S, Andresen BS et al. Identification of novel and known mutations in the genes for keratin 5 and 14 in Danish patients with epidermolysis bullosa simplex: correlation between genotype and phenotype. J Invest Dermatol 1999; 112: 184–190.

579 Sasaki Y, Shimizu H, Akiyama M et al. A recurrent keratin 14 mutation in Dowling-Meara epidermolysis bullosa simplex. Br J Dermatol 1999; 141: 747–748.

580 Stephens K, Sybert VP, Wijsman EM et al. A keratin 14 mutational hot spot for epidermolysis bullosa simplex, Dowling-Meara: implications for diagnosis. J Invest Dermatol 1993; 101: 240–243.

581 Irvine AD, McKenna KE, Bingham A et al. A novel mutation in the helix termination peptide of keratin 5 causing epidermolysis bullosa simplex Dowling-Meara. J Invest Dermatol 1997; 109: 815–816.

582 Takizawa Y, Shimizu H, Rouan F et al. Four novel plectin gene mutations in Japanese patients with epidermolysis bullosa with muscular dystrophy disclosed by heteroduplex scanning and protein truncation tests. J Invest Dermatol 1999; 112: 109–112.

583 Gache Y, Chavanas S, Lacour JP et al. Defective expression of plectin in epidermolysis bullosa simplex with muscular dystrophy. J Invest Dermatol 1996; 106: 842 (abstract).

584 Uitto J, Amano S, McGrath J et al. Absent expression of the hemidesmosomal inner plaque protein HD-1 and its cell biological consequences in epidermolysis bullosa with muscular dystrophy. J Invest Dermatol 1996; 106: 842 (abstract).

535 Eady RAJ, Leigh IM, McMillan JR et al. Epidermolysis bullosa simplex with muscular dystrophy: loss of plectin expression in skin and muscle. J Invest Dermatol 1996; 106: 842 (abstract).

586 Mellerio JE, Smith FJD, McMillan JR et al. Recessive epidermolysis bullosa simplex associated with plectin mutations: infantile respiratory complications in two unrelated cases. Br J Dermatol 1997; 137: 898–906.

587 Shimizu H, Takizawa Y, Pulkkinen L et al. Epidermolysis bullosa simplex associated with muscular dystrophy: Phenotype-genotype correlations and review of the literature. J Am Acad Dermatol 1999; 41: 950–956.

588 Kunz M, Rouan F, Pulkkinen L et al. Epidermolysis bullosa simplex associated with severe mucous membrane involvement and novel mutations in the plectin gene. J Invest Dermatol 2000; 114: 376–380.

589 Rouan F, Pulkkinen L, Meneguzzi G et al. Epidermolysis bullosa: novel and *de novo* premature termination codon and deletion mutations in the plectin gene predict late-onset muscular dystrophy. J Invest Dermatol 2000; 114: 381–387.

590 Bruckner-Tuderman L, Vogel A, Ruegger S et al. Epidermolysis bullosa simplex with mottled pigmentation. J Am Acad Dermatol 1989; 21: 425–432.

591 Coleman R, Harper JI, Lake BD. Epidermolysis bullosa simplex with mottled pigmentation. Br J Dermatol 1993; 128: 679–685.

592 Fine J-D, Johnson L, Wright T. Epidermolysis bullosa simplex superficialis. Arch Dermatol 1989; 125: 631–638.

593 Irvine AD, Rugg EL, Lane EB et al. Molecular confirmation of the unique phenotype of epidermolysis bullosa simplex with mottled pigmentation. Br J Dermatol 2001; 144: 40–45.

594 Medenica-Mojsilovic L, Fenske NA, Espinoza CG. Epidermolysis bullosa herpetiformis with mottled pigmentation and an unusual punctate keratoderma. Arch Dermatol 1986; 122: 900–908.

595 Eisenberg M, Shorey CD, de Chair-Baker W. Epidermolysis bullosa – a new subgroup. Australas J Dermatol 1986; 27: 15–18.

596 Niemi K-M, Sommer H, Kero M et al. Epidermolysis bullosa simplex associated with muscular dystrophy with recessive inheritance. Arch Dermatol 1988; 124: 551–554.

597 Bart BJ, Gorlin RJ, Anderson VE, Lynch FW. Congenital localized absence of skin and associated abnormalities resembling epidermolysis bullosa. Arch Dermatol 1966; 93: 296–304.

598 Fisher GB Jr, Greer KE, Cooper PH. Congenital self-healing (transient) mechanobullous dermatosis. Arch Dermatol 1988; 124: 240–243.

599 Amichai B, Metzker A. Bart's syndrome. Int J Dermatol 1994; 33: 161–163.

600 Kanzler MH, Smoller B, Woodley DT. Congenital localized absence of the skin as a manifestation of epidermolysis bullosa. Arch Dermatol 1992; 128: 1087–1090.

601 Zelickson B, Matsumura K, Kist D et al. Bart's syndrome. Ultrastructure and genetic linkage. Arch Dermatol 1995; 131: 663–668.

602 Duran-McKinster C, Rivera-Franco A, Tamayo L et al. Bart syndrome: the congenital localized absence of skin may follow the lines of Blaschko. Report of six cases. Pediatr Dermatol 2000; 17: 179–182.

603 Kero M, Peltonen L, Foidart JM, Savolainen E-R. Immunohistological localization of three basement membrane components in various forms of epidermolysis bullosa. J Cutan Pathol 1982; 9: 316–328.

604 Fine J-D, Gay S. LDA-1 monoclonal antibody. An excellent reagent for immunofluorescence mapping studies in patients with epidermolysis bullosa. Arch Dermatol 1986; 122: 48–51.

605 Prieto VG, McNutt NS. Immunohistochemical detection of keratin with the monoclonal antibody MNF116 is useful in the diagnosis of epidermolysis bullosa simplex. J Cutan Pathol 1994; 21: 118–122.

606 Haneke E, Anton-Lamprecht I. Ultrastructure of blister formation in epidermolysis bullosa hereditaria: V. Epidermolysis bullosa simplex localisata type Weber-Cockayne. J Invest Dermatol 1982; 78: 219–223.

607 Taylor G, Venning V, Wojnarowska F, Millard PR. Suction-induced basal cell cytolysis in the Weber-Cockayne variant of epidermolysis bullosa simplex. J Cutan Pathol 1993; 20: 389–392.

608 Hoffman MD, Fleming MG, Pearson RW. Acantholytic epidermolysis bullosa. Arch Dermatol 1995; 131: 586–589.

609 Anton-Lamprecht I, Schnyder UW. Epidermolysis bullosa herpetiformis Dowling-Meara. Dermatologica 1982; 164: 221–235.

610 Roth RR, Smith KJ, James WD. Eosinophilic infiltrates in epidermolysis bullosa. Arch Dermatol 1990; 126: 1191–1194.

611 Niemi K-M, Kero M, Kanerva L, Mattila R. Epidermolysis bullosa simplex. A new histologic subgroup. Arch Dermatol 1983; 119: 138–141.

612 Bourgault I, Prost C, André C et al. Transient intraepidermal bullous reaction after skin graft for toxic epidermal necrolysis. Arch Dermatol 1991; 127: 1369–1374.

613 Smith LT. Ultrastructural findings in epidermolysis bullosa. Arch Dermatol 1993; 129: 1578–1584.

614 Gil SG, Brown TA, Ryan MC, Carter WG. Junctional epidermolysis bullosis: defects in expression of epiligrin/nicein/kalinin and integrin β4 that inhibit hemidesmosome formation. J Invest Dermatol 1994; 103: 31S–38S.

615 McMillan JR, McGrath JA, Pulkkinen L et al. Immunohistochemical analysis of the skin in junctional epidermolysis bullosa using laminin 5 chain specific antibodies is of limited value in predicting the underlying gene mutation. Br J Dermatol 1997; 136: 817–822.

616 Heagerty AHM, Eady RAJ, Kennedy AR et al. Rapid prenatal diagnosis of epidermolysis bullosa letalis using GB3 monoclonal antibody. Br J Dermatol 1987; 117: 271–275.

617 Kennedy AR, Heagerty AHM, Ortonne J-P et al. Abnormal binding of an anti-amnion antibody to epidermal basement membrane provides a novel diagnostic probe for junctional epidermolysis bullosa. Br J Dermatol 1985; 113: 651–659.

618 Fine J-D. Changing clinical and laboratory concepts in inherited epidermolysis bullosa. Arch Dermatol 1988; 124: 523–526.

619 Ashton GHS, Sorelli P, Mellerio JE et al. α6β4 integrin abnormalities in junctional epidermolysis bullosa with pyloric atresia. Br J Dermatol 2001; 144: 408–414.

620 McGrath JA, Ashton GHS, Mellerio JE et al. Moderation of phenotypic severity in dystrophic and junctional forms of epidermolysis bullosa through in-frame skipping of exons containing non-sense or frameshift mutations. J Invest Dermatol 1999; 113: 314–321.

621 Thomas L, Faure M, Cambazard F et al. Cultured epithelia from junctional epidermolysis bullosa letalis keratinocytes express the main phenotypic characteristics of the disease. Br J Dermatol 1990; 122: 137–145.

622 Fine J-D, Horiguchi Y, Couchman JR. 19-DEJ-1, a hemidesmosome-anchoring filament complex-associated monoclonal antibody. Definition of a new skin basement membrane antigenic defect in junctional and dystrophic epidermolysis bullosa. Arch Dermatol 1989; 125: 520–523.

623 Inoue M, Tamai K, Shimizu H et al. A homozygous missense mutation in the cytoplasmic tail of β4 integrin, G931D, that disrupts hemidesmosome assembly and underlies non-Herlitz junctional epidermolysis bullosa without pyloric atresia? J Invest Dermatol 2000; 114: 1061–1064.

624 Matsumura Y, Horiguchi Y, Toda K et al. Mosaic expression of uncein and 180-kDa bullous pemphigoid antigen in generalized atrophic benign epidermolysis bullosa. Br J Dermatol 1997; 136: 757–761.

625 Stouthamer A, Nieboer C, van der Waal RIF, Jonkman MF. Normal expression of the 19-DEJ-1 epitope in two siblings with late-onset junctional epidermolysis bullosa. Br J Dermatol 2001; 144: 1054–1057.

626 Kirtschig G, Caux F, McMillan JR et al. Acquired junctional epidermolysis bullosa associated with IgG autoantibodies to the β subunit of laminin-5. Br J Dermatol 1998; 138: 125–130.

627 McMillan JR, McGrath JA, Tidman MJ, Eady RAJ. Hemidesmosomes show abnormal association with the keratin filament network in junctional forms of epidermolysis bullosa. J Invest Dermatol 1998; 110: 132–137.

628 Krueger JW, Lin AN, Leong I, Carter DM. Junctional epidermolysis bullosa keratinocytes in culture display adhesive, structural, and functional abnormalities. J Invest Dermatol 1991; 97: 849–861.

629 Chapman SJ, Leigh IM, Tidman MJ, Eady RAJ. Abnormal expression of hemidesmosome-like structures by junctional epidermolysis bullosa keratinocytes *in vitro*. Br J Dermatol 1990; 123: 137–144.

630 Turner TW. Two cases of junctional epidermolysis bullosa (Herlitz-Pearson). Br J Dermatol 1980; 102: 97–107.

631 Ashton GHS, Mellerio JE, Dunnill MGS et al. A recurrent laminin 5 mutation in British patients with lethal (Herlitz) junctional epidermolysis bullosa: evidence for a mutational hotspot rather than propagation of an ancestral allele. Br J Dermatol 1997; 136: 674–677.

632 Basarab T, Dunnill MGS, Eady RAJ, Russell-Jones R. Herlitz junctional epidermolysis bullosa: a case report and review of current diagnostic methods. Pediatr Dermatol 1997; 14: 307–311.

633 Schachner L, Lazarus GS, Dembitzer H. Epidermolysis bullosa hereditaria letalis. Br J Dermatol 1977; 96: 51–58.

634 Parsapour K, Reep MD, Mohammed L et al. Herlitz junctional epidermolysis bullosa presenting at birth with anonychia: a case report and review of H-JEB. Pediatr Dermatol 2001; 18: 217–222.

635 Takizawa Y, Shimizu H, Pulkkinen L et al. Novel mutations in the LAMB3 gene shared by two Japanese unrelated families with Herlitz junctional epidermolysis bullosa, and their application for prenatal testing. J Invest Dermatol 1998; 110: 174–178.

636 Takizawa Y, Pulkkinen L, Chao S-C et al. Complete paternal uniparental isodisomy of chromosome 1: a novel mechanism for Herlitz junctional epidermolysis bullosa. J Invest Dermatol 2000; 115: 307–311.

637 Cserhalmi-Friedman PB, Yeboa KA, Christiano AM. DNA based molecular analysis in the rapid diagnosis of Herlitz junctional epidermolysis bullosa. Clin Exp Dermatol 2001; 26: 205–207.

638 Pulkkinen L, Meneguzzi G, McGrath JA et al. Predominance of the recurrent mutation R635X in the LAMB3 gene in European patients with Herlitz junctional epidermolysis bullosa has implications for mutation detection strategy. J Invest Dermatol 1997; 109: 232–237.

639 Nakano A, Pfendner E, Pulkkinen L et al. Herlitz junctional epidermolysis bullosa: novel and recurrent mutations in the LAMB3 gene and the population carrier frequency. J Invest Dermatol 2000; 115: 493–498.

640 Takizawa Y, Pulkkinen L, Shimizu H et al. Maternal uniparental meroisodisomy in the LAMB3 region of chromosome 1 results in lethal junctional epidermolysis bullosa. J Invest Dermatol 1998; 110: 828–831.

641 Lim KK, Su WPD, McEvoy MT, Pittelkow MR. Generalized gravis junctional epidermolysis bullosa: case report, laboratory evaluation, and review of recent advances. Mayo Clin Proc 1996; 71: 863–868.

642 Paller AS, Fine J-D, Kaplan S, Pearson RW. The generalized atrophic benign form of junctional epidermolysis bullosa. Arch Dermatol 1986; 122: 704–710.

643 Hintner H, Wolff K. Generalized atrophic benign epidermolysis bullosa. Arch Dermatol 1982; 118: 375–384.

644 Newbould MJ, Harrison PV, Blewitt RW, Jones CJP. Junctional epidermolysis bullosa: a mild variant in two Indian sisters. Clin Exp Dermatol 1992; 17: 106–111.

645 Darling T, McGrath JA, Yee C et al. Mutations in the bullous pemphigoid antigen 2 (BPAG2) gene in five Austrian families with generalized atrophic benign epidermolysis bullosa (GABEB). J Invest Dermatol 1996; 106: 842 (abstract).

646 McGrath JA, Darling T, Gatalica B et al. A homozygous deletion mutation in the gene encoding the 180-kDa bullous pemphigoid antigen (BPAG2) in a family with generalized atrophic benign epidermolysis bullosa. J Invest Dermatol 1996; 106: 771–774.

647 Mellerio JE, Denyer JE, Atherton DJ et al. Prognostic implications of determining 180 kDa bullous pemphigoid antigen (BPAG2) gene/protein pathology in neonatal junctional epidermolysis bullosa. Br J Dermatol 1998; 138: 661–666.

648 Woo HJ, Lee JH, Kim SC et al. Generalized atrophic benign epidermolysis bullosa – poor prognosis associated with chronic renal failure. Clin Exp Dermatol 2000; 25: 212–214.

649 Swensson O, Christophers E. Generalized atrophic benign epidermolysis bullosa in 2 siblings complicated by multiple squamous cell carcinomas. Arch Dermatol 1998; 134: 199–203.

650 Darling TN, Yee C, Koh B et al. Cycloheximide facilitates the identification of aberrant transcripts resulting from a novel splice-site mutation in COL17A1 in a patient with generalized atrophic benign epidermolysis bullosa. J Invest Dermatol 1998; 110: 165–169.

651 Mazzanti C, Gobello T, Posteraro P et al. 180-kDa bullous pemphigoid antigen defective generalized atrophic benign epidermolysis bullosa: report of four cases with an unusually mild phenotype. Br J Dermatol 1998; 138: 859–866.

652 Darling TN, Koh BB, Bale SJ et al. A deletion mutation in COL17A1 in five Austrian families with generalized atrophic benign epidermolysis bullosa represents propagation of an ancestral allele. J Invest Dermatol 1998; 110: 170–173.

653 Pulkkinen L, Marinkovich MP, Tran HT et al. Compound heterozygosity for novel splice site mutations in the BPAG2/COL17A1 gene underlies generalized atrophic benign epidermolysis bullosa. J Invest Dermatol 1999; 113: 1114–1118.

654 Guerriero C, De Simone C, Venier A et al. Non-Herlitz junctional epidermolysis bullosa without hair involvement associated with BP180 deficiency. Dermatology 2001; 202: 58–62.

655 Mellerio JE, Eady RAJ, Atherton DJ et al. E210K mutation in the gene encoding the β3 chain of laminin-5 (LAMB3) is predictive of a phenotype of generalized atrophic benign epidermolysis bullosa. Br J Dermatol 1998; 139: 325–331.

656 Takizawa Y, Hiraoka Y, Takahashi H et al. Compound heterozygosity for a point mutation and a deletion located at splice acceptor sites in the LAMB3 gene leads to generalized atrophic benign epidermolysis bullosa. J Invest Dermatol 2000; 115: 312–315.

657 Floeth M, Bruckner-Tuderman L. Digenic junctional epidermolysis bullosa: mutations in COL17A1 and LAMB3 genes. Am J Hum Genet 2000; 65: 1530–1537.

658 Kim JN, Namgung R, Kim S-C et al. Pyloric atresia with junctional epidermolysis bullosa (PA-JEB) syndrome: absence of detectable β4 integrin and reduced expression of epidermal linear IgA dermatosis antigen. Int J Dermatol 1999; 38: 467–470.

659 Marinkovich MP, Tran HH, Rao SK et al. LAD-1 is absent in a subset of junctional epidermolysis bullosa patients. J Invest Dermatol 1997; 109: 356–359.

660 Shimizu H, Takizawa Y, Pulkkinen L et al. The 97 kDa linear IgA bullous dermatosis antigen is not expressed in a patient with generalized atrophic benign epidermolysis bullosa with a novel homozygous G258X mutation in COL17A1. J Invest Dermatol 1998; 111: 887–892.

661 Jonkman MF, Pas HH, Fine JD. Mosaic expression of uncein, linear IgA bullous dermatosis antigen and 180-kDa bullous pemphigoid antigen in generalized atrophic benign epidermolysis bullosa. Br J Dermatol 1998; 138: 904.

662 Holbrook KA. Extracutaneous epithelial involvement in inherited epidermolysis bullosa. Arch Dermatol 1988; 124: 726–731.

663 Lestringant GG, Akel SR, Qayed KI. The pyloric atresia–junctional epidermolysis bullosa syndrome. Arch Dermatol 1992; 128: 1083–1086.

664 Valari MD, Phillips RJ, Lake BD, Harper JI. Junctional epidermolysis bullosa and pyloric atresia: a distinct entity. Clinical and pathological studies in five patients. Br J Dermatol 1995; 133: 732–736.

665 Shimizu H, Fine J-D, Suzumori K et al. Prenatal exclusion of pyloric atresia–junctional epidermolysis bullosa syndrome. J Am Acad Dermatol 1994; 31: 429–433.

666 Wallerstein R, Klein ML, Genieser N et al. Epidermolysis bullosa, pyloric atresia, and obstructive uropathy: a report of two case reports with molecular correlation and clinical management. Pediatr Dermatol 2000; 17: 286–289.

667 Shaw DW, Fine J-D, Piacquadio DJ et al. Gastric outlet obstruction and epidermolysis bullosa. J Am Acad Dermatol 1997; 36: 304–310.

668 Mellerio JE, Pulkkinen L, McMillan JR et al. Pyloric atresia–junctional epidermolysis bullosa syndrome: mutations in the integrin β4 gene (ITGB4) in two unrelated patients with mild disease. Br J Dermatol 1998; 139: 862–871.

669 Shimizu H, Suzumori K, Hatta N, Nishikawa T. Absence of detectable α6 integrin in pyloric atresia–junctional epidermolysis bullosa syndrome. Application for prenatal diagnosis in a family at risk for recurrence. Arch Dermatol 1996; 132: 919–925.

670 Dank JP, Kim S, Parisi MA et al. Outcome after surgical repair of junctional epidermal bullosa–pyloric atresia syndrome. Arch Dermatol 1999; 135: 1243–1247.

671 Puvabanditsin S, Garrow E, Samransamraujkit R et al. Epidermolysis bullosa associated with congenital localized absence of skin, fetal abdominal mass, and pyloric atresia. Pediatr Dermatol 1997; 14: 359–362.

672 Puvabanditsin S, Garrow E, Kim DU et al. Junctional epidermolysis bullosa associated with congenital localized absence of skin, and pyloric atresia in two newborn siblings. J Am Acad Dermatol 2001; 44: 330–335.

673 Morrell DS, Rubenstein DS, Briggaman RA et al. Congenital pyloric atresia in a newborn with extensive aplasia cutis congenita and epidermolysis bullosa simplex. Br J Dermatol 2000; 143: 1342–1343.

674 Wasel N, Idikio H, Lees G et al. Junctional epidermolysis bullosa with pyloric stenosis presenting with electron microscopic findings suggestive of epidermolysis bullosa simplex. Pediatr Dermatol 2000; 17: 395–398.

675 Heng MCY, Barrascout CE, Rasmus W et al. Elevated serum chymotrypsin levels in a patient with junctional epidermolysis bullosa. Int J Dermatol 1987; 26: 385–388.

676 Floeth M, Fiedorowicz J, Schäcke H et al. Novel homozygous and compound heterozygous COL17A1 mutations associated with junctional epidermolysis bullosa. J Invest Dermatol 1998; 111: 528–533.

677 Haber RM, Hanna W. Epidermolysis bullosa progressiva. J Am Acad Dermatol 1987; 16: 195–200.

678 Bircher AJ, Lang-Muritano M, Pfaltz M, Bruckner-Tuderman L. Epidermolysis bullosa junctionalis progressiva in three siblings. Br J Dermatol 1993; 128: 429–435.

679 Haber RM, Hanna W, Ramsay CA, Boxall LBH. Cicatricial junctional epidermolysis bullosa. J Am Acad Dermatol 1985; 12: 836–844.

680 Peltier FA, Tschen EH, Raimer SS, Kuo T-t. Epidermolysis bullosa letalis associated with congenital pyloric atresia. Arch Dermatol 1981; 117: 728–731.

681 Oakley CA, Wilson N, Ross JA, Barnetson R St C. Junctional epidermolysis bullosa in two siblings: clinical observations, collagen studies and electron microscopy. Br J Dermatol 1984; 111: 533–543.

682 Heagerty AHM, Kennedy AR, Leigh IM et al. Identification of an epidermal basement membrane defect in recessive forms of dystrophic epidermolysis bullosa by LH 7:2 monoclonal antibody: use in diagnosis. Br J Dermatol 1986; 115: 125–131.

683 Hovnanian A, Christiano AM, Uitto J. The molecular genetics of dystrophic epidermolysis bullosa. Arch Dermatol 1993; 129: 1566–1570.

684 Dunhill MGS, Eady RAJ. The management of dystrophic epidermolysis bullosa. Clin Exp Dermatol 1995; 20: 179–188.

685 Bauer EA, Ludman MD, Goldberg JD et al. Antenatal diagnosis of recessive dystrophic epidermolysis bullosa: collagenase expression in cultured fibroblasts as a biochemical marker. J Invest Dermatol 1986; 87: 597–601.

686 Hovnanian A, Hilal L, Blanchet-Bardon C et al. DNA-based prenatal diagnosis of generalized recessive dystrophic epidermolysis bullosa in six pregnancies at risk for recurrence. J Invest Dermatol 1995; 104: 456–461.

687 McGrath JA, Dunnill MGS, Christiano AM et al. First trimester DNA-based exclusion of recessive dystrophic epidermolysis bullosa from chorionic villus sampling. Br J Dermatol 1996; 134: 734–739.

688 Uitto J, Eady R, Fine J-D et al. The DEBRA International Visioning/Consensus Meeting on Epidermolysis Bullosa: summary and recommendations. J Invest Dermatol 2000; 114: 734–737.

689 Dallinger G, Puttaraju M, Mitchell LG et al. Collagen 17A1 gene correction using spliceosome mediated RNA trans-splicing (SMaRT™) technology. J Invest Dermatol 2000; 115: 332 (abstract).

690 Dharma B, Moss C, McGrath JA et al. Dominant dystrophic epidermolysis bullosa presenting as familial nail dystrophy. Clin Exp Dermatol 2001; 26: 93–96.

691 Sehgal VN, Rege VL, Ghosh SK, Kamat SM. Dystrophic epidermolysis bullosa. Interesting gastro-intestinal manifestations. Br J Dermatol 1977; 96: 389–392.

692 Tidman MJ, Martin IR, Wells RS et al. Oesophageal web formation in dystrophic epidermolysis bullosa. Clin Exp Dermatol 1988; 13: 279–281.

693 Wojnarowska FT, Eady RAJ, Wells RS. Dystrophic epidermolysis bullosa presenting with congenital localized absence of skin: report of four cases. Br J Dermatol 1983; 108: 477–483.

694 McCarthy MA, Clarke T, Powell FC. Epidermolysis bullosa and aplasia cutis. Int J Dermatol 1991; 30: 481–484.

695 Fine J-D, Tamura T, Johnson L. Blood vitamin and trace metal levels in epidermolysis bullosa. Arch Dermatol 1989; 125: 374–379.

696 Lechner-Gruskay D, Honig PJ, Pereira G, McKinney S. Nutritional and metabolic profile of children with epidermolysis bullosa. Pediatr Dermatol 1988; 5: 22–27.

697 Monk BE, Pembroke AC. Epidermolysis bullosa with squamous cell carcinoma. Clin Exp Dermatol 1987; 12: 373–374.

698 McGrath JA, Schofield OMV, Mayou BJ et al. Epidermolysis bullosa complicated by squamous cell carcinoma: report of 10 cases. J Cutan Pathol 1992; 19: 116–123.

699 Smoller BA, McNutt NS, Carter DM et al. Recessive dystrophic epidermolysis bullosa skin displays a chronic growth-activated immunophenotype. Implications for carcinogenesis. Arch Dermatol 1990; 126: 78–83.

700 Slater SD, McGrath JA, Hobbs C et al. Expression of mutant p53 gene in squamous carcinoma arising in patients with recessive dystrophic epidermolysis bullosa. Histopathology 1992; 20: 237–241.

701 Hoss DM, McNutt NS, Carter DM et al. Atypical melanocytic lesions in epidermolysis bullosa. J Cutan Pathol 1994; 21: 164–169.

702 Yi S, Naito M, Takahashi K et al. Complicating systemic amyloidosis in dystrophic epidermolysis bullosa, recessive type. Pathology 1988; 20: 184–187.

703 Bourke JF, Browne G, Gaffney EF, Young M. Fatal systemic amyloidosis (AA type) in two sisters with dystrophic epidermolysis bullosa. J Am Acad Dermatol 1995; 33: 370–372.

704 Briggaman RA. Is there any specificity to defects of anchoring fibrils in epidermolysis bullosa dystrophica, and what does this mean in terms of pathogenesis? J Invest Dermatol 1985; 84: 371–373.

705 Tidman MJ, Eady RAJ. Evaluation of anchoring fibrils and other components of the dermal-epidermal junction in dystrophic epidermolysis bullosa by a quantitative ultrastructural technique. J Invest Dermatol 1985; 84: 374–377.

706 McGrath JA, Ishida-Yamamoto A, O'Grady A et al. Structural variations in anchoring fibrils in dystrophic epidermolysis bullosa: correlation with type VII collagen expression. J Invest Dermatol 1993; 100: 366–372.

707 Takamori K, Ikeda S, Naito K, Ogawa H. Proteases are responsible for blister formation in recessive dystrophic epidermolysis bullosa and epidermolysis bullosa simplex. Br J Dermatol 1985; 112: 533–538.

708 Takamori K, Naito K, Taneda A, Ogawa H. Increased neutral protease and collagenase activity in recessive dystrophic epidermolysis bullosa. Br J Dermatol 1983; 108: 687–694.

709 Kero M, Palotie A, Peltonen L. Collagen metabolism in two rare forms of epidermolysis bullosa. Br J Dermatol 1984; 110: 177–184.

710 Ikeda S, Manabe M, Muramatsu T et al. Protease inhibitor therapy for recessive dystrophic epidermolysis bullosa. J Am Acad Dermatol 1988; 18: 1246–1252.

711 Bauer EA, Tabas M. A perspective on the role of collagenase in recessive dystrophic epidermolysis bullosa. Arch Dermatol 1988; 124: 734–736.

712 Leigh IM, Eady RAJ, Heagerty AHM et al. Type VII collagen is a normal component of epidermal basement membrane, which shows altered expression in recessive dystrophic epidermolysis bullosa. J Invest Dermatol 1988; 90: 639–642.

713 Smith LT, Sybert VP. Intra-epidermal retention of type VII collagen in a patient with recessive dystrophic epidermolysis bullosa. J Invest Dermatol 1990; 94: 261–264.

714 Bruckner-Tuderman L, Mitsuhashi Y, Schnyder UW, Bruckner P. Anchoring fibrils and type VII collagen are absent from skin in severe recessive dystrophic epidermolysis bullosa. J Invest Dermatol 1989; 93: 3–9.

715 Rusenko KW, Gammon WR, Fine J-D, Briggaman RA. The carboxyl-terminal domain of type VII collagen is present at the basement membrane in recessive dystrophic epidermolysis bullosa. J Invest Dermatol 1989; 92: 623–627.

716 Fine J-D, Horiguchi Y, Stein DH et al. Intraepidermal type VII collagen. Evidence for abnormal intracytoplasmic processing of a major basement membrane protein in rare

717 Jenison M, Fine J-D, Gammon WR, O'Keefe EJ. Normal molecular weight of type VII collagen produced by recessive dystrophic epidermolysis bullosa keratinocytes. J Invest Dermatol 1993; 100: 93–96.

718 König A, Winberg J-O, Gedde-Dahl T Jr, Bruckner-Tuderman L. Heterogeneity of severe dystrophic epidermolysis bullosa: overexpression of collagen VII by cutaneous cells from a patient with mutilating disease. J Invest Dermatol 1994; 102: 155–159.

719 Bruckner-Tuderman L, Niemi K-M, Kero M et al. Type VII collagen is expressed but anchoring fibrils are defective in dystrophic epidermolysis bullosa inversa. Br J Dermatol 1990; 122: 383–390.

720 McGrath JA, Sakai LY, Eady RAJ. Fibrillin immunoreactivity is associated with normal or fragmented elastic microfibrils at the dermal-epidermal junction in recessive dystrophic epidermolysis bullosa. Br J Dermatol 1994; 131: 465–471.

721 Christiano AM, Morricone A, Paradisi M et al. A glycine-to-arginine substitution in the triple-helical domain of type VII collagen in a family with dominant dystrophic epidermolysis bullosa. J Invest Dermatol 1995; 104: 438–440.

722 Christiano AM, D'Alessio M, Paradisi M et al. A common insertion mutation in COL7A1 in two Italian families with recessive dystrophic epidermolysis bullosa. J Invest Dermatol 1996; 106: 679–684.

723 Kon A, Nomura K, Pulkkinen L et al. Novel glycine substitution mutations in COL7A1 reveal that the Pasini and Cockayne–Touraine variants of dominant dystrophic epidermolysis bullosa are allelic. J Invest Dermatol 1997; 109: 684–687.

724 Mellerio JE, Salas-Alanis JC, Talamantes ML et al. A recurrent glycine substitution mutation, G2043R, in the type VII collagen gene (COL7A1) in dominant dystrophic epidermolysis bullosa. Br J Dermatol 1998; 139: 730–737.

725 Wessagowit V, Ashton GHS, Mohammedi R et al. Three cases of de novo dominant dystrophic epidermolysis bullosa associated with the mutation G2043R in COL7A1. Clin Exp Dermatol 2001; 26: 97–99.

726 Kon A, Pulkkinen L, Ishida-Yamamoto A et al. Novel COL7A1 mutations in dystrophic forms of epidermolysis bullosa. J Invest Dermatol 1998; 111: 534–537.

727 Terracina M, Posteraro P, Schubert M et al. Compound heterozygosity for a recessive glycine substitution and a splice site mutation in the COL7A1 gene causes an unusually mild form of localized recessive dystrophic epidermolysis bullosa. J Invest Dermatol 1998; 111: 744–750.

728 Hammami-Hauasli N, Kalinke DU, Schumann H et al. A combination of a common splice site mutation and a frameshift mutation in the COL7A1 gene: absence of functional collagen VII in keratinocytes and skin. J Invest Dermatol 1997; 109: 384–389.

729 Mellerio JE, Dunnill MGS, Allison W et al. Recurrent mutations in the type VII collagen gene (COL7A1) in patients with recessive dystrophic epidermolysis bullosa. J Invest Dermatol 1997; 109: 246–249.

730 Christiano AM, Amano S, Eichenfield LF et al. Premature termination codon mutations in the type VII collagen gene in recessive dystrophic epidermolysis bullosa result in nonsense-mediated mRNA decay and absence of functional protein. J Invest Dermatol 1997; 109: 390–394.

731 Whittock NV, Ashton GHS, Mohammedi R et al. Comparative mutation detection screening of the type VII collagen gene (COL7A1) using the protein truncation test, fluorescent chemical cleavage of mismatch, and conformation sensitive gel electrophoresis. J Invest Dermatol 1999; 113: 673–686.

732 Salas-Alanis JC, Amaya-Guerra M, McGrath JA. The molecular basis of dystrophic epidermolysis bullosa in Mexico. Int J Dermatol 2000; 39: 436–442.

733 Salas-Alanis JC, Mellerio JE, Amaya-Guerra M et al. Frameshift mutations in the type VII collagen gene (COL7A1) in five Mexican cousins with recessive dystrophic epidermolysis bullosa. Br J Dermatol 1998; 138: 852–858.

734 Rouan F, Pulkkinen L, Jonkman MF et al. Novel and de novo glycine substitution mutations in the type VII collagen gene (COL7A1) in dystrophic epidermolysis bullosa: implications for genetic counseling. J Invest Dermatol 1998; 111: 1210–1213.

735 Ashton GHS, Mellerio JE, Dunnill MGS et al. Recurrent molecular abnormalities in type VII collagen in southern Italian patients with recessive dystrophic epidermolysis bullosa. Clin Exp Dermatol 1999; 24: 232–235.

736 Mohammedi R, Mellerio JE, Ashton GHS et al. A recurrent COL7A1 mutation, R2814X, in British patients with recessive dystrophic epidermolysis bullosa. Clin Exp Dermatol 1999; 24: 37–39.

737 Shimizu H, McGrath JA, Christiano AM et al. Molecular basis of recessive dystrophic epidermolysis bullosa: genotype/phenotype correlation in a case of moderate clinical severity. J Invest Dermatol 1996; 106: 119–124.

738 Christiano AM, McGrath JA, Uitto J. Influence of the second COL7A1 mutation in determining the phenotypic severity of recessive dystrophic epidermolysis bullosa. J Invest Dermatol 1996; 106: 766–770.

patients with dominant and possibly localized recessive forms of dystrophic epidermolysis bullosa. J Am Acad Dermatol 1990; 22: 188–195.

739 König A, Lauharanta J, Bruckner-Tuderman L. Keratinocytes and fibroblasts from a patient with mutilating dystrophic epidermolysis bullosa synthesize drastically reduced amounts of collagen VII: lack of effect of transforming growth factor-β. J Invest Dermatol 1992 99: 808–812.

740 Kalinke DU, Kalinke U, Winberg J-O et al. Collagen VII in severe recessive dystrophic epidermolysis bullosa: expression of mRNA but lack of intact protein product in skin and cutaneous cells in vitro. J Invest Dermatol 1994; 102: 260–262.

741 König A, Raghunath M, Steinmann B, Bruckner-Tuderman L. Intracellular accumulation of collagen VII in cultured keratinocytes from a patient with dominant dystrophic epidermolysis bullosa. J Invest Dermatol 1994; 102: 105–110.

742 Chan LS, Fine J-D, Hammerberg C et al. Defective in vivo expression and apparently normal in vitro expression of a newly identified 105-kDa lower lamina lucida protein in dystrophic epidermolysis bullosa. Br J Dermatol 1995; 132: 725–729.

743 Fine J-D. Epidermolysis bullosa. Clinical aspects, pathology, and recent advances in research. Int J Dermatol 1986; 25: 143–157.

744 Kero M, Niemi K-M. Epidermolysis bullosa. Int J Dermatol 1986; 25: 75–82.

745 Jonkman MF, Moreno G, Rouan F et al. Dominant dystrophic epidermolysis bullosa Pasini caused by a novel glycine substitution mutation in the type VII collagen gene (COL7A1). J Invest Dermatol 1999; 112: 815–817.

746 Furue M, Ando I, Inoue Y et al. Pretibial epidermolysis bullosa. Arch Dermatol 1986; 122: 310–313.

747 Lichtenwald DJ, Hanna W, Sauder DN et al. Pretibial epidermolysis bullosa: report of a case. J Am Acad Dermatol 1990; 22: 346–350.

748 Soriano L, Fariña C, Manzarbeitia F, Requena L. Pretibial epidermolysis bullosa Int J Dermatol 1999; 38: 536–538.

749 Lee JY-Y, Chen H-C, Lin S-J. Pretibial epidermolysis bullosa: a clinicopathologic study. J Am Acad Dermatol 1993; 29: 974–981.

750 Tang WYM, Lee KC, Chow TC, Lo KK. Three Hong Kong Chinese cases of pretibial epidermolysis bullosa: a genodermatosis that can masquerade as an acquired inflammatory disease. Clin Exp Dermatol 1999; 24: 149–153.

751 Naeyaert JM, Nuytinck L, De Bie S et al. Genetic linkage between the collagen type VII gene COL7A1 and pretibial epidermolysis bullosa with lichenoid features. J Invest Dermatol 1995; 104: 803–805.

752 Betts CM, Posteraro P, Costa AM et al. Pretibial dystrophic epidermolysis bullosa: a recessively inherited COL7A1 splice site mutation affecting procollagen VII processing. Br J Dermatol 1999; 141: 833–839.

753 Nordal EJ, Mecklenbeck S, Hausser I et al. Generalized dystrophic epidermolysis bullosa: identification of a novel, homozygous glycine substitution, G2031S, in exon 73 of COL7A1 in monozygous triplets. Br J Dermatol 2001; 144: 151–157.

754 McGrath JA, O'Grady A, Mayou BJ, Eady RAJ. Mitten deformity in severe generalized recessive dystrophic epidermolysis bullosa: histological, immunofluorescence, and ultrastructural study. J Cutan Pathol 1992; 19: 385–389.

755 Gryboski JD, Touloukian R, Campanella RA. Gastrointestinal manifestations of epidermolysis bullosa in children. Arch Dermatol 1988; 124: 746–752.

756 Gans LA. Eye lesions of epidermolysis bullosa. Arch Dermatol 1988; 124: 762–764.

757 Fine J-D, Osment LS, Gay S. Dystrophic epidermolysis bullosa. A new variant characterized by progressive symmetrical centripetal involvement with scarring. Arch Dermatol 1985; 121: 1014–1017.

758 Ishikawa O, Warita S, Ohnishi K, Miyachi Y. A scleroderma-like variant of dystrophic epidermolysis bullosa? Br J Dermatol 1993; 129: 602–605.

759 Tidman MJ, Eady RAJ. Structural and functional properties of the dermoepidermal junction in obligate heterozygotes for recessive forms of epidermolysis bullosa. Arch Dermatol 1986; 122: 278–281.

760 McGrath JA, Schofield OMV, Eady RAJ. Epidermolysis bullosa pruriginosa: dystrophic epidermolysis bullosa with distinctive clinicopathological features. Br J Dermatol 1994; 130: 617–625.

761 Cambiaghi S, Brusasco A, Restano L et al. Epidermolysis bullosa pruriginosa. Dermatology 1997; 195: 65–68.

762 Mellerio JE, Ashton GHS, Mohammedi R et al. Allelic heterogeneity of dominant and recessive COL7A1 mutations underlying epidermolysis bullosa pruriginosa. J Invest Dermatol 1999; 112: 984–987.

763 Pearson RW, Paller AS. Dermolytic (dystrophic) epidermolysis bullosa inversa. Arch Dermatol 1988; 124: 544–547.

764 Lin AN, Smith LT, Fine J-D. Dystrophic epidermolysis bullosa inversa: report of two cases with further correlation between electron microscopic and immunofluorescence studies. J Am Acad Dermatol 1995; 33: 361–365.

765 Bruckner-Tuderman L, Pfaltz M, Schnyder UW. Epidermolysis bullosa dystrophica inversa in a child. Pediatr Dermatol 1990; 7: 116–121.

766 Bruckner-Tuderman L, Winberg J-O, Anton-Lamprecht I et al. Anchoring fibrils collagen

767 Eng AM, Keegan CA, Hashimoto K et al. Transient bullous dermolysis of the newborn. J Cutan Pathol 1991; 18: 328–332.

768 Hashimoto K, Eng AM. Transient bullous dermolysis of the newborn. J Cutan Pathol 1992; 19: 496–501.

769 Phillips RJ, Harper JI, Lake BD. Intraepidermal collagen type VII in dystrophic epidermolysis bullosa: report of five new cases. Br J Dermatol 1992; 126: 222–230.

770 Fine J-D, Johnson LB, Cronce D et al. Intracytoplasmic retention of type VII collagen and dominant dystrophic epidermolysis bullosa: reversal of defect following cessation of or marked improvement in disease activity. J Invest Dermatol 1993; 101: 232–236.

771 Hanson SG, Fine J-D, Levy ML. Three new cases of transient bullous dermolysis of the newborn. J Am Acad Dermatol 1999; 40: 471–476.

772 Hatta N, Takata M, Shimizu H. Spontaneous disappearance of intraepidermal type VII collagen in a patient with dystrophic epidermolysis bullosa. Br J Dermatol 1995; 133: 619–624.

773 Hammami-Hauasli N, Raghunath M, Küster W, Bruckner-Tuderman L. Transient bullous dermolysis of the newborn associated with compound heterozygosity for recessive and dominant COL7A1 mutations. J Invest Dermatol 1998; 111: 1214–1219.

774 Christiano AM, Fine J-D, Uitto J. Genetic basis of dominantly inherited transient bullous dermolysis of the newborn: a splice site mutation in the type VII collagen gene. J Invest Dermatol 1997; 109: 811–814.

775 McGrath JA, Leigh IM, Eady RAJ. Intracellular expression of type VII collagen during wound healing in severe recessive dystrophic epidermolysis bullosa and normal human skin. Br J Dermatol 1992; 127: 312–317.

776 Grunwald MH, Amichai B, Avinoach I et al. Dystrophic epidermolysis bullosa associated with eosinophilic infiltrate and elevated serum IgE. Pediatr Dermatol 1999; 16: 16–18.

777 Bolte C, Gonzalez S. Rapid diagnosis of major variants of congenital epidermolysis bullosa using a monoclonal antibody against collagen type IV. Am J Dermatopathol 1995; 17: 580–583.

778 Eady RAJ. Fetoscopy and fetal skin biopsy for prenatal diagnosis of genetic skin disorders. Semin Dermatol 1988; 7: 2–8.

779 Woodley DT, Briggaman RA, Gammon WT. Review and update of epidermolysis bullosa acquisita. Semin Dermatol 1988; 7: 111–122.

780 Gammon WR. Epidermolysis bullosa acquisita. Semin Dermatol 1988; 7: 218–224.

781 Gammon WR, Briggaman RA. Epidermolysis bullosa acquisita and bullous systemic lupus erythematosus. Diseases of autoimmunity to type VII collagen. Dermatol Clin 1993; 11: 535–547.

782 Roenigk HH Jr, Ryan JG, Bergfeld WF. Epidermolysis bullosa acquisita. Report of three cases and review of all published cases. Arch Dermatol 1971; 103: 1–10.

783 Jappe U, Zillikens D, Bonnekoh B, Gollnick H. Epidermolysis bullosa acquisita with ultraviolet radiation sensitivity. Br J Dermatol 2000; 142: 517–520.

784 Gammon WR, Briggaman RA, Wheeler CE Jr. Epidermolysis bullosa acquisita presenting as an inflammatory bullous disease. J Am Acad Dermatol 1982; 7: 382–387.

785 Tokuda Y, Amagai M, Yaoita H et al. A case of an inflammatory variant of epidermolysis bullosa acquisita: chronic bullous dermatosis associated with nonscarring mucosal blisters and circulating IgG anti-type-VII- collagen antibody. Dermatology 1998; 197: 58–61.

786 Wieme N, Lambert J, Moerman M et al. Epidermolysis bullosa acquisita with combined features of bullous pemphigoid and cicatricial pemphigoid. Dermatology 1999; 198: 310–313.

787 Edwards S, Wakelin SH, Wojnarowska F et al. Bullous pemphigoid and epidermolysis bullosa acquisita: presentation, prognosis, and immunopathology in 11 children. Pediatr Dermatol 1998; 15: 184–190.

788 Lee CW, Jun KM. Epidermolysis bullosa acquisita presenting with localized facial blisters. Clin Exp Dermatol 1992; 17: 363–365.

789 Kurzhals G, Stolz W, Meurer M et al. Acquired epidermolysis bullosa with the clinical features of Brunsting-Perry cicatricial bullous pemphigoid. Arch Dermatol 1991; 127: 391–395.

790 Gammon WR, Briggaman RA, Woodley DT et al. Epidermolysis bullosa acquisita – a pemphigoid-like disease. J Am Acad Dermatol 1984; 11: 820–832.

791 Caux F, Kirtschig G, Lemarchand-Venencie F et al. IgA-epidermolysis bullosa acquisita in a child resulting in blindness. Br J Dermatol 1997; 137: 270–275.

792 Kazama T, Yamamoto Y, Hashimoto T et al. Application of confocal laser scanning microscopy to differential diagnosis of bullous pemphigoid and epidermolysis bullosa acquisita. Br J Dermatol 1998; 138: 593–601.

793 Luke MC, Darling TN, Hsu R et al. Mucosal morbidity in patients with epidermolysis bullosa acquisita. Arch Dermatol 1999; 135: 954–959.

794 Lang PG Jr, Tapert MJ. Severe ocular involvement in a patient with epidermolysis bullosa acquisita. J Am Acad Dermatol 1987; 16: 439–443.

VII, and neutral metalloproteases in recessive dystrophic epidermolysis bullosa inversa. J Invest Dermatol 1992; 99: 550–558.

795 Bauer JW, Schaeppi H, Metze D et al. Ocular involvement in IgA-epidermolysis bullosa acquisita. Br J Dermatol 1999; 141: 887–892.

796 Lee CW. Epidermolysis bullosa acquisita associated with vesicular cystitis. Br J Dermatol 1988; 119: 101–105.

797 Stewart MI, Woodley DT, Briggaman RA. Epidermolysis bullosa acquisita and associated symptomatic esophageal webs. Arch Dermatol 1991; 127: 373–377.

798 Medenica-Mojsilovic L, Fenske NA, Espinoza CG. Epidermolysis bullosa acquisita. Direct immunofluorescence and ultrastructural studies. Am J Dermatopathol 1987; 9: 324–333.

799 Taniuchi K, Inaoki M, Nishimura Y et al. Nonscarring inflammatory epidermolysis bullosa acquisita with esophageal involvement and linear IgG deposits. J Am Acad Dermatol 1997; 36: 320–322.

800 Rubenstein R, Esterly NB, Fine J-D. Childhood epidermolysis bullosa acquisita. Detection in a 5-year-old girl. Arch Dermatol 1987; 123: 772–776.

801 McCuaig CC, Chan LS, Woodley DT et al. Epidermolysis bullosa acquisita in childhood. Differentiation from hereditary epidermolysis bullosa. Arch Dermatol 1989; 125: 944–949.

802 Kirtschig G, Wojnarowska F, Marsden RA et al. Acquired bullous diseases of childhood: re-evaluation of diagnosis by indirect immunofluorescence examination on 1 M NaCl split skin and immunoblotting. Br J Dermatol 1994; 130: 610–616.

803 Lacour J-P, Bernard P, Rostain G et al. Childhood acquired epidermolysis bullosa. Pediatr Dermatol 1995; 12: 16–20.

804 Inauen P, Hunziker Th, Gerber H et al. Childhood epidermolysis bullosa acquisita. Br J Dermatol 1994; 131: 898–900.

805 Arpey CJ, Elewski BE, Moritz DK, Gammon WR. Childhood epidermolysis bullosa acquisita. Report of three cases and review of literature. J Am Acad Dermatol 1991; 24: 706–714.

806 Roger H, Machado P, Nicolas J-F et al. Epidermolysis bullosa acquisita in a 3½-year-old girl. J Am Acad Dermatol 1992; 27: 858–862.

807 Park SB, Cho KH, Youn JI et al. Epidermolysis bullosa acquisita in childhood – a case mimicking chronic bullous dermatosis of childhood. Clin Exp Dermatol 1997; 22: 220–222.

808 Callot-Mellot C, Bodemer C, Caux F et al. Epidermolysis bullosa acquisita in childhood. Arch Dermatol 1997; 133: 1122–1126.

809 Hayashi K, Ueda M, Sakai M et al. Epidermolysis bullosa acquisita in a 6-year-old Japanese boy. Int J Dermatol 1998; 37: 612–614.

810 Su JC, Varigos GA, Dowling J. Epidermolysis bullosa acquisita in childhood. Australas J Dermatol 1998; 39: 38–41.

811 Chorzelski T, Karczewska K, Dyduch A et al. Epidermolysis bullosa acquisita in a 4-year-old boy. Pediatr Dermatol 2000; 17: 157–158.

812 Briggaman RA, Gammon WR, Woodley DT. Epidermolysis bullosa acquisita of the immunopathological type (dermolytic pemphigoid). J Invest Dermatol 1985; 85: 79s–84s.

813 Miller JL, Stricklin GP, Fine JD et al. Remission of severe epidermolysis bullosa acquisita induced by extracorporeal photochemotherapy. Br J Dermatol 1995; 133: 467–471.

814 Dotson AD, Raimer SS, Pursley TV, Tschen J. Systemic lupus erythematosus occurring in a patient with epidermolysis bullosa acquisita. Arch Dermatol 1981; 117: 422–426.

815 Boh E, Roberts LJ, Lieu T-S et al. Epidermolysis bullosa acquisita preceding the development of systemic lupus erythematosus. J Am Acad Dermatol 1990; 22: 587–593.

816 Ray TL, Levine JB, Weiss W, Ward PA. Epidermolysis bullosa acquisita and inflammatory bowel disease. J Am Acad Dermatol 1982; 6: 242–252.

817 Livden JK, Nilsen R, Thunold S, Schjonsby H. Epidermolysis bullosa acquisita and Crohn's disease. Acta Derm Venereol 1978; 58: 241–244.

818 Chou K, Kauh YC, Jacoby RA, Webster GF. Autoimmune bullous disease in a patient with HIV infection. J Am Acad Dermatol 1991; 24: 1022–1023.

819 Palestine RF, Kossard S, Dicken CH. Epidermolysis bullosa acquisita: a heterogeneous disease. J Am Acad Dermatol 1981; 5: 43–53.

820 Krivo JM, Miller F. Immunopathology of epidermolysis bullosa acquisita. Association with mixed cryoglobulinemia. Arch Dermatol 1978; 114: 1218–1220.

821 Burke WA, Briggaman RA, Gammon WR. Epidermolysis bullosa acquisita in a patient with multiple endocrinopathies syndrome. Arch Dermatol 1986; 122: 187–189.

822 Modiano P, Prost C, Barbaud A et al. Epidermolysis bullosa acquisita and benign schwannoma. J Am Acad Dermatol 1996; 35: 472–473.

823 Kero M, Niemi K-M, Kanerva L. Pregnancy as a trigger of epidermolysis bullosa acquisita. Acta Derm Venereol 1983; 63: 353–356.

824 Reed RJ. The relationship of epidermolysis bullosa acquisita to cicatricial pemphigoid. Am J Dermatopathol 1981; 3: 69–72.

825 Caughman SW. Epidermolysis bullosa acquisita. The search for identity. Arch Dermatol 1986; 122: 159–161.

826 Furue M, Iwata M, Tamaki K, Ishibashi Y. Anatomical distribution and immunological characteristics of epidermolysis bullosa acquisita antigen and bullous pemphigoid antigen. Br J Dermatol 1986; 114: 651–659.

827 Woodley DT, Briggaman RA, Gammon WR et al. Epidermolysis bullosa acquisita antigen, a major cutaneous basement membrane component is synthesized by human dermal fibroblasts and other cutaneous tissues. J Invest Dermatol 1986; 87: 227–231.

828 Woodley DT, O'Keefe EJ, Reese MJ et al. Epidermolysis bullosa acquisita antigen, a new major component of cutaneous basement membrane, is a glycoprotein with collagenous domains. J Invest Dermatol 1986; 86: 668–672.

829 Gammon WR, Briggaman RA. Functional heterogeneity of immune complexes in epidermolysis bullosa acquisita. J Invest Dermatol 1987; 89: 478–483.

830 Tatnall FM, Whitehead PC, Black MM et al. Identification of the epidermolysis bullosa acquisita antigen by LH 7.2 monoclonal antibody: use in diagnosis. Br J Dermatol 1989; 120: 533–539.

831 Gammon WR. Autoimmunity to collagen VII: autoantibody-mediated pathomechanisms regulate clinical-pathological phenotypes of acquired epidermolysis bullosa and bullous SLE. J Cutan Pathol 1993; 20: 109–114.

832 Shimizu H, McDonald JN, Gunner DB et al. Epidermolysis bullosa acquisita antigen and the carboxy terminus of type VII collagen have a common immunolocalization to anchoring fibrils and lamina densa of basement membrane. Br J Dermatol 1990; 122: 577–585.

833 Tanaka T, Furukawa F, Imamura S. Epitope mapping for epidermolysis bullosa acquisita autoantibody by molecularly cloned cDNA for type VII collagen. J Invest Dermatol 1994; 102: 706–709.

834 Borradori L, Caldwell JB, Briggaman RA et al. Passive transfer of autoantibodies from a patient with mutilating epidermolysis bullosa acquisita induces specific alterations in the skin of neonatal mice. Arch Dermatol 1995; 131: 590–595.

835 Kawachi Y, Ikegami M, Hashimoto T et al. Autoantibodies to bullous pemphigoid and epidermolysis bullosa acquisita antigens in an infant. Br J Dermatol 1996; 135: 443–447.

836 Woodley DT, Sarret Y, Briggaman RA. Autoimmunity to type VII collagen. Semin Dermatol 1991; 10: 232–239.

837 McHenry PM, Dagg JH, Tidman MJ, Lever RS. Epidermolysis bullosa acquisita occurring in association with systemic lupus erythematosus. Clin Exp Dermatol 1993; 18: 378–380.

838 Prussick R, Gupta AK, Assaad DM et al. Epidermolysis bullosa acquisita with features of bullous lupus erythematosus. Int J Dermatol 1994; 33: 192–195.

839 Kofler H, Wambacher-Gasser B, Topar G et al. Intravenous immunoglobulin treatment in therapy-resistant epidermolysis bullosa acquisita. J Am Acad Dermatol 1996; 34: 331–335.

840 Engineer L, Ahmed AR. Emerging treatment for epidermolysis bullosa acquisita. J Am Acad Dermatol 2001; 44: 818–828.

841 Wilson BD, Birnkrant AF, Beutner EH, Maize JC. Epidermolysis bullosa acquisita: a clinical disorder of varied etiologies. J Am Acad Dermatol 1980; 3: 280–291.

842 Lacour J-P, Juhlin L, El Baze P, Ortonne J-P. Epidermolysis bullosa acquisita with negative direct immunofluorescence. Arch Dermatol 1985; 121: 1183–1185.

843 Barthelemy H, Kanitakis J, Cambazard F et al. Epidermolysis bullosa acquisita – mapping of antigenic determinants by an immunofluorescent technique. Clin Exp Dermatol 1986; 11: 378–386.

844 Pardo RJ, Penneys NS. Location of basement membrane type IV collagen beneath subepidermal bullous diseases. J Cutan Pathol 1990; 17: 336–341.

845 Mooney E, Falk RJ, Gammon WR. Studies on complement deposits in epidermolysis bullosa acquisita and bullous pemphigoid. Arch Dermatol 1992; 128: 58–60.

846 Unis ME, Pfau RG, Patel H et al. An acquired form of epidermolysis bullosa with immunoreactants. Report of a case. J Am Acad Dermatol 1985; 13: 377–380.

847 Smoller BR, Woodley DT. Differences in direct immunofluorescence staining patterns in epidermolysis bullosa acquisita and bullous pemphigoid. J Am Acad Dermatol 1992; 27: 674–678.

848 Nieboer C, Boorsma DM, Woerdeman MJ, Kalsbeek GL. Epidermolysis bullosa acquisita. Br J Dermatol 1980; 102: 383–392.

849 Zhu X, Niimi Y, Bystryn J-C. Epidermolysis bullosa acquisita. Incidence in patients with basement membrane zone antibodies. Arch Dermatol 1990; 126: 171–174.

850 Lee CW. Serum IgA autoantibodies in patients with epidermolysis bullosa acquisita: a high frequency of detection. Dermatology 2000; 200: 83–84.

851 Ghohestani RF, Nicolas JF, Rousselle P, Claudy AL. Diagnostic value of indirect immunofluorescence on sodium chloride-split skin in differential diagnosis of subepidermal autoimmune bullous dermatoses. Arch Dermatol 1997; 133: 1102–1107.

852 Mutasim DF. The accuracy of indirect immunofluorescence on sodium chloride-split skin in differentiating subepidermal bullous diseases. Arch Dermatol 1997; 133: 1158–1160.

853 Wakelin SH, Bhogal B, Black MM et al. Epidermolysis bullosa acquisita associated with epidermal-binding circulating antibodies. Br J Dermatol 1997; 136: 604–609.

854 Jonckman MF, Schuur J, Dijk F et al. Inflammatory variant of epidermolysis bullosa acquisita with IgG autoantibodies against type VII collagen and laminin α3. Arch Dermatol 2000; 136: 227–231.

855 De Jong MCJM, Bruins S, Heeres K et al. Bullous pemphigoid and epidermolysis bullosa acquisita. Arch Dermatol 1996; 132: 151–157.

856 Gibbs RB, Minus HR. Epidermolysis bullosa acquisita with electron microscopical studies. Arch Dermatol 1975; 111: 215–220.

857 Klein GF, Hintner H, Schuler G, Fritsch P. Junctional blisters in acquired bullous disorders of the dermal-epidermal junction zone: role of the lamina lucida as the mechanical *locus minoris resistentiae*. Br J Dermatol 1983; 109: 499–508.

858 Fine J-D, Tyring S, Gammon WR. The presence of intra-lamina lucida blister formation in epidermolysis bullosa acquisita: possible role of leukocytes. J Invest Dermatol 1989; 92: 27–32.

859 Yaoita H, Briggaman RA, Lawley TJ et al. Epidermolysis bullosa acquisita: ultrastructural and immunological studies. J Invest Dermatol 1981; 76: 288–292.

860 Kárpáti S, Stolz W, Meurer M et al. In situ localization of IgG in epidermolysis bullosa acquisita by immunogold technique. J Am Acad Dermatol 1992; 26: 726–730.

861 Ishiko A, Hashimoto T, Shimizu H, Nishikawa T. Epidermolysis bullosa acquisita: report of a case with comparison of immunogold electron microscopy using pre- and postembedding labelling. Br J Dermatol 1996; 134: 147–151.

862 Sajben FP, Gibbs NF, Friedlander SF. Transillumination blisters in a neonate. J Am Acad Dermatol 1999; 41: 264–265.

863 Bergman R, David R, Ramon Y et al. Delayed postburn blisters: an immunohistochemical and ultrastructural study. J Cutan Pathol 1997; 24: 429–433.

864 Chen DM, Fairley JA. A bullous pemphigoid-like skin eruption after a chemical burn. J Am Acad Dermatol 1998; 38: 337–340.

865 Azurdia RM, Guerin DM, Sharpe GR. Recurrent bullous dermatitis artefacta mimicking immunobullous disease. Br J Dermatol 2000; 143: 229–230.

866 Requena L, Requena C, Sanchez M et al. Chemical warfare. Cutaneous lesions from mustard gas. J Am Acad Dermatol 1988; 19: 529–536.

867 Smith KJ, Hurst CG, Moeller RB et al. Sulfur mustard: its continuing threat as a chemical warfare agent, the cutaneous lesions induced, progress in understanding its mechanism of action, its long-term health effects, and new developments for protection and therapy. J Am Acad Dermatol 1995; 32: 765–776.

868 Momeni A-Z, Enshaeih S, Meghdadi M, Amindjavaheri M. Skin manifestations of mustard gas. Arch Dermatol 1992; 128: 775–780.

869 Waltzer JF, Flowers FP. Bullous variant of chemotherapy-induced acral erythema. Arch Dermatol 1993; 129: 43–45.

870 Baran R, Juhlin L, Brun P. Bullae in skin grafts. Br J Dermatol 1984; 111: 221–225.

871 Winzer M, Ruppert M, Baretton G et al. Bullöse poikilodermatische Amyloidose der Haut mit junktionaler Blasenbildung bei einem IgG-Leichtketten-Plasmozytom vom Lambdatyp. Hautarzt 1992; 42: 199–204.

872 West NY, Fitzpatrick JE, David-Bajar KM, Bennion SD. Waldenström macroglobulinemia-induced bullous dermatosis. Arch Dermatol 1998; 134: 1127–1131.

873 Whittaker SJ, Bhogal BS, Black MM. Acquired immunobullous disease: a cutaneous manifestation of IgM macroglobulinaemia. Br J Dermatol 1996; 135: 283–286.

874 Brooke CP, Spiers EM, Omura EF. Noninflammatory bullae associated with ε-aminocaproic acid infusion. J Am Acad Dermatol 1992; 27: 880–882.

Subepidermal blisters with lymphocytes

875 Fried R, Lynfield Y, Vitale P, Anhalt G. Paraneoplastic pemphigus appearing as bullous pemphigoid-like eruption after palliative radiation therapy. J Am Acad Dermatol 1993; 29: 815–817.

876 Loucas E, Russo G, Millikan LE. Genetic and acquired cutaneous disorders associated with internal malignancy. Int J Dermatol 1995; 34: 749–758.

877 Camisa C, Helm TN. Paraneoplastic pemphigus is a distinct neoplasia-induced autoimmune disease. Arch Dermatol 1993; 129: 883–886.

878 Mutasim DF, Pelc NJ, Anhalt GJ. Paraneoplastic pemphigus. Dermatol Clin 1993; 11: 473–481.

879 Borradori L, Lombardi T, Samson J et al. Anti-CD20 monoclonal antibody (Rituximab) for refractory erosive stomatitis secondary to CD20⁺ follicular lymphoma-associated paraneoplastic pemphigus. Arch Dermatol 2001; 137: 269–272.

880 Gooptu C, Littlewood TJ, Frith P et al. Paraneoplastic pemphigus: an association with fludarabine? Br J Dermatol 2001; 144: 1255–1261.

881 Dega H, Laporte JL, Joly P et al. Paraneoplastic pemphigus associated with Hodgkin's disease. Br J Dermatol 1998; 138: 196–198.

882 Chiewchanvit S, Hashimoto T, Chaiwun B, Nishikawa T. A pemphigus case with long term survival, implicating the spectrum between paraneoplastic pemphigus and pemphigus vulgaris. Int J Dermatol 1997; 36: 957–958.

883 Leyn J, Degreef H. Paraneoplastic pemphigus in a patient with a thymoma. Dermatology 2001; 202: 151–154.

884 Caneppele S, Picart N, Bayle-Lebey P et al. Paraneoplastic pemphigus associated with Castleman's tumour. Clin Exp Dermatol 2000; 25: 219–221.

885 Kim S-C, Chang SN, Lee IJ et al. Localized mucosal involvement and severe pulmonary involvement in a young patient with paraneoplastic pemphigus associated with Castleman's tumour. Br J Dermatol 1998; 138: 667–671.

886 Wolff H, Kunte C, Messer G et al. Paraneoplastic pemphigus with fatal pulmonary involvement in a woman with a mesenteric Castleman tumour. Br J Dermatol 1999; 140: 313–316.

887 Chorzelski T, Hashimoto T, Maciejewska B et al. Paraneoplastic pemphigus associated with Castleman tumor, myasthenia gravis, and bronchiolitis obliterans. J Am Acad Dermatol 1999; 41: 393–400.

888 Lee I-J, Kim S-C, Kim HS et al. Paraneoplastic pemphigus associated with follicular dendritic cell sarcoma arising from Castleman's tumor. J Am Acad Dermatol 1999; 40: 294–297.

889 Mascaró JM Jr, Ferrando J, Solé MT et al. Paraneoplastic pemphigus: a case of long-term survival associated with systemic lupus erythematosus and polymyositis. Dermatology 1999; 199: 63–66.

890 Anhalt GJ. Paraneoplastic pemphigus: the role of tumours and drugs. Br J Dermatol 2001; 144: 1101–1104.

891 Su WPD, Oursler JR, Muller SA. Paraneoplastic pemphigus: a case with high titer of circulating anti-basement membrane zone autoantibodies. J Am Acad Dermatol 1994; 30: 841–844.

892 Rongioletti F, Truchetet F, Rebora A. Paraneoplastic pemphigoid-pemphigus? Subepidermal bullous disease with pemphigus-like direct immunofluorescence. Int J Dermatol 1993; 32: 48–51.

893 Musette P, Joly P, Gilbert D et al. A paraneoplastic mixed bullous skin disease: breakdown in tolerance to multiple epidermal antigens. Br J Dermatol 2000; 143: 149–153.

894 Wong KC, Ho KK. Pemphigus with pemphigoid-like presentation, associated with squamous cell carcinoma of the tongue. Australas J Dermatol 2000; 41: 178–180.

895 Sapadin AN, Anhalt GJ. Paraneoplastic pemphigus with a pemphigus vegetans-like plaque as the only cutaneous manifestation. J Am Acad Dermatol 1998; 39: 867–871.

896 Chorzelski TP, Hashimoto T, Amagai M et al. Paraneoplastic pemphigus with cutaneous and serological features of pemphigus foliaceus. Br J Dermatol 1999; 141: 357–359.

897 Reich K, Brinck U, Letschert M et al. Graft-versus-host disease-like immunophenotype and apoptotic keratinocyte death in paraneoplastic pemphigus. Br J Dermatol 1999; 141: 739–746.

898 Stevens SR, Griffiths CEM, Anhalt GJ, Cooper KD. Paraneoplastic pemphigus presenting as a lichen planus pemphigoides-like eruption. Arch Dermatol 1993; 129: 866–869.

899 Passeron T, Bahadoran P, Lacour J-P et al. Paraneoplastic pemphigus presenting as erosive lichen planus. Br J Dermatol 1999; 140: 552–553.

900 Nguyen VT, Ndoye A, Bassler KD et al. Classification, clinical manifestions, and immunopathologic mechanisms of the epithelial variant of paraneoplastic autoimmune multiorgan syndrome. A reappraisal of paraneoplastic pemphigus. Arch Dermatol 2001; 137: 193–206.

901 Hsiao C-J, Hsu MM-L, Lee JY-Y et al. Paraneoplastic pemphigus in association with a retroperitoneal Castleman's disease presenting with a lichen planus pemphigoides-like eruption. A case report and review of the literature. Br J Dermatol 2001; 144: 372–376.

902 Bystryn J-C, Hodak E, Gao S-Q et al. A paraneoplastic mixed bullous skin disease associated with anti-skin antibodies and a B-cell lymphoma. Arch Dermatol 1993; 129: 870–875.

903 Setterfield J, Shirlaw PJ, Lazarova Z et al. Paraneoplastic cicatricial pemphigoid. Br J Dermatol 1999; 141: 127–131.

904 Kirsner RS, Anhalt GJ, Kerdel FA. Treatment with alpha interferon associated with the development of paraneoplastic pemphigus. Br J Dermatol 1995; 132: 474–478.

905 Lee M-S, Kossard S, Ho KKL et al. Paraneoplastic pemphigus triggered by radiotherapy. Australas J Dermatol 1995; 36: 206–210.

906 Nousari HC, Kimyai-Asadi A, Anhalt GJ. Elevated serum levels of interleukin-6 in paraneoplastic pemphigus. J Invest Dermatol 1999; 112: 396–398.

907 Lemon MA, Weston WL, Huff JC. Childhood paraneoplastic pemphigus associated with Castleman's tumour. Br J Dermatol 1997; 136: 115–117.

908 Schoen H, Foedinger D, Derfler K et al. Immunoapheresis in paraneoplastic pemphigus. Arch Dermatol 1998; 134: 706–710.

909 Tankel M, Tannenbaum S, Parekh S. Paraneoplastic pemphigus presenting as an unusual bullous eruption. J Am Acad Dermatol 1993; 29: 825–828.

910 Ostezan LB, Fabré VC, Caughman SW et al. Paraneoplastic pemphigus in the absence of a known neoplasm. J Am Acad Dermatol 1995; 33: 312–315.

911 Gooptu C, Mendelsohn S, Amagai M et al. Unique immunobullous disease in a child with a predominantly IgA response to three desmosomal proteins. Br J Dermatol 1999; 141: 882–886.

912 Cordel N, Ringeisen F, Antoine M et al. Paraneoplastic pemphigus with constrictive bronchiolitis obliterans. Dermatology 2001; 202: 145.

913 Beele H, Claerhout I, Kestelyn P et al. Bilateral corneal melting in a patient with paraneoplastic pemphigus. Dermatology 2001; 202: 147–150.

914 Perniciaro C, Kuechle MK, Colón-Otero G et al. Paraneoplastic pemphigus: a case of prolonged survival. Mayo Clin Proc 1994; 69: 851–855.

915 Camisa C, Helm TN, Liu Y-C et al. Paraneoplastic pemphigus: a report of three cases including one long-term survivor. J Am Acad Dermatol 1992; 27: 547–553.

916 Kim S-C, Kwon YD, Lee IJ et al. cDNA cloning of the 210-kDa paraneoplastic pemphigus antigen reveals that envoplakin is a component of the antigen complex. J Invest Dermatol 1997; 109: 365–369.

917 de Bruin A, Müller E, Wyder M et al. Periplakin and envoplakin are target antigens in canine and human paraneoplastic pemphigus. J Am Acad Dermatol 1999; 40: 682–685.

918 Mahoney MG, Aho S, Uitto J, Stanley JR. The members of the plakin family of proteins recognized by paraneoplastic pemphigus antibodies include periplakin. J Invest Dermatol 1998; 111: 308–313.

919 Borradori L, Trüeb RM, Jaunin F et al. Autoantibodies from a patient with paraneoplastic pemphigus bind periplakin, a novel member of the plakin family. J Invest Dermatol 1998; 111: 338–340.

920 Ishii M, Izumi J, Fujiwara H et al. Immunoblotting detection of γ-catenin (plakoglobin) antibody in the serum of a patient with paraneoplastic pemphigus. Br J Dermatol 2001; 144: 377–379.

921 Proby C, Fujii Y, Owaribe K et al. Human autoantibodies against HD1/plectin in paraneoplastic pemphigus. J Invest Dermatol 1999; 112: 153–156.

922 Aho S, Mahoney MG, Uitto J. Plectin serves as an autoantigen in paraneoplastic pemphigus. J Invest Dermatol 1999; 113: 422–423.

923 Martel P, Gilbert D, Labeille B et al. A case of paraneoplastic pemphigus with antidesmoglein 1 antibodies as determined by immunoblotting. Br J Dermatol 2000; 142: 812–813.

924 Ohyama M, Amagai M, Hashimoto T et al. Clinical phenotype and anti-desmoglein autoantibody profile in paraneoplastic pemphigus. J Am Acad Dermatol 2001; 44: 593–598.

925 Bouloc A, Joly P, Saint-Leger E et al. Paraneoplastic pemphigus with circulating antibodies directed exclusively against the pemphigus vulgaris antigen desmoglein 3. J Am Acad Dermatol 2000; 43: 714–717.

926 Inaoki M, Kodera M, Fujimoto A et al. Paraneoplastic pemphigus without antidesmoglein 3 or antidesmoglein 1 autoantibodies. Br J Dermatol 2001; 144: 610–613.

927 Chan LS. Epitope spreading in paraneoplastic pemphigus. Autoimmune induction in antibody-mediated blistering skin diseases. Arch Dermatol 2000; 136: 663–664.

928 Bowen GM, Peters NT, Fivenson DP et al. Lichenoid dermatitis in paraneoplastic pemphigus. Arch Dermatol 2000; 136: 652–656.

929 Mehregan DR, Oursler JR, Leiferman KM et al. Paraneoplastic pemphigus: a subset of patients with pemphigus and neoplasia. J Cutan Pathol 1993; 20: 203–210.

930 Horn TD, Anhalt GJ. Histologic features of paraneoplastic pemphigus. Arch Dermatol 1992; 128: 1091–1095.

931 Nishibori Y, Hashimoto T, Ishiko A et al. Paraneoplastic pemphigus: the first case report from Japan. Dermatology 1995; 191: 39–42.

932 Joly P, Richard C, Gilbert D et al. Sensitivity and specificity of clinical, histologic, and immunologic features in the diagnosis of paraneoplastic pemphigus. J Am Acad Dermatol 2000; 43: 619–626.

933 Schaeppi H, Bauer JW, Hametner R et al. A localized variant of paraneoplastic pemphigus: acantholysis associated with malignant melanoma. Br J Dermatol 2001; 144: 1249–1254.

934 Rybojad M, Leblanc T, Flageul B et al. Paraneoplastic pemphigus in a child with a T-cell lymphoblastic lymphoma. Br J Dermatol 1993; 128: 418–422.

935 Hashimoto T, Amagai M, Watanabe K et al. Characterization of paraneoplastic pemphigus autoantigens by immunoblot analysis. J Invest Dermatol 1995; 104: 829–834.

936 Liu AY, Valenzuela R, Helm TN et al. Indirect immunofluorescence on rat bladder transitional epithelium: a test with high specificity for paraneoplastic pemphigus. J Am Acad Dermatol 1993; 28: 696–699.

937 Helou J, Allbritton J, Anhalt GJ. Accuracy of indirect immunofluorescence testing in the diagnosis of paraneoplastic pemphigus. J Am Acad Dermatol 1995; 32: 441–447.

Subepidermal blisters with eosinophils

938 Rosen LB, Frank BL, Rywlin AM. A characteristic vesiculobullous eruption in patients with chronic lymphocytic leukemia. J Am Acad Dermatol 1986; 15: 943–950.

939 Thivolet J, Barthelemy H. Bullous pemphigoid. Semin Dermatol 1988; 7: 91–103.

940 Korman NJ. Bullous pemphigoid. Dermatol Clin 1993; 11: 483–498.

941 Korman NJ. Bullous pemphigoid. The latest in diagnosis, prognosis, and therapy. Arch Dermatol 1998; 134: 1137–1141.

942 Korman N. Bullous pemphigoid. J Am Acad Dermatol 1987; 16: 907–924.

943 Fonseca E, Contreras F. Annular bullous pemphigoid in a child. J Am Acad Dermatol 1993; 29: 661–662.

944 Amato DA, Silverstein J, Zitelli J. The prodrome of bullous pemphigoid. Int J Dermatol 1988; 27: 560–563.

945 Alonso-Llamazares J, Rogers RS III, Oursler JR, Calobrisi SD. Bullous pemphigoid presenting as generalized pruritus: observations in six patients. Int J Dermatol 1998; 37: 508–514.

946 Gengoux P, Lachapelle J-M. Pemphigoid presenting as atypical excoriated prurigo: regarding 11 cases. Dermatology 1997; 194: 392–394.

947 Strohal R, Rappersberger K, Pehamberger H, Wolff K. Nonbullous pemphigoid: prodrome of bullous pemphigoid or a distinct pemphigoid variant? J Am Acad Dermatol 1993; 29: 293–299.

948 Wolf R, Ophir J, Dechner E. Nonbullous bullous pemphigoid. Int J Dermatol 1992; 31: 498–500.

949 Korman NJ, Woods SG. Erythrodermic bullous pemphigoid is a clinical variant of bullous pemphigoid. Br J Dermatol 1995; 133: 967–971.

950 Scrivener Y, Heid E, Grosshans E, Cribier B. Erythrodermic bullous pemphigoid. J Am Acad Dermatol 1999; 41: 658–659.

951 Alonso-Llamazares J, Dietrich SM, Gibson LE. Bullous pemphigoid presenting as exfoliative erythroderma. J Am Acad Dermatol 1998; 39: 827–830.

952 Gilmour E, Bhushan M, Griffiths CEM. Figurate erythema with bullous pemphigoid: a true paraneoplastic phenomenon? Clin Exp Dermatol 1999; 24: 446–448.

953 Hauschild A, Swensson O, Christophers E. Paraneoplastic bullous pemphigoid resembling erythema gyratum repens. Br J Dermatol 1999; 140: 550–552.

954 Van Joost T, Vuzevski VD, ten Kate F, Tank B. Localized bullous pemphigoid, a T cell-mediated disease? Electron microscopic and immunologic studies. Acta Derm Venereol 1989; 69: 341–344.

955 Guenther LC, Shum D. Localized childhood vulvar pemphigoid. J Am Acad Dermatol 1990; 22: 762–764.

956 Schumann H, Amann U, Tasanen K et al. A child with localized vulval pemphigoid and IgG autoantibodies targeting the C-terminus of collagen XVII/BP180. Br J Dermatol 1999; 140: 1133–1138.

957 Farrell AM, Kirtschig G, Dalziel KL et al. Childhood vulval pemphigoid: a clinical and immunopathological study of five patients. Br J Dermatol 1999; 140: 308–312.

958 Person JR. Hydrostatic bullae and pretibial pemphigoid. Int J Dermatol 1983; 22: 237–238.

959 Borradori L, Prost C, Wokenstein P et al. Localized pretibial pemphigoid and pemphigoid nodularis. J Am Acad Dermatol 1992; 27: 863–867.

960 Bull RH, Fallowfield ME, Marsden RA. Autoimmune blistering diseases associated with HIV infection. Clin Exp Dermatol 1994; 19: 47–50.

961 Soh H, Hosokawa H, Miyauchi H et al. Localized pemphigoid shares the same target antigen as bullous pemphigoid. Br J Dermatol 1991; 125: 73–75.

962 Long CC, Lever LR, Marks R. Unilateral bullous pemphigoid in a hemiplegic patient. Br J Dermatol 1992; 126: 614–616.

963 Salomon RJ, Briggaman RA, Wernikoff SY, Kayne AL. Localized bullous pemphigoid. A mimic of acute contact dermatitis. Arch Dermatol 1987; 123: 389–392.

964 Liu H-NH, Su WPD, Rogers RS III. Clinical variants of pemphigoid. Int J Dermatol 1986; 25: 17–27.

965 Duhra P, Ryatt KS. Haemorrhagic pompholyx in bullous pemphigoid. Clin Exp Dermatol 1988; 13: 342–343.

966 Barth JH, Fairris GM, Wojnarowska F, White JE. Haemorrhagic pompholyx is a sign of bullous pemphigoid and an indication for low-dose prednisolone therapy. Clin Exp Dermatol 1986; 11: 409–412.

967 Descamps V, Flageul B, Vignon-Pennamen D et al. Dyshidrosiform pemphigoid: report of three cases. J Am Acad Dermatol 1992; 26: 651–652.

968 Scola F, Telang GH, Swartz C. Dyshidrosiform pemphigoid. J Am Acad Dermatol 1995; 32: 516–517.

969 Bhushan M, Chalmers RJG, Cox NH. Acute oedema blisters: a report of 13 cases. Br J Dermatol 2001; 144: 580–582.

970 Eng TY, Hogan WJ, Jordon RE. Oesophageal involvement in bullous pemphigoid. Br J Dermatol 1978; 99: 207–210.

971 Kiyokawa C, Fujito S, Mori O et al. Bullous pemphigoid showing unusual ocular changes. Br J Dermatol 1998; 139: 693–696.

972 Kirtschig G, Venning VA, Wojnarowska F. Bullous pemphigoid: correlation of mucosal involvement and mucosal expression of autoantigens studied by indirect immunofluorescence and immunoblotting. Clin Exp Dermatol 1999; 24: 208–212.

973 Bushkell LL, Jordon RE. Bullous pemphigoid: a cause of peripheral blood eosinophilia. J Am Acad Dermatol 1983; 8: 648–651.

974 Caproni M, Palleschi GM, Falcos D et al. Serum eosinophil cationic protein (ECP) in bullous pemphigoid. Int J Dermatol 1995; 34: 177–180.

975 Czech W, Schaller J, Schöpf E, Kapp A. Granulocyte activation in bullous diseases: release of granular proteins in bullous pemphigoid and pemphigus vulgaris. J Am Acad Dermatol 1993; 29: 210–215.

976 Jung M, Kippes W, Messer G et al. Increased risk of bullous pemphigoid in male and very old patients: A population-based study on incidence. J Am Acad Dermatol 1999; 41: 266–268.

977 Miyagawa S, Ishii H, Kitamura W, Sakamoto K. Bullous pemphigoid in a man and his nephew. Arch Dermatol 1983; 119: 605–606.

978 Oranje AP, van Joost T. Pemphigoid in children. Pediatr Dermatol 1989; 6: 267–274.

979 Nemeth AJ, Klein AD, Gould EW, Schachner LA. Childhood bullous pemphigoid. Arch Dermatol 1991; 127: 378–386.

980 Oranje AP, Vuzevski VD, van Joost T et al. Bullous pemphigoid in children. Report of three cases with special emphasis on therapy. Int J Dermatol 1991; 30: 339–342.

981 Nagano T, Tani M, Adachi A et al. Childhood bullous pemphigoid: immunohistochemical, immunoelectron microscopic, and Western blot analysis. J Am Acad Dermatol 1994; 30: 884–888.

982 Chimanovitch I, Hamm H, Georgi M et al. Bullous pemphigoid of childhood. Autoantibodies target the same epitopes within the NC16A domain of BP180 as autoantibodies in bullous pemphigoid of adulthood. Arch Dermatol 2000; 136: 527–532.

983 Cunha PR, Thomazeski PVG, Hipólito E et al. Bullous pemphigoid in a 2-month-old infant. Int J Dermatol 1998; 37: 935–938.

984 Weston WL, Morelli JG, Huff JC. Misdiagnosis, treatments, and outcomes in the immunobullous diseases in children. Pediatr Dermatol 1997; 14: 264–272.

985 Banfield CC, Wojnarowska F, Allen J et al. The association of HLA-DQ7 with bullous pemphigoid is restricted to men. Br J Dermatol 1998; 138: 1085–1090.

986 Bernard P, Vaillant L, Labeille B et al. Incidence and distribution of subepidermal autoimmune bullous skin diseases in three French regions. Arch Dermatol 1995; 131: 48–52.

987 Vaillant L, Bernard P, Joly P et al. Evaluation of clinical criteria for diagnosis of bullous pemphigoid. Arch Dermatol 1998; 134: 1075–1080.

988 Shimizu H, Hayakawa K, Nishikawa T. A comparative immunoelectron microscopic study of typical and atypical cases of pemphigoid. Br J Dermatol 1988; 119: 717–722.

989 Domloge-Hultsch N, Utecht L, James W, Yancey KB. Autoantibodies from patients with localized and generalized bullous pemphigoid immunoprecipitate the same 230-kd keratinocyte antigen. Arch Dermatol 1990; 126: 1337–1341.

990 Gruber GG, Owen LG, Callen JP. Vesicular pemphigoid. J Am Acad Dermatol 1980; 3: 619–622.

991 Komine M, Nashiro K, Asahina A et al. Vesicular pemphigoid. Int J Dermatol 1992; 31: 868–870.

992 Satoh S, Seishima M, Izumi T et al. A vesicular variant of bullous pemphigoid with autoantibodies against unidentified 205- and 150-kDa proteins at the basement membrane zone. Br J Dermatol 1997; 137: 768–773.

993 Inoh Y, Nishikawa T, Hashimoto T. The vesicular pemphigoid phenotype may be related to antibodies to a 200 kDa antigen in the lower lamina lucida. Br J Dermatol 1998; 139: 738–739.

994 Ohnishi Y, Tajima S, Ishibashi A, Fujiwara S. A vesicular bullous pemphigoid with an autoantibody against plectin. Br J Dermatol 2000; 142: 813–815.

995 Okura M, Tatsuno Y, Sato M et al. Vesicular pemphigoid with antidesmoplakin autoantibodies. Br J Dermatol 1997; 136: 794–796.

996 Winkelmann RK, Su WPD. Pemphigoid vegetans. Arch Dermatol 1979; 115: 446–448.

997 Al-Najjar A, Reilly GD, Bleehen SS. Pemphigoid vegetans: a case report. Acta Derm Venereol 1984; 64: 450–452.

998 Ueda Y, Nashiro K, Seki Y et al. Pemphigoid vegetans. Br J Dermatol 1989; 120: 449–453.

999 Chan LS, Dorman MA, Agha A et al. Pemphigoid vegetans represents a bullous pemphigoid variant. J Am Acad Dermatol 1993; 28: 331–335.

1000 Ogasawara M, Matsuda S, Nishioka K, Asagami C. Pemphigoid vegetans. J Am Acad Dermatol 1994; 30: 649–650.

1001 Honeyman JF, Honeyman AR, de la Parra MA et al. Polymorphic pemphigoid. Arch Dermatol 1979; 115: 423–427.

1002 Tamaki K, Furuya T, Kubota Y et al. Seborrheic pemphigoid and polymorphic pemphigoid. J Am Acad Dermatol 1991; 25: 568–570.

1003 Jablonska S, Chorzelski TP, Beutner EH et al. Dermatitis herpetiformis and bullous pemphigoid. Intermediate and mixed forms. Arch Dermatol 1976; 112: 45–48.

1004 Sander HM, Utz MMP, Peters MS. Bullous pemphigoid and dermatitis herpetiformis: mixed bullous disease or coexistence of two separate entities? J Cutan Pathol 1989; 16: 370–374.

1005 Allan SJR, Tidman MJ. Pemphigoid excoriée: a further variant of bullous pemphigoid? Br J Dermatol 1999; 141: 585–586.

1006 Roenigk RK, Dahl MV. Bullous pemphigoid and prurigo nodularis. J Am Acad Dermatol 1986; 14: 944–947.

1007 Tani M, Murata Y, Masaki H. Pemphigoid nodularis. J Am Acad Dermatol 1989; 21: 1099–1104.

1008 Bourke JF, Berth-Jones J, Gawkrodger DJ, Burns DA. Pemphigoid nodularis: a report of two cases. Clin Exp Dermatol 1994; 19: 496–499.

1009 Kossard S. Prurigo papules with blisters. Australas J Dermatol 1996; 37: 104–105.

1010 Ross JS, McKee PH, Smith NP et al. Unusual variants of pemphigoid: from pruritus to pemphigoid nodularis. J Cutan Pathol 1992; 19: 212–216.

1011 Gawkrodger DJ, O'Doherty C StJ. Pemphigoid en cocarde. J Am Acad Dermatol 1989; 20: 1125.

1012 Ahmed AR, Hardy D. Bullous pemphigoid family of autoimmune diseases. Int J Dermatol 1981; 20: 541–543.

1013 Giannini JM, Callen JP, Gruber GG. Bullous pemphigoid and rheumatoid arthritis. J Am Acad Dermatol 1981; 4: 695–697.

1014 Szabo E, Husz S, Kovacs L. Coexistent atypical bullous pemphigoid and systemic lupus erythematosus. Br J Dermatol 1981; 104: 71–75.

1015 Loche F, Bernard P, Bazex J. Bullous pemphigoid associated with systemic lupus erythematosus. Br J Dermatol 1998; 139: 927–928.

1016 Huang C-Y, Chen T-C. Bullous pemphigoid associated with systemic lupus erythematosus: the discrimination of antibasement membrane zone antibody. Int J Dermatol 1997; 36: 40–42.

1017 Hamilton DV, McKenzie AW. Bullous pemphigoid and primary biliary cirrhosis. Br J Dermatol 1978; 99: 447–450.

1018 Barth JH, Kelly SE, Wojnarowska F et al. Pemphigoid and ulcerative colitis. J Am Acad Dermatol 1988; 19: 303–308.

1019 Lynfield YL, Green K, Gopal R. Bullous pemphigoid and multiple autoimmune diseases. J Am Acad Dermatol 1983; 9: 257–261.

1020 Chuang T-Y, Korkij W, Soltani K et al. Increased frequency of diabetes mellitus in patients with bullous pemphigoid: a case-control study. J Am Acad Dermatol 1984; 11: 1099–1102.

1021 How J, Bewsher PD, Stankler L. Bullous pemphigoid, polymyalgia rheumatica and thyroid disease. Br J Dermatol 1980; 103: 201–204.

1022 Smith WDF, Lewis Jones MS, Stewart TW, Fernando MU. Bullous pemphigoid occurring in psoriatic plaques in association with Hashimoto's thyroiditis. Clin Exp Dermatol 1991; 16: 389–391.

1023 Masouye I, Schmied E, Didierjean L et al. Bullous pemphigoid and multiple sclerosis: more than a coincidence? Report of three cases. J Am Acad Dermatol 1989; 21: 63–68.

1024 Chosidow O, Doppler V, Bensimon G et al. Bullous pemphigoid and amyotrophic lateral sclerosis. A new clue for understanding the bullous disease? Arch Dermatol 2000; 136: 521–524.

1025 Beer TW, Smith HR. Bullous pemphigoid associated with cutaneous leukocytoclastic vasculitis. Int J Dermatol 1998; 37: 940–942.

1026 Modiano P, Reichert S, Barbaud A et al. Bullous pemphigoid in association with cutaneous lesions specific to a myelodysplastic syndrome. Br J Dermatol 1997; 136: 402–405.

1027 Ueki H, Kohda M, Hashimoto T et al. Bullous pemphigoid associated with silicosis. Dermatology 2000; 201: 265–267.

1028 Yesudian PD, Wilson NJE, Parslew R. Bullous pemphigoid and neurofibromatosis – a chance association requiring special vigilance. Clin Exp Dermatol 2000; 25: 658–659.

1029 Shiraishi S, Ho T, Shirakata Y et al. Bullous pemphigoid in a patient with a C4 deficiency. Br J Dermatol 1991; 124: 296–298.

1030 Taylor G, Venning V, Wojnarowska F. Bullous pemphigoid and associated autoimmune thrombocytopenia: two case reports. J Am Acad Dermatol 1993; 29: 900–902.

1031 Razack EM, Premalatha S, Rao NR, Zahra A. Acanthosis palmaris in a patient with bullous pemphigoid. J Am Acad Dermatol 1987; 16: 217–219.

1032 Van Joost T, Muntendam J, Heule F et al. Subepidermal bullous autoimmune disease associated with immune nephritis. Immunomorphologic studies. J Am Acad Dermatol 1986; 14: 214–220.

1033 Simon CA, Winkelmann RK. Bullous pemphigoid and glomerulonephritis. J Am Acad Dermatol 1986; 14: 456–463.

1034 Barnadas MᵃA, Gelpi C, Rocamora V et al. Bullous pemphigoid associated with acute glomerulonephritis. Br J Dermatol 1998; 138: 867–871.

1035 Harrington CI, Sneddon IB. Coexistence of bullous pemphigoid and pemphigus foliaceus. Br J Dermatol 1979; 100: 441–445.

1036 Grattan CEH. Evidence of an association between bullous pemphigoid and psoriasis. Br J Dermatol 1985; 113: 281–283.

1037 Kirtschig G, Chow ETY, Venning VA, Wojnarowska FT. Acquired subepidermal bullous diseases associated with psoriasis: a clinical, immunopathological and immunogenetic study. Br J Dermatol 1996; 135: 738–745.

1038 Denli YG, Uslular C, Acar MA et al. Bullous pemphigoid in a psoriatic patient. J Eur Acad Dermatol Venereol 2000; 14: 316–317.

1039 Graham-Brown RAC. Bullous pemphigoid with figurate erythema associated with carcinoma of the bronchus. Br J Dermatol 1987; 117: 385–388.

1040 Jablonska S, Chorzelski TP, Blaszczyk M, Maciejowska E. Bullous diseases and malignancy. Semin Dermatol 1984; 3: 316–326.

1041 Tzemos N, Aravindan P, Chitoni M et al. Cholangiocarcinoma associated with bullous pemphigoid. Br J Dermatol 1999; 140: 1180–1181.

1042 Muramatsu T, Iida T, Tada H et al. Bullous pemphigoid associated with internal malignancies: identification of 180-kDa antigen by Western immunoblotting. Br J Dermatol 1996; 135: 782–784.

1043 Rub R, Avidor Y, Messer G, Schreiber L. Bullous pemphigoid as an initial presentation of renal oncocytoma. Dermatology 1999; 198: 322–323.

1044 Deguchi M, Tsunoda T, Tagami H. Resolution of bullous pemphigoid and improvement of vitiligo after successful treatment of squamous cell carcinoma of the skin. Clin Exp Dermatol 1999; 24: 14–15.

1045 Lindelof B, Islam N, Eklund G, Arfors L. Pemphigoid and cancer. Arch Dermatol 1990; 126: 66–68.

1046 Taylor G, Venning V, Wojnarowska F, Welch K. Bullous pemphigoid and autoimmunity. J Am Acad Dermatol 1993; 29: 181–184.

1047 Roujeau J-C, Lok C, Bastuji-Garin S et al. High risk of death in elderly patients with extensive bullous pemphigoid. Arch Dermatol 1998; 134: 465–469.

1048 Bernard P, Didierjean L, Denis F et al. Heterogeneous bullous pemphigoid antibodies: detection and characterization by immunoblotting when absent by indirect immunofluorescence. J Invest Dermatol 1989; 92: 171–174.

1049 Logan RA, Bhogal B, Das AK. Localization of bullous pemphigoid antibody – an indirect immunofluorescence study of 228 cases using a split-skin technique. Br J Dermatol 1987; 117: 471–478.

1050 Mutasim DF, Morrison LH, Takahashi Y et al. Definition of bullous pemphigoid antibody binding to intracellular and extracellular antigen associated with hemidesmosomes. J Invest Dermatol 1989; 92: 225–230.

1051 Meyer LJ, Taylor TB, Kadunce DP, Zone JJ. Two groups of bullous pemphigoid antigens are identified by affinity-purified antibodies. J Invest Dermatol 1990; 94: 611–616.

1052 Robledo MA, Kim S-C, Korman NJ et al. Studies of the relationship of the 230-kD and 180-kD bullous pemphigoid antigens. J Invest Dermatol 1990; 94: 793–797.

1053 Mueller S, Klaus-Kovtun V, Stanley JR. A 230-kD basic protein is the major bullous pemphigoid antigen. J Invest Dermatol 1989; 92: 33–38.

1054 Cook AL, Hanahoe THP, Mallett RB, Pye RJ. Recognition of two distinct major antigens by bullous pemphigoid sera. Br J Dermatol 1990; 122: 435–444.

1055 Hashimoto T, Ebihara T, Ishiko A et al. Comparative study of bullous pemphigoid antigens among Japanese, British, and U.S. patients indicates similar antigen profiles with the 170-kD antigen present both in the basement membrane and on the keratinocyte cell membrane. J Invest Dermatol 1993; 100: 385–389.

1056 Korman NJ. In situ-bound antibodies eluted from the skin of patients with bullous pemphigoid are preferentially directed against the 230-kD bullous pemphigoid antigen. J Invest Dermatol 1995; 105: 824–830.

1057 Klatte DH, Jones JCR. Purification of the 230-kD bullous pemphigoid antigen (BP230) from bovine tongue mucosa: structural analyses and assessment of BP230 tissue distribution using a new monoclonal antibody. J Invest Dermatol 1994; 102: 39–44.

1058 Miller JE, Rico MJ, Hall RP III. IgG antibodies from patients with bullous pemphigoid bind to fusion proteins encoded by BPAg1 cDNA. J Invest Dermatol 1993; 101: 779–782.

1059 Giudice GJ, Emery DJ, Diaz LA. Cloning and primary structural analysis of the bullous pemphigoid autoantigen BP180. J Invest Dermatol 1992; 99: 243–250.

1060 Hopkinson SB, Riddelle KS, Jones JCR. Cytoplasmic domain of the 180-kD bullous pemphigoid antigen, a hemidesmosomal component: molecular and cell biologic characterization. J Invest Dermatol 1992; 99: 264–270.

1061 Fairley JA, Heintz PW, Neuburg M et al. Expression pattern of the bullous pemphigoid-180 antigen in normal and neoplastic epithelia. Br J Dermatol 1995; 133: 385–391.

1062 Masunaga T, Shimizu H, Yee C et al. The extracellular domain of BPAG2 localizes to anchoring filaments and its carboxyl terminus extends to the lamina densa of normal human epidermal basement membrane. J Invest Dermatol 1997; 109: 200–206.

1063 Zillikens D, Mascaro JM, Rose PA et al. A highly sensitive enzyme-linked immunosorbent assay for the detection of circulating anti-BP180 autoantibodies in patients with bullous pemphigoid. J Invest Dermatol 1997; 109: 679–683.

1064 Zillikens D, Rose PA, Balding SD et al. Tight clustering of extracellular BP180 epitopes recognized by bullous pemphigoid autoantibodies. J Invest Dermatol 1997; 109: 573–579.

1065 Schmidt E, Obe K, Bröcker E-B, Zillikens D. Serum levels of autoantibodies to BP180 correlate with disease activity in patients with bullous pemphigoid. Arch Dermatol 2000; 136: 174–178.

1066 Egan CA, Taylor TB, Meyer LJ et al. Bullous pemphigoid sera that contain antibodies to BPAg2 also contain antibodies to LABD97 that recognize epitopes distal to the NC16A domain. J Invest Dermatol 1999; 112: 148–152.

1067 Jiao D, Bystryn J-C. Relation between antibodies to BP180 and gender in bullous pemphigoid. J Am Acad Dermatol 1999; 41: 269–270.

1068 Mainguy G, Ernø H, Montesinos ML et al. Regulation of epidermal bullous pemphigoid antigen 1 (BPAG1) synthesis by homeoprotein transcription factors. J Invest Dermatol 1999; 113: 643–650.

1069 Sato M, Shimizu H, Ishiko A et al. Precise ultrastructural localization of in vivo deposited IgG antibodies in fresh perilesional skin of patients with bullous pemphigoid. Br J Dermatol 1998; 138: 965–971.

1070 Skaria M, Jaunin F, Hunziker T et al. IgG autoantibodies from bullous pemphigoid patients recognize multiple antigenic reactive sites located predominantly within the B and C subdomains of the COOH-terminus of BP230. J Invest Dermatol 2000; 114: 998–1004.

1071 Gaucherand M, Nicolas J-F, Paranhos Baccala G et al. Major antigenic epitopes of bullous pemphigoid 230 kDa antigen map within the C-terminal end of the protein. Evidence using a 55 kDa recombinant protein. Br J Dermatol 1995; 132: 190–196.

1072 Zhu X-J, Niimi Y, Bystryn J-C. Molecular identification of major and minor bullous pemphigoid antigens. J Am Acad Dermatol 1990; 23: 876–880.

1073 Ghohestani R, Kanitakis J, Nicolas JF et al. Comparative sensitivity of indirect immunofluorescence to immunoblot assay for the detection of circulating antibodies to bullous pemphigoid antigens 1 and 2. Br J Dermatol 1996; 135: 74–79.

1074 Venning VA, Whitehead PH, Leigh IM et al. The clinical expression of bullous pemphigoid is not determined by the specificity of the target antigen. Br J Dermatol 1991; 125: 561–565.

1075 Tanaka M, Hashimoto T, Dykes PJ, Nishikawa T. Clinical manifestations in 100 Japanese bullous pemphigoid cases in relation to autoantigen profiles. Clin Exp Dermatol 1996; 21: 23–27.

1076 Bernard P, Bedane C, Bonnetblanc J-M. Anti-BP180 autoantibodies as a marker of poor prognosis in bullous pemphigoid: a cohort analysis of 94 elderly patients. Br J Dermatol 1997; 136: 694–698.

1077 Matasim DF. Levels of antibodies to BP180 correlate with disease activity in bullous pemphigoid. Arch Dermatol 2000; 136: 253–254.

1078 Döpp R, Schmidt E, Chimanovitch I et al. IgG4 and IgE are the major immunoglobulins targeting the NC16A domain of BP180 in bullous pemphigoid: Serum levels of these immunoglobulins reflect disease activity. J Am Acad Dermatol 2000; 42: 577–583.

1079 Laffitte E, Skaria M, Jaunin F et al. Autoantibodies to the extracellular and intracellular domain of bullous pemphigoid 180, the putative key autoantigen in bullous pemphigoid, belong predominantly to the IgG1 and IgG4 subclasses. Br J Dermatol 2001; 144: 760–768.

1080 Kirtschig G, Wojnarowska F. IgA basement membrane zone autoantibodies in bullous pemphigoid detect epidermal antigens of 270–280kDa, 230kDa, and 180kDa molecular weight by immunoblotting. Clin Exp Dermatol 1999; 24: 302–307.

1081 Fujisawa H, Ishii Y, Tateishi T et al. Pemphigoid nodularis with IgA autoantibodies against the intracellular domain of desmoglein 1. Br J Dermatol 2000; 142: 143–147.

1082 Nakatani C, Muramatsu T, Shirai T. Immunoreactivity of bullous pemphigoid (BP) autoantibodies against the NC16A and C-terminal domains of the 180 kDa BP antigen (BP180): immunoblot analysis and enzyme-linked immunosorbent assay using BP180 recombinant proteins. Br J Dermatol 1998; 139: 365–370.

1083 Ostlere LS, Stevens H, Black MM et al. Bullous pemphigoid in infancy – a case report including new immunoblotting observations. Clin Exp Dermatol 1993; 18: 483–485.

1084 Trüeb RM, Didierjean L, Fellas A et al. Childhood bullous pemphigoid: Report of a case with characterization of the targeted antigens. J Am Acad Dermatol 1999; 40: 338–344.

1085 Mori O, Hachisuka H, Kusuhara M et al. Bullous pemphigoid in a 19-year-old woman. A case with unusual target antigens. Br J Dermatol 1994; 130: 241–245.

1086 Gao S-Q, Bystryn J-C. A novel bullous pemphigoid antigen (BP125) located in the deeper layers of the basement membrane zone. Arch Dermatol 1994; 130: 873–878.

1087 Laffitte E, Favre B, Fontao L et al. Plectin, an unusual target antigen in bullous pemphigoid. Br J Dermatol 2001; 144: 136–138.

1088 Hashimoto T, Watanabe K, Ishiko A et al. A case of bullous pemphigoid with antidesmoplakin autoantibodies. Br J Dermatol 1994; 131: 694–699.

1089 Kanitakis J, Zambruno G, Vassileva S et al. Alpha-6 (CD 49f) integrin expression in genetic and acquired bullous skin diseases. J Cutan Pathol 1992; 19: 376–384.

1090 Sams WM Jr, Gammon WR. Mechanism of lesion production in pemphigus and pemphigoid. J Am Acad Dermatol 1982; 6: 431–449.

1091 Shrikhande M, Hunziker T, Braathen LR et al. Increased coexpression of eotaxin and interleukin 5 in bullous pemphigoid. Acta Derm Venereol 2000; 80: 277–280.

1092 Wakugawa M, Nakamura K, Hino H et al. Elevated levels of eotaxin and interleukin-5 in blister fluid of bullous pemphigoid: correlation with tissue eosinophilia. Br J Dermatol 2000; 143: 112–116.

1093 Takamori K, Yoshiike T, Morioka S, Ogawa H. The role of proteases in the pathogenesis of bullous dermatoses. Int J Dermatol 1988; 27: 533–539.

1094 Kitajima Y, Nojiri M, Yamada T et al. Internalization of the 180 kDa bullous pemphigoid antigen as immune complexes in basal keratinocytes: an important early event in blister formation in bullous pemphigoid. Br J Dermatol 1998; 138: 71–76.

1095 Perriard J, Jaunin F, Favre B et al. IgG autoantibodies from bullous pemphigoid (BP) patients bind antigenic sites on both the extracellular and the intracellular domains of the BP antigen 180. J Invest Dermatol 1999; 112: 141–147.

1096 Muramatsu T, Fukumoto T, Nakatani C et al. Bullous pemphigoid with circulating autoantibodies against the basal and apical-lateral surfaces of the basal keratinocytes. Br J Dermatol 1998; 139: 534–536.

1097 Brown LF, Harrist TJ, Yeo K-T et al. Increased expression of vascular permeability factor (vascular endothelial growth factor) in bullous pemphigoid, dermatitis herpetiformis, and erythema multiforme. J Invest Dermatol 1995; 104: 744–749.

1098 Schmidt E, Reimer S, Kruse N et al. Autoantibodies to BP180 associated with bullous pemphigoid release interleukin-6 and interleukin-8 from cultured human keratinocytes. J Invest Dermatol 2000; 115: 842–848.

1099 Lin M-S, Fu C-L, Giudice GJ et al. Epitopes targeted by bullous pemphigoid T lymphocytes and autoantibodies map to the same sites on the bullous pemphigoid 180 ectodomain. J Invest Dermatol 2000; 115: 955–961.

1100 Sun C-C, Wu J, Wong T-T et al. High levels of interleukin-8, soluble CD4 and soluble CD8 in bullous pemphigoid blister fluid. The relationship between local cytokine production and lesional T-cell activities. Br J Dermatol 2000; 143: 1235–1240.

1101 Rico MJ, Benning C, Weingart ES et al. Characterization of skin cytokines in bullous pemphigoid and pemphigus vulgaris. Br J Dermatol 1999; 140: 1079–1086.

1102 Alcalay J, David M, Ingber A et al. Bullous pemphigoid mimicking bullous erythema multiforme: an untoward side effect of penicillins. J Am Acad Dermatol 1988; 18: 345–349.

1103 Hodak E, Ben-Shetrit A, Ingber A, Sandbank M. Bullous pemphigoid – an adverse effect of ampicillin. Clin Exp Dermatol 1990; 15: 50–52.

1104 Miralles J, Barnadas MA, Baselga E et al. Bullous pemphigoid-like lesions induced by amoxicillin. Int J Dermatol 1997; 36: 42–47.

1105 Laing VB, Sherertz EF, Flowers FP. Pemphigoid-like eruption related to ibuprofen. J Am Acad Dermatol 1988; 19: 91–94.

1106 Kashihara M, Danno K, Miyachi Y et al. Bullous pemphigoid-like lesions induced by phenacetin. Arch Dermatol 1984; 120: 1196–1199.

1107 Smith EP, Taylor TB, Meyer LJ, Zone JJ. Antigen identification in drug-induced bullous pemphigoid. J Am Acad Dermatol 1993; 29: 879–882.

1108 Spivak D, Orion E, Brenner S. Bullous pemphigoid possibly triggered and exacerbated by ophthalmic preparations. Int J Dermatol 2000; 39: 554–555.

1109 Baykal C, Okan G, Sarica R. Childhood bullous pemphigoid developed after the first vaccination. J Am Acad Dermatol 2001; 44: 348–350.

1110 Fournier B, Descamps V, Bouscarat F et al. Bullous pemphigoid induced by vaccination. Br J Dermatol 1996; 135: 153–154.

1111 Lear JT, Tan BB, English JSC. Bullous pemphigoid following influenza vaccination. Clin Exp Dermatol 1996; 21: 392.

1112 Downs AMR, Lear JT, Bower CPR, Kennedy CTC. Does influenza vaccination induce bullous pemphigoid? A report of four cases. Br J Dermatol 1998; 138: 363.

1113 Amos B, Deng J-S, Flynn K, Suarez S. Bullous pemphigoid in infancy: case report and literature review. Pediatr Dermatol 1998; 15: 108–111.

1114 Shachar E, Bialy-Golan A, Srebrnik A, Brenner S. "Two-step" drug-induced bullous pemphigoid. Int J Dermatol 1998; 37: 938–939.

1115 Ameen M, Harman KE, Black MM. Pemphigoid nodularis associated with nifedipine. Br J Dermatol 2000; 142: 575–577.

1116 Shimizu H, Ueda M, Takai T et al. A case of serratiopeptidase-induced subepicdermal bullous dermatosis. Br J Dermatol 1999; 141: 1139–1140.

1117 Czechowicz RT, Reid CM, Warren LJ et al. Bullous pemphigoid induced by cephalexin. Australas J Dermatol 2001; 42: 132–135.

1118 Boulinguez S, Bernard P, Bedane C et al. Bullous pemphigoid induced by bumetanide. Br J Dermatol 1998; 138: 548–549.

1119 Rault S, Grosieux-Dauger C, Verraes S et al. Bullous pemphigoid induced by fluoxetine. Br J Dermatol 1999; 141: 755–756.

1120 Millard TP, Smith HR, Black MM, Barker JNWN. Bullous pemphigoid developing during systemic therapy with chloroquine. Clin Exp Dermatol 1999; 24: 263–265.

1121 Mehravaran M, Gyulai R, Husz S, Dobozy A. Drug-induced erythema multiforme-like bullous pemphigoid. Acta Derm Venereol 1999; 79: 233.

1122 Kimyai-Asadi A, Usman A, Nousari HC. Ciprofloxacin-induced bullous pemphigoid. J Am Acad Dermatol 2000; 42: 847.

1123 Castel T, Gratacos R, Castro J et al. Bullous pemphigoid induced by frusemide. Clin Exp Dermatol 1981; 6: 635–638.

1124 Parslew R, Verbov JL. Bullous pemphigoid at sites of trauma. Br J Dermatol 1997; 137: 825–826.

1125 Bastuji-Garin S, Joly P, Picard-Dahan C et al. Drugs associated with bullous pemphigoid. Arch Dermatol 1996; 132: 272–276.

1126 Weller R, White MI. Bullous pemphigoid and penicillamine. Clin Exp Dermatol 1996; 21: 121–122.

1127 Macfarlane AW, Verbov JL. Trauma-induced bullous pemphigoid. Clin Exp Dermatol 1989; 14: 245–249.

1128 Vassileva S, Mateev G, Balabanova M, Tsankov N. Burn-induced bullous pemphigoid. J Am Acad Dermatol 1994; 30: 1027–1028.

1129 Wagner GH, Ive FA, Paraskevopoulos S. Bullous pemphigoid and burns: the unveiling of the attachment plaque? Australas J Dermatol 1995; 36: 17–20.

1130 Balato N, Ayala F, Patruno C et al. Bullous pemphigoid induced by a thermal burn. Int J Dermatol 1994; 33: 55–56.

1131 Sacher C, König C, Scharffetter-Kochanek K et al. Bullous pemphigoid in a patient treated with UVA-1 phototherapy for disseminated morphea. Dermatology 2001; 202: 54–57.

1132 Duschet P, Schwarz T, Gschnait F. Bullous pemphigoid after radiation therapy. J Am Acad Dermatol 1988; 18: 441–444.

1133 Sheerin N, Bourke JF, Holder J et al. Bullous pemphigoid following radiotherapy. Clin Exp Dermatol 1995; 20: 80–82.

1134 Knoell KA, Patterson JW, Gampper TJ, Hendrix JD Jr. Localized bullous pemphigoid following radiotherapy for breast carcinoma. Arch Dermatol 1998; 134: 514–515.

1135 Ahmed AR. Diagnosis of bullous disease and studies in the pathogenesis of blister formation using immunopathological techniques. J Cutan Pathol 1984; 11: 237–248.

1136 Beer TW, Langtry JAA, Phillips WG, Wojnarowska F. Flame figures in bullous pemphigoid. Dermatology 1994; 188: 310–312.

1137 Nishioka K, Hashimoto K, Katayama I et al. Eosinophilic spongiosis in bullous pemphigoid. Arch Dermatol 1984; 120: 1166–1168.

1138 Saxe N, Kahn LB. Subepidermal bullous disease. A correlated clinico-pathologic study of 51 cases. J Cutan Pathol 1976; 3: 88–94.

1139 Redondo P, España A, Idoate M et al. Unusual bullous disorder with features of toxic epidermal necrolysis, bullous pemphigoid and cicatricial pemphigoid. Clin Exp Dermatol 1995; 20: 65–69.

1140 Barnadas MA, Pujol RM, Curell R et al. Generalized pruritic eruption with suprabasal acantholysis preceeding the development of bullous pemphigoid. J Cutan Pathol 2000; 27: 96–98.

1141 Ahmed AR, Maize JC, Provost TT. Bullous pemphigoid. Clinical and immunological follow-up after successful therapy. Arch Dermatol 1977; 113: 1043–1046.

1142 Weigand DA, Clements MK. Direct immunofluorescence in bullous pemphigoid: effects of extent and location of lesions. J Am Acad Dermatol 1989; 20: 437–440.

1143 Chaidemenos GC, Maltezos E, Chrysomallis F et al. Value of routine diagnostic criteria of bullous pemphigoid. Int J Dermatol 1998; 37: 206–210.

1144 Peters MS, Rogers RS III. Clinical correlations of linear IgA deposition at the cutaneous basement membrane zone. J Am Acad Dermatol 1989; 20: 761–770.

1145 Barnadas MA, González MJ, Planagumà M et al. Clinical, histopathologic, and therapeutic aspects of subepidermal autoimmune bullous diseases with IgG on the floor of salt-split skin. Int J Dermatol 2001; 40: 268–272.

1146 Wakelin SH, Allen J, Wojnarowska F. Childhood bullous pemphigoid – report of a case with dermal fluorescence on salt-split skin. Br J Dermatol 1995; 133: 615–618.

1147 Pang BK, Lee YS, Ratnam KV. Floor-pattern salt-split skin cannot distinguish bullous pemphigoid from epidermolysis bullosa acquisita. Arch Dermatol 1993; 129: 744–746.

1148 Barnadas MªA, Gelpí C, Curell R et al. Repeat direct immunofluorescence (DIF) test, using 1 M NaCl treated skin, in the subepidermal autoimmune bullous diseases that contain IgG at the dermal epidermal junction. J Cutan Pathol 1999; 26: 37–41.

1149 Onodera Y, Shimizu H, Hashimoto T et al. Difference in binding sites of autoantibodies against 230- and 170-kD bullous pemphigoid antigens on salt-split skin. J Invest Dermatol 1994; 102: 686–690.

1150 Yancey KB, Hintner H. Advances in the diagnosis of subepidermal bullous diseases. Arch Dermatol 1996; 132: 220–222.

1151 D'Ambra-Cabry K, Deng DH, Flynn KL et al. Antigen retrieval in immunofluorescent testing of bullous pemphigoid. Am J Dermatopathol 1995; 17: 560–563.

1152 Hodge L, Black MM, Ramnarain N, Bhogal B. Indirect complement immunofluorescence in the immunopathological assessment of bullous pemphigoid, cicatricial pemphigoid, and herpes gestationis. Clin Exp Dermatol 1978; 3: 61–67.

1153 Ghohestani R, Kanitakis J, Nicolas JF et al. Comparative sensitivity of indirect immunofluorescence to immunoblot assay for the detection of circulating antibodies to bullous pemphigoid antigens 1 and 2. Br J Dermatol 1996; 135: 74–79.

1154 Delmonte S, Cozzani E, Drosera M et al. Rat bladder epithelium: a sensitive substrate for indirect immunofluorescence of bullous pemphigoid. Acta Derm Venereol 2000; 80: 175–178.

1155 Hachisuka H, Kurose K, Karashima T et al. Serum from normal elderly individuals contains anti-basement membrane zone antibodies. Arch Dermatol 1996; 132: 1201–1205.

1156 Gomes MA, Dambuyant C, Thivolet J, Bussy R. Bullous pemphigoid: a correlative study of autoantibodies, circulating immune complexes and dermo-epidermal deposits. Br J Dermatol 1982; 107: 43–52.

1157 Machado P, Michalaki H, Roche P et al. Serological diagnosis of bullous pemphigoid (BP): comparison of the sensitivity of indirect immunofluorescence on salt-split skin to immunoblotting. Br J Dermatol 1992; 126: 236–241.

1153 Lazarova Z, Yancey KB. Reactivity of autoantibodies from patients with defined subepidermal bullous diseases against 1 mol/L salt-split skin. J Am Acad Dermatol 1996; 35: 398–403.

1159 Allen J, Shears E, Powell J, Wojnarowska F. Assessment of skin basement membrane zone antibodies in the urine of patients with acquired subepidermal immunobullous diseases. Br J Dermatol 2001; 144: 540–545.

1160 Giannotti B, Fabbri P, Panconesi E. Ultrastructural findings in bullous pemphigoid. J Cutan Pathol 1975; 2: 103–108.

1161 Schaumburg-Lever G, Orfanos CE, Lever WF. Electron microscopic study of bullous pemphigoid. Arch Dermatol 1972; 106: 662–667.

1162 Joly P, Gilbert D, Thomine E et al. Relationship between the in vivo localization and the immunoblotting pattern of anti-basement membrane zone antibodies in patients with bullous pemphigoid. Arch Dermatol 1997; 133: 719–724.

1163 Holmes RC, Black MM. The specific dermatoses of pregnancy. J Am Acad Dermatol 1983; 8: 405–412.

1164 Winton GB, Lewis CW. Dermatoses of pregnancy. J Am Acad Dermatol 1982; 6: 977–998.

1165 Shornick JK. Herpes gestationis. J Am Acad Dermatol 1987; 17: 539–556.

1166 Sasseville D, Wilkinson RD, Schnader JY. Dermatoses of pregnancy. Int J Dermatol 1981; 20: 223–241.

1167 Mayou SE, Black MM, Holmes RC. Pemphigoid 'herpes' gestationis. Semin Dermatol 1988; 7: 104–110.

1168 Shornick JK. Herpes gestationis. Dermatol Clin 1993; 11: 527–533.

1169 Lowe PM, Fryer J, Shumack S. Pemphigoid gestationis occurring in a patient with HELLP syndrome. Australas J Dermatol 1996; 37: 89–92.

1170 Jenkins RE, Hern S, Black MM. Clinical features and management of 87 patients with pemphigoid gestationis. Clin Exp Dermatol 1999; 24: 255–259.

1171 Tindall JG, Rea TH, Shulman I, Quismorio FP. Herpes gestationis in association with a hydatidiform mole. Immunopathologic studies. Arch Dermatol 1981; 117: 510–512.

1172 Kelly SE, Black MM. Pemphigoid gestationis: placental interactions. Semin Dermatol 1989; 8: 12–17.

1173 Jurecka W, Holmes RC, Black MM et al. An immunoelectron microscopy study of the relationship between herpes gestationis and polymorphic eruption of pregnancy. Br J Dermatol 1983; 108: 147–151.

1174 Fine J-D, Omura EF. Herpes gestationis. Persistent disease activity 11 years post partum. Arch Dermatol 1985; 121: 924–926.

1175 Castle SP, Mather-Mondrey M, Bennion S et al. Chronic herpes gestationis and antiphospholipid antibody syndrome successfully treated with cyclophosphamide. J Am Acad Dermatol 1996; 34: 333–336.

1176 Hern S, Harman K, Bhogal BS, Black MM. A severe persistent case of pemphigoid gestationis treated with intravenous immunoglobulins and cyclosporin. Clin Exp Dermatol 1998; 23: 185–188.

1177 Hertz KC, Katz SI, Maize J, Ackerman AB. Herpes gestationis. A clinicopathologic study. Arch Dermatol 1976; 112: 1543–1548.

1178 Jenkins RE, Vaughan Jones SA, Black MM. Conversion of pemphigoid gestationis to bullous pemphigoid – two refractory cases highlighting this association. Br J Dermatol 1996; 135: 595–598.

1179 Triffet MK, Gibson LE, Leiferman KM. Severe subepidermal blistering disorder with features of bullous pemphigoid and herpes gestationis. J Am Acad Dermatol 1999; 40: 797–801.

1180 Shornick JK, Bangert JL, Freeman RG, Gilliam JN. Herpes gestationis: clinical and histologic features of twenty-eight cases. J Am Acad Dermatol 1983; 8: 214–224.

1181 Shornick JK, Black MM. Fetal risks in herpes gestationis. J Am Acad Dermatol 1992; 26: 63–68.

1182 Powell J, Wojnarowska F, James M, Allott H. Pemphigoid gestationis with intra-uterine death associated with foetal cerebral haemorrhage in the mid-trimester. Clin Exp Dermatol 2000; 25: 452–453.

1183 Holmes RC, Black MM. The fetal prognosis in pemphigoid gestationis (herpes gestationis). Br J Dermatol 1984; 110: 67–72.

1184 Chen SH, Chopra K, Evans TY et al. Herpes gestationis in a mother and child. J Am Acad Dermatol 1999; 40: 847–849.

1185 Holmes RC, Black MM. Herpes gestationis. A possible association with autoimmune thyrotoxicosis (Graves' disease). J Am Acad Dermatol 1980; 3: 474–477

1186 Shornick JK, Black MM. Secondary autoimmune diseases in herpes gestationis (pemphigoid gestationis). J Am Acad Dermatol 1992; 26: 563–566.

1187 Holmes RC, Black MM, Jurecka W et al. Clues to the aetiology and pathogenesis of herpes gestationis. Br J Dermatol 1983; 109: 131–139.

1139 Holmes RC, Black MM, Dann J et al. A comparative study of toxic erythema of pregnancy and herpes gestationis. Br J Dermatol 1982; 106: 499–510.

1139 Shornick JK, Jenkins RE, Artlett CM et al. Class II MHC typing in pemphigoid gestationis. Clin Exp Dermatol 1995; 20: 123–126.

1190 Kelly SE, Black MM, Fleming S. Hypothesis. Pemphigoid gestationis: a unique mechanism of initiation of an autoimmune response by MHC class II molecules? J Pathol 1989; 158: 81–82.

1191 Kelly SE, Black MM, Fleming S. Antigen-presenting cells in the skin and placenta in pemphigoid gestationis. Br J Dermatol 1990; 122: 593–599.

1192 Kelly SE, Cerio R, Bhogal BS, Black MM. The distribution of IgG subclasses in pemphigoid gestationis: PG factor is an IgG1 autoantibody. J Invest Dermatol 1989; 92: 695–698.

1193 Kelly SE, Bhogal BS, Wojnarowska F, Black MM. Expression of a pemphigoid gestationis-related antigen by human placenta. Br J Dermatol 1988; 118: 605–611.

1194 Ortonne J-P, Hsi B-L, Verrando P et al. Herpes gestationis factor reacts with the amniotic epithelial basement membrane. Br J Dermatol 1987; 117: 147–154.

1195 Chimanovitch I, Schmidt E, Messer G et al. IgG$_1$ and IgG$_3$ are the major immunoglobulin subclasses targeting epitopes within the NC16A domain of BP180 in pemphigoid gestationis. J Invest Dermatol 1999; 113: 140–141.

1196 Haase C, Büdinger L, Borradori L et al. Detection of IgG autoantibodies in the sera of patients with bullous and gestational pemphigoid: ELISA studies utilizing a baculovirus-encoded form of bullous pemphigoid antigen 2. J Invest Dermatol 1998; 110: 282–286.

1197 Karvonen J, Ilonen J, Reunala T, Tiilikainen A. Immunity in herpes gestationis: inhibition of mixed lymphocyte culture by patients' sera. Br J Dermatol 1984; 111: 183–189.

1198 Eberst E, Tongio MM, Eberst B et al. Herpes gestationis and anti-HLA immunization. Br J Dermatol 1981; 104: 543–559.

1199 Shornick JK, Jenkins RE, Briggs DC et al. Anti-HLA antibodies in pemphigoid gestationis (herpes gestationis). Br J Dermatol 1993; 129: 257–259.

1200 Scheman AJ, Hordinsky MD, Groth DW et al. Evidence for eosinophil degranulation in the pathogenesis of herpes gestationis. Arch Dermatol 1989; 125: 1079–1083.

1201 Schaumburg-Lever G, Saffold OE, Orfanos CE, Lever WF. Herpes gestationis. Histology and ultrastructure. Arch Dermatol 1973; 107: 888–892.

1202 Harrington CI, Bleehen SS. Herpes gestationis: immunopathological and ultrastructural studies. Br J Dermatol 1979; 100: 389–399.

1203 Shornick JK, Artlett CM, Jenkins RE et al. Complement polymorphism in herpes gestationis: association with C4 null allele. J Am Acad Dermatol 1993; 29: 545–549.

1204 Cutler TP. Herpes gestationis. Clin Exp Dermatol 1982; 7: 201–207.

1205 Holubar K, Konrad K, Stingl G. Detection by immunoelectron microscopy of immunoglobulin G deposits in skin of immunofluorescence negative herpes gestationis. Br J Dermatol 1977; 96: 569–571.

1206 Vaughan Jones SA, Bhogal BS, Black MM et al. A typical case of pemphigoid gestationis with a unique pattern of intercellular immunofluorescence. Br J Dermatol 1997; 136: 245–248.

1207 Borrego L, Peterson EA, Diez LI et al. Polymorphic eruption of pregnancy and herpes gestationis: comparison of granulated cell proteins in tissue and serum. Clin Exp Dermatol 1999; 24: 213–225.

1208 Quimby SR, Xenias SJ, Perry HO. Herpes gestationis. Mayo Clin Proc 1982; 57: 520–526.

1209 Carruthers JA, Black MM, Ramnarain N. Immunopathological studies in herpes gestationis. Br J Dermatol 1977; 96: 35–43.

1210 Katz SI, Hertz KC, Yaoita H. Herpes gestationis. Immunopathology and characterization of the HG factor. J Clin Invest 1976; 57: 1434–1441.

1211 Karpati S, Stolz W, Meurer M et al. Herpes gestationis: ultrastructural identification of the extracellular antigenic sites in diseased skin using immunogold techniques. Br J Dermatol 1991; 125: 317–324.

1212 Walker GB, Harrison PV. Seasonal bullous eruption due to mosquitoes. Clin Exp Dermatol 1985; 10: 127–132.

1213 Correia O, Delgado L, Barros MA. Bullous photodermatosis after lomefloxacin. Arch Dermatol 1994; 130: 808–809.

Subepidermal blisters with neutrophils

1214 Magro CM, Crowson AN. A distinctive vesiculopustular eruption associated with hepatobiliary disease. Int J Dermatol 1997; 36: 837–844.

1215 Thiers BH. Dermatitis herpetiformis. J Am Acad Dermatol 1981; 5: 114–117.

1216 Faure M. Dermatitis herpetiformis. Semin Dermatol 1988; 7: 123–129.

1217 Smith EP, Zone JJ. Dermatitis herpetiformis and linear IgA bullous dermatosis. Dermatol Clin 1993; 11: 511–526.

1218 Gawkrodger DJ, Vestey JP, O'Mahony S, Marks JM. Dermatitis herpetiformis and established coeliac disease. Br J Dermatol 1993; 129: 694–695.

1219 Hall RP III. Dermatitis herpetiformis. J Invest Dermatol 1992; 99: 873–881.

1220 Greenberg RD. Laryngeal involvement in dermatitis herpetiformis: case report. J Am Acad Dermatol 1989; 20: 690–691.

1221 Fraser NG, Kerr NW, Donald D. Oral lesions in dermatitis herpetiformis. Br J Dermatol 1973; 89: 439–450.

1222 Lähteenoja H, Irjala K, Viander M et al. Oral mucosa is frequently affected in patients with dermatitis herpetiformis. Arch Dermatol 1998; 134: 756–758.

1223 Ermacora E, Prampolini L, Tribbia G et al. Long-term follow-up of dermatitis herpetiformis in children. J Am Acad Dermatol 1986; 15: 24–30.

1224 Woollons A, Darley CR, Bhogal BS et al. Childhood dermatitis herpetiformis: an unusual presentation. Clin Exp Dermatol 1999; 24: 283–385.

1225 Leitao EA, Bernhard JD. Perimenstrual nonvesicular dermatitis herpetiformis. J Am Acad Dermatol 1990; 22: 331–334.

1226 Meyer LJ, Zone JJ. Familial incidence of dermatitis herpetiformis. J Am Acad Dermatol 1987; 17: 643–647.

1227 Sachs JA, Leonard J, Awad J et al. A comparative serological and molecular study of linear IgA disease and dermatitis herpetiformis. Br J Dermatol 1988; 118: 759–764.

1228 Hall RP, Clark RE, Ward FE. Dermatitis herpetiformis in two American blacks: HLA type and clinical characteristics. J Am Acad Dermatol 1990; 22: 436–439.

1229 Hervonen K, Karell K, Holopainen P et al. Concordance of dermatitis herpetiformis and celiac disease in monozygous twins. J Invest Dermatol 2000; 115: 990–993.

1230 Garioch JJ, Lewis HM, Sargent SA et al. 25 years' experience of a gluten-free diet in the treatment of dermatitis herpetiformis. Br J Dermatol 1994; 131: 541–545.

1231 Lewis HM, Renaula TL, Garioch JJ et al. Protective effect of gluten-free diet against development of lymphoma in dermatitis herpetiformis. Br J Dermatol 1996; 135: 363–367.

1232 Reunala T. Incidence of familial dermatitis herpetiformis. Br J Dermatol 1996; 134: 394–398.

1233 Kumar V, Hemedinger E, Chorzelski TP et al. Reticulin and endomysial antibodies in bullous diseases. Comparison of specificity and sensitivity. Arch Dermatol 1987; 123: 1179–1182.

1234 Ciclitira PJ, Ellis HJ, Venning VA et al. Circulating antibodies to gliadin subfractions in dermatitis herpetiformis and linear IgA dermatosis of adults and children. Clin Exp Dermatol 1986; 11: 502–509.

1235 Karpati S, Torok E, Kosnai I. IgA class antibody against human jejunum in sera of children with dermatitis herpetiformis. J Invest Dermatol 1986; 87: 703–706.

1236 Buckley DB, English J, Molloy W et al. Dermatitis herpetiformis: a review of 119 cases. Clin Exp Dermatol 1983; 8: 477–487.

1237 Weetman AP, Burrin JM, Mackay D et al. The prevalence of thyroid autoantibodies in dermatitis herpetiformis. Br J Dermatol 1988; 118: 377–383.

1238 Chorzelski TP, Jablonska S, Chadzynska M et al. IgA endomysium antibody in children with dermatitis herpetiformis treated with gluten-free diet. Pediatr Dermatol 1986; 3: 291–294.

1239 Beutner EH, Chorzelski TP, Kumar V et al. Sensitivity and specificity of IgA-class antiendomysial antibodies for dermatitis herpetiformis and findings relevant to their pathogenic significance. J Am Acad Dermatol 1986; 15: 464–473.

1240 Peters MS, McEvoy MT. IgA antiendomysial antibodies in dermatitis herpetiformis. J Am Acad Dermatol 1989; 21: 1225–1231.

1241 Kumar V, Zane H, Kaul N. Serologic markers of gluten-sensitive enteropathy in bullous diseases. Arch Dermatol 1992; 128: 1474–1478.

1242 Reunala T, Chorzelski TP, Viander M et al. IgA anti-endomysial antibodies in dermatitis herpetiformis: correlation with jejunal morphology, gluten-free diet and anti-gliadin antibodies. Br J Dermatol 1987; 117: 185–191.

1243 Rose C, Dieterich W, Bröcker E-B et al. Circulating autoantibodies to tissue transglutaminase differentiate patients with dermatitis herpetiformis from those with linear IgA disease. J Am Acad Dermatol 1999; 41: 957–961.

1244 Chorzelski TP, Rosinska D, Beutner EH et al. Aggressive gluten challenge of dermatitis herpetiformis cases converts them from seronegative to seropositive for IgA-class endomysial antibodies. J Am Acad Dermatol 1988; 18: 672–678.

1245 Caproni M, Cardinali C, Renzi D et al. Tissue transglutaminase antibody assessment in dermatitis herpetiformis. Br J Dermatol 2001; 144: 196–197.

1246 Accetta P, Kumar V, Beutner EH et al. Anti-endomysial antibodies. A serologic marker of dermatitis herpetiformis. Arch Dermatol 1986; 122: 459–462.

1247 Dieterich W, Laag E, Bruckner-Tuderman L et al. Antibodies to tissue transglutaminase as serologic markers in patients with dermatitis herpetiformis. J Invest Dermatol 1999; 113: 133–136.

1248 Callen JP. Internal disorders associated with bullous disease of the skin. J Am Acad Dermatol 1980; 3: 107–119.

1249 Lambert D, Collet E, Foucher JL et al. Dermatitis herpetiformis associated with ulcerative colitis. Clin Exp Dermatol 1991; 16: 458–459.

1250 Reunala T, Collin P. Diseases associated with dermatitis herpetiformis. Br J Dermatol 1997; 136: 315–318.

1251 Dodd HJ. Dermatitis herpetiformis and ulcerative colitis: report of a case. Clin Exp Dermatol 1984; 9: 99–101.

1252 Fligiel A, Aronson PJ, Kitajima J, Payne RR. Dermatitis herpetiformis – bullous lupus erythematosus overlap syndrome of 27 years pre- and postdating discoid lupus and septal panniculitis. J Cutan Pathol 1988; 15: 307 (abstract).

1253 Fraser NG, Rennie AGR, Donald D. Dermatitis herpetiformis and Sjögren's syndrome. Br J Dermatol 1979; 100: 213–215.

1254 Reunala T, Salmi J, Karvonen J. Dermatitis herpetiformis and celiac disease associated with Addison's disease. Arch Dermatol 1987; 123: 930–932.

1255 Walton C, Walton S. Primary biliary cirrhosis in a diabetic male with dermatitis herpetiformis. Clin Exp Dermatol 1987; 12: 46–47.

1256 Isaac M, McNeely MC. Dermatitis herpetiformis associated with lichen planopilaris. J Am Acad Dermatol 1995; 33: 1050–1051.

1257 Davies MG, Fifield R, Marks R. Atopic disease and dermatitis herpetiformis. Br J Dermatol 1979; 101: 429–434.

1258 Reunala T, Helin H, Pasternack A et al. Renal involvement and circulating immune complexes in dermatitis herpetiformis. J Am Acad Dermatol 1983; 9: 219–223.

1259 Jenkins D, Lynde CW, Stewart WD. Histiocytic lymphoma occurring in a patient with dermatitis herpetiformis. J Am Acad Dermatol 1983; 9: 252–256.

1260 Katz SI, Strober W. The pathogenesis of dermatitis herpetiformis. J Invest Dermatol 1978; 70: 63–75.

1261 Mobacken H, Andersson H, Dahlberg E et al. Spontaneous remission of dermatitis herpetiformis: dietary and gastrointestinal studies. Acta Derm Venereol 1986; 66: 245–250.

1262 Griffiths CEM, Leonard JN, Fry L. Dermatitis herpetiformis exacerbated by indomethacin. Br J Dermatol 1985; 112: 443–445.

1263 Tousignant J, Lafontaine N, Rochette L, Rozenfarb E. Dermatitis herpetiformis induced by nonsteroidal anti-inflammatory drugs. Int J Dermatol 1994; 33: 199–203.

1264 Snider RL, Maize JC. Can chemicals precipitate dermatitis herpetiformis? J Am Acad Dermatol 1993; 28: 111–112.

1265 Burnie J. A possible immunological mechanism for the pathogenesis of dermatitis herpetiformis with reference to coeliac disease. Clin Exp Dermatol 1980; 5: 451–463.

1266 Hall RP. The pathogenesis of dermatitis herpetiformis: recent advances. J Am Acad Dermatol 1987; 16: 1129–1144.

1267 Dahlback K, Sakai L. IgA immunoreactive deposits collocal with fibrillin immunoreactive fibers in dermatitis herpetiformis skin. Acta Derm Venereol 1990; 70: 194–198.

1268 Lightner VA, Sakai LY, Hall RP. IgA-binding structures in dermatitis herpetiformis skin are independent of elastic-microfibrillar bundles. J Invest Dermatol 1991; 96: 88–92.

1269 Kárpáti S, Meurer M, Stolz W et al. Dermatitis herpetiformis bodies. Ultrastructural study on the skin of patients using direct preembedding immunogold labelling. Arch Dermatol 1990; 126: 1469–1474.

1270 Olbricht SM, Flotte TJ, Collins AB et al. Dermatitis herpetiformis. Cutaneous deposition of polyclonal IgA1. Arch Dermatol 1986; 122: 418–421.

1271 Wojnarowska F, Delacroix D, Gengoux P. Cutaneous IgA subclasses in dermatitis herpetiformis and linear IgA disease. J Cutan Pathol 1988; 15: 272–275.

1272 Graeber M, Baker BS, Garioch JJ et al. The role of cytokines in the generation of skin lesions in dermatitis herpetiformis. Br J Dermatol 1993; 129: 530–532.

1273 Caproni M, Feliciani C, Fuligni A et al. Th2-like cytokine activity in dermatitis herpetiformis. Br J Dermatol 1998; 138: 242–247.

1274 Karttunen T, Autio-Harmainen H, Rasanen O et al. Immunohistochemical localization of epidermal basement membrane laminin and type IV collagen in bullous lesions of dermatitis herpetiformis. Br J Dermatol 1984; 111: 389–394.

1275 Garioch JJ, Baker BS, Leonard JN, Fry L. T lymphocytes in lesional skin of patients with dermatitis herpetiformis. Br J Dermatol 1994; 131: 822–826.

1276 Kell DL, Glusac EJ, Smoller BR. T lymphocytes bearing the γ/δ T-cell receptor in cutaneous lesions of dermatitis herpetiformis. J Cutan Pathol 1994; 21: 413–418.

1277 Amerio P, Verdolini R, Giangacomi M et al. Expression of eotaxin, interleukin 13 and tumour necrosis factor-α in dermatitis herpetiformis. Br J Dermatol 2000; 143: 974–978.

1278 Blenkinsopp WK, Fry L, Haffenden GP, Leonard JN. Histology of linear IgA disease, dermatitis herpetiformis, and bullous pemphigoid. Am J Dermatopathol 1983; 5: 547–554.

1279 Williams BT, Hampton MT, Mitchell DF, Metcalf JS. Intracorneal nuclear dust aggregates in dermatitis herpetiformis. A clue to diagnosis. Am J Dermatopathol 1995; 17: 48–52.

1280 Marsden RA, McKee PH, Bhogal B et al. A study of benign chronic bullous dermatosis of childhood and comparison with dermatitis herpetiformis and bullous pemphigoid occurring in childhood. Clin Exp Dermatol 1980; 5: 159–172.

1281 Smith SB, Harrist TJ, Murphy GF et al. Linear IgA bullous dermatosis v dermatitis herpetiformis. Quantitative measurements of dermoepidermal alterations. Arch Dermatol 1984; 120: 324–328.

1282 De Mento FJ, Grover RW. Acantholytic herpetiform dermatitis. Arch Dermatol 1973; 107: 883–887.

1283 De Jong MCJM, van der Meer JB, de Nijs JAM, van der Putte SCJ. Concomitant immunohistochemical characteristics of pemphigoid and dermatitis herpetiformis in a patient with atypical bullous dermatosis. Acta Derm Venereol 1983; 63: 476–482.

1284 Jawitz J, Kumar V, Nigra TP, Beutner EH. Vesicular pemphigoid vs dermatitis herpetiformis. J Am Acad Dermatol 1984; 10: 892–896.

1285 Setterfield J, Bhogal B, Black MM, McGibbon DH. Dermatitis herpetiformis and bullous pemphigoid: a developing association confirmed by immunoelectronmicroscopy. Br J Dermatol 1997; 136: 253–256.

1236 Ameen M, Bhogal BS, Black MM. Dermatitis herpetiformis evolving into bullous pemphigoid: a probable example of 'epitope spreading'. Clin Exp Dermatol 2000; 25: 398–400.

1287 Haffenden G, Wojnarowska F, Fry L. Comparison of immunoglobulin and complement deposition in multiple biopsies from the uninvolved skin in dermatitis herpetiformis. Br J Dermatol 1979; 101: 39–45.

1288 Beutner EH, Chorzelski TP, Jablonska S. Immunofluorescence tests. Clinical significance of sera and skin in bullous diseases. Int J Dermatol 1985; 24: 405–421.

1289 Zone JJ, Meyer LJ, Petersen MJ. Deposition of granular IgA relative to clinical lesions in dermatitis herpetiformis. Arch Dermatol 1996; 132: 912–918.

1290 Kawana S, Segawa A. Confocal laser scanning microscopic and immunoelectron microscopic studies of the anatomical distribution of fibrillar IgA deposits in dermatitis herpetiformis. Arch Dermatol 1993; 129: 456–459.

1291 Karlsson IJ, Dahl MGC, Marks JM. Absence of cutaneous IgA in coeliac disease without dermatitis herpetiformis. Br J Dermatol 1978; 99: 621–625.

1292 Fry L, Walkden V, Wojnarowska F et al. A comparison of IgA positive and IgA negative dapsone responsive dermatoses. Br J Dermatol 1980; 102: 371–382.

1293 Seah PP, Fry L. Immunoglobulins in the skin in dermatitis herpetiformis and their relevance in diagnosis. Br J Dermatol 1975; 92: 157–166.

1294 Beutner EH, Baughman RD, Austin BM et al. A case of dermatitis herpetiformis with IgA endomysial antibodies but negative direct immunofluorescent findings. J Am Acad Dermatol 2000; 43: 329–332.

1295 Zaenglein AL, Hafer L, Helm KF. Diagnosis of dermatitis herpetiformis by an avidin-biotin-peroxidase method. Arch Dermatol 1995; 131: 571–573.

1296 Ljunghall K, Tjernlund U. Dermatitis herpetiformis: effect of gluten-restricted and gluten free diet on dapsone requirement and on IgA and C3 deposits in uninvolved skin. Acta Derm Venereol 1983; 63: 129–136.

1297 Smith JB, Taylor TB, Zone JJ. The site of blister formation in dermatitis herpetiformis is within the lamina lucida. J Am Acad Dermatol 1992; 27: 209–213.

1298 Pehamberger H, Konrad K, Holubar K. Juvenile dermatitis herpetiformis: an immunoelectron microscopic study. Br J Dermatol 1979; 101: 271–277.

1299 Wojnarowska F, Marsden RA, Bhogal B, Black MM. Chronic bullous disease of childhood, childhood cicatricial pemphigoid, and linear IgA disease of adults. A comparative study demonstrating clinical and immunopathologic overlap. J Am Acad Dermatol 1988; 19: 792–805.

1300 Wojnarowska F. Chronic bullous disease of childhood. Semin Dermatol 1988; 7: 58–65.

1301 Egan CA, Zone JJ. Linear IgA bullous dermatosis. Int J Dermatol 1999; 38: 818–827.

1302 Ajithkumar K, Kurian S, Jacob M, Pulimood S. Linear IgA bullous dermatosis in South India. Int J Dermatol 1997; 36: 191–193.

1303 Wojnarowska F. What's new in linear IgA disease? J Eur Acad Dermatol Venereol 2000; 14: 441–443.

1304 Leigh G, Marsden RA, Wojnarowska F. Linear IgA dermatosis with severe arthralgia. Br J Dermatol 1988; 119: 789–792.

1305 Bean SF, Jordon RE. Chronic nonhereditary blistering disease in children. Arch Dermatol 1974; 110: 941–944.

1306 Faber WR, Van Joost T. Juvenile pemphigoid. Br J Dermatol 1973; 89: 519–522.

1307 Marsden RA, Skeete MVH, Black MM. The chronic acquired bullous diseases of childhood. Clin Exp Dermatol 1979; 4: 227–240.

1308 Rogers M, Bartlett B, Walder B, Cains J. Chronic bullous disease of childhood – aspects of management. Australas J Dermatol 1982; 23: 62–69.

1309 Hruza LL, Mallory SB, Fitzgibbons J, Mallory GB Jr. Linear IgA bullous dermatosis in a neonate. Pediatr Dermatol 1993; 10: 171–176.

1310 Baldari U, Raccagni AA, Celli B, Righini MG. Chronic bullous disease of childhood following Epstein–Barr virus seroconversion: a case report. Clin Exp Dermatol 1996; 21: 123–126.

1311 Ratnam KV, Lee CT, Tan T. Chronic bullous dermatosis of childhood in Singapore. Int J Dermatol 1986; 25: 34–37.

1312 Surbrugg SK, Weston WL. The course of chronic bullous disease of childhood. Pediatr Dermatol 1985; 2: 213–215.

1313 Burge S, Wojnarowska F, Marsden A. Chronic bullous dermatosis of childhood persisting into adulthood. Pediatr Dermatol 1988; 5: 246–249.

1314 Wojnarowska F, Marsden RA, Bhogal B, Black MM. Childhood cicatricial pemphigoid with linear IgA deposits. Clin Exp Dermatol 1984; 9: 407–415.

1315 Leonard JN, Haffenden GP, Ring NP et al. Linear IgA disease in adults. Br J Dermatol 1982; 107: 301–316.

1316 Leonard JN, Griffiths CEM, Powles AV et al. Experience with a gluten free diet in the treatment of linear IgA disease. Acta Derm Venereol 1987; 67: 145–148.

1317 Wilson BD, Beutner EH, Kumar V et al. Linear IgA bullous dermatosis. An immunologically defined disease. Int J Dermatol 1985; 24: 569–574.

1318 Argenyi ZB, Bergfeld WF, Valenzuela R et al. Linear IgA bullous dermatosis mimicking erythema multiforme in adult. Int J Dermatol 1987; 26: 513–517.

1319 Mobacken H, Kastrup W, Ljunghall K et al. Linear IgA dermatosis: a study of ten adult patients. Acta Derm Venereol 1983; 63: 123–128.

1320 Tanita Y, Masu S, Kato T, Tagami H. Linear IgA bullous dermatosis clinically simulating pemphigus vulgaris. Arch Dermatol 1986; 122: 246–248.

1321 Ratnam KV. IgA dermatosis in an adult Chinese population. A 10-year study of linear IgA and dermatitis herpetiformis in Singapore. Int J Dermatol 1988; 27: 21–24.

1322 Dippel E, Orfanos CE, Zouboulis ChC. Linear IgA dermatosis presenting with erythema annulare centrifugum lesions: report of three cases in adults. J Eur Acad Dermatol Venereol 2001; 15: 167–170.

1323 Ansai S-I, Mitsuhashi Y. Linear IgA bullous dermatosis limited to the seborrhoeic regions. Br J Dermatol 1996; 135: 1006–1007.

1324 Porter WM, Hardman CM, Leonard JN, Fry L. Sarcoidosis in a patient with linear IgA disease. Clin Exp Dermatol 1999; 24: 67–70.

1325 Takagi Y, Sawada S, Yamauchi M et al. Coexistence of psoriasis and linear IgA bullous dermatosis. Br J Dermatol 2000; 142: 513–516.

1326 Handley J, Shields M, Dodge J et al. Chronic bullous disease of childhood and ulcerative colitis. Pediatr Dermatol 1993; 10: 256–258.

1327 Paige DG, Leonard JN, Wojnarowska F, Fry L. Linear IgA disease and ulcerative colitis. Br J Dermatol 1997; 136: 779–782.

1328 Swensson O, Stüber E, Nickel T et al. Linear IgA disease associated with lymphocytic colitis. Br J Dermatol 1999; 140: 317–321.

1329 Hayakawa K, Shiohara T, Yagita A, Nagashima M. Linear IgA bullous dermatosis associated with rheumatoid arthritis. J Am Acad Dermatol 1992; 26: 110–113.

1330 Barnadas MA, Moreno A, Brunet S et al. Linear IgA bullous dermatosis associated with Hodgkin's disease. J Am Acad Dermatol 1988; 19: 1122–1124.

1331 Godfrey K, Wojnarowska F, Leonard J. Linear IgA disease of adults: association with lymphoproliferative malignancy and possible role of other triggering factors. Br J Dermatol 1990; 123: 447–452.

1332 Russell Jones R, Goolamali SK. IgA bullous pemphigoid: a distinct blistering disorder. Case report and review of the literature. Br J Dermatol 1980; 102: 719–725.

1333 McEvoy MT, Connolly SM. Linear IgA dermatosis: association with malignancy. J Am Acad Dermatol 1990; 22: 59–63.

1334 Lacour J-P, Vitetta A, Ortonne J-P. Linear IgA dermatosis and thyroid cancer. J Am Acad Dermatol 1992; 26: 257–259.

1335 Ródenas JM, Herranz MT, Tercedor J, Concha A. Linear IgA disease in a patient with bladder carcinoma. Br J Dermatol 1997; 136: 257–259.

1336 van der Waal RIF, van de Scheur MR, Pas HH et al. Linear IgA bullous dermatosis in a patient with renal cell carcinoma. Br J Dermatol 2001; 144: 870–873.

1337 Chappe SG, Esterly NB, Furey NL et al. Subepidermal bullous disease and glomerulonephritis in a child. J Am Acad Dermatol 1981; 5: 280–289.

1338 Egan CL, Liu V, Harris RM et al. Linear IgA disease associated with membranous glomerulonephropathy. Int J Dermatol 2000; 39: 379–382.

1339 Khan IU, Bhol KC, Ahmed AR. Linear IgA bullous dermatosis in a patient with chronic renal failure: Response to intravenous immunoglobulin therapy. J Am Acad Dermatol 1999; 40: 485–488.

1340 Friedman IS, Rudikoff D, Phelps RG, Sapadin AN. Captopril-triggered linear IgA bullous dermatosis. Int J Dermatol 1998; 37: 608–612.

1341 Kuechle MK, Stegemeir E, Maynard B et al. Drug-induced linear IgA bullous dermatosis: report of six cases and review of the literature. J Am Acad Dermatol 1994; 30: 187–192.

1342 König C, Eickert A, Scharffetter-Kochanek K et al. Linear IgA bullous dermatosis induced by atorvastatin. J Am Acad Dermatol 2001; 44: 689–692.

1343 Cerottini J-P, Ricci C, Guggisberg D, Panizzon RG. Drug-induced linear IgA bullous dermatosis probably induced by furosemide. J Am Acad Dermatol 1999; 41: 103–105.

1344 Wakelin SH, Allen J, Zhou S, Wojnarowska F. Drug-induced linear IgA disease with antibodies to collagen VII. Br J Dermatol 1998; 138: 310–314.

1345 Tranvan A, Pezen DS, Medenica M et al. Interleukin-2 associated linear IgA bullous dermatosis. J Am Acad Dermatol 1996; 35: 865–867.

1346 Yawalkar N, Reimers A, Hari Y et al. Drug-induced linear IgA bullous dermatosis associated with ceftriaxone- and metronidazole-specific T cells. Dermatology 1999; 199: 25–30.

1347 McWhirter JD, Hashimoto K, Fayne S, Ito K. Linear IgA bullous dermatosis related to lithium carbonate. Arch Dermatol 1987; 123: 1120–1122.

1348 Primka E, Gay D, Bergfeld W. Drug-induced linear IgA disease (histopathologic features of three cases). J Cutan Pathol 1996; 23: 58 (abstract).

1349 Primka EJ III, Liranzo MO, Bergfeld WF, Dijkstra JW. Amiodarone-induced linear IgA disease. J Am Acad Dermatol 1994; 31: 809–811.

1350 Acostamadiedo JM, Perniciaro C, Rogers RS III. Phenytoin-induced linear IgA bullous disease. J Am Acad Dermatol 1998; 38: 352–356.

1351 Hughes AP, Callen JP. Drug-induced linear IgA bullous dermatosis mimicking toxic epidermal necrolysis. Dermatology 2001; 202: 138–139.

1352 Baden LA, Apovian C, Imber MJ, Dover JS. Vancomycin-induced linear IgA bullous dermatosis. Arch Dermatol 1988; 124: 1186–1188.

1353 Carpenter S, Berg D, Sidhu-Malik N et al. Vancomycin-associated linear IgA dermatosis. A report of three cases. J Am Acad Dermatol 1992; 26: 45–48.

1354 Whitworth JM, Thomas I, Peltz SA et al. Vancomycin-induced linear IgA bullous dermatosis (LABD). J Am Acad Dermatol 1996; 34: 890–891.

1355 Klein PA, Callen JP. Drug-induced linear IgA bullous dermatosis after vancomycin discontinuance in a patient with renal insufficiency. J Am Acad Dermatol 2000; 42: 316–323.

1356 Bitman LM, Grossman ME, Ross H. Bullous drug eruption treated with amputation. A challenging case of vancomycin-induced linear IgA disease. Arch Dermatol 1996; 132: 1289–1290.

1357 Danielsen AG, Thomsen K. Vancomycin-induced linear IgA bullous disease. Br J Dermatol 1999; 141: 756–757.

1358 Gabrielsen TO, Staerfelt F, Thune PO. Drug-induced bullous dermatosis with linear IgA deposits along the basement membrane. Acta Derm Venereol 1981; 61: 439–441.

1359 Bouldin MB, Clowers-Webb HE, Davis JL et al. Naproxen-associated linear IgA bullous dermatosis: case report and review. Mayo Clin Proc 2000; 75: 967–970.

1360 Pellicano R, Lomuto M, Cozzani E et al. Linear IgA bullous dermatosis after contact with sodium hypochlorite. Dermatology 1997; 194: 284–286.

1361 Girão L, Fiadeiro T, Rodrigues JC. Burn-induced linear IgA dermatosis. J Eur Acac Dermatol Venereol 2000; 14: 507–510.

1362 Kroiss MM, Vogt T, Landthaler M, Stolz W. High-dose intravenous immune globulin is also effective in linear IgA disease. Br J Dermatol 2000; 142: 582.

1363 Young HS, Coulson IH. Linear IgA disease: successful treatment with cyclosporin. Br J Dermatol 2000; 143: 204–205.

1364 Collier PM, Kelly SE, Wojnarowska F. Linear IgA disease and pregnancy. J Am Acad Dermatol 1994; 30: 407–411.

1365 Verhelst F, Demedts M, Verschakelen J et al. Adult linear IgA bullous dermatosis with bronchial involvement. Br J Dermatol 1987; 116: 587–590.

1366 Kelly SE, Frith PA, Millard PR et al. A clinicopathological study of mucosal involvement in linear IgA disease. Br J Dermatol 1988; 119: 161–170.

1367 Chan LS, Regezi JA, Cooper KD. Oral manifestations of linear IgA disease. J Am Acad Dermatol 1990; 22: 362–365.

1368 Leonard JN, Wright P, Williams DM et al. The relationship between linear IgA disease and benign mucous membrane pemphigoid. Br J Dermatol 1984; 110: 307–314.

1369 Webster GF, Raber I, Penne R et al. Cicatrizing conjunctivitis as a predominant manifestation of linear IgA bullous dermatosis. J Am Acad Dermatol 1994; 30: 355–357.

1370 Zambruno G, Manca V, Kanitakis J et al. Linear IgA bullous dermatosis with autoantibodies to a 290 kd antigen of anchoring fibrils. J Am Acad Dermatol 1994; 31: 884–888.

1371 Collier PM, Wojnarowska F, Welsh K et al. Adult linear IgA disease and chronic bullous disease of childhood: the association with human lymphocyte antigens Cw7, B8, DR3 and tumour necrosis factor influences disease expression. Br J Dermatol 1999; 141: 867–875.

1372 Wojnarowska F, Collier PM, Allen J, Millard PR. The localization of the target antigens and antibodies in linear IgA disease is heterogeneous, and dependent on the methods used. Br J Dermatol 1995; 132: 750–757.

1373 Hashimoto T, Ishiko A, Shimizu H et al. A case of linear IgA bullous dermatosis with IgA anti-type VII collagen autoantibodies. Br J Dermatol 1996; 134: 336–339.

1374 Haftek M, Zone JJ, Taylor TB et al. Immunogold localization of the 97-kD antigen of linear

1375 IgA bullous dermatosis (LABD) detected with patient's sera. J Invest Dermatol 1994; 103: 656–659.

1375 Harman KE, Bhogal BS, Eady RAJ et al. Defining target antigens in linear IgA disease using skin from subjects with inherited epidermolysis bullosa as a substrate for indirect immunofluorescence microscopy. Br J Dermatol 1999; 141: 475–480.

1376 Zhou S, Ferguson DJP, Allen J, Wojnarowska F. The localization of target antigens and autoantibodies in linear IgA disease is variable: correlation of immunogold electron microscopy and immunoblotting. Br J Dermatol 1998; 139: 591–597.

1377 Wojnarowska F, Allen J, Collier PM, Leigh IM. A comparison of the expression of known basement membrane components with the linear IgA disease antigens using the novel substrate cylindroma. Br J Dermatol 1999; 141: 62–70.

1378 Megahed M, Motoki K, McGrath J et al. Cloning of the human linear IgA disease gene (LADA) encoding a novel anchoring filament protein, ladinin. J Invest Dermatol 1996; 106: 832 (abstract).

1379 Marinkovich MP, Taylor TB, Keene DR et al. LAD-1, the linear IgA bullous dermatosis autoantigen, is a novel 120-kDa anchoring filament protein synthesized by epidermal cells. J Invest Dermatol 1996; 106: 734–738.

1380 Zillikens D, Herzele K, Georgi M et al. Autoantibodies in a subgroup of patients with linear IgA disease react with the NC16A domain of BP180. J Invest Dermatol 1999; 113: 947–953.

1381 Schmidt E, Herzele K, Schumann H et al. Linear IgA disease with circulating IgA antibodies against the NC16A domain of BP180. Br J Dermatol 1999; 140: 964–966.

1382 Nie Z, Nagata Y, Joubeh S et al. IgA antibodies of linear IgA bullous dermatosis recognize the 15th collagenous domain of BP180. J Invest Dermatol 2000; 115: 1164–1166.

1383 Roh JY, Yee C, Lazarova Z et al. The 120-kDa soluble ectodomain of type XVII collagen is recognized by autoantibodies in patients with pemphigoid and linear IgA dermatosis. Br J Dermatol 2000; 143: 104–111.

1384 Ishiko A, Shimizu H, Masunaga T et al. 97 kDa linear IgA bullous dermatosis antigen localizes in the lamina lucida between the NC16A and carboxyl terminal domains of the 180 kDa bullous pemphigoid antigen. J Invest Dermatol 1998; 111: 93–96.

1385 Zone JJ, Taylor TB, Meyer LJ, Petersen MJ. The 97 kDa linear IgA bullous disease antigen is identical to a portion of the extracellular domain of the 180 kDa bullous pemphigoid antigen, BPAg2. J Invest Dermatol 1998; 110: 207–210.

1386 Yomoda M, Komai A, Hashimoto T. Sublamina densa-type linear IgA bullous dermatosis successfully treated with oral tetracycline and niacinamide. Br J Dermatol 1999; 141: 608–609.

1387 Allen J, Zhou S, Wakelin SH et al. Linear IgA disease: a report of two dermal binding sera which recognize a pepsin-sensitive epitope (? NC-1 domain) of collagen type VII. Br J Dermatol 1997; 137: 526–533.

1388 Zambruno G, Kanitakis J. Linear IgA dermatosis with IgA antibodies to type VII collagen. Br J Dermatol 1996; 135: 1004.

1389 Yamane Y, Sato H, Higashi K, Yaoita H. Linear immunoglobulin A (IgA) bullous dermatosis of childhood: identification of the target antigens and study of the cellular sources. Br J Dermatol 1996; 135: 785–790.

1390 Fujimoto W, Ohtsu T, Toi Y et al. Linear IgA disease with IgA antibodies directed against 200- and 280-kDa epidermal antigens. Br J Dermatol 2000; 142: 1213–1218.

1391 Arechalde A, Braun RP, Calza AM et al. Childhood bullous pemphigoid associated with IgA antibodies against BP180 or BP230 antigens. Br J Dermatol 1999; 140: 112–118.

1392 Paul C, Wolkenstein P, Prost C et al. Drug-induced linear IgA disease: target antigens are heterogeneous. Br J Dermatol 1997; 136: 406–411.

1393 Wilsteed E, Bhogal BS, Black MM et al. Use of 1M NaCl split skin in the indirect immunofluorescence of the linear IgA bullous dermatoses. J Cutan Pathol 1990; 17: 144–148.

1394 Christophoridis S, Büdinger L, Borradori L et al. IgG, IgA and IgE autoantibodies against the ectodomain of BP180 in patients with bullous and cicatricial pemphigoid and linear IgA bullous dermatosis. Br J Dermatol 2000; 143: 349–355.

1395 Powell J, Kirtschig G, Allen J et al. Mixed immunobullous disease of childhood: a good response to antimicrobials. Br J Dermatol 2001; 144: 769–774.

1396 Hertl M, Büdinger L, Christophoridis S et al. IgG and IgA antibodies in linear IgA/IgG bullous dermatosis target the ectodomain of bullous pemphigoid antigen 2. Br J Dermatol 1999; 140: 750–752.

1397 Darling TN, Cardenas AA, Beard JS et al. A child with antibodies targeting both linear IgA bullous dermatosis and bullous pemphigoid antigens. Arch Dermatol 1995; 131: 1438–1442.

1398 Chan LS, Traczyk T, Taylor TB et al. Linear IgA bullous dermatosis. Characterization of a subset of patients with concurrent IgA and IgG anti-basement membrane autoantibodies. Arch Dermatol 1995; 131: 1432–1437.

1399 Adachi A, Tani M, Matsubayashi S et al. Immunoelectronmicroscopic differentiation of linear IgA bullous dermatosis of adults with coexistence of IgA and IgG deposition from bullous pemphigoid. J Am Acad Dermatol 1992; 27: 394–399.

1400 Caproni M, Rolfo S, Bernacchi E et al. The role of lymphocytes, granulocytes, mast cells and their related cytokines in lesional skin of linear IgA bullous dermatosis. Br J Dermatol 1999; 140: 1072–1078.

1401 Petersen MJ, Gammon WR, Briggaman RA. A case of linear IgA disease presenting initially with IgG immune deposits. J Am Acad Dermatol 1986; 14: 1014–1019.

1402 Tse Y, Lim HW. Chronic bullous dermatosis of childhood: differentiation from other autoimmune blistering diseases in children. Int J Dermatol 1994; 33: 507–509.

1403 Flotte TJ, Olbricht SM, Collins AB, Harrist TJ. Immunopathologic studies of adult linear IgA bullous dermatosis. Arch Pathol Lab Med 1985; 109: 457–459.

1404 Wojnarowska F, Bhogal BS, Black MM. Chronic bullous disease of childhood and linear IgA disease of adults are IgA1-mediated diseases. Br J Dermatol 1994; 131: 201–204.

1405 Egan CA, Martineau MR, Taylor TB et al. IgA antibodies recognizing LABD97 are predominantly IgA1 subclass. Acta Derm Venereol 1999; 79: 343–346.

1406 Collier PM, Wojnarowska F, Millard PR. Variation in the deposition of the antibodies at different anatomical sites in linear IgA disease of adults and chronic bullous disease of childhood. Br J Dermatol 1992; 127: 482–484.

1407 Blickenstaff RD, Perry HO, Peters MS. Linear IgA deposition associated with cutaneous varicella-zoster infection. J Cutan Pathol 1988; 15: 49–52.

1408 Saklayen MG, Schroeter AL, Nafz MA, Jalil K. IgA deposition in the skin of patients with alcoholic liver disease. J Cutan Pathol 1996; 23: 12–18.

1409 Horiguchi Y, Toda K, Okamoto H, Imamura S. Immunoelectron microscopic observations in a case of linear IgA bullous dermatosis of childhood. J Am Acad Dermatol 1986; 14: 593–599.

1410 Ortonne JP, Schmitt D, Jacquelin L. Chronic bullous dermatosis of childhood. Immunological and ultrastructural studies on the melanocyte-dermal junction. Acta Derm Venereol 1978; 58: 291–296.

1411 Chorzelski T, Jablonska S. Evolving concept of IgA linear dermatosis. Semin Dermatol 1988; 7: 225–232.

1412 Bhogal B, Wojnarowska F, Marsden RA et al. Linear IgA bullous dermatosis of adults and children: an immunoelectron microscopic study. Br J Dermatol 1987; 117: 289–296.

1413 Bhogal BS, Wojnarowska F, Black MM et al. Immunopathology of linear IgA bullous dermatosis. J Cutan Pathol 1988; 15: 298 (abstract).

1414 Prost C, Colonna de Leca A, Combemale P et al. Diagnosis of adult linear IgA dermatosis by immunoelectronmicroscopy in 16 patients with linear IgA deposits. J Invest Dermatol 1989; 92: 39–45.

1415 Roberts LJ, Sontheimer RD. Chronic bullous dermatosis of childhood: immunopathologic studies. Pediatr Dermatol 1987; 4: 6–10.

1416 Hardy KM, Perry HO, Pingree GC et al. Benign mucous membrane pemphigoid. Arch Dermatol 1971; 104: 467–475.

1417 Ahmed AR, Hombal SM. Cicatricial pemphigoid. Int J Dermatol 1986; 25: 90–96.

1418 Ahmed AR, Kurgis BS, Rogers RS III. Cicatricial pemphigoid. J Am Acad Dermatol 1991; 24: 987–1001.

1419 McKee PH. The diagnosis of auto-immune-mediated acquired sub-epidermal blisters: variations on a theme. Curr Diagn Pathol 1997; 4: 10–19.

1420 Thornhill M, Pemberton M, Buchanan J, Theaker E. An open clinical trial of sulphamethoxypyridazine in the treatment of mucous membrane pemphigoid. Br J Dermatol 2000; 143: 117–126.

1421 Rosenbaum MM, Esterly NB, Greenwald MJ, Gerson CR. Cicatricial pemphigoid in a 6-year-old child: report of a case and review of the literature. Pediatr Dermatol 1984; 2: 13–22.

1422 Rogers M, Painter D. Cicatricial pemphigoid in a four-year-old child: a case report. Australas J Dermatol 1981; 22: 21–23.

1423 Venning VA, Frith PA, Bron AJ et al. Mucosal involvement in bullous and cicatricial pemphigoid. A clinical and immunopathological study. Br J Dermatol 1988; 118: 7–15.

1424 Harrington CI, Sneddon IB. An unusual case of benign mucous membrane pemphigoid. Acta Derm Venereol 1977; 57: 459–467.

1425 Behlen CH II, Mackey DM. Benign mucous membrane pemphigus with a generalized eruption. Arch Dermatol 1965; 92: 566–567.

1426 Mallon E, Wojnarowska F. Cicatricial pemphigoid presenting with unusual palmar involvement, successfully treated with a combination of nicotinamide and tetracycline. Clin Exp Dermatol 1994; 19: 526–530.

1427 Ball S, Walkden V, Wojnarowska F. Cicatricial pemphigoid rarely involves the scalp. Australas J Dermatol 1998; 39: 258–260.

1428 Marren P, Walkden V, Mallon E, Wojnarowska F. Vulval cicatricial pemphigoid may mimic lichen sclerosus. Br J Dermatol 1996; 134: 522–524.

1429 Fisher I, Dahl MV, Christiansen TA. Cicatricial pemphigoid confined to the larynx. Cutis 1980; 25: 371–373.

1430 Gaspar ZS, Wojnarowska F. Cicatricial pemphigoid with severe laryngeal involvement necessitating tracheostomy (laryngeal cicatricial pemphigoid). Clin Exp Dermatol 1996; 21: 209–210.

1431 Nousari HC, Rencic A, Hsu R et al. Anti-epiligrin cicatricial pemphigoid with antibodies against the γ2 subunit of laminin 5. Arch Dermatol 1999; 135: 173–176.

1432 Warren LJ, Wojnarowska F, Wilkinson JD. Oesophageal involvement in cicatricial pemphigoid. Australas J Dermatol 1997; 38: 148–151.

1433 Thomson J, Lang W, Craig JA. Deafness complicating mucous membrane pemphigoid: a case report. Br J Dermatol 1975; 93: 337–339.

1434 Burge SM, Powell SM, Ryan TJ. Cicatricial pemphigoid with nail dystrophy. Clin Exp Dermatol 1985; 10: 472–475.

1435 Sabet HY, Davis JL, Rogers RS III. Mucous membrane pemphigoid, thymoma, and myasthenia gravis. Int J Dermatol 2000; 39: 701–704.

1436 Ostlere LS, Branfoot AC, Staughton RCD. Cicatricial pemphigoid and carcinoma of the pancreas. Clin Exp Dermatol 1992; 17: 67–68.

1437 Fujimoto W, Ishida-Yamamoto A, Hsu R et al. Anti-epiligrin cicatricial pemphigoid: a case associated with gastric carcinoma and features resembling epidermolysis bullosa acquisita. Br J Dermatol 1998; 139: 682–687.

1438 Gibson GE, Daoud MS, Pittelkow MR. Anti-epiligrin (laminin 5) cicatricial pemphigoid and lung carcinoma: coincidence or association? Br J Dermatol 1997; 137: 780–782.

1439 Spigel GT, Winkelmann RK. Cicatricial pemphigoid and rheumatoid arthritis. Arch Dermatol 1978; 114: 415–417.

1440 Redman RS, Thorne EG. Cicatricial pemphigoid in a patient with systemic lupus erythematosus. Arch Dermatol 1981; 117: 109–110.

1441 Nayar M, Wojnarowska F, Venning V, Taylor CJ. Association of autoimmunity and cicatricial pemphigoid: is there an immunogenetic basis? J Am Acad Dermatol 1991; 25: 1011–1015.

1442 Van Joost TH, Crone RA, Overdijk AD. Ocular cicatricial pemphigoid associated with practolol therapy. Br J Dermatol 1976; 94: 447–450.

1443 Van Joost TH, Faber WR, Manuel HR. Drug-induced anogenital cicatricial pemphigoid. Br J Dermatol 1980; 102: 715–718.

1444 Burgess MJA, Fivenson DP. Generalization of cicatricial pemphigoid during azathioprine therapy. Arch Dermatol 2000; 136: 1274.

1445 Egan CA, Lazarova A, Darling TN et al. Anti-epiligrin cicatricial pemphigoid and relative risk for cancer. Lancet 2001; 357: 1850–1851.

1446 Fine J-D, Neises GR, Katz SI. Immunofluorescence and immunoelectron microscopic studies in cicatricial pemphigoid. J Invest Dermatol 1984; 82: 39–43.

1447 Bernard P, Prost C, Lecerf V et al. Studies of cicatricial pemphigoid autoantibodies using direct immunoelectron microscopy and immunoblot analysis. J Invest Dermatol 1990; 94: 630–635.

1448 Bédane C, Prost C, Bernard P et al. Cicatricial pemphigoid antigen differs from bullous pemphigoid antigen by its exclusive extracellular localization: a study by indirect immunoelectronmicroscopy. J Invest Dermatol 1991; 97: 3–9.

1449 Chan LS, Yancey KB, Hammerberg C et al. Immune-mediated subepithelial blistering diseases of mucous membranes. Arch Dermatol 1993; 129: 448–455.

1450 Banfield CC, Papadavid E, Frith P et al. Bullous pemphigoid evolving into cicatricial pemphigoid? Clin Exp Dermatol 1997; 22: 30–33.

1451 Balding SD, Prost C, Diaz LA et al. Cicatricial pemphigoid autoantibodies react with multiple sites on the BP180 extracellular domain. J Invest Dermatol 1996; 106: 141–146.

1452 Hashimoto T, Murakimi H, Senboshi Y et al. Antiepiligrin cicatricial pemphigoid: the first case report from Japan. J Am Acad Dermatol 1996; 34: 940–942.

1453 Lish KM, Washenik K, Yancey KB et al. Anti-epiligrin cicatricial pemphigoid in a patient with HIV. J Am Acad Dermatol 1997; 36: 486–488.

1454 Leverkus M, Schmidt E, Lazarova Z et al. Antiepiligrin cicatricial pemphigoid. An underdiagnosed entity within the spectrum of scarring autoimmune subepidermal bullous diseases? Arch Dermatol 1999; 135: 1091–1098.

1455 Allbritton JI, Nousari HC, Anhalt GJ. Anti-epiligrin (laminin 5) cicatricial pemphigoid. Br J Dermatol 1997; 137: 992–996.

1456 Lazarova Z, Hsu R, Yee C, Yancey KB. Antiepiligrin cicatricial pemphigoid represents an autoimmune response to subunits present in laminin 5 (α3β3γ2). Br J Dermatol 1998; 139: 791–797.

1457 Lazarova Z, Hsu R, Yee C, Yancey KB. Human anti-laminin 5 autoantibodies induce subepidermal blisters in an experimental human skin graft model. J Invest Dermatol 2000; 114: 178–184.

1458 Hashimoto Y, Suga Y, Yoshiike T et al. A case of antiepiligrin cicatricial pemphigoid successfully treated by plasmapheresis. Dermatology 2000; 201: 58–60.

1459 Ghohestani R, Rousselle P, Nicolas JF, Claudy A. α and β subunits of laminin-5 are target antigens in a subset of patients with cicatricial pemphigoid. J Invest Dermatol 1996; 106: 846 (abstract).

1460 Ghohestani R, Rouselle P, Nicolas JF, Claudy A. Laminin-5, BPAg2, and a 168kD mucosal protein are recognized by the cicatricial pemphigoid auto-antibodies. Br J Dermatol (Suppl) 1996; 47: 13 (abstract).

1461 Seo SH, Kye Y-C, Kim SN, Kim S-C. Antiepiligrin cicatricial pemphigoid with autoantibodies to the beta subunit of laminin 5 and associated with severe laryngeal involvement necessitating tracheostomy. Dermatology 2001; 202: 63–66.

1462 Fujimoto W, Toi Y, Okazaki F et al. Anti-epiligrin cicatricial pemphigoid with IgG autoantibodies to the β and γ subunits of laminin 5. J Am Acad Dermatol 1999; 40: 637–639.

1463 Taniuchi K, Takata M, Matsui C et al. Antiepiligrin (laminin 5) cicatricial pemphigoid associated with an underlying gastric carcinoma producing laminin 5. Br J Dermatol 1999; 140: 696–700.

1464 Fleming TE, Korman NJ. Cicatricial pemphigoid. J Am Acad Dermatol 2000; 43: 571–591.

1465 Hsu RC-C, Lazarova Z, Lee H-G et al. Antiepiligrin cicatricial pemphigoid. J Am Acad Dermatol 2000; 42: 841–844.

1466 Kawahara Y, Amagai M, Ohata Y et al. A case of cicatricial pemphigoid with simultaneous IgG autoantibodies against the 180 kd bullous pemphigoid antigen and laminin 5. J Am Acad Dermatol 1998; 38: 624–627.

1467 Hsu R, Lazarova Z, Yee C, Yancey KB. Noncomplement fixing, IgG₄ autoantibodies predominate in patients with anti-epiligrin cicatricial pemphigoid. J Invest Dermatol 1997; 109: 557–561.

1468 Niimi Y, Zhu X-J, Bystryn J-C. Identification of cicatricial pemphigoid antigens. Arch Dermatol 1992; 128: 54–57.

1469 Shimizu H, Masunaga T, Ishiko A et al. Autoantibodies from patients with cicatricial pemphigoid target different sites in epidermal basement membrane. J Invest Dermatol 1995; 104: 370–373.

1470 Rao SK, Tran HH, Allen J et al. Identification of multiple, distinct cicatricial pemphigoid autoantigens. J Invest Dermatol 1996; 106: 812 (abstract).

1471 Ghohestani R, Rousselle P, Nicolas JF, Claudy A. A subset of patients with cicatricial pemphigoid have autoantibodies directed to a 168kD mucosal protein but not to laminin-5. J Invest Dermatol 1996; 106: 847 (abstract).

1472 Langeland T. Childhood cicatricial pemphigoid with linear IgA deposits: a case report. Acta Derm Venereol 1985; 65: 354–355.

1473 Kumar V, Rogozinski T, Yarbrough C et al. A case of cicatricial pemphigoid or cicatricial linear IgA bullous dermatosis. J Am Acad Dermatol 1980; 2: 327–331.

1474 Sarret Y, Hall R, Cobo LM et al. Salt-split human skin substrate for the immunofluorescent screening of serum from patients with cicatricial pemphigoid and a new method of immunoprecipitation with IgA antibodies. J Am Acad Dermatol 1991; 24: 952–958.

1475 Chan LS, Hammerberg C, Cooper KD. Cicatricial pemphigoid. Identification of two distinct sets of epidermal antigens by IgA and IgG class circulating autoantibodies. Arch Dermatol 1990; 126: 1466–1468.

1476 Kirtschig G, Mengel R, Mittag H et al. Desquamative gingivitis and balanitis – linear IgA disease or cicatricial pemphigoid? Clin Exp Dermatol 1998; 23: 173–177.

1477 Person JR, Rogers RS III. Bullous and cicatricial pemphigoid. Clinical, histopathologic, and immunopathologic correlations. Mayo Clin Proc 1977; 52: 54–66.

1478 Zelger B. Blue & pink, clue & think. An appreciation of the Editor. Dermatopathology: Practical & Conceptual 1999; 5: 32–36.

1479 Leonard JN, Hobday CM, Haffenden GP et al. Immunofluorescent studies in ocular cicatricial pemphigoid. Br J Dermatol 1988; 118: 209–217.

1480 Griffith MR, Fukuyama K, Tuffanelli D, Silverman S Jr. Immunofluorescent studies in mucous membrane pemphigoid. Arch Dermatol 1974; 109: 195–199.

1481 Venning VA, Allen J, Millard PR, Wojnarowska F. The localization of the bullous pemphigoid and cicatricial pemphigoid antigens: direct and indirect immunofluorescence of suction blisters. Br J Dermatol 1989; 120: 305–315.

1482 Fleming MG, Valenzuela R, Bergfeld WF, Tuthill RJ. Mucous gland basement membrane immunofluorescence in cicatricial pemphigoid. Arch Dermatol 1988; 124: 1407–1410.

1483 Bean SF. Cicatricial pemphigoid. Immunofluorescent studies. Arch Dermatol 1974; 110: 552–555.

1484 Korman NJ, Watson RD. Immune-mediated subepithelial blistering diseases of the mucous membranes. Improving the detection of circulating autoantibodies by the use of concentrated serum samples. Arch Dermatol 1996; 132: 1194–1198.

1485 Setterfield J, Shirlaw PJ, Bhogal BS et al. Cicatricial pemphigoid: serial titres of circulating IgG and IgA antibasement membrane antibodies correlate with disease activity. Br J Dermatol 1999; 140: 645–650.

1486 Egan CA, Hanif N, Taylor TB et al. Characterization of the antibody response in oesophageal cicatricial pemphigoid. Br J Dermatol 1999; 140: 859–864.

1487 Egan CA, Taylor TB, Meyer LJ et al. The immunoglobulin A antibody response in clinical subsets of mucous membrane pemphigoid. Dermatology 1999; 198: 330–335.

1488 Setterfield J, Shirlaw PJ, Kerr-Muir M et al. Mucous membrane pemphigoid: a dual circulating antibody response with IgG and IgA signifies a more severe and persistent disease. Br J Dermatol 1998; 138: 602–610.

1489 Kumar V, Yarbrough C, Beutner EH. Complement-fixing intercellular antibodies in a case of cicatricial pemphigoid. Arch Dermatol 1980; 116: 812–814.

1490 Brauner GJ, Jimbow K. Benign mucous membrane pemphigoid. An unusual case with electron microscopic findings. Arch Dermatol 1972; 106: 535–540.

1491 Prost C, Labeille B, Chaussade V et al. Immunoelectron microscopy in subepidermal autoimmune bullous diseases: a prospective study of IgG and C3 bound in vivo in 32 patients. J Invest Dermatol 1987; 89: 567–573.

1492 Smith EP, Taylor TB, Meyer LJ, Zone JJ. Identification of a basement membrane zone antigen reactive with circulating IgA antibody in ocular cicatricial pemphigoid. J Invest Dermatol 1993; 101: 619–623.

1493 Buhac J, Bhol K, Padilla T Jr et al. Coexistence of pemphigus vulgaris and ocular cicatricial pemphigoid. J Am Acad Dermatol 1996; 34: 884–886.

1494 Brunsting LA, Perry HO. Benign pemphigoid? A report of seven cases with chronic, scarring, herpetiform plaques about the head and neck. Arch Dermatol 1957; 75: 489–501.

1495 Michel B, Bean SF, Chorzelski T, Fedele CF. Cicatricial pemphigoid of Brunsting-Perry. Arch Dermatol 1977; 113: 1403–1405.

1496 Ahmed AR, Salm M, Larson R, Kaplan R. Localized cicatricial pemphigoid (Brunsting-Perry). A transplantation experiment. Arch Dermatol 1984; 120: 932–935.

1497 Leenutaphong V, von Kries R, Plewig G. Localized cicatricial pemphigoid (Brunsting-Perry): electron microscopic study. J Am Acad Dermatol 1989; 21: 1089–1093.

1498 Baldwin H, Lynfield Y. Brunsting-Perry cicatricial pemphigoid precipitated by trauma. Arch Dermatol 1991; 127: 911–912.

1499 Weedon D, Robertson I. Localized chronic pemphigoid. J Cutan Pathol 1976; 3: 41–44.

1500 Monihan JM, Nguyen TH, Guill MA. Brunsting-Perry pemphigoid simulating basal cell carcinoma. J Am Acad Dermatol 1989; 21: 331–334.

1501 Hanno R, Foster DR, Bean SF. Brunsting-Perry cicatricial pemphigoid associated with bullous pemphigoid. J Am Acad Dermatol 1980; 3: 470–473.

1502 Kurzhals G, Stolz W, Maciejewski W et al. Localized cicatricial pemphigoid of the Brunsting-Perry type with transition into disseminated cicatricial pemphigoid. Arch Dermatol 1995; 131: 580–585.

1503 Joly P, Ruto F, Thomine E et al. Brunsting-Perry cicatricial pemphigoid: a clinical variant of localized acquired epidermolysis bullosa? J Am Acad Dermatol 1993; 28: 89–92.

1504 Drummond A, Gupta G, Swan IRC, Thomson J. An inflammatory desquamative dermatosis of the ear with anti-180 kDa antibodies: localized cicatricial pemphigoid? Br J Dermatol 2000; 142: 815–816.

1505 Chan LS, Cooper KD. A novel immune-mediated subepidermal bullous dermatosis characterized by IgG autoantibodies to a lower lamina lucida component. Arch Dermatol 1994; 130: 343–347.

1506 Chan LS, Fine J-D, Briggaman RA et al. Identification and partial characterization of a novel 105-kDalton lower lamina lucida autoantigen associated with a novel immune-mediated subepidermal blistering disease. J Invest Dermatol 1993; 101: 262–267.

1507 Cotell SL, Lapiere JC, Chen JD et al. A novel 105-kDa lamina lucida autoantigen: association with bullous pemphigoid. J Invest Dermatol 1994; 103: 78–83.

1508 Kawahara Y, Matsuo Y, Hashimoto T, Nishikawa T. A case of unique subepidermal blistering disease with autoantibodies against a novel dermal 200-kD antigen. Dermatology 1998; 196: 213–216.

1509 Mascaró JM Jr, Zillikens D, Giudice GJ et al. A subepidermal bullous eruption associated with IgG autoantibodies to a 200 kd dermal antigen: The first case report from the United States. J Am Acad Dermatol 2000; 42: 309–315.

1510 Salmhofer W, Kawahara Y, Soyer HP et al. A subepidermal blistering disease with histopathological features of dermatitis herpetiformis and immunofluorescence characteristics of bullous pemphigoid: a novel subepidermal blistering disease or a variant of bullous pemphigoid? Br J Dermatol 1997; 137: 599–604.

1511 Zillikens D, Ishiko A, Jonkman MF et al. Autoantibodies in anti-p200 pemphigoid stain skin lacking laminin 5 and type VII collagen. Br J Dermatol 2000; 143: 1043–1049.

1512 Tyring SK, Lee PC. Hemorrhagic bullae associated with *Vibrio vulnificus* septicemia. Report of two cases. Arch Dermatol 1986; 122: 818–820.

1513 Fisher K, Berger BW, Keusch GT. Subepidermal bullae secondary to *Escherichia coli* septicemia. Arch Dermatol 1974; 110: 105–106.

1514 Bagel J, Grossman ME. Hemorrhagic bullae associated with *Morganella morganii* septicemia. J Am Acad Dermatol 1985; 12: 575–576.

1515 Elbaum DJ, Wood C, Abuabara F, Morhenn VB. Bullae in a patient with toxic shock syndrome. J Am Acad Dermatol 1984; 10: 267–272.

1516 Tani M, Shimizu R, Ban M et al. Systemic lupus erythematosus with vesiculobullous lesions. Immunoelectron microscopic studies. Arch Dermatol 1984; 120: 1497–1501.

Miscellaneous blistering diseases

1517 Roholt NS, Lapiere JC, Traczyk T et al. A nonscarring sublamina densa bullous drug eruption. J Am Acad Dermatol 1995; 32: 367–371.

1518 Goodheart HP. "Devotional dermatoses": A new nosologic entity? J Am Acad Dermatol 2001; 44: 543.

15 9 Izu K, Yamamoto O, Asahi M. Occupational skin injury by hydrogen peroxide. Dermatology 2000; 201: 61–64.

1520 Talanin NY, Shelley WB, Shelley ED. IgE bullous disease. Clin Exp Dermatol 1997; 22: 82–86.

1521 Feldman SR, Jones RS, Lesesne HR et al. A blistering eruption associated with Wilson's disease. J Am Acad Dermatol 1989; 21: 1030–1032.

1522 Webster GF, Iozzo RV, Schwartzman RJ et al. Reflex sympathetic dystrophy: occurrence of chronic edema and nonimmune bullous skin lesions. J Am Acad Dermatol 1993; 28: 29–32.

1523 Leavell UW, Farley CH, McIntyre JS. Cutaneous changes in a patient with carbon monoxide poisoning. Arch Dermatol 1969; 99: 429–433.

1524 Leavell UW. Sweat gland necrosis in barbiturate poisoning. Arch Dermatol 1969; 100: 218–221.

1525 Godden DJ, McPhie JL. Bullous skin eruption associated with carbamazepine overdosage. Postgrad Med J 1983; 59: 336–337.

1526 Herschthal D, Robinson MJ. Blisters of the skin in coma induced by amitryptyline and clorazepate dipotassium. Arch Dermatol 1979; 115: 499.

1527 Setterfield JF, Robinson R, MacDonald D, Calonje E. Coma-induced bullae and sweat gland necrosis following clobazam. Clin Exp Dermatol 2000; 25: 215–218.

1528 Arndt KA, Mihm MC Jr, Parrish JA. Bullae: a cutaneous sign of a variety of neurologic diseases. J Invest Dermatol 1973; 60: 312–320.

1529 Naeyaert JM, Derom E, Santosa S, Rubens R. Sweat-gland necrosis after beta-adrenergic antagonist treatment in a patient with pheochromocytoma. Br J Dermatol 1987; 117: 371–376.

1530 Mehregan DR, Daoud M, Rogers RS III. Coma blisters in a patient with diabetic ketoacidosis. J Am Acad Dermatol 1992; 27: 269–270.

1531 Mandy S, Ackerman AB. Characteristic traumatic skin lesions in drug-induced coma. JAMA 1970; 213: 253–256.

1532 Brehmer-Andersson E, Pedersen NB. Sweat gland necrosis and bullous skin changes in acute drug intoxication. Acta Derm Venereol 1969; 49: 157–162.

1533 Sánchez Yus E, Requena L, Simón P, Hospital M. Histopathology of cutaneous changes in drug-induced coma. Am J Dermatopathol 1993; 15: 208–216.

1534 Meawad OB, Assaf HM. Coma-induced epidermal necrolysis. Int J Dermatol 1995; 34: 801–803.

1535 Kato N, Ueno H, Mimura M. Histopathology of cutaneous changes in non-drug-induced coma. Am J Dermatopathol 1996; 18: 344–350.

1536 Henzemans-Boer M, Toonstra J, Meulenbelt J et al. Skin lesions due to exposure to methyl bromide. Arch Dermatol 1988; 124: 917–921.

1537 Smith KJ, Smith WJ, Hamilton T et al. Histopathologic and immunohistochemical features in human skin after exposure to nitrogen and sulfur mustard. Am J Dermatopathol 1998; 20: 22–28.

1538 Ramsay B, Bloxham C, Eldred A et al. Blistering, erosions and scarring in a patient on etretinate. Br J Dermatol 1989; 121: 397–400.

1539 Friedmann PS, Coburn P, Dahl MGC et al. PUVA-induced blisters, complement deposition, and damage to the dermoepidermal junction. Arch Dermatol 1987; 123: 1471–1477.

1540 Nagase T, Takanashi M, Takada H, Ohmori K. Extensive vesiculobullous eruption following limited ruby laser treatment for incontinentia pigmenti: a case report. Australas J Dermatol 1997; 38: 155–157.

1541 Saikia NK, Mackie RM, McQueen A. A case of bullous pemphigoid and figurate erythema in association with metastatic spread of carcinoma. Br J Dermatol 1973; 88: 331–334.

1542 Watsky KL, Orlow SJ, Bolognia JL. Figurate and bullous eruption in association with breast carcinoma. Arch Dermatol 1990; 126: 649–652.

1543 Vircendeau P, Claudy A, Thivolet J et al. Bullous dermatosis and myeloma. Arch Dermatol 1980; 116: 681–682.

1544 Wong DA, Hunt MJ, Stapleton K. IgA multiple myeloma presenting as an acquired bullous disorder. Australas J Dermatol 1999; 40: 31–34.

1545 Moranz JF, Siegle RJ, Barrett JL. Lymphatic bullae arising as a complication of second-intention healing. J Dermatol Surg Oncol 1989; 15: 874–877.

1546 Groff JW, White JW. Vesiculobullous cutaneous lymphatic reflux. Cutis 1988; 42: 31–32.

1547 Johnson WT. Cutaneous chylous reflux. 'The weeping scrotum'. Arch Dermatol 1979; 115: 464–466.

1548 Alora MB, Dover JS. Spontaneous bullae over laser resurfaced skin. J Am Acad Dermatol 2000; 42: 288–290.

1549 Ballo F, Maroon M, Millon SJ. Fracture blisters. J Am Acad Dermatol 1994; 30: 1033–1034.

The granulomatous reaction pattern

INTRODUCTION

The granulomatous reaction pattern is defined as a distinctive inflammatory pattern characterized by the presence of granulomas. Granulomas are relatively discrete collections of histiocytes or epithelioid histiocytes with variable numbers of admixed multinucleate giant cells of varying types and other inflammatory cells. Conditions in which there is a diffuse infiltrate of histiocytes within the dermis, such as lepromatous leprosy, are not included in this reaction pattern. The group is subdivided by way of:

- the arrangement of granulomas;
- the presence of accessory features such as central necrosis, suppuration or necrobiosis; and
- the presence of foreign material or organisms.

It is difficult to present a completely satisfactory classification of the granulomatous reactions.[1] As Hirsh and Johnson remark in their review of the subject, 'Sometimes a perfect fit can be achieved only with the help of an enlightened shove'.[2] Many conditions described within this group may show only non-specific changes in the early evolution of the inflammatory process and in a late or resolving stage show fibrosis and non-specific changes without granulomas. Occasionally a variety of granuloma types may be seen in one area, e.g. in reactions to foreign bodies or around ruptured hair follicles.

It is necessary in any granulomatous dermatitis to exclude an infectious cause. Culture of fresh tissue as well as histological search increases the chances of identifying a specific infectious agent. The time-consuming examination of multiple sections may be necessary to exclude such a cause. Special stains for organisms may be indicated. Occasionally fungi are shown only by silver stains, such as Grocott methenamine silver, and not by PAS staining. All granulomas should be examined under polarized light to detect or exclude birefringent foreign material.

Considerable advances have been made in the understanding of the formation and maintenance of granulomas in tissue reactions and the roles played by B and T lymphocytes and cytokines.[3–6] It is also clear that there are several types of macrophages in granulomas, particularly at an ultrastructural level.[7] The different forms of multinucleate giant cells seen in granulomas may simply reflect the types of cytokines being produced by the component cells.[8] This new information has not so far been shown to be useful in routine diagnostic problems. Polymerase chain reaction techniques (PCR) have proved useful in detecting infectious agents in tissue sections, particularly mycobacterial species.[9–13]

The following types of granulomas form the basis of the subclassification of diseases in this reaction pattern.

- *Sarcoidal* – granulomas composed of epithelioid histiocytes and giant cells with a paucity of surrounding lymphocytes and plasma cells ('naked' granulomas).
- *Tuberculoid* – granulomas composed of epithelioid histiocytes, giant cells of Langhans and foreign body type with a more substantial rim of lymphocytes and plasma cells and sometimes showing central 'caseation' necrosis. Granulomas have a tendency to confluence.
- *Necrobiotic* – granulomas are usually poorly formed and there are collections, and a more diffuse array, of histiocytes, lymphocytes and giant cells with associated 'necrobiosis'. The inflammatory component may be admixed with the 'necrobiosis' or form a palisade around it.
- *Suppurative* – granulomas composed of epithelioid histiocytes and multinucleate giant cells with central collections of neutrophils. Chronic inflammatory cells are usually present at the periphery of the granulomas.

- *Foreign body* – granulomas composed of epithelioid histiocytes, multinucleate (foreign body-type) giant cells and variable numbers of other inflammatory cells. There is identifiable foreign material, either exogenous or endogenous in origin.
- *Miscellaneous* – a category in which the granulomas may be variable in appearance or do not always fit neatly into one of the above categories.

Many of the conditions exhibiting a granulomatous tissue reaction have been discussed in other chapters; they will be mentioned only briefly.

The various granulomatous diseases will be discussed, in order, according to the classification listed above.

SARCOIDAL GRANULOMAS

Sarcoidal granulomas are found in sarcoidosis and in certain types of reaction to foreign materials and squames.

The prototypic condition in this group is sarcoidosis. Sarcoidal granulomas are discrete, round to oval, and composed of epithelioid histiocytes and multinucleate giant cells which may be of either Langhans or foreign body type. Generally, the type of multinucleate histiocyte present in a granuloma is not helpful in arriving at a specific histological diagnosis. Giant cells may contain asteroid bodies, conchoidal bodies (Schaumann bodies) or crystalline particles. Typical granulomas are surrounded by a sparse rim of lymphocytes and plasma cells, and only occasional lymphocytes are present within them. Consequently, they have been described as having a 'naked' appearance. Although the granulomas may be in close proximity to one another, their confluence is not commonly found. With reticulin stains, a network of reticulin fibers is seen surrounding and permeating the histiocytic cluster.

Sarcoidal granulomas can be found in the following circumstances:

- sarcoidosis
- Blau's syndrome
- foreign body reactions (see Table 7.1)
- secondary syphilis
- Sézary syndrome[14]
- herpes-zoster scars[15]
- systemic lymphomas[16]
- common variable immunodeficiency (see p. 211).

Sarcoidal granulomas are exceedingly rare in secondary syphilis (see p. 650), Sézary syndrome (see p. 1110), herpes-zoster scars (see p. 699) and systemic lymphomas. They will not be considered further in this section.

SARCOIDOSIS

Sarcoidosis is a multisystem disease which may involve any organ of the body but most commonly affects the lungs, lymph nodes (mediastinal and peripheral), skin, liver, spleen and eyes.[17–20] There is an increased incidence of sarcoidosis in people of Irish and Afro-Caribbean origin.[21]

Between 10% and 35% of patients with systemic sarcoidosis have cutaneous lesions.[22–24] Although sarcoidosis is usually a multiorgan disease, chronic cutaneous lesions may be the only manifestation.[25] The skin lesions may be specific, showing a granulomatous histology, or non-specific. The most common non-specific skin lesion is erythema nodosum which is said to occur in 3–25% of cases.[22] An erythema nodosum-like eruption with the histological changes of sarcoidosis has also been described.[26] Sarcoidosis predominantly affects adults; skin lesions are rarely seen in children.[27,28] There are reports of its occurrence in monozygotic twins.[29]

A diversity of clinical forms of cutaneous sarcoidosis occurs. These forms include:

- papules, plaques and nodules, which may be arranged in an annular or serpiginous pattern
- a maculopapular eruption associated with acute lymphadenopathy, uveitis or pulmonary involvement
- plaques with marked telangiectasia (angiolupoid sarcoidosis)
- lupus pernio, consisting of violaceous nodules, particularly on the nose, cheeks and ears[30,31]
- nodular subcutaneous sarcoidosis[32-37]
- a miscellaneous group which includes cicatricial alopecia,[38,39] an acral form,[40] ichthyosiform sarcoidosis,[41-43] ulcerative,[44] necrotizing, morpheaform and mutilating forms,[45-49] verrucous lesions[50,51] and erythroderma.[52]

This miscellaneous group represents rare cutaneous manifestations of sarcoidosis. Lupus pernio may resolve with fibrosis and scarring and is often associated with involvement of the upper respiratory tract and lungs.[53] Oral lesions may also occur.[54] The majority of skin lesions resolve without scarring. Hypopigmented macules without underlying granulomas have been described, particularly in patients of African descent.[55] Other rare presentations have included leonine facies,[56] faint erythema,[57] palmar erythema[58] and lesions confined to the vulva.[59]

It is generally considered that the presence of cutaneous lesions in association with systemic involvement is an indicator of more severe disease. Skin lesions may occur in scars[60] following trauma (including surgery and venepuncture),[61,62] radiation and chronic infection. In some cases these lesions may be the first manifestation of sarcoidosis.[63] Other cases do not appear to be related to systemic sarcoidosis and may be a sarcoidal reaction to a foreign body.

Various systemic diseases have been reported in association with cutaneous sarcoidosis. The association in many of these conditions is probably fortuitous. They include cutaneous lymphoma,[64] hypoparathyroidism,[65] auto-immune thyroiditis and/or vitiligo,[66-68] and HIV infection.[69] In one case of HIV infection, the sarcoidosis became manifest after the commencement of highly active antiretroviral therapy (HAART) and the restoration of some immune function.[69] The term 'immune restoration disease' has been used for this circumstance.

The etiology of sarcoidosis remains controversial although an infectious origin has long been suspected.[70] The main candidate is a cell-wall-deficient form of an acid-fast bacillus, similar, if not identical to, *Mycobacterium tuberculosis*.[71] In one study, DNA sequences coding for the mycobacterial 65 kd antigen were found in 11 of 35 cases of sarcoidosis,[72] while in a more recent study, using only cutaneous specimens, mycobacterial DNA was demonstrated by PCR in 16 of 20 cases.[73] Non-tuberculous (atypical) mycobacteria constitute the largest group of the species identified in this study.[73] Other findings supportive of a mycobacterial etiology are the beneficial effects of long-term tetracyclines[74] and the activation of a case following concurrent *M. marinum* infection of the skin.[75] A recent study concluded that there was no role for human herpesvirus type 8 (HHV-8) in the etiology, despite earlier reports suggesting a role.[76]

The exact relationship of **Blau's syndrome** to sarcoidosis is uncertain. It is characterized by the familial presentation of a sarcoid-like granulomatous disease involving the skin, uveal tract and joints, but not the lung.[77] Onset is in childhood and the mode of inheritance appears to be autosomal dominant. It has been regarded by some as a familial form of early-onset sarcoidosis but it is generally regarded as a unique condition.

Histopathology

There is a dermal infiltrate of granulomas of the type already described (Fig. 7.1). Granulomas may be present only in the superficial dermis or they may extend through the whole thickness of the dermis or subcutis, depending on the type of cutaneous lesion. There is no particular localization to skin appendages or nerves. Necrosis is not usually seen in granulomas but has been reported.[78] Small amounts of fibrinous or granular material may be seen in some granulomas.[17] Fibrinoid necrosis is said to be quite common in the cutaneous lesions of black South Africans.[21] Slight perigranulomatous fibrosis may be present but marked dermal scarring is unusual except in lupus pernio or necrotizing and ulcerating lesions.

Overlying epidermal hyperplasia occurs in verrucous lesions[50] and hyperkeratosis occurs in the rare ichthyosiform variant.[41] Otherwise, in most cases, the overlying epidermis is normal or atrophic.

Transepidermal elimination has been reported in sarcoidosis and the histology shows characteristic elimination channels.[79] In some cases the round cell infiltrate surrounding the granulomas is more intense and the granulomas less discrete. The diagnosis of sarcoidosis may then become one of exclusion.

Asteroid bodies and conchoidal bodies (Schaumann bodies) may be seen in multinucleate giant cells but are not specific for sarcoidosis and may occur

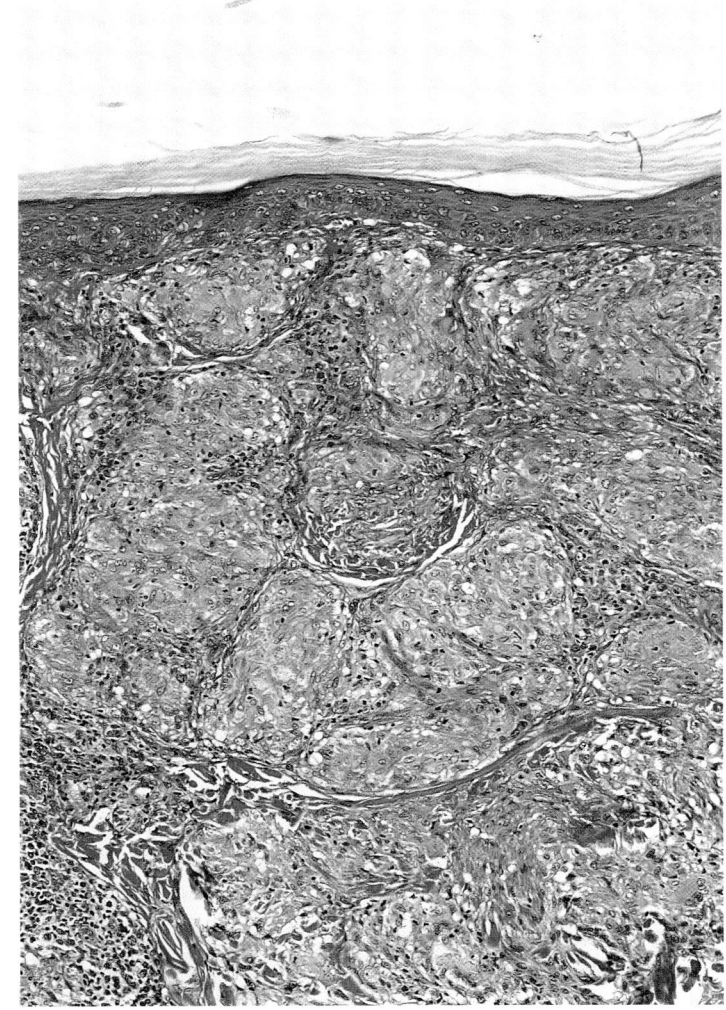

Fig. 7.1 **Sarcoidosis.** The granulomas in the dermis are composed of epithelioid histiocytes and multinucleate giant cells with only a sparse infiltrate of lymphocytes at the periphery ('naked' granulomas). (H & E)

in other granulomatous reactions including tuberculosis (Fig. 7.2). Schaumann bodies, which are shell-like calcium-impregnated protein complexes, are much more common in the granulomas of sarcoidosis than in those of tuberculosis.[80] Birefringent material was found in the granulomas in 12 of the 50 cases studied in a recent report.[81] Electron probe microanalysis identified calcium, phosphorus, silicon and aluminum. It is thought that the calcium salts are probably the precursors of Schaumann bodies. Another explanation for the material is that it represents foreign material inoculated during a previous episode of inapparent trauma leading to granuloma formation subsequently in a patient with sarcoidosis.[82,83] Asteroid bodies are said by some to be formed from trapped collagen bundles[84] or from components of the cytoskeleton, predominantly vimentin intermediate filaments.[85]

Biopsies taken from Kveim–Siltzbach skin test sites, sometimes used in the past for the diagnosis of sarcoidosis, show a variety of changes ranging from poorly formed granulomas with a heavy mononuclear cell infiltrate to small granulomas with few mononuclear cells. Measurement of the serum angiotensin-converting enzyme (ACE) level has now replaced this skin test.

Immunohistochemical marker studies have shown that the T lymphocytes expressing the suppressor/cytotoxic phenotype are found predominantly in the perigranulomatous mantle whereas those expressing the helper/inducer phenotype are present throughout the granuloma.[86] B lymphocytes are also present in the mantle zone.

Immunofluorescence studies in some cases have shown IgM at the dermo-epidermal junction, IgM within blood vessel walls, and IgG within and around the granuloma. A fibrin network is present within granulomas.[87]

REACTIONS TO FOREIGN MATERIALS

A number of foreign substances and materials when introduced into the skin may induce a granulomatous dermatitis which histologically resembles sarcoidosis. They are listed in Table 7.1.

Following some kind of trauma, silica may contaminate a wound in the form of dirt, sand, rock or glass (including windshield glass from motor vehicles).[88] Papules and nodules arise in the area of trauma. The granulomas seen in the dermal reaction contain varying numbers of Langhans or foreign body giant cells, some of which may contain clear colorless particles. These may be difficult to see with routine microscopy but are birefringent in polarized light. The differentiation from true sarcoidosis may be difficult, since granulomas

sometimes develop in scars in sarcoidosis and the granulomas can contain birefringent calcite crystals. A sarcoidal reaction to identifiable foreign material does not exclude sarcoidosis. It has been suggested that particulate foreign material may serve as a nidus for granuloma formation in sarcoidosis.[89] Silica-rich birefringent particles have also been described in lesions without a history of injury or silica exposure.[90] Energy-dispersive X-ray analysis techniques using scanning electron microscopy can be used to identify elements present in the crystalline material.[91] The granulomas are thought to develop as a response to colloidal silica particles and not as a result of a hypersensitivity reaction.[92]

A granulomatous dermatitis may occur in response to pigments used in tattooing (see p. 440).[93,94] The skin lesions are sometimes limited to certain areas of a tattoo where a particular pigment has been used.[94] Two patterns are seen, a foreign body type and a sarcoid type.[95] In the latter form there are aggregates of epithelioid histiocytes and giant cells with a sparse peri-granulomatous round cell infiltrate. The histiocytes and giant cells contain pigment particles. True sarcoidosis has also been reported in tattoos, in some cases associated with pulmonary hilar lymphadenopathy. Some of these cases may represent a generalized sarcoid-like reaction to tattoo pigments rather than true sarcoidosis.[96,97] Other granulomatous complications of tattoos include tuberculosis cutis and leprosy.[98]

Zirconium compounds used in under-arm deodorants and other skin preparations have been associated with a granulomatous skin reaction in sensitized individuals.[99,100] Histologically, the lesions are identical to sarcoidosis. Usually no birefringent material is seen in polarized light. In one case of a reaction to an aluminum–zirconium complex, foreign body granulomas and birefringent particles were seen as well as tuberculoid type granulomas.[101] Ophthalmic drops containing sodium bisulfite have been implicated in the formation of pigmented papules on the face. The papules were caused by sarcoidal granulomas with brown-black pigment in foreign body giant cells.[102]

Sarcoidal granulomas have been reported at the injection sites of interferon, both interferon β-1b used in the treatment of multiple sclerosis,[103] and interferon α-2a used in the treatment of hepatitis C.[104]

In the past, cutaneous granulomatous lesions with histology similar to sarcoidosis have been reported in persons exposed to beryllium compounds in industry.[105,106] Other foreign bodies capable of inducing sarcoidal granulomas include acrylic and nylon fibers, wheat stubble and sea urchin spines.[107–109] Sea urchin spines can produce all types of granuloma, not only sarcoidal ones.

Occasionally, keratin from ruptured cysts or hair follicles can induce sarcoidal granulomas rather than the more usual foreign body type of reaction.

Table 7.1 **Foreign material producing sarcoidal granulomas**

Silica (including windshield glass)
Tattoo pigments
Zirconium
Beryllium
Zinc
Acrylic or nylon fibers
Keratin from ruptured cysts (uncommon)
Exogenous ochronosis
Sea-urchin spines
Cactus
Wheat stubble
Desensitizing injections
Ophthalmic drops (sodium bisulfite)
Sulfonamides
Interferon injection sites

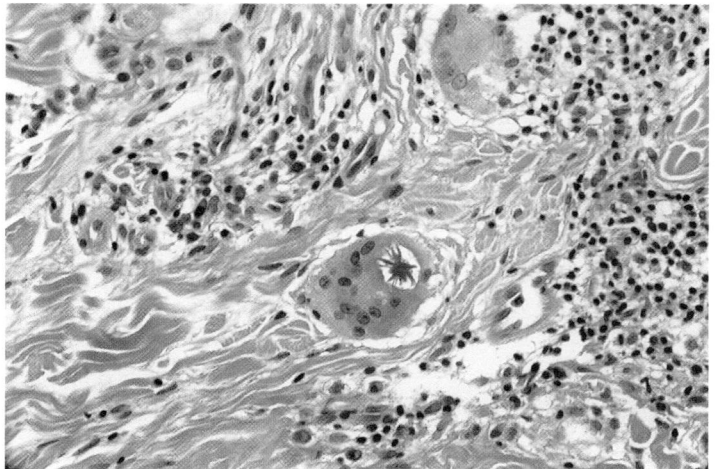

Fig. 7.2 **Sarcoidosis.** An asteroid body is present in the cytoplasm of a multinucleate giant cell. (H & E)

TUBERCULOID GRANULOMAS

While the granulomas in the tuberculoid group consist of collections of epithelioid histiocytes, including multinucleate forms, they tend to be less circumscribed than those in the sarcoidal group, have a greater tendency to confluence, and are surrounded by a substantial rim of lymphocytes and plasma cells. Langhans giant cells tend to be more characteristic of this group but foreign body type giant cells are also seen. There may be areas of caseation in the lesions of tuberculosis.

Tuberculoid granulomas are seen in the following conditions:

- tuberculosis
- tuberculids
- leprosy
- late syphilis
- leishmaniasis
- rosacea
- perioral dermatitis
- lupus miliaris disseminatus faciei
- Crohn's disease.

In addition to these diseases, tuberculoid granulomas, some with central necrosis, have been described at injection sites of protamine–insulin, as a hypersensitivity reaction to protamine.

TUBERCULOSIS

Typical tuberculoid granulomas can be seen in the dermal inflammatory reaction of late primary inoculation tuberculosis, late miliary tuberculosis, tuberculosis cutis orificialis, tuberculosis verrucosa cutis ('prosector's wart'), scrofuloderma and lupus vulgaris.[110] Cutaneous tuberculosis is discussed in detail with the bacterial infections (see p. 625). A similar pattern of inflammation can be seen after BCG vaccination and immunotherapy.[111,112]

Histopathology
Santa Cruz and Strayer have stressed the variety of histological changes seen in cutaneous tuberculosis.[113] In many forms, particularly in early lesions, there is a mixture of inflammatory cells within the dermis which includes histiocytes and multinucleate cells without well-formed epithelioid granulomas. The changes seen in the overlying epidermis are variable. In some forms inflammatory changes extend into the subcutis. Areas of caseation may or may not be present within granulomas. In some cases this may be difficult to distinguish from the necrobiosis seen in rheumatoid nodules (see p. 204). The number of acid-fast organisms varies in different lesions. In lesions with caseation, organisms are most frequently found in the centers of necrotic foci.[114] Generally, where there are well-formed granulomas without caseation necrosis, organisms are absent or difficult to find. Neutrophils may be a component of the inflammatory infiltrate, and abscesses form in some clinical subtypes. Both Schaumann bodies and asteroid bodies can occasionally be present in multinucleate giant cells.

In lesions with caseation and demonstrable acid-fast organisms, the histological diagnosis may be straightforward. In lupus vulgaris, however, caseation necrosis, if present, is minimal and organisms are rarely found. Evidence of mycobacterial infection may be determined by polymerase chain reaction techniques.[115]

Histological differential diagnosis
There is usually a heavier round cell infiltrate about tuberculous granulomas

than is seen in sarcoidosis. It is to be remembered that the small foci of fibrinous material that sometimes are seen in the granulomas of sarcoidosis may mimic and be mistaken for caseation. Epidermal changes and dermal fibrosis are not commonly part of the histopathology of sarcoidosis.

Lesions of other non-tuberculous mycobacterial infections of the skin, such as those due to *Mycobacterium marinum*, may be histologically indistinguishable from cutaneous tuberculosis. Organisms are usually difficult to find in *M. marinum* infections; they are described as being longer and broader than typical *M. tuberculosis*. Culture or PCR is required for species identification.

The combination of marked irregular epidermal hyperplasia, epidermal and dermal abscesses and dermal tuberculoid granulomas may be seen in tuberculosis verrucosa cutis, caused by *M. tuberculosis*, and in swimming pool granuloma due to *M. marinum* infection. This reaction pattern is also seen in cutaneous fungal infections such as sporotrichosis, chromomycosis and blastomycosis. Diagnosis depends on identification of the appropriate organism.

The lesions of tuberculosis cutis orificialis must be distinguished from those of oral or anal Crohn's disease and from the Melkersson–Rosenthal syndrome (see p. 208). This is not always possible on histological grounds and may depend on clinical history and associated lesions. Foci of caseation and acid-fast organisms may be seen in tuberculous lesions. Marked edema and granulomas related to or in the lumen of dilated lymphatic channels are present in the Melkersson–Rosenthal syndrome.

TUBERCULIDS

The tuberculids are a heterogeneous group of cutaneous disorders associated with tuberculous infections elsewhere in the body or in other parts of the skin (see p. 627). They include lichen scrofulosorum, papulonecrotic tuberculid and erythema induratum–nodular vasculitis. Although it has previously been thought that organisms are not found in tuberculids, recent PCR studies have demonstrated mycobacterial DNA in some cases (see p. 627).[115]

In *lichen scrofulosorum* there is a superficial inflammatory reaction about hair follicles and sweat ducts which may include tuberculoid granulomas. Acid-fast organisms are not usually seen or cultured from the lesions.[116] Caseation is rare.[117]

Histopathologic studies of *papulonecrotic tuberculid* have shown a subacute or granulomatous vasculitis and dermal coagulative necrosis with, in some cases, a surrounding palisading histiocytic reaction resembling granuloma annulare.[118] Acid-fast bacilli are not found in the lesions. Tuberculoid granulomas were not described in one study[119] but have been recorded in others.[110]

In *erythema induratum–nodular vasculitis* there is a lobular panniculitis, although tuberculoid granulomas usually extend into the deep dermis (see p. 524).

LEPROSY

Tuberculoid granulomas are seen in the tuberculoid (TT), borderline tuberculoid (BT) and borderline (BB) groups of the classification of leprosy introduced by Ridley and Jopling.[120] Leprosy is considered further on page 629.

Histopathology[121]
In tuberculoid leprosy (TT), single or grouped epithelioid granulomas with a peripheral rim of lymphocytes are distributed throughout the dermis and subcutis. Unlike lepromatous leprosy this infiltrate does not spare the upper papillary dermis (grenz zone) and it may extend into and destroy the basal layer and part of the stratum malpighii. The granulomas are characteristically arranged in and around neurovascular bundles and arrectores pilorum

muscles. Granulomas, particularly in the deeper parts of the infiltrate, tend to be oval and elongated along the course of the nerves and vessels (Fig. 7.3). Small cutaneous nerve bundles are infiltrated and enlarged by the inflammatory cells. There may be destruction of nerves, sometimes with caseation necrosis which may mimic cutaneous tuberculosis. In contrast, the infiltrate in tuberculosis is not particularly related to nerves. The granulomas in tuberculoid leprosy may contain well-formed Langhans-type giant cells and less well-formed multinucleate foreign body giant cells. The causative organism, *Mycobacterium leprae*, which is best demonstrated by modifications of the Ziehl–Neelsen stain such as the Wade–Fite method, is usually not found in the lesions of tuberculoid leprosy. Rare organisms may be present in nerve fibers. PCR has been used to demonstrate DNA of *M. leprae* in lesions.[13]

Granulomas in the *borderline tuberculoid form* (BT) are surrounded by fewer lymphocytes, contain more foreign body giant cells than Langhans cells, and may or may not extend up to the epidermis. Organisms may be found in small numbers or not at all. Nerve bundle enlargement is not so prominent and there is no caseation necrosis or destruction of the epidermis.

In the *borderline form* (BB) the granulomas are poorly formed and the epithelioid cells separated by edema. Scant lymphocytes are present about the granulomas and there are no giant cells. Nerve involvement is slight. Organisms are found, usually only in small numbers.

LATE SYPHILIS

Some lesions of late secondary syphilis and nodular lesions of tertiary syphilis show a superficial and deep dermal inflammatory reaction in which there are tuberculoid granulomas (see p. 650).[122] Plasma cells are generally but not always prominent in the inflammatory infiltrate and there may be swelling of endothelial cells.[123,124] One recent study has found that a plasma cell infiltrate and endothelial swelling, traditionally associated with syphilis of the skin, are in fact infrequently seen in biopsies.[125] Organisms are rarely demonstrable in these lesions.

LEISHMANIASIS

In chronic cutaneous leishmaniasis (see p. 721) and leishmaniasis recidivans, tuberculoid granulomas are present in the upper and lower dermis.[126] The overlying epidermal changes are variable. Occasionally the granulomas extend to the basal layer of the epidermis as in tuberculoid leprosy.[127] Necrosis is not usually seen in the granulomas.[128] Leishmaniae are usually scarce but may be found in histiocytes or, rarely, free in the dermis. The organisms have sometimes been mistaken for *Histoplasma capsulatum* but differ from the latter in having a kinetoplast.

ROSACEA

Rosacea is characterized by persistent erythema and telangiectasia, predominantly of the cheeks but also affecting the chin, nose and forehead (see p. 484). In the papular form, papules and papulopustules are superimposed on this background. Tuberculoid granulomas are seen in the granulomatous form. Granulomatous rosacea has been reported in children as well as adults, and in association with infection with the human immunodeficiency virus (HIV).[129–131] Granulomas may be a response to Demodex organisms or lipids.[132,133] Granulomas have also been described in the lesions of pyoderma faciale, thought to be an extreme form of rosacea.[134]

Histopathology[135]

The changes seen in biopsies of the papules are variable and relate to the age of the lesion. Early lesions may show only a mild perivascular lymphocytic infiltrate in the dermis. In older lesions there is a mixed inflammatory infiltrate related to the vessels or to vessels and pilosebaceous units. The infiltrate consists of lymphocytes and histiocytes with variable numbers of plasma cells and multinucleate giant cells of Langhans or foreign body type. In some lesions epithelioid histiocytes and giant cells are organized into tuberculoid granulomas (granulomatous rosacea) (Fig. 7.4).[136] An acute folliculitis with follicular and perifollicular pustules and destruction of the hair follicle is sometimes seen. Granulomatous inflammation may be centered on identifiable ruptured hair follicles. There is dermal edema and vascular dilatation. Epidermal changes, if present, are mild and non-specific.

In granulomatous rosacea, the granulomas are usually of tuberculoid type and not the 'naked' granulomas of sarcoidosis (see p. 195). Changes resembling caseous necrosis may be present, associated with a histiocytic reaction. In one series, necrosis was present in 11% of cases.[129] Differentiation from lupus vulgaris may be difficult. In some cases of rosacea the inflammatory changes may be related to damaged hair follicles. The presence of marked vascular dilatation is suggestive of rosacea.

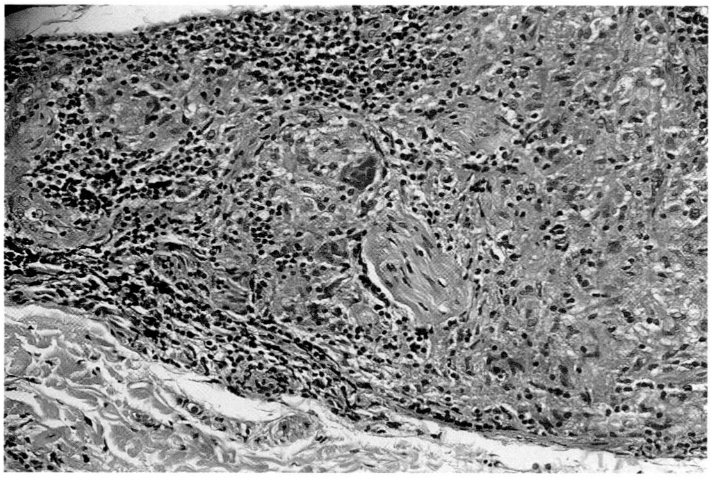

Fig. 7.3 **Leprosy.** The tuberculoid granuloma is elongated along the course of a nerve in the deep dermis. (H & E)

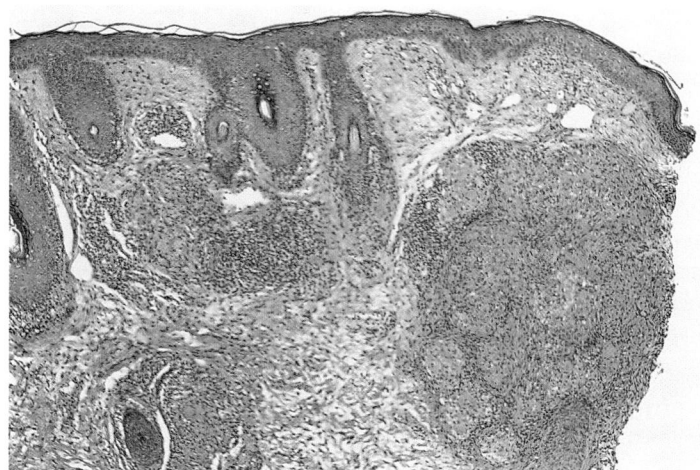

Fig. 7.4 **Granulomatous rosacea.** Tuberculoid granulomas are present in the dermis. There is some telangiectasia of vessels in the superficial dermis. (H & E)

PERIORAL DERMATITIS

Perioral dermatitis is regarded by some as a distinct entity[137] and by others as a variant of rosacea.[138] The histological changes seen in perioral dermatitis and acne rosacea overlap, and clinical features are often more important in separating these two conditions.[139]

Red papules, papulovesicles or papulopustules on a background of erythema are arranged symmetrically on the chin and nasolabial folds with a characteristic clear zone around the lips. Lesions may occur less commonly on the lower aspect of the cheeks and on the forehead.[140] A periocular variant has also been described.[141,142] Perioral dermatitis chiefly affects young women, but it has also been reported in children.[143–145] Granulomatous perioral dermatitis of childhood is particularly seen in children of Afro-Caribbean descent. This form has been given the acronym FACE – facial Afro-Caribbean childhood eruption.[146–148] In many cases the eruption appears to be related to the application of one or more cosmetic preparations which may act by occlusion.[149] The use of strong topical corticosteroids, particularly fluorinated ones, may also have an etiologic role.[150,151] Various types of toothpaste have been implicated.[152,153] Perioral dermatitis has been reported in renal transplant recipients maintained on oral corticosteroids and azathioprine.[154] It has also been associated with the wearing of the veil by Arab women.[155]

Histopathology

The histological changes in perioral dermatitis have been described as identical to those seen in rosacea.[138,143] Others have found the epidermal changes to be more prominent than in rosacea, consisting of parakeratosis, often related to hair follicle ostia, spongiosis, which sometimes involves the hair follicle, and slight acanthosis.[156] The changes in the dermis are similar to those in papular rosacea and consist of perivascular or perifollicular infiltrates of lymphocytes and histiocytes and vascular ectasia. Uncommonly, an acute folliculitis is present. Tuberculoid granulomas have been described in the dermis in some series, but not in others.[156]

LUPUS MILIARIS DISSEMINATUS FACIEI

Although the cause of lupus miliaris disseminatus faciei is unknown, it may be related to rosacea.[157] It has also been called acne agminata and acnitis. It is characterized by yellowish brown papules distributed over the central part of the face, including the eyebrows and eyelids. When widespread facial lesions are present, the appearances may mimic sarcoidosis.[158] Occasionally lesions occur elsewhere, including the axillae.[159,160] The lesions last for months and heal with scarring.[161] This condition occurs in both sexes, predominantly in adolescents and young adults and rarely in the elderly.[162,163] It has been suggested that as the currently used name is confusing, a new title should be substituted – FIGURE (*facial idiopathic granulomas with regressive evolution*).[164]

Studies using PCR techniques have failed to demonstrate the DNA of *M. tuberculosis* in lesional skin.[165]

Histopathology

There are few histopathological studies of this condition.[166] Biopsy appearances overlap those of both rosacea and perioral dermatitis. The characteristic lesion is an area of dermal necrosis, sometimes described as caseation necrosis, surrounded by epithelioid histiocytes, multinucleate giant cells and lymphocytes (Fig. 7.5). In many cases granulomas appear related to ruptured pilosebaceous units.[167] Nuclear fragments may be seen in the necrotic foci. Early lesions show superficial perivascular infiltrates of lymphocytes, histiocytes and occasional neutrophils. Late lesions have these changes

together with dermal fibrosis, particularly about follicles. Established lesions may show tuberculoid or suppurative granulomas. *Demodex folliculorum* were not seen in one study.[166] Small vessel changes with necrosis of blood vessel walls, thrombi and extravasated red blood cells have also been described.[159] Acid-fast bacilli are not found in the areas of necrosis and there is no evidence that this condition is related to tuberculosis (see above).

One study of lysozyme in these lesions suggests that there is an immunological mechanism involved in the pathogenesis of this condition rather than a foreign body reaction to an unidentified dermal agent.[168] Conversely, it has been suggested that the lesions represent a granulomatous reaction to damaged pilosebaceous units.[169]

CROHN'S DISEASE

Non-caseating granulomas of tuberculoid type may be found, rarely, in the dermis and subcutis in Crohn's disease (see p. 554). However, they are not uncommon in the wall of perianal sinuses and fistulas. A granulomatous cheilitis has also been reported (see p. 208).[170] It is important to exclude Crohn's disease in cases of apparent Melkersson–Rosenthal syndrome.[171]

There is even a report of cutaneous granulomas developing in a patient with histologically proven ulcerative colitis.[172]

NECROBIOTIC GRANULOMAS

The term 'necrobiosis' has been retained here because of common usage and refers to areas of altered dermal connective tissue in which, by light microscopy, there is blurring and loss of definition of collagen bundles, sometimes separation of fibers, a decrease in connective tissue nuclei and an alteration in staining by routine histological stains, often with increased basophilia or eosinophilia. Granular stringy mucin is sometimes seen in such areas in granuloma annulare, and fibrin may be seen in rheumatoid nodules. Necrobiotic areas are partially or completely surrounded by a histiocytic rim which may include multinucleate giant cells. In some cases histiocytes become more spindle-shaped and form a 'palisade'.

Necrobiotic granulomas[173] are found in the following conditions:

- granuloma annulare and its variants
- necrobiosis lipoidica

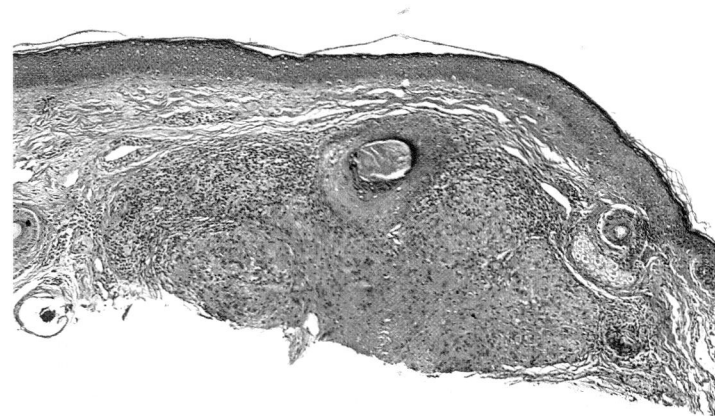

Fig. 7.5 **Lupus miliaris disseminatus faciei.** A shave biopsy of one of several papules near the lower eyelid. (H & E)

- necrobiotic xanthogranuloma
- rheumatoid nodules
- rheumatic fever nodules
- reactions to foreign materials and vaccines.

GRANULOMA ANNULARE

Granuloma annulare is a dermatosis of unknown etiology in which characteristic necrobiotic granulomas are seen in typical examples.[174] Either the skin or the subcutis, or both, may be involved. The clinical variants of granuloma annulare include localized, generalized, perforating[175] and subcutaneous or deep forms.[176,177] Rare types include a follicular pustulous variant and a patch form,[178] although the latter cases are probably examples of the interstitial granulomatous form of drug reaction (see p. 212). The linear variant reported some years ago would now be regarded as a variant of interstitial granulomatous dermatitis (see p. 211).[179]

In the *localized form*, one or more erythematous or skin-colored papules are found. Grouped papules tend to form annular or arciform plaques. The hands, feet, arms and legs are the sites of predilection in some 80% of cases.[180] A papular umbilicated form has been described in children in which grouped umbilicated flesh-colored papules are limited to the dorsum of the hands and fingers.[181] The *generalized form* accounts for approximately 15% of cases.[174,182] Multiple macules, papules or nodules are distributed over the trunk and limbs.[183] Rarely there may be confluent erythematous patches or plaques.[184,185] It has been reported as a side-effect of allopurinol.[186] Lesions in *perforating granuloma annulare* are grouped papules, some of which have a central umbilication with scale.[187] The extremities are the most common site. The generalized form may also have perforating lesions.[188] A high incidence of perforating granuloma annulare has been reported in Hawaii.[189] In *subcutaneous (or deep) granuloma annulare*, deep dermal or subcutaneous nodules are found on the lower legs, hands, head and buttocks. These lesions are associated with superficial papules in 25% of cases.[190] This group also includes those lesions described as pseudorheumatoid nodules, palisading subcutaneous granuloma and benign rheumatoid nodules.[191–193] Although arthritis does not usually occur in children with these nodular lesions IgM rheumatoid factor has been found in serum in some cases.[194,195] There is a report of one case occurring in association with juvenile rheumatoid arthritis.[193] Computed tomography (CT) scan changes of this variant have been described.[196] Rarely, the changes may involve deeper soft tissues and produce a destructive arthritis and limb deformity.[197] The author remains to be convinced that all cases previously reported as juxta-articular pseudo-rheumatoid nodules are synonymous with deep granuloma annulare. Some cases have an identical histological appearance to rheumatoid nodules and exhibit both fibrin and small amounts of mucin in the necrobiotic center.

Granuloma annulare has been reported as a seasonal eruption on the elbows or hands[198,199] and from unusual sites such as the penis,[200,201] palms,[202] about the eyes[203–206] and ear.[207] There has been one case of cutaneous granuloma annulare associated with histologically similar intra-abdominal visceral lesions in a male with insulin-dependent diabetes.[208]

Females are affected more than twice as commonly as males. The localized and deep forms are more common in children and young adults. Generalized granuloma annulare occurs most frequently in middle-aged to elderly adults. Most cases of granuloma annulare are sporadic but familial cases have occasionally been reported.[209] Patients with the generalized form of the disease show a significantly higher frequency of HLA-BW35 compared with controls and with those who have the localized form of the disease.[210]

Lesions of granuloma annulare have a tendency to regress spontaneously; however, about 40% of cases recur.[180] Spontaneous regression of localized lesions in children occurred, in one series, from 6 months to 7 years, with a mean of 2.5 years.[211] In the generalized form, the clinical course is chronic with infrequent spontaneous resolution and poor response to therapy.[183] Non-perforating lesions are usually asymptomatic.[212]

Although the etiology and pathogenesis of the skin lesions in granuloma annulare remain uncertain, possible triggering events include insect bites, trauma, the presence of viral warts, erythema multiforme and exposure to sunlight.[213–215] Lesions have occurred in the scars of herpes zoster, localized or generalized,[216–218] and at the sites of tuberculin skin tests.[219] The possible link between both the localized and generalized forms and diabetes mellitus remains controversial. There is more convincing evidence of this association with the generalized form than with the localized form although there may be a weak association with nodular as opposed to the annular type of localized lesion.[220–222] It has been reported in association with sarcoidosis,[223] Alagille syndrome,[224] autoimmune thyroiditis,[225] hepatitis C infection,[226] waxing-induced pseudofolliculitis,[227] tattoos,[228] granulomatous mycosis fungoides,[229] a monoclonal gammopathy,[230] myelodysplastic syndrome,[231] Hodgkin's lymphoma, non-Hodgkin's lymphoma and metastatic adenocarcinoma.[232–234] In these conditions, the clinical presentation may be atypical.[235] Localized, generalized and perforating forms of granuloma annulare have been reported in patients with AIDS; the generalized form is the most common clinical pattern.[236–242] It may, rarely, be the presenting complaint in AIDS.[243]

It has been suggested that the underlying cause of the necrobiotic granulomas is an immunoglobulin-mediated vasculitis.[244] In a recent study, neutrophils and neutrophil fragments were commonly present in early lesions but a true vasculitis was rare. Direct immunofluorescence studies did not demonstrate immune deposits in vessel walls.[245] Other studies have stressed the importance of cell-mediated immune mechanisms.[246] Collagen synthesis is increased in the lesions of granuloma annulare, probably representing a reparative phenomenon.[247]

Histopathology

Three histological patterns may be seen in granuloma annulare – necrobiotic granulomas, an interstitial or 'incomplete' form, and granulomas of sarcoidal or tuberculoid type. The third of these patterns is uncommon.[248] In most histopathological studies, the interstitial form is most common.[249]

In the form with *necrobiotic granulomas*, one or more areas of necrobiosis, surrounded by histiocytes and lymphocytes, are present in the superficial and mid dermis (Fig. 7.6). The peripheral rim of histiocytes may form a palisaded pattern (Fig. 7.7). Variable numbers of multinucleate giant cells are found in this zone. Some histiocytes have an epithelioid appearance. An increased mitotic rate is found in the histiocytes in some cases.[250] Surprisingly, in one series, the histiocytic component of the infiltrate stained only for vimentin and lysozyme and not the other common histiocyte markers (HAM56, CD68 (KP1), Mac-387 and factor XIIIa).[251] The intervening areas of the dermis between the necrobiotic granulomas are relatively normal compared with necrobiosis lipoidica, and there is no fibrosis. A perivascular infiltrate of lymphocytes and histiocytes is also present; eosinophils are found in 40–66% of cases but plasma cells are rare.[252,253] In contrast, plasma cells are not uncommon in necrobiosis lipoidica. The central necrobiotic areas contain increased amounts of connective tissue mucins which may appear as basophilic stringy material between collagen bundles. Special stains such as colloidal iron and alcian blue aid in the demonstration of mucin. Elastic fibers may be reduced, absent or unchanged in the involved skin.[254,255]

Occasionally, neutrophils or nuclear fragments are present in necrobiotic areas.[245] In the rare follicular-pustulous form there are neutrophils in the upper portion of the follicles leading to pustule formation. Palisading necrobiotic granulomas surround hair follicles.[256] An acute or subacute vasculitis

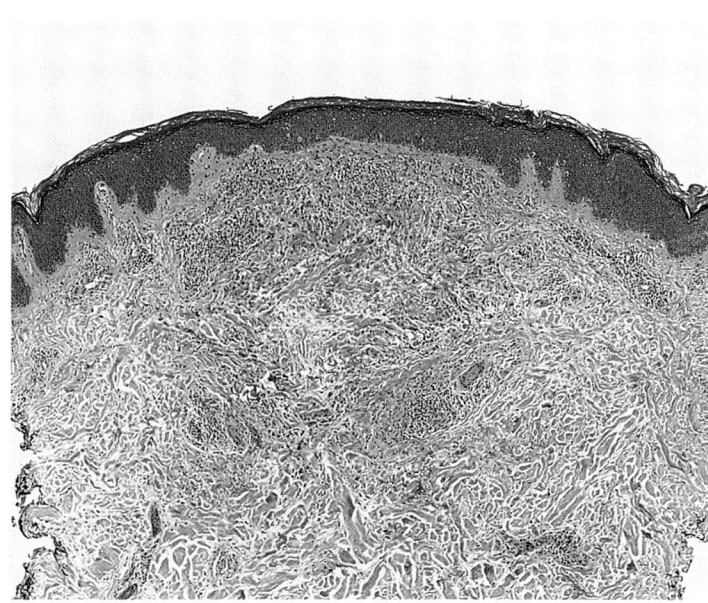

Fig. 7.6 **Granuloma annulare.** The inflammatory cell infiltrate surrounds the area of 'necrobiosis' on all sides. It is not 'open ended' as in necrobiosis lipoidica. (H & E)

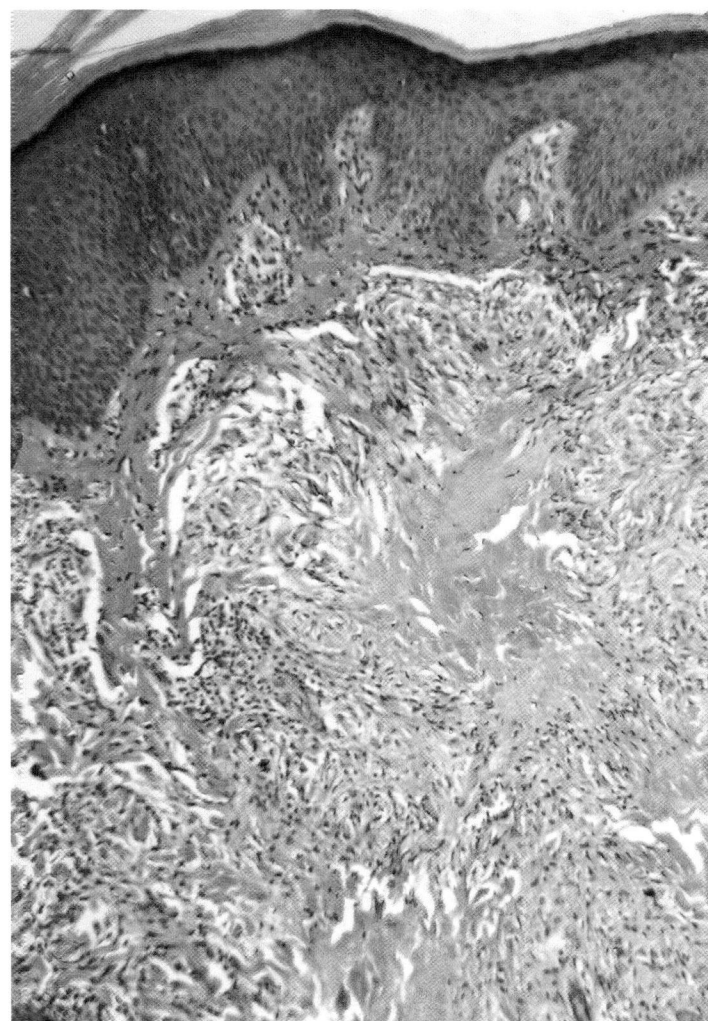

Fig. 7.7 **Granuloma annulare.** A palisade of inflammatory cells surrounds the central zone of 'necrobiosis'. (H & E)

has been described in or near foci of necrobiosis, associated with varying degrees of endothelial swelling, necrosis of vessel walls, fibrin exudation and nuclear dust.[244]

The lesions of subcutaneous or deep granuloma annulare have areas of necrobiosis which are often larger than in the superficial type (Fig. 7.8). These foci are distributed in the deep dermis, subcutis and, rarely, deep soft tissues.[197,257] There may be overlying superficial dermal lesions. Eosinophils are said to be more common in this variant than in the superficial lesions.

In the disseminated form of granuloma annulare, the granulomatous foci are often situated in the papillary dermis (Fig. 7.9). Necrobiosis may be inconspicuous. There is some superficial resemblance to lichen nitidus (see p. 39), although in disseminated granuloma annulare there are no acanthotic downgrowths of the epidermis at the periphery of the lesions.

In the *interstitial* or *'incomplete' form* of granuloma annulare, the histological changes are subtle and best assessed at lower power. The dermis has a 'busy' look due to increased numbers of inflammatory cells, mainly histiocytes and lymphocytes (Fig. 7.10). They are arranged about vessels and between collagen bundles which are separated by increased connective tissue mucin. There are no formed areas of necrobiosis. In some cases the interstitial component is minimal. A similar appearance can be seen in the interstitial

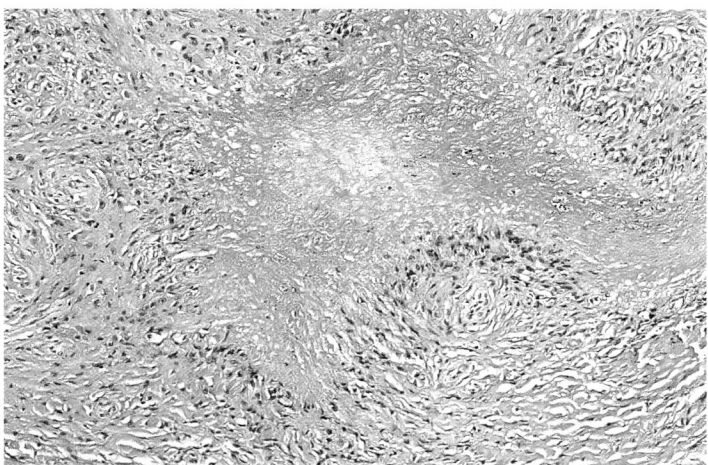

Fig. 7.8 **Subcutaneous granuloma annulare.** There are large areas of 'necrobiosis' surrounded by a palisade of lymphocytes and histiocytes. (H & E)

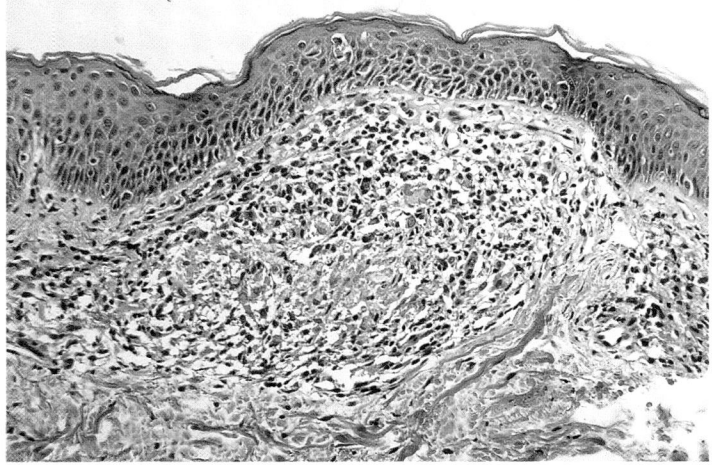

Fig. 7.9 **Disseminated granuloma annulare with involvement of the papillary dermis.** There are no acanthotic downgrowths of rete pegs at the margins of the inflammatory focus, as seen in lichen nitidus. 'Necrobiosis' may be subtle in this form of granuloma annulare. (H & E)

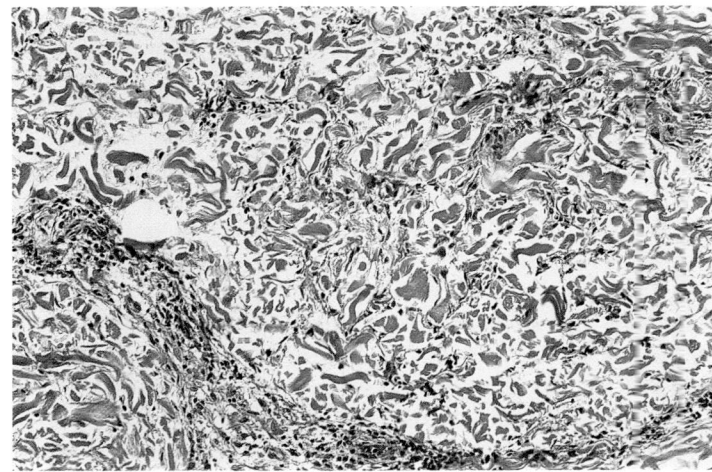

Fig. 7.10 **Granuloma annulare of 'incomplete' type.** The dermis is hypercellular (a so-called 'busy dermis') and there is an increased amount of interstitial mucin. (H & E)

granulomatous drug reaction (see p. 212) although in the latter condition true necrobiosis is uncommon, and, if present, localized. Furthermore, eosinophils are often present and there may be lichenoid changes at the dermal–epidermal interface. In interstitial granulomatous dermatitis there are both neutrophils and eosinophils in the infiltrate, although both cell types may be sparse. Another characteristic feature is the presence of a palisade of histiocytes around one or many collagen fibers, which often have a basophilic hue.

Cases of the non-necrobiotic *sarcoidal or tuberculoid type* of granuloma annulare are uncommon and pose a diagnostic problem. The presence of increased dermal mucin or eosinophils may be helpful distinguishing features. Eosinophils and obvious mucin are not seen in sarcoidosis.[252] However, granuloma annulare and sarcoidosis have been reported in the same patient.[258]

In most cases of granuloma annulare, the epidermal changes are minimal. Perforating lesions have a central epidermal perforation which communicates with an underlying necrobiotic granuloma (Fig. 7.11). At the edges of the perforation there are varying degrees of downward epidermal hyperplasia to form a channel. The channel contains necrobiotic material and cellular debris. There is surface hyperkeratosis.[175] The lesions sometimes perforate by way of a hair follicle.[259]

Immunofluorescence studies have shown fibrin in areas of necrobiosis.[258] IgM and C3 were present in blood vessel walls in one series.[244]

Immunoperoxidase techniques have demonstrated activated T lymphocytes with an excess of helper/inducer phenotype and CD1-positive dendritic cells related to Langerhans cells in the perivascular and granulomatous infiltrates.[246] A study of the staining pattern of lysozyme in the inflammatory cell infiltrate suggests that this may be useful in distinguishing granuloma annulare from other necrobiotic granulomas.[260] The distribution of the inhibitor of metalloproteinase-1 is different in granuloma annulare and necrobiosis lipoidica.[261]

Electron microscopy

Ultrastructural studies have confirmed the presence of histiocytes in the dermal infiltrate together with cellular debris and fibroblasts. Degenerative changes in collagen in areas of necrobiosis include swelling, loss of periodic banding and fragmentation of fibers. Elastic fibers also show degenerative changes. Fibrin and other amorphous material is present in interstitial areas.[262]

NECROBIOSIS LIPOIDICA

Necrobiosis lipoidica was originally called 'necrobiosis lipoidica diabeticorum' but, although some cases are associated with diabetes mellitus,[263,264] it is not peculiar to diabetes.[265] In one recent series only 11% of patients with necrobiosis lipoidica had diabetes mellitus at presentation, while a further 11% developed impaired glucose tolerance/diabetes in the succeeding 15 years.[266] The incidence in diabetics is low – approximately 3 cases per 1000.[263] It is even lower in childhood diabetes.[267]

The legs, particularly the shins, are overwhelmingly the commonest site of involvement, but lesions may also occur on the forearms, hands and trunk. Unusual sites include the nipple, penis and surgical scars.[268–271] Three-quarters of cases are bilateral at presentation and many more become bilateral later. Lesions may be single but are more often multiple. Diffuse disease is rare.[272] Females are affected more than males in a ratio of 3 to 1. The average age of onset in one series was 34 years, but the condition may be seen in children.[273]

The earliest lesions are red papules which enlarge radially to become patches or plaques with an atrophic, slightly depressed, shiny yellow-brown center and a well-defined raised red to purplish edge. Some lesions resolve spontaneously but many are persistent and chronic and may ulcerate;[274–276] this occurred in 13% of cases in one series.[277] Rarely, squamous cell carcinoma may arise in long-standing lesions.[278–280] The simultaneous occurrence of necrobiosis lipoidica with granuloma annulare[281] and with sarcoidosis has been reported.[282,283]

The association of these lesions with diabetes has already been referred to but the role of this metabolic disorder in the development of the cutaneous lesions is not understood. Diabetic vascular changes may be important: in some early lesions a necrotizing vasculitis has been described.[284] The finding in areas of sclerotic collagen of Glut-1, a protein responsible for glucose transport across epithelial and endothelial barrier tissue, raises the possibility that a disturbance in glucose transport by fibroblasts may contribute to the histological findings.[285] Adults and children with insulin-dependent diabetes mellitus and necrobiosis lipoidica are at high risk for diabetic nephropathy and retinopathy.[286]

Histopathology

The histopathological changes in necrobiosis lipoidica involve the full thickness of the dermis and often the subcutis (Fig. 7.12). Early lesions are not often biopsied. They are said to show a superficial and deep perivascular and interstitial mixed inflammatory cell infiltrate in the dermis. Similar changes are present in septa of adipose tissue. A necrotizing vasculitis with adjacent areas of necrobiosis and necrosis of adnexal structures is also seen.[284]

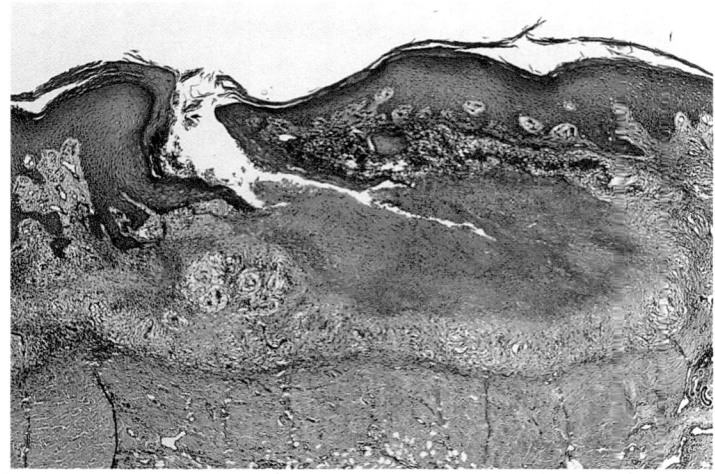

  Fig. 7.11 **Perforating granuloma annulare.** (H & E)

In active chronic lesions there is some variability between cases. The characteristic changes are seen at the edge of the lesions. These changes involve most of the dermis but particularly its lower two-thirds. Areas of

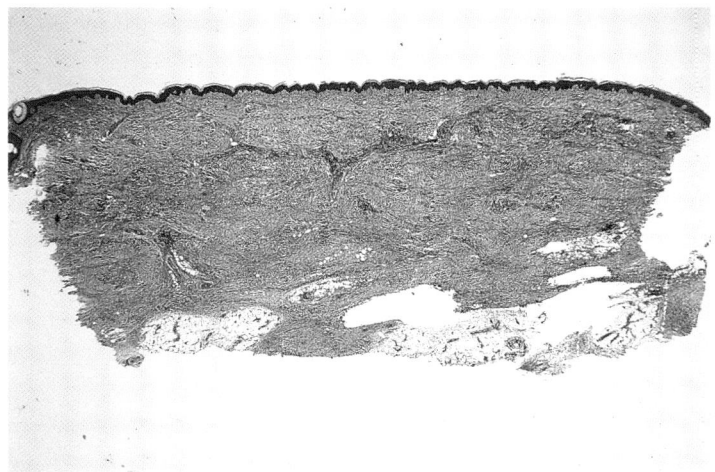

Fig. 7.12 **Necrobiosis lipoidica.** There is involvement of the full thickness of the dermis with extension into the subcutis. (H & E)

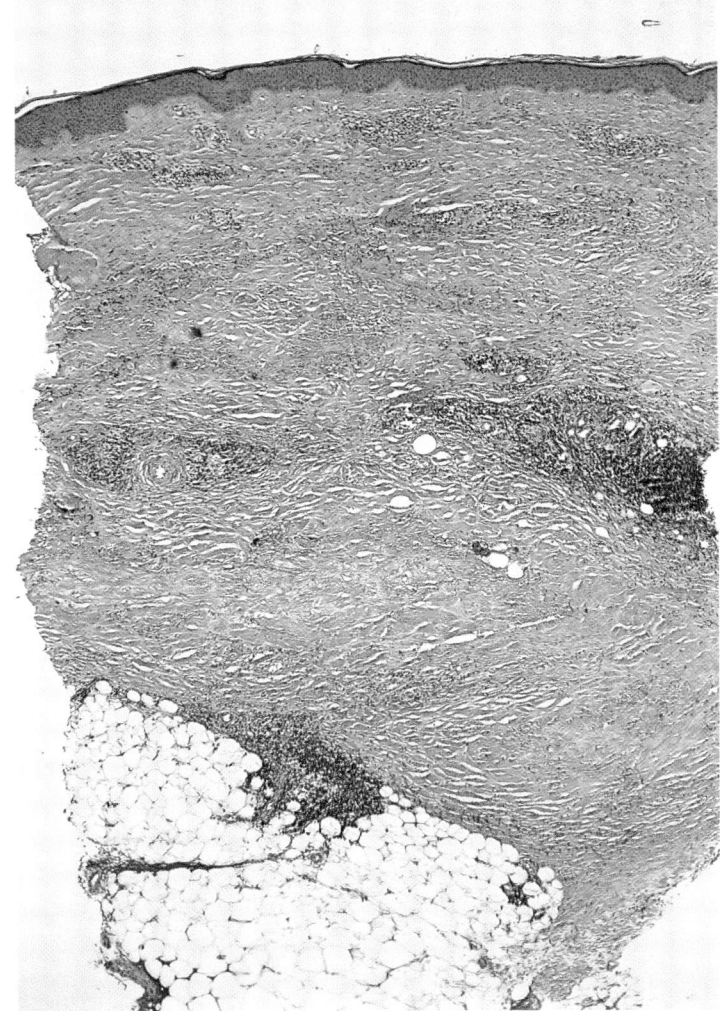

Fig. 7.13 **Necrobiosis lipoidica.** There are several layers of 'necrobiosis' within the dermis. (H & E)

necrobiosis may be extensive or slight: they are often more extensive and less well defined than in granuloma annulare (Fig. 7.13). The intervening areas of the dermis are also abnormal. Histiocytes, including variable numbers of multinucleate Langhans or foreign body giant cells, outline the areas of necrobiosis. The necrobiosis tends to be irregular and less complete than in granuloma annulare. There is a variable amount of dermal fibrosis and a superficial and deep perivascular inflammatory reaction which, in contrast to the usual picture in granuloma annulare, includes plasma cells (Fig. 7.14). Occasional eosinophils may be present.[252] In some cases necrobiotic areas are less frequent and there are collections of epithelioid histiocytes and multinucleate cells, particularly about dermal vessels. The dermal changes extend into the underlying septa of the subcutis and into the periphery of fat lobules. This septal panniculitis may resemble erythema nodosum but in that condition there are no significant dermal changes. Lymphoid cell aggregates, containing germinal centers, are present in the deep dermis or subcutis in approximately 10% of cases of necrobiosis lipoidica.[287]

In old atrophic lesions and in the center of plaques there is little necrobiosis and much dermal fibrosis. The underlying subcutis is also fibrotic. Elastic tissue stains demonstrate considerable loss of elastic tissue. Scattered histiocytes may be present.

The presence of lipid in necrobiotic areas (demonstrated by Sudan stains) has been used in the past to distinguish necrobiosis lipoidica from granuloma annulare, but subsequent studies have also shown lipid droplets in granuloma annulare.[255] Cholesterol clefts may be present, uncommonly, in areas of necrobiosis.[268,288] Rarely they are a conspicuous feature.[289] Fibrin can also be demonstrated in necrobiotic areas.[264] There may be small amounts of mucin in the affected dermis but the presence of large amounts in areas of necrobiosis favors a diagnosis of granuloma annulare.

Vascular changes are more prominent in necrobiosis lipoidica, particularly in the deeper vessels.[173] These range from endothelial swelling to a lymphocytic vasculitis and perivasculitis. Epithelioid granulomas may be present in the vessel wall or adjacent to it. In old lesions the wall may show fibrous thickening. The smaller, more superficial vessels are increased in number and telangiectatic. Apart from atrophy and ulceration, epidermal changes are unremarkable in necrobiosis lipoidica. Transepidermal elimination of degenerate collagen has been reported;[289,290] it may be associated with focal acanthosis or pseudo-epitheliomatous hyperplasia.

Although in most cases it is possible to distinguish necrobiosis lipoidica from granuloma annulare, there are cases in which this is difficult both clinically and

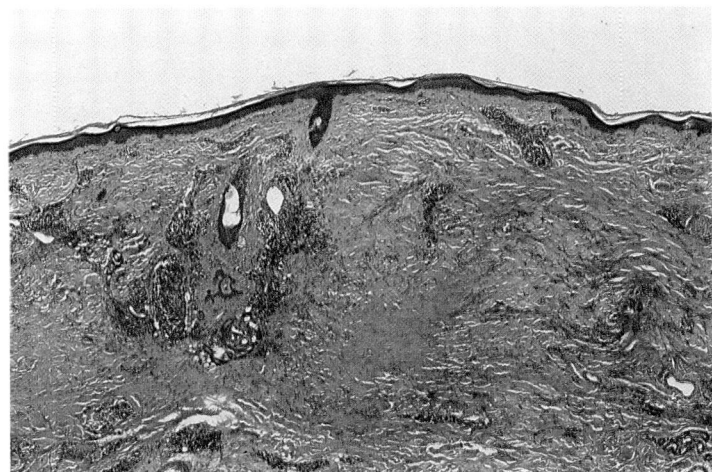

Fig. 7.14 **Necrobiosis lipoidica.** A perivascular inflammatory cell infiltrate is present in the dermis. There is 'necrobiosis' of the adjacent collagen. (H & E)

histologically.[264] There may also be difficulties distinguishing between necrobiosis lipoidica and necrobiotic xanthogranuloma (see below). Cholesterol clefts and transepidermal elimination may occur in both these conditions. Clinical features are usually distinctive in necrobiotic xanthogranuloma but not all cases are associated with paraproteinemia or a periorbital distribution of lesions.[288, 291]

Immunofluorescence studies have demonstrated IgM and C3 in the walls of blood vessels in the involved skin. Fibrin is seen in necrobiotic areas. IgM, C3 and fibrinogen may be present at the dermoepidermal junction.[292]

Ultrastructural studies have shown degeneration of collagen and elastin in the lesions.[293] Another study has shown a decreased number of S100-positive nerves in plaques, in conformity with the cutaneous anesthesia that may be a feature of these lesions.[294]

NECROBIOTIC XANTHOGRANULOMA

Necrobiotic xanthogranuloma is a rare condition characterized by the presence of violaceous to red, partly xanthomatous plaques and nodules; there is a predilection for the periorbital area. A paraproteinemia is often present. The clinical course is chronic. It is discussed further in Chapter 40, page 1073.

Histopathology

There are broad zones of hyaline necrobiosis as well as granulomatous foci composed of histiocytes, foam cells and multinucleate cells (Fig. 7.15). The amount of xanthomatization is variable. Distinction from necrobiosis lipoidica is sometimes difficult on a small biopsy, but the clinical features of these two conditions are quite different.

RHEUMATOID NODULES

Skin manifestations, including rheumatoid nodules, are relatively common in rheumatoid arthritis.[295] These nodules occur in approximately 20% of patients, usually in the vicinity of joints. Sited primarily in the subcutaneous tissue, they may involve the deep and even the superficial dermis. They vary from millimeters to centimeters in size and consist of fibrous white masses in which there are creamy yellow irregular areas of necrobiosis. Old lesions may have clefts and cystic spaces in these regions. It is most probable that rheumatoid nodules result from a vasculitic process; however, even in very early lesions such a change may be difficult to demonstrate.[296] Nodules usually persist for months to years. Rarely, similar lesions occur in systemic lupus erythematosus.[297–299]

Multiple small nodules may develop on the hands, feet and ears during methotrexate therapy.[300] This event is known as 'accelerated rheumatoid nodulosis'.

Histopathology

There are one or more irregular areas of necrobiosis in the subcutis and dermis (Fig. 7.16). These are surrounded by a well-developed palisade of elongated histiocytes, with occasional lymphocytes, neutrophils, mast cells and foreign body giant cells.[301] The central necrobiotic focus is usually homogeneous and eosinophilic.[302] There is sometimes obvious fibrin. In contrast, the areas of necrobiosis in the subcutaneous or deep variant of granuloma annulare are often pale and mucinous with a tendency to basophilia. Old rheumatoid nodules may show areas of dense fibrosis, clefts and 'cystic' degeneration of the necrobiotic foci. The dermis and subcutis surrounding the necrobiotic granulomas show a perivascular round cell infiltrate which includes plasma cells. Eosinophils may be present. Uncommonly, an acute vasculitis is seen in the surrounding vessels and sometimes a necrotic blood

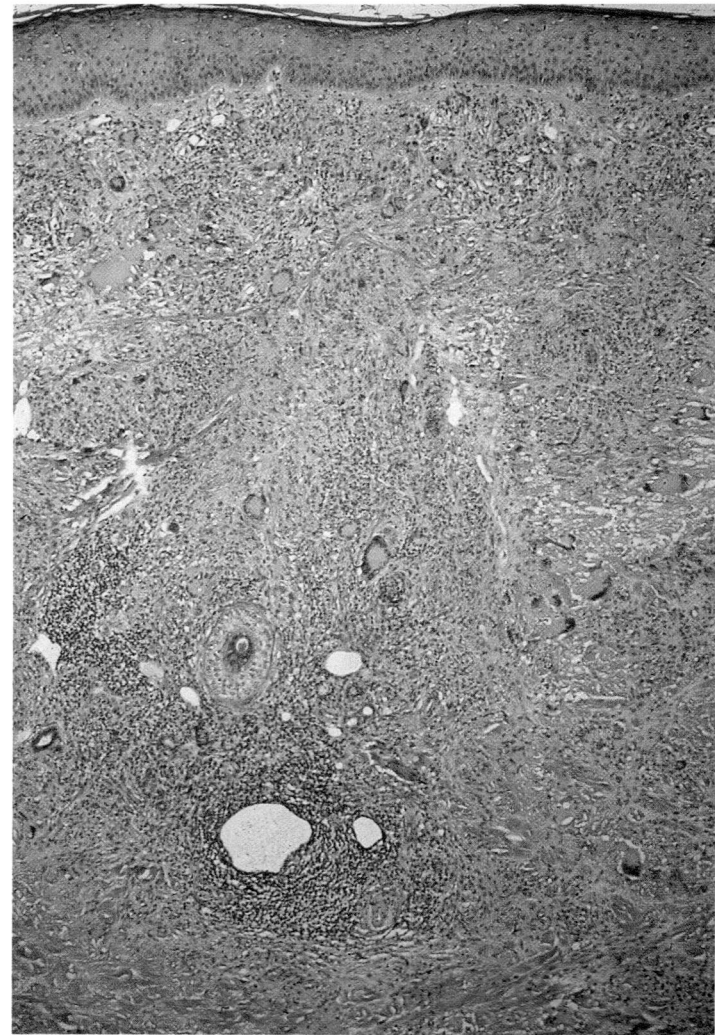

Fig. 7.15 **Necrobiotic xanthogranuloma.** The 'necrobiosis' is only focal. Numerous giant cells are present. (H & E)

vessel associated with nuclear fragments or sparse neutrophils may be seen in the center of areas of necrobiosis. Occasionally, a superficial nodule may perforate the epidermis.[303]

Fibrin is present in the center of the necrobiotic areas.[304] Rarely, immunoglobulins and complement have been demonstrated in vessels exhibiting a vasculitis. It is unusual to find mucin in necrobiotic foci in rheumatoid nodules, and this is the single most useful feature in distinguishing these lesions from the deep variant of granuloma annulare.[302] In some cases of deep granuloma annulare the changes are very similar to those of rheumatoid nodules; clinical information is most helpful in these instances.

RHEUMATIC FEVER NODULES

With the decline in the prevalence of rheumatic fever in developed countries, rheumatic nodules are now rarely seen or biopsied. Consequently, most histological studies are found in the older literature.[305] Nodules are more common in children than adults and are usually associated with acute rheumatic carditis. They are usually asymptomatic and are distributed symmetrically over bony prominences, particularly at the elbows.[306] Their size ranges from a few millimeters to 2–3 centimeters in diameter. The lesions, unlike rheumatoid nodules, last for only a short time and eventually involute.[305]

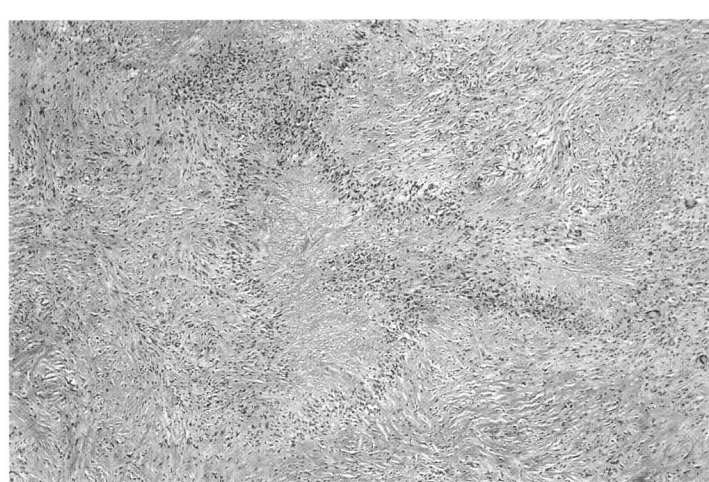
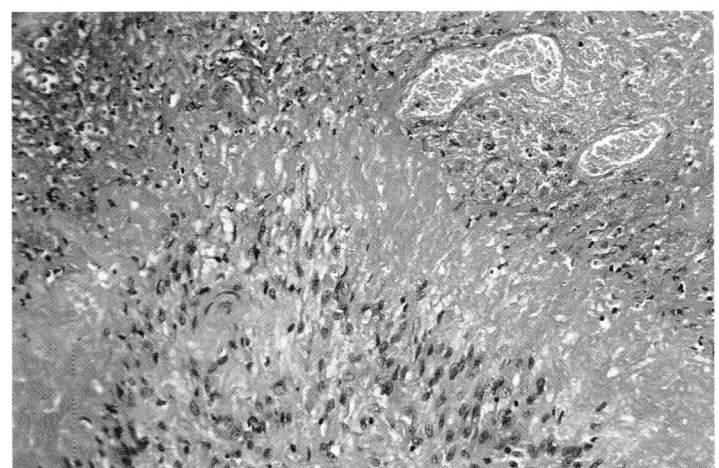

Fig. 7.16 **(A) Rheumatoid nodule. (B)** A palisade of elongate histiocytes surrounds a zone of 'necrobiosis'. (H & E)

Histopathology

Rheumatic nodules form in the subcutis or in the tissue deep to it. They include one or more foci of altered collagen (fibrinoid necrosis or fibrinoid change): this change is characterized by separation and swelling of the collagen bundles and increased eosinophilia. These foci may contain scattered inflammatory cells[306] or cell debris[305] and are surrounded by histiocytes, sometimes arranged in palisaded array.[305] Multinucleate histiocytes may be seen. A mixed inflammatory cell infiltrate is present at the periphery of these areas and around the vessels. Lipid may be seen in histiocytes about the altered collagen.[305] Apparent differences in the published histological description of these lesions may reflect differences in their age, early lesions being more exudative. A study of 40 rheumatic fever nodules, including ultrastructural features of two cases, has been published from India.[307]

REACTIONS TO FOREIGN MATERIALS AND VACCINES

Purified bovine collagen is currently being used, in the form of intracutaneous injections, to treat certain forms of superficial scarring (see p. 444). In some persons this results in a granulomatous reaction resembling granuloma annulare. There are irregular foci of eosinophilic necrobiosis surrounded by a palisading rim of multinucleate and mononuclear histiocytes, with lymphocytes and plasma cells.[308]

Areas of necrobiosis associated with a granulomatous reaction have also been described, rarely, in association with *Trichophyton rubrum* and with the presence of splinters of wood and suture material (Fig. 7.17).[309–311] Necrobiotic areas are also seen in cutaneous berylliosis. Changes which superficially resemble necrobiotic granulomas are also seen in injection sites of drugs of abuse.[312]

Necrobiotic palisaded granulomas have been reported at the sites of injection of hepatitis B vaccine and of disodium clodronate.[313,314]

SUPPURATIVE GRANULOMAS

The suppurative granulomas consist of collections of epithelioid histiocytes, with or without multinucleate giant cells, in the centers of which are collections of neutrophils (Fig. 7.18). Most of the conditions included in this group are

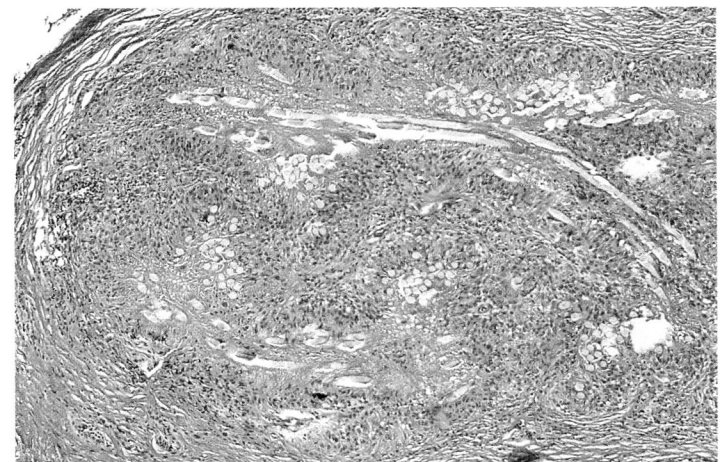

Fig. 7.17 **Suture granuloma.** There is a palisaded, centrally 'necrobiotic' granuloma to foreign material. (H & E)

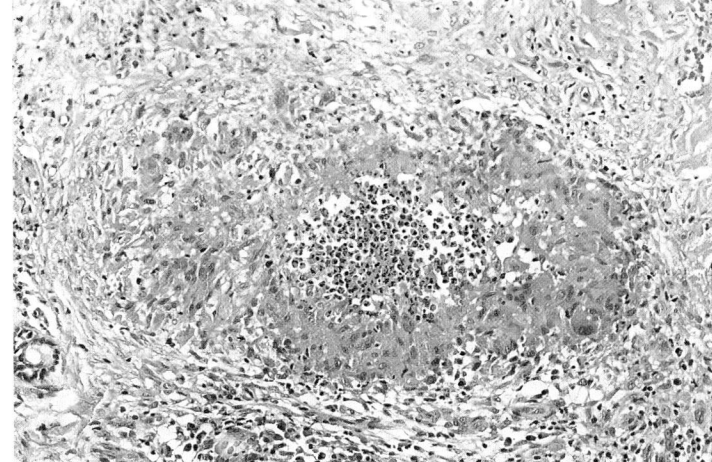

Fig. 7.18 **Sporotrichosis.** A suppurative granuloma is present. (H & E)

discussed in other chapters and only the major differential histological features will be noted here.

Suppurative granulomas are seen in the following conditions:

* chromomycosis and phaeohyphomycosis
* sporotrichosis
* non-tuberculous mycobacterial infections
* blastomycosis
* paracoccidioidomycosis
* coccidioidomycosis
* blastomycosis-like pyoderma
* mycetoma, nocardiosis and actinomycosis
* cat-scratch disease
* lymphogranuloma venereum
* pyoderma gangrenosum
* ruptured cysts and follicles.

Histopathology

The first seven conditions listed above show very similar histological changes. These include marked irregular epidermal hyperplasia ('pseudoepitheliomatous' hyperplasia), intraepidermal and dermal microabscesses, suppurative granulomas and a mixed inflammatory cell infiltrate which includes scattered multinucleate giant cells. Specific diagnosis depends on identification of the causative agent in tissue sections or by culture. Similar changes are seen in halogenodermas but granulomas and giant cells are not seen, except in relation to ruptured hair follicles. It is necessary to cut multiple sections and carefully examine them for microorganisms when such a histopathological pattern is seen. Most organisms can be seen in routine histological sections if care is taken, but stains for fungi (for example, the PAS and Grocott methenamine silver methods) and mycobacteria may reveal organisms that escape detection in hematoxylin and eosin preparations.

CHROMOMYCOSIS AND PHAEOHYPHOMYCOSIS

In chromomycosis the characteristic organisms are round to oval thick-walled brown cells about 6–12 μm in diameter (sclerotic bodies, Medlar bodies). Intracellular septation may be seen. Single organisms or small groups are found within multinucleate giant cells, within microabscesses, suppurative granulomas or surface crust. Tuberculoid granulomas are occasionally seen in the dermal infiltrate.[315] In phaeohyphomycosis, which is clinically distinct from chromomycosis, there are hyphal and yeast forms in suppurative granulomas. Species identification requires culture of the organism. Chromomycosis and phaeohyphomycosis are discussed further in Chapter 25, pages 672–673.

SPOROTRICHOSIS

The causative organism, *Sporothrix schenckii*, is present in the lesions of primary cutaneous sporotrichosis (see p. 673) in the yeast form; it is only rarely found in its hyphal form. The formation of sporothrix asteroids by the encasement of individual yeast cells by a deposit of immune complexes and fibrin is an occasional finding. These asteroids are seen infrequently in sporotrichotic lesions in some parts of the world, but are comparatively common in those seen in Australia and South Africa.[316] The yeast cells are small, round to oval structures, some of which show budding. They may be found within giant cells or in suppurative granulomas. They are difficult to see and may require PAS stains for recognition. The asteroids are found only in microabscesses and the centers of suppurative granulomas. They can be recognized in these locations on careful study of hematoxylin and eosin preparations. Generally, organisms are few in sporotrichosis.

NON-TUBERCULOUS MYCOBACTERIAL INFECTIONS

Tuberculoid or suppurative granulomas may be seen in infections caused by non-tuberculous mycobacteria, including *M. marinum* and *M. chelonae* (see p. 627). In *M. marinum* infections, caseation is not usually seen. Organisms are sparse; when found, they are usually within histiocytes. Organisms may be moderately plentiful in *M. chelonae* infections. They are frequently seen in and about round to oval clear spaces in the center of suppurative foci.

BLASTOMYCOSIS

In the disseminated form of blastomycosis the organisms are scarce and are found either within giant cells or free in the dermis (see p. 670). The organism (*Blastomyces dermatitidis*) is a thick-walled round cell, 8–15 μm in diameter. Multiple nuclei may be seen in the cell. Single broad-based buds are occasionally present on the surface. PAS or Grocott methenamine silver stains facilitate demonstration of the organism.

PARACOCCIDIOIDOMYCOSIS

Most cutaneous lesions in paracoccidioidomycosis ('South American blastomycosis') are secondary lesions seen in the course of the disseminated form of the disease (see p. 670). The causative agent, *Paracoccidioides brasiliensis*, is usually found in giant cells. The organisms vary more in size than *Blastomyces dermatitidis* and can be larger. Also, *P. brasiliensis* is thin walled, lacks multiple nuclei and often has multiple buds arranged round the mother cell.

COCCIDIOIDOMYCOSIS

The cutaneous lesions of coccidioidomycosis are almost always secondary to pulmonary disease (see p. 670). Areas of necrosis are sometimes present in the dermis. Sporangia of *Coccidioides immitis* are rounded structures, 10–80 μm in diameter, which contain multiple sporangiospores, 1–5 μm in diameter. Sporangia are usually easily identified in sections stained with hematoxylin and eosin. Spherules and sporangiospores stain with silver stains. Sporangiospores are PAS positive whereas spherules may be negative or only weakly positive.[317]

BLASTOMYCOSIS-LIKE PYODERMA

Marked epidermal hyperplasia and epidermal, follicular and dermal abscesses are seen in blastomycosis-like pyoderma (see p. 622). There is usually severe solar elastosis. In some cases a palisading rim of histiocytes is seen surrounding the suppurative foci in the dermis. Multinucleate giant cells are occasionally present in this zone but they are not as common as in the mycoses discussed above. Bacteria, particularly Gram-positive cocci, may be seen in suppurative foci. *Staphylococcus aureus* is often isolated from tissue samples but not from the skin surface.

MYCETOMAS, NOCARDIOSIS AND ACTINOMYCOSIS

In mycetomas, nocardiosis and actinomycosis, foci of suppuration may become surrounded by a histiocytic rim to form suppurative granulomas. Organisms are present within the suppurative foci. These conditions are discussed in Chapter 25, pages 675–677.

CAT-SCRATCH DISEASE

Suppurative granulomas and zones of necrosis surrounded by a palisade of epithelioid cells may be seen in the skin, at the site of injury, in cat-scratch disease (see p. 636). A variable number of lymphocytes, plasma cells, histiocytes and eosinophils are present in the adjacent tissues.[318]

LYMPHOGRANULOMA VENEREUM

The cutaneous lesions of lymphogranuloma venereum do not have a specific histopathological appearance (see p. 637). The characteristic suppurative and centrally necrotic granulomas are found in the regional lymph nodes.[318]

PYODERMA GANGRENOSUM

Superficial granulomatous pyoderma is a variant of pyoderma gangrenosum (see p. 251) which has a more indolent course than classic pyoderma gangrenosum.[319,320] One group has suggested that this condition would be better called 'pathergic granulomatous cutaneous ulceration'.[321] Unlike the typical pyoderma gangrenosum, there are suppurative granulomas and scattered multinucleate giant cells in the dermis associated with irregular epidermal hyperplasia, sinus formation, fibrosis and a heavy mixed inflammatory infiltrate which includes plasma cells and eosinophils.[320,322] The histological changes mimic an infectious process but the lesions respond to corticosteroid therapy and not antibiotics.

RUPTURED CYSTS AND FOLLICLES

Occasionally suppurative granulomas are seen adjacent to ruptured cysts (epidermal and dermoid cysts, in particular) and to inflamed hair follicles which rupture, liberating their contents into the dermis.

FOREIGN BODY GRANULOMAS

The essential feature of foreign body granulomas is the presence either of identifiable *exogenous* (foreign) material or of *endogenous* material which has become altered in some way so that it acts as a foreign body. Around this material are arranged histiocytes (including epithelioid histiocytes), multinucleate giant cells derived from histiocytes, and variable numbers of other inflammatory cells. Multinucleate giant cells are often of foreign body type, with nuclei scattered irregularly throughout the cytoplasm, but Langhans giant cells are also seen. In some cases the reaction consists almost entirely of multinucleate cells. Where there are moderate to large amounts of foreign material, histiocytes are sometimes arranged in an irregular palisade. Some foreign materials, e.g. tattoo pigment, induce granulomas of different types. The causative agent may or may not be birefringent when sections are examined in polarized light.

EXOGENOUS MATERIAL

Foreign body granulomas are formed around such disparate substances as starch,[323] talc,[324] tattoo material (Fig. 7.19),[95] cactus bristles,[325] wood splinters, suture material, retained epicardial pacing wires,[326] Bioplastique and Artecoll microimplants,[327,328] injected hyaluronic acid (Hylaform®),[329] pencil lead,[330] bovine collagen,[331] artificial hair,[332] golf club graphite[333] and insect mouth parts.[334] Some foreign materials such as glass, zirconium,[335] beryllium, acrylic

fibers and tattoo pigments may induce local sarcoidal granulomas (see p. 196). Tuberculoid granulomas have been reported in one patient at the site of injection of zinc-containing insulin.[336]

Talc particles are birefringent, as are starch granules; the latter exhibit a characteristic Maltese cross birefringence in polarized light. Incidentally, it is not well known that cryptococci may also be birefringent in polarized light. Materials used to 'cut' heroin and other addictive drugs and the filler materials in crushed tablets may produce cutaneous foreign body granulomas in intravenous drug abusers.[337] The elemental nature of unknown inorganic material can be determined using energy-dispersive X-ray analysis techniques if necessary. A granulomatous reaction has been recorded at the base of the penis following the injection of acyclovir (aciclovir) tablets dissolved in hydrogen peroxide, in the self-treatment of recurrent genital herpes infection.[338]

Plant material may be readily identified by its characteristic structure and may be PAS positive.[325] It is prudent to perform stains for bacteria and fungi to exclude contaminating organisms when foreign bodies such as wood splinters or bone fragments are found.

A granulomatous reaction at the site of an arthropod bite may be a reaction to insect fragments or introduced epidermal elements.[334] A florid granulomatous reaction producing an exophytic tumor has been reported following multiple bee stings used as a folk remedy.[339]

A granulomatous reaction is sometimes seen about certain types of suture material including nylon, silk and dacron.[340] Each type of suture material has a characteristic appearance and birefringence pattern in tissue sections.

Immunization with aluminum-adsorbed vaccines such as tetanus toxoid may produce an unusual foreign body reaction.[341,342] A central zone of granular debris containing aluminum and phosphate is surrounded by a rim of granular histiocytes (see p. 442). A marked lymphoid infiltrate with lymphoid follicles and eosinophils is present at the periphery. This may superficially resemble the changes of Kimura's disease.

A granulomatous reaction has been reported on the eyelids following the use of aluminum salts in blepharopigmentation, a process which attempts to produce a permanent line along the eyelid margin, simulating a cosmetic eyeliner.[343]

Granulomas have been described in the skin at the point of entry of acupuncture and venepuncture needles coated with silicone.[344] Particles of silicon were detected in macrophages by X-ray microanalysis. Silica granulomas of the elbow have been reported in a tennis player as a consequence of falls

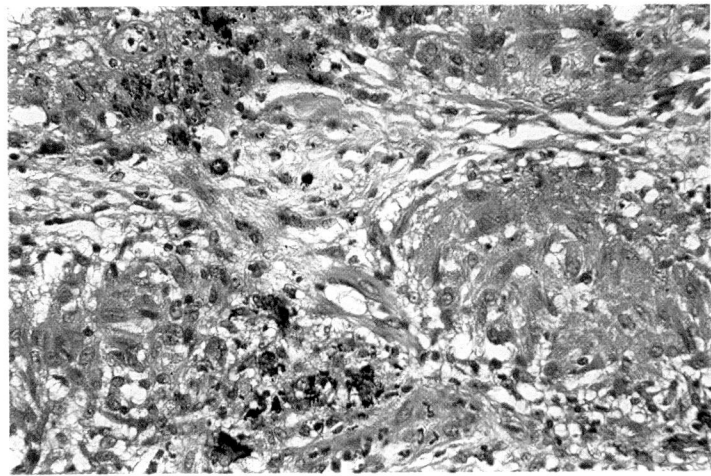

Fig. 7.19 **Foreign body granuloma.** There is tattoo pigment present. (H & E)

on a tennis court which was covered with an artificial silica/polypropylon grass surface.[345]

ENDOGENOUS MATERIAL

Endogenous materials include calcium deposits, urates, oxalate,[346,347] keratin and hair.

Both metastatic and dystrophic calcification may be associated with a granulomatous foreign body reaction. This is also seen in idiopathic calcinosis of the scrotum and subepidermal calcified nodules.

A granulomatous reaction to keratin and hair shafts occurs adjacent to ruptured epidermal, pilar and dermoid cysts, pilomatrixoma and any condition associated with rupture or destruction of a hair follicle. Granulomas have been reported as a reaction to autologous hairs incarcerated during hair transplantation.[348] A similar reaction is seen in the interdigital web spaces of barbers from implanted hair.[349] It is not uncommon for enlargement of a banal nevocellular nevus to be due to a granulomatous reaction following damage to a hair follicle. Fragments of keratin may or may not be found in these reactions. Occasional fine wavy eosinophilic squames may be identifiable within spaces in the dermis or within giant cells. Hair shafts are oval or rounded structures when cut in section and sometimes exhibit cortical and medullary layers: they are variably birefringent in polarized light and acid fast when stained by the Ziehl–Neelsen technique. Foreign body granulomas to keratin are also seen near squamous cell carcinomas and in recurrences. Their presence is an indication for a careful search for residual tumor.[350]

Cutaneous amyloid is usually inert but in nodular amyloidosis it may occasionally provoke a foreign body giant cell reaction.

MISCELLANEOUS GRANULOMAS

The miscellaneous category includes conditions which do not fit neatly into any of the more established categories of granulomatous disease.

This section will discuss the following conditions:

- Melkersson–Rosenthal syndrome
- elastolytic granulomas
- annular granulomatous lesions in ochronosis
- granulomas in immunodeficiency disorders
- interstitial granulomatous dermatitis
- interstitial granulomatous drug reaction
- granulomatous T-cell lymphomas.

MELKERSSON–ROSENTHAL SYNDROME

The Melkersson–Rosenthal syndrome is a rare condition of unknown etiology characterized by the triad of chronic orofacial swelling predominantly involving the lips, recurrent facial nerve palsy and a fissured tongue (lingua plicata).[351–356] The complete triad occurs in about 25% of cases. A monosymptomatic form, in which there is localized episodic swelling of the lip(s) has been called cheilitis granulomatosa of Miescher or granulomatous cheilitis.[357] The term 'oro-facial granulomatosis' was introduced by Wiesenfeld and colleagues in 1985 to cover both granulomatous cheilitis and Melkersson–Rosenthal syndrome.[351] It has not gained widespread acceptance.

The presenting complaint is usually swelling of the lips, but adjacent areas of the cheek are frequently involved.[356] The initial facial swelling may last only a few days and be soft and fluctuant, but it becomes firmer and persistent with time.[358] Facial nerve palsy, usually unilateral, occurs in 13–50% of cases.[351,359]

Facial swelling has also been reported in association with syringomyelia.[360] The median age at onset was 20 years in one series, and there was an equal sex incidence.[351]

The etiology is unknown but the syndrome has been considered to be a manifestation of sarcoidosis, a reaction to infection or to foreign material, such as silicates, and a delayed hypersensitivity to cow's milk protein or food additives.[361] *Borrelia burgdorferi* has been excluded as an etiological agent,[362] but the DNA of *Mycobacterium tuberculosis* has been identified by PCR in one case.[363] Elimination of odontogenic infections has produced remission in some cases.[364]

Occasional cases have been associated with other granulomatous skin lesions or granulomatous lymphadenopathy.[351,365] A granulomatous cheilitis may be a manifestation of Crohn's disease.[170,366] The lip sign may predate gastrointestinal symptoms by years.[367] There is one report of a patient with Crohn's disease and the full triad of lesions associated with the Melkersson–Rosenthal syndrome.[368]

Histopathology

There is marked edema in the dermis together with a perivascular inflammatory cell infiltrate consisting of lymphocytes, plasma cells, histiocytes and occasional eosinophils; the infiltrate may extend into underlying muscle. Small 'naked' collections of epithelioid cells, loose tuberculoid granulomas with a peripheral round cell infiltrate or isolated multinucleate giant cells are usually present. The inflammatory infiltrate is more consistently related to vessels than that in sarcoidosis (Fig. 7.20). Schaumann bodies and birefringent fragments may occasionally be seen in histiocytes and giant cells. Lymphatics are usually widely dilated and may contain collections of inflammatory cells. Alternatively, inflammatory cell collections may bulge into the lumen of vessels.[369] Older lesions may show dermal fibrosis. Collagenous nodules which represent fibrosed granulomas may be found after treatment with steroids.[370] Overlying epithelial changes are non-specific. There are no reliable features to allow distinction of those cases which represent a manifestation of Crohn's disease.

Similar histological changes are seen in association with chronic edema and swelling of the vulva and penis in some cases of recurrent infections of this region.[371] Squamous cell carcinoma of the vulva has been reported in long-standing vulvitis granulomatosa.[372]

The solitary violaceous lesions reported recently in patients with rheumatoid arthritis as **cutaneous histiocytic lymphangitis** and **angioendotheliomatosis** have some histological similarities to both Melkersson–Rosenthal syndrome and angioendotheliomatosis.[373,374] Both reports would appear to be describing the same entity. There were dilated lymphatics in the dermis containing aggregates of inflammatory cells, mainly histiocytes, with adjacent lymphoid aggregates, but no granulomas as seen in Melkersson–Rosenthal syndrome.

ELASTOLYTIC GRANULOMAS

The elastolytic granulomas predominantly affect the exposed skin of the head, neck and limbs. This group of granulomatous conditions includes actinic granuloma,[375] atypical necrobiosis lipoidica of the face and scalp[376] and Miescher's granuloma.[377] They are all characterized by annular lesions exhibiting a zonal histological pattern that includes a granulomatous response with giant cells at the annular rim and centrally a loss of elastic fibers or the presence of solar elastotic material. These conditions may represent a single diagnostic entity and have been grouped under the title 'annular elastolytic giant cell granuloma'.[378,379] The relationship, if any, of this group to the necrobiotic granulomas is controversial. Another lesion, granuloma multiforme,

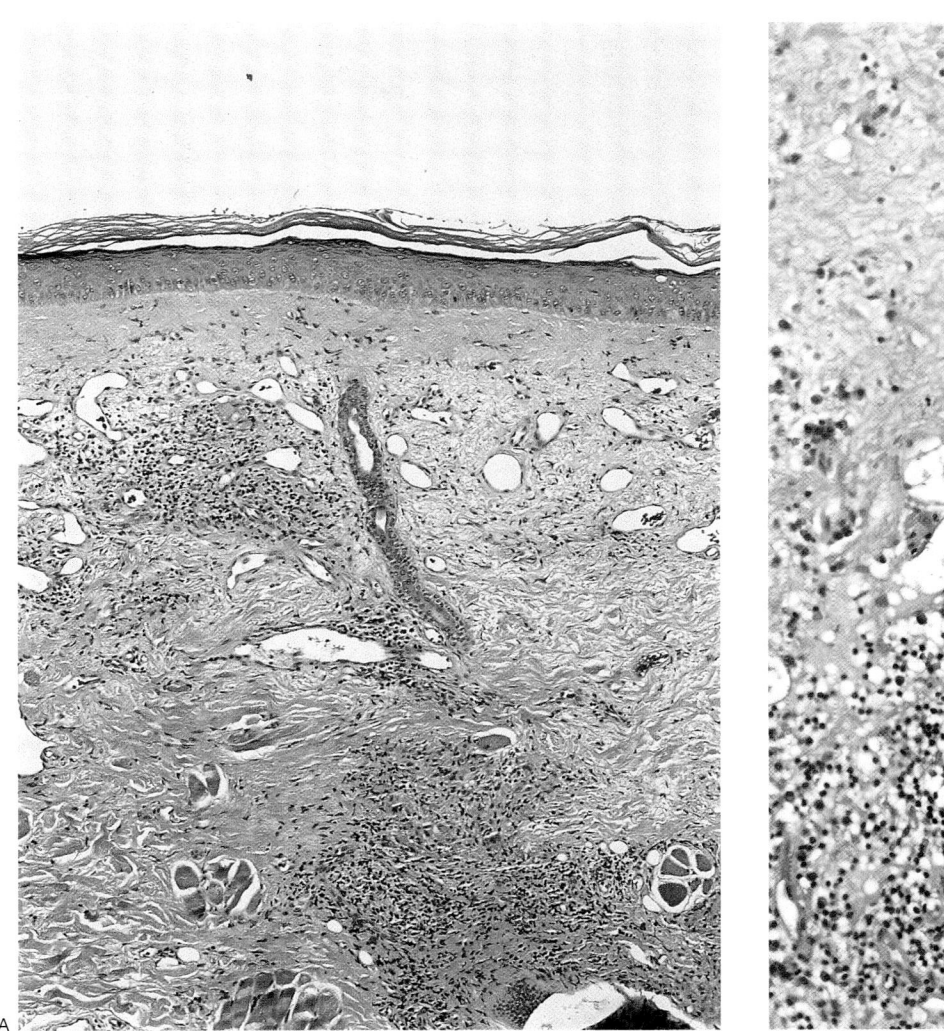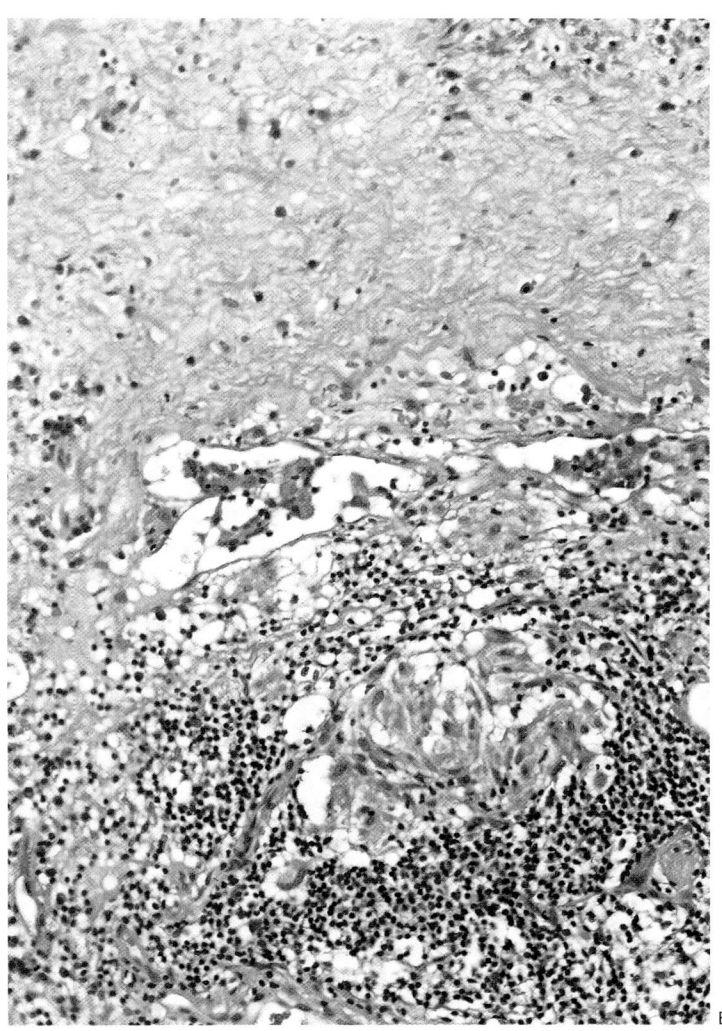

Fig. 7.20 **(A) Melkersson–Rosenthal syndrome. (B)** A granulomatous reaction is present adjacent to a vessel containing inflammatory cells. (H & E)

is also very similar clinically and histologically to these conditions and is discussed here.

Actinic granuloma

In 1975, O'Brien described annular skin lesions which occurred in sun-damaged skin and were characterized histologically by disappearance of solar elastotic fibers and, at the edge of the lesion, by a histiocytic and giant cell inflammatory reaction.[375] His concept of a granulomatous response to solar elastosis was challenged by some[380] and supported by others.[381,382] Some felt that this lesion was granuloma annulare in sun-damaged skin.[380] Others have proposed the term 'annular elastolytic giant cell granuloma' because of the absence of solar elastosis in some of their cases.[378] Lesions have also been reported in covered areas of the body.[383,384] In support of O'Brien, similar changes have been described in association with solar elastosis in pinguecula of the bulbar conjunctiva.[385,386] Temporal arteritis may arise in association with actinic granuloma. Both conditions have been regarded as a response to actinically damaged elastic tissue.[387]

As initially described, actinic granuloma begins as single or grouped pink papules which evolve to annular lesions in sun-exposed regions of the neck, face, chest and arms. Both sexes are affected equally and most of the patients are 40 years of age or older. Solitary cases have been reported in association

with relapsing polychondritis,[388] molluscum contagiosum[389] and cutaneous amyloidosis.[390] Elastolytic granulomas, not associated with solar elastosis but having a similar histological appearance, have been described in generalized and systemic forms.[391,392]

Actinic granuloma has been reported following prolonged sunbed usage.[393]

Histopathology

In annular lesions, the changes seen at the rim of the lesion differ from those in the center (Fig. 7.21). The dermis in the region of the rim is infiltrated by histiocytes and there are many foreign body giant cells. The latter are applied to, and engulf, elastotic fibers (elastoclasis; Fig. 7.22). There is also a variable component of lymphocytes, plasma cells and eosinophils. Within the central zone, there is complete or almost complete loss of both elastotic fibers and normal elastic fibers. The dermal collagen in this region is relatively normal or slightly increased. Unlike granuloma annulare and necrobiosis lipoidica, necrobiosis is not usually seen. The absence of increased dermal mucin also distinguishes most cases from granuloma annulare. Asteroid bodies are sometimes present in giant cells. In some cases mononuclear histiocytes may be more prominent than multinucleate giant cells, and occasionally tuberculoid granulomas form.[394]

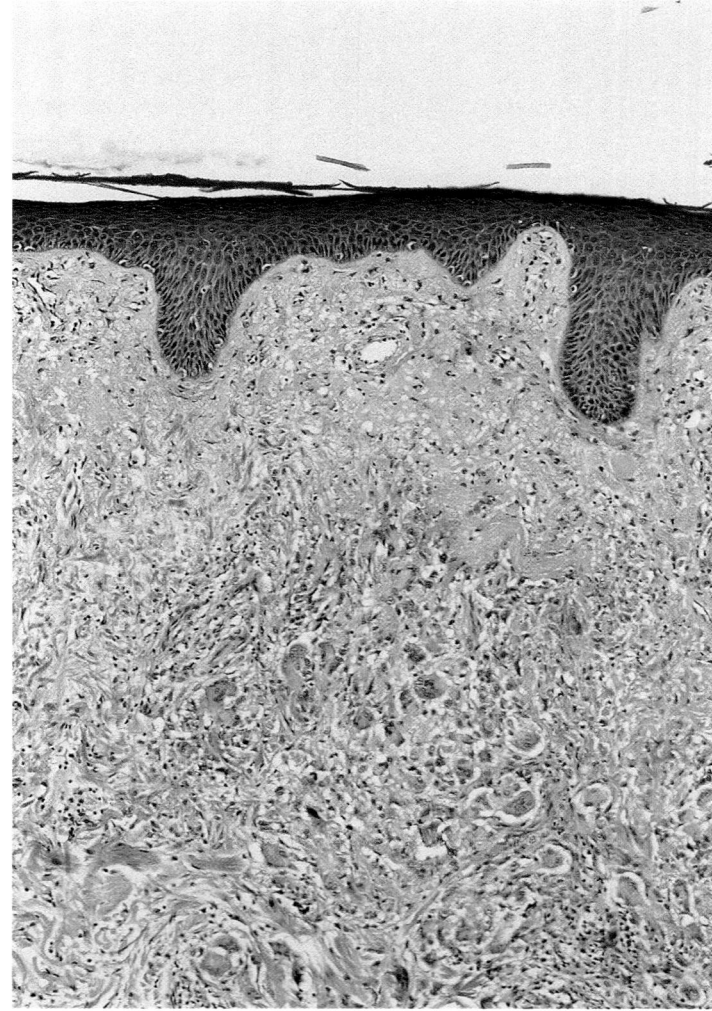

Fig. 7.21 **Actinic granuloma.** There are many foreign body giant cells arranged around elastotic fibers. Some fibers have been phagocytosed. (H & E)

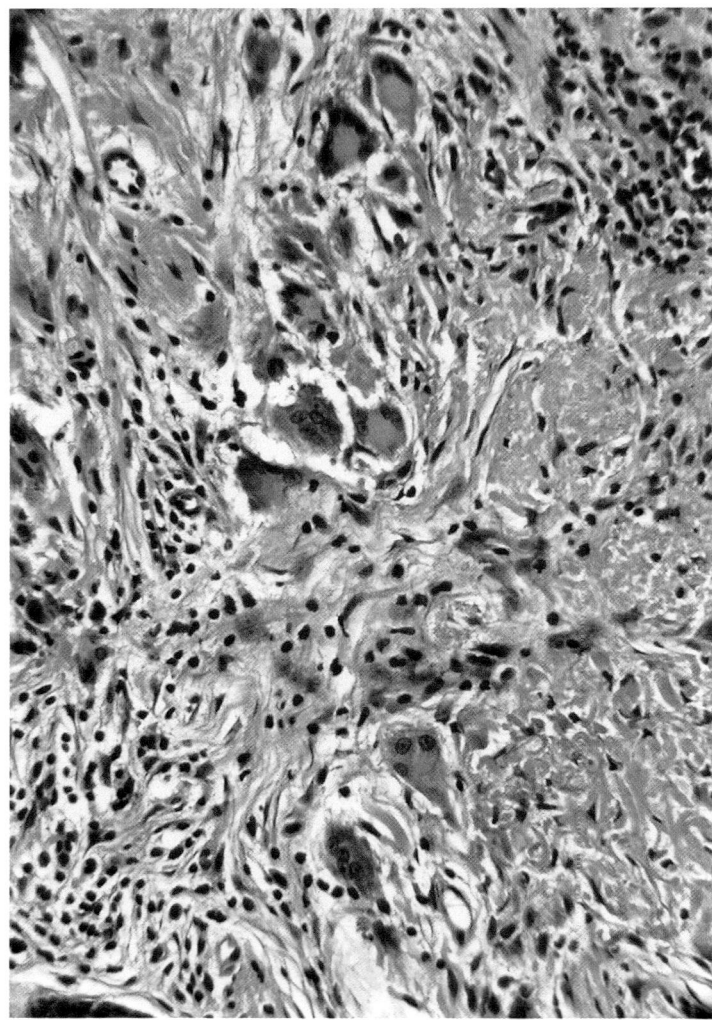

Fig. 7.22 **Actinic granuloma.** Multinucleate giant cells are engulfing elastotic fibers. (H & E)

A similar granulomatous response can occur in relation to some basal cell carcinomas and keratoacanthomas.[382] Elastoclasis has also been described in granuloma annulare,[395] elastosis perforans serpiginosa and other lesions occurring in sun-damaged skin.[380] In these cases, elastoclasis may represent a secondary response to elastotic fibers which have been altered in some as yet unknown way by the primary process, whereas in actinic granuloma there is no obvious provoking cause. It has been suggested that there is a cell-mediated immune response to antigenic determinants on actinically altered elastotic fibers.[396] Elastophagocytosis may also be seen in sun-protected skin in association with a variety of inflammatory conditions.[397]

In one study comparing actinic granuloma and granuloma annulare, absence of elastotic material in the center of the lesions and the presence of scarring and giant cells with up to 12 nuclei were characteristic of actinic granuloma. By comparison, granuloma annulare was characterized by moderate amounts of elastotic material within granulomas, scarring was absent and giant cells contained fewer nuclei.[398]

Immunohistochemical studies have shown the presence of lysozyme in giant cells and a predominance of helper T cells in the lymphocytic infiltrate.[396] One ultrastructural study has demonstrated both extracellular and intracellular digestion of elastotic fibers.[399]

Atypical necrobiosis lipoidica

A condition characterized by annular lesions of the upper face and scalp has been called 'atypical necrobiosis lipoidica'.[376] It occurs predominantly in females. The average age of onset is around 35 years. The lesions resolve spontaneously or persist for many years. Unlike necrobiosis lipoidica, they heal without scarring or alopecia. Some patients have necrobiosis lipoidica at other sites.

Lesions with similar clinical and histological features to those seen in atypical necrobiosis lipoidica have been described as Miescher's granuloma of the face.[377] It has been suggested that both conditions represent actinic granulomas although solar elastosis has not been a conspicuous feature in either.[375] The issue is further confused by reports of actinic granuloma with areas of necrobiosis.[394,400]

Histopathology

These lesions are characterized by a central healing zone, in which there is loss of elastic tissue, and a peripheral raised edge. In the latter region there is a lymphocytic and histiocytic dermal infiltrate which is distributed between collagen bundles. The infiltrate includes multinucleate giant cells, some of which contain asteroid bodies. Necrobiotic areas and increased dermal mucin have not been described.

Granuloma multiforme

The granulomatous dermatitis, granuloma multiforme, was originally recognized because of its potential importance in the differential diagnosis of tuberculoid leprosy, which it resembles clinically and, to some extent, histologically.[401,402] First reported in Nigeria, granuloma multiforme has also been reported in other central African countries, in Indonesia and in India.[401,403] Papular and annular lesions occur on exposed regions of the trunk and arms. Both sexes are affected and most of the patients are aged 40 years or more. There was a marked female predominance in one series.[404] It has been suggested that this is a variant of granuloma annulare or necrobiosis lipoidica.[404] Others consider it to be related to actinic granuloma.[375]

Histopathology

The zonal histology described in actinic granuloma is also seen in this condition (see above). There is destruction of dermal elastic tissue, with mild fibrosis in the center of annular lesions. In the raised active edge of the lesion there is a granulomatous reaction which includes histiocytes, multinucleate giant cells, lymphocytes, eosinophils and plasma cells. Elastoclasia (elastic fiber phagocytosis by histiocytes) is seen in this region. Areas of necrobiosis have been described, surrounded by a palisaded rim of histiocytes, in the middle and upper dermis in the annular rim.[404] Solar elastosis may occur in black-skinned people but it is not clear whether it is present in the lesions of granuloma multiforme in black patients.[405]

In one series of cases there was no evidence of fat within these lesions on special staining; mucin stains were inconclusive.[404]

ANNULAR GRANULOMATOUS LESIONS IN OCHRONOSIS

There have been several reports from South Africa of an annular eruption in ochronotic areas of the face in a group with hydroquinone-induced ochronosis.[406–408] The lesions clinically resemble actinic granuloma and have a zonal appearance with a peripheral hyperpigmented ochronotic zone, an elevated rim and a central hypopigmented area.

Histopathology

Sections of the rim show a granulomatous response with histiocytes, epithelioid histiocytes, giant cells, lymphocytes and plasma cells. Phagocytosis of ochronotic fibers is seen, these fibers representing pigmented swollen collagen fibers. There may be epidermal changes associated with trans-epidermal elimination of ochronotic material in this region. The central zone has an atrophic epidermis with underlying absence of elastotic material and ochronotic fibers together with mild fibrosis. Elastophagocytosis was not seen despite the absence of elastotic material. Sarcoidal granulomas have also been reported in these lesions.[406] It has been suggested that these lesions may represent a manifestation of sarcoidosis since some but not all cases are associated with systemic sarcoidosis.[408]

GRANULOMAS IN IMMUNODEFICIENCY DISORDERS

Granulomas of various types have been described in cutaneous lesions in persons with genetic and acquired immune deficiency disorders.[409] They are listed in Table 7.2. In those with non-AIDS-related immune deficiency, a variety of granuloma types have been described in cutaneous lesions.[410] Although, as might be expected, some are associated with a variety of infectious agents to which these patients are prone, many are not. Excellent

Table 7.2 **Immunodeficiency disorders with cutaneous granulomas**

Chronic granulomatous disease
X-linked hypogammaglobulinemia
Common variable immunodeficiency
Ataxia-telangiectasia
Severe combined immunodeficiency
Primary acquired hypogammaglobulinemia

reviews of the primary immunodeficiency disorders have recently been published.[411,412]

In *chronic granulomatous disease*, despite the name, true granulomas are not common in cutaneous lesions. There are a variety of reports of suppurative granulomas with organisms, foreign body granulomas with and without organisms and caseation necrosis.[410,413–418] Caseating granulomas have been described in *X-linked infantile hypogammaglobulinemia*. Lymphocytes in the granulomas were almost exclusively of CD8 phenotype.[419] Sarcoid-like and caseating granulomas have been reported in lesions of *common variable immunodeficiency*.[420–425] Tumor necrosis factor-α (TNF-α) is elevated in this condition, and specific inhibition of this cytokine has been successful in moderating the disease.[426] Cutaneous lesions in *ataxia-telangiectasia* have contained necrobiotic and tuberculoid granulomas.[427–429] Necrobiotic and tuberculoid granulomas have also been reported in *combined immuno-deficiency*.[430] Sarcoidosis with typical granulomas may also be associated with combined immunodeficiency.[431] In one case of *primary acquired agamma-globulinemia*, non-caseating granulomas were described.[432]

The association of granuloma annulare and HIV infection has been described previously.[433] Occasionally, granulomas with no apparent infectious agent are seen in the papular lesions of AIDS. As might be expected because of low levels of CD4+ T lymphocytes, organisms associated with granulomas in immunodeficient individuals usually proliferate without granuloma formation or with poor granuloma formation.[434] There are, however, reports of granuloma formation in Kveim tests in HIV-positive individuals[435] and granuloma formation without organism proliferation has been described in a series of patients with both borderline tuberculoid leprosy and HIV infection,[436] suggesting that factors other than CD4+ T lymphocytes are involved in granuloma formation. A study of foreign body reactions to ruptured cysts in HIV-infected individuals has shown some differences compared to the reaction in the immunocompetent. These included little tendency to form giant cells, macrophages phagocytosing lymphoid cells, and increased numbers of mast cells and eosinophils.[437]

INTERSTITIAL GRANULOMATOUS DERMATITIS

Interstitial granulomatous dermatitis is the preferred designation for a clinically heterogeneous entity that may present as linear cords (the 'rope sign'), papules or plaques.[438–444] The cords tend to be skin-colored and situated on the lateral trunk, while the papules are skin-colored or erythematous with umbilication, crusting or perforation in some lesions. The plaques, which are asymptomatic, are erythematous to violaceous and symmetrically distributed.[444]

A variety of systemic illnesses are associated with these lesions, particularly rheumatoid arthritis, although tests for rheumatoid factor are not always positive. Some patients present with arthralgias. The term '*interstitial granulomatous dermatitis with arthritis*' is often used for these cases to highlight the importance of the accompanying joint disease. Other terms used include '*rheumatoid papules*' and '*palisaded and neutrophilic granulomatous dermatitis*'.[439] Autoimmune thyroiditis, systemic lupus erythematosus, vasculitis, metastatic carcinoma, lymphoma and leukemia have been associated with these cutaneous lesions.[439,441,442,445] The papular eruption developing in some patients with rheumatoid disease treated with methotrexate has some histological similarities.

The etiology is unknown but the clinical associations would strongly support immune complex deposition.[439]

Histopathology[439,441,445]

There is some resemblance to the changes described in 1983 by Finan and Winkelmann as 'cutaneous extravascular necrotizing granuloma (Churg–Strauss granuloma)'.[445] Different patterns have been described but they probably represent different stages or variable expression of the disease. One pattern resembles incomplete granuloma annulare with an interstitial and perivascular dermal infiltrate of neutrophils, neutrophil fragments, histiocytes and lymphocytes. Eosinophils may be present. In some cases there is a leukocytoclastic vasculitis. Dermal collagen appears somewhat basophilic, possibly from nucleic acid staining. In the second pattern there are small granulomas composed of a palisade of histiocytes about a small number of basophilic collagen fibers (Fig. 7.23). There may be central neutrophils and neutrophil fragments. Changes may involve the full thickness of the dermis and sometimes the superficial subcutis or primarily the lower dermis.[438] Accentuation of the

process in the lower dermis is a characteristic feature. Some authors describe mucin within and around the granulomas but there is less mucin than occurs in granuloma annulare. Older lesions may have dermal fibrosis.

It is claimed by one group that the early lesions differ from conventional leukocytoclastic vasculitis by having broader fibrin cuffs about vessels, fewer extravasated erythrocytes and more neutrophils and neutrophil dust in the dermis.[439] There are more interstitial neutrophils in the dermis than are typically seen in either the incomplete or granulomatous forms of granuloma annulare. The author has seen several cases with relatively sparse neutrophils and eosinophils.

Some lesions have surface necrosis, scale crust or epidermal hyperplasia associated with perforation.

Immunofluorescence studies have demonstrated C3, IgM and fibrinogen in dermal blood vessels in some cases.[441,445]

INTERSTITIAL GRANULOMATOUS DRUG REACTION

Twenty cases were reported under the title 'interstitial granulomatous drug reaction' in 1998.[446] It has since received scant attention. Some dermatopathologists have expressed doubts about its validity. In the author's experience

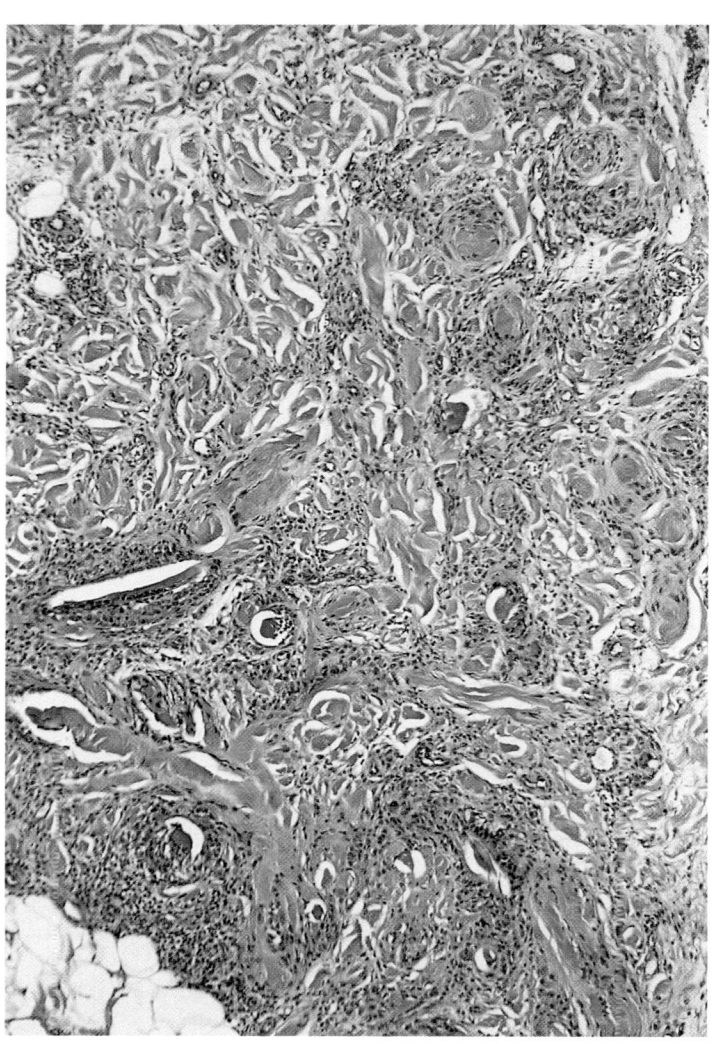

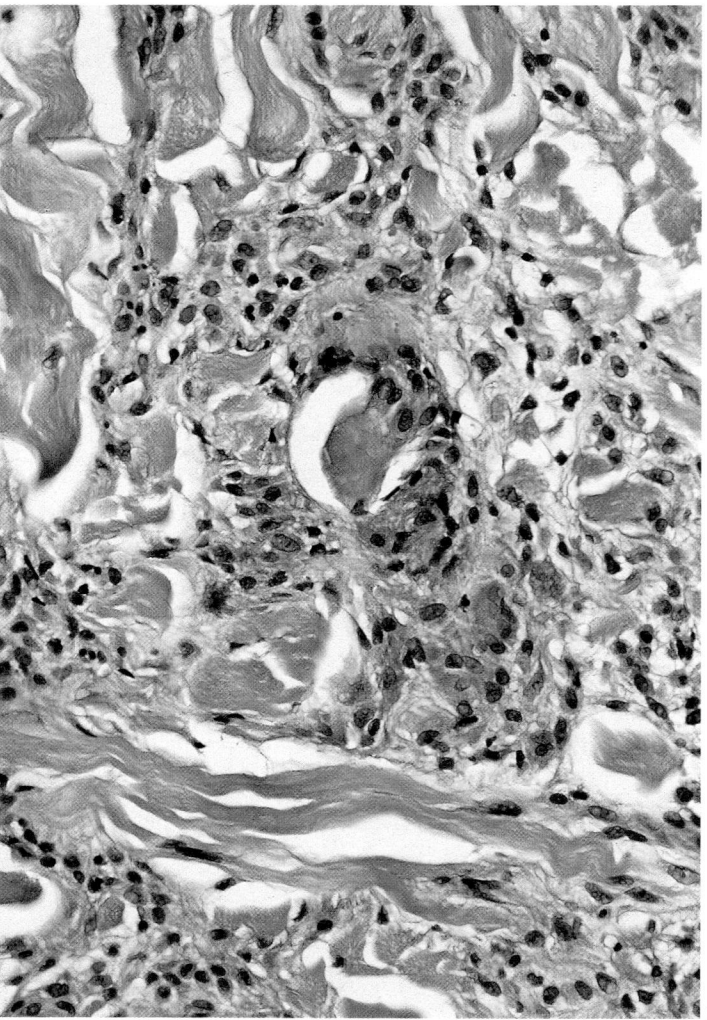

Fig. 7.23 **Interstitial granulomatous dermatitis in a patient with rheumatoid arthritis. (A)** The lower half of the dermis is thickened and involved. **(B)** Individual collagen bundles have a palisade of histiocytes and lymphocytes. Eosinophils are not obvious in this field. (H & E)

of 15 cases, the clinical and histological features have been consistent with those originally described.

Clinically the lesions are erythematous to violaceous, non-pruritic plaques, often having an annular configuration. There may be one or several plaques or widespread lesions. The inner aspects of the arms, medial thighs, intertriginous areas and the trunk are sites of predilection. The provisional clinical diagnosis usually includes such entities as granuloma annulare, mycosis fungoides, lupus erythematosus or erythema annulare centrifugum. A drug reaction is not usually suspected.[446]

Drugs implicated in the etiology of this eruption include calcium channel blockers, beta-blockers, angiotensin converting enzyme inhibitors, lipid-lowering agents, antihistamines, anticonvulsants and antidepressants.[446] Patients are often on one or more of these drugs. Several personally studied cases have been using the combination of a thiazide diuretic and hormone replacement therapy. The lesions resolve on cessation of the drug(s).

Histopathology[446]

The low-power impression is of the incomplete form of granuloma annulare (see p. 201) because of the hypercellular ('busy') dermis resulting from a diffuse interstitial infiltrate of lymphocytes and histiocytes with piecemeal fragmentation of collagen and elastic fibers (Fig. 7.24). The lymphocytes appear activated and mildly atypical. There may be focal epidermotropism. A few multinucleate giant cells may be present, but they are not a conspicuous

feature. Eosinophils are usually present in small numbers. Red cell extravasation is sometimes present. Mucin deposition is variable.

Another feature which is usually present is a mild interface (lichenoid) reaction with vacuolar change and occasional apoptotic keratinocytes.

This drug reaction differs from granuloma annulare by the absence of any significant necrobiosis, the general predominance of lymphocytes over histiocytes and the presence of eosinophils and interface change. It differs from interstitial granulomatous dermatitis (see above) by the lack of deep dermal accentuation and the less conspicuous rimming of isolated collagen bundles by histiocytes.

GRANULOMATOUS T-CELL LYMPHOMAS

Rare cases of mycosis fungoides have a granulomatous infiltrate in the dermis (see p. 1107). Granulomas are also present in granulomatous slack skin,[447–449] a variant of T-cell lymphoma (see p. 1110). In both conditions phagocytosis of elastic fibers and lymphocytes may occur.

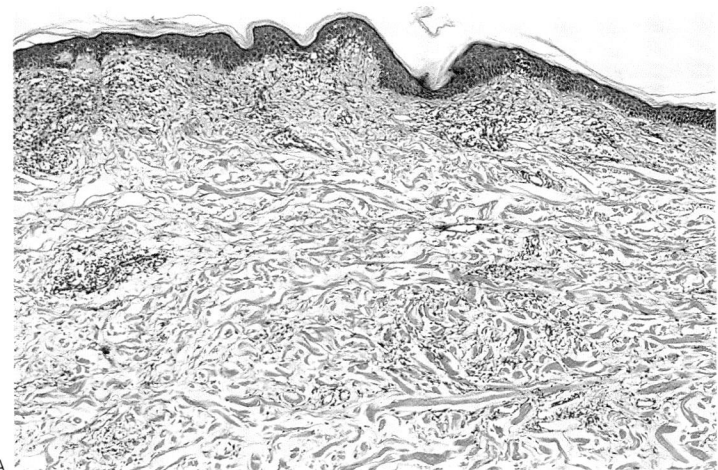

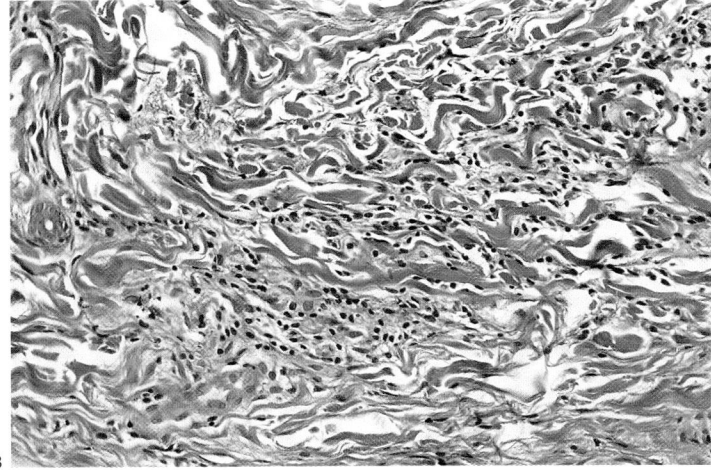

Fig. 7.24 **(A) Interstitial granulomatous drug reaction. (B)** There is a 'busy' (hypercellular) dermis mimicking the incomplete (interstitial) type of granuloma annulare. (H & E)

REFERENCES

Introduction

1 Rabinowitz LO, Zaim MT. A clinicopathologic approach to granulomatous dermatoses. J Am Acad Dermatol 1996; 35: 588–600.

2 Hirsh BC, Johnson WC. Concepts of granulomatous inflammation. Int J Dermatol 1984; 3: 90–100.

3 Kunkel SL, Chensue SW, Stricter RM et al. Cellular and molecular aspects of granulomatous inflammation. Am J Respir Cell Mol Biol 1989; 1: 439–447.

4 Ahmed AA, Nordlind K, Schultzberg M, Lidén S. Interleukin-1 alpha- and beta-, interleukin-6- and tumour necrosis factor-alpha-like immunoreactivities in chronic granulomatous skin conditions. Acta Derm Venereol 1994; 74: 435–440.

5 Epstein WL, Fukuyama K. Mechanisms of granulomatous inflammation. In: Norris DA, ed. Immune mechanisms in cutaneous disease. New York: Marcel Dekker, 1989; 687–719.

6 Editorial. Granulomas and cytokines. Lancet 1991; 337: 1067–1069.

7 Epste n WL. Ultrastructural heterogeneity of epithelioid cells in cutaneous organized granulomas of diverse etiology. Arch Dermatol 1991; 127: 821–826.

8 McNally AK, Anderson JM. Interleukin-4 induces foreign body giant cells from human monocytes/macrophages. Differential lymphokine regulation of macrophage fusion leads to morphological variants of multinucleated giant cells. Am J Pathol 1995; 147: 1487–1499.

9 Templeton NS. The polymerase chain reaction. History, methods, and applications. Diagn Mol Pathol 1992; 1: 58–72.

10 Lo AC, Feldman SR. Polymerase chain reaction: basic concepts and clinical applications in dermatology. J Am Acad Dermatol 1994; 30: 250–260.

11 Ghossein RA, Ros DG, Salomon RN, Rabson AR. Rapid detection and species identification of mycobacteria in paraffin-embedded tissues by polymerase chain reaction. Diagn Mol Pathol 1992; 1: 185–191.

12 Cook SM, Bartos RE, Pierson CL, Frank TS. Detection and characterization of atypical mycobacteria by the polymerase chain reaction. Diagn Mol Pathol 1994; 3: 53–58.

13 Fiallo P, Williams DL, Chan GP, Gillis TP. Effects of fixation on polymerase chain reaction detection of *Mycobacterium leprae*. J Clin Microbiol 1992; 30: 3095–3098.

Sarcoidal granulomas

14 Gregg PJ, Kantor GR, Telang GH et al. Sarcoidal reaction in Sézary syndrome. J Am Acad Dermatol 2000; 43: 372–376.

15 Corazza M, Bacilieri S, Strumia R. Post-herpes zoster scar sarcoidosis. Acta Derm Venereol 1999; 79: 95.

16 Farrell AM, Henry K, Woodrow D et al. Cutaneous granulomas associated with high-grade T-cell non-Hodgkin's lymphoma. Br J Dermatol 1999; 140: 145–149.

17 Mitchell DN, Scadding JG, Heard BE, Hinson KFW. Sarcoidosis: histopathological definition and clinical diagnosis. J Clin Pathol 1977; 30: 395–408.

18 Kerdel FA, Moschella SL. Sarcoidosis. An updated review. J Am Acad Dermatol 1984; 11: 1–19.

19 Chesnutt AN. Enigmas in sarcoidosis. West J Med 1995; 162: 519–526.

20 English JC III, Patel PJ, Greer KE. Sarcoidosis. J Am Acad Dermatol 2001; 44: 725–743.

21 Jacyk WK. Cutaneous sarcoidosis in black South Africans. Int J Dermatol 1999; 38: 841–845.

22 Hanno R, Callen JP. Sarcoidosis. A disorder with prominent cutaneous features and their interrelationship with systemic disease. Med Clin North Am 1980; 64: 847–866.

23 Samtsov AV. Cutaneous sarcoidosis. Int J Dermatol 1992; 31: 385–391.

24 Mañá J, Marcoval J, Graells J et al. Cutaneous involvement in sarcoidosis. Relationship to systemic disease. Arch Dermatol 1997; 133: 882–888.

25 Veien NK, Stahl D, Brodthagen H. Cutaneous sarcoidosis in Caucasians. J Am Acad Dermatol 1987; 16: 534–540.

26 Okamoto H, Mizuno K, Imamura S et al. Erythema nodosum-like eruption in sarcoidosis. Clin Exp Dermatol 1994; 19: 507–510.

27 O'Driscoll JB, Beck MH, Lendon M et al. Cutaneous presentation of sarcoidosis in an infant. Clin Exp Dermatol 1990; 15: 60–62.

28 Yotsumoto S, Takahashi Y, Takei S et al. Early onset sarcoidosis masquerading as juvenile rheumatoid arthritis. J Am Acad Dermatol 2000; 43: 969–971.

29 Swale VJ, Spector TD, Bataille VA. Sarcoidosis in monozygotic twins. Br J Dermatol 1998; 139: 350–352.

30 Spiteri MA, Matthey F, Gordon T et al. Lupus pernio: a clinico-radiological study of thirty-five cases. Br J Dermatol 1985; 112: 315–322.

31 Green JJ, Lawrence N, Heymann WR. Generalized ulcerative sarcoidosis induced by therapy with the flashlamp-pumped pulsed dye laser. Arch Dermatol 2001; 137: 507–508.

32 Vainsencher D, Winkelmann RK. Subcutaneous sarcoidosis. Arch Dermatol 1984; 120: 1028–1031.

33 Higgins EM, Salisbury JR, Du Vivier AWP. Subcutaneous sarcoidosis. Clin Exp Dermatol 1993; 18: 65–66.

34 Shidrawi RG, Paradinas F, Murray-Lyon IM. Sarcoidosis presenting as multiple subcutaneous nodules. Clin Exp Dermatol 1994; 19: 356–358.

35 Curco N, Pagerols X, Vives P. Subcutaneous sarcoidosis with dactylitis. Clin Exp Dermatol 1995; 20: 434–435.

36 Ruiz de Erenchun F, Vazquez-Doval FJ, Idoate M et al. Subcutaneous nodules as the first clinical manifestation of sarcoidosis. Clin Exp Dermatol 1992; 17: 192–194.

37 Carriere M, Loche F, Schwarze HP et al. Sarcoid panniculitis. Clin Exp Dermatol 2000; 25: 257–258.

38 Golitz LE, Shapiro L, Hurwitz E, Stritzler R. Cicatricial alopecia of sarcoidosis. Arch Dermatol 1973; 107: 758–760.

39 Katta R, Nelson B, Chen D, Roenigk H. Sarcoidosis of the scalp: A case series and review of the literature. J Am Acad Dermatol 2000; 42: 690–692.

40 Antony F, Layton AM. A case of cutaneous acral sarcoidosis with response to allopurinol. Br J Dermatol 2000; 142: 1052–1053.

41 Kauh YC, Goody HE, Luscombe HA. Ichthyosiform sarcoidosis. Arch Dermatol 1978; 114: 100–101.

42 Feind-Koopmans AG, Lucker GPH, van de Kerkhof PCM. Acquired ichthyosiform erythroderma and sarcoidosis. J Am Acad Dermatol 1996; 35: 826–828.

43 Cather JC, Cohen PR. Ichthyosiform sarcoidosis. J Am Acad Dermatol 1999; 40: 862–865.

44 Albertini JG, Tyler W, Miller OF III. Ulcerative sarcoidosis. Case report and review of the literature. Arch Dermatol 1997; 133: 215–219.

45 Neill SM, Smith NP, Eady RAJ. Ulcerative sarcoidosis: a rare manifestation of common disease. Clin Exp Dermatol 1984; 9: 277–279.

46 Verdegem TD, Sharma OP. Cutaneous ulcers in sarcoidosis. Arch Dermatol 1987; 123: 1531–1534.

47 Mitsuishi T, Nogita T, Kawashima M. Psoriasiform sarcoidosis with ulceration. Int J Dermatol 1992; 31: 339–340.

48 Lee JB, Koblenzer PS. Disfiguring cutaneous manifestation of sarcoidosis treated with thalidomide: A case report. J Am Acad Dermatol 1998; 39: 835–838.

49 Dumitrescu SM, Schwartz RA, Baredes S et al. Mutilating facial sarcoidosis. Dermatology 1999; 199: 265–267.

50 Herzlinger DC, Marland AM, Barr RJ. Verrucous ulcerative skin lesions in sarcoidosis. An unusual clinical presentation. Cutis 1979; 23: 569–572.

51 Smith HR, Black MM. Verrucous cutaneous sarcoidosis. Clin Exp Dermatol 2000; 25: 98–99.

52 Greer KE, Harman LE, Kayne AL. Unusual cutaneous manifestations of sarcoidosis. South Med J 1977; 70: 666–668.

53 Neville E, Mills RGS, Jash DK et al. Sarcoidosis of the upper respiratory tract and its association with lupus pernio. Thorax 1976; 31: 660–664.

54 Gold RS, Sager E. Oral sarcoidosis: review of the literature. J Oral Surg 1976; 34: 237–244.

55 Alexis JB. Sarcoidosis presenting as cutaneous hypopigmentation with repeatedly negative skin biopsies. Int J Dermatol 1994; 33: 44–45.

56 Ford PG, Jorizzo JL, Hitchcock MG. Previously undiagnosed sarcoidosis in a patient presenting with leonine facies and complete heart block. Arch Dermatol 2000; 136: 712–714.

57 Okano M, Nishimura H, Morimoto Y, Maeda H. Faint erythema. Another manifestation of cutaneous sarcoidosis? Int J Dermatol 1997; 36: 681–684.

58 Cliff S, Hart Y, Knowles G, Misch K. Sarcoidosis presenting as palmar erythema. Clin Exp Dermatol 1998; 23: 123–124.

59 Klein PA, Appel J, Callen JP. Sarcoidosis of the vulva: A rare cutaneous manifestation. J Am Acad Dermatol 1998; 39: 281–283.

60 James DG. Dermatological aspects of sarcoidosis. Q J Med 1959; 28: 109–124.

61 Burgdorf WHC, Hoxtell EO, Bart BJ. Sarcoid granulomas in venipuncture sites. Cutis 1979; 24: 52–53.

62 Lewis FM, Harrington CI. Lupus pernio following facial trauma. Clin Exp Dermatol 1993; 18: 476–477.

63 Girão L, Bajanca R, Barata Feio A, Apetato M. Systemic sarcoidosis revealed by the coexistence of scar and subcutaneous sarcoidosis. J Eur Acad Dermatol Venereol 2000; 14: 428–430.

64 Schmuth M, Prior C, Illersperger B et al. Systemic sarcoidosis and cutaneous lymphoma: is the association fortuitous? Br J Dermatol 1999; 140: 952–955.

65 Badell A, Servitje O, Graells J et al. Hypoparathyroidism and sarcoidosis. Br J Dermatol 1998; 138: 915–917.

66 Marzano AV, Gasparini LG, Cavicchini S et al. Scar sarcoidosis associated with vitiligo, autoimmune thyroiditis and autoimmune chronic hepatitis. Clin Exp Dermatol 1996; 21: 466–467.

67 Barnadas MA, Rodríguez-Arias JM, Alomar A. Subcutaneous sarcoidosis associated with vitiligo, pernicious anaemia and autoimmune thyroiditis. Clin Exp Dermatol 2000; 25: 55–56.

68 Terunuma A, Watabe A, Kato T, Tagami H. Coexistence of vitiligo and sarcoidosis in a patient with circulating autoantibodies. Int J Dermatol 2000; 39: 551–553.

69 Mirmirani P, Maurer TA, Herndier B et al. Sarcoidosis in a patient with AIDS: A manifestation of immune restoration syndrome. J Am Acad Dermatol 1999; 41: 285–286.

70 Toutous-Trellu L, Ninet B, Rohner P et al. Three cases of cutaneous sarcoidosis: search for bacterial agent by the 16S RNA gene analysis and treatment with antibiotics. Dermatology 2000; 200: 342–345.

71 Mitchell DN. Mycobacteria and sarcoidosis. Lancet 1996; 348: 768–769.

72 Popper HH, Klemen H, Hoefler G, Winter E. Presence of mycobacterial DNA in sarcoidosis. Hum Pathol 1997; 28: 796–800.

73 Li N, Bajoghli A, Kubba A, Bhawan J. Identification of mycobacterial DNA in cutaneous lesions of sarcoidosis. J Cutan Pathol 1999; 26: 271–278.

74 Bachelez H, Senet P, Cadranel J et al. The use of tetracyclines for the treatment of sarcoidosis. Arch Dermatol 2001; 137: 69–73.

75 Gudi VS, Campbell SM, Gould DJ et al. Activation of cutaneous sarcoidosis following *Mycobacterium marinum* infection of skin. J Eur Acad Dermatol Venereol 2000; 14: 296–297.

76 Lebbé C, Agbalika F, Flageul B et al. No evidence for a role of human herpesvirus type 8 in sarcoidosis: molecular and serological analysis. Br J Dermatol 1999; 141: 492–496.

77 Scerri L, Cook LJ, Jenkins EA, Thomas AL. Familial juvenile systemic granulomatosis (Blau's syndrome). Clin Exp Dermatol 1996; 21: 445–448.

78 Kuramoto Y, Shindo Y, Tagami H. Subcutaneous sarcoidosis with extensive caseation necrosis. J Cutan Pathol 1988; 15: 188–190.

79 Batres E, Klima M, Tschen J. Transepithelial elimination in cutaneous sarcoidosis. Cutan Pathol 1982; 9: 50–54.

80 Jones Williams W. The nature and origin of Schaumann bodies. J Path Bact 1960; 79: 193–201.

81 Kim YC, Triffet MK, Gibson LE. Foreign bodies in sarcoidosis. Am J Dermatopathol 2000; 22: 408–412.

82 Marcoval J, Mañá J, Moreno A et al. Foreign bodies in granulomatous cutaneous lesions of patients with systemic sarcoidosis. Arch Dermatol 2001; 137: 427–430.

83 Callen JP. The presence of foreign bodies does not exclude the diagnosis of sarcoidosis. Arch Dermatol 2001; 137: 485–486.

84 Azar HA, Lunardelli C. Collagen nature of asteroid bodies of giant cells in sarcoidosis. Am J Pathol 1969; 57: 81–92.

85 Cain H, Kraus B. Immunofluorescence microscopic demonstration of vimentin filaments in asteroid bodies of sarcoidosis. Virchows Arch (B) 1983; 42: 213–226.

86 Modlin RL, Gottlieb B, Hofman FM et al. Demonstration *in situ* of subsets of T-lymphocytes in sarcoidosis. Am J Dermatopathol 1984; 6: 423–427.

87 Quismorio FP, Sharma OP, Chandor S. Immunopathological studies on the cutaneous lesions in sarcoidosis. Br J Dermatol 1977; 97: 635–642.

88 Mowry RG, Sams WM Jr, Caulfield JB. Cutaneous silica granuloma. Arch Dermatol 1991; 127: 692–694.

89 Walsh NMG, Hanly JG, Tremaine R, Murray S. Cutaneous sarcoidosis and foreign bodies. Am J Dermatopathol 1993; 15: 203–207.

90 Val-Bernal JF, Sánchez-Quevedo MC, Corral J, Campos A. Cutaneous sarcoidosis and foreign bodies. An electron probe roentgenographic microanalytic study. Arch Pathol Lab Med 1995; 119: 471–474.

91 Schewach-Millet M, Ziv R, Trau H et al. Sarcoidosis versus foreign-body granulomas. Int J Dermatol 1987; 26: 582–583.

92 Shelley WB, Hurley HJ. The pathogenesis of silica granulomas in man: a non-allergic colloidal phenomenon. J Invest Dermatol 1960; 34: 107–123.

93 Weidman AI, Andrade R, Franks AG. Sarcoidosis. Report of a case of sarcoid lesions in a tattoo and subsequent discovery of pulmonary sarcoidosis. Arch Dermatol 1966; 94: 320–325.

94 Sowden JM, Cartwright PH, Smith AG et al. Sarcoidosis presenting with a granulomatous reaction confined to red tattoos. Clin Exp Dermatol 1992; 17: 446–448.

95 Goldstein AP. VII. Histologic reactions in tattoos. J Dermatol Surg Oncol 1979; 5: 896–900.

96 Dickinson JA. Sarcoidal reactions in tattoos. Arch Dermatol 1969; 100: 315–319.

97 Hanada K, Chiyoya S, Katabira Y. Systemic sarcoidal reaction in tattoo. Clin Exp Dermatol 1985; 10: 479–484.

98 Goldstein N. IV. Complications from tattoos. J Dermatol Surg Oncol 1979; 5: 869–878.

99 Shelley WB, Hurley HJ. Allergic origin of zirconium deodorant granuloma. Br J Dermatol 1958; 70: 75–101.

100 LoPresti PJ, Hambrick GW Jr. Zirconium granuloma following treatment of Rhus dermatitis. Arch Dermatol 1965; 92: 188–191.

101 Skelton HG III, Smith KJ, Johnson FB et al. Zirconium granuloma resulting from an aluminum zirconium complex: a previously unrecognized agent in the development of hypersensitivity granulomas. J Am Acad Dermatol 1993; 28: 874–876.

102 Carlson JA, Schutzer P, Pattison T et al. Sarcoidal foreign-body granulomatous dermatitis associated with ophthalmic drops. Am J Dermatopathol 1998; 20: 175–178.

103 Mehta CL, Tyler RJ, Cripps DJ. Granulomatous dermatitis with focal sarcoidal features associated with recombinant interferon β-1b injections. J Am Acad Dermatol 1998; 39: 1024–1028.

104 Eberlein-König B, Hein R, Abeck D et al. Cutaneous sarcoid foreign body granulomas developing in sites of previous skin injury after systemic interferon-alpha treatment for chronic hepatitis C. Br J Dermatol 1999; 140: 370–372.

105 Dutra FR. Beryllium granulomas of the skin. Arch Dermatol Syph 1949; 60: 1140–1147.

106 Helwig EB. Chemical (beryllium) granulomas of skin. Mil Surgeon 1951; 109: 540–558.

107 Pimentel JC. Sarcoid granulomas of the skin produced by acrylic and nylon fibres. Br J Dermatol 1977; 96: 673–677.

108 Pimentel JC. The 'wheat-stubble sarcoid granuloma': a new epithelioid granuloma of the skin. Br J Dermatol 1972; 87: 444–449.

109 Kinmont PDC. Sea-urchin sarcoidal granuloma. Br J Dermatol 1965; 77: 335–343.

Tuberculoid granulomas

110 Hirsh BC, Johnson WC. Pathology of granulomatous diseases. Epithelioid granulomas, Part I. Int J Dermatol 1984; 23: 237–246.

111 Shea C, Imber MJ, Cropley TG et al. Granulomatous eruption after BCG vaccine immunotherapy for malignant melanoma. J Am Acad Dermatol 1989; 21: 1119–1122.

112 Kuniyuki S, Asada M. An ulcerated lesion at the BCG vaccination site during the course of Kawasaki disease. J Am Acad Dermatol 1997; 37: 303–304.

113 Santa Cruz DJ, Strayer DS. The histologic spectrum of the cutaneous mycobacterioses. Hum Pathol 1982; 13: 485–495.

114 Ulbright TM, Katzenstein A-LA. Solitary necrotizing granulomas of the lung. Am J Surg Pathol 1980; 4: 13–28.

115 Degitz K. Detection of mycobacterial DNA in the skin. Etiologic insights and diagnostic perspectives. Arch Dermatol 1996; 132: 71–75.

116 Smith NP, Ryan TJ, Sanderson KV, Sarkany I. Lichen scrofulosorum. A report of four cases. Br J Dermatol 1976; 94: 319–325.

117 Hudson PM. Tuberculide (lichen scrofolosorum) secondary to osseous tuberculosis. Clin Exp Dermatol 1976; 1: 391–394.

118 Jordaan HF, Van Niekerk DJT, Louw M. Papulonecrotic tuberculid. A clinical, histopathological, and immunohistochemical study of 15 patients. Am J Dermatopathol 1994; 16: 474–485.

119 Wilson Jones E, Winkelmann RK. The histopathology of papulonecrotic tuberculid (PNT). J Cutan Pathol 1986; 13: 81 (abstract).

120 Ridley DS, Jopling WH. Classification of leprosy according to immunity. A five-group system. Int J Lepr 1966; 34: 255–273.

121 Ridley DS. Histological classification and the immunological spectrum of leprosy. Bull WHO 1974; 51: 451–465.

122 Lantis LR, Petrozzi JW, Hurley HJ. Sarcoid granuloma in secondary syphilis. Arch Dermatol 1969; 99: 748–752.

123 Abell E, Marks R, Wilson Jones E. Secondary syphilis: a clinico-pathological review. Br J Dermatol 1975; 93: 53–61.

124 Hirsh BC, Johnson WC. Pathology of granulomatous diseases. Epithelioid granulomas, Part II. Int J Dermatol 1984; 23: 306–313.

125 Pandhi RK, Singh N, Ramam M. Secondary syphilis: a clinicopathologic study. Int J Dermatol 1995; 34: 240–243.

126 Farah FS, Malak JA. Cutaneous leishmaniasis. Arch Dermatol 1971; 103: 467–474.

127 Hart M, Livingood CS, Goltz RW, Totonchy M. Late cutaneous leishmaniasis. Arch Dermatol 1969; 99: 455–458.

128 Paksoy N, Hekim E. Comparative analysis of the clinicopathological features in cutaneous leishmaniasis and lupus vulgaris in Turkey. Trop Med Parasitol 1993; 44: 37–39.

129 Helm KF, Menz J, Gibson LE, Dicken CH. A clinical and histopathologic study of granulomatous rosacea. J Am Acad Dermatol 1991; 25: 1038–1043.

130 Sanchez-Viera M, Hernanz JM, Sampelayo T et al. Granulomatous rosacea in a child infected with the human immunodeficiency virus. J Am Acad Dermatol 1992; 27: 1010–1011.

131 Vin-Christian K, Maurer TA, Berger TG. Acne rosacea as a cutaneous manifestation of HIV infection. J Am Acad Dermatol 1994; 30: 139–140.

132 Amichai B, Grunwald MH, Avinoach I, Halevy S. Granulomatous rosacea associated with *Demodex folliculorum*. Int J Dermatol 1992; 31: 718–719.

133 Basta-Juzbasic A, Marinovic T, Dobric I et al. The possible role of skin surface lipid in rosacea with epithelioid granulomas. Acta Med Croatica 1992; 46; 119–123.

134 Plewig G, Jansen T, Kligman AM. Pyoderma faciale. A review and report of 20 additional cases: is it rosacea? Arch Dermatol 1992; 128: 1611–1617.

135 Marks R, Harcourt-Webster JN. Histopathology of rosacea. Arch Dermatol 1969; 100: 683–691.

136 Mullanax MG, Kierland RR. Granulomatous rosacea. Arch Dermatol 1970; 101: 206–211.

137 Marks R, Wilkinson DS. Rosacea and perioral dermatitis. In: Rook A, Wilkinson DS, Ebling FJG et al, eds. Textbook of dermatology, 4th ed. Oxford: Blackwell Scientific Publications, 1986; 1605–1617.

138 Ackerman AB. Histologic diagnosis of inflammatory skin diseases. Philadelphia: Lea & Febiger, 1978; 658.

139 Rhodes LE, Parslew RAG, Ashworth J. Outcome of facial rashes with non-specific histological features: a long-term follow-up of 64 cases. J Cutan Pathol 1995; 22: 160–163.

140 Hjorth N, Osmundsen P, Rook AJ et al. Perioral dermatitis. Br J Dermatol 1968; 80: 307–313.

141 Fisher AA. Periocular dermatitis akin to the perioral variety. J Am Acad Dermatol 1986; 15: 642–644.

142 Velangi SS, Humphreys F, Beveridge GW. Periocular dermatitis associated with the prolonged use of a steroid eye ointment. Clin Exp Dermatol 1998; 23: 297–298.

143 Frieden IJ, Prose NS, Fletcher V, Turner ML. Granulomatous perioral dermatitis in children. Arch Dermatol 1989; 125: 369–373.

144 Hogan DJ. Perioral dermatitis. Curr Probl Dermatol 1995; 22: 98–104.

145 Manders SM, Lucky AW. Perioral dermatitis in childhood. J Am Acad Dermatol 1992; 27: 688–692.

146 Knautz MA, Lesher JL Jr. Childhood granulomatous periorificial dermatitis. Pediatr Dermatol 1996; 13: 131–134.

147 Hansen KK, McTigue MK, Esterly NB. Multiple facial, neck, and upper trunk papules in a black child. Arch Dermatol 1992; 128: 1396.

148 Sillevis Smitt JH, Das PK, Van Ginkel CJW. Granulomatous perioral dermatitis (facial Afro-Caribbean childhood eruption [FACE]). Br J Dermatol 1991; 125: 399.

149 Malik R, Quirk CJ. Topical applications and perioral dermatitis. Australas J Dermatol 2000; 41: 34–38.

150 Sneddon I. Perioral dermatitis. Br J Dermatol 1972; 87: 430–434.

151 Wells K, Brodell RT. Topical corticosteroid 'addiction'. A cause of perioral dermatitis. Postgrad Med 1993; 93 (5): 225–230.

152 Beacham BE, Kurgansky D, Gould WM. Circumoral dermatitis and cheilitis caused by tartar control dentifrices. J Am Acad Dermatol 1990; 22: 1029–1032.

153 Sainio EL, Kanerva L. Contact allergens in toothpastes and a review of their hypersensitivity. Contact Dermatitis 1995; 33: 100–105.

154 Adams SJ, Davison AM, Cunliffe WJ, Giles GR. Perioral dermatitis in renal transplant recipients maintained on corticosteroids and immunosuppressive therapy. Br J Dermatol 1982. 106: 589–592.

155 El-Rifaie ME. Perioral dermatitis with epithelioid granulomas in a woman: a possible new etiology. Acta Derm Venereol 1980; 60: 359–360.

156 Marks R, Black MM. Perioral dermatitis – a histopathological study of 26 cases. Br J Dermatol 1971; 84: 242–247.

157 Ackerman AB. Histologic diagnosis of inflammatory skin diseases. Philadelphia: Lea & Febiger, 1978; 407.

158 Simonart T, Lowy M, Rasquin F et al. Overlap of sarcoidosis and rosacea. Dermatology 1997; 194: 416–418.

159 Russell Jones R, Wilson Jones E. Disseminated acne agminata. Br J Dermatol (Suppl) 1981; 19: 76.

160 Bedlow AJ, Otter M, Marsden RA. Axillary acne agminata (lupus miliaris disseminatus faciei). Clin Exp Dermatol 1998; 23: 125–128.

161 Kumano K, Tani M, Murata Y. Dapsone in the treatment of miliary lupus of the face. Br J Dermatol 1983; 109: 57–62.

162 Dekio S, Jido J, Imaoka C. Lupus miliaris disseminatus faciei – report of a case in an elderly woman. Clin Exp Dermatol 1991; 16: 295–296.

163 Walchner M, Plewig G, Messer G. Lupus miliaris disseminatus faciei evoked during pregnancy in a patient with cutaneous lupus erythematosus. Int J Dermatol 1998; 37: 864–867.

164 Skowron F, Causeret A-S, Pabion C et al. F.I.G.U.R.E.: Facial Idiopathic GranUlomas with Regressive Evolution. Dermatology 2000; 201: 287–289.

165 Hodak E, Trattner A, Feuerman H et al. Lupus miliaris disseminatus faciei – the DNA of *Mycobacterium tuberculosis* is not detectable in active lesions by polymerase chain reaction. Br J Dermatol 1997; 137: 614–619.

166 El Darouti M, Zaher H. Lupus miliaris disseminatus faciei – pathologic study of early, fully developed, and late lesions. Int J Dermatol 1993; 32: 508–511.

167 Shitara A. Clinicopathological and immunological studies of lupus miliaris disseminatus faciei. J Dermatol 1982; 9: 383–395.

168 Mihara K, Isoda M. Immunohistochemical study of lysozyme in lupus miliaris disseminatus faciei. Br J Dermatol 1986; 115: 187–192.

169 Shitara A. Lupus miliaris disseminatus faciei. Int J Dermatol 1984; 23: 542–544.

170 Dummer W, Lurz C, Jeschke R et al. Granulomatous cheilitis and Crohn's disease in a 3-year-old boy. Pediatr Dermatol 1999; 16: 39–42.

171 Eveson JW. Granulomatous disorders of the oral mucosa. Semin Diagn Pathol 1996; 13: 118–127.

172 Shoji T, Ali S, Gateva E et al. A granulomatous dermatitis associated with idiopathic ulcerative colitis. Int J Dermatol 2000; 39: 215–217.

Necrobiotic granulomas

173 Johnson WC. Necrobiotic granulomas. J Cutan Pathol 1984; 12: 289–299.

174 Muhlbauer JE. Granuloma annulare. J Am Acad Dermatol 1980; 3: 217–230.

175 Owens DW, Freeman RG. Perforating granuloma annulare. Arch Dermatol 1971; 103: 64–67.

176 Salomon RJ, Gardepe SF, Woodley DT. Deep granuloma annulare in adults. Int J Dermatol 1986; 25: 109–112.

177 Rubin M, Lynch FW. Subcutaneous granuloma annulare. Comment on familial granuloma annulare. Arch Dermatol 1966; 93: 416–420.

178 Mutasim DF, Bridges AG. Patch granuloma annulare: Clinicopathologic study of 6 patients. J Am Acad Dermatol 2000; 42: 417–421.

179 Harpster EF, Mauro T, Barr RJ. Linear granuloma annulare. J Am Acad Dermatol 1989; 21: 1138–1141.

180 Wells RS, Smith MA. The natural history of granuloma annulare. Br J Dermatol 1963; 75: 199–205.

181 Lucky AW, Prose NS, Bove K et al. Papular umbilicated granuloma annulare. A report of four pediatric cases. Arch Dermatol 1992; 128: 1375–1378.

182 Setterfield J, Huilgol SC, Black MM. Generalised granuloma annulare successfully treated with PUVA. Clin Exp Dermatol 1999; 24: 458–460.

183 Dabski K, Winkelmann RK. Generalized granuloma annulare: clinical and laboratory findings in 100 patients. J Am Acad Dermatol 1989; 20: 39–47.

184 Guitart J, Zemtsov A, Bergfeld WF, Tomecki KJ. Diffuse dermal histiocytosis. A variant of generalized granuloma annulare. Am J Dermatopathol 1991; 13: 174–178.

185 Erkek E, Karaduman A, Bükülmez G et al. An unusual form of generalized granuloma annulare in a patient with insulin-dependent diabetes mellitus. Acta Derm Venereol 2001; 81: 48–50.

186 Becker D, Enk A, Brauninger W, Knop J. Granuloma annulare disseminatum as a rare side effect of allopurinol. Hautarzt 1995; 46: 343–345.

187 Peñas PF, Jones-Caballero M, Fraga J et al. Perforating granuloma annulare. Int J Dermatol 1997; 36: 340–348.

188 Delaney TJ, Gold SC, Leppard B. Disseminated perforating granuloma annulare. Br J Dermatol 1973; 89: 523–526.

189 Samlaska CP, Sandberg GD, Maggio KL, Sakas EL. Generalized perforating granuloma annulare. J Am Acad Dermatol 1992; 27: 319–322.

190 Draheim JH, Johnson LC, Helwig EB. A clinico-pathologic analysis of 'rheumatoid' nodules occurring in 54 children. Am J Pathol 1959; 35: 678.

191 Burrington JD. 'Pseudorheumatoid' nodules in children. Report of 10 cases. Pediatrics 1970; 45: 473–478.

192 Simons FER, Schaller JG. Benign rheumatoid nodules. Pediatrics 1975; 56: 29–33.

193 Medlock MD, McComb JG, Raffel C, Gonzalez-Gomez I. Subcutaneous palisading granuloma of the scalp in childhood. Pediatr Neurosurg 1994; 21: 113–116.

194 Berardinelli JL, Hyman CJ, Campbell EE, Fireman P. Presence of rheumatoid factor in ten children with isolated rheumatoid-like nodules. J Pediatr 1972; 81: 751–757.

195 Evans MJ, Blessing K, Gray ES. Pseudorheumatoid nodule (deep granuloma annulare) of childhood: clinicopathologic features of twenty patients. Pediatr Dermatol 1994; 11: 6–9.

196 Argent JD, Fairhurst JJ, Clarke NMP. Subcutaneous granuloma annulare: four cases and review of the literature. Pediatr Radiol 1994; 24: 527–529.

197 Dabski K, Winkelmann RK. Destructive granuloma annulare of the skin and underlying soft tissues – report of two cases. Clin Exp Dermatol 1991; 16: 218–221.

198 McLelland J, Young S, Marks JM, Lawrence CM. Seasonally recurrent granuloma annulare of the elbows. Clin Exp Dermatol 1991; 16: 129–130.

199 Uenotsuchi T, Imayama S, Furue M. Seasonally recurrent granuloma annulare on sun-exposed areas. Br J Dermatol 1999; 141: 367.

200 Kossard S, Collins AG, Wegman A, Hughes MR. Necrobiotic granulomas localised to the penis: a possible variant of subcutaneous granuloma annulare. J Cutan Pathol 1990; 17: 101–104.

201 Trap R, Wiebe B. Granuloma annulare localized to the shaft of the penis. Scand J Urol Nephrol 1993; 27: 549–551.

202 Hsu S, Lehner AC, Chang JR. Granuloma annulare localized to the palms. J Am Acad Dermatol 1999; 41: 287–288.

203 Burnstine MA, Headington JT, Reifler DM et al. Periocular granuloma annulare, nodular type. Occurrence in late middle age. Arch Ophthalmol 1994; 112: 1590–1593.

204 Moegelin A, Thalmann U, Haas N. Subcutaneous granuloma annulare of the eyelid. A case report. Int J Oral Maxillofac Surg 1995; 24: 236–238.

205 Sandwich JT, Davis LS. Granuloma annulare of the eyelid: a case report and review of the literature. Pediatr Dermatol 1999; 16: 373–376.

206 Cronquist SD, Stashower ME, Benson PM. Deep dermal granuloma annulare presenting as an eyelid tumor in a child, with review of pediatric eyelid lesions. Pediatr Dermatol 1999; 16: 377–380.

207 Mills A, Chetty R. Auricular granuloma annulare. A consequence of trauma? Am J Dermatopathol 1992; 14: 431–433.

208 Thomas DJB, Rademaker M, Munro DD et al. Visceral and skin granuloma annulare, diabetes, and polyendocrine disease. Br Med J 1986; 293: 977–978.

209 Friedman SJ, Winkelmann RK. Familial granuloma annulare. Report of two cases and review of the literature. J Am Acad Dermatol 1987; 16: 600–605.

210 Friedman-Birnbaum R, Haim S, Gideone O, Barzilai A. Histocompatibility antigens in granuloma annulare. Comparative study of the generalized and localized types. Br J Dermatol 1978; 98: 425–428.

211 Rapelanoro-Rabenja F, Maleville J, Taieb A. [Localized granuloma annulare in children: outcome in 30 cases]. Arch Pediatr 1995; 12: 1145–1148.

212 Weston WL, Morelli JG. "Painful and disabling granuloma annulare": a case of Munchausen by proxy. Pediatr Dermatol 1997; 14: 363–364.

213 Beer WE, Wayte DM, Morgan GW. Knobbly granuloma annulare (GA) of the fingers of a milkman – a possible relationship to his work. Clin Exp Dermatol 1992; 17: 63–64.

214 Smith MD, Downie JB, DiCostanzo D. Granuloma annulare. Int J Dermatol 1997; 36: 326–333.

215 Abraham Z, Feuerman EJ, Schafer I, Feinmesser M. Disseminated granuloma annulare following erythema multiforme minor. Australas J Dermatol 2000; 41: 238–241.

216 Friedman SJ, Fox BJ, Albert HL. Granuloma annulare arising in herpes zoster scars. Report of two cases and review of the literature. J Am Acad Dermatol 1986; 14: 764–770.

217 Zanolli MD, Powell BL, McCalmont T et al. Granuloma annulare and disseminated herpes zoster. Int J Dermatol 1992; 31: 55–57.

218 Krahl D, Hartschuh W, Tilgen W. Granuloma annulare perforans in herpes zoster scars. J Am Acad Dermatol 1993; 29: 859–862.

219 Beer WE, Wilson Jones E. Granuloma annulare following tuberculin Heaf tests. Trans St John's Hosp Dermatol Soc 1966; 52: 68.

220 Friedman-Birnbaum R. Generalized and localized granuloma annulare. Int J Dermatol 1986; 25: 364–366.

221 Muhlemann MF, Williams DRR. Localized granuloma annulare is associated with insulin-dependent diabetes mellitus. Br J Dermatol 1984; 111: 325–329.

222 Choudry K, Charles-Holmes R. Are patients with localized nodular granuloma annulare more likely to have diabetes mellitus? Clin Exp Dermatol 2000; 25: 451–452.

223 Ehrich EW, McGuire JL, Kim YH. Association of granuloma annulare with sarcoidosis. Arch Dermatol 1992; 128: 855–856.

224 Kibarian MA, Mallory SB, Keating J, Shitabata P. Papular umbilicated granuloma annulare in association with Alagille syndrome. Int J Dermatol 1997; 36: 207–209.

225 Vázquez-López F, González-López MA, Raya-Aguado C, Pérez-Oliva N. Localized granuloma annulare and autoimmune thyroiditis: A new case report. J Am Acad Dermatol 2000; 43: 943–945.

226 Granel B, Serratrice J, Rey J et al. Chronic hepatitis C virus infection associated with a generalized granuloma annulare. J Am Acad Dermatol 2000; 43: 918–919.

227 Young HS, Coulson IH. Granuloma annulare following waxing induced pseudofolliculitis – resolution with isotretinoin. Clin Exp Dermatol 2000; 25: 274–276.

228 Gradwell E, Evans S. Perforating granuloma annulare complicating tattoos. Br J Dermatol 1998; 138: 360–361.

229 Wong W-R, Yang L-J, Kuo T-t, Chan H-L. Generalized granuloma annulare associated with granulomatous mycosis fungoides. Dermatology 2000; 200: 54–56.

230 Guill C, Guillen D, Stricker J, Cockerell C. Monoclonal gammopathy associated with a granuloma annulare-like eruption. J Cutan Pathol 2000; 27: 558 (abstract).

231 Jones MA, Laing VB, Files B, Park HK. Granuloma annulare mimicking septic emboli in a child with myelodysplastic syndrome. J Am Acad Dermatol 1998; 38: 106–108.

232 Barksdale SK, Perniciaro C, Halling KC, Strickler TG. Granuloma annulare in patients with malignant lymphoma: clinicopathologic study of thirteen new cases. J Am Acad Dermatol 1994; 31: 42–48.

233 Lo JS, Guitart J, Bergfeld WF. Granuloma annulare associated with metastatic adenocarcinoma. Int J Dermatol 1991; 30: 281–283.

234 Ono H, Yokozeki H, Katayama I, Nishioka K. Granuloma annulare in a patient with malignant lymphoma. Dermatology 1997; 195: 46–47.

235 Magro CM, Crowson AN, Regauer S. Granuloma annulare and necrobiosis lipoidica tissue reactions as a manifestation of systemic disease. Hum Pathol 1996; 27: 50–56.

236 Ghadially R, Sibbald RG, Walter JB, Haberman HF. Granuloma annulare in patients with human immunodeficiency virus infections. J Am Acad Dermatol 1989; 20: 232–235.

237 Smith NP. AIDS, Kaposi's sarcoma and the dermatologist. J R Soc Med 1985; 78: 97–99.

238 Penneys NS, Hicks B. Unusual cutaneous lesions associated with acquired immunodeficiency syndrome. J Am Acad Dermatol 1985; 13: 845–852.

239 Huerter CJ, Bass J, Bergfeld WF, Tubbs RR. Perforating granuloma annulare in a patient with acquired immunodeficiency syndrome. Arch Dermatol 1987; 123: 1217–1220.

240 Cohen PR. Granuloma annulare. A mucocutaneous condition in human immunodeficiency virus-infected patients. Arch Dermatol 1999; 135: 1404–1407.

241 Toro JR, Chu P, Yen T-SB, LeBoit PE. Granuloma annulare and human immunodeficiency virus infection. Arch Dermatol 1999; 135: 1341–1346.

242 O'Moore EJ, Nandawni R, Uthayakumar S et al. HIV-associated granuloma annulare (HAGA): a report of six cases. Br J Dermatol 2000; 142: 1054–1056.

243 McGregor JM, McGibbon DH. Disseminated granuloma annulare as a presentation of acquired immunodeficiency syndrome (AIDS). Clin Exp Dermatol 1992; 17: 60–62.

244 Dahl MV, Ullman S, Goltz RW. Vasculitis in granuloma annulare: histopathology and direct immunofluorescence. Arch Dermatol 1977; 113: 463–467.

245 Bergman R, Pam Z, Lichtig C et al. Localized granuloma annulare. Histopathological and direct immunofluorescence study of early lesions, and the adjacent normal-looking skin of actively spreading lesions. Am J Dermatopathol 1993; 15: 544–548.

246 Modlin RL, Vaccaro SA, Gottlieb B et al. Granuloma annulare. Identification of cells in the cutaneous infiltrate by immunoperoxidase techniques. Arch Pathol Lab Med 1984; 108: 379–382.

247 Kallioinen M, Sandberg M, Kinnunen T, Oikarinen A. Collagen synthesis in granuloma annulare. J Invest Dermatol 1992; 98: 463–468.

248 Umbert P, Winkelmann RK. Histologic, ultrastructural and histochemical studies of granuloma annulare. Arch Dermatol 1977; 113: 1681–1686.

249 Friedman-Birnbaum R, Weltfriend S, Munichor M, Lichtig C. A comparative histopathologic study of generalized and localized granuloma annulare. Am J Dermatopathol 1989; 11: 144–148.

250 Trotter MJ, Crawford RI, O'Connell JX, Tron VA. Mitotic granuloma annulare: a clinicopathologic study of 20 cases. J Cutan Pathol 1996; 23: 537–545.

251 Mullans E, Helm KF. Granuloma annulare: an immunohistochemical study. J Cutan Pathol 1994; 21: 135–139.

252 Silverman RA, Rabinowitz AD. Eosinophils in the cellular infiltrate of granuloma annulare. J Cutan Pathol 1985; 12: 13–17.

253 Romero LS, Kantor GR. Eosinophils are not a clue to the pathogenesis of granuloma annulare. Am J Dermatopathol 1998; 20: 29–34.

254 Friedman-Birnbaum R, Weltfriend S, Kerner H, Lichtig C. Elastic tissue changes in generalized granuloma annulare. Am J Dermatopathol 1989; 11: 429–433.

255 Dabski K, Winkelmann RK. Generalized granuloma annulare: histopathology and immunopathology. Systematic review of 100 cases and comparison with localized granuloma annulare. J Am Acad Dermatol 1989; 20: 28–39.

256 Vargas-Díez E, Feal-Cortizas C, Fraga J et al. Follicular pustulous granuloma annulare. Br J Dermatol 1998; 138: 1075–1078.

257 Kossard S, Goellner JR, Su WPD. Subcutaneous necrobiotic granulomas of the scalp. J Am Acad Dermatol 1980; 3: 180–185.

258 Umbert P, Winkelmann RK. Granuloma annulare: direct immunofluorescence study. Br J Dermatol 1977; 97: 481–486.

259 Bardach HG. Granuloma annulare with transfollicular perforation. J Cutan Pathol 1977; 4: 99–104.

260 Pacilla RS, Mukai K, Dahl MV et al. Differential staining pattern of lysozyme in palisading granulomas: an immunoperoxidase study. J Am Acad Dermatol 1983; 8: 634–638.

261 Saarialho-Kere UK, Chang ES, Welgus HG, Parks WC. Expression of interstitial collagenase, 92-kDa gelatinase, and tissue inhibitor of metalloproteinases-1 in granuloma annulare and necrobiosis lipoidica diabeticorum. J Invest Dermatol 1993; 100: 335–342.

262 Friedman-Birnbaum R, Ludatscher RM. Comparative ultrastructural study of generalized and localized granuloma annulare. Am J Dermatopathol 1986; 8: 302–308.

263 Muller SA, Winkelmann RK. Necrobiosis lipoidica diabeticorum. A clinical and pathological investigation of 171 cases. Arch Dermatol 1966; 93: 272–281.

264 Muller SA, Winkelmann RK. Necrobiosis lipoidica diabeticorum. Histopathologic study of 98 cases. Arch Dermatol 1966; 94: 1–10.

265 Lowitt MH, Dover JS. Necrobiosis lipoidica. J Am Acad Dermatol 1991; 25: 735–748.

266 O'Toole EA, Kennedy U, Nolan JJ et al. Necrobiosis lipoidica: only a minority of patients have diabetes mellitus. Br J Dermatol 1999; 140: 283–286.

267 de Silva BD, Schofield OMV, Walker JD. The prevalence of necrobiosis lipoidica diabeticorum in children with type 1 diabetes. Br J Dermatol 1999; 141: 593–594.

268 Gebauer K, Armstrong M. Koebner phenomenon with necrobiosis lipoidica diabeticorum. Int J Dermatol 1993; 32: 895–896.

269 España A, Sánchez-Yus E, Serna MJ et al. Chronic balanitis with palisading granuloma: an atypical genital localization of necrobiosis lipoidica responsive to pentoxifylline. Dermatology 1994; 188: 222–225.

270 Sahl WJ Jr. Necrobiosis lipoidica diabeticorum. Localization in surgical scars. J Cutan Pathol 1978; 5: 249–253.

271 Velasco-Pastor AM, del Pino Gil-Mateo M, Martinez-Aparicio A, Aliaga-Boniche A. Necrobiosis lipoidica of the glans penis. Br J Dermatol 1996; 135: 154–155.

272 Imakado S, Satomi H, Iskikawa M et al. Diffuse necrobiosis lipoidica diabeticorum associated with non-insulin dependent diabetes mellitus. Clin Exp Dermatol 1998; 23: 271–273.

273 Muller SA. Dermatologic disorders associated with diabetes mellitus. Mayo Clin Proc 1966; 41: 689–703.

274 Darvay A, Acland KM, Russell-Jones R. Persistent ulcerated necrobiosis lipoidica responding to treatment with cyclosporin. Br J Dermatol 1999; 141: 725–727.

275 Patel GK, Harding KG, Mills CM. Severe disabling Köebnerizing ulcerated necrobiosis lipoidica successfully managed with topical PUVA. Br J Dermatol 2000; 143: 668–669.

276 Owen CM, Murphy H, Yates VM. Tissue-engineered dermal skin grafting in the treatment of ulcerated necrobiosis lipoidica. Clin Exp Dermatol 2001; 26: 176–178.

277 Dwyer CM, Dick D. Ulceration in necrobiosis lipoidica – a case report and study. Clin Exp Dermatol 1993; 18: 366–369.

278 Kossard S, Collins E, Wargon O, Downie D. Squamous carcinomas developing in bilateral lesions of necrobiosis lipoidica. Australas J Dermatol 1987; 28: 14–17.

279 Beljaards RC, Groen J, Starink TM. Bilateral squamous cell carcinomas arising in long-standing necrobiosis lipoidica. Dermatologica 1990; 180: 96–98.

280 Gudi VS, Campbell S, Gould DJ, Marshall R. Squamous cell carcinoma in an area of necrobiosis lipoidica diabeticorum: a case report. Clin Exp Dermatol 2000; 25: 597–599.

281 Schwartz ME. Necrobiosis lipoidica and granuloma annulare. Simultaneous occurrence in a patient. Arch Dermatol 1982; 118: 192–193.

282 Monk BE, Du Vivier AWP. Necrobiosis lipoidica and sarcoidosis. Clin Exp Dermatol 1987; 12: 294–295.

283 Gudmundsen K, Smith O, Dervan P, Powell FC. Necrobiosis lipoidica and sarcoidosis. Clin Exp Dermatol 1991; 16: 287–291.

284 Ackerman AB. Histologic diagnosis of inflammatory skin diseases. Philadelphia: Lea & Febiger, 1978; 424.

285 Holland C, Givens V, Smoller BR. Expression of the human erythrocyte glucose transporter glut-1 in areas of sclerotic collagen in necrobiosis lipoidica. J Cutan Pathol 2001; 28: 287–290.

286 Verrotti A, Chiarelli F, Amerio P, Morgese G. Necrobiosis lipoidica diabeticorum in children and adolescents: a clue for underlying renal and retinal disease. Pediatr Dermatol 1995; 12: 220–223.

287 Alerge VA, Winkelmann RK. A new histopathologic feature of necrobiosis lipoidica diabeticorum: lymphoid nodules. J Cutan Pathol 1988; 15: 75–77.

288 Gibson LE, Reizner GT, Winkelmann RK. Necrobiosis lipoidica diabeticorum with cholesterol clefts in the differential diagnosis of necrobiotic xanthogranuloma. J Cutan Pathol 1988; 15: 18–21.

289 De la Torre C, Losada A, Cruces MJ. Necrobiosis lipoidica. A case with prominent cholesterol clefting and transepithelial elimination. Am J Dermatopathol 1999; 21: 575–577.

290 Parra CA. Transepithelial elimination in necrobiosis lipoidica. Br J Dermatol 1977; 96: 83–86.

291 McGregor JM, Muller J, Smith NP, Hay RJ. Necrobiotic xanthogranuloma without periorbital lesions. J Am Acad Dermatol 1993; 29: 466–469.

292 Ullman S, Dahl MV. Necrobiosis lipoidica. An immunofluorescence study. Arch Dermatol 1977; 113: 1671–1673.

293 Oikarinen A, Mortenhumer M, Kallioinen M, Savolainen E-R. Necrobiosis lipoidica: ultrastructural and biochemical demonstration of a collagen defect. J Invest Dermatol 1987; 88: 227–232.

294 Boulton AJM, Cutfield RG, Abouganem D et al. Necrobiosis lipoidica diabeticorum: a clinicopathologic study. J Am Acad Dermatol 1988; 18: 530–537.

295 Yamamoto T, Ohkubo H, Nishioka K. Skin manifestations associated with rheumatoid arthritis. J Dermatol 1995; 22: 324–329.

296 Rasker JJ, Kuipers FC. Are rheumatoid nodules caused by vasculitis? A study of 13 early cases. Ann Rheum Dis 1983; 42: 384–388.

297 Hahn BH, Yardley JH, Stevens MB. 'Rheumatoid' nodules in systemic lupus erythematosus. Ann Intern Med 1970; 72: 49–58.

298 Schofield JK, Cerio R, Grice K. Systemic lupus erythematosus presenting with 'rheumatoid nodules'. Clin Exp Dermatol 1992; 17: 53–55.

299 Vachvanichsanong P, Dissaneewate P. Childhood systemic lupus erythematosus in Songklanagarind Hospital: a potential unique subgroup. Clin Rheumatol 1993; 12: 346–349.

300 Williams FM, Cohen PR, Arnett FC. Accelerated cutaneous nodulosis during methotrexate therapy in a patient with rheumatoid arthritis. J Am Acad Dermatol 1998; 39: 359–362.

301 Veys EM, De Keyser F. Rheumatoid nodules: differential diagnosis and immunohistological findings. Ann Rheum Dis 1993; 52: 625–626.

302 Patterson JW. Rheumatoid nodule and subcutaneous granuloma annulare. A comparative histologic study. Am J Dermatopathol 1988; 10: 1–8.

303 Patterson JW, Demos PT. Superficial ulcerating rheumatoid necrobiosis: a perforating rheumatoid nodule. Cutis 1985; 36: 323–328.

304 Aherne MJ, Bacon PA, Blake DR et al. Immunohistochemical findings in rheumatoid nodules. Virchows Arch (A) 1985; 407: 191–202.

305 Allen AC. The skin. St. Louis: C.V. Mosby, 1954; 146.

306 Bennett GA, Zeller JW, Bauer W. Subcutaneous nodules of rheumatoid arthritis and rheumatic fever. Arch Pathol 1940; 30: 70–89.

307 Chopra P, Narula JP, Tandon R. Ultrastructure of naturally occurring subcutaneous nodule in acute rheumatic fever. Int J Cardiol 1991; 30: 124–127.

308 Barr RJ, King DF, McDonald RM, Bartlow GA. Necrobiotic granulomas associated with bovine collagen test site injections. J Am Acad Dermatol 1982; 6: 867–869.

309 Graham JH. Superficial fungus infections. In: Graham JH, Johnson WC, Helwg EB. Dermal pathology. Hagerstown, Maryland: Harper & Row 1972; 176.

310 Alguacil-Garcia A. Necrobiotic palisading suture granulomas simulating rheumatoid nodule. Am J Surg Pathol 1993; 17: 920–923.

311 Kuhn C, Lima M, Hood A. Palisading granulomas caused by foreign bodies. J Cutan Pathol 1997; 24: 108.

312 Rosen VJ. Cutaneous manifestations of drug abuse by parenteral injections. Am J Dermatopathol 1985; 7: 79–83.

313 Ajithkumar K, Anand U, Pulimood S et al. Vaccine-induced necrobiotic granuloma. Clin Exp Dermatol 1998; 23: 222–224.

314 Lalinga AV, Pellegrino M, Laurini L, Miracco C. Necrobiotic palisading granuloma at injection site of disodium clodronate: a case report. Dermatology 1999; 198: 394–395.

Suppurative granulomas

315 Leslie DF, Beardmore GL. Chromoblastomycosis in Queensland: a retrospective study of 13 cases at the Royal Brisbane Hospital. Australas J Dermatol 1979; 20: 23–30.

316 Bullpitt P, Weedon D. Sporotrichosis: a review of 39 cases. Pathology 1978; 10: 249–256.

317 Hirsh BC, Johnson WC. Pathology of granulomatous diseases. Mixed inflammatory granulomas. Int J Dermatol 1984; 23: 585–597.

318 Reyes-Flores O. Granulomas induced by living agents. Int J Dermatol 1986; 25: 158–165.

319 Wilson-Jones E, Winkelmann RK. Superficial granulomatous pyoderma: a localized vegetative form of pyoderma gangrenosum. J Am Acad Dermatol 1988; 18: 511–521.

320 Lichter MD, Welykyj SE, Gradini R, Solomon LM. Superficial granulomatous pyoderma. Int J Dermatol 1991; 30: 418–421.

321 Hardwick N, Cerio R. Superficial granulomatous pyoderma. A report of two cases. Br J Dermatol 1993; 129: 718–722.

322 Quimby SR, Gibson LE, Winkelmann RK. Superficial granulomatous pyoderma: clinicopathologic spectrum. Mayo Clin Proc 1989; 64: 37–43.

Foreign body granulomas

323 Leonard DD. Starch granulomas. Arch Dermatol 1973; 107: 101–103.

324 Tye MJ, Hashimoto K, Fox F. Talc granulomas of the skin. JAMA 1966; 198: 1370–1372.

325 Snyder RA, Schwartz RA. Cactus bristle implantation. Report of an unusual case initially seen with rows of yellow hairs. Arch Dermatol 1983; 119: 152–154.

326 Matwiyoff GN, McKinlay JR, Miller CH, Graham BS. Transepidermal migration of external cardiac pacing wire presenting as a cutaneous nodule. J Am Acad Dermatol 2000; 42: 865–866.

327 Rudolph CM, Soyer HP, Schuller-Petrovic S, Kerl H. Foreign body granuloma due to bioplastique microimplants. Am J Dermatopathol 2000; 22: 358 (abstract).

328 Rudolph CM, Soyer HP, Schuller-Petrovic S, Kerl H. Foreign body granulomas due to injectable aesthetic microimplants. Am J Surg Pathol 1999; 23: 113–117.

329 Raulin C, Greve B, Hartschuh W, Soegding K. Exudative granulomatous reaction to hyaluronic acid (Hylaform®). Contact Dermatitis 2000; 43: 178–179.

330 Hatano Y, Asada Y, Komada S et al. A case of pencil core granuloma with an unusual temporal profile. Dermatology 2000; 201: 151–153.

331 Overholt MA, Tschen JA, Font RL. Granulomatous reaction to collagen implant: light and electron microscopic observations. Cutis 1993; 51: 95–98.

332 Peluso AM, Fanti PA, Monti M et al. Cutaneous complications of artificial hair implantation: a pathological study. Dermatology 1992; 184: 129–132.

333 Young PC, Smack DP, Sau P et al. Golf club granuloma. J Am Acad Dermatol 1995; 32: 1047–1048.

334 Allen AC. Persistent 'insect bites' (dermal eosinophilic granulomas) simulating lymphoblastomas, histiocytoses, and squamous cell carcinomas. Am J Pathol 1948; 24: 367–375.

335 Montemarano AD, Sau P, Johnson FB, James WD. Cutaneous granulomas caused by an aluminum-zirconium complex: An ingredient of antiperspirants. J Am Acad Dermatol 1997; 37: 496–498.

336 Jordaan HF, Sandler M. Zinc-induced granuloma – a unique complication of insulin therapy. Clin Exp Dermatol 1989; 14: 227–229.

337 Posner DI, Guill MA III. Cutaneous foreign body granulomas associated with intravenous drug abuse. J Am Acad Dermatol 1985; 13: 869–872.

338 Porter WM, Grabczynska S, Francis N, Staughton RCD. The perils and pitfalls of penile injections. Br J Dermatol 1999; 141: 736–738.

339 Park J-H, Kim JG, Cha S-H, Park SD. Eosinophilic foreign body granuloma after multiple self-administered bee stings. Br J Dermatol 1998; 139: 1102–1105.

340 Postlethwait RW, Willigan DA, Ulin AW. Human tissue reaction to sutures. Ann Surg 1975; 181: 144–150.

341 Fawcett HA, Smith NP. Injection-site granuloma due to aluminum. Arch Dermatol 1984; 120: 1318–1322.

342 Cominos D, Strutton G, Busmanis I. Granulomas associated with tetanus toxoid immunisation. Am J Dermatopathol 1993; 15: 114–117.

343 Schwarze HP, Giordano-Labadie F, Loche F et al. Delayed-hypersensitivity granulomatous reaction induced by blepharopigmentation with aluminum-silicate. J Am Acad Dermatol 2000; 42: 888–891.

344 Yanagihara M, Fujii T, Wakamatu N et al. Silicone granuloma on the entry points of acupuncture, venepuncture and surgical needles. J Cutan Pathol 2000; 27: 301–305.

345 Murphy M, Wiehe P, Barnes L. Silica granuloma: another cause of tennis elbow. Br J Dermatol 1997; 137: 477.

346 Sina B, Lutz LL. Cutaneous oxalate granuloma. J Am Acad Dermatol 1990; 22: 316–318.

347 Isonokami M, Nishida K, Okada N, Yoshikawa K. Cutaneous oxalate granulomas in a haemodialysed patient: report of a case with unique clinical features. Br J Dermatol 1993; 128: 690–692.

348 Altchek DD, Pearlstein HH. Granulomatous reaction to autologous hairs incarcerated during hair transplantation. J Dermatol Surg Oncol 1978; 4: 928–929.

349 Joseph HL, Gifford H. Barber's interdigital pilonidal sinus. Arch Dermatol 1954; 70: 616–624.

350 Leshin B, Prichard EH, White WL. Dermal granulomatous inflammation to cornified cells. Significance near cutaneous squamous cell carcinoma. Arch Dermatol 1992; 128: 649–652.

Miscellaneous granulomas

351 Wiesenfeld D, Ferguson MM, Mitchell DN et al. Oro-facial granulomatosis – a clinical and pathological analysis. Q J Med 1985; 54: 101–113.

352 Greene RM, Rogers RS III. Melkersson–Rosenthal syndrome: a review of 36 patients. J Am Acad Dermatol 1989; 21: 1263–1270.

353 Meisel-Stosiek M, Hornstein OP, Stosiek N. Family study on Melkersson–Rosenthal syndrome. Acta Derm Venereol 1990; 70: 221–226.

354 Armstrong DKB, Burrows D. Orofacial granulomatosis. Int J Dermatol 1995; 34: 830–833.

355 Allen CM, Camisa C, Hamzeh S, Stephens L. Cheilitis granulomatosa: report of six cases and review of the literature. J Am Acad Dermatol 1990; 23: 444–450.

356 Stein SL, Mancini AJ. Melkersson–Rosenthal syndrome in childhood: Successful management with combination steroid and minocycline therapy. J Am Acad Dermatol 1999; 41: 746–748.

357 Ziem PE, Pfrommer C, Goerdt S et al. Melkersson–Rosenthal syndrome in childhood: a challenge in differential diagnosis and treatment. Br J Dermatol 2000; 143: 860–863.

358 Levenson MJ, Ingerman M, Grimes C, Anand KV. Melkersson–Rosenthal syndrome. Arch Otolaryngol 1984; 110: 540–542.

359 Vistnes LM, Kernahan DA. The Melkersson–Rosenthal syndrome. Plast Reconstr Surg 1971; 48: 126–132.

360 Sabroe RA, Kennedy CTC. Facial granulomatous lymphoedema and syringomyelia. Clin Exp Dermatol 1996; 21: 72–74.

361 Levy FS, Bircher AJ, Büchner SA. Delayed-type hypersensitivity to cow's milk protein in Melkersson–Rosenthal syndrome: coincidence or pathogenetic role? Dermatology 1996; 192: 99–102.

362 Muellegger RR, Weger W, Zoechling N et al. Granulomatous cheilitis and *Borrelia burgdorferi*. Polymerase chain reaction and serologic studies in a retrospective case series of 12 patients. Arch Dermatol 2000; 136: 1502–1506.

363 Apaydin R, Bilen N, Bayramgürler D et al. Detection of *Mycobacterium tuberculosis* DNA in a patient with Melkersson–Rosenthal syndrome using polymerase chain reaction. Br J Dermatol 2000; 142: 1251–1252.

364 Rogers RS III. Granulomatous cheilitis, Melkersson–Rosenthal syndrome, and orofacial granulomatosis. Arch Dermatol 2000; 136: 1557–1558.

365 Nelson HM, Stevenson AG. Melkersson–Rosenthal syndrome with positive Kveim test. Clin Exp Dermatol 1988; 13: 49–50.

366 Thiriar S, Deroux E, Dourov N et al. Granulomatous vulvitis, granulomatous cheilitis: a single diagnosis? Dermatology 1998; 196: 455–458.

367 Carr D. Granulomatous cheilitis in Crohn's disease. Br Med J 1974; 4: 636.

368 De Aloe G, Rubegni P, Mazzatenta C, Fimiani M. Complete Melkersson–Rosenthal syndrome in a patient with Crohn's disease. Dermatology 1997; 195: 182.

369 Rhodes EL, Stirling GA. Granulomatous cheilitis. Arch Dermatol 1965; 92: 40–44.

370 Krutchkoff D, James R. Cheilitis granulomatosa. Successful treatment with combined local triamcinolone injections and surgery. Arch Dermatol 1978; 114: 1203–1206.

371 Westermark P, Henriksson T-G. Granulomatous inflammation of the vulva and penis, a genital counterpart to cheilitis granulomatosa. Dermatologica 1979; 158: 269–274.

372 Samaratunga H, Strutton G, Wright RG, Hill B. Squamous cell carcinoma arising in a case of vulvitis granulomatosa or vulval variant of Melkersson–Rosenthal syndrome. Gynaecol Oncol 1991; 41: 263–269.

373 Pruim B, Strutton G, Congdon S et al. Cutaneous histiocytic lymphangitis: an unusual manifestation of rheumatoid arthritis. Australas J Dermatol 2000; 41: 101–105.

374 Tomasini C, Soro E, Pippione M. Angioendotheliomatosis in a woman with rheumatoid arthritis. Am J Dermatopathol 2000; 22: 334–338.

375 O'Brien JP. Actinic granuloma. An annular connective tissue disorder affecting sun- and heat-damaged (elastotic) skin. Arch Dermatol 1975; 111: 460–466.

376 Wilson Jones E. Necrobiosis lipoidica presenting on the face and scalp. An account of 29 patients and a detailed consideration of recent histochemical findings. Trans St. John's Hosp Dermatol Soc 1971; 57: 202–220.

377 Mehregan AH, Altman J. Miescher's granuloma of the face. A variant of the necrobiosis lipoidica–granuloma annulare spectrum. Arch Dermatol 1973; 107: 62–64.

378 Hanke CW, Bailin PL, Roenigk HH. Annular elastolytic giant cell granuloma. A clinicopathologic study of five cases and a review of similar entities. J Am Acad Dermatol 1979; 1: 413–421.

379 Özkaya-Bayazit E, Büyükbabani N, Baykal C et al. Annular elastolytic giant cell granuloma: sparing of a burn scar and successful treatment with chloroquine. Br J Dermatol 1999; 140: 525–530.

380 Ragaz A, Ackerman AB. Is actinic granuloma a specific condition? Am J Dermatopathol 1979; 1: 43–50.

381 Wilson Jones E. Actinic granuloma. Am J Dermatopathol 1980; 2: 89–90.

382 Weedon D. Actinic granuloma: the controversy continues. Am J Dermatopathol 1980; 2: 90–91.

383 Ishibashi A, Yokoyama A, Hirano K. Annular elastolytic giant cell granuloma occurring in covered areas. Dermatologica 1987; 174: 293–297.

384 Revenga F, Rovira I, Pimentel J, Alejo M. Annular elastolytic giant cell granuloma – actinic granuloma? Clin Exp Dermatol 1996; 21: 51–53.

385 Proia AD, Browning DJ, Klintworth GK. Actinic granuloma of the conjunctiva. Am J Ophthalmol 1983; 96: 116–118.

386 Steffen C. Actinic granuloma of the conjunctiva. Am J Dermatopathol 1992; 14: 253–254.

387 O'Brien JP, Regan W. Actinically degenerate elastic tissue is the likely antigenic basis of actinic granuloma of the skin and of temporal arteritis. J Am Acad Dermatol 1999; 40: 214–222.

388 Pierard GE, Henrijean A, Foidart JM, Lapiere CM. Actinic granulomas and relapsing polychondritis. Acta Derm Venereol 1982; 62: 531–533.

389 Agarwal S, Takwale A, Bajallan N et al. Co-existing actinic granuloma and giant molluscum contagiosum. Clin Exp Dermatol 2000; 25: 401–403.

390 Lee Y-S, Vijayasingam S, Chan H-L. Photosensitive annular elastolytic giant cell granuloma with cutaneous amyloidosis. Am J Dermatopathol 1989; 11: 443–450.

391 Sina B, Wood C, Rudo K. Generalized elastophagocytic granuloma. Cutis 1992; 49: 355–357.

392 Kurose N, Nakagawa H, Iozumi K et al. Systemic elastolytic granulomatosis with cutaneous, ocular, lymph nodal, and intestinal involvement. J Am Acad Dermatol 1992; 26: 359–363.

393 Davies MG, Newman P. Actinic granulomata in a young woman following prolonged surbed usage. Br J Dermatol 1997; 136: 797–798.

394 O'Brien JP. Actinic granuloma: the expanding significance. Int J Dermatol 1985; 24: 473–490.

395 Burket JM, Zelickson AS. Intracellular elastin in generalized granuloma annulare. J Am Acad Dermatol 1986; 14: 975–981.

396 McGrae JD Jr. Actinic granuloma. A clinical, histopathologic, and immunocytochemical study. Arch Dermatol 1986; 122: 43–47.

397 Barnhill RL, Goldenhersh MA. Elastophagocytosis: a non-specific reaction pattern associated with inflammatory processes in sun-protected skin. J Cutan Pathol 1989; 16: 199–202.

398 Steffen C. Actinic granuloma (O'Brien). J Cutan Pathol 1988; 15: 66–74.

399 Yanagihara M, Kato F, Mori S. Extra- and intra-cellular digestion of elastic fibers by macrophages in annular elastolytic giant cell granuloma. J Cutan Pathol 1987; 14: 303–308.

400 Prendiville J, Griffiths WAD, Russell Jones R. O'Brien's actinic granuloma. Br J Dermatol 1985; 113: 353–358.

401 Meyers WM, Connor DH. In: Binford CH, Connor DH, eds. Pathology of tropical and extraordinary diseases, Volume 2. Washington, D.C.: Armed Forces Institute of Pathology, 1976; 676.

402 Leiker DL, Koh SH, Spaas JAJ. Granuloma multiforme. A new skin disease resembling leprosy. Int J Lepr 1964; 32: 368–376.

403 Cherian S. Is granuloma multiforme a photodermatosis? Int J Dermatol 1994; 33: 21–22.

404 Allenby CF, Wilson Jones E. Granuloma multiforme. Trans St. John's Hosp Dermatol Soc 1969; 55: 88–98.

405 Kligman AM. Early destructive effect of sunlight on human skin. JAMA 1969; 210: 2377–2380.

406 Dogiotti M, Leibowitz M. Granulomatous ochronosis – a cosmetic-induced disorder in blacks. S Afr Med J 1979; 56: 757–760.

407 Jordaan HF, Mulligan RP. Actinic granuloma-like change in exogenous ochronosis: case report. J Cutan Pathol 1990; 17: 236–240.

408 Jacyk WK. Annular granulomatous lesions in exogenous ochronosis are manifestations of sarcoidosis. Am J Dermatopathol 1995; 33: 18–22.

409 Berron-Ruiz A, Berron-Perez R, Ruiz-Maldonado R. Cutaneous markers of primary immunodeficiency diseases in children. Pediatr Dermatol 2000; 17: 91–96.

410 Arbiser JL. Genetic immunodeficiencies: cutaneous manifestations and recent progress. J Am Acad Dermatol 1995; 33: 82–89.

411 Ten RM. Primary immunodeficiencies. Mayo Clin Proc 1998; 73: 865–872.

412 Buckley RH. Primary immunodeficiency diseases due to defects in lymphocytes. N Engl J Med 2000; 343: 1313–1324.

413 Marques AR, Kwon-Chung KJ, Holland SM et al. Suppurative cutaneous granulomata caused by *Microascus cinereus* in a patient with chronic granulomatous disease. Clin Infect Dis 1995; 20: 110–114.

414 Windhorst DB, Good RA. Dermatologic manifestations of fatal granulomatous disease of childhood. Arch Dermatol 1971; 103: 351–357.

415 Tauber AI, Borregaard N, Simons E, Wright J. Chronic granulomatous disease: a syndrome of phagocyte oxidase deficiencies. Medicine 1983; 62: 286–309.

416 Dohil M, Prendiville JS, Crawford RI, Speert DP. Cutaneous manifestations of chronic granulomatous disease. A report of four cases and review of the literature. J Am Acad Dermatol 1997; 36: 899–907.

417 Mertens G, DeSmet D, Gielis M. A case of chronic granulomatous skin disease associated with deficient HLA class I expression. Br J Dermatol 2000; 143: 659–660.

418 Chowdhury MMU, Anstey A, Matthews CNA. The dermatosis of chronic granulomatous disease. Clin Exp Dermatol 2000; 25: 190–194.

419 Fleming MG, Gewurz AT, Pearson RW. Caseating cutaneous granulomas in a patient with X-linked infantile hypogammaglobulinemia. J Am Acad Dermatol 1991; 24: 629–633.

420 Torrelo A, Mediero IG, Zambrano A. Caseating cutaneous granulomas in a child with common variable immunodeficiency. Pediatr Dermatol 1995; 12: 170–173.

421 Levine TS, Price AB, Boyle S, Webster ADB. Cutaneous sarcoid-like granulomas in primary immunodeficiency disorders. Br J Dermatol 1994; 130: 118–120.

422 Cornejo P, Romero A, López S et al. Cutaneous and hepatic granulomas in a young woman with common variable immunodeficiency. Br J Dermatol 1999; 140: 546–547.

423 Ziegler EM, Seung LM, Soltani K, Medenica MM. Cutaneous granulomas with two clinical presentations in a patient with common variable immunodeficiency. J Am Acad Dermatol 1997; 37: 499–500.

424 Álvarez-Cuesta C, Molinos L, Cascante JA et al. Cutaneous granulomas in a patient with common variable immunodeficiency. Acta Derm Venereol 1999; 79: 334.

425 Pujol RM, Nadal C, Taberner R et al. Cutaneous granulomatous lesions in common variable immunodeficiency: complete resolution after intravenous immunoglobulin. Dermatology 1999; 198: 156–158.

426 Smith KJ, Skelton H. Common variable immunodeficiency treated with a recombinant human IgG, tumour necrosis factor-α receptor fusion protein. Br J Dermatol 2001. 144: 597–600.

427 Paller AS, Massey RB, Curtis A et al. Cutaneous granulomatous lesions in patients with ataxia-telangiectasia. J Pediatr 1991; 119: 917–922.

428 Joshi RK, Al Asiri RH, Haleem A et al. Cutaneous granuloma with ataxia telangiectasia – a case report and review of literature. Clin Exp Dermatol 1993; 18: 458–461.

429 Drolet BA, Drolet B, Zvulunov A et al. Cutaneous granulomas as a presenting sign in ataxia-telangiectasia. Dermatology 1997; 194: 273–275.

430 Siegfried EC, Prose NS, Friedman NJ, Paller AS. Cutaneous granulomas in children with combined immunodeficiency. J Am Acad Dermatol 1991; 25: 761–766.

431 Crofts MJ, Joyner MV, Sharp JC et al. Sarcoidosis associated with combined immunodeficiency. Postgrad Med J 1980; 56: 263–265.

432 Skinner MD, Masters R. Primary acquired agammaglobulinemia with granulomas of the skin and internal organs. Arch Dermatol 1970; 102: 109–110.

433 Cohen PR, Grossman ME, Silvers DN, DeLeo VA. Human immunodeficiency virus-associated granuloma annulare. Int J STD AIDS 1991; 2: 168–171.

434 Fischl MA, Daikos GL, Uttamchandani RB et al. Clinical presentation and outcome of patients with HIV infection and tuberculosis caused by multiple-drug-resistant bacilli. Ann Intern Med 1992; 117: 184–190.

435 Amin DN, Sperber K, Brown LK et al. Positive Kveim test in patients with coexisting sarcoidosis and human immunodeficiency virus infection. Chest 1992; 101: 1454–1456.

436 Sampaio EP, Caneshi JRT, Nerry JAC et al. Cellular immune response to *Mycobacterium leprae* infection in human immunodeficiency virus-infected individuals. Infect Immun 1995; 63: 1848–1854.

437 Smith KJ, Skelton HG III, Yeager J et al. Histologic features of foreign body reactions in patients with human immunodeficiency virus type 1. J Am Acad Dermatol 1993; 28: 470–476.

438 Gottlieb GJ, Duve RS, Ackerman AB. Interstitial granulomatous dermatitis with cutaneous cords and arthritis: linear subcutaneous bands in rheumatoid arthritis revisited. Dermatopathology: Practical and Conceptual 1995; 1: 3–6.

439 Chu P, Connolly MK, LeBoit PE. The histopathologic spectrum of palisaded neutrophilic and granulomatous dermatitis in patients with collagen vascular disease. Arch Dermatol 1994; 130: 1278–1283.

440 Dykman CJ, Galens GJ, Good AE. Linear subcutaneous bands in rheumatoid arthritis: an unusual form of rheumatoid granuloma. Ann Intern Med 1965; 63: 134–140.

441 Wilmoth GJ, Perniciaro C. Cutaneous extravascular necrotizing granuloma (Winkelmann granuloma): confirmation of the association with systemic disease. J Am Acad Dermatol 1996; 34: 753–759.

442 Higaki Y, Yamashita H, Sato K et al. Rheumatoid papules: a report on four patients with histopathologic analysis. J Am Acad Dermatol 1993; 28: 406–411.

443 Long D, Thiboutot DM, Majeski JT et al. Interstitial granulomatous dermatitis with arthritis. J Am Acad Dermatol 1996; 34: 957–961.

444 Aloi F, Tomasini C, Pippione M. Interstitial granulomatous dermatitis with plaques. Am J Dermatopathol 1999; 21: 320–323.

445 Finan MC, Winkelmann RK. The cutaneous extravascular necrotizing granuloma (Churg–Strauss granuloma) and systemic disease: a review of 27 cases. Medicine 1983; 62: 142–158.

446 Magro CM, Crowson AN, Schapiro BL. The interstitial granulomatous drug reaction: a distinctive clinical and pathological entity. J Cutan Pathol 1998; 25: 72–78.

447 van Haselen CW, Toonstra J, van der Putte SJC et al. Granulomatous slack skin. Report of three patients with an updated review of the literature. Dermatology 1998; 196: 382–391.

448 Camacho FM, Burg G, Moreno JC et al. Granulomatous slack skin in childhood. Pediatr Dermatol 1997; 14: 204–208.

449 Tsuruta D, Kono T, Kutsuna H et al. Granulomatous slack skin: an ultrastructural study. J Cutan Pathol 2001; 28: 44–48.

The vasculopathic reaction pattern

8

INTRODUCTION

Cutaneous blood supply

The skin is supplied by small segmental arteries that may reach the skin directly or after supplying the underlying muscle and soft tissue en route. These vessels branch to supply the subcutis with a meshwork of arteries and arterioles. In the dermis, there is a *deep (lower) horizontal plexus*, situated near the interface with the subcutis, and a *superficial (upper) horizontal plexus* at the junction of the papillary and reticular dermis. The two plexuses are joined by vertically oriented arterioles. These interconnecting arterioles also give rise to vessels that form an arborizing plexus around the hair follicles. The sweat g and plexus of vessels may also arise from the vertical arterioles or from arteries in the subcutis.

The superficial horizontal plexus is a band-like network of anastomosing small arterioles and postcapillary venules, connected by a capillary network. The bulk of the microcirculation of the skin resides in this plexus and the capillary loops that form from it and pass into the dermal papillae. The postcapillary venules are the important functional sites for disease processes in the skin. For example, they represent the site of immune complex deposition in acute vasculitis, the site of vascular permeability in urticaria, and an area for leukocyte recruitment and diapedesis in vasculitis.

The *arterioles* in the superficial plexus have a homogeneous basement membrane, a discontinuous subendothelial elastic lamina, and one or two layers of smooth muscle cells (in contrast to arterioles in the deep plexus which have 4–5 layers). The capillary wall contains a basement membrane which changes from homogeneous to multilayered as it changes from an *arteriolar capillary* to a venous capillary. The *postcapillary venule* is surrounded by veil cells rather than the smooth muscle cells seen in arterioles. The venules drain into large veins that accompany the vertically oriented arterioles. At the dermal–subcutaneous junction there are collecting veins with two cusped valves that are oriented to prevent the retrograde flow of blood.

In addition to the vessels listed above, there are *arteriovenous anastomoses* (shunts) which bypass the capillary network. They play a role in thermo-regulation. A special form of arteriovenous shunt, occurring in the periphery, is the *glomus apparatus*. The glomus is composed of an endothelial-lined channel surrounded by cuboidal glomus cells; it has a rich nerve supply.

The dermal lymphatic network has a similar pattern of distribution to that of the blood supply.

At a functional level, the endothelial adherens junction complex is an important mechanism in the control of leukocyte and macromolecule trans-migration. The adherens junction is formed by transmembrane molecules of the cadherin family linking to catenins, which anchor the adhesion plaque to the cytoskeleton of the endothelial cell.[2] The cadherin is cell-type specific and in the vessel is known as vascular endothelial (VE)-cadherin.[2] Interestingly, the VE-cadherin knockout mouse dies during embryonic development, indicating the importance of this substance in organogenesis.[2]

Categorization of diseases of blood vessels

Diseases of cutaneous blood vessels are an important cause of morbidity. In the case of the vasculitides, mortality may occasionally result. Blood vessels have a limited number of ways in which they can react to insults of various kinds, resulting in considerable morphological overlap between the various clinical syndromes that have been described.

The broad classifications used in this chapter are morphologically rather than etiologically based, as this is the most practical scheme to follow when confronted with a biopsy.

Excluding tumors and telangiectases, which are discussed in Chapter 38, there are six major groups of vascular diseases:

- non-inflammatory purpuras
- vascular occlusive diseases
- urticarias
- vasculitis
- neutrophilic dermatoses
- miscellaneous.

The *non-inflammatory purpuras* are characterized by the extravasation of erythrocytes into the dermis. There is no inflammation or occlusion of blood vessels.

The *vascular occlusive* diseases exhibit narrowing or obliteration of the lumina of small vessels by fibrin or platelet thrombi, cryoglobulins, cholesterol or other material. Purpura and sometimes ulceration and necrosis may be clinical features of this group.

The *urticarias* involve the leakage of plasma and some cells from dermal vessels. Some of the urticarias have overlapping features with the vasculitides, further justification for their inclusion in this chapter.

In *vasculitis* there is inflammation of the walls of blood vessels. In subsiding lesions there may only be an inflammatory infiltrate in close contact with vessel walls. The vasculitides are subclassified on the basis of the inflammatory process into acute, chronic lymphocytic and granulomatous forms. Fibrin-platelet thrombi may sometimes form, particularly in acute vasculitis, leading to some overlap with the vascular occlusive diseases.

The *neutrophilic dermatoses* are a group of conditions in which there is a prominent dermal infiltrate of neutrophils, but usually without the fibrinoid necrosis of vessel walls that typifies acute (leukocytoclastic) vasculitis.

The *miscellaneous group* of vascular disorders includes vascular calcification, pericapillary fibrin cuffs, vascular aneurysms and erythermalgia.

NON-INFLAMMATORY PURPURAS

Purpura is hemorrhage into the skin. Clinically, this may take the form of small lesions less than 3 mm in diameter (petechiae) or larger areas known as ecchymoses. There is a predilection for the limbs. The numerous causes of purpura may be broadly grouped into defects of blood vessels, platelets or coagulation factors.[3,4]

At the histopathological level, purpuras are characterized by an extravasation of red blood cells into the dermis from small cutaneous vessels. If the purpura is chronic or recurrent, hemosiderin or hematoidin pigment may be present.[5,6] Purpuras have traditionally been divided into an inflammatory group (vasculitis) and a non-inflammatory group when there is no inflammation of vessel walls.

The non-inflammatory purpuras include idiopathic thrombocytopenic purpura, senile purpura, the autoerythrocyte sensitization syndrome (psychogenic purpura), traumatic (including factitious) purpura and drug purpuras.[5,7–11] Sickle-cell disease is an unusual cause of purpura.[12] Only senile purpura will be considered in further detail in this volume.

SENILE PURPURA

Senile purpura is a common form of non-inflammatory purpura that occurs on the extensor surfaces of the forearms and hands of elderly individuals.[13,14] Usually large ecchymoses are present. It has been suggested that the bleeding results from minor shearing injuries to poorly supported cutaneous vessels.

Senile purpura tends to persist longer than other forms of purpura, indicating slower removal or breakdown of the erythrocytes. Furthermore, senile purpura does not usually show the color changes of bruising, as seen in purpura of other causes.

Histopathology
Senile purpura is characterized by extravasation of red blood cells into the dermis. This is most marked in the upper dermis and in a perivascular location. There is also marked solar elastosis and often some thinning of the dermis with atrophy of collagen bundles.

VASCULAR OCCLUSIVE DISEASES

Occlusion of cutaneous blood vessels is quite uncommon. The clinical picture that results is varied. It may include purpura, livedo reticularis,[15–17] erythromelalgia, ulceration or infarction. Cutaneous infarction only occurs when numerous vessels in the lower dermis and subcutis are occluded.

Complete or partial occlusion of cutaneous vessels usually results from the lodgment of fibrin-platelet thrombi. Other causes include platelet-rich thrombi in thrombocythemia and thrombotic thrombocytopenic purpura, cryoglobulins in cryoglobulinemia, cholesterol in atheromatous emboli, swollen endothelial cells containing numerous acid-fast bacilli in Lucio's phenomenon of leprosy, fungi in mucormycosis[18] and fibrous tissue producing intimal thickening in endarteritis obliterans.[19]

Excluding vasculitis, which is considered later, vascular occlusion may be seen in the following circumstances:

- warfarin necrosis
- atrophie blanche (livedoid vasculopathy)
- disseminated intravascular coagulation
- purpura fulminans
- thrombotic thrombocytopenic purpura
- thrombocythemia
- cryoglobulinemia
- cholesterol embolism
- antiphospholipid syndrome
- factor V Leiden mutation
- Sneddon's syndrome
- CADASIL
- miscellaneous conditions.

WARFARIN NECROSIS

Cutaneous infarction is a rare, unpredictable complication of anticoagulant therapy with the coumarin derivative warfarin sodium. It has a predilection for fatty areas such as the thighs, buttocks and breasts of obese, middle-aged women.[20,21] Lesions usually develop several days after the commencement of therapy. There are well-defined ecchymotic changes that rapidly progress to blistering and necrosis. Purpuric[22] and linear lesions[23] have been reported.

Warfarin necrosis is related to low levels of protein C, a vitamin K-dependent plasma protein with potent anticoagulant properties.[24] This deficiency in protein C may be induced by the anticoagulant therapy[25] or pre-exist in those who are heterozygous for protein C deficiency.[26] Homozygotes with absent protein C present with neonatal purpura fulminans (see below). Warfarin necrosis has recently been associated with the factor V Leiden mutation, indicating that several closely related factors may contribute to

warfarin-induced necrosis.[27] Rarely, widespread disseminated intravascular coagulation is associated with warfarin therapy.[28]

Histopathology
Fibrin-platelet thrombi are present in venules and arterioles in the deep dermis and subcutis. There is variable hemorrhage and subsequently the development of infarction. Large areas of the skin may be involved.

ATROPHIE BLANCHE (LIVEDOID VASCULOPATHY)

Although previously considered to be caused by a vasculitis, atrophie blanche (white atrophy) is best regarded as a manifestation of a thrombogenic vasculopathy in which occlusion of small dermal vessels by fibrin thrombi is the primary event.[29–31] It appears to result from decreased fibrinolytic activity of the blood with defective release of tissue plasminogen activator from vessel walls.[32–36] The platelets usually show an increased tendency to aggregate. An elevated level of fibrinopeptide A, suggestive of a thrombogenic state, has been found in patients with this condition.[30] Several cases with a lupus-type anticoagulant and an increased level of anticardiolipin antibodies have been reported.[37] This abnormality can alter fibrinolytic activity. Other associations of atrophie blanche include protein C deficiency,[38] factor V Leiden mutation[39] and homocysteinemia,[40] all of which can contribute to a hypercoagulable condition.

Atrophie blanche (synonyms: livedoid vasculopathy, livedo vasculitis, segmental hyalinizing vasculitis and painful purpuric ulcers with reticular patterning on the lower extremities – PURPLE)[41] is characterized by the development of telangiectatic, purpuric papules and plaques leading to the formation of small crusted ulcers, which heal after many months to leave white atrophic stellate scars.[42,43] The ulcers are painful and recurrent. Sometimes they are large and slow to heal. The lower parts of the legs, especially the ankles and the dorsum of the feet, are usually involved, although rarely the extensor surfaces of the arms below the elbows can be affected. Many patients also have livedo reticularis,[44] while some may have systemic diseases such as scleroderma, systemic lupus erythematosus and cryoglobulinemia.[45] The disorder has a predilection for middle-aged females, but all ages may be affected.[42]

Atrophie blanche-like scarring can occur uncommonly after pulsed dye laser treatment of vascular malformations.[46] A response to PUVA therapy has been reported.[47]

Histopathology[48]
The changes will depend on the age of the lesion which is biopsied. The primary event is the formation of hyaline thrombi in the lumen of small vessels in the upper and mid dermis.[45] Rarely, deeper vessels are involved.[42] Fibrinoid material is also present in the walls of these blood vessels and in perivascular stroma (Fig. 8.1). This material is PAS positive and diastase resistant. There is usually infarction of the superficial dermis, often with a small area of ulceration. Sometimes a thin parakeratotic layer is present overlying infarcted or atrophic epidermis. The epidermis adjacent to the ulceration may be spongiotic. A sparse perivascular lymphocytic infiltrate may be present, but there is no vasculitis. Neutrophils, if present, are usually sparse and confined to the infarcted upper dermis and ulcer base. There are often extravasated red cells in the upper dermis. Small blood vessels are often increased in the adjacent papillary dermis, but this is a common feature in biopsies from the lower parts of the legs and is therefore of no diagnostic value.

In older lesions there is thickening and hyalinization of vessels in the dermis with some endothelial cell edema and proliferation. Fibrinoid material may

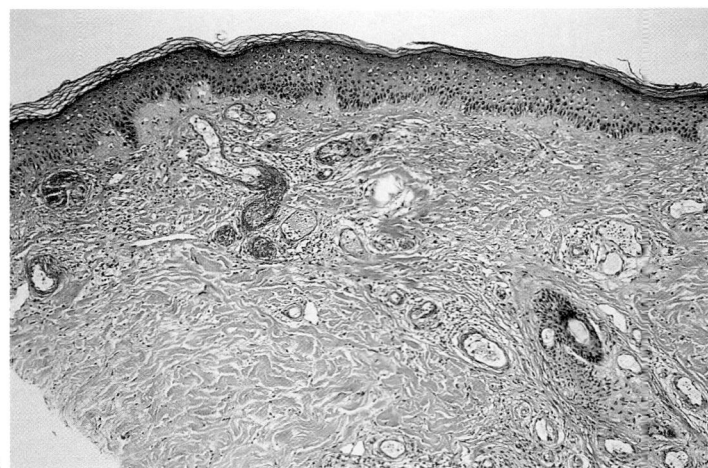
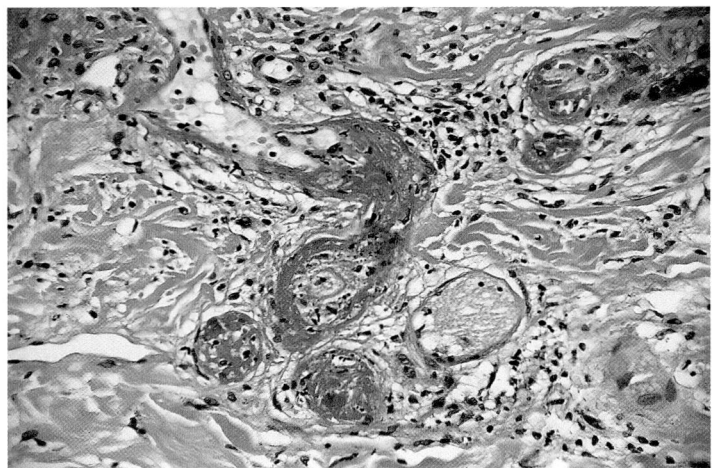

Fig. 8.1 **(A) Atrophie blanche in the pre-ulcerative stage. (B)** Fibrinoid material is present in the walls of small blood vessels in the upper dermis. (H & E)

also be present in vessel walls. It should be pointed out that fibrinoid material is almost invariably present in blood vessels in the base of ulcers, of many different causes, on the lower legs. In atrophie blanche the involved vessels are not only in the base of any ulcer, but also may be found at a distance beyond this.

In even later lesions, there is dermal sclerosis and scarring with some dilated lymphatics and epidermal atrophy. There may be a small amount of hemosiderin in the upper dermis. As these areas may become involved again, it is possible to find dermal sclerosis in some early lesions.

Immunofluorescence will demonstrate fibrin in vessel walls in early lesions, while in later stages there are also immunoglobulins and complement components in broad bands about vessel walls.[29,49]

Electron microscopy

This has confirmed the presence of luminal fibrin deposition with subsequent endothelial damage.[29]

DISSEMINATED INTRAVASCULAR COAGULATION

Disseminated intravascular coagulation (DIC) is an acquired disorder in which activation of the coagulation system leads to the formation of thrombi in the microcirculation of many tissues and organs.[50,51] As a consequence of the consumption of platelets and of fibrin and other factors during the coagulation process, hemorrhagic manifestations also occur. DIC may complicate infections, various neoplasms, certain obstetric incidents, massive tissue injury such as burns, and miscellaneous conditions such as liver disease, snake bite and vasculitis.[50]

Cutaneous changes are present in approximately 70% of cases and these may be the initial manifestations of DIC.[52,53] Petechiae, ecchymoses, hemorrhagic bullae, purpura fulminans, bleeding from wounds, acral cyanosis and frank gangrene have all been recorded.[52,54,55]

The formation of thrombi appears to be a consequence of the release of thromboplastins into the circulation and/or widespread injury to endothelial cells. Decreased levels of protein C have been reported; the level returns to normal with clinical recovery.[56]

Histopathology[53]

In early lesions, fibrin thrombi are present in capillaries and venules of the papillary dermis and occasionally in vessels in the reticular dermis and subcutis (Fig. 8.2). Hemorrhage is also present, but there is no vasculitis or inflammation.

In older lesions, of 2–3 days' duration, there may be epidermal necrosis, subepidermal bullae, extensive hemorrhage and patchy necrosis of eccrine glands, the pilosebaceous apparatus and the papillary dermis. Nearby blood vessels are thrombosed but there is only mild inflammation in the dermis. In chronic states, some vascular proliferation and ectasia may occur.

PURPURA FULMINANS

Purpura fulminans is a rare clinical manifestation of disseminated intravascular coagulation (DIC) in which there are large cutaneous ecchymoses and hemorrhagic necrosis of the skin resulting from thrombosis of the cutaneous microvasculature.[26] It is not known why only certain patients with DIC develop the full picture of purpura fulminans. Hypotension and fever are also present, but visceral manifestations are uncommon. Only a few cases have been reported in adults;[57–59] the majority arise in infancy and early childhood some days after an infectious illness,[60] usually of streptococcal, meningococcal,[61] pneumococcal[62] or viral[63] etiology. Rarely, purpura fulminans occurs in the neonatal period associated with severe congenital deficiency of protein C or protein S.[26,63,64] Protein S is a cofactor for protein C. Acquired deficiencies of

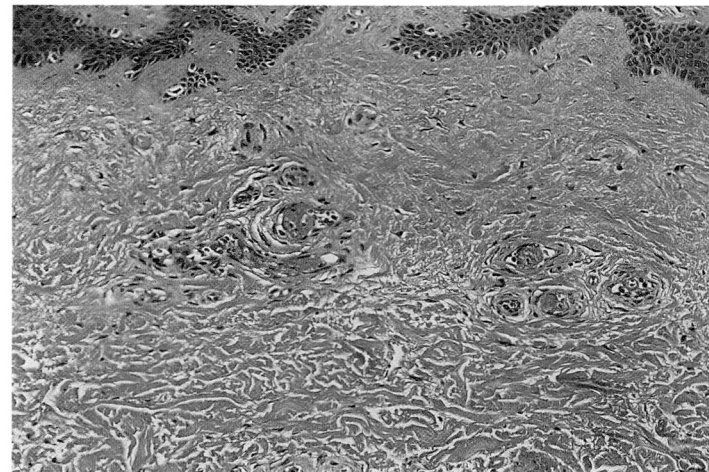

Fig. 8.2 **Disseminated intravascular coagulation.** Small vessels in the upper dermis contain fibrin-platelet thrombi. (H & E)

these proteins, probably due to the primary infectious process, appear to be responsible for cases in later life. The factor V Leiden mutation has been incriminated in a small number of adult and childhood cases.[59]

The cutaneous lesions can commence as erythematous macules which rapidly enlarge and develop central purpura. The central zone becomes necrotic, and the eventual removal of the resulting eschar leads to an area of ulceration.[26] There is a predilection for the lower extremities and the lateral aspect of the buttocks and thighs. Peripheral gangrene may sometimes develop. The use of fresh frozen plasma has considerably improved the prognosis of this disease.

Histopathology[26]
Fibrin thrombi fill most of the venules and capillaries in the skin. There is a mild perivascular infiltrate in some areas, but no vasculitis. Extensive hemorrhage is present with the subsequent development of epidermal necrosis. Occasionally, a subepidermal bulla develops.

THROMBOTIC THROMBOCYTOPENIC PURPURA

Thrombotic thrombocytopenic purpura is a rare syndrome characterized by the clinical picture of microangiopathic hemolytic anemia, thrombocytopenia, neurological symptoms, renal disease and fever.[65–67] Cutaneous hemorrhages in the form of petechiae and ecchymoses are quite common.[65] Prior to the introduction of plasmapheresis and antiplatelet agents, the disease was almost invariably fatal.

It appears to result from prostacyclin inhibition and impaired fibrinolysis. While drugs, infectious agents and obstetric incidents have been implicated in triggering this syndrome, in the majority of individuals there is no apparent causal event or underlying disease process.[65] Drugs incriminated include the antiplatelet drugs ticlopidine and clopidogrel.[68,69] Coagulation studies fail to show evidence of disseminated intravascular coagulation.

Histopathology
Platelet-rich thrombi admixed with a small amount of fibrin deposit in vessels at the level of the arteriolocapillary junction.[65] They may also involve small arteries.[67] There may be slight dilatation of vessels proximal to the thrombi. The material is PAS positive. There is no evidence of any associated vasculitis. Extravasation of red blood cells also occurs. In severe cases, necrosis of the epidermis may ensue.

THROMBOCYTHEMIA

Thrombocythemia is a rare, chronic myeloproliferative disorder characterized by a significant increase in the platelet count. Cutaneous manifestations, which include livedo reticularis, erythromelalgia and ischemic manifestations, occur in approximately 20% of patients.[70–72] Platelet plugging, leading to erythematous plaques, may develop in other myeloproliferative disorders.[73]

Histopathology
If biopsies are taken from areas of erythromelalgia, there is fibromuscular intimal proliferation involving arterioles and small arteries similar to the changes seen in Sneddon's syndrome.[74–77]

If ischemic areas are biopsied, there is vascular thrombosis, which may involve vessels of all sizes. Infarction of the dermis and/or epidermis may accompany these thrombosed vessels.

CRYOGLOBULINEMIA

Cryoglobulins are immunoglobulins that reversibly precipitate from the serum or plasma on cooling.[78,79] There are two distinct types of cryoglobulinemia, monoclonal (type I) and mixed (type II), which reflect the composition of the cryoglobulins involved.[80] In the monoclonal type intravascular deposits of cryoglobulins can be seen in biopsy specimens, while the mixed variant is a vasculitis. They are considered together for convenience.

Monoclonal cryoglobulinemia
The monoclonal variant, which accounts for approximately 25% of cases of cryoglobulinemia, is associated with the presence of IgG or IgM cryoglobulin or, rarely, of a cryoprecipitable light chain.[78,81] Monoclonal cryoglobulins, also known as type I cryoglobulins, are usually seen in association with multiple myeloma, Waldenström's macroglobulinemia[82] and chronic lymphatic leukemia.[78,83] Sometimes, no underlying disease is present (essential cryoglobulinemia). The condition may be asymptomatic or result in purpura, acral cyanosis or focal ulceration, which is usually limited to the lower extremities.[84]

Mixed cryoglobulinemia
In the mixed variant, the cryoglobulins are composed of either a monoclonal immunoglobulin which possesses antibody activity towards, and is attached to, polyclonal IgG (type II), or two or more polyclonal immunoglobulins (type III).[85] Mixed cryoglobulins usually take the form of immune complexes and interreact with complement. They are seen in autoimmune diseases such as rheumatoid arthritis, systemic lupus erythematosus and Sjögren's syndrome, as well as in various chronic infections resulting from the hepatitis and Epstein–Barr viruses.[85,86] Numerous cases associated with infection with the hepatitis C virus have been reported in recent years.[87–97] A mixed cryoglobulinemia may be the etiology of some cases of the 'red finger syndrome' seen in patients with HIV infection.[98] In approximately 50% of cases, no detectable autoimmune, lymphoproliferative or active infective disease is present.[99] These cases of *essential mixed cryoglobulinemia* are characterized by a chronic course with intermittent palpable purpura, polyarthralgia, Raynaud's phenomenon and occasionally glomerulonephritis.[86,99] Other cutaneous manifestations that may be present include ulcers, urticaria, digital necrosis and, rarely, pustular purpura.[100]

Histopathology[80]

Monoclonal cryoglobulinemia
Purpuric lesions will show extravasation of red blood cells into the dermis. Small vessels in the upper dermis may be filled with homogeneous, eosinophilic material which is also PAS positive.[81,84,101] These intravascular deposits are seen more commonly beneath areas of ulceration.[84] Although there is no vasculitis, there may be a perivascular infiltrate of predominantly mononuclear cells.[101]

Mixed cryoglobulinemia
The histological features are those of an acute vasculitis. There may be some variation from case to case in the extent of the infiltrate and the degree of leukocytoclasis, probably reflecting the stage of the lesion.[102] There are usually some extravasated red blood cells; in cases of long standing, hemosiderin may be present. Intravascular hyaline deposits are the exception, but they may be found beneath areas of ulceration.[85,100] A septal panniculitis is a rare association.[103] Immunoglobulins and complement are often found in vessel walls by immunofluorescence.[102]

Electron microscopy

The ultrastructural features depend on the involved immunoglobulins and on their respective quantities. There may be tubular microcrystals, filaments or cylindrical and annular bodies.[100] In a recently reported case of monoclonal cryoglobulinemia, immunoglobulin crystalloid structures were present within the small cutaneous vessels, admixed with fibrin and red blood cells.[104]

CUTANEOUS CHOLESTEROL EMBOLISM

Cutaneous involvement occurs in 35% of patients with cholesterol crystal embolization.[105–107] The source of the emboli is atheromatous plaques in major blood vessels, particularly the abdominal aorta. This material may dislodge spontaneously or following vascular procedures or anticoagulant therapy.[108] There is a high mortality. Cutaneous lesions are found particularly on the lower limbs and include livedo reticularis, gangrene, ulceration, cyanosis, purpura and cutaneous nodules.[105,109,110] Rare manifestations have included a hemorrhagic panniculitis on the chest[111] and an eschar on the ear.[112]

Histopathology[105,109,113]

Multiple sections are sometimes required to find the diagnostic acicular clefts indicating the site of cholesterol crystals in arterioles and small arteries in the lower dermis or subcutis. A fibrin thrombus often surrounds the cholesterol material. Foreign body giant cells and a few inflammatory cells may also be present. Cutaneous infarction and associated inflammatory changes sometimes develop.

Deposits of **atrial myxoma** in peripheral arterioles and small arteries may at first glance be mistaken for cholesterol emboli. However, a loose myxoid stroma and lack of cholesterol clefting should allow a confident diagnosis of 'metastatic' atrial myxoma.[114]

ANTIPHOSPHOLIPID SYNDROME

The antiphospholipid syndrome is characterized by the presence of autoantibodies directed against phospholipids and associated with repeated episodes of thrombosis, fetal loss and thrombocytopenia.[115–124] These antibodies can be detected as a lupus anticoagulant or as anticardiolipin antibodies. Antibodies can be found in 20–50% of patients with systemic lupus erythematosus (SLE), but only about half of these patients have the antiphospholipid syndrome. The syndrome may also occur in association with rheumatoid arthritis, infections, certain drugs and malignant disorders.[118] The term 'primary antiphospholipid syndrome' is used for those patients who do not have an associated disease.

Patients may be asymptomatic or develop thrombosis with systemic and/or cutaneous disease.[125] Skin lesions include livedo reticularis, Raynaud's phenomenon,[126] thrombophlebitis, cutaneous infarction and gangrene of the digits, ulceration, subungual splinter hemorrhages and painful skin nodules resembling vasculitis (but without vasculitis on biopsy).[118,127,128] Cutaneous necrosis can sometimes be quite extensive.[129,130] There are isolated reports of its association with atrophie blanche, malignant atrophic papulosis (Degos)[118] and factor V Leiden mutation.[131]

It is not known why only a minority of patients with the autoantibodies develop thrombotic complications.[132] Furthermore, the mechanisms by which the thromboses occur are poorly understood.[125,133]

Histopathology

In early cutaneous lesions there is prominent dermal edema and hemorrhage with thrombi in both arteries and veins.[134] Some endothelial cells may have pyknotic nuclei, while others are swollen and disrupted. There is usually a mild lymphocytic infiltrate around involved vessels and sometimes there are plasma cells as well. There is no vasculitis.

In later lesions there is organization of thrombi and subsequent recanalization. Reactive vascular proliferation develops. Some endothelial cells may be prominent and contain eosinophilic globules similar to those seen in Kaposi's sarcoma. Hemosiderin pigment is also present in late lesions.[134] Some vessels may show intimal hyperplasia. This may reflect organization of earlier mural thrombi.[135]

FACTOR V LEIDEN MUTATION

Resistance to activated protein C (APC), leading to a hypercoagulable state, occurs in 2–5% of the US population. It is more frequent in some parts of Europe.[59] In most patients this APC resistance is caused by a single point mutation (Leiden mutation) involving a substitution of glutamine for arginine in the gene encoding factor V.[131,136,137] This mutation makes the activated form of factor V relatively resistant to degradation by APC.[138] Other mutations causing APC resistance have been described.

The factor V Leiden mutation increases the risk of venous thrombosis up to tenfold. It is an important cause of venous leg ulcers.[131,139–142]

SNEDDON'S SYNDROME

Sneddon's syndrome is a rare neurocutaneous disorder of uncertain etiology, characterized by widespread livedo reticularis and ischemic cerebrovascular manifestations resulting from damage to small and medium-sized arteries.[74,143–150] It most commonly affects young and middle-aged females; it is rare in children.[151]

Detailed pathological studies by Zelger and Sepp have shown an 'endothelitis' in affected vessels, followed by a subendothelial proliferation of smooth muscle cells and fibrosis. Vascular occlusion may occur (see below). Antiendothelial cell antibodies have been demonstrated in 35% of patients with Sneddon's syndrome, but their significance in the pathogenesis is uncertain.[147] Possibly of greater relevance is the finding of similar intimal changes in thrombocythemia, suggesting that platelet-derived factors may also play a role in the pathogenesis of Sneddon's syndrome.[74] Other factors appear to be important as Sneddon's syndrome can occur in association with the antiphospholipid syndrome (see above) and with systemic lupus erythematosus.[152]

Histopathology

In the skin, small to medium-sized arteries near the dermal–subcutaneous junction are affected in a stage-specific sequence.[148,149] The initial phase involves attachment of lymphohistiocytic cells to the endothelium with detachment of the endothelium ('endothelitis'). This is followed by partial or complete occlusion of the lumen by a plug of fibrin admixed with the inflammatory cells. This plug is replaced by proliferating subendothelial cells, which have the markers of smooth muscle cells. A corona of dilated small capillaries usually develops in the adventitia. Fibrosis of the intima or the plug may occur. Shrinkage and atrophy of these vessels then occurs.[148,149]

CADASIL

CADASIL is the acronym used in preference to cerebral *a*utosomal *d*ominant *a*rteriopathy with *s*ubcortical *i*nfarcts and *l*eukoencephalopathy, a vascular disorder associated with migraines, recurrent ischemic strokes, and early-onset dementia.[153] There is luminal obliteration of small leptomeningeal and intracerebral arteries but no vascular occlusion in the skin. The defect involves a mutation in the *NOTCH3* gene on chromosome 19q12, which encodes a transmembrane receptor protein.[154]

Electron microscopic examination of skin biopsies is diagnostic.[153,154] A granular, electron-dense, osmiophilic material is present in the basement membrane of vascular smooth muscle cells. As the deposits may be patchy in superficial dermal vessels, several sections should be searched to avoid a false-negative result. Light microscopy is normal.

MISCELLANEOUS CONDITIONS CAUSING VASCULAR OCCLUSION

Rare causes of cutaneous microthrombi include the hypereosinophilic syndrome,[155] renal failure with hyperparathyroidism (the vascular calcification–cutaneous necrosis syndrome),[156–158] protein C and/or protein S deficiency,[159–161] as well as dopamine,[162] vasopressin,[163] Depo-Provera®[164] and heparin therapy (embolia cutis medicamentosa),[130,165–168] the intravascular injection of large amounts of cocaine,[169] temazepam or flunitrazepam,[170] the treatment of afibrinogenemia,[171] ulcerative colitis[172] and embolic processes, including bacterial endocarditis. The eschar found in some rickettsial infections is a cutaneous infarct with fibrin-platelet thrombi in marginal vessels. A lymphocytic vasculitis is usually present as well.

Vascular occlusion, either partial or complete, may occur in endarteritis obliterans as a result of fibrous thickening of the intima. It may be seen in a range of clinicopathological settings which include peripheral atherosclerosis, Raynaud's phenomenon, scleroderma, diabetes, hypertension and healed vasculitis.[19]

Obstruction of the vena cava may produce cutaneous symptoms. The superior vena cava syndrome, which occurs when extrinsic compression or intraluminal occlusion impedes blood flow through the vessels, may present as persistent erythematous edema of the face.[173] Obstruction of the inferior vena cava usually results from pelvic tumors, but a case related to factor V Leiden mutation has been reported.[138] The patient presented with varicose and thrombosed veins on her abdominal wall.[138]

Acrocyanosis of uncertain pathogenesis has been reported following the inhalation of butyl nitrite.[174] Vascular disturbances producing livedo reticularis have already been discussed. Additional causes include pancreatitis[175] and a latent infective endocarditis due to *Coxiella burnetii*.[176]

URTICARIAS

Urticaria is a cutaneous reaction pattern characterized clinically by transient, often pruritic, edematous, erythematous papules or wheals which may show central clearing.[177–179] Angioedema is a related process in which the edema involves the subcutaneous tissues and/or mucous membranes. It may coexist with urticaria.[180,181]

Urticaria is a common affliction, affecting 15% or more of the population on at least one occasion in their life. Most cases are transient (acute) and the etiology is usually detected.[182] The use of antibiotics for viral illnesses is an important cause of acute urticaria.[183] A variant of acute urticaria in infants and young children is the annular form which often results from the use of furazolidone in the treatment of diarrhea.[184] On the other hand, chronic urticaria, which is arbitrarily defined as urticaria persisting for longer than 6 weeks, is idiopathic in approximately 75% of cases.[178,185,186] It tends to involve middle-aged people, in contrast to acute urticaria which occurs more commonly in children and young adults. When chronic urticaria does occur in children, the etiological factors are more readily identifiable than in adults.[187] Chronic urticaria may be aggravated by salicylates, food additives and the like.[188–191] This has led to the suggestion that chronic urticaria results from an occult allergy to some everyday substance.

Papular urticaria is a clinical variant of urticaria in which the lesions are more persistent than the usual urticarial wheal.[192] It may result from a hypersensitivity reaction to the bites of arthropods such as fleas, lice, mites and bed bugs.[192–194] It usually occurs in crops on exposed skin.[186] Erosions are common. Rare clinical variants of urticaria include bullous and purpuric forms,[182] urticaria with anaphylaxis[182] and recurrent urticaria with fever and eosinophilia.[195] Schnitzler's syndrome combines chronic urticaria, fever, disabling bone pain and macroglobulinemia.[196–202] Monoclonal IgM and its autoantibody deposit in the epidermis and at the dermoepidermal junction in the region of the anchoring fibrils.[203]

Most of the literature on urticaria refers to the chronic form of the disease because this is often an important clinical problem. The remainder of this discussion will refer to chronic urticaria.

CHRONIC URTICARIA

Chronic urticaria is urticaria persisting longer than 6 weeks.[185] There are many variants of chronic urticaria, although they share in common the presence of erythematous papules or wheals. These variants are usually classified etiopathogenetically, as follows:[204]

- physical urticarias
- cholinergic urticaria
- angioedema
- urticarias due to histamine-releasing agents
- IgE-mediated urticarias
- immune complex-mediated urticarias
- idiopathic urticarias.

Some overlap exists between these various categories. For example, drugs and foodstuffs may produce chronic urticaria through more than one of the above mechanisms.

Physical urticarias

Physical stimuli such as heat, cold, pressure, light, water and vibration are the most commonly identified causes of chronic urticaria, accounting for approximately 15% of all cases.[205–208] The wheals are usually of short duration and limited to the area of the physical stimulus.[205] Accordingly, the physical urticarias tend to occur on exposed areas. Angioedema may coexist.[209] More than one of the physical agents listed above may induce urticaria in some individuals.[206] Some of the physical urticarias can be transferred passively.[209–211] *Cold urticaria*, which is produced at sites of localized cooling of the skin, is usually acquired, although a rare familial form has been reported.[212–215] A locus on chromosome 1q44 has been identified for the familial form, which is an autosomal dominant condition.[216] A variant with localized perifollicular lesions has been reported.[217] Cold urticaria may follow a viral illness[218] or the use of drugs such as penicillin and griseofulvin, although in most cases no underlying cause is found.[219] *Heat urticaria*, by contrast, is exceedingly rare.[220–222] *Solar urticaria* is another rare physical urticaria which results from exposure to sun and light.[223–232] An inhibition spectrum may be present, whereby activation occurs following exposure to a certain range of wavelengths, but not if re-irradiation with certain other wavelengths is immediately carried out.[233,234] Solar urticaria has a faster onset and shorter duration than polymorphous light eruption.[235] Progression to polymorphous light eruption has been reported.[236] A rare variant, limited to fixed skin sites, has been reported in three patients.[237] A similar fixed urticaria may rarely occur as a manifestation of a drug reaction. Solar urticaria has been induced by tetracycline therapy.[238] *Aquagenic urticaria* follows contact with water.[239,240] Sometimes there is an underlying disorder, the expression of which may coincide with the onset of the urticaria. Examples include the myelodysplastic syndrome, the hypereosinophilic syndrome, HIV infection and an underlying cancer.[241,242] Much more common is *aquagenic pruritus* in which prickly discomfort occurs in the absence of any cutaneous lesion.[243-248] It appears to be an entity distinct from aquagenic urticaria and may follow increased degranulation of a normal number of mast cells.[249] In *pressure urticaria*, deep wheals develop after a delay of several hours following the application of pressure.[250-253] It is probably more common than generally realized, being present in some patients who do not report pressure-related wheals.[254,255] It can affect quality of life.[256] Systemic symptoms, which include an influenza-like illness, may also develop.[257] Eosinophil granule major basic protein and neutrophil granule elastase are significantly increased in delayed pressure urticaria, in a similar manner to the IgE-mediated late phase reaction. There is no increase of these products in dermographism.[258] *Vibratory urticaria* is a related disorder resulting from vibratory stimuli.[206] *Dermographism*, which is the production of a linear wheal in response to a scratch, is an accentuation of the physiological whealing of the Lewis triple response.[259] Minor forms of dermographism are quite common, but only a small percentage of affected persons are symptomatic with pruritus. A delayed form, which is an entity similar to delayed pressure urticaria, also occurs.[252]

The physical urticaria which is least well understood is *contact urticaria*.[260-265] In this variant a wheal and flare response is usually elicited 30–60 minutes after skin contact with various chemicals in medicaments, cosmetics, foods and industrial agents.[260,266] It may follow exposure to the common stinging nettle (*Urtica dioica*)[267] and a long list of other substances including latex,[268] flavored toothpaste,[269] insect repellent,[270] formaldehyde,[271] tofu,[272] topical immunotherapy with diphenylcyclopropenone,[273] petrol and kerosene. Distinction from a contact irritant dermatitis may sometimes be difficult.[274] An IgE-mediated form and a non-immunological form have been delineated.[274,275] Contact urticaria may be superimposed on an 'eczematous dermatitis' of different types.[260] A recurrent urticaria has been reported at the previous injection sites of insulin.[276]

Cholinergic urticaria

Cholinergic urticaria is produced by exercise, heat and emotion, with general overheating of the body as the final common pathway.[207,277-280] Accordingly, it is sometimes included with the physical urticarias, with which it may coexist.[281,282] Young adults are mainly affected, but the condition is usually mild, not requiring medical attention.[283,284] We have seen several cases in medical practitioners, following a game of golf. Two further cases had an urticarial vasculitis. The lesions are distinctive and consist of 2–3 mm wheals surrounded by large erythematous flares.[207] There is a predilection for blush areas. Increased sympathetic activity may result in the release of acetylcholine at nerve endings, causing mast cells to degranulate.[285]

Angioedema

There is a special form of angioedema (hereditary angioedema) which may be associated with swelling of the face and limbs or involve the larynx with potentially life-threatening consequences.[286] It results from an absolute or functional deficiency of C1 esterase inhibitor.[287,288] Non-familial angioedema may occur in association with various urticarias.[209,289] It is often seen at the injection site of granulocyte-monocyte colony-stimulating factor. It may also be associated with the use of ACE inhibitors,[290,291] and intrauterine infection with parvovirus B19.[292]

Urticaria due to histamine-releasing agents

Histamine may be released by mast cells in response to certain drugs, such as opiates, and some foodstuffs, including strawberries, egg white and lobster.[178]

IgE-mediated urticarias

Antigen-specific IgE may be responsible for some of the urticarias due to certain foods, drugs[293] and pollens in addition to the urticaria related to parasitic infestations and stings. Over 300 causes have been identified. Mast cell degranulation is the final common pathway.[182]

Immune complex-mediated urticarias

Immune complexes may be involved in the pathogenesis of the chronic urticaria seen in infectious hepatitis, infectious mononucleosis, systemic lupus erythematosus and serum sickness-like illnesses.[294] They have also been implicated in the urticarial reactions that are an uncommon manifestation of various internal cancers. In some instances, fever, purpura and joint pains are also present. The urticaria is usually more persistent, particularly in those cases with an accompanying vasculitis. A serum sickness-like reaction has been seen as a complication of cefaclor, an oral cephalosporin.[295]

Idiopathic urticaria

Up to 75% of all chronic urticarias fall into the idiopathic category.[204,296]

Miscellaneous urticarias

An urticarial reaction is sometimes seen in individuals who are infected with *Candida albicans*;[204] the role of this organism in the causation of urticarias has been overstated in the past. Recently, *Helicobacter pylori* gastritis has been reported in some patients with chronic urticaria,[297-300] but its etiological significance has since been challenged.[301-303] Urticaria may be a manifestation of autoimmune progesterone dermatitis, a disorder which is usually manifest some days before the menses.[304-307] The mechanism is probably not an 'autoimmune' reaction, despite the title.[308] An estrogen-induced urticaria also occurs.[309]

Other recently published causes of urticaria have included hepatitis C infection,[310-312] interleukin-3 therapy,[313] gelatin in a vaccine,[314] hepatitis B immunization,[315] ethanol,[316,317] drugs such as non-steroidal anti-inflammatory agents,[318] methylprednisolone (intra-articular),[319] bleomycin,[320] cetirizine,[321,322] alendronate,[323] and minocycline,[324,325] nicotine in tobacco smoke,[326] ovarian cancer,[325] the parasite *Anisakis* sp.,[327,328] contact with hedgehogs[329] and caterpillars,[330] thyroid autoimmunity,[331,332] adult Still's disease[333,334] and chronic, infantile, neurological, cutaneous and articular syndrome (CINCA).[335]

Pathogenesis of urticaria

Urticaria results from vasodilatation and increased vascular permeability associated with the extravasation of protein and fluids into the dermis.[287] Angioedema results when a similar process occurs in the deep dermis and subcutis. Histamine has generally been regarded as the mediator of these changes, although other mediators such as prostaglandin D_2 and interleukin-1[336] are possibly involved in some circumstances.[251] Interleukin-1 and other cytokines can induce the expression of endothelial adhesion molecules which is upgraded in urticarial reactions.[337] Both immunological[338] (type I and type III) and non-immunological mechanisms can cause mast cells and basophils to degranulate, liberating histamine and other substances.[287,339] Although immediate (type I), IgE-mediated mast cell release is the classic underlying mechanism of urticarial reactions, there is evidence that delayed-type hypersensitivity reactions are often involved as well. For example, the cytokine interleukin-4 (IL-4) can upregulate IgE secretion, whereas the opposite occurs with interferon (IFN).[179] The neuropeptide substance P, derived from unmyelinated sensory nerve endings, can also evoke the release of histamine, but not prostaglandin D_2, from cutaneous mast cells.[179] Eosinophil degranulation occurs in most urticarias. The number of free eosinophil granules correlates with the duration of the wheal; granules are numerous in wheals of long duration.[340] The granules may provoke the persistent activation of the mast cells in the wheal.

Recent work has shown that approximately one-third of patients with chronic urticaria have circulating autoantibodies to $Fc\varepsilon RI\alpha$ (the high-affinity IgE receptor), resulting in the release of histamine from mast cells.[341–343] This subset of patients has more severe disease.[344] An association with HLA class II has been reported.[345] The beneficial effect of cyclosporine and intravenous immunoglobulin on chronic urticaria provides further support for the role of histamine-releasing autoantibodies in its pathogenesis.[346,347] Extensive laboratory investigations do not contribute substantially to the diagnosis of chronic urticaria or the detection of underlying disorders.[348]

In summary, several different mechanisms have now been elucidated that are capable of stimulating the release of histamine from mast cells and/or basophils.

Histopathology[349,350]

The cell type and the intensity of the inflammatory response in urticaria are quite variable.[251] There is increasing evidence to suggest that the age of the lesion biopsied and the nature of the evoking stimulus may both influence the type and the intensity of the inflammatory response.

Dermal edema, which is recognized by separation of the collagen bundles, is an important feature of urticaria. Mild degrees may be difficult to detect. Urticarial edema differs from the mucinoses by the absence of granular, stringy, basophilic material in the widened interstitium. There is also dilatation of small blood vessels and lymphatics, and swelling of their endothelium is often present (Fig. 8.3). The histopathological changes in urticaria are most marked in the upper dermis, but involvement of the deep dermis may be present, particularly in those with coexisting angioedema.[351]

The cellular infiltrate in urticaria is usually mild and perivascular in location. It consists of lymphocytes and, in most cases, a few eosinophils.[351] Occasional interstitial eosinophils and mast cells are also present. Eosinophil granule major basic protein has been identified in the dermis in several types of urticaria.[352] Neutrophils are often noted in early lesions but in most cases they are relatively sparse; there is some evidence to suggest that they are more prominent in the physical urticarias,[353–355] particularly delayed pressure urticaria.[350] An important diagnostic feature of many early urticarias is the presence of neutrophils and sometimes eosinophils in the lumen of small vessels in the upper dermis.[354] Further mention will be made below of the presence of neutrophils in other circumstances. Although mast cells are often increased in early lesions and even in non-stimulated skin of patients with chronic urticaria,[356] they appear to be decreased in late lesions, apparently due to the failure of histochemical methods to detect degranulated mast cells.[257,285]

Neutrophils have been described in urticaria in several different circumstances.[357–359] As already noted, a few intravascular and perivascular neutrophils are a common feature in early urticaria.[357] At times, there may be sufficient transmigration of neutrophils through vessel walls to give a superficial resemblance to 'vasculitis', but there is no fibrinoid change, hemorrhage or leukocytoclasis. A more diffuse dermal neutrophilia has also been described in nearly 10% of urticarias.[358,360] The term '*neutrophilic urticaria*' is used in these circumstances. In these cases, neutrophils are scattered among

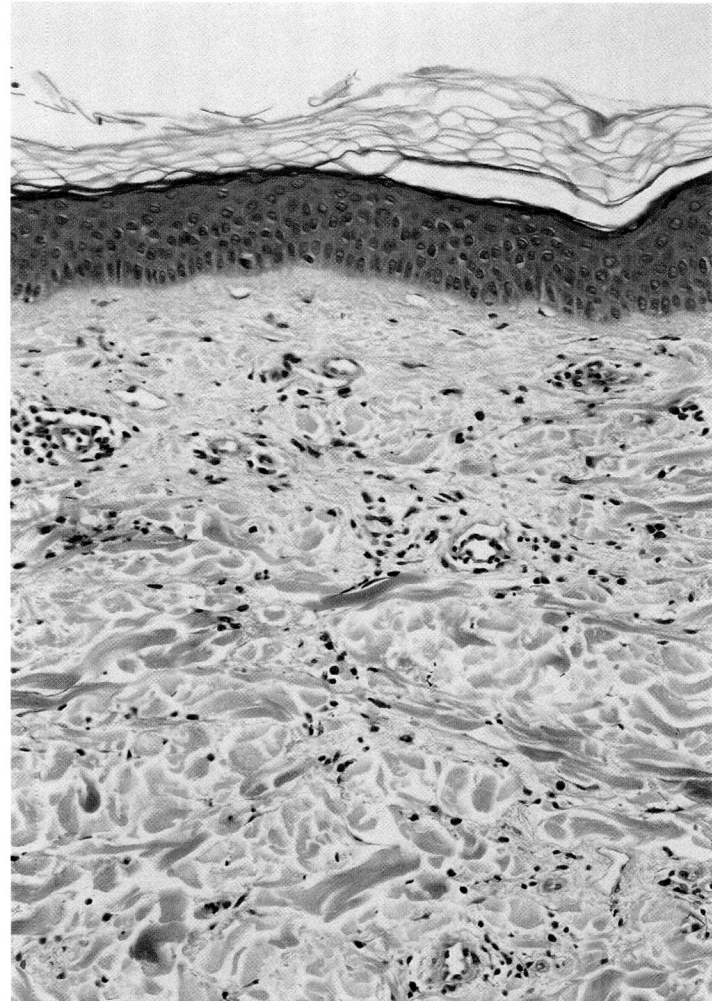

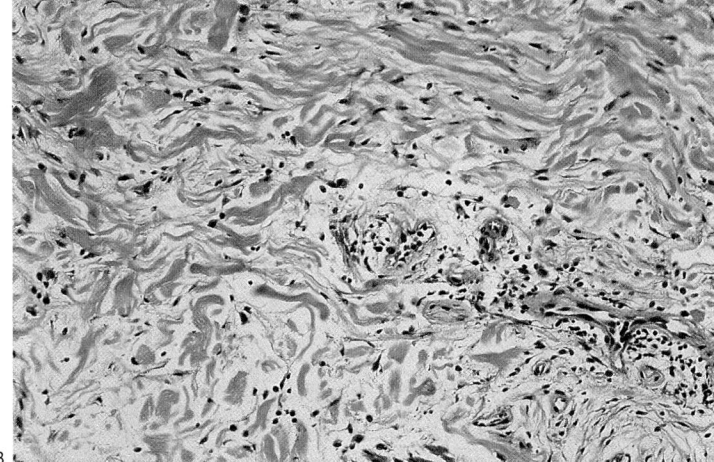

Fig. 8.3 **(A) Urticaria. (B)** There is mild dermal edema and a perivascular infiltrate of lymphocytes, mast cells and eosinophils. Occasional interstitial eosinophils are also present. (H & E)

the collagen bundles, usually in the upper dermis but sometimes throughout its thickness. The infiltrate is usually mild in intensity.[358] Rare nuclear 'dusting' may also be present. Interstitial eosinophils and perivascular eosinophils and lymphocytes are usually noted as well.[358] Neutrophils are also present in the leukocytoclastic vasculitis that sometimes accompanies chronic urticaria. The term 'urticarial vasculitis' has been applied to cases of this type in which the clinical picture is that of an urticaria and the histopathology is a vasculitis.[361–365] In urticarial vasculitis (see also p. 233) the urticarial lesions are usually of longer duration than in the 'usual' chronic urticaria and may be accompanied by systemic symptoms.[366–369] The incidence of vasculitis in chronic urticaria varies with the strictness of the criteria used for defining vasculitis.[370,371] There appears to be a continuum of changes with a few intravascular and perivascular neutrophils at one end of the spectrum and an established leukocytoclastic vasculitis at the other.

Other histopathological features have been described in several of the specific types of urticaria. In *dermographism*, perivascular mononuclear cells are increased, even prior to the initiation of a wheal.[372] In *contact urticaria*, subcorneal vesiculation and spongiosis have been reported, but this may simply reflect a concomitant allergic or irritant contact dermatitis.[260] In *papular urticaria* the inflammatory cell infiltrate is usually heavier than in other chronic urticarias and consists of a superficial and deep infiltrate of lymphocytes and eosinophils in a perivascular location.[192,373] The infiltrate is often wedge shaped.[374] Interstitial eosinophils may also be present and in lesions of less than 24 hours' duration there are also some neutrophils.[192] There is variable subepidermal edema. In *angioedema*, the edema and vascular dilatation involve the deep dermis and/or subcutis, although in the hereditary form there is usually no infiltrate of inflammatory cells.[209]

ACUTE VASCULITIS

The term 'vasculitis' refers to a heterogeneous group of disorders in which there is inflammation and damage of blood vessel walls.[375–377] It may be limited to the skin or some other organ or be a multisystem disorder with protean manifestations. Numerous classifications of vasculitis have been proposed but there is still no universally acceptable one.[375,378–383] Even the Chapel Hill Consensus Conference has failed to come up with a problem-free classification.[384]

Vasculitis can be classified on an etiological basis, although in approximately 50% of cases there is no discernible cause.[385] Furthermore, a single etiological agent can result in several clinical expressions of vasculitis. A modification of the etiological classification is a pathogenetic one, which is becoming more popular as more is known of the pathogenesis of the vasculitides (see Table 8.1). The major shortcoming of this classification is that it ignores the close interrelationship of the various components of the immune system, more than one of which is likely to be involved in some of the conditions. Another approach to the classification of the vasculitides has been on the basis of the size and type of blood vessel involved, as this correlates to some extent with the cutaneous manifestations. For example, small or medium-sized arteries are involved in polyarteritis nodosa, Kawasaki disease and nodular vasculitis, while large arteries are involved in giant cell (temporal) arteritis and Takayasu arteries and large veins are involved in thrombophlebitis. Both small and large vessels are involved in rheumatoid arthritis and certain 'collagen diseases'. However, most cases of cutaneous vasculitis involve small vessels, particularly venules. The classification to be adopted here is based on the nature of the inflammatory response, with three major categories: acute (neutrophilic) vasculitis, chronic lymphocytic vasculitis and vasculitis with granulomatosis (Fig. 8.4). A fourth category, the neutrophilic dermatoses, is included although most of the diseases in this group have been regarded at various times as instances of acute (neutrophilic) vasculitis. There is an infiltration of neutrophils in the dermis but there is usually no fibrin extravasation into the vessel wall, a cardinal feature of acute vasculitis.[387]

Table 8.1 **Classification of vasculitis based on pathogenesis** (modified from Jennette et al[386])

Direct infection

Bacterial
Rickettsial
Mycobacterial
Spirochetal
Fungal (e.g. mucormycosis)
Viral (e.g. herpes)

Immunological injury

Immune complex-mediated
Henoch–Schönlein purpura
Cryoglobulinemic vasculitis
Lupus vasculitis
Rheumatoid vasculitis
Serum sickness vasculitis
Infection-induced immune complex vasculitis:
- Viral (e.g. hepatitis B and C virus)
- Bacterial (e.g. streptococcal)
Paraneoplastic vasculitis
Some drug-induced vasculitis
Behçet's disease
Erythema elevatum diutinum
Hyperimmunoglobulinemia (Waldenström and D syndrome)

Direct antibody mediated/associated
Antiendothelial cell antibody (AECA):
- Kawasaki disease (?)
- Lupus vasculitis (some cases only)
Antineutrophil cytoplasmic antibody (ANCA):
- Wegener's granulomatosis (some cases have AECA)
- Microscopic polyangiitis (polyarteritis)
- Churg–Strauss syndrome
- Some drug-related vasculitis (e.g. thiouracil)

Cell-mediated
Allograft rejection

Unknown

Giant cell (temporal) arteritis
Takayasu arteritis
Polyarteritis nodosa (possibly immune complex mediated)
Granuloma faciale (possibly Arthus-type reaction)

The classification below has some shortcomings because vasculitis is a dynamic process, with the evolution of some acute lesions into a chronic stage.[388,389] Furthermore, lesions are sometimes seen in which there are features of both acute and chronic vasculitis. Whether this represents a stage in the evolution of the disease or a change de novo is debatable. Each category of vasculitis can be further subdivided into a number of clinicopathological entities.[390] In the case of acute vasculitis, they are as follows:

- leukocytoclastic (hypersensitivity) vasculitis
- Henoch–Schönlein purpura
- eosinophilic vasculitis
- rheumatoid vasculitis
- urticarial vasculitis
- mixed cryoglobulinemia
- hypergammaglobulinemic purpura
- hypergammaglobulinemia D syndrome
- septic vasculitis
- erythema elevatum diutinum
- granuloma faciale

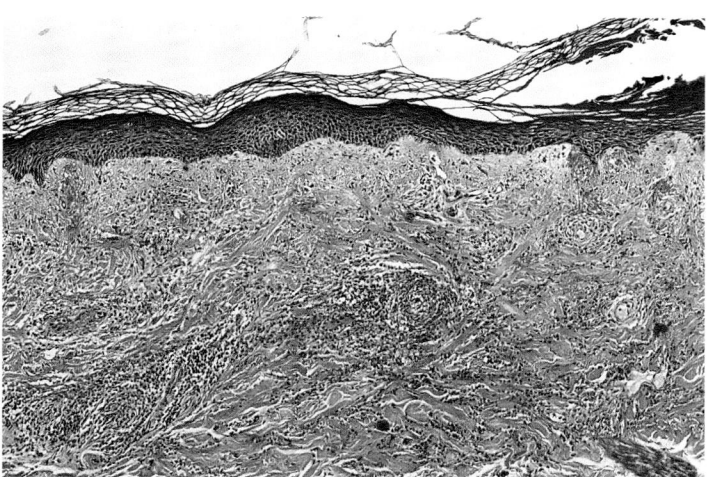
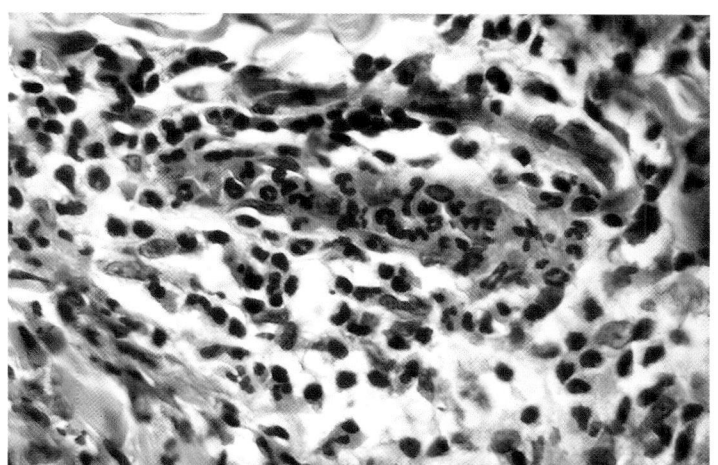

Fig. 8.4 **(A) Acute vasculitis. (B)** There is a neutrophilic infiltrate in the walls of small vessels and in their vicinity. (H & E)

- localized chronic fibrosing vasculitis
- microscopic polyangiitis (polyarteritis)
- polyarteritis nodosa
- Kawasaki syndrome
- superficial thrombophlebitis
- miscellaneous associations.

LEUKOCYTOCLASTIC (HYPERSENSITIVITY) VASCULITIS

The term 'leukocytoclastic vasculitis' has been chosen for this group of vasculitides in place of the equally unsatisfactory term 'hypersensitivity vasculitis'. Common usage has influenced the decision to make this change. To be cynical, if dermatomyositis can be diagnosed in the absence of myositis, then perhaps leukocytoclastic vasculitis can be diagnosed in the absence of leukocytoclasis, this being the situation in at least 20% of biopsies of otherwise typical cases. Other diagnoses that have been applied to this condition include allergic vasculitis,[391] hypersensitivity angiitis[392] and necrotizing vasculitis.[393] 'Necrotizing' is a particularly inappropriate group designation. Like leukocytoclasis, necrosis is not invariably present and is usually applied indiscriminately to cases with minimal fibrin extravasation.

Clinical manifestations

Leukocytoclastic vasculitis usually presents with erythematous macules or palpable purpura, with a predilection for dependent parts, particularly the lower parts of the legs.[394,395] Other lesions which may be present include hemorrhagic vesicles and bullae, nodules,[396] crusted ulcers[397,398] and, less commonly, livedo reticularis, pustules[399] or annular lesions.[400–403] Cases with urticarial lesions are classified separately as urticarial vasculitis (see below). Individual lesions vary from 1 mm to several centimeters in diameter. Large lesions are sometimes painful.[390] There may be a single crop of lesions that subside spontaneously after a few weeks or crops of lesions at different stages of evolution which may recur intermittently.[404]

Extracutaneous manifestations occur in approximately 20% of affected individuals and include arthralgia, myositis, low-grade fever and malaise.[394,405] Less commonly, there are renal, gastrointestinal, pulmonary or neurological manifestations.[391,394] The severity of the histopathological changes is not predictive of extracutaneous involvement.[406] Many of these cases with systemic manifestations would now be classified as microscopic polyangiitis

(polyarteritis) – see page 237. There is a low mortality in leukocytoclastic vasculitis; death, when due to the vasculitis, is related to involvement of systemic vessels. In one study of 160 patients with leukocytoclastic vasculitis, the mortality was 1.9%.[405]

Etiology

There are several different etiological groups, although in approximately 40% of cases there is no apparent cause. The recognized groups include infections, drugs and chemicals, cancers and systemic diseases.[390,394,407] *Miscellaneous causes* include certain arthropod bites, severe atherosclerosis,[408] prolonged exercise,[409] some coral ulcers[410] and coronary artery bypass surgery.[411]

Streptococcal infection of the upper respiratory tract is the most commonly implicated *infection*.[390] Others include influenza, *Mycobacterium tuberculosis*,[412] *M. haemophilum*, hepatitis B, herpes simplex,[413] herpes zoster/varicella,[413] human herpesvirus 6 (HHV-6),[414] cytomegalic inclusion disease,[415] parvovirus infection,[378] HIV infection[416,417] and malaria.[390]

Drug causes of leukocytoclastic vasculitis include penicillin,[385] ampicillin,[418] erythromycin,[419] clindamycin,[420] the cephalosporins,[394] sulfonamides,[418] griseofulvin,[418] furosemide (frusemide),[421] levamisole,[422,423] thiouracil,[424] propylthiouracil,[425–427] allopurinol,[418] aspirin,[394] amiodarone,[428] phenylbutazone,[418] cimetidine,[392] granulocyte colony-stimulating factor,[429] procainamide,[392] potassium iodide,[418] gold,[430] phenothiazines,[431] thiazides,[394] quinidine,[418] mefloquine,[432,433] disulfiram,[430] phenytoin (diphenylhydantoin),[418] indinavir,[434] haloperidol,[435] sotalol[436] and cytarabine (cytosine arabinoside).[437] Injection-site vasculitis has been reported following the use of interferon-α.[438] *Chemicals* used in industry, drug and food additives,[439,440] hyposensitizing antigens, nicotine patches,[441] protein A column pheresis[442] and intravenous drug abuse can be included in this etiological category.[431]

The *cancers* associated with leukocytoclastic vasculitis include lymphomas,[443,444] myelodysplastic syndrome,[445] mycosis fungoides,[446] hairy cell leukemia[447] and, very rarely, a visceral tumor.[448]

The *systemic diseases* include systemic lupus erythematosus, dermatomyositis,[449] Behçet's disease,[450] celiac disease,[443] inflammatory bowel disease,[451] cystic fibrosis,[452] Sjögren's disease,[453] subcorneal pustular dermatosis,[454] pyoderma gangrenosum,[455] sarcoidosis,[400] the Wiskott–Aldrich syndrome[452] and α_1-antitrypsin deficiency.[379]

Pathogenesis

The pathogenesis of leukocytoclastic vasculitis involves the deposition of immune complexes in vessel walls with activation of the complement system, particularly the terminal components.[456] This contrasts with microscopic polyangiitis in which immune complexes are often absent. Chemotaxis of neutrophils and injury to vessel walls with exudation of serum, erythrocytes and fibrin result. Cell adhesion molecules play a critical role in the interaction between the vascular endothelium and leukocytes.[457] These adhesion molecules are likely to be involved in the recruitment of the neutrophils.[458] Mast cells may also play a role.[459] The size of the immune complexes, which depends on the valence of the respective antigen and antibody and their relative concentrations (which is in part determined by the number of binding sites on the antigen), determines the likelihood of their deposition.[390] The complexes most likely to precipitate are those with antigens bearing 2–4 binding sites and in a concentration approximately equivalent with antibody.[390] These are the largest immune complexes that ordinarily remain soluble.[390]

Various antibodies have been detected in patients with acute vasculitis. They include antineutrophil cytoplasmic antibodies (ANCA) and IgA class anticardiolipin antibodies.[460,461] In one study, cryoglobulins were found in 25% of cases.[405]

Lymphokines also play an important role in the evolution of the vascular lesions. Interleukins (IL-1, IL-6, IL-8) are increased in the circulation, as is tumor necrosis factor (TNF). Both TNF and IL-1 may stimulate the endothelium to activate the intrinsic and extrinsic coagulation pathways and reduce its fibrinolytic activity. This may be the explanation for the thrombosis that occurs in vasculitis.[457]

Hemodynamic factors such as turbulence and increased venous pressure, as well as the reduced fibrinolytic activity that occurs in the legs, may explain why localization of lesions to this site is common.[462] Rarely, lesions may develop in areas of previously traumatized skin – the Koebner phenomenon.[463] The size and configuration of the complexes may also determine the class of vessel affected. The size of the affected vessels correlates with the clinical features. For example, involvement of small dermal vessels results in erythema or palpable purpura while lesions in larger arteries may lead to nodules, ulcers or livedo reticularis.[452] Deep venous involvement results in nodules without ulceration.[452]

Histopathology[464]

Acute vasculitis is a dynamic process. Accordingly, not all the features described below will necessarily be present at a particular stage in the evolution of the disease.[390] It is best to biopsy a lesion of 18–24 hours'

duration as this will show the most diagnostic features.[392] The changes to be described usually involve the small venules (postcapillary venules) in the dermis, although in severe cases arterioles may also be affected. Some of the cases involving arterioles would now be classified as microscopic polyangiitis (see p. 237). There is infiltration of vessel walls with neutrophils which also extend into the perivascular zone and beyond. These neutrophils undergo degeneration (leukocytoclasis) with the formation of nuclear dust (Fig. 8.5). The vessel walls are thickened by the exudate of inflammatory cells and edema fluid. There is also exudation of fibrin ('fibrinoid necrosis') which often extends into the adjacent perivascular connective tissue. Endothelial cells are usually swollen and some are degenerate. Thrombosis of vessels is sometimes present. The dermis shows variable edema and extravasation of red blood cells.

In some lesions, particularly those of longer duration, eosinophils and lymphocytes are also present, particularly in a perivascular location. Macrophages, which are scattered in the interstitium even in the early stages, show a time-dependent increase.[465] In vasculitis due to drugs, a mixed inflammatory cell infiltrate of eosinophils, lymphocytes and occasional neutrophils is commonly seen.[418]

In resolving lesions, there is usually only a mild perivascular infiltrate of lymphocytes and some eosinophils. A rare plasma cell may also be present. A striking feature of late resolving lesions is hypercellularity of the dermis with an increased number of interstitial fibroblasts and histiocytes, giving the appearance of a 'busy dermis' (Fig. 8.6). There is sometimes a mild increase in acid mucopolysaccharides imparting a vague 'necrobiotic' appearance.

Uncommonly, the subepidermal edema is so pronounced that vesiculobullous lesions result. Cutaneous infarction, usually involving only the epidermis and upper third of the dermis, may follow thrombosis of affected vessels. Presumptive ischemic changes are not uncommon in sweat glands, even in the absence of infarction.[466] They include apoptosis, necrosis and basal cell hyperplasia. Rare changes reported in leukocytoclastic vasculitis include subepidermal microabscess formation resembling dermatitis herpetiformis[467] and intraepidermal vesiculation with acantholytic cells containing vacuolated nuclei.[468]

Although previous studies have suggested that direct immunofluorescence is not particularly useful unless performed on lesions less than 6 hours old,[375,385] more recent studies have found fibrinogen, C3 and IgM in early lesions, albumin, fibrinogen and IgG in fully developed lesions, and mainly fibrinogen, with some C3, in late lesions.[469] Another study found vascular

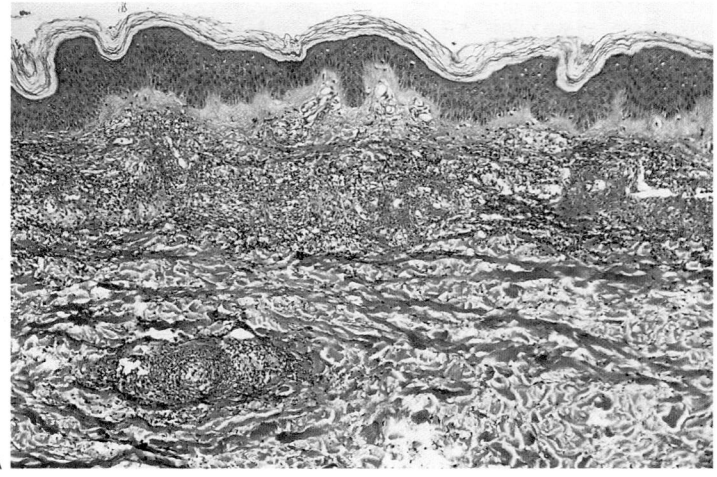
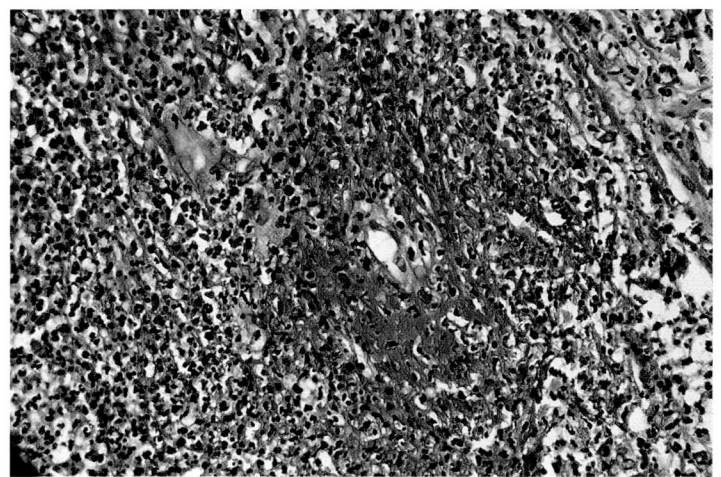

Fig. 8.5 **(A) Leukocytoclastic vasculitis. (B)** There is a heavy infiltrate of neutrophils with leukocytoclasis and marked fibrin extravasation. (H & E)

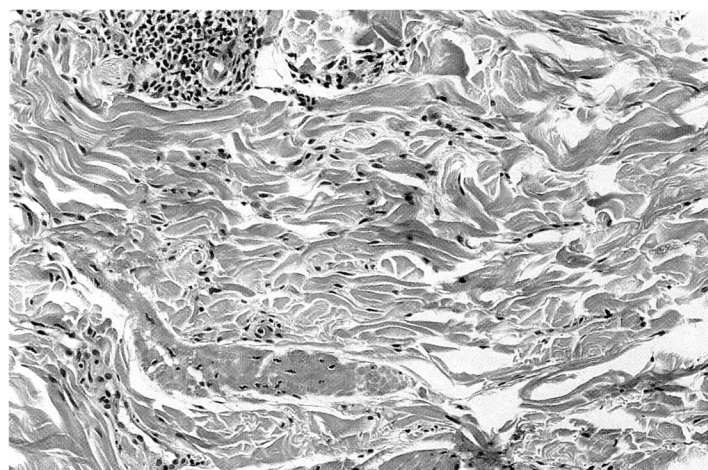

Fig. 8.6 Subsiding vasculitis. It is characterized by a perivascular infiltrate of lymphocytes, a hypercellular ('busy') dermis and some interstitial mucin. (H & E)

deposits of immunoglobulin in 81% of cases. The presence of immunoglobulin was seen more often in those patients who had at least one extracutaneous manifestation.[470] The presence of IgA was a strong predictor of renal disease.[470] E-selectin (ELAM-1) is present early in the course of vasculitis, but decreases as the lesion evolves.[465]

HENOCH–SCHÖNLEIN PURPURA

The Henoch–Schönlein variant of leukocytoclastic vasculitis is characterized by a purpuric rash, usually on the lower parts of the legs, which is often accompanied by one or more of the following: arthritis, abdominal pain, hematuria and, rarely, cardiac or neurological manifestations.[471–473] In adult cases there is a relatively high incidence of renal involvement.[474] The rash may be macular, papular, urticarial and, rarely, vesiculobullous.[475,476] The bullae may be hemorrhagic.[477] It is usually preceded by an upper respiratory tract infection or the ingestion of certain drugs or foods, with the formation of IgA-containing complexes, which may precipitate in vessels in the skin and certain other organs.[478,479] The alternate complement pathway is thereby activated. Anticardiolipin antibodies[480] and antineutrophil cytoplasmic antibodies (ANCA),[481] both of IgA class, have been reported in Henoch–Schönlein purpura. However, IgA ANCA are present in only 10% of cases. They can be detected in a wide variety of other cutaneous vasculitides.[482] Specific associations have included *Helicobacter pylori* infection of the stomach, other bacterial and viral infections,[483] vaccinations and drugs such as penicillin, ampicillin, clarithromycin,[484] erythromycin, chlorpromazine and aspirin (acetylsalicylic acid).[485] Henoch–Schönlein purpura has a predilection for children, although occurrence in adults is known.[479,486–488] It has been reported in two siblings who had simultaneous onset but no obvious underlying infection.[489]

The disease usually runs a self-limited course, although in a small percentage of patients persistent renal involvement occurs.

The condition reported as **infantile acute hemorrhagic edema** of the skin is a closely related condition.[490–494] The histopathology is the same, although IgA deposition is not a feature.[495] It has a benign course, leading to the suggestion that it be considered a separate entity.[496]

Histopathology

The appearances are usually indistinguishable from those seen in leukocytoclastic vasculitis. IgA, predominantly of the IgA1 subclass,[497] is

demonstrable in vessel walls in both involved and uninvolved skin in most cases, provided that the biopsy is taken early in the course of the disease.[478,479] Apoptotic dendrocytes (factor XIIIa positive) were noted around vessels in one case.[498]

Henoch–Schönlein purpura is not synonymous with IgA-associated vasculit s. Rather, it is one subcategory of it. An IgA vasculitis has been seen, without the usual clinical features of Henoch–Schönlein purpura, in a setting of prior infection, usually of the upper respiratory tract, in Wegener's granulomatosis, inflammatory bowel disease and malignancies.[499]

EOSINOPHILIC VASCULITIS

Eosinophilic vasculitis is a recently identified form characterized by an eosinophil-predominant necrotizing vasculitis affecting small dermal vessels.[500,501] It presents with pruritic, erythematous and purpuric papules and plaques. It may be idiopathic, or associated with connective tissue diseases or the hypereosinophilic syndrome.[500,502] It may show a good response to steroids, but recurrences are common.[503]

Histopathology

There is a necrotizing, eosinophil-rich vasculitis involving small vessels in the dermis and, sometimes, the subcutis (Fig. 8.7). It involves a smaller class of vessel than allergic granulomatosis. There is marked deposition of eosinophil granule major basic protein in the vessel walls.[501,504]

RHEUMATOID VASCULITIS

Rheumatoid vasculitis typically occurs in patients with seropositive, erosive rheumatoid arthritis of long standing.[505–507] A similar vasculitis may occur in some cases of systemic lupus erythematosus, mixed connective tissue disease, Sjögren's syndrome and, rarely, dermatomyositis and scleroderma. Rheumatoid vasculitis is an acute vasculitis which differs from leukocytoclastic vasculitis in its involvement of large as well as small blood vessels. This leads to varied clinical presentations which may include digital gangrene, cutaneous ulcers and digital nail fold infarction as well as palpable purpura.[508] Involvement of the vasa nervorum can result in a neuropathy.[508]

In rheumatoid vasculitis, lesions are often recurrent. The overall mortality may approach 30%.[505] Immune complexes appear to be involved in the pathogenesis.[508]

Histopathology[505,508]

As already mentioned, rheumatoid vasculitis is an acute vasculitis with involvement of several sizes of blood vessels. The involvement of medium-sized muscular arteries may be indistinguishable from that seen in polyarteritis nodosa. In the skin, vessels in the lower dermis are sometimes involved, while superficial vessels may be spared. Intimal proliferation and thrombosis of vessels also occur.

Rheumatoid vasculitis should be distinguished from rheumatoid neutrophilic dermatosis, which is one of the neutrophilic dermatoses and as such has no vasculitis.

URTICARIAL VASCULITIS

Urticarial vasculitis is another clinical variant of leukocytoclastic vasculitis; the cutaneous lesions comprise urticarial wheals and/or angioedema, rather than palpable purpura.[361,369,509] Erythematous papules and plaques may also occur. The wheals usually persist longer than is usual for chronic urticaria without vasculitis and they may resolve leaving an ecchymotic stain. Massive

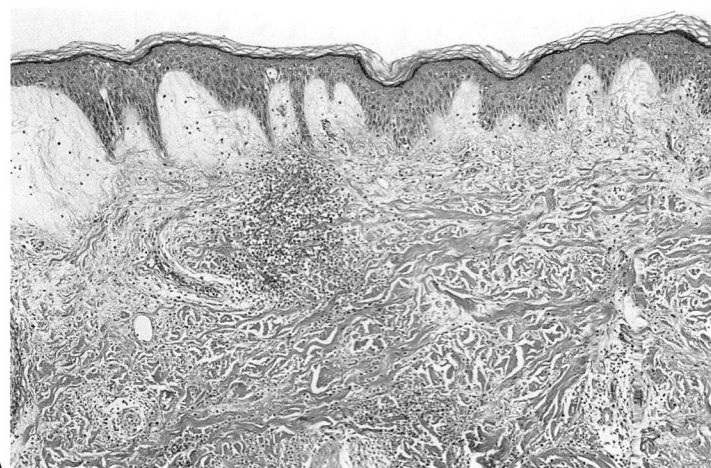
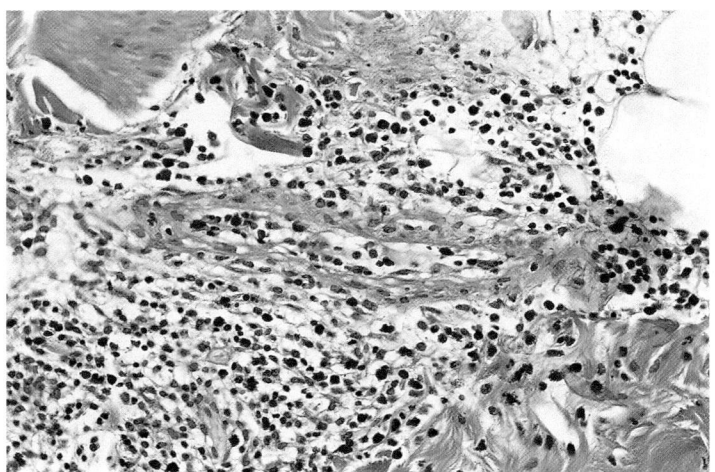

Fig. 8.7 **(A) Eosinophilic vasculitis. (B)** Eosinophils are a prominent component of the infiltrate. The patient had rheumatoid arthritis. (H & E)

subcutaneous hemorrhage has been reported.[510] The lesions are often generalized without any predilection for the lower legs. Systemic involvement, including renal failure, may occur and this is more likely in those with concurrent hypocomplementemia.[362,363,511,512] A lupus erythematosus-like syndrome is sometimes present.[513,514] Urticarial vasculitis has been reported in association with hepatitis B and C infection,[515,516] Sjögren's syndrome, IgA myeloma, an IgM gammopathy (Schnitzler's syndrome),[517] polycythemia rubra vera,[518] systemic lupus erythematosus, solar and cold urticaria,[367] exercise,[519] pregnancy,[520] visceral malignancy[521] and following the use of certain drugs,[522,523] including diltiazem[524] and cocaine.[525] Methotrexate may exacerbate the condition.[526]

The initial event is the deposition of immune complexes and C3 in the postcapillary venules. Complement activation ensues; its ongoing activation forms the membrane attack complex that may cause damage to the endothelial cell membranes.[527,528] At the cellular level, eosinophils appear at an early stage, at least in exercise-induced urticarial vasculitis.[519]

Histopathology[529]

The changes are similar to those seen in leukocytoclastic vasculitis, although there is usually prominent edema of the upper dermis. The inflammatory infiltrate is sometimes quite mild. A variant with a lymphocytic vasculitis has been reported.[368]

One study has found that the hypocomplementemic cases often have a more diffuse neutrophilia and the deposition of immunoreactants in a granular pattern along the basement membrane zone.[530] The authors suggested that these cases could represent a subset of systemic lupus erythematosus.[530]

MIXED CRYOGLOBULINEMIA

Mixed cryoglobulinemia has been discussed earlier in this chapter along with the monoclonal form (see p. 225). The histopathological changes are those of an acute vasculitis resembling leukocytoclastic vasculitis. In contrast to the monoclonal form, intravascular hyaline deposits are the exception, although they are sometimes found beneath areas of ulceration.

HYPERGAMMAGLOBULINEMIC PURPURA

Hypergammaglobulinemic purpura (Waldenström) is characterized by recurrent purpura, anemia, an elevated erythrocyte sedimentation rate and polyclonal hypergammaglobulinemia.[390,531] There is a significant association with autoimmune diseases, especially Sjögren's syndrome and lupus erythematosus.[532–534] Antibodies to Ro/SSA antigen are often present.[533]

Histopathology

The changes are similar to those occurring in leukocytoclastic vasculitis.

HYPERGAMMAGLOBULINEMIA D SYNDROME

The hypergammaglobulinemia (hyperimmunoglobulinemia) D syndrome presents in early childhood with recurrent febrile attacks with abdominal distress, headache and arthralgias.[535] Skin lesions are common during the attacks.[536] They may be erythematous macules, urticarial lesions or erythematous nodules.

The inheritance is autosomal recessive. The condition is caused by a mutation in the mevalonate kinase (*MVK*) gene on chromosome 12q24. The enzyme involved participates in the sterol biosynthesis pathway.[535] The mutation is common in northern Europe.

Histopathology

The usual cutaneous changes are those of a mild acute vasculitis, which may be leukocytoclastic.[536,537] The pattern may rarely mimic Sweet's syndrome or a cellulitis.

SEPTIC VASCULITIS

Septic vasculitis, also referred to (somewhat erroneously) as non-leukocytoclastic vasculitis,[538] is a variant of acute vasculitis seen in association with various septicemic states. These include meningococcal septicemia, gonococcal septicemia, *Pseudomonas* septicemia, streptococcal septicemia,[539] infective endocarditis, particularly that due to *Staphylococcus aureus*,[540] and some cases of secondary syphilis. Certain rickettsial infections can produce similar lesions.

Cutaneous lesions occur in 80% or more of cases of acute meningococcal infections.[541] There are erythematous macules, nodules, plaques and petechiae which may be surmounted with small pustules.[541,542] There is a predilection for the extremities and pressure sites. Features of disseminated intravascular coagulation are invariably present. Acute gonococcemia is exceedingly rare in comparison, although localized pustular lesions have been reported on the digits.[543,544] In *Pseudomonas* infections, hemorrhagic bullae, ulcers and eschars are seen.[545,546] These changes are discussed elsewhere as ecthyma gangrenosum (see p. 620). Acute pustular lesions also occur in infective endocarditis as Osler nodes and Janeway lesions.

Chronic infections with *Neisseria meningitidis* and *N. gonorrhoeae* are characterized by the triad of intermittent fever, arthralgia and vesiculopustular or hemorrhagic lesions.[547–549] In chronic gonococcal septicemia there is a marked female preponderance and lesions are fewer in number than in chronic meningococcal septicemia. Positive blood cultures have been obtained during febrile episodes.

Histopathology

In *acute meningococcal septicemia* there is widespread vascular damage characterized by endothelial swelling and focal necrosis, fibrinoid change in vessel walls, and occlusive thrombi composed of platelets, fibrin, red blood cells and neutrophils (Fig. 8.8).[550,551] There are neutrophils in and around vessel walls, as well as in the interstitium. Leukocytoclasis is often present, although it is usually quite mild.[541] There is also some perivascular hemorrhage. The adnexa may show degenerative changes.[550] Subepidermal edema and pustulation occur as well as intraepidermal pustules.[550] Large numbers of Gram-negative diplococci are seen in endothelial cells and neutrophils.[550,551]

In *chronic meningococcal septicemia* and *chronic gonococcal septicemia* there is a vasculitis which differs from hypersensitivity vasculitis in subtle ways. Arterioles are often affected in addition to venules, and deep vessels may show changes just as conspicuous as those in the superficial dermis. Extravasation of erythrocytes is often conspicuous. There is also an admixture of mononuclear cells in chronic septic vasculitis, and vascular thrombi are more regularly seen.[547,548] Leukocytoclasis is often present, but it is not a prominent feature.[552] Another distinguishing feature is the regular presence of subepidermal and intraepidermal pustules with partial destruction of the epidermis.[547,553] Organisms are usually not found with a Gram stain of tissue sections, although bacterial antigens are commonly identified using immunofluorescence techniques.[547,553]

There are conflicting reports on the histopathological findings in the Osler nodes and Janeway lesions of infective endocarditis. Osler nodes appear to be a septic vasculitis, involving in part the glomus apparatus,[554] while Janeway lesions have variously been regarded as a similar process[555,556] or as an embolic suppurative process with or without vasculitis.[557–559] Organisms have been found in the septic microemboli of Janeway lesions.[560,561] Similar lesions, but without organisms, can be seen in marantic endocarditis.[562]

ERYTHEMA ELEVATUM DIUTINUM

Erythema elevatum diutinum is a rare dermatosis in which there are persistent red, violaceous and yellowish papules, plaques and nodules that are usually distributed acrally and symmetrically on extensor surfaces, including the buttocks.[563] Pedunculated lesions[564,565] and nodules surmounted by vesicles and bullae have also been described.[566,567] Arthralgia,[563] peripheral ulcerative keratitis[568] and pulmonary infiltrates[569] may occur. An association with myelodysplastic syndrome,[570] lymphoma,[571] multiple myeloma, IgA monoclonal gammopathy,[572–575] hyperimmunoglobulinemia D syndrome[576] and cryoglobulinemia[577] has been documented. It has also been reported in association with celiac disease,[578,579] ulcerative colitis,[580] Crohn's disease,[581] mosquito bites,[582] relapsing polychondritis,[583] rheumatoid arthritis,[584] and HIV and HHV-6 infections.[585–591] Onset is usually in middle life. Lesions may involute after 5–10 years, but persistence for 20 years has been reported.

The etiology is unknown but erythema elevatum diutinum is thought to be a variant of leukocytoclastic vasculitis resulting from an Arthus-type reaction to bacterial and even viral antigens.[592] Various cytokines, such as IL-8, allow a selective recruitment of leukocytes to involved sites.[593] The formation of granulation tissue in lesions results in local perpetuation of the process as newly formed vessels are more vulnerable to injury.

Histopathology[563,594,595]

Erythema elevatum diutinum is typically characterized by acute histological features which contrast with the chronic clinical course.[596] Nevertheless, the histological appearances vary somewhat according to the age of the lesion.

In early lesions there is a moderately dense perivascular infiltrate of neutrophils, with deposits of fibrin ('toxic hyalin') within and around the walls of small dermal blood vessels.[563,565] These may also show endothelial swelling. Leukocytoclasis is also present. There are lesser numbers of histiocytes and lymphocytes and only a few eosinophils. Necrotizing granulomas were reported in one case.[582] Extravasation of red cells is uncommon.

In more established lesions the infiltrate of neutrophils involves the entire dermis. The epidermis is usually uninvolved, but there may be focal spongiosis. In vesiculobullous lesions there is subepidermal vesiculation and pustulation.[566] Focal epidermal necrosis is sometimes present.[566] Basophilic nuclear dust may encrust collagen bundles in some cases.[594] Capillary proliferation is usually present in established lesions. In one instance, this resembled a pyogenic granuloma.[582]

In late lesions there is variable fibrosis and in some instances a fascicled proliferation of spindle cells.[584,594] The low-power picture resembles a dermatofibroma. Small foci of neutrophilic vasculitis are scattered through the fibrotic areas.[565] Capillary proliferation is also present. *Extracellular cholesterosis* of the older literature[596] is now regarded as a variant in which lipids are secondarily deposited within macrophages and other cellular elements and possibly between the collagen.[597,598] Since the introduction of dapsone in the treatment of this entity, cholesterol deposits no longer seem to be recorded.

Although immunoglobulins and complement have been reported in the vicinity of small vessels in the dermis, this has not been an invariable finding.[563] Factor XIIIa-positive dendrocytes are present in the dermis, but in similar numbers to that seen in ordinary acute leukocytoclastic vasculitis.[599]

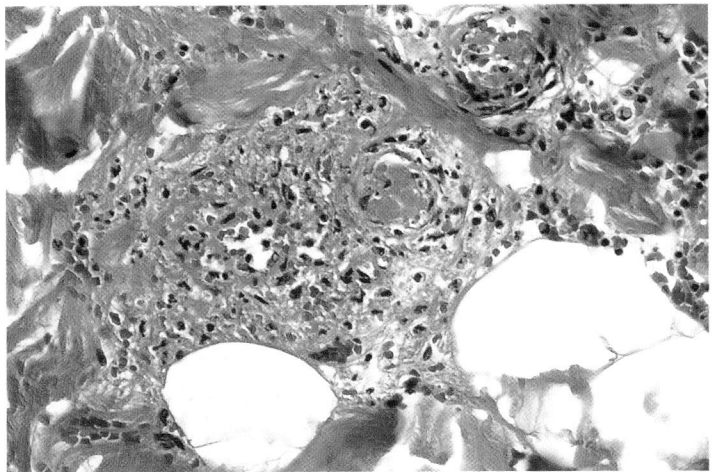

Fig. 8.8 **Meningococcal septicemia.** A vessel is occluded by a fibrin thrombus. There are some neutrophils in the surrounding dermis. (H & E)

Although the clinical features are quite distinct, the histological features of early lesions may be indistinguishable from the neutrophilic dermatoses – Sweet's syndrome, rheumatoid neutrophilic dermatosis, the bowel-associated dermatosis-arthritis syndrome and Behçet's disease. Erythema elevatum ciutinum differs from granuloma faciale in the predominance of neutrophils rather than eosinophils and the involvement of the adventitial dermis which is spared in granuloma faciale (see below).[594]

Electron microscopy

In addition to the fibrin deposition and neutrophil fragmentation, there are histiocytes present which contain fat droplets and myelin figures.[594] Cholesterol crystals have been present in some cases, both intracellular and extracellular in position.[594] Langerhans cells are increased in the dermis in both early and late lesions.[600]

GRANULOMA FACIALE

Granuloma faciale is a rare dermatosis which manifests as one or several brown-red plaques, nodules or sometimes papules on the face.[601–604] There is a predilection for white males of middle age.[605] Childhood cases occur.[606] Extrafacial involvement is quite uncommon.[607–610] The lesions are usually persistent and essentially asymptomatic.

The etiology is unknown, but a form of vasculitis, mediated by a localized Arthus-like process, has been postulated.[611] The lymphocytic component of the infiltrate is thought to be attracted to the skin by IFN-γ-induced mechanisms.[612]

Histopathology[601,613]

There is usually a dense, polymorphous, inflammatory cell infiltrate in the upper two-thirds of the dermis, with a narrow, uninvolved grenz zone beneath the epidermis and often around pilosebaceous follicles (Fig. 8.9). Occasionally the entire dermis and even the upper subcutis are involved.[614] Sometimes the infiltrate is less dense and then tends to show perivascular accentuation. The infiltrate consists of eosinophils, usually quite numerous, together with neutrophils, lymphocytes, histiocytes and a few mast cells and plasma cells (Fig. 8.10). Neutrophils are usually localized around the blood vessels and there may be mild leukocytoclasis. There is controversy as to whether neutrophils are related to the intensity of the inflammation or the stage of the disease.[601,613] A few foam cells and foreign body giant cells may be present.[611] In lesions of long standing there is usually some fibrosis.

Blood vessels in the upper dermis are usually dilated, often with some endothelial swelling. Eosinophilic fibrinoid material, so-called 'toxic hyalin', may be deposited around some vessels, but many cases do not show this feature. The material is PAS positive and diastase resistant. Extravasated red blood cells are often present and hemosiderin is present in over half of all biopsies. A true vasculitis may be present, but this presumably depends on the timing of the biopsy with respect to the course of the disease process.[614]

Immunoglobulins, particularly IgG, and complement are often present along the basement membrane and around blood vessels.[615] Fibrin is usually present around the vessels, even when toxic hyalin is not present on light microscopy.[615] Abundant eosinophilic cationic protein can be demonstrated in the dermis using immunohistochemistry.[616]

Erythema elevatum diutinum (see above) has many histological similarities, but in this condition the proportion of neutrophils to eosinophils is higher than in granuloma faciale and there is usually no well-defined grenz zone.[613] Toxic hyalin is more abundant and often intimately related to the vessel wall in erythema elevatum diutinum.[617]

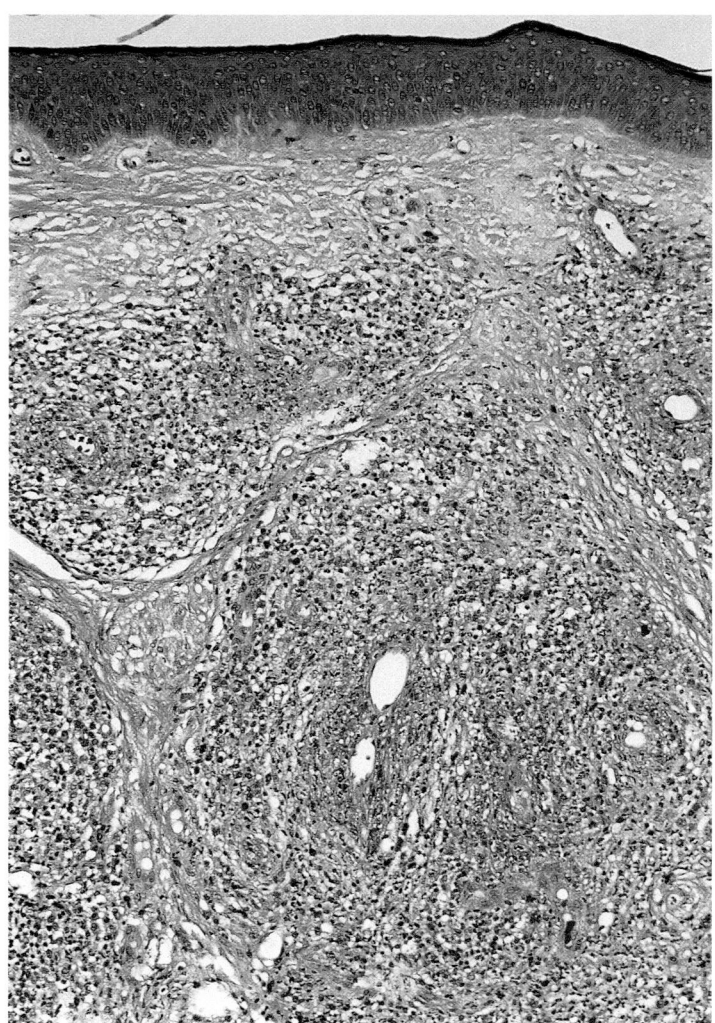

Fig. 8.9 **Granuloma faciale.** A grenz zone of uninvolved dermis overlies a mixed inflammatory cell infiltrate. A small amount of fibrin is present in vessel walls. The dermal infiltrate is more widespread than in most cases of hypersensitivity vasculitis. (H & E)

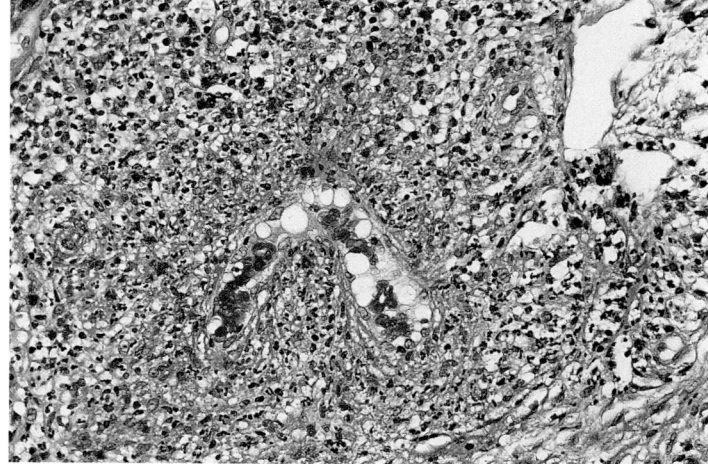

Fig. 8.10 **Granuloma faciale.** A mixed infiltrate, which includes neutrophils, eosinophils and lymphocytes, surrounds a dermal blood vessel. (H & E)

Electron microscopy

Electron microscopy reveals abundant eosinophils, often with cytoplasmic degenerative changes.[618] Charcot–Leyden crystals are commonly seen.

LOCALIZED CHRONIC FIBROSING VASCULITIS

The term 'localized chronic fibrosing vasculitis' was used by Carlson and LeBoit for a solitary lesion whose histology resembled late-stage erythema elevatum diutinum or granuloma faciale, but with a clinical picture that resembled neither.[619] The lesions were red-brown, violaceous papules, plaques and nodules that had been present for several months.

Histopathology[619]

The lesions combined variable amounts of patterned fibrosis (storiform, concentric or lamellar) and inflammation which was nodular or diffuse (Fig. 8.11).

Focal leukocytoclastic vasculitis was usually present. Both neutrophils and eosinophils were present in varying numbers with admixed lymphocytes and aggregates of plasma cells. In some parts, the lesion resembled inflammatory pseudotumor and in other areas a sclerotic fibroma.

MICROSCOPIC POLYANGIITIS (POLYARTERITIS)

Microscopic polyangiitis is a systemic small-vessel vasculitis associated with focal and segmental glomerulonephritis and the presence of circulating antibodies to one of the antineutrophil cytoplasmic antibodies (p-ANCA). There are few, if any, immune complexes deposited in vessel walls.[620] It affects predominantly middle-aged males. Constitutional symptoms are usually present and pulmonary involvement is not uncommon.[621,622]

Cutaneous lesions are present in 30–50% of cases. They are usually purpuric lesions on the lower limbs; necrotic ulcers are uncommon and nodules are rare.[621]

Similar cases have been classified in the past as hypersensitivity vasculitis with systemic involvement or included with polyarteritis nodosa.

Histopathology[620]

There is an acute (neutrophilic) vasculitis with variable leukocytoclasis, accompanied by extravasation of red blood cells and patchy fibrinoid degeneration of vessels. Characteristically the process involves arterioles but capillaries and postcapillary venules may also be involved. It spares medium-sized muscular arteries. The uncommon nodular lesions show a heavy mixed inflammatory cell infiltrate, particularly in the lower dermis and upper subcutis, and an accompanying vasculitis. Such cases may be difficult to distinguish from Wegener's granulomatosis but granulomas and upper airways involvement are absent in microscopic polyarteritis. Furthermore, Wegener's granulomatosis is usually associated with c-ANCA, although p-ANCA is sometimes found. These two conditions are part of a spectrum of ANCA-associated disease.[623] The specificity of ANCA in defining a subset of patients with leukocytoclastic vasculitis has been challenged.[624] Despite these reservations, a cutaneous-limited variant associated with antimyeloperoxidase autoantibodies has been suggested.[625]

POLYARTERITIS NODOSA

Polyarteritis nodosa is a rare inflammatory disease of small and medium-sized muscular arteries. It usually involves multiple organs,[626–628] including the

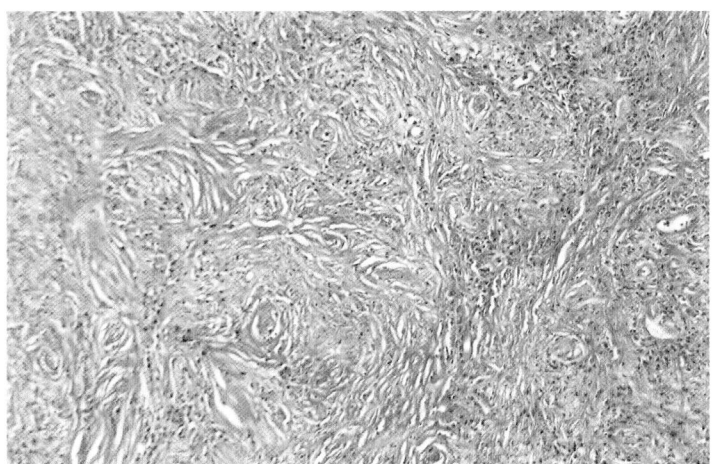

Fig. 8.11 **Localized chronic fibrosing vasculitis.** There is patterned fibrosis and only mild diffuse inflammation. (H & E) (Microscopic slide kindly provided by Dr Philip LeBoit)

kidneys, liver, gastrointestinal tract and nervous system. The skin is involved in approximately 10–15% of cases, resulting in palpable purpura and sometimes ulceration of the lower extremities.[629] There are usually constitutional symptoms such as fever, weight loss, fatigue, arthralgia and myalgia.[626] No age is exempt, but there is a predilection for adult males.

The course is variable, but it is not possible to predict those likely to develop progressive disease.[626] The 5-year survival rate is approximately 50%; death is usually the result of involvement of the kidneys or gastrointestinal tract.[626]

A *cutaneous form* of polyarteritis nodosa, with a chronic relapsing course but usually no evidence of systemic disease, has been reported.[630–632] Renal involvement was reported in one series.[633] This variant usually presents with nodules, often painful, livedo reticularis or ulceration involving the lower limbs.[634] There may be mild constitutional symptoms but the prognosis is nevertheless good.[635] An unusual complication has been the formation of periosteal new bone beneath the cutaneous lesions.[636] A variant localized to the breast has been reported.[637]

There are probably many causes of polyarteritis nodosa. Immune complexes appear to play an important role in the pathogenesis. Hepatitis B surface antigen has been detected in up to 50% of systemic cases[638] but this figure is much higher than has been recorded in most series.[639] The antigen has also been reported in the localized cutaneous form.[633,640,641] Hepatitis C infection has been present in some cases.[642] Preceding bacterial infections, particularly streptococcal, have been documented in both types and it appears to be a frequent association in childhood cutaneous cases.[643–645] Most of the cutaneous cases reviewed at the Mayo Clinic were idiopathic.[634]

Polyarteritis nodosa-like lesions have been reported in association with Crohn's disease,[646] B-cell lymphoma,[647] Kawasaki syndrome (see below), rheumatoid arthritis, angioimmunoblastic lymphadenopathy and following the repair of coarctation of the aorta.[648] They have also been noted following the intravenous injection of methamphetamine (metamfetamine, 'speed')[649] and following the prolonged use of minocycline in the treatment of acne.[650]

Histopathology[651]

In the early stages there is marked thickening of the wall of the vessel, particularly the intima, as a result of edema and a fibrinous and cellular exudate. The infiltrate is composed of neutrophils, with some eosinophils and lymphocytes. Leukocytoclasis is sometimes present. In older lesions there is a greater proportion of mononuclear cells, particularly lymphocytes. Luminal thrombi and aneurysms may form. Initially the lesions are segmental but the infiltrate expands to involve the full circumference of the artery. The changes are often localized to the region of a bifurcation of the vessel. At a still later stage there is intimal and mural fibrosis leading to obliteration of the vessel. A characteristic feature of polyarteritis nodosa is the presence of lesions at all stages of development.

In the *cutaneous form* small and medium-sized arteries in the subcutis and occasionally the deep dermis are involved. The inflammation is localized to the vessel and its immediate vicinity, allowing a distinction to be made from the various panniculitides (Fig. 8.12). There may be a mild perivascular lymphocytic infiltrate in the overlying dermis.

Immunofluorescence of the cutaneous form has shown IgM and sometimes C3 in the vessel walls.[630]

KAWASAKI SYNDROME

Kawasaki syndrome (Kawasaki disease, mucocutaneous lymph node syndrome) is an acute, multisystem, febrile illness of unknown cause that occurs predominantly in infancy and early childhood.[652–656] Adult cases have been reported,[657] but some of these may represent erythema multiforme or the toxic shock syndrome.[658] In addition to the prolonged fever, clinical features include non-exudative conjunctivitis, cervical lymphadenopathy, oropharyngeal inflammation, thrombocytosis and a vasculitis which predominantly involves the coronary arteries, leading to coronary artery aneurysms or ectasias in 20% or more of cases.[653,659,660] The disease is usually self-limited although 1% may end fatally, almost exclusively from the cardiac involvement.

Cutaneous manifestations include a polymorphous, exanthematous rash, accompanied by brawny edema and erythema of the palms and soles.[653,659] This is followed by desquamation which particularly involves the tips of the fingers and toes. Recurrent skin peeling may continue for several years.[661] An erythematous, desquamating perineal eruption is a distinctive feature in many cases.[662] A pustular rash resembling miliaria pustulosa also occurs in some patients.[663]

Although the etiology is unknown, a microbial cause, possibly involving a bacterial superantigen,[657] is suggested by the clinical features, by the occurrence of epidemic outbreaks and by the amelioration of coronary artery abnormalities by the use of gamma globulin.[664] A retrovirus and

Propionibacterium acnes have been suggested at one time or another, but no agent has been consistently demonstrable.[665] Infection with HIV has rarely been present.[666] Antiendothelial antibodies have been detected in some cases.[386]

Histopathology

Biopsies of the skin lesions are infrequently performed. They have shown non-specific features which include edema of the papillary dermis and a mild perivascular infiltrate of lymphocytes and mononuclear cells.[659,667] Subtle vascular changes, including subendothelial edema, focal endothelial cell necrosis and vascular deposition of small amounts of fibrinoid material, were noted in one report.[667] The pustular lesions are small intraepidermal and subcorneal abscesses; they are not related to eccrine ducts.[663]

Although autopsies on fatal cases have shown a polyarteritis nodosa-like involvement of the coronary and some other visceral arteries, no cutaneous vasculitis has been reported.[652]

SUPERFICIAL THROMBOPHLEBITIS

Superficial thrombophlebitis presents with tender, erythematous swellings or cord-like thickenings of the subcutis, usually on the lower parts of the legs. Multiple segments of a vein may be involved over time, hence the use of the term 'migratory' in the older literature to describe this process. Superficial thrombophlebitis may occur in association with Behçet's disease, Buerger's disease (thromboangiitis obliterans) or an underlying cancer, most often a carcinoma of the pancreas or stomach.[668,669] It may be associated with various hypercoagulable states.[670,671]

Mondor's disease is a variant of superficial thrombophlebitis occurring in relation to the breast or anterolateral chest wall.[672–674] A history of preceding trauma, including breast surgery, is obtained in a number of cases.

Histopathology

Superficial thrombophlebitis involves veins in the upper subcutis. In early lesions, the inflammatory cell infiltrate is composed of numerous neutrophils, although at a later stage there are lymphocytes and occasional multinucleate giant cells. Intramural microabscesses are commonly present in the vein in the thrombophlebitis which accompanies Buerger's disease; there is some controversy whether this finding is specific for this disease (Fig. 8.13). The inflammatory cell infiltrate extends only a short distance into the surrounding fat, in contrast to the more extensive panniculitis seen in erythema induratum–nodular vasculitis.

Thrombus is often present in the lumen of the affected veins and this eventually undergoes recanalization.

MISCELLANEOUS ASSOCIATIONS

An acute vasculitis is a feature of erythema nodosum leprosum (see p. 632). It has also been reported in the rose spots of paratyphoid fever[675] and in the Jarisch–Herxheimer reaction which may follow therapy for syphilis.[676] In this latter condition, the acute inflammatory changes are superimposed on a background of chronic inflammation in which plasma cells are usually prominent.[676]

The condition known as erythema induratum–nodular vasculitis is also an acute vasculitis. It results in a panniculitis and accordingly is discussed with the panniculitides on page 524.

Rarely, a fixed drug eruption will present as a localized area of acute vasculitis. As in erythema elevatum diutinum, the upper dermis may contain

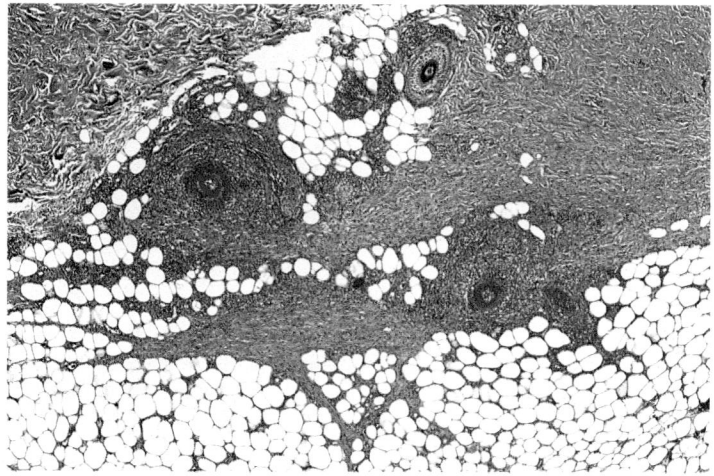

Fig. 8.12 **Cutaneous polyarteritis nodosa.** The affected small arteries in the upper subcutis show marked fibrin extravasation into their walls. (H & E)

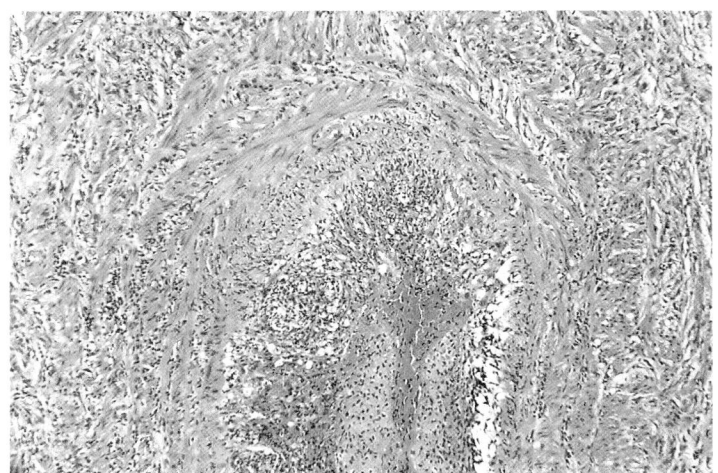

Fig. 8.13 **Superficial thrombophlebitis in Buerger's disease.** There is focal suppuration of the vein wall and a luminal thrombus. There is some controversy as to the specificity of this finding. (H & E)

many neutrophils despite the lesion being of some weeks duration. There are no lichenoid features present.

NEUTROPHILIC DERMATOSES

The neutrophilic dermatoses are a clinically heterogeneous group of entities characterized histopathologically by the presence of a heavy dermal infiltrate of neutrophils and variable leukocytoclasis.[677] On casual examination of tissue sections the appearances suggest an acute vasculitis, although on closer inspection there is no significant fibrinoid necrosis of vessel walls. Further-more, the neutrophilic infiltrate is usually much heavier in the neutrophilic dermatoses than in leukocytoclastic vasculitis. Limited vascular damage in the form of endothelial swelling may be present, and in some biopsies fibrinoid necrosis of some vessel walls may be found. The term 'pustular vasculitis' has been proposed as an alternative designation, particularly for those cases in which there is evidence of a vasculitis, a sign of the confusion which surrounds the nosological classification of this group.[678,679]

Circulating immune complexes with heightened chemotaxis of neutrophils are thought to have an important pathogenetic role.[679] The immune complexes appear to be of diverse origin. Cytokines such as interleukin-1 (IL-1) may play a contributory role.[680]

The following diseases will be considered in this category, although it should be noted that the lesions in some stages of Behçet's syndrome do not qualify for inclusion:

- Sweet's syndrome
- bowel-associated dermatosis-arthritis syndrome
- rheumatoid neutrophilic dermatosis
- acute generalized pustulosis
- Behçet's syndrome
- abscess-forming neutrophilic dermatosis.

Although it has many histopathological features in common with this group, erythema elevatum diutinum has prominent fibrinoid change in vessel walls and is best included with the acute vasculitides. Pyoderma gangrenosum has also been included in this group by some authorities.[387]

Familial Mediterranean fever, an autosomal recessive disease that tends to affect certain ethnic groups, may present with a cutaneous vasculitis.

More often, there is an erysipelas-like erythema, which is the pathognomonic skin manifestation.[681] It rapidly resolves. This is not due to a vasculitis but a very mild neutrophilic dermatosis with nuclear dust and admixed lymphocytes. The infiltrate is predominantly perivascular.

Another periodic fever syndrome is **TRAPS**, tumor necrosis factor receptor-associated periodic syndrome (see p. 253).

SWEET'S SYNDROME

Sweet's syndrome (acute febrile neutrophilic dermatosis) is a rare dermatosis. It is characterized by the abrupt onset of tender or painful erythematous plaques and nodules on the face[682–684] and extremities and, less commonly, on the trunk, in association with fever, malaise and a neutrophil leukocytosis.[685,686] A variant with raised annular lesions and another with palmoplantar pustulosis have been reported.[687,688] The skin lesions are sometimes studded with small vesicles or pustules, but ulceration is unusual and true bullae are uncommon.[689] Lesions usually heal without scarring although there may be residual pigmentation attributed to hemosiderin. There is a predilection for females; the patients may be of any age.[690,691] Other clinical features may include polyarthritis, conjunctivitis and episcleritis.[686,692] Intestinal involvement has been reported.[693]

In 10–15% of cases an associated leukemia,[694] usually of acute myelomonocytic type, is present, or develops later.[695–703] In some of these cases, features of atypical pyoderma gangrenosum may be present and it has been suggested that Sweet's syndrome and pyoderma gangrenosum may be at opposite ends of the spectrum of one process.[704–707] Both Sweet's syndrome and pyoderma gangrenosum have resulted from the use of leukocyte colony-stimulating factors.[708–711] Other associations have included polycythemia vera,[712–714] chemotherapy-induced granulocytopenia,[706,715] lymphoma,[716–718] myeloma,[719] solid cancers,[636,720–723] relapsing polychondritis,[724] Behçet's syndrome,[725,726] pregnancy,[683,727] sarcoidosis,[728] rheumatoid arthritis, lupus erythematosus,[729,730] ulcerative colitis,[685,731] Crohn's disease,[732] sensorineural hearing loss,[733] subacute thyroiditis,[734] erythema nodosum,[735] chronic granulomatous disease,[736] T-cell immunodeficiency,[737] and chlamydial,[738] *Salmonella enteritidis*,[739] *Capnocytophaga canimorsus*,[740] *Helicobacter pylori*,[741] streptococcal, mycobacterial,[742] hepatitis B[743] and HIV infection.[744–746] BCG vaccination[747] and the ingestion of furosemide (frusemide),[748] minocycline,[749] trimethoprim-sulfamethoxazole,[750] hydralazine,[751] diazepam[752] or the oral contraceptive pill[753] are further associations.

A case of Sweet's syndrome with a clonal neutrophilic dermatosis has been reported in a patient with CD34-positive acute myelogenous leukemia treated with granulocyte colony-stimulating factor.[754]

The etiology is unknown, but the syndrome is assumed to represent an immunological hypersensitivity reaction triggered by some antecedent process. There is sometimes a history of a preceding upper respiratory tract infection. Enhanced chemotaxis for neutrophils has been reported in several cases.[755–757] One study concluded that the pathogenesis is mediated through helper T-cell type 1 cytokines (IL-2, IFN-γ).[758] Antibodies to neutrophil cytoplasmic antigens (ANCA) have also been found.[759]

Histopathology[686,760]

There is a dense infiltrate of mature neutrophils in the upper half of the dermis. Neutrophils may extend throughout the dermis and even into the subcutis. The epidermis is usually spared, although it may be pale staining. Neutrophils may be so dense in the center of the lesion that the appearances simulate an incipient abscess. A neutrophil-poor variant is rare.[761] Leukocytoclasis with the formation of nuclear dust is usually present but there is no true vasculitis or fibrinoid extravasation (Fig. 8.14). However, the vessels often show endothelial swelling. Lymphocytes are present in older lesions but are usually perivascular and few in number. One report has suggested that early lesions contain numerous histiocytes that may morphologically mimic neutrophils,[762] but this has not been confirmed by a subsequent study[680] or by the author's own experience. Early forms of neutrophils, with bilobed nuclei, are often present and may be mistaken for other cell types. A few eosinophils may be present in the infiltrate. In later lesions, macrophages containing phagocytosed neutrophils are sometimes prominent in the upper dermis.

Varying numbers of atypical leukemic cells may be seen in the infiltrate in the rare cases of Sweet's syndrome precipitated by transretinoic acid treatment of a leukemia.[763,764] There are reports of their presence in other cases of leukemia and myelodysplastic syndrome.[765,766]

There is often marked edema of the papillary dermis which may lead to the appearance of subepidermal vesiculation (Fig. 8.15). Delicate strands of dermal collagen usually stretch across this pseudobullous space.[686] Dilated vessels and extravasated red blood cells may be found in this zone.

Destruction of dermal elastic tissue producing acquired cutis laxa **(Marshall's syndrome)** is a rare complication. It may be related to a coexistent deficiency of α_1-antitrypsin which has recently been reported in this condition.[767]

The appearances resemble erythema elevatum diutinum, except for the absence of fibrinoid material in Sweet's syndrome. A case with clinical and histological overlap has been reported.[768] In granuloma faciale there are more eosinophils, even in early lesions, and there is a well-defined grenz zone.

A neutrophilic dermatosis resembling Sweet's syndrome was present in a case with different clinical features and reported as **neutrophilic figurate erythema of infancy**.[769] An exceedingly rare neutrophilic dermatosis which also includes vesiculation and erosions is **congenital erosive and vesicular dermatosis healing with reticulated supple scarring**.[770]

Pustular vasculitis of the hands

We have seen a distinctive variant of Sweet's syndrome characterized by hemorrhagic and edematous papules and large plaques limited to the dorsum of the radial side of the hands and the first three digits.[771–775] In contrast to the usual appearances of Sweet's syndrome, a severe leukocytoclastic vasculitis was present in all cases.[771]

BOWEL-ASSOCIATED DERMATOSIS-ARTHRITIS SYNDROME

The use of intestinal bypass surgery for the treatment of morbid obesity is complicated in 10–20% of patients by an influenza-like illness with malaise, fever, polyarthritis and the development of small pustular lesions in the skin of the upper extremities and trunk.[776] Erythema nodosum-like lesions are sometimes present.[777] A similar clinicopathological syndrome has been reported rarely in patients with other bowel conditions,[778] such as ulcerative colitis, Crohn's disease and intestinal diverticula, and following partial gastrectomy.[779,780] This has prompted the new designation used above, in place of the previous term, the 'bowel bypass syndrome'. There have been no recent reports of this condition.

The deposition of immune complexes containing the bacterial antigen peptidoglycan, derived from an overgrowth of bacteria in a blind loop or abnormal segment of bowel, may be responsible for this syndrome.[776,781] Cryoglobulins are also often present.[781]

Histopathology

The changes resemble those of Sweet's syndrome with subepidermal edema and a heavy infiltrate of neutrophils in the upper and mid dermis which is both perivascular and diffuse in distribution.[780] There is variable leukocytoclasis. In older lesions, lymphocytes, eosinophils and macrophages containing neutrophil debris are also present. Although signs of vascular damage are usually limited to some endothelial swelling, fibrin deposition around vessels can be present. A purulent folliculitis has also been reported, but this is more common in the pustular lesions, particularly on the face, in patients with ulcerative colitis.[782] Septal and lower dermal inflammation is present in the erythema nodosum-like lesions.[777]

Immunofluorescence findings have not been consistent. Immunoglobulins and complement have been noted at the dermoepidermal junction and even in vessel walls.[777,781]

RHEUMATOID NEUTROPHILIC DERMATOSIS

Rheumatoid neutrophilic dermatosis is a rare cutaneous manifestation of severe rheumatoid arthritis. It has received scant attention in the literature.[783–789] Clinically, it presents with plaques and nodules overlying joints of the extremities, particularly the hands, resembling erythema elevatum

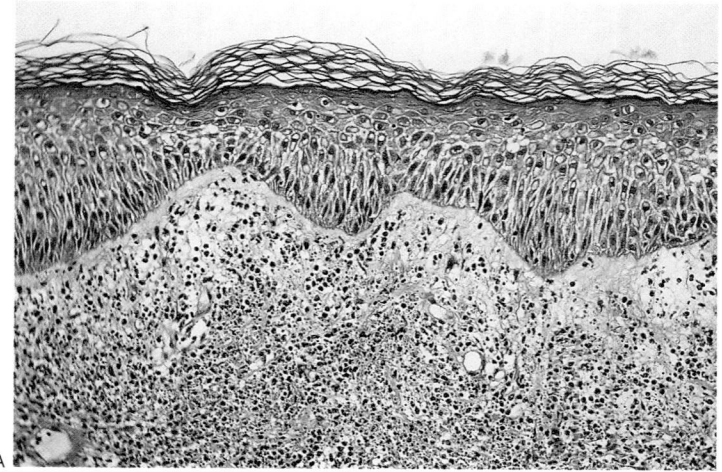
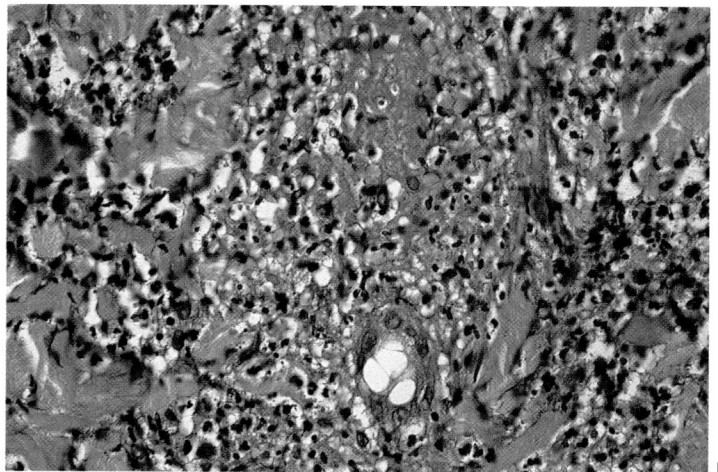

Fig. 8.14 **(A) Sweet's syndrome. (B)** There are numerous neutrophils surrounding a dermal blood vessel which is devoid of fibrin in its wall. (H & E)

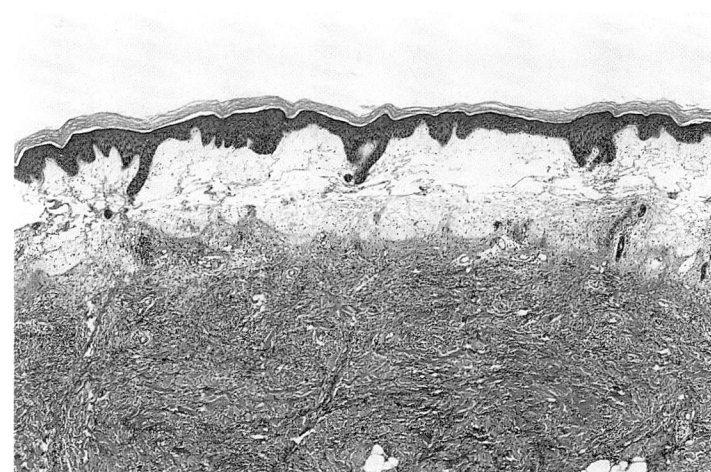

Fig. 8.15 **Sweet's syndrome with marked subepidermal edema.** The underlying dermis contains a heavy infiltrate of neutrophils. (H & E)

diutinum.[783,790] At other times the lesions are flat, erythematous plaques, more widely distributed on the extremities and sometimes on the trunk.[784] It has also been reported in a patient with seronegative rheumatoid arthritis.

Histopathology

There is a dense neutrophilic infiltrate throughout the dermis, but particularly in the upper and middle levels. There is variable leukocytoclasis. In late lesions lymphocytes, plasma cells and macrophages containing neutrophilic debris are also present (Fig. 8.16). There is no vasculitis. Sometimes the neutrophils collect in the papillary dermis, forming microabscesses similar to those seen in dermatitis herpetiformis.[783] Intraepidermal spongiotic blisters containing a few neutrophils may also be present.[791]

The author has seen a case with overlap features with interstitial granulomatous dermatitis (see p. 211).

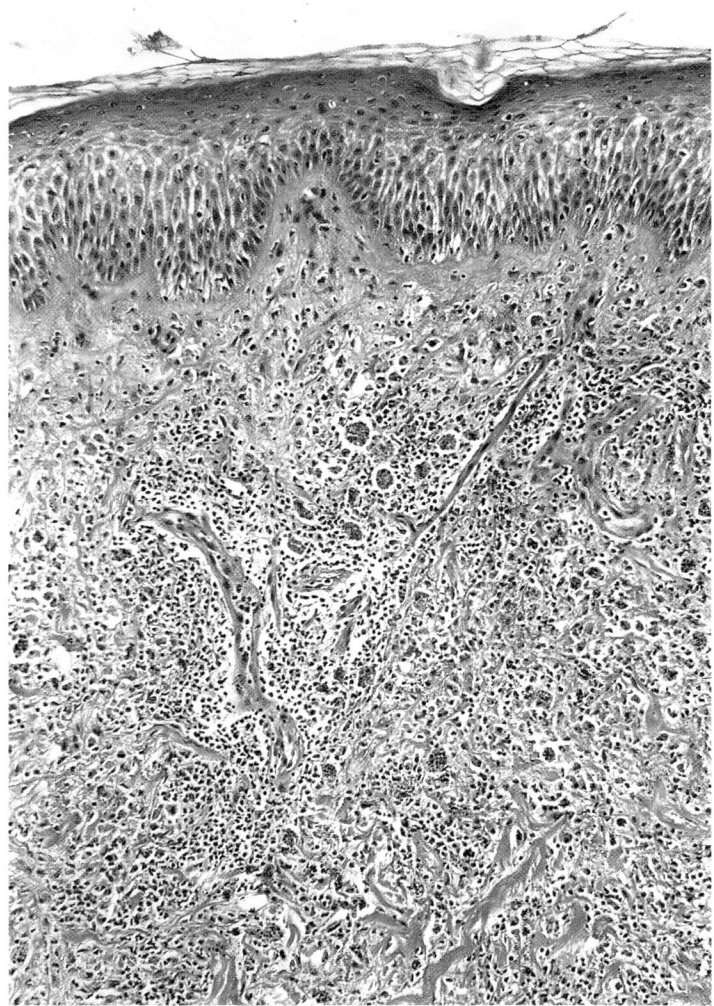

Fig. 8.16 **Rheumatoid neutrophilic dermatosis.** A late lesion is shown. Macrophages have neutrophil debris in their cytoplasm. (H & E)

ACUTE GENERALIZED PUSTULOSIS

There have been several reports of the occurrence of a widespread pustular purpura following an infection or occurring as an idiopathic phenomenon.[792–794] The terms 'acute generalized pustular bacterid'[792] and 'primary idiopathic cutaneous pustular vasculitis'[794] refer to the same condition. Most of these cases would now be regarded as variants of acute generalized exanthematous pustulosis (see p. 136). Accordingly, the continued use of this diagnosis is of doubtful validity.

Histopathology[792–795]

There is a large subcorneal or intraepidermal pustule overlying a massive perivascular and interstitial infiltrate of neutrophils in the upper and mid dermis. There is some exocytosis of neutrophils through the epidermis. Leukocytoclasis is variable. Vessel walls may show 'fibrinoid necrosis'. In older lesions there are perivascular collections of lymphocytes and some eosinophils in addition to the neutrophils.

BEHÇET'S DISEASE

Behçet's disease is a multisystem disorder in which the presence of recurrent aphthous ulcers in the oral cavity is an almost universal feature.[796,797] The ulcers are painful, measure 2–10 mm in diameter and heal within 7–14 days, only to recur subsequently.[798] Other characteristic signs include genital ulceration, ocular abnormalities such as uveitis, hypopyon and iridocyclitis, and cutaneous lesions.[799] Complex aphthosis (oral and genital aphthae) in the absence of other features is probably a forme fruste of Behçet's disease.[800,801] Less frequent manifestations include synovitis, neurological lesions including meningoencephalitis, and epididymitis.[799] The clinical course is variable; death may result from central nervous system involvement or arterial aneurysms.[802]

The most characteristic cutaneous lesions are erythema nodosum-like nodules on the legs,[803] superficial and/or deep thrombophlebitis, acral purpuric papulonodular lesions,[804] papulopustular lesions[796,805,806] and the development of self-healing, sterile pustules at sites of trauma ('pathergy').[807] Pathergic lesions, which may be induced by a needle prick, are commonly seen in cases reported from Turkey, but are less common in the United Kingdom.[808] Lesions resembling those seen in Sweet's syndrome have also been a presenting feature.[809,810]

Behçet's disease occurs most often in young adult males.[811] It is uncommon in children.[812,813] There are different prevalence rates in different geographical areas: the highest incidence has been reported in Japan, Korea, China and eastern Mediterranean countries.[814] A strong association with certain HLA types, particularly Bw51 and B12, has been reported.[799] Familial cases occur.[815] Juvenile onset is more likely in these familial cases.[816]

Numerous causes have been proposed and may be grouped into viral, bacterial, immunological and environmental.[799,814,817,818] An immunological basis is most favored because of the wide variety of immunological disturbances that have been identified.[819] These include the presence of circulating immune complexes,[820,821] enhanced chemotactic activity of neutrophils,[820] alteration of T-cell subsets,[822] lymphocytotoxicity to oral epithelial cells or dermal microvascular endothelial cells[823] and evidence of delayed hypersensitivity to certain streptococcal antigens.[824] The common denominator in all systems appears to be a vasculitis with early infiltration by mononuclear cells and the later presence of neutrophils in some sites.[825]

The serum interleukin-8 (IL-8) levels are a reliable marker of disease activity.[826]

Histopathology

In *aphthous ulcers* there is a variable infiltrate of lymphocytes, macrophages and neutrophils in the base of the ulcer.[822] The infiltrate is accentuated around small vessels and also extends into the epithelium at the margins of the ulcer.[824,827] Some of the intraepithelial lymphocytes appear activated with large indented nuclei.[828] Degenerating prickle cells may be present in the marginal epithelium. There is a virtual absence of plasma cells in early lesions, but these may be quite prominent in older lesions.[827]

The *erythema nodosum-like lesions* show a perivascular infiltrate of lymphocytes and other mononuclear cells in the deep dermis and the septa of the subcutaneous fat.[829] Lymphocytes may extend into vessel walls in the manner of a lymphocytic vasculitis. Endothelial cells are often enlarged and sometimes show degenerative features, particularly on ultrastructural examination.[829] Subsequently neutrophils are found in the perivascular collections and in some cases are quite numerous.[829] Kim and LeBoit believe that vasculitis is an important event in the pathogenesis of the lesions.[330] The lesions lack the histiocytic granulomas of the usual type of erythema nodosum.[799] A lobular panniculitis has also been described in lesions of Behçet's disease.[803] Polyp-like structures, composed of lipophages, have been found protruding into cavities resulting from lysis of fat cells in the lobular panniculitis of Behçet's disease.[831]

In *pathergic lesions* there is a heavy neutrophil infiltrate, without fibrinoid changes, in the vessel walls. This has been called pustular vasculitis or 'Sweet's-like vasculitis' to distinguish it from leukocytoclastic vasculitis in which fibrinoid change and leukocytoclasis are prominent features.[832] Intraepidermal pustules may occur at the point of impact of the pathergic stimulus.[833] Despite the attention given to the neutrophilic infiltration, recent detailed studies of pathergic lesions have found a significant mononuclear cell infiltrate in the dermis, around vessels and appendages and extending into the deep dermis.[834]

In some lesions of Behçet's disease the pattern is that of a tight superficial and deep perivascular infiltrate of mononuclear cells. A lymphocytic or leukocytoclastic vasculitis may be present,[835,836] leading to the suggestion that Behçet's disease should be set aside from the neutrophilic dermatoses and classified as a true vasculitis.[837] Usually a few perivascular or interstitial neutrophils will be found.[796] Skin biopsy specimens are often nonspecific.[838]

The thrombophlebitic lesions are rarely biopsied. Folliculitis, acneiform lesions,[839] dermal abscesses, polyarteritis nodosa[840] and a necrotizing vasculitis[449] have all been described in Behçet's disease.[841]

Immunofluorescence studies have shown IgM and C3 in aphthous lesions, often diffusely distributed.[824] Immunoreactants are a less constant feature in the erythema nodosum-like lesions.

ABSCESS-FORMING NEUTROPHILIC DERMATOSIS

Some patients with hematologic malignancies present with pustules and abscesses which do not clinically resemble Sweet's syndrome or pyoderma gangrenosum.[774] This group appears to represent another type of neutrophilic dermatosis.

Histopathology

There is a dense dermal infiltrate of neutrophils with the formation of dermal abscesses. There is usually subepidermal edema. Extensive leukocytoclasis is seen in older lesions.

CHRONIC LYMPHOCYTIC VASCULITIS

Lymphocytic vasculitis is not a disease sui generis, but rather a group term for a number of clinically heterogeneous diseases which on histopathological examination have evidence of a lymphocytic vasculitis; that is, there is a predominantly lymphocytic infiltrate involving and surrounding the walls of small vessels in the dermis.[842] Often there is associated endothelial cell swelling and some extravasation of erythrocytes, but nuclear dusting is uncommon. While there may be an extravasation of fibrin into vessel walls, this feature should *not* be a requirement for the diagnosis of lymphocytic vasculitis. After all, exudative phenomena are not usually a feature of chronic inflammation.

The above definition of lymphocytic vasculitis has been criticized as 'failing to provide objective criteria that would enable a pathologist to determine whether an infiltrate "involves" a vessel rather than merely exiting through it at the time that the biopsy specimen is taken'.[843] The phenomenon of 'exiting' (diapedesis) does not occur in arteries or veins, nor is it such a widespread or prominent phenomenon in smaller vessels (such as postcapillary venules) that it is likely to be mistaken for lymphocytic vasculitis. If the criteria are made too rigid and problems associated with sampling and evolution of the disease not acknowledged, then lymphocytic vasculitis becomes a rare diagnosis and 'lymphocytic perivasculitis' and 'perivascular dermatitides' assume an importance they do not deserve. The article referred to above defined cutaneous lymphocytic vasculitis as '...requiring the presence of either acute or chronic damage to the walls of small vessels (e.g. fibrin deposition, lamination by pericytes). In the case of muscular vessels, the presence of lymphocytes within the vessel wall is sufficient, because diapedesis of lymphocytes does not occur in arteries or veins.'[843] In the authors' view, the pigmented purpuric dermatoses did not meet these criteria, yet atrophie blanche and Sneddon's syndrome did.[843]

Kossard has defined three forms of lymphocytic vasculitis: an *angiodestructive form* seen in association with Behçet's disease, acute lupus erythematosus, lupus panniculitis, late stages of acute vasculitis and in cases that may clinically mimic acute vasculitis with palpable purpura; *lichenoid lymphocytic vasculitis*, as defined below; and *lymphocytic endovasculitis* in which there is intimal hyperplasia with vessel wall mucinosis or segmental hyalinosis and a variable lymphocytic infiltrate.[844] Kossard states that these three major patterns are not mutually exclusive.[844]

The following clinical conditions may be regarded as lymphocytic vasculitides:

- toxic erythema
- collagen vascular disease

- PUPPP (polymorphic eruption of pregnancy)
- prurigo of pregnancy
- gyrate and annular erythemas
- pityriasis lichenoides
- pigmented purpuric dermatoses
- malignant atrophic papulosis (Degos)
- perniosis
- rickettsial and viral infections
- pyoderma gangrenosum
- polymorphous light eruption (one variant)
- TRAPS
- sclerosing lymphangitis of the penis
- leukemic vasculitis.

Sneddon's syndrome could also be included but it has been discussed earlier in this chapter (see p. 226). It should be noted at the outset that the inclusion of several of these entities is controversial; this will be considered further in the discussion that follows. A lymphocytic vasculitis has also been reported in the toxic shock syndrome, which results from a toxin produced by *Staphylococcus aureus*,[845] but it is not an invariable finding in this condition. Some drugs, such as aspirin, acetaminophen (paracetamol, Panadol), lipid-lowering agents and herbal medicines, may give this pattern. A localized lymphocytic vasculitis has been reported at the site of injection of etanercept.[846] It may also occur in connective tissue diseases.[847] Behçet's syndrome can also be included as a lymphocytic vasculitis.

Lymphocytic vasculitis is a rare manifestation of leukemia.[848] More common is leukemic vasculitis, a manifestation of leukemia cutis in which atypical blast cells, rather than inflammatory cells, infiltrate vessel walls.

Lichenoid lymphocytic vasculitis (Fig. 8.17) is a specific variant of lymphocytic vasculitis, characterized by the additional feature of a lichenoid tissue reaction (interface dermatitis), often mild. It is seen as a disordered cellular immune reaction to some viruses and putative viruses and in some drug reactions. Pityriasis lichenoides, some cases of erythema multiforme and variants of Gianotti–Crosti syndrome may have this histological pattern. Combinations of an interface dermatitis, several patterns of vasculitis and a diffuse histiocytic infiltrate have been reported by Magro and Crowson as a 'superantigen ID reaction' associated with various microbial pathogens.[849] The author does not recall ever seeing such a pattern.

TOXIC ERYTHEMA

Toxic erythema is a poorly defined clinical entity in which there is a macular or blotchy erythema, sometimes with a small purpuric component. It is usually present on the trunk and proximal extremities. The histopathological term 'lymphocytic vasculitis' is sometimes given clinical connotations and used in place of toxic erythema: this should be avoided because the histological picture that this term describes is common to several clinically distinct conditions.

Toxic erythema may result from the ingestion of various drugs, including antibiotics, oral contraceptives,[850] aspirin and, rarely, acetaminophen (paracetamol), as well as various preservatives and dyes added to foods.[851] Viral infections are sometimes implicated. On many occasions the etiology of toxic erythema is unknown or at best presumptive.

Histopathology
The appearances are those of a lymphocytic vasculitis, as described above (Fig. 8.18). A small amount of nuclear dust is sometimes present, although fibrin extravasation is quite uncommon.

COLLAGEN VASCULAR DISEASE

The term 'collagen vascular disease' is still widely used for a group of related diseases in which the skin, soft tissues, muscles, joints and various other organs may be involved. Sometimes, the clinical features do not fulfil the criteria for the diagnosis of a named disease such as lupus erythematosus, rheumatoid arthritis or dermatomyositis. Cutaneous manifestations are variable and may be intermittent. There may be widespread erythematous lesions resembling toxic erythema (see above).

Histopathology
There is a lymphocytic vasculitis that usually involves both the superficial and deep plexuses (Fig. 8.19). There is sometimes mild fibrin extravasation in scattered vessels. In recurrent lesions and those of long duration, mild thickening of the walls of venules and capillaries, indicative of previous fibrin extravasation, may be seen.

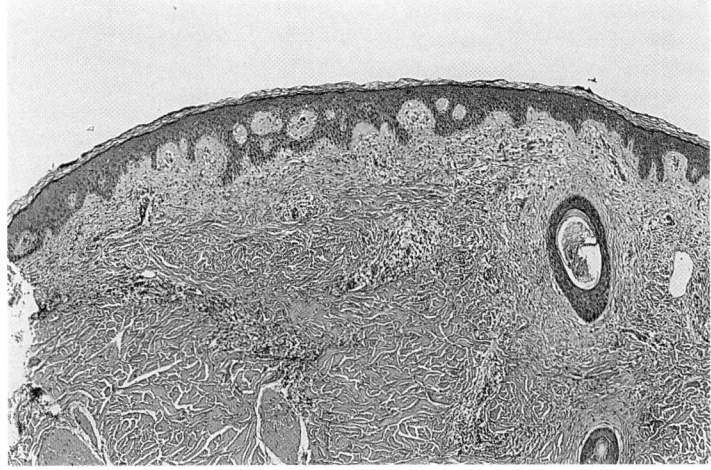
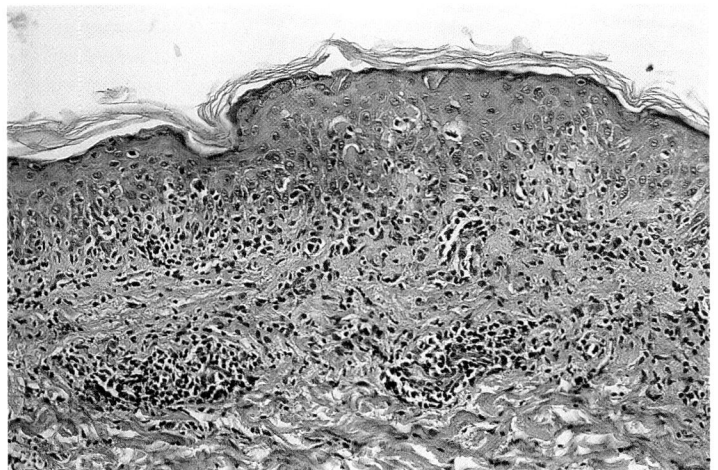

Fig. 8.17 **(A) Lichenoid lymphocytic vasculitis. (B)** There are prominent interface changes. This patient had a persistent dermatosis following a viral-ike illness. It did not resemble any named dermatosis. (H & E)

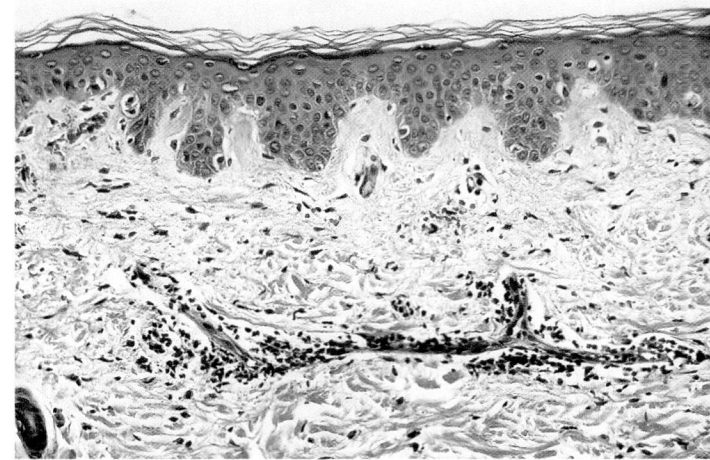

Fig. 8.18 **Toxic erythema with a lymphocytic vasculitis.** There is no fibrin in vessel walls. Fibrin is often absent in the lymphocytic vasculitides. (H & E)

PRURITIC URTICARIAL PAPULES AND PLAQUES OF PREGNANCY (PUPPP)

PUPPP (polymorphic eruption of pregnancy),[852–859] which occurs in approximately one in 200 pregnancies, has other synonyms, such as toxic erythema of pregnancy[860] and late onset prurigo of pregnancy.[861,862] PUPPP is the usual designation in the United States, while PEP (polymorphic eruption of pregnancy) is used in Europe and the United Kingdom.[863] It presents as an intensely pruritic eruption of papules and urticarial plaques, sometimes studded with small vesicles. The lesions develop in and around the abdominal striae in the last few weeks of pregnancy.[860,864] Subsequently they may become widespread on the trunk and limbs, but in contrast to pemphigoid gestationis (herpes gestationis) there is usually sparing of the periumbilical region.[860] The rash usually resolves spontaneously or with delivery.[865] There are no adverse effects on fetal outcome.[866] Only occasionally does it recur in subsequent pregnancies.[854] Recurrence of similar lesions much later in life has been reported in one patient.[867] The finding of increased maternal weight gain, increased neonatal birth weight (not always) and increased twin and triplet rate suggests that abdominal distension or a reaction to it may play a role in the development of this condition.[868–875] The occurrence of familial cases (in which sisters were married to brothers of another family) raises the possibility of a paternal influence such as a circulating paternal factor.[876]

One large study gives some perspective to the relative incidence of the various pruritic lesions of pregnancy.[877] Fifty-one cases were identified in 3192 pregnancies. Of these, 2 cases were herpes gestationis, 17 were pruritus gravidarum (pruritus with normal skin, apart from excoriations), 15 were PUPPP, 7 were prurigo of pregnancy (of Besnier), one was pruritic folliculitis of pregnancy, 2 were intercurrent disease (scabies and exfoliative dermatitis), and 7 were not diagnosed.[877]

Histopathology[860]

There is a lymphocytic vasculitis with a varying admixture of eosinophils and variable edema of the papillary dermis.[862] The infiltrate may only involve the superficial plexus, although at other times it extends to a deeper level. A variant with interstitial eosinophils, resembling an arthropod bite reaction, is sometimes seen. However, this variant differs from a bite reaction by the absence of a wedge-shaped infiltrate and no deep extension of the infiltrate. There is sometimes perivascular edema in the dermis. Nuclear dust has been present in a few cases,[878] but there is no fibrin extravasation. Epidermal

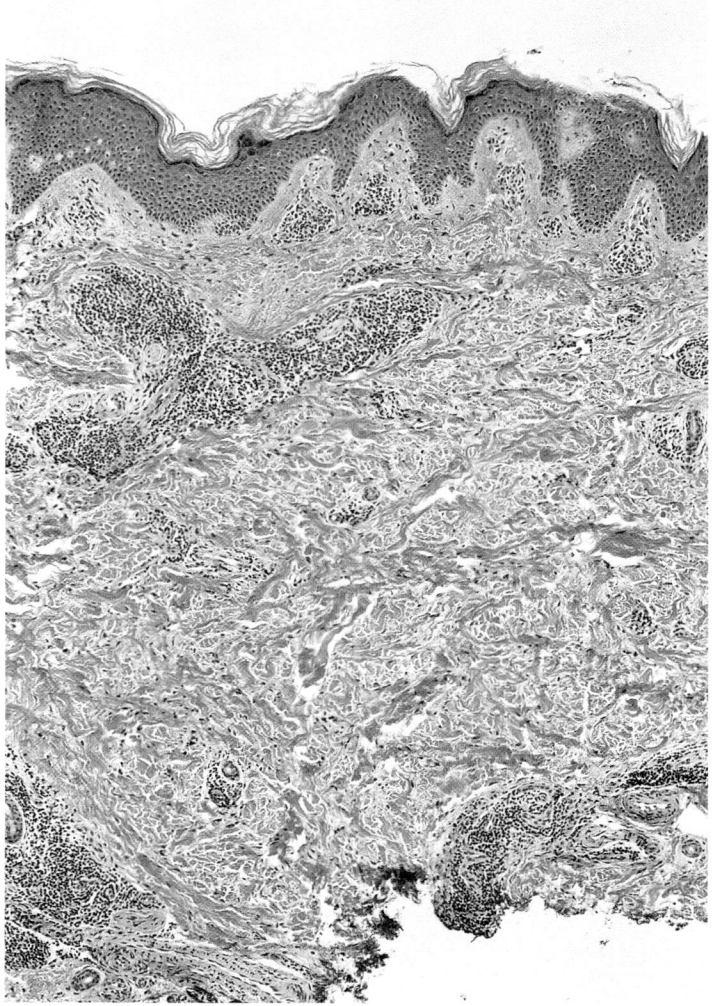

Fig. 8.19 **Collagen vascular disease.** The patient had arthralgia, mild muscle weakness and an erythematous maculopapular eruption. (H & E)

changes are present in about one-third of cases and include focal spongiosis and parakeratosis (Fig. 8.20).[879] Exocytosis of inflammatory cells is sometimes present.

Immunofluorescence studies are usually negative, in contrast to the finding of C3 in the basement membrane zone in pemphigoid gestationis.[852] However, nonspecific immunoreactants may be found in dermal blood vessels and near the dermoepidermal junction.[880] A possible subset, with circulating IgM antibodies to the basement membrane zone, has been suggested;[881] a subsequent study has shown that normal pregnancy may be associated with low levels of IgM autoreactivity against epidermal proteins.[882]

PRURIGO OF PREGNANCY

The term 'prurigo of pregnancy' has been proposed for another pruritic eruption of pregnancy characterized by widely scattered acral papules, usually arising earlier in pregnancy than toxic erythema.[883–885] The onset in one study was at 22 (±9) weeks of gestation.[877] It is possibly a heterogeneous entity that includes prurigo gestationis of Besnier, early onset prurigo of Nurse,[861] pruritic papules of pregnancy[886] and papular dermatitis of pregnancy.[879] It has been suggested recently that many cases of prurigo of pregnancy may in fact have been cases of 'eczema', which appears to be increased in pregnancy.[866]

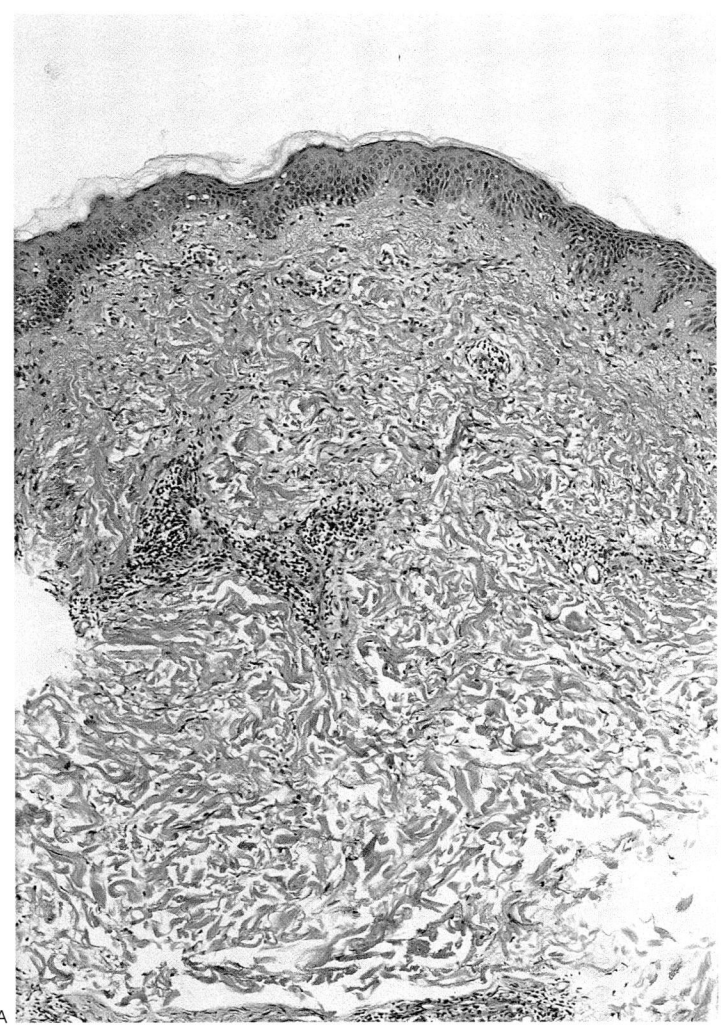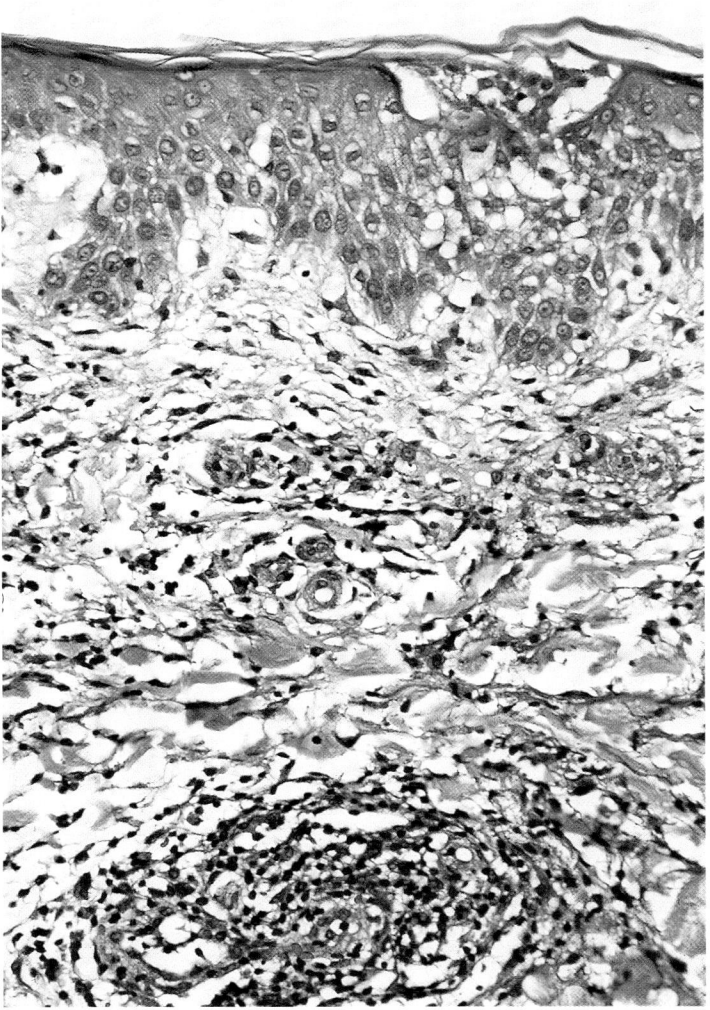

Fig. 8.20 **(A) PUPPP (B)** Focal spongiosis overlies a lymphocytic vasculitis. (H & E)

Histopathology

There are few descriptions of the histopathological changes. A lymphocytic vasculitis similar to that of toxic erythema of pregnancy is present, with the additional features of focal parakeratosis, acanthosis and sometimes excoriations.[886] In some cases the infiltrate is only loosely arranged around vessels and there is then no evidence of vasculitis.[877]

GYRATE AND ANNULAR ERYTHEMAS

The gyrate and annular erythemas are a heterogeneous group of dermatoses which are akin to toxic erythema[887] in having a tight perivascular lymphohistiocytic infiltrate, which at times involves the vessel walls in the manner of a lymphocytic vasculitis. Clinically, there are one or more circinate, arcuate or polycyclic lesions which may be fixed or migratory.[887–889] The term 'palpable migratory arciform erythema' has been used for the variant with arcuate lesions.[890]

Histopathologically, the gyrate and annular erythemas have been divided on the basis of the distribution of the perivascular infiltrate into a superficial type and a deep type.[891] The superficial erythemas are usually accompanied by slight spongiosis and focal parakeratosis, which corresponds to the peripheral scale noted clinically; in the deep type there is no spongiosis or parakeratosis and clinically the lesions have a firm cord-like border but no scale. Both types have been included within the entity known as erythema annulare centrifugum, suggesting that it is a heterogeneous entity.[892] The various clinical forms of gyrate and annular erythema fall into one or other of these pathological groups.

The following conditions will be considered:

- erythema annulare centrifugum
- erythema gyratum repens
- erythema marginatum
- annular erythemas of infancy
- erythema chronicum migrans.

Erythema annulare centrifugum

Erythema annulare centrifugum is characterized by the presence of one or more annular, erythematous lesions which may spread outwards or remain stationary.[887,888] A fine scale is sometimes present inside the advancing edge. The lesions may be pruritic. They are found most commonly on the trunk and proximal parts of the limbs.

A variety of agents have been implicated in the etiology of erythema annulare centrifugum, but in a significant number of cases no etiological agent can be found.[888] The condition has been associated with infections by bacteria,[893] rickettsia,[894] viruses[895] and fungi and with infestation by parasites.[896] Malignant tumors,[897,898] foods[888] and drugs[899] have also been blamed. The drugs have included penicillin, cimetidine,[900] gold,[901] salicylates, thiazides,[902] estrogen-progesterone in oil and antimalarials.[903] The recurrent annular erythema which is occasionally seen in patients with anti-Ro/SSA antibodies, in association with systemic lupus erythematosus or with Sjögren's syndrome, has a wide, elevated border.[904-910] Other immunological associations of this variant of annular erythema have been reported.[911]

The pathogenetic mechanism is unknown; a hypersensitivity reaction to one or other of the agents mentioned above has been suggested.[902]

Histopathology[888,892]

As mentioned above, two distinct patterns – a superficial type and a deep type – may be found. In the superficial variant there is a moderately dense infiltrate of lymphocytes, histiocytes and, rarely, eosinophils around vessels of the superficial vascular plexus. The infiltrate is well demarcated and has a 'coat-sleeve' distribution. Cells may extend into the walls of the small vessels, but there is never any fibrin extravasation. There may be slight edema of the papillary dermis. At the advancing edge there is slight spongiosis and focal parakeratosis. In some cases, the appearances are indistinguishable from pityriasis rosea.

In the deep type a similar infiltrate involves both the superficial and deep vascular plexuses. The epidermis is normal.

Erythema gyratum repens

Erythema gyratum repens is rare and is the most distinctive of the gyrate erythemas.[888,889,912] There are broad erythematous bands arranged in an arcuate or polycyclic pattern, often accompanied by a trailing scale and likened to wood grain or marble.[913] The eruption, which is often pruritic, may migrate up to 1 cm per day. It is usually confined to the trunk and proximal parts of the limbs; the face is not affected.[887]

Erythema gyratum repens is usually associated with an internal cancer, particularly of pulmonary origin.[914,915] It has been reported in association with pulmonary tuberculosis,[916] ichthyosis[917] and in the resolving stage of pityriasis rubra pilaris.[918] It also occurs in otherwise healthy individuals.[919,920]

It has been suggested that lymphokines produced by the tumor, such as epidermal growth factor, may play a role in the pathogenesis.[915]

Histopathology[888]

There is usually mild spongiosis with focal parakeratosis and mild to moderate acanthosis. A sparse to moderately heavy lymphohistiocytic infiltrate is present around vessels of the superficial plexus, often associated with mild edema of the papillary dermis. Sometimes the infiltrate includes variable numbers of eosinophils. Its extension to involve the deep vascular plexus has also been reported.[892] Unusual accumulations of Langerhans cells were present in the upper epidermis in one case.[921]

Direct immunofluorescence often reveals the presence of granular deposits of IgG and/or C3 along the basement membrane zone, usually in a less regular pattern than occurs in bullous pemphigoid.[922] The deposits are beneath the lamina densa.[915]

Erythema marginatum

Erythema marginatum is a diagnostic manifestation of rheumatic fever, seen in less than 10% of cases.[923] It may develop at any time during the course of the disease and is more likely to occur in children than in adults. The annular eruption is macular or slightly raised, with a pink or red border and a paler center.[924] Lesions are asymptomatic, transient and migratory.

Histopathology[923,924]

Erythema marginatum is included here because of its clinical appearances. The histopathological changes are not usually those of a lymphocytic vasculitis.[925] Rather, there is a perivascular infiltrate in the upper dermis which includes many neutrophils in addition to a few lymphocytes and eosinophils. It is often said that there is no vasculitis, although mild leukocytoclasis was noted in earlier accounts of the disease.

Annular erythemas of infancy

The term 'annular erythemas of infancy' refers to a rare, heterogeneous group of non-pruritic, annular erythemas reported under various titles, including familial annular erythema,[926] annular erythema of infancy,[927,928] persistent annular erythema of infancy,[929,930] erythema gyratum atrophicans transiens neonatale[931] and infantile epidermodysplastic erythema gyratum.[932] Clinical differences exist between all these entities. Several cases have been associated with maternal lupus erythematosus.[933] A hypersensitivity response to unrecognized antigens is suspected.[934] Intestinal colonization with *Candida albicans* has been incriminated.[930]

Histopathology

Most annular erythemas of infancy show a superficial and deep lymphohistiocytic infiltrate in a perivascular distribution, as seen in the so-called 'deep gyrate erythemas'.[929] They differ by the presence usually of eosinophils and sometimes of neutrophils in the infiltrate. Occasional interstitial eosinophils, resembling the pattern of an arthropod bite reaction, are sometimes present. Epidermal atrophy was present in one variant,[931] while bowenoid features were recorded in the epidermis in another.[932]

Erythema chronicum migrans

Erythema chronicum migrans, caused by *Borrelia burgdorferi*, has been discussed in detail with the spirochetal infections (see p. 654). The histopathological changes are those of a deep gyrate erythema.

PITYRIASIS LICHENOIDES

Pityriasis lichenoides is an uncommon, self-limiting dermatosis of disputed histogenesis with a spectrum of clinical changes. At one end is a relatively acute disorder with hemorrhagic papules which resolve to leave varioliform scars – pityriasis lichenoides et varioliformis acuta (PLEVA); at the other end of the spectrum is a less severe disease with small, scaly, red-brown maculopapules, known as pityriasis lichenoides chronica.[935,936] The distinction between the acute and chronic forms is not always clearcut.[936,937] Pityriasis lichenoides may develop at all ages, but there is a predilection for males in the second and third decades of life. Lesions, which vary in number from 20 or so to several hundred, are most common on the anterior aspect of the trunk and the flexor surfaces of the proximal parts of the extremities. In a review of 22 pediatric cases of pityriasis lichenoides, 72% were of the chronic type.[938] No cases in this study or another large series[939] progressed to lymphoma although occasional cases of this complication have been recorded.[940] Monoclonal populations of T cells can be found in both the acute and chronic variants in a significant number of cases (see below).[941,942]

PLEVA

The acute form of pityriasis lichenoides (sometimes called Mucha–Habermann disease) is a papular eruption in which the lesions may become hemorrhagic or crusted before healing to leave a superficial varioliform scar. The lesions appear in crops which heal in several weeks; new lesions may continue to appear for many months or even years, with varying periods of remission. A severe form with ulceronecrotic lesions and constitutional symptoms has been described.[943–946] Fortunately it is quite rare. PLEVA has been reported in patients with HIV infection.[947]

Pityriasis lichenoides chronica

The chronic form is more scaly and less hemorrhagic and consists of red-brown inflammatory papules and macules with a characteristic, centrally adherent, 'mica' scale which is easily detached. Postinflammatory hypopigmentation is quite common in dark-skinned individuals.[948] Rare presentations have included an acral and a segmental type.[949,950]

The pathogenesis of pityriasis lichenoides is unknown: cell-mediated immune mechanisms, possibly related to viral[951,952] or other infections,[953–955] may be important.[956] It is usually regarded as a lymphocytic vasculitis. Its relationship to lymphomatoid papulosis is controversial. The favored view is that the two diseases are pathogenetically distinct,[957] although both are part of the spectrum of clonal T-cell lymphoproliferative disorders.[941,958]

Histopathology[957,959]

Pityriasis lichenoides is essentially a lymphocytic vasculitis in which the associated inflammatory cell infiltrate shows exocytosis into the epidermis with obscuring of the dermoepidermal interface.[960] There is variable death of epidermal keratinocytes which may involve scattered single cells or sheets of cells, resulting in confluent necrosis of the epidermis.[961] Some of the keratinocytes undergo apoptosis. The inflammatory infiltrate and the degree of epidermal changes are more prominent in PLEVA than in pityriasis lichenoides chronica. Cases anywhere along this spectrum can occur. In summary, both are lichenoid (interface) dermatitides with lymphocytic vasculitis (lichenoid lymphocytic vasculitis).

In *PLEVA* there is a sharply delimited, sparse to moderately dense inflammatory cell infiltrate involving the superficial vascular plexus. Sometimes this extends in a wedge-shaped pattern to involve the lower dermis also. The infiltrate is composed of lymphocytes and some macrophages; in florid cases there may be some perivascular neutrophils as well and even a leukocytoclastic vasculitis.[945] A few atypical lymphoid cells may be found in a small number of cases. There is endothelial swelling involving small vessels and extravasation of red blood cells. Only occasionally do the vessels show 'fibrinoid necrosis'. The papillary dermis is variably edematous.

Lymphocytes and some erythrocytes extend into the epidermis (Fig. 8.21). This is associated with some basal vacuolar change and spongiosis.[959] Degenerate keratinocytes are not restricted to the basal layer and they are often more prominent in the upper layers of the epidermis. In advanced lesions there is often extensive epidermal necrosis. Overlying parakeratosis is quite common and there may be some neutrophils forming a parakeratotic crust.

In *pityriasis lichenoides chronica*[962] the infiltrate is less dense and more superficial than in PLEVA and the epidermal changes are much less pronounced.[963] There is a relatively sparse perivascular infiltrate with only subtle features of a lymphocytic vasculitis. A few extravasated erythrocytes may be present. There are small areas of basal vacuolar change associated with minimal exocytosis of lymphocytes and occasional degenerate keratinocytes.

The epidermis shows variable acanthosis and is sometimes vaguely psoriasiform. Pallor of the upper epidermis may be noted, with overlying parakeratosis. Late lesions may show mild fibrosis of the papillary dermis and the presence of some melanophages, changes which are also found in late lesions of PLEVA.

Immunofluorescence reveals the presence of immunoreactants, particularly IgM and C3, along the basement membrane zone and in vessels of the papillary dermis in a small number of cases.[964] Immunoperoxidase studies have shown that the lymphocytes in the dermal infiltrate are T cells, particularly of the cytotoxic/suppressor (CD8) type in PLEVA, although CD4+ cells appear to predominate in the chronic form.[941] Approximately 5% of the perivascular cells are Langerhans or indeterminate cells.[956] Cases with CD30+ cells have been reported.[965] The epidermis in the lesions is HLA-DR positive.[963]

PIGMENTED PURPURIC DERMATOSES

The pigmented purpuric dermatoses (PPD) are a group of chronic skin disorders with overlapping clinical and histopathological features.[966–968] The lesions are purpuric, with variable pigmentation resulting from the deposition of hemosiderin, which is, in turn, a consequence of the extravasation of red blood cells from capillaries in the papillary dermis. There is a predilection for the lower extremities of young adults but cases have also been reported in children.[969] Six clinical variants have been recognized. Some cases defy classification into one of these groups, such as the unilateral linear cases first reported some years ago.[970,971]

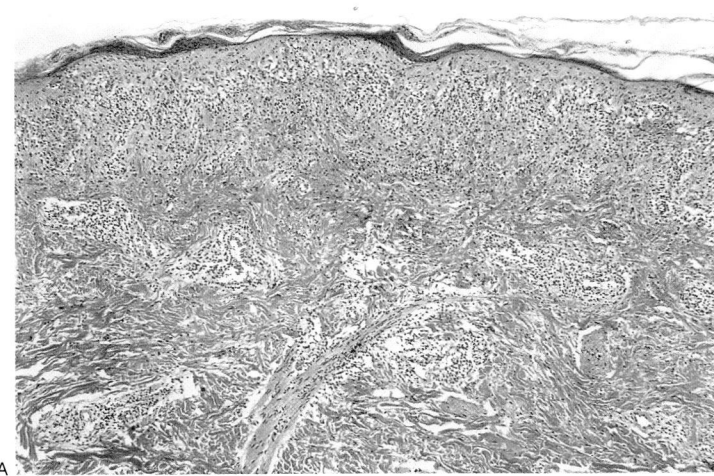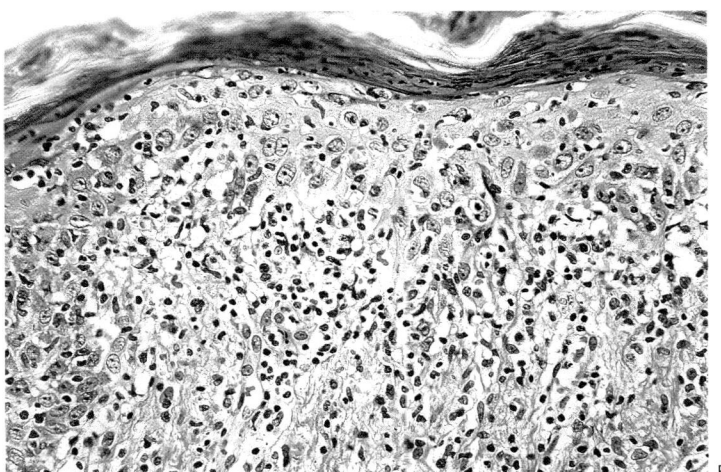

Fig. 8.21 **(A) Pityriasis lichenoides. (B)** In this acute variant there is a lichenoid reaction pattern with 'interface obscuring'. (H & E)

Progressive pigmentary dermatosis (Schamberg's disease)

Progressive pigmentary dermatosis is the most common type.[968] There are numerous punctate purpuric macules forming confluent patches. These are usually symmetrically distributed in the pretibial region. Familial cases[972,973] and a unilateral distribution have been described.[974,975] The eczematid-like purpura of Doucas and Kapetanakis,[976] the itching purpura of Loewenthal[977] and disseminated pruriginous angiodermatitis[978] are now regarded as variants of Schamberg's disease. These pruritic forms usually have an acute onset and a self-limited course.

Purpura annularis telangiectodes of Majocchi

There are annular patches with perifollicular, red punctate lesions and telangiectasias.[967] A familial case has been reported.[979]

Pigmented purpuric lichenoid dermatosis of Gougerot and Blum

Pigmented purpuric lichenoid dermatosis of Gougerot and Blum consists of lichenoid papules which may coalesce to give plaque-like lesions. They are often symmetrically distributed on the lower legs.[967] If unilateral, the plaque may mimic Kaposi's sarcoma.[980] Hepatitis C infection is a rare association.[981]

Lichen aureus

Lichen aureus is closely related to the Gougerot and Blum variant (see above). There are grouped macules or lichenoid papules having a rusty, golden or even purplish color.[982,983] Lesions may occur on the trunk or upper extremity, although the lower parts of the legs are the site of predilection.[984,985] Involvement of the glans penis has been reported.[986] Lichen aureus is usually unilateral.[983,987] Slow, spontaneous resolution occurs over a period ranging from 1 to 12 years.[969]

Purpuric contact dermatitis

Purpuric contact dermatitis is not well known. It is a form of allergic contact dermatitis to textile dyes and resins in personal clothing.[988] Sometimes an impressive pattern of purpura and hemosiderotic pigmentation will occur in the distribution of clothing. The dyes Disperse Blue and Disperse Red have been incriminated on many occasions.[988,989]

PPD/mycosis fungoides overlap

There appears to be a relationship between some cases of persistent PPD and mycosis fungoides. LeBoit[990] summarized the dilemma in the title of a paper in 1997 – 'simulant, precursor, or both?'. His group reported patients with a PPD that presented clinically as mycosis fungoides as well as patients who had features of both conditions.[990] Clonal populations of lymphocytes were present in 8 of 12 specimens that were typical of the lichenoid patterns of PPD.[990] Others have reported cases of mycosis fungoides that presented clinically as PPD.[991,992] Crowson and colleagues found that several classes of drugs, including calcium channel blockers, ACE inhibitors, lipid-lowering agents, β-blockers, antihistamines, antidepressants and analgesics could produce a histologically atypical pigmentary purpura (including clonality in two cases) which resolved on cessation of the drug.[992]

Three different pathogenetic mechanisms have been proposed for the PPDs.[993] They include disturbed humoral immunity, cellular immune reactions (delayed hypersensitivity) related to the dermal infiltrate of lymphocytes, macrophages and Langerhans cells,[993,994] and weakness of blood vessels with increased capillary fragility.[995] Perforator vein incompetence was present in one series of cases of lichen aureus.[996] There is increased expression of cellular adhesion molecules in lesional skin; a similar pattern can be seen in delayed hypersensitivity reactions.[997,998] There are isolated reports implicating sensitivity to oils used in wool processing, exposure to dyes (see above)[999]

and treatment with thiamine,[999] carbromal, meprobamate, diuretics, ampicillin, non-steroidal anti-inflammatory drugs,[968] acetaminophen (paracetamol),[1000] herbal remedies, glipizide,[1001] and medroxyprogesterone acetate.[1002] Other drug classes have been incriminated in producing so-called 'atypical pigmentary purpura' (see above).

Bioflavonoids and ascorbic acid, both of which increase capillary resistance, have been shown to have a beneficial effect.[1003]

Histopathology

There is a variable infiltrate of lymphocytes and macrophages in the upper dermis. This is band-like and heavy in lichen aureus, and less dense and with perivascular accentuation in the other variants (Figs 8.22, 8.23). A lymphocytic vasculitis involving vessels in the papillary dermis is often present in active cases (Fig. 8.24). Some authors do not accept this condition as a lymphocytic vasculitis, because of the absence of fibrin.[968] However, fibrin is not a prerequisite for the diagnosis of chronic inflammation in other organ systems. The infiltrate is composed predominantly of T lymphocytes, a majority of which are CD4[+], admixed with some reactive CD1a[+] dendritic cells.[993,998,1004] Plasma cells are sometimes present in lichen aureus, while a

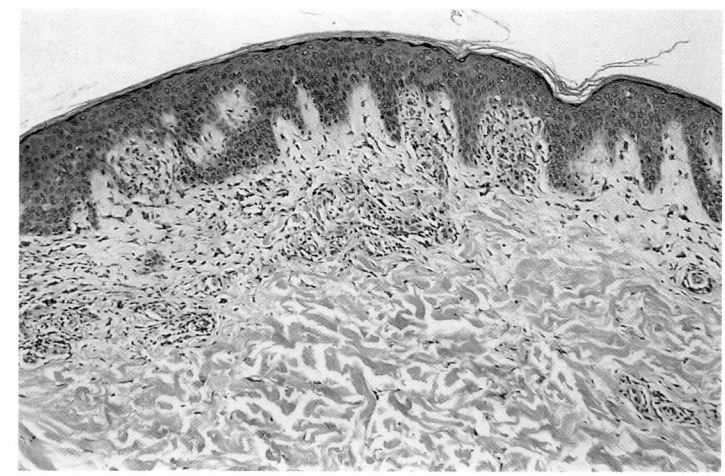

Fig. 8.22 **Pigmented purpuric dermatosis.** This condition is characterized by an infiltrate which fills the papillary dermis. Tight lymphocytic cuffing of vessels in the papillary dermis is often present. (H & E)

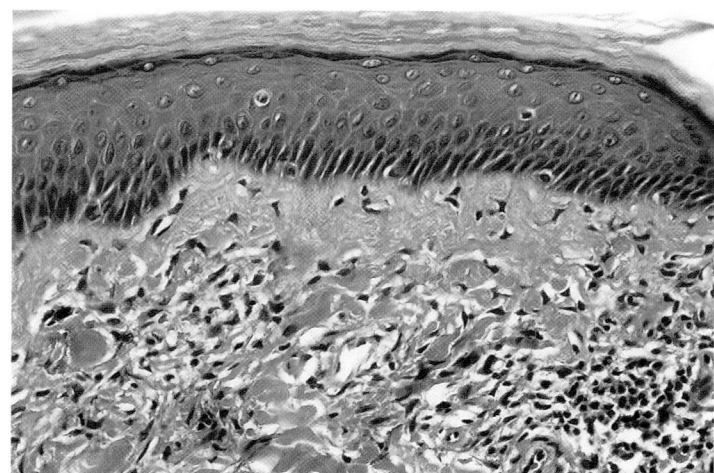

Fig. 8.23 **Pigmented purpuric dermatosis.** The infiltrate is less heavy in this case. Hemosiderin pigment can just be discerned. (H & E)

few neutrophils are usually seen in the infiltrate in the lesions of itching purpura (Fig. 8.25). There is often exocytosis of lymphocytes and associated spongiosis of the epidermis in all variants except lichen aureus; in the latter a thin layer of uninvolved collagen separates the undersurface of the epidermis from the inflammatory infiltrate below.[1005] When spongiosis is present, there is often focal parakeratosis as well.

There is variable extravasation of red blood cells into the papillary dermis. Hemosiderin is present, predominantly in macrophages, although small amounts are sometimes found lying free in the papillary dermis and even in the epidermis. Sometimes the macrophages containing the hemosiderin are at or below the lower margin of the inflammatory infiltrate, but the hemosiderin is never as deep in the dermis as in stasis dermatitis.[966] Hemosiderin is usually absent in early lesions of itching purpura. Blood vessels in the papillary dermis may be dilated, but more often there is endothelial swelling causing luminal narrowing. Occasionally, there is hyaline thickening of blood vessel walls or pericapillary fibrosis.

The histological overlap between mycosis fungoides and PPDs, particularly those with lichenoid features, is well known. Both are part of the LUMP mnemonic that lists diseases with infiltrates filling the papillary dermis — lichenoid disease, urticaria pigmentosa, mycosis fungoides and precursors, and the pigmented purpuric dermatoses. Features favoring PPD in these overlap cases and simulants include lack of atypia and papillary dermal fibrosis and the presence of mild edema in the papillary dermis. Both can show epidermotropism but in mycosis fungoides this usually extends higher than the basal layer of cells.[990] Furthermore in mycosis fungoides the intraepidermal lymphocytes appear more atypical than the dermal-based ones.[992] In some cases, a diagnosis of mycosis fungoides/PPD overlap is the best that can be given in our current state of knowledge (Fig. 8.26).

Immunofluorescence studies have usually been negative, except for the presence of perivascular fibrin. In one study C3, and sometimes immunoglobulins, were present in vessel walls.[1006]

Electron microscopy

Ultrastructural studies have not contributed in any way to our understanding of these dermatoses.[1007] Langerhans cells have been identified in the inflammatory infiltrate.

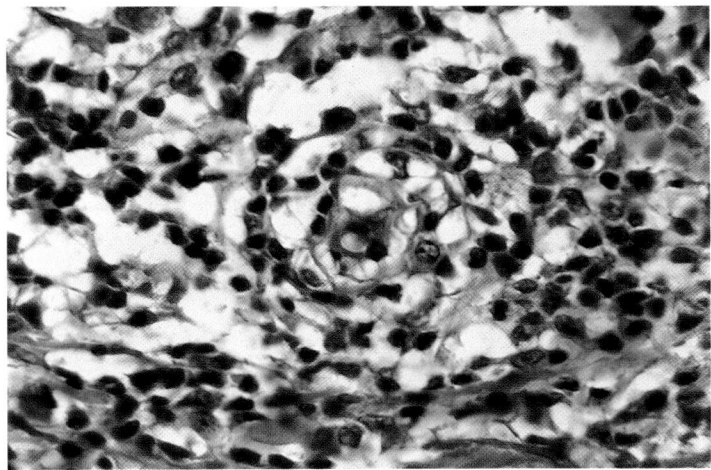

Fig. 8.24 **Pigmented purpuric dermatosis.** A lymphocytic vasculitis is present. It is not always as obvious as in this case. (H & E)

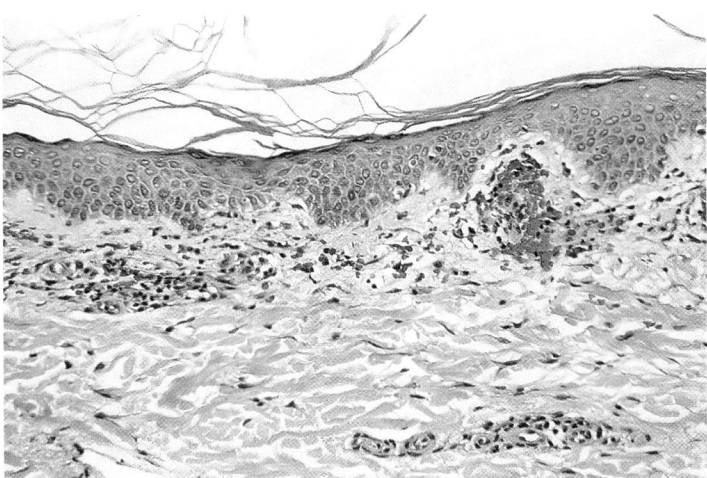

Fig. 8.25 **Itching purpura.** There is extravasation of erythrocytes and mild cuffing of small vessels in the papillary dermis by lymphocytes. (H & E)

MALIGNANT ATROPHIC PAPULOSIS

Malignant atrophic papulosis (Degos' disease) is a rare, often fatal, multi-system disorder in which pathognomonic skin lesions are frequently associated with infarctive lesions of other viscera, particularly the gastrointestinal tract.[1008,1009] Patients develop crops of papules, approximately 0.5–1 cm in diameter, which evolve slowly to become umbilicated with a porcelain white center and a telangiectatic rim and finally leave an atrophic scar.[1010] There are approximately 10–40 lesions at any time, in different stages of evolution. Penile ulceration was the mode of presentation in one case.[1011] In 60% of cases, gastrointestinal involvement supervenes, usually within a year but sometimes after a long interval.[1009] Some patients have only cutaneous lesions and a relatively benign course.[1012–1015] Involvement of the central nervous system may also occur;[1016] less commonly, other viscera also develop infarcts.[1017] There are several reports of familial involvement,[1018–020] including one in which the mother and five children were affected.[1021] It has been reported in a patient with AIDS.[1022]

Malignant atrophic papulosis has been regarded as an 'endovasculitis' or primary endothelial defect,[1023] with secondary thrombosis leading to infarctive lesions.[1024] Impaired fibrinolytic activity and alterations in platelet function have been detected,[1025,1026] but there are no circulating immune complexes[1023] or antiendothelial cell antibodies. Anticardiolipin antibodies were present in one case.[1027] Most authors agree that the condition is not a vasculitis in the sense that allergic vasculitis and polyarteritis nodosa are;[1023] however, a study of ultrathin sections led to the conclusion that it is a lymphocyte-mediated necrotizing vasculitis.[1028] Malignant atrophic papulosis has also been regarded as a mucinosis (see p. 414)[1008] but the deposition of mucin is only a secondary phenomenon.

Histopathology[1009,1028]

A well-developed lesion shows epidermal atrophy with overlying hyperkeratosis and an underlying wedge-shaped area of cutaneous ischemia, the apex of which extends into the deep dermis (Fig. 8.27). This dermal area is uniformly hypereosinophilic and relatively acellular. A mild to moderately dense lymphocytic infiltrate is present at the edge of the ischemic wedge, particularly in the mid and lower dermis.[1012,1028] The infiltrate has a perivenular and intervenular distribution. There is marked endothelial swelling of venules and, to a lesser extent, arterioles, sometimes with obliteration of the lumen. There are fibrin-platelet thrombi in some small vessels and there is some perivenular distribution of fibrin in the dermis.[1028] A study using thin

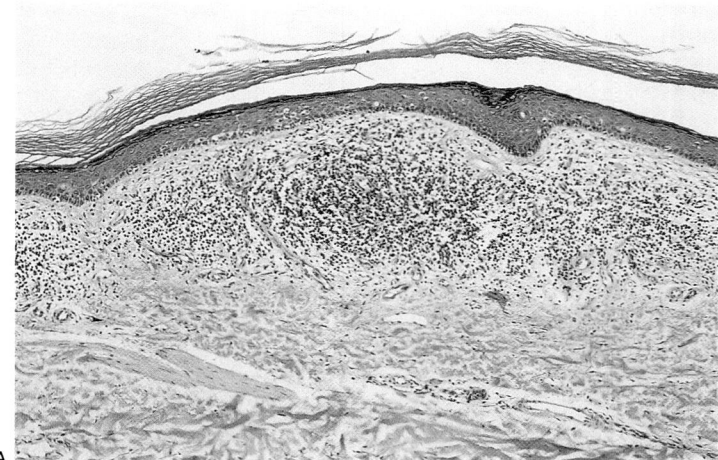

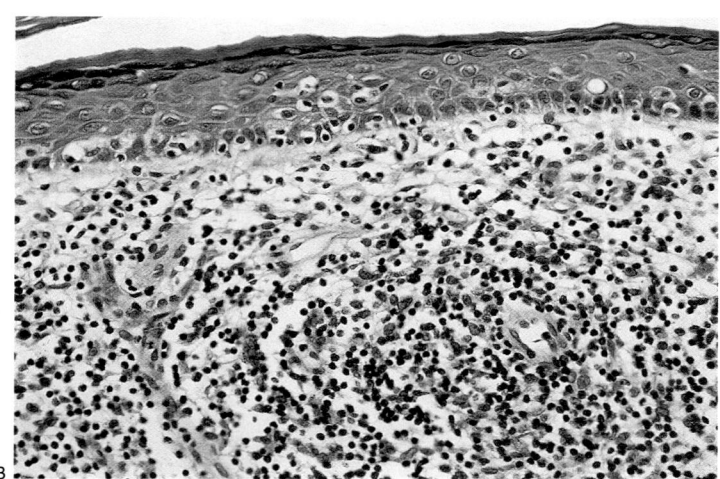

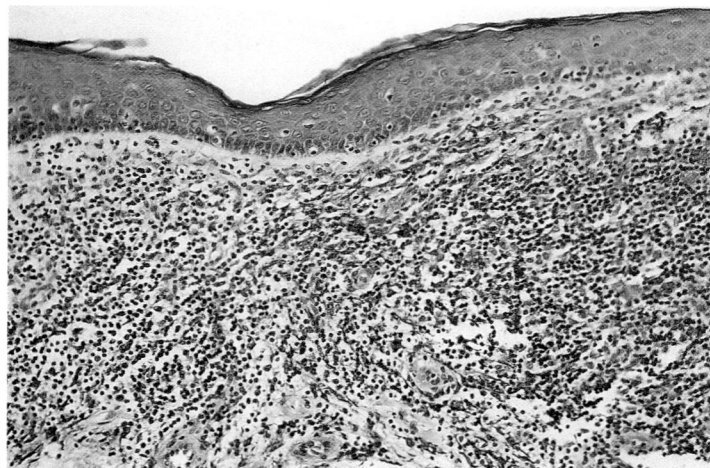

Fig. 8.26 **(A) Mycosis fungoides/pigmented purpuric dermatosis overlap.**
(B) Epidermotropism is quite marked (H & E). **(C)** The same case showing abundant hemosiderin pigment. (Perls stain)

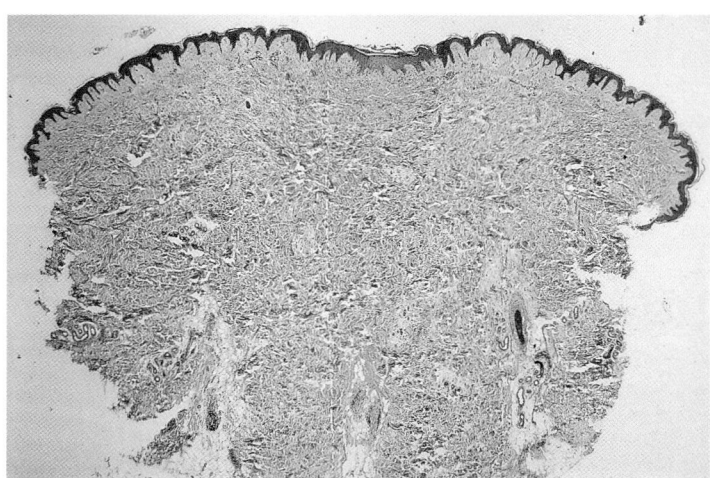

Fig. 8.27 **Malignant atrophic papulosis.** There is a wedge-shaped area of altered epidermis and dermis with a lymphocytic vasculitis at the apex near the dermal–subcutaneous junction. (H & E)

A prominent feature is the presence of abundant acid mucopolysaccharides in the dermis.[1008] Initially these are localized to the ischemic zone, but in older lesions the material is confined to the margins of this zone. They stain with the colloidal iron or alcian blue methods.

Immunofluorescence studies have given conflicting results. Fibrin is always demonstrated, and sometimes immunoglobulins and complement may be found around small dermal vessels or near the basement membrane.[1028]

Electron microscopy
There is swelling of endothelial cells with various degenerative changes[1028] and sometimes luminal occlusion by endothelial cells and cell fragments. Tubular aggregates are often seen in the endothelial cells.[1029]

PERNIOSIS

Perniosis is a localized inflammatory lesion which develops in certain individuals exposed to cold temperatures.[1030–1033] Classic perniosis (chilblains) occurs on the fingers and toes, and sometimes the ears, but plaques have also been described on the thighs.[1031] Lupus erythematosus is uncommonly complicated by lesions mimicking perniosis (chilblain lupus).[1034] An association with chronic myelomonocytic leukemia,[1035] viral hepatitis, HIV infection and rheumatoid arthritis has been reported.[1036]

Equestrian perniosis is the term used for a particular form of perniosis that occurs on the buttocks and lateral thighs of female horseriders in the winter.[1037] Cryoproteins may be present in these horseriders and in children with perniosis.[1037,1038]

A perniotic-like reaction has been reported following the use of the amphetamine analogues fenfluramine and phentermine for weight reduction.[1039]

Histopathology[1031]
Perniosis is a lymphocytic vasculitis in which there is edema and thickening of vessel walls associated with a mural and perivascular infiltrate of lymphocytes (Fig. 8.28). Fibrin is not always present, but as stated earlier it is not a prerequisite for the diagnosis of a lymphocytic vasculitis. A few neutrophils and eosinophils may be present in early lesions; the presence of a leukocytoclastic vasculitis is rare.[1040] The term 'fluffy edema' has been used to describe the vessel wall changes.[1031] Usually vessels at all levels of the dermis

sections has also shown ghost-like infarcted small vessels and demyelination of cutaneous nerves.[1028] Red cells fill the lumen of some small vessels.

Sometimes the epidermis shows focal infarction or scattered necrotic keratinocytes in addition to the atrophy. There may also be some basal vacuolar change. The late-stage changes closely resemble a miniaturized version of lichen sclerosus et atrophicus.[1015]

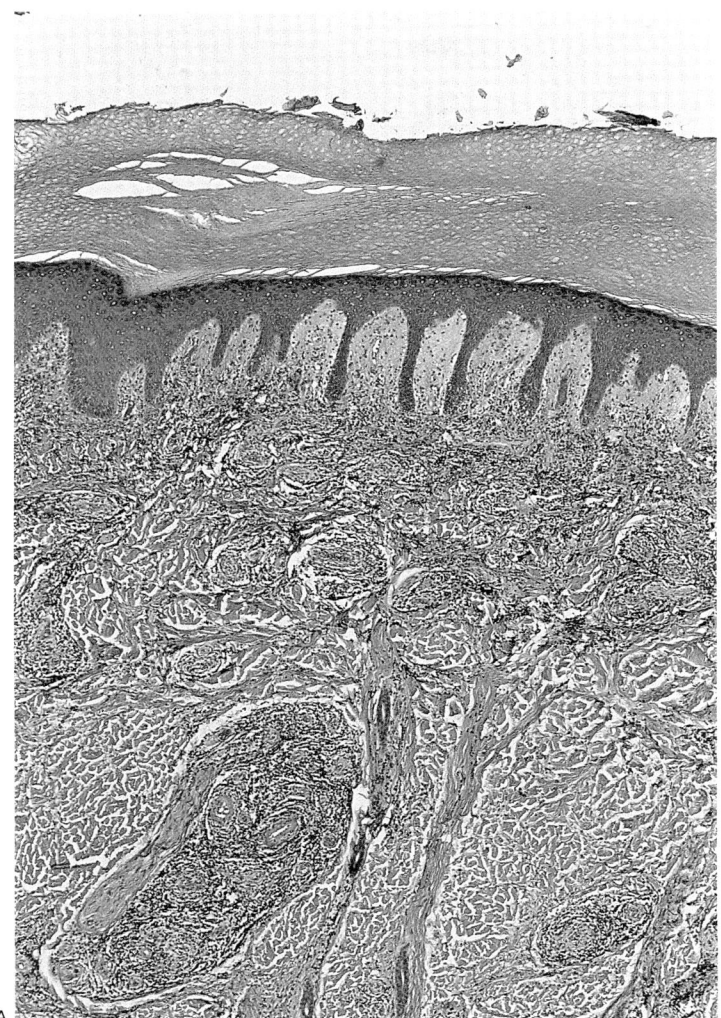

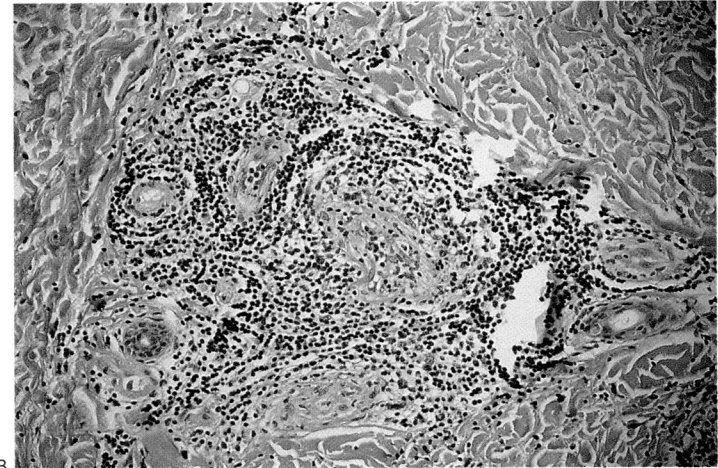

Fig. 8.28 **(A) Perniosis. (B)** There is a lymphocytic vasculitis. Fibrin was present in a larger vessel in the upper subcutis. (H & E)

RICKETTSIAL AND VIRAL INFECTIONS

A lymphocytic vasculitis, often associated with fibrin extravasation, is characteristic of the maculopapular rash of the various rickettsial infections. If an eschar is present, necrosis of the epidermis and upper dermis will be found, with a vasculitis at the periphery of the lesion. Fibrin thrombi are often present in these vessels.

Herpesvirus and other viral infections may be associated with a lymphocytic vasculitis.[1041] A lichenoid lymphocytic vasculitis can be seen in some recurrent and persistent herpesvirus infections and in persistent reactions to certain viruses (see p. 692).

PYODERMA GANGRENOSUM

Pyoderma gangrenosum is a clinically distinctive disorder characterized by the development of an erythematous pustule or nodule which rapidly progresses to become a necrotic ulcer with a ragged, undermined, violaceous edge.[1042–1044] Lesions may be single or multiple.[1045] Although most ulcers are less than 3 cm in diameter, large lesions up to 20 cm or more in diameter may result from coalescence of smaller ulcers.[1045] Not infrequently, minor trauma may initiate the onset of a lesion, a process known as pathergy.[1046,1047]

Pyoderma gangrenosum has a predilection for the lower extremities[1043] although sometimes the trunk, and rarely the head and neck,[1048,1049] may also be involved. The penis is a rare site of involvement.[1050,1051] Extracutaneous manifestations include sterile pyoarthrosis,[1052] oropharyngeal involvement,[1053] neutrophilic myositis[1054] and pulmonary inflammatory infiltrates.[1055] Onset is usually in mid-adult life, but childhood onset has been recorded.[1049,1056–1062] Familial occurrence is exceedingly rare.[1063]

In cases associated with hematological malignancies, the lesions may develop bullae at the advancing edge – *bullous pyoderma gangrenosum*.[1064–1067] This clinical variant is histogenetically similar to Sweet's syndrome, and cases with overlap features have been recorded. A case of bullous pyoderma gangrenosum has been recorded after granulocyte colony-stimulating factor (GCSF) treatment.[1068] This group of patients usually has a poor prognosis.[1066] Another clinical variant is *malignant pyoderma*, a rare, ulcerating, destructive condition of the skin of the head, neck and upper part of the trunk, but which has a predilection for the preauricular region.[1046,1069–1071] Individual lesions lack the undermined, violaceous border of pyoderma gangrenosum and there is usually no associated systemic disease.[1069,1072] It has been suggested that malignant pyoderma is a variant of Wegener's granulomatosis rather than pyoderma gangrenosum.[1073] The cANCA has been positive in several cases.[1073] It has also been positive in the more usual form of pyoderma gangrenosum.[1074] Another clinicopathological variant has been reported as *superficial granulomatous pyoderma* (vegetative pyoderma gangrenosum).[1075–1081] It is characterized by a superficial ulcer, usually solitary and on the trunk. It may arise at sites of surgical incision or other pathergic stimuli. Draining sinuses may be present.[1075] It runs a chronic course, although it usually responds to topical therapy.[1076]

Pyoderma gangrenosum can occur in an autosomal dominant condition known as the PAPA syndrome – *pyogenic sterile arthritis, pyoderma gangrenosum and acne*.[1082] It can also occur in association with chronic multifocal osteomyelitis.[1083]

In more than half of the cases of pyoderma gangrenosum there is an associated systemic illness such as ulcerative colitis,[1084] Crohn's disease,[150,1084–1086] rheumatoid arthritis,[1043] seronegative polyarthritis, or a monoclonal gammopathy, particularly of IgA type.[1087] Parastomal lesions are an important complication of inflammatory bowel disease.[1088,1089] Rare clinical associations[1090] have included chronic active hepatitis,[1091] chronic

are involved, while at other times the process is confined to the more superficial vessels. Vascular ectasia may be present. There is variable edema of the papillary dermis, which is sometimes quite intense.[1031] Basal vacuolar change is present in lupus pernio[1034] but it is usually more widespread than the focal interface change that can be seen in idiopathic perniosis.

persistent hepatitis,[1092] hepatitis C infection,[1093] thyroid disease,[1043] sarcoidosis, systemic lupus erythematosus,[1094] anticardiolipin antibodies,[1095] hidradenitis suppurativa,[1043] Behçet's disease,[1096] Cogan's syndrome,[1097] Cushing's disease,[1098] Takayasu's arteritis,[1099] *Chlamydia pneumoniae* infection,[1100] subcorneal pustular dermatosis,[1101,1102] isotretinoin therapy for acne,[1103] internal cancer,[1104,1105] diabetes mellitus,[1106] polycythemia rubra vera,[1107] myelofibrosis,[1108] autoimmune hemolytic anemia,[1109] IgA paraproteinemia,[1053] paroxysmal nocturnal hemoglobinuria[1110] and postoperative[1111–1113] and immunosuppressed states,[1114,1115] including HIV infection.[1116] Pyoderma gangrenosum-like lesions may be a presenting sign of Wegener's granulomatosis.[1117] Pyoderma gangrenosum may mimic cutaneous tuberculosis.[1118]

Pyoderma gangrenosum may run an acute progressive course with rapidly expanding lesions which require systemic treatment to arrest their growth.[1119,1120] Other cases pursue a more chronic course with slow extension and sometimes spontaneous regression after weeks or months.[1119] Lesions eventually heal leaving a parchment or cribriform scar. Responses have been reported to thalidomide,[1121,1122] clofazimine,[1123] mycophenolate mofetil[1124,1125] and immunosuppression combined with bioengineered-skin grafting.[1126]

Multiple abnormalities of humoral immunity, cell-mediated immunity and neutrophil function have been reported, although the pathogenetic significance of these findings remains an enigma.[1042,1127–1130] Some of these abnormalities may be nothing more than epiphenomena. The role, if any, of a vasculitis in the pathogenesis of pyoderma gangrenosum is debatable (see below).

Histopathology[1042,1043,1131]

The findings are quite variable and depend on the age of the lesion and the site biopsied. The most controversial aspect of the histopathology relates to the presence (or absence) of a vasculitis.[1092] A lymphocytic and/or leukocytoclastic vasculitis has been reported at the advancing erythematous edge in 73% of cases,[1044] although Ackerman has written, 'I now believe that all cases of pyoderma gangrenosum begin as folliculitides and that vasculitis is not a primary event in pyoderma gangrenosum'.[1132]

The earliest lesion shows follicular and perifollicular inflammation with intradermal abscess formation.[1057,1132,1133] In later lesions there is necrosis of the superficial dermis and epidermis forming an ulcer, the base of which shows a mixed inflammatory cell infiltrate with abscess formation.[1131] The process may extend into the underlying subcutis (Fig. 8.29). Giant cells are sometimes present, particularly in cases associated with Crohn's disease.[1134]

At the advancing edge there is a tight perivascular infiltrate of lymphocytes and plasma cells with endothelial swelling and fibrinoid extravasation representing a lymphocytic vasculitis.[1131] This finding has been disputed by some authors.[1120] A leukocytoclastic vasculitis is sometimes present.[1133,1135,1136] There is often subepidermal edema at the advancing edge. This is prominent and associated with intraepidermal bullae with pustulation in those variants with bullous changes at the advancing edge. Acanthosis is a prominent change in the perilesional erythematous zone.

In the variant known as *superficial granulomatous pyoderma*, there are superficial dermal abscesses surrounded by a narrow zone of histiocytes and some giant cells of foreign body type.[1075,1076,1078,1137] Necrotizing granulomas are rarely seen in other forms of pyoderma gangrenosum.[1138] Beyond the zone of histiocytes there is a mixed inflammatory cell infiltrate which usually includes plasma cells and eosinophils. There is often pseudoepitheliomatous hyperplasia. The follicular infundibula may be enlarged, possibly in association with transepidermal elimination of inflammatory debris. There is some resemblance to the changes seen in blastomycosis-like pyoderma, although in this latter condition the inflammatory process is usually much deeper in the

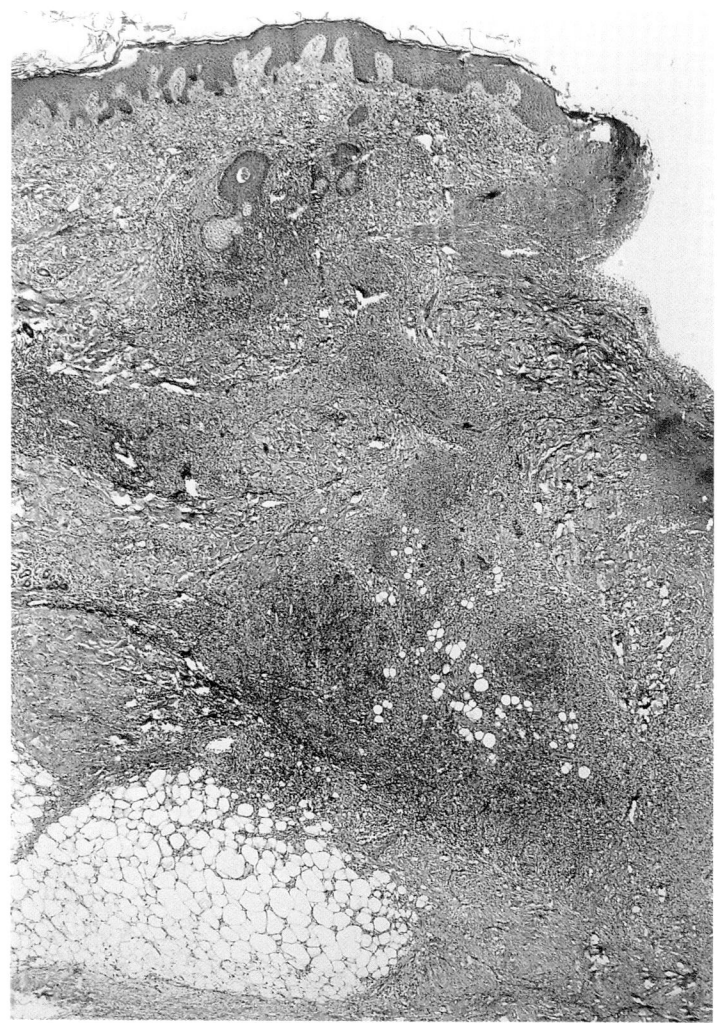

Fig. 8.29 **Pyoderma gangrenosum.** A deep ulcer is present, as is tight lymphocytic cuffing of vessels in the margin of the ulcer. (H & E)

dermis and palisading histiocytes are not usually prominent; furthermore, the two processes usually occur at different sites.

It has been suggested that pyoderma gangrenosum has four distinctive clinical and histological variants – ulcerative, pustular, bullous and vegetative.[1139] In part, these 'variants' represent stages in the evolution of the lesions and, not surprisingly, overlap exists. The *ulcerative* lesions are said to be characterized by central neutrophilic abscesses and 'peripheral lymphocytic angiocentric' infiltrates (lymphocytic vasculitis?), the *pustular* lesions by subcorneal pustules with subepidermal edema and dense dermal neutrophilia, the *bullous* lesions by subepidermal bullae with dermal neutrophilia, and the *vegetative* form (previously reported from the same institution as superficial granulomatous pyoderma) by pseudoepitheliomatous hyperplasia, dermal abscesses, sinus tracts and a palisading granulomatous reaction (Fig. 8.30).[1139]

Immunoreactants have been reported around blood vessels in the dermis in over 50% of cases of pyoderma gangrenosum in one series.[1140] They have not been detected by others.[1120]

POLYMORPHOUS LIGHT ERUPTION

In some cases of polymorphous light eruption, particularly the papulovesicular variant, the tight perivascular lymphocytic infiltrate mimics closely the picture

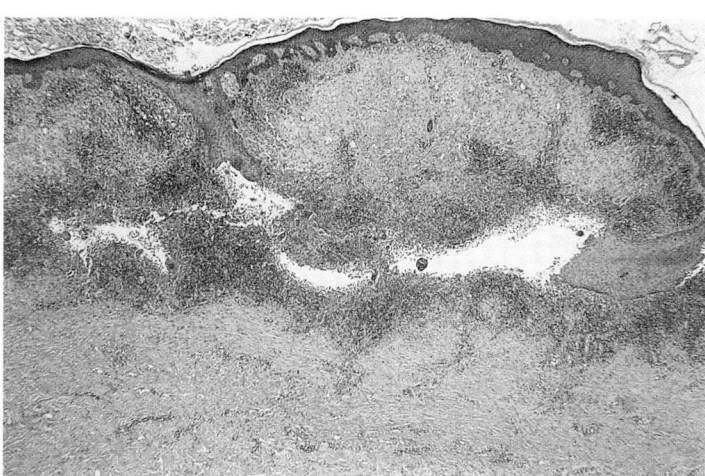

Fig. 8.30 **Pyoderma gangrenosum, superficial granulomatous type.** There is a dermal abscess which drains into an overlying follicle. (H & E)

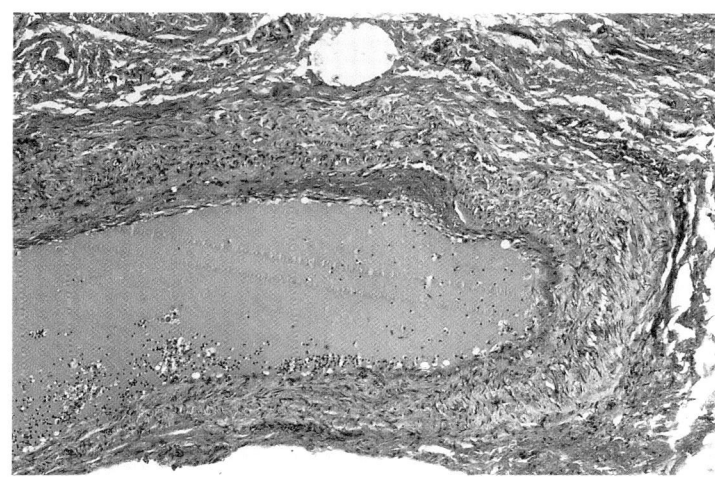

Fig. 8.31 **Sclerosing lymphangitis of the penis.** Condensed eosinophilic material fills the lumen of a vessel, most likely a vein. (H & E)

seen in lymphocytic vasculitis, although there is never any fibrinoid change in the vessels. Red cell extravasation is invariably present in the papulovesicular variant. Polymorphous light eruption is discussed further on page 602.

TRAPS

TRAPS is the acronym for *tumor necrosis factor receptor-associated periodic syndrome*, a periodic fever syndrome resulting from mutations in the *TNFRSF1A* gene, which encodes the tumor necrosis factor receptor.[535] It is on chromosome 12p13.3.

The skin eruption consists of migratory macules and patches and edematous dermal plaques beginning in the first few years of life. Fever is always present and there may be abdominal pain, myalgia, arthralgia, pleuritic chest pain and headache.[535] It must be distinguished from two other familial fever syndromes, hypergammaglobulinemia (hyperimmunoglobulinemia) D syndrome (see p. 234) and familial Mediterranean fever (see p. 239).

Histopathology

There is a superficial and deep perivascular and interstitial infiltrate of lymphocytes and monocytes. The photomicrographs in a large series of 25 patients suggest a lymphocytic vasculitis without fibrin.[535]

SCLEROSING LYMPHANGITIS OF THE PENIS

Sclerosing lymphangitis of the penis is characterized by the sudden appearance of a firm, cord-like, nodular lesion in the coronal sulcus or on the dorsum of the shaft of the penis.[1141] It is usually asymptomatic and subsides after several weeks. Recurrences are documented. The etiology is unknown, but sexual intercourse,[1142,1143] herpes infection[1144] and secondary syphilis[1145] have been incriminated in some cases.

Histopathology[1146,1147]

Established lesions show a dilated vessel, the lumen of which contains condensed eosinophilic material or a fibrin thrombus in the process of recanalization (Fig. 8.31). Lymphocytes and macrophages are often present within the thrombus. The wall of the vessel shows prominent fibrous thickening.[1141] There is usually a mild inflammatory cell infiltrate and some

edema around the involved channel. The vessel is usually said to be a lymphatic but the suggestion has been made that it is in fact a vein and that the condition may be likened to Mondor's phlebitis.[1148]

Electron microscopy

Small lymphatic capillaries containing lymphocytes form within the luminal thrombus.[1146] Newly formed collagen fibrils are present in the vessel walls.

LEUKEMIC VASCULITIS

A leukocytoclastic vasculitis may occur in patients with leukemia secondary to sepsis and medications, or as a rare paraneoplastic phenomenon. A specific form of vasculitis, mediated by leukemic blast cells rather than reactive inflammatory cells, has been reported recently as leukemic vasculitis.[1149,1150] It is a manifestation of leukemia cutis, particularly in the setting of acute myelomonocytic leukemia. Leukemic vasculitis is usually an indicator of poor prognosis.[1151]

Atypical (angiocentric) infiltrates can also be seen in angiocentric lymphoma, its variant lymphomatoid granulomatosis, some cutaneous lymphomas of natural killer cells (CD56+) and in the reversible cutaneous lymphoma associated with methotrexate therapy for rheumatoid arthritis.[1152]

VASCULITIS WITH GRANULOMATOSIS

The term 'vasculitis with granulomatosis' is the preferred designation for those diseases which show varying degrees of granulomatosis, both angiocentric and unrelated to vessels, in combination with a vasculitis which may be necrotizing.[1153,1154] The term 'granulomatous vasculitis', although often used interchangeably, is more limited in its meaning[1155] and, strictly interpreted, refers to granulomatous involvement of vessel walls[1156] without the formation of extravascular granulomas.

The important clinical entities showing vasculitis with granulomatosis include Wegener's granulomatosis, lymphomatoid granulomatosis, allergic granulomatosis (Churg–Strauss syndrome) and midline granuloma.[1153] Temporal arteritis and Takayasu's arteritis are usually considered with this group, although the granulomatous inflammation is restricted to the vessel

253

walls. Granulomatous involvement of vessel walls and/or perivascular granulomas may also be seen in a wide range of clinical settings which include lymphoma,[1157] angioimmunoblastic lymphadenopathy, sarcoidosis, systemic vasculitis,[1157] Crohn's disease,[1158] drug reactions,[1159] the site of previous herpes zoster[1160–1162] or herpes simplex,[1163] rheumatoid arthritis, infectious granulomatous diseases such as tuberculosis and tertiary syphilis, and less well defined circumstances.[1164] The important entities will be considered below.

WEGENER'S GRANULOMATOSIS

Wegener's granulomatosis is a rare systemic disease with necrotizing vasculitis and granulomas involving the upper and lower respiratory tracts, accompanied usually by a focal necrotizing glomerulitis.[1165] A vasculitis involving both arteries and veins may involve other organs, including the skin.[1166] The disease usually presents in the fourth and fifth decades of life with symptoms related to the upper respiratory tract such as persistent rhinorrhea and sinus pain.[1166,1167] Childhood cases are uncommon.[1168,1169] Other clinical features may include a cough, hemoptysis, otitis media, ocular signs, gingival hyperplasia, arthralgia and constitutional symptoms.[1170–1172] Several cases have been associated with vasculitis of the temporal artery; only one was of giant-cell type.[1173]

Cutaneous manifestations occur in 30–50% of cases and may occasionally be the presenting complaint.[1174–1176] They often take the form of papulonecrotic lesions distributed symmetrically over the elbows, knees and sometimes the buttocks. Other reported clinical lesions[1177] include purpura,[1167] vesicular and urticarial eruptions, large ulcers resembling pyoderma gangrenosum,[1178,1179] subcutaneous nodules, necrotizing granulomas in scars and, in two cases,[1180,1181] breast involvement.

An important clinical variant is the so-called '*limited form*' in which pulmonary lesions predominate and a glomerulitis is absent.[1182,1183] Cutaneous lesions are less frequent and may take the form of subcutaneous nodules. The limited form has a better prognosis. Another clinical variant, characterized by protracted mucosal and cutaneous lesions, is known as *protracted superficial Wegener's granulomatosis*.[1156,1184]

Wegener's granulomatosis is almost uniformly fatal if not treated; deaths may occur despite treatment.

The etiology and pathogenesis are unknown, but it appears to result from an immunological disturbance, possibly following an infective trigger.[623] A clinical response to antibiotics is sometimes demonstrated, although this does not necessarily imply an infective etiology.[1185]

Of interest is the finding in the serum of antibodies, usually of IgG class, which react against cytoplasmic components of neutrophils. Two types of these antineutrophil cytoplasmic antibodies (ANCA) are found – cytoplasmic ANCA (c-ANCA), which are mostly directed against granular enzyme proteinase 3 (PR3), and perinuclear ANCA (p-ANCA) which have multiple antigenic specificities, the best defined being myeloperoxidase (MPO).[623,1074,1186–1188] In Wegener's granulomatosis, approximately 80% of patients have ANCA, mostly of c-ANCA type.[1179,1189] The myeloperoxidase subtype of p-ANCA tends to occur in patients with renal-limited disease but it is seen in some patients with Wegener's granulomatosis; no patient has had both subtypes.[481,1189] The titer of ANCA reflects disease activity.[481]

A new disease complex has been proposed – ANCA-associated systemic vasculitis.[1190] It includes what is now known as Wegener's granulomatosis, as well as microscopic polyangiitis (polyarteritis) and renal-limited disease (crescentic glomerulonephritis).[623] In these conditions, the pathogenesis may be an autoimmune inflammatory response, characterized by specific mediators, in which the endothelium is both target and active participant.[457]

Histopathology[1156,1174,1191,1192]

The full picture of a necrotizing vasculitis with granulomatosis is seen in the skin in 20% or less of cases of Wegener's granulomatosis.[1153] Sometimes the findings are quite non-specific, with only a chronic inflammatory cell infiltrate in the dermis. In specifically diagnostic lesions, vascular and extravascular changes are present in varying proportions.

Extravascular changes include small foci of necrosis and fibrinoid degeneration, usually without vascular participation. There may be some neutrophil infiltration and nuclear dusting in these foci. Rarely, the pattern mimics a neutrophilic dermatosis.[1193] Palisading, which varies from minimal to well defined, may develop in older lesions. Poorly formed granulomas, unrelated to necrotic areas, may also be present. Giant cells are almost invariably present in the palisading margins of the granulomas, in granulation tissue lining ulcerated surfaces, or scattered irregularly in the chronic inflammation which forms a background to the entire process.[1156] Rarely, eosinophils are prominent in the infiltrate.[1194] No atypical mononuclear cells are present. Granulomas resembling those seen in allergic granulomatosis (Churg–Strauss syndrome) have been reported in several cases.[1195]

Vascular changes may take the form of a necrotizing angiitis involving small and medium-sized dermal vessels. Fibrin extends around the vessel walls and sometimes there is a fibrin thrombus in the lumen. A small vessel leukocytoclastic vasculitis is sometimes present.[1196] Red cell extravasation accompanies either type of vasculitis. Less commonly, a granulomatous vasculitis with angiocentric granulomas is present.[1174] In a recent study of 46 patients, no examples of granulomatous vasculitis were found. Extravascular granulomatous inflammation was found in 19% of cases.[1197] Patients with leukocytoclastic vasculitis (31%) had onset of the disease at an earlier age and more rapidly progressive and widespread disease.[1197]

Special stains are non-contributory, although specific infective causes of granulomas should always be kept in mind in the differential diagnosis. Immunofluorescence microscopy will sometimes show C3 and immunoglobulins related to vessels in early lesions.

LYMPHOMATOID GRANULOMATOSIS

Lymphomatoid granulomatosis was first described in 1972[1198] as a unique form of pulmonary angiitis and granulomatosis which frequently had extrapulmonary manifestations.[1199] It is now regarded as an angiocentric lymphoma (see p. 1101).[1200–1202] Skin lesions have been noted in 40–60% of cases and these may be the presenting complaint.[1203–1208] They take the form of erythematous or violaceous nodules and plaques which may be widely distributed on the trunk and lower extremities.[1204] Rarely, paranasal or ulcerated palatal lesions are present. Any of the lesions may become ulcerated, with surface eschar formation, but this is more common with nodules on the leg.

Other clinical features include fever, cough, malaise, weight loss, dyspnea and pulmonary infiltrates.[1199] Onset is usually in early middle age; the illness runs a rapid course with a median survival of 14 months.[1199] Death may result from respiratory failure or the effects of the diffuse peripheral lymphoma that may develop.[1209–1217]

Histopathology[1204]

There is a polymorphous infiltrate in the dermis, with perivascular, periappendageal and perineural accentuation.[1203,1210] Sweat glands are particularly involved.[1206] The infiltrate often extends into the subcutis, although the epidermis and papillary dermis are usually spared.[1218]

The infiltrate is composed of a mixture of lymphocytes, histiocytes and 'lymphohistiocytoid' cells, some of which may show plasmacytoid features.[1203]

Occasional giant cells impart a vague granulomatous aura. However, granulomas are less conspicuous and much less distinct than in Wegener's granulomatosis.[1153] Occasional eosinophils may be present in the infiltrate but neutrophils are rare, except beneath ulcerated surfaces. There may be atypical cells and scattered mitoses but the degree of atypia, which is never as great in the skin as in other organs, varies from case to case.[1219] An attempt has been made to grade the atypia of the infiltrate seen in lymphomatoid granulomatosis and other angiocentric immunoproliferative lesions.[1220] The grading is of more value in extracutaneous lesions.

As well as being angiocentric, the infiltrate is frequently angioinvasive (Fig. 8.32). Sometimes an endothelium-lined lumen in the center of a lymphohistiocytic aggregate is the only sign of a residual vessel.[1218] Both arteries and veins may be affected. Fibrinoid necrosis of vessel walls and infarction are not usually prominent features in the skin. Marked fibroblastic proliferation may be present in some lesions.

Sometimes the histology of the skin lesions is not diagnostic, despite the presence of typical changes in other organs of the body.

A related histological picture has been reported in a patient with an EBV-associated lymphoproliferative disorder of granular lymphocytes.[1221] This condition, which has a common T-cell subset (CD3⁺, CD8⁺) and a rarer NK-cell subset, has some similarities to the 'angiocentric immunoproliferative lesions', of which lymphomatoid granulomatosis is a member. Similar cases have been reported in young adult males, who presented with necrotic papulovesicles on the face.[1222] Three of these four cases eventually developed lymphoma.[1222]

ALLERGIC GRANULOMATOSIS

Allergic granulomatosis (Churg–Strauss syndrome) is a clinically distinctive, idiopathic disease in which systemic vasculitis and hypereosinophilia develop in individuals with pre-existing asthma and allergic rhinitis.[1223–1226] Tissue eosinophilia, peripheral neuropathy, cardiac lesions and mild renal disease may also be present. A limited form of the disease, in which not all of the above features are present, has been described.[1227] Rare associations include a temporal arteritis of non-giant cell type[1228] and Wells' syndrome.[1229]

Cutaneous lesions are common and include purpura, erythema or urticarial lesions and distinctive nodules.[1230] These nodules, which are often tender, arise on the scalp or symmetrically on the extremities. They may involve the dermis or subcutis. Ulceration may occur secondary to the arteritis and thrombosis of dermal vessels.[1231]

The prognosis is variable, but most patients appear to have a good response to corticosteroid therapy.

The etiology of allergic granulomatosis is unknown. Whether it is best categorized as an allergic disorder or a vascular disease is unclear.[1231]

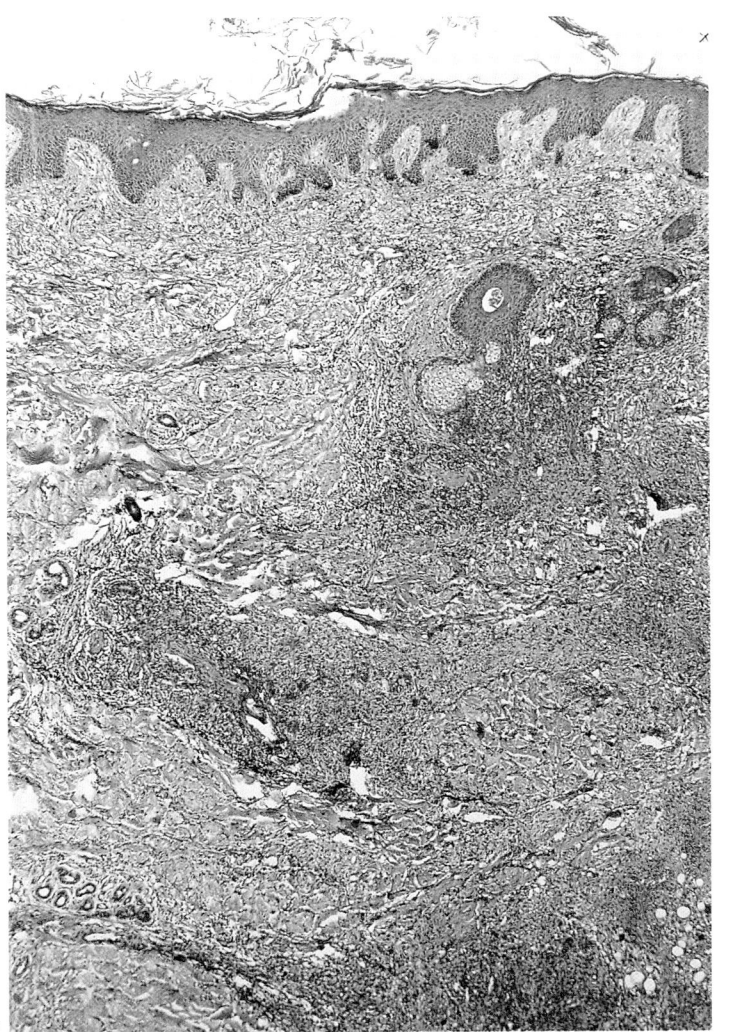
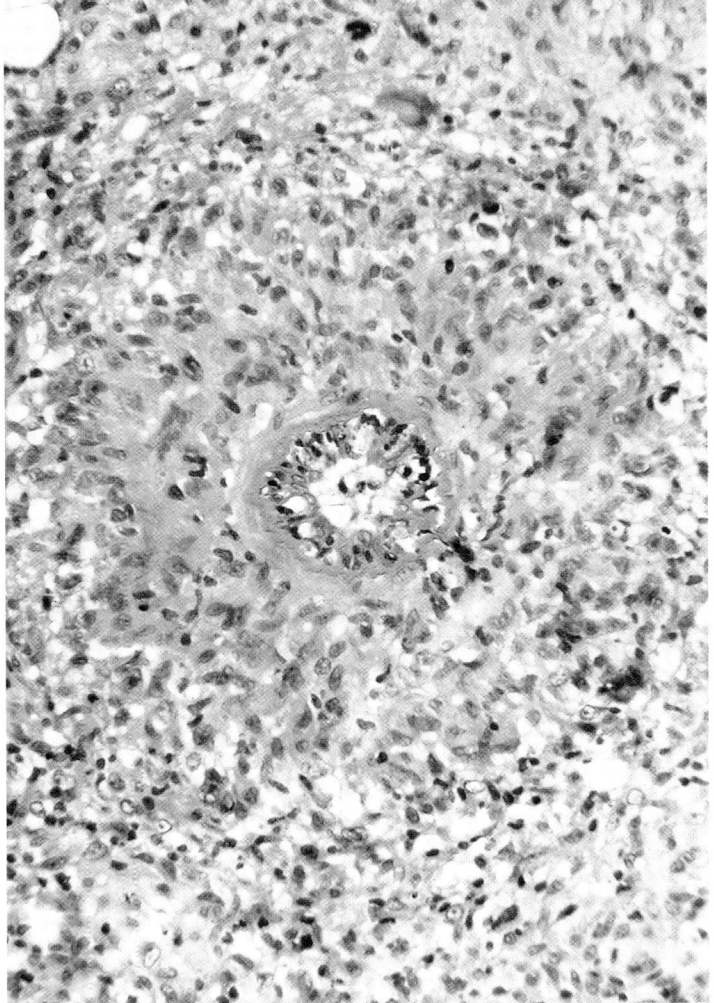

Fig. 8.32 **(A) Lymphomatoid granulomatosis. (B)** An atypical infiltrate involves the wall of a small artery in the deep dermis from this same case. (H & E)

Antibodies to hepatitis B virus and to the human immunodeficiency virus have been reported in only one case.[1232] Antibodies to p-ANCA are often present.[1231] Requena and colleagues believe that degeneration of collagen bundles, resulting from lysosomal enzymes released from granulocytes, is the primary event. This is followed by the infiltration of histiocytes that become arranged in a palisade.[1233]

Histopathology

The three major histological features are a necrotizing vasculitis, tissue infiltration by eosinophils, and extravascular granulomas.[1224] The vasculitis involves small arteries and veins, but it may also affect larger arteries and resemble polyarteritis nodosa. It may take the form of a leukocytoclastic vasculitis.[1234,1235] Older lesions show healing with scarring. The tissue infiltration with eosinophils is accompanied by destruction of some of these cells, leading to release of their granules and increased eosinophilia of the collagen (Fig. 8.33).[1224] The extravascular granulomas, which result in the cutaneous nodules found in some patients, show central necrosis which may be fibrinoid or partly basophilic, with interspersed eosinophils, some neutrophils and also debris.[1230] This area is surrounded by a granulomatous proliferation of histiocytes, lymphocytes and giant cells, often in palisaded

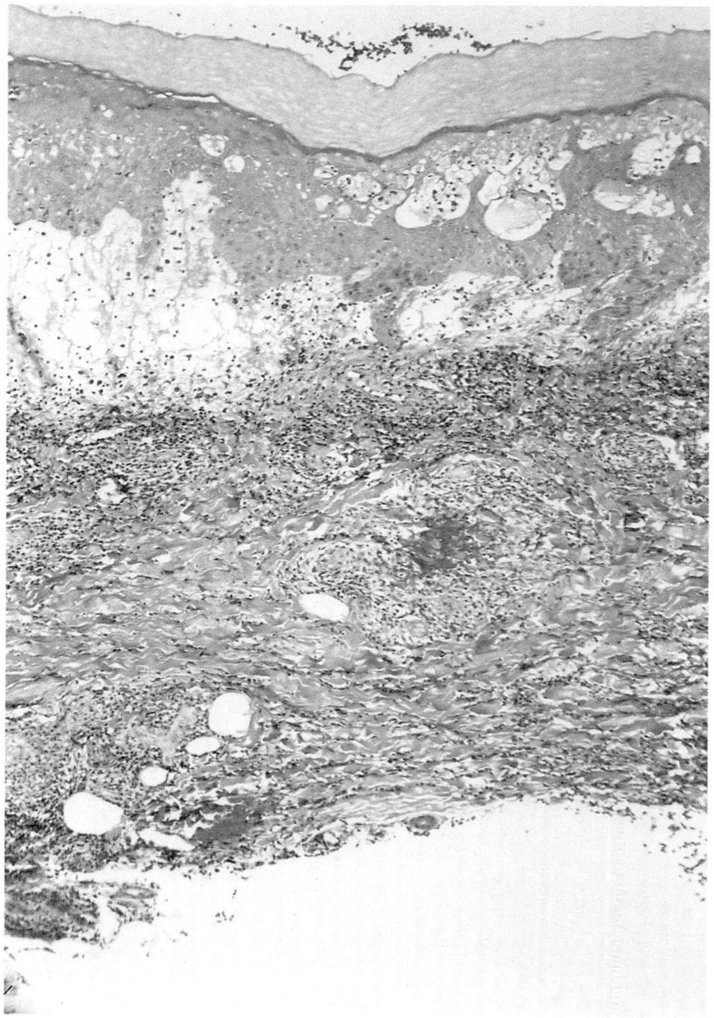

Fig. 8.33 **Allergic granulomatosis.** A flame figure is present in an area of numerous eosinophils. There is prominent subepidermal edema. (H & E)

array.[1230] Granulomas were present in less than half the autopsy cases included in one review.[1224] Non-necrotizing granulomas were present in a case of limited allergic granulomatosis.[1227]

It should be noted that the three components mentioned above do not always coexist temporally or spatially.[1224] Furthermore, similar extravascular granulomas, initially referred to as Churg–Strauss granulomas, have been described in association with circulating immune complexes:[1195,1236–1239] these associated conditions include systemic lupus erythematosus, rheumatoid arthritis, Wegener's granulomatosis, polyarteritis nodosa, Takayasu's aortitis,[1240] various lymphoproliferative disorders[1241] and some other conditions.[1242,1243] Other terms used for these unique, palisaded granulomatous lesions include 'rheumatoid papules', 'superficial ulcerating rheumatoid necrobiosis', 'interstitial granulomatous dermatitis with arthritis' and, recently, 'palisaded neutrophilic and granulomatous dermatitis of immune complex disease'.[1236] The term 'interstitial granulomatous dermatitis' is used here. The lesions present as papules, linear cords or plaques on the trunk or extremities. In the granulomas found in these circumstances, the central necrotic area is invariably basophilic.[1244] Furthermore, there is an absence of the tissue eosinophilia within and around the granulomas that is seen in allergic granulomatosis.

LETHAL MIDLINE GRANULOMA

Lethal midline granuloma (Stewart type of non-healing necrotizing granuloma) is a controversial disease category, now of historical interest only, which was regarded by some as a distinct clinicopathological entity[1245] and by others as merely a clinical term to describe any rapidly evolving, destructive lesion of the nose and deep facial tissues.[1246,1247] This term is now being discarded but the suggested replacements – 'angiocentric lymphoma' and 'angiocentric immunoproliferative lesion (AIL)' – are not without problems.[1248] The latter term also includes lymphomatoid granulomatosis. Some cases originate as polyclonal proliferations of lymphoid cells from which a clonal population (usually T cell, but sometimes B cell) may arise. Epstein–Barr virus (EBV) has been detected in many cases.[1216,1249]

Histopathology[1245]

Lethal midline granuloma, as originally defined, could be included here because granulomas and vasculitis sometimes occurred.[1153] The usual picture was of a dense polymorphic infiltrate composed of lymphocytes, plasma cells and some polygonal and spindle-shaped histiocytes in a background of granulation and fibrous tissue. Necrosis was usually prominent. Vasculitis was uncommon but endarteritis obliterans was often seen. Clearcut granulomas were present in 4 of the 10 cases in one series.[1245]

GIANT CELL (TEMPORAL) ARTERITIS

Giant cell arteritis is a granulomatous vasculitis involving large or medium-sized elastic arteries, with a predilection for the superficial temporal and ophthalmic arteries and to a lesser extent other extracranial branches of the carotid arteries.[1250–1253] The onset is usually late in life. The protean clinical manifestations include severe headache, jaw claudication and visual and neurological disturbances.[1254] Its relationship to polymyalgia rheumatica is controversial.

Cutaneous manifestations are uncommon, the most frequent being necrosis of the scalp with ulceration.[255–1258] This may be localized to one side or bitemporal with large areas of necrosis.[1259] Actinic granuloma is a rare association.[1260] Alopecia, hyperpigmentation and scalp tenderness may occur.[1261] Giant cell arteritis is rarely associated with other forms of systemic vasculitis.[1262]

The etiology is unknown. It has been suggested that the condition results from inflammation and elastolysis (with resorption), involving actinically damaged fibers of the internal elastic lamina of the temporal artery.[1263] Another suggestion is that cell-mediated immunity, especially a T-cell-regulated granulomatous reaction, may play a role in the pathogenesis of temporal arteritis.[1264] The antigen in such cases may be actinically degenerate elastic tissue in the vessel wall.[1265]

The rare form of temporal arteritis that occurs in children and young adults is not the same as classic giant cell (temporal) arteritis. It presents as a lump on the forehead which may be non-tender or painful.[1266] The erythrocyte sedimentation rate is normal, in contrast to the usually elevated rate in the giant cell form.[1266,1267] A similar case, but with accompanying systemic vasculitis, has been reported in an adult.[1268]

Histopathology[1269]

It has been suggested that as a significant number of patients with clinical temporal arteritis have negative biopsies, a trial of corticosteroid therapy would be a better indicator of this diagnosis than temporal artery biopsy.[1270] Corticosteroid therapy is not without risk, however. The percentage of positive biopsies depends on the number of sections examined, as skip lesions do occur.[1271] In a recent retrospective study, the incidence of skip lesions was 8.5%, although a previous study recorded skip lesions in 28.3% of cases.[1272] Another study examined further levels on 132 biopsies initially reported as normal and found one additional case of temporal arteritis, while 2 of 14 cases diagnosed initially as periarterial lymphocytic infiltration (see below) revealed giant cell arteritis on further levels.[1273]

The classic findings are a granulomatous arteritis involving the inner media, with prominent giant cells of both Langhans and 'foreign body' type (Figs 8.34, 8.35). This is associated with fragmentation and focal destruction of the internal elastic lamina. A non-specific inflammatory cell infiltrate which includes variable numbers of lymphocytes, histiocytes and even eosinophils is often present. Giant cells are not mandatory for the diagnosis.[1274] Granulomatous inflammation may persist despite prolonged corticosteroid treatment and clinical resolution of the symptoms.[1275]

A recent study attempted to assess the significance of small foci of perivascular inflammation without any intimal or medial involvement **(periarterial lymphocytic infiltration)**. The authors concluded that, while this change may be a marker of associated vasculitis in a small number of cases (see above), in the majority of cases it had no significance.[1276] It may be an age-related change.

Some biopsies show intimal thickening with a proliferation of fibroblasts and myointimal cells, but little or no change in the media.[1269] There is usually an abundant myxomatoid stroma and a scattering of inflammatory cells. The internal elastic lamina is fragmented or thickened, with some loss of staining with elastic stains. The lumen is narrowed. These changes appear to represent an active process and not a healed stage, as once thought.[1269] If there is no inflammation at all, however, reliable distinction from arteriosclerotic changes is impossible.[1277] In old lesions, there may be evidence of recanalization of the lumen.

A much more florid inflammatory reaction is present in the exceedingly rare cases of Buerger's disease (thromboangiitis obliterans) of the temporal artery.[1278]

In juvenile temporal arteritis, there is an eosinophilic panarteritis and thrombosis, with or without microaneurysmal disruption of the artery. Lymphocytes and plasma cells are also present, but there are no giant cells.[1266]

TAKAYASU'S ARTERITIS

Takayasu's arteritis (aortic arch syndrome, pulseless disease) is an uncommon large vessel granulomatous vasculitis, with a predilection for young females.[1279] It results in fibrosis, leading to constriction or occlusion of the aorta and its main branches. Associated skin lesions include erythema nodosum, pyodermatous ulcers, non-specific erythematous rashes, urticaria and necrotizing vasculitis involving small blood vessels of the skin.[1240,1279,1280]

MISCELLANEOUS VASCULAR DISORDERS

There are several vascular disorders which do not fit into any of the other major categories. One such example, which will not be considered further, is the development of stasis dermatitis of the hand secondary to an iatrogenic arteriovenous fistula.[1281] Some of these conditions are mentioned in other sections; they are included here for completeness.

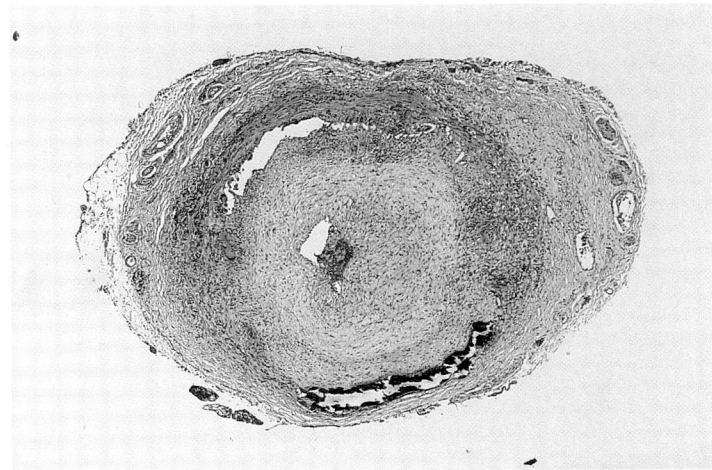

Fig. 8.34 **Temporal arteritis.** An inflammatory cell infiltrate is present in relation to the internal elastic lamina. (H & E)

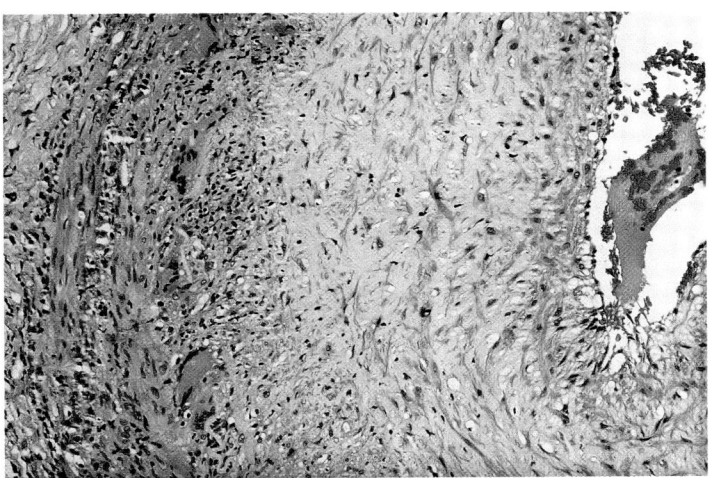

Fig. 8.35 **Temporal arteritis.** A few multinucleate giant cells and some lymphocytes are present in the wall of the temporal artery adjacent to the internal elastic lamina. (H & E)

VASCULAR CALCIFICATION

Calcification of the media of muscular arteries is a well-known complication of the aging process (Mönckeberg's sclerosis). It may also occur in cutaneous and deeper vessels in chronic renal failure, affecting predominantly small arteries. In these circumstances, the calcification may be accompanied by intimal hyperplasia, vascular thrombosis and cutaneous ulceration and necrosis.[156–158,1282–1284] There is usually an elevated calcium-phosphate product and secondary hyperparathyroidism. The term 'calciphylaxis' has been used for this process, although it has also been used for a subgroup of patients with renal failure with vascular and soft tissue calcification without an elevated calcium-phosphate product.[157] Calciphylaxis has been reported in patients without renal failure.[1285]

Histopathology

The calcification involves the media of small arteries in the lower dermis and subcutis. It is often circumferential and accompanied by intimal fibrosis and thickening. Superimposed thrombi may be present and recanalization may subsequently occur.

PERICAPILLARY FIBRIN CUFFS

Fibrin cuffs are a common finding around capillary blood vessels in venous leg ulcers. Initially they were thought to be of pathogenetic significance in the formation of the ulcer and the accompanying lipodermatosclerosis.[1286] Incidentally, it is now thought that leukocyte binding to endothelial cells, as a result of their expression of adhesion molecules, contributes to the pathogenesis of venous ulcers.[1287] Recent studies have shown pericapillary fibrin cuffs (caps) in leg ulcers of non-venous origin and adjacent to ulcers.[1288,1289] They can also be seen in association with venous stasis without ulceration and in venous hypertension of the hand caused by hemodialysis shunts.[1290] This indicates a role for venous hypertension in their pathogenesis.

VASCULAR ANEURYSMS

Pulsatile cutaneous aneurysms have been reported in several patients with arterial fibromuscular dysplasia.[1291]

A large vessel, which may at first glance appear to be aneurysmal, is also seen in the condition known as caliber-persistent artery (see p. 1006).

ERYTHERMALGIA

Erythermalgia and erythromelalgia both refer to a symptom complex characterized by recurrent, red, warm extremities accompanied by burning pain.[1292,1293] Michiels and colleagues have defined erythromelalgia as the symptom complex which accompanies thrombocythemia, and erythermalgia as an independent disease process which may arise at a young age (primary erythermalgia) or be associated with various underlying disorders (but not thrombocythemia) in adults (secondary erythermalgia).[76,77,1294,1295]

Erythromelalgia may be broader than the definition proposed above.[1296,1297] The final common pathway may be microvascular arteriovenous shunting,[1298] although small-fiber neuropathy has been suggested as another contributing factor.[1299] It has been reported as a paraneoplastic phenomenon[1300] and following the use of ticlopidine, an inhibitor of platelet aggregation.[1301] It has also been reported in a patient with HIV infection.[1302]

Histopathology

Recent studies of primary erythermalgia have shown thickening of the basement membrane of capillaries, moderate endothelial swelling, perivascular edema and a scant perivascular infiltrate of mononuclear cells.[76] There is usually mild dilatation of capillaries in the superficial dermis.

CUTANEOUS NECROSIS AND ULCERATION

There are many causes of cutaneous *necrosis*, most of which have been covered in the section on vascular occlusive diseases at the beginning of this chapter. Additional causes include severe vasculitis,[423] septic vasculitis, angiotropic lymphoma, calciphylaxis,[1283] oxalosis, thromboemboli, some arthropod bites, including wasp stings, and certain drugs and injections such as cisplatin in systemic scleroderma,[1303] triple vaccine (DTP) injection[1304] and recombinant interferon.[1305] It has been reported as a paraneoplastic phenomenon, an example being the occurrence of digital necrosis associated with ovarian cancer.[1306] Some of the most striking examples are seen in association with purpura fulminans.

Chronic *ulcers*, particularly on the legs, are frequently biopsied, often to exclude malignancy. It is sometimes difficult to offer an etiologic diagnosis because of the superficial nature of the biopsy material. The common causes of chronic leg ulcers are venous and/or arterial insufficiency and neuropathic factors. Despite the presence of small vessel disease in diabetics, it is stated that 70% of diabetic foot ulcers have adequate vascularity and are neuropathic in nature.[1307]

Of leg ulcers in general, 10% are thought to be due to arterial insufficiency and a further 10% to combined arterial and venous disease.[1308] Such ulcers will not usually heal with conservative measures.[1308] In about 50% of patients with leg ulcers, there is a history of previous deep vein thrombosis (DVT).[141] The deep vein thrombosis may be a consequence of protein S deficiency,[1309] the antiphospholipid syndrome or factor V Leiden mutation.[137,139–141] The risk of a previous DVT being followed by a chronic leg ulcer is about 5%.[137] Venous ulcers usually show neovascularization of the upper dermis beneath the ulcer base, as well as hemosiderin pigment and mild fibrosis.

Other causes of leg ulcers include atrophie blanche, prolidase deficiency, hyper-IgM syndrome,[1310] hydroxyurea therapy[1311,1312] and thrombocytosis.[72] Decubitus ulcers are considered elsewhere (see p. 594).

Experimentally, venous leg ulcers have increased plasminogen activation. This influences the activity of metalloproteinase (MMP)-2, which appears to play a role in their pathogenesis.[1313] Trauma is sometimes an initiating event. If ulcers are treated with laboratory cultured skin products then the site often shows mucin deposition, myofibroblastic proliferation, and foreign body giant cells in up to 25% of cases. The presence of granulomas does not result in an adverse outcome.[1314]

REFERENCES

Introduction

1 Braverman IM. The cutaneous microcirculation. J Invest Dermatol (Symposium Proceedings) 2000; 5: 3–9.

2 Petzelbauer P, Halama T, Gröger M. Endothelial adherens junctions. J Invest Dermatol (Symposium Proceedings) 2000; 5: 10–13.

Non-inflammatory purpuras

3 Lotti T, Ghersetich I, Panconesi E. The purpuras. Int J Dermatol 1994; 33: 1–10.

4 Baselga E, Drolet BA, Esterly NB. Purpura in infants and children. J Am Acad Dermatol 1997; 37: 673–705.

5 Rasmussen JE. Puzzling purpuras in children and young adults. J Am Acad Dermatol 1982; 6: 67–72.

6 Ackerman Z, Michaeli J, Gorodetsky R. Skin discoloration in chronic idiopathic thrombocytopenic purpura: detection of local iron deposition by X-ray spectrometry. Dermatologica 1986; 172: 222–224.

7 Yates VM. Factitious purpura. Clin Exp Dermatol 1992; 17: 238–239.

8 Berman DA, Roenigk HH, Green D. Autoerythrocyte sensitization syndrome (psychogenic purpura). J Am Acad Dermatol 1992; 27: 829–832.

9 Lotti T, Benci M, Sarti MG et al. Psychogenic purpura with abnormally increased tPA dependent cutaneous fibrinolytic activity. Int J Dermatol 1993; 32: 521–523.

10 Sudy E, Urbina F, Vasquez P. Autoerythrocyte sensitization syndrome with positive anticardiolipin antibodies. Br J Dermatol 1998; 138: 367–368.

11 Regazzini R, Malagoli PG, Zerbinati N et al. Diamond–Gardner syndrome: a case report. Pediatr Dermatol 1998; 15: 43–45.

12 Wu SJ, Pellegrini AE. Purpura as a cutaneous association of sickle cell disease. Am J Dermatopathol 1999; 21: 384–386.

13 Feinstein RJ, Halprin KM, Penneys NS et al. Senile purpura. Arch Dermatol 1973; 108: 229–232.

14 Haboubi NY, Haboubi NAA, Gyde O et al. Zinc deficiency in senile purpura. J Clin Pathol 1985; 38: 1189–1191.

Vascular occlusive diseases

15 Copeman PWM. Livedo reticularis. Signs in the skin of disturbance of blood viscosity and of blood flow. Br J Dermatol 1975; 93: 519–529.

16 Champion RH. Livedo reticularis. A review. Br J Dermatol 1965; 77: 167–179.

17 Bruce S, Wolf JE Jr. Quinidine-induced photosensitive livedo reticularis-like eruption. J Am Acad Dermatol 1985; 12: 332–336.

18 Kramer BS, Hernandez AD, Reddick RL, Levine AS. Cutaneous infarction. Manifestation of disseminated mucormycosis. Arch Dermatol 1977; 113: 1075–1076.

19 Kossard S, Spigel GT, Winkelmann RK. Cutaneous and subcutaneous endarteritis obliterans. Arch Dermatol 1978; 114: 1652–1658.

20 Schleicher SM, Fricker MP. Coumarin necrosis. Arch Dermatol 1980; 116: 444–445.

21 Bauer KA. Coumarin-induced skin necrosis. Arch Dermatol 1993; 129: 766–768.

22 Stone MS, Rosen T. Acral purpura: an unusual sign of coumarin necrosis. J Am Acad Dermatol 1986; 14: 797–802.

23 Schwartz RA, Moore C III, Lambert WC. Linear localized coumarin necrosis. Dermatologica 1984; 168: 31–34.

24 Rose VL, Kwaan HC, Williamson K et al. Protein C antigen deficiency and warfarin necrosis. Am J Clin Pathol 1986; 86: 653–655.

25 Teepe RGC, Broekmans AW, Vermeer BJ et al. Recurrent coumarin-induced skin necrosis in a patient with an acquired functional protein C deficiency. Arch Dermatol 1986; 122: 1408–1412.

26 Auletta MJ, Headington JT. Purpura fulminans. A cutaneous manifestation of severe protein C deficiency. Arch Dermatol 1988; 124: 1387–1391.

27 Freeman BD, Schmieg RE Jr, McGrath S et al. Factor V Leiden mutation in a patient with warfarin-associated skin necrosis. Surgery 2000; 127: 595–596.

28 Norris PG. Warfarin skin necrosis treated with prostacyclin. Clin Exp Dermatol 1987; 12: 370–372.

29 Shornick JK, Nicholas BK, Bergstresser PR, Gilliam JN. Idiopathic atrophie blanche. J Am Acad Dermatol 1983; 8: 792–798.

30 McCalmont CS, McCalmont TH, Jorizzo JL et al. Livedo vasculitis: vasculitis or thrombotic vasculopathy? Clin Exp Dermatol 1992; 17: 4–8.

31 Jorizzo JL. Livedoid vasculopathy. What is it? Arch Dermatol 1998; 134: 491–493.

32 Pizzo SV, Murray JC, Gonias SL. Atrophie blanche. A disorder associated with defective release of tissue plasminogen activator. Arch Pathol Lab Med 1986; 110: 517–519.

33 Margolis DJ, Kruithof EKO, Barnard M et al. Fibrinolytic abnormalities in two different cutaneous manifestations of venous disease. J Am Acad Dermatol 1996; 34: 204–208.

34 Klein KL, Pittelkow MR. Tissue plasminogen activator for treatment of livedoid vasculitis. Mayo Clin Proc 1992; 67: 923–933.

35 Papi M, Didona B, De Pità O et al. Livedo vasculopathy vs small vessel cutaneous vasculitis. Arch Dermatol 1998; 134: 447–452.

36 Hsiao G-H, Chiu H-C. Livedoid vasculitis. Response to low-dose danazol. Arch Dermatol 1996; 132: 749–751.

37 Grob JJ, Bonerandi JJ. Thrombotic skin disease as a marker of the anticardiolipin syndrome. J Am Acad Dermatol 1989; 20: 1063–1069.

38 Boyvat A, Kundakçi N, Babikir MOA, Gürgey E. Livedoid vasculopathy associated with heterozygous protein C deficiency. Br J Dermatol 2000; 143: 840–842.

39 Biedermann T, Flaig MJ, Sander CA. Livedoid vasculopathy in a patient with factor V mutation (Leiden). J Cutan Pathol 2000; 27: 410–412.

40 Gibson GE, Li H, Pittelkow MR. Homocysteinemia and livedoid vasculitis. J Am Acad Dermatol 1999; 40: 279–281.

41 Milstone LM, Braverman IM. PURPLE (Oops! atrophie blanche) revisited. Arch Dermatol 1998; 134: 1634.

42 Suster S, Ronnen M, Bubis JJ, Schewach-Millet M. Familial atrophie blanche-like lesions with subcutaneous fibrinoid vasculitis. The Georgian ulcers. Am J Dermatopathol 1986; 8: 386–391.

43 Maessen-Visch MB, Koedam MI, Hamulyák K, Neumann HAM. Atrophie blanche. Int J Dermatol 1999; 38: 161–172.

44 Choi H-J, Hann S-K. Livedo reticularis and livedoid vasculitis responding to PUVA therapy. J Am Acad Dermatol 1999; 40: 204–207.

45 Milstone LM, Braverman IM, Lucky P, Fleckman P. Classification and therapy of atrophie blanche. Arch Dermatol 1983; 119: 963–969.

46 Sommer S, Sheehan-Dare RA. Atrophie blanche-like scarring after pulsed dye laser treatment. J Am Acad Dermatol 1999; 41: 100–102.

47 Lee JH, Choi H-J, Kim SM et al. Livedoid vasculitis responding to PUVA therapy. Int J Dermatol 2001; 40: 153–157.

48 Gray HR, Graham JH, Johnson W, Burgoon CF. Atrophie blanche: periodic painful ulcers of lower extremities. Arch Dermatol 1966; 93: 187–193.

49 Schroeter AL, Diaz-Perez JL, Winkelmann RK, Jordon RE. Livedo vasculitis (the vasculitis of atrophie blanche). Immunohistopathologic study. Arch Dermatol 1975; 111: 188–193.

50 Bell WR. Disseminated intravascular coagulation. Johns Hopkins Med J 1980; 146: 289–299.

51 Camilleri JP, Finlay AY, Douglas-Jones AG et al. Transient epidermal necrosis associated with disseminated intravascular coagulation in a patient with urticaria. Br J Dermatol 1991; 125: 380–383.

52 Colman RW, Minna JD, Robboy SJ. Disseminated intravascular coagulation: a dermatologic disease. Int J Dermatol 1977; 16: 47–51.

53 Robboy SJ, Colman RW, Minna JD. Pathology of disseminated intravascular coagulation (DIC). Analysis of 26 cases. Hum Pathol 1972; 3: 327–343.

54 Robboy SJ, Mihm MC, Colman RW, Minna JD. The skin in disseminated intravascular coagulation. Br J Dermatol 1973; 88: 221–229.

55 Davis MDP, Byrd J, Lior T et al. Symmetrical peripheral gangrene due to disseminated intravascular coagulation. Arch Dermatol 2001; 137: 139–140.

56 Marlar RA, Endres-Brooks J, Miller C. Serial studies of protein C and its plasma inhibitor in patients with disseminated intravascular coagulation. Blood 1985; 66: 59–63.

57 Silverman RA, Rhodes AR, Dennehy PH. Disseminated intravascular coagulation and purpura fulminans in a patient with candida sepsis. Am J Med 1986; 80: 679–684.

58 Guccione JL, Zemtsov A, Cobos E et al. Acquired purpura fulminans induced by alcohol and acetaminophen. Arch Dermatol 1993; 129: 1267–1269.

59 Patel GK, Morris E, Rashid MR, Anstey AV. Severe digital necrosis in an elderly patient with heterozygous factor V Leiden mutation. Br J Dermatol 2000; 143: 1302–1305.

60 Herbst JS, Raffanti S, Pathy A, Zaiac MN. Dysgonic fermenter type 2 septicemia with purpura fulminans. Dermatologic features of a zoonosis acquired from household pets. Arch Dermatol 1989; 125: 1380–1382.

61 Powars DR, Rogers ZR, Patch MJ et al. Purpura fulminans in meningococcemia: association with acquired deficiencies of proteins C and S. N Engl J Med 1987; 317: 571–572.

62 Hautekeete ML, Berneman ZN, Bieger R et al. Purpura fulminans in pneumococcal sepsis. Arch Intern Med 1986; 146: 497–499.

63 Phillips WG, Marsden JR, Hill FG. Purpura fulminans due to protein S deficiency following chickenpox. Br J Dermatol 1992; 127: 30–32.

64 Yuen P, Cheung A, Lin HJ et al. Purpura fulminans in a Chinese boy with congenital protein C deficiency. Pediatrics 1986; 77: 670–676.

65 Ridolfi RL, Bell WR. Thrombotic thrombocytopenic purpura. Report of 25 cases and review of the literature. Medicine (Baltimore) 1981; 60: 413–428.

66 Amorosi EL, Ultmann JE. Thrombotic thrombocytopenic purpura: report of 16 cases and review of the literature. Medicine (Baltimore) 1966; 45: 139–159.

67 Burruss JB, Cohen LM, Thomas HA, Callen JP. Unilateral emboli in a patient with thrombotic thrombocytopenic purpura. J Am Acad Dermatol 1993; 29: 838–840.

68 Bennett CL, Connors JM, Carwile JM et al. Thrombotic thrombocytopenic purpura associated with clopidogrel. N Engl J Med 2000; 342: 1773–1777.

69 Sallière D, Kassler-Taub KB. Clopidogrel and thrombotic thrombocytopenic purpura. N Engl J Med 2000; 343: 1191.

70 Itin PH, Winkelmann RK. Cutaneous manifestations in patients with essential thrombocythemia. J Am Acad Dermatol 1991; 24: 59–63.

71 Velasco JA, Santos JC, Bravo J, Santana J. Ulceronecrotic lesions in a patient with essential thrombocythaemia. Clin Exp Dermatol 1991; 16: 53–54.

72 Wirth K, Schoepf E, Mertelsmann R, Lindemann A. Leg ulceration with associated thrombocytosis: healing of ulceration associated with treatment of the raised platelet count. Br J Dermatol 1998; 138: 533–535.

73 Stone MS, Robson KJ, Piette WW. Erythematous plaques due to platelet plugging: A clue to underlying myeloproliferative disorder. J Am Acad Dermatol 2000; 43: 355–357.

74 Tamm E, Jungkunz W, Wolter M, Marsch WCh. Immunohistochemical characterization of the 'intimal proliferation' phenomenon in Sneddon's syndrome and essertial thrombocythaemia. Br J Dermatol 1994; 131: 814–821.

75 Michiels JJ, Ten Kate FWJ, Vuzevski VD, Abels J. Histopathology of erythromelalgia in thrombocythaemia. Histopathology 1984; 8: 669–678.

76 Drenth JPH, Vuzevski V, Van Joost T et al. Cutaneous pathology in primary erythermalgia. Am J Dermatopathol 1996; 18: 30–34.

77 Michiels JJ, Drenth JPH, van Genderen PJJ. Classification and diagnosis of erythromelalgia and erythermalgia. Int J Dermatol 1995; 34: 97–100.

78 Heim LR. Cryoglobulins: Characterization and classification. Cutis 1979; 23 259–266.

79 Davis MDP, Su WPD. Cryoglobulinemia: recent findings in cutaneous and extracutaneous manifestations. Int J Dermatol 1996; 35: 240–248.

80 Cohen SJ, Pittelkow MR, Su WPD. Cutaneous manifestations of cryoglobulinemia: Clinical and histopathologic study of seventy-two patients. J Am Acad Dermatol 1991; 25: 21–27.

81 Beightler E, Diven DG, Sanchez RL, Solomon AR. Thrombotic vasculopathy associated with cryofibrinogenemia. J Am Acad Dermatol 1991; 24: 342–345.

82 Appenzeller P, Leith CP, Foucar K et al. Cutaneous Waldenstrom macroglobulinemia in transformation. Am J Dermatopathol 1999; 21: 151–155.

83 Revenga F, Aguilar C, González R et al. Cryofibrinogenaemia with a good response to stanozolol. Clin Exp Dermatol 2000; 25: 621–623.

84 Baughman RD, Sommer RG. Cryoglobulinemia presenting as 'factitial ulceration'. Arch Dermatol 1966; 94: 725–731.

85 Brouet J-C, Clauvel J-P, Danon F et al. Biologic and clinical significance of cryoglobulins. Am J Med 1974; 57: 775–788.

86 Boom BW, Brand A, Bavinck J-NB et al. Severe leukocytoclastic vasculitis of the skin in a patient with essential mixed cryoglobulinemia treated with high-dose gamma-globulin intravenously. Arch Dermatol 1988; 124: 1550–1553.

87 Lin RY, Caren CB, Menikoff H. Hypocomplementaemic urticarial vasculitis, interstitial lung disease and hepatitis C. Br J Dermatol 1995; 132: 821–823.

88 Daoud MS, El-Azhary RA, Gibson LE et al. Chronic hepatitis C, cryoglobulinemia, and cutaneous necrotizing vasculitis. Clinical, pathologic, and immunopathologic study of twelve patients. J Am Acad Dermatol 1996; 34: 219–223.

89 Sepp NT, Umlauft F, Illersperger B et al. Necrotizing vasculitis associated with hepatitis C infection: successful treatment of vasculitis with interferon-alpha despite persistence of mixed cryoglobulinemia. Dermatology 1995; 191: 43–45.

90 Buezo GF, García-Buey M, Rios-Buceta L et al. Cryoglobulinemia and cutaneous leukocytoclastic vasculitis with hepatitis C virus infection. Int J Dermatol 1996 35: 112–115.

91 Dupin N, Chosidow O, Lunel F et al. Essential mixed cryoglobulinemia. Arch Dermatol 1995; 131: 1124–1127.

92 Karlsberg PL, Lee WM, Casey DL et al. Cutaneous vasculitis and rheumatoid factor positivity as presenting signs of hepatitis C virus-induced mixed cryoglobulinemia. Arch Dermatol 1995; 131: 1119–1123.

93 Pakula AS, Garden JM, Roth SI. Cryoglobulinemia and cutaneous leukocytoclastic vasculitis associated with hepatitis C virus infection. J Am Acad Dermatol 1993; 28: 850–853.

94 Romani J, Puig L, de Moragas JM. Detection of antineutrophil cytoplasmic antibodies in patients with hepatitis C virus-induced cutaneous vasculitis with mixed cryoglobulinemia. Arch Dermatol 1996; 132: 974–975.

95 Abe Y, Tanaka Y, Takenaka M et al. Leucocytoclastic vasculitis associated with mixed cryoglobulinaemia and hepatitis C virus infection. Br J Dermatol 1997; 136: 272–274.

96 von Kobyletzki G, Stücker M, Hoffman K et al. Severe therapy-resistant necrotizing vasculitis associated with hepatitis C virus infection: successful treatment of the vasculitis with extracorporeal immunoadsorption. Br J Dermatol 1998; 138: 718–719.

97 Güngör E, Cirit A, Alli N et al. Prevalence of hepatitis C virus antibodies and cryoglobulinemia in patients with leukocytoclastic vasculitis. Dermatology 1998; 198: 26–28.

98 Abajo P, Porras-Luque JI, Buezo GF et al. Red finger syndrome associated with necrotizing vasculitis in an HIV-infected patient with hepatitis B. Br J Dermatol 1998; 139 154–155.

99 Solinas A, Cottoni F, Tanda F, Tocco A. Toxic epidermal necrolysis in a patient affected by mixed essential cryoglobulinemia. J Am Acad Dermatol 1988; 18: 1165–1169.

100 Berliner S, Weinberger A, Ben-Bassat M et al. Small skin blood vessel occlusions by cryoglobulin aggregates in ulcerative lesions in IgM-IgG cryoglobulinemia. J Cutan Pathol 1982; 9: 96–103.

101 Koda H, Kanaide A, Asahi M, Urabe H. Essential IgG cryoglobulinemia with purpura and cold urticaria. Arch Dermatol 1978; 114: 784–786.

102 Gorevic PD, Kassab HJ, Levo Y et al. Mixed cryoglobulinemia: clinical aspects and long-term follow-up of 40 patients. Am J Med 1980; 69: 287–308.

103 Buchsbaum M, Werth V. Erythema nodosum-like nodules associated with vasculitis resulting from mixed cryoglobulinemia. J Am Acad Dermatol 1994; 31: 493–495.

104 Armin AR, Rosenbaum L, Chapman-Winokur R, Hawkins ET. Intravascular immunoglobulin crystalloids in monoclonal cryoglobulinemia-associated dermatitis: ultrastructural findings. J Cutan Pathol 1993; 20: 74–78.

105 Falanga V, Fine MJ, Kapoor WN. The cutaneous manifestations of cholesterol crystal embolization. Arch Dermatol 1986; 122: 1194–1198.

106 Sklar J, Taira JW. Cholesterol emboli syndrome. Int J Dermatol 1993; 32: 607–609.

107 Borrego L, Gil R, Mazuecos A et al. Cholesterol embolism to the skin. Clin Exp Dermatol 1992; 17: 424–426.

108 Dupont PJ, Lightstone L, Clutterbuck EJ et al. Cholesterol emboli syndrome. BMJ 2000; 321: 1065–1066.

109 Kalter DC, Rudolph A, McGavran M. Livedo reticularis due to multiple cholesterol emboli. J Am Acad Dermatol 1985; 13: 235–242.

110 Finch TM, Ryatt KS. Livedo reticularis caused by cholesterol embolization may improve with simvastatin. Br J Dermatol 2000; 143: 1319–1320.

111 Day LL, Aterman K. Hemorrhagic panniculitis caused by atheromatous embolization. A case report and brief review. Am J Dermatopathol 1984; 6: 471–478.

112 Chesney TMcC. Atheromatous embolization to the skin. Am J Dermatopathol 1982; 4: 271–273.

113 Karg K, Botella R, White CR Jr. Subtle clues to the diagnosis of cholesterol embolism. Am J Dermatopathol 1996; 18: 380–384.

114 McAllister SM, Bornstein AM, Callen JP. Painful acral purpura. Arch Dermatol 1998; 134: 789–791.

115 Alegre VA, Winkelmann RK. Histopathologic and immunofluorescence study of skin lesions associated with circulating lupus anticoagulant. J Am Acad Dermatol 1988; 19: 117–124.

116 O'Neill A, Gatenby PA, McGaw B et al. Widespread cutaneous necrosis associated with cardiolipin antibodies. J Am Acad Dermatol 1990; 22: 356–359.

117 Alegre VA, Gastineau DA, Winkelmann RK. Skin lesions associated with circulating lupus anticoagulant. Br J Dermatol 1989; 120: 419–429.

118 Asherson RA, Cervera R. Antiphospholipid syndrome. J Invest Dermatol 1993; 100: 21S–27S.

119 Stephens CJM. The antiphospholipid syndrome. Clinical correlations, cutaneous features, mechanism of thrombosis and treatment of patients with the lupus anticoagulant and anticardiolipin antibodies. Br J Dermatol 1991; 125: 199–210.

120 Gantcheva M. Dermatologic aspects of antiphospholipid syndrome. Int J Dermatol 1998; 37: 173–180.

121 Del Castillo LF, Soria C, Schoendorff C et al. Widespread cutaneous necrosis and antiphospholipid antibodies: Two episodes related to surgical manipulation and urinary tract infection. J Am Acad Dermatol 1997; 36: 872–875.

122 Gibson GE, Su WPD, Pittelkow MR. Antiphospholipid syndrome and the skin. J Am Acad Dermatol 1997; 36: 970–982.

123 Aronoff DM, Callen JP. Necrosing livedo reticularis in a patient with recurrent pulmonary hemorrhage. J Am Acad Dermatol 1997; 37: 300–302.

124 Nahass GT. Antiphospholipid antibodies and the antiphospholipid antibody syndrome. J Am Acad Dermatol 1997; 36: 149–168.

125 Hill VA, Whittaker SJ, Hunt BJ et al. Cutaneous necrosis associated with the antiphospholipid syndrome and mycosis fungoides. Br J Dermatol 1994; 130: 92–96.

126 Vayssairat M, Abuaf N, Baudot N et al. Abnormal IgG cardiolipin antibody titers in patients with Raynaud's phenomenon and/or related disorders: Prevalence and clinical significance. J Am Acad Dermatol 1998; 38: 555–558.

127 Asherson RA, Jacobelli S, Rosenberg H et al. Skin nodules and macules resembling vasculitis in the antiphospholipid syndrome – a report of two cases. Clin Exp Dermatol 1992; 17: 266–269.

128 Ishikawa O, Takahashi A, Tamura A, Miyachi Y. Cutaneous papules and nodules in the diagnosis of the antiphospholipid syndrome. Br J Dermatol 1999; 140: 725–729.

129 Creamer D, Hunt BJ, Black MM. Widespread cutaneous necrosis occurring in association with the antiphospholipid syndrome: a report of two cases. Br J Dermatol 2000; 142: 1199–1203.

130 Gibson GE, Gibson LE, Drage LA et al. Skin necrosis secondary to low-molecular weight heparin in a patient with antiphospholipid antibody syndrome. J Am Acad Dermatol 1997; 37: 855–859.

131 Grossman D, Heald PW, Wang C, Rinder HM. Activated protein C resistance and anticardiolipin antibodies in patients with venous leg ulcers. J Am Acad Dermatol 1997; 37: 409–413.

132 Piette WW. Antiphospholipid antibody syndrome: the problems and the promise. Br J Dermatol 2000; 142: 1080–1083.

133 Ogawa H, Zhao D, Dlott JS et al. Elevated anti-annexin V antibody levels in antiphospholipid syndrome and their involvement in antiphospholipid antibody specificities. Am J Clin Pathol 2000; 114: 619–628.

134 Smith KJ, Skelton HG III, James WD et al. Cutaneous histopathologic findings in 'antiphospholipid syndrome'. Arch Dermatol 1990; 126: 1176–1183.

135 Hughson MD, McCarty GA, Brumback RA. Spectrum of vascular pathology affecting patients with the antiphospholipid syndrome. Hum Pathol 1995; 26: 716–724.

136 Depaire-Duclos F, Gris JC, Dandurand M, Guillot B. Thrombotic Klinefelter syndrome associated with factor V Leiden mutation. Arch Dermatol 1997; 133: 1051–1052.

137 Gaber Y, Siemens H-J, Schmeller W. Resistance to activated protein C due to factor V Leiden mutation: high prevalence in patients with post-thrombotic leg ulcers. Br J Dermatol 2001; 144: 546–548.

138 García-Doval I, Losada A, de la Torre C et al. Abdominal nodules as a presentation of obstruction of the inferior vena cava and factor V Leiden mutation. J Am Acad Dermatol 2000; 42: 862–864.

139 Peus D, von Schmiedeberg S, Pier A et al. Coagulation factor V gene mutation associated with activated protein C resistance leading to recurrent thrombosis, leg ulcers, and lymphedema: successful treatment with intermittent compression. J Am Acad Dermatol 1996; 35: 306–309.

140 Feus D, Heit JA, Pittelkow MR. Activated protein C resistance caused by factor V gene mutation: Common coagulation defect in chronic venous leg ulcers? J Am Acad Dermatol 1997; 36: 616–620.

141 Maessen-Visch MB, Hamulyak K, Tazelaar DJ et al. The prevalence of factor V Leiden mutation in patients with leg ulcers and venous insufficiency. Arch Dermatol 1999; 135: 41–44.

142 Hafner J, Kühne A, Schär B et al. Factor V Leiden mutation in postthrombotic and non-postthrombotic venous ulcers. Arch Dermatol 2001; 137: 599–603.

143 Deffer TA, Berger TG, Gelinas-Sorell D. Sneddon's syndrome. A case report. J Am Acad Dermatol 1987; 16: 1084–1087.

144 Marsch WC, Muckelmann R. Generalized racemose livedo with cerebrovascular lesions (Sneddon syndrome): an occlusive arteriolopathy due to proliferation and migration of medial smooth muscle cells. Br J Dermatol 1985; 112: 703–708.

145 Grattan CEH, Burton JL, Boon AP. Sneddon's syndrome (livedo reticularis and cerebral thrombosis) with livedo vasculitis and anticardiolipin antibodies. Br J Dermatol 1989; 120: 441–447.

146 Zelger B, Sepp N, Stockhammer G et al. Sneddon's syndrome. A long-term follow-up of 21 patients. Arch Dermatol 1993; 129: 437–447.

147 Francès C, Le Tonquèze M, Salohzin KV et al. Prevalence of anti-endothelial cell antibodies in patients with Sneddon's syndrome. J Am Acad Dermatol 1995; 33: 64–68.

148 Sepp N, Zelger B, Schuler G et al. Sneddon's syndrome – an inflammatory disorder of small arteries followed by smooth muscle proliferation. Am J Surg Pathol 1995; 19: 448–453.

149 Zelger B, Sepp N, Schmid KW et al. Life history of cutaneous vascular lesions in Sneddon's syndrome. Hum Pathol 1992; 23: 668–675.

150 Lipsker D, Piette JC, Laporte JL et al. Annular atrophic lichen planus and Sneddon's syndrome. Dermatology 1997; 195: 402–403.

151 Gottlöber P, Bezold G, Schaer A et al. Sneddon's syndrome in a child. Br J Dermatol 2000; 142: 374–376.

152 Francès C, Piette JC. The mystery of Sneddon syndrome: relationship with antiphospholipid syndrome and systemic lupus erythematosus. J Autoimmun 2000; 15: 139–143.

153 Walsh JS, Perniciaro C, Meschia JF. CADASIL (cerebral autosomal dominant arteriopathy with subcortical infarcts and leukoencephalopathy): Diagnostic skin biopsy changes determined by electron microscopy. J Am Acad Dermatol 2000; 43: 1125–1127.

154 Rumbaugh JA, LaDuca JR, Shan Y, Miller CA. CADASIL: The dermatologic diagnosis of a neurologic disease. J Am Acad Dermatol 2000; 43: 1128–1130.

155 Fitzpatrick JE, Johnson C, Simon P, Owenby J. Cutaneous microthrombi: a histologic clue to the diagnosis of hypereosinophilic syndrome. Am J Dermatopathol 1987; 9: 419–422.

156 Miller JA, Machin SJ, Dowd PM. Cutaneous gangrene with hyperparathyroidism. Clin Exp Dermatol 1988; 13: 204–206.

157 Dahl PR, Winkelmann RK, Connolly SM. The vascular calcification-cutaneous necrosis syndrome. J Am Acad Dermatol 1995; 33: 53–58.

158 Hafner J, Keusch G, Wahl C et al. Uremic small-artery disease with medial calcification and intimal hyperplasia (so-called calciphylaxis): a complication of chronic renal failure and benefit from parathyroidectomy. J Am Acad Dermatol 1995; 33: 954–962.

159 Miller SJ. The dermatologist and protein C. J Am Acad Dermatol 1988; 19: 904–907.

160 Marlar RA, Adcock DM. Clinical evaluation of protein C: a comparative review of antigenic and functional assays. Hum Pathol 1989; 20: 1040–1047.

161 Weir NU, Snowden JA, Greaves M, Davies-Jones GAB. Livedo reticularis associated with hereditary protein C deficiency and recurrent thromboembolism. Br J Dermatol 1995; 132: 283–285.

162 Park JY, Kanzler M, Swetter SM. Dopamine-associated symmetric peripheral gangrene. Arch Dermatol 1997; 133: 247–249.

163 Lin R-Y, Du S-L, Yeh H-S, Wang W-M. Vasopressin-induced amber-like skin necrosis. Dermatology 1997; 195: 271–273.

164 Clark SM, Lanigan SW. Acute necrotic skin reaction to intramuscular Depo-Provera®. Br J Dermatol 2000; 143: 1356–1357.

165 Yates P, Jones S. Heparin skin necrosis – an important indicator of potentially fatal heparin hypersensitivity. Clin Exp Dermatol 1993; 18: 138–141.

166 Mar AW-Y, Dixon B, Ibrahim K, Parkin JD. Skin necrosis following subcutaneous heparin injection. Australas J Dermatol 1995; 36: 201–203.

167 Santamaria A, Romani J, Souto JC et al. Skin necrosis at the injection site induced by low-molecular-weight heparin: case report and review. Dermatology 1998; 196: 264–265.

168 Köhler LD, Schwedler S, Worret WI. Embolia cutis medicamentosa. Int J Dermatol 1997; 36: 197.

169 Heng MCY, Haberfeld G. Thrombotic phenomena associated with intravenous cocaine. J Am Acad Dermatol 1987; 16: 462–468.

170 Menni S, Boccardi D, Coggi A. Skin necrosis caused by flunitrazepam abuse. Acta Derm Venereol 1999; 79: 171.

171 Rupec RA, Kind P, Ruzicka T. Cutaneous manifestations of congenital afibrinogenaemia. Br J Dermatol 1996; 134: 548–550.

172 Stapleton SR, Curley RK, Simpson WA. Cutaneous gangrene secondary to focal thrombosis – an important cutaneous manifestation of ulcerative colitis. Clin Exp Dermatol 1989; 14: 387–389.

173 Jansen T, Romiti R, Messer G et al. Superior vena cava syndrome presenting as persistent erythematous oedema of the face. Clin Exp Dermatol 2000; 25: 198–200.

174 Hoegl L, Thoma-Greber E, Poppinger J, Röcken M. Butyl nitrite-induced acrocyanosis in an HIV-infected patient. Arch Dermatol 1999; 135: 90–91.

175 Goulc JW, Helms SE, Schulz SM, Stevens SR. Relapsing livedo reticularis in the setting of chronic pancreatitis. J Am Acad Dermatol 1998; 39: 1035–1036.

176 Granel B, Genty I, Serratrice J et al. Livedo reticularis revealing a latent infective endocarditis due to Coxiella burnetti. J Am Acad Dermatol 1999; 41: 842–844.

Urticarias

177 Synkowski D, Dore N, Provost TT. Urticaria and urticaria-like lesions. Clin Rheum Dis 1982; 8: 383–395.

178 Monroe EW. Urticaria. Int J Dermatol 1981; 20: 32–41.

179 Black AK, Greaves MW, Champion RH, Pye RJ. The urticarias 1990. Br J Dermatol 1991; 124: 100–108.

180 Juhlin L. Recurrent urticaria: clinical investigation of 330 patients. Br J Dermatol 1981; 104: 369–381.

181 Grattan C, Powell S, Humphreys F. Management and diagnostic guidelines for urticaria and angio-oedema. Br J Dermatol 2001; 144: 708–714.

182 Champion RH. Acute and chronic urticaria. Semin Dermatol 1987; 6: 286–291.

183 Mortureux P, Léauté-Labrèze C, Legrain-Lifermann V et al. Acute urticaria in infancy and early childhood. Arch Dermatol 1998; 134: 319–323.

184 Tamayo-Sanchez L, Ruiz-Maldonado R, Laterza A. Acute annular urticaria in infants and children. Pediatr Dermatol 1997; 14: 231–234.

185 Sibbald RG, Cheema AS, Lozinski A, Tarlo S. Chronic urticaria. Int J Dermatol 1991; 30: 381–386.

186 Bindslev-Jensen C, Finzi A, Greaves M et al. Chronic urticaria: diagnostic recommendations. J Eur Acad Dermatol Venereol 2000; 14: 175–180.

187 Ghosh S, Kanwar AJ, Kaur S. Urticaria in children. Pediatr Dermatol 1993; 10: 107–110.

188 Michaelsson G, Juhlin L. Urticaria induced by preservatives and dye additives in food and drugs. Br J Dermatol 1973; 88: 525–532.

189 Ohnishi-Inoue Y, Mitsuya K, Horio T. Aspirin-sensitive urticaria: provocation with a leukotriene receptor antagonist. Br J Dermatol 1998; 138: 483–485.

190 Irion R, Gall H, Werfel T, Peter R-U. Delayed-type hypersensitivity rash from paracetamol. Contact Dermatitis 2000; 43: 60–61.

191 Wright AL, Minford A. Urticaria and hidden salicylates. Pediatr Dermatol 1999; 16: 463–464.

192 Heng MCY, Kloss SG, Haberfelde GC. Pathogenesis of papular urticaria. J Am Acad Dermatol 1984; 10: 1030–1034.

193 Hannuksela M. Urticaria in children. Semin Dermatol 1987; 6: 321–325.

194 Monroe EW. Urticaria and urticarial vasculitis. Med Clin North Am 1980; 64: 867–883.

195 Gleich GJ, Schroeter AL, Marcoux JP et al. Episodic angioedema associated with eosinophilia. N Engl J Med 1984; 310: 1621–1626.

196 Baty V, Hoen B, Hudziak H et al. Schnitzler's syndrome: two case reports and review of the literature. Mayo Clin Proc 1995; 70: 570–572.

197 Lebbe C, Rybojad M, Klein F et al. Schnitzler's syndrome associated with sensorimotor neuropathy. J Am Acad Dermatol 1994; 30: 316–318.

198 Welsh B, Tate B. Schnitzler's syndrome: report of a case with progression to Waldenström's macroglobulinaemia. Australas J Dermatol 1999; 40: 201–203.

199 Husak R, Nestoris S, Goerdt S, Orfanos CE. Severe course of chronic urticaria, arthralgia, fever and elevation of erythrocyte sedimentation rate: Schnitzler's syndrome without monoclonal gammopathy? Br J Dermatol 2000; 142: 581–582.

200 Saurat JH, Masouyé I, Aractingi S. Schnitzler's syndrome. Clin Exp Dermatol 2000; 25: 336 (abstract).

201 Cianchini G, Bergamo F, Scala E et al. Schnitzler's syndrome: a report of three cases. Clin Exp Dermatol 2000; 25: 341 (abstract).

202 Gallo R, Sabroe RA, Black AK, Greaves MW. Schnitzler's syndrome: no evidence for autoimmune basis in two patients. Clin Exp Dermatol 2000; 25: 281–284.

203 Lipsker D, Spehner D, Drillien R et al. Schnitzler syndrome: heterogeneous immunopathological findings involving IgM-skin interactions. Br J Dermatol 2000; 142: 954–959.

204 Champion RH. Urticaria: then and now. Br J Dermatol 1988; 119: 427–436.

205 Gorevic PD, Kaplan AP. The physical urticarias. Int J Dermatol 1980; 19: 417–435.

206 Sibbald RG. Physical urticaria. Dermatol Clin 1984; 3: 57–69.

207 Jorizzo JL, Smith EB. The physical urticarias. An update and review. Arch Dermatol 1982; 118: 194–201.

208 Briganti S, Cristaudo A, D'Argento V et al. Oxidative stress in physical urticarias. Clin Exp Dermatol 2001; 26: 284–288.

209 Soter NA. Physical urticaria/angioedema. Semin Dermatol 1987; 6: 302–312.

210 Duschet P, Leyen P, Schwarz T et al. Solar urticaria – effective treatment by plasmapheresis. Clin Exp Dermatol 1987; 12: 185–188.

211 Kojima M, Horiko T, Nakamura Y, Aoki T. Solar urticaria. The relationship of photoallergen and action spectrum. Arch Dermatol 1986; 122: 550–555.

212 Neittaanmaki H. Cold urticaria. Clinical findings in 220 patients. J Am Acad Dermatol 1985; 13: 636–644.

213 Lawlor F, Kobza Black A, Breathnach AS et al. A timed study of the histopathology, direct immunofluorescence and ultrastructural findings in idiopathic cold-contact urticaria over a 24-h period. Clin Exp Dermatol 1989; 14: 416–420.

214 Ormerod AD, Smart L, Reid TMS, Milford-Ward A. Familial cold urticaria. Investigation of a family and response to stanozolol. Arch Dermatol 1993; 129: 343–346.

215 Zip CM, Ross JB, Greaves MW et al. Familial cold urticaria. Clin Exp Dermatol 1993; 18: 338–341.

216 Hoffman HM, Wright FA, Broide DH et al. Identification of a locus on chromosome 1q44 for familial cold urticaria. Am J Hum Genet 2000; 66: 1693–1698.

217 Baxter DL Jr, Utecht LM, Yeager JK, Cobb MW. Localized, perifollicular cold urticaria. J Am Acad Dermatol 1992; 26: 306–308.

218 Doeglas HMG, Rijnten WJ, Schroder FP, Schirm J. Cold urticaria and virus infections: a clinical and serological study in 39 patients. Br J Dermatol 1986; 114: 311–318.

219 Black AK. Cold urticaria. Semin Dermatol 1987; 6: 292–301.

220 Freeman PA, Watt GC. Localized heat urticaria (heat contact urticaria). Australas J Dermatol 1988; 29: 43–46.

221 Chang A, Zic JA. Localized heat urticaria. J Am Acad Dermatol 1999; 41: 354–356.

222 Baba T, Nomura K, Hanada K, Hashimoto I. Immediate-type heat urticaria report of a case and study of plasma histamine release. Br J Dermatol 1998; 138: 326–328.

223 Armstrong RB, Horan DB, Silvers DN. Leukocytoclastic vasculitis in urticaria induced by ultraviolet irradiation. Arch Dermatol 1985; 121: 1145–1148.

224 Armstrong RB. Solar urticaria. Dermatol Clin 1986; 4: 253–259.

225 Horio T, Fujigaki K. Augmentation spectrum in solar urticaria. J Am Acad Dermatol 1988; 18: 1189–1193.

226 Farr PM. Solar urticaria. Br J Dermatol 2000; 142: 4–5.

227 Uetsu N, Miyauchi-Hashimoto H, Okamoto H, Horio T. The clinical and photobiological characteristics of solar urticaria in 40 patients. Br J Dermatol 2000; 142: 32–38.

228 Alora MBT, Taylor CR. Solar urticaria: Case report and phototesting with lasers. J Am Acad Dermatol 1998; 38: 341–343.

229 Harris A, Burge SM, George SA. Solar urticaria in an infant. Br J Dermatol 1997; 136: 105–107.

230 Roelandts R, Ryckaert S. Solar urticaria: the annoying photodermatosis. Int J Dermatol 1999; 38: 411–418.

231 Horio T. Solar urticaria. Clin Exp Dermatol 2000; 25: 332–333 (abstract).

232 Beissert S, Ständer H, Schwarz T. UVA rush hardening for the treatment of solar urticaria. J Am Acad Dermatol 2000; 42: 1030–1032.

233 Leenutaphong V. Solar urticaria induced by UVA and inhibited by visible light. J Am Acad Dermatol 1993; 29: 337–340.

234 Watanabe M, Matsunaga Y, Katayama I. Solar urticaria: a consideration of the mechanism of inhibition spectra. Dermatology 1999; 198: 252–255.

235 Ryckaert S, Roelandts R. Solar urticaria. A report of 25 cases and difficulties in phototesting. Arch Dermatol 1998; 134: 71–74.

236 Patel GK, Gould DJ, Hawk JLM, McGregor JM. A complex photodermatosis: solar urticaria progressing to polymorphic light eruption. Clin Exp Dermatol 1998; 23: 77–78.

237 Reinauer S, Leenutaphong V, Hölzle E. Fixed solar urticaria. J Am Acad Dermatol 1993; 29: 161–165.

238 Yap LM, Foley PA, Crouch RB, Baker CS. Drug-induced solar urticaria due to tetracycline. Australas J Dermatol 2000; 41: 181–184.

239 Bonnetblanc JM, Andrieu-Pfahl F, Meraud JP, Roux J. Familial aquagenic urticaria. Dermatologica 1979; 158: 468–470.

240 Hide M, Yamamura Y, Sanada S, Yamamoto S. Aquagenic urticaria: a case report. Acta Derm Venereol 2000; 80: 148–149.

241 Ferguson JE, August PJ, Guy AJ. Aquagenic pruritus associated with metastatic squamous cell carcinoma of the cervix. Clin Exp Dermatol 1994; 19: 257–258.

242 Fearfield LA, Gazzard B, Bunker CB. Aquagenic urticaria and human immunodeficiency virus infection: treatment with stanozolol. Br J Dermatol 1997; 137: 620–622.

243 Archer CB, Greaves MG. Aquagenic pruritus. Semin Dermatol 1988; 7: 301–303.

244 Bircher AJ, Meier-Ruge W. Aquagenic pruritus. Water-induced activation of acetylcholinesterase. Arch Dermatol 1988; 124: 84–89.

245 Wolf R, Krakowski A. Variations in aquagenic pruritus and treatment alternatives. J Am Acad Dermatol 1988; 18: 1081–1083.

246 Shelley WB, Shelley ED. Aquadynia: Noradrenergic pain induced by bathing and responsive to clonidine. J Am Acad Dermatol 1998; 38: 357–358.

247 Spelman L, Dicker T. Aquagenic pruritus relieved by tight fitting clothing. Australas J Dermatol 2001; 42: 146.

248 Ho me SA, Anstey AV. Aquagenic pruritus responding to intermittent photochemotherapy. Clin Exp Dermatol 2001; 26: 40–41.

249 Steinman HK, Greaves MW. Aquagenic pruritus. J Am Acad Dermatol 1985; 13: 91–96.

250 Lawlor F, Black AK, Ward AM et al. Delayed pressure urticaria, objective evaluation of a variable disease using a dermographometer and assessment of treatment using colchicine. Br J Dermatol 1989; 120: 403–408.

251 Lawlor F, Barr R, Kobza-Black A et al. Arachidonic acid transformation is not stimulated in delayed pressure urticaria. Br J Dermatol 1989; 121: 317–321.

252 Dover JS, Black AK, Ward AM, Greaves MW. Delayed pressure urticaria. Clinical features, laboratory investigations, and response to therapy of 44 patients. J Am Acad Dermatol 1988; 18: 1289–1298.

253 Warin RP. Clinical observations on delayed pressure urticaria. Br J Dermatol 1989; 121: 225–228.

254 Barlow RJ, Warburton F, Watson K et al. Diagnosis and incidence of delayed pressure urticaria in patients with chronic urticaria. J Am Acad Dermatol 1993; 29: 954–958.

255 Mijailović BB, Karadaglić DM, Ninković MP et al. Bullous delayed pressure urticaria; pressure testing may produce a systemic reaction. Br J Dermatol 1997; 136: 434–436.

256 Poon E, Seed PT, Greaves MW, Kobza-Black A. The extent and nature of disability in different urticarial conditions. Br J Dermatol 1999; 140: 667–671.

257 Czarnetzki BM, Meentken J, Kolde G, Brocker E-B. Morphology of the cellular infiltrate in delayed pressure urticaria. J Am Acad Dermatol 1985; 12: 253–259.

258 McEvoy MT, Peterson EA, Kobza-Black A et al. Immunohistological comparison of granulated cell proteins in induced immediate urticarial dermographism and delayed pressure urticaria lesions. Br J Dermatol 1995; 133: 853–860.

259 Lawlor F, Kobza-Black A, Murdoch RD, Greaves MW. Symptomatic dermographism: wealing, mast cells and histamine are decreased in the skin following long-term application of a potent topical corticosteroid. Br J Dermatol 1989; 121: 629–634.

260 Burdick AE, Mathias CGT. The contact urticaria syndrome. Dermatol Clin 1985; 3: 71–84.

261 Turjanmaa K, Reunala T, Rasanen L. Comparison of diagnostic methods in latex surgical glove contact urticaria. Contact Dermatitis 1988; 19: 241–247.

262 Kligman AM. The spectrum of contact urticaria. Wheals, erythema and pruritus. Dermatol Clin 1990; 8: 57–60.

263 Pecquet C, Leynadier F, Dry J. Contact urticaria and anaphylaxis to natural latex. J Am Acad Dermatol 1990; 22: 631–633.

264 Wakelin S. Contact urticaria. Clin Exp Dermatol 2000; 25: 332 (abstract).

265 Wakelin SH. Contact urticaria. Clin Exp Dermatol 2001; 26: 132–136.

266 Kanerva L, Estlander T, Jolanki R. Long-lasting contact urticaria from castor bean. J Am Acad Dermatol 1990; 23: 351–355.

267 Oliver F, Amon EU, Breathnach A et al. Contact urticaria due to the common stinging nettle (Urtica dioica) – histological, ultrastructural and pharmacologic studies. Clin Exp Dermatol 1991; 16: 1–7.

268 Valsecchi R, Leghissa P, Cortinovis R et al. Contact urticaria from latex in healthcare workers. Dermatology 2000; 201: 127–131.

269 Holmes G, Freeman S. Cheilitis caused by contact urticaria to mint flavoured toothpaste. Australas J Dermatol 2001; 42: 43–45.

270 Wantke F, Focke M, Hemmer W et al. Generalized urticaria induced by a diethyltoluamide-containing insect repellent in a child. Contact Dermatitis 1996; 35: 186–187.

271 Torresani C, Periti I, Beski L. Contact urticaria syndrome from formaldehyde with multiple physical urticarias. Contact Dermatitis 1996; 35: 174–175.

272 Ikeda I, Ogawa T, Ono T. Tofu-induced urticarial contact dermatitis. Arch Dermatol 2000; 136: 127–128.

273 Alam M, Gross EA, Savin RC. Severe urticarial reaction to diphenyl cylopropenone therapy for alopecia areata. J Am Acad Dermatol 1999; 40: 110–112.

274 Lahti A, Maibach HI. Immediate contact reactions: contact urticaria syndrome. Semin Dermatol 1987; 6: 313–320.

275 Von Krogh G, Maibach HI. The contact urticaria syndrome – an updated review. J Am Acad Dermatol 1981; 5: 328–342.

276 Sackey AH. Recurrent generalised urticaria at insulin injection sites. BMJ 2000; 321: 1449.

277 Jorizzo JL. Cholinergic urticaria. Arch Dermatol 1987; 123: 455–457.

278 Berth-Jones J, Graham-Brown RAC. Cholinergic pruritus, erythema and urticaria: a disease spectrum responding to danazol. Br J Dermatol 1989; 121: 235–237.

279 Hanakawa Y, Tohyama M, Shirakata Y et al. Food-dependent exercise-induced anaphylaxis: a case related to the amount of food allergen ingested. Br J Dermatol 1998; 138: 898–900.

280 Itakura E, Urabe K, Yasumoto S et al. Cholinergic urticaria associated with acquired generalized hypohidrosis: report of a case and review of the literature. Br J Dermatol 2000; 143: 1064–1066.

281 Mayou SC, Kobza-Black A, Eady RAJ, Greaves MW. Cholinergic dermographism. Br J Dermatol 1986; 115: 371–377.

282 Ormerod AD, Kobza-Black A, Milford-Ward A, Greaves MW. Combined cold urticaria and cholinergic urticaria – clinical characterization and laboratory findings. Br J Dermatol 1988; 118: 621–627.

283 Zuberbier T, Althaus C, Chantraine-Hess S, Czarnetzki BM. Prevalence of cholinergic urticaria in young adults. J Am Acad Dermatol 1994; 31: 978–981.

284 Casale TB, Keahey TM, Kaliner M. Exercise-induced anaphylactic syndromes. JAMA 1986; 255: 2049–2053.

285 Hirschmann JV, Lawlor F, English JSC et al. Cholinergic urticaria. A clinical and histologic study. Arch Dermatol 1987; 123: 462–467.

286 Warin RP, Cunliffe WJ, Greaves MW, Wallington TB. Recurrent angioedema: familial and oestrogen-induced. Br J Dermatol 1986; 115: 731–734.

287 Jorizzo JL. Classification of urticaria and the reactive inflammatory vascular dermatoses. Dermatol Clin 1985; 3: 3–28.

288 Agostoni A. Hereditary angioedema. Clin Exp Dermatol 2000; 25: 337–338 (abstract).

289 Heymann WR. Acquired angioedema. J Am Acad Dermatol 1997; 36: 611–615.

290 Sabroe RA, Kobza Black A. Angiotensin-converting enzyme (ACE) inhibitors and angio-oedema. Br J Dermatol 1997; 136: 153–158.

291 Sabroe RA, Black AK. Drug-induced angioedema. Clin Exp Dermatol 2000; 25: 338 (abstract).

292 Miyagawa S, Takahashi Y, Nagai A et al. Angio-oedema in a neonate with IgG antibodies to parvovirus B19 following intrauterine parvovirus B19 infection. Br J Dermatol 2000; 143: 428–430.

293 Gammon WR. Manifestations of drug reactions: urticaria and cutaneous necrotizing venulitis. Clin Dermatol 1986; 4: 50–57.

294 Bielory L, Yancey KB, Young NS et al. Cutaneous manifestations of serum sickness in patients receiving antithymocyte globulin. J Am Acad Dermatol 1985; 13: 411–417.

295 Hebert AA, Sigman ES, Levy ML. Serum sickness-like reactions from cefaclor in children. J Am Acad Dermatol 1991; 25: 805–808.

296 Humphreys F, Hunter JAA. The characteristics of urticaria in 390 patients. Br J Dermatol 1998; 138: 635–638.

297 Tebbe B, Geilen CC, Schulzke J-D et al. *Helicobacter pylori* infection and chronic urticaria. J Am Acad Dermatol 1996; 34: 685–686.

298 Liutu M, Kalimo K, Uksila J, Kalimo H. Etiologic aspects of chronic urticaria. Int J Dermatol 1998; 37: 515–519.

299 Hizal M, Tüzün B, Wolf R, Tüzün Y. The relationship between Helicobacter pylori IgG antibody and autologous serum test in chronic urticaria. Int J Dermatol 2000; 39: 443–445.

300 Radenhausen M, Schulzke J-D, Geilen CC et al. Frequent presence of *Helicobacter pylori* infection in chronic urticaria. Acta Derm Venereol 2000; 80: 48–49.

301 Wustlich S, Brehler R, Luger TA et al. *Helicobacter pylori* as a possible bacterial focus of chronic urticaria. Dermatology 1999; 198: 130–132.

302 Daudén E, Jiménez-Alonso I, García-Díez A. *Helicobacter pylori* and idiopathic chronic urticaria. Int J Dermatol 2000; 39: 446–452.

303 Höök-Nikanne J, Varjonen E, Harvima RJ, Kosunen TU. Is *Helicobacter pylori* infection associated with chronic urticaria? Acta Derm Venereol 2000; 80: 425–426.

304 Stephens CJM, Black MM. Perimenstrual eruptions: autoimmune progesterone dermatitis. Semin Dermatol 1989; 8: 26–29.

305 Miura T, Matsuda M, Yanbe H, Sugiyama S. Two cases of autoimmune progesterone dermatitis. Immunohistochemical and serological studies. Acta Derm Venereol 1989; 69: 308–310.

306 Yee KC, Cunliffe WJ. Progesterone-induced urticaria: response to buserelin. Br J Dermatol 1994; 130: 121–123.

307 Shahar E, Bergman R, Pollack S. Autoimmune progesterone dermatitis: effective prophylactic treatment with danazol. Int J Dermatol 1997; 36: 708–711.

308 Wilkinson SM, Beck MH, Kingston TP. Progesterone-induced urticaria – need it be autoimmune? Br J Dermatol 1995; 133: 792–794.

309 Lee A-Y, Lee K-H, Kim Y-G. Oestrogen urticaria associated with pregnancy. Br J Dermatol 1999; 141: 774.

310 Kanazawa K, Yaoita H, Tsuda F, Okamoto H. Hepatitis C virus infection in patients with urticaria. J Am Acad Dermatol 1996; 35: 195–198.

311 Smith R, Caul EO, Burton JL. Urticaria and hepatitis C. Br J Dermatol 1997; 136: 980.

312 Cribier BJ, Santinelli F, Schmitt C et al. Chronic urticaria is not significantly associated with hepatitis C or hepatitis G infection. Arch Dermatol 1999; 135: 1335–1339.

313 Bridges AG, Helm TN, Bergfeld WF et al. Interleukin-3-induced urticaria-like eruption. J Am Acad Dermatol 1996; 34: 1076–1078.

314 Worm M, Sterry W, Zuberbier T. Gelatin-induced urticaria and anaphylaxis after tick-borne encephalitis vaccine. Acta Derm Venereol 2000; 80: 232.

315 Barbaud A, Tréchot P, Reichert-Pénétrat S et al. Allergic mechanisms and urticaria/angioedema after hepatitis B immunization. Br J Dermatol 1998; 139: 925–926.

316 Emonet S, Hogendijk S, Voegeli J et al. Ethanol-induced urticaria: elevated tryptase levels after double-blind, placebo-controlled challenge. Dermatology 1998; 197: 181–182.

317 Smith KE, Fenske NA. Cutaneous manifestations of alcohol abuse. J Am Acad Dermatol 2000; 43: 1–16.

318 Kimura M, Kawada A, Hiruma M, Ishibashi A. A case of urticarial drug eruption from loxoprofen sodium. Clin Exp Dermatol 1997; 22: 303–304.

319 Pollock B, Wilkinson SM, MacDonald Hull SP. Chronic urticaria associated with intra-articular methylprednisolone. Br J Dermatol 2001; 144: 1228–1230.

320 Rubeiz NG, Salem Z, Dibbs R, Kibbi A-G. Bleomycin-induced urticarial flagellate drug hypersensitivity drug reaction. Int J Dermatol 1999; 38: 140–141.

321 Karamfilov T, Wilmer A, Hipler U-C, Wollina U. Cetirizine-induced urticarial reaction. Br J Dermatol 1999; 140: 979–980.

322 Calista D, Schianchi S, Morri M. Urticaria induced by cetirizine. Br J Dermatol 2001; 144: 196.

323 Kontoleon P, Ilias I, Stavropoulos PG, Papapetrou PD. Urticaria after administration of alendronate. Acta Derm Venereol 2000; 80: 398.

324 Landau M, Schachar E, Brenner S. Minocycline-induced serum sickness-like reaction. J Eur Acad Dermatol Venereol 2000; 14: 67–68.

325 Reinhold U, Bruske T, Schupp G. Paraneoplastic urticaria in a patient with ovarian carcinoma. J Am Acad Dermatol 1996; 35: 988–989.

326 Lee IW, Ahn SK, Choi EH, Lee SH. Urticarial reaction following the inhalation of nicotine in tobacco smoke. Br J Dermatol 1998; 138: 486–488.

327 Pirrotta L, Scala E, Giani M et al. Occupational chronic urticaria by Anisakis simplex. A case report. Clin Exp Dermatol 2000; 25: 341 (abstract).

328 Daschner A, Alonso-Gómez A, Caballero T et al. Gastric anisakiasis: an underestimated cause of acute urticaria and angio-oedema? Br J Dermatol 1998; 139: 822–828.

329 Fairley JA, Suchniak J, Paller AS. Hedgehog hives. Arch Dermatol 1999; 135: 561–563.

330 Dunlop K, Freeman S. Caterpillar dermatitis. Australas J Dermatol 1997; 38: 193–195.

331 Heymann WR. Chronic urticaria and angioedema associated with thyroid autoimmunity: Review and therapeutic implications. J Am Acad Dermatol 1999; 40: 229–232.

332 Turktas I, Gokcora N, Demirsoy S et al. The association of chronic urticaria and angioedema with autoimmune thyroiditis. Int J Dermatol 1997; 36: 187–190.

333 Cohen C, Geller B, Whang EJ et al. Adult Still's disease presenting as serum sickness. Int J Dermatol 1997; 36: 928–931.

334 Setterfield JF, Hughes GRV, Kobza Black A. Urticaria as a presentation of adult Still's disease. Br J Dermatol 1998; 138: 906–908.

335 Ramet J, Desprechins B, Otten J, De Raeve L. Chronic, infantile, neurological, cutaneous, and articular syndrome in a neonate: a case report. Arch Dermatol 2000; 136: 431–433.

336 Shelley WB, Shelley ED. Delayed pressure urticaria syndrome: a clinical expression of interleukin 1. Acta Derm Venereol 1987; 67: 438–441.

337 Barlow RJ, Ross EL, MacDonald D et al. Adhesion molecule expression and the inflammatory cell infiltrate in delayed pressure urticaria. Br J Dermatol 1994; 131: 341–347.

338 Leenutaphong V, Holzle E, Plewig G. Pathogenesis and classification of solar urticaria: a new concept. J Am Acad Dermatol 1989; 21: 237–240.

339 Czarnetzki BM. Mechanisms and mediators in urticaria. Semin Dermatol 1987; 6: 272–285.

340 Toyoda M, Maruyama T, Morohashi M, Bhawan J. Free eosinophil granules in urticaria. A correlation with the duration of wheals. Am J Dermatopathol 1996; 18: 49–57.

341 Niimi N, Francis DM, Kermani F et al. Dermal mast cell activation by autoantibodies against the high affinity IgE receptor in chronic urticaria. J Invest Dermatol 1996; 106: 1001–1006.

342 Sabroe RA, Greaves MW. The pathogenesis of chronic idiopathic urticaria. Arch Dermatol 1997; 133: 1003–1008.

343 Sabroe RA, Grattan CEH, Francis DM et al. The autologous serum skin test: a screening test for autoantibodies in chronic idiopathic urticaria. Br J Dermatol 1999; 140: 446–452.

344 Sabroe RA, Seed PT, Francis DM et al. Chronic idiopathic urticaria: Comparison of the clinical features of patients with and without anti-FcεRI or anti-IgE autoantibodies. J Am Acad Dermatol 1999; 40: 443–450.

345 O'Donnell BF, O'Neill CM, Francis DM et al. Human leucocyte antigen class II associations in chronic idiopathic urticaria. Br J Dermatol 1999; 140: 853–858.

346 O'Donnell BF, Barr RM, Kobza Black A et al. Intravenous immunoglobulin in autoimmune chronic urticaria. Br J Dermatol 1998; 138: 101–106.

347 Grattan CEH, O'Donnell BF, Francis DM et al. Randomized double-blind study of cyclosporin in chronic 'idiopathic' urticaria. Br J Dermatol 2000; 143: 365–372.

348 Kozel MMA, Mekkes JR, Bossuyt PMM, Bos JD. The effectiveness of a history-based diagnostic approach in chronic urticaria and angioedema. Arch Dermatol 1998; 134: 1575–1580.

349 Synkowski DR, Levine MI, Rabin BS, Yunis EJ. Urticaria. An immunofluorescence and histopathology study. Arch Dermatol 1979; 115: 1192–1194.

350 Haas N, Toppe E, Henz BM. Microscopic morphology of different types of urticaria. Arch Dermatol 1998; 34: 41–46.

351 Sánchez JL, Benmamán O. Clinicopathological correlation in chronic urticaria. Am J Dermatopathol 1992; 14: 220–223.

352 Leiferman KM, Norris PG, Murphy GM et al. Evidence for eosinophil degranulation with deposition of granule major basic protein in solar urticaria. J Am Acad Dermatol 1989; 21: 75–80.

353 Winkelmann RK, Black AK, Dover J, Greaves MW. Pressure urticaria – histopathological study. Clin Exp Dermatol 1986; 11: 139–147.

354 Norris PG, Murphy GM, Hawk JLM, Winkelmann RK. A histological study of the evolution of solar urticaria. Arch Dermatol 1988; 124: 80–83.

355 Winkelmann RK. The histology and immunopathology of dermographism J Cutan Pathol 1985; 12: 486–492.

356 Rantanen T, Suhonen R. Solar urticaria: a case with increased skin mast cells and good therapeutic response to an antihistamine. Acta Derm Venereol 1980; 60: 363–365.

357 Peters MS, Winkelmann RK. Neutrophilic urticaria. Br J Dermatol 1985; 113: 25–30.

358 Winkelmann RK, Reizner GT. Diffuse dermal neutrophilia in urticaria. Hum Pathol 1988; 19: 389–393.

359 Winkelmann RK, Wilson-Jones E, Smith NP et al. Neutrophilic urticaria. Acta Derm Venereol 1988; 68: 129–133.

360 Toppe E, Haas N, Henz BM. Neutrophilic urticaria: clinical features, histological changes and possible mechanisms. Br J Dermatol 1998; 138: 248–253.

361 Gammon WR, Wheeler CE Jr. Urticarial vasculitis. Report of a case and review of the literature. Arch Dermatol 1979; 115: 76–80.

362 Callen JP, Kalbfleisch S. Urticarial vasculitis: a report of nine cases and review of the literature. Br J Dermatol 1982; 107: 87–94.

363 Sanchez NP, Winkelmann RK, Schroeter AL, Dicken CH. The clinical and histopathologic spectrums of urticarial vasculitis: study of forty cases. J Am Acad Dermatol 1982; 7: 599–605.

364 Russell Jones R, Eady RAJ. Endothelial cell pathology as a marker for urticaria vasculitis: a light microscopic study. Br J Dermatol 1984; 110: 139–149.

365 Monroe EW. Urticarial vasculitis. Semin Dermatol 1987; 6: 328–333.

366 Wanderer AA, Nuss DD, Tormey AD, Giclas PC. Urticarial leukocytoclastic vasculitis with cold urticaria. Arch Dermatol 1983; 119: 145–151.

367 Eady RAJ, Keahey TM, Sibbald RG, Black AK. Cold urticaria with vasculitis: report of a case with light and electron microscopic, immunofluorescence and pharmacological studies. Clin Exp Dermatol 1981; 6: 355–366.

368 Aboobaker J, Greaves MW. Urticarial vasculitis. Clin Exp Dermatol 1986; 11: 436–444.

369 Monroe EW. Urticarial vasculitis: an updated review. J Am Acad Dermatol 1981; 5: 88–95.

370 Monroe EW, Schulz CI, Maize JC, Jordon RE. Vasculitis in chronic urticaria: an immunopathologic study. J Invest Dermatol 1981; 76: 103–107.

371 Peteiro C, Toribio J. Incidence of leukocytoclastic vasculitis in chronic idiopathic urticaria. Study of 100 cases. Am J Dermatopathol 1989; 11: 528–533.

372 English JSC, Murphy GM, Winkelmann RK, Bhogal B. A sequential histopathological study of dermographism. Clin Exp Dermatol 1988; 13: 314–317.

373 Jordaan HF, Schneider JW. Papular urticaria: a histopathologic study of 30 patients. Am J Dermatopathol 1997; 19: 119–126.

374 DiLeonardo M. Urticaria vs. urticarial lesions of bullous pemphigoid vs. papular urticaria. Dermatopathology: Practical & Conceptual 1996; 2: 39–40.

Acute vasculitis

375 Sams WM Jr. Necrotizing vasculitis. J Am Acad Dermatol 1980; 3: 1–13.

376 Ryan TJ. Cutaneous vasculitis. J Cutan Pathol 1985; 12: 381–387.

377 Mooney EE, Shea CR. Cutaneous vasculitis. Curr Diagn Pathol 1997; 4: 1–9.

378 Conn DL. Update on systemic necrotizing vasculitis. Mayo Clin Proc 1989; 64: 535–543.

379 Dowd SK, Rodgers GC, Callen JP. Effective treatment with α_1-protease inhibitor of chronic cutaneous vasculitis associated with α_1-antitrypsin deficiency. J Am Acad Dermatol 1995; 33: 913–916.

380 Parums DV. The arteritides. Histopathology 1994; 25: 1–20.

381 Kelly RI. Cutaneous vasculitis and cutaneous vasculopathies. Australas J Dermatol 1995; 36: 109–119.

382 Cavallo T. Pathologic approach to the diagnosis of vasculitis. Curr Diagn Pathol 1998; 5: 73–81.

383 Magro CM, Crowson AN. The cutaneous neutrophilic vascular injury syndromes. Semin Diagn Pathol 2001; 18: 47–58.

384 Callen JP. Cutaneous vasculitis. What have we learned in the past 20 years? Arch Dermatol 1998; 134: 355–357.

385 Mackel SE, Jordon RE. Leukocytoclastic vasculitis. A cutaneous expression of immune complex disease. Arch Dermatol 1982; 118: 296–301.

386 Jennette CJ, Milling DM, Falk RJ. Vasculitis affecting the skin. Arch Dermatol 1994; 130: 899–906.

387 Jorizzo JL, Solomon AR, Zanolli MD, Leshin B. Neutrophilic vascular reactions. J Am Acad Dermatol 1988; 19: 983–1005.

388 Zax RH, Hodge SJ, Callen JP. Cutaneous leukocytoclastic vasculitis. Serial histopathologic evaluation demonstrates the dynamic nature of the infiltrate. Arch Dermatol 1990; 126: 69–72.

389 Smoller BR, McNutt NS, Contreras F. The natural history of vasculitis. What the histology tells us about pathogenesis. Arch Dermatol 1990; 126: 84–89.

390 Sams WM Jr. Immunologic aspects of cutaneous vasculitis. Semin Dermatol 1988; 7: 140–148.

391 Ramsay C, Fry L. Allergic vasculitis: clinical and histological features and incidence of renal involvement. Br J Dermatol 1969; 81: 96–102.

392 Sams WM Jr. Hypersensitivity angiitis. J Invest Dermatol 1989; 93: 78s–81s.

393 Lotti T, Comacchi C, Ghersetich I. Cutaneous necrotizing vasculitis. Int J Dermatol 1996; 35: 457–474.

394 Ekenstam EA, Callen JP. Cutaneous leukocytoclastic vasculitis. Clinical and laboratory features of 82 patients seen in private practice. Arch Dermatol 1984; 120: 484–489.

395 Hodge SJ, Callen JP, Ekenstam E. Cutaneous leukocytoclastic vasculitis: correlation of histopathological changes with clinical severity and course. J Cutan Pathol 1987; 14: 279–284.

396 Gougerot H, Duperrat B. The nodular allergides of Gougerot. Br J Dermatol 1954; 66: 283–286.

397 Ratnam KV, Boon YH, Pang BK. Idiopathic hypersensitivity vasculitis: clinicopathologic correlation of 61 cases. Int J Dermatol 1995; 34: 786–789.

398 Hafeez ZH. Unusual presentation of cutaneous vasculitis. Int J Dermatol 1998; 37: 687–690.

399 Diaz LA, Provost TT, Tomasi TB Jr. Pustular necrotizing angiitis. Arch Dermatol 1973; 108: 114–118.

400 Branford WA, Farr PM, Porter DI. Annular vasculitis of the head and neck in a patient with sarcoidosis. Br J Dermatol 1982; 106: 713–716.

401 Kelly FI, Cook MG, Marsden RA. Annular vasculitis associated with pregnancy. Br J Dermatol 1993; 129: 599–601.

402 Cribier B, Cuny JF, Schubert B et al. Recurrent annular erythema with purpura: a new variant of leucocytoclastic vasculitis responsive to dapsone. Br J Dermatol 1996; 135: 972–975.

403 Nousari HC, Kimyai-Asadi A, Stone JH. Annular leukocytoclastic vasculitis associated with monoclonal gammopathy of unknown significance. J Am Acad Dermatol 2000; 43: 955–957.

404 Fauci AS. The spectrum of vasculitis. Clinical, pathologic, immunologic, and therapeutic considerations. Ann Intern Med 1978; 89: 660–676.

405 Sais G, Vidaller A, Jucglà A et al. Prognostic factors in leukocytoclastic vasculitis. A clinicopathologic study of 160 patients. Arch Dermatol 1998; 134: 309–315.

406 Cribier B, Couilliet D, Meyer P, Grosshans E. The severity of histopathological changes of leukocytoclastic vasculitis is not predictive of extracutaneous involvement. Am J Dermatopathol 1999; 21: 532–536.

407 Lotti T, Ghersetich I, Comacchi C, Jorizzo JL. Cutaneous small-vessel vasculitis. J Am Acad Dermatol 1998; 39: 667–687.

408 Alegre VA, Winkelmann RK. Necrotizing vasculitis and atherosclerosis. Br J Dermatol 1988; 119: 381–384.

409 Prins M, Veraart JCJM, Vermeulen AHM et al. Leucocytoclastic vasculitis induced by prolonged exercise. Br J Dermatol 1996; 134: 915–918.

410 Bianchini G, Lotti T, Campolmi P et al. Coral ulcer as a vasculitis. Int J Dermatol 1988; 27: 506–507.

411 George J, Levy Y, Afec A et al. Leucocytoclastic vasculitis after coronary bypass artery grafting. Br J Dermatol 1996; 135: 1015–1016.

412 Lee A-Y, Jang J-H, Lee K-H. Two cases of leukocytoclastic vasculitis with tuberculosis. Clin Exp Dermatol 1998; 23: 225–226.

413 Cohen C, Trapuckd S. Leukocytoclastic vasculitis associated with cutaneous infection by herpesvirus. Am J Dermatopathol 1984; 6: 561–565.

414 Drago F, Rampini P, Brusati C, Rebora A. Leukocytoclastic vasculitis in a patient with HHV-6 infection. Acta Derm Venereol 2000; 80: 68.

415 Curtis JL, Egbert BM. Cutaneous cytomegalovirus vasculitis: an unusual clinical presentation of a common opportunistic pathogen. Hum Pathol 1982; 13: 1138–1141.

416 Chren M-M, Silverman RA, Sorensen RU, Elmets CA. Leukocytoclastic vasculitis in a patient infected with human immunodeficiency virus. J Am Acad Dermatol 1989; 21: 1161–1164.

417 Weimer CE Jr, Sahn EE. Follicular accentuation of leukocytoclastic vasculitis in an HIV-seropositive man. Report of a case and review of the literature. J Am Acad Dermatol 1991; 24: 898–902.

418 Mullick FG, McAllister HA Jr, Wagner BM, Fenoglio JJ Jr. Drug related vasculitis. Clinicopathologic correlations in 30 patients. Hum Pathol 1979; 10: 313–325.

419 Roenigk HH Jr. Vasculitis. Int J Dermatol 1976; 15: 395–404.

420 Lambert WC, Kolber LR, Proper SA. Leukocytoclastic angiitis induced by clindamycin. Cutis 1982; 30: 615–619.

421 Hendricks WM, Ader RS. Furosemide-induced cutaneous necrotizing vasculitis. Arch Dermatol 1977; 113: 375.

422 Rongioletti F, Ghio L, Ginevri F et al. Purpura of the ears: a distinctive vasculopathy with circulating autoantibodies complicating long-term treatment with levamisole in children. Br J Dermatol 1999; 140: 948–951.

423 Menni S, Pistritto G, Gianotti R et al. Ear lobe bilateral necrosis by levamisole-induced occlusive vasculitis in a pediatric patient. Pediatr Dermatol 1997; 14: 477–479.

424 Cox NH, Dunn LK, Williams J. Cutaneous vasculitis associated with long-term thiouracil therapy. Clin Exp Dermatol 1985; 10: 292–295.

425 Otsuka S, Kinebuchi A, Tabata H et al. Myeloperoxidase-antineutrophil cytoplasmic antibody-associated vasculitis following propylthiouracil therapy. Br J Dermatol 2000; 142: 828–830.

426 Chastain MA, Russo GG, Boh EE et al. Propylthiouracil hypersensitivity: Report of two patients with vasculitis and review of the literature. J Am Acad Dermatol 1999; 41: 757–764.

427 Miller RM, Savige J, Nassis L, Cominos BI. Antineutrophil cytoplasmic antibody (ANCA)-positive cutaneous leucocytoclastic vasculitis associated with antithyroid therapy in Graves' disease. Australas J Dermatol 1998; 39: 96–99.

428 Dootson G, Byatt C. Amiodarone-induced vasculitis and a review of the cutaneous side-effects of amiodarone. Clin Exp Dermatol 1994; 19: 422–424.

429 Jain KK. Cutaneous vasculitis associated with granulocyte colony-stimulating factor. J Am Acad Dermatol 1994; 31: 213–215.

430 Sanchez NP, van Hale HM, Su WPD. Clinical and histopathologic spectrum of necrotizing vasculitis. Report of findings in 101 cases. Arch Dermatol 1985; 121: 220–224.

431 Bickley LK, Schwartz RA, Lambert WC. Localized cutaneous leukocytoclastic vasculitis in an intravenous drug abuser. Int J Dermatol 1988; 27: 512–513.

432 Scerri L, Pace JL. Mefloquine-associated cutaneous vasculitis. Int J Dermatol 1993; 32: 517–518.

433 Smith HR, Croft AM, Black MM. Dermatological adverse effects with the antimalarial drug mefloquine: a review of 74 published case reports. Clin Exp Dermatol 1999; 24: 249–254.

434 Rachline A, Lariven S, Descamps V et al. Leucocytoclastic vasculitis and indinavir. Br J Dermatol 2000; 143: 1112–1113.

435 Lee A-Y. A case of leukocytoclastic vasculitis associated with haloperidol. Clin Exp Dermatol 1999; 24: 430.

436 Rustmann WC, Carpenter MT, Harmon C, Botti CF. Leukocytoclastic vasculitis associated with sotalol therapy. J Am Acad Dermatol 1998; 38: 111–112.

437 Ahmed I, Chen K-R, Nakayama H, Gibson LE. Cytosine arabinoside-induced vasculitis. Mayo Clin Proc 1998; 73: 239–242.

438 Christian MM, Diven DG, Sanchez RL, Soloway RD. Injection site vasculitis in a patient receiving interferon alfa for chronic hepatitis C. J Am Acad Dermatol 1997; 37: 118–120.

439 Lowry MD, Hudson CF, Callen JP. Leucocytoclastic vasculitis caused by drug additives. J Am Acad Dermatol 1994; 30: 854–855.

440 Vogt T, Landthaler M, Stolz W. Sodium benzoate-induced acute leukocytoclastic vasculitis with unusual clinical appearance. Arch Dermatol 1999; 135: 726–727.

441 Van der Klauw MM, van Hillo E, van den Berg WHHW et al. Vasculitis attributed to the nicotine patch (Nicotinell). Br J Dermatol 1996; 134: 361–364.

442 Arbiser JL, Dzieczkowski JS, Harmon JV, Duncan LM. Leukocytoclastic vasculitis following staphylococcal protein A column immunoadsorption therapy. Arch Dermatol 1995; 131: 707–709.

443 Alegre VA, Winkelmann RK, Diez-Martin JL, Banks PM. Adult celiac disease, small and medium vessel cutaneous necrotizing vasculitis, and T cell lymphoma. J Am Acad Dermatol 1988; 19: 973–978.

444 Farrell AM, Stern SCM, El-Ghariani K et al. Splenic lymphoma with villous lymphocytes presenting as leucocytoclastic vasculitis. Clin Exp Dermatol 1999; 24: 19–22.

445 O'Donnell BF, Williams HC, Carr R. Myelodysplastic syndrome presenting as cutaneous vasculitis. Clin Exp Dermatol 1995; 20: 439–442.

446 Granstein RD, Soter NA, Haynes HA. Necrotizing vasculitis with cutaneous lesions of mycosis fungoides. J Am Acad Dermatol 1983; 9: 128–133.

447 Spann CR, Callen JP, Yam LT, Apgar JT. Cutaneous leukocytoclastic vasculitis complicating hairy cell leukemia (leukemic reticuloendotheliosis). Arch Dermatol 1986; 122: 1057–1059.

448 Stashower ME, Rennie TA, Turiansky GW, Gilliland WR. Ovarian cancer presenting as leukocytoclastic vasculitis. J Am Acad Dermatol 1999; 40: 287–289.

449 Hunger RE, Dürr C, Brand CU. Cutaneous leukocytoclastic vasculitis in dermatomyositis suggests malignancy. Dermatology 2001; 202: 123–126.

450 Lee SH, Chung KY, Lee WS, Lee S. Behçet's syndrome associated with bullous necrotizing vasculitis. J Am Acad Dermatol 1989; 21: 327–330.

451 Newton JA, McGibbon DH, Marsden RA. Leucocytoclastic vasculitis and angio-oedema associated with inflammatory bowel disease. Clin Exp Dermatol 1984; 9: 618–623.

452 Resnick AH, Esterly NB. Vasculitis in children. Int J Dermatol 1985; 24: 139–146.

453 Alexander E, Provost TT. Sjögren's syndrome. Association of cutaneous vasculitis with central nervous system disease. Arch Dermatol 1987; 123: 801–810.

454 Barlow RJ, Schulz EJ. Chronic subcorneal pustulosis with vasculitis: a variant of generalized pustular psoriasis in black South Africans. Br J Dermatol 1991; 124: 470–474.

455 Thompson DM, Main RA, Beck JS, Albert-Recht F. Studies on a patient with leucocytoclastic vasculitis 'pyoderma gangrenosum' and paraproteinaemia. Br J Dermatol 1973; 88: 117–125.

456 Boom BW, Out-Luiting CJ, Baldwin WM et al. Membrane attack complex of complement in leukocytoclastic vasculitis of the skin. Arch Dermatol 1987; 123: 1192–1195.

457 Savage COS, Bacon PA. Overview of vasculitis: classification and pathogenesis. Curr Diagn Pathol 1995; 2: 256–265.

458 Sais G, Vidaller A, Jucglà A et al. Adhesion molecule expression and endothelial cell activation in cutaneous leukocytoclastic vasculitis. An immunohistologic and clinical study in 42 patients. Arch Dermatol 1997; 133: 443–450.

459 Tosca N, Stratigos JD. Possible pathogenetic mechanisms in allergic cutaneous vasculitis. Int J Dermatol 1988; 27: 291–296.

460 Sais G, Vidaller A, Peyri J. Anticardiolipin antibodies in leukocytoclastic vasculitis. J Am Acad Dermatol 1997; 37: 805–806.

461 Burden AD, Tillman DM, Foley P, Holme E. IgA class anticardiolipin antibodies in cutaneous leukocytoclastic vasculitis. J Am Acad Dermatol 1996; 35: 411–415.

462 Cunliffe WJ. Fibrinolysis and vasculitis. Clin Exp Dermatol 1976; 1: 1–16.

463 Chan LS, Cooper KD, Rasmussen JE. Koebnerization as a cutaneous manifestation of immune complex-mediated vasculitis. J Am Acad Dermatol 1990; 22: 775–781.

464 Jones RE Jr (ed). Questions to the Editorial Board and other authorities. Am J Dermatopathol 1985; 7: 181–187.

465 Bielsa I, Carrascosa JM, Hausmann G, Ferrándiz C. An immunohistopathologic study in cutaneous necrotizing vasculitis. J Cutan Pathol 2000; 27: 130–135.

466 Akosa AB, Lampert IA. The sweat gland in cutaneous vasculitis. Histopathology 1991; 18: 553–558.

467 Russell Jones R, Bhogal B. Dermatitis herpetiformis-like changes in cutaneous leucocytoclastic vasculitis with IgA deposition. Clin Exp Dermatol 1981; 6: 495–501.

468 Minkowitz S, Adler M, Alderete MN. Nuclear vacuolar acantholytic vesicular dermatitis associated with leukocytoclastic vasculitis. J Am Acad Dermatol 1986; 15: 1083–1089.

469 Grunwald MH, Avinoach I, Amichai B, Halevy S. Leucocytoclastic vasculitis – correlation between different histologic stages and direct immunofluorescence results. Int J Dermatol 1997; 36: 349–352.

470 Lerner LH, Lio P, Flotte TJ. The prognostic significance of vascular immunoglobulin deposits in 94 cases of cutaneous leukocytoclastic vasculitis. J Cutan Pathol 2000; 27: 562 (abstract).

471 Heng MCY. Henoch–Schönlein purpura. Br J Dermatol 1985; 112: 235–240.

472 Raimer SS, Sanchez RL. Vasculitis in children. Semin Dermatol 1992; 11: 48–56.

473 Nussinovitch M, Prais D, Finkelstein Y, Varsano I. Cutaneous manifestations of Henoch–Schönlein purpura in young children. Pediatr Dermatol 1998; 15: 426–428.

474 Tancrede-Bohin E, Ochonisky S, Vignon-Pennamen M-D et al. Schönlein–Henoch purpura in adult patients. Arch Dermatol 1997; 133: 438–442.

475 Wananukul S, Pongprasit P, Korkij W. Henoch–Schonlein purpura presenting as hemorrhagic vesicles and bullae: case report and literature review. Pediatr Dermatol 1995; 12: 314–317.

476 Kobayashi T, Sakuraoka K, Iwamoto M, Kurihara S. A case of anaphylactoid purpura with multiple blister formation: possible pathophysiological role of gelatinase (MMP-9). Dermatology 1998; 197: 62–64.

477 Saulsbury FT. Hemorrhagic bullous lesions in Henoch–Schönlein purpura. Pediatr Dermatol 1998; 15: 357–359.

478 Van Hale HM, Gibson LE, Schroeter AL. Henoch–Schönlein vasculitis: direct immunofluorescence study of uninvolved skin. J Am Acad Dermatol 1986; 15: 665–670.

479 Piette WW, Stone MS. A cutaneous sign of IgA-associated small dermal vessel leukocytoclastic vasculitis in adults (Henoch–Schönlein purpura). Arch Dermatol 1989; 125: 53–56.

480 Burden AD, Gibson IW, Rodger RSC, Tillman DM. IgA anticardiolipin antibodies associated with Henoch–Schönlein purpura. J Am Acad Dermatol 1994; 31: 857–860.

481 Burrows NP, Lockwood CM. Antineutrophil cytoplasmic antibodies and their relevance to the dermatologist. Br J Dermatol 1995; 132: 173–181.

482 Rovel-Guitera P, Diemert M-C, Charuel J-L et al. IgA antineutrophil cytoplasmic antibodies in cutaneous vasculitis. Br J Dermatol 2000; 143: 99–103.

483 Egan CA, O'Reilly MA, Meadows KP, Zone JJ. Relapsing Henoch–Schönlein purpura associated with Pseudomonas aeruginosa pyelonephritis. J Am Acad Dermatol 1999; 41: 381–383.

484 Goldberg EI, Shoji T, Sapadin AN. Henoch–Schönlein purpura induced by clarithromycin. Int J Dermatol 1999; 38: 706–708.

485 Reinauer S, Megahed M, Goerz G et al. Schönlein–Henoch purpura associated with gastric Helicobacter pylori infection. J Am Acad Dermatol 1995; 33: 876–879.

486 Bansal AS, Dwivedi N, Adsett M. Serum and blister fluid cytokines and complement proteins in a patient with Henoch Schönlein purpura associated with a bullous skin rash. Australas J Dermatol 1997; 38: 190–192.

487 Piette WW. What is Schönlein–Henoch purpura, and why should we care? Arch Dermatol 1997; 133: 515–518.

488 McCarthy R, Rosen T, Chen S-H et al. Adult Henoch–Schönlein purpura with fatal complications. Arch Dermatol 2001; 137: 19–21.

489 Levy-Khademi F, Korman SH, Amitai Y. Henoch–Schönlein purpura: simultaneous occurrence in two siblings. Pediatr Dermatol 2000; 17: 139–140.

490 Legrain V, Lejean S, Taïeb A et al. Infantile acute hemorrhagic edema of the skin: study of ten cases. J Am Acad Dermatol 1991; 24: 17–22.

491 Dubin BA, Bronson DM, Eng AM. Acute hemorrhagic edema of childhood: an unusual variant of leukocytoclastic vasculitis. J Am Acad Dermatol 1990; 23: 347–350.

492 Ince E, Mumcu Y, Suskan E et al. Infantile acute hemorrhagic edema: a variant of leukocytoclastic vasculitis. Pediatr Dermatol 1995; 12: 224–227.

493 Cunningham BB, Caro WA, Eramo LR. Neonatal acute hemorrhagic edema of childhood: case report and review of the English-language literature. Pediatr Dermatol 1996; 13: 39–44.

494 Tomaç N, Saraçlar Y, Türktas I, Kalayci Ö. Acute haemorrhagic oedema of infancy: a case report. Clin Exp Dermatol 1996; 21: 217–219.

495 Millard T, Harris A, MacDonald D. Acute infantile hemorrhagic oedema. J Am Acad Dermatol 1999; 41: 837–839.

496 Gonggryp LA, Todd G. Acute hemorrhagic edema of childhood (AHE). Pediatr Dermatol 1998; 15: 91–96.

497 Egan CA, Taylor TB, Meyer LJ et al. IgA1 is the major IgA subclass in cutaneous blood vessels in Henoch–Schönlein purpura. Br J Dermatol 1999; 141: 859–862.

498 Arrese Estrada J, Goffin F, Cornil F et al. Dendrocytoclasis in Henoch–Schönlein purpura. Acta Derm Venereol 1991; 71: 358–359.

499 Magro CM, Crowson AN. A clinical and histologic study of 37 cases of immunoglobulin A-associated vasculitis. Am J Dermatopathol 1999; 21: 234–240.

500 Jang K-A, Lim Y-S, Choi J-H et al. Hypereosinophilic syndrome presenting as cutaneous necrotizing eosinophilic vasculitis and Raynaud's phenomenon complicated by digital gangrene. Br J Dermatol 2000; 143: 641–644.

501 Chen K-R, Pittelkow MR, Su WPD et al. Recurrent cutaneous necrotizing eosinophilic vasculitis. Arch Dermatol 1994; 130: 1159–1166.

502 Yomoda M, Inoue M, Nakama T et al. Cutaneous eosinophilic vasculitis associated with rheumatoid arthritis. Br J Dermatol 1999; 140: 754–756.

503 Launay D, Delaporte E, Gillot J-M et al. An unusual cause of vascular purpura: recurrent cutaneous eosinophilic necrotizing vasculitis. Acta Derm Venereol 2000; 80: 394–395.

504 Chen K-R, Su WPD, Pittelkow MR et al. Eosinophilic vasculitis in connective tissue disease. J Am Acad Dermatol 1996; 35: 173–182.

505 Scott DGI, Bacon PA, Tribe CR. Systemic rheumatoid vasculitis: a clinical and laboratory study of 50 cases. Medicine (Baltimore) 1981; 60: 288–297.

506 Houck HE, Kauffman CL, Casey DL. Minocycline treatment for leukocytoclastic vasculitis associated with rheumatoid arthritis. Arch Dermatol 1997; 133: 15–16.

507 Nousari HC, Kimyai-Asadi A, Stebbing J, Stone JH. Purple toes in a patient with end-stage rheumatoid arthritis. Arch Dermatol 1999; 135: 648–650.

508 Gordon GV. Rheumatoid vasculitis. Int J Dermatol 1981; 20: 546–547.

509 Mehregan DR, Hall MJ, Gibson LE. Urticarial vasculitis: a histopathologic and clinical review of 72 cases. J Am Acad Dermatol 1992; 26: 441–448.

510 Wollenberg A, Hänel S, Spannagl M et al. Urticaria haemorrhagica profunda. Br J Dermatol 1997; 136: 108–111.

511 Asherson RA, Buchanan N, Kenwright S et al. The normocomplementemic urticarial vasculitis syndrome – report of a case and response to colchicine. Clin Exp Dermatol 1991; 16: 424–427.

512 Worm M, Muche M, Schulze P et al. Hypocomplementaemic urticarial vasculitis: successful treatment with cyclophosphamide-dexamethasone pulse therapy. Br J Dermatol 1998; 139: 704–707.

513 Gammon WR. Urticarial vasculitis. Dermatol Clin 1985; 3: 97–105.

514 Bisaccia E, Adamo V, Rozan SW. Urticarial vasculitis progressing to systemic lupus erythematosus. Arch Dermatol 1988; 124: 1088–1090.

515 Lin RY. Urticarial vasculitis. Br J Dermatol 1996; 135: 1016.

516 Hamid S, Cruz PD Jr, Lee WM. Urticarial vasculitis caused by hepatitis C virus infection: Response to interferon alfa therapy. J Am Acad Dermatol 1998; 39: 278–280.

517 Borradori L, Rybojad M, Puissant A et al. Urticarial vasculitis associated with a monoclonal IgM gammopathy: Schnitzler's syndrome. Br J Dermatol 1990; 123: 113–118.

518 Farell AM, Sabroe RA, Bunker CB. Urticarial vasculitis associated with polycythaemia rubra vera. Clin Exp Dermatol 1996; 21: 302–304.

519 Kano Y, Orihara M, Shiohara T. Cellular and molecular dynamics in exercise-induced urticarial vasculitis lesions. Arch Dermatol 1998; 134: 62–67.

520 Kwon CW, Lee CW, Kim YT, Kim JH. Urticarial vasculitis developed on the striae distensae during pregnancy. Int J Dermatol 1993; 32: 751–752.

521 Lewis JE. Urticarial vasculitis occurring in association with visceral malignancy. Acta Derm Venereol 1990; 70: 345–347.

522 Berg RE, Kantor GR, Bergfeld WF. Urticarial vasculitis. Int J Dermatol 1988; 27 468–472.

523 Sozer NA. Urticarial vasculitis. Clin Exp Dermatol 2000; 25: 335–336 (abstract).

524 Wittal RA, Fischer GO, Georgouras KE, Baird PJ. Skin reactions to diltiazem. Australas J Dermatol 1992; 33: 11–18.

525 Hofbauer GFL, Hafner J, Trüeb RM. Urticarial vasculitis following cocaine use. Br J Dermatol 1999; 141: 600–601.

526 Borcea A, Greaves MW. Methotrexate-induced exacerbation of urticarial vasculitis: an unusual adverse reaction. Br J Dermatol 2000; 143: 203–204.

527 Mehregan DR, Gibson LE. Pathophysiology of urticarial vasculitis. Arch Dermatol 1998; 134: 88–89.

528 Sais G, Vidaller A. Pathogenesis of exercise-induced urticarial vasculitis lesions: can the changes be extrapolated to all leukocytoclastic vasculitis lesions? Arch Dermatol 1999; 135: 87–88.

529 Russell Jones R, Bhogal B, Dash A, Schifferli J. Urticaria and vasculitis: a continuum of histological and immunopathological changes. Br J Dermatol 1983; 108: 695–703.

530 Davis MDP, Daoud MS, Kirby B et al. Clinicopathologic correlation of hypocomplementemic and normocomplementemic urticarial vasculitis. J Am Acad Dermatol 1998; 38: 899–905.

531 Tan E, Ng SK, Tan SH, Wong GC. Hypergammaglobulinaemic purpura presenting as reticulate purpura. Clin Exp Dermatol 1999; 24: 469–472.

532 Finder KA, McCollough ML, Dixon SL et al. Hypergammaglobulinemic purpura of Waldenström. J Am Acad Dermatol 1990; 23: 669–676.

533 Miyagawa S, Fukumoto T, Kanauchi M et al. Hypergammaglobulinaemic purpura of Waldenström and Ro/SSA autoantibodies. Br J Dermatol 1996; 134: 919–923.

534 Miller RM, Weedon D, Robertson IM. Benign hypergammaglobulinaemic purpura of Waldenström associated with lymphoid interstitial pneumonitis. Australas J Dermatol 1998; 39: 238–240.

535 Toro JR, Aksentijevich I, Hull K et al. Tumor necrosis factor receptor-associated periodic syndrome. A novel syndrome with cutaneous manifestations. Arch Dermatol 2000; 136: 1487–1494.

536 Drenth JPH, Boom BW, Toonstra J et al. Cutaneous manifestations and histologic findings in the hyperimmunoglobulinemia D syndrome. Arch Dermatol 1994; 130: 59–65.

537 Boom BW, Daha MR, Vermeer B-J, van der Meer JWM. IgD immune complex vasculitis in a patient with hyperimmunoglobulinemia D and periodic fever. Arch Dermatol 1990; 126: 1621–1624.

538 Ackerman AB. Histologic diagnosis of inflammatory skin diseases. Philadelphia: Lea & Febiger, 1978; 356–362.

539 O'Brien TJ, Mcdonald MI, Reid BF, Trethewie D. Streptococcal septic vasculitis. Australas J Dermatol 1995; 36: 211–213.

540 Plaut ME. Staphylococcal septicemia and pustular purpura. Arch Dermatol 1969; 99: 82–85.

541 Hill WR, Kinney TD. The cutaneous lesions in acute meningococcemia. A clinical and pathologic study. JAMA 1947; 134: 513–518.

542 Drolet BA, Baselga E, Esterly NB. Painful, purpuric plaques in a child with fever. Arch Dermatol 1997; 133: 1500–1501.

543 Scott MJ Jr, Scott MJ Sr. Primary cutaneous *Neisseria gonorrhoeae* infections. Arch Dermatol 1982; 118: 351–352.

544 Rosen T. Unusual presentations of gonorrhea. J Am Acad Dermatol 1982; 6: 369–372.

545 Hurwitz RM, Leaming RD, Horine RK. Necrotic cellulitis. A localized form of septic vasculitis. Arch Dermatol 1984; 120: 87–92.

546 Mandell IN, Feiner HD, Price NM, Simberkoff M. *Pseudomonas cepacia* endocarditis and ecthyma gangrenosum. Arch Dermatol 1977; 113: 199–202.

547 Shapiro L, Teisch JA, Brownstein MH. Dermatohistopathology of chronic gonococcal sepsis. Arch Dermatol 1973; 107: 403–406.

548 Nielsen LT. Chronic meningococcemia. Arch Dermatol 1970; 102: 97–101.

549 Ackerman AB. Hemorrhagic bullae in gonococcemia. N Engl J Med 1970; 282: 793–794.

550 Sotto MN, Langer B, Hoshino-Shimizu S, de Brito T. Pathogenesis of cutaneous lesions in acute meningococcemia in humans: light, immunofluorescent, and electron microscopic studies of skin biopsy specimens. J Infect Dis 1976; 133: 506–514.

551 Dalldorf FG, Jennette JC. Fatal meningococcal septicemia. Arch Pathol Lab Med 1977; 101: 6–9.

552 Scherer R, Braun-Falco O. Alternative pathway complement activation: a possible mechanism inducing skin lesions in benign gonococcal sepsis. Br J Dermatol 1976; 95: 303–309.

553 Ackerman AB, Miller RC, Shapiro L. Gonococcemia and its cutaneous manifestations. Arch Dermatol 1965; 91: 227–232.

554 Von Gemmingen GR, Winkelmann RK. Osler's node of subacute bacterial endocarditis. Focal necrotizing vasculitis of the glomus body. Arch Dermatol 1967; 95: 91–94.

555 Alpert JS, Krous HF, Dalen JE et al. Pathogenesis of Osler's nodes. Ann Intern Med 1976; 85: 471–473.

556 Rubenfeld S, Min K-W. Leukocytoclastic angiitis in subacute bacterial endocarditis. Arch Dermatol 1977; 113: 1073–1074.

557 Kerr A Jr, Tan JS. Biopsies of the Janeway lesion of infective endocarditis. J Cutan Pathol 1979; 6: 124–129.

558 Cardullo AC, Silvers DN, Grossman ME. Janeway lesions and Osler's nodes: a review of histopathologic findings. J Am Acad Dermatol 1990; 22: 1088–1090.

559 Pinogh M, Velasco M, Botella R et al. Janeway lesions: differential diagnosis with Osler's nodes. Int J Dermatol 1993; 32: 673–674.

560 Vinson RP, Chung A, Elston DM, Keller RA. Septic microemboli in a Janeway lesion of bacterial endocarditis. J Am Acad Dermatol 1996; 35: 984–985.

561 Parikh SK, Lieberman A, Colbert DA et al. The identification of methicillin-resistant *Staphylococcus aureus* in Osler's nodes and Janeway lesions of acute bacterial endocarditis. J Am Acad Dermatol 1996; 35: 767–768.

562 Kimyai-Asadi A, Usman A, Milani F. Cutaneous manifestations of marantic endocarditis. Int J Dermatol 2000; 39: 290–292.

563 Katz SI, Gallin JI, Hertz KC et al. Erythema elevatum diutinum: skin and systemic manifestations, immunologic studies, and successful treatment with dapsone. Medicine (Baltimore) 1977; 56: 443–455.

564 English JSC, Smith NP, Kersy PJW, Levene GM. Erythema elevatum diutinum – an unusual case. Clin Exp Dermatol 1985; 10: 577–580.

565 Caputo R, Alessi E. Unique aspects of a lesion of erythema elevatum diutinum. Am J Dermatopathol 1984; 6: 465–469.

566 Vollum DI. Erythema elevatum diutinum – vesicular lesions and sulphone response. Br J Dermatol 1968; 80: 178–183.

567 Shanks JH, Banerjee SS, Bishop PW et al. Nodular erythema elevatum diutinum mimicking cutaneous neoplasms. Histopathology 1997; 31: 91–96.

568 Takiwaki H, Kubo Y, Tsuda H et al. Peripheral ulcerative keratitis associated with erythema elevatum diutinum and a positive rheumatoid factor: a report of three cases. Br J Dermatol 1998; 138: 893–897.

569 Creus L, Salleras M, Sola MA et al. Erythema elevatum diutinum associated with pulmonary infiltrates. Br J Dermatol 1997; 137: 652–653.

570 Aractingi S, Bachmeyer C, Dombret H et al. Simultaneous occurrence of two rare cutaneous markers of poor prognosis in myelodysplastic syndrome: erythema elevatum diutinum and specific lesions. Br J Dermatol 1994; 131: 112–117.

571 Futei Y, Konohana I. A case of erythema elevatum diutinum associated with B-cell lymphoma: a rare distribution involving palms, soles and nails. Br J Dermatol 2000; 142: 116–119.

572 Yiannias JA, El-Azhary RA, Gibson LE. Erythema elevatum diutinum: a clinical and histopathologic study of 13 patients. J Am Acad Dermatol 1992; 26: 38–44.

573 Kavanagh GM, Colaco CB, Bradfield JW, Archer CB. Erythema elevatum diutinum associated with Wegener's granulomatosis and IgA paraproteinemia. J Am Acad Dermatol 1993; 28: 846–849.

574 Wayte JA, Rogers S, Powell FC. Pyoderma gangrenosum, erythema elevatum diutinum and IgA monoclonal gammopathy. Australas J Dermatol 1995; 36: 21–23.

575 Chow RKP, Benny WB, Coupe RL et al. Erythema elevatum diutinum associated with IgA paraproteinemia successfully controlled with intermittent plasma exchange. Arch Dermatol 1996; 132: 1360–1364.

576 Miyagawa S, Kitamura W, Morita K et al. Association of hyperimmunoglobulinaemia D syndrome with erythema elevatum diutinum. Br J Dermatol 1993; 128: 572–574.

577 Morrison JGL, Hull PR, Fourie E. Erythema elevatum diutinum, cryoglobulinaemia, and fixed urticaria on cooling. Br J Dermatol 1977; 97: 99–104.

578 Rodriguez-Serna M, Fortea J-M, Perez A et al. Erythema elevatum diutinum associated with celiac disease: response to a gluten-free diet. Pediatr Dermatol 1993; 10: 125–128.

579 Tasanen K, Raudasoja R, Kallioinen M, Ranki A. Erythema elevatum diutinum in association with coeliac disease. Br J Dermatol 1997; 136: 624–627.

580 Buahene K, Hudson M, Mowat A et al. Erythema elevatum diutinum – an unusual association with ulcerative colitis. Clin Exp Dermatol 1991; 16: 204–206.

581 Ortel CH, McGregor JM, Whittaker SJ et al. Erythema elevatum diutinum and Crohn disease: a common pathogenic role for measles virus? Arch Dermatol 1996; 132: 1523–1525.

582 Sangüeza OP, Pilcher B, Sangüeza JM. Erythema elevatum diutinum: A clinicopathological study of eight cases. Am J Dermatopathol 1997; 19: 214–222.

583 Bernard P, Bedane C, Debrous J-L et al. Erythema elevatum diutinum in a patient with relapsing polychondritis. J Am Acad Dermatol 1992; 26: 312–315.

584 Collier PM, Neill SM, Branfoot AC, Staughton RCD. Erythema elevatum diutinum – a solitary lesion in a patient with rheumatoid arthritis. Clin Exp Dermatol 1990; 15: 394–395.

585 Requena L, Sánchez Yus E, Martín L et al. Erythema elevatum diutinum in a patient with acquired immunodeficiency syndrome. Arch Dermatol 1991; 127: 1819–1822.

586 LeBoit PE, Cockerell CJ. Nodular lesions of erythema elevatum diutinum in patients infected with the human immunodeficiency virus. J Am Acad Dermatol 1993; 28: 919–922.

587 Muratori S, Carrera C, Gorani A, Alessi E. Erythema elevatum diutinum and HIV infection: a report of five cases. Br J Dermatol 1999; 141: 335–338.

588 Dronda F, González-López A, Lecona M, Barros C. Erythema elevatum diutinum in human immunodeficiency virus-infected patients – report of a case and review of the literature. Clin Exp Dermatol 1996; 21: 222–225.

589 Sanz-Trelles A, Ayala-Carbonero A, Ojeda-Mertos A. Erythema elevatum diutinum in an HIV + hemophilic patient. Am J Dermatopathol 1999; 21: 587–588.

590 Revenga F, Vera A, Muñoz A et al. Erythema elevatum diutinum and AIDS: are they related? Clin Exp Dermatol 1997; 22: 250–251.

591 Drago F, Semino M, Rampini P et al. Erythema elevatum diutinum in a patient with human herpesvirus 6 infection. Acta Derm Venereol 1999; 79: 91–92.

592 Da Cunha Bang F, Weismann K, Ralfkiær E et al. Erythema elevatum diutinum and pre-AIDS. Acta Derm Venereol 1986; 66: 272–274.

593 Grabbe J, Haas N, Möller A, Henz BM. Erythema elevatum diutinum – evidence for disease-dependent leucocyte alterations and response to dapsone. Br J Dermatol 2000; 143: 415–420.

594 LeBoit PE, Yen TSB, Wintroub B. The evolution of lesions in erythema elevatum diutinum. Am J Dermatopathol 1986; 8: 392–402.

595 Wilkinson SM, English JSC, Smith NP. Erythema elevatum diutinum: a clinicopathological study. Clin Exp Dermatol 1992; 17: 87–93.

596 Haber H. Erythema elevatum diutinum. Br J Dermatol 1955; 67: 121–145.

597 Mrez JP, Newcomer VD. Erythema elevatum diutinum. Arch Dermatol 1967; 96: 235–246.

598 Kanitakis J, Cozzani E, Lyonnet S, Thivolet J. Ultrastructural study of chronic lesions of erythema elevatum diutinum: 'Extracellular cholesterosis' is a misnomer. J Am Acad Dermatol 1993; 29: 363–367.

599 Pacheco LS, Sotto MN. Factor XIIIa⁺ dermal dendrocytes in erythema elevatum diutinum and ordinary cutaneous leukocytoclastic vasculitis lesions. J Cutan Pathol 2000; 27: 136–140.

600 Lee AY, Nakagawa H, Nogita T, Ishibashi Y. Erythema elevatum diutinum: an ultrastructural case study. J Cutan Pathol 1989; 16: 211–217.

601 Pedace FJ, Perry HO. Granuloma faciale. A clinical and histopathologic review. Arch Dermatol 1966; 94: 387–395.

602 Dowlati B, Firooz A, Dowlati Y. Granuloma faciale: successful treatment of nine cases with a combination of cryotherapy and intralesional corticosteroid injection. Int J Dermatol 1997; 36: 548–551.

603 Gómez-de la Fuente E, de Rio R, Rodriguez M et al. Granuloma faciale mimicking rhinophyma: response to clofazimine. Acta Derm Venereol 2000; 80: 144.

604 Scott DM, Carlson JA, Ball N. Granuloma faciale associated with basal cell carcinoma. J Cutan Pathol 2000; 27: 571 (abstract).

605 Jacyk WK. Facial granuloma in a patient treated with clofazimine. Arch Dermato 1981; 117: 597–598.

606 Welsh JH, Schroeder TL, Levy ML. Granuloma faciale in a child successfully treated with the pulsed dye laser. J Am Acad Dermatol 1999; 41: 351–353.

607 Rusin LJ, Dubin HV, Taylor WB. Disseminated granuloma faciale. Arch Dermatol 976; 112: 1575–1577.

608 Sears JK, Gitter DG, Stone MS. Extrafacial granuloma faciale. Arch Dermatol 1991; 127: 742–743.

609 Castaño E, Segurado A, Iglesias L et al. Granuloma faciale entirely in an extrafacial location. Br J Dermatol 1997; 136: 978–979.

610 Roustan G, Sánchez Yus E, Salas C, Simón A. Granuloma faciale with extrafacial lesions. Dermatology 1999; 198: 79–82.

611 Guill MA, Aton JK. Facial granuloma responsive to dapsone therapy. Arch Dermatol 1982; 118: 332–335.

612 Smoller BR, Bortz J. Immunophenotypic analysis suggests that granuloma faciale is a γ-interferon-mediated process. J Cutan Pathol 1993; 20: 442–446.

613 Lever WF, Leeper RW. Eosinophilic granuloma of the skin. Arch Dermatol 1950; 62: 85–96.

614 Frost FA, Heenan PJ. Facial granuloma. Australas J Dermatol 1984; 25: 121–124.

615 Nieboer C, Kalsbeek GL. Immunofluorescence studies in granuloma eosinophilicum faciale. J Cutan Pathol 1978; 5: 68–75.

616 Selvaag E, Roald B. Immunohistochemical findings in granuloma faciale. The role of eosinophilic granulocytes. J Eur Acad Dermatol Venereol 2000; 14: 517–513.

617 Johnson WC, Higdon RS, Helwig EB. Granuloma faciale. Arch Dermatol 1959; 79: 42–52.

618 Schnitzler L, Verret JL, Schubert B. Granuloma faciale. Ultrastructural study of three cases. J Cutan Pathol 1977; 4: 123–133.

619 Carlson JA, LeBoit PE. Localized chronic fibrosing vasculitis of the skin: an inflammatory reaction that occurs in settings other than erythema elevatum diutinum and granuloma faciale. Am J Surg Pathol 1997; 21: 698–705.

620 Jennette JC, Thomas DB, Falk RJ. Microscopic polyangiitis (microscopic polyarteritis). Semin Diagn Pathol 2001; 18: 3–13.

621 Peñas PF, Porras JI, Fraga J et al. Microscopic polyangiitis. A systemic vasculitis with a positive P-ANCA. Br J Dermatol 1996; 134: 542–547.

622 Savage COS, Harper L, Cockwell P et al. ABC of arterial and vascular disease. Vasculitis. BMJ 2000; 320: 1325–1328.

623 Irvine AD, Bruce IN, Walsh M et al. Dermatological presentation of disease associated with antineutrophil cytoplasmic antibodies: a report of two contrasting cases and a review of the literature. Br J Dermatol 1996; 134: 924–928.

624 Sais G, Vidaller A, Jucglà A et al. Antineutrophil cytoplasmic antibodies in leukocytoclastic vasculitis. Arch Dermatol 1998; 134: 239.

625 Irvine AD, Bruce IN, Walsh MY, Bingham EA. Microscopic polyangiitis. Delineation of a cutaneous-limited variant associated with antimyeloperoxidase autoantibody. Arch Dermatol 1997; 133: 474–477.

626 Cohen RD, Conn DL, Ilstrup DM. Clinical features, prognosis, and response to treatment in polyarteritis. Mayo Clin Proc 1980; 55: 146–155.

627 Goodless DR, Dhawan SS, Alexis J, Wiszniak J. Cutaneous periarteritis nodosa. Int J Dermatol 1990; 29: 611–615.

628 Bonsib SM. Polyarteritis nodosa. Semin Diagn Pathol 2001; 18: 14–23.

629 Vertzman L. Polyarteritis nodosa. Clin Rheum Dis 1980; 6: 297–317.

630 Diaz-Perez JL, Schroeter AL, Winkelmann RK. Cutaneous periarteritis nodosa. Immunofluorescence studies. Arch Dermatol 1980; 116: 56–58.

631 Cvancara JL, Meffert JJ, Elston DM. Estrogen-sensitive cutaneous polyarteritis nodosa: Response to tamoxifen. J Am Acad Dermatol 1998; 39: 643–646.

632 Ginarte M, Pereiro M, Toribio J. Cutaneous polyarteritis nodosa in a child. Pediatr Dermatol 1998; 15: 103–107.

633 Minkowitz G, Smoller BR, McNutt NS. Benign cutaneous polyarteritis nodosa. Relationship to systemic polyarteritis nodosa and to hepatitis B infection. Arch Dermatol 1991; 127: 1520–1523.

634 Daoud MS, Hutton KP, Gibson LE. Cutaneous periarteritis nodosa: a clinicopathological study of 79 cases. Br J Dermatol 1997; 136: 706–713.

635 Siberry GK, Cohen BA, Johnson B. Cutaneous polyarteritis nodosa. Reports o two cases in children and review of the literature. Arch Dermatol 1994; 130: 884–889.

636 Brandrup F, Petersen EM, Hansen BF. Localized polyarteritis nodosa in the lower limb with new bone formation. Acta Derm Venereol 1980; 60: 182–184.

637 Trüeb RM, Scheidegger EP, Pericin M et al. Periarteritis nodosa presenting as a breast lesion: report of a case and review of the literature. Br J Dermatol 1999; 141: 1117–1121.

638 Trepo CG, Zuckerman AJ, Bird RC, Prince AM. The role of circulating hepatitis B antigen/antibody immune complexes in the pathogenesis of vascular and hepatic manifestations in polyarteritis nodosa. J Clin Pathol 1974; 27: 863–868.

639 Gocke DJ, Hsu K, Morgan C et al. Association between polyarteritis and Australia antigen. Lancet 1970; 2: 1149–1153.

640 Whittaker SJ, Dover JS, Greaves MW. Cutaneous polyarteritis nodosa associated with hepatitis B surface antigen. J Am Acad Dermatol 1986; 15: 1142–1145.

641 Van de Pette JEW, Jarvis JM, Wilton JMA, MacDonald DM. Cutaneous periarteritis nodosa. Arch Dermatol 1984; 120: 109–111.

642 Soufir N, Descamps V, Crickx B et al. Hepatitis C virus infection in cutaneous polyarteritis nodosa: a retrospective study of 16 cases. Arch Dermatol 1999; 135: 1001–1002.

643 Sheth AP, Olson JC, Esterly NB. Cutaneous polyarteritis nodosa of childhood. J Am Acad Dermatol 1994; 31: 561–566.

644 Choonhakarn C, Jirarattanapochai K. Cutaneous polyarteritis nodosa: a report of a case associated with melioidosis (Burkholderia pseudomallei). Int J Dermatol 1998; 37: 433–436.

645 Albornoz MA, Benedetto AV, Korman M et al. Relapsing cutaneous polyarteritis nodosa associated with streptococcal infections. Int J Dermatol 1998; 37: 664–666.

646 Goslen JB, Graham W, Lazarus GS. Cutaneous polyarteritis nodosa. Report of a case associated with Crohn's disease. Arch Dermatol 1983; 119: 326–329.

647 Mizutani H, Asahi K, Shimizu M. Complete remission of recalcitrant polyarteritis nodosa after combination chemotherapy for accompanying B-cell non-Hodgkin lymphoma. Int J Dermatol 1998; 37: 397–399.

648 Fernandez-Diaz J. General pathology of necrotizing vasculitis. Clin Rheum Dis 1980; 6: 279–295.

649 Citron BP, Halpern M, McCarron M et al. Necrotizing angiitis associated with drug abuse. N Engl J Med 1970; 283: 1003–1011.

650 Schaffer JV, Davidson DM, McNiff JM, Bolognia JL. Perinuclear antineutrophilic cytoplasmic antibody-positive cutaneous polyarteritis nodosa associated with minocycline therapy for acne vulgaris. J Am Acad Dermatol 2001; 44: 198–206.

651 Rose GA, Spencer H. Polyarteritis nodosa. Q J Med 1957; 26: 43–81.

652 Kawasaki T, Kosaki F, Okawa S et al. A new infantile acute febrile mucocutaneous lymph node syndrome (MLNS) prevailing in Japan. Pediatrics 1974; 54: 271–276.

653 Hicks RV, Melish ME. Kawasaki syndrome. Pediatr Clin North Am 1986; 33: 1151–1175.

654 Melish ME. Kawasaki syndrome: a 1992 update. Pediatr Dermatol 1992; 9: 335–337.

655 Wortmann DW. Kawasaki syndrome. Semin Dermatol 1992; 11: 37–47.

656 Han RK, Sinclair B, Newman A et al. Recognition and management of Kawasaki disease. CMAJ 2000; 162: 807–812.

657 Phillips WG, Marsden JR. Adult Kawasaki syndrome. Br J Dermatol 1993; 129: 330–333.

658 Butler DF, Hough DR, Friedman SJ, Davis HE. Adult Kawasaki syndrome. Arch Dermatol 1987; 123: 1356–1361.

659 Weston WL, Huff JC. The mucocutaneous lymph node syndrome: a critical re-examination. Clin Exp Dermatol 1981; 6: 167–178.

660 Bell DM, Brink EW, Nitzkin JL et al. Kawasaki syndrome: description of two outbreaks in the United States. N Engl J Med 1981; 304: 1568–1575.

661 Michie C, Kinsler V, Tulloh R, Davidson S. Recurrent skin peeling following Kawasaki disease. Arch Dis Child 2000; 83: 353–355.

662 Friter BS, Lucky AW. The perineal eruption of Kawasaki syndrome. Arch Dermatol 1988; 124: 1805–1810.

663 Kimura T, Miyazawa H, Watanabe K, Moriya T. Small pustules in Kawasaki disease. A clinicopathological study of four patients. Am J Dermatopathol 1988; 10: 218–223.

664 Newburger JW, Takahashi M, Burns JC et al. The treatment of Kawasaki syndrome with intravenous gamma globulin. N Engl J Med 1986; 315: 341–347.

665 Rauch AM. Kawasaki syndrome: review of new epidemiologic and laboratory developments. Pediatr Infect Dis 1987; 6: 1016–1021.

666 Martinez-Escribano JA, Redondo C, Galera C et al. Recurrent Kawasaki syndrome in an adult with HIV-1 infection. Dermatology 1998; 197: 96–97.

667 Hirose S, Hamashima Y. Morphological observations on the vasculitis in the mucocutaneous lymph node syndrome. A skin biopsy study of 27 cases. Eur J Pediatr 1978; 129: 17–27.

668 Giblin WJ, James WD, Benson PM. Buerger's disease. Int J Dermatol 1989; 28: 638–642.

669 Abdullah AN, Keczkes K. Thromboangiitis obliterans (Bürger's disease) in a woman – a case report and review of the literature. Clin Exp Dermatol 1990; 15: 46–49.

670 Samlaska CP, James WD. Superficial thrombophlebitis I. Primary hypercoagulable states. J Am Acad Dermatol 1990; 22: 975–989.

671 Samlaska CP, James WD. Superficial thrombophlebitis II. Secondary hypercoagulable states. J Am Acad Dermatol 1990; 23: 1–18.

672 Aloi FG, Tomasini CF, Moliners A. Railway track-like dermatitis: an atypical Mondor's disease? J Am Acad Dermatol 1989; 20: 920–923.

673 Hacker SM. Axillary string phlebitis in pregnancy: a variant of Mondor's disease. J Am Acad Dermatol 1994; 30: 636–638.

674 Mayor M, Burón I, Calvo de Mora J et al. Mondor's disease. Int J Dermatol 2000; 39: 922–925.

675 Fine JD, Harrist TJ. Cutaneous leukocytoclastic vasculitis in the rose spot of paratyphoid fever. Int J Dermatol 1982; 21: 216–217.

676 Rosen T, Rubin H, Ellner K et al. Vesicular Jarisch–Herxheimer reaction. Arch Dermatol 1989; 125: 77–81.

Neutrophilic dermatoses

677 Hunt SJ, Santa Cruz DJ. Neutrophilic dermatoses. Semin Dermatol 1989; 8: 266–275.

678 Jorizzo JL. Pustular vasculitis: an emerging disease concept. J Am Acad Dermatol 1983; 9: 160–162.

679 Jorizzo JL, Schmalstieg FC, Dinehart SM et al. Bowel-associated dermatosis-arthritis syndrome. Immune complex-mediated vessel damage and increased neutrophil migration. Arch Intern Med 1984; 144: 738–740.

680 Bourke JF, Jones JL, Fletcher A, Graham-Brown RAC. An immunohistochemical study of the dermal infiltrate and epidermal staining for interleukin 1 in 12 cases of Sweet's syndrome. Br J Dermatol 1996; 134: 705–709.

681 Barzilai A, Langevitz P, Goldberg I et al. Erysipelas-like erythema of familial Mediterranean fever: Clinicopathologic correlation. J Am Acad Dermatol 2000; 42: 791–795.

682 Fitzgerald RL, McBurney EI, Nesbitt LT Jr. Sweet's syndrome. Int J Dermatol 1996; 35: 9–15.

683 Von den Driesch P. Sweet's syndrome (acute febrile neutrophilic dermatosis). J Am Acad Dermatol 1994; 31: 535–556.

684 Bulengo-Ransby SM, Brown MD, Dubin HV et al. Sweet's syndrome presenting as an unusual periorbital eruption. J Am Acad Dermatol 1991; 24: 140–141.

685 Sweet RD. An acute febrile neutrophilic dermatosis. Br J Dermatol 1964; 76: 349–356.

686 Greer KE, Cooper PH. Sweet's syndrome (acute febrile neutrophilic dermatosis). Clin Rheum Dis 1982; 8: 427–441.

687 Christensen OB, Holst R, Svensson A. Chronic recurrent annular neutrophilic dermatosis. An entity? Acta Derm Venereol 1989; 69: 415–418.

688 Sommer S, Wilkinson SM, Merchant WJ, Goulden V. Sweet's syndrome presenting as palmoplantar pustulosis. J Am Acad Dermatol 2000; 42: 332–334.

689 Ahn S-J, Choi J-H, Sung K-J et al. Sweet's syndrome presenting with lesions resembling eruptive xanthoma. Br J Dermatol 2000; 143: 449–450.

690 Collins P, Rogers S, Keenan P, McCabe M. Acute febrile neutrophilic dermatosis in childhood (Sweet's syndrome). Br J Dermatol 1991; 124: 203–206.

691 Dunn TR, Saperstein HW, Biederman A, Kaplan RP. Sweet syndrome in a neonate with aseptic meningitis. Pediatr Dermatol 1992; 9: 288–292.

692 Wilson DM, John GR, Callen JP. Peripheral ulcerative keratitis – an extracutaneous neutrophilic disorder: Report of a patient with rheumatoid arthritis, pustular vasculitis, pyoderma gangrenosum, and Sweet's syndrome with an excellent response to cyclosporine therapy. J Am Acad Dermatol 1999; 40: 331–334.

693 Fain O, Mathieu E, Feton N et al. Intestinal involvement in Sweet's syndrome. J Am Acad Dermatol 1996; 35: 989–990.

694 Castanet J, Lacour JP, Garnier G et al. Neutrophilic dermatosis associated with chronic neutrophilic leukemia. J Am Acad Dermatol 1993; 29: 290–292.

695 Gisser SD. Acute febrile neutrophilic dermatosis (Sweet's syndrome) in a patient with hairy-cell leukemia. Am J Dermatopathol 1983; 5: 283–288.

696 Ilchyshyn A, Smith AG, Phaure TAJ. Sweet's syndrome associated with chronic lymphatic leukaemia. Clin Exp Dermatol 1987; 12: 277–279.

697 Clemmensen OJ, Menne T, Brandrup F et al. Acute febrile neutrophilic dermatosis – a marker of malignancy? Acta Derm Venereol 1989; 69: 52–58.

698 Fett DL, Gibson LE, Su WPD. Sweet's syndrome: systemic signs and symptoms and associated disorders. Mayo Clin Proc 1995; 70: 234–240.

699 Bourke JF, Keohane S, Long CC et al. Sweet's syndrome and malignancy in the U.K. Br J Dermatol 1997; 137: 609–613.

700 Probert C, Ehmann WC, Al-Mondhiry H et al. Sweet's syndrome without granulocytosis. Int J Dermatol 1998; 37: 108–112.

701 Cho K-H, Han K-H, Kim S-W et al. Neutrophilic dermatoses associated with myeloid malignancy. Clin Exp Dermatol 1997; 22: 269–273.

702 Delmonte S, Brusati C, Parodi A, Rebora A. Leukemia-related Sweet's syndrome elicited by pathergy to arnica. Dermatology 1998; 197: 195–196.

703 Mégarbane B, Bodemer C, Valensi F et al. Association of acute neutrophilic dermatosis and myelodysplastic syndrome with (6;9) chromosome translocation: a case report and review of the literature. Br J Dermatol 2000; 143: 1322–1324.

704 Caughman W, Stern R, Haynes H. Neutrophilic dermatosis of myeloproliferative disorders. J Am Acad Dermatol 1983; 9: 751–758.

705 Callen JP. Acute febrile neutrophilic dermatosis (Sweet's syndrome) and the related conditions of 'bowel bypass' syndrome and bullous pyoderma gangrenosum. Dermatol Clin 1985; 3: 153–163.

706 Suzuki Y, Kuroda K, Kojima T et al. Unusual cutaneous manifestations of myelodysplastic syndrome. Br J Dermatol 1995; 133: 483–486.

707 Davies MG, Hastings A. Sweet's syndrome progressing to pyoderma gangrenosum – a spectrum of neutrophilic skin disease in association with cryptogenic cirrhosis. Clin Exp Dermatol 1991; 16: 279–282.

708 Johnson ML, Grimwood RE. Leucocyte colony-stimulating factors. A review of associated neutrophilic dermatoses and vasculitides. Arch Dermatol 1994; 130: 77–81.

709 Scott GA. Report of three cases of cutaneous reactions to granulocyte macrophage-colony-stimulating factor and a review of the literature. Am J Dermatopathol 1995; 17: 107–114.

710 Richard MA, Grob JJ, Laurans R et al. Sweet's syndrome induced by granulocyte colony-stimulating factor in a woman with congenital neutropenia. J Am Acad Dermatol 1996; 35: 629–631.

711 Prevost-Blank PL, Shwayder TA. Sweet's syndrome secondary to granulocyte colony-stimulating factor. J Am Acad Dermatol 1996; 35: 995–997.

712 Horan MP, Redmond J, Gehle D et al. Postpolycythemic myeloid metaplasia, Sweet's syndrome, and acute myeloid leukemia. J Am Acad Dermatol 1987; 16: 458–462.

713 Watanabe Y, Miki Y. Neutrophilic dermatosis with polycythemia vera. J Am Acad Dermatol 1995; 32: 672–673.

714 Wong GAE, Guerin DM, Parslew R. Sweet's syndrome and polycythaemia rubra vera. Clin Exp Dermatol 2000; 25: 296–298.

715 Aractingi S, Mallet V, Pinquier L et al. Neutrophilic dermatoses during granulocytopenia. Arch Dermatol 1995; 131: 1141–1145.

716 Krolikowski FJ, Reuter K, Shultis EW. Acute febrile neutrophilic dermatosis (Sweet's syndrome) associated with lymphoma. Hum Pathol 1985; 16: 520–522.

717 Schwartz RA, French SW, Rubenstein DJ, Lambert WC. Acute neutrophilic dermatosis with diffuse histiocytic lymphoma. J Am Acad Dermatol 1984; 10: 350–354.

718 Woodrow SL, Munn SE, Basarab T, Russell Jones R. Sweet's syndrome in association with non-Hodgkin's lymphoma. Clin Exp Dermatol 1996; 21: 357–359.

719 Berth-Jones J, Hutchinson PE. Sweet's syndrome and malignancy: a case associated with multiple myeloma and review of the literature. Br J Dermatol 1989; 121: 123–127.

720 Mali-Gerrits MGH, Rampen FHJ. Acute febrile neutrophilic dermatosis (Sweet's syndrome) and adenocarcinoma of the rectum. Clin Exp Dermatol 1988; 13: 105–106.

721 Dyall-Smith D, Billson V. Sweet's syndrome associated with adenocarcinoma of the prostate. Australas J Dermatol 1988; 29: 25–27.

722 Char H-L, Lee Y-S, Kuo T-T. Sweet's syndrome: clinicopathologic study of eleven cases. Int J Dermatol 1994; 33: 425–432.

723 Inomata N, Sasaki T, Nakajima H. Sweet's syndrome with gastric cancer. J Am Acad Dermatol 1999; 41: 1033–1034.

724 Fujimoto N, Tajima S, Ishibashi A et al. Acute febrile neutrophilic dermatosis (Sweet's syndrome) in a patient with relapsing polychondritis. Br J Dermatol 1998; 139: 930–931.

725 Mizoguchi M, Chikakane K, Goh K et al. Acute febrile neutrophilic dermatosis (Sweet's syndrome) in Behçet's disease. Br J Dermatol 1987; 116: 727–734.

726 Mizoguchi M, Matsuki K, Mochizuki M et al. Human leukocyte antigen in Sweet's syndrome and its relationship to Behçet's disease. Arch Dermatol 1988; 124: 1069–1073.

727 Satra K, Zalka A, Cohen PR, Grossman ME. Sweet's syndrome and pregnancy. J Am Acad Dermatol 1994; 30: 297–300.

728 Wilkinson SM, Heagerty AHM, English JSC. Acute febrile neutrophilic dermatosis in association with erythema nodosum and sarcoidosis. Clin Exp Dermatol 1993; 18: 47–49.

729 Servitje O, Ribera M, Juanola X, Rodriguez-Moreno J. Acute neutrophilic dermatosis associated with hydralazine-induced lupus. Arch Dermatol 1987; 123: 1435–1436.

730 Choi JW, Chung KY. Sweet's syndrome with systemic lupus erythematosus and herpes zoster. Br J Dermatol 1999; 140: 1174–1175.

731 Sitjas D, Puig L, Cuatrecasas M, de Moragas JM. Acute febrile neutrophilic dermatosis (Sweet's syndrome). Int J Dermatol 1993; 32: 261–268.

732 Beitner H, Nakatani T, Hammar H. A case report of acute febrile neutrophilic dermatosis (Sweet's syndrome) and Crohn's disease. Acta Derm Venereol 1991; 71: 360–363.

733 Phars DB, Cerenko D, Caughman SW. Sweet's syndrome in a patient with idiopathic progressive bilateral sensorineural hearing loss. J Am Acad Dermatol 2000; 42: 932–935.

734 Kalmus Y, Kovatz S, Shilo L et al. Sweet's syndrome and subacute thyroiditis. Postgrad Med J 2000; 76: 229–230.

735 Waltz KM, Long D, Marks JG Jr, Billingsley EM. Sweet's syndrome and erythema nodosum. The simultaneous occurrence of 2 reactive dermatoses. Arch Dermatol 1999; 135: 62–66.

736 Lyon CC, Griffiths CEM. Chronic granulomatous disease and acute neutrophilic dermatosis. Clin Exp Dermatol 1999; 24: 368–371.

737 Lipp KE, Shenefelt PD, Nelson RP Jr et al. Persistent Sweet's syndrome occurring in a child with a primary immunodeficiency. J Am Acad Dermatol 1999; 40: 838–841.

738 Rubegni P, Marano MR, De Aloe G et al. Sweet's syndrome and *Chlamydia pneumoniae* infection. J Am Acad Dermatol 2001; 44: 862–864.

739 Flórez A, Sánchez-Aguilar D, Rosón E et al. Sweet's syndrome associated with *Salmonella enteritidis* infection. Clin Exp Dermatol 1999; 24: 239–240.

740 Bang B, Zachariae C. *Capnocytophaga canimorsus* sepsis causing Sweet's syndrome. Acta Derm Venereol 2001; 81: 73–74.

741 Kürkçüoğlu N, Aksoy F. Sweet's syndrome associated with *Helicobacter pylori* infection. J Am Acad Dermatol 1997; 37: 123–124.

742 Choonhakarn C, Chetchotisakd P, Jirarattanapochai K, Mootsikapun P. Sweet's syndrome associated with non-tuberculous mycobacterial infection: a report of five cases. Br J Dermatol 1998; 139: 107–110.

743 Tan E, Yosipovitch G, Giam Y-C, Tan SH. Bullous Sweet's syndrome associated with acute hepatitis B infection: a new association. Br J Dermatol 2000; 143: 914–916.

744 Amichai B, Lazarov A, Cagnano M, Halevy S. Sweet's syndrome and chlamycial infection. Australas J Dermatol 1993; 34: 31–33.

745 Berger TG, Dhar A, McCalmont TH. Neutrophilic dermatoses in HIV infection. J Am Acad Dermatol 1994; 31: 1045–1047.

746 Kemmett D, Hunter JAA. Sweet's syndrome: a clinicopathologic review of twenty-nine cases. J Am Acad Dermatol 1990; 23: 503–507.

747 Radeff B, Harms M. Acute febrile neutrophilic dermatosis (Sweet's syndrome) following BCG vaccination. Acta Derm Venereol 1986; 66: 357–358.

748 Cobb MW. Furosemide-induced eruption simulating Sweet's syndrome. J Am Acad Dermatol 1989; 21: 339–343.

749 Thibault M-J, Billick RC, Srolovitz H. Minocycline-induced Sweet's syndrome. J Am Acad Dermatol 1992; 27: 801–804.

750 Walker DC, Cohen PR. Trimethoprim-sulfamethoxazole-associated acute febrile neutrophilic dermatosis: case report and review of drug-induced Sweet's syndrome. J Am Acad Dermatol 1996; 34: 918–923.

751 Gilmour E, Chalmers RJG, Rowlands DJ. Drug-induced Sweet's syndrome (acute febrile neutrophilic dermatosis) associated with hydralazine. Br J Dermatol 1995; 133: 490–491.

752 Guimerá FJ, García-Bustínduy M, Noda A et al. Diazepam-associated Sweet's syndrome. Int J Dermatol 2000; 39: 795–798.

753 Tefany FJ, Georgouras K. A neutrophilic reaction of Sweet's syndrome type associated with the oral contraceptive. Australas J Dermatol 1991; 32: 55–59.

754 Magro CM, De Moraes E, Burns F. Sweet's syndrome in the setting of CD34-positive acute myelogenous leukemia treated with granulocyte colony stimulating factor: evidence for a clonal neutrophilic dermatosis. J Cutan Pathol 2001; 28: 90–96.

755 Kaplan SS, Wechsler HL, Basford RE et al. Increased plasma chemoattractant in Sweet's syndrome. J Am Acad Dermatol 1985; 12: 1013–1021.

756 Keefe M, Wakeel RA, Kerr REI. Sweet's syndrome, plantar pustulosis and vulval pustules. Clin Exp Dermatol 1988; 13: 344–346.

757 von den Driesch P, Simon M Jr, Djawari D, Wassmuth R. Analysis of HLA antigens in Caucasian patients with acute febrile neutrophilic dermatosis (Sweet's syndrome). J Am Acad Dermatol 1997; 37: 276–278.

758 Giasuddin ASM, El-Orfi AHAM, Ziu MM, El-Barnawi NY. Sweet's syndrome: is the pathogenesis mediated by helper T cell type 1 cytokines? J Am Acad Dermatol 1998; 39: 940–943.

759 Kemmett D, Harrison DJ, Hunter JAA. Antibodies to neutrophil cytoplasmic antigens: a serologic marker for Sweet's syndrome. J Am Acad Dermatol 1991; 24: 967–969.

760 Jordaan HF. Acute febrile neutrophilic dermatosis. A histopathological study of 37 patients and a review of the literature. Am J Dermatopathol 1989; 11: 99–111.

761 Smith HR, Ashton RE, Beer TW, Theaker JM. Neutrophil-poor Sweet's syndrome with response to potassium iodide. Br J Dermatol 1998; 139: 555–556.

762 Delabie J, de Wolf-Peeters C, Morren M et al. Histiocytes in Sweet's syndrome. Br J Dermatol 1991; 124: 348–353.

763 Piette WW, Trapp JF, O'Donnell MJ et al. Acute neutrophilic dermatosis with myeloblastic infiltrate in a leukemia patient receiving all-*trans*-retinoic acid therapy. J Am Acad Dermatol 1994; 30: 293–297.

764 Cox NH, O'Brien HAW. Sweet's syndrome associated with trans-retinoic acid treatment in acute promyelocytic leukaemia. Clin Exp Dermatol 1994; 19: 51–52.

765 Urano Y, Miyaoka Y, Kosaka M et al. Sweet's syndrome associated with chronic myelogenous leukemia: Demonstration of leukemic cells within a skin lesion. J Am Acad Dermatol 1999; 40: 275–279.

766 Tomasini C, Aloi F, Osella-Abate S et al. Immature myeloid precursors in chronic neutrophilic dermatosis associated with myelodysplastic syndrome. Am J Dermatopathol 2000; 22: 429–433.

767 Hwang ST, Williams ML, McCalmont TH, Frieden IJ. Sweet's syndrome leading to acquired cutis laxa (Marshall's syndrome) in an infant with α1-antitrypsin deficiency. Arch Dermatol 1995; 131: 1175–1177.

768 Evans AV, Sabroe RA, Setterfield J, Greaves MW. Erythema elevatum diutinum/Sweet's syndrome overlap with gastrointestinal and oral involvement. Br J Dermatol 1999; 141: 766–767.

769 Annessi G, Signoretti S, Angelo C et al. Neutrophilic figurate erythema of infancy. Am J Dermatopathol 1997; 19: 403–406.

770 Sidhu-Malik NK, Resnick SD, Wilson BB. Congenital erosive and vesicular dermatosis healing with reticulated supple scarring: report of three new cases and review of the literature. Pediatr Dermatol 1998; 15: 214–218.

771 Strutton G, Weedon D, Robertson I. Pustular vasculitis of the hands. J Am Acad Dermatol 1995; 32: 192–198.

772 Von den Driesch P. Sweet's syndrome and vasculitis. J Am Acad Dermatol 1996; 34: 539.

773 Hall AP, Goudge RJ, Ireton HJC, Burrell LM. Pustular vasculitis of the hands. Australas J Dermatol 1999; 40: 204–207.

774 Galaria NA, Junkins-Hopkins JM, Kligman D, James WD. Neutrophilic dermatosis of the dorsal hands: Pustular vasculitis revisited. J Am Acad Dermatol 2000; 43: 870–874.

775 Curcó N, Pagerols X, Tarroch X, Vives P. Pustular vasculitis of the hands. Report of two men. Dermatology 1998; 196: 346–347.

776 Ely PH. The bowel bypass syndrome: a response to bacterial peptidoglycans. J Am Acad Dermatol 1980; 2: 473–487.

777 Kennedy C. The spectrum of inflammatory skin disease following jejuno-ileal bypass for morbid obesity. Br J Dermatol 1981; 105: 425–436.

778 Kemp DR, Gin D. Bowel-associated dermatosis-arthritis syndrome. Med J Aust 1990; 152: 43–45.

779 Dicken CH. Bowel-associated dermatosis-arthritis syndrome: bowel bypass syndrome without bowel bypass. Mayo Clin Proc 1984; 59: 43–46.

780 Dicken CH. Bowel-associated dermatosis-arthritis syndrome: bowel bypass syndrome without bowel bypass. J Am Acad Dermatol 1986; 14: 792–796.

781 Utsinger PD. Systemic immune complex disease following intestinal bypass surgery: bypass disease. J Am Acad Dermatol 1980; 2: 488–495.

782 O'Loughlin S, Perry HO. A diffuse pustular eruption associated with ulcerative colitis. Arch Dermatol 1978; 114: 1061–1064.

783 Ackerman AB. Histologic diagnosis of inflammatory skin diseases. Philadelphia: Lea & Febiger, 1978; 449–451.

784 Scherbenske JM, Benson PM, Lupton GP, Samlaska CP. Rheumatoid neutrophilic dermatitis. Arch Dermatol 1989; 125: 1105–1108.

785 Delaporte E, Graveau DJ, Piette FA, Bergoend HA. Acute febrile neutrophilic dermatosis (Sweet's syndrome). Association with rheumatoid vasculitis. Arch Dermatol 1989; 125: 1101–1104.

786 Sánchez JL, Cruz A. Rheumatoid neutrophilic dermatitis. J Am Acad Dermatol 1990; 22: 922–925.

787 Hughes JR, Erhardt CC, Clement M. Neutrophilic dermatosis in association with rheumatoid arthritis. Clin Exp Dermatol 1995; 20: 168–170.

788 Mashek HA, Pham CT, Helm TN, Klaus M. Rheumatoid neutrophilic dermatitis. Arch Dermatol 1997; 133: 757–760.

789 Macaya A, Servitje O, Jucglà A, Peyri J. Rheumatoid neutrophilic dermatitis associated with pyoderma gangrenosum. Br J Dermatol 2000; 142: 1246–1248.

790 Hassab-el-Naby HMM, Alsaleh QA, Khalifa MA. Rheumatoid neutrophilic dermatitis. Int J Dermatol 1996; 35: 207–208.

791 Lowe L, Kornfeld B, Clayman J, Golitz LE. Rheumatoid neutrophilic dermatitis. J Cutan Pathol 1992; 19: 48–53.

792 Tan RS-H. Acute generalized pustular bacterid. An unusual manifestation of leukocytoclastic vasculitis. Br J Dermatol 1974; 91: 209–215.

793 Miyachi Y, Danno K, Yanase K, Imamura S. Acute generalized pustular bacterid and immune complexes. Acta Derm Venereol 1980; 60: 66–69.

794 McNeely MC, Jorizzo JL, Solomon AR Jr et al. Primary idiopathic cutaneous pustular vasculitis. J Am Acad Dermatol 1986; 14: 939–944.

795 Rustin MHA, Robinson TWE, Dowd PM. Toxic pustuloderma: a self-limiting eruption. Br J Dermatol 1990; 123: 119–124.

796 Jorizzo JL, Abernethy JL, White WL et al. Mucocutaneous criteria for the diagnosis of Behçet's disease: an analysis of clinicopathologic data from multiple international centers. J Am Acad Dermatol 1995; 32: 968–976.

797 Mangelsdorf HC, White WL, Jorizzo JL. Behçet's disease. Report of twenty-five patients from the United States with prominent mucocutaneous involvement. J Am Acad Dermatol 1996; 34: 745–750.

798 Jorizzo JL, Taylor RS, Schmalstieg FC et al. Complex aphthosis: a forme fruste of Behçet's syndrome? J Am Acad Dermatol 1985; 13: 80–84.
799 Arbesfeld SJ, Kurban AK. Behçet's disease. New perspectives on an enigmatic syndrome. J Am Acad Dermatol 1988; 19: 767–779.
800 Ghate JV, Jorizzo JL. Behçet's disease and complex aphthosis. J Am Acad Dermatol 1999; 40: 1–18.
801 Verpilleux M-P, Bastuji-Garin S, Revuz J. Comparative analysis of severe aphthosis and Behçet's disease: 104 cases. Dermatology 1999; 198: 247–251.
802 Matsumoto T, Uekusa T, Fukuda Y. Vasculo-Behçet's disease: a pathologic study of eight cases. Hum Pathol 1991; 22: 45–51.
803 Chun SI, Su WPD, Lee S, Rogers RS III. Erythema nodosum-like lesions in Behçet's syndrome: a histopathologic study of 30 cases. J Cutan Pathol 1989; 16: 259–265.
804 King R, Crowson AN, Murray E, Magro CM. Acral purpuric papulonodular lesions as a manifestation of Behçet's disease. Int J Dermatol 1995; 34: 190–192.
805 Jacyk WK. Behçet's disease in South African blacks: report of five cases. J Am Acad Dermatol 1994; 30: 869–873.
806 Alpsoy E, Aktekin M, Er H et al. A randomized, controlled and blinded study of papulopustular lesions in Turkish Behçet's patients. Int J Dermatol 1998; 37: 839–842.
807 Gilhar A, Winterstein G, Turani H et al. Skin hyperreactivity response (pathergy) in Behçet's disease. J Am Acad Dermatol 1989; 21: 547–552.
808 Wong RC, Ellis CN, Diaz LA. Behçet's disease. Int J Dermatol 1984; 23: 25–32.
809 Cho KH, Shin KS, Sohn SJ et al. Behçet's disease with Sweet's syndrome-like presentation – a report of six cases. Clin Exp Dermatol 1989; 14: 20–24.
810 Lee M-S, Barnetson RStC. Sweet's syndrome associated with Behçet's disease. Australas J Dermatol 1996; 37: 99–101.
811 Rakover Y, Adar H, Tal I et al. Behçet's disease: long-term follow-up of three children and review of the literature. Pediatrics 1989; 83: 986–992.
812 Kim D-K, Chang SN, Bang D et al. Clinical analysis of 40 cases of childhood-onset Behçet's disease. Pediatr Dermatol 1994; 11: 95–101.
813 Sarica R, Azizlerli G, Köse A et al. Juvenile Behçet's disease among 1784 Turkish Behçet's patients. Int J Dermatol 1996; 35: 109–111.
814 Jorizzo JL. Behçet's disease. An update based on the 1985 international conference in London. Arch Dermatol 1986; 122: 556–558.
815 Dundar SV, Gencalp U, Simsek H. Familial cases of Behçet's disease. Br J Dermatol 1985; 113: 319–321.
816 Treudler R, Orfanos CE, Zouboulis ChC. Twenty-eight cases of juvenile-onset Adamantiades–Behçet's disease in Germany. Dermatology 1999; 199: 15–19.
817 Avci O, Ellidokuz E, Şimşek İ et al. *Helicobacter pylori* and Behçet's disease. Dermatology 1999; 199: 140–143.
818 İlter N, Şenol E, Gürer MA, Öztaş MO. Behçet's disease and HCV infection. Int J Dermatol 2000; 39: 396–397.
819 Örem A, Çimşit G, Değer O et al. Autoantibodies against oxidatively modified low-density lipoprotein in patients with Behçet's disease. Dermatology 1999; 198: 243–246.
820 Jorizzo JL, Hudson RD, Schmalstieg FC et al. Behçet's syndrome: immune regulation, circulating immune complexes, neutrophil migration, and colchicine therapy. J Am Acad Dermatol 1984; 10: 205–214.
821 Abdallah MA, Ragab N, Khalil R, Kamel N. Circulating immune complexes in various forms of Behçet's disease. Int J Dermatol 1995; 34: 841–845.
822 Kaneko F, Takahashi Y, Muramatsu R et al. Natural killer cell numbers and function in peripheral lymphoid cells in Behçet's disease. Br J Dermatol 1985; 113: 313–318.
823 Treudler R, Zouboulis CC, Büttner P et al. Enhanced interaction of patients' lymphocytes with human dermal microvascular endothelial cell cultures in active Adamantiades–Behçet's disease. Arch Dermatol 1996; 132: 1323–1329.
824 Kaneko F, Takahashi Y, Muramatsu Y, Miura Y. Immunological studies on aphthous ulcer and erythema nodosum-like eruptions in Behçet's disease. Br J Dermatol 1985; 113: 303–312.
825 James DG. Behçet's syndrome. N Engl J Med 1979; 301: 431–432.
826 Katsantonis J, Adler Y, Orfanos CE, Zouboulis CC. Adamantiades–Behçet's disease: serum IL-8 is a more reliable marker for disease activity than C-reactive protein and erythrocyte sedimentation rate. Dermatology 2000; 201: 37–39.
827 Muller W, Lehner T. Quantitative electron microscopical analysis of leukocyte infiltrate in oral ulcers of Behçet's syndrome. Br J Dermatol 1982; 106: 535–544.
828 Honma T, Saito T, Fujioka Y. Intraepithelial atypical lymphocytes in oral lesions of Behçet's syndrome. Arch Dermatol 1981; 117: 83–85.
829 Bang D, Honma T, Saito T et al. The pathogenesis of vascular changes in erythema nodosum-like lesions of Behçet's syndrome: an electron microscopic study. Hum Pathol 1987; 18: 1172–1179.
830 Kim B, LeBoit PE. Histopathologic features of erythema nodosum-like lesions in Behçet's disease. Am J Dermatopathol 2000; 22: 379–390.
831 Ohtake N, Kanekura T, Kawamura K, Kanzaki T. Unusual polyp-like structures in lobular panniculitis of a patient with Behçet's disease. Am J Dermatopathol 1997; 19: 185–188.
832 Jorizzo JL, Solomon AR, Cavallo T. Behçet's syndrome. Arch Pathol Lab Med 1985; 109: 747–751.
833 Ergun T, Gürbüz O, Harvell J et al. The histopathology of pathergy: a chronologic study of skin hyperreactivity in Behçet's disease. Int J Dermatol 1998; 37: 929–933.
834 Gül A, Esin S, Dilsen N et al. Immunohistology of skin pathergy reaction in Behçet's disease. Br J Dermatol 1995; 132: 901–907.
835 Magro CM, Crowson AN. Cutaneous manifestations of Behçet's disease. Int J Dermatol 1995; 34: 159–165.
836 Ibbotson SH, McLelland J. Episodic vasculitis of the hands and feet in association with Behçet's disease. Clin Exp Dermatol 1996; 21: 465–466.
837 Chen K-R, Kawahara Y, Miyakawa S, Nishikawa T. Cutaneous vasculitis in Behçet's disease: A clinical and histopathologic study of 20 patients. J Am Acad Dermatol 1997; 36: 689–696.
838 Balabanova M, Calamia KT, Perniciaro C et al. A study of the cutaneous manifestations of Behçet's disease in patients from the United States. J Am Acad Dermatol 1999; 41: 540–545.
839 Ergun T, Gürbüz O, Doğusoy G et al. Histopathologic features of the spontaneous pustular lesions of Behçet's syndrome. Int J Dermatol 1998; 37: 194–196.
840 Liao Y-H, Hsiao G-H, Hsiao C-H. Behçet's disease with cutaneous changes resembling polyarteritis nodosa. Br J Dermatol 1999; 140: 368–369.
841 Toroko Y, Seto T, Abe Y et al. Skin lesions in Behçet's disease. Int J Dermatol 1977; 16: 227–244.

Chronic lymphocytic vasculitis
842 Massa MC, Su WPD. Lymphocytic vasculitis: is it a special clinicopathologic entity? J Cutan Pathol 1984; 11: 132–139.
843 Carlson JA, Mihm MC Jr, LeBoit PE. Cutaneous lymphocytic vasculitis: a definition, a review, and a proposed classification. Semin Diagn Pathol 1996; 13: 72–90.
844 Kossard S. Defining lymphocytic vasculitis. Australas J Dermatol 2000; 41: 149–155.
845 Vuzevski VD, van Joost T, Wagenvoort JHT, Day JJM. Cutaneous pathology in toxic shock syndrome. Int J Dermatol 1989; 28: 94–97.
846 Murphy FT, Enzenauer RJ, Battafarano DF, David-Bajar K. Etanercept-associated injection-site reactions. Arch Dermatol 2000; 136: 556–557.
847 Oh CW, Lee SH. A case suggesting lymphocytic vasculitis as a presenting sign of early undifferentiated connective tissue disease. J Cutan Pathol 2000; 27: 567 (abstract).
848 Farrell AM, Gooptu C, Woodrow D et al. Cutaneous lymphocytic vasculitis in acute myeloid leukaemia. Br J Dermatol 1996; 135: 471–474.
849 Magro CM, Crowson AN. A distinctive cutaneous reaction pattern indicative of infection by reactive arthropathy-associated microbial pathogens: the superantigen ID reaction. J Cutan Pathol 1998; 25: 538–544.
850 Coskey RJ. Eruptions due to oral contraceptives. Arch Dermatol 1977; 113: 333–334.
851 Gupta G, Holmes SC, Spence E, Mills PR. Capillaritis associated with interferon-alfa treatment of chronic hepatitis C infection. J Am Acad Dermatol 2000; 43: 937–938.
852 Jurecka W, Holmes RC, Black MM et al. An immunoelectron microscopy study of the relationship between herpes gestationis and polymorphic eruption of pregnancy. Br J Dermatol 1983; 108: 147–151.
853 Charles-Holmes R. Polymorphic eruption of pregnancy. Semin Dermatol 1989; 8: 18–22.
854 Yancey KB, Hall RP, Lawley TJ. Pruritic urticarial papules and plaques of pregnancy. Clinical experience in twenty-five patients. J Am Acad Dermatol 1984; 10: 473–480.
855 Uhl n SR. Pruritic urticarial papules and plaques of pregnancy. Involvement in mother and infant. Arch Dermatol 1981; 117: 238–239.
856 Borradori L, Saurat J-H. Specific dermatoses of pregnancy. Toward a comprehensive view? Arch Dermatol 1994; 130: 778–780.
857 Bos JD. Reappraisal of dermatoses of pregnancy. Lancet 1999; 354: 1140.
858 Tarocchi S, Carli P, Caproni M, Fabbri P. Polymorphic eruption of pregnancy. Int J Dermatol 1997; 36: 448–450.
859 García-González E, Ahued-Ahued R, Arroyo E et al. Immunology of the cutaneous disorders of pregnancy. Int J Dermatol 1999; 38: 721–729.
860 Holmes RC, Black MM, Dann J et al. A comparative study of toxic erythema of pregnancy and herpes gestationis. Br J Dermatol 1982; 106: 499–510.
861 Nurse DS. Prurigo of pregnancy. Australas J Dermatol 1968; 9: 258–267.
862 Faber WR, van Joost T, Hausman R, Weenink GH. Late prurigo of pregnancy. Br J Dermatol 1982; 106: 511–516.
863 Borrego L. Follicular lesions in polymorphic eruption of pregnancy. J Am Acad Dermatol 2000; 42: 146.
864 Vaughan Jones SA, Black MM. Pregnancy dermatoses. J Am Acad Dermatol 1999; 40: 233–241.

865 Beltrani VP, Beltrani VS. Pruritic urticarial papules and plaques of pregnancy: a severe case requiring early delivery for relief of symptoms. J Am Acad Dermatol 1992; 26: 266–267.

866 Vaughan Jones SA, Hern S, Nelson-Piercy C et al. A prospective study of 200 women with dermatoses of pregnancy correlating clinical findings with hormonal and immunopathological profiles. Br J Dermatol 1999; 141: 71–81.

867 Saraswat A, Rai R, Kumar B. Lesions resembling polymorphic eruption of pregnancy several years after pregnancy. Dermatology 2001; 202: 82.

868 Cohen LM, Capeless EL, Krusinski PA, Maloney ME. Pruritic urticarial papules and plaques of pregnancy and its relationship to maternal-fetal weight gain and twin pregnancy. Arch Dermatol 1989; 125: 1534–1536.

869 Bunker CB, Erskine K, Rustin MHA, Gilkes JJH. Severe polymorphic eruption of pregnancy occurring in twin pregnancies. Clin Exp Dermatol 1990; 15: 228–231.

870 Pauwels C, Bucaille-Fleury L, Recanati G. Pruritic urticarial papules and plaques of pregnancy: relationship to maternal weight gain and twin or triplet pregnancies. Arch Dermatol 1994; 130: 801–802.

871 Vaughan Jones SA, Dunnill MGS, Black MM. Pruritic urticarial papules and plaques of pregnancy (polymorphic eruption of pregnancy): two unusual cases. Br J Dermatol 1996; 135: 102–105.

872 Lawley TJ, Hartz KC, Wade TR et al. Pruritic urticarial papules and plaques of pregnancy. JAMA 1979; 241: 1696–1699.

873 Goldberg NS. Pruritic urticarial papules and plaques of pregnancy in triplet pregnancy. Br J Dermatol 1997; 137: 161.

874 Powell FC. Pruritic urticarial papules and plaques of pregnancy and multiple pregnancies. J Am Acad Dermatol 2000; 43: 730–731.

875 Elling SV, McKenna P, Powell FC. Pruritic urticarial papules and plaques of pregnancy in twin and triplet pregnancies. J Eur Acad Dermatol Venereol 2000; 14: 378–381.

876 Weiss R, Hull P. Familial occurrence of pruritic urticarial papules and plaques of pregnancy. J Am Acad Dermatol 1992; 26: 715–717.

877 Roger D, Vaillant L, Fignon A et al. Specific pruritic diseases of pregnancy. A prospective study of 3192 pregnant women. Arch Dermatol 1994; 130: 734–739.

878 Callen JP, Hanno R. Pruritic urticarial papules and plaques of pregnancy (PUPPP). A clinicopathologic study. J Am Acad Dermatol 1981; 5: 401–405.

879 Winton GB, Lewis CW. Dermatoses of pregnancy. J Am Acad Dermatol 1982; 6: 977–998.

880 Aronson IK, Bond S, Fiedler VC et al. Pruritic urticarial papules and plaques of pregnancy: Clinical and immunopathologic observations in 57 patients. J Am Acad Dermatol 1998; 39: 933–939.

881 Zurn A, Celebi CR, Bernard P et al. A prospective immunofluorescence study of 11 cases of pruritic dermatoses of pregnancy: IgM anti-basement membrane zone antibodies as a novel finding. Br J Dermatol 1992; 126: 474–478.

882 Borradori L, Didierjean L, Bernard P et al. IgM autoantibodies to 180- and 230- to 240-kd human epidermal proteins in pregnancy. Arch Dermatol 1995; 131: 43–47.

883 Holmes RC, Black MM. The specific dermatoses of pregnancy: a reappraisal with specific emphasis on a proposed simplified clinical classification. Clin Exp Dermatol 1982; 7: 65–73.

884 Holmes RC, Black MM. The specific dermatoses of pregnancy. J Am Acad Dermatol 1983; 8: 405–412.

885 Black MM. Prurigo of pregnancy, papular dermatitis of pregnancy, and pruritic folliculitis of pregnancy. Semin Dermatol 1989; 8: 23–25.

886 Rahbari H. Pruritic papules of pregnancy. J Cutan Pathol 1978; 5: 347–352

887 Harrison PV. The annular erythemas. Int J Dermatol 1979; 18: 282–290.

888 Hurley HJ, Hurley JP. The gyrate erythemas. Semin Dermatol 1984; 3: 327–336.

889 White JW Jr. Gyrate erythema. Dermatol Clin 1985; 3: 129–139.

890 Abech D, Ollert MW, Eckert F et al. Palpable migratory arciform erythema. Clinical morphology, histopathology, immunohistochemistry, and response to treatment. Arch Dermatol 1997; 133: 763–766.

891 Ackerman AB. Histologic diagnosis of inflammatory skin diseases. Philadelphia: Lea & Febiger, 1978; 231–233.

892 Bressler GS, Jones RE Jr. Erythema annulare centrifugum. J Am Acad Dermatol 1981; 4: 597–602.

893 Burkhart CG. Erythema annulare centrifugum. A case due to tuberculosis. Int J Dermatol 1982; 21: 538–539.

894 Betlloch I, Amador C, Chiner E et al. Erythema annulare centrifugum in Q fever. Int J Dermatol 1991; 30: 502.

895 Vasily DB, Bhatia SG. Erythema annulare centrifugum and molluscum contagiosum. Arch Dermatol 1978; 114: 1853.

896 Hendricks AA, Lu C, Elfenbein GJ, Hussain R. Erythema annulare centrifugum associated with ascariasis. Arch Dermatol 1981; 117: 582–585.

897 Dodd HJ, Kirby JDT, Chambers TJ, Stansfeld AG. Erythema annulare centrifugum and malignant histiocytosis – report of a case. Clin Exp Dermatol 1984; 9: 608–613.

898 Yaniv R, Shpielberg O, Shpiro D et al. Erythema annulare centrifugum as the presenting sign of Hodgkin's disease. Int J Dermatol 1993; 32: 59–60.

899 Mahood JM. Erythema annulare centrifugum: a review of 24 cases with special reference to its association with underlying disease. Clin Exp Dermatol 1983; 8: 383–387.

900 Merrett AC, Marks R, Dudley FJ. Cimetidine-induced erythema annulare centrifugum: no cross-sensitivity with ranitidine. Br Med J 1981; 283: 698.

901 Tsuji T, Nishimura M, Kimura S. Erythema annulare centrifugum associated with gold sodium thiomalate therapy. J Am Acad Dermatol 1992; 27: 284–287.

902 Goette DK, Beatrice E. Erythema annulare centrifugum caused by hydrochlorothiazide-induced interstitial nephritis. Int J Dermatol 1988; 27: 129–130.

903 Ashurst PJ. Erythema annulare centrifugum; due to hydroxychloroquine sulfate and chloroquine sulfate. Arch Dermatol 1967; 95: 37–39.

904 Teramoto N, Katayama I, Arai H et al. Annular erythema: a possible association with primary Sjögren's syndrome. J Am Acad Dermatol 1989; 20: 596–601.

905 Miyagawa S, Dohi K, Shima H, Shirai T. HLA antigens in anti-Ro(SS-A)-positive patients with recurrent annular erythema. J Am Acad Dermatol 1993; 28: 185–188.

906 Miyagawa S, Iida T, Fukimoto T et al. Anti-Ro/SSA-associated annular erythema in childhood. Br J Dermatol 1995; 133: 779–782.

907 Ostlere LS, Harris D, Rustin MHA. Urticated annular erythema: a new manifestation of Sjögren's syndrome. Clin Exp Dermatol 1993; 18: 50–51.

908 Watanabe T, Tsuchida T, Furue M, Yoshinoya S. Annular erythema, dermatomyositis, and Sjögren's syndrome. Int J Dermatol 1996; 35: 235–287.

909 McCauliffe DP, Faircloth E, Wang L et al. Similar Ro/SS-A autoantibody epitope and titer responses in annular erythema of Sjögren's syndrome and subacute cutaneous lupus erythematosus. Arch Dermatol 1996; 132: 528–531.

910 Kawakami T, Saito R. The relationship between facial annular erythema and anti-SS-A/Ro antibodies in three East Asian women. Br J Dermatol 1999; 140: 136–140.

911 Hoshino Y, Hashimoto T, Mimori T et al. Recurrent annular erythema associated with anti-SS-B/La antibodies: analysis of the disease-specific epitope. Br J Dermatol 1992; 127: 608–613.

912 Boyd AS, Neldner KH, Menter A. Erythema gyratum repens: a paraneoplastic eruption. J Am Acad Dermatol 1992; 26: 757–762.

913 Olsen TG, Milroy SK, Jones-Olsen S. Erythema gyratum repens with associated squamous cell carcinoma of the lung. Cutis 1984; 34: 351–355.

914 Appell ML, Ward WQ, Tyring SK. Erythema gyratum repens. A cutaneous marker of malignancy. Cancer 1988; 62: 548–550.

915 Caux F, Lebbe C, Thomine E et al. Erythema gyratum repens. A case studied with immunofluorescence, immunoelectron microscopy and immunohistochemistry. Br J Dermatol 1994; 131: 102–107.

916 Barber PV, Doyle L, Vickers DM, Hubbard H. Erythema gyratum repens with pulmonary tuberculosis. Br J Dermatol 1978; 98: 465–468.

917 Juhlin L, Lacour JP, Larrouy JC et al. Episodic erythema gyratum repens with ichthyosis and palmoplantar hyperkeratosis without signs of internal malignancy. Clin Exp Dermatol 1989; 14: 223–226.

918 Cheesbrough MJ, Williamson DM. Erythema gyratum repens, a stage in the resolution of pityriasis rubra pilaris? Clin Exp Dermatol 1985; 10: 466–471.

919 Langlois JC, Shaw JM, Odland GF. Erythema gyratum repens unassociated with internal malignancy. J Am Acad Dermatol 1985; 12: 911–913.

920 Garrett SJ, Roenigk HH Jr. Erythema gyratum repens in a healthy woman. J Am Acad Dermatol 1992; 26: 121–122.

921 Wakeel RA, Ormerod AD, Sewell HF, White MI. Subcorneal accumulation of Langerhans cells in erythema gyratum repens. Br J Dermatol 1992; 126: 189–192.

922 Albers SE, Fenske NA, Glass LF. Erythema gyratum repens: direct immunofluorescence microscopic findings. J Am Acad Dermatol 1993; 29: 493–494.

923 Willis WF. The gyrate erythemas. Int J Dermatol 1978; 17: 698–702.

924 Troyer C, Grossman M, Silvers DN. Erythema marginatum in rheumatic fever: early diagnosis by skin biopsy. J Am Acad Dermatol 1983; 8: 724–728.

925 Sahn EE, Maize JC, Silver RM. Erythema marginatum: an unusual histopathologic manifestation. J Am Acad Dermatol 1989; 21: 145–147.

926 Beare JM, Froggatt P, Jones JH, Neill DW. Familial annular erythema. An apparently new dominant mutation. Br J Dermatol 1966; 78: 59–68.

927 Cox NH, McQueen A, Evans TJ, Morley WN. An annular erythema of infancy. Arch Dermatol 1987; 123: 510–513.

928 Hebert AA, Esterly NB. Annular erythema of infancy. J Am Acad Dermatol 1986; 14: 339–343.

929 Toonstra J, de Wit RFE. 'Persistent' annular erythema of infancy. Arch Dermatol 1984; 120: 1069–1072.

930 Stachowitz S, Abeck D, Schmidt T, Ring J. Persistent annular erythema of infancy associated with intestinal Candida colonization. Clin Exp Dermatol 2000; 25: 404–405.

931 Gianotti F, Ermacora E. Erythema gyratum atrophicans transiens neonatale. Arch Dermatol 1975; 111: 615–616.

932 Saurat JH, Janin-Mercier A. Infantile epidermodysplastic erythema gyratum responsive to imidazoles. A new entity? Arch Dermatol 1984; 120: 1601–1603.

933 Miyagawa S, Kitamura W, Yoshioka J, Sakamoto K. Placental transfer of anticytoplasmic antibodies in annular erythema of newborns. Arch Dermatol 1981; 117: 569–572.

934 Helm TN, Bass J, Chang LW, Bergfeld WF. Persistent annular erythema of infancy. Pediatr Dermatol 1993; 10: 46–48.

935 Marks R, Black M, Wilson Jones E. Pityriasis lichenoides: a reappraisal. Br J Dermatol 1972; 86: 215–225.

936 Rogers M. Pityriasis lichenoides and lymphomatoid papulosis. Semin Dermatol 1992; 11: 73–79.

937 Truhan AP, Hebert AA, Esterly NB. Pityriasis lichenoides in children: therapeutic response to erythromycin. J Am Acad Dermatol 1986; 15: 66–70.

938 Romani J, Puig L, Fernández-Figueras MT, de Moragas JM. Pityriasis lichenoides in children: clinicopathologic review of 22 patients. Pediatr Dermatol 1998; 15: 1–6.

939 Gelmetti C, Rigoni C, Alessi E et al. Pityriasis lichenoides in children: a long-term follow-up of eighty-nine cases. J Am Acad Dermatol 1990; 23: 473–478.

940 Fortson JS, Schroeter AL, Esterly NB. Cutaneous T-cell lymphoma (parapsoriasis en plaque). An association with pityriasis lichenoides et varioliformis acuta in young children. Arch Dermatol 1990; 126: 1449–1453.

941 Shieh S, Mikkola DL, Wood GS. Differentiation and clonality of lesional lymphocytes in pityriasis lichenoides chronica. Arch Dermatol 2001; 137: 305–308.

942 Hermanns-Lê T, Piérard GE. Medullary CD30+ T cell lymphoma with eosinophilia and hyper-IgE supervening during the relentless course of pityriasis lichenoides. Dermatology 2000; 200: 170–172.

943 Luberti AA, Rabinowitz LG, Ververeli KO. Severe febrile Mucha–Habermann's disease in children: case report and review of the literature. Pediatr Dermatol 1991; 8: 51–57.

944 López-Estebaranz JL, Vanaclocha F, Gil R et al. Febrile ulceronecrotic Mucha–Habermann disease. J Am Acad Dermatol 1993; 29: 903–906.

945 Fink-Puches R, Soyer HP, Kerl H. Febrile ulceronecrotic pityriasis lichenoides et varioliformis acuta. J Am Acad Dermatol 1994; 30: 261–263.

946 Puddu P, Cianchini G, Colonna L et al. Febrile ulceronecrotic Mucha–Habermann's disease with fatal outcome. Int J Dermatol 1997; 36: 691–694.

947 Smith KJ, Nelson A, Skelton H et al. Pityriasis lichenoides et varioliformis acuta in HIV-1+ patients: a marker of early stage disease. Int J Dermatol 1997; 36: 104–109.

948 Clayton R, Warin A. Pityriasis lichenoides chronica presenting as hypopigmentation. Br J Dermatol 1979; 100: 297–302.

949 Chung HG, Kim S-C. Pityriasis lichenoides chronica with acral distribution mimicking palmoplantar syphilid. Acta Derm Venereol 1999; 79: 239.

950 Cliff S, Cook MG, Ostlere LS, Mortimer PS. Segmental pityriasis lichenoides chronica. Clin Exp Dermatol 1996; 21: 464–465.

951 Auster BI, Santa Cruz DJ, Eisen AZ. Febrile ulceronecrotic Mucha–Habermann's disease with interstitial pneumonitis. J Cutan Pathol 1979; 6: 66–76.

952 Almagro M, Del Pozo J, Martínez W et al. Pityriasis lichenoides-like exanthem and primary infection by Epstein–Barr virus. Int J Dermatol 2000; 39: 156–159.

953 Zlatkov NB, Andreev VC. Toxoplasmosis and pityriasis lichenoides. Br J Dermatol 1972; 87: 114–116.

954 English JC III, Collins M, Bryant-Bruce C. Pityriasis lichenoides et varioliformis acuta and group A-beta hemolytic streptococcal infection. Int J Dermatol 1995; 34: 642–644.

955 Rongioletti F, Delmonte S, Rebora A. Pityriasis lichenoides and acquired toxoplasmosis. Int J Dermatol 1999; 38: 372–374.

956 Muhlbauer JE, Bhan AK, Harrist TJ et al. Immunopathology of pityriasis lichenoides acuta. J Am Acad Dermatol 1984; 10: 783–795.

957 Willemze R, Scheffer E. Clinical and histologic differentiation between lymphomatoid papulosis and pityriasis lichenoides. J Am Acad Dermatol 1985; 13: 418–428.

958 Niemczyk UM, Zollner TM, Wolter M et al. The transformation of pityriasis lichenoides chronica into parakeratosis variegata in an 11-year-old girl. Br J Dermatol 1997; 137: 983–987.

959 Hood AF, Mark EJ. Histopathologic diagnosis of pityriasis lichenoides et varioliformis acuta and its clinical correlation. Arch Dermatol 1982; 118: 478–482.

960 Szymanski FJ. Pityriasis lichenoides et varioliformis acuta: histopathological evidence that it is an entity distinct from parapsoriasis. Arch Dermatol 1959; 79: 7–16.

961 Longley J, Demar L, Feinstein RP et al. Clinical and histologic features of pityriasis lichenoides et varioliformis acuta in children. Arch Dermatol 1987; 123: 1335–1339.

962 Benmaman O, Sanchez JL. Comparative clinicopathological study on pityriasis lichenoides chronica and small plaque parapsoriasis. Am J Dermatopathol 1988; 10: 189–196.

963 Wood GS, Strickler JG, Abel EA et al. Immunohistology of pityriasis lichenoides et varioliformis acuta and pityriasis lichenoides chronica. Evidence for their interrelationship with lymphomatoid papulosis. J Am Acad Dermatol 1987; 16: 559–570.

964 Clayton R, Haffenden G. An immunofluorescence study of pityriasis lichenoides. Br J Dermatol 1978; 99: 491–493.

965 Panhans A, Bodemer C, Macinthyre E et al. Pityriasis lichenoides of childhood with atypical CD30-positive cells and clonal T-cell receptor gene rearrangements. J Am Acad Dermatol 1996; 35: 489–490.

966 Graham RM, English JS, Emmerson RW. Lichen aureus – a study of twelve cases. Clin Exp Dermatol 1984; 9: 393–401.

967 Newton RC, Raimer SS. Pigmented purpuric eruptions. Dermatol Clin 1985; 3: 165–169.

968 Ratnam KV, Su WPD, Peters MS. Purpura simplex (inflammatory purpura without vasculitis): a clinicopathologic study of 174 cases. J Am Acad Dermatol 1991; 25: 642–647.

969 Gelmetti C, Cerri D, Grimalt R. Lichen aureus in childhood. Pediatr Dermatol 1991; 8: 280–283.

970 Riordan CA, Darley C, Markey AC et al. Unilateral linear capillaritis. Clin Exp Dermatol 1992; 17: 182–185.

971 Filo V, Galbavy Š, Filová A et al. Unilateral progressive pigmented capillaropathy (Schamberg's disease?) of the arm. Br J Dermatol 2001; 144: 190–191.

972 Baden HP. Familial Schamberg's disease. Arch Dermatol 1964; 90: 400.

973 Kanwar AJ, Thami GP. Familial Schamberg's disease. Dermatology 1999; 198: 175–176.

974 Hersh CS, Shwayder TA. Unilateral progressive pigmentary purpura (Schamberg's disease) in a 15-year-old boy. J Am Acad Dermatol 1991; 24: 651.

975 Mar A, Fergin P, Hogan P. Unilateral pigmented purpuric eruption. Australas J Dermatol 1999; 40: 211–214.

976 Doucas C, Kapetanakis J. Eczematid-like purpura. Dermatologica 1953; 106: 86–95.

977 Pravda DJ, Moynihan GD. Itching purpura. Cutis 1980; 25: 147–151.

978 Mosto SJ, Casala AM. Disseminated pruriginous angiodermatitis (itching purpura). Arch Dermatol 1965; 91: 351–356.

979 Honda M, Saijo S, Tagami H. Majocchi's disease in a newborn baby: a familial case. Br J Dermatol 1997; 137: 655–656.

980 Wong RC, Solomon AR, Field SI, Anderson TF. Pigmented purpuric lichenoid dermatitis of Gougerot–Blum mimicking Kaposi's sarcoma. Cutis 1983; 31: 406–410.

981 Rao BK, Igwegbe I, Wiederkehr M et al. Gougerot–Blum disease as a manifestation of hepatitis C infection. J Cutan Pathol 2000; 27: 569 (abstract).

982 Ayala F, Donofrio P. Lichen aureus vel purpuricus: report of a case. Clin Exp Dermatol 1984; 9: 205–208.

983 Price ML, Wilson Jones E, Calnan CD, MacDonald DM. Lichen aureus: a localized persistent form of pigmented purpuric dermatitis. Br J Dermatol 1985; 112: 307–314.

984 English J. Lichen aureus. J Am Acad Dermatol 1985; 12: 377–378.

985 Rudolph RI. Lichen aureus. J Am Acad Dermatol 1983; 8: 722–724.

986 Kossard S, Shumack S. Lichen aureus of the glans penis as an expression of Zoon's balanitis. J Am Acad Dermatol 1989; 21: 804–806.

987 Mishra D, Maheshwari V. Segmental lichen aureus in a child. Int J Dermatol 1991; 30: 654–655.

988 Lazarov A, Cordoba M. Purpuric contact dermatitis in patients with allergic reaction to textile dyes and resins. J Eur Acad Dermatol Venereol 2000; 14: 101–105.

989 van der Veen JPW, Neering H, de Haan P, Bruynzeel DP. Pigmented purpuric clothing dermatitis due to Disperse Blue 85. Contact Dermatitis 1985; 13: 222–223.

990 Toro JR, Sander CA, LeBoit PE. Persistent pigmented purpuric dermatitis and mycosis fungoides: simulant, precursor, or both? Am J Dermatopathol 1997; 19: 108–118.

991 Puddu P, Ferranti G, Frezzolini A et al. Pigmented purpura-like eruption as cutaneous sign of mycosis fungoides with autoimmune purpura. J Am Acad Dermatol 1999; 40: 298–299.

992 Crowson AN, Magro CM, Zahorchak R. Atypical pigmentary purpura: a clinical, histopathologic, and genotypic study. Hum Pathol 1999; 30: 1004–1012.

993 Aiba S, Tagami H. Immunohistologic studies in Schamberg's disease. Evidence for cellular immune reaction in lesional skin. Arch Dermatol 1988; 124: 1058–1062.

994 Simon M Jr, Heese A, Gotz A. Immunopathological investigations in purpura pigmentosa chronica. Acta Derm Venereol 1989; 69: 101–104.

995 Reinhardt L, Wilkin JK, Tausend R. Vascular abnormalities in lichen aureus. J Am Acad Dermatol 1983; 8: 417–420.

996 Shelley WB, Swaminathan R, Shelley ED. Lichen aureus: a hemosiderin tattoo associated with perforator vein incompetence. J Am Acad Dermatol 1984; 11: 260–264.

997 Von den Driesch P, Simon M Jr. Cellular adhesion antigen modulation in purpura pigmentosa chronica. J Am Acad Dermatol 1994; 30: 193–200.

998 Ghersetich I, Lotti T, Bacci S et al. Cell infiltrate in progressive pigmented purpura (Schamberg's disease): immunophenotype, adhesion receptors, and intercellular relationships. Int J Dermatol 1995; 34: 846–850.

999 Nishioka K, Sarashi C, Katayama I. Chronic pigmented purpura induced by chemical substances. Clin Exp Dermatol 1980; 5: 213–218.

1000 Abeck D, Gross GE, Kuwert C et al. Acetaminophen-induced progressive pigmentary purpura (Schamberg's disease). J Am Acad Dermatol 1992; 27: 123–124.

1001 Adams BB, Gadenne A-S. Glipizide-induced pigmented purpuric dermatosis. J Am Acad Dermatol 1999; 41: 827–829.

1002 Tsao H, Lerner LH. Pigmented purpuric eruption associated with injection medroxyprogesterone acetate. J Am Acad Dermatol 2000; 43: 308–310.

1003 Reinhold U, Seiter S, Ugurel S, Tilgen W. Treatment of progressive pigmented purpura with oral bioflavonoids and ascorbic acid: An open pilot study in 3 patients. J Am Acad Dermatol 1999; 41: 207–208.

1004 Smoller BR, Kamel OW. Pigmented purpuric eruptions: immunopathologic studies supportive of a common immunophenotype. J Cutan Pathol 1991; 18: 423–427.

1005 Waisman M. Lichen aureus. Int J Dermatol 1985; 24: 645–646.

1006 Iwatsuki K, Aoshima T, Tagami H et al. Immunofluorescence study in purpura pigmentosa chronica. Acta Derm Venereol 1980; 60: 341–345.

1007 Geiger JM, Grosshans E, Hanau D. Lichen aureus: ultrastructural study. J Cutan Pathol 1981; 8: 150.

1008 Magrinat G, Kerwin KS, Gabriel DA. The clinical manifestations of Degos' syndrome. Arch Pathol Lab Med 1989; 113: 354–362.

1009 Degos R. Malignant atrophic papulosis. Br J Dermatol 1979; 100: 21–35.

1010 Güven FO, Bozdağ KE, Ermete M, Karaman A. Degos' disease. Int J Dermatol 2000; 39: 361–362.

1011 Thomson KF, Highet AS. Penile ulceration in fatal malignant atrophic papulosis (Degos' disease). Br J Dermatol 2000; 143: 1320–1322.

1012 Roenigk HH, Farmer RG. Degos' disease (malignant papulosis). Report of three cases with clues to etiology. JAMA 1968; 206: 1508–1514.

1013 Willa-Craps C, Zala LB, Nievergelt H et al. Malignant atrophic papulosis. Dermatology 1997; 195: 89–90.

1014 D'Avino M, Schiavo AL, Baroni A et al. Degos' disease: a case with cutaneous lesions only: absence of paramyxovirus by PCR. Dermatology 2000; 201: 278–279.

1015 Harvell JD, Williford PL, White WL. Benign cutaneous Degos' disease. A case report with emphasis on histopathology as papules chronologically evolve. Am J Dermatopathol 2001; 23: 116–123.

1016 Barlow RJ, Heyl T, Simson IW, Schulz EJ. Malignant atrophic papulosis (Degos' disease) – diffuse involvement of brain and bowel in an African patient. Br J Dermatol 1988 118: 117–123.

1017 Mauad T, de Fátima Lopes Calvo Tiberio I, Baba E et al. Malignant atrophic papulosis (Degos' disease) with extensive cardiopulmonary involvement. Histopathology 1996; 28: 84–86.

1018 Newton JA, Black MM. Familial malignant atrophic papulosis. Clin Exp Dermatol 1984; 9: 298–299.

1019 Katz SK, Mudd LJ, Roenigk HH Jr. Malignant atrophic papulosis (Degos' disease) involving three generations of a family. J Am Acad Dermatol 1997; 37: 480–484.

1020 Powell J, Bordea C, Wojnarowska F et al. Benign familial Degos disease worsening during immunosuppression. Br J Dermatol 1999; 141: 524–527.

1021 Kisch LS, Bruynzeel DP. Six cases of malignant atrophic papulosis (Degos' disease) occurring in one family. Br J Dermatol 1984; 111: 469–471.

1022 Requena L, Fariña MC, Barat A. Degos disease in a patient with acquired immunodeficiency syndrome. J Am Acad Dermatol 1998; 38: 852–856.

1023 Tribble K, Archer ME, Jorizzo JL et al. Malignant atrophic papulosis: absence of circulating immune complexes or vasculitis. J Am Acad Dermatol 1986; 15: 365–369.

1024 Muller SA, Landry M. Exchange autografts in malignant atrophic papulosis (Degos' disease). Mayo Clin Proc 1974; 49: 884–888.

1025 Black MM, Nishioka K, Levene GM. The role of dermal blood vessels in the pathogenesis of malignant atrophic papulosis (Degos' disease). Br J Dermatol 1973; 88: 213–219.

1026 Vázquez-Doval FJ, Ruiz de Erenchun F, Páramo JA, Quintanilla E. Malignant atrophic papulosis. A report of two cases with altered fibrinolysis and platelet function. Clin Exp Dermatol 1993; 18: 441–444.

1027 Farrell AM, Moss J, Costello C et al. Benign cutaneous Degos' disease. Br J Dermatol 1998; 139: 708–712.

1028 Soter NA, Murphy GF, Mihm MC. Lymphocytes and necrosis of the cutaneous microvasculature in malignant atrophic papulosis: a refined light microscope study. J Am Acad Dermatol 1982; 7: 620–630.

1029 Bleehen SS. Intra-endothelial tubular aggregates in malignant atrophic papulosis (Degos' disease). Clin Exp Dermatol 1977; 2: 73–74.

1030 Coskey RJ, Mehregan AH. Shoe boot pernio. Arch Dermatol 1974; 109: 56–57.

1031 Wall LM, Smith NP. Perniosis: a histopathological review. Clin Exp Dermatol 1981; 6: 263–271.

1032 Goette DK. Chilblains (perniosis). J Am Acad Dermatol 1990; 23: 257–262.

1033 Wessagowit P, Asawanonda P, Noppakun N. Papular perniosis mimicking erythema multiforme: the first case report in Thailand. Int J Dermatol 2000; 39: 527–529.

1034 Millard LG, Rowell NR. Chilblain lupus erythematosus (Hutchinson). Br J Dermatol 1978; 98: 497–506.

1035 Kelly JW, Dowling JP. Pernio. A possible association with chronic myelomonocytic leukemia. Arch Dermatol 1985; 121: 1048–1052.

1036 Crowson AN, Magro CM. Idiopathic perniosis and its mimics: a clinical and histological study of 38 cases. Hum Pathol 1997; 28: 478–484.

1037 De Silva BD, McLaren K, Doherty VR. Equestrian perniosis associated with cold agglutinins: a novel finding. Clin Exp Dermatol 2000; 25: 285–288.

1038 Weston WL, Morelli JG. Childhood pernio and cryoproteins. Pediatr Dermatol 2000; 17: 97–99.

1039 Quinn TR, Lewtas J, From L. Perniotic-like lymphocytic vascular reaction with anorectic agent use. J Cutan Pathol 1997; 24: 118 (abstract).

1040 Klapman MH, Johnston WH. Localized recurrent postoperative pernio associated with leukocytoclastic vasculitis. J Am Acad Dermatol 1991; 24: 811–813.

1041 Uhoda I, Piérard-Franchimont C, Piérard GE. Varicella-zoster virus vasculitis: a case of recurrent varicella without epidermal involvement. Dermatology 2000; 200: 173–175.

1042 Schwaegerle SM, Bergfeld WF, Senitzer D, Tidrick RT. Pyoderma gangrenosum: a review. J Am Acad Dermatol 1988; 18: 559–568.

1043 Powell FC, Schroeter AL, Su WPD, Perry HO. Pyoderma gangrenosum: a review of 86 patients. Q J Med 1985; 55: 173–186.

1044 von den Driesch P. Pyoderma gangrenosum: a report of 44 cases with follow-up. Br J Dermatol 1997; 137: 1000–1005.

1045 Prystowsky JH, Kahn SN, Lazarus GS. Present status of pyoderma gangrenosum. Review of 21 cases. Arch Dermatol 1989; 125: 57–64.

1046 Malkinson FD. Pyoderma gangrenosum vs malignant pyoderma. Arch Dermatol 1987; 123: 333–337.

1047 Sassolas B, Le Ru Y, Plantin P et al. Pyoderma gangrenosum with pathergic phenomenon in pregnancy. Br J Dermatol 2000; 142: 827–828.

1048 Snyder RA. Pyoderma gangrenosum involving the head and neck. Arch Dermatol 1986; 122: 295–302.

1049 Samlaska CP, Smith RA, Myers JB et al. Pyoderma gangrenosum and cranial osteolysis: case report and review of the paediatric literature. Br J Dermatol 1995; 133: 972–977.

1050 Sánchez MH, Sánchez SR, del Cerro Heredero M et al. Pyoderma gangrenosum of penile skin. Int J Dermatol 1997; 36: 638–639.

1051 Farrell AM, Black MM, Bracka A, Bunker CB. Pyoderma gangrenosum of the penis. Br J Dermatol 1998; 138: 337–340.

1052 Darben T, Savige J, Prentice R et al. Pyoderma gangrenosum with secondary pyarthrosis following propylthiouracil. Australas J Dermatol 1999; 40: 144–146.

1053 Setterfield JF, Shirlaw PJ, Challacombe SJ, Black MM. Pyoderma gangrenosum associated with severe oropharyngeal involvement and IgA paraproteinaemia. Br J Dermatol 2001; 144: 393–396.

1054 Marie I, Levesque H, Joly P et al. Neutrophilic myositis as an extracutaneous manifestation of neutrophilic dermatosis. J Am Acad Dermatol 2001; 44: 137–139.

1055 Brown TS, Marshall GS, Callen JP. Cavitating pulmonary infiltrate in an adolescent with pyoderma gangrenosum: A rarely recognized extracutaneous manifestation of a neutrophilic dermatosis. J Am Acad Dermatol 2000; 43: 108–112.

1056 Powell FC, Perry HO. Pyoderma gangrenosum in childhood. Arch Dermatol 1984; 120: 757–761.

1057 Barnes L, Lucky AW, Bucuvalas JC, Suchy FJ. Pustular pyoderma gangrenosum associated with ulcerative colitis in childhood. J Am Acad Dermatol 1986; 15: 608–614.

1058 Merke DP, Honig PJ, Potsic WP. Pyoderma gangrenosum of the skin and trachea in a 9-month-old boy. J Am Acad Dermatol 1996; 34: 681–682.

1059 Graham JA, Hansen KK, Rabinowitz LG, Esterly NB. Pyoderma gangrenosum in infants and children. Pediatr Dermatol 1994; 11: 10–17.

1060 Vadillo M, Jucgla A, Podzamczer D et al. Pyoderma gangrenosum with liver, spleen and bone involvement in a patient with chronic myelomonocytic leukaemia. Br J Dermatol 1999; 141: 541–543.

1061 Beele H, Verhaeghe E, Stockman A et al. Pyoderma gangrenosum as an early revelator of acute leukemia. Dermatology 2000; 200: 176–178.

1062 Asai M, Aragane Y, Kawada A et al. Pyoderma gangrenosum associated with biphenotypic acute leukemia. J Am Acad Dermatol 2001; 44: 530–531.

1063 Shands JW Jr, Flowers FP, Hill HM, Smith JO. Pyoderma gangrenosum in a kindred. J Am Acad Dermatol 1987; 16: 931–934.

1064 Horton JJ, Trounce JR, MacDonald DM. Bullous pyoderma gangrenosum and multiple myeloma. Br J Dermatol 1984; 110: 227–230.

1065 Duguid CM, O'Loughlin S, Otridge B, Powell FC. Paraneoplastic pyoderma gangrenosum. Australas J Dermatol 1993; 34: 17–22.

1066 Koester G, Tarnower A, Levisohn D, Burgdorf W. Bullous pyoderma gangrenosum. J Am Acad Dermatol 1993; 29: 875–878.

1067 Grattan CEH, McCann BG, Lockwood CM. Pyoderma gangrenosum, polyarthritis and lung cysts with novel antineutrophil cytoplasmic antibodies to azurocidin. Br J Dermatol 1998; 139: 352–353.

1068 Ross HJ, Moy LA, Kaplan R, Figlin RA. Bullous pyoderma gangrenosum after granulocyte colony-stimulating factor treatment. Cancer 1991; 68: 441–443.

1069 Dicken CH. Malignant pyoderma. J Am Acad Dermatol 1985; 13: 1021–1025.

1070 Wernikoff S, Merritt C, Briggaman RA, Woodley DT. Malignant pyoderma or pyoderma gangrenosum of the head and neck? Arch Dermatol 1987; 123: 371–375.

1071 Erdi H, Anadolu R, Pişkin G, Gürgey E. Malignant pyoderma: a clinical variant of pyoderma gangrenosum. Int J Dermatol 1996; 35: 811–813.

1072 Novice FM, Hacker P, Unger WP, Keystone EC. Malignant pyoderma. Int J Dermatol 1987; 26: 42–44.

1073 Gibson LE, Daoud MS, Muller SA, Perry HO. Malignant pyodermas revisited. Mayo Clin Proc 1997; 72: 734–736.

1074 Hoffman MD. Pyoderma gangrenosum associated with c-ANCA (h-lamp-2). Int J Dermatol 2001; 40: 135–137.

1075 Wilson-Jones E, Winkelmann RK. Superficial granulomatous pyoderma: a localized vegetative form of pyoderma gangrenosum. J Am Acad Dermatol 1988; 18: 511–521.

1076 Quimby SR, Gibson LE, Winkelmann RK. Superficial granulomatous pyoderma: clinicopathologic spectrum. Mayo Clin Proc 1989; 64: 37–43.

1077 Lichter MD, Welykyj SE, Gradini R, Solomon LM. Superficial granulomatous pyoderma. Int J Dermatol 1991; 30: 418–421.

1078 Hardwick N, Cerio R. Superficial granulomatous pyoderma. A report of two cases. Br J Dermatol 1993; 129: 718–722.

1079 Peretz E, Cagnano E, Grunwald MH et al. Vegetative pyoderma gangrenosum: an unusual presentation. Int J Dermatol 1999; 38: 703–706.

1080 Çalikoğlu E. Superficial granulomatous pyoderma of the scrotum: an extremely rare cause of genital ulcer. Acta Derm Venereol 2000; 80: 311–312.

1081 Lachapelle J-M, Marot L, Jablonska S. Superficial granulomatous pyoderma gangrenosum of the face, successfully treated by ciclosporine: a long-term follow-up. Dermatology 2001; 202: 155–157.

1082 Lindor NM, Arsenault TM, Solomon H et al. A new autosomal dominant disorder of pyogenic sterile arthritis, pyoderma gangrenosum, and acne: PAPA syndrome. Mayo Clin Proc 1997; 72: 611–615.

1083 Nurre LD, Rabalais GP, Callen JP. Neutrophilic dermatosis-associated sterile chronic multifocal osteomyelitis in pediatric patients: case report and review. Pediatr Dermatol 1999; 16: 214–216.

1084 Levitt MD, Ritchie JK, Lennard-Jones JE, Phillips RKS. Pyoderma gangrenosum in inflammatory bowel disease. Br J Surg 1991; 78: 676–678.

1085 Burgdorf W. Cutaneous manifestations of Crohn's disease. J Am Acad Dermatol 1981; 5: 689–695.

1086 Keltz M, Lebwohl M, Bishop S. Peristomal pyoderma gangrenosum. J Am Acad Dermatol 1992; 27: 360–364.

1087 Powell FC, Schroeter AL, Su WPD, Perry HO. Pyoderma gangrenosum and monoclonal gammopathy. Arch Dermatol 1983; 119: 468–472.

1088 Sheldon DG, Sawchuk LL, Kozarck RA, Thirlby RC. Twenty cases of peristomal pyoderma gangrenosum. Arch Surg 2000; 135: 564–569.

1089 Lyon CC, Smith AJ, Beck MH et al. Parastomal pyoderma gangrenosum: Clinical features and management. J Am Acad Dermatol 2000; 42: 992–1002.

1090 Hickman JG, Lazarus GS. Pyoderma gangrenosum: a reappraisal of associated systemic diseases. Br J Dermatol 1980; 102: 235–237.

1091 Burns DA, Sarkany I. Active chronic hepatitis and pyoderma gangrenosum: report of a case. Clin Exp Dermatol 1979; 4: 465–469.

1092 Green LK, Hebert AA, Jorizzo JL et al. Pyoderma gangrenosum and chronic persistent hepatitis. J Am Acad Dermatol 1985; 13: 892–897.

1093 Keane FM, MacFarlane CS, Munn SE, Higgins EM. Pyoderma gangrenosum and hepatitis C virus infection. Br J Dermatol 1998; 139: 924–925.

1094 Pinto GM, Cabeças MA, Riscado M, Gonçalves H. Pyoderma gangrenosum associated with systemic lupus erythematosus: Response to pulse steroid therapy. J Am Acad Dermatol 1991; 24: 818–821.

1095 Freedman AM, Phelps RG, Lebwohl M. Pyoderma gangrenosum associated with anticardiolipin antibodies in a pregnant patient. Int J Dermatol 1997; 36: 205–207.

1096 Munro CS, Cox NH. Pyoderma gangrenosum associated with Behçet's syndrome – response to thalidomide. Clin Exp Dermatol 1988; 13: 408–410.

1097 Boulinguez S, Bernard P, Bedane C et al. Pyoderma gangrenosum complicating Cogan's syndrome. Clin Exp Dermatol 1998; 23: 286–289.

1098 De Silva B, Doherty VR. Coexistence of pyoderma gangrenosum and Cushing's disease: a paradoxical association? Br J Dermatol 2000; 142: 1051–1052.

1099 Fearfield LA, Ross JR, Farrell AM et al. Pyoderma gangrenosum associated with Takayasu's arteritis responding to cyclosporin. Br J Dermatol 1999; 141: 339–343.

1100 Vannucci SA, Mitchell WM, Stratton CW, King LE Jr. Pyoderma gangrenosum and Chlamydia pneumoniae infection in a diabetic man: Pathogenic role or coincidence? J Am Acad Dermatol 2000; 42: 295–297.

1101 Venning VA, Ryan TJ. Subcorneal pustular dermatosis followed by pyoderma gangrenosum. Br J Dermatol 1986; 115: 117–118.

1102 Kohl PK, Hartschuh W, Tilgen W, Frosch PJ. Pyoderma gangrenosum followed by subcorneal pustular dermatosis in a patient with IgA paraproteinemia. J Am Acad Dermatol 1991; 24: 325–328.

1103 Hughes BR, Cunliffe WJ. Development of folliculitis and pyoderma gangrenosum in association with abdominal pain in a patient following treatment with isotretinoin. Br J Dermatol 1990; 122: 683–687.

1104 Mahood JM, Sneddon IB. Pyoderma gangrenosum complicating non-Hodgkin's lymphoma. Br J Dermatol 1980; 102: 223–225.

1105 Cartwright PH, Rowell NR. Hairy-cell leukaemia presenting with pyoderma gangrenosum. Clin Exp Dermatol 1987; 12: 451–452.

1106 Philpott JA Jr, Goltz RW, Park RK. Pyoderma gangrenosum, rheumatoid arthritis, and diabetes mellitus. Arch Dermatol 1966; 94: 732–738.

1107 Cox NH, White SI, Walton S et al. Pyoderma gangrenosum associated with polycythaemia rubra vera. Clin Exp Dermatol 1987; 12: 375–377.

1108 Assady S, Bergman R, Finkelstein R, Edoute Y. Pyoderma gangrenosum associated with myelofibrosis. Br J Dermatol 1998; 139: 163–164.

1109 Coors EA, von den Driesch P. Pyoderma gangrenosum in a patient with autoimmune haemolytic anaemia and complement deficiency. Br J Dermatol 2000; 143: 154–156.

1110 Goulden V, Bond L, Highet AS. Pyoderma gangrenosum associated with paroxysmal nocturnal haemoglobinuria. Clin Exp Dermatol 1994; 19: 271–273.

1111 Esnault P, Dompmartin A, Moreau A et al. Recurring postoperative pyoderma gangrenosum. Int J Dermatol 1995; 34: 647–650.

1112 Sotillo-Gago I, Muñoz-Pérez MA, Camacho-Martinez F. Pyoderma gangrenosum after augmentation mammoplasty. Acta Derm Venereol 1999; 79: 486.

1113 Stone N, Harland C, Ross L, Holden C. Pyoderma gangrenosum complicating Caesarian section. Clin Exp Dermatol 1996; 21: 468.

1114 Haim S, Friedman-Birnbaum R. Pyoderma gangrenosum in immunosuppressed patients. Dermatologica 1976; 153: 44–48.

1115 Van de Kerkhof PCM, de Vaan GAM, Holland R. Pyoderma gangrenosum in acute myeloid leukaemia during immunosuppression. Eur J Pediatr 1988; 148: 34–36.

1116 Clark HH, Cohen PR. Pyoderma gangrenosum in an HIV-infected patient. J Am Acad Dermatol 1995; 32: 912–914.

1117 Micali G, Cook B, Ronan S et al. Cephalic pyoderma gangrenosum (PG)-like lesions as a presenting sign of Wegener's granulomatosis. Int J Dermatol 1994; 33: 477–480.

1118 Matsui M, Ohtoshi E, Yamaoka J et al. Cutaneous tuberculosis and pyoderma gangrenosum. Int J Dermatol 2000; 39: 38–40.

1119 Holt PJA. The current status of pyoderma gangrenosum. Clin Exp Dermatol 1979; 4: 509–516.

1120 Holt PJA, Davies MG, Saunders KC, Nuki G. Pyoderma gangrenosum. Clinical and laboratory findings in 15 patients with special reference to polyarthritis. Medicine (Baltimore) 1980; 59: 114–133.

1121 Hecker MS, Lebwohl MG. Recalcitrant pyoderma gangrenosum: Treatment with thalidomide. J Am Acad Dermatol 1998; 38: 490–491.

1122 Federman GL, Federman DG. Recalcitrant pyoderma gangrenosum treated with thalidomide. Mayo Clin Proc 2000; 75: 842–844.

1123 Pari T, George S, Jacob M et al. Malignant pyoderma responding to clofazimine. Int J Dermatol 1996; 35: 757–758.

1124 Wollina U, Karamfilov T. Treatment of recalcitrant ulcers in pyoderma gangrenosum with mycophenolate mofetil and autologous keratinocyte transplantation on a hyaluronic acid matrix. J Eur Acad Dermatol Venereol 2000; 14: 187–190.

1125 Gilmour E, Stewart DG. Severe recalcitrant pyoderma gangrenosum responding to a combination of mycophenolate mofetil with cyclosporin and complicated by a mononeuritis. Br J Dermatol 2001; 144: 397–400.

1126 de Imus G, Golomb C, Wilkel C et al. Accelerated healing of pyoderma gangrenosum treated with bioengineered skin and concomitant immunosuppression. J Am Acad Dermatol 2001; 44: 61–66.

1127 Breathnach SM, Wells GC, Valdimarsson H. Idiopathic pyoderma gangrenosum and impaired lymphocyte function: failure of azathioprine and corticosteroid therapy. Br J Dermatol 1981; 104: 567–573.

1128 Berbis P, Mege JL, Capo C et al. Hyperimmunoglobulin E and impaired neutrophil functions in a case of pyoderma gangrenosum: effect of clofazimine. J Am Acad Dermatol 1988; 18: 574–576.

1129 Shaya S, Kindzelskii AL, Minor J et al. Aberrant integrin (CR4; $\alpha_x\beta_2$; CD11c/CD13) oscillations on neutrophils in a mild form of pyoderma gangrenosum. J Invest Dermatol 1998; 111: 154–158.

1130 Adachi Y, Kindzelskii AL, Cookingham G et al. Aberrant neutrophil trafficking and metabolic oscillations in severe pyoderma gangrenosum. J Invest Dermatol 1998; 111: 259–268.

1131 Su WPD, Schroeter AL, Perry HO, Powell FC. Histopathologic and immunopathologic study of pyoderma gangrenosum. J Cutan Pathol 1986; 13: 323–330.

1132 Ackerman AB. Questions to the Editorial Board. Am J Dermatopathol 1983; 5: 409–410.

1133 Hurwitz RM, Haseman JH. The evolution of pyoderma gangrenosum: a clinicopathologic correlation. Am J Dermatopathol 1993; 15: 28–33.

1134 Sanders S, Tahan SR, Kwan T, Magro CM. Giant cells in pyoderma gangrenosum. J Cutan Pathol 2001; 28: 97–100.

1135 English JSC, Fenton DA, Barth J et al. Pyoderma gangrenosum and leucocytoclastic vasculitis in association with rheumatoid arthritis – report of two cases. Clin Exp Dermatol 1984; 9: 270–276.

1136 Wong E, Greaves MW. Pyoderma gangrenosum and leucocytoclastic vasculitis. Clin Exp Dermatol 1985; 10: 68–72.

1137 del Cerro Heredero M, Sánchez Yus E, Gómez-Calcerrada MR et al. Superficial granulomatous pyoderma. Dermatology 1998; 196: 358–360.

1138 Park H-J, Kim Y-C, Cinn Y-W, Yoon T-Y. Granulomatous pyoderma gangrenosum: two unusual cases showing necrotizing granulomatous inflammation. Clin Exp Dermatol 2000; 25: 617–620.

1139 Powell FC, Su WPD, Perry HO. Pyoderma gangrenosum: classification and management. J Am Acad Dermatol 1996; 34: 395–409.

1140 Powell FC, Schroeter AL, Perry HO, Su WPD. Direct immunofluorescence in pyoderma gangrenosum. Br J Dermatol 1983; 108: 287–293.

1141 Nickel WR, Plumb RT. Nonvenereal sclerosing lymphangitis of penis. Arch Dermatol 1962; 86: 761–763.

1142 Fiumara NJ. Nonvenereal sclerosing lymphangitis of the penis. Arch Dermatol 1975; 111: 902–903.

1143 Greenberg RD, Perry TL. Nonvenereal sclerosing lymphangitis of the penis. Arch Dermatol 1972; 105: 728–729.

1144 Van Der Staak WJBM. Non-venereal sclerosing lymphangitis of the penis following herpes progenitalis. Br J Dermatol 1977; 96: 679–680.

1145 Baden HP, Provan J, Tanenbaum L. Circular indurated lymphangitis of the penis. Arch Dermatol 1976; 112: 1146.

1146 Marsch WC, Stuttgen G. Sclerosing lymphangitis of the penis: a lymphangiofibrosis thrombotica occlusiva. Br J Dermatol 1981; 104: 687–695.

1147 Kandil E, Al-Kashlan IM. Non-venereal sclerosing lymphangitis of the penis. A clinicopathologic treatise. Acta Derm Venereol 1970; 50: 309–312.

1148 Findlay GH, Whiting DA. Mondor's phlebitis of the penis. A condition miscalled 'non-venereal sclerosing lymphangitis'. Clin Exp Dermatol 1977; 2: 65–67.

1149 Jones D, Dorfman DM, Barnhill RL, Granter SR. Leukemic vasculitis. A feature of leukemia cutis in some patients. Am J Clin Pathol 1997; 107: 637–642.

1150 Smoller BR. Leukemic vasculitis: a newly described pattern of cutaneous involvement. Am J Clin Pathol 1997; 107: 627–629.

1151 Paydaş S, Zorludemir S. Leukaemia cutis and leukaemic vasculitis. Br J Dermatol 2000; 143: 773–779.

1152 LeBoit PE. A vessel runs through it. Am J Dermatopathol 2000; 22: 285–287.

Vasculitis with granulomatosis

1153 Chanda JJ, Callen JP. Necrotizing vasculitis (angiitis) with granulomatosis. Int J Dermatol 1984; 23: 101–107.

1154 Yevich I. Necrotizing vasculitis with granulomatosis. Int J Dermatol 1988; 27: 540–546.

1155 Hoekstra JA, Fauci AS. The granulomatous vasculitides. Clin Rheum Dis 1980; 6: 373–388.

1156 Fienberg R. The protracted superficial phenomenon in pathergic (Wegener's) granulomatosis. Hum Pathol 1981; 12: 458–467.

1157 Gibson LE, El-Azhary RA, Smith TF, Reda AM. The spectrum of cutaneous granulomatous vasculitis: histopathologic report of eight cases with clinical correlation. J Cutan Pathol 1994; 21: 437–445.

1158 Chalvardjian A, Nethercott JR. Cutaneous granulomatous vasculitis associated with Crohn's disease. Cutis 1982; 30: 645–648.

1159 Eeckhout E, Willemsen M, Deconinck A, Somers G. Granulomatous vasculitis as a complication of potassium iodide treatment for Sweet's syndrome. Acta Derm Venereol 1987; 67: 362–364.

1160 Langenberg A, Yen TSB, LeBoit PE. Granulomatous vasculitis occurring after cutaneous herpes zoster despite absence of viral genome. J Am Acad Dermatol 1991; 24: 429–433.

1161 Baalbaki SA, Malak JA, Al-Khars MAA, Natarajan S. Granulomatous vasculitis in herpes zoster scars. Int J Dermatol 1994; 33: 268–269.

1162 Rodríguez-Pereira C, Suárez-Peñaranda JM, Del Río E, Forteza-Vila J. Cutaneous granulomatous vasculitis after herpes zoster infection showing polyarteritis nodosa-like features. Clin Exp Dermatol 1997; 22: 274–276.

1163 Snow JL, el-Azhary RA, Gibson LE et al. Granulomatous vasculitis associated with herpes virus: a persistent, painful, postherpetic papular eruption. Mayo Clin Proc 1997; 72: 851–853.

1164 Gibson LE, Winkelmann RK. Cutaneous granulomatous vasculitis. Its relationship to systemic disease. J Am Acad Dermatol 1986; 14: 492–501.

1165 Yi ES, Colby TV. Wegener's granulomatosis. Semin Diagn Pathol 2001; 18: 34–46.

1166 Godman GC, Churg J. Wegener's granulomatosis. Pathology and review of the literature. Arch Pathol 1954; 58: 533–553.

1167 Chyu JYH, Hagstrom WJ, Soltani K et al. Wegener's granulomatosis in childhood: cutaneous manifestations as the presenting signs. J Am Acad Dermatol 1984; 10: 341–346.

1168 Stein SL, Miller LC, Konnikov N. Wegener's granulomatosis: case report and literature review. Pediatr Dermatol 1998; 15: 352–356.

1169 Brazzelli V, Vassallo C, Baldini F et al. Wegener granulomatosis in a child: cutaneous findings as the presenting signs. Pediatr Dermatol 1999; 16: 277–280.

1170 Fauci AS, Wolff SM. Wegener's granulomatosis: studies in eighteen patients and a review of the literature. Medicine (Baltimore) 1973; 52: 535–561.

1171 Dias BM, Nahass GT. Palpable purpura and respiratory failure. Arch Dermatol 1997; 133: 435–437.

1172 Knight JM, Hayduk MJ, Summerlin D-J, Mirowski GW. "Strawberry" gingival hyperplasia. A pathognomonic mucocutaneous finding in Wegener granulomatosis. Arch Dermatol 2000; 136: 171–173.

1173 Nishino H, DeRemee RA, Rubino FA, Parisi JE. Wegener's granulomatosis associated with vasculitis of the temporal artery: report of five cases. Mayo Clin Proc 1993; 68: 115–121.

1174 Hu C-H, O'Loughlin S, Winkelmann RK. Cutaneous manifestations of Wegener granulomatosis. Arch Dermatol 1977; 113: 175–182.

1175 Francès C, Du LTH, Piette J-C et al. Wegener's granulomatosis. Dermatological manifestations in 75 cases with clinicopathologic correlation. Arch Dermatol 1994; 130: 861–867.

1176 Patten SF, Tomecki KJ. Wegener's granulomatosis: cutaneous and oral mucosal disease. J Am Acad Dermatol 1993; 28: 710–718.

1177 Kesseler ME. Wegener's granulomatosis. Clin Exp Dermatol 1982; 7: 103–108.

1178 Handfield-Jones SE, Parker SC, Fenton DA et al. Wegener's granulomatosis presenting as pyoderma gangrenosum. Clin Exp Dermatol 1992; 17: 197–200.

1179 Daoud MS, Gibson LE, DeRemee RA et al. Cutaneous Wegener's granulomatosis: clinical, histopathologic, and immunopathologic features of thirty patients. J Am Acad Dermatol 1994; 31: 605–612.

1180 Elsner B, Harper FB. Disseminated Wegener's granulomatosis with breast involvement. Arch Pathol 1969; 87: 544–547.

1181 Goulart RA, Mark EJ, Rosen S. Tumefactions as an extravascular manifestation of Wegener's granulomatosis. Am J Surg Pathol 1995; 19: 145–153.

1182 Cassan SM, Coles DT, Harrison EG Jr. The concept of limited forms of Wegener's granulomatosis. Am J Med 1970; 49: 366–379.

1183 Burke AP, Virmani R. Localized vasculitis. Semin Diagn Pathol 2001; 18: 59–66.

1184 Kihiczak D, Nychay SG, Schwartz RA et al. Protracted superficial Wegener's granulomatosis. J Am Acad Dermatol 1994; 30: 863–866.

1185 De Remee RA, McDonald TJ, Weiland LH. Wegener's granulomatosis: observations on treatment with antimicrobial agents. Mayo Clin Proc 1985; 60: 27–32.

1186 Specks U, Wheatley CL, McDonald TJ et al. Anticytoplasmic autoantibodies in the diagnosis and follow-up of Wegener's granulomatosis. Mayo Clin Proc 1989; 64: 28–36.

1187 Cross CE, Lillington GA. Serodiagnosis of Wegener's granulomatosis: pathobiologic and clinical implications. Mayo Clin Proc 1989; 64: 119–122.

1188 Specks U, Homburger HA. Anti-neutrophil cytoplasmic antibodies. Mayo Clin Proc 1994; 69: 1197–1198.

1189 Fienberg R, Mark EJ, Goodman M et al. Correlation of antineutrophil cytoplasmic antibodies with the extrarenal histopathology of Wegener's (pathergic) granulomatosis and related forms of vasculitis. Hum Pathol 1993; 24: 160–168.

1190 Jayne DRW, Rasmussen N. Treatment of antineutrophil cytoplasm autoantibody-associated systemic vasculitis: initiatives of the European Community Systemic Vasculitis Clinical Trials Study Group. Mayo Clin Proc 1997; 72: 737–747.

1191 Le T, Pierard GE, Lapière CM. Granulomatous vasculitis of Wegener. J Cutan Pathol 1981; 8: 34–39.

1192 Devaney KO, Travis WD, Hoffman G et al. Interpretation of head and neck biopsies in Wegener's granulomatosis. A pathologic study of 126 biopsies in 70 patients. Am J Surg Pathol 1990; 14: 555–564.

1193 Gürses L, Yücelten D, Cömert A et al. Wegener's granulomatosis presenting as neutrophilic dermatosis: a case report. Br J Dermatol 2000; 143: 207–209.

1194 Yousem SA, Lombard CM. The eosinophilic variant of Wegener's granulomatosis. Hum Pathol 1988; 19: 682–688.

1195 Finan MC, Winkelmann RK. The cutaneous extravascular necrotizing granuloma (Churg–Strauss granuloma) and systemic disease: a review of 27 cases. Medicine (Baltimore) 1983; 62: 142–158.

1196 Mangold MC, Callen JP. Cutaneous leukocytoclastic vasculitis associated with active Wegener's granulomatosis. J Am Acad Dermatol 1992; 26: 579–584.

1197 Barksdale SK, Hallahan CW, Kerr GS et al. Cutaneous pathology in Wegener's granulomatosis. A clinicopathologic study of 75 biopsies in 46 patients. Am J Surg Pathol 1995; 19: 161–172.

1198 Liebow AA, Carrington CRB, Friedman PJ. Lymphomatoid granulomatosis. Hum Pathol 1972; 3: 457–533.

1199 Katzenstein A-LA, Carrington CB, Liebow AA. Lymphomatoid granulomatosis. A clinicopathologic study of 152 cases. Cancer 1979; 43: 360–373.

1200 McNiff JM, Cooper D, Howe G et al. Lymphomatoid granulomatosis of the skin and lung. An angiocentric T-cell-rich B-cell lymphoproliferative disorder. Arch Dermatol 1996; 132: 1464–1470.

1201 Nicholson AG, Wotherspoon AC, Diss TC et al. Lymphomatoid granulomatosis: evidence that some cases represent Epstein–Barr virus-associated B-cell lymphoma. Histopathology 1996; 29: 317–324.

1202 Lin BT-Y. Lymphomatoid granulomatosis. Am J Surg Pathol 1999; 23: 1162.

1203 Jambrosic J, From L, Assaad DA et al. Lymphomatoid granulomatosis. J Am Acad Dermatol 1987; 17: 621–631.

1204 James WD, Odom RB, Katzenstein A-LA. Cutaneous manifestations of lymphomatoid granulomatosis. Report of 44 cases and a review of the literature. Arch Dermatol 1981; 117: 196–202.

1205 Camisa C. Lymphomatoid granulomatosis: two cases with skin involvement. J Am Acad Dermatol 1989; 20: 571–578.

1206 Wood ML, Harrington CI, Slater DN et al. Cutaneous lymphomatoid granulomatosis: a rare cause of recurrent skin ulceration. Br J Dermatol 1984; 110: 619–625.

1207 Tawfik NH, Magro CMJ, Crowson AN, Maxwell I. Lymphomatoid granulomatosis presenting as a solitary cutaneous lesion. Int J Dermatol 1994; 33: 188–189.

1208 Tong MM, Cooke B, Barnetson RStC. Lymphomatoid granulomatosis. J Am Acad Dermatol 1992; 27: 872–876.

1209 Font RL, Rosenbaum PS, Smith JL Jr. Lymphomatoid granulomatosis of eyelid and brow with progression to lymphoma. J Am Acad Dermatol 1990; 23: 334–337.

1210 Brodell RT, Miller CW, Eisen AZ. Cutaneous lesions of lymphomatoid granulomatosis. Arch Dermatol 1986; 122: 303–306.

1211 Chan JKC, Ng CS, Ngan KC et al. Angiocentric T-cell lymphoma of the skin. An aggressive lymphoma distinct from mycosis fungoides. Am J Surg Pathol 1988; 12: 861–876.

1212 Foley JF, Linder J, Koh J et al. Cutaneous necrotizing granulomatous vasculitis with evolution to T cell lymphoma. Am J Med 1987; 82: 839–844.

1213 Carlson KC, Gibson LE. The cutaneous signs of lymphomatoid granulomatosis. J Cutan Pathol 1989; 16: 298.

1214 Norton AJ. Angiocentric lymphoma. Curr Diagn Pathol 1994; 1: 158–166.

1215 Medeiros LJ, Peiper SC, Elwood L et al. Angiocentric immunoproliferative lesions: a molecular analysis of eight cases. Hum Pathol 1991; 22: 1150–1157.

1216 Angel CA, Slater DN, Royds JA et al. Epstein–Barr virus in cutaneous lymphomatoid granulomatosis. Histopathology 1994; 25: 545–548.

1217 Madison JF, Crotty PL, Howe G et al. Lymphomatoid granulomatosis: a T cell rich B cell lymphoproliferative disorder. J Cutan Pathol 1996; 23: 55 (abstract).

1218 Kessler S, Lund HZ, Leonard DD. Cutaneous lesions of lymphomatoid granulomatosis. Comparison with lymphomatoid papulosis. Am J Dermatopathol 1981; 3: 115–127.

1219 Kay S, Fu Y-S, Minars N, Brady JW. Lymphomatoid granulomatosis of the skin: light microscopic and ultrastructural studies. Cancer 1974; 34: 1675–1682.

1220 Magro CMJ, Tawfik NH, Crowson AN. Lymphomatoid granulomatosis. Int J Dermatol 1994; 33: 157–160.

1221 Tsai T-F, Chen R-L, Su I-J et al. Epstein–Barr virus-associated lymphoproliferative disorder of granular lymphocytes presenting initially as cutaneous vasculitis. J Am Acad Dermatol 1994; 30: 339–344.

1222 Cho KH, Kim CW, Lee DY et al. An Epstein–Barr virus-associated lymphoproliferative lesion of the skin presenting as recurrent necrotic papulovesicles of the face. Br J Dermatol 1996; 134: 791–796.

1223 Churg J, Strauss L. Allergic granulomatosis, allergic angiitis, and periarteritis nodosa. Am J Pathol 1951; 27: 277–301.

1224 Lanham JG, Elkon KB, Pusey CD, Hughes GR. Systemic vasculitis with asthma and eosinophilia: a clinical approach to the Churg–Strauss syndrome. Medicine (Baltimore) 1984; 63: 65–81.

1225 Lie JT. The classification of vasculitis and a reappraisal of allergic granulomatosis and angiitis (Churg–Strauss syndrome). Mt Sinai J Med (NY) 1986; 53: 429–439.

1226 Morita H, Kitano Y. Allergic granulomatosis and angiitis of Churg–Strauss syndrome. Int J Dermatol 1996; 35: 726–728.

1227 Nissim F, von der Valde J, Czernobilsky B. A limited form of Churg–Strauss syndrome. Ocular and cutaneous manifestations. Arch Pathol Lab Med 1982; 106: 305–307.

1228 Endo T, Katsuta Y, Kimura Y et al. A variant form of Churg–Strauss syndrome: initial temporal non-giant cell arteritis followed by asthma – is this a distinct clinicopathologic entity? Hum Pathol 2000; 31: 1169–1171.

1229 Lee S-C, Shin S-S, Lee J-B et al. Wells syndrome associated with Churg–Strauss syndrome. J Am Acad Dermatol 2000; 43: 556–557.

1230 Crotty CP, De Remee RA, Winkelmann RK. Cutaneous clinicopathologic correlation of allergic granulomatosis. J Am Acad Dermatol 1981; 5: 571–581.

1231 Schwartz RA, Churg J. Churg–Strauss syndrome. Br J Dermatol 1992; 127: 199–204.

1232 Cooper LM, Patterson JAK. Allergic granulomatosis and angiitis of Churg–Strauss. Case report in a patient with antibodies to human immunodeficiency virus and hepatitis B virus. Int J Dermatol 1989; 28: 597–599.

1233 Requena L, Sarasa JL, Martin L et al. Churg–Strauss syndrome: diagnosis suspected by cutaneous biopsy. Dermatopathology: Practical & Conceptual 1996; 2: 21–24.

1234 Davis MDP, Daoud MS, McEvoy MT, Su WPD. Cutaneous manifestations of Churg–Strauss syndrome: A clinicopathologic correlation. J Am Acad Dermatol 1997; 37: 199–203.

1235 Sanchez J. Allergic granulomatosis of Churg and Strauss is a distinctive expression of leukocytoclastic vasculitis. Dermatopathology: Practical & Conceptual 1996; 2: 25–26.

1236 Chu P, Connolly MK, LeBoit PE. The histopathologic spectrum of palisaded neutrophilic and granulomatous dermatitis in patients with collagen vascular disease. Arch Dermatol 1994; 130: 1278–1283.

1237 Wilmoth GJ, Perniciaro C. Cutaneous extravascular necrotizing granuloma (Winkelmann granuloma): confirmation of the association with systemic disease. J Am Acad Dermatol 1996; 34: 753–759.

1238 Hantich B, Ackerman AB. Churg–Strauss granuloma? Dermatopathology: Practical & Conceptual 1996; 2: 27–31.

1239 Lee M-W, Jang K-A, Lim Y-S et al. Cutaneous extravascular necrotizing granuloma (Churg Strauss granuloma). Clin Exp Dermatol 1999; 24: 193–195.

1240 Perniciaro C, Winkelmann RK. Cutaneous extravascular necrotizing granuloma in a patient with Takayasu's aortitis. Arch Dermatol 1986; 122: 201–204.

1241 Finan MC, Winkelmann RK. Cutaneous extravascular necrotizing granuloma and lymphocytic lymphoma. Arch Dermatol 1983; 119: 419–422.

1242 Chumbley LC, Harrison EG Jr, De Remee RA. Allergic granulomatosis and angiitis (Churg–Strauss syndrome). Report and analysis of 30 cases. Mayo Clin Proc 1977; 52: 477–484.

1243 Magro CM, Crowson AN, Regauer S. Granuloma annulare and necrobiosis lipoidica tissue reactions as a manifestation of systemic disease. Hum Pathol 1996; 27: 50–56.

1244 Dicken CH, Winkelmann RK. The Churg–Strauss granuloma. Cutaneous necrotizing, palisading granuloma in vasculitis syndromes. Arch Pathol Lab Med 1978; 102: 576–580.

1245 Fauci AS, Johnson RE, Wolff SM. Radiation therapy of midline granuloma. Ann Intern Med 1976; 84: 140–147.

1246 Ishii Y, Yamanaka N, Ogawa K et al. Nasal T-cell lymphoma as a type of so-called 'lethal midline granuloma'. Cancer 1982; 50: 2336–2344.

1247 Kassel SH, Echevarria RA, Guzzo FP. Midline malignant reticulosis (so-called lethal midline granuloma). Cancer 1969; 23: 920–935.

1248 Friedmann I. Ulcerative/necrotizing diseases of the nose and paranasal sinuses. Curr Diagn Pathol 1995; 2: 236–255.

1249 Lee PY, Freeman NJ, Khorsand J, Weinstock MA. Angiocentric T-cell lymphoma presenting as lethal midline granuloma. Int J Dermatol 1997; 36: 419–427.

1250 Bunker CB, Dowd PM. Giant cell arteritis and systemic lupus erythematosus. Br J Dermatol 1988; 119: 115–120.

1251 Thielen KR, Wijdicks EFM, Nichols DA. Giant cell (temporal) arteritis: involvement of the vertebral and internal carotid arteries. Mayo Clin Proc 1998; 73: 444–446.

1252 Keung Y-K, Yung C, Wong JW et al. Association of temporal arteritis, retinal vasculitis, and xanthomatosis with multiple myeloma: case report and literature review. Mayo Clin Proc 1998; 73: 657–660.

1253 Weidner N. Giant-cell vasculitides. Semin Diagn Pathol 2001; 18: 24–33.

1254 Healey LA, Wilske KR. Manifestations of giant cell arteritis. Med Clin North Am 1977; 61: 261–270.

1255 Berth-Jones J, Holt PJA. Temporal arteritis presenting with scalp necrosis and a normal erythrocyte sedimentation rate. Clin Exp Dermatol 1988; 13: 200–201.

1256 Abdullah AN, Keczkes K, Wyatt EH. Skin necrosis in giant cell (temporal) arteritis: report of three cases. Br J Dermatol 1989; 120: 843–846.

1257 Dummer W, Zillikens D, Schulz A et al. Scalp necrosis in temporal (giant cell) arteritis: implications for the dermatologic surgeon. Clin Exp Dermatol 1996; 21: 154–158.

1258 Botella-Estrada R, Sammartín O, Martínez V et al. Magnetic resonance angiography in the diagnosis of a case of giant cell arteritis manifesting as scalp necrosis. Arch Dermatol 1999; 135: 769–771.

1259 Kinmont PDC, McCallum DI. Skin manifestations of giant-cell arteritis. Br J Dermatol 1964; 76: 299–308.

1260 Lau H, Reid BJ, Weedon D. Actinic granuloma in association with giant cell arteritis: are both caused by sunlight? Pathology 1997; 29: 260–262.

1261 Baum EW, Sams WM Jr, Payne RR. Giant cell arteritis: a systemic disease with rare cutaneous manifestations. J Am Acad Dermatol 1982; 6: 1081–1088.

1262 Nitta Y. Temporal arteritis with systemic vasculitis. Br J Dermatol 1999; 140: 549–550.

1263 O'Brien JP, Regan W. A study of elastic tissue and actinic radiation in 'aging', temporal arteritis, polymyalgia rheumatica, and atherosclerosis. J Am Acad Dermatol 1991 24: 765–776.

1264 Shiki H, Shimokama T, Watanabe T. Temporal arteritis: cell composition and the possible pathogenetic role of cell-mediated immunity. Hum Pathol 1989; 20: 1057–1064.

1265 O'Brien JP, Regan W. Actinically degenerate elastic tissue: The prime antigen in the giant cell (temporal) arteritis syndrome? New data from the posterior ciliary arteries. Clin Exp Rheumatol 1998; 16: 39–48.

1266 Tomlinson FH, Lie JT, Nienhuis BJ et al. Juvenile temporal arteritis revisited. Mayo Clin Proc 1994; 69: 445–447.

1267 Fujimoto M, Sato S, Hayashi N et al. Juvenile temporal arteritis with eosinophilia: a distinct clinicopathological entity. Dermatology 1996; 192: 32–35.

1268 Grishman E, Wolfe D, Spiera H. Eosinophilic temporal and systemic arteritis. Hum Pathol 1995; 26: 241–244.

1269 Mambo NC. Temporal (granulomatous) arteritis: a histopathological study of 32 cases. Histopathology 1979; 3: 209–221.

1270 Allsop CJ, Gallagher PJ. Temporal artery biopsy in giant-cell arteritis. A reappraisal. Am J Surg Pathol 1981; 5: 317–323.

1271 Klein RG, Campbell RJ, Hunder GG, Carney JA. Skip lesions in temporal arteritis. Mayo Clin Proc 1976; 51: 504–510.

1272 Poller DN, van Wyk Q, Jeffrey MJ. The importance of skip lesions in temporal arteritis. J Clin Pathol 2000; 53: 137–139.

1273 Chakrabarty A, Franks AJ. Temporal artery biopsy: is there any value in examining biopsies at multiple levels? J Clin Pathol 2000; 53: 131–136.

1274 Goodman BW Jr. Temporal arteritis. Am J Med 1979; 67: 839–852.

1275 Evans JM, Batts KP, Hunder GG. Persistent giant cell arteritis despite corticosteroid treatment. Mayo Clin Proc 1994; 69: 1060–1061.

1276 Corcoran GM, Prayson RA, Herzog KM. The significance of perivascular inflammation in the absence of arteritis in temporal artery biopsy specimens. Am J Clin Pathol 2001; 115: 342–347.

1277 Cox M, Gilks B. Healed or quiescent temporal arteritis versus senescent changes in temporal artery biopsy specimens. Pathology 2001; 33: 163–166.

1278 Lie JT, Michet CJ Jr. Thromboangiitis obliterans with eosinophilia (Buerger's disease) of the temporal arteries. Hum Pathol 1988; 19: 598–602.

1279 Hall S, Barr W, Lie JT et al. Takayasu arteritis. A study of 32 North American patients. Medicine (Baltimore) 1985; 64: 89–99.

1280 Skaria AM, Ruffieux P, Piletta P et al. Takayasu arteritis and cutaneous necrotizing vasculitis. Dermatology 2000; 200: 139–143.

Miscellaneous vascular disorders

1281 Bilen N, Apaydin R, Harova G et al. Stasis dermatitis of the hand associated with an iatrogenic arteriovenous fistula. Clin Exp Dermatol 1998; 23: 208–210.

1282 Török L, Középessy L. Cutaneous gangrene due to hyperparathyroidism secondary to chronic renal failure (uraemic gangrene syndrome). Clin Exp Dermatol 1996; 21: 75–77.

1283 Whittam LR, McGibbon DH, MacDonald DM. Proximal cutaneous necrosis in association with chronic renal failure. Br J Dermatol 1996; 135: 778–781.

1284 Walsh JS, Fairley JA. Calciphylaxis. J Am Acad Dermatol 1996; 35: 786.

1285 Fader DJ, Kang S. Calciphylaxis without renal failure. Arch Dermatol 1996; 132: 837–838.

1286 Gross EA, Wood CR, Lazarus GS, Margolis DJ. Venous leg ulcers: an analysis of underlying venous disease. Br J Dermatol 1993; 129: 270–274.

1287 Weyl A, Vanscheidt W, Weiss JM et al. Expression of the adhesion molecules ICAM-1, VCAM-1, and E-selectin and their ligands VLA-4 and LFA-1 in chronic venous leg ulcers. J Am Acad Dermatol 1996; 34: 418–423.

1288 Balslev E, Thomsen HK, Danielsen L, Warburg F. The occurrence of pericapillary fibrin in venous hypertension and ischaemic leg ulcers: a histopathological study. Br J Dermatol 1992; 126: 582–585.

1289 Vanscheidt W, Laaff H, Wokalek H et al. Pericapillary fibrin cuff: a histological sign of venous leg ulceration. J Cutan Pathol 1990; 17: 266–268.

1290 Brakman M, Faber WR, Zeegelaar JE et al. Venous hypertension of the hand caused by hemodialysis shunt: immunofluorescence studies of pericapillary cuffs. J Am Acad Dermatol 1994; 31: 23–26.

1291 Kanzaki T, Kobayashi T, Shimizu H et al. Aneurysm in the skin: arterial fibromuscular dysplasia. J Am Acad Dermatol 1992; 27: 883–885.

1292 Davis MDP, O'Fallon WM, Rogers RS III, Rooke TW. Natural history of erythromelalgia. Presentation and outcome in 168 patients. Arch Dermatol 2000; 136: 330–336.

1293 Rudikoff D, Jaffe IA. Erythromelalgia: Response to serotonin reuptake inhibitors. J Am Acad Dermatol 1997; 37: 281–283.

1294 Drenth JPH, Michiels JJ. Erythromelalgia and erythermalgia: diagnostic differentiation. Int J Dermatol 1994; 33: 393–397.

1295 Seishima M, Kanoh H, Izumi T et al. A refractory case of secondary erythermalgia successfully treated with lumbar sympathetic ganglion block. Br J Dermatol 2000; 143: 868–872.

1296 Cohen JS. Erythromelalgia: New theories and new therapies. J Am Acad Dermatol 2000; 43: 841–847.

1297 Mørk C, Kvernebo K. Erythromelalgia – a mysterious condition? Arch Dermatol 2000; 136: 406–409.

1298 Mørk C, Asker CL, Salerud EG, Kvernebo K. Microvascular arteriovenous shunting is a probable pathogenetic mechanism in erythromelalgia. J Invest Dermatol 2000; 114: 643–646.

1299 Davis MDP, Rooke TW, Sandroni P. Mechanisms other than shunting are likely contributing to the pathophysiology of erythromelalgia. J Invest Dermatol 2000; 115: 1166–1167.

1300 Mørk C, Kalgaard OM, Kvernebo K. Erythromelalgia as a paraneoplastic syndrome in a patient with abdominal cancer. Acta Derm Venereol 1999; 79: 394.

1301 Yosipovitch G, Rechavia E, Feinmesser M, David M. Adverse cutaneous reactions to ticlopidine in patients with coronary stents. J Am Acad Dermatol 1999; 41: 473–476.

1302 Mørk C, Kalgaard OM, Myrvang B, Kvernebo K. Erythromelalgia in a patient with AIDS. J Eur Acad Dermatol Venereol 2000; 14: 498–500.

1303 Marie I, Levesque H, Plissonnier D et al. Digital necrosis related to cisplatin in systemic sclerosis. Br J Dermatol 2000; 142: 833–834.

1304 Nagore E, Torrelo A, González-Mediero I, Zambrano A. Livedoid skin necrosis (Nicolau syndrome) due to triple vaccine (DTF) injection. Br J Dermatol 1997; 137: 1030–1031.

1305 Weinberg JM. Cutaneous necrosis associated with recombinant interferon injection. J Am Acad Dermatol 1998; 39: 807.

1306 Legrain S, Raguin G, Piette J-C. Digital necrosis revealing ovarian cancer. Dermatology 1999; 199: 183–184.

1307 Valencia IC, Falabella A, Kirsner RS, Eaglstein WH. Chronic venous insufficiency and venous leg ulceration. J Am Acad Dermatol 2001; 44: 401–421.

1308 Hafner J, Schaad I, Schneider E et al. Leg ulcers in peripheral arterial disease (arterial leg ulcers): Impaired wound healing above the threshold of chronic critical limb ischemia. J Am Acad Dermatol 2000; 43: 1001–1008.

1309 Kulthanan K, Krudum T, Pintadit P et al. Chronic leg ulcers associated with hereditary protein S deficiency. Int J Dermatol 1997; 36: 210–212.

1310 Uğuz A, Yilmaz E, Çiflçioğlu MA, Yeğin O. An unusual presentation of immunodeficiency with hyper-IgM. Pediatr Dermatol 2001; 18: 48–50.

1311 Sirieix M-E, Debure C, Baudot N et al. Leg ulcers and hydroxyurea. Forty-one cases. Arch Dermatol 1999; 135: 818–820.

1312 Chaine B, Neonato M-G, Girot R, Aractingi S. Cutaneous adverse reactions to hydroxyurea in patients with sickle cell disease. Arch Dermatol 2001; 137: 467–470.

1313 Herouy Y, Trefzer D, Hellstern MO et al. Plasminogen activation in venous leg ulcers. Br J Dermatol 2000; 143: 930–936.

1314 Badiavas EV, Wilkel C, Golomb C et al. Histologic findings in chronic wounds grafted with bioengineered skin. J Cutan Pathol 2000; 27 548 (abstract).

The epidermis

Disorders of epidermal maturation and keratinization

INTRODUCTION

This chapter deals with a heterogeneous group of diseases in which an abnormality of maturation, of keratinization or of structural integrity of the epidermis is present. Most of these conditions are genetically determined, although a few are acquired diseases of adult life. An understanding of these disorders requires a knowledge of the structure of the epidermis and the process of normal keratinization.

Structure of the epidermis

The epidermis is a stratified squamous epithelial sheet covering the external surface of the body. It is continuously regenerating with the cells undergoing terminal differentiation and death. Folds of the epidermis (the *rete ridges*) extend into the dermis while the dermis projects upwards between these ridges, the so-called '*dermal papillae*'. The epidermis is separated from the dermis by the basement membrane, a complex, multilayered structure that contributes to the structural framework of the epidermis (see p. 143).

Resting on the basement membrane is the *basal layer* of the epidermis, which contains the proliferating cells of the epidermis. Normally, only about 17% of the basal cells make up the dividing cell population. Cells leave this layer to undergo terminal differentiation, whereas some immediately die by apoptosis as a result of an intrinsic program or imbalance of signaling factors.[1] Cells destined to differentiate enter the *prickle cell layer*, where they acquire more cytoplasm and well-formed bundles of keratin intermediate filaments (tonofilaments). The major function of the keratin filaments is to endow epithelial cells with the mechanical resilience they need to withstand stress.[2] The intercellular attachments, the prickles or *desmosomes*, develop here. There is also a change in the keratin composition of the keratin intermediate filaments; the keratins K1 and K10 are expressed in suprabasal cells, in contrast to K5 and K14 in the basal layer (see below). The prickle cell layer varies in thickness from 4 to 10 cells. As the cells are pushed outwards they begin synthesizing the proteins that eventually constitute the keratohyaline granules and cell envelope of the granular layer and stratum corneum respectively. The *granular layer* or *stratum granulosum* is identified by the presence of the keratohyaline granules. This layer is 1–3 cells thick. The cells lose their cytoplasmic organelles and metabolic activity. They flatten further and become compacted into a dense keratinous layer known as the *stratum corneum*. The superficial flake-like squames are eventually cast off (desquamate).

The total epidermal renewal time is approximately 2 months. The cells take 26–42 days to transit from the basal layer to the granular layer and a further 14 days to pass through the keratin layer.

Keratinization

Keratinization refers to the cytoplasmic events that occur in the cytoplasm of epidermal keratinocytes during their terminal differentiation. It involves the formation of keratin polypeptides and their polymerization into keratin intermediate filaments (tonofilaments). It is estimated that each keratin intermediate filament contains 20 000–30 000 keratin polypeptides. More than thirty different keratins have been identified – more than 20 epithelial keratins and 10 hair keratins.[3] The epithelial keratins are divided by molecular weight and isoelectric points into two types – type I keratins, which are acidic and of lower molecular weight, and type II keratins which are neutral basic. The type I keratins are further subdivided numerically from K10 to K20 and the type II keratins from K1 to K9. As a general rule, the epithelial keratins are coexpressed in specific pairings with one from each type.[3] For example, in the basal layer the keratins are K5 and K14 and in the suprabasal layers K1 and K10. K15 has no defined type II partner.[4] Keratins additional to a pair are

sometimes found. For example, K6, K16 and K17 are found in the nail bed epithelium.

Keratins exhibit a high degree of tissue specificity. The primary location of each of the keratin types is shown in Table 9.1, which is based on Irvine and McLean's work.[5] Keratin mutations can cause epithelial fragility syndromes, such as epidermolysis bullosa simplex, in addition to some of the ichthyoses and keratodermas.[5] The various disorders of keratin and their corresponding keratin mutation are listed in Table 9.2.

The keratin intermediate filaments aggregate into bundles (tonofilaments) which touch the nuclear membrane and extend through the cytoplasm to interconnect with adjacent cells, indirectly, via the desmosomal plaques.[3,6]

The keratohyaline granules which give the identifying features to the granular layer result from the accumulation of newly synthesized proteins. One of these is *profilaggrin*. It undergoes dephosphorylation to form *filaggrin*, a histidine-rich protein which acts as a matrix glue and facilitates filament aggregation into even larger bundles. Trichohyalin, found primarily in the inner root sheath cells, is sometimes coexpressed with filaggrin.[7] The keratin filaments are stabilized by disulfide crosslinks which make this intracytoplasmic structural mesh highly insoluble. A second polypeptide, *loricrin*, is localized to the keratohyaline granules. It contributes to the formation of a stable, intracytoplasmic, insoluble barrier known as the *cell envelope* (*cornified envelope*) – see below.

The granular layer also contains small, lipid-rich lamellated granules (100–500 nm in diameter), known as *Odland bodies* or *membrane-coating*

Table 9.1 **Cellular location of the various keratins**

Keratin type	Primary location
K1, K10	Suprabasal cells
K2e	Late suprabasal cells
K2p*	Hard palate
K3, K12	Cornea
K4, K13	Mucosa
K5, K14	Basal keratinocytes
K6a, K16	Palmoplantar, mucosa, appendages
K7*	Myoepithelia, simple epithelia
K8*, K18	Simple epithelia
K9	Palmoplantar
K15*	Basal keratinocytes, outer root sheath
K17, K6b	Epidermal appendages
K19*	Simple epithelia, epidermal appendages
K20*	Gastrointestinal tract
hHb6, hHb1	Cortical trichocytes

* Indicates that mutations causing human disease have not so far been identified

Table 9.2 **Disorders of keratin**

Disease	Keratin mutation
Bullous congenital ichthyosiform erythroderma	K1, K10
Ichthyosis bullosa of Siemens	K2e
Epidermolytic palmoplantar keratoderma	K9
Nonepidermolytic palmoplantar keratoderma	K1 (one family), type II keratin cluster (not yet clarified)
Palmoplantar keratosis with anogenital leukokeratosis	K6, K16
Focal nonepidermolytic palmoplantar keratoderma	K1, K16
Unilateral palmoplantar verrucous nevus	K16
Pachyonychia congenita	K6a, K16, K17
White sponge nevus	K4, K13
Monilethrix	hHb6, hHb1
Epidermolysis bullosa simplex	K5, K14

granules. They are secreted into the intercellular space in this region. Their lipid-rich nature contributes to the permeability barrier (see below).[8]

The *cell envelope (cornified envelope)* forms just beneath the cell membrane. It is 7–15 nm wide and composed of crosslinked proteins. Several proteins are involved in the formation of the cell envelope including loricrin, involucrin, keratolinin and small proline-rich proteins.[3,9] Polymerization and crosslinking of these proteins requires the action of calcium-dependent epidermal transglutaminases, of which three have been identified in the skin.

Keratinocytes in the stratum corneum (corneocytes) are dead. They eventually undergo desquamation, an orderly process in which individual corneocytes detach from their neighbors at the skin surface and are swept away.[10] This occurs, in part, because the desmosomes are degraded (presumably by proteases) during transit through the stratum corneum.[11] However, the process of desquamation (dyshesion) is more complex than simple desmosomal degeneration.[12] It is known that cholesterol esters are important components of cell adhesion. For example, in X-linked ichthyosis, there is an accumulation of cholesterol sulfate associated with a deficiency in aryl sulfatase, which results in decreased desquamation and keratin accumulation. It is thought that cholesterol sulfate inhibits proteases that are involved in desquamation.[13] Lipids also play a role in the permeability barrier of the skin, a function which resides in the region of the granular layer.[14,15] Lipids secreted by the Odland bodies (see above) are an important component of the permeability barrier. In addition to the structures already described, there is a skin surface lipid film produced by secreted sebum mixed with lipid from the keratinizing epithelium.[16] It contributes to barrier function.

The chromosomal localizations of the various genes encoding the various polypeptides involved in keratinization have been elucidated – type I keratins on chromosome 17, type II on chromosome 12, transglutaminases on chromosome 14, and profilaggrin, trichohyalin, loricrin, involucrin and the small proline-rich proteins on chromosome 1q21.[3] Because this latter gene complex controls the structural proteins of cornification, the term 'epidermal differentiation complex' has been proposed for this region.[9] The expression of these genes is controlled by proteins called transcription factors.[17,18]

The abnormal process, where known, for each of the disorders of keratinization is shown in Table 9.3. This is based on a publication by Hohl.[19]

ICHTHYOSES

The ichthyoses are a heterogeneous group of hereditary and acquired disorders of keratinization characterized by the presence of visible scales on the skin surface.[20–23] The word is derived from the Greek root for fish – *ichthys*. There are four major types of ichthyosis: ichthyosis vulgaris, X-linked ichthyosis, ichthyosis congenita and epidermolytic hyperkeratosis (bullous ichthyosiform erythroderma). In addition, there are several rare syndromes in which ichthyosis is a major feature. It has been estimated that nearly 1 million Americans have either ichthyosis vulgaris or X-linked recessive ichthyosis, the most common forms.[24]

Kinetic studies have shown that lamellar ichthyosis and epidermolytic hyperkeratosis are characterized by hyperproliferation of the epidermis with transit times of 4–5 days, whereas the scale in ichthyosis vulgaris and X-linked ichthyosis is related to prolonged retention of the stratum corneum (retention hyperkeratoses).[11,20,21] This may be related to a persistence of desmosomes in the stratum corneum.[25]

Although the mode of inheritance was originally used as a major criterion in the delineation of the various forms of ichthyosis, recent studies have shown some evidence of genetic heterogeneity in the various groups.[26,27]

Table 9.3 **Disorders of keratinization**

Abnormal process	Diseases with this abnormal process
Calcium pump	Darier's disease Hailey–Hailey disease
Sulfatase disorders	X-linked ichthyosis Kallmann's syndrome (ichthyosis and hypogonadism) Multiple sulfatase deficiency X-linked recessive chondrodysplasia punctata
Keratin disorders	See Table 9.2
Desmosomal defects (desmoplakin; cadherins)	Striate palmoplantar keratoderma
Processing of filaggrin	Granular parakeratosis Ichthyosis vulgaris (AGL variant)
Loricrin	Progressive symmetrical erythrokeratodermia (PSEK)-loricrin variant Vohwinkel's syndrome (ichthyotic variant)
Precursor proteins of cell envelope	Camisa keratoderma PSEK (loricrin variant)
Connexin	Erythrokeratodermia variabilis Vohwinkel's syndrome (keratoderma variant) Hidrotic ectodermal dysplasia
Abnormal lipid metabolism	Sjögren–Larsson syndrome (fatty aldehyde dehydrogenase gene) Conradi's syndrome (included as peroxisomal by some) CHILD syndrome (included as peroxisomal by some)
Peroxisomes	Refsum disease (increased phytanic acid) Chondrodysplasia punctata (two variants)
Cell envelope (transglutaminase-1)	Lamellar ichthyosis Congenital ichthyosiform erythroderma (50%)
Proteinase disorders	Netherton's syndrome Papillon–Lefèvre syndrome (cathepsin C gene)

ICHTHYOSIS VULGARIS

Ichthyosis vulgaris is the most common type of ichthyosis (incidence 1:250), with an onset in early childhood and an autosomal dominant inheritance.[20] It may have only very mild expression and be misdiagnosed as dry skin. The disorder is lifelong. It is characterized by fine, whitish scales involving particularly the extensor surfaces of the arms and legs, as well as the scalp. Flexures are spared. There may be accentuation of palmar and plantar markings, keratosis pilaris and features of atopy.

In ichthyosis vulgaris, there is a deficiency in profilaggrin which is converted into filaggrin, the major protein of keratohyalin.[11,28] There are quantitative decreases in filaggrin, related to the severity of the disease.[29]

There is a subset of patients with ichthyosis vulgaris in whom the granular layer is consistently absent.[30] They exhibit reduced or absent profilaggrin mRNA. Linkage to chromosome 1q21 has been found in one family.[30] This variant, known as ichthyosis vulgaris AGL, may be either autosomal dominant or recessive in its inheritance. Its exact relationship to the other type is somewhat confused, as this distinction has not always been made.

Histopathology

The epidermis may be of normal thickness or slightly thinned with some loss of the rete ridges.[31] There is mild to moderate hyperkeratosis, associated paradoxically with diminution or absence of the granular layer (Fig. 9.1). The

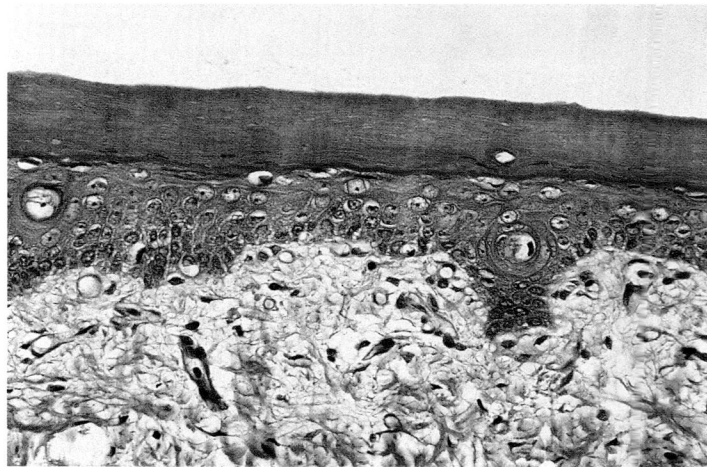

Fig. 9.1 **Ichthyosis vulgaris.** There is a thickened layer of compact orthokeratosis overlying a diminished granular layer. (H & E)

thickened stratum corneum is often laminated in appearance. The hyperkeratosis may extend into the hair follicles. The sebaceous and sweat glands are often reduced in size and number.

Electron microscopy
Electron microscopy shows defective keratohyaline synthesis with small granules having a crumbled or spongy appearance.[28]

X-LINKED ICHTHYOSIS

This form of ichthyosis, which is inherited as an X-linked recessive trait, is present at birth or develops in the first few months of life. It is characterized by large polygonal scales which are dirty brown in color and adherent. X-linked ichthyosis may involve the entire body in varying degree, although there is sparing of the palms and soles. The preauricular region is characteristically involved in this variant of ichthyosis; in contrast, this site is usually spared in ichthyosis vulgaris.[32] Corneal opacities and mental retardation may also occur in X-linked ichthyosis.[33,34] Other rare associations include Poland's syndrome (unilateral absence of the pectoralis major muscle)[35] and Kallmann's syndrome (hypogonadism, renal agenesis, anosmia and synkinesis).[36] Interestingly, X-linked ichthyosis and Kallmann's syndrome result from abnormalities in contiguous genes.[36] Ichthyosis vulgaris and X-linked ichthyosis have been reported in the same family.[37] Male-pattern baldness does occur, despite earlier claims to the contrary.[38,39]

Its incidence is approximately one in 6000 males, but occasionally female heterozygotes have mild scaling of the legs.

This condition is characterized by a deficiency of steroid sulfatase in a wide range of tissues, including leukocytes and fibroblasts. As a result there is an accumulation of cholesterol sulfate in the pathological scales and in serum and leukocytes.[10,40–43] Accumulation in the skin interferes with normal barrier function[44,45] and with proteases involved in the dissolution of desmosomes required for desquamation of the stratum corneum.[12] There are elevated levels of cholesterol sulfate and dehydroepiandrosterone in the serum.[46] The deficiency in placental sulfatase which is also present results in decreased maternal urinary estrogens and a failure to initiate labor in some cases.[33] The steroid sulfatase gene is on the distal short arm of the X chromosome (Xp22.3).[34] Most cases involve complete or partial deletion of the *STS* gene.[47–53] The defect is usually inherited and it is not due to a *de novo* mutation.[54]

Histopathology
There is usually conspicuous acanthosis with thickening of the stratum corneum and a normal to thickened granular layer. Thinning of the granular layer is sometimes present.[55] There is often hyperkeratosis of follicular and sweat duct orifices.[56] There may be a few lymphocytes around the vessels in the superficial dermis.

ICHTHYOSIS CONGENITA

In recent years there has been an attempt to reclassify the autosomal recessive ichthyoses previously known as lamellar ichthyosis (LI) and non-bullous congenital ichthyosiform erythroderma (CIE) as ichthyosis congenita on the basis of ultrastructural findings suggesting that there are at least four types.[57–59] This new classification has not yet been widely accepted by clinicians; furthermore, inheritance and ultrastructure have not always proven to be a reliable basis for classifications. A defect in keratinocyte transglutaminase has been detected in about 50% of the families studied.[60] The four subtypes of ichthyosis congenita are as follows.

Type I
Type I is the largest group and corresponds to CIE of the older classification (see below). There is erythroderma with fine scaling. About 40% present as a 'collodion baby', in which the infant is encased in a tight membrane.[59] Most have palmoplantar keratoderma. Clear ultrastructural criteria are lacking but numerous lipid droplets are usually present in the horny cells.[58] It has been suggested that the diagnosis be made by exclusion of the other three types. This group may still be heterogeneous.

Type II
Type II is characterized by cholesterol clefts in the horny cells. It corresponds to lamellar ichthyosis (see below).

Type III
There is generalized lamellar scaling with a pronounced reticulate pattern. There is erythroderma and pruritus. This group usually presents as a collodion baby. There are perinuclear, elongated membrane structures in the granular and horny cells.[58,61]

Type IV
There is a variable clinical phenotype. Types III and IV were both previously included with CIE.[62] There are masses of lipid membranes in the granular and horny cells. A case that clinically resembled diffuse cutaneous mastocytosis has been reported.[63]

Lamellar ichthyosis

Lamellar ichthyosis (LI) is characterized by large plate-like scales of ichthyosis.[64] It corresponds to ichthyosis congenita type II (see above). It may present as a 'collodion baby'.[21,65–67] The palms and soles are often involved.[21] An increased incidence of skin cancers has been reported in this variant of ichthyosis.[68]

Some cases have been shown to have mutations in the keratinocyte transglutaminase-1 gene on chromosome 14q11.[69–72] This defect interferes with the crosslinkage of loricrin and involucrin and the formation of the cornified cell envelope.[73] A second locus has been mapped to chromosome 2q33–q35; other loci are suspected.[74,75]

Congenital ichthyosiform erythroderma

Congenital ichthyosiform erythroderma (CIE) was known in the past as non-bullous congenital ichthyosiform erythroderma. It has also been included within the category of lamellar ichthyosis. CIE is known to be a heterogeneous entity; variants have been reclassified as ichthyosis congenita types I, III and IV (see above). Variants include a pustular form[76] and a reticulated pigmented form (ichthyosis variegata).[77,78] A patient with associated ocular albinism and Noonan's syndrome has been reported.[79] CIE differs from lamellar ichthyosis (LI) by the erythroderma and finer, pale scales which have a high content of n-alkanes.[41,80,81] A subset of patients with CIE has abnormal expression of keratinocyte transglutaminase-1.[82] Several cases of CIE have been linked to a defect on chromosome 3.[74]

Histopathology

Some of the reports in the literature have not distinguished between lamellar ichthyosis and congenital ichthyosiform erythroderma or the various subtypes of ichthyosis congenita; a composite description therefore follows.

There is hyperkeratosis, focal parakeratosis and a normal or thickened granular layer.[83] The hyperkeratosis is more marked in lamellar ichthyosis than other variants, and there is easily discernible parakeratosis in CIE.[80] There is often some acanthosis and occasionally there is irregular psoriasiform epidermal hyperplasia (Figs 9.2, 9.3).[27] Vacuolation of cells in the granular layer is a rare finding.[84] Keratotic plugging of follicular orifices may also be present. The dermis often shows a mild superficial perivascular infiltrate of lymphocytes.

The case presented recently with ichthyosiform erythroderma, onset in adolescence, and a lichenoid tissue reaction on histology probably represents a new entity.[85]

Electron microscopy

The ultrastructural features of the various types of ichthyosis congenita (including LI and CIE) have been outlined above.

BULLOUS ICHTHYOSIS

The term 'bullous ichthyosis' is preferred to bullous congenital ichthyosiform erythroderma and to epidermolytic hyperkeratosis (which merely describes a histological reaction pattern).[86–88] Bullous ichthyosis is a rare, autosomal dominant condition which is usually severe and characterized at birth by widespread erythema and some blistering.[21] Coarse, verrucous scales, particularly in the flexures, develop as the disposition to blistering subsides during childhood. Annular plaques, of late onset, have been reported.[89]

Bullous ichthyosis is a clinically heterogeneous condition.[90–94] Six subtypes were recently defined, the presence or absence of palmoplantar keratoderma being used as a major feature in defining the subtypes.[95] There is some evidence to suggest that cases with severe palmoplantar keratoderma have abnormalities in keratin 1, while those without have abnormalities in keratin 10.[96] In cases of palmoplantar keratoderma without diffuse cutaneous lesions, defects in keratin 9 are usual. The commonest abnormality in keratin 10 involves an arginine to histidine substitution at one point.[97,98] Other substitutions have been reported.[99,100] No abnormality in keratin 1 or 10 has been detected in some cases, suggesting that other genes may be involved. Keratin 1 and 10 are coexpressed to form keratin intermediate filaments in the suprabasal layers of the epidermis.[94,95,101–104] The keratin 1 and 10 genes are located on chromosome 12 in the type II keratin cluster. Clinical variants of bullous ichthyosis include a rare *acral group* (not included in the six subtypes mentioned above),[6] an *annular* form,[102,105] *ichthyosis hystrix of Curth–Macklin* (which may involve keratin 10 and is characterized ultrastructurally by perinuclear shells of unbroken tonofilaments),[106] *ichthyosis hystrix of Lambert*[107] and *ichthyosis bullosa of Siemens* (which lacks erythroderma and appears to result from a mutation in keratin 2e).[108–117] *Ichthyosis exfoliativa* is said to have a similar genetic defect and clinical features to ichthyosis bullosa of Siemens, but one report has suggested that there is no epidermolytic hyperkeratosis on histology.[118,119]

Prenatal diagnosis can be made at approximately 19 weeks by fetal skin biopsy examined by light and electron microscopy;[120] it can be made earlier by direct gene sequencing.[121]

Histopathology

The histological pattern is that of epidermolytic hyperkeratosis, characterized by marked hyperkeratosis and granular and vacuolar change in the upper spinous and granular layers (Fig. 9.4).[122] The keratohyaline granules appear coarse and basophilic with clumping. There is moderate acanthosis. The histological features of blistering can sometimes be subtle, with only slight separation of the markedly vacuolar cells in the mid and upper epidermis. There is usually a mild perivascular inflammatory cell infiltrate in the upper dermis.

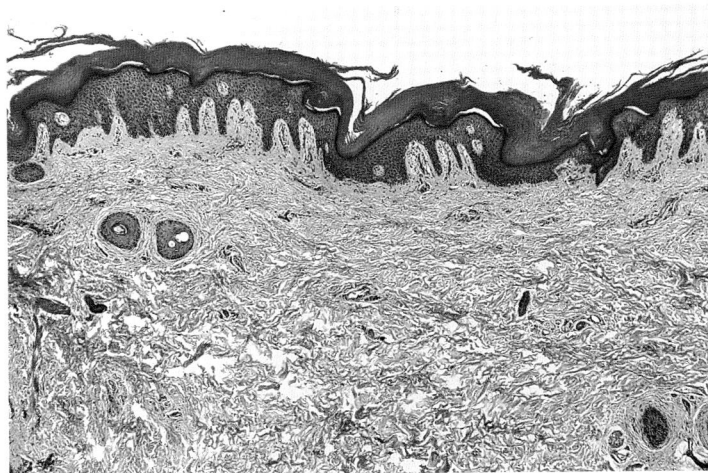

Fig. 9.2 **Lamellar ichthyosis.** There is compact orthokeratosis and mild psoriasiform hyperplasia of the epidermis. (H & E)

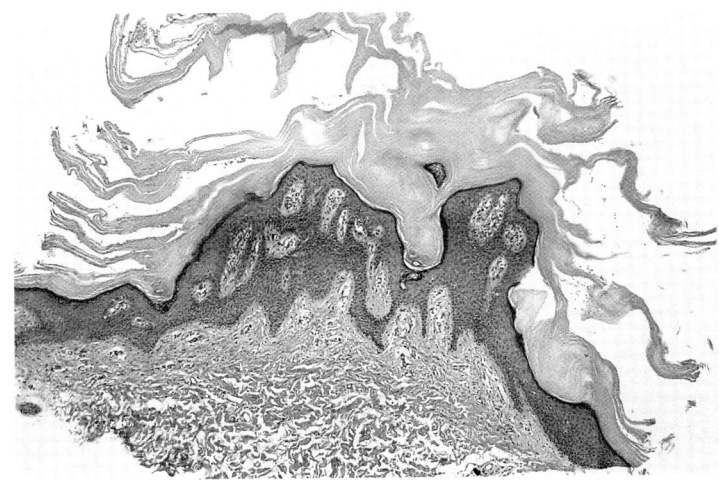

Fig. 9.3 **Lamellar ichthyosis.** Another case with more orthokeratosis and a less regular outline. (H & E)

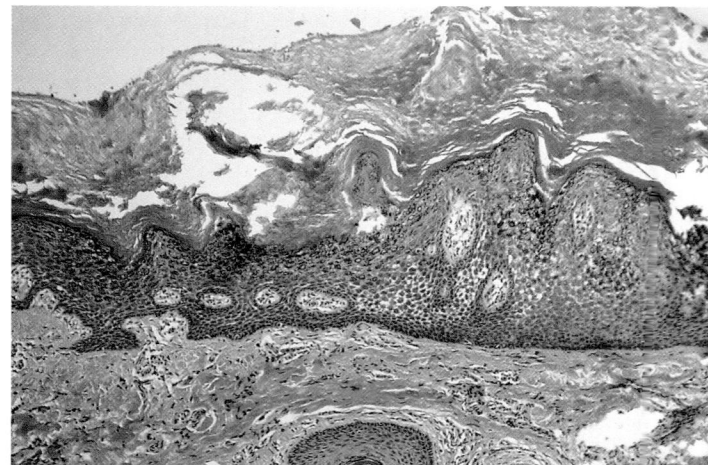

Fig. 9.4 **Bullous ichthyosis** with hyperkeratosis and granular and vacuolar change of the keratinocytes in the upper layers of the epidermis. Blistering is not shown in this field. (H & E)

Electron microscopy

There is aggregation of tonofilaments at the cell periphery with perinuclear areas free of tonofilaments and containing endoplasmic reticulum.[123,124] In the upper granular layer there are numerous keratohyaline granules, sometimes embedded in clumped tonofilaments. Although desmosomes appear normal, there is often an abnormality in the association of tonofilaments and desmosomes.

ICHTHYOSIS LINEARIS CIRCUMFLEXA

Ichthyosis linearis circumflexa is a rare autosomal recessive condition characterized by migratory annular and polycyclic erythema with scaling borders distributed on the trunk and extremities. Some patients have hair shaft abnormalities.[125-127] *Netherton's syndrome* is the term used for the triad of ichthyosis linearis circumflexa, trichorrhexis invaginata and an atopic diathesis.[128-131] Initially, most infants with Netherton's syndrome display a generalized erythroderma.[132] Intermittent aminoaciduria and mental retardation may also be present. Other hair shaft abnormalities such as pili torti, trichorrhexis nodosa and monilethrix have also been reported in Netherton's syndrome.[133,134] The hair shaft abnormalities are more common in eyebrow than scalp hair.[135] Hair shaft changes may not appear until 18 months of age.[136] The ichthyosiform component may, rarely, be of another type.[128]

Disturbances in the immune system have been reported in several patients with Netherton's syndrome.[137] This may be the explanation for the finding of HPV infection superimposed on the ichthyotic lesions.[138,139] A case with phenotypic overlap with the peeling skin syndrome (see p. 304) has been reported.[140] The gene responsible for Netherton's syndrome maps to chromosome 5q32 which is telomeric to the cytokine gene cluster in 5q31.[141]

The keratin filaments from the scales in this condition are composed of reduced amounts of high molecular subunits and increased amounts of low molecular subunits.[125]

Histopathology

The skin lesions show hyperkeratosis, a well-developed granular layer and acanthosis. The margin shows focal parakeratosis with absence of the granular layer and more obvious psoriasiform epidermal hyperplasia (Fig. 9.5).[125,142] In erythrodermic cases, the parakeratosis is more prominent; sometimes it constitutes the entire stratum corneum. In all cases, the outermost nucleated

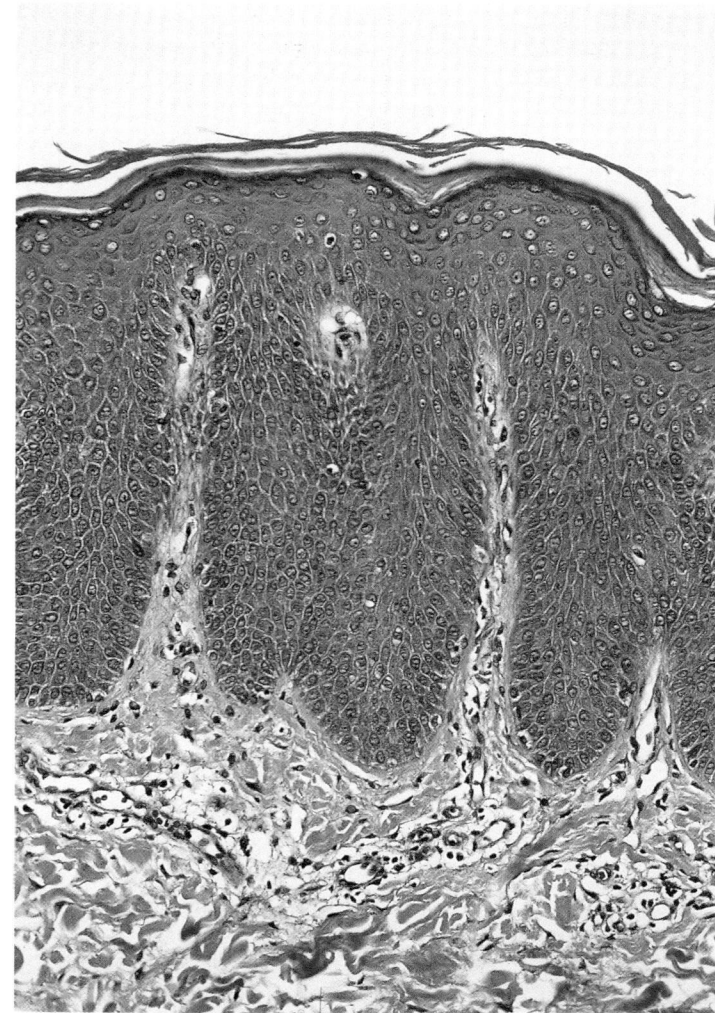

Fig. 9.5 **Ichthyosis linearis circumflexa.** This biopsy from a neonate shows a striking resemblance to psoriasis, but there are no mounds of parakeratosis containing neutrophils. (H & E)

layers do not flatten normally.[132] Pustules are sometimes seen in the erythrodermic stage. Epidermal mitoses are increased. In some cases PAS-positive, diastase-resistant granules can be found in the prickle cells. There is often a mild perivascular inflammatory cell infiltrate in the superficial dermis.

Electron microscopy

Electron microscopy shows an increase in mitochondria and numerous round or oval opaque (lipoid) bodies in the stratum corneum.[125] A distinctive feature is premature secretion of lamellar body contents.[132]

ERYTHROKERATODERMIA VARIABILIS

Erythrokeratodermia variabilis is a rare, usually autosomal dominant form of ichthyosis that develops in infancy; uncommonly it is present at birth.[143] An autosomal recessive variant is now recognized.[144] There are transient erythematous patches and erythematous hyperkeratotic plaques which are often polycyclic or circinate.[20,145,146] A targetoid appearance is seen in the rare cocarde variant.[147,148] Follicular hyperkeratosis has been described.[149] There is retention hyperkeratosis associated with a basal cell type of keratin.[150] In one study the region was localized to 1p34–p35, the site of a cluster of connexin genes.[151] At least 14 connexin genes have been described.[152] A more recent study has found a mutation in the gap junction protein β-3 (encoding connexin 31) in one family.[153] Mutations in the nearby gene for connexin 30.3 have also been described, indicating the heterogeneity of this entity.[148,152]

Progressive symmetrical erythrokeratodermia, thought at one time to be the same condition, appears to be a variant with its own specific abnormality, a mutant loricrin gene.[19,154] Profilaggrin N-terminal domains are aggregated with mutant loricrin within condensed nuclei. These nuclei persist in the cornified layer as parakeratosis.[155] The ichthyotic variant of Vohwinkel's syndrome also has this abnormality.

Histopathology

The findings are not distinctive. There is hyperkeratosis, irregular acanthosis, very mild papillomatosis in some biopsies, and a mild superficial perivascular infiltrate of lymphocytes. Dyskeratotic, grain-like cells may be seen in the lower stratum corneum.[156]

There may be parakeratosis and some vacuolation in the lower horny cells and in the granular layer.[149]

Electron microscopy

There is a reduction in keratinosomes in the stratum granulosum.[156] The dyskeratotic cells have clumped tonofilaments.[156]

HARLEQUIN FETUS

Harlequin fetus is a severe disorder of cornification. It is usually incompatible with extrauterine life and is of autosomal recessive inheritance.[21,157] There appears to be genetic heterogeneity.[158–160] It is characterized by thick, plate-like scales with deep fissures.[161] Prenatal diagnosis can be made by skin biopsy of the intrauterine fetus at about 17 weeks.[162,163] Harlequin ichthyosis is a disorder of epidermal keratinization in which there are altered lamellar granules and a variation in the expression of keratin and filaggrin.[159,164] Lipid levels may be increased in the stratum corneum.[165] In some cases, a defect of protein phosphatase has been demonstrated.[160] This enzyme may alter the processing of profilaggrin to filaggrin.[160]

Patients who survive the neonatal period develop a severe exfoliative erythroderma consistent with nonbullous congenital ichthyosiform erythroderma (CIE).[166] However, transglutaminase-1 levels have been normal in harlequin ichthyosis, and it is ultrastructurally distinct.[167,168]

Histopathology

There is massive hyperkeratosis in all biopsies. Some cases have parakeratosis with a thin or absent granular layer[169] while others have had persistence of the granular layer.[165]

Electron microscopy[170]

The stratum corneum is thickened and contains lipid and vacuolar inclusions.[171] Lamellar granules are abnormal or absent;[159,172,173] instead, dense core granules are produced.[170] The marginal band (cellular envelope of cornified cells) is present at birth, in contrast to collodion baby in which it is absent at birth, but may develop later.[174]

FOLLICULAR ICHTHYOSIS

Follicular ichthyosis is a rare, distinctive form in which the abnormal epidermal differentiation occurs mainly in hair follicles.[175,176] Its onset is at birth or in early childhood. The hyperkeratosis is more prominent on the head and neck. Photophobia and alopecia are often present.[177] Three of the patients reported have also had acanthosis nigricans-like lesions.[175]

Histopathology

There is marked follicular hyperkeratosis which is compact and extends deep within the follicle. There is a prominent granular layer.[175] In keratosis pilaris the hyperkeratosis has a more open basket-weave pattern and is confined to the infundibular region of the follicle.

ACQUIRED ICHTHYOSIS

Acquired ichthyosis, which occurs in adult life, is similar to ichthyosis vulgaris both clinically and histologically.[178] It is usually associated with an underlying malignant disease, particularly a lymphoma,[179] but it usually appears some time after other manifestations of the malignant process. Ichthyosis has also been associated with malnutrition, sympathectomy,[180] hypothyroidism, leprosy, HIV infection,[181] sarcoidosis,[182,183] eosinophilic fasciitis[184] and drugs such as clofazimine and nafoxidine.[185] An ichthyosiform contact dermatitis may follow the repeated application of antiseptic solutions containing cetrimide.[186] There is compact orthokeratosis and/or parakeratosis without spongiosis. Cetrimide appears to act on the lipids and enzymes of the lamellar bodies.[186] Acquired ichthyosis is sometimes seen in the recipients of bone marrow transplants.[187] Acquired ichthyosis must be distinguished from asteatosis (dry skin). It may be related to an essential fatty acid deficiency in some cases.[183]

Pityriasis rotunda, which is manifested by sharply demarcated, circular, scaly patches of variable diameter and number, is probably a variant of acquired ichthyosis. It is more common in black and oriental patients than in whites. An underlying malignant neoplasm or systemic illness is often present.[188–193] Pityriasis rotunda may also occur as a familial disease, suggesting that there are two types with significant prognostic differences.[194,195]

REFSUM'S SYNDROME

Refsum's syndrome, a rare autosomal recessive disorder, is characterized by ichthyosis, cerebellar ataxia, peripheral neuropathy and retinitis pigmentosa.[21] The skin most resembles ichthyosis vulgaris but the onset of scale is often delayed until adulthood. There is an inability to oxidize phytanic acid, and improvement occurs when the patient adheres to a diet free from chlorophyll, which contains phytol, the precursor of this fatty acid.[21]

Histopathology

A biopsy will show hyperkeratosis, a granular layer that may be increased or decreased in amount, and some acanthosis. Basal keratinocytes are vacuolated and these stain for neutral lipid.[196] Lipid vacuoles are also present in keratinocytes in the rare Dorfman–Chanarin syndrome in which congenital ichthyosis is present (see below).[197]

Electron microscopy

There are non-membrane-bound vacuoles in the basal and suprabasal keratinocytes.[195]

OTHER ICHTHYOSIS-RELATED SYNDROMES

There are a number of rare syndromes in which ichthyosis is a feature. As their histopathology resembles one of the already described forms of ichthyosis, they will be discussed only briefly.

Sjögren–Larsson syndrome

The Sjögren–Larsson syndrome is an autosomal recessive disorder characterized by the triad of congenital ichthyosis (most resembling lamellar ichthyosis), spastic paralysis and mental retardation.[198,199] Sometimes the ichthyosis does not develop until the first few months of life. An enzymatic defect in fatty alcohol oxidation has been identified.[200,201] This is due to a mutation in the fatty aldehyde dehydrogenase gene (*FALDH*). Various mutations have been described, including one leading to partial reduction in enzyme activity.[202–205] A prenatal diagnosis can be made by fetal skin biopsy.[206] The thickened keratin layer may still retain its basket-weave appearance.[207] There is also acanthosis, mild papillomatosis and a mildly thickened granular layer.

'KID' syndrome

The 'KID' syndrome comprises *keratitis*, *ichthyosis* and *deafness*.[208–218] Different modes of inheritance seem likely.[219] The ichthyosis is usually of the hyperorthokeratotic type but a variant with features of epidermolytic hyperkeratosis (ichthyosis hystrix) has been reported.[220] The term '*HID*' syndrome has been proposed for this variant (*hystrix ichthyosis* and *deafness*).[220] It has been suggested that the KID syndrome should be reclassified as an ectodermal dysplasia.[221]

Conradi's syndrome

Conradi's syndrome (Conradi–Hünermann syndrome) combines chondrodysplasia with ichthyosis and palmar and plantar hyperkeratosis.[20,222] At least three variants of chondrodysplasia and ichthyosis exist, reflecting genetic heterogeneity and incomplete gene penetrance.[223] In a recently reported X-linked variant, there were ichthyotic and psoriasiform lesions along Blaschko's lines,[224,225] in keeping with the distribution of cutaneous lesions in other X-linked dominant diseases.[225] Unilateral lesions are a rare occurrence.[223] Deficiency of a peroxisomal enzyme has been reported.[226] This is probably related to cholesterol biosynthesis.[225] A skin biopsy shows hyperkeratosis, a prominent granular layer, dilated ostia of pilosebaceous follicles with keratotic plugging, dilated acrosyringia and calcium in the stratum corneum.[227,228] Parakeratosis with a diminished granular layer sometimes occurs.[223] Dyskeratotic cells may be present in the hair follicles.[225]

'CHILD' syndrome

The 'CHILD' syndrome includes *congenital hemidysplasia*, *ichthyosiform erythroderma* and *limb defects*.[20,229–233] There is a lack of expression of epidermal differentiation markers in lesional ichthyotic skin.[234] As in Conradi's syndrome, there is also an abnormality in peroxisomal function, indicating the close relationship of these two conditions.[223,225] It is an X-linked recessive disorder that is lethal in males.[66] Variations include linear lesions, lesions along Blaschko's lines and verruciform xanthomas.[66]

Tay's syndrome

Tay's syndrome is associated with closeset eyes, a beaked nose and sunken cheeks.[20]

'IBIDS'

'IBIDS' combines *ichthyosis* with *brittle hair*, *impaired intelligence*, *decreased fertility* and *short stature*.[235,236]

Multiple sulfatase deficiency

Multiple sulfatase deficiency includes severe neurodegenerative disease, similar to metachromatic leukodystrophy, ichthyosis and signs of mucopolysaccharidosis.[21] It is an extremely rare autosomal recessive disorder affecting the activity of many sulfatases (arylsulfatase A, steroid sulfatase and several mucopolysaccharide sulfatases), an explanation for the various clinical manifestations of this disease.[237] The ichthyosis, not surprisingly, has some features of X-linked ichthyosis.

'MAUIE' syndrome

The 'MAUIE' syndrome consists of *micropinnae*, *alopecia universalis*, *congenital ichthyosis*, and *ectropion*. The early development of skin cancer has been reported in this syndrome.[238]

Neutral lipid storage disease

Neutral lipid storage disease (Dorfman–Chanarin syndrome), in which neutral lipid accumulates in the cytoplasm of many cells of the body, combines fatty liver with muscular dystrophy and ichthyosis.[21,239,240] It is an autosomal recessive disorder in which a defect of acylglycerol recycling from triacylglycerol to phospholipid has recently been identified in fibroblasts.[241] An excess of triacylglycerol accumulates in most cells.[242] Lipid droplets are found within leukocytes (Jordans' anomaly). A skin biopsy shows hyperkeratosis, mild acanthosis and discrete vacuolation of basal keratinocytes, sweat glands and sweat ducts.[243] The vacuoles contain lipid.

Shwachman syndrome

Shwachman syndrome combines pancreatic insufficiency and bone marrow dysfunction with xerosis and/or ichthyosis.[232,244]

Other unnamed associations have been described.[20,245–247]

PALMOPLANTAR KERATODERMAS AND RELATED CONDITIONS

In addition to the group of disorders usually categorized as the palmoplantar keratodermas, there are several rare genodermatoses that are usually regarded as discrete entities, in which palmoplantar keratoderma is a major clinicopathological feature. These disorders include hidrotic ectodermal dysplasia (see p. 291), acrokeratoelastoidosis (see p. 291), pachyonychia congenita (see p. 292), tyrosinosis (see p. 291) and pachydermoperiostosis (see p. 352). Keratoderma may also occur as a manifestation of certain inflammatory dermatoses, such as pityriasis rubra pilaris, Reiter's disease, psoriasis, Darier's disease and as a paraneoplastic manifestation.[248] These conditions will not be considered further in this chapter.

PALMOPLANTAR KERATODERMAS

The palmoplantar keratodermas are a heterogeneous group of congenital and acquired disorders of keratinization, characterized by diffuse or localized hyperkeratosis of the palms and soles, sometimes accompanied by other ectodermal abnormalities.[249,250] Another classification system has also been proposed: the four major categories include diffuse, focal and punctate palmoplantar keratodermas and the palmoplantar ectodermal dysplasias. Nineteen subtypes have been described in this latter category.[251] Categorization has been made on the basis of their mode of inheritance, sites of involvement and associated abnormalities.[252] The autosomal recessive types are usually the most severe and include mal de Meleda, Papillon–Lefèvre syndrome, some mutilating variants and a variant associated with generalized ichthyosis.[253] The other hereditary forms are autosomal dominant, although sporadic cases of most syndromes occur.[254]

Another feature used to distinguish the various subtypes of keratoderma is the presence of hyperkeratosis beyond the palms and soles. These 'transgrediens' lesions occur in the Olmsted, Greither, Vohwinkel and mal de Meleda types.[255] Onset of most keratodermas is at birth or in early infancy, but later onset is seen in the punctate and acquired forms. New syndromes continue to be reported.[256,257] In one of these, *papulotranslucent acrokeratoderma* (aquagenic palmoplantar keratoderma), already thickened palmar skin develops whitish papules after exposure to water. The eccrine ostia are dilated.[258–260] In another, a non-epidermolytic palmoplantar keratoderma is associated with sensorineural deafness and a mutation in the mitochondrial genome (mtDNA).[261] In *palmoplantar keratoderma with anogenital leukokeratosis*, an absence of K6 and K16 has been detected.[262] In the *Schöpf–Schulz–Passarge* syndrome there are associated apocrine hidrocystomas, hypodontia, hypotrichosis and hypoplastic nails.[263]

Brief mention will be made of the important clinical features of the various keratodermas.

Unna–Thost syndrome

Unna–Thost syndrome usually presents in the first few months of life.[264,265] Deafness is sometimes present,[266] while acrocyanosis and total anomalous pulmonary venous drainage are rare associations.[267,268] Verrucous carcinoma has been reported in one case.[269] The syndrome may not be as common as once thought, because of the inclusion of cases of Vörner's syndrome with which it is clinically, but not histologically, identical.[270] The disorder maps to the type II keratin cluster on chromosome 12q11–13.[271] A mutation in the K1 gene has been reported in a single family.[272]

Greither's syndrome

In this 'transgrediens' form (hyperkeratosis beyond the palms and soles), the elbows and knees may be more involved than the palms and soles.[249,273] It is associated with hyperhidrosis. The inheritance is autosomal dominant with reduced penetrance.[274]

Olmsted's syndrome

Periorificial keratoderma and oral leukokeratosis accompany the palmoplantar keratoderma.[255,275–279] This syndrome has been reported in twins.[280] A closely related entity with corneal epithelial dysplasia has been reported.[281] Abnormal expression of keratins 5 and 14 appears to be the underlying disorder.[282]

Vohwinkel's syndrome

There is a honeycombing pattern of keratoderma with starfish-shaped keratoses on the dorsa of the digits and linear keratoses on the knees and elbows.[283–286] Ainhum-like constriction bands develop, leading to gangrene of the digits in adolescence.[284,287–289] A recessive variant is associated with ectodermal dysplasia.[290] Congenital deaf-mutism is a rare association.[291] The subset of patients with mutilating keratoderma and sensorineural hearing loss appears to have a mutation in the *GJB2* gene which encodes the gap junction protein connexin26.[292] A subset of patients with Vohwinkel's keratoderma has an associated ichthyosiform dermatosis. It is in this group that a mutation in the loricrin gene on chromosome 1q21 is consistently present.[293,294] The mutant loricrin is translocated into the nucleus of the keratinocyte and not into the cornified cell envelope as might be expected.[154]

Epidermolytic palmoplantar keratoderma (Vörner's syndrome)

The term 'epidermolytic palmoplantar keratoderma' is widely used for this variant, reflecting the histological changes.[295–302] It is clinically indistinguishable from the Unna–Thost variant. It has early onset and thick yellowish hyperkeratosis.[303] Kindreds with associated internal malignancy,[304] and with woolly hair and dilated cardiomyopathy[305] have been reported. Mutations of keratin 9, which is specifically found in palmoplantar epidermis and outer root sheath epithelium, have been found in this variant.[303,306–312] It is linked to chromosome 17q11–q23.[313]

This type of keratoderma has occurred in several members of a family with Ehlers–Danlos syndrome, type III.[314] The genes for these two conditions are not closely linked.

Howel–Evans syndrome

The palmoplantar keratoderma begins early in life and affected family members develop a squamous cell carcinoma of the esophagus in middle adult life.[315] The gene has been linked to chromosome 17q24, which is distal to the type I keratin gene cluster.[251] Squamous cell carcinoma sometimes develops in the thickened skin of the palms.[316] Interestingly, palmoplantar keratoderma has been reported in one patient with postcorrosive stricture of the esophagus.[317]

Papillon–Lefèvre syndrome

In Papillon–Lefèvre syndrome, an autosomal recessive condition, there is periodontosis accompanied by premature loss of the deciduous and permanent teeth.[318–322] Involvement of the elbows and knees and calcification of the choroid plexus may occur.[323] This condition is caused by a mutation in the cathepsin C gene located at chromosome 11q14–q21.[324,325] The phenotypically related *Haim–Munk syndrome* is an allelic mutation.[326]

Mal de Meleda

Mal de Meleda, a rare, autosomal recessive variant, was first described in families living on the small island of Meleda in the Adriatic Sea.[327,328] The responsible gene has been localized to 8qter.[329,330] Onset is at birth or in infancy. Lesions may extend from the palms and soles on to the dorsum of the hands and feet respectively, although there is a sharp 'cut-off' at the wrists and ankles.[327,331–334] Pseudoainhum is a rare complication.[335] Hyperhidrosis leads to severe maceration.[252] *Palmoplantar keratoderma of Sybert* is clinically similar but its inheritance is autosomal dominant; only one family has been reported.[270]

Gamborg Nielsen keratoderma

Two Swedish families have been reported with very thick hyperkeratotic plaques on the dorsal aspect of the fingers.[270]

Palmoplantar keratoderma with sclerodactyly (Huriez syndrome)

In addition to the keratoderma and sclerodactyly, nail anomalies and malignant degeneration of affected skin may occur.[270,336,337] Additional features include telangiectasia of the lips, flexor contractures of the little finger, and poikiloderma-like lesions on the nose.[338] There are only seven families affected by this condition worldwide. It is autosomal dominant.[337,339]

Punctate keratoderma

Punctate keratoderma, a localized variant, is characterized by discrete, hard, keratotic plugs arising in normal skin.[340,341] A subset with verrucoid lesions has been reported.[342] Another variant is confined to the palmar and digital creases.[343] The plugs form again if removed. Onset is usually in adolescence, but it may be much later.[344] Sometimes the lesions are confined to the palmar creases,[345] particularly in black people.[346-348] An underlying malignancy has been present or developed subsequently in a few cases.[349,350] Punctate lesions, which are characterized histologically by a cornoid lamella, are best classified as punctate porokeratotic keratoderma;[351] they are clinically indistinguishable from the other punctate forms.[342,346-349,352,353] The term 'spiny keratoderma' has also been used for this type.[354,355]

Circumscribed keratoderma

Focal areas of thickening, sometimes tender, may develop on the palms and soles.[356] Some have an autosomal recessive inheritance. This is a clinically heterogeneous group,[356] which includes the conditions of *hereditary painful callosities (keratosis palmoplantaris nummularis)*[357-359] and *keratoderma palmoplantaris striata*.[360] In this latter condition, also known as *striate palmoplantar keratoderma*,[361] linkages to both chromosome 6p21 (the desmoplakin gene) and 18q12 (near the desmosomal cadherin glycoprotein genes) have been reported.[362] Corneal dystrophy has been present in some circumscribed variants.[356] Localized hypertrophy of the skin of the soles and palms can occur in the *Proteus syndrome*, a rare disorder in which the major manifestations are skeletal overgrowth, digital hypertrophy, exostoses of the skull, subcutaneous lipomas and, sometimes, epidermal nevi.[363] Tyrosinemia type II (Richner–Hanhart syndrome) also has localized lesions (see below). All of these circumscribed variants have been classified recently as 'nummular hereditary palmoplantar keratodermas',[270] a term which appears unsuitable with regard to the morphological diversity of the lesions. Recently, a variant of epidermolytic palmoplantar keratoderma, localized to the palm and sole of one side of the body and following Blaschko's lines, has been reported. The term 'unilateral palmoplantar verrucous nevus' was suggested for this mosaic mutation in K16.[364]

Acquired keratoderma

Palmoplantar keratoderma or discrete keratotic lesions may rarely develop in cases of myxedema,[365-367] mycosis fungoides,[368] lymphoma,[369] multiple myeloma[370] and internal cancers,[371] following exposure to arsenic and after the menopause or following bilateral oophorectomy (keratoderma climactericum).[372] Rugose lesions of the palms may occur in association with acanthosis nigricans, so-called 'tripe palms' (pachydermatoglyphy);[373] in a few instances, this condition has been reported in association with a cancer, without concurrent acanthosis nigricans.[374,375] TGF-α has been incriminated in the pathogenesis of this paraneoplastic change.[376] Keratoderma has been described in patients with AIDS, following the infusion of glucan, which was used as an immunostimulant.[377] Palmoplantar keratoderma has also followed the use of tegafur, in the treatment of an adenocarcinoma of the colon[378] and one of the gallbladder.[379] There was a preceding acral erythema. Similar side-effects have been reported with fluorouracil, a closely related drug.[378] Exposure to herbicides was implicated in another case.[380] Acquired punctate lesions on the palms and soles may follow dioxin intoxication.[381] The unusual acquired condition characterized by burning and edema after brief immersion in water has already been mentioned (see p. 289). Aquagenic palmoplantar keratoderma is an appropriate designation for this condition.[260] Keratoderma can also occur in patients with papulosquamous conditions such as lichen planus and pityriasis rubra pilaris.[382]

Interdigital keratoderma

The rare interdigital variant is characterized by a symmetrical keratoderma localized to the interdigital spaces of the fingers.[383]

Histopathology

The *diffuse forms* show prominent orthokeratotic hyperkeratosis, with variable amounts of focal parakeratosis. The granular layer is often thickened. There is also some acanthosis of the epidermis and a sparse, superficial, perivascular infiltrate of chronic inflammatory cells. In Greither's syndrome there are circumscribed foci of orthokeratotic hyperkeratosis located on delled areas of the epidermis.[274] In a case of Olmsted's syndrome reported recently, there was massive hyperkeratosis and a reduced to absent granular layer.[384] In the Huriez syndrome there is massive hyperkeratosis, marked acanthosis and hypergranulosis.[385] The scleroatrophic areas show thickening of the dermal collagen bundles.[385]

The *epidermolytic form* shows epidermolytic hyperkeratosis. This tissue reaction is described on page 294.

The *punctate forms* show a dense, homogeneous keratin plug which often results in an undulating appearance in the epidermis.[344,352] There is usually a slight depression in the epidermis beneath the plug (Fig. 9.6).[352] Those punctate cases with a parakeratotic plug are best classified as punctate porokeratotic keratoderma (Figs 9.7, 9.8).[386] Focal acantholytic dyskeratosis was present in the punctate lesions in one reported case.[387]

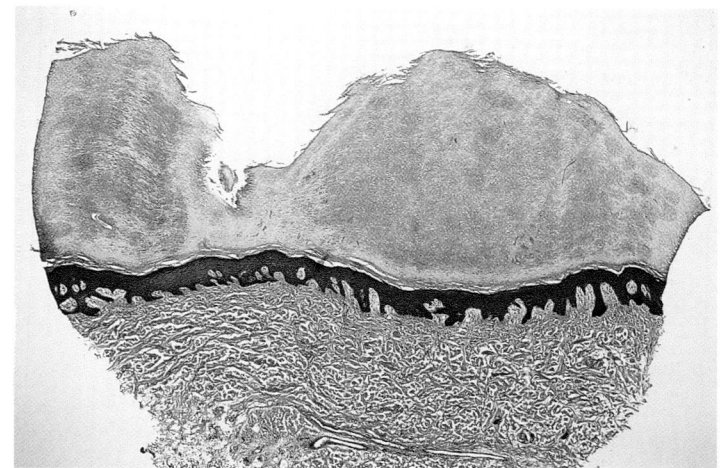

Fig. 9.6 **Punctate keratoderma.** There is slight depression of the epidermis beneath a keratin plug. There is a pit in the adjacent stratum corneum. (H & E)

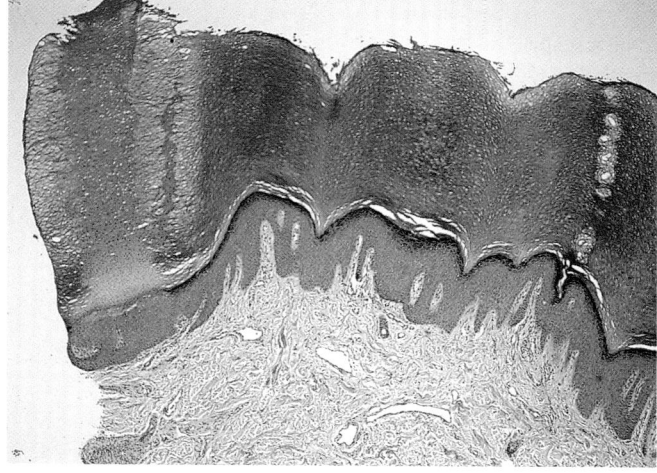

Fig. 9.7 **Punctate porokeratotic (spiny) keratoderma.** A wide cornoid lamella is present towards one edge of the field. (H & E) (Photograph kindly supplied by Dr JJ Sullivan)

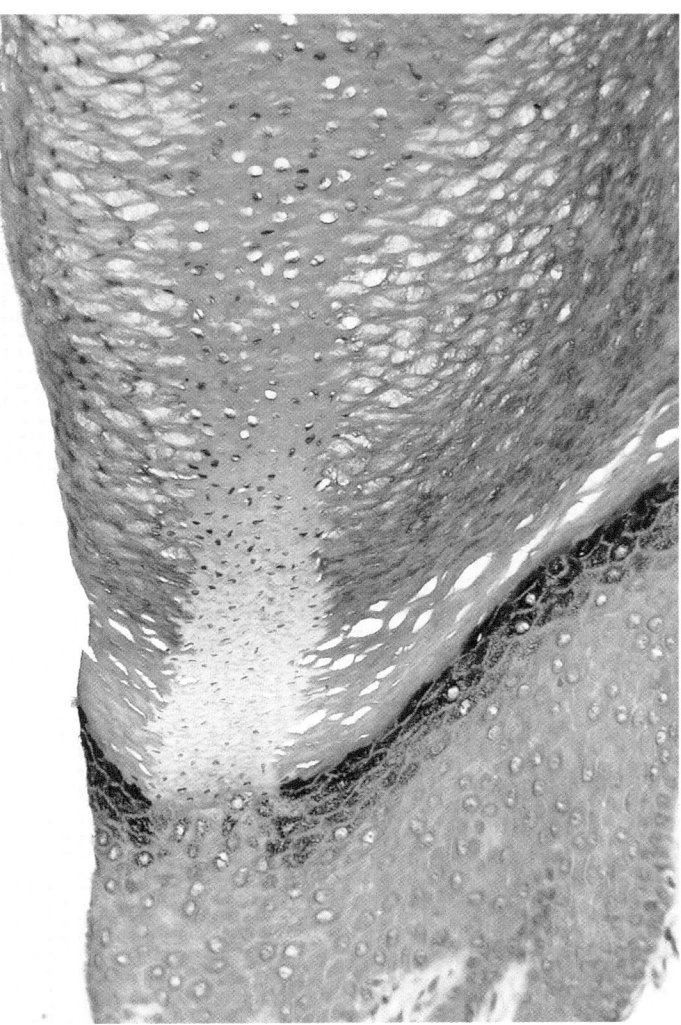

Fig. 9.8 Punctate porokeratotic (spiny) keratoderma. The granular layer is absent beneath the parakeratotic zone. (H & E) (Photograph kindly supplied by Dr JJ Sullivan)

In *hereditary callosities with blisters*, there is intraepidermal vesiculation with cytolysis of keratinocytes and clumping of tonofilaments.[357] The changes resemble those seen in pachyonychia congenita (see p. 292). In other cases, epidermolytic hyperkeratosis has been present.[359]

Electron microscopy

Ultrastructural studies have not shown consistent abnormalities. It seems that the normal association of filaggrin and keratin filaments does not occur in the stratum corneum.[249] Nucleolar hypertrophy has been noted in the punctate form.[352] Ultrastructural studies of the Papillon–Lefèvre syndrome have shown lipid-like vacuoles in corneocytes, abnormally shaped keratohyaline granules and a reduction in tonofilaments.[388] Vacuoles and many membrane-coating granules were seen in corneocytes in Vohwinkel's syndrome.[286]

OCULOCUTANEOUS TYROSINOSIS

Oculocutaneous tyrosinosis, also known as tyrosinemia II and the Richner–Hanhart syndrome, is an extremely rare, autosomal recessive genodermatosis caused by a deficiency of hepatic tyrosine aminotransferase.[389–394] The gene is located at 16q22.1–q22.3. It is usually characterized by corneal ulcerations and painful keratotic lesions on the palms and soles, but ocular

lesions have been absent in some kindreds.[395] The palmoplantar lesions vary from fine 1–2 mm keratoses to linear or diffuse keratotic thickenings.[393] Erosions and blisters have also been reported.[396] Mental retardation is often present. The condition is treated by a dietary restriction of tyrosine and phenylalanine.

Histopathology[390]

The palmoplantar lesions show prominent hyperkeratosis and parakeratosis with variable epidermal hyperplasia. Scattered mitoses and multinucleate keratinocytes may be present.[397,398] Epidermolytic hyperkeratosis and intra-epidermal bulla formation have been present in some families.[396]

Electron microscopy

Lipid-like granules have been noted in the upper epidermis.[399] An increase in tonofibrils and keratohyalin has also been seen in affected skin.[397]

HIDROTIC ECTODERMAL DYSPLASIA

The hidrotic, autosomal dominant variant of ectodermal dysplasia (see p. 303 for a discussion of the ectodermal dysplasias) is characterized by the triad of alopecia, dystrophic nails and palmoplantar keratoderma.[400–402] Dental abnormalities may also be present but sweating is normal, in contrast to many other ectodermal dysplasias.

Histopathology

The palms and soles show prominent hyperkeratosis of orthokeratotic type. There is some acanthosis. The granular layer is of normal thickness.

ACROKERATOELASTOIDOSIS

Acrokeratoelastoidosis (Costa's papular acrokeratosis)[403] is a variant of palmoplantar keratoderma which occurs both sporadically and as an autosomal dominant genodermatosis.[404–406] There appears to be some variability in the morphological expression of the disease.[407] Its onset is in childhood or early adult life and there is a female predominance. There are multiple, small (2–5 mm in diameter), firm, translucent papules which are most numerous along the junction of the dorsal and palmar or plantar surfaces of the hands and feet respectively.[408] They may be localized to the sides of the fingers, particularly the inner side of the thumb and the adjoining index finger. In this situation, they resemble clinically the lesions seen in collagenous and elastotic plaques of the hands (see p. 392), an entity which is found predominantly in males over the age of 50 and which results from trauma and actinic damage.[403] In acrokeratoelastoidosis there may also be a mild diffuse hyperkeratosis of the palms and soles; this was a prominent feature in one report.[409] There may also be isolated lesions over inter-phalangeal joints and elsewhere on the dorsum of the hands and feet.[410]

Histopathology[411]

There may be slight hyperkeratosis with a shallow depression in the underlying epidermis, which shows a prominent granular layer and mild acanthosis. The dermis may be normal or slightly thickened. The elastic fibers are decreased in number, thin and somewhat fragmented in the mid and deep reticular dermis.[412] In some cases the elastic fibers are coarse and fragmented.[410] Cases have been reported with no light microscopic changes in the dermis.[404] The group which lacks elastorrhexis has been designated 'focal acral hyperkeratosis'.[413–415]

Electron microscopy

In acrokeratoelastoidosis there is disaggregation of elastic fibers with fragmentation of the microfibrils.[404] In one report the fibroblasts contained dense granules in the cytoplasm and there was an absence of extracellular fibers, leading to the hypothesis that there was a block in the synthesis of elastic fibers by the fibroblasts.[416]

PACHYONYCHIA CONGENITA

Pachyonychia congenita is a rare genodermatosis in which symmetrical, hard thickening of the nails of the fingers and toes is the most striking and consistent feature.[417–419] Various other abnormalities of keratinization are usually present.[420] These include palmar and plantar keratoderma, follicular keratoses on the extensor surfaces of the knees and elbows, keratosis pilaris, blister formation on the feet and sometimes on the palms, callosities of the feet, leukokeratosis of the oral mucosa (often complicated by candidosis),[421] hair abnormalities and hyperhidrosis of the palms and soles. These clinical features typify the so-called 'type I' (Jadassohn–Lewandowsky) cases.[420,422] Patients with the type II variant (Jackson–Lawler type) have the addition of natal teeth (teeth erupted prior to birth) and multiple cutaneous cysts, either epidermal cysts or steatocystomas,[423] but no oral leukokeratosis.[424] In type III, the features of type I are accompanied by leukokeratosis of the cornea. Type IV combines the clinical features of the other types with laryngeal lesions, mental retardation and alopecia.[425]

There is some variability in the age of onset of the various manifestations, but nail changes are usually present at birth or soon afterwards and become progressively more disfiguring over the first year of life. Nail dystrophy of late onset (pachyonychia congenita tarda) has been reported.[426–429]

Pachyonychia congenita is usually inherited as an autosomal dominant trait with incomplete penetrance, although several cases with autosomal recessive inheritance have been reported.[417] Type II pachyonychia congenita is due to an abnormality in keratin 17 (K17) and in its expression partner keratin 6,[430] the former resulting from a gene mutation in the type I keratin cluster on chromosome 17q.[431] Similar mutations in the K17 gene can cause steatocystoma multiplex with little or no nail dystrophy.[432] Type I disease results from a mutation in the helix initiation peptide of keratin 16 (K16).[433,434]

Mention is made here for completeness of **ectopic nails**. They have been reported on the volar surface of fingers and toes and elsewhere.[435] Ectopic nails are most frequently caused by traumatic inoculation of nail matrix.

Histopathology

The involved mucous membranes and skin, including the nail bed, show marked intracellular edema involving cells in the upper malpighian layer and in the thickened stratum corneum.[417,420,436–439] There is sometimes rupture of cell walls, particularly with lesions on plantar surfaces, with the formation of intraepidermal vesicles. The epidermis is markedly thickened as a consequence of the edema and the accompanying hyperkeratosis and focal parakeratosis.

The hyperkeratotic papules on the knees and elbows show hyperkeratosis, a prominent granular layer and acanthosis.[417,440] There is usually a thick horny plug extending above the infundibulum of the hair follicle. In one case, the plug resembled a cornoid lamella;[441] in another, the plug, which was not related to a follicle, penetrated into the dermis in the manner seen in Kyrle's disease (see p. 301).[442] Horny plugs have also been described in sweat pores.[440]

The plantar callosities show hyperkeratosis, focal parakeratosis and sometimes mild papillomatosis and acanthosis. The granular layer is thick except for the area overlying any papillomatous foci.[420]

Two kindreds have been reported with pigment incontinence and amyloid in the papillary dermis.[443]

CORNOID LAMELLATION

The cornoid lamella is a thin column of parakeratotic cells with an absent or decreased underlying granular zone and vacuolated or dyskeratotic cells in the spinous layer. It is the key histological feature of porokeratosis and its clinical variants, but like some of the other minor 'tissue reaction patterns' (see Ch. 1, p. 10) can be found as an incidental phenomenon in a range of inflammatory, hyperplastic and neoplastic conditions of the skin. The cornoid lamella represents a localized area of faulty keratinization and is manifest clinically as a raised keratotic or thin thread-like border to an annular, gyrate or linear lesion.

Cornoid lamellation has been regarded as a clonal disease[444] and as a morphological expression of disordered epithelial metabolism.[445] Abnormal DNA ploidy and abnormalities of keratinocyte maturation have been demonstrated in the epidermis in some lesions of porokeratosis.[446–449] Overexpression of p53 has been detected in the nuclei of keratinocytes in the basal layers of the epidermis beneath the cornoid lamella.[450,451] This is accompanied by a reduction in mdm2 and p21.[452,453]

POROKERATOSIS AND VARIANTS

Porokeratosis is a genodermatosis with many different clinical expressions.[454] Lesions may be solitary or numerous, inconspicuous or prominent, small or large,[455] atrophic or hyperkeratotic[456] and asymptomatic or pruritic.[457] The lip,[458] mouth,[459] face,[460,461] penis,[462,463] scrotum,[464] genitocrural and perianal regions[465,466] and natal cleft[467] are sites that are rarely involved. Involvement of a burn scar has been reported.[468] Other rare clinical associations include Crohn's disease,[469] chronic renal failure,[470] hepatitis C virus-related hepatocellular carcinoma,[471] previous renal transplant,[472–475] myelodysplastic syndrome,[476] systemic lupus erythematosus,[477] microsatellite instability in association with hereditary non-polyposis colorectal cancer,[478] lesions localized to the access region for hemodialysis[479] and onset after electron beam radiation,[480,481] PUVA,[482] tanning salon use[483] and furosemide (frusemide).[484] Although it was originally regarded as a familial disease with autosomal dominant inheritance,[485] numerous non-familial cases have now been reported.

The most important clinical forms are porokeratosis of Mibelli (characterized by one or more round, oval or gyrate plaques with an atrophic center and a thin, elevated, guttered, keratotic rim which may show peripheral expansion) and disseminated superficial actinic porokeratosis[486–488] (DSAP) consisting of multiple, annular, keratotic lesions less than 1 cm in diameter, with a hyperkeratotic, thread-like border and occurring particularly on the exposed extremities. A locus for this variant has been found at 12q23.2–24.1.[489]

Rare clinical variants include a linear[490–496] or systematized[497,498] variant, a reticulate form,[499] porokeratosis plantaris discreta[500,501] (painful plantar lesions), porokeratotic palmoplantar keratoderma discreta,[502] punctate porokeratotic keratoderma, also known as punctate porokeratosis[503–507] and porokeratosis punctata palmaris et plantaris – spiny keratoderma[354,508,509] (asymptomatic pits or plugs, usually on the palms, digits or soles and not universally accepted as a variant of porokeratosis),[510] linear palmoplantar porokeratotic hamartoma (the cornoid lamellae are not related to eccrine ostia),[511] porokeratosis plantaris, palmaris et disseminata[512–519] (annular and serpiginous lesions on the palms and soles with later involvement of other areas), and the related superficial disseminated eruptive form.[520,521] Other rare variants of porokeratosis are a hyperkeratotic verrucous type[522–524] and a facial variant.[525,526] Closely related are the cases with cornoid lamellae in eccrine and hair follicle ostia, described as 'porokeratotic eccrine ostial and dermal duct nevus',[527–535] 'porokeratotic eccrine duct and hair follicle nevus'[536,537] and 'reticular erythema with ostial porokeratosis'.[538]

The disseminated superficial actinic variant coexists rarely with other types of porokeratosis, particularly the linear type.[492,496,539,540] The association of these two forms is an example of type 2 segmental involvement, occurring in an autosomal dominant skin disorder.[541] DSAP may be exacerbated by exposure to ultraviolet light.[542,543] Both DSAP and porokeratosis of Mibelli have developed in immunosuppressed patients.[544–550] Age-related immunosuppression has been used to explain the occurrence of disseminated porokeratosis in the elderly.[551]

Porokeratotic lesions are usually persistent although clearance with subsequent recurrence has been reported.[552] Ulceration is another complication.

The development of squamous cell carcinoma[553–557] or intraepidermal carcinoma[558,559] is a rare clinical complication of several of the variants of porokeratosis. The linear type is particularly prone to malignant change.[560] The term 'malignant disseminated porokeratosis' has been applied to several cases in which the porokeratotic lesions had a significant potential to undergo malignant degeneration.[561,562] Allelic loss has been suggested as a possible pathogenetic mechanism for these tumors.[560]

Histopathology

It is important that the biopsy is taken across the edge of the peripheral rim in order to show the typical cornoid lamella, the features of which have been described above. Multiple cornoid lamellae will usually be seen in biopsies from the linear and reticulate form. There may be two cornoid lamellae, one on each side of a keratotic plug, at either edge of a lesion of DSAP (Fig. 9.9).[563] In porokeratosis of Mibelli there is invagination of the epidermis at the site of the cornoid lamella with adjacent mild papillomatosis. A PAS stain reveals that the cornoid lamella contains numerous purple granules, representing intracellular glycogen and glycoproteins.[564] Beneath the lamella there is absence or diminution of the granular layer, sometimes only several cells in width (Fig. 9.10). However, in the solitary palmar or plantar lesions the cornoid lamella is quite broad with a corresponding wide zone where the underlying granular zone is absent or markedly reduced. Sometimes one or

more dyskeratotic cells are present in the spinous layer. Basal vacuolar change and vacuolated cells in the spinous layer are other changes found beneath the cornoid lamella.[565]

Beneath the lamella there are often dilated capillaries in the papillary dermis, associated with a lymphocytic infiltrate. The most prominent inflammatory changes are seen in DSAP, in which a superficial band-like infiltrate with lichenoid qualities (including Civatte bodies) is usually present. The infiltrate is usually present inside the porokeratotic rim.[565] In addition, the epidermis between the lamellae is often atrophic in this form, with overlying hyperkeratosis, and the dermis may show solar elastotic changes. Focal epidermal necrosis and ulceration have been reported at the periphery of a lesion of porokeratosis.[566,567] Subepidermal blistering is a rare event.[568] Amyloid has been found in the papillary dermis in several cases.[569–572]

Electron microscopy

Scanning electron microscopy has shown bud-like spreading of the active edge,[573] while transmission electron microscopy has demonstrated that the basophilic granular material in the cornoid lamella consists of degenerate cells with pyknotic nuclei.[574] Langerhans cells are in close contact with degenerating keratinocytes.[575] The granular layer is inconspicuous with only small amounts of keratohyalin. Vacuolated cells and others showing filamentous degeneration

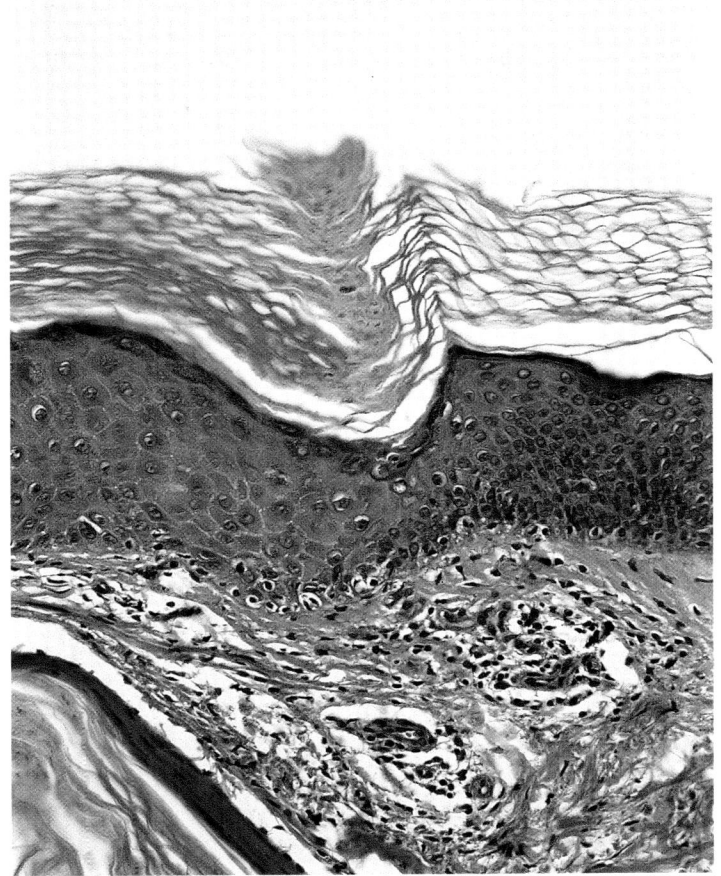

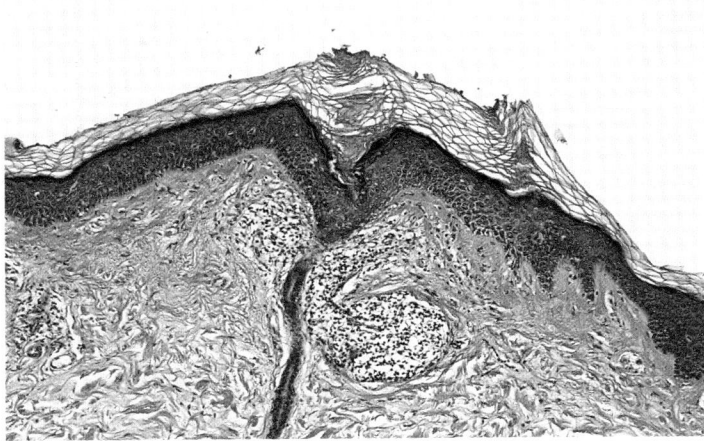

Fig. 9.9 **Porokeratosis.** There are two cornoid lamellae close together. One overlies an acrosyringium. Follicular infundibula may also be involved. (H & E)

Fig. 9.10 **Porokeratosis.** The parakeratotic column (cornoid lamella) overlies an area several cells in width, in which the granular layer is absent. (H & E)

('dyskeratotic' cells) are often present. Apoptotic bodies may be seen in the basal layer and in the dermal papillae.[576]

EPIDERMOLYTIC HYPERKERATOSIS

Epidermolytic hyperkeratosis is an abnormality of epidermal maturation characterized by compact hyperkeratosis, accompanied by granular and vacuolar degeneration of the cells of the spinous and granular layers (Fig. 9.11). It may be a congenital or an acquired defect. This histological pattern may be seen in a number of different clinical settings, some of which will be considered in other sections of this chapter. It may be:

- *generalized*: bullous ichthyosis (see p. 285)
- *systematized or linear*: epidermal nevus variant (see below and p. 754)
- *palmoplantar*: palmoplantar keratoderma variant (see p. 289)
- *solitary*: epidermolytic acanthoma (see below)
- *multiple discrete*: disseminated epidermolytic acanthoma (see below)
- *incidental*: focal epidermolytic hyperkeratosis (see below)
- *solar keratosis related*: a rare variant of solar keratosis (see p. 761)
- *follicular*: nevoid follicular epidermolytic hyperkeratosis (see below)
- *mucosal*: epidermolytic leukoplakia.

Epidermolytic hyperkeratosis is a relatively uncommon histological pattern in epidermal nevi, being present in only 8 of 160 cases reported from the Mayo Clinic (the clinical appearance of the lesions in this series is not described).[577] There are reports of cases with a systematized pattern (ichthyosis hystrix)[578,579] and with a linear pattern (Fig. 9.12).[579] Bullous ichthyosis (generalized epidermolytic hyperkeratosis) has been reported in the offspring of patients with the linear form of the disease.[87,580] This is an example of the reverse of type 2 segmental involvement occurring in an autosomal dominant skin condition. It is unusual for those with segmental disease to pass on the generalized form.

Focal epidermolytic hyperkeratosis has been found incidentally in a range of circumstances, including the wall of a pilar cyst, in a seborrheic keratosis, in a cutaneous horn and a skin tag, overlying an intradermal nevus and even in association with dermatoses.[122] It may be found adjacent to any lesion as an incidental phenomenon.[581,582] It may also involve the intraepidermal eccrine sweat duct[583,584] and oral mucosa.[585]

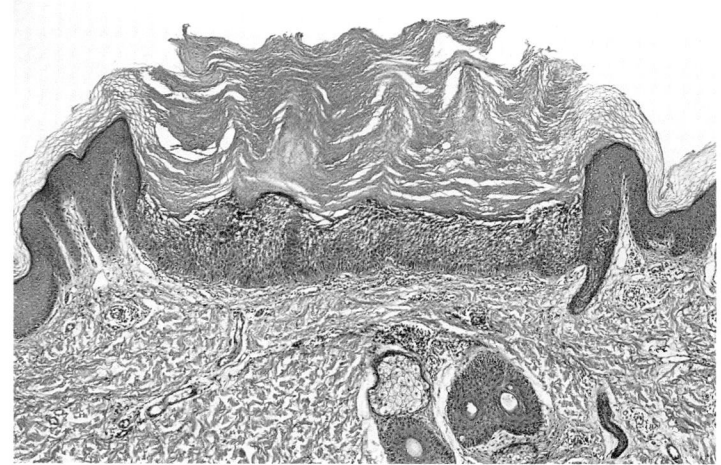

Fig. 9.12 **Linear nevus of epidermolytic hyperkeratotic type.** (H & E)

The nevoid follicular variant[586] presents as comedo-like follicular papules that may have the appearance of nevus comedonicus.[587,588]

Epidermolytic hyperkeratosis has also been found rarely in solar keratoses[589] and in leukoplakic lesions of the lips[589,590] and prepuce.[591] It has been found adjacent to atypical nevocellular nevi, although it has no diagnostic significance in this situation.[592]

Electron microscopy

There are similar ultrastructural changes in the different variants of epidermolytic hyperkeratosis.[593] There is clumping of tonofilaments and cytoplasmic vacuolation.[594] Keratohyaline granules are of variable size.

EPIDERMOLYTIC ACANTHOMA

Epidermolytic acanthoma is an uncommon lesion which presents clinically as a wart in patients of all ages.[595,596] A disseminated form has also been reported;[597–600] in one report of four cases, the lesions developed after sun exposure.[601] Trauma has also been incriminated.[600]

Histopathology

The lesions show the typical features of epidermolytic hyperkeratosis. The entire thickness of the epidermis may be involved or only the upper part of the nucleated epidermis (Fig. 9.13). There is a diminution in the expression of K1 and K10 in the altered granular layer of lesional skin.[596]

ACANTHOLYTIC DYSKERATOSIS

Acantholytic dyskeratosis is a histological reaction pattern characterized by suprabasilar clefting with acantholytic and dyskeratotic cells at all levels of the epidermis (Fig. 9.14).[602] It may also be regarded as a special subdivision of the vesiculobullous tissue reaction, but it is considered in this chapter because the vesiculation is not usually apparent clinically and the primary abnormality involves the tonofilament–desmosome complex with disordered epidermal maturation.

Like epidermolytic hyperkeratosis, acantholytic dyskeratosis may be found in a number of different clinical settings.[602] The two histological patterns have even been found in the same biopsy.[603] Acantholytic dyskeratosis may be:

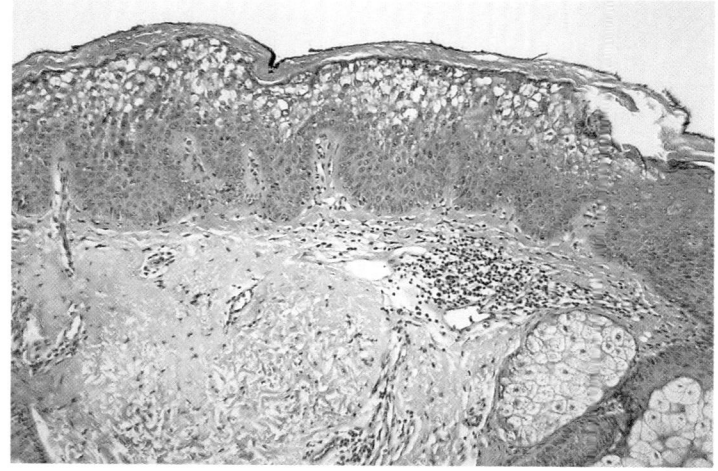

Fig. 9.11 **Epidermolytic hyperkeratosis.** Compact orthokeratosis overlies an epidermis showing granular and vacuolar change in its upper layers. (H & E)

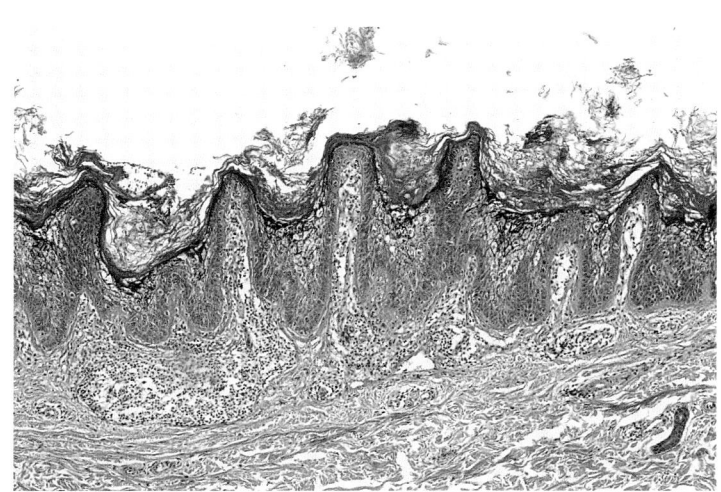

Fig. 9.13 **Epidermolytic acanthoma.** Clinically this was a solitary, keratotic lesion. (H & E)

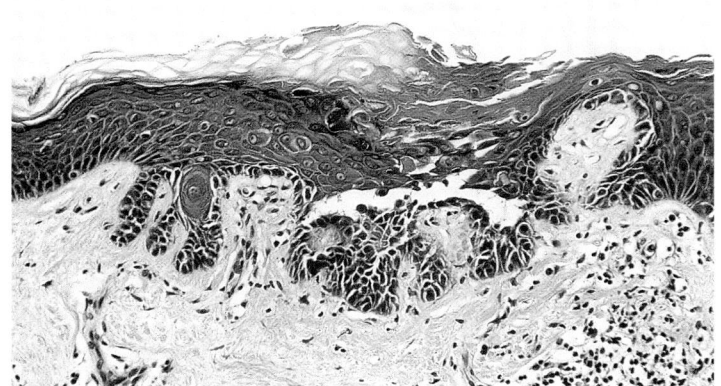

Fig. 9.14 **Acantholytic dyskeratosis** with suprabasal clefting and occasional acantholytic and dyskeratotic cells. (H & E)

- *generalized*: Darier's disease (see p. 296)
- *systematized or linear*: zosteriform (segmental) Darier's disease or linear nevus (see below and p. 296)
- *transient*: Grover's disease (see p. 297)
- *palmoplantar*: a very rare form of keratoderma (see p. 290)
- *solitary*: warty dyskeratoma (see p. 299)
- *incidental*: focal acantholytic dyskeratosis (see below)
- *solar keratosis-related*: acantholytic solar keratosis (see p. 142)
- *mucosal*: vulval and anal acantholytic dyskeratosis (see below).

Of the various clinical settings listed above, focal acantholytic dyskeratosis, Darier's disease, Grover's disease and warty dyskeratoma will be considered separately. Hailey–Hailey disease (familial benign chronic pemphigus) is also included in this section because of some overlap features with Darier's disease. However, in Hailey–Hailey disease the acantholysis is more extensive and dyskeratosis is not a prominent feature. Only brief mention will be made of the other clinical settings because of their rarity or because they belong more appropriately to another section of this volume.

The occurrence of acantholytic dyskeratosis in lesions with a linear or systematized distribution is best regarded as an example of segmental Darier's disease induced by postzygotic mosaicism,[604–608] and not as an example of

epidermal nevus as previously thought.[609–612] It is now well known that autosomal dominant skin disorders may sometimes become manifest in a mosaic form, involving the body in a linear, patchy or circumscribed arrangement.[613,614] The segmental disease usually shows the same degree of severity as that found in the corresponding nonmosaic trait.[613] Loss of heterozygosity for the same allele causes more severe changes.[613,615] Acantholytic dyskeratosis is an uncommon finding in 'epidermal nevi', being present in only 2 of a series of 167 epidermal nevi reported from the Mayo Clinic.[577] Such lesions would have followed Blaschko's lines, reflecting as it does genetic mosaicism.[616] The sole of the foot is a rare site for segmental disease.[617]

Acantholytic dyskeratosis has also been reported as a rare pattern in familial dyskeratotic comedones, a condition with some features in common with nevus comedonicus (see p. 755).[618]

Acantholytic dyskeratosis appears to affect cells within the germinative cellular pool of the epidermis.[619] The dyskeratosis that occurs within the acantholytic cells is probably a secondary phenomenon as the acantholytic cells are metabolically inert.[619]

FOCAL ACANTHOLYTIC DYSKERATOSIS

Although the term 'focal acantholytic dyskeratosis' is often used both for clinically inapparent incidental foci and for clinically apparent solitary lesions with the histological pattern of acantholytic dyskeratosis,[620] some authors restrict its use to its incidental finding in histological sections. This is not an uncommon event.[621,622] The term 'papular acantholytic dyskeratoma' has been applied to the clinically apparent solitary lesions,[623] and 'papular acantholytic dyskeratosis' to the exceedingly rare cases in which multiple lesions have developed on the vulva,[624–628] perianal area[629–631] or penis.[632] A clinically apparent lesion has also been reported on the lip.[620]

Histopathology

There is acantholytic dyskeratosis, as already defined (see above). Hyperkeratosis is less prominent in incidental lesions than in Darier's disease. Warty dyskeratomas differ from focal acantholytic dyskeratomas by having more prominent villi, clefting and corps ronds. Some of the genital and crural cases, mentioned above, have a histological resemblance to Hailey–Hailey disease, with marked acantholysis and little dyskeratosis. They belong to the recently recognized acantholytic subset of acantholytic dyskeratosis; another subset features dyskeratosis alone (see below).

Acantholytic subset

Acantholysis, with little or no dyskeratosis, can be seen as an incidental phenomenon[633] or as a solitary tumor of the skin – acantholytic acanthoma (see p. 757).[634] This pattern has also been found in multiple papules[635] and as a variant of epidermal nevus with horn-like processes. This latter case was reported as 'nevus corniculatus'.[636]

A high proportion of the rare genital, crural and perineal cases referred to as papular acantholytic dyskeratosis (see above) have had a histological resemblance to Hailey–Hailey disease, with prominent acantholysis and little or no dyskeratosis.[626,637–639] An appropriate designation for these cases would seem to be *'acantholytic dermatosis of the genitocrural/perineal region'*.[640] The exact classification of the recently reported vulval case with histological resemblance to pemphigus vegetans remains to be determined.[641]

Generalized acantholysis is seen in Hailey–Hailey disease. It is discussed on page 298. A peculiar form of acantholysis, localized to the acrosyringium, has been reported in several febrile patients. The clinical picture resembled Grover's disease.[642] The authors proposed the name 'sudoriferous acrosyringeal acantholytic disease'.[642]

Finally, acantholysis with minimal dyskeratosis can be seen, as an incidental phenomenon, in other disease processes such as pityriasis rubra pilaris[643] and seborrheic keratoses.

Dyskeratotic subset

Although regarded as a variant of epidermolytic acanthoma, the isolated lesion reported as 'isolated dyskeratotic acanthoma' is best classified here.[644] It combined dyskeratotic cells throughout the epidermis with a parakeratotic horn containing large rounded cells at all levels.[644]

The term 'acquired dyskeratotic acanthosis' has recently been applied to a case in which multiple maculopapules, 3–8 mm in diameter, developed in sun-exposed areas. There were clusters of parakeratotic cells which appeared eosinophilic to 'ghostlike'. The epidermis was papillomatous and acanthotic with foci of dyskeratotic keratinocytes.[645]

DARIER'S DISEASE

Darier's disease is a rare, autosomal dominant genodermatosis in which greasy, yellow to brown, crusted papular lesions develop, mainly in the seborrheic areas of the head, neck and trunk.[646–649] A rare acral variant exists.[650] The coalescence of papules produces plaques, which may at times become papillomatous. Onset is usually in adolescence and the disease runs a chronic course. Verrucous lesions resembling acrokeratosis verruciformis may be present on the dorsum of the hands and feet in approximately 70% of cases.[648,651]

Punctate keratoses are sometimes found on the palms and soles.[651] Longitudinal striations are usually present in the nails.[652] Rare clinical variants include a bullous,[653,654] a comedonal[655–657] and a hypertrophic (cornifying) form.[658,659] Cutaneous depigmentation,[660–663] secondary eczematization,[664] cutis verticis gyrata,[665] mucosal lesions,[666,667] ocular disorders,[568] bone cysts[669] and mental deficiency[670] have also been recorded. Darier's disease has been exacerbated and initiated by lithium carbonate therapy[671] and by UVB radiation.[672] Localized (segmental) disease has been precipitated by the administration of menotropin[673] and it has been associated with Gardner's syndrome in one case.[674]

There is a predisposition to bacterial, fungal and viral infections, although no consistent and specific immunological abnormality has been demonstrated.[646,675,676] Infection with herpes simplex virus, vaccinia[677] and even Coxsackievirus A16[678] may produce the features of Kaposi's varicelliform eruption[679–681] (see Ch. 26, p. 692). An HPV-related subungual squamous cell carcinoma has been reported.[682]

The mechanism of acantholysis in Darier's disease is still the subject of controversy.[646] It is usually ascribed to a defect in the synthesis, organization or maturation of the tonofilament–desmosome complexes.[683] It appears that the proteins of the desmosomal attachment plaque are primarily affected.[684,685] There is a loss of desmoplakin I and II and plakoglobin from the desmosomes.[684] The pathogenetic significance of the finding that there is a delay in the expression of the suprabasal skin-specific keratins is uncertain.[686] This may, in some way, contribute to the formation of dyskeratotic cells; their presence has not been satisfactorily explained. All these changes may be secondary to other events. The adherens junction is another site of abnormality.[687] The genetic defect has been mapped to chromosome 12q23–24.1.[688–691] Very recently, *ATP2A2*, which encodes the sarco/endoplasmic reticulum Ca²⁺-ATPase type 2 isoform (SERCA2), a keratinocyte Ca^{2+} pump, has been identified as the gene responsible.[687] Variable clinical severity may occur in different members of the same family.[692]

Histopathology

An individual papule of Darier's disease shows suprabasal acantholysis with the formation of a small cleft (lacuna). Irregular projections of the papillary dermis covered by a single layer of basal cells, the so-called 'villi', extend into the lacunae (Fig. 9.15).[646] A thick orthokeratotic plug, often showing focal parakeratosis, overlies each lesion. Mild papillomatosis is often present.

Two characteristic types of dyskeratotic cell are present – *corps ronds* and *grains*. The *corps ronds* are found as solitary cells or sometimes small groups of separated cells in the upper malpighian layer and stratum corneum.[693] They have a small pyknotic nucleus, a clear perinuclear halo and brightly eosinophilic cytoplasm. The *grains* are small cells with elongated nuclei and scant cytoplasm in the upper layers of the epidermis. They resemble parakeratotic cells but are somewhat larger (Fig. 9.16).

The keratotic papules on the dorsum of the hands resemble those seen in acrokeratosis verruciformis, but small foci of suprabasal acantholytic dyskeratosis may be seen if serial sections are examined.

The cases reported as comedonal Darier's disease have had multiple lesions resembling warty dyskeratoma (Fig. 9.17).[655,656]

Immunoglobulins and C3 have been found in the intercellular areas of affected skin by direct immunofluorescence;[694] this finding has not been confirmed in other studies.[695]

Confocal reflectance microscopy has been used to make the diagnosis.[696]

Electron microscopy

The *corps ronds* have a vacuolated perinuclear halo surrounded by a ring of tonofilaments aggregated with keratohyaline granules.[697–699] The *grains* show premature aggregation of tonofilaments.[699] The synthesis of keratohyalin in association with clumped tonofilaments is peculiar to Darier's disease.[699] It is not seen in Hailey–Hailey disease. As already mentioned, there is controversy over whether the withdrawal of the tonofilaments from the attachment plate of the desmosomes is the primary event in the acantholytic process or merely secondary to the splitting of the desmosomes.[700] Another ultrastructural finding in Darier's disease is the presence of cytoplasmic processes projecting from the basal keratinocytes into the underlying dermis through small defects in the basal lamina.[701]

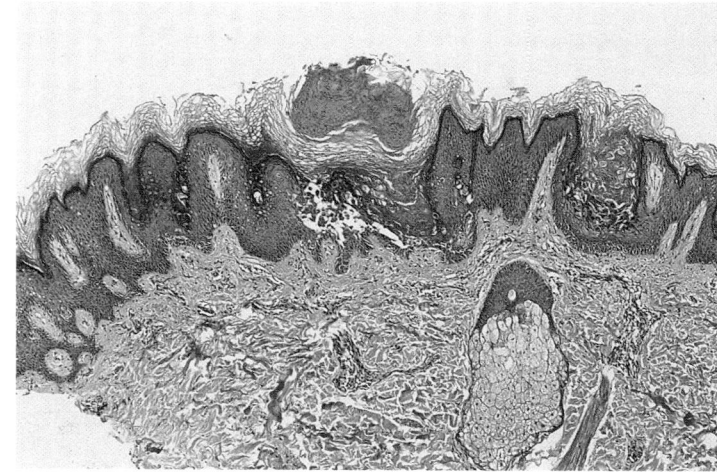

Fig. 9.15 **Darier's disease.** There is suprabasal clefting with a thickened stratum corneum and some dyskeratotic cells in the epidermis. (H & E)

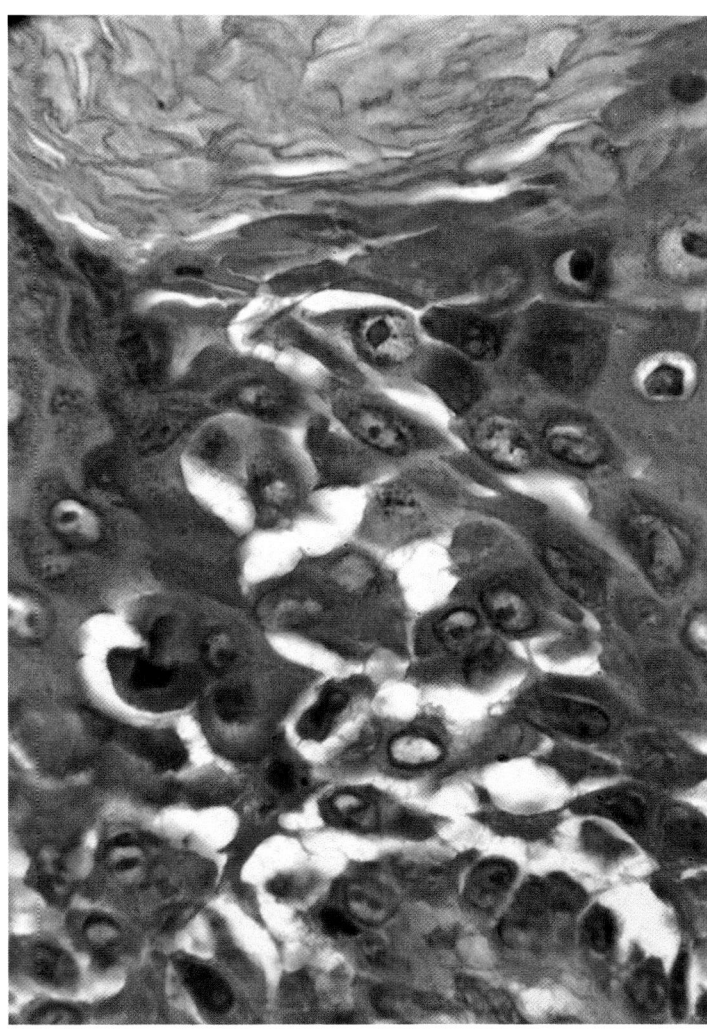

Fig. 9.16 **Darier's disease.** Dyskeratotic cells (corps ronds) are present above the suprabasal cleft. (H & E)

GROVER'S DISEASE

The eponymous designation Grover's disease is the preferred title for several closely related dermatoses characterized by the sudden onset of small,

discrete, sometimes crusted, erythematous papules and papulovesicles.[702–704] They usually develop on the upper trunk of older men. A zosteriform variant has been reported.[705] Lesions may be transient, lasting for weeks or several months[702] (transient acantholytic dermatosis) or they may persist for several years[706] (persistent acantholytic dermatosis[707–709] or papular acantholytic dermatosis[710]). Intense pruritus is often present. Oral involvement has been reported,[711] as has the coexistence of other dermatoses such as asteatotic eczema,[712,713] allergic contact dermatitis,[713] atopic eczema,[713] psoriasis,[712] pemphigus foliaceus[714] and a neutrophilic dermatosis in association with Waldenström's macroglobulinemia.[715]

Some cases of Grover's disease have followed or been exacerbated by exposure to ultraviolet light.[708,710] A few are associated with chronic renal failure.[716,717] One case involved a febrile postoperative patient.[718] The role of heat, persistent fever and sweating has been postulated in the etiology of this condition.[719–722] The cytokine interleukin-4, the synthetic guanosine analog ribavirin,[723] and D-penicillamine therapy[724] have all precipitated Grover's disease.[725] Several mechanisms are theoretically possible as explanations for the occurrence of Grover's disease in cancer patients. Several cases appear to have followed induction therapy, and one followed the use of 2-chlorodeoxyadenosine in the treatment of hairy cell leukemia.[726] Other cases have been in patients who underwent high-dose chemotherapy followed by bone marrow transplantation or autologous stem cell infusion.[727]

Despite the histological similarity to Darier's disease, Grover's disease does not share an abnormality in the *ATP2A2* gene.[728] Its pathogenesis is unknown. Loss of syndecan-1 expression occurs, but this is seen in other bullous diseases. Syndecan-1 is a heparan sulfate proteoglycan present on the keratinocyte membrane; it functions in intercellular adhesion.[729]

Histopathology

Four histological patterns may be seen[712] – Darier-like, Hailey–Hailey-like, pemphigus vulgaris-like and spongiotic (Figs 9.18, 9.19). The Darier pattern was the most common in one series.[706] In a recent review of 72 cases from the Mayo Clinic, however, the acantholysis resembled pemphigus vulgaris in 40, Darier's disease in 16, pemphigus foliaceus in 2, Hailey–Hailey disease in 2, and it was spongiotic in 12.[730] In the spongiotic type there are a few acantholytic cells within and contiguous with spongiotic foci.[707,712] More than one of these histological patterns may be present. In some reports, the persistent cases have tended to have either a Darier-like[708] or pemphigus pattern.[710] In addition to the epidermal changes, there is usually a superficial dermal infiltrate of lymphocytes and sometimes eosinophils.[706,707] The

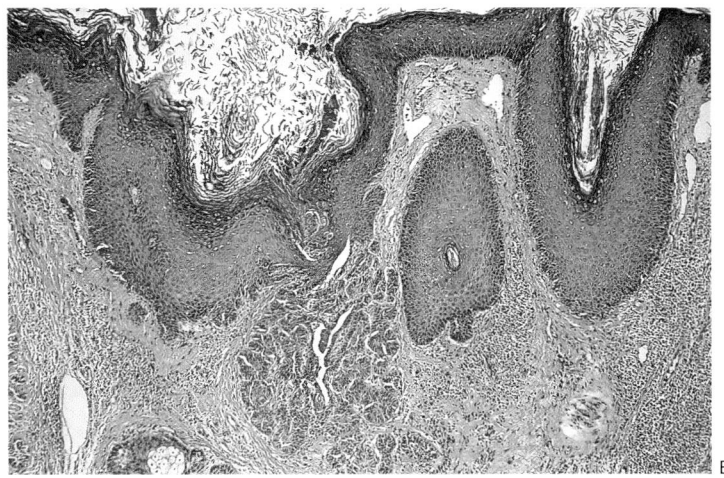

A   B

Fig. 9.17 **(A) Comedonal Darier's disease. (B)** There are basal layer downgrowths with villi, resembling those seen in warty dyskeratoma. (H & E)

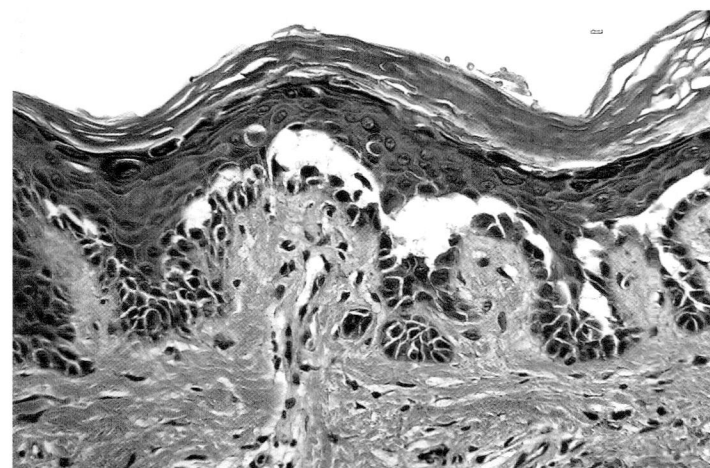

Fig. 9.18 **Grover's disease.** A few acantholytic cells are present within the suprabasal cleft. There is a mild inflammatory infiltrate in the dermis. (H & E)

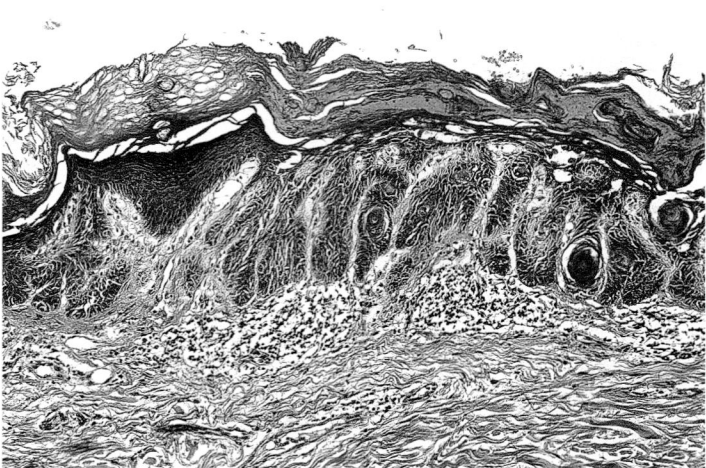

Fig. 9.20 **Grover's disease.** This lesion was of some duration and accordingly there is conspicuous acanthosis. Clefting is just visible in the upper layers of the epidermis. Biopsies of lesions such as this are often misdiagnosed as a solar keratosis. (H & E)

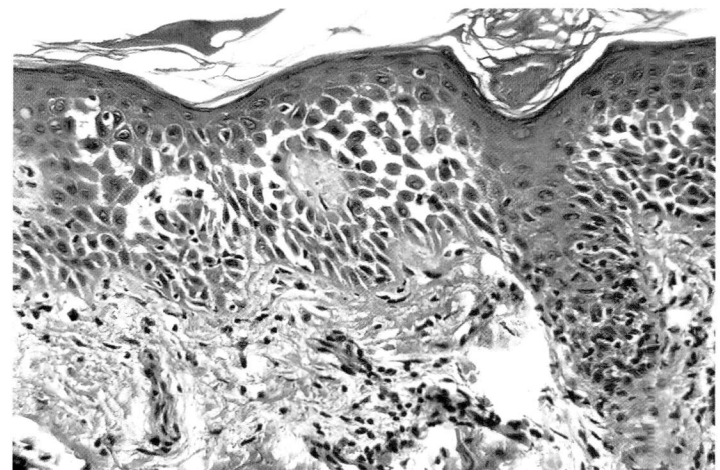

Fig. 9.19 **Grover's disease.** There is prominent acantholysis resembling Hailey–Hailey disease. (H & E)

HAILEY–HAILEY DISEASE

Hailey–Hailey disease (familial benign chronic pemphigus) is an uncommon genodermatosis with recurrent, erythematous, vesicular plaques, which progress to small flaccid bullae with subsequent rupture and crusting.[737,738] The plaques are well demarcated and spread peripherally, often with a circinate border. Rare clinical forms include papular,[739] verrucous,[740,741] annular and vesiculopustular variants.[742] Nikolsky's sign may be positive. There is a predilection for the neck, axillae and intertriginous areas such as the genitocrural, perianal and inframammary region. Occasionally large areas of the skin are involved.[743] There are rare reports of involvement of oral, ocular, esophageal[744] and vaginal[745] mucous membranes or of lesions limited to the vulva[625,746,747] or perianal[748] region. These latter cases are best included with the cases that are now classified as 'acantholytic dermatosis of the genitocrural region' (see p. 295).

Another condition with the histological features of Hailey–Hailey disease and unique clinical features is relapsing linear acantholytic dermatosis, in which there are lesions, following the lines of Blaschko, that wax and wane in a systematic pattern.[749]

Hailey–Hailey disease is inherited as an autosomal dominant condition with incomplete gene penetrance. The responsible gene, *ATP2C1*, has been mapped to chromosome 3q21–q24.[750] It encodes a novel Ca^{2+} pump, indicating the critical role of Ca^{2+} signaling in maintaining epidermal integrity.[751] Nearly one-third of cases are sporadic. Onset is usually in the late teens and there is a tendency for the disease to improve in late adulthood.[752]

The chronic course is punctuated by periods of spontaneous remission with subsequent exacerbations. Lesions may be induced in genetically predisposed tissues by trauma,[753,754] heat, ultraviolet light,[755] perspiration and infection with scabies,[756] bacteria, herpes virus[757] or yeasts. Lesions are often mildly pruritic or burning. They are also malodorous.

Rare associations have included psoriasis,[753,758,759] Darier's disease,[760,761] localized bullous pemphigoid,[762] syringomas of the vulva[763] and squamous and basal cell carcinomas.[764–766] Selected cases that have been refractory to other forms of treatment have benefited by excision of affected skin and split-skin grafting using uninvolved skin.[767] Conversely, if suspensions of keratinocytes from affected skin are placed onto healthy heterologous dermis, devoid of its epidermis, the morphological features of the disease are reproduced *in vitro*.[768] Dermabrasion and laser therapy have also been used with success.[769–771]

presence of eosinophils in Grover's disease serves as a distinguishing feature from Darier's disease, in which they are usually absent.

Older lesions may have considerable acanthosis and only subtle clefting and acantholysis (Fig. 9.20). They may be misdiagnosed as a solar keratosis or non-specific lesion. Small, non-pigmented seborrheic keratoses seem to be increased in number[731] and are sometimes biopsied instead of the lesions of Grover's disease. The transient, vesiculobullous variant with a pemphigus foliaceus pattern on histology is best regarded as a variant of pemphigus foliaceus and not of Grover's disease.[732] Another histological variant, with acantholysis localized to the acrosyringium, has been reported.[642]

Direct immunofluorescence is usually negative,[719] although there are several reports describing variable patterns of immunoglobulin and complement deposition.[707,733,734]

Electron microscopy

Ultrastructural changes reflect the light microscopic features with variable degrees of acantholysis, dyskeratosis and cytoplasmic vacuolization.[735,736] The dyskeratosis is represented by an increase in tonofilaments with some clumping.[736] There is some loss of desmosomes in the affected area, but the hemidesmosomes of the basal layer are preserved.[731]

The mechanism of the acantholysis in Hailey–Hailey disease appears to be localized in the adherens junction region.[687,772] Initially, the defect was thought to be related to a deficiency in one of the intracellular desmosomal proteins, but recent work has shown that they are all biochemically intact.[773] However, there is dissociation of intra- and extracellular domains of desmosomal cadherin and E-cadherin (an adherens junction-associated protein).[687] This occurs in both Hailey–Hailey and Darier's disease, but not in pemphigus.[687] There is normal expression of the gap junction proteins connexins 26 and 43 in non-lesional skin.[774] During acantholysis there is internalization of gap junctions, but this appears to be a secondary process.[774] In contrast to Darier's disease, in which abnormal cell adhesion is only demonstrable in clinically involved skin, Hailey–Hailey disease is characterized by a widespread subclinical abnormality in keratinocyte adhesion.[772,775]

Histopathology

In early lesions, there are lacunae formed by suprabasilar clefting, with acantholytic cells either singly or in clumps lining the clefts and lying free within them. The lacunae progress to broad, acantholytic vesicles and bullae (Fig. 9.21). Intercellular edema leading to partial acantholysis gives rise to areas with a characteristic 'dilapidated brick wall' appearance (Fig. 9.22).[776]

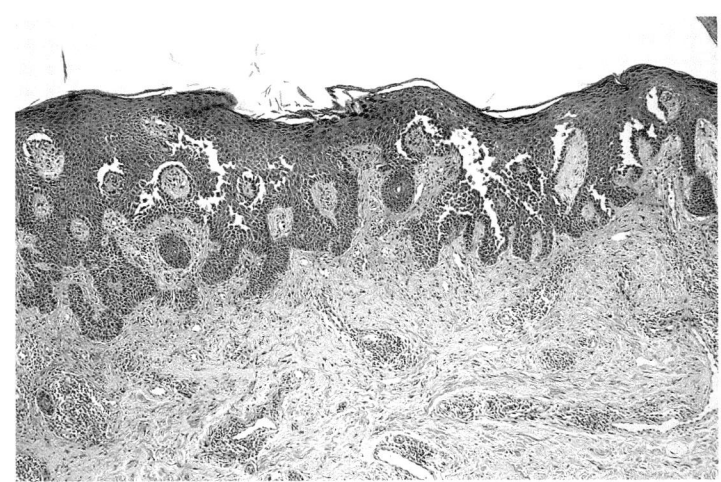

Fig. 9.21 **Hailey–Hailey disease.** There is suprabasal clefting with pronounced acantholysis. (H & E)

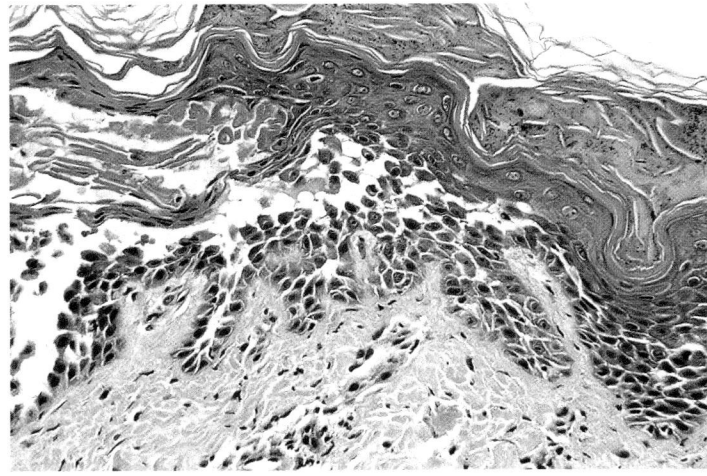

Fig. 9.22 **Hailey–Hailey disease** with many acantholytic keratinocytes. (H & E)

Epidermal hyperplasia is commonly seen and this is formed, in part, by downward elongation of the rete ridges. Elongated papillae covered by one or several layers of keratinocytes ('villi') may protrude up into the bullae.

Some acantholytic cells are dyskeratotic but they have a well-defined nucleus and preserved cytoplasm in contrast to the degenerating dyskeratotic cells of pemphigus. Corps ronds are infrequent and grains are rare.

Neutrophils are sometimes numerous within the vesicles or in the surface parakeratotic crust. Bacteria may also be present in the crust.[737] The dermis shows a variable, superficial chronic inflammatory cell infiltrate.

The Hailey–Hailey variant of Grover's disease has only a narrow vesicle involving no more than a few rete ridges, in contrast to the broad lesions of Hailey–Hailey disease.[776] Although pemphigus vulgaris usually has less acantholysis and some of its cells show more pronounced dyskeratosis, it can be difficult sometimes to distinguish between it and Hailey–Hailey disease without recourse to immunofluorescence.

Electron microscopy

Although earlier ultrastructural studies reported that detachment of tonofilaments from desmosomes with the subsequent disruption and disappearance of the latter was the primary event leading to acantholysis,[777] subsequent studies have shown that the initial event is a series of changes in the microvilli leading to loss of cellular adhesions.[778,779] Desmosomes are then separated and invaginated into cells. Thickened bundles of tonofilaments, sometimes in whorls, are found in cells of the prickle cell and granular layers.[778]

WARTY DYSKERATOMA

Warty dyskeratomas are rare, usually solitary, papules or nodules with an umbilicated or pore-like center.[780,781] They have a predilection for the head and neck of middle-aged and elderly individuals.[782,783] A subungual and an oral lesion have also been reported.[784–786] Warty dyskeratomas average 5 mm in diameter, although an unusually large example, 3 cm in diameter, has been described.[787] They occasionally bleed or intermittently discharge cheesy material.[781]

The lesions in comedonal Darier's disease have the histological features of warty dyskeratoma.[655,656]

Histopathology[781,782]

There is a circumscribed, cup-shaped, invaginating lesion extending into the underlying dermis (Fig. 9.23). The central depression is filled with a plug of keratinous material containing some grains. These keratin plugs have sometimes been dislodged, particularly in oral lesions.[785] The epidermal component shows suprabasilar clefting with numerous acantholytic and dyskeratotic cells within the lacuna. Protruding into the lacuna are villi, which are dermal papillae covered by a layer of basal cells. The papillae contain dilated vessels, occasional melanophages and a few inflammatory cells; inflammatory cells are also present in the underlying dermis. Pilosebaceous follicles may open into the lesion.

Corps ronds and grains are better developed in the skin lesions than in those in the mouth.[785]

HYPERGRANULOTIC DYSCORNIFICATION

Hypergranulotic dyscornification is a newly recognized pattern of epidermal dysmaturation. It is analogous to other epithelial patterns of disordered

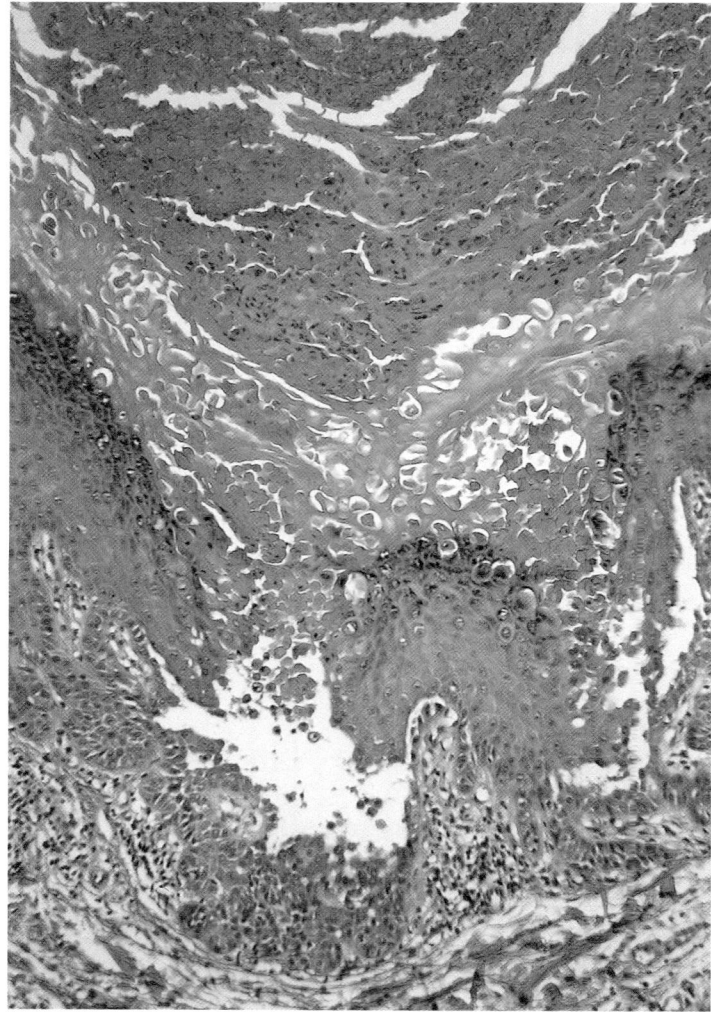

Fig. 9.23 **Warty dyskeratoma.** A cup-shaped invagination is filled with a keratinous plug which in turn overlies an area of suprabasal clefting. (H & E)

keratinization such as epidermolytic hyperkeratosis and acantholytic dyskeratosis.[788] To date, the lesions reported have been solitary, scaly papules or nodules on the extremity or trunk.

The nature of this process is uncertain. The following possibilities were considered in the original article – a variant of epidermolytic hyperkeratosis, a variant of maturation in a verruca vulgaris, or a variant of the epidermolytic-like changes seen in ichthyosis hystrix of Curth–Macklin and related disorders (see p. 285).[788,789] It would not be surprising to find incidental, segmental and generalized variants of this abnormality.

Histopathology[788]

The lesions are exoendophytic with digitate epidermal hyperplasia with hypergranulosis. There are some similarities to a verruca vulgaris. Overlying the thickened granular layer, at the tips of the epidermal papillations, are orthokeratotic mounds of large, eosinophilic corneocytes. Keratohyalin granules are retained within these cells. There is often some basket-weave orthokeratin overlying thick and compacted orthokeratin. A pale basophilic substance is present in the higher spinous layer and granular zone. This appears to be in an intercellular location.

There is a variable lymphocytic infiltrate in the upper dermis.

COLLOID KERATOSIS

Colloid keratosis is characterized by the presence of homogeneous eosinophilic masses of variable size and number within the upper layers of squamous epithelia.[790] It has been seen as an incidental finding in neoplastic and non-neoplastic lesions in the skin and respiratory tract,[791] as well as in pachyonychia congenita and other onychoses.[790] Reports have appeared mainly in the non-English and dental literature.

It appears to result from a defect in keratinization with the accumulation of cytokeratin precursors or related protein products. Colloid keratosis has no clinical significance and it is a reaction pattern rather than a disease entity.

Histopathology[790]

Homogeneous and rounded pools of eosinophilic material are found in the upper layers of the epidermis. The material is PAS positive and diastase resistant. Ultrastructurally, it is amorphous and devoid of any filaments.

Colloid keratosis must be distinguished from **pagetoid dyskeratosis**, which is another incidental histological finding (Fig. 9.24). It is characterized by cells with a pyknotic nucleus with a clear halo and a rim of pale cytoplasm.[792,793] Both entities must be distinguished from clear cell papulosis (see p. 760) in which clear cells containing mucin and keratin are present in the epidermis.[794] It has been suggested that the clear cells might be precursor cells for cutaneous Paget's disease.[794]

DISCRETE KERATOTIC LESIONS

There is a group of rare genodermatoses of late onset in which multiple, discrete, keratotic lesions develop as a result of abnormal keratinization. This group includes hyperkeratosis lenticularis perstans, Kyrle's disease, multiple minute digitate keratoses and waxy keratoses. Discrete keratotic lesions associated with palmar-plantar involvement or cornoid lamellation are considered elsewhere in this chapter. Certain acquired lesions such as warts, cutaneous horns, callosities, corns, stucco keratoses, solar keratoses, seborrheic keratoses and lesions produced by tar may present as discrete keratotic lesions. They are not included in this section, which is concerned essentially with keratotic genodermatoses.

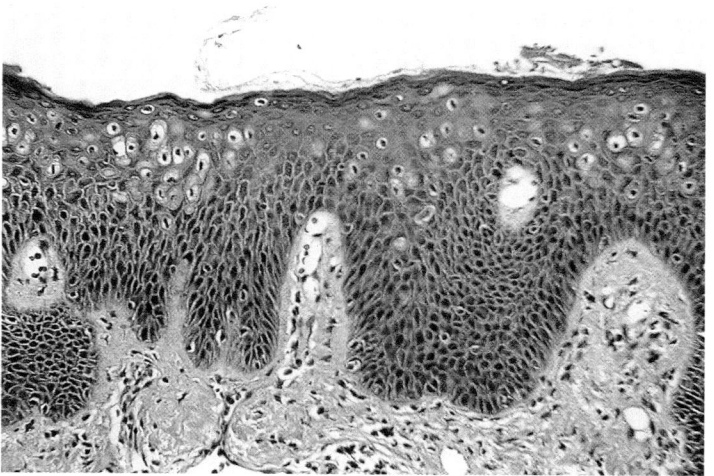

Fig. 9.24 **Pagetoid dyskeratosis.** Clear cells are scattered through the upper epidermis. (H & E)

HYPERKERATOSIS LENTICULARIS PERSTANS

Hyperkeratosis lenticularis perstans (Flegel's disease)[795] is a rare genodermatosis of late onset in which an abnormality in keratinization results in the development of multiple, discrete, 1–5 mm keratoses.[796–798] An autosomal dominant inheritance is sometimes present.[799–801] The lesions are most prominent on the dorsum of the feet and the anterior aspect of the lower legs, but they may also develop on the thighs, upper limbs and pinnae.[797,802] The keratoses develop in mid to late adult life and persist. Removal of the spiny scale causes slight bleeding.[803] A unilateral variant has been described.[804] This may be a manifestation of the postzygotic mosaicism seen in autosomal dominant skin disease.

Several reports, but not all,[802,805] have documented a decrease in or qualitative defects of the membrane-coating granules (lamellar or Odland bodies) in affected areas of epidermis.[806–810] It has been suggested that these abnormalities are the basis for the defect in keratinization.[807]

Histopathology[797,802,807]

There is a discrete zone of compact, deeply eosinophilic hyperkeratosis, with patchy areas of parakeratosis.[801] There is some acanthosis at the margins of the lesions but the epidermis at the base of the plaque of keratin is thinned with effacement of the rete ridge pattern.[797] The malpighian layer may eventually be only three cells thick. The granular layer is usually less prominent in this area. There may be some basal vacuolar change[811] and occasional apoptotic cells.[797] They were prominent in a case reported by Hunter and Donald.[812] The superficial dermis has a dense band-like infiltrate of lymphocytes, some of which appear activated.[808] Some of the small lymphocytes have a nucleus with deep infoldings, resembling Sézary cells.[813] Many of the cells are CD8+.[810] Capillary proliferation is sometimes present.

It is tempting to speculate that the inflammatory infiltrate is an immunological reaction directed against emerging clones of abnormal epidermal cells, in much the same way that this occurs in some cases of porokeratosis.[814]

Electron microscopy

Studies have shown a reduction in keratohyaline granules and some persistence of desmosomal components in the stratum corneum.[805,813] The disparate findings with regard to membrane-coating granules (lamellar bodies) have been referred to above.[805] Vesicular bodies, lacking an internal lamellate structure, have been described.[810]

KYRLE'S DISEASE

The eponymous designation Kyrle's disease is preferable to the original designation of hyperkeratosis follicularis et parafollicularis in cutem penetrans.[815] This controversial entity is regarded by some as a late-onset genodermatosis in which abnormal clones of epidermal cells lead to premature keratinization at the expense of epidermal thickness, with the subsequent introduction of keratinous material into the dermis.[816,817] Others regard it as a variant of perforating folliculitis, a view which is supported by the finding of perforating lesions in patients with chronic renal failure on dialysis, with clinical and histological overlap features between Kyrle's disease, perforating folliculitis and even reactive perforating collagenosis.[818–820] It has also been suggested that Kyrle's disease and Flegel's disease (hyperkeratosis lenticularis perstans – see above) may be different manifestations of the same disease process.[821,822]

Kyrle's disease, as traditionally described, consists of hyperkeratotic papules 2–8 mm in diameter, containing a central, cone-shaped plug.[815,823] The papules may be follicular or extrafollicular in location and they may coalesce to form a verrucous plaque.[824] There is a predilection for the lower limbs, but lesions may also occur on the upper limbs and less often on the head and neck.[823,825] Palmar and plantar surfaces are rarely involved.[826] A female preponderance has been noted in some series.[817] Onset is usually in the fourth decade. A family history has been present in a few cases.[817] Kyrle's disease has been associated with chronic renal failure[827–829] and with diabetes mellitus[823] and more rarely with hepatic dysfunction.[823,830]

Histopathology[831,832]

There is a keratotic plug overlying an invaginated atrophic epidermis. Focal parakeratosis is present in part of the plug; often there is some basophilic cellular debris, which does not stain for elastin. If serial sections are studied, a focus where the epidermal cells are absent and the keratotic plug is in contact with the dermis will often be seen. An inflammatory infiltrate which includes lymphocytes, occasional neutrophils and sometimes a few foreign body giant cells will be present in these areas. Follicular involvement may be present, particularly in those with chronic renal failure where overlap with perforating folliculitis occurs. Eccrine duct involvement was present in one atypical case reported in the literature.[826]

In Flegel's disease, in contrast, there is massive orthokeratosis and only focal parakeratosis, but no basophilic debris in the keratin layer.[817] Also, the inflammatory infiltrate is more conspicuous and usually band-like in distribution.

MULTIPLE MINUTE DIGITATE KERATOSES

Multiple minute digitate keratosis is a rare non-follicular disorder of keratinization, also known as disseminated spiked hyperkeratosis. It can occur in four different clinical settings: a familial type with autosomal dominant inheritance,[833–835] a sporadic type,[836,837] a paraneoplastic variant[838] and a postinflammatory type.[839,840] Hundreds of minute keratotic spikes develop, usually in early adult life. Cases localized to the palms and soles[841,842] are probably best classified with the palmoplantar keratodermas. There is a predilection for the upper parts of the trunk and for the proximal parts of the limbs.[843,844]

A closely related entity, **minute aggregate keratoses**,[845] has dome-shaped papules and crateriform or annular lesions in addition to the spicular lesions seen in multiple minute digitate keratoses.

Minute keratotic spikes have been reported as an acquired phenomenon following X-irradiation,[846] in Crohn's disease[847] and following the use of etretinate.[848]

A solitary spiked lesion, representing a vertically growing ectopic nail, may occur on a finger tip.[849]

Histopathology

The spicules are composed of densely compacted, thin stacks of orthokeratotic material, often arising from a finely pointed epidermal elevation. The keratinous spicules are 1–3 mm in height. They are not related to hair follicles. There may be mild underlying epidermal hyperplasia. The dermis is normal. The digitate keratoses that develop following irradiation are characterized by parakeratotic plugs and underlying epidermal invaginations.[846,850] Parakeratotic horns were also present in the patient with Crohn's disease, referred to above.

The digitate keratoses reported from the scalp as **'congenital trichoid keratosis'** consisted of a column of corneocytes with shadow cells suggesting matrical differentiation.[851]

Electron microscopy

Electron microscopy shows a thickened stratum corneum and a reduced keratohyalin content in the superficial epidermis.[852] Odland bodies are present.[833,852]

WAXY KERATOSES

Waxy keratoses are easily detachable, hyperkeratotic papules with a shiny yellowish 'waxy' appearance and an onset in childhood.[853] The distribution is predominantly truncal and the condition may be familial.[853] The associated presence of confluent hyperkeratosis at other sites is a variable feature.

Larger papules with a mosaic pattern and acral distribution have been reported under the title **'mosaic acral keratosis'**.[854]

Histopathology

Waxy keratoses of childhood are characterized by marked orthokeratotic hyperkeratosis, tenting/papillomatosis of the epidermis and some acanthosis. There is some resemblance to confluent and reticulated papillomatosis (Gougerot and Carteaud), see page 575; however, waxy keratoses have more prominent hyperkeratosis.

MISCELLANEOUS EPIDERMAL GENODERMATOSES

The group of miscellaneous epidermal genodermatoses includes such disparate conditions as acrokeratosis verruciformis, xeroderma pigmentosum, the ectodermal dysplasias, cutaneous and mucosal dyskeratosis, nevoid hyperkeratosis of the areola, and the peeling skin syndrome.

ACROKERATOSIS VERRUCIFORMIS

Acrokeratosis verruciformis is an autosomal dominant genodermatosis in which multiple papules, resembling plane warts, develop on the dorsum of the hands and fingers and to a lesser extent on the feet, forearms and legs.[855–859] Onset is usually before puberty, but late onset has been recorded.[855–858] It is more common in males.[858]

Lesions identical to those of acrokeratosis verruciformis develop in a significant number of patients with Darier's disease (see p. 296). Such lesions may precede, follow or develop concurrently with the onset of the more usual lesions of Darier's disease.[860] Acrokeratosis verruciformis has been reported in the relatives of individuals with Darier's disease.[861] There is considerable controversy as to the nature of the relationship of these two conditions and also about their relationship to the palmar and plantar keratoses which may accompany either disease. One view is that the acral lesions of Darier's disease and acrokeratosis verruciformis are separate entities.[858] This is based on the finding of small foci of acantholytic dyskeratosis in some acral lesions of Darier's disease if multiple sections are examined. The contrary view is that both diseases result from a single autosomal dominant genetic defect with variable expressivity of the gene.[860,862,863]

Histopathology[855,858]

Sections show hyperkeratosis, regular acanthosis and low papillomatosis, imparting a regular undulating appearance to the surface (Figs 9.25, 9.26). These changes have been likened to 'church spires'. There is no parakeratosis, no epidermal vacuolation and no significant dermal inflammatory infiltrate.

Squamous cell carcinomas have been reported in two cases of long standing.[858]

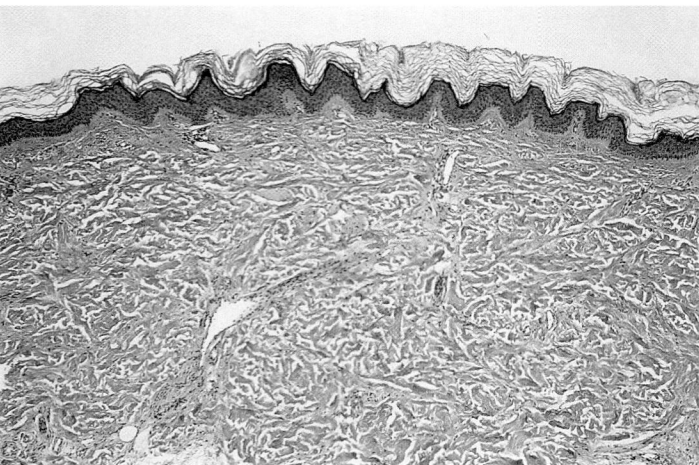

Fig. 9.25 **Acrokeratosis verruciformis.** There is low papillomatosis ('church spiring'). Multiple lesions were present, but there were no features of Darier's disease. (H & E)

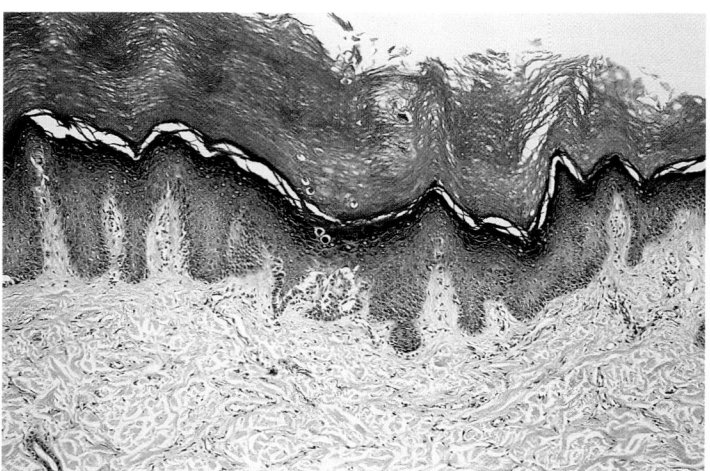

Fig. 9.26 **Acrokeratosis verruciformis in a patient with Darier's disease.** There is compact orthokeratosis and low papillomatosis imparting an undulating appearance to the epidermis. There is a small focus of acantholytic dyskeratosis. (H & E)

XERODERMA PIGMENTOSUM

Xeroderma pigmentosum is a rare, autosomal recessive genodermatosis characterized by deficient DNA repair, photophobia, severe solar sensitivity, cutaneous pigmentary changes, xerosis and the early development of mucocutaneous and ocular cancers, particularly in sun-exposed areas.[864–870] Neurological abnormalities are present in up to 20%[871] and these are most severe in the De Sanctis–Cacchione syndrome (microcephaly, dwarfism, choreoathetosis and mental deficiency).[864,866,872] The earliest changes usually develop before the age of 2 with a severe sunburn reaction and the development of multiple freckles with variable intensity of melanin pigmentation and interspersed hypopigmented macules.[873] Pigmentation often develops on the palms and soles and mucous membranes. Later there is dry, scaly skin (xerosis) with poikilodermatous features. Skin tumors, which include solar keratoses, cutaneous horns, keratoacanthomas, squamous and basal cell carcinomas, basosquamous carcinoma, atypical fibroxanthoma,[874] malignant melanomas[875] and angiomas, may develop in late childhood; patients may ultimately die from the consequences of their tumors.[871] The development of the cutaneous lesions can be retarded by protection from the sun from birth.[616,876] Immunological abnormalities have been present in some patients.[877]

Xeroderma pigmentosum involves both sexes and all races with an incidence of 1:250 000 and a gene frequency of 1:200.[864] There is a high incidence of consanguinity.[878] Heterozygotes could not, until recently, be reliably demonstrated in the laboratory.[879] They are asymptomatic, although there is one report of an increased incidence of malignant skin tumors in these individuals.[864] Prenatal diagnosis of xeroderma pigmentosum can be made by an analysis of DNA repair in cells cultured from the amniotic fluid of women at risk.[880]

There is genetic heterogeneity with at least nine different groups recognized by somatic cell fusion studies – so-called 'complementation groups'.[864,881] Seven of these groups (labeled A to G) have deficient excision repair of ultraviolet radiation-induced DNA damage (particularly nucleotide excision repair),[882] while in one (the so-called 'XP variant') there is defective ability to convert newly synthesized DNA from low to high molecular weight after UV irradiation (postreplication repair).[864,883–885] These different complementation groups have different clinical correlations, including differing susceptibility to the various cutaneous tumors.[886] For example, XP-A is the most severe form and some of this group have the De Sanctis–Cacchione syndrome (see above). The severity of the neurological abnormalities in Japanese patients in this group correlates with the sites of non-sense mutations in the XP-A gene.[887] XP-E is the mildest form, with late onset and a higher residual capacity to repair UV-induced DNA damage in in vitro studies.[888,889] XP-F,[890–892] XP-G[893] and XP-B are extremely rare; the latter group has been associated with the Cockayne syndrome (short stature, photosensitivity, deafness, mental deficiency, large ears and nose and sunken eyes).[864,867,894–899] A gene responsible for the Cockayne syndrome is located on chromosome 10q11–21, but others have also been listed. XP-C is the most prevalent form among North Americans and Europeans.[900] Squamous cell carcinomas are commonly found in group A, basal cell carcinomas in groups C and E and in the variant form and malignant melanomas in groups C and D and also in the variant form.[864,901–903]

In one study, a skin fibroblast cell strain from a patient with xeroderma pigmentosum was reported to have shown spontaneous morphological transformation to an anchorage-independent form after serial passage.[904] This presumably has some significance in the development of tumors in vivo; the finding of reduced natural killer cell activity may have a similar significance.[905]

It is now well established that cultured fibroblasts from patients with xeroderma pigmentosum show defective DNA repair following ultraviolet radiation. This abnormality is also present in keratinocytes and melanocytes cultured from affected patients.[906] Cultured keratinocytes from patients with xeroderma pigmentosum are more sensitive than normal cells to UVB-induced apoptosis.[882]

The gene responsible for xeroderma pigmentosum group A (XP-A) has been cloned and designated the XPA gene. At least three mutations of this gene exist, resulting in a different clinical severity for each mutation group.[879,907,908] Chromosomes 1 and 9 appear to be involved. All the genes for xeroderma pigmentosa have now been cloned except that for XP-E, the mildest form.[889] The gene for XP-D maps to chromosome 19q13.2–q13.3. The defect in xeroderma pigmentosum is thought to involve the initial, endonucleolytic step of excision repair.[909] In the case of the XPC gene, it is thought to be involved in the repair of damage to bulk nontranscribed DNA.[900] The XP variant gene has been cloned and identified as DNA polymerase.[889]

Histopathology[865]
In the initial stages there are no diagnostically specific features. There may be variability in epidermal melanin concentration, telangiectasia of superficial vessels and a mild perivascular inflammatory cell reaction. With time, the pigmentary changes are more marked, with areas of prominent melanin pigmentation of the basal, malpighian and spinous layers and pigmentary incontinence. Areas of hypopigmentation, sometimes with epidermal atrophy, may be seen. There is eventually prominent solar elastosis and the development of areas of hyperkeratosis. Keratoses and the other tumors already mentioned eventually develop. Tumors of the anterior part of the tongue have also been reported.[910]

Electron microscopy
Various changes have been noted. They include irregular nuclear morphology, melanosomes with a high degree of polymorphism and dilated rough endoplasmic reticulum, vacuoles and disrupted desmosomes in basal keratinocytes.[911] Fibroblast-like cells may show melanophagic activity.[911] Structures resembling anchoring fibrils and the basal lamina have been noted in the dilated endoplasmic reticulum of these cells.[912]

ECTODERMAL DYSPLASIAS

The ectodermal dysplasias are an expanding but nevertheless rare group of genodermatoses characterized by a diffuse, non-progressive disorder of the epidermis and at least one of its appendages.[400,913] The epidermal component may involve keratinocytes, melanocytes[914] or Langerhans cells or any combination thereof; the 'appendageal' component may affect the hair, sebaceous or eccrine glands, the nails or the teeth.[915] The ectodermal dysplasias comprise over 100 clinically distinct syndromes and the limits of this entity are not clearly defined.[916,917] Abnormalities of non-ectodermal structures may also be present.

The traditional classification of the ectodermal dysplasias into hidrotic and anhidrotic types is not appropriate for the broad range of abnormalities that may occur in this group. They are now classified on the basis of the presence or absence of trichodysplasia,[918] dental abnormalities, onychodysplasia and dyshidrosis. The Naegeli–Franceschetti–Jadassohn syndrome affects sweat glands, nails, teeth and skin. It includes reticulate pigmentation of the skin as an important component and is therefore discussed with other disorders of pigmentation (see p. 332). The gene maps to chromosome 17q21 in the region of the type I keratin gene cluster.[919] Most of the syndromes are extremely rare and of little dermatopathological importance.[920] Four of them merit further discussion.

Anhidrotic ectodermal dysplasia
In anhidrotic ectodermal dysplasia, an X-linked recessive disorder also known as the Christ–Siemens–Touraine syndrome, there is anhidrosis or marked hypohidrosis, complete or partial anodontia, hypotrichosis and a characteristic facies.[420,921–923] Less frequent manifestations include nail dystrophy, genital anomalies, absence of mammary glands, impaired immunity[924] and mental retardation.[925,926] A prenatal diagnosis can be made by an examination of fetal skin.[927] Female carriers may show reduced sweating and faulty dentition.[928] The gene responsible is localized at Xq12–q13.1.[929,930] It affects a transmembrane protein expressed by keratinocytes, hair follicles and sweat glands.[931] The gene responsible for the less frequent autosomal recessive form maps to chromosome 2q11–q13.[931] A related autosomal recessive disorder combining hypohidrotic ectodermal dysplasia and skin fragility, resulting from absence of the desmosomal plaque protein plakophilin 1, has been reported.[932,933]

Hidrotic ectodermal dysplasia
In hidrotic ectodermal dysplasia, also known as Clouston's syndrome, there is a normal ability to perspire.[402,934,935] Palmar-plantar keratoderma is usually a prominent feature. The finding of an increased number of desmosomal disks

in the thickened stratum corneum suggests that the hyperkeratosis in this disorder is caused by delayed desquamation of the stratum corneum.[934] Linkage to chromosome 13q11–q12.1 has been reported in several families.[936–938]

Orofaciodigital syndrome

Orofaciodigital syndrome is an X-linked dominant disorder which is usually lethal in males.[400,939] There is a marked reduction in sebaceous glands on the scalp or face, dental dysplasia, evanescent facial milia, cleft lip and palate and malformation of the digits. Mental retardation may be present.

Ectodermal dysplasias with clefting

There are several clinical syndromes characterized by ectoderma dysplasia in association with clefting of the lip and/or palate. They include the EEC syndrome (ectodermal dysplasia, ectodactyly, cleft lip/palate), the Rapp–Hodgkin syndrome (the additional clinical feature is facial hypoplasia) and the Hay–Wells or AEC syndrome (the additional clinical feature is ankyloblepharon).[940–945] The EEC syndrome is due to a mutation in the *p63* gene on chromosome 3p27–29.[946]

Histopathology

The histological features will obviously vary according to which epidermal and appendageal components are involved.

In *anhidrotic ectodermal dysplasia* the epidermis is thinned. Eccrine glands are absent or rudimentary, although poorly formed intraepidermal eccrine ducts may be present.[947] Apocrine glands may also be hypotrophic. There is a reduction in pilosebaceous follicles although, paradoxically, foci of sebaceous hyperplasia have sometimes been noted on the upper cheeks.[948] Other reported features include a reduction in seromucous glands in the respiratory tract,[949] a reduction in epidermal Langerhans cells, and fragmentation of dermal elastic fibers. As eccrine glands do not develop until 20–24 weeks of gestation, whereas hair follicles should be present at this time, it is the absence of pilar units which is used to make the diagnosis on fetal skin biopsies taken at this period of gestation.[927]

In *hidrotic ectodermal dysplasia* there is pronounced hyperkeratosis, particularly of the palms and soles, and a normal number of sweat glands. The sweat glands are also normal in number in the *orofaciodigital syndrome*, but sebaceous glands are diminished or absent.[939] The epidermis may be somewhat atrophic.

In *ectodermal dysplasias with clefting* the pilosebaceous follicles are reduced in size and small vellus follicles are present.[941] A scalp dermatitis with variable histological changes may be present.

CUTANEOUS AND MUCOSAL DYSKERATOSIS

There has been a report describing a father and son with brownish papules with central keratotic plugs.[950] Single cell keratinization (dyskeratosis) was present in the epidermis, as well as in the epithelium of the mouth and the conjunctiva.[950] In another case, numerous dyskeratotic cells were present in epithelium of the lips, palate and gums and on the labial surfaces of the genitalia, as an acquired phenomenon: this condition was referred to as acquired dyskeratotic leukoplakia.[951] Dyskeratotic cells were also a feature of the cases reported as hereditary mucoepithelial dysplasia.[952]

NEVOID HYPERKERATOSIS OF THE NIPPLE

The rare condition nevoid hyperkeratosis of the nipple is manifest by hyperpigmentation of the areola with accompanying verrucous thickening.[953]

It may be unilateral or bilateral.[954,955] Similar, but usually milder, changes may be seen in Darier's disease, acanthosis nigricans, pregnancy and, rarely, in men receiving estrogen therapy for prostatic adenocarcinoma.[956] Cases unrelated to estrogen therapy have been reported in males.[957,958]

Histopathology

There is hyperkeratosis, papillomatosis and acanthosis, the latter often having a filiform interconnecting pattern. Keratin-filled ostia are also present.[956] There is a superficial resemblance to a seborrheic keratosis, but with a more delicate, interconnecting acanthosis.

PEELING SKIN SYNDROME

The peeling skin syndrome is a rare autosomal recessive disorder characterized by spontaneous, continual peeling of the skin.[959] Variants in which the peeling has been localized to the palm[960] or acral regions[961,962] have been reported. A keratohyaline abnormality has been found.[963] A variant, related to an alteration of epidermal retinoic acid metabolism with splitting occurring in the desmosomal plaque, has recently been reported.[964] Azathioprine has been associated with a clinical simulant.

Histopathology

There is hyperkeratosis, parakeratosis, reduction of the granular layer and acanthosis. There is separation of the stratum corneum from the underlying granular layer.[959,965]

In **erythrokeratolysis hiemalis**, a rare autosomal dominant genodermatosis which is common in South Africa and related to an abnormality in chromosome 8p22–p23, there is 'necrobiosis' of keratinocytes in the malpighian layer.[960] It is also characterized by skin peeling.

Electron microscopy

Keratohyaline granules are poorly formed and keratin filaments are incompletely aggregated below the level of the split.[962]

MISCELLANEOUS DISORDERS

GRANULAR PARAKERATOSIS

Granular parakeratosis is an acquired abnormality of keratinization first described in 1991 as axillary granular parakeratosis.[965,967] It has since been described in other intertriginous areas such as the inguinal region,[968] inter- and submammary region,[969] the vulva and perianal region.[967,969] Rare cases involving the abdomen and the knee have been seen, indicating that the adjectives 'axillary' and 'intertriginous' are both inappropriate in the title. The lesions are red to hyperpigmented patches that are often pruritic. Axillary lesions can resemble acanthosis nigricans.

There appears to be a defect in the processing of profilaggrin to filaggrin that results in a failure to degrade keratohyaline granules.[967] The etiology is unknown. Suggestions that the condition may result from excess use of topical antiperspirants seem difficult to sustain in cases occurring outside the axilla.[970] A response to retinoids has been noted.[971]

Histopathology

There is a thick parakeratotic layer with retention of keratohyaline granules in this region (Fig. 9.27). The stratum granulosum is also preserved. The underlying epidermis may be normal, mildly atrophic or show psoriasiform acanthosis.

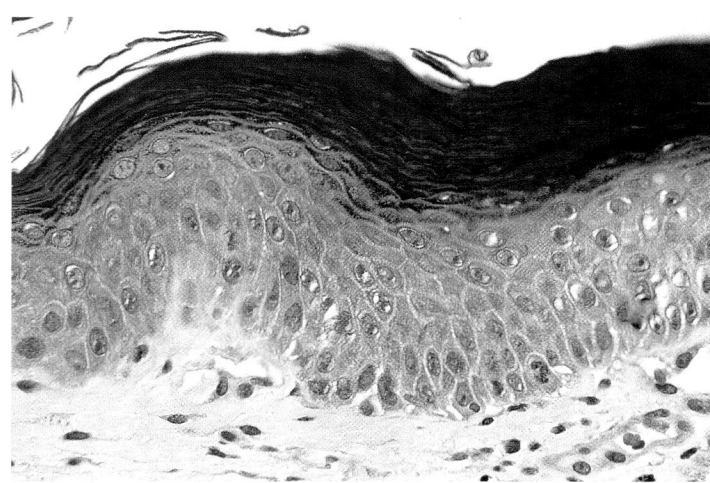

Fig. 9.27 **Granular parakeratosis.** This biopsy, from the axilla, shows a thick parakeratotic layer with retention of keratohyaline granules.

REFERENCES

Introduction

1 Haake AR, Polakowska RR. Cell death by apoptosis in epidermal biology. J Invest Dermatol 1993; 101: 107–112.

2 McGowan KM, Coulombe PA. Keratin 17 expression in the hard epithelial context of the hair and nail, and its relevance for the pachyonychia congenita phenotype. J Invest Dermatol 2000; 114: 1101–1107.

3 Smack DP, Korge BP, James WD. Keratin and keratinization. J Am Acad Dermatol 1994; 30: 85–102.

4 Waseem A, Dogan B, Tidman N et al. Keratin 15 expression in stratified epithelia: downregulation in activated keratinocytes. J Invest Dermatol 1999; 112: 362–369.

5 Irvine AD, McLean WHI. Human keratin diseases: the increasing spectrum of disease and subtlety of the phenotype-genotype correlation. Br J Dermatol 1999; 140: 815–828.

6 Mills CM, Marks R. Acral epidermolytic hyperkeratosis. Br J Dermatol 1993; 128: 342–347.

7 Ishida-Yamamoto A, Hashimoto Y, Manabe M et al. Distinctive expression of filaggrin and trichohyalin during various pathways of epithelial differentiation. Br J Dermatol 1997; 137: 9–16.

8 Odland GF, Holbrook KA. The lamellar granules of epidermis. Curr Probl Dermatol 1981; 9: 29–49.

9 Mischke D, Korge BP, Marenholz I et al. Genes encoding structural proteins of epidermal cornification and S100 calcium-binding proteins form a gene complex ('epidermal differentiation complex') on human chromosome 1q21. J Invest Dermatol 1996; 106: 989–992.

10 Williams ML. Epidermal lipids and scaling diseases of the skin. Semin Dermatol 1992; 11: 169–175.

11 Williams ML. Ichthyosis: mechanisms of disease. Pediatr Dermatol 1992; 9: 365–368.

12 Ekholm IE, Brattsand M, Egelrud T. Stratum corneum tryptic enzyme in normal epidermis: a missing link in the desquamation process? J Invest Dermatol 2000; 114: 56–63.

13 Sato J, Denda M, Nakanishi J et al. Cholesterol sulfate inhibits proteases that are involved in desquamation of stratum corneum. J Invest Dermatol 1998; 111: 189–193.

14 Squier CA. The permeability of keratinized and nonkeratinized oral epithelium to horseradish peroxidase. J Ultrastr Res 1973; 43: 160–177.

15 Norlén L, Nicander I, Rozell BL et al. Inter- and intra-individual differences in human stratum corneum lipid content related to physical parameters of skin barrier function *in vivo*. J Invest Dermatol 1999; 112: 72–77.

16 Sheu H-M, Chao S-C, Wong T-W et al. Human skin surface lipid film: an ultrastructural study and interaction with corneocytes and intercellular lipid lamellae of the stratum corneum. Br J Dermatol 1999; 140: 385–391.

17 Rossi A, Jang S-I, Ceci R et al. Effect of AP1 transcription factors on the regulation of transcription in normal human epidermal keratinocytes. J Invest Dermatol 1998; 110: 34–40.

18 Eckert RL, Crish JF, Banks EB, Welter JF. The epidermis: genes on – genes off. J Invest Dermatol 1997; 109: 501–509.

19 Hohl D. Towards a better classification of erythrokeratodermias. Br J Dermatol 2000; 143: 1133–1137.

Ichthyoses

20 Rand RE, Baden HP. The ichthyoses – a review. J Am Acad Dermatol 1983; 8: 285–305.

21 Williams ML. The ichthyoses – pathogenesis and prenatal diagnosis: a review of recent advances. Pediatr Dermatol 1983; 1: 1–24.

22 Williams ML, Elias PM. Genetically transmitted, generalized disorders of cornification. The ichthyoses. Dermatol Clin 1987; 5: 155–178.

23 Kumar S, Sehgal VN, Sharma RC. Common genodermatoses. Int J Dermatol 1996; 35: 685–694.

24 Bale SJ, Doyle SZ. The genetics of ichthyosis: a primer for epidemiologists. J Invest Dermatol 1994; 102: 49S–50S.

25 Elsayed-Ali H, Barton S, Marks R. Serological studies of desmosomes in ichthyosis vulgaris. Br J Dermatol 1992; 126: 24–28.

26 Williams ML, Elias PM. Ichthyosis. Genetic heterogeneity, genodermatoses, and genetic counseling. Arch Dermatol 1986; 122: 529–531.

27 Bernhardt M, Baden HP. Report of a family with an unusual expression of recessive ichthyosis. Report of 42 cases. Arch Dermatol 1986; 122: 428–433.

28 Sybert VP, Dale BA, Holbrook KA. Ichthyosis vulgaris: identification of a defect in synthesis of filaggrin correlated with an absence of keratohyaline granules. J Invest Dermatol 1985; 84: 191–194.

29 Peña Penabad C, Pérez Arellano JL, Becker E et al. Differential patterns of filaggrin expression in lamellar ichthyosis. Br J Dermatol 1998; 139: 958–964.

30 Presland RB, Boggess D, Lewis SP et al. Loss of normal profilaggrin and filaggrin in flaky tail *(ft/ft)* m ce: an animal model for the filaggrin-deficient skin disease ichthyosis vulgaris. J Invest Dermatol 2000; 115: 1072–1081.

31 DiLeonardo M. Ichthyosis vulgaris vs. X-linked ichthyosis vs. lamellar ichthyosis. Dermatopathology: Practical & Conceptual 1997; 2: 132.

32 Okano M, Kitano Y, Yoshikawa K et al. X-linked ichthyosis and ichthyosis vulgaris: comparison of their clinical features based on biochemical analysis. Br J Dermatol 1988; 119: 777–783.

33 Honour JW, Goolamali SK, Taylor NF. Prenatal diagnosis and variable presentation of recessive X-linked ichthyosis. Br J Dermatol 1985; 112: 423–430.

34 Paige DG, Emilion GG, Bouloux PMG, Harper JI. A clinical and genetic study of X-linked recessive ichthyosis and contiguous gene defects. Br J Dermatol 1994; 131: 622–629.

35 Vélez A, Moreno J-C. Poland's syndrome and recessive X-linked ichthyosis in two brothers. Clin Exp Dermatol 2000; 25: 308–311.

36 Quinton R, Schofield JK, Duke VM et al. X-linked ichthyosis with hypogonadism: not always Kallmann's syndrome. Clin Exp Dermatol 1997; 22: 201–204.

37 Cuevas-Covarrubias SA, Valdes-Flores M, Rivera-Vega MR et al. Ichthyosis vulgaris and X-linked ichthyosis: simultaneous segregation in the same family. Acta Derm Venereol 1999; 79: 494–495.

38 Trüeb RM, Meyer JC. Male-pattern baldness in men with X-linked recessive ichthyosis. Dermatology 2000; 200: 247–249.

39 Happle R, Hoffmann R. Absence of male-pattern baldness in men with X-linked recessive ichthyosis? A hypothesis to be challenged. Dermatology 1999; 198: 231–232.

40 Yoshiike T, Matsui T, Ogawa H. Steroid sulphatase deficiency in patients initially diagnosed as ichthyosis vulgaris or recessive X-linked ichthyosis. Br J Dermatol 1985; 112: 431–433.

41 Brown BE, Williams ML, Elias PM. Stratum corneum lipid abnormalities in ichthyosis. Detection by a new lipid microanalytical method. Arch Dermatol 1984; 120: 204–209.

42 Jobsis AC, de Groot WP, Meijer AEFH, van der Loos CM. A new method for the determination of steroid sulphatase activity in leukocytes in X-linked ichthyosis. Br J Dermatol 1983; 108: 567–572.

43 Dijkstra AC, Vermeesch-Markslag AMG, Vromans EWM et al. Substrate specific sulfatase activity from hair follicles in recessive X-linked ichthyosis. Acta Derm Venereol 1987; 67: 369–376.

44 Zettersten E, Man M-Q, Sato J et al. Recessive x-linked ichthyosis: role of cholesterol-sulfate accumulation in the barrier abnormality. J Invest Dermatol 1998; 111: 784–790.

45 Öhman H, Vahlquist A. The pH gradient over the stratum corneum differs in X-linked recessive and autosomal dominant ichthyosis: a clue to the molecular origin of the "acid skin mantle"? J Invest Dermatol 1998; 111: 674–677.

46 Delfino M, Procaccini EM, Pilliano GM, Milone A. X-linked ichthyosis: relation between cholesterol sulphate, dehydroepiandrosterone sulphate and patient's age. Br J Dermatol 1998; 138: 655–657.

47 Hernández-Martin A, González-Sarmiento R, De Unamuno P. X-linked ichthyosis: an update. Br J Dermatol 1999; 141: 617–627.

48 Saeki H, Kuwata S, Nakagawa H et al. Deletion pattern of the steroid sulphatase gene in Japanese patients with X-linked ichthyosis. Br J Dermatol 1998; 139: 96–98.

49 Valdes-Flores M, Kofman-Alfaro SH, Jimenez Vaca AL, Cuevas-Covarrubias SA. A novel partial deletion of exons 2–10 of the STS gene in recessive X-linked ichthyosis. J Invest Dermatol 2000; 114: 591–593.

50 Morita E, Katoh O, Shinoda S et al. A novel point mutation in the steroid sulfatase gene in X-linked ichthyosis. J Invest Dermatol 1997; 109: 244–245.

51 Aviram-Goldring A, Goldman B, Netanelov-Shapira I et al. Deletion patterns of the STS gene and flanking sequences in Israeli X-linked ichthyosis patients and carriers: analysis by polymerase chain reaction and fluorescence in situ hybridization techniques. Int J Dermatol 2000; 39: 182–187.

52 Oyama N, Satoh M, Iwatsuki K, Kaneko F. Novel point mutations in the steroid sulfatase gene in patients with X-linked ichthyosis: transfection analysis using the mutated genes. J Invest Dermatol 2000; 114: 1195–1199.

53 Valdes-Flores M, Jimenez Vaca AL, Kofman-Alfaro SH, Cuevas-Covarrubias SA. Characterization of a novel point mutation (Arg432His) in X-linked ichthyosis. Acta Derm Venereol 2001; 81: 54–55.

54 Cuevas-Covarrubias SA, Valdes-Flores M, Orozco Orozco E et al. Most "sporadic" cases of X-linked ichthyosis are not de novo mutations. Acta Derm Venereol 1999; 79 143–144.

55 Piccirillo A, Auricchio L, Fabbrocini G et al. Ocular findings and skin histology in a group of patients with X-linked ichthyosis. Br J Dermatol 1988; 119: 185–188.

56 De Unamuno P, Martin-Pascual A, Garcia-Perez A. X-linked ichthyosis. Br J Dermatol 1977; 97: 53–58.

57 Finlay AY. Major autosomal recessive ichthyoses. Semin Dermatol 1988; 7: 26–35.

58 De Wolf K, Gourdain JM, de Dobbeleer G, Song M. A particular subtype of ichthyosis congenita type III. Am J Dermatopathol 1995; 17: 606–611.

59 Niemi K-M, Kanerva L, Kuokkanen K, Ignatius J. Clinical, light and electron microscopic features of recessive congenital ichthyosis type I. Br J Dermatol 1994; 130: 626–633.

60 Hohl D, Aeschlimann D, Huber M. In vitro and rapid in situ transglutaminase assays for congenital ichthyoses – a comparative study. J Invest Dermatol 1998; 110: 268–271.

61 Patrizi A, Neri I, Di Lernia V et al. Lamellar ichthyosis with laminated membrane structures. Br J Dermatol 1993; 128: 348–351.

62 Niemi K-M, Kuokkanen K, Kanerva L, Ignatius J. Recessive ichthyosis congenita type IV. Am J Dermatopathol 1993; 15: 224–228.

63 Brusasco A, Gelmetti C, Tadini G, Caputo R. Ichthyosis congenita type IV: a new case resembling diffuse cutaneous mastocytosis. Br J Dermatol 1997; 136: 377–379.

64 Akiyama M. Severe congenital ichthyosis of the neonate. Int J Dermatol 1998; 37: 722–728.

65 Frenk E, de Techtermann F. Self-healing collodion baby: evidence for autosomal recessive inheritance. Pediatr Dermatol 1992; 9: 95–97.

66 Hashimoto K, Prada S, Lopez AP et al. CHILD syndrome with linear eruptions, hypopigmented bands, and verruciform xanthoma. Pediatr Dermatol 1998; 15: 360–366.

67 Bergers M, Traupe H, Dunnwald SC et al. Enzymatic distinction between two subgroups of autosomal recessive lamellar ichthyosis. J Invest Dermatol 1990; 94: 407–412.

68 Elbaum DJ, Kurz G, MacDuff M. Increased incidence of cutaneous carcinomas in patients with congenital ichthyosis. J Am Acad Dermatol 1995; 33: 884–886.

69 Huber M, Rettler I, Bernasconi K et al. Lamellar ichthyosis is genetically heterogeneous – cases with normal keratinocyte transglutaminase. J Invest Dermatol 1995; 105: 653–654.

70 Bichakjian CK, Nair RP, Wu WW et al. Prenatal exclusion of lamellar ichthyosis based on identification of two new mutations in the transglutaminase 1 gene. J Invest Dermatol 1998; 110: 179–182.

71 Hashimoto K, Gee S, Tanaka K. Lamellar ichthyosis: response to etretinate with transglutaminase 1 recovery. Am J Dermatopathol 2000; 22: 277–280.

72 Cserhalmi-Friedman PB, Milstone LM, Christiano AM. Diagnosis of autosomal recessive lamellar ichthyosis with mutations in the TGM1 gene. Br J Dermatol 2001; 144 726–730.

73 Hohl D, Huber M, Frenk E. Analysis of the cornified cell envelope in lamellar ichthyosis. Arch Dermatol 1993; 129: 618–624.

74 Fischer J, Faure A, Bouadjar B et al. Two new loci for autosomal recessive ichthyosis on chromosomes 3p21 and 19p12–q12 and evidence for further genetic heterogeneity. Am J Hum Genet 2000; 66: 904–913.

75 Akiyama M, Takizawa Y, Kokaji T, Shimizu H. Novel mutations of TGM1 in a child with congenital ichthyosiform erythroderma. Br J Dermatol 2001; 144: 401–407.

76 Langtry JAA, Carr MM, Ive FA et al. Ichthyosiform erythroderma associated with generalized pustulosis. Br J Dermatol 1998; 138: 502–505.

77 Brusasco A, Cambiaghi S, Tadini G et al. Unusual hyperpigmentation developing in congenital reticular ichthyosiform erythroderma (ichthyosis variegata). Br J Dermatol 1998; 139: 893–896.

78 Metze D, Traupe H. Explaining clinical features and histopathological findings by electron microscopy: congenital reticular ichthyosiform erythroderma. Dermatopathology: Practical & Conceptual 1999; 5: 130–131.

79 Hill VA, Griffiths WAD, Kerr-Muir MG, Hardman-Lea S. Non-bullous congenital ichthyosiform erythroderma, with ocular albinism and Noonan syndrome. Clin Exp Dermatol 2000; 25: 611–614.

80 Hazell M, Marks R. Clinical, histologic, and cell kinetic discriminants between lamellar ichthyosis and nonbullous congenital ichthyosiform erythroderma. Arch Dermatol 1985; 121: 489–493.

81 Dover R, Burge S, Ralfs I, Ryan TJ. Congenital non-bullous ichthyosiform erythroderma – cell kinetics before and after treatment with etretinate. Clin Exp Dermatol 1986; 11: 431–435.

82 Choate KA, Williams ML, Khavari PA. Abnormal transglutaminase 1 expression pattern in a subset of patients with erythrodermic autosomal recessive ichthyosis. J Invest Dermatol 1998; 110: 8–12.

83 Schnyder UW. Inherited ichthyosis. Arch Dermatol 1970; 102: 240–251.

84 Niemi K-M, Kanerva L. Ichthyosis with laminated membrane structures. Am J Dermatopathol 1989; 11: 149–156.

85 Mevorah B, Landau M, Gat A et al. Adolescent-onset ichthyosiform-like erythroderma with lichenoid tissue reaction: a new entity? Br J Dermatol 2001; 144: 1063–1066.

86 Kumar S, Sehgal VN, Sharma RC. Epidermolytic hyperkeratosis. Int J Dermatol 1999; 38: 914–915.

87 Reddy BSN, Thadeus J, Kumar SKA et al. Generalized epidermolytic hyperkeratosis in a child born to a parent with systematized epidermolytic linear epidermal nevus. Int J Dermatol 1997; 36: 198–200.

88 Khatri ML, Shafi M, Ben-Ghazeil M. Epidermolytic hyperkeratosis (bullous ichthyosis). J Eur Acad Dermatol Venereol 2000; 14: 324–325.

89 Sahn EE, Weimer CE Jr, Garen PD. Annular epidermolytic ichthyosis: a unique phenotype. J Am Acad Dermatol 1992; 27: 348–355.

90 McGrath J, Cerio R, Wilson-Jones E. The phenotypic heterogenicity of bullous ichthyosis – a case report of three family members. Clin Exp Dermatol 1991; 16: 25–27.

91 Yang J-M, Chipev CC, DiGiovanna JJ et al. Mutations in the H1 and 1A domains in the keratin 1 gene in epidermolytic hyperkeratosis. J Invest Dermatol 1994; 102: 17–23.

92 Huber M, Scaletta C, Benathan M et al. Abnormal keratin 1 and 10 cytoskeleton in cultured keratinocytes from epidermolytic hyperkeratosis caused by keratin 10 mutations. J Invest Dermatol 1994; 102: 691–694.

93 McLean WHI, Eady RAJ, Dopping-Hepenstal PJC et al. Mutations in the rod 1A domain of keratins 1 and 10 in bullous congenital ichthyosiform erythroderma (BCIE). J Invest Dermatol 1994; 102: 24–30.

94 DiGiovanna JJ, Bale SJ. Epidermolytic hyperkeratosis: applied molecular genetics. J Invest Dermatol 1994; 102: 390–394.

95 DiGiovanna JJ, Bale SJ. Clinical heterogeneity in epidermolytic hyperkeratosis. Arch Dermatol 1994; 130: 1026–1035.

96 Steijlen PM, Maessen E, Kresse H et al. Expression of tenascin, biglycan and decorin in disorders of keratinization. Br J Dermatol 1994; 130: 564–568.

97 Chipev CC, Steinert PM, Woodworth CD. Characterization of an immortalized cell line from a patient with epidermolytic hyperkeratosis. J Invest Dermatol 1996; 106; 385–390.

98 Mayuzumi N, Shigihara T, Ikeda S, Ogawa H. Recurrent R156H mutation of KRT10 in a Japanese family with bullous congenital ichthyosiform erythroderma. J Eur Acad Dermatol Venereol 2000; 14: 304–306.

99 Yang J-M, Yoneda K, Morita E et al. An alanine to proline mutation in the 1A rod domain of the keratin 10 chain in epidermolytic hyperkeratosis. J Invest Dermatol 1997; 109: 692–694.

100 Yang J-M, Nam K, Kim H-C et al. A novel glutamic acid to aspartic acid mutation near the end of the 2B rod domain in the keratin 1 chain in epidermolytic hyperkeratosis. J Invest Dermatol 1999; 112: 376–379.

101 Kremer H, Lavrijsen APM, McLean WHI et al. An atypical form of bullous congenital ichthyosiform erythroderma is caused by a mutation in the L12 linker region of keratin 1. J Invest Dermatol 1998; 111: 1224–1226.

102 Suga Y, Duncan KO, Heald PW, Roop DR. A novel helix termination mutation in keratin 10 in annular epidermolytic ichthyosis, a variant of bullous congenital ichthyosiform erythroderma. J Invest Dermatol 1998; 111: 1220–1223.

103 Arin MJ, Longley MA, Anton-Lamprecht I et al. A novel substitution in keratin 10 in epidermolytic hyperkeratosis. J Invest Dermatol 1999; 112: 506–508.

104 Cserhalmi-Friedman PB, Squeo R, Gordon D et al. Epidermolytic hyperkeratosis in a Hispanic family resulting from a mutation in the keratin 1 gene. Clin Exp Dermatol 2000; 25: 241–243.

105 Yoneda K, Morita E, Akiyama M et al. Annular epidermolytic ichthyosis. Br J Dermatol 1999; 141: 748–750.

106 Brusasco A, Cavalli R, Cambiaghi S et al. Ichthyosis Curth–Macklin: a new sporadic case with immunohistochemical study of keratin expression. Arch Dermatol 1994; 130: 1077–1079.

107 Kriner J, Montes LF. Gigantic ichthyosis hystrix. J Am Acad Dermatol 1997; 36: 646–647.

108 Traupe H, Kolde G, Hamm H, Happle R. Ichthyosis bullosa of Siemens: a unique type of epidermolytic hyperkeratosis. J Am Acad Dermatol 1986; 14: 1000–1005.

109 Murdoch ME, Leigh IM. Ichthyosis bullosa of Siemens and bullous ichthyosiform erythroderma – variants of the same disease? Clin Exp Dermatol 1990; 15: 53–56.

110 Kramer H, Zeeuwen P, McLean WHI et al. Ichthyosis bullosa of Siemens is caused by mutations in the keratin 2e gene. J Invest Dermatol 1994; 103: 286–289.

111 McLean WHI, Morley SM, Lane EB et al. Ichthyosis bullosa of Siemens – a disease involving keratin 2e. J Invest Dermatol 1994; 103: 277–281.

112 Moraru R, Cserhalmi-Friedman PB, Grossman ME et al. Ichthyosis bullosa of Siemens resulting from a novel missense mutation near the helix termination motif of the keratin 2e gene. Clin Exp Dermatol 1999; 24: 412–415.

113 Smith FJD, Maingi C, Covello SP et al. Genomic organization and fine mapping of the keratin 2e gene (KRT2E): K2e VI domain polymorphism and novel mutations in ichthyosis bullosa of Siemens. J Invest Dermatol 1998; 111: 817–821.

114 Basarab T, Smith FJD, Jolliffe VML et al. Ichthyosis bullosa of Siemens: report of a family with evidence of a keratin 2e mutation, and a review of the literature. Br J Dermatol 1999; 140: 689–695.

115 Arin MJ, Longley MA, Epstein EH Jr et al. A novel mutation in the 1A domain of keratin 2e in ichthyosis bullosa of Siemens. J Invest Dermatol 1999; 112: 380–382.

116 Takizawa Y, Akiyama M, Nagashima M, Shimizu H. A novel asparagine → aspartic acid mutation in the rod 1A domain in keratin 2e in a Japanese family with ichthyosis bullosa of Siemens. J Invest Dermatol 2000; 114: 193–195.

117 Irvine AD, Smith FJD, Shum KW et al. A novel mutation in the 2B domain of keratin 2e causing ichthyosis bullosa of Siemens. Clin Exp Dermatol 2000; 25: 648–651.

118 Steijlen PM, Kramer H, Vakilzadeh F et al. Genetic linkage of the keratin type II gene cluster with ichthyosis bullosa of Siemens and with autosomal dominant ichthyosis exfoliativa. J Invest Dermatol 1994; 103: 282–285.

119 Vakilzadeh F, Kolde G. Autosomal dominant ichthyosis exfoliativa. Br J Dermatol 1991; 124: 191–194.

120 Holbrook KA. Progress in prenatal diagnosis of bullous congenital ichthyosiform erythroderma (epidermolytic hyperkeratosis). Semin Dermatol 1984; 3: 216–220.

121 Rothnagel JA, Longley MA, Holder RA et al. Prenatal diagnosis of epidermolytic hyperkeratosis by direct gene sequencing. J Invest Dermatol 1994; 102: 13–16.

122 Ackerman AB. Histopathologic concept of epidermolytic hyperkeratosis. Arch Dermatol 1970; 102: 253–259.

123 Wilgram GF, Caulfield JB. An electron microscopic study of epidermolytic hyperkeratosis. Arch Dermatol 1966; 94: 127–143.

124 Ishida-Yamamoto A, Eady RAJ, Underwood RA et al. Filaggrin expression in epidermolytic ichthyosis (epidermolytic hyperkeratosis). Br J Dermatol 1994; 131: 767–779.

125 Yoshiike T, Manabe M, Negi M, Ogawa H. Ichthyosis linearis circumflexa: morphological and biochemical studies. Br J Dermatol 1985; 112: 277–283.

126 Suga Y, Tsuboi R, Hashimoto Y et al. A case of ichthyosis linearis circumflexa successfully treated with topical tacrolimus. J Am Acad Dermatol 2000; 42: 520–522.

127 Gambichler T, Senger E, Altmeyer P, Hoffmann K. Clearance of ichthyosis linearis circumflexa with balneophototherapy. J Eur Acad Dermatol Venereol 2000; 14: 397–399.

128 Greene SL, Muller SA. Netherton's syndrome. Report of a case and review of the literature. J Am Acad Dermatol 1985; 13: 329–337.

129 Judge MR, Morgan G, Harper JI. A clinical and immunological study of Netherton's syndrome. Br J Dermatol 1994; 131: 615–621.

130 Cockayne SE, Lee JA, Harrington CI. Oleogranulomatous response in lymph nodes associated with emollient use in Netherton's syndrome. Br J Dermatol 1999; 141: 562–564.

131 Van Gysel D, Koning H, Baert MRM et al. Clinico-immunological heterogeneity in Comèl–Netherton syndrome. Dermatology 2001; 202: 99–107.

132 Fartasch M, Williams ML, Elias PM. Altered lamellar body secretion and stratum corneum membrane structure in Netherton syndrome. Arch Dermatol 1999; 135: 823–832.

133 Caputo R, Vanotti P, Bertani E. Netherton's syndrome in two adult brothers. Arch Dermatol 1984; 120: 220–222.

134 De Felipe I, Vázquez-Doval FJ, Vicente J. Comèl–Netherton syndrome. A diagnostic challenge. Br J Dermatol 1997; 137: 468–469.

135 Powell J, Dawber RPR, Ferguson DJP, Griffiths WAD. Netherton's syndrome: increased likelihood of diagnosis by examining eyebrow hairs. Br J Dermatol 1999; 141: 544–546.

136 Ansai S, Mitsuhashi Y, Sasaki K. Netherton's syndrome in siblings. Br J Dermatol 1999; 141: 1097–1100.

137 Stryk S, Siegfried EC, Knutsen AP. Selective antibody deficiency to bacterial polysaccharide antigens in patients with Netherton syndrome. Pediatr Dermatol 1999; 16: 19–22.

138 Föster-Holst R, Swensson O, Stockfleth E et al. Comèl–Netherton syndrome complicated by papillomatous skin lesions containing human papillomaviruses 51 and 52 and plane warts containing human papillomavirus 16. Br J Dermatol 1999; 140: 1139–1143.

139 Weber F, Fuchs PG, Pfister HJ et al. Human papillomavirus infection in Netherton's syndrome. Br J Dermatol 2001; 144: 1044–1049.

140 Schneider I, Sebök B, Kosztolányi G, Szekeres G. Comel–Netherton syndrome: evolution of manifestation in a 20-year follow-up and phenotypic overlap with peeling skin syndrome type B. Acta Derm Venereol 2000; 80: 209–210.

141 Chavanas S, Garner C, Bodemer C et al. Localization of the Netherton syndrome gene to chromosome 5q32, by linkage analysis and homozygosity mapping. Am J Hum Genet 2000; 66: 914–921.

142 Altman J, Stroud J. Netherton's syndrome and ichthyosis linearis circumflexa. Arch Dermatol 1969; 100: 550–558.

143 Hendrix JD Jr, Greer KE. Erythrokeratodermia variabilis present at birth: case report and review of the literature. Pediatr Dermatol 1995; 12: 351–354.

144 Armstrong DKB, Hutchinson TH, Walsh MY, McMillan JC. Autosomal recessive inheritance of erythrokeratoderma variabilis. Pediatr Dermatol 1997; 14: 355–358.

145 Gewirtzman GB, Winkler NW, Dobson RL. Erythrokeratodermia variabilis. A family study. Arch Dermatol 1978; 114: 259–261.

146 Knipe RC, Flowers FP, Johnson FR Jr et al. Erythrokeratodermia variabilis: case report and review of the literature. Pediatr Dermatol 1995; 12: 21–23.

147 Rajagopalan B, Pulimood S, George S, Jacob M. Erythrokeratoderma en cocardes. Clin Exp Dermatol 1999; 24: 173–174.

148 Ishida-Yamamoto A, Kelsell D, Common J et al. A case of erythrokeratoderma variabilis without mutations in connexin 31. Br J Dermatol 2000; 143: 1283–1287.

149 Niemi K-M, Kanerva L. Histological and ultrastructural study of a family with erythrokeratodermia progressiva symmetrica. J Cutan Pathol 1993; 20: 242–249.

150 McFadden N, Oppedal BR, Ree K, Brandtzaeg P. Erythrokeratodermia variabilis: immunohistochemical and ultrastructural studies of the epidermis. Acta Derm Venereol 1987; 67: 284–288.

151 Richard G, Lin J-P, Smith L et al. Linkage studies in erythrokeratodermias: fine mapping, genetic heterogeneity, and analysis of candidate genes. J Invest Dermatol 1997; 109: 666–671.

152 Macari F, Landau M, Cousin P et al. Mutation in the gene for connexin 30.3 in a family with erythrokeratodermia variabilis. Am J Hum Genet 2000; 67: 1296–1301.

153 Wilgoss A, Leigh IM, Barnes MR et al. Identification of a novel mutation R42P in the gap junction protein β-3 associated with autosomal dominant erythrokeratoderma variabilis. J Invest Dermatol 1999; 113: 1119–1122.

154 Ishida-Yamamoto A, Kato H, Kiyama H et al. Mutant loricrin is not crosslinked into the cornified cell envelope but is translocated into the nucleus in loricrin keratoderma. J Invest Dermatol 2000; 115: 1088–1094.

155 Ishida-Yamamoto A, Tanaka H, Nakane H et al. Programmed cell death in normal epidermis and loricin keratoderma. Multiple functions of profilaggrin in keratinization. J Invest Dermatol (Symposium Proceedings) 1999; 4: 145–149.

156 Rappaport IP, Goldes JA, Goltz RW. Erythrokeratodermia variabilis treated with isotretinoin. A clinical, histologic, and ultrastructural study. Arch Dermatol 1986; 122: 441–445.

157 Roberts LJ. Long-term survival of a harlequin fetus. J Am Acad Dermatol 1989; 21: 335–339.

158 Baden HP, Kubilus J, Rosenbaum K, Fletcher A. Keratinization in the harlequin fetus. Arch Dermatol 1982; 118: 14–18.

159 Dale BA, Holbrook KA, Fleckman P et al. Heterogeneity in harlequin ichthyosis, an inborn error of epidermal keratinization: variable morphology and structural protein expression and a defect in lamellar granules. J Invest Dermatol 1990; 94: 6–18.

160 Dale BA, Kam E. Harlequin ichthyosis. Variability in expression and hypothesis for disease mechanism. Arch Dermatol 1993; 129: 1471–1477.

161 Unamuno P, Pierola JM, Fernandez E et al. Harlequin foetus in four siblings. Br J Dermatol 1987; 116: 569–572.

162 Blanchet-Bardon C, Dumez Y. Prenatal diagnosis of a harlequin fetus. Semin Dermatol 1984; 3: 225–228.

163 Akiyama M, Kim D-K, Main DM et al. Characteristic morphologic abnormality of harlequin ichthyosis detected in amniotic fluid cells. J Invest Dermatol 1994; 102: 210–213.

164 Elias PM, Fartasch M, Crumrine D et al. Origin of the corneocyte lipid envelope (CLE): observations in harlequin ichthyosis and cultured human keratinocytes. J Invest Dermatol 2000; 115: 765–769.

165 Buxman MM, Goodkin PE, Fahrenbach WH, Dimond RL. Harlequin ichthyosis with epidermal lipid abnormality. Arch Dermatol 1979; 115: 189–193.

166 Haftek M, Cambazard F, Dhouailly D et al. A longitudinal study of a harlequin infant presenting clinically as non-bullous congenital ichthyosiform erythroderma. Br J Dermatol 1996; 135: 448–453.

167 Choate KA, Williams ML, Elias PM, Khavari PA. Transglutaminase 1 expression in a patient with features of harlequin ichthyosis: Case report. J Am Acad Dermatol 1998; 38: 325–329.

168 Akiyama M, Yoneda K, Kim S-Y et al. Cornified cell envelope proteins and keratins are normally distributed in harlequin ichthyosis. J Cutan Pathol 1996; 23: 571–575.

169 Dahlstrom JE, McDonald T, Maxwell L, Jain S. Harlequin ichthyosis – a case report. Pathology 1995; 27: 289–292.

170 Hashimoto K, Khan S. Harlequin fetus with abnormal lamellar granules and giant mitochondria. J Cutan Pathol 1992; 19: 247–252.

171 Fleck RM, Barnadas M, Schulz WW et al. Harlequin ichthyosis: an ultrastructural study. J Am Acad Dermatol 1989; 21: 999–1006.

172 Milner ME, O'Guin WM, Holbrook KA, Dale BA. Abnormal lamellar granules in harlequin ichthyosis. J Invest Dermatol 1992; 99: 824–829.

173 Hashimoto K, de Dobbeleer G, Kanzaki T. Electron microscopic studies of harlequin fetuses. Pediatr Dermatol 1993; 10: 214–223.

174 Sandler B, Hashimoto K. Collodion baby and lamellar ichthyosis. J Cutan Pathol 1998; 25: 116–121.

175 Hazell M, Marks R. Follicular ichthyosis. Br J Dermatol 1984; 111: 101–109.

176 Rothe MJ, Weiss DS, Dubner BH et al. Ichthyosis follicularis in two girls: an autosomal dominant disorder. Pediatr Dermatol 1990; 7: 287–292.

177 Eramo LR, Esterly NB, Zieserl EJ et al. Ichthyosis follicularis with alopecia and photophobia. Arch Dermatol 1985; 121: 1167–1174.

178 Dykes PJ, Marks R. Acquired ichthyosis: multiple causes for an acquired generalized disturbance in desquamation. Br J Dermatol 1977; 97: 327–334.

179 Yokote R, Iwatsuki K, Hashizume H, Takigawa M. Lymphomatoid papulosis associated with acquired ichthyosis. J Am Acad Dermatol 1994; 30: 889–892.

180 Lowenstein EJ, Gordon RE, Phelps RG. Sympathectomy-induced ichthyosis-like eruption. Int J Dermatol 2000; 39: 146–151.

181 Kaplan MH, Sadick NS, McNutt NS et al. Acquired ichthyosis in concomitant HIV-I and HTLV-II infection: a new association with intravenous drug abuse. J Am Acad Dermatol 1993; 29: 701–708.

182 Kauh YC, Goody HE, Luscombe HA. Ichthyosiform sarcoidosis. Arch Dermatol 1978; 114: 100–101.

183 Banse-Kupin L, Pelachyk JM. Ichthyosiform sarcoidosis. Report of two cases and a review of the literature. J Am Acad Dermatol 1987; 17: 616–620.

184 De la Cruz-Álvarez J, Allegue F, Oliver J. Acquired ichthyosis associated with eosinophilic fasciitis. J Am Acad Dermatol 1996; 34: 1079–1080.

185 Aram H. Acquired ichthyosis and related conditions. Int J Dermatol 1984; 23: 458–461.

186 Lee JY-Y. Pathogenesis of abnormal keratinization in ichthyosiform cetrimide dermatitis: an ultrastructural study. Am J Dermatopathol 1997; 19: 162–167.

187 Spelman LJ, Strutton GM, Robertson IM, Weedon D. Acquired ichthyosis in bone marrow transplant recipients. J Am Acad Dermatol 1996; 35: 17–20.

188 Kahana M, Levy A, Ronnen M et al. Pityriasis rotunda in a white patient. Report of the second case and review of the literature. J Am Acad Dermatol 1986; 15: 362–365.

189 Rubin MG, Mathes B. Pityriasis rotunda: two cases in black Americans. J Am Acad Dermatol 1986; 14: 74–78.

190 DiBisceglie AM, Hodkinson HJ, Berkowitz I, Kew MC. Pityriasis rotunda. A cutaneous marker of hepatocellular carcinoma in South African blacks. Arch Dermatol 1986; 122: 802–804.

191 Berkowitz I, Hodkinson HJ, Kew MC, DiBisceglie AM. Pityriasis rotunda as a cutaneous marker of hepatocellular carcinoma: a comparison with its prevalence in other diseases. Br J Dermatol 1989; 120: 545–549.

192 Segal R, Hodak E, Sandbank M. Pityriasis rotunda in a Caucasian woman from the Mediterranean area. Clin Exp Dermatol 1989; 14: 325–327.

193 Gibbs S. Pityriasis rotunda in Tanzania. Br J Dermatol 1996; 135: 491–492.

194 Grimalt R, Gelmetti C, Brusasco A et al. Pityriasis rotunda: report of a familial occurrence and review of the literature. J Am Acad Dermatol 1994; 31: 866–871.

195 Aste N, Pau M, Aste N, Biggio P. Pityriasis rotunda: a survey of 42 cases observed in Sardinia, Italy. Dermatology 1997; 194: 32–35.

196 Davies MG, Marks R, Dykes PJ, Reynolds D. Epidermal abnormalities in Refsum's disease. Br J Dermatol 1977; 97: 401–406.

197 Srebrnik A, Tur E, Perluk C et al. Dorfman–Chanarin syndrome. A case report and a review. J Am Acad Dermatol 1987; 17: 801–808.

198 Liden S, Jagell S. The Sjögren–Larsson syndrome. Int J Dermatol 1984; 23: 247–253.

199 Nigro JF, Rizzo WB, Esterly NB. Redefining the Sjögren–Larsson syndrome: Atypical findings in three siblings and implications regarding diagnosis. J Am Acad Dermatol 1996; 35: 678–684.

200 Levisohn D, Dintiman B, Rizzo WB. Sjögren–Larsson syndrome: case reports. Pediatr Dermatol 1991; 8: 217–220.

201 Taube B, Billeaud C, Labrèze C et al. Sjögren–Larsson syndrome: early diagnosis, dietary management and biochemical studies in two cases. Dermatology 1999; 198: 340–345.

202 Willemsen MAAP, Steijlen PM, de Jong JGN et al. A novel 4 bp deletion mutation in the FALDH gene segregating in a Turkish family with Sjögren–Larsson syndrome. J Invest Dermatol 1999; 112: 827–828.

203 Aoki N, Suzuki H, Ito K, Ito M. A novel point mutation of the *FALDH* gene in a Japanese family with Sjögren–Larsson syndrome. J Invest Dermatol 2000; 114: 1065–1066.

204 Kawakami T, Saito R, Fujikawa Y et al. Incomplete Sjögren–Larsson syndrome in two Japanese siblings. Dermatology 1999; 198: 93–96.

205 Rizzo WB, Carney G, Lin Z. The molecular basis of Sjögren–Larsson syndrome: mutation analysis of the fatty aldehyde dehydrogenase gene. Am J Hum Genet 1999; 65: 1547–1560.

206 Trepeta R, Stenn KS, Mahoney MJ. Prenatal diagnosis of Sjögren–Larsson syndrome. Semin Dermatol 1984; 3: 221–224.

207 Hofer PA, Jagell S. Sjögren–Larsson syndrome: a dermato-histopathological study. J Cutan Pathol 1982; 9: 360–376.

208 Harms M, Gilardi S, Levy PM, Saurat JH. KID syndrome (keratitis, ichthyosis, and deafness) and chronic mucocutaneous candidiasis: case report and review of the literature. Pediatr Dermatol 1984; 2: 1–7.

209 Grob JJ, Breton A, Bonafe JL et al. Keratitis, ichthyosis, and deafness (KID) syndrome. Vertical transmission and death from multiple squamous cell carcinomas. Arch Dermatol 1987; 123: 777–782.

210 Mallory SB, Haynie LS, Williams ML, Hall W. Ichthyosis, deafness, and Hirschsprung's disease. Pediatr Dermatol 1989; 6: 24–27.

211 Singh K. Keratitis, ichthyosis and deafness (KID syndrome). Australas J Dermatol 1987; 28: 38–41.

212 McGrae JD Jr. Keratitis, ichthyosis, and deafness (KID) syndrome with adult onset of keratitis component. Int J Dermatol 1990; 29: 145–146.

213 McGrae JD Jr. Keratitis, ichthyosis, and deafness (KID) syndrome. Int J Dermatol 1990; 29: 89–93.

214 Hazen PG, Walker AE, Stewart JJ et al. Keratitis, ichthyosis, and deafness (KID) syndrome: management with chronic oral ketoconazole therapy. Int J Dermatol 1992; 31: 58–59.

215 Langer K, Konrad K, Wolff K. Keratitis, ichthyosis and deafness (KID)-syndrome: report of three cases and a review of the literature. Br J Dermatol 1990; 122: 689–697.

216 De Berker D, Branford WA, Soucek S, Michaels L. Fatal keratitis ichthyosis and deafness syndrome (KIDS): aural, ocular, and cutaneous histopathology. Am J Dermatopathol 1993; 15: 64–69.

217 Caceres-Rios H, Tamayo-Sanchez L, Duran-Mckinster C et al. Keratitis, ichthyosis, and deafness (KID syndrome): review of the literature and proposal of a new terminology. Pediatr Dermatol 1996; 13: 105–113.

218 Alli N, Güngör E. Keratitis, ichthyosis and deafness (KID) syndrome. Int J Dermatol 1997; 36: 37–39.

219 Koné-Paut I, Hesse S, Palix C et al. Keratitis, ichthyosis, and deafness (KID) syndrome in half sibs. Pediatr Dermatol 1998; 15: 219–221.

220 Nousari HC, Kimyai-Asadi A, Pinto JL. KID syndrome associated with features of ichthyosis hystrix. Pediatr Dermatol 2000; 17: 115–117.

221 Chastain MA, Russo GG, Boh EE. KID syndrome: report of a case and support for its reclassification as an ectodermal dysplasia. Pediatr Dermatol 2000; 17: 244–245.

222 Kalter DC, Atherton DJ, Clayton PT. X-linked dominant Conradi–Hünermann syndrome presenting as congenital erythroderma. J Am Acad Dermatol 1989; 21: 248–256.

223 Corbi MR, Conejo-Mir JS, Linares M et al. Conradi–Hünermann syndrome with unilateral distribution. Pediatr Dermatol 1998; 15: 299–303.

224 Bruch D, Megahed M, Majewski F, Ruzicka T. Ichthyotic and psoriasiform skin lesions along Blaschko's lines in a woman with X-linked dominant chondrodysplasia punctata. J Am Acad Dermatol 1995; 33: 356–360.

225 DiPreta EA, Smith KJ, Skelton H. Cholesterol metabolism defect associated with Conradi–Hunerman–Happle syndrome. Int J Dermatol 2000; 39: 846–850.

226 Emami S, Hanley KP, Esterly NB. X-linked dominant ichthyosis with peroxisomal deficiency. Arch Dermatol 1994; 130: 325–336.

227 Hamaguchi T, Bondar G, Siegfried E, Penneys NS. Cutaneous histopathology of Conradi–Hunermann syndrome. J Cutan Pathol 1995; 22: 38–41.

228 Yanagihara M, Ueda K, Asano N et al. Usefulness of histopathologic examination of thick scales in the diagnosis of X-linked dominant chondrodysplasia punctata (Happle). Pediatr Dermatol 1996; 13: 1–4.

229 Hebert AA, Esterly NB, Holbrook KA, Hall JC. The CHILD syndrome. Histologic and ultrastructural studies. Arch Dermatol 1987; 123: 503–509.

230 Hashimoto K, Topper S, Sharata H, Edwards M. CHILD syndrome: analysis of abnormal keratinization and ultrastructure. Pediatr Dermatol 1995; 12: 116–129.

231 Emami S, Rizzo WB, Hanley KP et al. Peroxisomal abnormality in fibroblasts from involved skin of CHILD syndrome. Arch Dermatol 1992; 128: 1213–1222.

232 Mortureux P, Taieb A, Surlève Bazeille J-E. Shwachman syndrome: a case report. Pediatr Dermatol 1992; 9: 57–61.

233 Fink-Puches R, Soyer HP, Pierer G et al. Systematized inflammatory epidermal nevus with symmetrical involvement: An unusual case of CHILD syndrome? J Am Acad Dermatol 1997; 36: 823–826.

234 Dale BA, Kimball JR, Fleckman P et al. CHILD syndrome: lack of expression of epidermal differentiation markers in lesional ichthyotic skin. J Invest Dermatol 1992; 98: 442–449.

235 Jorizzo JL, Atherton DJ, Crounse RG, Wells RS. Ichthyosis, brittle hair, impaired intelligence, decreased fertility and short stature (IBIDS syndrome). Br J Dermatol 1982; 106: 705–710.

236 Rebora A, Crovato F. PIBI(D)S syndrome – trichothiodystrophy with xeroderma pigmentosum (group D) mutation. J Am Acad Dermatol 1987; 16: 940–947.

237 Castaño Suárez E, Segurado Rodriguez A, Guerra Tapia A et al. Ichthyosis: the skin manifestation of multiple sulfatase deficiency. Pediatr Dermatol 1997; 14: 369–372.

238 Hendrix JD Jr, Patterson JW, Greer KE. Skin cancer associated with ichthyosis: The MAUIE syndrome. J Am Acad Dermatol 1997; 37: 1000–1002.

239 Bañuls J, Betlloch I, Botella R et al. Dorfman–Chanarin syndrome (neutral lipid storage disease). A case report. Clin Exp Dermatol 1994; 19: 434–437.

240 Srebrnik A, Brenner S, Ilie B, Messer G. Dorfman–Chanarin syndrome: morphologic studies and presentation of new cases. Am J Dermatopathol 1998; 20: 79–85.

241 Wollenberg A, Geiger E, Schaller M, Wolff H. Dorfman–Chanarin syndrome in a Turkish kindred: conductor diagnosis requires analysis of multiple eosinophils. Acta Derm Venereol 2000; 80: 39–43.

242 Peña-Penabad C, Almagro M, Martinez W et al. Dorfman–Chanarin syndrome (neutral lipid storage disease): new clinical features. Br J Dermatol 2001; 144: 430–432.

243 Judge MR, Atherton DJ, Salvayre R et al. Neutral lipid storage disease. Case report and lipid studies. Br J Dermatol 1994; 130: 507–510.

244 Goeteyn M, Oranje AP, Vuzevski VD et al. Ichthyosis, exocrine pancreatic insufficiency, impaired neutrophil chemotaxis, growth retardation, and metaphyseal dysplasia (Shwachman syndrome). Arch Dermatol 1991; 127: 225–230.

245 Bacen HP, Bronstein BR. Ichthyosiform dermatosis and deafness. Report of a case and review of the literature. Arch Dermatol 1988; 124: 102–106.

246 Hoeger PH, Adwani SS, Whitehead BF et al. Ichthyosiform erythroderma and cardiomyopathy: report of two cases and review of the literature. Br J Dermatol 1998; 139: 1055–1059.

247 Yos povitch G, Mevorah B, David M et al. Migratory ichthyosiform dermatosis with type 2 diabetes mellitus and insulin resistance. Arch Dermatol 1999; 135: 1237–1242.

Palmoplantar keratodermas and related conditions

248 Zemtsov A, Veitschegger M. Keratodermas. Int J Dermatol 1993; 32: 493–501.

249 Sybert VP, Dale BA, Holbrook KA. Palmar-plantar keratoderma. A clinical, ultrastructural, and biochemical study. J Am Acad Dermatol 1988; 18: 75–86.

250 Paller AS. The molecular bases for the palmoplantar keratodermas. Pediatr Dermatol 1999; 16: 483–486.

251 Stevens HP, Kelsell DP, Bryant SP et al. Linkage of an American pedigree with palmoplantar keratoderma and malignancy (palmoplantar ectodermal dysplasia type III) to 17q24. Arch Dermatol 1996; 132: 640–651.

252 Bergfeld WF, Derbes VJ, Elias PM et al. The treatment of keratosis palmaris et plantaris with isotretinoin. J Am Acad Dermatol 1982; 6: 727–731.

253 Pujol RM, Moreno A, Alomar A, de Moragas JM. Congenital ichthyosiform dermatosis with linear keratotic flexural papules and sclerosing palmoplantar keratoderma. Arch Dermatol 1989; 125: 103–106.

254 Thomas JR III, Greene SL, Su WPD. Epidermolytic palmo-plantar keratoderma. Int J Dermatol 1984; 23: 652–655.

255 Poulin Y, Perry HO, Muller SA. Olmsted syndrome – congenital palmoplantar and periorificial keratoderma. J Am Acad Dermatol 1984; 10: 600–610.

256 Steijlen PM, Neumann HAM, der Kinderen DJ et al. Congenital atrichia, palmoplantar hyperkeratosis, mental retardation, and early loss of teeth in four siblings: a new syndrome? J Am Acad Dermatol 1994; 30: 893–898.

257 Barlag KE, Goerz G, Ruzicka T, Schürer NY. Palmoplantar keratoderma with an unusual composition of stratum corneum and serum sterol derivatives: a new entity? Br J Dermatol 1995; 133: 639–643.

258 English JC III, McCollough ML. Transient reactive papulotranslucent acrokeratoderma. J Am Acad Dermatol 1996; 34: 686–687.

259 Lowes MA, Khaira GS, Holt D. Transient reactive papulotranslucent acrokeratoderma associated with cystic fibrosis. Australas J Dermatol 2000; 41: 172–174.

260 Yan AC, Aasi SZ, Alms WJ et al. Aquagenic palmoplantar keratoderma. J Am Acad Dermatol 2001; 44: 696–699.

261 Martin L, Toutain A, Guillen C et al. Inherited palmoplantar keratoderma and senscrineural deafness associated with A7445G point mutation in the mitochondrial genome. Br J Dermatol 2000; 143: 876–883.

262 Lautenschlager S, Pittelkow MR. Palmoplantar keratoderma and leukokeratosis anogenitalis: the second case of a new disease. Dermatology 1998; 197: 300–302.

263 Verplancke P, Driessen L, Wynants P, Naeyaert JM. The Schöpf–Schulz–Passarge syndrome. Dermatology 1998; 196: 463–466.

264 Menni S, Saleh F, Piccinno R et al. Palmoplantar keratoderma of Unna–Thost: response to biotin in one family. Clin Exp Dermatol 1992; 17: 337–338.

265 Sehgal VN, Kumar S, Narayan S. Hereditary palmoplantar keratoderma (four cases in three generations). Int J Dermatol 2001; 40: 130–132.

266 Hatamochi A, Nakagawa S, Ueki H et al. Diffuse palmoplantar keratoderma with deafness. Arch Dermatol 1982; 118: 605–607.

267 Gamborg Nielsen P. Diffuse palmoplantar keratoderma associated with acrocyanosis. A family study. Acta Derm Venereol 1989; 69: 156–161.

268 Hoeger PH, Yates RW, Harper JI. Palmoplantar keratoderma associated with congenital heart disease. Br J Dermatol 1998; 138: 506–509.

269 Rogozinski TT, Schwartz RA, Towpik E. Verrucous carcinoma in Unna–Thost hyperkeratosis of the palms and soles. J Am Acad Dermatol 1994; 31: 1061–1062.

270 Lucker GPH, van de Kerkhof PCM, Steijlen PM. The hereditary palmoplantar keratoses: an updated review and classification. Br J Dermatol 1994; 131: 1–14.

271 Ratnavel RC, Griffiths WAD. The inherited palmoplantar keratodermas. Br J Dermatol 1997; 137: 485–490.

272 Kimonis V, DiGiovanna JJ, Yang J-M et al. A mutation in the V1 end domain of keratin 1 in non-epidermolytic palmar-plantar keratoderma. J Invest Dermatol 1994; 103: 764–769.

273 Kansky A, Arzensek J. Is palmoplantar keratoderma of Greither's type a separate nosologic entity? Dermatologica 1979; 158: 244–248.

274 Grilli R, Aguilar A, Escalonilla P et al. *Transgrediens et progrediens* palmoplantar keratoderma (Greither's disease) with particular histopathologic findings. Cutis 2000; 65: 141–145.

275 Atherton DJ, Sutton C, Jones BM. Mutilating palmoplantar keratoderma with periorificial keratotic plaques (Olmsted's syndrome). Br J Dermatol 1990; 122: 245–252.

276 Kress DW, Seraly MP, Falo L et al. Olmsted syndrome. Case report and identification of a keratin abnormality. Arch Dermatol 1996; 132: 797–800.

277 Harms M, Bergues JP, Saurat J-H. Syndrome de Olmsted (keratodermia palmoplantaire et periorificielle congenitale). Ann Dermatol Venereol 1985; 112: 479.

278 Santos OLR, Amorim JH, Voloch K et al. The Olmsted syndrome. Int J Dermatol 1997; 36: 359–360.

279 Frias-Iniesta J, Sanchez-Pedreño P, Martinez-Escribano JA, Jimenez-Martinez A. Olmsted syndrome: report of a new case. Br J Dermatol 1997; 136: 935–938.

280 Cambiaghi S, Tadini G, Barbareschi M, Caputo R. Olmsted syndrome in twins. Arch Dermatol 1995; 131: 738–739.

281 Judge MR, Misch K, Wright P, Harper JI. Palmoplantar and periorificial keratoderma with corneal epithelial dysplasia: a new syndrome. Br J Dermatol 1991; 125: 186–188.

282 Fonseca E, Peña C, del Pozo J et al. Olmsted syndrome. J Cutan Pathol 2001; 28: 271–275.

283 Camisa C, Rossana C. Variant of keratoderma hereditaria mutilans (Vohwinkel's syndrome). Arch Dermatol 1984; 120: 1323–1328.

284 Goldfarb MT, Woo TY, Rasmussen JE. Keratoderma hereditaria mutilans (Vohwinkel's syndrome): a trial of isotretinoin. Pediatr Dermatol 1985; 2: 216–218.

285 Gibbs RC, Frank SB. Keratoderma hereditaria mutilans (Vohwinkel). Differentiating features of conditions with constriction of digits. Arch Dermatol 1966; 94: 619–625.

286 Palungwachira P, Iwahara K, Ogawa H. Keratoderma hereditaria mutilans. Etretinate treatment and electron microscope studies. Australas J Dermatol 1992; 33: 19–30.

287 Chang Sing Pang AFI, Oranje AP, Vuzevki VD, Stolz E. Successful treatment of keratoderma hereditaria mutilans with an aromatic retinoid. Arch Dermatol 1981; 117: 225–228.

288 Reddy BSN, Gupta SK. Mutilating keratoderma of Vohwinkel. Int J Dermatol 1983; 22: 530–533.

289 Singh K. Mutilating palmo-plantar keratoderma. Int J Dermatol 1986; 25: 436–439.

290 Gamborg Nielsen P. Mutilating palmo-plantar keratoderma. Acta Derm Venereol 1983; 63: 365–367.

291 Peris K, Salvati EF, Torlone G, Chimenti S. Keratoderma hereditarium mutilans (Vohwinkel's syndrome) associated with congenital deaf-mutism. Br J Dermatol 1995; 132: 617–620.

292 Solis RR, Diven DG, Trizna Z. Vohwinkel's syndrome in three generations. J Am Acad Dermatol 2001; 44: 376–378.

293 Armstrong DKB, McKenna KE, Hughes AE. A novel insertional mutation in loricrin in Vohwinkel's keratoderma. J Invest Dermatol 1998; 111: 702–704.

294 Korge BP, Ishida-Yamamoto A, Pünter C et al. Loricrin mutation in Vohwinkel's keratoderma is unique to the variant with ichthyosis. J Invest Dermatol 1997; 109: 604–610.

295 Fritsch P, Honigsman H, Jaschke E. Epidermolytic hereditary palmoplantar keratoderma. Br J Dermatol 1978; 99: 561–568.

296 Blas k LG, Dimond RL, Baughman RD. Hereditary epidermolytic palmoplantar keratoderma. Arch Dermatol 1981; 117: 229–231.

297 Camisa C, Williams H. Epidermolytic variant of hereditary palmoplantar keratoderma. Br J Dermatol 1985; 112: 221–225.

298 Kanitakis J, Tsoitis G, Kanitakis C. Hereditary epidermolytic palmoplantar keratoderma (Vörner type). J Am Acad Dermatol 1987; 17: 414–422.

299 Moriwaki S, Tanaka T, Horiguchi Y et al. Epidermolytic hereditary palmoplantar keratoderma. Arch Dermatol 1988; 124: 555–559.

300 Requena L, Schoendorff C, Sanchez Yus E. Hereditary epidermolytic palmo-plantar keratoderma (Vörner type) — report of a family and review of the literature. Clin Exp Dermatol 1991; 16: 383–388.

301 Weavers A, Kuhn A, Mahrle G. Palmoplantar keratoderma with tonotubular keratin. J Am Acad Dermatol 1991; 24: 638–642.

302 Ghali FE, Groben PA. Thickened palms and soles in a toddler. Pediatr Dermatol 1998; 15: 477–479.

303 Covello SP, Irvine AD, McKenna KE et al. Mutations in keratin K9 in kindreds with epidermolytic palmoplantar keratoderma and epidemiology in Northern Ireland. J Invest Dermatol 1998; 111: 1207–1209.

304 Blanchet-Bardon C, Nazzaro V, Chevrant-Breton J et al. Hereditary epidermolytic palmoplantar keratoderma associated with breast and ovarian cancer in a large kindred. Br J Dermatol 1987; 117: 363–370.

305 Carvajal-Huerta L. Epidermolytic palmoplantar keratoderma with woolly hair and dilated cardiomyopathy. J Am Acad Dermatol 1998; 39: 418–421.

306 Navsaria HA, Swensson O, Ratnavel RC et al. Ultrastructural changes resulting from keratin-9 gene mutations in two families with epidermolytic palmoplantar keratoderma. J Invest Dermatol 1995; 104: 425–429.

307 Bonifas JM, Matsumura K, Chen MA et al. Mutations of keratin 9 in two families with palmoplantar epidermolytic hyperkeratosis. J Invest Dermatol 1994; 103: 474–477.

308 Rothnagel JA, Wojcik S, Liefer KM et al. Mutations in the 1A domain of keratin 9 in patients with epidermolytic palmoplantar keratoderma. J Invest Dermatol 1995; 104: 430–433.

309 Mayuzumi N, Shigihara T, Ikeda S, Ogawa H. R162W mutation of keratin 9 in a family with autosomal dominant palmoplantar keratoderma with unique histologic features. J Invest Dermatol (Symposium Proceedings) 1999; 4: 150–152.

310 Coleman CM, Munro CS, Smith FJD et al. Epidermolytic palmoplantar keratoderma due to a novel type of keratin mutation, a 3-bp insertion in the keratin 9 helix termination motif. Br J Dermatol 1999; 140: 486–490.

311 Morgan VA, Byron K, Paiman L, Varigos GA. A case of spontaneous mutation in the keratin 9 gene associated with epidermolytic palmoplantar keratoderma. Australas J Dermatol 1999; 40: 215–216.

312 Szalai S, Szalai C, Becker K, Török E. Keratin 9 mutations in the coil 1A region in epidermolytic palmoplantar keratoderma. Pediatr Dermatol 1999; 16: 430–435.

313 Warmuth I, Cserhalmi-Friedman PB, Schneiderman P et al. Epidermolytic palmoplantar keratoderma in a Hispanic kindred resulting from a mutation in the keratin 9 gene. Clin Exp Dermatol 2000; 25: 244–246.

314 Mofid MZ, Costarangos C, Gruber SB, Koch SE. Hereditary epidermolytic palmoplantar keratoderma (Vörner type) in a family with Ehlers–Danlos syndrome. J Am Acad Dermatol 1998; 38: 825–830.

315 Howel-Evans W, McConnell RB, Clarke CA, Sheppard PM. Carcinoma of the oesophagus with keratosis palmaris et plantaris (tylosis). A study of two families. Q J Med 1958; 27: 413–429.

316 Yesudian P, Premalatha S, Thambiah AS. Genetic tylosis with malignancy: a study of a South Indian pedigree. Br J Dermatol 1980; 102: 597–600.

317 Thambiah AS, Yesudian P, Augustine SM et al. Tylosis following post-corrosive stricture of the oesophagus. Br J Dermatol 1975; 92: 219–221.

319 Nguyen TQ, Greer KE, Fisher GB Jr, Cooper PH. Papillon–Lefèvre syndrome. Report of two patients treated successfully with isotretinoin. J Am Acad Dermatol 1986; 15: 46–49.

319 Puliyel JM, Iyer KSS. A syndrome of keratosis palmo-plantaris congenita, pes planus, onychogryphosis, periodontosis, arachnodactyly and a peculiar acro-osteolysis. Br J Dermatol 1986; 115: 243–248.

320 Singh R, Nor M, Ghazali W. Atypical Papillon–Lefèvre syndrome: keratosis palmoplantaris with periodontopathy. Int J Dermatol 1993; 32: 450–452.

321 Reyes VO, King-Ismael D, Abad-Venida L. Papillon–Lefèvre syndrome. Int J Dermatol 1998; 37: 268–270.

322 Khandpur S, Reddy BSN. Papillon–Lefèvre syndrome with pyogenic hepatic abscess: a rare association. Pediatr Dermatol 2001; 18: 45–47.

323 Bach JN, Levan NE. Papillon–Lefèvre syndrome. Arch Dermatol 1968; 97: 154–158.

324 Nakano A, Nomura K, Nakano H et al. Papillon–Lefèvre syndrome: mutations and polymorphisms in the cathepsin C gene. J Invest Dermatol 2001; 116: 339–343.

325 Zhang Y, Lundgren T, Renvert S et al. Evidence of a founder effect for four cathepsin C gene mutations in Papillon–Lefèvre syndrome patients. J Med Genet 2001; 38: 96–101.

326 Hart TC, Hart PS, Michalec MD et al. Haim–Munk syndrome and Papillon–Lefèvre syndrome and allelic mutations in cathepsin C. J Med Genet 2000; 37: 88–94.

327 Reed ML, Stanley J, Stengel F et al. Mal de Meleda treated with 13-cis retinoic acid. Arch Dermatol 1979; 115: 605–608.

328 Lestringant GG, Frossard PM, Adeghate E, Qayed KI. Mal de Meleda: a report of four cases from the United Arab Emirates. Pediatr Dermatol 1997; 14: 186–191.

329 Bouadjar B, Benmazouzia S, Prud'homme J-F et al. Clinical and genetic studies of 3 large, consanguineous, Algerian families with mal de Meleda. Arch Dermatol 2000; 136: 1247–1252.

330 Patel H, Nardelli M, Fenn T et al. Homozygosity at chromosome 8qter in individuals affected by mal de Meleda (Meleda disease) originating from the island of Meleda. Br J Dermatol 2001; 144: 731–734.

331 Jee S-H, Lee Y-Y, Wu Y-C et al. Report of a family with mal de Meleda in Taiwan: a clinical, histopathological and immunological study. Dermatologica 1985; 171: 30–37.

332 Salamon T, Plavsic B, Nikulin A. Electron microscopic study of fingernails in the disease of Mljet (Mal de Meleda). Acta Derm Venereol 1984; 64: 302–307.

333 Chotzen VA, Starr JC, Mauro TM. Mal de Meleda in a Laotian family. Int J Dermatol 1993; 32: 602–604.

334 Rajashekhar N, Moideen R. Palmoplantar keratoderma – Mal de Meleda syndrome. Int J Dermatol 1997; 36: 854–856.

335 Bergman R, Bitterman-Deutsch O, Fartasch M et al. Mal de Meleda keratoderma with pseudoainhum. Br J Dermatol 1993; 128: 207–212.

336 Patrizi A, Di Lernia V, Patrone P. Palmoplantar keratoderma with sclerodactyly (Huriez syndrome). J Am Acad Dermatol 1992; 26: 855–857.

337 Guerriero C, Albanesi C, Girolomoni G et al. Huriez syndrome: case report with a detailed analysis of skin dendritic cells. Br J Dermatol 2000; 143: 1091–1096.

338 Kavanagh GM, Jardine PE, Peachey RD et al. The scleroatrophic syndrome of Huriez. Br J Dermatol 1997; 137: 114–118.

339 Downs AMR, Kennedy CTC. Scleroatrophic syndrome of Huriez in an infant. Pediatr Dermatol 1998; 15: 207–209.

340 Rustad OJ, Corwin Vance J. Punctate keratoses of the palms and soles and keratotic pits of the palmar creases. J Am Acad Dermatol 1990; 22: 468–476.

341 Stanimirović A, Kansky A, Basta-Juzbašić A et al. Hereditary palmoplantar keratoderma, type papulosa, in Croatia. J Am Acad Dermatol 1993; 29: 435–437.

342 Baran R, Juhlin L. Keratodermia palmoplantare papuloverrucoides progressiva: successful treatment with etretinate. J Am Acad Dermatol 1983; 8: 700–702.

343 Just M, Ribera M, Bielsa I et al. Keratosis punctata of the palmar creases: report of two cases associated with ichthyosis vulgaris. Br J Dermatol 1999; 141: 551–553.

344 Buchanan RN Jr. Keratosis punctata palmaris et plantaris. Arch Dermatol 1963; 88: 644–650.

345 Del-Rio E, Vázquez-Veiga H, Aquilar A et al. Keratosis punctata of the palmar creases. A report on three generations, demonstrating an association with ichthyosis vulgaris and evidence of involvement of the acrosyringium. Clin Exp Dermatol 1994; 19: 165–167.

346 Anderson WA, Elam MD, Lambert WC. Keratosis punctata and atopy. Report of 31 cases with a prospective study of prevalence. Arch Dermatol 1984; 120: 884–890.

347 Kalter DC, Stone MS, Kettler A et al. Keratosis punctata of the palmar creases: extremely uncommon? J Am Acad Dermatol 1986; 14: 510–511.

348 Ortega M, Quintana J, Camacho F. Keratosis punctata of the palmar creases. J Am Acad Dermatol 1985; 13: 381–382.

349 Bennion SD, Patterson JW. Keratosis punctata palmaris et plantaris and adenocarcinoma of the colon. J Am Acad Dermatol 1984; 10: 587–591.

350 Stevens HP, Kelsell DP, Leigh IM et al. Punctate palmoplantar keratoderma and malignancy in a four-generation family. Br J Dermatol 1996; 134: 720–726.

351 Stone OJ, Mullins JF. Nail changes in keratosis punctata. Arch Dermatol 1965; 92: 557–558.

352 Rubenstein DJ, Schwartz RA, Hansen RC, Payne CM. Punctate hyperkeratosis of the palms and soles. An ultrastructural study. J Am Acad Dermatol 1980; 3: 43–49.

353 Friedman SJ, Herman PS, Pittelkow MR, Su WPD. Punctate porokeratotic keratoderma. Arch Dermatol 1988; 124: 1678–1682.

354 Hashimoto K, Toi Y, Horton S, Sun T-T. Spiny keratoderma – a demonstration of hair keratin and hair type keratinization. J Cutan Pathol 1999; 26: 25–30.

355 Bernal AI, González A, Aragoneses H et al. A patient with spiny keratoderma of the palms and a lymphoproliferative syndrome: an unrelated paraneoplastic condition? Dermatology 2000; 201: 379–380.

356 Callan NJ. Circumscribed palmoplantar keratoderma. Aust J Dermatol 1970; 11: 76–81.

357 Baden HP, Bronstein BR, Rand RE. Hereditary callosities with blisters. Report of a family and review. J Am Acad Dermatol 1984; 11: 409–415.

358 Wachters DHJ, Frensdorf EL, Hausman R, van Dijk E. Keratosis palmoplantaris nummularis ('hereditary painful callosities'). Clinical and histopathologic aspects. J Am Acad Dermatol 1983; 9: 204–209.

359 Nogita T, Furue M, Nakagawa H, Ishibashi Y. Keratosis palmoplantaris nummularis. J Am Acad Dermatol 1991; 25: 113–114.

360 Casado M, Jimenez-Acosta F, Borbujo J et al. Keratoderma palmoplantaris striata. Clin Exp Dermatol 1989; 14: 240–242.

361 Sidhu GS, Cassai ND, Rico MJ. Composite keratohyaline granules in striate keratoderma. Ultrastruct Pathol 2000; 24: 391–397.

362 Whittock NV, Ashton GHS, Dopping-Hepenstal PJC et al. Striate palmoplantar keratoderma resulting from desmoplakin haploinsufficiency. J Invest Dermatol 1999; 113: 940–946.

363 Viljoen DL, Saxe N, Temple-Camp C. Cutaneous manifestations of the Proteus syndrome. Pediatr Dermatol 1988; 5: 14–21.

364 Terrinoni A, Puddu P, Didona B et al. A mutation in the V1 domain of K16 is responsible for unilateral palmoplantar verrucous nevus. J Invest Dermatol 2000; 114: 1136–1140.

365 Tan OT, Sarkany I. Severe palmar keratoderma in myxoedema. Clin Exp Dermatol 1977; 2: 287–288.

366 Hodak E, David M, Feuerman EJ. Palmoplantar keratoderma in association with myxedema. Acta Derm Venereol 1986; 66: 354–357.

367 Miller JJ, Roling D, Spiers E et al. Palmoplantar keratoderma associated with hypothyroidism. Br J Dermatol 1998; 139: 741–742.

368 Aram H, Zeidenbaum M. Palmoplantar hyperkeratosis in mycosis fungoides. J Am Acad Dermatol 1985; 13: 897–899.

369 Trattner A, Katzenelson V, Sandbank M. Palmoplantar keratoderma in a noncutaneous T-cell lymphoma. Int J Dermatol 1991; 30: 871–872.

370 Smith CH, Barker JNWN, Hay RJ. Diffuse plane xanthomatosis and acquired palmoplantar keratoderma in association with myeloma. Br J Dermatol 1995; 132: 286–289.

371 Murata Y, Kumano K, Tani M et al. Acquired diffuse keratoderma of the palms and soles with bronchial carcinoma: report of a case and review of the literature. J Am Acad Dermatol 1988; 124: 497–498.

372 Wachtel TJ. Plantar and palmar hyperkeratosis in young castrated women. Int J Dermatol 1981; 20: 270–271.

373 Breathnach SM, Wells GC. Acanthosis palmaris: tripe palms. A distinctive pattern of palmar keratoderma frequently associated with internal malignancy. Clin Exp Dermatol 1980; 5: 181–189.

374 Pujol RM, Puig L, Garcia-Marques JM, de Moragas JM. Acquired pachydermatoglyphy. A cutaneous sign of internal malignancy. Int J Dermatol 1988; 27: 688–689.

375 Cohen PR, Kurzrock R. Malignancy-associated tripe palms. J Am Acad Dermatol 1992; 27: 271–272.

376 Chosidow O, Bécherel P-A, Piette J-C et al. Tripe palms associated with systemic mastocytosis: the role of transforming growth factor-α and efficacy of interferon-alfa. Br J Dermatol 1998; 138: 698–703.

377 Duvic M, Reisman M, Finley V et al. Glucan-induced keratoderma in acquired immunodeficiency syndrome. Arch Dermatol 1987; 123: 751–756.

378 Jucglà A, Sais G, Navarro M, Peyri J. Palmoplantar keratoderma secondary to chronic acral erythema due to tegafur. Arch Dermatol 1995; 131: 364–365.

379 Won Y-H, Seo J-J, Kim S-J et al. Knuckle pad-like keratoderma: a new cutaneous side reaction induced by tegafur. Int J Dermatol 1998; 37: 315–317.

380 Poskitt LB, Duffill MB, Rademaker M. Chloracne, palmplantar keratoderma and localized scleroderma in a weed sprayer. Clin Exp Dermatol 1994; 19: 264–267.

381 Geusau A, Jurecka W, Nahavandi H et al. Punctate keratoderma-like lesions on the palms and soles in a patient with chloracne: a new clinical manifestation of dioxin intoxication? Br J Dermatol 2000; 143: 1067–1071.

382 Reed WB, Porter PS. Keratosis. Arch Dermatol 1971; 104: 99–100.

383 Di Lernia V, Cavazza A, Bisighini G. Symmetrical interdigital keratoderma of the hands. Clin Exp Dermatol 1995; 20: 240–241.

384 Lucker GPH, Steijlen PM. The Olmsted syndrome: mutilating palmoplantar and periorificial keratoderma. J Am Acad Dermatol 1994; 31: 508–509.

385 Delaporte E, N'Guyen-Mailfer C, Janin A et al. Keratoderma with scleroatrophy of the extremities or sclerotylosis (Huriez syndrome): a reappraisal. Br J Dermatol 1995; 133: 409–416.

386 Herman PS. Punctate porokeratotic keratoderma. Dermatologica 1973; 147: 206–213.

387 Caputo R, Carminati G, Ermacora E, Menni S. Keratosis punctata palmaris et plantaris as an expression of focal acantholytic dyskeratosis. Am J Dermatopathol 1989; 11: 574–576.

388 Nazzaro V, Blanchet-Bardon C, Mimoz C et al. Papillon–Lefèvre syndrome. Ultrastructural study and successful treatment with acitretin. Arch Dermatol 1988; 124: 533–539.

389 Goldsmith LA. Tyrosinemia II. Arch Intern Med 1985; 145: 1697–1700.

390 Goldsmith LA. Tyrosinemia II: lesions in molecular pathophysiology. Pediatr Dermatol 1983; 1: 25–34.

391 Hurziker N. Richner–Hanhart syndrome and tyrosinemia type II. Dermatologica 1980; 160: 180–189.

392 Fraser NG, MacDonald J, Griffiths WAD, McPhie JL. Tyrosinaemia type II (Richner–Hanhart syndrome) – report of two cases treated with etretinate. Clin Exp Dermatol 1987; 12: 440–443.

393 Goldsmith LA. Tyrosine-induced skin disease. Br J Dermatol 1978; 98: 119–123.

394 Benoldi D, Orsoni JB, Allegra F. Tyrosinemia type II: a challenge for ophthalmologists and dermatologists. Pediatr Dermatol 1997; 14: 110–112.

395 Rehak A, Selim MM, Yadav G. Richner–Hanhart syndrome (tyrosinaemia-II) (report of four cases without ocular involvement). Br J Dermatol 1981; 104: 469–475.

396 Zaleski WA, Hill A, Kushniruk W. Skin lesions in tyrosinosis: response to dietary treatment. Br J Dermatol 1973; 88: 335–340.

397 Machino H, Miki Y, Kawatsu T et al. Successful dietary control of tyrosinemia II. J Am Acad Dermatol 1983; 9: 533–539.

398 Shimizu N, Ito M, Ito K et al. Richner–Hanhart's syndrome. Electron microscopic study of the skin lesion. Arch Dermatol 1990; 126: 1342–1346.

399 Goldsmith LA, Kang E, Bienfang DC et al. Tyrosinemia with plantar and palmar keratosis and keratitis. J Pediatr 1973; 83: 798–805.

400 Solomon LM, Cook B, Klipfel W. The ectodermal dysplasias. Dermatol Clin 1987; 5 231–237.

401 McNaughton PZ, Pierson DL, Rodman OG. Hidrotic ectodermal dysplasia in a black mother and daughter. Arch Dermatol 1976; 112: 1448–1450.

402 Rajagopalan K, Tay CH. Hidrotic ectodermal dysplasia. Study of a large Chinese pedigree. Arch Dermatol 1977; 113: 481–485.

403 Rahbari H. Acrokeratoelastoidosis and keratoelastoidosis marginalis – any relation? J Am Acad Dermatol 1981; 5: 348–350.

404 Johansson EA, Kariniemi AL, Niemi KM. Palmoplantar keratoderma of punctate type: acrokeratoelastoidosis Costa. Acta Derm Venereol 1980; 60: 149–153.

405 Costa OG. Akrokerato-elastoidosis (a hitherto undescribed skin disease). Dermatologica 1953; 107: 164–168.

406 Nelson-Adesokan P, Mallory SB, Lombardi C, Lund R. Acrokeratoelastoidosis of Costa. Int J Dermatol 1995; 34: 431–433.

407 Highet AS, Rook A, Anderson JR. Acrokeratoelastoidosis. Br J Dermatol 1982; 106: 337–344.

408 Shbaklo Z, Jamaleddine NF, Kibbi A-G et al. Acrokeratoelastoidosis. Int J Dermatol 1990; 29: 333–336.

409 Matthews CNA, Harman RRM. Acrokerato-elastoidosis in a Somerset mother and her two sons. Br J Dermatol (Suppl) 1977; 15: 42–43.

410 Korc A, Hansen RC, Lynch PJ. Acrokeratoelastoidosis of Costa in North America. A report of two cases. J Am Acad Dermatol 1985; 12: 832–836.

411 Abulafia J, Vignale RA. Degenerative collagenous plaques of the hands and acrokeratoelastoidosis: pathogenesis and relationship with knuckle pads. Int J Dermatol 2000; 39: 424–432.

412 Jung EG, Beil FU, Anton-Lamprecht I et al. Akrokeratoelastoidosis. Hautarzt 1974; 25: 127–133.

413 Dowd PM, Harman RRM, Black MM. Focal acral hyperkeratosis. Br J Dermatol 1983; 109: 97–103.

414 Handfield-Jones S, Kennedy CTC. Acrokeratoelastoidosis treated with etretinate. J Am Acad Dermatol 1987; 17: 881–882.

415 Satoh T, Yokozeki H, Katayama I, Nishioka K. A new variant of punctate acrokeratoderma associated with a pigmentary disorder. Br J Dermatol 1993; 128: 693–695.

416 Masse R, Quillard A, Hery B et al. Acrokerato-elastoidose de Costa. Ann Dermatol Venereol 1977; 104: 441–445.

417 Haber RM, Rose TH. Autosomal recessive pachyonychia congenita. Arch Dermatol 1986; 122: 919–923.

418 Su WPD, Chun SI, Hammond DE, Gordon H. Pachyonychia congenita: a clinical study of 12 cases and review of the literature. Pediatr Dermatol 1990; 7: 33–38.

419 Munro CS. Pachyonychia congenita: mutations and clinical presentations. Br J Dermatol 2001; 144: 929–930.

420 Schönfeld PHIR. The pachyonychia congenita syndrome. Acta Derm Venereol 1980; 60: 45–49.

421 Mawhinney H, Creswell S, Beare JM. Pachyonychia congenita with candidiasis. Clin Exp Dermatol 1981; 6: 145–149.

422 Smith FJD, Del Monaco M, Steijlen PM et al. Novel proline substitution mutations in keratin 16 in two cases of pachyonychia congenita type 1. Br J Dermatol 1999; 141: 1010–1016.

423 Vineyard WR, Scott RA. Steatocystoma multiplex with pachyonychia congenita. Arch Dermatol 1961; 84: 824–827.

424 Soderquist NA, Reed WB. Pachyonychia congenita with epidermal cysts and other congenital dyskeratoses. Arch Dermatol 1968; 97: 31–33.

425 Feinstein A, Friedman J, Schewach-Millet M. Pachyonychia congenita. J Am Acad Dermatol 1988; 19: 705–711.

426 Iraci S, Bianchi L, Gatti S et al. Pachyonychia congenita with late onset of nail dystrophy – a new clinical entity? Clin Exp Dermatol 1993; 18: 478–480.

427 Lucker GPH, Steijlen PM. Pachyonychia congenita tarda. Clin Exp Dermatol 1995; 20: 226–229.

428 Mouaci-Midoun N, Cambiaghi S, Abimelec P. Pachyonychia congenita tarda. J Am Acad Dermatol 1996; 35: 334–335.

429 Hannaford RS, Stapleton K. Pachyonychia congenita tarda. Australas J Dermatol 2000; 41: 175–177.

430 Çelebi JT, Tanzi EL, Yao YJ et al. Identification of a germline mutation in keratin 7 in a family with pachyonychia congenita type 2. J Invest Dermatol 1999; 113: 848–850.

431 Fujimoto W, Nakanishi G, Hirakawa S et al. Pachyonychia congenita type 2: Keratin 17 mutation in a Japanese case. J Am Acad Dermatol 1998; 38: 1007–1009.

432 Covello SP, Smith FJD, Sillevis Smitt JH et al. Keratin 17 mutations cause either steatocystoma multiplex or pachyonychia congenita type 2. Br J Dermatol 1998; 139: 475–480.

433 McLean WHI, Rugg EL, Lunny DP et al. Keratin 16 and keratin 17 mutations cause pachyonychia congenita. Nat Genet 1995; 9: 273–278.

434 Connors JB, Rahil AK, Smith FJD et al. Delayed-onset pachyonychia congenita associated with a novel mutation in the central 2B domain of keratin 16. Br J Dermatol 2001; 144: 1058–1062.

435 Kopera D, Soyer HP, Kerl H. Ectopic calcaneal nail. J Am Acad Dermatol 1996; 35: 484–485.

436 Forslind B, Nylen B, Swanbeck G et al. Pachyonychia congenita. A histologic and microradiographic study. Acta Derm Venereol 1973; 53: 211–216.

437 Anneroth G, Isacsson G, Lagerholm B et al. Pachyonychia congenita. Acta Derm Venereol 1975; 55: 387–394.

438 Kelly EW Jr, Pinkus H. Report of a case of pachyonychia congenita. Arch Dermatol 1958; 77: 724–726.

439 Witkop CJ, Gorlin RJ. Four hereditary mucosal syndromes. Arch Dermatol 1961; 84: 762–771.

440 Thormann J, Kobayasi T. Pachyonychia congenita Jadassohn–Lewandowsky: a disorder of keratinization. Acta Derm Venereol 1977; 57: 63–67.

441 Wilkin JK, Rosenberg EW, Kanzaki T. Cornoid lamella in pachyonychia congenita. Arch Dermatol 1978; 114: 1795–1796.

442 Ruiz-Maldonado R, Tamayo L. Pachyonychia congenita (Jadassohn–Lewandowsky) and Kyrle's disease in the same patient. Int J Dermatol 1977; 16: 675–678.

443 Tidman MJ, Wells RS, MacDonald DM. Pachyonychia congenita with cutaneous amyloidosis and hyperpigmentation – a distinct variant. J Am Acad Dermatol 1987; 16: 935–940.

Cornoid lamellation

444 Reed RJ, Leone P. Porokeratosis – a mutant clonal keratosis of the epidermis. . Histogenesis. Arch Dermatol 1970; 101: 340–347.

445 Wade TR, Ackerman AB. Cornoid lamellation. A histologic reaction pattern. Am J Dermatopathol 1980; 2: 5–15.

446 Otsuka F, Shima A, Ishibashi Y. Porokeratosis as a premalignant condition of the skin. Cytologic demonstration of abnormal DNA ploidy in cells of the epidermis. Cancer 1989; 63: 891–896.

447 Otsuka F, Shima A, Ishibashi Y. Porokeratosis has neoplastic clones in the epidermis: microfluorometric analysis of DNA content of epidermal cell nuclei. J Invest Dermatol 1989; 92: 231s–233s.

448 Gray MH, Smoller BS, McNutt NS. Carcinogenesis in porokeratosis. Evidence for a role relating to chronic growth activation of keratinocytes. Am J Dermatopathol 1991; 13: 438–444.

449 Ito M, Fujiwara H, Maruyama T et al. Morphogenesis of the cornoid lamella: histochemical, immunohistochemical, and ultrastructural study of porokeratosis. J Cutan Pathol 1991; 18: 247–256.

450 Magee JW, McCalmont TH, LeBoit PE. Overexpression of p53 tumor suppressor protein in porokeratosis. Arch Dermatol 1994; 130: 187–190.

451 Puig L, Alegre M, Costa I et al. Overexpression of p53 in disseminated superficial actinic porokeratosis with and without malignant degeneration. Arch Dermatol 1995; 131: 353–354.

452 Quinn AG. p21[Waf1/Cip1] and p53 expression in the skin – intertwined but not inseparable. Br J Dermatol 1999; 141: 614–616.

453 Nelson C, Cowper S, Morgan M. p53, mdm-2, and p21[waf-1] in the porokeratoses. Am J Dermatopathol 1999; 21: 420–425.

454 Chernosky ME. Porokeratosis. Arch Dermatol 1986; 122: 869–870.

455 Otsuka F, Watanabe R, Kawashima M et al. Porokeratosis with large skin lesions. Acta Derm Venereol 1991; 71: 437–440.

456 Jacyk WK, Esplin L. Hyperkeratotic form of porokeratosis of Mibelli. Int J Dermatol 1993; 32: 902–903.

457 Mikhail GR, Wertheimer FW. Clinical variants of porokeratosis (Mibelli). Arch Dermatol 1968; 98: 124–131.

458 Dupre A, Christol B. Mibelli's porokeratosis of the lips. Arch Dermatol 1978; 114: 1841–1842.

459 Rosón E, García-Doval I, De La Torre C et al. Disseminated superficial porokeratosis with mucosal involvement. Acta Derm Venereol 2001; 81: 64–65.

460 Enk A, Bork K, Hoede N, Knop J. Atypical facial porokeratosis of Mibelli. Br J Dermatol 1991; 125: 596–598.

461 Ranbari H, Fazel Z, Mehregan AH. Destructive facial porokeratosis. J Am Acad Dermatol 1995; 33: 1049–1050.

462 Tangoren IA, Weinberg JM, Ioffreda M et al. Penile porokeratosis of Mibelli. J Am Acad Dermatol 1997; 36: 479–481.

463 Porter WM, Menagé HDuP, Philip G, Bunker CB. Porokeratosis of the penis. Br J Dermatol 2001; 144: 643–644.

464 Levell NJ, Bewley AP, Levene GM. Porokeratosis of Mibelli on the penis, scrotum and natal cleft. Clin Exp Dermatol 1994; 19: 77–78.

465 Stone N, Ratnavel R, Wilkinson JD. Bilateral perianal inflammatory verrucous porokeratosis (porokeratosis ptychotropica). Br J Dermatol 1999; 140: 553–555.

466 Trcka J, Pettke-Rank CV, Bröcker E-B, Hamm H. Genitoanocrural porokeratosis following chronic exposure to benzene. Clin Exp Dermatol 1998; 23: 28–31.

467 Lucker GPH, Happle R, Steijlen PM. An unusual case of porokeratosis involving the natal cleft: porokeratosis ptychotropica? Br J Dermatol 1995; 132: 150–151.

468 Nova MP, Goldberg LJ, Mattison T, Halperin A. Porokeratosis arising in a burn scar. J Am Acad Dermatol 1991; 25: 354–356.

469 Morton CA, Shuttleworth D, Douglas WS. Porokeratosis and Crohn's disease. J Am Acad Dermatol 1995; 32: 894–897.

470 Hernandez MH, Lai C-H, Mallory SB. Disseminated porokeratosis associated with chronic renal failure: a new type of disseminated porokeratosis? Arch Dermatol 2000; 136: 1568–1569.

471 Kono T, Kobayashi H, Ishii M et al. Synchronous development of disseminated superficial porokeratosis and hepatitis C virus-related hepatocellular carcinoma. J Am Acad Dermatol 2000; 43: 966–968.

472 Herranz P, Pizarro A, De Lucas R et al. High incidence of porokeratosis in renal transplant recipients. Br J Dermatol 1997; 136: 176–179.

473 Knoell KA, Patterson JW, Wilson BB. Sudden onset of disseminated porokeratosis of Mibelli in a renal transplant patient. J Am Acad Dermatol 1999; 41: 830–832.

474 Kanitakis J, Euvrard S, Claudy A. Porokeratosis in organ transplant recipients. J Am Acad Dermatol 2001; 44: 144–145.

475 Mizukawa Y, Shiohara T. Onset of porokeratosis of Mibelli in organ transplant recipients: Lack of a search for transmissible agents in these patients. J Am Acad Dermatol 2001; 44: 143–144.

476 Levin RM, Heymann WR. Superficial disseminate porokeratosis in a patient with myelodysplastic syndrome. Int J Dermatol 1999; 38: 138–139.

477 Robak E, Woźniacka A, Sysa-Jedrzejowska A et al. Disseminated superficial actinic porokeratosis in a patient with systemic lupus erythematosus. Br J Dermatol 1999; 141: 759–761.

478 Takata M, Shirasaki F, Nakatani T, Takehara K. Hereditary non-polyposis colorectal cancer associated with disseminated superficial porokeratosis. Microsatellite instability in skin tumours. Br J Dermatol 2000; 143: 851–855.

479 Nakazawa A, Matsuo I, Ohkido M. Porokeratosis localized to the access region for hemodialysis. J Am Acad Dermatol 1991; 25: 338–340.

480 Halper S, Medinica M. Porokeratosis in a patient treated with total body electron beam radiation. J Am Acad Dermatol 1990; 23: 754–755.

481 Romani J, Pujol RM, Cassanova JM, De Moragas JM. Disseminated superficial porokeratosis developing after electron-beam total skin irradiation for mycosis fungoides. Clin Exp Dermatol 1996; 21: 310–312.

482 Allen AL, Glaser DA. Disseminated superficial actinic porokeratosis associated with topical PUVA. J Am Acad Dermatol 2000; 43: 720–722.

483 Fleischer AB Jr, Donahue MJ, Feldman SR. Tanning salon porokeratosis. J Am Acad Dermatol 1993; 29: 787–788.

484 Kroiss MM, Stolz W, Hohenleutner U, Landthaler M. Disseminated superficial porokeratosis induced by furosemide. Acta Derm Venereol 2000; 80: 52–53.

485 Pirozzi DJ, Rosenthal A. Disseminated superficial actinic porokeratosis. Analysis of an affected family. Br J Dermatol 1976; 95: 429–432.

486 Schwarz T, Seiser A, Gschnait F. Disseminated superficial 'actinic' porokeratosis. J Am Acad Dermatol 1984; 11: 724–730.

487 Shumack SP, Commens CA. Disseminated superficial actinic porokeratosis: a clinical study. J Am Acad Dermatol 1989; 20: 1015–1022.

488 Böhm M, Luger TA, Bonsmann G. Disseminated superficial actinic porokeratosis: Treatment with topical tacalcitol. J Am Acad Dermatol 1999; 40: 479–480.

489 Xia J-H, Yang Y-F, Deng H et al. Identification of a locus for disseminated superficial actinic porokeratosis at chromosome 12q23.2–24.1. J Invest Dermatol 2000; 114: 1071–1074.

490 McMillan GL, Krull EA, Mikhail GR. Linear porokeratosis with giant cornoid lamella. Arch Dermatol 1976; 112: 515–516.

491 Rahbari H, Cordero AA, Mehregan AH. Linear porokeratosis. A distinctive clinical variant of porokeratosis of Mibelli. Arch Dermatol 1974; 109: 526–528.

492 Commens CA, Shumack SP. Linear porokeratosis in two families with disseminated superficial actinic porokeratosis. Pediatr Dermatol 1987; 4: 209–214.

493 Hunt SJ, Sharra G, Abell E. Linear and punctate porokeratosis associated with end-stage liver disease. J Am Acad Dermatol 1991; 25: 937–939.

494 Fisher CA, LeBoit PE, Frieden IJ. Linear porokeratosis presenting as erosions in the newborn period. Pediatr Dermatol 1995; 12: 318–322.

495 Goldman GD, Milstone LM. Generalized linear porokeratosis treated with etretinate. Arch Dermatol 1995; 131: 496–497.

496 Suh DH, Lee HS, Kim SD et al. Coexistence of disseminated superficial porokeratosis in childhood with congenital linear porokeratosis. Pediatr Dermatol 2000; 17: 466–468.

497 Razack EMA, Natarajan M. Ulcerative systematized porokeratosis (Mibelli). Arch Dermatol 1977; 113: 1583–1584.

498 Karadaglic DL, Berger S, Jankovic D, Stefanovic Z. Zosteriform porokeratosis of Mibelli. Int J Dermatol 1988; 27: 589–590.

499 Helfman RJ, Poulos EG. Reticulated porokeratosis. A unique variant of porokeratosis. Arch Dermatol 1985; 121: 1542–1543.

500 Mandojana RM, Katz R, Rodman OG. Porokeratosis plantaris discreta. J Am Acad Dermatol 1984; 10: 679–682.

501 Kang WH, Chun SI. Porokeratosis plantaris discreta. A case showing transepidermal elimination. Am J Dermatopathol 1988; 10: 229–233.

502 Korstanje MJ, Vrints LWMA. Porokeratotic palmoplantar keratoderma discreta – a new entity or a variant of porokeratosis plantaris discreta? Clin Exp Dermatol 1996; 21: 451–453.

503 Sakas EL, Gentry RH. Porokeratosis punctata palmaris et plantaris (punctate porokeratosis). Case report and literature review. J Am Acad Dermatol 1985; 13: 908–912.

504 Rahbari H, Cordero AA, Mehregan AH. Punctate porokeratosis. A clinical variant of porokeratosis of Mibelli. J Cutan Pathol 1977; 4: 338–341.

505 Roberts LC, de Villez RL. Congenital unilateral punctate porokeratosis. Am J Dermatopathol 1984; 6: 57–61.

506 Kondo S, Shimoura T, Hozumi Y, Aso K. Punctate porokeratotic keratoderma: some pathogenetic analyses of hyperproliferation and parakeratosis. Acta Derm Venereol 1990; 70: 478–482.

507 Bianchi L, Orlandi A, Iraci S et al. Punctate porokeratotic keratoderma – its occurrence with internal neoplasia. Clin Exp Dermatol 1994; 19: 139–141.

508 Lestringant GG, Berge T. Porokeratosis punctata palmaris et plantaris. A new entity? Arch Dermatol 1989; 125: 816–819.

509 Anderson D, Cohen DE, Lee HS, Thellman C. Spiny keratoderma in association with autosomal dominant polycystic kidney disease with liver cysts. J Am Acad Dermatol 1996; 34: 935–936.

510 Osman Y, Daly TJ, Don PC. Spiny keratoderma of the palms and soles. J Am Acad Dermatol 1992; 26: 879–881.

511 Fimiani M, Rubegni P, Andreassi L. Linear palmo-plantar porokeratotic hamartoma. Br J Dermatol 1996; 135: 492–494.

512 McCallister RE, Estes SA, Yarbrough CL. Porokeratosis plantaris, palmaris, et disseminata. Report of a case and treatment with isotretinoin. J Am Acad Dermatol 1985; 13: 598–603.

513 Shaw JC, White CR Jr. Porokeratosis plantaris palmaris et disseminata. J Am Acad Dermatol 1984; 11: 454–460.

514 Marschalko M, Somlai B. Porokeratosis plantaris, palmaris, et disseminata. Arch Dermatol 1986; 122: 890–891.

515 Neumann RA, Knobler RM, Gebhart W. Unusual presentation of porokeratosis palmaris, plantaris et disseminata. J Am Acad Dermatol 1989; 21: 1131–1133.

516 Patrizi A, Passarini B, Minghetti G, Masina M. Porokeratosis palmaris et plantaris disseminata: an unusual clinical presentation. J Am Acad Dermatol 1989; 21: 415–418.

517 Beers B, Jaszcz W, Sheetz K et al. Porokeratosis palmaris et plantaris disseminata. Report of a case with abnormal DNA ploidy in lesional epidermis. Arch Dermatol 1992; 128: 236–239.

518 Lucke TW, Fallowfield M, Kemmett D. A sporadic case of porokeratosis plantaris palmaris et disseminata. Br J Dermatol 1998; 138: 556–557.

519 Özkan Ş, Fetil E, Aydoğan T et al. Lack of TP53 mutations in a case of porokeratosis palmaris, plantaris and disseminata. Dermatology 2000; 201: 158–161.

520 Eng AM, Kolton B. Generalized eruptive porokeratosis of Mibelli with associated psoriasis. J Cutan Pathol 1975; 2: 203–213.

521 Štork J, Kodetová D. Disseminated superficial porokeratosis: an eruptive pruritic papular variant. Dermatology 1997; 195: 304–305.

522 Sato A, Bohm W, Bersch A. Hyperkeratotic form of porokeratosis Mibelli. Dermatologica 1977; 155: 340–349.

523 Schaller M, Korting HC, Kollmann M, Kind P. The hyperkeratotic variant of porokeratosis Mibelli is a distinct entity: clinical and ultrastructural evidence. Dermatology 1996; 192: 255–258.

524 Jang K-A, Choi J-H, Sung K-J et al. The hyperkeratotic variant of disseminated superficial actinic porokeratosis (DSAP). Int J Dermatol 1999; 38: 204–206.

525 Mehregan AH, Khalili H, Fazel Z. Mibelli's porokeratosis of the face. A report of seven cases. J Am Acad Dermatol 1980; 3: 394–396.

526 Navarro V, Pinazo I, Martínez E et al. Facial superficial porokeratosis. Dermatology 2000; 201: 361.

527 Abell E, Read SI. Porokeratotic eccrine ostial and dermal duct naevus. Br J Dermatol 1980; 103: 435–441.

528 Aloi FG, Pippione M. Porokeratotic eccrine ostial and dermal duct nevus. Arch Dermatol 1986; 122: 892–895.

529 Driban NE, Cavicchia JC. Porokeratotic eccrine ostial and dermal duct nevus. J Cutan Pathol 1987; 14: 118–121.

530 Bergman R, Lichtig C, Cohen A, Friedman-Birnbaum R. Porokeratotic eccrine ostial and dermal duct nevus. Am J Dermatopathol 1992; 14: 319–322.

531 Jiménez J, Gómez I, González C et al. Porokeratotic eccrine ostial and dermal duct naevus. Br J Dermatol 1995; 132: 490–492.

532 Del Pozo J, Martínez W, Verea MM et al. Porokeratotic eccrine ostial and dermal duct naevus: treatment with carbon dioxide laser. Br J Dermatol 1999; 141: 1144–1145.

533 Leung CS, Tang WYM, Lam WY et al. Porokeratotic eccrine ostial and dermal duct naevus with dermatomal trunk involvement: literature review and report on the efficacy of laser treatment. Br J Dermatol 1998; 138: 684–688.

534 Soloeta R, Yanguas I, Lozano M et al. Immunohistochemical study of porokeratotic eccrine nevus. Int J Dermatol 1996; 35: 881–883.

535 Sassmannshausen J, Bogomilsky J, Chaffins M. Porokeratotic eccrine ostial and dermal duct nevus: A case report and review of the literature. J Am Acad Dermatol 2000; 43: 364–367.

536 Coskey RJ, Mehregan AH, Hashimoto K. Porokeratotic eccrine duct and hair follicle nevus. J Am Acad Dermatol 1982; 6: 940–943.

537 Kroumpouzos G, Stefanato CM, Wilkel CS et al. Systematized porokeratotic eccrine and hair follicle naevus: report of a case and review of the literature. Br J Dermatol 1999; 141: 1092–1096.

538 Kossard S, Freeman S. Reticular erythema with ostial porokeratosis. J Am Acad Dermatol 1990; 22: 913–916.

539 Dover JS, Phillips TJ, Burns DA, Krafchik BR. Disseminated superficial actinic porokeratosis. Coexistence with other porokeratotic variants. Arch Dermatol 1986; 122: 887–889.

540 Gautam RK, Bedi GK, Sehgal VN, Singh N. Simultaneous occurrence of disseminated superficial actinic porokeratosis (DSAP), linear, and punctate porokeratosis. Int J Dermatol 1995; 34: 71–72.

541 Freyschmidt-Paul P, Hoffmann R, König A, Happle R. Linear porokeratosis superimposed on disseminated superficial actinic porokeratosis: Report of two cases exemplifying the concept of type 2 segmental manifestation of autosomal dominant skin disorders. J Am Acad Dermatol 1999; 41: 644–647.

542 Neumann RA, Knobler RM, Jurecka W, Gebhart W. Disseminated superficial actinic porokeratosis: experimental induction and exacerbation of skin lesions. J Am Acad Dermatol 1989; 21: 1182–1188.

543 Ibbotson SH. Disseminated superficial porokeratosis: what is the association with ultraviolet radiation? Clin Exp Dermatol 1996; 21: 48–50.

544 Bencini PL, Crosti C, Sala F. Porokeratosis: immunosuppression and exposure to sunlight. Br J Dermatol 1987; 116: 113–116.

545 Neumann RA, Knobler RM, Metze D, Jurecka W. Disseminated superficial porokeratosis and immunosuppression. Br J Dermatol 1988; 119: 375–380.

546 Komorowski RA, Clowry LJ. Porokeratosis of Mibelli in transplant recipients. Am J Clin Pathol 1989; 91: 71–74.

547 Bencini PL, Tarantino A, Grimalt R et al. Porokeratosis and immunosuppression. Br J Dermatol 1995; 132: 74–78.

548 Wilkinson SM, Cartwright PH, English JSC. Porokeratosis of Mibelli and immunosuppression. Clin Exp Dermatol 1991; 16: 61–62.

549 Kanitakis J, Misery L, Nicolas JF et al. Disseminated superficial porokeratosis in a patient with AIDS. Br J Dermatol 1994; 131: 284–289.

550 Rodríguez EA, Jakubowicz S, Chinchilla DA et al. Porokeratosis of Mibelli and HIV-infection. Int J Dermatol 1996; 35: 402–404.

551 Patrizi A, D'Acunto C, Passarini B, Neri I. Porokeratosis in the elderly: a new subtype of disseminated superficial actinic porokeratosis. Acta Derm Venereol 2000; 80: 302–304.

552 Adriaans B, Salisbury JR. Recurrent porokeratosis. Br J Dermatol 1991; 124: 383–386.

553 Shrum JR, Cooper PH, Greer KE, Landes HB. Squamous cell carcinoma in disseminated superficial actinic porokeratosis. J Am Acad Dermatol 1982; 6: 58–62.

554 Chernosky ME, Rapini RP. Squamous cell carcinoma in lesions of disseminated superficial actinic porokeratosis: a report of two cases. Arch Dermatol 1986; 122: 853–855.

555 James WD, Rodman OG. Squamous cell carcinoma arising in porokeratosis of Mibelli. Int J Dermatol 1986; 25: 389–391.

556 Lozinski AZ, Fisher BK, Walter JB, Fitzpatrick PJ. Metastatic squamous cell carcinoma in linear porokeratosis of Mibelli. J Am Acad Dermatol 1987; 16: 448–451.

557 Sawai T, Hayakawa H, Danno K et al. Squamous cell carcinoma arising from giant porokeratosis: a case with extensive metastasis and hypercalcemia. J Am Acad Dermatol 1996; 34: 507–509.

558 Coskey RJ, Mehregan A. Bowen disease associated with porokeratosis of Mibelli. Arch Dermatol 1975; 111: 1480–1481.

559 Otsuka F, Huang J, Sawara K et al. Disseminated porokeratosis accompanying multicentric Bowen's disease. J Am Acad Dermatol 1990; 23: 355–359.

560 Happle R. Cancer proneness of linear porokeratosis may be explained by allelic loss. Dermatology 1997; 195: 20–25.

561 Brodkin RH, Rickert RR, Fuller FW, Saporito C. Malignant disseminated porokeratosis. Arch Dermatol 1987; 123: 1521–1526.

562 Waldman JS, Barr RJ. Familial disseminated malignant porokeratosis. J Cutan Pathol 1988; 15: 349 (abstract).

563 Rapini RP, Chernosky ME. Histologic changes in early lesions of disseminated superficial actinic porokeratosis. J Cutan Pathol 1988; 15: 340 (abstract).

564 Kutzner H, Rütten A, Hügel H. Peppered pattern of cornoid lamellation: a clue to porokeratosis. Dermatopathology: Practical & Conceptual 1996; 2: 55–56.

565 Shumack S, Commens C, Kossard S. Disseminated superficial actinic porokeratosis. A histological review of 61 cases with particular reference to lymphocytic inflammation. Am J Dermatopathol 1991; 13: 26–31.

566 Burge SM, Ryan TJ. Punched-out porokeratosis. A histological variant of disseminated superficial actinic porokeratosis. Am J Dermatopathol 1987; 9: 240–242.

567 Watanabe T, Murakami T, Okochi H et al. Ulcerative porokeratosis. Dermatology 1998; 196: 256–259.

568 Ricci C, Rosset A, Panizzon RG. Bullous and pruritic variant of disseminated superficial actinic porokeratosis: successful treatment with grenz rays. Dermatology 1999; 199: 328–331.

569 Piamphongsant T, Sittapairoachana D. Localized cutaneous amyloidosis in disseminated superficial actinic porokeratosis. J Cutan Pathol 1974; 1: 207–210.

570 Lee JYY, Lally M, Abell E. Disseminated superficial porokeratosis with amyloid deposits in a Chinese man. J Cutan Pathol 1988; 15: 323 (abstract).

571 Amantea A, Giuliano MC, Balus L. Disseminated superficial porokeratosis with dermal amyloid deposits. Am J Dermatopathol 1998; 20: 86–88.

572 Kuno Y, Sato K, Tsuji T. Porokeratosis of Mibelli associated with dermal amyloid deposits. Br J Dermatol 1999; 141: 949–950.

573 Menter MA, Fourie PB. A surface impression and scanning electron microscopy study of porokeratosis of Mibelli. Br J Dermatol 1977; 96: 393–397.

574 Mann PR, Cort DF, Fairburn EA, Abdel-Aziz A. Ultrastructural studies on two cases of porokeratosis of Mibelli. Br J Dermatol 1974; 90: 607–617.

575 Jurecka W, Neumann RA, Knobler RM. Porokeratoses: immunohistochemical, light and electron microscopic evaluation. J Am Acad Dermatol 1991; 24: 96–101.

576 Sato A, Masu S, Seiji M. Electron microscopic studies of porokeratosis Mibelli – Civatte bodies and amyloid deposits in the dermis. J Dermatol 1980; 7: 323–333.

Epidermolytic hyperkeratosis

577 Su WPD. Histopathologic varieties of epidermal nevus. A study of 160 cases. Am J Dermatopathol 1982; 4: 161–170.

578 Adam JE, Richards R. Ichthyosis hystrix. Epidermolytic hyperkeratosis; discordant in monozygotic twins. Arch Dermatol 1973; 107: 278–282.

579 Zeligman I, Pomeranz J. Variations of congenital ichthyosiform erythroderma. Arch Dermatol 1965; 91: 120–125.

580 Nazzaro V, Ermacora E, Santucci B, Caputo R. Epidermolytic hyperkeratosis: generalized form in children from parents with systematized linear form. Br J Dermatol 1990; 122: 417–422.

581 Mahaisavariya P, Cohen PR, Rapini RP. Incidental epidermolytic hyperkeratosis. Am J Dermatopathol 1995; 17: 23–28.

582 Sánchez Yus E, Martin-Dorado E, López-Negrete E et al. Incidental epidermolytic hyperkeratosis (IEH). An epidemiologic study. Am J Dermatopathol 2000; 22: 352 (abstract).

583 Mehregan AH. Epidermolytic hyperkeratosis. Incidental findings in the epidermis and in the intraepidermal eccrine sweat duct units. J Cutan Pathol 1978; 5: 76–80.

584 Zina AM, Bundino S, Pippione MG. Acrosyringial epidermolytic papulosis neviformis. Dermatologica 1985; 171: 122–125.

585 Goette DK, Lapins NA. Epidermolytic hyperkeratosis as an incidental finding in normal oral mucosa. Report of two cases. J Am Acad Dermatol 1984; 10: 246–249.

586 Plewig G, Christophers E. Nevoid follicular epidermolytic hyperkeratosis. Arch Dermatol 1975; 111: 223–226.

587 Barsky S, Doyle JA, Winkelmann RK. Nevus comedonicus with epidermolytic hyperkeratosis. A report of four cases. Arch Dermatol 1981; 117: 86–88.

588 Lookingbill DP, Ladda RL, Cohen C. Generalized epidermolytic hyperkeratosis in the child of a parent with nevus comedonicus. Arch Dermatol 1984; 120: 223–226.

589 Ackerman AB, Reed RJ. Epidermolytic variant of solar keratosis. Arch Dermatol 1973; 107: 104–106.

590 Vakilzadeh F, Happle R. Epidermolytic leukoplakia. J Cutan Pathol 1982; 9: 267–270.

591 Kolde G, Vakilzadeh F. Leukoplakia of the prepuce with epidermolytic hyperkeratosis: a case report. Acta Derm Venereol 1983; 63: 571–573.

592 Williams BT, Barr RJ. Epidermolytic hyperkeratosis in nevi. A possible marker for atypia. Am J Dermatopathol 1996; 18: 156–158.

593 Haneke E. Epidermolytic hyperkeratosis. J Cutan Pathol 1983; 10: 289–290.

594 Wilgram GF, Caulfield JB. An electron microscopic study of epidermolytic hyperkeratosis. Arch Dermatol 1966; 94: 127–143.

595 Shapiro L, Baraf CS. Isolated epidermolytic acanthoma. A solitary tumor showing granular degeneration. Arch Dermatol 1970; 101: 220–223.

596 Cohen PR, Ulmer R, Theriault A et al. Epidermolytic acanthomas: clinical characteristics and immunohistochemical features. Am J Dermatopathol 1997; 19: 232–241.

597 Miyamoto Y, Ueda K, Sato M, Yasuno H. Disseminated epidermolytic acanthoma. J Cutan Pathol 1979; 6: 272–279.

598 Hirone T, Fukushiro R. Disseminated epidermolytic acanthoma. Acta Derm Venereol 1973; 53: 393–402.

599 Knipper JE, Hud JA, Cockerell CJ. Disseminated epidermolytic acanthoma. Am J Dermatopathol 1993; 15: 70–72.

600 Sánchez-Carpintero I, España A, Idoate MA. Disseminated epidermolytic acanthoma probably related to trauma. Br J Dermatol 1999; 141: 728–730.

601 Suzuki H, Takahashi H, Miyashita M, Takemura T. Persistent actinic epidermolytic hyperkeratosis. J Am Acad Dermatol 1995; 32: 63–66.

Acantholytic dyskeratosis

602 Ackerman AB. Focal acantholytic dyskeratosis. Arch Dermatol 1972; 106: 702–706.

603 Ackerman AB, Goldman G. Combined epidermolytic hyperkeratosis and focal acantholytic dyskeratosis. Arch Dermatol 1974; 109: 385–386.

604 Munro CS, Cox NH. An acantholytic dyskeratotic epidermal naevus with other features of Darier's disease on the same side of the body. Br J Dermatol 1992; 127: 168–171.

605 Cambiaghi S, Brusasco A, Grimalt R, Caputo R. Acantholytic dyskeratotic epidermal nevus as a mosaic form of Darier's disease. J Am Acad Dermatol 1995; 32: 284–286.

606 O'Malley MP, Haake A, Goldsmith L, Berg D. Localized Darier disease. Implications for genetic studies. Arch Dermatol 1997; 133: 1134–1138.

607 Sakuntabhai A, Dhitavat J, Burge S, Hovnanian A. Mosaicism for ATP2A2 mutations causes segmental Darier's disease. J Invest Dermatol 2000; 115: 1144–1147.

608 Cox NH. Unilateral Darier disease with contralateral renal agenesis. Arch Dermatol 1998; 134: 634–635.

609 Starink TM, Woerdeman MJ. Unilateral systematized keratosis follicularis. A variant of Darier's disease or an epidermal naevus (acantholytic dyskeratotic epidermal naevus)? Br J Dermatol 1981; 105: 207–214.

610 Demetree JW, Lang PG, St Clair JT. Unilateral, linear, zosteriform epidermal nevus with acantholytic dyskeratosis. Arch Dermatol 1979; 115: 875–877.

611 Youn M, Hann S-K, Moon T-K, Lee M-G. Acantholytic dyskeratotic epidermal nevus induced by ultraviolet B radiation. J Am Acad Dermatol 1998; 39: 301–304.

612 Cottoni F, Masala MV, Cossu S. Acantholytic dyskeratotic epidermal naevus localized unilaterally in the cutaneous and genital areas. Br J Dermatol 1998; 138: 875–878.

613 Happle R. A rule concerning the segmental manifestation of autosomal dominant skin disorders. Arch Dermatol 1997; 133: 1505–1509.

614 Elston DM. Zosteriform distribution of acantholytic dyskeratotic epidermal nevus? J Am Acad Dermatol 1999; 40: 647.

615 Itin PH, Büchner SA, Happle R. Segmental manifestation of Darier disease. What is the genetic background in type 1 and type 2 mosaic phenotypes? Dermatology 2000; 200: 254–257.

616 Slor H, Batko S, Khan SG et al. Clinical, cellular, and molecular features of an Israeli xeroderma pigmentosum family with a frameshift mutation in the XPC gene: sun protection prolongs life. J Invest Dermatol 2000; 115: 974–980.

617 Micali G, Nasca MR, De Pasquale R. Linear acantholytic dyskeratotic epidermal nevus of the sole. Pediatr Dermatol 1999; 16: 166–168.

618 Hall JR, Holder W, Knox JM et al. Familial dyskeratotic comedones. Report of three cases and review of the literature. J Am Acad Dermatol 1987; 17: 808–814.

619 Pierard-Franchimont C, Pierard GE. Suprabasal acantholysis. A common biological feature of distinct inflammatory diseases. Am J Dermatopathol 1983; 5: 421–426.

620 Ahn SK, Chang SN, Lee SH. Focal acantholytic dyskeratosis on the lip. Am J Dermatopathol 1995; 17: 189–191.

621 Kolbusz RV, Fretzin DF. Focal acantholytic dyskeratosis in condyloma acuminata. J Cutan Pathol 1989; 16: 44–47.

622 DiMaio DJM, Cohen PR. Incidental focal acantholytic dyskeratosis. J Am Acad Dermatol 1998; 38: 243–247.

623 O'Connell BM, Nickoloff BJ. Solitary labial papular acantholytic dyskeratoma in an immunocompromised host. Am J Dermatopathol 1987; 9: 339–342.

624 Coppola G, Muscardin LM, Piazza P. Papular acantholytic dyskeratosis. Am J Dermatopathol 1986; 8: 364.

625 Chorzelski TP, Kudejko J, Jablonska S. Is papular acantholytic dyskeratosis of the vulva a new entity? Am J Dermatopathol 1984; 6: 557–560.

626 Cooper PH. Acantholytic dermatosis localized to the vulvocrural area. J Cutan Pathol 1989; 16: 81–84.

627 Salopek TG, Krol A, Jimbow K. Case report of Darier disease localized to the vulva in a 5-year-old girl. Pediatr Dermatol 1993; 10: 146–148.

628 Van Joost Th, Vuzevski VD, Tank B, Menke HE. Benign persistent papular acantholytic and dyskeratotic eruption: a case report and review of the literature. Br J Dermatol 1991; 124: 92–95.

629 Warkel RL, Jager RM. Focal acantholytic dyskeratosis of the anal canal. Am J Dermatopathol 1986; 8: 362–363.

630 Grossin M, Battin-Bertho R, Belaich S. Another case of focal acantholytic dyskeratosis of the anal canal. Am J Dermatopathol 1993; 15: 194–195.

631 Schepers C, Soler J, Palou J, Mascaró JM. Papular acantholytic dyskeratosis of the genitocrural area simulating molluscum contagiosum. J Cutan Pathol 1997; 24: 122 (abstract).

632 Van der Putte SCJ, Oey HB, Storm I. Papular acantholytic dyskeratosis of the penis. Am J Dermatopathol 1986; 8: 365–366.

633 Sánchez Yus E, Requena L, Simón P, de Hijas CM. Incidental acantholysis. J Cutan Pathol 1993; 20: 418–423.

634 Brownstein MH. Acantholytic acanthoma. J Am Acad Dermatol 1988; 19: 783–786.

635 Van Joost T, Vuzevski VD, Menke HE. Benign papular acantholytic non-dyskeratotic eruption: a new paraneoplastic syndrome? Br J Dermatol 1989; 121: 147–148.

636 Happle R, Steijlen PM, Kolde G. Naevus corniculatus: a new acantholytic disorder. Br J Dermatol 1990; 122: 107–112.

637 Weedon D. Papular acantholytic dyskeratosis of vulva. Am J Dermatopathol 1986; 8: 363.

638 Wieselthier JS, Pincus SH. Hailey–Hailey disease of the vulva. Arch Dermatol 1993; 129: 1344–1345.

639 Metze D. Hailey–Hailey-like pattern of acantholysis – a new histopathologic pattern. Am J Dermatopathol 2000; 22: 345 (abstract).

640 Wong T-Y, Mihm MC Jr. Acantholytic dermatosis localized to genitalia and crural areas of male patients: a report of three cases. J Cutan Pathol 1994; 21: 27–32.

641 Wong KT, Wong KK. A case of acantholytic dermatosis of the vulva with features of pemphigus vegetans. J Cutan Pathol 1994; 21: 453–456.

642 Hashimoto K, Moiin A, Chang MW, Tada J. Sudoriferous acrosyringeal acantholytic disease. A subset of Grover's disease. J Cutan Pathol 1996; 23: 151–164.

643 Howe K, Foresman P, Griffin T, Johnson W. Pityriasis rubra pilaris with acantholysis. J Cutan Pathol 1996; 23: 270–274.

644 Roten SV, Bhawan J. Isolated dyskeratotic acanthoma. A variant of isolated epidermolytic acanthoma. Am J Dermatopathol 1995; 17: 63–66.

645 Sedivy SA. Acquired dyskeratotic acanthosis. J Cutan Pathol 1996; 23: 60 (abstract).

646 Rand R, Baden HP. Commentary: Darier–White disease. Arch Dermatol 1983; 119: 81–83.

647 Burge SM, Wilkinson JD. Darier–White disease: a review of the clinical features in 163 patients. J Am Acad Dermatol 1992; 27: 40–50.

648 Munro CS. The phenotype of Darier's disease: penetrance and expressivity in adults and children. Br J Dermatol 1992; 127: 126–130.

649 Burge S. Darier's disease – the clinical features and pathogenesis. Clin Exp Dermatol 1994; 19: 193–205.

650 Romano C, Massai L, Alessandrini C et al. A case of acral Darier's disease. Dermatology 1999; 199: 365–368.

651 Beck AL Jr, Finocchio AF, White JP. Darier's disease: a kindred with a large number of cases. Br J Dermatol 1977; 97: 335–339.

652 Zaias N, Ackerman AB. The nail in Darier–White disease. Arch Dermatol 1973; 107: 193–199.

653 Telfer NR, Burge SM, Ryan TJ. Vesiculo-bullous Darier's disease. Br J Dermatol 1990; 122: 831–834.

654 Speight EL. Vesiculobullous Darier's disease responsive to oral prednisolone steroids. Br J Dermatol 1998; 139: 934–935.

655 Hayakawa K, Nagashima M. A rare presentation of acantholytic dyskeratosis. Br J Dermatol 1995; 133: 487–489.

656 Derrick EK, Darley CR, Burge S. Comedonal Darier's disease. Br J Dermatol 1995; 132: 453–455.

657 Nakagawa T, Masada M, Moriue T, Takaiwa T. Comedo-like acantholytic dyskeratosis of the face and scalp: a new entity? Br J Dermatol 2000; 142: 1047–1048.

658 Peck GL, Kraemer KH, Wetzel B et al. Cornifying Darier disease – a unique variant. Arch Dermatol 1976; 112: 495–503.

659 Katta R, Reed J, Wolf JE. Cornifying Darier's disease. Int J Dermatol 2000; 39: 844–845.

660 Berth-Jones J, Hutchinson PE. Darier's disease with peri-follicular depigmentation. Br J Dermatol 1989; 120: 827–830.

661 Rowley MJ, Nesbitt LT Jr, Carrington PR, Espinoza CG. Hypopigmented macules in acantholytic disorders. Int J Dermatol 1995; 34: 390–392.

662 Bleiker TO, Burns DA. Darier's disease with hypopigmented macules. Br J Dermatol 1998; 138: 913–914.

663 Peterson CM, Lesher JL Jr, Sangueza OP. A unique variant of Darier's disease. Int J Dermatol 2001; 40: 278–280.

664 Shahidullah H, Humphreys F, Beveridge GW. Darier's disease: severe eczematization successfully treated with cyclosporin. Br J Dermatol 1994; 131: 713–716.

665 Parlak M, Erdem T, Karakuzu A et al. Darier's disease seen with cutis verticis gyrata. Acta Derm Venereol 2001; 81: 75.

666 Klein A, Burns L, Leyden JJ. Rectal mucosa involvement in keratosis follicularis. Arch Dermatol 1974; 109: 560–561.

667 Weathers DR, Olansky S, Sharpe LO. Darier's disease with mucous membrane involvement. A case report. Arch Dermatol 1969; 100: 50–53.

668 Itin P, Buchner SA, Gloor B. Darier's disease and retinitis pigmentosa; is there a pathogenetic relationship? Br J Dermatol 1988; 119: 397–402.

669 Crisp AJ, Rowland Payne CME, Adams J et al. The prevalence of bone cysts in Darier's disease: a survey of 31 cases. Clin Exp Dermatol 1984; 9: 78–83.

670 Getzler NA, Flint A. Keratosis follicularis. A study of one family. Arch Dermatol 1966; 93: 545–549.

671 Rubin MB. Lithium-induced Darier's disease. J Am Acad Dermatol 1995; 32: 674–675.

672 Otley CC, Momtaz K. Induction of Darier–White disease with UVB radiation in a clinically photo-insensitive patient. J Am Acad Dermatol 1996; 34: 931–934.

673 Telang GH, Atillasoy E, Stierstorfer M. Localized keratosis follicularis associated with menotropin treatment and pregnancy. J Am Acad Dermatol 1994; 30: 271–272.

674 Romiti R, Arnone M, Sotto MN. Epidermal naevus with Darier's disease-like changes in a patient with Gardner's syndrome. J Am Acad Dermatol 2000; 43: 380–382.

675 Henry JC, Padilla RS, Becker LE, Bankhurst AD. Cell-mediated immunity in Darier's disease. J Am Acad Dermatol 1979; 1: 348–351.

676 Halevy S, Weltfriend S, Pick AI et al. Immunologic studies in Darier's disease. Int J Dermatol 1988; 27: 101–105.

677 Salo OP, Valle MJ. Eczema vaccinatum in a family with Darier's disease. Br J Dermatol 1973; 89: 417–422.

678 Higgins PG, Crow KD. Recurrent Kaposi's varicelliform eruption in Darier's disease. Br J Dermatol 1973; 88: 391–394.

679 Toole JWP, Hofstader SL, Ramsay CA. Darier's disease and Kaposi's varicelliform eruption. J Am Acad Dermatol 1979; 1: 321–324.

680 Carney JF, Caroline NL, Nankervis GA, Pomeranz JR. Eczema vaccinatum and eczema herpeticum in Darier disease. Arch Dermatol 1973; 107: 613–614.

681 Hur W, Lee WS, Ahn SK. Acral Darier's disease: report of a case complicated by Kaposi's varicelliform eruption. J Am Acad Dermatol 1994; 30: 860–862.

682 Downs AMR, Ward KA, Peachey RDG. Subungual squamous cell carcinoma in Darier's disease. Clin Exp Dermatol 1997; 22: 277–279.

683 Caulfield JB, Wilgram GF. An electron-microscopic study of dyskeratosis and acantholysis in Darier's disease. J Invest Dermatol 1963; 41: 57–65.

684 Hashimoto K, Fujiwara K, Tada J et al. Desmosomal dissolution in Grover's disease, Hailey–Hailey's disease and Darier's disease. J Cutan Pathol 1995; 22: 488–501.

685 Tada J, Hashimoto K. Ultrastructural localization of cell junctional components (desmoglein, plakoglobin, E-cadherin, and β-catenin) in Hailey–Hailey disease, Darier's disease, and pemphigus vulgaris. J Cutan Pathol 1998; 25: 106–115.

686 Burge SM, Fenton DA, Dawber RPR, Leigh IM. Darier's disease: an immunohistochemical study using monoclonal antibodies to human cytokeratins. Br J Dermatol 1988; 118: 629–640.

687 Hakuno M, Shimizu H, Akiyama M et al. Dissociation of intra- and extracellular domains of desmosomal cadherins and E-cadherin in Hailey–Hailey disease and Darier's disease. Br J Dermatol 2000; 142: 702–711.

688 Richard G, Wright AR, Harris S et al. Fine mapping of the Darier's disease locus on chromosome 12q. J Invest Dermatol 1994; 103: 665–668.

689 Ikeda S, Wakem P, Haake A et al. Localization of the gene for Darier disease to a 5-cM interval on chromosome 12q. J Invest Dermatol 1994; 103: 478–481.

690 Ikeda S, Shigihara T, Ogawa H et al. Narrowing of the Darier disease gene interval on chromosome 12q. J Invest Dermatol 1998; 110: 847–848.

691 Burge S. Management of Darier's disease. Clin Exp Dermatol 1999; 24: 53–56.

692 Inada M, Shimizu H, Yamada S et al. Three cases of Darier's disease in a family showing marked heterogeneous clinical severity. Dermatology 1999; 198: 167–170.

693 Steffen C. Dyskeratosis and the dyskeratoses. Am J Dermatopathol 1988; 10: 356–363.

694 Vedtofte P, Joensen HD, Dabelsteen E, Veien N. Intercellular and circulating antibodies in patients with dyskeratosis follicularis, Darier's disease. Acta Derm Venereol 1978; 58: 51–55.

695 Hori Y, Tsuru N, Niimura M. Bullous Darier's disease. Arch Dermatol 1982; 118: 278–279.

696 González S, Rubinstein G, Mordovtseva V et al. In vivo abnormal keratinization in Darier–White's disease as viewed by real-tissue confocal imaging. J Cutan Pathol 1999; 26: 504–508.

697 De Panfilis G, Manara GC, Ferrari C et al. Darier's keratosis follicularis: an ultrastructural study during and after topical treatment with retinoic acid alone or in combination with 5-fluorouracil. J Cutan Pathol 1981; 8: 214–218.

698 Gottlieb SK, Lutzner MA. Darier's disease. An electron microscopic study. Arch Dermatol 1973; 107: 225–230.

699 Sato A, Anton-Lamprecht I, Schnyder UW. Ultrastructure of dyskeratosis in morbus Darier. J Cutan Pathol 1977; 4: 173–184.

700 Mann PR, Haye KR. An electron microscope study on the acantholytic and dyskeratotic processes in Darier's disease. Br J Dermatol 1970; 82: 561–566.

701 El-Gothamy Z, Kamel MM. Ultrastructural observations in Darier's disease. Am J Dermatopathol 1988; 10: 306–310.

702 Grover RW. Transient acantholytic dermatosis. Arch Dermatol 1970; 101: 426–434.

703 Helfman RJ. Grover's disease treated with isotretinoin. Report of four cases. J Am Acad Dermatol 1985; 12: 981–984.

704 Parsons JM. Transient acantholytic dermatosis (Grover's disease): A global perspective. J Am Acad Dermatol 1996; 35: 653–666.

705 Liss WA, Norins AL. Zosteriform transient acantholytic dermatosis. J Am Acad Dermatol 1993; 29: 797–798.

706 Heenan PJ, Quirk CJ. Transient acantholytic dermatosis. Br J Dermatol 1980; 102: 515–520.

707 Simon RS, Bloom D, Ackerman AB. Persistent acantholytic dermatosis. A variant of transient acantholytic dermatosis (Grover disease). Arch Dermatol 1976; 112: 1429–1431.

708 Fawcett HA, Miller JA. Persistent acantholytic dermatosis related to actinic damage. Br J Dermatol 1983; 109: 349–354.

709 Dodd HJ, Sarkany I. Persistent acantholytic dermatosis. Clin Exp Dermatol 1984; 9: 431–434.

710 Heaphy MR, Tucker SB, Winkelmann RK. Benign papular acantholytic dermatosis. Arch Dermatol 1976; 112: 814–821.

711 Kanzaki T, Hashimoto K. Transient acantholytic dermatosis with involvement of oral mucosa. J Cutan Pathol 1978; 5: 23–30.

712 Chalet M, Grover R, Ackerman AB. Transient acantholytic dermatosis. A reevaluation. Arch Dermatol 1977; 113: 431–435.

713 Grover RW, Rosenblaum R. The association of transient acantholytic dermatosis with other skin diseases. J Am Acad Dermatol 1984; 11: 253–256.

714 Fleckman P, Stenn K. Transient acantholytic dermatosis associated with pemphigus foliaceus. Coexistence of two acantholytic diseases. Arch Dermatol 1983; 119: 155–156.

715 Roger M, Valence C, Bressieux JM et al. Grover's disease associated with Waldenström's macroglobulinemia and neutrophilic dermatosis. Acta Derm Venereol 2000; 80: 145–146.

716 Chua SH, Giam YC. Acantholytic dermatosis in chronic renal failure. Int J Dermatol 1997; 36: 200–202.

717 Casanova JM, Pujol RM, Taberner R et al. Grover's disease in patients with chronic renal failure receiving hemodialysis: Clinicopathologic review of 4 cases. J Am Acad Dermatol 1999; 41: 1029–1033.

718 Quarterman MJ, Davis LS. Transient acantholytic dermatosis in a postoperative febrile patient. Int J Dermatol 1995; 34: 113.

719 Hu C-H, Michel B, Farber EM. Transient acantholytic dermatosis (Grover's disease). A skin disorder related to heat and sweating. Arch Dermatol 1985; 121: 1439–1441.

720 Horn TD, Groleau GE. Transient acantholytic dermatosis in immunocompromised febrile patients with cancer. Arch Dermatol 1987; 123: 238–240.

721 Zelickson BD, Tefferi A, Gertz MA et al. Transient acantholytic dermatosis associated with lymphomatous angioimmunoblastic lymphadenopathy. Acta Derm Venereol 1989; 69: 445–448.

722 French LE, Piletta P-A, Etienne A et al. Incidence of transient acantholytic dermatosis (Grover's disease) in a hospital setting. Dermatology 1999; 198: 410–411.

723 Antunes I, Azevedo F, Mesquita-Guimarães J et al. Grover's disease secondary to ribavirin. Br J Dermatol 2000; 142: 1257–1258.

724 Zvulunov A, Grunwald MH, Avinoach I, Halevy S. Transient acantholytic dermatosis (Grover's disease) in a patient with progressive systemic sclerosis treated with D-penicillamine. Int J Dermatol 1997; 36: 476–477.

725 Mahler SJ, de Villez RL, Pulitzer DR. Transient acantholytic dermatosis induced by recombinant human interleukin 4. J Am Acad Dermatol 1993; 29: 206–209.

726 Cohen PR, Kurzrock R. 2-chlorodeoxyadenosine-associated transient acantholytic dermatosis in hairy cell leukemia patients. Am J Dermatopathol 1999; 21: 106–107.

727 Harvell JD, Hashem C, Williford PL, White WL. Grover's-like disease in the setting of bone marrow transplantation and autologous peripheral blood stem cell infusion. Am J Dermatopathol 1998; 20: 179–184.

728 Powell J, Sakuntabhai A, James M et al. Grover's disease, despite histological similarity to Darier's disease, does not share an abnormality in the ATP2A2 gene. Br J Dermatol 2000; 143: 658.

729 Bayer-Garner IB, Dilday BR, Sanderson RD, Smoller BR. Acantholysis and spongiosis are associated with loss of syndecan-1 expression. J Cutan Pathol 2001; 28: 135–139.

730 Davis MDP, Dinneen AM, Landa N, Gibson LE. Grover's disease: clinicopathologic review of 72 cases. Mayo Clin Proc 1999; 74: 229–234.

731 Kennedy C, Moss R. Transient acantholytic dermatosis. Br J Dermatol (Suppl) 1979; 17: 67–69.

732 Waisman M, Stewart JJ, Walker AE. Bullous transient acantholytic dermatosis. Arch Dermatol 1976; 112: 1440–1441.

733 Bystryn J-C. Immunofluorescence studies in transient acantholytic dermatosis (Grover's disease). Am J Dermatopathol 1979; 1: 325–327.

734 Millns JL, Doyle JA, Muller SA. Positive cutaneous immunofluorescence in Grover's disease. Arch Dermatol 1980; 116: 515.

735 Grover RW. Transient acantholytic dermatosis. Electron microscope study. Arch Dermatol 1971; 104: 26–37.

736 Grover RW, Duffy JL. Transient acantholytic dermatosis. Electron microscopic study of the Darier type. J Cutan Pathol 1975; 2: 111–127.

737 Palmer DD, Perry HO. Benign familial chronic pemphigus. Arch Dermatol 1962; 86: 493–502.

738 Michel B. Commentary: Hailey–Hailey disease. Familial benign chronic pemphigus. Arch Dermatol 1982; 118: 781–783.

739 Witkowski JA, Parish LC. Familial benign chronic pemphigus. A papular variant. Arch Dermatol 1973; 108: 842–843.

740 Barron DR, Estes SA. Papuloverrucoid Hailey–Hailey disease: an unusual presentation. J Cutan Pathol 1989; 16: 296 (abstract).

741 Langenberg A, Berger TG, Cardelli M et al. Genital benign chronic pemphigus (Hailey–Hailey disease) presenting as condylomas. J Am Acad Dermatol 1992; 26: 951–955.

742 Lyles TW, Knox JM, Richardson JB. Atypical features in familial benign chronic pemphigus. Arch Dermatol 1958; 78: 446–453.

743 Marsch WC, Stuttgen G. Generalized Hailey–Hailey disease. Br J Dermatol 1978; 99: 553–560.

744 Kahn D, Hutchinson E. Esophageal involvement in familial benign chronic pemphigus. Arch Dermatol 1974; 109: 718–719.

745 Vaclavinkova V, Neumann E. Vaginal involvement in familial benign chronic pemphigus (morbus Hailey–Hailey). Acta Derm Venereol 1982; 62: 80–81.

746 Evron S, Leviatan A, Okon E. Familial benign chronic pemphigus appearing as leukoplakia of the vulva. Int J Dermatol 1984; 23: 556–557.

747 Hazelrigg DE, Stoller LJ. Isolated familial benign chronic pemphigus. Arch Dermatol 1977; 113: 1302.

748 Cooper DL. Familial benign chronic pemphigus of perianal skin. Arch Dermatol 1971; 103: 219–220.

749 Duschet P, Happle R, Schwarz T, Gschnait F. Relapsing linear acantholytic dermatosis. J Am Acad Dermatol 1995; 33: 920–922.

750 Richard G, Korge BP, Wright AR et al. Hailey–Hailey disease maps to a 5 cM interval on chromosome 3q21–q24. J Invest Dermatol 1995; 105: 357–360.

751 Sudbrak R, Brown J, Dobson-Stone C et al. Hailey–Hailey disease is caused by mutations in ATP2C1 encoding a novel Ca²⁺ pump. Hum Mol Genet 2000; 12: 1131–1140.

752 Burge SM. Hailey–Hailey disease: the clinical features, response to treatment and prognosis. Br J Dermatol 1992; 126: 275–282.

753 Morales A, Livingood CS, Hu F. Familial benign chronic pemphigus. Arch Dermatol 1966; 93: 324–328.

754 Izumi AK, Shmunes E, Wood MG. Familial benign chronic pemphigus. The role of trauma including contact sensitivity. Arch Dermatol 1971; 104: 177–181.

755 Cram DL, Muller SA, Winkelmann RK. Ultraviolet-induced acantholysis in familial benign chronic pemphigus. Detection of the forme fruste. Arch Dermatol 1967; 96: 636–641.

756 Gerdsen R, Hartl C, Christ S et al. Hailey–Hailey disease: exacerbation by scabies. Br J Dermatol 2001; 144: 211–212.

757 Leppard B, Delaney TJ, Sanderson KV. Chronic benign familial pemphigus. Induction of lesions by Herpesvirus hominis. Br J Dermatol 1973; 88: 609–613.

758 Heaphy MR, Winkelmann RK. Coexistence of benign familial pemphigus and psoriasis vulgaris. Arch Dermatol 1976; 112: 1571–1574.

759 Hayakawa K, Shiohara T. Coexistence of psoriasis and familial benign chronic pemphigus: efficacy of ultraviolet B treatment. Br J Dermatol 1999; 140: 374–375.

760 Nicolis G, Tosca A, Marouli O, Stratigos J. Keratosis follicularis and familial benign chronic pemphigus in the same patient. Dermatologica 1979; 159: 346–351.

761 Ganor S, Sagher F. Keratosis follicularis (Darier) and familial benign chronic pemphigus (Hailey–Hailey) in the same patient. Br J Dermatol 1965; 77: 24–29.

762 Mehregan DA, Umbert IJ, Peters MS. Histologic findings of Hailey–Hailey disease in a patient with bullous pemphigoid. J Am Acad Dermatol 1989; 21: 1107–1112.

763 King DT, Hirose FM, King LA. Simultaneous occurrence of familial benign chronic pemphigus (Hailey–Hailey disease) and syringoma of the vulva. Arch Dermatol 1978; 114: 801.

764 Furue M, Seki Y, Oohara K, Ishibashi Y. Basal cell epithelioma arising in a patient with Hailey–Hailey's disease. Int J Dermatol 1987; 26: 461–462.

765 Cockayne SE, Rassl DM, Thomas SE. Squamous cell carcinoma arising in Hailey–Hailey disease of the vulva. Br J Dermatol 2000; 142: 540–542.

766 Holst VA, Fair KP, Wilson BB, Patterson JW. Squamous cell carcinoma arising in Hailey–Hailey disease. J Am Acad Dermatol 2000; 43: 368–371.

767 Berger RS, Lynch PJ. Familial benign chronic pemphigus. Surgical treatment and pathogenesis. Arch Dermatol 1971; 104: 380–384.

768 De Dobbeleer G, de Graef C, M'Poudi E et al. Reproduction of the characteristic morphologic changes of familial benign chronic pemphigus in cultures of lesional keratinocytes onto dead deepidermized dermis. J Am Acad Dermatol 1989; 21: 961–965.

769 Hamm H, Metze D, Bröcker E-B. Hailey–Hailey disease. Eradication by dermabrasion. Arch Dermatol 1994; 130: 1143–1149.

770 Kartamaa M, Reitamo S. Familial benign chronic pemphigus (Hailey–Hailey disease). Treatment with carbon dioxide laser vaporization. Arch Dermatol 1992; 128: 646–648.

771 Kruppa A, Korge B, Lasch J et al. Successful treatment of Hailey–Hailey disease with a scanned carbon dioxide laser. Acta Derm Venereol 2000; 80: 53–54.

772 Metze D, Hamm H, Schorat A, Luger T. Involvement of the adherens junction–actin filament system in acantholytic dyskeratosis of Hailey–Hailey disease. J Cutan Pathol 1996; 23: 211–222.

773 Berrards M, Korge BP. Desmosome assembly and keratin network formation after Ca²⁺/serum induction and UVB radiation in Hailey–Hailey keratinocytes. J Invest Dermatol 2000; 114: 1058–1061.

774 Haftek M, Kowalewski C, Mesnil M et al. Internalization of gap junctions in benign familial pemphigus (Hailey–Hailey disease) and keratosis follicularis (Darier's disease). Br J Dermatol 1999; 141: 224–230.

775 Burge SM, Millard PR, Wojnarowska F. Hailey–Hailey disease: a widespread abnormality of cell adhesion. Br J Dermatol 1991; 124: 329–332.

776 Steffen CG. Familial benign chronic pemphigus. Am J Dermatopathol 1987; 9: 58–73.

777 Wilgram GF, Caulfield JB, Lever WF. An electronmicroscopic study of acantholysis and dyskeratosis in Hailey and Hailey's disease. J Invest Dermatol 1962; 39: 373–381.

778 Gottlieb SK, Lutzner MA. Hailey–Hailey disease – an electron microscopic study. J Invest Dermatol 1970; 54: 368–376.

779 De Dobbeleer G, Achten G. Disrupted desmosomes in induced lesions of familial benign chronic pemphigus. J Cutan Pathol 1979; 6: 418–424.

780 Szymanski FJ. Warty dyskeratoma. A benign cutaneous tumor resembling Darier's disease microscopically. Arch Dermatol 1957; 75: 567–572.

781 Graham JH, Helwig EB. Isolated dyskeratosis follicularis. Arch Dermatol 1958; 77: 377–389.

782 Tanay A, Mehregan AH. Warty dyskeratoma. Dermatologica 1969; 138: 155–164.

783 Griffiths TW, Hashimoto K, Sharata HH, Ellis CN. Multiple warty dyskeratomas of the scalp. Clin Exp Dermatol 1997; 22: 189–191.

784 Gorlin RJ, Peterson WC. Warty dyskeratoma. A note concerning its occurrence on the oral mucosa. Arch Dermatol 1967; 95: 292–293.

785 Harrist TJ, Murphy GF, Mihm MC. Oral warty dyskeratoma. Arch Dermatol 1980; 116: 929–931.

786 Baran R, Perrin C. Focal subungual warty dyskeratoma. Dermatology 1997; 195: 278–280.

787 Panja RK. Warty dyskeratoma. J Cutan Pathol 1977; 4: 194–200.

Hypergranulotic dyscornification

788 Reichel M. Hypergranulotic dyscornification. A distinctive histologic pattern of maturation of epidermal epithelium present in solitary keratoses. Am J Dermatopathol 1999; 21: 21–24.

789 Magro CM, Baden LA, Crowson AN et al. A novel nonepidermolytic palmoplantar keratoderma: A clinical and histopathologic study of six cases. J Am Acad Dermatol 1997; 37: 27–33.

Colloid keratosis

790 Gonzalez SB. Colloid keratosis. Morphologic characterization of a nonspecific reaction pattern of squamous epithelium. Am J Dermatopathol 1986; 8: 194–201.

791 Gardner DG, Hyams VJ, Heffner DK. Eosinophilic pooling. Am J Surg Pathol 1983; 7: 502–503.

792 Tschen JA, McGavran MH, Kettler AH. Pagetoid dyskeratosis: a selective keratinocytic response. J Am Acad Dermatol 1988; 19: 891–894.

793 Val-Bernal JF, Garijo MF. Pagetoid dyskeratosis of the prepuce. An incidental histologic finding resembling extramammary Paget's disease. J Cutan Pathol 2000; 27: 387–391.

794 Kuo T-T, Chan H-L, Hsueh S. Clear cell papulosis of the skin. A new entity with histogenetic implications for cutaneous Paget's disease. Am J Surg Pathol 1987; 11: 827–834.

Discrete keratotic lesions

795 Flegel H. Hyperkeratosis lenticularis perstans. Hautarzt 1958; 9: 362–364.

796 Kocsard E, Bear CL, Constance TJ. Hyperkeratosis lenticularis perstans (Flegel). Dermatologica 1968; 136: 35–42.

797 Price ML, Wilson Jones E, MacDonald DM. A clinicopathological study of Flegel's disease (hyperkeratosis lenticularis perstans). Br J Dermatol 1987; 116: 681–691.

798 Cooper SM, George S. Flegel's disease treated with psoralen ultraviolet A. Br J Dermatol 2000; 142: 340–342.

799 Bean SF. Hyperkeratosis lenticularis perstans. A clinical, histopathologic, and genetic study. Arch Dermatol 1969; 99: 705–709.

800 Bean SF. The genetics of hyperkeratosis lenticularis perstans. Arch Dermatol 1972; 106: 72.

801 Beveridge GW, Langlands AO. Familial hyperkeratosis lenticularis perstans associated with tumours of the skin. Br J Dermatol 1973; 88: 453–458.

802 Pearson LH, Smith JG Jr, Chalker DK. Hyperkeratosis lenticularis perstans. J Am Acad Dermatol 1987; 16: 190–195.

803 Raffle EJ, Rogers J. Hyperkeratosis lenticularis perstans. Arch Dermatol 1969; 100: 423–428.

804 Miranda-Romero A, Sánchez Sambucety P, Bajo del Pozo C et al. Unilateral hyperkeratosis lenticularis perstans (Flegel's disease). J Am Acad Dermatol 1998; 39: 655–657.

805 Tidman MJ, Price ML, MacDonald DM. Lamellar bodies in hyperkeratosis lenticularis perstans. J Cutan Pathol 1987; 14: 207–211.

806 Ikai K, Murai T, Oguchi M et al. An ultrastructural study of the epidermis in hyperkeratosis lenticularis perstans. Acta Derm Venereol 1978; 58: 363–365.

807 Frenk E, Tapernoux B. Hyperkeratosis lenticularis perstans (Flegel). A biological model for keratinization occurring in the absence of Odland bodies? Dermatologica 1976; 153: 253–262.

808 Kuokkanen K, Alavaikko M, Pitkanen R. Hyperkeratosis lenticularis perstans (Flegel's disease). Acta Derm Venereol 1983; 63: 357–360.

809 Van de Staak WJBM, Bergers AMG, Bongaarts P. Hyperkeratosis lenticularis perstans (Flegel). Dermatologica 1980; 161: 340–346.

810 Jang K-A, Choi J-H, Sung K-J et al. Hyperkeratosis lenticularis perstans (Flegel's disease): histologic, immunohistochemical, and ultrastructural features in a case. Am J Dermatopathol 1999; 21: 395–398.

811 Ikada J. Hyperkeratosis lenticularis perstans. Arch Dermatol 1974; 110: 464–465.

812 Hunter GA, Donald GF. Hyperkeratosis lenticularis perstans (Flegel) or dyskeratotic psoriasiform dermatosis. A single dermatosis or two? Arch Dermatol 1968; 98: 239–247.

813 Langer K, Zonzits E, Konrad K. Hyperkeratosis lenticularis perstans (Flegel's disease). J Am Acad Dermatol 1992; 27: 812–816.

814 Buchner SA. Hyperkeratosis lenticularis perstans (Flegel's disease). In situ characterization of T cell subsets and Langerhans' cells. Acta Derm Venereol 1988; 68: 341–345.

815 Holubar K. Hyperkeratosis follicularis et parafollicularis in cutem penetrans. Josef Kyrle and 'his' disease. Am J Dermatopathol 1985; 7: 261–263.

816 Woo TY, Rasmussen JE. Disorders of transepidermal elimination. Part 2. Int J Dermatol 1985; 24: 337–348.

817 Cunningham SR, Walsh M, Matthews R et al. Kyrle's disease. J Am Acad Dermatol 1987; 16: 117–123.

818 Patterson JW. The perforating disorders. J Am Acad Dermatol 1984; 10: 561–581.

819 White CR Jr. The dermatopathology of perforating disorders. Semin Dermatol 1986; 5: 359–366.

820 Price ML, Wilson Jones E, MacDonald DM. Flegel's disease, not Kyrle's disease. J Am Acad Dermatol 1988; 18: 1366.

821 Kocsard E, Palmer G, Constance TJ. Coexistence of hyperkeratosis lenticularis perstans (Flegel) and hyperkeratosis follicularis et parafollicularis in cutem penetrans (Kyrle) in a patient. Acta Derm Venereol 1970; 50: 385–390.

822 Walsh M, Cunningham SR, Burrows D. Flegel's disease, not Kyrle's disease. Reply. J Am Acad Dermatol 1988; 18: 1366–1367.

823 Carter VH, Constantine VS. Kyrle's disease. I. Clinical findings in five cases and review of the literature. Arch Dermatol 1968; 97: 624–632.

824 Woodrow SL, Rytina ERC, Norris PG. Kyrle's-en-plaque. Clin Exp Dermatol 1999; 24: 48–49.

825 Baer RL. Kyrle's disease (hyperkeratosis follicularis et parafollicularis in cutem penetrans). Arch Dermatol 1967; 96: 351–352.

826 Schamroth JM, Kellen P, Grieve TP. Atypical Kyrle's disease. Int J Dermatol 1986; 25: 310–313.

827 Gupta AK, Gupta MA, Cardella CJ, Haberman HF. Cutaneous associations of chronic renal failure and dialysis. Int J Dermatol 1986; 25: 498–504.

828 Hood AF, Hardegen GL, Zarate AR et al. Kyrle's disease in patients with chronic renal failure. Arch Dermatol 1982; 118: 85–88.

829 Stone RA. Kyrle-like lesions in two patients with renal failure undergoing dialysis. J Am Acad Dermatol 1981; 5: 707–709.

830 Aram H, Szymanski FJ, Bailey WE. Kyrle's disease. Hyperkeratosis follicularis et parafollicularis in cutem penetrans. Arch Dermatol 1969; 100: 453–456.

831 Constantine VS, Carter VH. Kyrle's disease. II. Histopathologic findings in five cases and review of the literature. Arch Dermatol 1968; 97: 633–639.

832 Moss HV. Kyrle's disease. Cutis 1979; 23: 463–466.

833 Balus L, Donati P, Amantea A, Breathnach AS. Multiple minute digitate hyperkeratosis. J Am Acad Dermatol 1988; 18: 431–436.

834 Nedwich JA, Sullivan JJ. Disseminated spiked hyperkeratosis. Int J Dermatol 1987; 26: 358–361.

835 Takagawa S, Satoh T, Yokozeki H, Nishioka K. Multiple minute digitate hyperkeratoses. Br J Dermatol 2000; 142: 1044–1046.

836 Wilkinson SM, Wilkinson N, Chalmers RJG. Multiple minute digitate keratoses: a transient, sporadic variant. J Am Acad Dermatol 1994; 31: 802–803.

837 Rubegni P, De Aloe G, Pianigiani E et al. Two sporadic cases of idiopathic multiple minute digitate hyperkeratosis. Clin Exp Dermatol 2001; 26: 53–55.

838 Paul C, Fermand J-P, Flageul B et al. Hyperkeratotic spicules and monoclonal gammopathy. J Am Acad Dermatol 1995; 33: 346–351.

839 Benoldi D, Zucchi A, Allegra F. Multiple minute digitate hyperkeratoses. Clin Exp Dermatol 1993; 18: 261–262.

840 Cox NH, Ince P. Transient post-inflammatory digitate keratoses. Clin Exp Dermatol 1989; 14: 170–172.

841 Knobler EH, Grossman ME, Rabinowitz AD. Multiple minute palmar-plantar digitate hyperkeratoses. Br J Dermatol 1989; 121: 239–242.

842 Kaddu S, Soyer HP, Kerl H. Palmar filiform hyperkeratosis: a new paraneoplastic syndrome? J Am Acad Dermatol 1995; 33: 337–340.

843 Goldstein N. Multiple minute digitate hyperkeratoses. Arch Dermatol 967; 96: 692–693.

844 Yoon SW, Gibbs RB. Multiple minute digitate hyperkeratoses. Arch Dermatol 1975; 111: 1176–1177.

845 Shuttleworth D, Graham-Brown RAC, Hutchinson PE. Minute aggregate keratoses – a report of three cases. Clin Exp Dermatol 1985; 10: 566–571.

846 Mizuno K, Okamoto H, Imamura S. Postirradiation multiple minute digitate hyperkeratoses. Clin Exp Dermatol 1995; 20: 425–427.

847 Aloi FG, Molinero A, Pippione M. Parakeratotic horns in a patient with Crohn's disease. Clin Exp Dermatol 1989; 14: 79–81.

848 Carmichael AJ, Tan CY. Digitate keratoses – a complication of etretinate used in the treatment of disseminated superficial actinic porokeratosis. Clin Exp Dermatol 1990; 15: 370–371.

849 Kato N. Vertically growing ectopic nail. J Cutan Pathol 1992; 19: 445–447.

850 Burns DA. Post-irradiation digitate keratoses. Clin Exp Dermatol 1986; 11: 646–649.

851 Timpatanapong P, Jerasutus S, Sriprachya-anunt S, Hotrakitya S. Congenital trichoid keratosis of the scalp. Arch Dermatol 1992; 128: 1549–1550.

852 Frenk E, Mevorah B, Leu F. Disseminated spiked hyperkeratosis. An unusual discrete nonfollicular keratinization disorder. Arch Dermatol 1981; 117: 412–414.

853 Coleman R, Malone M, Handfield-Jones S et al. Waxy keratoses of childhood. Clin Exp Dermatol 1994; 19: 173–176.

854 Jacyk WK, Smith A. Mosaic acral keratosis. Clin Exp Dermatol 1990; 15: 361–362.

Miscellaneous epidermal genodermatoses

855 Waisman M. Verruciform manifestations of keratosis follicularis. Arch Dermatol 1960; 81: 1–14.

856 Niedelman ML, McKusick VA. Acrokeratosis verruciformis (Hopf). A follow-up study. Arch Dermatol 1962; 86: 779–782.

857 Rook A, Stevanovic D. Acrokeratosis verruciformis. Br J Dermatol 1957; 69: 450–451.

858 Panja RK. Acrokeratosis verruciformis (Hopf) – a clinical entity? Br J Dermatol 1977; 96: 643–652.

859 Schueller WA. Acrokeratosis verruciformis of Hopf. Arch Dermatol 1972; 106: 81–83.

860 Herndon JH, Wilson JD. Acrokeratosis verruciformis (Hopf) and Darier's disease. Genetic evidence for a unitary origin. Arch Dermatol 1966; 93: 305–310.

861 Niordson AM, Sylvest B. Bullous dyskeratosis follicularis and acrokeratosis verruciformis. Report of a case. Arch Dermatol 1965; 92: 166–168.

862 Verbov J. Acrokeratosis verruciformis of Hopf with steatocystoma multiplex and hypertrophic lichen planus. Br J Dermatol 1972; 86: 91–94.

863 Penrod JN, Everett MA, McCreight WG. Observations on keratosis follicularis. Arch Dermatol 1960; 82: 367–370.

864 Jung EG. Xeroderma pigmentosum. Int J Dermatol 1986; 25: 629–633.

865 Kraemer KH, Slor H. Xeroderma pigmentosum. Clin Dermatol 1985; 3: 33–69.

866 Kraemer KH, Lee MM, Scotto J. Xeroderma pigmentosum. Cutaneous ocular, and neurologic abnormalities in 830 published cases. Arch Dermatol 1987; 123: 241–250.

867 Lambert WC. Genetic diseases associated with DNA and chromosomal instability. Dermatol Clin 1987; 5: 85–108.

868 Cleaver JE, Thomas GH. Clinical syndromes associated with DNA repair deficiency and enhanced sun sensitivity. Arch Dermatol 1993; 129: 348–350.

869 Tessari G, D'Onghia FS, Stefanini M, Barba A. Discordance between DNA analysis and the clinical picture in a case of xeroderma pigmentosum. Acta Derm Venereol 1999; 79: 94–95.

870 Itoh T, Mori T, Ohkubo H, Yamaizumi M. A newly identified patient with clinical xeroderma pigmentosum phenotype has a non-sense mutation in the DDB2 gene and incomplete repair in (6-4) photoproducts. J Invest Dermatol 1999; 113: 251–257.

871 English JSC, Swerdlow AJ. The risk of malignant melanoma, internal malignancy and mortality in xeroderma pigmentosum patients. Br J Dermatol 1987; 117: 457–461.

872 Hessel A, Siegle RJ, Mitchell DL, Cleaver JE. Xeroderma pigmentosum variant with multisystem involvement. Arch Dermatol 1992; 128: 1233–1237.

873 Nishigori C, Miyachi Y, Takebe H, Imamura S. A case of xeroderma pigmentosum with clinical appearance of dyschromatosis symmetrica hereditaria. Pediatr Dermatol 1986; 3: 410–413.

874 Youssef N, Vabres P, Buisson T et al. Two unusual tumors in a patient with xeroderma pigmentosum: atypical fibroxanthoma and basosquamous carcinoma. J Cutan Pathol 1999; 26: 430–435.

875 Spicer MS, Stampien TM, Lambert WC et al. Severe xeroderma pigmentosum associated with numerous melanomas, no other skin tumors, high natural killer cell activity, normal interferon production, and a benign course. J Cutan Pathol 1997; 24: 126 (abstract).

876 Kondoh M, Ueda M, Nakagawa K, Ichihashi M. Siblings with xeroderma pigmentosum complementation group A with different skin cancer development: importance of sun protection at an early age. J Am Acad Dermatol 1994; 31: 993–996.

877 Wysenbeek AJ, Weiss H, Duczyminer-Kahana M et al. Immunologic alterations in xeroderma pigmentosum patients. Cancer 1986; 58: 219–221.

878 Bhutani LK. The photodermatoses as seen in tropical countries. Semin Dermatol 1982; 1: 175–181.

879 Kondoh M, Ueda M, Ichihashi M. Correlation of the clinical manifestations and gene mutations of Japanese xeroderma pigmentosum Group A patients. Br J Dermatol 1995; 133: 579–585.

880 Auerbach AD. Diagnosis of diseases of DNA synthesis and repair that affect the skin using cultured amniotic fluid cells. Semin Dermatol 1984; 3: 172–184.

881 Han Z-B, Hara R, Ayaki H et al. Assignment of three Chinese xeroderma pigmentosum patients to complementation group C and one to group E. Br J Dermatol 1998; 138: 131–136.

882 Petit-Frère C, Capulas E, Lowe JE et al. Ultraviolet-B-induced apoptosis and cytokine release in xeroderma pigmentosum keratinocytes. J Invest Dermatol 2000; 115: 687–693.

883 Cleaver JE. Xeroderma pigmentosum: genetic and environmental influences in skin carcinogenesis. Int J Dermatol 1978; 17: 435–444.

884 Friedberg EC. Xeroderma pigmentosum. Recent studies on the DNA repair defects. Arch Pathol Lab Med 1978; 102: 3–7.

885 Stone N, Reed J, Mahood J et al. Xeroderma pigmentosum: the role of phototesting. Br J Dermatol 2000; 143: 595–597.

886 Fischer E, Jung EG. Photosensitivity and the genodermatoses. Semin Dermatol 1982; 1: 169–174.

887 Maeda T, Sato K, Tanaka T et al. Compound heterozygous group A xeroderma pigmentosum patient with a novel mutation and an inherited reciprocal translocation. Br J Dermatol 2000; 143: 174–179.

888 Kondo S, Fukuro S, Mamada A et al. Assignment of three patients with xeroderma pigmentosum to complementation group E and their characteristics. J Invest Dermatol 1988; 90: 152–157.

889 Itoh T, Linn S, Ono T, Yamaizumi M. Reinvestigation of the classification of five cell strains of xeroderma pigmentosum group E with reclassification of three of them. J Invest Dermatol 2000; 114: 1022–1029.

890 Norris PG, Hawk JLM, Avery JA, Giannelli F. Xeroderma pigmentosum complementation group F in a non-Japanese patient. J Am Acad Dermatol 1988; 18: 1185–1188.

891 Yamamura K, Ichihashi M, Hiramoto T et al. Clinical and photobiological characteristics of xeroderma pigmentosum complementation group F: a review of cases from Japan. Br J Dermatol 1989; 121: 471–480.

892 Sijbers AM, van Voorst Vader PC, Snoek JW et al. Homozygous R788W point mutation in the *XPF* gene of a patient with xeroderma pigmentosum and late-onset neurologic disease. J Invest Dermatol 1998; 110: 832–836.

893 Norris PG, Hawk JLM, Avery JA, Giannelli F. Xeroderma pigmentosum complementation group G – report of two cases. Br J Dermatol 1987; 116: 861–866.

894 Otsuka F, Robbins JH. The Cockayne syndrome – an inherited multisystem disorder with cutaneous photosensitivity and defective repair of DNA. Comparison with xeroderma pigmentosum. Am J Dermatopathol 1985; 7: 387–392.

895 Norris PG, Arlett CF, Cole J et al. Abnormal erythemal response and elevated T lymphocyte HRPT mutant frequency in Cockayne's syndrome. Br J Dermatol 1991; 124: 453–460.

896 Scott RJ, Itin P, Kleijer WJ et al. Xeroderma pigmentosum–Cockayne syndrome complex in two patients: absence of skin tumors despite severe deficiency of DNA excision repair. J Am Acad Dermatol 1993; 29: 883–889.

897 Miyauchi H, Horio T, Akaeda T et al. Cockayne syndrome in two adult siblings. J Am Acad Dermatol 1994; 30: 329–335.

898 Miyauchi-Hashimoto H, Akaeda T, Maihara T et al. Cockayne syndrome without typical clinical manifestations including neurologic abnormalities. J Am Acad Dermatol 1998; 39: 565–570.

899 Bartenjev I, Rogl Butina M, Potočnik M. Rare case of Cockayne syndrome with xeroderma pigmentosum. Acta Derm Venereol 2000; 80: 213–214.

900 Khan SG, Levy HL, Legerski R et al. Xeroderma pigmentosum group C splice mutation associated with autism and hypoglycinemia. J Invest Dermatol 1998; 111: 791–796.

901 Lynch HT, Fusaro RM, Johnson JA. Xeroderma pigmentosum. Complementation group C and malignant melanoma. Arch Dermatol 1984; 120: 175–179.

902 Chi H-I, Kawachi Y, Otsuka F. Xeroderma pigmentosum variant: DNA ploidy analysis of various skin tumors and normal-appearing skin in a patient. Int J Dermatol 1994; 33: 775–778.

903 Anstey AV, Arlett CF, Cole J et al. Long-term survival and preservation of natural killer cell activity in a xeroderma pigmentosum patient with spontaneous regression and multiple deposits of malignant melanoma. Br J Dermatol 1991; 125: 272–278.

904 Nagasawa H, Zamansky GB, McCone EF et al. Spontaneous transformation to anchorage-independent growth of a xeroderma pigmentosum fibroblast cell strain. J Invest Dermatol 1987; 88: 149–153.

905 Norris PG, Limb GA, Hamblin AS et al. Immune function, mutant frequency, and cancer risk in the DNA repair defective genodermatoses xeroderma pigmentosum, Cockayne's syndrome, and trichothiodystrophy. J Invest Dermatol 1990; 94: 94–100.

906 Kraemer KH, Herlyn M, Yuspa SH et al. Reduced DNA repair in cultured melanocytes and nevus cells from a patient with xeroderma pigmentosum. Arch Dermatol 1989; 125: 263–268.

907 Nishigori C, Moriwaki S, Takebe H et al. Gene alterations and clinical characteristics of xeroderma pigmentosum Group A patients in Japan. Arch Dermatol 1994; 130: 191–197.

908 Kore-eda S, Tanaka T, Moriwaki S et al. A case of xeroderma pigmentosum group A diagnosed with a polymerase chain reaction (PCR) technique. Arch Dermatol 1992; 128: 971–974.

909 Kraemer KH, Levy DD, Parris CN et al. Xeroderma pigmentosum and related disorders: examining the linkage between defective DNA repair and cancer. J Invest Dermatol 1994; 103: 96–101.

910 Wade MH, Plotnick H. Xeroderma pigmentosum and squamous cell carcinoma of the tongue. Identification of two black patients as members of complementation group C. J Am Acad Dermatol 1985; 12: 515–521.

911 Plotnick H, Lupulescu A. Ultrastructural studies of xeroderma pigmentosum. J Am Acad Dermatol 1983; 9: 876–882.

912 Tsuji T. Electron microscopic studies of xeroderma pigmentosum: unusual changes in the keratinocyte. Br J Dermatol 1974; 91: 657–666.

913 Friere-Maia N, Pinheiro M. Ectodermal dysplasias: a clinical and genetic syndrome. New York: Alan R Liss, 1984.

914 Lucky AW, Esterly NB, Tunnessen WW Jr. Ectodermal dysplasia and abnormal thumbs. J Am Acad Dermatol 1980; 2: 379–384.

915 Solomon LM, Keuer EJ. The ectodermal dysplasias. Problems of classification and some newer syndromes. Arch Dermatol 1980; 116: 1295–1299.

916 Tsakalakos N, Jordaan FH, Taljaard JJF, Hough SF. A previously undescribed ectodermal dysplasia of the tricho-odonto-onychial subgroup in a family. Arch Dermatol 1986; 122: 1047–1053.

917 Bartstra HLJ, Hulsmans RFHJ, Steijlen PM et al. Mosaic expression of hypohidrotic ectodermal dysplasia in an isolated affected female child. Arch Dermatol 1994; 130: 1421–1424.

918 Argenziano G, Monsurrò MR, Pazienza R, Delfino M. A case of probable autosomal recessive ectodermal dysplasia with corkscrew hairs and mental retardation in a family with tuberous sclerosis. J Am Acad Dermatol 1997; 37: 341–348.

919 Whittock NV, Coleman CM, McLean WHI et al. The gene for Naegeli–Franceschetti–Jadassohn syndrome maps to 17q21. J Invest Dermatol 2000; 115: 694–698.

920 Yotsumoto S, Setoyama M, Hozumi H et al. A novel point mutation affecting the tyrosine kinase domain of the *TRKA* gene in a family with congenital insensitivity to pain with anhidrosis. J Invest Dermatol 1999; 112: 810–814.

921 Martin-Pascual A, de Unamuno P, Aparicio M, Herreros V. Anhidrotic (or hypohidrotic) ectodermal dysplasia. Dermatologica 1977; 154: 235–243.

922 Sybert VP. Hypohidrotic ectodermal dysplasia: argument against an autosomal recessive form clinically indistinguishable from X-linked hypohidrotic ectodermal dysplasia (Christ–Siemens–Touraine syndrome). Pediatr Dermatol 1989; 6: 76–81.

923 Hizli Ş, Özdemir S, Bakkaloğlu A. Anhidrotic ectodermal dysplasia (Christ–Siemens–Touraine syndrome) presenting as a fever of unknown origin in an infant. Int J Dermatol 1998; 37: 132–134.

924 Davis JR, Solomon LM. Cellular immunodeficiency in anhidrotic ectodermal dysplasia. Acta Derm Venereol 1976; 56: 115–120.

925 Reed WB. Lopez DA, Landing B. Clinical spectrum of anhidrotic ectodermal dysplasia. Arch Dermatol 1970; 102: 134–143.

926 Reddy BSN, Chandra S, Jha PK, Singh G. Anhidrotic ectodermal dysplasia. Int J Dermatol 1978; 17: 139–141.

927 Arnold M-L, Rauskolb R, Anton-Lamprecht I et al. Prenatal diagnosis of anhidrotic ectodermal dysplasia. Prenatal Diagnosis 1984; 4: 85–98.

928 Verbov J. Hypohidrotic (or anhidrotic) ectodermal dysplasia – an appraisal of diagnostic methods. Br J Dermatol 1970; 83: 341–348.

929 Martinez F, Millán JM, Orellano C, Prieto F. X-linked anhidrotic (hypohidrotic) ectodermal dysplasia caused by a novel mutation in EDA1 gene: 406T>G (Leu55Arg). J Invest Dermatol 1999; 113: 285–286.

930 Aoki N, Ito K, Tachibana T, Ito M. A novel arginine → serine mutation in *EDA1* in a Japanese family with X-linked anhidrotic ectodermal dysplasia. J Invest Dermatol 2000; 115: 329–330.

931 Cambiaghi S, Restano L, Pääkkönen K et al. Clinical findings in mosaic carriers of hypohidrotic ectodermal dysplasia. Arch Dermatol 2000; 136: 217–224.

932 McGrath JA, Hoeger PH, Christiano AM et al. Skin fragility and hypohidrotic ectodermal dysplasia resulting from ablation of plakophilin 1. Br J Dermatol 1999; 140: 297–307.

933 Whittock NV, Haftek M, Angoulvant N et al. Genomic amplification of the human *plakophilin* 1 gene and detection of a new mutation in ectodermal dysplasia/skin fragility syndrome. J Invest Dermatol 2000; 115: 368–374.

934 Ando Y, Tanaka T, Horiguchi Y et al. Hidrotic ectodermal dysplasia: a clinical and ultrastructural observation. Dermatologica 1988; 176: 205–211.

935 Tan E, Tay Y-K. What syndrome is this? Pediatr Dermatol 2000; 17: 65–67.

936 Stevens HP, Choon SE, Hennies HC, Kelsell DP. Evidence for a single genetic locus in Clouston's hidrotic ectodermal dysplasia. Br J Dermatol 1999; 140: 963–964.

937 Taylor TD, Hayflick SJ, McKinnon W et al. Confirmation of linkage of Clouston syndrome (hidrotic ectodermal dysplasia) to 13q11–q12.1 with evidence for multiple independent mutations. J Invest Dermatol 1998; 111: 83–85.

938 Lamartine J, Laoudj D, Blanchet-Bardon C et al. Refined localization of the gene for Clouston syndrome (hidrotic ectodermal dysplasia) in a large French family. Br J Dermatol 2000; 142: 248–252.

939 Solomon LM, Fretzin D, Pruzansky S. Pilosebaceous dysplasia in the oral-facial-digital syndrome. Arch Dermatol 1970; 102: 598–602.

940 Arbesfeld D. Thomas I, Janniger CK et al. Ectrodactyly, ectodermal dysplasia, and cleft palate syndrome: report of a case with generalized telangiectasias. J Am Acad Dermatol 1993; 29: 347–350.

941 Fosko SW, Stenn KS, Bolognia JL. Ectodermal dysplasias associated with clefting: significance of scalp dermatitis. J Am Acad Dermatol 1992; 27: 249–256.

942 O'Donnell BP, James WD. Rapp–Hodgkin ectodermal dysplasia. J Am Acad Dermatol 1992; 27: 323–326.

943 Cambiaghi S, Tadini G, Barbareschi M et al. Rapp–Hodgkin syndrome and AEC syndrome: are they the same entity? Br J Dermatol 1994; 130: 97–101.

944 Bertola DR, Kim CA, Sugayama SMM et al. AEC syndrome and CHAND syndrome: further evidence of clinical overlapping in the ectodermal dysplasias. Pediatr Dermatol 2000; 17: 218–221.

945 Zenteno JC, Venegas C, Kofman-Alfaro S. Evidence that AEC syndrome and Bowen–Armstrong syndrome are variable expressions of the same disease. Pediatr Dermatol 1999; 16: 103–107.

946 Wessagowit W, Mellerio JE, Pembroke AC, McGrath JA. Heterozygous germline missense mutation in the *p63* gene underlying EEC syndrome. Clin Exp Dermatol 2000; 25: 441–443.

947 Lambert WC, Bilinski DL. Diagnostic pitfalls in anhidrotic ectodermal dysplasia: indications for palmar skin biopsy. Cutis 1983; 31: 182–187.

948 Katz SI, Penneys NS. Sebaceous gland papules in anhidrotic ectodermal dysplasia. Arch Dermatol 1971; 103: 507–509.

949 Frix CD III, Bronson DM. Acute miliary tuberculosis in a child with anhidrotic ectodermal dysplasia. Pediatr Dermatol 1986; 3: 464–467.

950 From E, Philipsen HP, Thormann J. Dyskeratosis benigna intraepithelialis mucosae et cutis hereditaria. A report of this disorder in father and son. J Cutan Pathol 1978; 5: 105–115.

951 James WD, Lupton GP. Acquired dyskeratotic leukoplakia. Arch Dermatol 1988; 124: 117–120.

952 Scheman AJ, Ray DJ, Witkop CJ Jr, Dahl MV. Hereditary mucoepithelial dysplasia. Case report and review of the literature. J Am Acad Dermatol 1989; 21: 351–357.

953 Xifra M, Lagodin C, Wright D et al. Nevoid keratosis of the nipple. J Am Acad Dermatol 1999; 41: 325–326.

954 Toros P, Önder M, Gürer MA. Bilateral nipple hyperkeratosis treated successfully with topical isotretinoin. Australas J Dermatol 1999; 40: 220–222.

955 Busse A, Peschen M, Schöpf E, Vanscheidt W. Treatment of hyperkeratosis areolae mammae naeviformis with the carbon dioxide laser. J Am Acad Dermatol 1999; 41: 274–276.

956 Revert A, Bañuls J, Montesinos E et al. Nevoid hyperkeratosis of the areola. Int J Dermatol 1993; 32: 745–746.

957 Kubota Y, Koga T, Nakayama J, Kiryu H. Naevoid hyperkeratosis of the nipple and areola in a man. Br J Dermatol 2000; 142: 382–384.

958 Mitxelena J, Ratón JA, Bilbao I, Díaz-Perez JL. Nevoid hyperkeratosis of the areola in men: response to cryotherapy. Dermatology 1999; 199: 73–74.

959 Aras N, Sutman K, Tastan HB et al. Peeling skin syndrome. J Am Acad Dermatol 1994; 30: 135–136.

960 Brusasco A, Veraldi S, Tadini G, Caputo R. Localized peeling skin syndrome: case report with ultrastructural study. Br J Dermatol 1998; 139: 492–495.

961 Shwayder T, Lowe L. Acral peeling skin syndrome. Arch Dermatol 1997; 133: 535–536.

962 Hashimoto K, Hamzavi I, Tanaka K, Shwayder T. Acral peeling skin syndrome. J Am Acad Dermatol 2000; 43: 1112–1119.

963 Mevorah B, Frenk E, Saurat JH, Siegenthaler G. Peeling skin syndrome: a clinical, ultrastructural and biochemical study. Br J Dermatol 1987; 116: 117–125.

964 Mevorah B, Salomon D, Siegenthaler G et al. Ichthyosiform dermatosis with superficial blister formation and peeling: evidence for a desmosomal anomaly and altered epidermal vitamin A metabolism. J Am Acad Dermatol 1996; 34: 379–385.

965 Tastan HB, Akar A, Gür AR, Deveci S. Peeling skin syndrome. Int J Dermatol 1999; 38: 208–210.

Miscellaneous disorders

966 Northcutt AD, Nelson DM, Tschen JA. Axillary granular parakeratosis. J Am Acad Dermatol 1991; 24: 541–544.

967 Metze D, Rütten A. Granular parakeratosis – a unique acquired disorder of keratinization. J Cutan Pathol 1999; 26: 339–352.

968 Mehregan DA, Thomas JE, Mehregan DR. Intertriginous granular parakeratosis. J Am Acad Dermatol 1998; 39: 495–496.

969 Wohlrab J, Lüftl M, Wolter M, Marsch WC. Submammary granular parakeratosis: An acquired punctate hyperkeratosis of exogenous origin. J Am Acad Dermatol 1999; 40: 813–814.

970 Kossard S, White A. Axillary granular parakeratosis. Australas J Dermatol 1998; 39: 186–187.

971 Webster CG, Resnik KS, Webster GF. Axillary granular parakeratosis: Response to isotretinoin. J Am Acad Dermatol 1997; 37: 789–790.

Disorders of pigmentation

INTRODUCTION

This chapter deals with the various disorders of cutaneous pigmentation, excluding those entities in which there is an obvious lentiginous proliferation of melanocytes in sections stained with hematoxylin and eosin; it also excludes tumors of the nevus-cell–melanocyte system. Both of the excluded categories are discussed in Chapter 32. Cutaneous pigmentation may also result from the deposition of drug complexes in the dermis. This category of pigmentation is discussed among other cutaneous deposits in Chapter 14. A related condition is the excessive dietary intake of carotenoid-containing foods, which may cause yellow-orange discoloration of the skin.[1]

Cutaneous pigmentary disorders can be divided into two major categories: disorders with hypopigmentation and those with hyperpigmentation. The dyschromatoses, in which areas both of hypopigmentation and hyperpigmentation are present, have been arbitrarily included with the disorders of hyperpigmentation.

The pigmentary system

The pigmentary system involves a complex set of reactions with numerous potential sites for dysfunction.[2] Melanin is produced in melanosomes in the cytoplasm of melanocytes by the action of tyrosinase on tyrosine. A number of intermediate steps involving the formation of dopa and dopaquinone take place prior to the synthesis of melanin. The melanin synthesized in any one melanocyte is then transferred to an average of 36 keratinocytes by the phagocytosis of the melanin-laden dendritic tips of the melanocytes.[3] The protease-activated receptor 2 (PAR-2), which is expressed on keratinocytes, is a key receptor involved in melanosome transfer.[4] Other important participants in this process include kinesin and actin-associated myosin V. The latter protein secures the peripheral melanosomes, preparing them for transfer to surrounding keratinocytes.[5] This transfer of melanin can be disrupted by any inflammatory process involving the basal layer of the epidermis. Specific enzyme defects and destruction of melanocytes are other theoretical causes of hypopigmentation.

The pathogenesis of hyperpigmentation is not as well understood. Prominent pigment incontinence is an obvious cause of hyperpigmentation. Ultrastructural examination in some disorders of hyperpigmentation has shown an increase in size or melanization of the melanosomes, although in others the reasons for the basal hyperpigmentation have not been determined.

The disorders of hypopigmentation will be discussed first.

DISORDERS CHARACTERIZED BY HYPOPIGMENTATION

There are multiple potential sites for dysfunction in the formation of melanin pigment in basal melanocytes.[3] Attempts have been made to categorize the various diseases with hypopigmentation on the basis of their presumed pathogenesis. The following categories may be considered.

1. *Abnormal migration/differentiation of melanoblasts*: piebaldism, Waardenburg's and Woolf's syndromes.
2. *Destruction of melanocytes*: vitiligo, Vogt–Koyanagi–Harada syndrome, chemical leukoderma.
3. *Reduced tyrosinase activity*: oculocutaneous albinism type IA, phenylketonuria(?).
4. *Abnormal structure of melanosomes*: 'ash leaf spots' of tuberous sclerosis, Chédiak–Higashi syndrome, progressive macular hypomelanosis.
5. *Reduced melanization and/or numbers of melanosomes*: albinism (other tyrosinase-positive variants), Griscelli syndrome, Elejalde syndrome, idiopathic guttate hypomelanosis, hypomelanosis of Ito, 'ash leaf spots', pityriasis versicolor (tinea versicolor), nevus depigmentosus.
6. *Reduced transfer to keratinocytes*: nevus depigmentosus, pityriasis alba, postinflammatory leukoderma, pityriasis versicolor (tinea versicolor), Chédiak–Higashi syndrome. Increased degradation of melanosomes within melanocytes may also apply in some conditions listed in this section.
7. *Abnormal vasculature*: nevus anemicus.

In addition to the conditions listed above, there are isolated reports of one or more cases in which the hypopigmentation does not correspond neatly to any of the named diseases.[6–8] These cases will not be considered further.

Phenylketonuria, an autosomal recessive disorder with a deficiency of the enzyme L-phenylalanine hydroxylase, is characterized by oculocutaneous pigmentary dilution in addition to neurological abnormalities.[3,9] There are several steps in the biosynthesis of melanin that may be affected by this enzyme deficiency. As biopsies are rarely taken, this condition will not be discussed further.

PIEBALDISM

In piebaldism (partial albinism), an autosomal dominant disorder, there are non-progressive, discrete patches of leukoderma present from birth.[3] The chalk-white areas of hypomelanosis involve the anterior part of the trunk, the mid-region of the extremities, the forehead and the mid-frontal area of the scalp beneath a white forelock.[3] This hair change is present in up to 90% of those with piebaldism and it is sometimes found as an isolated change in the absence of cutaneous leukoderma.[10] Within the areas of hypomelanosis there are hyperpigmented and normally pigmented macules of various sizes.[11]

There are several rare syndromes in which extracutaneous manifestations, such as Hirschsprung's disease, accompany the piebaldism.[3,12–14] Other examples include *Waardenburg's syndrome*, in which piebaldism is associated with neurosensory hearing loss and other abnormalities,[15–18] and *Woolf's syndrome* in which the hearing loss is the only associated feature.[3] Two variants of Waardenburg's syndrome have been described, due to the involvement of two different, but interrelated genes. *PAX3*, the gene responsible for type 1, regulates *MITF*, the gene responsible for type 2. The *MITF* gene (microphthalmia-associated transcription factor) is assigned to chromosome 3p14.1–p12.3.[19] Neurofibromatosis 1 (NF-1) has also been associated with piebaldism.[20]

Piebaldism results from mutations of the *kit* proto-oncogene, which encodes a cell-surface receptor, tyrosine kinase, whose ligand is the stem/mast cell growth factor.[21,22] In humans, the *kit* proto-oncogene has been mapped to the proximal long arm of chromosome 4 (4q11–q12).[14,22] Variations in the phenotype relate to the site of the *kit* gene mutation. A novel *kit* mutation, Val620Ala, results in piebaldism with progressive depigmentation.[23] In mice, *kit*-mediated signal transduction is required in embryogenesis for the proliferation and migration of melanoblasts from the neural crest. It appears to be required, in humans, for melanocyte proliferation.[10,21,22] The successful use of autologous grafts to repigment the affected areas is not inconsistent with these theories.[24,25]

Histopathology

There are usually no melanocytes and no melanin in the leukodermic areas. Sometimes a small number of morphologically abnormal melanocytes is present, particularly near the margins of hypopigmentation. These melanocytes may have spherical melanosomes. Some clear cells, representing Langerhans cells, are usually present in the epidermis.[26]

The hyperpigmented islands contain normal numbers of melanocytes: there are abundant melanosomes in the melanocytes and in keratinocytes. There are no dopa-positive melanocytes in the hair bulbs of the white forelock.[16]

VITILIGO

Vitiligo is an acquired, idiopathic disorder in which there are depigmented macules of variable size which enlarge and coalesce to form extensive areas of leukoderma.[27–30] An erythematous border is occasionally present in the initial stages.[3,31–33] Repigmentation may lead to several shades of color in a particular lesion,[34] as may transitional stages in depigmentation (trichrome vitiligo).[35] The incidence in Caucasians is approximately 1%. This condition may develop at any age, although in 50% of affected persons it appears before the age of 20 years.[36,37] A family history is present in up to 25% of cases; the inheritance appears to be polygenic.[28,38–40] Vitiligo does not appear to be caused by mutations in the GTP-cyclohydrolase I gene, which regulates melanin biosynthesis.[41]

There is a predilection for the face, back of the hands, axillae, groins, umbilicus and genitalia, and for the skin overlying bony areas such as the knees and elbows.[28] Sometimes the depigmented area is segmental or dermatomal in distribution (type B); more often it is more generalized (type A).[42,43] Repigmentation seldom occurs in type B, which is also resistant to treatment and more common in children.[43–46]

Approximately 20–30% of individuals with vitiligo (usually those with bilateral/generalized disease)[44] have an associated autoimmune and/or endocrine disorder[3] such as Hashimoto's disease, hyperthyroidism, pernicious anemia, Addison's disease,[47] insulin-dependent diabetes mellitus[48–50] and alopecia areata.[51,52] Less frequent associations include various lympho-proliferative diseases, morphea,[53] chronic actinic dermatitis,[54] the mitochondrial encephalomyopathy, lactic acidosis and stroke-like episodes syndrome (MELAS),[55] Crohn's disease,[56,57] prior infection with cytomegalovirus[58,59] and chronic mucocutaneous candidosis.[60] The reported association of vitiligo with psoriasis and erythema dyschromicum perstans[61] is probably fortuitous. Depigmentation resembling vitiligo has been reported following contact with hydroquinones, certain phenolic agents,[28] cinnamic aldehyde in toothpaste,[62] topical minoxidil,[63] and PUVA therapy.[64,65] Ganciclovir, used in the treatment of graft-versus-host disease (GVHD), produced extensive vitiligo in one patient.[66]

Vitiligo may be accompanied by a variety of ocular pigmentary disturbances.[67] The best known of these is the *Vogt–Koyanagi–Harada* syndrome, which includes uveitis, poliosis, dysacusis, alopecia, vitiligo and signs of meningeal irritation.[68,69] Not all these features are present in all cases. An immunologic etiology has been suggested.[70] A rare variant of this syndrome with inflammatory vitiligo has been described.[71]

Sometimes there is a history in the patient or the patient's immediate family of premature graying of the hair (poliosis), a halo nevus or even a malignant melanoma.[72] It is interesting to note that individuals with metastatic melanoma who develop vitiligo-like depigmentation have a better prognosis than those who do not.[73,74] Both lesions have clonally expanded T cells with identical BV regions.[75]

The onset of vitiligo is usually insidious with no precipitating cause. In approximately 20% of cases it develops after severe sunburn or some severe emotional or physical stress.[28] The majority of cases have a progressive clinical course.[76,77] In generalized forms the depigmentation may eventually involve large areas of skin. Some repigmentation may occur but it is usually incomplete and short lived.[28,68] Repigmentation probably involves melanocytes from hair follicles.[78,79] Eventually the process of depigmentation ceases. Vitiligo may have a significant effect on the psychological well-being of some patients.[80]

Pathogenesis

Three hypotheses have been proposed to explain the destruction of melanocytes which results in the depigmentation.[30,68,81,82] These may be summarized as the neural, the self-destructive and the immune theories. They are not mutually exclusive.[47] The *neural hypothesis* suggests that a neurochemical mediator released at nerve endings results in destruction of melanocytes. It has been proposed that the segmental form (type B) of vitiligo results from dysfunction of sympathetic nerves in the affected areas.[43] Support for this hypothesis comes from the finding of increased neuropeptide Y activity in vitiligo.[83] The *self-destruction hypothesis* (autocytotoxicity) is based on the known toxicity of melanin precursors for melanocytes. It is assumed that affected individuals have an intrinsic inability to eliminate or handle these toxic precursors, such as free radicals, which accumulate and result in the destruction of melanocytes.[29,84] Experimental studies suggest that early cell death of vitiligo melanocytes is related to their increased sensitivity to oxidative stress, which may in some way be linked to the abnormal expression of tyrosinase-related protein (TRP-1).[85] The *immune hypothesis*, which is currently most favored, particularly for the generalized forms, proposes that antibody-dependent, cell-mediated cytotoxicity utilizing natural killer cells is responsible for the loss of melanocytes.[86] Infiltrating T cells and macrophages have been observed adjacent to the remaining perilesional melanocytes in generalized vitiligo.[87] However, other studies have suggested that antibodies to melanocytes in the IgG fraction of patient's serum may be the effector mechanism for melanocyte destruction;[88–91] the level of the antibodies correlates with disease activity.[92] The antibodies do not appear to be directed against tyrosinase, despite some reports to the contrary.[93–96] Other experiments also downplay the role of natural killer and lymphokine-activated killer cells in the pathogenesis.[97–99] Various other abnormalities in the immune system have been recorded in vitiligo.[100] These include a decrease in T-helper cells,[101–103] an increase in natural killer cells,[102,104] circulating antibodies to surface antigens on melanocytes[105–108] and to certain melanoma cell lines,[109,110] an increase in met-enkephalin secretion,[111] a decrease in the expression of c-*kit* protein by melanocytes adjacent to lesional skin,[112,113] abnormal expression of MHC class II molecules and ICAM-1 by perilesional melanocytes,[114] and possible functional impairment of Langerhans cells.[115,116]

Grafting studies have until recently shown variable results;[117,118] localized vitiligo has now been successfully treated using autologous grafts, although non-surgical treatments such as corticosteroids and UVB therapy continue to be used with some success.[119–124] Generalized vitiligo is more difficult to treat, although some success has been achieved with autologous minigrafting.[120,125–129] Plaques of verruca vulgaris have been seen in grafted skin of a vitiligo patient.[130] Laser therapy can be used to remove disfiguring residual pigmentation in patients with generalized disease.[131]

Histopathology

Vitiliginous skin shows a complete loss of melanin pigment from the epidermis and an absence of melanocytes (Fig. 10.1). At the advancing border the melanocytes may be increased in size with an increased number of dendrites (Fig. 10.2).[28] Occasional lymphocytes may be present in this region;[132] these cells are invariably present if there is an inflammatory border clinically. In these instances there is also a perivascular infiltrate of mononuclear cells

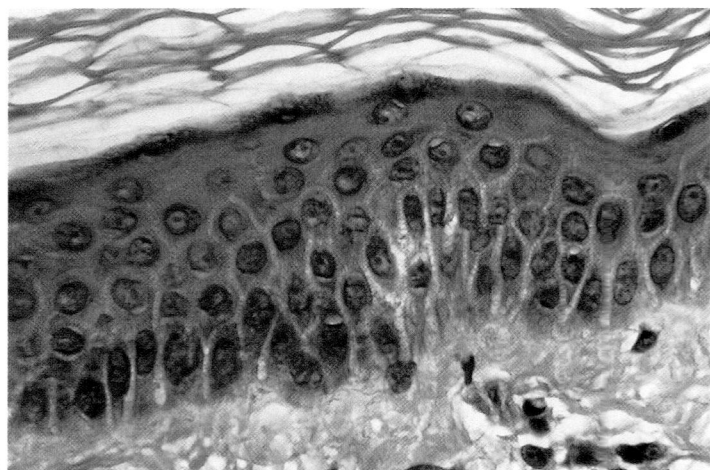 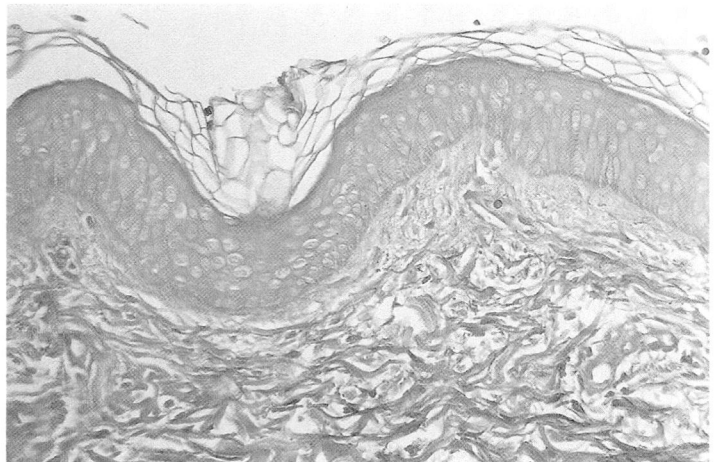

Fig. 10.1 **Vitiligo. (A)** Melanocytes and melanin are absent from the basal layer (H & E). **(B)** No melanin can be seen in the basal layer or dermis in this stain for melanin. (Masson–Fontana)

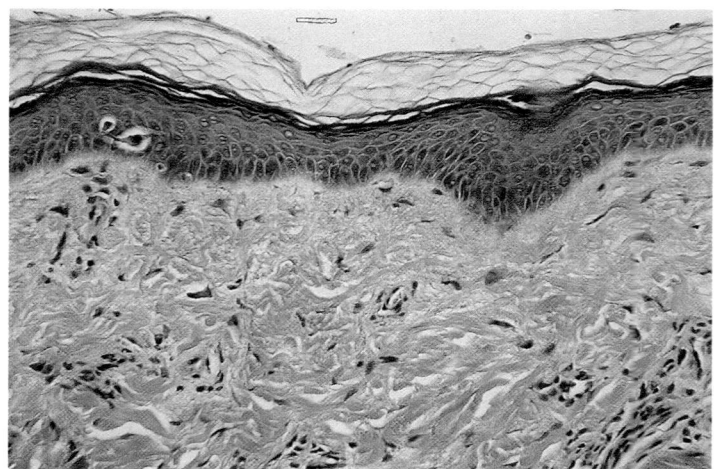

Fig. 10.2 **Vitiligo.** A melanocyte with a giant melanosome is present at the edge of the depigmented area. (H & E)

involving the superficial plexus, as well as some superficial edema.[133] A heavy lymphocytic infiltrate in the upper dermis is a rare finding.[134] Ultrathin sections will often show vacuolated keratinocytes and extracellular granular material in the basal layer of the normal skin adjacent to areas of vitiligo.[135] If serial sections are examined, a lymphocyte will sometimes be found in close apposition to a melanocyte at the advancing edge (Fig. 10.3). Degenerative changes have also been reported in nerves and sweat glands.[136] Merkel cells were absent from lesional skin in one study.[137]

The incidence of actinic damage and various skin cancers is surprisingly low in vitiligo patients, possibly because they practise sun-protection strategies.[138]

Electron microscopy

Melanocytes are absent from lesions of long standing.[139] Melanocytes and keratinocytes adjacent to the vitiliginous areas show degenerative changes in the form of intracellular edema and vacuolar formation.[135,139–141] Extracellular material derived from degenerating keratinocytes is sometimes present.[135] Fibrillar masses similar to colloid bodies may also be present in the upper dermis and in the basal layer.[135] Numerous nerve endings may be seen in

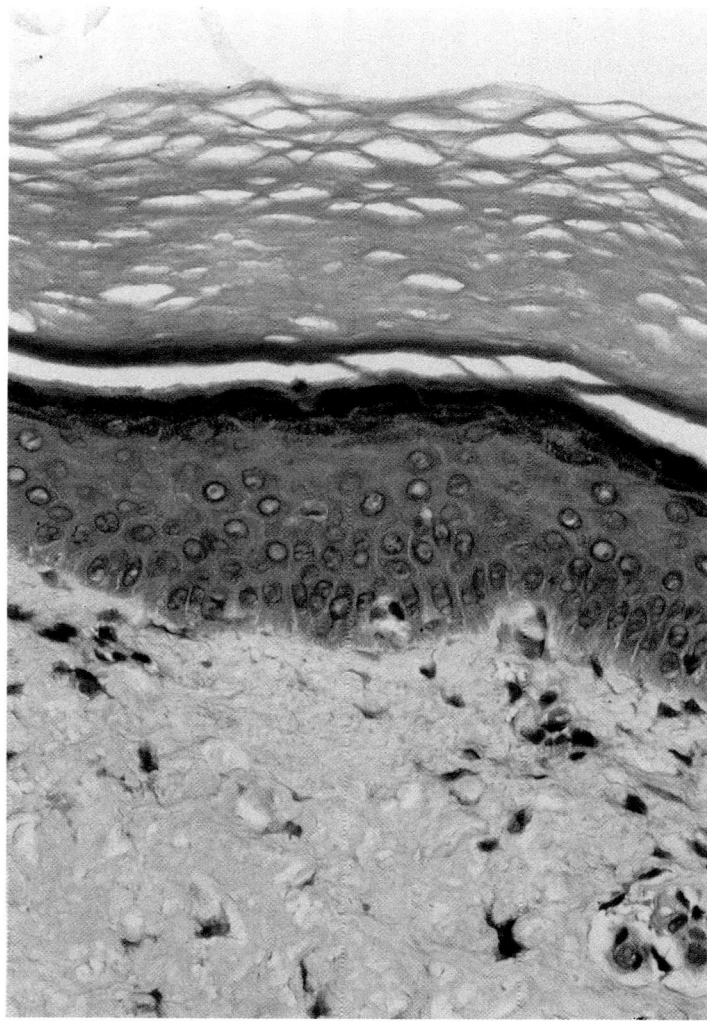

Fig. 10.3 **Vitiligo.** A lymphocyte is present next to a melanocyte showing early apoptosis. Melanocytes are absent elsewhere in the basal layer. (H & E)

close contact with the basal lamina.[40] There may be increased thickness of the basement membrane of Schwann cells and features of both axonal degeneration and nerve regeneration.[142]

OCULOCUTANEOUS ALBINISM

Oculocutaneous albinism is a genetically heterogeneous group of disorders in which there is a generalized decrease or absence of melanin pigment in the eyes, hair and skin.[143] At least 10 forms of this condition have been identified, each presumably resulting from a different biochemical block in the synthesis of melanin.[3]

Type IA oculocutaneous albinism

In type IA, the classic type, the defect is a complete absence of tyrosinase activity in melanocytes.[144] The tyrosinase gene has been cloned. It is present on chromosome 11q14–q21.[145–147] Many different mutations of type IA have been described.[145,148,149] Prenatal diagnosis of type IA can be made by performing a dopa test on the hair bulbs of fetuses, obtained by scalp biopsy.[150] This technique has been superseded by analysis of the fetal tyrosinase gene.[151] Inheritance is autosomal recessive in type. The clinical presentation at birth is white hair and skin and blue eyes.

Ocular disorders include photophobia, nystagmus, strabismus and reduced visual acuity. In the skin there is accelerated photoaging and an increased incidence of keratoses and squamous and basal cell carcinomas.[152,153] Malignant melanomas develop occasionally.[154] The dysplastic nevus syndrome has also been reported in individuals with oculocutaneous albinism.[155] Lentigines and nevi do not form in type IA, the tyrosinase-negative phenotype.[3]

In all phenotypes except type IA, there is some increase in pigment with age, the amount depending on the ethnic background of the individual and the particular subtype of the disorder.[143] Red-yellow pheomelanin is the first to form; black-brown eumelanin is synthesized only after a long period of pheomelanin formation.[143]

Yellow mutant oculocutaneous albinism (type IB)

In yellow mutant oculocutaneous albinism (type IB), tyrosinase activity and melanin biosynthesis are greatly reduced.[149] There is extreme hypopigmentation at birth with the eventual development of yellow or blond hair. A splicing mutation of the tyrosinase gene on chromosome 11q14–q21 has been reported.[156]

Oculocutaneous albinism type 2

In oculocutaneous albinism type 2, an autosomal recessive disease, there is defective melanin production in the skin, hair and eyes.[157] It is caused by mutations of the *P* gene, located on chromosome 15q11–q13, and thought to act as a transporter in the melanosomal membrane. The *P* gene is deleted in the majority of patients with Angelman syndrome and Prader–Willi syndrome.[157]

Tyrosinase-positive oculocutaneous albinism

In tyrosinase-positive oculocutaneous albinism, one of the commonest genetic conditions in Africa, there is also a defect in chromosome 15q11–q13. It appears to be a phenotypic variant of type 2. Palmoplantar freckles and melanocytic nevi occur in a significant number of subjects with this form of the disease.[158]

Hermansky–Pudlak syndrome

In the Hermansky–Pudlak syndrome, one of the clinical variants of oculocutaneous albinism, there is also a defect in platelets.[3,159] Lipid and ceroid pigment are present in macrophages in various organs, including the skin.[160] Pulmonary ceroid deposition leading to respiratory failure is a common cause of death.[161] The *HPS1* gene, mutations of which are responsible for the Hermansky–Pudlak syndrome, maps to chromosome 10q23.[162,163] Mutations cause lysosomal dysfunction in platelets and melanocytes, possibly by affecting calcium channel integrity in the cells.[164,165] Other cutaneous findings, most often related to a specific 16-base pair duplication of the *HPS1* gene, include dysplastic nevi, acanthosis nigricans-like lesions in the neck and axilla, and trichomegaly.[162]

The Chédiak–Higashi syndrome, the Griscelli syndrome and the Elejalde syndrome (see below) are sometimes regarded as other clinical variants. They have in common the presence of silvery hair and mild skin coloration which is not strictly albinism.

Generalized cutaneous depigmentation resembling albinism has been reported in a patient treated with a sulfonamide. However, the absence of melanocytes on electron microscopy was more in keeping with vitiligo or chemical leukoderma.[166]

Histopathology

There is a complete or partial reduction in melanin pigment in the skin and hair bulbs. Melanocytes are normal in number and morphology (Fig. 10.4). Tyrosinase activity is lacking in melanocytes in freshly plucked anagen hair bulbs in type IA;[167] it is reduced in heterozygotes with this phenotype and variably reduced in some of the other types. Tyrosinase activity is normal in type II.[144]

Electron microscopy

Melanocytes and melanosomes are normal in configuration. There are no stage III or IV melanosomes in type IA. Macromelanosomes have been found in the basal layers of the epidermis in the Hermansky–Pudlak syndrome.[165,168] The melanocytes have shortened dendritic processes.[169]

CHÉDIAK–HIGASHI SYNDROME

The Chédiak–Higashi syndrome is a rare, autosomal recessive disorder in which there is partial oculocutaneous albinism associated with frequent pyogenic infections and the presence of abnormal, large granules in leukocytes and some other cells.[170–172] The disease usually enters an accelerated phase in childhood, with pancytopenia, hepatosplenomegaly and lymphohistiocytic

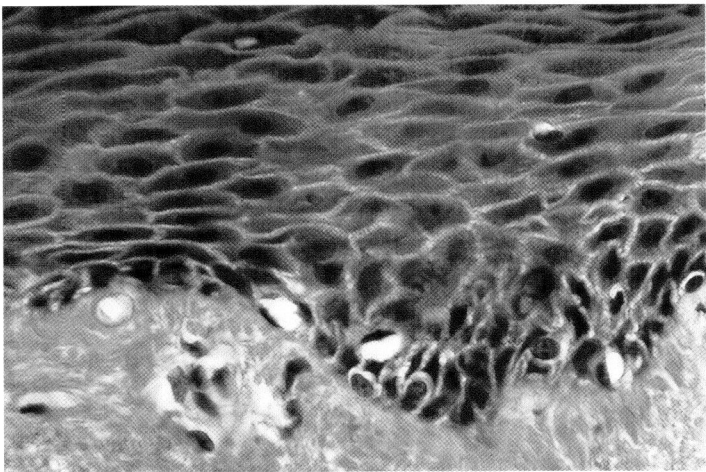

Fig. 10.4 **Albinism.** Melanin is absent from the basal layer but melanocytes are normal in number and morphology. (H & E)

infiltrates in various organs.[173] This phase, which resembles the virus-associated hemophagocytic syndrome, is usually followed by death.[173]

The pigmentary dilution involves at least one and often all three of the following – skin, hair and eyes.[170,174] There is increased susceptibility to burning. The hair is usually blond or light brown in color.

The increased susceptibility to infection is related to impaired function of leukocytes and natural killer cells associated with lysosomal defects while the reduced skin pigmentation is related to similar defects in melanocytes.[173,175] The inclusions found in these and other cells are massive secondary lysosomal structures formed through a combined process of fusion, cytoplasmic injury and phagocytosis.[173,175]

The gene responsible for this condition maps to chromosome 1q42–1q43. The gene has been designated *LYST* (lysosomal trafficking regulator).

Histopathology

There is a striking reduction or even absence of melanin pigment in the basal layer and in hair follicles.[170] A few large pigment granules corresponding to giant melanosomes are present.[176] In less affected individuals and in some heterozygotes, clumps of enlarged pigment granules may also be present in the dermis in macrophages and endothelial cells and lying free in the interstitium.[174]

Staining with toluidine blue demonstrates large cytoplasmic inclusions in cutaneous mast cells.[176]

Electron microscopy

Giant melanosomes and degenerating cytoplasmic residues are found in melanocytes.[177] The pigment granules passed to keratinocytes are bigger than normal.[177] The giant melanosomes appear to arise from defective premelanosomes.[177] Giant cytoplasmic granules have also been found in Langerhans cells.[178] They are believed to be derived from the fusion of lysosomes or some portion of Birbeck granules.[178]

GRISCELLI SYNDROME

The Griscelli syndrome is characterized by reduced skin pigmentation, often regarded as partial albinism, and silvery-gray hair combined with immunodeficiency.[179] It has an autosomal recessive mode of inheritance with the gene mapping to chromosome 15q21; more loci probably exist.[180] There are no abnormal cytoplasmic granules in leukocytes as found in the Chédiak–Higashi syndrome (see above).

Histopathology

There is some pigment in melanocytes but none in adjacent keratinocytes.

Electron microscopy

There are some type IV melanosomes in basal melanocytes and shortened dendritic processes. The hair shafts show uneven clusters of aggregated melanin pigment, mainly in the medulla.[179]

ELEJALDE SYNDROME

The Elejalde syndrome has the triad of silvery hair, hypopigmented skin (sometimes referred to as partial albinism) and severe dysfunction of the central nervous system (hypotonia, seizures and mental retardation).[181] There is no immunodeficiency.

Histopathology

Melanin granules in the basal layer are of irregular size and distribution with overall reduced pigmentation. Hair shafts are similar to those seen in the Griscelli syndrome (see above).

PROGRESSIVE MACULAR HYPOMELANOSIS

Progressive macular hypomelanosis of the trunk is an acquired form of hypopigmentation with a predisposition to affect the back of young adult females of Caribbean origin.[182] The hypopigmented macules, which measure 1–3 cm in diameter, coalesce into large patches. The disease may remit in 3–4 years. A recent study has suggested that idiopathic guttate hypomelanosis (see below) is a related disorder along a spectrum of disorders of depigmentation.[183]

Histopathology[182]

There is a decrease in melanin pigment within the epidermis. Melanocytes are normal in number.

Electron microscopy

There is a reduction in stage IV (negroid) melanosomes which are replaced by small type I–III melanosomes in an aggregated (caucasoid) pattern.

TUBEROUS SCLEROSIS

Tuberous sclerosis is characterized by the triad of epilepsy, mental retardation and multiple angiofibromas ('adenoma sebaceum') (see p. 918). In addition, circumscribed macules of hypopigmentation known as 'ash leaf spots' can be present at birth on the trunk and lower extremities.[3,184] They vary in diameter from mm to 12 cm. The more common shapes are oval, polygonal or ash leaf-like. The basic abnormality appears to be an arrest in the maturation of melanosomes.[3]

Histopathology

Epidermal melanin is reduced, but not absent.

Electron microscopy[3,185]

Electron microscopy has shown a normal number of melanocytes and a reduction in the number, size and melanization of the melanosomes.[184] The small melanosomes often form aggregates within the keratinocytes.

IDIOPATHIC GUTTATE HYPOMELANOSIS

Idiopathic guttate hypomelanosis is a common leukodermic dermatosis of unknown etiology in which multiple achromic or hypochromic macules, 2–5 mm in diameter, develop over many years.[186–189] They are usually found on the sun-exposed extremities of elderly individuals, but scattered lesions may occur on the trunk.[190,191] Repigmentation does not occur. The author and colleagues have seen this pattern of pigmentation in patients who have received bone marrow transplants (unpublished observation).

Histopathology[188,189,192]

There is a decrease in melanin pigment in the basal layer of the epidermis and a reduction in the number of dopa-positive melanocytes, although these cells are never completely absent. The epidermis usually shows some atrophy, with flattening of the rete pegs. There may be basket-weave hyperkeratosis.

Electron microscopy

Some of the melanocytes remaining in affected areas of skin show a reduction in dendritic processes and melanosomes.[193,194]

HYPOMELANOSIS OF ITO

Hypomelanosis of Ito (incontinentia pigmenti achromians) presents at birth or in infancy with sharply demarcated, hypopigmented macular lesions on the trunk and extremities, with a distinctive linear or whorled pattern distributed along the lines of Blaschko.[195–200] The pattern resembles a negative image of the pigmentation seen in incontinentia pigmenti (see p. 333).[201] The co-existence of hypomelanosis of Ito and incontinentia pigmenti in the same family, even though disputed by a subsequent author,[202] and the report of several patients with a preceding erythematous or verrucous stage[203,204] have led several authorities to postulate a link between these two conditions.[196,203]

Other features of hypomelanosis of Ito include a female preponderance, a tendency for lesions to become somewhat pigmented in late childhood, a family history in a few cases[205] and the coexistence in a high percentage of patients of abnormalities of the central nervous system (particularly seizures and mental retardation), eyes, hair, teeth and musculoskeletal system.[195,196,206–208]

Many different chromosomal abnormalities have been recorded in this condition, leading to a suggestion that this is not a discrete diagnostic condition.[198,207]

Histopathology

The hypopigmented areas show a reduction in melanin pigment in the basal layer, but this is usually not discernible in hematoxylin and eosin-stained sections and requires a Masson–Fontana stain for confirmation. Dopa stains show a reduction in staining of melanocytes and sometimes shortening of their dendrites.[209] A reduction in the number of melanocytes[210] and vacuolization of basal keratinocytes have been mentioned in some reports but specifically excluded in most.[211]

Electron microscopy

Electron microscopy has shown a reduction in melanosomes in melanocytes in the hypopigmented areas and a decrease in the number of melanin granules in keratinocytes.[195] There are isolated reports of aggregation of melanosomes, vacuolization of melanocytes[140] and an increase in the number of Langerhans cells in the epidermis.[212]

NEVUS DEPIGMENTOSUS

Nevus depigmentosus (achromic nevus) is a little-studied entity consisting of isolated, circular or rectangular, hypopigmented macules with a predisposition for the trunk and proximal parts of the extremities.[3] It may also occur along Blaschko's lines or in a systematized pattern, the latter having some clinical resemblance to the pattern seen in hypomelanosis of Ito.[185,213] In the majority of cases the lesions are present at birth or appear in early childhood.[214] Systemic lesions are uncommon[215] but an association with unilateral lentiginosis and ILVEN (see p. 755) has been reported.[216,217]

One study found a selective defect in eumelanogenesis in nevus depigmentosus, although this remains to be confirmed.[218]

Histopathology

Melanocytes are said to be normal or slightly reduced in number, although there is reduced dopa activity.[3,214]

Electron microscopy[185]

Melanosomes are normal in size but there may be abnormal aggregation of them within melanocytes.[218] One study showed a reduction of melanosomes in melanocytes.[214] Degradation of melanosomes within autophagosomes of melanocytes has been noted. Melanosomes are decreased in number in keratinocytes, suggesting impaired transfer.[215]

PITYRIASIS ALBA

Pityriasis alba consists of variably hypopigmented, slightly scaly patches with a predilection for the face, neck and shoulders of dark-skinned atopic individuals.[219–221] The etiology is unknown although it has been regarded as postinflammatory hypopigmentation following eczema.[219]

A supposed variant with extensive non-scaling macules involving the lower part of the trunk has been reported, but there is no real evidence that this is the same process.[220,221] It is not related to atopy.

Another suggested clinical variant is *pigmenting pityriasis alba*, in which a central zone of bluish hyperpigmentation develops in a scaly, hypopigmented patch.[222] A dermatophyte was present in 65% of these cases.[222]

Histopathology

There are no detailed studies of the usual facial type of pityriasis alba. In a personally studied case there was mild hyperkeratosis, focal parakeratosis and focal mild spongiosis with prominent exocytosis of lymphocytes.[223] There was also a mild superficial perivascular inflammatory cell infiltrate in the dermis. Melanin pigmentation of the basal layer was markedly reduced, but there was no melanin incontinence.[223] Melanocytes were normal in number. This conforms with one other reported case.[224] A reduced number of melanocytes with smaller melanosomes is another suggested finding.[222]

A study of the 'extensive' variant showed reduced basal pigmentation, a decreased number of functional melanocytes on the dopa preparation, and a reduction in the number and size of melanosomes.[220]

A study of 39 Mexican patients showed follicular spongiosis and keratotic follicular plugging as a prominent feature, a change usually associated with the follicular papules of atopic dermatitis (see p. 103).[225] There was irregular melanization of the basal layer.[225]

POSTINFLAMMATORY LEUKODERMA

Hypopigmented areas may develop during the course of a number of inflammatory diseases of the skin, usually during the resolving phases.[3] Examples include the various eczematous dermatitides, psoriasis, discoid lupus erythematosus, pityriasis rosea, variants of parapsoriasis, lichen sclerosus et atrophicus, syphilis and the viral exanthems.[3] Uncommonly, hypopigmentation may follow lichen planus and other lichenoid eruptions. Hypomelanotic lesions occur in an early stage of the disease, albeit uncommonly, in some of the following lesions – alopecia mucinosa, sarcoidosis, mycosis fungoides, pityriasis lichenoides chronica, pityriasis versicolor (tinea versicolor), onchocerciasis, yaws and leprosy.[3]

The mechanism in many of these conditions is thought to be a block in the transfer of melanosomes from melanocytes to keratinocytes; in the lichenoid dermatoses damage to melanocytes may also contribute. In pityriasis versicolor, melanosomes are poorly melanized; impaired transfer is also present.

Various mechanisms have been proposed for the hypopigmentation of lesions in indeterminate and tuberculoid leprosy (see p. 631).

Histopathology

There is a reduction in melanin pigment in the basal layer, although not a complete absence. Melanocytes are usually normal in number. Pigment-containing melanophages are sometimes present in the upper dermis, particularly in black patients. Residual features of the preceding or concurrent inflammatory dermatosis may also be present.

NEVUS ANEMICUS

Nevus anemicus is an uncommon congenital disorder in which there is usually a solitary asymptomatic patch that is paler than the surrounding normal skin.[226] Its margin is irregular and there may be islands of sparing within the lesion.[227] The pale area averages 5–10 cm in diameter. There is a predilection for the upper trunk, although involvement of the face and extremities occurs.[228] A variant with multiple lesions on the arms has been reported.[229] Nevus anemicus sometimes occurs in association with neurofibromatosis,[230] phakomatosis pigmentovascularis, or port wine stains.[231]

Nevus anemicus is regarded as a pharmacological nevus in which the pallor is attributable to increased sensitivity of the blood vessels in the area to catecholamines.[232] It has been found that the vessels do not respond normally to proinflammatory cytokines, at least at the level of E-selectin expression.[233] **Nevus oligemicus** is a related entity in which there is livid erythema rather than pallor.[234,235]

Histopathology

No abnormalities have been shown by light or electron microscopy.

DISORDERS CHARACTERIZED BY HYPERPIGMENTATION

The disorders characterized by hyperpigmentation constitute a heterogeneous group of diseases comprising a bewildering number of rare conditions. Japanese people are predisposed to many of the entities to be discussed below. Several factors are taken into consideration in the clinical categorization of these various disorders, including the distribution, arrangement and morphology of individual lesions as well as the presence or absence of hypopigmented areas.[236,237] Four clinical categories of hyperpigmentation can be recognized.

1. *Diffuse hyperpigmentation*: generalized hyperpigmentary disorders (scleroderma, Addison's disease, myxedema, Graves' disease, malnutrition including pellagra, chronic liver disease including hemochromatosis and Wilson's disease, porphyria, folate and vitamin B_{12} deficiency, heavy metal toxicity and the ingestion of certain drugs and chemicals), universal acquired melanosis and the generalized melanosis that may develop in malignant melanoma.

2. *Localized (patchy) hyperpigmentation*: ephelis (freckle), café-au-lait spots, macules of Albright's syndrome, macules of Peutz–Jeghers syndrome, macules of Laugier–Hunziker syndrome, Becker's nevus, acromelanosis, melasma, fixed drug eruption, frictional melanosis, notalgia paresthetica, familial progressive hyperpigmentation and idiopathic eruptive macular pigmentation.

3. *Punctate, reticulate hyperpigmentation (including whorls and streaks)*: Dowling–Degos disease, Kitamura's disease, Naegeli–Franceschetti–Jadassohn syndrome, dermatopathia pigmentosa reticularis, macular amyloidosis, 'ripple neck' in atopic dermatitis, hereditary diffuse hyperpigmentation, incontinentia pigmenti, prurigo pigmentosa, confluent and reticulated papillomatosis, patterned hypermelanosis and chimerism.

4. *Dyschromatosis (hyperpigmentation and hypopigmentation)*: dyskeratosis congenita, dyschromatosis symmetrica hereditaria (Dohi), dyschromatosis universalis, heterochromia extremitarum[237] and hereditary congenital hypopigmented and hyperpigmented macules.[238]

Theoretically, the hyperpigmentation observed in these various conditions could result from increased basal pigmentation and/or melanin incontinence. Alterations in the epidermal configuration can also produce apparent pigmentation of the skin.

Although there is some variability in the histopathological features reported in some of the disorders of hyperpigmentation, the following subclassification provides a useful approach to a biopsy from such a disease.

Disorders with basal hyperpigmentation (mild melanin incontinence is sometimes present also): generalized hyperpigmentary disorders, universal acquired melanosis, acromelanosis (increased melanocytes were noted in one report), familial progressive hyperpigmentation, idiopathic eruptive macular pigmentation, dyschromatosis symmetrica hereditaria, dyschromatosis universalis, patterned hypermelanosis, chimerism, melasma, acquired brachial dyschromatosis, ephelis (freckle), café-au-lait spots, macules of Albright's syndrome, Laugier–Hunziker syndrome, Ruvalcaba–Myhre–Smith syndrome and Peutz–Jeghers syndrome, and Becker's nevus (melanosis).

Disorders with epidermal changes: Dowling–Degos disease (the epidermal changes resemble those of solar lentigo), Kitamura's disease (the epidermal changes resembling Dowling–Degos disease but with intervening epidermal atrophy also) and confluent and reticulated papillomatosis of Gougerot–Carteaud (the epidermal changes are those of papillomatosis).

Disorders with striking melanin incontinence: postinflammatory melanosis, prurigo pigmentosa, generalized melanosis in malignant melanoma, dermatopathia pigmentosa reticularis, Naegeli–Franceschetti–Jadassohn syndrome, incontinentia pigmenti and late fixed drug eruptions.

Disorders with melanin incontinence and epidermal atrophy or 'dyskeratotic' cells: dyskeratosis congenita, frictional melanosis, notalgia paresthetica, 'ripple neck' in atopic dermatitis, active fixed drug eruptions and active prurigo pigmentosa.

Fixed drug eruptions and dyskeratosis congenita are discussed with the lichenoid reaction pattern on pages 42 and 55 respectively. Confluent and reticulated papillomatosis is considered on page 575.

GENERALIZED HYPERPIGMENTARY DISORDERS

As mentioned above, generalized cutaneous hyperpigmentation can be seen in a number of metabolic, endocrine,[239] hepatic and nutritional disorders, as well as following the application of topical calcipotriene (calcipotriol),[240] and the intake of certain drugs[241] and heavy metals.[242] Hyperpigmentation may follow sympathectomy.[243] It may also occur in the Crow–Fukase (POEMS) syndrome[244] (see p. 1063).

Histopathology

Biopsies of the pigmented skin are not often taken from individuals with these conditions. There is an increase in melanin in the lower layers of the epidermis and sometimes a small amount of pigment in the dermis. Of interest is the finding of large nuclei in the keratinocytes of the pigmented skin in some megaloblastic anemias.[245,246]

Hemosiderin pigment was present around dermal capillaries and sweat glands in two cases of hyperpigmentation associated with hyperthyroidism.[247]

UNIVERSAL ACQUIRED MELANOSIS

Universal acquired melanosis is an extremely rare condition, also known as the 'carbon baby' syndrome. It is characterized by progressive pigmentation of the skin during childhood, resembling that seen in black races.[248]

Histopathology

In the reported case there was hyperpigmentation of the epidermis and an increase in type III and IV (negroid pattern) melanosomes in melanocytes.[248]

ACROMELANOSIS

Acromelanosis refers to the presence of pigmented patches and macules on the dorsal surface of the phalanges, usually in colored people.[236,237] Several clinical variants have been recognized on the basis of the distribution of the pigment and the progression of the disorder.[237,249]

Histopathology

Basal hyperpigmentation is the usual finding, although an increase in basal melanocytes with associated acanthosis has also been reported.[249]

FAMILIAL PROGRESSIVE HYPERPIGMENTATION

Patches of hyperpigmentation are present at birth in this rare genodermatosis.[250] They increase in size and number with age. Eventually a large percentage of the skin and mucous membranes becomes hyperpigmented.[250]

Histopathology[250]

The most striking change is an increase in melanin pigment within the epidermis, especially in the basal layer. There is some concentration at the tips of the rete ridges.

IDIOPATHIC ERUPTIVE MACULAR PIGMENTATION

Idiopathic eruptive macular pigmentation is an exceedingly rare condition characterized by asymptomatic, pigmented macules involving the neck, trunk and proximal extremities.[251] This idiopathic disorder involves children and adolescents. Spontaneous resolution can be expected within several months to a few years.[251]

Histopathology

There is increased pigmentation of the basal layer, pigmentary incontinence with many melanophages in the upper dermis, and a sparse perivascular lymphohistiocytic infiltrate.

DYSCHROMATOSIS SYMMETRICA HEREDITARIA

Dyschromatosis symmetrica hereditaria, also known as reticulate acro-pigmentation of Dohi, consists of freckle-like lesions on the dorsum of the hands and feet with scattered depigmented macules in between.[236,237,252–254] Cases from Japan and Korea generally have an autosomal dominant pattern of inheritance. Several cases reported recently from the Middle East had autosomal recessive inheritance.[255]

Histopathology

The epidermis shows increased pigmentation, mainly basal, in the hyper-pigmented areas, and reduced pigmentation, sometimes accompanied by a reduction in the number of melanocytes, in hypopigmented areas.[237]

DYSCHROMATOSIS UNIVERSALIS

Dyschromatosis universalis is the prototype condition for a group of dyschromatoses characterized by areas of hypopigmentation and hyperpigmentation.[236] The absence of atrophy and telangiectasia distinguishes this group from the poikilodermas.[236] Onset is in early childhood, with involvement being most prominent on the trunk and extremities. Clinical variants have been described.[256–260]

Histopathology

There is variable epidermal pigmentation which may be accompanied by some pigment incontinence. The number of melanocytes is sometimes reduced in the hypopigmented areas.[256]

PATTERNED HYPERMELANOSIS

The term 'patterned hypermelanosis' is proposed for several rare dermatoses with overlapping features which have been reported in the past by different names. They are characterized by linear, whorled or reticulate areas of hyperpigmentation.[237] Although the term 'zosteriform' has been used to describe the pattern of the pigmentation in some of these cases, it has been pointed out that this term has not always been used correctly; the hyper-pigmentation usually follows Blaschko's lines (the boundary lines separating areas of the skin subserved by different peripheral nerves) and not the courses of the nerves themselves as in a zosteriform pattern.[261–263] A review of 54 children with segmental, linear or swirled hyper- and/or hypo-pigmentation along the lines of Blaschko revealed that 16 had extracutaneous manifestations.[200]

Included in the patterned hypermelanoses are cases reported as 'linear and whorled nevoid hypermelanosis',[261,263–269] 'reticulate hyperpigmentation distributed in a zosteriform fashion',[270] 'progressive cribriform and zosteriform hyperpigmentation',[271,272] 'zebra-like hyperpigmentation',[273] 'progressive zosteriform macular pigmented lesions',[274] 'dyschromia in confetti' (following topical immunotherapy with diphenylcyclopropenone)[275] and 'infant with abnormal pigmentation'.[276] The term 'patterned hypermelanosis' is not applicable to well-defined entities such as incontinentia pigmenti and the reticulate acral pigmentations of Kitamura and of Dowling and Degos (see p. 332). Streaks of hyper- and hypopigmentation can be seen in the Killian–Teschler–Nicola syndrome associated with tetrasomy of chromosome 12p.[277]

Histopathology

In all cases there has been an increase in melanin pigment in the basal layer. Pigment incontinence has been present in several cases.[274] A mild increase in the number of melanocytes, usually demonstrable only when quantitative studies are made, has been reported in a few cases.[261,273,276]

CHIMERISM

Chimerism results from double fertilization of an ovum, producing an individual (a chimera) with differing sets of chromosomes.[278] Abnormalities of skin pigmentation, usually in the form of irregular areas of hyperpigmentation, are a rare manifestation of the chimeric state.[278]

Histopathology

Melanin is increased in the basal layers of the epidermis in the hyper-pigmented lesions.[278]

MELASMA

Melasma (chloasma) refers to the symmetrical hyperpigmentation of the forehead and cheeks which develops in some women who are pregnant or taking oral contraceptives.[279–281] It has also been reported in women taking isotretinoin[282] or hormone replacement therapy;[283] the forearms are sometimes involved in this latter group.[284,285] The hormonal basis for melasma is not understood.

Histopathology

There is increased melanin in the epidermis, particularly in the basal layers. Mild pigment incontinence is sometimes present.

ACQUIRED BRACHIAL DYSCHROMATOSIS

Acquired brachial (cutaneous) dyschromatosis was applied recently to the asymptomatic, gray-brown patches of pigmentation, occasionally interspersed with hypopigmented macules, found predominantly on the dorsum of the forearms, mostly bilateral, of middle-aged patients.[286] There was a predilection for women, many of whom had been taking antihypertensive drugs, especially angiotensin-converting enzyme (ACE) inhibitors.[286] Many patients also had Civatte's poikiloderma of the neck.

Histopathology[286]

The pigmented lesions showed epidermal atrophy, increased basal layer pigmentation, superficial telangiectases and actinic elastosis. There was no pigmentary incontinence or amyloid.

The hypopigmented macules showed a decrease in pigmentation of the basal layer.

EPHELIS (FRECKLES)

Ephelides (freckles) are small, well-defined, pigmented macules 1–2 mm in diameter with a predilection for the face, arms and shoulder regions of fair-skinned individuals. They appear at an early age and may follow an episode of severe sunburn.

Histopathology

The epidermis appears normal in structure. The basal cells in the affected areas are more heavily pigmented with melanin than those in the surrounding skin and there is usually sharp delimitation of the abnormal areas from the normal (Fig. 10.5). There are normal numbers of melanocytes.[287]

CAFÉ-AU-LAIT SPOTS

Café-au-lait spots are uniformly pigmented, tan to dark brown macules which vary in size from small, freckle-like lesions to large patches 20 cm or more in diameter.[288] They may be present at birth or develop within the first few years of life.[289] They are found in approximately 15% of individuals.[290–292] They are not increased in patients with tuberous sclerosis, contrary to common belief.[293] Multiple café-au-lait spots are a feature of neurofibromatosis;[289,292,294] axillary freckling is often also present in these cases (see p. 983). Café-au-lait spots have also been reported in Bloom's syndrome, Cowden's disease, Fanconi's anemia, ring chromosome syndromes and ataxia-telangiectasia.[292,295] Familial, multiple café-au-lait spots have also been reported without any evidence of coexisting disease.[296]

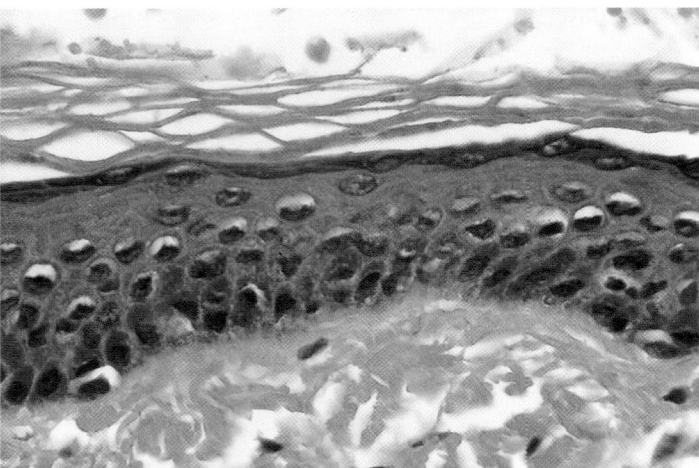

Fig. 10.5 **Freckle (ephelis).** Melanin is increased in the basal layers of the epidermis but melanocytes are normal in number and morphology. (H & E)

Histopathology

In hematoxylin and eosin preparations, the lesions resemble freckles, with basal hyperpigmentation but no apparent increase in the number of melanocytes. However, quantitative studies have shown a slight increase in melanocytes, which are accommodated in focally elongated rete ridges.[297,298] Giant melanin granules (macromelanosomes), measuring up to 6 μm in diameter and recognizable on light microscopy, can be seen in café-au-lait spots in many patients with neurofibromatosis.[299] The diagnostic significance of macromelanosomes is diminished by their absence in some children with neurofibromatosis and their presence in normal skin and other pigmented macular lesions.[300–303]

Electron microscopy

There are many subepidermal and intraepidermal nerves present in lesional skin.[298] Macromelanosomes are present in some melanocytes.

MACULES OF ALBRIGHT'S SYNDROME

Albright's syndrome is characterized by the triad of polyostotic fibrous dysplasia, sexual precocity, especially in the female, and pigmented macules. These macules are large, often unilateral, and related to the side of the bone lesions. The outline of the macules is very irregular, in contrast to that of café-au-lait spots. The macules may follow Blaschko's lines.[304]

The syndrome is associated with a somatic mutation of the gene encoding the α subunit of the G protein.

Histopathology

The lesions resemble freckles, showing hyperpigmentation of the basal layer. Rarely, macromelanosomes can be identified.[301]

LAUGIER–HUNZIKER SYNDROME

The Laugier–Hunziker syndrome is characterized by melanotic pigmentation of the mouth and lips which is frequently accompanied by longitudinal melanonychia.[305–307] In a small number of cases, there are dark palmoplantar and interdigital lesions. Pigmented macules may also develop about the nails. There are no associated internal disorders or familial association. Onset occurs between 20 and 50 years of age.[307]

Histopathology

The changes are similar in all lesions with acanthosis, basal hypermelanosis and some melanin incontinence with scattered melanophages in the upper dermis.[307] Some large melanosomes have been noted on electron microscopy.[306]

PEUTZ–JEGHERS SYNDROME

The autosomal dominant Peutz–Jeghers syndrome is characterized by the association of gastrointestinal polyposis with the presence of pigmented macules on the buccal mucosa, lips, perioral skin and sometimes the digits.[308] Patients with this syndrome have an increased risk of developing cancer at a relativey young age. There appears to be genetic heterogeneity, although many cases involve the *STK11/LKB1* gene on chromosome 19p13.3.[309] A case associated with primary melanoma of the rectum has been reported.[310] The **Cronkhite–Canada syndrome** is also characterized by intestinal polyposis and lentigo-like macules, commonly on the face, extremities and the palms.[311]

Histopathology

There is basal hyperpigmentation in the pigmented macules. There are conflicting views as to whether the melanocytes are quantitatively increased.[312,313] Basal hyperpigmentation, without an increase in melanocytes, is seen in the Cronkhite–Canada syndrome.[311]

RUVALCABA–MYHRE–SMITH SYNDROME

Ruvalcaba–Myhre–Smith syndrome combines juvenile polyposis coli, macrocephaly and pigmented macules limited to the shaft and glans of the penis.[314] It appears to be associated with loss of chromatin between 10q22.3 and 10q24.1.[314]

BECKER'S NEVUS

Becker's nevus (melanosis) is usually found in the region of the shoulder girdle of young men as unilateral, hyperpigmented areas of somewhat thickened skin.[302,315] Hypertrichosis may develop after the pigmentation but is not invariable. A Becker's nevus is usually acquired in adolescence, but a congenital onset has been recorded,[316] as have familial cases.[317,318] Occasionally, lesions have been said to follow severe sunburn. Lesional tissue has been found to have an increased level of androgen receptors, suggesting that heightened local androgen sensitivity may result in the hypertrichosis.[319] Various skeletal malformations have been reported in individuals with a Becker's nevus.[320,321] Other associations have included a connective tissue nevus,[322,323] an accessory scrotum,[324] limb deformities and areolar hypoplasia.[325,326]

Histopathology

The epicermal changes are variable but usually there is acanthosis and sometimes mild papillomatous hyperplasia (Fig. 10.6). The changes may resemble those seen in an epidermal nevus (see p. 754), although in Becker's nevus the elongated rete ridges tend to have flat, rather than pointed tips. There is variable hyperpigmentation of the basal layer with some melanophages in the dermis. Melanocyte proliferation is usually mild and not always obvious in routine sections; special studies have shown a quantitative increase.[327] There is sometimes an increase in the number and size of hair follicles and sebaceous glands. There may be smooth muscle hypertrophy of the arrectores pilorum as well as smooth muscle bundles in the dermis which are not related to cutaneous adnexa.[328,329] Controversy exists about the relationship of these cases to smooth muscle hamartoma (see p. 970).[330,331]

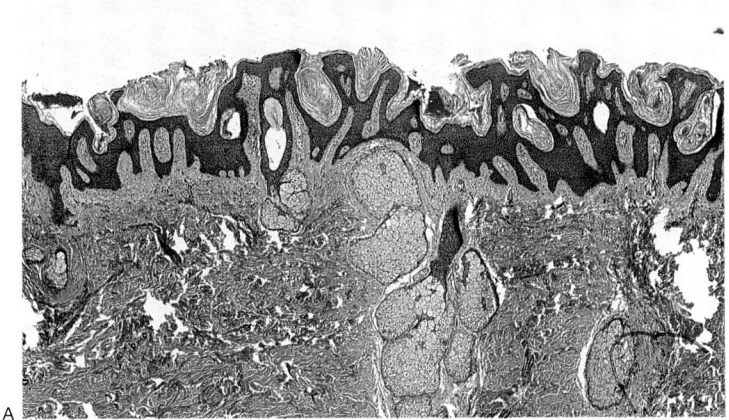

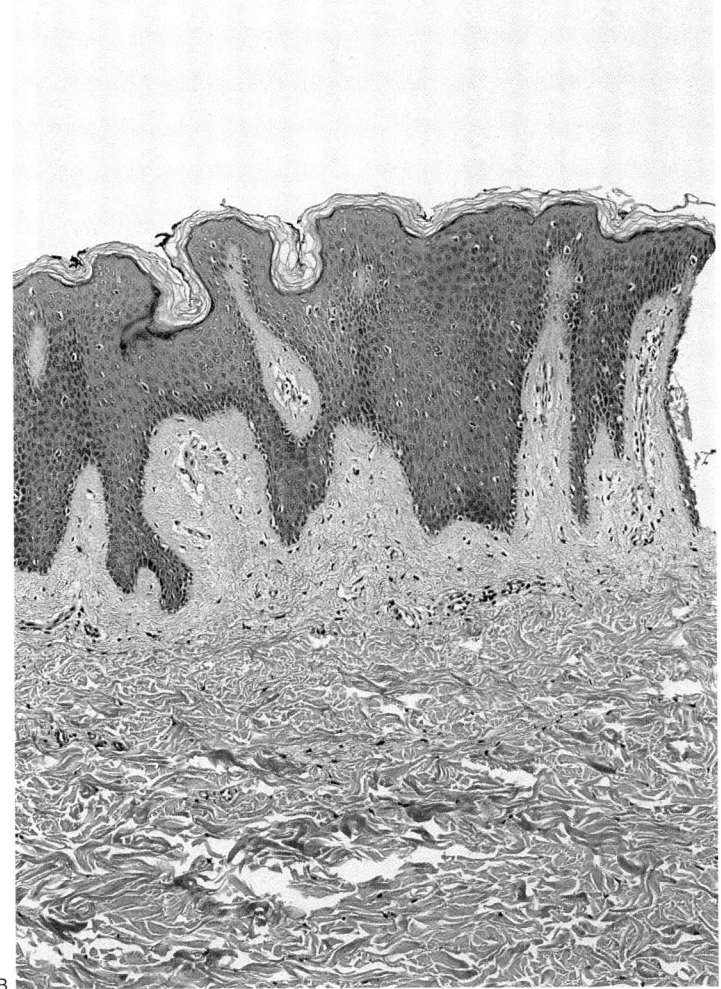

Fig. 10.6 **Becker's nevus. (A)** The epidermis shows mild papillomatosis and basal hyperpigmentation. **(B)** The bottom of some of the rete pegs is straight. (H & E)

Electron microscopy

There is an increase in the number and size of melanosome complexes in the basal and prickle cells of the epidermis with an increase in the number of melanosomes in the complexes.[332] There are also many single collagen fibrils in the dermis.

DOWLING–DEGOS DISEASE

Dowling–Degos disease, also known as reticulate pigmented anomaly of the flexures, is a rare autosomal dominant genodermatosis in which there are spotted and reticulate pigmented macules of the flexures.[333,334] Less constant features include pigmented pits in the perioral area, scattered comedo-like lesions,[335,336] keratoacanthomas,[337] hidradenitis suppurativa[338] and seborrheic keratoses.[333,339,340] The condition usually develops in early adult life and is slowly progressive.[333] Patients with achromic macules and papules probably constitute a variant of Dowling–Degos disease.[341]

It is now considered that *Haber's disease*,[342,343] in which there are rosacea-like facies and seborrheic keratosis-like lesions, and *reticulate ccropigmentation of Kitamura*,[344–351] in which there are reticulate, slightly depressed, pigmented macules on the extensor surface of the hands and feet in association with palmar 'pits', are different phenotypic expressions of the same genodermatosis.[352–358] A further related entity, characterized by reticulate pigmentation on the face and neck and epidermal cysts on the trunk, has been reported.[359]

Histopathology[333,336]

There are filiform downgrowths of the epidermis and also of the variably dilated pilosebaceous follicles.[333,360] Small horn cysts and comedo-like lesions are also present. Hyperpigmentation is quite pronounced at the tips of the rete ridges. There is a superficial resemblance to the adenoid form of seborrheic keratosis (see p. 757) although the downgrowths are more digitate than in seborrheic keratosis and there is no papillomatosis. In Kitamura's disease the appearances resemble those seen in a solar lentigo, with club-shaped elongations of the rete ridges but with intervening epidermal atrophy.[353,361,362] Dopa-positive melanocytes are increased.[361] Other features include melanin incontinence and a mild to moderate superficial perivascular infiltrate of lymphocytes.

Electron microscopy

Melanosomes are markedly increased in keratinocytes and these may be dispersed through the cytoplasm or loosely aggregated.[364,365] They are of normal size. Melanocytes are increased in number in Kitamura's variant.[361] There are many melanosomes in melanocytes, keratinocytes and melanophages.[363]

POSTINFLAMMATORY MELANOSIS

Hyperpigmentation may follow a number of inflammatory dermatoses, particularly those involving damage to the basal layer. Thus, it may follow various disorders that present a lichenoid reaction pattern, such as lichen planus, lichenoid drug eruptions and fixed drug eruptions. Prominent hyperpigmentation is almost invariable in the resolving phases of a phytophotodermatitis (see p. 600).

Histopathology

In addition to prominent melanin incontinence there may be normal or increased amounts of melanin in the basal layer of the epidermis. Basal pigmentation is prominent in phytophotodermatitis. If basal pigmentation is markedly reduced, the clinical appearance will be of hypopigmentation. There may also be occasional lymphocytes around vessels in the papillary dermis and a mild increase in fibroblasts and even collagen in the papillary dermis. There is usually no evidence of the underlying dermatosis that resulted in the area of pigmentation.

PRURIGO PIGMENTOSA

Prurigo pigmentosa is a pruritic dermatosis in which erythematous papules, characteristically on the back, neck and chest, coalesce to form a reticulate pattern. This stage resolves within days, leaving a mottled or reticulate hyperpigmentation.[366–369] Most cases have been reported from Japan, leading to the suggestion that an environmental factor is responsible.[370] Ketosis has also been implicated.[371–373] Prurigo pigmentosa may be classed as a post-inflammatory melanosis.[374]

Histopathology[366–368,375]

In the papular stage there is acanthosis, mild spongiosis and exocytosis of lymphocytes, resulting in the death of isolated keratinocytes. That is, there is a lichenoid reaction pattern (interface dermatitis) although the changes are not confined to the basal layer. The dermal infiltrate is predominantly perivascular and involves the superficial and mid dermis. A few eosinophils are included in the infiltrate. The published descriptions suggest a florid lichenoid drug reaction, but with a bizarre pattern.

In the late stages there is prominent melanin incontinence with numerous melanophages in the dermis.

GENERALIZED MELANOSIS IN MALIGNANT MELANOMA

Cutaneous pigmentation which is slate gray or bluish black in color may rarely develop in patients with disseminated malignant melanoma (see p. 830).[376,377] Although generalized, the pigmentation is often accentuated in areas exposed to the light.

The pathogenesis of the pigmentation is controversial.[377] It has been attributed to epidermal hyperpigmentation, the deposition of melanophages that have circulated in the blood, the presence of scattered melanoma cells within the dermis[378] and the regression of dermal tumor cells (see p. 830).

Histopathology[377]

The usual finding is the presence of melanin pigment throughout the dermis in perivascular and interstitial melanophages and as free granules. A scant perivascular infiltrate of lymphocytes and sometimes plasma cells may be present. Individual melanoma cells are not usually present.

DERMATOPATHIA PIGMENTOSA RETICULARIS

Dermatopathia pigmentosa reticularis combines reticulate pigmentation with nail dystrophy and partial alopecia.[379,380] Macules of hypopigmentation may develop at a later stage. There are similarities to the Naegeli–Franceschetti–Jadassohn syndrome, although the associated features are different.

An autosomal dominant inheritance was present in one family.[381]

Histopathology

The hyperpigmented areas show conspicuous melanin incontinence.[379] The epidermis appears normal.

NAEGELI–FRANCESCHETTI–JADASSOHN SYNDROME

Naegeli–Franceschetti–Jadassohn syndrome is an extremely rare, autosomal dominant ectodermal dysplasia combining dark brown, reticulate pigmentation of the trunk and limbs with diffuse or punctate hyperkeratosis of the palms and soles.[382,383] Hypohidrosis, enamel hypoplasia and nail dystrophy may also be present. Incomplete forms or variations have been reported;[384,385] the term 'hereditary diffuse hyperpigmentation' was used for one such case.[386] The gene for this syndrome maps to chromosome 17q21.[387]

This genodermatosis is one of the many that may present with reticulate, patchy and mottled pigmentation of the neck. A review of all such dermatoses, congenital and acquired, was published a few years ago.[388,389]

Histopathology
Melanin is increased in the basal layers of the epidermis and there is prominent melanin incontinence.[382]

Numerous milia were present in one case.[385]

INCONTINENTIA PIGMENTI

Incontinentia pigmenti is an uncommon, multisystem genodermatosis with cutaneous, skeletal, ocular, neurological, dental and other abnormalities.[390–393] The cutaneous lesions evolve through vesiculobullous, verrucous and pigmentary stages, but in a small number of individuals pigmentation is the first manifestation. The vesiculobullous lesions, accompanied by erythematous areas, are present at birth or soon after, in a linear arrangement on the extremities and lateral aspects of the trunk. Vesicular recurrences, later in life, are rare.[394] The verrucous lesions evolve some weeks or months later and resolve spontaneously to give atrophy, depigmentation or both. In the third stage, which has a peak onset around 3–6 months, there are streaks and whorls of brown to slate gray pigmentation, often asymmetrically distributed on the trunk and sometimes on the extremities.[391,395] The pigmentation, which is not necessarily in areas of the earlier lesions, progressively fades at about puberty. Areas of hyperpigmentation may remain. Uncommonly, streaks of hypopigmentation are the predominant feature;[396–399] they are usually found in adulthood but may develop earlier.[400,401]

Other cutaneous manifestations include alopecia, woolly hair nevus,[402] nail dystrophy and painful subungual tumors which may involve several fingers and sometimes toes. These keratotic tumors have an onset in late adolescence and may involute spontaneously.[403,404] Several cases of incontinentia pigmenti have been associated with cancer in childhood.[405] One case was associated with neonatal herpes simplex infection.[406]

Incontinentia pigmenti is a chromosomal instability disorder which is inherited as an X-linked dominant gene that usually causes the death in utero of affected males.[398,402,405,407] Two gene loci have been identified for this disease: Xp11.21 and Xq28.[394] The small number of males reported with the condition[408] may represent gene mutations.[391] Father-to-daughter transmission has been recorded.[409]

Several patients have had defects in neutrophil chemotaxis and lymphocyte function.[410–413] Leukotriene B₄ has been demonstrated in extracts of the crusted scales from vesiculobullous lesions and this may have an important role in the chemotaxis of eosinophils into the epidermis.[414]

It has been postulated that the manifestations of incontinentia pigmenti can be explained as an autoimmune attack on ectodermal clones expressing an abnormal surface antigen[415] or as premature (programmed) cell death in defective ectodermal clones.[416]

Histopathology
The first stage of incontinentia pigmenti is characterized by eosinophilic spongiosis; that is, spongiosis progressing to intraepidermal vesicle formation with prominent exocytosis of eosinophils into and around them (Fig. 10.7). A few basophils are also present.[417] The erythematous areas show only minimal spongiosis, but there is still prominent exocytosis of eosinophils. There are

occasional dyskeratotic cells with eosinophilic hyaline cytoplasm in the epidermis adjacent to the vesicles.[402] The superficial dermis contains an infiltrate of eosinophils and some mononuclear cells. Eosinophil granule major basic protein is also present.[418]

In the verrucous stage, there are hyperkeratosis, acanthosis, mild irregular papillomatosis and numerous dyskeratotic cells (Fig. 10.8). Some macrophages migrate into the epidermis; on electron microscopy, these have been shown to phagocytose the dyskeratotic cells as well as melanosomes. Inflammatory cells are quite sparse. In the third stage there is pronounced melanin incontinence. Pale scarred areas may be found on the lower part of the legs; these show a reduction in the number of melanocytes and some increase in dermal collagen.[419]

The subungual lesions show hyperkeratosis, verrucous or pseudo-epitheliomatous hyperplasia and dyskeratotic cells at all levels of the epidermis.[403,404] Neighboring keratinocytes may form whorls around the dyskeratotic cells.

Electron microscopy
On electron microscopy, some of the dyskeratotic cells have masses of loosely arranged tonofilaments, although most have clumped, electron-dense

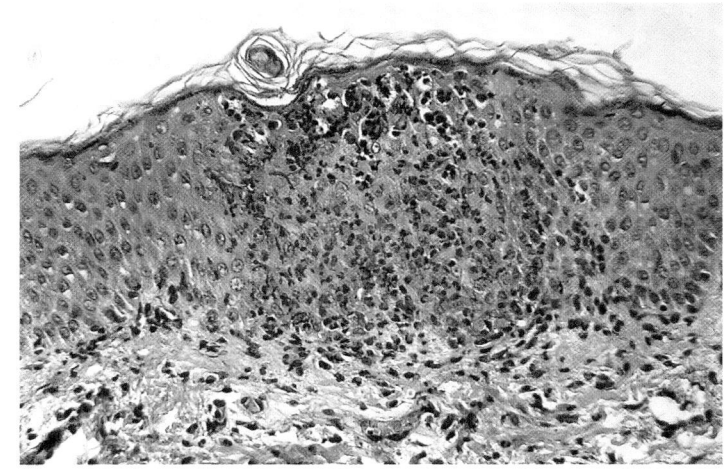

Fig. 10.7 **Incontinentia pigmenti (first stage).** Numerous eosinophils extend into the epidermis. Spongiosis is mild in this field. (H & E)

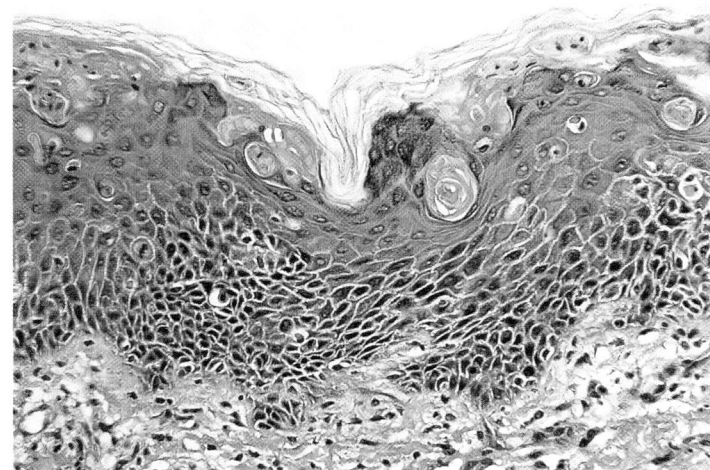

Fig. 10.8 **Incontinentia pigmenti (verrucous stage).** There are many dyskeratotic cells within the epidermis. (H & E)

tonofilaments.[420] Pigment incontinence appears to result from phagocytosis of melanosomes by macrophages.[421,422]

FRICTIONAL MELANOSIS

Localized hyperpigmentation may develop at sites of chronic friction.[423,424] This condition must be distinguished from macular amyloidosis, which clinically it resembles.

Histopathology

A prominent feature is the presence in the upper dermis of melanin, most of which is contained in melanophages.[423] Vacuolar change and scattered degenerate keratinocytes have also been noted in some cases.[423]

NOTALGIA PARESTHETICA

Notalgia paresthetica is a sensory neuropathy involving the posterior primary rami of thoracic nerves T2 to T6 and presenting as a localized area of pruritus of the back.[425,426] The affected region is sometimes lightly pigmented and composed of groups of small tan macules. Similar cases have been reported in the literature as 'peculiar spotty pigmentation'[427] and 'idiopathic pigmentation of the upper back'.[428] Clinically, notalgia paresthetica resembles macular amyloidosis, a condition which in one report required ultrastructural examination to confirm the presence of amyloid, as histochemical tests were negative.[429]

The symptoms may result from an increase in sensory epidermal innervation in affected skin.[430] More likely is the role played by degenerative changes in the spine, leading to spinal nerve impingement.[431,432]

Histopathology

There is melanin pigment in macrophages in the upper dermis sometimes accompanied by mild hyperpigmentation of the basal layer (Fig. 10.9).[428,433] In several reported cases, scattered degenerate keratinocytes were present within the epidermis.[425,430] Although no amyloid was seen in a recent series of 10 cases, it is often present.[432] It is possible that amyloid forms in chronic lesions as a consequence of prolonged scratching.

'RIPPLE' PIGMENTATION OF THE NECK

Although 'ripple' pigmentation is usually regarded as a feature of macular amyloidosis, it has also been described on the neck in almost 2% of individuals with atopic dermatitis of long standing.[434,435]

Histopathology

The most prominent feature is the presence of melanin in the upper dermis, both free and in macrophages.[434] An increase in melanocytes with associated mild vacuolar change in the basal layer has been an inconstant feature.[435]

'TERRA FIRMA-FORME' DERMATOSIS

'Terra firma-forme' dermatosis is a relatively common condition that usually affects the neck of children. It has also been reported as *dermatitis neglecta* (see p. 594). It has the appearance of a dirty brown mark that cannot be washed off with soap but is easily removed with alcohol.[436] It can often be mistaken for acanthosis nigricans and other conditions. It appears to be caused by disordered keratinization.

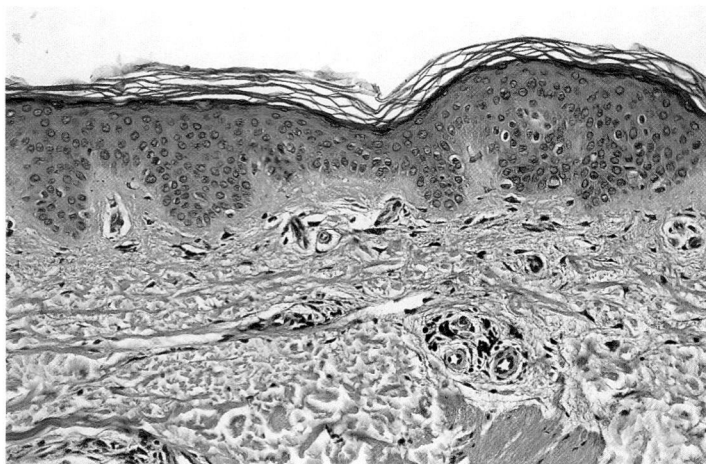

Fig. 10.9 **Notalgia paresthetica.** There are numerous melanophages, particularly around vessels in the superficial plexus. No amyloid was present. (H & E)

Histopathology

There is mild acanthosis and orthokeratosis with numerous keratin globules in the stratum corneum.

REFERENCES

Introduction

1 La Placa M, Pazzaglia M, Tosti A. Lycopenaemia. J Eur Acad Dermatol Venereol 2000; 14: 311–312.

2 Grichnik JM, Burch JA, Burchette J, Shea CR. The SCF/KIT pathway plays a critical role in the control of normal human melanocyte homeostasis. J Invest Dermatol 1998; 111: 233–238.

3 Bolognia JL, Pawelek JM. Biology of hypopigmentation. J Am Acad Dermatol 1988; 9: 217–255.

4 Hermanns JF, Petit L, Martalo O et al. Unraveling the patterns of subclinical pheomelanin-enriched facial hyperpigmentation: effect of depigmenting agents. Dermatology 2000; 201: 118–122.

5 Hara M, Yaar M, Byers HR et al. Kinesin participates in melanosomal movement along melanocyte dendrites. J Invest Dermatol 2000; 114: 438–443.

Disorders characterized by hypopigmentation

6 Cole GW, Barr RJ. Hypomelanosis associated with a colonic abnormality. A possible result of defective development of the neural crest. Am J Dermatopathol 1987; 9: 45–50.

7 Cole LA. Hypopigmentation with punctate keratosis of the palms and soles. Arch Dermatol 1976; 112: 998–1000.

8 Orecchia G, Stock J. Diphenylcyclopropenone: an important agent known to cause depigmentation. Dermatology 1999; 199: 277.

9 Jablonska S, Stachow A, Suffczynska M. Skin and muscle indurations in phenylketonuria. Arch Dermatol 1967; 95: 443–450.

10 Mosher DB, Fitzpatrick TB. Piebaldism. Arch Dermatol 1988; 124: 364–365.

11 Fukai K, Hamada T, Ishii M et al. Acquired pigmented macules in human piebald lesions. Ultrastructure of melanocytes in hypomelanotic skin. Acta Derm Venereol 1989; 69: 524–527.

12 Mahakrishnan A, Srinivasan MS. Piebaldism with Hirschsprung's disease. Arch Dermatol 1980; 116: 1102.

13 Reed WB, Stone VM, Boder E, Ziprkowski L. Pigmentary disorders in association with congenital deafness. Arch Dermatol 1967; 95: 176–186.

14 Sijmons RH, Kristoffersson U, Tuerlings JHAM et al. Piebaldism in a mentally retarded girl with rare deletion of the long arm of chromosome 4. Pediatr Dermatol 1993; 10: 235–239.

15 Perrot H, Ortonne J-P, Thivolet J. Ultrastructural study of leukodermic skin in Waardenburg–Klein syndrome. Acta Derm Venereol 1977; 57: 195–200.

16 Ortonne J-P. Piebaldism, Waardenburg's syndrome, and related disorders. 'Neural crest depigmentation syndromes'? Dermatol Clin 1988; 6: 205–216.

17 Mancini AJ. Waardenburg syndrome type II in a Taiwanese woman with a family history of pseudoxanthoma elasticum. Int J Dermatol 1997; 36: 933–935.

18 Dourmishev AL, Dourmishev LA, Schwartz RA, Janniger CK. Waardenburg syndrome. Int J Dermatol 1999; 38: 656–663.

19 Tachibana M. A cascade of genes related to Waardenburg syndrome. J Invest Dermatol (Symposium Proceedings) 1999; 4: 126–129.

20 Chang T, McGrae JD Jr, Hashimoto K. Ultrastructural study of two patients with both piebaldism and neurofibromatosis 1. Pediatr Dermatol 1993; 10: 224–234.

21 Spritz RA. Molecular basis of human piebaldism. J Invest Dermatol 1994; 103: 137s–140s.

22 Ward KA, Moss C, Sanders DSA. Human piebaldism: relationship between phenotype and site of *kit* gene mutation. Br J Dermatol 1995; 132: 929–935.

23 Richards KA, Fukai K, Oiso N, Paller AS. A novel *KIT* mutation results in piebaldism with progressive depigmentation. J Am Acad Dermatol 2001; 44: 288–292.

24 Selmanowitz VJ. Pigmentary correction of piebaldism by autografts. II. Pathomechanism and pigment spread in piebaldism. Cutis 1979; 24: 66–73.

25 Njoo MD, Nieuweboer-Krobotova L, Westerhof W. Repigmentation of leucodermic defects in piebaldism by dermabrasion and thin split-thickness skin grafting in combination with minigrafting. Br J Dermatol 1998; 139: 829–833.

26 Comings DE, Odland GF. Partial albinism. JAMA 1966; 195: 519–523.

27 Koranne RV, Sachdeva KG. Vitiligo. Int J Dermatol 1988; 27: 676–681.

28 Nordlund JJ, Lerner AB. Vitiligo. It is important. Arch Dermatol 1982; 118: 5–8.

29 Sharquie KE. Vitiligo. Clin Exp Dermatol 1984; 9: 117–126.

30 Kovacs SO. Vitiligo. J Am Acad Dermatol 1998; 38: 647–666.

31 Lee D, Lazova R, Bolognia JL. A figurate papulosquamous variant of inflammatory vitiligo. Dermatology 2000; 200: 270–274.

32 Baran R, Ortonne JP, Perrin Ch. Vitiligo associated with a lichen planus border. Dermatology 1997; 194: 199.

33 Cribier B, Santinelli F, Lipsker D, Grosshans E. Vitiligo with inflammatory raised border mimicking mycosis fungoides: a clinicopathological study of 4 cases. Am J Dermatopathol 2000; 22: 349 (abstract).

34 Fargnoli MC, Bolognia JL. Pentachrome vitiligo. J Am Acad Dermatol 1995; 33: 853–856.

35 Hann SK, Kim Y-S, Yoo JH, Chun Y-S. Clinical and histopathologic characteristics of trichrome vitiligo. J Am Acad Dermatol 2000; 42: 589–596.

36 Halder RM, Grimes PE, Cowan CA et al. Childhood vitiligo. J Am Acad Dermatol 1987; 16: 948–954.

37 Jaisankar TJ, Baruah MC, Garg BR. Vitiligo in children. Int J Dermatol 1992; 31: 621–623.

38 Ando I, Chi H-I, Nakagawa H, Otsuka F. Difference in clinical features and HLA antigens between familial and non-familial vitiligo of non-segmental type. Br J Dermatol 1993; 129: 408–410.

39 Majumder PP, Nordlund JJ, Nath SK. Pattern of familial aggregation of vitiligo. Arch Dermatol 1993; 129: 994–998.

40 Kim SM, Chung HS, Hann S-K. The genetics of vitiligo in Korean patients. Int J Dermatol 1998; 38: 908–910.

41 Bandyopadhyay D, Lawrence E, Majumder PP, Ferrell RE. Vitiligo is not caused by mutations in GTP-cyclohydrolase I gene. Clin Exp Dermatol 2000; 25: 152–153.

42 Koga M. Vitiligo: a new classification and therapy. Br J Dermatol 1977; 97: 255–261.

43 Koga M, Tango T. Clinical features and course of type A and type B vitiligo. Br J Dermatol 1988; 118: 223–228.

44 Barona MI, Arrunátegui A, Falabella R, Alzate A. An epidemiologic case-control study in a population with vitiligo. J Am Acad Dermatol 1995; 33: 621–625.

45 Cho S, Kang H-C, Hahm J-H. Characteristics of vitiligo in Korean children. Pediatr Dermatol 2000; 17: 189–193.

46 Hann SK, Lee HJ. Segmental vitiligo: Clinical findings in 208 patients. J Am Acad Dermatol 1996; 35: 671–674.

47 Kemp EH, Ajjan RA, Waterman EA et al. Analysis of microsatellite polymorphism of the cytotoxic T-lymphocyte antigen-4 gene in patients with vitiligo. Br J Dermatol 1999; 140: 73–78.

48 Gould IM, Gray RS, Urbaniak SJ et al. Vitiligo in diabetes mellitus. Br J Dermatol 1985; 113: 153–155.

49 Macaron C, Winter RJ, Traisman HS et al. Vitiligo and juvenile diabetes mellitus. Arch Dermatol 1977; 113: 1515–1517.

50 Mandry RC, Ortiz LJ, Lugo-Somolinos A, Sánchez JL. Organ-specific antibodies in vitiligo patients and their relatives. Int J Dermatol 1996; 35: 18–21.

51 Grimes PE, Halder RM, Jones C et al. Autoantibodies and their clinical significance in a black vitiligo population. Arch Dermatol 1983; 119: 300–303.

52 Adams BB, Lucky AW. Colocalization of alopecia areata and vitiligo. Pediatr Dermatol 1999; 16: 364–366.

53 Saihan EM, Peachey RDG. Vitiligo and morphoea. Clin Exp Dermatol 1979; 4: 103–106.

54 Von den Driesch P, Fartasch M, Hornstein OP. Chronic actinic dermatitis with vitiligo-like depigmentation. Clin Exp Dermatol 1992; 17: 38–43.

55 Karvonen S-L, Haapasaari K-M, Kallioinen M et al. Increased prevalence of vitiligo, but no evidence of premature ageing, in the skin of patients with bp 3243 mutation in mitochondrial DNA in the mitochondrial encephalomyopathy, lactic acidosis and stroke-like episodes syndrome (MELAS). Br J Dermatol 1999; 140: 634–639.

56 Monroe EW. Vitiligo associated with regional enteritis. Arch Dermatol 1976; 112: 833–834.

57 McPoland PR, Moss RL. Cutaneous Crohn's disease and progressive vitiligo. J Am Acad Dermatol 1988; 19: 421–425.

58 Grimes F, Sevall JS, Vojdani A et al. Demonstration of cytomegalovirus (CMV) DNA and CMV ant body responses in the peripheral blood of vitiligo patients and matched controls. J Invest Dermatol 1996; 106: 912 (abstract).

59 Grimes PE, Sevall JS, Vojdani A. Cytomegalovirus DNA identified in skin biopsy specimens of patients with vitiligo. J Am Acad Dermatol 1996; 35: 21–26.

60 Howanitz N, Nordlund JL, Lerner AB, Bystryn J-C. Antibodies to melanocytes. Occurrence in patients with vitiligo and chronic mucocutaneous candidiasis. Arch Dermatol 1981; 117: 705–708.

61 Henderson CD, Tschen JA, Schaefer DG. Simultaneously active lesions of vitiligo and erythema dyschromicum perstans. Arch Dermatol 1988; 124: 1258–1260.

62 Mathias CGT, Maibach HI, Conant MA. Perioral leukoderma simulating vitiligo from use of a toothpaste containing cinnamic aldehyde. Arch Dermatol 1980; 116: 1172–1173.

63 Malakar S, Dhar S. Leucoderma associated with the use of topical minoxidil: a report of two cases. Dermatology 2000; 201: 183–184.

64 Todes-Taylor N, Abel EA, Cox AJ. The occurrence of vitiligo after psoralens and ultraviolet A therapy. J Am Acad Dermatol 1983; 9: 526–532.

65 Falabella R, Escobar CE, Carrascal E, Arroyave JA. Leukoderma punctata. J Am Acad Dermatol 1988; 18: 485–494.

66 Aubin F, Cahn JY, Ferrand C et al. Extensive vitiligo after ganciclovir treatment of GvHD in a patient who had received donor T cells expressing herpes simplex virus thymidine kinase. Lancet 2000; 355: 626–627.

67 Cowan CL Jr, Halder RM, Grimes PE et al. Ocular disturbances in vitiligo. J Am Acad Dermatol 1986; 15: 17–24.

68 Barnes L. Vitiligo and the Vogt–Koyanagi–Harada syndrome. Dermatol Clin 1988; 6: 229–239.

69 Ravikumar BC, Balachandram C, Sabita L, Acharya S. Vogt–Koyanagi–Harada syndrome: the useful role of punch grafting. Int J Dermatol 2000; 39: 460–462.

70 Wong SS, Ng SK, Lee HM. Vogt–Koyanagi–Harada disease: extensive vitiligo with prodromal generalized erythroderma. Dermatology 1999; 198: 65–68.

71 Tsuruta D, Hamada T, Teramae H et al. Inflammatory vitiligo in Vogt–Koyanagi–Harada disease. J Am Acad Dermatol 2001; 44: 129–131.

72 Lerner AB, Kirkwood JM. Vitiligo and melanoma: can genetically abnormal melanocytes result in both vitiligo and melanoma within a single family? J Am Acad Dermatol 1984; 11: 696–701.

73 Bystryn J-C, Rigel D, Friedman RJ, Kopf A. Prognostic significance of hypopigmentation in malignant melanoma. Arch Dermatol 1987; 123: 1053–1055.

74 Nordlund JJ. Hypopigmentation, vitiligo, and melanoma. New data, more enigmas. Arch Dermatol 1987; 123: 1005–1008.

75 Becker JC, Guldberg P, Zeuthen J et al. Accumulation of identical T cells in melanoma and vitiligo-like leukoderma. J Invest Dermatol 1999; 113: 1033–1038.

76 Hann S-K, Chun WH, Park Y-K. Clinical characteristics of progressive vitiligo. Int J Dermatol 1997; 36: 353–355.

77 Chun WH, Hann S-K. The progression of non-segmental vitiligo: clinical analysis of 318 patients. Int J Dermatol 1997; 36: 908–910.

78 Arrunátegui A, Arroyo C, Garcia L et al. Melanocyte reservoir in vitiligo. Int J Dermatol 1994; 33: 484–487.

79 Cui J, Shen L-Y, Wang G-C. Role of hair follicles in the repigmentation of vitiligo. J Invest Dermatol 1991; 97: 410–416.

80 Kent G, Al'Abadie M. Psychologic effects of vitiligo: A critical incident analysis. J Am Acad Dermatol 1996; 35: 895–898.

81 Le Poole IC, van den Wijngaard RMJGJ, Westerhof W et al. Presence or absence of melanocytes in vitiligo lesions: an immunohistochemical investigation. J Invest Dermatol 1993; 100: 816–822.

82 Westerhof W. Vitiligo – a window in the darkness. Dermatology 1995; 190: 181–182.

83 Al'Abadie MSK, Senior HJ, Bleehen SS, Gawkrodger DJ. Neuropeptide and neuronal marker studies in vitiligo. Br J Dermatol 1994; 131: 160–165.

84 Maresca V, Roccella M, Roccella F et al. Increased sensitivity to peroxidative agents as a possible pathogenic factor of melanocyte damage in vitiligo. J Invest Dermatol 1997; 109: 310–313.

85 Jimbow K, Chen H, Park J-S, Thomas PD. Increased sensitivity of melanocytes to oxidative stress and abnormal expression of tyrosinase-related protein in vitiligo. Br J Dermatol 2001; 144: 55–65.

86 Al Badri AMT, Todd PM, Garioch JJ et al. An immunohistological study of cutaneous lymphocytes in vitiligo. J Pathol 1993; 170: 149–155.

87 Van Den Wijngaard RMJGJ, Aten J, Scheepmaker A et al. Expression and modulation of apoptosis regulatory molecules in human melanocytes: significance in vitiligo. Br J Dermatol 2000; 143: 573–581.

88 Cui J, Arita Y, Bystryn J-C. Cytolytic antibodies to melanocytes in vitiligo. J Invest Dermatol 1993; 100: 812–815.

89 Gilhar A, Zelickson B, Ulman Y, Etzioni A. In vivo destruction of melanocytes by the IgG fraction of serum from patients with vitiligo. J Invest Dermatol 1995; 105: 683–686.

90 Yu H-S, Kao C-H, Yu C-L. Coexistence and relationship of antikeratinocyte and antimelanocyte antibodies in patients with non-segmental-type vitiligo. J Invest Dermatol 1993; 100: 823–828.

91 Li Y-L, Yu C-L, Yu H-S. IgG anti-melanocyte antibodies purified from patients with active vitiligo induce HLA-DR and intercellular adhesion molecule-1 expression and an increase in interleukin-8 release by melanocytes. J Invest Dermatol 2000; 115: 969–973.

92 Park KC, Lee YS, Youn SW et al. Flow cytometric analysis of cytotoxic antibodies to melanocytes in vitiligo. J Invest Dermatol 1996; 106: 930 (abstract).

93 Kemp EH, Waterman EA, Gawkrodger DJ et al. Autoantibodies to tyrosinase-related protein-1 detected in the sera of vitiligo patients using a quantitative radiobinding assay. Br J Dermatol 1998; 139: 798–805.

94 Kemp EH, Waterman EA, Gawkrodger DJ et al. Identification of epitopes on tyrosinase which are recognized by autoantibodies from patients with vitiligo. J Invest Dermatol 1999; 113: 267–271.

95 Xie Z, Chen D, Jiao D, Bystryn J-C. Vitiligo antibodies are not directed to tyrosinase. Arch Dermatol 1999; 135: 417–422.

96 Rocha IM, Oliveira LJN, Miranda de Castro LC et al. Recognition of melanoma cell antigens with antibodies present in sera from patients with vitiligo. Int J Dermatol 2000; 39: 840–843.

97 Durham-Pierre DG, Walters CS, Halder RM et al. Natural killer cell and lymphokine-activated killer cell activity against melanocytes in vitiligo. J Am Acad Dermatol 1995; 33: 26–30.

98 Torres-Alvarez B, Moncada B, Fuentes-Ahumada C et al. The immunopathogenesis of vitiligo. Arch Dermatol 1994; 130: 387–388.

99 Behrens-Williams SC, Peters EM, Schallreuter KU. In vivo delayed-type hypersensitivity in 109 patients with vitiligo. Int J Dermatol 2000; 39: 593–598.

100 Ghoneum M, Grimes PE, Gill G, Kelly AP. Natural cell-mediated cytotoxicity in vitiligo. J Am Acad Dermatol 1987; 17: 600–605.

101 Grimes PE, Ghoneum M, Stockton T et al. T cell profiles in vitiligo. J Am Acad Dermatol 1986; 14: 196–201.

102 Halder RM, Walters CS, Johnson BA et al. Aberrations in T lymphocytes and natural killer cells in vitiligo: a flow cytometric study. J Am Acad Dermatol 1986; 14: 733–737.

103 Mozzanica N, Frigerio U, Finzi AF et al. T cell subpopulations in vitiligo: a chronobiologic study. J Am Acad Dermatol 1990; 22: 223–230.

104 Mozzanica N, Frigerio U, Negri M et al. Circadian rhythm of natural killer cell activity in vitiligo. J Am Acad Dermatol 1989; 20: 591–596.

105 Naughton GK, Eisinger M, Bystryn J-C. Detection of antibodies to melanocytes in vitiligo by specific immunoprecipitation. J Invest Dermatol 1983; 81: 540–542.

106 Naughton GK, Reggiardo D, Bystryn J-C. Correlation between vitiligo antibodies and extent of depigmentation in vitiligo. J Am Acad Dermatol 1986; 15: 978–981.

107 Harning R, Cui J, Bystryn J-C. Relation between the incidence and level of pigment cell antibodies and disease activity in vitiligo. J Invest Dermatol 1991; 97: 1078–1080.

108 Cui J, Harning R, Henn M, Bystryn J-C. Identification of pigment cell antigens defined by vitiligo antibodies. J Invest Dermatol 1992; 98: 162–165.

109 Takei M, Mishima Y, Uda H. Immunopathology of vitiligo vulgaris, Sutton's leukoderma and melanoma-associated vitiligo in relation to steroid effects. I. Circulating antibodies for cultured melanoma cells. J Cutan Pathol 1984; 11: 107–113.

110 Cui J, Bystryn J-C. Melanoma and vitiligo are associated with antibody responses to similar antigens on pigment cells. Arch Dermatol 1995; 131: 314–318.

111 Mozzanica N, Villa ML, Foppa S et al. Plasma α-melanocyte-stimulating hormone, β-endorphin, met-enkephalin, and natural killer cell activity in vitiligo. J Am Acad Dermatol 1992; 26: 693–700.

112 Norris A, Todd C, Graham A et al. The expression of the c-kit receptor by epidermal melanocytes may be reduced in vitiligo. Br J Dermatol 1996; 134: 299–306.

113 Dippel E, Haas N, Grabbe J et al. Expression of the c-kit receptor in hypomelanosis: a comparative study between piebaldism, nevus depigmentosus and vitiligo. Br J Dermatol 1995; 132: 182–189.

114 Al Badri AMT, Foulis AK, Todd PM et al. Abnormal expression of MHC class I and ICAM-1 by melanocytes in vitiligo. J Pathol 1993; 169: 203–206.

115 Uehara M, Miyauchi H, Tanaka S. Diminished contact sensitivity response in vitiliginous skin. Arch Dermatol 1984; 120: 195–198.

116 Hatchome N, Aiba S, Kato T et al. Possible functional impairment of Langerhans' cells in vitiliginous skin. Arch Dermatol 1987; 123: 51–54.

117 Beck H-I, Schmidt H. Graft exchange in vitiligo. Acta Derm Venereol 1986; 66: 311–315.

118 Falabella R, Escobar C, Borrero I. Transplantation of in vitro-cultured epidermis bearing melanocytes for repigmenting vitiligo. J Am Acad Dermatol 1989; 21: 257–264.

119 Lerner AB. Repopulation of pigment cells in patients with vitiligo. Arch Dermatol 1988; 124: 1701–1702.

120 Falabella R, Arrunategui A, Barona MI, Alzate A. The minigrafting test for vitiligo: detection of stable lesions for melanocyte transplantation. J Am Acad Dermatol 1995; 32: 228–232.

121 Hann SK, Im S, Bong HW, Park Y-K. Treatment of stable vitiligo with autologous epidermal grafting and PUVA. J Am Acad Dermatol 1995; 32: 943–948.

122 Löntz W, Olsson MJ, Moellmann G, Lerner AB. Pigment cell transplantation for treatment of vitiligo: a progress report. J Am Acad Dermatol 1994; 30: 591–597.

123 Njoo MD, Spuls PI, Bos JD et al. Nonsurgical repigmentation therapies in vitiligo. Arch Dermatol 1998; 134: 1532–1540.

124 Njoo MD, Bos JD, Westerhof W. Treatment of generalized vitiligo in children with narrow-band (TL-01) UVB radiation therapy. J Am Acad Dermatol 2000; 42: 245–253.

125 Boersma BR, Westerhof W, Bos JD. Repigmentation in vitiligo vulgaris by autologous minigrafting: results in nineteen patients. J Am Acad Dermatol 1995; 33: 990–995.

126 Olsson MJ, Juhlin L. Transplantation of melanocytes in vitiligo. Br J Dermatol 1995; 132: 587–591.

127 Njoo MD, Westerhof W, Bos JD, Bossuyt PMM. A systematic review of autologous transplantation methods in vitiligo. Arch Dermatol 1998; 134: 1543–1549.

128 Kim HY, Kang KY. Epidermal grafts for treatment of stable and progressive vitiligo. J Am Acad Dermatol 1999; 40: 412–417.

129 Yaar M, Gilchrest BA. Vitiligo. The evolution of cultured epidermal autografts and other surgical treatment modalities. Arch Dermatol 2001; 137: 348–349.

130 Kang HY, Song J, Im S. Verruca vulgaris following treatment of vitiligo with epidermal grafting. Br J Dermatol 2000; 143: 645–646.

131 Njoo MD, Vodegel RM, Westerhof W. Depigmentation therapy in vitiligo universalis with topical 4-methoxyphenol and the Q-switched ruby laser. J Am Acad Dermatol 2000; 42: 760–769.

132 Gopinathan T. A study of the lesion of vitiligo. Arch Dermatol 1965; 91: 397–404.

133 Kumakiri M, Kimura T, Miura Y, Tagawa Y. Vitiligo with an inflammatory erythema in Vogt–Koyanagi–Harada disease: demonstration of filamentous masses and amyloid deposits. J Cutan Pathol 1982; 9: 258–266.

134 Horn TD, Abanmi A. Analysis of the lymphocytic infiltrate in a case of vitiligo. Am J Dermatopathol 1997; 19: 400–402.

135 Bhawan J, Bhutani LK. Keratinocyte damage in vitiligo. J Cutan Pathol 1983; 10: 207–212.

136 Gokhale BB, Mehta LN. Histopathology of vitiliginous skin. Int J Dermatol 1983; 22: 477–480.

137 Bose SK. Absence of Merkel cells in lesional skin. Int J Dermatol 1994; 33: 481–483.

138 Saarinen KA, Lestringant GG, Masouye I, Frossard PM. Actinic damage and squamous cell carcinoma in sun-exposed skin affected by vitiligo. Br J Dermatol 2000; 143: 219–221.

139 Galadari E, Mehregan AH, Hashimoto K. Ultrastructural study of vitiligo. Int J Dermatol 1993; 32: 269–271.

140 Morohashi M, Hashimoto K, Goodman TF Jr et al. Ultrastructural studies of vitiligo, Vogt–Koyanagi syndrome, and incontinentia pigmenti achromians. Arch Dermatol 1977; 13: 755–766.

141 Moellmann G, Klein-Angerer S, Scollay DA et al. Extracellular granular material and degeneration of keratinocytes in the normally pigmented epidermis of patients with vitiligo. J Invest Dermatol 1982; 79: 321–330.

142 Al'Abadie MSK, Warren MA, Bleehen SS, Gawkrodger DJ. Morphologic observations on the dermal nerves in vitiligo: an ultrastructural study. Int J Dermatol 1995; 34: 837–840.

143 King RA, Summers CG. Albinism. Dermatol Clin 1988; 6: 217–228.

144 King RA, Olds DP. Hairbulb tyrosinase activity in oculocutaneous albinism: suggestions for pathway control and block location. Am J Med Genet 1985; 20: 49–55.

145 Tomita Y. Tyrosinase gene mutations causing oculocutaneous albinisms. J Invest Dermatol 1993; 100: 186s–190s.

146 Oetting WS, King RA. Molecular basis of oculocutaneous albinism. J Invest Dermatol 1994; 103: 131s–136s.

147 Schnur RE, Sellinger BT, Holmes SA et al. Type I oculocutaneous albinism associated with a full-length deletion of the tyrosinase gene. J Invest Dermatol 1996; 106: 1137–1140.

148 Tomita Y. The molecular genetics of albinism and piebaldism. Arch Dermatol 1994; 130: 355–358.

149 Matsunaga J, Dakeishi-Hara M, Miyamura Y et al. Sequence-based diagnosis of tyrosinase-related oculocutaneous albinism: successful sequence analysis of the tyrosinase gene from blood spots dried on filter paper. Dermatology 1998; 196: 189–193.

150 Gershoni-Baruch R, Benderly A, Brandes JM, Gilhar A. Dopa reaction test in hair bulbs of fetuses and its application to the prenatal diagnosis of albinism. J Am Acad Dermatol 1991; 24: 220–222.

151 Shimizu H, Niizeki H, Suzumori K et al. Prenatal diagnosis of oculocutaneous albinism by analysis of the fetal tyrosinase gene. J Invest Dermatol 1994; 103: 104–106.

152 Okoro AN. Albinism in Nigeria. A clinical and social study. Br J Dermatol 1975; 92: 485–492.

153 Lookingbill DP, Lookingbill GL, Leppard B. Actinic damage and skin cancer in albinos in northern Tanzania: findings in 164 patients enrolled in an outreach skin care program. J Am Acad Dermatol 1995; 32: 653–658.

154 Dargent JL, Lespagnard L, Heenen M, Verhest A. Malignant melanoma occurring in a case of oculocutaneous albinism. Histopathology 1992; 21: 74–76.

155 Levin DL, Roth DE, Muhlbauer JE. Sporadic dysplastic nevus syndrome in a tyrosinase-positive oculocutaneous albino. J Am Acad Dermatol 1988; 19: 393–396.

156 Matsunaga J, Dakeishi-Hara M, Tanita M et al. A splicing mutation of the tyrosinase gene causes yellow oculocutaneous albinism in a Japanese patient with a pigmented phenotype. Dermatology 1999; 199: 124–129.

157 Saitoh S, Oiso N, Wada T et al. Oculocutaneous albinism type 2 with a P gene missense mutation in a patient with Angelman syndrome. J Med Genet 2000; 37: 392–394.

158 Bothwell JE. Pigmented skin lesions in tyrosinase-positive oculocutaneous albinos: a study in black South Africans. Int J Dermatol 1997; 36: 831–836.

159 Dimson O, Drolet BA, Esterly NB. Hermansky–Pudlak syndrome. Pediatr Dermatol 1999; 16: 475–477.

160 Schachne JP, Glaser N, Lee S et al. Hermansky–Pudlak syndrome: case report and clinicopathologic review. J Am Acad Dermatol 1990; 22: 926–932.

161 Hussain S, Heftler N, Reed JA, McNutt NS. Hermansky–Pudlak syndrome: a report of two cases. J Cutan Pathol 1997; 24: 104 (abstract).

162 Toro J, Turner M, Gahl WA. Dermatologic manifestations of Hermansky–Pudlak syndrome in patients with and without a 16-base pair duplication in the HPS1 gene. Arch Dermatol 1999; 135: 774–780.

163 Wildenberg SC, Fryer JP, Gardner JM et al. Identification of a novel transcript produced by the gene responsible for the Hermansky–Pudlak syndrome in Puerto Rico. J Invest Dermatol 1998; 110: 777–781.

164 Schallreuter KU, Beazley WD, Hibberts NA et al. Perturbed epidermal pterin metabolism in Hermansky–Pudlak syndrome. J Invest Dermatol 1998; 111: 511–516.

165 Horikawa T, Araki K, Fukai K et al. Heterozygous HPS1 mutations in a case of Hermansky–Pudlak syndrome with giant melanosomes. Br J Dermatol 2000; 143: 635–640.

166 Martínez-Ruiz E, Ortega C, Calduch L et al. Generalized cutaneous depigmentation following sulfamide-induced drug eruption. Dermatology 2000; 201: 252–254.

167 King RA, Olds DP, Witkop CJ. Characterization of human hair bulb tyrosinase: properties of normal and albino enzyme. J Invest Dermatol 1978; 71: 136–139.

168 Vanhooteghem O, Courtens W, Andre J et al. Hermansky–Pudlak syndrome: a case report and discussion. Pediatr Dermatol 1998; 15: 374–377.

169 Husain S, Marsh E, Saenz-Santamaria MC, McNutt NS. Hermansky–Pudlak syndrome: report of a case with histological, immunohistochemical and ultrastructural findings. J Cutan Pathol 1998; 25: 380–385.

170 Blume RS, Wolff SM. The Chediak–Higashi syndrome: studies in four patients and a review of the literature. Medicine (Baltimore) 1972; 51: 247–280.

171 Anderson LL, Paller AS, Malpass D et al. Chediak–Higashi syndrome in a black child. Pediatr Dermatol 1992; 9: 31–36.

172 Arbiser JL. Genetic immunodeficiencies: cutaneous manifestations and recent progress. J Am Acad Dermatol 1995; 33: 82–89.

173 Barak Y, Nir E. Chediak–Higashi syndrome. Am J Pediatr Hematol Oncol 1987; 9: 42–55.

174 Bedoya V. Pigmentary changes in Chediak–Higashi syndrome. Microscopic study of 12 homozygous and heterozygous subjects. Br J Dermatol 1971; 85: 336–347.

175 White JG, Clawson CC. The Chediak–Higashi syndrome: the nature of the giant neutrophil granules and their interactions with cytoplasm and foreign particulates. Am J Pathol 1980; 98: 151–196.

176 Moran TJ, Estevez JM. Chediak–Higashi disease. Morphologic studies of a patient and her family. Arch Pathol 1969; 88: 329–339.

177 Zelickson AS, Windhorst DB, White JG, Good RA. The Chediak–Higashi syndrome: formation of giant melanosomes and the basis of hypopigmentation. J Invest Dermatol 1967; 49: 575–581.

178 Carrillo-Farga J, Gutierrez-Palomera G, Ruiz-Maldonado R et al. Giant cytoplasmic granules in Langerhans cells in Chediak–Higashi syndrome. Am J Dermatopathol 1990; 12: 81–87.

179 Mancini AJ, Chan LS, Paller AS. Partial albinism with immunodeficiency: Griscelli syndrome: Report of a case and review of the literature. J Am Acad Dermatol 1998; 38: 295–300.

180 Lambert J, Naeyaert JM, De Paepe A et al. Arg-Cys substitution at codon 1246 of the human myosin Va gene is not associated with Griscelli syndrome. J Invest Dermatol 2000; 114: 731–733.

181 Duran-McKinster C, Rodriguez-Jurado R, Ridaura C et al. Elejalde syndrome – a melanolysosomal neurocutaneous syndrome. Clinical and morphological findings in 7 patients. Arch Dermatol 1999; 135: 182–186.

182 Guillet G, Helenon R, Gauthier Y et al. Progressive macular hypomelanosis of the trunk: primary acquired hypopigmentation. J Cutan Pathol 1988; 15: 286–289.

183 Pagnoni A, Kligman AM, Sadiq I, Stoudemayer T. Hypopigmented macules of photodamaged skin and their treatment with topical tretinoin. Acta Derm Venereol 1999; 79: 305–310.

184 Fitzpatrick TB, Szabo G, Hori Y et al. White leaf-shaped macules. Earliest visible sign of tuberous sclerosis. Arch Dermatol 1968; 98: 1–6.

185 Jimbow K, Fitzpatrick TB, Szabo G, Hori Y. Congenital circumscribed hypomelanosis: a characterization based on electron microscopic study of tuberous sclerosis, nevus depigmentosus, and piebaldism. J Invest Dermatol 1975; 64: 50–62.

186 Whitehead WJ, Moyer DG, Vander Ploeg DE. Idiopathic guttate hypomelanosis. Arch Dermatol 1966; 94: 279–281.

187 Hamada T, Saito T. Senile depigmented spots (idiopathic guttate hypomelanosis). Arch Dermatol 1967; 95: 665.

188 Fabella R, Escobar C, Giraldo N et al. On the pathogenesis of idiopathic guttate hypomelanosis. J Am Acad Dermatol 1987; 16: 35–44.

189 Falabella R. Idiopathic guttate hypomelanosis. Dermatol Clin 1988; 6: 241–247.

190 Wilson PD, Lavker RM, Kligman AM. On the nature of idiopathic guttate hypomelanosis. Acta Derm Venereol 1982; 62: 301–306.

191 Cummings KI, Cottel WI. Idiopathic guttate hypomelanosis. Arch Dermatol 1966; 93: 184–186.

192 Wallace ML, Grichnik JM, Prieto VG, Shea CR. Numbers and differentiation status of melanocytes in idiopathic guttate hypomelanosis. J Cutan Pathol 1998; 25: 375–379.

193 Ortonne J-P, Perrot H. Idiopathic guttate hypomelanosis. Arch Dermatol 1980; 116: 664–668.

194 Savall R, Ferrandiz C, Ferrer I, Peyri J. Idiopathic guttate hypomelanosis. Br J Dermatol 1980; 103: 635–642.

195 Buzas JW, Sina B, Burnett JW. Hypomelanosis of Ito. Report of a case and review of the literature. J Am Acad Dermatol 1981; 4: 195–204.

196 Takematsu H, Sato S, Igarashi M, Seiji M. Incontinentia pigmenti achromians (Ito). Arch Dermatol 1983; 119: 391–395.

197 Sybert VP. Hypomelanosis of Ito. Pediatr Dermatol 1990; 7: 74–76.

198 Sybert VP. Hypomelanosis of Ito: a description, not a diagnosis. J Invest Dermatol 1994; 103: 141s–143s.

199 Finkelstein E, Shinwell E, Avinoach I et al. Hypomelanosis of Ito: report of two cases. Australas J Dermatol 1992; 33: 97–101.

200 Nehal KS, PeBenito R, Orlow SJ. Analysis of 54 cases of hypopigmentation and hyperpigmentation along the lines of Blaschko. Arch Dermatol 1996; 132: 1167–1170.

201 Hamada T, Saito T, Sugai T, Morita Y. 'Incontinentia pigmenti achromians (Ito)'. Arch Dermatol 1967; 96: 673–676.

202 Jelinek JE, Bart RS, Schiff GM. Hypomelanosis of Ito ('Incontinentia pigmenti achromians'). Report of three cases and review of the literature. Arch Dermatol 1973; 107: 596–601.

203 Griffiths A, Payne C. Incontinentia pigmenti achromians. Arch Dermatol 1975; 111: 751–752.

204 Mittal R, Handa F, Sharma SC. Incontinentia pigmenti et achromians. Dermatologica 1975; 150: 355–359.

205 Rubin MB. Incontinentia pigmenti achromians. Multiple cases within a family. Arch Dermatol 1972; 105: 424–425.

206 Ruiz-Malconado R, Toussaint S, Tamayo L et al. Hypomelanosis of Ito: diagnostic criteria and report of 41 cases. Pediatr Dermatol 1992; 9: 1–10.

207 Pulimood S, Rajagopalan B, Jacob M et al. Hypomelanosis of Ito with unusual associations. Clin Exp Dermatol 1997; 22: 295–296.

208 Haenen I, Vancuickenborne L, Kerre S, Degreef H. Hypomelanosis of Ito. Dermatology 1993; 196: 467–469.

209 Nordlund JJ, Klaus SN, Gino J. Hypomelanosis of Ito. Acta Derm Venereol 1977; 57: 261–264.

210 Hellgren L. Incontinentia pigmenti achromians (Ito). Acta Derm Venereol 1975; 55: 237–240.

211 Maize JC, Headington JT, Lynch PJ. Systematized hypochromic nevus. Incontinentia pigmenti achromians of Ito. Arch Dermatol 1972; 106: 884–885.

212 Peña L, Ruiz-Maldonado R, Tamayo L et al. Incontinentia pigmenti achromians (Ito's hypomelanosis). Int J Dermatol 1977; 16: 194–202.

213 Coupe RL. Unilateral systematized achromic naevus. Dermatologica 1967; 134: 19–35.

214 Lee H-S, Chun Y-S, Hann S-K. Nevus depigmentosus: Clinical features and histopathologic characteristics in 67 patients. J Am Acad Dermatol 1999; 40: 21–26.

215 Di Lernia V. Segmental nevus depigmentosus: analysis of 20 patients. Pediatr Dermatol 1999; 16: 349–353.
216 Alkemade H, Juhlin L. Unilateral lentiginosis with nevus depigmentosus on the other side. J Am Acad Dermatol 2000; 43: 361–363.
217 Ogunbiyi AO, Ogunbiyi JO. Nevus depigmentosus and inflammatory linear epidermal nevus – an unusual combination with a note on histology. Int J Dermatol 1998; 37: 600–602.
218 Fukai K, Ishii M, Kadoya A et al. Naevus depigmentosus systematicus with partial yellow scalp hair due to selective suppression of eumelanogenesis. Pediatr Dermatol 1993; 10: 205–208.
219 Hanifin JM. Clinical and basic aspects of atopic dermatitis. Semin Dermatol 1983; 2: 5–19.
220 Zaynoun ST, Aftimos BG, Tenekjian KK et al. Extensive pityriasis alba: a histological histochemical and ultrastructural study. Br J Dermatol 1983; 108: 83–90.
221 Zaynoun S, Jaber LAA, Kurban AK. Oral methoxsalen photochemotherapy of extensive pityriasis alba. J Am Acad Dermatol 1986; 15: 61–65.
222 Du Toit MJ, Jordaan HF. Pigmenting pityriasis alba. Pediatr Dermatol 1993; 10: 1–5.
223 Weedon D. Unpublished observations.
224 Wells BT, Whyte HJ, Kierland RR. Pityriasis alba. A ten-year survey and review of the literature. Arch Dermatol 1960; 82: 183–189.
225 Vargas-Ocampo F. Pityriasis alba: a histologic study. Int J Dermatol 1993; 32: 870–873.
226 Mountcastle EA, Diestelmeier MR, Lupton GP. Nevus anemicus. J Am Acad Dermatol 1986; 14: 628–632.
227 Daniel RH, Hubler WR Jr, Wolf JE Jr, Holder WR. Nevus anemicus. Donor-dominant defect. Arch Dermatol 1977; 113: 53–56.
228 Mandal SB, Dutta AK. Pathophysiology of nevus anemicus. JCE Dermatol 1978; 16(4): 13–18.
229 Miura Y, Tajima S, Ishibashi A, Hata Y. Multiple anemic macules on the arms: a variant form of nevus anemicus? Dermatology 2000; 201: 180–182.
230 Fleisher TL. Nevus anemicus. Arch Dermatol 1969; 100: 750–755.
231 Katugampola GA, Lanigan SW. The clinical spectrum of naevus anaemicus and its association with port wine stains: report of 15 cases and a review of the literature. Br J Dermatol 1996; 134: 292–295.
232 Greaves MW, Birkett D, Johnson C. Nevus anemicus: a unique catecholamine-dependent nevus. Arch Dermatol 1970; 102: 172–176.
233 Mizutani H, Ohyanagi S, Umeda Y et al. Loss of cutaneous delayed hypersensitivity reactions in nevus anemicus. Arch Dermatol 1997; 133: 617–620.
234 Davies MG, Greaves MW, Coutts A, Black AK. Nevus oligemicus. A variant of nevus anemicus. Arch Dermatol 1981; 117: 111–113.
235 Plantin P, Leroy JP, Guillet G. Nevus oligemicus: a new case. J Am Acad Dermatol 1992; 26: 268–269.

Disorders characterized by hyperpigmentation

236 Fulk CS. Primary disorders of hyperpigmentation. J Am Acad Dermatol 1984 10: 1–16.
237 Griffiths WAD. Reticulate pigmentary disorders – a review. Clin Exp Dermatol 1984; 9: 439–450.
238 Westerhof W, Beemer FA, Cormane RH et al. Hereditary congenital hypopigmented and hyperpigmented macules. Arch Dermatol 1978; 114: 931–936.
239 Jones D, Kay M, Craigen W et al. Coal-black hyperpigmentation at birth in a child with congenital adrenal hypoplasia. J Am Acad Dermatol 1995; 33: 323–326.
240 Glässer R, Röwert J, Mrowietz U. Hyperpigmentation due to topical calcipotriol and photochemotherapy in two psoriatic patients. Br J Dermatol 1998; 139: 148–151.
241 Kanwar AJ, Jaswal R, Thami GP, Bedi GK. Acquired acromelanosis due to phenytoin. Dermatology 1997; 194: 373–374.
242 Hendrix JD Jr, Greer KE. Cutaneous hyperpigmentation caused by systemic drugs. Int J Dermatol 1992; 31: 458–466.
243 Samuel C, Bird DR, Burton JL. Hyperpigmentation after sympathectomy. Clin Exp Dermatol 1980; 5: 349–350.
244 Shelley WB, Shelley ED. The skin changes in the Crow–Fukase (POEMS) syndrome. Arch Dermatol 1987; 123: 85–87.
245 Marks VJ, Briggaman RA, Wheeler CE Jr. Hyperpigmentation in megaloblastic anaemia. J Am Acad Dermatol 1985; 12: 914–917.
246 Lee SH, Lee WS, Whang KC et al. Hyperpigmentation in megaloblastic anemia. Int J Dermatol 1988; 27: 571–575.
247 Banba K, Tanaka N, Fujioka A, Tajima S. Hyperpigmentation caused by hyperthyroidism: differences from the pigmentation of Addison's disease. Clin Exp Dermatol 1999; 24: 196–198.
248 Ruiz-Maldonado R, Tamayo L, Fernández-Diez J. Universal acquired melanosis. The carbon baby. Arch Dermatol 1978; 114: 775–778.
249 González JR, Botet MV. Acromelanosis. A case report. J Am Acad Dermatol 1980; 2: 128–131.
250 Chernosky ME, Anderson DE, Chang JP. Familial progressive hyperpigmentation. Arch Dermatol 1971; 103: 581–598.
251 Jang K-A, Choi J-H, Sung K-J et al. Idiopathic eruptive macular pigmentation: Report of 10 cases. J Am Acad Dermatol 2001; 44: 351–353.
252 Danese P, Zanca A, Bertazzoni MG. Familial reticulate acropigmentation of Dohi. J Am Acad Dermatol 1997; 37: 884–886.
253 Tan H-H, Tay Y-K. Neurofibromatosis and reticulate acropigmentation of Dohi: a case report. Pediatr Dermatol 1997; 14: 296–298.
254 Ohtoshi E, Matsumura Y, Nishigori C et al. Useful applications of DNA repair tests for differential diagnosis of atypical dyschromatosis symmetrica hereditaria from xeroderma pigmentosum. Br J Dermatol 2001; 144: 162–168.
255 Alfadley A, Al Ajlan A, Hainau B et al. Reticulate acropigmentation of Dohi: A case report of autosomal recessive inheritance. J Am Acad Dermatol 2000; 43: 113–117.
256 Foldes C, Wallach D, Launay J-M, Chirio R. Congenital dyschromia with erythrocyte, platelet, and tryptophan metabolism abnormalities. J Am Acad Dermatol 1988; 19: 642–655.
257 Petrozzi JW. Unusual dyschromia in a malnourished infant. Arch Dermatol 1971; 103: 515–519.
258 Rycroft RJG, Calnan CD, Wells RS. Universal dyschromatosis, small stature and high-tone deafness. Clin Exp Dermatol 1977; 2: 45–48.
259 Hara M, Kumasaka K, Tomita Y, Tagami H. Unilateral dermatomal pigmentary dermatosis: a variant dyschromatosis? J Am Acad Dermatol 1992; 27: 763–764.
260 Yang J-H, Wong C-K. Dyschromatosis universalis with X-linked ocular albinism. Clin Exp Dermatol 1991; 16: 436–440.
261 Kalter DC, Griffiths WA, Atherton DJ. Linear and whorled nevoid hypermelanosis. J Am Acad Dermatol 1988; 19: 1037–1044.
262 Kubota Y, Shimura Y, Shimada S et al. Linear and whorled nevoid hypermelanosis in a child with chromosomal mosaicism. Int J Dermatol 1992; 31: 345–347.
263 Alvarez J, Peteiro C, Toribio J. Linear and whorled nevoid hypermelanosis. Pediatr Dermatol 1993; 10: 156–158.
264 Harre J, Millikan LE. Linear and whorled pigmentation. Int J Dermatol 1994; 33: 529–537.
265 Kanwar AJ, Dhar S, Ghosh S, Kaur S. Linear and whorled nevoid hypermelanosis. Int J Dermatol 1993; 32: 385–386.
266 Akiyama M, Aranami A, Sasaki Y et al. Familial linear and whorled nevoid hypermelanosis. J Am Acad Dermatol 1994; 30: 831–833.
267 Hassab-El-Naby HMM, Alsaleh QA, Fathallah MA. Linear and whorled nevoid hypermelanosis: report of a case associated with cerebral palsy. Pediatr Dermatol 1996; 13: 148–150.
268 Schepis C, Siragusa M, Alberti A, Cavallari V. Linear and whorled nevoid hypermelanosis in a boy with mental retardation and congenital defects. Int J Dermatol 1996; 35: 654–655.
269 Quecedo E, Febrer I, Aliaga A. Linear and whorled nevoid hypermelanosis. A spectrum of pigmentary disorders. Pediatr Dermatol 1997; 14: 247–248.
270 Iijima S, Naito Y, Naito S, Uyeno K. Reticulate hyperpigmentation distributed in a zosteriform fashion: a new clinical type of hyperpigmentation. Br J Dermatol 1987; 117: 503–510.
271 Rower JM, Carr RD, Lowney ED. Progressive cribriform and zosteriform hyperpigmentation. Arch Dermatol 1978; 114: 98–99.
272 Schepis C, Alberti A, Siragusa M, Romano C. Progressive cribriform and zosteriform hyperpigmentation: the late-onset feature of linear and whorled nevoid hypermelanosis associated with congenital neurological, skeletal and cutaneous anomalies. Dermatology 1999; 199: 72–73.
273 Alimurung FM, Lapenas D, Willis I, Lang P. Zebra-like hyperpigmentation in an infant with multiple congenital defects. Arch Dermatol 1979; 115: 878–881
274 Simoes GA. Progressive zosteriform macular pigmented lesions. Arch Dermatol 1980; 116: 20.
275 Van der Steen P, Happle R. 'Dyschromia in confetti' as a side effect of topical immunotherapy with diphenylcyclopropenone. Arch Dermatol 1992; 128: 518–520.
276 Ment L, Alper J, Sirota RL, Holmes LB. Infant with abnormal pigmentation, malformations, and immune deficiency. Arch Dermatol 1978; 114: 1043–1044.
277 Ohman AB Jr, Pride HB, Papa CA. What syndrome is this? Pediatr Dermatol 2000; 17: 151–153.
278 Findlay GH, Moores PP. Pigment anomalies of the skin in the human chimaera: their relation to systematized naevi. Br J Dermatol 1980; 103: 489–498.
279 Kovacs G, Marks R. Contraception and the skin. Australas J Dermatol 1987; 28: 86–92.
280 Jelinek JE. Cutaneous side effects of oral contraceptives. Arch Dermatol 1970; 101: 181–186.
281 Grimes PE. Melasma. Etiologic and therapeutic considerations. Arch Dermatol 1995; 131: 1453–1457.
282 Burke H, Carmichael AJ. Reversible melasma associated with isotretinoin. Br J Dermatol 1996; 135: 862.

283 O'Brien TJ, Dyall-Smith D, Hall AP. Melasma of the arms associated with hormone replacement therapy. Br J Dermatol 1999; 141: 592–593.

284 Johnston GA, Sviland L, McLelland J. Melasma of the arms associated with hormone replacement therapy. Br J Dermatol 1998; 139: 932.

285 O'Brien TJ, Dyall-Smith D, Hall AP. Melasma of the forearms. Australas J Dermatol 1997; 38: 35–37.

286 Rongioletti F, Rebora A. Acquired brachial cutaneous dyschromatosis: A common pigmentary disorder of the arm in middle-aged women. J Am Acad Dermatol 2000; 42: 680–684.

287 Breathnach AS. Melanocyte distribution in forearm epidermis of freckled human subjects. J Invest Dermatol 1957; 29: 253–261.

288 Erdi H, Boyvat A, Çalikoğlu E. Giant café au lait spot in a patient with neurofibromatosis. Acta Derm Venereol 1999; 79: 496.

289 Riccardi VM. Von Recklinghausen neurofibromatosis. N Engl J Med 1981; 305: 1617–1627.

290 Kopf AW, Levine LJ, Rigel DS et al. Prevalence of congenital-nevus-like nevi, nevi spili, and café-au-lait spots. Arch Dermatol 1985; 121: 766–769.

291 McLean DI, Gallagher RP. 'Sunburn' freckles, café-au-lait macules, and other pigmented lesions of schoolchildren: the Vancouver Mole Study. J Am Acad Dermatol 1995; 32: 565–570.

292 Landau M, Krafchik BR. The diagnostic value of café-au-lait macules. J Am Acad Dermatol 1999; 40: 877–890.

293 Bell SD, MacDonald DM. The prevalence of café-au-lait patches in tuberous sclerosis. Clin Exp Dermatol 1985; 10: 562–565.

294 Kestler HA, Haschka M. A model for the emergence of café-au-lait macules. J Invest Dermatol 1999; 113: 858–859.

295 Khumalo NP, Joss DV, Huson SM, Burge S. Pigmentary anomalies in ataxia-telangiectasia: a clue to diagnosis and an example of twin spotting. Br J Dermatol 2001; 144: 369–371.

296 Arnsmeier SL, Riccardi VM, Paller AS. Familial multiple cafe au lait spots. Arch Dermatol 1994; 130: 1425–1426.

297 Johnson BL, Charneco DR. Café au lait spot in neurofibromatosis and in normal individuals. Arch Dermatol 1970; 102: 442–446.

298 Mihara M, Nakayama H, Aki T et al. Cutaneous nerves in cafe au lait spots with white halos in infants with neurofibromatosis. Electron microscopic study. Arch Dermatol 1992; 128: 957–961.

299 Jimbow K, Szabo G, Fitzpatrick TB. Ultrastructure of giant pigment granules (macromelanosomes) in the cutaneous pigmented macules of neurofibromatosis. J Invest Dermatol 1973; 61: 300–309.

300 Silvers DN, Greenwood RS, Helwig EB. Café au lait spots without giant pigment granules. Occurrence in suspected neurofibromatosis. Arch Dermatol 1974; 110: 87–88.

301 Benedict PH, Szabo G, Fitzpatrick TB, Sinesi SJ. Melanotic macules in Albright's syndrome and in neurofibromatosis. JAMA 1968; 205: 618–626.

302 Bhawan J, Chang WH. Becker's melanosis. Dermatologica 1979; 159: 221–230.

303 Bhawan J, Purtilo DT, Riordan JA et al. Giant and 'granular melanosomes' in leopard syndrome: an ultrastructural study. J Cutan Pathol 1976; 3: 207–216.

304 Rieger E, Kofler R, Borkenstein M et al. Melanotic macules following Blaschko's lines in McCune–Albright syndrome. Br J Dermatol 1994; 130: 215–220.

305 Gerbig AW, Hunziker T. Idiopathic lenticular mucocutaneous pigmentation or Laugier–Hunziker syndrome with atypical features. Arch Dermatol 1996; 132: 844–845.

306 Porneuf M, Dandurand M. Pseudo-melanoma revealing Laugier–Hunziker syndrome. Int J Dermatol 1997; 36: 138–141.

307 Yamamoto O, Yoshinaga K, Asahi M, Murata I. A Laugier–Hunziker syndrome associated with esophageal melanocytosis. Dermatology 1999; 199: 162–164.

308 Gregory B, Ho VC. Cutaneous manifestations of gastrointestinal disorders. Part 1. J Am Acad Dermatol 1992; 26: 153–166.

309 Entius MM, Keller JJ, Westerman AM et al. Molecular genetic alterations in hamartomatous polyps and carcinomas of patients with Peutz–Jeghers syndrome. J Clin Pathol 2001; 54: 126–131.

310 Wong SS, Rajakulendran S. Peutz–Jeghers syndrome associated with primary malignant melanoma of the rectum. Br J Dermatol 1996; 135: 439–442.

311 Bruce A, Ng CS, Wolfsen HC et al. Cutaneous clues to Cronkhite–Canada syndrome: a case report. Arch Dermatol 1999; 135: 212.

312 Blank AA, Schneider BV, Panizzon R. Pigmentfleckenpolypose (Peutz–Jeghers-Syndrom). Hautarzt 1981; 32: 296–300.

313 Yamada K, Matsukawa A, Hori Y, Kukita A. Ultrastructural studies on pigmented macules of Peutz–Jeghers syndrome. J Dermatol 1981; 8: 367–377.

314 Bishop PR, Nowicki MJ, Parker PH. What syndrome is this? Pediatr Dermatol 2000; 17: 319–321.

315 Becker SW. Concurrent melanosis and hypertrichosis in distribution of nevus unius lateris. Arch Dermatol Syph 1949; 60: 155–160.

316 Picascia DD, Esterly NB. Congenital Becker's melanosis. Int J Dermatol 1989; 28: 127–128.

317 Jain HC, Fisher BK. Familial Becker's nevus. Int J Dermatol 1989; 28: 263–264.

318 Book SE, Glass AT, Laude TA. Congenital Becker's nevus with a familial association. Pediatr Dermatol 1997; 14: 373–375.

319 Person JR, Longcope C. Becker's nevus: an androgen-mediated hyperplasia with increased androgen receptors. J Am Acad Dermatol 1984; 10: 235–238.

320 Glinick SE, Alper JC, Bogaars H, Brown JA. Becker's melanosis: associated abnormalities. J Am Acad Dermatol 1983; 9: 509–514.

321 Moore JA, Schosser RH. Becker's melanosis and hypoplasia of the breast and pectoralis major muscle. Pediatr Dermatol 1985; 3: 34–37.

322 Fenske NA, Donelan PA. Becker's nevus coexistent with connective-tissue nevus. Arch Dermatol 1984; 120: 1347–1350.

323 Kim D-H, Kim C-W, Kim T-Y. Becker's naevus associated with connective tissue naevus. Acta Derm Venereol 1999; 79: 393–394.

324 Szylit J-A, Grossman ME, Luyando Y et al. Becker's nevus and an accessory scrotum. A unique occurrence. J Am Acad Dermatol 1986; 14: 905–907.

325 Sharma R, Mishra A. Becker's naevus with ipsilateral areolar hypoplasia in three males. Br J Dermatol 1997; 136: 471–472.

326 Crone AM, James MP. Giant Becker's naevus with ipsilateral areolar hypoplasia and limb asymmetry. Clin Exp Dermatol 1997; 22: 240–241.

327 Tate PR, Hodge SJ, Owen LG. A quantitative study of melanocytes in Becker's nevus. J Cutan Pathol 1980; 7: 404–409.

328 Urbanek RW, Johnson WC. Smooth muscle hamartoma associated with Becker's nevus. Arch Dermatol 1978; 114: 104–106.

329 Haneke E. The dermal component of melanosis naeviformis Becker. J Cutan Pathol 1979; 6: 53–58.

330 Glinick SE, Alper JA. Spectrum of Becker's melanosis changes is greater than believed. Arch Dermatol 1986; 122: 375.

331 Ferreira MJ, Bajanca R, Fiadeiro T. Congenital melanosis and hypertrichosis in a bilateral distribution. Pediatr Dermatol 1998; 15: 290–292.

332 Frenk E, Delacretaz J. Zur Ultrastruktur der Becker schen Melanose. Hautarzt 1970; 21: 397–400.

333 Wilson Jones E, Grice K. Reticulate pigmented anomaly of the flexures. Dowling Degos disease, a new genodermatosis. Arch Dermatol 1978; 114: 1150–1157.

334 Crovato F, Nazzari G, Rebora A. Dowling–Degos disease (reticulate pigmented anomaly of the flexures) is an autosomal dominant condition. Br J Dermatol 1983; 108: 473–476.

335 Kershenovich J, Langenberg A, Odom RB, LeBoit PE. Dowling–Degos' disease mimicking chloracne. J Am Acad Dermatol 1992; 27: 345–348.

336 Kim YC, Davis MDP, Schanbacher CF, Su WPD. Dowling–Degos disease (reticulate pigmented anomaly of the flexures): A clinical and histopathologic study of 6 cases. J Am Acad Dermatol 1999; 40: 462–467.

337 Fenske NA, Groover CE, Lober CW, Espinoza CG. Dowling–Degos disease, hidradenitis suppurativa, and multiple keratoacanthomas. J Am Acad Dermatol 1991; 24: 888–892.

338 Bedlow AJ, Mortimer PS. Dowling–Degos disease associated with hidradenitis suppurativa. Clin Exp Dermatol 1996; 21: 305–306.

339 Boyle J, Burton JL. Reticulate pigmented anomaly of the flexures and seborrhoeic warts. Clin Exp Dermatol 1985; 10: 379–383.

340 Cliff S, Otter M, Cook MG, Marsden RA. Dowling Degos disease in association with multiple seborrhoeic warts. Clin Exp Dermatol 1997; 22: 34–36.

341 Lestringant GG, Masouyé I, Frossard PM et al. Co-existence of leukoderma with features of Dowling–Degos disease: reticulate acropigmentation of Kitamura spectrum in five unrelated patients. Dermatology 1997; 195: 337–343.

342 Seiji M, Otaki N. Haber's syndrome. Familial rosacea-like dermatosis with keratotic plaques and pitted scars. Arch Dermatol 1971; 103: 452–455.

343 Kikuchi I, Saita B, Inoue S. Haber's syndrome. Report of a new family. Arch Dermatol 1981; 117: 321–324.

344 Woodley DT, Caro I, Wheeler CE Jr. Reticulate acropigmentation of Kitamura. Arch Dermatol 1979; 115: 760–761.

345 Griffiths WAD. Reticulate acropigmentation of Kitamura. Br J Dermatol 1976; 95: 437–443.

346 Kanwar AJ, Kaur S, Rajagopalan M. Reticulate acropigmentation of Kitamura. Int J Dermatol 1990; 29: 217–219.

347 Griffiths WAD. Reticulate pigmentary disorders – a review. Clin Exp Dermatol 1984; 9: 439–450.

348 Berth-Jones J, Graham-Brown RAC. A family with Dowling Degos disease showing features of Kitamura's reticulate acropigmentation. Br J Dermatol 1989; 120: 463–466.

349 Cox NH, Long E. Dowling–Degos disease and Kitamura's reticulate acropigmentation: support for the concept of a single disease. Br J Dermatol 1991; 125: 169–171.

350 Oriba HA, Lo JS, Dijkstra JWE, Bergfeld WF. Reticulate nonmelanocytic hyperpigmentation anomaly. A probable variant of Dowling–Degos disease. Int J Dermatol 1991; 30: 39–42.

351 Sharma R, Chandra M. Pigmentation and pits at uncommon sites in a case with reticulate acropigmentation of Kitamura. Dermatology 2000; 200: 57–58.

352 Crovato F, Desirello G, Rebora A. Is Dowling–Degos disease the same disease as Kitamura's reticulate acropigmentation? Br J Dermatol 1983; 109: 105–110.

353 Rebora A, Crovato F. The spectrum of Dowling–Degos disease. Br J Dermatol 1984; 110: 627–630.

354 Crovato F, Rebora A. Reticulate pigmented anomaly of the flexures associating reticulate acropigmentation: one single entity. J Am Acad Dermatol 1986; 14: 359–361.

355 Kikuchi I, Crovato F, Rebora A. Haber's syndrome and Dowling–Degos disease. Int J Dermatol 1988; 27: 96–97.

356 Wallis MS, Mallory SB. Reticulate acropigmentation of Kitamura with localized alopecia. J Am Acad Dermatol 1991; 25: 114–116.

357 Ostlere L, Holden CA. Dowling–Degos disease associated with Kitamura's reticulate acropigmentation. Clin Exp Dermatol 1994; 19: 492–495.

358 Thami GP, Jaswal R, Kanwar AJ et al. Overlap of reticulate acropigmentation of Kitamura, acropigmentation of Dohi and Dowling–Degos disease in four generations. Dermatology 1998; 196: 350–351.

359 Hori Y, Kubota Y. Pigmentatio reticularis faciei et colli with multiple epithelial cysts. Arch Dermatol 1985; 121: 109–111.

360 Howell JB, Freeman RG. Reticular pigmented anomaly of the flexures. Arch Dermatol 1978; 114: 400–403.

361 Mizoguchi M, Kukita A. Behavior of melanocytes in reticulate acropigmentation of Kitamura. Arch Dermatol 1985; 121: 659–661.

362 Erel A, Gurer MA, Edali N. Reticulate acropigmentation of Kitamura: two case reports. Int J Dermatol 1993; 32: 726–727.

363 Kameyama K, Morita M, Sugaya K et al. Treatment of reticulate acropigmentation of Kitamura with azelaic acid. An immunohistochemical and electron microscopic study. J Am Acad Dermatol 1992; 26: 817–820.

364 Grosshans E, Geiger JM, Hanau D et al. Ultrastructure of early pigmentary changes in Dowling–Degos' disease. J Cutan Pathol 1980; 7: 77–87.

365 Brown WG. Reticulate pigmented anomaly of the flexures. Case reports and genetic investigation. Arch Dermatol 1982; 118: 490–493.

366 Cox NH. Prurigo pigmentosa. Br J Dermatol 1987; 117: 121–124.

367 Joyce AP, Horn TD, Anhalt GJ. Prurigo pigmentosa. Report of a case and review of the literature. Arch Dermatol 1989; 125: 1551–1554.

368 Shimizu H, Yamasaki Y, Harada T, Nishikawa T. Prurigo pigmentosa. Case report with an electron microscopic observation. J Am Acad Dermatol 1985; 12: 165–169.

369 Yazawa N, Ihn H, Yamane K et al. The successful treatment of prurigo pigmentosa with macrolide antibiotics. Dermatology 2001; 202: 67–69.

370 Schepis C, Siragusa M, Palazzo R et al. Prurigo pigmentosa treated with minocycline. Br J Dermatol 1996; 135: 158–159.

371 Teraki Y, Teraki E, Kawashima M et al. Ketosis is involved in the origin of prurigo pigmentosa. J Am Acad Dermatol 1996; 34: 509–511.

372 Nakada T, Sueki H, Iijima M. Prurigo pigmentosa (Nagashima) associated with anorexia nervosa. Clin Exp Dermatol 1998; 23: 25–27.

373 Ohnishi T, Kisa H, Ogata E, Watanabe S. Prurigo pigmentosa associated with diabetic ketoacidosis. Acta Derm Venereol 2000; 80: 447–448.

374 Teraki Y, Shiohara T, Nagashima M, Nishikawa T. Prurigo pigmentosa: role of ICAM-1 in the localization of the eruption. Br J Dermatol 1991; 125: 360–363.

375 Yanguas I, Goday JJ, González-Güemes M et al. Prurigo pigmentosa in a white woman. J Am Acad Dermatol 1996; 35: 473–475.

376 Silverberg I, Kopf AW, Gumport SL. Diffuse melanosis in malignant melanoma. Arch Dermatol 1968; 97: 671–677.

377 Sexton M, Snyder CR. Generalized melanosis in occult primary melanoma. J Am Acad Dermatol 1989; 20: 261–266.

378 Schuler G, Honigsman H, Wolff K. Diffuse melanosis in metastatic melanoma. Further evidence for disseminated single cell metastases in the skin. J Am Acad Dermatol 1980; 3: 363–369.

379 Rycroft RJG, Calnan CD, Allenby CF. Dermatopathia pigmentosa reticularis. Clin Exp Dermatol 1977; 2: 39–44.

380 Maso MJ, Schwartz RA, Lambert WC. Dermatopathia pigmentosa reticularis Arch Dermatol 1990; 126: 935–939.

381 Heimer WL II, Brauner G, James WD. Dermatopathia pigmentosa reticularis a report of a family demonstrating autosomal dominant inheritance. J Am Acad Dermatol 1992; 26: 298–301.

382 Sparrow GP, Samman PD, Wells RS. Hyperpigmentation and hypohidrosis (the Naegeli–Franceschetti–Jadassohn syndrome): report of a family and review of the literature. Clin Exp Dermatol 1976; 1: 127–140.

383 Itin PH, Lautenschlager S, Meyer R et al. Natural history of the Naegeli–Franceschetti–Jadassohn syndrome and further delineation of its clinical manifestations. J Am Acad Dermatol 1993; 28: 942–950.

384 Kudo Y, Fujiwara S, Takayasu S et al. Reticulate pigmentary dermatosis associated with hypohydrosis and short stature: a variant of Naegeli–Franceschetti–Jadassohn syndrome? Int J Dermatol 1995; 34: 30–31.

385 Tzermias C, Zioga A, Hatzis I. Reticular pigmented genodermatosis with milia – a special form of Naegeli–Franceschetti–Jadassohn syndrome or a new entity? Clin Exp Dermatol 1995; 20: 331–335.

386 Verbov J. Hereditary diffuse hyperpigmentation. Clin Exp Dermatol 1980; 5: 227–234.

387 Whittock NV, Coleman CM, McLean WHI et al. The gene for Naegeli–Franceschetti–Jadassohn syndrome maps to 17q21. J Invest Dermatol 2000; 115: 694–698.

388 Itin PH, Lautenschlager S. Genodermatosis with reticulate, patchy and mottled pigmentation of the neck – a clue to rare dermatologic disorders. Dermatology 1998; 197: 281–290.

389 Lautenschlager S, Itin PH. Reticulate, patchy and mottled pigmentation of the neck. Acquired forms. Dermatology 1998; 197: 291–296.

390 Carney RG, Carney RG Jr. Incontinentia pigmenti. Arch Dermatol 1970; 102: 157–162.

391 Carney RG Jr. Incontinentia pigmenti. A world statistical analysis. Arch Dermatol 1976; 112: 535–542.

392 Yell JA, Walshe M, Desai SN. Incontinentia pigmenti associated with bilateral cleft lip and palate. Clin Exp Dermatol 1991; 16: 49–50.

393 Miteva L, Nikolova A. Incontinentia pigmenti: a case associated with cardiovascular anomalies. Pediatr Dermatol 2001; 18: 54–56.

394 van Leeuwen RL, Wintzen M, van Praag MCG. Incontinentia pigmenti: an extensive second episode of a "first-stage" vesiculobullous eruption. Pediatr Dermatol 2000; 17: 70.

395 Di Landro A, Marchesi L, Reseghetti A, Cainelli T. Warty linear streaks of the palm and sole: possible late manifestations of incontinentia pigmenti. Br J Dermatol 2000; 143: 1102–1103.

396 Moss C, Ince P. Anhidrotic and achromians lesions in incontinentia pigmenti. Br J Dermatol 1987; 116: 839–849.

397 Nazzaro V, Brusasco A, Gelmetti C et al. Hypochromic reticulated streaks in incontinentia pigmenti: an immunohistochemical and ultrastructural study. Pediatr Dermatol 1990; 3: 174–178.

398 Dutheil P, Vabres P, Hors Cayla MC, Enjolras O. Incontinentia pigmenti: late sequelae and genotypic diagnosis: a three-generation study of four patients. Pediatr Dermatol 1995; 12: 107–111.

399 Abe Y, Seno A, Tada J, Arata J. Incontinentia pigmenti achromians-like depigmentation in the mother of a baby with typical incontinentia pigmenti. Arch Dermatol 1994; 130: 936–938.

400 Zillikens D, Mehringer A, Lechner W, Burg G. Hypo- and hyperpigmented areas in incontinentia pigmenti. Light and electron microscopic studies. Am J Dermatopathol 1991; 13: 57–62.

401 Sahn EE, Davidson LS. Incontinentia pigmenti: three cases with unusual features. J Am Acad Dermatol 1994; 31: 852–857.

402 Wiklund DA, Weston WL. Incontinentia pigmenti. A four-generation study. Arch Dermatol 1980; 116: 701–703.

403 Mascaro JM, Palou J, Vives P. Painful subungual keratotic tumors in incontinentia pigmenti. J Am Acad Dermatol 1985; 13: 913–918.

404 Simmons DA, Kegel MF, Scher RK, Hines YC. Subungual tumors in incontinentia pigmenti. Arch Dermatol 1986; 122: 1431–1434.

405 Roberts WM, Jenkins JJ, Moorhead EL II, Douglass EC. Incontinentia pigmenti, a chromosomal instability syndrome, is associated with childhood malignancy. Cancer 1988; 62: 2370–2372.

406 Stitt WZD, Scott GA, Caserta M, Goldsmith LA. Coexistence of incontinentia pigmenti and neonatal herpes simplex virus infection. Pediatr Dermatol 1998; 15: 112–115.

407 Bjellerup M. Incontinentia pigmenti with dental anomalies: a three-generation study. Acta Derm Venereol 1982; 62: 262–264.

408 Bargman HB, Wyse C. Incontinentia pigmenti in a 21-year-old man. Arch Dermatol 1975; 111: 1606–1608.

409 Emery MM, Siegfried EC, Stone MS et al. Incontinentia pigmenti: transmission from father to daughter. J Am Acad Dermatol 1993; 29: 368–372.

410 Jessen RT, van Epps DE, Goodwin JS, Bowerman J. Incontinentia pigmenti. Evidence for both neutrophil and lymphocyte dysfunction. Arch Dermatol 1978; 114: 1182–1186.

411 Dahl MV, Matula G, Leonards R, Tuffanelli DL. Incontinentia pigmenti and defective neutrophil chemotaxis. Arch Dermatol 1975; 111: 1603–1605.

412 Menni S, Piccinno R, Biolchini A et al. Incontinentia pigmenti and Behçet's syndrome: an unusual combination. Acta Derm Venereol 1986; 66: 351–354.

413 Menni S, Piccinno R, Biolchini A, Plebani A. Immunologic investigations in eight patients with incontinentia pigmenti. Pediatr Dermatol 1990; 7: 275–277.

414 Takematsu H, Terui T, Torinuki W, Tagami H. Incontinentia pigmenti: eosinophil chemotactic activity of the crusted scales in the vesiculobullous stage. Br J Dermatol 1986; 115: 61–66.

415 Person JR. Incontinentia pigmenti: a failure of immune tolerance? J Am Acad Dermatol 1985; 13: 120–124.

416 Wilkin JK. Response. J Am Acad Dermatol 1985; 13: 123–124.

417 Schmalstieg FC, Jorizzo JL, Tschen J, Subrt P. Basophils in incontinentia pigmenti. J Am Acad Dermatol 1984; 10: 362–364.

418 Thyresson NH, Goldberg NC, Tye MJ, Leiferman KM. Localization of eosinophil granule major basic protein in incontinentia pigmenti. Pediatr Dermatol 1991; 8: 102–106.

419 Ashley JR, Burgdorf WHC. Incontinentia pigmenti: pigmentary changes independent of incontinence. J Cutan Pathol 1987; 14: 248–250.

420 Schamburg-Lever G, Lever WF. Electron microscopy of incontinentia pigmenti. J Invest Dermatol 1973; 61: 151–158.

421 Caputo R, Gianotti F, Innocenti M. Ultrastructural findings in incontinentia pigmenti. Int J Dermatol 1975; 14: 46–55.

422 Guerrier CJW, Wong CK. Ultrastructural evolution of the skin in incontinentia pigmenti (Bloch–Sulzberger). Dermatologica 1974; 149: 10–22.

423 Magaña-García M, Carrasco E, Herrera-Goepfert R, Pueblitz-Peredo S. Hyperpigmentation of the clavicular zone: a variant of friction melanosis. Int J Dermatol 1989; 28: 119–122.

424 Naimer SA, Trattner A, Biton A et al. Davener's dermatosis: A variant of friction hypermelanosis. J Am Acad Dermatol 2000; 42: 442–445.

425 Weber PJ, Poulos EG. Notalgia paresthetica. Case reports and histologic appraisal. J Am Acad Dermatol 1988; 18: 25–30.

426 Layton AM, Cotterill JA. Notalgia paraesthetica – report of three cases and their treatment. Clin Exp Dermatol 1991; 16: 197–198.

427 Gibbs RC, Frank SB. A peculiar, spotty pigmentation: report of five cases. Dermatol Int 1969; 8: 14–16.

428 El Zawahry M. Idiopathic pigmentation of the upper back. Arch Dermatol 1974; 109: 101–102.

429 Black MM, Maibach HI. Macular amyloidosis simulating naevoid hyperpigmentation. Br J Dermatol 1974; 90: 461–464.

430 Springall DR, Karanth SS, Kirkham N et al. Symptoms of notalgia paresthetica may be explained by increased dermal innervation. J Invest Dermatol 1991; 97: 555–561.

431 Eisenberg E, Barmeir E, Bergman R. Notalgia paresthetica associated with nerve root impingement. J Am Acad Dermatol 1997; 37: 998–1000.

432 Şavk E, Şavk ŞO, Bolukbasi O et al. Notalgia paresthetica: a study on pathogenesis. Int J Dermatol 2000; 39: 754–759.

433 Marcusson JA, Lundh B, Sidén A, Persson A. Notalgia paresthetica – puzzling posterior pigmented pruritic patch. Report on two cases. Acta Derm Venereol 1990; 70: 452–454.

434 Colver GB, Mortimer PS, Millard PR et al. The 'dirty neck' – a reticulate pigmentation in atopics. Clin Exp Dermatol 1987; 12: 1–4.

435 Manabe T, Inagaki Y, Nakagawa S et al. Ripple pigmentation of the neck in atopic dermatitis. Am J Dermatopathol 1987; 9: 301–307.

436 O'Brien TJ, Hall AP. Terra firma-forme dermatosis. Australas J Dermatol 1997; 38: 163–164.

The dermis and subcutis

4

Disorders of collagen   345
Disorders of elastic tissue   381
Cutaneous mucinoses   405
Cutaneous deposits   423
Diseases of cutaneous appendages 455
Cysts, sinuses and pits   503
Panniculitis   521

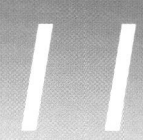
Disorders of collagen

INTRODUCTION

Collagen is the major structural constituent of mammalian connective tissues.[1] It accounts for well over 70% of the dry weight of the skin.[2] There are at least 10 genetically distinct types of collagen and it is the relative content of these different collagen types, as well as the amount of elastic tissue and non-structural constituents such as the proteoglycans, that determines the specific biomechanical properties of the various connective tissues.[3,4]

Normal collagen

Before discussing the disorders of collagen in the skin, a brief account will be given of the composition, types and metabolism of collagen.

Composition of collagen[1]

The structural collagens – types I, II and III – are composed of three poly-peptide chains, called alpha chains, each of which contains approximately 1000 amino acid residues, one-third of which are glycine. Proline and hydroxyproline are other important amino acids, constituting up to 20% of the amino acids. The sequence and composition of amino acids differ in the alpha chains of the various collagens.[4] Each of the alpha chains is coiled in a helix, and the three chains which together constitute a collagen molecule are in turn coiled on each other to form a triple helical structure. Short non-helical extensions are found at both ends of the molecule at the time it is secreted into the tissues. These extensions are soon cleaved from the procollagen molecules by two different proteases. This produces a shorter molecule which, by lateral and longitudinal association with others, produces collagen fibrils. At the same time, oxidation of lysyl and hydroxylysine residues results in the formation of stable crosslinks that give tensile strength to the collagen.

Types of collagen[3–6]

As mentioned above, at least 10 genetically distinct collagens have now been characterized, and at least 20 distinct genes encode the subunits of the various types of collagen.[7] Two of the three structural collagens types I and III, are important constituents of the skin, while type IV collagen is an important constituent of the basement membrane (see p. 143). Only small amounts of the other collagen types are found in the skin.[3]

Type I collagen is the most abundant collagen in the dermis.[3] It is composed of two identical alpha chains and a third chain of different amino acid composition. The genes for these different chains are thought to be on chromosomes 17 and 7 respectively.

Type III collagen constitutes approximately 50% of fetal skin but less than 20% of adult skin.[2] It is also present in internal organs. This collagen type is composed of three identical alpha chains. Type III collagen is believed to accommodate the expansion and contraction of tissues such as blood vessels and viscera.[8] Reticulin fibers may represent type III collagen. The synthesis of type III collagen is controlled by the COL3A1 gene on chromosome 2q31–q32.

Type IV collagen has a honeycomb or reticular pattern in contrast to the fibrillar pattern of the other major collagen types.[9,10] It is an important constituent of the lamina densa of the basement membrane.[9,10] Type V collagen is a low-abundance fibrillar collagen that is coexpressed with collagen I in many tissues and forms with it heterotypic fibrils.[11] Collagen V appears to play a crucial role in the assembly of these heterotypic fibers and in regulating their diameter.[11] An abnormality has been found in some patients with Ehlers–Danlos syndrome type I. Type VII collagen is found in the sublamina densa region of the basement membrane zone forming the anchoring filaments (see p. 143). Type XVI collagen, a member of the fibril-associated

collagens with interrupted triple helices, localizes preferentially in the papillary dermis. It is also found in some sclerotic processes, such as scleroderma.[12] Type XVII collagen is the bullous pemphigoid antigen.

Metabolism of collagen

The metabolism of collagen is a complex process involving a balance between its synthesis and its degradation.[13] There are numerous steps involved in the synthesis of collagen, and the regulatory mechanisms are not fully understood. Procollagen is formed in the rough endoplasmic reticulum of fibroblasts. After passing through the Golgi apparatus it is transported to the cell surface and secreted into the interstitium of the connective tissue.[13] Here occur cleavage of the terminal extensions of procollagen and the subsequent crosslinking of molecules to form stable collagen.[14] Collagen appears to be turned over continuously; its degradation is brought about by collagenase. It is remarkably resistant to proteolysis by most tissue proteinases.[13]

Various substances can interfere with the synthesis of collagen: the most important are the corticosteroids, which appear to act at several levels in the biosynthetic pathway.[14]

Categorization of collagen disorders

Although the various disorders of connective tissue have been assigned to a particular chapter of this volume on the basis of which element is most affected, it must be emphasized that an alteration in one component of connective tissue may influence the synthesis, deposition and structure of other components.[15] For instance, alterations in the elastic tissue and proteoglycan composition of the dermis may be found in some of the primary disorders of collagen.

The following categories will be considered, although it is acknowledged that the allocation of some of the disorders to a particular section is some-what arbitrary:

- scleroderma
- sclerodermoid disorders
- other hypertrophic collagenoses
- atrophic collagenoses
- perforating collagenoses
- variable collagen changes
- syndromes of premature aging.

It should be noted that diseases such as systemic lupus erythematosus and polyarteritis nodosa, which have been regarded in the past as 'collagen diseases', are not included in this chapter as they are not disorders of collagen in the strict sense. They are discussed with their appropriate tissue reaction pattern.

SCLERODERMA

The term 'scleroderma' refers to a group of diseases in which there is deposition of collagen in the skin and sometimes other organs as well. It may occur as a localized cutaneous disease in which the disorder of connective tissue is limited to the skin and sometimes structures beneath the affected skin, or it may occur as a systemic disease in which cutaneous lesions are accompanied by Raynaud's phenomenon and variable involvement of other organs.[16–19]

This classification of scleroderma will be used in the account that follows:

1. *localized scleroderma*
   morphea and variants

linear scleroderma
2. *systemic scleroderma*
   diffuse form (progressive systemic sclerosis)
   limited form (includes acrosclerosis and the 'CREST' syndrome)
3. *mixed connective tissue disease*
4. *eosinophilic fasciitis.*

LOCALIZED SCLERODERMA

Localized scleroderma is the most common form of scleroderma.[20] It generally occurs in children and young adults and there is a female preponderance.[21] Neonatal onset has been recorded.[22] There is no visceral involvement or Raynaud's phenomenon and it usually has a self-limiting course. Progression to or coexistence of the systemic form is rare.[21,23] Antinuclear antibodies are uncommon except in the linear form;[24] antibodies to single-stranded DNA are sometimes present, particularly in generalized morphea.[25,26] Antihistone antibodies are present in nearly 50% of cases;[27] this figure is higher in generalized morphea.[28] Increased levels of circulating ICAM-1 are present; the levels correlate with the number of lesions and the area involved.[29]

Morphea

Morphea is the commonest form of scleroderma. Usually it presents on the trunk or extremities as one or several indurated plaques with an ivory center and a violaceous border (the 'lilac ring'). Irregular areas of hyperpigmentation or hypopigmentation may be present within the lesion.[30] Other clinical forms include guttate, generalized, subcutaneous, keloidal and bullous types.[21,31,32] Occasionally, more than one type is present in the same individual.

Guttate morphea consists of small, pale, slightly indurated lesions on the upper part of the trunk which may resemble lichen sclerosus et atrophicus.[33] In the rare *generalized morphea* there are large plaque-like lesions, often with vague symmetry, involving the trunk and extremities.[34] Atrophy and fibrosis of the deep tissues may lead to crippling deformities. Ulceration and calcification may also develop in some of the lesions.[33] *Disabling pansclerotic morphea* is an aggressive variant of the generalized type and is of early onset.[35,36] Lesions may extend circumferentially on an extremity leading to massive pansclerosis and atrophy.[33] Peripheral eosinophilia and mild non-progressive visceral changes are sometimes present in this variant.[36] Cutaneous squamous cell carcinoma is a rare complication of long-standing lesions.[37] *Subcutaneous morphea* (morphea profunda) consists of one or more ill-defined, deep sclerotic plaques on the abdomen, sacral area or extremities; its progression is slow but relentless.[38–42] Rarely, the lesions have a linear arrangement.[43] *Keloidal (nodular) morphea* may be part of this spectrum, although the nodules may also be in the dermis, clinically resembling a keloid.[21,44,45] Nodules are a rare finding in systemic and linear scleroderma.[46–50] *Bullous lesions* may rarely complicate both localized and systemic scleroderma.[51] In some cases, bullous morphea represents the secondary appearance of bullous lichen sclerosus et atrophicus on a lesion of morphea.[52]

Lesions of morphea may coexist with lichen sclerosus et atrophicus (see p. 354)[53] and there are isolated reports of localized sclerodermatous lesions occurring in association with elastosis perforans serpiginosa ('perforating morphea'),[54] granuloma annulare,[55] xanthomatosis,[56] discoid lupus erythematosus,[57] subacute lupus erythematosus[58] and the presence of the so-called 'lupus anticoagulant' (see p. 226).[59] Generalized morphea has been reported in a patient with Felty's syndrome.[60]

The etiology of morphea is controversial. Antibodies and lymphoproliferative responses[61] to *Borrelia burgdorferi*, the cause of Lyme disease, have been detected in a significant number of patients with morphea in

Austria and some other parts of Europe.[62–64] Spirochetes have been demonstrated in tissue sections in some cases using a modified silver stain,[65] an avidin-biotin immunoperoxidase system[66,67] or techniques using the polymerase chain reaction (PCR).[68] However, these findings have not been confirmed in most other countries[69–71] and this leads to the view that in most instances there is no association between *B. burgdorferi* infection and morphea.[72–78] Another explanation is that certain genotypes of *Borrelia* found only in parts of Europe and Japan are responsible, as is the situation with lichen sclerosus et atrophicus.[79] However, this explanation is not confirmed by a recent study from Germany which found no evidence of *Borrelia* by PCR in lesional skin of 33 patients with morphea.[80] The increased collagen synthesis by fibroblasts in morphea may result from lymphokines released by the inflammatory cell infiltrate.[81] Serum levels of procollagen type I carboxyterminal propeptide are increased in patients with localized and systemic scleroderma.[82]

Morphea has developed, in a few instances, at the site of previous radiotherapy (radiation port scleroderma).[83–86] There is a marked upregulation of collagen synthesis following radiotherapy.[87] Morphea has also been reported in a patient taking the semisynthetic ergot alkaloid bromocriptine, a drug that has been associated with pulmonary fibrosis.[88] It has also developed adjacent to the site of a leaking silicone-gel breast implant.[89]

Therapy using various PUVA-related protocols has been used with some success.[90,91]

Linear scleroderma

Linear scleroderma is a variant of localized scleroderma in which sclerotic areas of skin develop in a linear pattern.[92,93] It may occur on the head, trunk or extremities; on the limbs it may extend the full length, leading to contractures of the joints that it crosses.[94] A familial case has been recorded.[95]

Linear scleroderma involving the frontoparietal area is referred to as *en coup de sabre* from its supposed likeness to the scar of a saber cut.[96–98] This variant, which is more likely to be bilateral than the other forms of linear scleroderma,[99,100] may be associated with various degrees of facial hemiatrophy (Romberg's disease).[101,102] Rarely, linear scleroderma has been observed overlying the sclerosing bone dystrophy known as melorheostosis,[103,104] or in association with hypertrichosis[105,106] or systemic lupus erythematosus.[107] In some cases the lesions appear to have followed Blaschko's lines.[108,109]

The onset of linear scleroderma is sometimes abrupt and occasionally follows trauma.[92] Its mean duration is longer than that of plaque-type morphea and it is less likely to resolve as completely.

Histopathology[21]

Localized scleroderma is characterized by three outstanding features – the deposition of collagen in the dermis and subcutis, vascular changes, and an inflammatory cell infiltrate, particularly in early lesions.[110] These changes are now considered in detail.

The epidermis may be normal, somewhat atrophic, or even slightly thicker than usual.[111]

The dermis is increased in thickness and composed of broad sclerotic collagen bundles which stain strongly with the trichrome stain. Collagen also replaces the fat around the sweat glands and extends into the subcutis. In the latter site the collagen is homogenized and less compact than in the dermis (Fig. 11.1) and it shows only weak birefringence and trichrome staining;[112] there is an increased number of fibroblasts. However, the collagen in the subcutis stains strongly with the PAS stain in contrast to the very weak staining of that in the dermis. Mucopolysaccharides are present in the early lesions, particularly in the subcutis. Rarely, a secondary cutaneous mucinosis, with significant interstitial mucin, is present. In most cases of morphea the

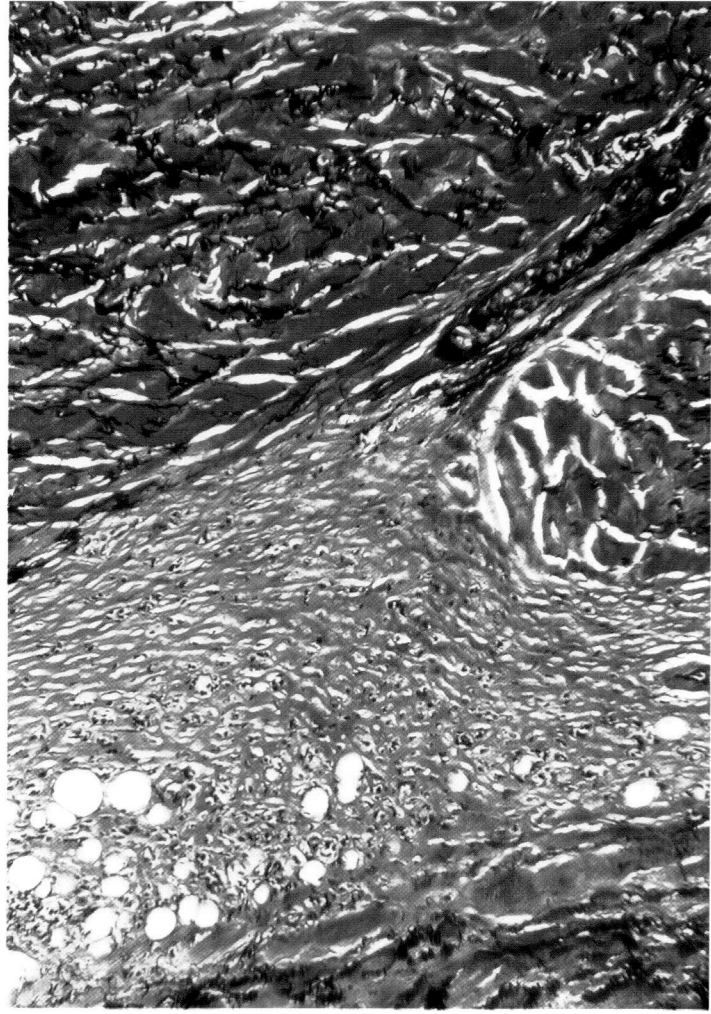

Fig. 11.1 Localized scleroderma (morphea). The recently deposited collagen stains weakly with the usual collagen stains and is devoid of elastic tissue. (Verhoeff van Gieson)

thickened collagen bundles are in the mid and deep reticular dermis. There is a variant, however, in which the histological features of collagen deposition and inflammation are restricted to the superficial dermis.[113,114] There are no features of lichen sclerosus et atrophicus. Dermal elastic fibers are not appreciably diminished, but there is some loss of CD34-positive spindle cells.[113] This variant has been called *superficial morphea*.[114]

There is atrophy of adnexal structures, particularly the pilosebaceous units. Eccrine glands are situated at a relatively high level in the dermis as a result of the collagen deposited below them (Fig. 11.2). The arrectores pilorum are often hypertrophied. The mesenchymal elements of peripheral nerves are involved in the sclerotic process.[115]

The vascular changes are thickening of the walls of small blood vessels and narrowing of their lumen. In small arteries there is fibromucinous thickening of the intima.

The inflammatory cell infiltrate is composed of lymphocytes with some macrophages and plasma cells. It is distributed around blood vessels or more diffusely through the lower dermis and subcutis, particularly at the border of early lesions. The infiltrate is more marked in localized scleroderma than systemic scleroderma and in early rather than late lesions. The infiltrate is rarely heavy.[116]

In *guttate lesions* the changes are more superficial with less collagen sclerosis but with subepidermal edema, resembling this feature of lichen sclerosus et atrophicus. *Linear lesions* may show a deeper and more diffuse inflammatory cell infiltrate extending into the underlying muscle. Vascular changes are usually prominent. Ossification of the dermis has been recorded.[117] The inflammation in the subcutis is also marked in the *generalized form*[118] and in subcutaneous morphea; in both there may be marked fibrosis in the subcutis.[33]

In *subcutaneous morphea* there is thickening and hyalinization of collagen in the deep dermis and in the septa and fascia.[119–121] There is a mixed inflammatory cell infiltrate which includes some multinucleate giant cells. Lipomembranous (membranocystic) changes may be present. Some confusion has arisen because of the variable use of the term 'subcutaneous morphea'. One group has suggested that the term 'morphea profunda' be used as an all-embracing one to include cases with dermal, subcutaneous and fascial involvement, while 'subcutaneous morphea' should be used for cases in which the subcutaneous fat is mainly affected.[119] According to this concept, eosinophilic fasciitis refers to the fascial component of morphea profunda.[119] The concept has not gained wide acceptance.

In *keloidal nodules* there are hyalinized thick collagen bundles associated with an increase in fibroblasts and mucin.[46] *Bullous lesions* show subepidermal edema with dilated lymphatics in the underlying dermis.[31,119,122] Erythrocytes are often present in the blister.[122]

The differentiation of morphea from the fibrotic lesions of acrodermatitis chronica atrophicans (see p. 654) can sometimes be difficult.[123] Although morphea and systemic scleroderma share many histological features, the lesions of morphea are usually more inflammatory than in systemic scleroderma. Furthermore, there may be some collagen deposition in the papillary dermis in morphea;[124] it is, of course, a feature of the superficial variant.

Immunofluorescence is usually negative in the lesions of localized scleroderma although a few deposits of IgM may be found in the basement membrane zone and in small dermal blood vessels.[33] An increased number of cells in the dermis express factor XIIIa and vimentin, with a reduced number expressing CD34 in established lesions.[125,126]

The cases reported as **'self-involuting atrophoderma'** occurred as non-indurated, slightly depressed lesions on the lateral upper arm that disappeared spontaneously within a year.[127] There was some fibrosis of the lower dermis, but not the subcutis. This is best regarded as a variant of morphea.

Electron microscopy

There is disarray and variable thickness of collagen at the advancing border.[128] Endothelial cells in blood vessels contain vacuoles and there is widening of the gap between the cells.[110] Collagen fibrils in the subcutis have a reduced diameter.[129]

SYSTEMIC SCLERODERMA

Systemic scleroderma (systemic sclerosis) is an uncommon connective tissue disease characterized by symmetrical tightness, thickening and induration of the skin, Raynaud's phenomenon and sometimes involvement of one or more internal organs.[130–132] The spectrum of systemic scleroderma ranges from a relatively mild form with limited acral skin involvement to a more rapidly progressive diffuse form with early and significant involvement of various internal organs.[17,130]

Diffuse systemic scleroderma

The diffuse form accounts for 20–40% of cases of systemic scleroderma. There is usually truncal and acral skin involvement of abrupt onset, associated

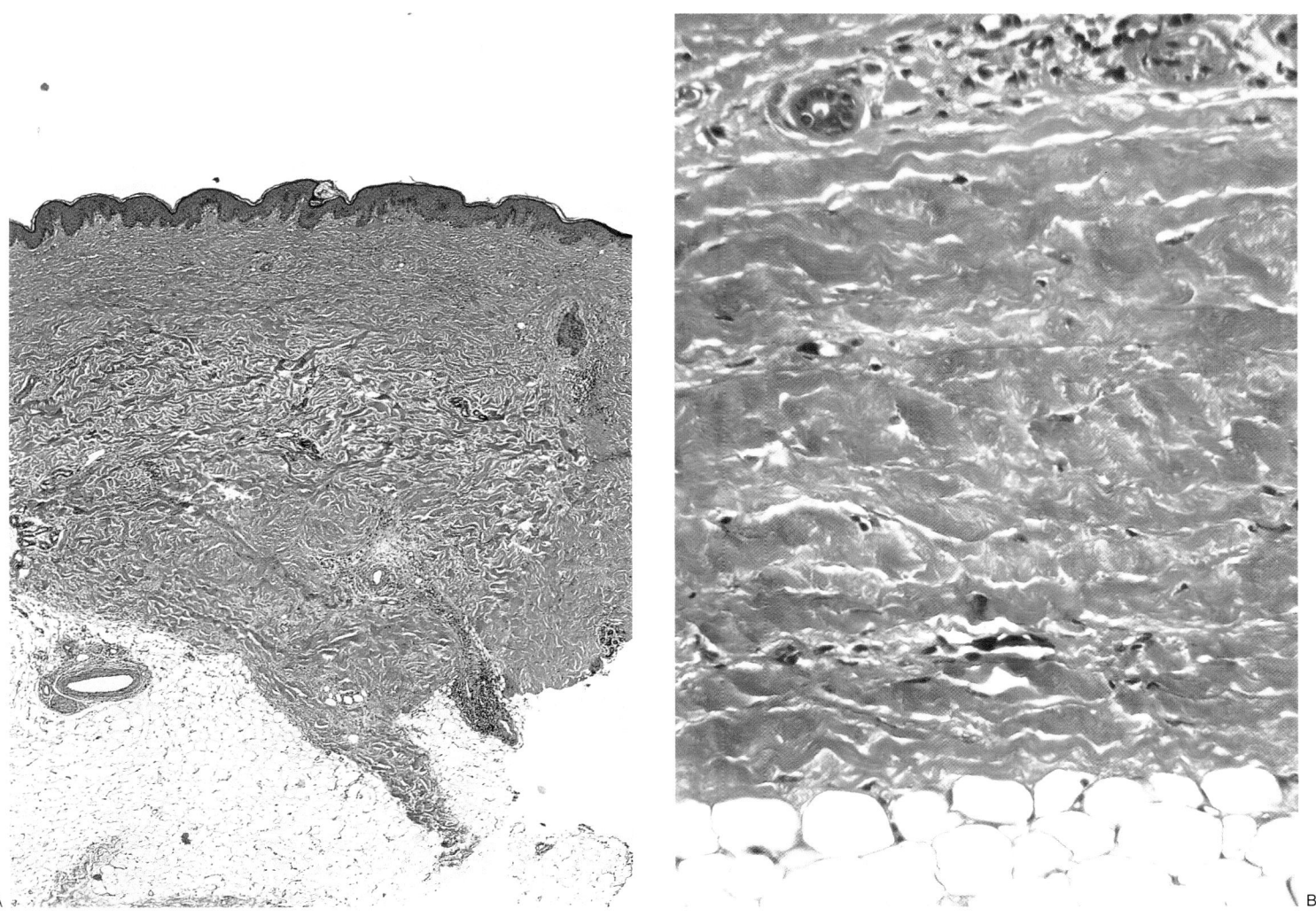

Fig. 11.2 **(A) Localized scleroderma (morphea). (B)** Note the swollen collagen bundles, the atrophic sweat glands and the straight edge of the dermal–subcutaneous interface. (H & E)

with the appearance of Raynaud's phenomenon and constitutional symptoms.[130] Synovitis is common. Other features include esophageal hypomotility and strictures, rectal prolapse, sigmoid volvulus, nodular regenerative hyperplasia of the liver, primary biliary cirrhosis, idiopathic pulmonary fibrosis, pulmonary hypertension, Sjögren's disease, thrombosis of major vessels,[133,134] intrauterine fetal death[135] and renal failure.[130] Neurotropic ulceration secondary to peripheral neuropathy is a rare occurrence.[136]

Limited systemic scleroderma

The limited variant of systemic scleroderma typically affects older women. Raynaud's phenomenon often precedes the onset of cutaneous thickening, which is usually limited to the digits. Hair loss and anhidrosis are present in affected areas. Facial telangiectasia and cutaneous calcification often develop and there is an increased incidence of late-onset pulmonary hypertension. Anticentromere antibodies are present in up to 70–80% of patients.[137–142]

Limited systemic scleroderma includes the condition referred to as the CREST syndrome,[143,144] which derives its name from the clinical features of calcinosis, Raynaud's phenomenon, esophageal dysfunction, sclerodactyly and telangiectasia.[145] Not all of these features are invariably present, leading to suggestions that this term should be dropped in favor of the term 'limited systemic scleroderma'.[19] Another variant combines Raynaud's phenomenon, anticentromere antibodies, and digital necrosis without sclerodactyly.[146]

Pigmentary changes may be found in both the diffuse and the limited forms of systemic scleroderma.[147] They may take the form of vitiligo-like areas with perifollicular and sometimes supravascular sparing, diffuse hyperpigmentation with accentuation in sun-exposed areas, or pigmentary changes in areas of sclerosis.[148] Livedo reticularis and livedoid vasculitis with ulcers occur uncommonly.[134]

Other clinical features of systemic scleroderma include a weak association with certain HLA antigen types, particularly DR5 and DR1,[149] and rare familial cases.[150–152] Antinuclear antibodies are present in almost all patients, usually with a speckled or nucleolar pattern.[139,153–155] Further characterization of these antibodies is possible now that specific nuclear macromolecules have been identified.[139] Autoantibodies to the Fc receptor are present in about 50% of cases,[156] while antibodies to Scl-70 (antitopoisomerase) are present in approximately 30% of patients.[130,157,158] A patient with systemic lupus erythematosus and topoisomerase I antibody has been reported.[159] A subset of patients with lupus-like features has anticardiolipin antibodies.[160] Antibodies to the cytoplasmic antigen Ro/SSA are present in approximately one-third of cases.[161] Antineutrophil cytoplasmic antibodies of perinuclear type (p-ANCA) are present in a small number of patients.[162] Systemic angiitis has been reported as a rare complication of systemic sclerosis, but the p-ANCA status has been reported in only one of these cases.[162,163] The serum levels of various enzymes and substrates involved in the sclerotic process have been used as an indicator of disease activity. They include xylosyltransferase (involved in proteoglycan metabolism),[164,165] tissue inhibitors of metalloproteinase-2,[166] soluble vascular adhesion molecule 1 and E-selectin,[167] type I collagen degradation products[168] and hyaluronan.[169]

Pathogenesis of scleroderma

Although the pathogenetic basis for the fibrosis in scleroderma is still not elucidated, theories relate this to changes in the vascular system, immune disturbances or alterations of fibroblast function.[130,170–73] It is probable that these three factors will prove to be interdependent and interrelated.[172]

Vascular changes include the formation of gaps between endothelial cells, alterations in the composition of type IV collagen in vascular basement membrane,[174] reduplication of the basal lamina and disruption of endothelial cells.[171] It has been suggested that the endothelial cell is the principal target;[175] endothelial dysfunction precedes other cutaneous changes in systemic scleroderma.[176,177] Cutaneous hypoxia, which results from the fibromucinous intimal change in larger vessels, may play a role in the modulation of dermal fibroblast activity.[178]

Alterations in the *immune system* include the presence of autoantibodies and circulating immune complexes[137,179] as well as an increase in the T-helper/T-suppressor cell ratio.[171,180] There is also an association with other autoimmune diseases and a similarity to chronic graft-versus-host disease. It has been suggested that lymphokines and monokines produced by cells in the inflammatory infiltrate may play a role in fibroblast regulation;[171,180,181] transforming growth factor-β (TGF-β) appears to be one of the most important (see below). Endothelin-1, derived from keratinocytes, appears to play an important role in the pathogenesis of the skin hyperpigmentation seen in patients with systemic scleroderma.[182] Monocytes may be responsible for the release of toxic free oxygen radicals, long thought to be involved in the pathogenesis of systemic sclerosis.[183] Their role in the pathogenesis of bleomycin-induced sclerosis is discussed elsewhere (see p. 353).

Numerous studies have attempted to elucidate the mechanisms controlling *fibroblast activity* in scleroderma.[171] There is an increase in the synthesis, deposition and degradation of collagen, proteoglycans and fibronectin. The increased collagen may result from the accumulation of a distinct sub-population of fibroblasts with an activated transcriptional level of collagen gene expression.[184,185] As mentioned above, it seems that the increased fibroblast activity in scleroderma results from the activity of cytokines, the most important of which are interleukin-4 (IL-4)[186] and TGF-β.[187,188] This growth factor can, in turn, induce the production of three interrelated substances – connective tissue growth factor (CTGF), platelet-derived growth factor (PDGF) and tissue inhibitor of metalloproteinase-3 (TIMP-3)[189] – which influence the mitogenic activity and function of fibroblasts resulting in increased collagen production.[185,190] Collagen deposition may also be enhanced by the release of cytokines and polyamines from epidermal keratinocytes.[191] Lysyl oxidase, which initiates crosslinkage of collagen and elastin, is increased in amount.[192] Furthermore, the increased deposition of collagen is enhanced by reduced collagenase activity.[193,194] It is possible that endothelial damage followed by platelet aggregation initiates the release of PDGF and the subsequent cascade of events.[195] Some of the type III collagen that is initially produced retains the aminopeptide on its surface, resulting in the formation of thin collagen fibrils, 30–40 nm in diameter.[196,197] These fibrils may form bundles in the subcutis or at the advancing edge or be mixed with larger diameter fibrils.[196] In the later stages, the ratio of type III to type I collagen is normal.[198]

Histopathology[130,199–201]

The histopathological changes in systemic scleroderma are similar to those described above in the localized forms, although minor differences exist (Fig. 11.3). The inflammatory changes are less marked in systemic lesions and the deposition of collagen can be quite subtle in the early stages, particularly on the fingers. Edema fluid is present in the papillary and reticular dermis of early lesions.[202] Vascular changes are sometimes more prominent, particularly severe intimal fibrosis in small arteries and arterioles (Fig. 11.4).[203] These vessels may show evidence of recent or old thrombosis and adventitial fibrosis.[133] Sclerosis of the papillary dermis can be seen in morphea but it is absent in systemic scleroderma.[124]

Other changes described include calcification,[204] an increase in mast cells in the dermis of early lesions[202,205] and of clinically uninvolved skin,[206] and pigmentary changes corresponding to the clinical changes. For example, the vitiligo-like areas show an absence of melanocytes and of melanin in the basal layer.[147,148] Amyloid is a rare finding.[207] Digital lesions with the histology of focal mucinosis have been described.[208]

Direct immunofluorescence is usually negative, although a few cases have been described with a speckled nuclear pattern in epidermal cells similar to that seen in mixed connective tissue disease (see below).[209,210] Immunoperoxidase techniques show a reduced number of CD34-positive cells.[211]

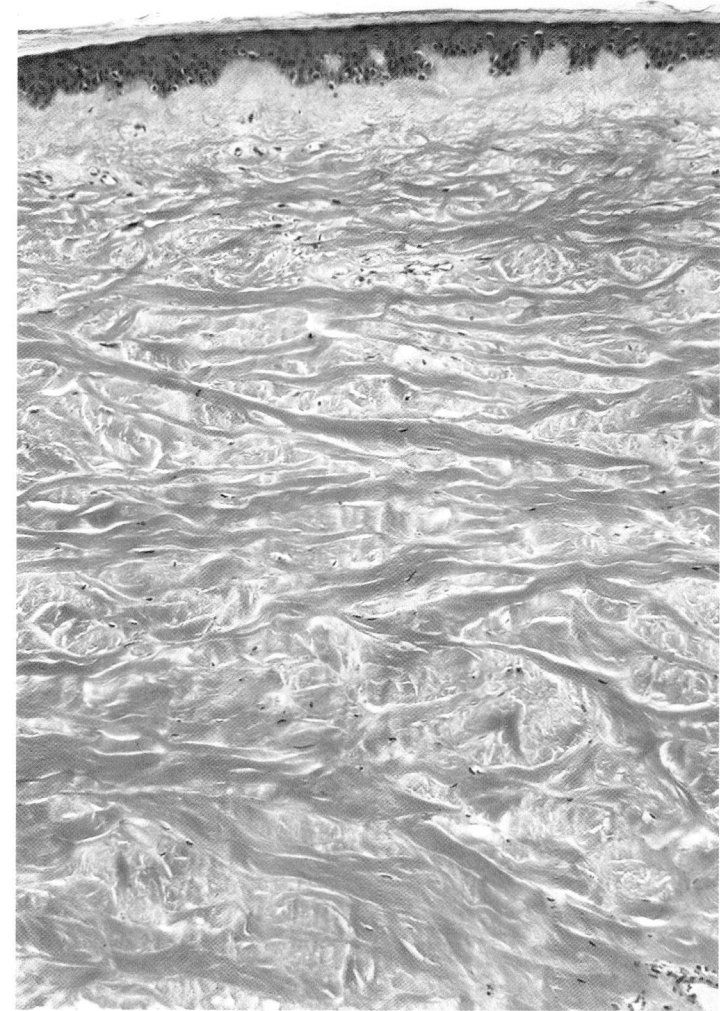

Fig. 11.3 **Systemic scleroderma** with thick collagen bundles in the dermis. Inflammation is absent. (H & E)

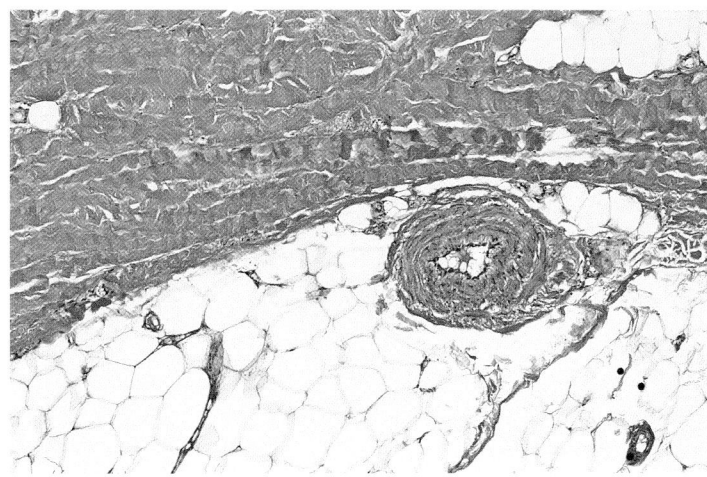

Fig. 11.4 **Systemic scleroderma.** There is fibromuscular thickening of the wall of a small artery with luminal narrowing. (H & E)

Electron microscopy
The changes are similar to those described for the localized form.[212] Fragmented elastic fibers and irregular arrangement of microfibrils have been noted in systemic scleroderma.[213]

MIXED CONNECTIVE TISSUE DISEASE

Mixed connective tissue disease (MCTD) is a distinct clinical syndrome sharing some clinical features of systemic lupus erythematosus, scleroderma and polymyositis. It is associated with the presence of circulating antibody to ribonucleoprotein.[214] Antibodies to the Sm antigen and to native DNA are usually absent.[215] Swollen or sclerotic fingers, Raynaud's phenomenon and arthritis are important clinical features, leading to a suggestion that the acronym SRA is more appropriate than MCTD.[216] Less constant clinical features include muscle tenderness and proximal weakness, lymphadenopathy, alopecia, esophageal hypomotility and pigmentary disturbances.[216–218] Approximately 20% develop restrictive lung disease.[216]

MCTD usually runs a chronic and benign course and shows a good response to systemic corticosteroids.

The terms **scleromyositis** and **sclerodermatomyositis** have been used for cases with overlap features of scleroderma and dermatomyositis.[219,220] The sera of these patients often show a homogeneous nucleolar pattern.[155]

Histopathology
If lupus-like lesions are present clinically, then a biopsy from such an area will show the features of cutaneous lupus erythematosus. Even in lesions that are not clinically typical of lupus erythematosus, the histological changes may resemble subacute lupus erythematosus.[221] In the early stages, a biopsy from a swollen finger reveals marked dermal edema with separation of collagen bundles.[217] In later lesions, dermal sclerosis resembling that seen in scleroderma may be present. The walls of vessels in the subcutis may be thickened with luminal narrowing.

Direct immunofluorescence of uninvolved skin shows a characteristic pattern of speckled epidermal nuclear staining, with specificity for IgG.[222]

EOSINOPHILIC FASCIITIS

In eosinophilic fasciitis (Shulman syndrome) there is a sudden onset, sometimes following strenuous physical activity, of symmetrical induration of the skin and subcutaneous tissues of the limbs.[223,224] There is usually sparing of the fingers. Localized variants, with involvement of part of a limb, have been reported.[225] The disease usually begins in mid-adult life, but no age is exempt.[226] Other clinical features include peripheral eosinophilia[227,228] and hypergammaglobulinemia,[224] although rare cases with specific immunoglobulin deficiencies have been reported.[229] Visceral involvement and Raynaud's phenomenon are usually absent.[230] An association with cutaneous T-cell lymphoma has been reported.[231,232] The majority of affected patients experience a complete or near complete recovery after 2–4 years, usually following steroid or PUVA-bath therapy but sometimes occurring spontaneously.[233,234]

Eosinophilic fasciitis is regarded as a variant of scleroderma.[235–237] As in scleroderma, fibroblasts in the involved skin of patients with eosinophilic fasciitis exhibit an activated phenotype.[238] Progression to scleroderma has been documented in several circumstances,[239] including a group of patients with the Spanish toxic oil syndrome (see p. 353). Patchy lesions of morphea are sometimes present on the trunk, further evidence of the close association between eosinophilic fasciitis and the various scleroderma syndromes.[226,240] The spirochete *Borrelia burgdorferi* has been implicated in the etiology of some cases of eosinophilic fasciitis.[241,242] Similar changes have also resulted from exposure to trichloroethylene,[243] and from radiation,[244] the subcutaneous injection of phytonadione (phytomenadione) in the treatment of hypoprothrombinemia[245] and the ingestion of products containing L-tryptophan. A virtual epidemic of the eosinophilia–myalgia syndrome occurred in the USA and Japan in 1989 following alterations in the manufacturing techniques of L-tryptophan. This condition is likely to become of historical interest only.[246–251]

Histopathology[226,252]
The earliest changes occur in the interlobular fibrous septa of the subcutis and the deep fascia. There is edema and an infiltration of lymphocytes, histiocytes, plasma cells and eosinophils.[252] Eosinophils are sometimes quite prominent, but in most instances there are only focal collections of these cells.[253] Lymphoid nodules may also be present.

Eventually, there is striking thickening of the deep fascia and septa of the subcutis with fibrosis and hyalinization of the collagen.[252,254] This process extends into the deep dermis where there is atrophy of appendages associated with the sclerosis of the lower dermis. Inflammatory changes may also extend into the fibrous septa of the underlying muscle,[255] but this process is not the same as eosinophilic myositis/perimyositis.[256] Similar changes were seen in the L-tryptophan-related cases[257] although there was greater dermal involvement in this condition; mucin and dermal sclerosis were often seen.[258–260]

Immunoglobulins and C3 have been present in the walls of vessels in the fascia and subcutis in some cases.

Thickening and fibrosis of the fascia may also be seen in scleroderma but there is usually a notable lack of inflammatory cells in the fascia in contrast to the more conspicuous inflammation found in eosinophilic fasciitis.[261,262]

SCLERODERMOID DISORDERS

The sclerodermoid disorders are a heterogeneous group of diseases in which lesions develop that may mimic clinically and/or histopathologically the changes found in scleroderma.[16,263,264] The sclerodermoid disorders, some of which are discussed elsewhere, as indicated below, include:

- sclerodermoid graft-versus-host disease
- stiff-skin syndrome

- Winchester's syndrome
- GEMSS syndrome
- pachydermoperiostosis
- pachydermodactyly
- acro-osteolysis
- chemical- and drug-related disorders
- paraneoplastic pseudoscleroderma
- nephrogenic fibrosing dermopathy
- lichen sclerosus et atrophicus
- scleredema (p. 410)
- scleromyxedema (p. 408)
- porphyria cutanea tarda (p. 559)
- chronic graft-versus-host disease (p. 46)
- chronic radiation dermatitis (p. 595)
- Werner's syndrome (p. 366)
- progeria (p. 367).

No detailed mention need be made of the carcinoid syndrome[265] and of phenylketonuria,[266,267] both of which are exceedingly rare causes of sclerodermatous skin lesions.

It should be noted that squeezing the skin with forceps, during a biopsy procedure, can produce an artifactual change locally in the dermis which resembles scleroderma somewhat on histopathological examination. Separation of the collagen bundles at the margins of this zone or artifactual changes in the overlying epidermis may also be present.

SCLERODERMOID GRAFT-VERSUS-HOST DISEASE

Scleroderma-like lesions may develop in chronic graft-versus-host disease (see p. 46). Most patients who develop this uncommon complication of GVHD have disseminated sclerosis of the trunk and the proximal extremities.[268] Atrophy of the skin is associated with a severe clinical evolution. Rarely, only localized lesions are present.[269] Antinucleolar, anticentromere and anti-Scl-70 antibodies are usually not present in patients with sclerodermatous GVHD.[268]

Histopathology
The sclerodermatous lesions of chronic GVHD show similar features, although the papillary and upper reticular dermis is involved at an earlier stage and there may be extension of the fibrosis into the subcutis.[270] The lichenoid changes of GVHD may also be present.[268] Secondary mucinosis is a rare finding.[271] In early lesions, the histological changes can be quite subtle despite the clinical features being quite overt.

STIFF-SKIN SYNDROME

The stiff-skin syndrome is characterized by stony-hard skin and limitation of joint mobility.[272,273] It differs from restrictive dermopathy (see p. 363), but has similarities to *congenital fascial dystrophy*.[274] Both appear to be genetically determined abnormalities of dermal and fascial collagen. Abortive forms have been described.[275]

Histopathology
In the cases reported as stiff-skin syndrome there has been mild fibrosis of the dermis and subcutis, but no inflammation.[273] An increase in dermal mucin was noted in some of the earlier cases but this is not a consistent feature. In cases reported as *fascial dystrophy*, the deep fascia is thickened 4–6 fold.[274] Again, there is no inflammation.[274]

WINCHESTER'S SYNDROME

The Winchester syndrome is an exceedingly rare inherited disorder of connective tissue which consists of dwarfism, carpal-tarsal osteolysis, rheumatoid-like small joint destruction and corneal opacities.[276,277] Cutaneous manifestations include a thick, leathery skin with areas of hypertrichosis and hyperpigmentation.[278]

Although the biochemical defect has not been elucidated, one study reported an abnormal oligosaccharide in the urine of two unrelated patients with this condition.[279] It is possible that this and another case[279,280] are examples of infantile systemic hyalinosis (see p. 438) and not the Winchester syndrome.

Histopathology
There is increased pigmentation of the basal layer and some thickening of the dermis. Fibroblasts are markedly increased in number, although in late lesions there are only a few fibroblasts in the thickened masses of amorphous collagen.[277] A perivascular lymphocytic infiltrate is also present. There is no increase in mucopolysaccharides in the dermis.

Electron microscopy
Dilated and vacuolated mitochondria are seen in dermal fibroblasts.[277] Cytoplasmic myofilaments, a prominent fibrous nuclear lamina and some dilatation of the rough endoplasmic reticulum have also been noted.[278]

GEMSS SYNDROME

GEMSS syndrome, a rare, autosomal dominant disorder, features glaucoma, lens ectopia, microspherophakia, stiffness of the joints and shortness. Sclerosis of the skin is sometimes present. This appears to be due to enhanced gene expression of TGF-β_1.[281]

Histopathology
The changes resemble those seen in systemic scleroderma.

PACHYDERMOPERIOSTOSIS

The clinical manifestations of this rare syndrome include digital clubbing, thickening of the legs and forearms resulting primarily from periosteal new bone formation at the distal ends of the long bones, and progressive coarsening of facial features with deeply furrowed, thickened skin on the cheeks, forehead and scalp (cutis verticis gyrata).[282,283] Pachydermoperiostosis has an insidious onset, usually in adolescence, and a self-limited course. There is a predilection for males.[284] A familial incidence is sometimes present and in these cases the inheritance is thought to be autosomal dominant with incomplete penetrance and variable expressivity of the gene.[285,286]

This condition has also been referred to as primary hypertrophic osteoarthropathy to distinguish it from a secondary form which is usually associated with an intrathoracic neoplasm.[287,288] Facial and scalp changes, usually less severe than in pachydermoperiostosis, have been reported in some individuals with the secondary form.[282 289–291] Finger clubbing may be the sole manifestation in some relatives of patients with pachydermoperiostosis, indicating the overlap between these conditions.[282,287,292]

The pathogenesis is unknown, although many mechanisms have been postulated for the secondary form. Increased peripheral blood flow is found in secondary hypertrophic osteoarthropathy, but not in the primary variant.[293] One study has shown an increased tissue sensitivity to circulating sex hormones, and this could induce enhanced tissue epidermal growth factor/TGF-α production and utilization.[294] Another study has found that fibroblasts from affected skin synthesize decreased amounts of collagen but increased amounts of the small dermatan sulfate-containing proteoglycan decorin.[295]

Histopathology[284,296]

The epidermis may be normal or mildly acanthotic. There is a diffuse thickening of the dermis with closely packed, broad collagen bundles. Some hyalinization of the collagen is usually present. Fibroblasts are increased in number in some areas. The subcutis may also participate in the fibrosing reaction. Elastic fibers are usually normal, although variations have been recorded. Acid mucopolysaccharides are sometimes increased in the dermis.[286] In late stages there is some thickening of capillary walls with an increase in pericapillary collagen.[293]

Other changes include a variable, usually mild, perivascular and peri-appendageal chronic inflammatory cell infiltrate and prominence of sebaceous and eccrine glands.[297]

PACHYDERMODACTYLY

Pachydermodactyly is characterized by fibrous thickening of the lateral aspects of the proximal interphalangeal joints of the fingers.[298,299] In contrast, knuckle pads, which have similar histological appearances, involve the dorsal aspect of the finger joints.

Pachydermodactyly and knuckle pads are usually regarded as localized forms of superficial fibromatosis. Accordingly, they are considered with the fibromatoses in Chapter 34, page 923.

ACRO-OSTEOLYSIS

Acro-osteolysis refers to lytic changes in the distal phalanges. There is a familial form, an idiopathic form with onset in early adult life, and an occupational variant related to exposure to vinyl chloride.[300] Cutaneous lesions have been described in only some idiopathic cases;[300] in contrast, they are a characteristic feature of occupational acro-osteolysis.[301] There are sclerodermoid plaques on the hands accompanied by Raynaud's phenomenon.[263] With altered work practices, occupational acro-osteolysis should become a historical disease.[302]

Histopathology[300]

The dermis is thickened, with swollen collagen bundles and decreased cellularity. There is usually no significant inflammation and there is no calcinosis. Elastic fibers are often fragmented.

CHEMICAL- AND DRUG-RELATED DISORDERS

Sclerodermoid lesions may develop in the skin following occupational exposure to polyvinyl chloride (acro-osteolysis, see above), vinyl chloride monomer,[303] trichlorethylene,[304] perchlorethylene, aromatic hydrocarbon solvents, herbicides,[305] certain epoxy resins and silica.[302,306–310] Silica has also been implicated in the etiology of scleroderma itself.[306,311] In recent years, there has been considerable controversy about the relationship between scleroderma and other connective tissue diseases and the use of breast prostheses containing silicone gel.[309,312–315] Notwithstanding this debate about the possible *systemic* effects of extravasated silicone, it is acknowledged that

a *localized*, dense collagenous reaction may ensue following such an event (see p. 444).

The injection of phytonadione (phytomenadione, vitamin K_1)[316–320] polyvinylpyrrolidone (a former plasma expander)[321] or pentazocine[16] will result in a localized sclerodermatous reaction.

The ingestion of an olive oil substitute – rapeseed oil, denatured with aniline – produced a multisystem disease of epidemic proportions in Spain some years ago.[322] Sclerodermoid lesions developed in the skin.[323] A similar multisystem illness followed the ingestion of products containing L-tryptophan following alterations in the manufacture of this product in 1989.[246] In both conditions, the tissue fibrosis may result from the stimulation of fibroblasts by cytokines such as TGF-β and platelet-derived growth factor.[246]

The chemotherapeutic agent bleomycin will produce cutaneous sclerosis, particularly involving the fingers, in addition to its other complications of alopecia, cutaneous pigmentation and pulmonary toxicity.[324–326] The cutaneous lesions produced by bleomycin in particular, and to a lesser extent by some of the other agents listed above, are self-limiting, with some resolution of the lesions after withdrawal of the offending agent. Experimentally, mice with bleomycin-induced dermal sclerosis had a reduction in this sclerosis following injection of superoxide dismutase, supporting a role for superoxide radicals in the pathogenesis of the fibrosis.[327] The second-generation anticancer drug uracil-tegafur (UFT) has been associated with a sclerodermatous reaction.[328]

Histopathology

The changes resemble quite closely those found in systemic scleroderma. In bleomycin-induced lesions, the homogenized collagen is often most prominent around blood vessels and adnexal structures.

PARANEOPLASTIC PSEUDOSCLERODERMA

Sclerotic skin lesions resembling systemic scleroderma are a rare complication of malignancies. This paraneoplastic syndrome is most often seen with lung cancer, plasmacytoma and carcinoids.[329,330] Marked expression of α1(I)-collagen and connective tissue growth factor (CTGF) mRNA, but not TGF-$β_1$, was found in fibroblasts.[329]

Histopathology

The changes in the dermis resemble those seen in systemic scleroderma. The fibrosis sometimes extends into the subcutis.[330]

NEPHROGENIC FIBROSING DERMOPATHY

Nephrogenic fibrosing dermopathy is the suggested title for a recently described cutaneous disease seen in renal dialysis patients, which is characterized by thickening and hardening of the skin on the trunk and limbs.[331] Rippled pigmentation may be present. The dialysis was usually being done following renal transplant, but in one case the dialysis was for acute tubular necrosis. The abnormality was initially regarded as being scleromyxedema-like.[332] The pathogenesis is currently unknown.

Histopathology[331,332]

The dermis is thickened with haphazardly arranged collagen bundles throughout the dermis and subcutaneous septa. Fibrocytes are increased in number. There is also an increase in interstitial mucin. Multinucleated histiocytes, usually of small size, are scattered throughout the dermis. They are sometimes few in number.

LICHEN SCLEROSUS ET ATROPHICUS

Lichen sclerosus et atrophicus (LSA) is a chronic disorder with a predilection for the anogenital region of middle-aged and elderly women.[333–337] Cases in childhood are uncommon.[338–340] About 20% of the patients have extragenital lesions, these sometimes occurring without coexisting genital involvement.[341] Extragenital sites which are affected include the upper part of the trunk, the neck, the upper part of the arms, the flexor surfaces of the wrists, and the forehead. Very rarely, palmar,[342] plantar[343,344] and digital[345] skin, the face,[346] scalp,[347] mouth[348] and even a surgical[349] or burn scar,[350] stoma[351] and a vaccination site[352] have been involved. Extragenital lesions may rarely follow Blaschko's lines.[353,354]

LSA may involve the glans, prepuce or external urethral meatus of uncircumcized prepubertal or adolescent males, resulting in phimosis.[355–360] These lesions, also known in the past as balanitis xerotica obliterans, are not associated with extragenital involvement,[355] although isolated extragenital lesions may be seen in other males.[361,362] HPV is present in a significant number of penile lesions in children.[363,364] A case has followed the use of alprostadil as an intracavernous injection for penile dysfunction.[365]

LSA commences as flat, ivory to white papules that coalesce to form plaques of varying size and shape. These develop follicular plugging and progressive atrophy leading to a parchment-like, wrinkled, flat or slightly depressed scar ('cigarette paper atrophy'). Vulval lesions may have secondary lichenification from the pruritus-related scratching or they may coexist with hypertrophic areas, the so-called 'mixed vulval dystrophy'.[334] Infrequently, hemorrhagic bullae form[366–371] and these may be complicated by the subsequent development of milia.[372] Small nodules have been recorded as an unusual clinical manifestation.[373] Pigmentation due to massive melanin incontinence is another rare finding.[374]

Usually, the disorder is slowly progressive with periods of quiescence. Spontaneous involution may occur, particularly in girls[375] at or about the menarche.[376–380]

There is controversy concerning the relationship of LSA to morphea.[381,382] Ackerman believes that LSA is a superficial variant of morphea. Although many authors have reported small numbers of cases of LSA coexisting with or superimposed upon morphea,[53,383] it is suggested, but not universally accepted,[384] that these patients have morphea with secondary lymphedema and sclerosis of the superficial dermis mimicking LSA both clinically and pathologically.[382] In most, but not all instances, there have been no genital lesions.[385] Some patients with LSA have had coexisting autoimmune diseases.[386–389] Other rare associations include glucose intolerance or diabetes mellitus,[390] vitiligo[391] and sclerodermatous GVHD.[392]

Extragenital lesions never undergo malignant degeneration, although in the genital region there may, uncommonly, be coexisting or subsequent squamous cell carcinoma.[336,393–396] In these circumstances, the tumor usually arises in the hyperplastic areas of what is a mixed vulval dystrophy.[378] Interestingly, there is increased p53 but not Ki67 expression in vulval lesions of lichen sclerosus et atrophicus when compared to non-vulval lesional skin.[397,398] The p53 changes may be of etiological significance in the development of some squamous cell carcinomas of the vulva arising in LSA.[399] Malignant change has been recorded in 5.8% of penile LSA.[400,401] Most of these cases had concomitant HPV infection.[400]

Although the etiology of LSA is unknown, attention has been directed at the role of *Borrelia burgdorferi*, which has been detected by a modified silver stain and immunoperoxidase techniques in lesional skin.[65–67] It has also been demonstrated by PCR-based techniques and serology. Most of the studies have been from Austria or nearby European countries.[402,403] Some *Borrelia*-associated cases have been reported from Japan.[404] Attempts at detecting this

organism in UK, USA and Australian cases have been unsuccessful.[76,404,405] It is possible that this geographical association is related to the presence of the genotypes *B. garinii* and *B. afzelii* in Europe, but not in the USA, where *B. burgdorferi sensu stricto* is the usual species of *Borrelia* found. This particular strain does not appear to be associated with LSA. *B. burgdorferi* can also be detected in cases of morphea, Lyme disease and atrophoderma of Pasini and Pierini; this latter condition has been reported in patients with LSA.[406]

In LSA there are numerous epidermotropic and dermal lymphocytes that are CD8+, CD57+. This profile is usually associated with viral diseases, autoimmune diseases and malignancies.[407] Morphea also exhibits CD57+ lymphocytes. Clonally expanded populations of T cells have been reported in the infiltrate. This probably represents a response to an antigen, as yet unidentified.[408] Immunological changes appear to occur at all levels of the skin.[409] The histological changes suggest that significant alteration of the extracellular matrix is occurring.[410,411] This may, in part, be mediated by the decreased epidermal expression of CD44, which can produce increased hyaluronate accumulation in the superficial dermis.[412]

Another finding in LSA is a loss of androgen receptors in lesional skin with disease progression.[413] This may be a secondary effect rather than of etiological significance.

Certain HLA types (particularly DQ7 but also DQ8 and DQ9) are more frequent in patients with LSA.[389,414,415] Familial cases are rare.[416]

Histopathology[417]

Established lesions show hyperkeratosis, follicular plugging, thinning of the epidermis and vacuolar alteration of the basal layer (Fig. 11.5). There is a broad zone of subepidermal edema with homogenization of collagen and poor staining in hematoxylin and eosin preparations. In later lesions, this zone becomes more sclerotic in appearance and shows more eosinophilia. Basement membrane thickening also occurs.[418] Expression of collagen IV and VII is increased.[419] There is dilatation of thin-walled vessels in the zone and sometimes hemorrhage. Beneath the edema there is a diffuse, perivascular infiltrate of lymphocytes, predominantly of T-cell type in the mid dermis. This infiltrate is sometimes quite sparse in established vulval lesions and it may contain a few plasma cells and histiocytes. Mast cells and liberated mast cell granules are also present.[405] In vulval lesions there is also more diversity of epidermal changes, with hyperplastic areas in mixed dystrophies.[420] The appendages are usually preserved. Two cases with a lymphohistiocytic and granulomatous phlebitis have been reported.[421]

In the early stages, elastic fibers are pushed downwards by the edematous zone and subsequently destroyed.[422] In contrast, elastic fibers are normal or increased in morphea.[423] Small amounts of acid mucopolysaccharide may be found in this zone. The basement membrane may focally fragment and PAS-positive material may be found in the subjacent dermis, partially as homogeneous clumps.[422]

In early lesions, the inflammatory infiltrate is quite heavy and is superficial and band-like, mimicking lichen planus (Fig. 11.6). Basal apoptosis and vacuolar change (Fig. 11.7) accompany the infiltrate; that is, there are features of the lichenoid tissue reaction (interface dermatitis). Overlap syndromes with lichen planus have also been suggested.[424,425] Features favoring a diagnosis of LSA over lichen planus include basilar epidermotropism, basement membrane thickening, epidermal atrophy, loss of papillary dermal elastic fibers, paucity of cytoid bodies and a lack of wedge-shaped hypergranulosis.[426] As the edematous zone broadens, the infiltrate is pushed downwards and becomes more dispersed and usually less intense.

In presumptive cases with coexisting morphea, the absence of vacuolar alteration, the lack of a well-defined inflammatory infiltrate beneath the

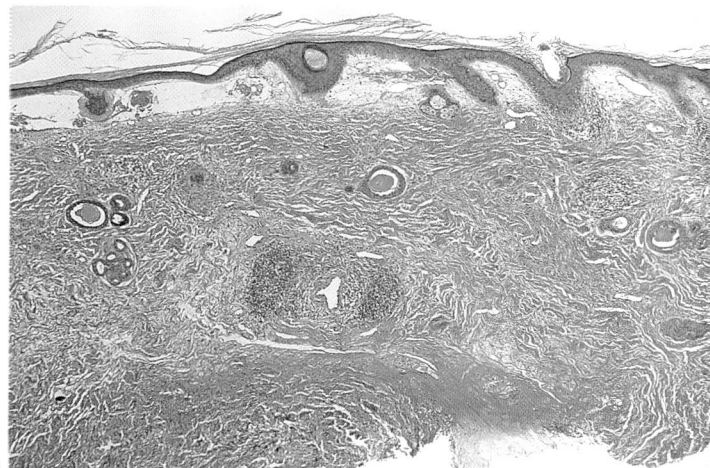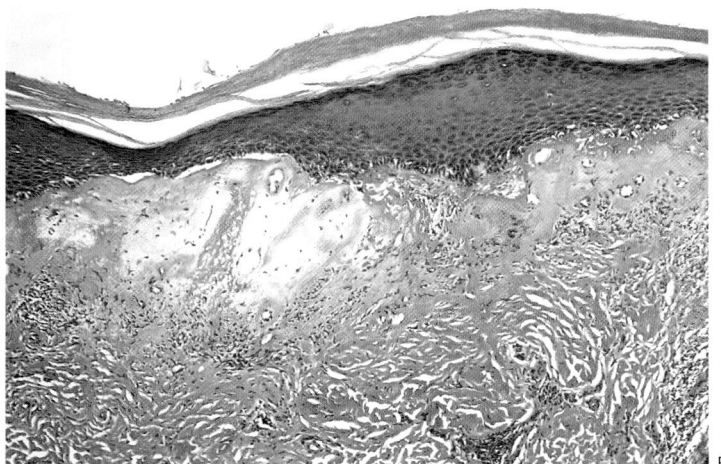

Fig. 11.5 **(A) Lichen sclerosus et atrophicus. (B)** There is orthokeratotic hyperkeratosis, some basal vacuolar change and subepidermal edema and homogenization of collagen. In established lesions the infiltrate is deeper and more dispersed. (H & E)

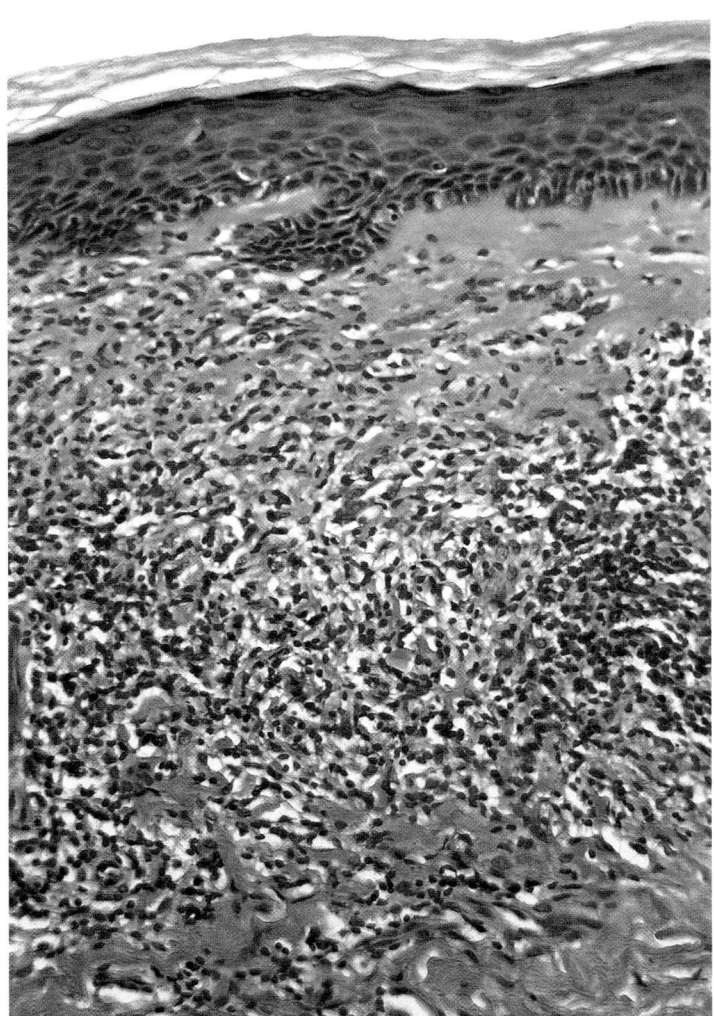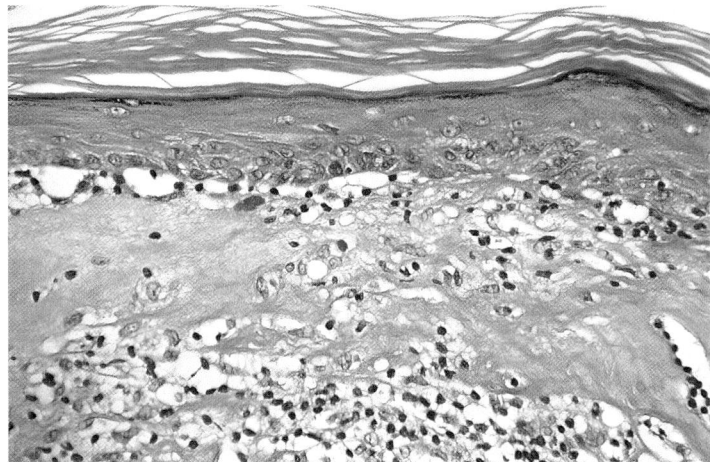

Fig. 11.7 **Lichen sclerosus et atrophicus.** Interface changes with vacuolar change can be seen. (H & E)

Microscopic features of LSA have been recorded, as an incidental finding, in acrochordons[427] and in the skin tag/folds of the perineum known as infantile pyramidal (perineal) protrusion.[428] Another study of this protrusion showed no histological evidence of LSA.[429]

Electron microscopy
Electron microscopy has shown degeneration and regeneration of superficial dermal collagen, the presence of collagen in intercellular spaces in the epidermis, abnormalities of the basement membrane zone and condensation of tonofilaments in the basal epidermal cells.[430,431]

POST-STRIPPING CUTANEOUS SCLEROSIS

The term 'post-stripping cutaneous sclerosis' is preferred to the rather cumbersome title of the original report – 'post-stripping sclerodermiform dermatitis'.[432] The condition presents as multiple hypopigmented and indurated plaques distributed in a linear arrangement along the path of a previously stripped saphenous vein.[432]

Fig. 11.6 **Lichen sclerosus et atrophicus.** Early lesion with a heavy lymphocytic infiltrate in the upper dermis. (H & E)

thickened dermis, and the presence of deep dermal changes of morphea are features supporting a diagnosis of morphea without coexisting LSA.[382]

Histopathology

There is diffuse dermal sclerosis, sometimes extending into the subcutis. There is superficial telangiectasia and/or lymphangiectasia with mild epidermal atrophy. There is often a mild deep perivascular infiltrate of lymphocytes but this was not present in two cases seen by the author. Inflammation may not be present in older lesions.

OTHER HYPERTROPHIC COLLAGENOSES

Collagen is increased in several conditions, but not necessarily in the manner seen in scleroderma and the sclerodermoid disorders. Connective tissue nevi and hypertrophic scars and keloids have been arbitrarily included in this section; they could also be regarded as tumor-like proliferations of fibrous tissue, other examples of which are discussed in Chapter 34.

The dermis is usually thickened and somewhat sclerotic in lipodermatosclerosis. It has been considered with the panniculitides (see Ch. 17, p. 532).

CONNECTIVE TISSUE NEVI

Connective tissue nevi are cutaneous hamartomas in which one of the components of the extracellular connective tissue – collagen, elastic fibers or glycosaminoglycans – is present in abnormal amounts.[433] They can be sub-classified on the basis of the component predominantly involved:

- *collagen type*
  collagenoma
  shagreen patch
- *elastin type*
  elastoma
- *proteoglycan type*
  nodules in Hunter's syndrome.

Sometimes there are alterations in more than one component of connective tissue, and these lesions may simply be categorized as connective tissue nevi.[434] Only the connective tissue nevi of collagen type will be discussed in this section.

Collagenoma

Collagenomas (connective tissue nevi of collagen type) are rare hamartomas of the skin in which there is an increase in dermal collagen. They usually present as asymptomatic, firm, flesh-colored plaques and nodules, 0.5–5.0 cm in diameter, on the trunk and upper part of the arms.[433] The ear[435] and vulva[436] are rare sites of involvement. There may be several lesions[437] or up to a hundred or more, with an onset in adolescence.[438,439] A family history is sometimes present (familial cutaneous collagenoma) and in these cases there is autosomal dominant inheritance.[438,440,441]

Associated clinical features have included a cardiomyopathy[433] and Down syndrome.[442,443] Uncommonly, the connective tissue nevi associated with the Buschke–Ollendorff syndrome (see p. 383) are of collagenous composition rather than of the usual elastic tissue type.[444–447] A connective tissue nevus of collagen type has been reported in association with pseudo-Hurler polydystrophy (mucolipidosis III).[448]

Solitary collagenomas are sometimes quite large, as seen with the cerebriform or 'paving stone' variants on the sole of the foot.[449,450] Sometimes a connective tissue nevus is associated with cutis verticis gyrata, a descriptive term for a condition of the scalp in which deep furrows and convolutions are present. The folds of skin may, however, have normal morphology.[451,452] Other pathological associations of cutis verticis gyrata include lymphedema,[453] adipocyte proliferation, acromegaly, myxedema, tumors and the insulin resistance syndrome.[454]

Collagenomas must be distinguished from sclerotic fibromas (see p. 922) which present as tumor-like nodules. They have a characteristic histological appearance with dense collagen bundles, often in a storiform arrangement. **Athlete's nodules** are related to, but different from, collagenomas. One such example is the dermal nodule found in the sacrococcygeal region of bicycle riders.[455]

Histopathology

The epidermis is usually normal, although an overlying epidermal nevus has been reported.[456] There is thickening of the dermis, sometimes with partial replacement of the subcutis. The collagen bundles are broad and have a haphazard arrangement.[457] Elastic fibers are more widely spaced, but this may represent a dilution phenomenon.[457] Sometimes the elastic fibers are thin and fragmented. There is no increase in mucopolysaccharides. Dermal dendrocytes are reduced using antibodies against factor XIIIa.[458] Calcification was present in one reported case.[459]

As the collagen in collagenomas is less well packed than normal, differences in polarization colors can be seen with picrosirius red staining followed by polarization microscopy.[460] The fibers appear green to yellow, in contrast to the orange to red color of normal dermal collagen.[460]

Shagreen patch

The shagreen patch is a distinct clinical variant of collagenoma, found exclusively in those with tuberous sclerosis. It consists of a slightly elevated, flesh-colored plaque of variable size, usually on the lower part of the trunk.[461] It has the appearance of untanned leather. Smaller 'goose flesh' papules may form as satellite lesions.

Histopathology[461]

There are dense sclerotic bundles of collagen, with an interwoven pattern, in the reticular dermis.[462] Fibroblasts appear hypertrophied.[462] There is no inflammatory infiltrate or increase in vascularity. The overlying epidermis is usually flat, although sometimes it has the pattern of acanthosis nigricans.[461]

WHITE FIBROUS PAPULOSIS OF THE NECK

White fibrous papulosis consists of multiple, pale, discrete, non-follicular lesions on the lateral and posterior neck.[463–466] The lesions are asymptomatic and gradually increase in number; eventually there may be 10–100 papules, measuring 1–3 mm in diameter. There is some clinical resemblance to pseudoxanthoma elasticum, but there are no angioid streaks. Most of the reported cases have been from Japan and Italy.[467]

There is significant overlap between cases reported as white fibrous papulosis of the neck and those reported as papillary-dermal elastolysis (acquired elastolysis of the papillary dermis simulating pseudoxanthoma elasticum) – see page 395. Accordingly, it has been suggested that both entities be combined under the term 'fibroelastolytic papulosis of the neck'.[467]

The etiology is unknown, but in view of the onset late in life, the condition may be the result of an age-related change in dermal collagen.[464] Cultured fibroblasts express increased amounts of collagen type I mRNA.[468]

Histopathology

White fibrous papulosis has some resemblance to a connective tissue nevus. There is a circumscribed area of thickened collagen bundles, involving the papillary and mid dermis.[464] Elastic fibers are usually reduced in areas of fibrosis.[467]

HYPERTROPHIC SCARS AND KELOIDS

Hypertrophic scars and keloids are a variation of the optimal wound healing process.[469–471] Keloids have been defined as cutaneous scars that extend beyond the confines of the original wound, and hypertrophic scars as raised scars that remain within the boundaries of the wound.[472] As the clinical distinction may be blurred, the usefulness of these definitions has been questioned.[473] Equally, the histopathological definitions proposed below have been criticized on the grounds that they do not always correlate with the above clinical definitions.[469] The differences between keloids, hyperplastic scars and the optimal (normal) wound healing process are of degree only, and it is not surprising that cases with overlap features exist. Keloids may be quite disfiguring and have therefore attracted much more attention than hypertrophic scars.

Keloids are firm, variably pruritic masses, usually at the site of injury. They may be unevenly contoured. Early lesions are erythematous, while older lesions are usually pale, although occasionally they may be pigmented.[473] Sites of predilection are the upper part of the back, the deltoid and presternal areas and the ear lobes. Rare sites include the genitalia, eyelids and even palms and soles.[473] They usually develop over a period of weeks or months. Attempted surgical excision of a keloid results in regrowth of a larger lesion unless some concurrent effective therapeutic measures, such as radiation therapy, or the use of cultured epithelial autografts are adopted.[473–477] Recurrence is significantly less frequent in hypertrophic scars.[474,478]

Factors leading to the formation of keloids and hypertrophic scars include race, increased skin tension in a wound, age of the patient, wound infection, site, as already mentioned, the use of isotretinoin therapy and a precisposition to scar hypertrophy.[469,472,479] Keloids are more common in black races. They have a predilection for individuals under 30 years of age.

Numerous experimental studies have been designed to identify the etiology and pathogenesis of keloids. Fibroblasts isolated from keloids often synthesize normal amounts of collagen,[480] although proline hydroxylase activity, a marker of collagen synthesis, is higher in keloids than in hypertrophic scars or normal wounds.[481] A lower rate of apoptosis and of mutations in p53 occurs in keloid fibroblasts.[482,483] Other studies suggest an important role for various cytokines, particularly TGF-β which is a potent chemotactic factor for fibroblasts[484–488] and stimulates them to produce major matrix components including collagen.[484] Interleukin-15 (IL-15) also appears to be involved.[489] The relative amounts of type III collagen are increased. There is also increased expression of type I and III collagen mRNA.[488,490,491] There is a major suppression of pro-α1(I) type I collagen gene expression in the dermis after excision of a keloid followed immediately by intrawound injection of triamcinolone acetonide, an explanation for the beneficial action of corticosteroid injections.[492] Collagenase activity may be normal or increased in keloids;[493] decreased levels have been found in hypertrophic scars.[494,495] Changes in the extracellular matrix proteins occur in keloids.[496] Their interaction with TGF-β may explain their mode of action. Tenascin C, biglycan and decorin are increased in some hypertrophic scars and keloids.[497–499] Expression of dermatopontin (a multifunctional protein of the extracellular matrix which influences collagen assembly), is decreased.[500] It appears that collagen accumulates in keloids and hypertrophic scars because there are more fibroblasts present, making more collagen than in normal wound healing, and this collagen may be protected from degradation by proteoglycan and specific protease inhibitors.[473,501]

Histopathology[478,502]

Early *keloids* show abundant fibrillary collagen (Fig. 11.8). Mature keloids have a characteristic appearance with broad, homogeneous, brightly eosinophilic collagen bundles in haphazard array (Fig. 11.9). Fibroblasts are increased and are found along the collagen bundles with an orientation similar to the accompanying collagen. The AgNOR count of the fibroblasts is significantly increased.[503] There is also abundant mucopolysaccharide, particularly chondroitin-4-sulfate, between the bundles. Keloids have reduced vascularity when compared with hypertrophic scars and normal healing wounds.[504]

Keloids are usually elevated above the surrounding skin surface. The overlying epidermis may be thin and beneath it there are often some telangiectatic vessels. A sparse, chronic inflammatory cell infiltrate may surround these peripheral vessels.

In contrast, *hypertrophic scars* are only slightly elevated, if at all, above the surrounding skin. The collagen bundles are characteristically oriented parallel to the skin surface, as are the accompanying fibroblasts (Fig. 11.10). They are markedly increased in number, although there is some reduction in number with time. Capillaries are generally oriented perpendicular to the skin surface and these may be surrounded by a sparse inflammatory cell infiltrate within the scar itself. There is little mucin except in early lesions. Elastic tissue is sparse or absent. Subepidermal clefting sometimes develops overlying a scar;[505] bullae are rare.[506]

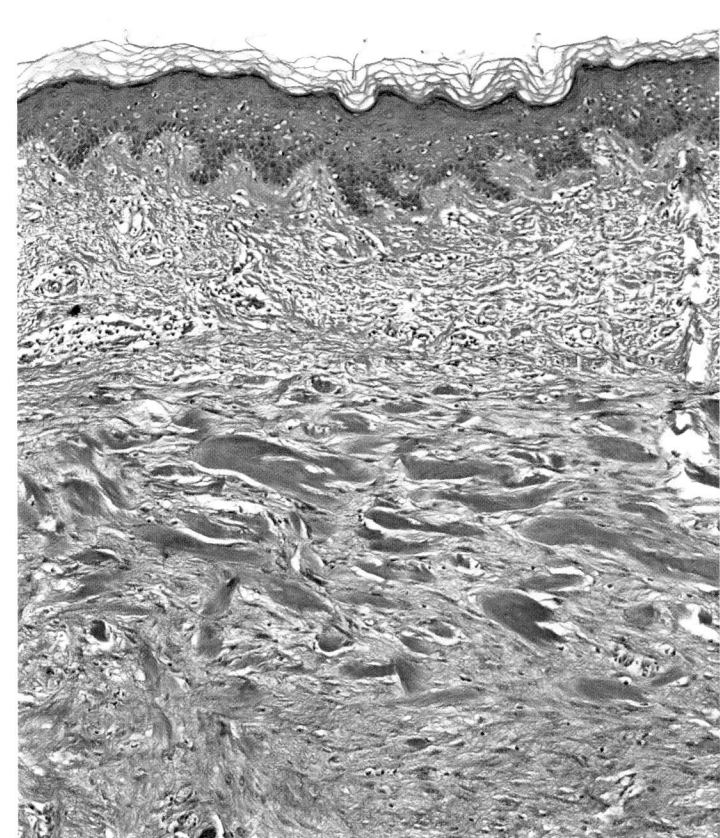

Fig. 11.8 **An early keloid** with thick hyaline collagen replacing the scar tissue. (H & E)

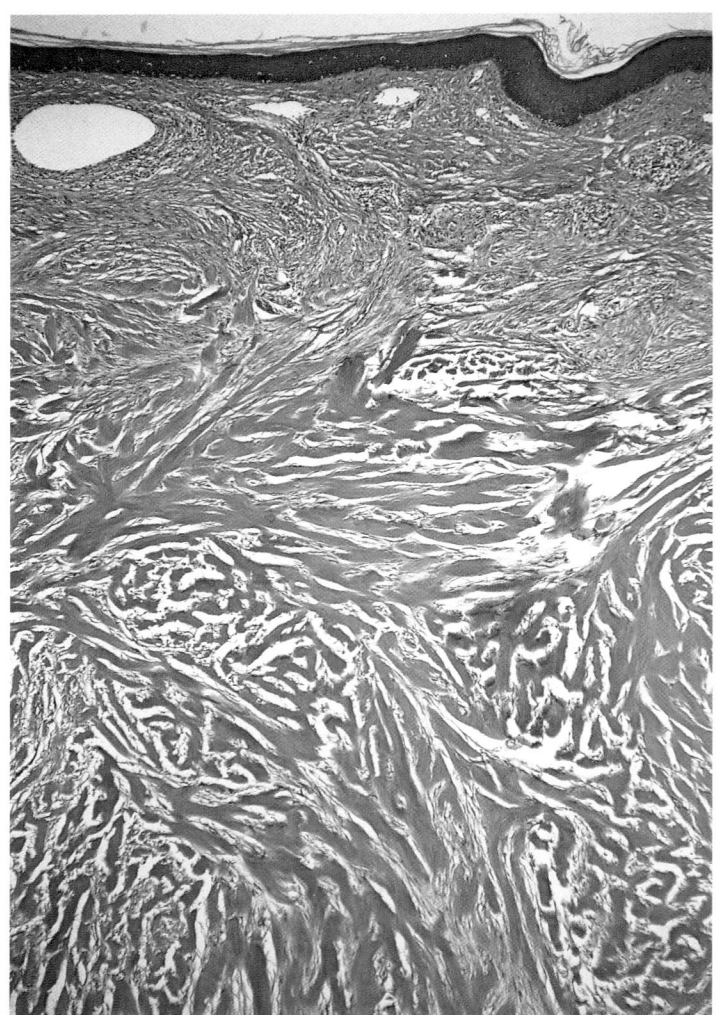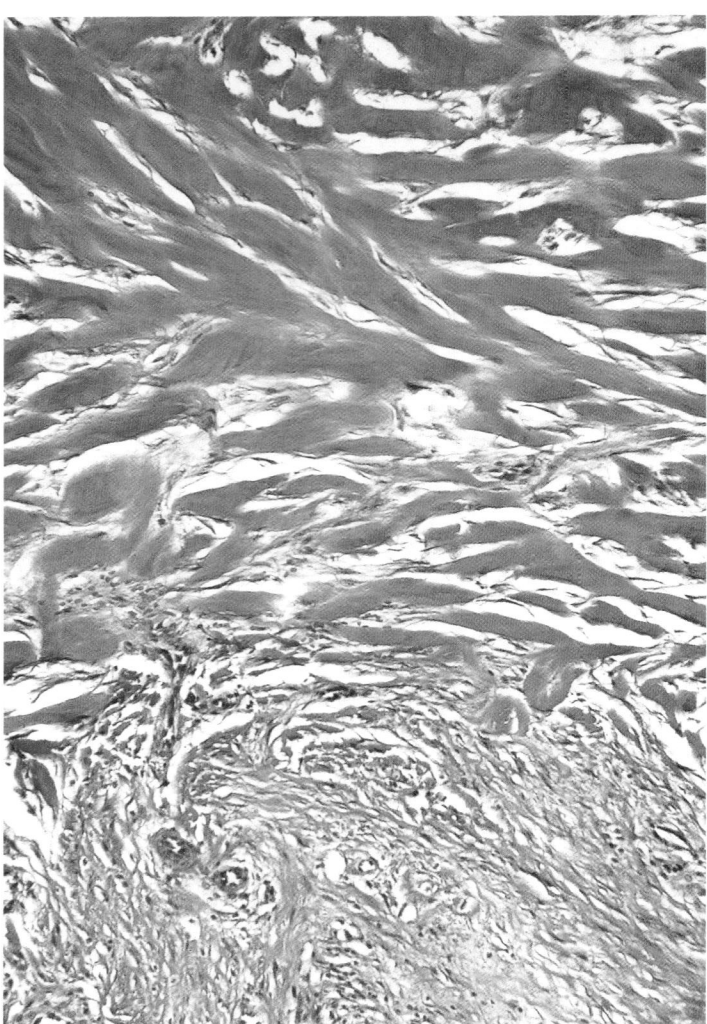

Fig. 11.9 **(A) Established keloid. (B)** The thick hyaline bundles of collagen contrast with the more normal ones below. (H & E)

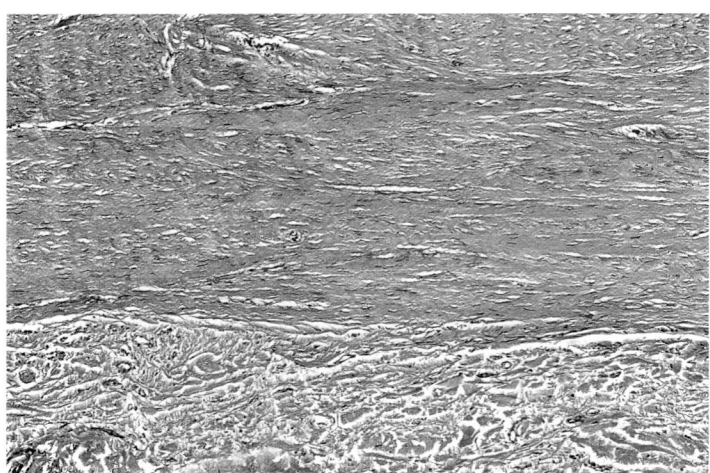

Fig. 11.10 **Hypertrophic scar.** There are parallel bundles of cellular collagen contrasting with those of the dermis below the scar. (H & E)

Mast cells are increased in both hypertrophic scars and keloids. Dystrophic calcification and bone may occasionally develop, particularly in abdominal scars.[507]

Attention has been drawn recently to the presence of S100-positive cells, including spindle cells with mild atypia, in cutaneous scars.[508] Care needs to be taken in these circumstances to avoid overdiagnosis of desmoplastic melanoma. Conversely, desmoplastic melanomas can also be misdiagnosed as scars.

Electron microscopy

Keloids exhibit numerous fibroblasts with prominent Golgi complexes and abundant rough endoplasmic reticulum.[509] Myofibroblasts have usually not been demonstrated,[509] although it has been speculated that they may be present in early lesions.[510] Very fine elastic fibers can be seen in hypertrophic scars on electron microscopy, although they cannot be demonstrated by light microscopy.[511]

STRIAE DISTENSAE

Striae distensae are a common finding in adolescents of both sexes,[512,513] particularly females, and in pregnancy (striae gravidarum).[514-516] They are also found following prolonged heavy lifting.[517,518] Striae form in association with the excess corticosteroid of Cushing's disease, with systemic steroid therapy and with prolonged topical use of steroid preparations.[519,520] They develop on the abdomen, lower part of the back, buttocks, thighs and female breasts.

Striae may also occur in HIV-positive persons receiving protease inhibitors, such as indinavir.[521]

Striae show a progression of clinical appearances, commencing as flat, pink lesions which broaden and lengthen and assume a violaceous color.[519] This gradually fades to leave a white, depressed scar. The direction of the striae is conditioned by the mechanical forces responsible, but they are usually linear. They have been attributed to the stretching of corticosteroid-conditioned skin.[517] It is possible that only minimal stress is required in some circumstances, such as adolescence.[522] This continuous strain on the dermal extracellular matrix may remodel the elastic fiber network in susceptible individuals.[523] The proportion of crosslinked to unlinked collagen may also be of critical pathogenetic importance.[522]

Histopathology[524–526]

Striae distensae are basically scars. The epidermis is flat with loss of the normal rete ridge pattern. The dermis may be thinned, suggesting that this condition would be better considered with the atrophic collagenoses.[527] Dermal collagen bundles are arranged in parallel array, resembling a scar.[524] There is an increase in glycosaminoglycan content in striae.[523] The Verhoeff van Gieson stain for elastic tissue will usually show a reduction in elastic fibers, but the orcein and Luna stains will often show many additional fine fibers.[525] Using specific markers, it has been shown that the numbers of vertical fibrillin fibers beneath the dermal–epidermal junction and elastin fibers in the papillary dermis are significantly reduced. The elastin and fibrillin fibers in the deep dermis show realignment parallel to the skin surface.[523] In older lesions, thicker elastic fibers can be seen in the affected skin.[526] Early lesions (striae rubrae) are rarely biopsied. They have been reported to show vascular dilatation and a mild perivascular inflammatory cell infiltrate. Another study has suggested that the early stages consist of mast cell degranulation, followed by an influx of activated macrophages that envelop fragmented elastic fibers.[528] The increase in elastic fibers noted in advanced lesions is presumably a later stage of repair.

FIBROBLASTIC RHEUMATISM

Only a few cases of fibroblastic rheumatism have been described since the initial report in 1980.[529–534] There is a sudden onset of symmetrical polyarthritis and Raynaud's phenomenon and the development of cutaneous nodules, 0.2–2 cm in diameter, which are found mainly on the hands. The cutaneous lesions resolve spontaneously after several months.[534] The nature of the disease is unknown.

Histopathology

The cutaneous nodules show a proliferation of plump spindle cells, as well as fibroblasts, set in a background of thickened collagen bundles having a whorled pattern.[531] The plump cells are myofibroblasts.[532] There is some loss of elastic tissue, but there is preservation of the vasculature. A mild, perivascular, chronic inflammatory cell infiltrate is sometimes present.

COLLAGENOSIS NUCHAE

Collagenosis nuchae (nuchal fibroma) is a recently delineated entity which presents clinically with diffuse induration and swelling, usually of the back of the neck, accompanied by features suggesting low-grade inflammation.[535–538] Extranuchal involvement has been recorded.[538] There is a male predominance. Non-destructive recurrences occasionally develop after excision.[538] Collagenosis nuchae has been reported in association with scleredema,[539]

diabetes[538] and Gardner's syndrome.[540] In Gardner's syndrome, the lesions may occur in multiple sites and in unusual locations.[541] The term '**Gardner-associated fibroma**' has been suggested for these lesions.[541]

Histopathology

Thick, disorganized collagen bundles partly replace the subcutaneous fat. The collagen merges almost imperceptibly with the lower dermis and the ligamentum nuchae. There are no inflammatory cells present, despite the clinical impression of inflammation (Fig. 11.11). Furthermore, there are very few fibroblasts, distinguishing the lesion from a fibromatosis. However, there has been a report of a desmoid fibromatosis having areas resembling collagenosis nuchae.[542] Many of the cells express CD34; a few contain factor XIIIa.[540] There is no increase in mucin, as seen in scleredema (see p. 410). Nerve entrapment is a frequent occurrence.[536]

LIPODERMATOSCLEROSIS

Lipodermatosclerosis is characterized by circumscribed, indurated inflammatory plaques on the lower extremities. Sometimes the plaques are quite large. The erythema and woody induration are often misdiagnosed as cellulitis. The condition is mentioned here because of the dermal thickening and fibrosis. There is considerable involvement of the subcutis, and this entity is therefore considered in more detail with the panniculitides (see Ch. 17, p. 532).

WEATHERING NODULES OF THE EAR

Weathering nodules are asymptomatic, white or skin-colored nodules measuring 2–3 mm in diameter. They have a gritty texture.[543] The lesions are usually bilateral and multiple with small chains of lesions producing a scalloped appearance of the helix. Reported cases have all been in elderly males with an outdoor occupation or hobby.[543] The lesions appear to be more common than is currently recognized.

Histopathology[543]

The lesions are composed of a spur of fibrous tissue in which there is a focus of metaplastic cartilage which is sometimes in continuity with the cartilage of the ear. The fibrous tissue sometimes extends to the undersurface of the

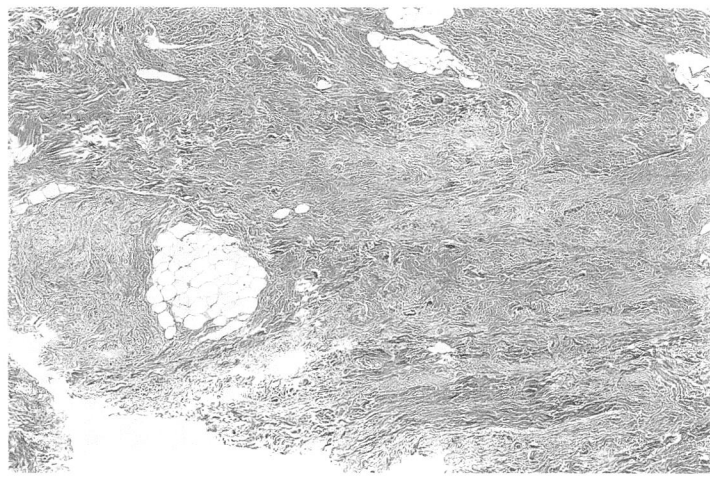

Fig. 11.11 **Collagenosis nuchae (nuchal fibroma).** Fibrous tissue replaces the subcutaneous fat. There is no inflammation. (H & E)

epidermis. It is relatively acellular but it may contain spindle-shaped cells that are negative for S100 protein and factor XIIIa.

ATROPHIC COLLAGENOSES

The microscopical assessment of dermal atrophy can be difficult in the early stages. It requires a knowledge of the regional variability in skin thickness. The age of the patient is also relevant, since there is some atrophy of the skin in the elderly. Technical artifacts in the preparation of histological sections can also influence dermal thickness.

The following conditions, discussed below, can be associated with a decrease in dermal thickness:

- aplasia cutis congenita
- focal dermal hypoplasia
- focal facial dermal dysplasia
- pseudoainhum constricting bands
- keratosis pilaris atrophicans
- corticosteroid atrophy
- atrophoderma of Pasini and Pierini
- linear atrophoderma of Moulin
- acrodermatitis chronica atrophicans
- restrictive dermopathy.

In addition, dermal thinning can be seen in type IV Ehlers–Danlos syndrome (see p. 365) and also in some forms of Marfan's syndrome (see p. 397). The dermis is usually thinned in striae distensae (see p. 358) but, because of the scar-like features, this condition has been considered with the hypertrophic collagenoses. The unique case with membranocystic degeneration of collagen fibers, associated with some deposition of fat, and with the clinical appearance of xanthomatosis, defies classification.[544]

APLASIA CUTIS CONGENITA

Aplasia cutis congenita is the term applied to a heterogeneous group of disorders in which localized or widespread areas of skin are absent at birth. The defect is most often limited to the vertex of the scalp,[545,546] but other parts of the body such as the trunk or limbs may be affected, often symmetrically, with or without accompanying scalp lesions.[547–550] Other recorded associations include limb defects,[551–554] mental retardation,[555] epidermal and organoid nevi,[556–558] epidermolysis bullosa,[559–563] chromosomal abnormalities,[548] fetus papyraceus[556,564] and focal dermal hypoplasia.[548,555,565] The Adams–Oliver syndrome refers to the combination of aplasia cutis congenita and transverse limb defects. Other systemic abnormalities may be present.[566]

The MIDAS (microphthalmia, dermal aplasia sclerocornea) syndrome is another distinct variant of aplasia cutis congenita presenting as linear facial skin defects. The Xp deletion syndrome, MLS syndrome and Gazali–Temple syndrome are similar conditions. It is lethal in males. There is usually a microdeletion at Xp22.[567] This syndrome is distinct from focal dermal hypoplasia, but it could be included with focal facial dermal dysplasia (see below).

Two publications have attempted to define distinct clinical subtypes, based on the location of the skin defects and the presence of associated malformations.[548,556] Some cases have an autosomal dominant inheritance with reduced penetrance of the gene;[568] others appear to be the result of gene mutation.[548] The condition has been reported in one of monozygotic twins.[569] Other factors that may be etiologically significant in individual cases

include amniotic adhesions, intrauterine trauma, drugs, particularly the antithyroid drug methimazole (thiamazole),[570,571] biomechanical forces from the hemispheric growth of the brain[572] and ischemia resulting from placental infarcts[573] or associated with the condition fetus papyraceus.[556,564] A case mimicking aplasia cutis congenita, but resulting from a congenital nevus, has been reported.[574]

The defect in the skin presents as an ulcer, a membranous lesion or an area of atrophic scarring. Sometimes there is a ring of coarse, long hair surrounding the scalp defect (the 'hair collar sign').[575,576] Lesions on the scalp usually heal with cicatricial alopecia.[577] An abnormal tendency to cutaneous scarring has been reported in two siblings with this condition.[578]

Skin dimpling, which may be confused with aplasia cutis congenita, has been reported as a complication of second trimester amniocentesis.[579]

Histopathology[556]

The epidermis may be absent or thin, with only two or three layers of flattened cells. The underlying dermis is usually thin and composed of loosely arranged connective tissue in which there is some disarray of collagen fibers (Fig. 11.12).[580] The dermis may resemble a scar.[581] Elastic fibers may be reduced, increased or fragmented.[582] Appendages are absent or rudimentary.[583] The subcutis is usually thin.

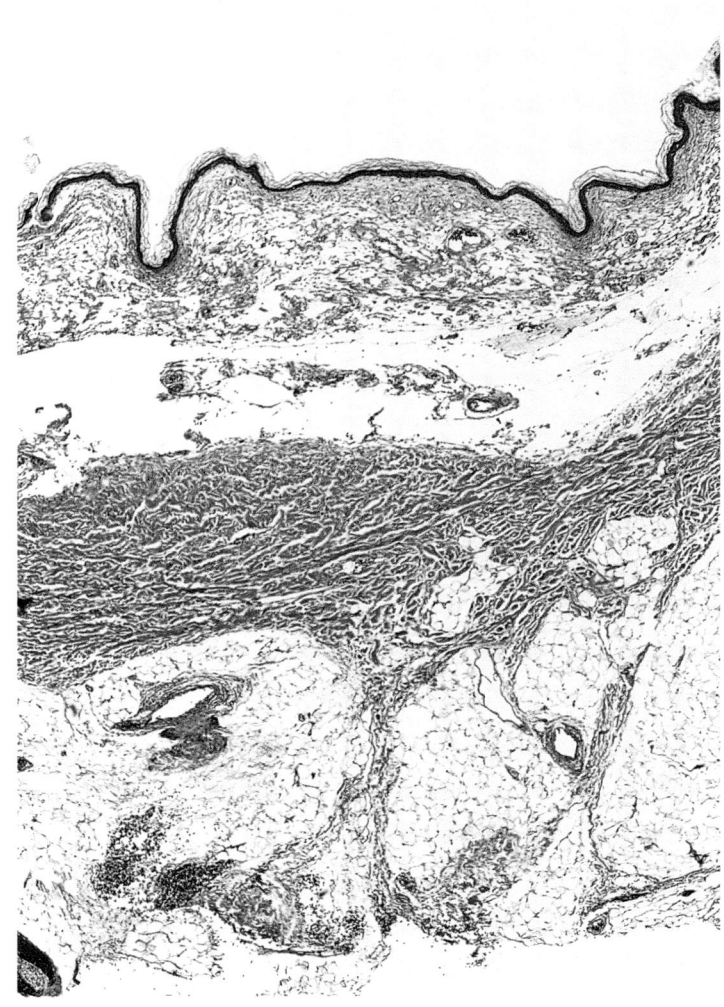

Fig. 11.12 **Aplasia cutis congenita of the scalp.** Appendages are lost and the dermis is composed of thin, widely-spaced bundles of collagen. (H & E)

FOCAL DERMAL HYPOPLASIA

Focal dermal hypoplasia (Goltz or Goltz–Gorlin syndrome) is a rare syndrome with multiple congenital malformations of mesoderm and ectoderm, affecting particularly the skin, bones, eyes and teeth.[584–588] It is thought to be inherited as an X-linked dominant trait, which usually is lethal in the male;[589] however, this is not absolute as some male cases have been reported.[590,591] Father-to-daughter transmission is a rare event.[592]

Cutaneous manifestations include widespread areas of dermal thinning in a reticular, cribriform and linear pattern, soft yellowish nodules representing either herniations of subcutaneous fat through an underdeveloped dermis or heterotopic fat (a fat nevus)[593] and linear or reticular areas of hyper- or hypo-pigmentation, often following Blaschko's lines.[584,594,595] Focal loss of hair, nail changes, total absence of skin from various sites, apocrine hidrocystomas,[59] lichenoid hyperkeratotic papules, giant papillomas[596] and periorificial tag-like lesions may also occur.[584,594] Skeletal abnormalities include syndactyly, polydactyly and longitudinal striations of the metaphyseal region of long bones (osteopathia striata).[595,597–600] Dermal hypoplasia may be a manifestation of the Proteus syndrome.[601] Rarely, only cutaneous abnormalities are present in focal dermal hypoplasia.

Experimental studies using fibroblasts from affected skin have shown that synthesis of collagen by individual fibroblasts is normal, but that there is an abnormality in cell kinetics with reduced proliferative activity of fibroblasts.[602] An absence of collagen type IV from the basement membrane zone has been reported.[591,603]

Histopathology[584,593,602]

The epidermis is usually normal. There is a marked reduction in the thickness of the dermis, with some thin, loosely arranged collagen fibers in the papillary dermis. Adipose tissue continuous with the subcutaneous fat extends almost to the undersurface of the epidermis in some areas. Clusters of adipocytes may be anywhere in the dermis or in a perivascular location.[604] The extreme degree of attenuation of the collagen seen in focal dermal hypoplasia is not present in nevus lipomatosus, in which mature fat also replaces part of the dermis; furthermore, the clinical presentations of the two conditions are quite distinct.

Inflammatory cells, sometimes quite numerous, have been present in biopsies of focal dermal hypoplasia taken in the neonatal period.[589,605] Other findings have included the presence of increased numbers of blood vessels and of some elastic tissue within the fat, a feature not present in normal subcutaneous fat.[606]

Electron microscopy

One study has shown fine filamentous tropocollagen within and between collagen bundles.[607] Rough endoplasmic reticulum and Golgi complexes are not prominent in dermal fibroblasts.[607] Multilocular fat cells, which are regarded as young fat cells, are often seen.[607] Disruption of the basement membrane zone is also present.[603]

FOCAL FACIAL DERMAL DYSPLASIA

Focal facial dermal dysplasia is a rare genodermatosis also known as congenital ectodermal dysplasia of the face. It is characterized by congenital, usually symmetrical, scar-like lesions of the temple.[608–610] Lesions may extend onto the face. There is often a spectrum of associated facial anomalies.[608] The tetralogy of Fallot was present in one case.[611] Inheritance is usually as an autosomal dominant trait with incomplete penetrance;[612] other patterns of inheritance have been reported in what are probably clinical variants.[613] A

'hair collar' may surround the defect.[614,615] This entity has been regarded in the past as a variant of aplasia cutis congenita[582] or as an ectodermal dysplasia.[616]

A specific variant of facial lesion that indicates the close relationship between focal facial dermal dysplasia and aplasia cutis congenita is the preauricular skin defect characterized by oval, atrophic patches distributed in a linear pattern on the preauricular region of the face.[617] It is thought to be the result of a persistent ectodermal groove in the region of the fusion between the maxillary and mandibular facial prominences.[617]

Histopathology

The epidermis is thin and usually depressed. There is more prominent thinning of the dermis and this is usually associated with some decrease in elastic tissue and absence of adnexal structures.[608,616] Small bundles of striated muscle are sometimes present within the dermis.[582,612]

PSEUDOAINHUM CONSTRICTING BANDS

The term 'pseudoainhum' refers to congenital constriction bands which may take the form of shallow depressions in the skin or deep constrictions associated with gross deformity or even amputation of a limb or digit.[618] The term 'ainhum' is a West African name for similar constrictive lesions, usually of the fifth toe, that lead eventually to spontaneous amputation and that probably result from the effects of repeated trauma in the genetically predisposed African patients.

Acquired lesions developing later in life may occur in association with scleroderma, syringomyelia, leprosy and pachyonychia congenita.[619]

Histopathology[618]

There is marked thinning of the dermis with finger-like projections of fibrous tissue extending into the underlying subcutis. Elastic tissue may be increased in this region.

KERATOSIS PILARIS ATROPHICANS

The term 'keratosis pilaris atrophicans' refers to a group of three related disorders in which keratosis pilaris is associated with mild perifollicular inflammation and subsequent atrophy, particularly involving the face. Differences in the location and the degree of atrophy have been used to categorize these three conditions – *keratosis pilaris atrophicans faciei (ulerythema ophryogenes), keratosis follicularis spinulosa decalvans* and *atrophoderma vermiculata (folliculitis ulerythematosa reticulata)*. All three conditions are regarded as congenital follicular dystrophies with abnormal keratinization of the superficial part of the follicles, and are therefore considered with other follicular abnormalities in Chapter 15, page 483. Dermal atrophy is an inconstant and disputed feature.

Histopathology

In all three variants of keratosis pilaris atrophicans there is follicular hyperkeratosis with atrophy of the underlying follicle and sebaceous gland. There is variable perifollicular fibrosis which may extend into the surrounding reticular dermis as horizontal lamellar fibrosis. The dermis may be reduced in thickness.

CORTICOSTEROID ATROPHY

Cutaneous atrophy is an important complication of the long-term topical application of corticosteroids, especially if occlusive dressings are used or the steroids are fluorinated preparations.[620–622] The injection of corticosteroids into the skin will also produce local atrophy;[623,624] rarely, atrophic linear streaks develop along the lines of the overlying lymphatic vessels draining the injection site.[625–628] Telangiectasia and striae are other complications that may develop.[629,630]

Profound digital collagen atrophy has been reported in a patient with Cushing's syndrome.[631] Elevated plasma cortisol levels were present secondary to an adrenal adenoma.

The pathogenesis of corticosteroid atrophy is not completely understood. It appears to involve diminished synthesis and enhanced degradation of collagen.[632–634]

Histopathology[629,635]

Epidermal thinning with loss of the rete ridges is an early change. The superficial dermis often has a loose texture and there may be telangiectasia of superficial vessels. The reticular dermis is reduced in thickness only after prolonged topical therapy. If atrophy is present the collagen bundles may appear thin and lightly stained.[636] At other times the collagen appears homogenized.[637] In some areas fibroblasts are decreased in number. Elastic fibers are focally crowded. There may also be a reduction in the size of the dermal appendages.[638]

Electron microscopy

There is disorganization of the collagen bundles and a variable thickness of the fibers.[636] Globular masses of microfibrils are also seen.

ATROPHODERMA

Atrophoderma (of Pasini and Pierini) is an uncommon yet distinctive form of dermal atrophy consisting of one or more sharply demarcated, depressed and pigmented patches.[639–641] The color varies from bluish to slate gray or brown.[642] There is no induration or wrinkling.[642] Individual lesions are round or ovoid and may coalesce to give large patches of involvement. There is a predilection for the trunk, particularly the back.[640] In one report, the lesions had a zosteriform distribution.[643] The onset, which is insidious, usually occurs in adolescence.[639] Lesions may slowly progress over many years or they may persist unchanged.

Atrophoderma is regarded by some as an abortive variant of morphea,[644,645] an opinion favored by some overlapping clinical and histopathological features and by isolated reports of progression to either morphea or systemic sclerosis.[646] Ackerman believes it is morphea, unqualified.[647] Others regard it as a distinct disease entity on the basis of the dermal atrophy, the usual absence of sclerosis,[639] and the unique glycosaminoglycan metabolism.[648] Unfortunately, this controversy is based on a small spectrum of clinical experience.[649]

The etiology and pathogenesis are unknown, but it has been suggested that macrophages and T lymphocytes that are present around the vessels in the dermis may play some role.[644] In one report, 10 of the 26 patients studied had elevated serum antibodies to *Borrelia burgdorferi*.[640] Twenty of the 25 patients treated with antibiotics showed clinical improvement.[640]

Histopathology

There is dermal atrophy but this may not be apparent unless adjacent normal skin is included in the biopsy for comparison (Fig. 11.13).[642,650] The collagen bundles in the mid and deep dermis are sometimes edematous or slightly homogenized in appearance.[639,645] Elastic fibers are usually normal, although there may be some clumping and loss of fibers in the deep dermis.[639] Adnexal

structures are usually preserved. There is a perivascular infiltrate of lymphocytes and a few macrophages; rarely, plasma cells are prominent.[640] The infiltrate is usually mild in the upper dermis and somewhat heavier around vessels in the deep dermis. Some superficial vessels may be mildly dilated.

The epidermis is usually normal, apart from hyperpigmentation of the basal layer. There may be a few melanophages in the superficial dermis.

Electron microscopy

In the one study known to the author, the collagen and elastic fibers were normal.[644]

LINEAR ATROPHODERMA OF MOULIN

Linear atrophoderma of Moulin was first described in 1992 and is characterized by a hyperpigmented atrophoderma that follows Blaschko's lines.[651] Onset is usually during childhood or adolescence. The absence of sclerosis and a lilac color are distinguishing features from linear scleroderma. The lesions are similar to atrophoderma of Pasini and Pierini but lesions in this latter entity do not follow Blaschko's lines.

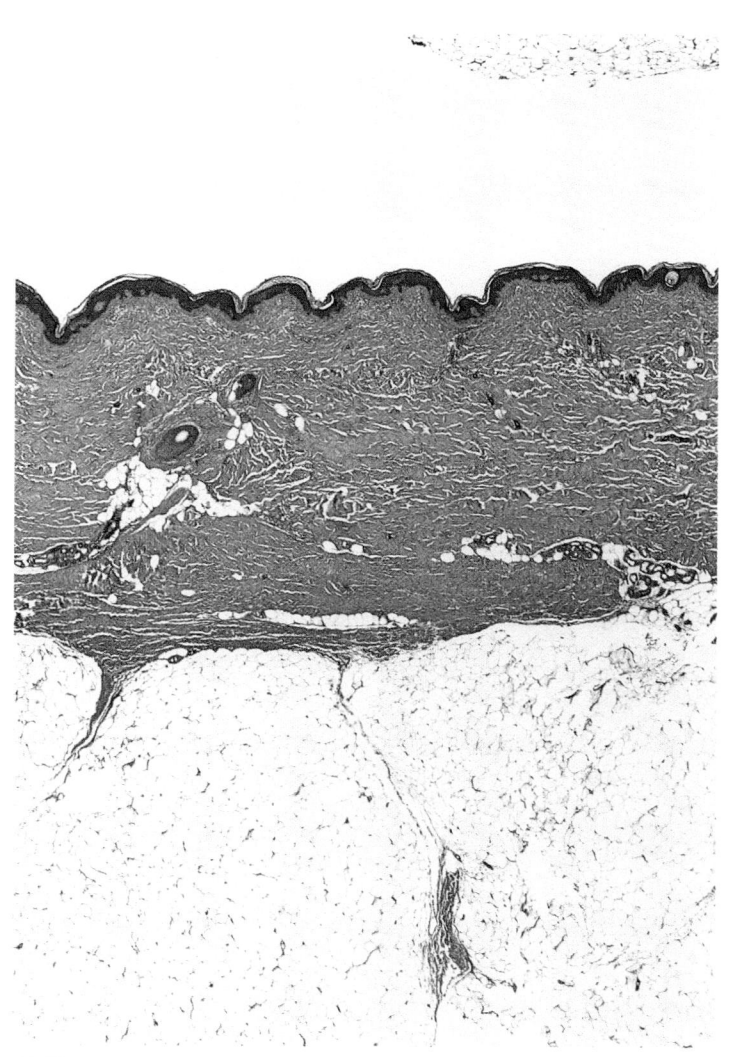

Fig. 11.13 **Atrophoderma.** There is some thinning of the dermis (on the back). Collagen bundles are slightly thickened and homogenized. (H & E)

Histopathology

The appearances are similar to those described for atrophoderma. The exact relationship of the case described recently with dermal inflammation and a psoriasiform epidermis is uncertain.[652]

ACRODERMATITIS CHRONICA ATROPHICANS

Acrodermatitis chronica atrophicans is a spirochete-induced disease (see p. 654) characterized by atrophy of the dermis to about half its normal thickness or less. The pilosebaceous follicles and subcutis also undergo atrophy.

Acrodermatitis chronica atrophicans may coexist with juxta-articular fibrotic nodules and morphea-like lesions.[653–655]

RESTRICTIVE DERMOPATHY

Restrictive dermopathy is a recently delineated, lethal, autosomal recessive disorder characterized by taut and shiny skin with facial dysmorphism, arthrogryposis multiplex and bone dysplasia.[656–662]

Fibroblasts show poor growth in culture, suggesting that restrictive dermopathy results from a primary abnormality in fibroblast growth and function.[656]

Histopathology

There is thinning of the dermis with the collagen bundles arranged parallel to the skin surface.[656] Elastic tissue may be normal or reduced in amount. Rudimentary hair follicles are usually present. There is also a reduction in adnexal structures and factor XIIIa-positive dendrocytes. The overlying epidermis is often hyperplastic with hyperkeratosis.[661]

Electron microscopy

The collagen fibrils are reduced in size with irregular interfibrillary spaces and some granulofilamentous deposits.[657,658] Degenerating fibroblasts have also been noted.

PERFORATING COLLAGENOSES

The perforating collagenoses are a group of dermatoses in which altered collagen is eliminated from the dermis through the epidermis.[663] Included in this group are reactive perforating collagenosis, the closely related entity of perforating verruciform 'collagenoma' (collagénome perforant verruciforme) and also chondrodermatitis nodularis helicis.

Collagen elimination is also found as a secondary event in some cases of granuloma annulare (perforating granuloma annulare) and of necrobiosis lipoidica. It has also been seen in healing wounds, in resolving keratoacanthomas and following the intradermal injection of corticosteroid.[664,665] Some cases do not fit neatly into any of the categories listed above.[666]

REACTIVE PERFORATING COLLAGENOSIS

Reactive perforating collagenosis, first described in 1967, is a rare condition in which collagen is eliminated from the dermis.[667] There are two distinct clinical variants.[668] In the usual form, in which the onset is in childhood, there are recurrent, umbilicated papules up to 6 mm or so in diameter which spontaneously disappear after 6–8 weeks, leaving a hypopigmented, some-

times scarred area.[669] New lesions develop as older lesions are involuting and this may continue into adult life.[670] The papules are found on the extremities, particularly the dorsum of the hands and forearms. The sole of the foot is a rare site.[671] There is often a history of superficial trauma, such as a scratch or insect bite.[672,673] Lesions have been induced experimentally by trauma.[668,674] An association with Down syndrome has been reported.[675] An autosomal recessive inheritance has been proposed for some cases.[663,676]

The other clinical variant is acquired in adult life and occurs especially in diabetics with chronic renal failure.[677–684] In patients with chronic renal failure there is sometimes clinical and histological overlap with other perforating disorders such as perforating folliculitis and Kyrle's disease.[685–688] The finding that both collagen and elastic fibers undergo transepithelial elimination in these circumstances suggests that a single disease process is present.[689] The term 'acquired perforating dermatosis' has been suggested for the different expressions of transepithelial elimination associated with renal disease and/or diabetes mellitus.[689–691] Reactive perforating collagenosis has also been reported in association with Hodgkin's disease,[692] internal cancers,[693,694] herpes zoster,[695–697] the Treacher Collins syndrome,[698] the red dye in a tattoo,[699] lichen amyloidosus, Wegener's granulomatosis, rheumatoid arthritis, Henoch–Schönlein purpura[663] and the acquired immunodeficiency syndrome associated with end-stage renal disease.[700]

It has been suggested that the acquired variant may be precipitated by the deposition of crystal-like microdeposits in the upper dermis, close to the site of the transepidermal channel.[691] Such material is possibly a byproduct of the chronic renal failure.

An attempt has been made to elucidate a common mechanism for the various perforating disorders. It has been suggested that elevated serum and tissue concentrations of fibronectin (a component of the extracellular matrix) may incite epithelial proliferation and migration, culminating in perforation.[701] TGF-β has also been implicated in this process.[702]

Histopathology[663,667,672]

The appearances vary with the stage of evolution of the lesion. In early lesions, there is acanthosis of the epidermis and an accumulation of basophilic collagen in the dermal papillae. In established lesions, there is a cup-shaped depression of the epidermis which is filled with a plug consisting of parakeratotic keratin, some collagen and inflammatory debris. The underlying epidermis is thin with fine slits through which basophilic collagen fibers in vertical orientation are extruded. Sometimes there is a complete break in the epidermis.[703] A few studies have shown elastic fibers in the extruded material and granulation tissue in the superficial dermis.[704] Immunohistochemical and ultrastructural studies have shown that the extruded collagen is normal.[691,704] One study has shown that the extruded collagen is type IV, suggesting origin from basement membrane.[705] Nuclear material derived from neutrophils, and neutrophils themselves, are present in the extruded material.[706,707] There is also absence of the basal lamina at the site of the perforation.[686]

PERFORATING VERRUCIFORM 'COLLAGENOMA'

Perforating verruciform 'collagenoma', also known as collagénome perforant verruciforme, is closely related to reactive perforating collagenosis. Traumatically altered collagen is eliminated in a single, self-limited episode.[665,708,709] The episode of trauma is usually more substantial than in reactive perforating collagenosis and the lesion that results is more verrucous. The author has seen a large plaque develop on the chest, following trauma from an automobile seat belt, with the histological features outlined below.[710]

Histopathology[709]

There is prominent epithelial hyperplasia with some acanthotic downgrowths encompassing necrobiotic collagen and debris (Fig. 11.14). Elastic fibers are partly preserved in the central plug.[687]

CHONDRODERMATITIS NODULARIS HELICIS

Chondrodermatitis nodularis helicis is a chronic, intermittently crusted, painful or tender nodule found primarily on the upper part of the helix of the ear of males over 50 years of age. The lesions are usually solitary and average 4–6 mm in diameter. There is a predilection for the right ear in some series.[711] The condition is infrequent in females, in whom it is more common on the antihelix.[692] The recurrence rate after treatment, which is usually curettage and cautery, can be as high as 20%.[712,713] Lesions are now being seen as a result of chronic pressure from cell (mobile) phones.[714] The location of the lesions correlates with the point of pressure of the phone.

The etiology and pathogenesis are speculative, but it has been suggested that the primary event is localized degeneration of dermal collagen with its subsequent partial extrusion through a central ulcer or by actual trans-epidermal elimination. The collagen degeneration possibly results from a combination of factors which include minor trauma or pressure (during sleep),[715] poor vascularity and sometimes solar damage.[712] An association with the limited form of systemic sclerosis and with dermatomyositis is a rare occurrence.[716,717] Goette has called chondrodermatitis nodularis helicis an 'actinically induced perforating necrobiotic granuloma', but this statement appears to be an overgeneralization.[718] It has also been suggested that the infundibular portion of the hair follicle is primarily involved, with perforation of follicular contents into the dermis.[719,720]

Histopathology[721,722]

The characteristic changes are a central area of ulceration or erosion or a more or less tight funnel-shaped defect in the epidermis overlying an area of dermal collagen which shows variable edema and fibrinoid degeneration (Fig. 11.15). Some inflammatory, keratinous and collagen debris caps the area of degenerate collagen, forming the crust noted clinically.

At the margins of the central defect there is variable epidermal acanthosis, which rarely assumes the proportions of pseudoepitheliomatous hyperplasia.[720] It extends peripherally over 3–5 rete pegs and there is usually a prominent granular layer with some overlying hyperkeratotic and parakeratotic scale.[722] Richly vascularized granulation tissue borders the necrobiotic material peripherally and sometimes the vessels have some glomus-like features. This area usually contains a mild, but sometimes moderately heavy inflammatory cell infiltrate. The infiltrate is predominantly lymphocytic with an admixture of plasma cells, histiocytes and sometimes a few neutrophils. Rarely, the histiocytes may assume a palisaded arrangement at the margins of the necrobiotic zone.[722] Irregular slit-like spaces may extend into the degenerate collagen, and other spaces containing fibrin may be found at the dermoepidermal junction above the peripheral granulation tissue. Uncommonly, degenerate collagen will be seen in slits within the epidermis, representing true transepidermal elimination.

Beyond the lesion itself there may be some telangiectatic vessels in the upper dermis and variable solar elastosis.[718] Elastic fibers are diminished and focally absent in the area of degenerate collagen.

In nearly all cases there are changes in the perichondrium which are most marked directly beneath the degenerate collagen. These changes include fibrous thickening and very mild chronic inflammation. Degenerative changes may also be found in the cartilage, with alterations in its staining qualities,

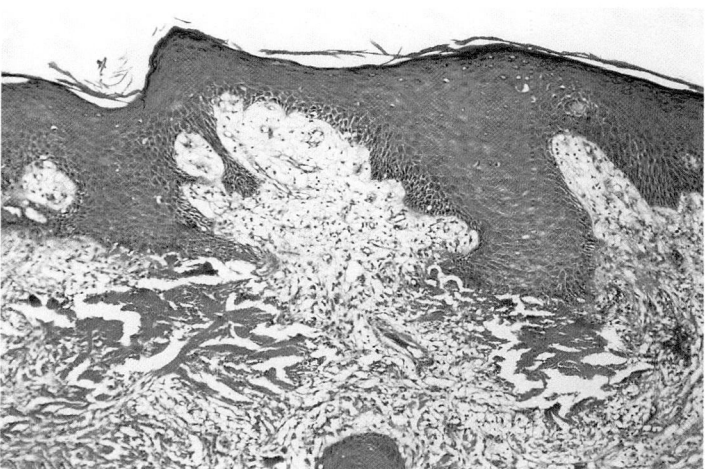

Fig. 11.14 **A variant of perforating collagenosis** following trauma from a seat belt in an automobile. Damaged collagen is being eliminated through the epidermal downgrowths. (H & E)

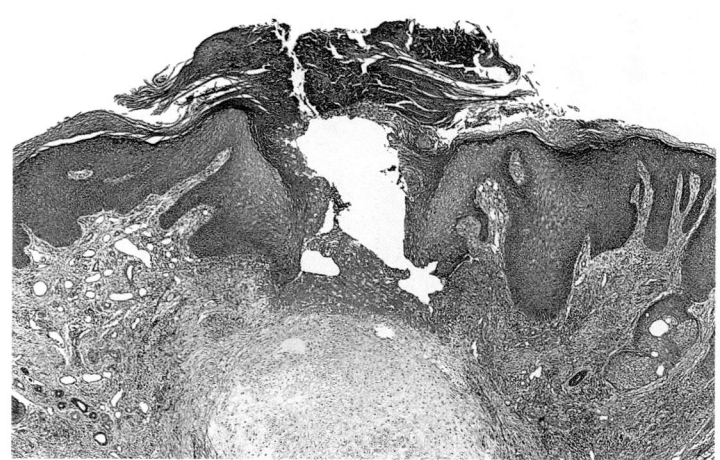

Fig. 11.15 **Chondrodermatitis nodularis helicis.** Fibrinoid material is present in the base of an ulcer which overlies the cartilage of the ear. (H & E)

patchy hyalinization and, uncommonly, partial destruction with necrosis.[722] Calcification and even ossification have been noted in the distal part of the chondral lamina.[723] In healed lesions there is dermal fibrosis which also involves the perichondrium (Fig. 11.16).

VARIABLE COLLAGEN CHANGES

Variable changes in dermal collagen are found in Ehlers–Danlos syndrome, osteogenesis imperfecta and Marfan's syndrome. Marked thinning of the dermis can occur in some forms of all three disorders, although in other clinical variants it may appear quite normal. Defects in the biosynthesis of collagen have been detected in a number of patients with osteogenesis imperfecta and Ehlers–Danlos syndrome, although in the majority of cases the defect has not been defined.[1]

EHLERS–DANLOS SYNDROME

Ehlers–Danlos syndrome is a heterogeneous disorder of connective tissue which combines hyperextensible fragile skin and loose-jointedness with a

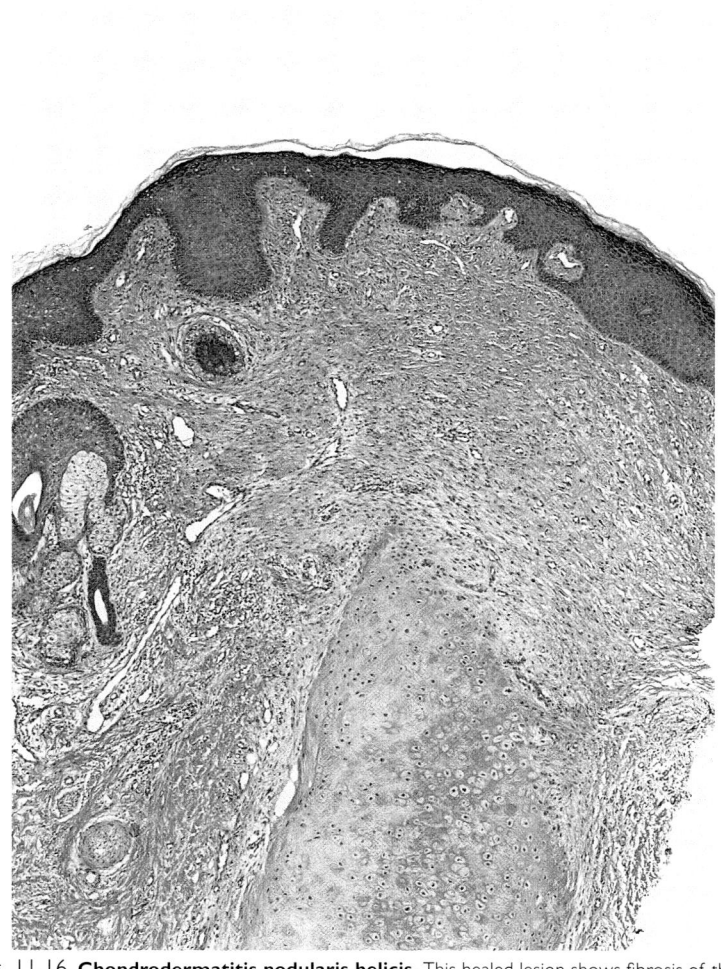

Fig. 11.16 **Chondrodermatitis nodularis helicis.** This healed lesion shows fibrosis of the dermis and perichondrium. (H & E)

tendency to bruising and bleeding.[724–729] Absence of the inferior labial and lingual frenula is associated with the classical and hypermobile types.[730] At least 11 types are now recognized, each with a characteristic clinical expression, inheritance pattern and, in some cases, a defined defect.[8,731] Paradoxically, specific defects in collagen biosynthesis have not been elucidated in the common forms of this disease.[732] Syndrome delineation is still proceeding and many cases do not fit neatly into any category.[733] In 1997, a revision of the traditional classification used below was proposed, based primarily on the cause of each type.[734] This new classification, which has not yet gained wide acceptance, is shown in Table 11.1.

Histopathology

Contradictory results have been published on the histopathology of this condition.[735,736] More recent reports have generally stated that the dermis is normal on light microscopy.[735] Marked thinning of the dermis has been reported in some variants of type IV[15] and also in type VI, while solar elastotic changes have been documented in type IV disease.[735] Elastosis perforans serpiginosa has been reported in several cases of the syndrome, again particularly type IV.[663] Similarly, ultrastructural studies have been contradictory, with some authors reporting normal fiber diameter and others observing some variability in size.[15,737,738] A distorted arrangement of fibrils has been

noted in several reports.[737] Scanning electron microscopy may offer further information in the future, as preliminary studies have shown disordered fibril aggregation and orientation.[726] Other ultrastructural findings will be mentioned below in the discussion of the specific types of the syndrome.

Subtypes of Ehlers–Danlos syndrome (traditional classification)

Type I (gravis)

Clinical features are usually severe in this common, autosomal dominant form of the disease.[4] Herniation of fat into the dermis, with subsequent calcification, may occur at pressure points.[739] Increased fiber diameter and loosely assembled fibrils have been reported.[740] The biochemical defect is not known, although reduced type III collagen production has been reported in one case.[740] Mutations have been found in the *COL5A1*, *COL5A2* and tenascin X genes in a limited number of patients/families.[11,741,742] Failure to detect a defect in many patients with types I/II may be due to so-called 'haploinsufficiency' (loss of expression of one allele) which is present in up to one-third of individuals with this classical type.[743] An arginine → cysteine substitution in type I collagen has also been reported in a family. This finding, which implicates another fibrillar collagen, confirms the genetic heterogeneity of this type.[744]

Type II (mitis)

The molecular defect in this mild, autosomal dominant form is unknown.[4] Partial deletion of the C-terminal end of the procollagen molecule has been demonstrated in one case.[6] Minor variations in fibril diameter have been noted ultrastructurally, and in one case there was lateral fusion of fibrils.[738] It has been suggested that mild variants of the mitis form are not uncommon in the general population.[745,746]

Type III (benign hypermobile)

There is marked joint hypermobility but only minor skin changes.[4,747] Inheritance is autosomal dominant. The molecular defect is unknown.

Type IV (arterial, ecchymotic)

Type IV is a heterogeneous group with at least four subtypes.[748,749] Both autosomal dominant and recessive variants occur.[748,750] There is a reduced life expectancy because of a propensity for rupture of large arteries and internal hollow viscera, particularly the colon.[8,751] Thin, translucent skin on the face and distal parts of the limbs in several subtypes gives the appearance of premature aging (acrogeria – p. 367).[749,752,753] Type IV results from a mutation in the *COL3A1* gene that controls type III collagen synthesis.[732,754] It is located in the region of chromosome 2q31.[755] A decreased amount of type III procollagen is recovered from cultured skin fibroblasts.[8,756,757] Defective type III collagen is sometimes found.[8] However, a case with type III collagen deficiency but with a normal phenotype has been documented.[758]

Ultrastructural changes have included the finding of collagen fibrils with reduced diameter, the presence of dilated rough endoplasmic reticulum in fibroblasts, and fragmentation of elastic fibers.[752]

Immunofluorescence of cultured skin fibroblasts has shown abnormal amounts of type III collagen retained in their cytoplasm.[759] This is not a feature in normal subjects or in other connective tissue diseases.

The presence of thin skin can be confirmed by ultrasound.[760]

Type V (X-linked)
The rare type V form shows marked cutaneous extensibility.[4,725,751] A defect in lysyl oxidase was found in one kindred, but this has not been confirmed in others.[761]

Type VI (ocular)
This autosomal recessive variant is characterized by ocular fragility, kyphoscoliosis and prominent cutaneous and joint signs.[4,762] There is a deficiency in peptidyl lysyl hydroxylase and an absence of hydroxylysine in dermal collagen.[724,763] This results in abnormal crosslinks in both type I and type III collagen.[764] This variant of the syndrome is probably a biochemically heterogeneous entity, as normal levels of enzyme have been found in some individuals.[4]

Type VII (arthrochalasis congenita)
There is gross joint instability leading to multiple dislocations at birth.[765] There are three subtypes, all of which are characterized by defects in the conversion of type I procollagen to collagen.[732] In types A and B, there are abnormalities in the N-terminal procollagen peptidase cleavage sites.[757,766] A deletion in chromosome 6q has been reported in one patient with type VII-B.[767] A third subgroup, type VII-C, results from deficient procollagen I N-protease.[768] It is similar to dermatosparaxis in cattle.[768–771] On electron microscopy there are small, irregular, and circular collagen fibers in the skin.[768]

Type VIII (periodontal)
The type VIII autosomal dominant form is marked by easy bruising, pretibial hyperpigmented scars and the early onset of periodontal disease.[724,772] There may be loose-jointedness of the fingers. The biochemical defect is unknown.[773]

Type IX
The type IX variant is X-linked and characterized by the presence of occipital horns and other skeletal abnormalities and a propensity to bladder diverticula and to hernias.[761,774] Cutaneous changes are mild. There is defective activity of lysyl oxidase. It has been suggested that all disorders with deficient lysyl oxidase, including Menkes' syndrome (see p. 396), should be classified as type IX disease,[775,776] but this ignores the absence of the usual clinical features of Ehlers–Danlos syndrome in patients with Menkes' syndrome.

Type X (fibronectin)
Some cases of the type X variant were originally classified as type IX disease.[777] There are moderately severe skin and joint changes and a defect in platelet aggregation.[777] The platelet defect can be corrected by fibronectin, which is an important adhesive glycoprotein that crosslinks to collagen.[777]

Type XI (familial joint instability syndrome)
Joint changes are prominent in this autosomal dominant variant.[733,738]

Other types
Many cases of Ehlers–Danlos syndrome defy classification, such as the case reported with abnormalities localized to the shoulder region[778] and another with intracellular degradation of alpha 2 chains of type I procollagen.[779] This same defect is found in some cases of osteogenesis imperfecta and of Marfan's syndrome.[779]

OSTEOGENESIS IMPERFECTA

Bone fragility is the cardinal manifestation of osteogenesis imperfecta, a genetically heterogeneous entity in which various defects in type I collagen have been detected.[7,780] Other clinical manifestations include short stature, joint laxity, blue sclerae and otosclerosis. The skin may be thin in the severe variants.

Histopathology
The dermis is markedly reduced in thickness in those with clinically thin skin.[15] The fine collagen bundles which constitute the dermis are often argyrophilic.

MARFAN'S SYNDROME

The clinical features of Marfan's syndrome include tall stature, skeletal malformations, arachnodactyly and dislocation of the lens.[781] Cutaneous manifestations are relatively insignificant. Marfan's syndrome is discussed further in Chapter 12, page 397.

Histopathology[15]
In some cases, thinning of the dermis, resulting from a diminished quantity of collagen and thinner collagen bundles, has been reported. This has been confirmed ultrastructurally. An increase in matrix material and fragmentation of elastic fibers have also been reported.

SYNDROMES OF PREMATURE AGING

The syndromes of premature aging can be a very small or quite large disease group, depending on the criteria used.[782] There are five conditions with prominent cutaneous findings that are usually included in any discussion on this subject – Werner's syndrome (adult progeria), progeria (Hutchinson–Gilford syndrome), acrogeria, Rothmund–Thomson syndrome (poikiloderma congenitale) and Cockayne's syndrome.[782,783] The Rothmund–Thomson syndrome includes poikiloderma as a major feature and is accordingly discussed with the lichenoid reaction pattern (see p. 54), while in Cockayne's syndrome photosensitivity and sensitivity of cultured fibroblasts to ultraviolet light is a major feature. The other three syndromes show changes in dermal collagen and accordingly they will be considered further in this chapter. In the two types of progeria this takes the form of sclerodermoid lesions, while in acrogeria the dermis is almost always atrophic.

WERNER'S SYNDROME (ADULT PROGERIA)

Werner's syndrome is an autosomal recessive disorder in which evidence of premature aging becomes manifest between the ages of 15 and 30 years.[782,784] It is common in Japan.[785] The clinical features include short stature, bird-like facies, juvenile cataracts, a tendency to diabetes mellitus, trophic ulcers of the legs, premature graying of the hair and balding, an increased incidence of neoplasms, and acral sclerodermoid changes.[782,786,787] Diffuse lentiginosis has been recorded in one case.[788] Death usually occurs in the fifth decade from the complications of arteriosclerosis.

Skin fibroblasts from patients with Werner's syndrome are difficult to culture, with a slow growth rate and short life span,[789,790] although in one study they produced more collagen but less glycosaminoglycans than normal.[791] Studies have confirmed that cultured fibroblasts produce increased amounts of some collagen, but not type VI;[792] the levels of type I and III collagen mRNA are increased, suggesting an alteration in the control of collagen synthesis at the transcriptional level.[793] Fibroblasts appear to become hyporesponsive in vitro to a stimulator of collagen synthesis that has been found in the serum of patients with Werner's syndrome.[794] The pathogenetic significance of these disparate findings remains to be elucidated. Cells in Werner's syndrome may have subtle defects in DNA repair.[795]

The responsible gene (*WRN*) has been mapped to chromosome 8p12–p21, the same location as the gene encoding for DNA polymerase β.[750] Chromosomal analyses on cultured fibroblasts reveal that aberrations occur frequently and randomly.[796]

Histopathology

There is usually some epidermal atrophy, although there may be hyperkeratosis over bony prominences.[786] In the scleroderma-like areas there s variable hyalinization of the thickened dermal collagen. There may be replacement of subcutaneous fat by connective tissue. The pilosebaceous structures and sweat glands become atrophic. Calcinosis cutis may also develop.[794]

In other areas, the dermis is thinned with a decrease in the size of the collagen bundles[794,797] and degenerative changes in the elastic fibers.

PROGERIA

Progeria (Hutchinson–Gilford syndrome) is a rare disease with markedly accelerated aging, clinical features becoming apparent in the first year of life. These features include growth retardation, alopecia, craniofacial disproportion, loss of subcutaneous fat and atrophy of muscle.[782, 798–800] The skin is generally thin as a result of the loss of subcutaneous fat, except for areas with scleroderma-like plaques.[801] Acral hyperplastic scars and keloid-like nodules composed of type IV collagen have also been described.[802] Although an autosomal recessive mode of inheritance has been postulated, the majority of cases are sporadic.

The biochemical basis of this disease is unknown, but it has been shown that skin fibroblasts are difficult to culture and tropoelastin production by fibroblasts is markedly increased.[798]

Histopathology[799,803]

The scleroderma-like plaques show a diffusely thickened dermis with hyalinization of collagen.[803] This may assume a homogenized appearance in the lower dermis. Fibrous tissue often extends into the subcutis. Hair follicles are atrophic and eventually lost.[804] There are variable changes in the elastic tissue. In other areas of the body there is loss of subcutaneous fat and some atrophy of the dermis.[803]

ACROGERIA

Acrogeria (Gottron's syndrome) is an exceedingly rare disease with onset in early childhood.[805] There is atrophy, dryness and wrinkling of the skin which is most severe on the face and extremities.[782,783,805] Interesting associations include bony abnormalities and disorders of dermal elastic tissue in the form of elastosis perforans serpiginosa and perforating elastomas.[805–807] Inheritance is probably autosomal recessive. A mutation in the *COL3A1* gene, located at chromosome 2q31–q32, has been reported in several cases.[755,808] A syndrome described as metageria has features that overlap with those of acrogeria.[732,783] Acrogeria is regarded by some as a distinct subgroup of type IV Ehlers–Danlos syndrome.[809]

Histopathology[782,805,806]

There is atrophy of the dermis with degenerative changes in the collagen. Fibers may be swollen and present a 'boiled' appearance. The subcutaneous fat is often replaced by connective tissue which is indistinguishable from the dermal collagen. Elastic fibers are disrupted and irregular, with some clumping. Changes of elastosis perforans serpiginosa may be present.

REFERENCES

Introduction

1 Spranger J. The developmental pathology of collagens in humans. Birth Defects 1987; 23: 1–16.
2 Uitto J, Lichtenstein JR. Defects in the biochemistry of collagen in diseases of connective tissue. J Invest Dermatol 1976; 66: 59–79.
3 Burgeson RE. Genetic heterogeneity of collagen. J Invest Dermatol 1982; 79: 25s–30s.
4 Krieg T, Ihme A, Weber L et al. Molecular defects of collagen metabolism in the Ehlers Danlos syndrome. Int J Dermatol 1981; 20: 415–425.
5 Prockop DJ, Kivirikko KI. Heritable diseases of collagen. N Engl J Med 1984; 311: 376–386.
6 Pope FM, Dorling J, Nicholls AC, Webb J. Molecular abnormalities of collagen: a review. J R Soc Med 1983; 76: 1050–1062.
7 Tsipouras P, Ramirez F. Genetic disorders of collagen. J Med Genet 1987; 24: 2–8.
8 Stolle CA, Pyeritz RE, Myers JC, Prockop DJ. Synthesis of an altered type III procollagen in a patient with type IV Ehlers–Danlos syndrome. J Biol Chem 1985; 260: 1937–1944.
9 Stanley JR, Woodley DT, Katz SI, Martin GR. Structure and function of basement membrane. J Invest Dermatol 1982; 79: 69s–72s.
10 Sage H. Collagens of basement membrane. J Invest Dermatol 1982; 79: 51s–59s.
11 Giunta C, Steinmann B. Compound heterozygosity for a disease-causing G1489D and disease-modifying G530S substitution in COL5A1 of a patient with the classical type of Ehlers–Danlos syndrome: an explanation of intrafamilial variability? Am J Med Genet 2000; 90: 72–79.
12 Akagi A, Tajima S, Ishibashi A et al. Expression of type XVI collagen in human skin fibroblasts: enhanced expression in fibrotic skin diseases. J Invest Dermatol 1999; 113: 246–250.
13 Uitto J, Tan EML, Ryhanen L. Inhibition of collagen accumulation in fibrotic processes: review of pharmacologic agents and new approaches with amino acids and their analogues. J Invest Dermatol 1982; 79: 113s–120s.
14 Prockop DJ, Kivirikko KI, Tuderman L, Guzman NA. The biosynthesis of collagen and its cisorders. N Engl J Med 1979; 301: 13–23.
15 Holbrook KA, Byers PH. Structural abnormalities in the dermal collagen and elastic matrix from the skin of patients with inherited connective tissue disorders. J Invest Dermatol 1982; 79: 7s–16s.

Scleroderma

16 Young EM Jr, Barr RJ. Sclerosing dermatoses. J Cutan Pathol 1985; 12: 426–441.
17 Rodnan GP, Jablonska S, Medsger TA Jr. Classification and nomenclature of progressive systemic sclerosis. Clin Rheum Dis 1979; 5: 5–12.
18 Callen JP, Provost TT, Tuffanelli DL. Periodic synopsis on collagen vascular disease. J Am Acad Dermatol 1985; 13: 809–815.
19 LeRoy EC, Black C, Fleischmajer R et al. Scleroderma (systemic sclerosis): classification, subsets and pathogenesis. J Rheumatol 1988; 15: 202–205.
20 Krafchik BR. Localized cutaneous scleroderma. Semin Dermatol 1992; 11: 65–72.
21 Jablonska S, Rodnan GP. Localized forms of scleroderma. Clin Rheum Dis 1979; 5: 215–241.
22 Barba A, Rosina P, Chieregato C, D'Onghia FS. Morphoea in a newborn boy. Br J Dermatol 1999; 140: 365–366.
23 Maricq HR. Capillary abnormalities, Raynaud's phenomenon, and systemic sclerosis in patients with localized scleroderma. Arch Dermatol 1992; 128: 630–632.

24 Ruffatti A, Peserico A, Glorioso S et al. Anticentromere antibody in localized scleroderma. J Am Acad Dermatol 1986; 15: 637–642.

25 Falanga V, Medsger TA Jr, Reichlin M. Antinuclear and anti-single-stranded DNA antibodies in morphea and generalized morphea. Arch Dermatol 1987; 123: 350–353.

26 Ruffatti A, Peserico A, Rondinone R et al. Prevalence and characteristics of anti single-stranded DNA antibodies in localized scleroderma. Arch Dermatol 1991; 127: 180–1183.

27 Sato S, Fujimoto M, Ihn H et al. Antigen specificity of antihistone antibodies in localized scleroderma. Arch Dermatol 1994; 130: 1273–1277.

28 Sato S, Fujimoto M, Ihn H et al. Clinical characteristics associated with antihistone antibodies in patients with localized scleroderma. J Am Acad Dermatol 1994; 3 : 567–571.

29 Ihn H, Fujimoto M, Sato S et al. Increased levels of circulating intercellular adhesion molecule-1 in patients with localized scleroderma. J Am Acad Dermatol 1994; 31: 591–595.

30 Serup J. Clinical appearance of skin lesions and disturbances of pigmentation in localized scleroderma. Acta Derm Venereol 1984; 64: 485–492.

31 Synkowski DR, Lobitz WC Jr, Provost TT. Bullous scleroderma. Arch Dermatol 981; 117: 135–137.

32 Peterson LS, Nelson AM, Su WPD. Classification of morphea (localized scleroderma). Mayo Clin Proc 1995; 70: 1068–1076.

33 Winkelmann RK. Localized cutaneous scleroderma. Semin Dermatol 1985; 4: 9C–103.

34 Leibovici V, Zlotogorski A, Kanner A, Shinar E. Generalized morphea and idiopathic thrombocytopenia. J Am Acad Dermatol 1988; 18: 1194–1196.

35 Cantwell AR Jr, Jones JE, Kelso DW. Pleomorphic, variably acid-fast bacteria in an adult patient with disabling pansclerotic morphea. Arch Dermatol 1983; 120: 656–66 .

36 Diaz-Perez JL, Connolly SM, Winkelmann RK. Disabling pansclerotic morphea of children. Arch Dermatol 1980; 116: 169–173.

37 Parodi PC, Riberti C, Draganic Stinco D et al. Squamous cell carcinoma arising in a patient with long-standing pansclerotic morphea. Br J Dermatol 2001; 144: 417–419.

38 Doyle JA, Connolly SM, Winkelmann RK. Cutaneous and subcutaneous inflammatory sclerosis syndromes. Arch Dermatol 1982; 118: 886–890.

39 Whittaker SJ, Smith NP, Russell Jones R. Solitary morphoea profunda. Br J Dermatol 1989; 120: 431–440.

40 Su WPD, Person JR. Morphea profunda. A new concept and a histopathologic study of 23 cases. Am J Dermatopathol 1981; 3: 251–260.

41 Kobayashi KA, Lui H, Prendiville JS. Solitary morphea profunda in a 5-year-old girl: case report and review of the literature. Pediatr Dermatol 1991; 8: 292–295.

42 Kirsner RS, Pardes JB, Falanga V. Solitary fibrosing paraspinal plaque: solitary morphoea profunda? Br J Dermatol 1993; 128: 99–101.

43 Blaszczyk M, Krysicka-Janiger K, Jabłońska S. Primary atrophic profound linear scleroderma. Dermatology 2000; 200: 63–66.

44 Akintewe TA, Alabi GO. Scleroderma presenting with multiple keloids. Br Med J 985; 291: 448–449.

45 Micalizzi C, Parodi A, Rebora A. Morphoea with nodular lesions. Br J Dermatol 1994; 131: 298–300.

46 Kennedy C, Leigh IM. Systemic sclerosis with subcutaneous nodules. Br J Dermatol 1979; 101: 93–96.

47 James WD, Berger TG, Butler DF, Tuffanelli DL. Nodular (keloidal) scleroderma. J Am Acad Dermatol 1984; 11: 1111–1114.

48 Perez-Wilson J, Pujol RM, Alejo M et al. Nodular (keloidal) scleroderma. Int J Dermatol 1992; 31: 422–423.

49 Krell JM, Solomon AR, Glavey CM, Lawley TJ. Nodular scleroderma. J Am Acad Dermatol 1995; 32: 343–345.

50 Hsu S, Lee M-WC, Carlton S, Kramer EM. Nodular morphea in a linear pattern. Int J Dermatol 1999; 38: 529–530.

51 Synkowski DR, Lobitz WC Jr, Provost TT. Bullous scleroderma. Arch Dermatol 1981; 117: 135–137.

52 Trattner A, David M, Sandbank M. Bullous morphea: a distinct entity? Am J Dermatopathol 1994; 16: 414–417.

53 Uitto J, Santa Cruz DJ, Bauer EA, Eisen AZ. Morphea and lichen sclerosus et atrophicus. J Am Acad Dermatol 1980; 3: 271–279.

54 Barr RJ, Siegel JM, Graham JH. Elastosis perforans serpiginosa associated with morphea. An example of 'perforating morphea'. J Am Acad Dermatol 1980; 3: 19–22.

55 Ben-Amitai D, Hodak E, Lapidoth M, David M. Coexisting morphoea and granuloma annulare – are the conditions related? Clin Exp Dermatol 1999; 24: 86–89.

56 Reed JR, De Luca N, McIntyre AS, Wilkinson JD. Localized morphoea, xanthomatosis and primary biliary cirrhosis. Br J Dermatol 2000; 143: 652–653.

57 Umbert P, Winkelmann RK. Concurrent localized scleroderma and discoid lupus erythematosus. Cutaneous 'mixed' or 'overlap' syndrome. Arch Dermatol 1978; 114: 1473–1478.

58 Rao BK, Coldiron B, Freeman RG, Sontheimer RD. Subacute cutaneous lupus erythematosus lesions progressing to morphea. J Am Acad Dermatol 1990; 23: 1019–1022.

59 Freeman WE, Lesher JL Jr, Smith JG Jr. Connective tissue disease associated with sclerodermoid features, early abortion, and circulating anticoagulant. J Am Acad Dermatol 1988; 19: 932–936.

60 Robertson LP, Davies MG, Hickling P. Generalized morphoea in a patient with Felty's syndrome. J Eur Acad Dermatol Venereol 2000; 14: 191–193.

61 Breier F, Klade H, Stanek G et al. Lymphoproliferative responses to Borrelia burgdorferi in circumscribed scleroderma. Br J Dermatol 1996; 134: 285–291.

62 Buechner SA, Winkelmann RK, Lautenschlager S et al. Localized scleroderma associated with Borrelia burgdorferi infection. J Am Acad Dermatol 1993; 29: 190–196.

63 Breier FH, Aberer E, Stanek G et al. Isolation of Borrelia afzelii from circumscribed scleroderma. Br J Dermatol 1999; 140: 925–930.

64 Özkan Ş, Atabey N, Fetil E et al. Evidence for Borrelia burgdorferi in morphea and lichen sclerosus. Int J Dermatol 2000; 39: 278–283.

65 Ross SA, Sanchez JL, Taboas JO. Spirochetal forms in the dermal lesions of morphea and lichen sclerosus et atrophicus. Am J Dermatopathol 1990; 12: 357–362.

66 Aberer E, Kollegger H, Kristoferitsch W, Stanek G. Neuroborreliosis in morphea and lichen sclerosus et atrophicus. J Am Acad Dermatol 1988; 19: 820–825.

67 Aberer E, Stanek G. Histological evidence of spirochetal origin of morphea and lichen sclerosus et atrophicans. Am J Dermatopathol 1987; 9: 374–379.

68 Schempp C, Bocklage H, Lange R et al. Further evidence for Borrelia burgdorferi infection in morphea and lichen sclerosus et atrophicus confirmed by DNA amplification. J Invest Dermatol 1993; 100: 717–720.

69 Tuffanelli D. Do some patients with morphea and lichen sclerosus et atrophicans have a Borrelia infection? Am J Dermatopathol 1987; 9: 371–373.

70 Lecerf V, Bagot M, Revuz J et al. Borrelia burgdorferi and localized scleroderma. Arch Dermatol 1989; 125: 297.

71 DeVito JR, Merogi AJ, Vo T et al. Role of Borrelia burgdorferi in the pathogenesis of morphea/scleroderma and lichen sclerosus et atrophicus: a PCR study of thirty-five cases. J Cutan Pathol 1996; 23: 350–358.

72 Hoesly JM, Mertz LE, Winkelmann RK. Localized scleroderma (morphea) and antibody to Borrelia burgdorferi. J Am Acad Dermatol 1987; 17: 455–458.

73 Halkier-Sorensen L, Kragballe K, Hansen K. Antibodies to the Borrelia burgdorferi flagellum in patients with scleroderma, granuloma annulare and porphyria cutanea tarda. Acta Derm Venereol 1989; 69: 116–119.

74 Garioch JJ, Rashid A, Thomson J, Seywright M. The relevance of elevated Borrelia burgdorferi titres in localized scleroderma. Clin Exp Dermatol 1989; 14: 439–441.

75 Meis JF, Koopman R, van Bergen B et al. No evidence for a relation between Borrelia burgdorferi infection and old lesions of localized scleroderma (morphea). Arch Dermatol 1993; 129: 386–387.

76 Dillon WI, Saed GM, Fivenson DP. Borrelia burgdorferi DNA is undetectable by polymerase chain reaction in skin lesions of morphea, scleroderma, or lichen sclerosus et atrophicus of patients from North America. J Am Acad Dermatol 1995; 33: 617–620.

77 Wienecke R, Schlüpen E-M, Zöchling N et al. No evidence for Borrelia burgdorferi-specific DNA in lesions of localized scleroderma. J Invest Dermatol 1995; 104: 23–26.

78 Raguin G, Boisnic S, Souteyrand P et al. No evidence for a spirochaetal origin of localized scleroderma. Br J Dermatol 1992; 127: 218–220.

79 Weide B, Walz T, Garbe C. Is morphoea caused by Borrelia burgdorferi? A review. Br J Dermatol 2000; 142: 636–644.

80 Weide B, Schittek B, Klyscz T et al. Morphoea is neither associated with features of Borrelia burgdorferi infection, nor is this agent detectable in lesional skin by polymerase chain reaction. Br J Dermatol 2000; 143: 780–785.

81 Hatamochi A, Ono M, Arakawa M et al. Analysis of collagen gene expression by cultured fibroblasts in morphoea. Br J Dermatol 1992; 126: 216–221.

82 Kikuchi K, Sato S, Kadono T et al. Serum concentration of procollagen type I carboxyterminal propeptide in localized scleroderma. Arch Dermatol 1994; 130: 1269–1272.

83 Colver GB, Rodger A, Mortimer PS et al. Post-irradiation morphoea. Br J Dermatol 1989; 120: 831–835.

84 Bleasel NR, Stapleton KM, Commens C, Ahern VA. Radiation-induced localized scleroderma in breast cancer patients. Australas J Dermatol 1999; 40: 99–102.

85 Davis DA, Cohen PR, McNeese MD, Duvic M. Localized scleroderma in breast cancer patients treated with supervoltage external beam radiation: Radiation port scleroderma. J Am Acad Dermatol 1996; 35: 923–927.

86 Schaffer JV, Carroll C, Dvoretsky I et al. Postirradiation morphea of the breast. Presentation of two cases and review of the literature. Dermatology 2000; 200: 67–71.

87 Riekki R, Jukkola A, Sassi M-L et al. Modulation of skin collagen metabolism by irradiation: collagen synthesis is increased in irradiated human skin. Br J Dermatol 2000; 142: 874–880.

88 Leshin B, Piette WW, Caplan RM. Morphea after bromocriptine therapy. Int J Dermatol 1989; 28: 177–179.

89 Granel B, Serratrice J, Gaudy C et al. Localized morphea after silicone-gel-filled breast implant. Dermatology 2001; 202: 143–144.

90 Morison WL. Psoralen UVA therapy for linear and generalized morphea. J Am Acad Dermatol 1997; 37: 657–659.

91 Grundmann-Kollmann M, Ochsendorf F, Zollner TM et al. PUVA-cream photochemotherapy for the treatment of localized scleroderma. J Am Acad Dermatol 2000; 43: 675–678.

92 Falanga V, Medsger TA Jr, Reichlin M, Rodnan GP. Linear scleroderma. Clinical spectrum, prognosis, and laboratory abnormalities. Ann Intern Med 1986; 104: 849–857.

93 Piette WW, Dorsey JK, Foucar E. Clinical and serologic expression of localized scleroderma. Case report and review of the literature. J Am Acad Dermatol 1985; 13: 342–350.

94 Long PR, Miller OF III. Linear scleroderma. Report of a case presenting as persistent unilateral eyelid edema. J Am Acad Dermatol 1982; 7: 541–544.

95 Patrizi A, Marzaduri S, Marini R. A familial case of scleroderma en coup de sabre. Acta Derm Venereol 2000; 80: 237.

96 Hulsmans RFHJ, Asghar SS, Siddiqui AH, Cormane RH. Hereditary deficiency of C2 in association with linear scleroderma 'en coup de sabre'. Arch Dermatol 1986; 122: 76–79.

97 Serup J, Serup L, Sjo O. Localized scleroderma 'en coup de sabre' with external eye muscle involvement at the same line. Clin Exp Dermatol 1984; 9: 196–200.

98 Eubanks LE, McBurney EI, Galen W, Reed R. Linear scleroderma in children. Int J Dermatol 1996; 35: 330–336.

99 Dilley JJ, Perry HO. Bilateral linear scleroderma en coup de sabre. Arch Dermatol 1968; 97: 688–689.

100 Rai R, Handa S, Gupta S, Kumar B. Bilateral en coup de sabre – a rare entity. Pediatr Dermatol 2000; 17: 222–224.

101 Lakhani PJ, David TJ. Progressive hemifacial atrophy with scleroderma and ipsilateral limb wasting (Parry–Romberg syndrome). J R Soc Med 1984; 77: 138–139.

102 Dintiman BJ, Shapiro RS, Hood AF, Guba AM. Parry–Romberg syndrome in association with contralateral Poland syndrome. J Am Acad Dermatol 1990; 22: 371–373.

103 Miyachi Y, Horio T, Yamada A, Ueo T. Linear melorheostotic scleroderma with hypertrichosis. Arch Dermatol 1979; 115: 1233–1234.

104 Wagers LT, Young AW Jr, Ryan SF. Linear melorheostotic scleroderma. Br J Dermatol 1972; 86: 297–301.

105 Fimiani M, Rubegni P, de Aloe G, Andreassi L. Linear melorheostotic scleroderma with hypertrichosis sine melorheostosis. Br J Dermatol 1999; 141: 771–772.

106 Juhn B-J, Cho Y-H, Lee M-H. Linear scleroderma associated with hypertrichosis in the absence of melorheostosis. Acta Derm Venereol 2000; 80: 62–63.

107 Majeed M, Al-Mayouf SM, Al-Sabban E, Bahabri S. Coexistent linear scleroderma and juvenile systemic lupus erythematosus. Pediatr Dermatol 2000; 17: 456–459.

108 Soma Y, Fujimoto M. Frontoparietal scleroderma (en coup de sabre) following Blaschko's lines. J Am Acad Dermatol 1998; 38: 366–368.

109 McKenna DB, Benton EC. A tri-linear pattern of scleroderma 'en coup de sabre' following Blaschko's lines. Clin Exp Dermatol 1999; 24: 467–468.

110 Serup J. Localized scleroderma (morphoea). Acta Derm Venereol (Suppl) 1986; 122: 1–61.

111 Morley SM, Gaylarde PM, Sarkany I. Epidermal thickness in systemic sclerosis and morphoea. Clin Exp Dermatol 1985; 10: 51–57.

112 Reed RJ, Clark WH, Mihm MC. The cutaneous collagenoses. Hum Pathol 1973; 4: 165–186.

113 McNiff JM, Glusac EJ, Lazova RZ, Carroll CB. Morphea limited to the superficial reticular dermis: an underrecognized histologic phenomenon. Am J Dermatopathol 1999; 21: 315–319.

114 Jacobson L, Jaworsky C. Superficial morphea. J Cutan Pathol 2000; 27: 542 (abstract).

115 Kobayasi T, Serup J. Nerve changes in morphea. Acta Derm Venereol 1983; 63: 321–327.

116 Brazzelli V, Vassallo C, Ardigò M et al. Unusual histologic presentation of morphea. Am J Dermatopathol 2000; 22: 359 (abstract).

117 Handfield-Jones SE, Peachey RDG, Moss ALH, Dawson A. Ossification in linear morphoea with hemifacial atrophy – treatment by surgical excision. Clin Exp Dermatol 1988; 13: 385–388.

118 Fleischmajer R, Nedwich A. Generalized morphea. I. Histology of the dermis and subcutaneous tissue. Arch Dermatol 1972; 106: 509–514.

119 Su WPD, Greene SL. Bullous morphea profunda. Am J Dermatopathol 1986; 8: 144–147.

120 Person JR, Su WPD. Subcutaneous morphoea: a clinical study of sixteen cases. Br J Dermatol 1979; 100: 371–380.

121 Sayama K, Chen M, Shiraishi S, Miki Y. Morphea profunda. Int J Dermatol 1991; 30: 873–875.

122 Daoud MS, Su WPD, Leiferman KM, Perniciaro C. Bullous morphea: clinical, pathologic, and immunopathologic evaluation of thirteen cases. J Am Acad Dermatol 1994; 30: 937–943.

123 Aberer E, Klade H, Hobisch G. A clinical, histological, and immunohistochemical comparison of acrodermatitis chronica atrophicans and morphea. Am J Dermatopathol 1991; 13: 334–341.

124 Torres JE, Sánchez JL. Histopathologic differentiation between localized and systemic scleroderma. Am J Dermatopathol 1998; 20: 242–245.

125 Skobieranda K, Helm KF. Decreased expression of the human progenitor cell antigen (CD34) in morphea. Am J Dermatopathol 1995; 17: 471–475.

126 Gilmour TK, Wilkinson B, Breit SN, Kossard S. Analysis of dendritic cell populations using a revised histological staging of morphoea. Br J Dermatol 2000; 143: 1183–1192.

127 Inazumi T, Kawashima J, Tajima S, Nishikawa T. Self-involuting atrophoderma of the lateral-upper arm. A new benign variant of morphea? Dermatology 1997; 194: 147–150.

128 Kobayasi T, Asboe-Hansen G. Ultrastructural changes in the inflammatory zone of localized scleroderma. Acta Derm Venereol 1974; 54: 105–112.

129 Fleischmajer R, Prunieras M. Generalized morphea. II. Electron microscopy of collagen, cells, and the subcutaneous tissue. Arch Dermatol 1972; 106: 515–524.

130 Krieg T, Meurer M. Systemic scleroderma. Clinical and pathophysiologic aspects. J Am Acad Dermatol 1988; 18: 457–481.

131 Chanda JJ. Scleroderma and other diseases associated with cutaneous sclerosis. Med Clin North Am 1980; 64: 969–983.

132 Perez MI, Kohn SR. Systemic sclerosis. J Am Acad Dermatol 1993; 28: 525–547.

133 Furey NL, Schmid FR, Kwaan HC, Friederici HHR. Arterial thrombosis in scleroderma. Br J Dermatol 1975; 93: 683–693.

134 Thomas JR III, Winkelmann RK. Vascular ulcers in scleroderma. Arch Dermatol 1983; 119: 803–807.

135 Doss BJ, Jacques SM, Mayes MD, Qureshi F. Maternal scleroderma: placental findings and perinatal outcome. Hum Pathol 1998; 28: 1524–1530.

136 Sant SM, Murphy GM. Neurotropic ulceration in systemic sclerosis. Clin Exp Dermatol 1994; 19: 65–66.

137 Chen Z, Virella G, Tung HE et al. Immune complexes and antinuclear, antinucleolar, and anticentromere antibodies in scleroderma. J Am Acad Dermatol 1984; 11: 461–467.

138 Chen Z, Fedrick JA, Pandey JP et al. Anticentromere antibody and immunoglobulin allotypes in scleroderma. Arch Dermatol 1985; 121: 339–344.

139 Tuffanelli DL, McKeon F, Kleinsmith DM et al. Anticentromere and anticentriole antibodies in the scleroderma spectrum. Arch Dermatol 1983; 119: 560–566.

140 Chorzelski TP, Jablonska S, Beutner EH et al. Anticentromere antibody: an immunological marker of a subset of systemic sclerosis. Br J Dermatol 1985; 113: 381–389.

141 Fritzler MJ, Arlette JP, Behm AR, Kinsella TD. Hereditary hemorrhagic telangiectasia versus CREST syndrome: can serology aid diagnosis? J Am Acad Dermatol 1984; 10: 192–196.

142 Valeski JE, Kumar V, Mattina G et al. Significance of in vivo pepper-dot epidermal nuclear reactions: correlation with anticentromere antibodies and CREST syndrome. J Am Acad Dermatol 1994; 30: 280–283.

143 Carr RD, Heisel EB, Stevenson TD. CREST syndrome. A benign variant of scleroderma. Arch Dermatol 1965; 92: 519–525.

144 Velayos EE, Masi AT, Stevens MB, Shulman LE. The 'CREST' syndrome. Comparison with systemic sclerosis (scleroderma). Arch Intern Med 1979; 139: 1240–1244.

145 Asboe-Hansen G. Scleroderma. J Am Acad Dermatol 1987; 17: 102–108.

146 Sachsenberger-Studer EM, Prins C, Saurat J-H, Salomon D. Raynaud's phenomenon, anticentromere antibodies, and digital necrosis without sclerodactyly: An entity independent of scleroderma? J Am Acad Dermatol 2000; 43: 631–634.

147 Sánchez JL, Vázquez M, Sánchez NP. Vitiligolike macules in systemic scleroderma. Arch Dermatol 1983; 119: 129–133.

148 Jawitz JC, Albert MK, Nigra TP, Bunning RD. A new skin manifestation of progressive systemic sclerosis. J Am Acad Dermatol 1984; 11: 265–268.

149 Luderschmidt C, Scholz S, Mehlhaff E et al. Association of progressive systemic scleroderma to several HLA-B and HLA-DR alleles. Arch Dermatol 1987; 123: 1188–1191.

150 Rendall JR, McKenzie AW. Familial scleroderma. Br J Dermatol 1974; 91: 517–522.

151 Greger RE. Familial progressive systemic scleroderma. Arch Dermatol 1975; 111: 81–85.

152 Black C, Briggs D, Welsh K. The immunogenetic background of scleroderma – an overview. Clin Exp Dermatol 1992; 17: 73–78.

153 Kleinsmith DM, Heinzerling RH, Burnham TK. Antinuclear antibodies as immunologic markers for a benign subset and different clinical characteristics of scleroderma. Arch Dermatol 1982; 118: 882–885.

154 McCarty GA. Autoantibodies in scleroderma and polymyositis: an update. Semin Dermatol 1991; 10: 206–216.

155 Blaszczyk M, Jarzabek-Chorzelska M, Jablońska S et al. Autoantibodies to nucleolar antigens in systemic scleroderma: clinical correlations. Br J Dermatol 1990; 123: 421–430.

156 Davis K, Boros P, Keltz M et al. Circulating Fcγ receptor-specific autoantibodies in localized and systemic scleroderma. J Am Acad Dermatol 1995; 33: 612–616.

157 Livingston JZ, Scott TE, Wigley FM et al. Systemic sclerosis (scleroderma): clinical, genetic, and serologic subsets. J Rheumatol 1987; 14: 512–518.

158 Reimer G, Steen VD, Penning CA et al. Correlates between autoantibodies to nucleolar antigens and clinical features in patients with systemic sclerosis (scleroderma). Arthritis Rheum 1988; 31: 525–532.

159 Katsumi S, Kobayashi N, Yamamoto Y et al. Development of systemic sclerosis in a patient with systemic lupus erythematosus and topoisomerase I antibody. Br J Dermatol 2000; 142: 1030–1033.

160 Katayama I, Otoyama K, Kondo S et al. Clinical manifestations in anticardiolipin antibody-positive patients with progressive systemic sclerosis. J Am Acad Dermatol 1990; 23: 198–201.

161 Bell S, Krieg T, Meurer M. Antibodies to Ro/SSA detected by ELISA: correlation with clinical features in systemic scleroderma. Br J Dermatol 1989; 121: 35–41.

162 Akimoto S, Ishikawa O, Tamura T, Miyachi Y. Antineutrophil cytoplasmic autoantibodies in patients with systemic sclerosis. Br J Dermatol 1996; 134: 407–410.

163 Ishikawa O, Tamura T, Ohnishi K et al. Systemic sclerosis terminating as systemic necrotizing angiitis. Br J Dermatol 1993; 129: 736–738.

164 Götting C, Sollberg S, Kuhn J et al. Serum xylosyltransferase: a new biochemical marker of the sclerotic process in systemic sclerosis. J Invest Dermatol 1999; 112: 919–924.

165 Götting C, Kuhn J, Sollberg S et al. Elevated serum xylosyltransferase activity correlates with a high level of hyaluronate in patients with systemic sclerosis. Acta Derm Venereol 2000; 80: 60–61.

166 Yazawa N, Kikuchi K, Ihn H et al. Serum levels of tissue inhibitor of metalloproteinases 2 in patients with systemic sclerosis. J Am Acad Dermatol 2000; 42: 70–75.

167 Yamane K, Ihn H, Kubo M et al. Increased serum levels of soluble vascular cell adhesion molecule 1 and E-selectin in patients with localized scleroderma. J Am Acad Dermatol 2000; 42: 64–69.

168 Hunzelmann N, Risteli J, Risteli L et al. Circulating type I collagen degradation products: a new serum marker for clinical severity in patients with scleroderma? Br J Dermatol 1998; 139: 1020–1025.

169 Søndergaard K, Heickendorff L, Risteli L et al. Increased levels of type I and III collagen and hyaluronan in scleroderma skin. Br J Dermatol 1997; 136: 47–53.

170 Fleischmajer R, Perlish JS, Duncan M. Scleroderma. A model for fibrosis. Arch Dermatol 1983; 119: 957–962.

171 Haustein UF, Herrmann K, Bohme HJ. Pathogenesis of progressive systemic sclerosis. Int J Dermatol 1986; 25: 286–293.

172 Lee EB, Anhalt GJ, Voorhees JJ, Diaz LA. Pathogenesis of scleroderma. Current concepts. Int J Dermatol 1984; 23: 85–89.

173 Murrell DF. A radical proposal for the pathogenesis of scleroderma. J Am Acad Dermatol 1993; 28: 78–85.

174 Hoyland JA, Newson L, Jayson MIV, Freemont AJ. The vascular basement membrane in systemic sclerosis skin: heterogeneity of type IV collagen. Br J Dermatol 1993; 129: 384–388.

175 LeRoy EC. Pathogenesis of scleroderma (systemic sclerosis). J Invest Dermatol 1982; 79: 87s–89s.

176 Freemont AJ, Hoyland J, Fielding P et al. Studies of the microvascular endothelium in uninvolved skin of patients with systemic sclerosis: direct evidence for a generalized microangiopathy. Br J Dermatol 1992; 126: 561–568.

177 Prescott RJ, Freemont AJ, Jones CJP et al. Sequential dermal microvascular and perivascular changes in the development of scleroderma. J Pathol 1992; 166: 255–263.

178 Silverstein JL, Steen VD, Medsger TA Jr, Falanga V. Cutaneous hypoxia in patients with systemic sclerosis (scleroderma). Arch Dermatol 1988; 128: 1379–1382.

179 Dowd PM, Kirby JD, Holborow EJ et al. Detection of immune complexes in systemic sclerosis and Raynaud's phenomenon. Br J Dermatol 1981; 105: 179–188.

180 Bruns M, Herrmann K, Haustein U-F. Immunologic parameters in systemic sclerosis. Int J Dermatol 1994; 33: 25–32.

181 Reitamo S, Remitz A, Varga J et al. Demonstration of interleukin 8 and autoantibodies to interleukin 8 in the serum of patients with systemic sclerosis and related disorders. Arch Dermatol 1993; 129: 189–193.

182 Tabata H, Hara N, Otsuka S et al. Correlation between diffuse pigmentation and keratinocyte-derived endothelin-1 in systemic sclerosis. Int J Dermatol 2000; 39: 899–902.

183 Sambo P, Jannino L, Candela M et al. Monocytes of patients with systemic sclerosis (scleroderma) spontaneously release in vitro increased amounts of superoxide anion. J Invest Dermatol 1999; 112: 78–84.

184 Kahari V-M, Sandberg M, Kalimo H et al. Identification of fibroblasts responsible for increased collagen production in localized scleroderma by in situ hybridization. J Invest Dermatol 1988; 90: 664–670.

185 Kikuchi K, Kadono T, Ihn H et al. Growth regulation in scleroderma fibroblasts: increased response to transforming growth factor-β1. J Invest Dermatol 1995; 105: 128–132.

186 Salmon-Ehr V, Serpier H, Nawrocki B et al. Expression of interleukin-4 in scleroderma skin specimens and scleroderma fibroblast cultures. Potential role in fibrosis. Arch Dermatol 1996; 132: 802–806.

187 Kawakami T, Ihn H, Xu W et al. Increased expression of TGF-β receptors by scleroderma fibroblasts: evidence for contribution of autocrine TGF-β signaling to scleroderma phenotype. J Invest Dermatol 1998; 110: 47–51.

188 Herzhoff K, Sollberg S, Huerkamp C et al. Fibroblast expression of collagen integrin receptors α1β1 and α2β1 is not changed in systemic scleroderma. Br J Dermatol 1999; 141: 218–223.

189 Mattila L, Airola K, Ahonen M et al. Activation of tissue inhibitor of metalloproteinases-3 (TIMP-3) mRNA expression in scleroderma skin fibroblasts. J Invest Dermatol 1998; 110: 416–421.

190 Igarashi A, Nashiro K, Kikuchi K et al. Significant correlation between connective tissue growth factor gene expression and skin sclerosis in tissue sections from patients with systemic sclerosis. J Invest Dermatol 1995; 105: 280–284.

191 Ohtsuka T, Koibuchi N, Matsuzaki S et al. Elevated expression of epidermal ornithine decarboxylase mRNA in scleroderma. Br J Dermatol 1998; 139: 1047–1048.

192 Chanoki M, Ishii M, Kobayashi H et al. Increased expression of lysyl oxidase in skin with scleroderma. Br J Dermatol 1995; 133: 710–715.

193 Takeda K, Hatamochi A, Ueki H et al. Decreased collagenase expression in cultured systemic sclerosis fibroblasts. J Invest Dermatol 1994; 103: 359–363.

194 Kikuchi K, Kubo M, Sato S et al. Serum tissue inhibitor of metalloproteinases in patients with systemic sclerosis. J Am Acad Dermatol 1995; 33: 973–978.

195 Falanga V, Alstadt SP. Effect of a platelet release fraction on glycosaminoglycan synthesis by cultured dermal fibroblasts from patients with progressive systemic sclerosis. Br J Dermatol 1988; 118: 339–345.

196 Perlish JS, Lemlich G, Fleischmajer R. Identification of collagen fibrils in scleroderma skin. J Invest Dermatol 1988; 90: 48–54.

197 Zachariae H, Halkier-Sørensen L, Heickendorff L. Serum aminoterminal propeptide of type III procollagen in progressive systemic sclerosis and localized scleroderma. Acta Derm Venereol 1989; 69: 66–70.

198 Lovell CR, Nicholls AC, Duance VC, Bailey AJ. Characterization of dermal collagen in systemic sclerosis. Br J Dermatol 1979; 100: 359–369.

199 Fleischmajer R, Damiano V, Nedwich A. Alteration of subcutaneous tissue in systemic scleroderma. Arch Dermatol 1972; 105: 59–66.

200 Fleischmajer R. The pathophysiology of scleroderma. Int J Dermatol 1977; 16: 310–318.

201 Fleischmajer R, Perlish JS, Shaw KV, Pirozzi DJ. Skin capillary changes in early systemic scleroderma. Arch Dermatol 1976; 112: 1553–1557.

202 Akimoto S, Ishikawa O, Igarashi Y et al. Dermal mast cells in scleroderma: their skin density, tryptase/chymase phenotypes and degranulation. Br J Dermatol 1998; 138: 399–406.

203 Rodnan GP, Myerowitz RL, Justh GO. Morphologic changes in the digital arteries of patients with progressive systemic sclerosis (scleroderma) and Raynaud phenomenon. Medicine (Baltimore) 1980; 59: 393–408.

204 Bottomley WW, Goodfield MJD, Sheehan-Dare RA. Digital calcification in systemic sclerosis: effective treatment with good tissue preservation using the carbon dioxide laser. Br J Dermatol 1996; 135: 302–304.

205 Nishioka K, Kobayashi Y, Katayama I, Takijiri C. Mast cell numbers in diffuse scleroderma. Arch Dermatol 1987; 123: 205–208.

206 Claman HN. Mast cell changes in a case of rapidly progressive scleroderma – ultrastructural analysis. J Invest Dermatol 1989; 92: 290–295.

207 Chanoki M, Suzuki S, Hayashi Y et al. Progressive systemic sclerosis associated with cutaneous amyloidosis. Int J Dermatol 1994; 33: 648–649.

208 Marzano AV, Berti E, Gasparini G et al. Unique digital skin lesions associated with systemic sclerosis. Br J Dermatol 1997; 136: 598–600.

209 Connolly SM, Winkelmann RK. Direct immunofluorescent findings in scleroderma syndromes. Acta Derm Venereol 1981; 61: 29–36.

210 Reimer G, Huschka U, Keller J et al. Immunofluorescence studies in progressive systemic sclerosis (scleroderma) and mixed connective tissue disease. Br J Dermatol 1983; 109: 27–36.

211 Aiba S, Tabata N, Ohtani H, Tagami H. CD34+ spindle-shaped cells selectively disappear from the skin lesion of scleroderma. Arch Dermatol 1994; 130: 593–597.

212 Fleischmajer R, Perlish JS, West WP. Ultrastructure of cutaneous cellular infiltrates in scleroderma. Arch Dermatol 1977; 113: 1661–1666.

213 Tabata H, Ohtsuka S, Yamakage A, Yamazaki S. Cutaneous electron microscopic study of sclerodermia diffusa in childhood. Int J Dermatol 1997; 36: 764–766.

214 Sharp GC, Irvin WS, Tan EM et al. Mixed connective tissue disease: an apparently distinct rheumatic disease syndrome associated with a specific antibody to an extractable nuclear antigen (ENA). Am J Med 1972; 52: 148–159.

215 Sharp GC, Anderson PC. Current concepts in the classification of connective tissue diseases. Overlap syndromes and mixed connective tissue disease. J Am Acad Dermatol 1980; 2: 269–279.

216 Rasmussen EK, Ullman S, Hoier-Madsen M et al. Clinical implications of ribonucleoprotein antibody. Arch Dermatol 1987; 123: 601–605.

217 Chubick A, Gilliam JN. A review of mixed connective tissue disease. Int J Dermatol 1978; 17: 123–133.

218 Gilliam JN, Prystowsky SD. Mixed connective tissue disease syndrome. Arch Dermatol 1977; 113: 583–587.

219 Blaszczyk M, Jablońska S, Szymańska-Jagiello W et al. Childhood scleromyositis: an overlap syndrome associated with PM-Scl antibody. Pediatr Dermatol 1991; 8: 1–8.

220 García-Patos V, Bartralot R, Fonollosa V et al. Childhood sclerodermatomyositis: report of a case with the anti-PM/Scl antibody and mechanic's hands. Br J Dermatol 1996; 135: 613–616.

221 Magro CM, Crowson AN, Regauer S. Mixed connective tissue disease. A clinical, histologic, and immunofluorescence study of eight cases. Am J Dermatopathol 1997; 19: 206–213.

222 Bentley-Phillips CB, Geake TMS. Mixed connective tissue disease characterized by speckled epidermal nuclear IgG deposition in normal skin. Br J Dermatol 1980; 102: 529–533.

223 Chanda JJ, Callen JP, Taylor WB. Diffuse fasciitis with eosinophilia. Arch Dermatol 1978; 114: 1522–1524.

224 Golitz LE. Fasciitis with eosinophilia: the Shulman syndrome. Int J Dermatol 1980; 19: 552–555.

225 Lupton GP, Goette DK. Localized eosinophilic fasciitis. Arch Dermatol 1979; 115: 85–87.

226 Michet CJ Jr, Doyle JA, Ginsburg WW. Eosinophilic fasciitis. Report of 15 cases. Mayo Clin Proc 1981; 56: 27–34.

227 Falanga V, Medsger TA Jr. Frequency, levels, and significance of blood eosinophilia in systemic sclerosis, localized scleroderma, and eosinophilic fasciitis. J Am Acad Dermatol 1987; 17: 648–656.

228 Fleischmajer R, Jacotot AB, Binnick SA. Scleroderma, eosinophilia, and diffuse fasciitis. Arch Dermatol 1978; 114: 1320–1325.

229 Ormerod AD, Grieve JHK, Rennie JAN, Edward N. Eosinophilic fasciitis – a case with hypogammaglobulinaemia. Clin Exp Dermatol 1984; 9: 416–418.

230 Bennett RM, Herron A, Keogh L. Eosinophilic fasciitis. Case report and review of the literature. Ann Rheum Dis 1977; 36: 354–359.

231 Chan LS, Hanson CA, Cooper KD. Concurrent eosinophilic fasciitis and cutaneous T-cell lymphoma. Arch Dermatol 1991; 127: 862–865.

232 Masuoka H, Kikuchi K, Takahashi S et al. Eosinophilic fasciitis associated with low-grade T-cell lymphoma. Br J Dermatol 1998; 139: 928–930.

233 Lee P. Eosinophilic fasciitis – new associations and current perspectives (Editorial). J Rheumatol 1981; 8: 6–8.

234 Schiener R, Behrens-Williams SC, Gottlöber P et al. Eosinophilic fasciitis treated with psoralen-ultraviolet A bath photochemotherapy. Br J Dermatol 2000; 142: 804–807.

235 Torres VM, George WM. Diffuse eosinophilic fasciitis. A new syndrome or a variant of scleroderma. Arch Dermatol 1977; 113: 1591–1593.

236 Jarratt M, Bybee JD, Ramsdell W. Eosinophilic fasciitis: an early variant of scleroderma. J Am Acad Dermatol 1979; 1: 221–226.

237 Cramer SF, Kent L, Abramowsky C, Moskowitz RW. Eosinophilic fasciitis. Arch Pathol Lab Med 1982; 106: 85–91.

238 Kahari V-M, Heino J, Niskanen L et al. Eosinophilic fasciitis. Increased collagen production and type I procollagen messenger RNA levels in fibroblasts cultured from involved skin. Arch Dermatol 1990; 126: 613–617.

239 Frayha RA, Atiyah F, Karam P et al. Eosinophilic fasciitis terminating as progressive systemic sclerosis in a child. Dermatologica 1985; 171: 291–294.

240 Coyle E, Chapman RS. Eosinophilic fasciitis (Shulman syndrome) in association with morphoea and systemic sclerosis. Acta Derm Venereol 1980; 60: 181–182.

241 Stanek G, Konrad K, Jung M, Ehringer H. Shulman syndrome, a scleroderma subtype caused by *Borrelia burgdorferi*? Lancet 1987; 1: 1490.

242 Sepp N, Schmutzhard E, Fritsch P. Shulman syndrome associated with *Borrelia burgdorferi* and complicated by carpal tunnel syndrome. J Am Acad Dermatol 1988; 18: 1361–1362.

243 Hayashi N, Igarashi A, Matsuyama T, Harada S. Eosinophilic fasciitis following exposure to trichloroethylene: successful treatment with cyclosporin. Br J Dermatol 2000; 142: 830–832.

244 Desruelles F, Lacour J-P, Chevallier P et al. Radiation myo-fasciitis. Acta Derm Venereol 2000; 80: 310–311.

245 Janin-Mercier A, Mosser C, Souteyrand P, Bourges M. Subcutaneous sclerosis with fasciitis and eosinophilia after phytonadione injections. Arch Dermatol 1985; 121: 1421–1423.

246 Kaufman LD, Gruber BL, Gomez-Reino JJ, Miller F. Fibrogenic growth factors in the eosinophilia–myalgia syndrome and the toxic oil syndrome. Arch Dermatol 1994; 130: 41–47.

247 Mizutani T, Mizutani H, Hashimoto K et al. Simultaneous development of two cases of eosinophilia–myalgia syndrome with the same lot of L-tryptophan in Japan. J Am Acad Dermatol 1991; 25: 512–517.

248 Blauvelt A, Falanga V. Idiopathic and L-tryptophan-associated eosinophilic fasciitis before and after L-tryptophan contamination. Arch Dermatol 1991; 127: 1159–1166.

249 Varga J, Jimenez SA, Uitto J. L-tryptophan and the eosinophilia–myalgia syndrome: current understanding of the etiology and pathogenesis. J Invest Dermatol 1993; 100: 97S–105S.

250 Kaufman LD, Seidman RJ, Phillips ME, Gruber BL. Cutaneous manifestations of the L-tryptophan-associated eosinophilia–myalgia syndrome: a spectrum of sclerodermatous skin disease. J Am Acad Dermatol 1990; 23: 1063–1069.

251 Greenberg AS, Takagi H, Hill RH et al. Delayed onset of skin fibrosis after the ingestion of eosinophilia–myalgia syndrome-associated L-tryptophan. J Am Acad Dermatol 1996; 35: 264–266.

252 Barnes L, Rodnan GP, Medsger TA Jr, Short D. Eosinophilic fasciitis. A pathologic study of twenty cases. Am J Pathol 1979; 96: 493–518.

253 Weinstein D, Schwartz RA. Eosinophilic fasciitis. Arch Dermatol 1978; 114: 1047–1049.

254 Keczkes K, Goode JD. The Shulman syndrome: report of a further case. Br J Dermatol 1979; 100: 381–384.

255 Kent LT, Cramer SF, Moskowitz RW. Eosinophilic fasciitis. Clinical, laboratory, and microscopic considerations. Arthritis Rheum 1981; 24: 677–683.

256 Trüeb RM, Pericin M, Winzeler B et al. Eosinophilic myositis/perimyositis: Frequency and spectrum of cutaneous manifestations. J Am Acad Dermatol 1997; 37: 385–391.

257 Martin RW, Duffy J, Lie JT. Eosinophilic fasciitis associated with use of L-tryptophan: a case-control study and comparison of clinical and histopathologic features. Mayo Clin Proc 1991; 66: 892–898.

258 Winkelmann RK, Connolly SM, Quimby SR et al. Histopathologic features of the L-tryptophan-related eosinophilia–myalgia (fasciitis) syndrome. Mayo Clin Proc 1991; 66: 457–463.

259 Feldman SR, Silver RM, Maize JC. A histopathologic comparison of Shulman's syndrome (diffuse fasciitis with eosinophilia) and the fasciitis associated with the eosinophilia–myalgia syndrome. J Am Acad Dermatol 1992; 26: 95–100.

260 Guerin SB, Schmidt JJ, Kulik JE, Golitz LE. L-tryptophan syndrome: histologic features of scleroderma-like skin changes. J Cutan Pathol 1992; 19: 207–211.

261 Tamura T, Saito Y, Ishikawa H. Diffuse fasciitis with eosinophilia: histological and electron microscopic study. Acta Derm Venereol 1979; 59: 325–331.

262 Botet MV, Sánchez JL. The fascia in systemic scleroderma. J Am Acad Dermatol 1980; 3: 36–42.

Sclerodermoid disorders

263 Fleischmajer R, Pollock JL. Progressive systemic sclerosis: pseudoscleroderma. Clin Rheum Dis 1979; 5: 243–261.

264 Uitto J, Jimenez S. Fibrotic skin diseases. Clinical presentations, etiologic considerations, and treatment options. Arch Dermatol 1990; 126: 661–664.

265 Ratnavel RC, Burrows NP, Pye RJ. Scleroderma and the carcinoid syndrome. Clin Exp Dermatol 1994; 19: 83–85.

266 Jablonska S, Stachow A, Suffczynska M. Skin and muscle indurations in phenylketonuria. Arch Dermatol 1967; 95: 443–450.

267 Nova MP, Kaufman M, Halperin A. Scleroderma-like skin indurations in a child with phenylketonuria: a clinicopathologic correlation and review of the literature. J Am Acad Dermatol 1992; 26: 329–333.

268 Chosidow O, Bagot M, Vernant J-P et al. Sclerodermatous chronic graft-versus-host disease. Analysis of seven cases. J Am Acad Dermatol 1992; 26: 49–55.

269 Aractingi S, Socie G, Devergie A et al. Localized scleroderma-like lesions on the legs in bone marrow transplant recipients: association with polyneuropathy in the same distribution. Br J Dermatol 1993; 129: 201–203.

270 Tabata H, Yamakage A, Yamazaki S. Electron-microscopic study of sclerodermatous chronic graft-versus-host disease. Int J Dermatol 1996; 35: 862–866.

271 Ameen M, Russell-Jones R. Macroscopic and microscopic mucinosis in chronic sclerodermoid graft-versus-host disease. Br J Dermatol 2000; 142: 529–532.

272 Jablonska S, Schubert H, Kikuchi I. Congenital facial dystrophy: stiff skin syndrome – a human counterpart of the tight-skin mouse. J Am Acad Dermatol 1989; 21: 943–950.

273 Richard MA, Grob JJ, Philip N et al. Physiopathogenic investigations in a case of familial stiff-skin syndrome. Dermatology 1998; 197: 127–131.

274 Fidzianska A, Jablonska S. Congenital fascial dystrophy: Abnormal composition of the fascia. J Am Acad Dermatol 2000; 43: 797–802.

275 Jablonska S, Blaszczyk M. Scleroderma-like indurations involving fascias: an abortive form of congenital fascial dystrophy (stiff skin syndrome). Pediatr Dermatol 2000; 17: 105–110.

276 Winchester P, Grossman H, Lim WN, Danes BS. A new acid mucopolysaccharidosis with skeletal deformities simulating rheumatoid arthritis. Am J Roentgenol 1969; 106: 121–128.

277 Hollister DW, Rimoin DL, Lachman RS et al. The Winchester syndrome: a nonlysosomal connective tissue disease. J Pediatr 1974; 84: 701–709.

278 Cohen AH, Hollister DW, Reed WB. The skin in the Winchester syndrome. Histologic and ultrastructural studies. Arch Dermatol 1975; 111: 230–236.

279 Dunger DB, Dicks-Mireaux C, O'Driscoll P et al. Two cases of Winchester syndrome: with increased urinary oligosaccharide excretion. Eur J Pediatr 1987; 146: 615–619.

280 Nabai H, Mehregan AH, Mortezai A et al. Winchester syndrome: report of a case from Iran. J Cutan Pathol 1977; 4: 281–285.

281 Kunz M, Paulus W, Sollberg S et al. Sclerosis of the skin in the GEMMS syndrome. An overproduction of normal collagen. Arch Dermatol 1995; 131: 1170–1174.

282 Mackenzie CR. Pachydermoperiostosis: a paraneoplastic syndrome. N Y State J Med 1986; 86: 153–154.

283 Venencie PY, Boffa GA, Delmas PD et al. Pachydermoperiostosis with gastric hypertrophy, anemia, and increased serum bone Gla-protein levels. Arch Dermatol 1988; 124: 1831–1834.

284 Vogl A, Goldfischer S. Pachydermoperiostosis. Primary or idiopathic hypertrophic osteoarthropathy. Am J Med 1962; 33: 166–187.

285 Rimoin DL. Pachydermoperiostosis (idiopathic clubbing and periostosis). N Engl J Med 1965; 272: 923–931.

286 Oikarinen A, Palatsi R, Kylmäniemi M et al. Pachydermoperiostosis: analysis of the connective tissue abnormality in one family. J Am Acad Dermatol 1994; 31: 947–953.

287 Stone OJ. Clubbing and koilonychia. Dermatol Clin 1985; 3: 485–490.

288 Lee S-C, Moon H-J, Cho D et al. Pachydermoperiostosis with cutaneous squamous cell carcinomas. Int J Dermatol 1998; 37: 693–696.

289 Gray RG, Gottlieb NL. Pseudoscleroderma in hypertrophic osteoarthropathy. JAMA 1981; 246: 2062–2063.

290 Marmelzat WL. Secondary hypertrophic osteoarthropathy and acanthosis nigricans. Arch Dermatol 1964; 89: 328–333.

291 Brenner S, Srebrnik A, Kisch ES. Pachydermoperiostosis with new clinical and endocrinologic manifestations. Int J Dermatol 1992; 31: 341–342.

292 Curth HO, Firschein IL, Alpert M. Familial clubbed fingers. Arch Dermatol 1961; 83: 828–836.

293 Matucci-Cerinic M, Lotti T, Jajic I et al. Cutaneous fibrinolytic activity in primary hypertrophic osteoarthropathy. Scand J Rheumatol 1987; 16: 205–212.

294 Bianchi L, Lubrano C, Carrozzo AM et al. Pachydermoperiostosis: study of epidermal growth factor and steroid receptors. Br J Dermatol 1995; 132: 128–133.

295 Wegrowski Y, Gillery P, Serpier H et al. Alteration of matrix macromolecule synthesis by fibroblasts from a patient with pachydermoperiostosis. J Invest Dermatol 1996; 106: 70–74.

296 Hambrick GW Jr, Carter DM. Pachydermoperiostosis. Arch Dermatol 1966; 94: 594–608.

297 Shawarby K, Ibrahim MS. Pachydermoperiostosis. A review of literature and report on four cases. Br Med J 1962; 1: 763–766.

298 Kapera D, Soyer HP, Kerl H. Pachydermodactyly. Int J Dermatol 1999; 38: 237.

299 Kang BD, Hong SH, Kim IH et al. Two cases of pachydermodactyly. Int J Dermatol 1997; 36: 768–772.

300 Meyerson LB, Meier GC. Cutaneous lesions in acroosteolysis. Arch Dermatol 1972; 106: 224–227.

301 Markowitz SS, McDonald CJ, Fethiere W, Kerzner MS. Occupational acroosteolysis. Arch Dermatol 1972; 106: 219–223.

302 Haustein UF, Ziegler V. Environmentally induced systemic sclerosis-like disorders. Int J Dermatol 1985; 24: 147–151.

303 Ostlere LS, Harris D, Buckley C et al. Atypical systemic sclerosis following exposure to vinyl chloride monomer. A case report and review of the cutaneous aspects of vinyl chloride disease. Clin Exp Dermatol 1992; 17: 208–210.

304 Saihan EM, Burton JL, Heaton KW. A new syndrome with pigmentation, scleroderma, gynaecomastia, Raynaud's phenomenon and peripheral neuropathy. Br J Dermatol 1978; 99: 437–440.

305 Dunnill MGS, Black MM. Sclerodermatous syndrome after occupational exposure to herbicides – response to systemic steroids. Clin Exp Dermatol 1994; 19: 518–520.

306 Haustein U-F, Ziegler V, Herrmann K et al. Silica-induced scleroderma. J Am Acad Dermatol 1990; 22: 444–448.

307 Fishman SJ, Russo GG. The toxic pseudosclerodermas. Int J Dermatol 1991; 30: 837–842.

308 Varga J, Jimenez SA. Chemical exposure-induced cutaneous fibrosis. Arch Dermatol 1994; 130: 97–100.

309 Ishikawa O, Warita S, Tamura A, Miyachi Y. Occupational scleroderma. A 17-year follow-up study. Br J Dermatol 1995; 133: 786–789.

310 Bottomley WW, Sheehan-Dare RA, Hughes P, Cunliffe WJ. A sclerodermatous syndrome with unusual features following prolonged occupational exposure to organic solvents. Br J Dermatol 1993; 128: 203–206.

311 Rustin MHA, Bull HA, Ziegler V et al. Silica-associated systemic sclerosis is clinically, serologically and immunologically indistinguishable from idiopathic systemic sclerosis. Br J Dermatol 1990; 123: 725–734.

312 Fenske NA, Vasey FB. Silicone-associated connective-tissue disease. The debate rages. Arch Dermatol 1993; 129: 97–98.

313 Silver RM, Sahn EE, Allen JO et al. Demonstration of silicon in sites of connective-tissue disease in patients with silicone-gel breast implants. Arch Dermatol 1993; 129: 63–68.

314 Sahn EE, Garen PD, Silver RM, Maize JC. Scleroderma following augmentation mammoplasty. Arch Dermatol 1990; 126: 1198–1202.

315 Varga J, Jimenez SA. Augmentation mammoplasty and scleroderma. Is there an association? Arch Dermatol 1990; 126: 1220–1222.

316 Brunskill NJ, Berth-Jones J, Graham-Brown RAC. Pseudosclerodermatous reaction to phytomenadione injection (Texier's syndrome). Clin Exp Dermatol 1988; 13: 276–278.

317 Robison JW, Odom RB. Delayed cutaneous reaction to phytonadione. Arch Dermatol 1978; 114: 1790–1792.

318 Morell A, Betlloch I, Sevila A et al. Morphea-like reaction from vitamin K$_1$. Int J Dermatol 1995; 34: 201–202.

319 Lemlich G, Green M, Phelps R et al. Cutaneous reactions to vitamin K$_1$ injections. J Am Acad Dermatol 1993; 28: 345–347.

320 Pang BK, Munro V, Kossard S. Pseudoscleroderma secondary to phytomenadione (vitamin K1) injections: Texier's disease. Australas J Dermatol 1996; 37: 44–47.

321 Kuo T-t, Hu S, Huang C-L et al. Cutaneous involvement in polyvinylpyrrolidone storage disease: a clinicopathologic study of five patients, including two patients with severe anemia. Am J Surg Pathol 1997; 21: 1361–1367.

322 Iglesias JL, de Moragas JM. The cutaneous lesions of the Spanish toxic oil syndrome. J Am Acad Dermatol 1983; 9: 159–160.

323 Martinez-Tello FJ, Navas-Palacios JJ, Ricoy JR et al. Pathology of a new toxic syndrome caused by ingestion of adulterated oil in Spain. Virchows Arch (A) 1982; 397: 261–285.

324 Cohen IS, Mosher MB, O'Keefe EJ et al. Cutaneous toxicity of bleomycin therapy. Arch Dermatol 1973; 107: 553–555.

325 Mountz JD, Downs Minor MB, Turner R et al. Bleomycin-induced cutaneous toxicity in the rat: analysis of histopathology and ultrastructure compared with progressive systemic sclerosis (scleroderma). Br J Dermatol 1983; 108: 679–686.

326 Yamamoto T, Takagawa S, Katayama I et al. Animal model of sclerotic skin. I: local injections of bleomycin induce sclerotic skin mimicking scleroderma. J Invest Dermatol 1999; 112: 456–462.

327 Yamamoto T, Takagawa S, Katayama I et al. Effect of superoxide dismutase on bleomycin-induced dermal sclerosis: implications for the treatment of systemic sclerosis. J Invest Dermatol 1999; 113: 843–847.

328 Kono T, Ishii M, Negoro N, Taniguchi S. Scleroderma-like reaction induced by uracil-tegafur (UFT), a second-generation anticancer agent. J Am Acad Dermatol 2000; 42: 519–520.

329 Querfeld C, Sollberg S, Huerkamp C et al. Pseudoscleroderma associated with lung cancer: correlation of collagen type I and connective tissue growth factor gene expression. Br J Dermatol 2000; 142: 1228–1233.

330 Cox NH, Ramsay B, Dobson C, Comaish JS. Woody hands in a patient with pancreatic carcinoma: a variant of cancer-associated fasciitis–panniculitis syndrome. Br J Dermatol 1996; 135: 995–998.

331 Cowper SE, Su LD, Bhawan J et al. Nephrogenic fibrosing dermopathy. Am J Dermatopathol 2001; 23: 383–393.

332 Cowper SE, Robin HS, Steinberg SM et al. Scleromyxoedema-like cutaneous diseases in renal-dialysis patients. Lancet 2000; 356: 1000–1001.

333 Wallace HJ. Lichen sclerosus et atrophicus. Trans St John's Hosp Dermatol Soc 1971; 57: 9–30.

334 Ridley CM. Lichen sclerosus et atrophicus. Semin Dermatol 1989; 8: 54–63.

335 Tremaine RDL, Miller RAW. Lichen sclerosus et atrophicus. Int J Dermatol 1989; 28: 10–16.

336 Meffert JJ, Davis BM, Grimwood RE. Lichen sclerosus. J Am Acad Dermatol 1995; 32: 393–416.

337 Powell JJ, Wojnarowska F. Lichen sclerosus. Lancet 1999; 353: 1777–1783.

338 Gibbon KL, Bewley AP, Salisbury JA. Labial fusion in children: a presenting feature of genital lichen sclerosus? Pediatr Dermatol 1999; 16: 388–391.

339 Powell J, Wojnarowska F, Dawber R et al. Childhood vulval lichen sclerosus in a patient with ectodermal dysplasia and uncombable hair. Pediatr Dermatol 1993; 15: 446–449.

340 Powell J, Wojnarowska F. Childhood vulvar lichen sclerosus: An increasingly common problem. J Am Acad Dermatol 2001; 44: 803–806.

341 Sanchez NP, Mihm MC Jr. Reactive and neoplastic alterations of the vulva. J Am Acad Dermatol 1982; 6: 378–388.

342 Purres J, Krull EA. Lichen sclerosus et atrophicus involving the palms. Arch Dermatol 1971; 104: 68–69.

343 Petrozzi JW, Wood MG, Tisa V. Palmar-plantar lichen sclerosus et atrophicus. Arch Dermatol 1979; 115: 884.

344 Hammar H. Plantar lesions of lichen sclerosus et atrophicus accompanied by erythermalgia. Acta Derm Venereol 1978; 58: 91–92.

345 Kossard S, Cornish N. Localized lichen sclerosus with nail loss. Australas J Dermatol 1998; 39: 119–120.

346 Dalziel K, Reynolds AJ, Holt PJA. Lichen sclerosus et atrophicus with ocular and maxillary complications. Br J Dermatol 1987; 116: 735–737.

347 Foulds IS. Lichen sclerosus et atrophicus of the scalp. Br J Dermatol 1980; 103: 197–200.

348 Miller RF. Lichen sclerosus et atrophicus with oral involvement. Arch Dermatol 1957; 76: 43–55.

349 Allan A, Andersen W, Rosenbaum M, Bhawan J. Histologic features of lichen sclerosus et atrophicus in a surgical scar. Am J Dermatopathol 1999; 21: 387–391.

350 Meffert JJ, Grimwood RE. Lichen sclerosus et atrophicus appearing in an old burn scar. J Am Acad Dermatol 1994; 31: 671–673.

351 Ah-Weng A, Charles-Holmes R. Peristomal lichen sclerosus affecting colostomy sites. Br J Dermatol 2000; 142: 177–178.

352 Anderton RL, Abele DC. Lichen sclerosus et atrophicus in a vaccination site. Arch Dermatol 1976; 112: 1787.

353 Libow LF, Coots NV. Lichen sclerosus following the lines of Blaschko. J Am Acad Dermatol 1998; 38: 831–833.

354 Choi SW, Yang JE, Park HJ, Kim CW. A case of extragenital lichen sclerosus following Blaschko's lines. J Am Acad Dermatol 2000; 43: 903–904.

355 Chalmers RJG, Burton PA, Bennett RF et al. Lichen sclerosus et atrophicus. A common and distinctive cause of phimosis in boys. Arch Dermatol 1984; 120: 1025–1027.

356 Rickwood AMK, Hemalatha V, Batcup G, Spitz L. Phimosis in boys. Br J Urol 1980; 52: 147–150.

357 Clemmensen OJ, Krogh J, Petri M. The histologic spectrum of prepuces from patients with phimosis. Am J Dermatopathol 1988; 10: 104–108.

358 Aynaud O, Piron D, Casanova J-M. Incidence of preputial lichen sclerosus in adults: Histologic study of circumcision specimens. J Am Acad Dermatol 1999; 41: 923–926.

359 Lipscombe TK, Wayte J, Wojnarowska F et al. A study of clinical and aetiological factors and possible associations of lichen sclerosus in males. Australas J Dermatol 1997; 38: 132–136.

360 Dahlman-Ghozlan K, Hedblad M-A, von Krogh G. Penile lichen sclerosus et atrophicus treated with clobetasol dipropionate 0.05% cream: A retrospective clinical and histopathologic study. J Am Acad Dermatol 1999; 40: 451–457.

361 Apisarnthanarax P, Osment LS, Montes LF. Extensive lichen sclerosus et atrophicus in a 7-year-old boy. Arch Dermatol 1972; 106: 94–96.

362 Meyrick Thomas RH, Ridley CM, Black MM. Clinical features and therapy of lichen sclerosus et atrophicus affecting males. Clin Exp Dermatol 1987; 12: 126–128.

363 Drut RM, Gómez MA, Drut R, Lojo MM. Human papillomavirus is present in some cases of childhood penile lichen sclerosus: an in situ hybridization and SP-PCR study. Pediatr Dermatol 1998; 15: 85–90.

364 Carlson JA, Rohwedder A. Genital and epidermodysplasia verruciformis-associated HPV types are frequently found in lichen sclerosus. J Cutan Pathol 2000; 27: 552 (abstract).

365 English JC, King DHC, Foley JP. Penile shaft hypopigmentation: Lichen sclerosus occurring after the initiation of alprostadil intracavernous injections for erectile dysfunction. J Am Acad Dermatol 1998; 39: 801–803.

366 Klein LE, Cohen SR, Weinstein M. Bullous lichen sclerosus et atrophicus: treatment by tangential excision. J Am Acad Dermatol 1984; 10: 346–350.

367 Di Silverio A, Serri F. Generalized bullous and haemorrhagic lichen sclerosus et atrophicus. Br J Dermatol 1975; 93: 215–217.

368 Wakelin SH, James MP. Extensive lichen sclerosus et atrophicus with bullae and ulceration – improvement with hydroxychloroquine. Clin Exp Dermatol 1994; 19: 332–334.

369 Marren P, de Berker D, Millard P, Wojnarowska F. Bullous and haemorrhagic lichen sclerosus with scalp involvement. Clin Exp Dermatol 1992; 17: 354–356.

370 Hallel-Halevy D, Grunwald MH, Yerushalmi J, Halevy S. Bullous lichen sclerosus et atrophicus. J Am Acad Dermatol 1998; 39: 500–501.

371 Boulinguez S, Bernard P, Lacour JP et al. Bullous lichen sclerosus with chronic hepatitis C virus infection. Br J Dermatol 1997; 137: 474–475.

372 Leppard B, Sneddon IB. Milia occurring in lichen sclerosus et atrophicus. Br J Dermatol 1975; 92: 711–714.

373 Kossard S, Pang B. Nodular lichen sclerosus. J Am Acad Dermatol 1994; 31: 817–818.

374 Farris DR, Hardy D, Kagen MH et al. Extragenital pigmented lichen sclerosus. J Eur Acad Dermatol Venereol 2000; 14: 322–324.

375 Clark JA, Muller SA. Lichen sclerosus et atrophicus in children. A report of 24 cases. Arch Dermatol 1967; 95: 476–482.

376 Shirer JA, Ray MC. Familial occurrence of lichen sclerosus et atrophicus. Arch Dermatol 1987; 123: 485–488.

377 Ridley CM. Lichen sclerosus et atrophicus. Arch Dermatol 1987; 123: 457–460.

378 Murphy FR, Lipa M, Haberman HF. Familial vulvar dystrophy of lichen sclerosus type. Arch Dermatol 1982; 118: 329–331.

379 Berth-Jones J, Graham-Brown RAC, Burns DA. Lichen sclerosus et atrophicus – a review of 15 cases in young girls. Clin Exp Dermatol 1991; 16: 14–17.

380 Helm KF, Gibson LE, Muller SA. Lichen sclerosus et atrophicus in children and young adults. Pediatr Dermatol 1991; 8: 97–101.

381 Goltz R. Questions to the Editorial Board and other authorities. Am J Dermatopathol 1980; 2: 283.

382 Patterson JAK, Ackerman AB. Lichen sclerosus et atrophicus is not related to morphea. Am J Dermatopathol 1984; 6: 323–335.

383 Tremaine R, Adam JE, Orizaga M. Morphea coexisting with lichen sclerosus et atrophicus. Int J Dermatol 1990; 29: 486–489.

384 Shono S, Imura M, Ota M et al. Lichen sclerosus et atrophicus, morphea, and coexistence of both diseases. Arch Dermatol 1991; 127: 1352–1356.

385 Farrell AM, Marren PM, Wojnarowska F. Genital lichen sclerosus associated with morphoea or systemic sclerosis: clinical and HLA characteristics. Br J Dermatol 2000; 143: 598–603.

386 Meyrick Thomas RH, Ridley CM, Black MM. The association of lichen sclerosus et atrophicus and autoimmune-related disease in males. Br J Dermatol 1983; 109: 661–664.

387 Meyrick Thomas RH, Ridley CM, McGibbon DH, Black MM. Lichen sclerosus et atrophicus and autoimmunity – a study of 350 women. Br J Dermatol 1988; 118: 41–46.

388 Fitzgerald EA, Connelly CS, Purcell SM, Kantor GR. Familial lichen sclerosus et atrophicus in association with CREST syndrome: a case report. Br J Dermatol 1996; 134: 1144–1146.

389 Azurdia RM, Luzzi GA, Byren I et al. Lichen sclerosus in adult men: a study of HLA associations and susceptibility to autoimmune disease. Br J Dermatol 1999; 140: 79–83.

390 Garcia-Bravo B, Sánchez-Pedreño P, Rodriguez-Pichardo A, Camacho F. Lichen sclerosus et atrophicus. A study of 76 cases and their relation to diabetes. J Am Acad Dermatol 1988; 19: 482–485.

391 Osborne GEN, Francis ND, Bunker CB. Synchronous onset of penile lichen sclerosus and vitiligo. Br J Dermatol 2000; 143: 218–219.

392 Córdoba S, Vargas E, Fraga J et al. Lichen sclerosus et atrophicus in sclerodermatous chronic graft-versus-host disease. Int J Dermatol 1999; 38: 708–711.

393 Leighton PC, Langley FA. A clinico-pathological study of vulval dermatoses. J Clin Pathol 1975; 28: 394–402.

394 Sloan PJM, Goepel J. Lichen sclerosus et atrophicus and perianal carcinoma: a case report. Clin Exp Dermatol 1981; 6: 399–402.

395 Hart WR, Norris HJ, Helwig EB. The malignant potential of lichen sclerosus et atrophicus of the vulva. Am J Clin Pathol 1975; 63: 758 (abstract).

396 Pride HP, Miller OF III, Tyler WB. Penile squamous cell carcinoma arising from balanitis xerotica obliterans. J Am Acad Dermatol 1993; 29: 469–473.

397 Tan S-H, Derrick E, McKee PH et al. Altered p53 expression and epidermal cell proliferation is seen in vulval lichen sclerosus. J Cutan Pathol 1994; 21: 316–323.

398 Scurry J, Beshay V, Cohen C, Allen D. Ki67 expression in lichen sclerosus of vulva in patients with and without associated squamous cell carcinoma. Histopathology 1998; 32: 399–404.

399 Carlson JA, Ambros R, Malfetano J et al. Vulvar lichen sclerosus and squamous cell carcinoma: a cohort, case control, and investigational study with historical perspective; implications for chronic inflammation and sclerosis in the development of neoplasia. Hum Pathol 1998; 29: 932–948.

400 Nasca MR, Innocenzi D, Micali G. Penile cancer among patients with genital lichen sclerosus. J Am Acad Dermatol 1999; 41: 911–914.

401 Simonart Th, Noel JC, De Dobbeleer G, Simonart JM. Carcinoma of the glans penis arising 20 years after lichen sclerosus. Dermatology 1998; 196: 337–338.

402 Aberer E, Schmidt BL, Breier F et al. Amplification of DNA of *Borrelia burgdorferi* in urine samples of patients with granuloma annulare and lichen sclerosus et atrophicus. Arch Dermatol 1999; 135: 210–212.

403 Breier F, Khanakah G, Stanek G et al. Isolation and polymerase chain reaction typing of *Borrelia afzelii* from a skin lesion in a seronegative patient with generalized ulcerating bullous lichen sclerosus et atrophicus. Br J Dermatol 2001; 144: 387–392.

404 Fujiwara H, Fujiwara K, Hashimoto K et al. Detection of *Borrelia burgdorferi* DNA (*B garinii* or *B afzelii*) in morphea and lichen sclerosus et atrophicus tissues of German and Japanese but not of US patients. Arch Dermatol 1997; 133: 41–44.

405 Farrell AM, Millard PR, Schomberg KH, Wojnarowska F. An infective aetiology for vulval lichen sclerosus re-addressed. Clin Exp Dermatol 1999; 24: 479–483.

406 Heymann WR. Coexistent lichen sclerosus et atrophicus and atrophoderma of Pasini and Pierini. Int J Dermatol 1994; 33: 133–134.

407 Carlson JA, Grabowski R, Chichester P et al. Comparative immunophenotypic study of lichen sclerosus. Epidermotropic CD57+ lymphocytes are numerous – implications for pathogenesis. Am J Dermatopathol 2000; 22: 7–16.

408 Lukowsky A, Muche JM, Sterry W, Audring H. Detection of expanded T cell clones in skin biopsy samples of patients with lichen sclerosus et atrophicus by T cell receptor-γ polymerase chain reaction assays. J Invest Dermatol 2000; 115: 254–259.

409 Farrell AM, Marren P, Dean D, Wojnarowska F. Lichen sclerosus: evidence that immunological changes occur at all levels of the skin. Br J Dermatol 1999; 140: 1087–1092.

410 Farrell AM, Dean D, Charnock FM, Wojnarowska F. Do plasminogen activators play a role in lichen sclerosus? Clin Exp Dermatol 2000; 25: 432–435.

411 Farrell AM, Dean D, Charnock FM, Wojnarowska F. Alterations in distribution of tenascin, fibronectin and fibrinogen in vulval lichen sclerosus. Dermatology 2000; 201: 223–229.

412 Kaya G, Augsburger E, Stamenkovic I, Saurat J-H. Decrease in epidermal CD44 expression as a potential mechanism for abnormal hyaluronate accumulation in superficial dermis in lichen sclerosus et atrophicus. J Invest Dermatol 2000; 115: 1054–1058.

413 Clifton MM, Bayer Garner IB, Kohler S, Smoller BR. Immunohistochemical evaluation of androgen receptors in genital and extragenital lichen sclerosus: Evidence for loss of androgen receptors in lesional epidermis. J Am Acad Dermatol 1999; 41: 43–36.

414 Marren P, Yell J, Charnock FM et al. The association between lichen sclerosus and antigens of the HLA system. Br J Dermatol 1995; 132: 197–203.

415 Powell J, Wojnarowska F, Winsey S et al. Lichen sclerosus premenarche: autoimmunity and immunogenetics. Br J Dermatol 2000; 142: 481–484.

416 Sahn EE, Bluestein EL, Oliva S. Familial lichen sclerosus et atrophicus in childhood. Pediatr Dermatol 1994; 11: 160–163.

417 Barker LP, Gross P. Lichen sclerosus et atrophicus of the female genitalia. Arch Dermatol 1962; 85: 362–373.

418 LeBoit PE. A thickened basement membrane is a clue to ... lichen sclerosus! Am J Dermatopathol 2000; 22: 457–458.

419 Marren P, Dean D, Charnock M, Wojnarowska F. The basement membrane zone in lichen sclerosus: an immunohistochemical study. Br J Dermatol 1997; 136: 508–514.

420 Suurmond D. Lichen sclerosus et atrophicus of the vulva. Arch Dermatol 1964; 90: 143–152.

421 Cabaleiro P, Drut RM, Drut R. Lymphohistiocytic and granulomatous phlebitis in penile lichen sclerosus. Am J Dermatopathol 2000; 22: 316–320.

422 Steigleder GK, Raab WP. Lichen sclerosus et atrophicus. Arch Dermatol 1961; 84: 219–226.

423 Rahbari H. Histochemical differentiation of localized morphea-scleroderma and lichen sclerosus et atrophicus. J Cutan Pathol 1989; 16: 342–347.

424 Marren P, Millard P, Chia Y, Wojnarowska F. Mucosal lichen sclerosus/lichen planus overlap syndromes. Br J Dermatol 1994; 131: 118–123.

425 Holmes SC, Burden AD. Lichen sclerosus and lichen planus: a spectrum of disease? Report of two cases and review of the literature. Clin Exp Dermatol 1998; 23: 129–131.

426 Fung MA, LeBoit PE. Light microscopic criteria for the diagnosis of early vulvar lichen sclerosus. A comparison with lichen planus. Am J Surg Pathol 1998; 22: 473–478.

427 Weigand DA. Microscopic features of lichen sclerosus et atrophicus in acrochordons: a clue to the cause of lichen sclerosus et atrophicus? J Am Acad Dermatol 1993; 28: 751–754.

428 Cruces MJ, De La Torre C, Losada A et al. Infantile pyramidal protrusion as a manifestation of lichen sclerosus et atrophicus. Arch Dermatol 1998; 134: 1118–1120.

429 Konta R, Hashimoto I, Takahashi M, Tamai K. Infantile perineal protrusion: a statistical, clinical, and histopathologic study. Dermatology 2000; 201: 316–320.

430 Mann PR, Cowan MA. Ultrastructural changes in four cases of lichen sclerosus et atrophicus. Br J Dermatol 1973; 89: 223–231.

431 Kint A, Geerts ML. Lichen sclerosus et atrophicus. An electron microscopic study. J Cutan Pathol 1975; 2: 30–34.

432 French LE, Braun R, Masouyé I et al. Post-stripping sclerodermiform dermatitis. Arch Dermatol 1999; 135: 1387–1391.

Other hypertrophic collagenoses

433 Uitto J, Santa Cruz DJ, Eisen AZ. Connective tissue nevi of the skin. J Am Acad Dermatol 1980; 3: 441–461.

434 Rocha G, Winkelmann RK. Connective tissue nevus. Arch Dermatol 1962; 85: 722–729.

435 Betti R, Inselvini E, Pazzini C et al. Symmetrical, papular, eruptive auricular collagenomas. J Am Acad Dermatol 1998; 39: 363–364.

436 Basarab T, Kobza Black A, Neill S, Russell-Jones R. A solitary collagenoma presenting in the labium majus. Br J Dermatol 1998; 139: 1135–1136.

437 Cohen EL. Connective tissue naevus of the palm. Clin Exp Dermatol 1979; 4: 543–544.

438 Uitto J, Santa Cruz DJ, Eisen AZ. Familial cutaneous collagenoma: genetic studies on a family. Br J Dermatol 1979; 101: 185–195.

439 Downs AMR, Lear JT, Condon CA et al. Eruptive collagenomas of the skin: a case history. Pediatr Dermatol 1998; 15: 269–270.

440 Henderson RR, Wheeler CE Jr, Abele DC. Familial cutaneous collagenoma. Report of cases. Arch Dermatol 1968; 98: 23–27.

441 Phillips JC, Knautz MA, Sangueza OP, Davis LS. Familial cutaneous collagenoma. J Am Acad Dermatol 1999; 40: 255–257.

442 Kopec AV, Levine N. Generalized connective tissue nevi and ichthyosis in Down's syndrome. Arch Dermatol 1979; 115: 623–624.

443 Smith JB, Hogan DJ, Glass LF, Fenske NA. Multiple collagenomas in a patient with Down syndrome. J Am Acad Dermatol 1995; 33: 835–837.

444 Morrison JGL, Wilson Jones E, MacDonald DM. Juvenile elastoma and osteopoikilosis (the Buschke–Ollendorff syndrome). Br J Dermatol 1977; 97: 417–422.

445 Ledoux-Corbusier M, Achten G, de Dobbeleer G. Juvenile elastoma (Weidman). An ultrastructural study. J Cutan Pathol 1981; 8: 219–227.

446 Trattner A, David M, Rothem A et al. Buschke–Ollendorff syndrome of the scalp: histologic and ultrastructural findings. J Am Acad Dermatol 1991; 24: 822–824.

447 Giro MG, Duvic M, Smith LT et al. Buschke–Ollendorff syndrome associated with elevated elastin production by affected skin fibroblasts in culture. J Invest Dermatol 1992; 99: 129–137.

448 Shinkai H, Katagiri K, Ishii Y, Takayasu S. Connective tissue naevus with pseudo-Hurler polydystrophy. Br J Dermatol 1994; 130: 528–533.

449 Uitto J, Bauer EA, Santa Cruz DJ et al. Decreased collagenase production by regional fibroblasts cultured from skin of a patient with connective tissue nevi of the collagen type. J Invest Dermatol 1982; 78: 136–140.

450 Botella-Estrada R, Alegre V, Sanmartin O et al. Isolated plantar cerebriform collagenoma. Arch Dermatol 1991; 127: 1589–1590.

451 Diven DG, Tanus T, Raimer SS. Cutis verticis gyrata. Int J Dermato 1991; 30: 710–712.

452 Del-Rio E, Vélez A, Martin N et al. Localized familial redundant scalp: atypical cutis verticis gyrata? Clin Exp Dermatol 1992; 17: 349–350.

453 Larralde M, Gardner SS, Torrado MdV et al. Lymphedema as a postulated cause of cutis verticis gyrata in Turner syndrome. Pediatr Dermatol 1998; 15: 18–22.

454 Woollons A, Darley CR, Lee PJ et al. Cutis verticis gyrata of the scalp in a patient with autosomal dominant insulin resistance syndrome. Clin Exp Dermatol 2000; 25: 125–128.

455 Kawaura K, Yano K, Takama H et al. Nodular lesion on the sacrococcygeal area in a bicycle rider. Br J Dermatol 2000; 143: 1124–1126.

456 Herbst VP, Kauh YC, Luscombe HA. Connective tissue nevus masquerading as a localized linear epidermal nevus. J Am Acad Dermatol 1987; 16: 264–266.

457 Pierard GE, Lapiere CM. Nevi of connective tissue. A reappraisal of their classification. Am J Dermatopathol 1985; 7: 325–333.

458 Stewart MI, Smoller BR. Dermal dendrocytes are decreased in collagenomas. J Cutan Pathol 1993; 20: 504–507.

459 Smith LR, Bernstein BD. Eruptive collagenoma. Arch Dermatol 1978; 114: 1710–1711.

460 Trau H, Dayan D, Hirschberg A et al. Connective tissue nevi collagens. Am J Dermatopathol 1991; 13: 374–377.

461 Nickel WR, Reed WB. Tuberous sclerosis. Special reference to the microscopic alterations in the cutaneous hamartomas. Arch Dermatol 1962; 85: 209–224.

462 Reed RJ. Cutaneous manifestations of neural crest disorders (neurocristopathies). Int J Dermatol 1977; 16: 807–826.

463 Vermersch-Langlin A, Delaporte E, Pagniez D et al. White fibrous papulosis of the neck. Int J Dermatol 1993; 32: 442–443.

464 Joshi RK, Abanmi A, Haleem A. White fibrous papulosis of the neck. Br J Dermatol 1992; 127: 295–296.

465 Cerio R, Gold S, Wilson Jones E. White fibrous papulosis of the neck. Clin Exp Dermatol 1991; 16: 224–225.

466 Zanca A, Contri MB, Carnevali C, Bertazzoni MG. White fibrous papulosis of the neck. Int J Dermatol 1996; 35: 720–722.

467 Balus L, Amantea A, Donati P et al. Fibroelastolytic papulosis of the neck: a report of 20 cases. Br J Dermatol 1997; 137: 461–466.

468 Sapacin A, Truter S, Rosenbaum J et al. Increased expression of type I collagen in cultured fibroblasts of white fibrous papulosis patients. J Invest Dermatol 1996; 106: 898 (abstract).

469 Ketchum LD. Hypertrophic scars and keloids. Clin Plast Surg 1977; 4: 301–310.

470 Sahl WJ Jr, Clever H. Cutaneous scars: Part I. Int J Dermatol 1994; 33: 681–691.

471 Sahl WJ Jr, Clever H. Cutaneous scars: Part II. Int J Dermatol 1994; 33: 763–769.

472 Ketchum LD, Cohen IK, Masters FW. Hypertrophic scars and keloids. A collective review. Plast Reconstr Surg 1974; 53: 140–154.

473 Murray JC, Pollack SV, Pinnell SR. Keloids: a review. J Am Acad Dermatol 1981; 4: 461–470.

474 Cosman B, Crikelair GF, Gaulin JC, Lattes R. The surgical treatment of keloids. Plast Reconstr Surg 1961; 27: 335–358.

475 Klumpar DI, Murray JC, Anscher M. Keloids treated with excision followed by radiation therapy. J Am Acad Dermatol 1994; 31: 225–231.

476 Berman B, Flores F. Recurrence rates of excised keloids treated with postoperative triamcinolone acetonide injections or interferon alfa-2b injections. J Am Acad Dermatol 1997; 37: 755–757.

477 Haas AF, Reilly DA. Cultured epithelial autografts in the treatment of extensive recalcitrant keloids. Arch Dermatol 1998; 134: 549–552.

478 Blackburn WR, Cosman B. Histologic basis of keloid and hypertrophic scar differentiation. Arch Pathol 1966; 82: 65–71.

479 Ginarte M, Peteiro C, Toribio J. Keloid formation induced by isotretinoin therapy. Int J Dermatol 1999; 38: 228–229.

480 Ala-Kokko L, Rintala A, Savolainen E-R. Collagen gene expression in keloids: analysis of collagen metabolism and type I, III, IV and V procollagen mRNAs in keloid tissue and keloid fibroblast cultures. J Invest Dermatol 1987; 89: 238–244.

481 Cohen IK, Keiser HR, Sjoerdsma A. Collagen synthesis in human keloid and hypertrophic scar. Surg Forum 1971; 22: 488–489.

482 Saed GM, Ladin D, Olson J et al. Analysis of p53 gene mutations in keloids using polymerase chain reaction-based single-strand conformational polymorphism and DNA sequencing. Arch Dermatol 1998; 134: 963–967.

483 Ishihara H, Yoshimoto H, Fujioka M et al. Keloid fibroblasts resist ceramide-induced apoptosis by overexpression of insulin-like growth factor I receptor. J Invest Dermatol 2000; 115: 1065–1071.

484 Varedi M, Tredget EE, Scott PG et al. Alteration in cell morphology triggers transforming growth factor-β1, collagenase, and tissue inhibitor of metalloproteinases-1 expression in normal and hypertrophic scar fibroblasts. J Invest Dermatol 1995; 104: 118–123.

485 Haisa M, Okochi H, Grotendorst GR. Elevated levels of PDGF α receptors in keloid fibroblasts contribute to an enhanced response to PDGF. J Invest Dermatol 1994; 103: 560–563.

486 Hammar H. Wound healing. Int J Dermatol 1993; 32: 6–15.

487 Babu M, Diegelmann R, Oliver N. Keloid fibroblasts exhibit an altered response to TGF-β. J Invest Dermatol 1992; 99: 650–655.

488 Zhang L-Q, Laato M, Muona P et al. Normal and hypertrophic scars: quantification and localization of messenger RNAs for type I, III and VI collagens. Br J Dermatol 1994; 130: 453–459.

489 Castagnoli C, Trombotto C, Ariotti S et al. Expression and role of IL-15 in post-burn hypertrophic scars. J Invest Dermatol 1999; 113: 238–245.

490 Zhang K, Garner W, Cohen L et al. Increased types I and III collagen and transforming growth factor-β1 mRNA and protein in hypertrophic burn scar. J Invest Dermatol 1995; 104: 750–754.

491 Sato M, Ishikawa O, Miyachi Y. Distinct patterns of collagen gene expression are seen in normal and keloid fibroblasts grown in three-dimensional culture. Br J Dermatol 1998; 138: 938–943.

492 Kauh YC, Rouda S, Mondragon G et al. Major suppression of pro-α1(I) type I collagen gene expression in the dermis after keloid excision and immediate intrawound injection of triamcinolone acetonide. J Am Acad Dermatol 1997; 37: 586–589.

493 Milsom JP, Craig RDP. Collagen degradation in cultured keloid and hypertrophic scar tissue. Br J Dermatol 1973; 89: 635–644.

494 Arakawa M, Hatamochi A, Mori Y et al. Reduced collagenase gene expression in fibroblasts from hypertrophic scar tissue. Br J Dermatol 1996; 134: 863–868.

495 Ghahary A, Shen YJ, Nedelec B et al. Collagenase production is lower in post-burn hypertrophic scar fibroblasts than in normal fibroblasts and is reduced by insulin-like growth factor-I. J Invest Dermatol 1996; 106: 476–481.

496 Meyer LJM, Russell SB, Russell JD et al. Reduced hyaluronan in keloid tissue and cultured keloid fibroblasts. J Invest Dermatol 2000; 114: 953–959.

497 Hunzelmann N, Anders S, Sollberg S et al. Co-ordinate induction of collagen type I and biglycan expression in keloids. Br J Dermatol 1996; 135: 394–399.

498 Dalkowski A, Schuppan D, Orfanos CE, Zouboulis CC. Increased expression of tenascin C by keloids in vivo and in vitro. Br J Dermatol 1999; 141: 50–56.

499 Sayani K, Dodd CM, Nedelec B et al. Delayed appearance of decorin in healing burn scars. Histopathology 2000; 36: 262–272.

500 Kuroda K, Okamoto O, Shinkai H. Dermatopontin expression is decreased in hypertrophic scar and systemic sclerosis skin fibroblasts and is regulated by transforming growth factor-β1, interleukin-4, and matrix collagen. J Invest Dermatol 1999; 112: 706–710.

501 Abergel RP, Pizzurro D, Meeker CA et al. Biochemical composition of the connective tissue in keloids and analysis of collagen metabolism in keloid fibroblast cultures. J Invest Dermatol 1985; 84: 384–390.

502 Ackerman AB, Ragaz A. The lives of lesions. Chronology in dermatopathology. New York: Masson Publishing USA, 1984: 58–61.

503 Ghazizadeh M, Miyata N, Sasaki Y et al. Silver-stained nucleolar organizer regions in hypertrophic and keloid scars. Am J Dermatopathol 1997; 19: 468–472.

504 Beer TW, Baldwin HC, Goddard JR et al. Angiogenesis in pathological and surgical scars. Hum Pathol 1998; 29: 1273–1278.

505 Pedragosa R, Serrano S, Carol-Murillo J et al. Blisters over burn scars in a child. Br J Dermatol 1986; 115: 501–506.

506 Pranteda G, Bottoni U, De Simone P et al. Bullous keloid: a distinct entity? Br J Dermatol 1999; 141: 375–377.

507 Redmond WJ, Baker SR. Keloidal calcification. Arch Dermatol 1983; 119: 270–272.

508 Robson A, Allen P, Hollowood K. S100 expression in cutaneous scars: a potential diagnostic pitfall in the diagnosis of desmoplastic melanoma. Histopathology 2001; 38: 135–140.

509 Matsuoka LY, Uitto J, Wortsman J et al. Ultrastructural characteristics of keloid fibroblasts. Am J Dermatopathol 1988; 10: 505–508.

510 James WD, Besanceney CD, Odom RB. The ultrastructure of a keloid. J Am Acad Dermatol 1980; 3: 50–57.

511 Tsuji T, Sawabe M. Elastic fibers in scar tissue: scanning and transmission electron microscopic studies. J Cutan Pathol 1987; 14: 106–113.

512 Elton RF, Pinkus H. Striae in normal men. Arch Dermatol 1966; 94: 33–34.

513 Nigam PK. Striae cutis distensae. Int J Dermatol 1989; 28: 426–428.

514 Wong RC, Ellis CN. Physiologic skin changes in pregnancy. J Am Acad Dermatol 1984; 10: 929–940.

515 Henry F, Piérard-Franchimont C, Pans A, Piérard GE. Striae distensae of pregnancy. An in vivo biomechanical evaluation. Int J Dermatol 1997; 36: 506–508.

516 Prebtani APH, Donat D, Ezzat S. Worrisome striae in pregnancy. Lancet 2000; 355: 1692.

517 Shelley WB, Cohen W. Stria migrans. Arch Dermatol 1964; 90: 193–194.

518 Carr RD, Hamilton JF. Transverse striae of the back. Arch Dermatol 1969; 99: 26–30.

519 Arem AJ, Kischer CW. Analysis of striae. Plast Reconstr Surg 1980; 65: 22–29.

520 Chernosky ME, Knox JM. Atrophic striae after occlusive corticosteroid therapy. Arch Dermatol 1964; 90: 15–19.

521 Darvay A, Acland K, Lynn W, Russell-Jones R. Striae formation in two HIV-positive persons receiving protease inhibitors. J Am Acad Dermatol 1999; 41: 467–469.

522 Shuster S. The cause of striae distensae. Acta Derm Venereol (Suppl) 1979; 85: 161–169.

523 Watson REB, Parry EJ, Humphries JD et al. Fibrillin microfibrils are reduced in skin exhibiting striae distensae. Br J Dermatol 1998; 138: 931–937.

524 Zheng P, Lavker RM, Kligman AM. Anatomy of striae. Br J Dermatol 1985; 112: 185–193.

525 Pinkus H, Keech MK, Mehregan AH. Histopathology of striae distensae with special reference to striae and wound healing in the Marfan syndrome. J Invest Dermatol 1966; 46: 283–292.

526 Tsuji T, Sawabe M. Elastic fibers in striae distensae. J Cutan Pathol 1988; 15: 215–222.

527 Lee KS, Rho YJ, Jang SI et al. Decreased expression of collagen and fibronectin genes in striae distensae tissue. Clin Exp Dermatol 1994; 19: 285–288.

528 Sheu H-M, Yu H-S, Chang C-H. Mast cell degranulation and elastolysis in the early stage of striae distensae. J Cutan Pathol 1991; 18: 410–416.

529 Chaouat Y, Aron-Brunetiere R, Faures B et al. Une nouvelle entité: le rhumatisme fibroblastique. A propos d'une observation. Rev Rhum Mal Osteoartic 1980; 47: 345–351.

530 Crouzet J, Amouroux J, Duterque M et al. Reumatisme fibroblastique. Un cas avec étude de l'histologie synoviale. Rev Rhum Mal Osteoartic 1982; 49: 469–472.

531 Vignon-Pennamen M-D, Naveau B, Foldes C et al. Fibroblastic rheumatism. J Am Acad Dermatol 1986; 14: 1086–1088.

532 Lacour JPh, Maquart FX, Bellon G et al. Fibroblastic rheumatism: clinical, histological, immunohistological, ultrastructural and biochemical study of a case. Br J Dermatol 1993; 128: 194–202.

533 Ostlere LS, Stevens HP, Jarmulowicz M et al. Fibroblastic rheumatism. Clin Exp Dermatol 1994; 19: 268–270.

534 Karzler MH, Dhillon I, Headington JT. Fibroblastic rheumatism. Arch Dermatol 1995; 131: 710–712.

535 Lister DM, Graham-Brown RAC, Burns DA et al. Collagenosis nuchae – a new entity? Clin Exp Dermatol 1988; 13: 263–264.

536 Balachandram K, Allen PW, MacCormac LB. Nuchal fibroma. A clinicopathological study of nine cases. Am J Surg Pathol 1995; 19: 313–317.

537 Weedon D (1989). Unpublished observations.

538 Michal M, Fetsch JF, Hes O, Miettinen M. Nuchal-type fibroma. A clinicopathologic study of 52 cases. Cancer 1999; 85: 156–163.

539 Banney LA, Weedon D, Muir JB. Nuchal fibroma associated with scleredema, diabetes mellitus and organic solvent exposure. Australas J Dermatol 2000; 41: 39–41.

540 Diwan AH, Graves ED, King JAC, Horenstein MG. Nuchal-type fibroma in two related patients with Gardner's syndrome. Am J Surg Pathol 2000; 24: 1563–1567.

541 Wehrli BM, Weiss SW, Yandow S, Coffin CM. Gardner-associated fibromas (GAF) in young patients. Am J Surg Pathol 2001; 25: 645–651.

542 Allen PW, Hasan N, Thorburn M. Nuchal-type fibroma appearance in a desmoid fibromatosis. Am J Surg Pathol 2001; 25: 828–829.

543 Kavanagh GM, Bradfield JWB, Collins CMP, Kennedy CTC. Weathering nodules of the ear: a clinicopathological study. Br J Dermatol 1996; 135: 550–554.

Atrophic collagenoses

544 Yasaka N, Otake N, Furue M, Tamaki K. Pseudoxanthomatous lesions with membranocystic changes of collagen fibers in an SLE patient receiving long-term steroid treatment. Dermatology 1997; 194: 162–165.

545 Guillen PS, Pichardo AR, Martinez FC. Aplasia cutis congenita. J Am Acad Dermatol 1985; 13: 429–433.

546 Pap GS. Congenital defect of scalp and skull in three generations of one family. Plast Reconstr Surg 1970; 46: 194–196.

547 Rauschkolb RR, Enriquez SI. Aplasia cutis congenita. Arch Dermatol 1962; 86: 54–57.

548 Sybert VP. Aplasia cutis congenita: a report of 12 new families and review of the literature. Pediatr Dermatol 1985; 3: 1–14.

549 Lane W, Zanol K. Duodenal atresia, biliary atresia, and intestinal infarct in truncal aplasia cutis congenita. Pediatr Dermatol 2000; 17: 290–292.

550 Tekinalp G, Yurdakök M, Kara A et al. Bilateral abdominal aplasia cutis congenita associated with atrial septal defect: a case report. Pediatr Dermatol 1997; 14: 117–119.

551 Irons GB, Olson RM. Aplasia cutis congenita. Plast Reconstr Surg 1980; 66: 199–203.

552 Scribanu N, Temtamy SA. The syndrome of aplasia cutis congenita with terminal, transverse defects of limbs. J Pediatr 1975; 87: 79–82.

553 Fryns JP, Corbeel L, van den Berghe H. Congenital scalp defect with distal limb reduction anomalies. Eur J Pediatr 1977; 126: 289–295.

554 Lin Y-J, Chen H-C, Jee S-H, Huang F-Y. Familial aplasia cutis congenita associated with limb anomalies and tetralogy of Fallot. Int J Dermatol 1993; 32: 52–53.

555 Ruiz-Maldonado R, Tamayo L. Aplasia cutis congenita, spastic paralysis, and mental retardation. Am J Dis Child 1974; 128: 699–701.

556 Frieden IJ. Aplasia cutis congenita: a clinical review and proposal for classification. J Am Acad Dermatol 1986; 14: 646–660.

557 Mimouni F, Han BK, Barnes L et al. Multiple hamartomas associated with intracranial malformation. Pediatr Dermatol 1986; 3: 219–225.

558 Högler W, Sidoroff A, Weber F et al. Aplasia cutis congenita, uvula bifida and bilateral retinal dystrophy in a girl with naevus sebaceous syndrome. Br J Dermatol 1999; 140: 542–543.

559 Bart BJ, Gorlin RJ, Anderson VE, Lynch FW. Congenital localized absence of skin and associated abnormalities resembling epidermolysis bullosa. Arch Dermatol 1966; 93: 296–304.

560 Wojnarowska FT, Eady RAJ, Wells RS. Dystrophic epidermolysis bullosa presenting with congenital localized absence of skin: report of four cases. Br J Dermatol 1983; 108: 477–483.

561 Skoven I, Drzewiecki KT. Congenital localized skin defect and epidermolysis bullosa hereditaria letalis. Acta Derm Venereol 1979; 59: 533–537.

562 Smith SZ, Cram DL. A mechanobullous disorder of the newborn: Bart's syndrome. Arch Dermatol 1978; 114: 81–84.

563 Jones EM, Hersh JH, Yusk JW. Aplasia cutis congenita, cleft palate, epidermolysis bullosa, and ectrodactyly: a new syndrome? Pediatr Dermatol 1992; 9: 293–297.

364 Léauté-Labrèze C, Depaire-Duclos F, Sarlangue J et al. Congenital cutaneous defects as complications in surviving co-twins. Aplasia cutis congenita and neonatal Volkmann ischemic contracture of the forearm. Arch Dermatol 1998; 134: 1121–1124.

565 Deeken JH, Caplan RM. Aplasia cutis congenita. Arch Dermatol 1970; 102: 386–389.

566 Mempel M, Abeck D, Lange I et al. The wide spectrum of clinical expression in Adams–Oliver syndrome: a report of two cases. Br J Dermatol 1999; 140: 1157–1160.

567 Zvulunov A, Kachko L, Manor E et al. Reticulolinear aplasia cutis congenita of the face and neck: a distinctive cutaneous manifestation in several syndromes linked to Xp22 Br J Dermatol 1998; 138: 1046–1052.

568 Fisher M, Schneider R. Aplasia cutis congenita in three successive generations. Arch Dermatol 1973; 108: 252–253.

569 Yagupsky P, Reuveni H, Karplus M, Moses S. Aplasia cutis congenita in one of monozygotic twins. Pediatr Dermatol 1986; 3: 403–405.

570 Kalb RE, Grossman ME. The association of aplasia cutis congenita with therapy of maternal thyroid disease. Pediatr Dermatol 1986; 3: 327–330.

571 Vogt T, Stolz W, Landthaler M. Aplasia cutis congenita after exposure to methimazole: a causal relationship? Br J Dermatol 1995; 133: 994–996.

572 Stephan MJ, Smith DW, Ponzi JW, Alden ER. Origin of scalp vertex aplasia cutis. J Pediatr 1982; 101: 850–853.

573 Levin DL, Nolan KS, Esterly NB. Congenital absence of skin. J Am Acad Dermatol 1980; 2: 203–206.

574 Mastruserio DN, Cobb MA, Ross VE. Nevocellular nevus associated with alopecia presenting as aplasia cutis congenita. Int J Dermatol 1998; 37: 37–39.

575 Drolet B, Prendiville J, Golden J et al. 'Membranous aplasia cutis' with hair collars. Congenital absence of skin or neuroectodermal defect? Arch Dermatol 1995; 131: 1427–1431.

576 Cambiaghi S, Gelmetti C, Nicolini U. Prenatal findings in membranous aplasia cutis. J Am Acad Dermatol 1998; 39: 638–640.

577 Munkvad JM, Nielsen AO, Asmussen T. Aplasia cutis congenita. A follow-up evaluation after 25 years. Arch Dermatol 1981; 117: 232–233.

578 Leung RSC, Beer WE, Mehta HK. Aplasia cutis congenita presenting as a familial triad of atrophic alopecia, ocular defects and a peculiar scarring tendency of the skin. Br J Dermatol 1988; 118: 715–720.

579 Cambiaghi S, Restano L, Cavalli R, Gelmetti C. Skin dimpling as a consequence of amniocentesis. J Am Acad Dermatol 1998; 39: 888–890.

580 Croce EJ, Purohit RC, Janovski NA. Congenital absence of skin (aplasia cutis congenita). Arch Surg 1973; 106: 732–734.

581 Harari Z, Pasmanik A, Dvoretzky I et al. Aplasia cutis congenita with dystrophic nail changes. Dermatologica 1976; 153: 363–368.

582 Rudolph RI, Schwartz W, Leyden JJ. Bitemporal aplasia cutis congenita. Occurrence with other cutaneous abnormalities. Arch Dermatol 1974; 110: 615–618.

583 Fukamizu H, Matsumoto K, Inoue K, Moriguchi T. Familial occurrence of aplasia cutis congenita. J Dermatol Surg Oncol 1982; 8: 1068–1070.

584 Goltz RW, Henderson RR, Hitch JM, Ott JE. Focal dermal hypoplasia syndrome. A review of the literature and report of two cases. Arch Dermatol 1970; 101: 1–11.

585 Ishibashi A, Kurihara Y. Goltz's syndrome: focal dermal dysplasia syndrome (focal dermal hypoplasia). Dermatologica 1972; 144: 156–167.

586 Lever WF. Hypoplasia cutis congenita. Arch Dermatol 1964; 90: 340.

587 Goltz RW. Focal dermal hypoplasia syndrome. An update. Arch Dermatol 1992; 128: 1108–1111.

588 Crutchfield CE III, Geiger J, Gorlin RJ, Ahmed I. What syndrome is this? Pediatr Dermatol 2000; 17: 484–486.

589 Prentice FM, Mackie RM. A case of focal dermal hypoplasia. Clin Exp Dermatol 1982; 7: 149–153.

590 Staughton RCD. Focal dermal hypoplasia (Goltz's syndrome) in a male. Proc R Soc Med 1976; 69: 232–233.

591 Buchner SA, Itin P. Focal dermal hypoplasia syndrome in a male patient. Arch Dermatol 1992; 128: 1078–1082.

592 Mahé A, Couturier J, Mathé C et al. Minimal focal dermal hypoplasia in a man: a case of father-to-daughter transmission. J Am Acad Dermatol 1991; 25: 879–881.

593 Howell JB, Freeman RG. Cutaneous defects of focal dermal hypoplasia: an ectomesodermal dysplasia syndrome. J Cutan Pathol 1989; 16: 237–258.

594 Gottlieb SK, Fisher BK, Violin GA. Focal dermal hypoplasia. A nine-year follow-up study. Arch Dermatol 1973; 108: 551–553.

595 Landa N, Oleaga JM, Ratón JA et al. Focal dermal hypoplasia (Goltz syndrome): an adult case with multisystemic involvement. J Am Acad Dermatol 1993; 28: 86–89.

596 Kore-eda S, Yoneda K, Ohtani T et al. Focal dermal hypoplasia (Goltz syndrome) associated with multiple giant papillomas. Br J Dermatol 1995; 133: 997–999.

597 Larrègue M, Duterque M. Striated osteopathy in focal dermal hypoplasia. Arch Dermatol 1975; 111: 1365.

598 Happle R, Lenz W. Striation of bones in focal dermal hypoplasia: manifestation of functional mosaicism? Br J Dermatol 1977; 96: 133–138.

599 Champion RH. Focal dermal hypoplasia. Br J Dermatol (Suppl) 1975; 11: 70–71.

600 Hardman CM, Garioch JJ, Eady RAJ, Fry L. Focal dermal hypoplasia: report of a case with cutaneous and skeletal manifestations. Clin Exp Dermatol 1998; 23: 281–285.

601 Happle R, Steijlen PM, Theile U et al. Patchy dermal hypoplasia as a characteristic feature of Proteus syndrome. Arch Dermatol 1997; 133: 77–80.

602 Uitto J, Bauer EA, Santa Cruz DJ et al. Focal dermal hypoplasia: abnormal growth characteristics of skin fibroblasts in culture. J Invest Dermatol 1980; 75: 170–175.

603 Lee IJ, Cha MS, Kim SC, Bang D. Electronmicroscopic observation of the basement membrane zone in focal dermal hypoplasia. Pediatr Dermatol 1996; 13: 5–9.

604 Ishii N, Baba N, Kanaizuka I et al. Histopathological study of focal dermal hypoplasia (Goltz syndrome). Clin Exp Dermatol 1992; 17: 24–26.

605 Atherton DJ, Hall M. Focal dermal hypoplasia syndrome. Clin Exp Dermatol 1979; 5: 249–252.

606 Howell JB. Nevus angiolipomatosus Vs focal dermal hypoplasia. Arch Dermatol 1965; 92: 238–248.

607 Tsuji T. Focal dermal hypoplasia syndrome. An electron microscopical study of the skin lesions. J Cutan Pathol 1982; 9: 271–281.

608 Magid ML, Prendiville JS, Esterly NB. Focal facial dermal dysplasia: bitemporal lesions resembling aplasia cutis congenita. J Am Acad Dermatol 1988; 18: 1203–1207.

609 Di Lernia V, Neri I, Patrizi A. Focal facial dermal dysplasia: two familial cases. J Am Acad Dermatol 1991; 25: 389–391.

610 Ward KA, Moss C. Evidence for genetic homogeneity of Setleis' syndrome and focal facial dermal dysplasia. Br J Dermatol 1994; 130: 645–649.

611 Tay Y-K, Morelli JG, Weston WL. Focal facial dermal dysplasia: report of a case with associated cardiac defects. Br J Dermatol 1996; 135: 607–608.

612 McGeoch AH, Reed WB. Familial focal facial dermal dysplasia. Arch Dermatol 1973; 107: 59 –595.

613 Kowalski DC, Fenske NA. The focal facial dermal dysplasias: report of a kindred and a proposed new classification. J Am Acad Dermatol 1992; 27: 575–582.

614 Stone N, Burge S. Focal facial dermal dysplasia with a hair collar. Br J Dermatol 1998; 139: 1136–1137.

615 Wells JM, Weedon D. Focal facial dermal dysplasia or aplasia cutis congenita: a case with a hair collar. Australas J Dermatol 2001; 42: 129–131.

616 Jensen NE. Congenital ectodermal dysplasia of the face. Br J Dermatol 1971; 84: 410–416.

617 Drolet BA, Baselga E, Gosain AK et al. Preauricular skin defects. A consequence of a persistent ectodermal groove. Arch Dermatol 1997; 133: 1551–1554.

618 Raque CJ, Stein KM, Lane JM, Reese EC Jr. Pseudoainhum constricting bands of the extremities. Arch Dermatol 1972; 105: 434–438.

619 Wollina U, Graefe T, Oelzner P et al. Pseudoainhum of all fingers associated with Reynold's syndrome and breast cancer: Report of a case and review of the literature. J Am Acad Dermatol 2001; 44: 381–384.

620 Snyder DS, Greenberg RA. Evaluation of atrophy production and vasoconstrictor potency in humans following intradermally injected corticosteroids. J Invest Dermatol 1974; 63: 461–463.

621 Stevanovic DV. Corticosteroid-induced atrophy of the skin with telangiectasia. Br J Dermatol 1972; 87: 548–556.

622 Sneddon IB. Atrophy of the skin. The clinical problems. Br J Dermatol (Suppl) 1976; 12: 121–123.

623 Fritsch WC. Deep atrophy of the skin of the deltoid area. Arch Dermatol 1970; 101: 585–587.

624 Goldman L. Reactions following intralesional and sublesional injections of corticosteroids. JAMA 1962; 182: 613–616.

625 Kikuchi I, Horikawa S. Perilymphatic atrophy of the skin. A side effect of topical corticosteroid injection therapy. Arch Dermatol 1974; 109: 558–559.

626 Gottlieb NL, Penneys NS, Brown HE Jr. Periarticular perilymphatic skin atrophy. JAMA 1978; 240: 559–560.

627 Gupta AK, Rasmussen JE. Perilesional linear atrophic streaks associated with intralesional corticosteroid injections in a psoriatic plaque. Pediatr Dermatol 1987; 4: 259–260.

628 Friedman SJ, Butler DF, Pittelkow MR. Perilesional linear atrophy and hypopigmentation after intralesional corticosteroid therapy. J Am Acad Dermatol 1988; 19: 537–541.

629 James MP, Black MM, Sparkes CG. Measurement of dermal atrophy induced by topical steroids using a radiographic technique. Br J Dermatol 1977; 96: 303–305.

630 Dykes PJ, Marks R. An appraisal of the methods used in the assessment of atrophy from topical corticosteroids. Br J Dermatol 1979; 101: 599–609.

631 Groves RW, MacDonald LM, MacDonald DM. Profound digital collagen atrophy: a new cutaneous presentation of adrenal-dependent Cushing's syndrome. Br J Dermatol 1990; 123: 667–671.

632 Cohen IK, Diegelmann RF, Johnson ML. Effect of corticosteroids on collagen synthesis. Surgery 1977; 82: 15–20.

633 Oikarinen A, Autio P. New aspects of the mechanism of corticosteroid-induced dermal atrophy. Clin Exp Dermatol 1991; 16: 416–419.

634 Oikarinen A. Dermal connective tissue modulated by pharmacologic agents. Int J Dermatol 1992; 31: 149–156.

635 Wilson Jones E. Steroid atrophy – a histological appraisal. Dermatologica (Suppl) 1976; 152: 107–115.

636 Jablonska S, Groniowska M, Dabrowski J. Comparative evaluation of skin atrophy in man induced by topical corticoids. Br J Dermatol 1979; 100: 193–206.

637 Fulop E. Mechanism of local skin atrophy caused by intradermally injected corticosteroids. Dermatologica (Suppl) 1976; 152: 139–146.

638 Schetman D, Hambrick GW Jr, Wilson CE. Cutaneous changes following local injection of triamcinolone. Arch Dermatol 1963; 88: 820–828.

639 Canizares O, Sachs PM, Jaimovich L, Torres VM. Idiopathic atrophoderma of Pasini and Pierini. Arch Dermatol 1958; 77: 42–59.

640 Buechner SA, Rufli T. Atrophoderma of Pasini and Pierini. Clinical and histopathologic findings and antibodies to Borrelia burgdorferi in thirty-four patients. J Am Acad Dermatol 1994; 30: 441–446.

641 Ramos-Caro FA, Podnos S, Ford M et al. Annular atrophic plaques of the skin (Christianson's disease). Int J Dermatol 1997; 36: 518–521.

642 Pullara TJ, Lober CW, Fenske NA. Idiopathic atrophoderma of Pasini and Pierini. Int J Dermatol 1984; 23: 643–645.

643 Wakelin SH, James MP. Zosteriform atrophoderma of Pasini and Pierini. Clin Exp Dermatol 1995; 20: 244–246.

644 Berman A, Berman GD, Winkelmann RK. Atrophoderma (Pasini–Pierini). Findings on direct immunofluorescent, monoclonal antibody, and ultrastructural studies. Int J Dermatol 1988; 27: 487–490.

645 Miller RF. Idiopathic atrophoderma. Report of a case and nosologic study. Arch Dermatol 1965; 92: 653–660.

646 Bisaccia EP, Scarborough DA, Lowney ED. Atrophoderma of Pasini and Pierini and systemic scleroderma. Arch Dermatol 1982; 118: 1–2.

647 Gatt P, Ackerman AB. Abortive morphea, abortive dermatofibroma, and abortive cutaneous T-cell lymphoma? Dermatopathology: Practical & Conceptual 1997; 3: 80–85.

648 Yokoyama Y, Akimoto S, Ishikawa O. Disaccharide analysis of skin glycosaminoglycans in atrophoderma of Pasini and Pierini. Clin Exp Dermatol 2000; 25: 436–440.

649 Perry HO. Diseases that present as cutaneous sclerosis. Australas J Dermatol 1982; 23: 45–52.

650 Franck J-M, MacFarlane D, Silvers DN et al. Atrophoderma of Pasini and Pierini: atrophy of dermis or subcutis? J Am Acad Dermatol 1995; 32: 122–123.

651 Wollenberg A, Baumann L, Plewig G. Linear atrophoderma of Moulin: a disease which follows Blaschko's lines. Br J Dermatol 1996; 135: 277–279.

652 Browne C, Fisher BK. Atrophoderma of Moulin with preceding inflammation. Int J Dermatol 2000; 39: 850–852.

653 Coulson IH, Smith NP, Holden CA. Acrodermatitis chronica atrophicans with coexisting morphoea. Br J Dermatol 1989; 121: 263–269.

654 Buechner SA, Rufli T, Erb P. Acrodermatitis chronica atrophicans: a chronic T-cell-mediated immune reaction against Borrelia burgdorferi? Clinical, histologic, and immunohistochemical study of five cases. J Am Acad Dermatol 1993; 28: 399–405.

655 Marsch WCh, Mayet A, Wolter M. Cutaneous fibroses induced by Borrelia burgdorferi. Br J Dermatol 1993; 128: 674–678.

656 Paige DG, Lake BD, Bailey AJ et al. Restrictive dermopathy: a disorder of fibroblasts. Br J Dermatol 1992; 127: 630–634.

657 Piérard-Franchimont C, Piérard GE, Arrese Estrada TH-LJ et al. Dermatopathological aspects of restrictive dermopathy. J Pathol 1992; 167: 223–228.

658 Welsh KM, Smoller BR, Holbrook KA, Johnston K. Restrictive dermopathy. Arch Dermatol 1992; 128: 228–231.

659 Happle R, Schuurmans Stekhoven JH, Hamel BCJ et al. Restrictive dermopathy in two brothers. Arch Dermatol 1992; 128: 232–235.

660 Sillevis Smitt JH, van Asperen CJ, Niessen CM et al. Restrictive dermopathy. Report of 12 cases. Arch Dermatol 1998; 134: 577–579.

661 Graham J, Esterly NB. What syndrome is this? Pediatr Dermatol 1999; 16: 151–153.

662 Wesche WA, Cutlan RT, Khare V et al. Restrictive dermopathy: report of a case and review of the literature. J Cutan Pathol 2001; 28: 211–218.

Perforating collagenoses

663 Woo TY, Rasmussen JE. Disorders of transepidermal elimination. Part 1. Int J Dermatol 1985; 24: 267–279.

664 Goette DK. Transepithelial elimination of altered collagen after intralesional adrenal steroid injections. Arch Dermatol 1984; 120: 539–540.

665 Delacretaz J, Gattlen JM. Transepidermal elimination of traumatically altered collagen. Dermatologica 1976; 152: 65–71.

666 Ardigò M, Brazzelli V, Vassallo C et al. Solitary perforating collagenosis: a case report. Am J Dermatopathol 2000; 22: 359 (abstract).

667 Mehregan AH, Schwartz OD, Livingood CS. Reactive perforating collagenosis. Arch Dermatol 1967; 96: 277–282.

668 Yusuk S, Trau H, Stempler D et al. Reactive perforating collagenosis. Int J Dermatol 1985; 24: 584–586.

669 Fretzin DF, Beal DW, Jao W. Light and ultrastructural study of reactive perforating collagenosis. Arch Dermatol 1980; 116: 1054–1058.

670 Weiner AL. Reactive perforating collagenosis. Arch Dermatol 1970; 102: 540–544.

671 Jang K-A, Lee H-K, Choi J-H et al. Perforating disorder on the sole of the foot. Br J Dermatol 1999; 140: 176–177.

672 Cerio R, Jones EW. Reactive perforating collagenosis: a clinicopathological review of 10 cases. J Cutan Pathol 1988; 15: 301 (abstract).

673 Kurschat P, Kröger A, Scharffetter-Kochanek K, Hunzelmann N. Acquired reactive perforating collagenosis triggered by scabies infection. Acta Derm Venereol 2000; 80: 384–385.

674 Bovenmyer DA. Reactive perforating collagenosis. Experimental production of the lesion. Arch Dermatol 1970; 102: 313–317.

675 De Berker DAR, Wilson CL, Millard PR. Reactive perforating collagenosis and Down's syndrome. Br J Dermatol 1992; 126: 71–73.

676 Nair BKH, Sarojini PA, Basheer AM, Nair CHK. Reactive perforating collagenosis. Br J Dermatol 1974; 91: 399–403.

677 Poliak SC, Lebwohl MG, Parris A, Prioleau PG. Reactive perforating collagenosis associated with diabetes mellitus. N Engl J Med 1982; 306: 81–84.

678 Cochran RJ, Tucker SB, Wilkin JK. Reactive perforating collagenosis of diabetes mellitus and renal failure. Cutis 1983; 31: 55–58.

679 Tang WYM, Chong LY, Lam SY, Yue CS. Acquired reactive perforating collagenosis in two Chinese patients. Int J Dermatol 1995; 34: 196–198.

680 Faver IR, Daoud MS, Su WPD. Acquired reactive perforating collagenosis. J Am Acad Dermatol 1994; 30: 575–580.

681 Kawakami T, Saito R. Acquired reactive perforating collagenosis associated with diabetes mellitus: eight cases that meet Faver's criteria. Br J Dermatol 1999; 140: 521–524.

682 Morton CA, Henderson IS, Jones MC, Lowe JG. Acquired perforating dermatosis in a British dialysis population. Br J Dermatol 1996; 135: 671–677.

683 Maurice PDL, Neild GH. Acquired perforating dermatosis and diabetic nephropathy – a case report and review of the literature. Clin Exp Dermatol 1997; 22: 291–294.

684 Robinson-Bostom L, DiGiovanna JJ. Cutaneous manifestations of end-stage renal disease. J Am Acad Dermatol 2000; 43: 975–986.

685 Gupta AK, Gupta MA, Cardella CJ, Haberman HF. Cutaneous associations of chronic renal failure and dialysis. Int J Dermatol 1986; 25: 498–504.

686 Beck H-I, Brandrup F, Hagdrup HK et al. Adult acquired reactive perforating collagenosis. Report of a case including ultrastructural findings. J Cutan Pathol 1988; 15: 124–128.

687 Patterson JW. The perforating disorders. J Am Acad Dermatol 1984; 10: 561–581.

688 Chang P, Fernández V. Acquired perforating disease: report of nine cases. Int J Dermatol 1993; 32: 874–876.

689 Rapini RP, Hebert AA, Drucker CR. Acquired perforating dermatosis. Evidence for combined transepidermal elimination of both collagen and elastic fibers. Arch Dermatol 1989; 125: 1074–1078.

690 Patterson JW. Progress in the perforating dermatoses. Arch Dermatol 1989; 125: 1121–1123.

691 Haftek M, Euvrard S, Kanitakis J et al. Acquired perforating dermatosis of diabetes mellitus and renal failure: further ultrastructural clues to its pathogenesis. J Cutan Pathol 1993; 20: 350–355.

692 Pedragosa R, Knobel HJ, Huguet P et al. Reactive perforating collagenosis in Hodgkin's disease. Am J Dermatopathol 1987; 9: 41–44.

693 Chae KS, Park YM, Cho SH, Cho BK. Reactive perforating collagenosis associated with periampullary carcinoma. Br J Dermatol 1998; 139: 548–550.

694 Bong JL, Fleming CJ, Kemmett D. Reactive perforating collagenosis associated with underlying malignancy. Br J Dermatol 2000; 142: 390–391.

695 Bang S-W, Kim Y-K, Whang K-U. Acquired reactive perforating collagenosis: unilateral umbilicated papules along the lesions of herpes zoster. J Am Acad Dermatol 1997; 36: 778–779.

696 Nakanishi G, Tsunemitsu R, Akagi O. Reactive perforating collagenosis occurring in a zosteriform distribution. Br J Dermatol 1999; 141: 367–369.

697 Lee HN, Lee DW, Lee JY, Cho BK. Two cases of reactive perforating collagenosis arising at the site of healed herpes zoster. Int J Dermatol 2001; 40: 191–192.

698 Tay Y-K, Weston WL, Aeling JL. Reactive perforating collagenosis in Treacher Collins syndrome. J Am Acad Dermatol 1996; 35: 982–983.

699 Bedlow AJ, Wong E, Cook MG, Marsden RA. Perforating collagenosis due to red dye in a tattoo. Br J Dermatol 1998; 139: 926–927.

700 Bank DE, Cohen PR, Kohn SR. Reactive perforating collagenosis in a setting of double disaster: acquired immunodeficiency syndrome and end-stage renal disease. J Am Acad Dermatol 1989; 21: 371–374.

701 Morgan MB, Truitt CA, Taira J et al. Fibronectin and the extracellular matrix in the perforating disorders of the skin. Am J Dermatopathol 1998; 20: 147–154.

702 Kawakami T, Soma Y, Mizoguchi M, Saito R. Immunohistochemical analysis of transforming growth factor-β3 expression in acquired reactive perforating collagenosis. Br J Dermatol 2001; 144: 197–199.

703 Yanagihara M, Fujita T, Shirasaki A et al. The pathogenesis of the transepithelial elimination of the collagen bundles in acquired reactive perforating collagenosis. A light and electron microscopical study. J Cutan Pathol 1996; 23: 398–403.

704 Millard PR, Young E, Harrison DE, Wojnarowska F. Reactive perforating collagenosis: light, ultrastructural and immunohistological studies. Histopathology 1986; 10: 1047–1056.

705 Herzinger T, Schirren CG, Sander CA et al. Reactive perforating collagenosis – transepidermal elimination of type IV collagen. Clin Exp Dermatol 1996; 21: 279–282.

706 Zelger B, Hintner H, Auböck J, Fritsch PO. Acquired perforating dermatosis. Arch Dermatol 1991; 127: 695–700.

707 Patterson JW, Brown PC. Ultrastructural changes in acquired perforating dermatosis. Int J Dermatol 1992; 31: 201–205.

708 Laugier P, Woringer F. Reflexions au sujet d'un collagènome perforant verruciforme. Ann Dermatol Syph 1963; 90: 29–36.

709 Detlefs RL, Goette DK. Collagènome perforant verruciforme. Arch Dermatol 1986; 122: 1044–1046.

710 Weedon D. Unpublished observation.

711 Burns DA, Calnan CD. Chondrodermatitis nodularis antihelicis. Clin Exp Dermatol 1978; 3: 207–208.

712 Bard JW. Chondrodermatitis nodularis chronica helicis. Dermatologica 1981; 163: 376–384.

713 Lawrence CM. The treatment of chondrodermatitis nodularis with cartilage removal alone. Arch Dermatol 1991; 127: 530–535.

714 Elgart ML. Cell phone chondrodermatitis. Arch Dermatol 2000; 136: 1568.

715 Dean E, Bernhard JD. Bilateral chondrodermatitis nodularis antihelicis. An unusual complication of cardiac pacemaker insertion. Int J Dermatol 1988; 27: 122.

716 Bottomley WW, Goodfield MDJ. Chondrodermatitis nodularis helicis occurring with systemic sclerosis – an under-reported association? Clin Exp Dermatol 1994; 19: 219–220.

717 Sasaki T, Nishizawa H, Sugita Y. Chondrodermatitis nodularis helicis in childhood dermatomyositis. Br J Dermatol 1999; 141: 363–365.

718 Goette DK. Chondrodermatitis nodularis helicis: a perforating necrobiotic granuloma. J Am Acad Dermatol 1980; 2: 148–154.

719 Hurwitz RM. Painful papule of the ear: a follicular disorder. J Dermatol Surg Oncol 1987; 13: 270–274.

720 Hurwitz RM. Pseudocarcinomatous or infundibular hyperplasia. Am J Dermatopathol 1989; 11: 189–191.

721 Shuman R, Helwig EB. Chondrodermatitis helicis. Am J Clin Pathol 1954; 24: 126–144.

722 Santa Cruz DJ. Chondrodermatitis nodularis helicis: a transepidermal perforating disorder. J Cutan Pathol 1980; 7: 70–76.

723 Garcia E, Silva L, Martins O et al. Bone formation in chondrodermatitis nodularis helicis. J Dermatol Surg Oncol 1980; 6: 582–585.

Variable collagen changes

724 Nelson DL, King RA. Ehlers–Danlos syndrome type VIII. J Am Acad Dermatol 1981; 5: 297–303.

725 Pinnell SR. Molecular defects in the Ehlers–Danlos syndrome. J Invest Dermatol 1982; 79: 90s–92s.

726 Black CM, Gathercole LJ, Bailey AJ, Beighton P. The Ehlers–Danlos syndrome: an analysis of the structure of the collagen fibres of the skin. Br J Dermatol 1980; 102: 85–96.

727 Burrows NP. The molecular genetics of the Ehlers–Danlos syndrome. Clin Exp Dermatol 1999; 24: 99–106.

728 Reichel JL, Weston WL, Bellus G, Morelli J. What syndrome is this [Ehlers–Danlos syndrome]? Pediatr Dermatol 2001; 18: 156–158.

729 Handa S, Sethuraman G, Mohan A, Sharma VK. Ehlers–Danlos syndrome with bladder diverticula. Br J Dermatol 2001; 144: 1084–1085.

730 De Felice C, Toti P, Di Maggio G et al. Absence of the inferior labial and lingual frenula in Ehlers–Danlos syndrome. Lancet 2001; 357: 1500–1502.

731 Pyeritz RE. Ehlers–Danlos syndrome. N Engl J Med 2000; 342: 730–732.

732 Byers PH. Ehlers–Danlos syndrome: recent advances and current understanding of the clinical and genetic heterogeneity. J Invest Dermatol 1994; 103: 47S–52S.

733 Maroteaux P, Frezal J, Cohen-Solal L. The differential symptomatology of errors of collagen metabolism. A tentative classification. Am J Med Genet 1986; 24: 219–230.

734 Beighton P, De Paepe A, Steinmann B et al. Ehlers–Danlos syndromes: revised nosology, Villefranche, 1997. Am J Med Genet 1998; 77: 31–37.

735 Sulica VI, Cooper PH, Pope FM et al. Cutaneous histologic features in Ehlers–Danlos syndrome. Arch Dermatol 1979; 115: 40–42.

736 Wechsler HL, Fisher ER. Ehlers–Danlos syndrome. Pathologic, histochemical, and electron microscopic observations. Arch Pathol 1964; 77: 613–619.

737 Kobayasi T, Oguchi M, Asboe-Hansen G. Dermal changes in Ehlers–Danlos syndrome. Clin Genet 1984; 25: 477–484.

738 Rizzo R, Contri MB, Micali G et al. Familial Ehlers–Danlos syndrome type II: abnormal fibrillogenesis of dermal collagen. Pediatr Dermatol 1987; 4: 197–204.

739 Pinnell SR. The skin in Ehlers–Danlos syndrome. J Am Acad Dermatol 1987; 16: 399–400.

740 De Paepe A, Nicholls A, Narcisi P et al. Ehlers–Danlos syndrome type I: a clinical and ultrastructural study of a family with reduced amounts of collagen type III. Br J Dermatol 1987; 117: 89–97.

741 Burrows NP, Nicholls AC, Yates JRW et al. Genetic linkage to the collagen α1 (V) gene (COL5A1) in two British Ehlers–Danlos syndrome families with variable type I and II phenotypes. Clin Exp Dermatol 1997; 22: 174–176.

742 Schwarze U, Atkinson M, Hoffman GG et al. Null alleles of the COL5A1 gene of type V collagen are a cause of the classical forms of Ehlers–Danlos syndrome (types I and II). Am J Hum Genet 2000; 66: 1757–1765.

743 Wenstrup RJ, Florer JB, Willing MC et al. COL5A1 haploinsufficiency is a common molecular mechanism underlying the classical form of EDS. Am J Hum Genet 2000; 66: 1766–1776.

744 Nuytinck L, Freund M, Lagae L et al. Classical Ehlers–Danlos syndrome caused by a mutation in type I collagen. Am J Hum Genet 2000; 66: 1398–1402.

745 Holzberg M, Hewan-Lowe KO, Olansky AJ. The Ehlers–Danlos syndrome: recognition, characterization and importance of a milder variant of the classic form. A preliminary study. J Am Acad Dermatol 1988; 19: 656–666.

746 Stanford DG, Georgouras KE. Ehlers–Danlos syndrome type II: importance of recognition. Australas J Dermatol 1995; 36: 153–155.

747 Iurassich S, Rocco D, Aurilia A. Type III Ehlers–Danlos syndrome: correlations among clinical signs, ultrasound, and histologic findings in a study of 35 cases. Int J Dermatol 2001; 40: 175–178.

748 Sulh HMB, Steinmann B, Rao VH et al. Ehlers–Danlos syndrome type IV D: an autosomal recessive disorder. Clin Genet 1984; 25: 278–287.

749 Pope FM, Jones PM, Wells RS et al. EDS IV (acrogeria): new autosomal dominant and recessive types. J R Soc Med 1980; 73: 180–186.

750 Pope FM, Martin GR, McKusick VA. Inheritance of Ehlers–Danlos type IV syndrome. J Med Genet 1977; 14: 200–204.

751 McFarland W, Fuller DE. Mortality in Ehlers–Danlos syndrome due to spontaneous rupture of large arteries. N Engl J Med 1964; 271: 1309–1310.

752 Hernandez A, Aguirre-Negrette MG, Gonzalez-Flores S et al. Ehlers–Danlos features with progeroid facies and mild mental retardation. Clin Genet 1986; 30: 456–461.

753 Jansen T, De Paepe A, Nuytinck L, Altmeyer P. Acrogeric phenotype in Ehlers–Danlos syndrome type IV attributed to a missense mutation in the COL3A1 gene. Br J Dermatol 2001; 144: 1086–1087.

754 Pepin M, Schwarze U, Superti-Furga A, Byers PH. Clinical and genetic features of Ehlers–Danlos syndrome type IV, the vascular type. N Engl J Med 2000; 342: 673–680.

755 Jansen T, de Paepe A, Luytinck N, Plewig G. COL3A1 mutation leading to acrogeria (Gottron type). Br J Dermatol 2000; 142: 178–180.

756 Kuivaniemi H, Tromp G, Bergfeld WF et al. Ehlers–Danlos syndrome type IV: a single base substitution of the last nucleotide of exon 34 in COL3A1 leads to exon skipping. J Invest Dermatol 1995; 105: 352–356.

757 Byers PH. Ehlers–Danlos syndrome type IV: a genetic disorder in many guises. J Invest Dermatol 1995; 105: 311–313.

758 Pope FM, Nicholls AC, Dorrance DE et al. Type III collagen deficiency with normal phenotype. J R Soc Med 1983; 76: 518–520.

759 Temple AS, Hinton P, Narcisi P, Pope FM. Detection of type III collagen in skin fibroblasts from patients with Ehlers–Danlos syndrome type IV by immunofluorescence. Br J Dermatol 1988; 118: 17–26.

760 Autio P, Turpeinen M, Risteli J et al. Ehlers–Danlos type IV: non-invasive techniques as diagnostic support. Br J Dermatol 1997; 137: 653–655.

761 Beighton P, Curtis D. X-linked Ehlers Danlos syndrome type V; the next generation. Clin Genet 1985; 27: 472–478.

762 Açil Y, Vetter U, Brenner R et al. Ehlers–Danlos syndrome type VI: cross-link pattern in tissue and urine sample as a diagnostic marker. J Am Acad Dermatol 1995; 33: 522–524.

763 Pinnell SR, Krane SM, Kenzora JE, Glimcher MJ. A heritable disorder of connective tissue. Hydroxylysine-deficient collagen disease. N Engl J Med 1972; 286: 1013–1020.

764 Ihme A, Krieg T, Nerlich A et al. Ehlers–Danlos syndrome type VI: collagen type specificity of defective lysyl hydroxylation in various tissues. J Invest Dermatol 1984; 83: 161–165.

765 Pope FM, Nicholls AC, Palan A et al. Clinical features of an affected father and daughter with Ehlers–Danlos syndrome type VIIB. Br J Dermatol 1992; 126: 77–82.

766 Cole WG, Evans R, Sillence DO. The clinical features of Ehlers–Danlos type VII due to a deletion of 24 amino acids from the pro α 1 (1) chain of type I procollagen. J Med Genet 1987; 24: 698–701.

767 Flórez A, Gómez Centeno P, Fernández-Redondo V, Toribio J. Clinical features of Ehlers–Danlos syndrome type VII in chromosome 6q deletion. Acta Derm Venereol 2000; 80: 58–59.

768 Petty EM, Seashore MR, Braverman IM et al. Dermatosparaxis in children. A case report and review of the newly recognized phenotype. Arch Dermatol 1993; 129: 1310–1315.

769 Lapiere CM, Nusgens BV. Ehlers–Danlos type VII-c, or human dermatosparaxis. Arch Dermatol 1993; 129: 1316–1319.

770 Piérard GE, Hermanns-Lê T, Arrese-Estrada J et al. Structure of the dermis in Type VII C Ehlers–Danlos syndrome. Am J Dermatopathol 1993; 15: 127–132.

771 Colige A, Sieron AL, Li S-W et al. Human Ehlers–Danlos syndrome type VIIC and bovine dermatosparaxis are caused by mutations in the procollagen I N-proteinase gene. Am J Hum Genet 1999; 65: 308–317.

772 Karrer S, Landthaler M, Schmalz G. Ehlers–Danlos syndrome type VIII with severe periodontitis and apical root resorption after orthodontic treatment. Acta Derm Venereol 2000; 80: 56–57.

773 Dyne KM, Vitellaro-Zuccarello L, Bacchella L et al. Ehlers–Danlos syndrome type VIII: biochemical, stereological and immunohistochemical studies on dermis from a child with clinical signs of Ehlers–Danlos syndrome and a family history of premature loss of permanent teeth. Br J Dermatol 1993; 128: 458–463.

774 Zalis EG, Roberts DC. Ehlers–Danlos syndrome. Arch Dermatol 1967; 96: 540–544.

775 Prockop DJ, Kivirikko KI, Tuderman L, Guzman NA. The biosynthesis of collagen and its disorders. N Engl J Med 1979; 301: 77–85.

776 Peltonen L, Kuivaniemi H, Palotie A et al. Alterations in copper and collagen metabolism in the Menkes syndrome and a new subtype of the Ehlers–Danlos syndrome. Biochemistry 1983; 22: 6156–6163.

777 Arneson MA, Hammerschmidt DE, Furcht LT, King RA. A new form of Ehlers–Danlos syndrome. Fibronectin corrects defective platelet function. JAMA 1980; 244: 144–147.

778 Cullen SI. Localized Ehlers–Danlos syndrome. Arch Dermatol 1979; 115: 332–333.

779 Sasaki T, Arai K, Ono M et al. Ehlers–Danlos syndrome. Arch Dermatol 1987; 123: 76–79.

780 Pope FM, Nicholls AC, McPheat J et al. Collagen genes and proteins in osteogenesis imperfecta. J Med Genet 1985; 22: 466–478.

781 Cohen PR, Schneiderman P. Clinical manifestations of the Marfan syndrome. Int J Dermatol 1989; 28: 291–299.

Syndromes of premature aging

782 Beauregard S, Gilchrest BA. Syndromes of premature aging. Dermatol Clin 1987; 5: 109–121.

783 Gilkes JJH, Sharvill DE, Wells RS. The premature ageing syndromes. Report of eight cases and description of a new entity named metageria. Br J Dermatol 1974; 91: 243–262.

784 Goldsmith LA. Genetic skin diseases with altered aging. Arch Dermatol 1997; 133: 1293–1295.

785 Satoh M, Imai M, Sugimoto M et al. Prevalence of Werner's syndrome heterozygotes in Japan. Lancet 1999; 353: 1766.

786 Hrabko RP, Milgrom H, Schwartz RA. Werner's syndrome with associated malignant neoplasms. Arch Dermatol 1982; 118: 106–108.

787 Poole S, Fenske NA. Cutaneous markers of internal malignancy. 1. Malignant involvement of the skin and genodermatoses. J Am Acad Dermatol 1993; 28: 1–13.

788 Lazarov A, Finkelstein E, Avinoach I et al. Diffuse lentiginosis in a patient with Werner's syndrome – a possible association with incomplete leopard syndrome. Clin Exp Dermatol 1995; 20: 46–50.

789 Iijima S, Arinami T, Otsuka F. Possible Werner syndrome. Arch Dermatol 1992; 128: 1238–1242.

790 Rünger TM, Bauer C, Dekant B et al. Hypermutable ligation of plasmid DNA ends in cells from patients with Werner syndrome. J Invest Dermatol 1994; 102: 45–48.

791 Gawkrodger DJ, Priestley GC, Vijayalaxmi et al. Werner's syndrome. Biochemical and cytogenetic studies. Arch Dermatol 1985; 121: 636–641.

792 Hatamochi A, Mori K, Takeda K et al. Decreased type VI collagen gene expression in cultured Werner's syndrome fibroblasts. J Invest Dermatol 1993; 100: 771–774.

793 Arakawa M, Hatamochi A, Takeda K, Ueki H. Increased collagen synthesis accompanying elevated m-RNA levels in cultured Werner's syndrome fibroblasts. J Invest Dermatol 1990; 94: 187–190.

794 Bauer EA, Uitto J, Tan EML, Holbrook KA. Werner's syndrome. Evidence for preferential regional expression of a generalized mesenchymal cell defect. Arch Dermatol 1988; 124: 90–101.

795 Bohr VA, Dianov G, Balajee A et al. DNA repair and transcription in human premature aging disorders. J Invest Dermatol (Symposium Proceedings) 1998; 3: 11–13.

796 Morita K, Nishigori C, Sasaki MS et al. Werner's syndrome – chromosome analyses of cultured fibroblasts and mitogen-stimulated lymphocytes. Br J Dermatol 1997; 136: 620–623.

797 Higuchi T, Ishikawa O, Hayashi H et al. Disaccharide analysis of the skin glycosaminoglycans in patients with Werner's syndrome. Clin Exp Dermatol 1994; 19: 487–491.

798 Sephal GC, Sturrock A, Giro MG, Davidson JM. Increased elastin production by progeria skin fibroblasts is controlled by the steady-state levels of elastin mRNA. J Invest Dermatol 1988; 90: 643–647.

799 Badame AJ. Progeria. Arch Dermatol 1989; 125: 540–544.

800 Gillar PJ, Kaye CI, McCourt JW. Progressive early dermatologic changes in Hutchinson–Gilford progeria syndrome. Pediatr Dermatol 1991; 8: 199–206.

801 Jansen T, Romiti R. Progeria infantum (Hutchinson–Gilford syndrome) associated with scleroderma-like lesions and acro-osteolysis: a case report and brief review of the literature. Pediatr Dermatol 2000; 17: 282–285.

802 Jimbow K, Kobayashi H, Ishii M et al. Scar and keloidlike lesions in progeria. Arch Dermatol 1988; 124: 1261–1266.

803 Fleischmajer R, Nedwich A. Progeria (Hutchinson–Gilford). Arch Dermatol 1973; 107: 253–258.

804 Ramesh V, Jain RK. Progeria in two brothers. Australas J Dermatol 1987; 28: 33–35.

805 De Groot WP, Tafelkruyer J, Woerdeman MJ. Familial acrogeria (Gottron). Br J Dermatol 1980; 103: 213–223.

806 Venencie PY, Powell FC, Winkelmann RK. Acrogeria with perforating elastoma and bony abnormalities. Acta Derm Venereol 1984; 64: 348–351.

807 Tajima S, Inazumi T, Kobayashi T. A case of acrogeria associated with late-onset focal dermal elastosis. Dermatology 1996; 192: 264–268.

808 Pope FM, Narcisi P, Nicholls AC et al. COL3A1 mutations cause variable clinical phenotypes including acrogeria and vascular rupture. Br J Dermatol 1996; 135: 163–181.

809 Pope FM, Nicholls AC, Narcici P et al. Type III collagen mutations in Ehlers Danlos syndrome type IV and other related disorders. Clin Exp Dermatol 1988; 13: 285–302.

Disorders of elastic tissue

INTRODUCTION

Normal elastic tissue

Elastic fibers are the important resilient component of mammalian connective tissue, and their presence is necessary for the proper structure and function of the cardiovascular, pulmonary and intestinal systems.[1,2] They constitute less than 4% of the dry weight of the skin, forming a complex and extensive network in the dermis which imparts elasticity to the skin.[3]

Structure and composition

Mature elastic fibers are composed of structural glycoproteins, which contribute to the formation of 10–12 nm microfibrils, and elastin, a fibrous protein with a molecular weight of 72 000 kd.[3] Elastin forms an amorphous core to the elastic fibers and this is surrounded by the microfibrils. Approximately 90% of the mature elastic fiber is elastin. It has a high concentration of alanine and valine, but less hydroxyproline than is present in collagen. Elastin-producing cells secrete tropoelastin, a 70 kd precursor of elastin, which becomes highly crosslinked by the action of lysyl oxidase to form mature elastin.[4] It is the product of a single copy gene, located in the chromosomal locus 7q11.23, in the human genome.[5] Mutations in this gene cause Williams' syndrome and some cases of cutis laxa. The microfibrils consist of several distinct proteins including fibrillin; abnormalities of the microfibrils occur in Marfan's syndrome (see p. 397). The fibrillin-1 gene (FBN1), identified in 1991, is located on chromosome 15q15–21.[4] There is a second fibrillin gene on chromosome 5 (FBN2), mutations of which cause congenital contractural arachnodactyly.[6]

The papillary dermis contains fine fibers which run perpendicular to the dermoepidermal junction and connect the basal lamina to the underlying dermal elastic tissue.[7] These oxytalan fibers, as they are called, consist of microfibrils without a core of elastin.[8] They branch to form a horizontal plexus in the upper reticular dermis, where they are known as elaunin fibers. They contain a small amount of elastin. The mature elastic fibers with their full composition of elastin are found below this in the reticular dermis. These three types of fibers probably correspond to consecutive stages of normal elastogenesis.[8]

Formation of elastic fibers

The formation of elastic fibers by fibroblasts, and in some circumstances by smooth muscle cells and chondroblasts, entails several different steps which are still poorly understood. Theoretically, these stages would include the expression of genes coding for elastin polypeptides, various intracellular processes, secretion of the precursor components, and extracellular modifications leading to the assembly of the fibers.[3]

Elastin is secreted in the form of a precursor, tropoelastin. This is ultimately crosslinked with desmosine to form stable elastin.[9] The formation of desmosine requires the copper-dependent enzyme lysyl oxidase.[9] Defects in this enzyme can result from a spectrum of mutations in the ATPase gene (ATP7A), as seen in Menkes' syndrome (see p. 397). Impaired elastinogenesis can also result from other altered transport mechanisms important to elastic fiber assembly.[6] One such example is a deficiency in elastin binding protein (EBP) which transports tropoelastin from its site of synthesis in the cell to the cell membrane. Costello syndrome (see p. 395) results from a functional deficiency in EBP.

Degrading of elastic tissue

Very few enzymes can degrade crosslinked elastin.[10] One of these is elastase, which is found in the pancreas and in neutrophils, macrophages, platelets, certain bacteria and cultured human fibroblasts.[9,10] Elastases exhibit a broad specificity. They are found in all classes of proteinases. Elastase activity is present in neutrophil elastase, cathepsin G, proteinase 3 and metalloproteinases 2 and 9 (gelatinases A and B).[11] The exact role of elastase in normal skin is uncertain; it plays a part in the elastolysis seen in anetoderma and in acquired cutis laxa associated with inflammatory skin lesions. Elastase inhibitors also exist; these include α_1-antitrypsin, α_2-macroglobulin and lysozyme.[12] There are two factors, vitronectin and delay-accelerating factor, which appear to prevent damage to elastic fibers by complement.[13] Further work is needed to clarify the role of these substances.

Age-related changes

There is evidence of continuing synthesis of elastic fibers throughout life, but after the age of 50 the new fibers are loosely rather than closely assembled.[14] With age, there is some loss of the superficial dermal fibers and a slow, progressive degradation of mature fibers.[9,15] This is accompanied by changes in collagen and extracellular matrix.[16,17] Ultrastructural changes include the formation of cystic spaces and lacunae, imparting a porous look to the fibers;[18,19] they may fragment or develop a fuzzy indistinct border.[18] The changes are quite distinct from those seen in solar elastosis.

Another age-related change is the deposition on elastic fibers of terminal complement complexes and vitronectin. This latter substance is a multi-functional glycoprotein that is hypothetically involved in the prevention of tissue damage in proximity to local complement activation.[20]

Staining of elastic tissue

Elastic tissue can be demonstrated in hematoxylin and eosin-stained sections if appropriate modifications, as described by O'Brien, are made.[21] Notwithstanding this method, the commonly used stains for elastic tissue are the orcein, aldehyde–fuchsin, Verhoeff and Weigert methods. However, the superficial fine elastic fibers do not stain with most of these methods, although they will with a modified orcein stain[9] and the Luna stain, which incorporates aldehyde–fuchsin and Weigert's iron hematoxylin.[22] The Luna stain also demonstrates a fibrillary component in solar elastosis. Elastic fibers stain a brilliant purple against a pale lavender background with this stain.[22] Miller's modification of Weigert's resorcin fuchsin has been suggested as the best method for demonstrating new elastic fibers.[23]

A monoclonal antibody, HB8, has been described as a stain for elastic fibers.[24] It has no advantages over the modified orcein, Luna or Miller stains.

Categorization of elastic tissue disorders

A simple classification of disorders of cutaneous elastic tissue divides them into those in which the elastic tissue is increased and those in which it is reduced.[25] The solar elastotic syndromes are best considered as a discrete group. Minor alterations in elastic tissue may occur in the various collagen disorders, in line with the observation that alterations in one component of the connective tissue matrix may influence the structure and function of others.[26] This group will not be considered in great detail here.

Although not categorized separately in this chapter, it should be remembered that elastic fibers are the most important structure to undergo transepidermal elimination. This can occur in elastosis perforans serpiginosa, perforating folliculitis, perforating pseudoxanthoma elasticum, solar elastosis, keratoacanthoma, healing wounds and hypertrophic discoid lupus erythematosus.

The clinical and pathological features of the major disorders of elastic tissue are summarized in Table 12.1.

Table 12.1 **Summary of the major disorders of elastic tissue**

Diagnosis	Clinical features	Pathology
Elastoma	Solitary or multiple; papules and disks; sometimes osteopoikilosis; linear variant reported	Increased, thick, branching elastic fibers
Linear focal elastosis	Palpable stria-like yellow lines; lumbosacral region	Numerous elongated wavy fibers, some with 'paintbrush' ends
Focal dermal elastosis	Late onset, PXE-like lesions	Increase in normal elastic fibers; no PXE changes
Elastoderma	Localized lax, wrinkled skin	Increased, pleomorphic elastic tissue in upper dermis
Elastofibroma	Deep scapular region; older age	Proliferation of collagen and elastic tissue
Elastosis perforans serpiginosa	Hyperkeratotic papules on face and neck	Papillary accumulation and transepidermal elimination of elastic tissue
Pseudoxanthoma elasticum (PXE)	Yellowish papules and plaques; angioid streaks	Fragmented and calcified elastic fibers in mid dermis; may perforate
Elastic globes	Asymptomatic	Basophilic cytoid bodies in the upper dermis
Solar elastosis	Thickened, furrowed skin	Accumulation of curled basophilic elastic fibers and elastic masses in upper dermis
Nodular elastosis	Usually periorbital with cysts and comedones	Comedones and usually solar elastosis
Elastotic nodules of the ears	Asymptomatic papules on the ear	Clumped masses of elastotic material
Collagenous and elastotic plaques	Waxy, linear plaques at juncture of palmar and dorsal skin	Thick collagen, some perpendicular; admixed granular, elastotic material; basophilic elastotic masses
Erythema ab igne	Follows repeated heat exposure	Elastotic material in dermis
Nevus anelasticus	Papular lesions on lower trunk; early onset, no inflammation	A 'minus nevus' with reduced, fragmented elastic tissue in reticular dermis
Perifollicular elastolysis	Common; face and back; often associated acne vulgaris	Loss of elastic tissue around follicles
Anetoderma	Well-circumscribed areas of soft, wrinkled skin; may have preceding inflammation or be secondary to some other disease	Loss of elastic fibers, particularly in mid dermis
Papillary-dermal elastolysis	Papules and cobblestone plaques on neck and upper trunk, resembling PXE	Loss of elastic tissue in papillary dermis; no calcification of remaining fibers
Mid-dermal elastolysis	Widespread patches of fine wrinkling; additional perifollicular papules in some cases; may have preceding inflammatory phase	Loss of elastic tissue from mid dermis
Cutis laxa	Widespread, large folds of pendulous skin; often involves internal organs; congenital or acquired	Fragmentation and loss of elastic fibers
Menkes' syndrome	Copper storage disease; brittle, 'steel wool' hair; vascular and neurological changes	Pili torti, often with monilethrix and trichorrhexis nodosa
'Granulomatous slack skin'	Pendulous skin in flexural areas; T-cell lymphoma	Lymphoid cells; granulomas with multinucleate giant cells; absence of elastic fibers

INCREASED ELASTIC TISSUE

Very little is known about the mechanisms which lead to an increase in dermal elastic tissue. Besides the conditions to be considered below, a mild increase in elastic tissue has been reported in osteogenesis imperfecta,[27] chronic acidosis,[28] amyotrophic lateral sclerosis[29] and some stages of radiation dermatitis.[30,31] The solar elastotic syndromes are also characterized by increased elastic tissue and they will be considered after this section.

ELASTOMA (ELASTIC NEVUS)

Elastoma (elastic nevus, juvenile elastoma,[32] nevus elasticus, connective tissue nevus of Lewandowsky type)[33] is a variant of connective tissue nevus (see p. 356) in which the predominant abnormality is an increase in dermal elastic

tissue.[34] The lesions may be solitary or multiple[32,35] and in the latter circumstance they are often associated with multiple small foci of sclerosis of bone (osteopoikilosis). This association is known as the Buschke–Ollendorf syndrome[36,37] and the cutaneous lesions as dermatofibrosis lenticularis disseminata. In several instances, the cutaneous lesions have shown abnormalities in collagen rather than elastic tissue (collagenomas)[38–40] and for this reason dermatofibrosis lenticularis disseminata is not entirely synonymous with the term 'elastoma'.[35]

The Buschke–Ollendorf syndrome is inherited as an autosomal dominant trait with variable expressivity.[36] Some family members have only cutaneous lesions or only bony lesions, but not both.[38,41,42]

Elastomas are usually small, flesh-colored or yellowish papules or disks, usually in asymmetric distribution on the lower trunk or extremities.[43] A large, multilobulated, exophytic variant has been reported.[44] They develop at an early age. Studies of the desmosine content of elastomas indicate a 3–7-fold increase in elastin.[45] There appears to be an abnormality of elastogenesis with faulty aggregation of elastin units associated with the overall increase in elastin.

Histopathology

Examination of hematoxylin and eosin-stained sections usually shows a normal dermis,[36] although sometimes there is an increase in its thickness. The epidermis may have a slight wavy pattern. Elastic tissue stains show an accumulation of broad, branching and interlacing elastic fibers in the mid and lower dermis (Fig. 12.1).[39] The papillary dermis is unaffected. Sometimes the elastic fibers encase the collagen in a marble-vein configuration.[32,46] Clumped elastic fibers have been reported;[47] they are a regular feature in linear focal elastosis.[48]

Uncommon changes include an increase in acid mucopolysaccharides,[39] slight thickening of collagen bundles or a well-developed vascular component.[49] Two cases have been reported with facial plaques and increased dermal elastic tissue;[50,51] in one, there was also perifollicular mucin.[51]

Electron microscopy

Ultrastructural findings have been variable.[45,52] Usually there are branched elastic fibers of variable diameter, without fragmentation. Elastic microfibrils may be replaced by granular or lucent material.[32,53] Collagen fibers are sometimes increased in diameter[52] and some fibroblasts may have dilated rough endoplasmic reticulum.[45] In linear focal elastosis, sequential maturation of elastic fibers can be seen, suggesting active elastogenesis.[54]

LINEAR FOCAL ELASTOSIS

Linear focal elastosis (elastotic striae) is a distinctive acquired lesion composed of palpable, stria-like, yellow lines that typically occur in the lumbosacral region.[48,54–60] There is a predilection for males. This condition, which has been likened to a keloid of elastic fibers, may be an unusual form of striae distensae (see p. 358).[58]

Histopathology

Numerous elongated, wavy elastic fibers are present in the mid dermis. At their ends, some fibers are split into a 'paintbrush formation'.[57] Fragmented fibers are also present. The elastic fibers have been reported as thickened[58] or thinned.

FOCAL DERMAL ELASTOSIS

Focal dermal elastosis is a distinct entity of late onset, characterized by a pseudoxanthoma elasticum-like eruption.[61,62] The elastin content of the skin is significantly increased.[63]

Histopathology

There is an increase in normal-appearing elastic fibers in the mid and deep dermis.[61] There are no changes of pseudoxanthoma elasticum.

ELASTODERMA

Elastoderma, an exceedingly rare condition, is an acquired, localized laxity of skin resembling cutis laxa with lax, extensible, wrinkled skin.[64,65] The lesions are not indurated. The clinical presentation differs, therefore, from nevus elasticus.

Histopathology

Elastoderma has an excessive accumulation of pleomorphic elastic tissue within the dermis, particularly the upper dermis. There are masses of thin, intertwined fibers.[64]

ELASTOFIBROMA

Elastofibroma (elastofibroma dorsi) is a slowly growing proliferation of collagen and abnormal elastic fibers with a predilection for the subscapular fascia of older individuals.[66–68] It is rarely found at other sites. Most elastofibromas are unilateral and asymptomatic. Nearly two-thirds of the 300 or more cases so far reported have been from Southern Japan.[69] Elastofibromas are gray-white or tan in color and measure 5–10 cm in diameter. The pathogenesis is unknown, but they may represent a reaction to prolonged mechanical stress, possibly involving disturbed elastic fibrillogenesis by periosteal-derived cells.[70] Subclinical elastofibromas have been found at autopsy.[71]

Histopathology

Elastofibromas are non-encapsulated lesions which blend with the surrounding fat and connective tissue.[67] They are composed of swollen collagen bundles admixed with numerous, irregular, lightly eosinophilic fibers and some

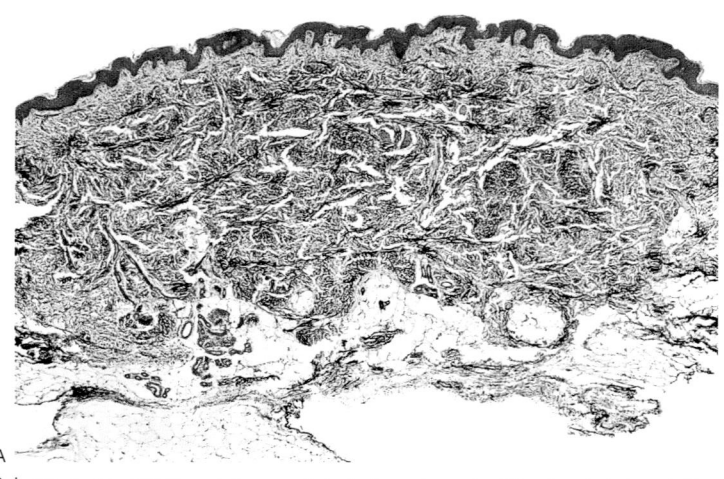
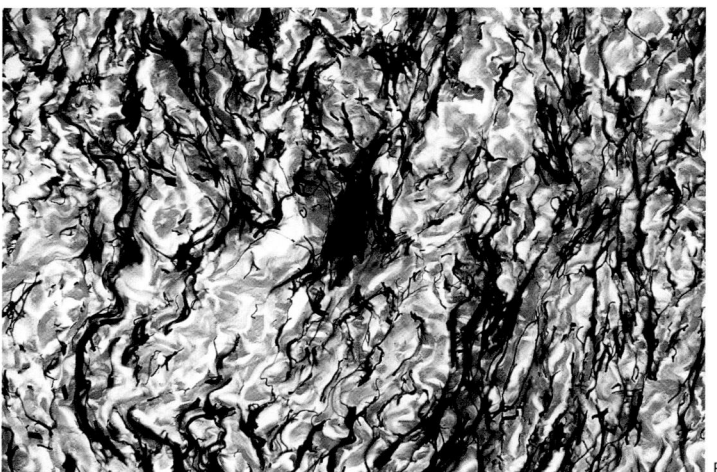

Fig. 12.1 **Elastoma. (A)** There is increased elastic tissue in much of the dermis, but excluding either end (Orcein). **(B)** There are coarse irregular clumps of elastic tissue within the reticular dermis. (Verhoeff van Gieson)

mature fat (Fig. 12.2). The fibers, which account for almost 50% of the tissue, stain black with the Verhoeff elastic stain. Some fibers are branched while others show a serrated edge.

Electron microscopy

Electron microscopy confirms the presence of abnormal elastic fibers, which result from a proliferation of elastic fibrils around the original elastic fibers.[71] Large ('active') fibroblasts[66] and cells with the features of myofibroblasts[72] have both been described.

ELASTOSIS PERFORANS SERPIGINOSA

Elastosis perforans serpiginosa (also known as perforating elastosis) presents as small papules, either grouped or in a circinate or serpiginous arrangement, on the neck, upper extremities, upper trunk or face.[73-78] Rarely, the lesions are generalized.[79,80] There is a predilection for males, with the onset usually in the second decade. Familial cases have been reported.[81-83] An autosomal dominant mode of inheritance with variable expressivity of the trait has been suggested.[84] In up to a third of cases there is an associated systemic condition or connective tissue disorder: these include Down syndrome,[80,85,86]

osteogenesis imperfecta,[87] cutis laxa,[88] Ehlers–Danlos syndrome, Marfan's syndrome, acrogeria, scleroderma,[89,90] an abnormal 47,XYY karyotype,[91] diabetes mellitus[92] and chronic renal failure.[93]

Similar cutaneous lesions have been reported in patients with Wilson's disease and cystinuria receiving long-term penicillamine therapy.[88,94-98] In these patients, a local copper depletion or a direct effect of penicillamine on elastin synthesis may be responsible for the formation of the abnormal elastic fibers, which are then eliminated transepidermally.[94,99] Elastic tissue damage appears to occur in other organs as well, a feature generally lacking in the usual idiopathic form of the disease.[99,100] The nature of the defect in the idiopathic form is unknown, but it is possible that perforating elastosis is the final common pathway for more than one abnormality of elastic fibers.[74,101] This theory is compatible with the recent finding of an elastin receptor in keratinocytes immediately surrounding the elastic materials being eliminated in lesions of elastosis perforans serpiginosa.[102] The elastin receptor may be involved in the interaction between keratinocytes and elastin.[102]

Histopathology[73-76]

In fully developed lesions there is a localized area of hyperplastic epidermis, associated with a channel through which the basophilic nuclear debris and brightly eosinophilic fragmented elastic fibers are being eliminated (Fig.12.3).

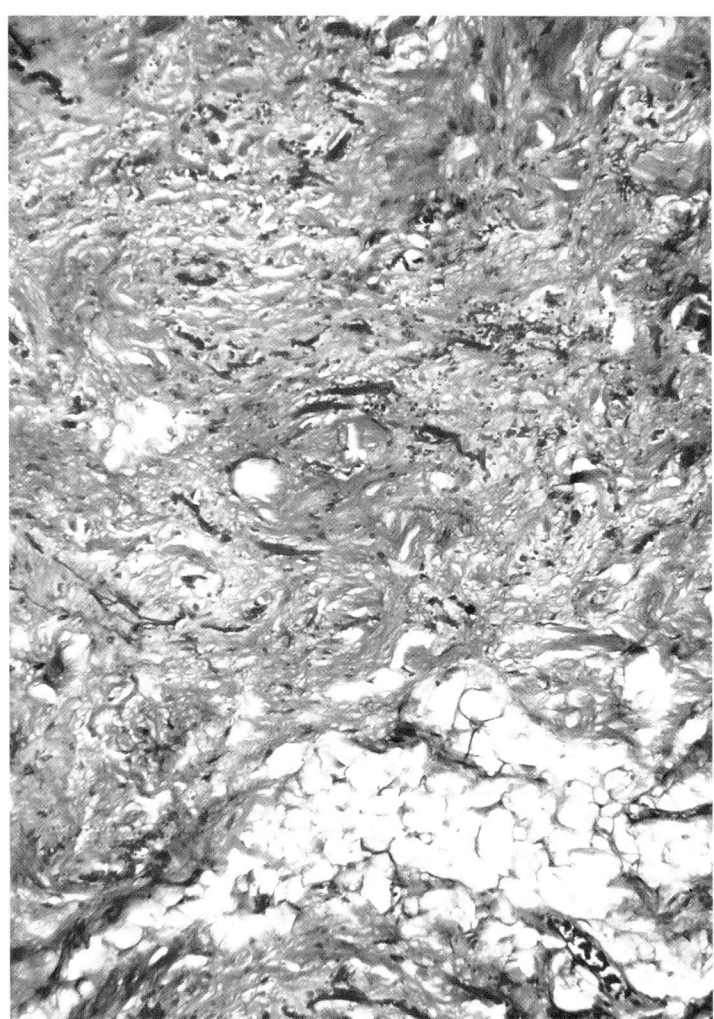

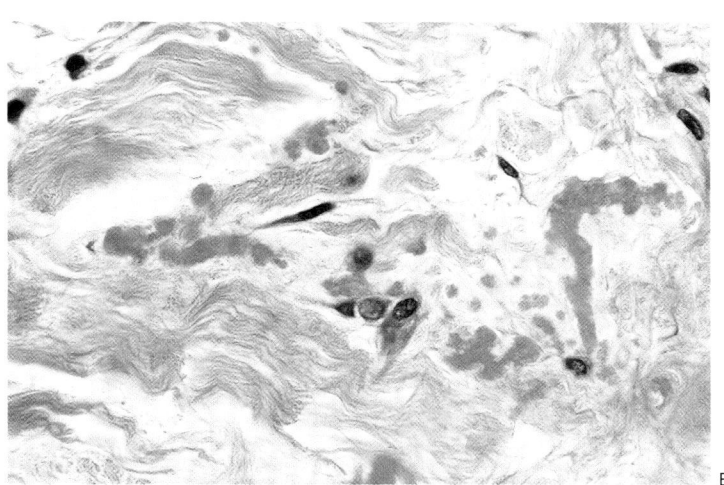

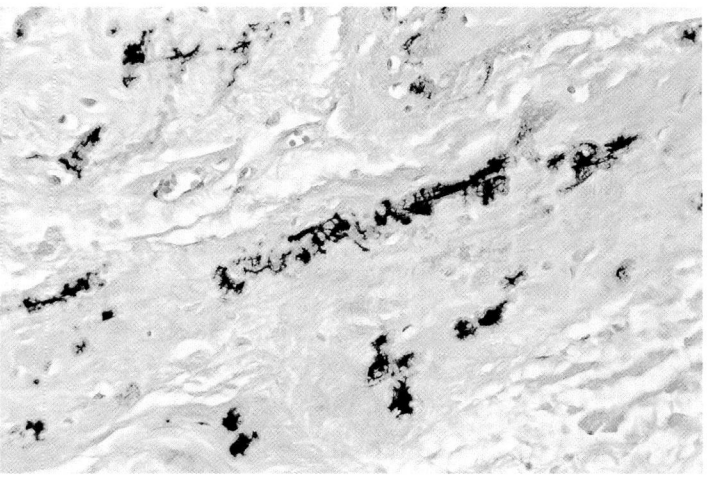

Fig. 12.2 **Elastofibroma dorsi. (A)** Coarse elastic fibers are admixed with collagen and adipose tissue. **(B)** The fibers have an irregular outline (H & E). **(C)** An elastic tissue stain confirms the irregular outline. (Verhoeff van Gieson)

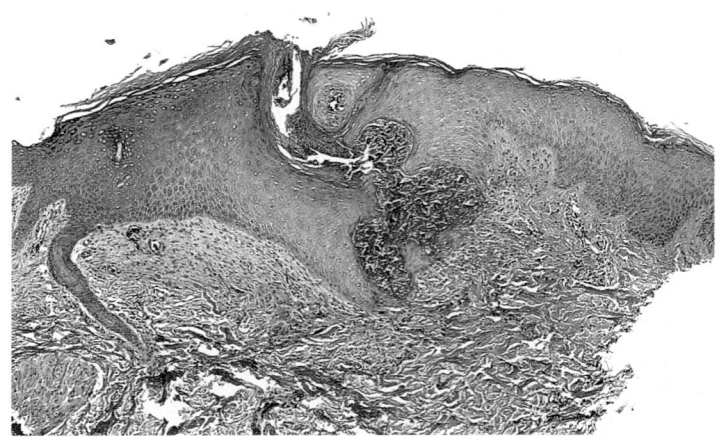

Fig. 12.3 **Elastosis perforans serpiginosa.** Debris is entering a channel within the epidermis. (H & E)

A keratinous plug usually overlies this channel, which may take the form of a dilated infundibular structure or a more oblique canal coursing through hyperplastic epidermis, follicular epithelium or the acrosyringium (Figs 12.4,

12.5). When the canal is oblique, sections may only show a surface plug of keratinous debris and a localized area of hyperplastic epidermis which in its lower portion forms a bulbous protrusion into the dermis. This appears to envelop an area of the papillary dermis containing basophilic debris and some refractile eosinophilic elastic fibers.

Elastic tissue stains show increased numbers of coarse elastic fibers in the papillary dermis. Some of these appear to overlap the basal epidermal cells. In the region of their transepidermal elimination, the elastic fibers lose their staining properties as they enter the canal and become brightly eosinophilic. They will stain with the Giemsa method. A few foreign body giant cells and inflammatory cells are often present in the dermis adjacent to the channel. In older lesions, there is focal dermal scarring and usually an absence of elastic fibers.

IgM, C3 and C4 were demonstrated on the abnormal elastic fibers in the papillary dermis in one of two cases studied by immunofluorescence.[103]

In *penicillamine-related cases*, there is an increased number of thickened elastic fibers in the reticular dermis and less hyperplasia of elastic fibers in the papillary dermis, except in the areas of active transepidermal elimination.[104] The elastic fibers are irregular in outline with buds and serrations. This may be discerned in hematoxylin and eosin-stained preparations, but it is well shown by elastic tissue stains[105] or in Epon-embedded thin sections stained with toluidine blue.[99]

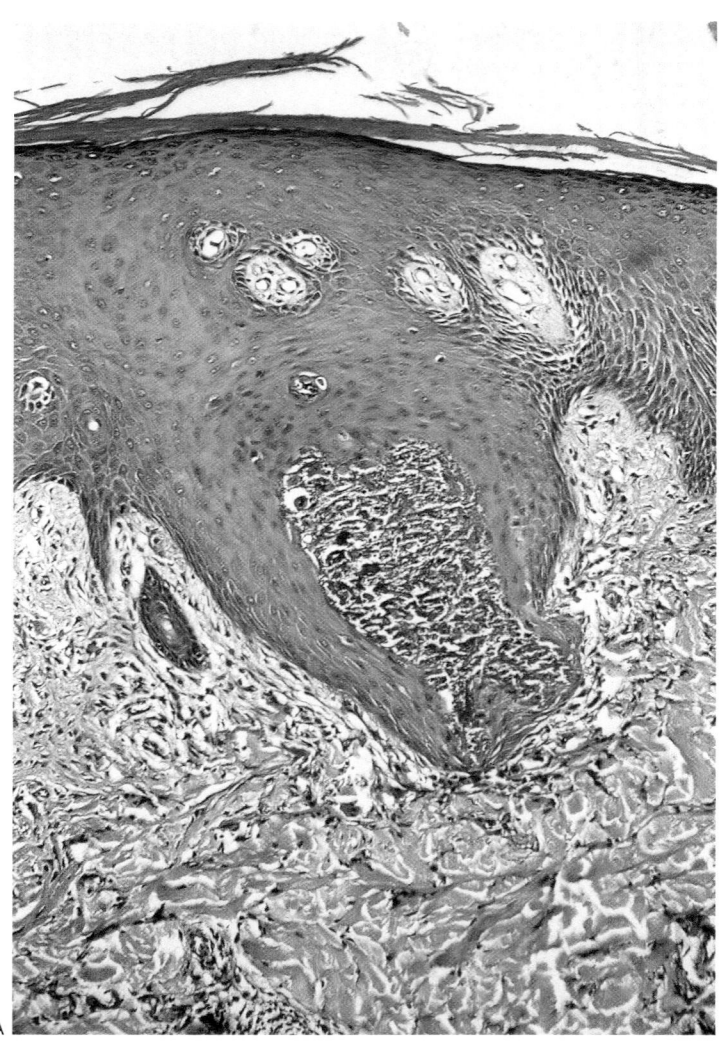
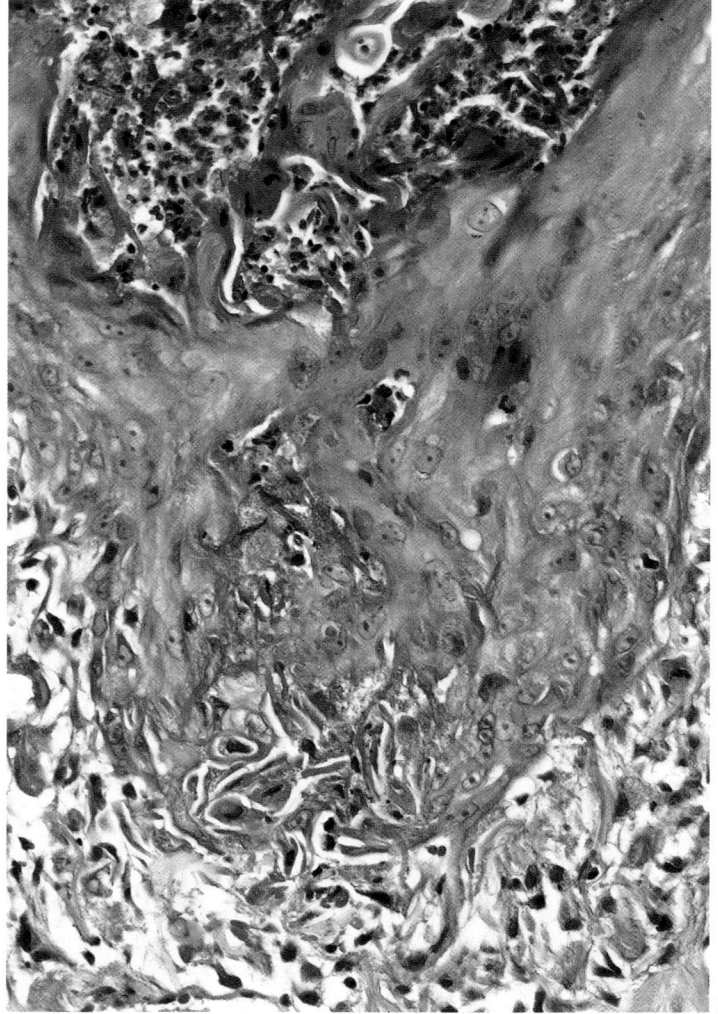

Fig. 12.4 **(A) Elastosis perforans serpiginosa. (B)** Debris and elastic fibers are being enveloped by a bulbous protrusion of the epidermis. (H & E)

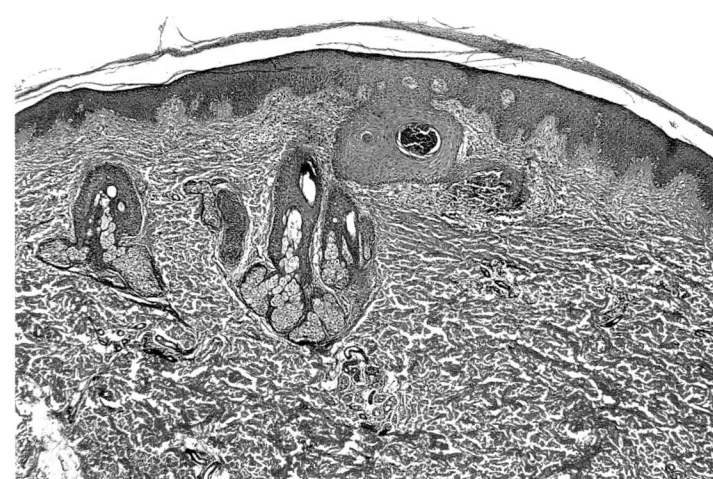

Fig. 12.5 **Elastosis perforans serpiginosa.** Another case with a less obvious epidermal channel. (H & E)

Electron microscopy

Ultrastructural examination of the dermis in penicillamine-related cases shows that the elastic fibers have a normal core and an irregular coat with thorn-like protrusions at regular intervals, the so-called 'lumpy bumpy' or 'bramble-bush' fibers.[104–107] Collagen fibers are also abnormal with extreme variations in thickness.[107,108] Electron microscopy of *idiopathic cases* has shown increased numbers of large elastic fibers which are convoluted and branching.[109] Fine filaments, similar to those in embryonic elastic fibers, are present on the surface of the fibers.[109,110]

PSEUDOXANTHOMA ELASTICUM

Pseudoxanthoma elasticum is an inherited disorder of connective tissue in which calcification of elastic fibers occurs in certain areas of the skin, eyes and cardiovascular system.[111–116] Skin changes are usually evident by the second decade and consist of closely set yellowish papules with a predilection for flexural creases, particularly in the neck and axillae and less commonly in the groins, periumbilical area and the cubital and popliteal fossae.[112–114] Oral lesions may occur.[115] The skin becomes wrinkled and thickened and eventually may become lax and redundant, resembling cutis laxa.[117–119] The calcium content of affected skin may be up to several hundred times normal.[120] Eye changes include angioid streaks and a degenerative choroidoretinitis which may lead to blindness. Calcification of elastic fibers in arteries and intimal and endocardial fibroelastosis develop. The vascular changes may lead to hypertension, sudden cardiac death,[121] cerebrovascular accidents and gastrointestinal hemorrhage.[122–124]

Genetic studies have shown a heterogeneous pattern.[125] There are two variants with autosomal dominant inheritance and two with autosomal recessive inheritance. In dominant type 1, there are cutaneous changes and often vascular complications and severe choroidoretinitis. In dominant type 2, there is an atypical yellowish macular rash, only mild retinal changes and no vascular complications. Recessive type 1, which appears to be the most common form, is of intermediate severity with classic skin changes.[126,127] Recessive type 2 is exceedingly rare and has generalized cutaneous laxity but no systemic complications.[125,128] Genetic studies are made difficult by the limited phenotypic expression of the disease in some parents of affected offspring.[129] The candidate gene underlying the majority of cases with pseudoxanthoma elasticum has been mapped to a distinct region in the short

arm of chromosome 16, at 16p13.1.[126] Recently, mutations in the *MRP6* gene, a member of the ABC transporter gene family, have been implicated in the etiology.[130] The exact location of this gene was not mentioned in the report.[130]

There has been one report of spontaneous resolution and repair of elastic tissue calcification.[131] Hyperphosphatasia has been present in several cases.[132] The administration of vitamin D_3 results in the further deposition of calcium salts.[133] Urinary glycosaminoglycan levels are elevated early in the disease.[134] Patients purported to have coexisting elastosis perforans serpiginosa and pseudoxanthoma elasticum have been reported; they are now regarded as having perforating pseudoxanthoma elasticum.[135–137] Many of these patients have so-called 'acquired pseudoxanthoma elasticum' (see below).

The factors that lead to the calcification of initially normal elastic fibers in pseudoxanthoma elasticum are not known.[138] Polyanionic material is deposited in association with the calcified material. Cultured fibroblasts from patients with this condition release a proteolytic substance and it has been postulated that this may cause selective damage to elastin, leading to calcification.[139] Fibrillin appears to be abnormal in only isolated cases (unlike the findings in Marfan's syndrome).[140] Decreased deposition of fibrillin 2 has been reported in pseudoxanthoma elasticum.[141]

Acquired pseudoxanthoma elasticum

Acquired pseudoxanthoma elasticum refers to an etiologically and clinically diverse group of patients with late onset of the disease, no family history, absence of vascular and retinal stigmata and identical dermal histology.[116,142,143] The term 'perforating calcific elastosis' has been suggested for some of these cases.[144] Included in this group are individuals exposed to calcium salts, including farmers exposed to Norwegian saltpeter (calcium and ammonium nitrate),[145,146] and obese, usually multiparous black women who develop reticulated and atrophic plaques and some discrete papules around the umbilicus[137,144,147] or lower chest.[148] Perforation is common in this latter group.[149] Patients with chronic renal failure on dialysis have also been reported with this acquired variant.[142,150,151] Approximately 10% of patients with β-thalassemia exhibit both ocular and skin alterations of pseudoxanthoma elasticum.[152]

Pseudo-pseudoxanthoma elasticum refers to the development of the systemic changes of pseudoxanthoma elasticum in a patient on long-term penicillamine therapy for Wilson's disease. However, it has also been used for the cases referred to above as acquired pseudoxanthoma elasticum.[153]

Histopathology[114]

There are short, curled, frayed, basophilic elastic fibers in the reticular dermis, particularly in the upper and mid parts (Fig. 12.6). The papillary dermis is spared except at sites of transepidermal elimination (perforation). The elastic fibers in affected skin are stained black with the von Kossa method (Fig. 12.7). They stain with the Verhoeff method and there is intense blue staining with phosphotungstic acid hematoxylin (PTAH). Calcinosis cutis[154] and osteoma cutis[119] are rare complications.

If perforation is present, there is a focal central erosion or tunnel with surrounding pseudoepitheliomatous hyperplasia or prominent acanthosis (Fig. 12.8). Basophilic elastic fibers are extruded through this defect. Sometimes foreign body giant cells, histiocytes and a few chronic inflammatory cells are present when there is perforation or traumatic ulceration.[155,156] The giant cells may then engulf some elastic fibers.

Electron microscopy

Calcification occurs initially in the central zones of the elastic fibers.[157] There

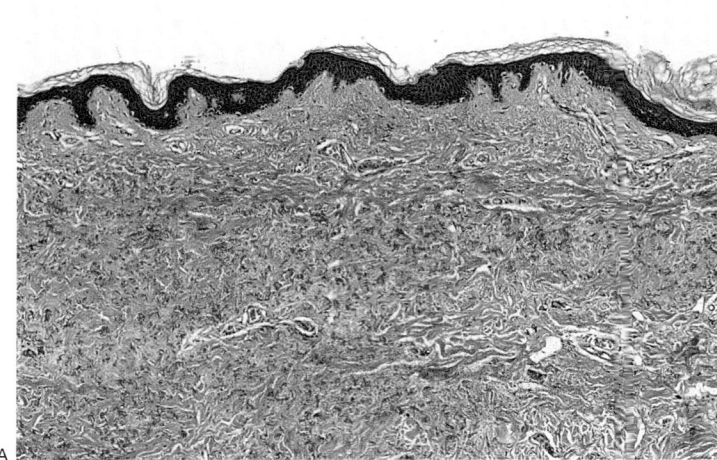 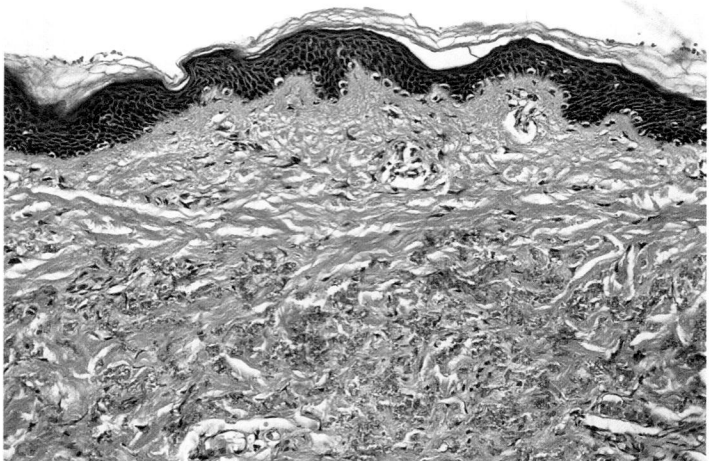

Fig. 12.6 **(A) Pseudoxanthoma elasticum. (B)** Note the short, curled elastic fibers in the reticular dermis. (H & E)

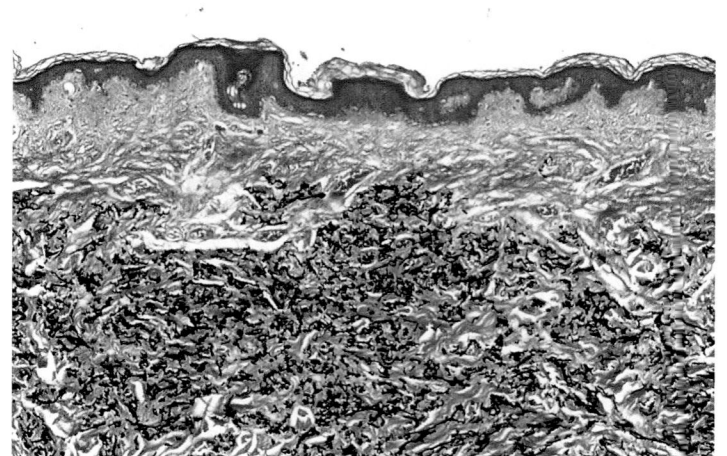

Fig. 12.7 **Pseudoxanthoma elasticum.** Calcium salts are deposited on the abnormal elastic fibers. (von Kossa)

is also some calcification of intercellular spaces and occasionally also of collagen fibers; the latter change may be reversible.[132,148] There is continuing elastogenesis with some normal elastic fibers.[132] Twisted collagen fibrils and thready material,[158] which has been found to contain fibrinogen, collagenous protein and glycoprotein, are also present.[159] This indicates that the abnormality is not limited to the elastic fibers.

ELASTIC GLOBES

Elastic globes are small basophilic bodies, found in the upper dermis of clinically normal skin, which stain positively for elastic fibers (Fig. 12.9). They are considered with the other dermal cytoid bodies on page 438. Numerous elastic globes have been reported in a patient with epidermolysis bullosa whose skin was wrinkled[160] and in a patient with the cartilage–hair hypoplasia syndrome, whose skin was hyperextensible.[161]

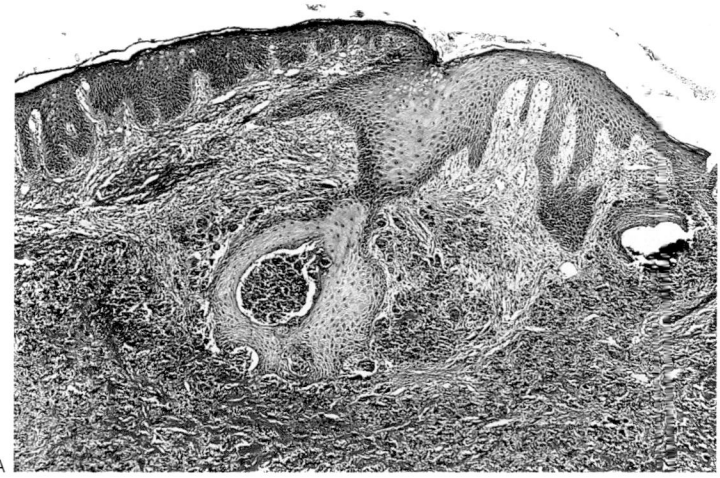 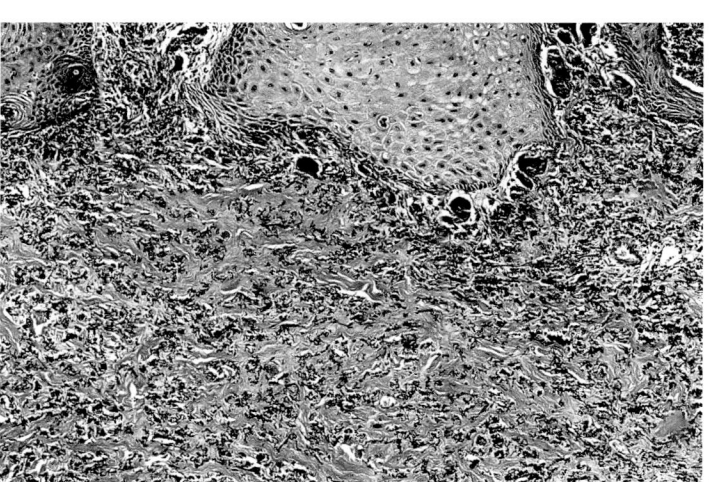

Fig. 12.8 **(A) Perforating pseudoxanthoma elasticum. (B)** The elastic fibers which are about to undergo transepithelial elimination are short, curled and frayed. Clumped elastic fibers are also present. (Verhoeff van Gieson)

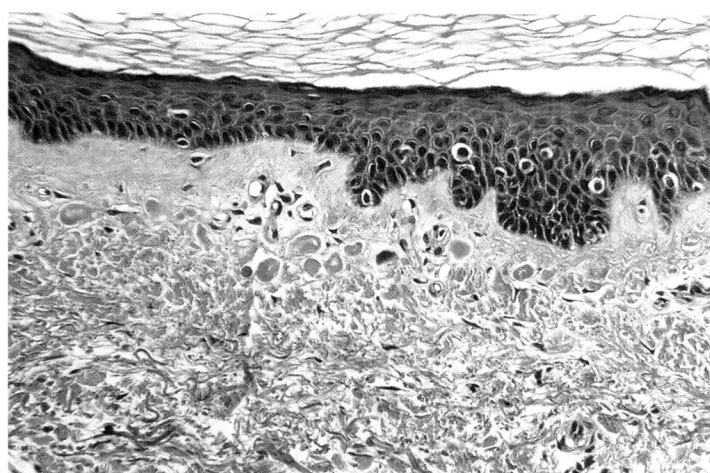
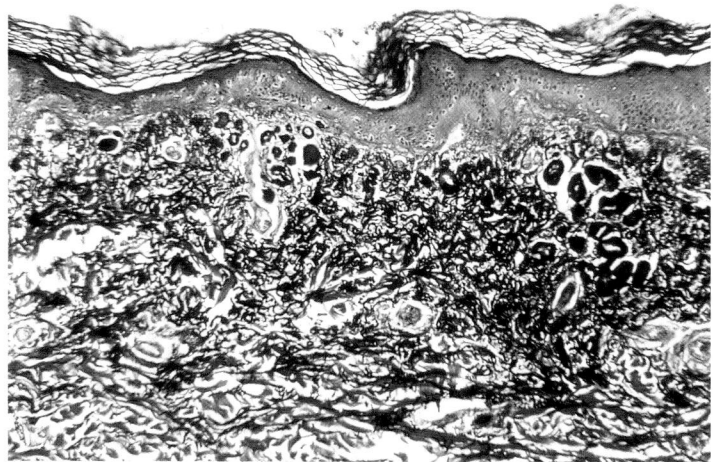

Fig. 12.9 **Elastic globes. (A)** There are multiple, round and ovoid deposits in the papillary dermis. Solar elastosis is also present (H & E). **(B)** An elastic tissue stain of the same case. (Verhoeff van Gieson)

SOLAR ELASTOTIC SYNDROMES

The term 'solar elastosis' refers to the accumulation of abnormal elastic tissue in the dermis in response to long-term sun exposure. Photoaging is a process distinct from the changes taking place due to chronological aging, although photoaging does increase in severity with chronological aging.[162,163] The cosmetic effects of photodamage are assuming increasing importance in society. There are many different clinical patterns of solar elastosis, some of which form distinct clinicopathological entities.[164,165] Other clinical patterns are histologically indistinguishable from one another and they are usually grouped together under the umbrella term 'solar elastosis'.

The following entities are regarded as solar elastotic syndromes:

- solar elastosis
- nodular elastosis with cysts and comedones
- elastotic nodules of the ears
- collagenous and elastotic plaques of the hands.

Colloid milium can also be regarded as a solar elastotic syndrome, as it appears that the colloid substance derives, at least in major part, from elastic fibers through actinic degeneration.[166] Colloid degeneration (paracolloid, colloid milium-like solar elastosis) has overlapping features histologically with both colloid milium and solar elastosis. These topics are considered with the cutaneous deposits in Chapter 14 (pp. 434 and 435).

Solar elastotic skin is more susceptible than normal skin to chronic infections with *Staphylococcus aureus* and several other bacteria. This results from a decline in the adaptive capabilities of the immune system.[167] Uncommonly, this results in a chronic suppurative process, variants of which have been reported as 'coral reef granuloma' and blastomycosis-like pyoderma (see p. 622). Actinic comedonal plaque, in which fibrous tissue and comedones are present with some residual elastosis at the periphery, can be the end-stage picture of this inflammatory process.

Another secondary change that may occur in sun-damaged skin is the formation of actinic granulomas in which there is a granulomatous response to solar elastotic material and its resorption by macrophages and giant cells (elastophagocytosis, elastoclasis).[168] Actinic granulomas present clinically as one or more annular lesions with an atrophic center and an elevated border. They are considered with the granulomatous tissue reaction (see p. 209).

Elastophagocytosis has also been reported in association with various inflammatory processes in sun-protected skin.[169]

Ultraviolet light is usually incriminated in the etiology of the degenerative changes.[170] Human studies have demonstrated that small amounts of UVA or solar-simulated UV are capable of producing cutaneous photodamage.[171,172] However, it has been suggested that infrared radiation may also contribute, as changes characteristic of solar elastosis are seen in erythema ab igne.[173] Although not usually regarded as one of the elastotic syndromes, this condition will be considered in this section because of its similar histological appearances. Two further causes of heightened elastosis are cigarette smoking[174] and photosensitivity resulting from the therapeutic use of hydroxyurea.[175]

SOLAR ELASTOSIS (ACTINIC ELASTOSIS)

The usual clinical appearance of solar elastosis is thickened, dry, coarsely wrinkled skin with loss of skin tone.[176] Sometimes there is a yellowish hue. There may be some telangiectasia and pigmentary changes (poikilodermatous changes) in severe cases.[177,178] The best recognized clinical variant is cutis rhomboidalis in which there is thickened, deeply fissured skin on the back of the neck. Other clinical patterns include citrine skin, Dubreuilh's and other elastomas[179] and solar elastotic bands of the forearm.[180] Bullous lesions are extremely rare.[181]

The origin of the elastotic material has been the subject of much debate. It has been attributed to the degradation of collagen or elastic fibers or both.[182,183] Alternatively, it has been suggested by others that the material results from the actinic stimulation of fibroblasts.[184] More recent work indicates that the elastotic material is primarily derived from elastic fibers.[185] The increased elastin appears to result from transcriptional activation of the elastin gene.[186,187] A small amount of type I and VI collagen and procollagen type III are present, but the significance of this finding remains uncertain.[185] Photoaging results in the accumulation of glycosaminoglycans on the elastotic material in the upper dermis and not between collagen and elastic fibers as in normal skin.[188] Collagen VII is reduced and this may contribute to the formation of wrinkles by weakening the bond between the dermis and the epidermis.[189] Matrix metalloproteinases 7 and 12 are increased in photodamaged skin; they may contribute to remodeling of elastotic areas.[190,191]

Metalloproteinase-1 may be responsible for the degeneration and reduction in collagen.[192–194] Other consequences of photoaging are mutations in p53 and the partial loss of the ability of epidermal cells to differentiate normally.[195] The changes are qualitatively quite different from those seen in chronological aging,[196,197] contrary to the assertion of some.[198]

Various therapies have been used in recent times to improve the clinical appearance of photoaged skin. One such technique, dermabrasion, produces clinical improvement by the synthesis of type I collagen.[199] Another technique, the prolonged application of topical tretinoin (retinoic acid), produces epidermal thickening,[200–203] hypergranulosis, an increase in epidermal Langerhans cells,[168] the deposition of collagen in the papillary dermis[204] and, sometimes, an increase in fine elastic fibers in the papillary dermis.[205] These changes may result in an improved clinical appearance,[206] although this has not occurred in all studies.[207] The prolonged use of sunscreens results in a significant reduction in the amount of solar elastosis and other harmful effects.[208,209]

Histopathology

In mild actinic damage there is a proliferation of elastic fibers in the papillary dermis. These are normal or slightly increased in thickness. In established cases the papillary and upper reticular dermis is replaced by accumulations of thickened, curled and serpiginous fibers forming tangled masses which are basophilic in hematoxylin and eosin-stained sections (Fig. 12.10).[14] Sometimes there are amorphous masses of elastotic material in which the outline of fibers is lost except at the periphery. These masses are thought to form from the tangled fibers, as transitions can be seen on electron microscopy. A thin grenz zone of normal-appearing collagen is present in the subepidermal zone.[210] This may have lost its network of fine vertical fibers. Collagen is reduced in amount in the reticular dermis. Transepidermal elimination of elastotic material can occur.[211] This process is not uncommon following cryotherapy to severely damaged skin, which seems to trigger it in some individuals (Fig. 12.11). The elastotic material stains black with the Verhoeff stain (Fig. 12.12). Sometimes the homogeneous deposits are less well stained. Melanocytes and Merkel cells are both increased in number.[212,213]

Biopsies from individuals with chronic sunlight exposure, some of whom had persistent erythema, have been described as showing a 'perivenular histiocytic-lymphocytic infiltrate in which numerous mast cells, often in close apposition to fibroblasts, were observed': this condition has been termed **'chronic heliodermatitis'**.[214]

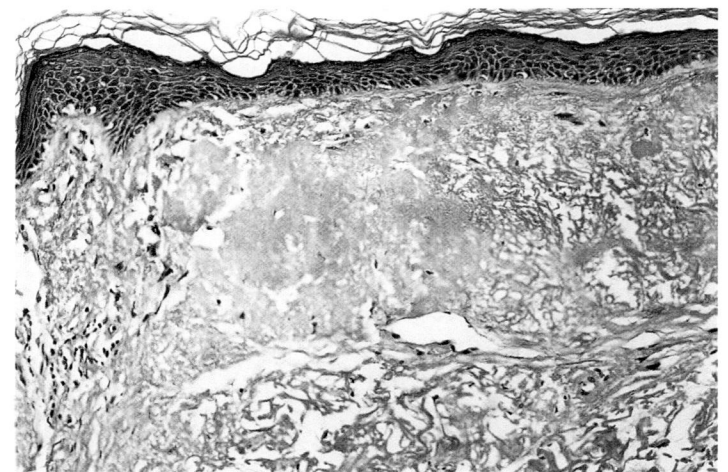

Fig. 12.10 **Solar elastosis** with amorphous and fibrillary material in the upper dermis. (H & E)

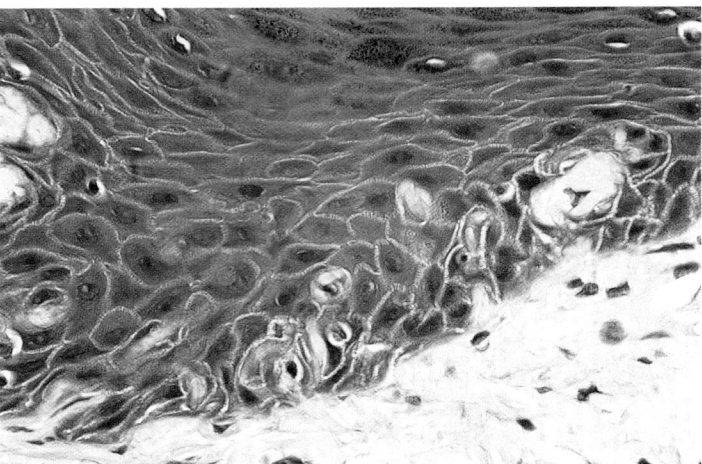

Fig. 12.11 **Solar elastosis.** Curled elastotic fibers are insinuating between basal keratinocytes. This represents the early stages of the transepidermal elimination of these damaged fibers. (H & E)

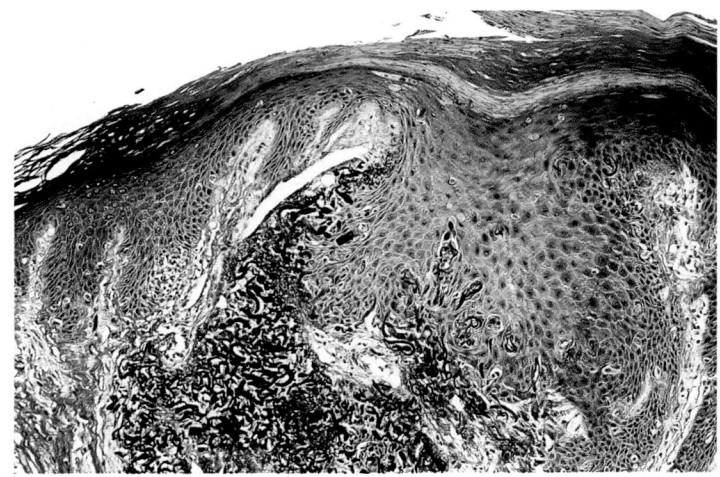

Fig. 12.12 **Perforating solar elastosis.** The elastic fibers being eliminated are thick, curled and serpiginous in morphology. (Verhoeff van Gieson)

Epidermal changes also occur in severely damaged skin. The stratum corneum may be compact and laminated or gelatinous; it sometimes contains vesicles full of proteinaceous material.[215] In the malpighian layer, cell heterogeneity, vacuolization and dysplasia may be found.[215]

Electron microscopy

A spectrum of ultrastructural changes is found which parallels the clinical degree of damage.[14,216,217] In mild cases, the elastic fibers in the papillary dermis are increased in number. The microfibrillar dense zones become irregular in outline, more electron dense and many times larger. In severe cases the elastin matrix becomes granular and develops lucent areas around the microfibrillar dense zones.[14] Some fibers become disrupted and show a moth-eaten appearance or become transformed into finely granular bodies.[14] Similar ultrastructural findings have been reported in chronic radiodermatitis.[218] Deformed collagen fibers, of various diameters, are found in the papillary dermis.[219] Following PUVA therapy, the elastic fiber changes include a breakdown of the microfibrils and subsequent fragmentation of the elastic fibers.[220] Melanocytes show degenerative changes with the development of large intracytoplasmic vacuoles.[212]

Scanning electron microscopy of solar elastosis shows some normal fibers, some thick damaged cylindrical fibers and large masses of markedly changed fibers, which probably correspond to the amorphous deposits seen in severe cases.[221]

NODULAR ELASTOSIS WITH CYSTS AND COMEDONES

The solar degenerative condition, nodular elastosis with cysts and comedones, is also known as the Favre–Racouchot syndrome. It occurs as thickened yellowish plaques studded with cysts and open comedones.[222–224] It involves the head and neck, but particularly the skin around the eyes. Lesions may extend to the temporal and zygomatic areas. A case involving the shoulder region has been reported.[225] There is a predilection for males who have a history of prolonged solar exposure. Smoking may act in conjunction with solar damage to potentiate the development of this condition.[226]

Histopathology[222,223]
In addition to the marked solar elastosis, there are dilated follicles and comedones which contain keratinous debris in the lumen. The sebaceous glands are often atrophic. A recent study of patients without much solar exposure showed multiple comedones without significant solar elastosis, suggesting that the two processes might be independent.[227]

ELASTOTIC NODULES OF THE EARS

Elastotic nodules are small, usually asymptomatic, pale papules and nodules found predominantly on the anterior crus of the antihelix in response to actinic damage.[228–230] They are often bilateral. There is a marked predilection for elderly white males. Rare cases develop on the helix, where they may be painful, simulating chondrodermatitis nodularis helicis. They may be diagnosed clinically as basal cell carcinoma, amyloid or even small gouty tophi.

Histopathology[229]
There is marked elastotic degeneration of the dermis with the formation of irregular, coarse elastotic fibers and larger clumped masses of elastotic material (Figs 12.13, 12.14). These changes are best seen with the Verhoeff elastic stain. The overlying epidermis shows mild to moderate orthokeratosis and some irregular acanthosis. There is mild telangiectasia of vessels in the papillary dermis, and some new collagen is often present in this area.

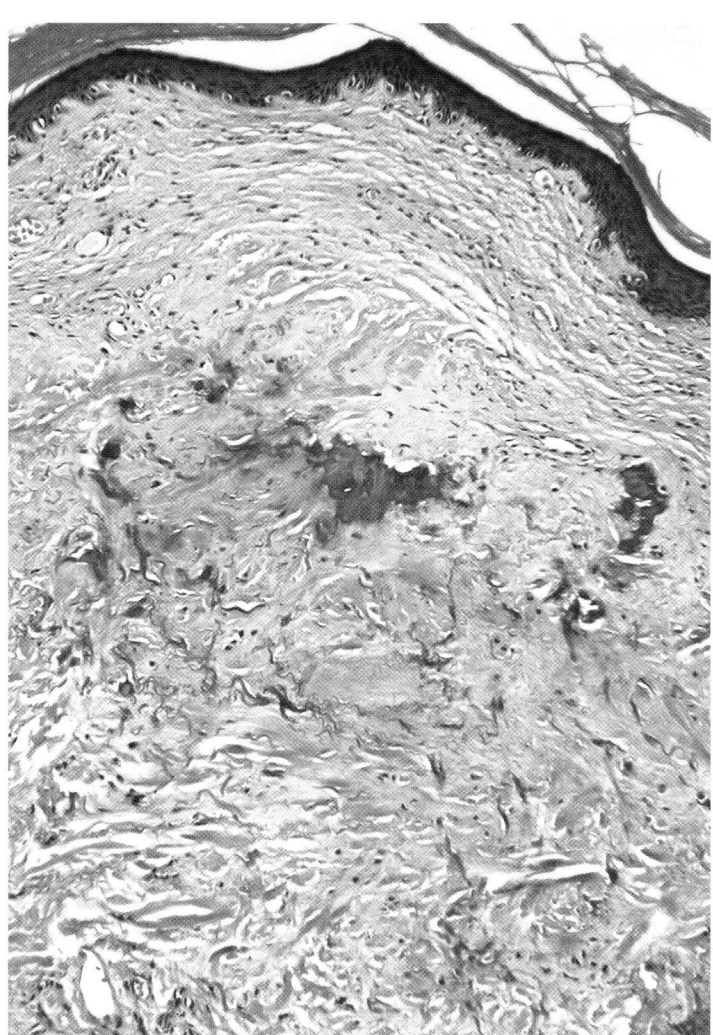
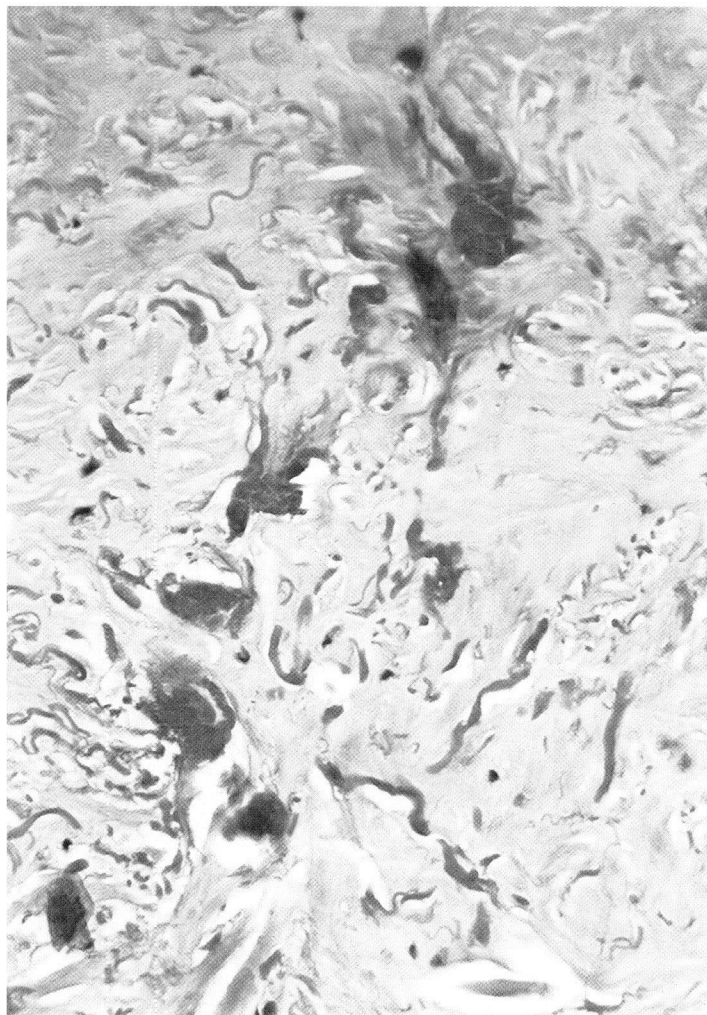

Fig. 12.13 **(A) Elastotic nodule of the ear. (B)** Clumped masses of elastotic material are present in the mid dermis. (H & E)

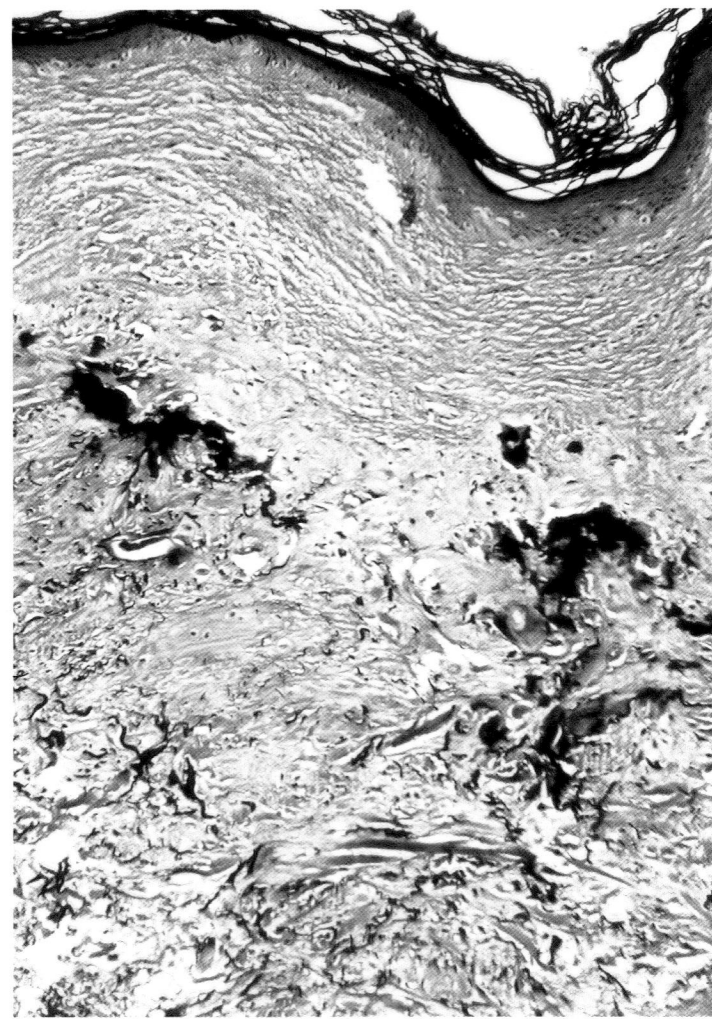

Fig. 12.14 **Elastotic nodule of the ear.** There are clumped masses of elastotic material. (Verhoeff van Gieson)

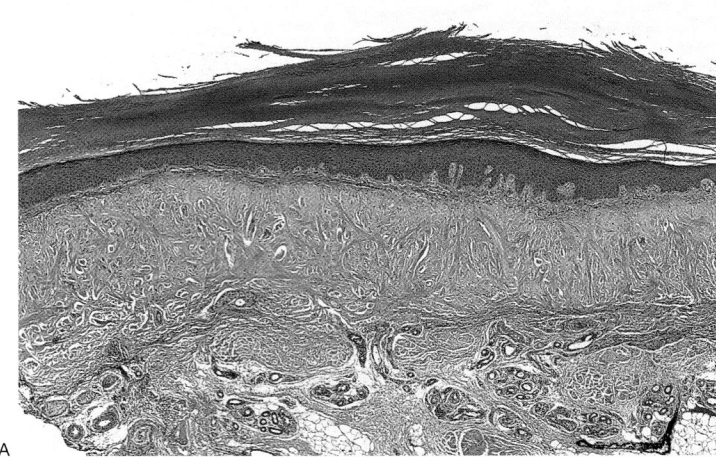

A

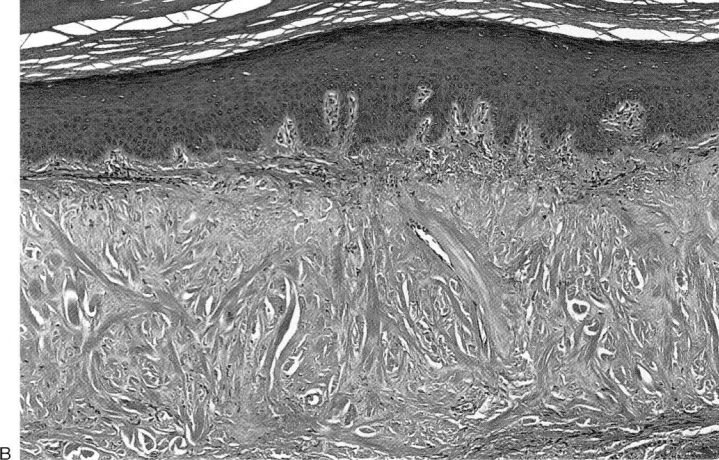

B

Fig. 12.15 **(A) Collagenous and elastotic plaque. (B)** The collagen bundles in the upper dermis have a characteristic haphazard arrangement with some bundles arranged vertically. Elastotic material is admixed. (H & E)

COLLAGENOUS AND ELASTOTIC PLAQUES OF THE HANDS

Also known as 'degenerative collagenous plaques of the hands', 'keratoelastoidosis marginalis' and 'digital papular calcific elastosis',[231] collagenous and elastotic plaques of the hands is a slowly progressive, degenerative condition found predominantly in older males.[232–235] There are waxy, linear plaques at the juncture of palmar and dorsal skin of the hands. The condition particularly involves the medial aspect of the thumbs and the lateral (radial) aspect of the adjacent index finger. In this respect the lesions resemble in part those seen in the genodermatosis acrokeratoelastoidosis (see p. 291).[232] Physical trauma of a repetitive nature and prolonged actinic exposure may play a role in the etiology of collagenous and elastotic plaques of the hand.[234,236]

Histopathology

The most noticeable changes are in the dermis where there are numerous thick collagen bundles having a haphazard arrangement, but with a proportion running perpendicular to the surface (Fig. 12.15).[237] There is often a slight basophilic tint to the dermis; elastotic fibers can be seen in the lower papillary dermis and intimately admixed with the collagen bundles in the reticular dermis. Basophilic elastotic masses are found in the upper dermis.[231] The dermis shows reduced cellularity with large areas devoid of fibroblasts.[235] Sweat ducts may be mildly dilated in the mid dermis and compressed in other areas.

In elastic tissue stains, the elastotic material in the lower papillary dermis is confirmed (Fig. 12.16). In the reticular dermis, granular and elastotic material can be seen in an intimate relationship within some of the larger collagen bundles.[232] In some cases, there are focal deposits of calcification in the dermis. The changes are distinct from those of solar elastosis.

The overlying epidermis may show mild hyperkeratosis and thickening of the granular layer. In some cases there is slight acanthosis, while in others there may be loss of the rete pattern.

ERYTHEMA AB IGNE

Erythema ab igne refers to the development of persistent areas of reticular erythema, with or without pigmentation, at the sites of repeated exposure to heat, usually from open hearths.[238,239] The lower legs are usually involved. Erythema ab igne is now seen only rarely.[240] Keratoses and, rarely, squamous cell carcinomas may develop in lesions of long standing.[241]

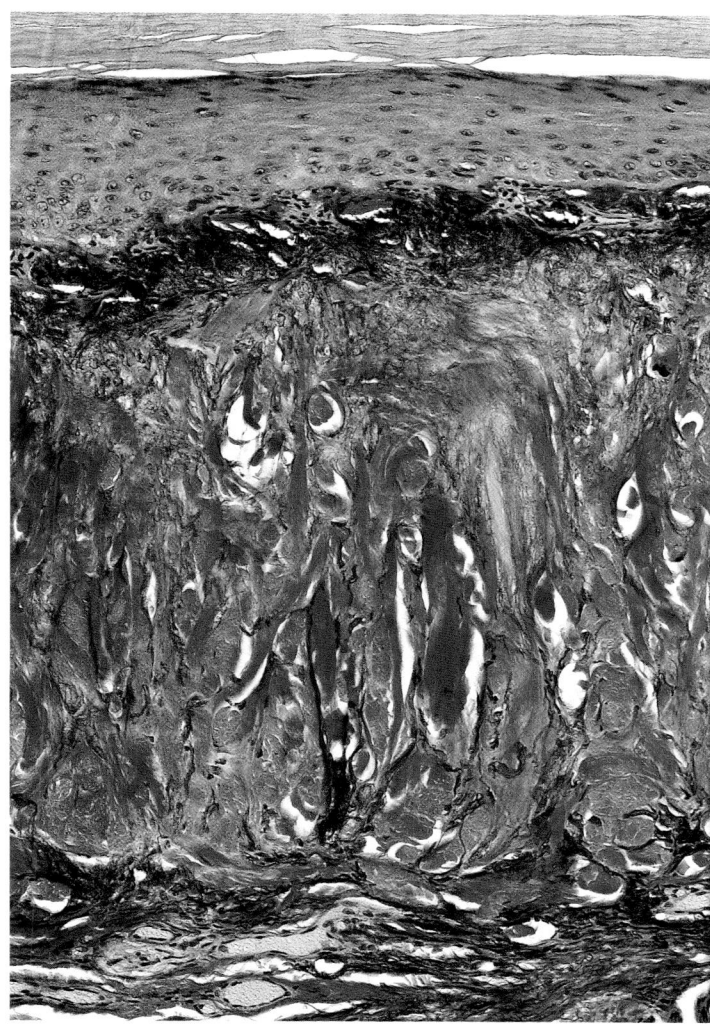

Fig. 12.16 **Collagenous and elastotic plaque.** Elastic tissue is reduced between the thickened vertical collagen. There are curled fibers in the papillary dermis. (Verhoeff van Gieson)

Histopathology[238,242]

There is thinning of the epidermis with effacement of the rete ridges and some basal vacuolar changes. Areas of epithelial atypia, resembling that seen in actinic keratoses, are sometimes present. There is usually prominent elastotic material in the mid dermis.[243] A small amount of hemosiderin and melanin may be present in the upper dermis.[238]

DECREASED ELASTIC TISSUE

There are several distinct levels in the biosynthesis of elastic fibers at which errors can be introduced. These can lead to reduced production of elastic fibers or to the appearance of abnormal ones. Breakdown of fibers (elastolysis) is another mechanism which can lead to a reduction in the elastic tissue content of the dermis. This probably results from increased elastase activity.

The reduction in dermal elastic tissue can be generalized, as in cutis laxa, or localized, as in anetoderma and blepharochalasis. Cases with features intermediate between these two types or with fine wrinkling of the skin occur. Sometimes the reduction in elastic fibers is subclinical or over-

shadowed by other features. This is the case in various granulomatous inflammatory disorders.

NEVUS ANELASTICUS

Nevus anelasticus is the term suggested by Staricco and Mehregan[49] for several cases reported in the earlier literature characterized by an absence or definite reduction and/or fragmentation of elastic fibers in cutaneous lesions of early onset.[244] Further cases have been reported in which multiple papular lesions have developed, particularly on the trunk.[244–247] The lesions are not perifollicular in distribution. Separation from the non-inflammatory type of anetoderma may be difficult (see below).

Histopathology

Sections show a localized reduction in elastic fibers, with normal collagen.[245] The elastic fibers may show intense fragmentation in some cases.[244] Fibers in the papillary dermis may be normal. There is no inflammation.

PERIFOLLICULAR ELASTOLYSIS

Perifollicular elastolysis is a not uncommon condition of the face and upper back in which 1–3 mm gray or white, finely wrinkled lesions develop in association with a central hair follicle.[248,249] Balloon-like bulging of larger lesions may develop.[248] The disorder is significantly associated with acne vulgaris.[249,250] An elastase-producing strain of *Staphylococcus epidermidis* was found in the hair follicles located within lesions in one report.[248]

Histopathology[248]

There is an almost complete loss of elastic fibers confined to the immediate vicinity of hair follicles (Fig. 12.17). There is no inflammation.

ANETODERMA

Anetoderma (macular atrophy) is a rare cutaneous disorder in which multiple, oval lesions with a wrinkled surface develop progressively over many years.[251,252] Individual lesions may bulge outwards or be slightly depressed. They usually herniate inwards with finger tip pressure. There is a predilection for the upper trunk and upper arms, but the neck and thighs may also be

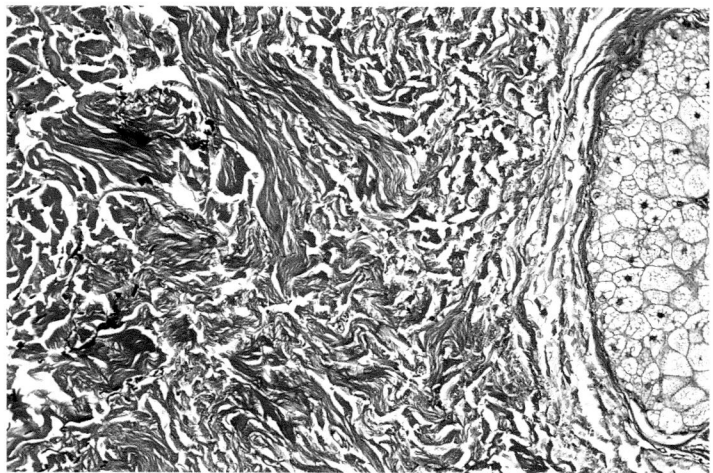

Fig. 12.17 **Perifollicular elastolysis.** There is absence of elastic tissue around the pilosebaceous follicle. A few thin fibers are present near the edge of the photomicrograph. (Verhoeff van Gieson)

involved. Facial involvement may lead to chalazodermia.[251] Onset of the lesions is in late adolescence and early adult life. Familial cases are quite rare.[253–257]

The onset of lesions may be preceded by an inflammatory stage with erythematous macules and papules (Jadassohn–Pellizzari type) or there may be no identifiable precursor inflammatory lesions (Schweninger–Buzzi type).[252] These two types have been classified as primary anetodermas to distinguish them from the secondary anetodermas[251,252] which may develop in the course of syphilis, leprosy, sarcoidosis, granuloma annulare,[258] tuberculosis, HIV infection,[259,260] folliculitis,[261] angular cheilitis,[262] acrodermatitis chronica atrophicans,[251] lupus erythematosus,[251] amyloidosis, lymphocytoma cutis,[263] cutaneous B-cell lymphoma,[264] juvenile xanthogranuloma,[265] immunocytoma[266] or following penicillamine therapy[267] or hepatitis B immunization.[268] Patches of anetoderma may develop in extremely premature infants,[269] usually at the sites of attachment of gel electrocardiographic electrodes.[270,271] Anetoderma-like changes have been reported in a patient with the clinical features of atrophoderma. The term 'atrophoderma elastolytica discreta' was used for these lesions.[272] The association with urticaria pigmentosa may be coincidental.[273] Rarely, secondary anetoderma overlies a pilomatrixoma.[274,275] The lesions of secondary anetoderma do not always correspond with those of the primary disease process.

A variety of ocular and skeletal defects have been reported in individuals with anetoderma. They have been chronicled in a review of the extensive European literature on this condition.[251]

Theoretically, anetoderma could result from increased degradation or reduced synthesis of elastic tissue.[276] It has been suggested that all cases have an inflammatory pathogenesis, which would tend to indicate that an elastolytic process is operative.[13,277] Increased expression of gelatinase A (metalloproteinase-2) and B (MMP-9) has been reported.[11] The concentration of elastin, as measured by the desmosine content of the skin, is markedly reduced.[276] Immunological abnormalities, the most common of which is a positive antinuclear factor, have been documented.[278–280]

Histopathology[277]

If a biopsy is taken from a clinically inflammatory lesion, the dermis will show a moderately heavy perivascular and even interstitial infiltrate, predominantly of lymphocytes. Plasma cells and eosinophils are occasionally present. Neutrophils have been noted sometimes in very early lesions.[277]

In established lesions, most reports have noted an essentially normal appearance in hematoxylin and eosin-stained sections. However, in one large series, a perivascular infiltrate of lymphocytes was found in all cases.[277] There was a predominance of helper T cells.[281] The authors of that account did not attempt to reconcile their findings with earlier reports in which inflammatory cells were noted to be absent.[252,276,277]

Scattered macrophages and giant cells, some showing elastophagocytosis, may also be present.[282] Non-caseating granulomas were present in one case, in association with Takayasu's arteritis.[283]

Elastic tissue stains show a normal complement of fibers in the early inflammatory lesions. In established lesions, elastic fibers are sparse in the superficial dermis and almost completely absent in the mid dermis (Fig. 12.18).

Direct immunofluorescence in some cases of primary anetoderma shows a pattern of immune deposits similar to that of lupus erythematosus.[284] There are no other manifestations of the latter disease in these cases.

Electron microscopy

The elastic fibers which remain are fragmented and irregular in appearance but the collagen is normal.[276,285] Occasionally, macrophages can be seen enveloping the fragmented fibers.[286]

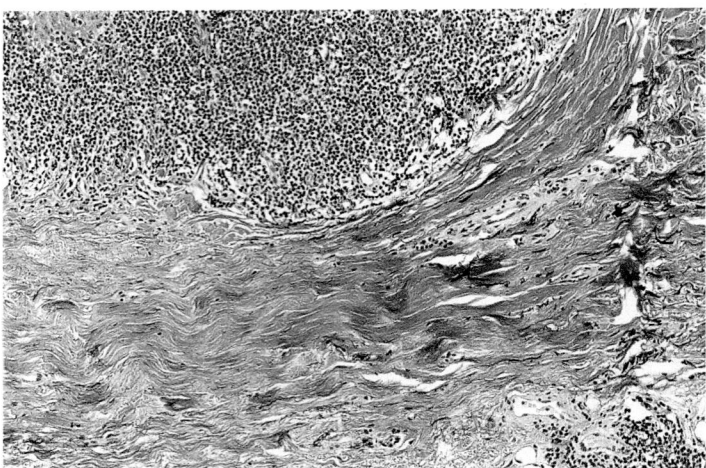

Fig. 12.18 **Anetoderma.** There is a heavy infiltrate of lymphocytes in the mid dermis. Beneath this the elastic fibers have almost completely disappeared. Five years after this biopsy was taken the patient developed cutaneous lupus erythematosus. (Verhoeff van Gieson)

CUTIS LAXA

The term 'cutis laxa' encompasses a group of rare disorders of elastic tissue in which the skin hangs in loose folds, giving the appearance of premature aging.[287] In many cases, there is a more generalized loss of elastic fibers involving the lungs, gastrointestinal tract and aorta, leading to emphysema, hernias, diverticula and aneurysms.[288–290] It is an etiologically heterogeneous disorder.

Congenital and acquired forms exist. *Congenital cutis laxa* is genetically heterogeneous: there are several different autosomal recessive forms of the disease, one of which is associated with growth retardation.[291,292] There is an autosomal dominant form which is less severe. The X-linked recessive variant,[293] in which there is a deficiency of lysyl oxidase, is now regarded as a variant of Ehlers–Danlos syndrome.[294,295] The congenital forms are associated with a characteristic facies, with a hooked nose and a long upper lip ('blood-hound' facies).[296]

More than 30 cases of *acquired cutis laxa* have been described. The changes may be generalized or localized.[297–300] Acquired cutis laxa may be of insidious onset[301] or develop after a prior inflammatory lesion of the skin[302] which may take the form of erythema, erythema multiforme, urticaria,[303,304] a vesicular eruption, including dermatitis herpetiformis,[305,306] or Sweet's syndrome.[307] Several cases have followed an allergic reaction to penicillin,[308,309] while others have been associated with isoniazid therapy,[310] myelomatosis,[311–314] cutaneous lymphoma,[315,316] systemic lupus erythematosus[317] or the nephrotic syndrome.[287] In two cases, associated with celiac disease, deposits of IgA were present on the dermal elastic fibers.[306,318] Cutis laxa may occur as a manifestation of an autosomal dominant form of pseudoxanthoma elasticum.

The congenital cases presumably result from a defect in the synthesis or assembly of the components of the elastic fiber. Possibly a different step is involved in the various genetic types. Mutations in exon 30 of the elastin gene (*ELN*) on chromosome 7q have been reported in two kindreds.[319] In those acquired cases associated with severe dermal inflammation, it has been suggested that granulocytic elastase may be involved. Cultured fibroblasts from one case showed increased elastase activity.[304] One report suggested that several factors, including high levels of cathepsin G, low lysyl oxidase activity and a reduction in circulating proteinase inhibitor(s) could all contribute to the loss of elastin.[320] Collagenase and gelatinase A and B expression is upregulated at the transcriptional level in cutis laxa.[321] This may explain the collagen abnormalities (see below) that are sometimes found.[322]

Localized areas of loose skin may develop in cutaneous lesions of sarcoidosis, syphilis and neurofibromatosis.[301] Loose skin localized to the hands, feet and neck is seen in **Costello syndrome** in which there are also characteristic facies, mental retardation, growth disorders and, sometimes, hypertrophic cardiomyopathy.[323] It results from a functional deficiency in elastin-binding protein.[6] Reduced elastic fibers were present in one case of the 'Michelin-tire' syndrome (see p. 970).[324]

Histopathology[325]

The fine elastic fibers in the papillary dermis are lost and there is a decrease in fibers elsewhere in the dermis (Fig. 12.19). Remaining fibers are often shortened and they vary greatly in diameter. The borders are sometimes indistinct and hazy. Fragmentation of fibers may be noted. Giant cells are rarely present, phagocytosing elastic fibers. A variable inflammatory reaction is present in the acquired cases with an associated clinical inflammatory component.[303] In several cases, the inflammatory infiltrate has been quite heavy, with neutrophils, eosinophils and lymphocytes in the superficial and deep dermis.[309] Deposits of immunoglobulins have been demonstrated on elastic fibers in the dermis in several cases.[306,314]

Shortening and rupture of elastic fibers are seen in Costello syndrome. There are decreased amounts of elastin.[323]

Electron microscopy[287]

The elastic tissue varies in content, appearance, and the proportion and manner by which elastin and the microfibrillar component associate.[326,327] The microfibrils are reduced in the papillary dermis.[328] There is some fragmentation of elastic fibers with accumulation of granular material.[311] Fragmented fibers are sometimes surrounded by fibroblasts or macrophages. Abnormalities of collagen structure have been noted in a few reports,[326,329] but specifically excluded in others.[311] An unusual case of acquired cutis laxa, associated with the cutaneous and systemic deposition of a fibrillar protein, has been reported.[330]

Elastolysis of the earlobes

Elastolysis of the earlobes may represent a variant of cutis laxa confined to the earlobes.[331] This is supported by cases with associated facial involvement.[304,331] *Blepharochalasis* is a similar lesion with eyelid and periorbital involvement.[317]

PAPILLARY-DERMAL ELASTOLYSIS

Papillary-dermal elastolysis is a rare disorder of elastic tissue characterized by clinical lesions resembling pseudoxanthoma elasticum, with small papules and cobblestone plaques on the neck and upper trunk.[17,332] Similar

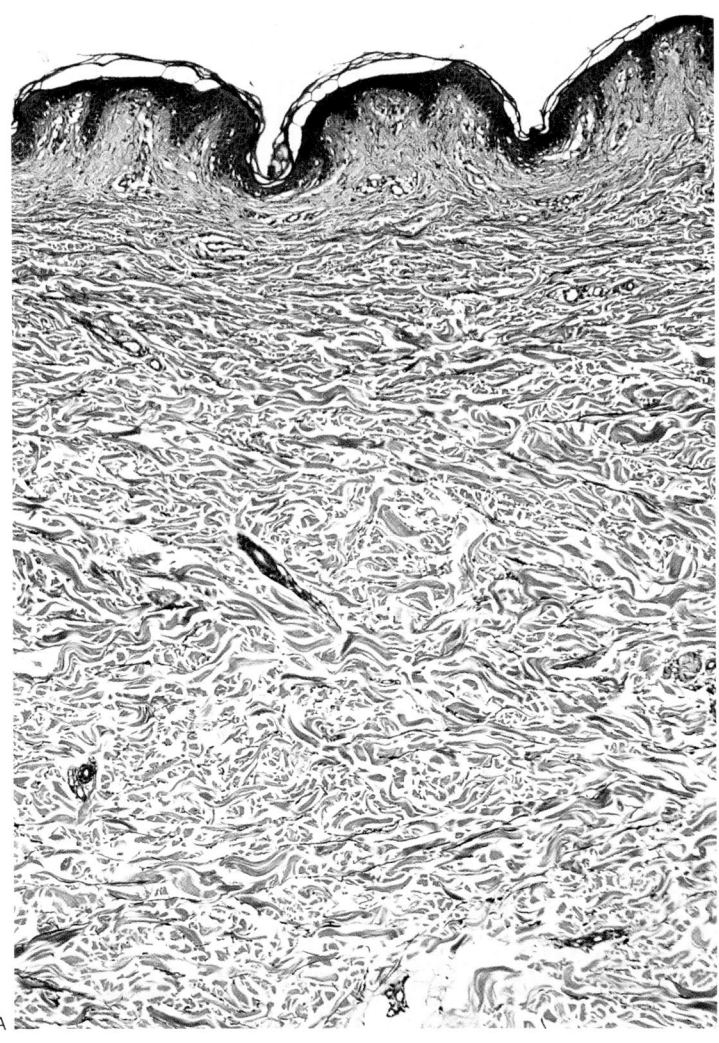 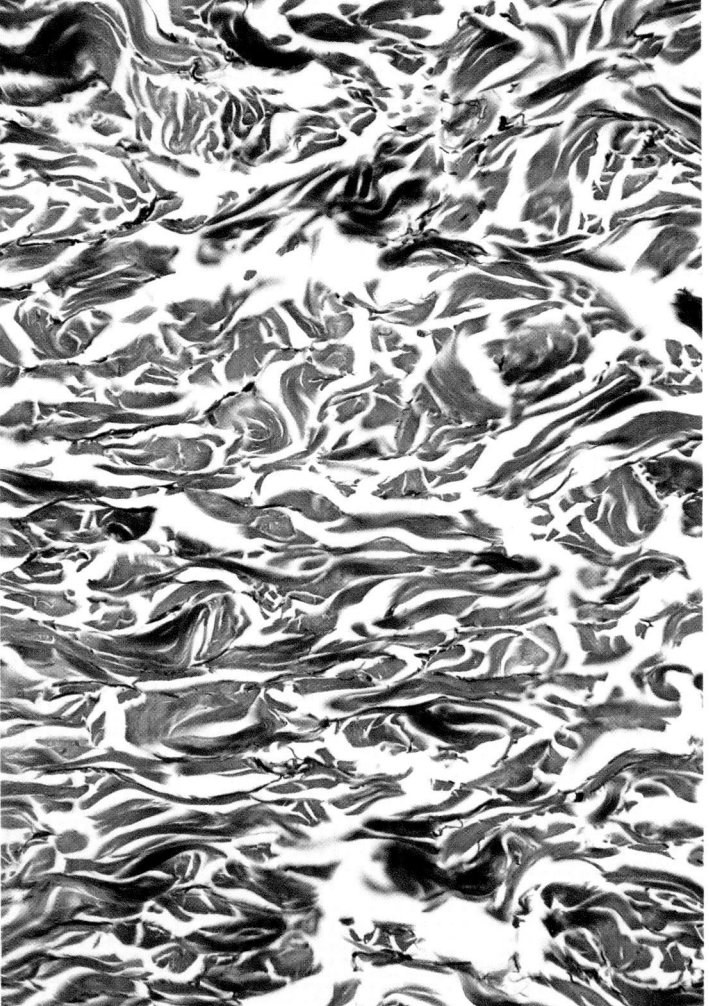

Fig. 12.19 **(A) Cutis laxa. (B)** There is an almost complete absence of elastic fibers. (Orcein)

histopathological changes were present in a case presenting as a small, hyperpigmented plaque.[333] It has been suggested recently that this condition is part of the spectrum of white fibrous papulosis of the neck (see p. 356), for which the term 'fibroelastolytic papulosis of the neck' has been suggested.

Histopathology

There is a complete loss of elastic fibers in the papillary dermis. The remaining fibers are not calcified or fragmented; that is, there are no histopathological features of pseudoxanthoma elasticum. Elastophagocytosis was present in one case, suggesting that this may be the mechanism for the loss of elastic fibers.[334] Immunohistochemical studies have demonstrated a disappearance of both elastin and fibrillin-1 from the papillary dermis, suggesting that this condition is more than an age-related state.[335,336]

MID-DERMAL ELASTOLYSIS

Mid-dermal elastolysis, first described by Shelley and Wood in 1977,[337] is characterized by widespread patches of fine wrinkling due to a loss of elastic fibers from the mid dermis.[337–342] A few cases have shown a second clinical feature with looseness of the skin around hair follicles.[343] Most cases have involved the upper extremities, neck and trunk of women. It may represent a variant of anetoderma.

In nearly 50% of cases, erythema, urticaria or burning precedes or coincides with the development of the lesions, suggesting that an inflammatory process may be involved in the pathogenesis. In some cases, the condition appears to be photoinduced or photoaggravated.[344,345] The onset has followed augmentation mammoplasty with silicone implants,[346] granuloma annulare[347] and lupus erythematosus.[348] Lesions may remain stable for many years.

There is some similarity to the cases reported from South Africa and South America, in young children, in whom wrinkling developed after a preceding inflammatory stage.[349–351]

Histopathology

Sections stained with hematoxylin and eosin may appear normal, although in the early inflammatory stage a mild infiltrate of lymphocytes is present around vessels and, to a lesser extent, in interstitial areas.[343,352] Phagocytosis of elastic fibers has been present in some cases,[341,353] but specifically excluded in others.[343,344] This may, of course, be related to the age of the lesion biopsied. Two cases of mid-dermal elastophagocytosis, presenting as persistent reticulate erythema, have been reported.[354]

Stains for elastic tissue show an absence of fibers in the mid dermis. Elastic tissue is usually preserved around appendages, even in the clinical subset with perifollicular involvement.[355] There is no involvement of the papillary dermis or the lower reticular dermis.[343]

Electron microscopy

Degeneration of elastic fibers has been recorded. Engulfment of elastic fibers by macrophages can be seen in those cases that have histological evidence of elastophagocytosis.[334,352]

WILLIAMS' SYNDROME

Williams' syndrome is a multisystem, congenital disorder characterized by cranio-facial, neurobehavioral, cardiovascular and metabolic changes.[356] It results from a microdeletion in the q11.23 region of chromosome 7, involving the elastin gene and several other genes. Despite a moderate reduction in elastin deposition in the skin, the clinical changes are relatively mild with increased softness and mobility of the skin.[356]

Histopathology

The overall appearances of the skin are normal. However, immunofluorescent studies show reduced elastin staining in the papillary dermis and some fragmentation of deep elastic fibers.[356]

MENKES' SYNDROME

Menkes' kinky hair syndrome is a rare multisystem disorder of elastic tissue transmitted as an X-linked recessive trait.[357–359] The defective gene (*ATP7A*) has been localized to chromosome Xp13.3.[360] Characteristically the hair is white, sparse, brittle and kinky. It looks and feels like steel wool. Pili torti and, occasionally, monilethrix are present. Neurodegenerative changes, vascular insufficiency, hypothermia and susceptibility to infections are other manifestations of this syndrome.[30,359] Mild forms occur.[361]

The finding of reduced serum copper levels led to the view that Menkes' syndrome was a simple copper deficiency state akin to that seen in copper-deficient sheep.[362,363] It is now thought to be due to a spectrum of mutations in the copper-transporting ATPase gene, *ATP7A*.[6] There is reduced activity of the copper-dependent enzyme lysyl oxidase in fibroblasts derived from the skin of patients with this syndrome.[364] This enzyme is necessary for the cross inking of elastin.[3] It has been suggested that this syndrome should be reclassified with Ehlers–Danlos syndrome type IX, in which a disorder of lysyl oxidase also occurs (see p. 366).

Histopathology

There are various hair shaft abnormalities which include pili torti, monilethrix and trichorrhexis nodosa.[359] The internal elastic lamina of vessels is fragmented and there is intimal proliferation. Dermal elastic tissue appears to be unaffected.

Electron microscopy

The elastic fibers in the reticular dermis show a paucity of the central amorphous component while retaining normal microfibrillary material.[360]

FRAGILE X SYNDROME

Fragile X syndrome, a rare X-linked form of mental retardation, is associated with a characteristic facies and connective tissue abnormalities which are clinically reminiscent of cutis laxa and the Ehlers–Danlos syndromes.[365] Most cases result from an increase in length of a stretch of CGG triplet repeats in the *FMR1* gene situated on the long arm of the X chromosome.[366,367] Rarely, the condition results from the deletion of all or part of this gene, or of the *FMR2* gene lying just distal to it.[367]

Histopathology[365]

There is a reduction in dermal elastic tissue. The fibers are fragmented and curled and lack arborization. There is a reduction in stromal acid mucopolysaccharides.

WRINKLY SKIN SYNDROME

Wrinkly skin syndrome is a rare autosomal recessive disorder characterized by wrinkled skin with poor elasticity over the abdomen and on the dorsum of the hands and feet.[368] Increased palmar and plantar creases, a prominent venous pattern on the chest, microcephaly and musculoskeletal abnormalities form part of the syndrome.

Histopathology

There is an irregular pattern of elastic fiber distribution. Oxytalan fibers are absent from the papillary dermis. Thickened and fragmented fibers are present in the mid dermis while there is a paucity of elastic fibers in the deep dermis; those present are in fragmented clumps.[368]

GRANULOMATOUS DISEASES

Rarely, anetoderma develops as a complication of sarcoidosis, leprosy or tuberculosis. Reduced numbers of elastic fibers, not necessarily leading to clinical manifestations, may occur in the course of several other granulomatous disorders. These include the closely related conditions of elastolytic giant cell granuloma, actinic granuloma, atypical necrobiosis lipoidica of the face and scalp, and Miescher's granuloma.[369,370] Elastic tissue is reduced in active lesions of granuloma annulare. Multinucleate giant cells and macrophages appear to be responsible for the digestion of the elastic fibers.[369] These conditions are discussed further in Chapter 7 (pp. 193–220).

'GRANULOMATOUS SLACK SKIN'

Granulomatous slack skin, a rare form of cutaneous T-cell lymphoma, is characterized by progressively pendulous skin folds in flexural areas and an abnormal cutaneous infiltrate.[371–375] The distinctive clinical appearance results from elastolysis, apparently mediated by giant cells in the infiltrate (see p. 1109).

Histopathology[371]

There is permeation of the entire dermis and subcutis by a heavy infiltrate of lymphocytes admixed with tuberculoid granulomas and giant cells with up to 30 nuclei. Foam cells may also be present.[373] There is almost complete absence of elastic tissue in the dermis, and elastic fibers may be seen within the giant cells. Loss of elastic fibers and subcutaneous granulomas are not present in the granulomatous form of mycosis fungoides which otherwise resembles this condition on histopathology (see p. 1107).[371]

MYXEDEMA

Elastic fibers are significantly reduced in the dermis in hypothyroid myxedema and in pretibial myxedema.[376] Ultrastructural examination shows wide variability of elastic fiber diameter and a decrease in microfibrils.[376]

ACROKERATOELASTOIDOSIS

Acrokeratoelastoidosis is a genodermatosis (see p. 291) in which the dermal elastic fibers are usually fragmented and decreased in number. Sometimes they are normal.[235] The epidermal changes are clinically more significant than the elastic tissue changes, although pathogenetically the elastorrhexis is probably the primary event and the accompanying keratoderma could be secondary to chronic trauma.[377]

VARIABLE OR MINOR ELASTIC TISSUE CHANGES

LEPRECHAUNISM

Leprechaunism is a rare disorder with characteristic facies, phallic enlargement and a deficiency of subcutaneous fat stores.[378] Cutaneous changes include hypertrichosis, acanthosis nigricans, wrinkled loose skin and prominent rugal folds around the body orifices.[378]

Histopathology

Loss and fragmentation of elastic fibers and decreased collagen were noted in one report of this condition.[379] In contrast, in a recent study it was noted that the elastic fibers were thick and extended into the widened septa of the subcutaneous fat.[378]

SYNDROMES OF PREMATURE AGING

The elastic tissue changes in the premature aging conditions are variable. They may be increased in Werner's syndrome (see p. 366) with granular and filamentous ultrastructural changes.[380] Elastosis perforans has been reported in acrogeria (see p. 367).[381] At other times there may be loss of elastic fibers in association with dermal atrophy or sclerosis.[382]

WRINKLES

Although of great cosmetic importance, wrinkles are of little dermatopathological interest. In general, wrinkles are bilateral and increased with aging and sun damage. One case of unilateral wrinkles has been reported.[383] Wrinkles are an important component of 'smoker's face', resulting from prolonged cigarette smoking.[174] Wrinkles may result from a reduction in collagen VII in photodamaged skin, with a consequent weakening of the bond between the dermis and epidermis.[189] Estrogen therapy appears to reduce the incidence of wrinkles.[384]

Histopathology[385–389]

It has been stated that wrinkles are a 'configurational change' with no distinguishing histological features.[385] In contrast, it has been reported that the dermis in a deep wrinkle shows substantially fewer elastotic changes than the surrounding areas and that the superficial elastic fibers appear slightly thickened and the overlying epidermis depressed.[388,389] Increased elastosis is found in biopsies from 'smoker's face'.

A recent study involving 157 skin biopsies has demonstrated numerous modifications in different structures of the skin: hypertrophied elastotic tissue on the flanks of the wrinkle and reduced or absent elastic fibers under the wrinkle, atrophy of the dermal collagen under the wrinkle, and a marked decrease in chondroitin sulfates and oxytalan fibers in the papillary dermis.[390]

Electron microscopy

Electron-dense inclusions have been noted in elastic fibers in the upper dermis of the wrinkled areas; these are thought to represent the earliest changes of solar elastosis.[388,389] More severe changes are present in the surrounding dermis.

SCAR TISSUE

There have been conflicting reports on the status of elastic fibers in scar tissue. If appropriate stains are used, fine elastic fibers can be demonstrated in scars that have been present for over 3 months.[23] They increase progressively over time, but they are always thinner than in normal skin.

MARFAN'S SYNDROME

Marfan's syndrome is a rare, autosomal dominant defect of connective tissue, with ocular, skeletal and cardiovascular manifestations.[391] Marfan's syndrome has an incidence of at least 1:10 000, and up to 30% of cases represent new mutations. Cutaneous manifestations are of little clinical importance; they include striae distensae and elastosis perforans serpiginosa.[392] Defects in the crosslinking and composition of collagen have been described, but abnormalities in elastic tissue (a mutation in the fibrillin-1 – *FBN1* – gene on chromosome 15q15–21) are the dominant feature.[5,393] Defects in the fibrillin-2 gene (*FBN2*) cause a phenotypically related disorder.[4] These various disorders have been called the microfibrillopathies.[4]

Histopathology

The striae distensae show the usual features of this lesion (see p. 358) with regeneration of elastic fibers.[394] The lesions of elastosis perforans serpiginosa resemble those already described for this entity (see p. 385).

Clinically normal skin shows no detectable abnormality, although one study suggested that the elastic fibers looked a little tortuous and fragmented.[392] In some cases, thinning of the dermis, resulting from a diminished quantity of collagen due to thinner collagen bundles, has been noted.

Electron microscopy

Electron microscopy shows an increase in fine elastic fibers, possibly resulting from incomplete fusion of elastic fibers.[392] Degenerative changes in elastic fibers have been observed in the lung.[395]

REFERENCES

Introduction

1 Sandberg LB, Soskel NT, Wolt TB. Structure of the elastic fiber: an overview. J Invest Dermatol 1982; 79 (Suppl 1): 128s–132s.

2 Davidson JM, Crystal RG. The molecular aspects of elastin gene expression. J Invest Dermatol 1982; 79 (Suppl 1): 133s–137s.

3 Uitto J, Rhyanen L, Abraham PA, Perejda AJ. Elastin in diseases. J Invest Dermatol 1982; 79 (Suppl 1): 160s–168s.

4 Robinson PN, Godfrey M. The molecular genetics of Marfan syndrome and related microfibrillopathies. J Med Genet 2000; 37: 9–25.

5 Christiano AM, Uitto J. Molecular pathology of the elastic fibers. J Invest Dermatol 1994; 103: 53s–57s.

6 Urbán Z, Boyd CD. Elastic-fiber pathologies: primary defects in assembly – and secondary disorders in transport and delivery. Am J Hum Genet 2000; 67: 4–7.

7 Tsuji T. Elastic fibers in the dermal papilla. Scanning and transmission electron microscopic studies. Br J Dermatol 1980; 102: 413–417.

8 Cotta-Pereira G, Rodrigo FG, Bittencourt-Sampaio S. Oxytalan, elaunin, and elastic fibers in the human skin. J Invest Dermatol 1976; 66: 143–148.

9 Frances C, Robert L. Elastin and elastic fibers in normal and pathologic skin. Int J Dermatol 1984; 23: 166–179.

10 Werb Z, Banda MJ, McKerrow JH, Sandhaus RA. Elastases and elastin degradation. J Invest Dermatol 1982; 79 (Suppl 1): 154s–159s.

11 Venencie PY, Bonnefoy A, Gogly B et al. Increased expression of gelatinases A and B by skin explants from patients with anetoderma. Br J Dermatol 1997; 137: 517–525.

12 Park PW, Biedermann K, Mecham L et al. Lysozyme binds to elastin and protects elastin from elastase-mediated degradation. J Invest Dermatol 1996; 106: 1075–1080.

13 Werth VP, Ivanov IE, Nussenzweig V. Decay-accelerating factor in human skin is associated with elastic fibers. J Invest Dermatol 1988; 91: 511–516.

14 Braverman IM, Fonferko E. Studies in cutaneous aging: 1. The elastic fiber network. J Invest Dermatol 1982; 78: 434–443.

15 Takema Y, Yorimoto Y, Kawai M, Imokawa G. Age-related changes in the elastic properties and thickness of human facial skin. Br J Dermatol 1994; 131: 641–648.

16 West MD. The cellular and molecular biology of skin aging. Arch Dermatol 1994; 130: 87–95.

17 Rongioletti F, Rebora A. Fibroelastolytic patterns of intrinsic skin aging: pseudoxanthoma-elasticum-like papillary dermal elastolysis and white fibrous papulosis of the neck. Dermatology 1995; 191: 19–24.

18 Tsuji T, Hamada T. Age-related changes in human dermal elastic fibres. Br J Dermatol 1981; 105: 57–63.

19 Herzberg AJ, Dinehart SM. Chronologic aging in black skin. Am J Dermatopathol 1989; 11: 319–328.

20 Dahlback K, Lofberg H, Alumets J, Dahlback B. Immunohistochemical demonstration of age-related deposition of vitronectin (S-protein of complement) and terminal complement complex on dermal elastic fibers. J Invest Dermatol 1989; 92: 727–733.

21 Grove GL, Grove MJ, Leyden JJ et al. Skin replica analysis of photodamaged skin after therapy with tretinoin emollient cream. J Am Acad Dermatol 1991; 25: 231–237.

22 Kligman LH. Luna's technique. A beautiful stain for elastin. Am J Dermatopathol 1981; 3: 199–201.

23 Roten SV, Bhat S, Bhawan J. Elastic fibers in scar tissue. J Cutan Pathol 1996; 23: 37–42.

24 Dawson JF, Brochier J, Schmitt D et al. Elastic fibres: histological correlation with orcein and a new monoclonal antibody, HB8. Br J Dermatol 1984; 110: 539–546.

25 Reed RJ, Clark WH, Mihm MC. The cutaneous elastoses. Hum Pathol 1973; 4: 187–199.

26 Holbrook KA, Byers PH. Structural abnormalities in the dermal collagen and elastic matrix from the skin of patients with inherited connective tissue disorders. J Invest Dermatol 1982; 79 (Suppl 1): 7s–16s.

Increased elastic tissue

27 Stadil P. Histopathology of the corium in osteogenesis imperfecta. Danish Med Bull 1961; 8: 131–134.

28 Olmstead EG, Lunseth JH. Skin manifestations of chronic acidosis. Arch Dermatol 1958; 77: 304–313.

29 Fullmer HM, Siedler HD, Krooth RS, Kurland LT. A cutaneous disorder of connective tissue in amyotrophic lateral sclerosis. A histochemical study. Neurology 1960; 10: 717–724.

30 Bader L. Disorders of elastic tissue: a review. Pathology 1973; 5: 269–289.

31 Fisher ER, Wechsler HL. The so-called collagen diseases and elastoses of skin. In: Helwig EB, Mostofi FK, eds. The skin. New York: Robert E Krieger, 1980; 366.

32 Ledoux-Corbusier M, Achten G, de Dobbeleer G. Juvenile elastoma (Weidman). An ultrastructural study. J Cutan Pathol 1981; 8: 219–227.

33 Raque CJ, Wood MG. Connective-tissue nevus. Arch Dermatol 1970; 102: 390–396.

34 Uitto J, Santa Cruz DJ, Eisen AZ. Connective tissue nevi of the skin. J Am Acad Dermatol 1980; 3: 441–461.

35 Verbov J. Buschke–Ollendorff syndrome (disseminated dermatofibrosis with osteopoikilosis). Br J Dermatol 1977; 96: 87–90.

36 Atherton DJ, Wells RS. Juvenile elastoma and osteopoikilosis (the Buschke–Ollendorf syndrome). Clin Exp Dermatol 1982; 7: 109–113.

37 Reinhardt LA, Rountree CB, Wilkin JK. Buschke–Ollendorff syndrome. Cutis 1983; 31: 94–96.

38 Schorr WF, Optiz JM, Reyes CN. The connective tissue nevus–osteopoikilosis syndrome. Arch Dermatol 1972; 106: 208–214.

39 Morrison JGL, Wilson Jones E, MacDonald DM. Juvenile elastoma and osteopoikilosis (the Buschke–Ollendorff syndrome). Br J Dermatol 1977; 97: 417–422.

40 Piette-Brion B, Lowy-Motulsky M, Ledoux-Corbusier M, Achten G. Dermatofibromas, elastomas and deafness: a new case of Buschke–Ollendorff syndrome? Dermatologica 1984; 168: 255–258.

41 Verbov J, Graham R. Buschke–Ollendorff syndrome – disseminated dermatofibrosis with osteopoikilosis. Clin Exp Dermatol 1986; 11: 17–26.

42 Woodrow SL, Pope FM, Handfield-Jones SE. The Buschke–Ollendorff syndrome presenting as familial elastic tissue naevi. Br J Dermatol 2001; 144: 890–893.

43 Huilgol SC, Griffiths WAD, Black MM. Familial juvenile elastoma. Australas J Dermatol 1994; 35: 87–90.

44 Fork HE, Sanchez RL, Wagner RF Jr, Raimer SS. A new type of connective tissue nevus: isolated exophytic elastoma. J Cutan Pathol 1991; 18: 457–463.

45 Uitto J, Santa Cruz DJ, Starcher BC et al. Biochemical and ultrastructural demonstration of elastin accumulation in the skin lesions of the Buschke–Ollendorff syndrome. J Invest Dermatol 1981; 76: 284–287.

46 Cole GW, Barr RJ. An elastic tissue defect in dermatofibrosis lenticularis disseminata. Arch Dermatol 1982; 118: 44–46.

47 Danielsen L, Midtgaard K, Christensen HE. Osteopoikilosis associated with dermatofibrosis lenticularis disseminata. Arch Dermatol 1969; 100: 465–470.

48 Moiin A, Hashimoto K. Linear focal elastosis in a young black man: a new presentation. J Am Acad Dermatol 1994; 30: 874–877.

49 Staricco RG, Mehregan AH. Nevus elasticus and nevus elasticus vascularis. Arch Dermatol 1961; 84: 943–947.

50 Sosis AC, Johnson WC. Connective tissue naevus. Dermatologica 1972; 144: 57–62.

51 Becke RFA, Musso LA. An unusual epithelial–connective tissue naevus with perifollicular mucinosis. Australas J Dermatol 1978; 19: 118–120.

52 Danielsen L, Kobayasi T, Jacobsen GK. Ultrastructural changes in disseminated connective tissue nevi. Acta Derm Venereol 1977; 57: 93–101.

53 Reymond JL, Stoebner P, Beani JC, Amblard P. Buschke–Ollendorf syndrome. An electron microscopic study. Dermatologica 1983; 166: 64–68.

54 Hagari Y, Mihara M, Morimura T, Shimao S. Linear focal elastosis. An ultrastructural study. Arch Dermatol 1991; 127: 1365–1368.

55 Burket JM, Zelickson AS, Padila RS. Linear focal elastosis (elastotic striae). J Am Acad Dermatol 1989; 20: 633–636.

56 Kirkegaard L, Goldsmith SM, Solomon AR. Linear focal elastosis. J Cutan Pathol 1996; 23: 53 (abstract).

57 Breier F, Trautinger F, Jurecka W, Hönigsmann H. Linear focal elastosis (elastotic striae): increased number of elastic fibres determined by a video measuring system. Br J Dermatol 1997; 137: 955–957.

58 Hashimoto K. Linear focal elastosis: Keloidal repair of striae distensae. J Am Acad Dermatol 1998; 39: 309–313.

59 Tamada Y, Yokochi K, Ikeya T et al. Linear focal elastosis: A review of three cases in young Japanese men. J Am Acad Dermatol 1997; 36: 301–303.

60 Choi SW, Lee JH, Woo HJ et al. Two cases of linear focal elastosis: different histopathologic findings. Int J Dermatol 2000; 39: 207–209.

61 Tajima S, Shimizu K, Izumi T et al. Late-onset focal dermal elastosis: clinical and histological features. Br J Dermatol 1995; 133: 303–305.

62 Limas C. Late onset focal dermal elastosis. A distinct clinicopathologic entity? Am J Dermatopathol 1999; 21: 381–383.

63 Tajima S, Tanaka N, Ohnishi Y et al. Analysis of elastin metabolism in patients with late-onset focal dermal elastosis. Acta Derm Venereol 1999; 79: 285–287.

64 Yen A, Wen J, Grau M et al. Elastoderma. J Am Acad Dermatol 1995; 33: 389–392.

65 Kornberg RL. Elastoderma. J Am Acad Dermatol 1996; 34: 1093.

66 Madri JA, Dise CA, LiVolsi VA et al. Elastofibroma dorsi: an immunochemical study of collagen content. Hum Pathol 1981; 12: 186–190.

67 Enzinger FM, Weiss SW. Soft tissue tumours. St Louis: Mosby, 1983; 33–37.

68 Schwarz T, Oppolzer G, Duschet P et al. Ulcerating elastofibroma dorsi. J Am Acad Dermatol 1989; 21: 1142–1144.

69 Ohtake N, Setoyama M, Kanzaki T. Elastofibroma dorsi. Dermatology 1998; 197: 74–77.

70 Kumaratilake JS, Krishnan R, Lomax-Smith J, Cleary EG. Elastofibroma: disturbed elastic fibrillogenesis by periosteal-derived cells? Hum Pathol 1991; 22: 1017–1029.

71 Jarvi OH, Lansimies PH. Subclinical elastofibromas in the scapular region in an autopsy series. Acta Path Microbiol Scand (A) 1975; 83: 87–108.

72 Ramos CV, Gillespie W, Narconis RJ. Elastofibroma. A pseudotumor of myofibroblasts. Arch Pathol Lab Med 1978; 102: 538–540.

73 Mehregan AH. Elastosis perforans serpiginosa. A review of the literature and report of 11 cases. Arch Dermatol 1968; 97: 381–393.

74 Patterson JW. The perforating disorders. J Am Acad Dermatol 1984; 10: 561–581.

75 Woo TY, Rasmussen JE. Disorders of transepidermal elimination. Part 1. Int J Dermatol 1985; 24: 267–279.

76 White CR. The dermatopathology of perforating disorders. Semin Dermatol 1986; 5: 359–366.

77 Weidman AI, Allyn B. Elastosis perforans serpiginosa. Two cases involving the ear. Arch Dermatol 1971; 103: 324–327.

78 Abdullah A, Colloby PS, Foulds IS, Whitcroft I. Localized idiopathic elastosis perforans serpiginosa effectively treated by the Coherent Ultrapulse 5000c Aesthetic Laser. Int J Dermatol 2000; 39: 719–720.

79 Pedro SD, Garcia RL. Disseminate elastosis perforans serpiginosa. Arch Dermatol 1974; 109: 84–85.

80 Rasmussen JE. Disseminated elastosis perforans serpiginosa in four mongoloids. Br J Dermatol 1972; 86: 9–13.

81 Woerdeman MJ, Bour DJH, Bijlsma JB. Elastosis perforans serpiginosa. Report of a family with a chromosomal investigation. Arch Dermatol 1965; 92: 559–560.

82 Ayala F, Donofrio P. Elastosis perforans serpiginosa. Report of a family. Dermatologica 1983; 166: 32–37.

83 Rios-Buceta L, Amigo-Echenagusia A, Sols-Candelas M et al. Elastosis perforans serpiginosa with simultaneous onset in two sisters. Int J Dermatol 1993; 32: 879–881.

84 Langeveld-Wildschut EG, Toonstra J, van Vloten WA, Beemer FA. Familial elastosis perforans serpiginosa. Arch Dermatol 1993; 129: 205–207.

85 Crotty G, Bell M, Estes SA, Kitzmiller KW. Cytologic features of elastosis perforans serpiginosa (EPS) associated with Down's syndrome. J Am Acad Dermatol 1983; 8: 255–256.

86 Siragusa M, Romano C, Cavallari V, Schepis C. Localized elastosis perforans serpiginosa in a boy with Down syndrome. Pediatr Dermatol 1997; 14: 244–246.

87 Carey TD. Elastosis perforans serpiginosa. Arch Dermatol 1977; 113: 1444–1445.

88 Hill VA, Seymour CA, Mortimer PS. Penicillamine-induced elastosis perforans serpiginosa and cutis laxa in Wilson's disease. Br J Dermatol 2000; 142: 560–561.

89 Barr RJ, Siegel JM, Graham JH. Elastosis perforans serpiginosa associated with morphea. An example of 'perforating morphea'. J Am Acad Dermatol 1980; 3: 19–22.

90 May NC, Lester RS. Elastosis perforans serpiginosa associated with systemic sclerosis. J Am Acad Dermatol 1982; 6: 945.

91 Armstrong DKB, Walsh MY, Allen GE. Elastosis perforans serpiginosa associated with unilateral atrophoderma of Pasini and Pierini in an individual with 47, XYY karyotype. Br J Dermatol 1997; 137: 158–160.

92 Wong KC, Fryer JA, Li M, Crosland G. Acquired perforating dermatosis in diabetes mellitus: an unusual case. Australas J Dermatol 1999; 40: 108–110.

93 Schamroth JM, Kellen P, Grieve TP. Elastosis perforans serpiginosa in a patient with renal disease. Arch Dermatol 1986; 122: 82–84.

94 Pass F, Goldfischer S, Sternlieb I, Scheinberg IH. Elastosis perforans serpiginosa during penicillamine therapy for Wilson disease. Arch Dermatol 1973; 108: 713–715.

95 Rosenblum GA. Liquid nitrogen cryotherapy in a case of elastosis perforans serpiginosa. J Am Acad Dermatol 1983; 8: 718–721.

96 Goldstein JB, McNutt NS, Hambrick GW Jr, Hsu A. Penicillamine dermatopathy with lymphangiectases. A clinical, immunohistologic, and ultrastructural study. Arch Dermatol 1989; 125: 92–97.

97 Levy RS, Fisher M, Alter JN. Penicillamine: review and cutaneous manifestations. J Am Acad Dermatol 1983; 8: 548–558.

98 Van Joost T, Vuzevski VD, ten Kate FJW et al. Elastosis perforans serpiginosa: clinical, histomorphological and immunological studies. J Cutan Pathol 1988; 15: 92–97.

99 Price RG, Prentice RSA. Penicillamine-induced elastosis perforans serpiginosa. Tip of the iceberg? Am J Dermatopathol 1986; 8: 314–320.

100 Eide J. Elastosis perforans serpiginosa with widespread arterial lesions: a case report. Acta Derm Venereol 1977; 57: 533–537.

101 Rapini RP, Hebert AA, Drucker CR. Acquired perforating dermatosis. Evidence for combined transepidermal elimination of both collagen and elastic fibers. Arch Dermatol 1989; 125: 1074–1078.

102 Fujimoto N, Tajima S, Ishibashi A. Elastin peptides induce migration and terminal differentiation of cultured keratinocytes via 67 kDa elastin receptor in vitro: 67 kDa elastin receptor is expressed in the keratinocytes eliminating elastic materials in elastosis perforans serpiginosa. J Invest Dermatol 2000; 115: 633–639.

103 Bergman R. Friedman-Birnbaum R, Hazaz B. A direct immunofluorescence study in elastosis perforans serpiginosa. Br J Dermatol 1985; 113: 573–579.

104 Bardach H, Gebhart W, Niebauer G. 'Lumpy-bumpy' elastic fibers in the skin and lungs of a patient with penicillamine-induced elastosis perforans serpiginosa. J Cutan Pathol 1979; 6: 243–252.

105 Gebhart W, Bardach H. The 'lumpy-bumpy' elastic fiber. A marker for long-term administration of penicillamine. Am J Dermatopathol 1981; 3: 33–39.

106 Kirsch N, Hukill PB. Elastosis perforans serpiginosa induced by penicillamine. Electron microscopic observations. Arch Dermatol 1977; 113: 630–635.

107 Hashimoto K, McEvoy B, Belcher R. Ultrastructure of penicillamine-induced skin lesions. J Am Acad Dermatol 1981; 4: 300–315.

108 Reymond JL, Stoebner P, Zambelli P et al. Penicillamine induced elastosis perforans serpiginosa: an ultrastructural study of two cases. J Cutan Pathol 1982; 9: 352–357.

109 Meves C, Vogel A. Electron microscopical studies in elastosis perforans serpiginosa. Dermatologica 1973; 145: 210–221.

110 Volpin D, Pasquali-Ronchetti I, Castellani I et al. Ultrastructural and biochemical studies on a case of elastosis perforans serpiginosa. Dermatologica 1978; 156: 209–223.

111 Hacker SM, Ramos-Caro FA, Beers BB, Flowers FP. Juvenile pseudoxanthoma elasticum: recognition and management. Pediatr Dermatol 1993; 10: 19–25.

112 Neldner KH. Pseudoxanthoma elasticum. Int J Dermatol 1988; 27: 98–100.

113 Woo TY, Rasmussen JE. Disorders of transepidermal elimination. Part 2. Int J Dermatol 1985; 24: 337–348.

114 Goodman RM, Smith EW, Paton D et al. Pseudoxanthoma elasticum: a clinical and histopathological study. Medicine (Baltimore) 1963; 42: 297–334.

115 Danielsen L, Kobayasi T. Pseudoxanthoma elasticum. An ultrastructural study of oral lesions. Acta Derm Venereol 1974; 54: 173–176.

116 Lebwohl M, Neldner K, Pope FM et al. Classification of pseudoxanthoma elasticum: report of a consensus conference. J Am Acad Dermatol 1994; 30: 103–107.

117 Rongioletti F, Bertamino R, Rebora A. Generalized pseudoxanthoma elasticum with deficiency of vitamin K-dependent clotting factors. J Am Acad Dermatol 1989; 21: 1150–1152.

118 Uenishi T, Uchiyama M, Sugiura H, Danno K. Pseudoxanthoma elasticum with generalized cutaneous laxity. Arch Dermatol 1997; 133: 664–666.

119 Choi GS, Kang D-S, Chung JJ, Lee M-G. Osteoma cutis coexisting with cutis laxa-like pseudoxanthoma elasticum. J Am Acad Dermatol 2000; 43: 337–339.

120 Reeve EB, Neldner KH, Subryan V, Gordon SG. Development and calcification of skin lesions in thirty-nine patients with pseudoxanthoma elasticum. Clin Exp Dermatol 1979; 4: 291–301.

121 Nolte KB. Sudden cardiac death owing to pseudoxanthoma elasticum: a case report. Hum Pathol 2000; 31: 1002–1004.

122 Mendelsohn G, Bulkley BH, Hutchins GM. Cardiovascular manifestations of pseudoxanthoma elasticum. Arch Pathol Lab Med 1978; 102: 298–302.

123 Dymock RB. Pseudoxanthoma elasticum: report of a case with reno-vascular hypertension. Australas J Dermatol 1979; 20: 82–84.

124 Akhtar M, Brody H. Elastic tissue in pseudoxanthoma elasticum. Ultrastructural study of endocardial lesions. Arch Pathol 1975; 99: 667–671.

125 Pope FM. Historical evidence for the genetic heterogeneity of pseudoxanthoma elasticum. Br J Dermatol 1975; 92: 493–509.

126 Uitto J, Boyd CD, Lebwohl MG et al. International Centennial Meeting on Pseudoxanthoma Elasticum: progress in PXE research. J Invest Dermatol 1998; 110: 840–842.

127 Sherer DW, Sapadin AN, Lebwohl MG. Pseudoxanthoma elasticum: an update. Dermatology 1999; 199: 3–7.

128 Macmillan DC. Pseudoxanthoma elasticum and a coagulation defect. Br J Dermatol 1971; 84: 182.

129 Sherer DW, Bercovitch L, Lebwohl M. Pseudoxanthoma elasticum: Significance of limited phenotypic expression in parents of affected offspring. J Am Acad Dermatol 2001; 44: 534–537.

130 Ringpfeil F, Lebwohl MG, Uitto J. Mutations in the MRP6 gene cause pseudoxanthoma elasticum. J Invest Dermatol 2000; 115: 332 (abstract).

131 Martinez-Hernandez A, Huffer WE, Neldner K et al. Resolution and repair of elastic tissue calcification in pseudoxanthoma elasticum. Arch Pathol Lab Med 1978; 102: 303–305.

132 Eng AM, Bryant J. Clinical pathologic observations in pseudoxanthoma elasticum. Int J Dermatol 1975; 14: 586–605.

133 Hamamoto Y, Nagai K, Yasui H, Muto M. Hyperreactivity of pseudoxanthoma elasticum-affected dermis to vitamin D3. J Am Acad Dermatol 2000; 42: 685–687.

134 Rodríguez-Cuartero A, García-Vera E. Pseudoxanthoma elasticum: a study of urinary glycosaminoglycan levels in two cases. Br J Dermatol 1997; 137: 473–474.

135 Schutt DA. Pseudoxanthoma elasticum and elastosis perforans serpiginosa. Arch Dermatol 1965; 91: 151–152.

136 Lund HZ, Gilbert CF. Perforating pseudoxanthoma elasticum. Its distinction from elastosis perforans serpiginosa. Arch Pathol Lab Med 1976; 100: 544–546.

137 Schwartz RA, Richfield DF. Pseudoxanthoma elasticum with transepidermal elimination. Arch Dermatol 1978; 114: 279–280.

138 Walker ER, Frederickson RG, Mayes MD. The mineralization of elastic fibers and alterations of extracellular matrix in pseudoxanthoma elasticum. Ultrastructure, immunocytochemistry, and x-ray analysis. Arch Dermatol 1989; 125: 70–76.

139 Gordon SG, Overland M, Foley J. Evidence for increased protease activity secreted from cultured fibroblasts from patients with pseudoxanthoma elasticum. Connect Tissue Res 1978; 6: 61–68.

140 Godfrey M, Cisler J, Geerts M-L et al. Fibrillin immunofluorescence in pseudoxanthoma elasticum. J Am Acad Dermatol 1995; 32: 589–594.

141 Truter S, Sapadin A, Rosenbaum J et al. Role of fibrillin-2 in pseudoxanthoma elasticum. J Invest Dermatol 1996; 106: 894 (abstract).

142 Nickoloff BJ, Noodleman FR, Abel EA. Perforating pseudoxanthoma elasticum associated with chronic renal failure and hemodialysis. Arch Dermatol 1985; 121: 1321–1322.

143 Dupre A, Bonafe JL, Christol B. Chequered localized pseudoxanthoma elasticum: a variety of Christensen's exogenous pseudoxanthoma elasticum? Acta Derm Venereol 1979; 59: 539–541.

144 Hicks J, Carpenter CL, Reed RJ. Periumbilical perforating pseudoxanthoma elasticum. Arch Dermatol 1979; 115: 300–303.

145 Christensen OB. An exogenous variety of pseudoxanthoma elasticum in old farmers. Acta Derm Venereol 1978; 58: 319–321.

146 Nielsen AO, Christensen OB, Hentzer B et al. Salpeter-induced dermal changes electron-microscopically indistinguishable from pseudoxanthoma elasticum. Acta Derm Venereol 1978; 58: 323–327.

147 Kazakis AM, Parish WR. Periumbilical perforating pseudoxanthoma elasticum. J Am Acad Dermatol 1988; 19: 384–388.

148 Neldner KH, Martinez-Hernandez A. Localized acquired cutaneous pseudoxanthoma elasticum. J Am Acad Dermatol 1979; 1: 523–530.

149 Pruzan D, Rabbin PE, Heilman ER. Periumbilical perforating pseudoxanthoma elasticum. J Am Acad Dermatol 1992; 26: 642–644.

150 Nikko AP, Dunningan M, Cockerell CJ. Calciphylaxis with histologic changes of pseudoxanthoma elasticum. Am J Dermatopathol 1996; 18: 396–399.

151 Sapadin AN, Lebwohl MG, Teich SA et al. Periumbilical pseudoxanthoma elasticum associated with chronic renal failure and angioid streaks – apparent regression with hemodialysis. J Am Acad Dermatol 1998; 39: 338–344.

152 Baccarani-Contri M, Bacchelli B, Boraldi F et al. Characterization of pseudoxanthoma elasticum-like lesions in the skin of patients with β-thalassemia. J Am Acad Dermatol 2001; 44: 33–39.

153 Sueki H, Amemiya M, Watanabe H et al. Spontaneous resolution in a case of pseudo-pseudoxanthoma elasticum. Br J Dermatol 2001; 144: 213–215.

154 Buka R, Wei H, Sapadin A et al. Pseudoxanthoma elasticum and calcinosis cutis. J Am Acad Dermatol 2000; 43: 312–315.

155 Heyl T. Pseudoxanthoma elasticum with granulomatous skin lesions. Arch Dermatol 1967; 96: 528–531.

156 Loche F, Raynal H, Bazex J. Acne-like eruption induced by pseudoxanthoma elasticum: effectiveness of liquid nitrogen cryotherapy. Eur J Dermatol 1998; 1: 63–65.

157 McKee PH, Cameron CHS, Archer DB, Logan WC. A study of four cases of pseudoxanthoma elasticum. J Cutan Pathol 1977; 4: 146–153.

158 Danielsen L, Kobayasi T. Pseudoxanthoma elasticum. An ultrastructural study of scar tissue. Acta Derm Venereol 1974; 54: 121–128.

159 Yamamura T, Sano S. Ultrastructural and histochemical analysis of thready material in pseudoxanthoma elasticum. J Cutan Pathol 1984; 11: 282–291.

160 Nakayama H, Hashimoto K, Kambe N, Eng A. Elastic globes: electron microscopic and immunohistochemical observations. J Cutan Pathol 1988; 15: 98–103.

161 Brennan TE, Pearson RW. Abnormal elastic tissue in cartilage–hair hypoplasia. Arch Dermatol 1988; 124: 1411–1414.

Solar elastotic syndromes

162 Gilchrest BA. A review of skin ageing and its medical therapy. Br J Dermatol 1996; 135: 867–875.

163 Malvy DJ-M, Guinot C, Preziosi P et al. Epidemiologic determinants of skin photoaging: Baseline data of the SU.VI.MAX. cohort. J Am Acad Dermatol 2000; 42: 47–55.

164 Salasche SJ, Clemons DE. Cutaneous manifestations of chronic solar exposure. J Assoc Milit Dermatol 1985; 11: 3–10.

165 Calderone DC, Fenske NA. The clinical spectrum of actinic elastosis. J Am Acad Dermatol 1995; 32: 1016–1024.

166 Hashimoto K, Black M. Colloid milium: a final degeneration product of actinic elastoid. J Cutan Pathol 1985; 12: 147–156.

167 Sunderkötter C, Kalden H, Luger TA. Aging and the skin immune system. Arch Dermatol 1997; 133: 1256–1262.

168 O'Brien JP, Regan W. Actinically degenerate elastic tissue is the likely antigenic basis of actinic granuloma of the skin and of temporal arteritis. J Am Acad Dermatol 1999; 40: 214–222.

169 Barnhill RL, Goldenhersh MA. Elastophagocytosis: a non-specific reaction pattern associated with inflammatory processes in sun-protected skin. J Cutan Pathol 1989; 16: 199–202.

170 Cockerell EG, Freeman RG, Knox JM. Changes after prolonged exposure to sunlight. Arch Dermatol 1961; 84: 467–472.

171 Lowe NJ, Meyers DP, Wieder JM et al. Low doses of repetitive ultraviolet A induce morphologic changes in human skin. J Invest Dermatol 1995; 105: 739–743.

172 Lavker RM, Gerberick GF, Veres D et al. Cumulative effects from repeated exposures to suberythemal doses of UVB and UVA in human skin. J Am Acad Dermatol 1995; 32: 53–62.

173 O'Brien JP. Solar and radiant damage to elastic tissue as a cause of internal vascular damage. Australas J Dermatol 1980; 21: 1–8.

174 Boyd AS, Stasko T, King LE Jr et al. Cigarette smoking-associated elastotic changes in the skin. J Am Acad Dermatol 1999; 41: 23–26.

175 Vélez A, López-Rubio F, Moreno J-C. Chronic hydroxyurea-induced dermatomyositis-like eruption with severe dermal elastosis. Clin Exp Dermatol 1998; 23: 94–95.

176 Castanet J, Ortonne J-P. Pigmentary changes in aged and photoaged skin. Arch Dermatol 1997; 133: 1296–1299.

177 Kocsard E. Senile elastosis: central phenomenon of aging of exposed skin. Geriatrics Digest 1970; 7: 10–18.

178 Taylor CR, Stern RS, Leyden JJ, Gilchrest BA. Photoaging/photodamage and photoprotection. J Am Acad Dermatol 1990; 22: 1–15.

179 Degos R, Touraine R, Civatte J, Belaich S. Elastome en nappe du nez. Bull Soc Franc Derm Syph 1966; 73: 123–124.

180 Raimer SS, Sanchez RL, Hubler WR Jr, Dodson RF. Solar elastotic bands of the forearm: an unusual clinical presentation of actinic elastosis. J Am Acad Dermatol 1986; 15: 650–656.

181 Williams BT, Barr RJ, Dutta B. Bullous solar elastosis. J Am Acad Dermatol 1996; 34: 836–858.

182 Mitchell RE. Chronic solar dermatosis: a light and electron microscopic study of the dermis. J Invest Dermatol 1967; 48: 203–220.

183 Stevanovic DV. Elastotic degeneration. A light and electron microscopic study. Br J Dermatol 1976; 94: 23–29.

184 Bouissou H, Pieraggi M-T, Julian M, Savit T. The elastic tissue of the skin. A comparison of spontaneous and actinic (solar) aging. Int J Dermatol 1988; 27: 327–335.

185 Chen VL, Fleischmajer R, Schwartz E et al. Immunochemistry of elastotic material in sun-damaged skin. J Invest Dermatol 1986; 87: 334–337.

186 Bernstein EF, Chen YQ, Tamai K et al. Enhanced elastin and fibrillin gene expression in chronically photodamaged skin. J Invest Dermatol 1994; 103: 182–186.

187 Miyachi Y, Ishikawa O. Dermal connective tissue metabolism in photoageing. Australas J Dermatol 1998; 39: 19–23.

188 Bernstein EF, Underhill CB, Hahn PJ et al. Chronic sun exposure alters both the content and distribution of dermal glycosaminoglycans. Br J Dermatol 1996; 135: 255–262.

189 Craven NM, Watson REB, Jones CJP et al. Clinical features of photodamaged human skin are associated with a reduction in collagen VII. Br J Dermatol 1997; 137: 344–350.

190 Saarialho-Kere U, Kerkelä E, Jeskanen L et al. Accumulation of matrilysin (MMP-7) and macrophage metalloelastase (MMP-12) in actinic damage. J Invest Dermatol 1999; 113: 664–672.

191 Fisher GJ, Datta SC, Talwar HS et al. Molecular basis of sun-induced premature skin ageing and retinoid antagonism. Nature 1996; 379: 335–339.

192 Fisher GJ, Wang ZQ, Datta SC et al. Pathophysiology of premature skin aging induced by ultraviolet light. N Engl J Med 1997; 337: 1419–1428.

193 Varani J, Warner RL, Gharaee-Kermani M et al. Vitamin A antagonizes decreased cell growth and elevated collagen-degrading matrix metalloproteinases and stimulates collagen accumulation in naturally aged human skin. J Invest Dermatol 2000; 114: 480–486.

194 Hase T, Shinta K, Murase T et al. Histological increase in inflammatory infiltrate in sun-exposed skin of female subjects: the possible involvement of matrix metalloproteinase-1 produced by inflammatory infiltrate on collagen degradation. Br J Dermatol 2000; 142: 267–273.

195 Yaar M, Gilchrest BA. Aging *versus* photoaging: postulated mechanisms and effectors. J Invest Dermatol (Symposium Proceedings) 1998; 3: 47–51.

196 Bhawan J, Andersen W, Lee J et al. Photoaging versus intrinsic aging: a morphologic assessment of facial skin. J Cutan Pathol 1995; 22: 154–159.

197 Warren R, Gartstein V, Kligman AM et al. Age, sunlight, and facial skin: a histologic and quantitative study. J Am Acad Dermatol 1991; 25: 751–760.

198 Montagna W, Carlisle K. Structural changes in aging human skin. J Invest Dermatol 1979; 73: 47–53.

199 Nelson BR, Majmudar G, Griffiths CEM et al. Clinical improvement following dermabrasion of photoaged skin correlates with synthesis of collagen 1. Arch Dermatol 1994; 130: 1136–1142.

200 Kossard S, Anderson P, Davies A, Cooper A. Histological evaluation of the effect of 0.05% tretinoin in the treatment of photodamaged skin. Australas J Dermatol 1993; 34: 89–95.

201 Weinstein GD, Nigra TP, Pochi PE et al. Topical tretinoin for treatment of photodamaged skin. A multicenter study. Arch Dermatol 1991; 127: 659–665.

202 Rosenthal DS, Roop DR, Huff CA et al. Changes in photo-aged human skin following topical application of All-trans retinoic acid. J Invest Dermatol 1990; 95: 510–515.

203 Bhawan J, Gonzalez-Serva A, Nehal K et al. Effects of tretinoin on photodamaged skin. A histologic study. Arch Dermatol 1991; 127: 666–672.

204 Kang S, Fisher GJ, Voorhees JJ. Photoaging and topical tretinoin. Therapy, pathogenesis, and prevention. Arch Dermatol 1997; 133: 1280–1284.

205 Ellis CN, Weiss JS, Hamilton TA et al. Sustained improvement with prolonged topical tretinoin (retinoic acid) for photoaged skin. J Am Acad Dermatol 1990; 23: 629–637.

206 Uitto J. Understanding premature skin aging. N Engl J Med 1997; 337: 1463–1465.

207 Green C, Orchard G, Cerio R, Hawk JLM. A clinicopathological study of the effects of topical retinyl propionate cream in skin photoageing. Clin Exp Dermatol 1998; 23: 162–167.

208 Boyd AS, Naylor M, Cameron GS et al. The effects of chronic sunscreen use on the histologic changes of dermatoheliosis. J Am Acad Dermatol 1995; 33: 941–946.

209 Phillips TJ, Bhawan J, Yaar M et al. Effect of daily versus intermittent sunscreen application on solar simulated UV radiation-induced skin response in humans. J Am Acad Dermatol 2000; 43: 610–618.

210 Lavker RM. Structural alterations in exposed and unexposed aged skin. J Invest Dermatol 1979; 73: 59–66.

211 Goette DK. Transepidermal elimination of actinically damaged connective tissue. Int J Dermatol 1984; 23: 669–672.

212 Toyoda M, Morohashi M. Morphological alterations of epidermal melanocytes in photoageing: an ultrastructural and cytomorphometric study. Br J Dermatol 1998; 139: 444–452.

213 Hartschuh W, Schulz T. Merkel cell hyperplasia in chronic radiation-damaged skin: its possible relationship to fibroepithelioma of Pinkus. J Cutan Pathol 1997; 24: 477–483.

214 Lavker RM, Kligman AM. Chronic heliodermatitis: a morphologic evaluation of chronic actinic dermal damage with emphasis on the role of mast cells. J Invest Dermatol 1988; 90: 325–330.

215 Montagna W, Kirchner S, Carlisle K. Histology of sun-damaged human skin. J Am Acad Dermatol 1989; 21: 907–918.

216 Ledoux-Corbusier M, Danis P. Pinguecula and actinic elastosis. An ultrastructural study. J Cutan Pathol 1979; 6: 404–413.

217 Danielsen L, Kobayasi T. Degeneration of dermal elastic fibres in relation to age and light-exposure. Preliminary report on electron microscopic studies. Acta Derm Venereol 1972; 52: 1–10.

218 Ledoux-Corbusier M, Achten G. Elastosis in chronic radiodermatitis. An ultrastructural study. Br J Dermatol 1974; 91: 287–295.

219 Bernstein EF, Chen YQ, Kopp JB et al. Long-term sun exposure alters the collagen of the papillary dermis. J Am Acad Dermatol 1996; 34: 209–218.

220 Zelickson AS, Mottaz JH, Zelickson BD, Muller SA. Elastic tissue changes in skin following PUVA therapy. J Am Acad Dermatol 1980; 3: 186–192.

221 Tsuji T. The surface structural alterations of elastic fibers and elastotic material in solar elastosis: a scanning electron microscopic study. J Cutan Pathol 1984; 11: 300–308.

222 Cuce LC, Paschoal LHC, Curban GV. Cutaneous nodular elastoidosis with cysts and comedones Arch Dermatol 1964; 89: 798–802.

223 Helm F. Nodular cutaneous elastosis with cysts and comedones (Favre–Racouchot syndrome). Arch Dermatol 1961; 84: 666–668.

224 Sharkey MJ, Keller RA, Grabski WJ et al. Favre–Racouchot syndrome. A combined therapeutic approach. Arch Dermatol 1992; 128: 615–616.

225 Siragusa M, Maglioli E, Batolo D, Schepis C. An unusual location of nodular elastosis with cysts and comedones (Favre–Racouchot's disease). Acta Derm Venereol 2000; 80: 452.

226 Keough GC, Laws RA, Elston DM. Favre–Racouchot syndrome: a case for smokers' comedones. Arch Dermatol 1997; 133: 796–797.

227 Hassounah A, Pierard GE. Kerosis and comedos without prominent elastosis in Favre–Racouchot disease. Am J Dermatopathol 1987; 9: 15–17.

228 Carter VH, Constantine VS, Poole WL. Elastotic nodules of the antihelix. Arch Dermatol 1969; 100: 282–285.

229 Weedon D. Elastotic nodules of the ear. J Cutan Pathol 1981; 8: 429–433.

230 Kocsard E, Ofner F, Turner B. Elastotic nodules of the antihelix. Arch Dermatol 1970; 101: 37C.

231 Jordaan HF, Rossouw DJ. Digital papular calcific elastosis: a histopathological, histochemical and ultrastructural study of 20 patients. J Cutan Pathol 1990; 17: 358–370.

232 Rahbari H. Acrokeratoelastoidosis and keratoelastoidosis marginalis – any relation? J Am Acad Dermatol 1981; 5: 348–350.

233 Burks JW, Wise LJ, Clark WH. Degenerative collagenous plaques of the hands. Arch Dermatol 1960; 82: 362–366.

234 Kocsard E. Keratoelastoidosis marginalis of the hands. Dermatologica 1964; 131: 169–175.

235 Abulafia J, Vignale RA. Degenerative collagenous plaques of the hands and acrokeratoelastoidosis: pathogenesis and relationship with knuckle pads. J Invest Dermatol 2000; 39: 424–432.

236 Todd D, Al-Aboosi M, Hameed O et al. The role of UV light in the pathogenesis of digital papular calcific elastosis. Arch Dermatol 2001; 137: 379–381.

237 Ritchie EB, Williams HM. Degenerative collagenous plaques of the hands. Arch Dermatol 1966; 93: 202–203.

238 Shahrad P, Marks R. The wages of warmth: changes in erythema ab igne. Br J Dermatol 1977; 97: 179–186.

239 Milligan A, Graham-Brown RAC. Erythema ab igne affecting the palms. Clin Exp Dermatol 1989; 14: 168–169.

240 Wilson NJE, Sharpe GR. Erythema ab igne in a child with atopic eczema. Clin Exp Dermatol 1999; 24: 337–338.

241 Arrington JH III, Lockman DS. Thermal keratoses and squamous cell carcinoma in situ associated with erythema ab igne. Arch Dermatol 1979; 115: 1226–1228.

242 Finlayson GR, Sams WM Jr, Smith JG Jr. Erythema ab igne: a histopathological study. J Invest Dermatol 1966; 46: 104–108.

243 Johnson WC, Butterworth T. Erythema ab igne elastosis. Arch Dermatol 1971; 104: 128–131.

Decreased elastic tissue

244 Bordas X, Ferrandiz C, Ribera M, Galofre E. Papular elastorrhexis: a variety of nevus anelasticus? Arch Dermatol 1987; 123: 433–434.

245 Crivellato E. Disseminated nevus anelasticus. Int J Dermatol 1986; 25: 171–173.

246 Sears JK, Stone MS, Argenyi Z. Papular elastorrhexis: a variant of connective tissue nevus. Case reports and review of the literature. J Am Acad Dermatol 1988; 19: 409–414.

247 Schirren H, Schirren CG, Stolz W et al. Papular elastorrhexis: a variant of dermatofibrosis lenticularis disseminata (Buschke–Ollendorff syndrome)? Dermatology 1994; 189: 368–372.

248 Varadi DP, Saqueton AC. Perifollicular elastolysis. Br J Dermatol 1970; 83: 143–150.

249 Taaffe A, Cunliffe WJ, Clayden AD. Perifollicular elastolysis – a common condition. Br J Dermatol (Suppl) 1983; 24: 20.

250 Wilson BB, Dent CH, Cooper PH. Papular acne scars. A common cutaneous finding. Arch Dermatol 1990; 126: 797–800.

251 Venencie PY, Winkelmann RK, Moore BA. Anetoderma. Clinical findings, associations, and long-term follow-up evaluations. Arch Dermatol 1984; 120: 1032–1039.

252 Miller WN, Ruggles CW, Rist TE. Anetoderma. Int J Dermatol 1979; 18: 43–45.

253 Friedman SJ, Venencie PY, Bradley RR, Winkelmann RK. Familial anetoderma. J Am Acad Dermatol 1987; 16: 341–345.

254 Aberer E, Weissenbacher G. Congenital anetoderma induced by intrauterine infection? Arch Dermatol 1997; 133: 526–527.

255 Peterman A, Scheel M, Sams WM Jr, Pandya AG. Hereditary anetoderma. J Am Acad Dermatol 1996; 35: 999–1000.

256 Zellman GL, Levy ML. Congenital anetoderma in twins. J Am Acad Dermatol 1997; 36: 483–485.

257 Gerritsen MJP, de Rooij MJM, Sybrandy-Fleuren BAM, van de Kerkhof PCM. Familial anetoderma. Dermatology 1999; 198: 321–322.

258 Özkan Ş, Fetil E, İzler F et al. Anetoderma secondary to generalized granuloma annulare. J Am Acad Dermatol 2000; 42: 335–338.

259 Ruiz-Rodriguez R, Longaker M, Berger TG. Anetoderma and human immunodeficiency virus infection. Arch Dermatol 1992; 128: 661–662.

260 Lindstrom J, Smith KJ, Skelton HG et al. Increased anticardiolipin antibodies associated with the development of anetoderma in HIV-1 disease. Int J Dermatol 1995; 34: 408–415.

261 Schepis C, Siragusa M. Secondary anetoderma in people with Down's syndrome. Acta Derm Venereol 1999; 79: 245.

262 Crone AM, James MP. Acquired linear anetoderma following angular cheilitis. Br J Dermatol 1998; 138: 923–924.

263 Jubert C, Cosnes A, Wechsler J et al. Anetoderma may reveal cutaneous plasmacytoma and benign cutaneous lymphoid hyperplasia. Arch Dermatol 1995; 131: 365–366.

264 Kasper RC, Wood GS, Nihal M, LeBoit PE. Anetoderma arising in cutaneous B-cell lymphoproliferative disease. Am J Dermatopathol 2001; 23: 124–132.

265 Ang P, Tay YK. Anetoderma in a patient with juvenile xanthogranuloma. Br J Dermatol 1999; 140: 541–542.

266 Child FJ, Woollons A, Price ML et al. Multiple cutaneous immunocytoma with secondary anetoderma: a report of two cases. Br J Dermatol 2000; 143: 165–170.

267 Davis W. Wilson's disease and penicillamine-induced anetoderma. Arch Dermatol 1977; 113: 976.

268 Daoud MS, Dicken CH. Anetoderma after hepatitis B immunization in two siblings. J Am Acad Dermatol 1997; 36: 779–780.

269 Prizant TL, Lucky AW, Frieden IJ et al. Spontaneous atrophic patches in extremely premature infants. Anetoderma of prematurity. Arch Dermatol 1996; 132: 671–674.

270 Todd DJ. Anetoderma of prematurity. Arch Dermatol 1997; 133: 789.

271 Colditz PB, Dunster KR, Joy GJ, Robertson IM. Anetoderma of prematurity in association with electrocardiographic electrodes. J Am Acad Dermatol 1999; 41: 478–481.

272 Carrington PR, Altick JA, Sanusi ID. Atrophoderma elastolytica discreta. Am J Dermatopathol 1996; 18: 212–217.

273 Carr RD. Urticaria pigmentosa associated with anetoderma. Acta Derm Venereol 1971; 51: 120–122.

274 Shames BS, Nassif A, Bailey CS, Saltzstein SL. Secondary anetoderma involving a pilomatricoma. Am J Dermatopathol 1994; 16: 557–560.

275 Kelly SE, Humphreys F, Aldridge RD. The phenomenon of anetoderma occurring over pilomatricomas. J Am Acad Dermatol 1993; 28: 511.

276 Oikarinen AI, Palatsi R, Adomian GE et al. Anetoderma: biochemical and ultrastructural demonstration of an elastin defect in the skin of three patients. J Am Acad Dermatol 1984; 11: 64–72.

277 Venencie PY, Winkelmann RK. Histopathologic findings in anetoderma. Arch Dermatol 1984; 120: 1040–1044.

278 Hodak E, Shamai-Lubovitz O, David M et al. Immunologic abnormalities associated with primary anetoderma. Arch Dermatol 1992; 128: 799–803.

279 Hodak E, Shamai-Lubovitz O, David M et al. Primary anetoderma associated with a wide spectrum of autoimmune abnormalities. J Am Acad Dermatol 1991; 25: 415–418.

280 Disdier P, Harlé J-R, Andrac L et al. Primary anetoderma associated with the antiphospholipid syndrome. J Am Acad Dermatol 1994; 30: 133–134.

281 Venencie PY, Winkelmann RK. Monoclonal antibody studies in the skin lesions of patients with anetoderma. Arch Dermatol 1985; 121: 747–749.

282 Zaki I, Scerri L, Nelson H. Primary anetoderma: phagocytosis of elastic fibres by macrophages. Clin Exp Dermatol 1994; 19: 388–390.

283 Taïeb A, Dufillot D, Pellegrin-Carloz B et al. Postgranulomatous anetoderma associated with Takayasu's arteritis in a child. Arch Dermatol 1987; 123: 796–800.

284 Bergman R, Friedman-Birnbaum R, Hazaz B et al. An immunofluorescence study of primary anetoderma. Clin Exp Dermatol 1990; 15: 124–130.

285 Venencie PY, Winkelmann RK, Moore BA. Ultrastructural findings in the skin lesions of patients with anetoderma. Acta Derm Venereol 1984; 64: 112–120.

286 Kossard S, Kronman KR, Dicken CH, Schroeter AL. Inflammatory macular atrophy: immunofluorescent and ultrastructural findings. J Am Acad Dermatol 1979; 1: 325–334.

287 Tsuji T, Imajo Y, Sawabe M et al. Acquired cutis laxa concomitant with nephrotic syndrome. Arch Dermatol 1987; 123: 1211–1216.

288 Schreiber MM, Tilley JC. Cutis laxa. Arch Dermatol 1961; 84: 266–272.

289 Ledoux-Corbusier M. Cutis laxa, congenital form with pulmonary emphysema: an ultrastructural study. J Cutan Pathol 1983; 10: 340–349.

290 Mehregan AH, Lee SC, Nabai H. Cutis laxa (generalized elastolysis). A report of four cases with autopsy findings. J Cutan Pathol 1978; 5: 116–126.

291 Sakati NO, Nyhan WL. Congenital cutis laxa and osteoporosis. Am J Dis Child 1983; 137: 452–454.

292 Agha A, Sakati NO, Higginbottom MC et al. Two forms of cutis laxa presenting in the newborn period. Acta Paediatr Scand 1978; 67: 775–780.

293 Byers PH, Siegel RC, Holbrook KA et al. X-linked cutis laxa. N Engl J Med 1980; 303: 61–65.

294 Brown FR III, Holbrook KA, Byers PH et al. Cutis laxa. Johns Hopkins Med J 1982; 150: 148–153.

295 Ostlere LS, Pope FM, Holden CA. Cutis laxa complicating Ehlers–Danlos syndrome type II. Clin Exp Dermatol 1996; 21: 135–137.

296 George S, Jacob M, Pulimood S, Chandi SM. Cutis laxa. Clin Exp Dermatol 1998; 23: 211–213.

297 Fisher BK, Page E, Hanna W. Acral localized acquired cutis laxa. J Am Acad Dermatol 1989; 21: 33–40.

298 Greenbaum SS, Krull EA, Rubin MG, Lee R. Localized acquired cutis laxa in one of identical twins. Int J Dermatol 1989; 28: 402–406.

299 Ghigliotti G, Parodi A, Borgiani L et al. Acquired cutis laxa confined to the face. J Am Acad Dermatol 1991; 24: 504–505.

300 Martin L, Requena L, Yus ES et al. Acrolocalized acquired cutis laxa. Br J Dermatol 1996; 134: 973–976.

301 Reed WB, Horowitz RE, Beighton P. Acquired cutis laxa. Primary generalized elastolysis. Arch Dermatol 1971; 103: 661–669.

302 Nanko H, Jepsen LV, Zachariae H, Sogaard H. Acquired cutis laxa (generalized elastolysis): light and electron microscopic studies. Acta Derm Venereol 1979; 59: 315–324.

303 Chun SI, Yoon J. Acquired cutis laxa associated with chronic urticaria. J Am Acad Dermatol 1995; 33: 896–899.

304 Boulec A, Godeau G, Zeller J et al. Increased fibroblast elastase activity in acquired cutis laxa. Dermatology 1999; 198: 346–350.

305 Lewis FM, Lewis-Jones S, Gipson M. Acquired cutis laxa with dermatitis herpetiformis and sarcoidosis. J Am Acad Dermatol 1993; 29: 846–848.

306 Garcia-Patos V, Pujol RM, Barnadas MA et al. Generalized acquired cutis laxa associated with coeliac disease: evidence of immunoglobulin A deposits on the dermal elastic fibres. Br J Dermatol 1996; 135: 130–134.

307 Muster AJ, Bharati S, Herman JJ et al. Fatal cardiovascular disease and cutis laxa following acute febrile neutrophilic dermatosis. J Pediatr 1983; 102: 243–248.

308 Harris RB, Heaphy MR, Perry HO. Generalized elastolysis (cutis laxa). Am J Med 1978; 65: 815–822.

309 Kerl H, Burg G, Hashimoto K. Fatal, penicillin-induced, generalized postinflammatory elastolysis (cutis laxa). Am J Dermatopathol 1983; 5: 267–276.

310 Koch SE, Williams ML. Acquired cutis laxa: case report and review of disorders of elastolysis. Pediatr Dermatol 1985; 2: 282–288.

311 Hashimoto K, Kanzaki T. Cutis laxa. Ultrastructural and biochemical studies. Arch Dermatol 1975; 111: 861–873.

312 Scott MA, Kauh YC, Luscombe HA. Acquired cutis laxa associated with multiple myeloma. Arch Dermatol 1976; 112: 853–855.

313 Ting HC, Foo MH, Wang F. Acquired cutis laxa and multiple myeloma. Br J Dermatol 1984; 110: 363–367.

314 Nikko A, Dunnigan M, Black A, Cockerell CJ. Acquired cutis laxa associated with a plasma cell dyscrasia. Am J Dermatopathol 1996; 18: 533–537.

315 Machet MC, Machet L, Vaillant L et al. Acquired localized cutis laxa due to cutaneous lymphoplasmacytoid lymphoma. Arch Dermatol 1995; 131: 110–111.

316 Chartier S, Faucher L, Tousignant J, Rochette L. Acquired cutis laxa associated with cutaneous angiocentric T-cell lymphoma. Int J Dermatol 1997; 36: 772–776.

317 Randle HW, Muller S. Generalized elastolysis associated with systemic lupus erythematosus. J Am Acad Dermatol 1983; 8: 869–873.

318 García-Patos V, Pujol RM, Barnadas MA et al. Generalized acquired cutis laxa associated with coeliac disease: evidence of immunoglobulin A deposits on the dermal elastic fibres. Br J Dermatol 1996; 135: 130–134.

319 Zhang M-C, He L, Giro MG et al. Cutis laxa arising from frameshift mutations in exon 30 of the elastin gene (ELN). J Biol Chem 1999; 274: 981–986.

320 Fornieri C, Quaglino D, Lungarella G et al. Elastin production and degradation in cutis laxa acquisita. J Invest Dermatol 1994; 103: 583–588.

321 Hatamochi A, Kuroda K, Shinkai H et al. Regulation of matrix metalloproteinase (MMP) expression in cutis laxa fibroblasts: upregulation of MMP-1, MMP-3 and MMP-9 genes but not of the MMP-2 gene. Br J Dermatol 1998; 138: 757–762.

322 Hatamochi A, Mori K, Arakawa M et al. Collagenase gene expression in cutis laxa fibroblasts is upregulated by transcriptional activation of the promoter gene through a 12-O-tetradecanoyl-phorbol-13-acetate (TPA)-responsive element. J Invest Dermatol 1996; 106: 631–636.

323 Hatamochi A, Nagayama H, Kuroda K et al. Costello syndrome with decreased gene expression of elastin in cultured dermal fibroblasts. Dermatology 2000; 201: 366–369.

324 Sato M, Ishikawa O, Miyachi Y et al. Michelin tyre syndrome: a congenital disorder of elastic fibre formation? Br J Dermatol 1997; 136: 583–586.

325 Goltz RW, Hult A-M, Goldfarb M, Gorlin RJ. Cutis laxa. A manifestation of generalized elastolysis. Arch Dermatol 1965; 92: 373–387.

326 Sephel GC, Byers PH, Holbrook KA, Davidson JM. Heterogeneity of elastin expression in cutis laxa fibroblast strains. J Invest Dermatol 1989; 93: 147–153.

327 Kitano Y, Nishida K, Okada N et al. Cutis laxa with ultrastructural abnormalities of elastic fiber. J Am Acad Dermatol 1989; 21: 378–380.

328 Lebwohl MG, Schwartz E, Jacobs L et al. Abnormalities of fibrillin in acquired cutis laxa. J Am Acad Dermatol 1994; 30: 950–954.

329 Marchase P, Holbrook K, Pinnell SR. A familial cutis laxa syndrome with ultrastructural abnormalities of collagen and elastin. J Invest Dermatol 1980; 75: 399–403.

330 Niemi K-M, Anton-Lamprecht I, Virtanen I et al. Fibrillar protein deposits with tubular substructure in a systemic disease beginning as cutis laxa. Arch Dermatol 1993; 129: 757–762.

331 Barker SM, Dicken CH. Elastolysis of the earlobes. J Am Acad Dermatol 1986; 14: 145–147.

332 El-Charif MA, Mousawi AM, Rubeiz NG, Kibbi A-G. Pseudoxanthoma elasticum-like papillary dermal elastolysis: a report of two cases. J Cutan Pathol 1994; 21: 252–255.

333 Ramos-Caro FA, Sevigny G, Mullins D. Solitary hyperpigmented island in a sea of elastosis (anelastosis). Int J Dermatol 1998; 37: 699–700.

334 Hashimoto K, Tye MJ. Upper dermal elastolysis: a comparative study with mid-dermal elastolysis. J Cutan Pathol 1994; 21: 533–540.

335 Ohnishi Y, Tajima S, Ishibashi A et al. Pseudoxanthoma elasticum-like papillary dermal elastolysis: report of four Japanese cases and an immunohistochemical study of elastin and fibrillin-1. Br J Dermatol 1998; 139: 141–144.

336 Tajima S, Ohnishi Y, Akagi A et al. Elastotic change in the subpapillary and mid-dermal layers in pseudoxanthoma elasticum-like papillary dermal elastolysis. Br J Dermatol 2000; 142: 586–588.

337 Shelley WB, Wood MG. Wrinkles due to idiopathic loss of mid-dermal elastic tissue. Br J Dermatol 1977; 97: 441–445.

338 Brenner W, Gschnait F, Konrad K et al. Non-inflammatory dermal elastolysis. Br J Dermatol 1978; 99: 335–338.

339 Rudolph RI. Mid dermal elastolysis. J Am Acad Dermatol 1990; 22: 203–206.

340 Rae V, Falanga V. Wrinkling due to middermal elastolysis. Report of a case and review of the literature. Arch Dermatol 1989; 125: 950–951.

341 Ortel B, Rappersberger K, Konrad K. Middermal elastolysis in an elderly man with evidence of elastic fiber phagocytosis. Arch Dermatol 1992; 128: 88–90.

342 Kim JM, Su WPD. Mid dermal elastolysis with wrinkling. Report of two cases and review of the literature. J Am Acad Dermatol 1992; 26: 169–173.

343 Sterling JC, Coleman N, Pye RJ. Mid-dermal elastolysis. Br J Dermatol 1994; 130: 502–506.

344 Snider RL, Lang PG, Maize JC. The clinical spectrum of mid-dermal elastolysis and the role of UV light in its pathogenesis. J Am Acad Dermatol 1993; 28: 938–942.

345 Harmon CB, Su WPD, Gagne EJ et al. Ultrastructural evaluation of mid-dermal elastolysis. J Cutan Pathol 1994; 21: 233–238.

346 Kirsner RS, Falanga V. Features of an autoimmune process in mid-dermal elastolysis. J Am Acad Dermatol 1992; 27: 832–834.

347 Yen A, Tschen J, Raimer SS. Mid-dermal elastolysis in an adolescent subsequent to lesions resembling granuloma annulare. J Am Acad Dermatol 1997; 37: 870–872.

348 Boyd AS, King LE Jr. Middermal elastolysis in two patients with lupus erythematosus. Am J Dermatopathol 2001; 23: 136–138.

349 Marshall J, Heyl T, Weber HW. Post-inflammatory elastolysis and cutis laxa. S Afr Med J 1966; 40: 1016–1022.

350 Verhagen AR, Woerdeman MJ. Post-inflammatory elastolysis and cutis laxa. Br J Dermatol 1975; 92: 183–190.

351 Lewis PG, Hood AF, Barnett NK, Holbrook KA. Postinflammatory elastolysis and cutis laxa. J Am Acad Dermatol 1990; 22: 40–48.

352 Neri I, Patrizi A, Fanti P et al. Mid-dermal elastolysis: a pathological and ultrastructural study of five cases. J Cutan Pathol 1996; 23: 165–169.

353 Brod BA, Rabkin M, Rhodes AR, Jegasothy BV. Mid-dermal elastolysis with inflammation. J Am Acad Dermatol 1992; 26: 882–884.

354 Bannister MJ, Rubel DM, Kossard S. Mid-dermal elastophagocytosis presenting as a persistent reticulate erythema. Australas J Dermatol 2001; 42: 50–54.

355 Maghrooui S, Grossin M, Crickx B et al. Mid dermal elastolysis. Report of a case with a predominant perifollicular pattern. J Am Acad Dermatol 1992; 26: 490–492.

356 Urbán Z, Peyrol S, Plauchu H et al. Elastin gene deletions in Williams syndrome patients result in altered deposition of elastic fibers in skin and a subclinical dermal phenotype. Pediatr Dermatol 2000; 17: 12–20.

357 Menkes JH, Alter M, Steigleder GK et al. A sex-linked recessive disorder with retardation of growth, peculiar hair, and focal cerebral and cerebellar degeneration. Pediatrics 1962; 29: 764–779.

358 Hockey A, Masters CL. Menkes' kinky (steely) hair disease. Australas J Dermatol 1977; 18: 77–80.

359 Hart DB. Menkes' syndrome: an updated review. J Am Acad Dermatol 1983; 9: 145–152.

360 Martins C, Gonçalves C, Moreno A et al. Menkes' kinky hair syndrome: ultrastructural cutaneous alterations of the elastic fibers. Pediatr Dermatol 1997; 14: 347–350.

361 Procopis P, Camakaris J, Danks DM. A mild form of Menkes' steely hair syndrome. J Pediatr 1981; 98: 97–99.

362 Danks DM, Stevens BJ, Campbell PE et al. Menkes' kinky hair syndrome. Lancet 1972; 1: 1100–1102.

363 Oakes BW, Danks DM, Campbell PE. Human copper deficiency: ultrastructural studies of the aorta and skin in a child with Menkes' syndrome. Exp Mol Pathol 1976; 25: 82–98.

364 Royce PM, Camakaris J, Danks DM. Reduced lysyl oxidase activity in skin fibroblasts from patients with Menkes' syndrome. Biochem J 1980; 192: 579–586.

365 Waldstein G, Mierau G, Ahmad R et al. Fragile X syndrome: skin elastin abnormalities. Birth Defects 1987; 23: 103–114.

366 Willemsen R, Olmer R, Otero YDD, Oostra BA. Twin sisters, monozygotic with the fragile X mutation, but with a different phenotype. J Med Genet 2000; 37: 603–604.

367 Moore SJ, Strain L, Cole GF et al. Fragile X syndrome with FMR1 and FMR2 deletion. J Med Genet 1999; 36: 565–566.

368 Boente MdC, Winik BC, Asial RA. Wrinkly skin syndrome: ultrastructural alterations of the elastic fibers. Pediatr Dermatol 1999; 16: 113–117.

369 Yanagihara M, Kato F, Mori S. Extra and intracellular digestion of elastic fibers by macrophages in annular elastolytic giant cell granuloma. An ultrastructural study. J Cutan Pathol 1987; 14: 303–308.

370 Boneschi V, Brambilla L, Fossati S et al. Annular elastolytic giant cell granuloma. Am J Dermatopathol 1988; 10: 224–228.

371 LeBoit PE, Zackheim HS, White CR Jr. Granulomatous variants of cutaneous T-cell lymphoma. The histopathology of granulomatous mycosis fungoides and granulomatous slack skin. Am J Dermatopathol 1988; 12: 83–95.

372 Alessi E, Crosti C, Sala F. Unusual case of granulomatous dermohypodermitis with giant cells and elastophagocytosis. Dermatologica 1986; 172: 218–221.

373 Balus L, Bassetti F, Gentili G. Granulomatous slack skin. Arch Dermatol 1985; 121: 250–252.

374 Convit J, Kerdel F, Goihman M et al. Progressive, atrophying, chronic granulomatous dermohypodermitis. Arch Dermatol 1973; 107: 271–274.

375 LeBoit PE, Beckstead JH, Bond B et al. Granulomatous slack skin: clonal rearrangement of the T-cell receptor β gene is evidence for the lymphoproliferative nature of a cutaneous elastolytic disorder. J Invest Dermatol 1987; 89: 183–186.

376 Matsuoka LY, Wortsman J, Uitto J et al. Altered skin elastic fibers in hypothyroid myxedema and pretibial myxedema. Arch Intern Med 1985; 145: 117–121.

377 Fiallo P, Pesce C, Brusasco A, Nunzi E. Acrokeratoelastoidosis of Costa: a primary disease of the elastic tissue? J Cutan Pathol 1998; 25: 580–582.

Variable or minor elastic tissue changes

378 Roth SI, Schedewie HK, Herzberg VK et al. Cutaneous manifestations of leprechaunism. Arch Dermatol 1981; 117: 531–535.

379 Patterson JH, Watkins WL. Leprechaunism in a male infant. J Pediatr 1962; 60: 730–739.

380 Bauer EA, Uitto J, Tan EML, Holbrook KA. Werner's syndrome. Evidence for preferential regional expression of a generalized mesenchymal cell defect. Arch Dermatol 1988; 124: 90–101.

381 Venencie PY, Powell FC, Winkelmann RK. Acrogeria with perforating elastoma and bony abnormalities. Acta Derm Venereol 1984; 64: 348–351.

382 Beauregard S, Gilchrest BA. Syndromes of premature aging. Dermatol Clin 1987; 5: 109–121.

383 Shelley WB, Wood MG. Unilateral wrinkles. Manifestation of unilateral elastic tissue defect. Arch Dermatol 1974; 110: 775–778.

384 Dunn LB, Damesyn M, Moore AA et al. Does estrogen prevent skin aging? Arch Dermatol 1997; 133: 339–342.

385 Kligman AM, Zheng P, Lavker RM. The anatomy and pathogenesis of wrinkles. Br J Dermatol 1985; 113: 37–42.

386 Wright ET, Shellow LR. The histopathology of wrinkles. Journal of the Society of Cosmetic Chemists 1965; 24: 81.

387 Montagna W, Carlisle K. Structural changes in aging human skin. J Invest Dermatol 1979; 73: 47–53.

388 Tsuji T. Ultrastructure of deep wrinkles in the elderly. J Cutan Pathol 1987; 14: 158–164.

389 Tsuji T, Yorifuji T, Hayashi Y, Hamada T. Light and scanning electron microscopic studies on wrinkles in aged persons' skin. Br J Dermatol 1986; 114: 329–335.

390 Contet-Audonneau JL, Jeanmaire C, Pauly G. A histological study of human wrinkle structures: comparison between sun-exposed areas of the face, with or without wrinkles, and sun-protected areas. Br J Dermatol 1999; 140: 1038–1047.

391 Pyeritz RE, McKusick VA. The Marfan syndrome: diagnosis and management. N Engl J Med 1979; 300: 772–777.

392 Tsuji T. Marfan syndrome: demonstration of abnormal elastic fibers in skin. J Cutan Pathol 1986; 13: 144–153.

393 Berteretche M-V, Hornebeck W, Pellat B et al. Histomorphometric parameters and susceptibility to neutrophil elastase degradation of skin elastic fibres from healthy individuals and patients with Marfan syndrome, Ehlers–Danlos type IV, and pseudoxanthoma elasticum. Br J Dermatol 1995; 133: 836–841.

394 Pinkus H, Keech MK, Mehregan AH. Histopathology of striae distensae with special reference to striae and wound healing in the Marfan syndrome. J Invest Dermatol 1966; 46: 283–292.

395 Sayers CP, Goltz RW, Mottaz J. Pulmonary elastic tissue in generalized elastolysis (cutis laxa) and Marfan's syndrome. A light and electron microscopic study. J Invest Dermatol 1975; 65: 451–457.

Cutaneous mucinoses

INTRODUCTION

The mucinoses are a diverse group of disorders which have in common the deposition of basophilic, finely granular and stringy material (mucin) in the connective tissues of the dermis (dermal mucinoses),[1,2] in the pilosebaceous follicles (follicular mucinoses), or in the epidermis and tumors derived therefrom (epithelial mucinoses).[3] The most important mucinoses are the dermal ones where glycosaminoglycans, also known as acid mucopolysaccharides, accumulate in the dermis.[4,5] These may be free, as in the case of hyaluronic acid, or fixed to proteins (proteoglycans). Glycosaminoglycans are produced by fibroblasts and they are able to bind very large amounts of water and minerals.[5] The loss of this water during paraffin processing results in residual basophilic strands and granules in widened dermal spaces in sections stained with hematoxylin and eosin. Fragmentation of the dermal collagen is quite common in the dermal mucinoses. Collagen type III is often reduced although there is a compensatory increase in type I collagen.[6]

The pathogenetic mechanisms involved in the accumulation of mucin in the skin are poorly understood. In many of the mucinoses there appears to be an increased production of acid mucopolysaccharides by fibroblasts, although in myxedema it has been suggested that impaired degradation leads to accumulation of mucin in the dermis (see below). Several of the cutaneous mucinoses have been reported in patients with HIV infection, although only the association with papular mucinosis (lichen myxedematosus) seems to be statistically significant.[7] The relationship between the infection and the mucin deposition is unclear.[7]

In the mucopolysaccharidoses, which are best considered separately from the other mucinoses, the predominant dermal mucin is chondroitin sulfate, rather than hyaluronic acid.

The two most common methods used for demonstrating mucin in the skin are the alcian blue technique at pH 2.5 and the colloidal iron stain, with which acid mucopolysaccharides are blue-green. Metachromasia of mucin is usually demonstrated with the toluidine blue or Giemsa methods. It has been suggested that fixation in a 1% solution of cetylpyridinium chloride in formalin, followed by colloidal iron staining of the paraffin sections, gives the best definition of glycosaminoglycans in the skin.[8]

The histological features of the various mucinoses are summarized in Table 13.1.

DERMAL MUCINOSES

The distribution of the glycosaminoglycans is said to differ in the various dermal mucinoses. However, in a comparative study some years ago, Matsuoka and colleagues found that the distribution of these substances is generally not diagnostically specific.[8] Accordingly, clinicopathological correlation is important in this group. Scleredema and scleromyxedema differ from the other dermal mucinoses by the presence of collagen deposition and fibroblast hypertrophy and/or hyperplasia, in addition to the deposition of mucin.

Alajlan and Ackerman have recently questioned the legitimacy of the concept of the dermal mucinoses.[9] They claim that the term has not yet been defined meaningfully and that each of the 'so-called dermal mucinoses can be identified on the basis of distinctive clinical and histopathological features.'[9]

Table 13.1 **Mucinoses – key histological features**

Disease	Histological features
Generalized myxedema	Subtle changes: mucin deposition often only perivascular or perifollicular; no fibroblast changes
Pretibial myxedema	Increased mucin often localized to mid and lower dermis; fibroblasts sometimes stellate, but not increased
Reticular erythematous mucinosis	Superficial and characteristic mid-dermal perivascular lymphocytic infiltrate; sometimes deeper extension around eccrine coils; mucin usually prominent
Scleredema	Thickening of reticular dermis due to swelling and separation of collagen bundles; no significant hyperplasia of fibroblasts; variable interstitial mucin, sometimes minimal in late stages; no deep inflammatory infiltrate as in morphea
Scleromyxedema	Prominent fibroblastic proliferation and increased collagen; variable mucin increase
Papular mucinosis	Discrete form resembles focal mucinosis; slight proliferation of fibroblasts in generalized form
Acral persistent papular mucinosis	Resembles papular mucinosis but mucin deposition and fibroblast proliferation less pronounced
Cutaneous mucinosis of infancy	May be a variant of scleromyxedema
Focal mucinosis	Dome-shaped solitary nodule with prominent mucin in upper or entire dermis with variable collagen replacement
Digital mucous cyst	Mucinous pool with stellate fibroblasts resembling focal mucinosis, or a cavity with a myxoid connective tissue wall
Mucocele	Pseudocystic space with surrounding macrophages and vascular loose fibrous tissue or granulation tissue with mucin, muciphages and inflammatory cells
Nevus mucinosus	Mucin in expanded papillary dermis; few fibroblasts present
Secondary dermal mucinoses	Mucin and changes of underlying disease such as lupus erythematosus, Degos' disease, Jessner's lymphocytic infiltrate, granuloma annulare and dermatomyositis
Follicular mucinosis (alopecia mucinosa)	Mucin in hair follicles and attached sebaceous gland with some dissolution of cellular attachments; variable inflammatory infiltrate; infiltrate is dense and atypical in secondary follicular mucinosis complicating lymphoma or mycosis fungoides
Mucopolysaccharidoses	Metachromatic granules in fibroblasts and sometimes eccrine glands and keratinocytes; extracellular mucin in maculopapular lesions of Hunter's syndrome

GENERALIZED MYXEDEMA

Myxedema is one of several cutaneous changes in hypothyroidism.[4,10–12] The changes are most pronounced around the eyes, nose and cheeks, often giving a characteristic facies, and also on the distal extremities. A diffuse, non-scarring alopecia may be present.[13] Cutis verticis gyrata is a rare presentation.[14]

Palmoplantar keratoderma is a poorly recognized presentation of myxedema.[15] Glycosaminoglycans are deposited in other organs of the body as well as the skin and it has been suggested that there is impaired degradation, rather than increased synthesis, of these substances.[5,16]

Generalized and pretibial myxedema have been grouped together as 'dysthyroidotic mucinoses' in the excellent review of the cutaneous mucinoses by Rongioletti and Rebora.[17]

Histopathology

In most cases, the changes are subtle with only small amounts of mucin in the dermis.[5] This is predominantly hyaluronic acid. Sometimes this material is deposited only focally around vessels and hair follicles.[5] There may be mild hyperkeratosis and keratotic follicular plugging. Elastic fibers are sometimes fragmented and reduced in amount.

PRETIBIAL MYXEDEMA

Pretibial myxedema is found in 1–4% of patients with Graves' disease, particularly those with exophthalmos, but it may not develop until after the correction of the hyperthyroidism.[18] It may also occur in patients with non-thyrotoxic Graves' disease[19] and occasionally in association with autoimmune thyroiditis. Pretibial myxedema has been reported in euthyroid patients with stasis dermatitis.[20]

It presents as sharply circumscribed nodular lesions, diffuse non-pitting edema or elephantiasis-like thickening of the skin.[21] There may be overlap of these lesions or progression from nodular to more diffuse plaques.[18] The anterior aspect of the lower legs, sometimes with spread to the dorsum of the feet, is the most usual site of involvement, although, rarely, the upper trunk, upper extremities and even the face, neck or ears have been involved.[22–24] Localization to scar tissue and to the toes has been reported.[25–29] Slow resolution of the lesions often occurs after many years. Hyperhidrosis, limited to areas of pretibial myxedema, has been reported.[30]

The theory that pretibial myxedema results from the stimulation of fibroblasts by LATS (long-acting thyroid stimulator) is no longer tenable, although one or multiple other substances or autoantibodies are presumably involved.[22,31] A circulating factor that stimulates increased synthesis of glycosaminoglycans by normal skin fibroblasts is present in increased amounts in patients with pretibial myxedema.[32,33] Furthermore, fibroblasts from pretibial skin cultured in the presence of serum from patients with pretibial myxedema produce increased amounts of hyaluronic acid.[34] The response of refractory cases of pretibial myxedema to octreotide (a somatostatin analogue with insulin-like growth factor 1 (IGF-1) antagonist properties) suggests that expression of IGF-1 receptor on fibroblasts may be upregulated in this condition, leading to increased secretion of hyaluronic acid.[35] Other explanations for this effect are possible. There is no primary lymphatic abnormality.[18] Hydrostatic forces appear to play a role in the localization of the pretibial mucinosis.[36]

Histopathology

There are large amounts of mucin deposited in the dermis, particularly in the mid and lower thirds (Figs 13.1, 13.2). This manifests as basophilic threads and granular material with wide separation of collagen bundles.[4] There is no

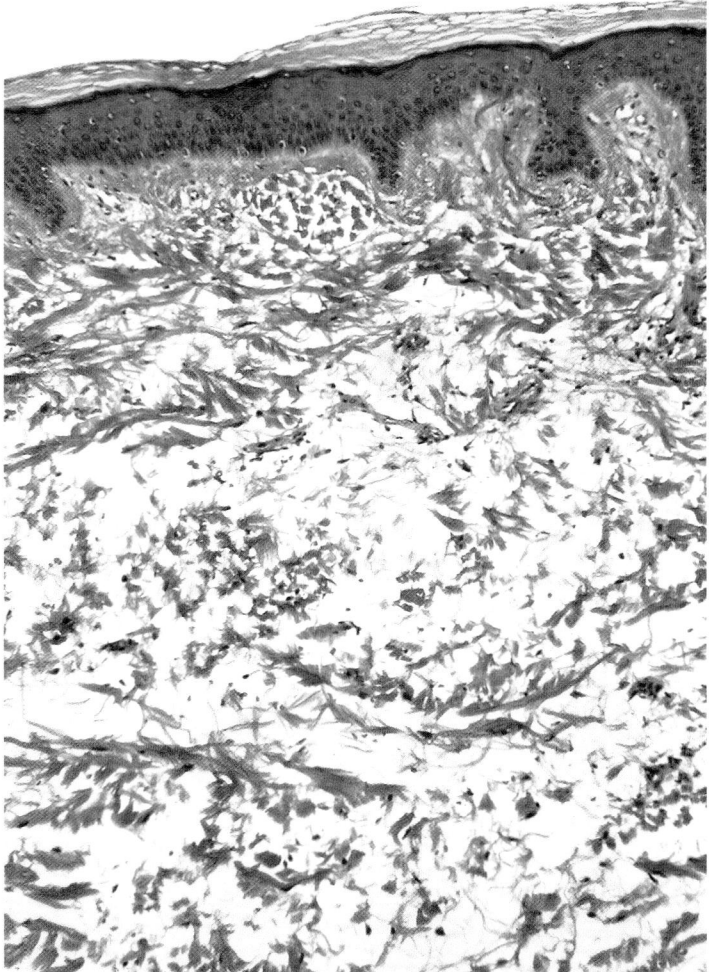

Fig. 13.1 **Pretibial myxedema.** The collagen bundles in the dermis are widely spaced, a consequence of the increased amount of interstitial mucin. (H & E)

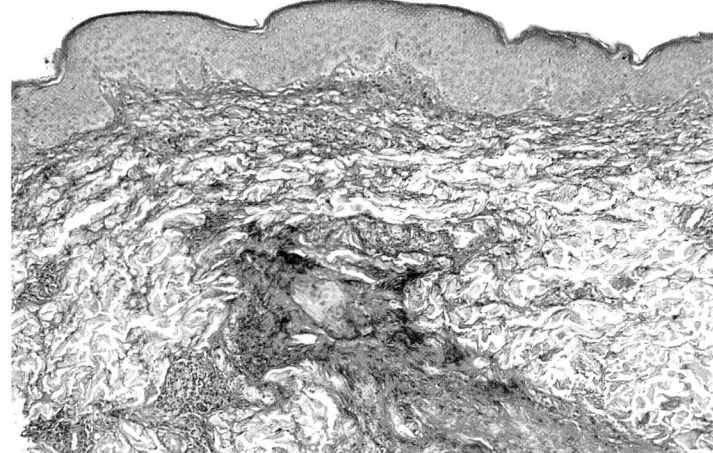

Fig. 13.2 **Pretibial myxedema.** There are large amounts of dermal mucin. (Alcian blue)

increase in fibroblasts although a few stellate forms may be present. There may be overlying hyperkeratosis which can be quite marked in clinically verrucous lesions.[37] A mild superficial perivascular chronic inflammatory cell infiltrate is often present.[16] In patients with underlying stasis dermatitis, the deposition of mucin is within the papillary dermis with sparing of the reticular dermis.[20] Angioplasia and hemosiderin deposition are additional features in the dermis.

Elastic tissue stains show fragmentation and a reduction in elastic tissue, a finding confirmed on electron microscopy[38] which also shows microfibrils with knobs (glycosaminoglycans)[39] or amorphous material (glycoproteins)[40] on the surface of fibroblasts that have dilated endoplasmic reticulum.[39,40]

PAPULAR MUCINOSIS AND SCLEROMYXEDEMA

Papular mucinosis (lichen myxedematosus) is a rare cutaneous mucinosis in which multiple, asymptomatic, pale or waxy papules, 2–3 mm in diameter, develop on the hands, forearms, face, neck and upper trunk.[41] A discrete papular variant also occurs.[42] It has been reported, rarely, in patients with hepatitis C[43] and with HIV infection[7,44–48] and also in the L-tryptophan-induced eosinophilia–myalgia syndrome[49] and in generalized morphea.[50] *Scleromyxedema* is a variant in which lichenoid papules and plaques are accompanied by skin thickening involving almost the entire body.[51–53] Involvement of the glabella region may give rise to bovine facies.[51] A paraproteinemia, particularly of IgG lambda type, is almost invariably present in scleromyxedema and sometimes in papular mucinosis.[4,54,55] Other classes of immunoglobulins are sometimes present;[56] a few patients have a normal immunoglobulin profile.[57] Multiple myeloma and Waldenström's macroglobulinemia are rare associations.[58,59] Bizarre neurological symptoms,[60] underlying carcinoma,[41,61,62] chronic hepatitis C,[63] pachydermoperiostosis,[41] dermatomyositis,[64] scleroderma,[59,65] atherosclerosis,[66] esophageal aperistalsis[67] and multiple keratoacanthomas[56] have all been reported in association with scleromyxedema.[59]

Scleromyxedema is usually progressive, but spontaneous resolution has been reported.[68] Mucin has been noted in other organs in a few autopsy cases, but it has been specifically excluded in others.[41,69–71] Rarely, hypothyroidism has been present.[72,73] Response to high-dose intravenous immunoglobulin, interferon alfa, prednisone and extracorporeal photopheresis has been reported.[74–77]

In 2001, Rongioletti and Rebora provided an updated classification of papular mucinosis/lichen myxedematosus/scleromyxedema.[78] They include acral persistent papular mucinosis, self-healing papular mucinosis (juvenile and adult variants), papular mucinosis of infancy and nodular lichen myxedematosus as variants, despite the absence of fibrosis in some of these conditions.

It has been postulated that a serum factor stimulates fibroblast proliferation and increased production of glycosaminoglycans.[65,79] Whether this factor is identical to the monoclonal immunoglobulin is controversial.[59,80] In one study, cultured skin fibroblasts from a patient with scleromyxedema produced an IgG immunoglobulin.[81]

An unusual scleromyxedema-like disease has been reported in renal dialysis patients. The term 'nephrogenic fibrosing dermopathy' has recently been applied to this condition. Accordingly, it is considered further in Chapter 11, page 353.

Histopathology

The histopathological features of *scleromyxedema* are the most precise of any of the mucinoses.[16,51] In addition to the dermal deposits of mucin, there is a marked proliferation of fibroblasts and increased collagen deposition in the upper and mid dermis (Figs 13.3, 13.4).[16] The fibroblasts are irregularly arranged and the collagen, which is most pronounced in older lesions, has a

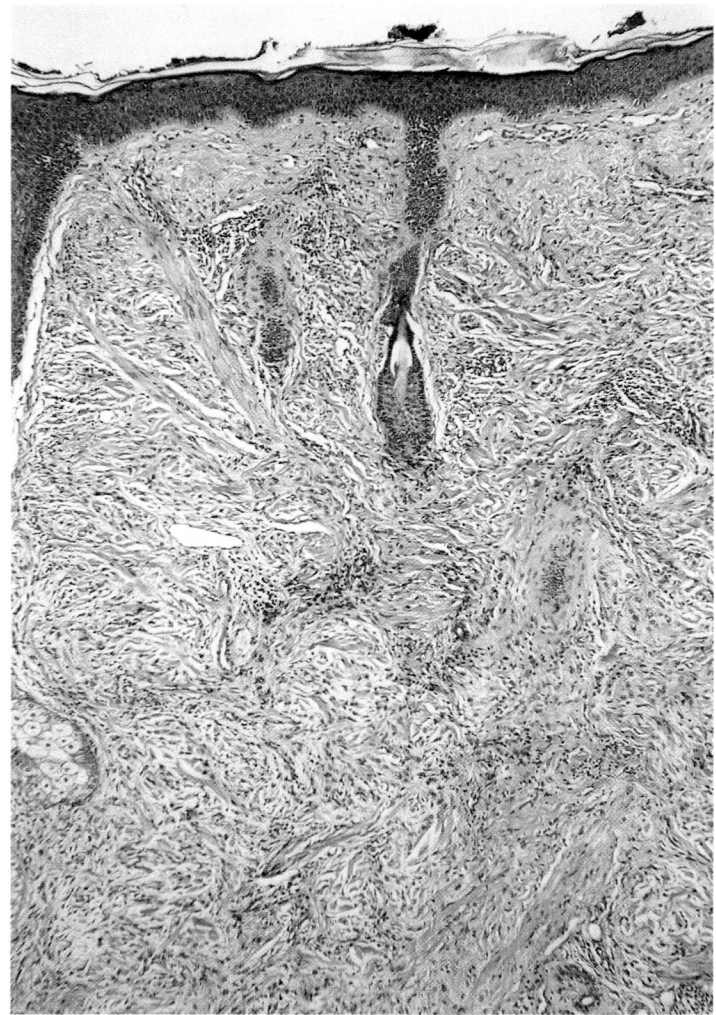

Fig. 13.3 **Scleromyxedema.** The dermis contains an increase in fibroblasts, collagen and interstitial mucin. (H & E)

whorled pattern. Flattening of the epidermis and atrophy of pilosebaceous follicles are secondary changes. Sweat duct proliferation is rare.[82] Elastic fibers are often fragmented.[81] A sparse perivascular infiltrate of lymphocytes is often present. Occasionally, eosinophils[67,69] or mast cells[83] are prominent. In one case there was a prominent perivascular infiltrate of plasma cells which were monotypic for λ light chain.[84]

Ultrastructurally, the fibroblasts have prominent rough endoplasmic reticulum. Proteoglycans are present between the collagen bundles.[85]

The changes in *papular mucinosis* are not as characteristic. In the discrete form, the changes may be indistinguishable from focal mucinosis,[86] although in the more generalized cases a slight proliferation of fibroblasts is often present in addition to the mucin deposition in the upper dermis.[72]

ACRAL PERSISTENT PAPULAR MUCINOSIS

Acral persistent papular mucinosis, which affects mainly women, is characterized by discrete, flesh-colored papules 2–5 mm in diameter on the back of the hands and, less commonly, on the forearms[87–94] and calves.[95] The lesions increase in number with the years. There is usually no associated disease. It is best regarded as a variant of papular mucinosis.[78]

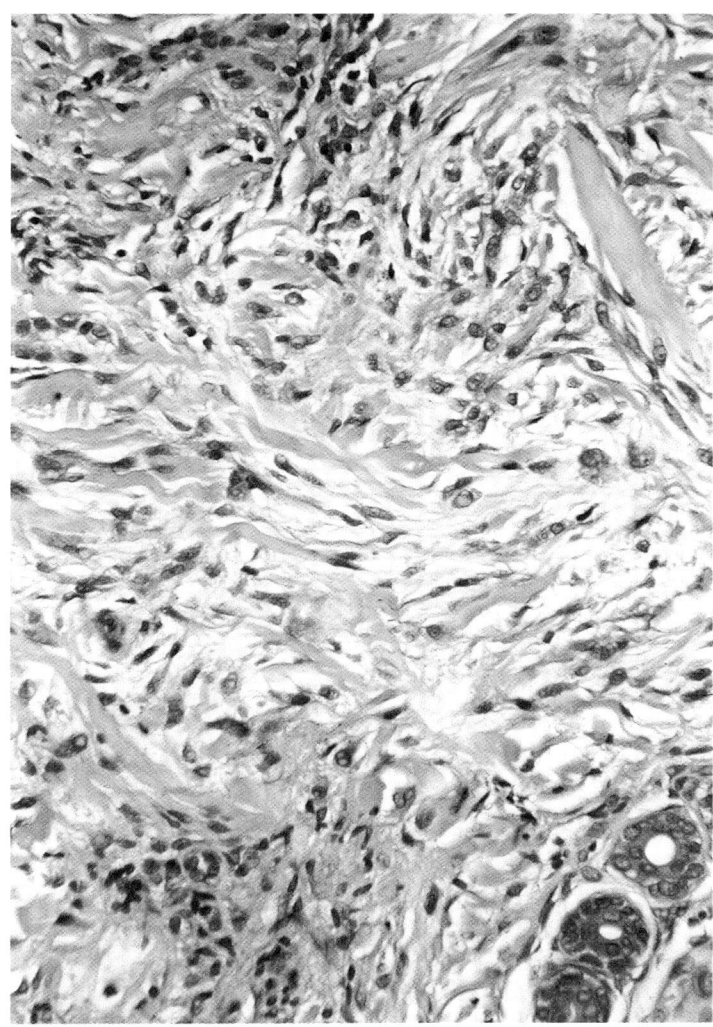

Fig. 13.4 **Scleromyxedema.** The characteristic triad of an increase in fibroblasts, collagen and mucin is present. (H & E)

A patient with a self-healing plaque on the dorsum of one hand has been reported as **self-healing localized cutaneous mucinosis**.[96] This case does not fit neatly into any of the current classifications of the mucinoses.

Histopathology

This condition shares some histological features with papular mucinosis by having mucin deposition and a proliferation of fibroblasts. However, the mucin is usually confined to the upper and mid dermis, in contrast to the more widespread distribution in the dermis in papular mucinosis. Furthermore, fibroblastic proliferation is not as pronounced as in papular mucinosis.[94]

Electron microscopy

Altered fibroblasts with concentric lysosomal structures in their cytoplasm have been reported.[90]

CUTANEOUS MUCINOSIS OF INFANCY

There have been several reports of infants presenting with multiple, small, papular lesions on the upper extremities or trunk.[2,97–100] The distribution of the lesions and their early onset raise the possibility that the lesions reported are connective tissue nevi of proteoglycan type (nevus mucinosus).[101,102]

There has been abundant mucin in the papillary dermis, no significant increase in fibroblasts, and a few chronic inflammatory cells in a perivascular distribution. In a recently reported case, however, there was both fibrosis and fibroblast proliferation, leading the authors to suggest that cutaneous mucinosis of infancy could be a pediatric form of lichen myxedematosus.[103]

SELF-HEALING JUVENILE CUTANEOUS MUCINOSIS

There have been several reports of a cutaneous mucinosis characterized by the rapid onset in childhood of infiltrated plaques on the head and torso and deep nodules on the face and periarticular region, with spontaneous resolution in weeks or months.[104–109] Recent reports have described a familial variant[110] and a case in an adult.[111] This mucinosis is thought to represent a reactive or reparative response to some antigenic stimulation, such as inflammation or a viral infection. It has developed in a child with a nephroblastoma who was undergoing chemotherapy.[108]

Histopathology

Biopsies of this condition have shown a normal epidermis overlying an 'edematous' dermis resulting from mucin separating collagen bundles in the dermis. An increase in fibroblasts was reported in one case.[108] A sparse perivascular inflammatory cell infiltrate is sometimes present.

RETICULAR ERYTHEMATOUS MUCINOSIS (REM)

This dermal mucinosis presents with erythematous maculopapules and infiltrated plaques, often with a reticulated or net-like pattern, in the mid-line of the back or chest, sometimes spreading to the upper abdomen.[112–116] Rarely, the face and arms[117] are involved and one case is said to have involved the gums.[118] There is a predilection for young to middle-aged females. Sunlight and hormonal influences may cause exacerbations and induce mild pruritus.[4,116,119] The lesions may subside after many years. Progression to cutaneous lupus erythematosus sometimes occurs, one of the reasons why Ackerman regards this condition as a variant of lupus erythematosus.

One study has shown that fibroblasts from lesional skin exhibit an abnormal response to exogenous interleukin-1β.[120]

Histopathology

There is a mild superficial and mid-dermal perivascular infiltrate with variable deep perivascular extension, the latter sometimes being restricted to the region of the eccrine glands (Fig. 13.5).[112] There may be some perifollicular infiltrate as well. This infiltrate is predominantly lymphocytic (helper T cells),[121] with a few admixed mast cells and histiocytes. There is slight vascular dilatation and, sometimes, focal mild hemorrhage in the upper dermis.[117]

There is separation of dermal collagen bundles, and variable amounts of stringy basophilic mucin can be seen predominantly in the upper and mid dermis (Fig. 13.6). The mucin is most conspicuous around the infiltrate and appendages and within the upper dermis.[116] A few stellate fibroblasts may be present, but this is not an obvious feature. The epidermis is usually normal, although mild exocytosis with spongiosis and focal lichenoid inflammation have been reported.[116]

The mucin gives variable staining reactions. Colloidal iron staining is superior to alcian blue, which on occasions has failed to demonstrate mucin.[122,123] The material is not usually metachromatic with toluidine blue.[123]

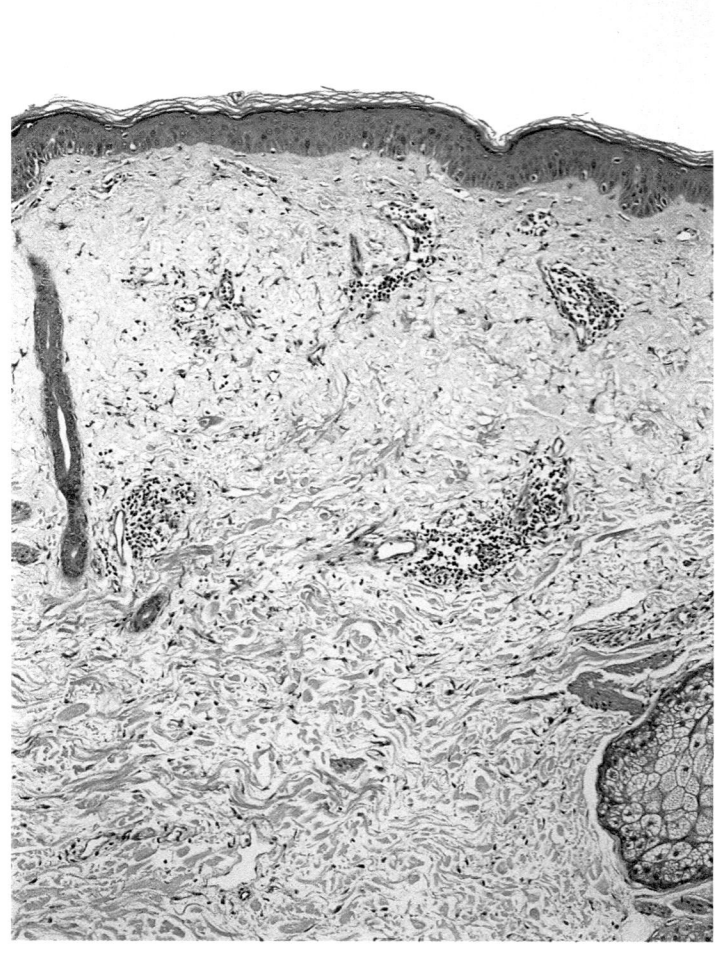

Fig. 13.5 **Reticular erythematous mucinosis.** There is a superficial and deep infiltrate of lymphocytes and an increase in interstitial mucin. (H & E)

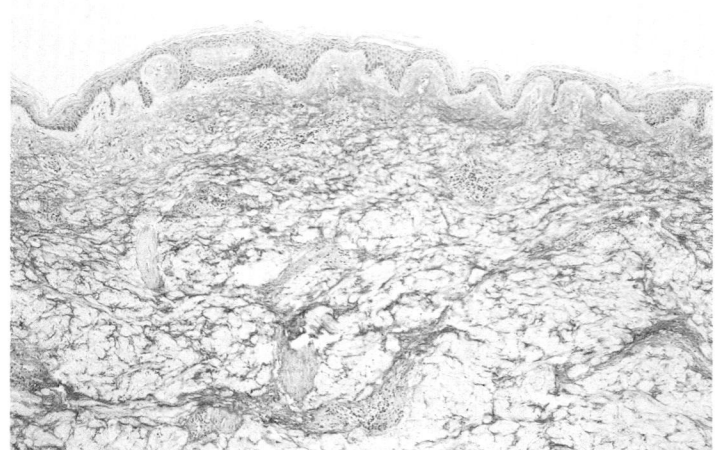

Fig. 13.6 **Reticular erythematous mucinosis.** There is increased mucin throughout the dermis. (Alcian blue)

Staining with colloidal iron and alcian blue will be negative following digestion with hyaluronidase. There may be focal fragmentation of elastic fibers.[122]

Direct immunofluorescence has shown the deposition of immunoglobulins, particularly IgM, along the basal layer in several cases.[124]

Electron microscopy

Electron microscopy shows widening of the intercollagenous spaces, focal fragmentation of elastic fibers, and some active fibroblasts.[125] Numerous tubular aggregates have also been seen in endothelial cells, pericytes and some dermal macrophages.[122,126] In one report, lesional skin showed granular basement membrane deposits of IgM, IgA and C3.[127]

SCLEREDEMA

Scleredema (scleredema adultorum of Buschke) is characterized by the development of non-pitting induration of the skin with a predilection for symmetrical involvement of the posterior neck, the shoulders, the upper trunk and the face.[128,129] Localization to the thighs has been reported.[130] In cases of more widespread involvement, the upper part of the body is always involved much more than the lower part, and the feet are spared. The condition occurs at all ages, although nearly 50% of cases develop in children and adolescents.[131] There is a predilection for females.

There are several different clinical settings.[132,133] In one group the onset is sudden and follows days to weeks after an acute febrile illness caused by streptococci or viruses. A case occurring in association with HIV infection has been reported.[7] Spontaneous resolution occurs in approximately one-third of the post-infectious group after 6–18 months. This group is now seen less frequently than previously. Another clinical group has an insidious onset, without any predisposing illness, and a protracted course. The third group is associated with insulin-dependent, maturity onset diabetes, which is difficult to control.[134–137] Vascular complications of diabetes are common.[138] A fourth group is associated with a monoclonal gammopathy.[139–149] Extracorporeal photopheresis has been used to treat one such case.[150] Scleredema is insidious in onset and prolonged in its course.

Systemic manifestations such as ECG changes, serosal effusions and involvement of skeletal, ocular and tongue musculature may develop. Rheumatoid arthritis has been present in a few patients.[151] Cutaneous abscesses or cellulitis may precede or follow the onset of the condition.[152,153] Rarely, there is erythema at sites of skin thickening.[154]

Scleredema is characterized by the accumulation of glycosaminoglycans, particularly hyaluronic acid, in the dermis with concurrent dermal sclerosis. The etiology is unknown, although fibroblasts from the fibrotic skin of patients with scleredema show enhanced collagen production and elevated type I procollagen messenger RNA levels in the cultured fibroblasts.[141] This suggests that fibroblasts from involved skin have a biosynthetically activated phenotype.[155]

Histopathology[128,139]

The epidermis is usually unaffected except for some effacement of the rete ridge pattern and occasionally mild basal hyperpigmentation.[156] There is thickening of the reticular dermis, with collagen extending also into the subcutis. The collagen fibers are swollen and separated from one another. The extent of this separation, which mirrors the amount of interstitial mucopolysaccharide present, depends on the stage of the disease (Fig. 13.7). This material may only be present in noticeable amounts at the onset of the disease.[133] Multiple biopsies and the use of several stains may be necessary to demonstrate the dermal mucin.[157] Sometimes it is most prominent in the lower dermis.[158] Cetylpyridinium has been proposed as a superior fixative to formalin for the preservation of the interstitial mucopolysaccharides.[131] These

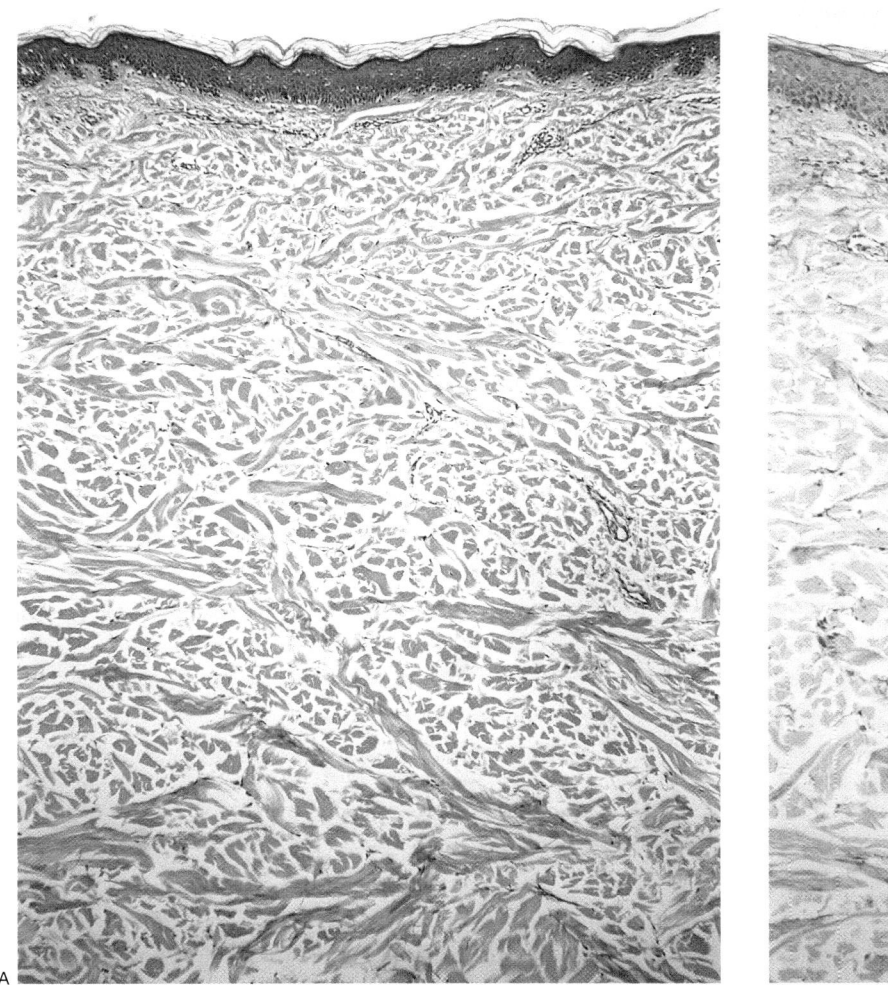
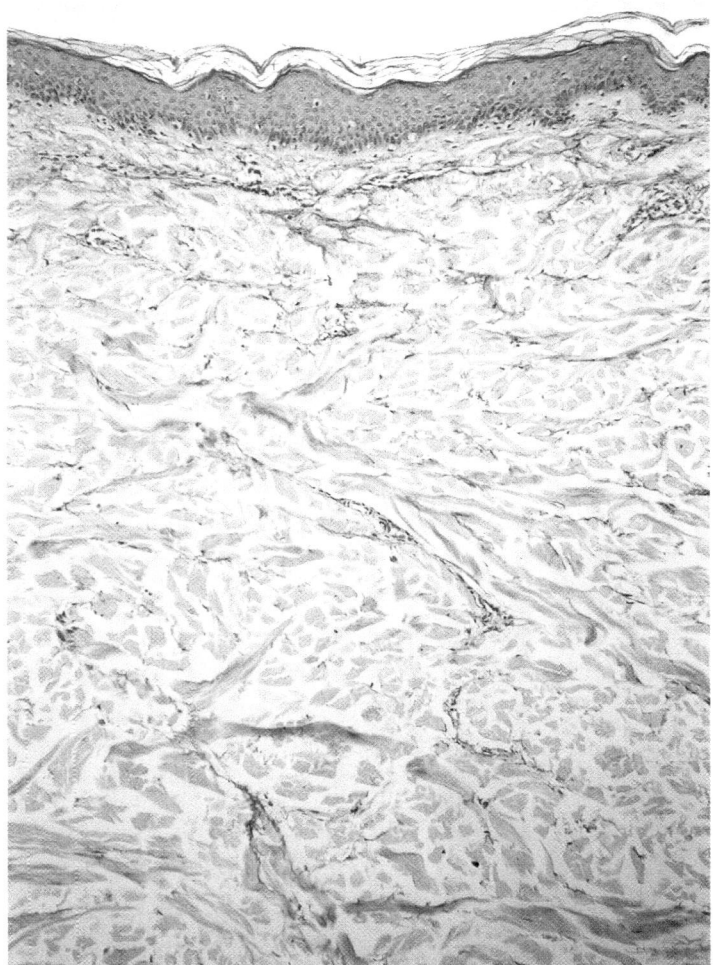

Fig. 13.7 **Scleredema. (A)** The collagen bundles are slightly swollen and separated from one another. Cellularity of the dermis is normal with no increase in fibroblasts (H & E). **(B)** Mucin deposits are present on the surface of the collagen. (Colloidal iron)

may subsequently be stained with alcian blue or toluidine blue (pH 5.0 or 7.0) or with colloidal iron. Cryostat sections of unfixed material usually result in the optimal preservation of the interstitial hyaluronic acid.

Other features of scleredema include preservation of the appendages and an increase in mast cells.[159] Other inflammatory cells are sparse. Elastic fibers are reduced and may be fragmented.[156]

The acellular fibrosis of the dermis in scleredema contrasts with the marked fibroblastic proliferation seen in scleromyxedema and the patchy deep inflammatory cell infiltrate seen at the advancing edge of plaques of morphea.

Electron microscopy

Electron microscopy shows thickened collagen fibers with widening of the interfibrillar spaces.[139] The fibroblasts have prominent rough endoplasmic reticulum.[139]

FOCAL MUCINOSIS

Focal mucinosis usually presents as a solitary, asymptomatic, flesh-colored papule or nodule on the face, trunk or proximal and mid extremities of adults.[160–162] The nodules average 1 cm in diameter. There has been a report of multiple nodules localized to a 'palm-wide area' of the right leg[163] and also a report of multiple lesions in a patient with hypothyroidism, which responded to thyroxine.[72] Digital lesions with the histology of focal mucinosis have been described in scleroderma (see p. 348). It has been reported in association with other cutaneous mucinoses.[164]

It is thought that increased amounts of hyaluronic acid are produced by fibroblasts at the expense of the connective tissue elements.[165]

Histopathology[165]

There is a slightly elevated or dome-shaped dermal nodule with separation and variable replacement of collagen bundles by mucinous deposits (Fig. 13.8). These deposits may be localized to the upper dermis or extend through the full thickness of the dermis. The subcutis is rarely involved.[166] Slit-like spaces occasionally develop. The margins of the mucinous deposition are not sharply demarcated. Spindle-shaped fibroblasts are present within the mucinous areas and there may be an increase in small blood vessels. The appearances resemble the early stages of a digital mucous cyst (see below) and an individual lesion of papular mucinosis. The material stains with colloidal iron and alcian blue at pH 2.5 and is metachromatic with toluidine

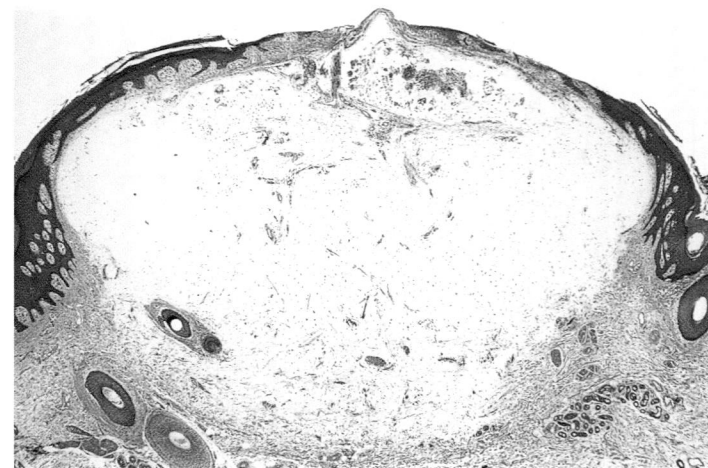

Fig. 13.8 **Focal mucinosis.** There is a large 'pool' of mucin dispersed through much of the dermis. This is the nodular variant. (H & E)

blue at pH 3.0 (Fig. 13.9). Immunohistochemistry confirms that the spindle cells are predominantly fibroblasts with some factor XIIIa-positive dendritic cells.[162]

Electron microscopy

The fibroblasts have a well-developed rough endoplasmic reticulum. In addition, there are large macrophages and granular and amorphous material representing the mucinous deposits.[163]

DIGITAL MUCOUS (MYXOID) CYST

Digital mucous cysts occur as solitary, dome-shaped, shiny, tense cystic nodules on the dorsum of the fingers, usually involving the base of the nail.[167] The toes are uncommonly involved. The cysts are found in the middle aged or elderly and there is a slight female preponderance. A second type, overlying the distal interphalangeal joint, is related to a ganglion as injection studies have demonstrated a connection with the underlying joint cavity.[168]

Histopathology[169]

The variant developing at the base of the nail resembles focal mucinosis with a large myxoid area containing stellate fibroblasts, sometimes with microcystic spaces (Fig. 13.10). The overlying epidermis may be thinned by the expanding subepidermal collection of mucus. The mucin stains with the colloidal iron stain, as well as with alcian blue at pH 2.5, and it is digested by hyaluronidase.[169]

The ganglionic variant comprises a cystic space with a well-defined fibrous wall of variable thickness and density (Fig. 13.11). There are often small areas of myxoid change adjacent to the wall.[170] There may be an attenuated synovial lining.

MUCOCELE OF THE LIP

Mucoceles (mucous cysts) result from the rupture of a duct of a minor salivary gland with extravasation of mucus into the submucosal tissues, most commonly of the lower lip.[171] They may also develop in the buccal mucosa or tongue. They are found mostly in young adults.

Mucoceles are translucent, whitish or bluish nodules with a firm cystic consistency and vary in size up to 1 cm in diameter. They occasionally rupture spontaneously or after minor trauma.

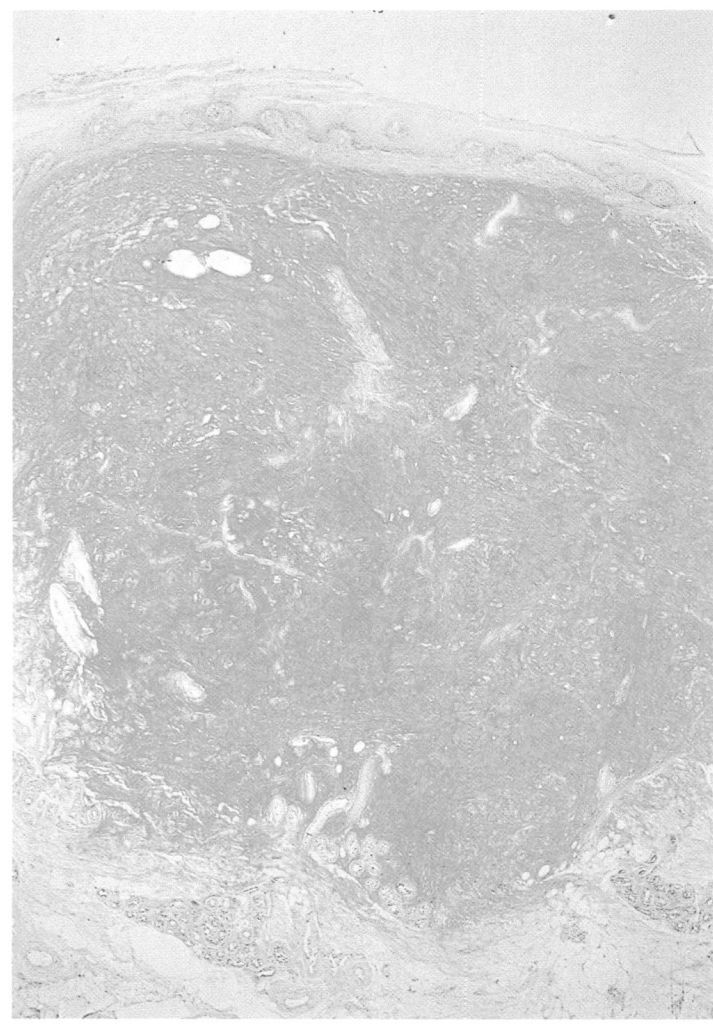

Fig. 13.9 **Focal mucinosis.** The abundant mucin is confirmed with a mucin stain. (Colloidal iron)

A superficial variant of mucocele, which results in vesicular lesions that may be mistaken for mucous membrane pemphigoid, has been reported.[172] They may be single or multiple and they arise on non-inflamed mucosa.

Histopathology

Two patterns may be seen, but there may be some overlap between them.[171] In one, there is a cystic space with a surrounding poorly defined lining of macrophages, fibroblasts and capillaries with variable amounts of connective tissue. In the other pattern, there is granulation and fibrous tissue containing mucin-filled spaces with variable numbers of muciphages (Fig. 13.12). Small cystic spaces may be present. Numerous neutrophils and some eosinophils are present in the cystic spaces or stroma of both types. There is no epithelial lining to the cyst, although occasionally a ruptured salivary duct may be seen at one edge of the cyst. Minor salivary gland tissue is present in the adjacent connective tissue.

The mucin is strongly PAS positive and diastase resistant and is positive with alcian blue at pH 2.5 and with colloidal iron.

Superficial mucoceles are subepithelial although there may be partial or complete epithelial regeneration across the vesicle floor. They contain sialomucin. Salivary gland ducts are present in the immediate vicinity of the lesions and are a clue to the diagnosis.[172]

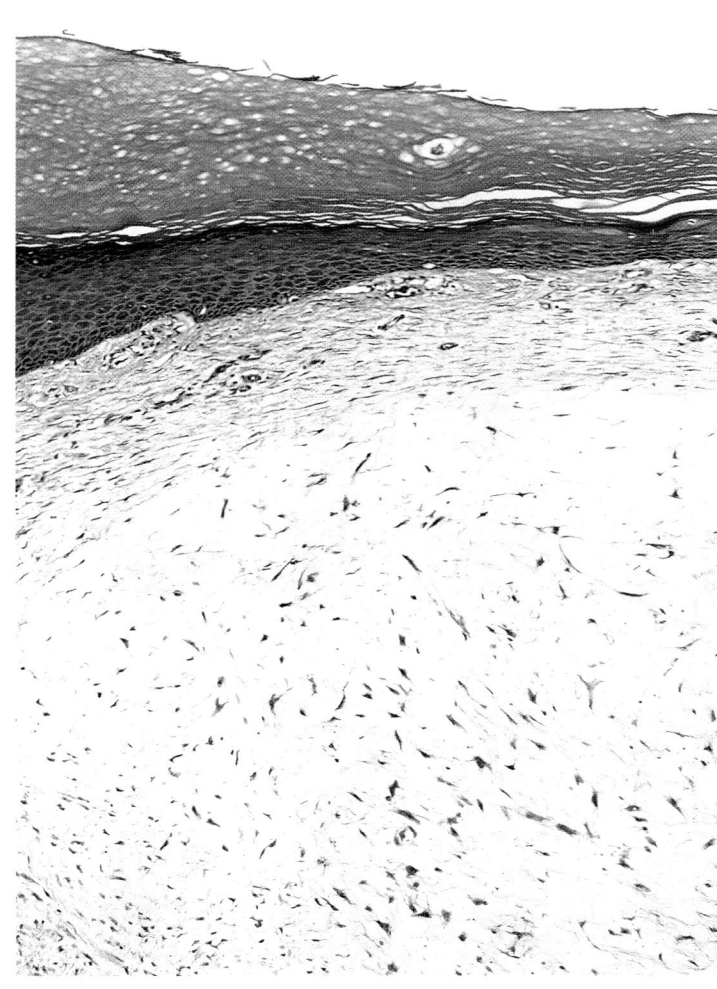

Fig. 13.10 **Digital mucous cyst.** There is a 'pool' of mucin containing many fibroblasts. This variant resembles focal mucinosis. (H & E)

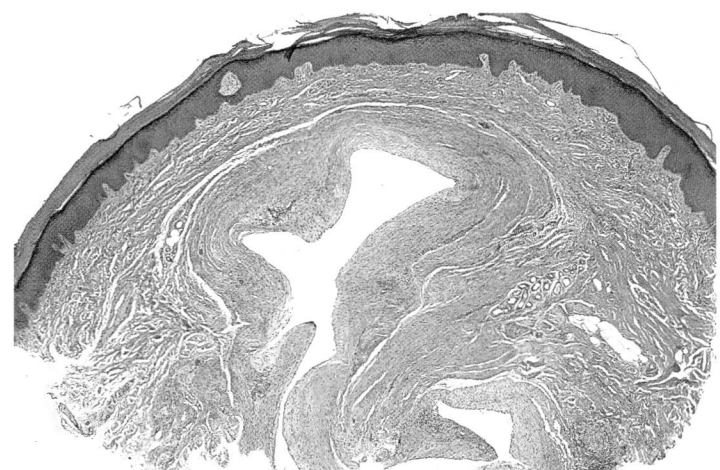

Fig. 13.11 **Digital mucous cyst.** This is the ganglionic variant. (H & E)

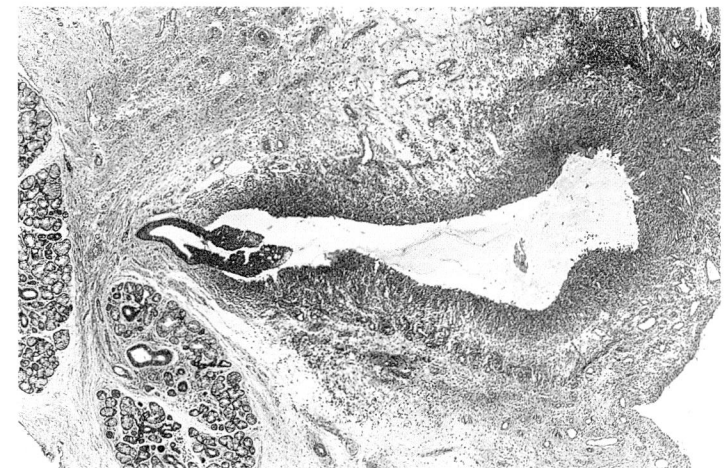

Fig. 13.12 **Mucocele.** A duct leads into a pseudocyst lined by granulation tissue and muciphages. (H & E)

CUTANEOUS MYXOMA

Cutaneous myxomas have been reported in approximately 50% of the patients with the complex of cardiac myxomas, spotty pigmentation (lentigines and blue nevi) and endocrine overactivity.[173–177] This combination of lesions is known as Carney's complex, an autosomal dominant condition which has been mapped to chromosome 2p16. It seems likely that a second genetic locus exists.[178] The cutaneous myxomas may be the earliest manifestation of the syndrome.[179] Similar cases have been reported as the NAME or LAMB syndrome (see Ch. 32, p. 804).

Solitary and disseminated myxomas unassociated with any systemic abnormalities may also occur.[180–184] They are benign neoplasms, but they are included here because of their prominent stromal mucin.

In one reported case, a patient with multiple periorbital myxomas progressed to a scleromyxedema-like dermatosis.[185]

Histopathology

The tumors are sharply circumscribed, non-encapsulated lesions which may be in the dermis or subcutis. They are composed of a prominent mucinous matrix containing variably shaped fibroblasts, prominent capillaries, mast cells, and a few collagen and reticulin fibers (Fig. 13.13). Sometimes an epithelial

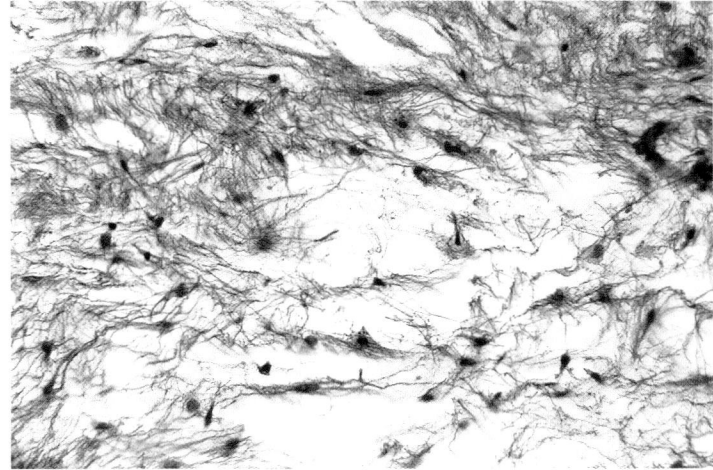

Fig. 13.13 **Myxoma.** There are thin collagen bundles and fibroblasts scattered through a mucinous matrix. (H & E)

component is present and this may take the form of a keratinous cyst or epithelial strands with trichoblastic features.[175] The lesions differ from focal mucinosis by their vascularity. If the vascular component is marked, the term 'angiomyxoma' is often used (see p. 942).[182] Nerve sheath myxomas are more cellular, often with a distinct patterned arrangement.

The designation 'fibromyxoma' has been applied to the lesions in a patient with multiple cutaneous tumors, resembling dermatofibromas clinically but containing more fibroblasts than the usual cutaneous myxomas and some histiocytes, in addition to the interstitial mucin.[186] Familial myxovascular fibroma is a morphologically related entity (see p. 920).

NEVUS MUCINOSUS

Nevus mucinosus is a variant of connective tissue nevus in which there is a deposition of acid mucopolysaccharides (proteoglycans) in the dermis.[101,187] The existence of such an entity has been postulated for some time in the light of the nevoid lesions of the other connective tissue elements – collagen and elastic tissue. Cases previously reported as cutaneous mucinosis of infancy (see above) may represent examples of nevus mucinosus.

The lesions are small papules, in a grouped, zosteriform or linear arrangement, on the extremities or trunk.[188] They are present at birth or appear in childhood or early adult life.[189]

Histopathology

The epidermis usually shows some acanthosis with thin, elongated rete ridges. There is a grossly thickened papillary dermis with an 'empty appearance' due to the deposition of abundant acid mucopolysaccharides. Fibroblasts are slightly increased in number, with occasional stellate forms.[101]

The mucin in nevus mucinosus is deposited in the upper dermis, in contrast to papular mucinosis where the mucin is at a lower level. Nevus mucinosus differs from acral persistent papular mucinosis on clinical grounds and also by having fewer fibroblasts within the lesions. Focal mucinosis differs by its larger size and solitary nature.

PROGRESSIVE MUCINOUS HISTIOCYTOSIS

Progressive mucinous histiocytosis, a rare, autosomal dominant histiocytosis of childhood, is characterized by multiple small papules composed of epithelioid and spindle-shaped histiocytes set in abundant stromal mucin. This entity is discussed in more detail with the histiocytoses (see p. 1071).

SECONDARY DERMAL MUCINOSES

Mucin deposition may be present in a wide variety of connective tissue diseases and in some tumors. These include dermatomyositis, lupus erythematosus (see below), scleroderma, linear morphea,[190] the toxic oil syndrome, hypertrophic scars, connective tissue nevi, granuloma annulare, malignant atrophic papulosis (Degos' disease), erythema annulare centrifugum, post-inflammatory hyperpigmentation,[191] mycosis fungoides[192] and Jessner's lymphocytic infiltrate.[4,5] Mucin is sometimes present in large amounts around the secretory coils of the eccrine glands of the lower leg when sweat excretion is blocked.[5] Tumors containing mucin include neurofibromas, neurilemmomas, nerve sheath myxomas, chondroid syringomas and some basal cell carcinomas. A diffuse dermal mucinosis can be found occasionally in biopsies of lesional skin from patients with discoid and systemic lupus erythematosus (SLE).[193,194] Rarely, patients with SLE can present with papulonodules or plaques due to a diffuse mucinous deposition in the skin (Fig. 13.14).[194–201] In these individuals, the deposition occurs in areas free from specific lesions of lupus erythematosus and it produces clinically distinct manifestations. A factor

(or factors) in the patient's serum appear(s) to stimulate fibroblasts to produce increased amounts of glycosaminoglycan.[98]

The case reported as 'plaque-like erythema with milia' occurred in a renal transplant recipient on cyclosporine, which was implicated in the pathogenesis. There were extensive mucin deposits in the dermis.[202]

FOLLICULAR MUCINOSES

Follicular mucinosis is a tissue reaction pattern in which hair follicles and the attached sebaceous gland accumulate mucin with some dissolution of cellular attachments (Fig. 13.15).[3] There is an accompanying perifollicular and perivascular inflammatory cell infiltrate of lymphocytes, histiocytes and a few eosinophils. Sometimes follicles are converted into cystic cavities with disruption of much of the external root sheath. These cysts contain mucin, inflammatory cells and keratinous debris. There is often a marked disparity between the amount of follicular mucin and the degree of follicular and perifollicular inflammation.[203] The material is stained by the alcian blue and colloidal iron methods. Follicular mucinosis is sometimes seen in arthropod bite reactions and in the exaggerated bite reactions that occur in some patients with chronic lymphocytic leukemia.[204]

The concept that follicular mucinosis is a tissue reaction pattern and not a disease sui generis is a relatively recent one[3] and, as a consequence, most reports in the literature use the term 'follicular mucinosis' for what Pinkus described as alopecia mucinosa in 1957.[205]

FOLLICULAR MUCINOSIS (ALOPECIA MUCINOSA)

Follicular mucinosis (alopecia mucinosa) is an uncommon inflammatory dermatosis with a predilection for adults in the third and fourth decades of life.[206] Three clinical types have traditionally been recognized:[207,208] a benign transient form with one or several plaques or grouped follicular papules, usually limited to the face or scalp and with accompanying alopecia;[209–212] a more widely distributed form with follicular papules, plaques and nodules on the extremities, face and trunk and a course often exceeding 2 years; and a third group, accounting for 15–30% of cases, with widespread lesions and associated with malignant lymphoma of the skin or mycosis fungoides.[213–217] Rarely, patients with leukemia cutis,[218] leukemia without skin lesions,[219] Hodgkin's disease,[220] familial reticuloendotheliosis,[221] Sézary syndrome,[222,223] squamous cell carcinoma of the tongue[224] and angiolymphoid hyperplasia[225,226] have also had this presentation. This third group was regarded by Hempstead and Ackerman[3] as belonging to the group of secondary follicular mucinoses because of the lack, at that time, of convincing examples of follicular mucinosis (alopecia mucinosa) progressing to mycosis fungoides or cutaneous lymphoma.[227,228] However, cases of follicular mucinosis progressing to mycosis fungoides have since been well documented.[229,230] A study of T-cell clonality in follicular mucinosis has shown a monoclonal T-cell population in all patients with associated cutaneous T-cell lymphoma and also in 9 of 16 patients with the primary form of the disease.[231] In another series of 4 cases, presenting as an acneiform eruption of the face in early adulthood, 2 cases have demonstrated a clonal rearrangement of the T-cell receptor within the cutaneous infiltrate.[232] A more recent study from Graz, Austria, has also cast doubt on the validity of the continued separation of the so-called 'primary form' of follicular mucinosis from the lymphoma-associated group. Not only was there some clinical overlap between the two groups, but histopathological examination did not allow differentiation of the two groups.[233]

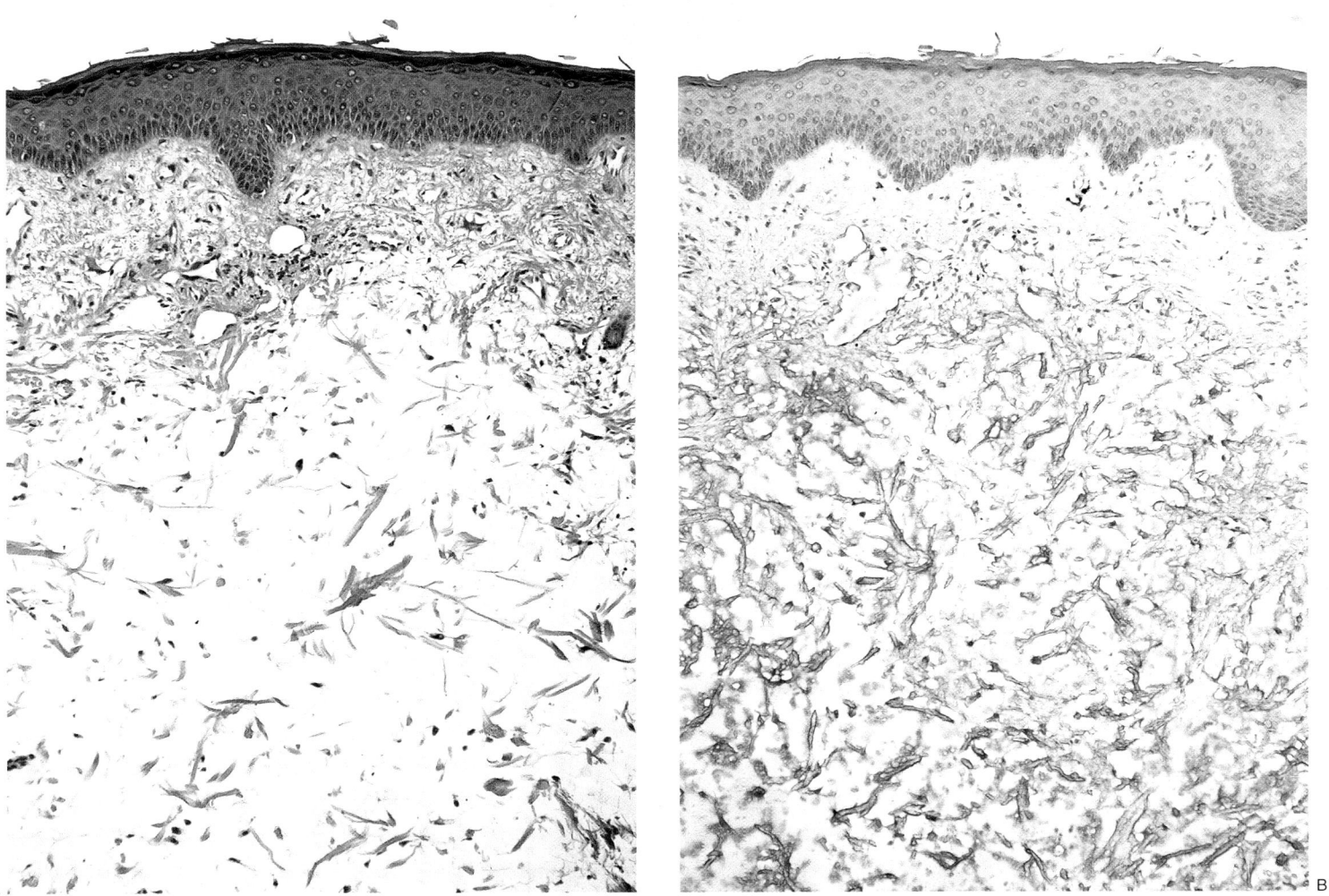

Fig. 13.14 **(A) Lupus mucinosis** (H & E). **(B)** There is wide separation of attenuated collagen bundles by mucin. (Colloidal iron) (Photographs kindly provided by Dr Geoffrey Strutton)

Furthermore, a monoclonal rearrangement of the TCR gene was demonstrated by PCR analysis in 4 of 10 cases from the primary group and 7 of 17 cases from the lymphoma-associated group. These authors postulate that even the primary form of follicular mucinosis may be a form of localized cutaneous T-cell lymphoma.[233] These cases raise the question – when does follicular mucinosis become mycosis fungoides?[234,235]

The protean clinical presentations attributed to follicular mucinosis, such as eczematous,[236] annular, pityriasis rosea-like[237] and folliculitis, are in many cases examples of specific dermatoses in which secondary follicular mucinosis is present.

Although it has been postulated that follicular keratinocytes are the source of the mucopolysaccharides,[3,238] this has not been confirmed in another study, which proposed a role for cell-mediated immune mechanisms in the etiology.[228]

Histopathology[208,239,240]

The major changes are those described above for the tissue reaction known as follicular mucinosis (Fig. 13.16). However, the inflammatory cell infiltrate is predominantly follicular, perifollicular and perivascular in location, in contrast to the follicular mucinosis secondary to lymphomas where the infiltrate is more dispersed, often heavier and nodular, and sometimes has more plasma cells and fewer eosinophils than in primary follicular mucinosis.[203] Further-

more, there is usually a milder mucinous change in follicular mucinosis related to lymphomas than in primary follicular mucinosis. However, as mentioned above, the study from Graz casts doubt on the validity of separating the primary form from the lymphoma-associated group.[233] Atypical cells and Pautrier microabscesses are not seen in follicular mucinosis,[203] but may be present in secondary follicular mucinosis with accompanying lymphoma or mycosis fungoides. Rarely, dermal mucinosis[220,241] or a proliferation of eccrine sweat duct epithelium is present.[242] The term **folliculotropic T-cell lymphocytosis** has been proposed for a case that clinically resembled follicular mucinosis, but in which there were minimal mucin deposits in the hair follicles.[243]

Electron microscopy
Electron microscopy shows disattached keratinocytes closely opposed to significant numbers of macrophages and Langerhans cells.[228] Some degeneration of keratinocytes has also been noted.[238,244] Fine granular and flocculent material is present between the keratinocytes.

SECONDARY FOLLICULAR MUCINOSES

Follicular mucinosis may be found as an incidental phenomenon in rare cases of lichen simplex chronicus, hypertrophic lichen planus, discoid lupus

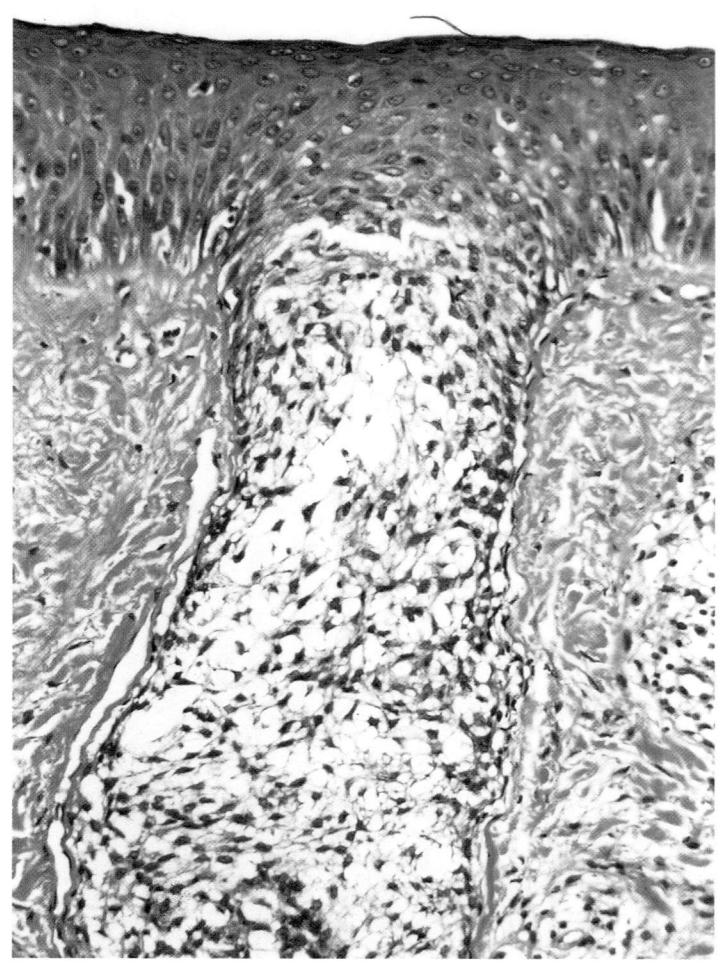

F g. 13.15 **Follicular mucinosis.** The accumulation of mucin within the hair follicle has resulted in the dissolution of many cellular attachments. (H & E)

erythematosus, acne vulgaris, pseudolymphoma, nevocellular nevi[245] and arthropod bite reactions.[3] The superficial follicular spongiosis seen in some cases of atopic dermatitis, Grover's disease and actinic prurigo,[246] as well as in infundibulofolliculitis, may contain small amounts of mucin.[247]

PERIFOLLICULAR MUCINOSIS

There is one report of an adolescent male who developed two plaques on the face characterized by prominent perifollicular mucin. The lesions were regarded as being of nevoid origin.[248] Perifollicular mucinosis has also been reported in a patient with HIV infection and an atypical pityriasis rubra pilaris-l ke eruption.[249]

EPITHELIAL MUCINOSES

Small foci of intercellular mucin are an inconstant and incidental finding in some spongiotic dermatoses, as well as in verrucae, seborrheic keratoses, basal cell and squamous cell carcinomas and keratoacanthomas.[3] Epidermal mucin is sometimes a conspicuous feature in mycosis fungoides (see p. 1104).

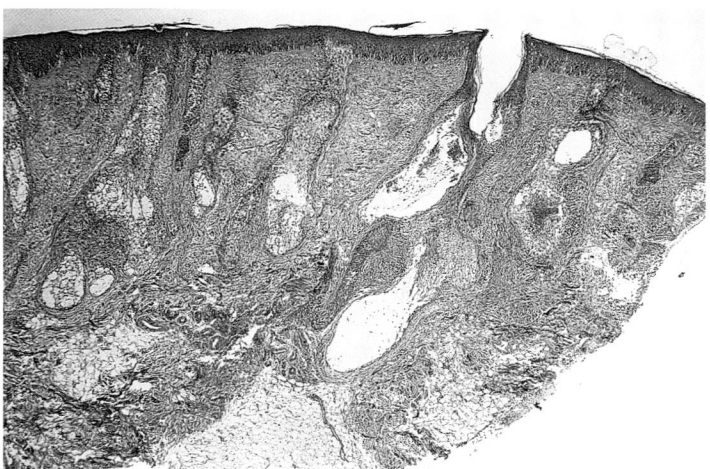

Fig. 13.16 **Alopecia mucinosa.** Multiple follicles show the reaction pattern of follicular mucinosis. (H & E)

Eccrine ductal mucinosis, in which there was mucin between the cells of the outer layer of the eccrine duct, has been reported in a patient with HIV infection and probable scabies. The significance of these related conditions and the nature of the mucinosis remain an enigma.[250]

MUCOPOLYSACCHARIDOSES

The mucopolysaccharidoses are a group of 10 lysosomal storage diseases which result from the deficiency of specific lysosomal enzymes involved in the degradation of dermatan sulfate, heparan sulfate or keratan sulfate, singly or in combination.[251-253] As a consequence, mucopolysaccharides accumulate in various tissues and are excreted in the urine.[254] Because of genetic variability, heterogeneity and pleiotropism, more than 10 clinical syndromes are associated with the 10 enzyme deficiencies.[251]

The specific enzyme defect can be identified using cultured fibroblasts, although in many instances a tentative diagnosis is possible on the clinical features alone. Analysis of the urine for certain mucopolysaccharides will also assist in the diagnosis. The urine contains heparan sulfate in the Sanfilippo syndrome (MPS III), keratan sulfate in the Morquio syndrome (MPS IV), dermatan sulfate in the Maroteaux–Lamy syndrome (MPS VI), and an excess of dermatan and heparan sulfates in varying ratios in the others.

The mucopolysaccharidoses share many clinical features.[251] These include skeletal abnormalities characterized as dysostosis multiplex (except in Morquio's syndrome), short stature (excluding Scheie's syndrome – MPS IS), corneal clouding (except in the Hunter – MPS II – and Sanfilippo – MPS III – syndromes), deafness, grotesque facies (gargoylism), hirsutism, premature arteriosclerosis, hepatosplenomegaly and severe mental retardation (excluding MPS VI and MPS IS).[251] The best known of the mucopolysaccharidoses are Hurler's syndrome (MPS I), which has the worst prognosis and is due to a deficiency of α-L-iduronidase,[255] and Hunter's syndrome (MPS II), which results from a deficiency of iduronate-2-sulfate sulfatase. Hunter's syndrome is the only X-linked mucopolysaccharidosis.[256] The genetic defect in Sanfilippo syndrome type A is situated on chromosome 17q25.3. To date, 46 different mutations have been identified.[257]

Cutaneous manifestations of the mucopolysaccharidoses include hirsutism and dryness of the skin. There may be mild thickening also; this is most marked in Hurler's syndrome where sclerodermoid thickening of the fingers and furrowing of the skin can occur.[258,259] Firm, flesh-colored to waxy papules and nodules can be found on the upper trunk, particularly in the scapular region, in Hunter's syndrome.[256,260–263]

Histopathology

Metachromatic granules are present in the cytoplasm of fibroblasts in all cases and are sometimes seen in eccrine sweat glands and epidermal keratinocytes.[258] Extracellular mucin of any significant amount is only found in the mid and lower dermis in the papulonodules of Hunter's syndrome.[260] The mucin is best seen in toluidine blue-stained sections of alcohol-fixed material, but it can also be demonstrated with the Giemsa and colloidal iron stains.[260] The fibroblasts are slightly more prominent than usual with an oval nucleus and a definable cytoplasmic outline, but these changes are quite subtle.

Electron microscopy

The ultrastructural features are characteristic with multiple membrane-bound vacuoles, containing some amorphous and granular material, within the cytoplasm of fibroblasts.[264,265] Vacuoles are also present, to a variable extent, in endothelial cells, Schwann cells,[264] mononuclear cells[266] and eccrine glands.[267] Lamellar inclusions are sometimes observed, particularly in Schwann cells.[268,269] A single large vacuole, indenting the nucleus of keratinocytes, has been seen in some cases.[270] Vacuoles may develop in some cells as an artifact of fixation; these should not be misinterpreted as features of a mucopolysaccharidosis.[271]

REFERENCES

Introduction

1 Reed RJ, Clark WH, Mihm MC. The cutaneous mucinoses. Hum Pathol 1973; 4: 201–205.
2 Rongioletti F, Rebora A. The new cutaneous mucinoses: a review with an up-to-date classification of cutaneous mucinoses. J Am Acad Dermatol 1991; 24: 265–270.
3 Hempstead RW, Ackerman AB. Follicular mucinosis. A reaction pattern in follicular epithelium. Am J Dermatopathol 1985; 7: 245–257.
4 Truhan AP, Roenigk HH. The cutaneous mucinoses. J Am Acad Dermatol 1986; 14: 1–18.
5 Steigleder GK, Kuchmeister B. Cutaneous mucinous deposits. J Cutan Pathol 1985; 12: 334–347.
6 Alves MFGS, Filgueira AL, Lorena DE, Porto LC. Type I and type III collagens in cutaneous mucinosis. Am J Dermatopathol 1998; 20: 41–47.
7 Rongioletti F, Ghigliotti G, De Marchi R, Rebora A. Cutaneous mucinoses and HIV infection. Br J Dermatol 1998; 139: 1077–1080.
8 Matsuoka LY, Wortsman J, Dietrich JG, Kupchella CE. Glycosaminoglycans in histologic sections. Arch Dermatol 1987; 123: 862.

Dermal mucinoses

9 Alajlan A, Ackerman AB. Illegitimacy of the concept of the "dermal mucinoses". Dermatopathology: Practical & Conceptual 2001; 7: 65–72.
10 Christianson HB. Cutaneous manifestations of hypothyroidism including purpura and ecchymoses. Cutis 1976; 17: 45–52.
11 Warin AP. Eczéma craquelé as the presenting feature of myxoedema. Br J Dermatol 1973; 89: 289–291.
12 Jabbour SA, Miller JL. Endocrinopathies and the skin. Int J Dermatol 2000; 39: 88–99.
13 Signore RJ, von Weiss J. Alopecia of myxedema: clinical response to levothyroxine sodium. J Am Acad Dermatol 1991; 25: 902–904.
14 Corbalán-Vélez R, Pérez-Ferriols A, Aliaga-Bouiche A. Cutis verticis gyrata secondary to hypothyroid myxedema. Int J Dermatol 1999; 38: 781–783.
15 Good JM, Neill SM, Rowland Payne CME, Staughton RCD. Keratoderma of myxoedema. Clin Exp Dermatol 1988; 13: 339–341.
16 Matsuoka LY, Wortsman J, Carlisle KS et al. The acquired cutaneous mucinoses. Arch Intern Med 1984; 144: 1974–1980.
17 Rongioletti F, Rebora A. Cutaneous mucinoses. Microscopic criteria for diagnosis. Am J Dermatopathol 2001; 23: 257–267.
18 Stewart G, Kinmonth JB, Browse NL. Pretibial myxedema. Ann R Coll Surg Engl 1984; 66: 391–395.
19 Lynch PJ, Maize JC, Sisson JC. Pretibial myxedema and nonthyrotoxic thyroid disease. Arch Dermatol 1973; 107: 107–111.
20 Somach SC, Helm TN, Lawlor KB et al. Pretibial mucin. Histologic patterns and clinical correlation. Arch Dermatol 1993; 129: 1152–1156.
21 Cho S, Choi J-H, Sung K-J et al. Graves' disease presenting as elephantiasic pretibial myxedema and nodules of the hands. Int J Dermatol 2001; 40: 276–277.
22 Noppakun N, Bancheun K, Chandraprasert S. Unusual locations of localized myxedema in Graves' disease. Arch Dermatol 1986; 122: 85–88.
23 Slater DN. Cervical nodular localized myxoedema in a thyroidectomy scar: light and electron microscopy and histochemical findings. Clin Exp Dermatol 1987; 12: 216–219.
24 Forgie JC, Highet AS, Kelly SA. Myxoedematous infiltrate of the forehead in treated hypothyroidism. Clin Exp Dermatol 1994; 19: 168–169.
25 Wright AL, Buxton PK, Menzies D. Pretibial myxedema localized to scar tissue. Int J Dermatol 1990; 29: 54–55.
26 Tong DW, Ho KK. Pretibial myxoedema presenting as a scar infiltrate. Australas J Dermatol 1998; 39: 255–257.
27 Missner SC, Ramsay EW, Houck HE, Kauffman CL. Graves' disease presenting as localized myxedema in a thigh donor graft site. J Am Acad Dermatol 1998; 39: 846–849.
28 Pujol RM, Monmany J, Bagué S, Alomar A. Graves' disease presenting as localized myxoedematous infiltration in a smallpox vaccination scar. Clin Exp Dermatol 2000; 25: 132–134.
29 Katsambas A, Pantazi V, Giannakopoulou H, Potouridou I. Localized myxedema in Grave's disease confined to the toes. Int J Dermatol 2000; 39: 953–954.
30 Gitter DG, Sato K. Localized hyperhidrosis in pretibial myxedema. J Am Acad Dermatol 1990; 23: 250–254.
31 Yeo PPB, Cheah JS, Sinniah R. Pretibial myxoedema: a clinical and pathological study. Aust N Z J Med 1978; 8: 60–62.
32 Jolliffe DS, Gaylarde PM, Brock AP, Sarkany I. Pretibial myxoedema: stimulation of mucopolysaccharide production of fibroblasts by serum. Br J Dermatol 1979; 100: 557–560.
33 Priestley GC, Aldridge RD, Sime PJ, Wilson D. Skin fibroblast activity in pretibial myxoedema and the effect of octreotide (Sandostatin ®) in vitro. Br J Dermatol 1994; 131: 52–56.
34 Cheung HS, Nicoloff JT, Kamiel MB et al. Stimulation of fibroblast biosynthetic activity by serum of patients with pretibial myxedema. J Invest Dermatol 1978; 71: 12–17.
35 Shinohara M, Hamasaki Y, Katayama I. Refractory pretibial myxoedema with response to intralesional insulin-like growth factor 1 antagonist (octreotide): downregulation of hyaluronic acid production by the lesional fibroblasts. Br J Dermatol 2000; 143: 1083–1086.
36 Scheicher SM, Milstein HJ. Treatment of pretibial mucinosis with gradient pneumatic compression. Arch Dermatol 1994; 130: 842–844.
37 Heymann WR. Cutaneous manifestations of thyroid disease. J Am Acad Dermatol 1992; 26: 885–902.
38 Matsuoka LY, Worstman J, Uitto J et al. Altered skin elastic fibers in hypothyroid myxedema and pretibial myxedema. Arch Intern Med 1985; 145: 117–121.
39 Kobayasi T, Danielsen L, Asboe-Hansen G. Ultrastructure of localized myxedema. Acta Derm Venereol 1976; 56: 173–185.
40 Konrad K, Brenner W, Pehamberger H. Ultrastructural and immunological findings in Graves' disease with pretibial myxedema. J Cutan Pathol 1980; 7: 99–108.
41 Farmer ER, Hambrick GW, Shulman LE. Papular mucinosis. A clinicopathologic study of four patients. Arch Dermatol 1982; 118: 9–13.
42 Poswig A, Hinrichs R, Megahed M et al. Discrete papular mucinosis – a rare subtype of lichen myxedematosus. Clin Exp Dermatol 2000; 25: 289–292.
43 Banno H, Takama H, Nitta Y et al. Lichen myxedematosus associated with chronic hepatitis C. Int J Dermatol 2000; 39: 212–215.
44 Ruiz-Rodriguez R, Maurer TA, Berger TG. Papular mucinosis and human immunodeficiency virus infection. Arch Dermatol 1992; 128: 995–996.
45 Tarantini G, Zerboni R, Muratori S et al. Lichen myxedematosus in a patient with AIDS. Br J Dermatol 1996; 134: 1122–1124.
46 Yen A, Sanchez RL, Raimer SS. Papular mucinosis associated with AIDS: Response to isotretinoin. J Am Acad Dermatol 1997; 37: 127–128.
47 Auñon JDD, Llorente CP, Martin RL et al. Lichen myxedematosus associated with human immunodeficiency virus infection – report of two cases and review of the literature. Clin Exp Dermatol 1997; 22: 265–268.
48 Azaña JM, De Misa RF, Casado J et al. Papular mucinosis associated with human-immunodeficiency-virus infection. Int J Dermatol 1996; 35: 652–654.
49 Valicenti JMK, Fleming MG, Pearson RW et al. Papular mucinosis in L-tryptophan-induced eosinophilia-myalgia syndrome. J Am Acad Dermatol 1991; 25: 54–58.
50 Rongioletti F, Rampini P, Parodi A, Rebora A. Papular mucinosis associated with generalized morphoea. Br J Dermatol 1999; 141: 905–908.
51 Chanda JJ. Scleromyxedema. Cutis 1979; 24: 549–552.

52 Milam CP, Cohen LE, Fenske NA, Ling NS. Scleromyxedema: therapeutic response to isotretinoin in three patients. J Am Acad Dermatol 1988; 19: 469–477.

53 Harris AO, Altman AR, Tschen JA, Wolf JE Jr. Scleromyxedema. Int J Dermatol 1989; 28: 661–667.

54 Boffa MJ, Ead RD. Spontaneous improvement of scleromyxoedema. Clin Exp Dermatol 1995; 20: 157–160.

55 Dinneen AM, Dicken CH. Scleromyxedema. J Am Acad Dermatol 1995; 33: 37–43.

56 Penmetcha M, Highet AS, Hopkinson JM. Failure of PUVA in lichen myxoedematosus: acceleration of associated multiple keratoacanthomas with development of squamous carcinoma. Clin Exp Dermatol 1987; 12: 220–223.

57 Howsden SM, Herndon JH, Freeman RG. Lichen myxedematosus. Dermal infiltrative disorder responsive to cyclophosphamide therapy. Arch Dermatol 1975; 111: 1325–1330.

58 Lang E, Zabel M, Schmidt H. Skleromyxödem Arndt-Gottron und assoziierte Phänomene. Dermatologica 1984; 169: 29–35.

59 Kantor GR, Bergfeld WF, Katzin WE et al. Scleromyxedema associated with scleroderma renal disease and acute psychosis. J Am Acad Dermatol 1986; 14: 879–888.

60 Gonzalez J, Palangio M, Schwartz J et al. Scleromyxedema with dermato-neuro syndrome. J Am Acad Dermatol 2000; 42: 927–928.

61 Lo P-Y, Tzung T-Y. Lichen myxedematosus in a patient with hepatocellular carcinoma. Br J Dermatol 2000; 143: 452–453.

62 Alfadley A, Al Hoqail I, Al Eisa A. Scleromyxedema: Possible association with seminoma. J Am Acad Dermatol 2000; 42: 875–878.

63 Montesu MA, Cottoni F, Sanna R, Cerimele D. Lichen myxedematosus associated with chronic hepatitis C: a case report. Acta Derm Venereol 2001; 81: 67–68.

64 Launay D, Hatron P-Y, Delaporte E et al. Scleromyxedema (lichen myxedematosus) associated with dermatomyositis. Br J Dermatol 2001; 144: 359–362.

65 Bata-Csorgo Z, Husz S, Foldes M et al. Scleromyxedema. J Am Acad Dermatol 1999; 40: 343–346.

66 Lowe NJ, Dufton PA, Hunter RD, Vickers CFH. Electron-beam treatment of scleromyxoedema. Br J Dermatol 1982; 106: 449–454.

67 Alligood TR, Burnett JW, Raines BL. Scleromyxedema associated with esophageal aperistalsis and dermal eosinophilia. Cutis 1981; 28: 60–66.

68 Hardie RA, Hunter JAA, Urbaniak S, Habeshaw JA. Spontaneous resolution of lichen myxoedematosus. Br J Dermatol 1979; 100: 727–730.

69 Rudner EJ, Mehregan A, Pinkus H. Scleromyxedema. A variant of lichen myxedematosus. Arch Dermatol 1966; 93: 3–12.

70 Godby A, Bergstresser PR, Chaker MB, Pandya AG. Fatal scleromyxedema: Report of a case and review of the literature. J Am Acad Dermatol 1998; 38: 289–294.

71 Morris-Jones R, Staughton RCD, Walker M et al. Lichen myxoedematosus with associated cardiac abnormalities. Br J Dermatol 2001; 144: 594–596.

72 Jakubovic HR, Salama SSS, Rosenthal D. Multiple cutaneous focal mucinoses with hypothyroidism. Ann Intern Med 1982; 96: 56–58.

73 Archibald GC, Calvert HT. Hypothyroidism and lichen myxedematosus. Arch Dermatol 1977; 113: 684.

74 Krasagakis K, Zouboulis ChC, Owsianowski M et al. Remission of scleromyxoedema following treatment with extracorporeal photopheresis. Br J Dermatol 1996; 135: 463–466.

75 Rayson D, Lust JA, Duncan A, Su WPD. Scleromyxedema: A complete response to prednisone. Mayo Clin Proc 1999; 74: 481–484.

76 Tschen JA, Chang JR. Scleromyxedema: treatment with interferon alfa. J Am Acad Dermatol 1999; 40: 303–307.

77 Lister RK, Jolles S, Whittaker S et al. Scleromyxedema: Response to high-dose intravenous immunoglobulin (hdIVIg). J Am Acad Dermatol 2000; 43: 403–408.

78 Rongioletti F, Rebora A. Updated classification of papular mucinosis, lichen myxedematosus, and scleromyxedema. J Am Acad Dermatol 2001; 44: 273–281.

79 Bergfeld WF, Lobur D, Cathcart M. Fibroblast studies in scleromyxedema: cellular proliferation and glycosaminoglycan metabolism. Arch Dermatol 1984; 120: 1609 (abstract).

80 Westheim AI, Lookingbill DP. Plasmapheresis in a patient with scleromyxedema. Arch Dermatol 1987; 123: 786–789.

81 Lai A, Fat RFM, Suurmond D, Radl J, van Furth R. Scleromyxoedema (lichen myxoedematosus) associated with a paraprotein IgG$_1$ of type kappa. Br J Dermatol 1973; 88: 107–116.

82 Stücker M, Nowack U, Röchling A et al. Sweat gland proliferations in scleromyxedema. Am J Dermatopathol 1999; 21: 259–264.

83 Abd El-Ad H, Salem SS, Salem A. Lichen myxedematosus: histochemical study. Dermatologica 1981; 162: 273–276.

84 Clark BJ, Mowat A, Fallowfield ME, Lee FD. Papular mucinosis: is the inflammatory cell infiltrate neoplastic? The presence of a monotypic plasma cell population demonstrated by in situ hybridization. Br J Dermatol 1996; 135: 467–470.

85 Ishii M, Furukawa M, Okada M, Hamada T. The use of improved ruthenium red staining for the ultrastructural detection of proteoglycan aggregates in normal skin and Lichen myxoedematosus. J Cutan Pathol 1984; 11: 292–295.

86 Coskey RJ, Mehregan A. Papular mucinosis. Int J Dermatol 1977; 16: 741–744.

87 Flowers SL, Cooper PH, Landes HB. Acral persistent papular mucinosis. J Am Acad Dermatol 1989; 21: 293–297.

88 Crovato F, Nazzari G, Desirello G. Acral persistent papular mucinosis. J Am Acad Dermatol 1990; 23: 121–122.

89 Stephens CJM, Ross JS, Charles-Holmes R et al. An unusual case of transient papular mucinosis associated with carpal tunnel syndrome. Br J Dermatol 1993; 129: 89–91.

90 Ahó HJ, Forsten Y, Hopsu-Havu VK. Ultrastructural signs of altered intracellular metabolism in acral persistent papular mucinosis. J Cutan Pathol 1991; 18: 347–352.

91 España A, Mosquera O, Idoate MA, Quintanilla E. Acral persistent papular mucinosis. Int J Dermatol 1993; 32: 600–601.

92 Fosko SW, Perez MI, Longley BJ. Acral persistent papular mucinosis. J Am Acad Dermatol 1992; 27: 1026–1029.

93 Coulson IH, Mallett RB, Holden CA. Acral persistent papular mucinosis. Br J Dermatol 1992; 126: 283–285.

94 Menni S, Cavicchini S, Brezzi A et al. Acral persistent papular mucinosis in two sisters. Clin Exp Dermatol 1995; 20: 431–433.

95 Abalde T, Ginarte M, Fernández-Redondo V, Toribio J. Aypical acral persistent papular mucinosis. Int J Dermatol 1999; 38: 470–473.

96 Cannata G, Gambini C, Ciaccio M. Self-healing localized cutaneous mucinosis. Dermatology 1994; 189: 93–94.

97 Lum D. Cutaneous mucinosis of infancy. Arch Dermatol 1980; 116: 198–200.

98 McGrae JD. Cutaneous mucinosis of infancy. A congenital and linear variant. Arch Dermatol 1983; 119: 272–273.

99 Calza A-M, Masouyé I, Saurat J-H. An unusual case of infantile dermal mucinosis. Pediatr Dermatol 1994; 11: 252–255.

100 Pattee SF, LeSueur BW, Bangert JL, Hansen RC. Persistent papules in an infant. Pediatr Dermatol 2001; 18: 159–161.

101 Brakman M, Starink ThM, Tafelkruyer J, Bos JD. Linear connective tissue naevus of the proteoglycan type ('naevus mucinosus'). Br J Dermatol 1994; 131: 368–370.

102 Stokes KS, Rabinowitz LG, Segura AD, Esterly NB. Cutaneous mucinosis of infancy. Pediatr Dermatol 1994; 11: 246–251.

103 Podda M, Rongioletti F, Greiner D et al. Cutaneous mucinosis of infancy: is it a real entity or the paediatric form of lichen myxedematosus (papular mucinosis)? Br J Dermatol 2001; 144: 590–593.

104 Bonerandi JJ, Andrac L, Follana J et al. Mucinose cutanée juvénile spontanément résolutive. Ann Dermatol Venereol 1980; 107: 51–57.

105 Pucevich MV, Latour DL, Bale GF, King LE. Self-healing juvenile cutaneous mucinosis. J Am Acad Dermatol 1984; 11: 327–332.

106 Caputo R, Grimalt R, Gelmetti C. Self-healing juvenile cutaneous mucinosis. Arch Dermatol 1995; 131: 459–461.

107 Kim YJ, Kim YT, Kim J-H. Self-healing cutaneous mucinosis. J Am Acad Dermatol 1994; 31: 815–816.

108 Wadee S, Roode H, Schulz EJ. Self-healing juvenile cutaneous mucinosis in a patient with nephroblastoma. Clin Exp Dermatol 1994; 19: 90–93.

109 Aydingöz İE, Candan İ, Dervent B. Self-healing juvenile cutaneous mucinosis. Dermatology 1999; 199: 57–59.

110 González-Enseñat MA, Vicente MA, Castellá N et al. Self-healing infantile familial cutaneous mucinosis. Pediatr Dermatol 1997; 14: 460–462.

111 Jang K-A, Han M-H, Choi J-H et al. Recurrent self-healing cutaneous mucinosis in an adult. Br J Dermatol 2000; 143: 650–652.

112 Quimby SR, Perry HO. Plaquelike cutaneous mucinosis: its relationship to reticular erythematous mucinosis. J Am Acad Dermatol 1982; 6: 856–861.

113 Kocsard E, Munro VF. Reticular erythematous mucinosis (REM syndrome) of Steigleder: its relationship to other mucinoses and to chronic erythemata. Aust J Dermatol 1978; 19: 121–124.

114 Cohen PR, Rabinowitz AD, Ruszkowski AM, DeLeo VA. Reticular erythematous mucinosis syndrome: review of the world literature and report of the syndrome in a prepubertal child. Pediatr Dermatol 1990; 7: 1–10.

115 Braddock SW, Davis CS, Davis RB. Reticular erythematous mucinosis and thrombocytopenic purpura. Report of a case and review of the world literature, including plaquelike cutaneous mucinosis. J Am Acad Dermatol 1988; 19: 859–868.

116 Triffet Treviño M, Ahmed I. Plaque-like cutaneous mucinosis (reticular erythematous mucinosis): a clinicopathologic analysis. J Cutan Pathol 1996; 23: 63 (abstract).

117 Morison WL, Shea CR, Parrish JA. Reticular erythematous mucinosis syndrome. Arch Dermatol 1979; 115: 1340–1342.

118 Keczkes K, Jadhav P. REM syndrome (reticular erythematous mucinosis). Report of a further case or variant of it. Arch Dermatol 1977; 113: 335–338.

119 Sidwell RU, Francis N, Bunker CB. Hormonal influence on reticular erythematous mucinosis. Br J Dermatol 2001; 144: 633–634.

120 Izumi T, Tajima S, Harada R, Nishikawa T. Reticular erythematous mucinosis syndrome: glycosaminoglycan synthesis by fibroblasts and abnormal response to interleukin-1β. Dermatology 1996; 192: 41–45.

121 Braddock SW, Kay HD, Maennle D et al. Clinical and immunologic studies in reticular erythematous mucinosis and Jessner's lymphocytic infiltrate of skin. J Am Acad Dermatol 1993; 28: 691–695.

122 Bleehen SS, Slater DN, Mahood J, Church RE. Reticular erythematous mucinosis: light and electron microscopy, immunofluorescence and histochemical findings. Br J Dermatol 1982; 106: 9–18.

123 Smith NP, Sanderson KV, Crow KD. Reticular erythematous mucinosis syndrome. Clin Exp Dermatol 1976; 1: 99–103.

124 Del Pozo J, Martinez W, Almagro M et al. Reticular erythematous mucinosis syndrome. Report of a case with positive immunofluorescence. Clin Exp Dermatol 1997; 22: 234–236.

125 Vanuytrecht-Henderickx D, Dewolf-Peeters C, Degreef H. Morphological study of the reticular erythematous mucinosis syndrome. Dermatologica 1984; 168: 163–169.

126 Chavaz P, Polla L, Saurat JH. Paramyxovirus-like inclusions and lymphocyte type in the REM syndrome. Br J Dermatol 1982; 106: 741.

127 Dodd HJ, Sarkany I, Sadrudin A. Reticular erythematous mucinosis syndrome. Clin Exp Dermatol 1987; 12: 36–39.

128 Carrington PR, Sanusi ID, Winder PR et al. Scleredema adultorum. Int J Dermatol 1984; 23: 514–522.

129 Burke MJ, Seguin J, Bove KE. Scleredema: an unusual presentation with edema limited to scalp, upper face, and orbits. J Pediatr 1982; 101: 960–963.

130 Farrell AM, Branfoot AC, Moss J et al. Scleredema diabeticorum of Buschke confined to the thighs. Br J Dermatol 1996; 134: 1113–1115.

131 Heilbron B, Saxe N. Scleredema in an infant. Arch Dermatol 1986; 122: 1417–1419.

132 Graff R. Scleredema adultorum (discussion). Arch Dermatol 1968; 98: 320.

133 Venencie PY, Powell FC, Su WPD, Perry HO. Scleredema: a review of thirty-three cases. J Am Acad Dermatol 1984; 11: 128–134.

134 Krakowski A, Covo J, Berlin C. Diabetic scleredema. Dermatologica 1973; 146: 193–198.

135 Cohn BA, Wheeler CE, Briggaman RA. Scleredema adultorum of Buschke and diabetes mellitus. Arch Dermatol 1970; 101: 27–35.

136 Parker SC, Fenton DA, Black MM. Scleredema. Clin Exp Dermatol 1989; 14: 385–386.

137 Tamburin LM, Pena JR, Meredith R, Soong VY. Scleredema of Buschke successfully treated with electron beam therapy. Arch Dermatol 1998; 134: 419–422.

138 McNaughton F, Keczkes K. Scleredema adultorum and diabetes mellitus (scleredema diutinum). Clin Exp Dermatol 1983; 8: 41–45.

139 Ohta A, Uitto J, Oikarinen AI et al. Paraproteinemia in patients with scleredema. Clinical findings and serum effects on skin fibroblasts in vitro. J Am Acad Dermatol 1987; 16: 96–107.

140 Pajarre S. Scleroedema adultorum Buschke. Acta Derm Venereol 1975; 55: 158–159.

141 Oikarinen A, Ala-Kokko L, Palatsi R et al. Scleredema and paraproteinemia. Arch Dermatol 1987; 123: 226–229.

142 McFadden N, Ree K, Soyland E, Larsen TE. Scleredema adultorum associated with a monoclonal gammopathy and generalized hyperpigmentation. Arch Dermatol 1987; 123: 629–632.

143 Hodak E, Tamir R, David M et al. Scleredema adultorum associated with IgG-kappa multiple myeloma – a case report and review of the literature. Clin Exp Dermatol 1988; 13: 271–274.

144 Salisbury JA, Shallcross H, Leigh IM. Scleredema of Buschke associated with multiple myeloma. Clin Exp Dermatol 1988; 13: 269–270.

145 Sansom JE, Sheehan AL, Kennedy CTC, Delaney TJ. A fatal case of scleredema of Buschke. Br J Dermatol 1994; 130: 669–670.

146 Schmidt KT, Gattuso P, Messmore H et al. Scleredema and smoldering myeloma. J Am Acad Dermatol 1992; 26: 319–321.

147 Basarab T, Burrows NP, Munn SE, Russell Jones R. Systemic involvement in scleredema of Buschke associated with IgG-kappa paraproteinaemia. Br J Dermatol 1997; 136: 939–942.

148 Ratip S, Akin H, Özdemirli M et al. Scleredema of Buschke associated with Waldenström's macroglobulinaemia. Br J Dermatol 2000; 143: 450–452.

149 Grudeva-Popova J, Dobrev H. Biomechanical measurement of skin distensibility in scleredema of Buschke associated with multiple myeloma. Clin Exp Dermatol 2000; 25: 247–249.

150 Stables GI, Taylor PC, Highet AS. Scleredema associated with paraproteinaemia treated by extracorporeal photophoresis. Br J Dermatol 2000; 142: 781–783.

151 Miyagawa S, Dohi K, Tsuruta S, Shirai T. Scleredema of Buschke associated with rheumatoid arthritis and Sjögren's syndrome. Br J Dermatol 1989; 121: 517–520.

152 Rees R, Moore A, Nanney L, King L. Scleredema adultorum: the surgical implications of a rare dermatologic disorder. Plast Reconstr Surg 1983; 72: 90–93.

153 Verghese A, Noble J, Diamond RD. Scleredema adultorum. A case of the recurrent cellulitis syndrome. Arch Dermatol 1984; 120: 1518–1519.

154 Millns JL, Fenske NA. Scleredema and persistent erythema. Arch Dermatol 1982; 118: 290–291.

155 Varga J, Gotta S, Li L et al. Scleredema adultorum: case report and demonstration of abnormal expression of extracellular matrix genes in skin fibroblasts in vivo and in vitro. Br J Dermatol 1995; 132: 992–999.

156 Holubar K, Mach KW. Scleredema (Buschke). Histological and histochemical investigations. Acta Derm Venereol 1967; 47: 102–110.

157 Cole HG, Winkelmann RK. Acid mucopolysaccharide staining in scleredema. J Cutan Pathol 1990; 17: 211–213.

158 Roupe G, Laurent TC, Malmstrom A et al. Biochemical characterization and tissue distribution of the scleredema in a case of Buschke's disease. Acta Derm Venereol 1987; 67: 193–198.

159 Fleischmajer R, Lara JV. Scleredema. A histochemical and biochemical study. Arch Dermatol 1965; 92: 643–652.

160 Nishiura S, Mihara M, Shimao S et al. Cutaneous focal mucinosis. Br J Dermatol 1989; 121: 511–515.

161 Yamamoto T, Katayama I, Nishioka K. Reactive nodular mucinosis: a variant of cutaneous focal mucinosis? Int J Dermatol 1996; 35: 73–74.

162 Wilk M, Schmoeckel C. Cutaneous focal mucinosis – a histopathological and immunohistochemical analysis of 11 cases. J Cutan Pathol 1994; 21: 446–452.

163 Suhonen R, Niemi K-M. Cutaneous focal mucinosis with spontaneous healing. J Cutan Pathol 1983; 10: 334–339.

164 Rongioletti F, Amantea A, Balus L, Rebora A. Cutaneous focal mucinosis associated with reticular erythematous mucinosis and scleromyxedema. J Am Acad Dermatol 1991; 24: 656–657.

165 Johnson WC, Helwig EB. Cutaneous focal mucinosis. Arch Dermatol 1966; 93: 13–20.

166 Terui T, Aiba S, Tagami H. Solitary subcutaneous mucinosis surrounded by bizarre-shaped, factor XIII-a positive cells with intranuclear vacuoles. J Cutan Pathol 1998; 25: 271–274.

167 Armijo M. Mucoid cysts of the fingers. J Dermatol Surg Oncol 1981; 7: 317–322.

168 Epstein E. A simple technique for managing digital mucous cysts. Arch Dermatol 1979; 115: 1315–1316.

169 Johnson WC, Graham JH, Helwig EB. Cutaneous myxoid cyst. JAMA 1965; 191: 109–114.

170 Hernández-Lugo AM, Domínguez-Cherit J, Vega-Memije ME. Digital mucoid cyst: the ganglion type. Int J Dermatol 1999; 38: 533–535.

171 Lattanand A, Johnson WC, Graham JH. Mucous cyst (mucocele). Arch Dermatol 1970; 101: 673–678.

172 Jensen JL. Superficial mucoceles of the oral mucosa. Am J Dermatopathol 1990; 12: 88–92.

173 Carney JA, Gordon H, Carpenter PC et al. The complex of myxomas, spotty pigmentation, and endocrine overactivity. Medicine (Baltimore) 1985; 64: 270–283.

174 Carney JA, Headington JT, Su WPD. Cutaneous myxomas. Arch Dermatol 1986; 122: 790–798.

175 Ferreiro JA, Carney JA. Myxomas of the external ear and their significance. Am J Surg Pathol 1994; 18: 274–280.

176 Gardner SS, Solomon AR. Cutaneous and cardiac myxomas: an important association. Semin Dermatol 1991; 10: 148–151.

177 Armstrong DKB, Irvine AD, Handley JM et al. Carney complex: report of a kindred with predominantly cutaneous manifestations. Br J Dermatol 1997; 136: 578–582.

178 Irvine AD, Armstrong DKB, Bingham EA et al. Evidence for a second genetic locus in Carney complex. Br J Dermatol 1998; 139: 572–576.

179 Murphy CM, Grau-Massanés M, Sánchez RL. Multiple cutaneous myxomas. J Cutan Pathol 1995; 22: 556–562.

180 Sanusi ID. Subungual myxoma. Arch Dermatol 1982; 118: 612–614.

181 Allen PW, Dymock RB, MacCormac LB. Superficial angiomyxomas with and without epithelial components. Report of 30 tumors in 28 patients. Am J Surg Pathol 1988; 12: 519–530.

182 Wilk M, Schmoeckel C, Kaiser HW et al. Cutaneous angiomyxoma: a benign neoplasm distinct from cutaneous focal mucinosis. J Am Acad Dermatol 1995; 33: 352–355.

183 Weinberg JM, Penczak RS, Don PC et al. Disseminated cutaneous myxomas in an adult. Int J Dermatol 1998; 37: 946–948.

184 Alaiti S, Nelson FP, Ryoo JW. Solitary cutaneous myxoma. J Am Acad Dermatol 2000; 43: 377–379.

185 Craig NM, Putterman AM, Roenigk RK et al. Multiple periorbital myxomas progressing to scleromyxedema. J Am Acad Dermatol 1996; 34: 928–930.

186 Zina AM, Bundino S. Multiple cutaneous fibromyxomas: a light and electron microscopic study. J Cutan Pathol 1980; 7: 335–341.

187 Bellón PR, Vázquez-Doval J, Idoate M, Quintanilla E. Mucinous nevus. J Am Acad Dermatol 1993; 28: 797–798.

188 Suhr K-B, Ro Y-W, Kim K-H et al. Mucinous nevus: Report of two cases and review of the literature. J Am Acad Dermatol 1997; 37: 312–313.

189 Rongioletti F, Rebora A. Mucinous nevus. Arch Dermatol 1996; 132: 1522–1523.

190 Chun SI, Cho NJ. Linear morphea with secondary cutaneous mucinosis. Am J Dermatopathol 1992; 14: 546–548.

191 Noto G, Pravatà G, Aricò M. Reticulate postinflammatory hyperpigmentation with band-like mucin deposition. Int J Dermatol 1998; 37: 829–832.

192 Vázquez-Doval FJ, Sola MA. Mucinosis of the mammary areolae and mycosis fungoides. Clin Exp Dermatol 1996; 21: 374–376.

193 Weigand DA, Burgdorf WHC, Gregg LJ. Dermal mucinosis in discoid lupus erythematosus. Report of two cases. Arch Dermatol 1981; 117: 735–738.

194 Rongioletti J, Rebora A. Papular and nodular mucinosis associated with systemic lupus erythematosus. Br J Dermatol 1986; 115: 631–636.

195 Gammon WR, Caro I, Long JC, Wheeler CE. Secondary cutaneous mucinosis with systemic lupus erythematosus. Arch Dermatol 1978; 114: 432–435.

196 Eskreis BD, Bronson DM. Cutaneous mucinosis in a child with systemic lupus erythematosus. Pediatr Dermatol 1992; 9: 259–263.

197 Choi EH, Hann SK, Chung K-Y, Park Y-K. Papulonodular cutaneous mucinosis associated with systemic lupus erythematosus. Int J Dermatol 1992; 31: 649–652.

198 Pandya AG, Sontheimer RD, Cockerell CJ et al. Papulonodular mucinosis associated with systemic lupus erythematosus: possible mechanisms of increased glycosaminoglycan accumulation. J Am Acad Dermatol 1995; 32: 199–205.

199 Kobayashi T, Shimizu H, Shimizu S et al. Plaquelike cutaneous lupus mucinosis. Arch Dermatol 1993; 129: 383–384.

200 Maruyama M, Miyauchi S, Hashimoto K. Massive cutaneous mucinosis associated with systemic lupus erythematosus. Br J Dermatol 1997; 137: 450–453.

201 Lee WS, Chung J, Ahn SK. Plaque and postauricular nodular mucinosis associated with lupus erythematosus. Int J Dermatol 1997; 36: 367–369.

202 Carrington PR, Nelson-Adesokan P, Smoller BR. Plaque-like erythema with milia: A noninfectious dermal mucinosis mimicking cryptococcal cellulitis in a renal transplant recipient. J Am Acad Dermatol 1998; 39: 334–337.

Follicular mucinoses

203 Nickoloff BJ, Wood C. Benign idiopathic versus mycosis-fungoides-associated follicular mucinosis. Pediatr Dermatol 1985; 2: 201–206.

204 Rongioletti F, Rebora A. Follicular mucinosis in exaggerated arthropod-bite reactions of patients with chronic lymphocytic leukemia. J Am Acad Dermatol 1999; 41: 500.

205 Pinkus H. Alopecia mucinosa. Arch Dermatol 1957; 76: 419–426.

206 Gibson LE, Muller SA, Peters MS. Follicular mucinosis of childhood and adolescence. Pediatr Dermatol 1988; 5: 231–235.

207 Coskey RJ, Mehregan AH. Alopecia mucinosa. A follow-up study. Arch Dermatol 1970; 102: 193–194.

208 Emmerson RW. Follicular mucinosis. A study of 47 patients. Br J Dermatol 1969; 81: 395–413.

209 Locker E, Duncan WC. Hypopigmentation in alopecia mucinosa. Arch Dermatol 1979; 115: 731–733.

210 Snyder RA, Crain WR, McNutt NS. Alopecia mucinosa. Report of a case with diffuse alopecia and normal-appearing scalp skin. Arch Dermatol 1984; 120: 496–498.

211 Roth DE, Owen LG, Hodge SJ, Callen JP. Follicular mucinosis associated with pregnancy. Int J Dermatol 1992; 31: 441–442.

212 Yotsumoto S, Uchimiya H, Kanzaki T. A case of follicular mucinosis treated successfully with minocycline. Br J Dermatol 2000; 142: 841–842.

213 Binnick AN, Wax FD, Clendenning WE. Alopecia mucinosa of the face associated with mycosis fungoides. Arch Dermatol 1978; 114: 791–792.

214 Plotnick H, Abbrecht M. Alopecia mucinosa and lymphoma. Report of two cases and review of literature. Arch Dermatol 1965; 92: 137–141.

215 Wilkinson JD, Black MM, Chu A. Follicular mucinosis associated with mycosis fungoides presenting with gross cystic changes on the face. Clin Exp Dermatol 1982; 7: 333–340.

216 Cottoni F, Massarelli G, Tedde G, Lissia A. Follicular mucinosis plus mycosis fungoides and acanthosis nigricans plus alveolar bronchiolar carcinoma. Int J Dermatol 1995; 34: 867–869.

217 Bonta MD, Tannous ZS, Demierre M-F et al. Rapidly progressing mycosis fungoides presenting as follicular mucinosis. J Am Acad Dermatol 2000; 43: 635–640.

218 Thomson J, Cochran REI. Chronic lymphatic leukemia presenting as atypical rosacea with follicular mucinosis. J Cutan Pathol 1978; 5: 81–87.

219 Sumner WT, Grichnik JM, Shea CR et al. Follicular mucinosis as a presenting sign of acute myeloblastic leukemia. J Am Acad Dermatol 1998; 39: 803–805.

220 Stankler L, Ewen SWB. Hodgkin's disease in a patient with follicular and dermal mucinosis and spontaneous ooze of mucin (mucinorrhoea). Br J Dermatol 1975; 93: 581–586.

221 Freeman RG. Familial reticuloendotheliosis with eosinophilia and follicular mucinosis. Arch Dermatol 1972; 105: 737–738.

222 Fairris GM, Kirkham N, Goodwin PG et al. Erythrodermic follicular mucinosis. Clin Exp Dermatol 1987; 12: 50–52.

223 Rivers JK, Norris PG, Greaves MW, Smith NP. Follicular mucinosis in association with Sézary syndrome. Clin Exp Dermatol 1987; 12: 207–210.

224 Walchner M, Messer G, Rust A et al. Follicular mucinosis in association with squamous cell carcinoma of the tongue. J Am Acad Dermatol 1998; 38: 622–624.

225 Wolff HH, Kinney J, Ackerman AB. Angiolymphoid hyperplasia with follicular mucinosis. Arch Dermatol 1978; 114: 229–232.

226 Bovet R, Delacrétaz J. Hyperplasie angio-lymphoïde avec mucinose folliculaire. Dermatologica 1979; 158: 343–347.

227 Kim R, Winkelmann RK. Follicular mucinosis (alopecia mucinosa). Arch Dermatol 1962; 85: 490–498.

228 Lancer HA, Bronstein BR, Nakagawa H et al. Follicular mucinosis: a detailed morphologic and immunopathologic study. J Am Acad Dermatol 1984; 10: 760–768.

229 Sentis HJ, Willemze R, Scheffer E. Alopecia mucinosa progressing into mycosis fungoides. A long-term follow-up of two patients. Am J Dermatopathol 1988; 10: 478–486.

230 Gibson LE, Muller SA, Leiferman KM, Peters MS. Follicular mucinosis: clinical and histopathologic study. J Am Acad Dermatol 1989; 20: 441–446.

231 Pujol RM, Alonso J, Gibson LE et al. Follicular mucinosis: clinicopathologic evaluation and genotypic analysis of 25 cases, with clonality evaluation by TCR gamma chain PCR amplification. J Cutan Pathol 1996; 23: 58 (abstract).

232 Witterberg GP, Gibson LE, Pittelkow MR, el-Azhary RA. Follicular mucinosis presenting as an acneiform eruption: Report of four cases. J Am Acad Dermatol 1998; 38: 849–851.

233 Cerroni L, Fink-Puches R, Bäck B, Kerl H. Follicular mucinosis: a reappraisal of clinico-pathologic features and association with mycosis fungoides and Sézary syndrome. Am J Dermatopathol 2000; 22: 358 (abstract).

234 Jackow CM, Papadopoulos E, Nelson B et al. Follicular mucinosis associated with scarring alopecia, oligoclonal T-cell receptor Vβ expansion, and *Staphylococcus aureus*: When does follicular mucinosis become mycosis fungoides? J Am Acad Dermatol 1997; 36: 828–831.

235 Tannous ZS, DaCosta-Bonta M, Longtine JA, Duncan LM. T-cell receptor γ gene rearrangement studies in follicular mucinosis. J Cutan Pathol 2000; 27: 574 (abstract).

236 Rustin MHA, Bunker CB, Levene GM. Follicular mucinosis presenting as acute dermatitis and response to dapsone. Clin Exp Dermatol 1989; 14: 382–384.

237 Kubba RK, Stewart TW. Follicular mucinosis responding to dapsone. Br J Dermatol 1974; 91: 217–220.

238 Ishibashi A. Histogenesis of mucin in follicular mucinosis. An electron microscopic study. Acta Derm Venereol 1976; 56: 163–171.

239 Pinkus H. Commentary: alopecia mucinosa. Arch Dermatol 1983; 119: 698–699.

240 Haber H. Follicular mucinosis (alopecia mucinosa. Pinkus). Br J Dermatol 1961; 73: 313–322.

241 Okun MR, Kay F. Follicular mucinosis (alopecia mucinosa). Arch Dermatol 1964; 89: 809–814.

242 Berger TG, Goette DK. Eccrine proliferation with follicular mucinosis. J Cutan Pathol 1987; 14: 188–190.

243 Kossard S, Rubel D. Folliculotropic T-cell lymphocytosis (mucin-poor follicular mucinosis). Australas J Dermatol 2000; 41: 120–123.

244 Ishibashi A, Chujo T. Ultrastructure of follicular mucinosis. J Cutan Pathol 1974; 1: 126–131.

245 Jordaan HF. Follicular mucinosis in association with a melanocytic nevus. A report of two cases. J Cutan Pathol 1987; 14: 122–126.

246 Weedon D. Unpublished observation.

247 Nickoloff BJ, Wood C, Farber EM. Follicular spongiosis with intercellular deposition of mucin: observations and speculations. Am J Dermatopathol 1985; 7: 302–303.

248 Becke RFA, Musso LA. An unusual epithelial-connective tissue naevus with perifollicular mucinosis. Australas J Dermatol 1978; 19: 118–120.

249 Perrin Ch, Durant JM, Lacour JPh et al. Horny perifollicular mucinosis. An atypical pityriasis rubra pilaris-like eruption associated with HIV infection. Am J Dermatopathol 1993; 15: 358–362.

Epithelial mucinoses

250 Daudén E, Martin R, Feal C et al. Eccrine ductal mucinosis in a human immunodeficiency virus-positive patient with probable scabies. Br J Dermatol 2000; 143: 1335–1336.

Mucopolysaccharidoses

251 McKusick VA, Neufeld EF. In: The metabolic basis of inherited disease, 5th ed. New York: McGraw-Hill, 1983; 751.

252 Gebhart W. Heritable metabolic storage diseases. J Cutan Pathol 1985; 12: 348–357.

253 Fluharty AL. The mucopolysaccharidoses: a synergism between clinical and basic investigation. J Invest Dermatol 1982; 79: 38s–44s.

254 McKusick VA. The nosology of the mucopolysaccharidoses. Am J Med 1969; 47: 730–747.

255 Schiro JA, Mallory SB, Demmer L et al. Grouped papules in Hurler-Scheie syndrome. J Am Acad Dermatol 1996; 35: 868–870.

256 Thappa DM, Singh A, Jaisankar TJ et al. Pebbling of the skin: a marker of Hunter's syndrome. Pediatr Dermatol 1998; 15: 370–373.

257 Beesley CE, Young EP, Vellodi A, Winchester BG. Mutational analysis of Sanfilippo syndrome type A (MPS IIIA): identification of 13 novel mutations. J Med Genet 2000; 37: 704–707.

258 Hambrick GW, Scheie HG. Studies of the skin in Hurler's syndrome. Arch Dermatol 1962; 85: 455–470.

259 Cole HN, Irving RC, Lund HZ et al. Gargoylism with cutaneous manifestations. Arch Dermatol 1952; 66: 371–383.

260 Freeman RG. A pathological basis for the cutaneous papules of mucopolysaccharidosis II (the Hunter syndrome). J Cutan Pathol 1977; 4: 318–328.

261 Prystowsky MD, Maumenee IH, Freeman RG et al. Cutaneous marker in the Hunter syndrome. Arch Dermatol 1977; 113: 602–605.

262 Finlayson LA. Hunter syndrome (mucopolysaccharidosis II). Pediatr Dermatol 1990; 7: 150–152.

263 Demitsu T, Kakurai M, Okubo Y et al. Skin eruption as the presenting sign of Hunter syndrome IIB. Clin Exp Dermatol 1999; 24: 179–182.

264 Lasser A, Carter DM, Mahoney MJ. Ultrastructure of the skin in mucopolysaccharidoses. Arch Pathol 1975; 99: 173–176.

265 Bioulac P, Mercier M, Beylot C, Fontan D. The diagnosis of mucopolysaccharidoses by electron microscopy of skin biopsies. J Cutan Pathol 1975; 2: 179–190.

266 Belcher RW. Ultrastructure and cytochemistry of lymphocytes in the genetic mucopolysaccharidoses. Arch Pathol 1972; 93: 1–7.

267 Belcher RW. Ultrastructure and function of eccrine glands in the mucopolysaccharidoses. Arch Pathol 1973; 96: 339–341.

268 O'Brien JS, Bernett J, Veath ML, Paa D. Lysosomal storage disorders: diagnosis by ultrastructural examination of skin biopsy specimens. Arch Neurol 1975; 32: 592–599.

269 Belcher RW. Ultrastructure of the skin in the genetic mucopolysaccharidoses. Arch Pathol 1972; 94: 511–518.

270 DeCloux RJ, Friederici HHR. Ultrastructural studies of the skin in Hurler's syndrome. Arch Pathol 1969; 88: 350–358.

271 Sipe JC, O'Brien JS. Ultrastructure of skin biopsy specimens: common sources of error in diagnosis. Clin Genet 1979; 15: 118–125.

Cutaneous deposits

INTRODUCTION

Cutaneous deposits are a heterogeneous group of substances which are not normal constituents of the skin. They are laid down, usually in the dermis, in a variety of different circumstances. There are five broad categories of deposits. The first group includes calcium salts, bone and cartilage.[1] The second category includes the hyaline deposits. These have an eosinophilic, somewhat glassy appearance in hematoxylin and eosin preparations. The third category includes various pigments, heavy metals (many of which are deposited in the form of a pigmented salt) and complex drug pigments. The fourth category, cutaneous implants, includes substances such as collagen and silicone which are inserted into the skin for cosmetic purposes. The fifth category includes miscellaneous substances such as oxalate crystals and fiberglass.

Some deposits evoke an inflammatory or foreign body reaction, although many of the hyaline and pigment deposits produce no significant response, except for some macrophages in the case of pigments. Hyaline deposits may blend imperceptibly with the surrounding collagen and require special histochemical staining for their positive identification.

CALCIUM, BONE AND CARTILAGE

CALCINOSIS CUTIS

The cutaneous deposition of calcium salts – calcinosis cutis – has historically been divided into a *dystrophic* variety, when the calcium is deposited in damaged or degenerate tissue, and a less common *metastatic* form associated with elevated serum levels of calcium or phosphate or both.[2,3] In many cases, the pathogenetic mechanism is unknown and these have been assigned to a third *idiopathic* group. Sometimes, several mechanisms are involved in the formation of the calcium deposits.[4,5] Rarely, no satisfactory explanation can be advanced for the calcium deposition.[6] The following classification is a modification of the historic one.[1]

Subepidermal calcified nodule
Subepidermal calcified nodule usually occurs as a solitary nodule on the head, particularly the ear, or the extremities of infants and young children, but it may develop in an older group of patients in whom it has a predilection for the upper extremities.[7–12] Subepidermal calcified nodule is one of the idiopathic calcinoses, although it has been suggested that the calcification occurs in a pre-existing nevus or hamartoma.[13] There is little evidence to support this view.

Idiopathic scrotal calcinosis
Single or multiple lesions, up to 3 cm or more in diameter, develop in the scrotal skin in children or young adults.[14–18] They may break down and discharge chalky material. It has been suggested that the lesions represent dystrophic calcification of eccrine duct milia[19] or of epidermal cysts,[17,20,21] although this has been disputed.[22,23]

A similar process involving the vulva and penis has been reported.[24–26]

Tumoral calcinosis
Tumoral calcinosis is an idiopathic condition consisting of massive subcutaneous deposits of calcium salts, often overlying the large joints in otherwise healthy patients.[27–30] There is a predilection for black races. Familial cases have been reported.[31] The pathogenesis remains an enigma,[31] although a small number of patients may have hyperphosphatemia.[32] Fibrohistiocytic nodules embedded in a dense collagenous stroma have been seen adjacent to early lesions of tumoral calcinosis.[33] Their role in the pathogenesis of this condition is uncertain.

Auricular calcinosis
Auricular calcinosis is a rare lesion of one or both ears that may be secondary to local factors such as inflammation, frost bite or trauma or be associated with systemic diseases such as Addison's disease, ochronosis or hypopituitarism.[34,35] The term 'petrified ear' is sometimes used.[36,37] Ossification rarely develops in auricular calcinosis.[38]

Infantile calcinosis of the heel
Calcinosis of the heel has been reported in infants who received multiple heel pricks for blood tests.[39,40] The deposits have been recognized at 10–12 months of age and they disappear about a year later. This group should probably be regarded as a clinical variant of dystrophic calcification; the nature of the underlying damage to the dermis which leads to the deposition of the calcium salts has not been elucidated.

Milia-like calcinosis
There have been several reports of children with pinhead-sized nodules, usually in the genital area, thighs or knees, which disappeared spontaneously, to recur a few weeks later.[41,42] This milia-like pattern of calcification may occur with Down syndrome.[43–46]

Dystrophic calcification
In dystrophic calcification there may be widespread large deposits (calcinosis universalis), such as occur in dermatomyositis[47–49] and rarely in lupus erythematosus,[50–54] or a few small deposits (calcinosis circumscripta), as seen in scleroderma[55,56] (see p. 349). Also included in the dystrophic group[1] are the calcium deposits that are found, rarely, in burns scars, keloids, acne scars, injection sites,[57–59] a violin pressure point,[60] and following calcium chloride or gluconate burns or infusions[61–64] and the use of calcium chloride-containing electrode pastes for electroencephalograms.[65–67] Cutaneous calcification of dystrophic type may follow the percutaneous penetration of calcium salts in those exposed to industrial drilling fluids containing calcium salts.[65] It has also been reported following neonatal herpes simplex infection[68] and in patients with the Ehlers–Danlos syndrome (see p. 364).

Metastatic calcification
Cutaneous involvement is a rare manifestation of the metastatic calcification that may accompany the hypercalcemia associated with primary or secondary hyperparathyroidism, destructive lesions of bone,[69] hypervitaminosis D and other rare causes.[5,70,71] The deposits are found in the deep dermis or subcutaneous tissue, particularly in the axillae, abdomen, medial aspect of the thighs and the flexural areas.[72,73] The term 'calciphylaxis' is used for a rare, often fatal, disease with progressive cutaneous necrosis and ulceration accompanied by widespread vascular calcification and thrombosis.[74–78] It occurs in some patients with chronic renal failure and secondary hyperparathyroidism, occasionally after initiation of dialysis.[79,80] It has also been reported with primary hyperparathyroidism,[81,82] presumptive functional protein C and protein S deficiency induced by chemotherapy,[83] and with metastatic breast carcinoma.[84]

Calcification of blood vessels
Calcification may involve blood vessels in the skin in metastatic and in dystrophic calcification.[85] It may be associated with cutaneous necrosis, particularly in calciphylaxis.[86–88]

Calcification of cysts and neoplasms

Calcification may occur in trichilemmal cysts, pilomatrixomas, trichoepitheliomas, syringomas,[89] basal cell carcinomas and hemangiomas.[1]

Histopathology

Calcium salts are easily recognized in hematoxylin and eosin sections by their intense, uniform basophilia; if necessary, their nature may be confirmed by von Kossa's silver stain which blackens the deposits. The subcutaneous deposits found in tumoral calcinosis (Fig. 14.1) and foci of metastatic and dystrophic calcification tend to be large and dense while those found in the dermis, as in subepidermal calcified nodule, are multiple, small and globular in type (Fig. 14.2). Scrotal deposits are more or less amorphous masses (Fig. 14.3). In subepidermal calcified nodule and in milia-like calcinosis there is often overlying pseudoepitheliomatous hyperplasia, associated with transepidermal elimination of some granules. Transepidermal elimination of calcium deposits is uncommon in the other forms.[71] Foreign body giant cells and peripheral condensation of connective tissue are other features often associated with the deposition of calcium salts. Chronic inflammation is mild or absent.

Epidermal and follicular calcification has been reported in the necrotic epithelium associated with toxic epidermal necrolysis in a patient who also had secondary hyperparathyroidism.[90] There were no dermal deposits of calcium present.

In calciphylaxis, there is usually epidermal ulceration, focal dermal necrosis and vascular calcification.[91] An acute and chronic calcifying panniculitis is the most common finding (Fig. 14.4).[92]

CUTANEOUS OSSIFICATION

Cutaneous ossification has traditionally been classified into a primary form (osteoma cutis), where there is an absence of a pre-existing or associated lesion, and a secondary type (metaplastic ossification), where ossification develops in association with or secondary to a wide range of inflammatory, traumatic and neoplastic processes.[3] There are several distinct clinical variants within the traditional primary group and several syndromes associated with cutaneous ossification. For this reason, the following classification is suggested to cover all circumstances in which bone is found in the skin.

Congenital plaque-like osteomatosis

Congenital plaque-like osteomatosis consists of the slow development of a large mass of bone in the lower dermis or subcutaneous tissues.[93–95] It is

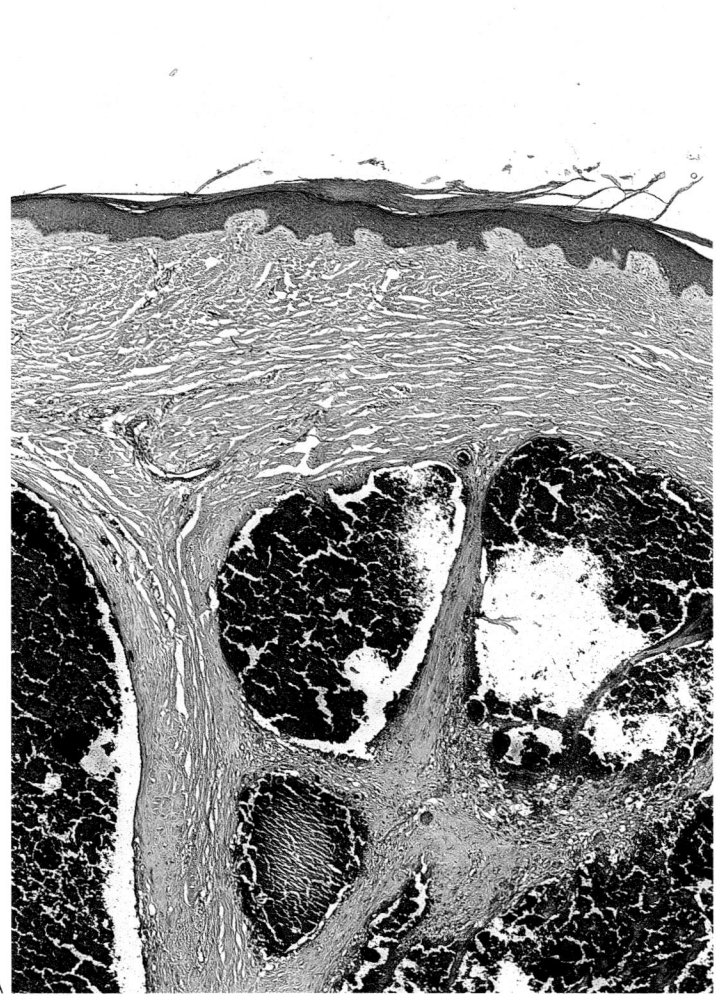

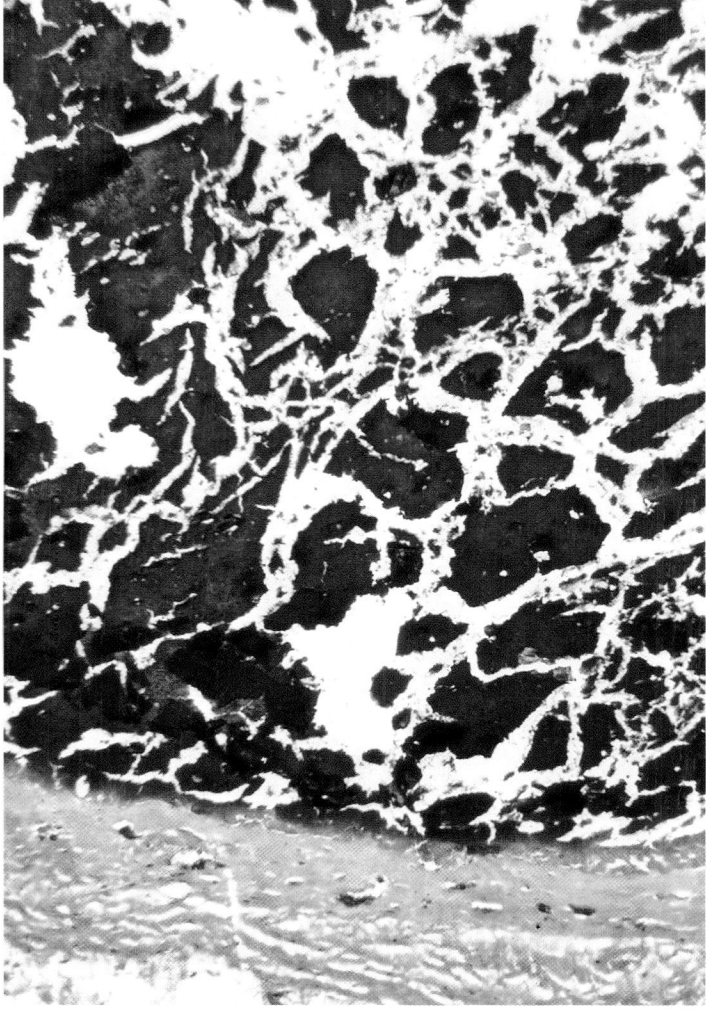

Fig. 14.1 **(A) Tumoral calcinosis. (B)** The calcium deposits are large and irregular in shape. (H & E)

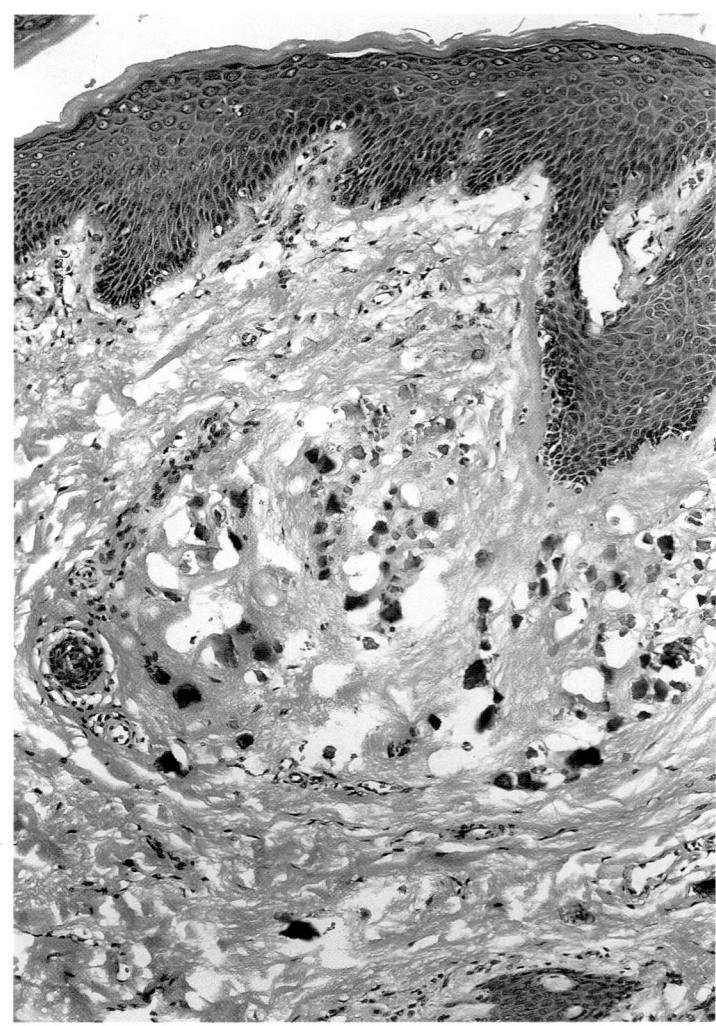

Fig. 14.2 **Subepidermal calcified nodule.** The calcium deposits are small and globular. (H & E)

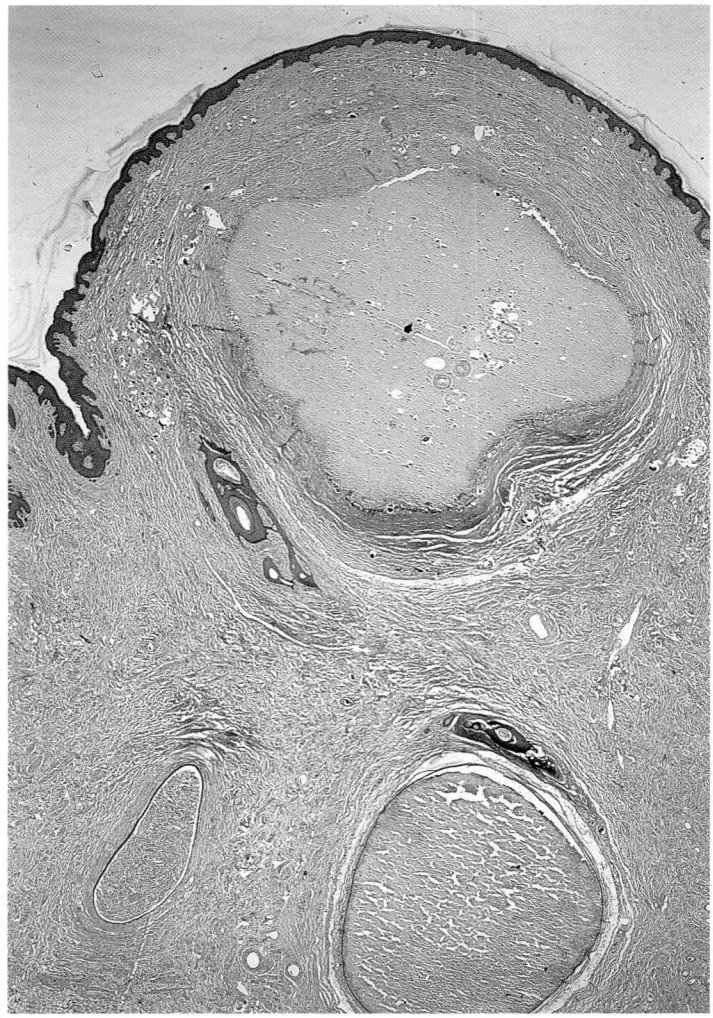

Fig. 14.3 **(A) Idiopathic scrotal calcinosis.**

present at birth or soon afterwards. It has been reported to involve the thigh,[96] scalp,[97–99] back[100] and calf.[101] Two cases reported as 'limited dermal ossification', although much more extensive in distribution than the typical plaque-like lesion just described, are best included in this category.[102,103]

Multiple osteomas

In this variant, multiple foci of cutaneous ossification are present at birth or develop in childhood.[104–108] A family history is sometimes present.[104,107] Albright's hereditary osteodystrophy should be excluded. An acquired, late-onset variant is mentioned in the literature.[94,109]

Multiple miliary osteomas of the face

Although there is usually a history of previous acne and/or dermabrasion of the face,[110–115] it appears that multiple miliary osteomas of the face may be found as a true primary condition.[116–118] Multiple, hard, flesh-colored papules, a few millimeters in diameter, develop on the face.

Osteomas of the distal extremities

Included in the osteomas of the distal extremities are the subungual exostoses, which are basically cartilage derived, and a rare group of bony

tumors of the digits in which no cartilage or bony connection can be demonstrated.

Albright's hereditary osteodystrophy

Cutaneous ossification at an early age may be a presenting feature of Albright's hereditary osteodystrophy, which includes the older clinical designations of pseudohypoparathyroidism and pseudopseudohypoparathyroidism.[119–124] The basic abnormality is a defect in tissue responsiveness to parathormone. Hypocalcemia may be present in some cases. The inheritance appears to be X-linked dominant in type. In addition to the ossification of dermal, subcutaneous or fascial tissues, there may also be a characteristic round facies, defective dentition, mental retardation, calcification of basal ganglia, cataracts, and characteristic short, thick-set fingers with stubby hands and feet attributable to early closure of the metacarpal and metatarsal epiphyses.[121,122]

Progressive osseous heteroplasia

Progressive osseous heteroplasia is an idiopathic disorder characterized by cutaneous calcification and ossification beginning in childhood.[125–128] There is both calcinosis cutis and ossification, the bone forming by endochondral and membranous ossification.

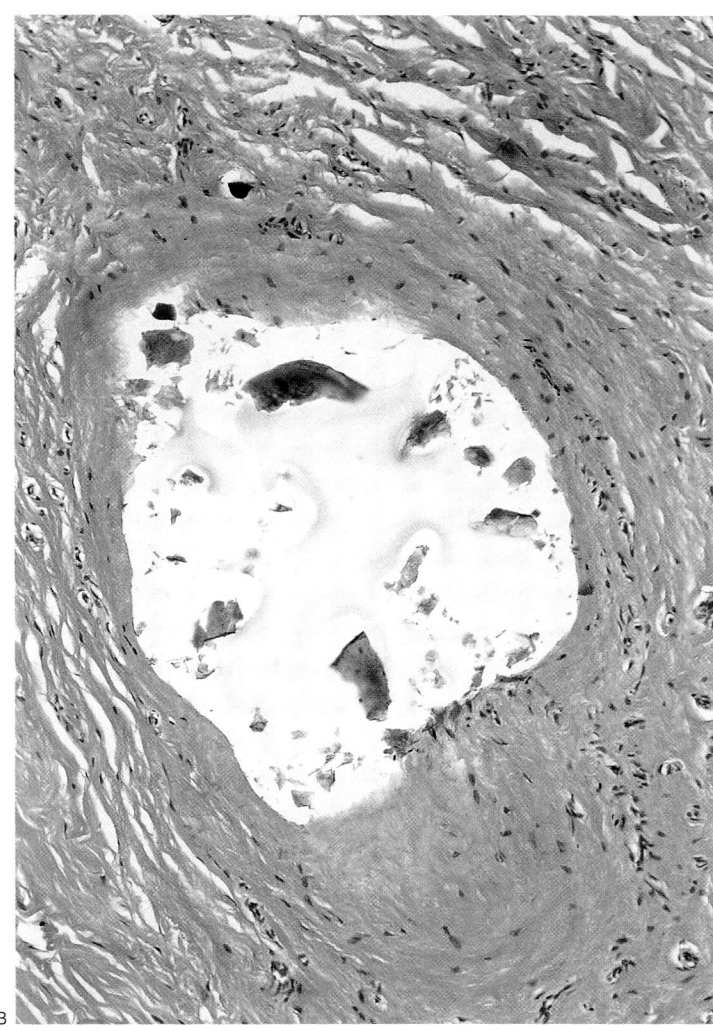

Fig. 14.3 *(Continued)* **(B)** The deposits are surrounded by hyaline fibrous tissue. (H & E)

Fig. 14.4 **(A) Calciphylaxis involving the subcutaneous fat** (H & E). **(B)** The small calcium deposits can be seen in vessels and thin collagenous septa. (von Kossa)

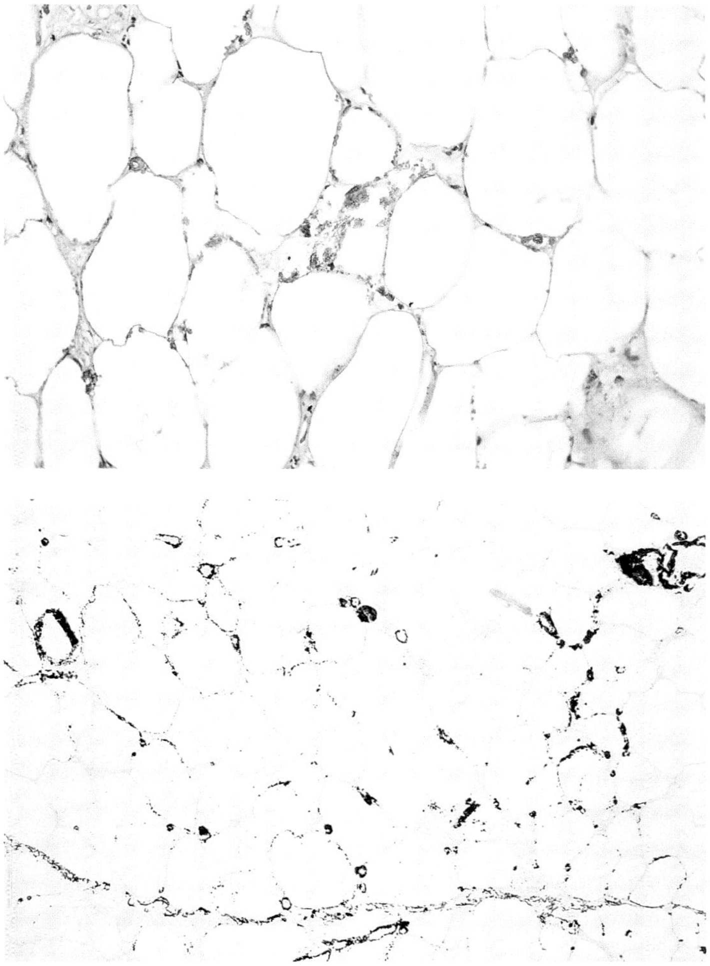

Fibrodysplasia ossificans progressiva

The extremely rare condition of fibrodysplasia ossificans progressiva is manifested by hallux valgus, shortening of the great toes and thumbs, and ossification in muscles and connective tissue.[129] Dermal ossification may precede or accompany these changes. Chondral elements may also be present. The muscles of the shoulder and axial skeleton are commonly involved.

Secondary ossification

This group accounts for the great majority of cases of cutaneous ossification.[93,94] Bone may be found in nevi, particularly on the face (osteonevus of Nanta), in basal cell carcinomas, in up to 20% of pilomatrixomas and less commonly in trichoepitheliomas, hemangiomas, pyogenic granulomas,[130] schwannomas, lipomas, chondroid syringomas, organoid nevi,[131] epidermal and dermoid cysts, dermatofibromas, desmoplastic melanomas[132] and some cutaneous metastases.[133] It may develop in sites of infection, trauma and scarring, such as acne scars,[134] injection sites, hematomas and surgical scars. Myositis ossificans and the related fibro-osseous pseudotumor of the digits[135] can also be included. Abdominal wounds are particularly involved and it seems that injury to the xiphoid process or pubis may liberate bone-forming cells into the wound with subsequent ossification which appears within the first 6 months after surgery.[136] Other circumstances include chronic venous insufficiency of the legs,[137] scrotal calcinosis,[94] auricular calcinosis,[38] scleroderma, morphea,[138,139] dermatomyositis and, rarely, gouty tophi. Secondary ossification has also been reported in neurological diseases associated with paralysis[140] and in a plaque of alopecia in a patient with polyostotic fibrous dysplasia.[141]

Histopathology

Cutaneous bone usually develops by membranous (mesenchymal) ossification without the presence of a cartilage precursor. There are small spicules or large masses of bone in the deep dermis and/or subcutaneous tissue (Fig. 14.5). Haversian systems and cement lines are usually present. Occasionally there is active osteoblastic activity, particularly in Albright's hereditary osteodystrophy, but this is unusual in the primary solitary lesion and secondary forms associated with acne scars. Osteoclasts are also uncommon. There is often a stromal component of fat, but occasionally hemopoietic cells are also present. In the congenital plaque-like osteomatosis, bone may extend around the dermal appendages (Fig. 14.6).[93] Pigmentation of the bone has been reported in acne patients receiving tetracycline or minocycline: clinically these nodules may have a bluish color.[142,143] The crystalline component of the bone is hydroxyapatite, as in skeletal bone.

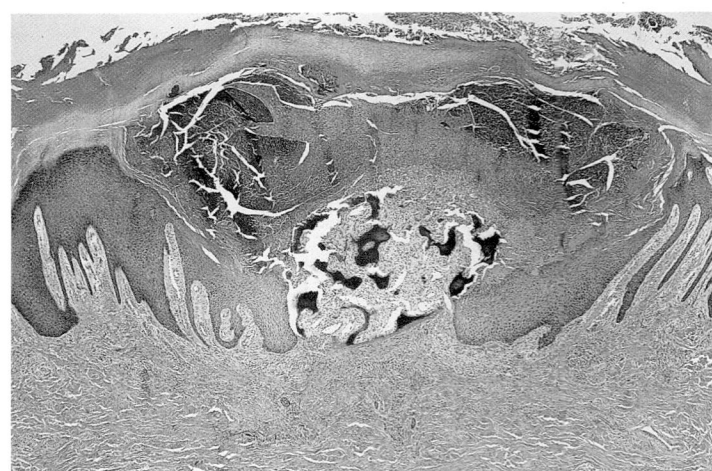

Fig. 14.5 **Osteoma cutis.** The spicules of bone are undergoing transepidermal elimination. Surface crusting is present. (H & E)

CARTILAGINOUS LESIONS OF THE SKIN

The term 'cartilaginous lesions of the skin' encompasses several different entities, which have in common the presence of cartilage of variable maturity. Some of these entities have been discussed in other sections. The following classification has been suggested by Hsueh and Santa Cruz.[144]

Chondromas

True cutaneous chondromas, without bony connection, are an exceedingly rare dermal tumor (see p. 973).

Hamartomas containing cartilage

The hamartomas containing cartilage include accessory tragi, the closely related Meckel's cartilage (cartilaginous rests in the neck, 'wattles'[145–147]), bronchogenic cysts and dermoid cysts. The lesions reported as elastic cartilage choristomas of the neck[148] were mid-line and suprasternal and therefore different from the usual laterally placed branchially derived remnants.

Soft tissue tumors with cartilaginous differentiation

These extraskeletal tumors arise most frequently in the soft tissues of the extremities, especially the fingers.[149] They may have varying degrees of cytological atypia in the chondrocytes, but despite this they invariably pursue a benign course.

Skeletal tumors with cartilaginous differentiation

This group includes osteochondromas, synovial chondromatosis and subungual exostoses (see p. 973).

Miscellaneous lesions

The eccrine tumor, chondroid syringoma, may have prominent cartilaginous differentiation which may at first glance obscure its sweat gland origin. Cartilage may develop in degenerated nuchal ligaments producing the **nuchal fibrocartilaginous pseudotumor**.[150,151]

The case described as 'cartilaginous papule of the ear' defies classification.[152] It may represent a reactive hyperplasia of auricular cartilage.

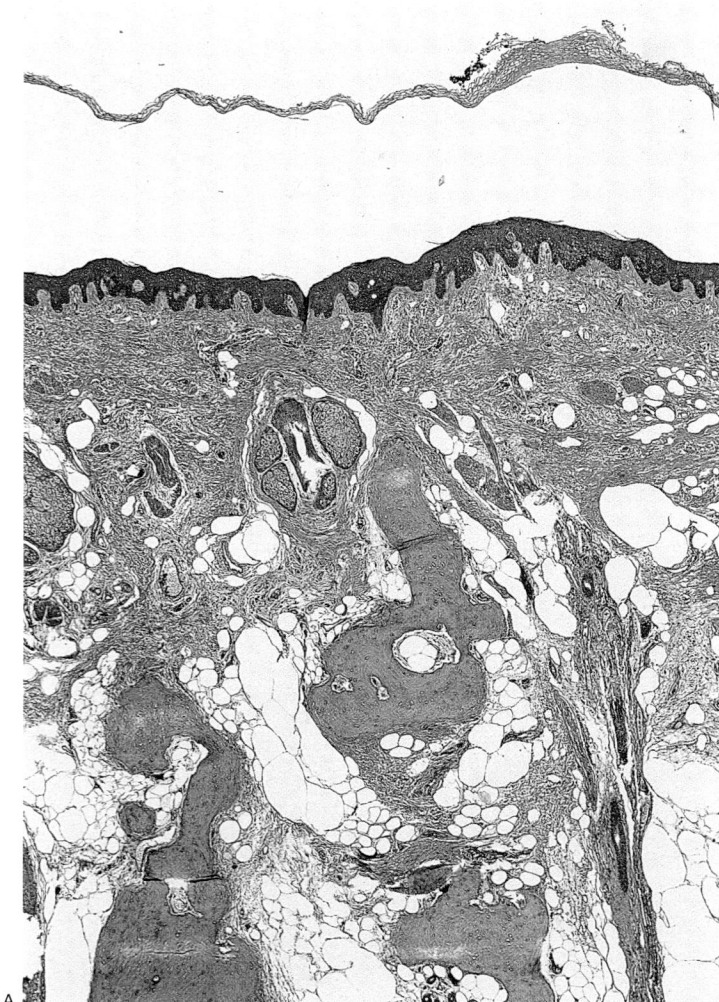

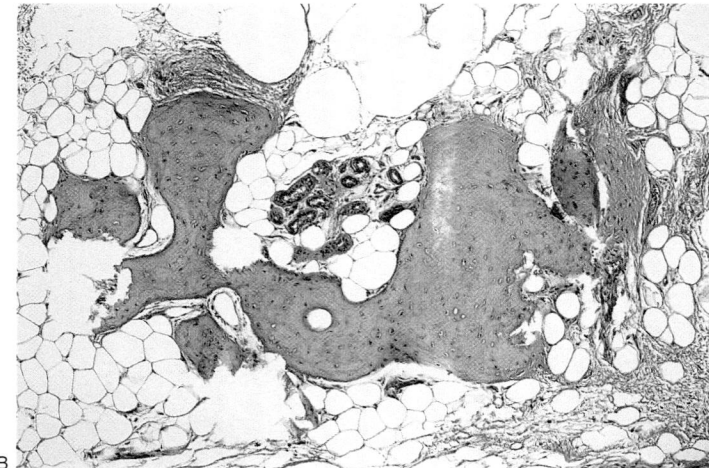

Fig. 14.6 **(A) Plaque-like osteoma cutis of the scalp. (B)** Bone extends around the eccrine glands. (H & E)

HYALINE DEPOSITS

Hyaline deposits may be seen in the dermis in several 'metabolic' disorders, including amyloidosis, erythropoietic protoporphyria and lipoid proteinosis and Waldenström's macroglobulinemia. In gouty tophi the deposits are of a crystalline nature, but when these are dissolved in an aqueous fixative the residual stromal tissue appears hyaline. Other causes of hyaline deposits are colloid milium and massive cutaneous hyalinosis; they may also occur following certain corticosteroid injections. Cytoid bodies are a heterogeneous group of hyaline deposits that are commonly overlooked in routine sections.

An unclassifiable deposit, of hyaline type, has been reported in a patient with IgG paraproteinemia and lesions resembling cutis laxa.[153] Eosinophilic homogeneous material was present in the dermis. The material had a tubular pattern on electron microscopy.[153]

GOUT

Although the prevalence of gout in the community is relatively constant, the proportion of gouty patients with cutaneous manifestations – tophi – shows a continuing decline.[3,154] This undoubtedly results from improved clinical management of these patients, particularly the use of allopurinol, a xanthine oxidase inhibitor that blocks uric acid production. Tophi, which are end-stage manifestations of primary gout, are deposits of monosodium urate crystals within and around joints, overlying the olecranon and prepatellar bursae and in the helix of the ears.[155] Sometimes chalky white material is extruded from tophi. Smaller nodular deposits have been described on the fingers and toes and there are reports of leg ulcers or a panniculitis with urate deposition, as the presenting manifestations of gout.[156–158] Tophi have been reported in a patient following the use of acitretin, an oral retinoid, in the treatment of erythrodermic psoriasis.[159]

Histopathology
Tophi are dermal and subcutaneous deposits of urate crystals.[160] If material is fixed in alcohol, they appear as well-demarcated deposits of closely arranged, brown, needle-shaped crystals (Fig. 14.7). The crystals are doubly refractile under polarized light. In formalin-fixed material, the crystals will usually have dissolved and there are characteristic, amorphous pink areas corresponding to the sites of crystal deposition (Fig. 14.8). Surrounding the deposits is a granulomatous reaction with macrophages and many foreign body giant cells.[161] There is usually only a sparse chronic inflammatory cell infiltrate. Often there is some fibrosis as well, and in old lesions calcification and even ossification may occasionally develop. Transepidermal elimination of crystals is rarely seen.[162]

It has been suggested that the primary event in the formation of a tophus is the accumulation of macrophages in an acinar arrangement followed by the centripetal transport of urate by the macrophages from the interstitial fluid to the central zone.[161] This expands progressively as more urate crystals are deposited. The corona of macrophages commonly disappears and adjacent deposits may fuse.[161]

AMYLOIDOSIS

Amyloidosis refers to the extracellular deposition of eosinophilic hyaline material of autologous origin which has characteristic staining properties and a fibrillar ultrastructure.[163–166]

The origin of amyloid is diverse: 16 different fibril proteins have been described so far.[167] Many of these are rare or have no relevance to the skin. Six amyloid proteins are of interest in cutaneous pathology: AA, ATTR, Aλ, Aκ, Aβ2M and AK.[167–169]

- AA (amyloid A protein) is associated with chronic inflammatory diseases, corresponding to secondary systemic amyloidosis of the traditional classification.
- ATTR (amyloid transthyretin protein) is found in cases of familial amyloidosis. It appears to be the same as FAP (familial amyloid polyneuropathy, type 1).
- Aλ and Aκ are usually grouped together as AL (amyloid light chain protein). These proteins are found in relation to myeloproliferative diseases, particularly multiple myeloma, or in cases with no known associated disease (idiopathic). Aλ is found much more commonly than Aκ. It is the type of amyloid usually found in nodular cutaneous amyloidosis.
- Aβ2M (amyloid β2 microglobulin protein) is found in amyloid deposits associated with long-term hemodialysis.[167] It deposits mainly in the osteo-articular system.[170]
- AK (amyloid keratin protein) is found in localized cutaneous amyloidosis, both lichen amyloidosus and macular amyloidosis. This protein will be discussed further below.

In addition to the specific fibrillar component, amyloid deposits have been shown to contain several associated and contaminating proteins such as amyloid P, apolipoprotein E and glycosaminoglycans.[167,171] Immunoglobulins may be non-specifically trapped within the fibrillar meshwork. Amyloid P,

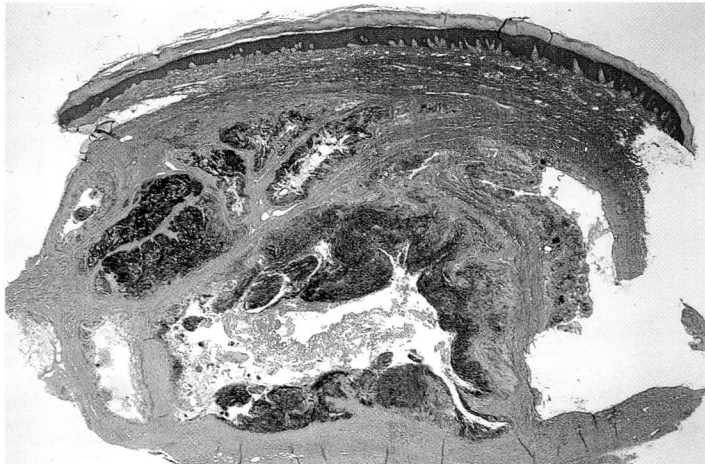

Fig. 14.7 **Gouty tophus.** There are brown, needle-shaped crystals forming large deposits in the dermis and subcutis. The biopsy was fixed in alcohol. (H & E)

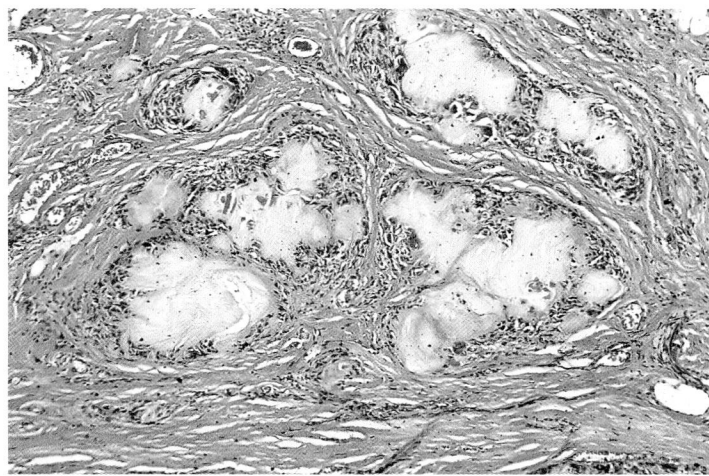

Fig. 14.8 **Gouty tophus.** The urate crystals have been dissolved in this formalin-fixed biopsy, leaving a pale hyaline area surrounded by macrophages and foreign body giant cells. (H & E)

which for a long time was used as a marker for amyloid, is a non-fibrillar glycoprotein which binds to all types of amyloid fibrils.

In primary cutaneous amyloidosis the amyloid is of keratinocyte origin, but how the keratin intermediate filaments transform into amyloid (AK) is speculative. Apoptosis of keratinocytes has been described, but this may simply be the method of cell death in basal keratinocytes that have accumulated an abnormal protein.[172] Another theory is that macrophages in the dermis 'process' the filament-rich colloid bodies, converting them into mature amyloid and in the process adopt a beta-pleated sheet pattern (as opposed to the usual alpha pattern of keratin). Active secretion of amyloid by basal keratinocytes is a less favored theory.[173,174] AK stains with general keratin antibodies, such as EKH4 and AE1.[172] Several subclasses of keratin are found, in particular K5, which is a constituent of normal basal keratinocytes.[169] However, the presence of K7, K17 and K19, not found in the interfollicular epidermis, suggests an appendageal contribution to the amyloid deposits.[169] Suggested etiological factors in the formation of this type of amyloid include prolonged friction, pruritus, genetic predisposition, Epstein–Barr virus and environmental factors.

The skin may be involved in the course of systemic (generalized) amyloidosis, but more commonly it is the only organ in the body to be involved – localized cutaneous (skin-limited) amyloidosis. Within each of these two major categories, several distinct clinical variants are found, as outlined in the traditional classification that follows.

- *Systemic amyloidosis*
  Primary and myeloma associated
  Secondary
  Heredofamilial
  Amyloid elastosis
- *Localized cutaneous amyloidosis*
  Lichen, macular and biphasic
  Nodular
  Poikilodermatous
  Anosacral
  Familial cutaneous
  Secondary localized.

The histochemical, immunofluorescence and ultrastructural properties of the various cutaneous amyloidoses will be discussed before the description of the individual clinical variants.

Histochemical properties

Amyloid stains pink with hematoxylin and eosin and metachromatically with crystal violet and methyl violet.[175] It stains selectively with Congo red; in addition, amyloid stained by Congo red gives an apple-green birefringence when viewed in polarized light. Amyloid gives a bright yellow-green fluorescence with thioflavine T.[176] We have found crystal violet to be more reliable than Congo red in sun-damaged skin, which sometimes gives false-positive staining with Congo red; false negatives also occur. The cotton dye pagoda red No. 9 (Dylon), used as a variant of the Congo red method, is said to be more specific for amyloid than Congo red, because it does not stain the material in paraffin sections of lipoid proteinosis, colloid milium or solar elastosis.[177–179] Congo red staining of the deposits in secondary systemic amyloidosis can be prevented by prior treatment of the sections with potassium permanganate.[180,181] In some cases of primary systemic amyloidosis the amyloid has relatively little affinity for Congo red. Early cases of localized cutaneous amyloidosis can also be negative using the Congo red method. The author has seen several cases of lichen amyloidosus missed because only a Congo red stain was performed.

Immunoperoxidase methods using monoclonal antisera can also be used to demonstrate amyloid P component (a non-fibrillar protein derived from a glycoprotein found in the blood of all normal persons) in all cutaneous deposits.[182–184] As already mentioned, the amyloid in lichen amyloidosus and macular amyloidosis, as well as in secondary localized cutaneous amyloidosis, stains with the monoclonal antibody EKH4 which recognizes 50 kd neutral and acidic keratin.[177] It also stains with the keratin antibody AE1. The antikeratin antibody EAB-903, which recognizes 57 kd and 66 kd keratin peptides, reacts with the amyloid deposits in both lichen amyloidosus and macular amyloidosis, but not with the amyloid in systemic amyloidosis.[185] Other keratin monoclonals have given mixed results.[185–188] Antisera are also available commercially against amyloid A (AA), amyloid L (AL), both anti-κ and anti-λ, islet amyloid polypeptide (IAPP) and amyloid β2 microglobulin (Aβ2M).

Immunofluorescence

Immunoglobulins, particularly IgM, and C3 complement are found in cutaneous amyloid deposits.[189,190] Most of the studies have been confined to the localized cutaneous forms. Amyloid is thought to act like a filamentous sponge with non-specific trapping of the immunoglobulins and complement.[191]

Ultrastructure[178]

Amyloid is composed of straight, non-branching filaments, 6–10 nm in diameter, of indefinite length and in random array (Fig. 14.9). A close association with elastic fibers is sometimes observed.[192–194] Intracellular amyloid has been noted in dermal fibroblasts[195,196] and in keratinocytes in lichen amyloidosus.[195]

The ultrastructural studies of Hashimoto and colleagues[197,198] and other groups[199–201] have shown that the basal epidermal cells are involved in the histogenesis of the amyloid in lichen amyloidosus and macular amyloidosis. Basal keratinocytes overlying dermal amyloid show degenerative changes with the accumulation of modified tonofilaments (thicker, but less electron-dense than normal) in the cytoplasm.[202]

Primary systemic amyloidosis

Cutaneous involvement is common in primary systemic amyloidosis and in the closely related myeloma-associated amyloidosis, with lesions in approximately one-third of patients.[163,203] There are non-pruritic, waxy papules on the scalp, face and neck and sometimes the genitalia.[181,204–206] There is a predilection for the periorbital areas. Plaque-like lesions may develop on the hands and flexural areas.[207] Hemorrhage into the lesions is quite common.[205,208] Rare presentations include alopecia,[209] occlusion of the external auditory canals,[210] chronic paronychia,[207] bullous lesions,[203,211–214] indurated cord-like lesions resulting from thick vascular deposits,[215] condyloma-like lesions in the perianal region[216] and elastolytic lesions.[217] As mentioned above, the fibrillar protein is derived from light chains of immunoglobulin (AL), either λ or κ.

Histopathology

Papular lesions result from deposits of amyloid in the papillary dermis; in plaques there is a more diffuse dermal infiltration, sometimes with extension into the subcutis (Fig. 14.10).[218] In this latter site, amyloid deposits around individual fat cells to form 'amyloid rings' (Fig. 14.11). Dermal blood vessels are usually involved in hemorrhagic lesions (Fig. 14.12) and pilosebaceous units are involved in areas of alopecia.[205,218] The rare bullous lesions are caused by intradermal cleavage within the amyloid deposits.[203,219] There is often clefting about and within the amyloid in the larger papular lesions. If the deposits are large, there is often attenuation of the overlying epidermis.[218] There are no pigmented cells, and inflammatory cells are scarce.[219]

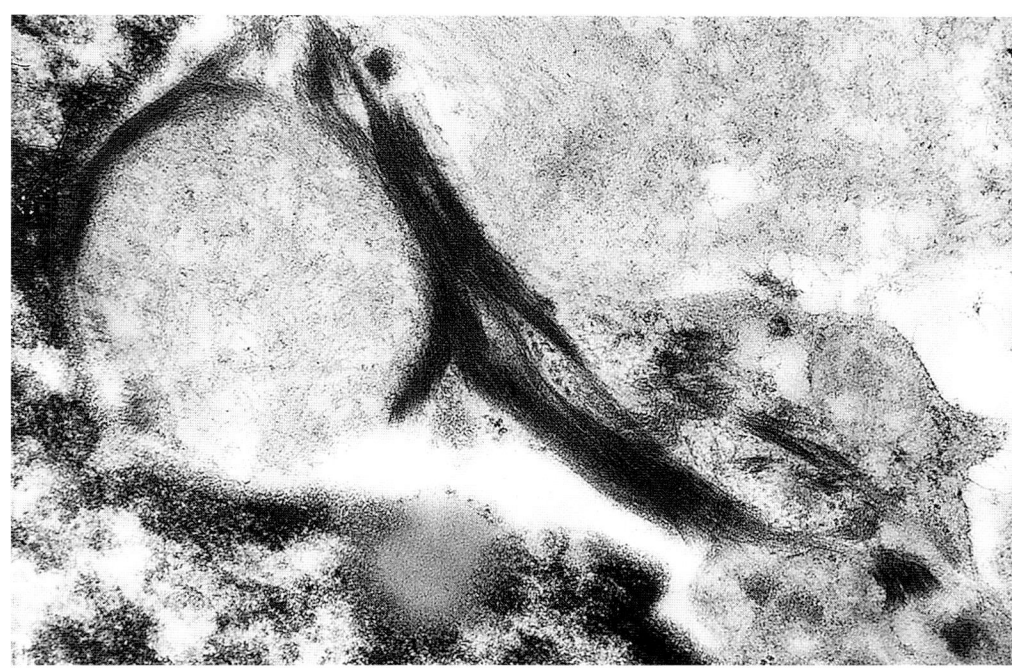

Fig. 14.9 **Lichen amyloidosus.** There are intracellular deposits and some dense tonofilament bundles in basal keratinocytes. The deposits appear to represent the earliest stages of amyloid formation. (×45 000)

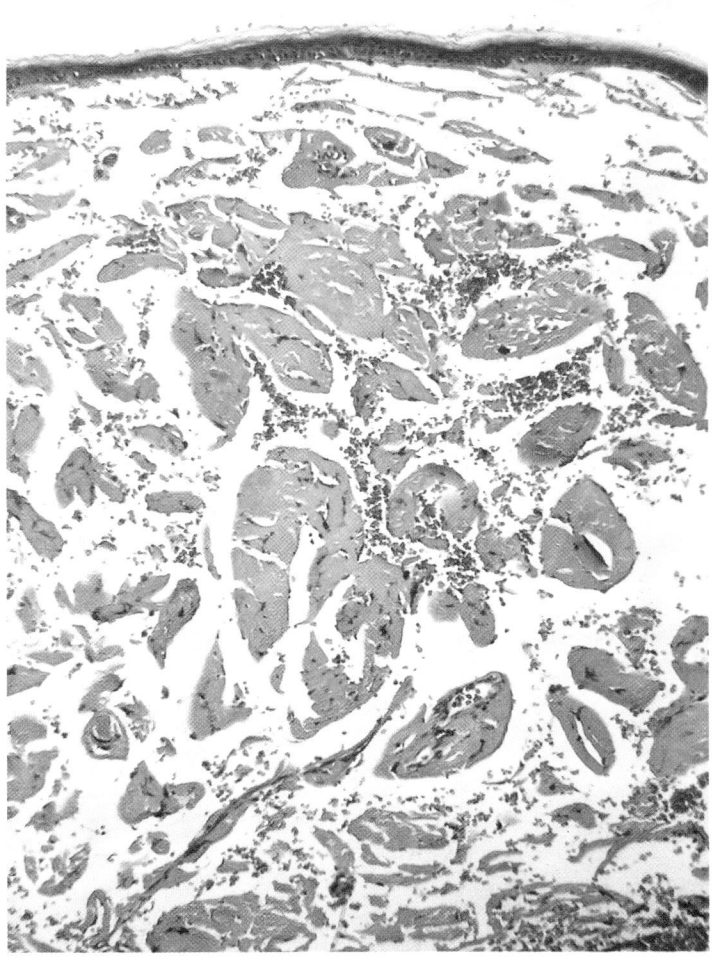

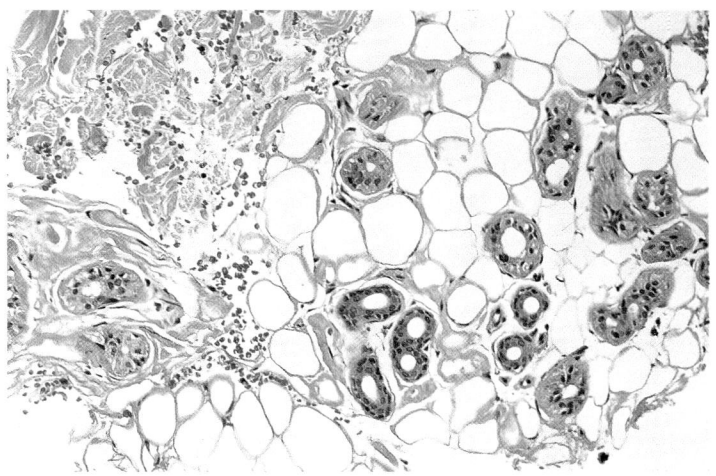

Fig. 14.11 **Amyloid rings.** There are fine deposits of amyloid surrounding individual fat cells. (H & E) (Photomicrograph kindly supplied by Dr G Strutton)

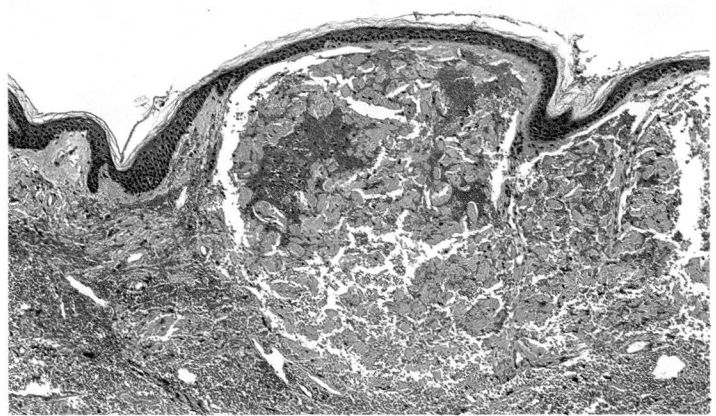

Fig. 14.10 **Primary amyloidosis.** The hyaline deposits in the dermis show some artifactual separation. (H & E)

Fig. 14.12 **Primary amyloidosis.** There is considerable hemorrhage between the hyaline deposits. (H & E)

Clinically normal skin will show deposits of amyloid in the dermis, usually in the walls of blood vessels, in more than 50% of biopsies in cases of primary systemic amyloidosis.[220] A recent study found cutaneous amyloid deposits in 97% of cases of systemic amyloidosis, making skin biopsy a preferred method of diagnosis of systemic amyloidosis.[168] Abdominal fat aspiration is another reliable procedure.[221]

Secondary systemic amyloidosis

Clinical involvement of the skin is rare in cases of secondary systemic amyloidosis.[163,218] Uncommonly, this form of amyloidosis is the result of an underlying chronic skin disease such as lepromatous leprosy, hidradenitis suppurativa, arthropathic psoriasis[180,222] or dystrophic epidermolysis bullosa.[223] It may occur following hemodialysis; in these circumstances the protein fibril deposited is β2-microglobulin.[170,224,225] In other circumstances the fibrillar component is amyloid A protein (AA).

Histopathology

Amyloid has been found in several sites in the clinically normal skin of some patients with secondary amyloidosis, including the papillary dermis, the subcutis, the walls of blood vessels and around eccrine sweat glands.[218–220]

Heredofamilial amyloidosis

There are skin manifestations in certain of the heredofamilial amyloidoses.[226] These include trophic changes and amyloid deposits in the arrector pili muscles in heredofamilial amyloid polyneuropathy[164,178,227] and urticaria in other forms such as the Muckle–Wells syndrome (urticaria, amyloidosis and deafness).[228,229]

Amyloid elastosis

Amyloid elastosis is a recently described entity with cutaneous lesions and progressive systemic disease.[230] The elastic fibers in the skin and serosae are coated with the amyloid material;[230] the amyloid is localized to the microfibrils of the elastic fibers.[231] Why amyloid is preferentially deposited on elastic fibers, resulting in clinically evident lesions, is unknown.

Lichen, macular and biphasic amyloidoses

Lichen amyloidosus and macular amyloidosis are clinical variants of the same process.[178,232,233] Patients with features of both variants, or transformation from one to the other (biphasic form), are well documented.[234–236] There is no visceral involvement in lichen amyloidosus or macular amyloidosis.[237] An association with multiple endocrine neoplasia syndrome 2A (MEN 2A) has been reported.[238] Other reported associations are possibly coincidental, although chronic pruritus could be implicated in two such associations.[239–242] The fibrillar component is derived from keratinocytes and designated AK (amyloid keratin).

Lichen amyloidosus presents as small, discrete, often pruritic, waxy papules with a predilection for the extensor surfaces of the lower extremities.[237] Rare clinical presentations have included similar distribution in identical twins[243] and involvement of the glans penis.[244] Lichen amyloidosus is not uncommon in South East Asia and some South American countries.[237,245] It has been associated with chronic Epstein–Barr virus (EBV) infection.[246,247] Others believe it is a consequence of chronic scratching.[248,249] This may be the explanation for its rare occurrence in HIV-associated papular pruritus[250] and in refractory atopic dermatitis.[251]

Macular amyloidosis is a less common variant. It occurs as poorly defined hyperpigmented and rippled patches on the trunk.[201,252] Rarely, there is widespread pigmentation.[253–255] There is a predilection for the interscapular region of adult females.[256] Lesions are often pruritic. Macular amyloidosis has been reported in Japanese following prolonged rubbing of the skin with nylon brushes and towels.[177,257,258] Other types of friction have sometimes been implicated.[259,260] Unusual presentations include involvement of the knees,[261] elbows[262] or auricular concha.[263]

Histopathology

Both lichen amyloidosus and macular amyloidosis are characterized by small globular deposits of amyloid in the papillary dermis (Fig. 14.13).[190] Sometimes a thin band of compressed collagen separates these deposits from the overlying epidermis;[237] at other times the deposits are in contact with the basal cells and sometimes interspersed between them. More extensive deposits are sometimes seen (Fig. 14.14). Transepidermal elimination of the amyloid sometimes occurs.[264] Pigmented cells are often seen within the dermal deposits.

In lichen amyloidosus (Fig. 14.15) the overlying epidermis shows hyperkeratosis and acanthosis, the changes sometimes resembling those of lichen simplex chronicus (see p. 86).[265]

In both types of amyloidosis occasional apoptotic bodies are present within the epidermis.[266] Basal vacuolar change also occurs.

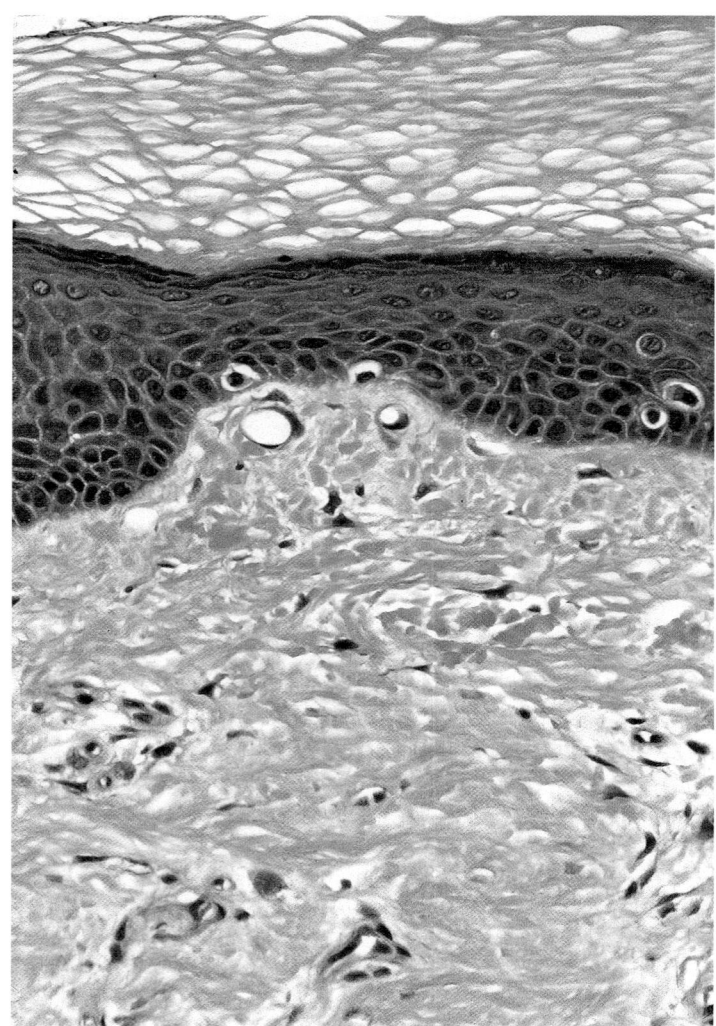

Fig. 14.13 **Macular amyloidosis.** Hyaline material, barely distinguishable from collagen, is present in the papillary dermis. The diagnosis can be easily missed. (H & E)

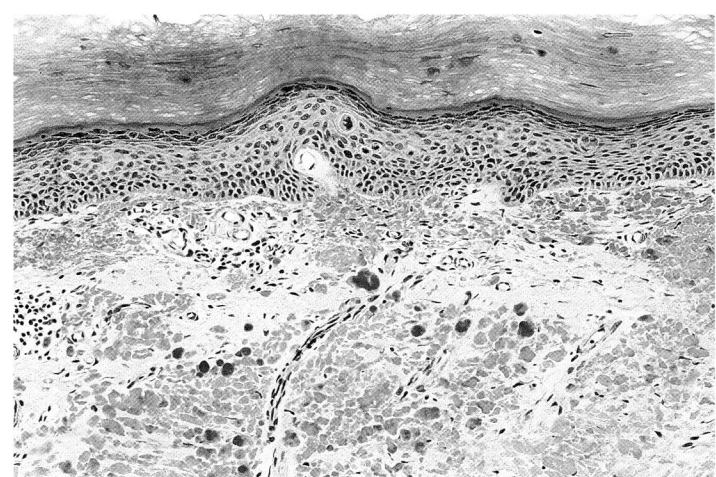

Fig. 14.14 **Macular amyloidosis.** There are more extensive deposits than usual. (Pagoda red)

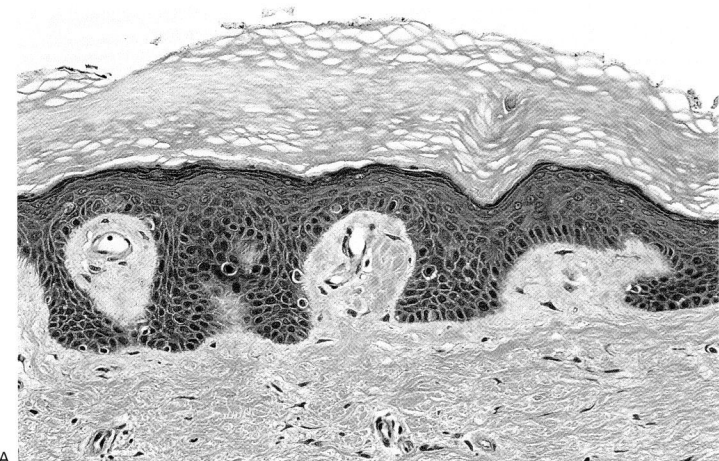

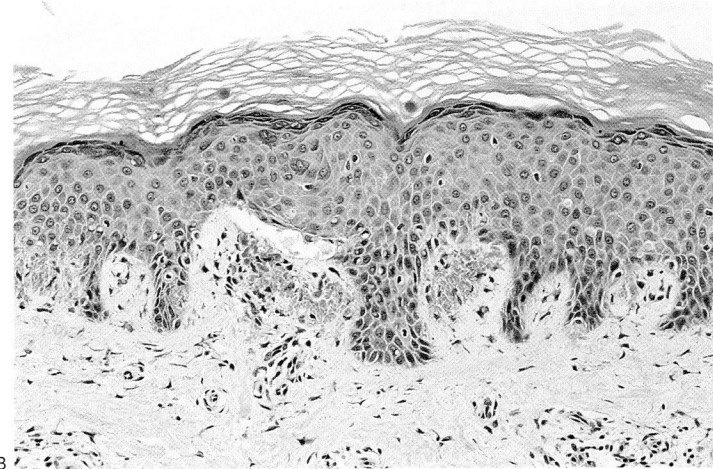

Fig. 14.15 **Lichen amyloidosus. (A)** Small, hyaline deposits of amyloid are situated in the papillary dermis. There is overlying epidermal hyperplasia (H & E). **(B)** The size of the deposits can be better appreciated on the special stain for amyloid. (Congo red)

Nodular amyloidosis

Nodular amyloidosis is an uncommon form of cutaneous amyloidosis which is manifested by solitary[267] or multiple waxy nodules, 0.5–7 cm in diameter,

on the lower extremities, face,[268,269] neck,[270] scalp or genital region.[271–275] In at least 15% of cases, the patient will subsequently develop systemic amyloidosis.[265,273,276] A light-chain origin of the amyloid (AL) has been proved in many cases.[271,275,277,278]

Nodular deposits of amyloid, derived mostly from β2-microglobulin, are a rare finding in the skin of patients with chronic renal failure on long-term hemodialysis.[170] 'Amyloidoma' refers to a rare tumor mass of amyloid that may be found in the subcutis.[279] It may be composed of AA, AL or IAPP (islet amyloid polypeptide) amyloid.[279]

Histopathology

There are large masses of amyloid in the dermis and subcutis, with accentuated deposition around deep vascular channels and adnexal structures.[205] Plasma cells, some with large Russell bodies, are usually quite prominent at the margins and within the amyloid islands.[219,273,280] Monoclonality of these cells has been confirmed.[281,282] The deposits do not stain with antikeratin antibodies.[169] They may stain for Aλ, Aκ or Aβ2M (see above). Foreign body giant cells and focal calcification are sometimes present.[273] The amyloid may be deposited in relation to the elastica.[192,283]

Poikilodermatous amyloidosis

Poikilodermatous lesions are rare.[284] A distinct subset of patients have short stature, early onset, light sensitivity and sometimes palmoplantar keratoderma – the *poikilodermatous cutaneous amyloidosis syndrome*.[284]

Included in this category are the cases reported as *amyloidosis cutis dyschromica*.[285]

Histopathology

There is amyloid in the dermal papillae and around dermal blood vessels, resembling the pattern of primary systemic amyloidosis.

Anosacral amyloidosis

Anosacral amyloidosis is a rare form of primary cutaneous amyloidosis that has been reported in Chinese persons.[286] It presents as a light brown lichenified plaque of the perianal region extending onto the lower sacrum. The amyloid is of keratinous origin (AK).

Histopathology

The amyloid deposits are situated in the papillary dermis. There is some overlying epidermal hyperkeratosis, acanthosis and melanin incontinence.[286]

Familial primary cutaneous amyloidosis

Familial primary cutaneous amyloidosis is an extremely rare, autosomal dominant genodermatosis with keratotic papules and/or swirled hyper- and hypopigmentation[287] on the extremities and sometimes the trunk.[205,288,289] The clinical features may resemble lichen amyloidosus.[290] Transepidermal elimination of the papillary dermal deposits has been a characteristic feature.[289]

Secondary localized cutaneous amyloidosis

Secondary localized cutaneous amyloidosis refers to the finding of amyloid in the stroma of various cutaneous tumors such as basal cell carcinoma (Fig. 14.16)[291,292] and, less commonly, squamous cell carcinomas,[293] nevocellular nevi,[294] trichoblastomas, cylindromas, pilomatrixomas and syringocystadenoma papilliferum.[295] Amyloid may underlie the epithelium in

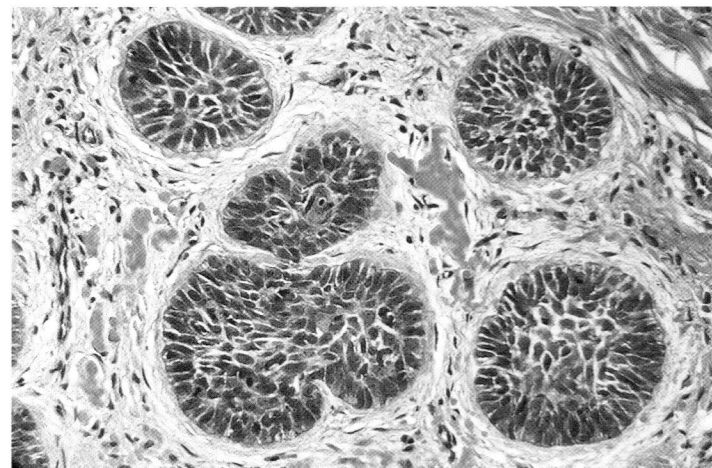

Fig. 14.16 **Secondary amyloidosis.** Hyaline deposits are present in the stroma of a basal cell carcinoma. (H & E)

seborrheic and actinic keratoses,[296] Bowen's disease,[297] porokeratosis, skin treated with ultraviolet A radiation after the ingestion of psoralens (PUVA),[298] and mycosis fungoides.[178,299,300] Amyloid has also been reported localized to areas of severe solar elastosis:[301] amyloid A protein was identified in this latter case. In all other circumstances, the amyloid appears to be of keratinocyte origin.

PORPHYRIA

Porphyria is a metabolic disorder with varied cutaneous manifestations. It is considered in detail in Chapter 18, page 557.

The characteristic histological feature of the cutaneous porphyrias is the deposition of lightly eosinophilic, hyaline material in and around small blood vessels in the upper dermis. In erythropoietic protoporphyria the hyaline material also forms an irregular cuff around these vessels but it does not encroach upon the adjacent dermis as much as the hyaline material does in lipoid proteinosis (see below). Furthermore, there is no involvement of the sweat glands in cutaneous porphyria. The hyaline material has similar staining characteristics in both diseases, although the hyaline material in porphyria tends to stain less intensely with Hale's colloidal iron method than it does in lipoid proteinosis.

LIPOID PROTEINOSIS

Lipoid proteinosis is a rare, autosomal recessive, multisystem genodermatosis which primarily affects the skin, oral cavity and larynx, with the deposition of an amorphous hyaline material.[302–309] The early clinical features are hoarseness and the development of recurrent skin infections, sometimes with vesiculobullous lesions which heal leaving atrophic pock-like scars.[310,311] Waxy papules and plaques develop progressively over several years on the face, scalp, neck and extremities.[312] Other features include beaded papules on the eyelid margins (blepharosis)[313] and verrucous lesions on the elbows, knees and hands. Although deposits have been found in many organs of the body, resulting dysfunction is rare.[314,315] Epilepsy may be associated with calcification of the hippocampus.

Two studies have suggested that lipoid proteinosis is a lysosomal storage disease,[316,317] with abnormalities in the degradative pathway of glycolipids or sphingolipids, leading to the storage of ceramide or more complex lipids.[317] Other work has shown the deposited material to be matrix glycoproteins with increased laminin and collagen of types IV and V and a relative decrease in collagen type I.[318–323] The selective increase in pro-α1(IV)mRNA in lipoid proteinosis may have relevance to the accumulation of this basement membrane component in the skin in this condition.[320]

Histopathology [324,325]

There is a progressive deposition of pale, eosinophilic, hyaline material in the superficial dermis, but this is initially localized around small blood vessels and at the periphery of eccrine sweat glands.[303] Small capillaries are sometimes increased in number. In advanced lesions, the deposits around blood vessels may have an 'onion-skin' appearance (Fig. 14.17). There is also progressive atrophy of secretory sweat glands associated with increasing hyaline deposition. This material is also deposited in arrector pili muscles and around pilosebaceous units. The epidermis may show hyperkeratosis and some acanthosis in the verrucous lesions.

The hyaline deposits are PAS positive and diastase resistant (Fig. 14.18). They stain positively with colloidal iron and alcian blue at pH 2.5 and also with Sudan black and oil red O on frozen sections.[326,327] The accumulation of lipid is usually a late and presumably secondary phenomenon.[326,328]

Although histologically and histochemically similar material is found in erythropoietic protoporphyria, the deposits in the latter condition are more limited in distribution, being perivascular only.[329] Sweat glands are not involved in porphyria.

Electron microscopy

In lipoid proteinosis there are fine collagen fibrils embedded in an amorphous, granular matrix.[312,330–332] There is prominent reduplication of the basal lamina at the dermoepidermal junction and concentrically around vessels.[318,321,332,333] Calcium deposits may be seen. Cytoplasmic inclusions have been noted in the fibroblasts; their exact significance is unknown.[316,321]

WALDENSTRÖM'S MACROGLOBULINEMIA

Translucent papules, formed by deposits of monoclonal IgM, are an uncommon manifestation of Waldenström's macroglobulinemia (see p. 151). The hyaline deposits that fill the papillary and upper reticular dermis are strongly PAS positive (Fig. 14.19). Ultrastructurally, they are composed of fibrillar and granular material.[334]

COLLOID MILIUM AND COLLOID DEGENERATION

There are at least four distinct clinicopathological conditions that can be included under the umbrella term of 'colloid milium and colloid degeneration'.[335] Regrettably, our knowledge of these conditions is limited by the paucity of reports in the literature. The four variants are:

1. colloid milium – classic adult type[308,336–339]
2. juvenile colloid milium[340]
3. pigmented colloid milium (hydroquinone related)[341]
4. colloid degeneration (paracolloid).[342]

The *adult type* develops in early to mid-adult life with numerous yellow-brown, semitranslucent, dome-shaped papules, 1–4 mm or more in diameter.

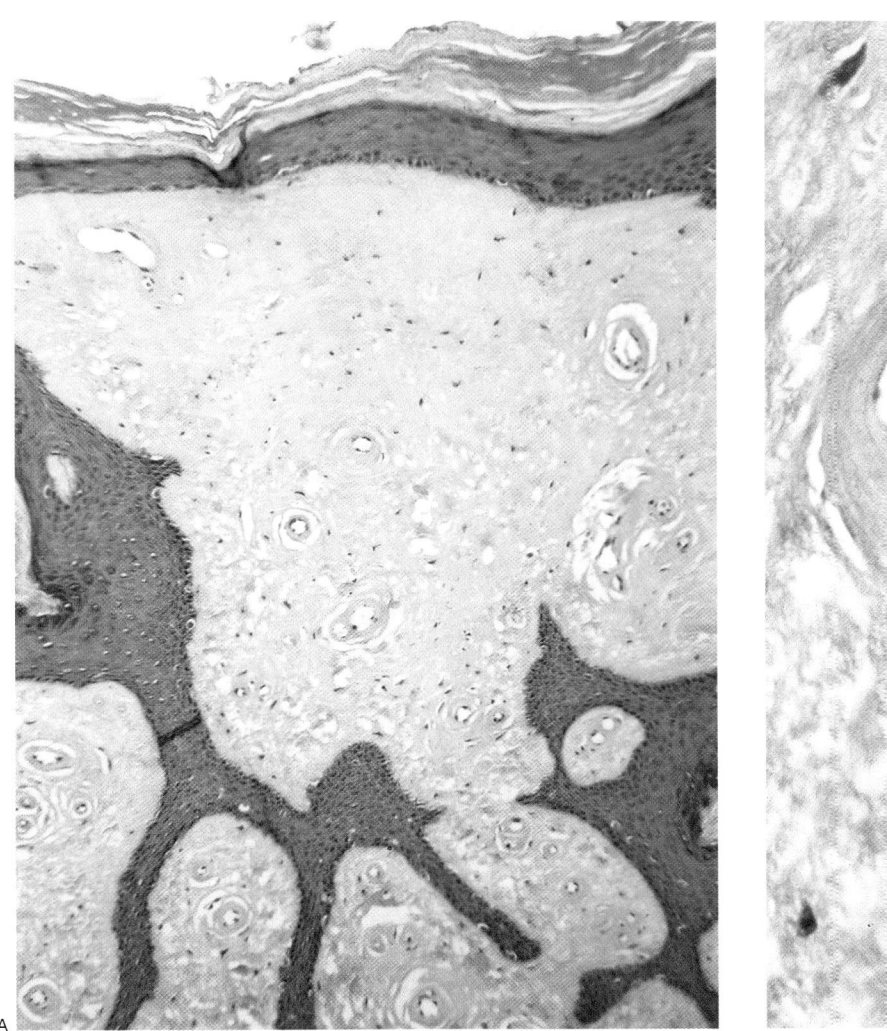
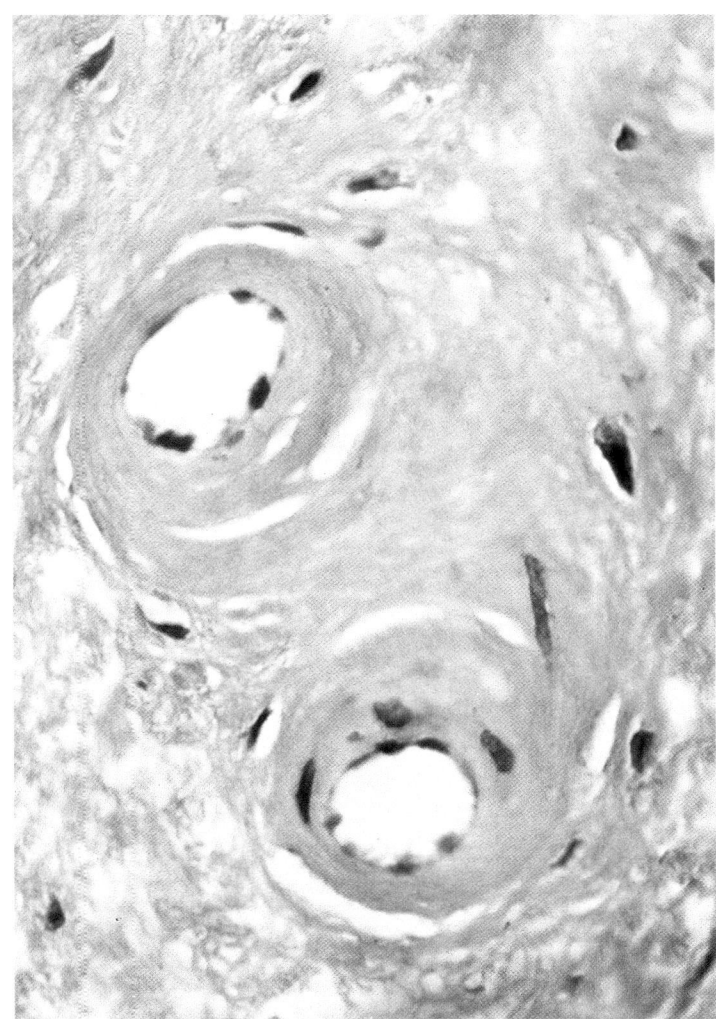

Fig. 14.17 **(A) Lipoid proteinosis. (B)** Hyaline material is arranged around blood vessels in the papillary dermis in an onion-skin pattern. (H & E)

They may be discrete or clustered to form plaques. Verrucous lesions are rare.[343] The cheeks, ears, neck and dorsum of the hands are sites of predilection. Often there is a history of exposure to petroleum products and/or excessive sunlight,[339,344] but obviously there is some underlying predisposition as well.[345] Unilateral involvement of the sun-exposed arm of taxi drivers has been reported.[346] The material in the dermis is thought to represent a degeneration product of elastic fibers induced by solar radiation (actinic elastoid).[347,348]

Juvenile colloid milium is exceedingly rare.[340,349–351] Papules or plaques develop, usually on the face and neck, prior to puberty. Some purported cases probably represent examples of erythropoietic protoporphyria.

Pigmented colloid milium[341] is found as gray to black clustered or confluent papules on the face, following the excessive use of hydroquinone bleaching creams (see ochronosis, p. 439).

Colloid degeneration (paracolloid) presents as nodular, plaque-like areas, usually on the face.[342,352] This is probably a heterogeneous group.

Histopathology

In the *adult form*, there are nodular masses of homogeneous, eosinophilic material expanding the papillary dermis and extending into the mid dermis (Fig. 14.20).[337] Fissures and clefts divide this material into smaller islands and

fibroblasts are commonly aligned along the lines of fissuring (Fig. 14.21). A thin grenz zone of uninvolved collagen usually separates the colloid material from the overlying epidermis, which is thinned.[353] Some clumped elastotic fibers are often present in this grenz zone and also between and below the colloid masses, but the colloid material itself stains only lightly or not at all with elastic stains.[348] This material has been reported to stain positively with crystal violet and Congo red and to give fluorescence with thioflavine T; such reactions are more likely to be positive on frozen than paraffin sections.[337,353] Our own material (including a few cases using frozen sections) has not shown these reactions. In contrast to lipoid proteinosis and primary cutaneous amyloidosis, colloid milium does not contain laminin or type IV collagen.[349]

In the *juvenile form*, hypocellular material is present in the broadened dermal papillae; this shows some clefting with intervening spindle or stellate fibroblasts.[340] In most areas there is no grenz zone and the basal layer may show hyaline transformation with a transition towards the dermal material. The colloid is PAS positive and sometimes methyl violet positive, but it is usually Congo red negative.[350]

In the *pigmented form*,[341] there are lightly pigmented colloid islands in the upper dermis (see p. 439).

In the *plaque type of colloid degeneration*,[342] there is amorphous, homogenized, dermal collagen with small fissures and clefts extending deeply

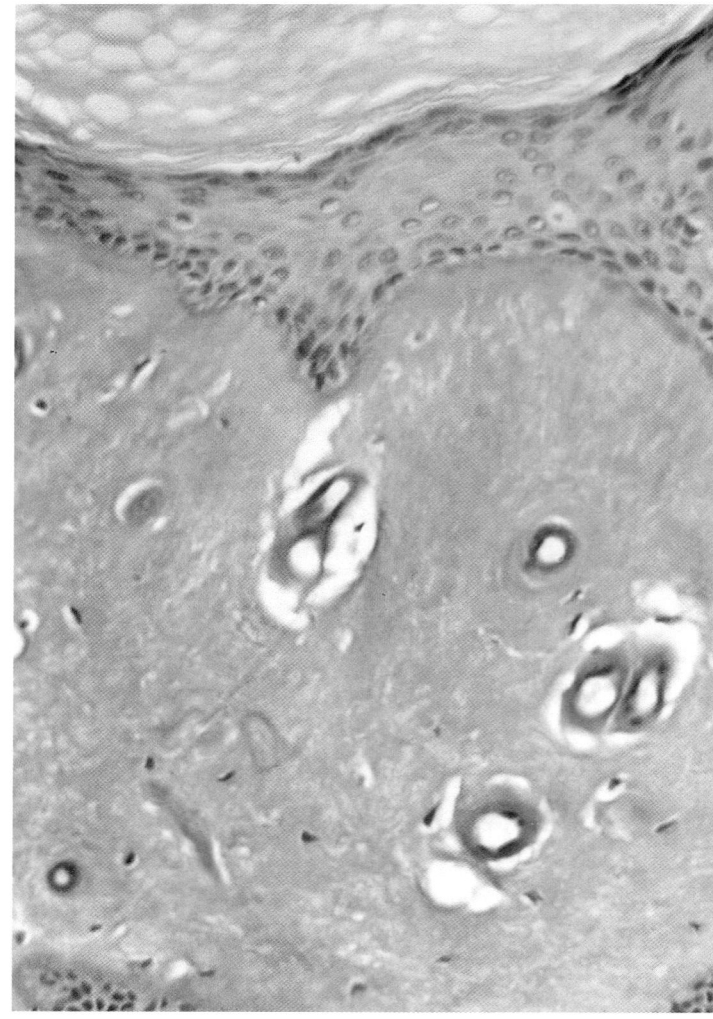

Fig. 14.18 **Lipoid proteinosis.** The hyaline material involving the papillary dermis and wall of blood vessels is PAS positive. (Periodic acid–Schiff)

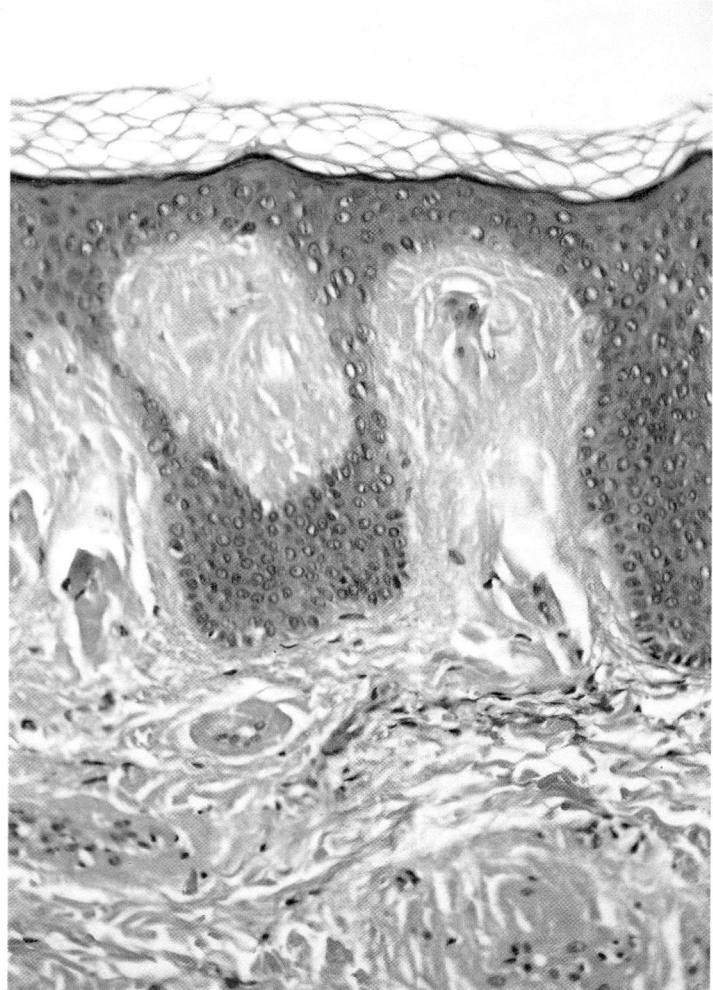

A

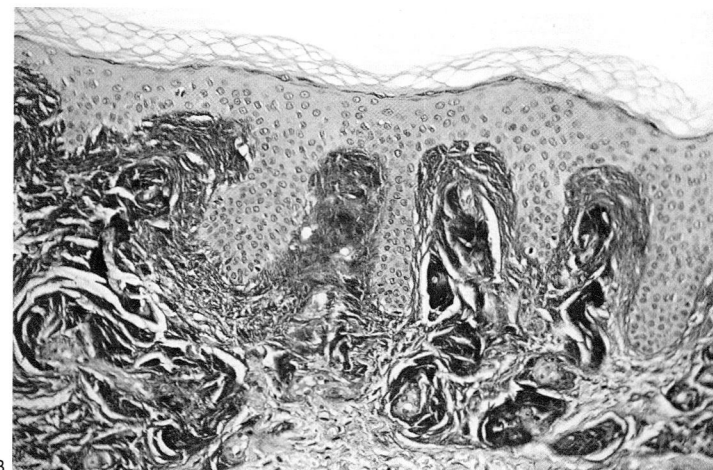

B

Fig. 14.19 **(A) Waldenström's macroglobulinemia.** Hyaline deposits fill the papillary dermis (H & E). **(B)** They appear to be more extensive on special stains. (Periodic acid–Schiff) (Slides kindly provided by Dr Richard Williamson)

into the dermis (Fig. 14.22). The material is relatively acellular. It is weakly PAS positive, but negative with Congo red and crystal violet. There is patchy staining with elastic tissue stains, but other areas are negative.

Electron microscopy
The ultrastructural features are different in the various types. In the *adult form*, there are large amounts of amorphous and granular material with some wavy, ill-defined, short and branching filaments.[353,354] Some components of actinic elastoid are present at the margins of the islands.[178] There are active fibroblasts. In the *juvenile form*, there are fibrillary masses with some whorling, rare nuclear remnants and some melanosomes and desmosomes.[340] Fibrillary transformation of keratinocytes has been observed, leading to the concept that the dermal tonofilament-like material is of epidermal origin.[340,350] This has been confirmed by positive staining using a polyclonal antikeratin antibody.[349] *Colloid degeneration* has shown microfilaments admixed with collagen, but more studies are needed before definite conclusions are reached.

MASSIVE CUTANEOUS HYALINOSIS

The term 'massive cutaneous hyalinosis' has been used to describe the condition of a patient with massive amorphous deposits of hyaline material in the deep dermis and subcutis of the face and upper trunk.[355] The material was PAS positive, Congo red negative and ultrastructurally non-fibrillary.[355] Subsequent investigations have shown that there are three major components of this hyaline material: kappa light chains, a mannose-rich glycoprotein, and type 1 collagen.[356]

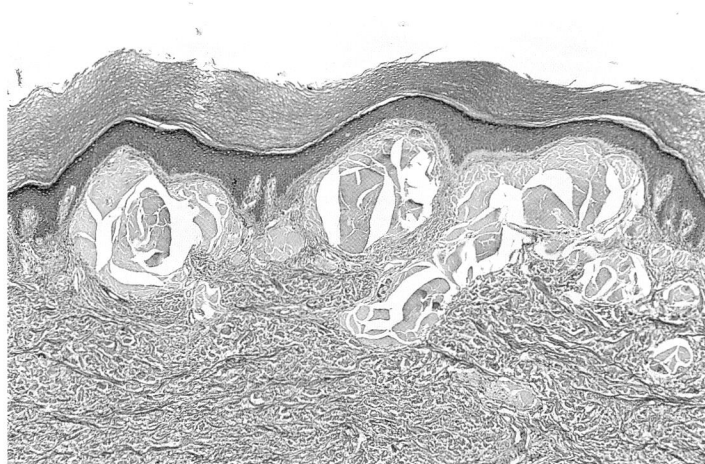

Fig. 14.20 **Colloid milium.** The clefted, hyaline material in the papillary dermis forms a papular lesion. (H & E)

CORTICOSTEROID INJECTION SITES

The local injection of corticosteroids into keloids or various soft tissue lesions results in a characteristic histological appearance should this site subsequently be biopsied.[357–360]

Histopathology

There are usually well-defined, irregularly contoured lakes of lightly staining material in the dermis or deeper tissues.[358] The material is finely granular or amorphous and is surrounded by a variable histiocytic response, sometimes with a few admixed foreign body giant cells and lymphocytes (Fig. 14.23).[360] On low power, the material resembles to some extent that seen in gouty tophi after the crystals have been dissolved by formalin fixation. Crystal-shaped empty spaces may be seen within the material and occasionally birefringent crystals have been present.[360] Sometimes there is no discernible reaction, while at other times a few neutrophils may be present. There is some controversy whether these differing appearances are time related.[360]

The material may be weakly PAS positive but, although superficially resembling mucin, it does not stain for it.[359]

A rheumatoid nodule-like appearance has been reported following corticosteroid injection.[358,360] Transepidermal elimination of altered collagen has followed the intralesional injection of triamcinolone in areas of psoriasis.

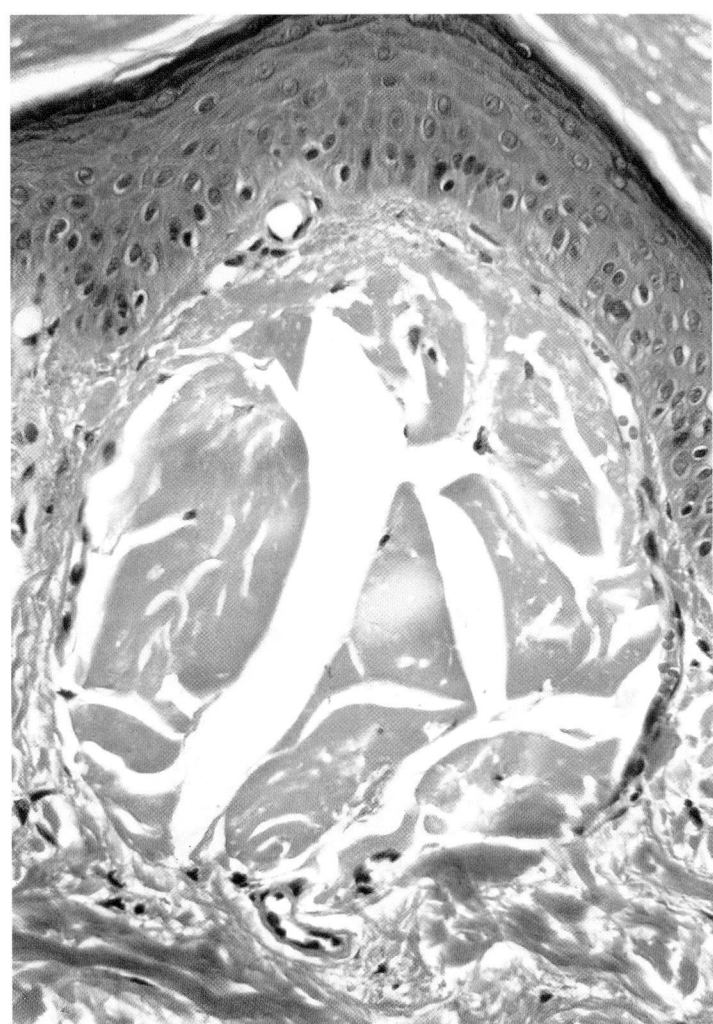

Fig. 14.21 **Colloid milium.** The clefted, hyaline material is hypocellular. (H & E)

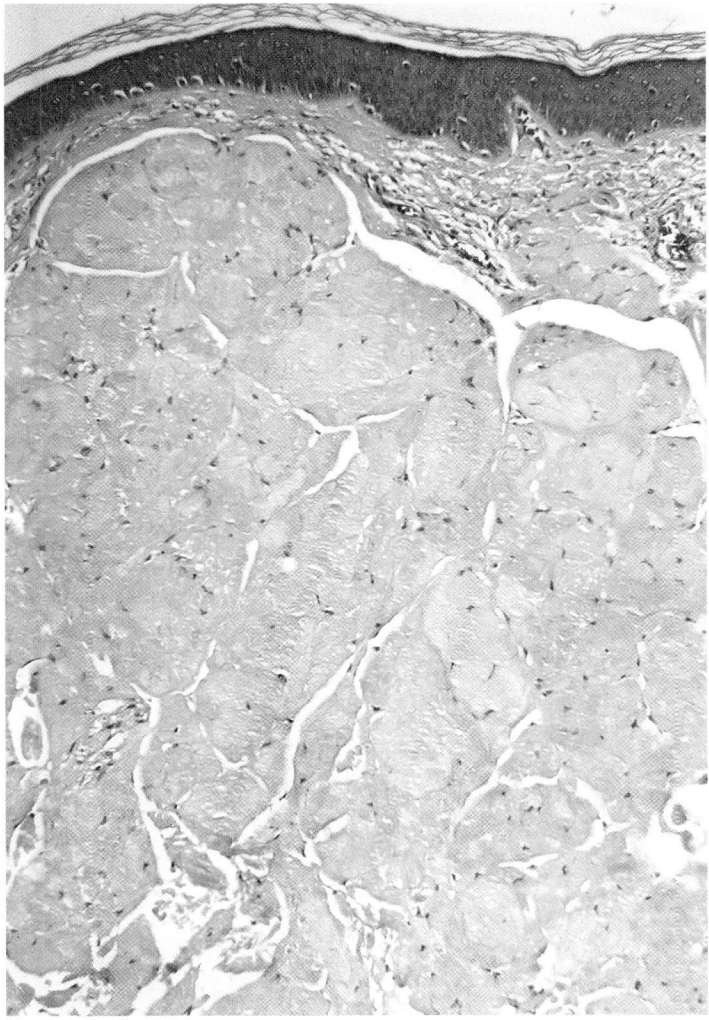

Fig. 14.22 **Colloid degeneration (paracolloid).** The deposits extend more deeply than in colloid milium and clefting is often less conspicuous. (H & E)

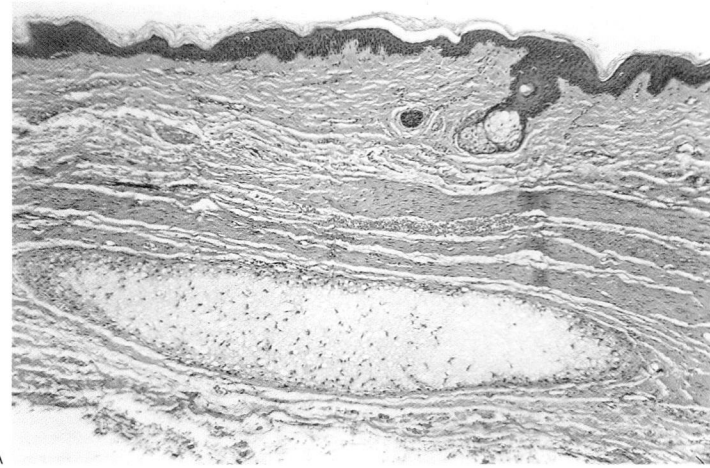
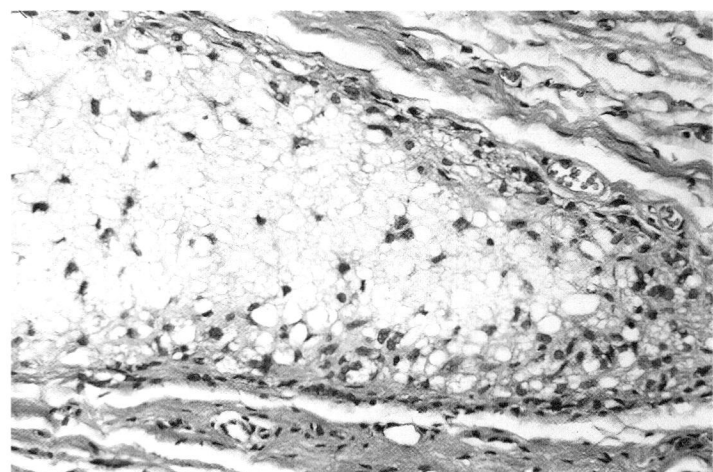

Fig. 14.23 **(A) Triamcinolone injection site. (B)** There is pale, foamy material surrounded by a palisade of macrophages. (H & E)

HYALIN ANGIOPATHY

Hyalin angiopathy is an unusual histological change that has been reported in the oral cavity and skin.[361] It is characterized by amorphous, eosinophilic material within and around blood vessels associated with acute or chronic inflammation. As the presence of giant cells is not always a conspicuous feature in the surrounding inflammatory reaction, it seems best not to refer to this condition as 'giant cell hyalin angiopathy'.[361]

INFANTILE SYSTEMIC HYALINOSIS

Infantile systemic hyalinosis is an autosomal recessive disorder of connective tissue in which hyaline material, as yet uncharacterized, is deposited in the skin as well as various organs.[362,363] There is failure to thrive; death occurs in early childhood.

The skin appears sclerodermatous. Velvety, hyperpigmented plaques develop over bony prominences.

Juvenile hyaline fibromatosis differs from infantile systemic hyalinosis by the presence of large tumor-like nodules and dermal involvement.[364] These features have led juvenile hyaline fibromatosis to be arbitrarily considered with the tumor-like conditions of fibrous tissue (see Ch. 34, p. 928).

Histopathology

Hyaline material, lacking elastic fibers, is deposited in the papillary dermis. Ultrastructurally, the material is fibrillogranular.[362]

CYTOID BODIES

Cytoid bodies are ovoid, round or polygonal, discrete deposits which vary in size from 5 to 20 μm or more in diameter. The term has been applied to a heterogeneous group of deposits which include amyloid, colloid bodies, Russell bodies and elastic globes.[365] With the exception of Russell bodies, which are derived from plasma cells, cytoid bodies are usually found in the papillary dermis. *Colloid bodies* are derived from degenerate keratinocytes, usually associated with the lichenoid reaction pattern. They represent tonofilament-rich bodies extruded into the dermis, but they are sometimes trapped in the epidermis and are carried upwards with normal epidermal maturation. They are considered with the lichenoid tissue reaction in Chapter 3, page 32.

Elastic globes were first described in the 19th century and were for a time regarded as a diagnostic sign in cutaneous lupus erythematosus or scleroderma.[365] In 1965, Pinkus and colleagues described them in normal skin and suggested that they are a structural variant of elastic fibers.[366] They can be found regularly in clinically normal skin from the face and extremities, particularly the calf. It has been suggested that elastic globes in some circumstances may represent the end stage of degenerated colloid bodies; this has not been confirmed by immunohistochemistry, which shows that elastic globes have an immunological profile close to elastic fiber microfibrils.[367]

Histopathology[365,368]

Elastic globes are usually amphophilic, PAS-positive structures found in the papillary dermis (see p. 388). They may have a slight basophilic tint in sun-damaged skin. They are usually larger than cell size (Fig. 14.24), stain strongly with elastic tissue stains and are weakly autofluorescent.

Electron microscopy

Electron microscopy shows electron-dense, granular, amorphous and filamentous material.

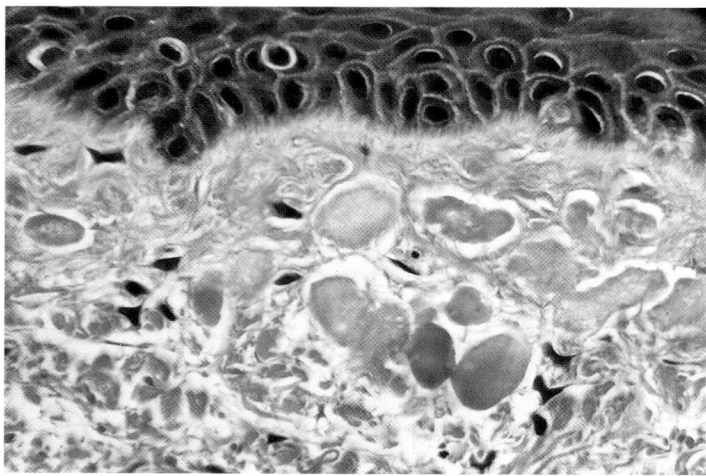

Fig. 14.24 **Elastic globes** in the papillary dermis. (H & E)

PIGMENT AND RELATED DEPOSITS

A heterogeneous group of exogenous and endogenous pigments may be found in the skin. For convenience, the various heavy metals and drugs that produce deposits and/or pigmentary changes are discussed here as well.

OCHRONOSIS

Ochronosis refers to the yellow-brown or ocher pigment (homogentisic acid) deposited in collagen-containing tissues in alkaptonuria. This is an autosomal recessive disorder in which the hepatic and renal enzyme homogentisic acid oxidase is absent.[3,369–374] The term is also used for the deposition of similar hydroquinone derivatives in certain exogenously induced conditions which sometimes followed the topical use of phenol in the treatment of leg ulcers and of picric acid in the treatment of burns (both procedures have now been abandoned) and which are still seen as a complication of the oral administration[375–377] or intramuscular injection[378] of antimalarial drugs and the topical use of hydroquinone bleaching creams in black races.[379–387] The author has also seen it in a patient who consumed large quantities of quinine-containing tonic water.

There is some clinical variability in the presentation of the various types. In alkaptonuria, there is bluish and bluish-black pigmentation of the face, neck, dorsum of the hands and palmoplantar region[388,389] and bluish discoloration of the sclerae and of the cartilage of the ears and sometimes of the nose.[390] In the pigmentation associated with antimalarial therapy, the pretibial, palatal, facial and subungual areas have been involved.[375] In hydroquinone-induced lesions, the face (particularly the malar areas), neck and sometimes the ears, corresponding to sites of application of the cream, are involved. There is hyperpigmentation, with variable development of finely papular and even colloid milium-like areas.[379–382] Of interest is the complete absence of hydroquinone-induced ochronosis in areas of vitiligo.[391] This suggests that melanocytes are necessary for the deposition of the pigment, which is presumably derived from a melanin-hydroquinone precursor.[391]

Histopathology[380,390]

There is a marked similarity between the ochronotic deposits in alkaptonuria and hydroquinone-induced ochronosis.[381] In the earliest stages, there is some basophilia of the collagen fibers in the upper dermis, followed by the appearance of stout, sharply defined, ocher-colored fibers which may be crescentic, vermiform or banana-shaped (Fig. 14.25).[380] Fragmented fibers and small pigmented deposits may also be present, the latter lying free in the dermis or in macrophages. Pigment granules are also found in the endothelial cells of blood vessels and the basement membrane of sweat glands.[370] Colloid milium-like foci often develop in the hydroquinone-induced lesions, and these foci may show no visible ochronotic material or only partial staining of the fibers.[380,382] Transepidermal elimination of ochronotic fibers has been observed.[382,392] There is a variable number of macrophages present, but they are usually infrequent in alkaptonuria. Rarely, foreign body giant cells surround the fibers, but this occurs more often in extracutaneous sites.[371] Actinic granuloma-like changes have also been reported (see p. 209).[393]

In hydroquinone-induced pigmentation there is usually diminution in basal melanin, but prominent melanin in macrophages in the papillary dermis. In lesions induced by antimalarial drugs, the changes are usually different, with small pigment granules which are predominantly in macrophages in a perivascular position and around appendages.[375,376] Small ocher-colored fibers can be present throughout the dermis, but large fibers in the upper dermis are not a feature. The pigment in the antimalarial-induced cases usually

stains positively for melanin and hemosiderin,[376] while in the other forms the fibers and smaller deposits are usually negative with these stains and also with elastic tissue stains.[380] They do, however, stain darkly with methylene blue.[381]

Electron microscopy

The ochronotic deposits are electron dense. They are usually homogeneous[381] but may be fibrillar.[369] There is granular, less electron-dense material at the periphery with fibroblasts investing and ramifying through it.[380] Active phagocytosis of electron-dense material is present.[381]

TATTOOS

Tattoos are produced by the mechanical introduction of insoluble pigments into the dermis. Most are decorative in type, but occasionally carbon or some other pigment is traumatically implanted in an industrial or firearm accident.[394,395] The incidence of complications is becoming quite rare with the declining use of mercury salts (although other red tattoo pigments may cause reactions)[396,397] and a greater emphasis on hygiene in tattoo parlors.

The complications have been well reviewed.[398–400] They may be grouped into several broad categories: infections introduced at the time of tattooing; cutaneous diseases that localize in tattoos, often in a Koebner-type phenomenon; allergic reactions to the tattoo pigments;[401] photosensitivity reactions;[400,402] tumors; and miscellaneous reactions. The infections reported have included pyogenic infections, syphilis, leprosy, tuberculosis,[403] tetanus, chancroid, verruca vulgaris,[399,404] vaccinia, herpes simplex and zoster, molluscum contagiosum,[405] viral hepatitis and a dermatophyte infection.[406] Cutaneous diseases that may localize in tattoos include psoriasis, lichen planus,[407] Darier's disease and discoid lupus erythematosus, the latter in the red areas.[400] Allergic reactions can occur to mercury,[408] chromium,[409,410] manganese,[411] aluminum,[412] cobalt and cadmium salts.[400,413,414] Photosensitivity reactions may be photoallergic or phototoxic, the latter reaction being quite common with cadmium sulfide, a yellow pigment.[413] The development of tumors such as basal cell[415] and squamous cell carcinomas, melanoma, keratoacanthoma, lymphoma[416] and reticulohistiocytoma may well be coincidental.[398] Miscellaneous lesions include keloids,[399] regional lymphadenopathy and a sarcoidal reaction which may be localized or systemic.[417–419]

Recent experimental work with guinea pigs suggests that the lightening of tattoos after laser therapy results more from widespread necrosis and

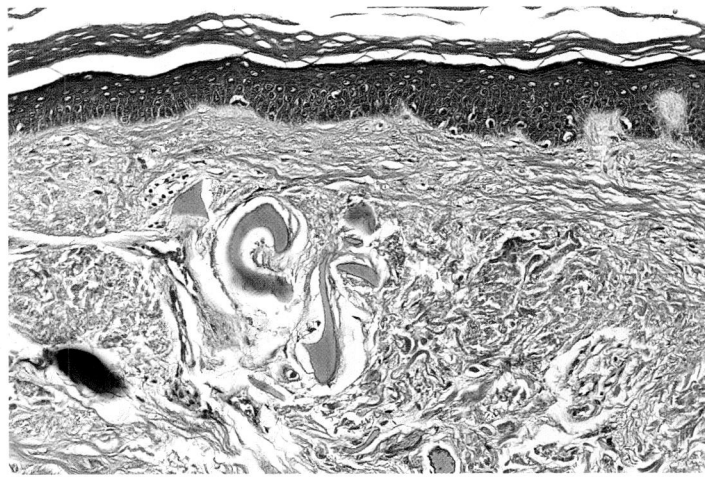

Fig. 14.25 **Ochronosis.** An irregularly shaped deposit is present in the mid dermis. (H & E)

subsequent tissue sloughing and dermal fibrosis than from any specific changes in the pigment or its handling by macrophages.[420] Other mechanisms appear to be involved with some of the newer lasers.[421] Some tattoo inks can be difficult to remove.[422,423] The presence of titanium dioxide in the inks is associated with a poor response to laser therapy.[424]

Histopathology[425]

Tattoo pigments are easily visualized in tissue sections. After several weeks they localize around vessels in the upper and mid dermis in macrophages and fibroblasts (Fig. 14.26). Extracellular deposits of pigment are also found between collagen bundles. The pigment is generally refractile, but not doubly refractile. A foreign body granulomatous reaction has not been recorded except in the presence of other severe reactions.

Hypersensitivity reactions in tattoos vary from a diffuse lymphohistiocytic infiltrate in the dermis (Fig. 14.27), with an admixture of some plasma cells and eosinophils, to a lichenoid reaction,[426–428] sometimes with associated epithelial hyperplasia.[414,429,430] Other reactions include the development of sarcoidal granulomas or of a pseudolymphomatous pattern.[429,431] Epidermal spongiosis has been reported.[425]

Recently, attempts have been made to correlate the ultrastructural features with the pigment used, as determined by X-ray microanalysis techniques.[432] The pigment present in macrophages may be granular or crystalline.[432] It is sometimes membrane bound. Tattoo pigment has also been found in dermal fibroblasts.[433]

HEMOCHROMATOSIS

Hemochromatosis is a multisystem disorder of iron metabolism in which cutaneous pigmentation is a manifestation in up to 90% of patients ('bronzed diabetes').[434,435] Although generalized, the pigmentation is most obvious on the face, especially the forehead and malar areas.[435] Some patients have been reported to have a slate-gray color, rather than the typical bronze pigmentation.[435] Cutaneous pigmentation fades slowly with venesection of the patient.

The bronze color results from increased melanin in the basal layers of the epidermis and, to a lesser extent, some coexisting thinning of the epidermis.[434] Patients with a slate-gray color have been reported to show hemosiderin deposits in the epidermis as well as the dermis, and it is assumed that the epidermal hemosiderin contributes to the skin color in these patients.[435] The absence of pigmentation in the vitiliginous areas of patients with both vitiligo and hemochromatosis indicates that hemosiderin in the usual dermal sites does not contribute significantly to the bronze color in patients with hemochromatosis.[436] Pigment changes are not as apparent in dark-skinned races, although the darkening of pre-existing epidermal cysts, due to increased melanin in their walls, or of keloids may be a useful marker.[437]

The increased melanin production is thought to result from the deposition of hemosiderin in the skin, as other heavy metals will produce a similar response. The mechanism by which the heavy metals stimulate melanin production is uncertain.

Histopathology[434,438]

There may be some thinning of the epidermis and increased melanin pigment in the basal layer. Golden brown granules of hemosiderin are present in the basement membrane region of the sweat glands and in macrophages in the loose connective tissue stroma of these glands. A small amount can often be seen associated with sebaceous glands and their stroma. In some cases, small specks of hemosiderin can be seen in the epidermis with the Perls' stain.[435,439]

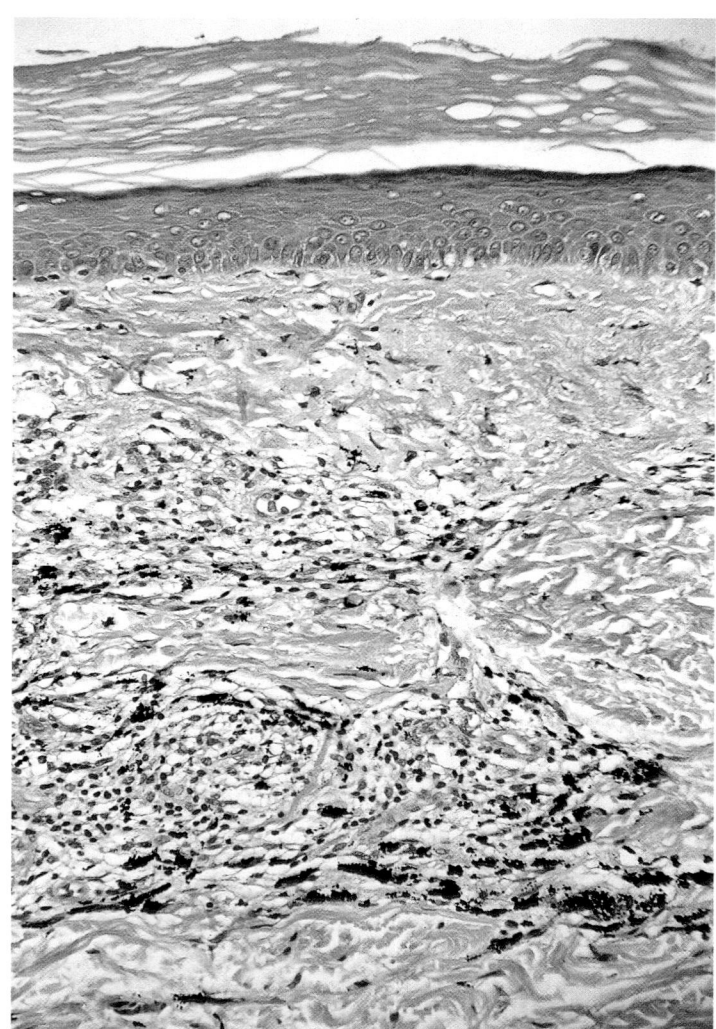

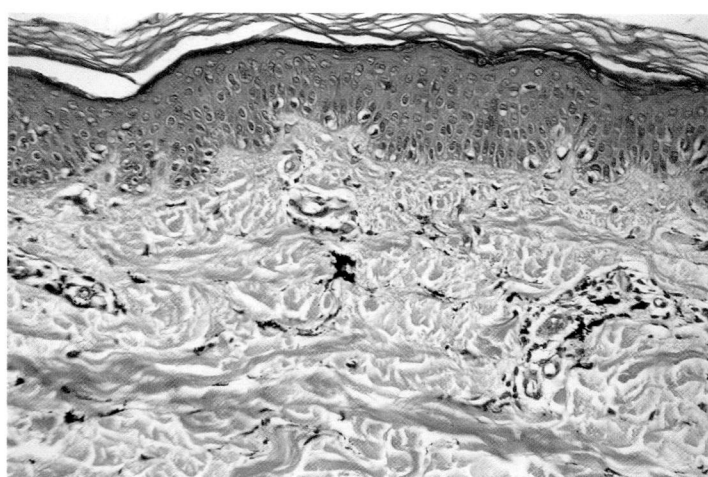

Fig. 14.26 **Tattoo.** Black pigment is seen in macrophages and lying free in a predominantly perivascular location. (H & E)

Fig. 14.27 **Tattoo pigment with an associated inflammatory reaction**, the result of an allergic reaction to one of the pigments. (H & E)

HEMOSIDERIN FROM OTHER SOURCES

Hemosiderin has also been noted in the skin following the application of Monsel's solution (20% aqueous ferric subsulfate) for hemostasis in minor surgical procedures[440–442] and the use of iron sesquioxide on a skin ulcer.[443] In both circumstances there has been ferrugination of collagen fibers with numerous siderophages[441,442] and sometimes multinucleate giant cells[443] in the interstitial tissues of the dermis. Perls' stain has been strongly positive in these areas.

Hemosiderin is conspicuous in venous stasis of the lower legs.[444] It is found in the pigmented purpuric dermatoses, Zoon's balanitis and Zoon's vulvitis, granuloma faciale and the pigmented pretibial patches of diabetes mellitus. Impregnation of iron from earrings has been reported.[445] Hemosiderin is also present around glass fragments in the dermis (Fig. 14.28), and in dermatofibromas and various tumors of blood vessels.

'BRONZE BABY' SYNDROME

'Bronze baby' syndrome refers to the transient bronze discoloration of the skin, serum and urine which is a relatively uncommon complication of phototherapy for neonatal hyperbilirubinemia.[446,447] The pigment is thought to be either a photo-oxidation product of bilirubin or a copper-bound porphyrin; it may even be biliverdin.[447] No histological studies have been undertaken.

Localized green discoloration of the palms and soles has been reported in an adult with hyperbilirubinemia.[448]

SILVER DEPOSITION (ARGYRIA)

Argyria, which refers to the systemic deposition of silver salts, is an iatrogenic disease resulting from the indiscriminate ingestion of silver-containing compounds or their application to mucous membranes or burnt skin.[449,450] Now that the availability of these preparations is restricted, argyria is very rare and is seen only in relation to industrial exposure[451] or bizarre dietary fads.[452–456]

Cutaneous changes of argyria consist of permanent blue-gray pigmentation, resembling cyanosis, which is most marked in sun-exposed areas.[457] The nail lunulae may be azure blue.[457,458] The pigmentation is thought to result from the photoactivated reduction of the absorbed silver salts to metallic silver.[452,459] There is probably some contribution from increased melanin production as well.

Localized argyria has been reported after prolonged topical exposure,[460] at the site of implanted acupuncture needles,[461,462] and from the wearing of silver earrings in pierced ears.[463]

Histopathology[449]
There are multiple, minute, brown-black granules deposited in a band-like fashion in relation to the basement membranes of sweat glands. They are also found in elastic fibers in the papillary dermis and to a lesser extent in the connective tissue sheaths around the pilosebaceous follicles, in the arrector pili muscles and in arteriolar walls. On dark-field examination, the deposits are more easily detected, giving a 'stars in heaven' pattern.[464] In one case of localized argyria the deposits were in the papillary dermis adjacent to the intraepidermal sweat duct.[460] There is usually an increase in melanin pigment in the basal layer of the epidermis, and melanophores are present in the papillary dermis.

Scanning electron microscopy has shown that the granules are larger and more abundant in exposed than non-exposed skin.[452] Transmission electron microscopy shows electron-dense bodies 13–1000 μm in diameter in relation

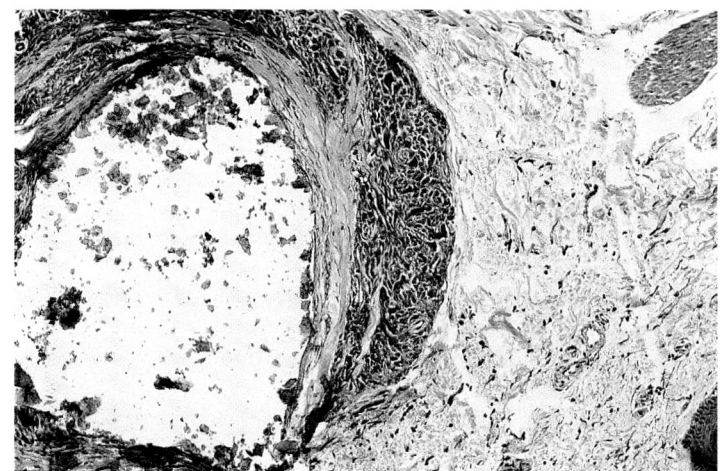

Fig. 14.28 **Hemosiderin deposits** around fragments of glass in the dermis. (H & E)

to sweat glands and the microfibrils of elastic fibers.[453,464–466] The granules are found in macrophages in membrane-bound aggregates.[452,453] Histochemical studies suggested that the deposits were in the form of silver sulfide;[467] the recent use of X-ray probe microanalysis has confirmed the presence of silver and sulfur, with the addition of selenium and other metals in trace amounts.[449,453]

GOLD DEPOSITION (CHRYSIASIS)

Chrysiasis refers to the permanent blue-gray pigmentation of the skin, most pronounced in sun-exposed areas, which results from the deposition of gold salts in the dermis, following gold injections for the treatment of rheumatoid arthritis and pemphigus.[449,468–471] Its development is, in part, dose related, but light exposure and even laser therapy appear to favor its deposition.[472–474]

Besides chrysiasis, gold injections may produce a non-specific eczematous or urticarial reaction, eruptions resembling lichen planus and pityriasis rosea and, rarely, erythema nodosum or erythroderma.[475,476]

Histopathology[449,472,477]
Small round or oval black granules, irregular in size, are present in dermal macrophages which tend to localize around blood vessels in the upper and mid dermis. Similar pigment may be in elongated, fibroblast-like cells in the upper dermis.[469] The gold is well visualized on dark-field examination. A striking orange-red birefringence can be demonstrated under polarized light.[478] The granules are larger than silver granules and, unlike argyria, there is no deposition of gold on membranes.

Electron microscopy
Electron microscopy shows electron-dense particles in phagolysosomes of macrophages.[469,479] The appearances vary with the method of staining used.[480]

MERCURY

Now that mercury-containing ointments are no longer commonly used, the slate gray pigmentation of the skin related to the topical application of mercury salts is rarely seen.[468,481–483] Another manifestation of mercury intoxication which is rarely seen is acrodynia (pink disease), a condition of early childhood attributed to chronic mercury ingestion in teething powders.[484] Acral parts assume a dusky pink color. Serious systemic symptoms and even death sometimes ensue. Cutaneous nodules containing globules of mercury have been reported in one patient, as a reaction to oral mercury.[485]

A widespread allergic reaction (mercury exanthem) may follow exposure to high concentrations of mercury vapor[486] or the topical application of mercury-containing ointments.[487] Local sclerosing granulomatous lesions may follow the implantation of mercury associated with skin trauma from a broken thermometer[488] or self-injection.[489]

Histopathology[482,489,490]

The pigmentation from topical applications of mercurial preparations results from the deposition of brown-black mercury granules in aggregates of up to 300 μm in macrophages around blood vessels in the upper dermis and in linear bands following the course of elastic fibers.[449] The particles are refractile. There may be a contribution from increased melanin in the basal layer.[491]

The mercury exanthem shows subcorneal neutrophilic microabscesses with a variable perivascular neutrophilic and lymphocytic infiltrate around vessels in the upper dermis.

The accidental or deliberate implantation of mercury into the skin results in a granulomatous foreign body giant cell reaction.[489,492] A zone of degenerate collagen often surrounds the black spherules of mercury in the tissues.[488,489,493] In older lesions there may be fibrosis around the deposits.[488] Ulceration or pseudoepitheliomatous hyperplasia may overlie dermal deposits of mercury.

Electron microscopy
Particles averaging 14 nm in diameter, but forming larger aggregates, are present in the dermis.

ARSENIC

Prolonged ingestion of arsenic may result in a diffuse, macular, bronze pigmentation, most pronounced on the trunk with 'raindrop' areas of normal or depigmented skin.[449] The color is said to arise partly from increased melanin in the basal layer and partly from the metal itself. Other manifestations of chronic arsenical poisoning include keratoses, hyperkeratosis of the palms and soles and carcinomas of the skin.

LEAD

Lead poisoning may result in a blue line at the gingival margin due to the subepithelial deposit of lead sulfide granules.[449,494]

ALUMINUM

Persistent subcutaneous nodules are a rare complication of the use of aluminum-adsorbed vaccines in immunization procedures.[495–497] The nodules may be painful or pruritic.[495,496] Aluminum salts used in tattooing rarely cause a granulomatous reaction in the skin.[412] An aluminum 'tattoo' can also result from the use of topical aluminum chloride in the cauterization of biopsy sites.[498]

Histopathology[497,499]

The nodular lesions show a heavy lymphoid infiltrate in the lower dermis and subcutis with well-formed lymphoid follicles, complete with germinal centers. The infiltrate around the follicles includes lymphocytes, plasma cells and sometimes eosinophils. Macrophages with slightly granular cytoplasm which stains purple-gray with hematoxylin and eosin are usually present.[496] Giant cells and small areas of necrosis are sometimes seen. The aluminum can be confirmed by X-ray microanalysis[496] or by the solochrome-azurine stain in which crystals of aluminum salts stain a deep gray-blue color.

Aluminum 'tattoos', following the topical application of aluminum chloride, contain variable numbers of macrophages with ample stippled cytoplasm, resembling the parasitized macrophages of certain infectious diseases. The particles are, however, larger and more variable in size than parasites.[498] An underlying scar is usually present.

BISMUTH

Generalized pigmentation resembling argyria may follow systemic use of bismuth. Metallic granules are present in the dermis.[449] Crops of small black carbon-like particles have been reported on the skin after prolonged ingestion of a bismuth subsalicylate preparation.[500] It has been suggested that prurigo pigmentosa, a condition seen mostly in Japan, is a persistent lichenoid reaction to bismuth with postinflammatory melanin incontinence and pigmentation of the skin.[501]

TITANIUM

Exposure to titanium dioxide may produce cutaneous lesions.[502,503] There is one report of a patient developing small papules on the penis following the application of an ointment containing titanium dioxide for the treatment of herpetic lesions.[502] Another report of occupational exposure documents involvement of the lungs, skin and synovium.[503] In the case involving the topical application, numerous brown granules, confirmed as titanium by electron probe microanalysis, were present in the upper dermis, both free and in macrophages.[502] In another case, a necrotizing lesion involving the subcutis, with extension into muscle, was present.[503]

DRUG DEPOSITS AND PIGMENTATION

A number of mechanisms are involved in the cutaneous pigmentation induced by certain drugs. These include an increased formation of melanin, the deposition of the drug or complexes derived therefrom in the dermis, and postinflammatory pigmentation, with melanin incontinence, usually following a lichenoid reaction.[468,504] The exact mechanism is still unknown in many cases. Drugs, therefore, share many features with the heavy metals already considered. This subject has been well reviewed.[449]

Antimalarial drugs
The long-term use of antimalarial drugs, either for malarial prophylaxis or in the treatment of various collagen diseases and dermatoses, can result in cutaneous pigmentation. Several patterns are seen.[449] Yellow pigmentation is sometimes seen with quinacrine (mepacrine), although the histopathology has not been described. Small ochronosis-like deposits are a rare finding. Pretibial pigmentation is more common and this is slate gray to blue-black in color. Pigment granules – some staining for hemosiderin, some for melanin and some for both – can be seen in macrophages and extracellularly.[505]

Phenothiazines
Prolonged use of phenothiazines produces a progressive gray-blue pigmentation in sun-exposed areas.[506] Slow fading occurs with cessation of the drug.[507] Similar cutaneous pigmentation has been reported in patients taking imipramine[508–511] and in one taking desipramine.[512] Refractile, golden-brown pigment with the staining properties of melanin is found in the dermis along collagen bundles and in macrophages, especially around vessels in the superficial vascular plexus.[449,510] The Perls' method for iron is negative.

Electron microscopy shows melanin granules in macrophages but also other bodies of varying electron densities which may represent metabolites or complexes of the drug.[513,514]

Tetracycline
Bluish pigmentation of cutaneous osteomas has resulted from the use of tetracycline.[515]

Methacycline
The prolonged use of the antibiotic methacycline produces gray-black pigmentation of light-exposed areas and some conjunctival pigmentation in a small percentage of patients.[449] In addition to increased melanin in the basal layer of the epidermis there is extracellular pigment in the elastotic sun-damaged areas which stains positively with the Masson–Fontana method for melanin.[516] Some of this pigment is in macrophages.

Minocycline
Three different patterns[517,518] of cutaneous pigmentation may follow long-term therapy with the antibiotic minocycline:

1. a generalized muddy brown pigmentation due to increased melanin in the basal layer[519]
2. bluish-black pigmentation of scars[520,521] and old inflammatory foci, including sites of immunobullous diseases,[522] related to hemosiderin or an iron chelate of minocycline
3. blue-gray pigmentation of the lower legs and arms due to a pigment which is probably a drug metabolite–protein complex chelated with iron and calcium.

A case involving the lips and one involving the tongue have been reported.[523,524] The sclerae may be involved in severe cases.[525] The pigmentation in all cases gradually fades after cessation of the drug.[522,526] Laser therapy has been used in cases of incomplete disappearance of the pigmentation.[527]

Histopathology[449,518]
The pigment in the localized types is present in macrophages, often aggregated in perivascular areas, in dermal dendrocytes[528] and in eccrine myoepithelial cells.[529] In other cases the pigment may deposit on elastic fibers (Fig. 14.29). This complex pigment is positive with both the Perls' method for iron and the Masson–Fontana method for melanin, but is negative with the PAS stain.[530] It is non-birefringent and non-fluorescent.

Electron microscopy
There are intracytoplasmic granules of dark homogeneous material and small fine particles containing iron.[518,531–533]

Amiodarone
Dermal lipofuscin is responsible for the blue-gray pigmentation of light-exposed skin that is an uncommon complication of the long-term use of amiodarone, an iodinated drug used in the treatment of cardiac arrhythmias.[534–537] The cutaneous pigmentation slowly disappears after cessation of the drug.[535]

Polyene antibiotics such as nystatin may also produce local lipofuscinosis.[534,536] The mechanism responsible for the production and deposition of the lipofuscin is unknown for both these drugs.

Localized lipofuscinosis has also been reported as an incidental phenomenon.[538] There was no history of trauma or the application of topical agents.

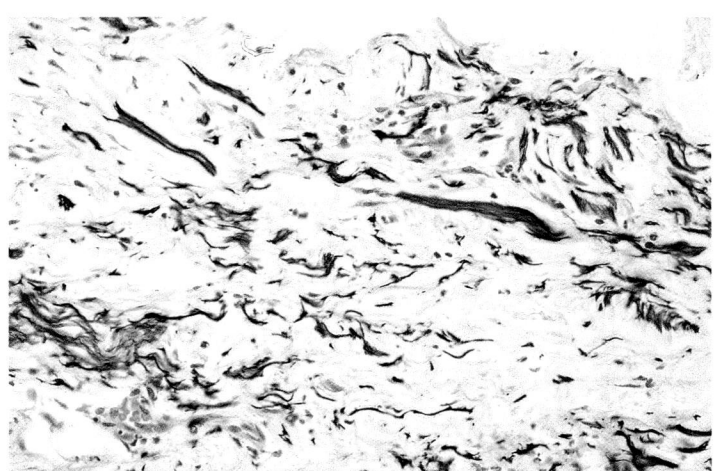

Fig. 14.29 **Minocycline pigment** deposited on dermal elastic fibers. (Masson–Fontana)

Histopathology[534,536]
Yellow-brown granules of lipofuscin are found in macrophages, which tend to accumulate around blood vessels at the junction of the papillary and reticular dermis. The granules stain positively with the PAS, prolonged Ziehl–Neelsen, Fontana and Sudan black methods.[534]

Electron microscopy
There are electron-dense, membrane-bound bodies in the cytoplasm of macrophages.[534,536] Melanosomal maturation may be blocked in some cases.[539]

Clofazimine
The substituted phenazine dye clofazimine is used in the treatment of leprosy, discoid lupus erythematosus and other dermatoses. A not uncommon side-effect is the development of cutaneous and conjunctival pigmentation which has a reddish blue hue.[468,540] Although light microscopy of routine hematoxylin and eosin-stained sections fails to show the pigment, birefringent red clofazimine crystals can be seen in fresh frozen sections.[540] These deposits, which are concentrated around larger vessels in the dermis, are vivid red on fluorescence microscopy.[540]

Chemotherapeutic agents
Pigmentation of the skin may follow the prolonged use of several anti-neoplastic chemotherapeutic agents including busulfan, bleomycin, doxorubicin, daunorubicin,[541] fluorouracil,[542] cyclophosphamide and the topical application of mechlorethamine (chlormethine, mustine) and carmustine (BCNU).[449,543] That following the use of bleomycin takes the form of 'flagellate streaks'.[544–548] Localization in striae distensae and in supravenous skin following venous infusions has been reported.[549–551] The pigmentation appears to result from increased melanin in the basal layer of the skin and in macrophages in the upper dermis.

CUTANEOUS IMPLANTS

Over the years, various agents have been injected or surgically implanted into the dermis and subcutaneous tissue as a cosmetic procedure to correct defects and scars and to augment tissues.[552] Paraffin was one such substance, although its complication, 'paraffinoma' (see p. 533), is rarely seen these days.[553,554] Bovine collagen and silicone are the agents used most frequently for these purposes. Other substances, such as gelatin matrix, Bioplastique, Artecoll and Dermalive have been introduced recently and it can be expected that others will be marketed in the future.[552,555] Adverse reactions to these substances in their current form is uncommon, but granulomatous inflammation has been reported.[555]

Suture material, another implant, produces a fairly stereotyped reaction with macrophages, foreign body giant cells and some lymphocytes. In the case of absorbable sutures, collections of macrophages with brown, foamy cytoplasm often remain after absorption is complete.[556] The morphological appearances of various suture materials in tissue sections were reviewed some time ago.[556] A brief account of the reactions to silicone and to bovine collagen follows.

SILICONE IMPLANTS

The term 'silicone' is used to designate certain polymeric organosilicon compounds which may be in liquid, gel or solid form.[552] A liquid form, dimethicone (dimethylpolysiloxane), is used to augment soft tissues. Little reaction is produced if only small amounts (less than 1 ml at each treatment session) are used;[552] severe reactions with granulomas and ulceration have been reported.[557] In an attempt to reduce the side-effects that result from the use of large amounts of the liquid or gel forms, 'bag-gel' implants were introduced for augmentation of the breasts.[558] Leakage of silicone can occasionally occur following trauma to the site of implantation, producing a local reaction; uncommonly, the silicone gel can migrate to distant sites where it may result in induration or a discharging wound.[558–562] Ulceration has also been recorded overlying areas of subcutaneous injection of liquid silicone.[563] Silicone has also been used to construct auricular prostheses.[564]

Controversy surrounds the development of systemic manifestations, such as scleroderma, in patients who have received silicone implants (see p. 347). Some of these cases have been the subject of litigation.

Histopathology[565]
Silicones can produce a range of histological reactions, depending mainly on the form of the silicone (liquid, gel or solid elastomer type) and the amount in the tissues.[558] Liquid silicone results in round to oval vacuoles of varying size surrounded usually by histiocytes, some with foamy cytoplasm (Fig. 14.30). A

few multinucleate giant cells may be present.[566] Small amounts of the gel form may remain in tissue sections after processing but the liquid forms are usually removed during paraffin processing, leading to the appearance of empty vacuoles.[558] A variable fibroblastic response ensues.[552] Artecoll and Dermalive, two new injectable esthetic microimplants, can also produce a granulomatous reaction.[555]

The reaction to silicone elastomer (silicone rubber), as used in joint prostheses, is strikingly different from that to liquid and gel forms of silicone and takes the form of foreign body granulomas.[558] The implant is sometimes extruded.[567]

Although earlier reports suggested that silicone is doubly refractile when examined with polarized light,[568] it is now thought that this property results from adulteration of the silicone with other material.[558] Talc deposition is sometimes seen with polarized light in these cases.[569] It is possibly introduced at the time of the implant surgery.

COLLAGEN IMPLANTS

The injection of bovine collagen (Zyderm®) is a relatively safe procedure used to correct defects caused by acne scars, trauma and aging.[552,570] Adverse reactions in the form of erythema, urticaria, abscess formation and induration of the injection site are relatively uncommon.[570,571] Granulomatous reactions are rare (see below).[572,573]

The mechanism of action of the implant appears to be to stimulate the deposition of new collagen by fibroblasts, which are increased in the vicinity of the implant.

Bovine collagen matrix, another bovine collagen product, is used to promote hemostasis in surgical wounds. It promotes the migration and attachment of stromal and epithelial cells, thereby accelerating wound healing.[574] Other implant materials are constantly being evaluated.[575]

Histopathology[552,576–579]
The bovine collagen commercially available as Zyderm® is composed mainly of type I collagen of relatively small fiber diameter. It can be recognized in tissues for several weeks after its injection as finely fibrillar material between the larger bundles of native collagen. In contrast to native collagen, which is birefringent under polarized light and which stains green with Masson's trichrome stain, bovine collagen fails to refract polarized light, stains a pale gray-violet color with Masson's trichrome stain and is only lightly eosinophilic in hematoxylin and eosin preparations.[576] Bovine collagen is apparently absorbed as it can no longer be detected by light microscopy or immunofluorescence techniques once several months have passed.[577]

Following injection of the material, a mild lymphocytic and histiocytic infiltrate is found around blood vessels in the vicinity. This is followed by a slight increase in the numbers of fibroblasts and the subsequent deposition of native collagen. Calcification, which is not uncommon at the site of injection of bovine collagen into animals, has not been recorded in humans. Rare reactions include the formation of foreign body granulomas[576,578] and abscesses[571] or of necrobiotic granulomas resembling granuloma annulare.[572]

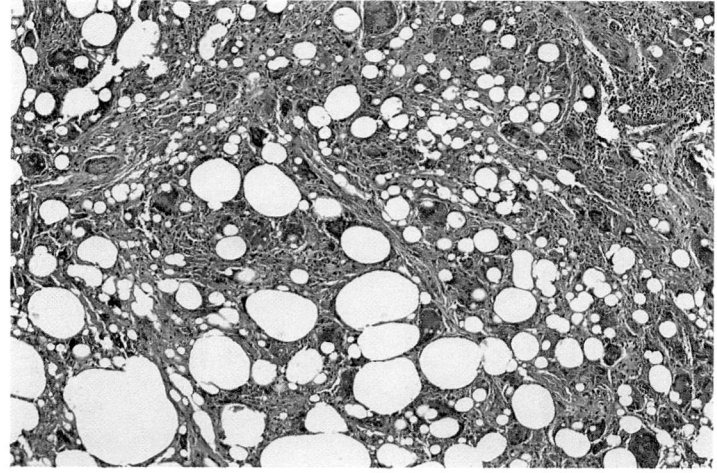

Fig. 14.30 **Silicone deposits** with characteristic vacuoles of varying size surrounded by macrophages and foreign body giant cells. (H & E)

MISCELLANEOUS DEPOSITS

OXALATE CRYSTALS

Oxalate crystals can be found in the skin in some cases of primary oxalosis, a genetically transmitted disorder of oxalate metabolism characterized by hyperoxaluria, nephrolithiasis, nephrocalcinosis and renal failure at an early age.[580,581] Cutaneous deposits are unusual in secondary oxalosis, which is seen most often in patients with chronic renal failure on long-term hemodialysis.[581] Such patients usually present with miliary deposits in the fingers, particularly on the palmar surface. A patient with multiple subcutaneous nodules has been reported.[582] Vascular deposition of oxalate crystals in either the primary or secondary form can produce livedo reticularis[583,584] or cutaneous necrosis.[585,586]

Histopathology[580–582]

Oxalate crystals, which are light yellow to brown in sections stained with hematoxylin and eosin, are birefringent. They are rhomboid in shape. They are deposited in the dermis and, rarely, as large nodular deposits in the subcutis. There may be a mild inflammatory reaction with some foreign body giant cells.

As the crystals usually contain calcium salts, they can be stained by the von Kossa method.[581]

In cases with livedo reticularis or cutaneous necrosis, oxalate crystals may be found in blood vessels in the subcutis.[583,585]

FIBERGLASS

Fiberglass dermatitis is rarely seen these days. Fiberglass can be identified in the stratum corneum and sometimes in the dermis after contact with this agent.[587]

MYOSPHERULOSIS

Myospherulosis refers to the histopathological changes of 'sac-like structures with endobodies'.[588,589] It is an incidental finding. In some instances, myospherulosis has followed the topical application of lanolin and petrolatum. The spherules are derived from erythrocytes altered by foreign lipids and human fat.[588]

REFERENCES

Introduction

1 Mehregan AH. Calcinosis cutis: a review of the clinical forms and report of 75 cases. Semin Dermatol 1984; 3: 53–61.

Calcium, bone and cartilage

2 Walsh JS, Fairley JA. Calcifying disorders of the skin. J Am Acad Dermatol 1995; 33: 693–706.
3 Touart DM, Sau P. Cutaneous deposition diseases. Part II. J Am Acad Dermatol 1998; 39: 527–544.
4 Rodriguez-Cano L, García-Patos V, Creus M et al. Childhood calcinosis cutis. Pediatr Dermatol 1996; 13: 114–117.
5 Lestringant GG, Masouyé I, El-Hayek M et al. Diffuse calcinosis cutis in a patient with congenital leukemia and leukemia cutis. Dermatology 2000; 200: 147–150.
6 Guberman D, Gilead LT, Nagler A. Skin calcinosis following allogenic bone marrow transplantation in an acute lymphoblastic leukaemia patient. Acta Derm Venereol 1999; 79: 324–325.
7 Shmunes E, Wood MG. Subepidermal calcified nodules. Arch Dermatol 1972; 105: 593–597.
8 Azón-Masoliver A, Ferrando J, Navarra E, Mascaro JM. Solitary congenital nodular calcification of Winer located on the ear: report of two cases. Pediatr Dermatol 1989; 6: 191–193.
9 Weigand DA. Subepidermal calcified nodule. Report of a case with apparent hair follicle origin. J Cutan Pathol 1976; 3: 109–115.
10 Butt KI, Tsuboi R, Takimoto R et al. Multiple subepidermal calcified nodules on the eyelids. Br J Dermatol 1995; 133: 664–665.
11 Evans MJ, Blessing K, Gray ES. Subepidermal calcified nodule in children: a clinicopathologic study of 21 cases. Pediatr Dermatol 1995; 12: 307–310.
12 Hansen KK, Segura AD, Esterly NB. Solitary congenital nodule on the ear of an infant. Pediatr Dermatol 1993; 10: 88–90.
13 Won JH, Ahn SK, Lee SH. Subepidermal calcified nodule of the ear in a child with hair follicle nevus. Int J Dermatol 1994; 33: 505–506.
14 Shapiro L, Platt N, Torres-Rodriguez VM. Idiopathic calcinosis of the scrotum. Arch Dermatol 1970; 102: 199–204.
15 Dekio S, Tsukazaki N, Jidoi J. Idiopathic calcinosis of the scrotum presenting as a solitary pedunculated tumour. Clin Exp Dermatol 1989; 14: 60–61.
16 Moss RL, Shewmake SW. Idiopathic calcinosis of the scrotum. Int J Dermatol 1981; 20: 134–136.
17 Song DH, Lee KH, Kang WH. Idiopathic calcinosis of the scrotum: histopathologic observations of fifty-one nodules. J Am Acad Dermatol 1988; 19: 1095–1101.
18 Swinehart JM, Golitz LE. Scrotal calcinosis. Dystrophic calcification of epidermoid cysts. Arch Dermatol 1982; 118: 985–988.
19 Dare AJ, Axelsen RA. Scrotal calcinosis: origin from dystrophic calcification of eccrine duct milia. J Cutan Pathol 1988; 15: 142–149.
20 Dini M, Colafranceschi M. Should scrotal calcinosis still be termed idiopathic? Am J Dermatopathol 1998; 20: 399–402.
21 Ito A, Sakamoto F, Ito M. Dystrophic scrotal calcinosis originating from benign eccrine epithelial cysts. Br J Dermatol 2001; 144: 146–150.
22 Gormally S, Dorman T, Powell FC. Calcinosis of the scrotum. Int J Dermatol 1992; 31: 75–79.
23 Wright S, Navsaria H, Leigh IM. Idiopathic scrotal calcinosis is idiopathic. J Am Acad Dermatol 1991; 24: 727–730.
24 Balfour PJT, Vincenti AC. Idiopathic vulvar calcinosis. Histopathology 1991; 18: 183–184.
25 Cecchi R, Giomi A. Idiopathic calcinosis cutis of the penis. Dermatology 1999; 198: 174–175.
26 Lucke T, Fallowfield M, McHenry P. Idiopathic calcinosis cutis of the penis. Br J Dermatol 1997; 137: 1025–1026.
27 Whiting DA, Simson IW, Kallmeyer JC, Dannheimer IPL. Unusual cutaneous lesions in tumoral calcinosis. Arch Dermatol 1970; 102: 465–473.
28 Pursley TV, Prince MJ, Chausmer AB, Raimer SS. Cutaneous manifestations of tumoral calcinosis. Arch Dermatol 1979; 115: 1100–1102.
29 McKee PH, Liomba NG, Hutt MSR. Tumoral calcinosis: a pathological study of fifty-six cases. Br J Dermatol 1982; 107: 669–674.
30 Harwood CA, Cook MG, Mortimer PS. Tumoral calcinosis: an unusual cause of cutaneous calcification. Clin Exp Dermatol 1996; 21: 163–166.
31 Slavin RE, Wen J, Kumar D, Evans EB. Familial tumoral calcinosis. Am J Surg Pathol 1993; 17: 788–802.
32 Smack DP, Norton SA, Fitzpatrick JE. Proposal for a pathogenesis-based classification of tumoral calcinosis. Int J Dermatol 1996; 35: 265–271.
33 Pakasa NM, Kalengayi RM. Tumoral calcinosis: a clinicopathological study of 111 cases with emphasis on the earliest changes. Histopathology 1997; 31: 18–24.
34 Chadwick JM, Downham TF. Auricular calcification. Int J Dermatol 1978; 17: 799–801.
35 Lautenschlager S, Itin PH, Rufli T. The petrified ear. Dermatology 1994; 189: 435–436.
36 Strumia R, Lombardi AR, Altieri E. The petrified ear – a manifestation of dystrophic calcification. Dermatology 1997; 194: 371–373.
37 Keane FM, Muller B, Murphy GM. Petrified ears. Clin Exp Dermatol 1997; 22: 242–243.
38 Yeatman JM, Varigos GA. Auricular ossification. Australas J Dermatol 1998; 39: 268–270.
39 Sell EJ, Hansen RC, Struck-Pierce S. Calcified nodules on the heel: a complication of neonatal intensive care. J Pediatr 1980; 96: 473–475.
40 Williamson D, Holt PJA. Calcified cutaneous nodules on the heels of children: a complication of heel sticks as a neonate. Pediatr Dermatol 2001; 18: 138–140.
41 Eng AM, Mandrea E. Perforating calcinosis cutis presenting as milia. J Cutan Pathol 1981; 8: 247–250.
42 Neild VS, Marsden RA. Pseudomilia – widespread cutaneous calculi. Clin Exp Dermatol 1985; 10: 398–401.
43 Sais G, Jucgla A, Moreno A, Peyri J. Milia-like idiopathic calcinosis cutis and multiple connective tissue nevi in a patient with Down syndrome. J Am Acad Dermatol 1995; 32: 129–130.
44 Schepis C, Siragusa M, Palazzo R et al. Milia-like idiopathic calcinosis cutis: an unusual dermatosis associated with Down syndrome. Br J Dermatol 1996; 134: 143–146.
45 Schepis C, Siragusa M, Palazzo R et al. Perforating milia-like idiopathic calcinosis cutis and periorbital syringomas in a girl with Down syndrome. Pediatr Dermatol 1994; 11: 258–260.
46 Kim D-H, Kang H, Cho S-H, Park Y-M. Solitary milialike idiopathic calcinosis cutis unassociated with Down's syndrome: two case reports. Acta Derm Venereol 2000; 80: 15–16.
47 Nielsen AO, Johnson E, Hentzer B, Kobayasi T. Dermatomyositis with universal calcinosis. J Cutan Pathol 1979; 6: 486–491.
48 Kawakami T, Nakamura C, Hasegawa H et al. Ultrastructural study of calcinosis universalis with dermatomyositis. J Cutan Pathol 1986; 13: 135–143.

49 Wananukul S, Pongprasit P, Wattanakrai P. Calcinosis cutis presenting years before other clinical manifestations of juvenile dermatomyositis: Report of two cases. Australas J Dermatol 1997; 38: 202–205.

50 Kabir DI, Malkinson FD. Lupus erythematosus and calcinosis cutis. Arch Dermatol 1969; 100: 17–22.

51 Johansson E, Kanerva L, Niemi K-M, Välimäki MM. Diffuse soft tissue calcifications (calcinosis cutis) in a patient with discoid lupus erythematosus. Clin Exp Dermatol 1988; 13: 193–196.

52 Rothe MJ, Grant-Kels JM, Rothfield NF. Extensive calcinosis cutis with systemic lupus erythematosus. Arch Dermatol 1990; 126: 1060–1063.

53 Nomura M, Okada N, Okada M, Yoshikawa K. Large subcutaneous calcification in systemic lupus erythematosus. Arch Dermatol 1990; 126: 1057–1059.

54 Marzano AV, Kolesnikova LV, Gasparini G, Alessi E. Dystrophic calcinosis cutis in subacute lupus. Dermatology 1999; 198: 90–92.

55 Brazzelli V, Dell'Orbo C, Borroni G et al. The role of the intercellular matrix in dermal calcinosis of the CRST syndrome. Am J Dermatopathol 1992; 14: 42–49.

56 Kawakami T, Soma Y, Mizoguchi M, Saito R. Immunohistochemical expression of transforming growth factor β3 in calcinosis in a patient with systemic sclerosis and CREST syndrome. Br J Dermatol 2000; 143: 1098–1100.

57 Magee KL, Schauder CS, Drucker CR, Rapini RP. Extensive calcinosis as a late complication of pentazocine injections: response to therapy with steroids and aluminum hydroxide. Arch Dermatol 1991; 127: 1591–1592.

58 Firooz A, Tehranchi-nia Z, Ahmed AR. Benefits and risks of intralesional corticosteroid injection in the treatment of dermatological diseases. Clin Exp Dermatol 1995; 20: 363–370.

59 Carruthers J, Jevon G, Prendiville J. Localized dystrophic periocular calcification: a complication of intralesional corticosteroid therapy for infantile periocular hemangiomas. Pediatr Dermatol 1998; 15: 23–26.

60 Oga A, Kadowaki T, Hamanaka S, Sasaki K. Dystrophic calcinosis cutis in the skin below the mandible of a violinist. Br J Dermatol 1998; 139: 940–941.

61 Jucglà A, Sais G, Curco N et al. Calcinosis cutis following liver transplantation: a complication of intravenous calcium administration. Br J Dermatol 1995; 132: 275–278.

62 Sahn EE. Annular dystrophic calcinosis cutis in an infant. J Am Acad Dermatol 1992; 26: 1015–1017.

63 Ahn SK, Kim KT, Lee SH et al. The efficacy of treatment with triamcinolone acetonide in calcinosis cutis following extravasation of calcium gluconate: a preliminary study. Pediatr Dermatol 1997; 14: 103–109.

64 Millard TP, Harris AJ, MacDonald DM. Calcinosis cutis following intravenous infusion of calcium gluconate. Br J Dermatol 1999; 140: 184–186.

65 Wheeland RG, Roundtree JM. Calcinosis cutis resulting from percutaneous penetration and deposition of calcium. J Am Acad Dermatol 1985; 12: 172–175.

66 Goldminz D, Barnhill R, McGuire J, Stenn KS. Calcinosis cutis following extravasation of calcium chloride. Arch Dermatol 1988; 124: 922–925.

67 Puig L, Rocamora V, Romaní J et al. Calcinosis cutis following calcium chloride electrode paste application for auditory-brainstem evoked potentials recording. Pediatr Dermatol 1998; 15: 27–30.

68 Beers BB, Flowers FP, Sherertz EF, Selden S. Dystrophic calcinosis cutis secondary to intrauterine herpes simplex. Pediatr Dermatol 1986; 3: 208–211.

69 Chaves Alvarez AJ, Herrera Saval A, Marquez Enriquez J, Camacho Martinez F. Metastatic calcinosis cutis in multiple myeloma. Br J Dermatol 2000; 142: 820–822.

70 Grattan CEH, Buist L, Hubscher SG. Metastatic calcification and cytomegalovirus infection. Br J Dermatol 1988; 119: 785–788.

71 Lázaro TE, Hernández-Cano N, Rubio FA et al. Cutaneous calcinosis with transepithelial elimination in a patient with sarcoidosis. Int J Dermatol 1998; 37: 41–43.

72 Cochran RJ, Wilkin JK. An unusual case of calcinosis cutis. J Am Acad Dermatol 1983; 8: 103–106.

73 Grob JJ, Legre R, Bertocchio P et al. Calcifying panniculitis and kidney failure. Considerations on pathogenesis and treatment of calciphylaxis. Int J Dermatol 1989; 28: 129–131.

74 Zouboulis ChC, Blume-Peytavi U, Lennert Th et al. Fulminant metastatic calcinosis with cutaneous necrosis in a child with end-stage renal disease and tertiary hyperparathyroidism. Br J Dermatol 1996; 135: 617–622.

75 Oh DH, Eulau D, Tokugawa DA et al. Five cases of calciphylaxis and a review of the literature. J Am Acad Dermatol 1999; 40: 979–987.

76 Wong JJ, Laumann A, Martinez M. Calciphylaxis and antiphospholipid antibody syndrome. J Am Acad Dermatol 2000; 42: 849.

77 Streit M, Paredes BE, Rüegger S, Brand CU. Typical features of calciphylaxis in a patient with end-stage renal failure, diabetes mellitus and oral anticoagulation. Dermatology 2000; 200: 356–359.

78 Robinson-Bostom L, DiGiovanna JJ. Cutaneous manifestations of end-stage renal disease. J Am Acad Dermatol 2000; 43: 975–986.

79 Cockerell CJ, Dolan ET. Widespread cutaneous and systemic calcification (calciphylaxis) in patients with the acquired immunodeficiency syndrome and renal disease. J Am Acad Dermatol 1992; 26: 559–562.

80 Ivker RA, Woosley J, Briggaman RA. Calciphylaxis in three patients with end-stage renal disease. Arch Dermatol 1995; 131: 63–68.

81 Pollock B, Cunliffe WJ, Merchant WJ. Calciphylaxis in the absence of renal failure. Clin Exp Dermatol 2000; 25: 389–392.

82 Buxtorf K, Cerottini J-P, Panizzon RG. Lower limb skin ulcerations, intravascular calcifications and sensorimotor polyneuropathy: calciphylaxis as part of a hyperparathyroidism? Dermatology 1999; 198: 423–425.

83 Goyal S, Huhn KM, Provost TT. Calciphylaxis in a patient without renal failure or elevated parathyroid hormone: possible aetiological role of chemotherapy. Br J Dermatol 2000; 143: 1087–1090.

84 Mastruserio DN, Nguyen EQ, Nielsen T et al. Calciphylaxis associated with metastatic breast carcinoma. J Am Acad Dermatol 1999; 41: 295–298.

85 Kossard S, Winkelmann RK. Vascular calcification in dermatopathology. Am J Dermatopathol 1979; 1: 27–34.

86 Yoong AKH, Smallman LA. Cutaneous gangrene, metastatic calcification and secondary hyperparathyroidism. Histopathology 1991; 18: 92–93.

87 Török L, Középessy L. Uraemic gangrene syndrome. Acta Derm Venereol 1991; 71: 455–457.

88 Tada J, Torigoe R, Shimoe K et al. Calcium deposition in the skin of a hemodialysis patient with widespread skin necrosis. Am J Dermatopathol 1991; 13: 605–610.

89 Maroon M, Tyler W, Marks VJ. Calcinosis cutis associated with syringomas: a transepidermal elimination disorder in a patient with Down syndrome. J Am Acad Dermatol 1990; 23: 372–375.

90 Solomon AR, Comite SL, Headington JT. Epidermal and follicular calciphylaxis. J Cutan Pathol 1988; 15: 282–285.

91 Mehta S, Crawford R. Three-dimensional analysis of a calciphylaxis lesion – clues to pathogenesis. J Cutan Pathol 2000; 27: 542 (abstract).

92 Essary LR, Wick MR. Cutaneous calciphylaxis. An underrecognized clinicopathologic entity. Am J Clin Pathol 2000; 113: 280–287.

93 Roth SI, Stowell RE, Helwig EB. Cutaneous ossification. Arch Pathol 1963; 76: 44–54.

94 Burgdorf W, Nasemann T. Cutaneous osteomas: a clinical and histopathologic review. Arch Derm Res 1977; 260: 121–135.

95 Sanmartin O, Alegre V, Martinez-Aparicio A et al. Congenital platelike osteoma cutis: case report and review of the literature. Pediatr Dermatol 1993; 10: 182–186.

96 Worret WI, Burgdorf W. Congenital plaque-like cutaneous osteoma. Hautarzt 1978; 29: 590–596.

97 Combes FC, Vanina R. Osteosis cutis. Arch Dermatol 1954; 69: 613–615.

98 Alegre VA, Pujol C, Martinez A, Aliaga A. Cutaneous ossification: report of three cases. J Cutan Pathol 1989; 16: 293 (abstract).

99 Fiedler E, Fellner F, Mahler V, Dobritz M. Cutaneous osteoma of the scalp. Br J Dermatol 1999; 140: 547–549.

100 Takato T, Yanai A, Tanaka H, Nagata S. Primary osteoma cutis of the back. Plast Reconstr Surg 1986; 77: 309–311.

101 Voncina D. Osteoma cutis. Dermatologica 1974; 148: 257–261.

102 Foster CM, Levin S, Levine M et al. Limited dermal ossification: clinical features and natural history. J Pediatr 1986; 109: 71–76.

103 Lim MO, Mukherjee AB, Hansen JW. Dysplastic cutaneous osteomatosis. Arch Dermatol 1981; 117: 797–799.

104 Maclean GD, Main RA, Anderson TE, Best PV. Connective tissue ossification presenting in the skin. Arch Dermatol 1966; 94: 168–174.

105 Gardner RJM, Yun K, Craw SM. Familial ectopic ossification. J Med Genet 1988; 25: 113–117.

106 O'Donnell TF, Geller SA. Primary osteoma cutis. Arch Dermatol 1971; 104: 325–326.

107 Peterson WC, Mandel SL. Primary osteomas of skin. Arch Dermatol 1963; 87: 626–632.

108 Gorman A, Rich P, White C. Multiple atrophic osteoma cutis in a newborn: a new entity? J Cutan Pathol 2000; 27: 542 (abstract).

109 Goldminz D, Greenberg RD. Multiple miliary osteoma cutis. J Am Acad Dermatol 1991; 24: 878–881.

110 Rossman RE, Freeman RG. Osteoma cutis, a stage of preosseous calcification. Arch Dermatol 1964; 89: 68–73.

111 Monteiro MR, Koblenzer CS. Multiple osteoma cutis lesions associated with acne. Int J Dermatol 2000; 39: 553–554.

112 Lo Scocco G, Di Lernia V, Bisighini G. Multiple miliary osteoma of the face. Clin Exp Dermatol 1997; 22: 152–153.

113 Novak C, Siller G, Wood D. Idiopathic multiple miliary osteomas of the face. Australas J Dermatol 1998; 39: 109–111.

114 Ochsendorf FR, Kaufmann R. Erbium: YAG laser ablation of osteoma cutis: modifications of the approach. Arch Dermatol 1999; 135: 1416.

115 Altman JF, Nehal KS, Busam KJ, Halpern AC. Treatment of primary miliary osteoma cutis with incision, curettage, and primary closure. J Am Acad Dermatol 2001; 44: 96–99.

116 Helm F, de la Pava S, Klein E. Multiple miliary osteomas of the skin. Arch Dermatol 1967; 96: 681–682.

117 Boneschi V, Alessi E, Brambilla L. Multiple miliary osteomas of the face. Am J Dermatopathol 1993; 15: 268–271.

118 Saluja A, McCall CO. Firm papules on the face: multiple miliary osteoma cutis. J Cutan Pathol 2000; 27: 542 (abstract).

119 Piesowicz AT. Pseudo-pseudo-hypoparathyroidism with osteoma cutis. Proc R Soc Med 1965; 58: 126–128.

120 Brook CGD, Valman HB. Osteoma cutis and Albright's hereditary osteodystrophy. Br J Dermatol 1971; 85: 471–475.

121 Barranco VP. Cutaneous ossification in pseudohypoparathyroidism. Arch Dermatol 1971; 104: 643–647.

122 Eyre WG, Reed WB. Albright's hereditary osteodystrophy with cutaneous bone formation. Arch Dermatol 1971; 104: 634–642.

123 Prendiville JS, Lucky AW, Mallory SB et al. Osteoma cutis as a presenting sign of pseudohypoparathyroidism. Pediatr Dermatol 1992; 9: 11–18.

124 Goeteyn V, De Potter CR, Naeyaert JM. Osteoma cutis in pseudohypoparathyroidism. Dermatology 1999; 198: 209–211.

125 Miller ES, Esterly NB, Fairley JA. Progressive osseous heteroplasia. Arch Dermatol 1996; 132: 787–791.

126 Jang K-A, Choi J-H, Sung K-J et al. Progressive osseous heteroplasia: a case report. Pediatr Dermatol 1999; 16: 74–75.

127 Miller ES, Esterly NB, Fairley JA. Progressive osseous heteroplasia. Arch Dermatol 1996; 132: 787–791.

128 Kaplan FS. Skin and bones. Arch Dermatol 1996; 132: 815–818.

129 Rogers JG, Geho WB. Fibrodysplasia ossificans progressiva. A survey of forty-two cases. J Bone Joint Surg 1979; 61A: 909–914.

130 Fulton RA, Smith GD, Thomson J. Bone formation in a cutaneous pyogenic granuloma. Br J Dermatol 1980; 102: 351–352.

131 Wilson Jones E, Heyl T. Naevus sebaceus. A report of 140 cases with special regard to the development of secondary malignant tumours. Br J Dermatol 1970; 82: 99–117.

132 Moreno A, Lamarca J, Martinez R, Guix M. Osteoid and bone formation in desmoplastic malignant melanoma. J Cutan Pathol 1986; 13: 128–134.

133 Fletcher CDM. Calcifying and ossifying soft tissue lesions presenting in the skin. J Cutan Pathol 1996; 23: 297.

134 Basler RSW, Watters JH, Taylor WB. Calcifying acne lesions. Int J Dermatol 1977; 16: 755–758.

135 Dupree WB, Enzinger FM. Fibro-osseous pseudotumor of the digits. Cancer 1986; 58: 2103–2109.

136 Marteinsson BTH, Musgrove JE. Heterotopic bone formation in abdominal incisions. Am J Surg 1975; 130: 23–25.

137 Lippmann HI, Goldin RR. Subcutaneous ossification of the legs in chronic venous insufficiency. Radiology 1960; 74: 279–288.

138 Monroe AB, Burgdorf WHC, Sheward S. Platelike cutaneous osteoma. J Am Acad Dermatol 1987; 16: 481–484.

139 Ahn SK, Won JH, Choi EH et al. Perforating plate-like osteoma cutis in a man with solitary morphoea profunda. Br J Dermatol 1996; 134: 949–952.

140 Kewalramani LD, Orth MS. Ectopic ossification. Am J Phys Med 1977; 56: 99–121.

141 Shelley WB, Wood MG. Alopecia with fibrous dysplasia and osteomas of skin. A sign of polyostotic fibrous dysplasia. Arch Dermatol 1976; 112: 715–719.

142 Walter JF, Macknet KD. Pigmentation of osteoma cutis caused by tetracycline. Arch Dermatol 1979; 115: 1087–1088.

143 Moritz DL, Elewski B. Pigmented postacne osteoma cutis in a patient treated with minocycline: report and review of the literature. J Am Acad Dermatol 1991; 24: 851–853.

144 Hsueh S, Santa Cruz DJ. Cartilaginous lesions of the skin and superficial soft tissue. J Cutan Pathol 1982; 9: 405–416.

145 Hogan D, Wilkinson RD, Williams A. Congenital anomalies of the head and neck. Int J Dermatol 1980; 19: 479–486.

146 Clarke JA. Are wattles of auricular or branchial origin? Br J Plast Surg 1976; 29: 238–244.

147 Vaughan TK, Sperling LC. Diagnosis and surgical treatment of congenital cartilaginous rests of the neck. Arch Dermatol 1991; 127: 1309–1310.

148 Rachman R, Heffernan AH. Elastic cartilage choristoma of the neck. Plast Reconstr Surg 1979; 63: 424–425.

149 Dahlin DC, Salvador AH. Cartilaginous tumors of the soft tissues of the hands and feet. Mayo Clin Proc 1974; 49: 721–726.

150 Schiffman R. Nuchal fibrocartilagenous pseudotumor. Am J Surg Pathol 1997; 22: 776.

151 O'Connell JX, Janzen DL, Hughes TR. Nuchal fibrocartilaginous pseudotumor: a distinctive soft-tissue lesion associated with prior neck injury. Am J Surg Pathol 1997; 21: 836–840.

152 Paslin DA. Cartilaginous papule of the ear. J Cutan Pathol 1991; 18: 60–63.

Hyaline deposits

153 Niemi K-M, Anton-Lamprecht I, Virtanen I et al. Fibrillar protein deposits with tubular substructure in a systemic disease beginning as cutis laxa. Arch Dermatol 1993; 129: 757–762.

154 O'Duffy JD, Hunder GG, Kelly PJ. Decreasing prevalence of tophaceous gout. Mayo Clin Proc 1975; 50: 227–228.

155 Lichtenstein L, Scott HW, Levin MH. Pathologic changes in gout. Survey of eleven necropsied cases. Am J Pathol 1956; 32: 871–886.

156 Niemi K-M. Panniculitis of the legs with urate crystal deposition. Report of a case. Arch Dermatol 1977; 113: 655–656.

157 Le Boit PE, Schneider S. Gout presenting as lobular panniculitis. Am J Dermatopathol 1987; 9: 334–338.

158 Sharma A. Baethge BA, Smith EB et al. Gout masquerading as rheumatoid vasculitis. J Rheumatol 1994; 21: 368–369.

159 Vanhooteghem O, Andre J, Pochet JM et al. Occurrence of gouty tophi following acitretin therapy. Clin Exp Dermatol 1998; 23: 274–276.

160 Fam AG, Assaad D. Intradermal urate tophi. J Rheumatol 1997; 24: 1126–1131.

161 Palmer DG, Highton J, Hessian PA. Development of the gout tophus. An hypothesis. Am J Clin Pathol 1989; 91: 190–195.

162 Lucke TW, Fallowfield ME, Evans A et al. Transepidermal elimination of urate-like crystals: a new perforating disorder? Br J Dermatol 1999; 141: 310–314.

163 Breathnach SM, Black MM. Systemic amyloidosis and the skin: a review with special emphasis on clinical features and therapy. Clin Exp Dermatol 1979; 4: 517–536.

164 Breathnach SM. The cutaneous amyloidoses. Pathogenesis and therapy. Arch Dermatol 1985; 121: 470–475.

165 Breathnach SM. Amyloid and amyloidosis. J Am Acad Dermatol 1988; 18: 1–16.

166 Tan SY, Pepys MB. Amyloidosis. Histopathology 1994; 25: 403–414.

167 Röcken C, Schwotzer EB, Linke RP, Saeger W. The classification of amyloid deposits in clinicopathological practice. Histopathology 1996; 29: 325–335.

168 Lee D-D, Huang C-Y, Wong C-K. Dermatopathologic findings in 20 cases of systemic amyloidosis. Am J Dermatopathol 1998; 20: 438–442.

169 Huilgol SC, Ramnarain N, Carrington P et al. Cytokeratins in primary cutaneous amyloidosis. Australas J Dermatol 1998; 39: 81–85.

170 Manabe T, Sugihara K. β2-microglobulin type cutaneous nodular amyloidosis in patients on long-term hemodialysis. Dermatopathology: Practical & Conceptual 1998; 4: 34–38.

171 Furumoto H, Shimizu T, Asagami C et al. Apolipoprotein E is present in primary localized cutaneous amyloidosis. J Invest Dermatol 1998; 111: 417–421.

172 Chang YT, Wong CK, Chow KC, Tsai CH. Apoptosis in primary cutaneous amyloidosis. Br J Dermatol 1999; 140: 210–215.

173 Horiguchi Y, Fine J-D, Leigh IM et al. Lamina densa malformation involved in histogenesis of primary localized cutaneous amyloidosis. J Invest Dermatol 1992; 99: 12–18.

174 Lee Y-S, Fong P-H. Macular and lichenoid amyloidosis: a possible secretory product of stimulated basal keratinocytes. An ultrastructural study. Pathology 1991; 23: 322–326.

175 Ebner H, Gebhart W. Light and electron microscopic differentiation of amyloid and colloid or hyaline bodies. Br J Dermatol 1975; 92: 637–645.

176 Shapiro L, Kurban AK, Azar HA. Lichen amyloidosus. A histochemical and electron microscopic study. Arch Pathol 1970; 90: 499–508.

177 Hashimoto K, Ito K, Kumakiri M, Headington J. Nylon brush macular amyloidosis. Arch Dermatol 1987; 123: 633–637.

178 Hashimoto K. Diseases of amyloid, colloid, and hyalin. J Cutan Pathol 1985; 12: 322–333.

179 Yanagihara M, Mehregan AH, Mehregan DR. Staining of amyloid with cotton dyes. Arch Dermatol 1984; 120: 1184–1185.

180 Sharma SC, Mortimer G, Kennedy S, Thomson J. Secondary amyloidosis affecting the skin in arthropathic psoriasis. Br J Dermatol 1983; 108: 205–210.

181 Wright JR. Clinical-pathologic differentiation of common amyloid syndromes. Medicine (Baltimore) 1981; 69: 429–448.

182 Noren P, Westermark P, Cornwell GG, Murdoch W. Immunofluorescence and histochemical studies of localized cutaneous amyloidosis. Br J Dermatol 1983; 108: 277–285.

183 Hintner H, Booker J, Ashworth J et al. Amyloid P component binds to keratin bodies in human skin and to isolated keratin filament aggregates in vitro. J Invest Dermatol 1988; 91: 22–28.

184 Breathnach SM, Bhogal B, Dyck RF et al. Immunohistochemical demonstration of amyloid P component in skin of normal subjects and patients with cutaneous amyloidosis. Br J Dermatol 1981; 105: 115–124.

185 Ishii M, Asai Y, Hamada T. Evaluation of cutaneous amyloid employing anti-keratin antibodies and the immunoperoxidase technique (PAP method). Acta Derm Venereol 1984; 64: 281–285.

186 Kobayashi H, Hashimoto K. Amyloidogenesis in organ-limited cutaneous amyloidosis: an antigenic identity between epidermal keratin and skin amyloid. J Invest Dermatol 1983; 80: 66–72.

187 Maeda H, Ohta S, Saito Y et al. Epidermal origin of the amyloid in localized cutaneous amyloidosis. Br J Dermatol 1982; 106: 345–351.

188 Masu S, Hosokawa M, Seiji M. Amyloid in localized cutaneous amyloidosis: immunofluorescence studies with anti-keratin antiserum especially concerning the difference between systemic and localized cutaneous amyloidosis. Acta Derm Venereol 1981; 61: 381–384.

189 MacDonald DM, Black MM, Ramnarain N. Immunofluorescence studies in primary localized cutaneous amyloidosis. Br J Dermatol 1977; 96: 635–641.

190 Habermann MC, Montenegro MR. Primary cutaneous amyloidosis: clinical, laboratory and histopathological study of 25 cases. Dermatologica 1980; 160: 240–248.

191 Mukai H, Eto H, Nishiyama S, Hashimoto K. Differential staining of skin-limited amyloid and colloid bodies with immunofluorescence after pretreatments. J Invest Dermatol 1988; 90: 520–525.

192 Danielsen L, Kobayasi T. An ultrastructural study of cutaneous amyloidosis. Acta Derm Venereol 1973; 53: 13–21.

193 Yanagihara M, Kato F, Shikano Y et al. Intimate structural association of amyloid and elastic fibers in systemic and cutaneous amyloidoses. J Cutan Pathol 1985; 12: 110–116.

194 Kobayasi T, Asboe-Hansen G. Ultrastructure of skin in primary systemic amyloidosis. Acta Derm Venereol 1979; 59: 407–413.

195 Hashimoto K, Onn LLY. Lichen amyloidosus. Electron microscopic study of a typical case and a review. Arch Dermatol 1971; 104: 648–666.

196 Runne U, Orfanos CE. Amyloid production by dermal fibroblasts. Br J Dermatol 1977; 97: 155–166.

197 Kumakiri M, Hashimoto K. Histogenesis of primary localized cutaneous amyloidosis: sequential change of epidermal keratinocytes to amyloid via filamentous degeneration. J Invest Dermatol 1979; 73: 150–162.

198 Hashimoto K, Kobayashi H. Histogenesis of amyloid in the skin. Am J Dermatopathol 1980; 2: 165–171.

199 Jambrosic J, From L, Hanna W. Lichen amyloidosus. Ultrastructure and pathogenesis. Am J Dermatopathol 1984; 6: 151–158.

200 Black MM. The role of the epidermis in the histopathogenesis of lichen amyloidosus. Br J Dermatol 1971; 85: 524–530.

201 Black MM, Wilson Jones E. Macular amyloidosis. A study of 21 cases with special reference to the role of the epidermis in its histogenesis. Br J Dermatol 1971; 84: 199–209.

202 Hashimoto K. Progress on cutaneous amyloidoses. J Invest Dermatol 1984; 82: 1–3.

203 Bluhm JF, Johnson SC, Norback DH. Bullous amyloidosis. Case report with ultrastructural studies. Arch Dermatol 1980; 115: 1164–1168.

204 Franklin EC. Amyloid and amyloidosis of the skin. J Invest Dermatol 1976; 67: 451–456.

205 Ratz JL, Bailin PL. Cutaneous amyloidosis. J Am Acad Dermatol 1981; 4: 21–26.

206 Taylor SC, Baker E, Grossman ME. Nodular vulvar amyloid as a presentation of systemic amyloidosis. J Am Acad Dermatol 1991; 24: 139.

207 Ahmed I, Cronk JS, Crutchfield CE III, Dahl MV. Myeloma-associated systemic amyloidosis presenting as chronic paronychia and palmodigital erythematous swelling and induration of the hands. J Am Acad Dermatol 2000; 42: 339–342.

208 Fairrie G, McKenzie AW. An unusual presentation of systemic amyloidosis. Br J Dermatol 1981; 105: 469–470.

209 Bedlow AJ, Sampson SA, Holden CA. Primary systemic amyloidosis of the hair and nails. Clin Exp Dermatol 1998; 23: 298–299.

210 Noojin RO, Arrington TS. Unusual cutaneous findings in primary systemic amyloidosis. Arch Dermatol 1965; 92: 157–159.

211 Beacham BE, Greer KE, Andrews BS, Cooper PH. Bullous amyloidosis. J Am Acad Dermatol 1980; 3: 506–510.

212 Bieber T, Ruzicka T, Linke RP et al. Hemorrhagic bullous amyloidosis. Arch Dermatol 1988; 124: 1683–1686.

213 Pramatarov K, Lazarova A, Mateev G, Popov A. Bullous hemorrhagic primary systemic amyloidosis. Int J Dermatol 1990; 29: 211–213.

214 Westermark P, Ohman S, Domar M, Sletten K. Bullous amyloidosis. Arch Dermatol 1981; 117: 782–784.

215 Breathnach SM, Wells GC. Amyloid vascular disease: cord-like thickening of mucocutaneous arteries, intermittent claudication and angina in a case with underlying myelomatosis. Br J Dermatol 1980; 102: 591–595.

216 Buezo GF, Peñas PF, Firaga J et al. Condyloma-like lesions as the presenting sign of multiple myeloma associated amyloidosis. Br J Dermatol 1996; 135: 665–666.

217 Yoneda K, Kanoh T, Nomura S et al. Elastolytic cutaneous lesions in myeloma-associated amyloidosis. Arch Dermatol 1990; 126: 657–660.

218 Brownstein MH, Helwig EB. The cutaneous amyloidoses. II. Systemic forms. Arch Dermatol 1970; 102: 20–28.

219 Westermark P. Amyloidosis of the skin: comparison between localized and systemic amyloidosis. Acta Derm Venereol 1979; 59: 341–345.

220 Rubinow A, Cohen AS. Skin involvement in generalized amyloidosis. Ann Intern Med 1978; 88: 781–785.

221 Masouyé I. Diagnostic screening of systemic amyloidosis by abdominal fat aspiration: an analysis of 100 cases. Am J Dermatopathol 1997; 19: 41–45.

222 Wittenberg GP, Oursler JR, Peters MS. Secondary amyloidosis complicating psoriasis. J Am Acad Dermatol 1995; 32: 465–468.

223 Brownstein MH, Helwig EB. Systemic amyloidosis complicating dermatoses. Arch Dermatol 1970; 102: 1–7.

224 Albers SE, Fenske NA, Glass LF et al. Atypical β2-microglobulin amyloidosis following short-term hemodialysis. Am J Dermatopathol 1994; 16: 179–184.

225 Sato KC, Kumakiri M, Koizumi H et al. Lichenoid skin lesions as a sign of β2-microglobulin-induced amyloidosis in a long-term haemodialysis patient. Br J Dermatol 1993; 128: 686–689.

226 Cohen AS. An update of clinical, pathologic, and biochemical aspects of amyloidosis. Int J Dermatol 1981; 20: 515–530.

227 Ramsey B, Terenghi G, Polak JM et al. Depleted cutaneous innervation in familial amyloid. Clin Exp Dermatol 1996; 21: 449–450.

228 Muckle TJ. The 'Muckle–Wells' syndrome. Br J Dermatol 1979; 100: 87–92.

229 Lieberman A, Grossman ME, Silvers DN. Muckle–Wells syndrome: Case report and review of cutaneous pathology. J Am Acad Dermatol 1998; 39: 290–291.

230 Winkelmann RK, Peters MS, Venencie PY. Amyloid elastosis. A new cutaneous and systemic pattern of amyloidosis. Arch Dermatol 1985; 121: 498–502.

231 Sepp N, Pichler E, Breathnach SM et al. Amyloid elastosis: analysis of the role of amyloid P component. J Am Acad Dermatol 1990; 22: 27–34.

232 Kibbi A-G, Rubeiz NG, Zaynoun ST, Kurban AK. Primary localized cutaneous amyloidosis. Int J Dermatol 1992; 31: 95–98.

233 Al-Ratrout JT, Satti MB. Primary localized cutaneous amyloidosis: a clinicopathologic study from Saudi Arabia. Int J Dermatol 1997; 36: 428–434.

234 Brownstein MH, Hashimoto K, Greenwald G. Biphasic amyloidosis: link between macular and lichenoid forms. Br J Dermatol 1973; 88: 25–29.

235 Toribio J, Quinones PA, Vigil TR, Santa Cruz CS. Mixed (lichenoid and macular) cutaneous amyloidoses. Acta Derm Venereol 1975; 55: 221–226.

236 Bourke JF, Berth-Jones J, Burns DA. Diffuse primary cutaneous amyloidosis. Br J Dermatol 1992; 127: 641–644.

237 Tay CH, Dacosta JL. Lichen amyloidosis. Clinical study of 40 cases. Br J Dermatol 1970; 82: 129–136.

238 De Argila D, Ortiz-Romero PL, Ortiz-Frutos J et al. Cutaneous macular amyloidosis associated with multiple endocrine neoplasia 2A. Clin Exp Dermatol 1996; 21: 313–314.

239 Soler-Carrillo J, Alsina-Gibert MM, Mascaró JM. Lichen amyloidosus universalis associated with long-term drug intake. Dermatology 1997; 195: 286–288.

240 Fujiwara K, Kono T, Ishii M et al. Primary localized cutaneous amyloidosis associated with autoimmune cholangitis. Int J Dermatol 2000; 39: 768–771.

241 Hongcharu W, Baldassano M, Gonzalez E. Generalized lichen amyloidosis associated with chronic lichen planus. J Am Acad Dermatol 2000; 43: 346–348.

242 Apaydin R, Bilen N, Bayramgürler D et al. Lichen amyloidosis, ankylosing spondylitis and autoimmune thyroiditis: coincidence or association? J Eur Acad Dermatol Venereol 2000; 14: 135–137.

243 Le Boit PE, Greene I. Primary cutaneous amyloidosis: identically distributed lesions in identical twins. Pediatr Dermatol 1986; 3: 244–246.

244 Weitzner S, Keen PE, Doughty WE. Primary localized amyloidosis of glans penis. Arch Dermatol 1970; 102: 463–464.

245 Wong C-K. Cutaneous amyloidoses. Int J Dermatol 1987; 26: 273–277.

246 Drago F, Ranieri E, Pastorino A et al. Epstein–Barr virus-related primary cutaneous amyloidosis. Successful treatment with acyclovir and interferon-alpha. Br J Dermatol 1996; 134: 170–174.

247 Chang YT, Liu HN, Wong CK et al. Detection of Epstein–Barr virus in primary cutaneous amyloidosis. Br J Dermatol 1997; 136: 823–826.

248 Weyers W, Weyers I, Bonczkowitz M et al. Lichen amyloidosus: A consequence of scratching. J Am Acad Dermatol 1997; 37: 923–928.

249 Drago F, Rebora A. Lichen amyloidosus: A consequence of scratching? J Am Acad Dermatol 1999; 41: 501.

250 Goller MM, Cohen PR, Duvic M. Lichen amyloidosis presenting as a papular pruritus syndrome in a human-immunodeficiency-virus-infected man. Dermatology 1997; 194: 62–64.

251 Behr FD, Levine N, Bangert J. Lichen amyloidosis associated with atopic dermatitis. Clinical resolution with cyclosporine. Arch Dermatol 2001; 137: 553–555.

252 Black MM, Maibach HI. Macular amyloidosis simulating naevoid hyperpigmentation. Br J Dermatol 1974; 90: 461–464.

253 Wang CK, Lee JY-Y. Macular amyloidosis with widespread diffuse pigmentation. Br J Dermatol 1996; 135: 135–138.

254 An HT, Han KH, Cho KH. Macular amyloidosis with an incontinentia pigmenti-like pattern. Br J Dermatol 2000; 142: 371–373.

255 Wang C-K, Lee JY-Y. Macular amyloidosis with widespread diffuse pigmentation. Br J Dermatol 1996; 135: 135–138.

256 Shanon J, Sagher F. Interscapular cutaneous amyloidosis. Arch Dermatol 1970; 102: 195–198.

257 Wong C-K, Lin C-S. Friction amyloidosis. Int J Dermatol 1988; 27: 302–307.

258 MacSween RM, Saihan EM. Nylon cloth amyloidosis. Clin Exp Dermatol 1997; 22: 28–29.

259 Goulden V, Highet AS, Shamy HK. Notalgia paraesthetica – report of an association with macular amyloidosis. Clin Exp Dermatol 1994; 19: 346–349.

260 Sumitra S, Yesudian P. Friction amyloidosis: a variant or an etiologic factor in amyloidosis cutis? Int J Dermatol 1993; 32: 422–423.

261 Ishii M, Terao Y, Asai Y, Hamada T. Macular amyloidosis with patchy filamentous degeneration of collagen islands. J Cutan Pathol 1981; 8: 421–428.

262 Okamoto H, Danno K, Horio T. Macular amyloidosis in unusual distribution. Dermatologica 1981; 163: 476–479.

263 Mahalingam M, Steinberg-Benjes L, Goldberg LJ. Primary amyloidosis of the auricular concha – a case report and review. J Cutan Pathol 2000; 27: 564 (abstract).

264 Maddox JL, Goette DK. Transepithelial elimination of amyloid. Arch Dermatol 1984; 120: 679–680.

265 Kyle RA. Amyloidosis: Part 3. Int J Dermatol 1981; 20: 75–80.

266 Kibbi AG, Bubetz NG, Shukrallah TA, Kuban AK. Macular and lichen amyloidosis: a clinicopathologic study of 57 patients. J Cutan Pathol 1989; 16: 312 (abstract).

267 Clement MI, Honavar M, Salisbury J, Neill S. Nodular localized primary cutaneous amyloidosis. Clin Exp Dermatol 1987; 12: 460–462.

268 Vestey JP, Tidman MJ, McLaren KM. Primary nodular cutaneous amyloidosis – long-term follow-up and treatment. Clin Exp Dermatol 1994; 19: 159–162.

269 Lien MH, Railan D, Nelson BR. The efficacy of dermabrasion in the treatment of nodular amyloidosis. J Am Acad Dermatol 1997; 36: 315–316.

270 Nguyen TU, Oghalai JS, McGregor DK et al. Subcutaneous nodular amyloidosis: a case report and review of the literature. Hum Pathol 2001; 32: 346–348.

271 Kitajima Y, Seno J, Aoki S et al. Nodular primary cutaneous amyloidosis. Arch Dermatol 1986; 122: 1425–1430.

272 Grattan CEH, Burton JL, Dahl MGC. Two cases of nodular cutaneous amyloid with positive organ-specific antibodies, treated by shave excision. Clin Exp Dermatol 1988; 13: 187–189.

273 Northcutt AD, Vanover MJ. Nodular cutaneous amyloidosis involving the vulva. Arch Dermatol 1985; 121: 518–521.

274 Masuda C, Mohri S, Nakajima H. Histopathological and immunohistochemical study of amyloidosis cutis nodularis atrophicans – comparison with systemic amyloidosis. Br J Dermatol 1988; 119: 33–43.

275 Truhan AP, Garden JM, Roenigk HH. Nodular primary localized cutaneous amyloidosis: immunohistochemical evaluation and treatment with the carbon dioxide laser. J Am Acad Dermatol 1986; 14: 1058–1062.

276 Trau H, Shpiro D, Schewach-Millet M et al. Nodular cutaneous amyloidosis. Am J Dermatopathol 1991; 13: 414–417.

277 Ann C-C, Lin C-S, Wong C-K. Nodular amyloidosis. Clin Exp Dermatol 1988; 13: 20–23.

278 Ito K, Hashimoto K, Kambe N, Van S. Roles of immunoglobulins in amyloidogenesis in cutaneous nodular amyloidosis. J Invest Dermatol 1987; 89: 415–418.

279 Romagnoli S, Braidotti P, Di Nuovo F, Coggi G. Amyloid tumour (amyloidoma) of the leg: histology, immunohistochemistry and electron microscopy. Histopathology 1999; 35: 188–189.

280 Horiguchi Y, Takahashi C, Imamura S. A case of nodular cutaneous amyloidosis. Amyloid production by infiltrating plasma cells. Am J Dermatopathol 1993; 15: 59–63.

281 Hagari Y, Michara M, Hagari S. Nodular localized cutaneous amyloidosis: detection of monoclonality of infiltrating plasma cells by polymerase chain reaction. Br J Dermatol 1996; 135: 630–633.

282 Hagari Y, Michara M, Konohana I et al. Nodular localized cutaneous amyloidosis: further demonstration of monoclonality of infiltrating plasma cells in four additional Japanese patients. Br J Dermatol 1998; 138: 652–654.

283 Chapel TA, Birmingham DJ, Malinowski YE. Nodular primary localized cutaneous amyloidosis. Arch Dermatol 1977; 113: 1248–1249.

284 Ogino A, Tanaka S. Poikiloderma-like cutaneous amyloidosis. Dermatologica 1977; 155: 301–309.

285 Moriwaki S, Nishigori C, Horiguchi Y et al. Amyloidosis cutis dyschromica. Arch Dermatol 1992; 128: 966–970.

286 Wang W-J, Huang C-Y, Chang Y-T, Wong C-K. Anosacral cutaneous amyloidosis: a study of 10 Chinese cases. Br J Dermatol 2000; 143: 1266–1269.

287 Eng AM, Cogan L, Gunnar RM, Blekys I. Familial generalized dyschromic amyloidosis cutis. J Cutan Pathol 1976; 3: 102–108.

288 Vasily DB, Bhatia SG, Uhlin SR. Familial primary cutaneous amyloidosis. Arch Dermatol 1978; 114: 1173–1176.

289 Newton JA, Jagjivan A, Bhogal B et al. Familial primary cutaneous amyloidosis. Br J Dermatol 1985; 112: 201–208.

290 Hartshorne ST. Familial primary cutaneous amyloidosis in a South African family. Clin Exp Dermatol 1999; 24: 438–442.

291 Hashimoto K, Brownstein MH. Localized amyloidosis in basal cell epitheliomas. Acta Derm Venereol 1973; 53: 331–339.

292 Weedon D, Shand E. Amyloid in basal cell carcinomas. Br J Dermatol 1979; 101: 141–146.

293 Malak JA, Smith EW. Secondary localized cutaneous amyloidosis. Arch Dermatol 1962; 86: 465–477.

294 MacDonald DM, Black MM. Secondary localized cutaneous amyloidosis in melanocytic naevi. Br J Dermatol 1980; 103: 553–556.

295 Jennings RC, Ahmed E. An amyloid forming nodular syringocystadenoma. Arch Dermatol 1970; 101: 224–226.

296 Hashimoto K, King LE. Secondary localized cutaneous amyloidosis associated with actinic keratosis. J Invest Dermatol 1973; 61: 293–299.

297 Speight EL, Milne DS, Lawrence CM. Secondary localized cutaneous amyloid in Bowen's disease. Clin Exp Dermatol 1993; 18: 286–288.

298 Hashimoto K, Kumakiri M. Colloid-amyloid bodies in PUVA-treated human psoriatic patients. J Invest Dermatol 1979; 72: 70–80.

299 Brownstein MH, Helwig EB. The cutaneous amyloidoses. I. Localized forms. Arch Dermatol 1970; 102: 8–19.

300 Romero LS, Kantor GR, Levin MW, Vonderheid EC. Localized cutaneous amyloidosis associated with mycosis fungoides. J Am Acad Dermatol 1997; 37: 124–127.

301 Tsuji T, Asai Y, Hamada T. Secondary localized cutaneous amyloidosis in solar elastosis. Br J Dermatol 1982; 106: 469–476.

302 Caro I. Lipoid proteinosis. Int J Dermatol 1978; 17: 388–393.

303 Piérard GE, van Cauwenberge D, Budo J, Lapière CM. A clinicopathologic study of six cases of lipoid proteinosis. Am J Dermatopathol 1988; 10: 300–305.

304 Hey T. Lipoid proteinosis. I. The clinical picture. Br J Dermatol 1963; 75: 465–477.

305 Nagasaka T, Tanaka M, Ito D et al. Protean manifestations of lipoid proteinosis in a 16-year-old boy. Clin Exp Dermatol 2000; 25: 30–32.

306 Rizzo R, Ruggieri M, Micali G et al. Lipoid proteinosis: a case report. Pediatr Dermatol 1997; 14: 22–25.

307 Bozdağ KE, Gül Y, Karaman A. Lipoid proteinosis. Int J Dermatol 2000; 39: 203–204.

308 Touart DM, Sau P. Cutaneous deposition diseases. Part I. J Am Acad Dermatol 1998; 39: 149–171.

309 Nanda A, Alsaleh QA, Al-Sabah H et al. Lipoid proteinosis: report of four siblings and brief review of the literature. Pediatr Dermatol 2001; 18: 21–26.

310 Pursley TV, Apisarnthanarax P. Lipoid proteinosis. Int J Dermatol 1981; 20: 137–139.

311 Buchan NG, Harvey Kemble JV. Successful surgical treatment of lipoid proteinosis. Br J Dermatol 1974; 91: 561–566.

312 Konstantinov K, Kabakchiev P, Karchev T et al. Lipoid proteinosis. J Am Acad Dermatol 1992; 27: 293–297.

313 Barthelemy H, Mauduit G, Kanitakis J et al. Lipoid proteinosis with pseudomembranous conjunctivitis. J Am Acad Dermatol 1986; 14: 367–371.

314 Caplan RM. Visceral involvement in lipoid proteinosis. Arch Dermatol 1967; 95: 149–155.

315 Caccamo D, Jaen A, Telenta M et al. Lipoid proteinosis of the small bowel. Arch Pathol Lab Med 1994; 118: 572–574.

316 Bauer EA, Santa Cruz DJ, Eisen AZ. Lipoid proteinosis: in vivo and in vitro evidence for a lysosomal storage disease. J Invest Dermatol 1981; 76: 119–125.

317 Navarro C, Fachal C, Rodriguez C et al. Lipoid proteinosis. A biochemical and ultrastructural investigation of two new cases. Br J Dermatol 1999; 141: 326–331.

318 Fleischmajer R, Krieg T, Dziadek M et al. Ultrastructure and composition of connective tissue in hyalinosis cutis et mucosae skin. J Invest Dermatol 1984; 82: 252–258.

319 Harper JI, Duance VC, Sims TJ, Light ND. Lipoid proteinosis: an inherited disorder of collagen metabolism? Br J Dermatol 1985; 113: 145–151.

320 Olsen DR, Chu M-L, Uitto J. Expression of basement membrane zone genes coding for type IV procollagen and laminin by human skin fibroblasts in vitro: elevated α1(IV) collagen mRNA levels in lipoid proteinosis. J Invest Dermatol 1988; 90: 734–738.

321 Moy LS, Moy RL, Matsuoka LY et al. Lipoid proteinosis: ultrastructural and biochemical studies. J Am Acad Dermatol 1987; 16: 1193–1201.

322 Ishibashi A. Hyalinosis cutis et mucosae. Dermatologica 1982; 165: 7–15.

323 Gjersvik PJ, Thorsrud AK, Jellum E. Lipoid proteinosis: high-resolution two-dimensional protein electrophoresis of affected and non-affected skin. Acta Derm Venereol 2000; 80: 230–231.

324 Hofer P-A. Urbach–Wiethe disease. Acta Derm Venereol (Suppl) 1973; 71: 5–37.

325 Metze D. Explaining clinical features and histopathological findings by electron microscopy: hyalinosis cutis et mucosae (Urbach–Wiethe). Dermatopathology: Practical & Conceptual 1999; 5: 46–47.

326 Harper JI, Filipe MI, Staughton RCD. Lipoid proteinosis: variations in the histochemical characteristics. Clin Exp Dermatol 1983; 8: 135–141.

327 Farolan MJ, Ronan SG, Solomon LM, Loeff DS. Lipoid proteinosis: case report. Pediatr Dermatol 1992; 9: 264–267.

328 Shore RN, Howard BV, Howard WJ, Shelley WB. Lipoid proteinosis. Demonstration of normal lipid metabolism in cultured cells. Arch Dermatol 1974; 110: 591–594.

329 Van der Walt JJ, Heyl T. Lipoid proteinosis and erythropoietic protoporphyria: a histologic and histochemical study. Arch Dermatol 1971; 104: 501–507.

330 Hashimoto K, Klingmuller G, Rodermund O-E. Hyalinosis cutis et mucosae. An electron microscopic study. Acta Derm Venereol 1972; 52: 179–195.

331 Aubin F, Blanc D, Badet J-M, Chobaut J-C. Lipoid proteinosis: case report. Pediatr Dermatol 1989; 6: 109–113.

332 Fabrizi G, Porfiri B, Borgioli M, Serri F. Urbach–Wiethe disease. Light and electron microscopic study. J Cutan Pathol 1980; 7: 8–20.

333 Newton JA, Rasbridge S, Temple A et al. Lipoid proteinosis – new immunopathological observations. Clin Exp Dermatol 1991; 16: 350–354.

334 Lipsker D, Cribier B, Spehner D et al. Examination of cutaneous macroglobulinosis by immunoelectron microscopy. Br J Dermatol 1996; 135: 287–291.

335 Agius JRG. Colloid pseudomilium. Br J Dermatol 1963; 74: 55–59.

336 Zoon JJ, Jansen LH, Hovenkamp A. The nature of colloid milium. Br J Dermatol 1955; 67: 212–217.

337 Graham JH, Marques AS. Colloid milium: a histochemical study. J Invest Dermatol 967; 49: 497–507.

338 Guin JD, Seale ER. Colloid degeneration of the skin (colloid milium). Arch Dermatol 1959; 80: 533–537.

339 Gilbert TM, Cox CB. Colloid degeneration of the skin: report of eight cases. Med J Aust 1946; 2: 21–22.

340 Ebner H, Gebhart W. Colloid milium: light and electron microscopic investigations. Clin Exp Dermatol 1977; 2: 217–226.

341 Findlay GH, Morrison JGL, Simson IW. Exogenous ochronosis and pigmented colloid milium from hydroquinone bleaching creams. Br J Dermatol 1975; 93: 613–622.

342 Dupre A, Bonafe JF, Pieraggi MT, Perrot H. Paracolloid of the skin. J Cutan Pathol 1979; 6: 304–309.

343 Muscardin LM, Bellocci M, Balus L. Papuloverrucous colloid milium: an occupational variant. Br J Dermatol 2000; 143: 884–887.

344 Innocenzi D, Barduagni F, Cerio R, Wolter M. UV-induced colloid milium. Clin Exp Dermatol 1993; 18: 347–350.

345 Holzberger PC. Concerning adult colloid milium. Arch Dermatol 1960; 82: 711–716.

346 Mayer FE, Milburn PB. Unilateral colloid milium. J Am Acad Dermatol 1990; 23: 1166–1167.

347 Hashimoto K, Black M. Colloid milium: a final degeneration product of actinic elastoid. J Cutan Pathol 1985; 12: 147–156.

348 Kobayashi H, Hashimoto K. Colloid and elastic fibre: ultrastructural study on the histogenesis of colloid milium. J Cutan Pathol 1983; 10: 111–122.

349 Hashimoto K, Nakayama H, Chimenti S et al. Juvenile colloid milium. Immunohistochemical and ultrastructural studies. J Cutan Pathol 1989; 16: 164–174.

350 Handfield-Jones SE, Atherton DJ, Black MM et al. Juvenile colloid milium: clinical, histological and ultrastructural features. J Cutan Pathol 1992; 19: 434–438.

351 Chowdhury MMU, Blackford S, Williams S. Juvenile colloid milium associated with ligneous conjunctivitis: report of a case and review of the literature. Clin Exp Dermatol 2000; 25: 138–140.

352 Sullivan M, Ellis FA. Facial colloid degeneration in plaques. Arch Dermatol 1961; 84: 816–823.

353 Hashimoto K, Miller F, Bereston ES. Colloid milium. Histochemical and electron microscopic studies. Arch Dermatol 1972; 105: 684–694.

354 Hashimoto K, Katzman RL, Kang AH, Kanzaki T. Electron microscopical and biochemical analysis of colloid milium. Arch Dermatol 1975; 111: 49–59.

355 Niemi K-M, Stenman S, Borgström GH et al. Massive cutaneous hyalinosis. A newly recognized disease. Arch Dermatol 1980; 116: 580–583.

356 Maury CPJ, Teppo A-M. Massive cutaneous hyalinosis. Am J Clin Pathol 1984; 82: 543–551.

357 Santa Cruz DJ, Ulbright TM. Mucin-like changes in keloids. Am J Clin Pathol 1981; 75: 18–22.

358 Weedon D, Gutteridge BH, Hockly RG, Emmett AJJ. Unusual cutaneous reactions to injections of corticosteroids. Am J Dermatopathol 1982; 4: 199–203.

359 Bhawan J. Steroid-induced 'granulomas' in hypertrophic scar. Acta Derm Venereol 1983; 63: 560–563.

360 Balogh K. The histologic appearance of corticosteroid injection sites. Arch Pathol Lab Med 1986; 110: 1168–1172.

361 Martin RW III, Lumadue JA, Corio RL et al. Cutaneous giant cell hyalin angiopathy. J Cutan Pathol 1993; 20: 356–358.

362 Sahn EE, Salinas CF, Sens MA et al. Infantile systemic hyalinosis in a black infant. Pediatr Dermatol 1994; 11: 52–60.

363 Glover MT, Lake BD, Atherton DJ. Clinical, histologic, and ultrastructural findings in two cases of infantile systemic hyalinosis. Pediatr Dermatol 1992; 9: 255–258.

364 Horiuchi Y, Mukosaka K, Fujimaki T. Systemic hyalinosis of delayed onset. Dermatology 1999; 198: 83–85.

365 Ebner H, Gebhart W. Light and electron microscopic studies on colloid and other cytoid bodies. Clin Exp Dermatol 1977; 2: 311–322.

366 Pinkus H, Mehregan AH, Staricco RG. Elastic globes in human skin. J Invest Dermatol 1965; 45: 81–85.

367 Nakayama H, Hashimoto K, Kambe N, Eng A. Elastic globes: electron microscopic and immunohistochemical observations. J Cutan Pathol 1988; 15: 98–103.

368 Gebhart W. Zytoide Korperchen in der menschlichen Haut. Wien Klin Wschr (Suppl) 1976; 60: 3–24.

Pigment and related deposits

369 Cullison D, Abele DC, O'Quinn JL. Localized exogenous ochronosis. J Am Acad Dermatol 1983; 8: 882–889.

370 Lichtenstein L, Kaplan L. Hereditary ochronosis. Pathologic changes observed in two necropsied cases. Am J Pathol 1954; 30: 99–125.

371 Kutty MK, Iqbal QM, Teh E-C. Ochronotic arthropathy. Arch Pathol 1973; 96: 100–103.

372 Albers SE, Brozena SJ, Glass LF, Fenske NA. Alkaptonuria and ochronosis: case report and review. J Am Acad Dermatol 1992; 27: 609–614.

373 Gutzmer R, Herbst RA, Kiehl P et al. Alkaptonuric ochronosis: Report of two affected brothers. J Am Acad Dermatol 1997; 37: 305–307.

374 Carlesimo M, Bonaccorsi P, Tamburrano G et al. Alkaptonuria. Dermatology 1999; 199: 70–71.

375 Tuffanelli D, Abraham RK, Dubois EI. Pigmentation from antimalarial therapy. Arch Dermatol 1963; 88: 419–426.

376 Mahler R, Sissons W, Watters K. Pigmentation induced by quinidine therapy. Arch Dermatol 1986; 122: 1062–1064.

377 Egorin MJ, Trump DL, Wainwright CW. Quinacrine ochronosis and rheumatoid arthritis. JAMA 1976; 236: 385–386.

378 Bruce S, Tschen JA, Chow D. Exogenous ochronosis resulting from quinine injections. J Am Acad Dermatol 1986; 15: 357–361.

379 Hoshaw RA, Zimmerman KG, Menter A. Ochronosislike pigmentation from hydroquinone bleaching creams in American blacks. Arch Dermatol 1985; 121: 105–108.

380 Phillips JI, Isaacson C, Carman H. Ochronosis in black South Africans who used skin lighteners. Am J Dermatopathol 1986; 8: 14–21.

381 Tidman MJ, Horton JJ, MacDonald DM. Hydroquinone-induced ochronosis – light and electron microscopic features. Clin Exp Dermatol 1986; 11: 224–228.

382 Findlay GH, Morrison JGL, Simson IW. Exogenous ochronosis and pigmented colloid milium from hydroquinone bleaching creams. Br J Dermatol 1975; 93: 613–622.

383 Hardwick N, van Gelder LW, van der Merwe CA, van der Merwe MP. Exogenous ochronosis: an epidemiological study. Br J Dermatol 1989; 120: 229–238.

384 Lawrence N, Bligard CA, Reed R, Perret WJ. Exogenous ochronosis in the United States. J Am Acad Dermatol 1988; 18: 1207–1211.

385 Findlay GH. Ochronosis following skin bleaching with hydroquinone. J Am Acad Dermatol 1982; 6: 1092–1093.

386 Snider RL, Thiers BH. Exogenous ochronosis. J Am Acad Dermatol 1993; 28: 662–664.

387 Kramer KE, Lopez A, Stefanato CM, Phillips TJ. Exogenous ochronosis. J Am Acad Dermatol 2000; 42: 869–871.

388 Cherian S. Palmoplantar pigmentation: a clue to alkaptonuric ochronosis. J Am Acad Dermatol 1994; 30: 264–265.

389 Vijaikumar M, Thappa DM, Srikanth S et al. Alkaptonuric ochronosis presenting as palmoplantar pigmentation. Clin Exp Dermatol 2000; 25: 305–307.

390 Attwood HD, Clifton S, Mitchell RE. A histological, histochemical and ultrastructural study of dermal ochronosis. Pathology 1971; 3: 115–121.

391 Hull PR, Procter PR. The melanocyte: an essential link in hydroquinone-induced ochronosis. J Am Acad Dermatol 1990; 22: 529–531.

392 Jordaan HF, van Niekerk DJT. Transepidermal elimination in exogenous ochronosis. A report of two cases. Am J Dermatopathol 1991; 13: 418–424.

393 Jordaan HF, Mulligan RP. Actinic granuloma-like change in exogenous ochronosis: case report. J Cutan Pathol 1990; 17: 236–240.

394 Hanke CW, Conner AC, Probst EL, Fondak AA. Blast tattoos resulting from black powder firearms. J Am Acad Dermatol 1987; 17: 819–825.

395 Terasawa N, Kishimoto S, Kibe Y et al. Graphite foreign body granuloma. Br J Dermatol 1999; 141: 774–776.

396 Sowden JM, Byrne JPH, Smith AG et al. Red tattoo reactions: X-ray microanalysis and patch-test studies. Br J Dermatol 1991; 124: 576–580.

397 Bendsoe N, Hansson C, Sterner O. Inflammatory reactions from organic pigments in red tattoos. Acta Derm Venereol 1991; 71: 70–73.

398 Beerman H, Lane RAG. 'Tattoo'. A survey of some of the literature concerning the medical complications of tattooing. Am J Med Sci 1954; 227: 444–465.

399 Scutt RWB. The medical hazards of tattooing. Br J Hosp Med 1972; 8: 195–202.

400 Goldstein N. IV. Complications from tattoos. J Dermatol Surg Oncol 1979; 5: 869–878.

401 Tope WD, Arbiser JL, Duncan LM. Black tattoo reaction: The peacock's tale. J Am Acad Dermatol 1996; 35: 477–479.

402 Lamb JH, Jones PE, Morgan RJ et al. Further studies in light-sensitive eruptions. Arch Dermatol 1961; 83: 568–581.

403 Horney DA, Gaither JM, Lauer R et al. Cutaneous inoculation tuberculosis secondary to 'jailhouse tattooing'. Arch Dermatol 1985; 121: 648–650.

404 Watkins DB. Viral disease in tattoos: verruca vulgaris. Arch Dermatol 1961; 84: 306–309.

405 Hallam R, Foulds IS. Molluscum contagiosum: an unusual complication of tattooing. Br Med J 1982; 285: 607.

406 Brancaccio RR, Berstein M, Fisher AA, Shalita AR. Tinea in tattoos. Cutis 1981; 28: 541–542.

407 Taaffe A, Wyatt EH. The red tattoo and lichen planus. Int J Dermatol 1980; 19: 394–396.

408 McGrouther DA, Downie PA, Thompson WD. Reactions to red tattoos. Br J Plast Surg 1977; 30: 84–85.

409 Rostenberg A, Brown RA, Caro MR. Discussion of tattoo reactions with report of a case showing a reaction to a green color. Arch Dermatol 1950; 62: 540–547.

410 Cairns RJ, Calnan CD. Green tattoo reactions associated with cement dermatitis. Br J Dermatol 1962; 74: 288–294.

411 Nguyen LQ, Allen HB. Reactions to manganese and cadmium in tattoos. Cutis 1979; 23: 71–72.

412 McFadden N, Lyberg T, Hensten-Pettersen A. Aluminum-induced granulomas in a tattoo. J Am Acad Dermatol 1989; 20: 903–908.

413 Bjornberg A. Reactions to light in yellow tattoos from cadmium sulfide. Arch Dermatol 1963; 88: 267–271.

414 Goldstein N. Mercury-cadmium sensitivity in tattoos. A photoallergic reaction in red pigment. Ann Intern Med 1967; 67: 984–989.

415 Earley MJ. Basal cell carcinoma arising in tattoos: a clinical report of two cases. Br J Plast Surg 1983; 36: 258–259.

416 Hickey KL, Henneberry JM. Unusual cutaneous reactions in tattoos: a report of two cases. J Cutan Pathol 2000; 27: 560 (abstract).

417 Hanada K, Chiyoya S, Katabira Y. Systemic sarcoidal reaction in tattoo. Clin Exp Dermatol 1985; 10: 479–484.

418 Blobstein SH, Weiss HD, Myskowski PL. Sarcoidal granulomas in tattoos. Cutis 1985; 32: 423–424.

419 Dickinson JA. Sarcoidal reactions in tattoos. Arch Dermatol 1969; 100: 315–319.

420 Diette KM, Bronstein BR, Parrish JA. Histologic comparison of argon and tunable dye lasers in the treatment of tattoos. J Invest Dermatol 1985; 85: 368–373.

421 Herd RM, Alora MB, Smoller B et al. A clinical and histologic prospective controlled comparative study of the picosecond titanium:sapphire (795 nm) laser versus the Q-switched alexandrite (752 nm) laser for removing tattoo pigment. J Am Acad Dermatol 1999; 40: 603–606.

422 Timko AL, Miller CH, Johnson FB, Ross EV. In vitro quantitative chemical analysis of tattoo pigments. Arch Dermatol 2001; 137: 143–147.

423 Anderson RR. Regarding tattoos. Is that sunlight, or an oncoming train at the end of the tunnel? Arch Dermatol 2001; 137: 210–212.

424 Ross EV, Yashar S, Michaud N et al. Tattoo darkening and nonresponse after laser treatment. A possible role for titanium dioxide. Arch Dermatol 2001; 137: 33–37.

425 Goldstein AP. VII. Histologic reactions in tattoos. J Dermatol Surg Oncol 1979; 5: 896–900.

426 Taaffe A, Knight AG, Marks R. Lichenoid tattoo hypersensitivity. Br Med J 1978; 1: 616–618.

427 Clarke J, Black MM. Lichenoid tattoo reactions. Br J Dermatol 1979; 100: 451–454.

428 Winkelmann RK, Harris RB. Lichenoid delayed hypersensitivity reactions in tattoos. J Cutan Pathol 1979; 6: 59–65.

429 Blumental G, Okun MR, Ponitch JA. Pseudolymphomatous reaction to tattoos. J Am Acad Dermatol 1982; 6: 485–488.

430 Biro L, Klein WP. Unusual complication of mercurial (cinnabar) tattoo. Arch Dermatol 1957; 96: 165–167.

431 Zinberg M, Heilman E, Glickman F. Cutaneous pseudolymphoma resulting from a tattoo. J Dermatol Surg Oncol 1982; 8: 955–958.

432 Slater DN, Durrant TE. Tattoos: light and transmission electron microscopy studies with X-ray microanalysis. Clin Exp Dermatol 1984; 9: 167–173.

433 Lea PJ, Pawlowski A. Human tattoo. Int J Dermatol 1987; 26: 453–458.

434 Cawley EP, Hsu YT, Wood BT, Weary PE. Hemochromatosis and the skin. Arch Dermatol 1969; 100: 1–6.

435 Milder MS, Cook JD, Stray S, Finch CA. Idiopathic hemochromatosis, an interim report. Medicine (Baltimore) 1980; 59: 34–49.

436 Perdrup A, Poulsen H. Hemochromatosis and vitiligo. Arch Dermatol 1964; 90: 34–37.

437 Leyden JJ, Lockshin NA, Kriebel S. The black keratinous cyst. A sign of hemochromatosis. Arch Dermatol 1972; 106: 379–381.

438 Chevrant-Breton J, Simon M, Bourel M, Ferrand B. Cutaneous manifestations of idiopathic hemochromatosis. Study of 100 cases. Arch Dermatol 1977; 113: 161–165.

439 Weintraub LR, Demis DJ, Conrad ME, Crosby WH. Iron excretion by the skin. Selective localization of iron^{59} in epithelial cells. Am J Pathol 1965; 46: 121–126.

440 Olmstead PM, Lund HZ, Leonard DD. Monsel's solution: a histologic nuisance. J Am Acad Dermatol 1980; 3: 492–498.

441 Amazon K, Robinson MJ, Rywlin AM. Ferrugination caused by Monsel's solution. Am J Dermatopathol 1980; 2: 197–205.

442 Wood C, Severin GL. Unusual histiocytic reaction to Monsel's solution. Am J Dermatopathol 1980; 2: 261–264.

443 Hanau D, Grosshans E. Monsel's solution and histological lesions. Am J Dermatopathol 1981; 3: 418–419.

444 Ackerman Z, Seidenbaum M, Loewenthal E, Rubinow A. Overload of iron in the skin of patients with varicose ulcers. Arch Dermatol 1988; 124: 1376–1378.

445 Kurban RS, Goldstein JA, Bhawan J. Earring-induced localized iron tattoo. J Am Acad Dermatol 1991; 24: 788–789.

446 Ashley JR, Littler CM, Burgdorf WHC, Brann BS. Bronze baby syndrome. Report of a case. J Am Acad Dermatol 1985; 12: 325–328.

447 Purcell SM, Wians FH, Ackerman NB, Davis BM. Hyperbiliverdinemia in the bronze baby syndrome. J Am Acad Dermatol 1987; 16: 172–177.

448 Allegue F, Hermo JA, Fachal C, Alfonsin N. Localized green pigmentation in a patient with hyperbilirubinemia. J Am Acad Dermatol 1996; 35: 108–109.

449 Granstein RD, Sober AJ. Drug- and heavy metal-induced hyperpigmentation. J Am Acad Dermatol 1981; 5: 1–18.

450 Gaul LE, Staud AH. Clinical spectroscopy. Seventy cases of generalized argyrosis following organic and colloidal silver medication. JAMA 1935; 104: 1387–1388.

451 Kapur N, Landon G, Yu RC. Localized argyria in an antique restorer. Br J Dermatol 2001; 144: 191–192.

452 Shelley WB, Shelley ED, Burmeister V. Argyria: the intradermal 'photograph', a manifestation of passive photosensitivity. J Am Acad Dermatol 1987; 16: 211–217.

453 Bleehen SS, Gould DJ, Harrington CI et al. Occupational argyria; light and electron microscopic studies and X-ray microanalysis. Br J Dermatol 1981; 104: 19–26.

454 East BW, Boddy K, Williams ED et al. Silver retention, total body silver and tissue silver concentrations in argyria associated with exposure to an anti-smoking remedy containing silver acetate. Clin Exp Dermatol 1980; 5: 305–311.

455 Rongioletti F, Robert E, Buffa P et al. Blue nevi-like dotted occupational argyria. J Am Acad Dermatol 1992; 27: 1015–1016.

456 Sarsfield P, White JE, Theaker JM. Silverworker's finger: an unusual occupational hazard mimicking a melanocytic lesion. Histopathology 1992; 20: 73–75.

457 Pariser RJ. Generalized argyria. Clinicopathologic features and histochemical studies. Arch Dermatol 1978; 114: 373–377.

458 Koplon BS. Azure lunulae due to argyria. Arch Dermatol 1966; 94: 333–334.

459 Marshall JP, Schneider RP. Systemic argyria secondary to topical silver nitrate. Arch Dermatol 1977; 113: 1077–1079.

460 Buckley WR. Localized argyria. Arch Dermatol 1963; 88: 531–539.

461 Suzuki H, Baba S, Uchigasaki S, Murase M. Localized argyria with chrysiasis caused by implanted acupuncture needles. J Am Acad Dermatol 1993; 29: 833–837.

462 Sato S, Sueki H, Nishijima A. Two unusual cases of argyria: the application of an improved

tissue processing method for X-ray microanalysis of selenium and sulphur in silver-laden granules. Br J Dermatol 1999; 140: 158–163.

463 Morton CA, Fallowfield M, Kemmett D. Localized argyria caused by silver earrings. Br J Dermatol 1996; 135: 484–485.

464 Johansson EA, Kanerva L, Niemi K-M, Lakomaa E-L. Localized argyria with low ceruloplasmin and copper levels in the serum. A case report with clinical and microscopical findings and a trial of penicillamine treatment. Clin Exp Dermatol 1982; 7: 169–176.

465 Mehta AC, Dawson-Butterworth K, Woodhouse MA. Argyria. Electron microscopic study of a case. Br J Dermatol 1966; 78: 175–179.

466 Prose PH. An electron microscopic study of human generalized argyria. Am J Pathol 1963; 42: 293–297.

467 Buckley WR, Oster CF, Fassett DW. Localized argyria. II. Chemical nature of the silver containing particles. Arch Dermatol 1965; 92: 697–705.

468 Levantine A, Almeyda J. Drug induced changes in pigmentation. Br J Dermatol 1973; 89: 105–112.

469 Cox AJ, Marich KW. Gold in the dermis following gold therapy for rheumatoid arthritis. Arch Dermatol 1973; 108: 655–657.

470 Millard PR, Chaplin AJ, Venning VA et al. Chrysiasis: transmission electron microscopy, laser microprobe mass spectrometry and epipolarized light as adjuncts to diagnosis. Histopathology 1988; 13: 281–288.

471 Smith RW, Leppard B, Barnett NL et al. Chrysiasis revisited: a clinical and pathological study. Br J Dermatol 1995; 133: 671–678.

472 Beckett VL, Doyle JA, Hadley GA, Spear KL. Chrysiasis resulting from gold therapy in rheumatoid arthritis. Mayo Clin Proc 1982; 57: 773–777.

473 Trotter MJ, Tron VA, Hollingdale J, Rivers JK. Localized chrysiasis induced by laser therapy. Arch Dermatol 1995; 131: 1411–1414.

474 Fleming CJ, Salisbury ELC, Kirwan P et al. Chrysiasis after low-dose gold and UV light exposure. J Am Acad Dermatol 1996; 34: 349–351.

475 Penneys NS, Ackerman AB, Gottlieb NL. Gold dermatitis. A clinical and histopathological study. Arch Dermatol 1974; 109: 372–376.

476 Penneys NS. Gold therapy: dermatologic uses and toxicities. J Am Acad Dermatol 1979; 1: 315–320.

477 Keen CE, Brady K, Kirkham N, Levison DA. Gold in the dermis following chrysotherapy: histopathology and microanalysis. Histopathology 1993; 23: 355–360.

478 Al-Talib RK, Wright DH, Theaker JM. Orange-red birefringence of gold particles in paraffin wax embedded sections: an aid to the diagnosis of chrysiasis. Histopathology 1994; 24: 176–178.

479 Schultz Larsen F, Boye H, Hage E. Chrysiasis: electron microscopic studies and X-ray microanalysis. Clin Exp Dermatol 1984; 9: 174–180.

480 Culora GA, Barnett N, Theaker JM. Artefacts in electron microscopy: ultrastructural features of chrysiasis. J Pathol 1995; 176: 421–425.

481 Kern AB. Mercurial pigmentation. Arch Dermatol 1969; 99: 129–130.

482 Lamar LM, Bliss BO. Localized pigmentation of the skin due to topical mercury. Arch Dermatol 1966; 93: 450–453.

483 Boyd AS, Seger D, Vannucci S et al. Mercury exposure and cutaneous disease. J Am Acad Dermatol 2000; 43: 81–90.

484 Dinehart SM, Dillard R, Raimer SS et al. Cutaneous manifestations of acrodynia (Pink disease). Arch Dermatol 1988; 124: 107–109.

485 Jun JB, Min PK, Kim DW et al. Cutaneous nodular reaction to oral mercury. J Am Acad Dermatol 1997; 37: 131–133.

486 Rogers M, Goodhew P, Szafraniec T, McColl I. Mercury exanthem. Australas J Dermatol 1986; 27: 70–75.

487 Tschanz C, Prins C. Drug rash with eosinophilia and systemic symptoms caused by topical application of mercury. Dermatology 2000; 201: 381–382.

488 Rachman R. Soft-tissue injury by mercury from a broken thermometer. Am J Clin Pathol 1974; 61: 296–300.

489 Lupton GP, Kao GF, Johnson FB et al. Cutaneous mercury granuloma. A clinicopathologic study and review of the literature. J Am Acad Dermatol 1985; 12: 296–303.

490 Kennedy C, Molland EA, Henderson WJ, Whiteley AM. Mercury pigmentation from industrial exposure. Br J Dermatol 1977; 96: 367–374.

491 Burge KM, Winkelmann RK. Mercury pigmentation. An electron microscopic study. Arch Dermatol 1970; 102: 51–61.

492 Allen CC, Lund KA, Treadwell P. Elemental mercury foreign body granulomas. Int J Dermatol 1992; 31: 353–354.

493 Sau P, Solivan G, Johnson FB. Cutaneous reaction from a broken thermometer. J Am Acad Dermatol 1991; 25: 915–919.

494 Allan BR, Moore MR, Hunter JAA. Lead and the skin. Br J Dermatol 1975; 92: 715–719.

495 Pembroke AC, Marten RH. Unusual cutaneous reactions following diphtheria and tetanus immunization. Clin Exp Dermatol 1979; 4: 345–348.

496 Slater DN, Underwood JCE, Durrant TE et al. Aluminium hydroxide granulomas: light and electron microscopic studies and X-ray microanalysis. Br J Dermatol 1982; 107: 103–108.

497 Fawcett HA, Smith NP. Injection-site granuloma due to aluminum. Arch Dermatol 1984; 120: 1318–1322.

498 Elston DM, Bergfeld WF, McMahon JT. Aluminum tattoo: a phenomenon that can resemble parasitized histiocytes. J Cutan Pathol 1993; 20: 326–329.

499 García-Patos V, Pujol RM, Alomar A et al. Persistent subcutaneous nodules in patients hyposensitized with aluminum-containing allergen extracts. Arch Dermatol 1995; 131: 1421–1424.

500 Ruiz-Maldonado R, Contreras-Ruiz J, Sierra-Santoyo A et al. Black granules on the skin after bismuth subsalicylate ingestion. J Am Acad Dermatol 1997; 37: 489–490.

501 Dijkstra JWE, Bergfeld WF, Taylor JS, Ranchoff RE. Prurigo pigmentosa. A persistent lichenoid reaction to bismuth? Int J Dermatol 1987; 26: 379–381.

502 Dupre A, Touron P, Daste J et al. Titanium pigmentation. An electron probe microanalysis study. Arch Dermatol 1985; 121: 656–658.

503 Moran CA, Mullick FG, Ishak KG et al. Identification of titanium in human tissues: probable role in pathologic processes. Hum Pathol 1991; 22: 450–454.

504 Scherschun L, Lee MW, Lim HW. Diltiazem-associated photodistributed hyperpigmentation. A review of 4 cases. Arch Dermatol 2001; 137: 179–182.

505 Tuffanelli D, Abraham RK, Dubois EI. Pigmentation from antimalarial therapy. Arch Dermatol 1963; 88: 419–426.

506 Buckley C, Thomas V, Lewin J et al. Stelazine-induced pigmentation. Clin Exp Dermatol 1994; 19: 149–151.

507 Almeyda J. Cutaneous side effects of phenothiazines. Br J Dermatol 1971; 84: 605–607.

508 Hashimoto K, Joselow SA, Tye MJ. Imipramine hyperpigmentation: a slate-gray discoloration caused by long-term imipramine administration. J Am Acad Dermatol 1991; 25: 357–361.

509 Ming ME, Bhawan J, Stefanato CM et al. Imipramine-induced hyperpigmentation: Four cases and a review of the literature. J Am Acad Dermatol 1999; 40: 159–166.

510 Sicari MC, Lebwohl M, Baral J et al. Photoinduced dermal pigmentation in patients taking tricyclic antidepressants: Histology, electron microscopy, and energy dispersive spectroscopy. J Am Acad Dermatol 1999; 40: 290–293.

511 Atkin DH, Fitzpatrick RE. Laser treatment of imipramine-induced hyperpigmentation. J Am Acad Dermatol 2000; 43: 77–80.

512 Narurkar V, Smoller BR, Hu C-H, Bauer EA. Desipramine-induced blue-gray photosensitive pigmentation. Arch Dermatol 1993; 129: 474–476.

513 Hashimoto K, Weiner W, Albert J, Nelson RG. An electron microscopic study of chlorpromazine pigmentation. J Invest Dermatol 1966; 47: 296–306.

514 Benning TL, McCormack KM, Ingram P et al. Microprobe analysis of chlorpromazine pigmentation. Arch Dermatol 1988; 124: 1541–1544.

515 Basler RSW, Taylor WB, Peacor DR. Postacne osteoma cutis. X-ray diffraction analysis. Arch Dermatol 1974; 110: 113–114.

516 Dyster-Aas K, Hansson H, Miorner G et al. Pigment deposits in eyes and light-exposed skin during long-term methacycline therapy. Acta Derm Venereol 1974; 54: 209–222.

517 Basler RSW. Minocycline-related hyperpigmentation. Arch Dermatol 1985; 121: 606–608.

518 Argenyi ZB, Finelli L, Bergfeld WF et al. Minocycline-related cutaneous hyperpigmentation as demonstrated by light microscopy, electron microscopy and X-ray energy spectroscopy. J Cutan Pathol 1987; 14: 176–180.

519 Simons JJ, Morales A. Minocycline and generalized cutaneous pigmentation. J Am Acad Dermatol 1980; 3: 244–247.

520 Butler JM, Marks R, Sutherland R. Cutaneous and cardiac valvular pigmentation with minocycline. Clin Exp Dermatol 1985; 10: 432–437.

521 Dwyer CM, Cuddihy AM, Kerr REI et al. Skin pigmentation due to minocycline treatment of facial dermatoses. Br J Dermatol 1993; 129: 158–162.

522 Ozog DM, Gogstetter DS, Scott G, Gaspari AA. Minocycline-induced hyperpigmentation in patients with pemphigus and pemphigoid. Arch Dermatol 2000; 136: 1133–1138.

523 Chu P, Van SL, Yen TSB, Berger TG. Minocycline hyperpigmentation localized to the lips: an unusual fixed drug reaction? J Am Acad Dermatol 1994; 30: 802–803.

524 Tanzi EL, Hecker MS. Minocycline-induced hyperpigmentation of the tongue. Arch Dermatol 2000; 136: 427–428.

525 Sabroe RA, Archer CB, Harlow D et al. Minocycline-induced discolouration of the sclerae. Br J Dermatol 1996; 135: 314–316.

526 Fenske NA, Millns JL. Cutaneous pigmentation due to minocycline hydrochloride. J Am Acad Dermatol 1980; 3: 308–310.

527 Green D, Friedman KJ. Treatment of minocycline-induced cutaneous pigmentation with the Q-switched Alexandrite laser and a review of the literature. J Am Acad Dermatol 2001; 44: 342–347.

528 Altman DA, Fivenson DP, Lee MW. Minocycline hyperpigmentation: model for in situ phagocytic activity of factor XIIIa positive dermal dendrocytes. J Cutan Pathol 1992; 19: 340–345.

529 Gordon G, Sparano BM, Iatropoulos MJ. Hyperpigmentation of the skin associated with minocycline therapy. Arch Dermatol 1985; 121: 618–623.

530 Pepine M, Flowers FP, Ramos-Caro FA. Extensive cutaneous hyperpigmentation caused by minocycline. J Am Acad Dermatol 1993; 28: 292–295.

531 Sato S, Murphy GF, Bernhard JD et al. Ultrastructural and X-ray microanalytical observations of minocycline-related hyperpigmentation of the skin. J Invest Dermatol 1981; 77: 264–271.

532 Okada N, Moriya K, Nishida K et al. Skin pigmentation associated with minocycline therapy. Br J Dermatol 1989; 121: 247–254.

533 McCrae JD Jr, Zelickson AS. Skin pigmentation secondary to minocycline therapy. Arch Dermatol 1980; 116: 1262–1265.

534 Miller RAW, McDonald ATJ. Dermal lipofuscinosis associated with amiodarone therapy. Arch Dermatol 1984; 120: 646–649.

535 Rappersberger K, Honigsmann H, Ortel B et al. Photosensitivity and hyperpigmentation in amiodarone-treated patients: incidence, time course, and recovery. J Invest Dermatol 1989; 93: 201–209.

536 Alinovi A, Reverberi C, Melissari M, Gabrielli M. Cutaneous hyperpigmentation induced by amiodarone hydrochloride. J Am Acad Dermatol 1985; 12: 563–566.

537 Bahadır S, Apaydın R, Çobanoilu Ü et al. Amiodarone pigmentation, eye and thyroid alterations. J Eur Acad Dermatol Venereol 2000; 14: 194–195.

538 Mooney EE, Sweeney E. Localised histiocytic lipofuscinosis: an unusual pigmented lesion. Am J Dermatopathol 1993; 15: 368–371.

539 Haas N, Schadendorf D, Hermes B, Henz BM. Hypomelanosis due to block of melanosomal maturation in amiodarone-induced hyperpigmentation. Arch Dermatol 2001; 137: 513–514.

540 Kossard S, Doherty E, McColl I, Ryman W. Autofluorescence of clofazimine in discoid lupus erythematosus. J Am Acad Dermatol 1987; 17: 867–871.

541 Anderson LL, Thomas DE, Berger TG, Vukelja SJ. Cutaneous pigmentation after daunorubicin chemotherapy. J Am Acad Dermatol 1992; 26: 255–256.

542 Vukelja SJ, Bonner MW, McCollough M et al. Unusual serpentine hyperpigmentation associated with 5-fluorouracil. J Am Acad Dermatol 1991; 25: 905–908.

543 Singal R, Tunnessen WW Jr, Wiley JM, Hood AF. Discrete pigmentation after chemotherapy. Pediatr Dermatol 1991; 8: 231–235.

544 Rademaker M, Meyrick Thomas RH, Lowe DG, Munro DD. Linear streaking due to bleomycin. Clin Exp Dermatol 1987; 12: 457–459.

545 Fernandez-Obregon AC, Hogan KP, Bibro MK. Flagellate pigmentation from intrapleural bleomycin. J Am Acad Dermatol 1985; 13: 464–468.

546 Duhra P, Ilchyshyn A, Das RN. Bleomycin-induced flagellate erythema. Clin Exp Dermatol 1991; 16: 216–217.

547 Miori L, Vignini M, Rabbiosi G. Flagellate dermatitis after bleomycin. Am J Dermatopathol 1990; 12: 598–602.

548 Mowad CM, Nguyen TV, Elenitsas R, Leyden JJ. Bleomycin-induced flagellate dermatitis: a clinical and histopathological review. Br J Dermatol 1994; 131: 700–702.

549 Tsuji T, Sawabe M. Hyperpigmentation in striae distensae after bleomycin treatment. J Am Acad Dermatol 1993; 28: 503–505.

550 Schrijvers D, Van Den Brande J, Vermorken JB. Supravenous discoloration of the skin due to docetaxel treatment. Br J Dermatol 2000; 142: 1069–1070.

551 Marcoux D, Anex R, Russo P. Persistent serpentine supravenous hyperpigmented eruption as an adverse reaction to chemotherapy combining actinomycin and vincristine. J Am Acad Dermatol 2000; 43: 540–546.

Cutaneous implants

552 Clark DP, Hanke CW, Swanson NA. Dermal implants: safety of products injected for soft tissue augmentation. J Am Acad Dermatol 1989; 21: 992–998.

553 Morgan AM. Localized reactions to injected therapeutic materials. Part 1. Medical agents. J Cutan Pathol 1995; 22: 193–214.

554 Feldmann R, Harms M, Chavaz P et al. Orbital and palpebral paraffinoma. J Am Acad Dermatol 1992; 26: 833–835.

555 Requena C, Izquierdo MJ, Navarro M et al. Adverse reactions to injectable aesthetic microimplants. Am J Dermatopathol 2001; 23: 197–202.

556 Postlethwait RW, Willigan DA, Ulin AW. Human tissue reaction to sutures. Ann Surg 1975; 181: 144–150.

557 Mastruserio DN, Pesqueira MJ, Cobb MW. Severe granulomatous reaction and facial ulceration occurring after subcutaneous silicone injection. J Am Acad Dermatol 1996; 34: 849–852.

558 Travis WD, Balogh K, Abraham JL. Silicone granulomas: report of three cases and review of the literature. Hum Pathol 1985; 16: 19–27.

559 Anderson DR, Schwartz J, Cottrill CM et al. Silicone granulomas in acral skin in a patient with silicone-gel breast implants and systemic sclerosis. Int J Dermatol 1996; 35: 36–38.

560 Teuber SS, Ito LK, Anderson M, Gershwin ME. Silicone breast implant-associated scarring dystrophy of the arm. Arch Dermatol 1995; 131: 54–56.

561 Raso DS, Greene WB, Harley RA, Maize JC. Silicone deposition in reconstruction scars of women with silicone breast implants. J Am Acad Dermatol 1996; 35: 32–36.

562 Marcusson JA, Bjarnason B. Unusual skin reaction to silicone content in breast implants. Acta Derm Venereol 1999; 79: 136–138.

563 Rae V, Pardo RJ, Blackwelder PL, Falanga V. Leg ulcers following subcutaneous injection of a liquid silicone preparation. Arch Dermatol 1989; 125: 670–673.

564 Butler DF, Gion GG, Rapini RP. Silicone auricular prosthesis. J Am Acad Dermatol 2000; 43: 687–690.

565 Morgan AM. Localized reactions to injected therapeutic materials. Part 2. Surgical agents. J Cutan Pathol 1995; 22: 289–303.

566 Krayenbühl BH, Panizzon RG. Silicone granuloma. Dermatology 2000; 200: 360–362.

567 Graham BS, Thiringer JK, Barrett TL. Nasal tip ulceration from infection and extrusion of a nasal alloplastic implant. J Am Acad Dermatol 2001; 44: 362–364.

568 Symmers W St C. Silicone mastitis in topless waitresses and some other varieties of foreign body mastitis. Br Med J 1968; 3: 19–22.

569 Kasper CS, Chandler PJ. Talc deposition in skin and tissues surrounding silicone gel-containing prosthetic devices. Arch Dermatol 1994; 130: 48–53.

570 Charriere G, Bejot M, Schnitzler L et al. Reactions to a bovine collagen implant. Clinical and immunologic study in 705 patients. J Am Acad Dermatol 1989; 21: 1203–1208.

571 Hanke CW, Higley HR, Jolivette DM et al. Abscess formation and local necrosis after treatment with Zyderm or Zyplast collagen implant. J Am Acad Dermatol 1991; 25: 319–326.

572 Barr RJ, King DF, McDonald RM, Bartlow GA. Necrobiotic granulomas associated with bovine collagen test site injections. J Am Acad Dermatol 1982; 6: 867–869.

573 Brooks N. A foreign body granuloma produced by an injectable collagen implant at a test site. J Dermatol Surg Oncol 1982; 8: 111–114.

574 Smith KJ, Skelton HG, Barrett TL et al. Histologic and immunohistochemical features in biopsy sites in which bovine collagen matrix was used for hemostasis. J Am Acad Dermatol 1996; 34: 434–438.

575 Piacquadio D, Jarcho M, Goltz R. Evaluation of hylan b gel as a soft-tissue augmentation implant material. J Am Acad Dermatol 1997; 36: 544–549.

576 Robinson JK, Hanke CW. Injectable collagen implant: histopathologic identification and longevity of correction. J Dermatol Surg Oncol 1985; 11: 124–130.

577 Stegman SJ, Chu S, Bensch K, Armstrong R. A light and electron microscopic evaluation of Zyderm collagen and Zyplast implants in aging human facial skin. Arch Dermatol 1987; 123: 1644–1649.

578 Burke KE, Naughton G, Waldo E, Cassai N. Bovine collagen implant: histologic chronology in pig dermis. J Dermatol Surg Oncol 1983; 9: 889–895.

579 Picerno NA, Azmi FH, Hood AF. Dermal implants: histopathologic identification and comparison of four commercially available products. J Cutan Pathol 2000; 27: 569 (abstract).

Miscellaneous deposits

580 Spiers EM, Sanders DY, Omura EF. Clinical and histologic features of primary oxalosis. J Am Acad Dermatol 1990; 22: 952–956.

581 Ohtake N, Uchiyama H, Furue M, Tamaki K. Secondary cutaneous oxalosis: cutaneous deposition of calcium oxalate dihydrate after long-term hemodialysis. J Am Acad Dermatol 1994; 31: 368–372.

582 Isonokami M, Nishida K, Okada N, Yoshikawa K. Cutaneous oxalate granulomas in a haemodialysed patient: report of a case with unique clinical features. Br J Dermatol 1993; 128: 690–692.

583 Winship IM, Saxe NP, Hugel H. Primary oxalosis – an unusual cause of livedo reticularis. Clin Exp Dermatol 1991; 16: 367–370.

584 Shih HA, Kao DMF, Elenitsas R, Leyden JJ. Livedo reticularis, ulcers, and peripheral gangrene: cutaneous manifestations of primary hyperoxaluria. Arch Dermatol 2000; 136: 1272–1273.

585 Somach SC, Davis BR, Paras FA et al. Fatal cutaneous necrosis mimicking calciphylaxis in a patient with type 1 primary hyperoxaluria. Arch Dermatol 1995; 131: 821–823.

586 Galimberti RL, Parra IH, Imperiali N et al. Fatal cutaneous necrosis in a hemodialyzed patient with oxalosis. Int J Dermatol 1999; 38: 918–920.

587 Fisher BK, Warkentin JD. Fiber glass dermatitis. Arch Dermatol 1969; 99: 717–719.

588 Lazarov A, Avinoach I, Giryes H, Halevy S. Dermal spherulosis (myospherulosis) after topical treatment for psoriasis. J Am Acad Dermatol 1994; 30: 265–267.

589 Waldman JS, Barr RJ, Espinoza FP, Simmons GE. Subcutaneous myospherulosis. J Am Acad Dermatol 1989; 21: 400–403.

Diseases of cutaneous appendages

15

INTRODUCTION

This chapter covers the non-tumorous disorders of the cutaneous appendages, the great majority of which are inflammatory diseases of the pilosebaceous apparatus. Inflammation of the apocrine and eccrine glands is quite uncommon by comparison. Hamartomas and some related congenital malformations are included with the appendageal tumors in Chapter 33 (pp. 859–901).

The following categories of appendageal diseases will be considered in this chapter:

- inflammatory diseases of the pilosebaceous apparatus
- hair shaft abnormalities
- alopecias
- miscellaneous disorders.

Before considering these diseases, a brief account will be given of the normal hair follicle. As the changes that occur during the hair cycle are relevant to the alopecias, this aspect is discussed on page 471.

The normal hair follicle

Hair follicles are derived from the fetal epidermis as a downward-projecting epithelial bud, which is guided in its subsequent development by an accumulation of mesenchymal cells in the underlying dermis – the dermal papilla.[1] This process is under the control of various substances, one of which is the mesenchymal cell membrane protein known as epimorphin.[2]

Hair follicles are found in a variably dense population throughout the body, except for palmar-plantar skin. The follicle and its attached sebaceous gland and arrector pili muscle form a structural unit. In some parts of the body (axilla and genitocrural region) an apocrine gland is connected to the upper part of the sebaceous duct. Hair follicles produce a hair shaft, which arises from the deep portion of the follicle. Two distinct types of hair shaft are recognized: *terminal hair*, a heavily pigmented, thick shaft arising from a terminal hair follicle, which projects into the deep dermis and even into the subcutis; and *vellus hair*, a short, fine, lightly pigmented shaft which arises from a *vellus hair* follicle; it only extends into the upper reticular dermis. Both types of hair follicle go through a life cycle (see p. 471) but the length of the anagen phase is much shorter in vellus hair follicles.[3] A schematic representation of the hair follicle is shown in Figure 15.1.

The hair follicle is divided into four anatomical regions – the infundibulum, the isthmus, the suprabulbar zone and the hair bulb. The *infundibulum* extends from the skin surface to the point of entry of the sebaceous duct. Its lining cells show epidermal keratinization. Below this is the *isthmus*, the short portion between the entry of the sebaceous duct and the attachment of the arrector pili muscle. Between the isthmus and the hair bulb is the *suprabulbar region*. The *bulb* is the expanded lower end of the follicle which includes the *dermal papilla*; it is surrounded on its top and sides by the *hair matrix,* the part of the bulb which is the actively growing portion of the hair shaft.

The terminal hair shaft is composed of three layers – the medulla, the cortex and the inner root sheath. The *medulla* forms the central core of the hair shaft. It is not present in all human hairs, although it is an important structure of some animal hairs, such as wool.[3] The size and form of the medulla, at least in scalp hair, is regulated by the stage of the hair cycle and by the cross-sectional size of the hair shaft.[4] The *cortex* constitutes the bulk of the hair. It is composed of densely packed keratins, both epithelial keratins and keratins unique to 'hard' structures such as nails and hairs. There are 13 hair keratins. Like epithelial keratins, they are grouped into type I (acidic) and type II (neutral-basic) hair keratins. There are nine type I hair keratins and four

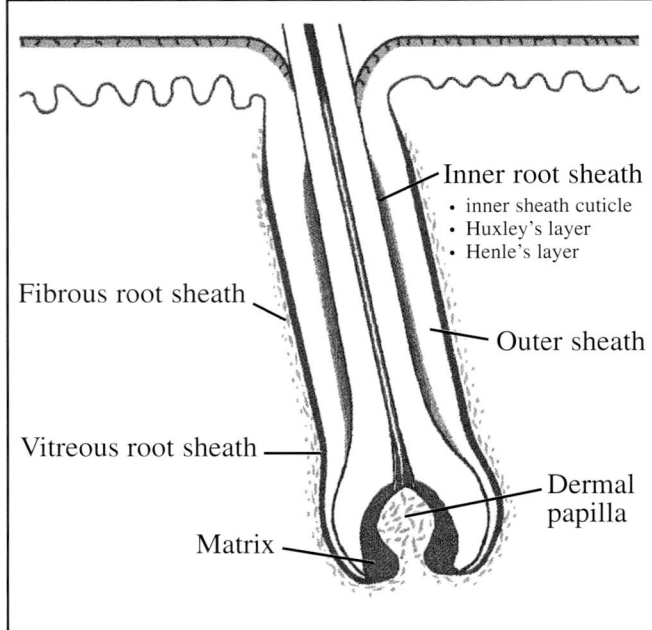

Fig. 15.1 **Schematic representation of the hair follicle.**

type II hair keratins (hHb1, 3, 5 and 6).[5] The hair cortex is covered by a single row of overlapping cells, the *shaft cuticle*. External to the shaft cuticle are the three layers forming the *inner (internal) root sheath* – an inner *sheath cuticle* (which intermeshes with the shaft cuticle), *Huxley's layer* and an outer *Henle's layer*, which keratinizes first. The three layers blend together with keratinization and are no longer distinct by the mid-follicle. Keratinization occurs through the formation of trichohyaline granules. Outside the inner root sheath is the *outer (external) root sheath*. It is composed of clear cells, rich in glycogen. It is only one cell thick at the level of the bulb; it is thickest at the isthmus, where it starts to keratinize, forming a narrow zone of tricholemmal keratinization. The single-cell inner layer of the outer root sheath undergoes specialized keratinization mediated by apoptosis.[6] Above the isthmus, the cells assume epidermal characteristics and line the infundibulum. Enclosing the hair follicle is a *vitreous ('glassy') layer*, which is PAS positive. It becomes thickened and wrinkled during catagen. Beyond this is the *fibrous root sheath* which is continuous below with the follicular papilla; it blends above with the collagen of the papillary dermis.

The adult hair follicle contains the following keratins: the basal layer keratinocytes of the infundibulum express K5/6 and 14, whereas those in the suprabasal layer show K1, 4, 10 and 14, similar to adult epidermis. The keratinocytes of the isthmus show K5/6, 14, 17 and 19. The cells of the inner root sheath stain for K4 and 18. All stain for involucrin, including the matrical cells which stain for nothing else.[7]

The arrector pili muscle attaches to the pilosebaceous apparatus, via elastic tendons, at the bulge area. Some muscle fibers can be found admixed with the connective tissue sheath encircling the follicle. The anchor between the distal arrector pili and the extracellular matrix includes both $\alpha 5\beta 1$ integrin and fibronectin.[8,9]

Attention has turned recently to the hair follicle immune system and its possible role in the causation of alopecia areata and the folliculitides that are a common problem in immunocompromised persons. The *distal* part of the human hair follicle appears to represent a specialized area of the skin immune system with interacting intraepithelial T cells and Langerhans cells. The sharply reduced numbers of T cells and Langerhans cells, and the virtual absence of

MHC class I expression all suggest that the anagen *proximal* hair follicle constitutes an area of immune privilege within the hair follicle immune system. Its collapse may be crucial to the pathogenesis of alopecia areata.[10]

Inflammatory diseases of the pilosebaceous apparatus

Inflammatory diseases of the pilosebaceous apparatus are a common problem in dermatological practice, although it is unusual for biopsies to be taken in many of the entities included in this category. It often assists in arriving at a specific diagnosis if the various inflammatory diseases are subdivided into six categories, although it should be recognized at the outset that this subdivision is somewhat arbitrary. These categories are as follows:

- acneiform lesions
- superficial folliculitides
- deep infectious folliculitides
- deep scarring folliculitides
- follicular occlusion triad
- miscellaneous folliculitides.

Acneiform lesions combine inflammation of the pilosebaceous apparatus with the presence of comedones and often scarring as well. Comedones are dilated and plugged hair follicles which may have a small infundibular orifice (closed comedo) or a wide patulous opening (open comedo). Comedones are not confined to acne, being found in senile skin and certain other circumstances (see below).

The other categories in this section are all folliculitides. The term *folliculitis* refers to the presence of inflammatory cells within the wall and lumen of a hair follicle, while *perifolliculitis* denotes their presence in the perifollicular connective tissue, sometimes extending into the adjacent reticular dermis. Folliculitis and perifolliculitis are often found together because an inflammatory process in the follicle spills over into the adjacent connective tissue. If the inflammatory process is severe enough, destruction of the hair follicle will ensue. Scarring may also result if the inflammatory process is severe and/or persistent. Five major categories of folliculitis, other than acneiform lesions, can be defined although, as already mentioned, this subdivision is somewhat arbitrary. They will be considered after the acneiform lesions have been discussed.

ACNEIFORM LESIONS

Acneiform lesions are characterized by the presence of comedones, as well as inflammation of the hair follicle. The inflammatory process frequently extends into the adjacent dermis with the formation of pustules, draining sinuses and subsequent scarring. The most important entity in this group is acne vulgaris.

ACNE VULGARIS

Acne vulgaris, an inflammatory disease of sebaceous follicles, is a common disorder that affects a large proportion of the teenage population.[11–15] It is usually a mild affliction which improves spontaneously after adolescence.[16] In a small proportion, it produces considerable disfigurement. Severity can impact on the quality of life of the affected individual.[17–19] Acne can also be found in some neonates, infants and adults.[20–24] Late-onset acne appears to be a special group in which endogenous factors play a major role.[25]

Acne is a polymorphic disorder with such diverse lesions as comedones, papules, pustules, cysts, sinuses and scars.[11] Scarring can be minimized by early effective treatment.[26,27] The comedones may take the form of tiny white papules known as 'whiteheads' (closed comedones) or small papules with a central core, the surface of which is black. These lesions are known as 'blackheads' (open comedones). Comedones are not confined to acne, being found in senile skin,[28] in a rare congenital form,[29] in nevus comedonicus and following exposure to certain chemicals such as coal tar.[30] Only a few inflammatory lesions are present at any one time in mild acne, although comedones may be present and dormant for years.[31]

Acne affects the face and, less frequently, the upper part of the trunk. These are sites of maximum density of sebaceous follicles.[12] In one report, acne presented in a zosteriform distribution ('acne nevus').[32] In another, the acneiform rash was localized to the site of previous herpes zoster infection.[33]

Etiology and pathogenesis

Acne vulgaris is of multifactorial origin with both intrinsic and extrinsic factors contributing to the final outcome.[34,35] There are four principal pathogenetic events: abnormal follicular keratinization with retention of keratinous material in the follicle, increased sebum production, the presence of the Gram-positive anaerobic diphtheroid *Propionibacterium acnes*, and inflammation.[12,36,37] These various factors are, in part, interrelated.

The initial event is abnormal keratinization of the infrainfundibular portion of sebaceous follicles, leading to the impaction of adherent horny lamellae within the follicle.[38,39] The cause of this retention hyperkeratosis is unknown although both the formation of free fatty acids and the follicular deficiency of the fatty acid linoleic acid[40] have been implicated at different times. Impacted follicles, which are the precursors of comedones and inflammatory lesions, are not detectable clinically.[38] They are termed 'microcomedones'.[41]

The role of sebum is poorly understood.[42] Acne patients have increased sebum secretion by the sebaceous follicles.[40] Sebum production is known to be under the influence of androgens,[43,44] which are increased in some patients, particularly females, with acne.[45–50] Dehydroepiandrosterone sulfate, the major adrenal androgen, is significantly higher in girls with acne than in age-matched controls.[20,51] Androgens also play a role in prepubertal acne in males.[52,53] Of interest is the finding that some women with acne have polycystic ovaries.[54,55] Furthermore, the injection of sebum into the skin produces inflammatory lesions that mimic those of acne.[56] Premenstrual acne flares may occur.[57]

P. acnes is the bacterial species most consistently isolated from lesions of acne,[58] although it is present in only 70% of early inflammatory lesions.[59] Bacteria are not essential for the formation of comedones.[60] *P. acnes* produces several factors which may be of pathogenetic importance.[61–64] These include lipases and proteases and chemotactic factors. *P. acnes* can, in some way, activate the complement system and it may stimulate the release of hydrolases from neutrophils.[62] These may in turn damage the follicular wall, leading to the liberation of the contents of the follicle into the dermis and the consequent inflammatory reaction. Recent studies suggest that an overly vigorous immune response to *P. acnes* may be the fundamental problem in patients with inflammatory acne.[65,66] The microflora of adolescent, persistent and late-onset acne is the same.[67] Antibiotic-resistant strains of *P. acnes* are present in some cases of recalcitrant acne vulgaris.[68,69] Phototherapy has been used to treat some of these antibiotic-resistant cases.[70]

Many external factors may influence the course of acne vulgaris.[71] These include drugs (halides, isoniazid, various hormones, barbiturates, lithium, etretinate, amineptine,[72] the recreational drug ecstasy,[73] and phenytoin (diphenylhydantoin)), cosmetics, soaps and shampoos, industrial chemicals, oils and tar,[74] ultraviolet light, infections such as infectious mononucleosis[75] and friction or trauma.[76,77]

Acneiform lesions are seen in Apert's syndrome (acrocephalo-syndactyly)[78,79] and pyoderma faciale, although in the latter there are cysts and draining sinuses but no comedones.[80] An acneiform eruption may complicate the use of topical and systemic corticosteroid therapy (*steroid acne*).[81,82] There is some suggestion that steroid acne is exacerbated or precipitated in some way by the presence of *Malassezia sp.*[83] Another form of acne is *aquagenic acne*, which occurs in some swimmers. It is probably of multifactorial origin, chlorine being only one of many contributing factors.[84]

Finally, **neonatal cephalic pustulosis**, said to be present in approximately 3% of neonates, is clinically similar to neonatal acne. It may be triggered by the yeast *Malassezia sympodialis*.[85]

Histopathology[11,86]

The three major components of acne vulgaris are comedones, inflammatory lesions and scars. A *comedo* is an impaction of horny cells in the lumen of a sebaceous follicle.[11,87] Preceding this is the microcomedo, a clinically invisible lesion in which there is only minimal distension of the infrainfundibular canal of a sebaceous follicle, accompanied by increased retention of horny cells and a prominent underlying granular layer.[37,38,88] There are two types of comedo: a closed comedo ('whitehead') with only a small orifice, and an open comedo ('blackhead') which in contrast has a wide patulous orifice.[86] Both consist of a cyst-like cavity filled with a compact mass of keratinous material and numerous bacteria.[86] In the closed comedo there are one or two hairs trapped in the lumen and atrophic sebaceous acini, while in the open comedo there are up to 10–15 hairs in the lumen and the sebaceous acini are atrophic or absent.[11,86] The epithelial lining of comedones is usually thin.

The source of the pigmentation in open comedones ('blackheads') is disputed. It has been attributed to the presence of active melanocytes in the uppermost follicle, but a more recent study failed to confirm this.[89] It is now suggested that densely packed, often concentric, horny material, interspersed with sebaceous material and bacterial breakdown products, may be responsible for the observed pigmentation.[89]

If comedones rupture, re-epithelialization may eventually occur, producing secondary comedones which may be distorted in shape as a consequence of the residual inflammation and dermal scarring.[11,86] Epidermal cysts may also form, particularly on the neck. They differ from comedones by their often larger size and the complete absence of sebaceous acini and a pilary unit.[86] Comedones of all types may be dormant for a long period. At any time they may become inflamed.

Inflammatory lesions have traditionally been attributed to the accumulation of neutrophils within microcomedones or comedones with subsequent rupture of the follicle and the formation of a pustule in the dermis. It now appears that there is an even earlier stage which involves the transmigration of lymphocytes into the wall of the follicle associated with increasing spongiosis of the follicular epithelium (Fig. 15.2).[88] This change has been likened to an allergic contact sensitivity reaction.[88] This is followed after 24–72 hours by the accumulation of neutrophils within the follicle, leading to its distension and subsequent rupture.[88] There may be a localized loss of the granular layer in the region of the eventual rupture, suggesting a defect in keratinization in this region. A perifollicular pustule develops following the rupture of the comedo (Fig. 15.3). Lymphocytes, plasma cells and foreign body giant cells subsequently appear. The follicular epithelium tends to encapsulate the inflammatory mass; sometimes this is followed by the formation of draining sinuses lined by remnants of the follicular epithelium.

When the inflammatory process subsides, distorted secondary comedones may result.

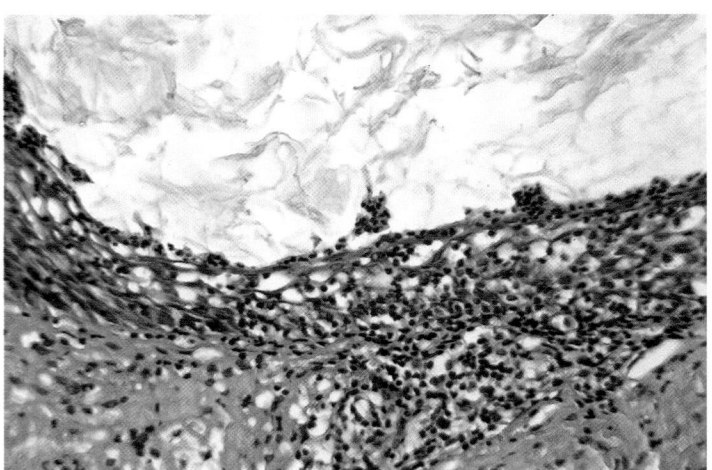

Fig. 15.2 **Acne vulgaris** (early lesion). There is transmigration of lymphocytes through the spongiotic epithelium lining a microcomedone. A few neutrophils are present along the inner edge. (H & E)

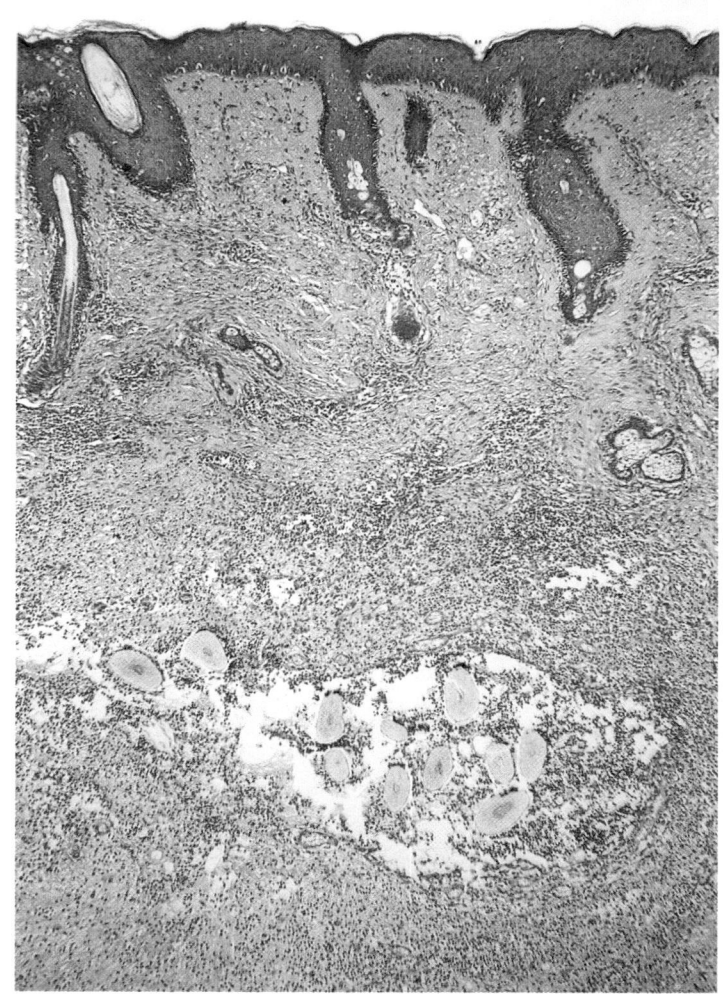

Fig. 15.3 **Acne vulgaris.** A perifollicular pustule is present in the dermis. It contains liberated hair shafts. (H & E)

Scars in acne vulgaris may take the form of localized dermal fibrosis or of hypertrophic scars, even with keloidal changes. Small atrophic pits are quite common.[86] A thin fibrotic dermis, devoid of appendages, is found directly beneath the epidermis-lined pit. Perifollicular fibrosis and elastolysis,[90] dystrophic calcification, osteoma cutis[91] and localized hemosiderosis[92] are other complications of inflammatory acne lesions.

Electron microscopy
Comedones contain keratinized cells, sebum, organisms and hairs.[93] Treatment with isotretinoin leads to a reduction in the quantity of this material and a loss of cohesion between the keratinized cells.[94] In early acne, the cells of the infrainfundibulum contain numerous tonofilaments and desmosomes, but fewer lamellar granules than usual.[37]

ACNE FULMINANS

Acne fulminans is a rare, acute form of acne, found usually in young adult males.[95,96] There is a sudden onset of painful, ulcerated and crusted lesions accompanied by fever, musculoskeletal pain and leukocytosis.[95,97] Lytic lesions of bone develop in 25% of cases.[95,98–100] A subgroup without systemic features has been reported.[101] Acne fulminans has been reported in association with Crohn's disease,[102] erythema nodosum[103,104] and the use of testosterone.[105] Familial cases have been reported.[106]

The etiology of this condition is unknown, although there is speculation that immune mechanisms are involved.[98] This is supported by the response that occurs to systemic corticosteroid therapy.[97,107]

Acne fulminans, or another pustular dermatosis such as acne conglobata, palmoplantar pustulosis, hidradenitis suppurativa or pustular psoriasis, may occur as the cutaneous manifestation of **SAPHO syndrome** (synovitis, *acne, pustulosis, hyperostosis and osteitis*).[108]

Histopathology[109]
Comedones are uncommon in acne fulminans. There are extensive inflammatory lesions in the dermis associated with necrosis of follicles and the overlying epidermis. Follicles distended with neutrophils are also present. Severe dermal scarring usually follows the subsidence of the inflammation.

CHLORACNE

Chloracne is an acneiform eruption caused by systemic poisoning by halogenated aromatic compounds.[110,111] Although the brominated compounds tend to be more toxic, the term 'chloracne' stems from the chlorinated version.[112] Industrial exposure is the usual source of the chloracnegens, although exposure to defoliants containing dioxin was encountered in the Vietnam War.[113–116] Cutaneous lesions may persist for long periods after the last exposure to the offending chemical.

Chloracne is distinct from other forms of acne.[110] It most often involves the malar crescent, the retroauricular region and the scrotum and penis. Erythema and pigmentation of the face may also occur.[110] The primary lesion is the comedo, which is intermingled with small cysts.[110] Inflammatory lesions are sparse. Dioxins have also produced areas resembling granuloma annulare and atrophoderma vermiculatum.[110]

Histopathology[110,113]
There is follicular hyperkeratosis with infundibular dilatation forming bottle-shaped and columnar funnels containing keratinous debris. Comedones and keratinous cysts with an attachment to the epidermis also form.[113] Small inflammatory foci may be present.

SUPERFICIAL FOLLICULITIDES

In the superficial folliculitides, the inflammatory infiltrate is found beneath the stratum corneum overlying a hair follicle and/or in the follicular infundibulum. Disruption of the follicle wall may lead to inflammation of the upper dermis adjacent to the affected hair follicle.

ACUTE SUPERFICIAL FOLLICULITIS

Acute superficial folliculitis, also known as impetigo of Bockhart, is characterized by small pustules developing around follicular ostia and frequently pierced by a hair.[117,118] *Staphylococcus aureus* has been implicated in the etiology.

Histopathology
There is a subcorneal pustule overlying the follicular infundibulum. In addition to neutrophils, there are also lymphocytes and macrophages in the infiltrate, which usually extends into the upper follicle and the surrounding dermis. A morphologically similar entity confined to the scalp and possibly related to infection with *Propionibacterium acnes* has been reported as chronic non-scarring folliculitis of the scalp.[119]

ACTINIC FOLLICULITIS

There have been several reports of a pustular folliculitis of the face and upper part of the trunk following exposure to sunlight.[120–123] The mechanism by which exposure to ultraviolet light results in folliculitic lesions remains to be elucidated, although the condition may be related to acne vulgaris and acne estivalis.[122]

Histopathology
The microscopic changes are those of an acute superficial folliculitis.[120,123] No organisms are seen and bacterial cultures have been negative.

ACNE NECROTICA

Acne necrotica (acne varioliformis) is a rare dermatosis of adults, consisting of crops of erythematous, follicle-based papules that become superficially necrotic, umbilicated and crusted, with subsequent healing which produces a depressed varioliform scar.[124–126] Only a small number of active lesions may be present at any time. They develop on the frontal hairline, forehead and face and sometimes on the upper part of the trunk.

Acne necrotica miliaris has been regarded as a pruritic, non-scarring variant of acne necrotica in which follicular vesiculopustules develop on the scalp.[124] This condition has been regarded as nothing more than neurotic excoriations superimposed on a bacterial folliculitis, an etiology that has also been proposed for acne necrotica itself.[127]

Histopathology[124]
Early lesions show an intense perivascular and perifollicular lymphocytic infiltrate extending to the mid dermis and associated with prominent sub-epidermal edema. The infiltrate also extends into the wall of the upper part of the follicle and into the epidermis, where there is associated spongiosis and death of individual keratinocytes. Later, there is confluent necrosis of the upper follicle, the epidermis and dermis. At this stage neutrophils are seen in

the upper follicle and the adjacent dermis. A florid superficial folliculitis and perifolliculitis are sometimes present (Fig. 15.4).

Biopsies of acne necrotica miliaris may show superficially inflamed excoriations, centered on hair follicles.[127] It is unusual to have an intact lesion biopsied; presumably a superficial folliculitis would be seen.

NECROTIZING FOLLICULITIS OF AIDS

A necrotizing folliculitis is a rare cutaneous manifestation of the acquired immunodeficiency syndrome (AIDS) or its prodromes.[128]

Histopathology

Although the folliculitis and perifolliculitis may not be confined to the superficial follicle, this condition is classified with the superficial folliculitides because the accompanying necrosis is confined to the upper part of the follicle and the adjacent epidermis and superficial dermis, characteristically in a wedge-shaped area.[128] There is fibrinoid necrosis of vessels at the apex of the wedge.

EOSINOPHILIC FOLLICULITIS

Eosinophilic folliculitis is a heterogeneous group of disorders with several clinical subsets:

- the classic form, eosinophilic pustular folliculitis (Ofuji's disease)
- HIV-associated eosinophilic folliculitis
- pediatric eosinophilic folliculitis
- fungal eosinophilic folliculitis
- a miscellaneous group.

The *classic form, eosinophilic pustular folliculitis (Ofuji's disease)*, is a rare, chronic dermatosis, first described in the Japanese[129–131] but now reported occasionally in Caucasians.[132–136] There are recurrent, sterile, follicular papules and pustules with a tendency to form circinate plaques.[137,138] These may show central clearing with residual hyperpigmentation. 'Seborrheic areas', such as the face, trunk and extensor surface of the proximal part of the limbs,[139] are usually involved but in 20% of cases the non-hair-bearing palms and soles may also be involved.[137] For this reason, the designations 'eosinophilic pustular

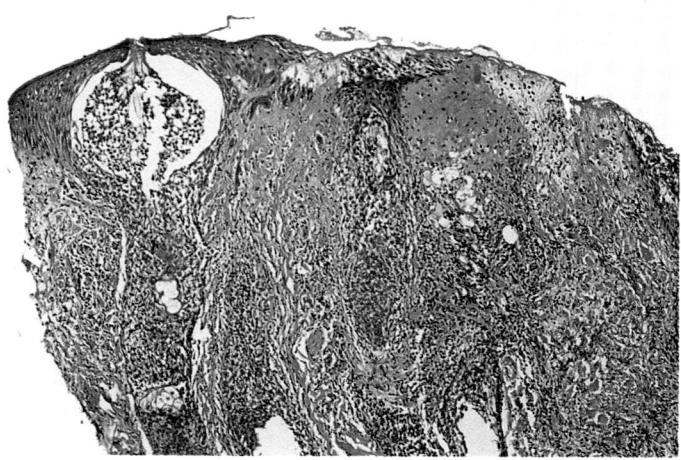

Fig. 15.4 **Acne necrotica.** Confluent necrosis involves the upper follicle and adjacent epidermis and papillary dermis. An adjacent follicle shows a superficial folliculitis. (H & E)

dermatosis'[140] and 'sterile eosinophilic pustulosis' have been suggested as more appropriate titles. A peripheral leukocytosis and eosinophilia are often present.

The condition reported in two brothers as circinate eosinophilic dermatosis has some similarities.[141]

The etiology of eosinophilic pustular folliculitis is unknown. Interestingly, a similar lesion has been reported in dogs.[142] Various immunological abnormalities have been reported in some patients, but this is not a constant feature.[143,144] Circulating antibodies to basal cell cytoplasm[145] and intercellular antigens have been noted.[146] Chemotactic factors have also been isolated from the skin.[147] More recently it has been suggested that the production of nitric oxide by eosinophils may have a pathogenetic role.[148]

HIV-associated eosinophilic folliculitis has been regarded as a subset of the pruritic papular eruption of human immunodeficiency virus infection.[149–155] It differs from the classic form (Ofuji's disease) by the severe pruritus, the absence of circinate and palmoplantar lesions, and the less frequent involvement of the face.[156] Coexisting follicular mucinosis has been reported in two patients.[157] It has been suggested that HIV-associated eosinophilic folliculitis is an autoimmune disease with the sebocyte or some constituent of sebum acting as the autoantigen.[158] In one patient, the eruption appeared to be related to the use of foscarnet therapy.[159]

Pediatric (childhood) eosinophilic folliculitis is usually confined to the scalp, although grouped aggregates of follicular pustules can occur on the face, extremities and trunk in some patients.[160–163] It usually has a self-limited course. This condition is no longer regarded as a variant of eosinophilic folliculitis as interfollicular inflammation is sometimes the predominant feature. Eosinophilic pustulosis appears to be an appropriate designation for these cases.

Fungal eosinophilic folliculitis is usually a localized disease, characterized by erosive and pustular plaques.[164,165]

The *miscellaneous group* includes patients in whom bacteria, such as *Pseudomonas*, have been isolated and patients with myeloproliferative or other hematological disorders.[166,167] Nine HIV-negative patients with an atopic diathesis have been reported with ulcerative and/or nodular plaques mainly on the face and/or extremities, sometimes in an annular configuration. The histology was that of a necrotizing eosinophilic folliculitis. These cases appear to be the 'eosinophilic equivalent' of sterile neutrophilic folliculitis with perifollicular vasculopathy (see p. 465). Drugs such as carbamazepine and minocycline have been associated with an eosinophilic folliculitis.[168] Rarely, pemphigus vegetans may present as an eosinophilic folliculitis.[169]

Histopathology[132,133,137,162]

The various clinical subsets of eosinophilic folliculitis have a similar histological appearance.[162] There is eosinophilic spongiosis and pustulosis involving particularly the infundibular region of the hair follicle. The infiltrate often extends into the attached sebaceous duct and sebaceous gland. Most follicles are preserved, but some show disruption or destruction of the wall by the inflammatory infiltrate.[132] Follicular necrosis and folliculocentric necrotizing eosinophilic vasculitis were features of the cases reported in association with an atopic diathesis (see above).[170] In addition to the eosinophils, there are variable numbers of neutrophils and some mononuclear cells; neutrophils are usually sparse.[162] There is also a moderately dense, perivascular and perifollicular inflammatory cell infiltrate composed of lymphocytes, eosinophils and macrophages. A PAS or silver methenamine preparation should always be examined, as dermatophyte infections occasionally give a similar appearance.[145,171]

Lesions on the palms and soles show subcorneal and intraepidermal pustules. There is a variable inflammatory infiltrate in the underlying dermis.

INFUNDIBULOFOLLICULITIS

Infundibulofolliculitis is mentioned here for completeness, although it is discussed in further detail with the spongiotic tissue reaction (see p. 102). The histopathological changes are those of follicular spongiosis. A few neutrophils may be found in the spongiotic infundibulum or in the keratin plug which is sometimes present in the involved follicle. A variable mononuclear cell infiltrate usually surrounds the upper dermal portion of the hair follicle.[172]

DEEP INFECTIOUS FOLLICULITIDES

In this group of folliculitides the inflammatory process involves the deep portion of the hair follicle, although both superficial and deep inflammation may be present (Fig. 15.5). The etiological agents include bacteria, fungi and viruses and are not always easily identified in routine tissue sections. A folliculitis is an uncommon presentation of secondary syphilis.

FURUNCLE

A furuncle (boil) is a deep-seated infection centered on the pilosebaceous unit.[173] Boils commonly occur at sites of friction by clothing such as the back of the neck, the buttocks and inner aspect of the thighs. The lesion begins as a painful, follicular papule with surrounding erythema and induration.[173] The center usually becomes yellow, softens and discharges pus. Healing takes place with minimal scarring. A carbuncle is a coalescence of multiple furuncles which may lead to multiple points of drainage on the skin surface. There are often constitutional symptoms.

Staphylococcus aureus is the organism most often involved.[174]

Histopathology[175]
A furuncle consists of a deep dermal abscess centered on a hair follicle. This is usually destroyed, although a residual hair shaft is sometimes present in the center of the abscess. There is often extension of the inflammatory process into the subcutis. The overlying epidermis is eventually destroyed and the surface is covered by an inflammatory crust.

PSEUDOMONAS FOLLICULITIS

Pseudomonas folliculitis is usually caused by *Pseudomonas aeruginosa*. It presents as an erythematous follicular eruption which may be maculopapular, vesicular, pustular or polymorphous.[176,177] It usually involves the trunk, axillae and proximal parts of the extremities. There may be constitutional symptoms.[178] Lesions develop 8–48 hours after recreational exposure to the organism, which is found in contaminated sponges, whirlpools and hot tubs.[179–181] Spontaneous clearing usually occurs within a week. Sporadic cases, without recreational exposure, also occur.[182]

Histopathology[176]
There is an acute suppurative folliculitis which may be both superficial and deep. If disruption of the follicular wall occurs, dermal suppuration may result. Attempts to demonstrate organisms in conventional histological preparations are usually unsuccessful.

OTHER BACTERIAL FOLLICULITIDES

A folliculitis caused by Gram-negative bacteria may occur as a complication of prolonged antibiotic therapy in patients with acne vulgaris.[183] Most of these

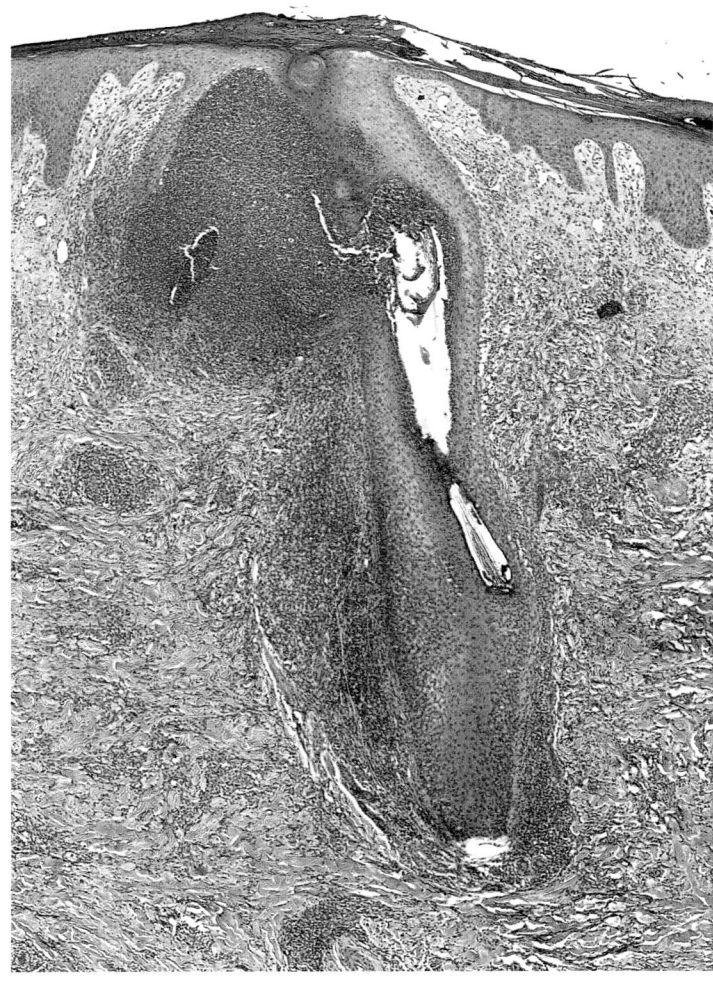

Fig. 15.5 **Acute folliculitis of fungal etiology** involving both the superficial and deep portion of the follicle. (H & E)

infections are caused by a subgroup of lactose-fermenting bacteria, resulting in superficial pustules grouped around the nose. *Pseudomonas aeruginosa* has also been implicated in this clinical setting.[184] In others, deep nodular and cystic lesions occur as a result of infection by species of *Proteus*.[183] *Citrobacter diversus*, *Klebsiella* sp., *Escherichia coli* and *Enterobacter* sp. have also been implicated.[185,186] In immunocompromised patients, organisms which are not usually pathogens, such as *Micrococcus*, have been involved.[187]

Bacteria, possibly complicating the application of various oils to the skin, have been implicated in a pustular eruption of the legs seen in parts of Africa and India and known as dermatitis cruris pustulosa et atrophicans.[188]

Salmonella dublin was isolated from one case of widespread folliculitis.[189]

Histopathology
Both a superficial and deep folliculitis may be present in these bacterial folliculitides. There is variable involvement of the perifollicular dermis.

VIRAL FOLLICULITIS

The pilosebaceous follicle may be infected with herpes simplex virus type I. Vesicular lesions may not be obvious clinically.[190]

An unidentified virus, possibly of the Papovaviridae family, has been implicated in the etiology of a folliculitis in an immunocompromised patient.[191] The term 'trichodysplasia spinulosa' was coined for this eruption which presented as erythematous, indurated papules with friable spinous processes and progressive alopecia.[191] The term 'pilomatrix dysplasia' has been used for a similar condition (see p. 870).

Histopathology

In herpes folliculitis there is partial or complete necrosis of the follicle with exocytosis of lymphocytes into the follicular wall and the attached sebaceous gland. Sometimes there is adjacent dermal necrosis. The epidermis sometimes shows the typical features of herpetic infection. At other times, a 'bottom heavy' perivascular and interstitial dermal inflammatory cell infiltrate, which may simulate a pseudolymphoma or lymphoma, is the only clue.[192] This finding necessitates the cutting of multiple deeper sections in search of an involved hair follicle. Inclusion bodies and multinucleate cells are not always found in the follicular epithelium. A syringitis may accompany the folliculitis.[193]

In the case reported as **trichodysplasia spinulosa** there was dilatation and keratotic plugging of the infundibula with marked dystrophy of the inner root sheath with enlarged, irregular, trichohyaline granules and numerous apoptotic cells. Inflammation was very mild.[191] As mentioned above, the changes have some similarities to those reported in another immunosuppressed patient as **pilomatrix dysplasia** (see p. 870).

DERMATOPHYTE FOLLICULITIS

Fungal elements may be seen on or within the hair shafts in certain dermatophyte infections, particularly tinea capitis. Various organisms may be involved, particularly *Trichophyton tonsurans*, *Microsporum canis* and *M. audouinii*.[194] Sometimes an inflamed boggy mass, known as a kerion, develops.

Histopathology

There is variable inflammation of the follicle and perifollicular dermis. If disruption of the hair follicle occurs, a few foreign body giant cells may be present. Hyphae and arthrospores may be found within the hair shaft or on the surface, depending on the nature of the infection. PAS or methenamine silver preparations are usually required in order to demonstrate the fungal elements.

Abscess formation with partial or complete destruction of hair follicles occurs in a kerion.

PITYROSPORUM FOLLICULITIS

Pityrosporum folliculitis, resulting from infection of the follicle by *Malassezia* sp. (Pityrosporum), has been described on page 668. The small oval yeast responsible can be seen within the inflamed follicle and may be found in the adjacent dermis following rupture of the follicle.

DEEP SCARRING FOLLICULITIDES

In the deep scarring group there is severe folliculitis involving the deep part of the follicle and often the upper part as well. Rupture of the follicle and its contents into the dermis leads to eventual scarring of variable severity. It is usually mild in folliculitis decalvans, but quite marked in folliculitis keloidalis nuchae. A similar picture can be seen following severe petrol burns of the skin.

FOLLICULITIS DECALVANS

Folliculitis decalvans is a chronic form of deep folliculitis that usually occurs on the scalp as oval patches of scarring alopecia at the expanding margins of which are follicular pustules.[117,195] Any or all of the hairy areas of the body may be involved. Folliculitis barbae (lupoid sycosis) is a related condition confined to the beard area, while epilating folliculitis of the glabrous skin is the name used in the earlier literature for a related condition involving the legs.[196] Folliculitis decalvans has been reported in identical twins.[197]

Folliculitis decalvans usually runs a prolonged course of variable severity. The etiology is unknown, although *Staphylococcus aureus* is sometimes cultured from the lesions.[198]

Tufted hair folliculitis (see p. 481) has been regarded as a clinicopathological variant of folliculitis decalvans,[199] but as it can be associated with other disease processes, it is best regarded as a distinct process.[200]

Histopathology[117,195]

Initially there is a folliculitis; this is followed by disruption of the follicular wall and liberation of the contents of the follicle into the dermis (Fig. 15.6). The dermis adjacent to the destroyed follicle contains a mixed inflammatory cell

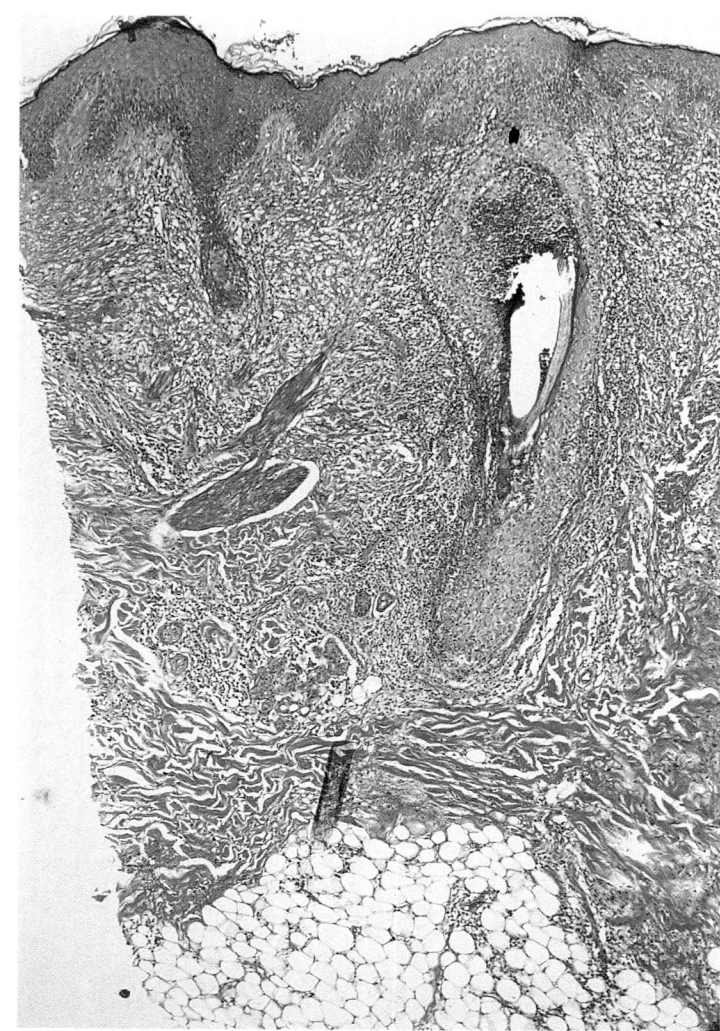

Fig. 15.6 **Folliculitis decalvans.** The patient had a scarring alopecia. There is early disruption of the wall of an inflamed follicle. (H & E)

infiltrate. Plasma cells are sometimes present in the infiltrate, particularly in resolving lesions. Foreign body giant cells may form around the hair shafts lying free in the dermis. Variable scarring results, but this is never as severe as in folliculitis keloidalis nuchae.

FOLLICULITIS KELOIDALIS NUCHAE

Folliculitis keloidalis nuchae, also known as acne keloidalis, is a rare, idiopathic, inflammatory condition of the nape of the neck, restricted to adult males.[201–203] It is a form of primary scarring alopecia of the occipital and nuchal region.[204] It is more common in blacks. There are follicular papules and pustules which enlarge, forming confluent, thickened plaques, sometimes with discharging sinuses.[201,205] Scarring results from this chronic inflammatory process. Surgery is sometimes required to manage the condition.[206]

The pathogenesis of this condition and the reasons for its occipital localization are not known. Postulated mechanisms include a seborrheic constitution, incurving hairs resulting from recurrent low-grade trauma (for example, by football helmets),[207] the use of antiepileptic drugs or cyclosporine[208,209] and an increase in mast cell numbers in the occipital region.[210–212]

Histopathology[201,202]

There is an initial folliculitis with subsequent rupture and destruction of the follicle and liberation of hair shafts into the dermis (Fig. 15.7).[202] Usually, by the time a biopsy is taken, there is already dense dermal fibrosis with a chronic inflammatory cell infiltrate which includes numerous plasma cells. Hair shafts are present in the dermis and these are surrounded by microabscesses and/or foreign body giant cells. Sinus tracts may lead to the surface. Sometimes there are claw-like epidermal downgrowths associated with the transepidermal elimination of hair shafts and inflammatory debris.[213] Involved follicles may show tufted hair folliculitis while intact follicles at the margins may show polytrichia.[201,214] Keloid fibers develop within the dense fibrous tissue in some cases.[201]

FOLLICULAR OCCLUSION TRIAD

The follicular occlusion triad refers to hidradenitis suppurativa, dissecting cellulitis of the scalp and acne conglobata. These three conditions constitute a form of deep scarring folliculitis: they are grouped together on the basis of their presumed common pathogenesis of poral occlusion followed by bacterial

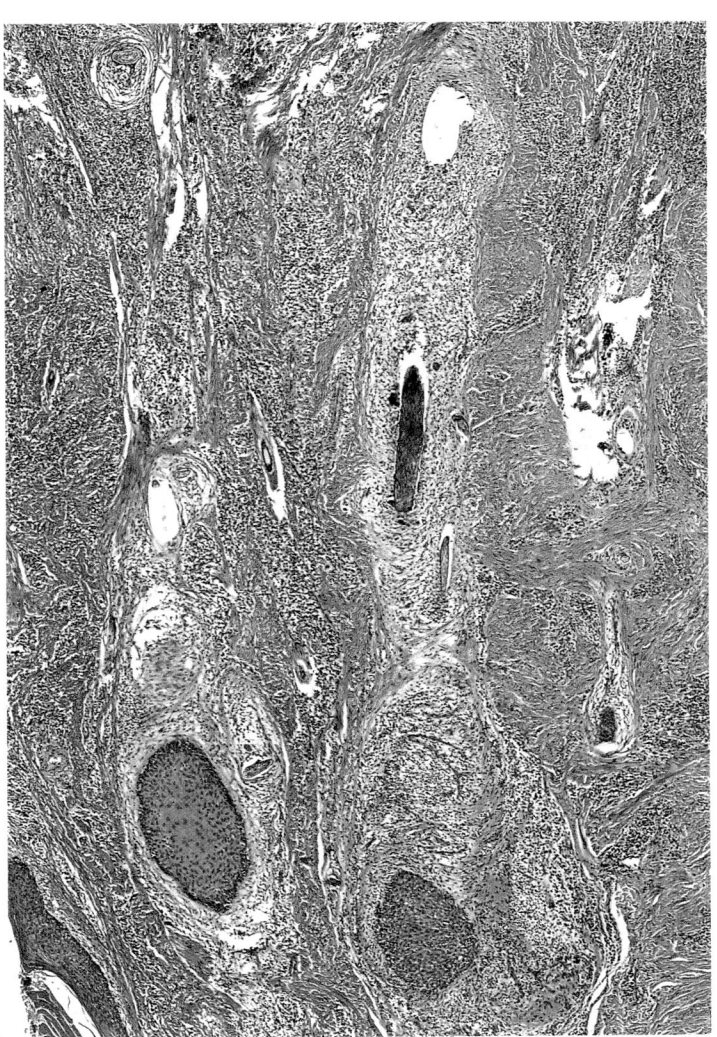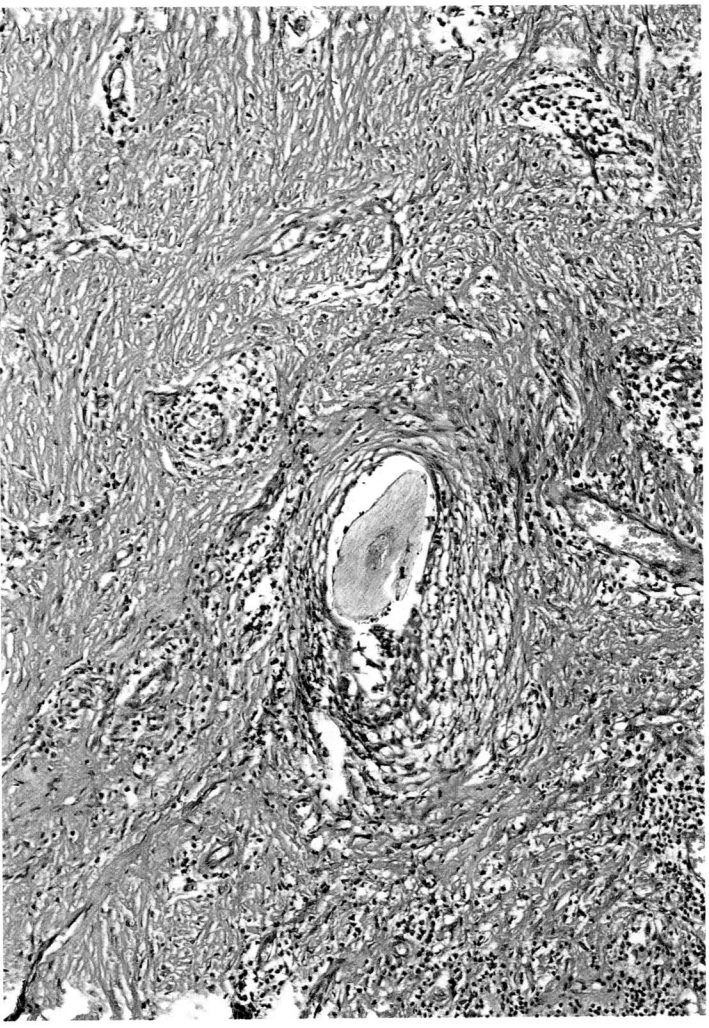

Fig. 15.7 **Folliculitis keloidalis. (A)** Hair shafts have been extruded into the dermis during the inflammatory destruction of the hair follicles. **(B)** Fibrosis of the dermis is also present. (H & E)

infection.[215] The presence of draining sinuses is a further characteristic feature of this group. It has been suggested that pilonidal sinus is a related entity. These follicular occlusion disorders may coexist.[216]

HIDRADENITIS SUPPURATIVA

Hidradenitis suppurativa (acne inversa, apocrine acne) is a chronic, relapsing, inflammatory disorder involving one or more apocrine gland-bearing areas, which include the axillae, groins, pubic region and perineum.[217–222] There are recurrent, deep-seated inflammatory nodules, complicated by draining sinuses and subsequent scarring. The disease causes a high degree of morbidity; pain is often a problem.[223] The development of squamous cell carcinoma is a late and rare complication.[224–227] Other clinical features include the presence of comedones in retroauricular and apocrine sites,[228] a female predominance[229,230] and a genetic predisposition.[231–233] Prepubertal onset is rare.[234] Associations with lithium therapy,[235] Dowling–Degos disease,[236] cigarette smoking,[237,238] and Crohn's disease have been reported.[239–241] Host defense mechanisms are usually normal, except in some severe cases, where a reduction in T lymphocytes has been documented.[242] There is now good evidence that hidradenitis suppurativa is an androgen-dependent disorder,[243–246] although how this relates to the poral occlusion by keratinous material is uncertain.[247] This occlusion is followed by an active folliculitis with an apocrinitis and apocrine destruction, whereas apoeccrine glands, which drain directly on to the epidermal surface, appear to be uninvolved.[248] Coagulase-negative staphylococci are the most common isolate;[249] however, the microbiological flora is not constant.[241]

Histopathology[250]

In established lesions, there is a heavy, mixed inflammatory cell infiltrate in the lower half of the dermis, usually with extension into the subcutis.[251] Chronic abscesses are present in active cases and these may connect with sinus tracts leading to the skin surface (Fig. 15.8). The sinuses are usually lined by stratified squamous epithelium in their outer part. They contain inflammatory and other debris.[252] Some of these tracts are probably residual follicular structures.[253,254]

Granulation tissue containing inflammatory cells and occasional foreign body giant cells is present in up to 25% of cases.[240] Epithelioid granulomas were present in one case with coexisting Crohn's disease.[240] Extensive fibrosis with destruction of pilosebaceous follicles and of apocrine and eccrine glands usually ensues. Inflammation of the apocrine glands may be present in the axillary region in about 20% of cases.[255] Perieccrine inflammation is seen in approximately one-third of cases, from all sites.[248]

In early lesions, there is folliculitis and perifolliculitis involving the lower part of the follicle.[256] The infundibulum is usually dilated and contains keratinous material and inflammatory debris.[257] These findings support the notion that hidradenitis suppurativa is primarily a follicular disease, but apocrine glands can be primarily involved in a minority of axillary lesions.[255]

DISSECTING CELLULITIS OF THE SCALP

Dissecting cellulitis of the scalp, also known as perifolliculitis capitis abscedens et suffodiens (Hoffmann's disease), is an extremely rare disease characterized by the appearance of tender, suppurative nodules with interconnecting draining sinuses and subsequent scarring.[258–260] Patchy alopecia usually overlies the lesions, which have a predilection for the vertex and occipital scalp. There is a predilection for young adult black males. Familial occurrence has been reported.[261] Dissecting cellulitis may occur alone or in association with the other follicular occlusion diseases – hidradenitis suppurativa and acne conglobata.[216]

The development of squamous cell carcinoma is a rare complication.[262]

Histopathology[263]

The earliest lesion is a folliculitis and perifolliculitis with a heavy infiltrate of neutrophils leading to abscess formation in the dermis. Draining sinuses may develop and in later lesions the infiltrate becomes mixed. Variable destruction of follicles ensues.

ACNE CONGLOBATA

Acne conglobata is an uncommon dermatosis, occurring almost exclusively in males and commencing after puberty. There are small and large, tender, inflamed nodules, cysts and discharging sinuses that eventually heal, leaving disfiguring scars.[264] Lesions may develop in any hair-bearing area, particularly the trunk, buttocks and proximal parts of the extremities.[265] The distribution is much wider than in hidradenitis suppurativa. Acne conglobata has been reported in association with lichen spinulosus in a man seropositive for the human immunodeficiency virus.[266] It has also followed pregnancy.[267]

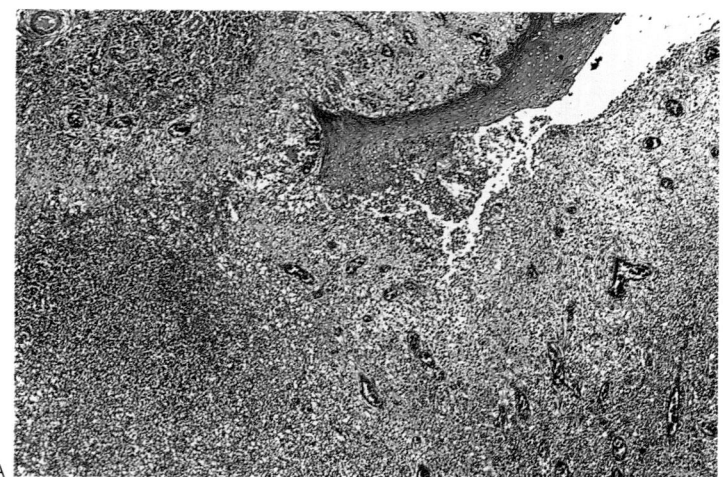
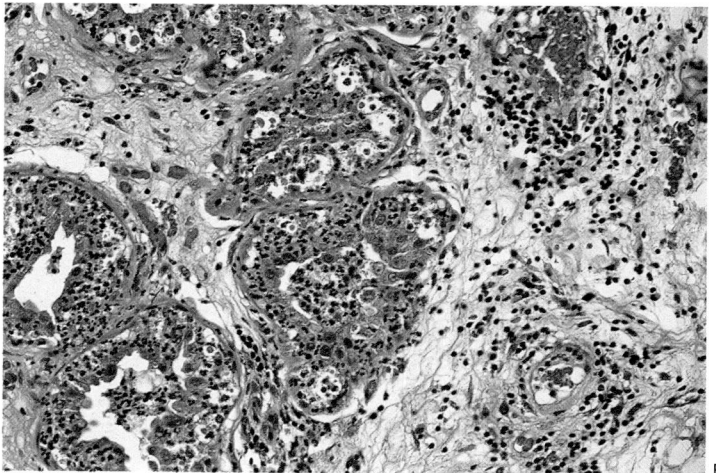

Fig. 15.8 **Hidradenitis suppurativa. (A)** There is acute and chronic inflammation in the dermis and an epithelial downgrowth (probably of follicular origin) 'draining' the area. There is hemorrhage at the deep edge. **(B)** Inflammation of the apocrine glands is present in this unusual case. (H & E)

Malignant degeneration can develop in lesions of acne conglobata of long standing.[264]

Histopathology

The appearances are similar to hidradenitis suppurativa, with deep abscesses and mixed inflammation, foreign body granulomas and discharging sinuses.[252] Comedones are often present.

MISCELLANEOUS FOLLICULITIDES

There are several folliculitides that do not fit appropriately into the categories already discussed. They include pseudofolliculitis, pruritic folliculitis of pregnancy and perforating folliculitis. Follicular pustules have also been reported in association with toxic erythema,[268] cyclosporine therapy,[269] C225 therapy (an antibody to epidermal growth factor receptor)[270] and in young individuals with acne treated with systemic steroids.[117] A lymphocytic folliculitis was present in a patient with an intensely pruritic eruption on the back, which developed after she stopped dieting.[271]

PSEUDOFOLLICULITIS

Pseudofolliculitis is a common disorder of adult black males. It is usually confined to the beard area of the face and neck,[272] but rarely the scalp,[273] pubic area[274] and legs[275] may be involved. It consists of papules and pustules in close proximity to hair follicles. Scarring and keloid formation sometimes result.[276]

Pseudofolliculitis is an inflammatory response to an ingrown hair. Hair shafts in black people have a tendency to form tight coils and, following shaving, the sharp ends may pierce the skin adjacent to the orifice of the follicles.[273]

Histopathology[272]

Surprisingly, little has been written about the histopathology of this common disorder. There are parafollicular inflammatory foci which are initially suppurative. Small foreign body granulomas and a mixed inflammatory cell infiltrate are present in older lesions. Variable scarring may ensue. In some instances, epithelium grows down from the surface to encase both the hair and the inflammatory response, assisting in their eventual transepithelial elimination.

PRURITIC FOLLICULITIS OF PREGNANCY

Pruritic folliculitis of pregnancy is a rare dermatosis in which pruritic, erythematous papules develop in a widespread distribution in the latter half of pregnancy.[277] The lesions clear spontaneously at delivery or in the postpartum period. There is no adverse effect on fetal well-being.[278] The etiology is unknown, but on the basis of a case with elevated androgens, it has been suggested that this condition is a 'form of hormonally induced acne'.[279] This finding has not been confirmed in a subsequent study.[278]

Histopathology[277]

The appearances are those of an acute folliculitis, sometimes resulting in destruction of follicular walls and abscess formation in the adjacent dermis. Perifollicular granulomas may be seen in late lesions.[280] No organisms have been noted in the cases reported so far.

PERFORATING FOLLICULITIS

Perforating folliculitis is manifested by discrete, keratotic, follicular papules with a predilection for the extensor surfaces of the extremities and the buttocks.[281] It may persist for months or years, although periods of remission often occur. Disease associations have included psoriasis,[282] juvenile acanthosis nigricans, HIV infection,[283] primary sclerosing cholangitis[284] and renal failure, often in association with hemodialysis.[281,285]

The features of perforating folliculitis associated with renal failure (see p. 363) may overlap those of reactive perforating collagenosis and Kyrle's disease[281] (the latter disease has been regarded by some as a variant of perforating folliculitis).[286] Lesions associated with renal failure are often pruritic, in contrast to the asymptomatic lesions of the majority of cases.[287]

The etiology of perforating folliculitis is unknown, although minor mechanical trauma may play a role. It has been suggested that perforation of the epithelium is the primary event and that it is not a disorder of transepithelial elimination.[287]

Histopathology[117,281]

There is a dilated follicular infundibulum filled with keratinous and cellular debris. A curled hair shaft is sometimes present. The follicular epithelium is disrupted in one or more areas in the infundibulum. The adjacent dermis shows degenerative changes involving the connective tissue, and sometimes collagen and elastic fibers are seen entering the perforation (Fig. 15.9). The elastic fibers are not increased as in elastosis perforans serpiginosa. A variable inflammatory reaction is present in the dermis in this region and sometimes a granulomatous perifolliculitis develops. Although a few neutrophils may be present in the infiltrate, they are never as plentiful as in pityrosporum folliculitis, which often ruptures into the dermis. Sometimes the follicular localization of perforating folliculitis is not appreciated unless serial sections are examined.

In chronic renal failure the lesion begins as a follicular pustule which perforates, resulting in a suppurative and granulomatous perifolliculitis.[288] Late lesions may develop epidermal features of prurigo nodularis.[288,289]

FOLLICULAR TOXIC PUSTULODERMA

The term 'follicular toxic pustuloderma' has been used for an acute pustular eruption with follicular localization. Most cases have been associated with the ingestion of drugs, particularly antibiotics, although in others an enterovirus infection has been incriminated.[290] As the lesions are not always follicle-based, the terms 'toxic pustuloderma' and 'acute generalized exanthematous pustulosis' are now used (see p. 136).

STERILE NEUTROPHILIC FOLLICULITIS WITH PERIFOLLICULAR VASCULOPATHY

The term 'sterile neutrophilic folliculitis with perifollicular vasculopathy' was coined by Magro and Crowson for a distinctive cutaneous reaction pattern, usually accompanying systemic diseases such as inflammatory bowel disease, Reiter's disease, Behçet's disease, hepatitis B and various connective tissue diseases.[291] It may present clinically as a folliculitis or a vasculitis or with vesiculopustular or acneiform lesions, predominantly on the legs, arms and upper back. Arthritis, fever and malaise are often present.

Histopathology

The reported cases showed a neutrophilic or suppurative and granulomatous folliculitis accompanied by a folliculocentric neutrophilic vascular reaction of Sweet's-like or leukocytoclastic vasculitis subtypes.[291]

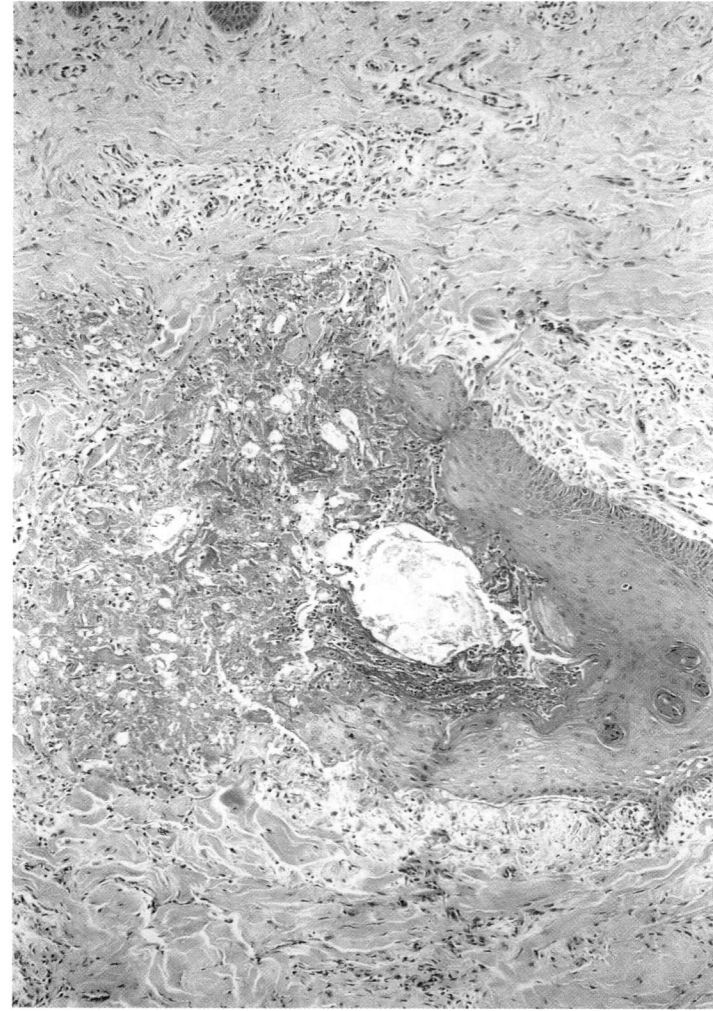

Fig. 15.9 **Perforating folliculitis.** Degenerate collagen and elastic tissue are entering the perforated follicle. The patient had chronic renal failure. (H & E)

PSEUDOLYMPHOMATOUS FOLLICULITIS

Pseudolymphomatous folliculitis is a subset of cutaneous lymphoid hyperplasia that is found at all ages and in both sexes.[292] It is almost exclusively a solitary lesion on the face measuring approximately 1 cm in diameter. The lesions often regress after incisional biopsy (see p. 1123).

Histopathology[292]

Pseudolymphomatous folliculitis has a dense dermal lymphocytic infiltrate simulating cutaneous lymphoma. The walls of the hair follicles are enlarged and irregularly deformed with their epithelial outline blurred by a lymphocytic infiltrate. Atypical lymphocytes are often present, leading to a misdiagnosis of lymphoma. Of the 15 cases reported in one series, 10 were composed predominantly of B cells and the remainder predominantly of T cells.[292] Increased numbers of dendritic cells expressing S100 and CD1a are present in the perifollicular region.

Hair shaft abnormalities

Hair shafts may be abnormal as a result of an intrinsic defect, either congenital or acquired, in the hair shaft itself or because of the deposition or attachment of extraneous matter such as fungi, bacteria or lacquer.[293] In either case, structural weakness of the hair shaft may occur; the resulting hair breakage and loss may be severe enough to produce alopecia.

Several clinical classifications of hair shaft abnormalities have been proposed.[293–296] One such classification distinguishes the structural defects with increased fragility from those without this characteristic, as only the cases in the former group (monilethrix, pili torti, trichorrhexis nodosa, trichothiodystrophy, Netherton's syndrome and Menkes' syndrome) present clinically with patchy or diffuse alopecia.[294] Another clinical approach has been to separate off those conditions associated with 'unruly hair', namely woolly hair, acquired progressive kinking of hair, pili torti and rare cases associated with brain growth deficiency.[297] One case that defies orderly classification has been called '**cutaneous pili migrans**'. In that case, a 7 cm long submerged hair extended as a blue line just below the skin surface.[298] There was no associated inflammation.

The classification to be followed here is morphologically based and is similar to the one proposed by Whiting.[293] Four major groups exist:

- fractures of hair shafts
- irregularities of hair shafts
- coiling and twisting abnormalities
- extraneous matter on hair shafts.

FRACTURES OF HAIR SHAFTS

The hair shaft fracture group of abnormalities is the most important because it may lead to alopecia. Sometimes, however, these abnormalities occur sporadically or intermittently,[299] involving only isolated hairs as an incidental phenomenon. This is particularly likely to occur in those who subject their hair to physical or chemical trauma. More than one type of fracture may be present in these cases.[300] The following types of fractures will be considered:

- trichorrhexis nodosa
- trichoschisis
- trichoclasis
- trichorrhexis invaginata
- tapered fracture
- trichoptilosis.

TRICHORRHEXIS NODOSA

Trichorrhexis nodosa is characterized by one or more small, beaded swellings along the hair shaft, corresponding to sites that fracture easily. Scalp hair is most often involved although the genital region may also be affected.[301] Trichorrhexis nodosa may be generalized or localized.[302] Alopecia may result because the hairs fracture easily.

The basic cause of trichorrhexis nodosa is prolonged mechanical trauma or chemical insults, although a contributing factor in some instances is an inherent weakness of the hair shaft. This weakness may result from a specific pilar dystrophy such as pili torti, monilethrix or trichorrhexis invaginata, or from an inborn error of metabolism affecting the hair such as arginosuccinic aminoaciduria, Menkes' syndrome[303] or trichothiodystrophy.[295,301,304–307] This latter group of abnormalities is quite rare but they usually form the basis of hereditary cases of trichorrhexis nodosa.[301]

Trichothiodystrophy refers to a rare group of autosomal recessive disorders that have in common short brittle hair with a sulfur content less than 50% of normal.[301,308–310] This results from a deficiency of the sulfur-containing aminoacid cystine in the cuticle and cortex.[311-313] A defect in excision repair of ultraviolet damage in fibroblasts has been detected in many patients. Unlike xeroderma pigmentosum, in which this defect also occurs, there is no increase in skin cancer.[314,315] Most patients exhibit mutations on the two alleles of the *XPD* gene, although rarely a mutated *XPB* gene or an unidentified gene may be present. Further information is provided in an excellent review by Itin and colleagues.[310] Trichothiodystrophy is often associated with *b*rittle hair, *i*mpaired intelligence, *d*ecreased fertility and *s*hort stature (BIDS syndrome), sometimes combined with *i*chthyosis (IBIDS syndrome),[311,316] osteosclerosis (SIBIDS syndrome)[317] or *p*hotosensitivity (PIBIDS syndrome).[318,319]

Histopathology

The expanded areas of the hair shaft are composed of frayed cortical fibers which usually remain attached.[300] This appearance has been likened to the splayed bristles of two paint brushes (or brooms) thrust into one another (Fig. 15.10).[308] The cuticular cells become disrupted prior to this splaying of the cortical fibers.

In black people, trauma-related cases of trichorrhexis nodosa usually affect the proximal part of the hair shaft, whereas in white and oriental races the distal part is more often affected.[293]

In those with underlying **trichothiodystrophy** striking bright and dark bands are seen with polarized light.[316,318] Lesions resembling trichorrhexis nodosa and trichoschisis may be present.[320] On scanning electron microscopy, the cuticle scales are often damaged or absent and there may be abnormal ridging of the surface.

TRICHOSCHISIS

Trichoschisis is a clean transverse fracture of the hair shaft through the cuticle and cortex.[293] It is usually seen in the brittle hair associated with trichothiodystrophy (see above).

Histopathology

Trichoschisis involves a clean transverse break in the shaft (Fig. 15.11).[293]

TRICHOCLASIS

There is a transverse or oblique fracture of the shaft with irregular borders and a cuticle which is partly intact.[293] As such it resembles a greenstick

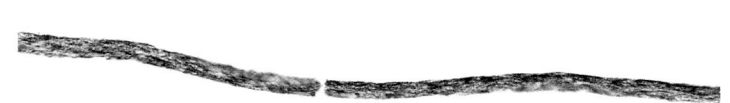

Fig. 15.11 **Trichoschisis.** There is a clean break in the shaft.

fracture.[293] It does not indicate any specific underlying systemic disease, but rather it may follow trauma to the hair or be associated with pili torti, monilethrix or other hair shaft abnormalities (see below).

TRICHORRHEXIS INVAGINATA

Trichorrhexis invaginata (bamboo hair) is a rare but unique abnormality of the hair shaft in which there are nodose swellings that give the hair an appearance reminiscent of a bamboo stem.[321] The scalp hair is usually short, dull and friable and the eyebrows and eyelashes may be sparse.[308] It is one of the hair anomalies associated with Netherton's syndrome, an autosomal recessive disorder in which there is also ichthyosis linearis circumflexa or some other ichthyosiform dermatosis (see p. 286).[315,321] This hair shaft anomaly is seen less characteristically as a sporadic change following trauma or in association with other hair shaft abnormalities.[293,321]

Trichorrhexis invaginata may result from a transient defect of keratinization of the hair shaft due to incomplete cystine linkages, leading to softness of the cortex at the point of disruption.[321]

Histopathology

There is a cup-like expansion of the proximal part of the hair shaft which surrounds the club-shaped distal segment in the manner of a ball and socket joint.[293] If only the proximal half of the invaginate node is present, the appearances have been described as 'golf-tee' hairs.[322]

Transmission electron microscopy shows cleavages and electron-dense depositions in the cortex.[321]

TAPERED FRACTURES

Tapered fractures refer to a progressive narrowing of the emerging hair shaft as a result of inhibition of protein synthesis in the hair root.[293] Fracture of the shaft may occur near the skin surface. Tapered fractures ('pencil-pointing') are seen in anagen effluvium caused by cytotoxic drugs.[293]

TRICHOPTILOSIS

Trichoptilosis refers to longitudinal splitting or fraying of the distal part of the hair shaft as a result of persistent trauma.[323] It results from separation of the longitudinal cortical fibers following loss of the cuticle from wear and tear.[293] A rare variant with the split in the center of the hair and reconstitution of the shaft distal to this has been reported.[324]

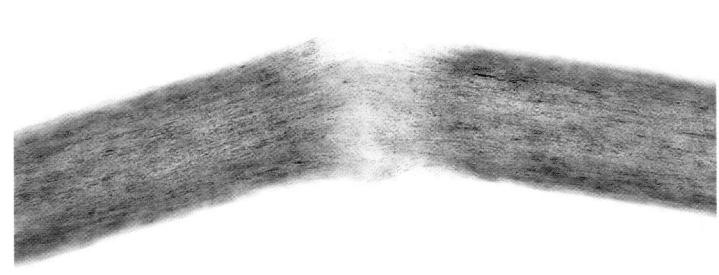

Fig. 15.10 **Trichorrhexis nodosa** with its characteristic fracturing of the hair shaft.

IRREGULARITIES OF HAIR SHAFTS

This group of hair shaft abnormalities is characterized by various morphological irregularities in the hair. A common change, which is sometimes classified as a discrete abnormality, is longitudinal grooving of the hair. It is usually an isolated phenomenon of no clinical importance, although rarely it is widespread and associated with a form of congenital hypotrichosis or with trichothiodystrophy.[293] It will not be considered further.

Included in this group are the following entities:

- pili canaliculati et trianguli
- pili bifurcati
- pili multigemini
- trichostasis spinulosa
- pili annulati
- monilethrix
- tapered hairs
- bubble hair.

Each of these entities will be considered in turn.

PILI CANALICULATI ET TRIANGULI

Pili canaliculati et trianguli, a rare disorder of the hair shaft, is also known as the uncombable hair syndrome, cheveux incoiffables,[325] and the spun-glass hair syndrome.[326–328] The hair is drier, glossier and lighter and it is unmanageable in that it does not lie flat when combed.[329,330] The condition derives its name from the longitudinal canalicular depression in one side of the shaft and its triangular or kidney shape in cross-section.[325,329] For clinical change to be apparent, approximately 50% of hairs must be affected with this abnormality.[331] It may result from a disorder of keratinization of the hair.[295] This hair shaft abnormality has been reported in patients with ectodermal dysplasia.[332,333]

Straight hair nevus, a localized disorder in which the involved hairs are short and straight, in contrast to the usual woolly hair of black people, in whom this condition has been described, has been regarded as a localized form of uncombable hair.[334] However, it should be noted that in straight hair nevus there may be an associated epidermal nevus; furthermore, the hairs are normal in cross-section, in contrast to pili canaliculati et trianguli.[335]

Histopathology

The hairs appear normal on light microscopy.[327] Under polarized light, however, they have a diagnostic homogeneous band on one edge.[327] Paraffin-blocked hairs have a triangular or kidney-shaped appearance on transverse section.[327] The shape is confirmed by scanning electron microscopy, which also shows the longitudinal depression of the shaft resembling a canal.[308,327]

PILI BIFURCATI

In the condition known as pili bifurcati, hairs show intermittent bifurcations of the shaft which subsequently rejoin further along the shaft to form a normal structure.[336] Unlike trichoptilosis, which it superficially resembles, each ramus of the bifurcated segments is invested by its own cuticle.[336] This abnormality has been regarded as a restricted form of pili multigemini.[293]

PILI MULTIGEMINI

Pili multigemini is a rare malformation of the pilary apparatus associated with the emergence of multiple hairs from a follicular canal which in turn is composed of as many papillae as there are hairs.[337] These multigeminate follicles may arise on the face or the scalp. It differs from *tufted-hair folliculitis* in which distinctive tufts of multiple hairs emerge from a single follicular orifice into which several complete follicles open (see p. 481).

TRICHOSTASIS SPINULOSA

Trichostasis spinulosa presents either as asymptomatic, comedone-like lesions on the nose[338] or as mildly pruritic hyperkeratotic papules on the upper trunk or arms.[293,339,340] With a hand lens, multiple vellus hairs can sometimes be seen protruding from the patulous follicles. There is retention of telogen hairs within the follicles, although the reason for this is unknown.[339]

Histopathology[340]

Multiple hairs are enveloped in a keratinous sheath within a dilated hair follicle. The keratin plug may protrude above the skin surface. There is only one hair matrix and papilla at the base of the follicle,[293] in contrast to pili multigemini. Sometimes there is mild perifollicular inflammation.

PILI ANNULATI

The condition of pili annulati (ringed hairs) is a rare, familial or sporadic anomaly in which there are alternating light and dark bands along the shaft, when viewed by reflected light.[307,341] Axillary hair is occasionally affected. An association with alopecia areata has been reported.[342]

The light bands are due to clusters of abnormal, air-filled cavities which appear to result from insufficient production of the interfibrillar matrix.[341,343]

The term '**pseudopili annulati**' refers to the presence of light and dark bands when slightly flattened or twisted hair is examined under reflected light.[344,345] It is thought to be a variant of normal hair and to have no clinical significance.[293]

Histopathology

The alternating light and dark bands occur approximately every 0.5 mm along the shaft when viewed by reflected light.[343,346] Scanning electron microscopy reveals the presence of many small holes within the cortex as well as an irregular arrangement of the cuticular scales.[343]

MONILETHRIX

In monilethrix the hairs have a beaded or moniliform appearance as a result of a periodic decrease in the diameter of the hair.[347,348] Inheritance is usually as an autosomal dominant trait with high gene penetrance but variable expressivity (see below).[293]

The hair is susceptible to fracture at the narrower internodal regions, leading to short hair and hair loss.[349] The occipital region is usually involved soon after birth and the affected area slowly extends.[295] Other hairy areas may also be involved. Some improvement occurs with age and occasionally there is spontaneous remission at puberty.[308]

The defect leading to monilethrix may result from a periodic dysfunction of the hair matrix.[347,350,351] Abnormalities also exist in the inner root sheath adjacent to the zones of abnormal shaft thinning. Transmission electron microscopy has shown an abnormal cortex with areas of homogeneous non-fibrillar material and a deviated axis of some microfibrils.[352]

The gene responsible for monilethrix maps to the region on chromosome 12 (12q11–q13) containing the type II keratin cluster, which includes the basic type II trichocyte keratins.[353,354] The defect may involve one of two type II keratin genes (hHb6) and (hHb1).[355,356] Several different mutations have been found.[357,358] Nail defects appear common with hHb1 defects.[356]

Pseudomonilethrix is now considered to be an artifact in which irregularly placed nodes develop at irregular intervals along the hair shaft as a result of the compression of normal or fragile hairs between glass slides, prior to their microscopic examination.[359]

Histopathology

The elliptical nodes of monilethrix, which are 0.7–1 mm apart, are separated by tapered internodes lacking a medulla (Fig. 15.12).[295] Scanning electron microscopy shows weathering changes with loss of cuticular cells and the presence of longitudinal grooves on the internodal shaft.[293,347]

Fractures and trichorrhexis nodosa may also be present.

TAPERED HAIRS

Tapered hairs can arise in the same way as tapered fractures and they may also occur in association with other abnormalities of the hair shaft.[293] Several distinct variants have been described. The *Pohl–Pinkus mark* is an isolated narrowing of the hair shaft which coincides with a surgical operation or some other traumatic episode.[293] This narrowing is not as abrupt in the *bayonet hair*, which may possibly be a form of the Pohl–Pinkus mark.[293] Newly growing anagen hairs often have a tapered, hypopigmented top.

BUBBLE HAIR

Bubble hair is a rare abnormality characterized by a large cavity in the shaft on scanning electron microscopy and an unusual 'bubble' appearance on light microscopy.[360] It presents with a localized area of brittle, easily broken hairs on the scalp.[361] The abnormality can be reproduced by heat, suggesting that hair dryers that overheat may be responsible.[362–364]

COILING AND TWISTING ABNORMALITIES

As the heading suggests, the hair shafts in this group of disorders adopt various configurations.[293] The following are involved:

- pili torti
- woolly hair
- acquired progressive kinking
- trichonodosis
- circle and rolled hair.

The condition of pili torti is the most important member of this group, while trichonodosis and circle hairs are of little consequence.

PILI TORTI

Pili torti result from a structural defect in which the hair shaft is twisted on its axis at irregular intervals, with flattening of the hair at the sites of twisting.[365] This leads to increased fragility, particularly in areas subjected to trauma.[297] There are several clinical settings in which pili torti can occur.[293]

The rare congenital (Ronchese) type presents at birth or soon after, with a localized area of alopecia or short hair which gradually spreads.[293] Sites other than the scalp may be affected. Pili torti may occur alone or in association with other syndromes, particularly of ectodermal type.[296] These include Bazex's, Crandall's and Bjornstad's syndromes[366,367] as well as

hypohidrotic ectodermal dysplasia.[297] They also occur in citrullinemia[365] and in Menkes' kinky hair syndrome.[295,308] Bjornstad's syndrome combines pili torti with congenital hearing loss.[368] The responsible gene maps to chromosome 2q34–36. In Menkes' syndrome the hair may show defects other than pili torti, including trichorrhexis nodosa, trichoclasis and irregular twisting.[369] The gene maps to chromosome Xq13.

Postpubertal onset has also been recorded (Beare type).[297] Involvement of multiple hair-bearing sites and mental retardation are usually features of this variant. An acquired form of pili torti has been described as a result of trauma, associated with cicatricial alopecia, following the use of synthetic retinoids (isotretinoin)[370] and on the abdomen and thighs of hirsute males and females.[371] Pili torti of early onset may improve with age.

'Corkscrew' hairs, an exaggeration of pili torti, have been reported in patients with ectodermal dysplasia.[372,373] The presence of a longitudinal groove on the hair shaft has led to 'corkscrew' hairs being called pili torti et canaliculi.[373] This abnormality can also be seen in hereditary congenital hypotrichosis of Marie–Unna (see p. 473).

Histopathology

The twisting of the shaft is easily appreciated on light microscopy (Fig. 15.13). Fractures and trichorrhexis nodosa are sometimes present as well.[349] *Corkscrew hairs* combine torsion and longitudinal grooving.

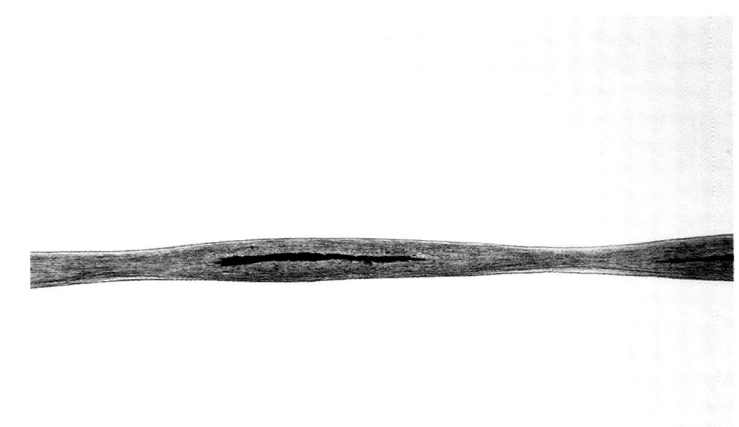

Fig. 15.12 **Monilethrix.** The tapered internodal regions lack a medulla.

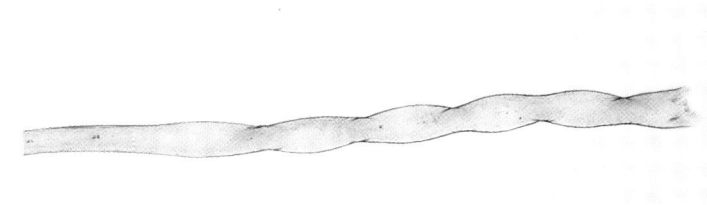

Fig. 15.13 **Pili torti.** Twisting of the hair shaft is present.

Curvatures and twisting have been recorded in the hair follicles that produce pili torti.[293,295]

WOOLLY HAIR

Woolly hair is very curly hair that is difficult to style. It is normal in most black races but in white races it occurs in several different clinical settings.[293,307,374,375] These include an autosomal dominant form which affects the entire scalp (the hereditary type), an autosomal recessive form (the familial type), a diffuse partial form where shorter, finer, curly hair is interspersed with normal hair[374] and a well-demarcated localized form (woolly hair nevus) which may be associated with an ipsilateral epidermal nevus.[376–379] Acquired progressive kinking of the hair (see below) is sometimes included as a variant of woolly hair.[295] Woolly hair has been reported in association with loose anagen hair.[380]

Histopathology

The hairs are usually normal on light microscopy, although on cross-section the shaft diameter is sometimes reduced.[293] In woolly hair nevus the hairs are more oval on cross-section than normal hairs;[374] a case with triangular hairs has been reported.[376] The follicles may be somewhat curved in woolly hair nevus.

ACQUIRED PROGRESSIVE KINKING

Acquired progressive kinking of the hair shaft is rare. It is sometimes considered to be a variant of woolly hair, but is best regarded as a distinct entity on the basis of its onset at or after puberty, the involvement of certain regions of the scalp rather than the entire scalp, and the tendency for affected hair to resemble pubic hair both in texture and color.[381–384] Acquired progressive kinking of the hair tends to occur in males who subsequently develop a male pattern alopecia of fairly rapid onset.[381,385,386] 'Whisker hair', which occurs not uncommonly about the ears, is probably a variant.[293,381,387]

Histopathology

There is usually some flattening of the hair shafts with partial twisting at irregular intervals.[385] Longitudinal canalicular grooves can be demonstrated on scanning electron microscopy.[385,388]

TRICHONODOSIS

Trichonodosis (knotted hair) is usually an incidental finding in individuals with various lengths and types of scalp hair, particularly those with curly or kinky hair.[389,390] There may be a single or a double knot. Various hair shaft abnormalities of a secondary nature may be present in and adjacent to the knots.[293]

Multiple large knots involving body hairs have been reported. The hairs show an unusual twisting and matting.[391]

Hair matting is a rare acquired condition characterized by irreversible tangling of hair. It has many causes other than trichonodosis. They include hair density and coiling, chemical and physical treatments to the hair, and neglect.[392]

CIRCLE AND ROLLED HAIR

Circle hair presents as a black circle related to hair follicles as the result of a hair shaft becoming coiled into a circle under a thin transparent roof of stratum corneum.[393,394] The cause of this abnormality is unknown but it may be seen in middle-aged men on the back, abdomen and thighs.[393] The case reported as pili migrans has some similarities (see p. 466).

Rolled hair (the term is sometimes used interchangeably with circle hair) refers to a common disorder of hair growth in which the hairs are irregularly coiled but do not form a perfect circle.[395] It is usually associated with some other disorder such as keratosis pilaris.

Histopathology

In circle hair there is no associated follicular abnormality or inflammatory component.[395]

Keratotic plugs containing a coiled or broken hair are a characteristic feature of keratosis pilaris (see p. 482).[393] Similar changes are seen in some cases of rolled hair, although keratotic follicular plugging is not always present.[393]

EXTRANEOUS MATTER ON HAIR SHAFTS

Hair shafts may be colonized by fungi (tinea capitis and piedra), bacteria (trichomycosis axillaris) and the eggs (nits) of the lice causing pediculosis capitis.[293] Casts resembling nits (hair casts, pseudo-nits) may occur in association with various scaly dermatoses of the scalp or as a rare, idiopathic phenomenon. Deposits such as lacquer, paint and glue form another category of extraneous matter.

TINEA CAPITIS

In tinea capitis, fungal elements may be found on the surface of the hair shaft (ectothrix) or within the substance of the hair (endothrix).[293] In both cases the affected hairs are fragile and break near the skin surface.

PIEDRA

The condition known as piedra occurs in two forms, white piedra and black piedra.[293] They are characterized by the formation of minute concretions on the affected hair (the Spanish word *piedra* means stone).

White piedra (trichosporonosis, trichosporosis)[396,397] is a rare superficial infection of the terminal part of the hair caused by the yeast-like fungus *Trichosporon beigelii (cutaneum)*. It occurs particularly in South America, parts of Europe, Japan, the Middle East and the USA.[398,399] There are numerous discrete or coalescing cream-colored nodules, just visible to the naked eye, forming sleeve-like concretions attached to the hair shaft.[400,401] White piedra may affect hairs on the face, scalp or scrotum.[400] Fracture of the hair shaft may result.

Black piedra, which is caused by the ascomycete *Piedraia hortae*, consists of gritty black nodules which are darker, firmer and more adherent than those found in white piedra.[401] Black piedra is prevalent in tropical climates.

Histopathology

In *white piedra*, a potassium hydroxide preparation of a hair shows that the concretions are composed of numerous fungal arthrospores in compact masses encasing the hair shaft.[401] In *black piedra*, the nodules are composed of brown hyphae with ovoid asci containing 2–8 ascospores.[401] The fungus shows strong keratinolytic activity with the capacity to destroy both the cuticle and the hair cortex.[402]

TRICHOMYCOSIS AXILLARIS

In trichomycosis axillaris, there are tiny, cream to yellow nodules attached to axillary or pubic hair (Fig. 15.14).[293] It is not a mycosis but the result of infection by a species of *Corynebacterium*.

PEDICULOSIS CAPITIS

Nits are small white to brown ovoid structures attached to the hair shaft.[293] They are the eggs of the lice responsible for pediculosis capitis (see p. 743).

Histopathology

The egg lies to one side of the hair shaft, to which it is attached by a sheath that envelops both the shaft and the base of the egg.[293]

HAIR CASTS

Hair casts (peripilar casts, pseudo-nits) are firmish, yellow-white concretions, 3–7 mm long, ensheathing hairs and movable along them.[403] Two types of hair casts exist.[404–408] The more common type (*parakeratotic hair cast*) is associated with various inflammatory scalp disorders such as psoriasis, seborrheic dermatitis and pityriasis capitis.[404] The second type (*peripilar keratin cast*), which is quite uncommon, occurs predominantly in female children without any underlying disease as a diffuse disorder of scalp hair.[405] Hair casts appear to be nothing more than portions of root sheath pulled out of the follicle by a hair shaft itself.[409] Tight plaiting of the hair, leading to local scalp ischemia and consequent damage to the root sheaths of the follicle, may be responsible for the formation of hair casts.[406–408]

Histopathology[409,410]

In both types of hair casts the follicular openings contain parakeratotic keratinous material which breaks off at intervals to form the hair casts. In casts associated with parakeratotic disorders it seems that only external sheath is present in the casts. In the uncommon peripilar casts, both inner and outer root sheaths are demonstrable on transverse section of the cast. Scanning electron microscopy has confirmed the presence of an inner, incomplete layer and an outer, thicker, but less compact layer.[409]

DEPOSITS

Various substances may become adherent to hair shafts, causing an unusual appearance on microscopy.[293] These include paint, hair spray, lacquer and glue. Hair lacquer and gel can produce hair beads.[411] Microscopy reveals that the deposits are not inherent parts of the hair shaft.[293]

Alopecias

There are several hundred disease states or events that may precipitate abnormal hair loss. As a consequence, any etiological classification of the alopecias is invariably composed of long lists of causative factors.[412,413] From a clinical viewpoint, alopecias are usually divided into those that are patterned and those that diffusely involve the scalp. Further subclassification into scarring and non-scarring types is usually made. Scarring alopecias are almost invariably irreversible and are therefore of great clinical importance. Biopsies are not often taken from alopecias which are diffuse and non-scarring as the

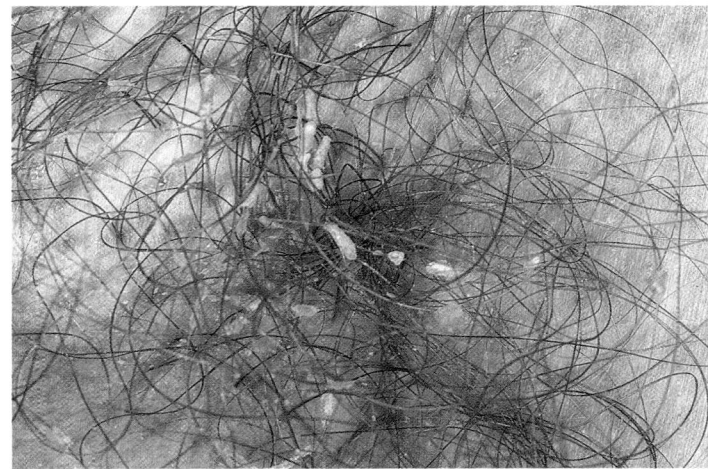

Fig. 15.14 **Trichomycosis.** Small pale nodules are attached to some of the hair shafts.

etiology is often apparent to the clinician or the alopecia is subclinical or not of cosmetic significance.

A more useful approach for the dermatopathologist is a classification based on the mechanisms involved in the hair loss.[414] This has some shortcomings in that our knowledge of these mechanisms is not complete, particularly in some of the congenital/hereditary alopecias. Furthermore, some of the early reports of this group lack histological descriptions of the skin and hair shafts. For this reason, the congenital/hereditary alopecias will be considered together until further knowledge allows a more accurate subdivision based on the mechanism involved.

The histological diagnosis of the alopecias is best made from transverse (horizontal) as opposed to the traditional vertical section (see Table 15.1).

Transverse (horizontal) sections allow all follicles in a biopsy to be visualized simultaneously.[415–417] The diagnostic yield can be maximized if both vertical and transverse sections are utilized.[418]

The following classification of alopecias will be used in the account which follows:

- congenital/hereditary alopecias
- premature catagen/telogen
- premature telogen with anagen arrest
- vellus follicle formation
- anagen defluvium
- scarring alopecias
- hair shaft abnormalities (see p. 466).

Before discussing the various mechanisms of hair loss, brief mention will be made of the normal hair cycle.

The normal hair cycle

The formation of hairs is a cyclical phenomenon which results from successive periods of growth, involution and rest by hair follicles.[419,420] The phase of active hair production is known as *anagen*. It lasts for a period of 2–6 years on the scalp, although the average duration is usually quoted as 1000 days.[293] At any one time, 85–90% of the 100 000 hair follicles on the scalp are in the anagen phase. There is regional variation in the duration of anagen. For example, anagen lasts for approximately 1 year in the beard region, while its duration in the axilla and pubic region is only a few months.[421]

The involutionary stage, *catagen*, is quite short, lasting for less than 2 weeks in each hair follicle on the scalp. There is very little regional variation in the duration of catagen, although in some animals this period may be as

Table 15.1 **The histological features of alopecias on horizontal (transverse) sections**

Infundibular level

Lichenoid reaction (interfollicular epidermis)	Lupus erythematosus Lichen planopilaris (one-third of cases)
Lymphocytic infiltrate ± fibrosis	Lupus erythematosus* Lichen planopilaris* (*Both have lichenoid features) Idiopathic scarring alopecia
Neutrophilic infiltrate ± fibrosis (also lymphocytes and plasma cells)	Dissecting cellulitis of the scalp Folliculitis decalvans Acne keloidalis Infectious folliculitis
Miniature hair shafts	Androgenic alopecia
Melanin casts	Trichotillomania/traumatic alopecia

Isthmus level

Lymphocytic infiltrate ± fibrosis	Lupus erythematosus Lichen planopilaris Idiopathic scarring alopecia
Miniature bulbs and follicles of varying diameter (non-inflamed)	Androgenic alopecia Alopecia areata (regrowth)
Miniature bulbs (inflamed ± apoptosis)	Alopecia areata Lupus erythematosus
Melanin casts/trichomalacia	Trichotillomania/traumatic alopecia

Hair bulb level

Fibrous tract and reduced number of follicles	Alopecia areata Lupus erythematosus } also pigment incontinence Lichen planus Androgenic alopecia Idiopathic scarring alopecia Traction alopecia
Inflamed hair bulbs ('swarm of bees')	Active alopecia areata
'Torn' catagen follicles ± hemorrhage	Trichotillomania/traumatic alopecia

short as 24 hours. Approximately 1% of scalp follicles are in the catagen phase at any time. In humans, the entry of follicles into catagen is a random process, in contrast to its synchronous onset in animals (molting). Seasonal factors, including temperature and light intensity, play some role in precipitating molting in certain animals. In other animals and in humans, the factors that normally precipitate catagen are not known.[422] Recent studies have addressed this issue of the 'hair cycle clock'.[423–425] The use of transgenic mice is providing valuable information.[426]

Transforming growth factor-β is expressed immediately before catagen and tumor necrosis factor-β during catagen.[423,427] The levels of c-*myc*, c-*myb*, *bax* and c-*jun* change immediately before or during early catagen, suggesting that they play a role in the induction of apoptosis.[423] The oncogene c-*myc* has the ability to induce both cell growth and apoptosis, depending on environmental conditions.[428] There are two clusters of c-*myc* expressing cells in anagen follicles.[429,430] A reduction in *bcl-2* expression also occurs during catagen.[431] It follows a set period of anagen which is presumably genetically determined in some way for each particular region. The mechanism by which hair follicles shorten during catagen was an enigma for a long time. It was in part attributed to the cessation of mitoses in the hair matrix and also to 'collapse', 'regression', 'disintegration' and 'involution' of the lower follicle.[432] It is now known that massive cell loss by apoptosis is the mechanism

responsible for catagen involution.[422,432,433] The apoptotic fragments are quickly phagocytosed by adjacent cells in the lower follicle and by macrophages.[422] With progressive retraction of the follicle resulting from this cell loss, there is wrinkling and thickening of the fibrous root sheath.

The resting phase, *telogen*, lasts for approximately 3–4 months. During this period, there is no active hair production.[421] At any one time, approximately 10–15% of scalp follicles are in this phase. Telogen is followed by regrowth of the hair follicle and a new anagen phase. The telogen hair (club hair) is extruded and shed at this time.

Each stage of the hair cycle has a characteristic morphological appearance.[419]

Catagen follicles are characterized by loss of mitotic activity in the matrix and the cessation of pigment production by melanocytes in the hair bulb. Scattered apoptotic cells develop in the outer root sheath, an easily recognizable sign of catagen (Fig. 15.15).[432] Some melanocytes also undergo apoptosis.[434] The inner root sheath disappears and there is progressive thickening and corrugation of the fibrous root sheath. The lower end of the follicle gradually retracts upwards with a trailing connective tissue streamer beneath it. It is possible that Langerhans cells play a role in the removal of melanin from the hair bulb in early catagen.[435]

Telogen follicles consist of a short protrusion of basaloid, undifferentiated cells below the epithelial sac which surrounds the club hair. This is situated not far below the entrance of the sebaceous duct. The telogen hair, if plucked,

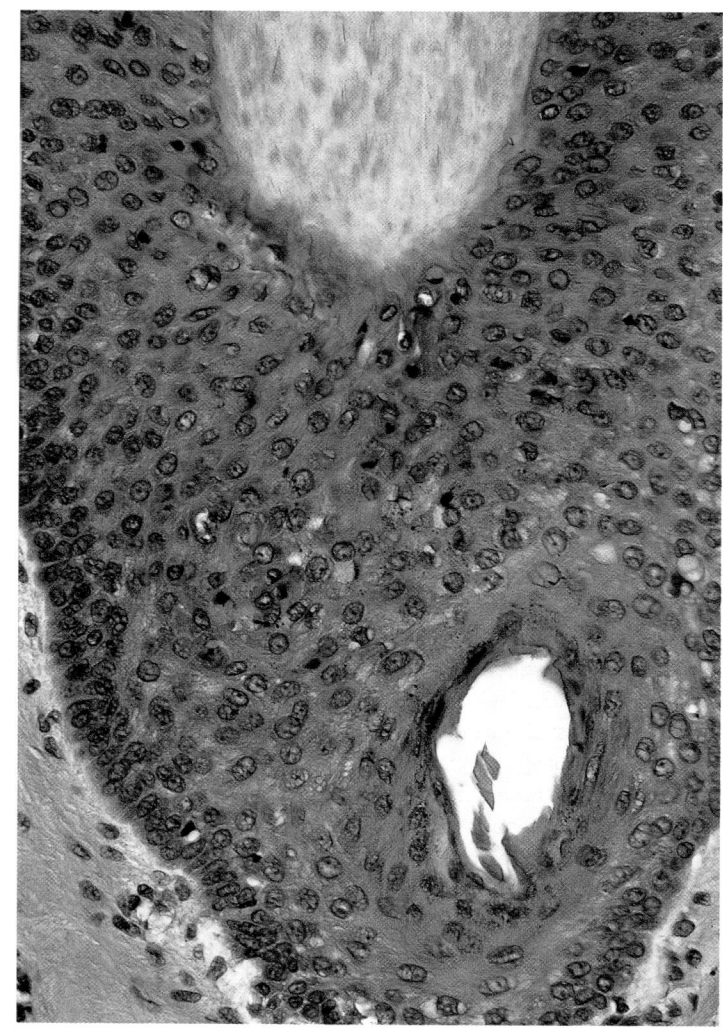

Fig. 15.15 **Early catagen follicle.** Note the numerous apoptotic cells. (H & E)

has a short, club-shaped root that lacks root sheaths and a keratogenous zone (Fig. 15.16). There is also depigmentation of the proximal part of the shaft.[293,421] The transition from anagen to telogen is marked by downregulation of hair cortex-specific keratins and the appearance of hK14 in the epithelial sac to which the telogen hair fiber is anchored.[436]

Anagen growth recapitulates to some extent the changes present in the original development of the follicle.[437] There is increased mitotic activity in the germinal cells at the base of the telogen follicle. This ball of cells extends downward, partly enclosing the dermal papilla.[438] Both descend into the dermis along the path of the connective tissue streamer that formed during the previous catagen phase. The matrix cells of the new anagen bulb form a new inner root sheath and hair.[438] Melanocytes lining the papillae form melanin again. The new hair eventually dislodges the club hair of the previous cycle. Plucked anagen hairs have long indented roots with intact inner and outer root sheaths and are fully pigmented.[421] Slowly plucked anagen roots are bare and show ruffling of the cuticle over a special segment of the root: quickly plucked anagen roots are usually covered by various sheath remnants, hence ruffling occurs only rarely.[439]

Fig. 15.16 **Telogen hairs with a short club-shaped root.**

CONGENITAL/HEREDITARY ALOPECIAS

The rare alopecias of the congenital/hereditary clinical grouping are considered together because the mechanisms involved in the pathogenesis of the hair loss are not known for some of the conditions.[438] Furthermore, biopsies have not been carried out on some of the entities listed, while in other instances the biopsy findings have not been consistent from one report to another. Several different clinical groups of congenital/hereditary alopecias (hypotrichosis) are usually recognized:[308,440]

- alopecias without associated defects
- alopecias in association with ectodermal dysplasia
- alopecias as a characteristic or inconstant feature of a named syndrome.

Alopecia or hypotrichosis occurs without any associated defect in alopecia congenitalis, hereditary hypotrichosis (Marie–Unna type) and atrichia with papular lesions and in keratosis pilaris atrophicans. These conditions are considered further below. Localized alopecia, possibly occurring as a nevoid state, has been reported.[441] Another localized form of alopecia, temporal triangular alopecia, involves the presence of vellus follicles and is discussed on page 478.

Alopecia is a characteristic feature of one subgroup of the ectodermal dysplasias, a heterogeneous group of congenital diseases involving the epidermis and at least one appendage. Absence or hypoplasia of hair follicles has been recorded in some of these rare syndromes,[442] while in others no detailed studies have been made. The ectodermal dysplasias have been discussed on page 303. They will not be considered further here.

There is a long list of rare syndromes in which alopecia is a characteristic or inconstant feature.[443,444] Skeletal abnormalities are present in one subgroup.[308,445] These have been reviewed elsewhere.[308] Little is known about the mechanism of the alopecia in this group. One entity, the Hallermann–Streiff syndrome, will be discussed briefly below because something is known of its pathology.

ALOPECIA CONGENITALIS

Alopecia congenitalis (alopecia universalis congenita, universal congenital alopecia) refers to cases of congenital alopecia without associated defects.[308,446] It is a heterogeneous group. Hair loss occurs at birth or shortly after in one subgroup with autosomal recessive inheritance, while in those with one form of autosomal dominant inheritance the hair is normal until mid childhood.[447,448] The autosomal recessive form is linked to the human hairless gene (*HR*).[449,450] Another autosomal dominant form has been called hypotrichosis simplex. It is of early onset and without associated abnormalities. A gene for this condition has been mapped to chromosome 6p21.3.[451] Yet another variant has been linked to a short anagen phase, but how it relates to the other variants already mentioned is unclear.[452]

Histopathology

Hair follicles are hypoplastic and reduced in number.[308] In one report, they were described as being of vellus type.[453] In one of the dominant forms, follicles are said to be normal in number initially, but they fail progressively to re-enter anagen.[438]

HEREDITARY HYPOTRICHOSIS

Hereditary hypotrichosis (Marie–Unna type) presents with short, sparse hair at birth and hair growth in childhood that is coarse and wiry. There is progressive loss of hair resembling androgenic alopecia, commencing during adolescence.[308] It is an autosomal dominant condition associated with a defect in chromosomal region 8p21. This is close to, but distinct from, the human hairless gene (*HR*) responsible for atrichia with papular lesions (see below).[454–456]

Histopathology

There are no specific features apart from a mild to moderate perifollicular inflammatory reaction, although progressive destruction of hair follicles is the probable mechanism.[308,457] Follicles are reduced in number. Milia, mild fibrosis and perifollicular granulomas have been recorded.[308,457]

ATRICHIA WITH PAPULAR LESIONS

Atrichia with papular lesions is a rare disorder in which progressive shedding of scalp and body hair occurs in the first few months of life.[458–460] The eyelashes are typically spared. Numerous small, milia-like cysts develop on the face, neck, scalp and extremities in childhood and early adult life.[458] It is an autosomal recessive condition in which mutations occur in the human hairless gene (*HR*), which has been mapped to chromosome 8p21–22.[449,461] Mutations in this gene are also responsible for alopecia congenitalis (universal congenital alopecia) which differs by having no papular lesions (see above).[449,462]

Histopathology[458]

The small follicular cysts resemble milia. They contain keratinous material, which is sometimes calcified, but there are no vellus hairs in the lumen. Scattered foreign body giant cells may be present around some of the cysts. In the scalp the infundibulum of the follicle is normally developed, although it often contains a keratin plug. There is a lack of development of the germinal end of the follicle, with no shaft formation.[463]

KERATOSIS PILARIS ATROPHICANS

Keratosis pilaris atrophicans refers to a group of clinically related syndromes in which inflammatory keratosis pilaris leads to atrophic scarring (see p. 483). This condition is mentioned here because it is regarded as a congenital follicular dystrophy.

HALLERMANN–STREIFF SYNDROME

The Hallermann–Streiff syndrome (mandibulo-oculofacial dyscephaly) is a branchial arch syndrome which combines a characteristic facies with ocular abnormalities and alopecia, which may have an unusual sutural distribution on the scalp.[464] Atrophic patches of skin, which may be limited to the areas of alopecia, also occur.[464] Most cases appear to occur as new mutations.[438]

Histopathology

Very little is known about the histological characteristics of the alopecia, although the atrophic areas are composed of loosely woven collagen.[438] The hair shafts show some cuticular weathering on scanning electron microscopy.[464] Circumferential grooving of the shaft has also been noted in some cases.[465]

PREMATURE CATAGEN/TELOGEN

At any one time, approximately 10–15% of the hair follicles of the scalp are in the resting (telogen) phase and, because of its shorter duration, only a small number of follicles are in the preceding involutionary stage of catagen. Under certain circumstances an abnormal number of hair follicles is in the telogen phase. This results from the premature termination of anagen.[466] After a latent period of approximately 3 months from the onset of catagen/telogen, club hairs are lost, leading to thinning of the hair.[466] It is surprising how much hair can be lost before this thinning becomes noticeable.[466]

Numerous telogen follicles are found in telogen effluvium (see below), a condition which results from various stressful circumstances and from some drugs, such as heparin.[466] Catagen hairs are not usually found because such conditions are not biopsied until the hair loss becomes noticeable, some 3 months after the onset.

In trichotillomania (see below) and certain traumatic alopecias, the insult is usually continuous and, accordingly, catagen follicles are seen in addition to telogen ones. Catagen follicles are sometimes prominent at the rapidly advancing edge of a patch of alopecia areata.

In summary, catagen follicles are prominent in trichotillomania and related traumatic alopecias resulting from traction associated with hairstyles and the like. They are often seen at the edge of a patch of alopecia areata. Telogen follicles are prominent in telogen effluvium, in alopecia areata and in a rare disorder with its onset in childhood, familial focal alopecia.[467] In this latter condition there is telogen arrest with prolonged persistence of telogen follicles, in contrast to the transient nature of the process in telogen effluvium.[467]

TRICHOTILLOMANIA AND TRAUMATIC ALOPECIA

Trichotillomania is a rare form of alopecia resulting from the deliberate, although at times unconscious, avulsion of hairs by patients who may be under psychosocial stress.[468] In adults it is more common in women; in children there has been no sex predilection in some series.

Although the crown and occipital scalp are primarily affected, other areas of the scalp, as well as the eyebrows, trunk and pubic areas, may also be involved. Similar features can result from traction of hair associated with hairstyles and from prolonged pressure.[469] Pressure appears to be involved in the occipital alopecia that occurs in children and some adults after surgery of prolonged duration.[470,471] The term 'traumatic alopecia' can be applied to such cases, including trichotillomania.[472,473] Clinical differentiation from alopecia areata can be difficult.

If trauma (such as traction) is repeated, prolonged and severe, then additional features, including scarring, will develop. This is best called traction alopecia with scarring, but it is also known as 'hot comb' alopecia and follicular degeneration syndrome (see p. 481).[474]

Histopathology[475–479]

The histological features are characteristic, but not all of the recognized features are present in every biopsy. There is a greater chance of observing them if multiple sections are examined. The two most specific features are the presence of increased numbers of catagen hairs, associated usually with the presence of early and late anagen hairs, and the presence of empty hair ducts. Other changes include dilated follicular infundibula which may contain melanin casts and keratin plugs, clefts around the lower end of hair follicles, distortion of the hair bulb with dissociation of cells in the hair matrix, the release of melanin pigment within the papilla and surrounding connective tissue sheaths, traumatized connective tissue sheaths, small areas of dermal hemorrhage and empty spaces in the sebaceous glands (Fig. 15.17).[476] The

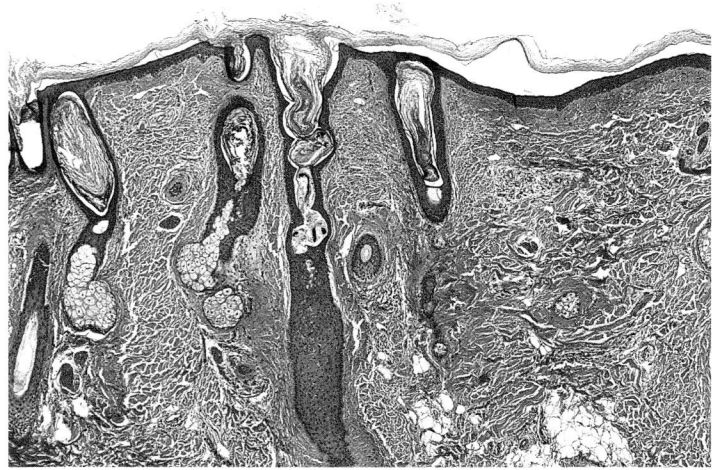

Fig. 15.17 **Trichotillomania.** Melanin casts and keratin plugs are present in the dilated follicular infundibula. (H & E)

pigment casts may not be the result of hair manipulation but rather a reflection of the sudden termination of the anagen phase of the hair cycle.[471] Sometimes there is even extrusion of sebaceous lobules. Only a very sparse inflammatory infiltrate is present.

TELOGEN EFFLUVIUM

Telogen effluvium has been regarded as a syndrome and as a non-specific reaction pattern, rather than as a disease sui generis.[466,480–482] It is nevertheless a useful term to apply to those cases of diffuse hair loss in which various stressful circumstances precipitate the premature termination of anagen. Telogen effluvium can follow febrile illness, parturition, systemic illnesses, chronic infections (including HIV infection),[483] allergic contact dermatitis of the scalp,[484] air travelers' 'jet lag', psychogenic illnesses, 'crash diets' and sudden severe stress.[485] It may also be associated with an internal cancer[414] and with the eosinophilia–myalgia syndrome.[486] Loss of hair in the newborn is a physiological example of this process.[466] Exceptionally, drugs such as heparin, clofibrate, gentamicin, niacin (nicotinic acid), nitrofurantoin, salicylates, oral contraceptives, anticonvulsants, excess vitamin A and the antihypertensive agent minoxidil[487] have been implicated in the etiology of telogen effluvium.[416,488,489] Headington has defined five different functional types of telogen effluvium.[489]

Telogen effluvium presents as a diffuse thinning of the scalp hair, although the hair loss is not always obvious clinically. Sometimes this hair loss unmasks small areas of alopecia, of other causes, which had previously gone unnoticed.

In *chronic* telogen effluvium (defined as shedding that persists beyond 3 months) there is hair shedding of abrupt onset followed by a fluctuating course in which there is diffuse thinning all over the scalp, frequently accompanied by bitemporal recession.[485,490] It is more common in postmenopausal women.[491] It must be distinguished from androgenic alopecia, which often has overlapping features.[492]

Histopathology
A biopsy of the affected scalp will show a proportionately greater number of normal telogen follicles than usual. There is no inflammation in the dermis. An examination of plucked hairs will reveal telogen counts greater than 25%.

In horizontal sections of *chronic* telogen effluvium the terminal/vellus-like hair ratio in one study was 9:1 compared to 1.9:1 in androgenic alopecia.[490] Inflammation is also more common in androgenic alopecia than in chronic telogen effluvium.[490]

PREMATURE TELOGEN WITH ANAGEN ARREST

Alopecia areata is the only type of hair loss in which the mechanism of premature telogen with anagen arrest applies. At the expanding edge, follicles in late catagen and telogen are characteristic findings, although in older lesions follicles in an arrested anagen phase are also present.

ALOPECIA AREATA

Alopecia areata is a relatively common condition affecting individuals of any age, but particularly those between the ages of 15 and 40.[493–495] Although mild cases may escape clinical detection, alopecia areata usually has a sudden onset with the development of one or more discrete, asymptomatic patches of non-scarring hair loss.[496] Exclamation mark hairs are found near the advancing margins.[496] The clinical course is variable.[497] There may be

spontaneous remission, sometimes followed by exacerbations, or there may be relentless progression to involve the entire scalp (alopecia totalis) and, uncommonly, all body hair (alopecia universalis).[498,499] Progression to alopecia totalis is more likely in children.[500,501] In one study 7% of patients with alopecia areata progressed to alopecia totalis or universalis.[502] HLA-DR11, HLA-DR4 and HLA-DQ7 are significantly increased in frequency in patients with alopecia totalis/alopecia universalis in contrast to patients with patchy alopecia areata.[503,504] Other HLA profiles may be increased in some ethnic groups.[505] Regeneration is heralded by the development of fine white or tan hair.[495] A family history of alopecia areata is present in 10–25% of affected individuals.[493,500,506,507] Inheritance is polygenic, but there appears to be an association with HLA class II genes.[461,508,509] There is a 55% concordance rate in identical twins.[510]

There are conflicting data on the clinical associations of alopecia areata. Many reports have documented an increased incidence of autoimmune diseases such as Hashimoto's thyroiditis, Addison's disease, vitiligo[511] and lupus erythematosus, but not others.[496,498,512] Autoantibodies to various thyroid antigens,[513–515] gastric parietal cells[506] and smooth muscle[516] have been reported,[517] although not all of these findings have been confirmed by others.[518] There are also conflicting results on the various cell-mediated functions in alopecia areata, but this may in part reflect the different techniques that have been used and the heterogeneous nature of this condition.[515,519] Other clinical associations have included atopic states,[520] Down syndrome,[521] the use of rifampin (rifampicin)[522] and interferon alpha,[523] HIV infection,[501] CMV infection,[510] pili annulati,[524] the sparing of a congenital nevus[525] and following vasectomy.[526] Various nail changes have been reported in 10% of patients.[527] Reduced sweating has also been documented.[528] Migratory poliosis may be a forme fruste of alopecia areata.[529]

Pathogenesis
Although the pathogenesis of alopecia areata is not understood, the evidence for an immunological basis comes from five sources:[498,530,531] the clinical association of other autoimmune diseases, the presence in some patients of circulating antibodies directed to a range of hair follicle antigens,[532–534] altered cellular immune functions,[535,536] the favorable effects of treatment with synthetic immunomodulators,[537,538] and the histopathological finding of activated and autoreactive T cells and HLA-DR expression[539,540] in the vicinity of the hair bulb.[541,542] Antibodies against hair follicles are present in patients with alopecia totalis occurring in association with the autoimmune polyendocrine syndrome type I.[543] The initial stages of the disease involve T lymphocytes and dendritic cells that are CD1a and CD36 positive.[544–546] The lymphocytes appear to be of oligoclonal origin.[547] Recent work suggests that CD8+ cells. even though they are less frequent than CD4+ cells in the infiltrate, play an important pathogenic role with the CD4+ cells in their classic helper/supporter role.[548–552] Adhesion molecule receptors are involved in the initial trafficking of leukocytes into the dermis.[544] The effect of psychological factors, which play an important role in some patients with alopecia areata, may be mediated by neuropeptide substance P which is increased in nerve fibers in areas of hair loss.[553]

The basic disturbance is the premature entry of anagen follicles into telogen, although some follicles survive for a time in a dystrophic anagen state.[554]

The term 'nanogen' has been proposed for the morphologically distorted telogen follicle that is produced in alopecia areata.[555] Follicles may re-enter anagen, but growth appears to be halted in anagen stage III and IV.[556] Interestingly, follicles producing non-pigmented hair are less susceptible to premature telogen.[493] Cell deletion by apoptosis, probably cell mediated, is the mechanism by which premature catagen and telogen come about.

Apoptosis may also play a role in the anagen arrest that occurs.[556] Graft experiments suggest that hair growth ability in situ is normal and the causation is mediated humorally.[557]

Histopathology[554]

The appearances vary according to the duration of the process at the biopsy site (Figs 15.18, 15.19). At the expanding edge the majority of the follicles are in late catagen and telogen. A few anagen follicles are in the subcutis while small mid-dermal ones may also be seen. The larger anagen follicles show a peribulbar infiltrate of lymphocytes (likened to a swarm of bees) and macrophages and sometimes a few eosinophils and plasma cells (Fig. 15.20).[554] Eosinophils were present in the fibrous tracts and near hair bulbs in 38 of 71 cases in one study,[558] and in 11 of 51 cases in another.[559] Mast cells are common in the fibrous tracts but they can also be found in androgenic alopecia. There is also exocytosis of inflammatory cells into the bulbar epithelium.[560] The majority of the lymphocytes are small and mature.[561] The small anagen follicles show a disproportionate reduction in the size of the epithelial matrix relative to that of the dermal papilla.

In established cases and in alopecia totalis there are many telogen follicles and some small anagen follicles with mid-dermal bulbs.[554] The anagen/telogen ratio is variable. Although routine sections give the impression of marked

follicle loss because of the absence of follicles in the subcutis, the use of transverse sections allows a better assessment of follicle density.[415] A quantitative study, using horizontal sections, found an average of 40 hairs in a 4 mm biopsy of normal scalp, but only 27 in alopecia areata.[562] The study also showed an increase in vellus follicles and also of telogen follicles in alopecia areata.[562] This has prognostic significance because it indicates that normal regrowth of hair is theoretically possible in these circumstances.[415] There is only a mild peribulbar inflammatory cell infiltrate around these small anagen follicles. Occasional apoptotic cells and mitoses can be seen. Atrophy of sebaceous glands is seen sometimes in long-standing cases.[563] Incidental follicular mucinosis has been reported.[564]

In regenerating areas, the number of melanocytes and the degree of pigmentation of the cells in the hair bulb are much less than in the normal pigmented follicle.[554,556]

In all stages, a non-sclerotic fibrous tract extends along the site of the previous follicle into the subcutis. This fibrous tract contains a few small vessels and small deposits of melanin. In cases of long standing there is widespread damage and fibrosis to the follicular sheath structures. There may be only a few lymphocytes and macrophages at the site of the previous hair bulb. There are no Arão–Perkins elastic bodies along this connective tissue tract, such as are seen in male pattern alopecia.[565]

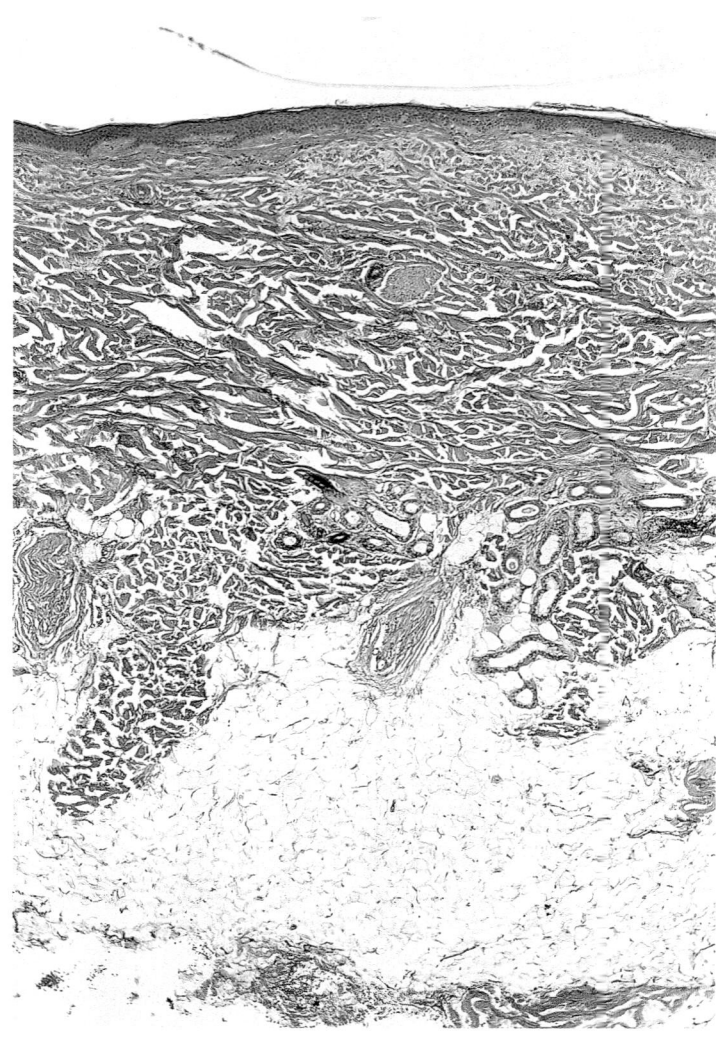

Fig. 15.18 **Alopecia areata.** This is a late stage lesion with a complete loss of follicles. (H & E)

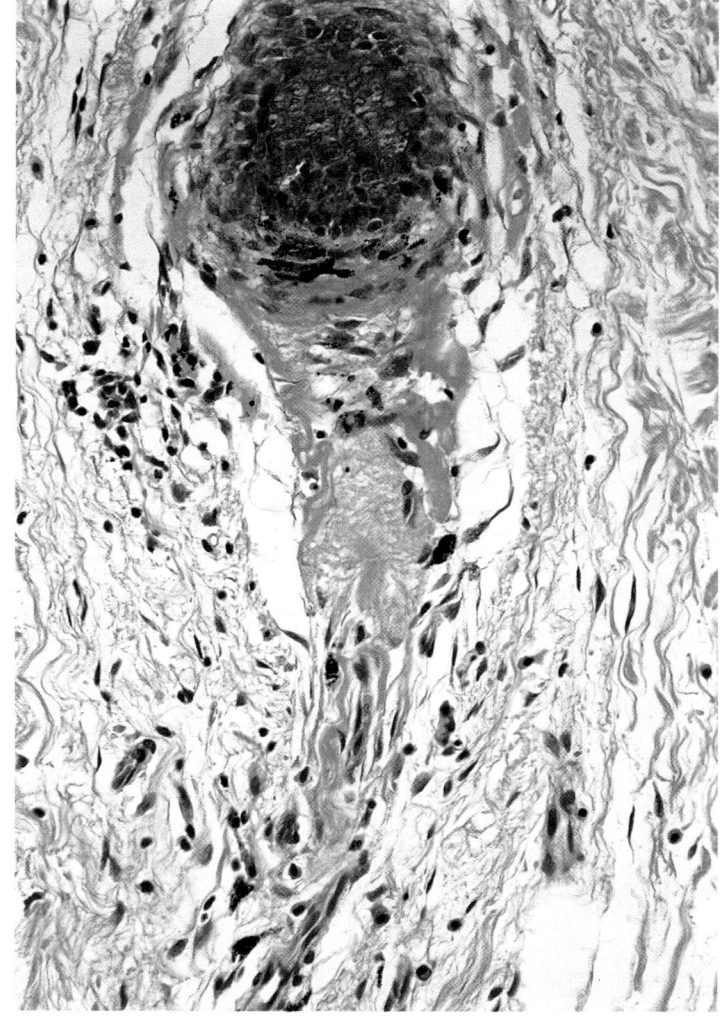

Fig. 15.19 **Alopecia areata.** A fibrous tract extends along the site of the previous follicle. A small, early anagen follicle is above. A few lymphocytes are also present. (H & E)

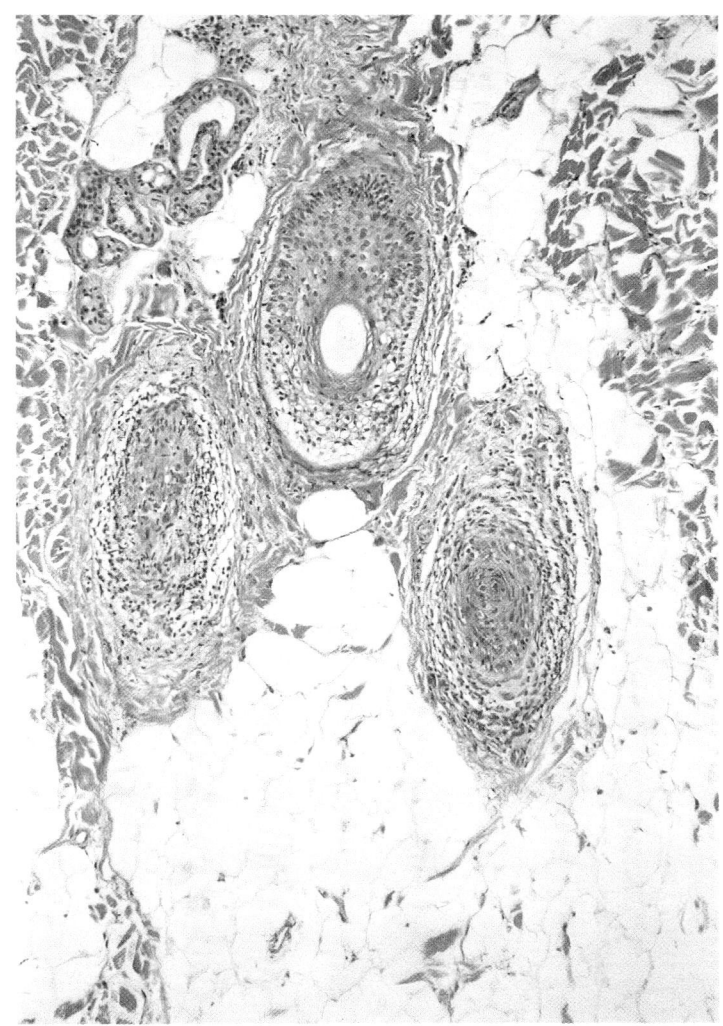

Fig. 15.20 **Alopecia areata.** Lymphocytes surround the bulbar region, giving the characteristic 'swarm of bees' sign. (H & E)

Assessments have been made of scalp biopsies from patients with long-standing alopecia totalis and universalis who did not respond to sensitizing therapies.[563] From a pathological viewpoint, non-responder patients constitute a heterogeneous population with early regrowth, telogen, scarring and early anagen arrest patterns present in different patients.[563]

Kossard has presented a case with miniaturized follicles and a heavy (non-lichenoid) lymphocytic infiltrate at the level of the stem-cell rich region near the entry of the sebaceous duct.[566] He considered that it might be a variant of alopecia areata and used the term 'diffuse alopecia with stem cell folliculitis'.[566]

Immunofluorescence shows deposits of C3 and occasionally of IgG and IgM along the basement zone of the inferior segment of hair follicles.[567] Careful ultrastructural studies are needed to assess the role of lymphocyte-mediated apoptosis in the pathogenesis of this disease.

Electron microscopy[568]
Apoptosis has been seen not only in the outer root sheath of catagen follicles but also in matrix keratinocytes and anagen hair bulbs. Dark cell transformation is also present. Ultrastructural studies of exclamation mark hairs show asymmetrical cortical disintegration below the frayed tip.[569] Cells in the dermal papilla show signs of injury and there are abnormal amounts of pigment.[570]

VELLUS FOLLICLE FORMATION

This group of alopecias is characterized by the presence of small vellus follicles in the dermis. In androgenic alopecia (common baldness), which is the most important member of this group, an early biopsy may only show a progressive diminution in the size of follicles which are not truly vellus. In established lesions typical vellus follicles will be seen. Vellus follicles are also a feature of temporal triangular alopecia but this presumably represents the development of vellus follicles in the affected site ab initio rather than the progressive reversion of terminal hair follicles to vellus follicles.

ANDROGENIC ALOPECIA (COMMON BALDNESS)

Androgenic alopecia (common baldness, androgenetic alopecia) is a physiological event which may commence in males soon after puberty.[571,572] It occurs less often in females and its onset is a decade or so later than in males. It has been said to affect at least 50% of men by the age of 50 years[573] and about 40% of women aged 70 years and over.[574] The hair loss is more obvious in men. Clinically there is progressive replacement of terminal hairs by fine, virtually unpigmented vellus hairs, with hair loss in distinct geographical areas of the scalp.[575] Hair diameter diversity is an important clinical sign that reflects the underlying follicular miniaturization characteristic of this condition.[576] Increased shedding of hairs is usually noted.[571] In females, there may be features of hyperandrogenism such as hirsutism and acne.[577] However, it has been reported in a female with hypopituitarism, indicating that it is not always androgen dependent.[578]

In males, the hair loss is patterned and involves the frontal, central and temporal regions. Various categories of male baldness have been defined, based on which of the above areas are involved.[571]

In females, three distinct patterns of hair loss have been recognized.[579,580] The most common type is a diffuse frontovertical thinning without temporal recession.[577] The second type is similar to that seen in the male (male pattern alopecia). It is often associated with virilism, although in one study it was found in a significant number of normal postmenopausal women.[581] The third pattern is diffuse thinning confined to the vertex and developing after the menopause.[579] A midline part will reveal a characteristic decrease in hair density from the vertex to the front of the scalp.[582] In endocrinologically normal females, the rate of progression of the alopecia is very slow. However, it should always be kept in mind that androgenic alopecia, in both sexes, may be accompanied or unmasked by other forms of hair loss such as alopecia areata, telogen effluvium or the hair loss associated with hypothyroidism and even with iron deficiency.[583]

Androgenic alopecia results from a progressive diminution in the size of terminal follicles with each successive cycle and their eventual conversion to vellus follicles.[571,584] This vellus conversion occurs under the influence of androgenic stimulation or in individuals with genetic predisposition.[577] The method of inheritance has not been clearly defined. It is probably polygenic. No relationship with the 5α-reductase gene or the human hairless gene has been found.[585–587] Androgenic alopecia is common in adrenoleukodystrophy, an X-linked recessive condition.[588] Racial influences also play a part.[577]

Elevated urinary[589] and sometimes serum dehydroepiandrosterone levels have been noted in male pattern alopecia.[590] Hair follicles from sites involved with baldness have shown altered levels in the activity of the enzyme responsible for the conversion of certain androgens to their more active metabolites.[591] Hyperandrogenism has been detected in approximately 40%

of females with the diffuse type of alopecia.[579,592] Polycystic ovaries are frequently the cause of this hyperandrogenic state.[592] Antiandrogen therapy will result in some improvement in up to 50% of patients, but this is usually confined to a decreased rate of hair loss.[593] Recent work suggests that the insulin growth factor 1 (IGF-1) axis may be important in the etiology of patterned hair loss in males.[594,595] Topical minoxidil and oral finasteride have been used with some success,[596–598] although the improvement is often not retained after cessation of treatment.[599] Furthermore, finasteride, a selective inhibitor of 5α-reductase 2, appears to be capable of reversing the miniaturization of follicles in androgenic alopecia of younger males, but not in postmenopausal women.[600,601]

Histopathology[602,603]

The earliest change in androgenic alopecia is focal basophilic degeneration of the connective tissue sheath of the lower one-third of otherwise normal anagen follicles.[571] The terminal follicles become progressively smaller and a proportion regress to the vellus state (Fig. 15.21). This progressive miniaturization of hair follicles and their shafts is best assessed on transverse sections.[560,604] Even the matrix and dermal papillae are reduced in size.[605] Only in very advanced stages do the vellus follicles disappear, leaving thin

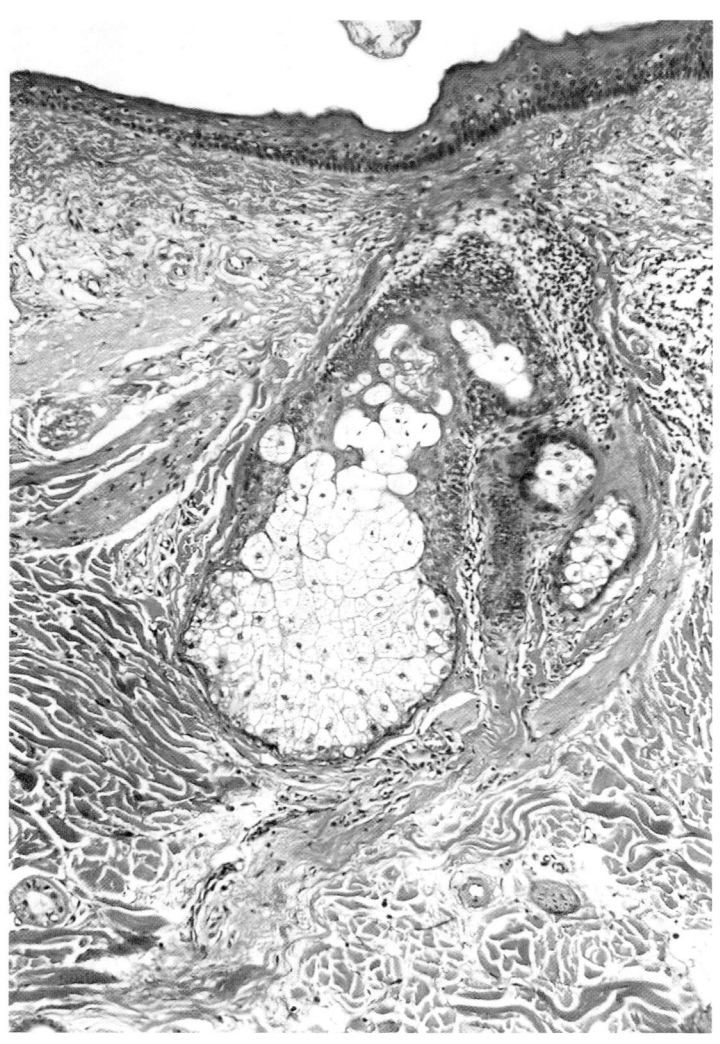

Fig. 15.21 Androgenic alopecia. A small vellus follicle is dwarfed by the adjacent sebaceous gland. (H & E)

hyaline strands in the dermis.[414] Some quiescent terminal follicles are present until a late stage and it is these which produce hairs under the influence of minoxidil.[606] Progressive fibroplasia of the perifollicular sheath appears to be a common process; this may result in the miniaturization of the follicle, rather than being a consequence of it.[607,608]

There is also an increase in the number of telogen and catagen hairs relative to the number of anagen hairs.[571] In one study, telogen hairs constituted 16% of the total, compared to 6.5% in normal subjects.[609] This results from a shortening of the anagen cycle. This altered telogen/anagen ratio cannot be appreciated in conventional sections because only a small number of follicles is present in the plane of section. However, if transverse sections are taken of the biopsy then a greater number of follicles is available for study.[415] The decreased hair diameter can also be quantified in these sections.

In the connective tissue streamers that lie beneath the vellus follicles, small elastin bodies can be seen. They are known as Arão–Perkins bodies and they indicate the sites of the papillae of each preceding generation of follicles.[412] They can be stained with the acid orcein method, but not the Verhoeff elastic stain.[412]

It is usually suggested that the sebaceous glands are increased in size, number and lobulation.[603] However, planimetric studies have shown that the total number of sebaceous glands is significantly decreased.[571] The arrectores eventually diminish in size, but this lags behind the follicles. Accordingly, relatively large arrectores can usually be seen attached to the connective tissue streamers (follicular stelae) below the small vellus follicles.

Other changes that may be present include mild vascular dilatation and a mild perivascular round cell infiltrate which often includes mast cells.[603] This has been called 'microinflammation'.[608] Multinucleate giant cells are present in up to one-third of biopsies.[610] Small nerve networks, resembling encapsulated end organs, may be seen. Solar elastosis and some thinning of the dermis may also be present in cases of long standing.

Female pattern alopecia is usually regarded as having similar morphological features to those seen in males.[602] One study showed frequent catagen follicles in the female type with a paucity of telogen follicles.[611] Numerous vellus follicles were also present.

TEMPORAL TRIANGULAR ALOPECIA

Temporal triangular alopecia consists of a triangular patch of alopecia with its base extending to the frontotemporal hairline.[612–614] Most cases develop during the first few years of life; the original designation 'congenital triangular alopecia' is a misnomer.[615,616] It is usually unilateral. Fine vellus hairs are often present in the area.[613]

It has been reported in association with colonic polyposis, eye defects, mental retardation and phakomatosis pigmentovascularis.[617,618]

Histopathology

There is replacement of the normal abundant terminal follicles of the scalp by vellus follicles. Sebaceous glands and the dermis appear normal.

ANAGEN DEFLUVIUM

Anagen defluvium (anagen effluvium) is the loss of anagen hairs, either because they are defective and break or, rarely, because they are easily detached from the hair follicles.[414] The hair loss may be patterned or diffuse and it appears 1 month or less after the causative event, much faster than the hair loss in telogen effluvium.[475]

Defective hairs that break easily occur in several hair shaft abnormalities such as pili torti, trichorrhexis nodosa and monilethrix.[414] They also develop following antimitotic agents, various drugs, thallium, arsenic, vitamin A intoxication and X-ray therapy.[414] Other causes include trauma, thyroid disease, hypopituitarism, deficiency states, infections of the follicle or hair shaft and alopecia areata.[414,475]

Easy detachment of anagen hairs is a rare cause of anagen defluvium, occurring in follicular mucinosis, lymphomatous infiltration of the hair follicles and the rare loose anagen syndrome (see below).

In most instances, the diagnosis is made on clinical grounds and scalp biopsies are rarely performed. Two disorders, the loose anagen syndrome and drug alopecia, will be considered in further detail. It should be noted that various mechanisms may be involved in drug alopecias.

LOOSE ANAGEN SYNDROME

Loose anagen syndrome is a recently delineated entity of childhood in which anagen hairs are easily pulled from the scalp of affected individuals, who present with diffuse hair loss.[619-623] It may sometimes be mimicked by alopecia areata.[624] Some improvement in the alopecia occurs with increasing age. Adult onset has been recorded.[625]

Histopathology

Abnormal keratinization of Huxley's and Henle's layers of the inner root sheath has been found in some samples.[620] The keratogenous zone of the follicle appears shorter than normal.[626] Marked cleft formation between hair shafts and regressively altered inner root sheaths were noted in another study.[619] The easily extracted hairs are misshapen anagen hairs without external root sheaths.[620]

DRUG-INDUCED ALOPECIA

Alopecia induced by drugs usually presents as diffuse, non-scarring hair loss that is reversible upon withdrawal of the drug.[627-629] It is a common complication of the various antimitotic agents used in the chemotherapy of cancer, but it may also occur as a rare complication of other therapeutic drugs.[630] A nationwide outbreak of alopecia has been reported recently in the USA, associated with the use of a commercial hair-straightening product.[631] The low pH of the product may have been responsible.

Drugs may interfere with hair growth in a number of different ways. For example, thallium, excess vitamin A, retinoids and certain cholesterol-lowering drugs interfere with the keratinization of the hair follicle.[627,632,633] The antimitotic drugs interfere with hair growth in the anagen phase by interrupting the normal replication of the hair matrix cells.[628] Other drugs induce telogen effluvium and the follicles remain in the resting phase.

Besides those already listed, drugs that may induce alopecia include anti-coagulants, antithyroid drugs, chemicals used in straightening hair,[631,634] anti-convulsants, hormone-related substances such as clomiphene, heavy metals such as lead, bismuth, arsenic, gold, mercury and lithium, antibacterial agents such as gentamicin, nitrofurantoin and ethambutol, and non-steroidal anti-inflammatory or antihyperuricemic agents such as naproxen, ibuprofen, allopurinol, probenecid and indomethacin.[627,628,635] Drugs that have been incriminated rarely include amphetamines, vasopressin,[636] beta-blocking agents, cimetidine, levodopa, methysergide, penicillamine, bromocriptine, borates,[637] quinacrine (mepacrine), selenium and tricyclic antidepressants.[628] Localized alopecia has been reported at the injection site of interferon alfa-2b.[638] A detailed listing is contained in the review article by Pillans and Woods.[629]

Histopathology

Those drugs producing telogen effluvium will induce catagen changes in many of the follicles. By the time a biopsy is taken, the follicles have usually entered the telogen phase. The antimitotic agents also induce premature catagen transformation. At a later stage the follicles enter anagen but their growth is then arrested at various stages of development.

SCARRING ALOPECIAS

The scarring (cicatricial) alopecias are an etiologically diverse group that share in common the destruction of hair follicles associated with atrophy and/or scarring of the affected area, usually leading to permanent hair loss.[639] They may result from intrinsic inflammation of the hair follicle (folliculitis) or destruction of follicles by an inflammatory or neoplastic process external to them.[640]

Recently, attention has focused on the role of the sebaceous gland in scarring alopecia. Stenn and colleagues have drawn attention to the fact that the sebaceous gland is lost in the early phases of scarring alopecia.[641] The mutant asebia mouse has hypoplastic sebaceous glands. It soon develops a scarring alopecia, support for the theory that primary sebaceous gland pathology may be involved in some scarring alopecias.[641]

The scarring alopecias may be classified on an etiological basis, as follows:[640]

- *developmental and related disorders*
  epidermal nevus
  aplasia cutis
  incontinentia pigmenti
  keratosis pilaris atrophicans
  porokeratosis of Mibelli
  ichthyosis vulgaris
  Darier's disease
  epidermolysis bullosa (recessive dystrophic)
  polyostotic fibrous dysplasia
- *physical injuries*
  mechanical trauma, including pressure/traction
  thermal, electric and petrol burns
  radiodermatitis
  therapeutic embolization[642]
- *specific infections*
  certain fungal infections (including kerion and favus)
  herpes zoster and varicella
  pyogenic folliculitides
  lupus vulgaris
  syphilis (late stages)
  leishmaniasis
- *specific dermatoses*
  lichen planus and variants
  lupus erythematosus
  scleroderma and morphea
  necrobiosis lipoidica
  necrobiotic xanthogranuloma
  lichen sclerosus et atrophicus
  sarcoidosis
  amyloidosis
  cicatricial pemphigoid
  follicular mucinosis

folliculitis decalvans
dissecting cellulitis of the scalp
- *neoplasms (alopecia neoplastica)*
basal and squamous cell carcinomas
angiosarcoma
lymphoma
secondary tumors
- *idiopathic*
idiopathic scarring alopecia (pseudopelade)
traction alopecia with scarring
postmenopausal frontal fibrosing alopecia
fibrosing alopecia in a pattern distribution
tufted-hair folliculitis.

With the exception of the idiopathic scarring alopecias, the above conditions have all been discussed in other sections of this volume.

Attention has been given in recent years to the regrouping of some of the scarring alopecias into an orderly classification. Sperling, Solomon and Whiting have looked at the central centrifugal scarring alopecias,[643] while Sullivan and Kossard have grouped together the pustular scarring alopecias.[644] These concepts are considered below. Readers are referred to the etiological classification above. It still provides a convenient checklist of the various scarring alopecias.

Different approaches to scarring alopecias

Two recent publications have attempted to bring some order to the confusing area of scarring alopecias. Although not followed here, they are worthy of some mention. Sullivan and Kossard have given a detailed classification of the scarring alopecias.[644] Their categorization of the *pustular scarring alopecias* is worth repeating (see Table 15.2).

The second publication, by Sperling, Solomon and Whiting, discussed the concept of *central centrifugal scarring alopecia*.[643] This term is a clinical one that includes patients with (1) hair loss centered on the crown or vertex, (2) chronic and progressive disease with eventual 'burnout', (3) symmetrical expansion, and (4) clinical and histological evidence of peripheral inflammation.[643] Their concept encompasses:

- follicular degeneration syndrome
- pseudopelade (idiopathic scarring alopecia)
- folliculitis decalvans
- tufted folliculitis

However, while fibrosing alopecia in a pattern distribution would seem to fit this definition, frontal fibrosing alopecia does not. Yet they would logically seem to fit together in any clinicopathological correlation. Furthermore, the above classification seems to include disorders with diverse etiologies, at least in our current state of 'knowledge'.[645,646] Another criticism of this concept has been provided by Ackerman and colleagues who point out that there is no such entity as the follicular degeneration syndrome, which is in reality a

Table 15.2 **Causes of pustular scarring alopecias**

Folliculitis decalvans
Tufted folliculitis
Erosive pustular dermatosis of the scalp
Acne keloidalis nuchae
Dissecting cellulitis of the scalp
Kerion
Traction alopecia

traction alopecia.[474] Interestingly, traction alopecia, fibrosing alopecia in a pattern distribution and postmenopausal frontal fibrosing alopecia all share a lichenoid perifolliculitis in the early stages. It may be that various stimuli are capable of altering the antigenicity of follicular cells, leading to a lichenoid (cell-mediated) reaction.

IDIOPATHIC SCARRING ALOPECIA (PSEUDOPELADE)

Idiopathic scarring alopecia (fibrosing alopecia,[412,565] alopecia cicatrisata, pseudopelade) is a rare, asymptomatic form of scarring alopecia in which there is patchy hair loss not accompanied by any clinical evidence of folliculitis, lichen planus, lupus erythematosus or any of the specific diseases listed above.[647] The term 'idiopathic scarring alopecia' is preferred to the more commonly employed name *pseudopelade*, which has been used in the past in a variety of contexts:[648-650] it has been applied to end-stage scarring alopecias following known dermatoses such as lichen planus and lupus erythematosus.[651] It is conceded that the term 'pseudopelade' has some use in a clinical setting to refer to a scarring alopecia, the cause of which is not yet known, but it should not be used to refer to a clinicopathological entity.[652]

Idiopathic scarring alopecia tends to affect females over the age of 40 years. It has an insidious onset and a chronic, usually slowly progressive course. It results in slightly depressed patches of irreversible hair loss which may occur singly or in groups that have been described as resembling 'footprints in the snow'.[414] The small patches may coalesce to form larger patches of scarring alopecia. Both the scalp and beard area were involved in one patient.[653] As the designation 'idiopathic' implies, the etiology is unknown.

Histopathology[412,565]

In established lesions there is loss of hair follicles and sebaceous glands and these are replaced by bands of fibrous tissue containing elastic fibers (Fig. 15.22). These bands extend above the level of the attachment of the arrectores pilorum, in contrast to normal telogen where the fibrous tissue replaces only the deeper part of the hair follicle. In transverse sections, a prominent perifollicular lamellar fibroplasia is usually seen.[416,654]

In early lesions, a moderately heavy infiltrate of lymphocytes surrounds the upper two-thirds of the follicle. It has been suggested that these may extend into the follicle, producing its massive apoptotic involution.[655] The epidermis is not involved by the inflammatory infiltrate. In late lesions the epidermis may show some atrophic changes with loss of the rete ridge pattern.

The orcein and Verhoeff van Gieson elastic stains may provide useful information in the scarring alopecias.[565,656] Whereas the fibrous tracts associated with the scarring alopecia of lichen planopilaris and lupus erythematosus are usually devoid of elastic fibers (this loss is more extensive in lupus erythematosus than in lichen planopilaris), there are elastic fibers in the fibrous tracts of idiopathic scarring alopecia and traction alopecia with scarring.[656] In a proportion of cases elastic fibers develop around the lower cyclic portion of the hair follicle.[565]

Direct immunofluorescence may also assist in the diagnosis of the scarring alopecias.[657] In idiopathic scarring alopecia immunofluorescence is negative, in contrast to lupus erythematosus in which a band of immunoglobulins and complement may be found along the basement membrane zone and surrounding hair follicles.[657] In lichen planus, colloid bodies containing IgM and often C3 are present beneath the epidermis and around hair follicles.[657] In 'burnt-out' lesions, direct immunofluorescence may be negative.

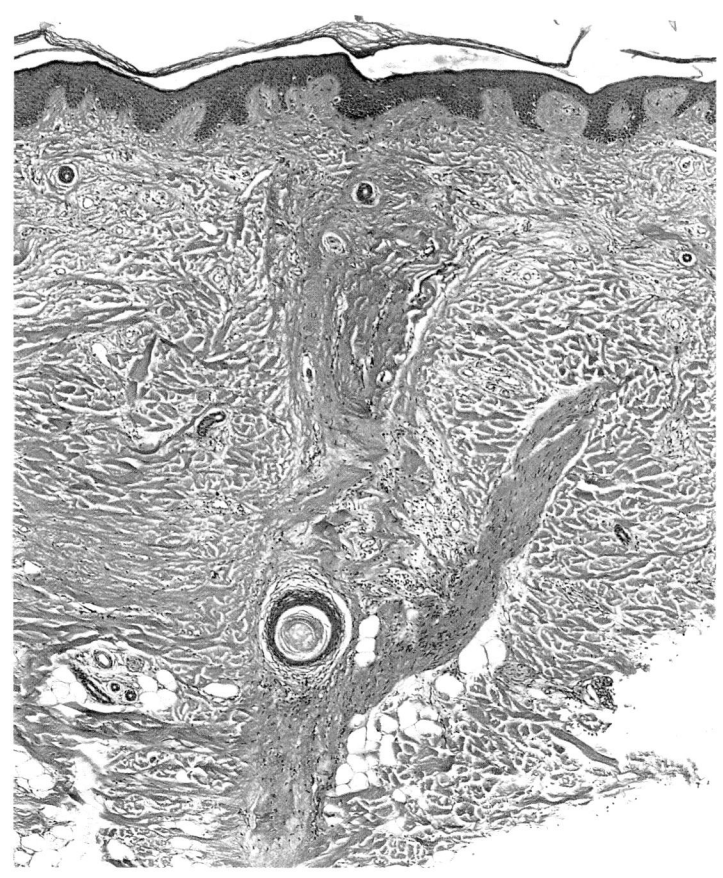

Fig 15.22 **Idiopathic scarring alopecia.** A band of fibrous tissue is present at the site of a destroyed hair follicle. (H & E)

TRACTION ALOPECIA WITH SCARRING

The term 'traction alopecia with scarring' is used in preference to 'hot comb' alopecia, central progressive alopecia in black females, and the follicular degeneration syndrome, for a form of scarring alopecia involving predominantly the crown of the scalp.[658,659] Hairs at the periphery of the scalp are spared. It primarily affects black women.

While minor degrees of traction can produce hair loss without significant scarring, as in trichotillomania (see p. 474), prolonged and recurrent severe traction can result in scarring. Recently, Ackerman and colleagues have presented a detailed study of this entity, pointing out that there is no follicular degeneration in these cases, and that the use of this term is no longer justified.[474]

Histopathology

As defined by Ackerman and colleagues, biopsies at an early stage show a lichenoid perifolliculitis in which infundibula are enveloped by lymphocytes with progressive perifollicular fibroplasia.[474] In fully developed lesions the infiltrate is sparse and the lower part of the infundibulum and isthmus are thinned, consequent to the fibroplasia. A granulomatous reaction to extravasated cornified material is present. This is followed by a loss of follicles and increased fibrosis with extension into the subcutis.

The Verhoeff van Gieson elastic stain shows a hyalinized dermis with markedly thickened elastic fibers. The elastin sheath is preserved at the periphery of the broad fibrous tracts.[656]

POSTMENOPAUSAL FRONTAL FIBROSING ALOPECIA

The term 'postmenopausal frontal fibrosing alopecia' has been used for a progressive frontal scarring alopecia associated with perifollicular erythema.[660,661] Kossard and colleagues have reported 16 cases, suggesting that it is more common than the paucity of reports would suggest.[662] The histological features are indistinguishable from those seen in lichen planopilaris. The absence of lesions of lichen planus elsewhere led to the suggestion that these cases might represent a unique follicular destruction syndrome mediated by lymphocytes and triggered by postmenopausal events.[660] It is best regarded as a frontal variant of lichen planopilaris (see p. 37).[662]

FIBROSING ALOPECIA IN A PATTERN DISTRIBUTION

Fibrosing alopecia in a pattern distribution appears to be another variant of lichen planopilaris in which the immune reaction is directed against miniaturized follicles of androgenic alopecia.[663] That is, these persons develop inflammatory scarring alopecia affecting only the balding central scalp.[643] The lichenoid infiltrate targets the upper follicle. Late lesions resemble end-stage lichen planopilaris.[663]

FOLLICULITIS DECALVANS

Folliculitis decalvans is sometimes considered to be a primary scarring alopecia. However, because inflammation of the follicle is a major feature. it has been considered with the folliculitides on page 462.

TUFTED-HAIR FOLLICULITIS

Tufted-hair folliculitis is characterized by areas of scarring alopecia with tufts of hair emerging from single follicular openings.[664–666] It is most likely a consequence of bacterial folliculitis involving the upper and mid follicle with rupture and scarring. It may complicate folliculitis decalvans,[199,200] folliculitis keloidalis nuchae (acne keloidalis) and pemphigus vulgaris.[667,668]

Histopathology

A biopsy is usually carried out at a late stage when there is folliculitis, perifolliculitis and scarring.[669] The characteristic feature is the presence of several closely set, complete follicles with a common follicular opening from which multiple hair shafts emerge.[666]

MISCELLANEOUS ALOPECIAS

There is one rare form of alopecia that does not fit neatly into any of the other categories. It is called lipedematous alopecia.

LIPEDEMATOUS ALOPECIA

Lipedematous alopecia, an acquired condition of unknown etiology, is characterized by a thick, boggy scalp with varying degrees of hair loss, occurring predominantly in adult black females.[670,671] There is doubling of the scalp thickness due to expansion of the subcutaneous fat layer. The term 'lipedematous scalp' has been used for cases without hair loss.[672]

Histopathology

There may be mild hyperkeratosis, acanthosis and keratinous follicular plugging. Hair follicles are usually reduced in number. The most noticeable feature is a thickening of the subcutis, which appears to encroach upon the dermis. The subcutis is edematous with disruption of fat architecture and cellular integrity. No inflammation or lipomembranous change has been described. Increased mucin was described in one case,[672] but specifically excluded in another.[670] The author has seen a case in which fat overgrowth without significant lymphedema produced a clinically similar condition. Fat overgrowth has been implied in some of the earlier reports of lipedematous alopecia.

Miscellaneous disorders

In this section, the following miscellaneous topics will be covered:

- pilosebaceous disorders
- apocrine disorders
- eccrine disorders
- vestibular gland disorders.

A brief account of the embryology and anatomy of the sebaceous, apocrine and eccrine glands will also be given.

PILOSEBACEOUS DISORDERS

The normal hair follicle has already been discussed earlier in this chapter. Its embryology and structure are considered on page 456, and the normal hair cycle on page 471.

The structure of the sebaceous gland will be considered here, followed by a discussion of various 'miscellaneous' disorders of the pilosebaceous unit, not previously considered.

The normal sebaceous gland

The sebaceous gland develops as a bud from the primordial hair follicle in the 13th to 15th week of fetal life. It is a multilobular gland connected by a short duct to the hair follicle at the junction of the infundibulum and isthmus. The gland is comprised of a peripheral zone of basal cells which accumulate lipid in the cytoplasm as they move towards the center of the gland. The sebocytes eventually disintegrate at the level of the duct, releasing the mature sebaceous product, known as sebum, which acts as an emollient, bacteriostat, insulator and pheromone.

Sebaceous glands are distributed throughout the body except for the palms and soles. They are largest and most numerous in the skin of the face and the upper part of the trunk (the so-called 'seborrheic areas'). The meibomian glands in the tarsus and the glands of Zeis at the lid margin are modified sebaceous glands.

The sebaceous glands increase in size at puberty. They atrophy in old age, particularly in females.

Miscellaneous disorders of the pilosebaceous unit

There are several diseases of the pilosebaceous unit which do not fit readily into any of the categories discussed above. They include hypertrichosis, keratosis pilaris, keratosis pilaris atrophicans, follicular spicules, lichen spinulosus, rosacea, pyoderma faciale and neutrophilic sebaceous adenitis.

Rosacea is traditionally included with the pilosebaceous disorders although there is increasing evidence that it is not a primary disease of the appendages.

HYPERTRICHOSIS

Hypertrichosis refers to the growth of hair on any part of the body in excess of the amount usually present in persons of the same age, race and sex.[673] Androgen-induced hair growth (hirsutism) is not included in this definition.[674] Several distinct clinical forms exist.

Congenital hypertrichosis lanuginosa

Congenital hypertrichosis lanuginosa is an exceedingly rare familial disorder, often inherited as an autosomal dominant trait, in which there is excessive growth of lanugo hair.[675] Dental and eye abnormalities may also be present.[676]

Acquired hypertrichosis lanuginosa

Acquired hypertrichosis lanuginosa is usually generalized, except for the palms and soles. An important cause is an underlying cancer, usually of epithelial type,[677] although rarely a lymphoma is present.[678] Hair growth may antedate the appearance of the tumor by months to several years.[679,680] The pathogenesis is unknown. Vellus hairs, intermediate forms and terminal hairs may be increased in cases of porphyria, malnutrition and brain injury and, usually reversibly, in patients taking streptomycin, phenytoin (diphenylhydantoin), corticosteroids, penicillamine, psoralens, benoxaprofen, the vasodilators diazoxide and minoxidil[681] and cyclosporin A.[673,682]

Congenital circumscribed hypertrichosis[673]

Localized areas of hypertrichosis can be seen in congenital pigmented nevi, Becker's nevus, nevoid hypertrichosis,[683] spinal dysraphism ('faun-tail')[684] and in depigmented hypertrichosis following Blaschko's lines.[685]

Moderate hypertrichosis of the lower extremities has been reported in a patient with mitochondrial encephalomyopathy with lactic acidosis and strokelike episodes (MELAS syndrome).[686]

Acquired circumscribed hypertrichosis[673]

Hypertrichosis may develop at sites of persistent friction and irritation in association with plaster casts and at sites of inflammation, including insect bites.[687]

Histopathology

Little has been written on the histopathology of hypertrichosis.[682] In the acquired form, the follicles have been reported to be small and deviated from their normal vertical position. They extend obliquely or even parallel to the epidermis and contain thin unmedullated hairs. The follicles are surrounded by small lipidized mantles representing sebaceous ducts showing early glandular differentiation.[688]

KERATOSIS PILARIS

Keratosis pilaris is a disorder of keratinization involving the infundibulum of the hair follicle. It is a common condition, being found in up to 5% of adult males and in 30% of females, particularly those showing hyperandrogenism and obesity.[689] It is also increased in patients with insulin-dependent diabetes mellitus.[690] The lesions, which vary from subtle follicular excrescences to more prominent follicular spikes, are found most often on the posterior aspect of the upper part of the arms and on the lateral aspect of the thighs and buttocks.[691] Follicular keratotic plugs resembling keratosis pilaris may be found in keratosis pilaris atrophicans (see below), lichen spinulosus (see p. 484), pityriasis rubra pilaris, ichthyosis, psoriasis, some eczemas, lithium therapy[692] and uremia.[689,693,694] Large follicular keratotic plugs are seen in the amputation stumps of some patients with lower limb amputations and ill-fitting prostheses;[695] they have also been seen as an idiopathic phenomenon.[696]

It is thought that adrogenic stimulation of the pilosebaceous follicle may result in the hyperkeratinization of the infundibulum.[689]

Histopathology

A keratin plug fills the infundibulum of the hair follicle and protrudes above the surface for a variable distance (Fig. 15.23). Serial sections are sometimes necessary to show the plug to best advantage. A very sparse lymphocytic infiltrate may be present in the dermis adjacent to the follicular infundibulum.

The follicular keratoses that sometimes form at amputation sites are composed of large parakeratotic plugs.[695]

In **keratosis follicularis squamosa (Dohi)**, a disorder of follicular keratinization reported from Japan, there is increased orthokeratin adjacent to the follicle, in addition to the follicular plug of keratin.[697] Clinically, there are asymptomatic small scaly patches with a central follicular plug.[697]

KERATOSIS PILARIS ATROPHICANS

The term 'keratosis pilaris atrophicans' refers to a group of three related disorders in which keratosis pilaris is associated with mild perifollicular inflammation and subsequent atrophy, particularly involving the face.[698] Differences in the location and the degree of atrophy have been used to categorize these three conditions.

Keratosis pilaris atrophicans faciei (ulerythema ophryogenes)

Keratosis pilaris atrophicans faciei is manifest soon after birth by follicular papules with an erythematous halo involving the lateral part of the eyebrows.[699,700] It may later involve the forehead and cheeks. Pitted scars and alopecia usually result.[700] Keratosis pilaris of the arms, buttocks and thighs is often present. Less common clinical associations include atopy, mental retardation,[700] woolly hair,[701] cardiofaciocutaneous syndrome,[702,703] Rubinstein–Taybi syndrome,[704] Noonan's syndrome[705–708] and a low serum vitamin A level.[700] Some reports suggest an autosomal dominant inheritance.[700] A gene in the 18p region may be involved.[709]

Keratosis follicularis spinulosa decalvans

Keratosis follicularis spinulosa decalvans is another exceedingly rare condition which begins in infancy with diffuse keratosis pilaris associated with scarring alopecia of the scalp and eyebrows.[710–712] 'Moth-eaten' scarring of the cheeks usually results. Associations include atopy, photophobia, corneal abnormalities, palmar-plantar keratoderma and other ectodermal defects.[713] The gene maps to Xp21.1–p22.2.[714] Some cases are sporadic. A variant with autosomal dominant inheritance and inflammation that begins at puberty has been called 'folliculitis spinulosa decalvans'.[698]

Atrophoderma vermiculata

Atrophoderma vermiculata (folliculitis ulerythematosa reticulata)[715,716] involves the preauricular region and cheeks.[717–720] It may follow Blaschko's lines.[721] It develops in late childhood with the formation of horny follicular plugs which are later shed. This is followed by a reticulate atrophy with some comedones and scattered milia. Inheritance is autosomal dominant in type. Rare clinical associations include Marfan's syndrome,[722] leukokeratosis oris[723] and trichoepitheliomas with basal cell carcinomas (ROMBO syndrome – see p. 862).[724,725] Keratosis pilaris of the limbs is quite commonly present. A condition described in the literature as *atrophia maculosa varioliformis cutis* affected a similar location on the cheeks[726–728] but there was no mention in these cases of a preceding stage with follicular plugging.[726] Another variant has been called 'hereditary perioral pigmented follicular atrophoderma'. It was associated with milia and epidermal cysts.[729]

All three conditions are regarded as congenital follicular dystrophies with abnormal keratinization of the superficial part of the follicles. A fourth condition, **erythromelanosis follicularis faciei et colli**, has minute follicular papules resulting from small keratin plugs associated with red-brown pigmentation and fine telangiectasias.[730–738] This rare disease appears to be another follicular dystrophy but is usually not considered with the other three conditions because it lacks any atrophy. A familial case has been reported.[739]

Histopathology

In all three variants of keratosis pilaris atrophicans there is follicular hyperkeratosis with atrophy of the underlying follicle and sebaceous gland.[716,740,741] Comedones and milia may also be present.[717] There is variable perifollicular fibrosis which may extend into the surrounding reticular dermis as horizontal lamellar fibrosis.[710] The dermis may be reduced in thickness. A mild perivascular and perifollicular infiltrate of lymphocytes and histiocytes is usually present.

In **erythromelanosis follicularis faciei et colli** there is follicular hyperkeratosis, mild basal pigmentation, dilatation of vessels in the papillary dermis, and a reduction in size of the hair shafts and the inner and outer root sheaths.[738]

FOLLICULAR SPICULES

Follicular spicules with a horny appearance have been reported on the face of patients with multiple myeloma and cryoglobulinemia.[742,743] The spicules are composed of eosinophilic, compact, homogeneous material which is largely the monoclonal protein of the underlying gammopathy.[743]

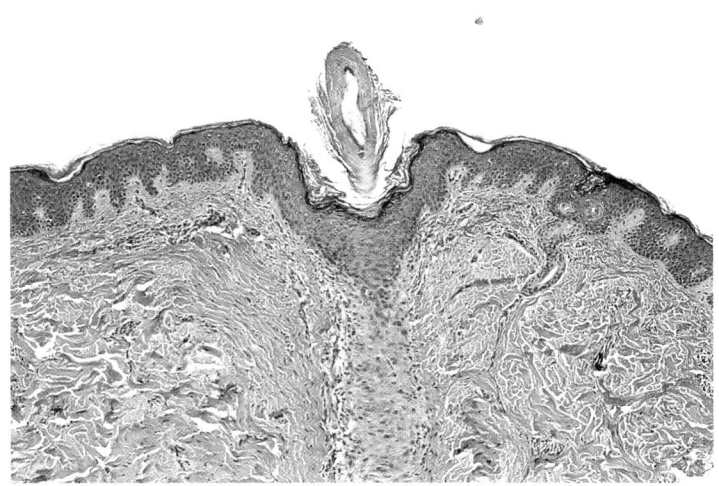

Fig. 15.23 **Keratosis pilaris.** A keratin plug fills the infundibulum of the follicle and protrudes above the surface. (H & E)

LICHEN SPINULOSUS

Lichen spinulosus is a rare dermatosis of unknown etiology characterized by follicular keratotic papules that are grouped into plaques, 2–6 cm in diameter.[744] The horny spines protrude 1–2 mm above the surface. Lesions are distributed symmetrically on the extensor surfaces of the arms and legs and on the back, chest, face and neck. Onset of the disease is in adolescence. It has been described in an HIV-positive man[745] and in an elderly female with Crohn's disease.[746]

Histopathology[744]

In lichen spinulosus, there is a keratotic plug in the follicular infundibulum as in keratosis pilaris. However, there is a heavier perifollicular infiltrate of lymphocytes in lichen spinulosus, particularly adjacent to the infundibulum of the follicle, which is often dilated. Less constant changes include perifollicular fibrosis and atrophy of the sebaceous glands.

Lichen spinulosus is best regarded as a variant of keratosis pilaris in which the lesions are more papular, a consequence of the more pronounced dermal inflammation.

ROSACEA

Rosacea (acne rosacea) is a fairly common disorder of adults, involving primarily the face.[747–752] Rarely, children are affected.[753] It exists in four clinical forms,[754] although cases with overlapping features are common:

1. an erythematous, telangiectatic type
2. a papulopustular type
3. a granulomatous type (see p. 198)
4. a hyperplastic glandular type which results in irregular, bulbous enlargement of the nose, the condition known as rhinophyma.[755]

Rosacea is a difficult entity to classify, not only because its pathogenesis is poorly understood but also because of the broad spectrum of histopathological changes found. Rosacea has been variously regarded as a folliculitis, a sebaceous gland disorder, a response to overabundant demodex mites, and a functional disorder of superficial dermal blood vessels associated with prominent flushing.[756,757] The last of these possibilities is currently the most favored, although some of the evidence supporting it is somewhat circumstantial.[751,758,759] Demodex mites may be increased secondary to these vascular changes.[760] Vasodilator drugs may also exacerbate rosacea.[761] Rosacea-like eruptions can be seen in response to heavy local infestations by *Demodex folliculorum* (rosacea-like demodicidosis – see p. 739),[762] following the topical application of potent fluorinated steroids[763] and the use of a halogenated steroid nasal spray.[764] Acne rosacea has been reported in patients with HIV infection.[765] There has been considerable interest in the role of *Helicobacter pylori* in the etiology of rosacea;[766,767] however, controlled trials offer no support for this association.[768–770] It is likely that the treatment used for *H. pylori* is beneficial for rosacea.[771–774]

Perioral dermatitis (see p. 199) is possibly a related entity.[775–780] **Periocular dermatitis** is considered to have a similar pathomechanism to perioral dermatitis.[781] Sometimes rosacea will present with periorbital edema.[782] This feature should not be confused with periocular dermatitis. Griffiths has drawn attention to a group of patients with lesions resembling what has been called perioral dermatitis which he calls the **MARSH syndrome**, combining as it does *m*elasma, *a*cne, *r*osacea, *s*eborrheic eczema and *h*irsutism.[783]

Histopathology[784]

Rosacea is characterized by a combination of several histopathological features. Sometimes the histopathological changes are non-diagnostic.[785] In the erythematous-telangiectatic group there is telangiectasia, sometimes prominent, of superficial dermal vessels (Fig. 15.24). There is a perivascular infiltrate of lymphocytes, usually mild to moderate in intensity. A small number of plasma cells is usually present and is an important clue to the diagnosis. Inconstant features include mild dermal edema, solar elastosis and mild perifolliculitis. The papulopustular lesions have a more pronounced inflammatory cell infiltrate which is both perivascular and peripilar, involving the superficial and mid dermis. The infiltrate may include a few neutrophils as well as lymphocytes and plasma cells. Active pustular lesions show a superficial folliculitis while in older lesions a granulomatous perifolliculitis is often present. Keratotic follicular plugging, but not comedones, may be present. Demodex mites are present in 20–50% of cases. The granulomatous form[786] is usually characterized by a tuberculoid reaction, often in the vicinity of damaged hair follicles (see p. 198). Necrosis, resembling caseation, was present in 11% of patients in one series (Fig. 15.25).[787]

Sebaceous gland hypertrophy and scattered follicular plugging are present in most cases of rhinophyma (Fig. 15.26).[788] In the less common fibrous variant of rhinophyma, there is telangiectasia, diffuse dermal fibrosis with abundant mucin, a virtual absence of pilosebaceous structures and an increase in factor XIIIa-positive cells in the dermis.[789,790] Telangiectasia of superficial dermal vessels is also quite common, a feature which is not present in senile sebaceous gland hyperplasia. Demodex may be present in the pilosebaceous follicles. Inconstant features include solar elastosis, dilatation of follicles, focal folliculitis and perifolliculitis. Sometimes, finger-like acanthotic downgrowths extend from the epidermis and follicular walls.[788] The infiltrate of lymphocytes

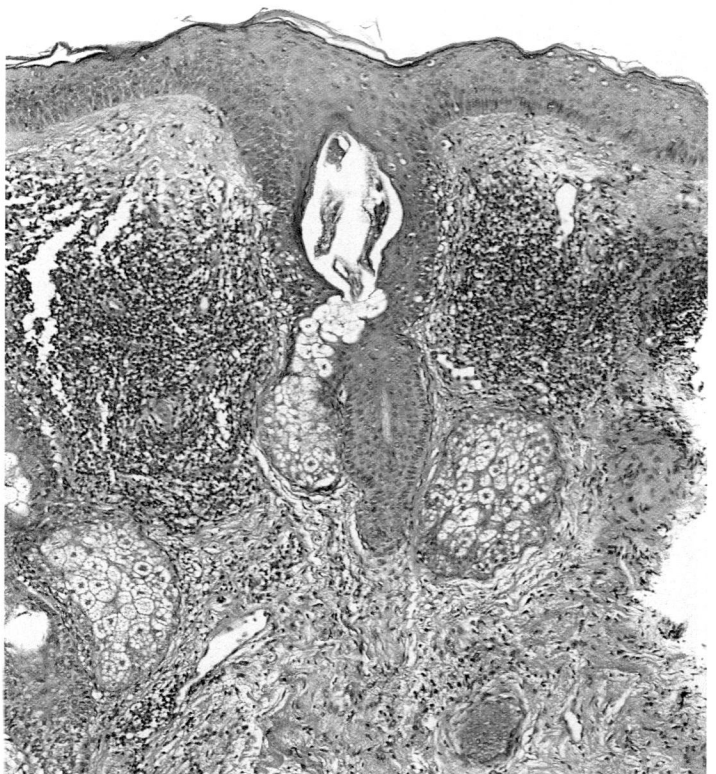

Fig. 15.24 **Rosacea.** A perivascular and perifollicular infiltrate of lymphocytes and plasma cells is present. Several demodex mites are present in the hair follicle. (H & E)

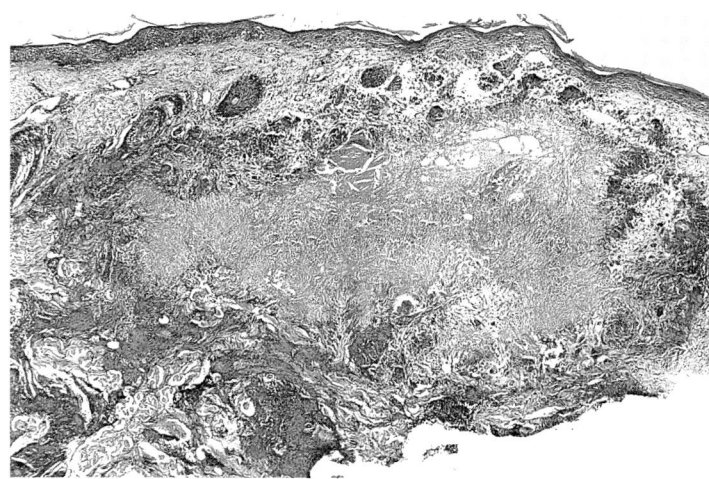

Fig. 15.25 **Granulomatous rosacea.** This florid case has extensive necrosis resembling caseation necrosis. (H & E)

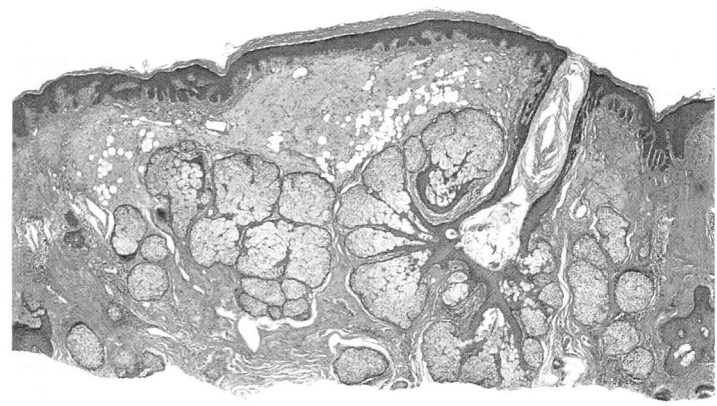

Fig. 15.26 **Rhinophyma.** There is sebaceous gland hyperplasia in this shave biopsy. (H & E)

and plasma cells around superficial vessels varies from sparse to moderately heavy in intensity.

Direct immunofluorescence has demonstrated the presence of immuno-globulins and complement in the region of the dermoepidermal junction in some cases.[791,792]

PYODERMA FACIALE (ROSACEA FULMINANS)

Pyoderma faciale is a rare disorder, now interpreted as a fulminant form of rosacea.[793–795] The term 'rosacea fulminans' has been suggested as a more appropriate designation.[796] It is characterized by the sudden onset of confluent nodules and papulopustules on the face, in women who are usually in their twenties.[793] Purulent material drains from many sinuses, which may be interconnecting. Pyoderma faciale may sometimes occur in association with inflammatory bowel disease.[796–798]

Histopathology[794]

Few cases have been biopsied. There is usually a heavy dermal infiltrate of neutrophils, lymphocytes and epithelioid cells with occasional granulomas with multinucleate giant cells. Perifollicular abscesses and sinus formation may be present.

SQUAMOUS METAPLASIA OF SEBACEOUS GLANDS

Squamous metaplasia has been reported at sites of pressure following cardiac surgery.[799] Ischemia appears to play a major role. The changes commence in the germinative outer layer of the sebaceous gland and advance in a centripetal manner, replacing sebocytes.[799]

NEUTROPHILIC SEBACEOUS ADENITIS

The term 'neutrophilic sebaceous adenitis' has been used for the circinate plaques on the face of a teenage male which were characterized histologically by neutrophilic infiltration of the sebaceous glands.[800] A case with similar clinical features, including spontaneous healing, has since been reported.[801] It differed from the original case by having few neutrophils and many lymphocytes

infiltrating sebaceous glands. This might have resulted from the age of the lesion, which had been present for 2 months at the time of the biopsy.

A **sebotropic drug reaction** has been reported following the ingestion of kava-kava extract, used as an antidepressant therapy.[802] The extract contains kavapyrones which are lipophilic. A dense lymphocytic infiltrate disrupted sebaceous glands, which were partly necrotic.[802]

A sebaceous adenitis (sebaceitis) can also be seen in herpes folliculitis.

FOLLICULAR SEBACEOUS CASTS

Multiple spiky lesions have been reported in the nasolabial region following isotretinoin therapy for acne. Microscopy revealed cast-like accumulations of holocrine secretion, derived from sebaceous glands (sebaceous casts), on the surface of the stratum corneum.[803] Subsequent correspondence suggested that this change had been reported earlier as follicular filaments (follicular casts).[804]

APOCRINE DISORDERS

The normal apocrine gland

Apocrine glands are found regularly in the axilla, anogenital region, the areola and nipple of the female breast, the eyelids (Moll's glands) and the external auditory canal. They are sometimes found in the skin of the scalp and the face. Apocrine glands are derived from the primary epithelial germ along with the hair follicle and sebaceous gland.

The apocrine gland consists of a secretory portion in the deep dermis or subcutis and a short duct which enters into the infundibulum of the hair follicle, above the entry of the sebaceous duct. Apocrine glands have a variable appearance in tissue sections, reflecting the functional state of the gland; secretions are stored in the gland. Both a 'budding type' (apocrine secretion) and a merocrine type of cytoplasmic secretion occur.

Disorders of apocrine glands

Diseases of the apocrine glands are exceedingly uncommon. Only apocrine miliaria and apocrine chromhidrosis have dermatopathological interest. Mucinous metaplasia of an apocrine duct is mentioned below, in the discussion of its eccrine equivalent.

APOCRINE MILIARIA (FOX–FORDYCE DISEASE)

Apocrine miliaria (Fox–Fordyce disease) presents as a chronic papular eruption limited to areas bearing apocrine glands.[805] There is intense pruritus which is sometimes intermittent.[806] The condition affects, almost exclusively, young adult females, although males are not exempt.[807,808] Axillary lesions have occasionally resulted from the prolonged use of topical antiperspirants.[809] It has been reported in two patients with Turner's syndrome under treatment with growth hormone.[810]

Apocrine miliaria results from rupture of the intraepidermal portion of the apocrine duct. This appears to result from keratotic plugging of the duct producing an outflow obstruction.

Histopathology[805,811]

Serial sections are often required to demonstrate the spongiosis and spongiotic vesiculation of the follicular infundibulum adjacent to the point of entry of the apocrine duct (Fig. 15.27). A keratotic plug is sometimes seen above this area.[806,811] There is an associated mild to moderate inflammatory cell infiltrate which may contain some neutrophils as well as chronic inflammatory cells.

Transverse sections, as used in the assessment of alopecias, demonstrate diagnostic features more effectively than conventional sections.[812]

APOCRINE CHROMHIDROSIS

Chromhidrosis refers to the production of colored sweat by apocrine or eccrine sweat glands.[813–815] Slight coloration of apocrine sweat is not uncommon. Pseudochromhidrosis refers to coloration of sweat on the surface of the skin by exogenous dyes or chromogenic organisms.[816]

Histopathology

Orange-brown cytoplasmic granules, predominantly in an apical location, are present in apocrine sweat glands in apocrine chromhidrosis (Fig. 15.28). The pigment may not always be lipofuscin, as originally believed.[813]

ECCRINE DISORDERS

The normal eccrine gland

The eccrine gland is derived from the primitive epidermal ridge. It is composed of a secretory coil (glandular portion) which leads into a coiled proximal duct and then a straight duct which eventually passes through the epidermis. The secretory coil is composed of glycogen-containing clear cells and dark cells which are surrounded by a layer of myoepithelial cells, outside which is the basement membrane. Eccrine glands are most numerous on the sole of the foot.

Eccrine sweat consists predominantly of water. The salt content of the secretions is reduced in the proximal duct, resulting in the release of hypotonic sweat on the skin surface. Sweating dissipates body heat by means of surface evaporation.

Disorders of eccrine glands

Functional disorders of the sweat gland, particularly hyperhidrosis (excessive sweating), are an important clinical problem but hyperhidrosis is not related to any morphological changes in the sweat glands.[817–822] Accordingly it will not be considered further. Obstruction of the eccrine duct produces small

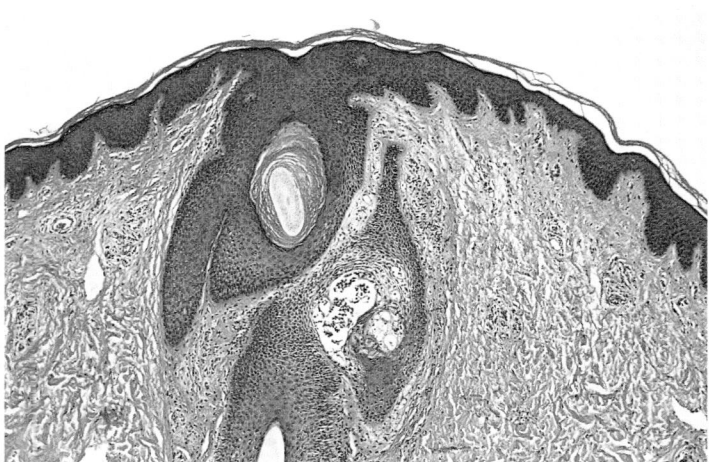

Fig. 15.27 **Apocrine miliaria (Fox–Fordyce disease).** There is spongiosis at the point of entry of the apocrine duct. (H & E)

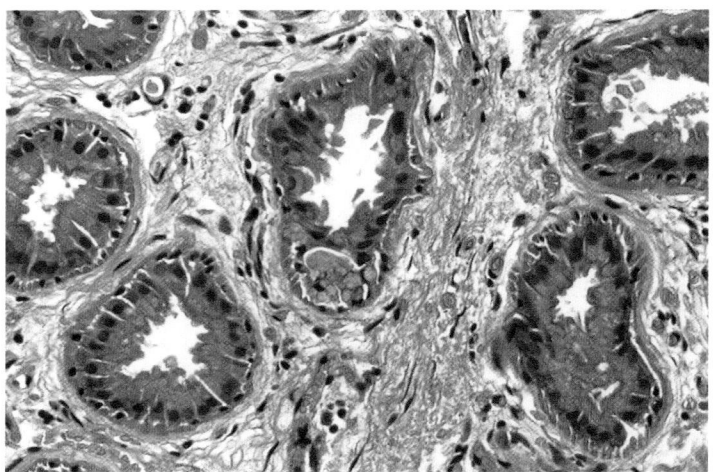

Fig. 15.28 **Apocrine chromhidrosis.** Granular material is present in the cytoplasm of some apocrine cells. (H & E)

vesicular lesions known as miliaria. The various types of miliaria are discussed on page 101. Eccrine glands may be absent in some types of ectodermal dysplasia and following radiation to the skin.

Six histopathological entities will be considered: eccrine duct hyperplasia, syringolymphoid hyperplasia, eccrine metaplasias, neutrophilic eccrine hidradenitis, palmoplantar eccrine hidradenitis and sweat gland necrosis.

ECCRINE DUCT HYPERPLASIA

The proliferation of eccrine ducts is not a distinct clinical entity but a histological reaction pattern that can be seen in a variety of circumstances.[823] The best documented of these is in keratoacanthomas,[824] in which the epithelium of the lower duct and of the secretory coil may show atypical hyperplasia or squamous metaplasia (see below). Rarely, eccrine ducts are prominent and presumably hyperplastic, overlying an intradermal nevus or adjacent to epithelial tumors on the dorsum of the hand and on the lower leg.[825] Branching ducts can also be seen in these circumstances. Some of these cases have been included, incorrectly, as variants of syringofibroadenoma (see p. 894).

Eruptive lesions resulting from eccrine duct hyperplasia have been reported following the use of benoxaprofen (Opren), a drug which has been withdrawn from the market.[826]

SYRINGOLYMPHOID HYPERPLASIA

Hyperplastic sweat ducts sleeved by a dense lymphocytic infiltrate (*syringolymphoid hyperplasia*) have been reported in patients with multiple reddish-brown papules, forming a plaque of alopecia.[827–829] Although this condition can be idiopathic, most cases represent a syringotropic cutaneous T-cell lymphoma.[830,831] Proliferation of ducts, without any inflammation, has been seen in a biopsy from the scalp of a patient with alopecia areata.[832]

Lymphocytic autoimmune hidradenitis is an exceedingly rare manifestation of Sjögren's syndrome in which an infiltrate of mature lymphocytes forms a sleeve around the eccrine glands. The sweat gland epithelium may be hyperplastic,[833] resembling eccrine syringolymphoid hyperplasia, or it can be atrophic.[834]

ECCRINE METAPLASIAS

Clear cell metaplasia, not due to glycogen or lipid, is occasionally an incidental finding in eccrine glands and, to a lesser extent, eccrine ducts.[835] This and other minor histological variations in the morphology of the eccrine apparatus have been reviewed on two occasions in the last 40 years.[26,836] Clear cell change was present in the eccrine ducts and to a lesser extent in the eccrine glands in a patient who presented with a miliaria-like papular eruption of the extremities.[837] The term '**eruptive clear cell hamartoma**' of sweat ducts was used.[837] A similar case has been reported as 'papular clear cell hyperplasia of the eccrine duct in a diabetic'.[838]

Squamous metaplasia of glandular and ductal epithelium (*squamous syringometaplasia*) is a not uncommon histological finding in areas of ischemia and adjacent to ulcers or healing surgical wounds;[839,840] it may follow radiation,[841,842] burns,[843] cryotherapy or curettage,[844,845] or present as a primary process.[846] This change has also been reported in pyoderma gangrenosum, annular elastolytic granuloma,[847] herpetic infection in HIV-positive patients,[848,849] cytomegalovirus infection,[850,851] phytophotodermatitis[852] and lobular panniculitis.[853] The occurrence of squamous metaplasia in patients receiving chemotherapy for various malignant tumors[854–858] has led to the suggestion that squamous syringometaplasia is at the non-inflammatory end of the spectrum of eccrine gland reactions induced by chemotherapy and neutrophilic eccrine hidradenitis (see below) is at the inflammatory end.[855] Squamous syringometaplasia may simulate squamous cell carcinoma because of the islands of atypical squamous epithelium in the dermis, but careful inspection will show a normal architectural pattern of sweat glands and the presence of a lumen with a hyaline inner cuticle. This condition is analogous to necrotizing sialometaplasia, an entity found in minor salivary glands.[859]

Mucinous syringometaplasia is a rare entity which presents as a verruca-like lesion on the sole of the foot or finger or as an ulcerated nodule in other sites.[860–862] Histologically, there is usually a shallow depression in the epidermis with one or several duct-like structures leading into the invagination. Deep invaginations have been reported.[863] The ducts and portions of the surface epithelium are lined by low columnar, mucin-containing cells admixed with squamous epithelium (Fig. 15.29). The goblet cells in one reported case also extended into the sweat glands in the deep dermis.[864] The staining characteristics suggest that a sialomucin is present. Positive staining for CEA, epithelial membrane antigen and CAM 5.2 has been reported.[860] The adjacent

dermis contains a variable chronic inflammatory cell infiltrate with lymphocytes and plasma cells.

Three other mucinous lesions of epithelium have been reported. **Eccrine ductal mucinosis** refers to the accumulation of mucin between the cells of the outer layers of the eccrine duct.[865] It has been reported in a patient with HIV infection.[865] **Benign mucinous metaplasia** affects the surface epithelium, which is replaced by mucin-containing cells and goblet cells. It has been reported on the vulva[866] and the penis.[867] It presents as an erythematous plaque. No ducts are involved as in mucinous syringometaplasia (see above). **Mucinous metaplasia of an apocrine duct** refers to a case in which a duct of presumptive apocrine origin was involved by this metaplastic process.[868]

NEUTROPHILIC ECCRINE HIDRADENITIS

Neutrophilic eccrine hidradenitis is a rare complication of induction chemotherapy used in the treatment of an underlying cancer.[840,869–872] The first reports concerned patients with acute myelogenous leukemia receiving cytarabine therapy,[869,873] but other cancers[874–876] and other chemotherapeutic agents[875,377] have now been implicated, as has granulocyte colony-stimulating

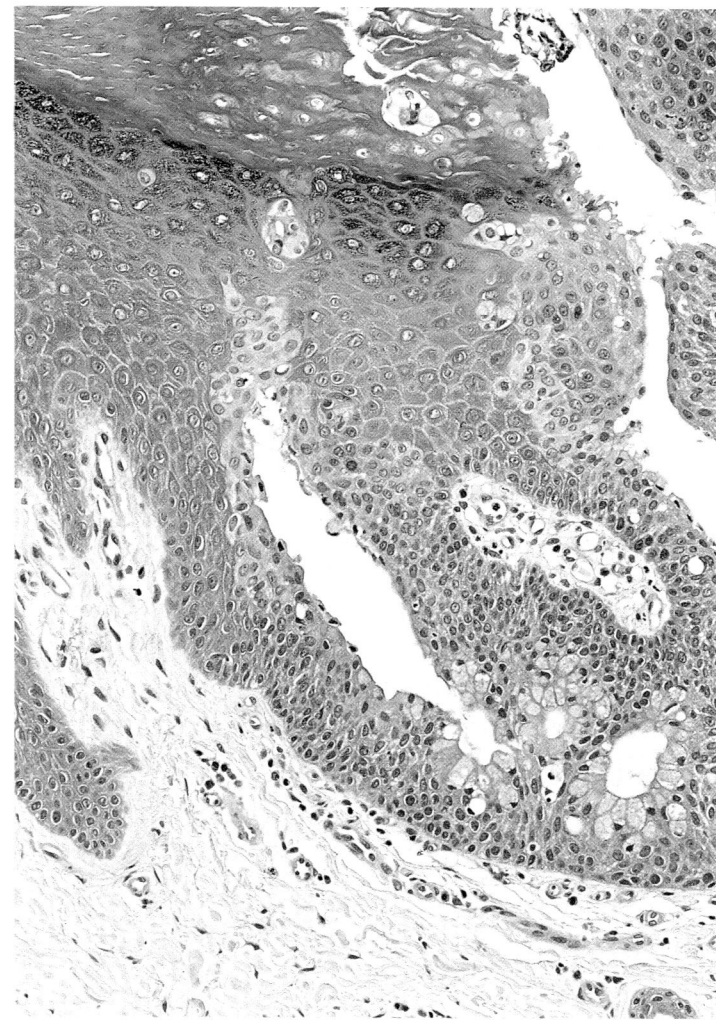

Fig. 15.29 **Mucinous syringometaplasia.** Mucin-containing cells are admixed with squamous epithelium in the duct-like structure which enters the epidermis from below. (H & E)

factor (G-CSF).[878] It has been reported in a patient with leukemia, unassociated with chemotherapy.[879] It has also been reported in HIV-infected patients.[880–882] It is rarely due to infection. *Serratia marcescens* has been implicated in two of these infective cases.[883] Clinically there are plaques and nodules, often on the trunk. Involvement of the ears has been reported.[884] The lesions may resolve after 2–3 weeks.

Histopathology[869,873–875]

There is an infiltrate of neutrophils around and within the eccrine secretory coils, associated with vacuolar degeneration and even necrosis of the secretory epithelium (Fig. 15.30). The neutrophilic infiltrate may be mild in patients with a neutropenia.[885] Squamous metaplasia is sometimes present. There may be edema and mucinous change in the loose connective tissue and fat surrounding the coils. Apocrine involvement has also been reported.[886] An epidermal lichenoid tissue reaction with prominent basal vacuolar change is sometimes present as well.

PALMOPLANTAR ECCRINE HIDRADENITIS

Palmoplantar eccrine hidradenitis is closely related to neutrophilic eccrine hidradenitis.[887–889] It was originally described in children presenting with tender, erythematous plantar nodules (idiopathic plantar hidradenitis);[887] patients with palmoplantar involvement have since been reported.[888,890,891] The lesions are self-limiting;[887] recurrences have been reported.[888] It has been suggested that plantar hidradenitis might be induced by exposure to a wet and cold milieu.[892] Certainly there is a seasonality in its occurrence.[890]

Histopathology

Dense neutrophilic infiltrates, localized to the eccrine units, are present. The infiltrate involves primarily the eccrine duct with partial sparing of the secretory segment. In contrast to neutrophilic eccrine hidradenitis (see above), squamous metaplasia is usually absent.[887]

SWEAT GLAND NECROSIS

Sweat gland necrosis occurs in association with vesiculobullous skin lesions in patients with drug-induced and carbon monoxide-induced coma. This entity is discussed in further detail on page 164.

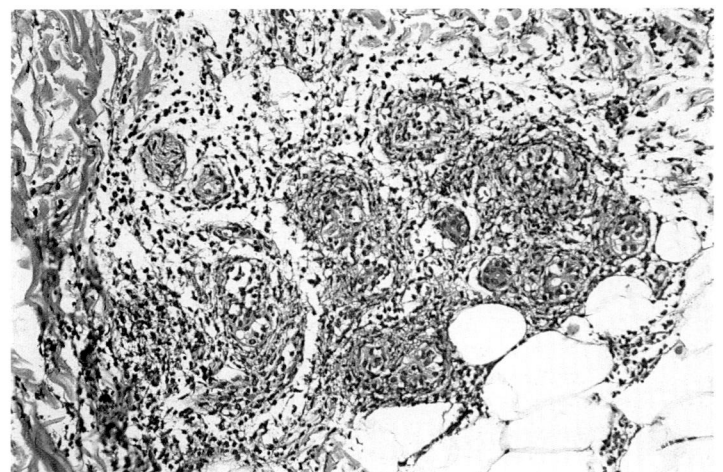

Fig. 15.30 **Eccrine hidradenitis.** Neutrophils surround and engulf the eccrine secretory glands. (H & E)

VESTIBULAR GLAND DISORDERS

VULVAR VESTIBULITIS

Vulvar vestibulitis (vestibular adenitis) is characterized by dyspareunia, point tenderness localized to the vulvar vestibule and varying degrees of erythema. There appears to be no association with human papillomavirus infection, as once thought.[893] Vulvar vestibulitis is just one of many causes of vulvodynia.[894]

Histopathology[893]

There is a chronic inflammatory cell infiltrate, composed predominantly of lymphocytes but with some plasma cells, involving mainly the mucosal lamina propria and periglandular/ periductal connective tissue. Squamous metaplasia of the minor vestibular glands is a consistent feature.[895] An adenomatous proliferation of mucous glands was present in one case with a similar clinical presentation.[893]

REFERENCES

Introduction

1 Messenger AG. The control of hair growth: an overview. J Invest Dermatol 1993; 101: 4S–9S.
2 Akiyama M, Amagai M, Smith LT et al. Epimorphin expression during human foetal hair follicle development. Br J Dermatol 1999; 141: 447–452.
3 Sperling LC. Hair anatomy for the clinician. J Am Acad Dermatol 1991; 25: 1–17.
4 Hutchinson PE, Thompson JR. The size and form of the medulla of human scalp hair is regulated by the hair cycle and cross-sectional size of the hair shaft. Br J Dermatol 1999; 140: 438–445.
5 Rogers MA, Winter H, Langbein L et al. Characterization of a 300 kbp region of human DNA containing the type II hair keratin gene domain. J Invest Dermatol 2000; 114: 464–472.
6 Tanaka T, Narisawa Y, Misago N, Hashimoto K. The innermost cells of the outer root sheath in human anagen hair follicles undergo specialized keratinization mediated by apoptosis. J Cutan Pathol 1998; 25: 316–321.
7 Schirren CG, Burgdorf WHC, Sander CA, Plewig G. Fetal and adult hair follicle. An immunohistochemical study of anticytokeratin antibodies in formalin-fixed and paraffin-embedded tissue. Am J Dermatopathol 1997; 19: 334–340.
8 Clifton MM, Mendelson JK, Mendelson B et al. Immunofluorescent microscopic investigation of the distal arrector pili: A demonstration of the spatial relationship between α5β1 integrin and fibronectin. J Am Acad Dermatol 2000; 43: 19–23.
9 Mendelson JK, Smoller BR, Mendelson B, Horn TD. The microanatomy of the distal arrector pili: possible role for α1β1 and α5β1 integrins in mediating cell-cell adhesion and anchorage to the extracellular matrix. J Cutan Pathol 2000; 27: 61–66.
10 Christoph T, Müller-Röver S, Audring H et al. The human hair follicle immune system: cellular composition and immune privilege. Br J Dermatol 2000; 142: 862–873.

Acneiform lesions

11 Kligman AM. An overview of acne. J Invest Dermatol 1974; 62: 268–287.
12 Cunliffe WJ, Clayden AD, Gould D, Simpson NB. Acne vulgaris – its aetiology and treatment. Clin Exp Dermatol 1981; 6: 461–469.
13 Kilkenny M, Merlin K, Plunkett A, Marks R. The prevalence of common skin conditions in Australian school students: 3. Acne vulgaris. Br J Dermatol 1998; 139: 840–845.
14 Stathakis V, Kilkenny M, Marks R. Descriptive epidemiology of acne vulgaris in the community. Australas J Dermatol 1997; 38: 115–123.
15 Chan JJ, Rohr JB. Acne vulgaris: yesterday, today and tomorrow. Australas J Dermatol 2000; 41 (Suppl): S69–S72.
16 Puhvel SM, Amirian D, Weintraub J, Reisner RM. Lymphocyte transformation in subjects with nodulo-cystic acne. Br J Dermatol 1977; 97: 205–211.
17 Kellett SC, Gawkrodger DJ. The psychological and emotional impact of acne and the effect of treatment with isotretinoin. Br J Dermatol 1999; 140: 273–282.
18 Lasek RJ, Chren M-M. Acne vulgaris and the quality of life of adult dermatology patients. Arch Dermatol 1998; 134: 454–458.
19 Aktan S, Özmen E, Şanli B. Anxiety, depression, and nature of acne vulgaris in adolescents. Int J Dermatol 2000; 39: 354–357.
20 Thiboutot DM, Lookingbill DP. Acne: acute or chronic disease? J Am Acad Dermatol 1995; 32: S2–S5.

21 Tabata N, Terui T, Watanabe M, Tagami H. Infantile acne associated with a high plasma testosterone level in a 21-month-old boy. J Am Acad Dermatol 1995; 33: 676–678.

22 Goulden V, Stables GI, Cunliffe WJ. Prevalence of facial acne in adults. J Am Acad Dermatol 1999; 41: 577–580.

23 Seukeran DC, Cunliffe WJ. Acne vulgaris in the elderly: the response to low-dose isotretinoin. Br J Dermatol 1998; 139: 99–101.

24 Katsambas AD, Katoulis AC, Stavropoulos P. Acne neonatorum: a study of 22 cases. Int J Dermatol 1999; 38: 128–130.

25 Goulden V, Clark SM, Cunliffe WJ. Post-adolescent acne: a review of clinical features. Br J Dermatol 1997; 136: 66–70.

26 Luther H, Altmeyer P. Eccrine sweat gland reaction. A histological and immunocytochemical study. Am J Dermatopathol 1988; 10: 390–398.

27 Goodman GJ. Post-acne scarring: a short review of its pathophysiology. Australas J Dermatol 2001; 42: 84–90.

28 Kumar P, Marks R. Sebaceous gland hyperplasia and senile comedones: a prevalence study in elderly hospitalized patients. Br J Dermatol 1987; 117: 231–236.

29 Piqué E, Olivares M, Fariña MC et al. Congenital nasal comedones – report of three cases. Clin Exp Dermatol 1996; 21: 220–221.

30 Adams BB, Chetty VB, Mutasim DF. Periorbital comedones and their relationship to pitch tar: A cross-sectional analysis and a review of the literature. J Am Acad Dermatol 2000; 42: 624–627.

31 Shalita AR, Lee W-L. Inflammatory acne. Dermatol Clin 1983; 1: 361–364.

32 Hughes BR, Cunliffe WJ. An acne naevus. Clin Exp Dermatol 1987; 12: 357–359.

33 Stubbings JM, Goodfield MJD. An unusual distribution of an acneiform rash due to herpes zoster infection. Clin Exp Dermatol 1993; 18: 92–93.

34 Goulden V, McGeown CH, Cunliffe WJ. The familial risk of adult acne: a comparison between first-degree relatives of affected and unaffected individuals. Br J Dermatol 1999; 141: 297–300.

35 Cunliffe WJ. The sebaceous gland and acne – 40 years on. Dermatology 1998; 196: 9–15.

36 Shalita AR, Leyden JE Jr, Pochi PE, Strauss JS. Acne vulgaris. J Am Acad Dermatol 1987; 16: 410–412.

37 Leyden JJ. New understandings of the pathogenesis of acne. J Am Acad Dermatol 1995; 32: S15–S25.

38 Heilman ER, Lavker RM. Abnormal follicular keratinization. Dermatol Clin 1983; 1: 353–359.

39 Cunliffe WJ, Holland DB, Clark SM, Stables GI. Comedogenesis: some new aetiological, clinical and therapeutic strategies. Br J Dermatol 2000; 142: 1084–1091.

40 Downing DT, Stewart ME, Wertz PW, Strauss JS. Essential fatty acids and acne. J Am Acad Dermatol 1986; 14: 221–225.

41 White GM. Recent findings in the epidemiologic evidence, classification, and subtypes of acne vulgaris. J Am Acad Dermatol 1998; 39: S34–S37.

42 Marsden JR, Middleton B, Mills C. Is remission of acne due to changes in sebum composition? Clin Exp Dermatol 1987; 12: 18–20.

43 Pochi PE. Hormones and acne. Semin Dermatol 1982; 1: 265–273.

44 Thiboutot D, Bayne E, Thorne J et al. Immunolocalization of 5α-reductase isozymes in acne lesions and normal skin. Arch Dermatol 2000; 136: 1125–1129.

45 Van der Meeren HLM, Thijssen JHH. Circulating androgens in male acne. Br J Dermatol 1984; 110: 609–611.

46 Lawrence D, Shaw M, Katz M. Elevated free testosterone concentration in men and women with acne vulgaris. Clin Exp Dermatol 1986; 11: 263–273.

47 Lookingbill DP, Horton R, Demers LM et al. Tissue production of androgens in women with acne. J Am Acad Dermatol 1985; 12: 481–487.

48 De Raeve L, de Schepper J, Smitz J. Prepubertal acne: a cutaneous marker of androgen excess. J Am Acad Dermatol 1995; 32: 181–184.

49 Thiboutot D, Gilliland K, Light J, Lookingbill D. Androgen metabolism in sebaceous glands from subjects with and without acne. Arch Dermatol 1999; 135: 1041–1045.

50 Cibula D, Hill M, Vohradnikova O et al. The role of androgens in determining acne severity in adult women. Br J Dermatol 2000; 143: 399–404.

51 Lucky AW, Biro FM, Huster GA et al. Acne vulgaris in premenarchal girls. Arch Dermatol 1994; 130: 308–314.

52 Shalita AR. Acne revisited. Arch Dermatol 1994; 130: 363–364.

53 Webster GF. Acne vulgaris. State of the science. Arch Dermatol 1999; 135: 1101–1102.

54 Bunker CB, Newton JA, Kilborn J et al. Most women with acne have polycystic ovaries. Br J Dermatol 1989; 121: 675–680.

55 Walton S, Cunliffe WJ, Keczkes K et al. Clinical, ultrasound and hormonal markers of androgenicity in acne vulgaris. Br J Dermatol 1995; 133: 249–253.

56 Strauss JS, Pochi PE. Intracutaneous injection of sebum and comedones. Histological observations. Arch Dermatol 1965; 92: 443–456.

57 Fisher DA. Desideratum dermatologicum – cause and control of premenstrual acne flare. Int J Dermatol 2000; 39: 334–336.

58 Kersey P, Sussman M, Dahl M. Delayed skin test reactivity to Propionibacterium acnes correlates with severity of inflammation in acne vulgaris. Br J Dermatol 1980; 103: 651–655.

59 Leeming JP, Holland KT, Cunliffe WJ. The microbial colonization of inflamed acne vulgaris lesions. Br J Dermatol 1988; 118: 203–208.

60 Lavker RM, Leyden JJ, McGinley KJ. The relationship between bacteria and the abnormal follicular keratinization in acne vulgaris. J Invest Dermatol 1981; 77: 325–330.

61 Webster GF, Leyden JJ. Mechanisms of Propionibacterium acnes-mediated inflammation in acne vulgaris. Semin Dermatol 1982; 1: 299–304.

62 Puhvel SM. Propionibacterium acnes and acne vulgaris. Semin Dermatol 1982; 1: 293–298.

63 Ingham E, Gowland G, Ward RM et al. Antibodies to P. acnes and P. acnes exocellular enzymes in the normal population at various ages and in patients with acne vulgaris. Br J Dermatol 1987; 116: 805–812.

64 Simpson N. Antibiotics in acne: time for a rethink. Br J Dermatol 2001; 144: 225–227.

65 Webster GF. Inflammation in acne vulgaris. J Am Acad Dermatol 1995; 33: 247–253.

66 Ashbee HR, Muir SR, Cunliffe WJ, Ingham E. IgG subclasses specific to Staphylococcus epidermidis and Propionibacterium acnes in patients with acne vulgaris. Br J Dermatol 1997; 136: 730–733.

67 Till AE, Goulden V, Cunliffe WJ, Holland KT. The cutaneous microflora of adolescent, persistent and late-onset acne patients does not differ. Br J Dermatol 2000; 142: 885–892.

68 Eady EA, Cove JH, Blake J et al. Recalcitrant acne vulgaris. Clinical, biochemical and microbiological investigation of patients not responding to antibiotic treatment. Br J Dermatol 1988; 118: 415–423.

69 Ross JI, Snelling AM, Eady EA et al. Phenotypic and genotypic characterization of antibiotic-resistant Propionibacterium acnes isolated from acne patients attending dermatology clinics in Europe, the U.S.A., Japan and Australia. Br J Dermatol 2001; 144: 339–346.

70 Cunliffe WJ, Goulden V. Phototherapy and acne vulgaris. Br J Dermatol 2000; 142: 855–856.

71 Mills OH Jr, Kligman AM. External factors aggravating acne. Dermatol Clin 1983; 1: 355–370.

72 Farella V, Sberna F, Knöpfel B et al. Acne-like eruption caused by amineptine. Int J Dermatol 1996; 35: 892–893.

73 Wollina U, Kammler H-J, Hesselbarth N et al. Ecstasy pimples – a new facial dermatosis. Dermatology 1998; 197: 171–173.

74 Finkelstein E, Lazarov A, Cagnano M, Halevy S. Oil acne: successful treatment with isotretinoin. J Am Acad Dermatol 1994; 30: 491–492.

75 Jansen T, Romiti R, Woitalla S, Plewig G. Eruptive acne vulgaris with infectious mononucleosis. Br J Dermatol 2000; 142: 837–838.

76 Kaminer MS, Gilchrest BA. The many faces of acne. J Am Acad Dermatol 1995; 32: S6–S14.

77 Plewig G, Jansen T. Acneiform dermatoses. Dermatology 1998; 196: 102–107.

78 Steffen C. The acneform eruption of Apert's syndrome is not acne vulgaris. Am J Dermatopathol 1984; 6: 213–220.

79 Henderson CA, Knaggs H, Clark A et al. Apert's syndrome and androgen receptor staining of the basal cells of sebaceous glands. Br J Dermatol 1995; 132: 139–143.

80 Massa MC, Su WPD. Pyoderma faciale: a clinical study of twenty-nine patients. J Am Acad Dermatol 1982; 6: 84–91.

81 Hurwitz RM. Steroid acne. J Am Acad Dermatol 1989; 21: 1179–1181.

82 Monk B, Cunliffe WJ, Layton AM, Rhodes DJ. Acne induced by inhaled corticosteroids. Clin Exp Dermatol 1993; 18: 148–150.

83 Yu H-J, Lee S-K, Son SJ et al. Steroid acne vs. Pityrosporum folliculitis: the incidence of Pityrosporum ovale and the effect of antifungal drugs in steroid acne. Int J Dermatol 1998; 37: 772–777.

84 Basler RSW, Basler GC, Palmer AH, Garcia MA. Special skin symptoms seen in swimmers. J Am Acad Dermatol 2000; 43: 299–305.

85 Niamba P, Weill FX, Sarlangue J et al. Is common neonatal cephalic pustulosis (neonatal acne) triggered by Malassezia sympodialis? Arch Dermatol 1998; 134: 995–998.

86 Plewig G. Morphologic dynamics of acne vulgaris. Acta Derm Venereol (Suppl) 1980; 89: 9–16.

87 Invitational Symposium on Comedogenicity. J Am Acad Dermatol 1989; 20: 272–277.

88 Norris JFB, Cunliffe WJ. A histological and immunocytochemical study of early acne lesions. Br J Dermatol 1988; 118: 651–659.

89 Zelickson AS, Mottaz JH. Pigmentation of open comedones. An ultrastructural study. Arch Dermatol 1983; 119: 567–569.

90 Wilson BB, Dent CH, Cooper PH. Papular acne scars. A common cutaneous finding. Arch Dermatol 1990; 126: 797–800.

91 Brodkin RH, Abbey AA. Osteoma cutis: a case of probable exacerbation following treatment of severe acne with isotretinoin. Dermatologica 1985; 170: 210–212.

92 Basler RSW, Kohnen PW. Localized hemosiderosis as a sequela of acne. Arch Dermatol 1978; 114: 1695–1697.

93 Wilborn WH, Montes LF, Lyons RE, Battista GW. Ultrastructural basis for the assay of topical acne treatments. Transmission and scanning electron microscopy of untreated comedones. J Cutan Pathol 1978; 5: 165–183.

94 Zelickson AS, Strauss JS, Mottaz J. Ultrastructural changes in open comedones following treatment of cystic acne with isotretinoin. Am J Dermatopathol 1985; 7: 241–244.

95 Nault P, Lassonde M, St-Antoine P. Acne fulminans with osteolytic lesions. Arch Dermatol 1985; 121: 662–664.

96 Jansen T, Plewig G. Acne fulminans. Int J Dermatol 1998; 37: 254–257.

97 Karvonen S-L. Acne fulminans: report of clinical findings and treatment of twenty-four patients. J Am Acad Dermatol 1993; 28: 572–579.

98 Pauli S-L, Kokko M-L, Suhonen R, Reunala T. Acne fulminans with bone lesions. Acta Derm Venereol 1988; 68: 351–355.

99 Jemec GBE, Rasmussen I. Bone lesions of acne fulminans. Case report and review of the literature. J Am Acad Dermatol 1989; 20: 353–357.

100 Gordon PM, Farr PM, Milligan A. Acne fulminans and bone lesions may present to other specialties. Pediatr Dermatol 1997; 14: 446–448.

101 Thomson KF, Cunliffe WJ. Acne fulminans 'sine fulminans'. Clin Exp Dermatol 2000; 25: 299–301.

102 McAuley D, Miller RA. Acne fulminans associated with inflammatory bowel disease. Arch Dermatol 1985; 121: 91–93.

103 Kellett JK, Beck MH, Chalmers RJG. Erythema nodosum and circulating immune complexes in acne fulminans after treatment with isotretinoin. Br Med J 1985; 290: 820.

104 Reizis Z, Trattner A, Hodak E et al. Acne fulminans with hepatosplenomegaly and erythema nodosum migrans. J Am Acad Dermatol 1991; 24: 886–888.

105 Traupe H, von Muhlendahl KE, Bramswig J, Happle R. Acne of the fulminans type following testosterone therapy in three excessively tall boys. Arch Dermatol 1988; 124: 414–417.

106 Wong SS, Pritchard MH, Holt PJA. Familial acne fulminans. Clin Exp Dermatol 1992; 17: 351–353.

107 Seukeran DC, Cunliffe WJ. The treatment of acne fulminans: a review of 25 cases. Br J Dermatol 1999; 141: 307–309.

108 Reith JD, Bauer TW, Schils JP. Osseous manifestations of SAPHO (Synovitis, Acne, Pustulosis, Hyperostosis, Osteitis) syndrome. Am J Surg Pathol 1996; 20: 1368–1377.

109 Goldschmidt H, Leyden JJ, Stein KH. Acne fulminans. Investigation of acute febrile ulcerative acne. Arch Dermatol 1977; 113: 444–449.

110 Tindall JP. Chloracne and chloracnegens. J Am Acad Dermatol 1985; 13: 539–558.

111 Scerri L, Zaki I, Millard LG. Severe halogen acne due to a trifluoromethylpyrazole derivative and its resistance to isotretinoin. Br J Dermatol 1995; 132: 144–148.

112 Coenraads P-J, Brouwer A, Olie K, Tang N. Chloracne. Some recent issues. Dermatol Clin 1994; 12: 569–576.

113 Crow KD. Chloracne. Semin Dermatol 1982; 1: 305–314.

114 Moses M, Prioleau PG. Cutaneous histologic findings in chemical workers with and without chloracne with past exposure to 2,3,7,8-tetrachlorodibenzo-p-dioxin. J Am Acad Dermatol 1985; 12: 497–506.

115 Vazquez ER, Macias PC, Tirado JGO et al. Chloracne in the 1990s. Int J Dermatol 1996; 35: 643–645.

116 Coenraads PJ, Olie K, Tang NJ. Blood lipid concentrations of dioxins and dibenzofurans causing chloracne. Br J Dermatol 1999; 141: 694–697.

Superficial folliculitides

117 Golitz L. Follicular and perforating disorders. J Cutan Pathol 1985; 12: 282–288.

118 Hsu S, Halmi BH. Bockhart's impetigo: complication of waterbed use. Int J Dermatol 1999; 38: 769–770.

119 Hersle K, Mobacken H, Möller A. Chronic non-scarring folliculitis of the scalp. Acta Derm Venereol 1979; 59: 249–253.

120 Nieboer C. Actinic superficial folliculitis; a new entity? Br J Dermatol 1985; 112: 603–606.

121 Verbov J. Actinic folliculitis. Br J Dermatol 1985; 112: 630–631.

122 Norris PG, Hawk JLM. Actinic folliculitis – response to isotretinoin. Clin Exp Dermatol 1989; 14: 69–71.

123 Labandeira J, Suarez-Campos A, Toribio J. Actinic superficial folliculitis. Br J Dermatol 1998; 138: 1070–1074.

124 Kossard S, Collins A, McCrossin I. Necrotizing lymphocytic folliculitis: the early lesion of acne necrotica (varioliformis). J Am Acad Dermatol 1987; 16: 1007–1014.

125 Rook A, Dawber R. Diseases of the hair and scalp. Oxford: Blackwell Scientific Publications, 1982; 475–477.

126 Maibach HI. Acne necroticans (varioliformis) versus *Propionibacterium acnes* folliculitis. J Am Acad Dermatol 1989; 21: 323.

127 Fisher DA. Acne necroticans (varioliformis) and *Staphylococcus aureus*. J Am Acad Dermatol 1988; 18: 1136–1137.

128 Barlow RJ, Schulz EJ. Necrotizing folliculitis in AIDS-related complex. Br J Dermatol 1987; 116: 581–584.

129 Ofuji S, Ogino A, Horio T et al. Eosinophilic pustular folliculitis. Acta Derm Venereol 1970; 50: 195–203.

130 Teraki Y, Konohana I, Shiohara T et al. Eosinophilic pustular folliculitis (Ofuji's disease). Immunohistochemical analysis. Arch Dermatol 1993; 129: 1015–1019.

131 Ota T, Hata Y, Tanikawa A et al. Eosinophilic pustular folliculitis (Ofuji's disease): indomethacin as a first choice of treatment. Clin Exp Dermatol 2001; 26: 179–181.

132 Jaliman HD, Phelps RG, Fleischmajer R. Eosinophilic pustular folliculitis. J Am Acad Dermatol 1986; 14: 479–482.

133 Dinehart SM, Noppakun N, Solomon AR, Smith EB. Eosinophilic pustular folliculitis. J Am Acad Dermatol 1986; 14: 475–479.

134 Moritz DL, Elmets CA. Eosinophilic pustular folliculitis. J Am Acad Dermatol 1991; 24: 903–907.

135 Kossard S, Saywell L. Pruritic follicular facial rash: eosinophilic folliculitis. Australas J Dermatol 1997; 38: 161–162.

136 Blume-Peytavi U, Chen W, Djemadji N et al. Eosinophilic pustular folliculitis (Ofuji's disease). J Am Acad Dermatol 1997; 37: 259–262.

137 Takematsu H, Nakamura K, Igarashi M, Tagami H. Eosinophilic pustular folliculitis. Report of two cases with a review of the Japanese literature. Arch Dermatol 1985; 121: 917–920.

138 Colton AS, Schachner L, Kowalczyk AP. Eosinophilic pustular folliculitis. J Am Acad Dermatol 1986; 14: 469–474.

139 Cutler TP. Eosinophilic pustular folliculitis. Clin Exp Dermatol 1981; 6: 327–332.

140 Saruta T, Nakamizo Y. Eosinophilic pustular folliculitis. Rinsho Dermatol 1979; 21: 689–697.

141 Beer WE, Emslie ES, Lanigan S. Circinate eosinophilic dermatosis. Int J Dermatol 1987; 26: 192–193.

142 Scott DW. Sterile eosinophilic pustulosis in dog and man. Comparative aspects. J Am Acad Dermatol 1987; 16: 1022–1026.

143 Lucky AW, Esterly NB, Heskel N et al. Eosinophilic pustular folliculitis in infancy. Pediatr Dermatol 1984; 1: 202–206.

144 Magro CMJ, Crowson AN. Eosinophilic pustular follicular reaction: a paradigm of immune dysregulation. Int J Dermatol 1994; 33: 172–178.

145 Nunzi E, Parodi A, Rebora A. Ofuji's disease: high circulating titers of IgG and IgM directed to basal cell cytoplasm. J Am Acad Dermatol 1985; 12: 268–273.

146 Vakilzadeh F, Suter L, Knop J, Macher E. Eosinophilic pustulosis with pemphigus-like antibody. Dermatologica 1981; 162: 265–272.

147 Takematsu H, Tagami H. Eosinophilic pustular folliculitis. Studies on possible chemotactic factors involved in the formation of pustules. Br J Dermatol 1986; 114: 209–215.

148 Maruo K, Kayashima K-I, Ono T. Expression of neuronal nitric oxide synthase in dermal infiltrated eosinophils in eosinophilic pustular folliculitis. Br J Dermatol 1999; 140: 417–420.

149 Bason MM, Berger TG, Nesbitt LT Jr. Pruritic papular eruption of HIV-disease. Int J Dermatol 1993; 32: 784–789.

150 Harris DWS, Ostlere L, Buckley C et al. Eosinophilic pustular folliculitis in an HIV-positive man: response to cetirizine. Br J Dermatol 1992; 126: 392–394.

151 Rosenthal D, LeBoit PE, Klumpp L, Berger TG. Human immunodeficiency virus-associated eosinophilic folliculitis. Arch Dermatol 1991; 127: 206–209.

152 Stell I, Leen E. HIV-associated eosinophilic pustular folliculitis: The first case reported in a woman. J Am Acad Dermatol 1996; 35: 106–108.

153 Ramdial PK, Morar N, Dlova NC, Aboobaker J. HIV-associated eosinophilic folliculitis in an infant. Am J Dermatopathol 1999; 21: 241–246.

154 Piantanida EW, Turiansky GW, Kenner JR et al. HIV-associated eosinophilic folliculitis: Diagnosis by transverse histologic sections. J Am Acad Dermatol 1998; 38: 124–126.

155 Rosatelli JB, Soares FA, Roselino AMF. Pruritic papular eruption of the acquired immunodeficiency syndrome: predominance of CD8+ cells. Int J Dermatol 2000; 39: 873–874.

156 Basarab T, Russell Jones R. HIV-associated eosinophilic folliculitis: case report and review of the literature. Br J Dermatol 1996; 134: 499–503.

157 Buezo GF, Fraga J, Abajo P et al. HIV-associated eosinophilic folliculitis and follicular mucinosis. Dermatology 1998; 197: 178–180.

158 Fearfield LA, Rowe A, Francis N et al. Itchy folliculitis and human immunodeficiency virus infection: clinicopathological and immunological features, pathogenesis and treatment. Br J Dermatol 1999; 141: 3–11.

159 Roos TC, Albrecht H. Foscarnet-associated eosinophilic folliculitis in a patient with AIDS. J Am Acad Dermatol 2001; 44: 546–547.

160 Giard F, Marcoux D, McCuaig C et al. Eosinophilic pustular folliculitis (Ofuji disease) in childhood: a review of four cases. Pediatr Dermatol 1991; 8: 189–193.

161 Dupond AS, Aubin F, Bourezane Y et al. Eosinophilic pustular folliculitis in infancy: report of two affected brothers. Br J Dermatol 1995; 132: 296–299.

162 McCalmont TH, Altemus D, Maurer T, Berger TG. Eosinophilic folliculitis. The histologic spectrum. Am J Dermatopathol 1995; 17: 439–446.

163 Larralde M, Morales S, Muñoz AS et al. Eosinophilic pustular folliculitis in infancy: report of two new cases. Pediatr Dermatol 1999; 16: 118–120.

164 Dyall-Smith D, Mason G. Fungal eosinophilic pustular folliculitis. Australas J Dermatol 1995; 36: 37–38.

165 Haupt HM, Stern JB, Weber CB. Eosinophilic pustular folliculitis: fungal folliculitis? J Am Acad Dermatol 1990; 23: 1012–1014.

166 Brenner S, Wolf R, Ophir J. Eosinophilic pustular folliculitis: a sterile folliculitis of unknown cause? J Am Acad Dermatol 1994; 31: 210–212.

167 Bull RH, Harland CA, Fallowfield ME, Mortimer PS. Eosinophilic folliculitis: a self-limiting illness in patients being treated for haematological malignancy. Br J Dermatol 1993; 129: 178–182.

168 Mizoguchi S, Setoyama M, Higashi Y et al. Eosinophilic pustular folliculitis induced by carbamazepine. J Am Acad Dermatol 1998; 38: 641–643.

169 Vassallo C, Brazzelli V, Ardigò M, Borroni G. Eosinophilic folliculitis: an histopathologic pattern common to different diseases. Am J Dermatopathol 2000; 22: 359 (abstract).

170 Magro CM, Crowson AN. Necrotizing eosinophilic folliculitis as a manifestation of the atopic diathesis. Int J Dermatol 2000; 39: 672–677.

171 Kuo T-T, Chen S-Y, Chan H-L. Tinea infection histologically simulating eosinophilic pustular folliculitis. J Cutan Pathol 1986; 13: 118–122.

172 Ravikumar BC, Balachandran C, Shenoi SD et al. Disseminate and recurrent infundibulofolliculitis: response to psoralen plus UVA therapy. Int J Dermatol 1999; 38: 75–76.

Deep infectious folliculitides

173 Tunnessen WW Jr. Practical aspects of bacterial skin infections in children. Pediatr Dermatol 1985; 2: 255–265.

174 Demirçay Z, Ekşioğlu-Demiralp E, Ergun T, Akoğlu T. Phagocytosis and oxidative burst by neutrophils in patients with recurrent furunculosis. Br J Dermatol 1998; 138: 1036–1038.

175 Pinkus H. Furuncle. J Cutan Pathol 1979; 6: 517–518.

176 Fox AB, Hambrick GW Jr. Recreationally associated *Pseudomonas aeruginosa* folliculitis. Report of an epidemic. Arch Dermatol 1984; 120: 1304–1307.

177 Chandrasekar PH, Rolston KVI, Kannangara DW et al. Hot tub-associated dermatitis due to *Pseudomonas aeruginosa*. Case report and review of the literature. Arch Dermatol 1984; 120: 1337–1340.

178 Feder HM Jr, Grant-Kels JM, Tilton RC. Pseudomonas whirlpool dermatitis. Report of an outbreak in two families. Clin Pediatr 1983; 22: 638–642.

179 Silverman AR, Nieland ML. Hot tub dermatitis: a familial outbreak of *Pseudomonas* folliculitis. J Am Acad Dermatol 1983; 8: 153–156.

180 Kitamura M, Kawai S, Horio T. *Pseudomonas aeruginosa* folliculitis: a sporadic case from use of a contaminated sponge. Br J Dermatol 1998; 139: 359–360.

181 Zichichi L, Asta G, Noto G. *Pseudomonas aeruginosa* folliculitis after shower/bath exposure. Int J Dermatol 2000; 39: 270–273.

182 Trüeb RM, Gloor M, Wüthrich B. Recurrent *Pseudomonas* folliculitis. Pediatr Dermatol 1994; 11: 35–38.

183 Blankenship ML. Gram-negative folliculitis. Follow-up observations in 20 patients. Arch Dermatol 1984; 120: 1301–1303.

184 Leyden JJ, McGinley KJ, Mills OH. *Pseudomonas aeruginosa* gram-negative folliculitis. Arch Dermatol 1979; 115: 1203–1204.

185 Neubert U, Jansen T, Plewig G. Bacteriologic and immunologic aspects of Gram-negative folliculitis: a study of 46 patients. Int J Dermatol 1999; 38: 270–274.

186 Chastain MA. A cycle: recurrent Gram-negative folliculitis with *Citrobacter diversus (koseri)* following eradication of recurrent staphylococcal pyoderma. Arch Dermatol 2000; 136: 803.

187 Smith KJ, Neafie R, Yeager J, Skelton HG. *Micrococcus* folliculitis in HIV-1 disease. Br J Dermatol 1999; 141: 558–561.

188 Jacyk WK. Clinical and pathologic observations in dermatitis cruris pustulosa et atrophicans. Int J Dermatol 1978; 17: 802–807.

189 Gillians JA, Palmer HW, Dyte PH. Follicular dermatitis caused by *Salmonella dublin*. Med J Aust 1982; 1: 390–391.

190 Jang K-A, Kim S-H, Choi J-H et al. Viral folliculitis on the face. Br J Dermatol 2000; 142: 555–559.

191 Haycox CL, Kim S, Fleckman P et al. Trichodysplasia spinulosa – a newly described folliculocentric viral infection in an immunocompromised host. J Invest Dermatol (Symposium Proceedings) 1999; 4: 268–271.

192 Sexton M. Occult herpesvirus folliculitis clinically simulating pseudolymphoma. Am J Dermatopathol 1991; 13: 234–240.

193 Brabek E, El Shabrawi-Caelen L, Woltsche-Kahr I et al. Herpetic folliculitis and syringitis simulating acne excoriée. Arch Dermatol 2001; 137: 97–98.

194 Tüzün Y, İşçimen A, Göksügür N et al. Wolf's isotopic response: *Trichophyton rubrum* folliculitis appearing on a herpes zoster scar. Int J Dermatol 2000; 39: 766–768.

Deep scarring folliculitides

195 Rook A, Dawber R. Diseases of the hair and scalp. Oxford: Blackwell Scientific Publications, 1982; 314–315.

196 Miller RF. Epilating folliculitis of the glabrous skin. Arch Dermatol 1961; 83: 777–784.

197 Douwes KE, Landthaler M, Szeimies R-M. Simultaneous occurrence of folliculitis decalvans capillitii in identical twins. Br J Dermatol 2000; 143: 195–197.

198 Walker SL, Smith HR, Lun K, Griffiths WAD. Improvement of folliculitis decalvans following shaving of the scalp. Br J Dermatol 2000; 142: 1245–1246.

199 Annessi G. Tufted folliculitis of the scalp: a distinctive clinicohistological variant of folliculitis decalvans. Br J Dermatol 1998; 138: 799–805.

200 Powell JJ, Dawber RPR, Gatter K. Folliculitis decalvans including tufted folliculitis: clinical, histological and therapeutic findings. Br J Dermatol 1999; 140: 328–333.

201 Cosman B, Wolff M. Acne keloidalis. Plast Reconstr Surg 1972; 50: 25–30.

202 Herzberg AJ, Dinehart SM, Kerns BJ, Pollack SV. Acne keloidalis. Transverse microscopy, immunohistochemistry, and electron microscopy. Am J Dermatopathol 1990; 12: 109–121.

203 Dinehart SM, Herzberg AJ, Kerns BJ, Pollack SV. Acne keloidalis: a review. J Dermatol Surg Oncol 1989; 15: 642–647.

204 Sperling LC, Homoky C, Pratt L, Sau P. Acne keloidalis is a form of primary scarring alopecia. Arch Dermatol 2000; 136: 479–484.

205 Rook A, Dawber R. Diseases of the hair and scalp. Oxford: Blackwell Scientific Publications, 1982; 477–478.

206 Gloster HM Jr. The surgical management of extensive cases of acne keloidalis nuchae. J Am Acad Dermatol 2000; 136: 1376–1379.

207 Knable AL Jr, Hanke CW, Gonin R. Prevalence of acne keloidalis nuchae in football players. J Am Acad Dermatol 1997; 37: 570–574.

208 Azurdia RM, Graham RM, Weismann K et al. Acne keloidalis in caucasian patients on cyclosporin following organ transplantation. Br J Dermatol 2000; 143: 465–467.

209 Carnero L, Silvestre JF, Guijarro J et al. Nuchal acne keloidalis associated with cyclosporin. Br J Dermatol 2001; 144: 429–430.

210 George AO, Akanji AO, Nduka EU et al. Clinical, biochemical and morphologic features of acne keloidalis in a black population. Int J Dermatol 1993; 32: 714–716.

211 Grunwald MH, Ben-Dor D, Livni E, Halevy S. Acne keloidalis-like lesions on the scalp associated with antiepileptic drugs. Int J Dermatol 1990; 29: 559–561.

212 Glenn MJ, Bennett RG, Kelly AP. Acne keloidalis nuchae: treatment with excision and second-intention healing. J Am Acad Dermatol 1995; 33: 243–246.

213 Goette DK, Berger TG. Acne keloidalis nuchae. A transepithelial elimination disorder. Int J Dermato 1987; 26: 442–444.

214 Luz Ramos M, Muñoz-Pérez MA, Pons A et al. Acne keloidalis nuchae and tufted hair folliculitis. Dermatology 1997; 194: 71–73.

Follicular occlusion triad

215 Highet AS, Warren RE, Weekes AJ. Bacteriology and antibiotic treatment of perineal suppurative hidradenitis. Arch Dermatol 1988; 124: 1047–1051.

216 Chicarilli ZN. Follicular occlusion triad: hidradenitis suppurativa, acne conglobata, and dissecting cellulitis of the scalp. Ann Plast Surg 1987; 18: 230–237.

217 Watson JD. Hidradenitis suppurativa – a clinical review. Br J Plast Surg 1985; 38: 567–569.

218 Broadwater JR, Bryant RL, Petrino RA et al. Advanced hidradenitis suppurativa. Review of surgical treatment in 23 patients. Am J Surg 1982; 144: 668–670.

219 Fearfield LA, Staughton RCD. Severe vulval apocrine acne successfully treated with prednisolone and isotretinoin. Clin Exp Dermatol 1999; 24: 189–192.

220 Jansen T, Plewig G. Acne inversa. Int J Dermatol 1998; 37: 96–100.

221 Endo Y, Tamura A, Ishikawa O, Miyachi Y. Perianal hidradenitis suppurativa: early surgical treatment gives good results in chronic or recurrent cases. Br J Dermatol 1998; 139: 906–910.

222 von der Werth JM, Williams HC. The natural history of hidradenitis suppurativa. J Eur Acad Dermatol Venereol 2000; 14: 389–392.

223 von der Werth JM, Jemec GBE. Morbidity in patients with hidradenitis suppurativa. Br J Dermatol 2001; 144: 809–813.

224 Mendonça H, Rebelo C, Fernandes A et al. Squamous cell carcinoma arising in hidradenitis suppurativa. J Dermatol Surg Oncol 1991; 17: 830–832.

225 Anstey AV, Wilkinson JD, Lord P. Squamous cell carcinoma complicating hidradenitis suppurativa. Br J Dermatol 1990; 123: 527–531.

226 Dufresne RG Jr, Ratz JL, Bergfeld WF, Roenigk RK. Squamous cell carcinoma arising from the follicular occlusion triad. J Am Acad Dermatol 1996; 35: 475–477.

227 Lapins J, Ye W, Nyrén O, Emtestam L. Incidence of cancer among patients with hidradenitis suppurativa. Arch Dermatol 2001; 137: 730–734.

228 Jemec GBE. The symptomatology of hidradenitis suppurativa in women. Br J Dermatol 1988; 119: 345–350.

229 Jemec GBE. Effect of localized surgical excisions in hidradenitis suppurativa. J Am Acad Dermatol 1988; 18: 1103–1107.

230 Jemec GBE, Heidenheim M, Nielsen NH. The prevalence of hidradenitis suppurativa and its potential precursor lesions. J Am Acad Dermatol 1996; 35: 191–194.

231 Fitzsimmons JS, Guilbert PR, Fitzsimmons EM. Evidence of genetic factors in hidradenitis suppurativa. Br J Dermatol 1985; 113: 1–8.

232 Fitzsimmons JS, Guilbert PR. A family study of hidradenitis suppurativa. J Med Genet 1985; 22: 367–373.

233 von der Werth JM, Williams HC, Raeburn JA. The clinical genetics of hidradenitis suppurativa revisited. Br J Dermatol 2000; 142: 947–953.

234 Mengesha YM, Holcombe TC, Hansen RC. Prepubertal hidradenitis suppurativa: two case reports and review of the literature. Pediatr Dermatol 1999; 16: 292–296.

235 Gupta AK, Knowles SR, Gupta MA et al. Lithium therapy associated with hidradenitis suppurativa: case report and a review of the dermatologic side effects of lithium. J Am Acad Dermatol 1995; 32: 382–386.

236 Li M, Hunt MJ, Commens CA. Hidradenitis suppurativa, Dowling Degos disease and perianal squamous cell carcinoma. Australas J Dermatol 1997; 38: 209–211.

237 König A, Lehmann C, Rompel R, Happle R. Cigarette smoking as a triggering factor of hidradenitis suppurativa. Dermatology 1999; 198: 261–264.

238 Jemec GBE. What's new in hidradenitis suppurativa? J Eur Acad Dermatol Venereol 2000; 14: 340–341.

239 Ostlere LS, Langtry JAA, Mortimer PS, Staughton RCD. Hidradenitis suppurativa in Crohn's disease. Br J Dermatol 1991; 125: 384–386.

240 Attanoos RL, Appleton MAC, Hughes LE et al. Granulomatous hidradenitis suppurativa and cutaneous Crohn's disease. Histopathology 1993; 23: 111–115.

241 Jansen T, Plewig G. What's new in acne inversa (alias hidradenitis suppurativa)? J Eur Acad Dermatol Venereol 2000; 14: 342–343.

242 O'Loughlin S, Woods R, Kirke PN et al. Hidradenitis suppurativa. Glucose tolerance, clinical, microbiologic, and immunologic features and HLA frequencies in 27 patients. Arch Dermatol 1988; 124: 1043–1046.

243 Ebling FJG. Hidradenitis suppurativa: an androgen-dependent disorder. Br J Dermatol 1986; 115: 259–262.

244 Mortimer PS, Dawber RPR, Gales MA, Moore RA. Mediation of hidradenitis suppurativa by androgens. Br Med J 1986; 292: 245–248.

245 Mortimer PS, Dawber RPR, Gales MA, Moore RA. A double-blind controlled cross-over trial of cyproterone acetate in females with hidradenitis suppurativa. Br J Dermatol 1986; 115: 263–268.

246 Farrell AM, Dawber RPR. Endocrine factors in pre- and postmenopausal women with hidradenitis suppurativa. Br J Dermatol 1997; 136: 802–803.

247 Jemec GBE, Heidenheim M, Nielsen NH. Hidradenitis suppurativa – characteristics and consequences. Clin Exp Dermatol 1996; 21: 419–423.

248 Attanoos RL, Appleton MAC, Douglas-Jones AG. The pathogenesis of hidradenitis suppurativa: a closer look at apocrine and apoeccrine glands. Br J Dermatol 1995; 133: 254–258.

249 Lapins J, Jarstrand C, Emtestam L. Coagulase-negative staphylococci are the most common bacteria found in cultures from the deep portions of hidradenitis suppurativa lesions, as obtained by carbon dioxide laser surgery. Br J Dermatol 1999; 140: 90–95.

250 Jemec GBE, Hansen U. Histology of hidradenitis suppurativa. J Am Acad Dermatol 1996; 34: 994–999.

251 Thomas R, Barnhill D, Bibro M, Hoskins W. Hidradenitis suppurativa: a case presentation and review of the literature. Obstet Gynecol 1985; 66: 592–595.

252 Hyland CH, Kheir SM. Follicular occlusion disease with elimination of abnormal elastic tissue. Arch Dermatol 1980; 116: 925–928.

253 Yu CC-W, Cook MG. Hidradenitis suppurativa: a disease of follicular epithelium, rather than apocrine glands. Br J Dermatol 1990; 122: 763–769.

254 Kurzen H, Jung EG, Hartschuh W et al. Forms of epithelial differentiation of draining sinus in acne inversa (hidradenitis suppurativa). Br J Dermatol 1999; 141: 231–239.

255 Jemec GBE, Hansen U. Histology of hidradenitis suppurativa. J Am Acad Dermatol 1996; 34: 994–999.

256 Jemec GBE, Gniadecka M. Ultrasound examination of hair follicles in hidradenitis suppurativa. Arch Dermatol 1997; 133: 967–970.

257 Boer J, Weltevreden EF. Hidradenitis suppurativa or acne inversa. A clinicopathological study of early lesions. Br J Dermatol 1996; 135: 721–725.

258 Berne B, Venge P, Ohman S. Perifolliculitis capitis abscedens et suffodiens (Hoffman). Complete healing associated with oral zinc therapy. Arch Dermatol 1985; 121: 1028–1030.

259 Glass LF, Berman B, Laub D. Treatment of perifolliculitis capitis abscedens et suffodiens with the carbon dioxide laser. J Dermatol Surg Oncol 1989; 15: 673–676.

260 Shaffer N, Billick RC, Srolovitz H. Perifolliculitis capitis abscedens et suffodiens. Arch Dermatol 1992; 128: 1329–1331.

261 Bjellerup M, Wallengren J. Familial perifolliculitis capitis abscedens et suffodiens in two brothers successfully treated with isotretinoin. J Am Acad Dermatol 1990; 23: 752–753.

262 Curry SS, Gaither DH, King LE Jr. Squamous cell carcinoma arising in dissecting perifolliculitis of the scalp. A case report and review of secondary squamous cell carcinomas. J Am Acad Dermatol 1981; 4: 673–678.

263 Moyer DG, Williams RM. Perifolliculitis capitis abscedens et suffodiens. A report of six cases. Arch Dermatol 1962; 85: 378–384.

264 Weinrauch L, Peled I, Hacham-Zadeh S, Wexler MR. Surgical treatment of severe acne conglobata. J Dermatol Surg Oncol 1981; 7: 492–494.

265 Darley CR. Acne conglobata of the buttocks aggravated by mechanical and environmental factors. Clin Exp Dermatol 1990; 15: 462–463.

266 Resnick SD, Murrell DF, Woosley J. Acne conglobata and a generalized lichen spinulosus-like eruption in a man seropositive for human immunodeficiency virus. J Am Acad Dermatol 1992; 26: 1013–1014.

267 van Pelt HPA, Juhlin L. Acne conglobata after pregnancy. Acta Derm Venereol 1999; 79: 169.

Miscellaneous folliculitides

268 Kushimoto H, Aoki T. Toxic erythema with generalized follicular pustules caused by streptomycin. Arch Dermatol 1981; 117: 444–445.

269 Lear J, Bourke JF, Burns DA. Hyperplastic pseudofolliculitis barbae associated with cyclosporin. Br J Dermatol 1997; 136: 132–133.

270 Busam KJ, Capodieci P, Motzer R et al. Cutaneous side-effects in cancer patients treated with the antiepidermal growth factor receptor antibody C225. Br J Dermatol 2001; 144: 1169–1176.

271 Hayakawa K, Shiohara T. An intensely pruritic eruption on the back occurring after stopping dieting. Acta Derm Venereol 2000; 80: 449–450.

272 Strauss JS, Kligman AM. Pseudofolliculitis of the beard. Arch Dermatol 1956; 74: 533–542.

273 Smith JD, Odom RB. Pseudofolliculitis capitis. Arch Dermatol 1977; 113: 328–329.

274 Alexander AM. Pseudofolliculitis diathesis. Arch Dermatol 1974; 109: 729–730.

275 Dilaimy M. Pseudofolliculitis of the legs. Arch Dermatol 1976; 112: 507–508.

276 Brauner GJ, Flandermeyer KL. Pseudofolliculitis barbae. 2. Treatment. Int J Dermatol 1977; 16: 520–525.

277 Zoberman E, Farmer ER. Pruritic folliculitis of pregnancy. Arch Dermatol 1981; 117: 20–22.

278 Vaughan Jones SA, Hern S, Black MM. Neutrophil folliculitis and serum androgen levels. Clin Exp Dermatol 1999; 24: 392–395.

279 Wilkinson SM, Buckler H, Wilkinson N et al. Androgen levels in pruritic folliculitis of pregnancy. Clin Exp Dermatol 1995; 20: 234–236.

280 Kroumpouzos G, Cohen LM. Pruritic folliculitis of pregnancy. J Am Acad Dermatol 2000; 43: 132–134.

281 Patterson JW. The perforating disorders. J Am Acad Dermatol 1984; 10: 561–581.

282 Patterson JW, Graff GE, Eubanks SW. Perforating folliculitis and psoriasis. J Am Acad Dermatol 1982; 7: 369–376.

283 Rubio FA, Herranz P, Robayna G et al. Perforating folliculitis: Report of a case in an HIV-infected man. J Am Acad Dermatol 1999; 40: 300–302.

284 Kahana M, Trau H, Delev E. Perforating folliculitis in association with primary sclerosing cholangitis. Am J Dermatopathol 1985; 7: 271–276.

285 Hurwitz RM, Melton ME, Creech FT III et al. Perforating folliculitis in association with hemodialysis. Am J Dermatopathol 1982; 4: 101–108.

286 Ackerman AB. Histologic diagnosis of inflammatory skin diseases. Philadelphia: Lea & Febiger, 1978; 685–687.

287 Burkhart CG. Perforating folliculitis. A reappraisal of its pathogenesis. Int J Dermatol 1981; 20: 597–599.

288 Hurwitz RM. The evolution of perforating folliculitis in patients with chronic renal failure. Am J Dermatopathol 1985; 7: 231–239.

289 White CR Jr, Heskel NS, Pokorny DJ. Perforating folliculitis of hemodialysis. Am J Dermatopathol 1982; 4: 109–116.

290 Fitzgerald DA, Heagerty AHM, Stephens M, Smith AG. Follicular toxic pustuloderma associated with allopurinol. Clin Exp Dermatol 1994; 19: 243–245.

291 Magro CM, Crowson AN. Sterile neutrophilic folliculitis with perifollicular vasculopathy: a distinctive cutaneous reaction pattern reflecting systemic disease. J Cutan Pathol 1998; 25: 215–221.

292 Arai E, Okubo H, Tsuchida T et al. Pseudolymphomatous folliculitis. A clinicopathologic study of 15 cases of cutaneous pseudolymphoma with follicular invasion. Am J Surg Pathol 1999; 23: 1313–1319.

Hair shaft abnormalities

293 Whiting DA. Structural abnormalities of the hair shaft. J Am Acad Dermatol 1987; 16: 1–25.

294 Rook A, Dawber R. Diseases of the hair and scalp. Oxford: Blackwell Scientific Publications, 1982; 179–232.

295 Camacho-Martinez F, Ferrando J. Hair shaft dysplasias. Int J Dermatol 1988; 27: 71–80.

296 Rogers M. Hair shaft abnormalities: Part 1. Australas J Dermatol 1995; 36: 179–185.

297 Mortimer PS. Unruly hair. Br J Dermatol 1985; 113: 467–473.

298 Thai K-E, Sinclair RD. Cutaneous pili migrans. Br J Dermatol 2001; 144: 219.

Fractures of hair shafts

299 Birnbaum PS, Baden HP, Bronstein BR et al. Intermittent hair follicle dystrophy. J Am Acad Dermatol 1986; 15: 54–60.

300 Chetty GN, Kamalam A, Thambiah AS. Acquired structural defects of the hair. Int J Dermatol 1981; 20: 119–121.

301 Leonard JN, Gummer CL, Dawber RPR. Generalized trichorrhexis nodosa. Br J Dermatol 1980; 103: 85–90.

302 Smith RA, Ross JS, Bunker CB. Localized trichorrhexis nodosa. Clin Exp Dermatol 1994; 19: 441–442.

303 Ricci MA, Tunnessen WW Jr, Pergolizzi JJ, Hellems MA. Menkes' kinky hair syndrome. Cutis 1982; 30: 55–58.

304 Papa CM, Mills OH Jr, Hanshaw W. Seasonal trichorrhexis nodosa. Arch Dermatol 1972; 106: 888–892.

305 Itin PH, Pittelkow MR. Trichothiodystrophy: review of sulfur-deficient brittle hair syndromes and association with the ectodermal dysplasias. J Am Acad Dermatol 1990; 22: 705–717.

306 Rushton DH, Norris MJ, James KC. Amino-acid composition in trichorrhexis nodosa. Clin Exp Dermatol 1990; 15: 24–28.

307 Rogers M. Hair shaft abnormalities: Part II. Australas J Dermatol 1996; 37: 1–11.

308 Birnbaum PS, Baden HP. Heritable disorders of hair. Dermatol Clin 1987; 5: 137–153.

309 Petrin JH, Meckler KA, Sybert VP. A new variant of trichothiodystrophy with recurrent infections, failure to thrive, and death. Pediatr Dermatol 1998; 15: 31–34.

310 Itin PH, Sarasin A, Pittelkow MR. Trichothiodystrophy: Update on the sulfur-deficient brittle hair syndromes. J Am Acad Dermatol 2001; 44: 891–920.

311 Price VH, Odom RB, Ward WH, Jones FT. Trichothiodystrophy. Sulfur-deficient brittle hair as a marker for a neuroectodermal symptom complex. Arch Dermatol 1980; 116: 1375–1384.

312 Gummer CL, Dawber RPR. Trichothiodystrophy: an ultrastructural study of the hair follicle. Br J Dermatol 1985; 113: 273–280.

313 Peter C, Tomczok J, Hoting E, Behrendt H. Trichothiodystrophy without associated neuroectodermal defects. Br J Dermatol 1998; 139: 137–140.

314 Chen E, Cleaver JE, Weber CA et al. Trichothiodystrophy: clinical spectrum, central nervous system imaging, and biochemical characterization of two siblings. J Invest Dermatol 1994; 103: 154S–158S.

315 Sarasin A, Blanchet-Bardon C, Renault G et al. Prenatal diagnosis in a subset of trichothiodystrophy patients defective in DNA repair. Br J Dermatol 1992; 127: 485–491.

316 Jorizzo JL, Atherton DJ, Crounse RG, Wells RS. Ichthyosis, brittle hair, impaired intelligence, decreased fertility and short stature (IBIDS syndrome). Br J Dermatol 1982; 106: 705–710.

317 Hersh JH, Klein LR, Joyce MR et al. Trichothiodystrophy and associated anomalies: a variant of SIBIDS or new symptom complex? Pediatr Dermatol 1993; 10: 117–122.

318 Calvieri S, Rossi A, Amorosi B et al. Trichothiodystrophy: ultrastructural studies of two patients. Pediatr Dermatol 1993; 10: 111–116.

319 McCuaig C, Marcoux D, Rasmussen JE et al. Trichothiodystrophy associated with photosensitivity, gonadal failure, and striking osteosclerosis. J Am Acad Dermatol 1993; 28: 820–826.

320 Price VH. Trichothiodystrophy: update. Pediatr Dermatol 1992; 9: 369–370.

321 Ito M, Ito K, Hashimoto K. Pathogenesis in trichorrhexis invaginata (bamboo hair). J Invest Dermatol 1984; 83: 1–6.

322 De Berker DAR, Paige DG, Ferguson DJP, Dawber RPR. Golf tee hairs in Netherton disease. Pediatr Dermatol 1995; 12: 7–11.

323 Yesudian P, Srinivas K. Ichthyosis with unusual hair shaft abnormalities in siblings. Br J Dermatol 1977; 96: 199–203.

324 Burkhart CG, Huttner JJ, Bruner J. Central trichoptilosis. J Am Acad Dermatol 1981; 5: 703–705.

Irregularities of hair shafts

325 Mallon E, Dawber RPR, de Berker D, Ferguson DJP. Cheveux incoiffables – diagnostic, clinical and hair microscopic findings, and pathogenic studies. Br J Dermatol 1994; 131: 608–614.

326 Matis WL, Baden H, Green R et al. Uncombable-hair syndrome. Pediatr Dermatol 1986; 4: 215–219.

327 Shelley WB, Shelley ED. Uncombable hair syndrome: observations on response to biotin and occurrence in siblings with ectodermal dysplasia. J Am Acad Dermatol 1985; 13: 97–102.

328 Ravella A, Pujoi RM, Noguera X, de Moragas JM. Localized pili canaliculi and trianguli. J Am Acad Dermatol 1987; 17: 377–380.

329 Zegpi M, Roa I. The uncombable hair syndrome. Arch Pathol Lab Med 1987; 111: 754–755.

330 Baden HP, Schoenfeld RJ, Stroud JO, Happle R. Physicochemical properties of 'spun glass' hair. Acta Derm Venereol 1981; 61: 441–444.

331 Rest EB, Fretzin DF. Quantitative assessment of scanning electron microscope defects in uncombable-hair syndrome. Pediatr Dermatol 1990; 7: 93–96.

332 Camacho F, Ferrando J, Pichardo AR et al. Rapp–Hodgkin syndrome with pili canaliculi. Pediatr Dermatol 1993; 10: 54–57.

333 Fritz TM, Trüeb RM. Uncombable hair syndrome with angel-shaped phalango-epiphyseal dysplasia. Pediatr Dermatol 2000; 17: 21–24.

334 Downham TF II, Chapel TA, Lupulescu AP. Straight-hair nevus syndrome: a case report with scanning electron microscopic findings of hair morphology. Int J Dermatol 1976; 15: 438–443.

335 Day TL. Straight-hair nevus, ichthyosis hystrix, leukokeratosis of the tongue. Arch Dermatol 1967; 96: 606.

336 Weary PE, Hendricks AA, Wawner F, Ajgaonkar G. Pili bifurcati. Arch Dermatol 1973; 108: 403–407.

337 Mehregan AH, Thompson WS. Pili multigemini. Br J Dermatol 1979; 100: 315–322.

338 Kailasam V, Kamalam A, Thambiah AS. Trichostasis spinulosa. Int J Dermatol 1979; 18: 297–300.

339 Sarkany I, Gaylarde PM. Trichostasis spinulosa and its management. Br J Dermatol 1971; 84: 311–315.

340 Young MC, Jorizzo JL, Sanchez RL et al. Trichostasis spinulosa. Int J Dermatol 1985; 24: 575–580.

341 Gummer CL, Dawber RPR. Pili annulati: electron histochemical studies on affected hairs. Br J Dermatol 1981; 105: 303–309.

342 Moffitt DL, Lear JT, de Berker DAR, Peachey RDG. Pili annulati coincident with alopecia areata. Pediatr Dermatol 1998; 15: 271–273.

343 Dini G, Casigliani R, Rindi L et al. Pili annulati. Optical and scanning electron microscopic studies. Int J Dermatol 1988; 27: 256–257.

344 Price VH, Thomas RS, Jones FT. Pseudopili annulati. An unusual variant of normal hair. Arch Dermatol 1970; 102: 354–358.

345 Lee S-SJ, Lee Y-S, Giam Y-C. Pseudopili annulati in a dark-haired individual: a light and electron microscopic study. Pediatr Dermatol 2001; 18: 27–30.

346 Dawber R, Comaish S. Scanning electron microscopy of normal and abnormal hair shafts. Arch Dermatol 1970; 101: 316–322.

347 Gummer CL, Dawber RPR, Swift JA. Monilethrix: an electron microscopic and electron histochemical study. Br J Dermatol 1981; 105: 529–541.

348 De Berker D, Dawber RPR. Variations in the beading configuration in monilethrix. Pediatr Dermatol 1992; 9: 19–21.

349 Dawber RPR. Weathering of hair in monilethrix and pili torti. Clin Exp Dermatol 1977; 2: 271–277.

350 Ito M, Hashimoto K, Yorder FW. Monilethrix: an ultrastructural study. J Cutan Pathol 1984; 11: 513–521.

351 Ito M, Hashimoto K, Katsuumi K, Sato Y. Pathogenesis of monilethrix: computer stereography and electron microscopy. J Invest Dermatol 1990; 95: 186–194.

352 De Berker DAR, Ferguson DJP, Dawber RPR. Monilethrix: a clinicopathological illustration of a cortical defect. Br J Dermatol 1993; 128: 327–331.

353 Stevens HP, Kelsell DP, Bryant SP et al. Linkage of monilethrix to the trichocyte and epithelial keratin gene cluster on 12q11–q13. J Invest Dermatol 1996; 106: 795–797.

354 Birch-Machin MA, Healy E, Turner R et al. Mapping of monilethrix to the type II keratin gene cluster at chrosome 12q13 in three new families, including one with variable expressivity. Br J Dermatol 1997; 137: 339–343.

355 Korge BP, Healy E, Munro CS et al. A mutational hotspot in the 2B domain of human hair basic keratin 6 (hHb6) in monilethrix patients. J Invest Dermatol 1998; 111: 896–899.

356 Korge BP, Hamm H, Jury CS et al. Identification of novel mutations in basic hair keratins hHb1 and hHb6 in monilethrix: implications for protein structure and clinical phenotype. J Invest Dermatol 1999; 113: 607–612.

357 Winter H, Clark RD, Tarras-Wahlberg C et al. Monilethrix: a novel mutation (Glu402Lys) in the helix termination motif and the first causative mutation (Asn114Asp) in the helix initiation motif of the Type II hair keratin hHb6. J Invest Dermatol 1999; 113: 263–266.

358 Pearce EG, Smith SK, Lanigan SW, Bowden PE. Two different mutations in the same codon of a type II hair keratin (hHb6) in patients with monilethrix. J Invest Dermatol 1999; 113: 1123–1127.

359 Zitelli JA. Pseudomonilethrix. An artifact. Arch Dermatol 1986; 122: 688–690.

360 Elston DM, Bergfeld WF, Whiting DA et al. Bubble hair. J Cutan Pathol 1992; 19: 439–444.

361 Brown VM, Crounse RG, Abele DC. An unusual new hair shaft abnormality: 'bubble hair'. J Am Acad Dermatol 1986; 15: 1113–1117.

362 Detwiler SP, Carson JL, Woosley JT et al. Bubble hair. Case caused by an overheating hair dryer and reproducibility in normal hair with heat. J Am Acad Dermatol 1994; 30: 54–60.

363 Gummer CL. Bubble hair: a cosmetic abnormality caused by brief, focal heating of damp hair fibres. Br J Dermatol 1994; 131: 901–903.
364 Krasnoff J, Glusac E, Bolognia JL. Bubble hair – a possible explanation for its distribution. Int J Dermatol 1998; 37: 380–382.

Coiling and twisting abnormalities

365 Patel HP, Unis ME. Pili torti in association with citrullinemia. J Am Acad Dermatol 1985; 12: 203–206.
366 Scott MJ Jr, Bronson DM, Esterly NB. Bjornstad syndrome and pili torti. Pediatr Dermatol 1983; 1: 45–50.
367 Petit A, Dontenwille MM, Blanchet Bardon C, Civatte J. Pili torti with congenital deafness (Bjornstad's syndrome) – report of three cases in one family, suggesting autosomal dominant transmission. Clin Exp Dermatol 1993; 18: 94–95.
368 Loche F, Bayle-Lebey P, Carriere JP et al. Pili torti with congenital deafness (Bjornstad syndrome): a case report. Pediatr Dermatol 1999; 16: 220–221.
369 Powell J, Ferguson DJP, Dawber RPR. Is kinky-hair disease a misnomer for Menkes syndrome? Arch Dermatol 2001; 137: 92–93.
370 Hays SB, Camisa C. Acquired pili torti in two patients treated with synthetic retinoids. Cutis 1985; 35: 466–468.
371 Barth JH, Dawber RPR. Pili torti and hirsuties: are twisted hairs a normal variant? Acta Derm Venereol 1987; 67: 455–457.
372 Abramovits-Ackerman W, Bustos T, Simosa-Leon V et al. Cutaneous findings in a new syndrome of autosomal recessive ectodermal dysplasia with corkscrew hairs. J Am Acad Dermatol 1992; 27: 917–921.
373 Argenziano G, Monsurrò MR, Pazienza R, Delfino M. A case of probable autosomal recessive ectodermal dysplasia with corkscrew hairs and mental retardation in a family with tuberous sclerosis. J Am Acad Dermatol 1997; 38: 344–348.
374 Ormerod AD, Main RA, Ryder ML, Gregory DW. A family with diffuse partial woolly hair. Br J Dermatol 1987; 116: 401–405.
375 Al-Harmozi SA, Mahmoud SF, Ejeckam GC. Woolly hair nevus syndrome. J Am Acad Dermatol 1992; 27: 259–260.
376 Hasper MF, Klokke AH. Woolly hair naevus with triangular hairs. Br J Dermatol 1983; 108: 111–113.
377 Peteiro C, Perez Oliva N, Zulaica A, Toribio J. Woolly-hair nevus: report of a case associated with a verrucous epidermal nevus in the same area. Pediatr Dermatol 1989; 6: 188–190.
378 Reda AM, Rogers RS III, Peters MS. Woolly hair nevus. J Am Acad Dermatol 1990; 22: 377–380.
379 Revenga F, Ferrando J, Grimalt R et al. Systematized, unilateral, velvety hyperpigmentation and homolateral patches of curled hairs. Pediatr Dermatol 2000; 17: 417–419.
380 García-Hernández M-J, Price VH, Camacho FM. Woolly hair associated with loose anagen hair. Acta Derm Venereol 2000; 80: 388–389.
381 Mortimer PS, Gummer C, English J, Dawber RPR. Acquired progressive kinking of hair. Arch Dermatol 1985; 121: 1031–1033.
382 English JSC, Mortimer PS. Acquired progressive kinking of the hair. Clin Exp Dermatol 1984; 9: 102–104.
383 Cullen SI, Fulghum DD. Acquired progressive kinking of the hair. Arch Dermatol 1989; 125: 252–255.
384 Boudou P, Reygagne P. Increased scalp skin and serum α-reductase reduced androgens in a man relevant to the acquired progressive kinky hair disorder and developing androgenetic alopecia. Arch Dermatol 1997; 133: 1129–1133.
385 Esterly NB, Lavin MP, Garancis JC. Acquired progressive kinking of the hair. Arch Dermatol 1989; 125: 813–815.
386 Tosti A, Piraccini BM, Pazzaglia M, Misciali C. Acquired progressive kinking of the hair. Clinical features, pathological study, and follow-up of 7 patients. Arch Dermatol 1999; 135: 1223–1226.
387 Norwood OT. Whisker hair. Arch Dermatol 1979; 115: 930–931.
388 Rebora A, Guarrera M. Acquired progressive kinking of the hair. J Am Acad Dermatol 1985; 12: 933–936.
389 English DT, Jones HE. Trichonodosis. Arch Dermatol 1973; 107: 77–79.
390 Dawber RPR. Knotting of scalp hair. Br J Dermatol 1974; 91: 169–173.
391 Itin PH, Bircher AJ, Lautenschlager S et al. A new clinical disorder of twisted and rolled body hairs with multiple, large knots. J Am Acad Dermatol 1994; 30: 31–35.
392 Al Ghani MA, Geilen CC, Blume-Peytavi U, Orfanos CE. Matting of hair: a multifactorial enigma. Dermatology 2000; 201: 101–104.
393 Levit F, Scott MJ Jr. Circle hairs. J Am Acad Dermatol 1983; 8: 423–425.
394 Contreras-Ruiz J, Duran-McKinster C, Tamayo-Sanchez L et al. Circle hairs: a clinical curiosity. J Eur Acad Dermatol Venereol 2000; 14: 495–497.
395 Smith JB, Hogan DJ. Circle hairs are not rolled hairs. J Am Acad Dermatol 1996; 35: 634–635.

Extraneous matter on hair shafts

396 Gold I, Sommer B, Urson S, Schewach-Millet M. White piedra. A frequently misdiagnosed infection of hair. Int J Dermatol 1984; 23: 621–623.
397 Benson PM, Lapins NA, Odom RB. White piedra. Arch Dermatol 1983; 119: 602–604.
398 Lassus A, Kanerva L, Stubb S, Salonen A. White piedra. Report of a case evaluated by scanning electron microscopy. Arch Dermatol 1982; 118: 208–211.
398 Kubec K, Dvorak R, Alsaleh QA. Trichosporosis (white piedra) in Kuwait. Int J Dermatol 1998; 37: 186–187.
400 Kalter DC, Tschen JA, Cernoch PL et al. Genital white piedra: epidemiology, microbiology, and therapy. J Am Acad Dermatol 1986; 14: 982–993.
401 Steinman HK, Pappenfort RB. White piedra – a case report and review of the literature. Clin Exp Dermatol 1984; 9: 591–598.
402 Figueras MJ, Guarro J, Zaror L. New findings in black piedra infection. Br J Dermatol 1996; 135: 157–158.
403 Dawber RPR. Hair casts. Arch Dermatol 1979; 100: 417–421.
404 Taïeb A, Surlève-Bazeille JE, Maleville J. Hair casts. A clinical and morphologic study. Arch Dermatol 1985; 121: 1009–1013.
405 Keipert JA. Hair casts. Review and suggestion regarding nomenclature. Arch Dermatol 1986; 122: 927–930.
406 Zhu W-Y, Xia M-Y, Wu J-H, Do D-A. Hair casts: a clinical and electron microscopic study. Pediatr Dermatol 1990; 7: 270–274.
407 Shieh X, Yi X. Hair casts: a clinical and morphologic control study. Arch Dermatol 1992; 128: 1553–1554.
408 Zhang W. Epidemiological and aetiological studies on hair casts. Clin Exp Dermatol 1995; 20: 202–207.
409 Fabbri P, Difonzo EM, Palleschi GM, Pacini P. Hair casts. Int J Dermatol 1988; 27: 319–321.
410 Scott MJ Jr, Roenigk HH Jr. Hair casts: classification, staining characteristics, and differential diagnosis. J Am Acad Dermatol 1983; 8: 27–32.
411 Itin PH, Schiller P, Mathys D, Guggenheim R. Cosmetically induced hair beads. J Am Acad Dermatol 1997; 36: 260–261.

Alopecias

412 Pinkus H. Alopecia. Clinicopathologic correlations. Int J Dermatol 1980; 19: 245–253.
413 Sullivan JR, Kossard S. Acquired scalp alopecia. Part I: A review. Australas J Dermatol 1998; 39: 207–221.
414 Ioannides G. Alopecia: a pathologist's view. Int J Dermatol 1982; 21: 316–328.
415 Headington JT. Transverse microscopic anatomy of the human scalp. A basis for a morphometric approach to disorders of the hair follicle. Arch Dermatol 1984; 120: 449–456.
416 Templeton SF, Santa Cruz DJ, Solomon AR. Alopecia: histologic diagnosis by transverse sections. Semin Diagn Pathol 1996; 13: 2–18.
417 Frishberg DP, Sperling LC, Guthrie VM. Transverse scalp sections: A proposed method for laboratory processing. J Am Acad Dermatol 1996; 35: 220–222.
418 Elston DM, McCollough ML, Angeloni VL. Vertical and transverse sections of alopecia biopsy specimens. Combining the two to maximise diagnostic yields. J Am Acad Dermatol 1995; 32: 454–457.
419 Montagna E, Parakkal PF. The structure and function of skin. New York: Academic Press, 1974.
420 Rook A, Dawber R. Diseases of the hair and scalp. Oxford: Blackwell Scientific Publications, 1982; 1–17.
421 Braun-Falco O, Heilgemeir GP. The trichogram. Structural and functional basis, performance, and interpretation. Semin Dermatol 1985; 4: 40–52.
422 Weedon D, Strutton G. Apoptosis as the mechanism of the involution of hair follicles in catagen transformation. Acta Derm Venereol 1981; 61: 335–339.
423 Seiberg M, Marthinuss J, Stenn KS. Changes in expression of apoptosis-associated genes in skin mark early catagen. J Invest Dermatol 1995; 104: 78–82.
424 Paus R, Müller-Röver S, Botchkarev VA. Chronobiology of the hair follicle: hunting the "hair cycle clock". J Invest Dermatol (Symposium Proceedings) 1999; 4: 338–345.
425 Malmusi M. How many cycles has a hair follicle? Dermatopathology: Practical & Conceptual 1999; 5: 255.
426 Paus R, Müller-Röver S, van der Veen C et al. A comprehensive guide for the recognition and classification of distinct stages of hair follicle morphogenesis. J Invest Dermatol 1999; 113: 523–532.
427 Soma T, Ogo M, Suzuki J et al. Analysis of apoptotic cell death in human hair follicles in vivo and in vitro. J Invest Dermatol 1998; 111: 948–954.
428 Müller-Röver S, Rossiter H, Lindner G et al. Hair follicle apoptosis and bcl-2. J Invest Dermatol (Symposium Proceedings) 1999; 4: 272–277.
429 Rumio C, Donetti E, Imberti A et al. c-Myc expression in human anagen hair follicles. Br J Dermatol 2000; 142: 1092–1099.

430 Barajon I, Rumio C, Donetti E et al. Pattern of expression of c-Myc, Max and BIN1 in human anagen hair follicles. Br J Dermatol 2001; 144: 1193–1203.

431 Stenn KS, Lawrence L, Veis D et al. Expression of the bcl-2 protooncogene in the cycling adult mouse hair follicle. J Invest Dermatol 1994; 103: 107–111.

432 Weedon D, Strutton G. The recognition of early stages of catagen. Am J Dermatopathol 1984; 6: 553–555.

433 Hollis DE, Chapman RE. Apoptosis in wool follicles during mouse epidermal growth factor (mEGF)-induced catagen regression. J Invest Dermatol 1987; 88: 455–458.

434 Tobin DJ, Hagen E, Botchkarev VA, Paus R. Do hair bulb melanocytes undergo apoptosis during hair follicle regression (catagen)? J Invest Dermatol 1998; 111: 941–947.

435 Tobin DJ. A possible role for Langerhans cells in the removal of melanin from early catagen hair follicles. Br J Dermatol 1998; 138: 795–798.

436 Bowden PE, Hainey SD, Parker G et al. Characterization and chromosomal localization of human hair-specific keratin genes and comparative expression during the hair growth cycle. J Invest Dermatol 1998; 110: 158–164.

437 Barth JH. Normal hair growth in children. Pediatr Dermatol 1987; 4: 173–184.

438 Rook A, Dawber R. Diseases of the hair and scalp. Oxford: Blackwell Scientific Publications, 1982; 146–178.

439 Chapman DM. The nature of cuticular "ruffles" on slowly plucked anagen hair roots. J Cutan Pathol 1997; 24: 434–439.

Congenital/hereditary alopecias

440 de Berker D. Congenital hypotrichiosis. Int J Dermatol 1999; 38 (Suppl 1): 25–33.

441 Barth JH, Dawber RPR. Focal naevoid hypotrichosis. Acta Derm Venereol 1987; 67: 178–179.

442 Vogt BR, Traupe H, Hamm H. Congenital atrichia with nail dystrophy, abnormal facies, and retarded psychomotor development in two siblings: a new autosomal recessive syndrome? Pediatr Dermatol 1988; 5: 236–242.

443 Blume-Peytavi U, Föhles J, Schulz R et al. Hypotrichosis, hair structure defects, hypercysteine hair and glucosuria: a new genetic syndrome? Br J Dermatol 1996; 134: 319–324.

444 Templeton SF, Wiegand SE. Pachyonychia congenita-associated alopecia. A microscopic analysis using transverse section technique. Am J Dermatopathol 1997; 19: 180–184.

445 Kulin P, Sybert VP. Hereditary hypotrichosis and localized morphea: a new clinical entity. Pediatr Dermatol 1986; 3: 333–338.

446 Baden HP, Kubilus J. Analysis of hair from alopecia congenita. J Am Acad Dermatol 1980; 3: 623–626.

447 Bentley-Phillips B, Grace HJ. Hereditary hypotrichosis. A previously undescribed syndrome. Br J Dermatol 1979; 101: 331–339.

448 Cambiaghi S, Barbareschi M. A sporadic case of congenital hypotrichosis simplex of the scalp: difficulties in diagnosis and classification. Pediatr Dermatol 1999; 16: 301–304.

449 Kruse R, Cichon S, Anker M et al. Novel *hairless* mutations in two kindreds with autosomal recessive papular atrichia. J Invest Dermatol 1999; 113: 954–959.

450 Rogaev EI, Zinchenko RA, Dvoryachikov G et al. Total hypotrichosis: genetic form of alopecia not linked to *hairless* gene. Lancet 1999; 354: 1097–1098.

451 Betz RC, Lee Y-A, Bygum A et al. A gene for hypotrichosis simplex of the scalp maps to chromosome 6p21.3. Am J Hum Genet 2000; 66: 1979–1983.

452 Barraud-Klenovsek MM, Trüeb RM. Congenital hypotrichosis due to short anagen. Br J Dermatol 2000; 143: 612–617.

453 Ibsen HHW, Clemmensen OJ, Brandrup F. Familial hypotrichosis of the scalp. Acta Derm Venereol 1991; 71: 349–351.

454 Sreekumar GP, Roberts JL, Wong C-Q et al. Marie Unna hereditary hypotrichosis gene maps to human chromosome 8p21 near *hairless*. J Invest Dermatol 2000; 114: 595–597.

455 Cichon S, Kruse R, Hillmer AM et al. A distinct gene close to the hairless locus on chromosome 8p underlies hereditary Marie Unna type hypotrichosis in a German family. Br J Dermatol 2000; 143: 811–814.

456 van Steensel M, Smith FJD, Steijlen PM et al. The gene for hypotrichosis of Marie Unna maps between D8S258 and D8S298: exclusion of the *hr* gene by cDNA and genomic sequencing. Am J Hum Genet 1999; 65: 413–419.

457 Roberts JL, Whiting DA, Henry D et al. Marie Unna congenital hypotrichosis: clinical description, histopathology, scanning electron microscopy of a previously unreported large pedigree. J Invest Dermatol (Symposium Proceedings) 1999; 4: 261–267.

458 Kanzler MH, Rasmussen JE. Atrichia with papular lesions. Arch Dermatol 1986; 122: 565–567.

459 Nomura K, Hashimoto I. Atrichia with papular lesions: successful genetic counselling about having a child. Br J Dermatol 1998; 139: 742–744.

460 Nomura K, Hashimoto I, Takahashi G, Ito M. Atrichia with papular lesions. Electron microscopic observations of cystic lesions. Am J Dermatopathol 2001; 23: 227–231.

461 Irvine AD, Christiano AM. Hair on a gene string: recent advances in understanding the molecular genetics of hair loss. Clin Exp Dermatol 2001; 26: 59–71.

462 Sprecher E, Lestringant GG, Szargel R et al. Atrichia with papular lesions resulting from a nonsense mutation within the human hairless gene. J Invest Dermatol 1999; 113: 687–690.

463 Del Castillo V, Ruiz-Maldonado R, Carnevale A. Atrichia with papular lesions and mental retardation in two sisters. Int J Dermatol 1974; 13: 261–265.

464 Grattan CEH, Liddle BJ, Willshaw HE. Atrophic alopecia in the Hallermann–Streiff syndrome. Clin Exp Dermatol 1989; 14: 250–252.

465 Golomb RS, Porter PS. A distinct hair shaft abnormality in the Hallermann–Streiff syndrome. Cutis 1975; 16: 122–128.

Premature catagen/telogen

466 Kligman AM. Pathologic dynamics of human hair loss. I. Telogen effluvium. Arch Dermatol 1961; 83: 175–198.

467 Headington JT, Astle N. Familial focal alopecia. A new disorder of hair growth clinically resembling pseudopelade. Arch Dermatol 1987; 123: 234–237.

468 Oranje AP, Peereboom-Wynia JDR, de Raeymaecker DMJ. Trichotillomania in childhood. J Am Acad Dermatol 1986; 15: 614–619.

469 Wiles JC, Hansen RC. Postoperative (pressure) alopecia. J Am Acad Dermatol 1985; 12: 195–198.

470 Ben-Amitai D, Garty BZ. Alopecia in children after cardiac surgery. Pediatr Dermatol 1993; 10: 32–33.

471 Hanly AJ, Jorda M, Badiavas E et al. Postoperative pressure-induced alopecia: report of a case and discussion of the role of apoptosis in non-scarring alopecia. J Cutan Pathol 1999; 26: 357–361.

472 Dawber R. Self-induced hair loss. Semin Dermatol 1985; 4: 53–57.

473 Whiting DA. Traumatic alopecia. Int J Dermatol 1999; 38 (Suppl 1): 34–44.

474 Ackerman AB, Walton NW III, Jones RE, Charissi C. "Hot comb alopecia"/"follicular degeneration syndrome" in African-American women is traction alopecia! Dermatopathology: Practical & Conceptual 2000; 6: 320–336.

475 Steck WD. The clinical evaluation of pathologic hair loss with a diagnostic sign in trichotillomania. Cutis 1979; 24: 293–301.

476 Lachapelle JM, Piérard GE. Traumatic alopecia in trichotillomania: a pathogenic interpretation of histologic lesions in the pilosebaceous unit. J Cutan Pathol 1977; 4: 51–67.

477 Mehregan AH. Trichotillomania. A clinicopathologic study. Arch Dermatol 1970; 102: 129–133.

478 Muller SA, Winkelmann RK. Trichotillomania. A clinicopathologic study of 24 cases. Arch Dermatol 1972; 105: 535–540.

479 Muller SA. Trichotillomania: a histopathologic study in sixty-six patients. J Am Acad Dermatol 1990; 23: 56–62.

480 Rook A, Dawber R. Diseases of the hair and scalp. Oxford: Blackwell Scientific Publications, 1982; 115–125.

481 Weedon D, Strutton G. Telogen effluvium. Arch Dermatol 1994; 130: 254.

482 Rebora A. Telogen effluvium: an etiopathogenetic theory. Int J Dermatol 1993; 32: 339–340.

483 Smith KJ, Skelton HG, DeRusso D et al. Clinical and histopathologic features of hair loss in patients with HIV-1 infection. J Am Acad Dermatol 1996; 34: 63–68.

484 Tosti A, Piraccini BM, van Neste DJJ. Telogen effluvium after allergic contact dermatitis of the scalp. Arch Dermatol 2001; 137: 187–190.

485 Sinclair R. Diffuse hair loss. Int J Dermatol 1999; 38 (Suppl 1): 8–18.

486 Benedict LM, Abell E, Jegasothy B. Telogen effluvium associated with eosinophilia–myalgia syndrome. J Am Acad Dermatol 1991; 25: 112.

487 Bardelli A, Rebora A. Telogen effluvium and minoxidil. J Am Acad Dermatol 1989; 21: 572–573.

488 Steck WD. Telogen effluvium. A clinically useful concept, with traction alopecia as an example. Cutis 1978; 21: 543–548.

489 Headington JT. Telogen effluvium. New concepts and review. Arch Dermatol 1993; 129: 356–363.

490 Whiting DA. Chronic telogen effluvium: increased scalp hair shedding in middle-aged women. J Am Acad Dermatol 1996; 35: 899–906.

491 García-Hernández M-J, Camacho FM. Chronic telogen effluvium: incidence, clinical and biochemical features, and treatment. Arch Dermatol 1999; 135: 1123–1124.

492 Rebora A. Telogen effluvium. Dermatology 1997; 195: 209–212.

Premature telogen with anagen arrest

493 Friedmann PS. Clinical and immunologic associations of alopecia areata. Semin Dermatol 1985; 4: 9–15

494 de Viragh PA, Gianadda B, Levy ML. Congenital alopecia areata. Dermatology 1997; 195: 96–98.

495 Bardazzi F, Neri I, Raone B, Patrizi A. Congenital alopecia areata: another case. Dermatology 1999; 199: 369.

496 Nelson DA, Spielvogel RL. Alopecia areata. Int J Dermatol 1985; 24: 26–34.

497 Shapiro J, Madani S. Alopecia areata: diagnosis and management. Int J Dermatol 1999; 38 (Suppl 1): 19–24.

498 Mitchell AJ, Krull EA. Alopecia areata: pathogenesis and treatment. J Am Acad Dermatol 1984; 11: 763–775.

499 Olsen E, Hordinsky M, McDonald-Hull S et al. Alopecia areata investigational assessment guidelines. J Am Acad Dermatol 1999; 40: 242–246.

500 Muller SA, Winkelmann RK. Alopecia areata. An evaluation of 736 patients. Arch Dermatol 1963; 88: 290–297.

501 Goldsmith LA. Summary of the Second International Research Workshop on Alopecia Areata. J Invest Dermatol 1995; 104: 2S–3S.

502 Safavi KH, Muller SA, Suman VJ et al. Incidence of alopecia areata in Olmsted County, Minnesota, 1975 through 1989. Mayo Clin Proc 1995; 70: 628–633.

503 Colombe BW, Price VH, Khoury EL et al. HLA class II antigen associations help to define two types of alopecia areata. J Am Acad Dermatol 1995; 33: 757–764.

504 Colombe BW, Lou CD, Price VH. The genetic basis of alopecia areata: HLA associations with patchy alopecia areata *versus* alopecia totalis and alopecia universalis. J Invest Dermatol (Symposium Proceedings) 1999; 4: 216–219.

505 Kavak A, Baykal C, Özarmağan G, Akar U. HLA in alopecia areata. Int J Dermatol 2000; 39: 589–592.

506 Friedman PS. Alopecia areata and auto-immunity. Br J Dermatol 1981; 105: 153–157.

507 Hordinsky MK, Hallgren H, Nelson D, Filipovich AH. Familial alopecia areata. HLA antigens and autoantibody formation in an American family. Arch Dermatol 1984; 120: 464–468.

508 Green J, Sinclair RD. Genetics of alopecia areata. Australas J Dermatol 2000; 41: 215–218.

509 de Andrade M, Jackow CM, Dahm N et al. Alopecia areata in families: association with the HLA locus. J Invest Dermatol (Symposium Proceedings) 1999; 4: 220–223.

510 Jackow C, Puffer N, Hordinsky M et al. Alopecia areata and cytomegalovirus infection in twins: Genes versus environment? J Am Acad Dermatol 1998; 38: 418–425.

511 Garcia-Hernández MJ, Rodríguez-Pichardo A. Multivariate analysis in alopecia areata: risk factors and validity of clinical forms. Arch Dermatol 1999; 135: 998–999.

512 Muller HK, Rook AJ, Kubba R. Immunohistology and autoantibody studies in alopecia areata. Br J Dermatol 1980; 102: 609–610.

513 Korkij W, Soltani K, Simjee S et al. Tissue-specific autoantibodies and autoimmune disorders in vitiligo and *alopecia areata*: a retrospective study. J Cutan Pathol 1984; 11: 522–530.

514 Galbraith GMP, Thiers BH, Vasily DB, Fudenberg HH. Immunological profiles in alopecia areata. Br J Dermatol 1984; 110: 163–170.

515 Hordinsky MK, Hallgren H, Nelson D, Filipovich AH. Suppressor cell number and function in alopecia areata. Arch Dermatol 1984; 120: 188–194.

516 Main RA, Robbie RB, Gray ES et al. Smooth muscle antibodies and alopecia areata. Br J Dermatol 1975; 92: 389–393.

517 Milgraum SS, Mitchell AJ, Bacon GE, Rasmussen JE. Alopecia areata, endocrine function, and autoantibodies in patients 16 years of age or younger. J Am Acad Dermatol 1987; 17: 57–61.

518 Cochran REI, Thomson J, MacSween RNM. An auto-antibody profile in alopecia totalis and diffuse alopecia. Br J Dermatol 1976; 95: 61–65.

519 Baadsgaard O, Lindskov R. Circulating lymphocyte subsets in patients with alopecia areata. Acta Derm Venereol 1986; 66: 266–268.

520 De Weert J, Temmerman L, Kint A. Alopecia: a clinical study. Dermatologica 1984; 168: 224–229.

521 Carter DM, Jegasothy BV. Alopecia areata and Down syndrome. Arch Dermatol 1976; 112: 1397–1399.

522 McMillen R, Duvic M. Alopecia areata occurring in sisters after administration of rifampicin. J Am Acad Dermatol 2001; 44: 142–143.

523 Kernland KH, Hunziker Th. Alopecia areata induced by interferon alpha? Dermatology 1999; 198: 418–419.

524 Smith SR, Kirkpatrick RC, Kerr JH, Mezebich D. Alopecia areata in a patient with pili annulati. J Am Acad Dermatol 1995; 32: 816–818.

525 Bon AM, Happle R, Itin PH. Renbök phenomenon in alopecia areata. Dermatology 2000; 201: 49–50.

526 Brown AC. Alopecia areata: a neuroendocrine disorder. Semin Dermatol 1985; 4: 16–28.

527 Shelley WB. The spotted lunula. A neglected nail sign associated with alopecia areata. J Am Acad Dermatol 1980; 2: 385–387.

528 Elieff D, Sundby S, Kennedy W, Hordinsky M. Decreased sweat-gland number and function in patients with alopecia areata. Br J Dermatol 1991; 125: 130–135.

529 Elston DM, Clayton AS, Meffert JJ, McCollough ML. Migratory poliosis: A forme fruste of alopecia areata? J Am Acad Dermatol 2000; 42: 1076–1077.

530 Perret CM, Steijlen PM, Happle R. Alopecia areata. Pathogenesis and topical immunotherapy. Int J Dermatol 1990; 29: 83–88.

531 Madani S, Shapiro J. Alopecia areata update. J Am Acad Dermatol 2000; 42: 549–566.

532 Tobin DJ, Orentreich N, Fenton DA, Bystryn J-C. Antibodies to hair follicles in alopecia areata. J Invest Dermatol 1994; 102: 721–724.

533 Goldsmith LA. Summary of the Third International Research Workshop on Alopecia Areata. J Invest Dermatol (Symposium Proceedings) 1999; 4: 200–201.

534 Tobin DJ, Hann S-K, Song M-S, Bystryn J-C. Hair follicle structures targeted by antibodies in patients with alopecia areata. Arch Dermatol 1997; 133: 57–61.

535 Majewski BBJ, Koh MS, Taylor DR et al. Increased ratio of helper to suppressor T cells in alopecia areata. Br J Dermatol 1984; 110: 171–175.

536 Lutz G, Niedecken H, Bauer R, Kreysel HW. Natural killer cell and cytotoxic/suppressor T cell deficiency in peripheral blood in subjects with alopecia areata. Australas J Dermatol 1988; 29: 29–32.

537 Galbraith GMP, Thiers BH, Jensen J, Hoehler F. A randomized double-blind study of inosiplex (Isoprinosine) therapy in patients with alopecia totalis. J Am Acad Dermatol 1987; 16: 977–983.

538 Swanson NA, Mitchell AJ, Leahy MS et al. Topical treatment of alopecia areata. Arch Dermatol 1981; 117: 384–387.

539 Baadsgaard O, Lindskov R, Clemmensen OJ. *In situ* lymphocyte subsets in alopecia areata before and during treatment with a contact allergen. Clin Exp Dermatol 1987; 12: 260–264.

540 Kalish RS, Johnson KL, Hordinsky MK. Alopecia areata. Autoreactive T cells are variably enriched in scalp lesions relative to peripheral blood. Arch Dermatol 1992; 128: 1072–1077.

541 Peereboom-Wynia JDR, van Joost T, Stolz E, Prins MEF. Markers of immunologic injury in progressive alopecia areata. J Cutan Pathol 1986; 13: 363–369.

542 Khoury EL, Price VH, Greenspan JS. HLA-DR expression by hair follicle keratinocytes in alopecia areata: evidence that it is secondary to the lymphoid infiltration. J Invest Dermatol 1988; 90: 193–200.

543 Hedstrand H, Perheentupa J, Ekwall O et al. Antibodies against hair follicles are associated with alopecia totalis in autoimmune polyendocrine syndrome type I. J Invest Dermatol 1999; 113: 1054–1058.

544 Ghersetich I, Campanile G, Lotti T. Alopecia areata: immunohistochemistry and ultrastructure of infiltrate and identification of adhesion molecule receptors. Int J Dermatol 1996; 35: 28–33.

545 Stewart MI, Smoller BR. Alopecia universalis in an HIV-positive patient: possible insight into pathogenesis. J Cutan Pathol 1993; 20: 180–183.

546 Hull SM, Nutbrown M, Pepall L et al. Immunohistologic and ultrastructural comparison of the dermal papilla and hair follicle bulb from 'active' and 'normal' areas of alopecia areata. J Invest Dermatol 1991; 96: 673–681.

547 Dressel D, Brütt CH, Manfras B et al. Alopecia areata but not androgenetic alopecia is characterised by a restricted and oligoclonal T-cell receptor-repertoire among infiltrating lymphocytes. J Cutan Pathol 1997; 24: 164–168.

548 McElwee KJ. Third International Research Workshop on Alopecia Areata. J Invest Dermatol 1999; 112: 822–824.

549 McElwee KJ, Spiers EM, Oliver RF. Partial restoration of hair growth in the DEBR model for alopecia areata after *in vivo* depletion of CD4+ T cells. Br J Dermatol 1999; 140: 432–437.

550 Bodemer C, Peuchmaur M, Fraitaig S et al. Role of cytotoxic T cells in chronic alopecia areata. J Invest Dermatol 2000; 114: 112–116.

551 Hoffmann R. The potential role of cytokines and T cells in alopecia areata. J Invest Dermatol (Symposium Proceedings) 1999; 4: 235–238.

552 McElwee KJ, Spiers EM, Oliver RF. *In vivo* depletion of CD8+ T cells restores hair growth in the DEBR model for alopecia areata. Br J Dermatol 1996; 135: 211–217.

553 Toyoda M, Makino T, Kagoura M, Morohashi M. Expression of neuropeptide-degrading enzymes in alopecia areata: an immunohistochemical study. Br J Dermatol 2001; 144: 46–54.

554 Messenger AG, Slater DN, Bleehen SS. Alopecia areata: alterations in the hair growth cycle and correlation with the follicular pathology. Br J Dermatol 1986; 114: 337–347.

555 Headington JT, Mitchell A, Swanson N. New histopathologic findings in alopecia areata studied in transverse sections. J Invest Dermatol 1981; 76: 325 (abstract).

556 Messenger AG, Bleehen SS. Alopecia areata: light and electron microscopic pathology of the regrowing white hair. Br J Dermatol 1984; 110: 155–162.

557 Gilhar A, Krueger GG. Hair growth in scalp grafts from patients with alopecia areata and alopecia universalis grafted onto nude mice. Arch Dermatol 1987; 123: 44–50.

558 Elston DM, McCollough ML, Bergfeld WF et al. Eosinophils in fibrous tracts and near hair bulbs: A helpful diagnostic feature of alopecia areata. J Am Acad Dermatol 1997; 37: 101–106.

559 El Darouti M, Marzouk SA, Sharawi E. Eosinophils in fibrous tracts and near hair bulbs: A helpful diagnostic feature of alopecia areata. J Am Acad Dermatol 2000; 42: 305–306.

560 Sperling LC, Lupton GP. Histopathology of non-scarring alopecia. J Cutan Pathol 1995; 22: 97–114.

561 Ranki A, Kianto U, Kanerva L et al. Immunohistochemical and electron microscopic characterization of the cellular infiltrate in alopecia (areata, totalis, and universalis). J Invest Dermatol 1984; 83: 7–11.

562 Whiting DA. Histopathology of alopecia areata in horizontal sections of scalp biopsies. J Invest Dermatol 1995; 105: 26S–27S.

563 Fanti PA, Tosti A, Bardazzi F et al. Alopecia areata. A pathological study of nonresponder patients. Am J Dermatopathol 1994; 16: 167–170.

564 Fanti PA, Tosti A, Morelli R et al. Follicular mucinosis in alopecia areata. Am J Dermatopathol 1992; 14: 542–545.

565 Pinkus H. Differential patterns of elastic fibers in scarring and non-scarring alopecias. J Cutan Pathol 1978; 5: 93–104.

566 Kossard S. Diffuse alopecia with stem cell folliculitis. Chronic diffuse alopecia areata or a distinct entity? Am J Dermatopathol 1999; 21: 46–50.

567 Igarashi R, Morohashi M, Takeuchi S, Sato Y. Immunofluorescence studies on complement components in the hair follicles of normal scalp and of scalp affected by alopecia areata. Acta Derm Venereol 1981; 61: 131–135.

568 Tobin DJ, Fenton DA, Kendall MD. Cell degeneration in alopecia areata. An ultrastructural study. Am J Dermatopathol 1991; 13: 248–256.

569 Tobin DJ, Fenton DA, Kendall MD. Ultrastructural study of exclamation-mark hair shafts in alopecia areata. J Cutan Pathol 1990; 17: 348–354.

570 Nutbrown M, Macdonald Hull SP, Baker TG et al. Ultrastructural abnormalities in the dermal papillae of both lesional and clinically normal follicles from alopecia areata scalps. Br J Dermatol 1996; 135: 204–210.

Vellus follicle formation

571 Rook A, Dawber R. Diseases of the hair and scalp. Oxford: Blackwell Scientific Publications, 1982; 90–114.

572 Tosti A, Piraccini BM. Androgenetic alopecia. Int J Dermatol 1999; 38 (Suppl 1): 1–7.

573 Whiting DA. Male pattern hair loss: current understanding. Int J Dermatol 1998; 37: 561–566.

574 Birch MP, Messenger JF, Messenger AG. Hair density, hair diameter and the prevalence of female pattern hair loss. Br J Dermatol 2001; 144: 297–304.

575 Rushton H, James KC, Mortimer CH. The unit area trichogram in the assessment of androgen-dependent alopecia. Br J Dermatol 1983; 109: 429–437.

576 de Lacharrière O, Deloche C, Misciali C et al. Hair diameter diversity. A clinical sign reflecting the follicle miniaturization. Arch Dermatol 2001; 137: 641–646.

577 Alexander S. Common baldness in women. Semin Dermatol 1985; 4: 1–3.

578 Orme S, Cullen DR, Messenger AG. Diffuse female hair loss: are androgens necessary? Br J Dermatol 1999; 141: 521–523.

579 De Villez RL, Dunn J. Female androgenic alopecia. Arch Dermatol 1986; 122: 1011–1015.

580 Ludwig E. Classification of the types of androgenetic alopecia (common baldness) occurring in the female sex. Br J Dermatol 1977; 97: 247–254.

581 Venning VA, Dawber RPR. Patterned alopecia in women. J Am Acad Dermatol 1988; 18: 1073–1077.

582 Olsen EA. The midline part: An important physical clue to the clinical diagnosis of androgenetic alopecia in women. J Am Acad Dermatol 1999; 40: 106–109.

583 Dawber RPR. Alopecia and hirsutism. Clin Exp Dermatol 1982; 7: 177–182.

584 Olsen EA, Buller TA, Weiner S, Delong ER. Natural history of androgenetic alopecia. Clin Exp Dermatol 1990; 15: 34–36.

585 Sreekumar GP, Pardinas J, Wong CQ et al. Serum androgens and genetic linkage analysis in early onset androgenetic alopecia. J Invest Dermatol 1999; 113: 277–279.

586 Ellis JA, Stebbing M, Harrap SB. Genetic analysis of male pattern baldness and the 5α-reductase genes. J Invest Dermatol 1998; 110: 849–853.

587 Sprecher E, Shalata A, Dabhah K et al. Androgenetic alopecia in heterozygous carriers of a mutation in the human hairless gene. J Am Acad Dermatol 2000; 42: 978–982.

588 König A, Happle R, Tchitcherina E et al. An X-linked gene involved in androgenetic alopecia: a lesson to be learned from adrenoleukodystrophy. Dermatology 2000; 200: 213–218.

589 Phillipou G, Kirk J. Significance of steroid measurements in male pattern alopecia. Clin Exp Dermatol 1981; 6: 53–56.

590 Pitts RL. Serum elevation of dehydroepiandrosterone sulfate associated with male pattern baldness in young men. J Am Acad Dermatol 1987; 16: 571–573.

591 Lucky AW. The paradox of androgens and balding: where are we now? J Invest Dermatol 1988; 91: 99–100.

592 Futterweit W, Dunaif A, Yeh H-C, Kingsley P. The prevalence of hyperandrogenism in 109 consecutive female patients with diffuse alopecia. J Am Acad Dermatol 1988; 19: 831–836.

593 Callan AW, Montalto J. Female androgenetic alopecia: an update. Australas J Dermatol 1995; 36: 51–57.

594 Signorello LB, Wuu J, Hsieh C-c et al. Hormones and hair patterning in men: A role for insulin-like growth factor 1? J Am Acad Dermatol 1999; 40: 200–203.

595 Platz EA, Pollak MN, Willett WC, Giovannucci E. Vertex balding, plasma insulin-like growth factor 1, and insulin-like growth factor binding protein 3. J Am Acad Dermatol 2000; 42: 1003–1007.

596 DeVilez RL, Jacobs JP, Szpunar CA, Warner ML. Androgenetic alopecia in the female. Arch Dermatol 1994; 130: 303–307.

597 Messenger AG. Medical management of male pattern hair loss. Int J Dermatol 2000; 39: 585–586.

598 Ramos-e-Silva M. Male pattern hair loss: prevention rather than regrowth. Int J Dermatol 2000; 39: 728–731.

599 Price VH, Menefee E, Strauss PC. Changes in hair weight and hair count in men with androgenetic alopecia, after application of 5% and 2% topical minoxidil, placebo, or no treatment. J Am Acad Dermatol 1999; 41: 717–721.

600 Whiting DA, Waldstreicher J, Sanchez M, Kaufman KD. Measuring reversal of hair miniaturization in androgenetic alopecia by follicular counts in horizontal sections of serial scalp biopsies: results of finasteride 1mg treatment of men and postmenopausal women. J Invest Dermatol (Symposium Proceedings) 1999; 4: 282–284.

601 Bayne EK, Flanagan J, Einstein M et al. Immunohistochemical localization of types 1 and 2 5α-reductase in human scalp. Br J Dermatol 1999; 141: 481–491.

602 Dawber RPR. Common baldness in women. Int J Dermatol 1981; 20: 647–650.

603 Lattarand A, Johnson WC. Male pattern alopecia. A histopathologic and histochemical study. J Cutan Pathol 1975; 2: 58–70.

604 Sperling LC, Winton GB. The transverse anatomy of androgenic alopecia. J Dermatol Surg Oncol 1990; 16: 1127–1133.

605 Alcaraz MV, Villena A, Pérez de Vargas I. Quantitative study of the human hair follicle in normal scalp and androgenetic alopecia. J Cutan Pathol 1993; 20: 344–349.

606 Pestana A, Olsen EA, Delong ER, Murray JC. Effect of ultraviolet light on topical minoxidil-induced hair growth in advanced male pattern baldness. J Am Acad Dermatol 1987; 16: 971–976.

607 Jaworsky C, Kligman AM, Murphy GF. Characterization of inflammatory infiltrates in male pattern alopecia: implications for pathogenesis. Br J Dermatol 1992; 127: 239–246.

608 Mahé YF, Michelet J-F, Billoni N et al. Androgenetic alopecia and microinflammation. Int J Dermatol 2000; 39: 576–584.

609 Whiting DA. Diagnostic and predictive value of horizontal sections of scalp biopsy specimens in male pattern androgenetic alopecia. J Am Acad Dermatol 1993; 28: 755–763.

610 Domnitz JM. Silvers DN. Giant cells in male pattern alopecia: a histologic marker and pathogenetic clue. J Cutan Pathol 1979; 6: 108–112.

611 Scott GS, Stenn KS, Savin R. Diffuse female pattern alopecia – a histological study of 40 cases. J Cutan Pathol 1988; 15: 341 (abstract).

612 Kubba R, Rook A. Congenital triangular alopecia. Br J Dermatol 1976; 95: 657–659.

613 Tosti A. Congenital triangular alopecia. Report of fourteen cases. J Am Acad Dermatol 1987; 16: 991–993.

614 García-Hernández MJ, Rodríquez-Pichardo A, Camacho F. Congenital triangular alopecia (Brauer nevus). Pediatr Dermatol 1995; 12: 301–303.

615 Trakimas C, Sperling LC, Skelton HG III et al. Clinical and histologic findings in temporal triangular alopecia. J Am Acad Dermatol 1994; 31: 205–209.

616 Trakimas CA, Sperling LC. Temporal triangular alopecia acquired in adulthood. J Am Acad Dermatol 1999; 40: 842–844.

617 Ruggieri M, Rizzo R, Pavone P et al. Temporal triangular alopecia in association with mental retardation and epilepsy in a mother and daughter. Arch Dermatol 2000; 136: 426–427.

618 Kim H, Park KB, Yang JM et al. Congenital triangular alopecia in phakomatosis pigmentovascularis: report of 3 cases. Acta Derm Venereol 2000; 80: 215–216.

Anagen defluvium

619 Hamm H, Traupe H. Loose anagen hair of childhood: the phenomenon of easily pluckable hair. J Am Acad Dermatol 1989; 20: 242–248.

620 Price VH, Gummer CL. Loose anagen syndrome. J Am Acad Dermatol 1989; 20: 249–256.

621 O'Donnell BP, Sperling LC, James WD. Loose anagen hair syndrome. Int J Dermatol 1992; 31: 107–109.

622 Baden HP, Kvedar JC, Magro CM. Loose anagen hair as a cause of hereditary hair loss in children. Arch Dermatol 1992; 128: 1349–1353.

623 Haskett M. Loose anagen syndrome. Australas J Dermatol 1995; 36: 35–36.

624 Nunez J, Grande K, Hsu S. Alopecia areata with features of loose anagen hair. Pediatr Dermatol 1999; 16: 460–462.

625 Tosti A, Peluso AM, Misciali C et al. Loose anagen hair. Arch Dermatol 1997; 133: 1089–1093.

626 Chapman DM, Miller RA. An objective measurement of the anchoring strength of anagen hair in an adult with the loose anagen hair syndrome. J Cutan Pathol 1996; 23: 288–292.

627 Rook A, Dawber R. Diseases of the hair and scalp. Oxford: Blackwell Scientific Publications, 1982; 133–145.

628 Stroud JD. Drug-induced alopecia. Semin Dermatol 1985; 4: 29–34.

629 Pillans PI, Woods DJ. Drug-associated alopecia. Int J Dermatol 1995; 34: 149–158.
630 Tran D, Sinclair RD, Schwarer AP, Chow CW. Permanent alopecia following chemotherapy and bone marrow transplantation. Australas J Dermatol 2000; 41: 106–108.
631 Swee W, Klontz KC, Lambert LA. A nationwide outbreak of alopecia associated with the use of a hair-relaxing formulation. Arch Dermatol 2000; 136: 1104–1108.
632 Feldman J, Levisohn DR. Acute alopecia: clue to thallium toxicity. Pediatr Dermatol 1993; 10: 29–31.
633 Tromme I, Van Neste D, Dobbelaere F et al. Skin signs in the diagnosis of thallium poisoning. Br J Dermatol 1998; 138: 321–325.
634 Nicholson AG, Harland CC, Bull RH et al. Chemically induced cosmetic alopecia. Br J Dermatol 1993; 128: 537–541.
635 Levantine A, Almeyda J. Drug induced alopecia. Br J Dermatol 1973; 89: 549–553.
636 Maceyko RF, Vidimos AT, Steck WD. Vasopressin-associated cutaneous infarcts, alopecia, and neuropathy. J Am Acad Dermatol 1994; 31: 111–113.
637 Beckett WS, Oskvig R, Gaynor ME, Goldgeier MH. Association of reversible alopecia with occupational topical exposure to common borax-containing solutions. J Am Acad Dermatol 2001; 44: 599–602.
638 Lang AM, Norland AM, Schuneman RL, Tope WD. Localized interferon alfa-2b-induced alopecia. Arch Dermatol 1999; 135: 1126–1128.

Scarring alopecias

639 Sehgal VN, Srivastva G, Bajaj P. Cicatricial (scarring) alopecia. Int J Dermatol 2001; 40: 241–248.
640 Rook A, Dawber R. Diseases of the hair and scalp. Oxford: Blackwell Scientific Publications, 1982; 307–341.
641 Stenn KS, Sundberg JP, Sperling LC. Hair follicle biology, the sebaceous gland, and scarring alopecias. Arch Dermatol 1999; 135: 973–974.
642 Toutos-Trellu L, Chavaz P, Piletta P. Cicatricial alopecia following therapeutic embolization. Acta Derm Venereol 1999; 79: 236–237.
643 Sperling LC, Solomon AR, Whiting DA. A new look at scarring alopecia. Arch Dermatol 2000; 136: 235–242.
644 Sullivan JR, Kossard S. Acquired scalp alopecia. Part II: A review. Australas J Dermatol 1999; 40: 61–72.
645 Mahé A. Scarring alopecia and ethnicity. Arch Dermatol 2001; 137: 374–375.
646 Powell J, Dawber RPR. Folliculitis decalvans and tufted folliculitis are specific infective diseases that may lead to scarring, but are not a subset of central centrifugal scarring alopecia. Arch Dermatol 2001; 137: 373.
647 Roenigk RK, Wheeland RG. Tissue expansion in cicatricial alopecia. Arch Dermatol 1987; 123: 641–646.
648 Collier PM, James MP. Pseudopelade of Brocq occurring in two brothers in childhood. Clin Exp Dermatol 1994; 19: 61–64.
649 Nayar M, Schomberg K, Dawber RPR, Millard PR. A clinicopathological study of scarring alopecia. Br J Dermatol 1993; 128: 533–536.
650 Sahl WJ. Pseudopelade: an inherited alopecia. Int J Dermatol 1996; 35: 715–719.
651 Ronchese F. Pseudopelade. Arch Dermatol 1960; 82: 336–343.
652 Dawber R. What is pseudopelade? Clin Exp Dermatol 1992; 17: 305–306.
653 Madani S, Trotter MJ, Shapiro J. Pseudopelade of Brocq in beard area. J Am Acad Dermatol 2000; 42: 895–896.
654 Templeton SF, Solomon AR. Scarring alopecia: a classification based on microscopic criteria. J Cutan Pathol 1994; 21: 97–109.
655 Piérard-Franchimont C, Piérard GE. Massive lymphocyte-mediated apoptosis during the early stage of pseudopelade. Dermatologica 1986; 172: 254–257.
656 Elston DM, McCollough ML, Warschaw KE, Bergfeld WF. Elastic tissue in scars and alopecia. J Cutan Pathol 2000; 27: 147–152.
657 Jordon RE. Subtle clues to diagnosis by immunopathology. Scarring alopecia. Am J Dermatopathol 1980; 2: 157–159.
658 Sperling LC, Skelton HG III, Smith KJ et al. Follicular degeneration syndrome in men. Arch Dermatol 1994; 130: 763–769.
659 Sperling LC, Sau P. The follicular degeneration syndrome in black patients. 'Hot comb alopecia' revisited and revised. Arch Dermatol 1992; 128: 68–74.
660 Kossard S. Postmenopausal frontal fibrosing alopecia. Scarring alopecia in a pattern distribution. Arch Dermatol 1994; 130: 770–774.
661 Camacho Martínez F, García-Hernández MJ, Mazuecos Blanca J. Postmenopausal frontal fibrosing alopecia. Br J Dermatol 1999; 140: 1181–1182.
662 Kossard S, Lee M-S, Wilkinson B. Postmenopausal frontal fibrosing alopecia: A frontal variant of lichen planopilaris. J Am Acad Dermatol 1997; 36: 59–66.
663 Zinkernagel MS, Trüeb RM. Fibrosing alopecia in a pattern distribution. Patterned lichen planopilaris or androgenetic alopecia with a lichenoid tissue reaction pattern? Arch Dermatol 2000; 136: 205–211.

664 Dalziel KL, Telfer NR, Wilson CL, Dawber RPR. Tufted folliculitis. A specific bacterial disease? Am J Dermatopathol 1990; 12: 37–41.
665 Tong AKF, Baden HP. Tufted folliculitis. J Am Acad Dermatol 1989; 21: 1096–1099.
666 Luelmo-Aguilar J, Gonzalez-Castro U, Castells-Rodellas A. Tufted hair folliculitis. A study of four cases. Br J Dermatol 1993; 128: 454–457.
667 Petronić-Rosić V, Krunić A, Mijušković M, Vesić S. Tufted hair folliculitis: A pattern of scarring alopecia? J Am Acad Dermatol 1999; 41: 112–114.
668 Saijyo S, Tagami H. Tufted hair folliculitis developing in a recalcitrant lesion of pemphigus vulgaris. J Am Acad Dermatol 1998; 39: 857–859.
669 Pujol RM, Matias-Guíu X, Garcia-Patos V, de Moragas JM. Tufted-hair folliculitis. Clin Exp Dermatol 1991; 16: 199–201.

Miscellaneous alopecias

670 Fair KP, Knoell KA, Patterson JW. Lipedematous alopecia: a clinicopathologic, histologic and ultrastructural study. J Cutan Pathol 2000; 27: 49–53.
671 Ikejima A, Yamashita M, Ikeda S, Ogawa H. A case of lipedematous alopecia occurring in a male patient. Dermatology 2000; 201: 168–170.
672 Kane KS, Kwan T, Baden HP. Woman with new-onset boggy scalp. Arch Dermatol 1998; 134: 499–504.

Pilosebaceous disorders

673 Fenton DA. Hypertrichosis. Semin Dermatol 1985; 4: 58–67.
674 Leung AKC, Robson WLM. Hirsutism. Int J Dermatol 1993; 32: 773–777.
675 Lee IJ, Im SB, Kim D-K. Hypertrichosis universalis congenita: a separate entity, or the same disease as gingival fibromatosis? Pediatr Dermatol 1993; 10: 263–266.
676 Judge MR, Khaw PT, Rice NSC et al. Congenital hypertrichosis lanuginosa and congenital glaucoma. Br J Dermatol 1991; 124: 495–497.
677 Sindhuphak W, Vibhagool A. Acquired hypertrichosis lanuginosa. Int J Dermatol 1982; 21: 599–601.
678 Jemec GBE. Hypertrichosis lanuginosa acquisita. Report of a case and review of the literature. Arch Dermatol 1986; 122: 805–808.
679 Goodfellow A, Calvert H, Bohn G. Hypertrichosis lanuginosa acquisita. Br J Dermatol 1980; 103: 431–433.
680 Pérez-Losada E, Pujol RM, Domingo P et al. Hypertrichosis lanuginosa acquisita preceding extraskeletal Ewing's sarcoma. Clin Exp Dermatol 2001; 26: 182–183.
681 González M, Landa N, Gardeazabal J et al. Generalized hypertrichosis after treatment with topical minoxidil. Clin Exp Dermatol 1994; 19: 157–158.
682 Kassis V, Sondergaard J. Hypertrichosis lanuginosa. Semin Dermatol 1984; 3: 282–286.
683 Cox NH, McClure JP, Hardie RA. Naevoid hypertrichosis – report of a patient with multiple lesions. Clin Exp Dermatol 1989; 14: 62–64.
684 Harris HW, Miller OF. Midline cutaneous and spinal defects. Midline cutaneous abnormalities associated with occult spinal disorders. Arch Dermatol 1976; 112: 1724–1728.
685 Schauder S, Hanefeld F, Noske UM, Zoll B. Depigmented hypertrichosis following Blaschko's lines associated with cerebral and ocular malformations: a new neurocutaneous, autosomal lethal gene syndrome from the group of epidermal naevus syndromes? Br J Dermatol 2000; 142: 1204–1207.
686 Kubota Y, Ishii T, Sugihara H et al. Skin manifestations of a patient with mitochondrial encephalomyopathy with lactic acidosis and strokelike episodes (MELAS syndrome). J Am Acad Dermatol 1999; 41: 469–473.
687 Tisocco LA, del Campo DV, Bennin B, Barsky S. Acquired localized hypertrichosis. Arch Dermatol 1981; 117: 127–128.
688 Hegedus SI, Schorr WF. Acquired hypertrichosis lanuginosa and malignancy. Arch Dermatol 1972; 106: 84–88.
689 Barth JH, Wojnarowska F, Dawber RPR. Is keratosis pilaris another androgen-dependent dermatosis? Clin Exp Dermatol 1988; 13: 240–241.
690 Yosipovitch G, Mevorah B, Mashiach J et al. High body mass index, dry scaly leg skin and atopic conditions are highly associated with keratosis pilaris. Dermatology 2000; 201: 34–36.
691 Poskitt L, Wilkinson JD. Natural history of keratosis pilaris. Br J Dermatol 1994; 130: 711–713.
692 Wakelin SH, Lipscombe T, Orton DI, Marren P. Lithium-induced follicular hyperkeratosis. Clin Exp Dermatol 1996; 21: 296–298.
693 Garcia-Bravo B, Rodriguez-Pichardo A, Camacho F. Uraemic follicular hyperkeratosis. Clin Exp Dermatol 1985; 10: 448–454.
694 Ostlere LS, Ashrafzadeh P, Harris D, Rustin MHA. Response of uremic follicular hyperkeratosis to peritoneal dialysis. J Am Acad Dermatol 1992; 26: 782–783.
695 Ibbotson SH, Simpson NB, Fyfe NCM, Lawrence CM. Follicular keratoses at amputation sites. Br J Dermatol 1994; 130: 770–772.

696 Kim TY, Park YM, Jang IG et al. Idiopathic follicular hyperkeratotic spicules. J Am Acad Dermatol 1997; 36: 476–477.

697 Shimizu S, Shimizu T, Tateishi Y, Shimizu H. Keratosis follicularis squamosa (Dohi): a follicular keratotic disorder well known in Japan. Br J Dermatol 2001; 144: 1070–1072.

698 Oranje AP, Molewaterplein Dr, van Osch LDM, Oosterwijk JC. Keratosis pilaris atrophicans. One heterogeneous disease or a symptom in different clinical entities? Arch Dermatol 1994; 130: 500–502.

699 Zouboulis ChC, Stratakis CA, Rinck G et al. Ulerythema ophryogenes and keratosis pilaris in a child with monosomy 18p. Pediatr Dermatol 1994; 11: 172–175.

700 Burnett JW, Schwartz MF, Berberian BJ. Ulerythema ophryogenes with multiple congenital anomalies. J Am Acad Dermatol 1988; 18: 437–440.

701 McHenry PM, Nevin NC, Bingham EA. The association of keratosis pilaris atrophicans with hereditary woolly hair. Pediatr Dermatol 1990; 7: 202–204.

702 Schepis C, Greco D, Romano C. Cardiofaciocutaneous (CFC) syndrome. Australas J Dermatol 1999; 40: 111–113.

703 Drolet BA, Baselga E, Esterly NB. What syndrome is this? [cardio-facio-cutaneous (CFC) syndrome]. Pediatr Dermatol 2000; 17: 231–234.

704 Centeno PG, Rosón E, Peteiro C et al. Rubinstein–Taybi syndrome and ulerythema ophryogenes in a 9-year-old boy. Pediatr Dermatol 1999; 16: 134–136.

705 Pierini DO, Pierini AM. Keratosis pilaris atrophicans faciei (ulerythema ophryogenes): a cutaneous marker in the Noonan syndrome. Br J Dermatol 1979; 100: 409–416.

706 Snell JA, Mallory SB. Ulerythema ophryogenes in Noonan syndrome. Pediatr Dermatol 1990; 7: 77–78.

707 Neild VS, Pegum JS, Wells RS. The association of keratosis pilaris atrophicans and woolly hair, with and without Noonan's syndrome. Br J Dermatol 1984; 110: 357–362.

708 Markey AC, Tidman MJ, Sharvill DE, Wells RS. Ulerythema ophryogenes in Noonan's syndrome. Br J Dermatol (Suppl) 1988; 33: 114.

709 Zouboulis CC, Stratakis CA, Gollnick HPM, Orfanos CE. Keratosis pilaris/ulerythema ophryogenes and 18p deletion: is it possible that the *LAMA1* gene is involved? J Med Genet 2001; 38: 127–128.

710 Rand R, Baden HP. Keratosis follicularis spinulosa decalvans. Report of two cases and literature review. Arch Dermatol 1983; 119: 22–26.

711 Drago F, Maietta G, Parodi A, Rebora A. Keratosis pilaris decalvans non-atrophicans. Clin Exp Dermatol 1993; 18: 45–46.

712 Herd RM, Benton EC. Keratosis follicularis spinulosa decalvans: report of a new pedigree. Br J Dermatol 1996; 134: 138–142.

713 Appell ML, Sherertz EF. A kindred with alopecia, keratosis pilaris, cataracts, and psoriasis. J Am Acad Dermatol 1987; 16: 89–95.

714 Kunte C, Loeser C, Wolff H. Folliculitis spinulosa decalvans: successful therapy with dapsone. J Am Acad Dermatol 1998; 39: 891–893.

715 Rozum LT, Mehregan AH, Johnson SAM. Folliculitis ulerythematosa reticulata. A case with unilateral lesions. Arch Dermatol 1972; 106: 388–389.

716 Nico MMS, Sakai Valente NY, Sotto MN. Folliculitis ulerythematosa reticulata (atrophoderma vermiculata): early detection of a case with unilateral lesions. Pediatr Dermatol 1998; 15: 285–286.

717 Frosch PJ, Brumage MR, Schuster-Pavlovic C, Bersch A. Atrophoderma vermiculatum. Case reports and review. J Am Acad Dermatol 1988; 18: 538–542.

718 Weightman W. A case of atrophoderma vermiculatum responding to isotretinoin. Clin Exp Dermatol 1998; 23: 89–91.

719 Hsu S, Nikko A. Unilateral atrophic skin lesion with features of atrophoderma vermiculatum: A variant of the epidermal nevus syndrome? J Am Acad Dermatol 2000; 43: 310–312.

720 Handrick C, Alster TS. Laser treatment of atrophoderma vermiculata. J Am Acad Dermatol 2001; 44: 693–695.

721 Cambiaghi S, Restano L, Tadini G. Atrophoderma vermiculata along Blaschko lines. Pediatr Dermatol 1999; 16: 165.

722 Sidwell RU, Harper JI. Vermiculate atrophoderma in a boy with Marfan syndrome. Br J Dermatol 1999; 141: 750–752.

723 Seville RH, Mumford PF. Congenital ectodermal defect. Atrophodermia vermicularis with leukokeratosis oris. Br J Dermatol 1956; 68: 310.

724 Michaelsson G, Olsson E, Westermark P. The ROMBO syndrome: a familial disorder with vermiculate atrophoderma, milia, hypotrichosis, trichoepitheliomas, basal cell carcinomas and peripheral vasodilation with cyanosis. Acta Derm Venereol 1981; 61: 497–503.

725 van Steensel MAM, Jaspers NGJ, Steijlen PM. A case of ROMBO syndrome. Br J Dermatol 2001; 144: 1215–1218.

726 Marks VJ, Miller OF. Atrophia maculosa varioliformis cutis. Br J Dermatol 1986; 115: 105–109.

727 Venencie PY, Foldes C, Cuny M et al. Atrophia maculosa varioliformis cutis with extrahepatic biliary atresia. J Am Acad Dermatol 1989; 21: 309.

728 Kolenik SA, Perez MI, Davidson DM et al. Atrophia maculosa varioliformis cutis. Report of two cases and review of the literature. J Am Acad Dermatol 1994; 30: 837–840.

729 Inoue Y, Ono T, Kayashima K, Johno M. Hereditary perioral pigmented follicular atrophoderma associated with milia and epidermoid cysts. Br J Dermatol 1998; 139: 713–718.

730 Andersen BL. Erythromelanosis follicularis faciei et colli. Br J Dermatol 1980; 102: 323–325.

731 Whittaker SJ, Griffiths WAD. Erythromelanosis follicularis faciei et colli. Clin Exp Dermatol 1987; 12: 33–35.

732 Watt TL, Kaiser JS. Erythromelanosis follicularis faciei et colli. J Am Acad Dermatol 1981; 5: 533–534.

733 Yañez S, Velasco JA, Gonzalez MP. Familial erythromelanosis follicularis faciei et colli – an autosomal recessive mode of inheritance. Clin Exp Dermatol 1993; 18: 283–285.

734 McGillis ST, Tuthill RJ, Ratz JL, Richards SW. Unilateral erythromelanosis follicularis faciei et colli in a young girl. J Am Acad Dermatol 1991; 25: 430–432.

735 Sodaify M, Baghestani S, Handjani F, Sotoodeh M. Erythromelanosis follicularis faciei et colli. Int J Dermatol 1994; 33: 643–644.

736 Warren FM, Davis LS. Erythromelanosis follicularis faciei in women. J Am Acad Dermatol 1995; 32: 863–866.

737 Juhlin L, Alkemade H. Erythrosis pigmentosa mediofacialis (Brocq) and erythromelanosis follicularis faciei et colli in the same patient. Acta Derm Venereol 1999; 79: 65–66.

738 Kim MG. Hong SJ, Son SJ et al. Quantitative histopathologic findings of erythromelanosis follicularis faciei et colli. J Cutan Pathol 2001; 28: 160–164.

739 Tüzün Y, Wolf R, Tüzün B et al. Familial erythromelanosis follicularis and chromosomal instability. J Eur Acad Dermatol Venereol 2001; 15: 150–152.

740 Davenport DD. Ulerythema ophryogenes. Arch Dermatol 1964; 89: 74–80.

741 Baden HP, Byers HR. Clinical findings, cutaneous pathology, and response to therapy in 21 patients with keratosis pilaris atrophicans. Arch Dermatol 1994; 130: 469–475.

742 Bork K, Bockers M, Pfeifle J. Pathogenesis of paraneoplastic follicular hyperkeratotic spicules in multiple myeloma. Arch Dermatol 1990; 126: 509–513.

743 Requena L, Sarasa JL, Masllorens FO et al. Follicular spicules of the nose: a peculiar cutaneous manifestation of multiple myeloma with cryoglobulinemia. J Am Acad Dermatol 1995; 32: 834–839.

744 Friedman SJ. Lichen spinulosus. Clinicopathologic review of thirty-five cases. J Am Acad Dermatol 1990; 22: 261–264.

745 Cohen SJ, Dicken CH. Generalized lichen spinulosus in an HIV-positive man. J Am Acad Dermatol 1991; 25: 116–118.

746 Kano Y, Orihara M, Yagita A, Shiohara T. Lichen spinulosus in a patient with Crohn's disease. Int J Dermatol 1995; 34: 670–671.

747 Ayres S Jr. Extrafacial rosacea is rare but does exist. J Am Acad Dermatol 1987; 16: 391–392.

748 Rebora A. Rosacea. J Invest Dermatol (Suppl) 1987; 88: 56s–60s.

749 Marks R, Wilson Jones E. Disseminated rosacea. Br J Dermatol 1969; 81: 16–28.

750 Wilkin JK. Rosacea. Int J Dermatol 1983; 22: 393–400.

751 Wilkin JK. Rosacea. Pathophysiology and treatment. Arch Dermatol 1994; 130: 359–362.

752 Quaterman MJ, Johnson DW, Abele DC et al. Ocular rosacea. Signs, symptoms, and tear studies before and after treatment with doxycycline. Arch Dermatol 1997; 133: 49–54.

753 Drolet B, Paller AS. Childhood rosacea. Pediatr Dermatol 1992; 9: 22–26.

754 Rosen T, Stone MS. Acne rosacea in blacks. J Am Acad Dermatol 1987; 17: 70–73.

755 Dotz W, Berliner N. Rhinophyma. A master's depiction, a patron's affliction. Am J Dermatopathol 1984; 6: 231–235.

756 Roihu T, Kariniemi A-L. *Demodex* mites in acne rosacea. J Cutan Pathol 1998; 25: 550–552.

757 Erbaĝci Z, Özgöztaşi O. The significance of *Demodex folliculorum* density in rosacea. Int J Dermatol 1998; 37: 421–425.

758 Findlay GH, Simson IW. Leonine hypertrophic rosacea associated with a benign bronchial carcinoid tumour. Clin Exp Dermatol 1977; 2: 175–176.

759 Sibenge S, Gawkrodger DJ. Rosacea: a study of clinical patterns, blood flow, and the role of *Demodex folliculorum*. J Am Acad Dermatol 1992; 26: 590–593.

760 Forton F, Seys B. Density of *Demodex folliculorum* in rosacea: a case-control study using standardized skin-surface biopsy. Br J Dermatol 1993; 128: 650–659.

761 Wilkin JK. Vasodilator rosacea. Arch Dermatol 1980; 116: 598.

762 Sanchez-Viera M, Hernanz JM, Sampelayo T et al. Granulomatous rosacea in a child infected with the human immunodeficiency virus. J Am Acad Dermatol 1992; 27: 1010–1011.

763 Leyden JJ, Thew M, Kligman AM. Steroid rosacea. Arch Dermatol 1974; 110: 619–622.

764 Egan CA, Rallis TM, Meadows KP, Krueger GG. Rosacea induced by beclomethasone dipropionate nasal spray. Int J Dermatol 1999; 38: 133–134.

765 Vin-Christian K, Maurer TA, Berger TG. Acne rosacea as a cutaneous manifestation of HIV infection. J Am Acad Dermatol 1994; 30: 139–140.

766 Rojo-García JM, Muñoz-Pérez MA, Escudero J et al. *Helicobacter pylori* in rosacea and chronic urticaria. Acta Derm Venereol 2000; 80: 156–157.

767 Rebora A, Drago F. *Helicobacter pylori* and rosacea. J Am Acad Dermatol 2000; 43: 884.

768 Bamford JTM, Tilden RL, Blankush JL, Gangeness DE. Effect of treatment of Helicobacter pylori infection on rosacea. Arch Dermatol 1999; 135: 659–663.

769 Son SW, Kim IH, Oh CH, Kim JG. The response of rosacea to eradication of *Helicobacter pylori*. Br J Dermatol 1999; 140: 984–985.

770 Bamford JTM, Tilden RL, Gangeness DE. Does *Helicobacter pylori* eradication treatment reduce the severity of rosacea? J Am Acad Dermatol 2000; 42: 535.

771 Utaş S, Özbakir Ö, Turasan A, Utaş C. *Helicobacter pylori* eradication treatment reduces the severity of rosacea. J Am Acad Dermatol 1999; 40: 433–435.

772 Powell FC. What's going on in rosacea? J Eur Acad Dermatol Venereol 2000; 14: 351–352.

773 Rebora AE. *Helicobacter pylori* and rosacea. J Eur Acad Dermatol Venereol 2000; 14: 344.

774 Strauss JS. Some thoughts on rosacea. J Eur Acad Dermatol Venereol 2000; 14: 345.

775 Marks R, Black MM. Perioral dermatitis. A histopathological study of 26 cases. Br J Dermatol 1971; 84: 242–247.

776 Cotterill JA. Perioral dermatitis. Br J Dermatol 1979; 101: 259–262.

777 Wilkinson DS, Kirton V, Wilkinson JD. Perioral dermatitis: a 12-year review. Br J Dermatol 1979; 101: 245–257.

778 Wilkinson D. What is perioral dermatitis? Int J Dermatol 1981; 20: 485–486.

779 Manders SM, Lucky AW. Perioral dermatitis in childhood. J Am Acad Dermatol 1992; 27: 688–692.

780 Boeck K, Abeck D, Werfel S, Ring J. Perioral dermatitis in children – clinical presentation, pathogenesis-related factors and response to topical metronidazole. Dermatology 1997; 195: 235–238.

781 Ward KA, Harris SC. Isolated periocular 'dermatitis'. Br J Dermatol 1999; 141: 593.

782 Chen DM, Crosby DL. Periorbital edema as an initial presentation of rosacea. J Am Acad Dermatol 1997; 37: 346–348.

783 Griffiths WAD. The red face – an overview and delineation of the MARSH syndrome. Clin Exp Dermatol 1999; 24: 42–47.

784 Marks R, Harcourt-Webster JN. Histopathology of rosacea. Arch Dermatol 1969; 100: 683–691.

785 Rhodes LE, Parslew RAG, Ashworth J. Outcome of facial rashes with non-specific histological features: a long-term follow-up of 64 cases. J Cutan Pathol 1995; 22: 160–163.

786 Mullanax MG, Kierland RR. Granulomatous rosacea. Arch Dermatol 1970; 101: 206–211.

787 Helm KF, Menz J, Gibson LE, Dicken CH. A clinical and histopathologic study of granulomatous rosacea. J Am Acad Dermatol 1991; 25: 1038–1043.

788 Acker DW, Helwig EB. Rhinophyma with carcinoma. Arch Dermatol 1967; 95: 250–254.

789 Tope WD, Sanguaza OP. Rhinophyma's fibrous variant. Histopathology and immunohistochemistry. Am J Dermatopathol 1994; 16: 307–310.

790 Aloi F, Tomasini C, Soro E, Pippione M. The clinicopathologic spectrum of rhinophyma. J Am Acad Dermatol 2000; 42: 468–472.

791 Nunzi E, Rebora A, Hamerlinck F, Cormane RH. Immunopathological studies on rosacea. Br J Dermatol 1980; 103: 543–551.

792 Manna V, Marks R, Holt P. Involvement of immune mechanisms in the pathogenesis of rosacea. Br J Dermatol 1982; 107: 203–208.

793 Jansen T, Plewig G. An historical note on pyoderma faciale. Br J Dermatol 1993; 129: 594–596.

794 Plewig G, Jansen T, Kligman AM. Pyoderma faciale. A review and report of 20 additional cases: is it rosacea? Arch Dermatol 1992; 128: 1611–1617.

795 Firooz A, Firoozabadi MR, Dowlati Y. Rosacea fulminans (pyoderma faciale): successful treatment of a 3-year-old girl with oral isotretinoin. Int J Dermatol 2001; 40: 203–205.

796 Romiti R, Jansen T, Heldwein W, Plewig G. Rosacea fulminans in a patient with Crohn's disease: a case report and review of the literature. Acta Derm Venereol 2000; 80: 127–129.

797 Dessoukey MW, Omar MF, Dayem HA. Pyoderma faciale: manifestation of inflammatory bowel disease. Int J Dermatol 1996; 35: 724–726.

798 Jansen T, Plewig G. Fulminating rosacea conglobata (rosacea fulminans) and ulcerative colitis. Br J Dermatol 1997; 137: 830–831.

799 Buezo GF, Fernández JF, Tello ED, Díez AG. Squamous metaplasia of sebaceous gland. J Cutan Pathol 2000; 27: 298–300.

800 Renfro L, Kopf AW, Gutterman A et al. Neutrophilic sebaceous adenitis. Arch Dermatol 1993; 129: 910–911.

801 Martins C, Tellechea O, Mariano A, Baptista AP. Sebaceous adenitis. J Am Acad Dermatol 1997; 36: 845–846.

802 Jappe U, Franke I, Reinhold D, Gollnick HPM. Sebotropic drug reaction resulting from kava-kava extract therapy: A new entity? J Am Acad Dermatol 1998; 38: 104–106.

803 Agarwal S, Charles-Holmes S. Nasolabial follicular sebaceous casts: a novel complication of isotretinoin therapy. Br J Dermatol 2000; 143: 228–229.

804 Plewig G. Nasolabial follicular sebaceous casts: a novel complication of isotretinoin therapy. Br J Dermatol 2001; 144: 919.

Apocrine disorders

805 MacMillan DC, Vickers HR. Fox–Fordyce disease. Br J Dermatol 1971; 84: 181.

806 Giacobetti R, Caro WA, Roenigk HH Jr. Fox–Fordyce disease. Control with tretinoin cream. Arch Dermatol 1979; 115: 1365–1366.

807 Graham JH, Shafer JC, Helwig EB. Fox–Fordyce disease in male identical twins. Arch Dermatol 1960; 82: 212–221.

808 Effendy I, Ossowski B, Happle R. Fox–Fordyce disease in a male patient – response to oral retinoid treatment. Clin Exp Dermatol 1994; 19: 67–69.

809 Carleton AB, Hall GS, Wigley JEM, Symmers W St C. Cited in Systemic pathology, 2nd ed. Edinburgh: Churchill Livingstone, 1980; 6: 26–36.

810 Patrizi A, Orlandi C, Neri I et al. Fox–Fordyce disease: two cases in patients with Turner syndrome. Acta Derm Venereol 1999; 79: 83–84.

811 Montes LF, Cortes A, Baker BL, Curtis AC. Fox–Fordyce disease. A report with endocrinological and histopathological studies, of a case which developed after surgical menopause. Arch Dermatol 1959; 80: 549–553.

812 Stashower ME, Krivda SJ, Turiansky GW. Fox–Fordyce disease: Diagnosis with transverse histologic sections. J Am Acad Dermatol 2000; 42: 89–91.

813 Mali-Gerrits MMG, van de Kerkhof PCM, Mier PD, Happle R. Axillary apocrine chromhidrosis. Arch Dermatol 1988; 124: 494–496.

814 Saff DM, Owens R, Kahn TA. Apocrine chromhidrosis involving the areolae in a 15-year-old amateur figure skater. Pediatr Dermatol 1995; 12: 48–50.

815 Cilliers J, de Beer C. The case of the red lingerie – chromhidrosis revisited. Dermatology 1999; 199: 149–152.

816 Thami GP, Kanwar AJ. Red facial pseudochromhidrosis. Br J Dermatol 2000; 142: 1219–1220.

Eccrine disorders

817 Ghali FE, Fine J-D. Idiopathic localized unilateral hyperhidrosis in a child. Pediatr Dermatol 2000; 17: 25–28.

818 Köse O, Baloglu H. Idiopathic unilateral circumscribed hyperhidrosis. Int J Dermatol 1997; 36: 209–210.

819 Naumann M, Hofmann U, Bergmann I et al. Focal hyperhidrosis. Effective treatment with intracutaneous botulinum toxin. Arch Dermatol 1998; 134: 301–304.

820 Leung AKC, Chan PYH, Choi MCK. Hyperhidrosis. Int J Dermatol 1999; 38: 561–567.

821 Boyvat A, Pişkin G, Erdi H. Idiopathic unilateral localized hyperhidrosis. Acta Derm Venereol 1999; 79: 404–405.

822 Kaddu S, Smolle J, Komericki P, Kerl H. Auriculotemporal (Frey) syndrome in late childhood: an unusual variant presenting as gustatory flushing mimicking food allergy. Pediatr Dermatol 2000; 17: 126–128.

823 Mehregan AH. Proliferation of sweat ducts in certain diseases of the skin. Am J Dermatopathol 1981; 3: 27–31.

824 Santa Cruz DJ, Clausen K. Atypical sweat duct hyperplasia accompanying keratoacanthoma. Dermatologica 1977; 154: 156–160.

825 Weedon D. Eccrine tumors: a selective review. J Cutan Pathol 1984; 11: 421–436.

826 Lerner TH, Barr RJ, Dolezal JF, Stagnone JJ. Syringomatous hyperplasia and eccrine squamous syringometaplasia associated with benoxaprofen therapy. Arch Dermatol 1987; 123: 1202–1204.

827 Vakilzadeh F, Brocker EB. Syringolymphoid hyperplasia with alopecia. Br J Dermatol 1984; 110: 95–101.

828 Kossard S, Munro V, King R. Syringolymphoid hyperplasia with alopecia. J Cutan Pathol 1988; 15: 322 (abstract).

829 Tomaszewski M-M, Lupton GP, Krishnan J et al. Syringolymphoid hyperplasia with alopecia. J Cutan Pathol 1994; 21: 520–526.

830 Tannous Z, Baldassano MF, Li VW et al. Syringolymphoid hyperplasia and follicular mucinosis in a patient with cutaneous T-cell lymphoma. J Am Acad Dermatol 1999; 41: 303–308.

831 Esche C, Sander CA, Zumdick M et al. Further evidence that syringolymphoid hyperplasia with alopecia is a cutaneous T-cell lymphoma. Arch Dermatol 1998; 134: 753–754.

832 Barnhill RL, Goldberg B, Stenn KS. Proliferation of eccrine sweat ducts associated with alopecia areata. J Cutan Pathol 1988; 15: 36–39.

833 Huang C-L, Kuo T-t, Chan H-L. Acquired generalized hypohidrosis/anhidrosis with subclinical Sjögren's syndrome: Report of a case with diffuse syringolymphoid hyperplasia and lymphocytic sialadenitis. J Am Acad Dermatol 1996; 35: 350–352.

834 Sais G, Admella C, Fantova MJ, Montero JC. Lymphocytic autoimmune hidradenitis, cutaneous leucocytoclastic vasculitis and primary Sjögren's syndrome . Br J Dermatol 1998; 139: 1073–1076.

835 Burket JM, Brooks R, Burket DA. Eccrine gland reticulated cytoplasm. J Am Acad Dermatol 1985; 13: 497–500.

836 Holyoke JB, Lobitz WC Jr. Histologic variations in the structure of human eccrine sweat glands. J Invest Dermatol 1952; 18: 147–167.

837 Izaki S, Kono E, Hirai A, Kitamura K. Eruptive clear cell hamartoma of sweat duct. J Cutan Pathol 1994; 21: 271–273.

838 Signoretti S, Annessi G, Occhiuto S et al. Papular clear cell hyperplasia of the eccrine duct in a diabetic. Br J Dermatol 1996; 135: 139–143.

839 Serrano T, Saez A, Moreno A. Eccrine squamous syringometaplasia. J Cutan Pathol 1993; 20: 61–65.

840 Wenzel FG, Horn TD. Nonneoplastic disorders of the eccrine glands. J Am Acad Dermatol 1998; 38: 1–17.

841 Leshin B, White WL, Koufman JA. Radiation-induced squamous sialometaplasia. Arch Dermatol 1990; 126: 931–934.

842 Rios-Buceta L, Peñas PF, Daudén-Tello E et al. Recall phenomenon with the unusual presence of eccrine squamous syringometaplasia. Br J Dermatol 1995; 133: 630–632.

843 Sommer B, Hagedorn M, Wood F, Heenan P. Eccrine squamous syringometaplasia in the skin of children after burns. J Cutan Pathol 1998; 25: 56–58.

844 Freeman RG. On the pathogenesis of pseudoepitheliomatous hyperplasia. J Cutan Pathol 1974; 1: 231–237.

845 King DT, Barr RJ. Syringometaplasia: mucinous and squamous variants. J Cutan Pathol 1979; 6: 284–291.

846 Jerasutus S, Laohabhan K, Suvanprakorn P. Primary squamous syringometaplasia with no underlying malignancy. Int J Dermatol 1999; 38: 375–376.

847 Helton JL, Metcalf JS. Squamous syringometaplasia in association with annular elastolytic granuloma. Am J Dermatopathol 1995; 17: 407–409.

848 Muñoz E, Valks R, Fernández-Herrera J, Fraga J. Herpetic syringitis associated with eccrine squamous syringometaplasia in HIV-positive patients. J Cutan Pathol 1997; 24: 425–428.

849 Choi SW, Yang JE, Kang SJ et al. Herpetic infection on the vulva associated with eccrine squamous syringometaplasia in malignant lymphoma. Acta Derm Venereol 1999; 79: 500–501.

850 Chetty R, Bramdev A, Govender D. Cytomegalovirus-induced syringosquamous metaplasia. Am J Dermatopathol 1999; 21: 487–490.

851 Daudén E, Porras JI, Buezo GF, García-Díez A. Eccrine squamous syringometaplasia and cytomegalovirus. Am J Dermatopathol 2000; 22: 559–560.

852 Vargas-Díez E, Valks R, Fraga J et al. Eccrine squamous syringometaplasia in a patient with phytophotodermatosis. Int J Dermatol 1998; 37: 715–717.

853 Metcalf JS, Maize JC. Squamous syringometaplasia in lobular panniculitis and pyoderma gangrenosum. Am J Dermatopathol 1990; 12: 141–149.

854 Bhawan J, Malhotra R. Syringosquamous metaplasia. A distinctive eruption in patients receiving chemotherapy. Am J Dermatopathol 1990; 12: 1–6.

855 Hurt MA, Halvorsen RD, Petr FC Jr et al. Eccrine squamous syringometaplasia. Arch Dermatol 1990; 126: 73–77.

856 Rongioletti F, Ballestrero A, Bogliolo F, Rebora A. Necrotizing eccrine squamous syringometaplasia presenting as acral erythema. J Cutan Pathol 1991; 18: 453–456.

857 Horn TD. Antineoplastic chemotherapy, sweat, and the skin. Arch Dermatol 1997; 133: 905–906.

858 Valks R, Fraga J, Porras-Luque J et al. Chemotherapy-induced eccrine squamous syringometaplasia. A distinctive eruption in patients receiving hematopoietic progenitor cells. Arch Dermatol 1997; 133: 873–878.

859 Kinney RB, Burton CS, Vollmer RT. Necrotizing sialometaplasia: a sheep in wolf's clothing. Arch Dermatol 1986; 122: 208–210.

860 Trotter MJ, Stevens PJ, Smith NP. Mucinous syringometaplasia – a case report and review of the literature. Clin Exp Dermatol 1995; 20: 42–45.

861 Kappel TJ, Abenoza P. Mucinous syringometaplasia. A case report with review of the literature. Am J Dermatopathol 1993; 15: 562–567.

862 Bergman R, David R, Friedman-Birnbaum R et al. Mucinous syringometaplasia. An immunohistochemical and ultrastructural study of a case. Am J Dermatopathol 1996; 18: 521–526.

863 Madison JF, Cooper PH, Burgdorf WHC. Mucinous syringometaplasia with prominent epithelial hyperplasia and deep dermal involvement. J Cutan Pathol 1990; 17: 220–224.

864 Scully K, Assaad D. Mucinous syringometaplasia. J Am Acad Dermatol 1984; 11: 503–508.

865 Daudén E, Martín R, Feal C et al. Eccrine ductal mucinosis in a human immunodeficiency virus-positive patient with probable scabies. Br J Dermatol 2000; 143: 1335–1336.

866 Coghill SB, Tyler X, Shaxted EJ. Benign mucinous metaplasia of the vulva. Histopathology 1990; 17: 373–375.

867 Val-Bernal JF, Hernández-Nieto E. Benign mucinous metaplasia of the penis. A lesion resembling extramammary Paget's disease. J Cutan Pathol 2000; 27: 76–79.

868 Bañuls J, Ramón R, Silvestre JF et al. Mucinous metaplasia of apocrine duct. Am J Dermatopathol 1998; 20: 189–193.

869 Harrist TJ, Fine JD, Berman RS et al. Neutrophilic eccrine hidradenitis. Arch Dermatol 1982; 118: 263–266.

870 Bernstein EF, Spielvogel RL, Topolsky DL. Recurrent neutrophilic eccrine hidradenitis. Br J Dermatol 1992; 127: 529–533.

871 Thorisdottir K, Tomecki KJ, Bergfeld WF, Andresen SW. Neutrophilic eccrine hidradenitis. J Am Acad Dermatol 1993; 28: 775–777.

872 Keane FM, Munn SE, Buckley DA et al. Neutrophilic eccrine hidradenitis in two neutropaenic patients. Clin Exp Dermatol 2001; 26: 162–165.

873 Flynn TC, Harrist TJ, Murphy GF et al. Neutrophilic eccrine hidradenitis: a distinctive rash associated with cytarabine therapy and acute leukemia. J Am Acad Dermatol 1984; 11: 584–590.

874 Beutner KR, Packman CH, Markowitch W. Neutrophilic eccrine hidradenitis associated with Hodgkin's disease and chemotherapy. Arch Dermatol 1986; 122: 809–811.

875 Fitzpatrick JE, Bennion SD, Reed OM et al. Neutrophilic eccrine hidradenitis associated with induction chemotherapy. J Cutan Pathol 1987; 14: 272–278.

876 Bailey DL, Barron D, Lucky AW. Neutrophilic eccrine hidradenitis: a case report and review of the literature. Pediatr Dermatol 1989; 6: 33–38.

877 Scallan PJ, Kettler AH, Levy ML, Tschen JA. Neutrophilic eccrine hidradenitis. Evidence implicating bleomycin as a causative agent. Cancer 1988; 62: 2532–2536.

878 Bachmeyer C, Chaibi P, Aractingi S. Neutrophilic eccrine hidradenitis induced by granulocyte colony-stimulating factor. Br J Dermatol 1998; 139: 354–355.

879 Roustan G, Salas C, Cabrera R, Simón A. Neutrophilic eccrine hidradenitis unassociated with chemotherapy in a patient with acute myelogenous leukemia. Int J Dermatol 2001; 40: 144–147.

880 Smith KJ, Skelton HG III, James WD et al. Neutrophilic eccrine hidradenitis in HIV-infected patients. J Am Acad Dermatol 1990; 23: 945–947.

881 Sevila A, Morell A, Bañuls J et al. Neutrophilic eccrine hidradenitis in an HIV-infected patient. Int J Dermatol 1996; 35: 651–652.

882 Bachmeyer C, Reygagne P, Aractingi S. Recurrent neutrophilic eccrine hidradenitis in an HIV-1-infected patient. Dermatology 2000; 200: 328–330.

883 Combemale P, Faisant M, Azoulay-Petit C et al. Neutrophilic eccrine hidradenitis secondary to infection with *Serratia marcescens*. Br J Dermatol 2000; 142: 784–788.

884 Ostlere LS, Wells J, Stevens HP et al. Neutrophilic eccrine hidradenitis with an unusual presentation. Br J Dermatol 1993; 128: 696–698.

885 Allegue F, Soria C, Rocamora A et al. Neutrophilic eccrine hidradenitis in two neutropenic patients. J Am Acad Dermatol 1990; 23: 1110–1113.

886 Brehler R, Reimann S, Bonsmann G, Metze D. Neutrophilic hidradenitis induced by chemotherapy involves eccrine and apocrine glands. Am J Dermatopathol 1997; 19: 73–78.

887 Stahr BJ, Cooper PH, Caputo RV. Idiopathic plantar hidradenitis: a neutrophilic eccrine hidradenitis occurring primarily in children. J Cutan Pathol 1994; 21: 289–296.

888 Rabinowitz LG, Cintra ML, Hood AF, Esterly NB. Recurrent palmoplantar hidradenitis in children. Arch Dermatol 1995; 131: 817–820.

889 Landau M, Metzker A, Gat A et al. Palmoplantar eccrine hidradenitis: three new cases and review. Pediatr Dermatol 1998; 15: 97–102.

890 Simon M Jr, Cremer H, von den Driesch P. Idiopathic recurrent palmoplantar hidradenitis in children. Report of 22 cases. Arch Dermatol 1998; 134: 76–79.

891 Buezo GF, Requena L, Fernández JF et al. Idiopathic palmoplantar hidradenitis. Am J Dermatopathol 1996; 18: 413–416.

892 Weigl L, Eberlein-König B, Ring J, Abeck D. Is recurrent plantar hidradenitis in children induced by exposure to a wet and cold milieu? Br J Dermatol 2000; 142: 1048–1050.

Vestibular gland disorders

893 Prayson RA, Stoler MH, Hart WR. Vulvar vestibulitis. A histopathologic study of 36 cases, including human papillomavirus in situ hybridization analysis. Am J Surg Pathol 1995; 19: 154–160.

894 Mroczkowski TF. Vulvodynia – a dermatovenereologist's perspective. Int J Dermatol 1998; 37: 567–569.

895 Lerner LH, Bell DA, Flotte TJ. Vulvar vestibulitis: a clinicopathologic study of 30 cases. J Cutan Pathol 1997; 24: 109 (abstract).

Cysts, sinuses and pits

16

INTRODUCTION

A *cyst* is an enclosed space within a tissue, usually containing fluid and lined by epithelium. Cysts are usually classified on the basis of their pathogenesis. In the skin, the most important cysts are derived from the dermal appendages as retention cysts. The developmental cysts, which result from the persistence of vestigial remnants, are much less common. The term 'pseudocyst' is sometimes applied to cyst-like structures without an epithelial lining. The important histological features of the various cutaneous cysts are shown in Table 16.1.

A *sinus* is a tract or recess lined by epithelium or granulation tissue. In contrast, a cutaneous *pit* is a small depression in the epidermal surface.

APPENDAGEAL CYSTS

EPIDERMAL (INFUNDIBULAR) CYST

Epidermal cysts are solitary, slowly growing cysts with a predilection for the trunk, neck and face. They measure 1–4 cm or more in diameter, although larger variants have been reported.[1,2] Epidermal cysts are usually located in the mid and lower dermis but they do not shell out like the tricholemmal cyst. There is often a surface punctum.

They are thought to be derived from the pilosebaceous follicle, but they may arise from implantation of the epidermis,[3] particularly on the palms and soles[4] and in the subungual region.[5] Eccrine ducts may rarely give rise to epidermal cysts,[6,7] particularly on the soles,[8] in association with HPV-60 infection (see below). Epidermal cysts have also developed following chronic dermabrasion.[9] Multiple cysts may be found, sometimes in association with Gardner's syndrome.[10–12] Epidermal cysts may become infected and this may be followed by rupture of the cyst, usually into the dermis. Cultures of infected cysts have grown *Staphylococcus aureus* or a mixed growth of organisms.[13] However, a recent study has shown that the microbiological milieu of inflamed and uninflamed cysts is the same, calling into question the traditional view that bacterial infection is the etiology of the inflammation in epidermal cysts.[14] There is a predominance of anaerobes in infected cysts in the genital and perineal regions.[13] Secondary infection by a dermatophyte has been reported.[15]

Histopathology

Epidermal cysts are lined by stratified squamous epithelium showing epidermal keratinization, that is, the formation of keratohyaline granules and flattened surface epithelium. As such, they are thought to be derived from or to mimic the infundibular portion of the hair follicle. Rupture of a non-inflamed cyst will produce a localized foreign body granulomatous reaction in the adjacent dermis, while rupture of an inflamed cyst usually results in a heavy inflammatory cell infiltrate in the adjacent dermis, sometimes with destruction of the cyst wall in the process. Fibrosis usually occurs subsequently.

Several histological variations in the epidermal lining have been reported. These include focal epidermal proliferation,[16] a seborrheic keratosis-like change,[17] basal hyperpigmentation (seen in black patients),[18] melanophagic proliferation,[19] focal pilomatrixoma-like changes (usually in kindreds with Gardner's syndrome),[11,20,21] clear cell change,[22] cornoid lamellation,[16] epidermolytic hyperkeratosis,[16] histological changes of Darier's disease,[23] pyogenic granuloma formation,[24] Paget's disease,[16] basal cell carcinoma,[16] mycosis fungoides and Bowen's disease.[25] Specific histological features are usually seen in HPV-related cysts (see below). Epidermal cysts express keratin

Table 16.1 **Histological features of various cysts**

Type	Important features
Epidermal	Epidermal keratinization; keratohyaline granules
HPV-related	Either intracytoplasmic inclusions and vacuolar keratinous changes or verrucous lining (papillated and/or digitated) with hypergranulosis
Tricholemmal	Tricholemmal keratinization; cholesterol clefts; sometimes calcification
Hybrid	Outer epidermal and inner tricholemmal keratinization; other combinations may occur
Hair matrix	Basaloid cells with luminal squamous maturation
Pigmented follicular	Epidermal-like; luminal pigmented hairs
Cutaneous keratocyst	Corrugated configuration; no granular layer; may contain vellus hairs
Vellus	Multiple; epidermal-like; luminal vellus hairs
Steatocystoma	Multiple; sebaceous glands in and adjoining wall; may contain vellus hairs
Milium	Small epidermal cyst with thinner wall
Eccrine hidrocystoma	Two layers of cuboidal epithelium
Apocrine cystadenoma	Columnar cells with decapitation secretion; basal myoepithelial cells
Bronchogenic	Mostly midline; respiratory epithelial lining; sometimes smooth muscle and mucous glands
Branchial	Lateral neck; stratified squamous and inner respiratory epithelial lining; heavy lymphoid tissue in wall
Thymic	Respiratory and/or squamous lining; Hassall's corpuscles in wall
Cutaneous ciliated	Lower limb of females; ciliated columnar or cuboidal lining
Median raphe	Ventral surface penis; pseudostratified columnar epithelium
Dermoid	Periorbital or midline; epidermal-like with attached pilosebaceous structures; sometimes smooth muscle in the wall

10 (K10).[26] Cases of malignant transformation,[27–29] reported in the older literature, have been questioned as some, at least, represent proliferating tricholemmal cysts (see p. 506) or proliferating epidermal cysts (see below). Despite the low risk of malignant transformation, it is generally agreed that all suspected cysts should be submitted for histological examination.[30]

HPV-RELATED EPIDERMAL CYSTS

Two distinctive, but rare, types of epidermal cyst have been reported in association with human papillomavirus infection. The first type, reported initially in Japan in 1986, usually involves pressure points on the plantar surface of the feet.[31,32] Lesions are usually solitary. HPV-60 has been demonstrated in most cases.[33] Eccrine ductal structures are sometimes noted in the cyst wall, suggesting that HPV infection of eccrine ducts may have a pathogenetic role in some cases.[33,34] However, immunostaining with monoclonal antibodies against various cytokeratins does not support this view.[35,36] Epidermal implantation may be involved in the pathogenesis.[35,36]

In the second type (verrucous epidermal cysts), an HPV genome of as yet uncharacterized type produces verrucous changes in the epithelial lining.[37–39] The cysts do not usually involve the palms or soles.[40]

Histopathology[31,33,37]

Epidermal cysts associated with HPV-60 infection are well-demarcated cysts in the dermis continuous with the overlying epidermis at the top of the cyst. Scattered keratinocytes in the upper layers of the epithelial lining contain intracytoplasmic, eosinophilic inclusions.[41,42] In addition, vacuolar structures are present in the keratinous (horny) material within the cyst. Parakeratotic nuclei are often present in this keratinous material. Ductal structures expressing carcinoembryonic antigen (CEA) may be found in the cyst walls.[34]

In the HPV-related *verrucous cysts*, there is an epidermal cyst lined by a papillated and/or digitated epithelium with focal, prominent hypergranulosis and irregular keratohyaline granules (Fig.16.1).[37] Squamous eddies, reminiscent of those seen in inverted follicular keratosis, are often present in the epithelial lining. Vacuolated keratinocytes, resembling koilocytes, have been present in some cases.[39]

PROLIFERATING EPIDERMAL CYST

In a recently published series of 96 cases of proliferating epithelial cysts, 63 were of tricholemmal type and 33 of epidermal type.[43] The tricholemmal variants had a predilection for females (71% of cases) and the scalp (78% of cases), while the proliferating epidermal cysts had a male preponderance

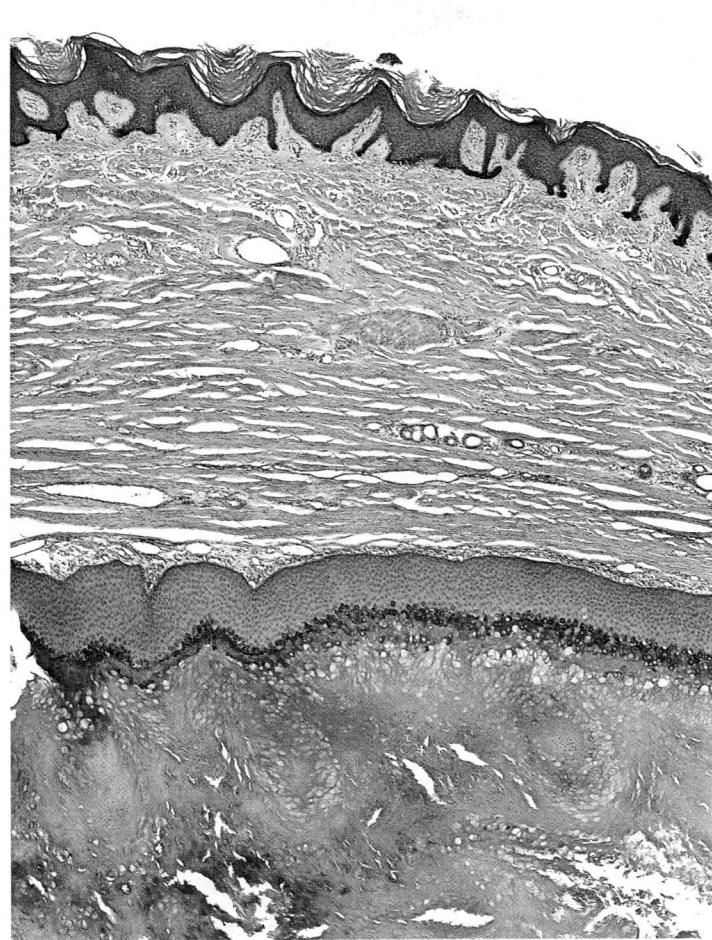

Fig. 16.1 **HPV-related epidermal cyst.** (H & E)

(64%) and a more widespread distribution involving the pelvic and anogenital region as well as the scalp, upper extremities and trunk.[43] Carcinomatous change developed in 20% of the proliferating epidermal cysts.

Histopathology

Proliferating epidermal cysts are subepidermal cystic tumors that often connect with the overlying epidermis by a narrow opening or through a dilated hair follicle.[43] An underlying epidermal cyst is often present, although this constitutes only a small part of the lesion. The lesion consists of multilocular cystic spaces containing keratinous material or proteinaceous fluid. The proliferating epithelium, which may show squamous eddies, extends into the adjacent stroma but there is usually still some circumscription. The squamous cells may have copious pale cytoplasm. Epidermal-type keratinization is a prerequisite for the diagnosis. The degree of cellularity and atypia is variable.[43] Carcinomatous change is characterized by infiltration into the surrounding dermis and subcutis, marked nuclear atypia, pleomorphism and frequent mitoses.

TRICHOLEMMAL (SEBACEOUS) CYST

Tricholemmal cysts are found as solitary or multiple intradermal or subcutaneous lesions with a predilection for the scalp. There is a female preponderance. There is no punctum and the cysts easily shell out at removal. Familial cases, often with multiple cysts, occur and some of these have an autosomal dominant inheritance.[44]

The cysts are smooth with a cream to white wall and similarly colored, semi-solid, cheesy contents.

Histopathology[45]

The cysts are lined by stratified squamous epithelium showing tricholemmal keratinization in which the individual cells increase in bulk and vertical diameter towards the lumen (Fig. 16.2). This usually occurs without the formation of keratohyaline granules and resembles that seen in the external root sheath in the region of the follicular isthmus.[46] There is an abrupt change into the eosinophilic-staining keratin within the lumen. Cholesterol clefts are common in this keratinous material and about one-quarter will show focal calcification of the contents. Tricholemmal cysts express both keratin 10 (K10) and 17 (K17).[26] About 10% have focal inflammation but this differs from that seen in

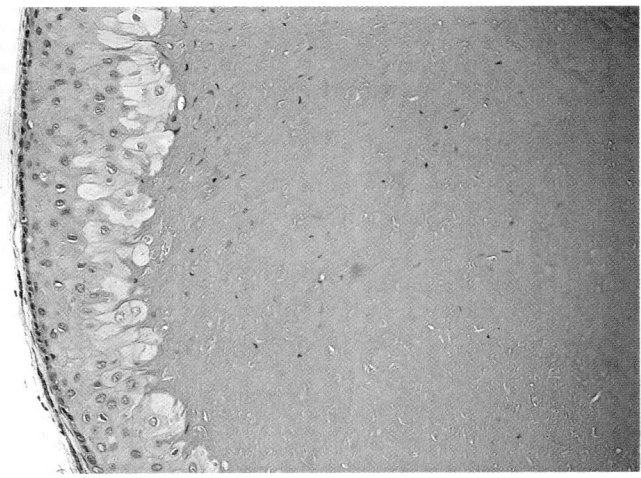

Fig. 16.2 **Tricholemmal cyst** (sebaceous cyst). It is lined by stratified squamous epithelium exhibiting tricholemmal keratinization. (H & E)

epidermal cysts. In tricholemmal cysts, there is a break in the wall with entry into the cysts of inflammatory cells and fibroblasts with subsequent organization (Fig. 16.3). Irregular hyperplasia of the epithelial lining may be a consequence of this. Sebaceous and apocrine differentiation have been reported in the wall.[47]

Under polarized light, the perpendicularly oriented bundles of tonofibrils can be seen in the lining epithelial cells, a feature of tricholemmal keratinization.[48] This mirrors the electron microscopic findings of an increase of filaments in the maturing cells which aggregate to form larger fibrillary bundles. Keratohyaline granules are not usually seen.

PROLIFERATING AND MALIGNANT TRICHOLEMMAL CYST

Although usually solid or only partly cystic, proliferating and malignant tricholemmal cyst is considered here because a spectrum of cases is observed, ranging from a tricholemmal cyst with minimal epithelial proliferation to a lesion with gross epithelial hyperplasia which is only minimally cystic and which may simulate a squamous cell carcinoma.[43,49] Ackerman and colleagues believe that a proliferating tricholemmal cyst (pilar tumor) is a variant of squamous cell carcinoma. They use the term 'proliferating tricholemmal cystic squamous-cell carcinoma' for such cases.[50,51] This view has not yet received wide acceptance.[52] This entity was first described by Wilson Jones as a proliferating epidermoid cyst.[53] Subsequent reports have not always made a distinction between proliferating tricholemmal cyst and proliferating epidermal cyst (see above).

The tumors are large, measuring 2–10 cm or more in diameter. They are sometimes exophytic and even ulcerated.[54] They are most commonly found on the scalp of middle-aged or elderly females.[43] The extremities are rarely involved.[43,55] Recurrence after excision and malignant transformation are both uncommon;[56–58] metastatic spread is very rare.[57,59–62] They may develop in organoid nevi,[63] but most arise de novo or in a pre-existing tricholemmal cyst.[54]

Histopathology

There is a lobular proliferation of squamous cells, often with some peripheral palisading and sometimes showing focal areas of vitreous membrane formation. There may be focal cystic areas or remnants of a more obvious

tricholemmal cyst at one margin (Fig. 16.4). The lesions are usually well circumscribed. Nests of squamous cells may extend into the adjacent connective tissue, simulating squamous cell carcinoma, but the proliferation of nests is mostly inwards into the cyst (Fig. 16.5). This contrasts with the outward extension of nests seen in proliferating epidermal cysts.

There are typical areas of tricholemmal keratinization and, in some cases, focal epidermal keratinization as well. There may also be vacuolated cells, variable cellular atypia,[64] focal necrosis, squamous eddies, individual cell keratinization and scattered mitoses. Sebaceous and acrosyringeal differentiation were noted in one case.[65] A spindle cell component has also been described.[66,67] Features favoring the diagnosis of proliferating tricholemmal cyst over squamous cell carcinoma include the presence of tricholemmal keratinization, cyst formation, calcification and the absence of a premalignant epidermal lesion.[68] Aneuploidy does not always assist in the assessment of malignancy as this feature can be present in proliferating tricholemmal cysts.[69–71] The diagnosis of a *malignant proliferating tricholemmal tumor* usually requires the identification in some areas of an underlying benign component.[56] It also requires the presence of extensive cellular atypia and invasion, sometimes focal, of adjacent structures.[57,72] Uncommonly, a spindle cell carcinoma forms the malignant component.[73] Stromal desmoplasia may be present in areas of

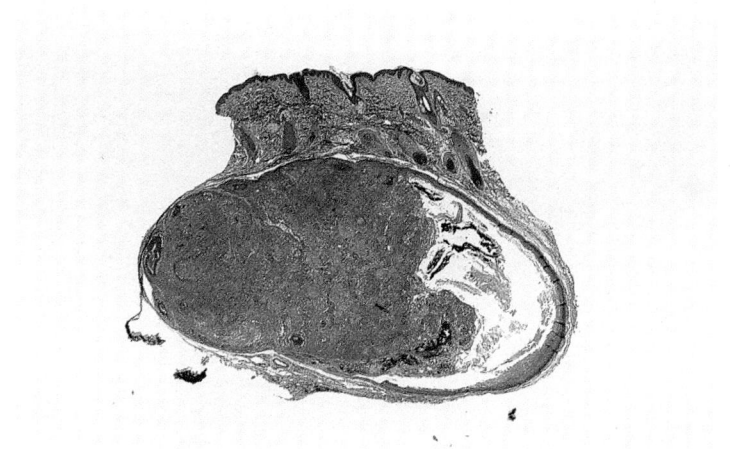

Fig. 16.4 **Proliferating tricholemmal cyst.** An early lesion with evidence of a pre-existing cyst at one edge. (H & E)

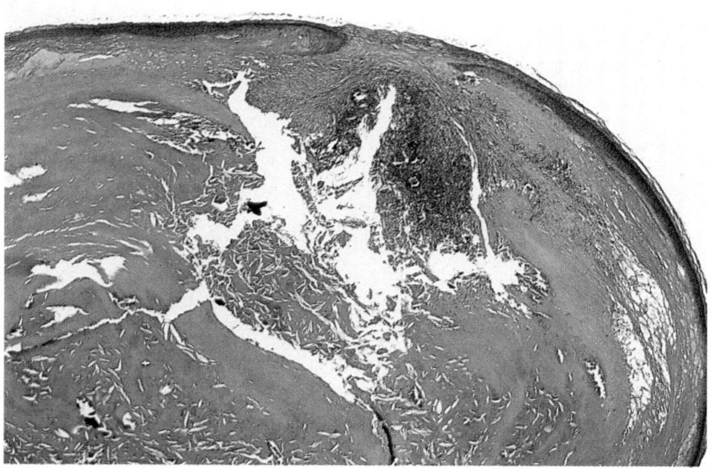

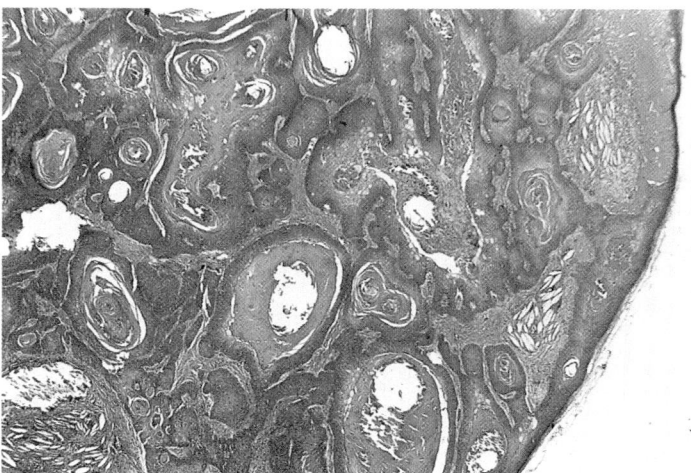

Fig. 16.5 **Proliferating tricholemmal cyst.** This is part of a large tumor in which nests of squamous epithelium extend into the adjacent dermis. (H & E)

Fig. 16.3 **Tricholemmal cyst** with 'rupture' and ingrowth of inflammatory cells and granulation tissue. (H & E)

malignant transformation. There is loss of CD34 immunostaining in malignant lesions.[71]

Electron microscopy has confirmed the presence of areas of tricholemmal keratinization.[74]

MALIGNANT ONYCHOLEMMAL CYST

The designation 'malignant proliferating onycholemmal cyst' was given, recently, to a slowly growing tumor of the nail unit in an elderly female.[75] It was thought to have arisen from a pre-existing subungual keratinous cyst. The lesion penetrated the underlying phalangeal bone.

Histopathology
The tumor was composed of small keratinous cysts with abrupt central keratinization and of solid nests and strands of atypical keratinocytes.[75]

HYBRID CYST

A hybrid cyst is one in which the lining of the upper portion shows epidermoid keratinization similar to an epidermal cyst, while the lower portion shows tricholemmal keratinization similar to that seen in a tricholemmal cyst.[76] There is a sharp transition between the two types of lining. A hybrid cyst should not be confused with a tricholemmal cyst showing very focal formation of a granular layer, which may be found in 10% of cases.[77]

The term 'hybrid cyst' has been expanded to include any follicular cyst with two different types of epithelial lining.[78] In addition to those just described with epidermal (infundibular) and tricholemmal differentiation, cysts may be found with epidermal and pilomatrical features (particularly in Gardner's syndrome), tricholemmal and pilomatrical differentiation, epidermal and apocrine changes,[79,80] and also eruptive vellus hair cyst features with either steatocystoma, epidermal or tricholemmal change.[78,81] A vellus hair cyst combined with an epidermal cyst and a benign melanocytic nevus has been reported.[82]

HAIR MATRIX CYST

The hair matrix variant of epidermal cyst is seen more often in children and young adults. There is some resemblance to the pattern of differentiation seen in pilomatrixomas.

Histopathology
The cyst wall is composed of several layers of basaloid cells that mature to squamoid cells near the lumen. This pattern recapitulates that seen in the normal hair matrix and cortex. Small cystic spaces are often present within the cyst wall. The lumen contains amorphous, keratinous material. If rupture occurs, a florid granulomatous reaction develops in the surrounding dermis.

PIGMENTED FOLLICULAR CYST

A rare, clinically pigmented cyst was first described in 1982.[83–86] There is one report of a patient with multiple pigmented cysts.[87]

Histopathology
The cyst is located in the dermis and has a narrow, pore-like opening to the surface. It contains laminated keratin as well as multiple, pigmented hair shafts (Fig. 16.6). Degenerating hair shafts may be present.[88] The cyst is lined by stratified squamous epithelium showing epidermal keratinization, but in addition the lining may show rete ridges and dermal papillae, features not seen in epidermal cysts. Both epidermal and tricholemmal keratinization were present in the cysts removed from the patient with multiple lesions.[87]

CUTANEOUS KERATOCYST

Cutaneous cysts are a feature of the basal cell nevus syndrome (see p. 771). Usually these cysts are of epidermal type, but there are rare reports of patients with this syndrome in whom the cutaneous cysts resembled keratocysts of the jaw.[89,90] They contained a thick brown fluid.

Histopathology[89]
The cysts had a corrugated or festooned configuration with a lining of several layers of squamous epithelium, but with no granular layer. Lanugo hairs were present in one cyst. There was a superficial resemblance to steatocystoma multiplex (see below), but there were no sebaceous lobules in the wall.

VELLUS HAIR CYST

Eruptive vellus hair cysts, first reported in 1977,[91] occur as multiple, small, asymptomatic papules with a predilection for the chest and axillae of children or young adults.[92,93] They are also found on the face,[94] neck and extremities.

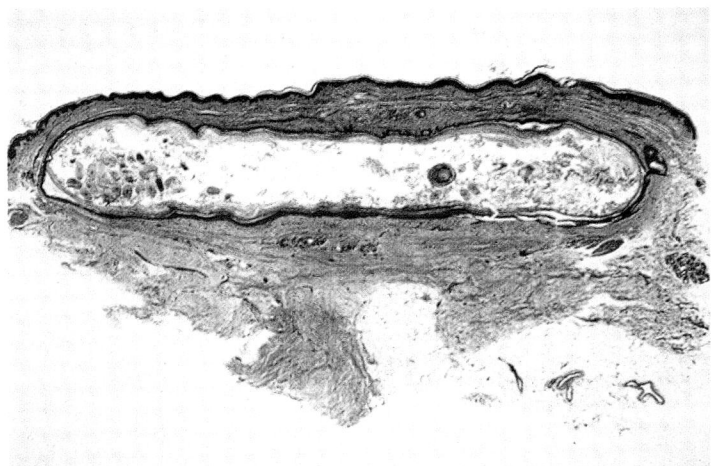

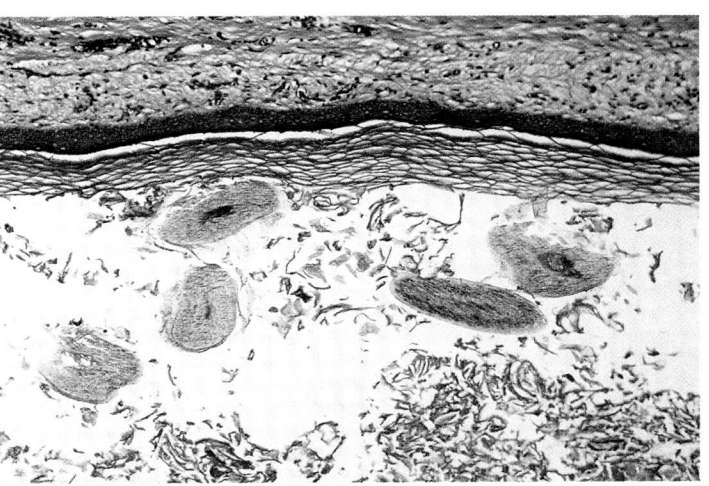

Fig. 16.6 **(A) Pigmented follicular cyst. (B)** The lumen of the cyst contains a number of pigmented hair shafts. (H & E)

They may have an autosomal dominant inheritance or occur sporadically.[95,96] Ectodermal dysplasia is a rare association.[97] Spontaneous regression of the cysts has been reported, probably following the transepidermal elimination of the cyst contents.[98]

Eruptive vellus hair cysts have been reported in patients with steatocystoma, suggesting that these two entities are in some way related;[99–102] both may be derived from the sebaceous duct.[103] However, their pattern of keratin expression is different: vellus hair cysts express keratin 17 (K17), while steatocystomas express both keratins 17 (K17) and 10 (K10).[26] Milia can also occur in association with these two entities.[104] Trichostasis spinulosa may rarely coexist with eruptive vellus hair cysts.[105]

Histopathology[91]

These small dermal cysts are lined by stratified squamous epithelium which may show focal tricholemmal as well as epidermoid keratinization. The lumen contains keratin and numerous transversely and obliquely sectioned vellus hair shafts (Fig. 16.7). These are doubly refractile with polarized light. A rudimentary hair follicle may be attached to the wall. Hybrid cysts with features of both vellus hair cysts and steatocystoma are sometimes seen.[78,101] There may be focal rupture of the cyst wall with a foreign body granulomatous reaction and associated dermal fibrosis and mild chronic inflammation.

Some cysts may show a connecting pore at the skin surface, the likely mechanism of the spontaneous regression mentioned above.

STEATOCYSTOMA MULTIPLEX

Steatocystoma multiplex is characterized by multiple yellowish to skin-colored papules or cysts measuring from less than 3 mm in diameter to 3 cm or more. They may be found on the face,[106–110] scalp,[111–113] trunk, axillae and the extremities,[114] but they have a predilection for the chest. Rarely, they have a linear distribution.[115] They are mostly sporadic, but familial cases with autosomal dominant inheritance are well documented. Other abnormalities may be present in the inherited cases.[107] The occurrence of steatocystoma multiplex in Alagille syndrome may be fortuitous,[116] but not their occurrence in association with trichoblastomas and trichoepitheliomas.[117] Patients with only a solitary lesion (steatocystoma simplex) are seen rarely.[118] The cysts usually present in adolescents as asymptomatic lesions, but infected cysts (steatocystoma multiplex suppurativum) may be painful.[119,120] Steatocystoma is thought to represent a nevoid malformation of the pilosebaceous duct.

Mutations in keratin 17, similar to those found in pachyonychia congenita, have been found in some patients with steatocystoma multiplex.[121,122]

Histopathology

The lining of the dermal cysts is usually undulating due to collapse of the cyst. It is composed of stratified squamous epithelium, only a few cells thick and without a granular layer. The characteristic feature is the presence of sebaceous glands of varying size in or adjacent to the wall (Fig. 16.8). A ribbon-like cord of epithelial cells connects the cyst with the epidermis, but this may not be seen in the plane of section. One pilar unit is associated with each cyst, and the cyst may contain one or more lanugo hairs. Large polygonal cells with abundant granular cytoplasm form part of the lining of the cyst on rare occasions. Such cells have the immunohistochemical characteristics of the macrophage/monocyte lineage.[113] Spherules ('myospherulosis'), formed by masses of erythrocytes in the presence of oil-containing substances, have been reported in the lumen.[123] Smooth muscle has been noted in the wall.[124]

Hybrid cysts with features of both steatocystoma and vellus hair cysts are sometimes seen;[78,101,125,126] epidermal cysts may form a third component.[81]

Electron microscopy

The keratinization takes place without the formation of keratohyaline granules, a feature which is characteristic of the sebaceous duct.[106]

MILIUM

A milium is a small (1 or 2 mm in diameter) dermal cyst which may arise from the pilosebaceous apparatus or eccrine sweat ducts.[127] Milia may be seen in the newborn as congenital lesions or they may develop later in life secondary to dermabrasion, to the topical application of corticosteroids[127] and to radiotherapy and as a consequence of subepidermal bullous disorders such as porphyria cutanea tarda, epidermolysis bullosa dystrophica and second-degree burns. They have also been reported in association with discoid lupus erythematosus,[128] pseudoxanthoma elasticum,[129] a congenital hemangioma,[130] and some inherited disorders.[131]

Milia most commonly occur as multiple lesions on the cheeks and forehead, but they may involve the genitalia or other sites, depending on the predisposing lesion.[132,133] A rare eruptive form[134] and an erythematous plaque variant (milia en plaque) have been reported.[131,135–144]

Histopathology

The small cysts are lined by several layers of stratified squamous epithelium with central keratinous material, resembling a small epidermal cyst. They may be connected to a vellus hair follicle or eccrine sweat duct, usually the latter.[145] Milia differ from comedones, which are keratinous plugs in dilated pilosebaceous orifices. Closed comedones, which may be particularly prominent in the condition known as nodular elastoidosis with cysts and comedones (Favre–Racouchot disease),[146,147] may superficially resemble milia. However, comedones are more likely to contain old hair shafts and laminated keratinous material containing numerous bacteria.[148]

ECCRINE HIDROCYSTOMA

Eccrine hidrocystomas are usually solitary lesions of the face, trunk or popliteal fossa, with a strong predilection for the periorbital area.[149,150] Cases with multiple (up to 200 or more) lesions are well documented.[151–154] There is a slight preponderance of adult females. Clinically, the lesions are usually

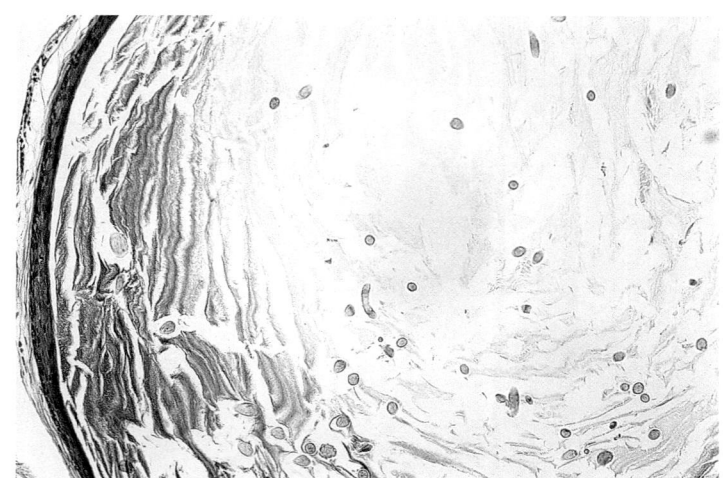

Fig. 16.7 **Vellus hair cyst.** The lumen of the cyst contains multiple small vellus hairs. (H & E)

translucent, pale blue, dome-shaped, cystic papules. The development of a squamous cell carcinoma in an eccrine hidrocystoma is a very rare complication.[155]

The existence of this entity has been challenged; many, if not all of these lesions are now regarded as being of apocrine type.

Histopathology

The cysts are unilocular and situated in the dermis, often in close proximity to eccrine glands. The wall is composed of two layers of cuboidal epithelium with eosinophilic cytoplasm (Fig. 16.9). Sometimes the lumen contains small amounts of pale eosinophilic secretions. There is no evidence of decapitation secretion but this may simply be a consequence of marked flattening of the lining cells by the intraluminal contents.

Electron microscopy

There are two cell layers with a peripheral basement membrane and extensive microvilli along the luminal border.[156] These findings are similar to those of the eccrine duct.

APOCRINE HIDROCYSTOMA

Apocrine hidrocystoma (apocrine gland cyst, apocrine cystadenoma) is regarded by some as an adenomatous cystic proliferation of apocrine glands and by others as a simple retention cyst.[157] Apocrine hidrocystomas are almost invariably solitary lesions, a few millimeters in diameter, on the head or neck of middle-aged to older adults.[158] A large variant has been described[159] and patients with multiple lesions have been observed.[160–162] Multiple cysts may be a marker of two rare inherited disorders, the Schöpf–Schulz–Passarge syndrome and a form of focal dermal hypoplasia.[162] Clinically, the lesions resemble eccrine hidrocystomas with a translucent or bluish hue.[163] Their contents are colorless or brown to black. Interestingly, they do not occur in the usual sites in which apocrine glands are found.[164] They may arise in an organoid nevus.[157] Cysts may also develop from the duct and secretory segment of Moll's gland, a modified apocrine gland of the eyelid.[162,165,166]

Histopathology

The cysts may be unilocular or multilocular with a lining of columnar epithelium with basal nuclei and an underlying flattened layer of elongated, basal myoepithelial cells. Characteristically, there is 'pinching off' ('decapitation') of the cytoplasm of the luminal border of the lining cells, typical of apocrine secretory activity (Fig. 16.10). Sometimes the epithelium is flattened, making distinction from eccrine hidrocystoma difficult.[167,168] It is now thought that most eccrine hidrocystomas are of apocrine origin. In nearly half the cases there are local areas of hyperplastic epithelium with microcysts in the lining

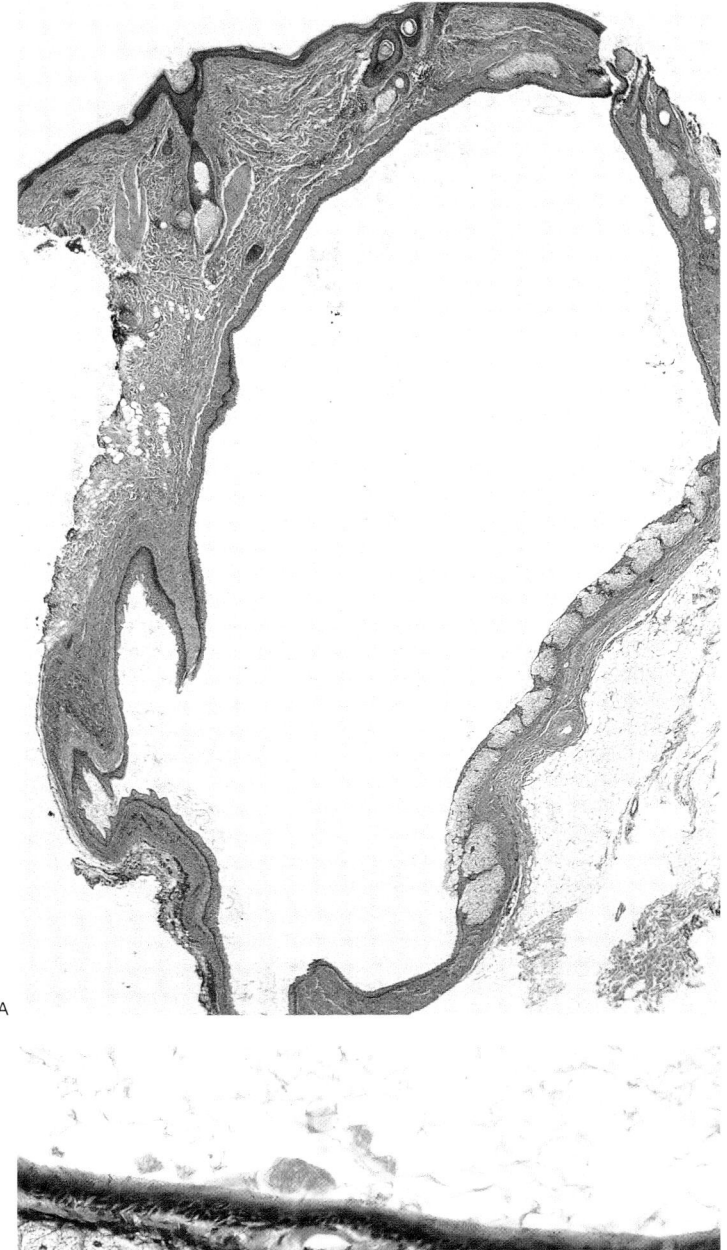

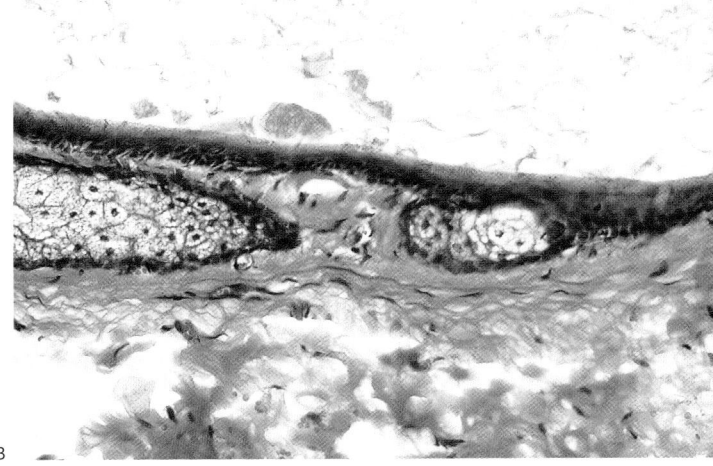

Fig. 16.8 **(A) Steatocystoma multiplex. (B)** Sebaceous glands are present within the cyst wall. (H & E)

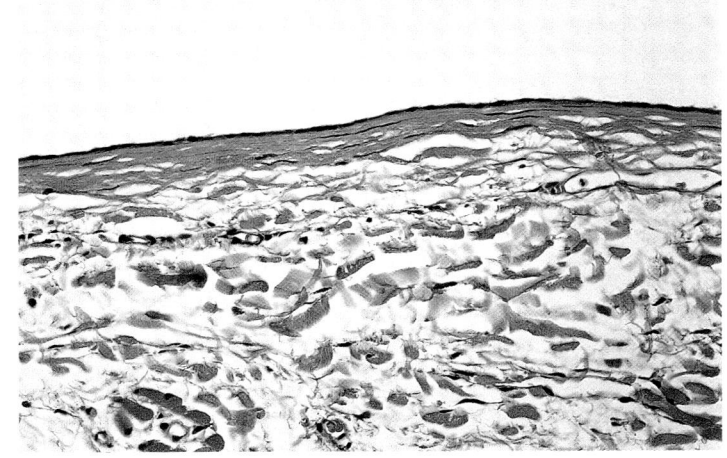

Fig. 16.9 **Eccrine hidrocystoma.** It has been suggested that such lesions are really of apocrine type. Attenuation of the lining may be responsible for loss of the 'decapitation' secretion. (H & E)

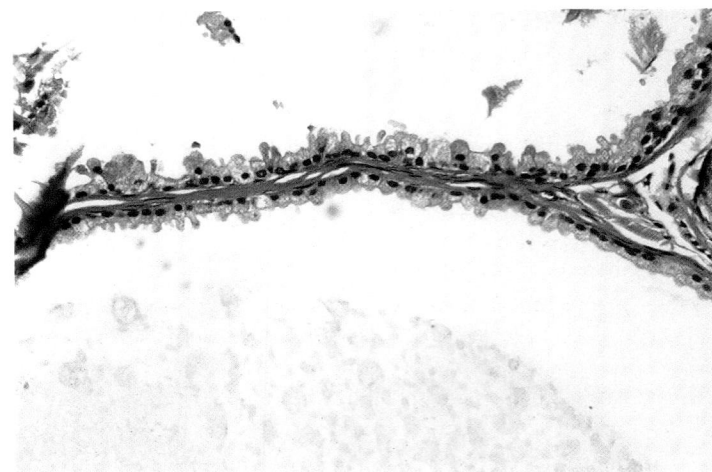

Fig. 16.10 **Apocrine cystadenoma.** This bilocular cyst is lined by apocrine epithelium showing 'decapitation' secretion. (H & E)

and intracystic papillary projections with a core of vascularized connective tissue. The presence of keratinizing squamous epithelium adjacent to apocrine epithelium occurs in one variant of hybrid cyst (see p. 507).

The secretory cells may contain PAS-positive diastase-resistant granules. Carcinoembryonic antigen (CEA) may also be present in both apocrine and eccrine cystadenomas.

Electron microscopy
The basal myoepithelial cells and the secretory cells show abundant secretory granules, decapitation secretion and usually annulate lamellae.[169]

DEVELOPMENTAL CYSTS

Included in this group are cysts derived from embryological vestiges such as the branchial cleft, thyroglossal duct, tracheobronchial bud, urogenital sinus and müllerian structures.[170] Others arise along lines of embryological closure. The term 'cutaneous ciliated cyst' has been applied to those which have in common a ciliated columnar epithelial lining, but which have been given different names according to their topographical localization.[171] Included in this concept are bronchogenic cysts, cutaneous ciliated cyst of the lower limbs, branchial and thyroglossal cysts, and cutaneous endosalpingiosis.[172] The term is best restricted to the cutaneous ciliated cyst of the lower limbs (see p. 511).

Cystic lesions devoid of an epithelial lining may occur in association with heterotopic brain tissue (see p. 988).[173]

BRONCHOGENIC CYST

A bronchogenic cyst is present at or soon after birth, most often in the midline near the manubrium sterni.[171,174–177] It has been reported on the chin,[178,179] the neck and even the shoulder and scapular region;[180,181] these latter examples are presumed to be derived from sequestrated cells of the tracheobronchial bud, although an equally valid argument can be made for a branchial origin for many of these cysts.[182,183] They present as a cyst or as a draining sinus. Bronchogenic cysts are four times more common in males than in females.[184]

The cysts are unilocular and situated in the dermis or subcutaneous tissues. They contain cloudy fluid.

Histopathology
The cysts are lined by ciliated and mucin-producing pseudostratified columnar or cuboidal epithelium (Fig. 16.11). Stratified squamous epithelium may be present in the outer part of the cyst in those presenting as a sinus on the skin surface.[185] Smooth muscle and even mucous glands are found commonly in

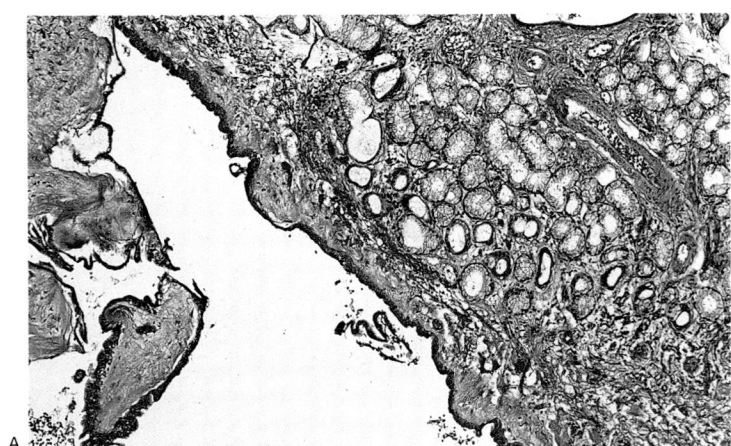

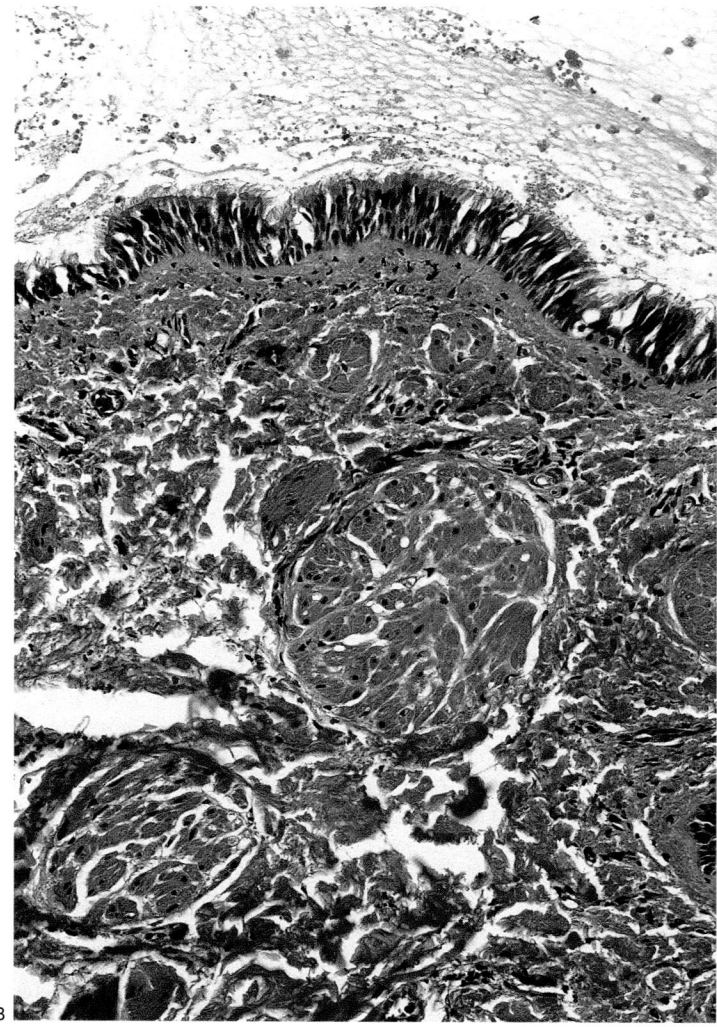

Fig. 16.11 **(A) Bronchogenic cyst** with a collection of mucous glands in the wall. **(B)** The lining is pseudostratified columnar with occasional goblet cells. There are smooth muscle bundles in the wall. (H & E)

the wall, but cartilage is present only occasionally. There may be some inflammation and fibrosis adjacent to the cyst, but lymphoid follicles, common in the wall of branchial cleft cysts (see below), are very rare in bronchogenic cysts.[186–188] **Ectopic respiratory mucosa**, without an associated cyst, is a rare finding in the skin.[189,190]

BRANCHIAL CLEFT CYST

Branchial cleft remnants present clinically as cysts, sinus tracts, skin tags or combinations of these lesions.[183,191,192] Those derived from the second branchial pouch are usually found along the anterior border of the sternomastoid muscle of children or young adults, while those of first pouch origin arise near the angle of the mandible. They may be found at any depth between the skin and pharynx. Secondary infection may cause sudden swelling of the lesions.

The cysts contain turbid fluid, rich in cholesterol crystals. Squamous cell carcinoma is a rare complication in lesions of long standing.[193,194]

Histopathology
The cysts are lined mostly by stratified squamous epithelium, but deeper parts may have a lining of ciliated columnar epithelium. A heavy lymphoid infiltrate invests the cyst or sinus wall, and this includes lymphoid follicles. Mucinous glands and cartilage are occasionally present in the wall;[182] thymic tissue has also been reported.[195]

Branchial cleft anomalies differ from bronchogenic cysts by their location, the common occurrence of lymphoid follicles and stratified squamous epithelium, and the rarity of smooth muscle.[187]

THYROGLOSSAL CYST

Most examples of thyroglossal cyst are deep lesions in the midline of the neck and therefore beyond the scope of this volume.[196,197] There is one report of a depressed lesion in the midline of the neck, present since birth, which consisted of tubular glands lined by respiratory epithelium, opening on to the skin surface.[182] Deeper branching tubules penetrated into the underlying striated muscle. The lesion was presumed to be of thyroglossal duct origin. A cyst reported in the lateral neck, attached to the thyroid gland, was most likely a foregut remnant. It resembled, in part, a bronchogenic cyst, but the wall also contained pancreatic tissue.[198]

THYMIC CYST

Thymic cysts are rare cysts found in the mediastinum or neck. The cervical lesions usually present as painless swellings in children or adolescents.[199–201] Thymic cysts are thought to arise from remnants of the thymopharyngeal duct, a derivative of the third pouch. They are most often found posterior to a lateral lobe of the thyroid, more often on the left-hand side.

The cysts are unilocular or multilocular and measure from 1 to 15 cm in diameter. The contents are variable, ranging from yellow-brown fluid to cloudy or gelatinous material. Cholesterol crystals may be present.

Histopathology
Thymic cysts are lined by one or more of the following epithelia: squamous, columnar, cuboidal or pseudostratified columnar. Occasionally, the cyst is devoid of an epithelial lining and has a fibrous tissue lining only. The wall characteristically contains Hassall's corpuscles and in addition there may be lymphoid tissue, cholesterol granulomas and sometimes parathyroid tissue.[199]

Thymic remnants, without cyst formation, have been reported in the skin of the neck.[202]

CUTANEOUS CILIATED CYST OF THE LOWER LIMBS

The term 'cutaneous ciliated cyst' is sometimes applied to several varieties of developmental cysts that, although lined by ciliated epithelium, are of quite different origin (see above). It is best restricted to a rare cyst which usually arises on the lower extremities of women in the second and third decade.[203–206] The cysts are less than 3 cm in diameter. They have been thought to be of müllerian origin, but the occurrence of rare cases in males has raised the possibility of an origin from an eccrine sweat gland.[207–209] A ciliated cyst reported in the perineal region of a male was thought to be derived from embryonic remnants of the cloacal membrane.[210] A perineal lesion has also been reported in a female.[211]

In a case of cutaneous ciliated cyst removed from the scalp, estrogen and progesterone receptors were demonstrated in the nuclei of the lining cells.[212]

Histopathology
The cyst is lined by ciliated cuboidal to columnar epithelium with pseudostratified areas (Fig. 16.12). Focal squamous metaplasia is sometimes present; mucinous cells are rare.[213] The cysts may be multilocular and there are often papillary projections into the lumen. Glandular and smooth muscle elements are absent.[214] Strong dynein positivity has been observed in the apical portion of the lining cells with immunohistochemistry.[211] This pattern is similar to normal salpingeal epithelium, support for a müllerian origin.

VULVAL MUCINOUS AND CILIATED CYSTS

Vulval mucinous and ciliated cysts are found in the vestibule of the vulva.[215,216] They vary in size from 0.5 to 3.0 cm or more. Included among the cases reported have been several instances of Bartholin's cyst. Vulval mucinous and ciliated cysts are presumed to be of urogenital sinus origin.

Histopathology
The cysts are lined by pseudostratified ciliated columnar epithelium and/or mucinous epithelium. There may be areas of squamous metaplasia.

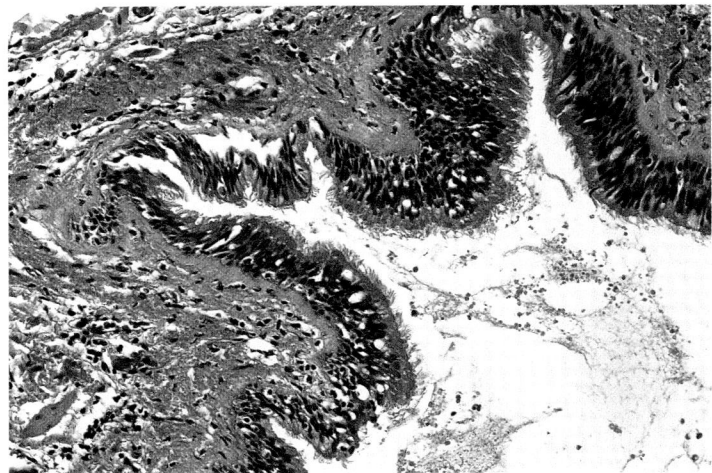

Fig. 16.12 **Cutaneous ciliated cyst.** The cyst is partly collapsed with some infolding of the wall. The lining is ciliated. (H & E)

MEDIAN RAPHE CYST

'Median raphe cyst' is the preferred term for midline developmental cysts found at any point from the external urethral meatus to the anus, including the ventral aspect of the penis, the scrotal raphe and the perineal raphe, but most commonly near the glans penis.[217–220] They are thought to arise as a result of defective embryological closure of the median raphe, but some may result from the anomalous outgrowth of the entodermal urethral lining (urethroid cyst).[221,222] They are most commonly diagnosed in the first three decades of life. Abrupt onset of a median raphe cyst may be precipitated by local trauma or secondary infection.[223] Canals coursing longitudinally in the line of the median raphe are sometimes found.[224]

Most raphe cysts are less than 1 cm in diameter. The contents are usually clear, but they may be turbid if there are abundant mucous glands in the wall.

Histopathology[217]

Median raphe cysts are situated in the dermis, but they do not connect with the overlying surface epithelium. They are lined by pseudostratified columnar epithelium, which may be quite attenuated in some areas. Occasionally, mucous glands are present in the wall, but ciliated cells are rare.[225] Pigmented cysts, resulting from the presence of melanocytes, have been reported.[226] In cysts situated near the meatus, the lining is usually of stratified squamous epithelium (Fig. 16.13).

DERMOID CYST

Dermoid cysts are rare subcutaneous cysts of ectodermal origin found along lines of embryonic fusion, particularly at the lateral angle of the eye or the midline of the forehead or neck.[227] Involvement of the scalp and penis is rare.[228,229] Dermoid cysts arising in the midline of the dorsum of the nose frequently have an overlying fistula communicating with the skin surface and the underlying cyst, which is sometimes quite deep.[230–233] The term **fistula of the dorsum of the nose** is used for this superficial component.[231] A tuft of hair usually protrudes from the central pit. A similar dermal 'sinus' has been reported in the occipital region of the scalp, overlying an intracranial dermoid cyst.[234]

Dermoid cysts are usually asymptomatic masses present at birth, but inflammation, often secondary to trauma, may draw attention to a pre-existing lesion in an older person.

The cysts are unilocular structures between 1 and 4 cm in diameter, containing fine hair shafts admixed with variable amounts of thick yellowish sebum.

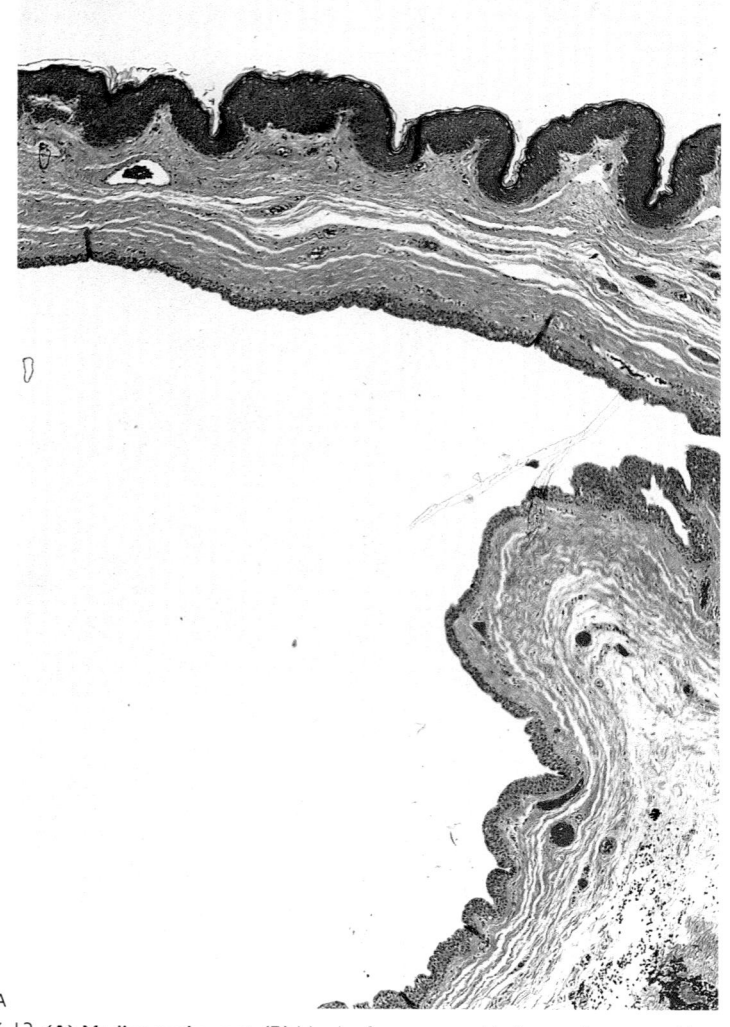
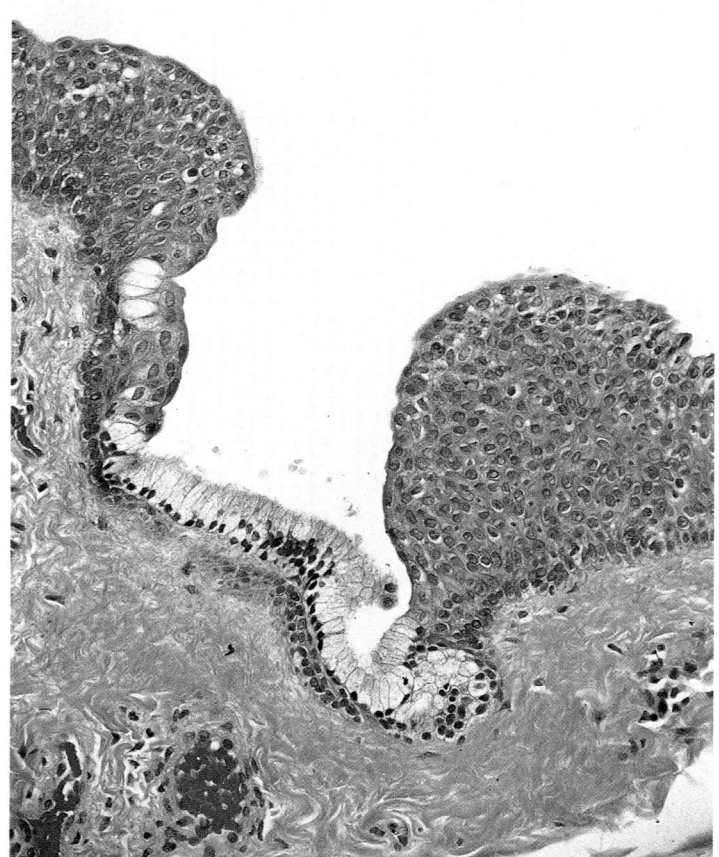

A   B

Fig. 16.13 **(A) Median raphe cyst. (B)** Islands of squamous epithelium are interspersed between mucin-secreting epithelium. (H & E)

The subcutaneous cyst on the back reported as a **cystic teratoma** had features of both a dermoid and bronchogenic cyst (see below).[235]

Histopathology[227]

Dermoid cysts are lined by keratinizing squamous epithelium with attached pilosebaceous structures (Fig.16.14). Non-keratinizing squamous epithelium with admixed goblet cells resembling conjunctival epithelium has been reported in orbital dermoid cysts.[236] Sebaceous glands may empty directly into the cyst, the lumen of which contains hair shafts and keratinous debris. Eccrine and apocrine glands, as well as smooth muscle, may be present in the wall of up to one-quarter of the cases. Partial rupture of the cyst, resulting in a local foreign body granulomatous reaction, may be found. Focal calcification is a rare finding.

The fistulous tract sometimes found in association with midline dermoids of the nose is lined by the same elements as are found in the cyst wall.[231]

CYSTIC TERATOMA

Several cases of cystic teratoma of the skin have been reported in the English language literature.[235,237,238] The lesions were present at birth. They have involved the glabellar region,[237] the back[235] and the knee.[238]

Histopathology

A diversity of tissue types may be present. One of the reported cases was composed of respiratory epithelium, thyroid and nervous tissue as well as striated and smooth muscle.[237] Another case was lined by gastrointestinal mucosa,[238] while another resembled a dermoid cyst with the addition of areas lined by pseudostratified, ciliated epithelium with goblet cells and occasional seromucinous glands and some surrounding smooth muscle.[235]

OMPHALOMESENTERIC DUCT CYST

Omphalomesenteric duct cysts arise in the periumbilical area.[239] They may be associated with a Meckel's diverticulum.

Histopathology

The cysts may be connected to the skin surface, with gastrointestinal mucosa adjoining the stratified squamous epithelium of the adjacent skin. The mucosa may be of gastric, colonic or small bowel type. Smooth muscle may be present in the wall.

MISCELLANEOUS CYSTS

PARASITIC CYSTS

Parasitic cysts are considered in Chapter 29. The most important is cysticercosis, the larval form of *Taenia solium*, which may present as one or more subcutaneous cysts[240] (see p. 732). Sparganosis may also present as a subcutaneous 'cyst' (see p. 732).

PHAEOMYCOTIC CYSTS

A phaeomycotic cyst (phaeohyphomycosis) is a subcutaneous cystic granuloma resulting from infection by hyphae with brown walls.[241] A wood splinter is sometimes present in the lumen and is the source of this opportunistic fungus (see p. 673).

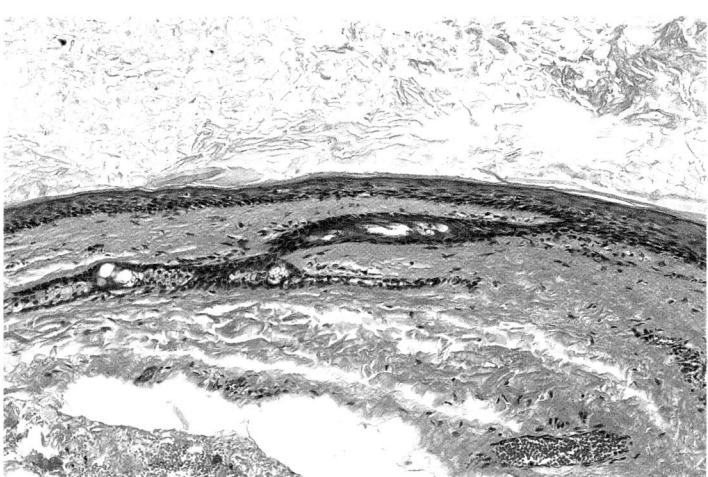

Fig. 16.14 **Dermoid cyst.** A pilosebaceous structure is attached to the cyst wall. (H & E)

DIGITAL MUCOUS CYST

A digital mucous cyst is usually found as a tense cystic nodule at the base of the nail of a finger or thumb. A second type (myxoid cyst) overlies a distal interphalangeal joint.[242] The latter type resembles a ganglion while the former resembles focal mucinosis. Digital mucous cysts are considered in detail with other mucinoses (see p. 412).

MUCOUS CYST (MUCOCELE)

Mucous cysts, found usually on the lower lip or buccal mucosa, result from the rupture of a duct of a minor salivary gland with extravasation of mucus. Large mucinous pools are formed with a variable inflammatory and fibroblastic response (Fig. 16.15). These lesions are considered with the mucinoses (see p. 412).

METAPLASTIC SYNOVIAL CYST

Metaplastic synovial cysts are intradermal cysts lined by a membrane that resembles hyperplastic synovium.[243,244] The lesions usually arise in surgical

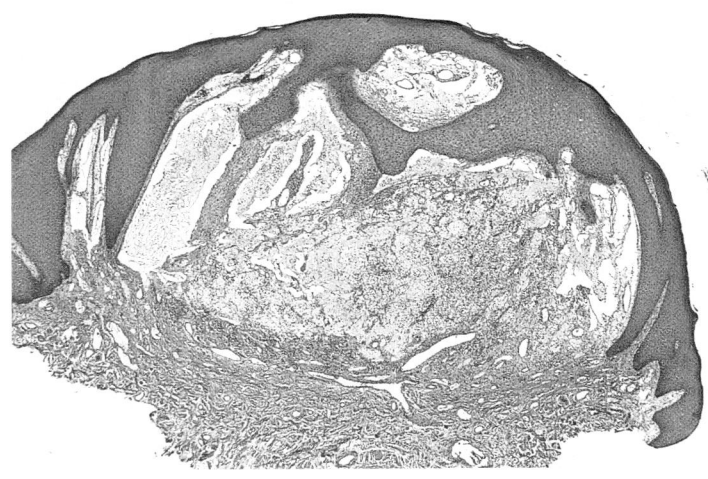

Fig. 16.15 **Mucocele.** There is a large mucinous pool. There is no epithelial lining in these cysts. (H & E)

scars or at sites of trauma,[245] unrelated to joints or other synovial structures.[244] Cutaneous fragility and anomalous scarring may be the explanation for the case that developed in a patient with Ehlers–Danlos syndrome.[246] They are usually solitary.[247]

Histopathology[243,244]

The cyst lining resembles hyperplastic synovium with partly hyalinized synovial villi. Sometimes only slit-like spaces lined by synovium are present (Fig. 16.16). The cystic cavities may communicate with the surface epidermis.

PSEUDOCYST OF THE AURICLE

Pseudocyst of the auricle is an uncommon, non-inflammatory, intra-cartilaginous lesion affecting the upper half or third of the ear, most often in young or middle-aged males.[248–251] Bilateral involvement has been reported.[252] There is usually no clearcut history of preceding trauma.[253] Ischemia has been suggested as a possible cause of the cartilaginous degeneration which is followed by the accumulation of yellowish fluid to form a pseudocyst.[254] The term 'seroma' has been used for a closely related entity in which the accumulation of fluid was thought on clinical grounds to be outside the cartilage.[255]

Histopathology

There is an intracartilaginous cavity without an epithelial lining.[248,250] The wall is composed of eosinophilic, amorphous material which may contain smaller clefts (Fig. 16.17). There is focal fibrosis within the cavity, particularly at the margins, and this probably increases with the duration of the lesion.

ENDOMETRIOSIS

Endometriosis may be found in the umbilicus, in operation scars of the lower abdomen, particularly those associated with cesarean sections, and, rarely, in the inguinal region, thighs and neck.[256–262] Cutaneous endometriosis accounts for less than 1% of cases of ectopic endometrial tissue. The endometrium in most lesions responds to the normal hormonal influences of the menstrual cycle.[263] It presents as a bluish-black tumor of the umbilicus that enlarges about the time of the menses. There may be an associated bloody discharge from the lesion. Most lesions measure from 1 to 3 cm in diameter.

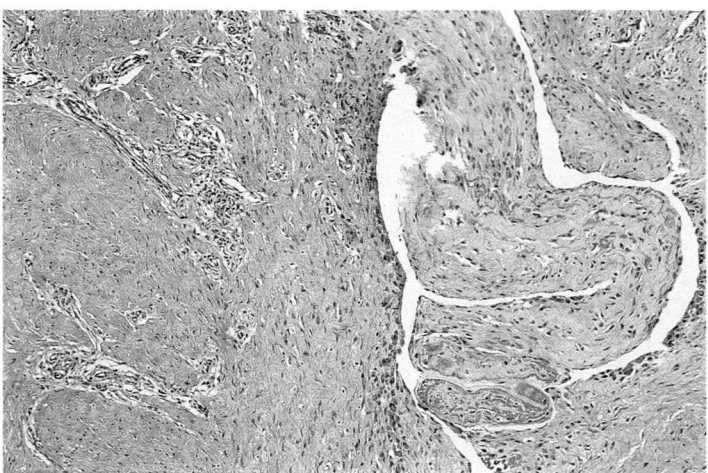

Fig. 16.16 **Metaplastic synovial cyst.** A slit-like cavity lined by synovium is present adjacent to an area of scar tissue in the dermis. (H & E)

Endometriosis arising in scars is usually less well delineated. Such lesions are only partly cystic.

Theories of etiology include implantation, coelomic metaplasia, lymphatic dissemination and hematogenous spread.

Histopathology[260]

There are multiple endometrial glands with surrounding endometrial stroma (Fig. 16.18). The glands may show the usual cyclical changes of the endometrium. Decidualization of the stroma is occasionally present.[264–266] The glands show variable cystic dilatation and may contain blood or debris. There is usually hemosiderin pigment in the functioning cases.[267] There may be dense fibrosis between the endometriotic foci. Adenocarcinoma has been reported as a very rare complication.[268]

CUTANEOUS ENDOSALPINGIOSIS

A patient has been reported with multiple papules around the umbilicus following salpingectomy.[172] The small dermal cysts were lined by tubal epithelium. This appears to be an example of endosalpingiosis, the aberrant growth of fallopian tube epithelium outside its normal location.

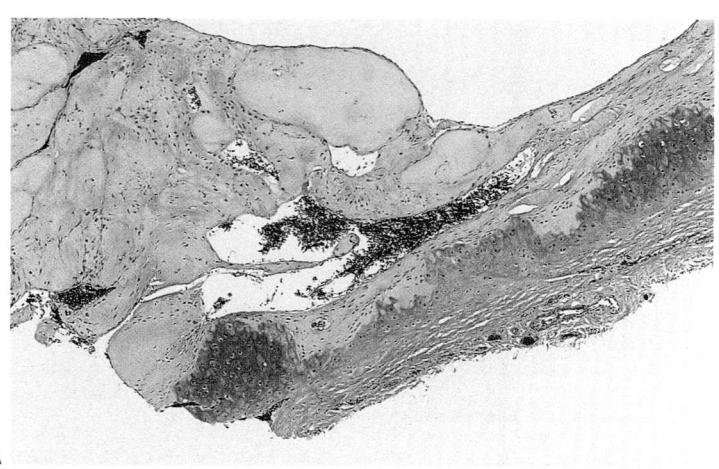

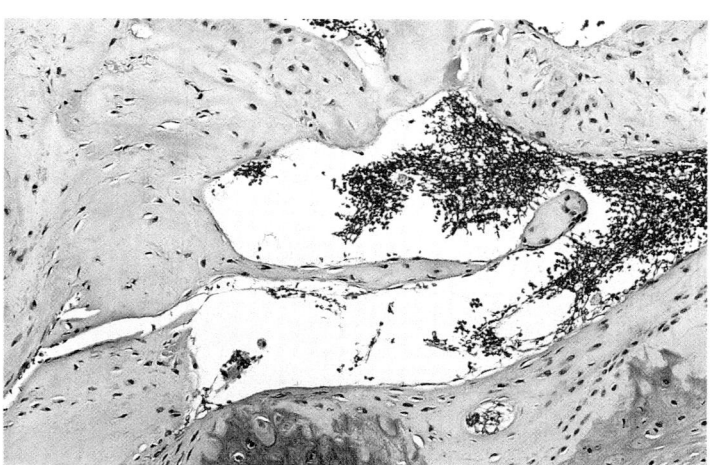

Fig. 16.17 **(A) Pseudocyst of the auricle. (B)** A cavity is present within the cartilage of the ear. Some operative hemorrhage is also present. (H & E)

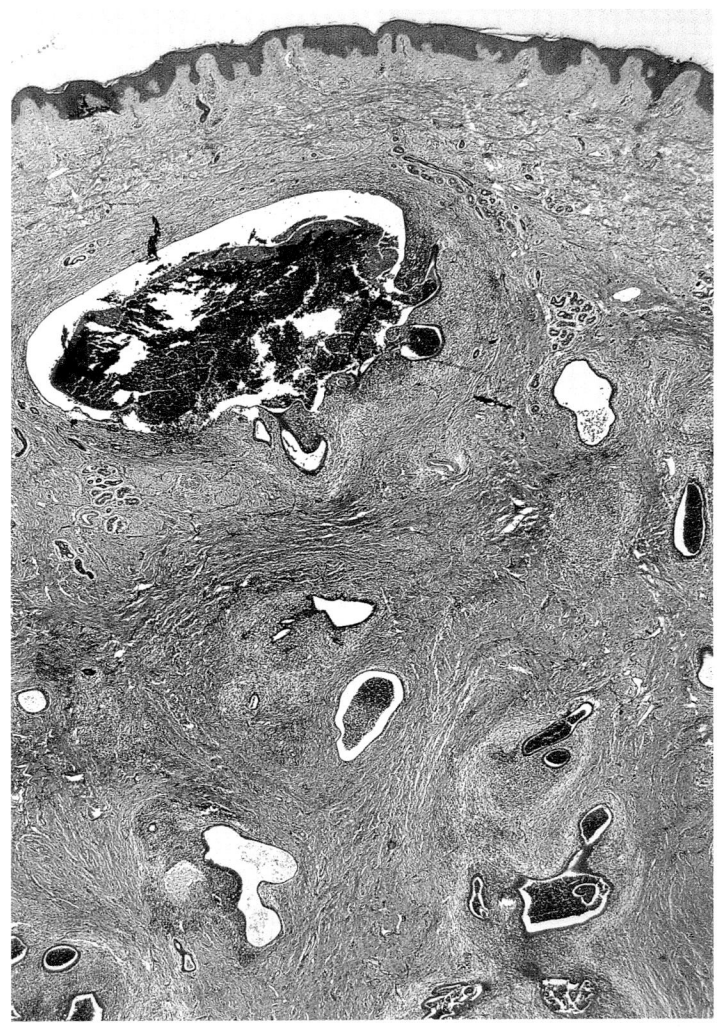

Fig. 16.18 Endometriosis of the umbilicus. Glands and stroma are set in fibrous tissue. The glands are functional with some luminal hemorrhage. (H & E)

Histopathology

The small cysts were unilocular and filled with granular material. There were some papillary projections into the cyst. The epithelium was composed of columnar, ciliated and secretory cells of endosalpingial type.

LYMPHATIC CYSTS

CYSTIC HYGROMA

Cystic hygroma usually presents as a cystic swelling of the subcutaneous tissue of the lower neck of neonates and infants. It is a variant of lymphangioma with large cavernous spaces in the subcutis lined by flattened endothelium (see p. 1004). Islands of connective tissue and sometimes smooth muscle are found between the channels.

SINUSES

Sinus tracts may develop in relation to infected wounds, acne,[269] inflamed and ruptured cysts, in association with thyroglossal or branchial cleft vestiges or defective closure of the neural tube,[270,271] chronic osteomyelitis and various chronic infections such as tuberculosis, mycetomas and actinomycosis. The sinuses reported in association with heterotopic salivary gland tissue in the lower neck were probably of branchial cleft origin.[272] Three sinuses of dermatopathological importance are the congenital midline cervical cleft, the cutaneous dental sinus and the pilonidal sinus.

CONGENITAL MIDLINE CERVICAL CLEFT

This rare anomaly of the ventral neck presents with a longitudinal opening along the midline which varies in length and width. The cleft is often weeping at birth; later there is scar formation if the cleft is not corrected surgically. There may be associated thyroglossal and branchial cleft anomalies. Its origin is disputed, although aberrant fusion of the branchial arches is favored.[273]

Histopathology

The cleft is covered by stratified squamous epithelium with overlying parakeratosis. The underlying dermis may be atrophic. Dense fibrous tissue may be present and often extends into the subcutis. The sinus tract associated with this condition (often at its caudal end) is usually lined with respiratory-type epithelium. Sometimes a fibrous cord overlies the defect. It may include interfasciculated bundles of skeletal muscle.[273]

CUTANEOUS DENTAL SINUS

An intermittently suppurating, chronic sinus tract may develop on the face or neck as a result of a chronic infection of dental origin.[274,275] This is usually an apical abscess.

Histopathology

The sinus tract is lined by heavily inflamed granulation and fibrous tissue. An epithelial lining is sometimes present in part of the tract in cases of long standing. There are no grains as seen in actinomycosis. Rarely, a squamous cell carcinoma may develop from this epithelium.[274]

PILONIDAL SINUS

Pilonidal sinus occurs most commonly as a sinus in the sacrococcygeal region of hirsute males.[276] Other sites include the umbilicus,[277] axilla, scalp,[278] genital region, eyelid, and the finger webs of barbers' hands. Sometimes small cysts may be found in the scalp following hair transplants.[279]

Malignancy, usually a squamous cell carcinoma, may develop as a rare complication in lesions of long standing.[280]

Histopathology

There is usually a sinus tract lined by granulation tissue, with areas of stratified squamous epithelium in the wall in about half the cases. This leads to a bulbous expansion in the lower dermis and subcutaneous tissues where there is a chronic abscess cavity. This contains one or more hair shafts which may be in the lumen, in branches of the main cavity or in the wall itself. There are usually foreign body granulomas in the vicinity of the hairs. There is variable fibrosis in the wall of the sinus and the deeper cavity.

Rarely, the glomus coccygeum, a glomus body lying close to the tip of the coccyx, may be an incidental finding in the tissue surrounding a pilonidal sinus removed from this region.[281]

PITS

Pits are depressions in the epidermal surface. They may be found on the palms in pitted keratolysis (see p. 623), punctate keratoderma (see p. 289), reticulate acropigmentation of Kitamura (see p. 332) and in chronic arsenicism. Pits can occur on the lip in the condition known as congenital lower lip pits (see below) and in type I orofaciodigital syndrome.[282] Pigmented pits may arise in the perioral region in Dowling–Degos disease (see p. 332).

CONGENITAL LOWER LIP PITS

Congenital lower lip pits (Van der Woude syndrome) is a rare autosomal dominant condition characterized by depressions and sometimes sinuses in the vermilion zone of the lower lip.[282,283] They are usually bilateral. There is a frequent association with cleft lip and/or cleft palate. The gene responsible has been mapped to the long arm of chromosome I (Iq32–41).[283]

Histopathology[282,283]

There is a depression/invagination in the epidermis with some thinning in the base. A zone of parakeratosis is often present at either side of the pit. Sometimes a small fistula leads from the base of the pit to underlying minor salivary glands. There is usually no significant inflammation.

REFERENCES

Appendageal cysts

1 Gupta S, Radotra BD, Kumar B et al. Multiple, large, polypoid infundibular (epidermoid) cysts in a cyclosporin-treated renal transplant recipient. Dermatology 2000; 201: 78.
2 Yamamoto T, Nishikawa T, Fujii T, Mizuno K. A giant epidermoid cyst demonstrated by magnetic resonance imaging. Br J Dermatol 2001; 144: 217–218.
3 Greer KE. Epidermal inclusion cyst of the sole. Arch Dermatol 1974; 109: 251–252.
4 Fisher BK, Macpherson M. Epidermoid cyst of the sole. J Am Acad Dermatol 1986; 15: 1127–1129.
5 Yung CW, Estes SA. Subungual epidermal cyst. J Am Acad Dermatol 1980; 3: 599–601.
6 Egawa K, Honda Y, Ono T. Epidermoid cyst with sweat ducts on the torso. Am J Dermatopathol 1995; 17: 71–74.
7 Egawa K, Kitasato H, Ono T. A palmar epidermoid cyst, showing histological features suggestive of eccrine duct origin, developing after a bee-sting. Br J Dermatol 2000; 143: 469–470.
8 Vasiloudes PE, Morelli JG, Weston WL. Plantar epidermal cysts in children. Arch Dermatol 1997; 133: 1465.
9 Ronnen M, Suster S, Shmuel Y et al. Development of epidermal cysts following chronic dermabrasion. Int J Dermatol 1987; 26: 465–466.
10 Leppard B, Bussey HJR. Epidermoid cysts, polyposis coli and Gardner's syndrome. Br J Surg 1975; 62: 387–393.
11 Narisawa Y, Kohda H. Cutaneous cysts of Gardner's syndrome are similar to follicular stem cells. J Cutan Pathol 1995; 22: 115–121.
12 Thewes M, Worret W-I, Abeck D. An unusual case of multiple epidermal finger cysts. Dermatology 1998; 196: 366–367.
13 Brook I. Microbiology of infected epidermal cysts. Arch Dermatol 1989; 125: 1658–1661.
14 Diven DG, Dozier SE, Meyer DJ, Smith EB. Bacteriology of inflamed and uninflamed epidermal inclusion cysts. Arch Dermatol 1998; 134: 49–51.
15 Pakzad SY, Snow JL, Su WPD. Dermatophytic epidermoid cyst. J Cutan Pathol 1997; 24: 116 (abstract).
16 Vicente J, Vázquez-Doval FJ. Proliferations of the epidermoid cyst wall. Int J Dermatol 1998; 37: 181–185.
17 Rahbari H. Epidermoid cysts with seborrheic verruca-like cyst walls. Arch Dermatol 1982; 118: 326–328.
18 Fieselman DW, Reed RJ, Ichinose H. Pigmented epidermal cyst. J Cutan Pathol 1974; 1: 256–259.

19 Vaideeswar P, Prabhat DP, Sivaraman A. Epidermal inclusion cyst with melanoma-like melanophagic proliferation. Acta Derm Venereol 1999; 79: 88.
20 Cooper PH, Fechner RE. Pilomatricoma-like changes in the epidermal cysts of Gardner's syndrome. J Am Acad Dermatol 1983; 8: 639–644.
21 Leppard BJ, Bussey HJR. Gardner's syndrome with epidermoid cysts showing features of pilomatrixomas. Clin Exp Dermatol 1976; 1: 75–82.
22 Satoh T, Mitho Y, Katsumata M et al. Follicular cyst derived from hair matrix and outer root sheath. J Cutan Pathol 1989; 16: 106–108.
23 Mittag H. Darier's disease involving an epidermoid cyst. J Cutan Pathol 1990; 17: 388–390.
24 Hunt SJ. Two pyogenic granulomas arising in an epidermoid cyst. Am J Dermatopathol 1989; 11: 360–363.
25 Shelley WB, Wood MG. Occult Bowen's disease in keratinous cysts. Br J Dermatol 1981; 105: 105–108.
26 Tomková H, Fujimoto W, Arata J. Expression of keratins (K10 and K17) in steatocystoma multiplex, eruptive vellus hair cysts, and epidermoid and trichilemmal cysts. Am J Dermatopathol 1997; 19: 250–253.
27 McDonald LW. Carcinomatous change in cysts of skin. Arch Dermatol 1963; 87: 208–211.
28 López-Ríos F, Rodriguez-Peralto JL, Castaño E, Benito A. Squamous cell carcinoma arising in a cutaneous epidermal cyst. Case report and literature review. Am J Dermatopathol 1999; 21: 174–177.
29 Malone JC, Sonnier GB, Hughes AP, Hood AF. Poorly differentiated squamous cell carcinoma arising within an epidermoid cyst. Int J Dermatol 1999; 38: 556–558.
30 Wade CL, Haley JC, Hood AF. The utility of submitting epidermoid cysts for histologic examination. Int J Dermatol 2000; 39: 314–315.
31 Kato N, Ueno H. Two cases of plantar epidermal cyst associated with human papillomavirus. Clin Exp Dermatol 1992; 17: 252–256.
32 Rios-Buceta LM, Fraga-Fernandez J, Fernandez-Herrera J. Human papillomavirus in an epidermoid cyst of the sole in a non-Japanese patient. J Am Acad Dermatol 1992; 27: 364–366.
33 Egawa K, Honda Y, Inaba Y et al. Detection of human papillomaviruses and eccrine ducts in palmoplantar epidermoid cysts. Br J Dermatol 1995; 132: 533–542.
34 Egawa K, Honda Y, Inaba Y et al. Multiple plantar epidermoid cysts harboring carcinoembryonic antigen and human papillomavirus DNA sequences. J Am Acad Dermatol 1994; 30: 494–496.
35 Abe H, Ohnishi T, Watanabe S. Does plantar epidermoid cyst with human papillomavirus infection originate from the eccrine dermal duct? Br J Dermatol 1999; 141: 161–162.
36 Ohnishi T, Watanabe S. Immunohistochemical observation of cytokeratins in keratinous cysts including plantar epidermoid cyst. J Cutan Pathol 1999; 26: 424–429.
37 Meyer LM, Tyring SK, Little WP. Verrucous cyst. Arch Dermatol 1991; 127: 1810–1812.
38 Soyer HP, Schadendorf D, Cerroni L, Kerl H. Verrucous cysts: histopathologic characterization and molecular detection of human papillomavirus-specific DNA. J Cutan Pathol 1993; 20: 411–417.
39 Aloi F, Tomasini C, Pippione M. HPV-related follicular cysts. Am J Dermatopathol 1992; 14: 37–41.
40 Elston DM, Parker LU, Tuthill RJ. Epidermoid cyst of the scalp containing human papillomavirus. J Cutan Pathol 1993; 20: 184–186.
41 Mihara M, Nishiura S, Aso M et al. Papillomavirus-infected keratinous cyst on the sole. A histologic, immunohistochemical, and electron microscopic study. Am J Dermatopathol 1991; 13: 293–299.
42 Egawa K, Inaba Y, Ono T, Arao T. 'Cystic papilloma' in humans? Demonstration of human papillomavirus in plantar epidermoid cysts. Arch Dermatol 1990; 126: 1599–1603.
43 Sau P, Graham JH, Helwig EB. Proliferating epithelial cysts. Clinicopathological analysis of 96 cases. J Cutan Pathol 1995; 22: 394–406.
44 Leppard BJ, Sanderson KV, Wells RS. Hereditary trichilemmal cysts. Clin Exp Dermatol 1977; 2: 23–32.
45 Leppard BJ, Sanderson KV. The natural history of trichilemmal cysts. Br J Dermatol 1976; 94: 379–390.
46 Pinkus H. 'Sebaceous cysts' are trichilemmal cysts. Arch Dermatol 1969; 99: 544–553.
47 Hanau D, Grosshans E. Trichilemmal cyst with intrinsic parietal sebaceous and apocrine structures. Clin Exp Dermatol 1980; 5: 351–355.
48 Headington JT. Tumors of the hair follicle. A review. Am J Pathol 1976; 85: 480–514.
49 Laing V, Knipe RC, Flowers FP et al. Proliferating trichilemmal tumor: report of a case and review of the literature. J Dermatol Surg Oncol 1991; 17: 295–298.
50 Noto G. 'Benign' proliferating trichilemmal tumour: does it really exist? Histopathology 1999; 35: 386–387.
51 Mones JM, Ackerman AB. Proliferating tricholemmal cyst is squamous-cell carcinoma. Dermatopathology: Practical & Conceptual 1998; 4: 295–310.
52 Noto G, Pravatà G, Aricò M. Proliferating tricholemmal cyst should always be considered as a low-grade carcinoma. Dermatology 1997; 194: 374–375.

53 Wilson Jones E. Proliferating epidermoid cysts. Arch Dermatol 1966; 94: 11–19.

54 Baptista AP, Silva LGE, Born MC. Proliferating trichilemmal cyst. J Cutan Pathol 1983; 10: 178–187.

55 Munro JM, Hall PA, Thompson HH. Proliferating trichilemmal cyst occurring on the skin. J Cutan Pathol 1986; 13: 246–249.

56 Mehregan AH, Lee KC. Malignant proliferating trichilemmal tumors – report of three cases. J Dermatol Surg Oncol 1987; 13: 1339–1342.

57 Weiss J, Heine M, Grimmel M, Jung EG. Malignant proliferating trichilemmal cyst. J Am Acad Dermatol 1995; 32: 870–873.

58 Takenaka H, Kishimoto S, Shibagaki R et al. Recurrent malignant proliferating trichilemmal tumour: local management with ethanol injection. Br J Dermatol 1998; 139: 726–729.

59 Batman PA, Evans HJR. Metastasising pilar tumour of scalp. J Clin Pathol 1986; 39: 757–760.

60 Amaral ALMP, Nascimento AG, Goellner JR. Proliferating pilar (trichilemmal) cyst. Report of two cases, one with carcinomatous transformation and one with distant metastases. Arch Pathol Lab Med 1984; 108: 808–810.

61 Noto G, Pravatà G, Aricò M. Malignant proliferating trichilemmal tumor. Am J Dermatopathol 1997; 19: 202–204.

62 Park BS, Yang SG, Cho KH. Malignant proliferating trichilemmal tumor showing distant metastases. Am J Dermatopathol 1997; 19: 536–539.

63 Rahbari H, Mehregan AH. Development of proliferating trichilemmal cyst in organoid nevus. J Am Acad Dermatol 1986; 14: 123–126.

64 Jaworski R. Unusual proliferating trichilemmal cyst. Am J Dermatopathol 1987;

65 Sakamoto F, Ito M, Nakamura A, Sato Y. Proliferating trichilemmal cyst with apocrine-acrosyringeal and sebaceous differentiation. J Cutan Pathol 1991; 18: 137–141.

66 Warner TFCS. Proliferating pilar cyst with spindle cell component. J Cutan Pathol 1979; 6: 310–316.

67 Mori O, Hachisuka H, Sasai Y. Proliferating trichilemmal cyst with spindle cell carcinoma. Am J Dermatopathol 1990; 12: 479–484.

68 Brownstein MH, Arluk DJ. Proliferating trichilemmal cyst: a simulant of squamous cell carcinoma. Cancer 1981; 48: 1207–1214.

69 Rutty GN, Richman PI, Laing JHE. Malignant change in trichilemmal cysts: a study of cell proliferation and DNA content. Histopathology 1992; 21: 465–468.

70 Sleater J, Beers B, Stefan M et al. Proliferating trichilemmal cyst. Report of four cases, two with nondiploid DNA content and increased proliferation index. Am J Dermatopathol 1993; 15: 423–428.

71 Herrero J, Monteagudo C, Ruiz A, Llombart-Bosch A. Malignant proliferating trichilemmal tumors: an histopathological and immunohistochemical study of three cases with DNA ploidy and morphometric evaluation. Histopathology 1998; 33: 542–546.

72 López-Rios F, Rodríguez-Peralto JL, Aguilar A et al. Proliferating trichilemmal cyst with focal invasion. Report of a case and a review of the literature. Am J Dermatopathol 2000; 22: 183–187.

73 Val-Bernal JF, Garijo MF, Fernández F. Malignant proliferating trichilemmal tumor. Am J Dermatopathol 1998; 20: 433.

74 Miyairi H, Takahashi S, Morohashi M. Proliferating trichilemmal cyst: an ultrastructural study. J Cutan Pathol 1984; 11: 274–281.

75 Alessi E, Zorgi F, Gianotti R, Parafioriti A. Malignant proliferating onycholemmal cyst. J Cutan Pathol 1994; 21: 183–188.

76 Brownstein MH. Hybrid cyst: A combined epidermoid and trichilemmal cyst. J Am Acad Dermatol 1983; 9: 872–875.

77 Brownstein MH. Combined epidermoid (epidermal) and trichilemmal (pilar) cyst. J Am Acad Dermatol 1984; 11: 141–142.

78 Requena L, Sánchez Yus E. Follicular hybrid cysts. An expanded spectrum. Am J Dermatopathol 1991; 13: 228–233.

79 Andersen WK, Rao BK, Bhawan J. The hybrid epidermoid and apocrine cyst. A combination of apocrine hydrocystoma and epidermal inclusion cyst. Am J Dermatopathol 1996; 18: 364–366.

80 Bourland AE. The hybrid epidermoid and apocrine cyst. Am J Dermatopathol 1997; 19: 619.

81 Ahn SK, Chung J, Lee WS et al. Hybrid cysts showing alternate combination of eruptive vellus hair cyst, steatocystoma multiplex, and epidermoid cyst, and an association among the three conditions. Am J Dermatopathol 1996; 18: 645–649.

82 Tsuruta D, Nakagawa K, Taniguchi S et al. Combined cutaneous hamartoma encompassing benign melanocytic naevus, vellus hair cyst and epidermoid cyst. Clin Exp Dermatol 2000; 25: 38–40.

83 Mehregan AH, Medenica M. Pigmented follicular cysts. J Cutan Pathol 1982; 9: 423–427.

84 Pavlidakey GP, Mehregan A, Hashimoto K. Pigmented follicular cysts. Int J Dermatol 1986; 25: 174–177.

85 Requena Caballero L, Sánchez Yus E. Pigmented follicular cyst. J Am Acad Dermatol 1989; 21: 1073–1075.

86 Sandoval R, Urbina F. Pigmented follicular cyst. Br J Dermatol 1994; 131: 130–131.

87 Salopek TG, Lee SK, Jimbow K. Multiple pigmented follicular cysts: a subtype of multiple pilosebaceous cysts. Br J Dermatol 1996; 134: 758–762.

88 Iwahara K, Koike M, Ogawa H. Pigmented follicular cyst showing degenerating pigmented hair shafts on histology. Br J Dermatol 1999; 140: 364–365.

89 Barr RJ, Headley JL, Jensen JL, Howell JB. Cutaneous keratocysts of nevoid basal cell carcinoma syndrome. J Am Acad Dermatol 1986; 14: 572–576.

90 Baselga E, Dzwierzynski WW, Neuburg M et al. Cutaneous keratocyst in naevoid basal cell carcinoma syndrome. Br J Dermatol 1996; 135: 810–812.

91 Esterly NB, Fretzin DF, Pinkus H. Eruptive vellus hair cysts. Arch Dermatol 1977; 113: 500–503.

92 Lee S, Kim J-G, Kang JS. Eruptive vellus hair cysts. Arch Dermatol 1984; 120: 1191–1195.

93 Grimalt R, Gelmetti C. Eruptive vellus hair cysts: case report and review of the literature. Pediatr Dermatol 1992; 9: 98–102.

94 Kumakiri M, Takashima I, Iju M et al. Eruptive vellus hair cysts – a facial variant. J Am Acad Dermatol 1982; 7: 461–467.

95 Piepkorn MW, Clark L, Lombardi DL. A kindred with congenital vellus hair cysts. J Am Acad Dermatol 1981; 5: 661–665.

96 Benoldi D, Allegra F. Congenital eruptive vellus hair cysts. Int J Dermatol 1989; 28: 340–341.

97 Romiti R, Neto CF. Eruptive vellus hair cysts in a patient with ectodermal dysplasia. J Am Acad Dermatol 1997; 36: 261–262.

98 Bovenmyer DA. Eruptive vellus hair cysts. Arch Dermatol 1979; 115: 338–339.

99 Sánchez-Yus E, Aguilar-Martinez A, Cristobal-Gil MC et al. Eruptive vellus hair cyst and steatocystoma multiplex: two related conditions? J Cutan Pathol 1988; 15: 40–42.

100 Moon SE, Lee YS, Youn JI. Eruptive vellus hair cyst and steatocystoma multiplex in a patient with pachyonychia congenita. J Am Acad Dermatol 1994; 30: 275–276.

101 Redondo P, Vázquel-Doval J, Idoate M et al. Multiple pilosebaceous cysts. Clin Exp Dermatol 1995; 20: 328–330.

102 Ohtake N, Kubota Y, Takayama O et al. Relationship between steatocystoma multiplex and eruptive vellus hair cysts. J Am Acad Dermatol 1992; 26: 876–878.

103 Sexton M, Murdock DK. Eruptive vellus hair cysts. A follicular cyst of the sebaceous duct (sometimes). Am J Dermatopathol 1989; 11: 364–368.

104 Patrizi A, Neri I, Guerrini V et al. Persistent milia, steatocystoma multiplex and eruptive vellus hair cysts: variable expression of multiple pilosebaceous cysts within an affected family. Dermatology 1998; 196: 392–396.

105 Lazarov A, Amichai B, Gagnano M, Halevy S. Coexistence of trichostasis spinulosa and eruptive vellus hair cysts. Int J Dermatol 1994; 33: 858–859.

106 Nishimura M, Kohda H, Urabe A. Steatocystoma multiplex. A facial papular variant. Arch Dermatol 1986; 122: 205–207.

107 Cole LA. Steatocystoma multiplex. Arch Dermatol 1976; 112: 1437–1439.

108 Holmes R, Black MM. Steatocystoma multiplex with unusually prominent cysts on the face. Br J Dermatol 1980; 102: 711–713.

109 Ahn SK, Hwang SM, Lee SH, Lee WS. Steatocystoma multiplex localized only in the face. Int J Dermatol 1997; 36: 372–373.

110 Lee YJ, Lee SH, Ahn SK. Sebocystomatosis: a clinical variant of steatocystoma multiplex. Int J Dermatol 1996; 35: 734–735.

111 Marley WM, Buntin DM, Chesney TM. Steatocystoma multiplex limited to the scalp. Arch Dermatol 1981; 117: 673–674.

112 Belinchón I, Mayol MJ, Onrubia JA. Steatocystoma multiplex confined to the scalp. Int J Dermatol 1995; 34: 429–430.

113 Setoyama M, Mizoguchi S, Usuki K, Kanzaki T. Steatocystoma multiplex. A case with unusual clinical and histological manifestation. Am J Dermatopathol 1997; 19: 89–92.

114 Rollins T, Levin RM, Heymann WR. Acral steatocystoma multiplex. J Am Acad Dermatol 2000; 43: 396–399.

115 Park YM, Cho SH, Kang H. Congenital linear steatocystoma multiplex of the nose. Pediatr Dermatol 2000; 17: 136–138.

116 Cambiaghi S, Riva S, Ramaccioni V et al. Steatocystoma multiplex and leuconychia in a child with Alagille syndrome. Br J Dermatol 1998; 138: 150–154.

117 Gianotti R, Cavicchini S, Alessi E. Simultaneous occurrence of multiple trichoblastomas and steatocystoma multiplex. Am J Dermatopathol 1997; 19: 294–298.

118 Brownstein MH. Steatocystoma simplex. A solitary steatocystoma. Arch Dermatol 1982; 118: 409–411.

119 Egbert BM, Price NM, Segal RJ. Steatocystoma multiplex. Report of a florid case and a review. Arch Dermatol 1979; 115: 334–335.

120 Apaydin R, Bilen N, Bayramgürler D et al. Steatocystoma multiplex suppurativum: oral isotretinoin treatment combined with cryotherapy. Australas J Dermatol 2000; 41: 98–100.

121 Smith FJD, Corden LD, Rugg EL et al. Mutations in keratin 17 cause steatocystoma multiplex. J Invest Dermatol 1996; 106: 843 (abstract).

122 Hohl D. Steatocystoma multiplex and oligosymptomatic pachyonychia congenita of the Jackson–Sertoli type. Dermatology 1997; 195: 86–88.

123 Patterson JW, Kannon GA. Spherulocystic disease ("myospherulosis") arising in a lesion of steatocystoma multiplex. J Am Acad Dermatol 1998; 38: 274–275.

124 Sabater-Marco V, Pérez-Ferriols A. Steatocystoma multiplex with smooth muscle. A hamartoma of the pilosebaceous apparatus. Am J Dermatopathol 1996; 18: 548–550.

125 Nogita T, Chi H-I, Nakagawa H, Ishibashi Y. Eruptive vellus hair cysts with sebaceous glands. Br J Dermatol 1991; 125: 475–476.

126 Sánchez Yus E, Simón RS, Herrera M et al. The many faces of steatocystoma-vellus hair cyst hamartoma. J Cutan Pathol 1997; 24: 121 (abstract).

127 Iacobelli D, Hashimoto K, Kato I et al. Clobetasol-induced milia. J Am Acad Dermatol 1989; 21: 215–217.

128 Boehm I, Schupp G, Bauer R. Milia en plaque arising in discoid lupus erythematosus. Br J Dermatol 1997; 137: 649–651.

129 Cho SH, Cho BK, Kim CW. Milia en plaque associated with pseudoxanthoma elasticum. J Cutan Pathol 1997; 24: 61–63.

130 Rositto A, Avila S, Carames C, Drut R. Congenital hemangioma with milialike structures: a case report. Pediatr Dermatol 1998; 15: 307–308.

131 Hubler WR Jr, Rudolph AH, Kelleher RM. Milia en plaque. Cutis 1978; 22: 67–70.

132 Ratnavel RC, Handfield-Jones SE, Norris PG. Milia restricted to the eyelids. Clin Exp Dermatol 1995; 20: 153–154.

133 Del-Río E, Pena J, Aguilar A. Milia cysts along the nasal groove in a child. Clin Exp Dermatol 1993; 18: 289–290.

134 Langley RGB, Walsh NMG, Ross JB. Multiple eruptive milia: Report of a case, review of the literature, and a classification. J Am Acad Dermatol 1997; 37: 353–356.

135 Samlaska CP, Benson PM. Milia en plaque. J Am Acad Dermatol 1989; 21: 311–313.

136 Lee DW, Choi SW, Cho BK. Milia en plaque. J Am Acad Dermatol 1994; 31: 107.

137 Keohane SG, Beveridge GW, Benton EC, Cox NH. Milia en plaque – a new site and novel treatment. Clin Exp Dermatol 1996; 21: 58–60.

138 Losada-Campa A, de la Torre-Fraga C, Cruces-Prado M. Milia en plaque. Br J Dermatol 1996; 134: 970–972.

139 García Sánchez MS, Gómez Centeno P, Rosón E et al. Milia en plaque in a bilateral submandibular distribution. Clin Exp Dermatol 1998; 23: 227–229.

140 Wong SS, Goh CL. Milia en plaque. Clin Exp Dermatol 1999; 24: 183–185.

141 Cairns ML, Knable AL. Multiple eruptive milia in a 15-year-old boy. Pediatr Dermatol 1999; 16: 108–110.

142 Bridges AG, Lucky AW, Haney G, Mutasim DF. Milia en plaque of the eyelids in childhood: case report and review of the literature. Pediatr Dermatol 1998; 15: 282–284.

143 Alsaleh QA, Nanda A, Sharaf A, Al-Sabah H. Milia en plaque: a new site. Int J Dermatol 2000; 39: 614–615.

144 Ergin Ş, Başak P, Sari A. Milia en plaque. J Eur Acad Dermatol Venereol 2000; 14: 47–49.

145 Tsuji T, Sugai T, Suzuki S. The mode of growth of eccrine duct milia. J Invest Dermatol 1975; 65: 388–393.

146 Hassounah A, Piérard G. Kerosis and comedos without prominent elastosis in Favre–Racouchot disease. Am J Dermatopathol 1987; 9: 15–17.

147 John SM, Hamm H. Actinic comedonal plaque – a rare ectopic form of the Favre–Racouchot syndrome. Clin Exp Dermatol 1993; 18: 256–258.

148 Sánchez-Yus E, del Río E, Simón P et al. The histopathology of closed and open comedones of Favre–Racouchot disease. Arch Dermatol 1997; 133: 743–745.

149 Smith JD, Chernosky ME. Hidrocystomas. Arch Dermatol 1973; 108: 676–679.

150 Sperling LC, Sakas EL. Eccrine hidrocystomas. J Am Acad Dermatol 1982; 7: 763–770.

151 Masri-Fridling GD, Elgart ML. Eccrine hidrocystomas. J Am Acad Dermatol 1992; 26: 780–782.

152 Fariña MC, Piqué E, Olivares M et al. Multiple hidrocystoma of the face: three cases. Clin Exp Dermatol 1995; 20: 323–327.

153 Bourke JF, Colloby P, Graham-Brown RAC. Multiple pigmented eccrine hidrocystomas. J Am Acad Dermatol 1996; 35: 480–482.

154 Alfadley A, Al Aboud K, Tulba A, Mourad MM. Multiple eccrine hidrocystomas of the face. Int J Dermatol 2001; 40: 125–129.

155 Theocharous C, Jaworski RC. Squamous cell carcinoma arising in an eccrine hidrocystoma. Pathology 1993; 25: 184–186.

156 Hassan MO, Khan MA. Ultrastructure of eccrine cystadenoma. A case report. Arch Dermatol 1979; 115: 1217–1221.

157 Mehregan AH. Apocrine cystadenoma. Arch Dermatol 1964; 90: 274–279.

158 Smith JD, Chernosky ME. Apocrine hidrocystoma (cystadenoma). Arch Dermatol 1974; 109: 700–702.

159 Holder WR, Smith JD, Mocega EE. Giant apocrine hidrocystoma. Arch Dermatol 1971; 104: 522–523.

160 Kruse TV, Khan MA, Hassan MO. Multiple apocrine cystadenomas. Br J Dermatol 1979; 100: 675–681.

161 Langer K, Konrad K, Smolle J. Multiple apocrine hidrocystomas on the eyelids. Am J Dermatopathol 1989; 11: 570–573.

162 Alessi E, Gianotti R, Coggi A. Multiple apocrine hidrocystomas of the eyelids. Br J Dermatol 1997; 137: 642–645.

163 Veraldi S, Gianotti R, Pabisch S, Gasparini G. Pigmented apocrine hidrocystoma – a report of two cases and review of the literature. Clin Exp Dermatol 1991; 16: 18–21.

164 Glusac EJ, Hendrickson MS, Smoller BR. Apocrine cystadenoma of the vulva. J Am Acad Dermatol 1994; 31: 498–499.

165 Hashimoto K, Zagula-Mally ZW, Youngberg G, Leicht S. Electron microscopic study of Moll's gland cyst. J Cutan Pathol 1987; 14: 23–26.

166 Combemale P, Kanitakis J, Dupin N et al. Multiple Moll's gland cysts (apocrine hidrocystomas) of the eyelids. Dermatology 1997; 194: 195–196.

167 Bures FA, Kotynek J. Differentiating between apocrine and eccrine hidrocystoma. Cutis 1982; 29: 616–620.

168 Sánchez Yus E, Simón RS. Eccrine, apocrine, or sebaceous duct cyst? J Cutan Pathol 1999; 26: 444–446.

169 Hassan MO, Khan MA, Kruse TV. Apocrine cystadenoma. An ultrastructural study. Arch Dermatol 1979; 115: 194–200.

Developmental cysts

170 Kurban RS, Bhawan J. Cutaneous cysts lined by nonsquamous epithelium. Am J Dermatopathol 1991; 13: 509–517.

171 Van der Putte SCJ, Toonstra J. Cutaneous 'bronchogenic' cyst. J Cutan Pathol 1985; 12: 404–409.

172 Doré N, Landry M, Cadotte M, Schürch W. Cutaneous endosalpingiosis. Arch Dermatol 1980; 116: 909–912.

173 Pryce DW, Khine M, Verbov JL, van Velzen D. Scalp cyst with heterotopic brain tissue. Br J Dermatol 1993; 129: 183–185.

174 Fraga S, Helwig EB, Rosen SH. Bronchogenic cysts in the skin and subcutaneous tissue. Am J Clin Pathol 1971; 56: 230–238.

175 Patterson JW, Pittman DL, Rich JD. Presternal ciliated cyst. Arch Dermatol 1984; 120: 240–242.

176 Kural YB, Ergün S, Büyükbabani N et al. Cutaneous bronchogenic cysts. Int J Dermatol 1998; 37: 137–140.

177 Ramón R, Betlloch I, Guijarro J et al. Bronchogenic cyst presenting as a nodular lesion. Pediatr Dermatol 1999; 16: 285–287.

178 Ambiavagar PC, Rosen Y. Cutaneous ciliated cyst of the chin. Probable bronchogenic cyst. Arch Dermatol 1979; 115: 895–896.

179 Calb IL, Haas E, Lewandowski MG, Maler L. Cutaneous bronchogenic cyst: an unusual localization and review of the literature. Br J Dermatol 2000; 143: 1353–1355.

180 Pul N, Pul M. Bronchogenic cyst of the scapular area in an infant: case report and review of the literature. J Am Acad Dermatol 1994; 31: 120–122.

181 Jona JZ. Extramediastinal bronchogenic cysts in children. Pediatr Dermatol 1995; 12: 304–306.

182 Shareef DS, Salm R. Ectopic vestigial lesions of the neck and shoulders. J Clin Pathol 1981; 34: 1155–1162.

183 Coleman WR, Homer RS, Kaplan RR. Branchial cleft heterotopia of the lower neck. J Cutan Pathol 1989; 16: 353–358.

184 Zvulunov A, Amichai B, Grunwald MH et al. Cutaneous bronchogenic cyst: delineation of a poorly recognized lesion. Pediatr Dermatol 1998; 15: 277–281.

185 Miller OF III, Tyler W. Cutaneous bronchogenic cyst with papilloma and sinus presentation. J Am Acad Dermatol 1984; 11: 367–371.

186 Beyer LG, English JC III, Halbach DP. Presternal bronchogenic sinus with pedunculated lymphoid aggregate. Am J Dermatopathol 2000; 22: 79–82.

187 Zvulunov A, Avinoach I. Branchial cleft anomalies and bronchogenic cysts are two unrelated disorders of embryogenesis. Pediatr Dermatol 2000; 17: 332–333.

188 Muezzinoglu B, Sozubir S, Tugay M, Guvenc BH. Histological and clinical overlapping. Am J Dermatopathol 2001; 23: 278–279.

189 Mahler V, Wurm J, von den Driesch P. Ectopic respiratory epithelium associated with multiple malformations. Br J Dermatol 1997; 136: 933–934.

190 Alfadley A, Hainau B, Al Aboud K et al. Ectopic respiratory mucosa in the skin associated with skeletal malformation and polydactyly. J Am Acad Dermatol 2000; 43: 939–942.

191 Foote JE, Anderson PC. Branchial cleft remnants suggesting tuberculous lymphadenitis. Arch Dermatol 1968; 97: 536–539.

192 Betti R, Lodi A, Palvarini M, Crosti C. Branchial cyst of the neck. Br J Dermatol 1992; 127: 195.

193 Bernstein A, Scardino PT, Tomaszewski M-M, Cohen MH. Carcinoma arising in a branchial cleft cyst. Cancer 1976; 37: 2417–2422.

194 Compagno J, Hyams VJ, Safavian M. Does branchiogenic carcinoma really exist? Arch Pathol Lab Med 1976; 100: 311–314.

195 Rizzo R, Micali G, Calvieri S et al. Branchio-oculo-facial syndrome and dermal thymus: case report and review of the literature. Pediatr Dermatol 1995; 12: 24–27.

196 Heymann WR. Advances in the cutaneous manifestations of thyroid disease. Int J Dermatol 1997; 36: 641–645.

197 Baek S-C, Houh D, Byun D-G, Cho B-K. Hürthle cell adenoma of the thyroglossal duct fistula. Int J Dermatol 1998; 37: 784–786.

198 Langlois NEI, Krukowski ZH, Miller ID. Pancreatic tissue in a lateral cervical cyst attached to the thyroid gland – a presumed foregut remnant. Histopathology 1997; 31: 378–380.

199 Sanusi ID, Carrington PR, Adams DN. Cervical thymic cyst. Arch Dermatol 1982; 118: 122–124.

200 Mikal S. Cervical thymic cyst. Case report and review of the literature. Arch Surg 1974; 109: 558–562.

201 Guba AM Jr, Adam AE, Jaques DA, Chambers RG. Cervical presentation of thymic cysts. Am J Surg 1978; 136: 430–436.

202 Barr RJ, Santa Cruz DJ, Pearl RM. Dermal thymus. A light microscopic and immunohistochemical study. J Cutan Pathol 1989; 125: 1681–1684.

203 Farmer ER, Helwig EB. Cutaneous ciliated cysts. Arch Dermatol 1978; 114: 70–73.

204 Al-Nafussi AI, Carder P. Cutaneous ciliated cyst: a case report and immunohistochemical comparison with fallopian tube. Histopathology 1990; 16: 595–598.

205 Osada A, Ohtake N, Furue M, Tamaki K. Cutaneous ciliated cyst on the sole of the foot. Br J Dermatol 1995; 132: 488–490.

206 Cortés-Franco R, Carrasco D, Teixeira F, Domínguez-Soto L. Cutaneous ciliated cyst. Int J Dermatol 1995; 34: 32–33.

207 Leonforte JF. Cutaneous ciliated cystadenoma in a man. Arch Dermatol 1982; 118: 1010–1012.

208 Ashton MA. Cutaneous ciliated cyst of the lower limb in a male. Histopathology 1995; 26: 467–469.

209 Trotter SE, Rassl DM, Saad M et al. Cutaneous ciliated cyst occurring in a male. Histopathology 1994; 25: 492–493.

210 Sidoni A, Bucciarelli E. Ciliated cyst of the perineal skin. Am J Dermatopathol 1997; 19: 93–96.

211 Dini M, Russo GL, Baroni G, Colafranceschi M. Cutaneous ciliated cyst. A case report with immunohistochemical evidence for dynein in ciliated cells. Am J Dermatopathol 2000; 22: 519–523.

212 Sickel JZ. Cutaneous ciliated cyst of the scalp. A case report with immunohistochemical evidence for estrogen and progesterone receptors. Am J Dermatopathol 1994; 16: 76–79.

213 Tachibana T, Sakamoto F, Ito M et al. Cutaneous ciliated cyst: a case report and histochemical, immunohistochemical, and ultrastructural study. J Cutan Pathol 1995; 22: 33–37.

214 True L, Golitz LE. Ciliated plantar cyst. Arch Dermatol 1980; 116: 1066–1067.

215 Robboy SJ, Ross JS, Prat J et al. Urogenital sinus origin of mucinous and ciliated cysts of the vulva. Obstet Gynecol 1978; 51: 347–351.

216 Kang IK, Kim YJ, Choi KC. Ciliated cyst of the vulva. J Am Acad Dermatol 1995; 32: 514–515.

217 Asarch RG, Golitz LE, Sausker WF, Kreye GM. Median raphe cysts of the penis. Arch Dermatol 1979; 115: 1084–1086.

218 LeVasseur JG, Perry VE. Perineal median raphe cyst. Pediatr Dermatol 1997; 14: 391–392.

219 Nagore E, Sánchez-Motilla JM, Febrer MI, Aliaga A. Median raphe cysts of the penis: a report of five cases. Pediatr Dermatol 1998; 15: 191–193.

220 Ohnishi T, Watanabe S. Immunohistochemical analysis of human milk fat globulin I and cytokeratin expression in median raphe cyst of the penis. Clin Exp Dermatol 2001; 26: 88–92.

221 Paslin D. Urethroid cyst. Arch Dermatol 1983; 119: 89–90.

222 Claudy AL, Dutoit M, Boucheron S. Epidermal and urethroid penile cyst. Acta Derm Venereol 1991; 71: 61–62.

223 Sharkey MJ, Grabski WJ, McCollough ML, Berger TG. Postcoital appearance of a median raphe cyst. J Am Acad Dermatol 1992; 26: 273–274.

224 Quiles DR, Mas IB, Martinez AJ et al. Gonococcal infection of the penile median raphe. Int J Dermatol 1987; 26: 242–243.

225 Romaní J, Barnadas MA, Miralles J et al. Median raphe cyst of the penis with ciliated cells. J Cutan Pathol 1995; 22: 378–381.

226 Urahashi J, Hara H, Yamaguchi Z-I, Morishima T. Pigmented median raphe cysts of the penis. Acta Derm Venereol 2000; 80: 297–298.

227 Brownstein MH, Helwig EB. Subcutaneous dermoid cysts. Arch Dermatol 1973; 107: 237–239.

228 Sinclair RD, Darley C, Dawber RPR. Congenital inclusion dermoid cysts of the scalp. Australas J Dermatol 1992; 33: 135–140.

229 Tomasini C, Aloi F, Puiatti P, Caliendo V. Dermoid cyst of the penis. Dermatology 1997; 194: 188–190.

230 Littlewood AHM. Congenital nasal dermoid cysts and fistulas. Plast Reconstr Surg 1961; 27: 471–488.

231 Brownstein MH, Shapiro L, Slevin R. Fistula of the dorsum of the nose. Arch Dermatol 1974; 109: 227–229.

232 Graham-Brown RAC, Shuttleworth D. Median nasal dermoid fistula. Int J Dermatol 1985; 24: 181–182.

233 Szalay GC, Bledsoe RC. Congenital dermoid cyst and fistula of the nose. Am J Dis Child 1972; 124: 392–394.

234 Saito H. Ogonuki R, Yanadori A et al. Congenital dermal sinus with intracranial dermoid cyst. Br J Dermatol 1994; 130: 235–237.

235 Moreno A, Muns R. A cystic teratoma in skin. Am J Dermatopathol 1985; 7: 383–386.

236 McCollough ML, Glover AT, Grabski WJ, Berger TG. Orbital dermoid cysts showing conjunctival epithelium. Am J Dermatopathol 1991; 13: 611–615.

237 Camacho F. Benign cutaneous cystic teratoma. J Cutan Pathol 1982; 9: 345–351.

238 Tsai T-F, Chuan M-T, Hsiao C-H. A cystic teratoma of the skin. Histopathology 1996; 29: 384–386.

239 Steck WD, Helwig EB. Cutaneous remnants of the omphalomesenteric duct. Arch Dermatol 1964; 90: 463–470.

Miscellaneous cysts

240 Raimer S, Wolf JE Jr. Subcutaneous cysticercosis. Arch Dermatol 1978; 114: 107–108.

241 Iwatsu T, Miyaji M. Phaeomycotic cyst. A case with a lesion containing a wood splinter. Arch Dermatol 1984; 120: 1209–1211.

242 de Berker D, Lawrence C. Ganglion of the distal interphalangeal joint (myxoid cyst). Therapy by identification and repair of the leak of joint fluid. Arch Dermatol 2001; 137: 607–610.

243 Gonzalez JG, Ghiselli RW, Santa Cruz DJ. Synovial metaplasia of the skin. Am J Surg Pathol 1987; 11: 343–350.

244 Stern DR, Sexton FM. Metaplastic synovial cyst after partial excision of nevus sebaceus. Am J Dermatopathol 1988; 10: 531–535.

245 Bhawan J, Dayal Y, Gonzales-Serva A, Eisen R. Cutaneous metaplastic synovial cyst. J Cutan Pathol 1990; 17: 22–26.

246 Nieto S, Buezo GF, Jones-Caballero M, Fraga J. Cutaneous metaplastic synovial cyst in an Ehlers–Danlos patient. Am J Dermatopathol 1997; 19: 407–410.

247 Singh SR, Ma ASP, Dixon A. Multiple cutaneous metaplastic synovial cysts. J Am Acad Dermatol 1999; 41: 330–332.

248 Glamb R, Kim R. Pseudocyst of the auricle. J Am Acad Dermatol 1984; 11: 58–63.

249 Fukamizu H, Imaizumi S. Bilateral pseudocysts of the auricles. Arch Dermatol 1984; 120: 1238–1239.

250 Heffner DK, Hyams VJ. Cystic chondromalacia (endochondral pseudocyst) of the auricle. Arch Pathol Lab Med 1986; 110: 740–743.

251 Devlin J, Harrison CJ, Whitby DJ, David TJ. Cartilaginous pseudocyst of the external auricle in children with atopic eczema. Br J Dermatol 1990; 122: 699–704.

252 Santos AD. Kelley PE. Bilateral pseudocyst of the auricle in an infant girl. Pediatr Dermatol 1995; 12: 152–155.

253 Grabski WJ, Salasche SJ, McCollough ML, Angeloni VL. Pseudocyst of the auricle associated with trauma. Arch Dermatol 1989; 125: 528–530.

254 Oliver M, Chopite M, Rondon A. Coexistence of pseudocyst of the auricle and preauricular fistula. Int J Dermatol 1994; 33: 135.

255 Lapins NA, Odom RB. Seroma of the auricle. Arch Dermatol 1982; 118: 503–505.

256 Michowitz M, Baratz M, Stavorovsky M. Endometriosis of the umbilicus. Dermatologica 1983; 167: 326–330.

257 Williams HE, Barsky S, Storino W. Umbilical endometrioma (silent type). Arch Dermatol 1976; 112: 435–1436.

258 Premalatha S, Augustine SM, Thambiah AS. Umbilical endometrioma. Clin Exp Dermatol 1978; 3: 35–37.

259 Beirne MF, Berkheiser SW. Umbilical endometriosis. A case report. Am J Obstet Gynecol 1955; 69: 895–897.

260 Tidman MJ. MacDonald DM. Cutaneous endometriosis: a histopathologic study. J Am Acad Dermatol 1988; 18: 373–377.

261 Symmers W StC. Endometriosis occurring in the neck. Personal communication, 1989.

262 Singh KK, Lessells AM, Adam DJ et al. Presentation of endometriosis to general surgeons: a 10-year experience. Br J Surg 1995; 82: 1349–1351.

263 Choi SW, Lee HN, Kang SJ, Kim HO. A case of cutaneous endometriosis developed in postmenopausal woman receiving hormonal replacement. J Am Acad Dermatol 1999; 41: 327–329.

264 Pellegrini AE. Cutaneous decidualized endometriosis. A pseudomalignancy. Am J Dermatopathol 1982; 4: 171–174.

265 Nogales FF, Martin F, Linares J et al. Myxoid change in decidualized scar endometriosis mimicking malignancy. J Cutan Pathol 1993; 20: 87–91.

266 Fair KP, Patterson JW, Murphy RJ, Rudd RJ. Cutaneous deciduosis. J Am Acad Dermatol 2000; 43: 102–107.

267 Albrecht LE, Tron V, Rivers JK. Cutaneous endometriosis. Int J Dermatol 1995; 34: 261–262.

268 Popoff L, Raitchev R, Andreev VC. Endometriosis of the skin. Arch Dermatol 1962; 85: 186–189.

Sinuses

269 Jansen T, Romiti R, Plewig G, Altmeyer P. Disfiguring draining sinus tracts in a female acne patient. Pediatr Dermatol 2000; 17: 123–125.

270 Hsu S-T, Lee JY-Y, Chao S-C et al. Congenital occipital dermal sinus with intracranial dermoid cyst complicated by recurrent *Escherichia coli* meningitis. Br J Dermatol 1998; 139: 922–924.

271 Anzai S, Yamaguchi T, Takasaki S et al. Tethered cord associated with intraspinal lipoma and a subcutaneous abscess secondary to a dermal sinus. Int J Dermatol 1998; 37: 77–78.

272 Sevila A, Morell A, Navas J et al. Orifices at the lower neck: heterotopic salivary glands. Dermatology 1997; 194: 360–361.

273 Eastlack JP, Howard RM, Frieden IJ. Congenital midline cervical cleft: case report and review of the English language literature. Pediatr Dermatol 2000; 17: 118–122.

274 Cioffi GA, Terezhalmy GT, Parlette HL. Cutaneous draining sinus tract. An odontogenic etiology. J Am Acad Dermatol 1986; 14: 94–100.

275 Lewin-Epstein J, Taicher S, Azaz B. Cutaneous sinus tracts of dental origin. Arch Dermatol 1978; 114: 1158–1161.

276 Matter I, Kunin J, Schein M, Eldar S. Total excision versus non-resectional methods in the treatment of acute and chronic pilonidal disease. Br J Surg 1995; 82: 752–753.

277 Eby CS, Jetton RL. Umbilical pilonidal sinus. Arch Dermatol 1972; 106: 893.

278 Moyer DG. Pilonidal cyst of the scalp. Arch Dermatol 1972; 105: 578–579.

279 Lepaw MI. Therapy and histopathology of complications from synthetic fiber implants for hair replacement. J Am Acad Dermatol 1980; 3: 195–204.

280 Kim YA, Thomas I. Metastatic squamous cell carcinoma arising in a pilonidal sinus. J Am Acad Dermatol 1993; 29: 272–274.

281 Albrecht S, Zbieranowski I. Incidental glomus coccygeum. When a normal structure looks like a tumor. Am J Surg Pathol 1990; 14: 922–924.

Pits

282 Nagore E, Sánchez-Motilla JM, Febrer MI et al. Congenital lower lip pits (Van der Woude syndrome): presentation of 10 cases. Pediatr Dermatol 1998; 15: 443–445.

283 Vignale R, Araujo J, Pascal G et al. Van der Woude syndrome. A case report. Pediatr Dermatol 1998; 15: 459–463.

Panniculitis

INTRODUCTION

The panniculus adiposus (subcutaneous fat) is a metabolic depot which also functions as a layer of insulation and as a buffer to trauma. It is composed of mature lipocytes, which are round to polygonal cells with an eccentric nucleus and a large cytoplasmic lipid vacuole. In contrast, fetal fat cells contain multiple small lipid vacuoles. The lipocytes are separated from their neighbors by an inconspicuous matrix.[1]

The panniculus adiposus is divided into lobules by fibrous septa, which are continuous with the dermis. Smaller microlobules have been described within the larger lobules, but these smaller units are not of pathological importance. Within the fibrous septa run the small arteries and arterioles, venules, lymphatics and nerves. The nutrient artery supplies the center of the lobule with drainage to venules in the fibrous septa.[1] As a consequence, interference with the arterial supply results in diffuse changes within the lobule (lobular panniculitis) while venous disorders are manifested by alterations in paraseptal regions (septal panniculitis).[1]

This chapter is concerned primarily with the inflammatory lesions of the subcutaneous fat – the panniculitides. Miscellaneous infiltrates and deposits will be mentioned briefly.

Inflammatory lesions of the subcutaneous fat can be classified into three distinct categories:

- septal panniculitis
- lobular panniculitis
- panniculitis associated with large vessel vasculitis.

Within each group, the histological appearances will depend on the stage of the disease at which the biopsy is taken. In early lesions there are often neutrophils in the inflammatory infiltrate, while later lesions have a chronic infiltrate composed predominantly of lymphocytes but with a variable admixture of giant cells and lipid-containing macrophages. At an even later stage there is some fibrosis. Accordingly, attempts at subclassifying the panniculitides on the basis of the predominant pattern of inflammation or cell type are largely unsuccessful, except for those with abundant eosinophils.

Inflammation of small venules will result in a *septal panniculitis* with some spillover of the inflammatory process into the lower dermis.[1] Involvement of the arterial supply, for example by vasculitis, will produce a *lobular panniculitis*. There are other mechanisms involved in some of the diseases that result in a lobular panniculitis. These will be considered in the appropriate sections. The *panniculitis associated with large vessel involvement*, such as polyarteritis nodosa and migratory thrombophlebitis, is usually localized to the immediate vicinity of the involved vessel. It often has mixed lobular and septal features.

Unless an adequate biopsy is received, it may be difficult to reach a specific diagnosis.[2,3] A diagnosis of 'lobular panniculitis ? type' may have to suffice in these cases. Another problem with the panniculitides is the considerable confusion that exists in the literature.[4] In some reports it would seem that a diagnosis has been made on purely clinical grounds and the pathological findings ignored. An excellent review of the panniculitides has recently been published.[5] It describes the diversity of histological appearances that can be seen during the evolution of an individual lesion of the various panniculitides.[5]

The histological features of the panniculitides are summarized in Table 17.1.

SEPTAL PANNICULITIS

In septal panniculitis the inflammatory reaction is centered on the connective tissue septa of the subcutaneous fat. If the lesions are of long standing or recurrent in the same area, the septa may be considerably widened with a corresponding reduction in the amount of intervening lobular fat. There is often some spillover of inflammatory cells and macrophages into the adjacent fat lobule. In small biopsies this spillover of inflammatory cells can be misinterpreted as a lobular panniculitis.

In addition to the diseases considered below, a septal panniculitis may be seen in some cases of factitial panniculitis (see p. 533), cellulitis (see p. 621), microscopic polyangiitis (see p. 237) and hydroa vacciniforme (see p. 601). It has also been recorded in a patient with cryoglobulinemia (see p. 225) and in patients receiving apomorphine infusion for Parkinson's disease.[6]

ERYTHEMA NODOSUM

Erythema nodosum is an acute, painful, erythematous, nodular eruption. The nodules, which range from 1 to 5 cm or more in diameter, are usually situated on the anterior aspect of the lower legs; more rarely, they occur on the arms, soles[7–9] or trunk. There may be associated fever, malaise and arthralgia. The lesions subside after a period of approximately 2–6 weeks or so. Erythema nodosum usually occurs in young adults, but childhood cases occur.[10] Encapsulated fat necrosis ('mobile encapsulated lipoma') is a rare complication (see p. 534).[11] Erythema nodosum may be associated with sarcoidosis,[3] Sweet's syndrome,[12,13] Behçet's disease,[14,15] inflammatory bowel disease, carcinomas,[16,17] leukemia,[18] lymphoma,[19,20] tularemia[21] or with streptococcal,[3] meningococcal,[22] campylobacter,[23] salmonella,[24] histoplasma,[3] mycoplasma,[25] chlamydial,[26] mycobacterial,[27] dermatophyte,[28] human immunodeficiency virus[29] or yersinia[30,31] infections. Various drugs have been incriminated,[32] including isotretinoin,[33] sulfonamides, penicillin, minocycline,[34] leukotriene-modifying drugs such as zileuton,[35] salicylates, iodides, gold salts, echinacea,[36] hepatitis B vaccine[25] and also oral contraceptives.[37] Radiotherapy may also trigger the onset of erythema nodosum.[38,39] In about one-third of cases the etiology is obscure. The pathogenesis of erythema nodosum is unknown but it may represent an allergic response to infection or systemic disease. Reactive oxygen intermediates, released by primed neutrophils, may play a role in the pathogenesis.[40]

In *erythema nodosum migrans* (subacute nodular migratory panniculitis), a centrifugally enlarging plaque with central clearing develops on the lower leg. It is usually solitary, but several lesions may exist.[41–44]

Histopathology

Erythema nodosum is a septal panniculitis with small foci of inflammatory cells extending into the adjacent lobular fat (Fig. 17.1). In some cases this spillover of cells is more marked and includes foam cells, sometimes associated with focal necrosis of fat cells adjacent to the septa. Lobular extension can be quite marked in the fasciitis–panniculitis associated with brucellosis.[45] The center of the lobule is spared, allowing a distinction to be made from lobular panniculitis. There is also some extension of inflammatory cells into the adjacent lower dermis. In most biopsies the septal infiltrate is predominantly lymphocytic, but there are variable numbers of giant cells, usually of foreign body type, as well as a few eosinophils and histiocytes (Fig. 17.2). Small nodules composed of spindle to oval histiocytes arranged around a minute slit may be found (Miescher's radial granulomas).[46] Well-formed tuberculoid granulomas are rare.

In early lesions neutrophils are usually present. They are numerous in the rare suppurative variant of erythema nodosum in which neutrophils extend into the adjacent lobule.[47,48] The fibrous septa are widened with edema and some fibrinoid change in the earlier stages. Later there are increased numbers of fibroblasts with some fibrosis.

Table 17.1 **Panniculitis: histopathological features**

Disease	Histopathological features
Erythema nodosum	Septal panniculitis with paraseptal inflammatory wedges; neutrophils early; septal giant cells; Miescher's radial granulomas
Necrobiosis lipoidica	Fibrous septal widening; dermal granulomas and necrobiosis
Scleroderma	Fibrous septal widening; dermal or fascial thickening with parallel coarse collagen
Erythema induratum–nodular vasculitis	Lobular and septolobular panniculitis; vasculitis and granulomas; necrosis common
Subcutaneous fat necrosis of the newborn	Lobular panniculitis; needle-shaped clefts in fat cells
Sclerema neonatorum	Similar needle-shaped clefts (crystals), but no inflammation
Weber–Christian disease	Doubtful entity; lobular panniculitis; neutrophils early; abundant foam cells
α_1-antitrypsin deficiency	Lobular panniculitis; dermal liquefaction; suppuration; septal collagenolysis
Cytophagic histiocytic panniculitis	Lobular panniculitis; numerous histiocytes showing cytophagocytosis ('bean bag' cells)
Panniculitis-like T-cell lymphoma	Lymphocytic lobular panniculitis; pleomorphic lymphocytes of variable size which rim adipocytes; karyorrhexis; necrosis; sometimes angioinvasion and cytophagocytosis
Pancreatic panniculitis	Lobular panniculitis; ghost-like necrotic fat cells; peripheral nuclear dusting
Lupus panniculitis	Lobular panniculitis with prominent lymphocytes (lymphocytic lobular panniculitis); paraseptal lymphoid follicles in 50%; often basal lichenoid tissue reaction
Lipodystrophy	Subcutaneous atrophy; sometimes early mild lobular panniculitis
HIV-associated lipodystrophy	Non-inflammatory except for scattered lymphocytes and lipophages; atrophy of fat
Gynoid lipodystrophy	Lipohypertrophy with variable thickness of septa; fat herniated into lower dermis (may be gender-related)
Membranous lipodystrophy	Microcysts with lipomembranous (membranocystic) change; dense fibrosis between islands of 'fatty microcysts'
Lipodermatosclerosis	Infarction of fat lobules; lipomembranous change; late fibrosis; hemosiderin; pericapillary fibrin caps; early inflammatory stage
Factitial panniculitis	Mixed septal and lobular panniculitis; sometimes suppurative; foreign body giant cells
Traumatic fat necrosis	Overlap with above; fat cysts, fibrosis and sometimes hemosiderin
Encapsulated fat necrosis	Lobules of necrotic fat; thin fibrous capsule which is usually hyaline; lipomembranous change common
Infective panniculitis	Suppuration or granulomas or numerous eosinophils depending on etiology
Non-infective neutrophilic panniculitis	Neutrophilic lobular panniculitis; necrosis sometimes present, admixture of cells with chronicity
Eosinophilic panniculitis	Numerous eosinophils in a lobular panniculitis; sometimes flame figures or parasite present
Miscellaneous	Urate crystals in gout; sarcoidal granulomas in sarcoidosis and Crohn's disease; necrobiotic granulomas in subcutaneous granuloma annulare or rheumatoid nodules
Panniculitis secondary to large vessel vasculitis	Vasculitis of artery or vein; panniculitis localized around vessel

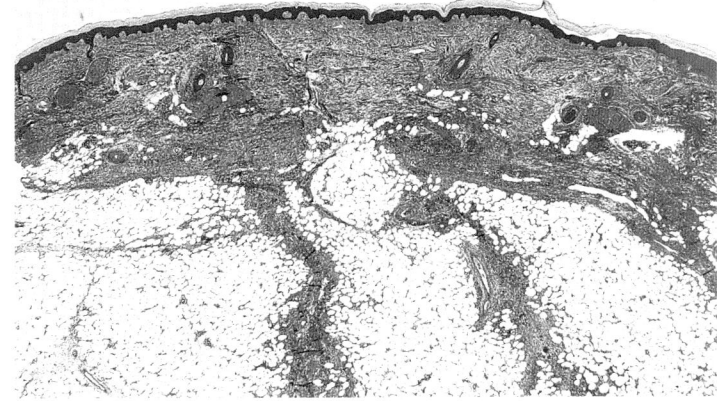

Fig. 17.1 **Erythema nodosum.** The inflammatory infiltrate is confined to the septa of the subcutis. (H&E)

Blood vessel changes are variable. There is usually prominent endothelial swelling of small septal vessels and sometimes of medium-sized veins. There is lymphocytic cuffing of septal venules. Sometimes a definite vasculitis is present, but by the time most biopsies are taken, only non-specific vascular changes are found. In the erythema nodosum-like lesions of Behçet's disease, a vasculitis is present in most cases. It may be of lymphocytic or leukocytoclastic type.[49] The lesions are not always confined to the septa.[49]

In a case reported as 'neoplastic erythema nodosum', a B-cell lymphoma produced both a lobular and a septal panniculitis.[20]

In *erythema nodosum migrans* (subacute nodular migratory panniculitis) the septa are markedly thickened and fibrotic. Inflammation is usually mild although multinucleated giant cells and granulomas may be conspicuous along the edge of the septa. Neovascularization is often present at the septal borders.

Electron microscopy
Ultrastructural examination has shown damage to endothelial cells of small vessels with some extension of inflammatory cells into the vessel walls.[15,50]

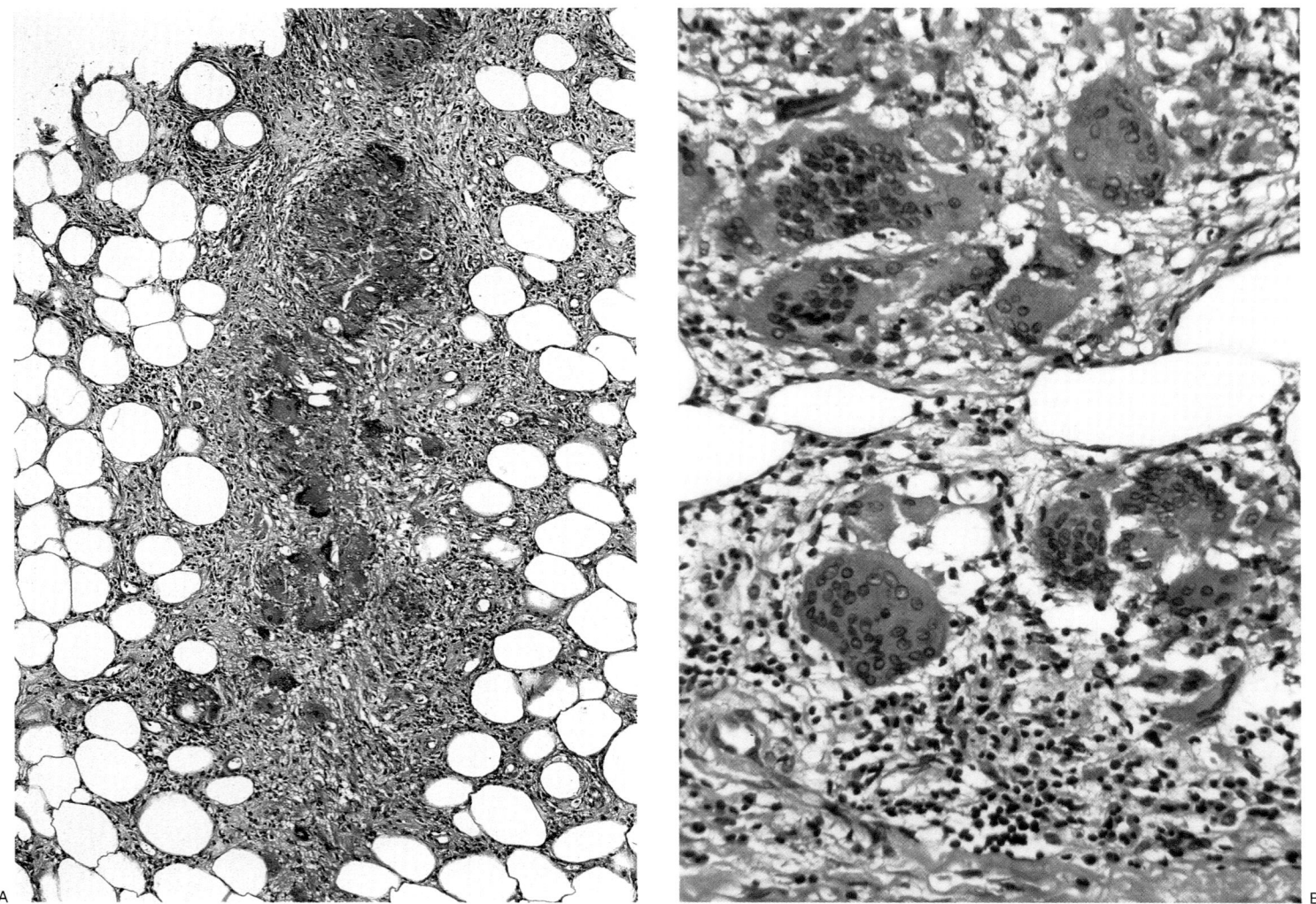

Fig. 17.2 **(A) Erythema nodosum. (B)** The inflamed septum contains a number of multinucleate giant cells in addition to lymphocytes and eosinophils. (H&E)

NECROBIOSIS LIPOIDICA

In necrobiosis lipoidica the necrobiotic and granulomatous process, followed by fibrosis, may extend from the dermis into the subcutaneous septa, producing marked widening of these structures, which encroach on the fat lobules. This condition is considered further in Chapter 7, page 202.

SCLERODERMA

In scleroderma and its localized cutaneous variants (morphea) there may be extension of the process from the dermis into the subcutaneous fat. There is marked fibrous thickening of the septa, and often lymphoid collections are present at the junction of the thickened septa and the fat lobules.[51]

There are variants of morphea in which only the subcutaneous fat and/or fascia are involved. The terms *subcutaneous morphea* and *morphea profunda* are often used interchangeably for these variants, although morphea profunda has been proposed as the appropriate diagnosis when both fat and fascia are involved and subcutaneous morphea for cases with involvement of fat only (see p. 348). Septal fibrosis and hyalinization are obvious features. There are often small lymphoid collections but not lymphoid follicles with germinal centers. Plasma cells are usually present.

A case of linear scleroderma with an intense plasma cell infiltrate in the dermis and subcutaneous fat has been reported.[52] Nodular aggregates of plasma cells were present in the fat lobules and the thickened interlobular septa. Scleroderma is considered further in Chapter 11 (pp. 346–351).

LOBULAR PANNICULITIS

In the lobular panniculitides, the inflammatory infiltrate is present throughout the lobule but there is often some septal involvement as well. There are many different causes of a lobular panniculitis and many of these are histologically distinct. However, sometimes it is not possible to distinguish between the various etiological groups, in which case the histological diagnosis may have to be simply 'lobular panniculitis'.

ERYTHEMA INDURATUM–NODULAR VASCULITIS

Erythema induratum and nodular vasculitis were originally regarded as one entity. However, it has been the practice for the last 50 years or so to recognize two variants – one of presumptive tuberculous origin (erythema induratum, Bazin-type) and the other of non-tuberculous origin, known as nodular vasculitis or erythema induratum, Whitfield-type.[2] The tuberculous group was regarded as a tuberculid (see p. 627) on the basis of the persistent failure to culture *Mycobacterium tuberculosis* from lesional tissue or to see organisms on acid-fast stains. The tuberculous origin of the Bazin subtype was assumed on the basis of strongly positive reactions with the Mantoux test, the presence of active tuberculosis in other organs in some cases, and the favorable response of the skin lesions to antituberculous therapy.[53–56]

The advent of PCR-based methods has led to the detection of mycobacterial DNA in from 30 to 80% of cases of erythema induratum–nodular vasculitis, defined on the basis of clinical presentation and a lobular granulomatous panniculitis on histology.[57–60] As no significant differences have been consistently demonstrated between cases with detectable mycobacterial DNA and those without, it does not seem tenable to continue the separation of erythema induratum and nodular vasculitis.[61] After all, erythema nodosum has multiple etiologies (including tuberculosis), and it is considered as one condition.[27,62] Thus the wheel has turned full circle and once again there is a single (composite) entity.

Erythema induratum–nodular vasculitis is characterized by recurrent crops of tender erythematous nodules, usually with a predilection for the calves, although the shins are sometimes involved as well. The nodules may coalesce to form one or more plaques. Uncommonly, lesions may develop in other sites such as the buttocks and arms. Although it was originally regarded as a disease of young adult females, a wide range of ages can be affected. Lesions occasionally ulcerate; they may heal with scarring.[63]

Erythema induratum–nodular vasculitis appears to be a disease of diverse etiologies, mycobacterial infection being one of them. Presumably other infections may be involved. To date, only hepatitis C has been incriminated.[64] The pathogenesis appears to involve a delayed hypersensitivity or Arthus-type reaction. Host responses may perpetuate the disease even after the infection has been cleared.[58]

Histopathology[58,62,65–67]

The inflammatory changes are usually restricted to the subcutis and the lower dermis. There is a lobular or septolobular panniculitis, usually diffuse, with varying combinations of granulomatous inflammation, vasculitis, focal necrosis and septal fibrosis (Fig. 17.3). As in other panniculitides the histological changes will vary with the duration of the lesions.

Granulomas may be well developed and tuberculoid; occasionally they show caseation necrosis. More often the granulomas are poorly developed. Lipophage collections are usually present. The inflammatory infiltrate includes neutrophils, lymphocytes and some plasma cells. Neutrophils predominate in areas of fat necrosis.

Vascular changes, which are present in approximately 90% of cases, involve all sizes of arteries and veins.[68] Involved vessels show endothelial swelling and a mixed inflammatory cell infiltrate in the wall and periadventitial tissues (Fig. 17.4). A necrotizing vasculitis is sometimes present, particularly in early lesions.

Although no histological feature consistently reflects a tuberculoid etiology, necrosis is slightly more common in this group. In the past, the presence of tuberculoid granulomas in the deep dermis, often around the eccrine glands, was regarded as suggestive of a tuberculous etiology.[69] However, it is the absence of consistent differences that has resulted in the concept of a unified entity.[69]

As a rule, erythema induratum–nodular vasculitis involves many contiguous lobules, whereas cutaneous polyarteritis nodosa produces a more localized panniculitis restricted to the vicinity of the involved vessels.

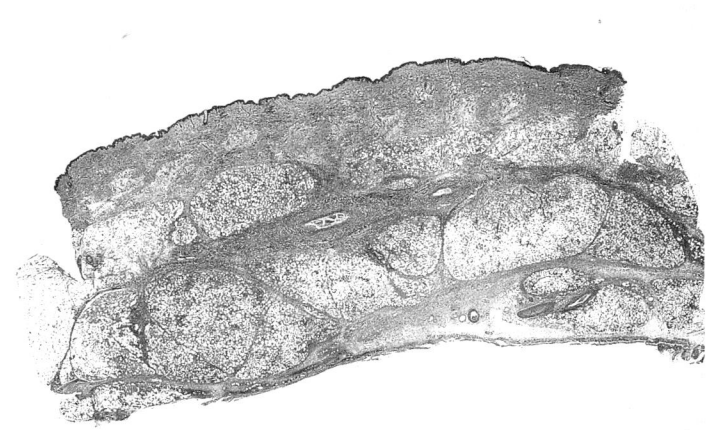

A

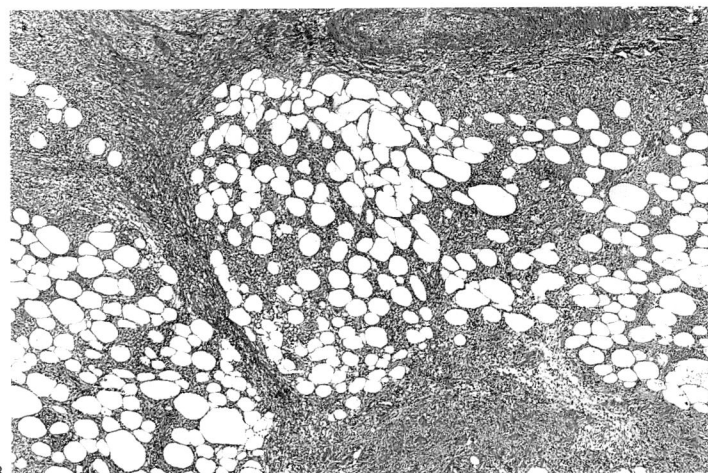

B

Fig. 17.3 **(A) Erythema induratum–nodular vasculitis. (B)** There is inflammation in the fat lobules and to a lesser extent in the septa. (H&E)

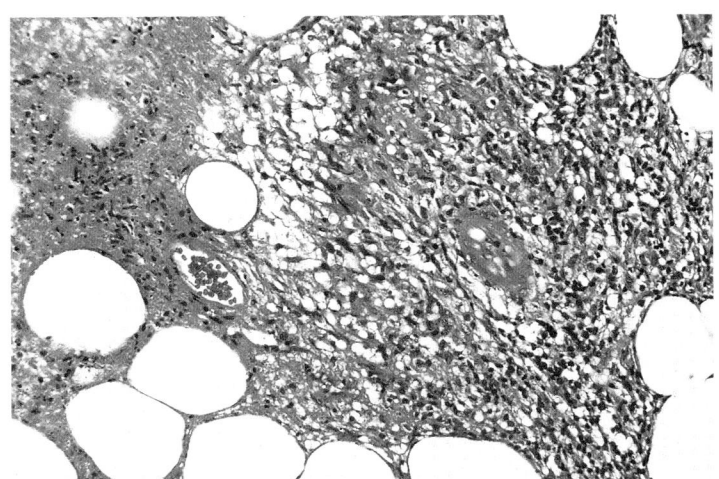

Fig. 17.4 **Erythema induratum–nodular vasculitis.** There is a lobular panniculitis with focal necrosis. A small blood vessel shows fibrinoid change. (H&E)

SUBCUTANEOUS FAT NECROSIS OF THE NEWBORN

Subcutaneous fat necrosis of the newborn is a self-limited condition, present at birth or appearing in the first few days of life.[70–72] It is characterized by indurated areas and distinct nodules with a predilection for the cheeks, shoulders, buttocks, thighs and calves.[73] Sometimes only solitary lesions are discernible. Hypercalcemia has been reported in some cases.[74–78] Obstetrical trauma, hypothermia, asphyxia and anemia have been incriminated in the etiology.[79] Cases have been reported after hypothermic cardiac surgery,[80,81] prostaglandin E administration and maternal exposure to cocaine or calcium channel blockers.[82,83] It has been suggested that trauma to fragile adipose tissue low in oleic acid and with a compromised circulation, followed by the release of hydrolases, leads to the breakdown of unsaturated fatty acids.[70] It should be remembered that infant fat already has a greater ratio of saturated to unsaturated fatty acids than exists in adult fat.

Histopathology[71,84,85]

There is a normal epidermis and dermis with an underlying lobular panniculitis. Focal fat necrosis is present and this may lead to fat cyst formation. There is an inflammatory infiltrate of lymphocytes, histiocytes, foreign body giant cells and sometimes a few eosinophils wedged between the fat cells (Fig. 17.5). Many of the fat cells retain their outline but contain fine, eosinophilic cytoplasmic strands, between which are narrow clefts radiating from a point near the periphery of the cell (Fig. 17.6). The clefts contain doubly refractile crystals, representing triglycerides, on frozen section. Similar fine, needle-like crystals can be seen in relation to some of the giant cells. Cases have been reported without the needle-like crystals.[86] In older lesions there is some fibrosis between the fat cells and there may be foci of calcification.

Electron microscopy[84,85]

There are intact and necrotic fat cells containing needle-shaped crystals arranged radially or in parallel. Dense granular material is also present in the necrotic fat cells, which are surrounded by macrophages.

SCLEREMA NEONATORUM

Sclerema neonatorum has a pathogenetic relationship to subcutaneous fat necrosis of the newborn and was at one stage regarded as a diffuse form of the latter.[87] It is also characterized by intracellular microcrystallization of

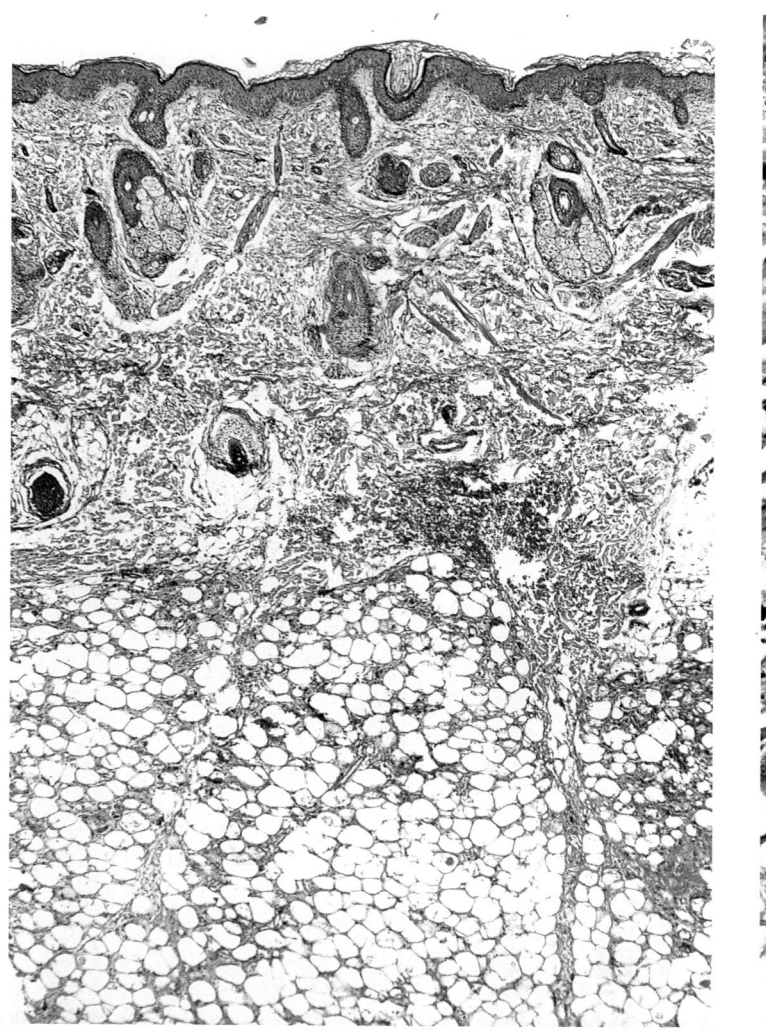

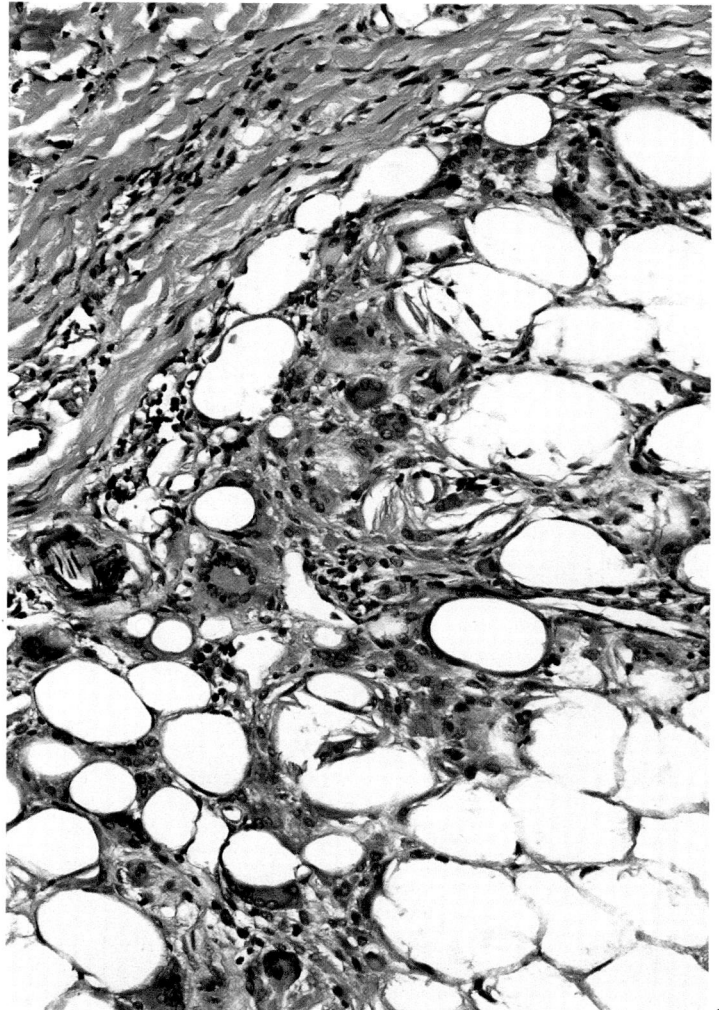

Fig. 17.5 **(A) Subcutaneous fat necrosis of the newborn. (B)** There is a lobular and paraseptal panniculitis with lymphocytes, macrophages and multinucleate giant cells wedged between the fat cells. (H&E)

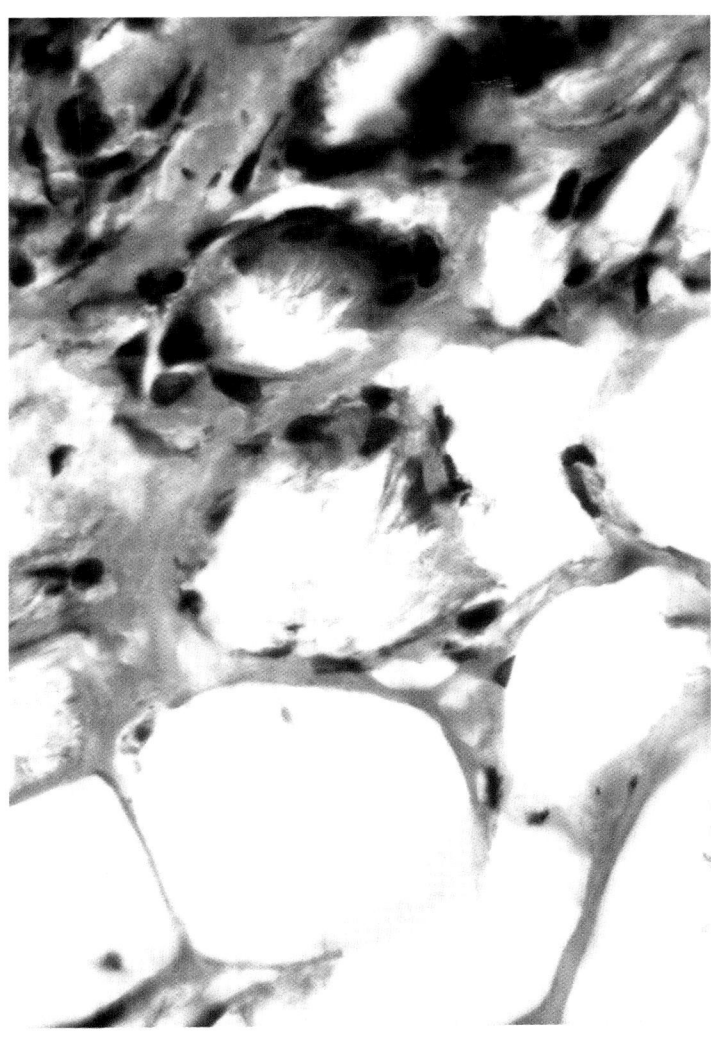

Fig. 17.6 **Subcutaneous fat necrosis of the newborn.** Narrow strands of tissue radiate from a point near the periphery of several of the fat cells. The intervening clefts represent the site of deposition of 'fat crystals'. (H&E)

triglyceride in the subcutaneous and sometimes also in the visceral fat of preterminal neonates. Sclerema neonatorum produces wax-like, hard skin which is also dry and cold. It is rarely seen these days, presumably because of improved neonatal care.

Histopathology

There are fine, needle-like crystals in the fat cells, but unlike subcutaneous fat necrosis of the newborn, there is very little inflammation, few giant cells and no calcification. The subcutaneous septa are often widened by edema which might explain the 'wide intersecting fibrous bands' formerly reported. Fat cells have been reported as increased in size, but a personally studied case showed small, immature fat cells.

COLD PANNICULITIS

Panniculitis may occur following exposure to severe cold, particularly in infants.[88–91] It has occurred in older children and on the thighs of women who have ridden horses in cold weather.[92,93] In the latter instance it has been suggested that tight pants may restrict the blood supply, contributing to the injury. The lesions are indurated, somewhat tender plaques and nodules.

Histopathology

There is a lobular panniculitis with a mixed inflammatory cell infiltrate. Changes are most marked near the dermosubcutaneous junction where the vessels show a perivascular infiltrate of lymphocytes and histiocytes. There is some thickening of vessel walls. There is overlap with the changes described in deep perniosis (see p. 250).[94]

WEBER–CHRISTIAN DISEASE

The diagnosis of Weber–Christian disease has engendered more confusion in dermatopathology than practically any other.[95–110] It has been applied by some to all cases of panniculitis with systemic symptoms or to all cases of fatal panniculitis with visceral involvement.[96] The term 'Weber–Christian disease' has been a convenient 'pigeon hole' for undiagnosable cases of panniculitis.[111]

Weber–Christian disease was defined in the past as a rare disorder with recurrent subcutaneous nodules and plaques with a predilection for the extremities and buttocks, commonly associated with fever.[107] It was said to have a short self-limited course or follow an unremitting course with a fatal outcome and visceral involvement.[104,108,109]

In a review of 30 cases diagnosed as Weber–Christian disease at the Mayo Clinic, White and Winkelmann were able to reclassify the cases as other entities, such as erythema nodosum, factitial panniculitis, cytophagic histiocytic panniculitis and post-phlebitic syndrome.[112] The diagnosis should no longer be used.

Histopathology

Weber–Christian disease was diagnosed in the past as a lobular panniculitis with numerous lipophages. It is this latter feature, now known to occur in other panniculitides, that often took precedence as a marker of the condition.

α₁-ANTITRYPSIN DEFICIENCY

α_1-Antitrypsin deficiency is a genetic disorder characterized by low serum levels of α_1-antitrypsin. There are at least 33 allelic variants of this condition. A nodular panniculitis is usually associated with the PiZ phenotype, but other phenotypes have been involved.[110,113] Panniculitis may be an early sign of this deficiency, but most cases present during the third and fourth decades.[114] The lesions begin as tender, erythematous, indurated, subcutaneous nodules that may be widely disseminated on the trunk or extremities.[100,102,114] They may be precipitated by trauma, including cryotherapy.[115] Spontaneous ulceration with discharge of an oily fluid may occur.

Histopathology

There is usually an acute panniculitis, sometimes septal as well as lobular, with masses of neutrophils and some necrosis of fat cells.[116,117] Neutrophils usually extend into the reticular dermis, producing a characteristic infiltrate between the collagen bundles (so-called 'splaying of neutrophils').[118] Dissolution of dermal collagen with transepidermal elimination of 'liquefied' dermis may occur. There may also be collagenolysis of the fibrous septa of the subcutis, resulting in isolated adipocyte lobules.[102] Destruction of elastic tissue may also be present.[100] Vasculitis is sometimes present in the subcutis. Later lesions show collections of histiocytic cells and lipophages and variable fibrosis. Dystrophic calcification may develop.[110]

CYTOPHAGIC HISTIOCYTIC PANNICULITIS

Winkelmann and colleagues coined the term 'cytophagic histiocytic panniculitis' over 20 years ago for a usually fatal syndrome which included a chronic and recurring panniculitis with an infiltrate of cytophagic histiocytes with eventual multisystem involvement, terminating usually with a hemorrhagic diathesis resulting from the hemophagocytic syndrome.[98,119-130] Other cases have been included in the past with systemic Weber–Christian disease.[97] The current status of this condition is controversial, but most dermatopathologists believe it is a form of cutaneous T-cell lymphoma.

A case has been made for the retention of cytophagic histiocytic panniculitis as an entity on the basis of several patients in whom the disease has not progressed to overt lymphoma after prolonged follow-up (41 years in one case).[131,132] Furthermore, monoclonal T-cell populations can not be detected in some of these cases, although parallels have been drawn with large plaque parapsoriasis in which this may also occur.[133] It is generally agreed that cytophagic histiocytic panniculitis and subcutaneous panniculitis-like T-cell lymphoma (see below) exist in a continuum, and that the former may precede the latter.[132] It is just possible that isolated cases represent a manifestation of a non-neoplastic, infection-associated hemophagocytic syndrome.[133-135]

The disease, as originally described, consists of ulcerating nodules or plaques, sometimes painful, with a predilection for the legs and forearms. Other sites are often involved in established cases. It affects mostly middle-aged or elderly individuals.

Histopathology

There is a lobular panniculitis, sometimes with extension into the lower dermis.[98] There may be fat necrosis, focal hemorrhage and a non-specific inflammatory infiltrate. The diagnostic feature is the presence of sheets and clusters of histiocytes showing prominent phagocytosis of red cells, white cells and nuclear debris. Cells stuffed with phagocytosed materials have been called 'bean bag' cells.[98] Occasional hyperchromatic cells and mitoses are seen; frank lymphoma may supervene (see below). Membranocystic change is uncommonly present.[136]

PANNICULITIS-LIKE T-CELL LYMPHOMA

Panniculitis-like T-cell lymphoma is a rare form of cutaneous lymphoma; fewer than 100 cases have been reported.[137-139] Affected individuals present with multiple subcutaneous tumors or plaques, often associated with constitutional symptoms. Sometimes a cytokine-induced hemophagocytic syndrome develops.[132,137] The disease is indolent in some,[138] but it may run a rapid course. Most cases have the phenotype of cytotoxic T cells.[140]

A panniculitis has also been reported in association with a lymphoma composed of natural killer cells. An association with Epstein–Barr virus is

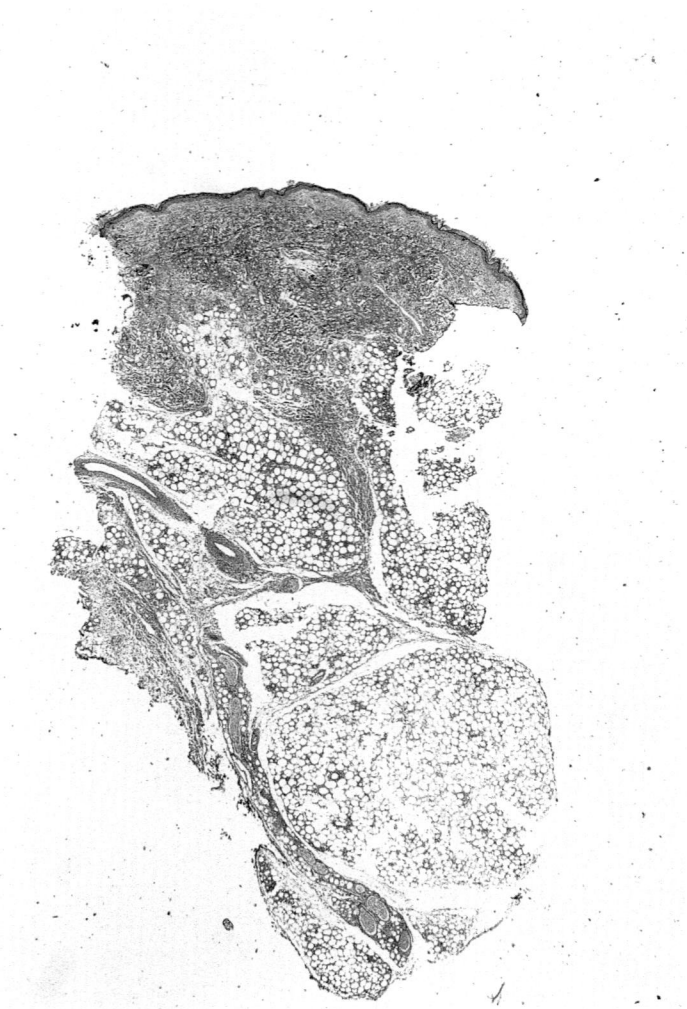

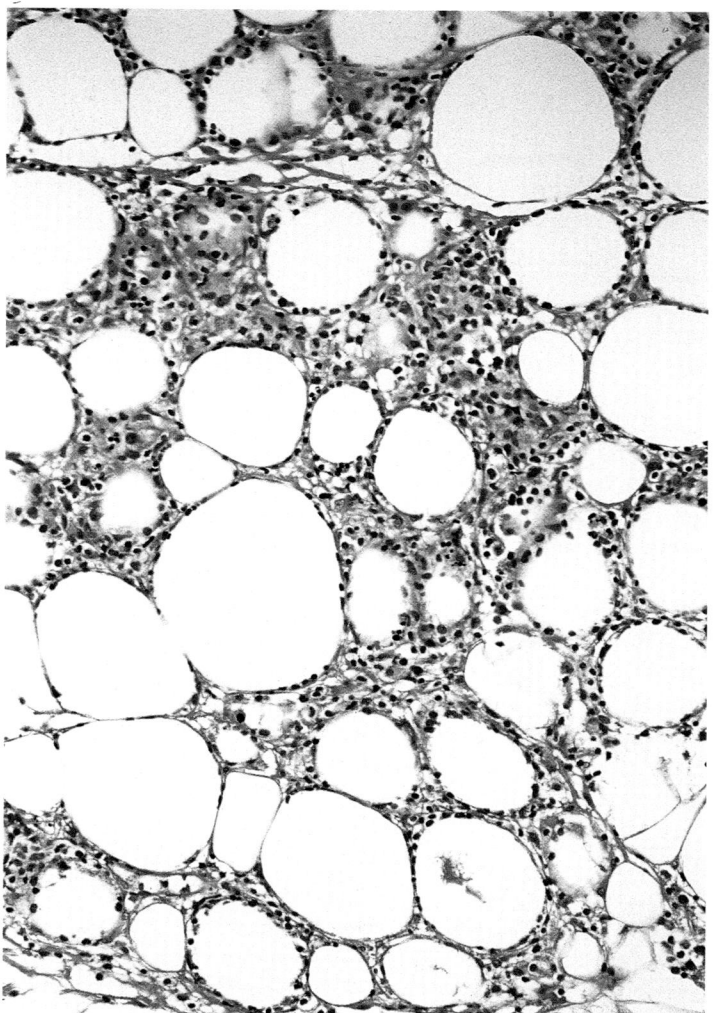

Fig. 17.7 **(A) Panniculitis-like T-cell lymphoma. (B)** There is a lobular panniculitis. There is atypia of lymphocytes but this diagnosis is often missed in early lesions. (H&E)

common in these CD56[+], nasal-type lymphomas.[137] They have an aggressive course, often terminating with a fatal hemophagocytic syndrome.

These two types of cutaneous lymphoma are considered further in Chapter 41 (pp. 1113–1114).

Histopathology

There is a variable admixture of pleomorphic small, medium or large lymphocytes and histiocytes infiltrating the subcutis in the pattern of a lobular panniculitis (Fig. 17.7).[141] Neoplastic cells rim individual adipocytes in a lace-like pattern.[140] Fat necrosis and karyorrhexis occur in all cases, while cytophagocytosis and angioinvasion are sometimes seen.

In the nasal-type lymphoma of CD56[+] natural killer cells, angioinvasion and necrosis are common.[137,142] Furthermore, they tend to be centered on the dermis with secondary involvement of the subcutis.

PANCREATIC PANNICULITIS

Pancreatic panniculitis manifests as painful or asymptomatic subcutaneous nodules or indurated plaques on the thighs, buttocks, lower trunk or distal extremities, usually the lower. The lesions are associated with acute pancreatitis[143–148] or, less commonly, pancreatic carcinoma,[149] either of which may be asymptomatic.[150–152] It has also been associated with low grade pancreatitis in a patient with a pancreas divisum.[153] There may also be polyserositis, arthritis, eosinophilia or rarely a leukemoid reaction. The pancreatic carcinoma, when present, is often of acinic type, although panniculitis has also been reported in association with an islet cell carcinoma.[154–157]

Lesions probably result from the local action of blood-borne pancreatic lipase and trypsin, although other factors may also be involved.[150,158] Cases have been reported without pancreatic disease, but with circulating lipase or amylase of uncertain origin.[159]

Histopathology

Sections of established lesions show a lobular panniculitis involving much of the fat of the affected lobule. Sometimes, contiguous lobules show a different stage in the histological evolution of the process. Early lesions show enzymatic fat necrosis, with the ghost-like outline of fat cells remaining (Fig. 17.8). It has been suggested, on the basis of one case, that at an even earlier stage (2-day-old lesions), there is a septal panniculitis.[160] Liquefaction with breakdown of fat cells will eventually occur. At the margins of the necrotic fat there is a variable neutrophil infiltrate, usually mild, associated with nuclear dusting, fine basophilic calcium deposits and some hemorrhage.[161] The necrotic fat cells may also have a pale basophilic hue due to the deposition of calcium salts. In older lesions there are giant cells, lipophages, lymphocytes, hemosiderin and other blood pigments, and eventual fibrosis. There may be some extension of the inflammatory process into the underlying dermis.

LUPUS PANNICULITIS

Lupus panniculitis (sometimes referred to as lupus erythematosus profundus) is a chronic, recurrent panniculitis with a predilection for the proximal extremities, trunk or lower back: it is a complication in approximately 1–3% of patients with cutaneous lupus erythematosus, both systemic and discoid forms.[162–166] The lesions present as subcutaneous nodules or indurated plaques, although large, painful, indolent ulcers may develop.[167,168] The panniculitis may precede, accompany or follow the development of the associated lupus erythematosus;[165] in nearly half of the cases no associated

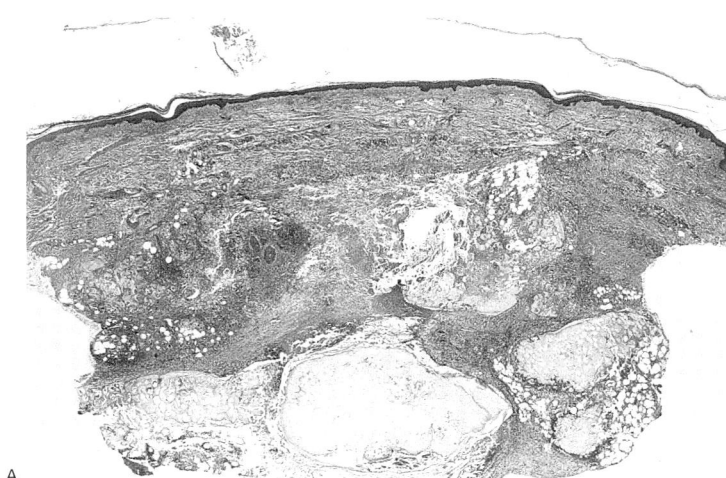

A

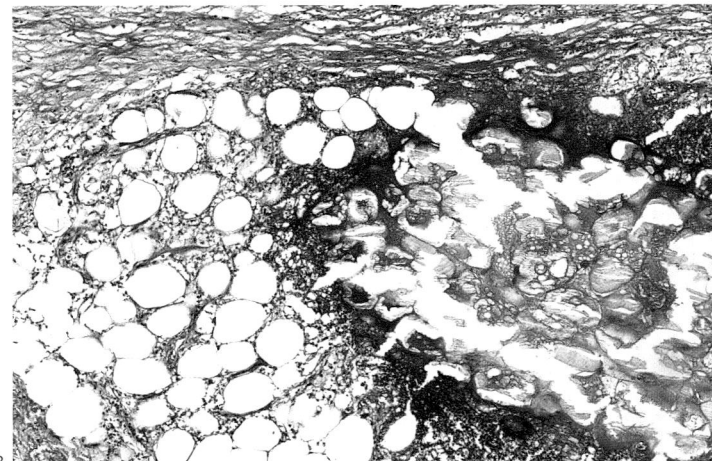

B

Fig. 17.8 **(A) Pancreatic fat necrosis** characterized by enzymatic fat necrosis surrounded by a zone containing nuclear dust and an inflammatory cell infiltrate. **(B)** The fat necrosis has a characteristic appearance. (H&E)

lupus subtype or autoimmune disease is present.[169,170] Accordingly, lupus panniculitis should be regarded as a unique entity within the lupus spectrum.[169] Onset in childhood has been reported.[171–173]

A panniculitis mimicking lupus panniculitis has been reported in a case of malignant atrophic papulosis (Degos disease).[174]

Histopathology

In up to half the cases there are epidermal and dermal changes of lupus erythematosus (particularly in those complicating discoid lupus erythematosus), with basal vacuolar change and a superficial and deep perivascular lymphocytic infiltrate with perifollicular involvement. There is a lobular panniculitis with a prominent lymphocytic infiltrate (lymphocytic lobular panniculitis).[139,163] A lymphocytic vasculitis with lymphocytic nuclear dust is sometimes present. A characteristic feature, found in 20–50% of cases, is the presence of lymphoid follicles, sometimes with germinal centers, adjacent to the fibrous septa (Fig. 17.9). Lymphoid follicles are uncommon in other panniculitides but they are occasionally seen in morphea, erythema nodosum and erythema induratum–nodular vasculitis.[175] Plasma cells are present in many cases while eosinophils may be seen in up to 25% of cases.[176] Lipophages may sometimes be quite numerous. Myxoid and hyaline change may be found in the connective tissue septa and lower dermis. Hyaline sclerosis may extend into

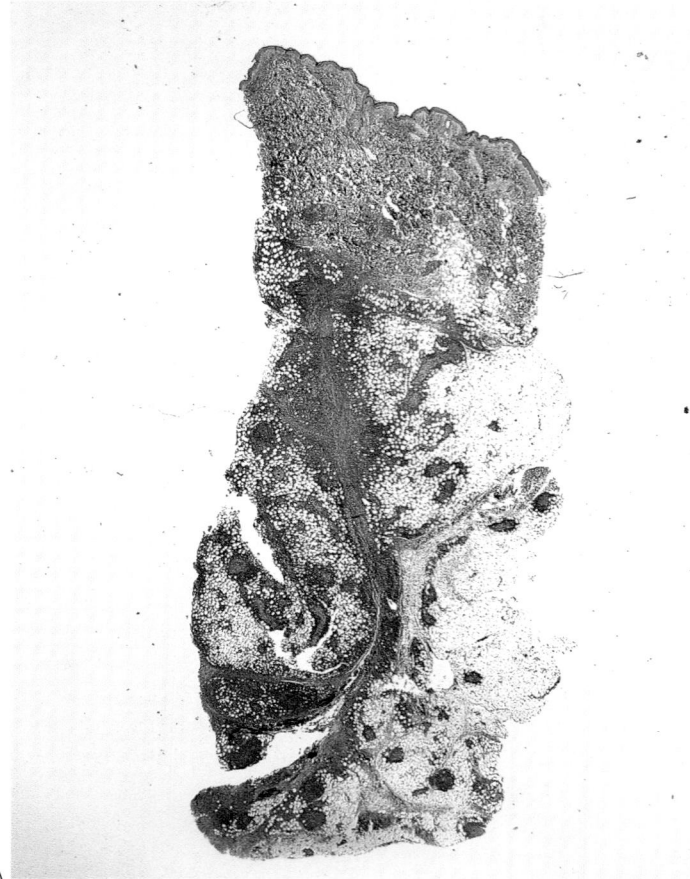

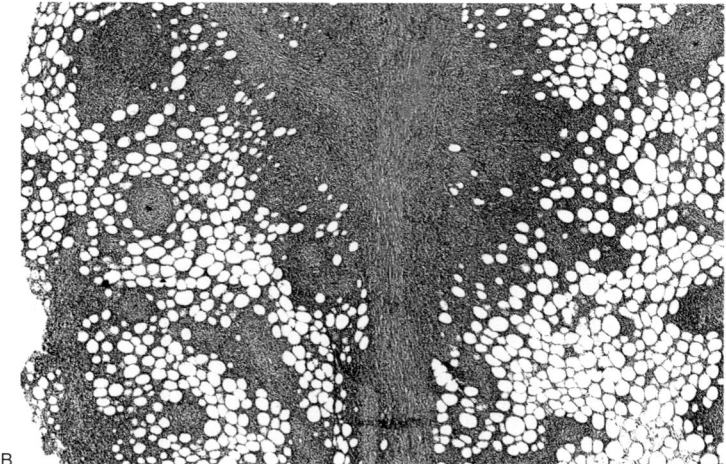

A

B

Fig. 17.9 **Lupus panniculitis. (A)** Paraseptal lymphoid follicles are characteristic. **(B)** Lymphocytes extend into the adjacent fat lobules. (H&E)

the lobules. Sometimes there are calcium deposits in older lesions. Membranocystic changes may be present.[169,177,178]

CONNECTIVE TISSUE PANNICULITIS

The diagnosis of connective tissue panniculitis has been applied to two patients with recurrent subcutaneous nodules with transient antinuclear antibody tests.[179] Cases followed by lipoatrophy have been included as a variant.[180–182] Connective tissue panniculitis may not represent a discrete entity.

Histopathology

The reported cases have shown a lobular panniculitis with some fat necrosis resembling the appearance in erythema induratum–nodular vasculitis but showing no vessel changes and no granulomas. There have been dense lymphocytic infiltrates (but no lymphoid follicles) and small foam cell collections.[179]

A pustular panniculitis has been reported in one patient with rheumatoid arthritis.[183]

POSTSTEROID PANNICULITIS

Poststeroid panniculitis consists of multiple subcutaneous nodules developing 1–35 days after the withdrawal of steroid therapy, particularly in children.[184]

Histopathology

There is a non-specific lobular panniculitis with lymphocytes, histiocytes, some foam cells and giant cells. Septal vessels are spared, distinguishing the lesions from those of erythema induratum–nodular vasculitis.

LIPODYSTROPHY SYNDROMES

The term 'lipodystrophy' has traditionally been used for primary, idiopathic atrophy of subcutaneous tissue, whether *total, partial* or *localized*.[185] It has been distinguished from the secondary lipoatrophy that may follow certain panniculitides such as lupus panniculitis, connective tissue panniculitis and subcutaneous morphea.[181,185,186] The term 'lipodystrophy' is also used for the lipoatrophy (and the rare lipohypertrophy) that may follow the repeated injection of insulin into the subcutis by diabetics.[187] It has been suggested that *lipedema*, characterized by the abnormal deposition of subcutaneous fat in the legs (associated with edema), is a lipodystrophy.[188] The three major categories of lipodystrophy will be considered further.

Total lipodystrophy

Total lipodystrophy may be congenital or acquired, the latter group being associated with metabolic disturbances such as diabetes or endocrine disorders.[164]

Partial lipodystrophy

Partial lipodystrophy begins usually with symmetrical loss of facial fat, often progressing to involve the upper trunk and arms.[189] Two variants of acquired partial lipodystrophy (Barraquer–Simons disease) have been described. In the Weir–Mitchell type there is loss of fat from the face, with or without atrophy of the arms and upper trunk, while in the Laignel–Lavastine type there is concomitant hypertrophy of the fat of the lower part of the body.[190] Unilateral variants of this have been described;[191,192] facial hemiatrophy is known as the Parry–Romberg syndrome.[191,193] Cases of partial lipodystrophy have been related to thyroid disease, acanthosis nigricans, dermatomyositis, myasthenia gravis, membranoproliferative glomerulonephritis[194–196] and recurrent infections.[164] Recently, an acquired lipodystrophy was reported in a 3-year-old girl in whom additional material was detected on chromosome 10 at the 10q26 location, at the site of the human pancreatic lipase gene.[197] However, most cases of partial lipodystrophy probably have an immunological mechanism.

Localized lipodystrophy

Localized lipodystrophy is characterized by annular or semicircular areas of atrophy, often solitary. It needs to be distinguished from morphea-related lipoatrophy.[198] Variants have been described near the ankles,[128,199,200] on the thighs,[129,201] over the sacrum[202] and on the abdomen (lipodystrophia centrifugalis abdominalis)[203–210] and in the form of a unilateral linear panatrophy of the extremities.[211] 'Post-injection' lipoatrophy is another variant of localized lipodystrophy. It can follow the injection of corticosteroids, iron dextran, vaccines, insulin and penicillin.[212] In one series of localized lipoatrophy, 9 of the 16 patients had received injections at the site.[213] Pressure appears to be involved in the causation of some other cases of the localized variant, particularly semicircular lipoatrophy.[201,214,215] Apoptosis of fat cells has been noted during the lipoatrophic process in one case of abdominal lipodystrophy.[216]

The histopathology of the three major categories of lipodystrophy will be considered together.

Histopathology

In *established* cases there is atrophy of subcutaneous fat and usually no evidence of inflammation. In some cases, biopsy of an early lesion shows a lobular panniculitis, often with some vascular involvement.[217–221] In one personally studied case there was a lobular panniculitis with numerous foam cells, small fat cysts and some lymphocytes; there was no vasculitis (Fig. 17.10). This patient had partial lipodystrophy with prominent facial involvement and a poorly characterized connective tissue disease. Her inflammatory lesions were transient.

It has been suggested that there are two histopathological types of lipodystrophy but whether this is always stage-related (see above) has not been clarified, as yet.[217] In one group there are prominent involutional changes to the subcutaneous fat with small lipocytes and intervening hyaline or myxoid connective tissue containing numerous capillaries. The second group has inflammatory changes characterized by a lobular panniculitis with lymphocytes, lipophages and plasma cells. This pattern was present in the young girl with abnormalities of chromosome 10 (see above). A dermal lymphocytic vasculitis has also been described.[190] The inflammatory type usually has multiple areas of lipoatrophy clinically and immunoreactants in blood vessels or the basement membrane on direct immunofluorescence.

The localized variants, such as semicircular and post-injection lipoatrophy, are infrequently biopsied. They show loss of fat with the deposition of new collagen. There is usually no evidence of panniculitis, although inflammation has been reported.[222] There are often scattered lipophages.[213,214] The appearances can resemble embryonic fat. Most cases correspond to the first group mentioned above.

HIV-ASSOCIATED LIPODYSTROPHY

A lipodystrophy can be seen in patients with the acquired immunodeficiency syndrome (AIDS). Three clinical settings appear to be involved. The most common variant, characterized by the presence of peripheral lipoatrophy and central adiposity, can develop following the use of protease inhibitor therapy.[223–227] Clinically evident lipodystrophy usually begins 2–14 months after the commencement of therapy. The changes include loss of fat from the arms, buttocks, thighs and legs, leading to prominence of veins and muscles, particularly on the legs.[228] Loss of the buccal fat pad gives a cachectic appearance.[225] The accompanying lipohypertrophy includes central obesity, enlargement of the dorsocervical fat pad ('buffalo hump') and deposition of abdominal fat. Indinavir is the protease inhibitor most often implicated. Resolution of the lipodystrophy usually occurs on discontinuation of the therapy.[223] It has been suggested that protease inhibitors bind to proteins that regulate lipid metabolism. Dysregulation of peroxisome function also occurs.[229]

A similar lipodystrophy has been reported with the use of reverse transcriptase inhibitors. It has been suggested that these cases may in some way be related to suppression of HIV replication.[226]

Finally, a third group of HIV-related cases appears to exist. Some patients with AIDS develop a facial lipoatrophy; not all have been on protease or reverse transcriptase inhibitor therapy.

Histopathology[225]

The lipoatrophy resembles the non-inflammatory variant of lipodystrophy (see above). There is atrophy of fat, sometimes accompanied by an alteration in the size and shape of adipocytes. The fat cells were reported as having a normal spherical shape in one report.[226] Focal collections of lymphocytes and lipophages are sometimes present, but they are not a prominent feature. A proliferation of small vessels may occur at the interface between the atrophic lobules and the septa, resembling immature (fetal) fat.

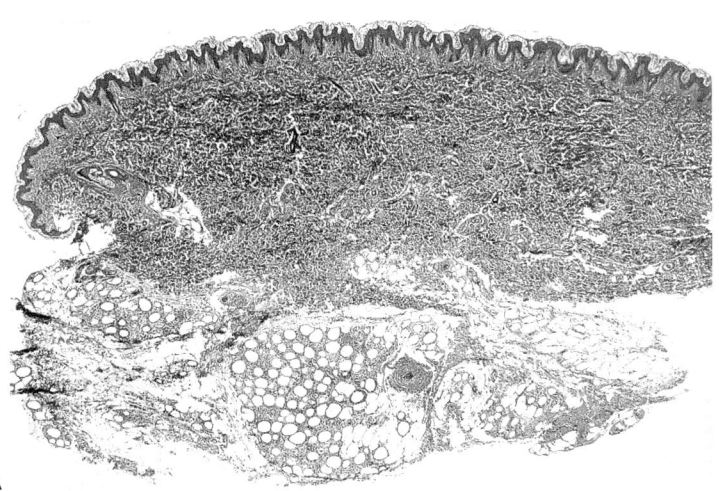
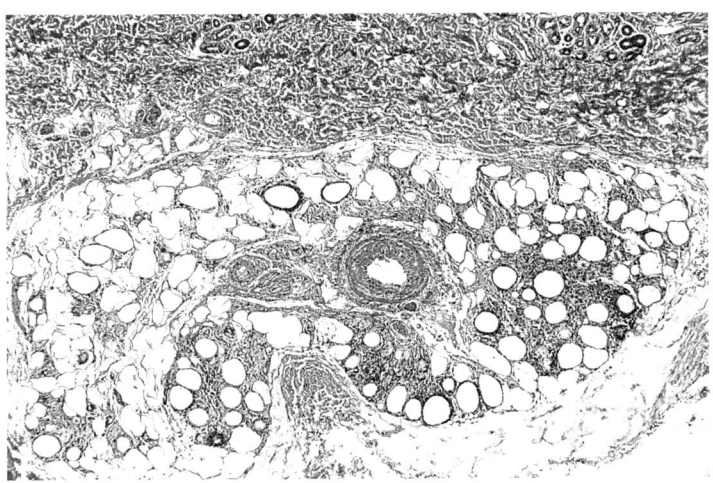

A B

Fig. 17.10 **(A) Partial lipodystrophy** at the stage of a lobular panniculitis. Atrophy developed subsequently. **(B)** Inflammatory changes are usually mild. (H&E)

GYNOID LIPODYSTROPHY (CELLULITE)

Gynoid lipodystrophy, better known as cellulite, is an alteration of the topography of the skin that occurs mainly in women on the buttocks, thighs and abdomen.[230] It gives the skin a dimpled ('orange peel', 'quilted', 'mattress') appearance.[231,232] It is very common in obese patients, although it differs from obesity both structurally and mechanistically.[230] Four grades of clinicopathological severity have been defined.[230]

The pathogenesis of gynoid lipodystrophy is complex and still being elucidated but it includes alterations in the composition and the amount of fat in adipocytes, changes in the microcirculation of the subcutis, and hyperpolymerization in the connective tissue of the fat septa.[230] These changes appear to be influenced by hormonal and psychosomatic factors as well as by race, sedentary lifestyle and an inherent predisposition.[230]

Histopathology[230,231]

There is no consensus on the histopathological features of gynoid lipodystrophy, possibly reflecting different stages of the disease process. Furthermore, there appears to be a physiological difference between the dermal–subcutaneous interface in men and women, with a smooth interface in males and a tendency to a 'lumpy' appearance in females as a consequence of the protrusion of superficial fat lobules into the dermis.[231]

In early stages, the superficial fat lobules are large. They may be squeezed between straightened fibrous septa, which are of variable thickness. This latter feature becomes more obvious in established cases when lumpy and loose swellings are interposed between thinner areas of the septa; a few myofibroblasts are present. The septa may come to resemble areas of stria distensa (see p. 358) with associated alterations in the elastic tissue which may consist of clumped and increased fibers and other areas with reduced elastic tissue.[231] Small collections of adipocytes may become encapsulated with fibrous strands.

Vascular changes are variable and may involve the dermis as well. There is often neovascularization, dilatation of vessels, intimal thickening of small arteries and microaneurysms with hemorrhage.[230]

MEMBRANOUS LIPODYSTROPHY

The term 'membranous lipodystrophy' was originally applied to a sudanophilic sclerosing leukoencephalopathy in which cystic degeneration of the marrow of long bones also occurred.[233] The fat showed a characteristic lipomembranous (membranocystic) change (see below). The term has since been applied to a varied group of panniculitides in which this same lipomembranous change occurs. There are several cases in the literature where this change has been found as a primary phenomenon in the subcutaneous fat of the skin; it has therefore been proposed that such cases should be designated *primary membranous lipodystrophy* to distinguish them from the cases in which it is merely an incidental histological feature – *secondary membranous lipodystrophy*.[234–236] Diseases in this latter category include erythema nodosum,[178,237] morphea profunda,[233] lupus panniculitis, traumatic fat necrosis, insulin lipoatrophy,[238] the panniculitis of Behçet's syndrome, encapsulated fat necrosis and the panniculitis of dermatomyositis.[239] Membranous lipodystrophy also occurs in association with circulatory disturbances, particularly diabetic microangiopathy and venous insufficiency; vasculitis-induced lesions are rare.[240] As lipodermatosclerosis also occurs in a setting of venous insufficiency, it is perhaps not surprising that lipomembranous change is common in lipodermatosclerosis.

It seems likely that membranous lipodystrophy will eventually be regarded as synonymous with lipomembranous (membranocystic) change – a histological change rather than a disease sui generis.

Histopathology[160,234–236]

Membranous lipodystrophy is characterized by lipomembranous (membranocystic) change. There are cysts of varying size, usually small, lined by amorphous, eosinophilic material having an arabesque architecture (Fig. 17.11). Sometimes the membranes form small pseudopapillae.[241] The material is stained by the PAS and Sudan black methods. Between groups of fat cysts there are dense, thick, fibrous septa. Myospherulosis (see p. 445) has been noted in one case.[242] In secondary membranous lipodystrophy, changes of the underlying process will, of course, be present as well.

LIPODERMATOSCLEROSIS

Criticisms not withstanding,[243] 'lipodermatosclerosis' is still the preferred term for an entity characterized by circumscribed, indurated, often inflammatory plaques on the lower extremities. The condition is usually associated with venous insufficiency, arterial ischemia or previous thrombophlebitis.[169,244] It may also complicate chronic lymphedema. There may also be mottled hyperpigmentation related to venous stasis.[245] Sometimes the clinical

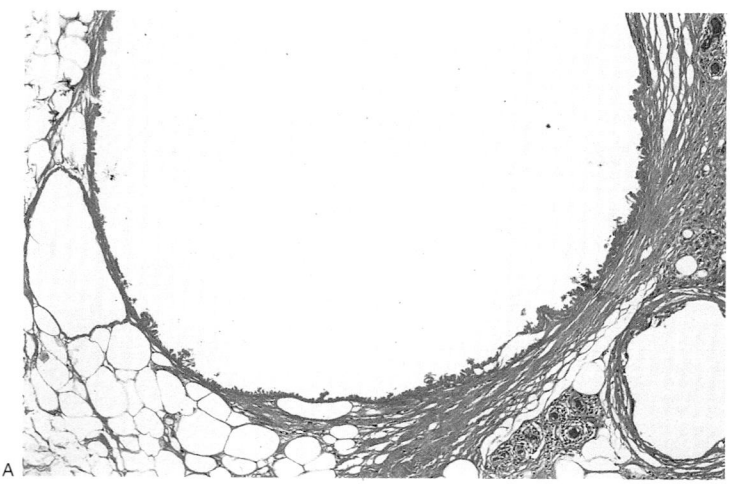
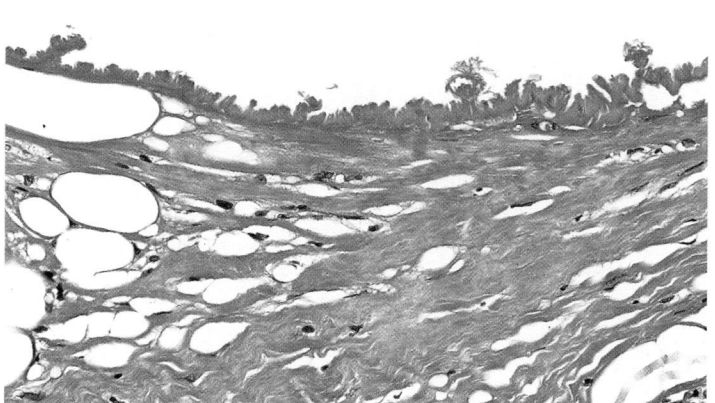

Fig. 17.11 **(A) Lipomembranous fat necrosis. (B)** There is some sclerosis in the wall of the fat cyst which is lined by hyaline eosinophilic material with an arabesque pattern. (H&E)

appearances mimic a cellulitis. Similar lesions have been reported as *sclerosing panniculitis*[246] and *hypodermitis sclerodermiformis*. So-called 'lipomembranous' (membranocystic) change is frequently seen on histology, thus this condition has also been regarded as a *membranous lipodystrophy* (see above) or simply called *lipomembranous (membranocystic) fat necrosis*.[178]

Lipodermatosclerosis appears to be a consequence of ischemia and venous stasis. There is abnormally low plasma fibrinolytic activity in these patients, as well as low levels of proteins C and S.[247] However, fibrinolytic activity is increased in affected tissues and this is associated with elevated levels of urokinase-type plasminogen activator (uPA).[248] In addition, there is elevated matrix turnover, although the significance of this finding is uncertain.[249] Ultrasound investigations have shown that the edema fluid in this condition is predominantly in the upper dermis in contrast to the deep dermal location of the fluid in chronic heart failure.[250] As light compression appears to enhance the removal of edema fluid, compression stockings have been used in the treatment of lipodermatosclerosis.[251]

Histopathology

Biopsies are usually obtained in the later stages of the disease when there is septal fibrosis and sclerosis and fatty microcysts with foci of membranocystic change. This consists of amorphous eosinophilic material, sometimes with a crenelated appearance, lining microcysts. This material is PAS positive and stains with Sudan black.[234] Microgranules may be present in macrophages. Hemosiderin pigment is often present in the dermis; it may also be in the subcutis. There is fibrosis of the dermis and pericapillary fibrin caps around small vessels in the upper dermis. The fibrous thickening of the lower dermis means that a punch biopsy of an involved area of skin may not include any subcutaneous fat (Fig. 17.12).

In early lesions (uncommonly biopsied as the site heals poorly), there is a septal and lobular panniculitis, with lymphocytes being the predominant cell. There is variable fat necrosis; sometimes an entire lobule is infarcted. Blood vessels appear prominent in the septa at all stages.

FACTITIAL PANNICULITIS

The clinical manifestations of self-induced panniculitis will depend on the nature and site of the insult. Factitial panniculitis may follow injections of all manner of substances, including milk, urine, feces, oils and drugs, into the subcutaneous fat. Reports have included the injection of procaine povidone,[252] meperidine (pethidine)[253] and pentazocine.[254] Sclerosing lipogranuloma (paraffinoma) is a special form of factitial panniculitis resulting from the injection of lipid, often paraffin, into the subcutaneous tissue,[255]

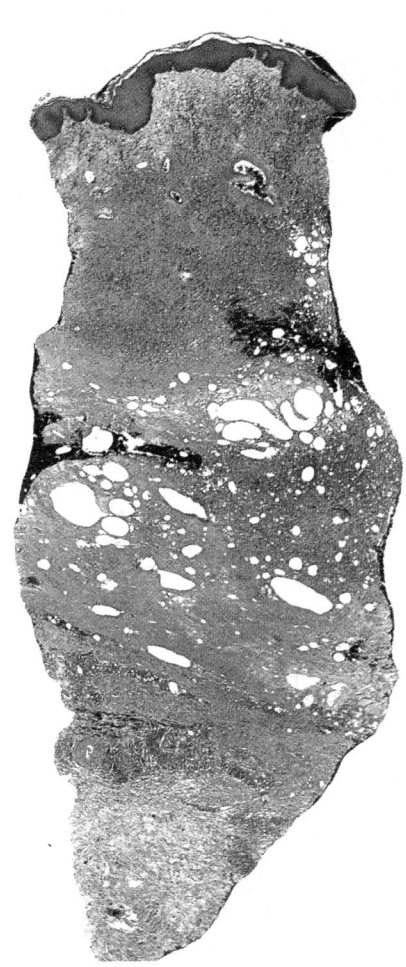
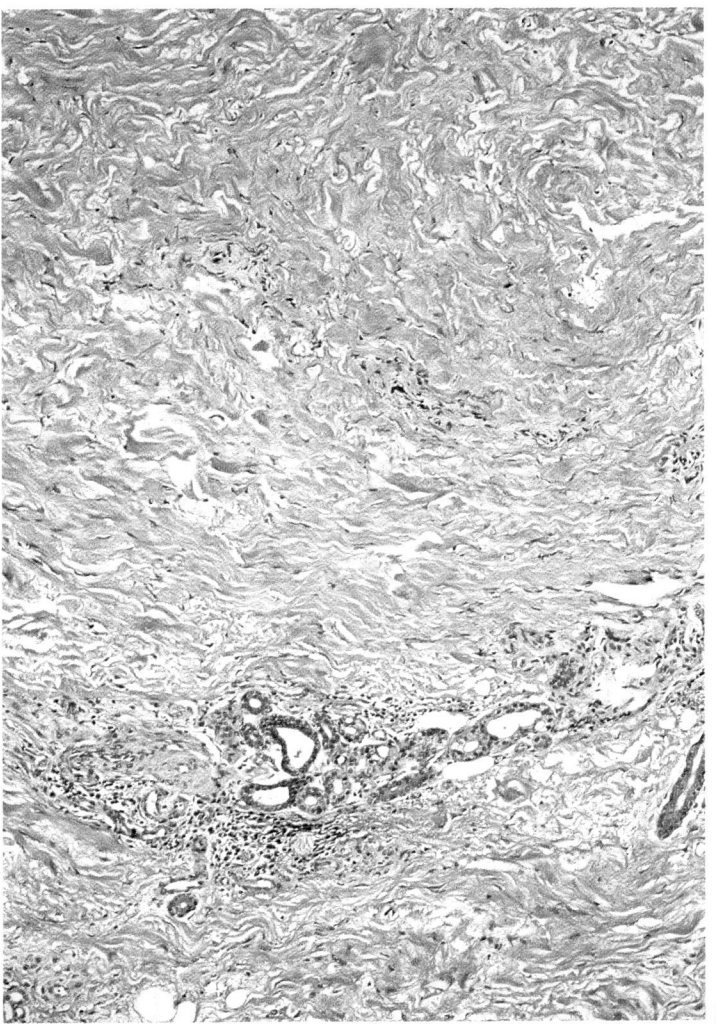

Fig. 17.12 **(A) Lipodermatosclerosis. (B)** Fibrous tissue replaces the subcutis. There is mild chronic inflammation at the level of the sweat glands. There is some hemosiderin pigment in the lower dermis. (H&E)

particularly in an attempt to produce enlargement of the penis and even the breasts.[256,257] Other oils and silicones have been involved.[258–260] The lesion presents as a painful rubbery induration of the involved area.

Histopathology

Although factitial panniculitis usually produces a lobular or mixed panniculitis or even a picture resembling Weber–Christian disease, other patterns such as a suppurative septal panniculitis can occur (Fig. 17.13). Foreign body giant cells with foreign material, sometimes doubly refractile, may be present. It is a good idea to examine by polarized light any unusual suppurative panniculitis or one with foreign body-type granulomas.

In paraffinomas and oleomas, there is a characteristic Swiss-cheese appearance with disruption of fat cells and their replacement by cystic spaces of variable size, some surrounded by attenuated foreign body giant cells containing lipid vacuoles.[257,260] There are bands of hyaline fibrous tissue between the fat cysts. The septa contain a scattering of lymphocytes and lipid-containing macrophages and foreign body giant cells. This pattern is referred to as sclerosing lipogranuloma.

TRAUMATIC FAT NECROSIS

Subcutaneous fat necrosis may follow trauma, particularly to the shins. Focal liquefaction of the injured fat often follows and this is sometimes discharged through a surface wound. Some cases of traumatic fat necrosis have a factitial origin, so there is obvious overlap with factitial panniculitis.[261]

Histopathology

Cases coming to biopsy usually show fat cysts of varying size with surrounding fibrosis. The microcysts sometimes show lipomembranous (membranocystic) change. There are often small collections of foam cells, a mild patchy lymphocytic infiltrate and some hemosiderin. In earlier lesions there is fat necrosis with cystic spaces and numerous neutrophils in the adjacent fat. A similar appearance follows surgical disruption of the subcutis.[262] Sometimes collections of fat cells, often necrotic, can be seen within the dermis, apparently in the process of being eliminated through a break in the epidermis.

ENCAPSULATED FAT NECROSIS

Encapsulated fat necrosis is the preferred designation for the small mobile nodules that may develop in the subcutis; they often follow trauma.[263] These lesions have also been called 'mobile encapsulated lipoma' and 'nodular-cystic fat necrosis'.[264]

The lesions, which are usually solitary, are whitish-yellow in color, and measure 3–20 mm in diameter.[263]

Histopathology

The lesions are composed of lobules of necrotic fat surrounded by a thin fibrous capsule which is usually hyaline (Fig. 17.14). Lipomembranous change (see above) is often present.[235,265] Small collections of lipophages and very focal inflammatory changes are sometimes seen, particularly near the capsule. Dystrophic calcification may be a late complication.

INFECTIVE PANNICULITIS

Various infections and infestations may result in a lobular or mixed lobular and septal panniculitis.[3,266] These include candidiasis,[234] cryptococcosis, mycetoma, actinomycosis, nocardiosis, chromomycosis, sporotrichosis and

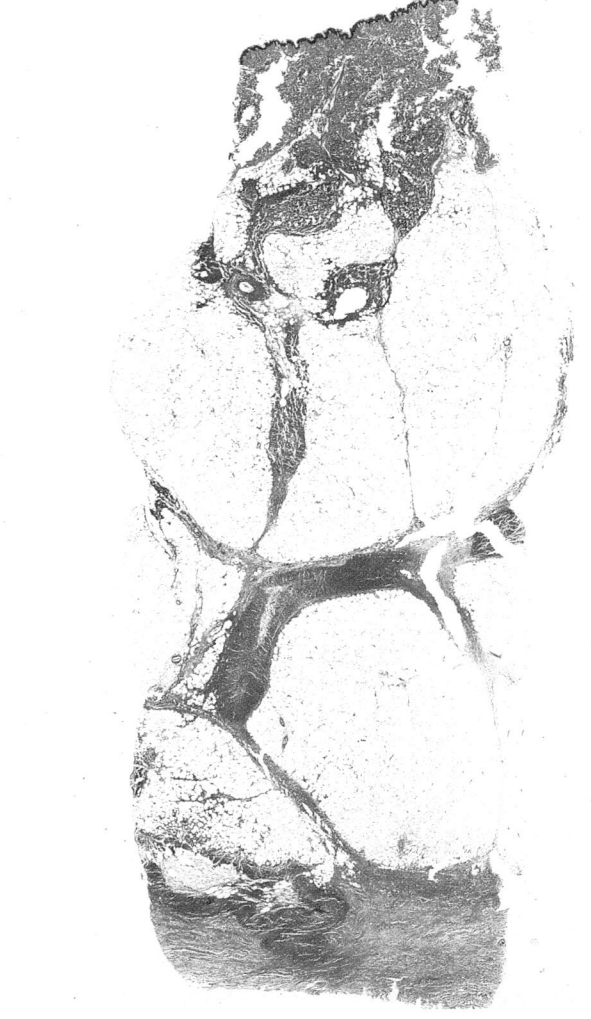

A

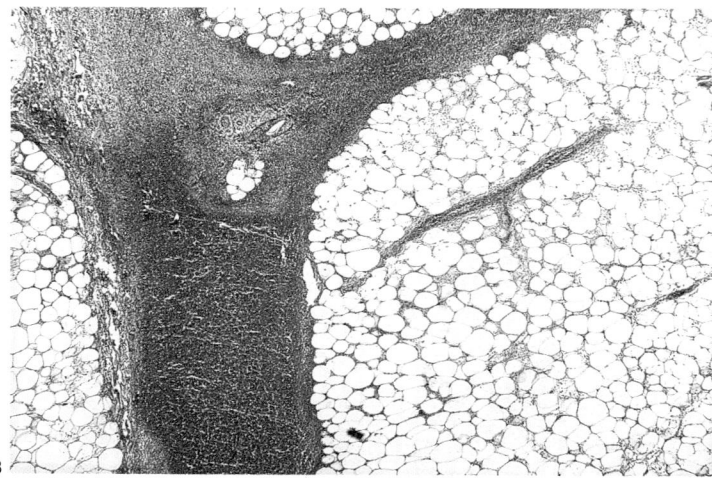

B

Fig. 17.13 **(A) An unusual case of factitial panniculitis. (B)** There is suppuration involving the interlobular septa. The deep fascia contains some doubly-refractile foreign material, the nature of which was not ascertained. (H&E)

histoplasmosis,[267,268] infections with *Mycobacterium marinum*,[269] *M. ulcerans*, *M. fortuitum, M. tuberculosis*,[270] *M. leprae* (erythema nodosum leprosum – see p. 632), *M. avium-intracellulare*[271] and other bacteria,[266] bites of ticks[272] and of the brown recluse spider (*Loxosceles reclusa*)[32] and metazoal infestations

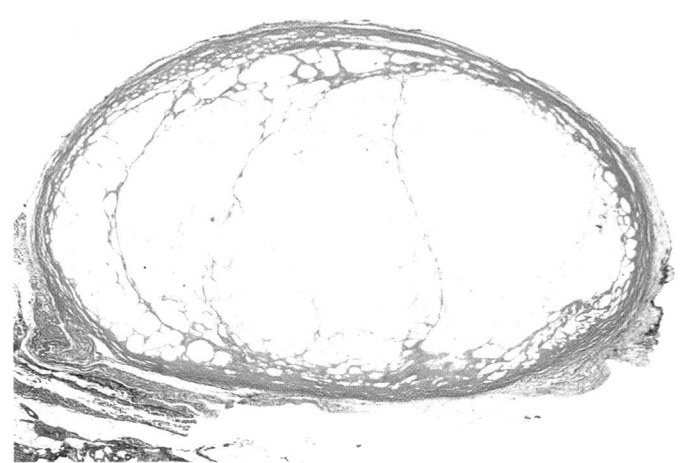

Fig. 17.14 Encapsulated fat necrosis. There is a hyaline capsule with central fat necrosis and cystic change. (H&E)

(myiasis, cysticercosis, sparganosis and infestations by some other helminths). Most cases of infection-induced panniculitis occur in patients who are immunosuppressed.[266]

Histopathology[266]

The presence of a lobular or mixed lobular and septal panniculitis in which there is a heavy infiltrate of neutrophils,[270] often with extension into the dermis, should raise the suspicion of an infective etiology (Fig. 17.15). Hemorrhage and necrosis are often present. In a case of neutrophilic lobular panniculitis due to acanthamebiasis, trophozoites measuring 20–30 µm in diameter were present.[273]

NON-INFECTIVE NEUTROPHILIC PANNICULITIS

While an infective cause should always be considered in the presence of a neutrophilic panniculitis, other etiologies do exist.[274,275] In the early stages of many of the panniculitides, neutrophilic infiltration occurs. Examples include erythema nodosum, Behçet's disease, pancreatic panniculitis and factitial panniculitis.

Rare causes of neutrophilic panniculitis include rheumatoid arthritis,[274] Sweet's syndrome, Crohn's disease,[276] and myelodysplastic syndromes.[277] In rheumatoid arthritis, fat necrosis, fat cyst formation and low grade vasculitis may also be present.

EOSINOPHILIC PANNICULITIS

The term 'eosinophilic panniculitis' has been applied to several different disease entities.[278] It has been used for a mixed lobular and septal panniculitis with numerous eosinophils and flame figures and features resembling those seen in the dermis in Wells' syndrome (see p. 1060):[279] in these cases, the panniculitis was thought to have followed inflammation or infection of the upper aerodigestive tract.[279,280] The term has been used for a panniculitis with numerous eosinophils in the infiltrate.[281] As such it is not a specific entity but a non-specific pattern seen in a diverse range of systemic diseases including erythema nodosum, vasculitis, parasitic infestation (Fig. 17.16), malignant lymphoma, atopy[282] and narcotic dependency with injection granulomas.[281] An eosinophilic panniculitis (septal or mixed septal and lobular) has been reported following the infusion of apomorphine for Parkinson's disease.[6] The term has also been used for a nodular migratory panniculitis which may accompany infestations with the larva of the nematode *Gnathostoma spinigerum* (deep larva migrans):[283,284] in this variety eosinophils make up 95% of the infiltrate. Finally, an eosinophilic panniculitis may rarely occur with other parasitic infestations, such as *Fasciola hepatica*.[249] Unlike *Gnasthostoma*-induced cases, no parasites are present in the panniculitis.

MISCELLANEOUS LESIONS

A focal non-specific panniculitis may be found in some cases of dermatomyositis, particularly in relation to underlying calcified deposits.[285,286] In a few cases tender, indurated plaques and nodules develop; they have the histological features of a lobular panniculitis.[287] A calcifying panniculitis resulting from calciphylaxis (see p. 258) has been reported in chronic renal failure.[288,289] Metastatic calcification in renal failure differs by its dermal localization and the absence of a panniculitis.[289]

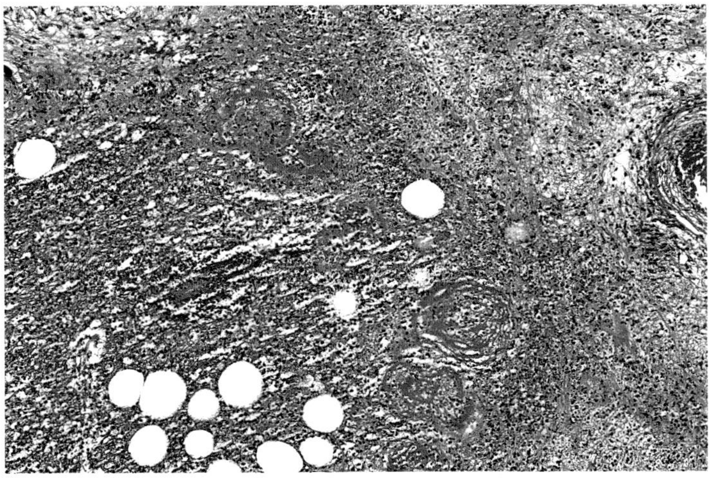

Fig. 17.15 *Mycobacterium ulcerans.* The presence of a widespread suppurative panniculitis, as shown here, warrants exclusion of an infective etiology. Numerous acid-fast bacilli were present. (H&E)

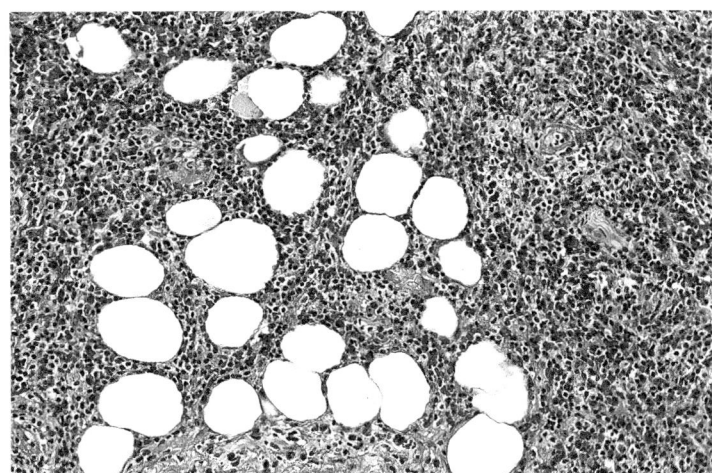

Fig. 17.16 Eosinophilic panniculitis. There is an almost pure infiltrate of eosinophils throughout the lobules of fat. A helminth was found nearby. (H&E)

Panniculitis with urate crystal deposition and necrosis of fat has been reported as the only cutaneous manifestation of gout.[290–292]

In the severe form of hydroa vacciniforme (see p. 601) a lobular or septal panniculitis and/or vasculitis are often present.[293]

A hemorrhagic panniculitis has followed atheromatous embolization of vessels of the skin.[294]

Non-caseating granulomas may be found in the subcutaneous tissue in sarcoidosis and, rarely, in Crohn's disease.[295,296] A neutrophilic lobular panniculitis with few granulomas has also been reported in Crohn's disease.[276]

The panniculitis found in about 5% of patients undergoing jejunoileal bypass for morbid obesity has been described as erythema nodosum-like[297] complicated by lobular fat necrosis and as Weber–Christian-like.[103] Published photomicrographs suggest a lobular panniculitis with some resemblance to erythema induratum–nodular vasculitis. A mixed septal and lobular panniculitis is a rare complication of the blind loop syndrome.[298]

Other rare causes of a panniculitis include malignancies,[299,300] particularly lymphomas.[3,301,302] Sometimes a florid granulomatous panniculitis accompanies the lymphomatous infiltrate; this may mask the correct diagnosis of lymphoma.[303,304] A lobular panniculitis is common in angiocentric immuno-proliferative lesions such as lymphomatoid granulomatosis (see p. 1101).[305] A lobular panniculitis with variable numbers of plasma cells has been reported in Sjögren's syndrome.[306,307] The erythema nodosum-like lesions in Behçet's disease may have either a septal or lobular panniculitis on histopathological examination.[49] Drugs such as phenytoin,[32] iodides and bromides and low-calorie diets and nutritional abnormalities[308] may produce a panniculitis. A necrotizing panniculitis, secondary to vascular thrombosis, may follow the use of recombinant human granulocytic colony-stimulating factor[309] or the injection of cocaine.[310] Granuloma annulare may also involve the subcutis. Radiation therapy for breast carcinoma may produce a pseudosclerodermatous panniculitis.[311]

Cases which defy an etiological classification are sometimes seen. Such a case was reported as 'suppressor-cytotoxic T-lymphocyte panniculitis'. The patient was febrile and had a lobular panniculitis with many CD8-positive lymphocytes in the infiltrate.[312]

PANNICULITIS SECONDARY TO LARGE VESSEL VASCULITIS

A localized area of panniculitis is almost invariable in the immediate vicinity of an inflamed large artery or vein, as it courses through the subcutaneous fat. There is no lobular panniculitis of contiguous lobules as is seen in erythema induratum–nodular vasculitis.

CUTANEOUS POLYARTERITIS NODOSA

There is a benign cutaneous form of polyarteritis nodosa that is distinct from the systemic form. It presents with painful subcutaneous nodules in crops, mainly on the lower limbs. There may be other associated cutaneous features. It is considered further in Chapter 8 (p. 237). In microscopic polyangiitis (see p. 237), there may be a septal panniculitis.

SUPERFICIAL MIGRATORY THROMBOPHLEBITIS

Superficial migratory thrombophlebitis presents as erythematous subcutaneous nodules or cord-like areas of induration, usually on the lower limbs. It may be associated with other conditions such as carcinoma of the pancreas, Behçet's disease and Buerger's disease. The panniculitis is limited to the area immediately adjacent to the involved vessel (Fig. 17.17). This entity is considered further in Chapter 8 (p.238).

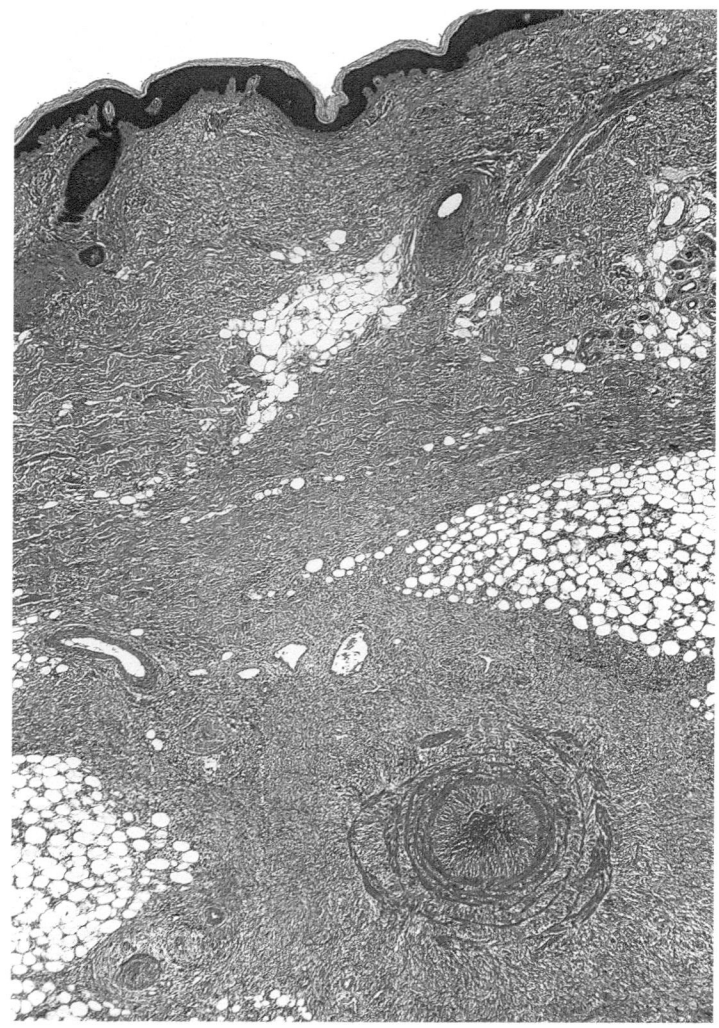

Fig. 17.17 **Superficial migratory thrombophlebitis** involving a small vein in the subcutis. Sometimes an elastic tissue stain is needed to distinguish between small arteries and arterialized veins in biopsies from the lower leg. (H&E)

REFERENCES

Introduction

1 Reed RJ, Clark WH, Mihm MC. Disorders of the panniculus adiposus. Hum Pathol 1973; 4: 219–229.

2 Niemi KM, Forstrom L, Hannuksela M et al. Nodules on the legs. Acta Derm Venereol 1977; 57: 145–154.

3 Black MM. Panniculitis. J Cutan Pathol 1985; 12: 366–380.

4 Pierini LE, Abulafia J, Wainfeld S. Idiopathic lipogranulomatous hypodermitis. Arch Dermatol 1968; 98: 290–298.

5 Diaz Cascajo C, Borghi S, Weyers W. Panniculitis. Definition of terms and diagnostic strategy. Am J Dermatopathol 2000; 22: 530–549.

Septal panniculitis

6 Acland KM, Churchyard A, Fletcher CL et al. Panniculitis in association with apomorphine infusion. Br J Dermatol 1998; 138: 480–482.

7 Hern AE, Shwayder TA. Unilateral plantar erythema nodosum. J Am Acad Dermatol 1992; 26: 259–260.

8 Suarez SM, Paller AS. Plantar erythema nodosum: cases in two children. Arch Dermatol 1993; 129: 1064–1065.

9 Ohtake N, Kawamura T, Akiyama C et al. Unilateral plantar erythema nodosum. J Am Acad Dermatol 1994; 30: 654–655.

10 Kakourou T, Drosatou P, Psychou F et al. Erythema nodosum in children: A prospective study. J Am Acad Dermatol 2001; 44: 17–21.

11 Ahn SK, Lee BJ, Lee SH, Lee WS. Nodular cystic fat necrosis in a patient with erythema nodosum. Clin Exp Dermatol 1995; 20: 263–265.

12 Blaustein A, Moreno A, Noguera J, de Moragas JM. Septal granulomatous panniculitis in Sweet's syndrome. Arch Dermatol 1985; 121: 785–788.

13 Ginarte M, Toribio J. Association of Sweet syndrome and erythema nodosum. Arch Dermatol 2000; 136: 673–674.

14 Kaneko F, Takahashi Y, Muramatsu Y, Miura Y. Immunological studies on aphthous ulcer and erythema nodosum-like eruptions in Behcet's disease. Br J Dermatol 1985; 113: 303–312.

15 Honma T, Bang D, Lee S, Saito T. Ultrastructure of endothelial cell necrosis in classical erythema nodosum. Hum Pathol 1993; 24: 384–390.

16 Altomare GF, Capella GL. Paraneoplastic erythema nodosum in a patient with carcinoma of the uterine cervix. Br J Dermatol 1995; 132: 667–668.

17 Durden FM, Variyam E, Chren M-M. Fat necrosis with features of erythema nodosum in a patient with metastatic pancreatic carcinoma. Int J Dermatol 1996; 35: 39–41.

18 Sumaya CV, Babu S, Reed RJ. Erythema nodosum-like lesions of leukemia. Arch Dermatol 1974; 110: 415–418.

19 Parodi A, Cestari R, Rebora A. Erythema nodosum as the presenting symptom of gastric centrofollicular lymphoma. Int J Dermatol 1989; 28: 336–337.

20 Matsuoka LY. Neoplastic erythema nodosum. J Am Acad Dermatol 1995; 32: 361–363.

21 Peter R, Banyai T. Erythema nodosum revealing oculoglandular tularemia. Dermatology 2001; 202: 79–80.

22 Whitton T, Smith AG. Erythema nodosum secondary to meningococcal septicaemia. Clin Exp Dermatol 1999; 24: 97–98.

23 Sanders CJG, Hulsmans R-FHJ. Persistent erythema nodosum and asymptomatic *Campylobacter* infection. J Am Acad Dermatol 1991; 24: 285–286.

24 Scott BB. Salmonella gastroenteritis – another cause of erythema nodosum. Br J Dermatol 1980; 102: 339–340.

25 Cribier B, Caille A, Heid E, Grosshans E. Erythema nodosum and associated diseases. A study of 129 cases. Int J Dermatol 1998; 37: 667–672.

26 Kousa M, Saikku P, Kanerva L. Erythema nodosum in chlamydial infections. Acta Derm Venereol 1980; 60: 319–322.

27 Boonchai W, Suthipinittharm P, Mahaisavariya P. Panniculitis in tuberculosis: a clinicopathologic study of nodular panniculitis associated with tuberculosis. Int J Dermatol 1998; 37: 361–363.

28 Calista D, Schianchi S, Morri M. Erythema nodosum induced by kerion celsi of the scalp. Pediatr Dermatol 2001; 18: 114–116.

29 Fegueux S, Maslo C, de Truchis P et al. Erythema nodosum in HIV-infected patients. J Am Acad Dermatol 1991; 25: 113.

30 Wantzin GL, Thomsen K. Panniculitis-like lesions in yersiniosis. Br J Dermatol 1982; 106: 481–484.

31 Debois J, Vandepitte J, Degreef H. Yersinia enterocolitica as a cause of erythema nodosum. Dermatologica 1978; 156: 65–78.

32 Eng AM, Aronson IK. Dermatopathology of panniculitis. Semin Dermatol 1984; 3: 1–13.

33 Tan BB, Lear JT, Smith AG. Acne fulminans and erythema nodosum during isotretinoin therapy responding to dapsone. Clin Exp Dermatol 1997; 22: 26–27.

34 Bridges AJ, Graziano FM, Calhoun W, Reizner GT. Hyperpigmentation, neutrophilic alveolitis, and erythema nodosum resulting from minocycline. J Am Acad Dermatol 1990; 22: 959–962.

35 Dellaripa PF, Wechsler ME, Roth ME, Drazen J. Recurrent panniculitis in a man with asthma receiving treatment with leukotriene-modifying agents. Mayo Clin Proc 2000; 75: 643–645.

36 Soon SL, Crawford RI. Recurrent erythema nodosum associated with echinacea herbal therapy. J Am Acad Dermatol 2001; 44: 298–299.

37 Salvatore MA, Lynch PJ. Erythema nodosum, estrogens, and pregnancy. Arch Dermatol 1980; 116: 557–558.

38 Takagawa S, Nakamura S, Yokozeki H, Nishioka K. Radiation-induced erythema nodosum. Br J Dermatol 1999; 140: 372–373.

39 Fearfield LA, Bunker CB. Radiotherapy and erythema nodosum. Br J Dermatol 2000; 142: 189.

40 Kunz M, Beutel S, Bröcker E-B. Leucocyte activation in erythema nodosum. Clin Exp Dermatol 1999; 24: 396–401.

41 Vilanova X, Piñol Aguadé J. Subacute nodular migratory panniculitis. Br J Dermatol 1959; 71: 45–50.

42 De Almeida Prestes C, Winkelmann RK, Su WPD. Septal granulomatous panniculitis: comparison of the pathology of erythema nodosum migrans (migratory panniculitis) and chronic erythema nodosum. J Am Acad Dermatol 1990; 22: 477–483.

43 Rostas A, Lowe D, Smout MS. Erythema nodosum migrans in a young woman. Arch Dermatol 1980; 116: 325–326.

44 Sanz Vico M-D, De Diego V, Sánchez Yus E. Erythema nodosum versus nodular vasculitis. Int J Dermatol 1993; 32: 108–112.

45 Zuckerman E, Naschitz JE, Yeshurun D et al. Fasciitis–panniculitis in acute brucellosis. Int J Dermatol 1994; 33: 57–59.

46 Sánchez Yus E, Sanz Vico MD, de Diego V. Miescher's radial granuloma. A characteristic marker of erythema nodosum. Am J Dermatopathol 1989; 11: 434–442.

47 Forstrom L, Winkelmann RK. Acute panniculitis. A clinical and histopathologic study of 34 cases. Arch Dermatol 1977; 113: 909–917.

48 Winkelmann RK, Forstrom L. New observations in the histopathology of erythema nodosum. J Invest Dermatol 1975; 65: 441–446.

49 Kim B, LeBoit PE. Histopathologic features of erythema nodosum-like lesions in Behçet disease. Comparison with erythema nodosum focusing on the role of vasculitis. Am J Dermatopathol 2000; 22: 379–390.

50 Haustein UF, Klug H. Ultrastrukturelle Untersuchungen der Blutgefässe beim Erythema nodosum. Dermatol Monatsschr 1977; 163: 13–22.

51 Su WPD, Person JR. Morphea profunda. A new concept and a histopathologic study of 23 cases. Am J Dermatopathol 1981; 3: 251–260.

52 Vincent F, Prokopetz R, Miller RAW. Plasma cell panniculitis: a unique clinical and pathologic presentation of linear scleroderma. J Am Acad Dermatol 1989; 21: 357–360.

Lobular panniculitis

53 Rademaker M, Lowe DG, Munro DD. Erythema induratum (Bazin's disease). J Am Acad Dermatol 1989; 21: 740–745.

54 Fernández del Moral R, Ereño C, Arrinda JM, Alvarez de Mon M. Erythema induratum of Bazin and active renal tuberculosis. J Am Acad Dermatol 1994; 31: 288–290.

55 Schneider JW, Jordaan HF, Geiger DH et al. Erythema induratum of Bazin. A clinicopathological study of 20 cases and detection of *Mycobacterium tuberculosis* DNA in skin lesions by polymerase chain reaction. Am J Dermatopathol 1995; 17: 350–356.

56 Ollert MW, Thomas P, Korting HC et al. Erythema induratum of Bazin. Evidence of T-lymphocyte hyperresponsiveness to purified protein derivative of tuberculin: report of two cases and treatment. Arch Dermatol 1993; 129: 469–473.

57 Yen A, Fearneyhough P, Rady P et al. Erythema induratum of Bazin as a tuberculid: Confirmation of *Mycobacterium tuberculosis* DNA polymerase chain reaction analysis. J Am Acad Dermatol 1997; 36: 99–101.

58 Baselga E, Margall N, Barnadas MA. Detection of *Mycobacterium tuberculosis* DNA in lobular granulomatous panniculitis (erythema induratum–nodular vasculitis). Arch Dermatol 1997; 133: 457–462.

59 Seckin D, Hizel N, Demirhan B, Tuncay C. The diagnostic value of polymerase chain reaction in erythema induratum of Bazin. Br J Dermatol 1997; 137: 1011–1012.

60 Yen A, Rady PL, Cortes-Franco R, Tyring SK. Detection of *Mycobacterium tuberculosis* in erythema induratum of Bazin using polymerase chain reaction. Arch Dermatol 1997; 133: 532–533.

61 Sánchez Yus E, Simón P. About the histopathology of erythema induratum–nodular vasculitis. Am J Dermatopathol 1999; 21: 301–303.

62 White WL. On Japanese baseball and erythema induratum of Bazin. Am J Dermatopathol 1997; 19: 318–322.

63 Kuramoto Y, Aiba S, Tagami H. Erythema induratum of Bazin as a type of tuberculid. J Am Acad Dermatol 1990; 22: 612–616.

64 Cardinali C, Gerlini G, Caproni M et al. Hepatitis C virus: a common triggering factor for both nodular vasculitis and Sjögren's syndrome? Br J Dermatol 2000; 142: 187–189.

65 Schneider JW, Jordaan HF. The histopathologic spectrum of erythema induratum of Bazin. Am J Dermatopathol 1997; 19: 323–333.

66 Cho K-H, Lee D-Y, Kim C-W. Erythema induratum of Bazin. Int J Dermatol 1996; 35: 802–808.

67 Hödl S. What is your diagnosis? Dermatopathology: Practical & Conceptual 2000; 6: 49–51.

68 Lee YS, Lee SW, Lee JR, Lee SC. Erythema induratum with pulmonary tuberculosis: histopathologic features resembling true vasculitis. Int J Dermatol 2001; 40: 193–196.

69 Forstrom L, Winkelmann RK. Granulomatous panniculitis in erythema nodosum. Arch Dermatol 1975; 111: 335–340.

70 Oswalt GC, Montes LF, Cassady G. Subcutaneous fat necrosis of the newborn. J Cutan Pathol 1985; 5: 193–199.

71 Friedman SJ, Winkelmann RK. Subcutaneous fat necrosis of the newborn: light, ultrastructural and histochemical microscopic studies. J Cutan Pathol 1989; 16: 99–105.

72 Mather MK, Sperling LC, Sau P. Subcutaneous fat necrosis of the newborn. Int J Dermatol 1997; 36: 450–452.

73 Chen TH, Shewmake SW, Hansen DD, Lacey HL. Subcutaneous fat necrosis of the newborn. Arch Dermatol 1981; 117: 36–37.

74 Thomsen RJ. Subcutaneous fat necrosis of the newborn and idiopathic hypercalcemia. Arch Dermatol 1980; 116: 1155–1158.

75 Norwood-Galloway A, Lebwohl M, Phelps RG, Raucher H. Subcutaneous fat necrosis of the newborn with hypercalcemia. J Am Acad Dermatol 1987; 16: 435–439.

76 Hicks MJ, Levy ML, Alexander J, Flaitz CM. Subcutaneous fat necrosis of the newborn and hypercalcemia: case report and review of the literature. Pediatr Dermatol 1993; 10: 271–276.

77 Lewis A, Cowen P, Rodda C, Dyall-Smith D. Subcutaneous fat necrosis of the newborn complicated by hypercalcaemia and thrombocytopenia. Australas J Dermatol 1992; 33: 141–144.

78 Burden AD, Krafchik BR. Subcutaneous fat necrosis of the newborn: a review of 11 cases. Pediatr Dermatol 1999; 16: 384–387.

79 Varan B, Gürakan B, Özbek N, Emir S. Subcutaneous fat necrosis of the newborn associated with anemia. Pediatr Dermatol 1999; 16: 381–383.

80 Glover MT, Catterall MD, Atherton DJ. Subcutaneous fat necrosis in two infants after hypothermic cardiac surgery. Pediatr Dermatol 1991; 8: 210–212.

81 Chuang S-D, Chiu H-C, Chang C-C. Subcutaneous fat necrosis of the newborn complicating hypothermic cardiac surgery. Br J Dermatol 1995; 132: 805–810.

82 Sharata H, Postellon DC, Hashimoto K. Subcutaneous fat necrosis, hypercalcemia, and prostaglandin E. Pediatr Dermatol 1995; 12: 43–47.

83 Rosbotham JL, Johnson A, Haque KN, Holden CA. Painful subcutaneous fat necrosis of the newborn associated with intra-partum use of a calcium channel blocker. Clin Exp Dermatol 1998; 23: 19–21.

84 Tsuji T. Subcutaneous fat necrosis of the newborn: light and electron microscopic studies. Br J Dermatol 1976; 95: 407–416.

85 Balazs M. Subcutaneous fat necrosis of the newborn with emphasis on ultrastructural studies. Int J Dermatol 1987; 26: 227–230.

86 Silverman AK, Michels EH, Rasmussen JE. Subcutaneous fat necrosis in an infant, occurring after hypothermic cardiac surgery. J Am Acad Dermatol 1986; 15: 331–336.

87 Moreno-Gumenez JC, Hérnandez-Aguado I, Arguisjuela MT, Camacho-Martinez F. Subcutaneous-fat necrosis of the newborn. J Cutan Pathol 1983; 10: 277–280.

88 Epstein EH Jr, Oren ME. Popsicle panniculitis. N Engl J Med 1970; 282: 966–967.

89 Rotman H. Cold panniculitis in children. Arch Dermatol 1966; 94: 720–721.

90 Duncan WC, Freeman RG, Heaton CL. Cold panniculitis. Arch Dermatol 1966; 94: 722–724.

91 Ter Poorten JC, Hebert AA, Ilkiw R. Cold panniculitis in a neonate. J Am Acad Dermatol 1995; 33: 383–385.

92 Solomon LM, Beerman H. Cold panniculitis. Arch Dermatol 1963; 88: 897–900.

93 Beacham BE, Cooper PH, Buchanan CS, Weary PE. Equestrian cold panniculitis in women. Arch Dermatol 1980; 116: 1025–1027.

94 Wall LM, Smith NP. Perniosis: a histopathological review. Clin Exp Dermatol 1981; 6: 263–271.

95 Panush RS, Yonker RA, Dlesk A et al. Weber–Christian disease. Analysis of 15 cases and review of the literature. Medicine (Baltimore) 1985; 64: 181–191.

96 Aronson IK, West DP, Variakojis D et al. Fatal panniculitis. J Am Acad Dermatol 1985; 12: 535–551.

97 Fayemi AO, Williams J, Cuttner J. Systemic Weber–Christian disease and thrombocythemia terminating in reticulum-cell sarcoma. Am J Clin Pathol 1974; 62: 88–93.

98 Crotty CP, Winkelmann RK. Cytophagic histiocytic panniculitis with fever, cytopenia, liver failure, and terminal hemorrhagic diathesis. J Am Acad Dermatol 1981; 4: 181–194.

99 Breit SN, Clark P, Robinson JP et al. Familial occurrence of α_1-antitrypsin deficiency and Weber–Christian disease. Arch Dermatol 1983; 119: 198–202.

100 Smith KC, Su WPD, Pittelkow MR, Winkelmann RK. Clinical and pathologic correlations in 96 patients with panniculitis, including 15 patients with deficient levels of α_1-antitrypsin. J Am Acad Dermatol 1989; 21: 1192–1196.

101 Bleumink E, Klokke HA. Protease-inhibitor deficiencies in a patient with Weber–Christian panniculitis. Arch Dermatol 1984; 120: 936–940.

102 Hendrick SJ, Silverman AK, Solomon AR, Headington JT. α_1-antitrypsin deficiency associated with panniculitis. J Am Acad Dermatol 1988; 18: 684–692.

103 Williams HJ, Samuelson CO, Zone JJ. Nodular nonsuppurative panniculitis associated with jejunoileal bypass surgery. Arch Dermatol 1979; 115: 1091–1093.

104 Ciclitira PJ, Wight DGD, Dick AP. Systemic Weber–Christian disease: a case report with lipoprotein profile and immunological evaluation. Br J Dermatol 1980; 103: 685–692.

105 Allen-Mersh TG. Weber–Christian panniculitis and auto-immune disease: a case report. J Clin Pathol 1976; 29: 144–149.

106 Iwatsuki K, Tagami H, Yamada M. Weber–Christian panniculitis with immunological abnormalities. Dermatologica 1982; 164: 181–188.

107 Albrectsen B. The Weber–Christian syndrome, with particular reference to etiology. Acta Derm Venereol 1960; 40: 474–484.

108 Wilkinson PJ, Harman RRM, Tribe CR. Systemic nodular panniculitis with cardiac involvement. J Clin Pathol 1974; 27: 808–812.

109 Stewart CA. Systemic form of Weber–Christian disease. Pathology 1978; 10: 165–168.

110 Gaillard M-C, Bothwell J, Dreyer L. A case of systemic nodular panniculitis associated with M1(Val213)Z phenotype of α_1-protease inhibitor. Int J Dermatol 1997; 36: 278–280.

111 Enk AH, Knop J. Treatment of relapsing idiopathic nodular panniculitis (Pfeifer–Weber–Christian disease) with mycophenolate mofetil. J Am Acad Dermatol 1998; 39: 508–509.

112 White JW Jr, Winkelmann RK. Weber–Christian panniculitis: A review of 30 cases with this diagnosis. J Am Acad Dermatol 1998; 39: 56–62.

113 Pinto AR, Maciel LS, Carneiro F et al. Systemic nodular panniculitis in a patient with alpha-1 antitrypsin deficiency (PiSS phenotype). Clin Exp Dermatol 1993; 18: 154–155.

114 Edmonds BK, Hodge JA, Rietschel RL. Alpha 1-antitrypsin deficiency-associated panniculitis: case report and review of the literature. Pediatr Dermatol 1991; 8: 296–299.

115 Linares-Barrios M, Conejo-Mir JS, Artola Igarza JL, Navarrete M. Panniculitis due to α_1-antitrypsin deficiency induced by cryosurgery. Br J Dermatol 1998; 138: 552–553.

116 Su WPD, Smith KC, Pittelkow MR, Winkelmann RK. α_1-antitrypsin deficiency panniculitis. A histopathologic and immunopathologic study of four cases. Am J Dermatopathol 1987; 9: 483–490.

117 Chng WJ, Henderson CA. Suppurative panniculitis associated with alpha 1-antitrypsin deficiency (PiSZ phenotype) treated with doxycycline. Br J Dermatol 2001; 144: 1282–1283.

118 Geller JD, Su WPD. A subtle clue to the histopathologic diagnosis of early α_1-antitrypsin deficiency panniculitis. J Am Acad Dermatol 1994; 31: 241–245.

119 Winkelmann RK, Bowie EJW. Hemorrhagic diathesis associated with benign histiocytic cytophagic panniculitis and systemic histiocytosis. Arch Intern Med 1980; 140: 1460–1463.

120 White JW Jr, Winkelmann RK. Cytophagic histiocytic panniculitis is not always fatal. J Cutan Pathol 1989; 16: 137–144.

121 Alegre VA, Winkelmann RK. Histiocytic cytophagic panniculitis. J Am Acad Dermatol 1989; 20: 177–185.

122 Alegre VA, Fortea JM, Camps C, Aliaga A. Cytophagic histiocytic panniculitis. Case report with resolution after treatment. J Am Acad Dermatol 1989; 20: 875–878.

123 Peters MS, Winkelmann RK. Cytophagic panniculitis and B cell lymphoma. J Am Acad Dermatol 1985; 13: 882–885.

124 Smith KJ, Skelton HG, Yeager J et al. Cutaneous histopathologic, immunohistochemical, and clinical manifestations in patients with hemophagocytic syndrome. Arch Dermatol 1992; 128: 193–200.

125 Perniciaro C, Winkelmann RK, Ehrhardt DR. Fatal systemic cytophagic histiocytic panniculitis: a histopathologic and immunohistochemical study of multiple organ sites. J Am Acad Dermatol 1994; 31: 901–905.

126 Aronson IK, West DP, Variakojis D et al. Panniculitis associated with cutaneous T-cell lymphoma and cytophagocytic histiocytosis. Br J Dermatol 1985; 112: 87–96.

127 Hytiroglou P, Phelps RG, Wattenberg DJ, Strauchen JA. Histiocytic cytophagic panniculitis: molecular evidence for a clonal T-cell disorder. J Am Acad Dermatol 1992; 27: 333–336.

128 Galende J, Vazquez ML, Almeida J et al. Histiocytic cytophagic panniculitis: a rare late complication of allogeneic bone marow transplantation. Bone Marrow Transplant 1994; 14: 637–639.

129 Ito M, Ohira H, Miyata M et al. Cytophagic histiocytic panniculitis improved by combined CHOP and cyclosporin A treatment. Intern Med 1999; 38: 296–301.

130 Harada H, Iwatsuki K, Kaneko F. Detection of Epstein–Barr virus genes in malignant lymphoma with clinical and histologic features of cytophagic histiocytic panniculitis. J Am Acad Dermatol 1994; 31: 379–383.

131 Craig AJ, Cualing H, Thomas G et al. Cytophagic histiocytic panniculitis – a syndrome associated with benign and malignant panniculitis: Case comparison and review of the literature. J Am Acad Dermatol 1998; 39: 721–736.

132 Marzano AV, Berti E, Paulli M, Caputo R. Cytophagic histiocytic panniculitis and subcutaneous panniculitis-like T-cell lymphoma. Report of 7 cases. Arch Dermatol 2000; 136: 889–896.

133 Wick MR, Patterson JW. Cytophagic histiocytic panniculitis – a critical reappraisal. Arch Dermatol 2000; 136: 922–924.

134 Huilgol SC, Fenton D, Pambakian H et al. Fatal cytophagic panniculitis and haemophagocytic syndrome. Clin Exp Dermatol 1998; 23: 51–55.

135 Zollner TM, Podda M, Ochsendorf FR et al. Monitoring of phagocytic activity in histiocytic cytophagic panniculitis. J Am Acad Dermatol 2001; 44: 120–123.

136 Ohtake N, Shimada S, Mizoguchi S et al. Membranocystic lesions in a patient with cytophagic histiocytic panniculitis associated with subcutaneous T-cell lymphoma. Am J Dermatopathol 1998; 20: 276–280.

137 Au WY, Ng WM, Choy C, Kwong YL. Aggressive subcutaneous panniculitis-like T-cell lymphoma: complete remission with fludarabine, mitoxantrone and dexamethasone. Br J Dermatol 2000; 143: 408–410.

138 Weenig RH, Ng CS, Perniciaro C. Subcutaneous panniculitis-like T-cell lymphoma. An elusive case presenting as lipomembranous panniculitis and a review of 72 cases in the literature. Am J Dermatopathol 2001; 23: 206–215.

139 Magro CM, Crowson AN, Kovatich AJ, Burns F. Lupus profundus, indeterminate lymphocytic lobular panniculitis and subcutaneous T-cell lymphoma: a spectrum of subcuticular T-cell lymphoid dyscrasia. J Cutan Pathol 2001; 28: 235–247.

140 Kumar S, Krenacs L, Medeiros J et al. Subcutaneous panniculitic T-cell lymphoma is a tumor of cytotoxic T lymphocytes. Hum Pathol 1998; 29: 397–403.

141 Salhany KE, Macon WR, Choi JK et al. Subcutaneous panniculitis-like T-cell lymphoma. Am J Surg Pathol 1998; 22: 881–893.

142 Bridges AG, Gibson LE. An unusual peripheral T-cell lymphoma presenting as a panniculitis. J Cutan Pathol 2000; 27: 550–551 (abstract).

143 Levine N, Lazarus GS. Subcutaneous fat necrosis after paracentesis. Report of a case in a patient with acute pancreatitis. Arch Dermatol 1976; 112: 993–994.

144 Detlefs RL. Drug-induced pancreatitis presenting as subcutaneous fat necrosis. J Am Acad Dermatol 1985; 13: 305–307.

145 Lee M-S, Lowe PM, Nevell DF et al. Subcutaneous fat necrosis following traumatic pancreatitis. Australas J Dermatol 1995; 36: 196–198.

146 Stanford AR, Mezebish DS, Cobb MW. Nodular fat necrosis associated with lupus-induced pancreatitis. Int J Dermatol 1997; 36: 856–858.

147 Cutlan RT, Wesche WA, Jenkins JJ III, Chesney TM. A fatal case of pancreatic panniculitis presenting in a young patient with systemic lupus. J Cutan Pathol 2000; 27: 466–471.

148 Riaz AA, Smith F, Phylactides L, Law NW. Panniculitis complicating gallstone pancreatitis with subsequent resolution after therapeutic endoscopic retrograde cholangiopancreatography. Br J Dermatol 2000; 143: 1332–1333.

149 Hughes PSH, Apisarnthanarax P, Mullins JF. Subcutaneous fat necrosis associated with pancreatic disease. Arch Dermatol 1975; 111: 506–510.

150 Berman B, Conteas C, Smith B et al. Fatal pancreatitis presenting with subcutaneous fat necrosis. J Am Acad Dermatol 1987; 17: 359–364.

151 Bennett RG, Petrozzi JW. Nodular subcutaneous fat necrosis. A manifestation of silent pancreatitis. Arch Dermatol 1975; 111: 896–898.

152 Dahl PR, Su WPD, Cullimore KC, Dicken CH. Pancreatic panniculitis. J Am Acad Dermatol 1995; 33: 413–417.

153 Haber RM, Assaad DM. Panniculitis associated with a pancreas divisum. J Am Acad Dermatol 1986; 14: 331–334.

154 Millns JL, Evans HL, Winkelmann RK. Association of islet cell carcinoma of the pancreas with subcutaneous fat necrosis. Am J Dermatopathol 1979; 1: 273–280.

155 Burdick C. Subcutaneous fat necrosis associated with pancreatic islet cell tumor. Am J Dermatopathol 1992: 14: 181.

156 Lewis CT III, Tschen JA, Klima M. Subcutaneous fat necrosis associated with pancreatic islet cell carcinoma. Am J Dermatopathol 1991; 13: 52–56.

157 Heykarts B, Anseeuw M, Degreef H. Panniculitis caused by acinous pancreatic carcinoma. Dermatology 1999; 198: 182–183.

158 Zellman GL. Pancreatic panniculitis. J Am Acad Dermatol 1996; 35: 282–283.

159 Forstrom L, Winkelmann RK. Acute, generalized panniculitis with amylase and lipase in skin. Arch Dermatol 1975; 111: 497–502.

160 Ball NJ, Adams SPA, Marx LH, Enta T. Possible origin of pancreatic fat necrosis as a septal panniculitis. J Am Acad Dermatol 1996; 34: 362–364.

161 Cannon JR, Pitha JV, Everett MA. Subcutaneous fat necrosis in pancreatitis. J Cutan Pathol 1979; 6: 501–506.

162 Tuffanelli DL. Lupus erythematosus panniculitis (profundus). Commentary and report on four cases. Arch Dermatol 1971; 103: 231–242.

163 Sanchez NP, Peters MS, Winkelmann RK. The histopathology of lupus erythematosus panniculitis. J Am Acad Dermatol 1981; 5: 673–680.

164 Winkelmann RK. Panniculitis in connective tissue disease. Arch Dermatol 1983; 119: 336–344.

165 Izumi AK, Takiguchi P. Lupus erythematosus panniculitis. Arch Dermatol 1983; 119: 61–64.

166 Tuffanelli DL. Lupus panniculitis. Semin Dermatol 1985; 4: 79–81.

167 Tamada Y, Arisawa S, Ikeya T et al. Linear lupus erythematosus profundus in a young man. Br J Dermatol 1999; 140: 177–178.

168 Kündig TM, Trüeb RM, Krasovec M. Lupus profundus/panniculitis. Dermatology 1997; 195: 99–101.

169 Ahmed I, Ahmed D. Lupus erythematosus panniculitis: a unique subset within the lupus erythematosus spectrum. Am J Dermatopathol 2000; 22: 352 (abstract).

170 Fujiwara K, Kono T, Ishii M et al. Lupus erythematosus panniculitis in a patient with autoimmune hepatitis. Acta Derm Venereol 2000; 80: 373–375.

171 Fox JN, Klapman MH, Rowe L. Lupus profundus in children: treatment with hydroxychloroquine. J Am Acad Dermatol 1987; 16: 839–844.

172 Burrows NP, Russell Jones R. Lupus erythematosus profundus with partial C4 deficiency. Br J Dermatol 1997; 137: 651.

173 Nousari HC, Kimyai-Asadi A, Santana HM et al. Generalized lupus panniculitis and antiphospholipid syndrome in a patient without complement deficiency. Pediatr Dermatol 1999; 16: 273–276.

174 Grilli R, Luisa Soriano M, José Izquierdo M et al. Panniculitis mimicking lupus erythematosus profundus. A new histopathologic finding in malignant atrophic papulosis (Degos disease). Am J Dermatopathol 1999; 21: 365–368.

175 Harris RB, Duncan SC, Ecker RI, Winkelmann RK. Lymphoid follicles in subcutaneous inflammatory disease. Arch Dermatol 1979; 115: 442–443.

176 Peters MS, Su WPD. Eosinophils in lupus panniculitis and morphea profunda. J Cutan Pathol 1991; 18: 189–192.

177 Kuwabara H, Uda H, Saito K. A light and electron microscopical study of membranocystic lesions in a case of lupus erythematosus profundus. Acta Pathol Jpn 1991; 41: 286–290.

178 Snow JL, Su WPD. Lipomembranous (membranocystic) fat necrosis. Clinicopathologic correlation of 38 cases. Am J Dermatopathol 1996; 18: 151–155.

179 Winkelmann RK, Padilha-Gonclaves A. Connective tissue panniculitis. Arch Dermatol 1980; 116: 291–294.

180 Moragon M, Jorda E, Ramon MD et al. Atrophic connective tissue panniculitis. Int J Dermatol 1988; 27: 185–186.

181 Handfield-Jones SE, Stephens CJM, Mayou BJ, Black MM. The clinical spectrum of lipoatrophic panniculitis encompasses connective tissue panniculitis. Br J Dermatol 1993; 129: 619–624.

182 Robinson-Bostom L, Fuller P, D'Ambra-Cabray K et al. Connective tissue panniculitis. J Cutan Pathol 1997; 24: 120 (abstract).

183 Newton J, Wojnarowska FT. Pustular panniculitis in rheumatoid arthritis. Br J Dermatol (Suppl) 1988; 30: 97–98.

184 Jaffe N, Hann HWL, Vawter GF. Post-steroid panniculitis in acute leukemia. N Engl J Med 1971; 284: 366–367.

185 Peters MS, Winkelmann RK. Localized lipoatrophy (atrophic connective tissue disease panniculitis). Arch Dermatol 1980; 116: 1363–1368.

186 Umbert IJ, Winkelmann RK. Adult lipophagic atrophic panniculitis. Br J Dermatol 1991; 124: 291–295.

187 Samadaei A, Hashimoto K, Tanay A. Insulin lipodystrophy, lipohypertrophic type. J Am Acad Dermatol 1987; 17: 506–507.

188 Harwood CA, Bull RH, Evans J, Mortimer PS. Lymphatic and venous function in lipoedema. Br J Dermatol 1996; 134: 1–6.

189 Gürbüz O, Yücelten D, Ergun T, Khalilazer R. Partial lipodystrophy. Int J Dermatol 1995; 34: 36–37.

190 Porter WM, O'Gorman-Lalor O, Lane RJM et al. Barraquer–Simons lipodystrophy, Raynaud's phenomenon and cutaneous vasculitis. Clin Exp Dermatol 2000; 25: 277–280.

191 Eadie MJ, Sutherland JM, Tyrer JH. The clinical features of hemifacial atrophy. Med J Aust 1963; 2: 177–180.

192 Akdeniz S, Harman M, Yaldiz M et al. Partial lipodystrophy with hemithoracic atrophy. Br J Dermatol 2000; 143: 665–666.

193 Bilen N, Efendi H, Apaydin R et al. Progressive facial hemiatrophy (Parry–Romberg syndrome). Australas J Dermatol 1999; 40: 223–225.

194 Chartier S, Buzzanga JB, Paquin F. Partial lipodystrophy associated with a type 3 form of membranoproliferative glomerulonephritis. J Am Acad Dermatol 1987; 16: 201–205.

195 Font J, Herrero C, Bosch X et al. Systemic lupus erythematosus in a patient with partial lipodystrophy. J Am Acad Dermatol 1990; 22: 337–340.

196 Lenane P, Murphy GM. Partial lipodystrophy and renal disease. Clin Exp Dermatol 2000; 25: 605–607.

197 Martinez A, Malone M, Hoeger P et al. Lipoatrophic panniculitis and chromosome 10 abnormality. Br J Dermatol 2000; 142: 1034–1039.

198 Rongioletti F, Rebora A. Annular and semicircular lipoatrophies. Report of three cases and review of the literature. J Am Acad Dermatol 1989; 20: 433–436.

199 Jablonska S, Szczepanski A, Gorkiewicz A. Lipo-atrophy of the ankles and its relation to other lipo-atrophies. Acta Derm Venereol 1987; 55: 135–140.

200 Nelson HM. Atrophic annular panniculitis of the ankles. Clin Exp Dermatol 1988; 13: 111–113.

201 Hodak E, David M, Sandbank M. Semicircular lipoatrophy – a pressure-induced lipoatrophy? Clin Exp Dermatol 1990; 15: 464–465.

202 Caputo R. Lipodystrophia centrifugalis sacralis infantilis. Acta Derm Venereol 1989; 69: 442–443.

203 Imamura S, Yamada M, Yamamoto K. Lipodystrophia centrifugalis abdominalis infantilis. J Am Acad Dermatol 1984; 11: 203–209.

204 Hiraiwa A, Takai K, Fukui Y et al. Nonregressing lipodystrophia centrifugalis abdominalis with angioblastoma (Nakagawa). Arch Dermatol 1990; 126: 206–209.

205 Zachary CB, Wells RS. Centrifugal lipodystrophy. Br J Dermatol 1984; 110: 107–110.

206 Giam YC, Rajan VS, Hock OB. Lipodystrophia centrifugalis abdominalis. Br J Dermatol 1982; 106: 461–464.

207 Furukawa F. Lipodystrophia centrifugalis abdominalis infantilis. A possible sequel to Kawasaki disease. Int J Dermatol 1989; 28: 338–339.

208 Franks A, Verbov JL. Unilateral localized idiopathic lipoatrophy. Clin Exp Dermatol 1993; 18: 468–469.

209 Müller S, Beissert S, Metze D et al. Lipodystrophia centrifugalis abdominalis infantilis in a 4-year-old caucasian girl: association with partial IgA deficiency and autoantibodies. Br J Dermatol 1999; 140: 1161–1164.

210 Llistosella E, Puig L, Pérez F. Lipodystrophia centrifugalis abdominalis infantilis: a case report. Pediatr Dermatol 1997; 14: 216–218.

211 Serup J, Weismann K, Kobayasi T et al. Local panatrophy with linear distribution: a clinical, ultrastructural and biochemical study. Acta Derm Venereol 1982; 62: 101–105.

212 Kuperman-Beade M, Laude TA. Partial lipoatrophy in a child. Pediatr Dermatol 2000; 17: 302–303.

213 Dahl PR, Zalla MJ, Winkelmann RK. Localized involutional lipoatrophy: A clinicopathologic study of 16 patients. J Am Acad Dermatol 1996; 35: 523–528.

214 De Groot AC. Is lipoatrophia semicircularis induced by pressure? Br J Dermatol 1994; 131: 887–890.

215 Nagore E, Sánchez-Motilla JM, Rodríquez-Serna M et al. Lipoatrophia semicircularis – a traumatic panniculitis: Report of seven cases and review of the literature. J Am Acad Dermatol 1998; 39: 879–881.

216 Okita H, Ohtsuka T, Yamakage A, Yamazaki S. Lipodystrophia centrifugalis abdominalis infantilis – immunohistochemical demonstration of an apoptotic process in the degenerating fatty tissue. Dermatology 2000; 201: 370–372.

217 Peters MS, Winkelmann RK. The histopathology of localized lipoatrophy. Br J Dermatol 1986; 114: 27–36.

218 Tsuji T, Kosaka K, Terao J. Localized lipodystrophy with panniculitis: light and electron microscopic studies. J Cutan Pathol 1989; 16: 359–364.

219 Aronson IK, Zeitz HJ, Variakojis D. Panniculitis in childhood. Pediatr Dermatol 1988; 5: 216–230.

220 Winkelmann RK, McEvoy MT, Peters MS. Lipophagic panniculitis of childhood. J Am Acad Dermatol 1989; 21: 971–978.

221 Hagari Y, Sasaoka R, Nishiura S et al. Centrifugal lipodystrophy of the face mimicking progressive lipodystrophy. Br J Dermatol 1992; 127: 407–410.

222 Kagoura M, Toyoda M, Matsui C et al. An ultrastructural study of lipodystrophia centrifugalis abdominalis infantilis, with special reference to fibrous long-spacing collagen. Pediatr Dermatol 2001; 18: 13–16.

223 Williamson K, Reboli AC, Manders SM. Protease inhibitor-induced lipodystrophy. J Am Acad Dermatol 1999; 40: 635–636.

224 Colebunders R, Bottieau E, de Mey I. Curly hair and lipodystrophy as a result of highly active antiretroviral treatment? Arch Dermatol 2000; 136: 1064–1065.

225 Pujol RM, Domingo P, Matias-Guiu X et al. HIV-1 protease inhibitor-associated partial lipodystrophy: Clinicopathologic review of 14 cases. J Am Acad Dermatol 2000; 42: 193–198.

226 Panse I, Vasseur E, Raffin-Sanson ML et al. Lipodystrophy associated with protease inhibitors. Br J Dermatol 2000; 142: 496–500.

227 Martinez E, Mocroft A, García-Viejo MA et al. Risk of lipodystrophy in HIV-1-infected patients treated with protease inhibitors: a prospective cohort study. Lancet 2001; 357: 592–598.

228 Rodwell GEJ, Maurer TA, Berger TG. Fat redistribution in HIV disease. J Am Acad Dermatol 2000; 42: 727–730.

229 Smith KJ, Skelton HG. Peroxisomal proliferator-activated ligand therapy for HIV lipodystrophy. Clin Exp Dermatol 2001; 26: 155–161.

230 Rossi ABR, Vergnanini AL. Cellulite: a review. J Eur Acad Dermatol Venereol 2000; 14: 251–262.

231 Piérard GE, Nizet JL, Piérard-Franchimont C. Cellulite. From standing fat herniation to hypodermal stretch marks. Am J Dermatopathol 2000; 22: 34–37.

232 Hexsel DM, Mazzuco R. Subcision: a treatment for cellulite. Int J Dermatol 2000; 39: 539–544.

233 Snow JL, Su WPD, Gibson LE. Lipomembranous (membranocystic) changes associated with morphea: a clinicopathologic review of three cases. J Am Acad Dermatol 1994; 31: 246–250.

234 Chun SI, Chung K-Y. Membranous lipodystrophy: secondary type. J Am Acad Dermatol 1994; 31: 601–605.

235 Pujol RM, Wang C-Y, Gibson LE, Su WPD. Lipomembranous changes in nodular-cystic fat necrosis. J Cutan Pathol 1995; 22: 551–555.

236 Chun SI, Ahn SK, Kim SC. Membranous lipodystrophy: primary idiopathic type. J Am Acad Dermatol 1991; 24: 844–847.

237 Ahn S, Yoo M, Lee S, Choi E. A clinical and histopathological study of 22 patients with membranous lipodystrophy. Clin Exp Dermatol 1996; 21: 269–272.

238 Kim KT, Ahn SK, Choi EH, Lee SH. Membranous lipodystrophy associated with insulin lipoatrophy. Int J Dermatol 1997; 36: 299–301.

239 Ishikawa O, Tamura A, Rijuzaki K et al. Membranocystic changes in the panniculitis of dermatomyositis. Br J Dermatol 1996; 134: 773–776.

240 Ramdial PK, Chetty R. Vasculitis-induced membranous fat necrosis. J Cutan Pathol 1999; 26: 405–410.

241 Ohtake N, Kanekura T, Kawamura K, Kanzaki T. Unusual polyp-like structures in lobular panniculitis of a patient with Behcet's disease. Am J Dermatopathol 1997; 19: 185–188.

242 Ono T, Kageshita T, Hirai S et al. Coexistence of spherulocytic disease (myospherulosis) and membranocystic degeneration. Arch Dermatol 1991; 127: 88–90.

243 Fisher DA. Desideration dermatologicum: eliminating lipodermatosclerosis; the term and the entities. Int J Dermatol 2000; 39: 490–492.

244 Sheth R, Poonevala V. Lipodermatosclerosis: a postphlebitic syndrome. Int J Dermatol 1997; 36: 931–932.

245 Demitsu T, Okada O, Yoneda K, Manabe M. Lipodermatosclerosis – report of three cases and review of the literature. Dermatology 1999; 199: 271–273.

246 Jorizzo JL, White WL, Zanolli MD et al. Sclerosing panniculitis. Arch Dermatol 1991; 127: 554–558.

247 Falanga V, Bontempo FA, Eaglstein WH. Protein C and protein S plasma levels in patients with lipodermatosclerosis and venous ulceration. Arch Dermatol 1990; 126: 1195–1197.

248 Herouy Y, Aizpurua J, Stetter C et al. The role of the urokinase-type plasminogen activator (UPA) and its receptor (CD87) in lipodermatosclerosis. J Cutan Pathol 2001; 28: 291–297.

249 Herouy Y, May AE, Pornschlegel G et al. Lipodermatosclerosis is characterized by elevated expression and activation of matrix metalloproteinases: implications for venous ulcer formation. J Invest Dermatol 1998; 111: 822–827.

250 Gniadecka M. Localization of dermal edema in lipodermatosclerosis, lymphedema, and cardiac insufficiency. J Am Acad Dermatol 1996; 35: 37–41.

251 Gniadecka M, Karlsmark T, Bertram A. Removal of dermal edema with class I and II compression stockings in patients with lipodermatosclerosis. J Am Acad Dermatol 1998; 39: 966–970.

252 Kossard S, Ecker RI, Dicken CH. Povidone panniculitis. Polyvinylpyrrolidone panniculitis. Arch Dermatol 1980; 116: 704–706.

253 Forstrom L, Winkelmann RK. Factitial panniculitis. Arch Dermatol 1974; 110: 747–750.

254 Parks DL, Perry HO, Muller SA. Cutaneous complications of pentazocine injections. Arch Dermatol 1971; 104: 231–235.

255 Klein JA, Cole G, Barr RJ et al. Paraffinomas of the scalp. Arch Dermatol 1985; 121: 382–385.

256 Oertel YC, Johnson FB. Sclerosing lipogranuloma of male genitalia. Arch Pathol 1977; 101: 321–326.

257 Claudy A, Garcier F, Schmitt D. Sclerosing lipogranuloma of the male genitalia: ultrastructural study. Br J Dermatol 1981; 105: 451–455.

258 Hirst AE, Heustis DG, Rogers-Neufeld B, Johnson FB. Sclerosing lipogranuloma of the scalp. A report of two cases. Am J Clin Pathol 1984; 82: 228–231.

259 Delage C, Shane JJ, Johnson FB. Mammary silicone granuloma. Arch Dermatol 1973; 108: 104–107.

260 Darsow U, Bruckbauer H, Worret W-I et al. Subcutaneous oleomas induced by self-injection of sesame seed oil for muscle augmentation. J Am Acad Dermatol 2000; 42: 292–294.

261 Winkelmann RK, Barker SM. Factitial traumatic panniculitis. J Am Acad Dermatol 1985; 13: 988–994.

262 Zelickson BD, Winkelmann RK. Lipophagic panniculitis in re-excision specimens. Acta Derm Venereol 1991; 71: 59–61.

263 Kiryu H, Rikihisa W, Furue M. Encapsulated fat necrosis – a clinicopathological study of 8 cases and a literature review. J Cutan Pathol 2000; 27: 19–23.

264 Hurt MA, Santa Cruz DJ. Nodular-cystic fat necrosis. A reevaluation of the so-called mobile encapsulated lipoma. J Am Acad Dermatol 1989; 21: 493–498.

265 Ohtake N, Gushi A, Matsushita S, Kanzaki T. Encapsulated fat necrosis in a patient with Ehlers–Danlos syndrome. J Cutan Pathol 1997; 24: 189–192.

266 Patterson JW, Brown PC, Broecker AH. Infection-induced panniculitis. J Cutan Pathol 1989; 16: 183–193.

267 Abildgaard WH Jr, Hargrove RH, Kalivas J. *Histoplasma* panniculitis. Arch Dermatol 1985; 121: 914–916.

268 Silverman AK, Gilbert SC, Watkins D et al. Panniculitis in an immunocompromised patient. J Am Acad Dermatol 1991; 24: 912–914.

269 Larson K, Glanz S, Bergfeld WF. Neutrophilic panniculitis caused by *Mycobacterium marinum*. J Cutan Pathol 1989; 16: 315 (abstract).

270 Langenberg A, Egbert B. Neutrophilic tuberculous panniculitis in a patient with polymyositis. J Cutan Pathol 1993; 20: 177–179.

271 Sanderson TL, Moskowitz L, Hensley GT et al. Disseminated *Mycobacterium avium-intracellulare* infection appearing as a panniculitis. Arch Pathol Lab Med 1982; 106: 112–114.

272 Cho BK, Kang H, Bang D et al. Tick bites in Korea. Int J Dermatol 1994; 33: 552–555.

273 Rosenberg AS, Morgan MB. Disseminated acanthamoebiasis presenting as lobular panniculitis with necrotizing vasculitis in a patient with AIDS. J Cutan Pathol 2001; 28: 307–313.

274 Tran T-AN, DuPree M, Carlson JA. Neutrophilic lobular (pustular) panniculitis associated with rheumatoid arthritis. A case report and review of the literature. Am J Dermatopathol 1999; 21: 247–252.

275 Kuniyuki S, Shindow K, Tanaka T. Pustular panniculitis in a patient with rheumatoid arthritis. Int J Dermatol 1997; 36: 292–293.

276 Yosipovitch G, Hodak E, Feinmesser M, David M. Acute Crohn's colitis with lobular panniculitis – metastatic Crohn's? J Eur Acad Dermatol Venereol 2000; 14: 405–406.

277 Matsumura Y, Tanabe H, Wada Y et al. Neutrophilic panniculitis associated with myelodysplastic syndromes. Br J Dermatol 1997; 136: 142–144.

278 Adame J, Cohen PR. Eosinophilic panniculitis: diagnostic considerations and evaluation. J Am Acad Dermatol 1996; 34: 229–234.

279 Burket JM, Burket BJ. Eosinophilic panniculitis. J Am Acad Dermatol 1985; 12: 161–164.

280 Glass LA, Zaghloul AB, Solomon AR. Eosinophilic panniculitis associated with chronic recurrent parotitis. Am J Dermatopathol 1989; 11: 555–559.

281 Winkelmann RK, Frigas E. Eosinophilic panniculitis: a clinicopathologic study. J Cutan Pathol 1986; 13: 1–12.

282 Samlaska CP, de Lorimier AJ, Heldman LS. Eosinophilic panniculitis. Pediatr Dermatol 1995; 12: 35–38.

283 Ollague W, Ollague J, Guevara de Veliz A, Peñaherrera S. Human gnathostomiasis in Ecuador (nodular migratory eosinophilic panniculitis). Int J Dermatol 1984; 23: 647–651.

284 Ruiz-Maldonado R, Mosqueda-Cabrera MA. Human gnathostomiasis (nodular migratory eosinophilic panniculitis). Int J Dermatol 1999; 38: 56–57.

285 Janis JF, Winkelmann RK. Histopathology of the skin in dermatomyositis. Arch Dermatol 1968; 97: 640–650.

286 Raimer SS, Solomon AR, Daniels JC. Polymyositis presenting with panniculitis. J Am Acad Dermatol 1985; 13: 366–369.

287 Ghali FE, Reed AM, Groben PA, McCauliffe DP. Panniculitis in juvenile dermatomyositis. Pediatr Dermatol 1999; 16: 270–272.

288 Richens G, Piepkorn MW, Krueger GG. Calcifying panniculitis associated with renal failure. A case of Selye's calciphylaxis in man. J Am Acad Dermatol 1982; 6: 537–539.

289 Lugo-Somolinos A, Sánchez JL, Méndez-Coll J, Joglar F. Calcifying panniculitis associated with polycystic kidney disease and chronic renal failure. J Am Acad Dermatol 1990; 22: 743–747.

290 Niemi K-M. Panniculitis of the legs with urate crystal deposition. Arch Dermatol 1977; 113: 655–656.

291 LeBoit PE, Schneider S. Gout presenting as lobular panniculitis. Am J Dermatopathol 1987; 9: 334–338.

292 Conejo-Mir J, Pulpillo A, Corbi MR et al. Panniculitis and ulcers in a young man. Arch Dermatol 1998; 134: 499–504.

293 Ruiz-Maldonado R, Parrilla FM, Orozco-Covarrubias ML et al. Edematous, scarring vasculitic panniculitis: a new multisystemic disease with malignant potential. J Am Acad Dermatol 1995; 32: 37–44.

294 Day LL. Aterman K. Hemorrhagic panniculitis caused by atheromatous embolization. A case report and brief review. Am J Dermatopathol 1984; 6: 471–478.

295 Vainsencher D, Winkelmann RK. Subcutaneous sarcoidosis. Arch Dermatol 1984; 120: 1028–1031.

296 Witkowski JA, Parish LC, Lewis JE. Crohn's disease – non-caseating granulomas on the legs. Acta Derm Venereol 1977; 57: 181–183.

297 Kennedy C. The spectrum of inflammatory skin disease following jejuno-ileal bypass for morbid obesity. Br J Dermatol 1981; 105: 425–436.

298 Caux F, Halimi C, Kevorkian J-P et al. Blind loop syndrome: An unusual cause of panniculitis. J Am Acad Dermatol 1997; 37: 824–827.

299 Piérard GE. Melanophagic dermatitis and panniculitis. A condition revealing an occult metastatic malignant melanoma. Am J Dermatopathol 1988; 10: 133–136.

300 Cotton J, Armstrong DJ, Wedig R, Hood AF. Melanoma-in-transit presenting as panniculitis. J Am Acad Dermatol 1998; 39: 876–878.

301 Ashworth J, Coady AT, Guy R, Breathnach SM. Brawny cutaneous induration and granulomatous panniculitis in large cell non-Hodgkin's (T suppressor/cytotoxic cell) lymphoma. Br J Dermatol 1989; 120: 563–569.

302 Tanaka K, Hagari Y, Sano Y et al. A case of T-cell lymphoma associated with panniculitis, progressive pancytopenia and hyperbilirubinaemia. Br J Dermatol 1990; 123: 649–652.

303 Wang C-YE, Su WPD, Kurtin PJ. Subcutaneous panniculitic T-cell lymphoma. Int J Dermatol 1996; 35: 1–8.

304 Prescott RJ, Banerjee SS, Cross PA. Subcutaneous T-cell lymphoma with florid granulomatous panniculitis. Histopathology 1992; 20: 535–537.

305 Takeshita M, Akamatsu M, Ohshima K et al. Angiocentric immunoproliferative lesions of the skin show lobular panniculitis and are mainly disorders of large granular lymphocytes. Hum Pathol 1995; 26: 1321–1328.

306 McGovern TW, Erickson AR, Fitzpatrick JE. Sjögren's syndrome plasma cell panniculitis and hidradenitis. J Cutan Pathol 1996; 23: 170–174.

307 Tait CP, Yu LL, Rohr J. Sjögren's syndrome and granulomatous panniculitis. Australas J Dermatol 2000; 41: 187–189.

308 Novick NL. Aspartame-induced granulomatous panniculitis. Ann Intern Med 1985; 102: 206–207.

309 Dereure O, Bessis D, Lavabre-Bertrand T et al. Thrombotic and necrotizing panniculitis associated with recombinant human granulocyte colony-stimulating factor treatment. Br J Dermatol 2000; 142: 834–836.

310 Scott DW, Morrell JI, Vernotica EM. Focal necrotizing panniculitis and vascular necrosis in rats given subcutaneous injections of cocaine hydrochloride. J Cutan Pathol 1997; 24: 25–29.

311 Winkelmann RK, Grado GL, Quimby SR, Connolly SM. Pseudosclerodermatous panniculitis after irradiation: an unusual complication of megavoltage treatment of breast carcinoma. Mayo Clin Proc 1993; 68: 122–127.

312 Solomon AR, Kantak AG, Ramirez JE et al. Suppressor-cytotoxic T-lymphocyte panniculitis. Pediatr Dermatol 1986; 3: 295–299.

The skin in systemic and miscellaneous diseases

543

Metabolic and storage diseases

18

INTRODUCTION

Three major disease categories will be considered in this chapter:

- vitamin and dietary disturbances
- lysosomal storage diseases
- miscellaneous metabolic and systemic diseases.

The various diseases included in these categories show a wide range of histopathological changes. They will be discussed in turn.

VITAMIN AND DIETARY DISTURBANCES

The skin and mucous membranes may be affected in various vitamin deficiency states. Usually multiple vitamins are involved, as the most common cause of deficiency is a nutritional disturbance. Nutritional deficiencies may result from alcoholism,[1] digestive tract disease (including cystic fibrosis,[2] resections and bypass surgery), dietary fads and anorexia nervosa.[3-5] The cutaneous manifestations of vitamin[6] and nutritional[7] deficiencies were reviewed some years ago. Cutaneous manifestations are particularly seen in vitamin C deficiency (scurvy), vitamin A deficiency (phrynoderma) and niacin (nicotinic acid) deficiency. These deficiencies are discussed further below.

Kwashiorkor, which results from protein malnutrition, is characterized by xerosis, patches of hypopigmentation, skin peeling, peripheral edema and thin hair shafts.[7-11] Deficiency of essential fatty acids, seen in some patients receiving parenteral nutrition, results in alopecia, xerosis and intertriginous erosions.[7]

Riboflavin and pyridoxine deficiency both lead to glossitis, angular stomatitis, cheilosis and a condition resembling seborrheic dermatitis.[7,12] In riboflavin deficiency there may be a scrotal dermatitis, while in pyridoxine deficiency there may be pellagra-like features.[7]

SCURVY

Scurvy results from a deficiency of vitamin C (ascorbic acid) which is a water-soluble vitamin necessary for proline hydroxylation in the formation of collagen.[6,13,14] It also plays a role in normal hair growth. Loss of the integrity of collagen leads to inadequate support for small vessels, resulting in hemorrhage from minor trauma.[15] This is characteristically perifollicular in distribution, but spontaneous petechiae and ecchymoses may also develop.[6,16] Other features include follicular hyperkeratosis, abnormal hair growth with the formation of corkscrew hairs, bleeding gums and poor wound healing.[6,17] Woody edema of the lower limbs with some surface scaling may be the only manifestation.[15] Scurvy may be seen in alcoholics and those with dietary fads and inadequacies[18,19] and, accordingly, associated deficiencies of other factors may contribute to the appearance of the cutaneous lesions. Rarely, there is no explanation for the deficiency.[20]

Histopathology

A characteristic feature is the presence of extravasated erythrocytes around vessels in the upper dermis (Fig. 18.1). This is often in a perifollicular distribution initially. Hemosiderin, a legacy of earlier hemorrhages, is sometimes found. There may also be follicular hyperkeratosis with coiled, fragmented, corkscrew-like hairs buried in the keratotic follicular material.[17] Ulceration of the skin is sometimes seen.

Electron microscopy

Affected skin may show alterations in fibroblasts, with defective collagen formation.[21] There may also be alterations in the endothelial cells of vessels and their junctions.[21]

VITAMIN A DEFICIENCY

Vitamin A is a fat-soluble vitamin; its active form is retinol. Deficiencies are rare and usually related to malabsorption states.[6,22] The skin becomes dry and scaly with follicular keratotic papules (phrynoderma).[23] Ocular changes include night blindness.[24,25]

Histopathology

Sections show hyperkeratosis and prominent keratotic follicular plugging.[24] Sweat glands may be atrophic; in severe cases they show squamous metaplasia.[23]

HYPERVITAMINOSIS A

Hypervitaminosis A is usually a result of self-administration of excess amounts of the vitamin.[26-28] Acute symptoms include vomiting, diarrhea and desquamation of skin. In the chronic form of vitamin A toxicity there is dry skin, cheilitis and patchy alopecia. Histological changes are non-specific.

VITAMIN K DEFICIENCY

Vitamin K is a fat-soluble vitamin which is necessary for the hepatic synthesis or secretion of various coagulation factors.[6] A deficiency may result from liver disease and from malabsorption; in infants it may be associated with diarrhea. Purpura is a common manifestation of vitamin K deficiency.

The parenteral injection of vitamin K may rarely give rise to an erythematous plaque at the site of injection, apparently due to a delayed hypersensitivity reaction.[29] A late sclerodermatous reaction is a rare complication (see p. 353).

VITAMIN B₁₂ DEFICIENCY

Vitamin B_{12} deficiency may be associated with poikilodermatous pigmentation. This clinical pattern results from basal pigmentation and some melanin

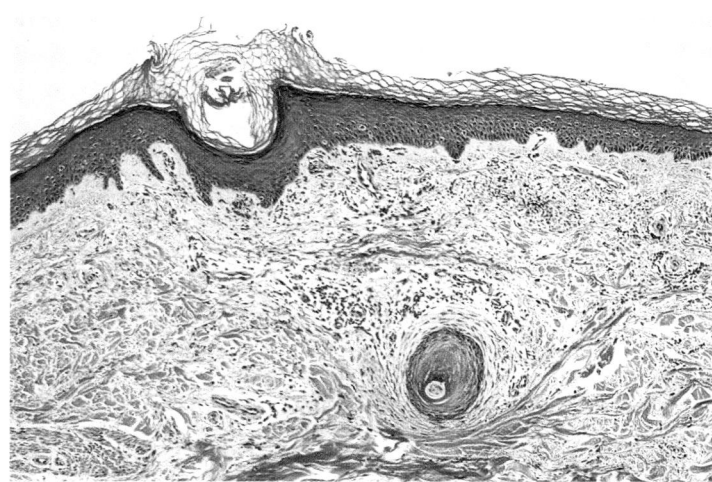

Fig. 18.1 **Scurvy.** The patient ate one brand of cookie as her only food. There is red cell extravasation, mild follicular hyperkeratosis and perifollicular fibrosis. (H & E)

incontinence. The nuclei of keratinocytes were reported to be larger than normal in one patient.[30]

PELLAGRA

Pellagra is a multisystem nutritional disorder caused by inadequate amounts of niacin (nicotinic acid) in the tissues.[31,32] This may result from a primary dietary deficiency,[33–35] malabsorption, certain chemotherapeutic agents such as isoniazid,[36,37] 6-mercaptopurine, 5-fluorouracil,[38] azathioprine,[39] 'alternative remedies'[40] and chloramphenicol, or from abnormalities of tryptophan metabolism.[6] In this latter category is the carcinoid syndrome, in which tumor cells divert tryptophan metabolism towards serotonin and away from nicotinic acid, and Hartnup disease, in which there is a congenital defect in tryptophan absorption and transfer[6] (see p. 554).

Pellagra is traditionally remembered as the 'disease of the four Ds': dermatitis, diarrhea, dementia and, if untreated, death.[41] The skin lesions commence as a burning erythema in sun-exposed areas, particularly the dorsum of the hands and the face and neck.[42] Blistering may occur. This is followed by intense hyperpigmentation with sharp margination and areas of epithelial desquamation.[6] There may also be glossitis, angular cheilitis and vulvitis.[41]

Histopathology[31]

The findings are not diagnostic. They include hyperkeratosis, parakeratosis, epidermal atrophy with pallor of the upper epidermis and hyperpigmentation of the basal layer (Fig. 18.2).[6,43] There is usually a mild, superficial dermal infiltrate of lymphocytes. Mild keratotic follicular plugging is sometimes seen in biopsies from the face.[36] Bullae may be either intraepidermal or subepidermal.[42] Hyperplasia of the sebaceous glands with follicular dilatation and plugging may occur.[31]

Similar histopathological changes are seen in Hartnup disease (see p. 554).

LYSOSOMAL STORAGE DISEASES

The lysosomal storage diseases are a specific subset of the inborn errors of metabolism: they are characterized by a deficiency in a specific lysosomal hydrolase or of a protein essential for the normal function of lysosomes.[44] As a consequence of this deficiency there is accumulation of the specific substrate in various organs of the body. The distribution of this stored material corresponds to the site where degradation of the substrate usually occurs. Lysosomes are particularly plentiful in macrophages and other cells of the mononuclear phagocyte system: organs rich in these cells, such as the liver and spleen, are frequently enlarged. In one subgroup of lysosomal storage diseases, the sphingolipidoses, there is an accumulation of certain glycolipids or phospholipids in various organs, particularly the brain.

The lysosomal storage diseases can be diagnosed by assaying for the specific enzyme thought to be deficient in serum, leukocytes or cultured fibroblasts.[44] In many of these diseases inclusions can be found on ultrastructural examination of the skin (Fig. 18.3). The inclusions are sometimes sufficiently distinctive to be diagnostic of a particular disease, although in many instances they are not. Accordingly, ultrastructural examination of the skin in the diagnosis of the lysosomal storage diseases is usually no more than a useful adjunct to enzyme assay.[45] Recently a fluorescent analogue of lactosylceramide has shown promise as a screening test for the sphingolipidoses and some other lysosomal storage diseases. It accumulates in the lysosomes of cultured fibroblasts from affected patients.[46]

With ultrastructural studies of the skin, care must be taken to avoid overdiagnosis.[45] Many cells in the skin may, at times, contain a few vacuoles, fat globules or other inclusions.[45] These must not be misinterpreted as indicating a lysosomal storage disease.

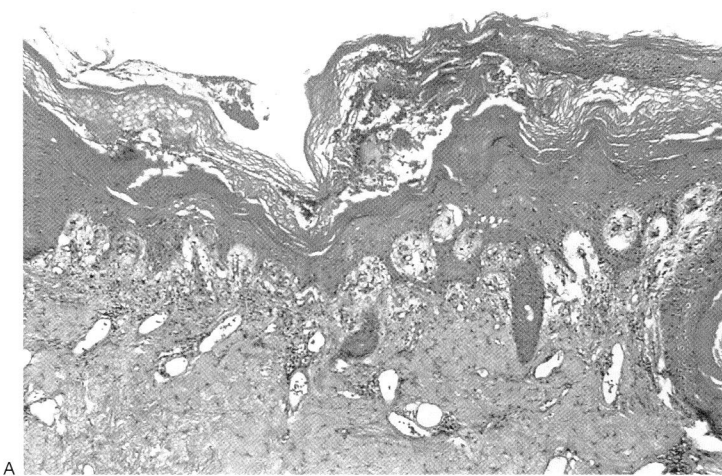

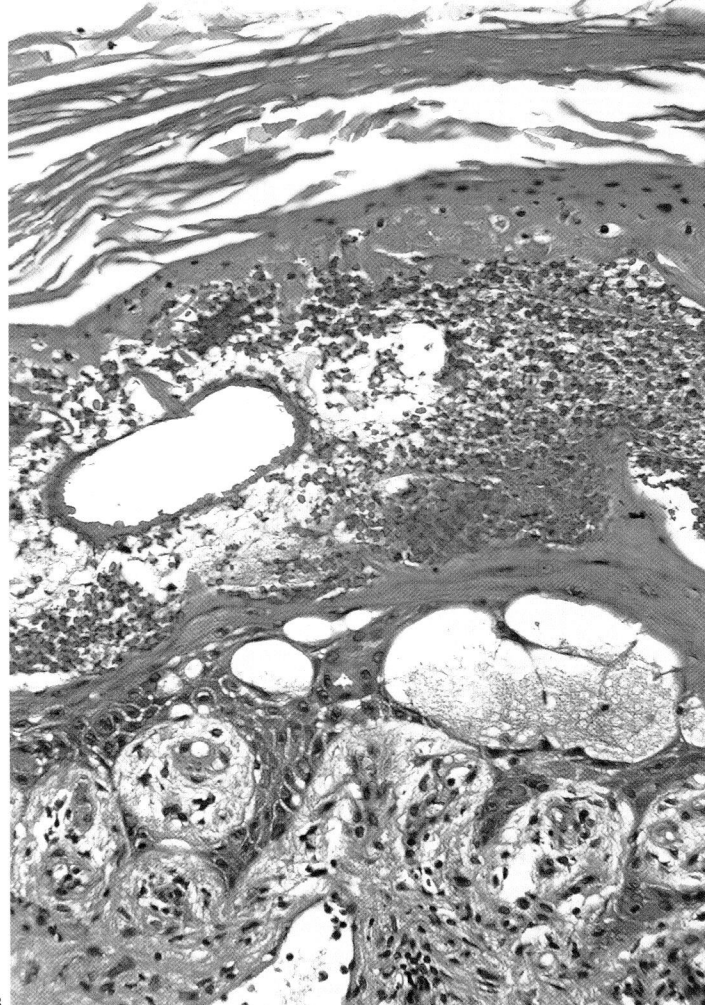

Fig. 18.2 **(A) Pellagra. (B)** There is partial necrosis and hemorrhage involving the superficial epidermis with underlying psoriasiform acanthosis. (H & E)

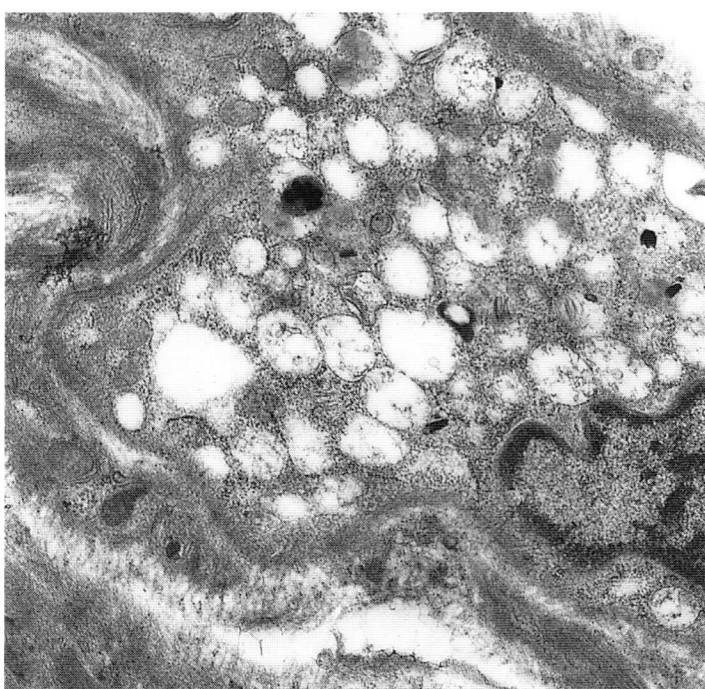

Fig. 18.3 **Vacuolated fibroblasts in the skin in a lysosomal storage disease.** The type of vacuole present is not diagnostic of a particular condition. (× 5000)

The lysosomal storage diseases, which have a prevalence of 1 in 7700 in the general Australian population, can be divided into several categories on the basis of the biochemical nature of the accumulated substrate:[47,48]

- sphingolipidoses
- oligosaccharidoses
- mucolipidoses
- mucopolysaccharidoses
- others.

SPHINGOLIPIDOSES

The sphingolipidoses are a heterogeneous group of lysosomal storage diseases that result from a variety of enzyme deficiencies affecting different levels in the metabolism of complex lipids. Certain glycolipids or phospholipids accumulate in various tissues of the body, particularly the brain.[49] Cutaneous changes are present in many of the sphingolipidoses.[45]

G_{M2}-gangliosidoses

The G_{M2}-gangliosidoses are a subgroup of sphingolipidoses in which there is an accumulation of the ganglioside G_{M2}, as a result of a defect in some aspect of the hexosaminidase system.[44,50] The most common clinical variant is Tay–Sachs disease in which there is progressive psychomotor deterioration and blindness. In Sandhoff's disease, which is phenotypically similar, the gangliosides are deposited in nearly all cells of the body, in contrast to Tay–Sachs disease in which deposits do not occur outside the nervous system.[45,51] The gene for Tay–Sachs disease maps to chromosome 15q23–q24.

Histopathology

Cytoplasmic inclusions can be seen in a number of cells in osmificated, semithin, Epon-embedded sections in Sandhoff's disease.[52]

Electron microscopy

Membrane-bound inclusions can be found in endothelial cells, smooth muscle cells, pericytes, Schwann cells and eccrine secretory cells. There are lamellar and vacuolar structures and 'zebra bodies' (vacuoles with transverse membranes). In Tay–Sachs disease, lesions are confined to nerve axons, which may be distended by residual bodies, a change also seen in Sandhoff's disease.[45]

Inclusion bodies are also found in cultured fibroblasts in Sandhoff's disease, but they are quite sparse in Tay–Sachs disease.[53]

G_{M1}-gangliosidoses

There are two major clinical variants of G_{M1}-gangliosidosis, of which Norman–Landing disease (pseudo-Hurler's syndrome) is the more severe.[50] This infantile form is characterized clinically by a gargoyle-like appearance, psychomotor regression, blindness, hirsutism, hepatosplenomegaly and deformities of the hands and feet.[45,54] As in G_{M2} gangliosidosis, a 'cherry-red spot' is often present.

The diagnosis can be made by measuring β-galactosidase activity in leukocytes or cultured skin fibroblasts.[44]

Histopathology

Vacuolation of fibroblasts, endothelial cells and eccrine secretory cells is sometimes discernible in sections stained with hematoxylin and eosin.[54]

Electron microscopy

There is vacuolation of fibroblasts, endothelial cells, smooth muscle cells and sweat gland epithelium. Schwann cells are less severely affected.[45] The vacuoles are empty or contain fine fibrillar or flocculent material.[55] Inclusions are also found in cultured fibroblasts.[53]

Gaucher's disease

In Gaucher's disease, glucocerebroside accumulates in the cells of the mononuclear macrophage system (reticuloendothelial system).[56,57] The gene for glucocerebrosidase is located on chromosome 1q21; many mutations are known.[58–60] This condition will not be discussed further as skin biopsies have consistently been negative, with no evidence of stored lipid in sweat ducts, fibroblasts or cutaneous nerves.[45,55]

Fabry's disease

Fabry's disease (angiokeratoma corporis diffusum) is an uncommon X-linked recessive disorder of glycosphingolipid metabolism in which there is a deficiency of the lysosomal hydrolase, α-galactosidase A (formerly called ceramide trihexosidase).[61,62] This leads to the accumulation of ceramide trihexoside in various tissues of the body, particularly the vascular and supporting elements.

The disease usually presents in late adolescence with recurrent fevers associated with pain in the fingers and toes and intermittent edema.[61,63,64] Characteristic whorled opacities are usually present in the cornea (cornea verticillata).[61,62] Cerebrovascular and cardiovascular disturbances are common, and progressive renal damage leading to renal failure in the fourth and fifth decades of life is almost invariable.[63] Heterozygous females are often asymptomatic, but they may show evidence of the disease to different degrees.[65,66]

The cutaneous lesions (angiokeratoma corporis diffusum) are multiple, deep red telangiectasias clustered on the lower part of the trunk, buttocks, thighs, scrotum and the shaft of the penis (see p. 1007).[61] Most sites can be involved, although the face and scalp are usually spared. Cutaneous lesions are occasionally absent.[62] There may be anhidrosis.[62]

Histopathology

There are large and small thin-walled vessels in the upper dermis (see p. 1008). The overlying epidermis is often thinned, with variable overlying hyperkeratosis. There are often acanthotic or elongated portions of rete ridge at the periphery of the lesions.[67] The vessels are angiectatic and not a new growth. Fibrin thrombi are sometimes present in the lumen.[68] There may be patchy vacuolization of the media of vessels in the deep dermis in both affected and normal skin. If frozen sections are examined, doubly refractile material may be seen in the vicinity of these vacuoles.[61] The material will also stain with Sudan black and the PAS stain.[69] The peroxidase-labeled lectins of *Ricinus communis* and *Bandeiraea simplicifolia* have been found to be strongly reactive with the material on frozen sections.[70] Fine PAS-positive granules are sometimes seen in the sweat glands.[68]

In semithin sections, fine intracytoplasmic granules can be seen in eccrine glands, vessel walls and fibroblasts in the dermis.

Electron microscopy[69,71]

Diagnostic intracytoplasmic inclusions having a lamellar structure can be found in endothelial cells, pericytes, fibroblasts, myoepithelial cells of sweat glands, and macrophages. Involvement of eccrine secretory cells is uncommon[62] and that of Schwann cells is rare.[52] The inclusions, which are sometimes membrane bound, may also be found in heterozygotes in skin biopsies[69] and cultured fibroblasts.[53]

Metachromatic leukodystrophy

Metachromatic leukodystrophy results from a deficiency in the activity of arylsulfatase A and the accumulation of metachromatic sulfatides in the nervous system and certain other organs.[44,50] Clinically, there is progressive psychomotor retardation. The gene maps to chromosome 22q13.31.

Histopathology

Vacuolated cells are sometimes seen in the endoneurium of cutaneous nerves. Brown metachromatic material can be seen in these nerves after cresyl violet staining of frozen sections.[72]

Electron microscopy[72]

The Schwann cells of myelinated nerves contain so-called 'tuff-stone' or 'herring bone' inclusions which are membrane bound.[45,52] Macrophages containing myelin breakdown products are found within the nerves. Inclusions with a concentric lamellar structure have been reported in cultured fibroblasts.[53]

Krabbe's disease

Krabbe's disease (globoid cell leukodystrophy) results from a deficiency of galactocerebroside-β-galactosidase.[44] There are progressive neurological symptoms, beginning usually in childhood.

Histopathology

Globoid cells with PAS-positive cytoplasm are found in the central nervous system, particularly in the white matter.[73] Cutaneous nerves appear normal on light microscopy.

Electron microscopy

Tubular and crystalloid inclusions have been reported in Schwann cells in cutaneous nerves,[52,73] but not consistently.[55] Cultured fibroblasts do not contain specific inclusions.[53]

Disseminated lipogranulomatosis (Farber's disease)

Disseminated lipogranulomatosis (Farber's disease) is a rare, autosomal recessive disorder of lipid metabolism in which there is a deficiency of acid ceramidase leading to an accumulation of ceramide and its degradation products.[74,75] The defect maps to chromosome 8p22–p21.3. The main clinical features usually appear at the age of 2–4 months and comprise progressive arthropathy, the development of subcutaneous, often periarticular nodules, hoarseness, irritability and pulmonary failure.[76] The disease is progressive, death usually occurring in early childhood.[76]

The diagnosis can be made by demonstrating a deficiency in ceramidase in cultured fibroblasts or in white blood cells.[77]

Histopathology[78]

There is extensive fibrosis of the reticular dermis and subcutis with collagen bundles of variable thickness traversing the nodules in various directions. Within the fibrotic areas are many histiocytes with distended, somewhat foamy cytoplasm.[75,79] Some cells are multinucleate. A few lymphocytes and plasma cells are often present. Histochemical stains have given variable results, depending on whether paraffin or frozen sections have been used. The oil red O stain and Baker's reaction for phospholipid may be positive.[78]

Electron microscopy[77,79]

There are characteristic curvilinear bodies (Farber bodies) within the cytoplasm of fibroblasts and occasionally of endothelial cells. They are also found within phagosomes of histiocytes at various stages of degradation. Banana-like bodies can be found within Schwann cells. 'Zebra bodies' (vacuoles with transverse membranes) may be seen in some endothelial cells. They represent gangliosides and may be found in other storage diseases.[77]

Niemann–Pick disease

Niemann–Pick disease is a rare autosomal recessive disorder in which sphingomyelin accumulates in many organs due to a deficiency of sphingomyelinase.[80] Recent work suggests that it is a heterogeneous entity with more than one enzyme defect probably involved.[81,82] The gene in some cases maps to chromosome 18q11.[83,84] The course is unremitting and death usually occurs in early childhood. Cutaneous lesions have been reported in a small number of cases and include diffuse tan brown hyperpigmentation, indurated brown plaques,[85] facial papules,[86] xanthomas[80] and juvenile xanthogranulomas.[87,88] A small number of cases have abnormalities in skin barrier function as a consequence of a marked reduction in sphingomyelin-derived ceramide.[89]

Histopathology

It is now thought that the lesions reported clinically as juvenile xanthogranulomas in Niemann–Pick disease are xanthomas associated with the basic phospholipid abnormality.[82,87] This view is based on the presence of cytoplasmic zebra bodies on electron microscopy of one case.[87] In the cutaneous lesions described there are large numbers of foamy histiocytes in the dermis admixed with a few lymphocytes. The foamy cells may have a pale brownish appearance in sections stained with hematoxylin and eosin.[86] The vacuoles may impart a mulberry appearance. The cytoplasmic lipids stain with oil red O and Sudan black;[80] they are metachromatic with toluidine blue.[86] Scattered multinucleate cells are present.

Electron microscopy

Cultured fibroblasts from patients with Niemann–Pick disease show characteristic membrane-bound myelin-like inclusions.[53] 'Washed-out' inclusions with a lamellar structure have been reported in endothelial cells and Schwann cells in the skin.[55]

OLIGOSACCHARIDOSES

The oligosaccharidoses (glycoproteinoses) are characterized by excess urinary excretion of oligosaccharides as a consequence of a deficiency in one of the lysosomal enzymes responsible for the degradation of the oligosaccharide portion of glycoproteins.[44] The four disorders included in this subgroup of lysosomal storage diseases are sialidosis, fucosidosis, mannosidosis and aspartyl-glycosaminuria. The cutaneous manifestations of this last condition have not been studied extensively and it will not be considered further.

Sialidosis

Sialidosis (mucolipidosis I) results from a deficiency of sialidase (neuraminidase).[90] Clinical features include coarse facies, ataxia, myoclonus and a cherry-red spot in the macula.[90]

Galactosialidosis is a slowly progressive neurodegenerative disease, with similar phenotypic features, which results from the combined deficiency of sialidase and β-galactosidase.[91,92] There is the lack of a 32 kd 'protective protein' that is crucial for the biological activity of these two enzymes. Angiokeratomas have been reported in patients with this combined deficiency state.[92]

Histopathology

Skin biopsies in sialidosis appear normal in sections stained with hematoxylin and eosin. In the combined deficiency, angiokeratomas may be present (see p. 1007): the endothelium of these vessels is sometimes vacuolated.[92]

Electron microscopy

Cultured fibroblasts from patients with sialidosis contain cytoplasmic vacuoles similar to those observed in various mucopolysaccharidoses and in mannosidosis.[93]

In *galactosialidosis*, vacuoles are seen in the endothelium of vessels and also in fibroblasts, sweat gland epithelium and the Schwann cells of non-myelinated nerves. The vacuoles are mostly empty, but some contain floccular material.[92] Lamellar inclusions also occur. Vacuolar and lamellar inclusions are present in cultured fibroblasts.[93]

Fucosidosis

Fucosidosis is a rare autosomal recessive disorder in which a deficiency of the lysosomal enzyme α-L-fucosidase leads to the accumulation of fucose-containing glycolipids and other substances in various tissues.[94,95] There is early onset of psychomotor retardation and other neurological signs. Three clinical variants have been reported, but only type 3 is associated with cutaneous lesions.[96] These are indistinguishable from the angiokeratomas seen in Fabry's disease (see p. 548).[97,98] Hypohidrosis may also be present.

Histopathology

The angiokeratomas are composed of dilated vessels in the papillary dermis (see p. 1008). The endothelial cells of these and other dermal vessels are vacuolated and somewhat swollen, leading to narrowing of the lumen of some small dermal vessels.[97] The eccrine secretory coils are lined by uniformly vacuolated cells.[97]

Electron microscopy[94,99]

There are membrane-bound vacuoles containing fine granular material in endothelial cells, fibroblasts, melanocytes, histiocytes, eccrine glands and occasional pericytes. Lamellated bodies representing complex lipids are present in myoepithelial cells of sweat glands and in Schwann cells.[97] Both types of cytosome are sparsely distributed in epidermal keratinocytes.[97,100] Smooth muscle cells are uninvolved.[97]

Mannosidosis

In mannosidosis, the deficiency of the lysosomal enzyme α-mannosidase leads to an accumulation of mannose-containing oligosaccharides in various tissues of the body, including the nervous system.[101] Patients have a gargoyle-like facies and mental retardation. The condition runs a relatively benign clinical course.

Histopathology

Biopsies from hyperplastic gingiva have shown vacuolated histiocytes in the lamina propria containing PAS-positive material.[101]

Electron microscopy

Membrane-bound vacuoles containing fine granular material are present in many different cells of the body, including cultures of skin fibroblasts.[93]

MUCOLIPIDOSES

The mucolipidoses are a group of lysosomal storage diseases that have clinical and biochemical features of both the mucopolysaccharidoses and the sphingolipidoses.[44] Glycolipids and glycosaminoglycans accumulate in the tissues. Type I mucolipidosis has been reclassified as sialidosis (see above), while type IV, which results from a deficiency of ganglioside sialidase, has not been extensively studied.[102] The most widely investigated of the mucolipidoses is I-cell disease (mucolipidosis II), so named because of the numerous inclusions seen in fibroblasts cultured from patients with the disease.[44] Type III mucolipidosis is regarded as a milder form of I-cell disease.

I-cell disease

I-cell disease is an autosomal recessive neurodegenerative disorder, characterized by a marked intracellular deficiency of a number of lysosomal hydrolases and by a significant elevation of these enzymes in plasma.[103] It is caused by a deficiency of uridine-diphosphate-N-acetylglucosamine 1-phosphotransferase, the enzyme that phosphorylates mannose residues of glycoproteins to allow their delivery to lysosomes.[104] The gene maps to chromosome 4q21–q23.

Clinically, there is short stature, facial dysmorphism, progressive mental and motor retardation and bony deformities.[105,106] The skin is generally pale and smooth.[105]

Histopathology

The dermis may have an increased number of oval or spindle-shaped cells, some with clear or foamy cytoplasm.[105] The cytoplasmic inclusions are PAS positive and metachromatic; they stain with oil red O in frozen sections.

Electron microscopy

There are membrane-bound vacuoles in the cytoplasm of various cells, including fibroblasts, pericytes, Schwann cells, secretory cells of the eccrine glands, and endothelial cells.[45,106] The vacuoles may contain a few dark rings. The inclusions in endothelial cells are more electron dense and multivesicular.[105] Cultured fibroblasts contain electron-dense inclusions.[93]

In *mucolipidosis IV*, there are small dense lipid and zebra bodies in addition to the vacuoles.[45]

OTHER LYSOSOMAL STORAGE DISEASES

Included in this group are glycogenosis type II and neuronal ceroid-lipofuscinosis, although no consistent enzyme defect has been elucidated in the latter condition.

The mucopolysaccharidoses are another major group of lysosomal storage diseases. They are considered with the mucinoses in Chapter 13 (see p. 416).

Glycogenosis (type II)

There are several different types of glycogen storage disease, but only in type II (Pompe's disease, generalized glycogenosis), characterized by a deficiency of acid maltase, is glycogen found in the skin.[44]

Histopathology

Glycogen is present in many cells in the skin and is best seen in biopsies fixed in Carnoy's solution and stained by the PAS method.

Electron microscopy

Clustered glycogen granules, enclosed within a limiting membrane, are found in many types of cell in the skin, including the arrector pili muscles.[45,52,55]

Neuronal ceroid-lipofuscinosis

Neuronal ceroid-lipofuscinosis is a progressive neurodegenerative disorder characterized by the accumulation of ceroid or lipofuscin-like substances in various organs, especially the nervous system.[107,108] No consistent enzyme deficiency has been demonstrated. Abnormal peroxidation of fatty acids may be the metabolic basis.[107]

Histopathology

Affected cells contain yellow-brown pigment which is autofluorescent.[52,107]

Electron microscopy[108,109]

Characteristic membrane-bound inclusions with a curvilinear or finger-print pattern have been reported in eccrine secretory cells, endothelial cells, smooth muscle cells and macrophages.[45] They are particularly prominent in endothelial cells.[55] Inclusions have not been found consistently in fibroblasts and Schwann cells.[110] In a recent case report only granular osmiophilic deposits were found; there were no curvilinear or finger-print inclusions in the cytoplasm of several cell types in the dermis.[111]

MISCELLANEOUS METABOLIC AND SYSTEMIC DISEASES

As the heading suggests, this section deals with a heterogeneous group of disorders with variable clinical and histopathological manifestations. The various cutaneous manifestations of **celiac disease** are considered in other sections. They include dermatitis herpetiformis, alopecia areata, chronic urticaria, vasculitis, Sjögren's syndrome, lupus erythematosus and linear IgA dermatosis.[112]

ACRODERMATITIS ENTEROPATHICA

Acrodermatitis enteropathica is a rare, recessively inherited disorder of zinc metabolism which usually presents in infancy, at the time of weaning, with the triad of alopecia, diarrhea and dermatitis.[113] The cutaneous lesions are periorificial and acral in distribution. There is a crusted eczematous eruption which is sometimes vesiculobullous or pustular.[114] Intercurrent infection with bacteria and yeasts, possibly related to impaired chemotaxis,[115] complicates the clinical picture.[114,116] Other features include photophobia, nail dystrophy, hair shaft abnormalities,[117] short stature, stomatitis and emotional disturbances. There are uncommon, mild forms of the disease,[118] some of which may not be diagnosed until adult life.[119,120]

Transient symptomatic zinc deficiency may also develop in advanced cancer[121] and in premature infants on artificial feeding[122] and rarely in breast-fed infants, both premature[123–126] and full-term,[127,128] associated with low or marginal levels of zinc in maternal milk.[129] Premature infants are more vulnerable to the development of zinc deficiency than full-term infants because they have low body stores of zinc and a poor capability to absorb zinc from the gut, despite their high zinc requirements.[130] Other rare causes of an acrodermatitis enteropathica-like eruption have included parenteral nutrition without zinc supplementation,[131–133] Crohn's disease,[134] intestinal bypass procedures,[135] gastrectomy,[136] advanced alcoholic cirrhosis,[137] the acquired immunodeficiency syndrome,[138] isoleucine deficiency,[139] anorexia nervosa[140] and cystic fibrosis.[141]

Although the pathogenetic mechanisms have not been fully elucidated, it appears that zinc transport and absorption in the gut are partially impaired. Acrodermatitis enteropathica is responsive to zinc therapy.[142,143] Several different factors may be implicated in transient symptomatic zinc deficiency. These include diminished tissue stores of zinc in premature infants, the decreased bioavailability of zinc in cow's milk when compared to human breast milk, and the rare, idiopathic occurrence of low zinc levels in breast milk, despite normal serum levels.[123]

A periorificial dermatitis resembling acrodermatitis enteropathica may occur in the rare aminoacidopathies, **methylmalonic and propionic acidemia**.[144,145] The histopathological changes have been variable.

Biotin deficiency can also mimic zinc deficiency clinically.[146] It can result from acquired deficiencies (such as from the consumption of raw egg whites) or from an inborn error in metabolism, such as biotinidase deficiency.[147]

An **amicrobial pustulosis of the flexures and scalp** has been reported in association with various autoimmune diseases.[148] It is mentioned here because of its response to zinc supplementation.

Histopathology[129,149]

The histological changes, which vary with the age of the lesion, are similar to those seen in the necrolytic migratory erythema of the glucagonoma syndrome (see below). In early lesions, there is confluent parakeratosis overlying a normal basket-weave stratum corneum.[149] The granular layer is absent and there is mild spongiosis and acanthosis. There is increasing pallor of the cells in the upper layers of the epidermis and variable psoriasiform epidermal hyperplasia.[150] Subcorneal or intraepidermal clefts may develop but established vesiculobullous lesions are intraepidermal in location and result from cytoplasmic vacuolar change with massive ballooning and reticular change producing cytolysis of keratinocytes.[151] Confluent necrosis leads to enlargement of the vesicles. Sometimes there is necrosis of the upper epidermis, but this was not encountered in one detailed study.[152]

In late lesions, there is confluent parakeratosis overlying psoriasiform epidermal hyperplasia, but there is no significant epidermal pallor (Fig. 18.4). Less common findings include apoptotic cells,[153] a few acantholytic cells in vesiculobullous lesions[154] and neutrophils within the epidermis. Secondary infection may complicate the picture.

Blood vessels in the papillary dermis are often dilated and there is a mild perivascular infiltrate of chronic inflammatory cells.

Pallor of the epidermal cells is also seen in the exceedingly rare **deficiency of the M-subunit of lactate dehydrogenase**, reported from Japan;[155,156]

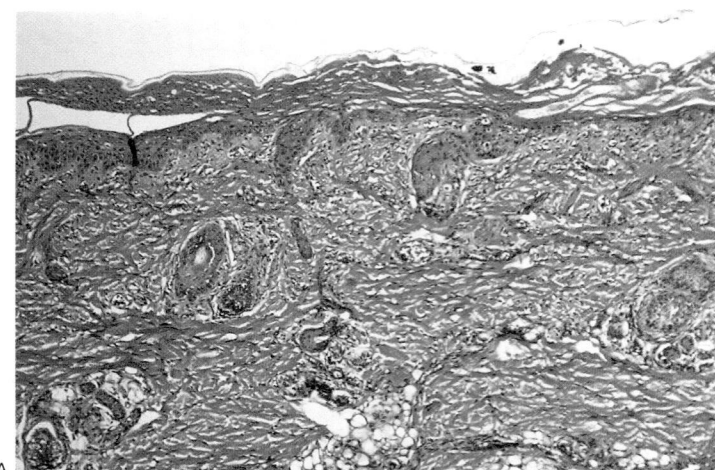
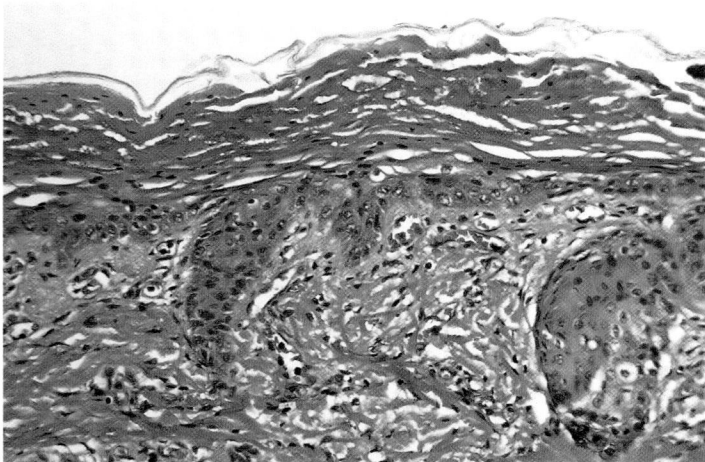

Fig. 18.4 **(A) Acrodermatitis enteropathica. (B)** This late lesion is characterized by confluent parakeratosis overlying an acanthotic epidermis. (H & E)

a similar disorder has been reported from Europe as 'annually recurring acroerythema'.[157]

Electron microscopy
Findings include lipid droplets and multiple cytoplasmic vacuoles in keratinocytes in the upper dermis.[131,149,158] Desmosomes may be diminished, associated often with widening of the intercellular space.[149]

GLUCAGONOMA SYNDROME

The clinical features of the rare glucagonoma syndrome include a distinctive cutaneous eruption (necrolytic migratory erythema), glossitis, stomatitis, diabetic type of glucose intolerance, scotoma, anemia, weight loss, venous thrombosis, elevated glucagon levels and decreased plasma amino acids.[159–162] A glucagon-secreting islet cell tumor of the pancreas is usually present and is malignant in the majority of cases.[159,163] The syndrome has also been reported in association with a jejunal adenocarcinoma,[164] in pancreatic insufficiency,[165] in association with a neuroendocrine tumor producing predominantly insulin,[166] in advanced cirrhosis of the liver,[167,168] in association with villous atrophy of the small intestine,[165] after intravenous glucagon for hypoglycemia resulting from an insulin-like tumor product,[169] and in a patient with elevated glucagon levels but no detectable tumor.[170] Impairment of hepatic function has been present in many of the cases of necrolytic migratory erythema without a glucagonoma.[171–173] Zinc deficiency is sometimes present as well in patients with cirrhosis of the liver.[173,174]

The cutaneous lesions, called *necrolytic migratory erythema* because of their similarities to both toxic epidermal necrolysis and annular erythema, are manifest by waves of extending annular or circinate erythema and superficial epidermal necrosis with shedding of the skin leading to flaccid bullae and crusted erosions. There is usually complete resolution of involved areas within 10–14 days.[175,176] The lesions primarily affect the trunk, groin, perineum, thighs and buttocks, but the legs, perioral skin[176] and sites of minor trauma may also be involved. Cutaneous lesions are not invariably present in the syndrome.

The pathogenesis of the skin lesions is uncertain, but their histological similarities to those seen in other deficiency states, such as pellagra and acrodermatitis enteropathica, and their disappearance with intravenous administration of supplemental amino acids suggest that profound amino acid deficiency induced by the catabolic effects of hyperglucagonemia may be

important.[176] Elevated levels of arachidonic acid, an inflammatory mediator, have been found in affected skin.[177]

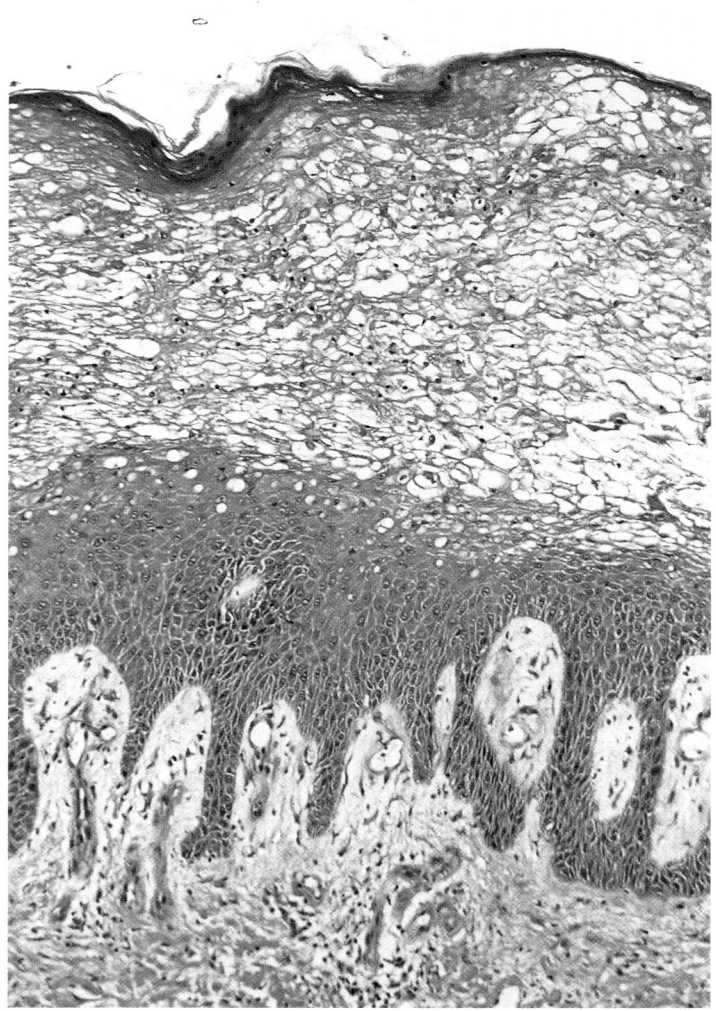

Fig. 18.5 **Glucagonoma syndrome.** This is an established lesion with a thick zone of pale, vacuolated keratinocytes in the upper epidermis. (H & E)

Histopathology[178]

Several histological patterns may be seen in necrolytic migratory erythema, depending on the stage of evolution of the lesion that is biopsied (Fig. 18.5). The most distinctive pattern is the presence of pale, vacuolated keratinocytes in the upper epidermis, leading to focal or confluent necrosis (Fig. 18.6).[170] This process has been termed 'necrolysis'.[175] Subcorneal or intraepidermal clefts may result; acantholytic cells are rarely found in these clefts.[179] Subcorneal pustules are sometimes found adjacent to the areas of necrosis, but they may also be the only manifestation of disease in the biopsy specimen.[178] Diffuse neutrophilic infiltration of the epidermis may accompany this pattern (Fig. 18.7).[180]

The least common histological pattern is psoriasiform hyperplasia of the epidermis with overlying confluent parakeratosis and vascular dilatation with some angioplasia in the papillary dermis (Fig. 18.8).[170,181]

In all biopsies there is usually a mild to moderate perivascular infiltrate of lymphocytes in the upper dermis. Sometimes there are occasional neutrophils as well, particularly if subcorneal pustules are present.

Uncommon histological findings include a suppurative folliculitis, the presence of concomitant candidosis,[182] suprabasal acantholysis[183] and scattered dyskeratotic cells in the upper epidermis.[184]

Electron microscopy

In one study, there was widening of the intercellular spaces in the upper epidermis and a reduction in the number of desmosomes.[185] The cytoplasm

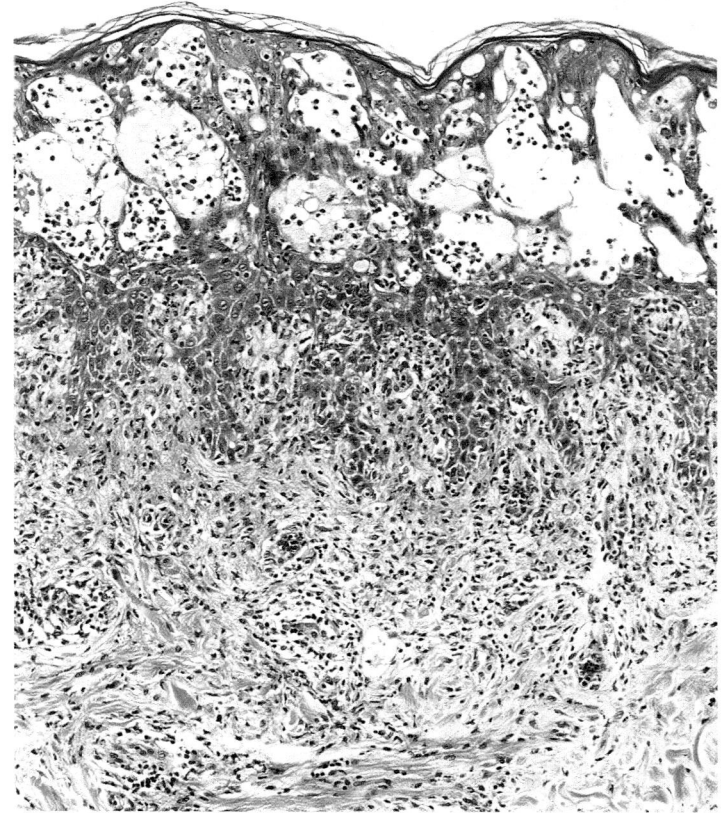

Fig. 18.7 **Glucagonoma syndrome.** A pustular lesion is present. (H & E)

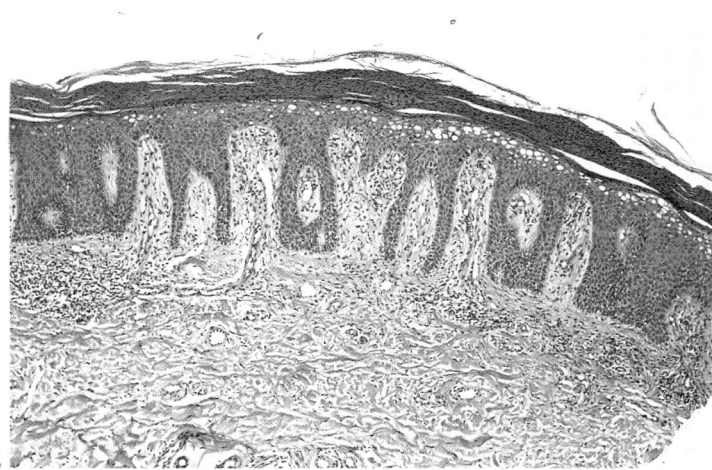

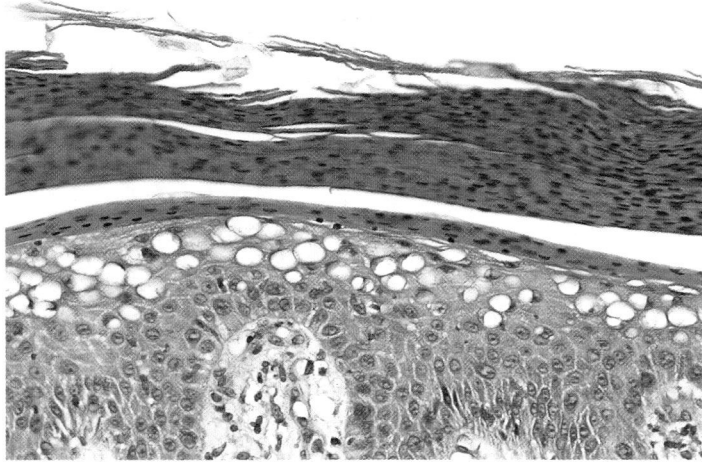

Fig. 18.6 **(A) Glucagonoma syndrome with psoriasiform hyperplasia. (B)** Vacuolated cells are quite conspicuous in the upper layers of the epidermis. (H & E)

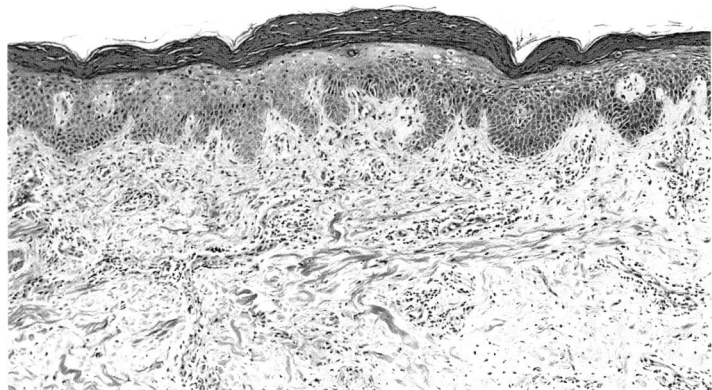

Fig. 18.8 **Glucagonoma syndrome.** Confluent parakeratosis overlies an epidermis in which there is mild psoriasiform hyperplasia. (H & E)

of affected cells showed vacuolar degeneration with lysis or absence of organelles.[185] Scattered dyskeratotic cells were noted.

NECROLYTIC ACRAL ERYTHEMA

Necrolytic acral erythema, first described in 1996, belongs to the family of necrolytic erythemas. This variant is unique in its acral location and its strong association with hepatitis C.[186,187] Clinically, there are eroded erythematous to violaceous patches and tender, flaccid blisters and erosions with hyperkeratotic plaques in older lesions. There is a predilection for the lower limbs. The condition responds to treatment with interferon alfa and oral zinc, although zinc levels are normal.[186]

Histopathology

The lesions resemble acrodermatitis enteropathica and necrolytic migratory erythema with hyperkeratosis, parakeratosis, superficial pallor of the epidermis, focal necrosis and spongiosis. There is a superficial mixed inflammatory cell infiltrate in the dermis.[186]

HARTNUP DISEASE

Hartnup disease, named after the first family to be described with this condition,[188] results from defective intestinal absorption of tryptophan and impaired renal tubular reabsorption of neutral amino acids.[189] There is a photosensitive, pellagra-like skin rash, cerebellar ataxia, mental disturbances, aminoaciduria and indicanuria.[190] Symptoms commence in childhood; there is often some improvement in later life. Sometimes the disease is inherited as an autosomal recessive condition. Other genetic defects of tryptophan metabolism, resulting in some symptoms in common with Hartnup disease, have been described.[191] In Hartnup disease, the defect is localized to chromosome 11q13.1–q13.3.

Histopathology

The changes in the skin are similar to those seen in pellagra (see p. 547).

PROLIDASE DEFICIENCY

Prolidase deficiency is an exceedingly rare, autosomal recessive, inborn error of metabolism in which recalcitrant leg ulcers are the most characteristic feature.[192–196] Other clinical features that may be present include mental retardation, splenomegaly, recurrent infections, a characteristic facies and premature graying of the hair.[197–199] Telangiectasias, photosensitivity, lymphedema and erosive cystitis[193] are rare manifestations.[192] The development of a squamous cell carcinoma in an ulcer is a surprisingly uncommon complication.[200] Onset of symptoms occurs in childhood. Large amounts of iminodipeptides are present in the urine.[201] The gene encoding this enzyme has been localized to chromosome 19 (19cen–q13.11).[195]

Histopathology

The cutaneous ulcers may show secondary infection and variable fibrosis in chronic cases. Two reports have mentioned the presence of amyloid-like material in vessel walls and in the immediately adjacent dermis.[202,203] Vascular wall thickening and infiltration of mononuclear cells and neutrophils have been observed in indurated lesions prior to their ulceration.[204] Although the dermal collagen in non-ulcerated areas appears normal on light microscopy, the fibers are seen to be smaller and irregularly patterned[199] on electron microscopy. Elastic fibers are fragmented.[199]

TANGIER DISEASE

Tangier disease is a rare disorder of plasma lipid transport in which there is a deficiency of normal high density lipoproteins in the plasma and an accumulation of cholesterol esters in many organs, particularly in the reticuloendothelial system.[205] The presence of enlarged yellowish tonsils and a low plasma cholesterol level is pathognomonic. The skin usually appears clinically normal, although small papular lesions have been described.[206] The gene responsible maps to chromosome 9q22–q31.

Histopathology

Biopsies from clinically normal skin show perivascular and interstitial nests of foam cells admixed with a few lymphocytes and plasma cells.[207] In frozen sections, the cytoplasm of the foam cells stains with oil red O and Sudan black.[207] Doubly refractile cholesterol esters are demonstrable in both an intracellular and extracellular location.[207] In semithin sections there is extensive vacuolization of the cytoplasm of Schwann cells in small, unmyelinated cutaneous nerves.[205]

Electron microscopy

The deposits are electron lucent and vary from spherical to crystalline in shape. They are not membrane bound. Lipid deposits are present in the cytoplasm of Schwann cells.[205]

LAFORA DISEASE

Lafora disease (Unverricht's disease, myoclonic epilepsy) is a familial, degenerative disorder with the clinical triad of seizures, myoclonus and dementia.[208] Cutaneous lesions are rarely present.[208] The enzyme defect is currently unknown, but the disease is usually regarded as an inborn error of carbohydrate metabolism.[209] The gene responsible maps to chromosome 6q23–25.[210] The intracytoplasmic inclusion bodies found in various organs, particularly in ganglion cells in parts of the brain, are glucose polymers;[208] they were first described by Lafora, who considered them to consist of amyloid.

Histopathology

The inclusion bodies (Lafora bodies, polyglucosan bodies) are well seen in the excretory ducts of eccrine and apocrine sweat glands of clinically normal skin.[209,211,212] They are PAS positive and diastase resistant. The number of inclusions may vary with the biopsy site;[208] axillary skin is favored.[210]

Electron microscopy

The inclusions are round or oval, non-membrane bound and often juxtanuclear in position.[209] They are composed of fine filamentous material, dark-staining granules and vacuoles.[208]

ULCERATIVE COLITIS AND CROHN'S DISEASE

Ulcerative colitis and Crohn's disease (regional enteritis) have many cutaneous manifestations in common.[213–217] Skin lesions occur in 10–20% of patients with either disease, but the incidence varies widely from one study to another, depending on the inclusion or otherwise of oral, perianal and non-specific lesions.[213,214] In the case of Crohn's disease, cutaneous manifestations are more common in patients with colonic rather than ileal disease. The onset of skin lesions occasionally precedes the symptoms and signs of the inflammatory bowel disease. There is no correlation, as a rule, with the severity or activity of the bowel disease.

Erythema nodosum and pyoderma gangrenosum are the most common and specific cutaneous manifestations of *both diseases*, although pyoderma gangrenosum is more frequent in ulcerative colitis.[218] Finger clubbing, aphthous ulcers of the mouth,[219] cutaneous polyarteritis nodosa,[220,221] psoriasis,[222] pyostomatitis vegetans,[223–225] erythema multiforme[226] and vitiligo[227,228] have been reported in both conditions.[213] Cutaneous complications of therapy sometimes develop.

In *Crohn's disease*, the perianal manifestations include skin tags, fistulas and abscesses.[229,230] They are found in up to 80% of individuals with colonic involvement.[231] Mucosal 'cobblestoning' and fissuring may occur in the mouth.[232–234] Intraepithelial IgA pustulosis is a rare oral disease occurring in Crohn's disease.[235] Cheilitis granulomatosa (see p. 208) may occur on the lips.[236] Other lesions described in Crohn's disease include erythema elevatum diutinum,[237] a vesiculopustular eruption,[238] a neutrophilic dermatosis of the malar regions,[239] epidermolysis bullosa acquisita,[240] acne fulminans,[241] pyoderma faciale,[242] a neutrophilic lobular panniculitis,[243] granulomatous vasculitis (Fig. 18.9),[244] porokeratosis and nutritional deficiency states related to zinc, niacin (nicotinic acid) and vitamin C.[213,232] The occurrence of granulomas in nodular, ulcerated or plaque-like lesions, at sites well removed from involved mucosal surfaces, has been called 'metastatic Crohn's disease'.[245–255] Some lesions are in intertriginous areas; the limbs are another favored site. The vulva, scrotum and penis are rarely involved.[256–260] Genital involvement appears to be more common in children than adults.[261,262] There are non-caseating granulomas, similar to those seen in the bowel, scattered through the dermis and sometimes the subcutis. Sometimes there are only occasional granulomas in a perivascular distribution (granulomatous perivasculitis).[263]

Uncommon manifestations of *ulcerative colitis* include thromboembolic phenomena, cutaneous vasculitis[218,264] and a vesiculopustular eruption.[265] Some of the pustular lesions described in ulcerative colitis probably represent evolving lesions of pyoderma gangrenosum, others resemble Sweet's syndrome,[266] while still others are non-specific pustular eruptions.[264,267–270] These may show either a suppurative folliculitis or intraepidermal or deeper abscesses. In short, a spectrum of neutrophilic dermatoses can occur.[266] Granulomas with admixed neutrophils were present in one proven case of ulcerative colitis.[271]

WHIPPLE'S DISEASE

Whipple's disease is a rare, multisystem, bacterial infection characterized by malabsorption, abdominal pain, arthritis and neurological manifestations. The organism responsible, *Tropheryma whippelii*, is related to the actinomycetes group of Gram-positive bacteria.[272] The cutaneous changes include hyperpigmentation of scars and sun-exposed skin, observed in approximately 40% of patients,[273] as well as erythema nodosum and, rarely, subcutaneous nodules.[274,275]

Histopathology[274,276]

The subcutaneous nodules show a non-specific panniculitis with pockets of foamy macrophages containing PAS-positive, diastase-resistant material and resembling those seen in small bowel biopsies.

CYSTIC FIBROSIS

Cutaneous manifestations of malnutrition are rarely seen in cystic fibrosis; they have been attributed to deficiencies of protein, zinc and fatty acids.[2,141,277] The lesions described include erythematous, desquamating papules and plaques, and scaling, sometimes annular, patches and plaques.[277] The lesions develop early in life.

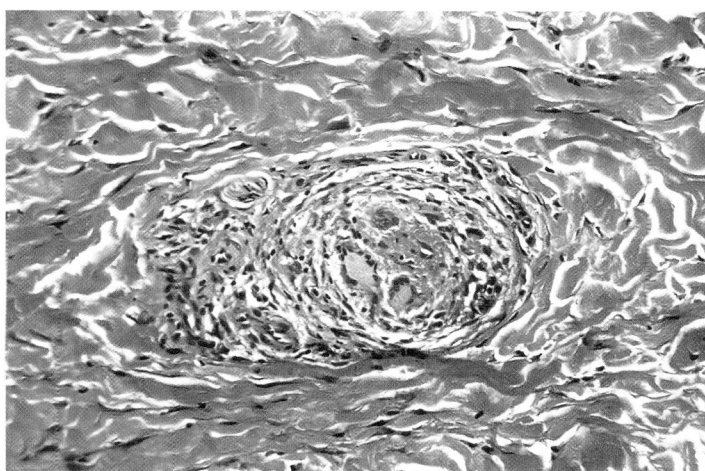

Fig. 18.9 **Crohn's disease.** A small, non-caseating granuloma is in intimate contact with a small blood vessel in the lower dermis. There is extravasation of fibrin into the vessel wall. (H & E)

Histopathology[277]

The changes are not diagnostically specific. They include acanthosis, a diminished granular layer with overlying parakeratosis, and a mild perivascular infiltrate of lymphocytes in the upper dermis. Mild spongiosis is sometimes present. The necrolysis and pallor seen in acrodermatitis enteropathica are absent.

DIABETES MELLITUS

Cutaneous manifestations are common in diabetics, occurring at some time in approximately 30% of all people who have the disease. Most of these skin complications and associations have been discussed elsewhere in this volume, but they are listed below for completeness. Three complications that have not been considered elsewhere – microangiopathic changes, pigmented pretibial patches (diabetic dermopathy), and bullous eruption of diabetes mellitus (bullosis diabeticorum) – are discussed in detail below.

There are many ways of subclassifying the cutaneous manifestations and associations of diabetes mellitus.[278–281] The one used here is based on the review published some years ago by Huntley.[282]

Vascular and neuropathic complications

Both large and small vessels are affected in diabetes.[282] Atherosclerosis of large vessels contributes to the ischemic complications, such as gangrene of the lower leg, but small vessel (microangiopathic) changes also play an important role. These latter changes are considered below. Other vascular-related phenomena include facial rubeosis[279] and the erysipelas-like areas of erythema sometimes seen on the lower parts of the legs, including the feet. Reduced sweating, loss of hair and glazed skin are, in part, related to vascular changes.

Sensory, motor and autonomic neuropathies may occur in diabetes. Autonomic dysfunction is sometimes associated with disturbances of sweating and vasomotor phenomena. Neuropathic ulcers may result from the sensory neuropathy.

Infections

Infections are seen less commonly than before, probably because there is better control of diabetes. Bacterial infections that may occur include furuncles, non-clostridial gas gangrene, *Pseudomonas* infections of the ears, and erythrasma (see p. 623). Infections with *Candida albicans* are still common in diabetics and may result in paronychia, stomatitis, vulvitis and balanitis (see p. 664). Dermatophyte infections may not be increased, as previously thought.[283] Rare mycotic infections in diabetics include nocardiosis (see p. 676), cryptococcosis (see p. 666) and the zygomycoses (see p. 677).

Distinct cutaneous manifestations

Diabetes mellitus may be associated with the following conditions: necrobiosis lipoidica (see p. 202), granuloma annulare of the disseminated type (see p. 200), scleredema (also known as diabetic thick skin[284] – see p. 410), pigmented pretibial patches (see below), bullous eruption of diabetes mellitus (see below), finger 'pebbles' which resemble knuckle pads histopathologically[285–287] (see p. 923) and eruptive xanthomas (see p. 1075). In some diabetics, the skin is waxy and thickened, particularly over the proximal interphalangeal joints of the hands, leading to stiffness of the joints.[282] Another manifestation is yellow skin, due in part to the carotenemia which is present in some diabetics.[279] A reduced threshold to suction-induced blisters has also been found in insulin-dependent diabetics.[288]

Less well documented associations[282] include skin tags (see p. 921), peripheral edema, yellow nails and perforating disorders associated with diabetic renal failure and hemodialysis (see p. 363).

Diabetes mellitus or an abnormal glucose tolerance test is present in a small number of patients with Werner's syndrome (see p. 366), scleroderma (see p. 346), vitiligo (see p. 323), lichen planus (see p. 33) and Cockayne's syndrome (see p. 303) and in relatives of patients with lipoid proteinosis (see p. 434).

Secondary diabetes mellitus[282]

Diabetes mellitus may occur as a secondary process in the course of a number of diseases, such as hemochromatosis (see p. 440), lipodystrophy (see p. 530), acanthosis nigricans (see p. 574), Cushing's syndrome, acromegaly and the hepatic porphyrias, particularly porphyria cutanea tarda (see p. 559). These disorders have their own cutaneous expressions, in addition to any related to the diabetic state.

Complications of therapy[282]

The use of oral hypoglycemic agents may be complicated by a maculopapular eruption, urticaria, photosensitivity and flushing when alcohol is consumed (with chlorpropamide) and very rarely by erythema multiforme, exfoliative dermatitis or a lichenoid eruption.

Localized reactions to the injection of insulin are not uncommon and include allergic reactions, localized induration, anesthetic nodules composed of hypertrophied fat and some fibrous tissue, focal dermal atrophy, ulceration and necrosis, brown hyperkeratotic papules, keloid formation and localized hyperpigmentation. Insulin-induced lipoatrophy is another complication which may develop 6–24 months after the onset of therapy.[289] It is more common in young females, particularly in areas of substantial fat deposition. The atrophy sometimes occurs at sites remote from injections.[278] Lipohypertrophy presents as a soft swelling resembling a lipoma. It is more common in males.[278] Generalized allergic reactions may also occur; these are more common with beef insulin than pork insulin.[289]

Diabetic microangiopathy

Diabetic microangiopathy refers to the abnormal small vessels found in many organs and tissues in diabetes mellitus. The kidneys, eyes, skin and muscles are particularly affected by this disease process, which is the principal factor determining the prognosis of individuals with diabetes mellitus.[278]

Microangiopathy may be involved in the pathogenesis of the pigmented pretibial patches, the erysipelas-like erythema and the necrobiosis lipoidica that may occur in diabetes mellitus. It may contribute to the neuropathy that sometimes occurs. Small vessel disease may be as important as atherosclerosis of large vessels in producing gangrene of the feet and lower limbs in diabetics. In many instances the microangiopathy is clinically silent.

Histopathology

There is thickening of the walls of small blood vessels in the dermis and subcutis and some proliferation of their endothelial cells. The thickening of the walls and subsequent luminal narrowing is caused by the deposition of PAS-positive material in the basement membrane region. This material is partially diastase labile, although most of it is not.[290] Membranocystic lesions, in which a thin hyaline zone surrounds a small 'cystic' space, have been reported in the subcutaneous fat (see p. 532).[291]

Electron microscopy

The walls of the small vessels are thickened by multiple layers of veil cells (a fibroblast-like cell) and of basement membrane material.[291,292] There may also be some deposition of collagen in the walls of small vessels in the dermis.[292]

Pigmented pretibial patches

Pigmented pretibial patches (diabetic dermopathy, skin spots) are the most common cutaneous finding in diabetes mellitus, although they are not specific to it.[282,293] They are found in up to 50% of diabetics, but as they are asymptomatic, they are usually overlooked.[294] They begin as flat-topped, dull-red papules that are round or oval, discrete or grouped and situated mainly on the pretibial areas.[278] Involvement of the forearms and thighs has been recorded.[295] As the lesions evolve they develop a thin scale and finally become variably atrophic and hyperpigmented.[279,289] They vary from 0.5 cm in diameter up to large patches covering much of the pretibial skin.

It has been suggested that the lesions represent an exaggerated response to trauma in skin overlying bony prominences[282] and that there may be an underlying diabetic angiopathy; the literature is replete with evidence to the contrary.[279,296]

Histopathology[297]

In the early lesions, which are infrequently biopsied, there is edema of the papillary dermis and a mild perivascular lymphocytic infiltrate with some extravasation of red blood cells.[282] There may be mild epidermal spongiosis and focal parakeratosis.

In atrophic lesions there is neovascularization of the papillary dermis, a sparse perivascular infiltrate of lymphocytes, and small amounts of hemosiderin, mostly in macrophages.

Bullous eruption of diabetes mellitus

Bullae, usually multiple and confined to the lower extremities, are a rare complication of long-standing diabetes mellitus.[298] They were originally reported in 1963 as 'phlyctenar lesions' because they become dark as they dry up, in the manner of a burn blister.[299] The bullae, which arise on a non-inflamed base, are tense and vary in diameter from 0.5 to 17 cm.[289,300] They heal in several weeks, usually without scarring.

It seems likely that cases reported under this title do not represent a homogeneous entity, some possibly representing the bullous dermopathy of chronic renal failure.[282,301] Furthermore, there is an increased frequency of diabetes in patients with bullous pemphigoid.[302]

Histopathology[298]

The majority of the bullae reported under this title have been intraepidermal in location, often with spongiotic changes in the surrounding epidermis.[303] It has been suggested that some of these may represent healing subepidermal blisters. In other cases the split has been subepidermal,[298,304–306] immediately beneath the lamina densa.[307] While it has been claimed that these have been early lesions and, as such, may more accurately reflect the true histological picture,[307] it should be noted that in the majority of cases with subepidermal blisters, diabetic nephropathy has been present.[301,307] The drugs being taken by these patients, a potentially important etiological aspect, have not been listed. In the author's experience, the bullae have been subepidermal in location.

The bullae contain fibrin and just a few inflammatory cells but there is no acantholysis. There may be diabetic microangiopathy with thickening of the walls of small dermal blood vessels, but there is usually only a sparse perivascular lymphocytic infiltrate.[304]

Direct immunofluorescence is negative.

PORPHYRIA

The porphyrias are a clinically and biochemically heterogeneous group of disorders in which there are abnormalities in the biosynthesis of heme, leading to the increased production of various porphyrin precursors.[308–318] The various enzyme deficiencies are not always accompanied by detectable increases in the relevant substrate, and overproduction of the precursors does not necessarily lead to symptomatic disease. However, the homozygous state for a particular enzyme deficiency is probably always clinically overt. The various enzyme deficiencies do not result in heme deficiency because a compensatory increase in substrate concentration is sufficient to restore the rate of heme synthesis to normal.[319]

Traditionally, the porphyrias have been classified on the basis of the primary site of overproduction of porphyrins.[320] In the *erythropoietic porphyrias* (congenital erythropoietic porphyria and erythropoietic protoporphyria) there is disordered synthesis of heme in the bone marrow.[321] In the *hepatic porphyrias* (acute intermittent porphyria, ALA-dehydratase deficiency, hereditary coproporphyria, variegate porphyria, porphyria cutanea tarda and hepatoerythropoietic porphyria) there is disordered synthesis of heme in the liver.[320] In some circumstances both sites are involved.

It is more appropriate to classify the porphyrias on the basis of their clinical manifestations. Three categories are then recognized.

1. *porphyrias with acute episodes and no cutaneous signs:*
   acute intermittent porphyria
   ALA-dehydratase deficiency
2. *porphyrias with acute episodes and cutaneous signs:*
   hereditary coproporphyria
   variegate porphyria
3. *porphyrias with cutaneous signs only:*
   congenital erythropoietic porphyria
   erythropoietic protoporphyria
   porphyria cutanea tarda
   hepatoerythropoietic porphyria.

In addition to these eight types of porphyria, there are rare variants that defy classification.[309] Such cases include neonates who develop a photosensitive eruption due to a transient porphyrinemia resulting from phototherapy for hemolytic disease of the newborn.[322,323]

The *acute episodes* referred to above are characterized by abdominal pain, neurological changes and psychiatric disturbances.[309,324] Sometimes these acute episodes are precipitated by exogenous factors such as drugs.[325] The *cutaneous manifestations* are of two types.[326] There may be an acute flare pattern with rapidly evolving, painful and burning lesions with some erythema and edema.[327] This pattern is typical of erythropoietic protoporphyria, although it occurs rarely in some of the other variants (see below). The other cutaneous pattern (seen in hereditary coproporphyria, variegate porphyria, congenital erythropoietic porphyria, porphyria cutanea tarda and hepatoerythropoietic porphyria) consists of slowly developing skin fragility with the development of blisters, erosions and scars.[327–329] These aspects are considered in further detail with each particular variant of porphyria (see below).

Biosynthesis of porphyrins

Glycine and succinyl coenzyme A react in the presence of ALA-synthase to form δ-aminolevulinic acid (ALA).[311] This is converted to porphobilinogen and subsequently to protoporphyrin IX by a series of enzymatic reactions (see Table 18.1). Protoporphyrin IX is chelated with iron in the presence of ferrochelatase to form heme.[330]

Acute intermittent porphyria

Acute intermittent porphyria is an autosomal dominant disorder resulting from a defect in porphobilinogen deaminase (uroporphyrinogen I synthase) which catalyzes the formation of uroporphyrinogen from four molecules of porphobilinogen.[331] The disorder is usually latent, but acute episodes consisting of neurological, psychiatric and abdominal symptoms may be precipitated by various factors, particularly drugs.[332] Barbiturates, sulfonamides and griseofulvin are most often incriminated.[325] There are no cutaneous manifestations.

Laboratory findings include greatly increased levels of porphobilinogen and ALA in the urine during, and usually between, attacks.

ALA-dehydratase deficiency porphyria

This very rare, autosomal recessive disorder results, as its name indicates, from a deficiency of ALA-dehydratase which was formerly known as porphobilinogen synthase (PBG-synthase). There are intermittent, acute episodes resembling those in acute intermittent porphyria; there are no cutaneous manifestations.[332]

The pattern of overproduction of heme precursors closely resembles that seen in severe lead poisoning. There is overproduction of ALA and of coproporphyrinogen III.

Hereditary coproporphyria

Hereditary coproporphyria is an autosomal dominant variant of acute porphyria which results from a deficiency of coproporphyrinogen oxidase.[327] Latent disease is more usual than the symptomatic form, which is characterized by episodic attacks of abdominal pain and neurological and psychiatric disturbances. These acute episodes are less severe than in acute intermittent porphyria. Cutaneous photosensitivity occurs in approximately 30% of cases and becomes manifest chiefly in association with the acute attacks.[327,333] The lesions resemble those seen in porphyria cutanea tarda (see below). There has been one report of a patient with porphyria-like photosensitivity following liver transplant. The coproporphyrin levels were only mildly elevated.[334] Acute coproporphyria has also been induced by the anabolic steroid methandrostenolone (methandienone).[335]

Laboratory findings include greatly elevated levels of urinary and fecal coproporphyrins. Porphobilinogen and ALA are increased, as in variegate porphyria (see below), during acute episodes.[333]

Table 18.1 **Summary of the biosynthesis of heme and the associated clinical disorders**

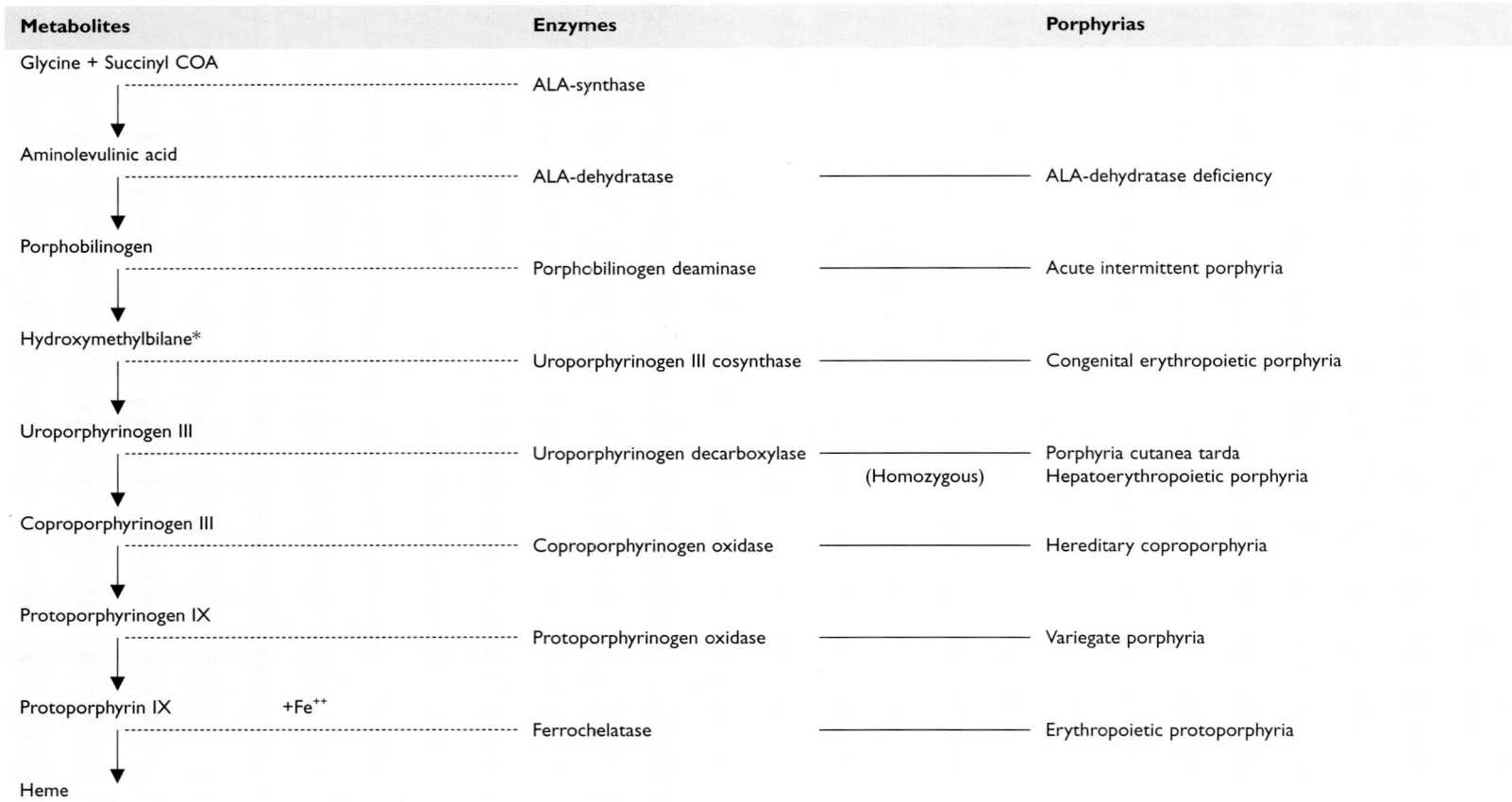

Metabolites	Enzymes	Porphyrias
Glycine + Succinyl COA	ALA-synthase	
Aminolevulinic acid	ALA-dehydratase	ALA-dehydratase deficiency
Porphobilinogen	Porphobilinogen deaminase	Acute intermittent porphyria
Hydroxymethylbilane*	Uroporphyrinogen III cosynthase	Congenital erythropoietic porphyria
Uroporphyrinogen III	Uroporphyrinogen decarboxylase	Porphyria cutanea tarda
	(Homozygous)	Hepatoerythropoietic porphyria
Coproporphyrinogen III	Coproporphyrinogen oxidase	Hereditary coproporphyria
Protoporphyrinogen IX	Protoporphyrinogen oxidase	Variegate porphyria
Protoporphyrin IX +Fe^{++}	Ferrochelatase	Erythropoietic protoporphyria
Heme		

*Hydroxymethylbilane may undergo spontaneous conversion to uroporphyrinogen I.

Variegate porphyria

Variegate porphyria, like hereditary coproporphyria, may be associated with acute episodes (as seen in acute intermittent porphyria) and with photocutaneous manifestations (as seen in porphyria cutanea tarda).[336,337] It is an autosomal dominant disorder in which the activity of the enzyme protoporphyrinogen oxidase is reduced by approximately 50%. This disorder is quite common in white Afrikaaners and much less so in other white people and in people of other races.[336] The *(PPOX)* gene, which controls the formation of the responsible enzyme, maps to chromosome 1q22–23.[338] Numerous mutations in this gene have been described in European patients, but in South Africa most patients have inherited the same mutation.[339–342]

Only a minority of people with the enzyme defect develop clinical manifestations, and only after puberty. Acute episodes are precipitated by exogenous factors such as the ingestion of various drugs.[325,343] Cutaneous changes include skin fragility, blistering and milia formation in sun-exposed areas, as in porphyria cutanea tarda, although very occasionally an acute phototoxic reaction (as seen in erythropoietic protoporphyria) may develop.[327] Variegate porphyria is not usually associated with liver dysfunction, although it has been reported in association with a hepatocellular carcinoma.[344,345] Dapsone, used in the treatment of dermatitis herpetiformis, has precipitated an acute attack of variegate porphyria.[346]

Laboratory findings are somewhat variable, depending on the activity of the disease.[327] There is usually an elevated plasma porphyrin level with plasma fluorescence that is maximal at a wavelength of 626 ± 1 nm.[347] In practice, the diagnosis is most often suggested by finding elevated levels of fecal proto-porphyrin and coproporphyrin.[343] Urinary ALA and porphobilinogen are usually increased during acute episodes.

It has been reported in one homozygote that the erythrocyte proto-porphyrin was raised and that this was predominantly zinc chelated.[348]

Congenital erythropoietic porphyria (Günther's disease)

Congenital erythropoietic porphyria is a rare, autosomal recessive disorder of heme synthesis resulting from a deficiency of uroporphyrinogen III cosynthase (URO-synthase) which leads to an accumulation of porphyrins, particularly uroporphyrinogen I and III, in the bone marrow, blood and other organs.[349–352] The URO-synthase gene has been localized to the narrow chromosomal region 10q25.3–q26.3.[350] Several different mutations have been described.[353] The defect leads to a chronic photobullous dermatosis, intermittent hemolysis and massive porphyrinuria.[349] Presentation is usually in infancy with red urine which stains diapers a pink color.[327] Late onset of the disease has been recorded.[354]

The severe photosensitivity leads to the formation of bullae within a day or two of exposure to the sun. Recurrent eruptions may lead to mutilating deformities of the hands and face and sclerodermoid thickening of affected parts.[355] Sunlight avoidance is the best therapy.[352] Other clinical features include the pathognomonic characteristic of erythrodontia (discoloration of the teeth under normal light and red fluorescence with ultraviolet light), hypertrichosis, patchy scarring alopecia, and nail changes.[349,356–358]

There are large amounts of uroporphyrins in the urine and coproporphyrins in the stool; these are predominantly type I isomers.[355] The plasma and erythrocytes contain increased levels of uroporphyrinogen and, to a lesser extent, coproporphyrinogen.[359] Heterozygotes have blood levels of URO-synthase activity intermediate between affected individuals and controls.[355]

Erythropoietic protoporphyria

Erythropoietic protoporphyria, more recently termed simply 'protoporphyria',[327,360] results from a defect in the terminal step of heme synthesis at which protoporphyrin IX and iron combine to form heme.[361-365] It is associated with a deficiency of ferrochelatase (heme synthase). Although originally regarded as autosomal dominant in inheritance, it is now known that autosomal recessive inheritance occurs in a few cases.[364,366] The gene for ferrochelatase has been cloned and mapped to the long arm of chromosome 18 (18q21.3). Numerous mutations have been described.[367,368]

It generally becomes manifest in early childhood with episodes of acute photosensitivity accompanied by a painful, burning sensation.[362] Often there is edema and erythema and rarely there may be urticaria and petechiae.[327,369] The changes develop within a few hours of exposure to the sun. In the chronic stages there is waxy scarring of the nose, radial scars around the lips and pits or scars on the forehead, nose and cheeks.[327,370] The skin on the dorsum of the hands has a leathery texture and it may also show 'cobblestone' thickening.[327] Deaths from cirrhosis accompanying heavy accumulation of protoporphyrin in the liver have been reported.[371-374]

Rare clinical presentations have included late onset,[370,375] the presence of scarring bullae and milia,[376] coexistence with lupus erythematosus,[377] a clinical picture resembling hydroa estivale[378] (see p. 601), and the presence of a fibrous band involving a digit (pseudoainhum).[379] In one group of patients with protoporphyria the disease appears to be exacerbated by the ingestion of iron;[361] exacerbation has also followed blood transfusion.[380] Clinical improvement, with lower erythrocyte porphyrin levels, occurs during pregnancy.[381,382]

Protoporphyria is the only disorder of porphyrin metabolism with normal urinary porphyrins.[327] There are markedly increased levels of protoporphyrin in the feces and blood. The erythrocytes show a red fluorescence which decays more rapidly than that in congenital erythropoietic porphyria (see above).[327]

Porphyria cutanea tarda

Porphyria cutanea tarda (PCT) is the commonest form of porphyria in Europe and North America.[327,383] It is not a single disorder but an etiologically diverse group that share in common reduced activity of uroporphyrinogen decarboxylase (URO-D), the enzyme which catalyzes the sequential decarboxylation of uroporphyrinogen to coproporphyrinogen in a two-stage process.[327,384,385] In most forms there is a reduction in hepatic URO-D, leading to overproduction of porphyrins in the liver.[386] In the uncommon familial form there is usually a deficiency of this enzyme in erythrocytes as well as in other tissues.

There are three major forms of PCT: familial, sporadic and toxic. In addition, the porphyria resulting from porphyrin-producing tumors of the liver[384,387] and that associated with chronic renal failure and URO-D deficiency are sometimes categorized as two further clinical variants of PCT.[386,388-392] Hepatoerythropoietic porphyria (see below) is regarded as the homozygous deficiency of URO-D.[386]

The *familial form* is inherited as an autosomal dominant trait.[386] The enzyme (URO-D) is located on chromosome 1p34.[393] The familial form was previously thought to be associated, invariably, with a deficiency of URO-D in erythrocytes as well as in the liver, but cases with a normal level of erythrocyte

URO-D have been documented.[394] Sometimes, overt disease is precipitated by some exogenous factor such as childbirth, exposure to ultraviolet radiation in tanning parlors, iron overload or excessive alcohol intake.[383,395] Its onset is usually earlier than that of the sporadic form.[396]

The *sporadic form* usually has its onset in mid-life. More than 70% of cases in the past were associated with alcohol abuse and liver damage.[386,397,398] Now, there is a virtual 'epidemic' of cases associated with hepatitis C virus, some of whom also develop hepatocellular carcinoma.[399-406] It has been suggested that the porphyria subtype should be called 'chronic hepatic porphyria'.[407] Estrogen therapy for carcinoma of the prostate[408,409] or for menopausal symptoms is sometimes the precipitating event. Oral contraceptives have also been incriminated.[410] Rare associations have included diabetes mellitus,[397] solar urticaria,[411] Wilson's disease,[412] hepatocellular carcinoma,[384,413] lymphoma,[414] HIV infection,[415-418] agnogenic myeloid metaplasia,[419] idiopathic myelofibrosis[420] and lupus erythematosus.[421-423] The sporadic form appears to result from inactivation of URO-D in the liver[385] although this appears to be independent of, rather than the consequence of, liver injury.[386] Mutations in the *HFE* gene associated with hereditary hemochromatosis have been associated with sporadic and familial PCT.[393,424] Co-inheritance of the genes for these two conditions appears to accelerate the onset of the porphyria.[425]

The *toxic form* results from exposure to polychlorinated aromatic hydrocarbons.[393,426] Other hepatotoxins have rarely been incriminated.

The cutaneous changes occur predominantly on light-exposed areas such as the face, arms and dorsum of the hands.[427] Their severity is highly variable. They include increased vulnerability to mechanical trauma and the formation of subepidermal vesicles or bullae measuring 0.5–3 cm in diameter.[397] Erosions, milia, scars and areas of hyperpigmentation are common.[397] Hypertrichosis, patchy alopecia, infections,[428] dystrophic calcification and sclerodermoid changes may occur but do so less frequently than the other cutaneous manifestations.[397] The sclerodermoid changes, which may be present in up to 20% of cases, do not always occur in light-exposed areas. They are not associated with sclerodactyly and they are not invariably permanent. It has been suggested that they are related to high levels of uroporphyrinogen.[429]

Hepatic changes are common in PCT. There is an increased risk of developing hepatocellular carcinoma.[384]

Laboratory findings include increased amounts of uroporphyrins in the urine and plasma and of coproporphyrins in the feces. The urine contains a predominance of 8-carboxyl and 7-carboxyl porphyrins, while the feces contain isocoproporphyrin, which is not found in significant amounts in other porphyrias.[385]

Hepatoerythropoietic porphyria

Hepatoerythropoietic porphyria is a rare, severe variant that is manifested clinically by photosensitivity commencing in early childhood.[430-433] As in porphyria cutanea tarda (PCT), there is a deficiency of uroporphyrinogen decarboxylase (URO-D), but the activity of this enzyme is much less than in PCT, reflecting a homozygous state.[434,435] To date, three different point mutations and/or a deletion in the URO-D gene have been reported.[436] Hepatic involvement is common. The cutaneous features resemble those of PCT.[437]

Laboratory findings are similar to those in PCT, but an additional feature is the presence of elevated levels of protoporphyrins in erythrocytes.[430]

Pseudoporphyria

The term 'pseudoporphyria' is used for a phototoxic bullous dermatosis which resembles porphyria cutanea tarda (PCT).[438,439] However, there are normal levels of porphyrins in the serum, urine and feces.[440] The term 'therapy-induced bullous photosensitivity' has been suggested as more appropriate[441] as this condition has been reported following the use of a number of drugs including tetracyclines,[442,443] sulfonamides, isotretinoin,[444] pravastatin,[445] furosemide (frusemide),[446,447] nalidixic acid,[448] naproxen,[449–452] oxaprozin,[453] mefenamic acid,[454] nabumetone,[455–459] pyridoxine,[460] chlorthalidone,[461] flutamide[462] and etretinate.[463] A few cases have followed the prolonged use of tanning beds.[464–466] Blistering has also been reported in patients with chronic renal failure undergoing hemodialysis.[467,468] In some patients pseudoporphyria has been associated with a deficiency of uroporphyrinogen decarboxylase with increased levels of porphyrins; in others, many of whom were also receiving furosemide (frusemide), the porphyrin levels have been normal.[467,469,470]

The lesions in pseudoporphyria, which consist of spontaneous blisters and skin fragility, usually involving the dorsum of the hands, may develop as early as 1 week or as late as several months after commencement of the drug.[449] In contrast to porphyria cutanea tarda, few patients with pseudoporphyria develop hypertrichosis, hyperpigmentation or sclerodermoid features.

The histopathology of the different variants of porphyria will be considered together.

Histopathology[471–473]

There are remarkable similarities in the cutaneous changes in the various porphyrias: the differences are quantitative rather than qualitative.[472] The hallmarks of porphyria are the presence of lightly eosinophilic hyaline material in and around small vessels in the upper dermis, reduplication of vascular and sometimes epidermal basement membrane, and the deposition of fibrillar and amorphous material around the superficial vessels and at the dermoepidermal junction.[471,472] The hyaline material seen on light microscopy is reduplicated basement membrane associated with the fibrillar and amorphous material just mentioned. Another distinctive feature seen in PCT, pseudoporphyria and erythropoietic protoporphyria are so-called 'caterpillar bodies'.[474,475] They represent basement membrane material and colloid bodies, akin to the Kamino bodies of Spitz nevi (see p. 811), deposited in the basal layer of the epidermis as elongated segmented bodies or globules. When blisters are present, these bodies are located in the roof.[474] The histological features of the various types of porphyria will be discussed in further detail.

In *erythropoietic protoporphyria* (EPP) the hyaline material not only involves the walls of small vessels in the papillary dermis, but also forms an irregular cuff around these vessels (Fig. 18.10). There is variable thickening of the vessel walls as a consequence of the presence of this hyaline material and this is sometimes associated with luminal narrowing. The hyaline material does not usually encroach on the adjacent dermis as much as it does in lipoid proteinosis (see p. 434) and furthermore, it does not involve the sweat glands.[476] The hyaline material is strongly PAS positive and diastase resistant. It stains with Sudan black in frozen sections and it is weakly positive with Hale's colloidal iron method.[477] It also stains, immunohistochemically, for laminin, collagen IV and immunoglobulin light chains.[478] Elastic fibers are pushed aside by the hyaline material.[477] Uninvolved areas of skin in EPP show minimal or undetectable changes, suggesting that the interaction of solar radiation is mandatory for the vascular changes.[478] Sometimes, a few neutrophils with foci of leukocytoclasis are present in the papillary dermis. A leukocytoclastic vasculitis has also been reported in a patient with prominent purpuric lesions.[369]

In *porphyria cutanea tarda* (PCT), the hyaline material is restricted to the vessel walls and their immediate vicinity. It does not form a significant cuff as in EPP. Again, the material is PAS positive and diastase resistant. In some cases, there is PAS-positive thickening of the basement membrane. These changes are not usually present in early lesions of pseudoporphyria, although some PAS-positive material is found in vessel walls. Small amounts of this material may be found in vessel walls in clinically uninvolved skin in PCT.[471] Solar elastosis is usually present in PCT, a change which is not often seen in patients with EPP, a reflection of their younger age.[472]

In *sclerodermoid lesions* there is thickening of the dermis which may be indistinguishable from that seen in scleroderma, although a looser arrangement of the collagen fibers is usually discernible in PCT.[471,472]

The *blisters* that form in the various forms of porphyria and in pseudoporphyria are subepidermal (dermolytic) with the dermal papillae projecting into the floor (festooning) (Fig. 18.11).[449,479,480] This latter change is not always prominent in pseudoporphyria.[449] There is only a very sparse inflammatory cell infiltrate, which in pseudoporphyria may sometimes include a rare eosinophil (Fig. 18.12). Focal hemorrhage is sometimes present in the upper dermis. The PAS-positive basement membrane is usually found in the roof of the blister.[449] Studies of laminin and type IV collagen suggest that the split in PCT and pseudoporphyria occurs in the lamina lucida.[481]

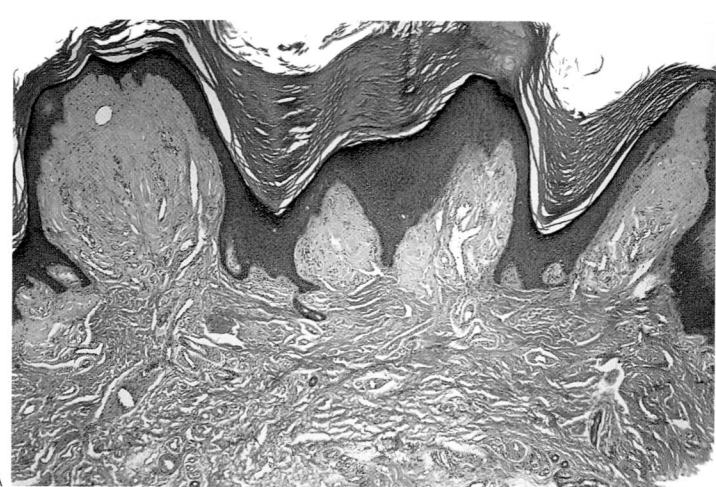
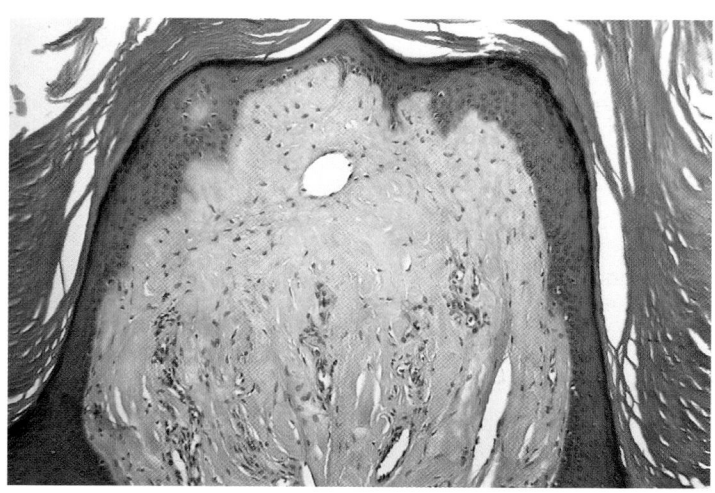

Fig. 18.10 **Erythropoietic protoporphyria. (A)** Hyaline material surrounds vessels in the papillary dermis. **(B)** This case was initially misdiagnosed as a variant of colloid milium because of the extensive involvement of the papillary dermis. (H & E)

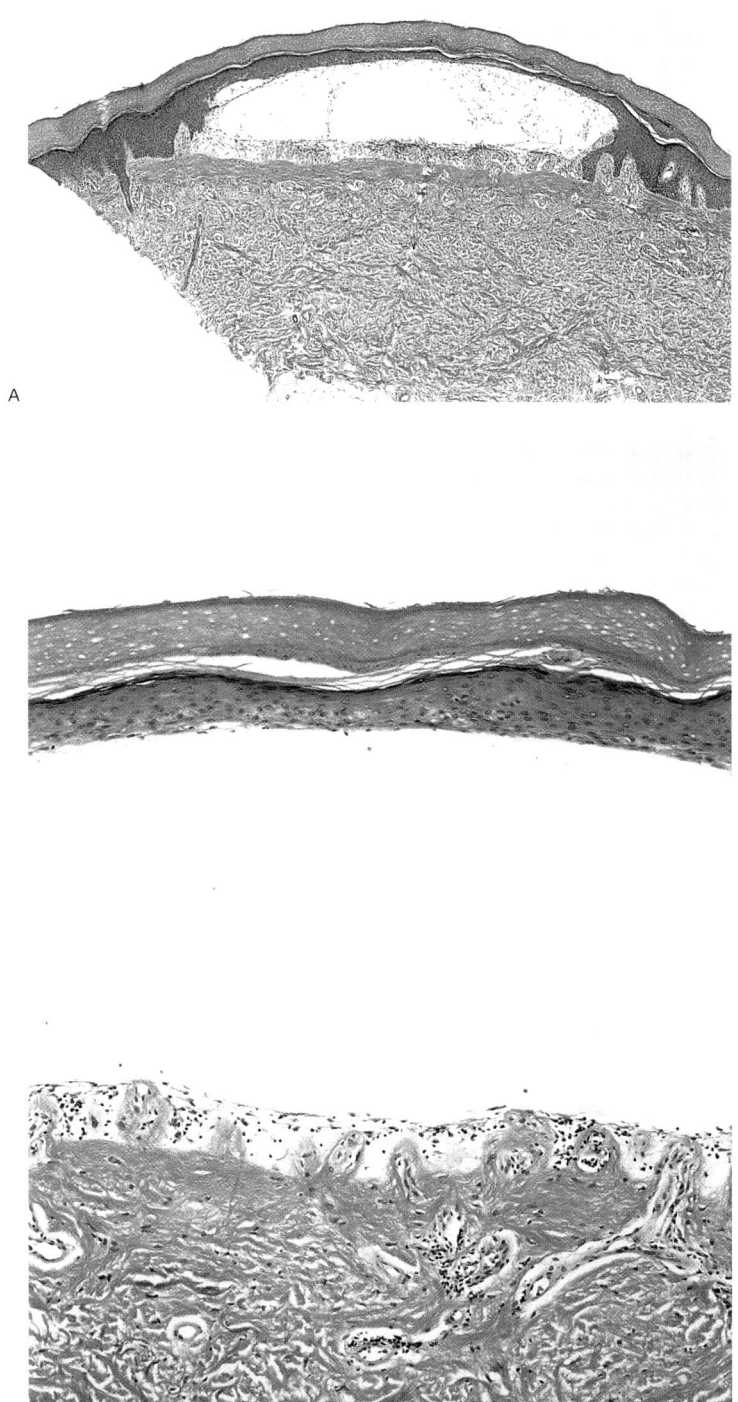

A

B

Fig. 18.11 **(A) Porphyria cutanea tarda. (B)** There is a cell-poor, subepidermal bulla with some 'festooning' in the base. (H & E)

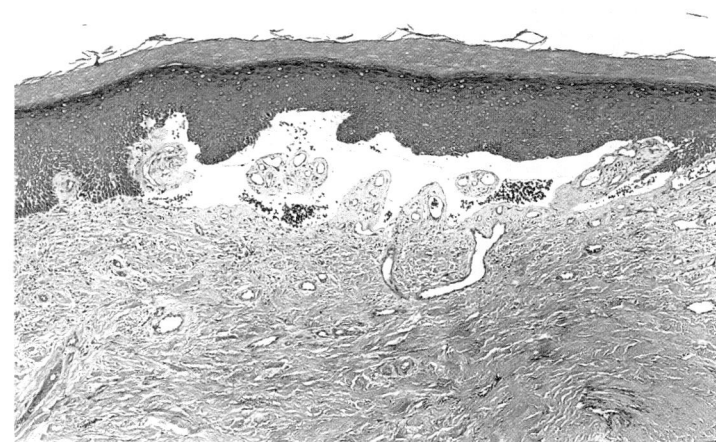

Fig. 18.12 **Pseudoporphyria.** There is some 'festooning' but the vessels within these areas have only thin walls. (H & E)

vessels.[482] Small deposits may also be found at the dermoepidermal junction.[362] Type IV collagen and laminin are additional components of the vascular and perivascular hyaline material which may be detected using monoclonal antibodies.[464,472]

Electron microscopy[471,472]

There is prominent reduplication of the basal laminae with encasement of the vessels in a concentric fashion. External to the laminae there is finely fibrillar material which also extends into the vessel wall.[471] Irregular clumps of amorphous material are also found in the perivascular regions.

Fine collagen fibrils are present within and around the vessels in the upper dermis, while the sclerodermoid lesions have fibrils with a bimodal size throughout the dermis.[483]

The 'caterpillar bodies' of PCT appear to be a combination of degenerating keratinocytes, colloid bodies and basement membrane bodies.[475]

Another ultrastructural finding in some of the porphyrias is reduplication of the basal lamina at the dermoepidermal junction. This is seen in PCT and variegate porphyria, but not usually in EPP.

In blisters the cleavage is usually dermolytic, with the roof containing a thin layer of dermal fibers still attached to the anchoring fibrils.[472] Early lesions appear to develop from the enlargement of membrane-limited vacuoles in the upper dermis.[484] Some of these appear to form in the pseudopodia of basal cells which protrude into the dermis.[484]

Finally, in one study of an acute flare reaction in EPP, endothelial cell damage was noted, leading to the suggestion that leakage of vascular contents contributes to the hyaline material.[485,486] The reduplication of the basal lamina may represent a reparative reaction to repeated endothelial injury.

Epidermal changes are usually mild in the various porphyrias. The epidermis in PCT may be normal, acanthotic or atrophic.[472] There is sometimes hyperkeratosis and mild hypergranulosis. In sclerodermoid lesions and in EPP there is sometimes effacement of the rete ridge pattern.

Direct immunofluorescence in the porphyrias reveals deposits of IgG and, less commonly, IgM and complement in and around the upper dermal

REFERENCES

Vitamin and dietary disturbances
1 Smith KE, Fenske NA. Cutaneous manifestations of alcohol abuse. J Am Acad Dermatol 2000; 43: 1–16.
2 Darmstadt GL, McGuire J, Ziboh VA. Malnutrition-associated rash of cystic fibrosis. Pediatr Dermatol 2000; 17: 337–347.
3 Gupta MA, Gupta AK, Haberman HF. Dermatologic signs in anorexia nervosa and bulimia nervosa. Arch Dermatol 1987; 123: 1386–1390.
4 Glorio R, Allevato M, De Pablo A et al. Prevalence of cutaneous manifestations in 200 patients with eating disorders. Int J Dermatol 2000; 39: 348–353.

5 Schulze UME, Pettke-Rank CV, Kreienkamp M et al. Dermatologic findings in anorexia and bulimia nervosa of childhood and adolescence. Pediatr Dermatol 1999; 16: 90–94.

6 Barthelemy H, Chouvet B, Cambazard F. Skin and mucosal manifestations in vitamin deficiency. J Am Acad Dermatol 1986; 15: 1263–1274.

7 Miller SJ. Nutritional deficiency and the skin. J Am Acad Dermatol 1989; 21: 1–30.

8 Prendiville JS, Manfredi LN. Skin signs of nutritional disorders. Semin Dermatol 1992; 11: 88–97.

9 Latham MC. The dermatosis of kwashiorkor in young children. Semin Dermatol 1991; 10: 270–272.

10 Eastlack JP, Grande KK, Levy ML, Nigro JF. Dermatosis in a child with Kwashiorkor secondary to food aversion. Pediatr Dermatol 1999; 16: 95–102.

11 Liu T, Howard RM, Mancini AJ et al. Kwashiorkor in the United States. Fad diets, perceived and true milk allergy, and nutritional ignorance. Arch Dermatol 2001; 137: 630–636.

12 Roe DA. Riboflavin deficiency: mucocutaneous signs of acute and chronic deficiency. Semin Dermatol 1991; 10: 293–295.

13 Hirschmann JV, Raugi GJ. Adult scurvy. J Am Acad Dermatol 1999; 41: 895–906.

14 Yalçin A, Ural AU, Beyan C et al. Scurvy presenting with cutaneous and articular signs and decrease in red and white blood cells. Int J Dermatol 1996; 35: 879–881.

15 Connelly TJ, Becker A, McDonald JW. Bachelor scurvy. Int J Dermatol 1982; 21: 209–211.

16 Chaine B, Cocheton J-J, Aractingi S. An odd case of abdominal purpura. Dermatology 2001; 202: 83.

17 Ellis CN, Vanderveen EE, Rasmussen JE. Scurvy. A case caused by peculiar dietary habits. Arch Dermatol 1984; 120: 1212–1214.

18 McKenna KE, Dawson JF. Scurvy occurring in a teenager. Clin Exp Dermatol 1993; 18: 75–77.

19 Ghorbani AJ, Eichler C. Scurvy. J Am Acad Dermatol 1994; 30: 881–883.

20 Shelton RM, Ryan MT. Scurvy: a case in a young healthy woman. J Am Acad Dermatol 1992; 27: 773–774.

21 Hashimoto K, Kitabchi AE, Duckworth WC, Robinson N. Ultrastructure of scorbutic human skin. Acta Derm Venereol 1970; 50: 9–21.

22 Bleasel NR, Stapleton KM, Lee M-S, Sullivan J. Vitamin A deficiency phrynoderma: Due to malabsorption and inadequate diet. J Am Acad Dermatol 1999; 41: 322–324.

23 Logan WS. Vitamin A and keratinization. Arch Dermatol 1972; 105: 748–753.

24 Wechsler HL. Vitamin A deficiency following small-bowel bypass surgery for obesity. Arch Dermatol 1979; 115: 73–75.

25 Welsh BM, Smith AL, Elder JE, Varigos GA. Night blindness precipitated by isotretinoin in the setting of hypovitaminosis A. Australas J Dermatol 1999; 40: 208–210.

26 Silverman AK, Ellis CN, Voorhees JJ. Hypervitaminosis A syndrome: a paradigm of retinoid side effects. J Am Acad Dermatol 1987; 16: 1027–1039.

27 Inkeles SB, Connor WE, Illingworth DR. Hepatic and dermatologic manifestations of chronic hypervitaminosis A in adults. Am J Med 1986; 80: 491–496.

28 Roe DA. Assessment of risk factors for carotenodermia and cutaneous signs of hypervitaminosis A in college-aged populations. Semin Dermatol 1991; 10: 303–308.

29 Sanders MN, Winkelmann RK. Cutaneous reactions to vitamin K. J Am Acad Dermatol 1988; 19: 699–704.

30 Gilliam JN, Cox AJ. Epidermal changes in vitamin B12 deficiency. Arch Dermatol 1973; 107: 231–236.

31 Hendricks WM. Pellagra and pellagralike dermatoses: etiology, differential diagnosis, dermatopathology, and treatment. Semin Dermatol 1991; 10: 282–292.

32 Isaac S. The "gauntlet" of pellagra. Int J Dermatol 1998; 37: 599.

33 Rapaport MJ. Pellagra in a patient with anorexia nervosa. Arch Dermatol 1985; 121: 255–257.

34 Judd LE, Poskitt BL. Pellagra in a patient with an eating disorder. Br J Dermatol 1991; 125: 71–72.

35 Kertesz SG. Pellagra in 2 homeless men. Mayo Clin Proc 2001; 76: 315–318.

36 Comaish JS, Felix RH, McGrath H. Topically applied niacinamide in isoniazid-induced pellagra. Arch Dermatol 1976; 112: 70–72.

37 Darvay A, Basarab T, McGregor JM, Russell-Jones R. Isoniazid induced pellagra despite pyridoxine supplementation. Clin Exp Dermatol 1999; 24: 167–170.

38 Stevens HP, Ostlere LS, Begent RHJ et al. Pellagra secondary to 5-fluorouracil. Br J Dermatol 1993; 128: 578–580.

39 Jarrett P, Duffill M, Oakley A, Smith A. Pellagra, azathioprine and inflammatory bowel disease. Clin Exp Dermatol 1997; 22: 44–45.

40 Wood B, Rademaker M, Oakley A, Wallace J. Pellagra in a woman using alternative remedies. Australas J Dermatol 1998; 39: 42–44.

41 Castiello RJ, Lynch PJ. Pellagra and the carcinoid syndrome. Arch Dermatol 1972; 105: 574–577.

42 El Zawahry M. Pellagra: notes and comments. Int J Dermatol 1973; 12: 158–162.

43 Findlay GH, Rein L, Mitchell D. Reactions to light on the normal and pellagrous Bantu skin. Br J Dermatol 1969; 81: 345–351.

Lysosomal storage diseases

44 Glewe RH, Basu A, Prence EM, Remaley AT. Biology of disease. Lysosomal storage diseases. Lab Invest 1985; 53: 250–269.

45 Dolman CL. Diagnosis of neurometabolic disorders by examination of skin biopsies and lymphocytes. Semin Diagn Pathol 1984; 1: 82–97.

46 Chen C-S, Patterson MC, Wheatley CL et al. Broad screening test for sphingolipid-storage diseases. Lancet 1999; 354: 901–905.

47 Agamanolis DP. The pathology of lysosomal storage diseases. Pathol Annu 1995; 30: 247–285.

48 Meikle PJ, Hopwood JJ, Clague AE, Carey WF. Prevalence of lysosomal storage disorders. JAMA 1999; 281: 249–254.

49 Brady RO. The sphingolipidoses. N Engl J Med 1966; 275: 312–318.

50 Volk DW, Adachi M, Schneck L. The gangliosidoses. Hum Pathol 1975; 6: 555–569.

51 Dolman CL, Chang E, Duke RJ. Pathologic findings in Sandhoff disease. Arch Pathol 1973; 96: 272–275.

52 Gebhart W. Heritable metabolic storage diseases. J Cutan Pathol 1985; 12: 348–357.

53 Takahashi K, Naito M, Suzuki Y. Lipid storage disease: Part III. Ultrastructural evaluation of cultured fibroblasts in sphingolipidoses. Acta Pathol Jpn 1987; 37: 261–272.

54 Drut R. Eccrine sweat gland involvement in GM1 gangliosidosis. J Cutan Pathol 1978; 5: 35–36.

55 O'Brien JS, Bernett J, Veath ML, Paa D. Lysosomal storage diseases. Diagnosis by ultrastructural examination of skin biopsy specimens. Arch Neurol 1975; 32: 592–599.

56 Peters SP, Lee RE, Glew RH. Gaucher's disease, a review. Medicine (Baltimore) 1977; 56: 425–442.

57 Lee RE, Robinson DB, Glew RH. Gaucher's disease. I. Modern enzymatic and anatomic methods of diagnosis. Arch Pathol Lab Med 1981; 105: 102–104.

58 Koprivica V, Stone DL, Park JK et al. Analysis and classification of 304 mutant alleles in patients with type 1 and type 3 Gaucher disease. Am J Hum Genet 2000; 66: 1777–1786.

59 Colombo R. Age estimate of the N370S mutation causing Gaucher disease in Ashkenazi Jews and European populations: a reappraisal of haplotype data. Am J Hum Genet 2000; 66: 692–697.

60 Diaz GA, Gelb BD, Risch N et al. Gaucher disease: the origins of the Ashkenazi Jewish N370S and 84GG acid β-glucosidase mutations. Am J Hum Genet 2000; 66: 1821–1832.

61 Wallace HJ. Anderson–Fabry disease. Br J Dermatol 1973; 88: 1–23.

62 Kang WH, Chun SI, Lee S. Generalized anhidrosis associated with Fabry's disease. J Am Acad Dermatol 1987; 17: 883–887.

63 Burkholder PM, Updike SJ, Ware RA, Reese OG. Clinicopathologic, enzymatic, and genetic features in a case of Fabry's disease. Arch Pathol Lab Med 1980; 104: 17–25.

64 Shelley ED, Shelley WB, Kurczynski TW. Painful fingers, heat intolerance, and telangiectases of the ear: easily ignored childhood signs of Fabry disease. Pediatr Dermatol 1995; 12: 215–219.

65 Voglino A, Paradisi M, Dompe G et al. Angiokeratoma corporis diffusum (Fabry's disease) with unusual features in a female patient. Light- and electron-microscopic investigation. Am J Dermatopathol 1988; 10: 343–348.

66 Handa Y, Yotsumoto S, Isobe E et al. A case of symptomatic heterozygous female Fabry's disease without detectable mutation in the alpha-galactosidase gene. Dermatology 2000; 200: 262–265.

67 Sagebiel RW, Parker F. Cutaneous lesions of Fabry's disease: glycolipid lipidosis. J Invest Dermatol 1968; 50: 208–213.

68 Nakamura T, Kaneko H, Nishino I. Angiokeratoma corporis diffusum (Fabry disease): ultrastructural studies of the skin. Acta Derm Venereol 1981; 61: 37–41.

69 Luderschmidt C, Wolff HH. Subtle clues to diagnosis of skin diseases by electron microscopy. Intracytoplasmic granules with lamellae as signs of heterozygous Fabry's disease. Am J Dermatopathol 1980; 2: 57–61.

70 Faraggiana T, Churg J, Grishman E et al. Light- and electron-microscopic histochemistry of Fabry's disease. Am J Pathol 1981; 103: 247–262.

71 Strayer DS, Santa Cruz D. Subtle clues to diagnosis of skin diseases by electron microscopy. Intracytoplasmic granules with lamellae in Fabry's disease. Am J Dermatopathol 1980; 2: 63–64.

72 Gebhart W, Lassmann H, Niebauer G. Demonstration of specific storage material within cutaneous nerves in metachromatic leukodystrophy. J Cutan Pathol 1978; 5: 5–14.

73 Takahashi K, Naito M. Lipid storage disease: Part II. Ultrastructural pathology of lipid storage cells in sphingolipidoses. Acta Pathol Jpn 1985; 35: 385–408.

74 Knobler RM, Becerano S, Gebhart W. Inborn errors of lipid metabolism – dermatological aspects. Clin Exp Dermatol 1988; 13: 365–370.

75 Chanoki M, Ishii M, Fukai K et al. Farber's lipogranulomatosis in siblings: light and electron microscopic studies. Br J Dermatol 1989; 121: 779–785.

76 Pavone L, Moser HW, Mollica F et al. Farber's lipogranulomatosis: ceramidase deficiency and prolonged survival in three relatives. Johns Hopkins Med J 1980; 147: 193–196.

77 Rauch HJ, Auböck L. 'Banana bodies' in disseminated lipogranulomatosis (Farber's disease). Am J Dermatopathol 1983; 5: 263–266.

78 Amirhakimi GH, Haghighi P, Ghalambor MA, Honari S. Familial lipogranulomatosis (Farber's disease). Clin Genet 1976; 9: 625–630.

79 Schmoeckel C. Subtle clues to diagnosis of skin diseases by electron microscopy. 'Farber bodies' in disseminated lipogranulomatosis (Farber's disease). Am J Dermatopathol 1980; 2: 153–156.

80 Crocker AC, Farber S. Niemann–Pick disease: a review of eighteen patients. Medicine (Baltimore) 1958; 37: 1–95.

81 Vanier MT, Wenger DA, Comly ME et al. Niemann–Pick disease group C: clinical variability and diagnosis based on defective cholesterol esterification. Clin Genet 1988; 33: 331–348.

82 Raddadi AA, Al Twaim AA. Type A Niemann–Pick disease. J Eur Acad Dermatol Venereol 2000; 14: 301–303.

83 Millat G, Marçais C, Rafi MA et al. Niemann–Pick C1 disease: the I1061T substitution is a frequent mutant allele in patients of Western European descent and correlates with a classic juvenile phenotype. Am J Hum Genet 1999; 65: 1321–1329.

84 Yamamoto T, Ninomiya H, Matsumoto M et al. Genotype-phenotype relationship of Niemann–Pick disease type C: a possible correlation between clinical onset and levels of NPC1 protein in isolated skin fibroblasts. J Med Genet 2000; 37: 707–711.

85 Mardini MK, Gergen P, Akhtar M, Ghandour M. Niemann–Pick disease: report of a case with skin involvement. Am J Dis Child 1982; 136: 650–651.

86 Toussaint M, Worret W-I, Drosner M, Marquardt K-H. Specific skin lesions in a patient with Niemann–Pick disease. Br J Dermatol 1994; 131: 895–897.

87 Wood WS, Dimmick JE, Dolman CL. Niemann–Pick disease and juvenile xanthogranuloma. Are they related? Am J Dermatopathol 1987; 9: 433–437.

88 Sibulkin D, Olichney JJ. Juvenile xanthogranuloma in a patient with Niemann–Pick disease. Arch Pathol 1973; 108: 829–831.

89 Schmuth M, Man M-Q, Weber F et al. Permeability barrier disorder in Niemann–Pick disease: sphingomyelin-ceramide processing required for normal barrier homeostasis. J Invest Dermatol 2000; 115: 459–466.

90 Young ID, Young EP, Mossman J et al. Neuraminidase deficiency: case report and review of the phenotype. J Med Genet 1987; 24: 283–290.

91 Sakuraba H, Suzuki Y, Akagi M et al. β-galactosidase-neuraminidase deficiency (galactosialidosis): clinical, pathological, and enzymatic studies in a postmortem case. Ann Neurol 1983; 13: 497–503.

92 Loonen MCB, Reuser AJJ, Visser P, Arts WFM. Combined sialidase (neuraminidase) and β-galactosidase deficiency. Clinical, morphological and enzymological observations in a patient. Clin Genet 1984; 26: 139–149.

93 Takahashi K, Naito M, Suzuki Y. Genetic mucopolysaccharidoses, mannosidosis, sialidosis, galactosialidosis, and I-cell disease. Ultrastructural analysis of cultured fibroblasts. Acta Pathol Jpn 1987; 37: 385–400.

94 Dvoretzky I, Fisher BK. Fucosidosis. Int J Dermatol 1979; 18: 213–216.

95 Willems PJ, Garcia CA, De Smedt MCH et al. Intrafamilial variability in fucosidosis. Clin Genet 1988; 34: 7–14.

96 Smith EB, Graham JL, Ledman JA, Snyder RD. Fucosidosis. Cutis 1977; 19: 195–198.

97 Kornfeld M, Snyder RD, Wenger DA. Fucosidosis with angiokeratoma. Electron microscopic changes in the skin. Arch Pathol Lab Med 1977; 101: 478–485.

98 Fleming C, Rennie A, Fallowfield M, McHenry PM. Cutaneous manifestations of fucosidosis. Br J Dermatol 1997; 136: 594–597.

99 Breier F, Hobisch G, Fang-Kircher S et al. Histology and electron microscopy of fucosidosis of the skin. Subtle clues to diagnosis by electron microscopy. Am J Dermatopathol 1995; 17: 379–383.

100 Epinette WW, Norins AL, Drew AL et al. Angiokeratoma corporis diffusum with α-L-fucosidase deficiency. Arch Dermatol 1973; 107: 754–757.

101 Dickersin GR, Lott IT, Kolodny EH, Dvorak AM. A light and electron microscopic study of mannosidosis. Hum Pathol 1980; 11: 245–256.

102 Slaugenhaupt SA, Acierno JS Jr, Helbling LA et al. Mapping of the mucolipidosis type IV gene to chromosome 19p and definition of founder haplotypes. Am J Hum Genet 1999; 65: 773–778.

103 Okada S, Kato T, Oshima T et al. Heterogeneity in mucolipidosis II (I-cell disease). Clin Genet 1983; 23: 155–159.

104 Ben-Yoseph Y, Mitchell DA, Nadler HL. First trimester prenatal evaluation for I-cell disease by N-acetyl-glucosamine 1-phosphotransferase assay. Clin Genet 1988; 33: 38–43.

105 Endo H, Miyazaki T, Asano S, Sagami S. Ultrastructural studies of the skin and cultured fibroblasts in I-cell disease. J Cutan Pathol 1987; 14: 309–317.

106 Kamiya M, Tada T, Kuhara H et al. I-cell disease. A case report and review of the literature. Acta Pathol Jpn 1986; 36: 1679–1692.

107 Dyken P, Krawiecki N. Neurodegenerative diseases of infancy and childhood. Ann Neurol 1983; 13: 351–364.

108 Carlesimo M, Giustini S, Rossodivita A et al. Late infantile ceroid-lipofuscinoses: an ultrastructural study. Am J Dermatopathol 1993; 15: 456–460.

109 Ishii M, Takahashi K, Hamada T et al. Cutaneous ultrastructural diagnosis of ceroid-lipofuscinosis. Br J Dermatol 1981; 104: 581–585.

110 Farrell DF, Sumi SM. Skin punch biopsy in the diagnosis of juvenile neuronal ceroid-lipofuscinosis. A comparison with leukocyte peroxidase assay. Arch Neurol 1977; 34: 39–44.

111 Manca V, Kanitakis J, Zambruno G et al. Ultrastructural study of the skin in a case of juvenile ceroid-lipofuscinosis. Am J Dermatopathol 1990; 12: 412–416.

Miscellaneous metabolic and systemic diseases

112 Poon E, Nixon R. Cutaneous spectrum of coeliac disease. Australas J Dermatol 2001; 42: 136–138.

113 Danbolt N. Acrodermatitis enteropathica. Br J Dermatol 1979; 100: 37–40.

114 Neldner KH, Hambidge KM, Walravens PA. Acrodermatitis enteropathica. Int J Dermatol 1978; 17: 380–387.

115 Weston WL, Huff JC, Humbert JR et al. Zinc correction of defective chemotaxis in acrodermatitis enteropathica. Arch Dermatol 1977; 113: 422–425.

116 Özkan Ş, Özkan H, Fetil E et al. Acrodermatitis enteropathica with *Pseudomonas aeruginosa* sepsis. Pediatr Dermatol 1999; 16: 444–447.

117 Traupe H, Happle R, Grobe H, Bertram HP. Polarization microscopy of hair in acrodermatitis enteropathica. Pediatr Dermatol 1986; 3: 300–303.

118 Sharma NL, Sharma RC, Gupta KR, Sharma RP. Self-limiting acrodermatitis enteropathica. A follow-up study of three interrelated families. Int J Dermatol 1988; 27: 485–486.

119 Bronson DM, Barsky R, Barsky S. Acrodermatitis enteropathica. Recognition at long last during a recurrence in a pregnancy. J Am Acad Dermatol 1983; 9: 140–144.

120 Owens CWI, Al-Khader AA, Jackson MJ, Prichard BNC. A severe 'stasis eczema', associated with low plasma zinc, treated successfully with oral zinc. Br J Dermatol 1981; 105: 461–464.

121 Stefanini M. Cutaneous bleeding related to zinc deficiency in two cases of advanced cancer. Cancer 1999; 86: 866–870.

122 Bonifazi E, Rigillo N, de Simone B, Meneghini CL. Acquired dermatitis to zinc deficiency in a premature infant. Acta Derm Venereol 1980; 60: 449–451.

123 Bilinski DL, Ehrenkranz RA, Cooley-Jacobs J, McGuire J. Symptomatic zinc deficiency in a breast-fed, premature infant. Arch Dermatol 1987; 123: 1221–1224.

124 Munro CS, Lazaro C, Lawrence CM. Symptomatic zinc deficiency in breast-fed premature infants. Br J Dermatol 1989; 121: 773–778.

125 Stapleton KM, O'Loughlin E, Relic JP. Transient zinc deficiency in a breast-fed premature infant. Australas J Dermatol 1995; 36: 157–159.

126 Buehning LJ, Goltz RW. Acquired zinc deficiency in a premature breast-fed infant. J Am Acad Dermatol 1993; 28: 499–501.

127 Glover MT, Atherton DJ. Transient zinc deficiency in two full-term breast-fed siblings associated with low maternal breast milk zinc concentration. Pediatr Dermatol 1988; 5: 10–13.

128 Bye AME, Goodfellow A, Atherton DJ. Transient zinc deficiency in a full-term breast-fed infant of normal birth weight. Pediatr Dermatol 1985; 2: 308–311.

129 Niemi KM, Anttila PH, Kanerva L, Johansson E. Histopathological study of transient acrodermatitis enteropathica due to decreased zinc in breast milk. J Cutan Pathol 1989; 16: 332–387.

130 Kuramoto Y, Igarashi Y, Tagami H. Acquired zinc deficiency in breast-fed infants. Semin Dermatol 1991; 10: 309–312.

131 Weismann K, Kvist N, Kobayasi T. Bullous acrodermatitis due to zinc deficiency during total parenteral nutrition: an ultrastructural study of the epidermal changes. Acta Derm Venereol 1983; 63: 143–146.

132 van Vloten WA, Bos LP. Skin lesions in acquired zinc deficiency due to parenteral nutrition. Dermatologica 1978; 156: 175–183.

133 Arlette JP, Johnston MM. Zinc deficiency dermatosis in premature infants receiving prolonged parenteral alimentation. J Am Acad Dermatol 1981; 5: 37–42.

134 McClain C, Soutor C, Zieve L. Zinc deficiency: a complication of Crohn's disease. Gastroenterology 1980; 78: 272–279.

135 Weismann K, Wadskov S, Mikkelsen HI et al. Acquired zinc deficiency dermatosis in man. Arch Dermatol 1978; 114: 1509–1511.

136 Jaffe AT, Heymann WR. Kwashiorkor/zinc deficiency overlap following partial gastrectomy. Int J Dermatol 1997; 37: 134–137.

137 Taniguchi S, Kaneto K, Hamada T. Acquired zinc deficiency associated with alcoholic liver cirrhosis. Int J Dermatol 1995; 34: 651–652.

138 Reichel M, Mauro TM, Ziboh VA et al. Acrodermatitis enteropathica in a patient with the acquired immunodeficiency syndrome. Arch Dermatol 1992; 128: 415–417.

139 Bosch AM, Sillevis Smitt JH, van Gennip AH et al. Iatrogenic isolated isoleucine deficiency as the cause of an acrodermatitis enteropathica-like syndrome. Br J Dermatol 1998; 139: 488–491.

140 Van Voorhees AS, Riba M. Acquired zinc deficiency in association with anorexia nervosa: case report and review of the literature. Pediatr Dermatol 1992; 9: 268–271.

141 Hansen RC, Lemen R, Revsin B. Cystic fibrosis manifesting with acrodermatitis enteropathica-like eruption. Arch Dermatol 1983; 119: 51–55.

142 Moynahan EJ. Acrodermatitis enteropathica: a lethal inherited human zinc-deficiency disorder. Lancet 1974; 2: 399–400.

143 Lynch WS, Roenigk HH Jr. Acrodermatitis enteropathica. Successful zinc therapy. Arch Dermatol 1976; 112: 1304–1307.

144 Bodemer C, de Prost Y, Bachollet B et al. Cutaneous manifestations of methylmalonic and propionic acidaemia: a description based on 38 cases. Br J Dermatol 1994; 131: 93–98.

145 Howard R, Frieden IJ, Crawford D et al. Methylmalonic acidemia, cobalamin C type, presenting with cutaneous manifestations. Arch Dermatol 1997; 133: 1563–1566.

146 Mock DM. Skin manifestions of biotin deficiency. Semin Dermatol 1991; 10: 296–302.

147 Navarro PC, Guerra A, Alvarez JG, Ortiz FJ. Cutaneous and neurologic manifestations of biotinidase deficiency. Int J Dermatol 2000; 39: 363–365.

148 Bénéton N, Wolkenstein P, Bagot M et al. Amicrobial pustulosis associated with autoimmune diseases: healing with zinc supplementation. Br J Dermatol 2000; 143: 1306–1310.

149 Gonzalez JR, Botet MV, Sanchez JL. The histopathology of acrodermatitis enteropathica. Am J Dermatopathol 1982; 4: 303–311.

150 Sjolin K-E. Zinc deficiency syndrome. J Cutan Pathol 1979; 6: 88–89.

151 Borroni G, Brazzelli V, Vignati G et al. Bullous lesions in acrodermatitis enteropathica. Histopathologic findings regarding two patients. Am J Dermatopathol 1992; 14: 304–309.

152 Brazin SA, Taylor Johnson W, Abramson LJ. The acrodermatitis enteropathica-like syndrome. Arch Dermatol 1979; 115: 597–599.

153 Mori H, Matsumoto Y, Tamada Y, Ohashi M. Apoptotic cell death in formation of vesicular skin lesions in patients with acquired zinc deficiency. J Cutan Pathol 1996; 23: 359–363.

154 Juljulian HH, Kurban AK. Acantholysis: a feature of acrodermatitis enteropathica. Arch Dermatol 1971; 103: 105–106.

155 Yoshikuni K, Tagami H, Yamada M et al. Erythematosquamous skin lesions in hereditary lactate dehydrogenase M-subunit deficiency. Arch Dermatol 1986; 122: 1420–1424.

156 Takayasu S, Fujiwara S, Waki T. Hereditary lactate dehydrogenase M-subunit deficiency: lactate dehydrogenase activity in skin lesions and in hair follicles. J Am Acad Dermatol 1991; 24: 339–342.

157 Nazzari G, Crovato F. Annually recurring acroerythema and hereditary lactate dehydrogenase M-subunit deficiency. J Am Acad Dermatol 1992; 27: 262–263.

158 Ginsburg R, Robertson A Jr, Michel B. Acrodermatitis enteropathica. Arch Dermatol 1976; 112: 653–660.

159 Leichter SB. Clinical and metabolic aspects of glucagonoma. Medicine (Baltimore) 1980; 59: 100–113.

160 Hashizume T, Kiryu H, Noda K et al. Glucagonoma syndrome. J Am Acad Dermatol 1988; 19: 377–383.

161 Schwartz RA. Glucagonoma and pseudoglucagonoma syndromes. Int J Dermatol 1997; 36: 81–89.

162 Alkemade JAC, van Tongeren JHM, van Haelst UJGM et al. Delayed diagnosis of glucagonoma syndrome. Clin Exp Dermatol 1999; 24: 455–457.

163 Vandersteen PR, Scheithauer BW. Glucagonoma syndrome. A clinicopathologic, immunocytochemical, and ultrastructural study. J Am Acad Dermatol 1985; 12: 1032–1039.

164 Walker NPJ. Atypical necrolytic migratory erythema in association with a jejunal adenocarcinoma. J R Soc Med 1982; 75: 134–135.

165 Thorisdottir K, Camisa C, Tomecki KJ, Bergfeld WF. Necrolytic migratory erythema: a report of three cases. J Am Acad Dermatol 1994; 30: 324–329.

166 Wilkinson SM, Cartwright PH, Allen C et al. Necrolytic migratory erythema: association with neuroendocrine tumour with predominant insulin secretion. Br J Dermatol 1990; 123: 801–805.

167 Doyle JA, Schroeter AL, Rogers RS III. Hyperglucagonaemia and necrolytic migratory erythema in cirrhosis – possible pseudoglucagonoma syndrome. Br J Dermatol 1979; 100: 581–587.

168 Blackford S, Wright S, Roberts DL. Necrolytic migratory erythema without glucagonoma: the role of dietary essential fatty acids. Br J Dermatol 1991; 125: 460–462.

169 Mullans EA, Cohen PR. Iatrogenic necrolytic migratory erythema: A case report and review of nonglucagonoma-associated necrolytic migratory erythema. J Am Acad Dermatol 1998; 38: 866–873.

170 Franchimont C, Piergard GE, Luyckx AS et al. Angioplastic necrolytic migratory erythema. Am J Dermatopathol 1982; 4: 485–495.

171 Marinkovich MP, Botella R, Datloff J, Sangueza OP. Necrolytic migratory erythema without glucagonoma in patients with liver disease. J Am Acad Dermatol 1995; 32: 604–609.

172 Kasper CS, McMurry K. Necrolytic migratory erythema without glucagonoma versus canine superficial necrolytic dermatitis: is hepatic impairment a clue to pathogenesis? J Am Acad Dermatol 1991; 25: 534–541.

173 Sinclair SA, Reynolds NJ. Necrolytic migratory erythema and zinc deficiency. Br J Dermatol 1997; 136: 783–785.

174 Delaporte E, Catteau B, Piette F. Necrolytic migratory erythema-like eruption in zinc deficiency associated with alcoholic liver disease. Br J Dermatol 1997; 137: 1027–1028.

175 Binnick AN, Spencer SK, Dennison WL Jr, Horton ES. Glucagonoma syndrome. Report of two cases and literature review. Arch Dermatol 1977; 113: 749–754.

176 Van der Loos TLJM, Lambrecht ER, Lambers JCCA. Successful treatment of glucagonoma-related necrolytic migratory erythema with decarbazine. J Am Acad Dermatol 1987; 16: 468–472.

177 Peterson LL, Shaw JC, Acott KM et al. Glucagonoma syndrome: in vitro evidence that glucagon increases epidermal arachidonic acid. J Am Acad Dermatol 1984; 11: 468–473.

178 Kheir SM, Omura EF, Grizzle WE et al. Histologic variation in the skin lesions of the glucagonoma syndrome. Am J Surg Pathol 1986; 10: 445–453.

179 Swenson KH, Amon RB, Hanifin JM. The glucagonoma syndrome. A distinctive cutaneous marker of systemic disease. Arch Dermatol 1978; 114: 224–228.

180 Parker CM, Hanke CW, Madura JA, Liss EC. Glucagonoma syndrome: case report and literature review. J Dermatol Surg Oncol 1984; 10: 884–889.

181 Kahan RS, Perez-Figaredo RA, Neimanis A. Necrolytic migratory erythema. Distinctive dermatosis of the glucagonoma syndrome. Arch Dermatol 1977; 113: 792–797.

182 Katz R, Fischmann AB, Galotto J et al. Necrolytic migratory erythema, presenting as candidiasis, due to a pancreatic glucagonoma. Cancer 1979; 44: 558–563.

183 Long CC, Laidler P, Holt PJA. Suprabasal acantholysis – an unusual feature of necrolytic migratory erythema. Clin Exp Dermatol 1993; 18: 464–467.

184 Hunt SJ, Narus VT, Abell E. Necrolytic migratory erythema: dyskeratotic dermatitis, a clue to early diagnosis. J Am Acad Dermatol 1991; 24: 473–477.

185 Ohyama K, Kitoh M, Arao T. Ultrastructural studies of necrolytic migratory erythema. Arch Dermatol 1982; 118: 679–682.

186 Khanna VJ, Shieh S, Benjamin J et al. Necrolytic acral erythema associated with hepatitis C. Effective treatment with interferon alfa and zinc. Arch Dermatol 2000; 136: 755–757.

187 El Darouti M, El Ela MA. Necrolytic acral erythema: a cutaneous marker of viral hepatitis C. Int J Dermatol 1996; 35: 252–256.

188 Baron DN, Dent CE, Harris H et al. Hereditary pellagra-like skin rash with temporary cerebellar ataxia, constant renal amino-aciduria, and other bizarre biochemical features. Lancet 1956; 2: 421–428.

189 Wong PWK, Pillai PM. Clinical and biochemical observations in two cases of Hartnup disease. Arch Dis Child 1966; 41: 383–388.

190 Oakley A, Wallace J. Hartnup disease presenting in an adult. Clin Exp Dermatol 1994; 19: 407–408.

191 Freundlich E, Statter M, Yatziv S. Familial pellagra-like skin rash with neurological manifestations. Arch Dis Child 1981; 56: 146–148.

192 Freij BJ, Der Kaloustian VM. Prolidase deficiency. A metabolic disorder presenting with dermatologic signs. Int J Dermatol 1986; 25: 431–433.

193 Milligan A, Graham-Brown RAC, Burns DA, Anderson I. Prolidase deficiency: a case report and literature review. Br J Dermatol 1989; 121: 405–409.

194 Bissonnette R, Friedmann D, Giroux J-M et al. Prolidase deficiency: a multisystemic hereditary disorder. J Am Acad Dermatol 1993; 29: 818–821.

195 Monafo V, Marseglia GL, Maghnie M et al. Transient beneficial effect of GH replacement therapy and topical GH application on skin ulcers in a boy with prolidase deficiency. Pediatr Dermatol 2000; 17: 227–230.

196 Dyne K, Zanaboni G, Bertazzoni M et al. Mild, late onset prolidase deficiency: another Italian case. Br J Dermatol 2001; 144: 635–636.

197 Der Kaloustian VM, Freij BJ, Kurban AK. Prolidase deficiency: an inborn error of metabolism with major dermatological manifestations. Dermatologica 1982; 164: 293–304.

198 Sheffield LJ, Schlesinger P, Faull K et al. Iminopeptiduria, skin ulcerations, and edema in a boy with prolidase deficiency. J Pediatr 1977; 91: 578–583.

199 Leoni A, Cetta G, Tenni R et al. Prolidase deficiency in two siblings with chronic leg ulcerations. Arch Dermatol 1987; 123: 493–499.

200 Fimiani M, Rubegni P, de Aloe G et al. Squamous cell carcinoma of the leg in a patient with prolidase deficiency. Br J Dermatol 1999; 140: 362–363.

201 Arata J, Umemura S, Yamamoto Y et al. Prolidase deficiency. Its dermatological manifestations and some additional biochemical studies. Arch Dermatol 1979; 115: 62–67.

202 Pierard GE, Cornil F, Lapiere CM. Pathogenesis of ulcerations in deficiency of prolidase. The role of angiopathy and of deposits of amyloid. Am J Dermatopathol 1984; 6: 491–497.

203 Ogata A, Tanaka S, Tomoda T et al. Autosomal recessive prolidase deficiency. Three patients with recalcitrant leg ulcers. Arch Dermatol 1981; 117: 689–694.

204 Yasuda K, Ogata K, Kariya K et al. Corticosteroid treatment of prolidase deficiency skin lesions by inhibiting iminodipeptide-primed neutrophil superoxide generation. Br J Dermatol 1999; 141: 846–851.

205 Ferrans VJ, Fredrickson DS. The pathology of Tangier disease. A light and electron microscopic study. Am J Pathol 1975; 78: 101–158.

206 Herbert PN, Forte T, Heinen RJ, Fredrickson DS. Tangier disease. One explanation of lipid storage. N Engl J Med 1978; 299: 519–521.

207 Waldorf DS, Levy RI, Fredrickson DS. Cutaneous cholesterol ester deposition in Tangier disease. Arch Dermatol 1967; 95: 161–165.

208 White JW Jr, Gomez MR. Diagnosis of Lafora disease by skin biopsy. J Cutan Pathol 1988; 15: 171–175.

209 Busard BLSM, Renier WO, Gabreels FJM et al. Lafora's disease. Arch Neurol 1986; 43: 296–299.

210 Karimipour D, Lowe L, Blaivas M et al. Lafora disease: Diagnosis by skin biopsy. J Am Acad Dermatol 1999; 41: 790–792.

211 Carpenter S, Karpati G. Sweat gland duct cells in Lafora disease: diagnosis by skin biopsy. Neurology 1981; 31: 1564–1568.

212 Idoate MA, Vazquez JJ, Soto J, de Castro P. Diagnosis of Lafora's disease in apocrine sweat glands of the axilla. Am J Dermatopathol 1991; 13: 410–413.

213 Paller AS. Cutaneous changes associated with inflammatory bowel disease. Pediatr Dermatol 1986; 3: 439–445.

214 Greenstein AJ, Janowitz HD, Sachar DB. The extra-intestinal complications of Crohn's disease and ulcerative colitis: a study of 700 patients. Medicine (Baltimore) 1976; 55: 401–412.

215 Verbov JL. The skin in patients with Crohn's disease and ulcerative colitis. Trans St John's Hosp Dermatol Soc 1973; 59: 30–36.

216 Gregory B, Ho VC. Cutaneous manifestations of gastrointestinal disorders. Part II. J Am Acad Dermatol 1992; 26: 371–383.

217 Apgar JT. Newer aspects of inflammatory bowel disease and its cutaneous manifestations: a selective review. Semin Dermatol 1991; 10: 138–147.

218 Johnson ML, Wilson HTH. Skin lesions in ulcerative colitis. Gut 1969; 10: 255–263.

219 Croft CB, Wilkinson AR. Ulceration of the mouth, pharynx, and larynx in Crohn's disease of the intestine. Br J Surg 1972; 59: 249–252.

220 Goslen JB, Graham W, Lazarus GS. Cutaneous polyarteritis nodosa. Report of a case associated with Crohn's disease. Arch Dermatol 1983; 119: 326–329.

221 Matsumura Y, Mizuno K, Ohta K et al. A case of cutaneous polyarteritis nodosa associated with ulcerative colitis. Br J Dermatol 2000; 142: 561–562.

222 Yates VM, Watkinson G, Kelman A. Further evidence for an association between psoriasis, Crohn's disease and ulcerative colitis. Br J Dermatol 1982; 106: 323–330.

223 Nevile BW, Laden SA, Smith SE et al. Pyostomatitis vegetans. Am J Dermatopathol 1985; 7: 69–77.

224 Ballo FS, Camisa C, Allen CM. Pyostomatitis vegetans. Report of a case and review of the literature. J Am Acad Dermatol 1989; 21: 381–387.

225 VanHale HM, Rogers RS III, Zone JJ, Greipp PR. Pyostomatitis vegetans. A reactive mucosal marker for inflammatory disease of the gut. Arch Dermatol 1985; 121: 94–98.

226 Brenner SM, Delany HM. Erythema multiforme and Crohn's disease of the large intestine. Gastroenterology 1972; 62: 479–482.

227 Monroe EW. Vitiligo associated with regional enteritis. Arch Dermatol 1976; 112: 833–834.

228 McPoland PR, Moss RL. Cutaneous Crohn's disease and progressive vitiligo. J Am Acad Dermatol 1988; 19: 421–425.

229 McCallum DI, Kinmont PDC. Dermatological manifestations of Crohn's disease. Br J Dermatol 1968; 80: 1–8.

230 Morales MS, Marini M, Caminero M, Caglio P. Perianal Crohn's disease. Int J Dermatol 2000; 39: 616–618.

231 Rankin GB, Watts HD, Melnyk CS, Kelley ML Jr. National Cooperative Crohn's Disease Study: extraintestinal manifestations and perianal complications. Gastroenterology 1979; 77: 914–920.

232 Burgdorf W. Cutaneous manifestations of Crohn's disease. J Am Acad Dermatol 1981; 5: 689–695.

233 Frankel DH, Mostofi RS, Lorincz AL. Oral Crohn's disease: report of two cases in brothers with metallic dysgeusia and a review of the literature. J Am Acad Dermatol 1985; 12: 260–268.

234 Dupuy A, Cosnes J, Revuz J et al. Oral Crohn disease. Clinical characteristics and long-term follow-up of 9 cases. Arch Dermatol 1999; 135: 439–442.

235 Borradori L, Saada V, Rybojad M et al. Oral intraepidermal IgA pustulosis and Crohn's disease. Br J Dermatol 1992; 126: 383–386.

236 Kano Y, Shiohara T, Yagita A, Nagashima M. Association between cheilitis granulomatosa and Crohn's disease. J Am Acad Dermatol 1993; 28: 801.

237 Walker KD, Badame AJ. Erythema elevatum diutinum in a patient with Crohn's disease. J Am Acad Dermatol 1990; 22: 948–952.

238 Matheson BK, Gilbertson EO, Eichenfield LF. Vesiculopustular eruption of Crohn's disease.

239 Smoller BR, Weishar M, Gray MH. An unusual cutaneous manifestation of Crohn's disease. Arch Pathol Lab Med 1990; 114: 609–610.

240 Ray TL, Levine JB, Weiss W, Ward PA. Epidermolysis bullosa acquisita and inflammatory bowel disease. J Am Acad Dermatol 1982; 6: 242–252.

241 McAuley D, Miller RA. Acne fulminans associated with inflammatory bowel disease. Report of a case. Arch Dermatol 1985; 121: 91–93.

242 McHenry PM, Hudson M, Smart LM et al. Pyoderma faciale in a patient with Crohn's disease. Clin Exp Dermatol 1992; 17: 460–462.

243 Berkowitz EZ, Lebwohl M. Cutaneous manifestations of inflammatory bowel disease. J Eur Acad Dermatol Venereol 2000; 14: 349–350.

244 Chalvardjian A, Nethercott JR. Cutaneous granulomatous vasculitis associated with Crohn's disease. Cutis 1982; 30: 645–655.

245 Levine N, Bangert J. Cutaneous granulomatosis in Crohn's disease. Arch Dermatol 1982; 118: 006–1009.

246 Lebwohl M, Fleischmajer R, Janowitz H et al. Metastatic Crohn's disease. J Am Acad Dermatol 1984; 10: 33–38.

247 Shum DT, Guenther L. Metastatic Crohn's disease. Case report and review of the literature. Arch Dermatol 1990; 126: 645–648.

248 Buckley C, Bayoumi A-HM, Sarkany I. Metastatic Crohn's disease. Clin Exp Dermatol 1990; 15: 131–133.

249 Peltz S, Vestey JP, Ferguson A et al. Disseminated metastatic cutaneous Crohn's disease. Clin Exp Dermatol 1993; 18: 55–59.

250 Kolansky G, Kimbrough-Green C, Dubin HV. Metastatic Crohn's disease of the face: an uncommon presentation. Arch Dermatol 1993; 129: 1348–1349.

251 Mooney EE, Sweeney E, Barnes L. Granulomatous leg ulcers: an unusual presentation of Crohn's disease in a young man. J Am Acad Dermatol 1993; 28: 115–117.

252 Cummins RE, Mullins D, Smith LJ, Ford MJ. Metastatic Crohn's disease: a case report. Pediatr Dermatol 1996; 13: 25–28.

253 Chen W, Blume-Peytavi U, Goerdt S, Orfanos CE. Metastatic Crohn's disease of the face. J Am Acad Dermatol 1996; 35: 986–988.

254 McLelland J, Griffin SM. Metastatic Crohn's disease of the umbilicus. Clin Exp Dermatol 1996; 21: 318–319.

255 Gilson RT, Elston D, Pruitt A. Metastatic Crohn's disease: Remission induced by mesalamine and prednisone. J Am Acad Dermatol 1999; 41: 476–479.

256 Vettraino IM, Merritt DF. Crohn's disease of the vulva. Am J Dermatopathol 1995; 17: 410–413.

257 Werlin SL, Esterly NB, Oechler H. Crohn's disease presenting as unilateral labial hypertrophy. J Am Acad Dermatol 1992; 27: 893–895.

258 Kim N-I, Eom J-Y, Sim W-Y, Haw C-R. Crohn's disease of the vulva. J Am Acad Dermatol 1992; 27: 764–765.

259 Urbanek M, Neill SM, McKee PH. Vulval Crohn's disease: difficulties in diagnosis. Clin Exp Dermatol 1996; 21: 211–214.

260 Acker SM, Sahn EE, Rogers HC et al. Genital cutaneous Crohn disease. Two cases with unusual clinical and histopathologic features in young men. Am J Dermatopathol 2000; 22: 443–446.

261 Ploysangam T, Heubi JE, Eisen D et al. Cutaneous Crohn's disease in children. J Am Acad Dermatol 1997; 36: 697–704.

262 Lin C, Bass J, Somach S. Cutaneous Crohn's disease in a child. J Cutan Pathol 2000; 27: 541 (abstract).

263 Burgdorf W, Orkin M. Granulomatous perivasculitis in Crohn's disease. Arch Dermatol 1981; 117: 674–675.

264 Callen JP. Severe cutaneous vasculitis complicating ulcerative colitis. Arch Dermatol 1979; 115: 226–227.

265 Basler RSW. Ulcerative colitis and the skin. Med Clin North Am 1980; 64: 941–954.

266 Salmon P, Rademaker M, Edwards L. A continuum of neutrophilic disease occurring in a patient with ulcerative colitis. Australas J Dermatol 1998; 39: 116–118.

267 Fenske NA, Gern JE, Pierce D, Vasey FB. Vesiculopustular eruption of ulcerative colitis. Arch Dermatol 1983; 119: 664–669.

268 O Loughlin S, Perry HO. A diffuse pustular eruption associated with ulcerative colitis. Arch Dermatol 1978; 114: 1061–1064.

269 Warin AP. The pustular eruption of ulcerative colitis. Br J Dermatol 1998; 139: 758.

270 Sarkany RPE, Burrows NP, Grant JW et al. The pustular eruption of ulcerative colitis: a variant of Sweet's syndrome? Br J Dermatol 1998; 138: 365–366.

271 Shoji T, Ali S, Gateva E et al. A granulomatous dermatitis associated with idiopathic ulcerative colitis. Int J Dermatol 2000; 39: 215–217.

272 Misbah SA, Mapstone NP. Whipple's disease revisited. J Clin Pathol 2000; 53: 750–755.

273 Comer GM, Brandt LJ, Abissi CJ. Whipple's disease: a review. Am J Gastroenterol 1983; 78: 107–114.

Pediatr Dermatol 1996; 13: 127–130.

274 Good AE, Beals TF, Simmons JL, Ibrahim MAH. A subcutaneous nodule with Whipple's disease: key to early diagnosis? Arthritis Rheum 1980; 23: 856–859.

275 Kwee D, Fields JP, King LE Jr. Subcutaneous Whipple's disease. J Am Acad Dermatol 1987; 16: 188–190.

276 Balestrieri GP, Villanacci V, Battocchio S et al. Cutaneous involvement in Whipple's disease. Br J Dermatol 1996; 135: 666–668.

277 Darmstadt GL, Schmidt CP, Wechsler DS et al. Dermatitis as a presenting sign of cystic fibrosis. Arch Dermatol 1992; 128: 1358–1364.

278 Haroon TS. Diabetes and skin – a review. Scott Med J 1974; 19: 257–267.

279 Gouterman IH, Sibrack LA. Cutaneous manifestations of diabetes. Cutis 1980; 25: 45–56.

280 Jelinek JE. Cutaneous manifestations of diabetes mellitus. Int J Dermatol 1994; 33: 605–617.

281 Perez MI, Kohn SR. Cutaneous manifestations of diabetes mellitus. J Am Acad Dermatol 1994; 30: 519–531.

282 Huntley AC. The cutaneous manifestations of diabetes. J Am Acad Dermatol 1982; 7: 427–455.

283 Lugo-Somolinos A, Sánchez JL. Prevalence of dermatophytosis in patients with diabetes. J Am Acad Dermatol 1992; 26: 408–410.

284 Hanna W, Friesen D, Bombardier C et al. Pathologic features of diabetic thick skin. J Am Acad Dermatol 1987; 16: 546–553.

285 Huntley AC. Finger pebbles: a common finding in diabetes mellitus. J Am Acad Dermatol 1986; 14: 612–617.

286 Cabo HA. Thick skin syndrome in diabetes mellitus. J Eur Acad Dermatol Venereol 2000; 14: 143–144.

287 Libecco JF, Brodell RT. Finger pebbles and diabetes: a case with broad involvement of the dorsal fingers and hands. Arch Dermatol 2001; 137: 510–511.

288 Bernstein JE, Levine LE, Medenica MM et al. Reduced threshold to suction-induced blister formation in insulin-dependent diabetics. J Am Acad Dermatol 1983; 8: 790–791.

289 Sibbald RG, Schachter RK. The skin and diabetes mellitus. Int J Dermatol 1984; 23: 567–584.

290 Cox NH, McCruden D, McQueen A et al. Histological findings in clinically normal skin of patients with insulin-dependent diabetes. Clin Exp Dermatol 1987; 12: 250–255.

291 Sueki H. Diabetic microangiopathy in subcutaneous fatty tissue. J Cutan Pathol 1987; 14: 217–222.

292 Cox NH, More IA, McCruden D et al. Electron microscopy of clinically normal skin of diabetic patients. Clin Exp Dermatol 1988; 13: 11–15.

293 Shemer A, Bergman R, Linn S et al. Diabetic dermopathy and internal complications in diabetes mellitus. Int J Dermatol 1998; 37: 113–115.

294 Danowski TS, Sabeh G, Sarver ME et al. Skin spots and diabetes mellitus. Am J Med Sci 1966; 251: 570–575.

295 Bauer M, Levan NE. Diabetic dermopathy. Br J Dermatol 1970; 83: 528–535.

296 Bauer MF, Levan NE, Frankel A, Bach J. Pigmented pretibial patches. A cutaneous manifestation of diabetes mellitus. Arch Dermatol 1966; 93: 282–286.

297 Fisher ER, Danowski TS. Histologic, histochemical, and electron microscopic features of the skin spots of diabetes mellitus. Am J Clin Pathol 1968; 50: 547–554.

298 Toonstra J. Bullosis diabeticorum. Report of a case with a review of the literature. J Am Acad Dermatol 1985; 13: 799–805.

299 Rocca FF, Pereyra E. Phlyctenar lesions in the feet of diabetic patients. Diabetes 1963; 12: 220–223.

300 Derighetti M, Hohl D, Krayenbühl BH, Panizzon RG. Bullosis diabeticorum in a newly discovered type 2 diabetes mellitus. Dermatology 2000; 200: 366–367.

301 Bernstein JE, Medenica M, Soltani K, Griem SF. Bullous eruption of diabetes mellitus. Arch Dermatol 1979; 115: 324–325.

302 Chuang T-Y, Korkij W, Soltani K et al. Increased frequency of diabetes mellitus in patients with bullous pemphigoid: a case-control study. J Am Acad Dermatol 1984; 11: 1099–1102.

303 Paltzik RL. Bullous eruption of diabetes mellitus. Bullosis diabeticorum. Arch Dermatol 1980; 116: 475–476.

304 James WD, Odom RB, Goette DK. Bullous eruption of diabetes mellitus. A case with positive immunofluorescence microscopy findings. Arch Dermatol 1980; 116: 1191–1192.

305 Kurwa A, Roberts P, Whitehead R. Concurrence of bullous and atrophic skin lesions in diabetes mellitus. Arch Dermatol 1971; 103: 670–675.

306 Basarab T, Munn SE, McGrath J, Russell Jones R. Bullosis diabeticorum. A case report and literature review. Clin Exp Dermatol 1995; 20: 218–220.

307 Goodfield MJD, Millard LG, Harvey L, Jeffcoate WJ. Bullosis diabeticorum. J Am Acad Dermatol 1986; 15: 1292–1294.

308 Magnus IA. The porphyrias. Semin Dermatol 1982; 1: 197–210.

309 Elder GH. Enzymatic defects in porphyria: an overview. Semin Liver Dis 1982; 2: 87–99.

310 Elder GH. The cutaneous porphyrias. Semin Dermatol 1990; 9: 63–69.

311 Moore MR, Disler PB. Chemistry and biochemistry of the porphyrins and porphyrias. Clin Dermatol 1985; 3: 7–23.

312 Mascaro JM. Porphyrias in children. Pediatr Dermatol 1992; 9: 371–372.

313 Paslin DA. The porphyrias. Int J Dermatol 1992; 31: 527–539.

314 Meola T, Lim HW. The porphyrias. Dermatol Clin 1993; 11: 583–596.

315 Young JW, Conte ET. Porphyrias and porphyrins. Int J Dermatol 1991; 30: 399–406.

316 Thadani H, Deacon A, Peters T. Diagnosis and management of porphyria. BMJ 2000; 320: 1647–1651.

317 Murphy GM. The cutaneous porphyrias: a review. Br J Dermatol 1999; 140: 573–581.

318 Elder GH. Update on enzyme and molecular defects in porphyria. Photodermatol Photoimmunol Photomed 1998; 14: 66–69.

319 Elder GH. Recent advances in the identification of enzyme deficiencies in the porphyrias. Br J Dermatol 1983; 108: 729–734.

320 Elder GH. Metabolic abnormalities in the porphyrias. Semin Dermatol 1986; 5: 88–98.

321 Thiers BH. The porphyrias. J Am Acad Dermatol 1981; 5: 621–625.

322 Mallon E, Wojnarowska F, Hope P, Elder G. Neonatal bullous eruption as a result of transient porphyrinemia in a premature infant with hemolytic disease of the newborn. J Am Acad Dermatol 1995; 33: 333–336.

323 Crawford RI, Lawlor ER, Wadsworth LD, Prendiville JS. Transient erythroporphyria of infancy. J Am Acad Dermatol 1996; 35: 833–834.

324 Tefferi A, Colgan JP, Solberg LA Jr. Acute porphyrias: diagnosis and management. Mayo Clin Proc 1994; 69: 991–995.

325 Targovnik SE, Targovnik JH. Cutaneous drug reactions in porphyrias. Clin Dermatol 1986; 4: 110–117.

326 Harber LC, Poh-Fitzpatrick M, Walther RR, Grossman ME. Cutaneous aspects of the porphyrias. Acta Derm Venereol (Suppl) 1982; 100: 9–15.

327 Poh-Fitzpatrick MB. Porphyrin-sensitized cutaneous photosensitivity. Pathogenesis and treatment. Clin Dermatol 1985; 3: 41–82.

328 Hunter GA. Clinical manifestations of the porphyrias: a review. Australas J Dermatol 1979; 20: 120–122.

329 Poh-Fitzpatrick MB. Pathogenesis and treatment of photocutaneous manifestations of the porphyrias. Semin Liver Dis 1982; 2: 164–176.

330 Batlle AM del C. Tetrapyrrole biosynthesis. Semin Dermatol 1986; 5: 70–87.

331 Mustajoki P. Acute intermittent porphyria. Semin Dermatol 1986; 5: 155–160.

332 Doss M. Enzymatic deficiencies in acute hepatic porphyrias: porphobilinogen synthase deficiency. Semin Dermatol 1986; 5: 161–168.

333 Roberts DT, Brodie MJ, Moore MR et al. Hereditary coproporphyria presenting with photosensitivity induced by the contraceptive pill. Br J Dermatol 1977; 96: 549–554.

334 Sheth AP, Esterly NB, Rabinowitz LG, Poh-Fitzpatrick MB. Cutaneous porphyrialike photosensitivity after liver transplantation. Arch Dermatol 1994; 130: 614–617.

335 Lane PR, Massey KL, Worobetz LJ et al. Acute hereditary coproporphyria induced by the androgenic/anabolic steroid methandrostenolone (Dianabol). J Am Acad Dermatol 1994; 30: 308–312.

336 Day RS. Variegate porphyria. Semin Dermatol 1986; 5: 138–154.

337 Corey TJ, DeLeo VA, Christianson H, Poh-Fitzpatrick MB. Variegate porphyria. Clinical and laboratory features. J Am Acad Dermatol 1980; 2: 36–43.

338 Frank J, Jugert FK, Kalka K et al. Variegate porphyria: Identification of a nonsense mutation in the protoporphyrinogen oxidase gene. J Invest Dermatol 1998; 110: 449–451.

339 Whatley SD, Puy H, Morgan RR et al. Variegate porphyria in Western Europe: identification of PPOX gene mutations in 104 families, extent of allelic heterogeneity, and absence of correlation between phenotype and type of mutation. Am J Hum Genet 1999; 65: 984–994.

340 Frank J, McGrath JA, Poh-Fitzpatrick MB et al. Mutations in the translation initiation codon of the protoporphyrinogen oxidase gene underlie variegate porphyria. Clin Exp Dermatol 1999; 24: 296–301.

341 Frank J, McGrath J, Lam HM et al. Homozygous variegate porphyria: identification of mutations on both alleles of the protoporphyrinogen oxidase gene in a severely affected proband. J Invest Dermatol 1998; 110: 452–455.

342 Palmer RA, Elder GH, Barrett DF, Keohane SG. Homozygous variegate porphyria: a compound heterozygote with novel mutations in the protoporphyrinogen oxidase gene. Br J Dermatol 2001; 144: 866–869.

343 Quiroz-Kendall E, Wilson FA, King LE Jr. Acute variegate porphyria following a Scarsdale Gourmet Diet. J Am Acad Dermatol 1983; 8: 46–49.

344 Tidman MJ, Higgins EM, Elder GH, MacDonald DM. Variegate porphyria associated with hepatocellular carcinoma. Br J Dermatol 1989; 121: 503–505.

345 Grabczynska SA, McGregor JM, Hawk JLM. Late onset variegate porphyria. Clin Exp Dermatol 1996; 21: 353–356.

346 Varma S, Lanigan SW. Management difficulties due to concurrent dermatitis herpetiformis and variegate porphyria. Br J Dermatol 2000; 143: 654–655.

347 Poh-Fitzpatrick MB. A plasma porphyrin fluorescence marker for variegate porphyria. Arch Dermatol 1980; 116: 543–547.

348 Norris PG, Elder GH, Hawk JLM. Homozygous variegate porphyria: a case report. Br J Dermatol 1990; 122: 253–257.

349 Nordmann Y, Deybach JC. Congenital erythropoietic porphyria. Semin Liver Dis 1982; 2: 154–163.

350 Warner CA, Poh-Fitzpatrick MB, Zaider EF et al. Congenital erythropoietic porphyria. Arch Dermatol 1992; 128: 1243–1248.

351 Huang J, Zaider E, Roth P et al. Congenital erythropoietic porphyria. Clinical, biochemical, and enzymatic profile of a severely affected patient. J Am Acad Dermatol 1996: 34: 924–927.

352 Fritsch C, Bolsen K, Ruzicka T, Goerz G. Congenital erythropoietic porphyria. J Am Acad Dermatol 1997; 36: 594–610.

353 Saval AH, Tirado AM. Congenital erythropoietic porphyria affecting two brothers. Br J Dermatol 1999; 141: 547–550.

354 Horiguchi Y, Horio T, Yamamoto M et al. Late onset erythropoietic porphyria. Br J Dermatol 1989; 121: 255–262.

355 Murphy GM, Hawk JLM, Nicholson DC, Magnus IA. Congenital erythropoietic porphyria (Günther's disease). Clin Exp Dermatol 1987; 12: 61–65.

356 Kaufman BM, Vickers HR, Rayne J, Ryan TJ. Congenital erythropoietic porphyria. Br J Dermatol 1966; 79: 210–220.

357 Bhutani LK, Sood SK, Das PK et al. Congenital erythropoietic porphyria. An autopsy report. Arch Dermatol 1974; 110: 427–431.

358 Stretcher GS. Erythropoietic porphyria. Two cases and the results of metabolic alkalinization. Arch Dermatol 1977; 113: 1553–1557.

359 Nordmann Y, Deybach JC. Congenital erythropoietic porphyria. Semin Dermatol 1986; 5: 106–114.

360 Bloomer JR. Protoporphyria. Semin Liver Dis 1982; 2: 143–153.

361 Milligan A, Graham-Brown RAC, Sarkany I, Baker H. Erythropoietic protoporphyria exacerbated by oral iron therapy. Br J Dermatol 1988; 119: 63–66.

362 Poh-Fitzpatrick MB. Erythropoietic protoporphyria. Int J Dermatol 1978; 17: 359–369.

363 Poh-Fitzpatrick MB. Erythropoietic protoporphyria. Semin Dermatol 1986; 5: 99–105.

364 Todd DJ. Erythropoietic protoporphyria. Br J Dermatol 1994; 131: 751–766.

365 Goerz G, Bunselmeyer S, Bolsen K, Schurer NY. Ferrochelatase activities in patients with erythropoietic protoporphyria and their families. Br J Dermatol 1996; 134: 880–885.

366 Norris PG, Nunn AV, Hawk JLM, Cox TM. Genetic heterogeneity in erythropoietic protoporphyria: a study of the enzymatic defect in nine affected families. J Invest Dermatol 1990; 95: 260–263.

367 Wang X, Piomelli S, Peacocke M et al. Erythropoietic protoporphyria: four novel frameshift mutations in the ferrochelatase gene. J Invest Dermatol 1997; 109: 688–691.

368 Wang X, Yang L, Kurtz L et al. Haplotype analysis of families with erythropoietic protoporphyria and novel mutations of the ferrochelatase gene. J Invest Dermatol 1999; 113: 87–92.

369 Patel GK, Weston J, Derrick EK, Hawk JLM. An unusual case of purpuric erythropoietic protoporphyria. Clin Exp Dermatol 2000; 25: 406–408.

370 Murphy GM, Hawk JLM, Magnus IA. Late-onset erythropoietic protoporphyria with unusual cutaneous features. Arch Dermatol 1985; 121: 1309–1312.

371 MacDonald DM, Germain D, Perrot H. The histopathology and ultrastructure of liver disease in erythropoietic protoporphyria. Br J Dermatol 1981; 104: 7–17.

372 Romslo I, Gadeholt HG, Hovding G. Erythropoietic protoporphyria terminating in liver failure. Arch Dermatol 1982; 118: 668–671.

373 Wells MM, Golitz LE, Bender BJ. Erythropoietic protoporphyria with hepatic cirrhosis. Arch Dermatol 1980; 116: 429–432.

374 Mercurio MG, Prince G, Weber FL Jr et al. Terminal hepatic failure in erythropoietic protoporphyria. J Am Acad Dermatol 1993; 29: 829–833.

375 Varma S, Haworth A, Keefe M, Anstey AV. Delayed onset of cutaneous symptoms in erythropoietic protoporphyria. Br J Dermatol 2000; 143: 221–223.

376 Schmidt H, Snitker G, Thomsen K, Lintrup J. Erythropoietic protoporphyria. A clinical study based on 29 cases in 14 families. Arch Dermatol 1974; 110: 58–64.

377 Mutasim DF, Pelc NJ. Erythropoietic protoporphyria and lupus erythematosus: case report and review of the literature. Arch Dermatol 1994; 130: 1330–1332.

378 Redeker AG, Bronow RS. Erythropoietic protoporphyria presenting as hydroa aestivale. Arch Dermatol 1964; 89: 104–109.

379 Christopher AP, Grattan CEH, Cowan MA. Pseudoainhum and erythropoietic protoporphyria. Br J Dermatol 1988; 118: 113–116.

380 Todd DJ, Callender ME, Mayne EE et al. Erythropoietic protoporphyria, transfusion therapy and liver disease. Br J Dermatol 1992; 127: 534–537.

381 Poh-Fitzpatrick MB. Human protoporphyria: Reduced cutaneous photosensitivity and lower erythrocyte porphyrin levels during pregnancy. J Am Acad Dermatol 1997; 36: 40–43.

382 Bewley AP, Keefe M, White JE. Erythropoietic protoporphyria improving during pregnancy. Br J Dermatol 1998; 139: 145–147.

383 Bleasel NR, Varigos GA. Porphyria cutanea tarda. Australas J Dermatol 2000; 41: 197–208.

384 O'Reilly K, Snape J, Moore MR. Porphyria cutanea tarda resulting from primary hepatocellular carcinoma. Clin Exp Dermatol 1988; 13: 44–48.

385 Mascaro JM, Herrero C, Lecha M, Muniesa AM. Uroporphyrinogen-decarboxylase deficiencies: porphyria cutanea tarda and related conditions. Semin Dermatol 1986; 5: 115–124.

386 Pimstone NR. Porphyria cutanea tarda. Semin Liver Dis 1982; 2: 132–142.

387 Keczkes K, Barker DJ. Malignant hepatoma associated with acquired hepatic cutaneous porphyria. Arch Dermatol 1976; 112: 78–82.

388 Lichtenstein JR, Babb EJ, Felsher BF. Porphyria cutanea tarda (PCT) in a patient with chronic renal failure on haemodialysis. Br J Dermatol 1981; 104: 575–578.

389 Stevens BR, Fleischer AB Jr, Piering F, Crosby DL. Porphyria cutanea tarda in the setting of renal failure. Response to renal transplantation. Arch Dermatol 1993; 129: 337–339.

390 Shieh S, Cohen JL, Lim HW. Management of porphyria cutanea tarda in the setting of chronic renal failure: A case report and review. J Am Acad Dermatol 2000; 42: 645–652.

391 Gibson GE, McGinnity E, McGrath P et al. Cutaneous abnormalities and metabolic disturbance of porphyrins in patients on maintenance haemodialysis. Clin Exp Dermatol 1997; 22: 124–127.

392 Kelly MA, O'Rourke KD. Treatment of porphyria cutanea tarda with phlebotomy in a patient on peritoneal dialysis. J Am Acad Dermatol 2001; 44: 336–338.

393 Kim JJ, Lim HW. Hexachlorobenzene and porphyria cutanea tarda. Arch Dermatol 1999; 135: 459–460.

394 Held JL, Sassa S, Kappas A, Harber LC. Erythrocyte uroporphyrinogen decarboxylase activity in porphyria cutanea tarda: a study of 40 consecutive patients. J Invest Dermatol 1989; 93: 332–334.

395 Malina L, Lim CK. Manifestation of familial porphyria cutanea tarda after childbirth. Br J Dermatol 1988; 118: 243–245.

396 Bruce AJ, Ahmed I. Childhood-onset porphyria cutanea tarda: Successful therapy with low-dose hydroxychloroquine (Plaquenil). J Am Acad Dermatol 1998; 38: 810–814.

397 Grossman ME, Bickers DR, Poh-Fitzpatrick MB et al. Porphyria cutanea tarda. Clinical features and laboratory findings in 40 patients. Am J Med 1979; 67: 277–286.

398 Topi GC, Amantea A, Griso D. Recovery from porphyria cutanea tarda with no specific therapy other than avoidance of hepatic toxins. Br J Dermatol 1984; 111: 75–82.

399 Conry-Cantilena C, Vilamidou L, Melpolder JC et al. Porphyria cutanea tarda in hepatitis C virus-infected blood donors. J Am Acad Dermatol 1995; 32: 512–514.

400 Cribier B, Petiau P, Keller F et al. Porphyria cutanea tarda and hepatitis C viral infection. Arch Dermatol 1995; 131: 801–804.

401 Lacour JPh, Bodokh I, Castanet J et al. Porphyria cutanea tarda and antibodies to hepatitis C virus. Br J Dermatol 1993; 128: 121–123.

402 Chuang T-Y, Brashear R, Lewis C. Porphyria cutanea tarda and hepatitis C virus: A case-control study and meta-analysis of the literature. J Am Acad Dermatol 1999; 41: 31–36.

403 Tsukazaki N, Watanabe M, Irifune H. Porphyria cutanea tarda and hepatitis C virus infection. Br J Dermatol 1998; 138: 1015–1017.

404 Cribier B, Rey D, Uhl G et al. Abnormal urinary coproporphyrin levels in patients infected by hepatitis C virus with or without human immunodeficiency virus. A study of 177 patients. Arch Dermatol 1996; 132: 1448–1452.

405 Brashear R, Began D, Petersen J, Chuang T-Y. An epidemic of porphyria cutanea tarda? Int J Dermatol 2000; 39: 154–156.

406 Blauvelt A. Hepatitis C virus and human immunodeficiency virus infection can alter porphyrin metabolism and lead to porphyria cutanea tarda. Arch Dermatol 1996; 132: 1503–1504.

407 Gomi H, Hatanaka K, Miura T, Matsuo I. Type of impaired porphyrin metabolism caused by hepatitis C virus is not porphyria cutanea tarda but chronic hepatic porphyria. Arch Dermatol 1997; 133: 1170–1171.

408 Roenigk HH Jr, Gottlob ME. Estrogen-induced porphyria cutanea tarda. Report of three cases. Arch Dermatol 1970; 102: 260–266.

409 Malina L, Chlumsky J. Oestrogen-induced familial porphyria cutanea tarda. Br J Dermatol 1975; 92: 707–709.

410 Urbanek RW, Cohen DJ. Porphyria cutanea tarda: pregnancy versus estrogen effect. J Am Acad Dermatol 1994; 31: 390–392.

411 Dawe RS, Clark C, Ferguson J. Porphyria cutanea tarda presenting as solar urticaria. Br J Dermatol 1999; 141: 590–591.

412 Chesney T McC, Wardlaw LL, Kaplan RJ, Chow JF. Porphyria cutanea tarda complicating Wilson's disease. J Am Acad Dermatol 1981; 4: 64–66.

413 Ochiai T, Morishima T, Kondo M. Symptomatic porphyria secondary to hepatocellular carcinoma. Br J Dermatol 1997; 136: 129–131.

414 Maughan WZ, Muller SA, Perry HO. Porphyria cutanea tarda associated with lymphoma. Acta Derm Venereol 1979; 59: 55–58.

415 Hogan D, Card RT, Ghadially R et al. Human immunodeficiency virus infection and porphyria cutanea tarda. J Am Acad Dermatol 1989; 20: 17–20.

416 Blauvelt A, Harris HR, Hogan DJ et al. Porphyria cutanea tarda and human immunodeficiency virus infection. Int J Dermatol 1992; 31: 474–479.

417 Nomura N, Zolla-Pazner S, Simberkoff M et al. Abnormal serum porphyrin levels in patients with the acquired immunodeficiency syndrome with or without hepatitis C virus infection. Arch Dermatol 1996; 132: 906–910.

418 O'Connor WJ, Murphy GM, Darby C et al. Porphyrin abnormalities in acquired immunodeficiency syndrome. Arch Dermatol 1996; 132: 1443–1447.

419 Fivenson DP, King AJ. Porphyria cutanea tarda in a patient with agnogenic myeloid metaplasia. Arch Dermatol 1984; 120: 538–539.

420 Lee SC, Yun SJ, Lee J-B et al. A case of porphyria cutanea tarda in association with idiopathic myelofibrosis and CREST syndrome. Br J Dermatol 2001; 144: 182–185.

421 Callen JP, Ross L. Subacute cutaneous lupus erythematosus and porphyria cutanea tarda. Report of a case. J Am Acad Dermatol 1981; 5: 269–273.

422 Clemmensen O, Thomsen K. Porphyria cutanea tarda and systemic lupus erythematosus. Arch Dermatol 1982; 118: 160–162.

423 Cram DL, Epstein JH, Tuffanelli DL. Lupus erythematosus and porphyria. Coexistence in seven patients. Arch Dermatol 1973; 108: 779–784.

424 Dereure O, Aguilar-Martinez P, Bessis D et al. HFE mutations and transferrin receptor polymorphism analysis in porphyria cutanea tarda: a prospective study of 36 cases from southern France. Br J Dermatol 2001; 144: 533–539.

425 Brady JJ, Jackson HA, Roberts AG et al. Co-inheritance of mutations in the uroporphyrinogen decarboxylase and hemochromatosis genes accelerates the onset of porphyria cutanea tarda. J Invest Dermatol 2000; 115: 868–874.

426 Crips DJ, Peters HA, Gocmen A, Dogramici I. Porphyria turcica due to hexachlorobenzene: a 20 to 30 year follow-up study on 204 patients. Br J Dermatol 1984; 111: 413–422.

427 Muhlbauer JE, Pathak MA. Porphyria cutanea tarda. Int J Dermatol 1979; 18: 767–780.

428 Kranz KR, Reed OM, Grimwood RE. Necrotizing fasciitis associated with porphyria cutanea tarda. J Am Acad Dermatol 1986; 14: 361–367.

429 Friedman SJ, Doyle JA. Sclerodermoid changes of porphyria cutanea tarda: possible relationship to urinary uroporphyrin levels. J Am Acad Dermatol 1985; 13: 70–74.

430 Lim HW, Poh-Fitzpatrick MB. Hepatoerythropoietic porphyria: a variant of childhood-onset porphyria cutanea tarda. Porphyrin profiles and enzymatic studies of two cases in a family. J Am Acad Dermatol 1984; 11: 1103–1111.

431 Smith SG. Hepatoerythropoietic porphyria. Semin Dermatol 1986; 5: 125–137.

432 Koszo F, Elder GH, Roberts A, Simon N. Uroporphyrinogen decarboxylase deficiency in hepatoerythropoietic porphyria: further evidence for genetic heterogeneity. Br J Dermatol 1990; 122: 365–370.

433 Simon N, Berko GY, Schneider I. Hepato-erythropoietic porphyria presenting as scleroderma and acrosclerosis in a sibling pair. Br J Dermatol 1977; 96: 663–668.

434 Bundino S, Topi GC, Zina AM, D'Allessandro Gandolfo L. Hepatoerythropoietic porphyria. Pediatr Dermatol 1987; 4: 229–233.

435 Day RS, Strauss PC. Severe cutaneous porphyria in a 12-year-old boy. Hepatoerythropoietic or symptomatic porphyria? Arch Dermatol 1982; 118: 663–667.

436 Meguro K, Fujita H, Ishida N et al. Molecular defects of uroporphyrinogen decarboxylase in a patient with mild hepatoerythropoietic porphyria. J Invest Dermatol 1994; 102: 681–685.

437 Czarnecki DB. Hepatoerythropoietic porphyria. Arch Dermatol 1980; 116: 307–311.

438 Green JJ, Manders SM. Pseudoporphyria. J Am Acad Dermatol 2001; 44: 100–108.

439 Schanbacher CF, Vanness ER, Daoud MS et al. Pseudoporphyria: a clinical and biochemical study of 20 patients. Mayo Clin Proc 2001; 76: 488–492.

440 Harber LC, Bickers DR. Porphyria and pseudoporphyria. J Invest Dermatol 1984; 82: 207–209.

441 Poh-Fitzpatrick MB. Porphyria, pseudoporphyria, pseudopseudoporphyria ...? Arch Dermatol 1986; 122: 403–404.

442 Hawk JLM. Skin changes resembling hepatic cutaneous porphyria induced by oxytetracycline photosensitization. Clin Exp Dermatol 1980; 5: 321–325.

443 Epstein JH, Tuffanelli DL, Siebert JS, Epstein WL. Porphyria-like cutaneous changes induced by tetracycline hydrochloride photosensitization. Arch Dermatol 1976; 112: 661–666.

444 Riordan CA, Anstey A, Wojnarowska F. Isotretinoin-associated pseudoporphyria. Clin Exp Dermatol 1993; 18: 69–71.

445 Schindl A, Trautinger F, Pernerstorfer-Schön H et al. Porphyria cutanea tarda induced by the use of pravastatin. Arch Dermatol 1998; 134: 1305–1306.

446 Burry JN, Lawrence JR. Phototoxic blisters from high frusemide dosage. Br J Dermatol 1976; 94: 495–499.

447 Breier F, Feldmann R, Pelzl M, Gschnait F. Pseudoporphyria cutanea tarda induced by furosemide in a patient undergoing peritoneal dialysis. Dermatology 1998; 197: 271–273.

448 Ramsay CA, Obreshkova E. Photosensitivity from nalidixic acid. Br J Dermatol 1974; 91: 523–528.

449 Judd LE, Henderson DW, Hill DC. Naproxen-induced pseudoporphyria. A clinical and ultrastructural study. Arch Dermatol 1986; 122: 451–454.

450 Burns DA. Naproxen pseudoporphyria in a patient with vitiligo. Clin Exp Dermatol 1987; 12: 296–297.

451 Rivers JK, Barnetson R St C. Naproxen-induced bullous photodermatitis. Med J Aust 1989; 151: 167–168.

452 De Silva B, Banney L, Uttley W et al. Pseudoporphyria and nonsteroidal antiinflammatory agents in children with juvenile idiopathic arthritis. Pediatr Dermatol 2000; 17: 480–483.

453 Ingrish G, Rietschel RL. Oxaprozin-induced pseudoporphyria. Arch Dermatol 1996; 132: 1519–1520.

454 O'Hagan AH, Irvine AD, Allen GE, Walsh M. Pseudoporphyria induced by mefenamic acid. Br J Dermatol 1998; 139: 1131–1132.

455 Krischer J, Scolari F, Kondo-Oestreicher M et al. Pseudoporphyria induced by nabumetone. J Am Acad Dermatol 1999; 40: 492–493.

456 Varma S, Lanigan SW. Pseudoporphyria caused by nabumetone. Br J Dermatol 1998; 138: 549–550.

457 Antony F, Layton AM. Nabumetone-associated pseudoporphyria. Br J Dermatol 2000; 142: 1067–1069.

458 Magro CM, Crowson AN. Pseudoporphyria associated with Relafen therapy. J Cutan Pathol 1999; 26: 42–47.

459 Meggitt SJ, Farr PM. Pseudoporphyria and propionic acid non-steroidal anti-inflammatory drugs. Br J Dermatol 1999; 141: 591–592.

460 Baer RL, Stillman MA. Cutaneous skin changes probably due to pyridoxine abuse. J Am Acad Dermatol 1984; 10: 527–528.

461 Baker EJ, Reed KD, Dixon SL. Chlorthalidone-induced pseudoporphyria: clinical and microscopic findings of a case. J Am Acad Dermatol 1989; 21: 1026–1029.

462 Borroni G, Brazzelli V, Baldini F et al. Flutamide-induced pseudoporphyria. Br J Dermatol 1998; 138: 711–712.

463 McDonagh AJG, Harrington CI. Pseudoporphyria complicating etretinate therapy. Clin Exp Dermatol 1989; 14: 437–438.

464 Murphy GM, Wright J, Nicholls DSH et al. Sunbed-induced pseudoporphyria. Br J Dermatol 1989; 120: 555–562.

465 Poh-Fitzpatrick MB, Ellis DL. Porphyrialike bullous dermatosis after chronic intense tanning bed and/or sunlight exposure. Arch Dermatol 1989; 125: 1236–1238.

466 Stenberg A. Pseudoporphyria and sunbeds. Acta Derm Venereol 1990; 70: 354–356.

467 Poh-Fitzpatrick MB, Masullo AS, Grossman ME. Porphyria cutanea tarda associated with chronic renal disease and hemodialysis. Arch Dermatol 1980; 116: 191–195.

468 Shelley WB, Shelley ED. Blisters of the fingertips: a variant of bullous dermatosis of hemodialysis. J Am Acad Dermatol 1989; 21: 1049–1051.

469 Rotstein H. Photosensitive bullous eruption associated with chronic renal failure. Australas J Dermatol 1978; 19: 58–64.

470 Keczkes K, Farr M. Bullous dermatosis of chronic renal failure. Br J Dermatol 1976; 95: 541–546.

471 Epstein JH, Tuffanelli DL, Epstein WL. Cutaneous changes in the porphyrias. A microscopic study. Arch Dermatol 1973; 107: 689–698.

472 Wolff K, Honigsmann H, Rauschmeier W et al. Microscopic and fine structural aspects of porphyrias. Acta Derm Venereol (Suppl) 1982; 100: 17–28.

473 Maynard B, Peters MS. Histologic and immunofluorescence study of cutaneous porphyrias. J Cutan Pathol 1992; 19: 40–47.

474 Egbert BM, LeBoit PE, McCalmont T et al. Caterpillar bodies: distinctive, basement membrane-containing structures in blisters of porphyria. Am J Dermatopathol 1993; 15: 199–202.

475 Raso DS, Greene WB, Maize JC et al. Caterpillar bodies of porphyria cutanea tarda ultrastructurally represent a unique arrangement of colloid and basement membrane bodies. Am J Dermatopathol 1996; 18: 24–29.

476 Van der Walt JJ, Heyl T. Lipoid proteinosis and erythropoietic protoporphyria. A histological and histochemical study. Arch Dermatol 1971; 104: 501–507.

477 Peterka ES, Fusaro RM, Goltz RW. Erythropoietic protoporphyria. II. Histological and histochemical studies of cutaneous lesions. Arch Dermatol 1965; 92: 357–361.

478 Timonen K, Kariniemi A-L, Niemi K-M et al. Vascular changes in erythropoietic protoporphyria: Histopathologic and immunohistochemical study. J Am Acad Dermatol 2000; 43: 489–497.

479 Cormane RH, Szabo E, Hoo TT. Histopathology of the skin in acquired and hereditary porphyria cutanea tarda. Br J Dermatol 1971; 85: 531–539.

480 Grossman ME, Poh-Fitzpatrick MB. Porphyria cutanea tarda. Diagnosis and management. Med Clin North Am 1980; 64: 807–827.

481 Dabski C, Beutner EH. Studies of laminin and type IV collagen in blisters of porphyria cutanea tarda and drug-induced pseudoporphyria. J Am Acad Dermatol 1991; 25: 28–32.

482 Ahmed AR. Diagnosis of bullous disease and studies in the pathogenesis of blister formation using immunopathological techniques. J Cutan Pathol 1984; 11: 237–248.

483 Parra CA, Pizzi de Parra N. Diameter of the collagen fibrils in the sclerodermatous skin of porphyria cutanea tarda. Br J Dermatol 1979; 100: 573–578.

484 Caputo R, Berti E, Gasparini G, Monti M. The morphologic events of blister formation in porphyria cutanea tarda. Int J Dermatol 1983; 22: 467–472.

485 Schnait FG, Wolff K, Konrad K. Erythropoietic protoporphyria – submicroscopic events during the acute photosensitivity flare. Br J Dermatol 1975; 92: 545–557.

486 Baart de la Faille H. Erythropoietic protoporphyria. A photodermatosis. Utrecht: Oosthoek, Scheltema and Holkema, 1975.

Miscellaneous conditions

ACCESSORY TRAGUS

Accessory tragi are usually found as solitary, dome-shaped papules and nodules, present at birth, usually in the preauricular region but sometimes in the neck, anterior to the sternomastoid muscle.[1–4] The cervical lesions have been regarded by some as a discrete but closely related entity, also of branchial origin:[5] they have been reported as cervical auricles, 'wattles' and congenital cartilaginous rests.[6–8]

Accessory tragi may be multiple and sometimes bilateral.[9] Rarely, they are associated with other syndromes of the first branchial arch, such as the oculo-auriculo-vertebral syndrome (Goldenhar's syndrome).[10] Clinically, accessory tragi, including the lower cervical variants, are usually diagnosed as skin tags.

Histopathology[1]

The lesions are polypoid elevations with a fibrovascular zone beneath the epidermis containing numerous hair follicles with small sebaceous glands sometimes attached (Figs 19.1, 19.2). Some of the follicles are of vellus type. Beneath this area, there is a zone of adipose tissue and usually a central core of cartilage. There is a prominent connective tissue framework in the fat, irrespective of the presence of cartilage.[11] Eccrine glands are often present and occasionally there are large nerve fibers and even Pacinian corpuscles.

In the cervical lesions there is mature cartilage embedded in fibrous tissue. Striated muscle in continuity with the underlying platysma muscle may also be present in the core. Telogen hairs are not always present in cervical lesions or at least their presence is not mentioned in the reports. Histological features of both hair follicle nevus (see p. 860) and accessory tragus can coexist in a single lesion. As a rule, the accessory tragus has abundant fat cells.[12]

The rare condition described as **dermatorynchus geneae** is a related first arch abnormality in which large amounts of striated muscle and sometimes bone form the central core of the elongated polypoid lesion.[13] The lesions reported as striated muscle hamartomas are closely related[14] morphologically; they were not in the preauricular region (see p. 972).

SUPERNUMERARY NIPPLE

Polythelia, as the presence of supernumerary nipples is sometimes called, is a developmental abnormality found in approximately 1% of the population.[15] There is a predilection for females. Familial cases have been recorded.[16] The supernumerary structure is usually a solitary, asymptomatic, slightly pigmented,

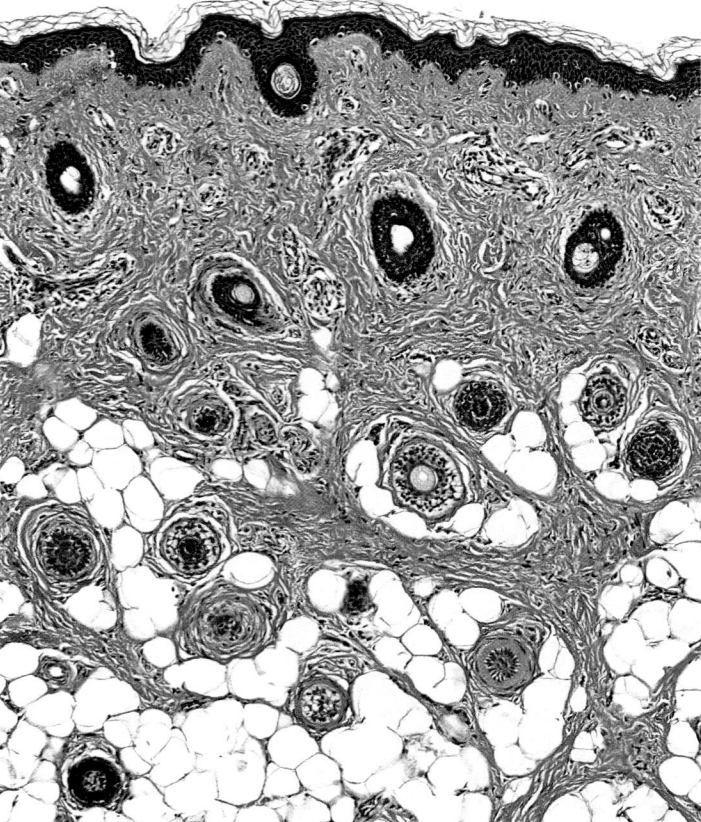

Fig. 19.2 **Accessory tragus.** Numerous hair follicles, some of vellus type, are present. Sebaceous glands are not well developed. (H & E)

nodular lesion, often with a small, central, nipple-like elevation. It may occur anywhere along the pathway of the embryonic milk line, particularly on the anterior aspect of the chest or the upper abdomen. Rarely, it is outside this line.[17,18] Clinically, it resembles a nevus or fibroma. There is said to be an increased incidence of renal abnormalities in patients with a supernumerary nipple,[19] although recent studies have failed to confirm this association.[20,21] Rarely, a small patch of hairs may be the only marker of underlying accessory breast tissue ('polythelia pilosa').[22] Accessory breast tissue is rarely seen in a Becker's nevus.[23]

Histopathology[15]

The appearances resemble those seen in the normal nipple and include epidermal thickening with mild papillomatosis and basal hyperpigmentation, the presence of pilosebaceous structures, variable amounts of smooth muscle, and mammary ducts which open into pilosebaceous ducts or enter the epidermis (Fig. 19.3). There may be underlying breast tissue, but complete supernumerary breasts are very rare.[19]

ACCESSORY SCROTUM

Accessory scrotum is the presence of scrotal skin outside of its normal location, but without testicular tissue. It is usually found in the perineal or

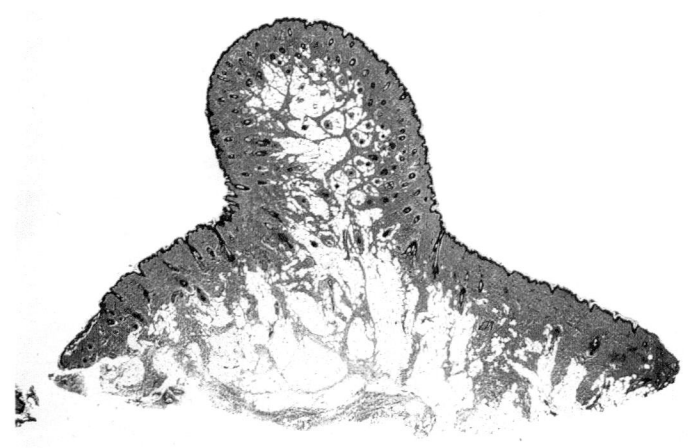

Fig. 19.1 **Accessory tragus.** In this case there is adipose tissue but no cartilage in the core. (H & E)

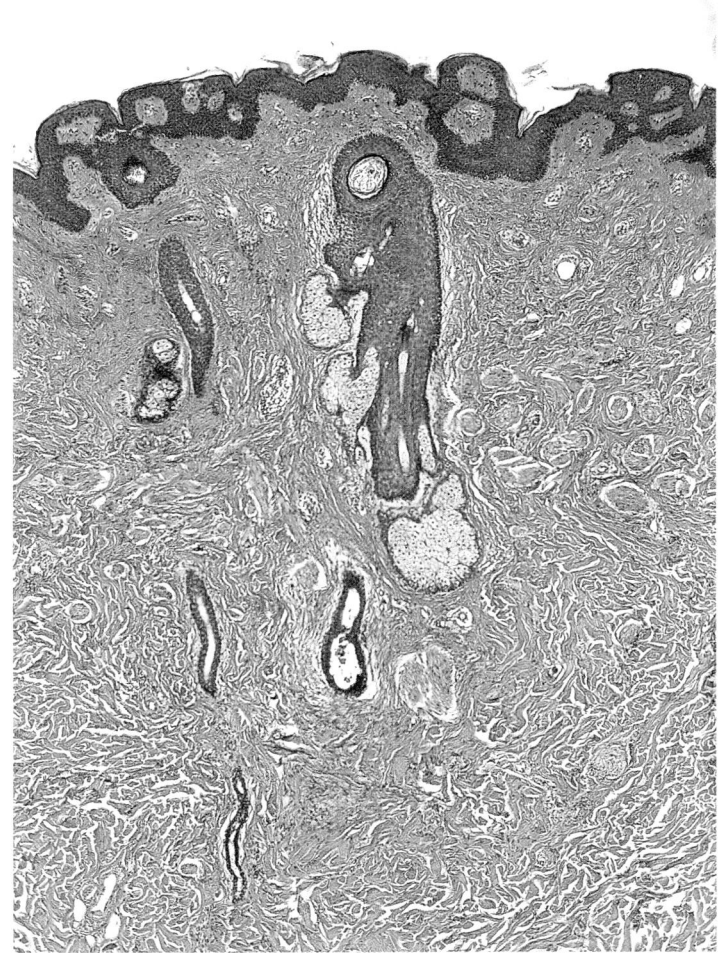

Fig. 19.3 **Supernumerary (accessory) nipple.** There is smooth muscle and a ductal structure. (H & E)

inguinal region.[24] A normal scrotum is also present. An accessory scrotum has been reported in a patient with a Becker's nevus (see p. 331).

Agenesis of the scrotum is an exceedingly rare event.[25]

ECTOPIC TISSUES

There are isolated reports of the occurrence in the skin of ectopic tissue. Most cases represent embryological vestiges, but trauma (surgery or a gunshot injury) is the explanation for splenic tissue in the subcutaneous tissues of the abdomen.[26,27]

Other ectopic tissues reported in the skin have included thymus (see p. 511), respiratory mucosa (see p. 511), salivary gland, brain (see p. 988) and pancreas (see p. 511).

CHEILITIS GLANDULARIS

Cheilitis glandularis appears to be a heterogeneous entity, which has been attributed in the past to hyperplasia of labial salivary glands.[28–30] However, a critical review of reported cases does not support this explanation[31] except in a few cases.[32] It has been suggested that the condition includes cases of factitious cheilitis,[33–35] premature and exaggerated actinic cheilitis, and cases

with a coexisting atopic diathesis in which mouth breathing may play a role.[31] It should be noted that only mild swelling of the lip is needed to produce eversion which in itself exaggerates the appearance of swelling.[31]

The patients present with macrocheilia, usually confined to the lower lip. There is often crusting and fissuring with a mucoid discharge. Salivary duct orifices may be prominent. Clinically, the lesions need to be distinguished from plasma cell cheilitis,[36] cheilitis granulomatosis (Melkersson–Rosenthal syndrome – see p. 208) and Ascher's syndrome, in which there is acute swelling of the lip and eyelids (usually the upper) resulting from edema, inflammation and a possible increase in size of labial and lacrimal glands respectively.[29,37–39]

Squamous cell carcinoma may sometimes supervene, further evidence that many cases have an actinic etiology.[28,30]

Histopathology

There is usually hyperkeratosis, focal parakeratosis and sometimes inflammatory crusting. There is underlying edema, variable but usually mild chronic inflammation, and variable solar elastosis.[31] Although the minor salivary glands are usually said to be hyperplastic, one study showed no increase in their size or appearance when compared to controls. Notwithstanding, enlargement of salivary glands with dilated ducts and some chronic inflammation have been present in some cases reported as cheilitis glandularis.[32]

UMBILICAL LESIONS

The umbilicus is an important embryological structure, into which the vitelline (omphalomesenteric) duct and urachus enter. Remnants of either structure may give rise to lesions at the umbilicus and, rarely, vestiges of both may coexist.[40]

The omphalomesenteric duct normally becomes obliterated early in embryonic life but remnants may persist, producing an enteric fistula, an umbilical sinus, a subcutaneous cyst or an umbilical polyp.[41,42] The latter presents as a bright red polyp or fleshy nodule, 0.5–2 cm in diameter;[43] it may discharge a mucoid secretion.

Urachal anomalies usually present at or shortly after birth.[40] A patent urachus will result in the passage of urine from the umbilicus. Urachal sinuses and deeper cysts result from partial obliteration of the urachus, with small persistent areas.

Other lesions presenting at the umbilicus include endometriosis (see p. 514), primary and secondary tumors (see p. 1046)[44] and inflammatory granulomas.[45] The granulomas result from inflammatory changes associated with persistent epithelialized tracts or simply from accumulation of debris in a deep umbilicus with resulting ulceration and inflammation.[40] Sometimes a pilonidal sinus is present.[46]

Histopathology

Umbilical (omphalomesenteric duct) polyps are covered by epithelium which is usually of small bowel or colonic type, but occasionally of gastric type. Ectopic pancreatic tissue has also been described.[41] There is usually an abrupt transition from epidermis to the intestinal or gastric type of epithelium. Urachal remnants are lined by transitional epithelium;[40] sometimes smooth muscle bundles are present in their wall. There may be a mild inflammatory cell infiltrate both in umbilical polyps and in urachal remnants.

Umbilical granulomas show variable inflammatory changes ranging from abscess formation to granulomatous areas.[40] Sometimes hair shafts or debris are present with associated foreign body giant cells. There is variable fibrosis.

Primary tumors of the umbilicus may take the form of adenocarcinoma, sarcoma, melanoma, squamous cell carcinoma or, rarely, basal cell carcinoma.[44] Rarely, umbilical adenocarcinomas assume a papillary pattern with psammoma bodies.[47]

RELAPSING POLYCHONDRITIS

Relapsing polychondritis is a rare disorder of unknown etiology manifesting with recurrent inflammation of the cartilaginous tissues of different organs, particularly the ear, but also the nasal septum and tracheobronchial cartilage.[48–51] A frequent presentation is with tenderness and reddening of one or both ears.[52,53] Onset is usually in middle age. Other manifestations include polyarthritis, ocular inflammation, audiovestibular damage, cardiac lesions and a vasculitis.[48,54,55] Relapsing polychondritis has been reported in association with psoriasis,[56] myelodysplastic syndromes,[57,58] acute febrile neutrophilic dermatosis (Sweet's syndrome),[59] and, in one case, pseudocyst of the auricle.[60] The course of the disease is variable, but there is usually progressive destruction of cartilage, with consequent deformities. Death ensues in up to 25% of patients as a result of respiratory and cardiovascular complications.

There are pointers to an immunological pathogenesis. These include the detection of cell-mediated immunity to cartilage, the presence of antibodies to type II collagen[61] and the demonstration by direct immunofluorescence of immunoglobulins and C3 in the chondrofibrous junction and around chondrocytes.[60,62] A case thought to have been precipitated by the use of the drug goserelin (Zoladex®) for the treatment of prostatic adenocarcinoma has been reported.[63]

Colchicine,[64] dapsone[65,66] and corticosteroids have been used in the management.

Histopathology[48]

The initial changes are a decrease in the basophilia of the involved cartilage, degeneration of marginal chondrocytes which become vacuolated with pyknotic nuclei, and a florid perichondritis with obscuring of the chondrofibrous interface. The inflammatory cell infiltrate initially contains many neutrophils, but there are progressively more lymphocytes, plasma cells and histiocytes in the infiltrate, with occasional eosinophils. With time there is derangement of the cartilaginous matrix and its replacement by fibrous tissue. Calcification and even metaplastic bone may develop in the late stages when only a scattering of chronic inflammatory cells remain.

Electron microscopy

A large number of dense granules and vesicles, compatible with matrix vesicles or lysosomes, surround the affected chondrocytes.[67]

ACANTHOSIS NIGRICANS

Acanthosis nigricans is a cutaneous manifestation of a diverse group of diseases which include internal cancers and various endocrine and congenital syndromes (see Table 19.1).[68–70] It may occur as an inherited disorder. It may also be related to the ingestion of certain drugs. In all these circumstances, acanthosis nigricans presents as symmetrical, pigmented, velvety plaques and verrucous excrescences confined usually to the flexural areas of the body, particularly the axillae.[68,69] It may also involve the back of the neck, the periumbilical and anogenital regions and the naso-facial sulcus.[71] Rarely, there is generalized involvement of the skin.[72] The oral mucosa, particularly that of the lips and tongue, is affected also in 25% or more of cases.[73] Involvement

Table 19.1 **Clinical associations of acanthosis nigricans**

Paraneoplastic
Carcinomas of alimentary tract, kidney, bladder, lung, cervix and lymphomas

Endocrine and congenital
Insulin resistance syndrome, hyperinsulinemia, lipoatrophy, Prader-Willi syndrome, leprechaunism, pineal hyperplasia

Familial

Drugs
Somatotrophin, corticosteroids, oral contraceptives, diethylstilbestrol (stilbestrol), methyltestosterone, niacin (nicotinic acid), triazinate, topical fusidic acid

of the esophagus has been reported.[74] Hyperkeratotic lesions may develop on the palms, soles and knuckles.[75,76]

The *paraneoplastic type* of acanthosis nigricans is a rare manifestation of an internal cancer, usually an adenocarcinoma of the stomach or other part of the alimentary tract.[77–82] Lymphomas,[83] renal carcinoma,[84] lung carcinoma,[85] bladder carcinoma[86] and squamous cell carcinomas[87] are occasionally associated. Acanthosis nigricans may precede or follow the diagnosis of the cancer but in most instances the two are diagnosed simultaneously.[78,88] There are some reports of the reversibility of the skin lesions upon removal or treatment of the accompanying malignant disease.[78,88]

The various *endocrine disorders* and *congenital syndromes* which may be complicated by acanthosis nigricans appear to have in common a resistance of the tissues to the action of insulin;[89–97] hyperinsulinemia may be present.[98,99] Insulin resistance is present in the case of lipoatrophy,[100–103] the Prader–Willi syndrome,[104] leprechaunism,[101] pineal hyperplasia and the so-called 'type A and B insulin resistance syndromes'.[89,90,105] Obesity is often present.[106,107] A combination of acanthosis nigricans and insulin resistance is found in approximately 5% of hyperandrogenic females, often in association with polycystic ovaries.[90,93,108,109]

Onset of the rare *familial cases* is in early childhood.[110–112] There may be accentuation of symptoms at puberty. This variant is inherited as an autosomal dominant trait, although there may be variable phenotypic expression.[110]

Drugs that have been incriminated in the causation of acanthosis nigricans include somatotrophin,[113] corticosteroids,[114] niacin (nicotinic acid),[115,116] oral contraceptives, diethylstilbestrol (stilbestrol), the folic acid antagonist triazinate[117] and methyltestosterone.[118] Acanthosis nigricans-like lesions have developed in ichthyotic skin following the topical application of fusidic acid.[119]

Although the molecular basis of acanthosis nigricans remains an enigma, the disease appears to represent an abnormal epidermal proliferation in response to various factors.[103] In the case of the paraneoplastic group, the factor may be a tumor-produced peptide, such as epidermal growth factor (EGF) or transforming growth factor (TGF-α),[85] while in the group related to tissue insulin resistance, the tissue growth factors may include insulin itself, which may be increased in some of these conditions.[93,103] The rare keratins, 18 and 19, have been reported in basal keratinocytes in acanthosis nigricans.[120]

Histopathology

There is hyperkeratosis, papillomatosis and mild acanthosis (Fig. 19.4).[69] The papillomatosis results from the upward projection of finger-like dermal papillae which are covered by thinned epidermis.[73] In the 'valleys' between these papillary projections the epithelium shows mild acanthosis with overlying hyperkeratosis (Fig. 19.5).[73] There may be some hyperpigmentation

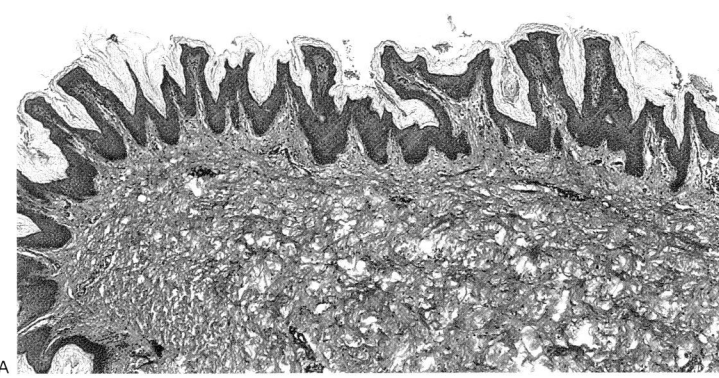

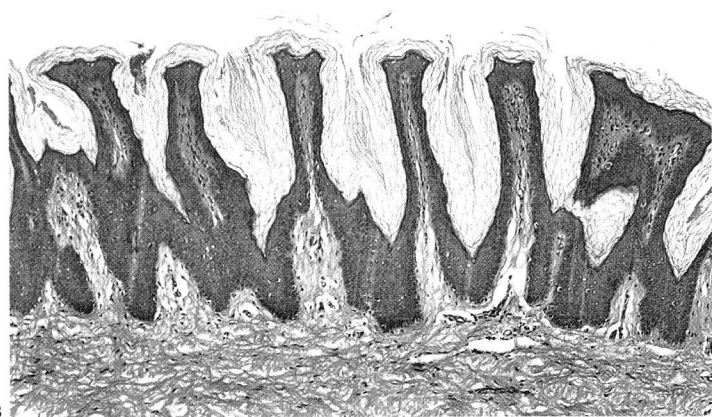

Fig. 19.4 **(A) Acanthosis nigricans. (B)** The papillomatosis and intervening 'valleys' are conspicuous in this case. (H & E)

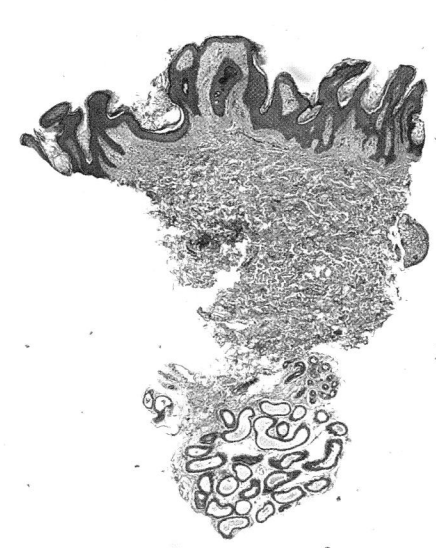

Fig. 19.5 **Acanthosis nigricans.** This biopsy taken from the axilla shows a less regular appearance than the previous case. (H & E)

of the basal layer, but it should be noted that the pigmentation of the lesions noted clinically results largely from the hyperkeratosis. In some instances, there is hypertrophy of all layers of the epidermis and the pattern resembles that seen in epidermal nevi. A resemblance to seborrheic keratoses has been noted in some cases. There is usually no dermal inflammation.

Oral lesions differ from the cutaneous ones by showing marked thickening of the epithelium with papillary hyperplasia and acanthosis.[73] There is a superficial resemblance to the lesions of condyloma acuminatum. There is usually mild chronic inflammation in the submucosal tissues.[73]

Finally, it is worth noting that a pattern resembling acanthosis nigricans has been reported at the site of repeated insulin injections.[121]

CONFLUENT AND RETICULATED PAPILLOMATOSIS

Confluent and reticulated papillomatosis (of Gougerot and Carteaud) is a rare form of papillomatosis characterized by the development of asymptomatic, small red to brown, slightly verrucous papules with a tendency to central confluence and a reticulate pattern peripherally.[122–125] It involves particularly the upper part of the chest and the intermammary region and back; the neck, chin, upper parts of the arms and the axillae may also be involved. It has been regarded as a variant of acanthosis nigricans, as a genodermatosis, as an unusual response to ultraviolet light[126] or to *Pityrosporum orbiculare* infection,[127–130] and as a result of some unidentified endocrine imbalance.[122,131] Response to calcipotriene (calcipotriol)[132,133] and isotretinoin[134] favors the theory that it is an abnormality of keratinization. On the other hand, response to various antibiotics has also been reported.[135–138] Familial occurrence has been documented.[139]

Histopathology[122,140]
The epidermis is undulating with hyperkeratosis, low papillomatosis and some acanthotic downgrowths from the bases of the 'valleys' between the papillomatous areas (Fig. 19.6). There may also be mild basal hyperpigmentation and focal atrophy of the malpighian layer. These changes resemble acanthosis nigricans,[141] although they are not usually as well developed as in this condition (Fig. 19.7). However, there may be mild dilatation of superficial dermal blood vessels and sometimes beading of elastic fibers, changes not usually attributed to acanthosis nigricans.

Electron microscopy
There is an alteration of cornified cell structures and an increase in the number of Odland bodies in the granular layer.[140,142]

ACROKERATOSIS PARANEOPLASTICA

Acrokeratosis paraneoplastica (Bazex's syndrome) is a skin condition associated with cancers which are usually supradiaphragmatic[143–145] in origin, although tumors at other sites have also been incriminated.[146,147] It commences with violaceous erythema and psoriasiform scaling on the fingers and toes with later extension to the ears and nose.[148,149] Violaceous keratoderma of the hands and feet develops, and ill-defined psoriasiform lesions eventually form at other sites on the arms and legs.[144] Bullous lesions are rare.[150] These changes in the skin usually precede the onset of symptoms related to the associated cancer.[151,152] This syndrome has been reported in association with acquired ichthyosis, another paraneoplastic disorder.[153] The pathogenesis of the condition is unknown, although transforming growth factor-α produced by tumor cells, may play a role.[153]

Histopathology[151]

The changes are somewhat variable and not diagnostically specific. There is hyperkeratosis, focal parakeratosis and acanthosis. Variable epidermal changes include spongiosis with associated exocytosis of lymphocytes, basal

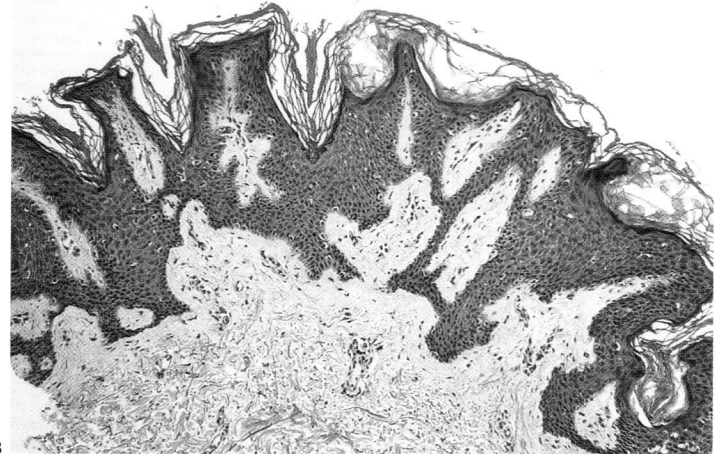

Fig. 19.6 **(A) Confluent and reticulated papillomatosis with papilloma formation.**
(B) The epidermis is undulating with acanthosis. (H & E)

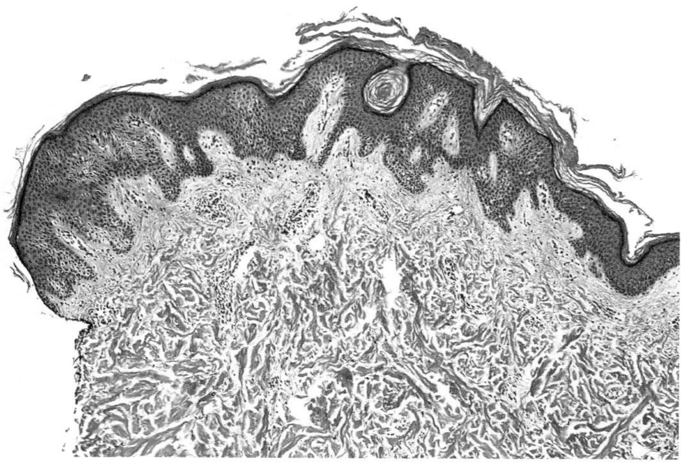

Fig. 19.7 **Another case of confluent and reticulated papillomatosis with less papillomatosis.** (H & E)

vacuolar change and scattered degenerate keratinocytes.[143,144] There is a mild perivascular lymphocytic infiltrate in the papillary dermis. Fibrinoid degeneration of small vessels and scattered 'pyknotic' neutrophils have been described in some reports, but specifically excluded in others.[143,151,154]

ERYTHRODERMA

Erythroderma (exfoliative dermatitis) is a cutaneous reaction pattern that can occur in a wide variety of benign and malignant diseases.[155–157] It is uncommon, with an incidence of 1–2 per 100 000 of the population.[155] Clinically, it is characterized by erythema and exfoliation which involve all or most of the skin surface.[156] Distressing pruritus is often present.[155] Other clinical features include fever, malaise, keratoderma, alopecia and a mild, generalized lymphadenopathy. Laboratory findings include blood eosinophilia, elevated levels of IgE and, in some, a polyclonal gammopathy.[155,158] The mean age at onset is approximately 60 years, although cases in infancy, often associated with ichthyosiform dermatoses (see p. 285) or immunodeficiency, have been reported.[159–161] There is a male predominance, particularly in the idiopathic group (see below).

Erythroderma is most often seen as an exacerbation of a pre-existing dermatological condition but it may also be drug related or be associated with cutaneous T-cell lymphoma or some other malignant tumors. Approximately 15% of cases are idiopathic (see Table 19.2). In one retrospective study, 62.5% were related to an underlying dermatosis, 16% were due to drug reactions, and 12.5% to cutaneous T-cell lymphoma.[162] In a more recent study, there was a pre-existing dermatosis in 74.4%, 14.6% were idiopathic, and drugs and malignancy each accounted for 5.5% of cases.[163]

A *pre-existing dermatosis* is present in more than 50% of cases. Psoriasis is the most common of these.[164] Various factors, including the use of systemic steroid therapy, have been incriminated in precipitating an erythrodermic crisis in psoriasis.[164] Other underlying dermatoses include atopic dermatitis, seborrheic dermatitis, allergic contact dermatitis, photosensitivity syndromes,[165] pityriasis rubra pilaris and, rarely, stasis dermatitis, dermatophytosis, pemphigus foliaceus and even bullous pemphigoid.[163,166–169] In some countries, there is a significant association with HIV infection.[170]

Drug-induced cases may follow topical sensitization to neomycin, ethylenediamine or clioquinol (Vioform®).[171] Usually, erythroderma follows the ingestion of a drug such as phenytoin, penicillin, isoniazid, trimethoprim and sulfonamides, antimalarials,[172] thiazide diuretics, gold, chlorpromazine, calcium carbimide (cyanamide),[173] nifedipine[174] or allopurinol.[166,175] There are

Table 19.2 **Etiologies of erythroderma**

Pre-existing dermatosis
Psoriasis, atopic dermatitis, seborrheic dermatitis, allergic contact dermatitis, photosensitivity syndromes, pityriasis rubra pilaris, stasis dermatitis, pemphigus foliaceus, bullous pemphigoid, HIV infection
Drugs
Phenytoin, penicillin, isoniazid, trimethoprim, sulfonamides, antimalarials, thiazides, gold, chlorpromazine, calcium carbimide (cyanamide), nifedipine, allopurinol, NSAIDs, timolol maleate eye drops, hypericum (St John's wort), recombinant cytokines
Lymphoma
Cutaneous T-cell lymphoma (mycosis fungoides and Sézary syndrome), extracutaneous lymphoma, rarely with solid tumors
Idiopathic

a few case reports of erythroderma following the use of certain non-steroidal anti-inflammatory drugs such as sulindac, meclofenamate sodium and phenylbutazone.[176] One case followed the use of β-blocker eye drops (timolol maleate)[177] and, another, the use of hypericum (St. John's wort).[178] The use of recombinant cytokine therapy may precipitate erythroderma (see p. 589).[179,180] Drug-related cases usually have a rapid onset and relatively quick resolution over 2–6 weeks, in contrast to the more prolonged course of the idiopathic and lymphoma-related cases.[166]

Approximately 10% of cases are associated with a *cutaneous T-cell lymphoma*, in the form of the Sézary syndrome or erythrodermic mycosis fungoides.[181] The erythroderma may precede or occur concurrently with the diagnosis of the cancer.[156,182] Uncommonly, erythroderma is associated with an extracutaneous lymphoma or some other tumor.[183]

The *idiopathic group*, also known as 'the red man syndrome', is associated more often with keratoderma and dermatopathic lymphadenitis than the other groups.[184] It is also more likely to persist than some of the other types. Some cases may progress to mycosis fungoides after many years.[184,185]

The pathogenetic mechanisms involved in erythroderma are not known. The erythema results from vascular dilatation and proliferation and it has been suggested that interreactions between lymphocytes and endothelium may play a role.[186] Circulating adhesion molecules are detectable in erythroderma but their values are not of differential diagnostic use.[187] A lymphocytopenia involving CD4[+] T cells is sometimes found, probably a consequence of the sequestration of these cells in the skin.[188]

Histopathology[189]

Skin biopsies in erythroderma have been regarded as 'largely unrewarding',[175] 'of variable usefulness',[166] 'of little value'[190] and 'misleading'.[190] However, in one series, an etiological diagnosis was made on the skin biopsy in 53% of cases[191] and, in another, in 66% of cases.[192] The diagnostic accuracy increases if multiple biopsies are taken simultaneously.[191] Biopsies are most often diagnostic in erythroderma associated with cutaneous T-cell lymphoma and, to a lesser extent, psoriasis and spongiotic dermatitis.[191] In cases related to an underlying dermatosis, the nature of this is not always discernible in the erythrodermic phase (Fig. 19.8).[189]

Usually, there is variable parakeratosis and hypogranulosis. The epidermis shows moderate acanthosis and, at times, there is psoriasiform hyperplasia, but this finding does not always correlate with the presence of underlying psoriasis.[190] Mild spongiosis is quite common even when there is underlying

psoriasis. Other features of psoriatic erythroderma resemble those seen in early lesions of psoriasis with only mild epidermal hyperplasia, mounds of parakeratosis with few neutrophils, and red cell extravasation in the papillary dermis.[193] Blood vessels in the upper dermis are usually dilated and sometimes there is endothelial swelling.[189]

There is a moderately heavy chronic inflammatory cell infiltrate in the upper dermis: this is sometimes perivascular in distribution and at other times more diffuse.[194] Atypical cells with cerebriform nuclei are present in the infiltrate in cases of erythroderma related to cutaneous T-cell lymphomas. Eosinophils may be present in the infiltrate and occasionally they are plentiful.[195] Exocytosis of lymphocytes is a frequent finding.

Drug-related cases may sometimes simulate the picture of mycosis fungoides, with prominent exocytosis and scattered atypical cells with cerebriform nuclei in the infiltrate.[15,195] In contrast to mycosis fungoides, however, Pautrier microabscesses are not present in the benign erythrodermas. Eosinophils are not always present in drug-related cases, as might be expected.[195] A very occasional apoptotic keratinocyte may be a clue to the drug etiology. Rarely, the picture is frankly lichenoid in type.[174,196]

Electron microscopy

One study showed a close association between lymphocytes and endothelial cells, although the significance of this finding remains to be evaluated.[186] Some lymphocytes were described as showing 'blastoid' transformation.[186]

PAPULOERYTHRODERMA

Papuloerythroderma of Ofuji is a rare entity, first reported from Japan, featuring widespread erythematous, flat-topped papules with a striking sparing of body folds (the so-called 'deck-chair' sign).[197–200] Eosinophilia and lymphopenia are sometimes present. It occurs most commonly in elderly males. It is often associated with underlying lymphoma or cancer.[201] It has developed in a patient with HIV infection[202] and in one with biliary sepsis.[203] Papuloerythroderma appears to be a distinct clinical entity, but its etiology is unknown. It has been suggested recently that it may be an early variant of mycosis fungoides.[204–206] Most cases run a chronic course.

Histopathology

The epidermis is usually normal, although it may show slight acanthosis, spongiosis and parakeratosis. There is a dense, predominantly perivascular infiltrate of lymphocytes, plasma cells and eosinophils in the upper and mid dermis.

S100-positive dendritic cells are abundant in the dermis.[199]

SCALP DYSESTHESIA

Scalp dysesthesia is characterized by symptoms of burning, stinging, or itching, which is often associated with psychological stress. The author has received biopsies (all normal) from at least 10 cases, and coined the term 'burning scalp syndrome'. Sometimes telogen effluvium may accompany this condition. Patients have benefited from low dose antidepressants.[207]

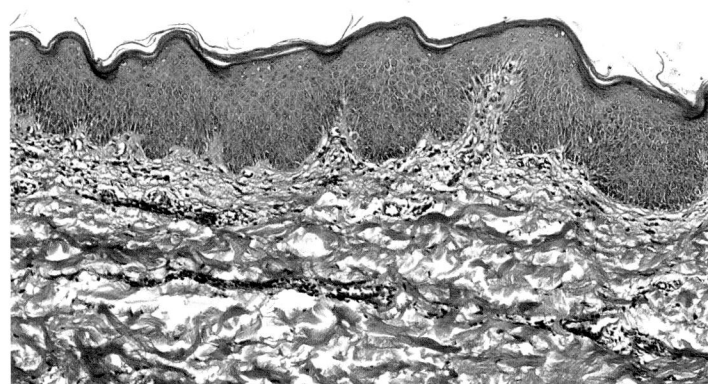

Fig. 19.8 **Erythroderma.** In this case of atopic dermatitis there is little spongiosis. The epidermal thickening with only mild psoriasiform folding is a feature of atopic dermatitis. (H & E)

REFERENCES

1 Brownstein MH, Wanger N, Helwig EB. Accessory tragi. Arch Dermatol 1971; 104: 625–631.
2 Sebben JE. The accessory tragus – no ordinary skin tag. J Dermatol Surg Oncol 1989; 15: 304–307.
3 Schissel DJ, Sartori C. An unusual papule. Arch Dermatol 1998; 134: 499–504.

4 Jansen T, Romiti R, Altmeyer P. Accessory tragus: report of two cases and review of the literature. Pediatr Dermatol 2000; 17: 391–394.

5 Hsueh S, Santa Cruz DJ. Cartilaginous lesions of the skin and superficial soft tissue. J Cutan Pathol 1982; 9: 405–416.

6 Sperling LC. Congenital cartilaginous rests of the neck. Int J Dermatol 1986; 25: 186–187.

7 Hogan D, Wilkinson RD, Williams A. Congenital anomalies of the head and neck. Int J Dermatol 1980; 19: 479–486.

8 Clarke JA. Are wattles of auricular or branchial origin? Br J Plast Surg 1976; 29: 238–244.

9 Tadini G, Cambiaghi S, Scarabelli G et al. Familial occurrence of isolated accessory tragi. Pediatr Dermatol 1993; 10: 26–28.

10 Resnick KI, Soltani K, Bernstein JE, Fathizadeh A. Accessory tragi and associated syndromes involving the first branchial arch. J Dermatol Surg Oncol 1981; 7: 39–41.

11 Satoh T, Tokura Y, Katsumata M et al. Histological diagnostic criteria for accessory tragi. J Cutan Pathol 1990; 17: 206–210.

12 Ban M, Kamiya H, Yamada T, Kitajima Y. Hair follicle nevi and accessory tragi: variable quantity of adipose tissue in connective tissue framework. Pediatr Dermatol 1997; 14: 433–436.

13 Drut R, Barletta L. Dermatorynchus geneae. J Cutan Pathol 1976; 3: 282–284.

14 Hendrick SJ, Sanchez RL, Blackwell SJ, Raimer SS. Striated muscle hamartoma: description of two cases. Pediatr Dermatol 1986; 3: 153–157.

15 Mehregan AH. Supernumerary nipple. A histologic study. J Cutan Pathol 1981; 8: 96–104.

16 Toumbis-Ioannou E, Cohen PR. Familial polythelia. J Am Acad Dermatol 1994; 30: 667–668.

17 Shewmake SW, Izuno GT. Supernumerary areolae. Arch Dermatol 1977; 113: 823–825.

18 Camisa C. Accessory breast on the posterior thigh of a man. J Am Acad Dermatol 1980; 3: 467–469.

19 Leung AKC, Robson WLM. Polythelia. Int J Dermatol 1989; 28: 429–433.

20 Armoni M, Filk D, Schlesinger M et al. Accessory nipples: any relationship to urinary tract malformation? Pediatr Dermatol 1992; 9: 239–240.

21 Camacho FM, Moreno-Gimenéz JC, García-Hernández MJ. Is aberrant mammary tissue a marker for chronic alcoholism or kidney-urinary tract malformations? Dermatology 1998; 197: 132–136.

22 Camacho F, González-Cámpora R. Polythelia pilosa: a particular form of accessory mammary tissue. Dermatology 1998; 196: 295–298.

23 Urbani CE, Betti R. Polythelia within Becker's naevus. Dermatology 1998; 196: 251–252.

24 Korkmaz A, Tekinalp G, Aygün C, Şahin S. Accessory scrotum: an unusual localization of scrotal skin. Pediatr Dermatol 1999; 16: 142–143.

25 Montero M, Méndez R, Tellado M et al. Agenesis of the scrotum. Pediatr Dermatol 2001; 18: 141–142.

26 Burvin R, Durst RY, Ben-Arieh Y, Barzilay A. Splenosis in exit gunshot wound. Br J Dermatol 1996; 135: 148–150.

27 Baack BR, Varsa EW, Burgdorf WHC, Blaugrund AC. Splenosis. A report of subcutaneous involvement. Am J Dermatopathol 1990; 12: 585–588.

28 Schweich L. Cheilitis glandularis simplex (Puente and Acevedo). Arch Dermatol 1964; 89: 301–302.

29 Findlay GH. Idiopathic enlargements of the lips: cheilitis granulomatosa, Ascher's syndrome and double lip. Br J Dermatol 1954; 66: 129–138.

30 Michalowski R. Cheilitis glandularis, heterotopic salivary glands and squamous cell carcinoma of the lip. Br J Dermatol 1962; 74: 445–449.

31 Swerlick RA, Cooper PH. Cheilitis glandularis: a re-evaluation. J Am Acad Dermatol 1984; 10: 466–472.

32 Weir TW, Johnson WC. Cheilitis glandularis. Arch Dermatol 1971; 103: 433–437.

33 Thomas JR III, Greene SL, Dicken CH. Factitious cheilitis. J Am Acad Dermatol 1983; 8: 368–372.

34 Crotty CP, Dicken CH. Factitious lip crusting. Arch Dermatol 1981; 117: 338–340.

35 Savage J. Localized crusting as an artefact. Br J Dermatol 1978; 99: 573–574.

36 Baughman RD, Berger P, Pringle WM. Plasma cell cheilitis. Arch Dermatol 1974; 110: 725–726.

37 Mathew MS, Srinivasan R, Goyal JL et al. Ascher's syndrome: an unusual case with entropion. Int J Dermatol 1992; 31: 710–712.

38 Navas J, Rodríguez-Pichardo A, Camacho F. Ascher syndrome: a case study. Pediatr Dermatol 1991; 8: 122–123.

39 Sanchez MR, Lee M, Moy JA, Ostreicher R. Ascher syndrome: a mimicker of acquired angioedema. J Am Acad Dermatol 1993; 29: 650–651.

40 Steck WD, Helwig EB. Umbilical granulomas, pilonidal disease and the urachus. Surg Gynecol Obstet 1965; 120: 1043–1057.

41 Steck WD, Helwig EB. Cutaneous remnants of the omphalomesenteric duct. Arch Dermatol 1964; 90: 463–470.

42 Armstrong DKB, Thornton C, Bingham EA. Infantile umbilical polyp: important diagnostic considerations. Dermatology 1998; 197: 94.

43 Hejazi N. Umbilical polyp: a report of two cases. Dermatologica 1975; 150: 111–115.

44 Barrow MV. Metastatic tumors of the umbilicus. J Chronic Dis 1966; 19: 1113–1117.

45 Powell FC, Su WPD. Dermatoses of the umbilicus. Int J Dermatol 1988; 27: 150–156.

46 Eby CS, Jetton RL. Umbilical pilonidal sinus. Arch Dermatol 1972; 106: 893.

47 Ross JE, Hill RB Jr. Primary umbilical adenocarcinoma. A case report and review of literature. Arch Pathol 1975; 99: 327–329.

48 McAdam LP, O'Hanlan MA, Bluestone R, Pearson CM. Relapsing polychondritis. Prospective study of 23 patients and a review of the literature. Medicine (Baltimore) 1976; 55: 193–215.

49 Cohen PR, Rapini RP. Relapsing polychondritis. Int J Dermatol 1986; 25: 280–285.

50 Hughes RAC, Berry CL, Seifert M, Lessof MH. Relapsing polychondritis. Three cases with a clinico-pathological study and literature review. Q J Med 1972; 41: 363–380.

51 White JW Jr. Relapsing polychondritis. South Med J 1985; 78: 448–451.

52 Thurston CS, Curtis AC. Relapsing polychondritis. Arch Dermatol 1966; 93: 664–669.

53 Khan JH, Ahmed I. A case of relapsing polychondritis involving the tragal and the conchal bowl areas with sparing of the helix and the antihelix. J Am Acad Dermatol 1999; 41: 299–302.

54 Hedfors E, Hammar H, Theorell H. Relapsing polychondritis. Presentation of 4 cases. Dermatologica 1982; 164: 47–53.

55 Weinberger A, Myers AR. Relapsing polychondritis associated with cutaneous vasculitis. Arch Dermatol 1979; 115: 980–981.

56 Borbujo J, Balsa A, Aguado P, Casado M. Relapsing polychondritis associated with psoriasis vulgaris. J Am Acad Dermatol 1989; 20: 130–131.

57 Enright H, Jacob HS, Vercellotti G et al. Paraneoplastic autoimmune phenomena in patients with myelodysplastic syndromes: response to immunosuppressive therapy. Br J Haematol 1995; 91: 403–408.

58 Diebold L, Rauh G, Jäger K, Löhrs U. Bone marrow pathology in relapsing polychondritis: high frequency of myelodysplastic syndromes. Br J Haematol 1995; 89: 820–830.

59 Fujimoto N, Tajima S, Ishibashi A et al. Acute febrile neutrophilic dermatosis (Sweet's syndrome) in a patient with relapsing polychondritis. Br J Dermatol 1998; 139: 930–931.

60 Helm TN, Valenzuela R, Glanz S et al. Relapsing polychondritis: a case diagnosed by direct immunofluorescence and coexisting with pseudocyst of the auricle. J Am Acad Dermatol 1992; 26: 315–318.

61 Anstey A, Mayou S, Morgan K et al. Relapsing polychondritis: autoimmunity to type II collagen and treatment with cyclosporin A. Br J Dermatol 1991; 125: 588–591.

62 Valenzuela R, Cooperrider PA, Gogate P et al. Relapsing polychondritis. Immunomicroscopic findings in cartilage of ear biopsy specimens. Hum Pathol 1980; 11: 19–22.

63 Labarthe M-P, Bayle-Lebey P, Bazex J. Cutaneous manifestations of relapsing polychondritis in a patient receiving goserelin for carcinoma of the prostate. Dermatology 1997; 195: 391–394.

64 Askari AD. Colchicine for treatment of relapsing polychondritis. J Am Acad Dermatol 1984; 10: 507–510.

65 Barranco VP, Minor DB, Solomon H. Treatment of relapsing polychondritis with dapsone. Arch Dermatol 1976; 112: 1286–1288.

66 Ridgway HB, Hansotia PH, Schorr WF. Relapsing polychondritis. Unusual neurological findings and therapeutic efficacy of dapsone. Arch Dermatol 1979; 115: 43–45.

67 Hashimoto K, Arkin CR, Kang AH. Relapsing polychondritis. An ultrastructural study. Arthritis Rheum 1977; 20: 91–99.

68 Flier JS. Metabolic importance of acanthosis nigricans. Arch Dermatol 1985; 121: 193–194.

69 Brown J, Winkelmann RK. Acanthosis nigricans: a study of 90 cases. Medicine (Baltimore) 1968; 47: 33–51.

70 Rogers DL. Acanthosis nigricans. Semin Dermatol 1991; 10: 160–163.

71 Akyol M, Polat M, Özçelik S et al. Acanthosis nigricans with atypical localization. Acta Derm Venereol 2000; 80: 399.

72 Andreev VC, Boyanov L, Tsankov N. Generalized acanthosis nigricans. Dermatologica 1981; 163: 19–24.

73 Hall JM, Moreland A, Cox GJ, Wade TR. Oral acanthosis nigricans: report of a case and comparison of oral and cutaneous pathology. Am J Dermatopathol 1988; 10: 68–73.

74 Kozlowski LM, Nigra TP. Esophageal acanthosis nigricans in association with adenocarcinoma from an unknown primary site. J Am Acad Dermatol 1992; 26: 348–351.

75 Hazen PG, Carney JF, Walker AE, Stewart JJ. Acanthosis nigricans presenting as hyperkeratosis of the palms and soles. J Am Acad Dermatol 1979; 1: 541–544.

76 Breathnach SM, Wells GC. Acanthosis palmaris: tripe palms. Clin Exp Dermatol 1980; 5: 181–189.

77 Andreev VC. Malignant acanthosis nigricans. Semin Dermatol 1984; 3: 265–272.

78 Rigel DS, Jacobs MI. Malignant acanthosis nigricans: a review. J Dermatol Surg Oncol 1980; 6: 923–927.

79 Hage E, Hage J. Malignant acanthosis nigricans – a para-endocrine syndrome? Acta Derm Venereol 1977; 57: 169–172.

80 Schmidt KT, Massa MC, Welykyj SE. Acanthosis nigricans and a rectal carcinoid. J Am Acad Dermatol 1991; 25: 361–365.

81 Anderson SHC, Hudson-Peacock M, Muller AF. Malignant acanthosis nigricans: potential role of chemotherapy. Br J Dermatol 1999; 141: 714–716.

82 Guo Y, Wieczorek R. Acanthosis nigricans. Dermatopathology: Practical & Conceptual 2000; 6: 157.

83 Schweitzer WJ, Goldin HM, Bronson DM, Brody PE. Acanthosis nigricans associated with mycosis fungoides. J Am Acad Dermatol 1988; 19: 951–953.

84 Moscardi JL, Macedo NA, Espasandin JA, Piñeyro MI. Malignant acanthosis nigricans associated with a renal tumor. Int J Dermatol 1993; 32: 893–894.

85 Bottoni U, Dianzani C, Pranteda G et al. Florid cutaneous and mucosal papillomatosis with acanthosis nigricans revealing a primary lung cancer. J Eur Acad Dermatol Venereol 2000; 14: 205–208.

86 Gohji K, Hasunuma Y, Gotoh A et al. Acanthosis nigricans associated with transitional cell carcinoma of the urinary bladder. Int J Dermatol 1994; 33: 433–435.

87 Mikhail GR, Fachnie DM, Drukker BH et al. Generalized malignant acanthosis nigricans. Arch Dermatol 1979; 115: 201–202.

88 Curth HO, Hilberg AW, Machacek GF. The site and histology of the cancer associated with malignant acanthosis nigricans. Cancer 1962; 15: 364–382.

89 Plourde PV, Marks JG Jr, Hammond JM. Acanthosis nigricans and insulin resistance. J Am Acad Dermatol 1984; 10: 887–891.

90 Barth JH, Ng LL, Wojnarowska F, Dawber RPR. Acanthosis nigricans, insulin resistance and cutaneous virilism. Br J Dermatol 1988; 118: 613–619.

91 Ober KP. Acanthosis nigricans and insulin resistance associated with hypothyroidism. Arch Dermatol 1985; 121: 229–231.

92 Dix JH, Levy WJ, Fuenning C. Remission of acanthosis nigricans, hypertrichosis, and Hashimoto's thyroiditis with thyroxine replacement. Pediatr Dermatol 1986; 3: 323–326.

93 Flier JS, Eastman RC, Minaker KL et al. Acanthosis nigricans in obese women with hyperandrogenism. Diabetes 1985; 34: 101–107.

94 Rendon MI, Cruz PD Jr, Sontheimer RD, Bergstresser PR. Acanthosis nigricans: a cutaneous marker of tissue resistance to insulin. J Am Acad Dermatol 1989; 21: 461–469.

95 Feingold KR, Elias PM. Endocrine–skin interactions. J Am Acad Dermatol 1988; 19: 1–20.

96 Esperanza LE, Fenske NA. Hyperandrogenism, insulin resistance, and acanthosis nigricans (HAIR-AN) syndrome: spontaneous remission in a 15-year-old girl. J Am Acad Dermatol 1996; 34: 892–897.

97 Harman M, Akdeniz S, Çetin H, Tuzcu A. Acanthosis nigricans with vitiligo and insulin resistance. Br J Dermatol 2000; 143: 899–900.

98 Brockow K, Steinkraus V, Rinninger F et al. Acanthosis nigricans: a marker for hyperinsulinemia. Pediatr Dermatol 1995; 12: 323–326.

99 Schwartz RA. Acanthosis nigricans. J Am Acad Dermatol 1994; 31: 1–19.

100 Brubaker MM, Levan NE, Collipp PJ. Acanthosis nigricans and congenital total lipodystrophy. Arch Dermatol 1965; 91: 320–325.

101 Reed WB, Dexter R, Corley C, Fish C. Congenital lipodystrophic diabetes with acanthosis nigricans. The Seip–Lawrence syndrome. Arch Dermatol 1965; 91: 326–334.

102 Janaki VR, Premalatha S, Rao NR, Thambiah AS. Lawrence–Seip syndrome. Br J Dermatol 1980; 103: 693–696.

103 Sherertz EF. Improved acanthosis nigricans with lipodystrophic diabetes during dietary fish oil supplementation. Arch Dermatol 1988; 124: 1094–1096.

104 Reed WB, Ragsdale W Jr, Curtis AC, Richards HJ. Acanthosis nigricans in association with various genodermatoses. Acta Derm Venereol 1968; 48: 465–473.

105 Kahn CR, Flier JS, Bar RS et al. The syndromes of insulin resistance and acanthosis nigricans. Insulin-receptor disorders in man. N Engl J Med 1976; 294: 739–745.

106 Hud JA Jr, Cohen JB, Wagner JM, Cruz PD. Prevalence and significance of acanthosis nigricans in an adult obese population. Arch Dermatol 1992; 128: 941–944.

107 Kuroki R, Sadamoto Y, Imamura M et al. Acanthosis nigricans with severe obesity, insulin resistance and hypothyroidism: improvement by diet control. Dermatology 1999; 198: 164–166.

108 Dunaif A, Hoffman AR, Scully RE et al. Clinical, biochemical, and ovarian morphologic features in women with acanthosis nigricans and masculinization. Obstet Gynecol 1985; 66: 545–552.

109 Panidis D, Skiadopoulos S, Rousso D et al. Association of acanthosis nigricans with insulin resistance in patients with polycystic ovary syndrome. Br J Dermatol 1995; 132: 936–941.

110 Tasjian D, Jarratt M. Familial acanthosis nigricans. Arch Dermatol 1984; 120: 1351–1354.

111 Dhar S, Dawn G, Kanwar AJ, Nada R. Familial acanthosis nigricans. Int J Dermatol 1996; 35: 126–127.

112 Nakanishi T, Hisa T, Hamada T et al. A case of acanthosis nigricans in obese siblings with a pedigree of familial polyposis coli. Clin Exp Dermatol 1997; 22: 99–100.

113 Downs AMR, Kennedy CTC. Somatotrophin-induced acanthosis nigricans. Br J Dermatol 1999; 141: 390–391.

114 Randle HW, Winkelmann RK. Steroid-induced acanthosis nigricans in dermatomyositis. Arch Dermatol 1979; 115: 587–588.

115 Elgart ML. Acanthosis nigricans and nicotinic acid. J Am Acad Dermatol 1981; 5: 709–710.

116 Coates P, Shuttleworth D, Rees A. Resolution of nicotinic acid-induced acanthosis nigricans by substitution of an analogue (acipimox) in a patient with type V hyperlipidaemia. Br J Dermatol 1992; 126: 412–414.

117 Greenspan AH, Shupack JL, Foo S-H, Wise AC. Acanthosis nigricans-like hyperpigmentation secondary to triazinate therapy. Arch Dermatol 1985; 121: 232–235.

118 Shuttleworth D, Weavind GP, Graham-Brown RAC. Acanthosis nigricans and diabetes mellitus in a patient with Klinefelter's syndrome: a reaction to methyltestosterone. Clin Exp Dermatol 1987; 12: 288–290.

119 Teknetzis A, Lefaki I, Joannides D, Minas A. Acanthosis nigricans-like lesions after local application of fusidic acid. J Am Acad Dermatol 1993; 28: 501–502.

120 Bonnekoh B, Wevers A, Spangenberger H et al. Keratin pattern of acanthosis nigricans in syndromelike association with polythelia, polycystic kidneys, and syndactyly. Arch Dermatol 1993; 129: 1177–1182.

121 Fleming MG, Simon SI. Cutaneous insulin reaction resembling acanthosis nigricans. Arch Dermatol 1986; 122: 1054–1056.

122 Hamilton D, Tavafoghi V, Shafer JC, Hambrick GW. Confluent and reticulated papillomatosis of Gougerot and Carteaud. Its relation to other papillomatoses. J Am Acad Dermatol 1980; 2: 401–410.

123 Thomsen K. Confluent and reticulated papillomatosis (Gougerot–Carteaud). Acta Derm Venereol (Suppl) 1979; 85: 185–187.

124 Fuller LC, Hay RJ. Confluent and reticulate papillomatosis of Gougerot and Carteaud clearing with minocycline. Clin Exp Dermatol 1994; 19: 343–345.

125 Lee MP, Stiller MJ, McClain SA et al. Confluent and reticulated papillomatosis: response to high-dose oral isotretinoin therapy and reassessment of epidemiologic data. J Am Acad Dermatol 1994; 31: 327–331.

126 Vassileva S, Pramatarov K, Popova L. Ultraviolet light-induced confluent and reticulated papillomatosis. J Am Acad Dermatol 1989; 21: 413–414.

127 Roberts SOB, Lachapelle JM. Confluent and reticulate papillomatosis (Gougerot–Carteaud) and Pityrosporum orbiculare. Br J Dermatol 1969; 81: 841–845.

128 Faergemann J. Lipophilic yeasts in skin diseases. Semin Dermatol 1985; 4: 173–184.

129 Broberg A, Faergemann J. A case of confluent and reticulate papillomatosis (Gougerot–Carteaud) with an unusual location. Acta Derm Venereol 1988; 68: 158–160.

130 Angel -Besson C, Koeppel MC, Jacquet P et al. Confluent and reticulated papillomatosis (Gougerot–Carteaud) treated with tetracyclines. Int J Dermatol 1995; 34: 567–569.

131 El-Tonsy MH, El-Benhawi MO, Mehregan AH. Confluent and reticulated papillomatosis. J Am Acad Dermatol 1987; 16: 893–894.

132 Carrozzo AM, Gatti S, Ferranti G et al. Calcipotriol treatment of confluent and reticulated papillomatosis (Gougerot–Carteaud syndrome). J Eur Acad Dermatol Venereol 2000; 14: 131–133.

133 Güleç AT, Seçkin D. Confluent and reticulated papillomatosis: treatment with topical calcipotriol. Br J Dermatol 1999; 141: 1150–1151.

134 Solomon BA, Laude TA. Two patients with confluent and reticulated papillomatosis: Response to oral isotretinoin and 10% lactic acid lotion. J Am Acad Dermatol 1996; 35: 645–646.

135 Raja Babu KK, Snehal S, Sudha Vani D. Confluent and reticulate papillomatosis: successful treatment with azithromycin. Br J Dermatol 2000; 142: 1252–1253.

136 Fung MA, Frieden IJ, LeBoit PE et al. Confluent and reticulate papillomatosis: successful treatment with minocycline. Arch Dermatol 1996; 132: 1400–1401.

137 Shimizu S, Han-Yaku H. Confluent and reticulated papillomatosis responsive to minocycline. Dermatology 1997; 194: 59–61.

138 Jang H-S, Oh C-K, Cha J-H et al. Six cases of confluent and reticulated papillomatosis alleviated by various antibiotics. J Am Acad Dermatol 2001; 44: 652–655.

139 Henning JPH, de Wit RFE. Familial occurrence of confluent and reticulated papillomatosis. Arch Dermatol 1981; 117: 809–810.

140 Jimbow M, Talpash O, Jimbow K. Confluent and reticulated papillomatosis: clinical, light, and electron microscopic studies. Int J Dermatol 1992; 31: 480–483.

141 Atherton DJ, Wells RS. Confluent and reticulate papillomatosis. Clin Exp Dermatol 1980; 5: 465–469.

142 Montemarano AD, Hengge M, Sau P, Welch M. Confluent and reticulated papillomatosis: response to minocycline. J Am Acad Dermatol 1996; 34: 253–256.

143 Bazex A, Griffiths A. Acrokeratosis paraneoplastica – a new cutaneous marker of malignancy. Br J Dermatol 1980; 103: 301–306.

144 Jacobsen FK, Abildtrup N, Laursen SO et al. Acrokeratosis paraneoplastica (Bazex' syndrome). Arch Dermatol 1984; 120: 502–504.

145 Poole S, Fenske NA. Cutaneous markers of internal malignancy. II. Paraneoplastic dermatoses and environmental carcinogens. J Am Acad Dermatol 1993; 28: 147–164.

146 Obasi OE, Garg SK. Bazex paraneoplastic acrokeratosis in prostate carcinoma. Br J Dermatol 1987; 117: 647–651.

147 Arregui MA, Ratón JA, Landa N et al. Bazex's syndrome (acrokeratosis paraneoplastica) – first case report of association with a bladder carcinoma. Clin Exp Dermatol 1993; 18: 445–448.

148 Rosner SA, Nurse DS, Dowling JP. Paraneoplastic acrokeratosis. Australas J Dermatol 1984; 25: 12–14.

149 Douglas WS, Bilsland DJ, Howatson R. Acrokeratosis paraneoplastica of Bazex – a case in the UK. Clin Exp Dermatol 1991; 16: 297–299.

150 Mutasim DF, Meiri G. Bazex syndrome mimicking a primary autoimmune bullous disorder. J Am Acad Dermatol 1999; 40: 822–825.

151 Richard M, Giroux J-M. Acrokeratosis paraneoplastica (Bazex' syndrome). J Am Acad Dermatol 1987; 16: 178–183.

152 Lomholt H, Thestrup-Pedersen K. Paraneoplastic skin manifestations of lung cancer. Acta Derm Venereol 2000; 80: 200–202.

153 Lucker GPH, Steijlen PM. Acrokeratosis paraneoplastica (Bazex syndrome) occurring with acquired ichthyosis in Hodgkin's disease. Br J Dermatol 1995; 133: 322–325.

154 Witkowski JA, Parish LC. Bazex's syndrome. Paraneoplastic acrokeratosis. JAMA 1982; 248: 2883–2884.

155 Hasan T, Jansen CT. Erythroderma: a follow-up of fifty cases. J Am Acad Dermatol 1983; 8: 836–840.

156 Callen JP. Skin signs of internal malignancy: fact, fancy, and fiction. Semin Dermatol 1984; 3: 340–357.

157 King LE Jr. Erythroderma. Who, where, when, why, and how.... Arch Dermatol 1994; 130: 1545–1547.

158 Asai T, Horiuchi Y. Senile erythroderma with serum hyper IgE. Int J Dermatol 1989; 28: 255–256.

159 Kalter DC, Atherton DJ, Clayton PT. X-linked dominant Conradi–Hünermann syndrome presenting as congenital erythroderma. J Am Acad Dermatol 1989; 21: 248–256.

160 Goodyear HM, Harper JI. Leiner's disease associated with metabolic acidosis. Clin Exp Dermatol 1989; 14: 364–366.

161 Pruszkowski A, Bodemer C, Fraitag S et al. Neonatal and infantile erythrodermas. A retrospective study of 51 patients. Arch Dermatol 2000; 136: 875–880.

162 Botella-Estrada R, Sanmartín O, Oliver V et al. Erythroderma. A clinicopathological study of 56 cases. Arch Dermatol 1994; 130: 1503–1507.

163 Pal S, Haroon TS. Erythroderma: a clinico-etiologic study of 90 cases. Int J Dermatol 1998; 37: 104–107.

164 Boyd AS, Menter A. Erythrodermic psoriasis. Precipitating factors, course, and prognosis in 50 patients. J Am Acad Dermatol 1989; 21: 985–991.

165 Sigurdsson V, Toonstra J, Hezemans-Boer M, van Vloten WA. Erythroderma. A clinical and follow-up study of 102 patients, with special emphasis on survival. J Am Acad Dermatol 1996; 35: 53–57.

166 King LE Jr, Dufresne RG Jr, Lovett GL, Rosin MA. Erythroderma: review of 82 cases. South Med J 1986; 79: 1210–1215.

167 Tappeiner G, Konrad K, Holubar K. Erythrodermic bullous pemphigoid. Report of a case. J Am Acad Dermatol 1982; 6: 489–492.

168 Wolf P, Müllegger R, Cerroni L et al. Photoaccentuated erythroderma associated with CD4+ T lymphocytopenia: Successful treatment with 5- methoxypsoralen and UVA, interferon alfa-2b, and extracorporeal photopheresis. J Am Acad Dermatol 1996; 35: 291–294.

169 Gupta R, Khera V. Erythroderma due to dermatophyte. Acta Derm Venereol 2001; 81: 70.

170 Morar N, Dlova N, Gupta AK et al. Erythroderma: a comparison between HIV positive and negative patients. Int J Dermatol 1999; 38: 895–900.

171 Petrozzi JW, Shore RN. Generalized exfoliative dermatitis from ethylenediamine. Sensitization and induction. Arch Dermatol 1976; 112: 525–526.

172 Slagel GA, James WD. Plaquenil-induced erythroderma. J Am Acad Dermatol 1985; 12: 857–862.

173 Kawana S. Drug eruption induced by cyanamide (carbimide): a clinical and histopathologic study of 7 patients. Dermatology 1997; 195: 30–34.

174 Reynolds NJ, Jones SK, Crossley J, Harman RRM. Exfoliative dermatitis due to nifedipine. Br J Dermatol 1989; 121: 401–404.

175 Sehgal VN, Srivastava G. Exfoliative dermatitis. A prospective study of 80 patients. Dermatologica 1986; 173: 278–284.

176 Bigby M, Stern R. Cutaneous reactions to nonsteroidal anti-inflammatory drugs. A review. J Am Acad Dermatol 1985; 12: 866–876.

177 Shelley WB, Shelley ED. Chronic erythroderma induced by β-blocker (timolol maleate) eyedrops. J Am Acad Dermatol 1997; 37: 799–800.

178 Holme SA, Roberts DL. Erythroderma associated with St. John's wort. Br J Dermatol 2000; 143: 1127–1128.

179 Asnis LA, Gaspari AA. Cutaneous reactions to recombinant cytokine therapy. J Am Acad Dermatol 1995; 33: 393–410.

180 Horn TD, Altomonte V, Vogelsang G, Kennedy MJ. Erythroderma after autologous bone marrow transplantation modified by administration of cyclosporine and interferon gamma for breast cancer. J Am Acad Dermatol 1996; 34: 413–417.

181 Duangurai K, Piamphongsant T, Himmungnan T. Sézary cell count in exfoliative dermatitis. Int J Dermatol 1988; 27: 248–252.

182 Winkelmann RK, Buecher SA, Diaz-Perez JL. Pre-Sézary syndrome. J Am Acad Dermatol 1984; 10: 992–999.

183 Leong ASY, Cowled PA, Zalewski PD et al. Erythroderma, an unusual manifestation of B cell lymphoma. Br J Dermatol 1978; 99: 99–106.

184 Thestrup-Pedersen K, Halkier-Sørensen L, Søgaard H, Zachariae H. The red man syndrome. Exfoliative dermatitis of unknown etiology: a description and follow–up of 38 patients. J Am Acad Dermatol 1988; 18: 1307–1312.

185 Sigurdsson V, Toonstra J, van Vloten VA. Idiopathic erythroderma: a follow-up study of 28 patients. Dermatology 1997; 194: 98–101.

186 Heng MCY, Heng CY, Kloss SG, Chase DG. Erythroderma associated with mixed lymphocyte–endothelial cell interaction and Staphylococcus aureus infection. Br J Dermatol 1986; 115: 693–705.

187 Groves RW, Kapahi P, Barker JNWN et al. Detection of circulating adhesion molecules in erythrodermic skin disease. J Am Acad Dermatol 1995; 32: 32–36.

188 Griffiths TW, Stevens SR, Cooper KD. Acute erythroderma as an exclusion criterion for idiopathic CD4+ T lymphocytopenia. Arch Dermatol 1994; 130: 1530–1533.

189 Nicolis GD, Helwig EB. Exfoliative dermatitis. A clinicopathologic study of 135 cases. Arch Dermatol 1973; 108: 788–797.

190 Abrahams I, McCarthy JT, Sanders SL. 101 cases of exfoliative dermatitis. Arch Dermatol 1963; 87: 96–101.

191 Walsh NMG, Prokopetz R, Tron VA et al. Histopathology in erythroderma: review of a series of cases by multiple observers. J Cutan Pathol 1994; 21: 419–423.

192 Zip C, Murray S, Walsh NMG. The specificity of histopathology in erythroderma. J Cutan Pathol 1993; 20: 393–398.

193 Tomasini C, Aloi F, Solaroli C, Pippione M. Psoriatic erythroderma: a histopathologic study of forty-five patients. Dermatology 1997; 194: 102–106.

194 Abel EA, Lindae ML, Hoppe RT, Wood GS. Benign and malignant forms of erythroderma: cutaneous and immunophenotypic characteristics. J Am Acad Dermatol 1988; 19: 1089–1095.

195 Sentis HJ, Willemze R, Scheffer E. Histopathologic studies in Sézary syndrome and erythrodermic mycosis fungoides: a comparison with benign forms of erythroderma. J Am Acad Dermatol 1986; 15: 1217–1226.

196 Patterson JW, Berry AD III, Darwin BS et al. Lichenoid histopathologic changes in patients with clinical diagnoses of exfoliative dermatitis. Am J Dermatopathol 1991; 13: 358–364.

197 Wakeel RA, Keefe M, Chapman RS. Papuloerythroderma. Another case of a new disease. Arch Dermatol 1991; 127: 96–98.

198 Nazzari G, Crovato F, Nigro A. Papuloerythroderma (Ofuji): two additional cases and review of the literature. J Am Acad Dermatol 1992; 26: 499–501.

199 Tay YK, Tan KC, Wong WK, Ong BH. Papuloerythroderma of Ofuji: a report of three cases and review of the literature. Br J Dermatol 1994; 130: 773–776.

200 Sommer S, Henderson CA. Papuloerythroderma of Ofuji responding to treatment with cyclosporin. Clin Exp Dermatol 2000; 25: 293–295.

201 Aste N, Fumo G, Conti B, Biggio P. Ofuji papuloerythroderma. J Eur Acad Dermatol Venereol 2000; 14: 55–57.

202 Lonnee ER, Toonstra J, van der Putte SCJ et al. Papuloerythroderma of Ofuji in a HIV-infected patient. Br J Dermatol 1996; 135: 500–501.

203 Azón-Masoliver A, Casadó J, Brunet J et al. Ofuji's papuloerythroderma following choledocholithiasis with secondary sepsis: complete resolution with surgery. Clin Exp Dermatol 1998; 23: 84–86.

204 Bech-Thomsen N, Thomsen K. Ofuji's papuloerythroderma: a study of 17 cases. Clin Exp Dermatol 1998; 23: 79–83.

205 Suh KS, Jang JG, Hur J et al. Is Ofuji papuloerythroderma a variant of mycosis fungoides? Am J Dermatopathol 2000; 22: 345 (abstract).

206 Tay YK, Tan KC, Ong BH. Papuloerythroderma of Ofuji and cutaneous T-cell lymphoma. Br J Dermatol 1997; 137: 160–161.

207 Hoss D, Segal S. Scalp dysethesia. Arch Dermatol 1998; 134: 327–330.

Cutaneous drug reactions

INTRODUCTION

A drug reaction can be defined as an undesirable response evoked by a medicinal substance. Any drug is a potential cause of an adverse reaction, although certain classes of drugs can be incriminated more often than others. Major offenders include antibiotics (particularly the newer ones and oral antifungal agents), non-steroidal anti-inflammatory drugs, psychotropic agents, beta blockers and gold.[1,2] Preservatives and coloring agents in foodstuffs, as well as chemicals used in industry, may sometimes produce cutaneous reactions that are indistinguishable from those produced by medicinal substances. These other agents should always be kept in mind in the etiology of an apparent drug reaction.

Although some drugs cause only one clinical pattern of reaction, most are capable of producing several different types of reaction.[3] While most of these adverse reactions involve the skin, other organs such as the lungs, kidneys, liver and lymph nodes may be affected singly or in various combinations.[4,5] Since the teratogenic effects of thalidomide received widespread coverage over 40 years ago, this potential complication receives considerable experimental attention in the early testing of new compounds.[6,7] Drug fever is another clinical manifestation of an adverse drug reaction.

Continuing advances in pharmacology have resulted in the introduction of an ever increasing number of drugs for therapeutic purposes with a consequent avalanche of case reports detailing adverse reactions.[8,9] The true prevalence of cutaneous drug reactions is difficult to determine as most studies have been based on hospital inpatients, many of whom are receiving several drugs simultaneously.[1,10] In these inpatient series, drug reactions have occurred in approximately 2% of patients;[11] this figure is probably not relevant to outpatients. If looked at in another way, drug reactions are relatively uncommon when the number of reactions per course of drug therapy is considered.[11] Another important facet is the drug interaction in which one drug affects the action of another, usually by causing increased or decreased plasma levels of that drug. This so-called 'pharmacokinetic reaction' usually results from the influence of one or more of the drugs on the cytochrome P-450 isoenzyme system in the liver.[12,13]

Diagnosing drug reactions

Attribution of a cutaneous reaction to a particular drug may be difficult since many patients receive many drugs simultaneously.[11] Furthermore, many drug reactions mimic various dermatoses, most of which may have other causes. Certain patterns are, however, frequently caused by drugs: these include exanthematous reactions, urticaria, photosensitive eruptions, fixed drug eruptions, erythema multiforme and toxic epidermal necrolysis.[1,3,14] Other factors that may be used to identify the offending drug include cessation of the suspected drug (dechallenge), rechallenge with the suspected drug at a later time (provocation),[15] the use of specifically designed computer algorithms,[16] a knowledge of drug reaction rates and the morphology of lesions produced by particular drugs.[8,17] Case reports, manufacturers' brochures and reporting systems have all contributed to our knowledge of the various reactions produced by particular drugs.[17-19] Another important factor in identifying an offending drug is the timing of events.[18] Most drug reactions occur within 10 days of receiving the offending agent, although longer periods have been recorded. Furthermore, some drug reactions may persist for weeks to months after use of the drug has ceased. This applies particularly to reactions to gold.[14]

Provocation tests, whereby the patient is challenged with the drug suspected of causing the reaction, may provide confirmation in over 50% of cases.[15] However, false-positive and false-negative reactions may occur, and there are also ethical considerations because in certain circumstances rechallenge may produce a severe anaphylaxis.[20] Withdrawal tests are time consuming if multiple drugs are involved.[9]

The shortcomings of in vivo testing and clinical observations have led to many studies being carried out to assess the reliability of various in vitro tests.[9] Most have involved immunological methods as drug allergy is one mechanism involved in the pathogenesis of drug reactions. Some, such as skin testing, radioallergosorbent tests (RAST) and lymphocyte transformation studies, have been of limited diagnostic value. Patch testing is usually of value only in allergic contact reactions, although positive patch tests have been found in 15% of patients with presumed drug reactions.[21] Prick and intradermal skin tests have also been used in the evaluation of drug reactions.[22]

The most sensitive test appears to be that for macrophage migration inhibition factor (MIF), a lymphokine which is released when sensitized T lymphocytes are challenged with the appropriate antigen.[8,9,23] It is seen with cell-mediated and some immediate-type reactions.[9] A positive MIF response to a variety of drugs has been found in 50–70% of patients with suspected drug eruptions but only in 5% of controls.[9] Accordingly, it is a useful adjunct to clinical observations in detecting the offending drug.

Mechanisms of drug reactions

Various mechanisms, including toxic, metabolic and allergic, have been implicated in the pathogenesis of cutaneous drug reactions.[24] Certain patient groups are at an increased risk of developing an adverse drug reaction, including women, patients with Sjögren's syndrome, and those with the acquired immunodeficiency syndrome.[25,26] It has been suggested that 'pharmacogenetic variability' may account for a susceptibility to certain serious drug reactions.[25] Examples include glutathione synthetase deficiency (particularly in patients with AIDS) predisposing to sulfonamide reactions, epoxide hydrolase deficiency leading to the anticonvulsant hypersensitivity syndrome (see p. 588), and defects in drug acetylation resulting in isoniazid reactions.[25] A 'toxic' hypothesis does not explain all the characteristics of drug reactions.[27] For many substances the mechanism is still uncertain. The term 'idiosyncratic drug reaction' has been used for unpredictable reactions that occur in only a small percentage of patients receiving the drug and which do not involve known pharmacological properties of the drug.[28] This term includes many of the reactions thought to have an immunological basis (see below).

Immunological (allergic) mechanisms are thought to account for less than 25% of all cutaneous drug reactions despite the fact that positive tests for MIF (see above) are found in over 50% of suspected cases.[4,9] This is because secondary immunological events may develop in the course of some drug reactions which basically are not of immunological pathogenesis.[8]

Immunological drug reactions have certain features that distinguish them from non-immunological reactions, although none is absolute.[29] They occur in only a small percentage of the population at risk; they may occur below the therapeutic range of the drug; and they appear after a latent period of several days, although this duration may be shorter on rechallenge.[29] Certain clinical patterns of drug reaction, such as systemic anaphylaxis, serum sickness, allergic and photoallergic contact dermatitis, fixed drug eruption, vasculitis and the systemic lupus erythematosus-like syndrome, are characteristic of the immunological types of drug reaction.[4,14,29,30] Urticaria may result from both immunological and non-immunological reactions, and some exanthematous reactions may have an immunological basis. The majority of allergic drug reactions are caused by antibiotics, blood products, anti-inflammatory agents and inhaled mucolytics.[10]

All four Coombs and Gell reactions may be involved in allergic reactions to drugs although cutaneous reactions have not been clearly shown to be cytotoxic (type II reaction) in nature.[4,30] The most significant drug reactions involve immediate hypersensitivity (type I reaction) and are IgE mediated.[24] The best studied of this class of reaction is penicillin allergy, in which IgE antibodies to penicillin have been detected in the serum of affected individuals. Clinical manifestations of type I reactions include anaphylaxis, urticaria and angioedema. Immune complexes (type III reaction) are involved in the pathogenesis of vasculitis, serum sickness, some urticarial and exanthematous reactions, systemic lupus erythematosus-like drug reactions and possibly erythema multiforme and erythema nodosum, when due to drugs.[24,30] Immunohistochemical analysis has identified CD8-positive T cells as the predominant epidermal T-cell subset in drug-induced maculopapular and bullous eruptions.[23] However, more recent studies have isolated a heterogeneous population of CD4+ lymphocytes which are drug specific.[31,32] The cells, when stimulated, produce interleukin-5. This cytokine may be responsible for the tissue eosinophilia often seen in drug reactions.[31] It seems that CD8+ cells are not the predominant cell type, as once thought. CD1a+ dendritic cells have been found in the dermis in eruptions caused by some antibiotics.[33] Delayed hypersensitivity (type IV reaction) is rarely the cause of drug reactions resulting from ingestion of a drug, although it is the usual mechanism involved following the topical application of a sensitizing drug.[24] Type IV reactions may be involved in fixed drug eruptions and in certain mixed reactions, as occur in erythema multiforme.

The offending drug, or a metabolite of it, acts as a hapten that combines with tissue or plasma protein to form a complete antigen, which in turn stimulates some part of the immune system.[14] If the drug is of high molecular weight, it may be antigenic in itself. The method of administration of the drug and even environmental factors, such as an underlying infection or the presence of light of a suitable wavelength, may all influence the outcome.[14]

Much less is known about the non-immunological mechanisms involved in drug reactions. These may involve activation of effector pathways (such as opiates releasing mast cell mediators and non-steroidal anti-inflammatory drugs altering arachidonic acid metabolism), overdosage (as seen with hemorrhage produced by an excess of anticoagulants), metabolic alterations (isotretinoin affecting lipid metabolism and certain drugs affecting porphyrin metabolism) and cumulative toxicity (as seen with color changes resulting from the deposition of drug metabolites in the skin).[14] Drugs may also exacerbate a pre-existing dermatological condition.[14]

CLINICOPATHOLOGICAL REACTIONS

Even though the skin can react in only a limited number of ways, there is still a bewildering number of clinicopathological presentations of drug reactions.[18,34] Usually, several drugs can produce any particular reaction, although certain drugs are more likely than others to give a particular pattern. The characteristics of the drug that determine which reaction is produced are largely unknown in the case of allergic drug reactions.

Although the important modifications of each of the major tissue reaction patterns induced by drugs are discussed in the respective chapters of this book, there are important clues common to a number of reaction patterns. They are shown in Table 20.1.

The most common reactions produced by drugs are exanthematous in type, followed by urticaria and angioedema.[1] Fixed drug eruptions have been the third most common pattern in some series, although they have been much less frequent in others.[1] The most severe drug reactions are exfoliative dermatitis, the Stevens–Johnson syndrome and toxic epidermal necrolysis. Sometimes, the clinical features of a drug reaction are difficult to characterize

into one of the named patterns. Many of these are maculopapular in nature. They are often included in the exanthematous reaction, even though they do not strictly resemble a viral exanthem. Included in this group is the maculopapular eruption that may develop in the course of the treatment of leukemia, corresponding to the stage of peripheral lymphocyte recovery.[35]

The various reactions produced by drugs have been discussed in other chapters with the exception of the exanthematous reactions and the vegetative lesions produced by halogens. These reactions will be discussed in detail below, followed by a brief summary of the other cutaneous patterns produced by drugs.

EXANTHEMATOUS DRUG REACTIONS

Exanthematous eruptions (also described as morbilliform and as erythematous maculopapular eruptions) are the most common type of drug reaction, accounting for approximately 40% of all reactions.[1,36] The rash develops 1 day to 3 weeks after the offending drug is first given, although the timing depends on previous sensitization.[18] Uncommonly, the onset is much later in the course of the drug therapy and rarely it may develop after administration of the drug has ended.

There are erythematous macules and papules that resemble a viral exanthem. Lesions usually appear first on the trunk or in areas of pressure or trauma.[14] They spread to involve the extremities, usually in a symmetrical fashion. A recent publication has drawn attention to a distinct pattern of involvement of the upper arms in exanthematous drug eruptions.[37] Such eruptions involve the T1 dermatome with a sharp linear margin of demarcation from the spared skin served by the C5 spinal nerves. In short, there is medial involvement and lateral sparing. This so-called 'drug line' corresponds to the dorsoventral pigmentary demarcation line seen in about 20% of individuals with black skin, but normally invisible in white skin and known as the Voigt–Futcher line.[37] Pruritus and fever are sometimes present. The eruption usually lasts for 1–2 weeks and clears with cessation of the drug.[14]

Exanthematous eruptions occur in 50–80% of patients who are given ampicillin while suffering from infectious mononucleosis, cytomegalovirus infection or chronic lymphatic leukemia or who are also taking allopurinol.[24] Amoxicillin may sometimes produce a similar reaction in the same circumstances. An exanthematous eruption also occurs commonly in patients with AIDS who are given co-trimoxazole (trimethoprim-sulfamethoxazole).[2,38] It appears that patients with lymphotrophic viral infections are at increased risk for cutaneous drug reactions.[39] Other drugs which cause an exanthematous reaction include penicillin, erythromycin, streptomycin, tetracyclines, bleomycin, amphotericin B, sulfonamides, oral hypoglycemic agents, thiazide diuretics, barbiturates, chloral hydrate, benzodiazepines, phenothiazines, ticlopidine,[40] codeine,[41] buserelin acetate,[42] allopurinol, thiouracil, quinine, quinidine, gold, captopril and the non-steroidal anti-inflammatory drugs.[18,43] Codeine and pseudoephedrine have produced an eruption resembling scarlet fever.[44]

Table 20.1 **Clues to a drug etiology**

- Eosinophils
- Plasma cells (with some reactions)
- Red cell extravasation (in 50% or more)
- Apoptotic keratinocytes
- Activated lymphocytes
- Urticarial edema (in some reactions)
- Endothelial swelling of vessels

The mechanisms involved in exanthematous reactions are unclear, although immunological mechanisms have been suggested.[24] The eruption does not always recur on rechallenge.[14]

Histopathology

At first glance, the histological changes in the exanthematous drug reactions appear non-specific, but they are in fact quite characteristic. There are small foci of spongiosis and vacuolar change involving the basal layer with mild spongiosis extending one or two cells above this (Fig. 20.1).[45] A few lymphocytes are usually present in these foci.[45] A characteristic feature is the presence of rare apoptotic keratinocytes (Civatte bodies) in the basal layer (Fig. 20.2). Very focal parakeratosis may be present in lesions of some duration.

The papillary dermis is usually mildly edematous and there may be vascular dilatation. The inflammatory cell infiltrate, which consists of lymphocytes (some with large nuclei suggesting activation), macrophages, mast cells, occasional eosinophils and, rarely, a few plasma cells, is usually mild and localized around the superficial vascular plexus.[45]

Epidermal changes may be minimal or even absent in scarlatiniform eruptions and in some non-specific maculopapular eruptions categorized as exanthematous for convenience.

HALOGENODERMAS

The term 'halogenoderma' includes iododerma, bromoderma[46] and the rare fluoroderma which result from the ingestion of iodides, bromides and fluorides.[47] Iododerma is an uncommon disorder, while the other two are now exceedingly rare.[48] Verrucous plaques resembling those seen in the halogenodermas have recently been reported in two patients receiving long-term lithium therapy.[49]

The usual source of the iodide is the potassium salt used in expectorants and some tonics.[50] Rarely, radiocontrast media[47,51] and amiodarone[52] have been implicated. The characteristic lesion is a papulopustule which progresses to a vegetating nodular lesion. This may be crusted and ulcerated. There are usually a number of lesions, 0.5–2 cm in diameter, on the face, neck, back or upper extremities.[47,50,53] The lesions clear with cessation of the halide. The mechanism involved in their pathogenesis is uncertain.[47]

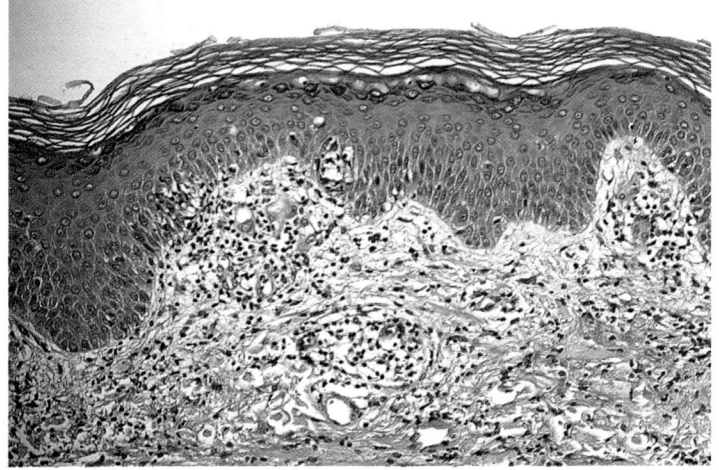

Fig. 20.1 **Exanthematous drug reaction** characterized by focal basal spongiosis, mild exocytosis of lymphocytes and a perivascular infiltrate of lymphocytes in the upper dermis. (H & E)

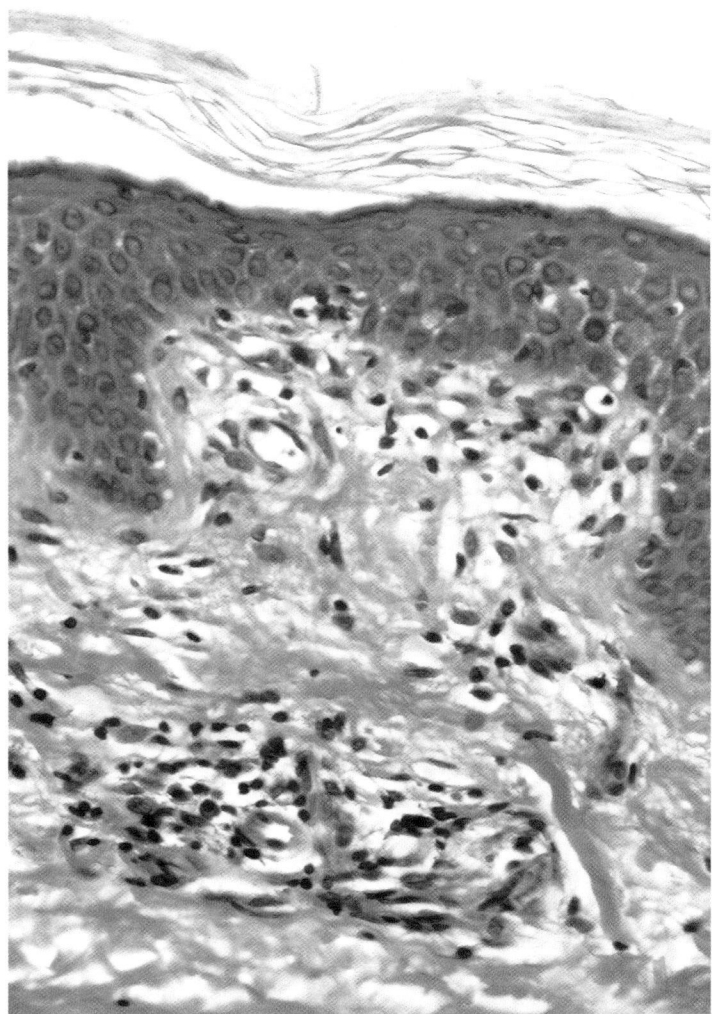

Fig. 20.2 **Exanthematous drug reaction.** A Civatte body (apoptotic keratinocyte) and a few lymphocytes are present in the basal layer. (H & E)

In addition to vegetating lesions, iodides may also produce erythematous papules, urticaria, vesicles, carbuncular lesions, erythema multiforme, vasculitis, polyarteritis nodosa and erythema nodosum-like lesions.[54] Iodides may also aggravate dermatitis herpetiformis, pyoderma gangrenosum, pustular psoriasis, erythema nodosum and blastomycosis-like pyoderma.[54,55]

Histopathology[54]

The vegetating lesions show pseudoepitheliomatous hyperplasia with intra-epidermal and some dermal abscesses.[56,57] The abscesses contain a few eosinophils and desquamated epithelial cells in addition to the neutrophils. There may be occasional multinucleate cells in the dermis, but this is never the prominent feature that it is in chromomycosis and sporotrichosis, which the reaction superficially resembles. In early lesions the 'intraepidermal' abscesses can be seen to be related to follicular infundibula.

OTHER CLINICOPATHOLOGICAL REACTIONS

The following account details in alphabetical order the various clinico-pathological patterns that have been associated with drugs.[14] The reader should refer to the appropriate page, listed for each reaction below, for an account of the clinical and histopathological features of each particular pattern and of the drugs that may be responsible.

Acanthosis nigricans

Various hormones and corticosteroids have been implicated in the etiology of some cases of acanthosis nigricans (see p. 574). There are no features that are specific for drug-induced lesions.

Acne

A number of drugs, cosmetics and industrial chemicals may precipitate and influence the course of acne vulgaris (see p. 457). Sometimes, pustular acneiform lesions develop without the presence of comedones.

Alopecia

Numerous drugs have been implicated in the etiology of alopecia. Several different mechanisms may be involved (see p. 479). The best understood of these is the alopecia produced by the various antimitotic agents that interfere with the replication of matrix cells during anagen.

Bullous reactions

Blisters are an integral part of erythema multiforme, toxic epidermal necrolysis and, often, fixed drug eruptions. Reactions resembling cicatricial pemphigoid (see p. 161), pemphigus[58,59] (see p. 132) and porphyria cutanea tarda (see p. 559) also occur. Bullae may develop in the course of drug-induced vasculitis or drug-induced coma (see p. 164). In addition to these circumstances, sub-epidermal bullae may also occur following the use of certain drugs (see p. 151).

Elastosis perforans serpiginosa

Lesions resembling elastosis perforans serpiginosa may be produced in patients receiving long-term penicillamine therapy (see p. 385).

Erythema multiforme

Drug-induced erythema multiforme is sometimes severe, with mucous membrane lesions and the clinical picture of the Stevens–Johnson syndrome (see p. 43). Target lesions are said to be less conspicuous in drug-related cases. The long-acting sulfonamides and various non-steroidal anti-inflammatory drugs are often implicated.[14]

Erythema nodosum

Drugs have sometimes been implicated in the etiology of erythema nodosum (see p. 522). There are no distinguishing features of drug-induced lesions.

Erythroderma (exfoliative dermatitis)

Drugs are a significant cause of erythroderma which usually commences some weeks after initiation of the drug (see p. 576). The rash often starts on the face and spreads over the rest of the body.

Fixed drug eruptions

There may be one or several sharply demarcated lesions, beginning as dusky patches, which fade, leaving an area of pigmentation (see p. 42). The lesion recurs in the same area after rechallenge with the drug. Urticarial and bullous forms have been described.

Granulomas

Rarely, a granulomatous tissue reaction is related to the ingestion of drugs, including the sulfonamides and allopurinol. Elastophagocytosis occasionally accompanies a drug reaction in sun-damaged skin. Granulomas may follow the local injection of various drugs, including toxoids containing aluminum salts. The interstitial granulomatous drug reaction is a distinctive clinico-pathological entity (see p. 212) which histologically resembles the incomplete form of granuloma annulare (Fig. 20.3).[60]

Hypersensitivity syndrome

A hypersensitivity reaction, characterized by fever, a generalized exanthem and multiorgan toxicity, has been reported following the ingestion of a number of drugs including phenytoin sodium and other anticonvulsants (see p. 588), sulfonamides, dapsone, calcium channel blockers, allopurinol and piroxicam.[61–65] It is an idiosyncratic reaction which is fortunately rare. It may occur after prolonged use of the drug. Infection with human herpesvirus-6 (HHV-6) and possibly HHV-7, as well as other viruses, may increase the risk of an individual developing this reaction (see p. 700).[66,67] A blood eosinophilia is often present and this appears to result from increased levels of interleukin-5.[68]

Hypertrichosis

Hypertrichosis, usually facial, may occur with certain drugs, of which minoxidil and oral contraceptives are the most familiar. Occasionally the hypertrichosis is permanent, although it usually subsides following cessation of the drug (see p. 482).

Infarction

Hemorrhagic infarction of the skin is an uncommon complication of anti-coagulant therapy (see p. 223). It usually occurs in the first week of therapy.[18]

Lichenoid drug eruption

The lichenoid reaction resembles lichen planus to a variable degree (see p. 41). Sometimes there is a slightly scaly ('eczematous') appearance to the lesions. Postinflammatory pigmentation is more prominent than in lichen planus.

Lipodystrophy

A lipodystrophy has been reported in patients infected with the human immunodeficiency virus (HIV), following treatment with protease inhibitors (see p. 531).

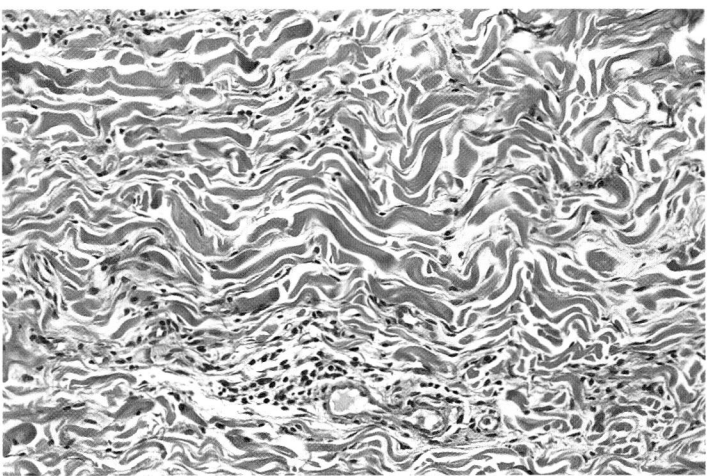

Fig. 20.3 **Interstitial granulomatous drug reaction.** There is a close resemblance to the incomplete form of granuloma annulare. (H & E)

Lupus erythematosus-like reaction

A disease resembling lupus erythematosus can be precipitated by several drugs (see p. 47). Procainamide-induced lupus erythematosus, which is the best studied, has a low incidence of renal involvement.

Neutrophilic eccrine hidradenitis

Neutrophilic eccrine hidradenitis is a rare complication of induction chemotherapy used in the treatment of certain types of cancer (see p. 487). Cytarabine has been the most frequently implicated drug.

Panniculitis

A panniculitis may result from the injection of certain drugs (see p. 533) and from the withdrawal of corticosteroids (see p. 530). Drugs including thiazides, sulfonamides, corticosteroids, oral contraceptives and sulindac may cause a pancreatitis which in turn may be associated with a panniculitis (see p. 529). Erythema nodosum (see above) is a specific pattern of panniculitis sometimes associated with drug ingestion.

Photosensitivity

Although the lesions in the various stages of photosensitivity are most marked in areas exposed to the sun (Fig. 20.4), they sometimes extend to areas protected from the sun.[69,70] Phototoxic and photoallergic variants have been recognized (see p. 599). Some persistent light reactions are drug induced (see p. 603).

Pigmentation

Several mechanisms are involved in the cutaneous pigmentation produced by drugs. These include an increased formation of melanin, melanin incontinence, and the deposition of drugs or drug complexes.[18] Antimalarials, phenothiazines, tetracycline and some of its derivatives, amiodarone, clofazimine and various antineoplastic chemotherapeutic agents may all produce cutaneous pigmentation. Coadministration of minocycline and amitriptyline may accelerate cutaneous pigmentation.[71]

Porphyria

Certain drugs may provoke attacks in those patients who have porphyria cutanea tarda or porphyria variegata, or in carriers of the genetic defect (see p. 559).

Pseudolymphoma

Drug-induced cutaneous pseudolymphoma is an uncommon reaction. It is seen most often with the anti-epileptic drugs,[72] such as phenytoin and carbamazepine. It has also been reported with valproate sodium, atenolol, griseofulvin, ACE inhibitors, allopurinol, cyclosporine, antihistamines and mexiletine (see p. 1122).

Psoriasiform drug reactions

Various drugs, particularly lithium, may precipitate or exacerbate psoriasis (Fig. 20.5) and pustular psoriasis (see p. 77). The withdrawal of steroids may also precipitate pustular psoriasis. Sometimes the beta blockers produce a clinical pattern resembling psoriasis although the histological picture is lichenoid or mixed lichenoid and psoriasiform in type.

Purpura

Purpura may result from damage to the vascular endothelium, thrombocytopenia, or both. Vasculitis is another association although this produces a so-called 'inflammatory purpura'; in the non-inflammatory purpuras there is simply an extravasation of red blood cells (see p. 222).

Pustular lesions

Pustules, usually resembling subcorneal pustular dermatosis on histopathological examination, have been reported with diltiazem, isoniazid and cephalosporins (see p. 134). Subcorneal, intraepidermal and even subepidermal pustules can be seen in acute generalized exanthematous pustulosis. Numerous drugs have been incriminated (see p. 136).

Sclerodermoid lesions

Sclerodermoid lesions may develop following occupational exposure to polyvinyl chloride and certain other chemicals, and following the use of bleomycin. Local sclerodermoid reactions may result from the injection of phytonadione (phytomenadione) or pentazocine (see p. 353).

Spongiotic reactions

Spongiotic reactions are seen with allergic and photoallergic contact reactions and in systemic contact dermatitis[73] (see p. 114). Uncommonly, drugs may exacerbate or precipitate a named spongiotic disorder such as seborrheic dermatitis or nummular dermatitis. The pityriasis rosea-like reactions (see p. 113) can also be included in this group. Certain drugs may produce a

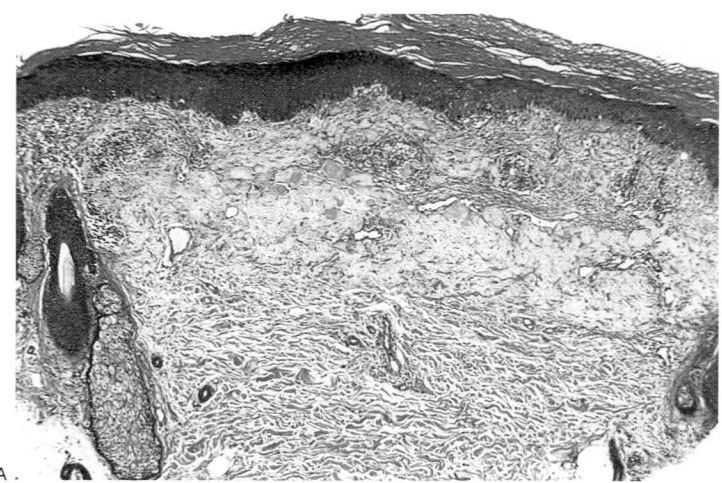
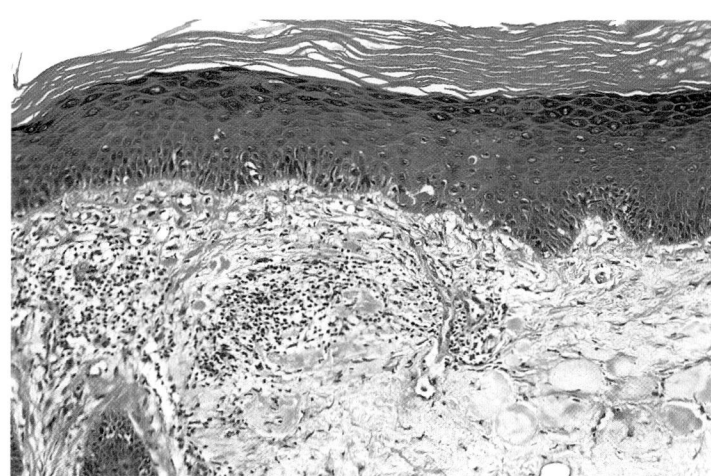

Fig. 20.4 **(A) Photosensitive drug eruption. (B)** There are solar elastosis, stellate 'fibroblasts' and occasional Civatte bodies. (H & E)

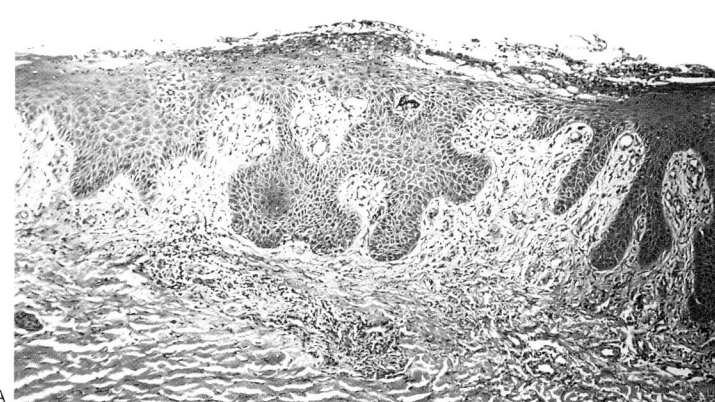

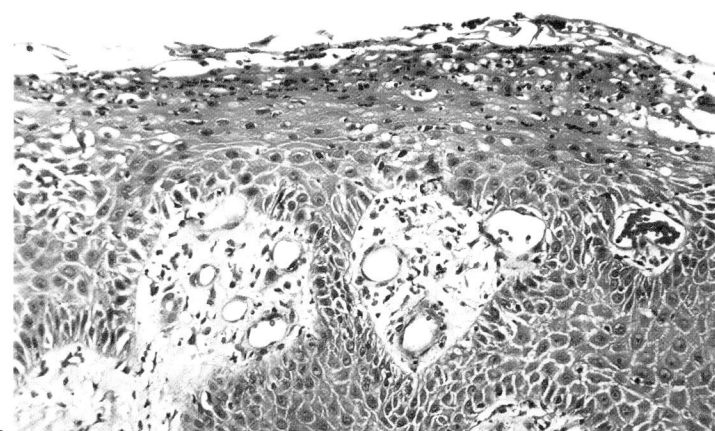

Fig. 20.5 **(A) Psoriasis precipitated by the ingestion of lithium carbonate. (B)** There is greater exocytosis of neutrophils and less regular psoriasiform hyperplasia than is usually seen in psoriasis. (H & E)

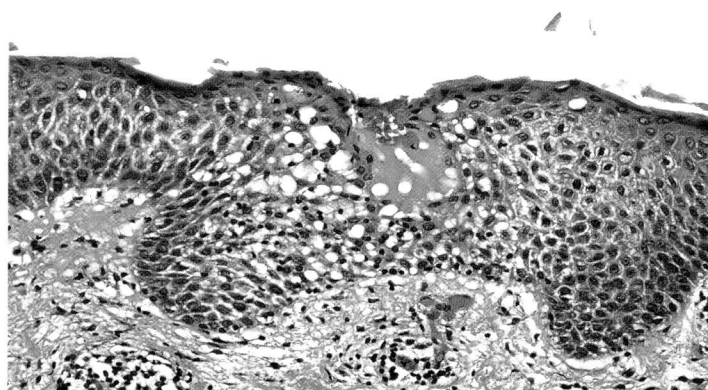

Fig. 20.6 **Spongiotic drug reaction following the ingestion of a thiazide diuretic.** Note the conspicuous exocytosis of lymphocytes associated with the focus of spongiosis. (H & E)

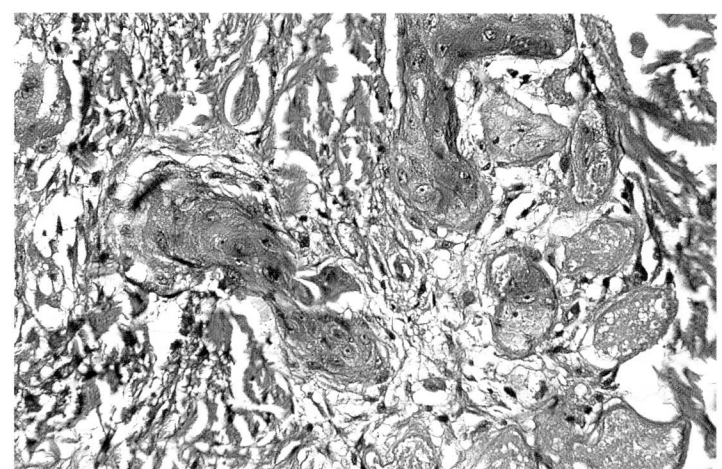

Fig. 20.7 **Sweat gland necrosis** in a comatose patient from a drug overdose. Squamous metaplasia is developing in several glands. (H & E)

spongiotic reaction with histopathological features (Fig. 20.6) that enable it to be distinguished from other spongiotic disorders (see p. 114).

Sweat gland necrosis

Sweat gland necrosis (Fig. 20.7) may occur in certain drug-induced comas (see p. 488).

Toxic epidermal necrolysis

Toxic epidermal necrolysis is the most serious cutaneous reaction to drugs. Large areas of the skin are sloughed and this is usually preceded by the development of large flaccid bullae[18] (see p. 45). Sulfonamides, allopurinol and the non-steroidal anti-inflammatory drugs are most often implicated.

Ulceration

Ulceration is an extremely rare complication of drugs. Allopurinol has been incriminated in the formation of a foot ulcer, resulting from a peripheral neuropathy.[74] Hydroxyurea is another cause of leg ulceration (see p. 258).

Urticaria

Urticaria is second only to drug exanthems as a manifestation of drug reactions. Numerous drugs have been responsible (see p. 227). The mechanisms involved include IgE-dependent reactions, immune complexes, and the non-immunological activation of effector pathways involved in mast cell degranulation.[14]

Vasculitis

The usual presentation of vasculitis is with 'palpable purpura' on the lower parts of the legs.[75] Immune mechanisms, particularly a type III reaction, are involved. Numerous drugs may produce a vasculitis (see p. 231).

Wound healing

Various drugs can influence wound healing. Adverse effects may be produced by corticosteroids, colchicine, cytotoxic drugs and antibiotics.[76]

OFFENDING DRUGS

The drugs which most often produce cutaneous reactions are the antibiotics, the non-steroidal anti-inflammatory drugs, psychotropic agents, the beta blockers and gold.[1,3,77] Other important drugs are the thiazide diuretics,[78] antimalarial drugs,[79,80] calcium channel blockers,[61,81] phenytoin and derivatives, recombinant cytokines[82] and anticancer chemotherapeutic agents.[83] Herbal remedies are an increasingly important cause of cutaneous reactions.[84]

Some drugs have a low incidence of reactions. Knowledge of these drugs may assist in determining the offending drug in patients receiving multiple therapeutic agents. Drugs in this category include antacids, antihistamines, atropine, digitalis glycosides,[78] insulin (regular), nystatin, potassium chloride, steroids, tetracycline, theophylline, thyroxine, vitamin preparations and warfarin.[18,24]

Brief mention will be made below of the major categories of offending drugs as well as the retinoids, recombinant cytokines, intravenous immunoglobulin and protease inhibitors, all emerging areas of importance.

Antibiotics

Antibiotics are the major cause of drug reactions, accounting for 42% of all reactions in one series involving hospital inpatients.[3] Co-trimoxazole (trimethoprim-sulfamethoxazole) produced the highest number of reactions in one study (59 reactions/1000 recipients) while the frequency for ampicillin was 52/1000 and for the semisynthetic penicillins 36/1000.[4] In another study, amoxicillin resulted in the highest number of reactions (51/1000 patients exposed).[10] In a recent study of 472 children with rashes following antibiotic exposure, the frequency of an eruption was 12.3% for cefaclor, 2.6% for other cephalosporins, 7.4% for penicillins and 8.5% for sulfonamides.[85] The macrolides (erythromycin, clarithromycin and azithromycin) have a low incidence of cutaneous side effects.[86]

The most common pattern of skin reaction caused by antibiotics is an exanthematous one, but most other clinicopathological patterns have been reported at some time.[87-92] In the case of the tetracyclines, photosensitivity and fixed drug eruptions are sometimes seen.[14] Skin and mucous membrane pigmentation, a lupus-like reaction and a hypersensitivity syndrome have been reported with minocycline.[93-96] The high incidence of reactions in patients taking ampicillin who also have infectious mononucleosis, cytomegalovirus infection or chronic lymphatic leukemia has been referred to above. In the case of co-trimoxazole (trimethoprim-sulfamethoxasole), two distinct eruptions have been recorded: an urticarial reaction with onset a few days after the onset of treatment and an exanthematous (morbilliform) reaction with its onset after 1 week of treatment.[38] Toxic epidermal necrolysis has also been reported with this drug.[97] There is a high incidence of reactions to this drug in patients infected with HIV.[98,99] It should be noted that celecoxib, a new cyclo-oxygenase (COX)2 inhibitor, contains a sulfonamide moiety and may give similar reactions.[100]

Other cutaneous reactions produced by antibiotics include an intertriginous eruption due to amoxicillin,[101] photosensitivity reactions with fluoroquinolones[102] and the 'red man/red neck' syndrome following the rapid infusion of vancomycin.[103]

Adverse reactions have been reported to the new oral antifungal agents. Cutaneous reactions including urticaria, erythema and pruritus have been reported in 2.3% of patients taking terbinafine.[104,105] Isolated reports of erythema multiforme, toxic epidermal necrolysis, fixed drug eruptions, acute generalized exanthematous pustulosis, an erythema annulare centrifugum-like psoriatic drug eruption, a hypersensitivity reaction and alopecia, resulting from terbinafine, have appeared.[106-108]

Many of these reactions have also been reported with the oral antifungal agents fluconazole and itraconazole.[104] In particular, itraconazole can produce acute generalized exanthematous pustulosis, a purpuric eruption and erythematous papules,[109-111] and fluconazole has been associated with erythema multiforme, toxic epidermal necrolysis, erythroderma, fixed drug eruption and angioedema.[104]

The antiviral agent foscarnet produces penile ulcers in a high proportion of those who take it. Erosions of the vulva have also been reported.[112]

Non-steroidal anti-inflammatory drugs

The non-steroidal anti-inflammatory drugs (NSAIDs) are a chemically heterogeneous group of compounds that can produce a variety of cutaneous reactions ranging from mild exanthematous eruptions to life-threatening toxic epidermal necrolysis.[113,114] They are among the most commonly prescribed class of drugs, accounting for approximately 5% of prescriptions dispensed in the USA.[43,114] Several drugs in this category have already been withdrawn from the market because of their cutaneous reactions.

The following categories of non-steroidal anti-inflammatory drugs are in use:[114]

- *salicylic acid derivatives*: aspirin and various compound analgesics
- *heterocyclic acetic acids*: indomethacin, sulindac and tolmetin
- *propionic acid derivatives*: ibuprofen, naproxen and fenoprofen
- *anthranilic acids*: mefenamic acid, flufenamic acid and meclofenamate sodium
- *pyrazole derivatives* (pyrazolones): phenylbutazone and oxyphenbutazone
- *oxicams*: piroxicam.

Drugs belonging to any given chemical group frequently share similar mechanisms of action and toxicity. The NSAIDs inhibit the enzyme cyclo-oxygenase and thus reduce production of prostaglandins and thromboxanes; this action is not solely responsible for their therapeutic actions.[43]

Exanthematous eruptions are commonly seen with phenylbutazone and indomethacin but they have been reported at some time or other with most of the other NSAIDs.[14] Aspirin is an important cause of acute urticaria; it also aggravates chronic urticaria.[114] Ibuprofen may produce a vasculitis, morbilliform eruption, urticaria, erythema multiforme, erythema nodosum, a bullous eruption or a lupus erythematosus-like eruption;[115] naproxen may produce a fixed drug eruption, a lichenoid reaction or a vesiculobullous reaction.[114] Piroxicam may result in a vesiculobullous eruption in areas exposed to the sun.[43] Most of the NSAIDs have been reported to cause toxic epidermal necrolysis and/or erythema multiforme at some time, although the substances most frequently responsible are the pyrazolones.[14,43]

Psychotropic drugs

The psychotropic drugs include the tricyclic antidepressants, antipsychotic drugs, lithium, and the hypnotic and anxiolytic (tranquilizer) agents.[116] This group of drugs produces the most diverse range of reactions, which include exacerbation of porphyria (chlordiazepoxide), blue-gray discoloration of the skin (chlorpromazine) and an acneiform eruption (lithium).[116,117] Further mention of the specific complications of the various drugs in this category is made in the description of the appropriate tissue reaction.

Phenytoin sodium

Phenytoin sodium is a widely prescribed anticonvulsant with a relatively low rate of side effects. Nevertheless, a broad spectrum of cutaneous reactions has been reported.[118] These include exanthematous eruptions, acneiform lesions, exfoliative dermatitis, erythema multiforme, toxic epidermal necrolysis, vasculitis, hypertrichosis, gingival hyperplasia, coarse facies, heel-pad thickening, a lupus erythematosus-like reaction, digital deformities[119] (the fetal hydantoin syndrome), a hypersensitivity syndrome[120,121] and a pseudolymphoma syndrome.[118] Carbamazepine, lamotrigine, phenobarbital (phenobarbitone) and primidone cause a similar hypersensitivity syndrome to that produced by phenytoin sodium – 'the anticonvulsant hypersensitivity syndrome'.[122–126] Generalized pustulation is one manifestation of the syndrome.[127] Phenytoin sodium has also resulted in cutaneous necrosis with multinucleate epidermal cells at the site of intravenous infusion.[128]

Gold

Gold produces a variety of cutaneous reactions which are most commonly 'eczematous' or maculopapular in type.[129] These reactions may occur as long as 2 years after the initiation of therapy.[14] The lesions may take months to resolve.[14] Other reactions produced by gold include cutaneous pigmentation, exfoliative dermatitis, vasomotor flushing, a lichenoid drug reaction, erythema nodosum and an eruption resembling pityriasis rosea.[130]

Retinoids

Retinoids are a group of compounds that produce their biologic responses via a specific receptor whose usual bindings are retinol and retinoic acid.[131] Synthetic retinoids such as etretinate, tretinoin and isotretinoin are of increasing importance in dermatologic therapy. They have received widespread media coverage because of their ability to improve photoaged skin.

Retinoids produce multiple changes, including a reduction in the keratin content of keratinocytes and in epidermal hyperplasia, and an increase in Langerhans cells, dermal collagen, tropoelastin and angiogenesis. They produce reduced collagenase and gelatinase activity and glycosaminoglycans.[131]

Retinoids appear to cause partial regression of established skin cancers and to inhibit the number of skin cancers that appear in susceptible individuals, such as those with xeroderma pigmentosum, as long as the treatment is continued.[131] The author was involved in an early clinical trial of retinoic acid, which was aborted when multilobate nuclei were found in the epidermis of individuals treated with topical retinoic acid for one year. This observation was never published.

Cutaneous side effects of synthetic retinoids include cheilitis, palmoplantar peeling, pyogenic granuloma-like lesions in acne, alopecia and paronychia.[131,132] Induction therapy with all-*trans*-retinoic acid in patients with acute promyelocytic leukemia can produce a range of scrotal lesions including ulceration, exfoliative dermatitis and Fournier's gangrene.[133]

Cytotoxic drugs

Cytotoxic drugs used in the treatment of cancer have many mucocutaneous complications. As combination chemotherapy is often used, it may be difficult to determine which drug is specifically responsible for a particular reaction. There is some evidence that some of the rashes attributed to drugs in the past may be examples of the eruption of lymphocyte recovery (see p. 47). It is still possible that a drug is responsible for these eruptions, in some cases, and that the reaction is only expressed when the number of immuno-competent cells returns to a sufficient level.[134] Their action on rapidly dividing cells means that cytotoxic drugs commonly produce alopecia, stomatitis, apoptotic keratinocytes and Beau's lines on the nails.[83,135] Chemical cellulitis, ulceration and phlebitis may result from local extravasation into the tissues of injected drugs.[136]

Other complications include alterations in cutaneous pigmentation (see p. 443), nail pigmentation,[137] neutrophilic eccrine hidradenitis (see p. 487), eccrine squamous syringometaplasia (see p. 487), an intertriginous eruption,[138] sclerodermoid reactions (see p. 353), urticaria, vasculitis, erythroderma, inflammation of keratoses (see p. 761), enlarged dermal macrophages[139] and exacerbation of porphyria (see p. 557).[83,135]

An acral erythema (chemotherapy-induced acral erythema) has been reported from the use of certain chemotherapeutic agents, such as fluorouracil, doxorubicin, cisplatin,[140] methotrexate,[141] and cytarabine (cytosine arabinoside).[142] The lesions subside within 1–2 weeks following dis-continuation of chemotherapy, with eventual desquamation. Acral erythema appears to be a common side effect of doxorubicin when it is encapsulated in liposomes (Doxil).[143] A bullous reaction is rare.[144] Microscopic examination reveals mild basal vacuolar change, scattered apoptotic keratinocytes, and a mild superficial perivascular infiltrate of lymphocytes.[145] Eccrine squamous syringometaplasia is not uncommon. It has been suggested that natural killer cells initially target keratinocytes in the eccrine apparatus, producing small spongiotic vesicles adjacent to the acrosyringium, apoptosis of cells at all levels of the eccrine apparatus and later squamous syringometaplasia.[146] Epidermal dysmaturation is sometimes produced.[147]

Intradermal bleomycin results in necrosis and apoptosis of epidermal keratinocytes and eccrine epithelium. There is an associated neutrophilic infiltrate around the sweat glands, resembling neutrophilic eccrine hidradenitis (see p. 487).[148]

A linear, serpentine erythematous eruption overlying the superficial veins of both arms has been reported following the intravenous use of 5-fluorouracil.[149] The changes have been called persistent supravenous erythematous eruption. The histological changes resemble erythema multiforme.

Subungual hemorrhages and abscesses have been reported as a side effect of docetaxel therapy.[150]

Mesna, a mercaptoalkane sulfonic compound used to lessen the urotoxic effects of drugs such as cyclophosphamide, produces urticarial reactions and a generalized fixed drug eruption.[151]

The various reactions to cytotoxic drugs have been reviewed by Fitzpatrick,[152] and more recently by Susser and colleagues.[153]

Recombinant cytokines

As a result of advances in recombinant DNA technology, recombinant cytokines are being used increasingly as therapeutic agents. An excellent review of this subject and the cutaneous reactions to this therapy was made by Asnis and Gaspari in 1995.[82]

Cutaneous reactions are more common with granulocyte–macrophage colony-stimulating factor (GMCSF) than with granulocyte colony-stimulating factor (GCSF). Reactions reported with GCSF include Sweet's syndrome, bullous pyoderma gangrenosum, acute vasculitis and an exacerbation of psoriasis. There are several reports describing the presence of numerous enlarged, plump macrophages in the dermal infiltrate of some eruptions.[154,155] Enlarged macrophages may also occur as a consequence of chemotherapy alone.[139] Irregularly shaped lymphocytes, with some mitoses, may also be found in some of these eruptions.[156] In the case of GMCSF, reported complications include widespread folliculitis, bullous pyoderma gangrenosum, a psoriasiform eruption, erythroderma and localized injection site reactions.[82,157,158]

Erythropoietin, used in the treatment of anemia of chronic renal failure, produces few reactions; they include hirsutism and a spongiotic reaction.

The interferons may produce injection site reactions, particularly interferon-β (IFN-β). Reactions include erythema, localized induration and necrosis, often with associated thrombosis.[159] A squamous cell carcinoma has been reported in one of many ulcers that developed in a patient following the injection of IFN-β.[160] If IFN-γ is used in the treatment of lepromatous leprosy, there is a high incidence of erythema nodosum leprosum. Alopecia is the most common side effect of IFN-α.

Interleukin-2 therapy has resulted in bullous disorders and erythema nodosum. An erythematous macular eruption, healing with desquamation, is very common. Other reactions include erythroderma, telogen effluvium, cutaneous ulcers, exacerbation of psoriasis and a persistent inflammatory reaction at the injection site.[161] Interleukin-3 use has been associated with an urticarial eruption.[162]

Finally, tumor necrosis factor-α produces a generalized erythematous eruption, vasculitis, alopecia and local reactions at the injection site.[82]

Intravenous immunoglobulin

High-dose intravenous immunoglobulin therapy (hdIVIg) has been used to treat various diseases including immunodeficiency states, autoimmune diseases, and hematological disorders. Adverse cutaneous reactions are uncommon and include reports of eczema, alopecia, erythema multiforme and a lichenoid dermatitis.[163,164]

Protease inhibitors

As mentioned earlier, patients infected with the human immunodeficiency virus have a higher incidence of drug hypersensitivity than individuals with normal immunity. Protease inhibitors have been used for several years in the treatment of HIV infection, often with dramatic effects on both the viral load and CD4 cell count. Adverse cutaneous reactions to protease inhibitors include a lipodystrophy (see p. 531), a maculopapular eruption,[165] stria formation and excess granulation tissue of the digits with paronychia.[166]

REFERENCES

Introduction

1 Kauppinen K, Stubb S. Drug eruptions: causative agents and clinical types. A series of in-patients during a 10-year period. Acta Derm Venereol 1984; 64: 320–324.
2 Mitsuyasu R, Groopman J. Cutaneous reaction to trimethoprim-sulfamethoxazole in patients with Kaposi's sarcoma. N Engl J Med 1983; 308: 1535–1536.
3 Alanko K, Stubb S, Kauppinen K. Cutaneous drug reactions: clinical types and causative agents. Acta Derm Venereol 1989; 69: 223–226.
4 Patterson R, Anderson J. Allergic reactions to drugs and biologic agents. JAMA 1982; 248: 2637–2645.
5 Mullick FG, Drake RM, Irey NS. Morphologic changes in adverse drug reactions in infants and children. Hum Pathol 1977; 8: 361–378.
6 Tseng S, Pak G, Washenik K et al. Rediscovering thalidomide: A review of its mechanism of action, side effects, and potential uses. J Am Acad Dermatol 1996; 35: 969–979.
7 Allen BR. Thalidomide. Br J Dermatol 2001; 144: 227–228.
8 Livni E, Halevy S, Stahl B, Joshua H. The appearance of macrophage migration-inhibition factor in drug reactions. J Allergy Clin Immunol 1987; 80: 843–849.
9 Halevy S, Grunwald MH, Sandbank M et al. Macrophage migration inhibition factor (MIF) in drug eruption. Arch Dermatol 1990; 126: 48–51.
10 Bigby M, Jick S, Jick H, Arndt K. Drug-induced cutaneous reactions. A report from the Boston Collaborative Drug Surveillance Program on 15438 consecutive inpatients, 1975 to 1982. JAMA 1986; 256: 3358–3363.
11 Arndt KA, Jick H. Rates of cutaneous reactions to drugs. A report from the Boston Collaborative Drug Surveillance Program. JAMA 1976; 235: 918–922.
12 Singer MI, Shapiro LE, Shear NH. Cytochrome P-450 3A: Interactions with dermatologic therapies. J Am Acad Dermatol 1997; 37: 765–771.
13 Barranco VP. Clinically significant drug interactions in dermatology. J Am Acad Dermatol 1998; 38: 599–612.
14 Wintroub BU, Stern R. Cutaneous drug reactions: pathogenesis and clinical classification. J Am Acad Dermatol 1985; 13: 167–179.
15 Kauppinen K, Alanko K. Oral provocation: uses. Semin Dermatol 1989; 8: 187–191.
16 Shear NH. Diagnosing cutaneous adverse reactions to drugs. Arch Dermatol 1990; 126: 94–97.
17 Stern RS. Epidemiologic assessment of adverse drug effects. Semin Dermatol 1989; 8: 136–140.
18 Swinyer LJ. Determining the cause of drug eruptions. Dermatol Clin 1983; 1: 417–431.
19 Kaufman DW, Shapiro S. Epidemiological assessment of drug-induced disease. Lancet 2000; 356: 1339–1343.

20 Girard M. Oral provocation: limitations. Semin Dermatol 1989; 8: 192–195.
21 Bruynzeel DP, van Ketel WG. Patch testing in drug eruptions. Semin Dermatol 1989; 8: 196–203.
22 Barbaud A, Reichert-Penetrat S, Tréchot P et al. The use of skin testing in the investigation of cutaneous adverse drug reactions. Br J Dermatol 1998; 139: 49–58.
23 Hertl M, Merk HF. Lymphocyte activation in cutaneous drug reactions. J Invest Dermatol 1995; 105: 95S–98S.
24 Dunagin WG, Millikan LE. Drug eruptions. Med Clin North Am 1980; 64: 983–1003.
25 Breathnach SM. Mechanisms of drug eruptions: Part 1. Australas J Dermatol 1995; 36: 121–127.
26 Smith KJ, Skelton HG, Yeager J et al. Increased drug reactions in HIV-1-postive patients: a possible explanation based on patterns of immune dysregulation seen in HIV-1 disease. Clin Exp Dermatol 1997; 22: 118–123.
27 Chosidow O, Bourgault I, Roujeau J-C. Drug rashes. What are the targets of cell-mediated cytotoxicity? Arch Dermatol 1994; 130: 627–629.
28 Sullivan JR, Shear NH. What are some of the lesions learnt from in vitro studies of severe unpredictable drug reactions? Br J Dermatol 2000; 142: 205–207.
29 Van Arsdel PP Jr. Allergy and adverse drug reactions. J Am Acad Dermatol 1982; 6: 833–845.
30 Millikan LE, Mroczkowski TF. Immunology of adverse drug eruptions. Clin Dermatol 1986; 4: 30–39.
31 Yawalkar N, Hari Y, Frutig K et al. T cells isolated from positive epicutaneous test reactions to amoxicillin and ceftriaxone are drug specific and cytotoxic. J Invest Dermatol 2000; 115: 647–652.
32 Barbaud AM, Béné M-C, Schmutz J-L et al. Role of delayed cellular hypersensitivity and adhesion molecules in amoxicillin-induced morbilliform rashes. Arch Dermatol 1997; 133: 481–486.
33 Barbaud AM, Béné MC, Reichert-Penetrat S et al. Immunocompetent cells and adhesion molecules in 14 cases of cutaneous drug reactions induced with the use of antibiotics. Arch Dermatol 1998; 134: 1040–1041.

Clinicopathological reactions

34 Stevens A, Dalziel K. The histopathology of drug rashes. Curr Diagn Pathol 1998; 5: 138–149.
35 Horn TD, Redd JV, Karp JE et al. Cutaneous eruptions of lymphocyte recovery. Arch Dermatol 1989; 125: 1512–1517.
36 Apaydin R, Bilen N, Dökmeci Ş et al. Drug eruptions: a study including all inpatients and outpatients at a dermatology clinic of a university hospital. J Eur Acad Dermatol Venereol 2000; 14: 518–520.
37 Shelley ED, Shelley WB, Pansky B. The drug line: The clinical expression of the pigmentary Voigt–Futcher line in turn derived from the embryonic ventral axial line. J Am Acad Dermatol 1999; 40: 736–740.
38 Roudier C, Caumes E, Rogeaux O et al. Adverse cutaneous reactions to trimethoprim-sulfamethoxazole in patients with the acquired immunodeficiency syndrome and Pneumocystis carinii pneumonia. Arch Dermatol 1994; 130: 1383–1386.
39 Cohen AD, Friger M, Sarov B, Halevy S. Which intercurrent infections are associated with maculopapular cutaneous drug reactions? A case-control study. Int J Dermatol 2001; 40: 41–44.
40 Yosipovitch G, Rechavia E, Feinmesser M, David M. Adverse cutaneous reactions to ticlopidine in patients with coronary stents. J Am Acad Dermatol 1999; 41: 473–476.
41 Möhrenschlager M, Glöckner A, Jessberger B et al. Codeine caused pruritic scarlatiniform exanthemata: patch test negative but positive to oral provocation test. Br J Dermatol 2000; 143: 663–664.
42 Kono T, Ishii M, Taniguchi S. Intranasal buserelin acetate-induced pigmented roseola-like eruption. Br J Dermatol 2000; 143: 658–659.
43 Bigby M. Nonsteroidal anti-inflammatory drug reactions. Semin Dermatol 1989; 8: 182–186.
44 Taylor BJ, Duffill MB. Recurrent pseudo-scarlatina and allergy to pseudoephedrine hydrochloride. Br J Dermatol 1988; 118: 827–829.
45 Fellner MJ, Prutkin L. Morbilliform eruptions caused by penicillin. A study by electron microscopy and immunologic tests. J Invest Dermatol 1970; 55: 390–395.
46 Smith SZ, Scheen SR. Bromoderma. Arch Dermatol 1978; 114: 458–459.
47 Boudoulas O, Siegle RJ, Grimwood RE. Iododerma occurring after orally administered iopanoic acid. Arch Dermatol 1987; 123: 387–388.
48 Alpay K, Kürçüoglu N. Iododerma: an unusual side effect of iodide ingestion. Pediatr Dermatol 1996; 13: 51–53.
49 Alagheband M, Engineer L. Lithium and halogenoderma. Arch Dermatol 2000; 136: 126–127.
50 Rosenberg FR, Einbinder J, Walzer RA, Nelson CT. Vegetating iododerma. An immunologic mechanism. Arch Dermatol 1972; 105: 900–905.
51 Chang MW, Miner JE, Moiin A, Hashimoto K. Iododerma after computed tomographic scan with intravenous radiopaque contrast media. J Am Acad Dermatol 1997; 36: 1014–1016.

CALCANEAL PETECHIAE ('BLACK HEEL')

'Black heel', which is usually bilateral and roughly symmetrical, consists of a painless, petechial eruption on the heels.[31,37–39] There is speckled, brownish-black pigmentation that may be mistaken for a plantar wart or even a melanoma.[40] It should not be forgotten that melanoma can occur on the heel.[41]

Calcaneal petechiae appear to be traumatic in origin. Their formation probably follows a pinching force imparted by shoes at the time of sudden stopping, such as occurs in the course of basketball, tennis and other sports.[40,42]

Lesions comparable in appearance, pathogenesis and pathology occur in other situations.[43] The term *post-traumatic punctate hemorrhage* has been proposed as a unifying term.[43]

Histopathology[39,44]

The pigmentation in calcaneal petechiae results from lakes of hemorrhage in the stratum corneum (Fig. 21.1). The red cells are extravasated into the lower epidermis from dilated vessels in the papillary dermis. They undergo trans-epidermal elimination during the progressive maturation of the epidermis and overlying stratum corneum.

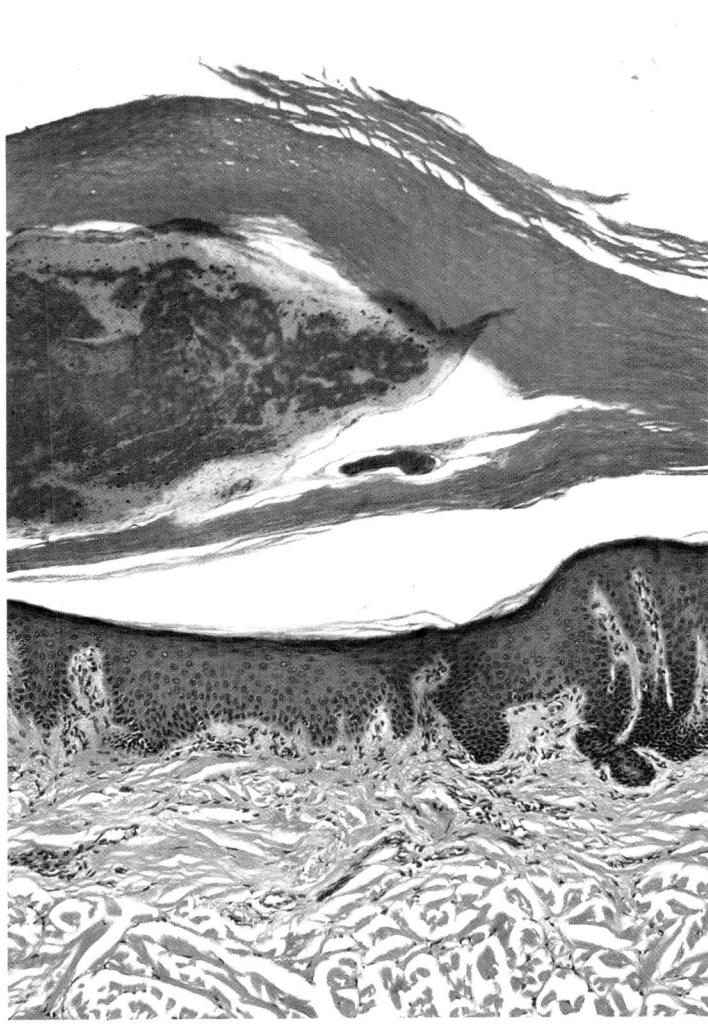

Fig. 21.1 **Traumatic hemorrhage involving the stratum corneum.** The lesion was removed because of a clinical suspicion that this was a melanoma. (H & E)

Red cells may also be found in the stratum corneum following trauma to the palms, soles and subungual region. Hemorrhage also occurs into the parakeratotic layer overlying the digitate papillomatous projections in warts. The hemoglobin in these deposits can be demonstrated with either the benzedine stain or the patent blue V stain.[45]

REACTIONS TO RADIATION

The early (acute) effects of *X-irradiation* differ markedly from those that develop many months or years later. In the skin, the terms 'acute radiodermatitis' and 'chronic radiodermatitis' have traditionally been used for these respective stages. Recently, a subacute form has been described with features resembling those of acute graft-versus-host disease.[46] All three stages are discussed below under the general heading of radiation dermatitis.

The effects of *ultraviolet radiation* are quite different. Ultraviolet-B radiation (UV-B) produces apoptosis of keratinocytes ('sunburn cells'), spongiosis and eventual parakeratosis. Endothelial cells in the superficial vascular plexus enlarge and there is some perivenular edema.[47] Langerhans cells in the epidermis are reduced in number for several days after the exposure. Ultraviolet-A radiation (UV-A) produces only mild swelling of keratinocytes and mild spongiosis but no sunburn cells.[47] Exposure to ultraviolet radiation, both UV-A and UV-B, in commercial tanning salons, has the potential to become a major public health problem in the future. Skin burns, which may predispose to the development of skin cancer later in life, have been reported in a significant number of users.[48]

Radiofrequency energy is used in a catheter ablation technique for the treatment of a variety of cardiac arrhythmias. If the procedure is prolonged, a localized acute radiodermatitis may result.[49] A tender or pruritic eythematous plaque develops several days later. Histologically, there are scattered apoptotic keratinocytes resembling a mild phototoxic dermatitis (see below).

RADIATION DERMATITIS

There is a common response to the different types of radiation that affect the skin, although the severity of the changes varies with the total dose, its fractionation and the depth of penetration of the radiation.[50–52] The use of megavoltage therapy for deep tumors has resulted in some sparing of the skin, although fibrosis in the deep subcutaneous tissues may result.[52,53]

The advent of coronary angioplasties and stenting has resulted in several cases of radiation dermatitis as a consequence of excessive radiation, usually associated with a prolonged procedure. Lesions are usually on the upper back.[54]

There is a well-defined progression of changes following irradiation of the skin.[52] These are usually divided into early changes (acute radiodermatitis) and chronic changes (chronic radiodermatitis) arising many months or years after the initial exposure.[55,56] An intermediate (subacute) stage is also recognized.

Early radiation dermatitis

In the weeks following irradiation there is variable erythema, accompanied by edema in the more severe cases.[52] This is followed by epilation and hyper-pigmentation. Severe changes such as vesiculation, erosion and ulceration are not seen very often in these days of more precisely controlled dosage; they may occur after accidental exposures.[57]

Subacute radiation dermatitis

Subacute radiation dermatitis, which occurs weeks to months after radiation exposure, was first described in 1989 by LeBoit.[46] A further case has been described as a consequence of radiation from fluoroscopy during coronary artery stenting.[58] It is a histological imitator of acute cutaneous graft-versus-host disease (see below).[46,58]

Eosinophilic, polymorphic, and pruritic eruption of radiotherapy (EPPER)

This complication of radiotherapy for cancer, particularly of the breast, has a unique clinicopathological profile. It has been diagnosed in the past as erythema multiforme and bullous pemphigoid following radiotherapy. It has received little attention in the literature, despite the ability of one institution to collect 14 cases.[59] The eruption is polymorphic and pruritic. The eruption usually occurs during radiation, but late onset has been recorded.[60] It is considered further with the spongiotic reaction pattern as this characterizes the histological pattern (see p. 100).

Late radiation changes

The chronic effects progress slowly and are usually subclinical in the early stages.[52] It seems that at least 1000 rads are required to produce chronic radiodermatitis.[61] The final changes resemble poikiloderma, with atrophy, telangiectasias, hypopigmentation with focal hyperpigmentation, and loss of appendages.[62] The affected skin is very susceptible to minor trauma, which may lead to persistent ulceration.[63]

A small proportion of patients develop squamous[64,65] or basal cell carcinoma 15 years or more after irradiation.[66,67] Rarely, fibrosarcomas have been reported: their diagnosis might not stand up to scrutiny with the immunoperoxidase markers available today. Basal cell carcinomas are more common following irradiation to the head and neck region.[68] Sometimes the tumors that develop are quite aggressive and there is a higher risk of metastasis with any squamous cell carcinoma that develops in the skin following irradiation than with cutaneous squamous cell carcinoma in general.[56] An absorbed dose of at least 2000 rads is required.[69] The risk of cutaneous cancer following superficial grenz therapy is very small indeed.[70,71]

Histopathology[52]

The *early changes* of radiation dermatitis are not commonly seen as there is usually little reason to perform a biopsy. There is some vacuolization of epidermal nuclei and cytoplasm with some degenerate keratinocytes. Inhibition of mitosis occurs in the germinal cells of the epidermis and pilosebaceous follicles. The follicles soon pass into the catagen phase. Later there is hyperpigmentation of the basal layer. The blood vessels in the papillary dermis are dilated and their endothelial cells are swollen. There is edema of the papillary dermis and extravasation of red blood cells and fibrin. Thrombi composed of fibrin and platelets may form in some vessels. Only a small number of inflammatory cells are present and these are usually dispersed and not perivascular in location.

In *subacute radiation dermatitis* there is a lichenoid tissue reaction (interface dermatitis) with basal vacuolar change and apoptotic keratinocytes. Lymphocytes, which are predominantly CD8+ and express TIA-1, are found in a superficial perivascular location in the dermis and also in the epidermis in close apposition with apoptotic keratinocytes ('satellitosis'). There may be a fibrinopurulent crust on the epidermal surface.[58]

In the *late stages* the epidermis may be atrophic with loss of the normal rete ridge pattern and the development of focal basal vacuolar change. Sometimes there is overlying hyperkeratosis. Dyskeratotic cells are usually present. The main changes are in the dermis where there is swollen, hyalinized collagen showing irregular eosinophilic staining (Fig. 21.2). This results from marked upregulation of collagen synthesis.[72] Atypical stellate cells with large nuclei containing clumped chromatin (radiation fibroblasts) are invariably

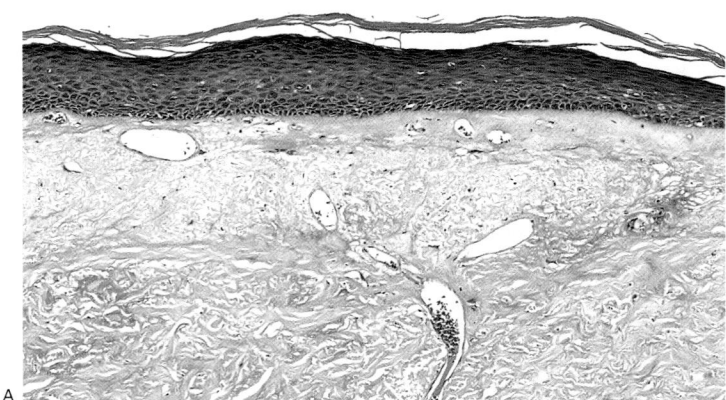

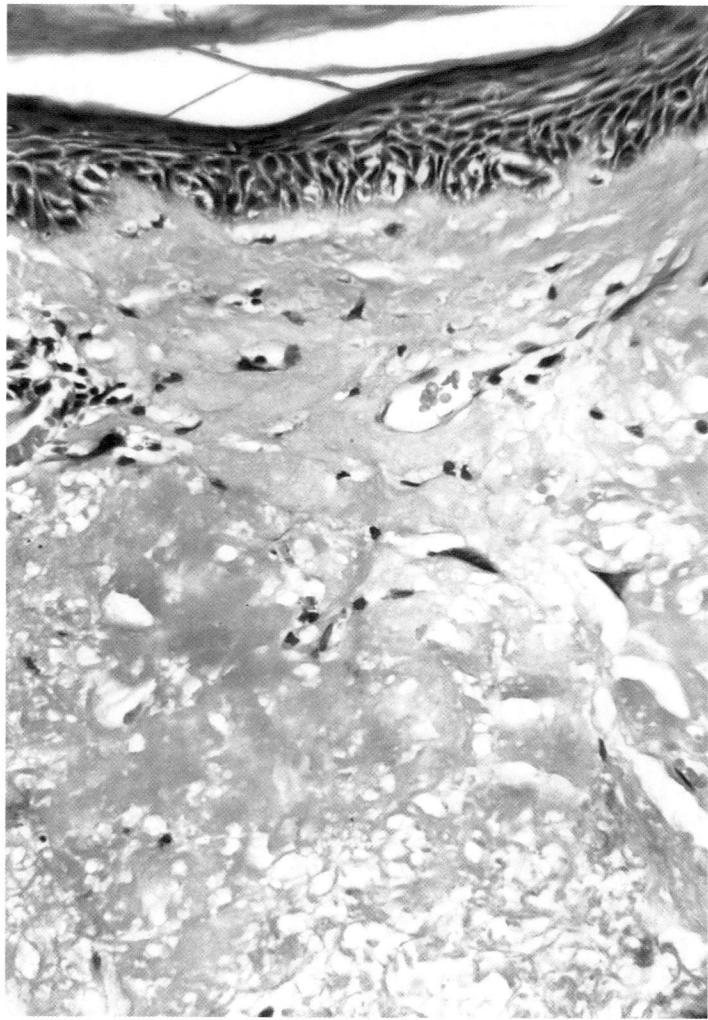

Fig. 21.2 **Radiation damage. (A)** There is loss of dermal appendages. Blood vessels are telangiectatic. **(B)** The dermal collagen is altered with several 'radiation fibroblasts' (dendrocytes). (H & E)

present.[73] Most of these cells express factor XIIIa;[74,75] a few express CD34.[74] There are telangiectatic vessels in the upper dermis with marked dilatation of their lumen and swelling of the endothelial cells. Vessels are generally reduced in number. Those near the dermal–subcutaneous junction may show varying degrees of myointimal proliferation. Small arterioles and venules often show hyaline change in their walls, with narrowing of the lumen.

Pilosebaceous structures are absent and there is some atrophy of eccrine sweat glands. The arrector pili muscles remain, in contrast to the changes following thermal burns, when they are lost. The surviving muscle fibers are often embedded in a pear-shaped mass of collagen, giving the appearance of a bulbous scar.

Less common findings include ulceration, secondary infection and inflammation, and dysplastic epidermal changes resembling an actinic keratosis. Basal or squamous cell carcinomas may supervene. The deep subcutaneous fibrosis that may follow megavoltage therapy overlies atrophic and degenerated skeletal muscle fibers.[53]

REACTIONS TO HEAT AND COLD

There are two broad groups of temperature-dependent skin disorders.[76] The first involves the physiological responses that occur in everyone subjected to extremes of temperature. This group includes thermal burns and cold-related disorders such as frostbite. The other group of disorders involves an abnormal response to heat and cold. Abnormal reactions to heat include erythema ab igne (see p. 392), cholinergic urticaria (see p. 228), heat urticaria (see p. 227) and erythermalgia.[76] There are numerous abnormal reactions to cold such as perniosis (see p. 250), livedo reticularis, cold urticaria (see p. 227), sclerema neonatorum (see p. 526), subcutaneous fat necrosis of the newborn (see p. 526), Raynaud's phenomenon (see p. 349) and cryoglobulinemia (see p. 225).[76]

The following reactions to heat and cold will be considered further:

- thermal burns
- electrical burns
- frostbite
- cryotherapy effects
- polymorphous cold eruption.

THERMAL BURNS

Thermal burns are an important cause of morbidity and mortality. In children, most burns are scalds from hot liquids, while in adults accidents with flammable liquids are more common.[77–80] Burns are sometimes a manifestation of child abuse.[81] Acute lesions have traditionally been classified into first-, second- and third-degree burns according to the extent of the damage.[82] However, some surgeons categorize burns into superficial and deep types. Unfortunately, even this simple classification is difficult to apply on the basis of physical findings alone.[83] A common but neglected phenomenon is the occurrence of blisters weeks to months following a burn, after initial successful healing of partial-thickness wounds. This 'delayed postburn blister' may occur for up to 12 months or more after injury.[84] Its mechanism is unknown but it may be due to shearing forces in an area with reduced numbers of anchoring fibrils.[84]

Secondary infections, usually due to Gram-negative bacteria, are an important complication in the acute stage. Alopecia may follow a deep burn to the scalp.[85] A late complication, occurring 20–40 years later, is the development of a squamous cell carcinoma.[86,87] These tumors have a higher risk of metastasis than the usual squamous cell carcinomas of the skin.[88] Basal

cell carcinomas and, rarely, malignant fibrous histiocytomas or malignant melanomas may likewise develop many years after the injury.[89–92] Dystrophic xanthomatosis is another rare complication (see p. 1075).

Histopathology[93]

Biopsy may be of assistance in evaluating the extent of the lesion and the presence of secondary infection, particularly if this is due to a fungus (e.g. *Aspergillus* or *Mucor*) or virus. It should be kept in mind that it may be difficult to assess the depth of dermal damage in the first 24 hours as the changes in the collagen are not always fully developed.

In first-degree burns there may be necrosis involving the upper part of the epidermis. Second-degree burns, also known as partial-thickness injury, vary greatly in their extent (Fig. 21.3). In superficial variants there is necrosis of the epidermis with an exudative crust of fibrin, neutrophils and epithelial cellular debris. Vertical elongation of epidermal keratinocytes usually occurs. Subepidermal blisters may also form. Dermal damage is mild and superficial, and there is only a sparse inflammatory cell infiltrate. In deep second-degree burns many of the pilosebaceous appendages are destroyed, together with much of the dermal collagen. There is fusion of collagen bundles, which show a refractile eosinophilic appearance. Similar changes may occur in vessel walls and there may be thrombosis. Granulation tissue forms at the interface

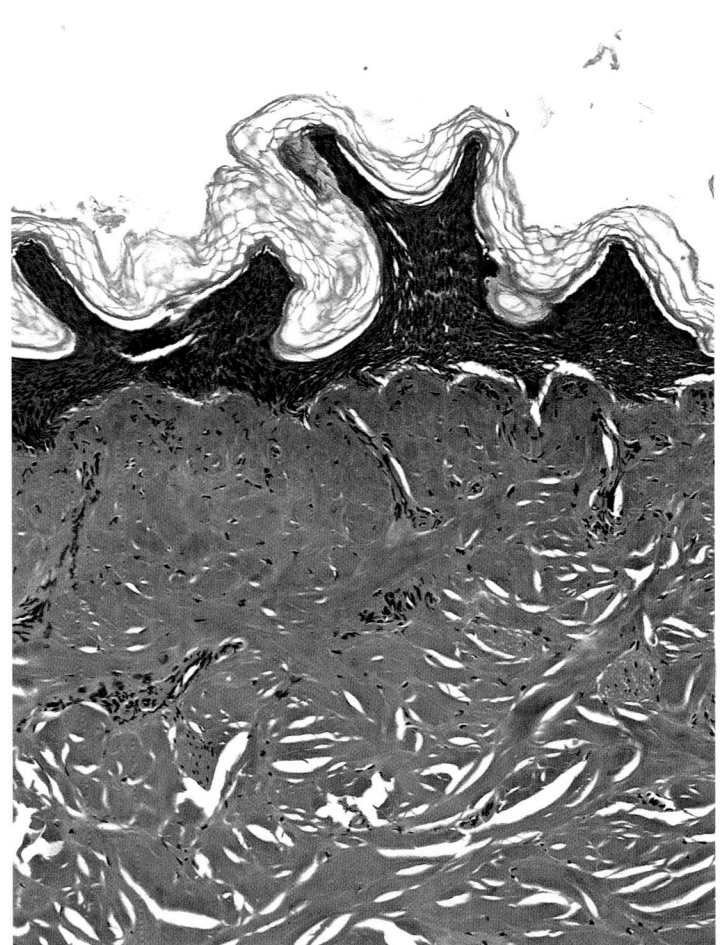

Fig. 21.3 **Thermal burn.** The dermal collagen is 'homogenous'. The epidermis is necrotic and there is focal subepidermal clefting. (H & E)

between damaged and viable tissues, resulting in scarring. Epidermal regeneration develops from surviving epithelial components, particularly the eccrine glands, which undergo squamous metaplasia.

In full-thickness (third-degree) burns the necrosis involves the entire thickness of the skin, including variable amounts of underlying fat. An inflammatory exudate forms at the junction of the viable and non-viable tissue and granulation tissue eventually forms. The necrotic eschar separates after about 3 weeks. As appendages have been destroyed, the only re-epithelialization that can occur is at the margins or by the application of a skin graft.

The scar that follows deep second-degree and third-degree burns is composed of hyalinized collagen. There is usually a decrease in the elastic fibers. Arrector pili muscles are generally lost, in contrast to their preservation in cases of chronic radiation damage, in which they become embedded in scar tissue (see p. 596).[94]

The delayed postburn blister that sometimes forms after initial healing is subepidermal in type.[84] There are no immune deposits.

ELECTRICAL BURNS

Electrical burns may be of variable severity, depending on the nature of the current, the voltage, and the extent of contact with the skin. They resemble third-degree thermal burns although in severe electrical burns there is deep vascular damage leading to cutaneous infarcts which are slow to heal.[82,95] Electrical burns in the mouth result in irregularly shaped ulcers covered by slough.[96]

Lightning strikes may be associated with full-thickness burns, linear charring, and branching or ferning marks known as Lichtenberg figures.[97,98]

Histopathology

The use of controlled electrical currents during diathermy and electrodesiccation produces epidermal necrosis resembling thermal burns. A similar picture results from the use of short-pulse, carbon dioxide laser.[99] It seems, based on animal experiments, that the energy required to vaporize the dermis is greater than that needed for the epidermis.[100] In electrical burns, elongated cytoplasmic processes extrude from the basal cells into the cavity that forms by dermoepidermal separation. More superficial keratinocytes in the epidermis may also show vertical elongation. There is also homogenization of the collagen in the upper dermis. In severe electrical burns there is infarction of the entire thickness of the dermis and subcutis, with necrosis of vessel walls in the deeper tissue.[95] Hemorrhage often accompanies this vessel damage.[95]

The Lichtenberg figures seen following lightning strikes show subcutaneous hemorrhage.[97]

FROSTBITE

Frostbite occurs when tissue freezes.[76] Usually, an acral part such as a finger, toe, ear or even the nose is involved. The affected part becomes white or bluish white.[76] A blister forms a day or so after rewarming and this is followed some days later by the formation of a hard eschar.[76] Autoamputation of the affected area eventually occurs. The terms 'chilblain' and 'perniosis' (see p. 250) are used for a specific lesion that may result from exposure to cold temperatures.

Histopathology

The affected area is necrotic and an inflammatory infiltrate is found at the periphery. Granulation tissue eventually forms at the junction between viable and necrotic tissue.

CRYOTHERAPY EFFECTS

Cryotherapy using carbon dioxide or liquid nitrogen is commonly used in the treatment of cutaneous tumors and premalignant keratoses. As cryotherapy involves rapid cooling it produces numerous intracellular ice crystals and hence more destruction than does the slow cooling of an area.[76]

The effects of cryotherapy on normal skin have been elucidated using volunteers and by studying the skin adjacent to lesions which are removed subsequent to cryotherapy. These studies have shown that different cells vary in their susceptibility to cold injury.[76] For example, melanocytes appear to be particularly sensitive to the effects of cold, an explanation for the hypopigmentation that may follow cryotherapy.

Histopathology[101]

The application of liquid nitrogen results in the loss of cellular outline in the epidermis, which appears homogenized. The upper dermis becomes edematous and a subepidermal bulla forms (Fig. 21.4). If the application is more prolonged, homogenization of the upper dermis also occurs. Similar changes occur in any tumor that is so treated.

New collagen is laid down in the papillary dermis over several weeks and this may be accompanied by blunting of the rete pegs. Sometimes excessive collagen forms, leading to scarring. In solar elastotic skin, new collagen fibers

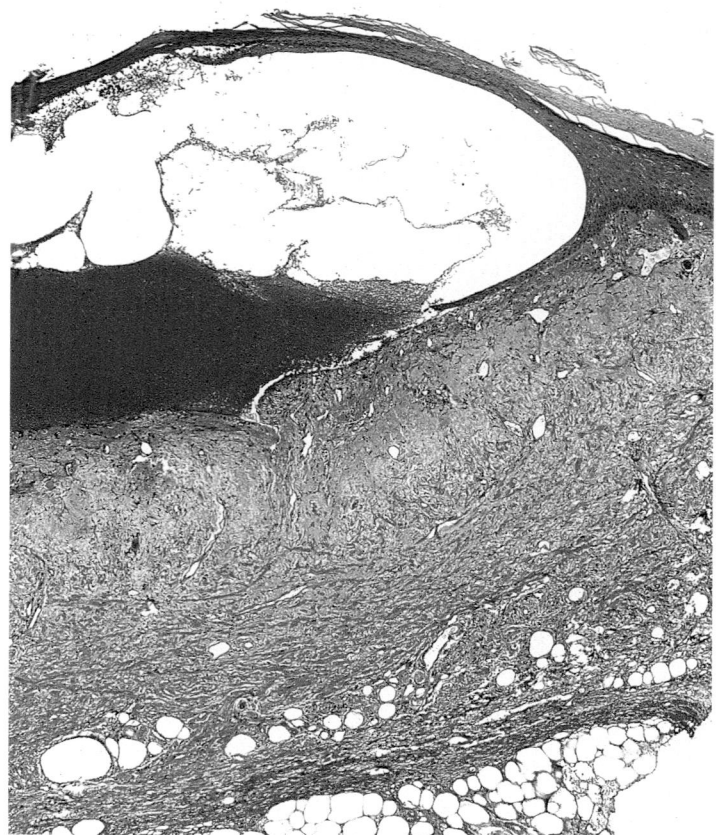

Fig. 21.4 **Cryotherapy blister.** The lesion is subepidermal with luminal hemorrhage. (H & E)

are often intermingled with elastotic fibers.[102] There may be small foci of giant cell elastoclasis, with multinucleate foreign body giant cells phagocytosing a few of the elastotic fibers.[102] Focal acanthosis or pseudoepitheliomatous hyperplasia may develop, often in relation to the transepidermal elimination of damaged collagen and elastic fibers.[102] These changes may lead to a clinical suspicion that the initial lesion has not responded to the cryotherapy.

Another change that follows cryotherapy is localized hypopigmentation, sometimes with a halo of hyperpigmentation.[103] In either case, there may be some melanin lying free, or in macrophages, in the upper dermis.

POLYMORPHOUS COLD ERUPTION

Polymorphous cold eruption, a rare, autosomal dominant disorder, is characterized by a non-pruritic erythematous eruption developing after generalized exposure to cold air.[104] The lesions are usually localized to the face and extremities. The eruption is often accompanied by fever, malaise and headache. It differs clinically and histologically from cold urticaria, with which it is often confused.

Histopathology[104]
There is a superficial and deep mixed inflammatory cell infiltrate composed of lymphocytes, neutrophils and eosinophils. An infiltrate composed predominantly of neutrophils is present around eccrine sweat glands. There is no vasculitis.

REACTIONS TO LIGHT (PHOTODERMATOSES)

The photodermatoses are a heterogeneous group of cutaneous disorders in which light plays a significant pathogenetic role.[105,106] This group is sometimes expanded by the inclusion of those conditions, both congenital and acquired, which are exacerbated in some way by light but which are not directly produced by it.[107–112] This expanded concept of light-sensitive dermatoses includes the following diseases.

- *Genodermatoses:*
  xeroderma pigmentosum
  Cockayne's syndrome
  Bloom's syndrome
  Hartnup disease
  Rothmund–Thomson disease
  Smith–Lemli–Opitz syndrome[113]
- *Metabolic/nutritional dermatoses:*
  porphyria
  disorders of tryptophan metabolism
  pellagra
- *Light-sensitive dermatoses:*
  lupus erythematosus
  lichen planus variants
  rosacea
  Hailey–Hailey disease
  Darier's disease
  seborrheic dermatitis
  atopic dermatitis
  erythema multiforme
  pityriasis rubra pilaris
  disseminated actinic porokeratosis
  herpes simplex infections

- *Photodermatoses:*
  phototoxic dermatitis
  photodynamic therapy
  photoallergic dermatitis
  hydroa vacciniforme
  polymorphous light eruption
  actinic prurigo
  solar urticaria
- *Chronic photodermatoses:*
  persistent light reaction
  photosensitive eczema
  actinic reticuloid
  brachioradial pruritus.

Before considering the various photodermatoses, a brief mention will be made of the complications of therapy using psoralens plus ultraviolet-A light (PUVA therapy). This therapy has been an effective treatment for psoriasis and some other dermatoses for many years. Several studies have shown an increased risk of skin cancers in these patients, particularly those who have received high doses.[114] For example, in one study of patients who had received cumulative ultraviolet-A doses greater than 2000 J/cm^2, 19% had developed squamous cell carcinomas and 46% solar keratoses.[115] Interestingly, none of the 13% of patients without PUVA lentigines (see p. 806) had developed keratoses or squamous cell carcinomas.[115] A Swedish study, published in 1999, found an increased incidence of squamous cell carcinoma in patients treated with PUVA, but no increased risk of melanoma, despite concern that melanomas might be a consequence.[116] However, trioxsalen bath PUVA and newer low-dose regimens may lower the risk of skin cancer developing.[117–119] Human papillomavirus was detected in some of the skin tumors that developed in one patient with PUVA-related lesions.[120]

In a study of 203 patients presenting with 'photosensitivity', the most frequent diagnoses were polymorphous light eruption (26% of cases), chronic actinic dermatitis (17%), photoallergic contact dermatitis (8%), systemic phototoxicity to therapeutic agents (7%) and solar urticaria 4%.[121] Of the remainder, 22% proved not to have photosensitivity, no diagnosis could be made in 12% because of failure of follow-up, and 4% had allergic contact dermatitis.[12]

The account that follows will be confined to the photodermatoses. Solar urticaria has been discussed with the urticarial reactions (see p. 227). The following entities will be discussed in turn:

- phototoxic dermatitis
- photodynamic therapy
- photoallergic dermatitis
- hydroa vacciniforme
- polymorphous light eruption
- actinic prurigo
- chronic photodermatoses:
  persistent light reaction
  photosensitive eczema
  actinic reticuloid
  brachioradial pruritus.

PHOTOTOXIC DERMATITIS

Phototoxicity is the damage induced by ultraviolet and/or visible radiation as a result of contact with or the ingestion of a photosensitizing substance.[122] It does not depend on an allergic reaction and is therefore akin to an irritant contact dermatitis.[123] Phytophotodermatitis is a photosensitivity reaction, usually phototoxic in type, which results from contact with plants containing psoralens and other furocoumarins.[124–126] The families Umbelliferae and Rutaceae contain many phototoxic species. They include celery,[124,127,128] parsnips, carrots, fennel, dill, limes and lemons.[129]

Clinically, phototoxic reactions resemble an exaggerated sunburn reaction with dusky erythema; when severe, vesiculation may occur, followed by desquamation and hyperpigmentation.[130–132] Two patterns of reaction are seen: an immediate reaction, which follows the ingestion of the photosensitizing agent and involves exposed areas such as the face, ears, V-area of the neck and dorsum of the hands;[133] and a delayed reaction, which follows contact with psoralens and peaks after 2 or 3 days. The reaction is limited to the site of contact with the photosensitizing agent. Prominent pigmentation lasting for weeks or months may follow phytophotodermatitis.[124] In some instances, the preceding erythematous phase may go unnoticed.[125] Chronic changes include wrinkling, atrophy, telangiectasia and the formation of keratoses.

Another presumed phototoxic reaction is the formation of subepidermal bullae, first reported in patients with chronic renal failure receiving high doses of furosemide (frusemide).[134] Other drugs which may produce this pseudoporphyria reaction (see p. 559) include naproxen,[135] oxaprozin, pravastatin, mefenamic acid, nabumetone, flutamide, dapsone, tetracycline, pyridoxine, nalidixic acid[136] and vinblastine.[137] A list of drugs producing photosensitivity reactions has recently been published.[138] Prolonged sunbed exposure of chronically sun-damaged skin has also been incriminated, although whether there is any phototoxic component remains to be seen.[139]

Ingested drugs capable of causing a phototoxic reaction include, in addition to those mentioned above, phenothiazines, thioxanthenes,[140] thiazides,[141,142] doxycycline,[143] fleroxacin,[144] ofloxacin,[145] tetrazepam,[146] non-steroidal anti-inflammatory drugs,[147] retinoids,[147] amiodarone,[148] carbamazepine and sulfonamides.[130,149] Topical agents associated with phototoxicity include coal tar and derivatives, psoralens[125] and textile dyes,[150] as well as some perfumes and sun barrier preparations.[151]

A phototoxic reaction requires the absorption of photons of specific wavelengths by the photosensitizing substance.[149] Energy is dissipated as it returns from an excited state to its ground state. Free radicals, peroxides and other substances are formed which may potentially damage cellular and subcellular membranes.[149,152] The action spectrum is usually in the ultraviolet-A range, although with some ingested substances (e.g. thiazides) it is in the shorter ultraviolet-B wavelengths.[130,141] The formation of apoptotic keratinocytes ('sunburn' cells) appears to require ultraviolet-B radiation; tumor necrosis factor-α, p53 protein and other factors are involved in some way.[153–155] There is some evidence that a p53-independent pathway can also be involved.[156]

Phototoxicity is more common than photoallergy, from which it differs by being dose related and by its subsidence on removal of the photosensitizer or the ultraviolet radiation. Some drugs produce both toxic and allergic reactions; in others, the mechanism has not been elucidated.

Histopathology

If the photosensitizing agent is applied to the skin there is some ballooning of keratinocytes in the upper dermis, with epidermal necrosis in severe reactions[123] and scattered apoptotic keratinocytes ('sunburn cells') in mild reactions (Figs 21.5, 21.6). There is variable spongiosis. A similar picture is seen in biopsies taken from photopatch test sites in phototoxic states.[157] If the chromophore reaches the skin through the vasculature there may be only minor epidermal changes.[158]

In both instances, there is a mild or moderate superficial inflammatory cell infiltrate in the dermis.[158] It is composed predominantly of lymphocytes, although a few neutrophils may be present in severe reactions. Eosinophils are sometimes seen. Although it is usually taught that the dermal infiltrate is both superficial and deep in the light-related dermatoses, this is not always so, particularly in acute lesions. Pigment incontinence is sometimes present,[141] while in late lesions of phytophotodermatitis there is also basal hyperpigmentation.

In bullous phototoxic reactions (pseudoporphyria) there is a subepidermal blister with only rare inflammatory cells in the base (see p. 560). A very occasional eosinophil is sometimes present. In cases of long standing, the blisters may heal with scarring and milia formation.[158] In chronic phototoxic states (bullous and non-bullous), basophilic elastotic fibers extend below the mid dermis (Fig. 21.7). There is also PAS-positive, diastase-resistant material in and around small blood vessels in the upper dermis. Fibroblasts and dendrocytes are also increased in photosensitivity reactions of some duration.

Small amounts of IgG and sometimes C3 are found adjacent to vessels and near the basement membrane zone in chronic states.[158]

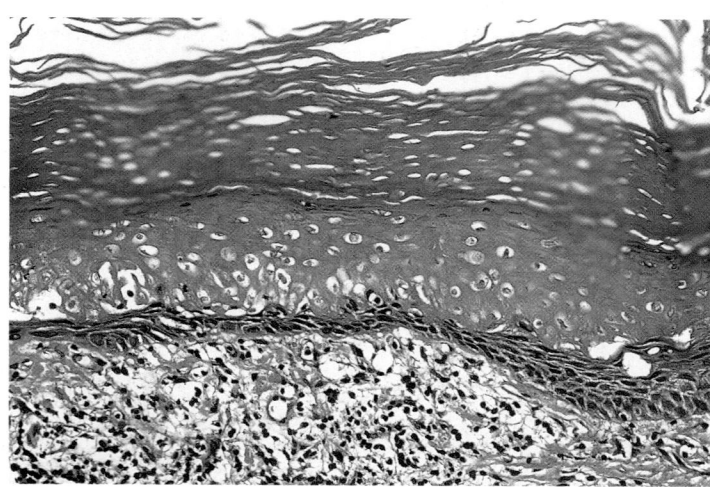

Fig. 21.5 Severe phototoxic reaction with epidermal necrosis. (H & E) (Photograph kindly provided by Dr JJ Sullivan)

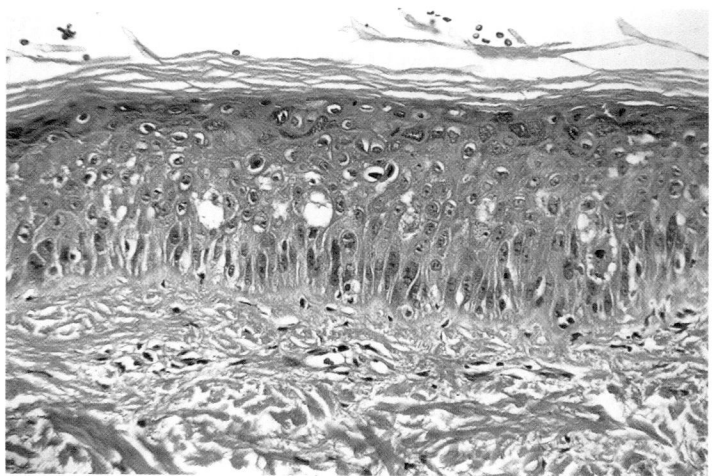

Fig. 21.6 Phototoxic reaction with scattered 'sunburn cells'. The reaction followed contact with a psoralen-containing plant (phytophotodermatitis). (H & E)

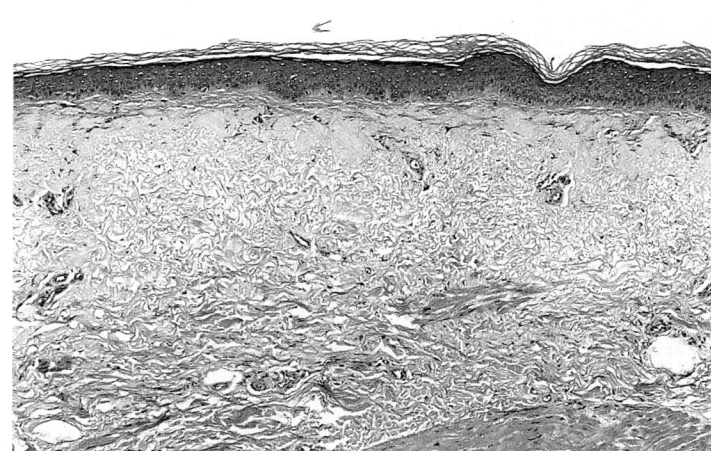

Fig. 21.7 **Chronic photosensitivity.** There are deeply extending basophilic elastotic fibers but no inflammation. (H & E)

Electron microscopy

In chronic phototoxicity there is reduplication of the basal lamina in dermal vessels and fine fibrillar deposits in their vicinity.[158]

PHOTODYNAMIC THERAPY

Photodynamic therapy is used, selectively, in the treatment of some cutaneous malignancies. It involves the use of a photosensitizing agent which is applied to, or accumulates in, malignant tissue, followed by the application of a light source that activates the photosensitizer. This results in the release of toxic oxygen radicals that destroy the malignant cells. Recently, partial-thickness burns have been reported following the ingestion of temoporfin, a second generation photosensitizer.[158a]

PHOTOALLERGIC DERMATITIS

Photoallergy is increased reactivity of the skin to ultraviolet and visible radiation and is brought about by a chemical agent on an immunological basis.[122,158] The photosensitizing chemical is usually applied topically to the skin; uncommonly, photoallergic reactions may follow ingestion of a drug.[122,159]

The usual photoallergic reaction develops 24–48 hours after sun exposure and is a pruritic, eczematous eruption.[160] Lichenification may occur in cases of long standing. Lichenoid papules have been reported in some thiazide-induced photoallergic reactions.[160] Photoallergic dermatitis occurs essentially on light-exposed areas, although there is a tendency for lesions to extend beyond the exposed areas. Regression usually occurs after 10–14 days, although in some cases the condition may persist for long periods and the patients become persistent light reactors (see below). Topical agents that have been implicated in photoallergic reactions include fragrances such as musk ambrette[161] and coumarin derivatives,[162] and sunscreens containing benzophenones[163–165] or para-aminobenzoic acid and its esters.[131,151,166] Benzocaine,[167] piroxicam gel,[168] plants in the *Compositae* family and, rarely, psoralens have been recorded as producing photoallergic reactions. The halogenated salicylanilides, which resulted in numerous cases of photoallergic dermatitis over two decades ago, have been withdrawn as topical antibacterial agents.[169] Systemically administered drugs which rarely produce photoallergy include quinine,[170,171] quinidine,[172,173] griseofulvin, possibly itraconazole,[174,175] ranitidine,[176,177] lomefloxacin,[178] chlorpromazine,[179] piroxicam,[180–182] ampiroxicam,[183]

droxicam,[184] piketoprofen,[185] ketoprofen,[186,187] pyridoxine hydrochloride (vitamin B_6),[188,189] tegafur,[190] flutamide,[191] alprazolam,[192] sertraline (Zoloft), triflusal,[193] amlodipine,[194] thiazides, sulfonamides,[195] celecoxib, certain tetracycline derivatives, diphenhydramine,[196] tolbutamide, ibuprofen,[197] fibric acid derivatives (such as fenofibrate and clofibrate),[198–200] chlordiazepoxide and cyclamates.[151,158] Drugs which may produce a lichenoid photoallergic reaction include, in addition to thiazide diuretics (see above), demeclocycline, enalapril, quinine, quinidine and chloroquine.[147] A flagellate dermatitis, resembling that produced by bleomycin (see p. 443), has been reported after the ingestion of raw shiitake mushrooms.[201]

Three factors are required in a photoallergic reaction: a photosensitizing agent, light (usually in the ultraviolet-A range), and a delayed hypersensitivity response.[122] The absorption of light energy appears to alter the photosensitizing chemical in some way to produce a hapten which attaches to a protein carrier and eventually stimulates immunocompetent cells, producing a hypersensitivity response.[149] Photopatch testing is used to elucidate the offending agent.[202]

Histopathology[123,149]

The changes resemble those seen in contact allergic dermatitis and include epidermal spongiosis, spotty parakeratosis and some acanthosis.[133,170] Spongiotic vesiculation occurs in severe cases. There is a moderately heavy infiltrate of lymphocytes, mainly in a perivascular location in the upper dermis. There is some exocytosis of these inflammatory cells. In some instances, the dermal reaction differs from that seen in contact allergic dermatitis by deeper extension of the infiltrate. This is particularly so in lesions of long standing. Prominent solar elastotic changes may also develop in chronic cases.

The lichenoid papules show a lichenoid tissue reaction with a superficial and mid-dermal inflammatory cell infiltrate. Spongiosis is sometimes present as well.[147]

HYDROA VACCINIFORME

Hydroa vacciniforme is a rare, debilitating photodermatosis of unknown pathogenesis.[203] It is manifested clinically by the development of erythema and vesicles, on uncovered skin, within 1–2 days of sun exposure.[203,204] The vesicles heal leaving varioliform scars. Ear mutilation has been reported as a consequence of recurrent lesions with scarring.[205,206] Rarely, there are crusted, non-vesicular lesions.[207] The disease usually begins in childhood and runs a chronic course before remitting in adolescence.[208] Late onset[209] and familial cases are exceedingly rare.[210,211] Coexistence with a malignant lymphoma has been documented.[212] Porphyrins are normal. Lesions may be reproduced in many instances by repeated exposures to ultraviolet-A radiation.[213–217] Dietary fish oil, which provides some systemic photoprotection, has produced variable clinical responses in this disease.[218]

Recently, attention has been drawn to a hydroa vacciniforme-like eruption associated with latent Epstein–Barr virus (EBV) infection, which has a high propensity to develop cutaneous lymphoma, usually of subcutaneous type.[219–221] Latent EBV infection has now been detected in the dermal infiltrate of children with typical manifestations of hydroa vacciniforme.[219] It has been suggested that both the typical and atypical forms are part of a spectrum, in which the atypical lesions have the potential to lead to an EBV-associated lymphoid malignancy.[219]

The exact status of **hydroa estivale** is uncertain.[222,223] It has been regarded in the past as a mild form of hydroa vacciniforme or a childhood form of polymorphous light eruption.[213] Some of the earlier reported cases may have been erythropoietic protoporphyria.[224,225]

Histopathology

The established lesions of hydroa vacciniforme show intraepidermal vesiculation with reticular degeneration and, later, confluent epidermal necrosis.[213] The vesicles are filled with serum, fibrin and inflammatory cells. Ulcerated lesions may be associated with superficial dermal necrosis.[224] Vascular thrombosis is sometimes present in these circumstances. Lymphocytes and neutrophils are present at the lower border of any necrotic zone. In addition, there is a superficial and deep perivascular infiltrate of lymphocytes and occasionally a few eosinophils. There are no PAS-positive deposits.[224] In some severe cases a lobular or septal panniculitis may also be present. Healed lesions show variable scarring in the upper dermis.[207]

Direct immunofluorescence sometimes shows scattered granular deposits of C3 at the dermoepidermal junction.[213]

POLYMORPHOUS LIGHT ERUPTION

Polymorphous light eruption (polymorphic light eruption) is an idiopathic photodermatosis in which lesions of varied morphology appear several hours or even days after exposure to the sun and subside in a further 7–10 days if further exposure is avoided.[226–229] Certain populations appear to be genetically predisposed: in Finland, cases with an autosomal dominant mode of inheritance, with reduced gene penetrance, have been reported.[230] Twin studies and genetic modeling have also established a clear genetic influence.[231,232] Polymorphous light eruption affects from 10% to 20% of those living in temperate climates;[228,233] it is much less common in populations living nearer to the equator.[234]

The lesions may take the form of small pruritic papules, papulovesicles or urticarial plaques.[235] The papulovesicular form has been regarded as a discrete subset.[236,237] Rarely, lesions may resemble those seen in erythema multiforme or insect bites.[235] Eczematous lesions and lesions resembling those of prurigo nodularis[238] have been described,[239,240] although these variants are not universally accepted as part of the spectrum of poly-morphous light eruption.[235] Lesions are usually monomorphous in the same individual. Sun-related pruritus may rarely precede the onset of the disease.[241] Contact and photocontact allergies are present, rarely, in patients with polymorphous light eruption.[242]

Lesions have a predilection for the dorsum of the hands and forearms, the upper part of the arms, the neck and the face.[243] The face is usually spared in the papulovesicular form. The photodermatosis known as 'juvenile spring eruption of the ears', a condition found predominantly in young boys, is a probable variant of polymorphous light eruption.[244] The mean age of onset of polymorphous light eruption is in the third decade of life.[245] In most series there has been a female preponderance.[235,246]

Various associations have been reported, some of which may be fortuitous. They include common variable hypogammaglobulinemia,[247] thyroid disease[248] and lupus erythematosus.[249,250] Lesions have rarely been limited to areas of vitiligo[251] or nevoid telangiectasia.[252]

The condition is chronic in nature, although in about half the cases there is diminished sensitivity to sunlight over time, with periods of total remission; light sensitivity increases in some patients.[245,253–255] The phenomenon of eventual tolerance to sunlight is known as 'hardening'.[256] Recent studies suggest that a delayed hypersensitivity reaction to sunlight-modified skin antigens is involved in the pathogenesis.[257–259] In normal subjects, ultraviolet exposure leads to a disappearance of Langerhans cells from healthy skin 48–72 hours later and an accumulation of CD11b+ macrophage-like cells, which reportedly produce interleukin-10. In patients with polymorphous light eruption, Langerhans cells do not disappear after ultraviolet exposure and

CD11b+ cells, already present at the time of exposure, further increase and invade the epidermis.[260] The action spectrum appears to be quite broad and may involve both the ultraviolet-A and ultraviolet-B range,[261–264] although ultraviolet-A radiation appears to be the more important.[234,265]

Histopathology[228,235,243]

There is marked variability in the histopathological changes in the various clinical subsets of polymorphous light eruption. However, a fairly constant feature (in keeping with the mnemonic mentioned on p. 13) is the presence of a dermal inflammatory cell infiltrate which is both superficial and deep, although if early lesions are biopsied it may not extend below the mid dermis. While the infiltrate is predominantly perivascular, there is sometimes a heavy interstitial infiltrate of lymphocytes in the upper dermis in those variants characterized by prominent subepidermal edema (Fig. 21.8). The lymphocytic infiltrate is composed of T cells[266,267] and there is evidence that these cells are CD4-positive in early lesions and predominantly CD8-positive in later lesions.[268] Various interleukins may act as lymphocyte attractants.[269] Eosinophils are sometimes present in the dermal infiltrate, while in the papulovesicular type a few neutrophils have sometimes been recorded. A rare neutrophil-rich variant occurs.

Edema of the upper dermis is often present and is quite prominent in plaque-like lesions. In the rare erythema multiforme-like lesions this may be so marked that subepidermal bullae form.[235] However, there is no lichenoid (interface) reaction as occurs in erythema multiforme. Extravasation of red cells is sometimes seen in the upper dermis, particularly in the papulovesicular form.[270] Unlike lupus erythematosus, there are no dermal deposits of acid mucopolysaccharides.[271]

The epidermal changes are variable depending on the clinical type. The epidermis may be normal or show slight changes such as very mild spongiosis, focal parakeratosis or acanthosis. In the papulovesicular form there is invariably spongiosis leading to spongiotic vesiculation.[270] There is often some basal vacuolation, but no cell death or basement membrane thickening. This may be accompanied by exocytosis of lymphocytes and erythrocytes.[270]

Direct immunofluorescence gives variable results. Focal perivascular and interstitial deposits of fibrin and perivascular C3 or IgM have all been recorded in a few cases.[272] The lupus band test is negative.[273]

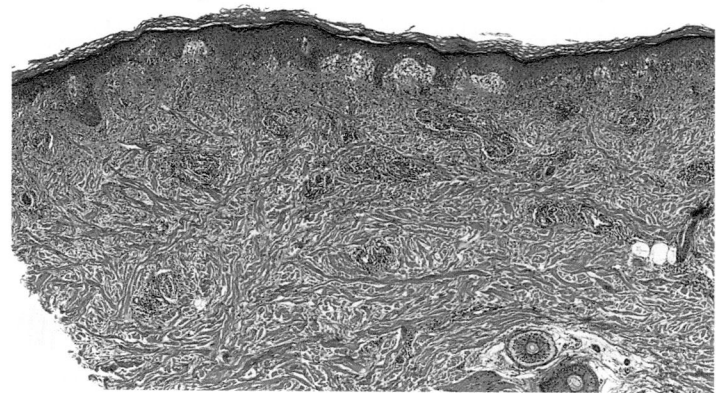

Fig. 21.8 **Polymorphous light eruption.** Note the superficial and deep perivascular infiltrate in the dermis. There is subepidermal edema and mild spongiosis. (H & E)

ACTINIC PRURIGO

Actinic prurigo (Hutchinson's summer prurigo,[274] hereditary polymorphous light eruption)[275,276] is a chronic photodermatitis occurring predominantly in North American Indians and in Central America, although Caucasians are not spared.[277–282] Actinic prurigo has been regarded as a variant of polymorphous light eruption,[277] although this has been challenged on the basis of its distinct HLA typing.[283] It is possible that the characteristic actinic prurigo phenotype is determined by this HLA type (DRB1*0407), found in 60% of patients. An association with DRB1*14 has been reported in an Inuit population.[284] Both actinic prurigo and polymorphous light eruption may share a common pathophysiological basis.[232,285,286] Families with members having either disease have been reported.[232,287] Light testing gives inconsistent results although the majority are sensitive to ultraviolet-A light.

Actinic prurigo is characterized by onset in childhood, female preponderance, a familial tendency, which is quite high in some communities, and severe pruritus.[277,278,288] It appears to be inherited as a dominant trait but with incomplete penetrance.[289] It commences as an eczematous eruption on exposed areas, particularly the face and forearms.[275] Papular, plaque-like and prurigo-like papulonodules develop.[278] Lichenification can be marked. Other features that may be present include an exudative and crusted cheilitis of the lower lip,[290] conjunctivitis[291] and alopecia of the eyebrows.[277]

One study found that those who developed actinic prurigo as children and teenagers were more often associated with cheilitis, acute eruptions and improvement over 5 years, while adults tended to have a milder and more persistent dermatosis.[292]

The pathogenesis may result from excessive tumor necrosis factor-α production by keratinocytes, triggered by ultraviolet light in genetically predisposed individuals.[293] The dermal infiltrate is composed of T-helper type I lymphocytes admixed with scattered B cells and dermal dendrocytes.[293]

Histopathology[277]

The findings are not diagnostically specific. There is usually hyperkeratosis, irregular acanthosis, prominent telangiectasia of superficial vessels, and a moderately heavy chronic inflammatory cell infiltrate which is predominantly lymphocytic and perivascular.[294] Lymphoid follicles may be present. The cellular infiltrate is usually confined to the superficial plexus, but extension around mid-dermal vessels may occur. Solar elastosis is not a consistent finding. In early eczematous lesions there is some epidermal spongiosis. Excoriation and changes of lichen simplex chronicus are present in the prurigo-like areas.[295]

The cheilitis is characterized by a dense lymphocytic infiltrate, often with well-formed lymphoid follicles – follicular cheilitis.[295,296] A similar follicular pattern is often present in the conjunctiva.[297]

CHRONIC PHOTODERMATOSES (CHRONIC ACTINIC DERMATITIS)

The terms 'chronic photodermatoses' and 'chronic actinic dermatitis' refer to a group of rare photodermatoses with overlapping clinical features that include persistent photosensitivity, a marked predominance in older males, and the presence of erythematous, edematous and lichenified plaques in areas exposed to light.[298–302] These conditions appear to be more common in Europe than in other parts of the world,[300,303–305] suggesting the possible etiological role of a photosensitizing agent. A report of the phototest results of 86 patients with this condition showed that 74% had a positive result: 36% of these positive patients were sensitive to sesquiterpene lactone mix (the main allergenic constituent of Compositae plants), 21% to fragrance compounds, 20% to colophony, and 14% to rubber chemicals.[302] Compositae appear to play no role in the United States.[306]

Included in the chronic photodermatoses are persistent light reaction, photosensitive eczema and actinic reticuloid.[307] The terms 'chronic actinic dermatitis'[308] and 'photosensitivity dermatitis – actinic reticuloid syndrome'[307] have also been used to embrace this group of photodermatoses, which differ from polymorphous light eruption in the age and sex of those involved and in the extreme photosensitivity. The term 'chronic actinic dermatitis' is being used increasingly for this group of chronic photodermatoses.[306,309,310] Actinic reticuloid and brachioradial pruritus have unique clinical and histopatnological features that distinguish them from the other chronic photodermatoses.[311]

There appears to be a weak association between chronic actinic dermatitis and infection with the human immunodeficiency virus (HIV); it may even be the presenting disorder.[312,313]

Abnormal phototest responses to ultraviolet-A and/or ultraviolet-B and/or increased sensitivity to visible light characterize this group of conditions.[310]

Persistent light reaction

The condition of persistent light reaction was first recognized in relation to the use of halogenated salicylanilides, when it was noticed that a photosensitive eczematous eruption continued after the withdrawal of the offending photosensitizer. The lesions may be confined to the area of application of the agent or be more generalized. Other features include a positive photopatch test to the agent and a sensitivity to ultraviolet-B radiation and sometimes other wavelengths as well.[314]

Other agents have now been incriminated; these may be used topically or systemically. Musk ambrette, which is used not only in after-shave lotions and various cosmetics but also in certain foodstuffs, is often involved.[314–316] Thiazide diuretics may also produce a photodermatosis which persists for many years after their withdrawal,[317] as may chlorpromazine, promethazine, pyrithione zinc, quinine, quinoxaline dioxide, furosemide (frusemide) and epoxy resins.[307] Contact with hexachlorophene rarely produces a persistent light reaction.[318]

Although the pathogenetic mechanisms are unknown, autosensitization of skin proteins with endogenous photosensitizers and a cellular hypersensitivity reaction to light have been suggested in preference to persistence of the initial photosensitizing agent.[307]

Histopathology[314]

There is epidermal spongiosis with focal parakeratosis and some acanthosis. Spongiotic vesiculation is present in florid cases. A moderately dense perivascular inflammatory cell infiltrate involves the upper and mid dermis. Superficially, the infiltrate may be more diffuse and there may be exocytosis of inflammatory cells, particularly in the thiazide-related cases.[317] The infiltrate is predominantly lymphocytic with occasional eosinophils, plasma cells and mast cells. In cases of long standing, basophilic fibers, resembling those seen in solar elastosis except for their lack of coiling, extend into the lower dermis.

A similar dermal infiltrate can be produced in clinically uninvolved skin by the application of ultraviolet-B radiation.[314]

Photosensitive eczema

Photosensitive eczema probably represents a photocontact allergic dermatitis in which the photoallergen is unrecognized, leading to persistence of the eczematous eruption.[298,319] The skin shows increased sensitivity to ultraviolet-B radiation. This entity should be distinguished from those eczematous processes that may be exacerbated by light, such as seborrheic dermatitis and some cases of atopic dermatitis. It appears that chronic actinic dermatitis is increased in patients with atopic dermatitis.[320,321]

Histopathology

The picture resembles photocontact allergic dermatitis with epidermal spongiosis and a superficial perivascular inflammatory cell infiltrate. The infiltrate extends deeper in the dermis than is usual in contact allergic dermatitis.

Actinic reticuloid

Actinic reticuloid has been separated from the other chronic photo-dermatoses on the basis of its histopathological picture, which shows a variable resemblance to a T-cell lymphoma.[311,322,323] Actinic reticuloid has clinical features that overlap with those of photosensitive eczema and persistent light reaction.[324] Differences include episodes of an erythroderma-like picture involving also non-exposed areas of the body and extreme sensitivity to ultraviolet-B and ultraviolet-A radiation and often to visible light as well.[325–327] A positive photopatch test is present in less than 10% of affected individuals, although contact allergic sensitivity without the involvement of radiation is sometimes present.[300] Offending agents in this category include oleoresins of various plants in the Compositae family and certain fragrances.[303,328,329] Persistent light reaction sometimes evolves into actinic reticuloid,[330,331] indicating that the chronic photodermatoses (chronic actinic dermatitis) are part of a spectrum. Avoidance of ultraviolet/visible light often leads to sustained improvement.[332]

The few reports of lymphoma developing in patients with actinic reticuloid appear to represent a chance occurrence, particularly as the patients with actinic reticuloid are usually elderly.[333,334] Furthermore, DNA aneuploidy has not been demonstrated using DNA flow cytometry.[335] More importantly, clonal T cells have not been identified.[336]

Although the pathogenesis of actinic reticuloid is unknown, theories similar to those advanced for persistent light reaction have been proposed. Of interest is the finding that cultured fibroblasts from the skin of individuals with actinic reticuloid show cytopathic changes and inhibition of RNA synthesis after exposure to ultraviolet-A radiation.[337,338]

Histopathology[304,311,339]

There is usually a dense, polymorphous infiltrate in the upper dermis which may be band-like or more diffuse with extension into the mid and lower dermis (Fig. 21.9). The infiltrate is composed of lymphocytes, a variable number of large lymphoid cells with hyperchromatic, convoluted nuclei, scattered stellate fibroblasts and a few plasma cells and sometimes eosinophils. Immunoperoxidase studies have shown that the infiltrate is composed of polyclonal T lymphocytes, Langerhans cells and HLA-DR-positive macrophages.[336,340–343] There is often exocytosis of lymphocytes and of the atypical mononuclear cells into the epidermis where they form small collections resembling the Pautrier microabscesses of mycosis fungoides. Although the dermal infiltrate contains a mixture of T-helper (Th) and T-suppressor-cytotoxic (Ts) cells, the epidermis contains a predominance of Ts cells, in contrast to cutaneous T-cell lymphoma.[344] There may be mild spongiosis, but this is not nearly as prominent as in the other chronic photosensitivity disorders.[339] A similar dermal infiltrate can be produced by irradiating uninvolved skin at certain wavelengths.[345]

The epidermis is usually acanthotic and sometimes there is psoriasiform epidermal hyperplasia associated with thickened collagen in the papillary dermis, representing superimposed changes of lichen simplex chronicus (Fig. 21.10).[339,346] Blood vessels may be increased in the papillary dermis and these are lined by plump endothelial cells.

Under lower power magnification the impression is often of a chronic eczematous dermatitis, but with minimal spongiosis and an excessive number

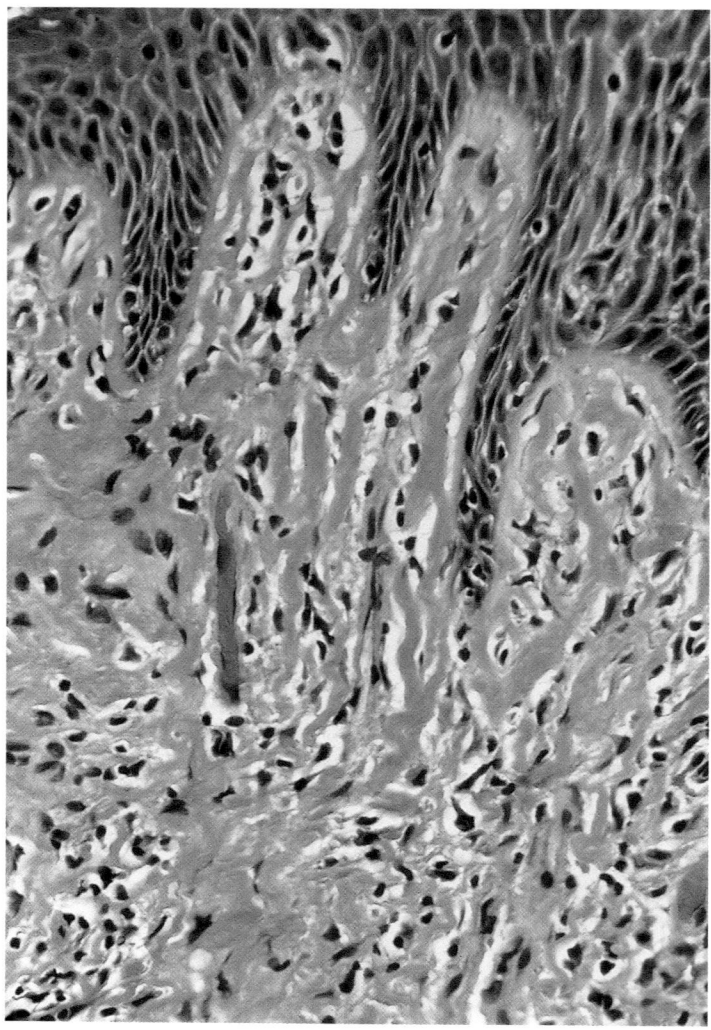

Fig. 21.10 **Actinic reticuloid.** Note the 'vertically-streaked' collagen in the papillary dermis, the stellate fibroblasts and occasional hyperchromatic lymphocyte. (H & E)

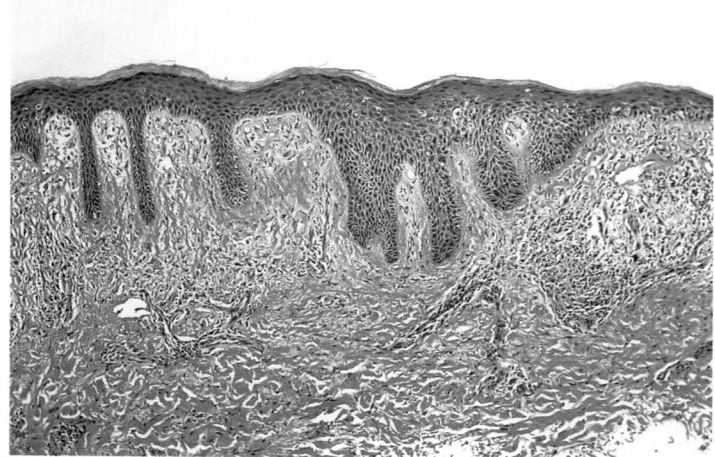

Fig. 21.9 **Actinic reticuloid.** There is variable acanthosis. The inflammatory infiltrate is heaviest in the upper dermis. (H & E)

of dermal cells for such a process. The finding of scattered hyperchromatic cells and stellate fibroblasts completes the picture.

Electron microscopy

The presence of Langerhans cells in the dermal infiltrate has been confirmed.[347] The atypical cells resemble the Sézary cell in having a hyper-convoluted nucleus.[348]

Brachioradial pruritus

Brachioradial pruritus is a rare and recurrent solar dermopathy which presents as a localized pruritic dermatosis involving the brachioradial region of the arm. In some patients, cervical spine disease has been incriminated. As there is usually a marginal increase in mast cells, many of which are enlarged, it is considered further with other mast cell disorders (see p. 1064).

REFERENCES

Introduction

1 Sutton RL Jr. Dermatoses due to physical agents. Cutis 1977; 19: 513–529.

Reactions to trauma and irritation

2 Basler RSW. Skin injuries in sports medicine. J Am Acad Dermatol 1989; 21: 1257–1262.
3 Foley S, Mallory SB. Air bag dermatitis. J Am Acad Dermatol 1995; 33: 824–825.
4 Metzker A, Brenner S, Merlob P. Iatrogenic cutaneous injuries in the neonate. Arch Dermatol 1999; 135: 697–703.
5 Griego RD, Rosen T, Orengo IF, Wolf JE. Dog, cat, and human bites: a review. J Am Acad Dermatol 1995; 33: 1019–1029.
6 Lyell A. Cutaneous artifactual disease. A review, amplified by personal experience. J Am Acad Dermatol 1979; 1: 391–407.
7 Lyell A. Dermatitis artefacta in relation to the syndrome of contrived disease. Clin Exp Dermatol 1976; 1: 109–126.
8 Stankler L. Factitious skin lesions in a mother and two sons. Br J Dermatol 1977; 97: 217–219.
9 Van Moffaert M, Vermander F, Kint A. Dermatitis artefacta. Int J Dermatol 1985; 24: 236–238.
10 Brodland DG, Staats BA, Peters MS. Factitial leg ulcers associated with an unusual sleep disorder. Arch Dermatol 1989; 125: 1115–1118.
11 Sneddon I, Sneddon J. Self-inflicted injury: a follow-up study of 43 patients. Br Med J 1975; 3: 527–530.
12 Somani VK. Witchcraft's syndrome: Munchausen's syndrome by proxy. Int J Dermatol 1998; 37: 229–230.
13 Lipp KE, Smith JB, Brandt TP, Messina JL. Reflex sympathetic dystrophy with mutilating ulcerations suspicious of a factitial origin. J Am Acad Dermatol 1996; 35: 843–845.
14 Shelley WB, Shelley ED. Keratoderma simplex: a novel entity simulating seborrhoeic keratosis. Br J Dermatol 1997; 136: 792.
15 Ruiz-Maldonado R, Durán-McKinster C, Tamayo-Sánchez L, Orozco-Covarrubias ML. Dermatosis neglecta: dirt crusts simulating verrucous nevi. Arch Dermatol 1999; 135: 728–729.
16 Cox NH, Wilkinson DS. Dermatitis artefacta as the presenting feature of auto-erythrocyte sensitization syndrome and naproxen-induced pseudoporphyria in a single patient. Br J Dermatol 1992; 126: 86–89.
17 Jackson RM, Tucker SB, Abraham JL, Millns JL. Factitial cutaneous ulcers and nodules: the use of electron-probe microanalysis in diagnosis. J Am Acad Dermatol 1984; 11: 1065–1069.
18 Tsuji T, Sawabe M. A new type of telangiectasia following trauma. J Cutan Pathol 1988; 15: 22–26.
19 Parish LC, Witkowski JA. The infected decubitus ulcer. Int J Dermatol 1989; 28: 643–647.
20 Yarkony GM, Kirk PM, Carlson C et al. Classification of pressure ulcers. Arch Dermatol 1990; 126: 1218–1219.
21 Phillips TJ. Chronic cutaneous ulcers: etiology and epidemiology. J Invest Dermatol 1994; 102: 38S–41S.
22 Witkowski JA, Parish LC. The decubitus ulcer: skin failure and destructive behavior. Int J Dermatol 2000; 39: 894–896.
23 Falanga V. Chronic wounds: pathophysiologic and experimental considerations. J Invest Dermatol 1993; 100: 721–725.
24 Kanj LF, Wilking SV, Phillips TJ. Pressure ulcers. J Am Acad Dermatol 1998; 38: 517–536.

25 Witkowski JA, Parish LC. Histopathology of the decubitus ulcer. J Am Acad Dermatol 1982; 6: 1014–1021.
26 Fader DJ, Kang S. Bedsore of an unknown primary site. Arch Dermatol 1995; 131: 1115–1116.
27 Bolton LL, Montagna W. Mast cells in human ulcers. Am J Dermatopathol 1993; 15: 133–138.
28 Vande Berg JS, Rudolph R. Pressure (decubitus) ulcer: variation in histopathology – a light and electron microscope study. Hum Pathol 1995; 26: 195–200.
29 Brehmer-Andersson E, Goransson K. Friction blisters as a manifestation of pathomimia. Acta Derm Venereol 1975; 55: 65–71.
30 Naylor PFD. Experimental friction blisters. Br J Dermatol 1955; 67: 327–342.
31 Pharis DB, Teller C, Wolf JE Jr. Cutaneous manifestations of sports participation. J Am Acad Dermatol 1997; 36: 448–459.
32 Epstein WL, Fukuyama K, Cortese TA. Autoradiographic study of friction blisters. Arch Dermatol 1969; 99: 94–106.
33 Sulzberger MB, Cortese TA Jr, Fishman L, Wiley HS. Studies on blisters produced by friction. I. Results of linear rubbing and twisting technics. J Invest Dermatol 1966; 47: 456–465.
34 Cortese TA Jr, Griffin TB, Layton LL, Hutsell TC. Experimental friction blisters in Macaque monkeys. J Invest Dermatol 1969; 53: 172–177.
35 Hunter JAA, McVittie E, Comaish JS. Light and electron microscopic studies of physical injury to the skin. I. Suction. Br J Dermatol 1974; 90: 481–490.
36 Hunter JAA, McVittie E, Comaish JS. Light and electron microscopic studies of physical injury to the skin. II. Friction. Br J Dermatol 1974; 90: 491–499.
37 Crissey JT, Peachey JC. Calcaneal petechiae. Arch Dermatol 1961; 83: 501.
38 Kirton V, Price MW. Black heel. Trans St John's Hosp Dermatol Soc 1965; 51: 80–84.
39 Mehregan AH. Black heel: a report of two cases. Can Med Assoc J 1966; 96: 584–585.
40 Ganpule M. Pinching trauma in 'black heel'. Br J Dermatol 1967; 79: 654–655.
41 Cho KH, Kim YG, Seo KI, Suh DH. Black heel with atypical melanocytic hyperplasia. Clin Exp Dermatol 1993; 18: 437–440.
42 Ayres S Jr, Mihan R. Calcaneal petechiae. Arch Dermatol 1972; 106: 262.
43 Garcia-Doval I, de la Torre C, Losada A, Cruces MJ. Disseminated punctate intraepidermal haemorrhage: a widespread counterpart of black heel. Acta Derm Venereol 1999; 79: 403.
44 Apted JH. Calcaneal petechiae (black heel). Australas J Dermatol 1973; 14: 132–135.
45 Hafner J, Haenseler E, Ossent P et al. Benzidine stain for the histochemical detection of hemoglobin in splinter hemorrhage (subungual hematoma) and black heel. Am J Dermatopathol 1995; 17: 362–367.

Reactions to radiation

46 LeBoit PE. Subacute radiation dermatitis: a histologic imitator of acute cutaneous graft-versus-host disease. J Am Acad Dermatol 1989; 20: 236–241.
47 Soter NA. Acute effects of ultraviolet radiation on the skin. Semin Dermatol 1990; 9: 11–15.
48 Rhainds M, De Guire L, Claveau J. A population-based survey on the use of artificial tanning devices in the Province of Québec, Canada. J Am Acad Dermatol 1999; 40: 572–576.
49 Nahass GT. Acute radiodermatitis after radiofrequency catheter ablation. J Am Acad Dermatol 1997; 36: 881–884.
50 Fajardo LF, Berthrong M. Radiation injury in surgical pathology. Part I. Am J Surg Pathol 1978; 2: 159–199.
51 Price NM. Radiation dermatitis following electron beam therapy. Arch Dermatol 1978; 114: 63–66.
52 Fajardo LF, Berthrong M. Radiation injury in surgical pathology. Part III. Salivary glands, pancreas and skin. Am J Surg Pathol 1981; 5: 279–296.
53 James WD, Odom RB. Late subcutaneous fibrosis following megavoltage radiotherapy. J Am Acad Dermatol 1980; 3: 616–618.
54 Kawakami T, Saito R, Miyazaki S. Chronic radiodermatitis following repeated percutaneous transluminal coronary angioplasty. Br J Dermatol 1999; 141: 150–153.
55 Young EM Jr, Barr RJ. Sclerosing dermatoses. J Cutan Pathol 1985; 12: 426–441.
56 Goldschmidt H, Sherwin WK. Reactions to ionizing radiation. J Am Acad Dermatol 1980; 3: 551–579.
57 Gottlöber P, Bezold G, Weber L et al. The radiation accident in Georgia: Clinical appearance and diagnosis of cutaneous radiation syndrome. J Am Acad Dermatol 2000; 42: 453–458.
58 Stone MS, Robson KJ, LeBoit PE. Subacute radiation dermatitis from fluoroscopy during coronary artery stenting: Evidence for cytotoxic lymphocyte mediated apoptosis. J Am Acad Dermatol 1998; 38: 333–336.
59 Rueda RA, Valencia IC, Covelli C et al. Eosinophilic, polymorphic, and pruritic eruption associated with radiotherapy. Arch Dermatol 1999; 135: 804–810.
60 Gallego H, Wilke MS, Lewis EJ. Delayed EPPER syndrome. Arch Dermatol 2001; 137: 821–822.
61 Goldschmidt H. Dermatologic radiotherapy. The risk-benefit ratio. Arch Dermatol 1986; 122: 1385–1388.

62   Peter RU, Braun-Falco O, Birioukov A et al. Chronic cutaneous damage after accidental exposure to ionizing radiation: the Chernobyl experience. J Am Acad Dermatol 1994; 30: 719–723.

63   Landthaler M, Hagspiel H-J, Braun-Falco O. Late irradiation damage to the skin caused by soft X-ray radiation therapy of cutaneous tumors. Arch Dermatol 1995; 131: 182–186.

64   Volden G, Larsen TE. Squamous cell carcinoma appearing in X-ray-treated mycosis fungoides. Acta Derm Venereol 1977; 57: 341–343.

65   Miller RAW, Aldrich JE. Radioactive gold ring dermatitis. J Am Acad Dermatol 1990; 23: 360–362.

66   Lazar P, Cullen SI. Basal cell epithelioma and chronic radiodermatitis. Arch Dermatol 1963; 88: 172–175.

67   Totten RS, Antypas PG, Dupertuis SM et al. Pre-existing roentgen-ray dermatitis in patients with skin cancer. Cancer 1957; 10: 1024–1030.

68   Sarkany I, Fountain RB, Evans CD et al. Multiple basal-cell epithelioma following radiotherapy of the spine. Br J Dermatol 1968; 80: 90–96.

69   Rowell NR. A follow-up study of superficial radiotherapy for benign dermatoses: recommendations for the use of X-rays in dermatology. Br J Dermatol 1973; 88: 583–590.

70   Brodkin RH, Bleiberg J. Neoplasia resulting from Grenz radiation. Arch Dermatol 1968; 97: 307–309.

71   Lindelof B, Eklund G. Incidence of malignant skin tumors in 14140 patients after grenz-ray treatment for benign skin disorders. Arch Dermatol 1986; 122: 1391–1395.

72   Riekki R, Jukkola A, Sassi M-L et al. Modulation of skin collagen metabolism by irradiation: collagen synthesis is increased in irradiated human skin. Br J Dermatol 2000; 142: 874–880.

73   Jacoby RA, Burgoon CF Jr. Atypical fibroblasts as a clue to radiation injury. Am J Dermatopathol 1985; 7: 53–56.

74   Moretto JC, Soslow RA, Smoller BR. Atypical cells in radiation dermatitis express factor XIIIa. Am J Dermatopathol 1998; 20: 370–372.

75   Meehan SA, LeBoit PE. An immunohistochemical analysis of radiation fibroblasts. J Cutan Pathol 1997; 24: 309–313.

Reactions to heat and cold

76   Page EH, Shear NH. Temperature-dependent skin disorders. J Am Acad Dermatol 1988; 18: 1003–1019.

77   Dembling RH. Burns. N Engl J Med 1985; 313: 1389–1398.

78   Schneider MS, Mani MM, Masters FW. Gasoline-induced contact burns. J Burn Care Rehabil 1991; 12: 140–143.

79   Wilson DI, Bailie FB. Petrol – something nasty in the woodshed? A review of gasoline-related burns in a British burns unit. Burns 1995; 21: 539–541.

80   Hunter GA. Chemical burns of the skin after contact with petrol. Br J Past Surg 1968; 21: 337–341.

81   Raimer BG, Raimer SS, Hebeler JR. Cutaneous signs of child abuse. J Am Acad Dermatol 1981; 5: 203–212.

82   Sutton RL Jr, Waisman M. Dermatoses due to physical agents. Cutis 1977; 19: 513–529.

83   Hendricks WM. The classification of burns. J Am Acad Dermatol 1990; 22: 838–839.

84   Compton CC. The delayed postburn blister. Arch Dermatol 1992; 128: 249–252.

85   Huang TT, Larson DL, Lewis SR. Burn alopecia. Plast Reconstr Surg 1977; 60: 763–767.

86   Novick M, Gard DA, Hardy SB, Spira M. Burn scar carcinoma: a review and analysis of 46 cases. Trauma 1977; 17: 809–817.

87   Abbas JS, Beecham JE. Burn wound carcinoma: case report and review of the literature. Burns 1988; 14: 222–224.

88   Lund HZ. How often does squamous cell carcinoma of the skin metastasize? Arch Dermatol 1965; 92: 635–637.

89   Goldberg NS, Robinson JK, Peterson C. Gigantic malignant melanoma in a thermal burn scar. J Am Acad Dermatol 1985; 12: 949–952.

90   Muhlemann MF, Griffiths RW, Briggs JC. Malignant melanoma and squamous cell carcinoma in a burn scar. Br J Plast Surg 1982; 35: 474–477.

91   Alconchel MD, Olivares C, Alvarez R. Squamous cell carcinoma, malignant melanoma and malignant fibrous histiocytoma arising in burn scars. Br J Dermatol 1997; 137: 793–798.

92   Yücel A, Yazar Ş, Demirkesen C et al. An unusual long-term complication of burn injury: malignant fibrous histiocytoma developed in chronic burn scar. Burns 2000; 26: 305–310.

93   Foley FD. Pathology of cutaneous burns. Surg Clin North Am 1970; 50: 1201–1210.

94   Warren S. Radiation effect on the skin. In: Helwig EB, Mostofi FK, eds. The skin. Huntington, New York: Robert E Krieger, 1980; 261–278.

95   Xuewei W, Wanrhong Z. Vascular injuries in electrical burns – the pathologic basis for mechanism of injury. Burns 1983; 9: 335–339.

96   Ackerman AB, Goldfaden GL. Electrical burns of the mouth in children. Arch Dermatol 1971; 104: 308–311.

97   Resnik BI, Wetli CV. Lichtenberg figures. Am J Forensic Med Pathol 1996; 17: 99–102.

98   Domart Y, Garet E. Lichtenberg figures due to a lightning strike. N Engl J Med 2000; 343: 1536.

99   Cotton J, Hood AF, Gonin R et al. Histologic evaluation of preauricular and postauricular human skin after high-energy, short-pulse carbon dioxide laser. Arch Dermatol 1996; 132: 425–428.

100   Smith KJ, Skelton HG, Graham JS et al. Depth of morphologic skin damage and viability after one, two, and three passes of a high-energy, short-pulse CO2 laser (Tru-Pulse) in pig skin. J Am Acad Dermatol 1997; 37: 204–210.

101   Kee CE. Liquid nitrogen cryotherapy. Arch Dermatol 1967; 96: 198–203.

102   Weedon D. Unpublished observations.

103   Kuflik EG, Lubritz RR, Torre D. Cryosurgery. Dermatol Clin 1984; 2: 319–332.

104   Urano Y, Shikiji T, Sasaki S et al. An unusual reaction to cold: a sporadic case of familial polymorphous cold eruption? Br J Dermatol 1998; 139: 504–507.

Reactions to light (photodermatoses)

105   Ledo E. Photodermatosis. Part I: photobiology, photoimmunology, and idiopathic photodermatoses. Int J Dermatol 1993; 32: 387–396.

106   Ledo E. Photodermatoses. Part II: chemical photodermatoses and dermatoses that can be exacerbated, precipitated, or provoked by light. Int J Dermatol 1993; 32: 480–492.

107   White HAD. The diagnosis of the photodermatoses: a review. Australas J Dermatol 1979; 20: 123–126.

108   Anstey AV, Taylor CR. Photosensitivity in the Smith–Lemli–Opitz syndrome: The US experience of a new congenital photosensitivity syndrome. J Am Acad Dermatol 1999; 41: 121–123.

109   Anstey AV, Ryan A, Rhodes LE et al. Characterization of photosensitivity in the Smith–Lemli–Opitz syndrome: a new congenital photosensitivity syndrome. Br J Dermatol 1999; 141: 406–414.

110   Charman CR, Ryan A, Tyrrell RM et al. Photosensitivity associated with the Smith–Lemli–Opitz syndrome. Br J Dermatol 1998; 138: 885–888.

111   Roelandts R. The diagnosis of photosensitivity. Arch Dermatol 2000; 136: 1152–1157.

112   González E, González S. Drug photosensitivity, idiopathic photodermatoses, and sunscreens. J Am Acad Dermatol 1996; 35: 871–885.

113   Azurdia RM, Anstey AV, Rhodes LE. Cholesterol supplementation objectively reduces photosensitivity in the Smith–Lemli–Opitz syndrome. Br J Dermatol 2001; 144: 143–145.

114   Chuang T-Y, Heinrich LA, Schultz MD et al. PUVA and skin cancer. A historical cohort study on 492 patients. J Am Acad Dermatol 1992; 26: 173–177.

115   Lever LR, Farr PM. Skin cancers or premalignant lesions occur in half of high-dose PUVA patients. Br J Dermatol 1994; 131: 215–219.

116   Lindelöf B, Sigurgeirsson B, Tegner E et al. PUVA and cancer risk: the Swedish follow-up study. Br J Dermatol 1999; 141: 108–112.

117   Morison WL, Baughman RD, Day RM et al. Consensus workshop on the toxic effects of long-term PUVA therapy. Arch Dermatol 1998; 134: 595–598.

118   Hobbs J, Lebwohl M, Lim HW. Improving the safety profile of long-term PUVA therapy. J Am Acad Dermatol 1999; 41: 496–497.

119   Hannuksela-Svahn A, Sigurgeirsson B, Pukkala E et al. Trioxsalen bath PUVA did not increase the risk of squamous cell skin carcinoma and cutaneous malignant melanoma in a joint analysis of 944 Swedish and Finnish patients with psoriasis. Br J Dermatol 1999; 141: 497–501.

120   Weinstock MA, Coulter S, Bates J et al. Human papillomavirus and widespread cutaneous carcinoma after PUVA photochemotherapy. Arch Dermatol 1995; 131: 701–704.

121   Fotiades J, Soter NA, Lim HW. Results of evaluation of 203 patients for photosensitivity in a 7.3-year period. J Am Acad Dermatol 1995; 33: 597–602.

122   Emmett EA. Drug photoallergy. Int J Dermatol 1978; 17: 370–379.

123   Epstein JH. Photoallergy. A review. Arch Dermatol 1972; 106: 741–748.

124   Seligman PJ, Mathias CGT, O'Malley MA et al. Phytophotodermatitis from celery among grocery store workers. Arch Dermatol 1987; 123: 1478–1482.

125   Stoner JG, Rasmussen JE. Plant dermatitis. J Am Acad Dermatol 1983; 9: 1–15.

126   Reynolds NJ, Burton JL, Bradfield JWB, Matthews CNA. Weed wacker dermatitis. Arch Dermatol 1991; 127: 1419–1420.

127   Ljunggren B. Severe phototoxic burn following celery ingestion. Arch Dermatol 1990; 126: 1334–1336.

128   Finkelstein E, Afek U, Gross E et al. An outbreak of phytophotodermatitis due to celery. Int J Dermatol 1994; 33: 116–118.

129   Pathak MA. Phytophotodermatitis. Clin Dermatol 1986; 4: 102–121.

130   Wintroub BU, Stern R. Cutaneous drug reactions: pathogenesis and clinical classification. J Am Acad Dermatol 1985; 13: 167–179.

131   Wennersten G, Thune P, Jansen CT, Brodthagen H. Photocontact dermatitis: current status with emphasis on allergic contact photosensitivity (CPS) occurrence, allergens, and practical phototesting. Semin Dermatol 1986; 5: 277–289.

132 Toback AC, Anders JE. Phototoxicity from systemic agents. Dermatol Clin 1986; 4: 223–230.

133 Willis I. Photosensitivity. Int J Dermatol 1975; 14: 326–337.

134 Rotstein H. Photosensitive bullous eruption associated with chronic renal failure. Australas J Dermatol 1987; 19: 58–64.

135 Rivers JK, Barnetson R St C. Naproxen-induced bullous photodermatitis. Med J Aust 1989; 151: 167–168.

136 Ramsay CA, Obreshkova E. Photosensitivity from nalidixic acid. Br J Dermatol 1974; 91: 523–528.

137 Breza TS, Halprin KM, Taylor JR. Photosensitivity reaction to vinblastine. Arch Dermatol 1975; 111: 1168–1170.

138 Bellaney GJ, Proby CM, Hawk JLM. Likely photosensitizing agents available in the United Kingdom – an update. Clin Exp Dermatol 1996; 21: 14–16.

139 Murphy GM, Wright J, Nicholls DSH et al. Sunbed-induced pseudoporphyria. Br J Dermatol 1989; 120: 555–562.

140 Eberlein-König B, Bindl A, Przybilla B. Phototoxic properties of neuroleptic drugs. Dermatology 1997; 194: 131–135.

141 Addo HA, Ferguson J, Frain-Bell W. Thiazide-induced photosensitivity: a study of 33 subjects. Br J Dermatol 1987; 116: 749–760.

142 Diffey BL, Langtry J. Phototoxic potential of thiazide diuretics in normal subjects. Arch Dermatol 1989; 125: 1355–1358.

143 Layton AM, Cunliffe WJ. Phototoxic eruptions due to doxycycline – a dose-related phenomenon. Clin Exp Dermatol 1993; 18: 425–427.

144 Kimura M, Kawada A, Kobayashi T et al. Photosensitivity induced by fleroxacin. Clin Exp Dermatol 1996; 21: 46–47.

145 Scheife RT, Cramer WR, Decker EL. Photosensitizing potential of ofloxacin. Int J Dermatol 1993; 32: 413–416.

146 Schwedler S, Mempel M, Schmidt T et al. Phototoxicity to tetrazepam – a new adverse reaction. Dermatology 1998; 197: 193–194.

147 Gould JW, Mercurio MG, Elmets CA. Cutaneous photosensitivity diseases induced by exogenous agents. J Am Acad Dermatol 1995; 33: 551–573.

148 Ferguson J, Addo HA, Jones S et al. A study of cutaneous photosensitivity induced by amiodarone. Br J Dermatol 1985; 113: 537–549.

149 Harber LC, Bickers DR, Armstrong RB, Kochevar IE. Drug photosensitivity: phototoxic and photoallergic mechanisms. Semin Dermatol 1982; 1: 183–195.

150 Hjorth N, Möller H. Phototoxic textile dermatitis ('bikini dermatitis'). Arch Dermatol 1976; 112: 1445–1447.

151 Hawk JLM. Photosensitizing agents used in the United Kingdom. Clin Exp Dermatol 1984; 9: 300–302.

152 Kochevar IE. Phototoxicity mechanisms: chlorpromazine photosensitized damage to DNA and cell membranes. J Invest Dermatol 1981; 76: 59–64.

153 Schwarz A, Bhardwaj R, Aragane Y et al. Ultraviolet-B-induced apoptosis of keratinocytes: evidence for partial involvement of tumor necrosis factor-α in the formation of sunburn cells. J Invest Dermatol 1995; 104: 922–927.

154 Lenane P, Murphy GM, Kay E et al. Hypothesis: does sunlight cause cell suicide? Curr Diagn Pathol 1998; 5: 204–207.

155 Shimizu H, Banno Y, Sumi N et al. Activation of p38 mitogen-activated protein kinase and caspases in UVB-induced apoptosis of human keratinocyte HaCaT cells. J Invest Dermatol 1999; 112: 769–774.

156 Gniadecki R, Hansen M, Wulf HC. Two pathways for induction of apoptosis by ultraviolet radiation in cultured human keratinocytes. J Invest Dermatol 1997; 109: 163–169.

157 Epstein S. Chlorpromazine photosensitivity. Phototoxic and photoallergic reactions. Arch Dermatol 1968; 98: 354–363.

158 Epstein JH. Phototoxicity and photoallergy in man. J Am Acad Dermatol 1983; 8: 141–147.

158a Hettiaratchy S, Clarke J, Taubel J, Besa C. Burns after photodynamic therapy. BMJ 2000; 320: 1245.

159 Elmets CA. Drug-induced photoallergy. Dermatol Clin 1986; 4: 231–241.

160 Horio T. Photoallergic reactions. Classification and pathogenesis. Int J Dermatol 1984; 23: 376–382.

161 Larsen WG, Maibach HI. Fragrance contact allergy. Semin Dermatol 1982; 1: 85–90.

162 Kaidbey KH, Kligman AM. Photosensitization by coumarin derivatives. Structure-activity relationships. Arch Dermatol 1981; 117: 258–263.

163 Knobler E, Almeida L, Ruzkowski AM et al. Photoallergy to benzophenone. Arch Dermatol 1989; 125: 801–804.

164 Collins P, Ferguson J. Photoallergic contact dermatitis to oxybenzone. Br J Dermatol 1994; 131: 124–129.

165 DeLeo VA, Suarez SM, Maso MJ. Photoallergic contact dermatitis. Arch Dermatol 1992; 128: 1513–1518.

166 Fernández De Corrès L, Diez JM, Audicana M et al. Photodermatitis from plant derivatives in topical and oral medicaments. Contact Dermatitis 1996; 35: 184–185.

167 Kaidbey KH, Allen H. Photocontact allergy to benzocaine. Arch Dermatol 1981; 117: 77–79.

168 Serrano G, Bonillo J, Aliaga A et al. Piroxicam-induced photosensitivity and contact sensitivity to thiosalicylic acid. J Am Acad Dermatol 1990; 23: 479–483.

169 Jarratt M. Drug photosensitization. Int J Dermatol 1976; 15: 317–325.

170 Ljunggren B, Sjovall P. Systemic quinine photosensitivity. Arch Dermatol 1986; 122: 909–911.

171 Diffey BL, Farr PM, Adams SJ. The action spectrum in quinine photosensitivity. Br J Dermatol 1988; 118: 679–685.

172 Armstrong RB, Leach EE, Whitman G et al. Quinidine photosensitivity. Arch Dermatol 1985; 121: 525–528.

173 Pariser DM, Taylor JR. Quinidine photosensitivity. Arch Dermatol 1975; 111: 1440–1443.

174 Hawk JLM. Photosensitivity induced by oral itraconazole. J Eur Acad Dermatol Venereol 2000; 14: 445.

175 Alvarez-Fernández JG, Castaño-Suárez E, Cornejo-Navarro P et al. Photosensitivity induced by oral itraconazole. J Eur Acad Dermatol Venereol 2000; 14: 501–503.

176 Todd P, Norris P, Hawk JLM, du Vivier AWP. Ranitidine-induced photosensitivity. Clin Exp Dermatol 1995; 20: 146–148.

177 Kondo S, Kagaya M, Yamada Y et al. UVB photosensitivity due to ranitidine. Dermatology 2000; 201: 71–73.

178 Poh-Fitzpatrick MB. Lomefloxacin photosensitivity. Arch Dermatol 1994; 130: 261.

179 Horio T. Chlorpromazine allergy. Coexistence of immediate and delayed type. Arch Dermatol 1975; 111: 1469–1471.

180 Serrano G, Bonillo J, Aliaga A et al. Piroxicam-induced photosensitivity. In vivo and in vitro studies of its photosensitizing potential. J Am Acad Dermatol 1984; 11: 113–120.

181 Kaidbey KH, Mitchell FN. Photosensitizing potential of certain nonsteroidal anti-inflammatory agents. Arch Dermatol 1989; 125: 783–786.

182 Serrano G, Fortea JM, Latasa JM et al. Oxicam-induced photosensitivity. J Am Acad Dermatol 1992; 26: 545–548.

183 Chishiki M, Kawada A, Fujioka A et al. Photosensitivity due to ampiroxicam. Dermatology 1997; 195: 409–410.

184 Ancnide A, Usiglio D, Pestarina A, Massone L. Droxicam photosensitivity with dyshidrotic hand dermatitis. Int J Dermatol 1997; 36: 318–320.

185 Goday Buján JJ, Oleaga Morante JM, González Güemes M et al. Photoallergic contact dermatitis from piketoprofen. Contact Dermatitis 2000; 43: 315.

186 Sugiura M, Hayakawa R, Kato Y et al. 4 cases of photocontact dermatitis due to ketoprofen. Contact Dermatitis 2000; 43: 16–19.

187 Albès B, Marguery MC, Schwarze HP et al. Prolonged photosensitivity following contact photoallergy to ketoprofen. Dermatology 2000; 201: 171–174.

188 Murata Y, Kumano K, Ueda T et al. Photosensitive dermatitis caused by pyridoxine hydrochloride. J Am Acad Dermatol 1998; 39: 314–317.

189 Morimoto K, Kawada A, Hiruma M, Ishibashi A. Photosensitivity from pyridoxine hydrochloride (vitamin B6). J Am Acad Dermatol 1996; 35: 304–305.

190 Revenga F, Paricio JF. Cutaneous side-effects caused by Tegafur. Int J Dermatol 1999; 38: 955–957.

191 Fujimoto M, Kikuchi K, Imakado S, Furue M. Photosensitive dermatitis induced by flutamide. Br J Dermatol 1996; 135: 496–497.

192 Watanabe Y, Kawada A, Ohnishi Y et al. Photosensitivity due to alprazolam with positive oral photochallenge test after 17 days administration. J Am Acad Dermatol 1999; 40: 832–833.

193 Nagore E, Pérez-Ferriols A, Sánchez-Motilla JM et al. Photosensitivity associated with treatment with triflusal. J Eur Acad Dermatol Venereol 2000; 14: 219–221.

194 Grabczynska SA, Cowley N. Amlodipine induced-photosensitivity presenting as telangiectasia. Br J Dermatol 2000; 142: 1255–1256.

195 Bouyssou-Gauthier M-L, Bédane C, Boulinguez S, Bonnetblanc J-M. Photosensitivity with sulfasalazopyridine hypersensitivity syndrome. Dermatology 1999; 198: 388–390.

196 Horio T. Allergic and photoallergic dermatitis from diphenhydramine. Arch Dermatol 1975; 112: 1124–1126.

197 Bergner T, Przybilla B. Photosensitization caused by ibuprofen. J Am Acad Dermatol 1992; 26: 114–116.

198 Serrano G, Fortea JM, Latasa JM et al. Photosensitivity induced by fibric acid derivatives and its relation to photocontact dermatitis to ketoprofen. J Am Acad Dermatol 1992; 27: 204–208.

199 Leenutaphong V, Manuskiatti W. Fenofibrate-induced photosensitivity. J Am Acad Dermatol 1996; 35: 775–777.

200 Machet L, Vaillant L, Jan V, Lorette G. Fenofibrate-induced photosensitivity: Value of photopatch testing. J Am Acad Dermatol 1997; 37: 808–809.

201 Hanada K, Hashimoto I. Flagellate mushroom (shiitake) dermatitis and photosensitivity. Dermatology 1998; 197: 255–257.

202 Neumann NJ, Hölzle E, Plewig G et al. Photopatch testing: The 12-year experience of the German, Austrian, and Swiss Photopatch Test Group. J Am Acad Dermatol 2000; 42: 183–192.

203 Sonnex TS, Hawk JLM. Hydroa vacciniforme: a review of ten cases. Br J Dermatol 1988; 118: 101–108.

204 Hwang LY, Hwong HK, Hsu S. Extensive hemorrhagic vesicles in a child. Pediatr Dermatol 2001; 18: 71–73.

205 Kim WS, Yeo UC, Chun HS, Lee ES. A case of hydroa vacciniforme with unusual ear mutilation. Clin Exp Dermatol 1998; 23: 70–72.

206 Blackwell VC, McGregor JM, Hawk JLM. Hydroa vacciniforme presenting in an adult successfully treated with cyclosporin A. Clin Exp Dermatol 1998; 23: 73–76.

207 Leenutaphong V. Hydroa vacciniforme: an unusual clinical manifestation. J Am Acad Dermatol 1991; 25: 892–895.

208 McGrae JD Jr, Perry HO. Hydroa vacciniforme. Arch Dermatol 1963; 87: 618–625.

209 Wong S-N, Tan SH, Khoo SW. Late-onset hydroa vacciniforme: two case reports. Br J Dermatol 2001; 144: 874–877.

210 Annamalai R. Hydroa vacciniforme in three alternate siblings. Arch Dermatol 1971; 103: 224–225.

211 Gupta G, Mohamed M, Kemmett D. Familial hydroa vacciniforme. Br J Dermatol 1999; 140: 124–126.

212 Oono T, Arata J, Masuda T, Ohtsuki Y. Coexistence of hydroa vacciniforme and malignant lymphoma. Arch Dermatol 1986; 122: 1306–1309.

213 Eramo LR, Garden JM, Esterly NB. Hydroa vacciniforme. Diagnosis by repetitive ultraviolet-A phototesting. Arch Dermatol 1986; 122: 1310–1313.

214 Halasz CLG, Leach EE, Walther RR, Poh-Fitzpatrick MB. Hydroa vacciniforme. Induction of lesions with ultraviolet A. J Am Acad Dermatol 1983; 8: 171–176.

215 Goldgeier MH, Nordlund JJ, Lucky AW et al. Hydroa vacciniforme. Diagnosis and therapy. Arch Dermatol 1982; 118: 588–591.

216 Hann SK, Im S, Park Y-K, Lee S. Hydroa vacciniforme with unusually severe scar formation: diagnosis by repetitive UVA phototesting. J Am Acad Dermatol 1991; 25: 401–403.

217 Gupta G, Man I, Kemmett D. Hydroa vacciniforme: A clinical and follow-up study of 17 cases. J Am Acad Dermatol 2000; 42: 208–213.

218 Rhodes LE, White SI. Dietary fish oil as a photoprotective agent in hydroa vacciniforme. Br J Dermatol 1998; 138: 173–178.

219 Iwatsuki K, Xu Z, Takata M et al. The association of latent Epstein–Barr virus infection with hydroa vacciniforme. Br J Dermatol 1999; 140: 715–721.

220 Iwatsuki K, Ohtsuka M, Akiba H, Kaneko F. Atypical hydroa vacciniforme in childhood: From a smoldering stage to Epstein–Barr virus-associated lymphoid malignancy. J Am Acad Dermatol 1999; 40: 283.

221 Cho K-H, Kim C-W, Heo D-S et al. Necrotizing papulovesicles in patients with hematologic malignant neoplasms. J Cutan Pathol 2000; 27: 553 (abstract).

222 Sullivan M. Hydroa aestivale. Arch Dermatol 1961; 83: 672.

223 Wheeler CE, Cawley EP, Whitmore CW. Hydroa aestivale in identical twins. Arch Dermatol 1960; 82: 590–594.

224 Bickers DR, Demar LK, DeLeo V et al. Hydroa vacciniforme. Arch Dermatol 1978; 114: 1193–1196.

225 Redeker AG, Bronow RS. Erythropoietic protoporphyria presenting as hydroa aestivale. Arch Dermatol 1964; 89: 104–109.

226 Epstein JH. Polymorphous light eruption. J Am Acad Dermatol 1980; 3: 329–343.

227 Norris PG, Hawk JLM. The acute idiopathic photodermatoses. Semin Dermatol 1990; 9: 32–38.

228 Epstein JH. Polymorphous light eruption. Dermatol Clin 1986; 4: 243–251.

229 Van Praag MCG, Boom BW, Vermeer BJ. Diagnosis and treatment of polymorphous light eruption. Int J Dermatol 1994; 33: 233–239.

230 Jansen CT. Heredity of chronic polymorphous light eruptions. Arch Dermatol 1978; 114: 188–190.

231 Millard TP, Bataille V, Snieder H et al. The heritability of polymorphic light eruption. J Invest Dermatol 2000; 115: 467–470.

232 McGregor JM, Grabczynska S, Vaughan R et al. Genetic modeling of abnormal photosensitivity in families with polymorphic light eruption and actinic prurigo. J Invest Dermatol 2000; 115: 471–476.

233 Morison WL, Stern RS. Polymorphous light eruption: a common reaction uncommonly recognized. Acta Derm Venereol 1982; 62: 237–240.

234 Pao C, Norris PG, Corbett M, Hawk JLM. Polymorphic light eruption: prevalence in Australia and England. Br J Dermatol 1994; 130: 62–64.

235 Holzle E, Plewig G, von Krias R, Lehmann P. Polymorphous light eruption. J Invest Dermatol 1987; 88: 32s–38s.

236 Jeanmougin M, Civatte J. Benign summer light eruption: a new entity? Arch Dermatol 1986; 122: 376.

237 Elpern DJ, Morison WL, Hood AF. Papulovesicular light eruption. A defined subset of polymorphous light eruption. Arch Dermatol 1985; 121: 1286–1288.

238 Stevanovic DV. Polymorphic light eruption. Br J Dermatol 1960; 72: 261–270.

239 Jansen CT. The morphologic features of polymorphous light eruptions. Cutis 1980; 26: 164–170.

240 Draelos ZK, Hansen RC. Polymorphic light eruption in pediatric patients with American Indian ancestry. Pediatr Dermatol 1986; 3: 384–389.

241 Dover JS, Hawk JLM. Polymorphic light eruption sine eruption. Br J Dermatol 1988; 118: 73–76.

242 Gudmundsen KJ, Murphy GM, O'Sullivan D et al. Polymorphic light eruption with contact and photocontact allergy. Br J Dermatol 1991; 124: 379–382.

243 Holzle E, Plewig G, Hofmann C, Roser-Maass E. Polymorphous light eruption. Experimental reproduction of skin lesions. J Am Acad Dermatol 1982; 7: 111–125.

244 Berth-Jones J, Norris PG, Graham-Brown RAC et al. Juvenile spring eruption of the ears: a probable variant of polymorphic light eruption. Br J Dermatol 1991; 124: 375–378.

245 Jansen CT. The natural history of polymorphous light eruptions. Arch Dermatol 1979; 115: 165–169.

246 Guarrera M, Micalizzi C, Rebora A. Heterogeneity of polymorphous light eruption: a study of 105 patients. Arch Dermatol 1993; 129: 1060–1061.

247 Creamer D, McGregor JM, Hawk JLM. Polymorphic light eruption occurring in common variable hypogammaglobulinaemia, and resolving with intravenous immunoglobulin therapy. Clin Exp Dermatol 1999; 24: 273–274.

248 Hasan T, Ranki A, Jansen CT, Karvonen J. Disease associations in polymorphous light eruption. A long-term follow-up study of 94 patients. Arch Dermatol 1998; 134: 1081–1085.

249 Nyberg F, Hasan T, Puska P et al. Occurrence of polymorphous light eruption in lupus erythematosus. Br J Dermatol 1997; 136: 217–221.

250 Millard TP, Lewis CM, Khamashta MA et al. Familial clustering of polymorphic light eruption in relatives of patients with lupus erythematosus: evidence of a shared pathogenesis. Br J Dermatol 2001; 144: 334–338.

251 Downs AMR, Lear JT, Dunnill MGS. Polymorphic light eruption limited to areas of vitiligo. Clin Exp Dermatol 1999; 24: 379–381.

252 Creamer D, Clement M, McGregor JM, Hawk JLM. Polymorphic light eruption occurring solely on an area of naevoid telangiectasia. Clin Exp Dermatol 1999; 24: 202–203.

253 Frain-Bell W, Mackenzie LA, Witham E. Chronic polymorphic light eruption (a study of 25 cases). Br J Dermatol 1969; 81: 885–896.

254 Jansen CT, Karvonen J. Polymorphous light eruption. A seven-year follow-up evaluation of 114 patients. Arch Dermatol 1984; 120: 862–865.

255 Petzelbauer P, Binder M, Nikolakis P et al. Severe sun sensitivity and the presence of antinuclear antibodies in patients with polymorphous light eruption-like lesions. J Am Acad Dermatol 1992; 26: 68–74.

256 Watanabe M, Yamanouchi H, Ogawa F, Katayama I. Polymorphous light eruption. A case report and consideration of the hardening mechanism. Dermatology 1999; 199: 158–161.

257 Horkay I, Krajczar J, Bodolay E et al. A study on cell-mediated immunity in polymorphic light eruption. Dermatologica 1983; 166: 75–80.

258 Verheyen AMF, Lambert JRMG, van Marck EAE, Dockx PFE. Polymorphic light eruption – an immunopathological study of provoked lesions. Clin Exp Dermatol 1995; 20: 297–303.

259 González-Amaro R, Baranda L, Salazar-Gonzalez JF et al. Immune sensitization against epidermal antigens in polymorphous light eruption. J Am Acad Dermatol 1991; 24: 70–73.

260 Kölgen W, Van Weelden H, Den Hengst S et al. CD11b+ cells and ultraviolet-B-resistant CD1a+ cells in skin of patients with polymorphous light eruption. J Invest Dermatol 1999; 113: 4–10.

261 Frain-Bell W, Dickson A, Herd J, Sturrock I. The action spectrum in polymorphic light eruption. Br J Dermatol 1973; 89: 243–249.

262 Ortel B, Tanew A, Wolff K, Honigmann H. Polymorphous light eruption: action spectrum and photoprotection. J Am Acad Dermatol 1986; 14: 748–753.

263 Ortel B, Wechdorn D, Tanew A, Honigmann H. Effect of nicotinamide on the phototest reaction in polymorphous light eruption. Br J Dermatol 1988; 118: 669–673.

264 Jansen C. The polymorphic phototest reaction. Arch Dermatol 1982; 118: 638–642.

265 Boonstra HE, van Weelden H, Toonstra J, van Vloten WA. Polymorphous light eruption: A clinical, photobiologic, and follow-up study of 110 patients. J Am Acad Dermatol 2000; 42: 199–207.

266 Moncada B, González-Amaro R, Baranda ML et al. Immunopathology of polymorphous light eruption. J Am Acad Dermatol 1984; 10: 970–973.

267 Muhlbauer JE, Bhan AK, Harrist TJ et al. Papular polymorphic light eruption: an immunoperoxidase study using monoclonal antibodies. Br J Dermatol 1983; 108: 153–162.

268 Norris PG, Morris J, McGibbon DM et al. Polymorphic light eruption: an immunopathological study of evolving lesions. Br J Dermatol 1989; 120: 173–183.

269 Norris P, Bacon K, Bird C et al. The role of interleukins 1, 6 and 8 as lymphocyte attractants in the photodermatoses polymorphic light eruption and chronic actinic dermatitis. Clin Exp Dermatol 1999; 24: 321–326.

270 Hood AF, Elpern DJ, Morison WL. Histopathologic findings in papulovesicular light eruption. J Cutan Pathol 1986; 13: 13–21.

271 Panet-Raymond G, Johnson WC. Lupus erythematosus and polymorphous light eruption. Differentiation by histochemical procedures. Arch Dermatol 1973; 108: 785–787.

272 Muhlbauer JE, Mihm MC Jr, Harrist TJ. Papular polymorphous light eruption. Arch Dermatol 1984; 120: 866–868.

273 Fisher DA, Epstein JH, Kay DN, Tuffanelli DL. Polymorphous light eruption and lupus erythematosus. Differential diagnosis by fluorescent microscopy. Arch Dermatol 1970; 101: 458–461.

274 Meara RH, Magnus IA, Grice K et al. Hutchinson's summer prurigo. Trans St John's Hosp Dermatol Soc 1971; 57: 87–97.

275 Birt AR, Davis RA. Hereditary polymorphic light eruption of American Indians. Int J Dermatol 1975; 14: 105–111.

276 Fusaro RM, Johnson JA. Topical photoprotection for hereditary polymorphic light eruption of American Indians. J Am Acad Dermatol 1991; 24: 744–746.

277 Scheen SR III, Connolly SM, Dicken CH. Actinic prurigo. J Am Acad Dermatol 1980; 5: 183–190.

278 Calnan CD, Meara RH. Actinic prurigo (Hutchinson's summer prurigo). Clin Exp Dermatol 1977; 2: 365–372.

279 Farr PM, Diffey BL. Treatment of actinic prurigo with PUVA: mechanism of action. Br J Dermatol 1989; 120: 411–418.

280 Durán MM, Ordoñez CP, Prieto JC, Bernal J. Treatment of actinic prurigo in Chimila Indians. Int J Dermatol 1996; 35: 413–416.

281 Fusaro RM, Johnson JA. Hereditary polymorphic light eruption of American Indians: occurrence in non-Indians with polymorphic light eruption. J Am Acad Dermatol 1996; 34: 612–617.

282 Batard M-L, Bonnevalle A, Ségard M et al. Caucasian actinic prurigo: 8 cases observed in France. Br J Dermatol 2001; 144: 194–196.

283 Lane PR, Sheridan DP, Hogan DJ, Moreland A. HLA typing in polymorphous light eruption. J Am Acad Dermatol 1991; 24: 570–573.

284 Wiseman MC, Orr PH, Macdonald SM et al. Actinic prurigo: Clinical features and HLA associations in a Canadian Innuit population. J Am Acad Dermatol 2001; 44: 952–956.

285 Grabczynska SA, McGregor JM, Kondeatis E et al. Actinic prurigo and polymorphic light eruption: common pathogenesis and the importance of HLA-DR4/DRB1*0407. Br J Dermatol 1999; 140: 232–236.

286 Hojyo-Tomoka T, Granados J, Vargas-Alarcón G et al. Further evidence of the role of HLA-DR4 in the genetic susceptibility to actinic prurigo. J Am Acad Dermatol 1997; 36: 935–937.

287 Dawe RS, Ferguson J. A family with actinic prurigo and polymorphic light eruption. Br J Dermatol 1997; 137: 827–829.

288 Bernal JE, Duran de Rueda MM, Ordonez CP et al. Actinic prurigo among the Chimila Indians in Colombia: HLA studies. J Am Acad Dermatol 1990; 22: 1049–1051.

289 Schnell AH, Elston RC, Hull PR, Lane PR. Major gene segregation of actinic prurigo among North American Indians in Saskatchewan. Am J Med Genet 2000; 92: 212–219.

290 Birt AR, Hogg GR. The actinic cheilitis of hereditary polymorphic light eruption. Arch Dermatol 1979; 115: 699–702.

291 Magaña M, Mendez Y, Rodriguez A, Mascott M. The conjunctivitis of solar (actinic) prurigo. Pediatr Dermatol 2000; 17: 432–435.

292 Lane PR, Hogan DJ, Martel MJ et al. Actinic prurigo: clinical features and prognosis. J Am Acad Dermatol 1992; 26: 683–692.

293 Arrese JE, Dominguez-Soto L, Hojyo-Tomoka MT et al. Effectors of inflammation in actinic prurigo. J Am Acad Dermatol 2001; 44: 957–961.

294 Hojyo-Tomoka MT, Dominguez-Soto L, Vargas-Ocampo F. Actinic prurigo: clinical-pathological correlation. Int J Dermatol 1978; 17: 706–710.

295 Lane PR, Murphy F, Hogan DJ et al. Histopathology of actinic prurigo. Am J Dermatopathol 1993; 15: 326–331.

296 Herrera-Geopfert R, Magaña M. Follicular cheilitis. A distinctive histopathologic finding in actinic prurigo. Am J Dermatopathol 1995; 17: 357–361.

297 Hojyo-Tomoka T, Vega-Memije E, Granados J et al. Actinic prurigo: an update. Int J Dermatol 1995; 34: 380–384.

298 Morison WL. Chronic photosensitivity. Dermatol Clin 1986; 4: 261–266.

299 Norris PG, Hawk JLM. Chronic actinic dermatitis. A unifying concept. Arch Dermatol 1990; 126: 376–378.

300 Lim HW, Baer RL, Gange RW. Photodermatoses. J Am Acad Dermatol 1987; 17: 293–299.

301 Lim HW, Buchness MR, Ashinoff R, Soter NA. Chronic actinic dermatitis. Study of the spectrum of chronic photosensitivity in 12 patients. Arch Dermatol 1990; 126: 317–323.

302 Menagé H du P, Ross JS, Norris PG et al. Contact and photocontact sensitization in chronic actinic dermatitis: sesquiterpene lactone mix is an important allergen. Br J Dermatol 1995; 132: 543–547.

303 Kingston TP, Lowe NJ, Sofen HL, Weingarten DP. Actinic reticuloid in a black man: successful therapy with azathioprine. J Am Acad Dermatol 1987; 16: 1079–1083.

304 Brody R, Bergfeld WF. Actinic reticuloid. Int J Dermatol 1981; 20: 374–379.

305 Lim HW, Cohen D, Soter NA. Chronic actinic dermatitis: Results of patch and photopatch tests with Compositae, fragrances, and pesticides. J Am Acad Dermatol 1998; 38: 108–111.

306 Menagé H du P, Hawk JLM. Chronic actinic dermatitis is not a viable concept. Arch Dermatol 1999; 135: 469–470.

307 Vandermaesen J, Roelandts R, Degreef H. Light on the persistent light reaction – photosensitivity dermatitis – actinic reticuloid syndrome. J Am Acad Dermatol 1986; 15: 685–692.

308 Hawk JLM, Magnus IA. Chronic actinic dermatitis – an idiopathic syndrome including actinic reticuloid and photosensitive eczema. Br J Dermatol (Suppl) 1979; 17: 24.

309 Roelandts R. Chronic actinic dermatitis. J Am Acad Dermatol 1993; 28: 240–249.

310 Lim HW, Morison WL, Kamide R et al. Chronic actinic dermatitis. Arch Dermatol 1994; 130: 1284–1289.

311 Ive FA, Magnus IA, Warin RP, Wilson Jones E. 'Actinic reticuloid'; a chronic dermatosis associated with severe photosensitivity and the histological resemblance to lymphoma. Br J Dermatol 1969; 81: 469–485.

312 Meola T, Sanchez M, Lim HW et al. Chronic actinic dermatitis associated with human immunodeficiency virus infection. Br J Dermatol 1997; 137: 431–436.

313 Smith KJ, Skelton HG, Yeager J et al. Histopathologic features seen in cutaneous photoeruptions in HIV-positive patients. Int J Dermatol 1997; 36: 745–753.

314 Kaidbey KH, Messenger JL. The clinical spectrum of the persistent light reactor. Arch Dermatol 1984; 120: 1441–1448.

315 Wojnarowska F, Calnan CD. Contact and photocontact allergy to musk ambrette. Br J Dermatol 1986; 114: 667–675.

316 Giovinazzo VJ, Harber LC, Armstrong RB, Kochevar IE. Photoallergic contact dermatitis to musk ambrette. Clinical report of two patients with persistent light reactor patterns. J Am Acad Dermatol 1980; 3: 384–393.

317 Robinson HN, Morison WL, Hood AF. Thiazide diuretic therapy and chronic photosensitivity. Arch Dermatol 1985; 121: 522–524.

318 Kalb RE. Persistent light reaction to hexachlorophene. J Am Acad Dermatol 1991; 24: 333–334.

319 Ramsay CA, Black AK. Photosensitive eczema. Trans St John's Hosp Dermatol Soc 1973; 52: 152–158.

320 Russell SC, Dawe RS, Collins P et al. The photosensitivity dermatitis and actinic reticuloid syndrome (chronic actinic dermatitis) occurring in seven young atopic dermatitis patients. Br J Dermatol 1998; 138: 496–501.

321 Ogboli MI, Rhodes LE. Chronic actinic dermatitis in young atopic dermatitis sufferers. Br J Dermatol 2000; 142: 845.

322 Frain-Bell W, Lakshmipathi T, Rogers J, Willock J. The syndrome of chronic photosensitivity dermatitis and actinic reticuloid. Br J Dermatol 1974; 91: 617–634.

323 Żak-Prelich M, Schwartz RA. Actinic reticuloid. Int J Dermatol 1999; 38: 335–342.

324 Toonstra J. Actinic reticuloid. Semin Diagn Pathol 1991; 8: 109–116.

325 Ferguson J. Photosensitivity dermatitis and actinic reticuloid syndrome (chronic actinic dermatitis). Semin Dermatol 1990; 9: 47–54.

326 Preesman AH, Schrooyen SJ, Toonstra J et al. The diagnostic value of morphometry on blood lymphocytes in erythrodermic actinic reticuloid. Arch Dermatol 1995; 131: 1298–1303.

327 Greaves K, Cripps AJ, Cripps DJ. Actinic reticuloid: action spectra and UVA protection factor sunscreens. Clin Exp Dermatol 1992; 17: 94–98.

328 Frain-Bell W, Hetherington A, Johnson BE. Contact allergic sensitivity to chrysanthemum and the photosensitivity dermatitis and actinic reticuloid syndrome. Br J Dermatol 1979; 101: 491–501.

329 Frain-Bell W, Johnson BE. Contact allergic sensitivity to plants and the photosensitivity dermatitis and actinic reticuloid syndrome. Br J Dermatol 1979; 101: 503–512.

330 Horio T. Actinic reticuloid via persistent light reaction from photoallergic contact dermatitis. Arch Dermatol 1982; 118: 339–342.

331 Frain-Bell W. Photosensitivity dermatitis and actinic reticuloid. Semin Dermatol 1982; 1: 161–168.

332 Dawe RS, Crombie IK, Ferguson J. The natural history of chronic actinic dermatitis. Arch Dermatol 2000; 136: 1215–1220.

333 Thomsen K. The development of Hodgkin's disease in a patient with actinic reticuloid. Clin Exp Dermatol 1977; 2: 109–113.

334 Bilsland D, Crombie IK, Ferguson J. The photosensitivity dermatitis and actinic reticuloid syndrome: no association with lymphoreticular malignancy. Br J Dermatol 1994; 131: 209–214.

335 Norris PG, Newton JA, Camplejohn RS, Hawk JLM. A flow cytometric study of actinic reticuloid. Clin Exp Dermatol 1989; 14: 128–131.

336 Bakels V, van Oostveen JW, Preesman AH et al. Differentiation between actinic reticuloid and cutaneous T cell lymphoma by T cell receptor γ gene rearrangement analysis and immunophenotyping. J Clin Pathol 1998; 51: 154–158.

337 Giannelli F, Botcherby PK, Marimo B, Magnus IA. Cellular hypersensitivity to UV-A: a clue to the aetiology of actinic reticuloid? Lancet 1983; 1: 88–91.

338 Applegate LA, Frenk E, Gibbs N et al. Cellular sensitivity to oxidative stress in the photosensitivity dermatitis/actinic reticuloid syndrome. J Invest Dermatol 1994; 102: 762–767.

339 Connors RC, Ackerman AB. Histologic pseudomalignancies of the skin. Arch Dermatol 1976; 112: 1767–1780.

340 Ralfkiaer E, Lange Wantzin G, Stein H, Mason DY. Photosensitive dermatitis with actinic reticuloid syndrome: an immunohistological study of the cutaneous infiltrate. Br J Dermatol 1986; 114: 47–56.

341 Norris PG, Morris J, Smith NP et al. Chronic actinic dermatitis: an immunohistologic and photobiologic study. J Am Acad Dermatol 1989; 21: 966–971.

342 Toonstra J, van der Putte SCJ, van Wichen DF et al. Actinic reticuloid: immunohistochemical analysis of the cutaneous infiltrate in 13 patients. Br J Dermatol 1989; 120: 779–786.

343 Toonstra J, Henquet CJM, van Weelden H et al. Actinic reticuloid. A clinical, photobiologic, histopathologic, and follow-up study of 16 patients. J Am Acad Dermatol 1989; 21: 205–214.

344 Heller P, Wieczorek R, Waldo E et al. Chronic actinic dermatitis. An immunohistochemical study of its T-cell antigenic profile, with comparison to cutaneous T-cell lymphoma. Am J Dermatopathol 1994; 16: 510–516.

345 Menter MA, McKerron RA, Amos HE. Actinic reticuloid: an immunological investigation providing evidence of basement membrane damage. Br J Dermatol 1974; 90: 507–515.

346 Guardiola A, Sanchez JL. Actinic reticuloid. Int J Dermatol 1980; 19: 154–158.

347 Schnitzler L, Verret JL, Schubert B, Picard MD. Langerhans cells in actinic reticuloid. J Cutan Pathol 1975; 2: 170–178.

348 Johnson SC, Cripps DJ, Norback DH. Actinic reticuloid. A clinical, pathologic, and action spectrum study. Arch Dermatol 1979; 115: 1078–1083.

Infections and infestations

Cutaneous infections and infestations – histological patterns

In this age of international travel it is necessary for dermatopathologists to be familiar with the appearances of all cutaneous infections, including those which are sometimes dismissed euphemistically as 'infections of other countries'. Unfortunately, there is a bewildering number of such infections, making it difficult to commit to memory the details of all of them. Further problems result from the variable morphological appearances which a particular infectious agent may produce. Factors that may influence the histopathological features of a cutaneous infection include the numbers and virulence of the organism, the host's immunological response, the stage of evolution of the disease, prior treatment, and the presence of secondary changes resulting from rubbing and scratching or superimposed further infection. Because certain infections may produce different histopathological changes under these various circumstances, it seems prudent to categorize the infections and infestations on an etiological rather than a morphological basis in the succeeding chapters. This traditional approach reduces unnecessary duplication.

Table 22.1 provides an outline of the morphological approach to infections of the skin and lists the various diseases that should be considered when a particular morphological feature is encountered in a biopsy. It does not include some of the very rare presentations of certain infections. These various infections and infestations are the subject of Chapters 23–30.

Table 22.1 **Histological patterns in infections and infestations**

Morphological feature	Diseases to be considered
Palisading granulomas	Phaeohyphomycosis (p. 673); mycobacteriosis (p. 625); treponematosis (p. 650); sporotrichosis (p. 673); cryptococcosis (p. 666); coccidioidomycosis (p. 670); cat-scratch disease (p. 636); lymphogranuloma venereum (p. 637); schistosomiasis (p. 732)
Tuberculoid granulomas	Tuberculosis (p. 625); tuberculids (p. 627); tuberculoid leprosy (p. 630); syphilis [late secondary or tertiary] (p. 650); dermatophytosis [Majocchi's granuloma] (p. 663); cryptococcosis (p. 666); alternariosis (p. 674); histoplasmosis (p. 670); keloidal blastomycosis (p. 679); prototphecosis (p. 679); leishmaniasis (p. 721); acanthamebiasis (p. 720); echinoderm injury (p. 729); *Vibrio* and *Rhodococcus* infection (p. 629)
Suppurative granulomas	Atypical mycobacterial infections (p. 627); lymphogranuloma venereum (p. 637); blastomycosis-like pyoderma* (p. 622); actinomycosis* (p. 677); nocardiosis* (p. 676); mycetoma* (p. 675); cryptococcosis (p. 666); aspergillosis (p. 678) and other deep fungal infections+ (p.671); prototphecosis (p. 679)
Histiocyte granulomas	Infections by atypical mycobacteria (p. 627); lepromatous leprosy (p. 630); leishmaniasis (p. 721); malakoplakia [Michaelis–Gutmann bodies in cytoplasm] (p. 637)
Histiocytes and plasma cells	Rhinoscleroma (p. 635); syphilis (p. 650); yaws (p. 653); granuloma inguinale [often abscesses also] (p. 633)
Plasma cells prominent	Syphilis (p. 650); yaws (p. 653); lymphogranuloma venereum (p. 637); chancroid (p. 634); visceral leishmaniasis (p. 723); trypanosomiasis (p. 721); arthropod bites [an uncommon pattern]; *Vibrio* infection (p. 621)
Eosinophils prominent	Arthropod bites (p. 738); helminth infestation (p. 732); cnidarian (coelenterate) contact (p. 728); subcutaneous phycomycosis (p. 678)
Neutrophils prominent	Impetigo [subcorneal neutrophils] (p. 618); ecthyma (p. 620); cellulitis (p. 621); erysipelas [prominent superficial edema also] (p. 620); granuloma inguinale [microabscesses] (p. 633); chancroid [superficial neutrophils] (p. 634); disseminated tuberculosis in AIDS patients (p. 627); erythema nodosum leprosum (p. 630); Lucio's phenomenon (p. 630); anthrax (p. 633); yaws (p. 653) and pinta (p. 653) [both have intraepidermal abscesses]; blastomycosis-like pyoderma (p. 622); actinomycosis (p. 677); nocardiosis (p. 676); mycetoma (p. 675); fungal kerion (p. 661); phaeohyphomycosis (p. 673); aspergillosis (p. 678); mucormycosis [also infarction present] (p. 677); flea bites (p. 745)
Parasitized macrophages	Rhinoscleroma (p. 635); granuloma inguinale (p. 633); lepromatous leprosy (p. 630); histoplasmosis (p. 670); leishmaniasis (p. 721); toxoplasmosis [pseudocysts present] (p. 723); *Penicillium* infection (p. 671)
Parasitized multinucleate giant cells or foreign body reaction	Various fungal infections; prototphecosis (p. 679); schistosomiasis (p. 732); demodex within tissues; some other mite infestations
Superficial and deep dermal perivascular lymphocytic inflammation	Leprosy [indeterminate stage] (p. 630); secondary syphilis [often plasma cells present] (p. 650); arthropod bites (p. 738) and coral reactions (p. 728) [usually interstitial eosinophils also]; onchocercal dermatitis [microfilariae in lymphatics] (p. 733)
Psoriasiform epidermal hyperplasia	Chronic candidosis (p. 665); tinea imbricata (p. 661); chronic dermatophytoses [rare] (p. 663)
Pseudoepitheliomatous or irregular epidermal hyperplasia	Amebiasis (p. 720); toxoplasmosis [rare] (p. 723); mucocutaneous leishmaniasis (p. 722); schistosomiasis (p. 732); chronic arthropod bite reactions [rare] (p. 745); yaws (p. 653); rhinoscleroma (p. 635); granuloma inguinale (p. 633); blastomycosis-like pyoderma [oblique follicles and draining sinuses] (p. 622); tuberculosis [tuberculosis verrucosa and some infections by atypical mycobacteria] (p. 626); *Vibrio* infection (p. 621); certain deep fungal infections+; human papilloma virus infections (p. 701); milker's nodule (p. 693) and orf (p. 694) [both of these may have thin, long rete pegs]; verrucous herpes/varicella lesions in HIV infection (p. 698)
Folliculitis and/or perifolliculitis	Syphilis [rare cases] (p. 650); dermatophytoses (p. 660); pityrosporum folliculitis (p. 663); pyogenic bacterial infections (p. 618); herpes simplex (p. 696); herpes zoster (p. 699); demodex infestations (p. 739); larva migrans [eosinophilic folliculitis] (p.734)
Vasculitis	Erythema nodosum leprosum (p. 630); Lucio's phenomenon (p. 630); ecthyma gangrenosum (p. 620); necrotizing fasciitis (p. 621); meningococcal and gonococcal septicemia (p. 624); recurrent herpes ['lichenoid lymphocytic vasculitis'] (p. 692); cytomegalovirus infection [endothelial cell inclusion bodies] (p. 699); rickettsial infections [lymphocytic vasculitis] (p. 637); spider bites (p. 738); papulonecrotic tuberculid
Tissue necrosis	Ecthyma gangrenosum (p. 620); necrotizing fasciitis (p. 621); diphtheria (p. 622); anthrax (p. 633); tularemia (p. 636); cat-scratch disease (p. 636); severe lepra reactional states (p. 630); scrofuloderma (p. 626); *Mycobacterium ulcerans* infections (p. 627); papulonecrotic tuberculid (p. 627); chancroid [superficial necrosis only] (p 634); rickettsial infections [eschar present] (p. 637); herpes folliculitis (p. 697); mucormycosis (p. 677); gnat, spider and beetle bites (p. 745); acute tick bites (p. 738); stonefish and stingray contact (p. 729); orf (p.694); amebiasis (p. 720)

Table 22.1 **Histological patterns in infections and infestations** *(Continued)*

Morphological feature	Diseases to be considered
Epidermal spongiosis	Dermatophytoses (p. 660); candidosis (p. 664); cercarial dermatitis [eosinophils and neutrophils also] (p. 732); larva migrans (p. 734); chigger bites (p. 742); other arthropod bites; contact with moths of the genus *Hylesia* (p. 745); contact with beetles; delayed reactions to cnidarians (p. 728); viral infections, including herpesvirus-6 and Coxsackievirus
Intraepidermal vesiculation	Herpes simplex, herpes zoster, varicella [all three have ballooning degeneration and intranuclear inclusions] (p. 696); orf (p. 694) and milker's nodule (p. 693) [both have pale superficial cytoplasm]; hand, foot and mouth disease (p. 705); erysipeloid [also superficial dermal edema] (p. 620); beetle bites (p. 745); certain other arthropod bites [may be bullous in hypersensitive persons]; dermatophytoses (p. 660); candidosis (p. 664)
Parasite in tissue sections	Helminth and arthropod infestations; certain injuries from forms of marine life
'Invisible dermatoses' (section stained with H&E appears normal at first glance)	Erythrasma (p. 623); pityriasis versicolor [spores and hyphae are usually easily seen] (p. 666); dermatophytoses [compact orthokeratosis, neutrophils in the stratum corneum or the 'Sandwich sign' often present] (p. 660); pitted keratolysis [crateriform defects, pits or pallor of the stratum corneum are usually obvious, as are bacteria] (p. 623)
Spindle cell pseudotumors	Atypical mycobacteria (p. 627); histoid leprosy (p. 630); acrodermatitis chronica atrophicans (p. 654)

* These infections are more suppurative than granulomatous; the latter component is not always present.
+ 'Deep fungal infections' is used here to include North American blastomycosis, sporotrichosis, chromomycosis, coccidioidomycosis, paracoccidioidomycosis, subcutaneous phycomycosis and phaeohyphomycosis.

Bacterial and rickettsial infections

23

INTRODUCTION

Various bacteria form part of the normal resident flora of the skin. In certain circumstances some of these may assume pathogenic importance. Other bacteria are present only in pathological circumstances. In this chapter the following categories of bacterial infections will be considered: pyogenic, corynebacterial, neisserial, mycobacterial, miscellaneous, chlamydial and rickettsial. **Pyogenic infections**, usually caused by *Staphylococcus aureus* and strains of *Streptococcus*, are numerically the most important bacterial infections of the skin. Two distinct groups (superficial and deep) can be distinguished on the basis of the anatomical level of involvement of the skin. The pyogenic infections, with the exception of the staphylococcal 'scalded skin' syndrome, which results from the effects of a bacterial exotoxin, are characterized histologically by a heavy infiltrate of neutrophils. These organisms may also infect hair follicles, resulting in folliculitis.

Corynebacterial infections, with the exception of diphtheria, are usually limited to the stratum corneum and, as a consequence, there is no significant inflammatory response: at first glance, the biopsy may appear normal.

Neisserial infections of the skin are rare, although they are an important cause of urethritis. Cutaneous lesions may occur in neisserial septicemias.

Mycobacterial infections usually result in a granulomatous tissue reaction, but this depends on the immune status of the individual, including the development of delayed hypersensitivity. Exceptions include lepromatous leprosy, in which a histiocytic response occurs, and some infections by atypical mycobacteria, in which suppurative granulomas, suppuration and even non-specific chronic inflammation may result at various times.

A variety of inflammatory reactions can be seen in the group of **miscellaneous bacterial infections** of the skin. The chapter closes with a brief discussion of chlamydial infections and rickettsial infections. Each group will be discussed in turn.

Although they are bacteria, infections by the **actinomycetes** are considered in Chapter 25 (pp. 675–677) because they produce lesions that are clinicopathologically similar in many respects to those produced by some fungi (mycetomas).

SUPERFICIAL PYOGENIC INFECTIONS

The superficial pyogenic infections of the skin (pyodermas) include impetigo and its variants and ecthyma. They also include the superficial infections of the hair follicles, which are dealt with in Chapter 15 (pp. 459–461). In addition, the staphylococcal 'scalded skin' syndrome can be included in this category, although the lesions result from the action of bacterial toxin rather than local infection itself.

IMPETIGO

Impetigo is an acute superficial pyoderma which heals without scar formation. It is the most common bacterial infection of the skin in childhood.[1–3] Adults are sometimes affected, particularly athletes, military personnel and those in institutions.[4] Minor trauma, especially from insect bites, as well as poor hygiene and a warm, humid climate, all predispose to this infection.[5]

There are two clinical forms of impetigo: a common, vesiculopustular type, and a bullous variant, which is considerably less frequent.[6,7] Recent studies have shown that *Staphylococcus aureus* is now the most common organism isolated from the non-bullous type of impetigo,[8–10] which in the past was caused mostly by a group A β-hemolytic streptococcus, sometimes with *Staph. aureus* as a secondary invader.[3,4] Anaerobes are now isolated in a number of cases.[10] The bullous form has always been related exclusively to *Staph. aureus*, usually of phage group II.[11]

Common impetigo

Common impetigo ('school sores') commences as thin-walled vesicles or pustules on an erythematous base: the lesions rapidly rupture to form a thick, golden crust.[12] Common impetigo occurs as a solitary lesion or a cluster of several lesions, which may coalesce. It is found on the face or extremities.[9] Local lymphadenopathy may be present.

Bullous impetigo

Bullous impetigo is composed of shallow erosions and flaccid bullae, 0.5–3 cm in diameter, with an erythematous rim.[4] The bulla has a thin roof which soon ruptures, resulting in a thin crust.[11] There may be a localized collection of a few bullae, or more generalized lesions.[13] Bullous impetigo is included with the staphylococcal epidermolytic toxin syndrome, as the lesions result from the production in situ of an epidermolytic toxin by staphylococci.[4]

Histopathology

Common impetigo is rarely biopsied, as the diagnosis can be made on clinical grounds. An early lesion will show a subcorneal collection of neutrophils, with exocytosis of these cells through the underlying epidermis. A few acantholytic cells are sometimes seen, but this is never a prominent feature. Established lesions show a thick surface crust composed of serum, neutrophils in various stages of breakdown, and some parakeratotic material. Gram-positive cocci can usually be found without difficulty in the surface crust.

In *bullous impetigo* the subcorneal bulla contains a few acantholytic cells, a small number of neutrophils, and some Gram-positive cocci (Fig. 23.1).[11] In contrast to the lesions of the staphylococcal 'scalded skin' syndrome, there is usually a mild to moderate mixed inflammatory cell infiltrate in the underlying papillary dermis.[11]

STAPHYLOCOCCAL 'SCALDED SKIN' SYNDROME (SSSS)

The staphylococcal 'scalded skin' syndrome results from the production of an epidermolytic toxin by certain strains of *Staph. aureus*, most notably type 71 of phage group II.[4,14] These organisms are responsible for a preceding upper

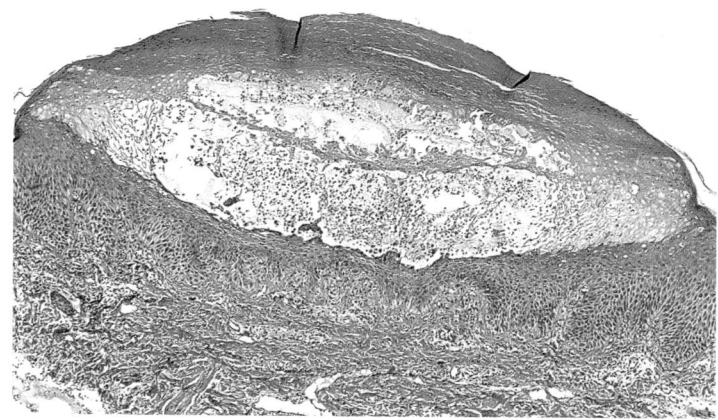

Fig. 23.1 **Bullous impetigo.** There is a subcorneal blister containing inflammatory cells and degenerate keratinocytes. Gram-positive cocci were found. (H & E)

respiratory tract infection, conjunctivitis or carrier state. Rarely, the syndrome follows a staphylococcal infection complicating varicella or measles.[15,16]

The SSSS predominantly affects healthy infants and children younger than 6 years, apparently reflecting an inability to handle and excrete the toxin.[17] Rarely, neonates are involved, a condition known in the past as Ritter's disease (Ritter von Rittershain's disease).[18] A few cases have been reported in adults, in whom there has usually been underlying immunosuppression (including the acquired immunodeficiency syndrome)[19] and/or renal insufficiency.[20–22] It occurs rarely in healthy adults.[23–25]

There is a sudden onset of skin tenderness and a scarlatiniform eruption which is followed by the development of large, easily ruptured, flaccid bullae and a positive Nikolsky sign.[18] Desquamation of large areas of the skin occurs in sheets and ribbons.[20] Occasionally, only the scarlatiniform eruption develops. The usual sites of involvement are the face, neck and trunk, including the axillae and groins. Mucous membranes are not involved.

The disease has a good prognosis in children, with spontaneous healing after several days as a consequence of the formation of neutralizing antibodies to the epidermolytic toxin.[26] In adults a staphylococcal septicemia may ensue and is sometimes fatal. A chronic case, evolving over two years, has been reported in an adult female patient.[27]

Desquamation results from the effects of an exotoxin of low molecular weight (exfoliatin), produced by certain strains of *Staph. aureus*. There are two forms of exfoliatin recognized – exfoliative toxin A (ETA), which is chromosomally encoded, and exfoliative toxin B (ETB), which is plasmid encoded.[28] Other toxins are sometimes found. The mechanism by which these toxins produce exfoliation is still disputed.[28] The condition can be reproduced in newborn mice by the subcutaneous or intraperitoneal injection of these organisms.[29]

Staphylococcal epidermolytic toxin syndrome
The SSSS, which was historically considered (incorrectly) to be a variant of toxic epidermal necrolysis (see p. 45), has been regarded as belonging to the staphylococcal epidermolytic toxin syndrome.[30–32] Also included in this concept are localized and generalized bullous impetigo, which result from the local production (as opposed to production at a distant site, as in SSSS) of a similar staphylococcal epidermolytic toxin.[15] Consequently, in bullous impetigo the organisms may be demonstrated within the lesion. Impetigo is discussed in further detail above.

Histopathology[33]
In the SSSS there is subcorneal splitting of the epidermis (Fig. 23.2). A few acantholytic cells and sparse neutrophils may be present within the blister, although often it is difficult to obtain an intact lesion. A sparse, mixed inflammatory cell infiltrate is present in the underlying dermis. This is in contrast to generalized bullous impetigo, and even pemphigus foliaceus, in which the dermal infiltrate is heavier.

Immunofluorescence is negative, in contrast to pemphigus foliaceus, in which intercellular immunoreactants are usually demonstrable.

Electron microscopy
There is widening of the intercellular spaces followed by disruption of desmosome attachments through their central density.[4,29] There are no cytotoxic changes.

STAPHYLOCOCCAL TOXIC SHOCK SYNDROME

The staphylococcal toxic shock syndrome was first recognized over a decade ago in healthy menstruating women who used tampons.[34,35] It results from a toxin produced by certain strains of *Staph. aureus* that proliferate in the vagina and cervix. The toxic shock syndrome can also complicate wound infections with *Staph. aureus*.[36] Currently, the incidence of non-menstrual disease exceeds that related to the female genital tract.[14] The clinical features of this syndrome include a fever, hypotension, inflammation of mucous membranes, vomiting and diarrhea, and cutaneous lesions that resemble viral exanthemata or erythema multiforme.[37,38] The skin lesions undergo desquamation in time.

A streptococcal toxic shock syndrome has also been reported (see below).

Histopathology[37]
The characteristic features of the toxic shock syndrome are small foci of epidermal spongiosis containing a few neutrophils, scattered degenerate keratinocytes, sometimes arranged in clusters, and a superficial perivascular and interstitial cell infiltrate.[37] The infiltrate contains lymphocytes, neutrophils and sometimes eosinophils.[37] Inflammatory cells often extend into the walls of the superficial dermal vessels, as seen in vasculitis, but there is no fibrin extravasation. Less constant features include irregular epidermal acanthosis, edema of the papillary dermis, extravasation of erythrocytes, and nuclear 'dust' in the vicinity of the blood vessels.[37] Focal parakeratosis, containing neutrophils and serum, may also be present.

STREPTOCOCCAL TOXIC SHOCK SYNDROME

The streptococcal toxic shock syndrome is caused by virulent strains of exotoxin-producing streptococci, almost always group A organisms such as *Streptococcus pyogenes*.[39] It often occurs in the setting of deep soft tissue infections, when the portal of entry of the organism appears to be through the skin, but it may complicate burns, surgical wounds or childbirth. Accordingly it can be seen in several clinical situations such as the young, the immunocompromised, the elderly and diabetics. Rarely, it has developed in patients taking non-steroidal anti-inflammatory drugs.[14]

Clinically there is fever, pain at the site of the deep tissue infection, and skin necrosis and bullae. A scarlatiniform rash may be present. A streptococcal bacteremia is present in 60% of cases, in contrast to the negative blood cultures in the staphylococcal toxic shock syndrome.[35]

Histopathology
The changes resemble those in ecthyma gangrenosum (see below). The deep soft tissue lesions, if present, are those of necrotizing fasciitis (see p. 621).

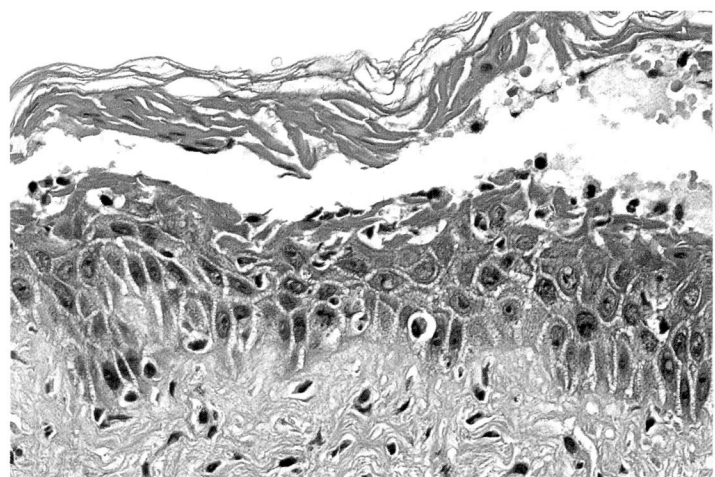

Fig. 23.2 **The staphylococcal scalded skin syndrome** with subcorneal splitting. (H & E)

PERIANAL STREPTOCOCCAL DERMATITIS

Perianal streptococcal dermatitis, caused by group A β-hemolytic streptococci, has been described almost exclusively in children, although a few adult cases have been reported.[40] It presents as perianal erythema with a clearly defined border followed by a desquamating scale and subsequent healing. Systemic symptoms, such as fever, are uncommon[41] in contrast to **toxin-mediated perineal erythema** which occurs abruptly after a bacterial pharyngitis due to *Staph. aureus* or *Streptococcus pyogenes*.[14]

ECTHYMA

Ecthyma is a deeper pyoderma than impetigo and much less frequent.[6] It has a predilection for the extremities of children, often at sites of minor trauma, which allow entry of the causative bacteria. Group A streptococci, particularly *Streptococcus pyogenes*, are usually implicated, although coagulase-positive staphylococci are sometimes isolated as well.[7,42] The lesions, which are sometimes multiple, consist of a dark crust adherent to a shallow ulcer and surrounded by a rim of erythema. Scarring usually results when the lesions heal.[7]

Ecthyma gangrenosum is a severe variant of ecthyma seen in 5% or more of immunosuppressed individuals who develop a septicemia with *Pseudomonas aeruginosa*.[43–48] It commences as an erythematous macule on the trunk or limbs: the lesion rapidly becomes vesicular, then pustular, and finally develops into a gangrenous ulcer with a dark eschar and an erythematous halo.[49,50] Annular lesions have been recorded.[51] Constitutional symptoms are usually present. Patients with solitary lesions have a better prognosis than those with multiple lesions. Similar necrotic ulcers have been reported in association with aspergillus infection, *Morganella morganii*,[52] candidosis, and following pseudomonas folliculitis (but usually without septicemia).[43] *Pseudomonas aeruginosa* septicemia may result in the development of bullae[53] or of a nodular cellulitis[54] rather than ecthyma gangrenosum.[55]

Histopathology

In ecthyma there is ulceration of the skin with an inflammatory crust on the surface. There is a heavy infiltrate of neutrophils in the reticular dermis, which forms the base of the ulcer. Gram-positive cocci may be seen within the inflammatory crust.

Ecthyma gangrenosum shows necrosis of the epidermis and the upper dermis, with some hemorrhage into the dermis.[49] The epidermis may separate from the dermis. A mixed inflammatory-cell infiltrate surrounds the infarcted region. In some cases there is a paucity of inflammation.[49,50] A necrotizing vasculitis with vascular thrombosis is present in the margins.[54] Numerous Gram-negative bacteria are usually present between the collagen bundles, and sometimes in the media and adventitia of small blood vessels.

DEEP PYOGENIC INFECTIONS (CELLULITIS)

Cellulitis is a diffuse inflammation of the connective tissue of the skin and/or the deeper soft tissues.[7,56,57] It is therefore a deeper pyoderma than impetigo and some cases of ecthyma, although ecthyma gangrenosum could be included in this category. Clinically, cellulitis presents as an expanding area of erythema, which is usually edematous and tender.[58] Necrosis sometimes supervenes.[59] In the past, these infections were usually caused by β-hemolytic streptococci and/or coagulase-positive staphylococci.[7,60] A diverse range of organisms is now implicated in the causation of cellulitis.[56,61–66] Neutropenic

and leukemic patients are now being seen with erythematous nodules on the leg caused by the opportunistic pathogen *Stenotrophomonas (Xanthomonas) maltophilia*.[67,68] Lower extremity cellulitis appears to be increased in patients who have undergone saphenous venectomy for coronary artery bypass graft surgery.[69]

Many different clinical variants of cellulitis have been reported, some with overlapping clinical features and causative bacteria.[58] This has led to a proliferation of terms for these different variants. The term 'gangrenous and crepitant cellulitis' has been used for a subset with prominent skin necrosis and/or the discernible presence of gas in the tissues.[59] The term 'hemorrhagic cellulitis' has also been used for this group, which includes progressive bacterial synergistic gangrene. It has been suggested that tumor necrosis factor-α is responsible for the damage to keratinocytes and vascular endothelium.[70]

The cellulitides are characterized histopathologically by an infiltrate of neutrophils throughout the dermis and/or the subcutaneous tissue, with variable subepidermal edema and vascular ectasia. In those variants with necrosis there is usually a necrotizing vasculitis, which may be associated with fibrin thrombi in the lumen.[71,72] Bacteria are often numerous in the group with necrosis, although usually only a few can be isolated in the other variants.[73]

ERYSIPELAS

Erysipelas is a distinctive type of cellulitis which has an elevated border and spreads rapidly.[7,74,75] Vesiculation may develop, particularly at the edge of the lesion. An uncommon bullous variant, usually confined to the lower legs, has recently been described.[76] The condition occurs particularly on the lower extremities, and less commonly on the face.[77,78] Underlying diabetes mellitus, peripheral vascular disease or lymphedema may be present.[77] The causative group A streptococci[57,79] or other organisms[80,81] gain entry through superficial abrasions. Bacteremia is common.[7]

An erysipelas-like erythema, usually on the lower legs, is seen in **familial Mediterranean fever**, an autosomal recessive disease affecting certain ethnic groups.[82] The histopathology has features more in keeping with a neutrophilic dermatosis than erysipelas.

Histopathology

There is marked subepidermal edema, which may lead to the formation of vesiculobullous lesions. Beneath this zone there is a diffuse and usually heavy infiltrate of neutrophils, but abscesses do not form. The infiltrate is sometimes accentuated around blood vessels. There is often vascular and lymphatic dilatation. In healing lesions the dermal infiltrate diminishes, and granulation tissue may form immediately below the zone of subepidermal edema (Fig. 23.3). Direct immunofluorescence has been used to confirm the streptococcal etiology of most cases of erysipelas.[79]

ERYSIPELOID

Erysipeloid is an uncommon infection, usually found on the hands, which clinically resembles erysipelas.[83] The causative organism, *Erysipelothrix rhusiopathiae*, is a contaminant of dead organic matter, and infection with this organism is an occupational hazard for fish and meat handlers. Less commonly, multiple cutaneous lesions or systemic spread of the organism may occur.

Histopathology[83]

There is usually massive edema of the papillary dermis overlying a diffuse and polymorphous infiltrate composed of lymphocytes, plasma cells and variable

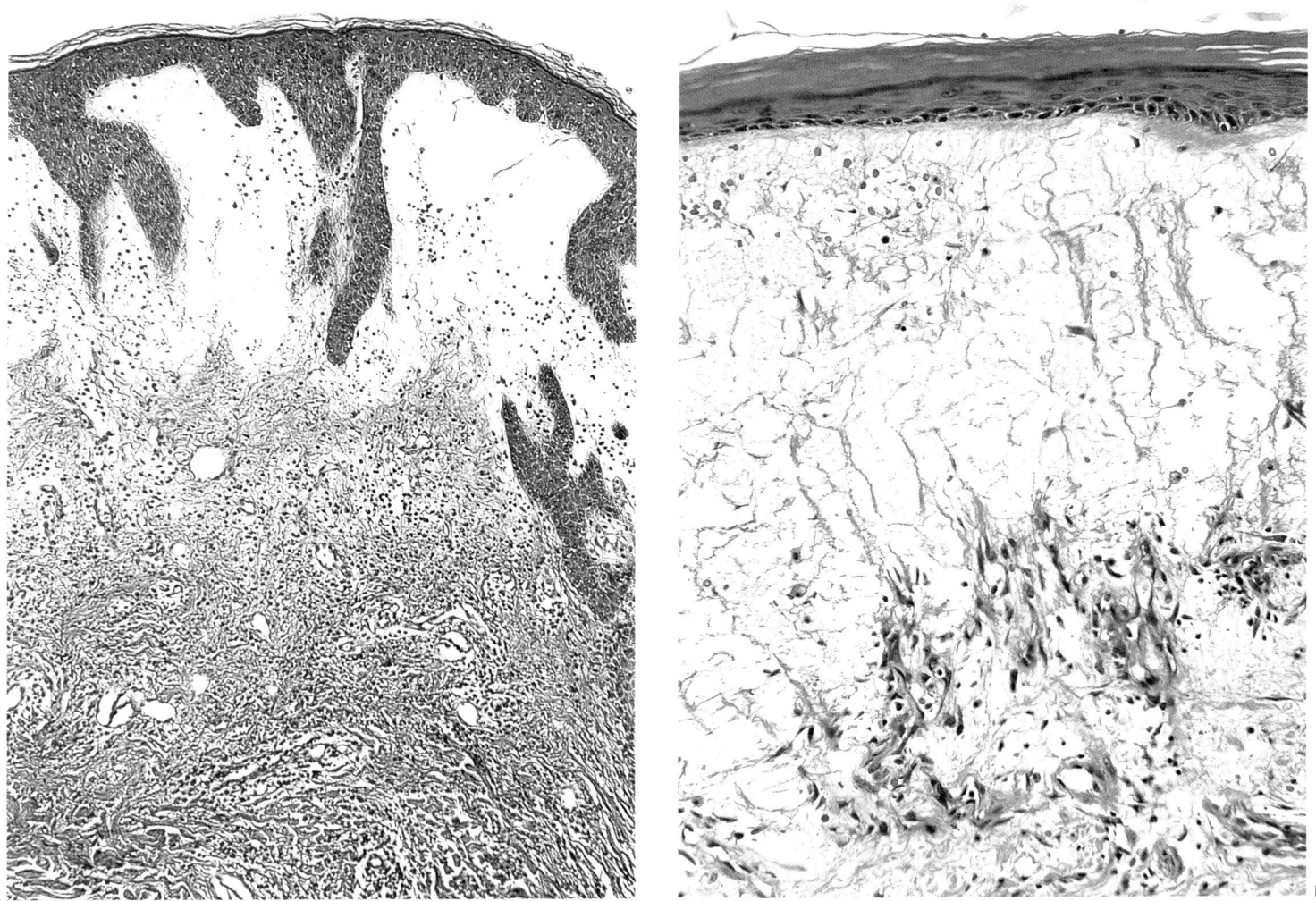

Fig. 23.3 **Erysipelas. (A)** Acute lesion with marked subepidermal edema. **(B)** This healing lesion shows little inflammation in the upper dermis. (H & E)

numbers of neutrophils. Sometimes there is spongiosis of the epidermis, leading to intraepidermal vesiculation. Organisms are not demonstrable in tissue sections, even with a Gram stain, possibly because they are present in the L form (without a cell wall).[83]

BLISTERING DISTAL DACTYLITIS

Blistering distal dactylitis is an uncommon yet distinctive infection localized to the volar fat pad of the distal phalanx of the fingers.[7,84–86] Group A streptococci are usually implicated, although rarely other organisms have been isolated.[87,88] The blistering results from massive subepidermal edema.

CELLULITIS

In addition to its use as a synonym for deep pyogenic infection (see above), the term 'cellulitis' is sometimes used in a more restricted sense for spreading inflammation of the cheek,[89–91] periorbital area[92] or the perianal region,[86,93–96] or in the margins of wounds.[7] The lesions lack the distinct border of erysipelas.[7] Various organisms have been implicated as the cause of this condition, including *Haemophilus influenzae* type B in the case of facial lesions[90] and *Vibrio vulnificus* in some infections of the extremities.[97–101] The

latter organism can produce various lesions, including hemorrhagic bullae,[102,103] cellulitis and necrotizing fasciitis.[104] *Pasteurella multocida* has been implicated in the wound infection and cellulitis that may follow animal bites.[105] *Vibrio cholerae* (non-01 type) can rarely produce a cellulitis or infect a pre-existing wound.[106,107] *Escherichia coli* has also been implicated, particularly in immunocompromised individuals.[108]

Histopathology

The appearances are similar to those of erysipelas; focal necrosis is sometimes present. Involvement of the subcutis may lead to a predominantly septal panniculitis.[71,97]

NECROTIZING FASCIITIS

Necrotizing fasciitis is a rare and distinct form of cellulitis that rapidly progresses to necrosis of the skin and underlying tissues.[109–114] The term 'flesh-eating bacteria' has appeared in the media, highlighting the progressive necrotizing nature of the disease.[115] It involves tissues at a deeper level than erysipelas, and may spread into the underlying muscle.[116] Necrotizing fasciitis commences as a poorly defined area of erythema, usually on the leg;[109] serosanguineous blisters develop and subsequently necrosis occurs at their center.[117,118] Uncommonly, the condition follows surgery.[119] Constitutional symptoms may be present, and there is a significant mortality.[116] The term 'streptococcal toxic shock syndrome' has been applied to this systemic illness,[120] although it more properly refers to a discrete entity with some similarity to the toxic shock syndrome of staphylococcal origin (see p. 619).[14] Various organisms have been isolated,[121] particularly group A streptococci.[118,122] Rapid diagnosis kits are available to confirm cases of streptococcal origin. Protein S deficiency may be responsible for the necrosis in some cases.[123] **Fournier's gangrene of the scrotum** is a closely related entity.[117] It is usually found in elderly men, with an underlying disease such as diabetes. Cases have been reported in younger persons.[124] It is a rare complication of the use of all-*trans*-retinoic acid as induction therapy in the treatment of acute promyelocytic leukemia. Its response to corticosteroids suggests that Fournier's gangrene is a localized vasculitis and represents a local Schwartzmann phenomenon.[125] Enterobacteria are common isolates, although a mixed growth is often seen.[126,127] In one recent series the mortality was nearly 10%.[126]

Histopathology[109,110]

Necrotizing fasciitis is a form of septic vasculitis with inflammation of the walls of vessels, sometimes associated with occlusion of the lumen by thrombi.[72] There is a mixed inflammatory cell infiltrate in the viable tissues bordering the areas of necrosis. The necrosis involves the epidermis, dermis and upper subcutis.

MISCELLANEOUS SYNDROMES

There are several rare but distinct clinicopathological entities that belong to the category of deep pyogenic infections. They include clostridial myonecrosis (gas gangrene), progressive bacterial synergistic gangrene and erosive pustular dermatosis of the scalp.[59]

Clostridial myonecrosis (gas gangrene)

Clostridial myonecrosis (gas gangrene) is associated with muscle and soft tissue necrosis. Cutaneous lesions, including bullae and necrosis, may overlie the deeper lesions. The usual causative organisms in gas gangrene are clostridial species; non-clostridial cases are infrequently reported.[128] Large Gram-positive bacilli are usually present in the affected tissues.[59] A bacterium related to the genus *Clostridium* – *Bacillus piloformis* – has produced localized verrucous lesions in a patient infected with HIV-1.[129] *Bacillus cereus* infection has been associated with a single necrotic bulla in a patient with a lymphoma.[130]

Progressive bacterial synergistic gangrene

Progressive bacterial synergistic gangrene is characterized by indurated ulcerated areas with a gangrenous margin, usually developing in operative wounds.[59,131] This condition, also known as Meleney's ulcer, is often associated with a mixed growth of peptostreptococci and *Staph. aureus* or enterobacteriaceae.[59]

Erosive pustular dermatosis

Erosive pustular dermatosis of the scalp consists of widespread erosions and crusted pustules, leading to scarring alopecia.[132–134] A clinically similar rash has been reported on the legs.[135] Its exact nosological position is uncertain, and there are some morphological similarities to blastomycosis-like pyoderma (see below). The inflammatory infiltrate is usually mixed, unless acute areas of pustulation are biopsied.[132] Trauma, previous herpes zoster infection, recent cryotherapy, radiation therapy and surgery have been implicated as predisposing factors.[136–140] *Staph. aureus* is sometimes isolated.[132]

BLASTOMYCOSIS-LIKE PYODERMA

Blastomycosis-like pyoderma is an unusual form of pyoderma that presents with large verrucous plaques studded with multiple pustules and draining sinuses.[141,142] There may be an underlying disturbance of immunological function in some cases.[142,143] A variant of this condition is found in subtropical areas of Australia in the actinically damaged skin of the elderly, particularly on the forearm.[144,145] This has been known as 'coral reef granuloma', on the basis of its clinical appearance.[146] Actinic comedonal plaque, in which plaques and nodules with a cribriform appearance develop in sun-damaged skin,[147] appears to be the end-stage of a similar but milder inflammatory process.[144,145] Similar lesions have been reported at the margins of tattoos.[144,148] Actinic comedonal plaque has also been regarded as an ectopic form of the Favre–Racouchot syndrome (see p. 391).[149]

Bacteria, particularly *Staph. aureus* and species of *Pseudomonas* and *Proteus*, have been isolated from biopsies.[142,144,150,151] Sun-damaged skin is known to diminish local immune responses, and this factor is probably important in the variant found in Australia.[152,153]

Histopathology

There is a heavy inflammatory infiltrate throughout the dermis, with multiple small abscesses set in a background of chronic inflammation (Fig. 23.4).[142] A few granulomas are occasionally present, but these are usually related to elastotic fibers. There is prominent pseudoepitheliomatous hyperplasia, which in some areas appears to result from hypertrophy of the follicular infundibulum. Intraepidermal microabscesses are present, and these probably represent the attempted transepidermal elimination of the dermal inflammatory process. Solar elastotic fibers are present in the variants known as 'coral reef granuloma' and 'actinic comedonal plaque'.[147] There may be some dermal fibrosis in healing lesions, although actinically damaged fibers usually persist in the upper dermis.

CORYNEBACTERIAL INFECTIONS

The corynebacteria are a diverse group of Gram-positive bacilli which include *Corynebacterium diphtheriae*, the causative organism of diphtheria, as well as a bewildering number of species that are found on the skin as part of the normal flora and which defy classification.[154] These latter organisms are usually referred to as diphtheroids or coryneforms. Certain strains have the ability to produce malodor of the axilla.[155] Three skin conditions appear to be related to an overabundance of these coryneforms: erythrasma, trichomycosis and pitted keratolysis.[154] Interestingly, the three have been reported to coexist in the same person.[156] Rarely, other species of corynebacteria have been incriminated as a source of infection in diabetics[157] or immunocompromised patients, the most important being the JK group (*C. jeikeium*).[158,159] These organisms have been found in patients with heart prostheses and endocarditis, and recently as a cause of cutaneous lesions in immunocompromised patients.[158] They may produce a histological picture mimicking botryomycosis (see p. 677).[159]

DIPHTHERIA

Cutaneous diphtheria is a rarely diagnosed entity which is still found very occasionally in tropical areas.[160–162] The typical lesion is an ulcer with a well-defined irregular margin; the base is covered with a gray slough. Systemic effects, from the absorption of exotoxin, and severe lymphadenitis may develop. Cutaneous carriers also occur.

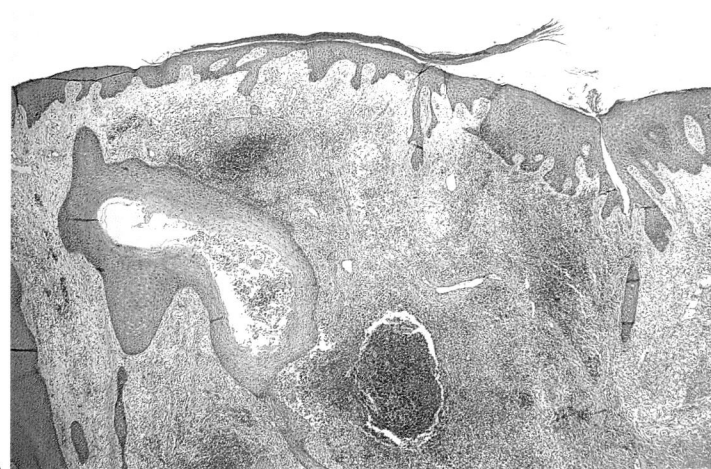 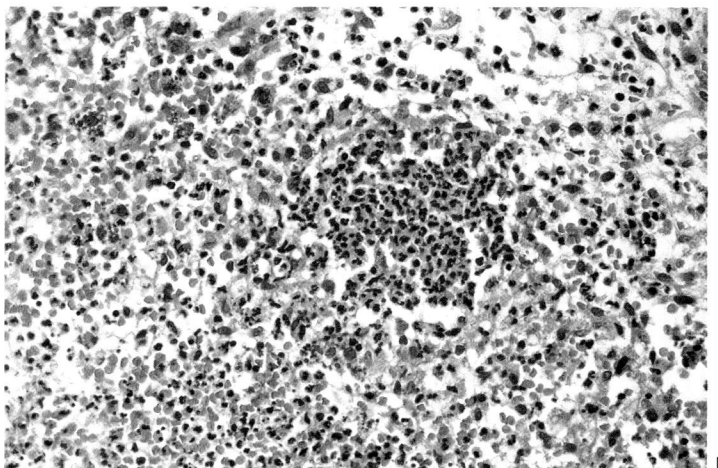

Fig. 23.4 **Blastomycosis-like pyoderma. (A)** There is dermal suppuration adjacent to enlarged follicular structures which become draining sinuses. **(B)** Suppurative granulomas are often present. (H & E)

Histopathology

There is necrosis of the epidermis and varying depths of the dermis. The base of the ulcer is composed of necrotic debris, fibrin and a mixed inflammatory infiltrate. The bacilli are often difficult to see in tissue sections.

ERYTHRASMA

Erythrasma, caused by a diphtheroid bacillus *Corynebacterium minutissimum*, presents as well-defined, red to brown finely scaling patches with a predilection for skin folds, particularly the inner aspect of the thigh just below the crural fold.[163–165] A rare generalized disciform variant has been reported.[165] Erythrasma is a not uncommon asymptomatic infection in the obese, and in diabetics and patients in institutions, particularly in humid climates.[163,164] Examination of affected skin under a Wood's ultraviolet lamp shows a characteristic coral-red fluorescence.

Erythrasma may coexist with a dermatophyte infection, particularly in the toe webs.[166,167]

Histopathology

The biopsy often appears normal when hematoxylin and eosin preparations are examined, erythrasma being an example of a so-called 'invisible dermatosis'. Small coccobacilli can be seen in the superficial part of the stratum corneum in Gram preparations. They are also seen in PAS (periodic acid–Schiff) and methenamine silver preparations (Fig. 23.5).

Electron microscopy

Electron microscopy has confirmed the bacterial nature of erythrasma. It has also shown decreased electron density in keratinized cells, with dissolution of normal keratin fibrils at sites of proliferation of organisms.[168,169]

TRICHOMYCOSIS

Trichomycosis is a bacterial infection of axillary hair (trichomycosis axillaris) and, uncommonly, pubic hair (trichomycosis pubis).[170,171] There are usually pale yellow concretions attached to the hair shaft: these are large bacterial colonies. Sometimes the casts are red, and rarely they are black.[171] They may be the source of an offensive odor. The causative organism was originally designated as *Corynebacterium tenuis*, but it now seems that at least three

species are involved.[171,172] The infecting bacteria are generally believed to produce a cement-like substance which they use to adhere to the hair shaft and to form the large concretions;[171] this traditional view has been challenged,[173] and it has now been suggested that the sheath substance in which the organisms are embedded is apocrine sweat.[173] Sometimes the bacteria invade the superficial hair cortex.[174] Trichomycosis must be distinguished from other extraneous substances attached to the hair shaft.

PITTED KERATOLYSIS

The condition known as pitted keratolysis takes the form of multiple asymptomatic pits and superficial erosions on the plantar surface of the feet, particularly in pressure areas.[175–180] Rarely, the palms are involved.[175,181,182] Sometimes there is brownish discoloration of involved areas, giving them a dirt-impregnated appearance.[183] Pitted keratolysis is more common if the feet are moist from hyperhidrosis or because the climate is hot.[184] Malodor is common.[180] The pits are thought to result from the keratolytic activity of species of *Corynebacterium*, but *Dermatophilus congolensis*[177,185] and *Micrococcus sedentarius*[186] have also been incriminated.

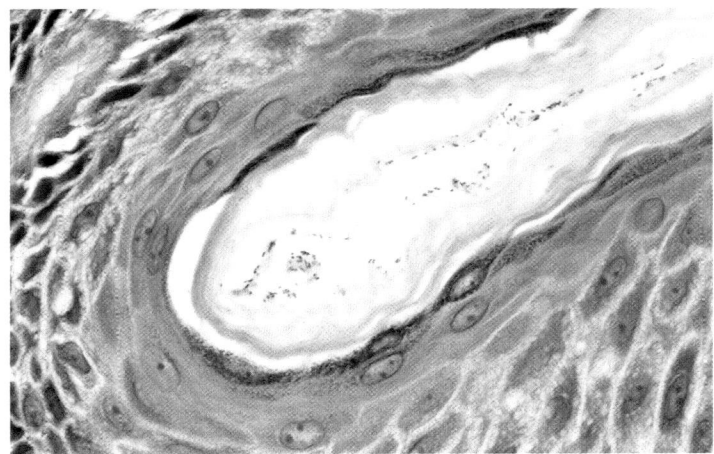

Fig. 23.5 **Erythrasma.** Minute organisms can be seen in the stratum corneum. There is no inflammatory response. (Periodic acid–Schiff)

Histopathology[176,183]

The pits appear as multiple crateriform defects in the stratum corneum. In early lesions there are areas of pallor within the stratum corneum (Fig. 23.6). In the base and margins of the pits there are fine filamentous and coccoid

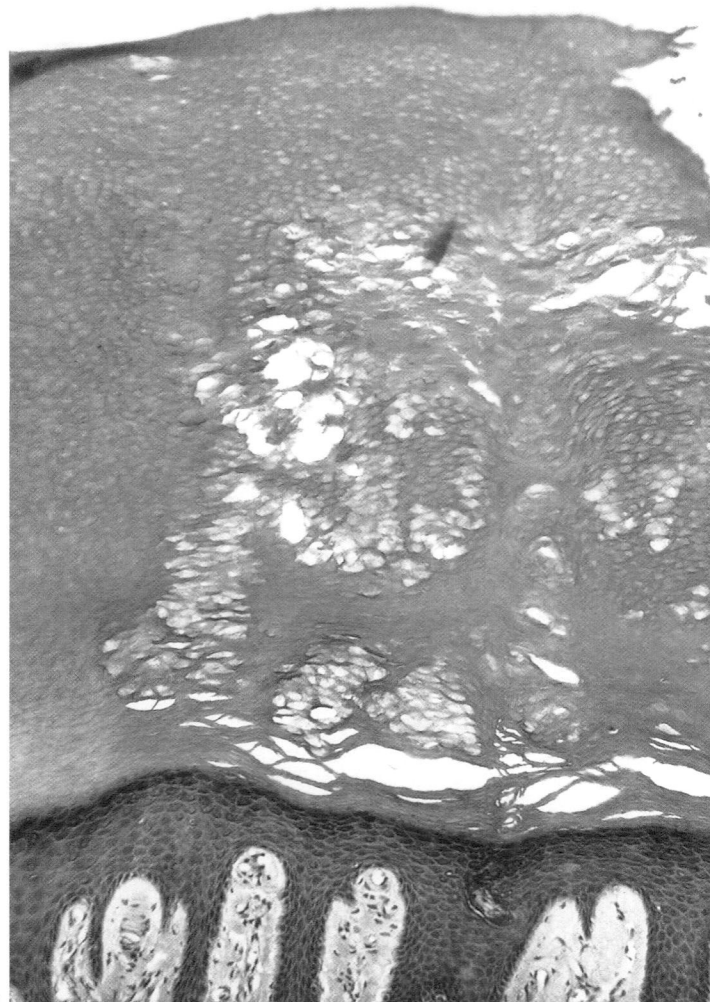

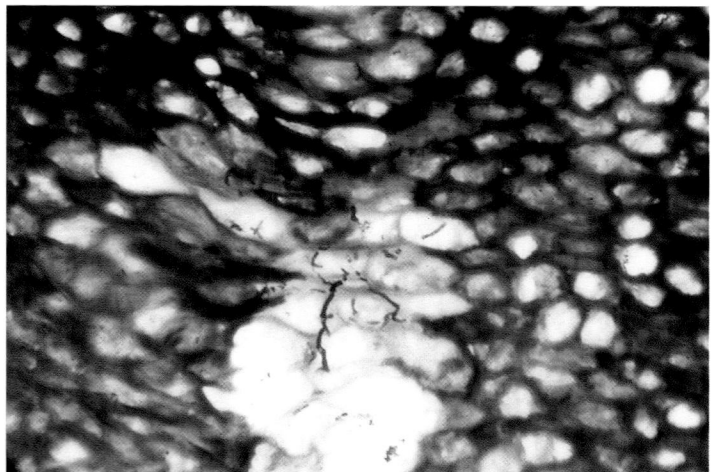

Fig. 23.6 **Pitted keratolysis. (A)** The stratum corneum adjacent to an area of pitting shows zones of pallor corresponding to foci containing the causative organisms (H & E). **(B)** They can be seen in the pale areas of the stratum corneum using silver stains. (Silver methenamine)

organisms that are Gram-positive and argyrophilic with the methenamine silver stain. It has been suggested that two types of pitted keratolysis can be distinguished histologically.[187] In the superficial or minor type there is only a small depression due to focal lysis. Coccoid bacteria are found on the surface of the stratum corneum. In the classical or major type the organisms exhibit dimorphism with septate 'hyphae' as well as coccoid forms, which extend into the stratum corneum forming more definite pits.[187]

Electron microscopy

Ultrastructural examination has confirmed the great variability in the morphology of the bacteria, with coccoid, diphtheroid and filamentous forms in the stratum corneum.[175]

Tunnel-like spaces form inside the horny layer, where the bacteria have a 'hairy' surface.[188]

NEISSERIAL INFECTIONS

Primary infections of the skin by *Neisseria meningitidis* and *N. gonorrheae* are rare because these organisms are unable to penetrate intact epidermis. However, cutaneous lesions do occur quite commonly in meningococcal and gonococcal septicemia; they take the form of a vasculitis (see Ch. 8, p. 234).

MENINGOCOCCAL INFECTIONS

Cutaneous lesions, which may take the form of erythematous macules, nodules, petechiae or small pustules, occur in 80% or more of acute meningococcal infections (see p. 234). Features of disseminated intravascular coagulation are invariably present. Chronic meningococcal septicemia is comparatively rare; it is characterized by the triad of intermittent fever, arthralgia and vesiculopustular or hemorrhagic lesions of the skin. The hemorrhagic lesions are usually a manifestation of purpura fulminans, which develops in 15–25% of those with meningococcemia.[189] It is a predictor of poor outcome.[189] Chronic meningococcemia is a rare complication in patients with the acquired immunodeficiency syndrome.[190]

Histopathology

The cutaneous lesions in meningococcal septicemia show an acute vasculitis, with fibrin thrombi in the small blood vessels of the dermis and extravasation of fibrin. There are neutrophils in and around the vessels, but the infiltrate is not as heavy as it is in hypersensitivity vasculitis. Leukocytoclasis is not usually a conspicuous feature.

In pustular lesions of chronic meningococcemia there are intraepidermal and subepidermal collections of neutrophils. A vasculitis is present in the dermis; the infiltrate contains some lymphocytes in addition to neutrophils.

GONOCOCCAL INFECTIONS

Urethritis (gonorrhea) is the usual manifestation of infection with *Neisseria gonorrhoeae*. This sexually transmitted disease may also infect the accessory glands of the vulva and the median raphe of the penis.[191] Primary infections of extragenital skin are very rare, although pustular lesions on the digits have been reported.[192]

Gonococcal septicemia, both acute and chronic, may result in a cutaneous vasculitis; the lesions resemble those seen in meningococcal septicemia (see above).

Histopathology

Primary pustular lesions on the penis or extragenital skin are usually ulcerated, with a heavy inflammatory cell infiltrate in the underlying dermis. There are numerous neutrophils, often forming small abscesses. Gram-negative intracellular diplococci can usually be found in tissue sections, but they are more easily found in smears made from the purulent exudate on the surface of the lesion.

In gonococcal septicemia the cutaneous lesions resemble those seen in meningococcal septicemia (see above); the appearances are those of a septic vasculitis (see p. 234).

MYCOBACTERIAL INFECTIONS

The cutaneous mycobacterioses include leprosy and tuberculosis, as well as a diverse group of infections caused by various environmental (atypical, non-tuberculous) mycobacteria. Within these three categories there are clinicopathological variants which are sometimes given the status of distinct entities; for example, infections by *Mycobacterium ulcerans* and *M. marinum* (Buruli ulcer and swimming pool granuloma, respectively) are often considered separately from infections caused by other non-tuberculous (atypical) mycobacteria.

Established mycobacterial infections generally give rise to a granulomatous tissue reaction, although considerable variability exists in the histopathological appearances of individual lesions.[193] These aspects will be considered further below.

TUBERCULOSIS

Tuberculosis of the skin has been declining in incidence all over the world, although it is still an important infective disorder in India and parts of Africa.[194–198] The epidemic of HIV/AIDS in parts of Africa has been followed by an epidemic of tuberculosis in its wake.[199] It has been estimated that nearly eight million new cases of tuberculosis occur in the world each year.[200] With the eradication of tuberculosis in cattle, human infections with *Mycobacterium bovis* are rarely seen these days.[201–203] Accordingly, cutaneous tuberculosis can be categorized into two major etiological groups: infections caused by *Mycobacterium tuberculosis*, and those caused by non-tuberculous (atypical) mycobacteria. Infections by non-tuberculous mycobacteria will be considered separately. In some of the so-called 'developed countries', such infections are more numerous than those caused by *M. tuberculosis*.

Not all individuals exposed to *M. tuberculosis* become infected. There is a complex interaction between the organism, the environment and the host.[204] Against this background researchers have attempted to identify a gene that may influence susceptibility to infection. One such gene maps to chromosome 2q35, which includes the *NRAMP1* gene (natural resistance-associated macrophage protein 1).[204] This study was based on susceptible individuals in a Canadian aboriginal population.[204]

Classification

Infections with *M. tuberculosis* have traditionally been classified into primary tuberculosis, when there has been no previous exposure to the organism, and secondary tuberculosis, resulting from reinfection with the tubercle bacillus.[194] Reinfection (secondary) tuberculosis of the skin is subdivided on the basis of various clinical features into lupus vulgaris, tuberculosis verrucosa, scrofuloderma, orificial tuberculosis and disseminated cutaneous tuberculosis.[205] The tuberculids are a further category and were thought to

represent a cutaneous reaction to a tuberculous infection elsewhere in the body, there being no detectable bacilli in the tuberculid skin lesions by conventional techniques.

This traditional classification has been disparaged somewhat, and a classification based on the presumed route of infection has been proposed.[206,207] Several modifications have already been suggested, but its basic format remains as follows:[208,209]

- infections due to inoculation from an *exogenous* source
- infections from an *endogenous* source, both contiguous (scrofuloderma in the traditional classification) and from autoinoculation (orificial tuberculosis)
- infections resulting from *hematogenous* spread.

The last of these three categories can be further subdivided into lupus vulgaris, acute disseminated tuberculosis, and the formation of cutaneous nodules or abscesses.

This relatively new system of classification has the advantage of applying to infections with atypical mycobacteria as well as those caused by *M. tuberculosis*. However, it still requires assumptions to be made when an attempt is made to classify an individual case. Furthermore, as infections with certain atypical mycobacteria (Buruli ulcer and swimming pool granuloma) are established clinical entities, it seems unlikely that this new classification will offer many advantages over the traditional one. Such has been the case. It should also be emphasized that cases occur which defy classification by any means, and it is quite appropriate to diagnose 'cutaneous tuberculosis' in these cases, pending the completion of cultural identification (if obtained).[205,210] Techniques using the polymerase chain reaction now provide a rapid and specific method for the identification of *M. tuberculosis* from tissue samples.[211–214] However, despite general enthusiasm for this technique,[215–219] a recent review concluded that PCR was not of much use in paucibacillary forms of cutaneous tuberculosis.[220] *M. tuberculosis* has also been identified by PCR in some cases of sarcoidosis.[221]

Any classification of cutaneous tuberculosis should also make provision for the complications of BCG vaccination.[222] These include local abscesses and secondary bacterial infections, lupus vulgaris,[223–225] lichen scrofulosorum,[226] lymphadenitis, scrofuloderma-like lesions and local keloid formation.[227] Fatalities have been recorded following BCG vaccination of individuals who are immunocompromised and develop disseminated disease.[228–231]

Of interest is the recent use of polyclonal anti-*Mycobacterium bovis* antibodies to detect bacterial and fungal microorganisms in paraffin-embedded tissue.[232] This technique is particularly useful in cases with only small numbers of organisms.

The following classification will be followed here:

- primary tuberculosis
- lupus vulgaris
- tuberculosis verrucosa
- scrofuloderma
- orificial tuberculosis
- disseminated cutaneous tuberculosis
- tuberculids.

Primary tuberculosis

Primary (inoculation) tuberculosis of the skin is the cutaneous analog of the pulmonary Ghon focus.[233] One to three weeks after introduction of the organism by way of a penetrating injury, a red indurated papule appears.[234–240] This subsequently ulcerates, forming a so-called 'tuberculoid chancre'. Ulcerated lesions may also be a manifestation of secondary (reinfection) tuberculosis,[241] when the source of infection may be endogenous or from inoculation, although secondary inoculation tuberculosis usually presents as tuberculosis verrucosa (see below).[242] Regional lymphadenopathy usually develops in primary tuberculosis.

Primary tuberculosis may be associated with tattooing,[234] ritual circumcision or injury by contaminated objects[243] to laboratory workers or to prosectors.[233,244] Sometimes no obvious source of infection can be identified, particularly in children.[245,246] Atypical mycobacteria are now implicated more often than *M. tuberculosis* in the etiology of primary tuberculous infection of the skin.

Histopathology[233]

Early lesions show a mixed dermal infiltrate of neutrophils, lymphocytes and plasma cells. This is followed by superficial necrosis and ulceration. After some weeks tuberculoid granulomas form, and these may be accompanied by caseation necrosis.[205] Acid-fast bacilli are usually easy to find in the early lesions, but there are very few bacilli once granulomas develop.

Lupus vulgaris

Lupus vulgaris is the most common form of reinfection tuberculosis, occurring predominantly in young adults.[247,248] It is caused almost exclusively by *M. tuberculosis* although rare reports implicating the *M. avium-intracellulare* complex and *M. bovis* have been published.[201,249,250] It has followed BCG vaccination.[225] Lupus vulgaris affects primarily the head and neck region, although in southeast Asia it appears to be more common on the extremities and buttocks.[251–254] Penile involvement can occur.[255] Lesions involving the nose and face can be destructive. The usual picture is of multiple erythematous papules forming a plaque, which on diascopy shows small 'apple jelly' nodules.[256,257] Crusted ulcers, local cellulitis[258] and dry verrucous plaques are sometimes seen.[251] The disease runs a chronic course and may result in significant scarring. Late complications include the development of contractures, lymphedema, squamous carcinoma[193,206,259,260] and, rarely, basal cell carcinoma,[261] malignant melanoma[262] and cutaneous lymphomas.[263,264]

Histopathology[251]

In lupus vulgaris there are tuberculoid granulomas with a variable mantle of lymphocytes in the upper and mid dermis.[247] The granulomas have a tendency to confluence (Fig. 23.7). Rarely they have a perifollicular arrangement.[265] Caseation is sometimes present. If prominent caseation is present in a facial lesion, granulomatous rosacea also needs consideration.[266] Multinucleate giant cells are not always numerous. Langerhans cells are present in moderate numbers in the granulomas.[267] The overlying epidermis may be atrophic or hyperplastic, but only rarely is there pseudoepitheliomatous hyperplasia. Transepidermal elimination of granulomas through a hyperplastic epidermis is rarely seen.[268] Bacilli are usually sparse and difficult to demonstrate in sections stained to show acid-fast organisms.[263] They can now be demonstrated using the polymerase chain reaction.[269,270] In one report, Michaelis–Gutmann bodies were present in macrophages in the infiltrate.[271]

Sometimes the histological appearances resemble sarcoidosis, with only a relatively sparse lymphocytic mantle around the granulomas: a consequent delay in making the correct diagnosis is common in such cases.[206,272]

Tuberculosis verrucosa

Tuberculosis verrucosa is an uncommon form of cutaneous tuberculosis resulting from inoculation of organisms into the skin in individuals with good immunity.[273] It may occur as an occupational hazard in the autopsy room. A verrucous plaque forms on the back of the hand or fingers.[205,274,275] The

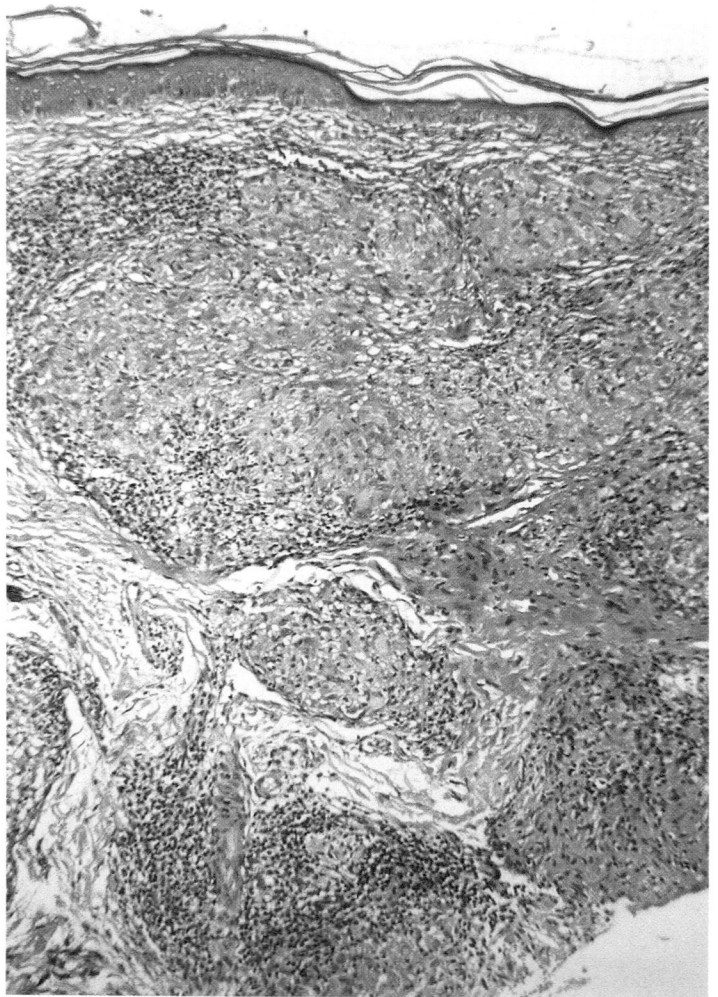

Fig. 23.7 **Lupus vulgaris.** There are tuberculoid granulomas, with a tendency to confluence, throughout the dermis. (H & E)

lower extremities are more often involved in cases occurring in India and Hong Kong.[194,276–279]

Histopathology[274]

There is hyperkeratosis and hyperplasia of the epidermis, often of pseudo-epitheliomatous proportions. In the mid dermis there are caseating granulomas.[195] Acid-fast bacilli can usually be found on careful examination of tissue sections.

Scrofuloderma

Scrofuloderma is tuberculous involvement of the skin resulting from direct extension from an underlying tuberculous lesion in lymph nodes or bone.[195,280] The term has also been used, incorrectly, for cases with presumptive cutaneous inoculation.[281] The neck and submandibular region are the most common sites.[282,283] Scrofuloderma usually presents as an undermined ulcer or discharging sinus, with surrounding induration and dusky red discoloration.[195,205,284,285] Non-tuberculous (atypical) mycobacteria are often responsible for this type of infection.

Histopathology[195]

The epidermis is usually atrophic or ulcerated, an underlying abscess and/or caseation necrosis involving the dermis and subcutis.[205] At the periphery of the necrotic tissue there are granulomas. They have fewer lymphocytes than is usual in tuberculosis, suggesting a weak cell-mediated immune response.[286] Acid-fast bacilli can usually be found in smears taken from the affected area, although they are not always demonstrable in tissue sections.[195]

Orificial tuberculosis

Orificial tuberculosis is a rare form of cutaneous tuberculosis that presents as shallow ulcers at mucocutaneous junctions in patients with advanced internal (usually pulmonary) tuberculosis.[214,287–290] It results from autoinoculation.[291] Perianal tuberculosis is a rare variant of orificial tuberculosis.[292]

Histopathology

There is ulceration with underlying caseating granulomas and numerous acid-fast bacilli.

Disseminated cutaneous tuberculosis

Disseminated cutaneous tuberculosis results from the dissemination of tubercle bacilli from pulmonary, meningeal or other tuberculous foci,[293] particularly in children.[283,294,295] There may be an underlying disturbance of the immune system predisposing to this widespread infection.[296] The usual presentation is with papules, pustules and vesicles that become necrotic, forming small ulcers.[205,296,297] Disseminated infection in patients with AIDS may take the form of multiple small pustules[203] or erythematous papules.[298]

Histopathology[299]

In early lesions there is focal necrosis and abscess formation, with numerous acid-fast bacilli, surrounded by a zone of non-specific chronic inflammation.[205,296] In older lesions granulomas usually develop in this outer zone. In the pustular lesions seen in patients with AIDS, there are numerous neutrophils in the papillary dermis, with rare Langhans giant cells.[203]

Tuberculids

Tuberculids are a heterogeneous group of cutaneous lesions which occur in association with tuberculous infections elsewhere in the body, or in other parts of the skin,[194,300–302] in patients with a high degree of immunity and allergic sensitivity to the organism.[303] Nevertheless, rare cases have been reported in patients with HIV infection.[304] Bacteria cannot be isolated from tuberculids, although *M. tuberculosis* DNA can be demonstrated in some cases using the polymerase chain reaction.[305] Response to antituberculous therapy has been recorded even in some cases in which no bacterial DNA could be detected.

The concept of tuberculids has been challenged from time to time, but they are usually considered to include erythema induratum–nodular vasculitis, lichen scrofulosorum and papulonecrotic tuberculid;[208] granulomatous phlebitis is possibly a fourth type (phlebitic tuberculid).[306,307] More than one type of tuberculid is sometimes present.[308,309]

Erythema induratum–nodular vasculitis. This is a panniculitis (see p. 524) which presents with bluish-red plaques and nodules, with a predilection for the lower part of the legs, particularly the calves.[310,311] The coexistence of this condition and papulonecrotic tuberculid has been reported.[312]

Lichen scrofulosorum. This tuberculid is characterized by asymptomatic, slightly scaly papules measuring 0.5–3 mm in diameter.[313–316] They are often follicular in distribution, mainly affecting the trunk of children and young adults.[314] Lichen scrofulosorum usually occurs in association with tuberculosis of bone or of lymph nodes, but it may be associated with tuberculous

infection in other sites;[313,314,317,318] rarely it may follow BCG vaccination[226] or infection with *M. avium*.[319]

Papulonecrotic tuberculid. This presents as dusky papules or nodules that sometimes undergo central necrosis and which leave varioliform scars on healing.[320–323] There is a predilection for the extremities, although the ears and genital region may also be involved.[324–326] It is uncommon in children.[327] In one study, a focus of tuberculosis was identified elsewhere in the body in 38% of cases.[310,328,329] The tuberculin test is usually strongly positive and the lesions respond to antituberculous drugs. In a number of cases *M. tuberculosis* DNA can be demonstrated in lesional skin by the polymerase chain reaction.[327,330] Non-tuberculous (atypical) mycobacteria have also been implicated.[331,332]

Histopathology

Erythema induratum–nodular vasculitis is a lobular panniculitis. It is not possible to diagnose which cases are due to tuberculosis on the histology alone (see p. 524). Traditionally, erythema induratum has been distinguished from nodular vasculitis on the basis of more prominent necrosis of the fat lobules and the extension of tuberculoid granulomas into the lower dermis.

Lichen scrofulosorum is characterized by non-caseating tuberculoid granulomas in the upper dermis;[333] the lesions have a perifollicular and eccrine localization.[314] Bacilli are not demonstrable.

Papulonecrotic tuberculid exhibits ulceration and V-shaped areas of necrosis, which include a variable thickness of dermis and the overlying epidermis. There is a surrounding palisade of histiocytes and chronic inflammatory cells, and an occasional well-formed granuloma.[320,327] Vessels in the vicinity show disruption and fibrinoid necrosis of their walls, sometimes with accompanying thrombosis or vasculitis.[202,334] Follicular necrosis or suppuration is present in approximately 20% of cases.[321] No bacilli can be demonstrated using routine staining methods.[320]

INFECTIONS BY NON-TUBERCULOUS (ATYPICAL) MYCOBACTERIA

The non-tuberculous (atypical, environmental) mycobacteria are a heterogeneous group of acid-fast bacteria which differ from *M. tuberculosis* in their clinical and cultural characteristics, as well as in their sensitivities to the various antimycobacterial drugs.[335,336] The traditional Runyon classification of the non-tuberculous (atypical) mycobacteria, which is based on colonial pigmentation, morphology and growth characteristics, is of no relevance to dermatopathology.

Non-tuberculous (atypical) mycobacteria can cause infections in the lungs, lymph nodes, meninges, synovium and skin.[335,337,338] Two species, *M. ulcerans* and *M. marinum*, result in well-defined clinicopathological entities known respectively as Buruli ulcer and swimming pool (fish tank) granuloma. They merit individual consideration. Cutaneous infections are rarely produced by the other non-tuberculous (atypical) mycobacteria; when they occur they are associated with a diversity of clinical and histopathological appearances that are not species specific.[193,339] Accordingly, they will be considered together after discussion of *M. ulcerans* and *M. marinum* infections.

Mycobacterium ulcerans infection (Buruli ulcer)

Infections with *Mycobacterium ulcerans* (Buruli ulcer, Bairnsdale ulcer) have been reported from many areas of central and west Africa,[340,341] as well as from New Guinea, Australia,[342] southeast Asia[343] and Mexico. The natural reservoir of the organism and the mode of transmission are unknown,[344] although current evidence suggests that infection is acquired through abraded skin after contact with contaminated water, soil or vegetation.[341] The organism grows preferentially at 32–33°C and produces an exotoxin which is responsible for tissue necrosis.[344]

M. ulcerans produces lesions that predominantly involve the skin and subcutaneous fat, and less commonly the underlying fascia, muscle and, rarely, bone. Systemic spread is exceedingly rare.[345] The initial lesion is usually a papule or pustule on the extremities, particularly on the lower part of the legs. Ulceration soon develops and may extend quite rapidly. The ulcer is painless and has a characteristic undermined edge.[346] Satellite lesions may develop.[344] Affected individuals are usually children or young adults.[341]

Histopathology[342,347]

The most striking feature is extensive 'coagulative' necrosis involving the dermis and subcutaneous fat, with remarkably little cellular infiltration (Figs 23.8, 23.9). The necrosis is probably caused by a macrolide toxin called mycolactone.[348] A septolobular panniculitis is present in some areas. In the viable margins there is a mixed inflammatory cell infiltrate. The epidermis at the margins of the ulceration shows variable changes; pseudoepitheliomatous hyperplasia may sometimes be present.[349] There is sometimes a vasculitis in-volving small vessels in the septa of the subcutaneous fat adjacent to areas of fat necrosis. There are usually numerous clumps of acid-fast bacilli, sometimes forming globular structures, in the necrotic tissue. These organisms are extracellular in location.

In long-standing or recurrent lesions there is usually a granulomatous response, although the granulomas are poorly defined. Caseation is absent. Organisms tend to be sparse in these lesions.

Calcification sometimes occurs in the necrotic tissues in cases of long standing.[350]

Mycobacterium marinum infection (swimming pool granuloma)

Mycobacterium marinum is a non-tuberculous (environmental, atypical) mycobacterium which has its natural habitat in brackish water, swimming pools and aquarium tanks.[351–354] In some areas it is the most common mycobacterial infection.[355] As it is unable to multiply at the temperature of the internal organs, the lesions that result from infection by it are usually confined to the skin. Involvement of the synovium and of the larynx[356] has been reported.

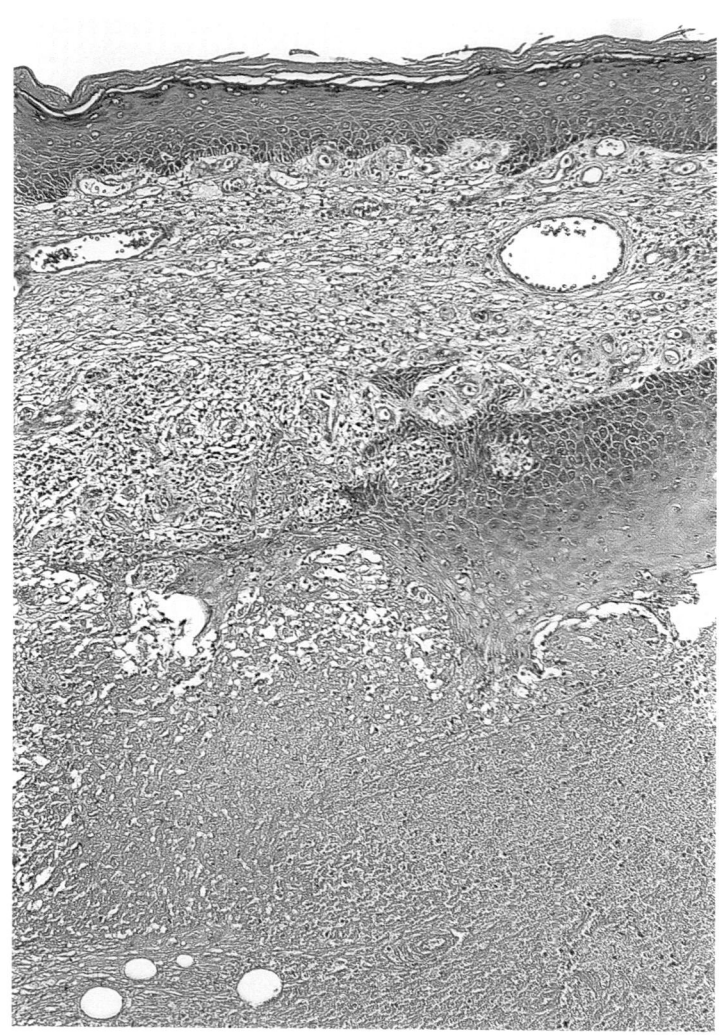

Fig. 23.8 *Mycobacterium ulcerans.* There is necrosis of the dermis with peripheral extension beyond the limits of the surface ulceration (so-called 'undermining'). An epidermal downgrowth is present at the edge of the ulcer. (H & E)

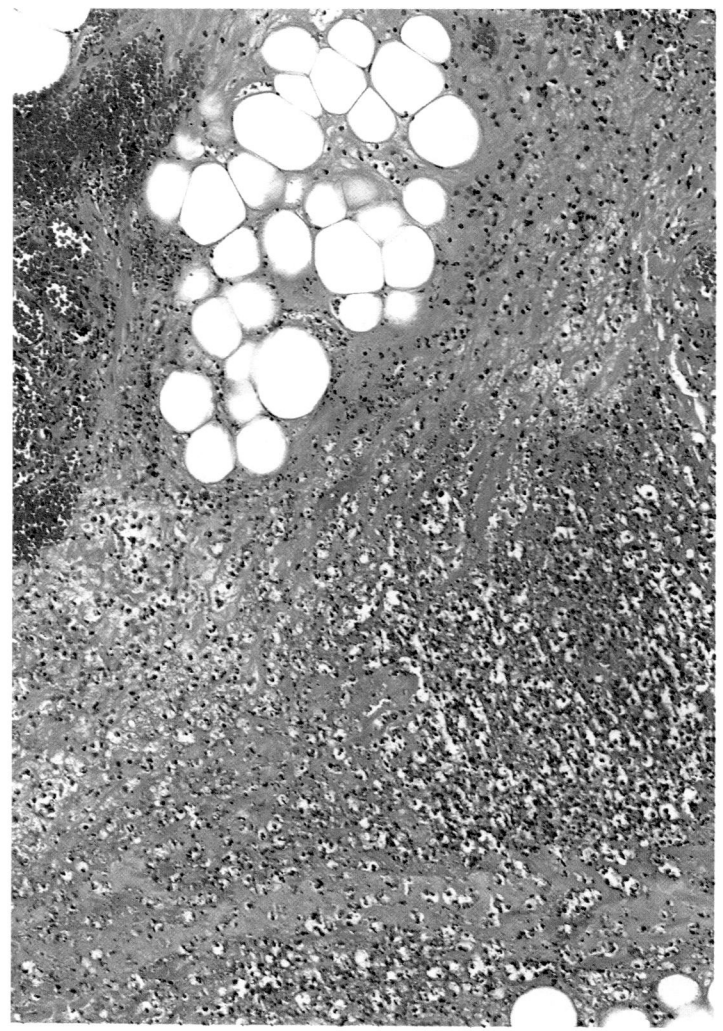

Fig. 23.9 *Mycobacterium ulcerans.* There is suppuration and necrosis in the subcutis. (H & E)

The cutaneous lesions are usually solitary verrucoid nodules or plaques on the elbows, hands or knees, which develop 1–2 weeks after superficial trauma, usually sustained in an aquatic environment.[357,358] Laboratory inoculation has also been reported.[359] Lesions may persist for months or years if untreated. Such cases have been seen among South Pacific Islanders, in whom untreated lesions have developed into extensive warty and ulcerated plaques.[360] Sometimes, in the so-called 'sporotrichoid' form of infection, there are multiple lesions along the course of the main superficial lymphatic vessels, reminiscent of the ascending lymphangitis of sporotrichosis.[351,361–364] More extensive cutaneous involvement has been reported in immunosuppressed individuals[355,365] and in a child.[366,367]

Histopathology[368–370]

The inflammatory process is usually confined to the dermis, although in the sporotrichoid form subcutaneous involvement is more common. The changes are quite variable, and range from a mostly acute process with suppuration to granuloma formation.[370] The granulomas are usually poorly formed; there is no evidence of caseation. Some neutrophils may be admixed, in places forming suppurative granulomas. A chronic inflammatory cell infiltrate is present between the granulomas and foci of suppuration. Epidermal changes are variable and include ulceration, acanthosis and sometimes even pseudoepitheliomatous hyperplasia.

Acid-fast bacilli are found in a minority of cases.[368] The organisms tend to be longer and fatter than *M. tuberculosis*, and sometimes they show transverse bands.[352] Rarely, organisms are abundant.[369] Isolation of the organism is readily achieved in culture at 30–33°C. PCR-based methods are now being used to confirm the diagnosis.[363]

Other non-tuberculous (atypical) mycobacteria

There is a miscellaneous group of non-tuberculous (atypical) mycobacteria that produce a diverse range of cutaneous lesions, including solitary verrucous nodules,[371] ulcers,[372,373] abscesses,[374] cellulitis,[375] rosacea-like lesions,[376] spindle-cell pseudotumors[348,377–379] and sporotrichoid nodules.[380,381] Infection may follow minor trauma,[382] injections,[383] biopsy and surgical procedures[384,385] and the implantation of prostheses, or occur in immunosuppressed individuals.[374,386] The species involved include *M. kansasii*,[240,332,374,375,387–392] *M. haemophilum*,[393–396] *M. scrofulaceum*,[397] *M. szulgai*,[398,399] *M. gordonae*,[371,377,400] the *M. avium-intracellulare* complex,[297,401–411] *M. fortuitum*,[385,412–414] *M. abscessus*[415–417] and *M. chelonae* (formerly *M. chelonei*).[382,383,386,418–422] The advent of PCR has allowed *M. avium* to be distinguished from *M. intracellulare* but few reports have appeared using this new technique for this purpose.[319] An increasing number of disseminated infections caused by the *M. avium-intracellulare* complex are being reported in patients with the acquired immunodeficiency syndrome (AIDS), although cutaneous lesions are uncommon in these cases.[403,423–426] They are sometimes seen after the initiation of highly active antiretroviral therapy (HAART). The appearance of skin lesions is thought to be a manifestation of partial immune restoration revealing a latent mycobacterial infection.[427,428] This organism has been reported, limited to the skin, in a patient with systemic lupus erythematosus.[429] It has also been isolated from lesional skin in a case of erythema multiforme.[430]

Histopathology[193]

The changes are not species specific. They include tuberculoid granulomas, poorly formed granulomas, non-specific chronic inflammation, suppuration and intermediate forms.[193] Less common patterns include a septal[431] or mixed lobular and septal panniculitis,[193] a necrotizing folliculitis[432] and a diffuse histiocytic infiltrate in the dermis resembling lepromatous leprosy[402,433] or the cells of Gaucher's disease.[434] The presence of poorly formed granulomas

with intervening chronic inflammation and foci of suppuration should always raise the suspicion of an infection by atypical mycobacteria. The location of the inflammation is inconstant, with no specific relationship to the organism or the type of inflammation.[193] The inflammation is mostly centered on the dermis, with some extension into the subcutis; the latter is more likely in immunosuppressed patients.[432]

Infections caused by *M. haemophilum* are posing an increasing diagnostic problem. They may present with non-granulomatous or pauci-granulomatous reactions without necrosis. A mixed suppurative and granulomatous reaction is still the most common pattern seen with this organism, but lichenoid (interface) and non-specific perivascular inflammation as well as necrotizing lymphocytic vasculitis are sometimes reported.[395]

In cases with spindle-cell pseudotumors there are plump to spindle-shaped cells with a histiocytic to myofibroblastic appearance.[377,379] The stroma contains collagen bundles of variable thickness.

Organisms are difficult to find, even in preparations stained to demonstrate acid-fast bacilli. They may be plentiful in cases with a histiocytoid pattern and in some infections with *M. avium* and *M. intracellulare*, although they are rarely as plentiful as in infections with *M. ulcerans*. The bacilli of *M. kansasii* are larger, broader and more coarsely beaded than other mycobacteria.[348] Grains formed of bacillary clumps and somewhat resembling those seen in mycetomas have been reported in a case of *M. chelonae* infection.[418] Intracellular non-tuberculous (atypical) mycobacteria have been said to be PAS positive, according to one report.[435] It should be noted that *Vibrio extorquens*, a rare cause of skin ulcers, is weakly acid fast in tissue sections;[436] granulomas may also be present. Also in this category (skin lesions with granulomas and acid-fast bacilli) are the lesions caused by *Rhodococcus*.[437]

LEPROSY

Leprosy (lepra) is a chronic infection caused by *Mycobacterium leprae*. It affects mainly the skin, nasal mucosa and peripheral nerves. Leprosy is most prevalent in tropical countries, particularly India, southeast Asia, central Africa and Central and South America. In India, which has two-thirds of the global leprosy burden, the case detection rate has remained stubbornly around 5 per 10 000 population.[438]

M. leprae is an obligate, intracellular, Gram-positive organism which is also acid fast, though less so than *M. tuberculosis*. The organism cannot be grown in vitro, although claims of successful cultivation are made from time to time.[439] *M. leprae* can be grown in the footpads of mice and in the nine-banded armadillo, an animal in which natural infection also occurs. *M. leprae* shares many antigens with other mycobacteria; it also possesses a unique antigen, phenolic glycolipid-1 (PGL-1).[440,441] Experimental studies are currently attempting to determine the exact role of the various components of the immune system in the defense against this organism.[442] *M. leprae* is found predominantly in three main cell types in the skin – Schwann cells, endothelial/perithelial cells and cells of the monocyte-macrophage system.[443]

The incubation period of leprosy is not known with certainty, but is thought to average 5 years.[440] This uncertainty and the long period make any study of the mode of transmission difficult. The organism is of low infectivity, and prolonged and/or close contact with patients who have the disease is considered necessary for transmission to occur.[444] The incidence of conjugal leprosy is low, further testimony to its low infectivity.[445] Contact with the armadillo may be an important source of infection in some countries.[446] There may also be a genetic predisposition to the disease.[447] The portal of entry of the organism is not known, but the skin and upper respiratory tract, particularly the nasal mucosa, are probable sites.[448] Droplet infection is the most likely mode of transmission, although rare cases of inoculation infection have been recorded.[448,449]

Concurrent infection with *M. tuberculosis* is rare, even in endemic countries.[450]

Clinical classification of leprosy

Leprosy exhibits a spectrum of clinical characteristics that correlate with the histopathological changes and the immunological status of the individual.[440,443,451–454] At one end of the spectrum is tuberculoid leprosy (TT), which is a highly resistant form with few lesions and a paucity of organisms (paucibacillary leprosy).[455] At the other end is lepromatous leprosy (LL), in which there are numerous lesions with myriad bacilli (multibacillary leprosy), and an associated defective cellular immune response.[455,456] In between these poles there are clinical forms which are classified as borderline-tuberculoid (BT), borderline (BB) and borderline-lepromatous (BL) leprosy. The clinical state of an individual may alter along this scale, although the polar forms (TT and LL) are the most stable and the borderline form (BB) the most labile. This categorization, known as the Ridley–Jopling classification,[452,457] is often modified by the addition of subpolar forms at either end of the spectrum (TTs and LLs), giving additional categories of subpolar lepromatous leprosy and subpolar tuberculoid leprosy. In the author's view this is taking 'splitting' to a level that is difficult to justify. There is also an indeterminate form of leprosy, which is classically the first lesion to develop although it may be overlooked clinically.

Indeterminate leprosy is most often recognized in endemic regions.[458] It presents as single or multiple slightly hypopigmented or faintly erythematous macules, usually on the limbs.[459] Sensation is normal or only slightly impaired. Indeterminate lesions often heal spontaneously, but in approximately 25% of cases this form develops into one of the determinate types, usually in the borderline region of the spectrum.[445] The clinical features of the determinate forms will now be considered in further detail.

Tuberculoid leprosy (TT) is a relatively stable form and the most common type in India and Africa.[445] There are one or several sharply defined reddish-brown anesthetic plaques which are distributed asymmetrically on the trunk or limbs.[460] An enlarged nerve may be seen entering and leaving the plaque; other superficial nerves, such as the ulnar and popliteal nerves, may also be enlarged, leading to nerve palsy.[460] Giant nerve 'abscesses' may occur.[461] The lepromin test is positive. This category is often divided into polar and subpolar forms.

Borderline-tuberculoid leprosy (BT) is usually associated with more numerous lesions than tuberculoid leprosy, and these are usually smaller. Daughter (satellite) patches may develop. Hypoesthesia and impairment of hair growth within the lesions are often present.[445]

Borderline leprosy (BB) is an unstable form with erythematous or copper-colored infiltrated patches which are often annular. Margins are often ill defined.

Borderline-lepromatous leprosy (BL) is associated with more numerous lesions that are less well defined, more shiny and less anesthetic than those at the tuberculoid end of the spectrum. Nodular lesions resembling those seen in lepromatous leprosy may be present. A rare subepidermal bullous form has been reported.[462] Nerve involvement, without cutaneous lesions other than hypoesthesia, has been seen.[463,464]

Lepromatous leprosy (LL) usually develops from borderline or borderline-lepromatous forms by a downgrading reaction. Polar and subpolar forms have been recognized. It is a systemic disease, although the primary clinical manifestations are in the skin.[465] Mucosal involvement may lead to ulceration of the nasal septum, whereas nerve lesions may result in acral anesthesia, claw hand and foot drop.[445] The cutaneous lesions, which are usually symmetrical, include multiple small macules, infiltrated plaques and nodules with poorly defined borders. Multiple facial nodules give a bovine appearance, and this is usually accompanied by sparse eyebrows.[445] Various autoantibodies have been demonstrated in this form of leprosy.[466] This may explain the increased incidence of vitiligo.[467]

Histoid leprosy is a rare variant of the nodular variety of lepromatous leprosy, and is characterized by the presence of cutaneous and/or sub-cutaneous nodules and plaques on apparently normal skin.[468–471] It may be caused by a drug-resistant strain of *M. leprae*, as it usually develops in cases of long standing.[469]

Although only a few instances of leprosy have been reported in patients with AIDS, the long incubation period and its occurrence in areas of central Africa where AIDS is also endemic suggest that leprosy complicating AIDS may be a problem in the future.[472–474]

Visceral leprosy is more common than would appear from the little attention it has received. A significant number of patients with internal organ involvement by *M. leprae* are asymptomatic. An excellent review of this topic has recently appeared.[475]

Reactional states in leprosy[445]

Reactional states are acute episodes that interrupt the usual chronic course and clinical stability of leprosy.[476,477] They are expressions of immunological instability. Pregnancy, which causes a relative decrease in cellular immunity, may precipitate a reactional state.[478] The reactions, which are major causes of tissue injury and morbidity, have been subdivided into three variants: the lepra reaction (type I), erythema nodosum leprosum (type II), and Lucio's phenomenon (sometimes included with type II reactions, at other times designated type III).[476,479] Not included in these categories, but nevertheless a manifestation of an upgrading reaction, is the rare sporotrichoid pattern caused by spread along peripheral nerves.[480]

Lepra (type I) reactions occur in borderline leprosy, and are usually associated with a shift toward the tuberculoid pole (upgrading) as a result of an increase in delayed hypersensitivity. Uncommonly the shift is toward the lepromatous pole (a downgrading reaction).[477,481] Lepra reactions are often seen in the first 6 months or so of therapy, but they may occur in untreated patients or be associated with pregnancy, stress or intercurrent infections. They are characterized by edema and increased erythema of skin lesions, sometimes accompanied by ulceration and the development of new lesions. Constitutional symptoms and neuritis may be present.

Erythema nodosum leprosum (type II reaction) occurs in 25–70% of all cases of lepromatous leprosy,[476,482] and occasionally in association with the borderline-lepromatous form.[483,484] There are crops of painful, erythematous and violaceous nodules, particularly involving the extremities.[485] Individual lesions last 7–20 days.[486] Severe constitutional symptoms may be present.[486] The pattern varies somewhat in severity in different ethnic groups,[479] necrotizing lesions sometimes developing.[487] Type II reactions are the result of an immune complex-mediated vasculitis,[483] although the participation of certain cytokines indicates that some cell-mediated components are involved.[488]

Lucio's phenomenon is seen mainly in Mexicans with the diffuse non-nodular form of lepromatous leprosy.[486,489] It is rare in other ethnic groups.[490] Hemorrhagic ulcers form as a result of the underlying necrotizing vasculitis[491] or of vascular occlusion due to endothelial swelling and thrombosis.[489]

Histopathology[445,457]

Skin biopsies should include the full thickness of the dermis and should be taken from the most active edge of a lesion. The bacilli may be detected in tissue sections using the Fite–Faraco staining method or an immunofluorescent technique.[492]

Two distinct types of histological changes are found in leprosy: the *lepromatous reaction*, in which large numbers of macrophages in the dermis are parasitized with acid-fast bacilli (Fig. 23.10), and the *tuberculoid reaction*, in which there are tubercle-like aggregates of epithelioid cells, multinucleate giant cells and lymphocytes, bacilli being difficult to find. These histological patterns are seen at either end of the clinical spectrum of leprosy; features overlapping with those of borderline forms may be present. Sometimes there is a disparity between the clinical and the histological subclassification of leprosy.[493] Early lesions are mostly of indeterminate or tuberculoid type.[494]

Indeterminate leprosy is characterized by a superficial and deep dermal infiltrate around blood vessels, dermal appendages and nerves, composed predominantly of lymphocytes with a few macrophages (Fig. 23.11).[452] Mast cells are markedly increased in number and they may extend into the small nerves in the deep dermis.[495] Less than 5% of the dermis is involved by the infiltrate.[495] Mild proliferation of Schwann cells may occur, but marked neural thickening is quite uncommon.[459] There may be a few lymphocytes in the epidermis; this is one of the earliest changes to occur in leprosy.[494] Bacilli are usually quite difficult to find,[494] but if serial sections are cut and a small dermal nerve is followed, sooner or later a single bacillus or a small group of bacilli will be discovered.[458] The mechanism of the hypopigmentation in this and other forms of leprosy is still not clear. There is a reduction in melanin in the basal layer; in some reports a decreased number of melanocytes has also been recorded.[496]

Tuberculoid leprosy (polar and subpolar) shows a tuberculoid reaction throughout the dermis, with non-caseating granulomas composed of epithelioid cells, some Langhans giant cells and lymphocytes (Fig. 23.12).[460] The predominant lymphocyte present is the T-helper cell, which is found throughout the granuloma, whereas T-suppressor cells predominate in the lymphocyte mantle that surrounds the granulomas.[497,498] There are said to be fewer lymphocytes in the *subpolar* form, a rather tenuous feature on which to base a distinct category. Granulomas may erode the undersurface of the epidermis and they may also extend into peripheral nerves and into the arrectores pilorum.[460] Inflammation often engulfs the sweat glands.[494] Bacilli are found in less than 50% of cases.[460]

Borderline-tuberculoid leprosy differs from tuberculoid leprosy in several ways.[445] Tubercle formation may be less evident and nerve destruction is not as complete. A subepidermal grenz zone is invariably present. Lymphocytes and Langhans cells are usually not as plentiful in the granulomas as in tuberculoid leprosy.

In *borderline leprosy* there are collections of epithelioid cells without the formation of well-defined granulomas. Langhans giant cells are absent and lymphocytes are more dispersed. Occasional bacilli can be found.

In *borderline-lepromatous leprosy* there are small collections of macrophages rather than epithelioid cells. These large cells have abundant granular cytoplasm, although a few may have foamy cytoplasm as seen in lepromatous leprosy.[445] A variable number of lymphocytes is present, and some of these are in the vicinity of small dermal nerves. A grenz zone is present in both borderline-lepromatous and true lepromatous leprosy. Bacilli are easily found.

Lepromatous leprosy (polar and subpolar) is characterized by collections and sheets of heavily parasitized macrophages with a sparse sprinkling of lymphocytes, the majority of which are of suppressor type (Fig. 23.13).[498] In older lesions the macrophages have a foamy appearance (lepra cells, Virchow cells). Numerous acid-fast bacilli are present in macrophages, sweat glands, nerves, Schwann cells and vascular endothelium,[499] a finding which has been confirmed by electron microscopy.[500] The macrophages express S100 protein.[501] The organisms in the macrophages may be arranged in parallel array, forming clusters, or in large masses known as globi (Fig. 23.14). In the *subpolar* form, there are fewer globi and a few more T lymphocytes than in the polar form.[501]

In *histoid leprosy* there are circumscribed nodular lesions consisting predominantly of spindle-shaped cells with some polygonal forms. The cells are arranged in an intertwining pattern.[468,469] Some cases may resemble a

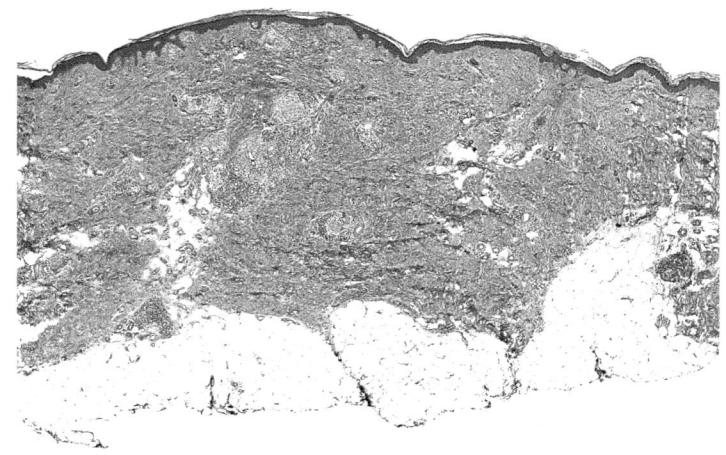

A

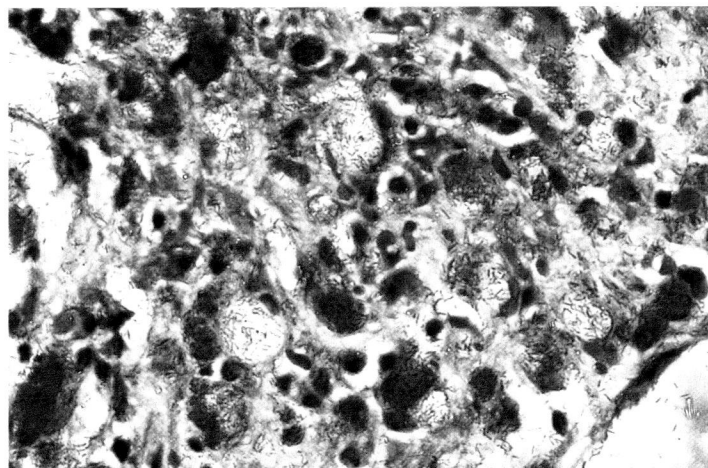

Fig. 23.10 **Lepromatous leprosy.** Numerous acid-fast bacilli are present within macrophages and lying free in the dermis. (Wade–Fite)

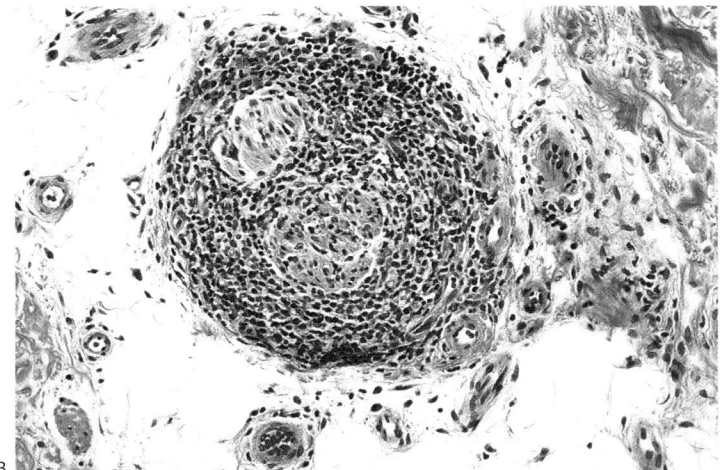

B

Fig. 23.11 **(A) Indeterminate leprosy. (B)** There is a superficial and deep infiltrate of lymphocytes with periappendageal and perineural extension. Epithelioid cells are present. (H & E)

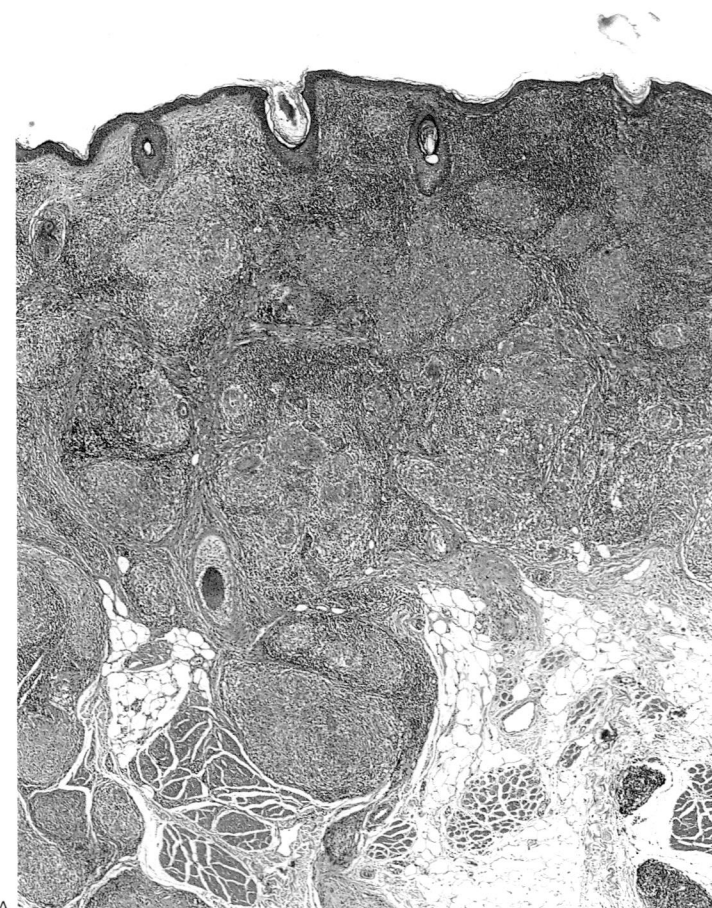

A

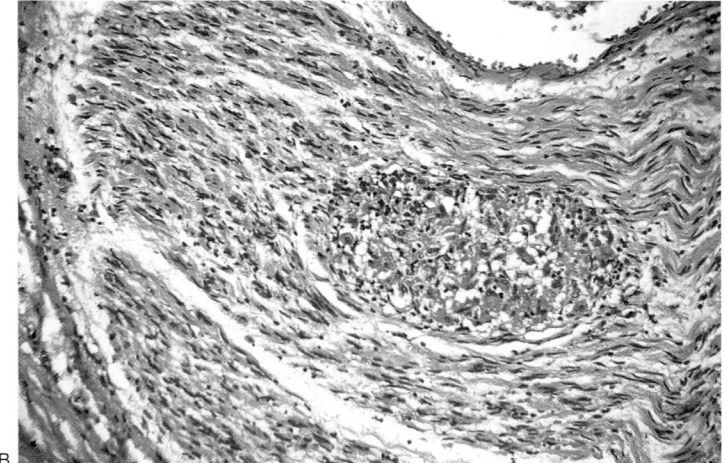

B

Fig. 23.12 **Tuberculoid leprosy. (A)** Non-caseating granulomas extend throughout the dermis. **(B)** A deep cutaneous nerve contains a granuloma. (H & E)

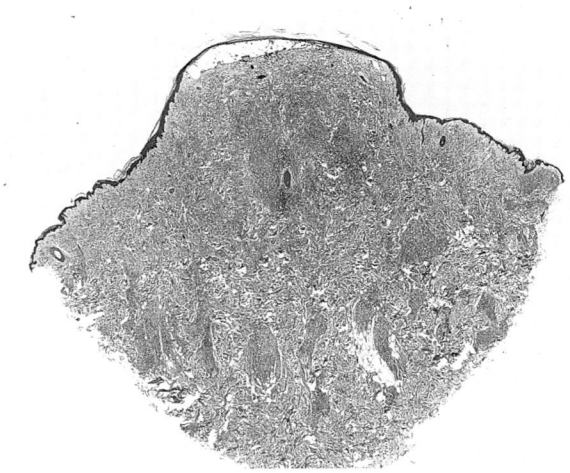

Fig. 23.13 **Lepromatous leprosy.** This case had numerous parasitized foamy macrophages with masses of organisms. (H & E)

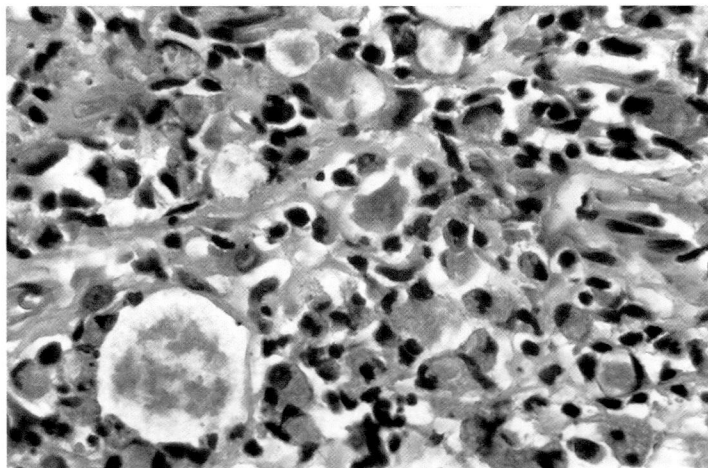

Fig. 23.14 **Lepromatous leprosy** with masses of organisms (globi) in the cytoplasm of macrophages. (H & E)

Lepra (type I) reactions show edema, an increase in lymphocytes and sometimes giant cells, as well as the formation of small clusters of epithelioid cells.[502,503] In severe cases fibrinoid necrosis may be present, and this is followed by scarring.[481] This is the picture seen in the usual upgrading reaction. In downgrading reactions there is replacement of lymphocytes and epithelioid cells by collections of macrophages, and there is a corresponding increase in the number of bacilli.[481]

Erythema nodosum leprosum is characterized by edema of the papillary dermis and a mixed dermal infiltrate of neutrophils and lymphocytes superimposed on collections of macrophages.[483] There are relatively more T lymphocytes of helper-inducer type than in non-reactive lepromatous leprosy.[497,504] This appears to be due to an absolute reduction in the number of T-suppressor (CD8⁺) cells.[505] A vasculitis may also be present.[483,486] There may be involvement of the subcutis, with the development of a mixed lobular and septal panniculitis; however, in the majority of cases involvement of the dermis is the primary and predominant finding.[487] Macrophages in the dermis contain fragmented organisms.[506] Direct immunofluorescence reveals the presence of C3 and IgG in the walls of dermal blood vessels.[483]

Lucio's phenomenon is usually the result of a necrotizing vasculitis of the small vessels in the upper and mid dermis, with associated infarction of the

fibrohistiocytic tumor (Fig. 23.15). Small collections of foamy macrophages may also be present. The component cells contain numerous acid-fast bacilli, which are longer than the usual bacilli of leprosy and are aligned along the long axis of the cell.[469] The spindle-shaped cells are dermal dendritic cells expressing factor XIIIa.[501]

dilated. Fibrin thrombi are sometimes present. Inflammatory cells are often surprisingly sparse, although sometimes a florid cellulitis is present with focal abscess formation.[508] Spongiosis and vesiculation may occur in the epidermis adjacent to the ulceration.

B. anthracis can be seen, usually in large numbers, in the exudate. It is easily recognized by its large size, square-cut ends and a tendency to be in chains. It is Gram positive. If antibiotic therapy has been given organisms are sparse and often do not stain positively by the Gram procedure.

BRUCELLOSIS

Cutaneous involvement occurs in 5–10% of patients with brucellosis.[511] It takes the form of a disseminated papulonodular eruption or a maculopapular rash.[511,512] Occasionally erythema nodosum-like nodules develop. Skin lesions may not develop for many weeks after the onset of symptoms of brucellosis.[511] A dermatitis has also been reported on the forearms of veterinarians involved in the manual removal of placentas from aborting cows infected with *Brucella abortus*.[512]

Histopathology[511,512]

The maculopapular lesions usually have a non-specific appearance with a mild perivascular infiltrate of lymphocytes in the upper dermis.[512] The papulonodules have an infiltrate of lymphocytes and histiocytes, which is both perivascular and periadnexal. There is also focal granulomatous change; multinucleate giant cells are uncommon. Focal exocytosis of inflammatory cells and keratinocyte necrosis may also be present. A leukocytoclastic vasculitis is exceedingly rare.[513]

The erythema nodosum-like lesions show a septal panniculitis, with considerable extension of the infiltrate into the fat lobules accompanied by focal necrosis. Plasma cells are also abundant. These features are not usually associated with lesions of typical erythema nodosum.

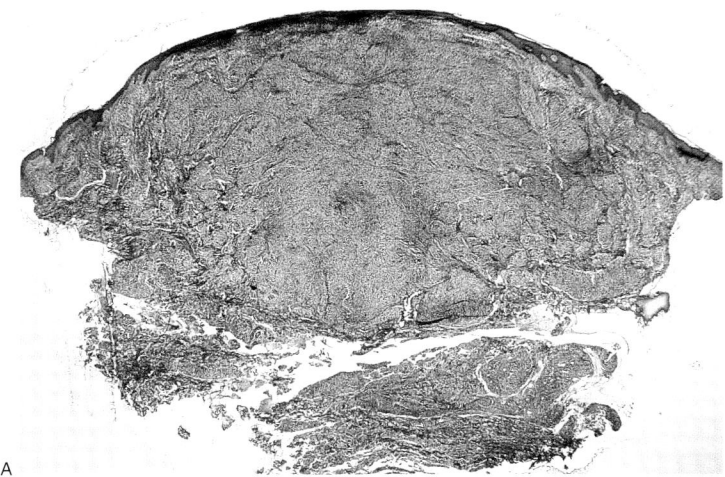

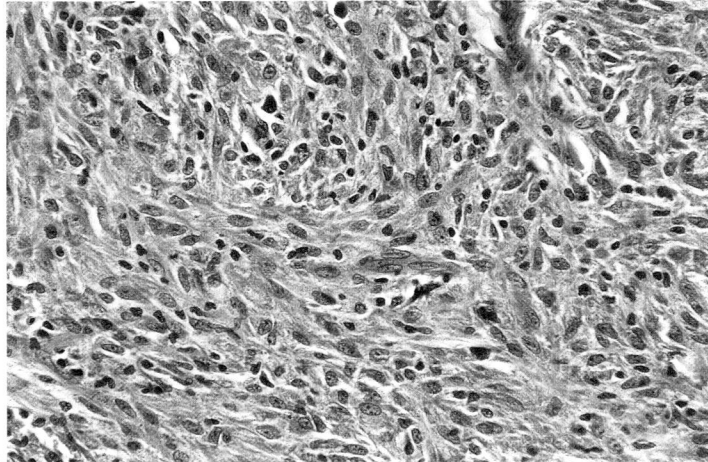

Fig. 23.15 **(A) Histoid leprosy. (B)** The cells mimic a fibrohistiocytic tumor. (H & E)

epidermis.[486] At other times there is prominent endothelial swelling and thrombosis of superficial vessels without a vasculitis.[489] The endothelial cells and macrophages in the dermis contain numerous bacilli.[486,490] There is usually only a mild inflammatory infiltrate, with fewer neutrophils than in erythema nodosum leprosum.[490]

YERSINIOSIS

Yersiniosis is a generally accepted term for diseases caused by *Yersinia pseudotuberculosis* and *Y. enterocolitica*. The incidence of cutaneous manifestations in yersiniosis is not known, although in some countries the disease is responsible for 10% or more of cases of erythema nodosum.[514,515] Erythema multiforme and figurate and non-specific erythemas may also occur.[514,516]

Histopathology

As in brucellosis, the erythema nodosum-like lesions may show some extension of the infiltrate into the fat lobules, as well as a necrotizing vasculitis and some necrosis.[514] The appearances in some cases are more in keeping with erythema induratum–nodular vasculitis than with erythema nodosum.

MISCELLANEOUS BACTERIAL INFECTIONS

ANTHRAX

Anthrax is mainly an occupational disease occurring in those who handle hair, wool, hide or the carcasses of infected animals.[507–509] The causative organism, *Bacillus anthracis*, may enter the body by the skin or by inhalation or ingestion. Anthrax is now an exceedingly rare infection.[510]

The initial cutaneous lesion is usually on an exposed site. It begins as a papule, which soon becomes bullous and then ulcerates, with the formation of a hemorrhagic crust (eschar). A ring of satellite vesicles may form. Hemorrhagic lymphadenopathy, constitutional symptoms and even a fatal septicemia may accompany the cutaneous lesion.

Histopathology[507,508]

There is necrosis of the epidermis and upper dermis, with surrounding edema, fibrin extravasation and hemorrhage. The blood vessels are conspicuously

GRANULOMA INGUINALE

Granuloma inguinale (granuloma venereum, donovanosis) is a sexually transmitted disease caused by a small Gram-negative bacillus, *Calymmatobacterium granulomatis*.[517] It has a relatively low level of infectivity. Clinically, the external genitalia are involved in most cases[518,519] but occasionally anal, vaginal, oral or extragenital cutaneous involvement is found.[520] The disease begins after an incubation period of from 2 to 4 weeks. The initial manifestation is a papule, which soon ulcerates. The lesion slowly spreads and may cause extensive destruction of the penis or vulva.[521–524] It may also spread to involve the adjacent parts of the thighs or lower abdomen.[520] An association with HIV infection has been recorded.[524] Squamous cell carcinoma may supervene, but care should be taken not to misinterpret the marginal pseudoepitheliomatous hyperplasia as carcinomatous.[520]

The diagnosis is easily made by examination of tissue smears stained by the Wright or Giemsa methods. Smears will show large mononuclear cells containing a number of the organisms, which appear as red-stained intracytoplasmic encapsulated ovoid structures with prominent polar granules. The organism can be cultured in an egg-yolk medium, and also by inoculation of the yolk sac of chick embryos.

Histopathology[520,525]

The center of the lesion is usually ulcerated, and at the margins there is often well-marked pseudoepitheliomatous hyperplasia. Plasma cells and macrophages predominate in the base of the ulcer, and there are often scattered neutrophil microabscesses as well. Blood vessels are prominent in the ulcer base, and sometimes endothelial swelling is present.[525] Transepithelial elimination of macrophages with cytoplasmic organisms has been reported through areas of pseudoepitheliomatous hyperplasia.[526] The diagnosis is made by finding parasitized macrophages. These are large cells, measuring 20 μm in diameter. Organisms are seldom numerous, but they can be recognized – if with some difficulty – in hematoxylin and eosin sections. They are more readily found in silver preparations, such as the Warthin–Starry method (Fig. 23.16), or when stained with Giemsa's solution. Plastic-embedded semithin sections enhance diagnosis.[527] In these sections, and in smears, the vacuolated nature of the cytoplasm of the parasitized macrophages can be appreciated. The organisms (Donovan bodies) are present singly or in clusters in the vacuoles (Fig. 23.17). They measure 1–2 μm in diameter, and show bipolar staining in silver preparations. For this reason they have been likened to minute safety pins. There may be up to several dozen in a macrophage.

Electron microscopy

The organism, which has a prominent capsule but no flagella, may be seen within phagosomes of macrophages.[528]

CHANCROID

Chancroid is a sexually transmitted disease caused by the Gram-negative bacillus *Haemophilus ducreyi*.[529–533] It has a short incubation period and presents as painful, irregular, non-indurated single or multiple ulcers, usually in the genital area or perineum.[534–536] Clinically, the ulcers may sometimes be difficult to distinguish from granuloma inguinale, or even herpes simplex.[536,537] Approximately half of the patients have tender inguinal lymphadenopathy, and occasionally draining sinuses arise from the suppurating nodes.

Chancroid is now seen less frequently than previously in Western countries, usually occurring as limited, but significant outbreaks.[538–541] However, it is a major cause of genital ulceration in Africa, where it appears to facilitate the heterosexual spread of the human immunodeficiency virus.[542] Gram-negative rods forming parallel chains ('school of fish' appearance) may be seen in smears. Selective agars are also available that facilitate the rapid isolation of *H. ducreyi*.[543,544]

Histopathology[529,540]

There is usually a broad area of ulceration, in the base of which three zones can be discerned. Superficially there is tissue necrosis, fibrin, red cells and neutrophils. Beneath this is a zone of vascular proliferation, with prominent endothelial cells and a mixed inflammatory infiltrate. In the deepest zone the

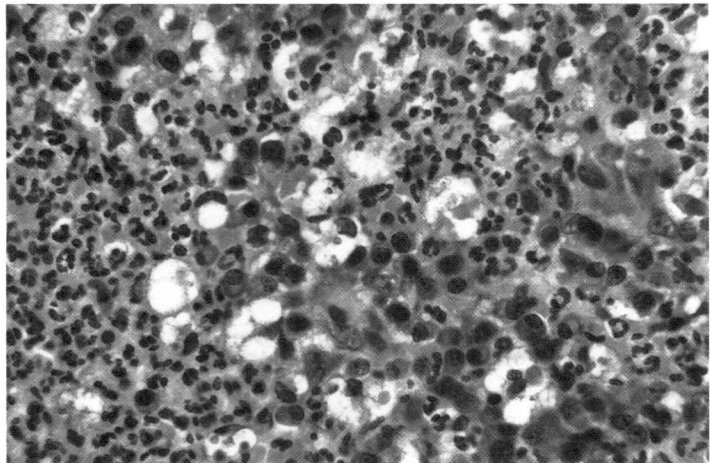
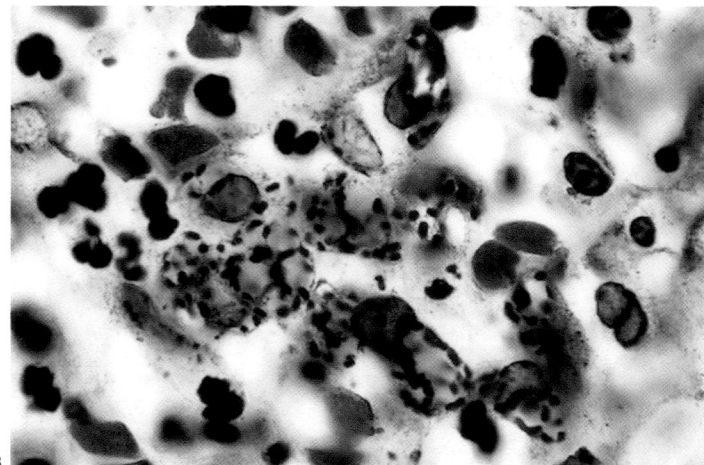

Fig. 23.16 **Granuloma inguinale. (A)** The infiltrate consists of neutrophils, plasma cells and parasitized macrophages (H & E). **(B)** The organisms can be seen in the cytoplasm of macrophages in this silver preparation. (Warthin–Starry)

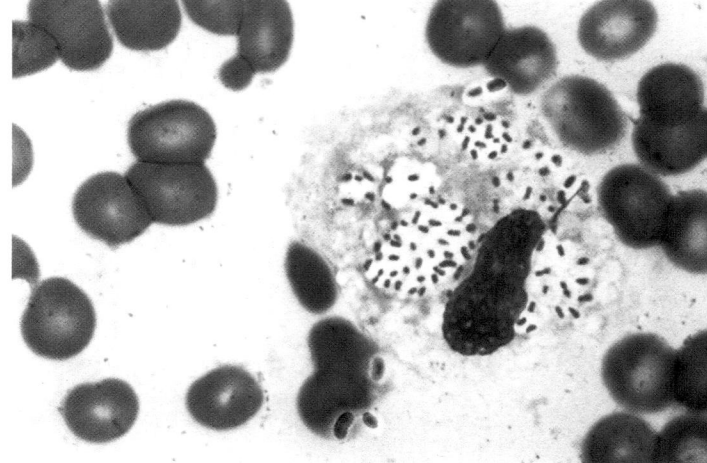

Fig. 23.17 **Imprint from a vulval lesion of granuloma inguinale.** Numerous organisms are present in vacuoles in the cytoplasm of a macrophage. (Giemsa)

infiltrate is more chronic, with plasma cells and lymphocytes predominating. The epidermis adjacent to the ulcer shows acanthosis, some overlying parakeratosis and occasional intraepidermal microabscesses.

A Giemsa stain or a silver impregnation method shows organisms both singly and in short chains, lying free and within histiocytes in the base of the ulcer.

RHINOSCLEROMA

Rhinoscleroma is a chronic inflammatory disease of the nasal and oral mucosa caused by the Gram-negative bacillus *Klebsiella rhinoscleromatis*.[545] In advanced cases it may spread to involve the larynx, trachea, bronchi and lips.[546] Rhinoscleroma is endemic in parts of Africa, Asia and Latin America. It is spread by direct or indirect contact. The incubation period is long.[545] Rhinoscleroma is an opportunistic infection that can occur in patients infected with the human immunodeficiency virus.[547]

Initially there is a non-specific rhinitis with the development of a purulent nasal discharge and some hypertrophy of the inflamed mucous membrane.[545] This is followed by an infiltrative and nodular stage, during which the involved tissues become swollen and eventually deformed.[546] Obstruction of the nasal cavity can be caused by the friable inflammatory masses. There is scarring and further deformity in the late stages.

Histopathology

In the fully developed lesions of rhinoscleroma the changes are diagnostic, with a variable admixture of plasma cells with conspicuous Russell bodies, and large mononuclear cells with vacuolated cytoplasm (Mikulicz cells) (Fig. 23.18). In addition there are some lymphocytes and foci of neutrophils. The Mikulicz cell, which varies from 10 to 100 μm in diameter, is a macrophage.[548] The causative organisms may be seen in the cytoplasm of these cells in PAS and Gram preparations. However, they are best visualized with silver impregnation methods, particularly the Warthin–Starry stain (Fig. 23.19).[549] The organisms can also be seen in smears from the lesions, and they are easily cultured.

The dense inflammatory infiltrate may cause ulceration or atrophy of the overlying mucosa. Sometimes the mucosa is hyperplastic, even to the extent of pseudoepitheliomatous hyperplasia.[549]

Electron microscopy

The vacuolated Mikulicz cells are macrophages with phagosomes containing bacterial mucopolysaccharide as well as some bacteria.[548] There is often fragmentation of the limiting membrane of some of the phagosomes.[548] Plasma cells are sometimes vacuolated to a limited extent. Russell bodies are readily seen in the plasma cells and extracellularly.

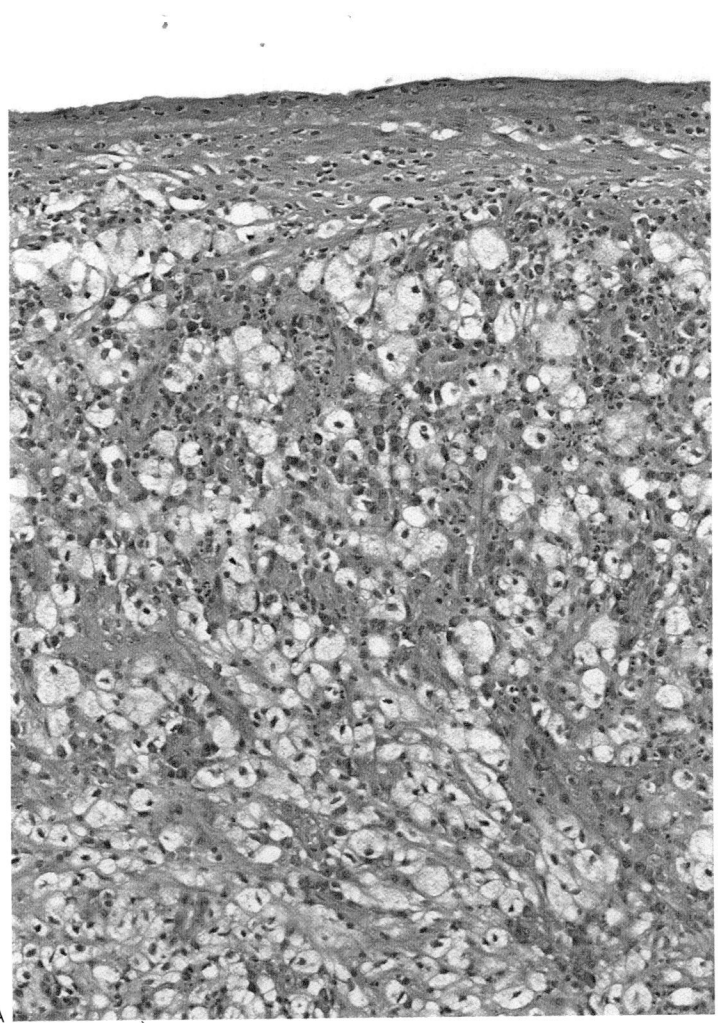 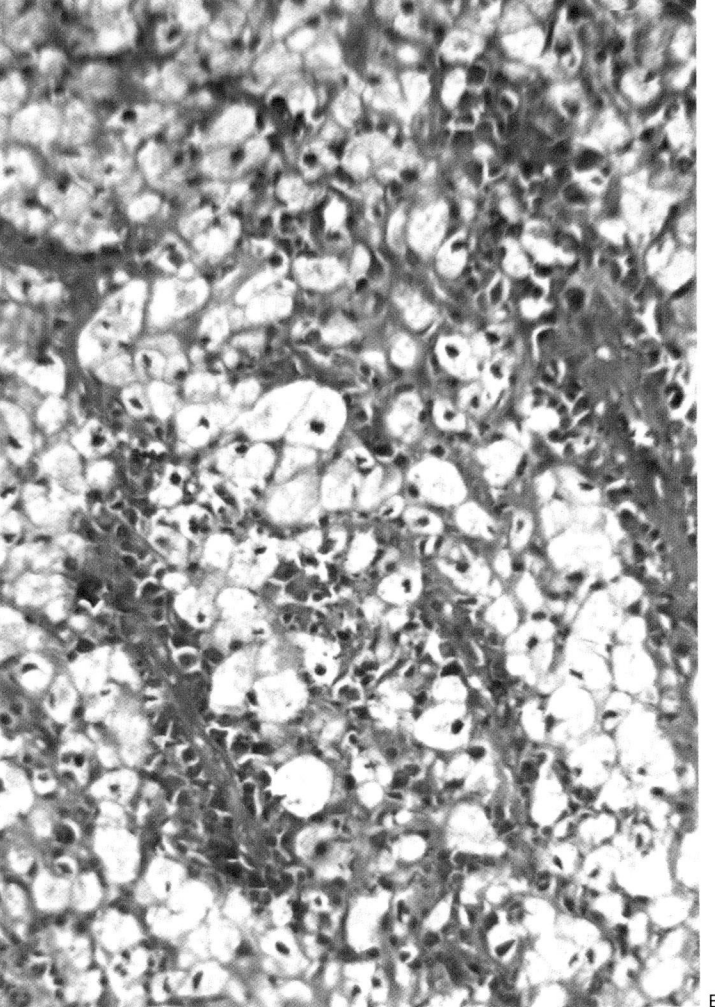

Fig. 23.18 **(A) Rhinoscleroma. (B)** The inflammatory infiltrate consists of an admixture of plasma cells and vacuolated macrophages (Mikulicz cells). (H & E)

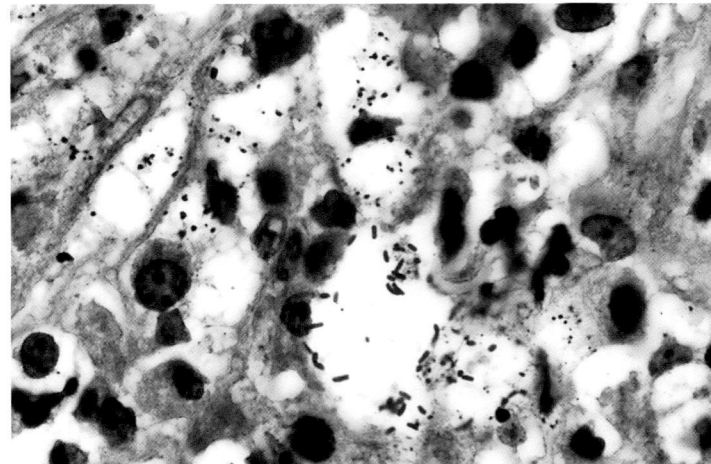

Fig. 23.19 **Rhinoscleroma.** The organisms can be seen on this silver stain. (Warthin–Starry)

TULAREMIA

Tularemia is named after Tulare County, California, where its occurrence was first recognized.[550] It is caused by *Francisella tularensis*, a minute Gram-negative coccobacillus which produces a fatal insect-borne septicemic infection in ground squirrels and other rodents. The disease is transmitted to man either by the bite of an infected vector, such as mosquitoes or ticks,[551] or by contact with an infected rodent or rabbit.[550,551] It has been recognized in parts of the United States of America,[552,553] Canada,[554] and the Soviet Union, and rarely in the British Isles and other parts of Europe. Skin lesions occur only in the ulceroglandular form of the disease.[555] This is characterized by a papule at the site of the initial inoculation, followed by an ascending lymphangitis. Nodules develop along the course of the affected lymphatics, as in the lymphangitic type of sporotrichosis.[550] The occurrence of erythema nodosum and erythema multiforme has been described.[556] Severe constitutional symptoms are usual.[557]

Histopathology

The primary lesion is an ulcer, with necrosis involving the epidermis and upper dermis. The adjacent epidermis is usually acanthotic with some spongiosis. In acute lesions there is focal necrosis and suppuration, whereas in more chronic lesions a granulomatous picture has been described around the necrotic focus in the dermis.

The causative organism cannot be seen in conventional histological preparations. It can be demonstrated in histological sections and in films of exudate by direct immunofluorescence, following treatment with fluorescein-labeled specific antiserum.[552] *F. tularensis* is a hazard to laboratory workers.[553]

LISTERIOSIS

Listeriosis is a rare infection of neonates, elderly patients and immuno-suppressed patients, including those with human immunodeficiency virus infection. It may also involve pregnant women. The organism, *Listeria monocytogenes*, is a Gram-positive coccobacillus that can replicate in macrophages. Bacteremia, with or without meningitis, is the usual clinical presentation.[558] Cutaneous lesions may be papular, pustular or purpuric.

Histopathology

The epidermis shows mild spongiosis with lymphocyte exocytosis.[558] In pustular lesions subcorneal and intraepidermal neutrophils are present. The dermis contains a mixed inflammatory cell infiltrate with many macrophages. Gram-positive coccobacilli are present in macrophages, in adnexal structures, and lying free in the dermis or in epidermal inflammatory cells.

CAT-SCRATCH DISEASE

Cat-scratch disease is a self-limited illness characterized by the development, at the site of a scratch by a cat, of a papule or crusted nodule, which is followed approximately 2 weeks later by regional lymphadenitis.[559–562] In 1–2% of patients severe systemic illness may develop: this may include an oculoglandular syndrome, pleurisy, encephalitis, osteomyelitis[563] and splenomegaly.[564] Other cutaneous manifestations have included erythema nodosum, urticaria, erythema marginatum, a Sweet's syndrome-like eruption[565] and purpura.[562,566]

Recently, small Gram-negative bacilli have been demonstrated in the skin[559,564] and lymph nodes[557,564,566–569] of most cases, using the Warthin–Starry silver stain or the Brown–Hopps modification of the Gram stain. The organism has been classified as *Bartonella henselae*. It is possible that the related bacillus *Afipia felis* may also be responsible (as originally reported), but there is a growing consensus that *B. henselae* is the predominant if not the sole pathogen.

The bacillus responsible for cat-scratch disease (*B. henselae*) has an etiological role in the causation of bacillary angiomatosis (epithelioid angiomatosis), a rare vascular proliferation seen in patients with the acquired immunodeficiency syndrome (see p. 1019).[570,571]

Another species of *Bartonella* (*B. quintana*) is the agent of trench fever, a disease transmitted from human to human by the body louse. There is a high prevalence of this infection in homeless persons.[572]

Histopathology [559,573]

The epidermal changes are variable and include acanthosis and ulceration. There is usually a zone of necrosis in the upper dermis, and this is surrounded by a mantle of macrophages and lymphocytes (Fig. 23.20). Neutrophils and eosinophils are often present around zones of necrosis. Multinucleate cells and well-defined granulomas may be present. Organisms are seen within macrophages and lying free, particularly in areas of necrosis and suppuration.[564] A rapid polymerase chain reaction-based detection of the causative organism can be carried out on fresh or paraffin-embedded samples.[574]

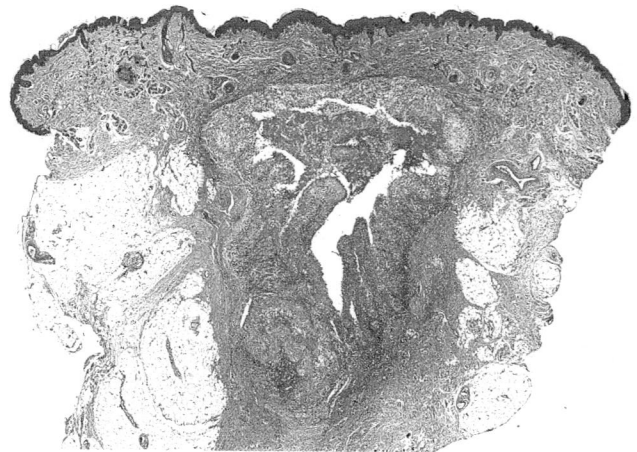

Fig. 23.20 **Cat-scratch disease.** There is a central zone of necrosis and a surrounding mantle of macrophages, lymphocytes and some granulomas. (H & E)

MALAKOPLAKIA

Malakoplakia is a rare chronic inflammatory disease which occurs predominantly in the urogenital tract, especially the bladder. More than 30 cases involving the skin and subcutaneous tissue have been reported.[575–579] Nearly one half of these patients were immunosuppressed;[580] occasionally this was due to the acquired immunodeficiency syndrome.[581,582] Cutaneous involvement is usually in the vulva[583] and perianal region,[584,585] where yellow-pink indurated or polypoid masses have been described. Less common sites are the axilla,[586] forehead[587] and an injection site.[588]

Although the pathogenesis of malakoplakia is uncertain, it appears to result from an acquired defect in the intracellular destruction of phagocytosed bacteria, usually *Escherichia coli*.[589] In the skin, *Staph. aureus* has also been isolated.[590]

Histopathology[575]

Malakoplakia is a chronic inflammatory process characterized by sheets of closely packed macrophages containing PAS-positive diastase-resistant inclusions (von Hansemann cells). A variable proportion of these cells contain calcospherites with a homogeneous or target-like appearance – the Michaelis–Gutmann bodies. These stain with the von Kossa method.[590] There is also a scattering of lymphocytes and plasma cells. Immunostaining with polyclonal anti-*Mycobacterium bovis* antibodies, a method for detecting bacterial organisms in low concentration, has been successful in demonstrating bacteria in malakoplakia.[586]

'SAGO PALM' DISEASE

'Sago palm' disease, also known as Sepik granuloma, is a rare condition that appears to be restricted to the Sepik district of New Guinea.[591] It appears to follow injury by the sago palm *(Metroxylon)*, but additional types of injury may also allow the entry of the causative organism, a Gram-positive bacillus. Affected individuals usually present with multiple cutaneous nodules on the extremities, but the face can also be involved. The organism has never been cultured.

Histopathology

There is a diffuse dermal infiltrate by large foamy histiocytes admixed with some plasma cells, lymphocytes and fibroblasts. A syncytium of amorphous pink material extends between the histiocytes. It is PAS positive. The material contains numerous gray, round to oval dots, representing Gram-positive organisms surrounded by ground substance.

CHLAMYDIAL INFECTIONS

Chlamydiae are obligate intracellular organisms that share many features with bacteria, including a discrete cell wall. There are two morphologically distinct species, *Chlamydia trachomatis* and *C. psittaci*. The latter is responsible for psittacosis, a pneumonia derived from infected birds, whereas different serotypes of *C. trachomatis* are responsible for trachoma, urethritis and lymphogranuloma venereum. The diagnosis can be confirmed by culture of the organism or by serology.

PSITTACOSIS

Psittacosis, caused by *Chlamydia psittaci*, usually presents as a pneumonic illness with various constitutional symptoms. Some patients develop a morbilliform rash or lesions resembling the rose spots of typhoid fever. Erythema nodosum,[592] erythema multiforme, erythema marginatum[593] and disseminated intravascular coagulation[594] with cutaneous manifestations have also been reported. The findings are not specific for psittacosis, either clinically or histopathologically.

LYMPHOGRANULOMA VENEREUM

Lymphogranuloma venereum (LGV), or lymphogranuloma inguinale, is a sexually transmitted disease caused by certain immunotypes (L1, L2 and L3) of *Chlamydia trachomatis*.[531,532] Worldwide in distribution,[595] it is most frequent in parts of Asia, Africa and South America. Clinically, three stages are recognized.[596] The initial lesion, which follows a few days or weeks after exposure to the organism, consists of a small papule, ulcer or herpetiform vesicle on the penis, labia or vaginal wall. Extragenital sites of involvement have been recorded.[597] The primary lesion is transient and often imperceptible. The secondary stage, which follows several weeks after the initial exposure, consists of regional lymphadenopathy. If the inguinal nodes are involved, enlarging buboes develop with draining sinuses. There may be constitutional symptoms at this stage. Erythema multiforme and erythema nodosum rarely develop. The tertiary stage, which is more common in women, encompasses the sequelae of the earlier inflammatory stages.[598] There may be rectal strictures, fistula formation, and rarely genital elephantiasis related to lymphedema.[599,600] The duration of the disease may be prolonged in HIV-positive patients.[532]

The organism can be isolated in a tissue culture system or in the yolk sac of eggs.[596] Serological methods are most commonly used to establish a diagnosis. A microimmunofluorescence test can detect antichlamydial antibodies to a range of serological variants of *C. trachomatis*.[596]

Histopathology

The primary lesion is not commonly biopsied. Ulceration is usually present, with a dense underlying infiltrate of plasma cells and lymphocytes.[601] There is thickening of vessel walls and some endothelial swelling. Small sinus tracts may lead to the surface. A few epithelioid cell collections may be present.[601]

The characteristic lesions occur in the lymph nodes in the second stage, with the development of stellate abscesses with a poorly formed palisade of epithelioid cells and histiocytes. Sinus formation also occurs. In later lesions there is variable fibrosis.

Direct immunofluorescence, using a fluorescein-labeled antibody to *C. trachomatis*, has been used to confirm the diagnosis.[602]

RICKETTSIAL INFECTIONS

Rickettsiae are small obligate intracellular bacteria which are transmitted in most instances by the bite of an arthropod. The various species of rickettsia are endemic in different geographical locations, and this has influenced the naming of some of the infections.[603,604] Table 23.1 lists the various rickettsial infections of humans, the corresponding etiological species and the mode of transmission. The organism for scrub typhus has been reclassified from the genus *Rickettsia* to *Orientia*.

Rickettsiae usually produce an acute febrile illness accompanied by headache, myalgia, malaise and morbidity. Rocky Mountain spotted fever has a mortality of approximately 5%.[35,605–608] A specific diagnosis is usually made by serological methods, as the attempted isolation of rickettsiae in the laboratory is potentially highly hazardous for the laboratory staff.[609] Human

Table 23.1 **Rickettsial infections**

Disease	Organism	Mode of transmission
Rocky Mountain spotted fever	*R. rickettsii*	Tick
Boutonneuse fever	*R. conorii*	Tick
Rickettsialpox	*R. akari*	Mite
Siberian tick typhus	*R. sibirica*	Tick
Queensland tick typhus	*R. australis*	Tick
Epidemic typhus	*R. prowazakii*	Louse feces
Murine typhus	*R. mooseri (typhi)*	Flea feces
Scrub typhus	*O. tsutsugamushi*	Mite
Q fever	*Coxiella burnetii*	Aerosol

granulocytic ehrlichiosis, caused by the tickborne rickettsia-like organism *Ehrlichia equi*, has some clinical similarities to Rocky Mountain spotted fever.[610] Having a similar vector, ehrlichiosis is usually found in the United States in areas where Lyme disease is prevalent.[611]

Cutaneous lesions are present in most rickettsial infections, with the exception of Q fever. Usually there is a macular or maculopapular rash; in rickettsialpox the rash may be papulovesicular.[612] A more characteristic lesion is the eschar (tache noire), a crusted ulcer 1 cm or more in diameter that develops at the site of the arthropod bite.[613] It is thought to result not from the bite but from the inoculation of rickettsiae, which invade vascular endothelial cells.[614] Eschars are characteristic of rickettsialpox,[612] scrub typhus,[615,616] boutonneuse fever,[617,618] Queensland tick typhus[619] and Siberian tick typhus.[613,617] An eschar is not found in epidemic typhus or in murine typhus, and only rarely in Rocky Mountain spotted fever.[603,613,617]

Rickettsia proliferate on the endothelium of small blood vessels, releasing cytokines which damage endothelial integrity. This leads to a cascade of events that may terminate in focal occlusive endangiitis.[620]

Histopathology

The pathological basis for the cutaneous lesions of rickettsial infections is a lymphocytic vasculitis. The eschars result from coagulative necrosis of the epidermis and underlying dermis.[621,622] A crust overlies this region. Bordering the area of necrosis there is a lymphocytic vasculitis, with some fibrinoid necrosis of vessels and related dermal hemorrhage.[617] Thrombosis of vessels is sometimes present.[617] There are often a few neutrophils in the inflammatory infiltrate. Numerous organisms can be demonstrated in vascular endothelium and vessel walls using fluorescein-labeled antisera to the appropriate rickettsial species.

The maculopapular lesions of Rocky Mountain spotted fever show a focal lymphocytic vasculitis with patchy fibrinoid necrosis of small vessels and extravasation of erythrocytes.[623,624] Progression to a leukocytoclastic vasculitis is common.[625,626] The most notable epidermal change is basal vacuolar degeneration with exocytosis of inflammatory cells.[625] *Rickettsia rickettsii* can be demonstrated in endothelium and vascular walls using fluorescein-labeled antisera[627] or with immunoperoxidase techniques using routine sections.[625]

The papulovesicular lesions of rickettsialpox show subepidermal edema associated with exocytosis of mononuclear cells into the epidermis.[612] These tend to obscure the dermoepidermal interface. There is a dense perivascular infiltrate in the underlying dermis, with prominence of the endothelial cells of the blood vessels and changes indicative of a mild vasculitis.[612] Fibrin thrombi are sometimes present, and there may be extravasation of red cells. The causative organism, *R. akari*, has not been identified in tissue sections other than by immunofluorescent techniques.[612]

REFERENCES

Superfical pyogenic infections

1 Hayden GF. Skin diseases encountered in a pediatric clinic. Am J Dis Child 1985; 139: 36–38.
2 Grossman KL, Rasmussen JE. Recent advances in pediatric infectious disease and their impact on dermatology. J Am Acad Dermatol 1991; 24: 379–389.
3 Darmstadt GL, Lane AT. Impetigo: an overview. Pediatr Dermatol 1994; 11: 293–303.
4 Melish ME. Staphylococci, streptococci and the skin. Review of impetigo and the staphylococcal scalded skin syndrome. Semin Dermatol 1982; 1: 101–109.
5 Maddox JS, Ware JC, Dillon HC Jr. The natural history of streptococcal skin infection: prevention with topical antibiotics. J Am Acad Dermatol 1985; 13: 207–212.
6 Tunnessen WW Jr. Cutaneous infections. Pediatr Clin North Am 1983; 30: 515–532.
7 Tunnessen WW Jr. Practical aspects of bacterial skin infections in children. Pediatr Dermatol 1985; 2: 255–265.
8 Barton LL, Friedman AD. Impetigo: a reassessment of etiology and therapy. Pediatr Dermatol 1987; 4: 185–188.
9 Coskey RJ, Coskey LA. Diagnosis and treatment of impetigo. J Am Acad Dermatol 1987; 17: 62–63.
10 Brook I, Frazier EH, Yeager JK. Microbiology of nonbullous impetigo. Pediatr Dermatol 1997; 14: 192–195.
11 Elias PM, Levy SW. Bullous impetigo. Occurrence of localized scalded skin syndrome in an adult. Arch Dermatol 1976; 112: 856–858.
12 El Zawahry M, Aziz AA, Soliman M. The aetiology of impetigo contagiosa. Br J Dermatol 1972; 87: 420–424.
13 Bronstein SW, Bickers DR, Lamkin BC. Bullous dermatosis caused by *Staphylococcus aureus* in locus minoris resistentiae. J Am Acad Dermatol 1984; 10: 259–263.
14 Manders SM. Toxin-mediated streptococcal and staphylococcal disease. J Am Acad Dermatol 1998; 39: 383–398.
15 Lyell A. Toxic epidermal necrolysis: the scalded skin syndrome. JCE Dermatol 1978; 16(11): 15–26.
16 Oranje AP, Vuzevski VD, Muntendam J, Rongen-Westerlaken C. Varicella complicated by staphylococcal scalded skin syndrome with unusual necrosis. Int J Dermatol 1988; 27: 38–39.
17 Fritsch P, Elias P, Varga J. The fate of staphylococcal exfoliatin in newborn and adult mice. Br J Dermatol 1976; 95: 275–284.
18 Rasmussen JE. Toxic epidermal necrolysis. A review of 75 cases in children. Arch Dermatol 1975; 111: 1135–1139.
19 Richard M, Mathieu-Serra A. Staphylococcal scalded skin syndrome in a homosexual adult. J Am Acad Dermatol 1986; 15: 385–389.
20 Borchers SL, Gomez EC, Isseroff RR. Generalized staphylococcal scalded skin syndrome in an anephric boy undergoing hemodialysis. Arch Dermatol 1984; 120: 912–918.
21 Cribier B, Piemont Y, Grosshans E. Staphylococcal scalded skin syndrome in adults. A clinical review illustrated with a new case. J Am Acad Dermatol 1994; 30: 319–324.
22 Hardwick N, Parry CM, Sharpe GR. Staphylococcal scalded skin syndrome in an adult. Influence of immune and renal factors. Br J Dermatol 1995; 132: 468–471.
23 Acland KM, Darvay A, Griffin C et al. Staphylococcal scalded skin syndrome in an adult associated with methicillin-resistant *Staphylococcus aureus*. Br J Dermatol 1999; 140: 518–520.
24 Patel GK, Varma S, Finlay AY. Staphylococcal scalded skin syndrome in healthy adults. Br J Dermatol 2000; 142: 1253–1255.
25 Oono T, Kanzaki H, Yoshioka T, Arata J. Staphylococcal scalded skin syndrome in an adult. Dermatology 1997; 195: 268–270.
26 Baker DH, Wuepper KD, Rasmussen JE. Staphylococcal scalded skin syndrome: detection of antibody to epidermolytic toxin by a primary binding assay. Clin Exp Dermatol 1978; 3: 17–24.
27 Shelley ED, Shelley WB, Talanin NY. Chronic staphylococcal scalded skin syndrome. Br J Dermatol 1998; 139: 319–324.
28 Farrell AM. Staphylococcal scalded-skin syndrome. Lancet 1999; 354: 880–881.
29 Dimond RL, Wolff HH, Braun-Falco O. The staphylococcal scalded skin syndrome. An experimental histochemical and electron microscopic study. Br J Dermatol 1977; 96: 483–492.
30 Lyell A. Toxic epidermal necrolysis (the scalded skin syndrome): a reappraisal. Br J Dermatol 1979; 100: 69–86.
31 Lyell A. The staphylococcal scalded skin syndrome in historical perspective: emergence of dermopathic strains of *Staphylococcus aureus* and discovery of the epidermolytic toxin. J Am Acad Dermatol 1983; 9: 285–294.
32 Falk DK, King LE Jr. Criteria for the diagnosis of staphylococcal scalded skin syndrome in adults. Cutis 1983; 31: 421–424.

33 Elias PM, Fritsch P, Epstein EH Jr. Staphylococcal scalded skin syndrome. Clinical features, pathogenesis, and recent microbiological and biochemical developments. Arch Dermatol 1977; 113: 207–219.

34 Tofte RW, Williams DN. Toxic shock syndrome: clinical and laboratory features in 15 patients. Ann Intern Med 1981; 94: 149–156.

35 Drage LA. Life-threatening rashes: dermatologic signs of four infectious diseases. Mayo Clin Proc 1999; 74: 68–72.

36 Huntley AC, Tanabe JL. Toxic shock syndrome as a complication of dermatologic surgery. J Am Acad Dermatol 1987; 16: 227–229.

37 Hurwitz RM, Ackerman AB. Cutaneous pathology of the toxic shock syndrome. Am J Dermatopathol 1985; 7: 563–578.

38 Resnick SD. Staphylococcal toxin-mediated syndromes in childhood. Semin Dermatol 1992; 11: 11–18.

39 Stanford DG, Georgouras KE, Konya J, Pang B. Toxic streptococcal syndrome. Australas J Dermatol 1997; 38: 158–160.

40 Neri I, Bardazzi F, Marzaduri S, Patrizi A. Perianal streptococcal dermatitis in adults. Br J Dermatol 1996; 135: 796–798.

41 Vélez A, Moreno J-C. Febrile perianal streptococcal dermatitis. Pediatr Dermatol 1999; 16: 23–24.

42 Kelly C, Taplin D, Allen AM. Streptococcal ecthyma. Arch Dermatol 1971; 103: 306–310.

43 El Baze P, Thyss A, Caldani C et al. *Pseudomonas aeruginosa* 0-11 folliculitis. Development into ecthyma gangrenosum in immunosuppressed patients. Arch Dermatol 1985; 121: 873–876.

44 Berger TG, Kaveh S, Becker D, Hoffman J. Cutaneous manifestations of *Pseudomonas* infections in AIDS. J Am Acad Dermatol 1995; 32: 278–280.

45 El Baze P, Thyss A, Vinti H et al. A study of nineteen immunocompromised patients with extensive skin lesions caused by *Pseudomonas aeruginosa* with and without bacteremia. Acta Derm Venereol 1991; 71: 411–415.

46 Sevinsky LD, Viecens C, Ballesteros DO, Stengel F. Ecthyma gangrenosum: a cutaneous manifestation of *Pseudomonas aeruginosa* sepsis. J Am Acad Dermatol 1993; 29: 104–106.

47 Boisseau AM, Sarlangue J, Perel Y et al. Perineal ecthyma gangrenosum in infancy and early childhood: septicemic and nonsepticemic forms. J Am Acad Dermatol 1992; 27: 415–418.

48 Güçlüer H, Ergun T, Demirçay Z. Ecthyma gangrenosum. Int J Dermatol 1999; 38: 299–302.

49 Greene SL, Su WPD, Muller SA. Ecthyma gangrenosum: report of clinical, histopathologic, and bacteriologic aspects of eight cases. J Am Acad Dermatol 1984; 11: 781–787.

50 Fast M, Woerner S, Bowman W et al. Ecthyma gangrenosum. Can Med Assoc J 1979; 120: 332–334.

51 Czechowicz RT, Warren LJ, Moore L, Saxon B. *Pseudomonas aeruginosa* infection mimicking erythema annulare centrifugum. Australas J Dermatol 2001; 42: 57–59.

52 Del Pozo J, García-Silva J, Almagro M et al. Ecthyma gangrenosum-like eruption associated with *Morganella morganii* infection. Br J Dermatol 1998; 139: 520–521.

53 Fleming MG, Milburn PB, Prose NS. *Pseudomonas* septicemia with nodules and bullae. Pediatr Dermatol 1987; 4: 18–20.

54 Schlossberg D. Multiple erythematous nodules as a manifestation of *Pseudomonas aeruginosa* septicemia. Arch Dermatol 1980; 116: 446–447.

55 Kim EJ, Foad M, Travers R. Ecthyma gangrenosum in an AIDS patient with normal neutrophil count. J Am Acad Dermatol 1999; 41: 840–841.

Deep pyogenic infections (cellulitis)

56 Fleisher G. Ludwig S, Campos J. Cellulitis: bacterial etiology, clinical features, and laboratory findings. J Pediatr 1980; 97: 591–593.

57 Leyden JJ. Cellulitis. Arch Dermatol 1989; 125: 823–824.

58 Hook EW III. Acute cellulitis. Arch Dermatol 1987; 123: 460–461.

59 Feingold DS. Gangrenous and crepitant cellulitis. J Am Acad Dermatol 1982; 6: 289–299.

60 Shelley WB, Talanin N, Shelley ED et al. Occult *Streptococcus pyogenes* in cellulitis: demonstration by immunofluorescence. Br J Dermatol 1995; 132: 989–991.

61 Grob JJ, Bollet C, Richard MA et al. Extensive skin ulceration due to EF-4 bacterial infection in a patient with AIDS. Br J Dermatol 1989; 121: 507–510.

62 Yanagi T, Kazagiri K, Sonoda T, Takayasu S. *Serratia marcescens* granuloma. Br J Dermatol 1997; 136: 289–290.

63 Nieves DS, James WD. Painful red nodules of the legs: A manifestation of chronic infection with gram-negative organisms. J Am Acad Dermatol 1999; 40: 319–321.

64 Huffam SE, Nowotny MJ, Currie BJ. *Chromobacterium violaceum* in tropical northern Australia. Med J Aust 1998; 168: 335–337.

65 Rosina P, Cunego S, Meloni G et al. Cutaneous and systemic infection by *Gemella morbillorum*. Acta Derm Venereol 1999; 79: 398.

66 Buckley DA, Murphy A, Dervan P et al. Persistent infection of the chin with an unusual skin pathogen (*Streptococcus milleri*): a sign of intraoral carcinoma. Clin Exp Dermatol 1998; 23: 35–37.

67 Moser C, Jønsson V, Thomsen K et al. Subcutaneous lesions and bacteraemia due to *Stenotrophomonas maltophilia* in three leukaemic patients with neutropenia. Br J Dermatol 1997; 136: 949–952.

68 Burns RL, Lowe L. *Xanthomonas maltophilia* infection presenting as erythematous nodules. J Am Acad Dermatol 1997; 37: 836–838.

69 Baddour LM, Googe PB, Stevens SL. Biopsy specimen findings in patients with previous lower extremity cellulitis after saphenous venectomy for coronary artery bypass graft surgery. J Am Acad Dermatol 1997; 37: 246–249.

70 Heng MCY, Khoo M, Cooperman A, Fallon-Friedlander S. Haemorrhagic cellulitis: a syndrome associated with tumour necrosis factor-α. Br J Dermatol 1994; 130: 65–74.

71 Beckman EN, Leonard GL, Castillo LE et al. Histopathology of marine vibrio wound infections. Am J Clin Pathol 1981; 76: 765–772.

72 Hurwitz RM, Leaming RD, Horine RK. Necrotic cellulitis. A localized form of septic vasculitis. Arch Dermatol 1984; 120: 87–92.

73 Musher DM. Cutaneous and soft-tissue manifestations of sepsis due to Gram-negative enteric bacilli. Rev Infect Dis 1980; 2: 854–866.

74 Chartier C, Grosshans E. Erysipelas. Int J Dermatol 1990; 29: 459–467.

75 Chartier C, Grosshans E. Erysipelas: an update. Int J Dermatol 1996; 35: 779–781.

76 Guberman D, Gilead LT, Zlotogorski A, Schamroth J. Bullous erysipelas: A retrospective study of 26 patients. J Am Acad Dermatol 1999; 41: 733–737.

77 Ronnen M, Suster S, Schewach-Millet M, Modan M. Erysipelas. Changing faces. Int J Dermatol 1985; 24: 169–172.

78 Keefe M, Wakeel RA, Kerr REI. Erysipelas complicating chronic discoid lupus erythematosus of the face – a case report and review of erysipelas. Clin Exp Dermatol 1989; 14: 75–78.

79 Bernard P, Bedane C, Mounier M et al. Streptococcal cause of erysipelas and cellulitis in adults. A microbiologic study using a direct immunofluorescence technique. Arch Dermatol 1989; 125: 779–782.

80 Shama S, Calandra GB. Atypical erysipelas caused by Group B streptococci in a patient with cured Hodgkin's disease. Arch Dermatol 1982; 118: 934–936.

81 Cox NH, Knowles MA, Porteus ID. Pre-septal cellulitis and facial erysipelas due to Moraxella species. Clin Exp Dermatol 1994; 19: 321–323.

82 Barzilai A, Langevitz P, Goldberg I et al. Erysipelas-like erythema of familial Mediterranean fever: Clinicopathologic correlation. J Am Acad Dermatol 2000; 42: 791–795.

83 Barnett JH, Estes SA, Wirman JA et al. Erysipeloid. J Am Acad Dermatol 1983; 9: 116–123.

84 McCray MK. Esterly NB. Blistering distal dactylitis. J Am Acad Dermatol 1981; 5: 592–594.

85 Telfer NR, Barth JH, Dawber RPR. Recurrent blistering distal dactylitis of the great toe associated with an ingrowing toenail. Clin Exp Dermatol 1989; 14: 380–381.

86 Barnett BO, Frieden IJ. Streptococcal skin diseases in children. Semin Dermatol 1992; 11: 3–10.

87 Frieden IJ. Blistering dactylitis caused by Group B streptococci. Pediatr Dermatol 1989; 6: 300–302.

88 Zemtsov A, Veitschegger M. *Staphylococcus aureus*-induced blistering distal dactylitis in an adult immunosuppressed patient. J Am Acad Dermatol 1992; 26: 784–785.

89 Hauger SB. Facial cellulitis: an early indicator of Group B streptococcal bacteremia. Pediatrics 1981; 67: 376–377.

90 Ginsburg CM. *Haemophilus influenzae* type B buccal cellulitis. J Am Acad Dermatol 1981; 4: 661–664.

91 Barton LL, Ramsey RA, Raval DS. Neonatal group B streptococcal cellulitis-adenitis. Pediatr Dermatol 1993; 10: 58–60.

92 Thirumoorthi MC, Asmar BI, Dajani AS. Violaceous discolouration in pneumococcal cellulitis. Pediatrics 1978; 62: 492–493.

93 Rehder PA, Eliezer ET, Lane AT. Perianal cellulitis. Cutaneous Group A streptococcal disease. Arch Dermatol 1988; 124: 702–704.

94 Montemarano AD, James WD. *Staphylococcus aureus* as a cause of perianal dermatitis. Pediatr Dermatol 1993; 10: 259–262.

95 Krol AL. Perianal streptococcal dermatitis. Pediatr Dermatol 1990; 7: 97–100.

96 Duhra P, Ilchyshyn A. Perianal streptococcal cellulitis with penile involvement. Br J Dermatol 1990; 123: 793–796.

97 Wickboldt LG, Sanders CV. *Vibrio vulnificus* infection. Case report and update since 1970. J Am Acad Dermatol 1983; 9: 243–251.

98 Park SD, Shon HS, Joh NJ. *Vibrio vulnificus* septicemia in Korea: clinical and epidemiologic findings in seventy patients. J Am Acad Dermatol 1991; 24: 397–403.

99 Wise KA, Newton PJ. A fatal case of *Vibrio vulnificus* septicemia. Pathology 1992; 24: 121–122.

100 Serrano-Jaen L, Vega-Lopez F. Fulminating septicaemia caused by *Vibrio vulnificus*. Br J Dermatol 2000; 142: 386–387.

101 Bisharat N, Agmon V, Finkelstein R et al. Clinical, epidemiological, and microbiological features of *Vibrio vulnificus* biogroup 3 causing outbreaks of wound infection and bacteraemia in Israel. Lancet 1999; 354: 1421–1424.

102 Tyring SK, Lee PC. Hemorrhagic bullae associated with *Vibrio vulnificus* septicemia. Report of two cases. Arch Dermatol 1986; 122: 818–820.

103 Nip-Sakamoto CJ, Pien FD. *Vibrio vulnificus* infection in Hawaii. Int J Dermatol 1989; 28: 313–316.

104 Woo ML, Patrick WGD, Simon MTP, French GL. Necrotising fasciitis caused by *Vibrio vulnificus*. J Clin Pathol 1984; 37: 1301–1304.

105 Acay MC, Oral ET, Yenigün M, Sahin A. *Pasteurella multocida* ulceration on the penis. Int J Dermatol 1993; 32: 519–520.

106 Chan H-L, Ho H-C, Kuo T-t. Cutaneous manifestations of non-01 *Vibrio cholerae* septicemia with gastroenteritis and meningitis. J Am Acad Dermatol 1994; 30: 626–628.

107 Newman C, Shepherd M, Woodard MD et al. Fatal septicemia and bullae caused by non-01 *Vibrio cholerae*. J Am Acad Dermatol 1993; 29: 909–912.

108 Yoon TY, Jung SK, Chang SH. Cellulitis due to *Escherichia coli* in three immunocompromised subjects. Br J Dermatol 1998; 139: 885–888.

109 Hammar H, Wanger L. Erysipelas and necrotizing fasciitis. Br J Dermatol 1977; 96: 409–419.

110 Umbert IJ, Winkelmann RK, Oliver GF, Peters MS. Necrotizing fasciitis: a clinical, microbiologic, and histopathologic study of 14 patients. J Am Acad Dermatol 1989; 20: 774–781.

111 Thomson H, Cartwright K. Streptococcal necrotizing fasciitis in Gloucestershire: 1994. Br J Surg 1995; 82: 1444–1445.

112 Morantes MC, Lipsky BA. 'Flesh-eating bacteria': return of an old nemesis. Int J Dermatol 1995; 34: 461–463.

113 Wall DB, de Virgilio C, Black S, Klein SR. Objective criteria may assist in distinguishing necrotizing fasciitis from nonnecrotizing soft tissue infection. Am J Surg 2000; 179: 17–21.

114 Andreasen TJ, Green SD, Childers BJ. Massive infectious soft-tissue injury: diagnosis and management of necrotizing fasciitis and purpura fulminans. Plast Reconstr Surg 2001; 107: 1025–1034.

115 Cox NH. Streptococcal necrotizing fasciitis and the dermatologist. Br J Dermatol 1999; 141: 613–616.

116 Goldberg GN, Hansen RC, Lynch PJ. Necrotizing fasciitis in infancy: report of three cases and review of the literature. Pediatr Dermatol 1984; 2: 55–63.

117 Tharakaram S, Keczkes K. Necrotizing fasciitis. A report of five patients. Int J Dermatol 1988; 27: 585–588.

118 Koehn GG. Necrotizing fasciitis. Arch Dermatol 1978; 114: 581–583.

119 Gibbon KL, Bewley AP. Acquired streptococcal necrotizing fasciitis following excision of malignant melanoma. Br J Dermatol 1999; 141: 717–719.

120 Wolf JE, Rabinowitz LG. Streptococcal toxic shock-like syndrome. Arch Dermatol 1995; 131: 73–77.

121 Leibowitz MR, Ramakrishnan KK. Necrotizing fasciitis: the role of *Staphylococcus epidermidis*, immune status and intravascular coagulation. Australas J Dermatol 1995; 36: 29–31.

122 Feingold DS, Weinberg AN. Group A streptococcal infections. An old adversary reemerging with new tricks? Arch Dermatol 1996; 132: 67–70.

123 Joly P, Chosidow O, Gouault-Heilmann M et al. Protein S deficiency in a patient with necrotizing cellulitis. Clin Exp Dermatol 1993; 18: 305–308.

124 Jiang T, Covington JA, Haile CA et al. Fournier gangrene associated with Crohn disease. Mayo Clin Proc 2000; 75: 647–649.

125 Schultz ES, Diepgen TL, von den Driesch P, Hornstein OP. Systemic corticosteroids are important in the treatment of Fournier's gangrene: a case report. Br J Dermatol 1995; 133: 633–635.

126 Eke N, Echem RC, Elenwo SN. Fournier's gangrene in Nigeria: a review of 21 consecutive patients. Int Surg 2000; 85: 77–81.

127 Folgaresi M, Simonetti V, Motolese A, Giannetti A. Fournier's gangrene: a case report. Acta Derm Venereol 1999; 79: 252–253.

128 Shimizu T, Harada M, Zempo N et al. Nonclostridial gas gangrene due to *Streptococcus anginosus* in a diabetic patient. J Am Acad Dermatol 1999; 40: 347–349.

129 Smith KJ, Skelton HG, Hilyard EJ et al. *Bacillus piliformis* infection (Tyzzer's disease) in a patient infected with HIV-1: Confirmation with 16S ribosomal RNA sequence analysis. J Am Acad Dermatol 1996; 34: 343–348.

130 Khavari PA, Bolognia JL, Eisen R et al. Periodic acid-Schiff-positive organisms in primary cutaneous *Bacillus cereus* infection. Arch Dermatol 1991; 127: 543–546.

131 Horgan-Bell C, From L, Ramsay C. Meleney's synergistic gangrene: pathological features. J Cutan Pathol 1989; 16: 307 (abstract).

132 Grattan CEH, Peachey RD, Boon A. Evidence for a role of local trauma in the pathogenesis of erosive pustular dermatosis of the scalp. Clin Exp Dermatol 1988; 13: 7–10.

133 Ikeda M, Arata J, Isaka H. Erosive pustular dermatosis of the scalp successfully treated with oral zinc sulphate. Br J Dermatol 1982; 106: 742–743.

134 Caputo R, Veraldi S. Erosive pustular dermatosis of the scalp. J Am Acad Dermatol 1993; 28: 96–98.

135 Bull RH, Mortimer PS. Erosive pustular dermatosis of the leg. Br J Dermatol 1995; 132: 279–282.

136 Layton AM, Cunliffe WJ. Erosive pustular dermatosis of the scalp following surgery. Br J Dermatol 1995; 132: 472–473.

137 Parodi A, Ciaccio M, Rebora A. Erosive pustular dermatosis of the scalp. Int J Dermatol 1990; 29: 517–518.

138 Rongioletti F, Delmonte S, Rossi ME et al. Erosive pustular dermatosis of the scalp following cryotherapy and topical tretinoin for actinic keratoses. Clin Exp Dermatol 1999; 24: 499–500.

139 Ena P, Lissia M, Doneddu GME, Campus GV. Erosive pustular dermatosis of the scalp in skin grafts: report of three cases. Dermatology 1997; 194: 80–84.

140 Trüeb RM, Krasovec M. Erosive pustular dermatosis of the scalp following radiation therapy for solar keratoses. Br J Dermatol 1999; 141: 763–765.

141 Williams HM Jr, Stone OJ. Blastomycosis-like pyoderma. Arch Dermatol 1966; 93: 226–228.

142 Su WPD, Duncan SC, Perry HO. Blastomycosis-like pyoderma. Arch Dermatol 1979; 115: 170–173.

143 Crowley JJ, Kim YH. Blastomycosis-like pyoderma in a man with AIDS. J Am Acad Dermatol 1997; 36: 633–634.

144 Weedon D. Actinic comedonal plaque. J Am Acad Dermatol 1981; 5: 611.

145 Kocsard E. Actinic comedonal plaque. J Am Acad Dermatol 1981; 5: 611–612.

146 Georgouras K. Coral reef granuloma. Cutis 1967; 3: 37–39.

147 Eastern JS, Martin S. Actinic comedonal plaque. J Am Acad Dermatol 1980; 3: 633–636.

148 Yaffee HS. Localized blastomycosis-like pyoderma occurring in a tattoo. Arch Dermatol 1960; 82: 99–100.

149 John SM, Hamm H. Actinic comedonal plaque – a rare ectopic form of the Favre–Racouchot syndrome. Clin Exp Dermatol 1993; 18: 256–258.

150 Trygg KJ, Madison KC. Blastomycosis-like pyoderma caused by *Pseudomonas aeruginosa*: report of a case responsive to ciprofloxacin. J Am Acad Dermatol 1990; 23: 750–752.

151 Rongioletti F, Semino M, Drago F et al. Blastomycosis-like pyoderma (pyoderma vegetans) responding to antibiotics and topical disodium chromoglycate. Int J Dermatol 1996; 35: 828–830.

152 O'Dell BL, Jessen T, Becker LE et al. Diminished immune response in sun-damaged skin. Arch Dermatol 1980; 116: 559–561.

153 Serre I, Cano JP, Picot M-C et al. Immunosuppression induced by acute solar-simulated ultraviolet exposure in humans: Prevention by a sunscreen with a sun protection factor of 15 and high UVA protection. J Am Acad Dermatol 1997; 37: 187–194.

Corynebacterial infections

154 Pitcher DG. Aerobic cutaneous coryneforms: recent taxonomic findings. Br J Dermatol 1978; 98: 363–370.

155 Leyden JJ, McGinley KJ, Holzle E et al. The microbiology of the human axilla and its relationship to axillary odor. J Invest Dermatol 1981; 77: 413–416.

156 Shelley WB, Shelley ED. Coexistent erythrasma, trichomycosis axillaris, and pitted keratolysis: an overlooked corynebacterial triad? J Am Acad Dermatol 1982; 7: 752–757.

157 Ceilley RI. Foot ulceration and vertebral osteomyelitis with *Corynebacterium haemolyticum*. Arch Dermatol 1977; 113: 646–647.

158 Jerdan MS, Shapiro RS, Smith NB et al. Cutaneous manifestations of *Corynebacterium* group JK sepsis. J Am Acad Dermatol 1987; 16: 444–447.

159 Jucglà A, Sais G, Carratala J et al. A papular eruption secondary to infection with *Corynebacterium jeikeium*, with histopathological features mimicking botryomycosis. Br J Dermatol 1995; 133: 801–804.

160 Bader M, Pedersen AHB, Spearman J, Harnisch JP. An unusual case of cutaneous diphtheria. JAMA 1978; 240: 1382–1383.

161 Höfler W. Cutaneous diphtheria. Int J Dermatol 1991; 30: 845–847.

162 Pandit N, Yeshwanth M. Cutaneous diphtheria in a child. Int J Dermatol 1999; 38: 298–305.

163 Cochran RJ, Rosen T, Landers T. Topical treatment for erythrasma. Int J Dermatol 1981; 20: 562–564.

164 Sinduphak W, MacDonald E. Smith EB. Erythrasma. Overlooked or misdiagnosed? Int J Dermatol 1985; 24: 95–96.

165 Engber PB, Mandel EH. Generalized disciform erythrasma. Int J Dermatol 1979; 18: 633–635.

166 Schlappner OLA, Rosenblum GA, Rowden G, Phillips TM. Concomitant erythrasma and dermatophytosis of the groin. Br J Dermatol 1979; 100: 147–151.

167 Svejgaard E, Christophersen J, Jelsdorf H-M. Tinea pedis and erythrasma in Danish recruits. J Am Acad Dermatol 1986; 14: 993–999.

168 Montes LF, Black SH. The fine structure of diphtheroids of erythrasma. J Invest Dermatol 1967; 48: 342–349.

169 Montes LF, Black SH, McBride ME. Bacterial invasion of the stratum corneum in erythrasma. J Invest Dermatol 1967; 49: 474–485.

170 White SW, Smith J. Trichomycosis pubis. Arch Dermatol 1979; 115: 444–445.

171 Shelley WB, Miller MA. Electron microscopy, histochemistry, and microbiology of bacterial adhesion in trichomycosis axillaris. J Am Acad Dermatol 1984; 10: 1005–1014.

172 McBride ME, Freeman RG, Knox JM. The bacteriology of trichomycosis axillaris. Br J Dermatol 1968; 80: 509–513.

173 Levit F. Trichomycosis axillaris: a different view. J Am Acad Dermatol 1988; 18: 778–779.

174 Orfanos CE, Schloesser E, Mahrle G. Hair destroying growth of *Corynebacterium tenuis* in the so-called trichomycosis axillaris. Arch Dermatol 1971; 103: 632–639.

175 Tilgen W. Pitted keratolysis (keratolysis plantare sulcatum). J Cutan Pathol 1979; 6: 18–30.

176 Zaias N. Pitted and ringed keratolysis. A review and update. J Am Acad Dermatol 1982; 7: 787–791.

177 Rubel LR. Pitted keratolysis and *Dermatophilus congolensis*. Arch Dermatol 1972; 105: 584–586.

178 Lamberg SI. Symptomatic pitted keratolysis. Arch Dermatol 1969; 100: 10–11.

179 Shah AS, Kamino H, Prose NS. Painful, plaque-like, pitted keratolysis occurring in childhood. Pediatr Dermatol 1992; 9: 251–254.

180 Takama H, Tamada Y, Yano K et al. Pitted keratolysis: clinical manifestations in 53 cases. Br J Dermatol 1997; 137: 282–285.

181 Emmerson RW, Wilson Jones E. Ringed keratolysis of the palms. Trans St John's Hosp Dermatol Soc 1967; 53: 165–167.

182 Lee H-J, Roh K-Y, Ha S-J, Kim J-W. Pitted keratolysis of the palm arising after herpes zoster. Br J Dermatol 1999; 140: 974–975.

183 Zaias N, Taplin D, Rebell G. Pitted keratolysis. Arch Dermatol 1965; 92: 151–154.

184 Gill KA, Buckels LJ. Pitted keratolysis. Arch Dermatol 1968; 98: 7–11.

185 Woodgyer AJ, Baxter M, Rush-Munro FM et al. Isolation of *Dermatophilus congolensis* from two New Zealand cases of pitted keratolysis. Australas J Dermatol 1985; 26: 29–35.

186 Nordstrom KM, McGinley KJ, Cappiello L et al. Pitted keratolysis. The role of *Micrococcus sedentarius*. Arch Dermatol 1987; 123: 1320–1325.

187 Wohlrab J, Rohrbach D, Marsch WC. Keratolysis sulcata (pitted keratolysis): clinical symptoms with different histological correlates. Br J Dermatol 2000; 143: 1348–1349.

188 de Almeida HL Jr, de Castro LAS, Rocha NEM, Abrantes VL. Ultrastructure of pitted keratolysis. Int J Dermatol 2000; 39: 698–701.

Neisserial infections

189 Darmstadt GL. Acute infectious purpura fulminans: pathogenesis and medical management. Pediatr Dermatol 1998; 15: 169–183.

190 Assier H, Chosidow O, Rekacewicz I et al. Chronic meningococcemia in acquired immunodeficiency infection. J Am Acad Dermatol 1993; 29: 793–794.

191 Rosen T. Unusual presentations of gonorrhea. J Am Acad Dermatol 1982; 6: 369–372.

192 Scott MJ Jr, Scott MJ Sr. Primary cutaneous *Neisseria gonorrhoeae* infections. Arch Dermatol 1982; 118: 351–352.

Mycobacterial infections

193 Santa Cruz DJ, Strayer DS. The histologic spectrum of the cutaneous mycobacterioses. Hum Pathol 1982; 13: 485–495.

194 Ramesh V, Misra RS, Jain RK. Secondary tuberculosis of the skin. Clinical features and problems in laboratory diagnosis. Int J Dermatol 1987; 26: 578–581.

195 Sehgal VN, Srivastava G, Khurana VK et al. An appraisal of epidemiologic, clinical, bacteriologic, histopathologic, and immunologic parameters in cutaneous tuberculosis. Int J Dermatol 1987; 26: 521–526.

196 Sehgal VN, Jain MK, Srivastava G. Changing pattern of cutaneous tuberculosis. A prospective study. Int J Dermatol 1989; 28: 231–236.

197 Sehgal VN. Cutaneous tuberculosis: the evolving scenario. Int J Dermatol 1994; 33: 97–104.

198 Grange JM, Zumla A. Paradox of the global emergency of tuberculosis. Lancet 1999; 353: 996.

199 Chintu C, Mwinga A. An African perspective on the threat of tuberculosis and HIV/AIDS – can despair be turned to hope? Lancet 1999; 353: 997.

200 Drobniewski FA, Watt B, Smith EG et al. A national audit of the laboratory diagnosis of tuberculosis and other mycobacterial diseases within the United Kingdom. J Clin Pathol 1999; 52: 334–337.

201 Hart V, Weedon D. Lupus vulgaris and *Mycobacterium bovis*: a case report. Australas J Dermatol 1977; 18: 86–87.

202 Iden DL, Rogers RS III, Schroeter AL. Papulonecrotic tuberculid secondary to *Mycobacterium bovis*. Arch Dermatol 1978; 114: 564–566.

203 Joly P, Picard-Dahan C, Bamberger N et al. Acute pustular eruption: an unusual clinical feature of disseminated mycobacterial infection in patients with acquired immunodeficiency syndrome. J Am Acad Dermatol 1993; 28: 264–266.

204 Abel L, Casanova J-L. Genetic predisposition to clinical tuberculosis: bridging the gap between simple and complex inheritance. Am J Hum Genet 2000; 67: 274–277.

205 Brown FS, Anderson RH, Burnett JW. Cutaneous tuberculosis. J Am Acad Dermatol 1982; 6: 101–106.

206 Beyt BE Jr, Ortbals DW, Santa Cruz DJ et al. Cutaneous mycobacteriosis: analysis of 34 cases with a new classification of the disease. Medicine (Baltimore) 1980; 60: 95–109.

207 Grange JM. Mycobacteria and the skin. Int J Dermatol 1982; 21: 497–503.

208 Saxe N. Mycobacterial skin infections. J Cutan Pathol 1985; 12: 300–312.

209 Grange JM, Noble WC, Yates MD, Collins CH. Inoculation mycobacterioses. Clin Exp Dermatol 1988; 13: 211–220.

210 Lantos G, Fisher BK, Contreras M. Tuberculous ulcer of the skin. J Am Acad Dermatol 1988; 19: 1067–1072.

211 Faizal M, Jimenez G, Burgos C et al. Diagnosis of cutaneous tuberculosis by polymerase chain reaction using a species-specific gene. Int J Dermatol 1996; 35: 185–188.

212 Degitz K. Detection of mycobacterial DNA in the skin. Arch Dermatol 1996; 132: 71–75.

213 Penneys NS, Leonardi CL, Cook S et al. Identification of *Mycobacterium tuberculosis* DNA in five different types of cutaneous lesions by the polymerase chain reaction. Arch Dermatol 1993; 129: 1594–1598.

214 Nachbar F, Classen V, Nachbar T et al. Orificial tuberculosis: detection by polymerase chain reaction. Br J Dermatol 1996; 135: 106–109.

215 Quirós E, Maroto MC, Bettinardi A et al. Diagnosis of cutaneous tuberculosis in biopsy specimens by PCR and Southern blotting. J Clin Pathol 1996; 49: 889–891.

216 Margall N, Baselga E, Coll P et al. Detection of *Mycobacterium tuberculosis* complex DNA by the polymerase chain reaction for rapid diagnosis of cutaneous tuberculosis. Br J Dermatol 1996; 135: 231–236.

217 Nenoff P, Rytter M, Schubert S et al. Multilocular inoculation tuberculosis of the skin after stay in Africa: detection of mycobacterial DNA using polymerase chain reaction. Br J Dermatol 2000; 143: 226–228.

218 Li JYW, Lo STH, Ng C-S. Molecular detection of *Mycobacterium tuberculosis* in tissues showing granulomatous inflammation without demonstrable acid-fast bacilli. Diagn Mol Pathol 2000; 9: 67–74.

219 Sanguinetti M, Posteraro B, Chinni LM et al. Polymerase chain reaction and reverse cross blot hybridization assay for detection of mycobacterial DNA in lupus vulgaris. Dermatology 1997; 195: 293–296.

220 Tan SH, Tan BH, Goh CL et al. Detection of *Mycobacterium tuberculosis* DNA using polymerase chain reaction in cutaneous tuberculosis and tuberculids. Int J Dermatol 1999; 38: 122–127.

221 Baselga E, Barnadas MA, Margall N, De Moragas JM. Detection of *M. tuberculosis* complex DNA in a lesion resembling sarcoidosis. Clin Exp Dermatol 1996; 21: 235–238.

222 Dostrovsky A, Sagher F. Dermatological complications of BCG vaccination. Br J Dermatol 1963; 75: 181–192.

223 Izumi AK, Matsunaga J. BCG vaccine-induced lupus vulgaris. Arch Dermatol 1982; 118: 171–172.

224 Stewart EJC, James MP. Lupus vulgaris-like reaction following BCG vaccination. Clin Exp Dermatol 1996; 21: 232–234.

225 Handjani F, Delir S, Sodaifi M, Kumar PV. Lupus vulgaris following bacille Calmette–Guérin vaccination. Br J Dermatol 2001; 144: 444–445.

226 Park YM, Kang H, Cho SH, Cho BK. Lichen scrofulosorum-like eruption localized to multipuncture BCG vaccination site. J Am Acad Dermatol 1999; 41: 262–264.

227 Kakakhel KU, Fritsch P. Cutaneous tuberculosis. Int J Dermatol 1989; 28: 355–362.

228 de la Monte SM, Hutchins GM. Fatal disseminated bacillus Calmette–Guérin infection and arrested growth of cutaneous malignant melanoma following intralesional immunotherapy. Am J Dermatopathol 1986; 8: 331–335.

229 Caplan SE, Kauffman CL. Primary inoculation tuberculosis after immunotherapy for malignant melanoma with BCG vaccine. J Am Acad Dermatol 1996; 35: 783–785.

230 McKenzie RHSB, Roux P. Disseminated BCG infection following bone marrow transplantation for X-linked severe combined immunodeficiency. Pediatr Dermatol 2000; 17: 208–212.

231 Ratón JA, Pocheville I, Vicente JM et al. Disseminated bacillus Calmette-Guerin infection in an HIV-infected child: a case with cutaneous lesions. Pediatr Dermatol 1997; 14: 365–368.

232 Kutzner H, Argenyi ZB, Requena L et al. A new application of BCG antibody for rapid screening of various tissue microorganisms. J Am Acad Dermatol 1998; 38: 56–60.

233 Goette DK, Jacobson KW, Doty RD. Primary inoculation tuberculosis of the skin. Prosector's paronychia. Arch Dermatol 1978; 114: 567–569.

234 Horney DA, Gaither JM, Lauer R et al. Cutaneous inoculation tuberculosis secondary to 'jailhouse tattooing'. Arch Dermatol 1985; 121: 648–650.

235 Hoyt EM. Primary inoculation tuberculosis. Report of a case. JAMA 1981; 245: 1556–1557.

236 Tham SN, Choong HL. Primary tuberculous chancre in a renal transplant patient. J Am Acad Dermatol 1992; 26: 342–344.

237 Konohana A, Noda J, Shoji K, Hanyaku H. Primary tuberculosis of the glans penis. J Am Acad Dermatol 1992; 26: 1002–1003.

238 Gil MP, Velasco M, Vilata JJ et al. Primary tuberculous chancre: An unusual kind of skin tuberculosis. J Am Acad Dermatol 1994; 31: 108–109.

239 Chowdhury MMU, Varma S, Howell S et al. Facial cutaneous tuberculosis: an unusual presentation. Clin Exp Dermatol 2000; 25: 48–50.

240 Chaves A, Torrelo A, Mediero IG et al. Primary cutaneous Mycobacterium kansasii infection in a child. Pediatr Dermatol 2001; 18: 131–134.

241 Vidal D, Barnadas M, Pérez M et al. Tuberculous gumma following venepuncture. Br J Dermatol 2001; 144: 601–603.

242 Sehgal VN, Srivastava G, Bajaj P, Sengal R. Re-infection (secondary) inoculation cutaneous tuberculosis. Int J Dermatol 2001; 40: 205–209.

243 Sahn SA, Pierson DJ. Primary cutaneous inoculation drug-resistant tuberculosis. Am J Med 1974; 57: 676–678.

244 Allen RK, Pierson DL, Rodman OG. Cutaneous inoculation tuberculosis: prosector's wart occurring in a physician. Cutis 1979; 23: 815–818.

245 Sah SP, AshokRaj G, Joshi A. Primary tuberculosis of the glans penis. Australas J Dermatol 1999; 40: 106–107.

246 Liang MG, Rooney JA, Rhodes KH, Calobrisi SD. Cutaneous inoculation tuberculosis in a child. J Am Acad Dermatol 1999; 41: 860–862.

247 McDaniel WR, Anderson ER. Lupus vulgaris in the United States. Occurrence in a Saudi-Arabian soldier. Int J Dermatol 1980; 19: 165–167.

248 Kumar B, Rai R, Kaur I et al. Childhood cutaneous tuberculosis: a study over 25 years from northern India. Int J Dermatol 2001; 40: 26–32.

249 Kullavanijaya P, Sirimachan S, Surarak S. Primary cutaneous infection with Mycobacterium avium intracellulare complex resembling lupus vulgaris. Br J Dermatol 1997; 136: 264–266.

250 Ara M, Seral C, Baselga C et al. Primary tuberculous chancre caused by Mycobacterium bovis after goring with a bull's horn. J Am Acad Dermatol 2000; 43: 535–537.

251 Warin AP, Wilson Jones E. Cutaneous tuberculosis of the nose with unusual clinical and histological features leading to a delay in the diagnosis. Clin Exp Dermatol 1977; 2: 235–242.

252 Sehgal VN, Srivastava G, Sharma VK. Lupus vulgaris, caries of the spine and lichen scrofulosorum – an intriguing association. Clin Exp Dermatol 1987; 12: 280–282.

253 Bilen N, Apaydin R, Harova G et al. Lupus vulgaris on the buttock: report of two cases. J Eur Acad Dermatol Venereol 2000; 14: 66–67.

254 Ramesh V, Misra RS, Beena KR, Mukherjee A. A study of cutaneous tuberculosis in children. Pediatr Dermatol 1999; 16: 264–269.

255 Jaisankar TJ, Garg BR, Reddy BS et al. Penile lupus vulgaris. Int J Dermatol 1994; 33: 272–274.

256 Drago F, Parodi A, Rebora A. Addison's disease and lupus vulgaris: report of a case. J Am Acad Dermatol 1988; 18: 581–583.

257 Munn SE, Basarab T, Russell Jones R. Lupus vulgaris – a case report. Clin Exp Dermatol 1995; 20: 56–57.

258 Lee NH, Choi EH, Lee WS, Ahn SK. Tuberculous cellulitis. Clin Exp Dermatol 2000; 25: 222–223.

259 Haim S, Friedman-Birnbaum R. Cutaneous tuberculosis and malignancy. Cutis 1978; 21: 643–647.

260 Yerushalmi J, Grunwald MH, Halevy DH et al. Lupus vulgaris complicated by metastatic squamous cell carcinoma. Int J Dermatol 1998; 37: 934–935.

261 Orfuss AJ. Lupus vulgaris and superimposed basal cell epitheliomas. Arch Dermatol 1971; 103: 555.

262 Sowden J, Paramsothy Y, Smith AG. Malignant melanoma arising in the scar of lupus vulgaris and response to treatment with topical azelaic acid. Clin Exp Dermatol 1988; 13: 353–356.

263 Duhra P, Grattan CEH, Ryatt KS. Lupus vulgaris with numerous tubercle bacilli. Clin Exp Dermatol 1988; 13: 31–33.

264 Harrison PV, Marks JM. Lupus vulgaris and cutaneous lymphoma. Clin Exp Dermatol 1980; 5: 73–77.

265 Hruza GJ, Posnick RB, Weltman RE. Disseminated lupus vulgaris presenting as granulomatous folliculitis. Int J Dermatol 1989; 28: 388–392.

266 Ferrara G, Cannone M, Scalvenzi M et al. Facial granulomatous diseases. A study of four cases tested for the presence of Mycobacterium tuberculosis DNA using nested polymerase chain reaction. Am J Dermatopathol 2001; 23: 8–15.

267 Ramesh V, Samuel B, Misra RS, Nath I. In situ characterization of cellular infiltrates in lupus vulgaris indicates lesional T-cell activation. Arch Dermatol 1990; 126: 331–335.

268 Goette DK, Odom RB. Transepithelial elimination of granulomas in cutaneous tuberculosis and sarcoidosis. J Am Acad Dermatol 1986; 14: 126–128.

269 Steidl M, Neubert U, Volkenandt M et al. Lupus vulgaris confirmed by polymerase-chain reaction. Br J Dermatol 1993; 129: 314–318.

270 Serfling U, Penneys NS, Leonardi CL. Identification of Mycobacterium tuberculosis DNA in a case of lupus vulgaris. J Am Acad Dermatol 1993; 28: 318–322.

271 Helander I, Aho HJ, Maki J. Lupus vulgaris with Michaelis–Gutmann-like bodies in an immunologically compromised patient – cutaneous malacoplakia of tuberculous origin? J Am Acad Dermatol 1988; 18: 577–579.

272 Marcoval J, Servitje O, Moreno A et al. Lupus vulgaris. Clinical, histopathologic, and bacteriologic study of 10 cases. J Am Acad Dermatol 1992; 26: 404–407.

273 Pereira MB, Gomes MK, Pereira F. Tuberculosis verrucosa cutis associated with tuberculous lymphadenitis. Int J Dermatol 2000; 39: 856–858.

274 Bordalo O, Garcia E, Silva L. Tuberculosis verrucosa cutis with liver involvement. Clin Exp Dermatol 1987; 12: 283–285.

275 Wortman PD. Pulmonary and cutaneous tuberculosis. J Am Acad Dermatol 1992; 27: 459–460.

276 Jaisankar TJ, Baruah MC, Garg BR. Tuberculosis verrucosa cutis arising from a trophic ulcer. Int J Dermatol 1992; 31: 503–504.

277 Pramatarov K, Balabanova M, Miteva L, Gantcheva M. Tuberculosis verrucosa cutis associated with lupus vulgaris. Int J Dermatol 1993; 32: 815–817.

278 Iizawa O, Aiba S, Tagami H. Tuberculosis verrucosa cutis in a tumour-like form. Br J Dermatol 1991; 125: 79–80.

279 Sehgal VN, Sehgal R, Bajaj P et al. Tuberculosis verrucosa cutis (TBVC). J Eur Acad Dermatol Venereol 2000; 14: 319–321.

280 Yates VM, Ormerod LP. Cutaneous tuberculosis in Blackburn district (U.K.): a 15-year prospective series, 1981–1995. Br J Dermatol 1997; 136: 483–489.

281 Özkan Ş, Gürler N, Fetil E et al. Scrofuloderma. Int J Dermatol 1998; 37: 606–608.

282 Sehgal VN, Jain S, Thappa DM, Logani K. Scrofuloderma and caries spine. Int J Dermatol 1992; 31: 505–506.

283 del Carmen Fariña M, Gegundez MI, Piqué E et al. Cutaneous tuberculosis: a clinical, histopathologic, and bacteriologic study. J Am Acad Dermatol 1995; 33: 433–440.

284 Tur E, Brenner S, Meiron Y. Scrofuloderma (tuberculosis colliquativa cutis). Br J Dermatol 1996; 134: 350–352.

285 Harris A, Burge S, Williams S, Desai S. Cutaneous tuberculosis abscess: a management problem. Br J Dermatol 1996; 135: 457–459.

286 Seghal VN, Gupta R, Bose M, Saha K. Immunohistopathological spectrum in cutaneous tuberculosis. Clin Exp Dermatol 1993; 18: 309–313.

287 Betlloch I, Bañuls J, Sevila A et al. Perianal tuberculosis. Int J Dermatol 1994; 33: 270–271.

288 Panzarelli A, Acosta M, Garrido L. Tuberculosis cutis orificialis. Int J Dermatol 1996; 35: 443–444.

289 Nachbar F, Classen V, Nachbar T et al. Orificial tuberculosis: detection by polymerase chain reaction. Br J Dermatol 1996; 135: 106–109.

290 Chen Y-J, Shieh P-P, Shen J-L. Orificial tuberculosis and Kaposi's sarcoma in an HIV-negative individual. Clin Exp Dermatol 2000; 25: 393–397.

291 Regan W, Harley W. Orificial and pulmonary tuberculosis: report of a case. Australas J Dermatol 1979; 20: 88–89.

292 Honig E, van der Meijden WI, van Zoelen ECG, De Waard-van der Spek FB. Perianal ulceration: a rare manifestation of tuberculosis. Br J Dermatol 2000; 142: 186–187.

293 Bateman DE, Makepeace W, Lesna M. Miliary tuberculosis in association with chronic cutaneous tuberculosis. Br J Dermatol 1980; 103: 557–560.

294 Munt PW. Miliary tuberculosis in the chemotherapy era: with a clinical review in 69 American adults. Medicine (Baltimore) 1971; 51: 139–155.

295 Rohatgi PK, Palazzolo JV, Sain NB. Acute miliary tuberculosis of the skin in acquired immunodeficiency syndrome. J Am Acad Dermatol 1992; 26: 356–359.

296 Lipper S, Watkins DL, Kahn LB. Nongranulomatous septic vasculitis due to miliary tuberculosis. Am J Dermatopathol 1980; 2: 71–74.

297 Inwald D, Nelson M, Cramp M et al. Cutaneous manifestations of mycobacterial infection in patients with AIDS. Br J Dermatol 1994; 130: 111–114.

298 Stack RJ, Bickley LK, Coppel IG. Miliary tuberculosis presenting as skin lesions in a patient with acquired immunodeficiency syndrome. J Am Acad Dermatol 1990; 23: 1031–1035.

299 Schermer DR, Simpson CG, Haserick JR, Van Ordstrand HS. Tuberculosis cutis miliaris acuta generalisata. Report of a case in an adult and review of the literature. Arch Dermatol 1969; 99: 64–69.

300 Jordaan HF, Schneider JW, Abdulla EAK. Nodular tuberculid: a report of four patients. Pediatr Dermatol 2000; 17: 183–188.

301 Choonhakarn C, Ackerman AB. Tuberculids. Dermatopathology: Practical & Conceptual 2000; 6: 138–143.

302 Kumar B, Parsad D. Is 'nodular tuberculid' a distinct entity? Pediatr Dermatol 2001; 18: 164–165.

303 Breathnach SM, Black MM. Atypical tuberculide (acne scrofulosorum) secondary to tuberculous lymphadenitis. Clin Exp Dermatol 1981; 6: 339–344.

304 Alsina M, Campo P, Toll A et al. Papulonecrotic tuberculide in a human immunodeficiency virus type I-seropositive patient. Br J Dermatol 2000; 143: 232–233.

305 Schneider JW, Jordaan HF, Geiger DH et al. Erythema induratum of Bazin. A clinicopathological study of 20 cases and detection of *Mycobacterium tuberculosis* DNA in skin lesions by polymerase chain reaction. Am J Dermatopathol 1995; 17: 350–356.

306 Parker SC. A new tuberculid? J Cutan Pathol 1989; 16: 319 (abstract).

307 Hara K, Tsuzuki T, Takagi N, Shimokata K. Nodular granulomatous phlebitis of the skin: a fourth type of tuberculid. Histopathology 1997; 30: 129–134.

308 Chuang YH, Kuo TT, Wang CM et al. Simultaneous occurrence of papulonecrotic tuberculide and erythema induratum and the identification of *Mycobacterium tuberculosis* DNA by polymerase chain reaction. Br J Dermatol 1997; 137: 276–281.

309 Park YM, Hong JK, Cho SH, Cho BK. Concomitant lichen scrofulosorum and erythema induratum. J Am Acad Dermatol 1998; 38: 841–843.

310 Morrison JGL, Fourie ED. The papulonecrotic tuberculide. From Arthus reaction to lupus vulgaris. Br J Dermatol 1974; 91: 263–270.

311 Chong L-Y, Lo K-K. Cutaneous tuberculosis in Hong Kong: a 10-year retrospective study. Int J Dermatol 1995; 34: 26–29.

312 Milligan A, Chen K, Graham-Brown RAC. Two tuberculides in one patient – a case report of papulonecrotic tuberculide and erythema induratum occurring together. Clin Exp Dermatol 1990; 15: 21–23.

313 Hudson PM. Tuberculide (lichen scrofulosorum) secondary to osseous tuberculosis. Clin Exp Dermatol 1976; 1: 391–394.

314 Smith NP, Ryan TJ, Sanderson KV, Sarkany I. Lichen scrofulosorum. A report of four cases. Br J Dermatol 1976; 94: 319–325.

315 Arianayagam AV, Ash S, Russell Jones R. Lichen scrofulosorum in a patient with AIDS. Clin Exp Dermatol 1994; 19: 74–76.

316 Beena KR, Ramesh V, Mukherjee A. Lichen scrofulosorum – a series of eight cases. Dermatology 2000; 201: 272–274.

317 Kakakhel K. Simultaneous occurrence of tuberculous gumma, tuberculosis verrucosis cutis, and lichen scrofulosorum. Int J Dermatol 1998; 37: 867–869.

318 Torrelo A, Valverde E, Mediero IG, Zambrano A. Lichen scrofulosorum. Pediatr Dermatol 2000; 17: 373–376.

319 Komatsu H, Terunuma A, Tabata N, Tagami H. *Mycobacterium avium* infection of the skin associated with lichen scrofulosorum: report of three cases. Br J Dermatol 1999; 141: 554–557.

320 Wilson-Jones E, Winkelmann RK. Papulonecrotic tuberculid: a neglected disease in Western countries. J Am Acad Dermatol 1986; 14: 815–826.

321 Jordaan HF, Van Niekerk DJT, Louw M. Papulonecrotic tuberculid. A clinical, histopathological, and immunohistochemical study of 15 patients. Am J Dermatopathol 1994; 16: 474–485.

322 Sloan JB, Medenica M. Papulonecrotic tuberculid in a 9-year-old American girl: case report and review of the literature. Pediatr Dermatol 1990; 7: 191–195.

323 Kullavanijaya P, Sirimachan S, Suwantaroj S. Papulonecrotic tuberculid. Necessity of long-term triple regimens. Int J Dermatol 1991; 30: 487–490.

324 Wong KO, Lee KP, Chiu SF. Tuberculosis of the skin in Hong Kong. Br J Dermatol 1968; 80: 424–429.

325 McCray MK, Esterly NB. Cutaneous eruptions in congenital tuberculosis. Arch Dermatol 1981; 117: 460–464.

326 Israelewicz S, Dharan M, Rosenman D et al. Papulonecrotic tuberculid of the glans penis. J Am Acad Dermatol 1985; 12: 1104–1106.

327 Jordaan HF, Schneider JW, Schaaf HS et al. Papulonecrotic tuberculid in children. A report of eight patients. Am J Dermatopathol 1996; 18: 172–185.

328 Almeida BM, Challacombe SJ, Hay RJ et al. Papulonecrotic tuberculide complicating scrofuloderma in a health-care worker. Br J Dermatol 1998; 139: 550–552.

329 Senol M, Ozcan A, Aydin A et al. Disseminated lupus vulgaris and papulonecrotic tuberculid: case report. Pediatr Dermatol 2000; 17: 133–135.

330 Victor T, Jordaan HF, Van Niekerk DJT et al. Papulonecrotic tuberculid. Identification of *Mycobacterium tuberculosis* DNA by polymerase chain reaction. Am J Dermatopathol 1992; 14: 491–495.

331 Williams JT, Pulitzer DR, DeVillez RL. Papulonecrotic tuberculid secondary to disseminated *Mycobacterium avium* complex. Int J Dermatol 1994; 33: 109–112.

332 Callahan EF, Licata AL, Madison JF. Cutaneous *Mycobacterium kansasii* infection associated with a papulonecrotic tuberculid reaction. J Am Acad Dermatol 1997; 36: 497–499.

333 Graham-Brown RAC, Sarkany I. Lichen scrofulosorum with tuberculous dactylitis. Br J Dermatol 1980; 103: 561–564.

334 Ramdial PK, Mosam A, Mallett R, Aboobaker J. Papulonecrotic tuberculid in a 2-year-old girl: with emphasis on extent of disease and presence of leucocytoclastic vasculitis. Pediatr Dermatol 1998; 15: 450–455.

335 Hanke CW, Temofeew RK, Slama SL. *Mycobacterium kansasii* infection with multiple cutaneous lesions. J Am Acad Dermatol 1987; 16: 1122–1128.

336 Lotti T, Hautmann G. Atypical mycobacterial infections: a difficult and emerging group of infectious dermatoses. Int J Dermatol 1993; 32: 499–501.

337 Escalonilla P, Esteban J, Soriano ML et al. Cutaneous manifestations of infection by nontuberculous mycobacteria. Clin Exp Dermatol 1998; 23: 214–221.

338 Palenque E. Skin disease and nontuberculous atypical mycobacteria. Int J Dermatol 2000; 39: 659–666.

339 Street ML, Umbert-Millet IJ, Roberts GD, Su WPD. Nontuberculous mycobacterial infections of the skin. Report of fourteen cases and review of the literature. J Am Acad Dermatol 1991; 24: 208–215.

340 Monson MH, Gybson DW, Connor DH et al. *Mycobacterium ulcerans* in Liberia: a clinicopathologic study of 6 patients with Buruli ulcer. Acta Trop (Basel) 1984; 41: 165–172.

341 van der Werf TS, van der Graaf WTA, Tappero JW, Asiedu K. *Mycobacterium ulcerans* infection. Lancet 1999; 354: 1013–1018.

342 Hayman J. Out of Africa: observations on the histopathology of *Mycobacterium ulcerans* infection. J Clin Pathol 1993; 46: 5–9.

343 Pettit JHS, Marchette NJ, Rees RJW. *Mycobacterium ulcerans* infection. Clinical and bacteriological study of the first cases recognized in South East Asia. Br J Dermatol 1966; 78: 187–197.

344 Ziefer A, Connor DH, Gybson DW. *Mycobacterium ulcerans*. Infection of two patients in Liberia. Int J Dermatol 1981; 20: 362–367.

345 Barker DJP. Mycobacterial skin ulcers. Br J Dermatol 1974; 91: 473–474.

346 Dawson JF, Allen GE. Ulcer due to *Mycobacterium ulcerans* in Northern Ireland. Clin Exp Dermatol 1985; 10: 572–576.

347 Hayman J, McQueen A. The pathology of *Mycobacterium ulcerans* infection. Pathology 1985; 17: 594–600.

348 Hale MJ. Mycobacterial infection: a histopathological chameleon. Curr Diagn Pathol 2000; 6: 93–102.

349 Hayman JA, Smith IM, Flood P. Pseudoepitheliomatous hyperplasia in *Mycobacterium ulcerans* infection. Pathology 1996; 28: 131–134.

350 Tomasini C, Grassi M, Soro E, Pippione M. Necrotizing panniculitis due to *Mycobacterium ulcerans*: an infection from Jurassic time. Am J Dermatopathol 2000; 22: 356 (abstract).

351 Huminer D, Pitlik SD, Block C et al. Aquarium-borne *Mycobacterium marinum* skin infection. Report of a case and review of the literature. Arch Dermatol 1986; 122: 698–703.

352 Philpott JA Jr, Woodburne AR, Philpott OS et al. Swimming pool granuloma. A study of 290 cases. Arch Dermatol 1963; 88: 158–162.

353 Kullavanijaya P, Sirimachan S, Bhuddhavudhikrai P. *Mycobacterium marinum* cutaneous infections acquired from occupations and hobbies. Int J Dermatol 1993; 32: 504–507.

354 Ang P, Rattana-Apiromyakij N, Goh C-L. Retrospective study of *Mycobacterium marinum* skin infections. Int J Dermatol 2000; 39: 343–347.

355 Wallace RJ Jr. Recent clinical advances in knowledge of the nonleprous environmental mycobacteria responsible for cutaneous disease. Arch Dermatol 1987; 123: 337–339.

356 Gould WM, McMeekin DR, Bright RD. *Mycobacterium marinum (balnei)* infection. Report of a case with cutaneous and laryngeal lesions. Arch Dermatol 1968; 97: 159–162.

357 Zeligman I. *Mycobacterium marinum* granuloma. Arch Dermatol 1972; 106: 26–31.

358 Papanaoum K, Marshmann G, Gordon LA et al. Concurrent infection due to *Shewanella putrefaciens* and *Mycobacterium marinum* acquired at the beach. Australas J Dermatol 1998; 39: 92–95.

359 Chappler RR, Hoke AW, Borchardt KA. Primary inoculation with *Mycobacterium marinum*. Arch Dermatol 1977; 113: 380.

360 Lee MW, Brenan J. *Mycobacterium marinum*: chronic and extensive infections of the lower limbs in South Pacific Islanders. Australas J Dermatol 1998; 39: 173–176.

361 Aria H, Nakajima K, Nagai R. *Mycobacterium marinum* infection of the skin in Japan. J Dermatol 1984; 11: 37–42.

362 Glickman FS. Sporotrichoid mycobacterial infections. Case report and review. J Am Acad Dermatol 1983; 8: 703–707.

363 Posteraro B, Sanguinetti M, Garcovich A et al. Polymerase chain reaction-reverse cross-blot hybridization assay in the diagnosis of sporotrichoid *Mycobacterium marinum* infection. Br J Dermatol 1998; 139: 872–876.

364 Speight EL, Williams HC. Fish tank granuloma in a 14-month-old girl. Pediatr Dermatol 1997; 14: 209–212.

365 Gombert ME, Goldstein EJC, Corrado ML et al. Disseminated *Mycobacterium marinum* infection after renal transplantation. Ann Intern Med 1981; 94: 486–487.

366 King AJ, Fairley JA, Rasmussen JE. Disseminated cutaneous *Mycobacterium marinum* infection. Arch Dermatol 1983; 119: 268–270.

367 Bleiker TO, Bourke JE, Burns DA. Fish tank granuloma in a 4-year-old boy. Br J Dermatol 1996; 135: 863–864.

368 Dickey RF. Sporotrichoid mycobacteriosis caused by *M. marinum (balnei)*. Arch Dermatol 1968; 98: 385–391.

369 Smith AG, Jiji RM. Cutaneous infection due to a rough variant of *Mycobacterium marinum*. Am J Clin Pathol 1975; 64: 263–270.

370 Travis WD, Travis LB, Roberts GD et al. The histopathologic spectrum in *Mycobacterium marinum* infection. Arch Pathol Lab Med 1985; 109: 1109–1113.

371 Shelley WB, Folkens AT. *Mycobacterium gordonae* infection of the hand. Arch Dermatol 1984; 120: 1064–1065.

372 Drabick JJ, Hoover DL, Roth RE et al. Ulcerative perineal lesions due to *Mycobacterium kansasii*. J Am Acad Dermatol 1988; 18: 1146–1147.

373 Fenske NA, Millns JL. Resistant cutaneous infection caused by *Mycobacterium chelonei*. Arch Dermatol 1981; 117: 151–153.

374 Bolivar R, Satterwhite TK, Floyd M. Cutaneous lesions due to *Mycobacterium kansasii*. Arch Dermatol 1980; 116: 207–208.

375 Rosen T. Cutaneous *Mycobacterium kansasii* infection presenting as cellulitis. Cutis 1983; 31: 87–89.

376 Nedorost ST, Elewski B, Tomford JW, Camisa C. Rosacea-like lesions due to familial *Mycobacterium avium-intracellulare* infection. Int J Dermatol 1991; 30: 491–497.

377 Perrin C, Michiels JF, Bernard E et al. Cutaneous spindle-cell pseudotumors due to *Mycobacterium gordonae* and *Leishmania infantum*. An immunophenotypic study. Am J Dermatopathol 1993; 15: 553–558.

378 Logani S, Lucas DR, Cheng JD et al. Spindle cell tumors associated with mycobacteria in lymph nodes of HIV-positive patients. Am J Surg Pathol 1999; 23: 656–661.

379 LeBoit PE. On the cover. Am J Dermatopathol 2001; 23: 158–159.

380 Higgins EM, Lawrence CM. Sporotrichoid spread of *Mycobacterium chelonei*. Clin Exp Dermatol 1988; 13: 234–236.

381 Murdoch ME, Leigh IM. Sporotrichoid spread of cutaneous *Mycobacterium chelonei* infection. Clin Exp Dermatol 1989; 14: 309–312.

382 Figuerora LD, Gonzalez JR. Primary inoculation complex of skin by *Mycobacterium chelonei*. J Am Acad Dermatol 1984; 10: 333–336.

383 Kelly SE. Multiple injection abscesses in a diabetic caused by *Mycobacterium chelonei*. Clin Exp Dermatol 1987; 12: 48–49.

384 Murillo J, Torres J, Bofill L et al. Skin and wound infection by rapidly growing mycobacteria. An unexpected complication of liposuction and liposculpture. Arch Dermatol 2000; 136: 1347–1352.

385 Buckley R, Cobb MW, Ghurani S et al. *Mycobacterium fortuitum* infection occurring after a punch biopsy procedure. Pediatr Dermatol 1997; 14: 290–292.

386 Heironimus JD, Winn RE, Collins CB. Cutaneous nonpulmonary *Mycobacterium chelonei* infection. Arch Dermatol 1984; 120: 1061–1063.

387 Owens DW, McBride ME. Sporotrichoid cutaneous infection with *Mycobacterium kansasii*. Arch Dermatol 1969; 100: 54–58.

388 Hirsh FS, Saffold OE. *Mycobacterium kansasii* infection with dermatologic manifestations. Arch Dermatol 1976; 112: 706–708.

389 Jarrett P, Ford G. *Mycobacterium kansasii* infection in a patient presenting with porphyria cutanea tarda. Clin Exp Dermatol 1996; 21: 286–287.

390 Czelusta A, Moore AY. Cutaneous *Mycobacterium kansasii* infection in a patient with systemic lupus erythematosus: Case report and review. J Am Acad Dermatol 1999; 40: 359–363.

391 Curcó N, Pagerols X, Gómez L, Vives P. *Mycobacterium kansasii* infection limited to the skin in a patient with AIDS. Br J Dermatol 1996; 135: 324–326.

392 Stengem J, Grande KK, Hsu S. Localized primary cutaneous *Mycobacterium kansasii* infection in an immunocompromised patient. J Am Acad Dermatol 1999; 41: 854–856.

393 Darling TN, Sidhu-Malik N, Corey GR et al. Treatment of *Mycobacterium haemophilum* infection with an antibiotic regimen including clarithromycin. Br J Dermatol 1994; 131: 376–379.

394 McGovern J, Bix BC, Webster G. *Mycobacterium haemophilum* skin disease successfully treated with excision. J Am Acad Dermatol 1994; 30: 269–270.

395 Busam KJ, Kiehn TE, Salob SP, Myskowski PL. Histologic reactions to cutaneous infections by *Mycobacterium haemophilum*. Am J Surg Pathol 1999; 23: 1379–1385.

396 Friedli A, Krischer J, Hirschel B et al. An annular plaque due to *Mycobacterium haemophilum* infection in a patient with AIDS. J Am Acad Dermatol 2000; 43: 913–915.

397 Murray-Leisure KA, Egan N, Weitekamp MR. Skin lesions caused by *Mycobacterium scrofulaceum*. Arch Dermatol 1987; 123: 369–370.

398 Cross GM, Guill MA, Aton JK. Cutaneous *Mycobacterium szulgai* infection. Arch Dermatol 1985; 121: 247–249.

399 Shimizu T, Kodama K, Kobayashi H et al. Successful treatment using clarithromycin for a cutaneous lesion caused by *Mycobacterium szulgai*. Br J Dermatol 2000; 142: 838–840.

400 Gengoux P, Portaels F, Lachapelle JM et al. Skin granulomas due to *Mycobacterium gordonae*. Int J Dermatol 1987; 26: 181–184.

401 Noel SB, Ray MC, Greer DL. Cutaneous infection with *Mycobacterium avium-intracellulare scrofulaceum intermediate*: a new pathogenic entity. J Am Acad Dermatol 1988; 19: 492–495.

402 Wood C, Nickoloff BJ, Todes-Taylor NR. Pseudotumor resulting from atypical mycobacterial infection. A 'histoid' variety of *Mycobacterium avium-intracellulare* complex infection. Am J Clin Pathol 1985; 83: 524–527.

403 Maurice PDL, Bunker C, Giles F et al. *Mycobacterium avium-intracellulare* infection associated with hairy-cell leukemia. Arch Dermatol 1988; 124: 1545–1549.

404 Cox SK, Strausbaugh LJ. Chronic cutaneous infection caused by *Mycobacterium intracellulare*. Arch Dermatol 1981; 117: 794–796.

405 Epps RE, el-Azhary RA, Hellinger WC et al. Disseminated cutaneous *Mycobacterium avium-intracellulare* resembling sarcoidosis. J Am Acad Dermatol 1995; 33: 528–531.

406 Sachs MK, Fraimow HF, Staros EB et al. *Mycobacterium intracellulare* soft tissue infection. J Am Acad Dermatol 1992; 27: 1019–1021.

407 Fujii K, Ohta K, Kuze F. Multiple primary *Mycobacterium avium* infection of the skin. Int J Dermatol 1997; 36: 54–56.

408 Hide M, Hondo T, Yonehara S et al. Infection with *Mycobacterium avium-intracellulare* with abscess, ulceration and fistula formation. Br J Dermatol 1997; 136: 121–123.

409 Ichiki Y, Hirose M, Akiyama T et al. Skin infection caused by *Mycobacterium avium*. Br J Dermatol 1997; 136: 260–263.

410 Satta R, Retanda G, Cottoni F. *Mycobacterium avium* complex: cutaneous infection in an immunocompetent host. Acta Derm Venereol 1999; 79: 249–250.

411 Sugita Y, Ishii N, Katsuno M et al. Familial cluster of cutaneous *Mycobacterium avium* infection resulting from use of a circulating, constantly heated bath water system. Br J Dermatol 2000; 142: 789–793.

412 Rotman DA, Blauvelt A, Kerdel FA. Widespread cutaneous infection with *Mycobacterium fortuitum*. Int J Dermatol 1993; 32: 512–514.

413 Beck A. *Mycobacterium fortuitum* in abscesses of man. J Clin Pathol 1965; 18: 307–313.

414 Retief CR, Tharp MD. *Mycobacterium fortuitum* panniculitis in a steroid-dependent asthmatic patient. J Am Acad Dermatol 1998; 39: 650–653.

415 Fitzgerald DA, Smith AG, Lees A et al. Cutaneous infection with *Mycobacterium abscessus*. Br J Dermatol 1995; 132: 800–804.

416 Rodríguez G, Ortegón M, Camargo D, Orozco LC. Iatrogenic *Mycobacterium abscessus* infection: histopathology of 71 patients. Br J Dermatol 1997; 137: 214–218.

417 Ozluer SM, De'Ambrosis BJ. *Mycobacterium abscessus* wound infection. Australas J Dermatol 2001; 42: 26–29.

418 Onate JM, Madero S, Vanaclocha F, Gil-Martin R. An unusual form of *Mycobacterium chelonei* infection. Am J Dermatopathol 1986; 8: 73–78.

419 Nelson BR, Rapini RP, Wallace RJ Jr, Tschen JA. Disseminated *Mycobacterium chelonae* sp. *abscessus* in an immunocompetent host and with a known portal of entry. J Am Acad Dermatol 1989; 20: 909–912.

420 Swetter SM, Kindel SE, Smoller BR. Cutaneous nodules of *Mycobacterium chelonae* in an immunosuppressed patient with preexisting pulmonary colonization. J Am Acad Dermatol 1993; 28: 352–355.

421 Valencia IC, Weiss E, Sukenik E, Kerdel FA. Disseminated cutaneous *Mycobacterium chelonae* infection after injection of bovine embryonic cells. Int J Dermatol 1999; 38: 770–773.

422 Nathan DL, Singh S, Kestenbaum TM, Casparian JM. Cutaneous *Mycobacterium chelonae* in a liver transplant patient. J Am Acad Dermatol 2000; 43: 333–336.

423 Bachelez H, Ducloy G, Pinquier L et al. Disseminated varioliform pustular eruption due to *Mycobacterium avium intracellulare* in an HIV-infected patient. Br J Dermatol 1996; 134: 801–803.

424 Alfandari S, Ajana F, Senneville E et al. Isolated cutaneous *Mycobacterium avium* complex infection in AIDS. Int J Dermatol 1997; 36: 294–295.

425 Paige DG, Price DA, Crook T et al. Isolated cutaneous non-tuberculous mycobacterial infection as a manifestation of AIDS. Clin Exp Dermatol 1996; 21: 226–229.

426 Esteban J, Gorgolas M, Fernandez-Guerrero ML, Soriano F. Localized cutaneous infection caused by *Mycobacterium avium* complex in an AIDS patient. Clin Exp Dermatol 1996; 21: 230–231.

427 Pelgrom J, Bastian I, Van den Enden E et al. Cutaneous ulcer caused by *Mycobacterium avium* and recurrent genital herpes after highly active antiretroviral therapy. Arch Dermatol 2000; 136: 129.

428 del Giudice P, Durant J, Counillon E et al. Mycobacterial cutaneous manifestations: a new sign of immune restoration syndrome in patients with acquired immunodeficiency syndrome. Arch Dermatol 1999; 135: 1129–1130.

429 Kakinuma H, Suzuki H. *Mycobacterium avium* complex infection limited to the skin in a patient with systemic lupus erythematosus. Br J Dermatol 1994; 130: 785–790.

430 Brown T, Yen A. Isolation of *Mycobacterium avium* complex from erythema multiforme. J Am Acad Dermatol 1998; 39: 493–495.

431 Hoss DM, McNutt NS, Kreuger JG et al. Cutaneous tuberculosis mimicking erythema nodosum. J Cutan Pathol 1989; 16: 307 (abstract).

432 Bartralot R, Pujol RM, Garcia-Patos V et al. Cutaneous infections due to nontuberculous mycobacteria: histopathological review of 28 cases. Comparative study between lesions

observed in immunosuppressed patients and normal hosts. J Cutan Pathol 2000; 27: 124–129.

433 Cole GW, Gebhard J. *Mycobacterium avium* infection of the skin resembling lepromatous leprosy. Br J Dermatol 1979; 101: 71–74.

434 Kahn H, Phelps RG. Pseudogaucher cells in cutaneous *Mycobacterium avium intracellulare* infection. Am J Dermatopathol 1999; 21: 51–54.

435 Pappolla MA, Mehta VT. PAS reaction stains phagocytosed atypical mycobacteria in paraffin sections. Arch Pathol Lab Med 1984; 108: 372–373.

436 Lambert WC, Pathan AK, Imaeda T et al. Culture of *Vibrio extorquens* from severe, chronic skin ulcers in a Puerto Rican woman. J Am Acad Dermatol 1983; 9: 262–268.

437 Martin T, Hogan DJ, Murphy F et al. *Rhodococcus* infection of the skin with lymphadenitis in a nonimmunocompromised girl. J Am Acad Dermatol 1991; 24: 328–332.

438 Young D. Leprosy and the genome – not yet a burnt-out case. Lancet 2001; 357: 1639–1640.

439 Hutchinson J. The *in vitro* cultivation of *Mycobacterium leprae*. In: Ryan TJ, McDougall AC, eds. Essays on leprosy. Oxford: St Francis Leprosy Guild, 1988; 30–51.

440 Modlin RL, Rea TH. Leprosy: new insight into an ancient disease. J Am Acad Dermatol 1987; 17: 1–13.

441 Rojas RE, Segal-Eiras Ciniba A. Characterization of circulating immune complexes in leprosy patients and their correlation with specific antibodies against *Mycobacterium leprae*. Clin Exp Dermatol 1997; 22: 223–229.

442 Kaminski MJ, Mroczkowski TF, Krotoski WA. Dendritic epidermal γ/δ T cells (DETC) activated *in vivo* proliferate *in vitro* in response to *Mycobacterium leprae* antigens. Int J Dermatol 2000; 39: 603–608.

443 Abulafia J, Vignale RA. Leprosy: pathogenesis updated. Int J Dermatol 1999; 38: 321–334.

444 Sehgal VN, Srivastava G. Leprosy in children. Int J Dermatol 1987; 26: 557–566.

445 Thangaraj RH, Yawalkar SJ. Leprosy for medical practitioners and paramedical workers. Basle: Ciba-Geigy, 1987; 15.

446 Bruce S, Schroeder TL, Ellner K et al. Armadillo exposure and Hansen's disease: An epidemiologic survey in southern Texas. J Am Acad Dermatol 2000; 43: 223–228.

447 Dessoukey MW, El-Shiemy S, Sallam T. HLA and leprosy: segregation and linkage study. Int J Dermatol 1996; 35: 257–264.

448 Machin M. The mode of transmission of human leprosy. In: Ryan TJ, McDougall AC, eds. Essays on leprosy. Oxford: St Francis Leprosy Guild, 1988; 1–29.

449 Sehgal VN. Inoculation leprosy. Current status. Int J Dermatol 1988; 27: 6–9.

450 Lee H, Vigeland K, White CR Jr. Concomitant pulmonary tuberculosis and leprosy: clinical, histological, and histochemical challenges. J Cutan Pathol 2000; 27: 541 (abstract).

451 Rea TH, Levan NE. Current concepts in the immunology of leprosy. Arch Dermatol 1977; 113: 345–352.

452 Ridley DS, Jopling WH. Classification of leprosy according to immunity. A five-group system. Int J Lepr 1966; 34: 255–273.

453 Rea TH, Modlin RL. Immunopathology of leprosy skin lesions. Semin Dermatol 1991; 10: 188–193.

454 Rea TH. Immune responses in leprosy, cytokines and new archetypes for dermatology. Clin Exp Dermatol 1995; 20: 89–97.

455 Narayanan RB. Immunopathology of leprosy granulomas – current status: a review. Lepr Rev 1988; 59: 75–82.

456 Grossman D, Rapini RP, Osborne B, Duvic M. Emergence of leprosy in a patient with mycosis fungoides. J Am Acad Dermatol 1994; 30: 313–315.

457 Ridley DS. Histological classification and the immunological spectrum of leprosy. Bull WHO 1974; 51: 451–465.

458 Browne SG. Indeterminate leprosy. Int J Dermatol 1985; 24: 555–559.

459 Murray KA, McLelland BA, Job CK. Early leprosy with perineural proliferation. Arch Dermatol 1984; 120: 360–361.

460 Ramasoota T, Johnson WC, Graham JH. Cutaneous sarcoidosis and tuberculoid leprosy. A comparative histopathologic and histochemical study. Arch Dermatol 1967; 96: 259–268.

461 Saxena U, Ramesh V, Misra RS, Mukherjee A. Giant nerve abscesses in leprosy. Clin Exp Dermatol 1990; 15: 349–351.

462 Singh K. An unusual bullous reaction in borderline leprosy. Lepr Rev 1987; 58: 61–67.

463 Jenkins D, Papp K, Jakubovic HR, Shiffman N. Leprotic involvement of peripheral nerves in the absence of skin lesions. J Am Acad Dermatol 1990; 23: 1023–1026.

464 Rodriguez G, Sánchez W, Chalela JG, Soto J. Primary neuritic leprosy. J Am Acad Dermatol 1993; 29: 1050–1052.

465 El-Shiemy S, El-Hefnawi H, Abdel-Fattah A et al. Testicular and epididymal involvement in leprosy patients, with special reference to gynecomastia. Int J Dermatol 1976; 15: 52–58.

466 Frey FLP, Gottlieb AB, Levis WR. A patient with lepromatous leprosy and anticytoskeletal antibodies. J Am Acad Dermatol 1988; 18: 1179–1184.

467 Boisseau-Garsaud A-M, Vezon G, Helenon R et al. High prevalence of vitiligo in lepromatous leprosy. Int J Dermatol 2000; 39: 837–839.

468 Mansfield RE. Histoid leprosy. Arch Pathol 1969; 87: 580–585.

469 Sehgal VN, Srivastava G. Histoid leprosy. Int J Dermatol 1985; 24: 286–292.

470 Kontochristopoulos GJ, Aroni K, Panteleos DN, Tosca AD. Immunohistochemistry in histoid leprosy. Int J Dermatol 1995; 34: 777–781.

471 Triscott JA, Nappi O, Ferrara G, Wick MR. 'Pseudoneoplastic' leprosy. Leprosy revisited. Am J Dermatopathol 1995; 17: 297–302.

472 Turk JL, Rees RJW. Aids and leprosy. Lepr Rev 1988; 59: 193–194.

473 Goodless DR, Viciana AL, Pardo RJ, Ruiz P. Borderline tuberculoid Hansen's disease in AIDS. J Am Acad Dermatol 1994; 30: 866–869.

474 Moreno-Giménez JC, Valverde F, Rios JJ et al. Lepromatous leprosy in an HIV-positive patient in Spain. J Eur Acad Dermatol Venereol 2000; 14: 290–292.

475 Klioze AM, Ramos-Caro FA. Visceral leprosy. Int J Dermatol 2000; 39: 641–658.

476 Sehgal VN. Reactions in leprosy. Clinical aspects. Int J Dermatol 1987; 26: 278–285.

477 Sehgal VN, Srivastava G, Sundharam JA. Immunology of reactions in leprosy. Current status. Int J Dermatol 1988; 27: 157–162.

478 Lyde CB. Pregnancy in patients with Hansen disease. Arch Dermatol 1997; 133: 623–627.

479 Kuo T-T, Chan H-L. Severe reactional state in lepromatous leprosy simulating Sweet's syndrome. Int J Dermatol 1987; 26: 518–520.

480 Ramesh V, Beena KR, Mukherjee A. Sporotrichoid presentations in leprosy. Clin Exp Dermatol 2000; 25: 227–230.

481 Ridley DS, Radia KB. The histological course of reactions in borderline leprosy and their outcome. Int J Lepr 1981; 49: 383–392.

482 Meyerson MS. Erythema nodosum leprosum. Int J Dermatol 1996; 35: 389–392.

483 Murphy GF, Sanchez NP, Flynn TC et al. Erythema nodosum leprosum: nature and extent of the cutaneous microvascular alterations. J Am Acad Dermatol 1986; 14: 59–69.

484 Modlin RL, Bakke AC, Vaccaro SA et al. Tissue and blood T-lymphocyte subpopulations in erythema nodosum leprosum. Arch Dermatol 1985; 121: 216–219.

485 Rea TH, Levan NE. Erythema nodosum leprosum in a general hospital. Arch Dermatol 1975; 111: 1575–1580.

486 Vázquez-Botet M, Sánchez JL. Erythema nodosum leprosum. Int J Dermatol 1987; 26: 436–437.

487 Ridley DS, Rea TH, McAdam KPWJ. The histology of erythema nodosum leprosum. Variant forms in New Guineans and other ethnic groups. Lepr Rev 1981; 52: 65–78.

488 Moraes MO, Sampaio EP, Nery JAC et al. Sequential erythema nodosum leprosum and reversal reaction with similar lesional cytokine mRNA patterns in a borderline leprosy patient. Br J Dermatol 2001; 144: 175–181.

489 Pursley TV, Jacobson RR, Apisarnthanarax P. Lucio's phenomenon. Arch Dermatol 1980; 116: 201–204.

490 Rea TH, Ridley DS. Lucio's phenomenon: a comparative histological study. Int J Lepr 1979; 47: 161–166.

491 Moschella SL. The lepra reaction with necrotizing skin lesions. A report of six cases. Arch Dermatol 1967; 95: 565–575.

492 Jariwala HJ, Kelkar SS. Fluorescence microscopy for detection of *M. leprae* in tissue sections. Int J Lepr 1979; 47: 33–36.

493 Sehgal VN, Koranne RV, Nayyar M, Saxena HMK. Application of clinical and histopathological classification of leprosy. Dermatologica 1980; 161: 93–96.

494 Nayar A, Narayanan JS, Job CK. Histopathological study of early skin lesions in leprosy. Arch Pathol 1972; 94: 199–204.

495 Tze-Chun L, Li-Zung Y, Gan-yun Y, Gu-Jing D. Histology of indeterminate leprosy. Int J Lepr 1982; 50: 172–176.

496 Parker M. Hypopigmentation in leprosy: its mechanism and significance. In: Ryan TJ, McDougall AC, eds. Essays on leprosy. Oxford: St Francis Leprosy Guild, 1988; 101–123.

497 Modlin RL, Gebhard JF, Taylor CR, Rea TH. *In situ* characterization of T lymphocyte subsets in the reactional states of leprosy. Clin Exp Immunol 1983; 53: 17–24.

498 Van Voorhis WC, Kaplan G, Sarno EN et al. The cutaneous infiltrates of leprosy. N Engl J Med 1982; 307: 1593–1597.

499 Coruh G, McDougall AC. Untreated lepromatous leprosy: histopathological findings in cutaneous blood vessels. Int J Lepr 1979; 47: 500–511.

500 Job CK. *Mycobacterium leprae* in nerve lesions in lepromatous leprosy. An electron microscopic study. Arch Pathol 1970; 89: 195–207.

501 Cuevas-Santos J, Contreras F, McNutt NS. Multibacillary leprosy: lesions with macrophages positive for S100 protein and dendritic cells positive for Factor 13a. J Cutan Pathol 1998; 25: 530–537.

502 Klenerman P. Aetiological factors in delayed-type hypersensitivity reactions in leprosy. In: Ryan TJ, McDougall AC, eds. Essays on leprosy. Oxford: St Francis Leprosy Guild, 1983; 52–63.

503 Moschella SL. Leprosy today. Australas J Dermatol 1983; 24: 47–54.

504 Modlin RL, Hofman FM, Taylor CR, Rea TH. T lymphocyte subsets in skin lesions of patients with leprosy. J Am Acad Dermatol 1983; 8: 182–189.

505 Mahaisavariya P, Kulthanan K, Khemngern S, Pinkaew S. Lesional T-cell subset in leprosy and leprosy reaction. Int J Dermatol 1999; 38: 345–347.

506 Jolliffe DS. Leprosy reactional states and their treatment. Br J Dermatol 1977; 97: 345–352.

Miscellaneous bacterial infections

507 Dutz W, Kohout-Dutz E. Anthrax. Int J Dermatol 1981; 20: 203–206.

508 Mallon E, McKee PH. Extraordinary case report: cutaneous anthrax. Am J Dermatopathol 1997; 19: 79–82.

509 Thappa DM, Karthikeyan K. Anthrax: an overview within the Indian subcontinent. Int J Dermatol 2001; 40: 216–222.

510 Morbidity and Mortality Report Centers for Disease Control, Atlanta. Human cutaneous anthrax – North Carolina, 1987. Arch Dermatol 1988; 124: 1324.

511 Ariza J, Servitje O, Pallares R et al. Characteristic cutaneous lesions in patients with brucellosis. Arch Dermatol 1989; 125: 380–383.

512 Berger TG, Guill MA, Goette DK. Cutaneous lesions in brucellosis. Arch Dermatol 1981; 117: 40–42.

513 Perez C, Hernandez R, Murie M et al. Relapsing leucocytoclastic vasculitis as the initial manifestation of acute brucellosis. Br J Dermatol 1999; 140: 1177–1178.

514 Niemi K-M, Hannuksela M, Salo OP. Skin lesions in human yersiniosis. A histopathological and immunohistological study. Br J Dermatol 1976; 94: 155–160.

515 Baldock NE, Catterall MD. Erythema nodosum from Yersinia enterocolitica. Br J Dermatol 1975; 93: 719–720.

516 Hannuksela M. Human yersiniosis: a common cause of erythematous skin eruptions. Int J Dermatol 1977; 16: 665–666.

517 Sehgal VN, Prasad ALS. Donovanosis. Current concepts. Int J Dermatol 1986; 25: 8–16.

518 Niemel PLA, Engelkens HJH, van der Meijden WI, Stolz E. Donovanosis (granuloma inguinale) still exists. Int J Dermatol 1992; 31: 244–246.

519 Hacker P, Fisher BK, Dekoven J, Shier RM. Granuloma inguinale: three cases diagnosed in Toronto, Canada. Int J Dermatol 1992; 31: 696–699.

520 Davis CM. Granuloma inguinale. A clinical, histological, and ultrastructural study. JAMA 1970; 211: 632–636.

521 Rosen T, Tschen JA, Ramsdell W et al. Granuloma inguinale. J Am Acad Dermatol 1984; 11: 433–437.

522 Fritz GS, Hubler WR Jr, Dodson RF, Rudolph A. Mutilating granuloma inguinale. Arch Dermatol 1975; 111: 1464–1465.

523 Bozbora A, Erbil Y, Berber E et al. Surgical treatment of granuloma inguinale. Br J Dermatol 1998; 138: 1079–1081.

524 Menders SM, Baxter JD. Granuloma inguinale and HIV: A unique presentation and novel treatment regimen. J Am Acad Dermatol 1997; 37: 494–496.

525 Sehgal VN, Shyamprasad AL, Beohar PC. The histopathological diagnosis of donovanosis. Br J Vener Dis 1984; 60: 45–47.

526 Ramdial PK, Kharsany ABM, Reddy R, Chetty R. Transepithelial elimination of cutaneous vulval granuloma inguinale. J Cutan Pathol 2000; 27: 493–499.

527 Dodson RF, Fritz GS, Hubler WR Jr et al. Donovanosis: a morphologic study. J Invest Dermatol 1974; 62: 611–614.

528 Kuberski T, Papadimitriou JM, Phillips P. Ultrastructure of Calymmatobacterium granulomatis in lesions of granuloma inguinale. J Infect Dis 1980; 142: 744–749.

529 Margolis RJ, Hood AF. Chancroid: Diagnosis and treatment. J Am Acad Dermatol 1982; 6: 493–499.

530 Ronald AR, Plummer F. Chancroid. A newly important sexually transmitted disease. Arch Dermatol 1989; 125: 1413–1414.

531 Buntin DM, Rosen T, Lesher JL Jr et al. Sexually transmitted diseases: bacterial infections. J Am Acad Dermatol 1991; 25: 287–299.

532 Czelusta A, Yen-Moore A, Van der Straten M et al. An overview of sexually transmitted diseases. Part III. Sexually transmitted diseases in HIV-infected patients. J Am Acad Dermatol 2000; 43: 409–432.

533 Trees DL, Morse SA. Chancroid and Haemophilus ducreyi: an update. Clin Microbiol Rev 1995; 8: 357–375.

534 Ronald AR. Chancroid. Recent advances in treatment and control. Int J Dermatol 1986; 25: 31–33.

535 Falk ES, Vorland LH, Bjorvatn B. A case of mixed chancre. Dermatologica 1984; 168: 47–49.

536 Salzman RS, Kraus SJ, Miller RG et al. Chancroidal ulcers that are not chancroid. Cause and epidemiology. Arch Dermatol 1984; 120: 636–639.

537 Werman BS, Herskowitz LJ, Olansky S et al. A clinical variant of chancroid resembling granuloma inguinale. Arch Dermatol 1983; 119: 890–894.

538 Fiumara NJ, Rothman K, Tang S. The diagnosis and treatment of chancroid. J Am Acad Dermatol 1986; 15: 939–943.

539 Hammond GW, Slutchuk M, Scatliff J et al. Epidemiologic, clinical, laboratory, and therapeutic features of an urban outbreak of chancroid in North America. Rev Infect Dis 1980; 2: 867–879.

540 McCarley ME, Cruz PD Jr, Sontheimer RD. Chancroid: clinical variants and other findings from an epidemic in Dallas County, 1986–1987. J Am Acad Dermatol 1988; 19: 330–337.

541 O'Farrell N. Chancroid in the United Kingdom. Sex Transm Infect 2000; 76: 67–68.

542 Magro CM, Crowson AN, Alfa M et al. A morphological study of penile chancroid lesions in human immunodeficiency virus (HIV)-positive and -negative African men with a hypothesis concerning the role of chancroid in HIV transmission. Hum Pathol 1996; 27: 1066–1070.

543 Kraus SJ, Werman BS, Biddle JW et al. Pseudogranuloma inguinale caused by Haemophilus ducreyi. Arch Dermatol 1982; 118: 494–497.

544 Jones CC, Rosen T. Cultural diagnosis of chancroid. Arch Dermatol 1991; 127: 1823–1827.

545 Tapia A. Rhinoscleroma: a naso-oral dermatosis. Cutis 1987; 40: 101–103.

546 Convit J, Kerdel-Vegas F, Gordon B. Rhinoscleroma. Review and presentation of a case. Arch Dermatol 1961; 84: 55–62.

547 Andraca R, Edson RS, Kern EB. Rhinoscleroma: a growing concern in the United States? Mayo Clinic experience. Mayo Clin Proc 1993; 68: 1151–1157.

548 Hoffmann EO, Loose LD, Harkin JC. The Mikulicz cell in rhinoscleroma. Light, fluorescent and electron microscopic studies. Am J Pathol 1973; 73: 47–58.

549 Fisher ER, Dimling C. Rhinoscleroma. Light and electron microscopic studies. Arch Pathol 1964; 78: 501–512.

550 Pullen RL, Stuart BM. Tularemia. Analysis of 225 cases. JAMA 1945; 129: 495–500.

551 Leggiadro RJ, Kenigsberg K, Annunziato D. Tick-borne ulceroglandular tularemia. NY State J Med 1983; 83: 1053–1054.

552 Young LS, Bicknell DS, Archer BG et al. Tularemia epidemic: Vermont, 1968. Forty-seven cases linked to contact with muskrats. N Engl J Med 1969; 280: 1253–1260.

553 Evans ME, Gregory DW, Schaffner W, McGee ZA. Tularemia: a 30-year experience with 88 cases. Medicine (Baltimore) 1985; 64: 251–269.

554 Martin T, Holmes IH, Wobeser GA et al. Tularemia in Canada with a focus on Saskatchewan. Can Med Assoc J 1982; 127: 279–282.

555 Cerny Z. Skin manifestations of tularemia. Int J Dermatol 1994; 33: 468–470.

556 Akdis AC, Kiliçturgay K, Helvaci S et al. Immunological evaluation of erythema nodosum in tularaemia. Br J Dermatol 1993; 129: 275–279.

557 Lewis JE. Suppurative inflammatory reaction occurring in septicemic tularemia. Cutis 1982; 30: 92–100.

558 Smith KJ, Skelton HG III, Angritt P et al. Cutaneous lesions of listeriosis in a newborn. J Cutan Pathol 1991; 18: 474–476.

559 Margileth AM, Wear DJ, Hadfield TL et al. Cat-scratch disease. Bacteria in skin at the primary inoculation site. JAMA 1984; 252: 928–931.

560 Margileth AM. Dermatologic manifestations and update of cat scratch disease. Pediatr Dermatol 1988; 5: 1–9.

561 Shinall EA. Cat-scratch disease: a review of the literature. Pediatr Dermatol 1990; 7: 11–18.

562 Carithers HA. Cat-scratch disease. An overview based on a study of 1,200 patients. Am J Dis Child 1985; 139: 1124–1133.

563 Gregory DW, Decker MD. Case report: cat scratch disease: an infection beyond the lymph node. Am J Med Sci 1986; 292: 389–390.

564 Margileth AM, Wear DJ, English CK. Systemic cat scratch disease: report of 23 patients with prolonged or recurrent severe bacterial infection. J Infect Dis 1987; 155: 390–402.

565 Landau M, Kletter Y, Avidor B et al. Unusual eruption as a presenting symptom of cat scratch disease. J Am Acad Dermatol 1999; 41: 833–836.

566 Sundaresh KV, Madjar DD, Camisa C, Carvallo E. Cat scratch disease associated with erythema nodosum. Cutis 1986; 38: 317–319.

567 Miller-Catchpole R, Variakojis D, Vardiman JW et al. Cat scratch disease. Identification of bacteria in seven cases of lymphadenitis. Am J Surg Pathol 1986; 10: 276–281.

568 Wear DJ, Margileth AM, Hadfield TL et al. Cat-scratch disease: a bacterial infection. Science 1983; 221: 1403–1405.

569 Gerber MA, Sedgwick AK, MacAlister TJ et al. The aetiological agent of cat scratch disease. Lancet 1985; 1: 1236–1239.

570 Walford N, van der Wouw PA, Das PK et al. Epithelioid angiomatosis in the acquired immunodeficiency syndrome: morphology and differential diagnosis. Histopathology 1990; 16: 83–88.

571 Nosal JM. Bacillary angiomatosis, cat-scratch disease, and bartonellosis: what's the connection? Int J Dermatol 1997; 36: 405–411.

572 Guibal F, de la Salmonière P, Rybojad M et al. High seroprevalence to Bartonella quintana in homeless patients with cutaneous parasitic infestations in downtown Paris. J Am Acad Dermatol 2001; 44: 219–223.

573 Johnson WT, Helwig EB. Cat-scratch disease. Histopathologic changes in the skin. Arch Dermatol 1969; 100: 148–154.

574 Mouritsen CL, Litwin CM, Maiese RL et al. Rapid polymerase chain reaction-based detection of the causative agent of cat scratch disease *(Bartonella henselae)* in formalin-fixed, paraffin-embedded samples. Hum Pathol 1997; 28: 820–826.

575 McLure J. Malakoplakia. J Pathol 1983; 140: 275–330.

576 Palazzo JP, Ellison DJ, Garcia IE et al. Cutaneous malakoplakia simulating relapsing malignant lymphoma. J Cutan Pathol 1990; 17: 171–175.

577 Sian CS, McCabe RE, Lattes CG. Malacoplakia of skin and subcutaneous tissue in a renal transplant recipient. Arch Dermatol 1981; 117: 654–655.

578 Lowitt MH, Kariniemi A-L, Niemi KM, Kao GF. Cutaneous malacoplakia: a report of two cases and review of the literature. J Am Acad Dermatol 1996; 34: 325–332.

579 Rémond B, Dompmartin A, Moreau A et al. Cutaneous malacoplakia. Int J Dermatol 1994; 33: 538–542.

580 Nieland ML, Borochovitz D, Silverman AR, Saferstein HL. Cutaneous malakoplakia. Am J Dermatopathol 1981; 3: 287–294.

581 Wittenberg GP, Douglass MC, Azam M et al. Cutaneous malacoplakia in a patient with the acquired immunodeficiency syndrome. Arch Dermatol 1998; 134: 244–245.

582 Barnard M, Chalvardjian A. Cutaneous malacoplakia in a patient with acquired immunodeficiency syndrome (AIDS). Am J Dermatopathol 1998; 20: 185–188.

583 Arul KJ, Emmerson RW. Malacoplakia of the skin. Clin Exp Dermatol 1977; 2: 131–135.

584 Almagro UA, Choi H, Caya JG, Norbach DH. Cutaneous malacoplakia. Report of a case and review of the literature. Am J Dermatopathol 1981; 3: 295–301.

585 Singh M, Kaur S, Vijpayee BK, Banerjee AK. Cutaneous malakoplakia with dermatomyositis. Int J Dermatol 1987; 26: 190–191.

586 Mehregan DR, Mehregan AH, Mehregan DA. Cutaneous malakoplakia: A report of two cases with the use of anti-BCG for the detection for micro-organisms. J Am Acad Dermatol 2000; 43: 351–354.

587 Feldman R, Breier F, Duschet P et al. Cutaneous malacoplakia on the forehead. Dermatology 1997; 194: 358–360.

588 Cespedes YP, Rockley PF, Eaglstein NF, Elgart GW. Cutaneous malacoplakia secondary to parenteral administration of gold and methotrexate in a patient with rheumatoid arthritis: routine and electron microscopic findings. J Cutan Pathol 2000; 27: 552 (abstract).

589 Sarkell B, Dannenberg M, Blaylock WK, Patterson JW. Cutaneous malacoplakia. J Am Acad Dermatol 1994; 30: 834–836.

590 Sencer O, Sencer H, Uluoglu O et al. Malakoplakia of the skin. Ultrastructure and quantitative X-ray microanalysis of Michaelis–Gutmann bodies. Arch Pathol Lab Med 1979; 103: 446–450.

591 Wilkey IS, Strano AJ. An unusual cutaneous infection from Papua New Guinea. Pathology 1973; 5: 335–340.

Chlamydial infections

592 Sarner M, Wilson RJ. Erythema nodosum and psittacosis: report of five cases. Br Med J 1965; 2: 1469–1470.

593 Green ST, Hamlet NW, Willocks L et al. Psittacosis presenting with erythema-marginatum-like lesions – a case report and a historical review. Clin Exp Dermatol 1990; 15: 225–227.

594 Semel JD. Cutaneous findings in a case of psittacosis. Arch Dermatol 1984; 120: 1227–1229.

595 Abrams AJ. Lymphogranuloma venereum. JAMA 1968; 205: 199–202.

596 Schachter J, Osoba AO. Lymphogranuloma venereum. Br Med Bull 1983; 39: 151–154.

597 de la Monte SM, Hutchins GM. Follicular proctocolitis and neuromatous hyperplasia with lymphogranuloma venereum. Hum Pathol 1985; 16: 1025–1032.

598 Sevinsky LD, Lambierto A, Casco R, Woscoff A. Lymphogranuloma venereum: tertiary stage. Int J Dermatol 1997; 36: 47–49.

599 Becker LE. Lymphogranuloma venereum. Int J Dermatol 1976; 15: 26–33.

600 Hopsu-Havu VK, Sonck CE. Infiltrative, ulcerative, and fistular lesions of the penis due to lymphogranuloma venereum. Br J Vener Dis 1973; 49: 193–202.

601 Smith EB, Custer RP. The histopathology of lymphogranuloma venereum. J Urol 1950; 63: 546–563.

602 Alacoque B, Cloppet H, Dumontel C, Moulin G. Histological, immunofluorescent, and ultrastructural features of lymphogranuloma venereum: a case report. Br J Vener Dis 1934; 60: 390–395.

Rickettsial infections

603 Boyd AS, Neldner KH. Typhus disease group. Int J Dermatol 1992; 31: 823–832.

604 Jayaseelan E, Rajendran SC, Shariff S et al. Cutaneous eruptions in Indian tick typhus. Int J Dermatol 1991; 30: 790–794.

605 Turner RC, Chaplinski TJ, Adams HG. Rocky Mountain spotted fever presenting as thrombotic thrombocytopenic purpura. Am J Med 1986; 81: 153–157.

606 Helmick CG, Bernard KW, D'Angelo LJ. Rocky Mountain spotted fever: clinical, laboratory, and epidemiological features of 262 cases. J Infect Dis 1984; 150: 480–488.

607 Zaki MH. Selected tickborne infections. A review of Lyme disease, Rocky Mountain spotted fever, and babesiosis. NY State J Med 1989; 89: 320–335.

608 Woodward TE. Rocky Mountain spotted fever: epidemiological and early clinical signs are keys to treatment and reduced mortality. J Infect Dis 1984; 150: 465–468.

609 Kaplan JE, Schonberger LB. The sensitivity of various serologic tests in the diagnosis of Rocky Mountain spotted fever. Am J Trop Med Hyg 1986; 35: 840–844.

610 Heymann WR. Human ehrlichiosis. Int J Dermatol 1995; 34: 618–619.

611 Ijdo JW, Meek JI, Cartter ML et al. The emergence of another tickborne infection in the 12-town area around Lyme, Connecticut: human granulocytic ehrlichiosis. J Infect Dis 2000; 181: 1388–1393.

612 Brettman LR, Lewin S, Holzman RS et al. Rickettsialpox: report of an outbreak and a contemporary review. Medicine (Baltimore) 1981; 60: 363–372.

613 Walker DH, Gay RM, Valdes-Dapena M. The occurrence of eschars in Rocky Mountain spotted fever. J Am Acad Dermatol 1981; 4: 571–576.

614 Silverman DJ. *Rickettsia rickettsii*-induced cellular injury of human vascular endothelium in vitro. Infect Immun 1984; 44: 545–553.

615 Brown GW. Recent studies in scrub typhus: a review. J Roy Soc Med 1978; 71: 507–510.

616 Taniguchi Y, Kanno Y, Ando K et al. Tsutsugamushi disease (scrub typhus). Int J Dermatol 1992; 31: 693–695.

617 Walker DH, Occhino C, Tringali GR et al. Pathogenesis of Rickettsial eschars: the tache noire of Boutonneuse fever. Hum Pathol 1988; 19: 1449–1454.

618 Raoult D, Jean-Pastor M-J, Xeridat B et al. La fièvre boutonneuse méditerranéenne: à propos de 154 cas récents. Ann Dermatol Venereol 1983; 110: 909–914.

619 Andrew R, Bonnin JM, Williams S. Tick typhus in North Queensland. Med J Aust 1946; 2: 253–258.

620 Cowan G. Rickettsial diseases: the typhus group of fevers – a review. Postgrad Med J 2000; 76: 269–272.

621 Herrero-Herrero JI, Walker DH, Ruiz-Beltran R. Immunohistochemical evaluation of the cellular immune response to *Rickettsia conorii* in *taches noires*. J Infect Dis 1987; 155: 802–805.

622 Montenegro MR, Mansueto S, Hegarty BC, Walker DH. The histology of 'taches noires' of boutonneuse fever and demonstration of *Rickettsia conorii* in them by immunofluorescence. Virchows Archiv (A) 1983; 400: 309–317.

623 Woodward TE, Pedersen CE Jr, Oster CN et al. Prompt confirmation of Rocky Mountain spotted fever: identification of Rickettsiae in skin tissues. J Infect Dis 1976; 134: 297–301.

624 Bradford WD, Hawkins HK. Rocky Mountain spotted fever in childhood. Am J Dis Child 1977; 131: 1228–1232.

625 Kao G, Ioffe O, Evancho C et al. Cutaneous histopathology of Rocky Mountain spotted fever. J Cutan Pathol 1996; 23: 53 (abstract).

626 Kao GF. Evancho CD, Ioffe O et al. Cutaneous histopathology of Rocky Mountain spotted fever. J Cutan Pathol 1997; 24: 604–610.

627 Walker DH, Cain BG, Olmstead PM. Laboratory diagnosis of Rocky Mountain spotted fever by immunofluorescent demonstration of *Rickettsia rickettsii* in cutaneous lesions. Am J Clin Pathol 1978; 69: 619–623.

Spirochetal infections

INTRODUCTION

The order *Spirochaetales* has two genera of medical importance, *Treponema* and *Borrelia*. Spirochetes are one of the few bacterial groups for which classical morphological criteria and RNA sequence analyses agree in predicting the phylogenetic relationships among the various members of the order.

TREPONEMATOSES

The treponematoses are caused by infection with the spirochete *Treponema pallidum* and its various subspecies. They include:

- syphilis
- endemic syphilis (bejel)
- yaws
- pinta.

The treponemes responsible for these different diseases are currently indistinguishable on morphological and serological grounds, although different names have been given to the various subspecies responsible for each condition; the various subspecies may differ by as little as a single nucleotide.

Syphilis is usually acquired by sexual (venereal) transmission, while the other conditions are contagious and endemic to various countries.

The clinical features of the treponematoses can usually be divided into distinct stages, reflecting initial local infection with the organism, followed by dissemination and the subsequent host response.

Other species of *Treponema* are found in humans: some species are found in the mouth and may be responsible for periodontal disease; others may be found in the sebaceous secretions of the genital region. There is no known clinical significance of these genital treponemes.

SYPHILIS

Syphilis is an infectious disease of worldwide distribution, caused by the spirochete *Treponema pallidum*.[1–4] The mode of infection is almost always by sexual contact and, consequently, seropositivity for human immunodeficiency virus (HIV) is sometimes present in individuals with active syphilis.[5–8] Non-sexual transmission (syphilis brephotropica) occurs, rarely, in children from infected parents.[9] Congenital infection is also quite rare, although its incidence appears to be increasing.[10–14] Acquired syphilis may be considered in four stages: primary, secondary, latent and tertiary.[15]

Primary syphilis

The initial lesion of syphilis – the primary chancre – is an indurated painless ulcer with a sharply defined edge that often is surrounded by an inflammatory zone. It is usually found on genital or perianal skin, although about 5% of chancres are extragenital.[16,17] In patients with HIV infection, multiple or more extensive chancres are sometimes present.[7] The serous exudate from the ulcer generally contains numerous treponemes, which can be identified by dark-ground microscopy.

In time the ulcer heals, leaving a small stellate or nondescript scar. The chancre is often accompanied by painless enlargement of the regional lymph nodes.

Secondary syphilis

In untreated cases the multiplication of the widely dispersed treponemes results in secondary syphilis, some 4–8 weeks after the chancre. Besides the mucocutaneous lesions there may be constitutional symptoms, which include fever, lymphadenitis and hepatitis.[18,19] A self-limited febrile reaction (the Jarisch–Herxheimer reaction), accompanied by systemic symptoms, may occur following the commencement of antibiotic therapy for syphilis.[20]

The cutaneous lesions of secondary syphilis[21] are usually maculopapular or erythematosquamous, somewhat psoriasiform lesions, but lichenoid, nodular,[22–24] corymbose,[25] annular,[26] bullous,[27] follicular,[28] pustular, rupial and ulcerative[29–32] lesions may develop. Atypical clinical presentations may occur in patients with coexisting HIV infection.[7,33–35] Furthermore, an accelerated progression through the various stages of syphilis can occur in these patients. The term 'lues maligna' has been applied to the noduloulcerative and necrotic lesions that can occur when there is concurrent HIV infection.[36–38] The lesions of secondary syphilis may mimic a wide variety of skin diseases. Pruritus is only occasionally present.[39] Large, fleshy, somewhat verrucous papules (condylomata lata) may develop in the anogenital region: these should not be confused with viral condylomata acuminata (see p. 704). A moth-eaten alopecia (alopecia syphilitica) is a characteristic manifestation of secondary syphilis.[40–42]

Latent syphilis

Even without treatment, the manifestations of secondary syphilis subside spontaneously. During this phase there are no signs or symptoms, although there is a tendency for cutaneous lesions to relapse in the first few years after the disappearance of the lesions of secondary syphilis. Serology is positive. Syphilis incognito is a variant of latent syphilis in which there has been no clinical evidence of a preceding primary or secondary stage.[43]

Tertiary syphilis

The manifestations of tertiary syphilis appear many years after the initial infection, reflecting the generalized nature of the disease. They involve predominantly the cardiovascular system, the central nervous system and the skeleton, but lesions also occur in the testes, lymph nodes and skin.

There are two types of cutaneous lesion in tertiary syphilis: one is nodular and the other a chronic gummatous ulcer.[44,45] They are usually solitary. The nodular form presents an undulating advancing border of red-brown scaly nodules, some of which may become ulcerated. Lesions may mimic granuloma annulare.[46] The gummatous form starts as a deep, firm swelling that eventually breaks down to form an ulcer.

Histopathology

Endothelial swelling of blood vessels and an inflammatory infiltrate which includes numerous plasma cells are the histological hallmarks of lesions of primary and secondary syphilis. Although great emphasis is placed on the presence of plasma cells, it should be noted that they are sometimes quite sparse in the lesions of secondary syphilis.

Primary syphilis

The epidermis at the periphery of the chancre shows marked acanthosis, but at the center it becomes thin and is eventually lost. The base of the ulcer is infiltrated with lymphocytes and plasma cells, particularly adjacent to the blood vessels, in which there is prominent endothelial swelling. The treponemes can usually be demonstrated by appropriate silver impregnation techniques, such as the Levaditi or Warthin–Starry stains. On dark-field examination of a smear from a chancre the *Treponema pallidum* can be seen as a thin, delicate spiral organism 4–15 μm in length and 0.25 μm in diameter. Electron microscopy has shown *T. pallidum* to be principally in the intercellular spaces in the vicinity of small blood vessels, as well as in macrophages, endothelial cells and even plasma cells.[47] Collagen fibers appear to be damaged by the treponeme.[48]

Secondary syphilis

There is considerable variation in the histological pattern.[19,49–51] Plasma cells may be absent or sparse in up to one-third of all biopsies, and the vascular changes may not be prominent. The infiltrate usually involves both the superficial and the deep dermis, except in the macular lesions, where it is more superficial (Fig. 24.1). Extension of the inflammatory infiltrate into the subcutis is uncommon.[19] The infiltrate is predominantly lymphocytic, with some histiocytes and variable numbers of plasma cells (Fig. 24.2). The histiocytic cells express both CD4 and CD14, while the majority of lymphocytes are CD8+.[52] Plasma cells are less numerous in macular lesions.[53] Early lesions often show a neutrophilic vascular reaction, which is presumed to be related to immune complex deposition.[54] A heavy neutrophil infiltrate resembling that in Sweet's syndrome has been reported.[55] Follicles and sweat glands may be sleeved by inflammatory cells.[49] In alopecia syphilitica, a lymphoid infiltrate around hair follicles and follicular keratotic plugging are almost invariable.[40,41] Peribulbar lymphoid aggregates may be present.[40] Sometimes the dermal infiltrate in secondary syphilis is dense and diffuse, and it has been likened to cutaneous lymphoma,[56,57] although its heterogeneous nature is against lymphoma. Epithelioid granulomas may be found in late secondary syphilis (Fig. 24.3), and there is a report of a palisading granuloma similar to that seen in granuloma annulare.[58] Sarcoidal granulomas are rare.[24] The epidermis is frequently involved. It may show acanthosis with spongiosis, psoriasiform hyperplasia and spongiform pustulation, with considerable exocytosis of neutrophils (Fig. 24.4).[50] A lichenoid tissue reaction may be present, particularly in late lesions (Fig. 24.5).[59] A granulomatous pattern may also be seen in secondary syphilis,[60] particularly after about 16 weeks of the disease.[49] In the rare ulcerative form there is necrosis of the upper dermis,[31] whereas in the follicular type there is microabscess formation in the outer

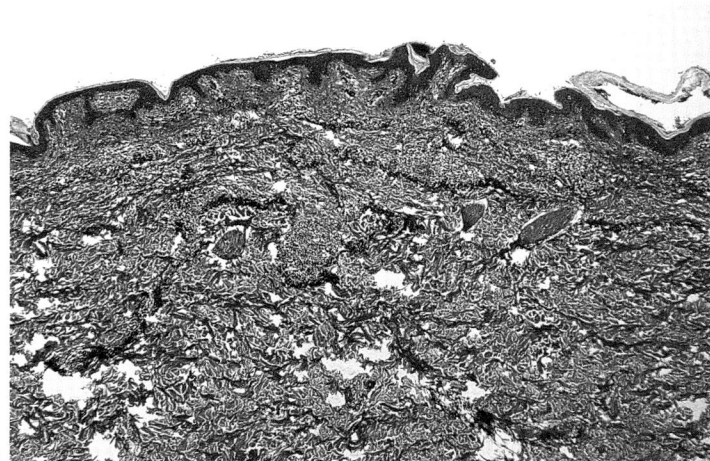
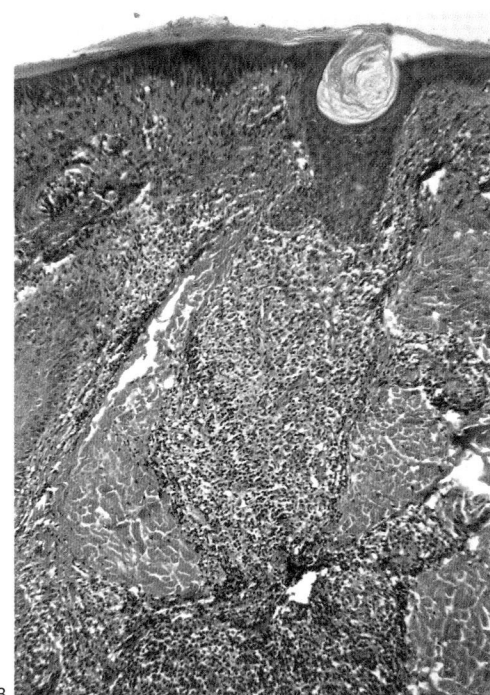

Fig. 24.1 **(A) Secondary syphilis. (B)** There is a superficial and deep perivascular infiltrate in the dermis. (H & E)

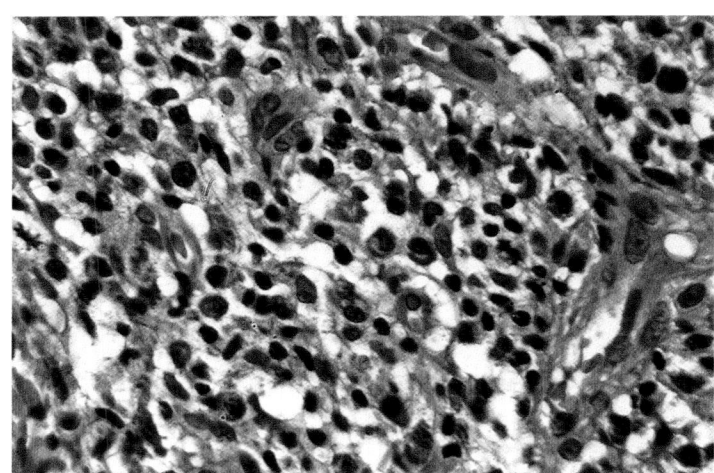

Fig. 24.2 **Secondary syphilis.** The perivascular infiltrate of inflammatory cells includes some plasma cells. (H & E)

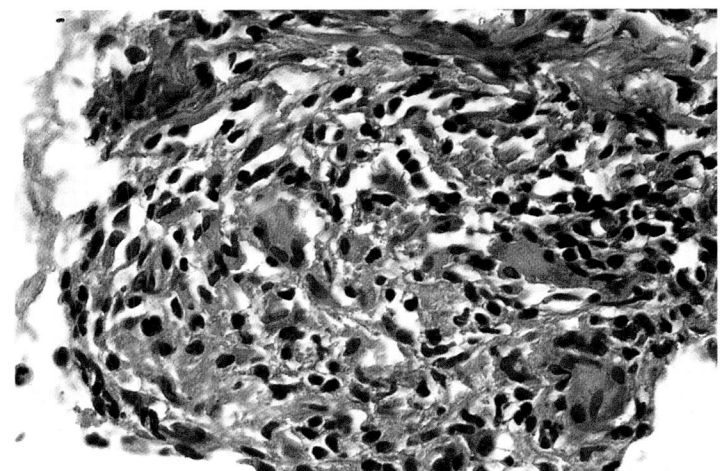

Fig. 24.3 **Late secondary syphilis.** A small, non-caseating granuloma is present in the dermis. (H & E)

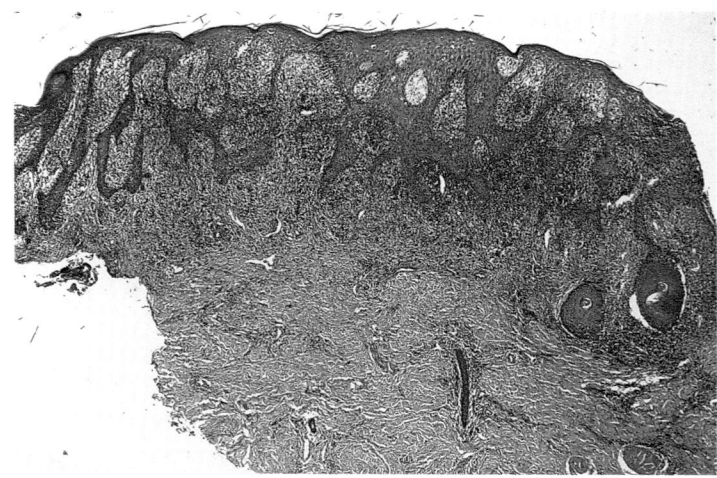

Fig. 24.4 **Late secondary syphilis.** There is psoriasiform hyperplasia and mild spongiosis. (H & E)

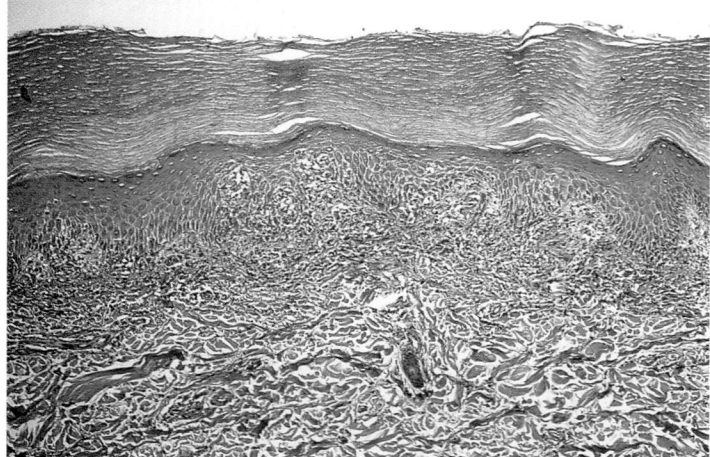

Fig. 24.5 **Late secondary syphilis.** A lichenoid (interface) reaction is present. (H & E)

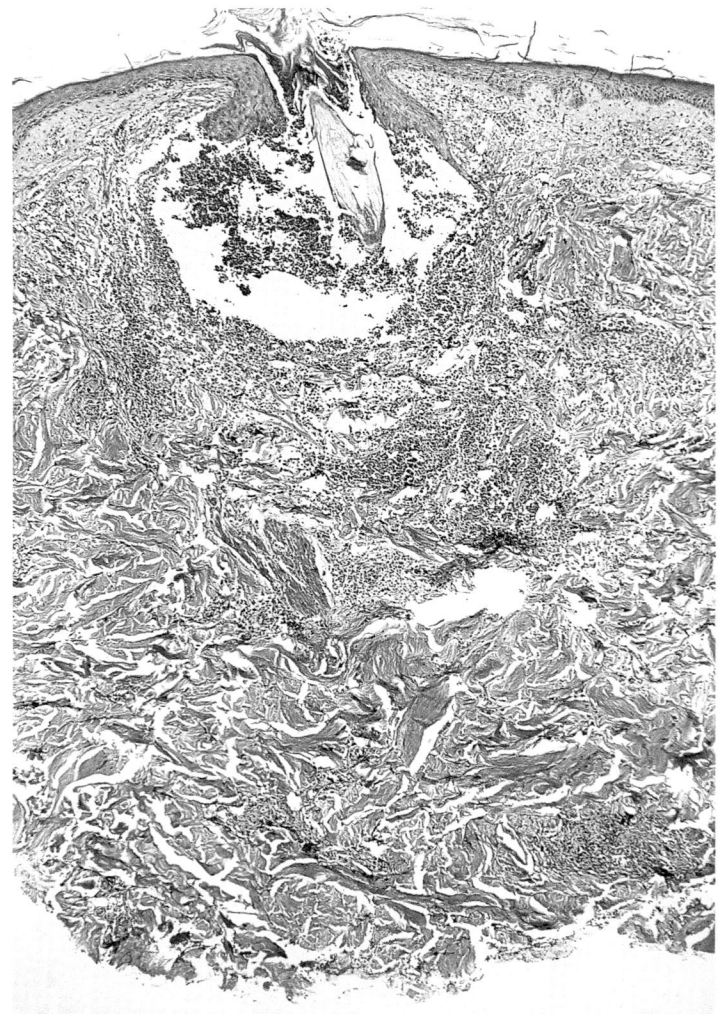

Fig. 24.6 **Secondary syphilis.** A follicular pustule of secondary syphilis. (H & E)

root sheath of the hair follicle, or a follicular pustule (Fig. 24.6). There may be perifollicular granulomas.[28] Condylomata lata have marked epidermal hyperplasia and a dermal infiltrate which is similar to that seen in other lesions of secondary syphilis. *T. pallidum* may be identified in tissue sections using silver stains such as the Warthin–Starry stain, or by immunoperoxidase techniques.[61] The latter are more sensitive than silver stains,[62] but the molecular detection of *Treponema pallidum*, using PCR-based techniques, is likely to become the 'gold standard'.[63]

Subepidermal vesicles have been reported, uncommonly, as a manifestation of the Jarisch–Herxheimer reaction.[20] The bullae reported in a case of bullous secondary syphilis were also subepidermal.[27]

Electron microscopy
Electron microscopy has shown only a modest number of treponemes; their outlines are less distinct than those found in primary chancres. The periplastic membrane (the outer envelope) is rarely intact.[64,55]

Tertiary syphilis
The gummas of tertiary syphilis have large areas of gummatous necrosis with a peripheral inflammatory cell infiltrate which includes lymphocytes, macrophages, giant cells, fibroblasts and plasma cells. There is usually

prominent endothelial swelling and sometimes proliferation involving small vessels. Attempts to demonstrate *T. pallidum* by silver staining techniques are usually unrewarding, although indirect immunofluorescence and PCR-based assays have been used with success.[63,66] The nodular or tuberculoid lesions show hyperkeratosis, often overlying an atrophic epidermis. There is a superficial and deep mixed inflammatory cell infiltrate, which usually includes plasma cells and tuberculoid granulomas.[67] Plasma cells may be sparse in an occasional case.[68]

ENDEMIC SYPHILIS (BEJEL)

Brief mention will be made of endemic syphilis (non-venereal syphilis, bejel), a contagious disease found in parts of the Middle East, particularly the Euphrates Valley.[69–71] This is caused by an organism indistinguishable from *Treponema pallidum*, and accordingly serological tests for syphilis are positive. The disease has virtually been eradicated following public health measures initiated by the World Health Organization. A primary lesion is rarely found, but otherwise the clinical and pathological manifestations resemble those of yaws in many respects (see below). The main features are 'mucous patches' in the mouth and pharynx, as well as cutaneous and bone lesions.

YAWS

Yaws, or frambesia, is a tropical non-venereal infection caused by *Treponema pertenue*, an organism that has hitherto been indistinguishable from *Treponema pallidum*.[72–75] Hybridization studies now suggest that the subspecies *pertenue* differs from the subspecies *pallidum* by a single nucleotide.[70] However, no serological test will differentiate yaws from syphilis, although slightly different lesions are produced when the respective organisms are inoculated into hamsters or rabbits.[75] The distinction is largely clinical, with some assistance from the histopathology. Yaws is contracted usually in childhood and spreads by direct contact, perhaps aided by an insect vector.[73] Despite successful eradication after World War Two, yaws is now returning in some tropical countries.[72,75–78] Reports of treatment failures using penicillin have been reported.[79]

The primary papule, usually on the legs or buttocks, develops into a chronic ulcerating papillomatous mass that may persist for months.[70] The secondary stage is characterized by similar, widespread exuberant lesions covered with a discharge. In warm moist areas, such as mucocutaneous junction areas, large condylomatous lesions may develop.[72] Periods of exacerbation and quiescence occur over the next few years, followed by a longer latent phase, which precedes the development of chronic gummatous ulcers. These occur on the central face or over long bones, often with involvement of the underlying bones. Hyperkeratosis and fissuring of the soles and palms may occur ('crab yaws'). Apart from the bone lesions there is no systemic involvement.

Histopathology

The appearances of the primary and secondary lesions are similar. There is usually prominent epidermal hyperplasia, which is usually of pseudo-epitheliomatous rather than psoriasiform type, with overlying scale crust and superficial epidermal edema (Fig. 24.7). There are intraepidermal abscesses and a heavy superficial and mid-dermal infiltrate of plasma cells, lymphocytes, macrophages, neutrophils, and often a few eosinophils. The neutrophils are more prominent superficially. Blood vessels show minimal endothelial swelling. The ulcerative lesions resemble those of syphilis.

The spirochete of yaws, like that of pinta, is most often demonstrated by silver techniques in the epidermis, in contrast to that of syphilis, which is found in the upper dermis (Fig. 24.8).

PINTA

Pinta (carate) is a contagious non-venereal treponematosis caused by *Treponema carateum*, which is morphologically identical to *Treponema pallidum*. The disease occurs in the Caribbean area, Central America and parts of tropical South America.[70,71,80] The lesions of pinta are confined to the skin and become very extensive. There is often overlap between the three clinical stages. Initial lesions are erythematous maculopapules, which grow by peripheral extension and often coalesce. The secondary lesions are widespread, long-lasting scaly plaques that show a striking variety of colors – red, pink, slate blue and purple. These lesions merge with the late stage, in which depigmentation resembling vitiligo occurs, and sometimes epidermal atrophy.

Histopathology[81]

Primary and secondary lesions are identical and show hyperkeratosis, parakeratosis and acanthosis. There is exocytosis of inflammatory cells, sometimes with intraepidermal abscesses. Hypochromic areas show loss of basal pigmentation with numerous melanophages in the upper dermis. The dermal infiltrate, like the other changes, is heavier in established than in early

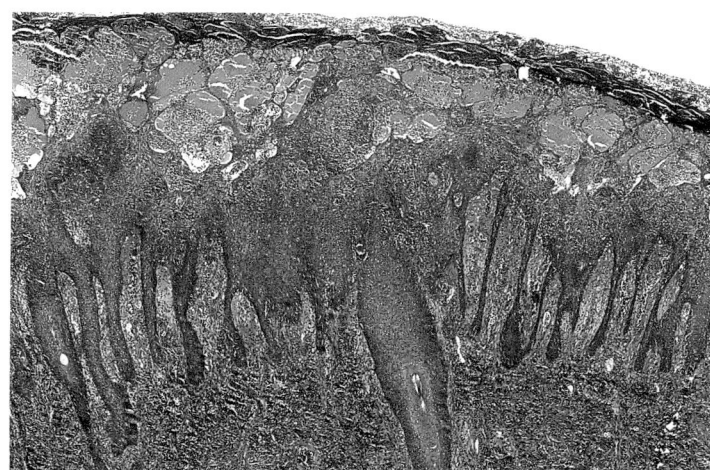

Fig. 24.7 **Yaws.** Note the epidermal hyperplasia and edema of the superficial epidermis. (H & E)

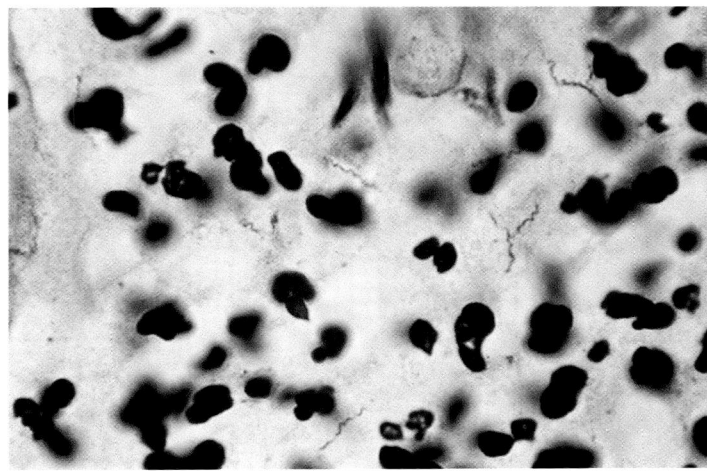

Fig. 24.8 **Yaws.** Numerous fine spirochetes are present. (Warthin–Starry ×1500)

lesions, and includes lymphocytes, plasma cells and sometimes neutrophils. The infiltrate is predominantly superficial and perivascular. The treponemes can be demonstrated by silver methods: they are present mainly in the upper epidermis and are seldom, if ever, found in the dermis.

BORRELIOSES

The borrelioses are an important group of spirochetal infections, found particularly in the temperate zones of Europe, North America and Asia. More than 100 000 cases have been recorded from the United States alone.[82] Unlike the treponematoses, which have no known animal reservoir, the borrelioses are an arthropod-borne infection, usually involving ticks of the genus *Ixodes*. Three genospecies of *Borrelia burgdorferi* have been identified as human pathogens: *B. burgdorferi* sensu stricto, *B. garinii* and *B. afzelii*. The genetic diversity of this species complex is considerable with more than 100 different strains identified in the United States and over 300 worldwide.[83] Although not known for certain, it is possible that different strains may be associated with different clinical manifestations.[83] *B. burgdorferi* is the only pathogenic genospecies in North America, explaining the rarity in that region of acrodermatitis chronica atrophicans, for which *B. afzelii* is the predominant, but not exclusive, etiological agent.[84]

Borrelia are involved in the following conditions:

- erythema chronicum migrans
- acrodermatitis chronica atrophicans
- Borrelia-associated B-cell lymphoma.

Borrelia burgdorferi has also been identified in several of the diseases of collagen, including eosinophilic fasciitis (borrelial fasciitis),[85] morphea, lichen sclerosus et atrophicus, and atrophoderma of Pasini and Pierini. These conditions appear to have other etiologies as well; accordingly, they are discussed in Chapter 11, pages 345–367. Orofacial granulomatosis and the Melkersson–Rosenthal syndrome do not appear to be caused by *Borrelia*.[85a,85b]

Although most borrelioses result from arthropod-borne infections, transplacental transmission of the organism can also occur; no distinct pattern of teratogenicity has been recorded.[86] Infection with *Borrelia* has been reported in a few HIV-infected individuals but it remains unknown whether the concurrent infection alters the disease as it does with another spirochetosis, syphilis.[87]

ERYTHEMA CHRONICUM MIGRANS

Erythema chronicum migrans is the distinctive cutaneous lesion of the multisystem tick-borne spirochetosis, Lyme disease (named after the community in Connecticut, USA, where many cases were originally recognized).[82,88–92] From 20% to 50% or more of the patients have extracutaneous signs or symptoms which may involve the joints, nervous system and heart.[93–96] The cutaneous lesion is a centrifugally spreading erythematous lesion at the site of the bite of the tick, *Ixodes scapularis* (*Ixodes dammini*), or other species such as *I. ricinus* in Great Britain.[97] The annular lesion, which measures 5–20 cm in diameter, develops within 3 months of the tick bite.[98] Uncommonly, the primary lesion may be vesicular.[99] The risk of infection appears to be low if the tick has been attached for less than 24 hours.[100] Lesions are multiple in about 25% of cases.[88] These other lesions (secondary erythema migrans) result from hematogenous dissemination of the organism.[101]

There has been recent debate on the appropriate nomenclature for the various manifestations of this borreliosis. 'Erythema chronicum migrans' should be used for the cutaneous lesion(s) and 'Lyme disease' for the multisystem disease, usually associated with multiple skin lesions, resulting from blood-borne disease.[102]

All three genospecies of *Borrelia burgdorferi* have been isolated from the vector and from some patients with Lyme disease,[103–106] and antibodies and lymphoproliferative responses to it have been found in the sera of patients with the disease.[107–109] Confirmation of *B. burgdorferi* infection is still only found in about 30% of the presumptive cases.[82] Even 40% of culture-positive cases remain seronegative.[110] The organism usually disappears from lesional skin after treatment with various antibiotics such as doxycycline and the synthetic penicillins.[111–113] The organisms may be isolated using BSK-II (Barbour–Stoenner–Kelly) medium.[98,114,115]

Further studies are required to determine the exact cause of the erythema migrans-like rashes associated with bites of the Lone Star tick (*Amblyomma americanum*). It is possible that the bites of this tick transmit other, as yet unidentified, spirochetes.[116]

Histopathology
There is a superficial and deep perivascular and interstitial infiltrate of lymphocytes, sometimes with abundant plasma cells and eosinophils.[117] Eosinophils are only prominent adjacent to the site of the initial tick bite.[82]

Rarely there are scattered neutrophils. With the Warthin–Starry silver stain a spirochete can be found in nearly half of the specimens in the papillary dermis near the dermoepidermal junction.[118–120] The diagnosis requires an index of suspicion based on the clinical features. The small size of the organism places some limits on its identification using conventional microscopic techniques.[115] The diagnosis has also been confirmed using an indirect immunofluorescence technique with a monoclonal antibody to the axial filaments of several *Borrelia* species.[121] Monoclonal antibodies can also be used in immunoperoxidase techniques. Recently, a technique that uses the polymerase chain reaction has been described which allows the molecular detection of *B. burgdorferi* in formalin-fixed paraffin-embedded lesions of this condition.[122,123]

ACRODERMATITIS CHRONICA ATROPHICANS

Acrodermatitis chronica atrophicans is a chronic/late manifestation of infection by a genospecies of *Borrelia burgdorferi*. *B. afzelii* is the predominant, but not exclusive, etiological agent.[84] The condition is most often reported from northern, central and eastern Europe, but not from North America, where *B. afzelii* is not endemic.[106,124–126] There are reports of this condition being preceded by erythema chronicum migrans.

Acrodermatitis chronica atrophicans usually occurs in the elderly and is rare in childhood.[127] Clinically, there is an initial inflammatory stage characterized by diffuse or localized erythema, which gradually spreads to involve the extensor surfaces of the extremities and areas around joints.[124,128] After some months there is gradual atrophy of the skin, with loss of appendages and often hypopigmentation. Areas resembling lichen sclerosus et atrophicus, sclerodermatous patches, and linear fibrotic bands over the ulna and tibia may also be found. In addition, juxta-articular fibrous nodules may develop in 10–25% of cases of acrodermatitis chronica atrophicans;[129,130] they regress rapidly under antibiotic therapy.[131]

B. afzelii DNA has been identified in cutaneous lesions, using the polymerase chain reaction and by culture.[132,133] The organisms are able to invade endothelial cells, fibroblasts and Langerhans cells and to survive in collagenous tissue causing tissue damage, resulting in acrodermatitis chronica atrophicans.[133]

Various mechanisms have been postulated to explain why borreliae can survive in the collagen for months or years despite the presence of high antibody titers against the organism and the presence of CD4-positive T lymphocytes. The significant downregulation of major histocompatibility complex class II molecules on epidermal Langerhans cells in both early and late stages of Lyme borreliosis indicates a poorly effective immune response and may partly explain the faulty elimination of the organisms from the skin.[133,134] A recent study has shown a restricted pattern of cytokine expression in this condition. Whereas interferon-γ is produced in lesions of erythema chronicum migrans, it is lacking in acrodermatitis chronica atrophicans.[135] This cytokine may play a role in spirochetal killing.[135]

Histopathology
The early stages of the disease show a superficial and deep chronic inflammatory cell infiltrate in the dermis which is moderately heavy and composed predominantly of lymphocytes with some histiocytes and plasma cells. There is often accentuation around blood vessels, which may show telangiectasia, and also around adnexae. Sometimes there is a superficial band-like infiltrate of inflammatory cells with a thin zone of collagen separating the inflammatory cells from the basal layer. Scattered vacuoles or groups of vacuoles that morphologically resemble fat cells (but which do not appear to stain for fat – pseudolipomatosis cutis) have been reported in the

upper dermis in some cases (see p. 957).[124] As the lesions progress there will be atrophy of the dermis to about half its normal thickness or less (Fig. 24.9). This is usually accompanied by loss of elastic fibers and pilosebaceous follicles, atrophy of the subcutis, and variable epidermal atrophy with loss of the rete pegs.[125]

Other changes that may be found include diffuse dermal edema, a sub-epidermal edematous or sclerotic zone, basal vacuolar change, hyperkeratosis, and changes resembling lichen sclerosus et atrophicus. Dense dermal sclerosis may be seen in the sclerodermatous patches. The juxta-articular fibrous nodules show broad bundles of homogeneous collagen in the upper subcutis enclosing islands of fatty tissue.[131] There is a perivascular and interstitial infiltrate of lymphocytes and plasma cells.[131]

Electron microscopy
Degenerative changes have been reported in collagen, elastic tissue and nerve fibers.[125]

BORRELIA-ASSOCIATED B-CELL LYMPHOMA

The occurrence of lymphoma in skin affected by acrodermatitis chronica atrophicans has been known for some time. More recently, *Borrelia burgdorferi*

has been identified by culture, or by detection of specific DNA, in up to 20% of cases of cutaneous B-cell lymphoma (see p. 1099).[136,137] Cases reported previously as pseudolymphoma and associated with *B. burgdorferi* are probably low-grade lymphomas akin to the marginal zone lymphomas associated with *Helicobacter pylori* infection.

REFERENCES

Treponematoses

1 Crissey JT, Denenholz DA. Syphilis – epidemiology. Clin Dermatol 1984; 2: 24–33.
2 Morbidity and Mortality Report Centers for Disease Control, Atlanta. Continuing increase in infectious syphilis – United States. Arch Dermatol 1988; 124: 509–510.
3 Rolfs RT, Cates W Jr. The perpetual lesions of syphilis. Arch Dermatol 1989; 125: 107–109.
4 Felman YM. Syphilis. From 1945 Naples to 1989 AIDS. Arch Dermatol 1989; 125: 1698–1700.
5 Radolf JD, Kaplan RP. Unusual manifestations of secondary syphilis and abnormal humoral immune response to *Treponema pallidum* antigens in a homosexual man with asymptomatic human immunodeficiency virus infection. J Am Acad Dermatol 1988; 18: 423–428.
6 Gregory N, Sanchez M, Buchness MR. The spectrum of syphilis in patients with human immunodeficiency virus infection. J Am Acad Dermatol 1990; 22: 1061–1067.
7 Czelusta A, Yen-Moore A, Van der Straten M et al. An overview of sexually transmitted diseases. Part III. Sexually transmitted diseases in HIV-infected patients. J Am Acad Dermatol 2000; 43: 409–432.
8 Adler MW, Meheus AZ. Epidemiology of sexually transmitted infections and human immunodeficiency virus in Europe. J Eur Acad Dermatol Venereol 2000; 14: 370–377.
9 Hofmann B, Schuppe H-C, Ruzicka T et al. Acquired syphilis II in early childhood: Reappearance of syphilis brephotrophica. J Am Acad Dermatol 1998; 38: 638–639.
10 Mascola C, Pelosi R, Blount JH et al. Congenital syphilis. Why is it still occurring? JAMA 1984; 252: 1719–1722.
11 Noppakun N, Hendrick SJ, Raimer SS, Sanchez RL. Palmoplantar milia: sequelae of early congenital syphilis. Pediatr Dermatol 1986; 3: 395–398.
12 Meštrović J, Krželj V, Balarin L et al. Congenital syphilis associated with hyperlipoproteinemia. Pediatr Dermatol 1997; 14: 226–228.
13 Bennett ML, Lynn AW, Klein LE, Balkowiec KS. Congenital syphilis: Subtle presentation of fulminant disease. J Am Acad Dermatol 1997; 36: 351–354.
14 Peihong J, Zhiyong L, Rengui C, Jian W. Early congenital syphilis. Int J Dermatol 2001; 40: 198–200.
15 Brown TJ, Yen-Moore A, Tyring SK. An overview of sexually transmitted diseases. Part I. J Am Acad Dermatol 1999; 41: 511–529.
16 Chapel T, Prasad P, Chapel J, Lekas N. Extragenital syphilitic chancres. J Am Acad Dermatol 1985; 13: 582–584.
17 Hædersdal M, Weismann K. Syphilitic chancre despite use of condoms: "condom chancre". Acta Derm Venereol 2000; 80: 235–236.
18 Longstreth P, Hoke AW, McElroy C. Hepatitis and bone destruction as uncommon manifestations of early syphilis. Report of a case. Arch Dermatol 1976; 112: 1451–1454.
19 Jordaan HF. Secondary syphilis. A clinicopathological study. Am J Dermatopathol 1988; 10: 399–409.
20 Rosen T, Rubin H, Ellner K et al. Vesicular Jarisch–Herxheimer reaction. Arch Dermatol 1989; 125: 77–81.
21 Rudolph AH. Acquired infectious syphilis. JCE Dermatology 1978; 16(8): 17–33.
22 Sapra S, Weatherhead L. Extensive nodular secondary syphilis. Arch Dermatol 1989; 125: 1666–1669.
23 Pavithran K. Nodular secondary syphilis. Int J Dermatol 1991; 30: 799–800.
24 Papini M, Bettacchi A, Guiducci A. Nodular secondary syphilis. Br J Dermatol 1998; 138: 704–705.
25 Kennedy CTC, Sanderson KV. Corymbose secondary syphilis. Arch Dermatol 1980; 116: 111–112.
26 Jain HC, Fisher BK. Annular syphilid mimicking granuloma annulare. Int J Dermatol 1988; 27: 340–341.
27 Lawrence P, Saxe N. Bullous secondary syphilis. Clin Exp Dermatol 1992; 17: 44–46.
28 Mikhail GR, Chapel TA. Follicular papulopustular syphilid. Arch Dermatol 1969; 100: 471–473.
29 Petrozzi JW, Lockshin NA, Berger BJ. Malignant syphilis. Severe variant of secondary syphilis. Arch Dermatol 1974; 109: 387–389.
30 Pariser H. Precocious noduloulcerative cutaneous syphilis. Arch Dermatol 1975; 111: 76–77.
31 Fisher DA, Chang LW, Tuffanelli DL. Lues maligna. Report of a case and a review of the literature. Arch Dermatol 1969; 99: 70–73.

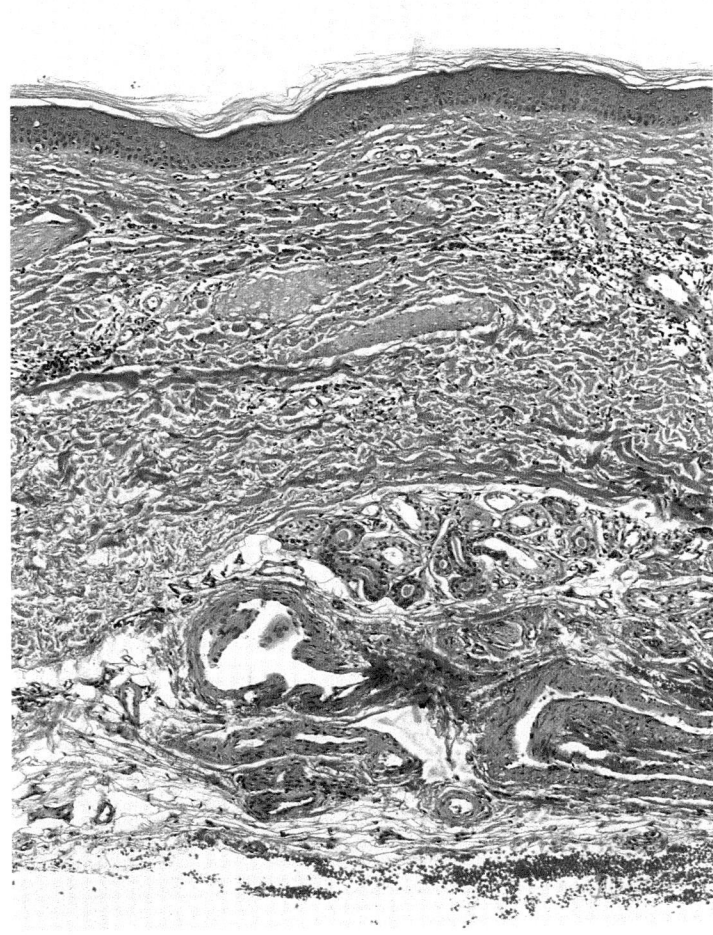

Fig. 24.9 **Acrodermatitis chronica atrophicans.** There is some atrophy of the dermis. (H & E)

32 Sharma VK, Sharma R, Kumar B, Radotra BD. Ulcerative secondary syphilis. Int J Dermatol 1990; 29: 585–586.

33 Glover RA, Piaquadio DJ, Kern S, Cockerell CJ. An unusual presentation of secondary syphilis in a patient with human immunodeficiency virus infection. Arch Dermatol 1992; 128: 530–534.

34 Tikjøb G, Russel M, Petersen CS et al. Seronegative secondary syphilis in a patient with AIDS: identification of Treponema pallidum in biopsy specimen. J Am Acad Dermatol 1991; 24: 506–508.

35 Fonseca E, García-Silva J, del Pozo J et al. Syphilis in an HIV infected patient misdiagnosed as leprosy. J Cutan Pathol 1999; 26: 51–54.

36 Don PC, Rubinstein R, Christie S. Malignant syphilis (lues maligna) and concurrent infection with HIV. Int J Dermatol 1995; 34: 403–407.

37 Tosca A, Stavropoulos PG, Hatziolou E et al. Malignant syphilis in HIV-infected patients. Int J Dermatol 1990; 29: 575–578.

38 Morar N, Ramdial PK, Naidoo DK et al. Lues maligna. Br J Dermatol 1999; 140: 1175–1177.

39 Cole GW, Amon RB, Russell PS. Secondary syphilis presenting as a pruritic dermatosis. Arch Dermatol 1977; 113: 489–490.

40 Lee JY-Y, Hsu M-L. Alopecia syphilitica, a simulator of alopecia areata: histopathology and differential diagnosis. J Cutan Pathol 1991; 18: 87–92.

41 Jordaan HF, Louw M. The moth-eaten alopecia of secondary syphilis. A histopathological study of 12 patients. Am J Dermatopathol 1995; 17: 158–162.

42 Cuozzo DW, Benson PM, Sperling LC, Skelton HG III. Essential syphilitic alopecia revisited. J Am Acad Dermatol 1995; 32: 840–844.

43 Stratigos JD, Katoulis AC, Hasapi V et al. An epidemiological study of syphilis incognito, an emerging public health problem in Greece. Arch Dermatol 2001; 137: 157–160.

44 Pembroke AC, Michell PA, McKee PH. Nodulo-squamous tertiary syphilide. Clin Exp Dermatol 1980; 5: 361–364.

45 Chung G, Kantor GR, Whipple S. Tertiary syphilis of the face. J Am Acad Dermatol 1991; 24: 832–835.

46 Wu SJ, Nguyen EQ, Nielsen TA, Pellegrini AE. Nodular tertiary syphilis mimicking granuloma annulare. J Am Acad Dermatol 2000; 42: 378–380.

47 Azar HA, Pham TD, Kurban AK. An electron microscopic study of a syphilitic chancre. Arch Pathol 1970; 90: 143–150.

48 Poulsen A, Kobayasi T, Secher L, Weismann K. Treponema pallidum in human chancre tissue: an electron microscopic study. Acta Derm Venereol 1986; 66: 423–430.

49 Abell E, Marks R, Wilson Jones E. Secondary syphilis: a clinico-pathological review. Br J Dermatol 1975; 93: 53–61.

50 Jeerapaet P, Ackerman AB. Histologic patterns of secondary syphilis. Arch Dermatol 1973; 107: 373–377.

51 Pandhi RK, Singh N, Ramam M. Secondary syphilis: a clinicopathologic study. Int J Dermatol 1995; 34: 240–243.

52 McBroom RL, Styles AR, Chiu MJ et al. Secondary syphilis in persons infected with and not infected with HIV-1. A comparative immunohistologic study. Am J Dermatopathol 1999; 21: 432–441.

53 Alessi E, Innocenti M, Ragusa G. Secondary syphilis. Clinical morphology and histopathology. Am J Dermatopathol 1983; 5: 11–17.

54 McNeely MC, Jorizzo JL, Solomon AR et al. Cutaneous secondary syphilis: preliminary immunohistopathologic support for a role for immune complexes in lesion pathogenesis. J Am Acad Dermatol 1986; 14: 564–571.

55 Jordaan HF, Cilliers J. Secondary syphilis mimicking Sweet's syndrome. Br J Dermatol 1986; 115: 495–496.

56 Cochran REI, Thomson J, Fleming KA, Strong AMM. Histology simulating reticulosis in secondary syphilis. Br J Dermatol 1976; 95: 251–254.

57 Hodak E, David M, Rothem A et al. Nodular secondary syphilis mimicking cutaneous lymphoreticular process. J Am Acad Dermatol 1987; 17: 914–917.

58 Green KM, Heilman E. Secondary syphilis presenting as a palisading granuloma. J Am Acad Dermatol 1985; 12: 957–960.

59 Carbia SG, Lagodin C, Abbruzzese M et al. Lichenoid secondary syphilis. Int J Dermatol 1999; 38: 53–55.

60 Kahn LB, Gordon WG. Sarcoid-like granulomas in secondary syphilis. Arch Pathol 1971; 92: 334–337.

61 Beckett JH, Bigbee JW. Immunoperoxidase localization of Treponema pallidum. Arch Pathol Lab Med 1979; 103: 135–138.

62 Phelps RG, Knispel J, Tu ES et al. Immunoperoxidase technique for detecting spirochetes in tissue sections: comparison with other methods. Int J Dermatol 2000; 39: 609–613.

63 Zoechling N, Schluepen EM, Soyer HP et al. Molecular detection of Treponema pallidum in secondary and tertiary syphilis. Br J Dermatol 1997; 136: 683–686.

64 Poulsen A, Kobayasi T, Secher L, Weismann K. Treponema pallidum in macular and papular secondary syphilitic skin eruptions. Acta Derm Venereol 1986; 66: 251–258.

65 Poulsen A, Kobayasi T, Secher L, Weismann K. Ultrastructural changes of Treponema pallidum isolated from secondary syphilitic skin lesions. Acta Derm Venereol 1987; 67: 289–294.

66 Handsfield HH, Lukehart SA, Sell S et al. Demonstration of Treponema pallidum in a cutaneous gumma by indirect immunofluorescence. Arch Dermatol 1983; 119: 677–680.

67 Matsuda-John SS, McElgunn PSJ, Ellis CN. Nodular late syphilis. J Am Acad Dermatol 1983; 9: 269–272.

68 Tanabe JL, Huntley AC. Granulomatous tertiary syphilis. J Am Acad Dermatol 1986; 15: 341–344.

69 Pace JL, Csonka GW. Endemic non-venereal syphilis (bejel) in Saudi Arabia. Br J Vener Dis 1984; 60: 293–297.

70 Koff AB, Rosen T. Nonvenereal treponematoses: yaws, endemic syphilis, and pinta. J Am Acad Dermatol 1993; 29: 519–535.

71 Engelkens HJH, Niemel PLA, van der Sluis JJ et al. Endemic treponematoses. Part II. Pinta and endemic syphilis. Int J Dermatol 1991; 30: 231–238.

72 Browne SG. Yaws. Int J Dermatol 1982; 21: 220–223.

73 Yaws or syphilis? Editorial. Br Med J 1979; 1: 912.

74 Engelkens HJH, Judanarso J, van der Sluis JJ et al. Disseminated early yaws: report of a child with a remarkable genital lesion mimicking venereal syphilis. Pediatr Dermatol 1990; 7: 60–62.

75 Green CA, Harman RRM. Yaws truly – a survey of patients indexed under "yaws" and a review of the clinical and laboratory problems of diagnosis. Clin Exp Dermatol 1986; 11: 41–48.

76 Sehgal VN, Jain S, Bhattacharya SN, Thappa DM. Yaws control/eradication. Int J Dermatol 1994; 33: 16–20.

77 Engelkens HJH, Niemel PLA, van der Sluis JJ, Stolz E. The resurgence of yaws. World-wide consequences. Int J Dermatol 1991; 30: 99–101.

78 Engelkens HJH, Judanarso J, Oranje AP et al. Endemic treponematoses. Part 1. Yaws. Int J Dermatol 1991; 30: 77–83.

79 Walker SL, Hay RJ. Yaws – a review of the last 50 years. Int J Dermatol 2000; 39: 258–260.

80 Woltsche-Kahr I, Schmidt B, Aberer W, Aberer E. Pinta in Austria (or Cuba?). Import of an extinct disease? Arch Dermatol 1999; 135: 685–688.

81 Binford CH, Connor DH. Pathology of tropical and extraordinary diseases. Vol 1. Washington DC: Armed Forces Institute of Pathology, 1976; 113.

Borrelioses

82 Felz MW, Chandler FW Jr, Oliver JH Jr et al. Solitary erythema migrans in Georgia and South Carolina. Arch Dermatol 1999; 135: 1317–1326.

83 Seinost G, Golde WT, Berger BW et al. Infection with multiple strains of Borrelia burgdorferi sensu stricto in patients with Lyme disease. Arch Dermatol 1999; 135: 1329–1333.

84 Picken RN, Strle F, Picken MM et al. Identification of three species of Borrelia burgdorferi sensu lato (B. burgdorferi sensu stricto, B. garinii, and B. afzelii) among isolates from acrodermatitis chronica atrophicans lesions. J Invest Dermatol 1998; 110: 211–214.

85 Granter SR, Barnhill RL, Duray PH. Borrelial fasciitis: diffuse fasciitis and peripheral eosinophilia associated with Borrelia infection. Am J Dermatopathol 1996; 18: 465–473.

85a Muellegger RR, Weger W, Zoechling N et al. Granulomatous cheilitis and Borrelia burgdorferi. Arch Dermato 2000; 136: 1502–1506.

85b Rogers RS III. Granulomatous cheilitis, Melkersson–Rosenthal syndrome, and orofacial granulomatosis. Arch Dermatol 2000; 136: 1557–1558.

86 Trevisan G, Stinco G, Cinco M. Neonatal skin lesions due to a spirochetal infection: a case of congenital Lyme borreliosis? Int J Dermatol 1997; 36: 677–680.

87 Cordoliani F, Vignon-Pennamen MD, Assous MV et al. Atypical Lyme borreliosis in an HIV-infected man. Br J Dermatol 1997; 137: 437–439.

88 Berger BW. Erythema chronicum migrans of Lyme disease. Arch Dermatol 1984; 120: 1017–1021.

89 Asbrink E, Hovmark A. Cutaneous manifestations in Ixodes-borne Borrelia spirochetosis. Int J Dermatol 1987; 26: 215–223.

90 Krafchik B. Lyme disease. Int J Dermatol 1989; 28: 71–74.

91 Trevisan G, Cinco M. Lyme disease. A general survey. Int J Dermatol 1990; 29: 1–8.

92 Berger BW, Johnson RC. Clinical and microbiologic findings in six patients with erythema migrans of Lyme disease. J Am Acad Dermatol 1989; 21: 1188–1191.

93 Steere AC, Malawista SE, Hardin JA et al. Erythema chronicum migrans and lyme arthritis. Ann Intern Med 1977; 86: 685–698.

94 Prose NS, Abson KG, Berg D. Lyme disease in children: diagnosis, treatment, and prevention. Semin Dermatol 1992; 11: 31–36.

95 Abele DC, Anders KH. The many faces and phases of borreliosis I. Lyme disease. J Am Acad Dermatol 1990; 23: 167–186.

96 Hashimoto Y, Takahashi H, Kishiyama K et al. Lyme disease with facial nerve palsy: rapid diagnosis using a nested polymerase chain reaction-restriction fragment length polymorphism analysis. Br J Dermatol 1998; 138: 304–309.

97 Muhlemann MF. Thirteen British cases of erythema chronicum migrans, a spirochaetal disease. Br J Dermatol 1984; 111: 335–339.

98 Kuiper H, Cairo I, Van Dam A et al. Solitary erythema migrans: a clinical, laboratory and epidemiological study of 77 Dutch patients. Br J Dermatol 1994; 130: 466–472.

99 Goldberg NS, Forseter G, Nadelman RB et al. Vesicular erythema migrans. Arch Dermatol 1992; 128: 1495–1498.

100 Berger BW, Johnson RC, Kodner C, Coleman L. Cultivation of Borrelia burgdorferi from human tick bite sites: a guide to the risk of infection. J Am Acad Dermatol 1995; 32: 184–187.

101 Melski JW, Reed KD, Mitchell PD, Barth GD. Primary and secondary erythema migrans in Central Wisconsin. Arch Dermatol 1993; 129: 709–716.

102 Melski JW. Language, logic, and lyme disease. Arch Dermatol 1999; 135: 1398–1400.

103 Steere AC, Grodzicki RL, Kornblatt AN et al. The spirochetal etiology of Lyme disease. N Engl J Med 1983; 308: 733–740.

104 Berger BW, Johnson RC, Kodner C, Coleman L. Failure of Borrelia burgdorferi to survive in the skin of patients with antibiotic-treated Lyme disease. J Am Acad Dermatol 1992; 27: 34–37.

105 Berger BW, Johnson RC, Kodner C, Coleman L. Cultivation of Borrelia burgdorferi from the blood of two patients with erythema migrans lesions lacking extracutaneous signs and symptoms of Lyme disease. J Am Acad Dermatol 1994; 30: 48–51.

106 Wienecke R, Zöchling N, Neubert U et al. Molecular subtyping of Borrelia burgdorferi in erythema migrans and acrodermatitis chronica atrophicans. J Invest Dermatol 1994; 103: 19–22.

107 Burgdorfer W, Barbour AG, Hayes SF et al. Lyme disease – a tick-borne spirochetosis? Science 1982; 216: 1317–1319.

108 Buechner SA, Lautenschlager S, Itin P et al. Lymphoproliferative responses to Borrelia burgdorferi in patients with erythema migrans, acrodermatitis chronica atrophicans, lymphadenosis benigna cutis, and morphea. Arch Dermatol 1995; 131: 673–677.

109 Agger WA, Case KL. Clinical comparison of borreliacidal-antibody test with indirect immunofluorescence and enzyme-linked immunosorbent assays for diagnosis of Lyme disease. Mayo Clin Proc 1997; 72: 510–514.

110 Lomholt H, Lebech AM, Hansen K et al. Long-term serological follow-up of patients treated for chronic cutaneous borreliosis or culture-positive erythema migrans. Acta Derm Venereol 2000; 80: 362–366.

111 Muellegger RR, Zoechling N, Soyer HP et al. No detection of Borrelia burgdorferi-specific DNA in erythema migrans lesions after minocycline treatment. Arch Dermatol 1995; 131: 678–682.

112 Hulshof MM, Vandenbroucke JP, Nohlmans LMKE et al. Long-term prognosis in patients treated for erythema chronicum migrans and acrodermatitis chronica atrophicans. Arch Dermatol 1997; 133: 33–37.

113 Feder HM Jr, Whitaker DL, Hoss DM. The truth about erythema migrans. Arch Dermatol 1997; 133: 93–94.

114 Berger BW, Kaplan MH, Rothenberg IR, Barbour AG. Isolation and characterization of the Lyme disease spirochete from the skin of patients with erythema chronicum migrans. J Am Acad Dermatol 1985; 13: 444–449.

115 Aberer E, Kersten A, Klade H et al. Heterogeneity of Borrelia burgdorferi in the skin. Am J Dermatopathol 1996; 18: 571–579.

116 Masters E, Granter S, Duray P, Cordes P. Physician-diagnosed erythema migrans and erythema migrans-like rashes following Lone Star tick bites. Arch Dermatol 1998; 134: 955–960.

117 Wu Y-S, Zhang W-F, Feng F-P et al. Atypical cutaneous lesions of Lyme disease. Clin Exp Dermatol 1993; 18: 434–436.

118 Berger BW, Clemmensen OJ, Gottlieb GJ. Spirochetes in lesions of erythema chronicum migrans. Am J Dermatopathol 1982; 4: 555–556.

119 Berger BW, Clemmensen OJ, Ackerman AB. Lyme disease is a spirochetosis. Am J Dermatopathol 1983; 5: 111–124.

120 Berg D, Abson KG, Prose NS. The laboratory diagnosis of Lyme disease. Arch Dermatol 1991; 127: 866–870.

121 Park HK, Jones BE, Barbour AG. Erythema chronicum migrans of Lyme disease: diagnosis by monoclonal antibodies. J Am Acad Dermatol 1986; 15: 406–410.

122 Wienecke R, Neubert U, Volkenandt M. Molecular detection of Borrelia burgdorferi in formalin-fixed, paraffin-embedded lesions of Lyme disease. J Cutan Pathol 1993; 20: 385–388.

123 Ranki A, Aavik E, Peterson P et al. Successful amplification of DNA specific for Finnish Borrelia burgdorferi isolates in erythema chronicum migrans but not in circumscribed scleroderma lesions. J Invest Dermatol 1994; 102: 339–345.

124 Asbrink E, Brehmer-Andersson E, Hovmark A. Acrodermatitis chronica atrophicans – a spirochetosis. Am J Dermatopathol 1986; 8: 209–219.

125 de Koning J, Tazelaar DJ, Hoogkamp-Korstanje JAA, Elema JD. Acrodermatitis chronica atrophicans: a light and electron microscopic study. J Cutan Pathol 1995; 22: 23–32.

126 Gellis SE, Stadecker MJ, Steere AC. Spirochetes in atrophic skin lesions accompanied by minimal host response in a child with Lyme disease. J Am Acad Dermatol 1991; 25: 395–397.

127 Muellegger RR, Schluepen EM, Millner MM et al. Acrodermatitis chronica atrophicans in an 11-year-old girl. Br J Dermatol 1996; 135: 609–612.

128 Burgdorf WHC, Worret W-I, Schultka O. Acrodermatitis chronica atrophicans. Int J Dermatol 1979; 18: 595–601.

129 Marsch WCh, Mayet A, Wolter M. Cutaneous fibroses induced by Borrelia burgdorferi. Br J Dermatol 1993; 128: 674–678.

130 España A, Torrelo A, Guerrero A et al. Periarticular fibrous nodules in Lyme borreliosis. Br J Dermatol 1991; 125: 68–70.

131 Marsch WCh, Wolter M, Mayet A. Juxta-articular fibrotic nodules in Borrelia infection – ultrastructural details of therapy-induced regression. Clin Exp Dermatol 1994; 19: 394–398.

132 Leslie TA, Levell NJ, Cutler SJ et al. Acrodermatitis chronica atrophicans: a case report and review of the literature. Br J Dermatol 1994; 131: 687–693.

133 Silberer M, Koszik F, Stingl G, Aberer E. Downregulation of class II molecules on epidermal Langerhans cells in Lyme borreliosis. Br J Dermatol 2000; 143: 786–794.

134 Buechner SA, Rufli T, Erb P. Acrodermatitis chronica atrophicans: a chronic T-cell-mediated immune reaction against Borrelia burgdorferi? J Am Acad Dermatol 1993; 28: 399–405.

135 Müllegger RR, McHugh G, Ruthazer R et al. Differential expression of cytokine mRNA in skin specimens from patients with erythema migrans or acrodermatitis chronica atrophicans. J Invest Dermatol 2000; 115: 1115–1123.

136 Slater DN. Borrelia burgdorferi-associated primary cutaneous B-cell lymphoma. Histopathology 2001; 38: 73–77.

137 Goodlad JR, Davidson MM, Hollowood K et al. Borrelia burgdorferi-associated cutaneous marginal zone lymphoma: a clinicopathological study of two cases illustrating the temporal progression of B. burgdorferi-associated B-cell proliferation in the skin. Histopathology 2000; 37: 501–508.

Mycoses and algal infections

INTRODUCTION

Fungi are an important cause of dermatological disease. Included in this chapter are the dermatophytes, which produce countless millions of skin infections each year, and the systemic and related mycoses whose clinical importance usually pertains to their involvement of organs other than the skin. This category assumes life-threatening importance in immunosuppressed individuals, a significant group being those suffering from HIV/AIDS. The mycoses are of global importance. The advent of new topical and systemic therapies in the last decade has been of great importance in the control of these infections.

The mycoses have long been a confusing area for anyone with only a peripheral interest in mycology. Classifications have been modified repeatedly and some fungi have undergone several changes in nomenclature in the space of a decade. The classification of the various fungal infections of the skin usually takes into account some of the morphological characteristics of the fungus concerned, as well as the distribution and nature of the infection that results. This approach has some shortcomings. For example, tinea nigra could be classified as either a superficial filamentous infection or as a dematiaceous fungal infection. Sporotrichosis is considered in this account with the dematiaceous fungi because of some clinical and histological overlap with chromomycosis. However, the yeast form in tissue sections is not pigmented, although the fungi are dematiaceous in culture. Members of the genus *Alternaria* are occasionally implicated as agents of phaeohyphomycosis; their colonies are gray to black, although they are not pigmented in tissues.[1] Against this background is the recent plea for a simplification of the nomenclature and the avoidance of fungal names as part of the clinical nomenclature to avoid confusion when the name of the organism is subject to change as a consequence of taxonomic reclassification.[2] This seems to occur not infrequently.

Fungal identification

Fungi grow slowly on laboratory media and their final identification, which is based on the appearance of their colonies and conidia in culture, as well as other characteristics, can take several weeks.[3] Accordingly, direct examination of tissue specimens is often undertaken in conjunction with histopathological examination of biopsy material in order to obtain a more rapid diagnosis.

The most widely used of these techniques, which is of most value in the examination of skin scrapings, is the application of a drop of 10% potassium hydroxide to a slide containing the material. This usually clears the tissues in 5 minutes or so, allowing fungi to be more easily visualized. It is our practice to use a solution that combines potassium hydroxide with glycerol (to prevent drying out) and calcofluor white, an agent that imparts a bright fluorescence to fungi when examined with a fluorescence microscope.

There are several methods of identifying fungi in paraffin-embedded material. Many fungi, particularly the dematiaceous and hyaline fungi, are readily visible in sections stained with hematoxylin and eosin. Some difficulty may be experienced with *Candida*, *Cryptococcus*, *Aspergillus*, *Blastomyces*, *Coccidioides* and *Mucor*.[4] Numerous sections may have to be examined in sporotrichosis to find fungal elements, and in most cases recourse to other stains (see below) is more practical. The dermatophytes are also difficult to see in sections stained with hematoxylin and eosin, but they can sometimes be made visible by racking down the condenser and reducing the light.

Various special stains can be used in an attempt to identify fungi in tissue sections. The PAS stain, sometimes combined with diastase digestion, is most frequently employed. It stains the cell walls of fungi a purple color of varying intensity. The silver methenamine stain, usually Grocott's modification, is a reliable method of detecting fungi: it stains them black against a green background. It is more reliable than the PAS stain for detecting degenerate fungal elements and the rare animal pathogens among the aquatic fungi, although it may be less reliable with zygomycetes.[5] *Cryptococcus neoformans* may be stained with the mucicarmine stain or a combined alcian blue–PAS stain, which shows the cell wall and capsule in contrasting colors.[6] It is usually doubly refractile under polarized light. Calcofluor white can be used to stain frozen or paraffin sections as well as tissue smears.[5] The sections must be viewed with a fluorescence microscope. Certain fungi are even auto-fluorescent when a section stained with hematoxylin and eosin is exposed to ultraviolet light.[4] These include *Blastomyces*, *Cryptococcus*, *Candida*, *Aspergillus*, *Coccidioides* and occasionally *Histoplasma*.[4,7]

An antiserum containing a polyclonal antibody to *Mycobacterium bovis* has been used with immunohistochemical techniques to identify a broad range of bacteria and fungi in paraffin-embedded tissue. This method seems to be particularly useful when organisms are sparse.[8]

The use of immunoperoxidase techniques and special fungal antibodies for the detection and diagnosis of fungi in smears and paraffin sections has been described.[9] The fungi stain a golden brown against a pale blue background. The technique is sensitive and specific. A major disadvantage is that most laboratories are unlikely to have available a comprehensive reference collection of fungal antibodies for use in this technique.

Polymerase chain reaction (PCR)-based techniques are now being used to identify specific species of fungi, including dermatophytes.[10–12] They have revealed marked genetic diversity among some fungi, particularly *Trichophyton mentagrophytes*.[13]

The majority of cutaneous mycoses are superficial infections caused by dermatophytes and various yeasts. The dermatophytoses will be considered first.

SUPERFICIAL FILAMENTOUS INFECTIONS

Two groups of fungal infections are included in this category, the dermatophytoses and the dermatomycoses. They are characterized by the presence of filamentous forms of the organism in tissue sections.

DERMATOPHYTOSES

The dermatophytes are a group of related filamentous fungi that have the ability to invade and colonize the keratinized tissues of man and animals.[14–16] Infections caused by these fungi, which account for 3–4% of dermatological consultations, are known as dermatophytoses (ringworm, tinea).[17,18]

The clinical appearances are quite variable and depend on a number of factors, including the species of fungus, the site of infection, the immunological status of the patient and the prior misuse of topical steroids.[19,20] The usual appearance on glabrous skin is an erythematous (and sometimes vesicular) annular centrifugally growing lesion, with peripheral scale and desquamation and central clearing.[17,21] Broken hairs and dystrophic nails occur with infections involving these structures. Less common presentations include subcutaneous and deep dermal infections[22–25] and abscesses,[26–29] verrucous lesions,[20] blastomycosis-like lesions,[30] and rarely lymphogenous or hematogenous extension.[31] Immunocompromised individuals are usually involved with these atypical presentations.[24,29,32,33] Lesions known as favus, kerion[34] and Majocchi's granuloma also occur, and these will be described later. The atypical presentations that may follow the use of topical steroids have been called 'tinea incognito'.[19,35,36]

Chronic persisting infections, defined on the basis of duration or treatment failure, also occur. Disturbed cellular immune functions have been found in many of these cases. Diabetes mellitus, palmoplantar keratoderma,[37] ichthyosis, atopic states, collagen diseases and Cushing's syndrome may all predispose to chronic and recurrent dermatophyte infections.[38]

A secondary allergic eruption ('id reaction') may develop, uncommonly, in patients with dermatophyte infections, particularly tinea pedis.[21] The id reaction (autoeczematization) is usually vesicular and on the palms (see p. 112). Erythema nodosum, vasculitis and erythema multiforme are other rare reactions to dermatophytes.[21]

Mycology

Dermatophytes belong to three genera, *Epidermophyton*, *Microsporum* and *Trichophyton*. There are three ecological groups of dermatophytes according to their natural habitats: anthropophilic, which preferentially affect humans; zoophilic, in which lower animals are the prime hosts; and geophilic, which live in the soil as saprophytes.[3,14] There is geographic variability in the distribution of fungi, although some species are widely distributed throughout the world.[39] The most common isolate is the anthropophilic fungus *T. rubrum*, which accounts for almost 40% of all dermatophyte infections worldwide.[38,40] Other common isolates include *T. violaceum*[41,42] (particularly in Africa and Europe, but not America), *T. mentagrophytes*, *T. tonsurans*, *E. floccosum*, *M. gypseum*,[43] *M. canis* and *M.audouinii*.[44] The last two species are declining in incidence, whereas infections caused by *T. rubrum* and *T. tonsurans* are on the increase.[39,45,46] The zoophilic fungi, such as *M. audouinii, M. canis, T. verrucosum*[47] and *T. tonsurans*, more commonly affect children and tend to evoke a more acute inflammatory response than do the anthropophilic fungi.[21]

Less common dermatophyte isolates of geographical or occupational interest include *T. soudanense*[48] (found in Africa and sometimes in travelers), *T. concentricum*[49,50] (the cause of tinea imbricata in the South Pacific and tropical America), *T. erinacei*[51] (from hedgehogs), *M. nanum*[52] (from swine), *T. simii*[53] (from monkeys), and *M. equinum*[54] and *T. equinum*[55] (from horses). Mixed isolates, sometimes including a yeast, occur.

The development of infection depends on exposure to an affected source and various factors diminishing host resistance. Associated diseases that predispose to dermatophyte infections have been mentioned above.[38] Local predisposing factors include abrasion, occlusive dressings, sweating, maceration and poor peripheral circulation.[38] The immunological mechanisms involved in eliminating dermatophytes are poorly understood. Acute infections are associated with good cell-mediated immunity, the short-term development of specific antibodies and the onset of delayed hypersensitivity.[21] Chronic infections, in which *T. rubrum* is commonly implicated,[56] are associated with poor in vitro cell-mediated immunity and sometimes elevated levels of IgE.[57–59] The dermatophyte itself may sometimes be the cause of the immunosuppression, which results from a serum factor found in widespread dermatophytosis.[60] There is no apparent HLA predilection to dermatophyte infections,[61] although it has been suggested that chronic *T. rubrum* infection (see above) occurs as a specific syndrome involving 'susceptible' hosts.[62]

Specific regional infections

Traditionally, dermatophyte infections of the skin have been considered on the basis of the site of involvement, because there are often some features unique to each. The subtypes considered are tinea capitis (including favus and kerion), tinea faciei, tinea barbae, tinea corporis, tinea cruris, tinea pedis and onychomycosis. Majocchi's granuloma is usually considered as a discrete entity. Tinea gladiatorum, found in wrestlers who have close body contact, will not be considered further.[63,64]

Tinea capitis

The regional variant tinea capitis was once almost exclusively an infection of children, and associated with either *M. canis* or *M. audouinii*.[65] Now, *T. tonsurans* and *T. violaceum* are the most common isolates in some geographical areas,[66–78] causing an endothrix type of hair invasion with the fungus entering the cortex just above the hair bulb and encircling the shaft beneath an intact cuticle.[79] Endothrix infections do not produce fluorescence with Wood's light, as opposed to ectothrix infections (*M. canis* and *M. audouinii*), which give a typical green fluorescence. *T. rubrum*, the commonest cause of tinea corporis, is not usually regarded as a scalp pathogen, although very occasional cases occur.[80] The effects vary from mild erythema with persistent scaliness and minimal hair loss through to inflammatory lesions with pustules and folliculitis and kerion formation.[81,82] Tinea capitis seems to be surprisingly rare in patients with HIV infection.[83,84] Transmission at the hairdresser has been recorded in two elderly women.[85]

Kerion

A kerion is a boggy violaceous inflammatory area of dermal suppuration and folliculitis.[34,86–89] It is most common on the scalp but can be produced in other sites,[90] as an occupational hazard, by zoophilic fungi. *T. verrucosum* and *T. tonsurans*, both endothrix fungi, are often implicated in the etiology of a kerion. *T. rubrum*[91–93] and *T. erinacei*[94] are rare isolates.

Favus

Favus is a chronic infection of the scalp, and more rarely of the glabrous skin, which is usually acquired in childhood.[95] It is still found in some developing countries,[74] although its incidence is decreasing in others.[96] The infection can persist for life. *T. schonleini* is most commonly involved, and rarely *T. violaceum*, *T. mentagrophytes* or *M. gypseum*.[95,97] It is characterized by yellow crusts (scutula) overlying an erythematous base. Localized alopecia often results.

Tinea faciei

Tinea faciei is an uncommon regional variant presenting as a facial erythema with scaling.[98,99] Diagnosis is often delayed. *T. rubrum*,[98] *T. mentagrophytes*[100] and *T. tonsurans*[101] have been implicated. One reported case had the histological appearance of granuloma faciale;[102] in another, abscess formation occurred.[103]

Tinea barbae, tinea corporis and tinea cruris

Tinea barbae, tinea corporis and tinea cruris have overlapping clinical features.[104] The usual organisms involved are *T. rubrum*,[105,106] *T. mentagrophytes* and *E. floccosum*.[38] The latter organism particularly involves the groin region and is common in closed communities because it is easily shed. It is unable to invade hair. Tinea cruris occurs almost exclusively in males, and unusual clinical appearances have been noted in patients with AIDS.[107] Penile involvement as an isolated lesion is exceedingly rare.[108] Diaper dermatitis is a variant that predominantly affects infants between 7 and 12 months of age.[109] Tinea imbricata is a special type of tinea corporis in which there are concentric rings of scale. It is a chronic infection that occurs in the West Pacific and South American regions; it is caused by *T. concentricum*.[49,110] The term 'radiation port dermatophytosis' is used for cases of tinea corporis localized to irradiated skin.[111]

Tinea pedis (athlete's foot)

Tinea pedis is the most common regional dermatophytosis in adolescents and adults. *T. rubrum* and *T. mentagrophytes* var. *interdigitale* are the most common isolates.[112,113] The appearances are often modified by maceration and fissuring, but the sharp scaling border is usually preserved. Pustular lesions are sometimes seen.[114] Tinea pedis is common in swimmers and in some male worshippers who practise communal ablution and subsequent prayer in bare feet.[115] Unilateral lesions of the sole have been reported in children.[116]

Majocchi's granuloma

The term 'Majocchi's granuloma' is given to nodular and plaque-like lesions of the lower leg, most common in females and showing a histological picture of a granulomatous perifolliculitis.[117,118] Various fungi have been implicated, including *T. rubrum*,[119] *M. canis*,[117] *T. violaceum*, *T. tonsurans*[120] and *T. mentagrophytes*. The terms 'nodular granulomatous perifoliculitis' and 'trichophytic granuloma' have been used for comparable lesions on the calf and scalp, respectively. Trichophytic granulomas, which are often nodular and in the subcutis, may occur in sites other than the scalp.[25] The condition often occurs in immunocompromised individuals.[121,122]

Onychomycosis

Onychomycosis is a generic term for any fungal infection of the nails. Some 40% or more cases of onychomycosis are caused by dermatophytes. The remainder result from yeasts, particularly *Candida albicans*, and various molds, such as *Scytalidium dimidiatum*, *Scopulariopsis brevicaulis*, *Fusarium* sp., *Acremonium* sp., *Alternaria* sp. and *Aspergillus* sp.[123–129] Dermatophytes mainly involve the toenails, with *T. rubrum* and, to a lesser extent, *T. mentagrophytes* var. *interdigitale* being the usual agents.[130] Various immunological disturbances and peripheral vascular disease may predispose to infection. Onychomycosis is a serious health burden, particularly in older persons and diabetics.[131,132] Extensive whitening of the nails due to *T. rubrum* has recently been reported in a patient with AIDS.[133]

The majority of infections caused by *Candida albicans* and other species of *Candida* involve the fingers. The soft tissues around the nail are involved first, producing a paronychia with secondary penetration of the keratin by the fungus.[134]

Clinically, dermatophyte infections of the nail have traditionally been divided into distal, lateral, proximal and white superficial variants according to the anatomical localization and appearances.[135] A new classification, expanding on this traditional one, has recently been proposed.[136] Its categories are distal and lateral subungual, superficial, proximal subungual, endonyx and total dystrophic.[136] Different combinations of these patterns may occur. The occurrence of these variants appears to reflect differing host–parasite relationships.

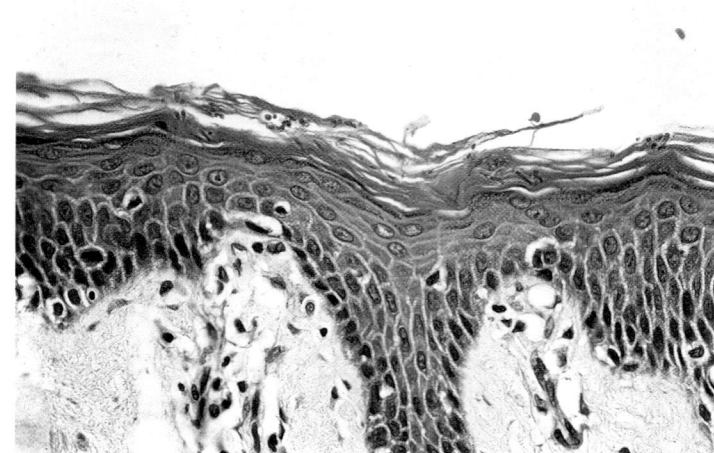

Fig. 25.1 **Dermatophyte infection.** Hyphae are present in the compact orthokeratotic layer. (H & E)

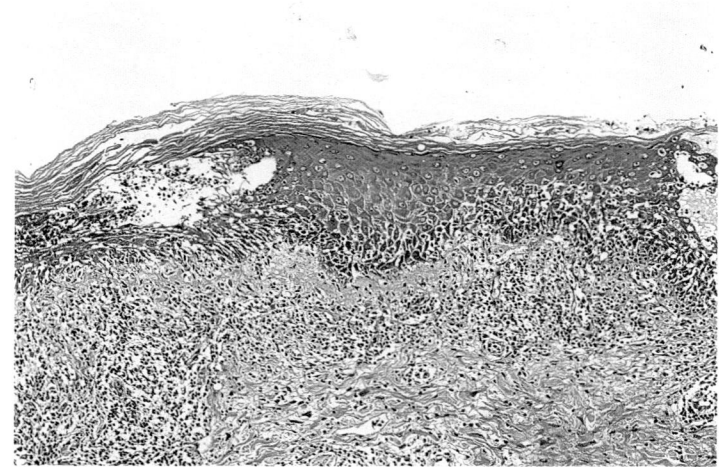

Fig. 25.2 **Dermatophyte infection.** Neutrophils are present within the spongiotic vesicle. (H & E)

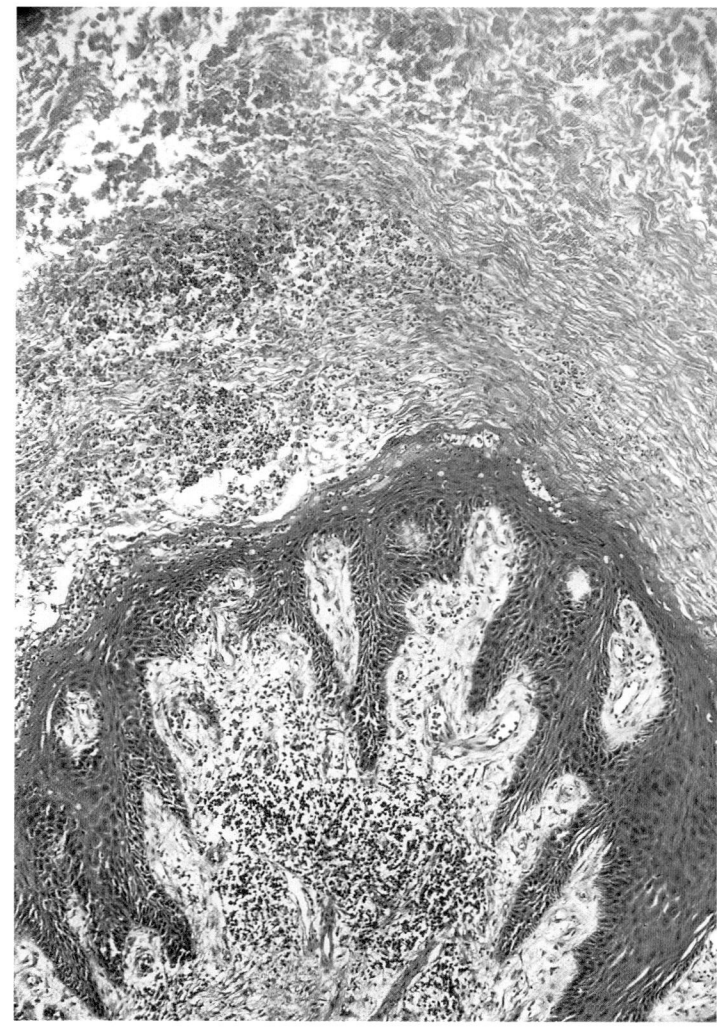

Fig. 25.3 **Tinea imbricata.** There are numerous hyphae and some spores in the thickened stratum corneum. The underlying epidermis shows psoriasiform hyperplasia. (H & E)

The fungal elements occur mostly in the deeper portions of the nail plate and in the hyperkeratotic nail bed, rather than on the surface of the nail plate.[137,138] Sometimes a thick hyperkeratotic nodule forms beneath the nail. This contains numerous clumped hyphae (dermatophytoma).[139] This is an explanation for the negative results obtained from scrapings in some cases of onychomycosis. Histopathological examination of the nail using the PAS stain is still the most sensitive diagnostic method.[140]

Histopathology of dermatophytoses

Biopsy material from dermatophyte infections can show a wide range of histological changes.[141] Ackerman has elaborated three different changes in the stratum corneum that can be associated with dermatophyte infections: the presence of neutrophils;[142] compact orthokeratosis (Fig. 25.1);[143] and the presence of the 'sandwich sign'.[144] The last refers to the presence of hyphae 'sandwiched in' between an upper but normal basket-weave stratum corneum, and a lower layer of recently produced stratum corneum which is abnormal in being compact orthokeratotic or parakeratotic in type.[144] Uncommonly, the stratum corneum retains its normal basket-weave pattern.

The epidermis is often mildly spongiotic; more florid spongiotic vesiculation is usually present when the palms and soles are involved. Subcorneal or intraepidermal pustulation is a less common pattern (Fig. 25.2).[141] Chronic lesions show variable acanthosis (Fig. 25.3). The dermis shows mild superficial edema and a sparse perivascular infiltrate, which includes lymphocytes and occasionally eosinophils or neutrophils.

At times the dermal infiltrate is much heavier, particularly if there is follicular involvement (Fig. 25.4). There may be perifollicular neutrophils or a mixed inflammatory infiltrate (Fig. 25.5). There is a heavy inflammatory infiltrate in a kerion, the proportion of the various cells depending on the duration of the lesion. In Majocchi's granuloma there are perifollicular and dermal granulomas and chronic inflammation; reactive lymphoid follicles may be present.[118] Fungal elements may take several forms: yeasts, bizarre hyphae and mucinous coatings.[118] Fungal elements are sometimes sparse.[145]

Rare patterns of inflammation include a resemblance to granuloma faciale, papular urticaria or eosinophilic pustular folliculitis.[146] In immunocompromised patients, large numbers of hyphae and pseudospores are present in areas of dermal necrosis.[20,147] The lesions often lack granulomas, a point of distinction from the usual Majocchi's granuloma (see above).

Dermatophytes exist in tissues in a parasitic form characterized by branched, septate hyphae and small spores. Methods for their identification have been mentioned above. Dermatophytes may invade the hair shaft (endothrix infection) or remain confined to its surface (ectothrix infection). *T. tonsurans*, *T. violaceum*, and *T. soudanense* are true endothrix parasites.[148]

DERMATOMYCOSES

The term 'dermatomycoses' encompasses infections of the hair, nails or skin caused by non-dermatophytes which have filamentous forms in tissues. It covers such infections as tinea nigra, piedra, pityriasis versicolor and candidosis.

Infections caused by the molds *Scytalidium dimidiatum* (previously known as *Hendersonula toruloidea*)[149,150] and *Scytalidium hyalinum*[151] are included as dermatomycoses. They are increasingly important as a cause of onychomycosis and tinea pedis.[152] They are being isolated with increasing frequency in the United Kingdom from individuals who have emigrated from tropical regions.[153]

Scopulariopsis brevicaulis, a widespread saprophytic fungus, is included here for completeness. It has been associated with onychomycosis and rarely chronic granulomatous skin infections.[154,155]

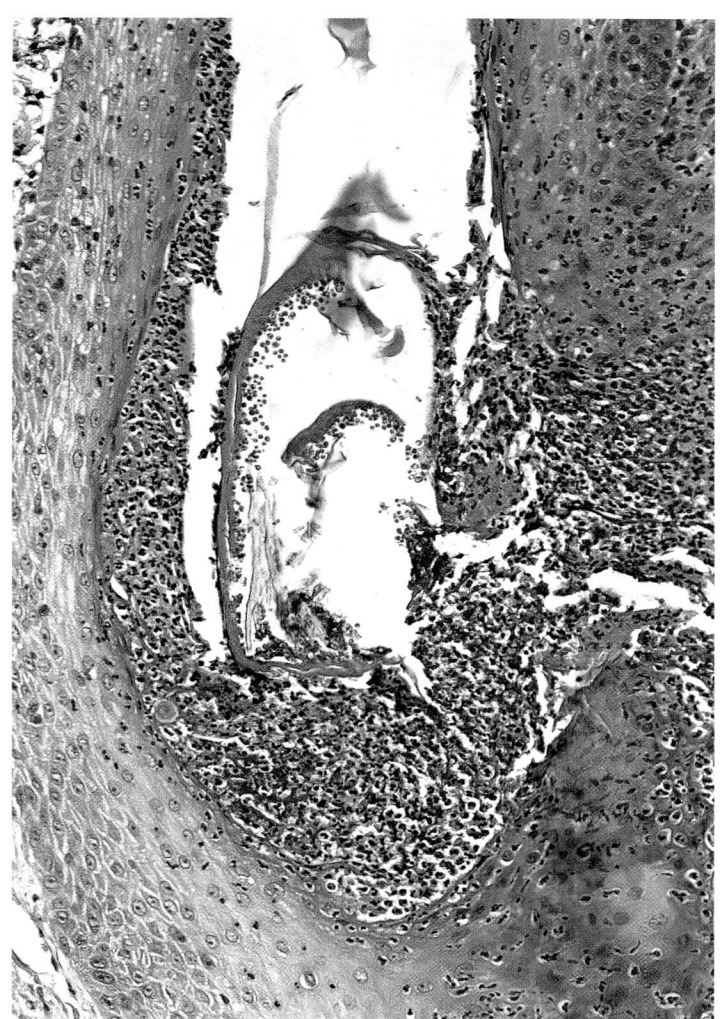

Fig. 25.4 **Folliculitis with suppuration resulting from a dermatophyte infection.** (H & E)

YEAST INFECTIONS

Yeasts are fungi of primarily unicellular growth habit.[156] The normal vegetative cells of yeasts are round or oval and measure 2.5–6 μm in diameter. Many yeasts can form hyphae or pseudohyphae in cutaneous infections. They are a regular constituent of the normal human flora, but most are potential pathogens. Opportunistic yeast infections increased with the advent of broad-spectrum antibiotics and immunosuppressive therapy.[157] They are now an important complication in patients with AIDS.

Candida albicans and *Cryptococcus neoformans* are the most important yeasts, producing, respectively, candidosis and cryptococcosis.

Malassezia globosa, previously known as *M. furfur* and *Pityrosporum orbiculare*, produces the cosmetically disfiguring condition pityriasis versicolor (tinea versicolor). *Malassezia* can also produce folliculitis. It has been incriminated in the etiology of confluent and reticulated papillomatosis, and of some cases of seborrheic dermatitis (including its occurrence in patients with the acquired immunodeficiency syndrome),[158] dandruff, psoriasis and atopic dermatitis.[159] It is likely that the organisms are present because of the favorable 'soil' in these conditions.

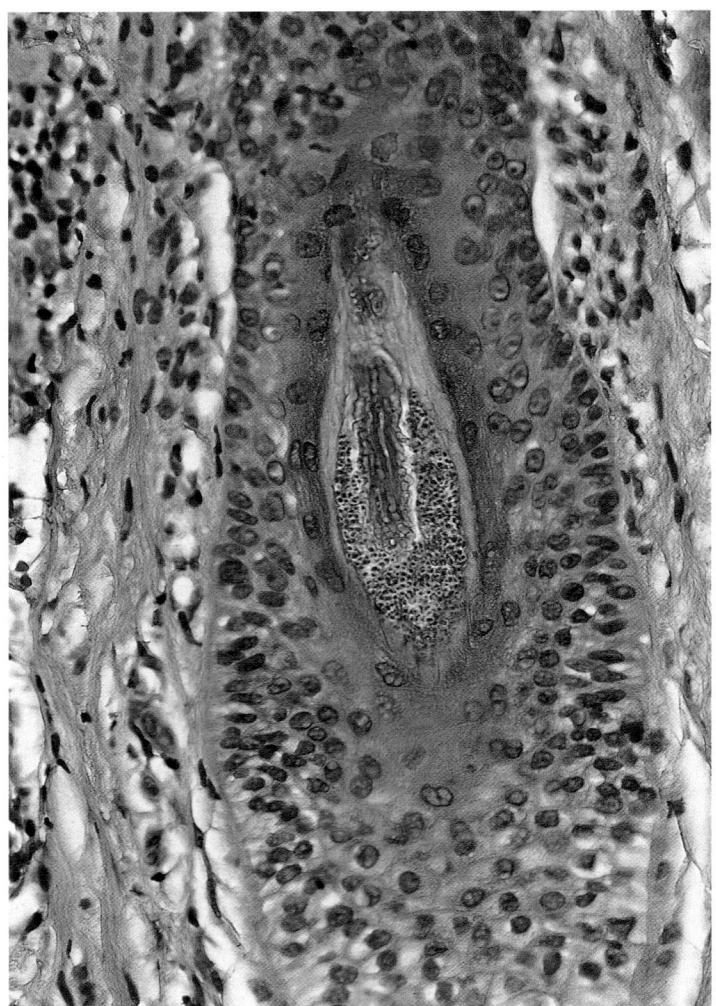 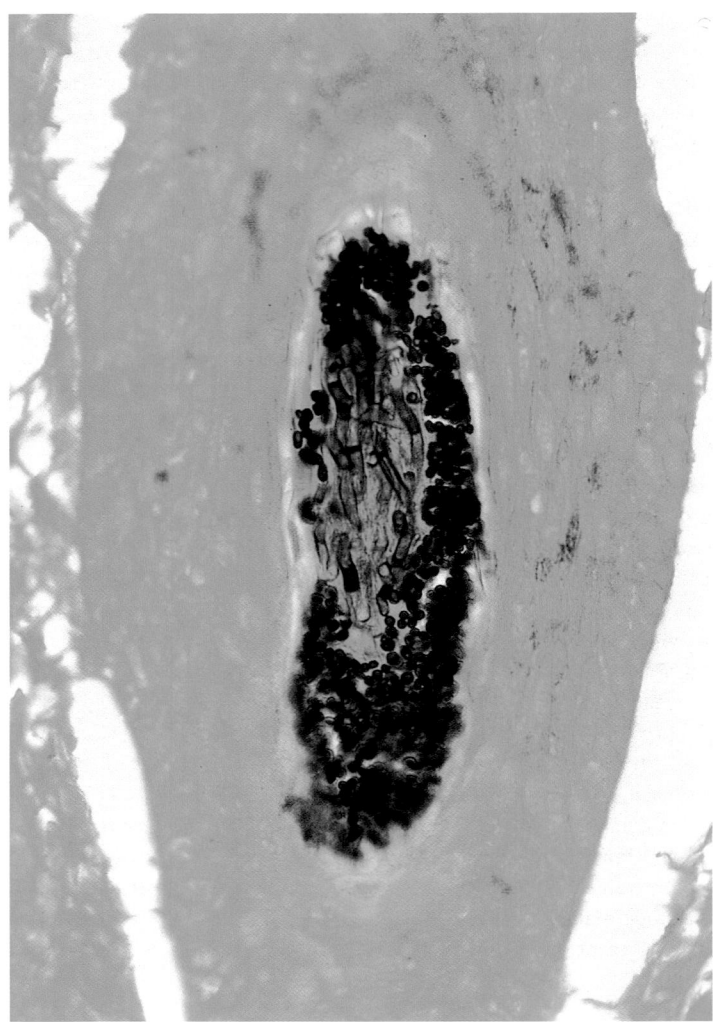

Fig. 25.5 **Tinea capitis. (A)** There is a sparse perifollicular inflammatory cell infiltrate and numerous fungal elements involving the hair (H & E). **(B)** Fungal elements can be seen within the hair shaft (endothrix infection). (Grocott stain)

Trichosporon sp. can produce both white piedra, a superficial infection of the hair, and a disseminated infection in immunosuppressed patients.

The genera *Rhodotorula*,[157] *Torulopsis*,[157] and *Sporobolomyces*[160] are of little importance in relation to the skin and will not be considered further.

CANDIDOSIS (CANDIDIASIS)

Candida albicans is the most frequent species of *Candida* implicated in human infections. These range from relatively trivial superficial infections to fatal disseminated disease.[161–163] *Candida albicans* is a normal inhabitant of the gastrointestinal tract and is found in the mouths of 40% of normal individuals. It is sometimes isolated from the skin surface, but it is not a usual constituent of the skin flora. There are many factors that predispose to clinical infection. These include pregnancy,[164] the neonatal period, immunological and endocrine dysfunction, antibiotic therapy, and immunocompromised and debilitating states.[161] Local factors such as increased skin moisture and heat also play a role. Recent studies have provided a better understanding of the various factors that contribute to the invasive properties of *Candida albicans*.[165] For example, the yeast can express at least three types of surface adhesion molecules to colonize epithelial surfaces, plus an aspartyl proteinase enzyme which facilitates penetration of keratinized cells.[165]

A number of clinical variants of candidosis occur: acute superficial candidosis, chronic mucocutaneous candidosis, systemic (disseminated) candidosis, and candidosis in the infant.[161] Oral, periungual and genital candidosis are best regarded as distinct entities that may occur alone or in association with other clinical forms of candidosis. Folliculitis and delayed surgical wound healing are rare manifestations of *Candida* infection.[166,167] *Candida* folliculitis may mimic tinea barbae.[168,169] Another species of *Candida*, *C. parapsilosis*, can sometimes cause localized and systemic infections in immunocompromised patients, and after extensive burns. It has also been responsible for a chondritis after surgery to the ear.[170]

Acute superficial candidosis

Acute superficial candidosis is the usual form of cutaneous infection with *Candida* species. There are vesicles, pustules and crusted erosions with a beefy-red appearance. These develop on skin folds and other areas, particularly in individuals living in a humid environment.[161] The condition may be self-limited; it responds well to treatment.

Histopathology

The characteristic histological feature is the presence of neutrophils in the stratum corneum. The infiltration may take the form of small collections of cells, spongiform pustulation or subcorneal pustulation resembling impetigo. The underlying epidermis may show focal spongiosis and mild acanthosis. Fungal elements may be sparse. They are best visualized with the PAS stain. Mycelia predominate over spores. Electron microscopy has shown that the majority of the fungal elements are inside the epithelial cells.[171,172]

Chronic mucocutaneous candidosis

The term 'chronic mucocutaneous candidosis' covers a heterogeneous group of disorders characterized by chronic and persistent infections of the mucous membranes, and infections of the skin and nails by various species of *Candida*, usually *C. albicans*.[173–175] The condition ranges in severity from a mild localized and persistent infection of the mouth, nails or vulva to a severe generalized condition.[161] It may be associated with a spectrum of cellular immunodeficiency states, including several defined syndromes that range from life-threatening to subtle.[174] A deficiency of the cytokine interleukin-2 was present in one case.[176] Other cytokines are also involved, and it now appears that the basic defect is altered cytokine production in response to candida antigens.[177] Other associations include endocrinopathies and nutritional deficiencies, the latter including disorders of iron metabolism.[161,174,178] On the basis of recent cases, it appears that there are two *Candida* endocrinopathy syndromes, one associated with hypoparathyroidism and/or hypoadrenalism[179] and the other associated with hypothyroidism. The former is inherited as an autosomal dominant trait and the latter syndrome as an autosomal recessive.[180] Late onset of chronic mucocutaneous candidosis in adults is rare and usually associated with cancer, particularly a thymoma.[174,181]

In all clinical groups, vaginitis, paronychia and oral thrush may also be present. The cutaneous lesions are asymptomatic plaques on the dorsum of the hands and feet and periorificial skin.[181] They are brown-red with sharp margins and a soft scale.[181] Sometimes a more extensive scaling eruption is present. Granulomatous lesions have been recorded.[182] In 20% of all cases there is a concurrent dermatophyte infection.[178,181]

Histopathology

There is some histological resemblance to the acute form, although the lesions tend to have more epidermal acanthosis, sometimes being vaguely psoriasiform in type (Fig. 25.6). There may be areas of compact orthokeratosis[183] and others of scale crust formation with degenerating neutrophils. This reflects the chronicity of the lesions. Spores and hyphae are usually found without difficulty in PAS preparations.

In granulomatous lesions there are vaguely formed granulomas in the dermis composed of lymphocytes, plasma cells, epithelioid cells and occasional Langhans giant cells. Occasional yeast forms and pseudohyphae may be found in the granulomas.

Disseminated candidosis

Disseminated (systemic) candidosis is increasingly being recognized in immunosuppressed and debilitated patients, particularly those with central venous catheters and those receiving broad-spectrum antibiotics.[161,184–186] Multisystem involvement occurs, although cutaneous lesions are present in only 15% of cases.[185] *C. tropicalis* is a frequent isolate from the cutaneous lesions in this type of candidosis.[187]

There is an erythematous papulonodular rash, with multiple lesions on the trunk and proximal parts of the extremities. Sometimes only isolated lesions are present. Another rare clinical presentation mimics that of ecthyma gangrenosum.[188,189]

Systemic candidosis is well recognized in heroin addicts, but only comparatively recently have cutaneous lesions, in the form of folliculitis, been reported in some addicts.[190,191]

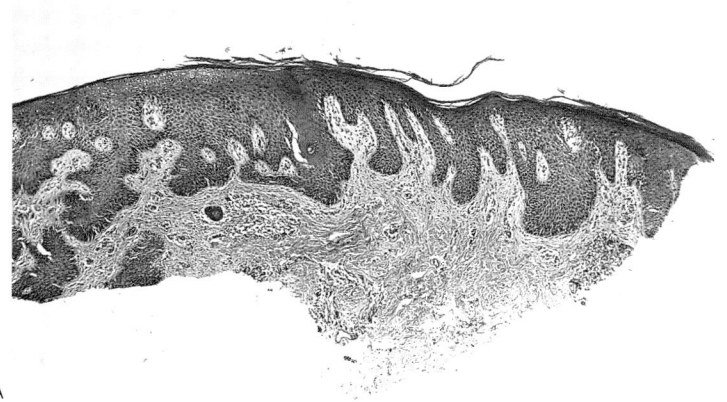
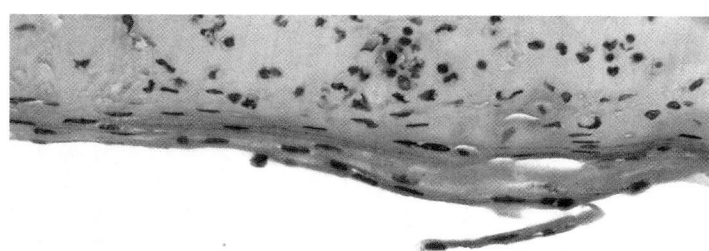
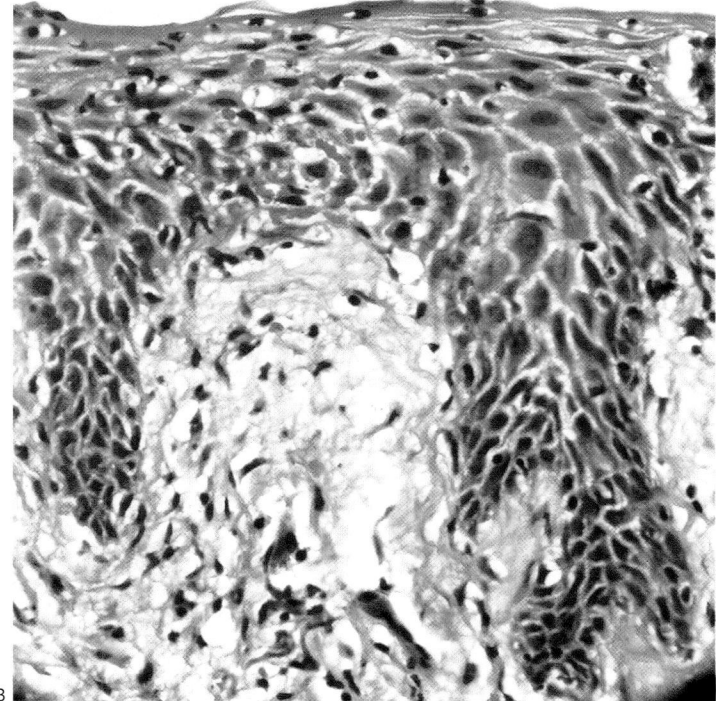

Fig. 25.6 **Chronic candidosis. (A)** There is mild psoriasiform hyperplasia of the epidermis. **(B)** There is overlying scale crust containing degenerate neutrophils. (H & E)

Histopathology

There are small microabscesses in the upper dermis, sometimes centered on blood vessels.[185] A few budding yeasts may be found in these areas on a PAS stain.[185] At other times the reaction is much milder, with only a perivascular mixed inflammatory cell infiltrate. A leukocytoclastic angiitis has been reported.[187] In lesions resembling ecthyma gangrenosum, the papillae are edematous and distended by numerous pseudohyphae, which may extend into vessel walls.[189] Ulceration is also present. In heroin addicts there is a suppurative folliculitis and perifolliculitis. Pseudohyphae are sometimes found within the hair.

Candidosis of the newborn

There are several distinct clinicopathological entities within this group: congenital cutaneous candidosis, neonatal candidosis and infantile gluteal granuloma.[161] Immunity is not impaired.

Congenital cutaneous candidosis presents at birth or in the first days of life with generalized erythematous macules and papulopustules.[192,193] It results from intrauterine infection.[194,195] Organisms may be demonstrated in the placenta and in the stratum corneum of the neonatal lesions.[192]

Neonatal candidosis presents with oral and perioral lesions in the first 2 weeks of life.[194] Infection is probably acquired during intravaginal passage at the time of delivery.[194] Sometimes there is involvement of the diaper area.[194]

Infantile gluteal granuloma is an etiologically controversial entity characterized by discrete granulomatous lesions in the diaper (napkin) area.[196] Diaper dermatitis is part of the spectrum.[197] The role of *Candida* is uncertain.[161,196,198] The use of topical fluorinated steroids and plastic pants in infants with diaper dermatitis has been incriminated.[196,199] Rarely, a similar entity has been reported in this region in adults, possibly as a consequence of *Candida* infection.[200]

Oral candidosis

Oral candidosis (thrush) is found mostly in infants as irregular white patches and plaques.[161,201] It can also be found as part of chronic mucocutaneous candidosis and in debilitated adults on long-term antibiotics or with a hematological malignancy. Rarely, thrush is related to poor oral hygiene and dentures.[202] Oral candidosis has been reported as an initial manifestation of the acquired immunodeficiency syndrome (AIDS).[203]

Other patterns of mucosal involvement occur on the tongue. These include median rhomboid glossitis[204] and black hairy tongue, although the latter has been attributed to species of *Candida* other than *C. albicans*.[161] A perioral pustular eruption has been ascribed to *Candida*.[205]

Epithelial hyperplasia is a characteristic feature of mucosal infection.

Genital candidosis

Vaginal candidosis is a common gynecological infection.[206] It tends to occur in the absence of other lesions. A thick creamy vaginal discharge is present. Sexual transmission of the infection sometimes occurs, but balanitis is much less common than vulvovaginitis.[206]

Periungual candidosis

Paronychia may occur as an isolated infection, particularly in women who frequently immerse their hands in water.[207] Minor mechanical trauma, diabetes and circulatory disturbances may also be incriminated.[161] The nail of the middle finger of the dominant hand is most frequently involved.[207] In chronic mucocutaneous candidosis there is usually onychodystrophy with nail bed deformity rather than onycholysis, which is more often a manifestation of acute infection.

CRYPTOCOCCOSIS

Cryptococcus neoformans (formerly known as *Torula histolytica*) is an encapsulated yeast-like fungus found in dried avian (particularly pigeon) and bat excreta, and in dust contaminated with such droppings.[208–211] Its usual portal of entry is the respiratory tract, leading to the formation of pulmonary granulomas. Meningoencephalitis is another clinical presentation of cryptococcosis. Hematogenous dissemination leading to cutaneous involvement occurs in about 10–15% of cases of cryptococcosis.

Skin lesions may be the first evidence of an occult systemic infection.[212,213] Although many cases have been reported as instances of primary cutaneous cryptococcosis,[214] probably only a few of these have resulted from primary inoculation of organisms into the skin, thereby fulfilling the criteria of a true primary cutaneous infection.[215–218] Most patients are immuno-compromised[219–222] and the infection is now a well-recognized occurrence in patients with AIDS.[223–231] The cutaneous presentations of cryptococcosis are protean and include papulonodules, ulcers, pustules, plaques, ecchymoses and cellulitis.[232–235] Lesions may rarely simulate pyoderma gangrenosum,[236] herpes,[223,237] keloids[238] or molluscum contagiosum.[225,226,237,239] Any site may be involved, but there is a predilection for the face, neck and forearms.[218]

A rapid diagnosis may be made by examination of India-ink preparations of aspirates or Tzanck smears. The organisms are readily isolated on Sabouraud's agar. Rarely, other species of *Cryptococcus* have been isolated from infected tissues.[240,241]

Histopathology[208,242]

The histology is variable, ranging from tuberculoid granulomas in the dermis and upper subcutis, with few organisms, to lesions in which large numbers of the yeast-like organisms, surrounded by their mucinous capsular material, form extensive mucoid masses (Figs 25.7, 25.8).[219] The organisms mostly range from 5 to 15 μm in diameter. A common pattern is a dense infiltrate of chronic inflammatory cells with multinucleate giant cells containing several organisms with refractile walls. Focal granulomas may be present, as may some small spaces containing numerous organisms, both free and in macrophages. Palisaded granulomas are rare.[243] A few neutrophils are often present; small microabscesses are less common. The overlying epidermis may show acanthosis, mild pseudoepitheliomatous hyperplasia or ulceration. Transepidermal elimination of organisms may be seen.[208]

The cell wall of *C. neoformans* will stain with the PAS or silver methenamine methods, and the capsule with mucicarmine or alcian blue.[208] A combined PAS–alcian blue stain which contrasts the cell wall and capsule is a useful method. Phagocytosed organisms often have an attenuated capsule that does not stain. Non-encapsulated tissue variants[244] and hyphal forms have been described in other sites. The latter are found only very rarely, and usually only in superficial ulcerated lesions at the body orifices. The organism is usually doubly refractile under polarized light. It may be confirmed by the use of indirect immunoperoxidase methods on routine paraffin sections.[245]

Electron microscopy

The organisms have an electron-dense wall and a surrounding clear space, beyond which is the capsule.[219] In some phagocytosed organisms the capsule has been destroyed and there is only a small amount of fibrillary material remaining.[242] Projecting buds may be seen, even on phagocytosed organisms.[242,246]

PITYRIASIS VERSICOLOR

Pityriasis versicolor (tinea versicolor) is a relatively common non-contagious superficial fungal infection, usually located on the upper trunk or upper arms.[247,248] It is both chronic and recurrent. Lesions are slightly scaly and may be macular, nummular or confluent. They vary in color from red-brown to white, and the scales show yellow fluorescence with Wood's light.[247] Infections are more common in patients with seborrheic dermatitis, dandruff[249] or hyperhidrosis, and in residents in the tropics.[246] In infants, a papulopustular eruption of the face (neonatal acne) may result from infection with the same fungus.[250] One subgroup of atopic dermatitis (head and neck dermatitis) can be aggravated by *Malassezia* sp.[251,252] Although affected patients have a normal cell-mediated immune response to the organism, they do not generate a protective response to mycelial antigens.[253]

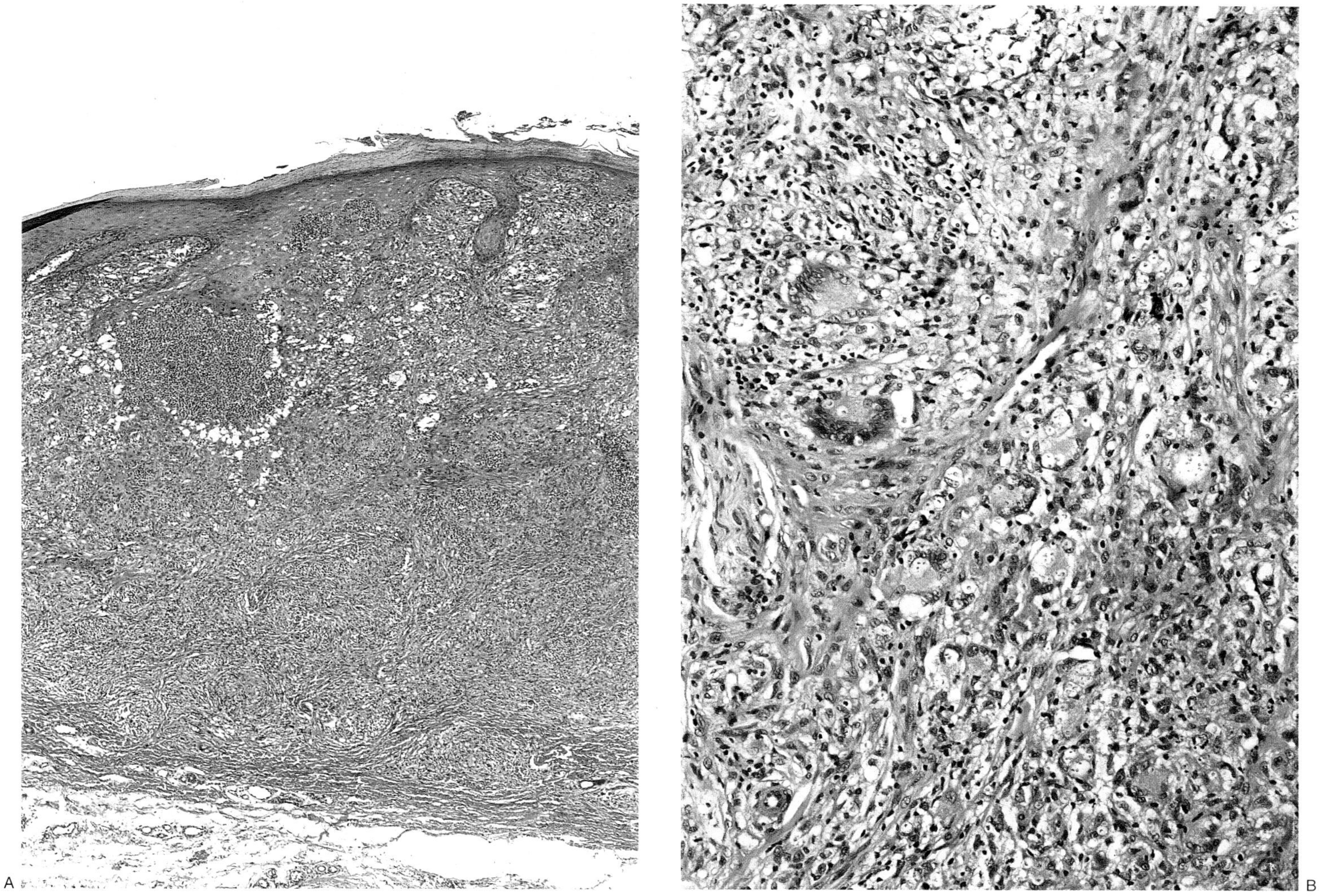

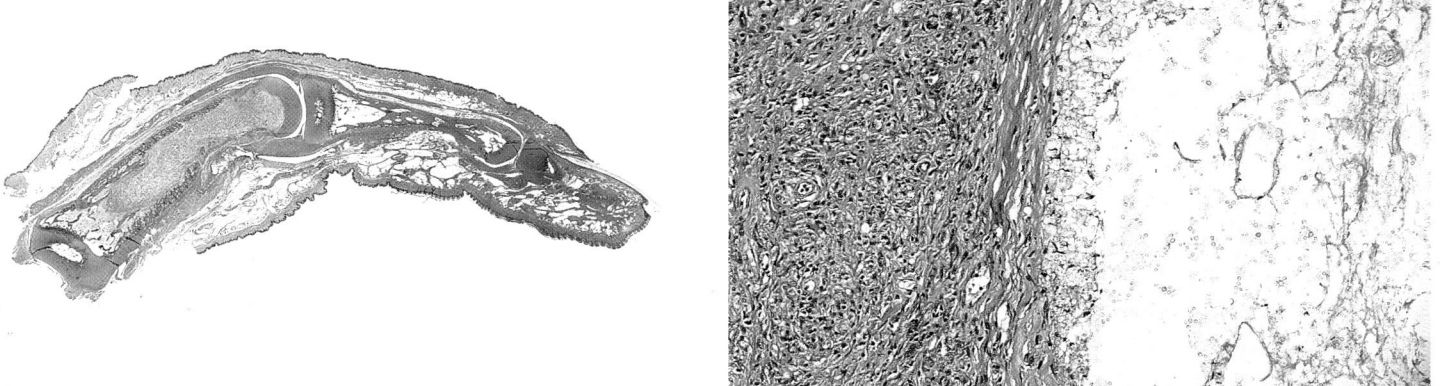

Fig. 25.7 **Cryptococcosis. (A)** There are granulomas and sheets of inflammatory cells in the dermis. **(B)** There are numerous yeasts in macrophages and giant cells. (H & E)

Fig. 25.8 **Cryptococcosis. (A)** Extension into bone and joint is occurring in this amputated finger. **(B)** There is a mucinous area with numerous organisms and a surrounding inflammatory palisade. (H & E)

The causative organism, previously called *Malassezia furfur*, is a dimorphic lipophilic fungus that is a normal inhabitant of the stratum corneum and infundibulum of the hair follicle.[254–256] The yeast phase of this organism has two morphologically discrete forms: an ovoid form, known for decades as *Pityrosporum ovale*, and a spherical form, *Pityrosporum orbiculare*.[257] Each form can transform into the other. A taxonomic revision of the genus *Malassezia* was carried out in 1996 with the description of four new species: *M. globosa*, *M. restricta*, *M. obtusa* and *M. slooffiae*. *M. sympodialis* and *M. pachydermatis* had been described earlier, the latter being regarded as a resident of animal skin.[258] The following summary details our current knowledge. It is likely to change as more studies accumulate from both tropical and temperate climates.

- *M. globosa* – pityriasis versicolor and healthy skin
- *M. sympodialis* – normal skin, particularly trunk
- *M. restricta* – seborrheic dermatitis and dandruff
- *M. pachydermatis* – cats and dogs, systemic infection in premature infants
- *M. slooffiae* – normal skin, low number of isolates
- *M. obtusa* – rare isolate, little known about it.

As a consequence of recent studies it now appears that pityriasis versicolor is caused by *M. globosa* in its mycelial phase.[258]

Hypopigmentation in pityriasis versicolor results from the production of dicarboxylic acids by the organisms. These have a tyrosinase inhibitor effect, thus interfering with the synthesis of melanin.[259,260] Hyperpigmentation may result in part from the production of large melanosomes, singly distributed,[261] but also from vascular hyperemia, orthokeratosis and the presence of organisms.[262,263]

Histopathology

There is slight to moderate hyperkeratosis and acanthosis. The dermis contains a mild, superficial perivascular inflammatory infiltrate which includes lymphocytes, histiocytes and occasional plasma cells. There may be mild melanin incontinence in some cases. In the stratum corneum there are numerous round budding yeasts (blastoconidia) and short septate hyphae (pseudomycelium), giving a so-called 'spaghetti and meat balls' appearance (Fig. 25.9). One study has shown that helper-inducer T cells dominate among the sparse dermal infiltrate.[264]

Electron microscopy

Fungi can be demonstrated at all levels of the stratum corneum, in follicles, and even intracellularly.[265]

PITYROSPORUM FOLLICULITIS

Pityrosporum folliculitis presents as erythematous follicular papules and pustules, 2–4 mm in diameter, with a predilection for the upper back, shoulders, chest and upper arms.[247,266,267] The lesions can be quite pruritic.[268] It is more common in females, and in those over the age of 30.[269] Sometimes there is associated seborrheic dermatitis or pityriasis versicolor.[266,270] It has been reported in Down syndrome,[271] pregnancy,[272] and in immuno-compromised patients,[273,274] in whom it may be confused clinically with more serious infections.[275] It has been reported as a nosocomial infection in three patients in the same intensive care unit.[276] *Malassezia furfur* can be cultured from lesions in about 75% of cases,[266] and affected individuals have serum antibody titers against this organism.[270] Little is known about the organism involved, using the most recent taxonomic classification, but it is likely that *M. globosa* will be the organism responsible. There is some evidence to suggest that follicular occlusion is the primary event in the pathogenesis of this condition, with yeast overgrowth being a secondary occurrence.[277]

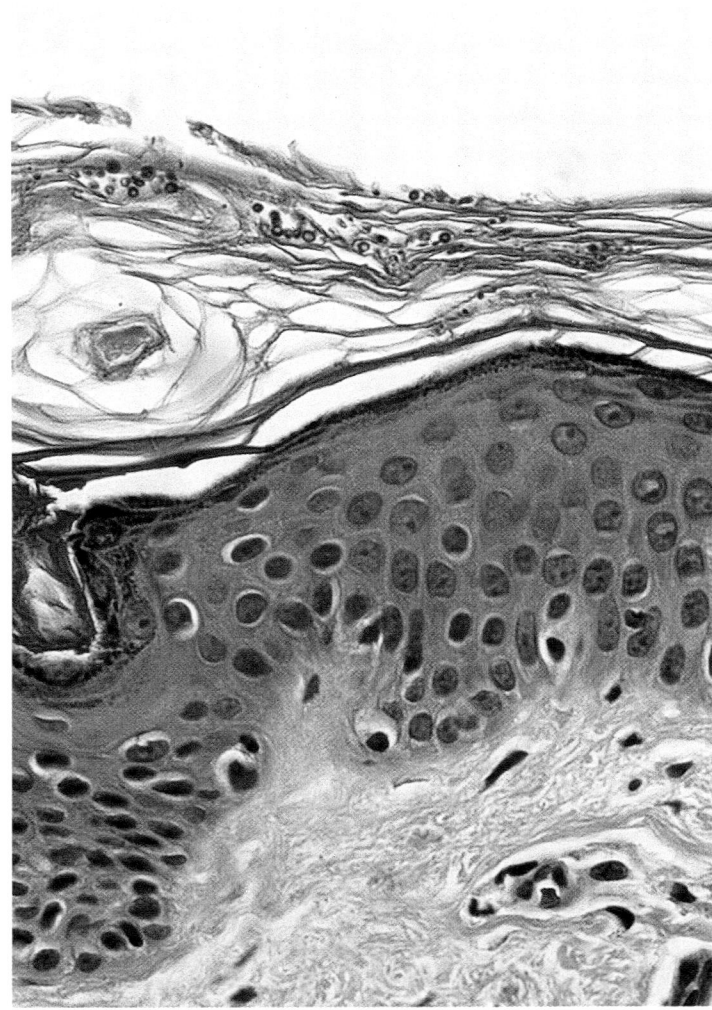

Fig. 25.9 **Pityriasis versicolor.** Numerous budding yeasts and short hyphae are present in the stratum corneum. (H & E)

Histopathology[278]

Involved follicles are dilated and often plugged with keratinous material and debris. There is a mild chronic inflammatory cell infiltrate around the infundibular portion of the follicle. Intrafollicular deposits of mucin are sometimes present.[279] If serial sections are examined disruption of the follicular epithelium is sometimes found, with basophilic granular debris, keratinous material, neutrophils and other inflammatory cells in the perifollicular dermis (Fig. 25.10).[278] A few foreign-body giant cells may also be present when rupture of the follicle has occurred. A PAS or silver methenamine stain will reveal spherical to oval yeast-like organisms, 2–4 μm in diameter. These are sometimes budding. They are found most often in the follicle, but following rupture they can also be found in the perifollicular inflammatory exudate.[280] Sometimes a few hyphae can also be seen.[266] Pseudoactinomycotic granules have been reported in two cases.[281]

TRICHOSPORONOSIS AND WHITE PIEDRA

The yeast *Trichosporon beigelii* (*T. cutaneum*) is a rare cause of a generalized blood-borne infection in immunosuppressed patients,[282] particularly those with leukemia or a lymphoma.[283,284] Trichosporonosis is frequently fatal in this clinical setting.[283] Cutaneous lesions occur in approximately 30% of patients

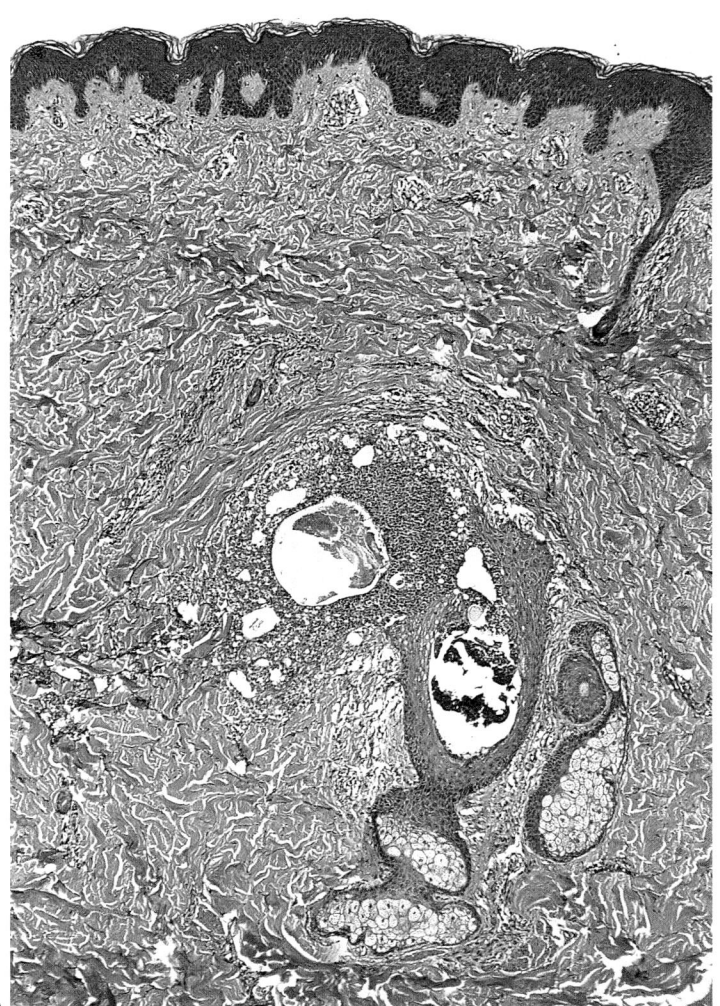

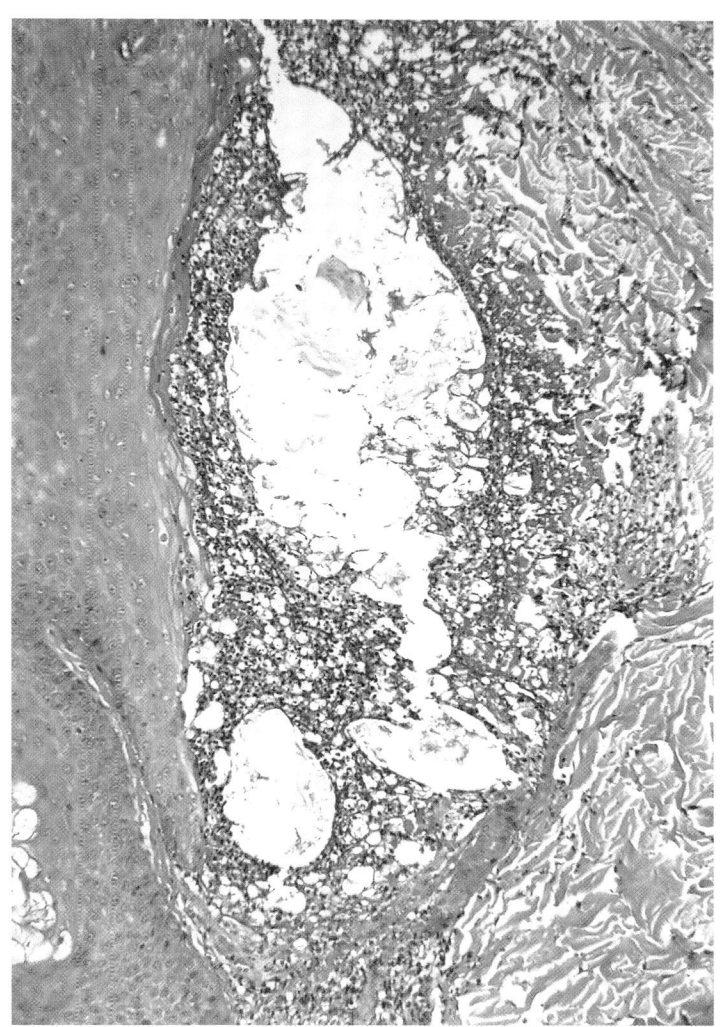

Fig. 25.10 **Pityrosporum folliculitis. (A)** Inflammatory cells and basophilic granular debris are present in the dermis adjacent to the point of rupture of the hair follicle. **(B)** The tiny yeasts are difficult to see at this magnification. (H & E)

with this infection; lesions take the form of purpuric papules and nodules with central necrosis or ulceration.[282] Isolated skin lesions and hand eczema are exceedingly rare.[285,286] *T. beigelii (cutaneum)* is a common cause of onychomycosis in some countries.[287]

A new classification for the genus Trichosporon has been proposed, *T. beigelii (cutaneum)* having been replaced by at least six species.[286] *T. ovoides* and *T. inkin* are the species now considered responsible for white piedra, a rare superficial infection of the hair resulting in white to tan-colored gritty nodules, just visible to the naked eye, along the hair shaft.[288,289] The scalp, face or pubic area may be involved. White piedra must be distinguished from black piedra, in which tightly adherent black nodules form on the hair, particularly on the scalp.[290] Black piedra is caused by infection with *Piedraia hortae*, which is not a yeast but an ascomycete. Piedra is discussed further in Chapter 15 (p. 470).

Histopathology

In fatal systemic infections numerous slender hyphae and budding yeasts can be seen in the deep dermis and in the walls of blood vessels.[283,291] The inflammatory response is usually poor because of the underlying neutropenia.[283]

In the localized cutaneous form, chronic inflammation with granuloma formation occurs in the mid and deep dermis, often with extension into the subcutis.[232,285] Numerous fungal elements can usually be seen on the PAS stain.

In white piedra, discrete nodules are found at intervals along the hair shaft. High-power light microscopy shows that the nodules consist of numerous spores. Scanning electron microscopy has shown hyphae perpendicular to the surface which are overlaid by budding arthrospores.[292] In black piedra, masses of brown hyphae with ovoid asci containing 2–8 single-celled ascospores are present along the hair shaft (see p. 470).[290]

SYSTEMIC MYCOSES

The term 'systemic mycoses' is used here to refer to infections caused by organisms in the following genera: *Blastomyces, Coccidioides, Paracoccidioides, Histoplasma* and *Cryptococcus*. In most cases the infection develops initially in the lungs; later, the skin and other organs may be involved. All these organisms except *Cryptococcus neoformans* are dimorphic, growing as mycelia in their natural state and assuming a yeast form in tissues. Cryptococcosis has already been considered with the infections caused by yeasts, and will not be considered further in this section. The dematiaceous fungi have also been excluded from this group.

NORTH AMERICAN BLASTOMYCOSIS

North American blastomycosis, caused by *Blastomyces dermatitidis*, occurs on the North American continent and in parts of Africa.[293,294] t has also been reported in India.[295] There are three clinical forms: pulmonary blastomycosis, disseminated blastomycosis and a primary cutaneous form that results from direct inoculation of organisms into the skin.[293,296,297] Most cutaneous lesions occur in the course of disseminated disease (secondary cutaneous blastomycosis); in this form the lesions may be restricted to the lungs, skin and subcutaneous tissue.[298] The rare primary inoculation form may be followed by lymphangitic lesions comparable to those of sporotrichosis.[293] The more usual lesion is a crusted verrucous nodule, sometimes with central healing and scarring, or an ulcerated plaque.[298] Multiple lesions are sometimes present. A widespread pustular eruption has been reported.[299] The disease is more frequent in adult males. It shows a predilection for exposed skin, particularly the face.

Histopathology[293]

An established verrucous lesion has many histological features in common with chromomycosis and sporotrichosis. There is pseudoepitheliomatous hyperplasia and a polymorphous dermal inflammatory cell infiltrate with scattered giant cells. Microabscesses are characteristic and occur in the dermis and in acanthotic downgrowths of the epidermis. Poorly formed granulomas and suppurative granulomas may be present.

The thick-walled yeasts measure 7–15 µm in diameter; they are found in the center of the abscesses and in some of the giant cells. A single bud is sometimes present on the surface of the organism. If organisms are difficult to find in hematoxylin and eosin-stained sections, a PAS or silver methenamine stain will usually demonstrate them.

The primary inoculation form shows less epidermal hyperplasia and a mixed dermal infiltrate containing numerous budding organisms. There are usually no giant cells or granulomas.

COCCIDIOIDOMYCOSIS

Infection with *Coccidioides immitis* is most frequently an acute self-limited pulmonary infection resulting from inhalation of dust-borne arthrospores.[300] The disease is endemic in the southwest of the USA, Mexico, and parts of Central and South America.[301] In less than 1% of cases, but particularly in immunocompromised patients,[302] dissemination of the infection occurs. The skin may be involved in disseminated disease, the cutaneous manifestations taking the form of a verrucous plaque, usually on the face,[303–305] or subcutaneous abscesses,[306] pustular lesions,[306] or rarely papules and plaques.[307,308] Primary cutaneous coccidioidomycosis is extremely rare and follows inoculation of the organisms at sites of minor trauma,[309] particularly in laboratory[310] or agricultural workers.[311] Rarely lymphangitic nodules develop, similar to those in sporotrichosis. Erythema nodosum occurs in up to 20% of patients with pulmonary infections, and erythema multiforme and a toxic erythema may also occur.[306] Hypercalcemia is a rare complication of systemic disease.[312]

DNA hybridization probe tests are now available commercially for the detection of coccidioidomycosis.[313]

Histopathology

Established lesions show non-caseating granulomas in the upper and mid dermis, with overlying pseudoepitheliomatous hyperplasia of the epidermis.[303] Thick-walled spherules of *C. immitis,* which usually range from 10 to 80 µm in diameter, are present within the granulomas, often in multinucleate giant cells.[304] Endospore (sporangiospore) formation is often seen in the largest spherules (sporangia).[304] The spherules can usually be seen without difficulty in hematoxylin and eosin-stained preparations. They are sometimes quite sparse.

Early lesions and subcutaneous abscesses show numerous neutrophils, with a variable admixture of lymphocytes, histiocytes and eosinophils.[311] Eosinophilic abscesses may form.[305] There are only occasional giant cells. Organisms are usually abundant in these lesions.

Collections of altered red blood cells can rarely mimic the appearances of an endosporulating fungus such as *C. immitis*. The term 'subcutaneous myospherulosis' has been applied to this artifact (see p. 445).[314]

PARACOCCIDIOIDOMYCOSIS

Paracoccidioidomycosis, also known as South American blastomycosis, is a systemic mycosis endemic in rural areas of Latin America.[315] It is caused by the dimorphic fungus *Paracoccidioides brasiliensis*.[316] The respiratory tract is the usual portal of entry, from where hematogenous dissemination to other parts of the body occurs.[317] Disseminated paracoccidioidomycosis with skin lesions has been reported in a patient with AIDS.[318] Transcutaneous (primary cutaneous) infection is less common.[319,320] Oral and mucosal involvement is frequently present in paracoccidioidomycosis, but cutaneous lesions are less common. There are usually several crusted ulcers when the skin is involved.[321] Over 90% of cases occur in males.[317] Terbinafine has been used successfully to treat the disease.[322]

Histopathology

Cutaneous lesions often show pseudoepitheliomatous hyperplasia overlying an acute and chronic inflammatory cell infiltrate in the dermis.[323] Granulomas are usually present and there may be foci of suppuration. The characteristic feature is the presence of small and large budding yeasts measuring 5–60 µm in diameter.[323] The buds are distributed on the surface in such a way as to give a 'steering wheel' appearance.[324] The organisms often have a thick wall with a double-contour appearance.[322] They can be found in macrophages and foreign-body giant cells and lying free in the tissues. They may be overlooked in hematoxylin and eosin-stained sections and are best seen with the Grocott silver methenamine stain.

HISTOPLASMOSIS

Histoplasmosis results from infection with *Histoplasma capsulatum*, a dimorphic soil fungus which is endemic in parts of America, Africa and Asia. The lung is the most usual primary focus of involvement, except in the African form (see below), and in 99% of cases the pulmonary infection is self-limited and asymptomatic.[325] Immunosuppression, including the acquired immunodeficiency syndrome,[326–335] old age and chronic disease states predispose to disseminated disease.[336–339] Cutaneous lesions occur in 5% or less of these patients.[325,337,340] This secondary cutaneous form presents as papules,[327] ulcerated nodules, cellulitis-like areas, acneiform lesions[328] or, rarely, as an erythroderma.[341] Erythema nodosum is an uncommon manifestation of histoplasmosis.[342] Rarely a cutaneous lesion is the only manifestation.[343] This primary cutaneous form usually presents as a solitary self-limited ulcerated nodule at the site of fungal inoculation.[344]

The African form of histoplasmosis usually presents with cutaneous granulomas or with skin lesions secondary to underlying osteomyelitis.[345,346] Disseminated disease can also occur. The causative organism, *H. capsulatum* var. *duboisii,* has much larger yeasts but is otherwise identical in laboratory characteristics to *H. capsulatum*.[345]

The laboratory diagnosis of histoplasmosis can be made by serological testing, positive cultures or histological visualization of organisms in affected tissue. The histoplasmin skin test is no longer considered useful because a positive reaction does not distinguish a current infection from a past one, and negative reactions often occur in disseminated disease.[337]

Histopathology

Usually there is a granulomatous infiltrate in the dermis, and sometimes the subcutis,[347,348] with numerous parasitized macrophages containing small ovoid yeast-like organisms, measuring $2–3 \times 3–5$ μm in diameter. There is often a surrounding clear halo. Langhans giant cells, lymphocytes and plasma cells are usually present, except in some acute disseminated cases in which parasitized macrophages predominate (Fig. 25.11). Extracellular organisms are sometimes found. Transepidermal elimination of macrophages has been reported. Healing lesions show progressive fibrosis. In patients with AIDS there may be only a sparse inflammatory cell infiltrate. Leukocytoclasis, dermal necrosis and cutaneous nerve parasitosis may be present in these cases.[332,349]

In the African form the organisms measure from 7 to 15 μm in diameter.[346] Suppuration is sometimes present,[345] but the characteristic tissue reaction is the formation of multinucleate giant cells of classic 'foreign-body' type, in the cytoplasm of which are usually 5–12 organisms.

Histoplasma must be distinguished from *Penicillium*, which also parasitizes macrophages. Whereas *Histoplasma* produces small surface buds, *Penicillium* divides by schizogony with the formation of septa within the organism.

Electron microscopy

The organism has a large eccentric nucleus, and a cell wall but no capsule.[346,350] The fungi are present in phagosomes in the cytoplasm of the macrophages.[350]

INFECTIONS BY DEMATIACEOUS FUNGI

The dematiaceous (pigmented) fungi are a clinically important group.[351] They are worldwide in distribution, although they are particularly prevalent in tropical and subtropical areas.[352] They are found in soil and decaying vegetable matter. The brown pigment of dematiaceous fungi is a melanin, which may be highlighted in tissue sections by the various stains for melanin.[353] They are capable of producing clinical diseases which range from a mild superficial cutaneous infection to life-threatening visceral disease.[354] Infection usually results from direct inoculation of infected material into the skin, but inhalation of organisms into the lungs may be the origin in some cases of systemic infection.

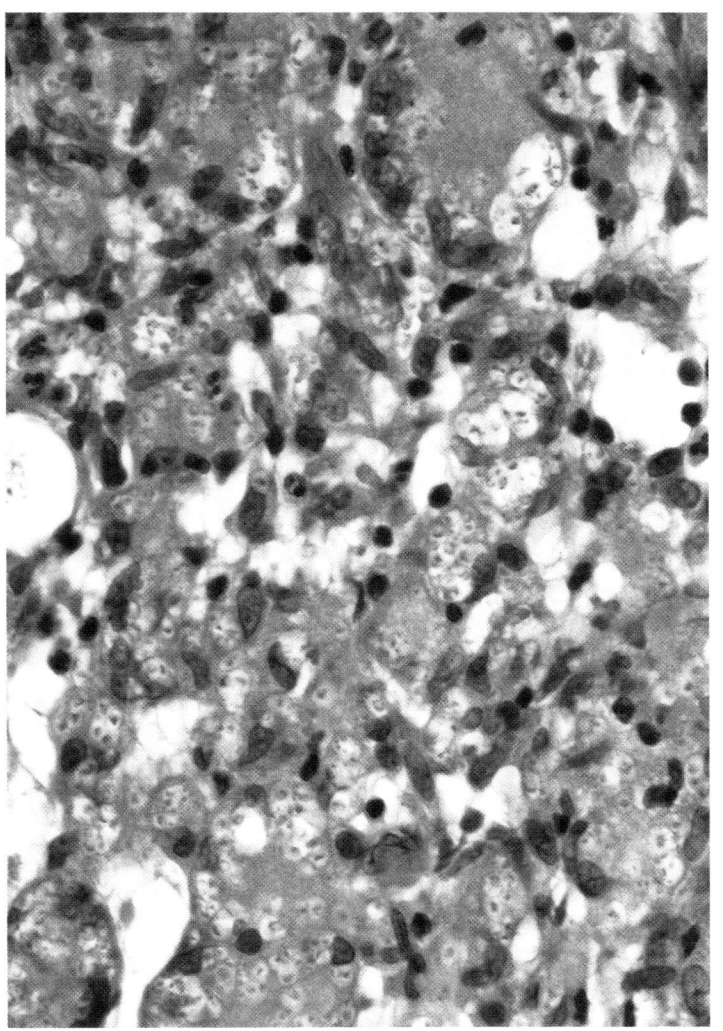
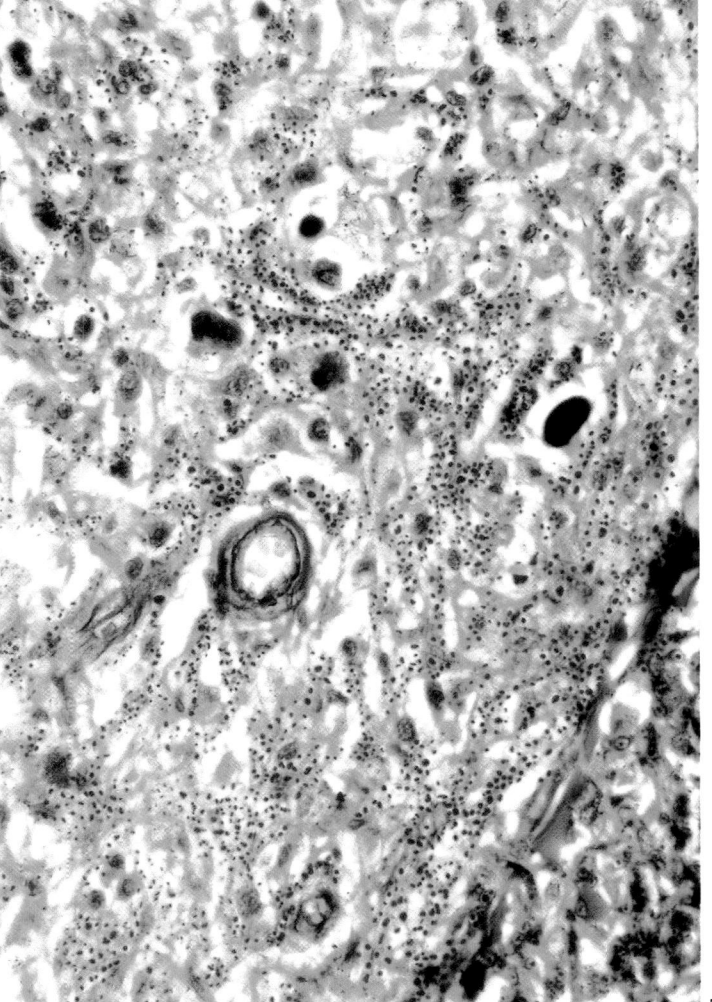

Fig. 25.11 **Histoplasmosis. (A)** There are parasitized macrophages and scant lymphocytes (H & E). **(B)** Numerous organisms can be seen in this silver preparation. (Grocott stain)

Various classifications have been proposed for the infections produced by dematiaceous fungi, with a proliferation of nomenclatures.[352,355,356] Some of the fungi have been reclassified several times in the past 20 years, resulting in taxonomic confusion. There are two clinicopathological groups, chromomycosis and phaeohyphomycosis,[356] which represent extremes of a continuum of infections.[357] Pigmented fungi may also produce mycetomas, which are tumefactive lesions with draining sinuses and the presence of grains in the tissue.[358] These cases are best considered with the mycetomas caused by other organisms (see p. 675).[356]

Chromomycosis is characterized by localized cutaneous infection and the presence in the tissues of thick-walled septate bodies (sclerotic bodies, muriform cells).[359] Phaeohyphomycosis[356,360] (phaeochromomycosis,[352] chromohyphomycosis[361]) is a collective term for a heterogeneous group of opportunistic infections that contain dematiaceous yeast-like cells and hyphae. These infections can be seen following direct implantation of infected material, or in immunosuppressed patients, in whom the portal of entry is not always evident.

CHROMOMYCOSIS

Chromomycosis (chromoblastomycosis) is a chronic fungal infection, usually localized to the distal parts of the extremities.[356,359,362,363] It starts as a scaly papule, often following superficial trauma, which slowly expands into a verrucous nodule or plaque.[364,365] In most series there has been a predilection for the lower legs, but in Australia the upper limbs are most often involved.[362] The face is rarely infected.[366] Also rare is dissemination with the formation of generalized cutaneous lesions,[367] lymphangitic nodules or hematogenous lesions.[354,359]

The six species that have been incriminated include *Fonsecaea pedrosoi*[368,369] (*Phialophora pedrosoi*), *Phialophora compacta* (*Fonsecaea compacta*),[370,371] *Phialophora verrucosa*, *Cladosporium carrionii*, *Aureobasidium pullulans*,[372] and rarely *Rhinocladiella aquaspersa* (*Acrotheca aquaspersa*).[354] Although sometimes cited as a cause,[352] *Wangiella dermatitidis* (*Phialophora dermatitidis*) is now no longer considered to be involved.[373] *F. pedrosoi* is the most commonly isolated organism, except in Australia, where *C. carrionii* is usually responsible.

Histopathology[356,359]

The appearances are similar to sporotrichosis, with hyperkeratosis, pseudoepitheliomatous hyperplasia and granulomas in the upper and mid dermis. The granulomas are mostly of tuberculoid type, although a few suppurative granulomas are usually present. Intraepidermal microabscesses are often present, but these are not as numerous as in sporotrichosis. There is a background infiltrate of chronic inflammatory cells, and sometimes a few eosinophils, in the upper dermis. Round, thick-walled, golden brown cells (sclerotic bodies, muriform cells, medlar bodies) 5–12 μm in diameter can be seen in giant cells and lying free in the intraepidermal microabscesses (Fig. 25.12).[374] These sclerotic bodies are thought to be an intermediate vegetative form, arrested between yeast and hyphal morphology.[356] They are usually seen readily in hematoxylin and eosin preparations, and particularly in sections stained with hematoxylin alone. Stains such as PAS and silver methenamine often obscure the natural pigmentation of the fungal cells, and this can result in misdiagnosis of the type of fungus. The fungal cells have a diversity of internal ultrastructure.[375,376] Hyphae have been reported in the stratum corneum in an otherwise typical case of chromomycosis.[377,378]

The pseudoepitheliomatous hyperplasia is probably the mechanism by which the transepithelial elimination of the fungal bodies and inflammatory

debris takes place.[379] There is progressive dermal fibrosis, and this is quite prominent in treated lesions.[380]

In sporotrichosis, foci of suppuration and suppurative granulomas are more obvious than in chromomycosis. Furthermore, the absence of organisms on a single hematoxylin and eosin section favors sporotrichosis as septate bodies are almost invariably found in a single section of chromomycosis.

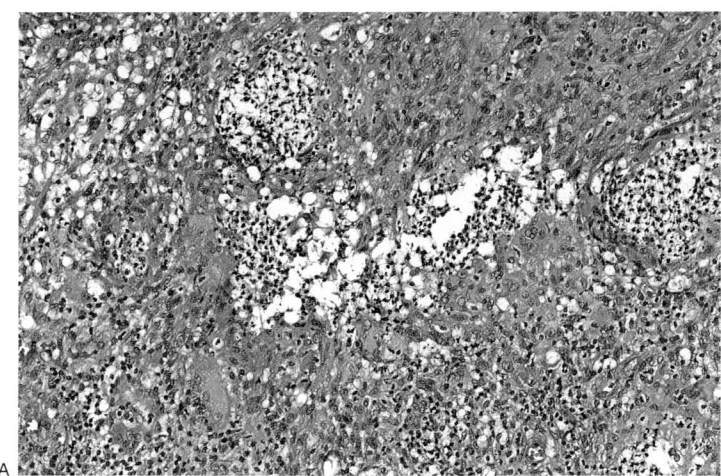

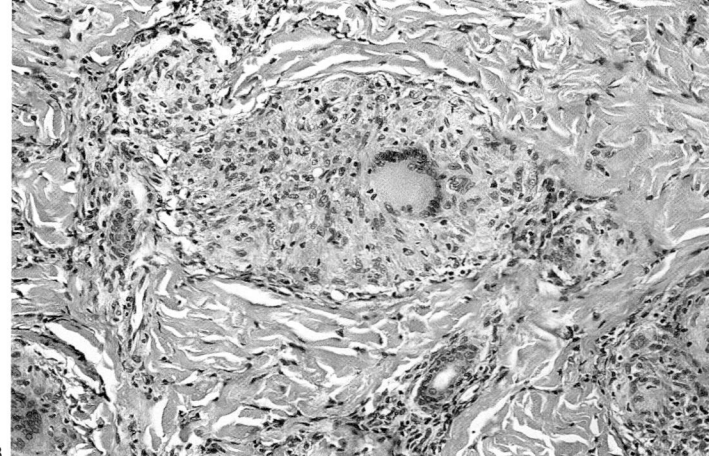

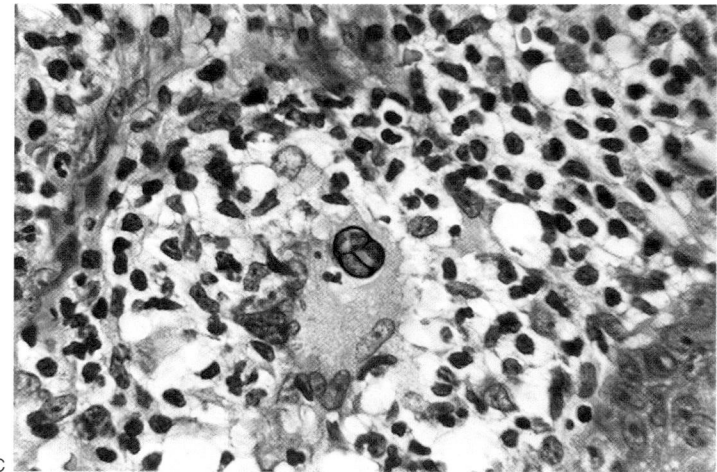

Fig. 25.12 **Chromomycosis. (A)** The granuloma is more suppurative than usual. **(B)** A septate body is present in the cytoplasm of a multinucleate giant cell. This granuloma is more typical. **(C)** High-power view of the septate body. (H & E)

Squamous cell carcinoma has been reported in extensive chromomycotic lesions of long standing.[381,382]

PHAEOHYPHOMYCOSIS

The term 'phaeohyphomycosis' is used for a diverse group of dematiaceous fungal infections[356,359] whose hallmark is the presence in tissues of pigmented hyphae. Four clinical categories are recognized: superficial (black piedra and tinea nigra), cutaneous or corneal, subcutaneous, and visceral (systemic).[356] Some overlap exists between the cutaneous and subcutaneous forms. Thirty-six different species of fungi were listed in one review article as being involved in the etiology of phaeohyphomycoses.[359] The most commonly isolated fungi in cutaneous and subcutaneous lesions are *Exophiala jeanselmei* (which some mycologists now consider to be identical with *Phialophora gougerotii*),[354,356,383–385] and *Wangiella dermatitidis*.[356] These fungi may also be isolated in the systemic forms involving the brain or other viscera. Cutaneous and/or subcutaneous lesions have also resulted from infection with *Exophiala spinifera*,[386] *E. dermatitidis*,[387] *Curvularia pallescens*,[388] *Hormonema dematioides*,[389] *Bipolaris spicifera*,[390,391] *Phoma* sp.,[392,393] *Geniculosporium* sp.,[394] *Cladophialophora bantiana*,[395,396] *Cladosporium cladosporioides*[397] and *Phialophora richardsiae*.[398] Other fungi involved in systemic infection include *Cladosporium trichoides*[352] and *Exserohilum* sp.[354,390,399–401] Patients with systemic infections are usually immunosuppressed.[390,399]

Cutaneous lesions may be nodular, cystic or verrucous.[402] They are usually solitary. Some patients are immunocompromised;[403–405] in others, the lesion follows a penetrating injury with implantation of a wood splinter or other vegetable matter.[406] The most common lesion is a subcutaneous cyst on the distal parts of the extremities.

Histopathology[406–409]

The characteristic lesion is a circumscribed cyst or chronic abscess situated in the subcutis or lower dermis (Fig. 25.13).[410] The wall is composed of dense fibrous tissue with a chronic granulomatous reaction adjacent to the cavity. The wall also contains chronic inflammatory cells and scattered giant cells. There is a central cystic space containing necrotic debris with some admixed neutrophils. A wood splinter or similar foreign body is sometimes present. Brown filamentous hyphae and yeast-like structures may be present in the wall, in giant cells, or in the debris. Sometimes the fungal elements can be seen in relation to the implanted foreign material.[411,412]

In some cases the lesions resemble those of cutaneous chromomycosis.[355] They may present simply as ulcerated, partly necrotic granulomas containing the characteristic pigmented hyphae.[413]

SPOROTRICHOSIS

Sporotrichosis is an uncommon fungal infection of worldwide distribution, caused by the dimorphic fungus *Sporothrix schenckii*.[414] Infection usually results from percutaneous implantation of infected vegetable matter, particularly wood splinters, or from injury by rose thorns or contamination of even minor skin wounds by infected hay and sphagnum moss.[415–417] Infection has also been acquired from animals[418,419] and in the laboratory.

There are two major cutaneous forms of sporotrichosis. The lymphangitic form (lymphocutaneous or sporotrichoid form) begins as a single nodule or ulcer and is followed by the development of subcutaneous nodules along the course of the local lymphatics. The initial and secondary nodules may ulcerate. This type accounts for 75% or more of all cases of sporotrichosis in many reports, but it is much less common in Australia and South Africa.[416,420–422]

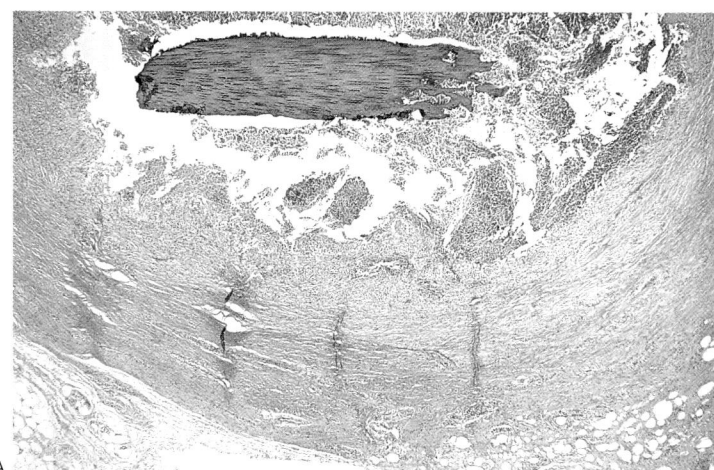

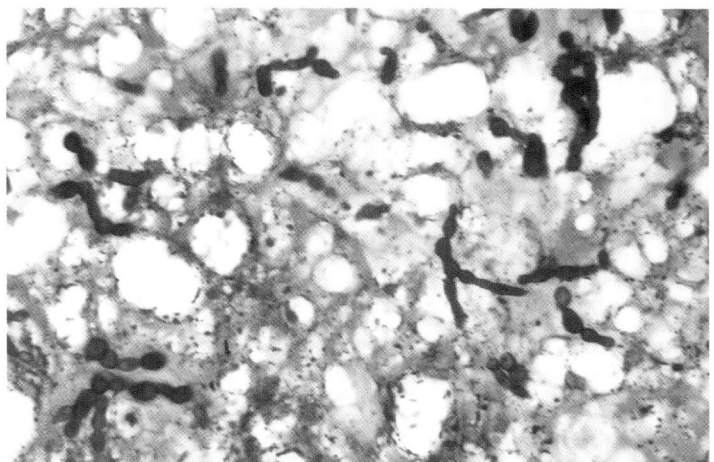

Fig. 25.13 **Phaeohyphomycosis. (A)** A small wood splinter is present in the 'cyst' (H & E). **(B)** The fungal elements are present in the inflammatory lining of the cavity. (PAS–tartrazine)

The localized form (fixed form) presents as an ulcerated nodule or verrucous plaque which measures 1–5 cm or more in diameter.[423,424] It has been suggested that this form is more likely to develop in patients previously sensitized to *Sporothrix schenckii*, but this does not explain why lesions in children,[425–428] and those on the face,[429,430] are often of this type. The temperature sensitivity of the particular strain of organism involved has also been suggested as influencing the clinical type of lesion.[431] The upper limbs are the most common site of involvement in both types of sporotrichosis. Spontaneous disappearance of lesions[432] and exogenous second infections[433] have also been documented.

Rarely, cutaneous lesions are erysipeloid[434] or generalized, the latter form usually occurring in association with visceral involvement.[435–437] Such lesions may clinically mimic pyoderma gangrenosum.[438] Visceral involvement may also occur without associated skin lesions.[439] The lungs, bones, joints and meninges are favored sites of extracutaneous involvement.[439–441] Disturbances in cell-mediated immunity (including AIDS),[442,443] cancer[440] and sarcoidosis[444] have been present in some patients with disseminated sporotrichosis.[445] Coinfection with leishmaniasis has been reported.[446]

Histopathology[420,447]

In the localized form there is usually prominent pseudoepitheliomatous hyperplasia with some overlying hyperkeratosis and focal parakeratosis (Fig. 25.14). Several types of granulomas are found within the dermis, including tuber-

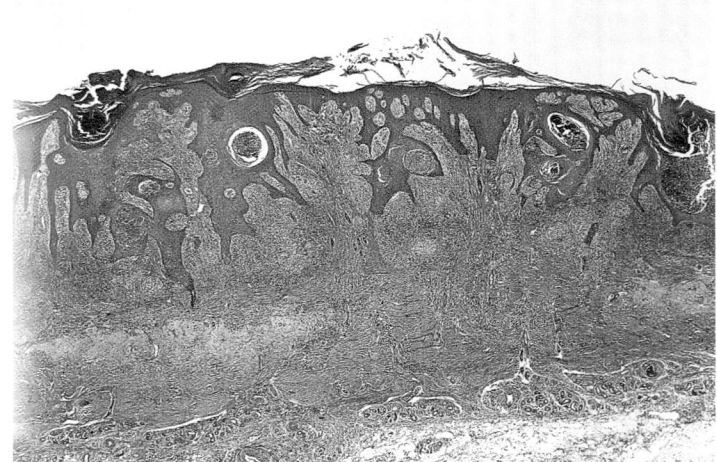

Fig. 25.14 **Sporotrichosis.** This localized lesion is characterized by pseudoepitheliomatous hyperplasia of the epidermis and suppurative granulomas in the upper dermis. (H & E)

culoid, histiocytic and suppurative granulomas. Multinucleate giant cells may be present at the periphery of the granulomas, and some of these are of foreign-body type. Intraepidermal microabscesses are not uncommon.

In the lymphangitic form the inflammatory nodules are situated in the lower dermis and there are usually no epidermal changes. There is often a more diffuse inflammatory infiltrate, and the granulomas are mostly of the suppurative type. Coalescence of abscesses may occur.

The traditional view has always been that fungal elements are infrequently demonstrated in human cases of sporotrichosis. In our study of 39 cases, only 2 of which were of lymphangitic type, fungal elements were found in all cases. This was achieved by examining multiple serial sections, some stained with hematoxylin and eosin and others with PAS.[447]

The sporothrix may be present in the tissues as yeast-like forms 2–8 μm in diameter, or as elongated cells ('cigar bodies') 2–4 × 4–10 μm, or as hyphae.[448] Hyphae are particularly rare.[448,449] A characteristic finding is the 'sporothrix asteroid': this is a yeast form (blastospore) surrounded by an intensely eosinophilic, hyaline material, ray-like processes of which extend for a short distance from the core (Fig. 25.15). The hyaline material stains faintly with PAS. This material represents deposits of immune complexes on the surface

of the fungal cell. The central yeast stains with anti-*Sporothrix* antibodies but the surrounding eosinophilic, ray-like processes do not.[450] Asteroids are found only in the center of suppurative granulomas and suppurative foci. In our experience each such focus will contain an asteroid, if examined by serial sections.[447] Spores can usually be demonstrated using a silver methenamine or PAS stain. Prior digestion with malt diastase has been suggested as a method to enhance recognition of spores in PAS preparations.[451] Numerous spores are sometimes present,[452] particularly if the lesion has been injected with steroids because of a mistaken clinical diagnosis (Fig. 25.16).[453]

TINEA NIGRA

Tinea nigra is a rare asymptomatic mycosis of the stratum corneum caused by *Exophiala (Phaeoannellomyces) werneckii*.[454,455] It presents as a slowly enlarging, brown to black macule, or large patch, involving the palms[456–458] or palmar surfaces of the fingers,[459] and less commonly the plantar[460,461] or lateral surfaces of the feet.[462] Lesions are sometimes bilateral.[460] Tinea nigra is more common in tropical areas. Clinically, it may mimic various melanocytic lesions.[462]

Histopathology[462]
The stratum corneum may be slightly more compact than usual. Numerous brown hyphae are present in its superficial layers and are easily seen in hematoxylin and eosin-stained sections. Spores may also be shown by the PAS stain. There is usually no inflammatory reaction (Fig. 25.17).

ALTERNARIOSIS

Members of the genus *Alternaria* are plant pathogens. They are a rare cause of infection in humans, affecting both healthy and, more usually, immunodeficient individuals.[463–468] The usual species, *A. alternata*, produces chronic crusted nodules, pustules or ulcers localized to an exposed area such as the face, forearms, hands and knees.[469–473] Sometimes, large ulcerated plaques intermingled with pustules form.[474,475] Subcutaneous nodules on the chest in association with *A. dianthicola*[463] and a nodule on the nasal septum caused by *A. chartarum*[476] have been reported. *A. chlamydospora* is another extremely rare human pathogen.[477] The rationale for including this group with the

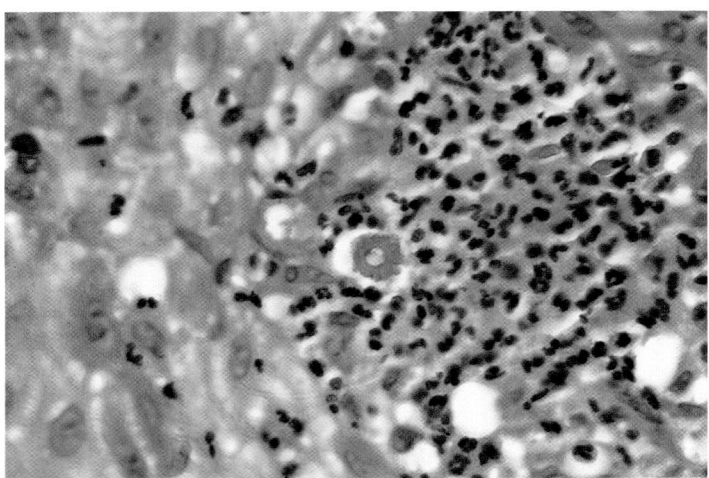

Fig. 25.15 **Sporotrichosis.** A *Sporothrix* asteroid is present at the center of a suppurative granuloma. (H & E)

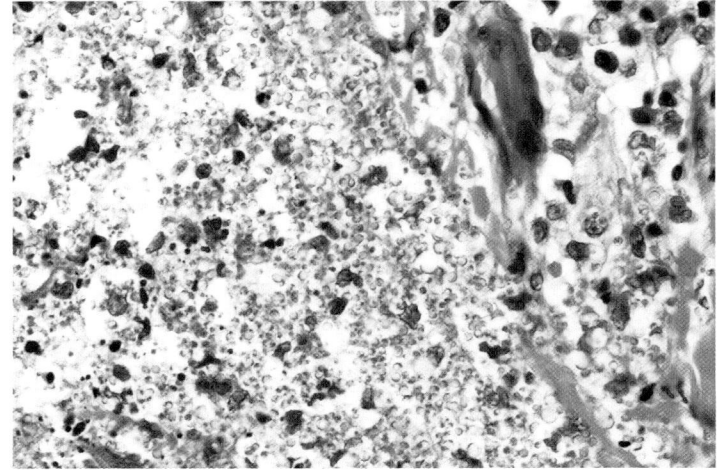

Fig. 25.16 **Sporotrichosis.** Numerous fungal elements are present. This lesion was injected with corticosteroids because of a mistaken clinical diagnosis of granuloma annulare. (H & E)

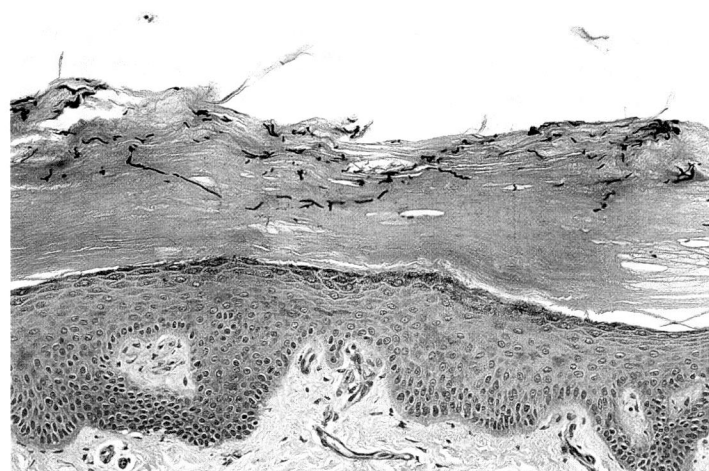

Fig. 25.17 **Tinea nigra.** Numerous hyphae are present in the superficial layers of the compact stratum corneum. (PAS stain)

dematiaceous fungi, in the absence of pigmented tissue elements, is the formation of gray to black colonies on culture.

Histopathology[469,478]

Usually there are non-caseating granulomas and chronic inflammation in the dermis, often with a few microabscesses. Sometimes the microabscesses are prominent.[479] Epidermal involvement may accompany the dermal inflammation, or occur as the only manifestation. It is characterized by intraepidermal abscesses and often a thick scale crust containing neutrophils. Septate hyphae and spores can be seen in the dermis and epidermis.[480]

The organisms often show degenerative changes on electron microscopic examination.[481]

MYCETOMA AND MORPHOLOGICALLY SIMILAR CONDITIONS

On a strict etiological basis, only the eumycetic mycetomas (mycetomas caused by true fungi) should be included in this chapter. As will be seen from the discussions that follow, a similar tissue reaction can be produced by filamentous bacteria of the order Actinomycetales (actinomycetic mycetoma) and certain other bacteria (botryomycosis). This is the rationale for the inclusion here of actinomycosis, nocardiosis and botryomycosis.

MYCETOMA

Mycetoma is an uncommon chronic infective disease of the skin and subcutaneous tissues, characterized by the triad of tumefaction, draining sinuses and the presence in the exudate of colonial grains.[482–485] The sinuses do not develop until relatively late in the course of the disease, discharging grains which are aggregates of the causal organism embedded in a matrix substance.[486,487] There are two main etiological groups of mycetoma: actinomycetic mycetomas, which are caused by aerobic filamentous bacteria of the order Actinomycetales, and eumycetic (maduromycotic) mycetomas caused by a number of species of true fungi.[488,489] The therapy of these two groups is quite different.[490] Similar clinical lesions can be produced by traditional bacteria (botryomycosis), and rarely by dermatophytes.[483,491,492]

Mycetoma is predominantly a disease of tropical countries, particularly West Africa, parts of India, and Central and South America.[493] There are only sporadic reports of cases in the USA,[494] Canada, Europe (including the United Kingdom)[495] and Australia.[496] Different species predominate in different countries.[493–497] Rural workers, particularly males, are most commonly infected. Over 70% of infections occur on the feet (Madura foot), with the hand the next most common site of involvement.

Repeated minor trauma or penetrating injury provides a portal of entry for the organism, which then produces a slowly progressive subcutaneous nodule after an incubation period of several weeks or months.[493] Sinuses develop after 6–12 months. Extension to involve the underlying fascia, muscle and bone is common. Rarely there is lymphatic dissemination to regional lymph nodes.[487] No unequivocal cases of visceral dissemination have been reported. Actinomycetic mycetomas often expand faster, are more invasive, and have more sinuses than eumycetic variants.[493]

Macroscopic features of the grains

The grains discharged from the sinuses vary in size, color and consistency, features that can be used for rapid provisional identification of the etiological agent.[493] Over 30 species have been identified as causes of mycetoma, and the grains of many of these have overlapping morphological features. Accordingly, culture is required for accurate identification of the causal agent.

The size of the grains varies from microscopic to 1–2 mm in diameter. Large grains are seen with madurellae (particularly *Madurella mycetomatosis*) and with *Actinomadura madurae* and *A. pelletieri*, whereas the granules of *Nocardia brasiliensis*, *N. cavae* and *N. asteroides* are small.

The colors of the grains of the most common species are shown in Table 25.1. Dark (black) grain mycetomas are found only among the eumycetic mycetomas.[498] The pigment is a melanoprotein or related substance.[499] The consistency of most grains is soft, but those of *Streptomyces somaliensis* and *Madurella mycetomatis* can be quite hard.[487]

Histopathology[482,487]

The characteristic grains are found in the center of zones of suppuration and in suppurative granulomas in the subcutis (Fig. 25.18). Neutrophils sometimes invade the grains. Surrounding the areas of suppuration there may be a palisade of histiocytes, beyond which is a mixed inflammatory infiltrate and progressive fibrosis. A few multinucleate giant cells are usually present. An eosinophilic fringe, resembling the Splendore–Hoeppli phenomenon found around some parasites, is sometimes present around the grains.

Several reviews have discussed the morphology of the grains on light microscopy.[487,493] Some of these features are highlighted in Table 25.2.[500–502]

Table 25.1 **Color of the grains (granules) in mycetomas**

Eumycetomas

Black grains: *Madurella mycetomatis, M. grisea, Leptosphaeria senegalensis, Exophiala jeanselmei, Pyrenochaeta romeroi, Curvularia lunata, Phialophora verrucosa, P. parasitica*

Pale grains: *Petriellidium boydii, Aspergillus nidulans, A. flavus, Fusarium sp., Acremonium sp., Neotestudina rosatii*, dermatophytes

Actinomycetomas

Red grains: *Actinomadura pelletieri*

Yellow grains: *Streptomyces somaliensis*

Pale grains: *Nocardia brasiliensis, N. cavae, N. asteroides, Actinomadura madurae*

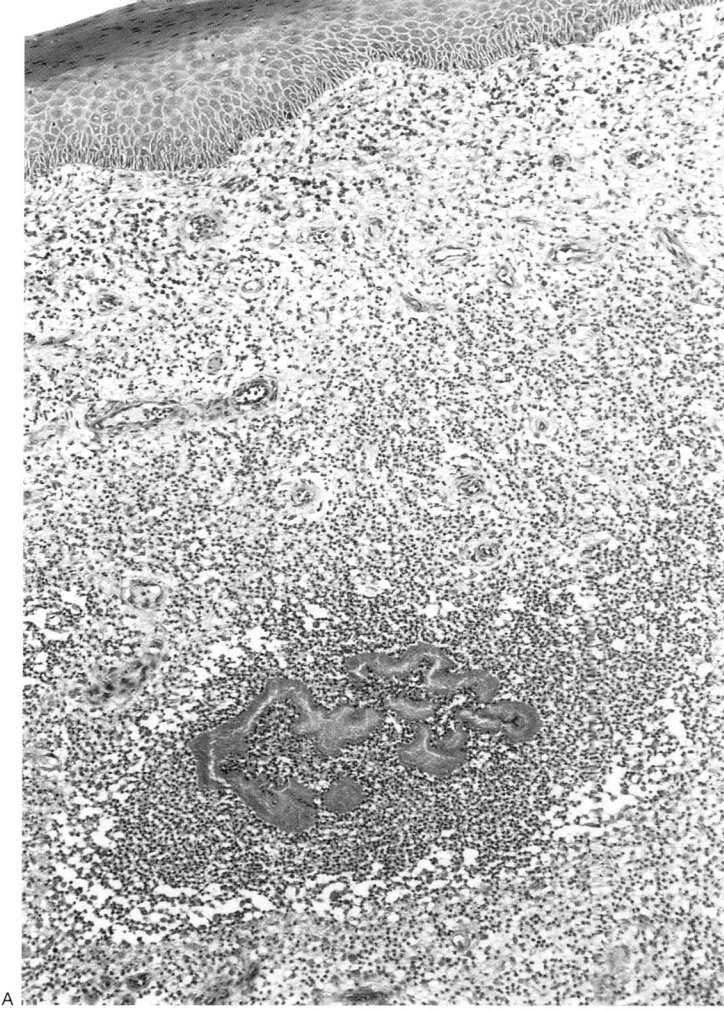

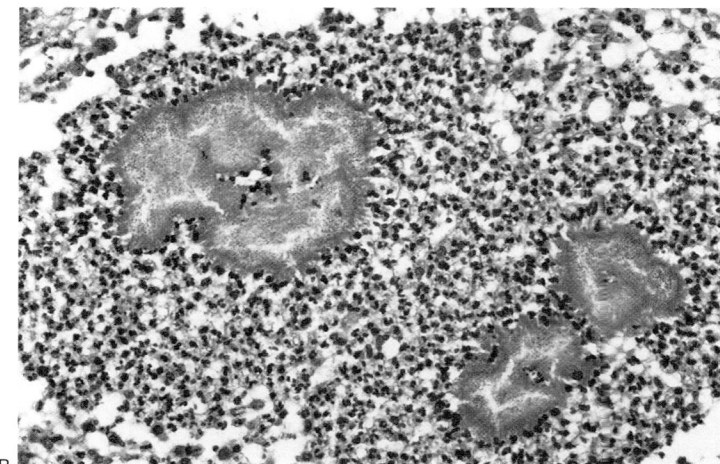

Fig. 25.18 **(A) Mycetoma. (B)** An irregularly-shaped grain is present in the center of a zone of suppuration. (H & E)

It should be noted that the granules in pale-grain eumycetomas are not morphologically distinctive and there is overlap between the various species.

The large segmented mycelial filaments (2–4 μm in diameter, with club-shaped hyphal swellings and chlamydospores) which characterize the fungi that cause eumycetomas (Fig. 25.19) contrast with the Gram-positive

Table 25.2 **Morphology of the grains (granules) in mycetomas**

Eumycetomas

Madurella mycetomatis: Large granules (up to 5 mm or more) with interlacing hyphae embedded in interstitial brownish matrix; hyphae at periphery arranged radially with numerous chlamydospores

Petriellidium boydii: Eosinophilic, lighter in the center; numerous vesicles or swollen hyphae; peripheral eosinophilic fringe; other pale eumycetomas have a minimal fringe and contain a dense mass of intermeshing hyphae

Actinomycetomas

Actinomadura madurae: Large (1–5 mm and larger) and multilobulate; peripheral basophilia and central eosinophilia or pale staining; filaments grow from the peripheral zone

Streptomyces somaliensis: Large (0.5–2 mm or more) with dense thin filaments; often stains homogeneously; transverse fracture lines

Nocardia brasiliensis: Small grains (approximately 1 mm); central purple zone; loose clumps of filaments; Gram-positive delicate branching filaments breaking up into bacillary and coccal forms; Gram-negative amorphous matrix (Brown and Benn method)

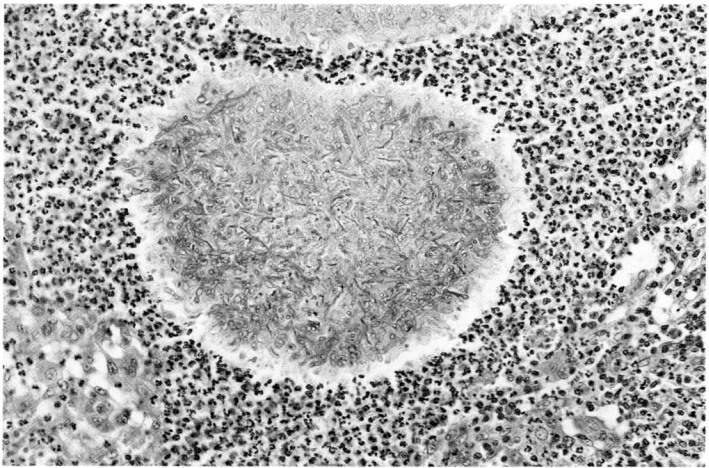

Fig. 25.19 **Eumycetoma.** The fungal elements comprising this grain are easily seen. (PAS stain)

thin filaments (1 μm or less in diameter) of the organisms that cause actinomycetomas.[482,496]

NOCARDIOSIS

Nocardiae are usually Gram-positive, partially acid-fast bacteria which are native to soil and decaying vegetable matter.[503] The common pathogenic species are *N. asteroides*,[504] *N. brasiliensis*[505,506] and *N. caviae*.[507,508] *N. farcinica*, now acknowledged to be a species distinct from *N. asteroides*, can produce severe systemic infections with subcutaneous abscesses. It is resistant to antibiotics.[509] Other species are rarely implicated.[510,511] The majority of cases of nocardiosis are septicemic infections, usually of pulmonary origin, in immunocompromised patients.[504,512] Cutaneous lesions develop in approximately 10% or more of hematogenous infections.[513,514] Primary cutaneous involvement can be of three different types: mycetoma, lymphocutaneous infection and superficial cutaneous infections, which may take the form of an abscess, an ulcer or cellulitis.[506,515–520] The lymphocutaneous (sporotrichoid,[521] chancriform) infection,[522] which includes a cervicofacial variant in children,[523] resembles sporotrichosis in having subcutaneous nodules along the course of the superficial lymphatics.[515,524,525] A history of trauma is often present in primary cutaneous lesions.[504,525–528]

Whereas *N. asteroides* is responsible for most pulmonary, cerebral and septicemic infections, *N. brasiliensis* is the most common nocardial pathogen in the skin.[503,529,530] There have been many exceptions to this generalization.[518,531–535] Both species of *Nocardia* have been isolated from a mycetoma on the forehead,[536] and both *N. asteroides* and *Sporothrix schenkii* have been isolated from a mycetoma of the forefoot.[537]

Histopathology

There is usually a dense infiltrate of neutrophils in the deep dermis and subcutis, with frank abscess formation.[538] In chronic lesions there is a thin fibrous capsule and many chronic inflammatory cells. Necrosis, hemorrhage and ulceration may all be present at times.[532]

The organisms are not readily visible in hematoxylin and eosin-stained sections. Special stains show them to be fine, branched filaments that are Gram positive, usually weakly acid fast, and which stain with the silver methenamine method.[539] Colonial grains are uncommon in cutaneous lesions other than mycetomas.[540]

ACTINOMYCOSIS

Actinomycosis is a chronic, sometimes fatal, infection that may involve any part of the body.[541–544] Its cutaneous manifestations include fluctuant swellings, which may progress to draining sinuses in the cervicofacial, thoracic or abdominal region.[545] In the latter site there is often underlying visceral involvement, or a history of previous surgery in the region. Multiple subcutaneous abscesses may result from hematogenous dissemination of a visceral infection.[546]

The causal organism is *Actinomyces israelii*, a filamentous bacterium which is isolated with difficulty by anerobic culture. It forms tiny, soft granules that may be detected in the pus ('sulfur granules'). *A. israelii* is a normal inhabitant of the oral cavity. Similar lesions can be caused by other actinomycetes, including species of *Streptomyces* and *Actinomadura*.[547,548]

Histopathology[541]

The usual cutaneous lesion is a subcutaneous abscess. There are often several locules, which are separated by areas of granulation tissue in which foamy macrophages are present.[541] There is an outer zone of granulation and fibrous tissue at the periphery of the abscess cavities, and this contains lymphocytes, plasma cells and some macrophages.

One or more colonial granules are present in the pus. These average about 300 μm in diameter, but may range up to 1–2 mm.[541] At the periphery of the granules, club-shaped bodies radiate in parallel fashion from the border. The clubs and matrix of the granules are Gram negative. The granules are composed of numerous slender beaded filaments that tend to be crowded at the periphery of the granules.[541] They are Gram positive but not acid fast.[549] They are usually PAS positive and stain gray or black with the silver methenamine stain. Free organisms are infrequently seen.

BOTRYOMYCOSIS

Botryomycosis (bacterial pseudomycosis) is an uncommon chronic bacterial infection of the skin or viscera in which small whitish granules composed of the causal bacteria are present in areas of suppuration.[550–552] In the skin they are often discharged through draining sinuses. As the lesions closely mimic clinically and histologically those of mycetoma, botryomycosis is included in this chapter.[553]

The cutaneous lesion is usually a large swollen tumor or plaque with nodular areas or ulcers, and discharging sinuses.[554–556] The hands, feet and head, and the inguinal and gluteal regions are most commonly involved.[557,558] Multiple cutaneous lesions in different parts of the body have been described.[559,560] Botryomycosis has sometimes been reported in patients with diabetes,[560] or with various abnormalities of the immune system,[557] including AIDS.[559,561] It has been documented in a patient with extensive follicular mucinosis,[562] and at the site of localized corticosteroid injections.[563]

Gram-positive organisms, particularly *Staphylococcus aureus*, are usually involved, but Gram-negative organisms, including *Actinobacillus lignieresi* and *Pseudomonas aeruginosa*,[564] have also been incriminated.[550,565] A mixed growth of organisms is rarely present.

Histopathology[550]

The lesion resembles mycetoma, with a small granule present in the center of a suppurative zone. The granules are basophilic, usually with a surrounding eosinophilic zone which is PAS positive.[550] The bacteria can be identified by a Gram stain. In contrast to mycetoma, there are no filaments present.[553] Transepidermal elimination of the granules has been reported.[566]

The matrix of the granules contains IgG and sometimes C3 complement.[559,567]

ZYGOMYCOSES

There is an increasing tendency to use the broader term 'zygomycoses', which covers infections caused by all fungi belonging to the class Zygomycetes,[568–571] rather than the older term 'mucormycosis (phycomycosis)', which is restricted to infections caused by various species in one family of the order Mucorales. However, as the infections caused by fungi within the order Entomophthorales, which is the other major group of Zygomycetes, are clinically quite different from mucormycosis, the two groups of infections will be considered separately.[572]

MUCORMYCOSIS

Mucormycosis refers to opportunistic infections by fungi within the family Mucoraceae, one of the many families in the order Mucorales.[573] There are three important genera responsible for human infections: *Rhizopus*, *Mucor* and *Absidia*. These fungi are widespread in nature, particularly in soil and decaying vegetable matter.[573] Several clinical categories of mucormycosis have been delineated: rhinocerebral, pulmonary, disseminated (hematogenous), gastrointestinal and cutaneous.[574] The cutaneous lesions may be further divided into primary and secondary types.

Primary cutaneous mucormycosis is rare and usually develops in diabetics, in patients with thermal burns and sometimes in those who are immunocompromised.[569,575–577] Lesions resulting from contaminated adhesive dressings were reported in the past.[578,579] Visceral dissemination may follow a primary lesion in the skin.[580–583]

Secondary cutaneous mucormycosis results from hematogenous seeding from a lesion elsewhere in the body.[584] Such patients may have underlying diabetes, leukemia, lymphoma, neutropenia, or be immunocompromised in some other way.[584,585] Premature infants and renal transplant recipients may be at risk.[586,587]

Cutaneous mucormycosis may present as a tender indurated large plaque with a dusky center, as an area of necrotizing cellulitis,[572] as an area of necrosis in a thermal burn, or as a lesion resembling ecthyma gangrenosum.[574,588] In one instance a large ulcer developed in a tattoo;[563] another report has documented involvement of the skin around the site of an intravenous catheter insertion.[589] Infection has also occurred at the site of an insect bite.[590]

Histopathology[591]

The appearances are quite variable. There may be suppuration or areas of necrosis. There may be a resemblance to superficial granulomatous pyoderma, although the presence of fungal elements assists in making a distinction.[592] Sometimes there is only a minimal inflammatory response. Hyphae often invade vessel walls, with subsequent thrombosis and infarction.[584,588] Subcutaneous granulomas have been reported with some species of *Absidia*.

The hyphae are broad and usually non-septate. They branch at right angles, in contrast to *Aspergillus*, which usually branches at an acute angle.[572] Sometimes the hyphae appear collapsed and twisted. They are often clearly seen in hematoxylin and eosin-stained sections.

SUBCUTANEOUS PHYCOMYCOSIS

Subcutaneous phycomycosis is the established, yet somewhat unsatisfactory, designation for infections caused by fungi of the order Entomophthorales.[593] Two genera, *Basidiobolus* and *Conidiobolus* (*Entomophthora*), are usually implicated in the infections, which typically are solitary and involve the subcutis of healthy individuals.[594–596] Spontaneous resolution of the lesions sometimes occurs. These infections have been mainly reported from Africa and southeast Asia.[597]

Phycomycoses have also been reported in animals, particularly horses ('swamp cancer').[598] In addition to fungi from this order, aquatic fungi (particularly *Pythium* sp.) from a totally unrelated 'class' have been incriminated in equine phycomycosis.[599] They are mentioned here because the author has seen two cases of a periorbital cellulitis in humans who had contact with horses, which were probably the source of these equine fungi.[600]

Histopathology[601–607]

There is granulomatous inflammation in the dermis and subcutis, with scattered abscesses and sometimes areas of necrosis.[602] The most striking feature is the presence of smudgy eosinophilic material surrounding the hyphae.[602,603] This resembles the Splendore–Hoeppli phenomenon seen in relation to certain metazoan parasites.[604,605] Eosinophils are also present in the inflammatory infiltrate.[606]

In the author's human cases of equine phycomycosis, foci resembling the flame figures of eosinophilic cellulitis were present (Fig. 25.20). The fungi were not visualized on hematoxylin and eosin or PAS preparations, but only with the silver methenamine stain.[600]

HYALOHYPHOMYCOSES

The term 'hyalohyphomycoses' has been applied to a heterogeneous group of opportunistic infections in which the pathogenic fungi grow in tissue in the form of hyphal elements that are unpigmented, septate and branched or unbranched.[356,608] Dematiaceous fungi are excluded. Examples of hyalo-hyphomycoses include infections caused by *Schizophyllum commune* and species of *Acremonium*,[609] *Pseudallescheria*,[610] *Paecilomyces*,[611–617] *Fusarium*,[618–626] *Penicillium*[627–630] and *Scedosporium*.[631–636] Infections caused by species of *Aspergillus* can also be accommodated in this group. Species of *Fusarium* have

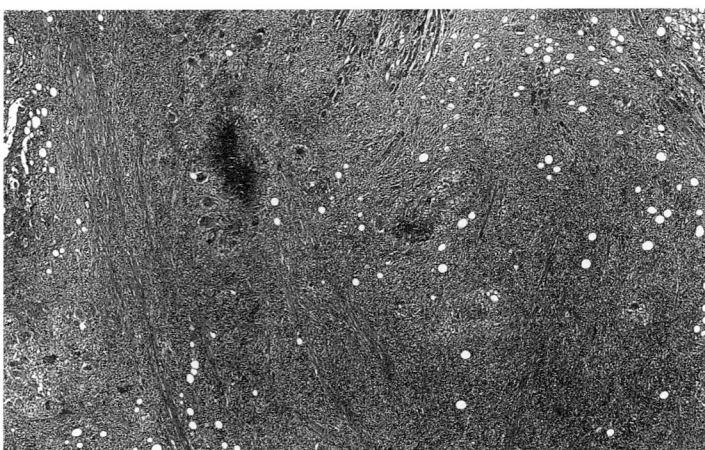

Fig. 25.20 **Equine phycomycosis in a human.** Multinucleate giant cells surround zones of necrosis. There are numerous eosinophils in the infiltrate. (H & E)

been associated with disseminated infection,[637,638] ecthyma gangrenosum-like lesions,[620] vasculitic lesions,[639] a lupus vulgaris-like lesion[626] and a facial granuloma.[640] Predisposing immunological disturbances are almost invariably present in individuals with these infections.[636] A contaminated skin lotion was the source of infection in one case.[612] Trauma is sometimes implicated,[623] but usually the precipitating factor is unknown.

ASPERGILLOSIS

Aspergillosis is an opportunistic infection second only to candidosis in frequency among patients with cancer.[641] It usually involves the lungs, and only rarely the skin.[642,643] Cutaneous lesions are usually part of a systemic infection in immunocompromised patients, although rarely they may be the only manifestation (primary cutaneous aspergillosis).[184,589,642,644–652] Many patients with primary cutaneous aspergillosis have leukemia, and lesions have developed at the sites of intravenous cannulae or of the associated dressings.[653–658] There are one or more violaceous plaques or nodules that rapidly progress to necrotic ulcers with a black eschar.[654,659,660] Plaques studded with pustules are sometimes seen.[648] *Aspergillus flavus* is the most common isolate;[653,661] *A. fumigatus*, *A. ustus*[662] and *A. niger* have also been responsible.[654,663] Rarely, burns or pyoderma gangrenosum are secondarily infected with *Aspergillus* species.[664,665]

Histopathology

Depending on the host response, there can be a variety of changes ranging from well-developed granulomas[644] to areas of suppuration and abscess formation,[655] or the presence of masses of fungi with a minimal mixed inflammatory cell response.[642] *Aspergillus* species are found as septate hyphae that branch dichotomously. They are best shown by the silver methenamine stain.

Overlying pseudoepitheliomatous hyperplasia of the epidermis has been reported.[666]

MISCELLANEOUS MYCOSES

Only two infections are of dermatopathological importance – keloidal blasto-mycosis and rhinosporidiosis. Both have a limited geographical distribution.

KELOIDAL BLASTOMYCOSIS (LÔBO'S DISEASE)

Keloidal blastomycosis is a rare, chronic fungal disease in which slowly growing keloid-like nodules or ulcerated verrucous plaques develop on exposed areas of the body.[667,668] Lymph node involvement occurs in up to 10% of patients.[669] The infection is caused by the fungus *Loboa loboi*, which is found almost exclusively in Central and South America.[670] The disease also affects dolphins.[671] Squamous cell carcinoma is a rare complication in chronic lesions.[672]

Histopathology[670,673]

There is an extensive granulomatous infiltrate in the dermis composed of histiocytes and giant cells of Langhans and foreign-body types, together with a few small collections of lymphocytes and plasma cells. There are numerous unstained fungal cells in hematoxylin and eosin-stained preparations, both free and in macrophages, giving a characteristic 'sieve-like' appearance (Fig. 25.21). They have a somewhat refractile wall and measure 6–12 μm in diameter. Some budding, with the formation of short chains, may be present. The organisms are PAS positive; they do not stain with mucicarmine.

RHINOSPORIDIOSIS

Rhinosporidiosis usually presents as polypoid lesions of the nasal and pharyngeal mucosa. Cutaneous lesions are rare, even in India, Sri Lanka and South America, where the fungus, *Rhinosporidium seeberi*, is endemic.[674-677] Several cases have been reported from rural Georgia in the USA.[678] The skin may be affected by contiguous spread from a mucosal lesion, by autoinoculation, and rarely through hematogenous dissemination.[679,680] The term 'rhinosporidioma' has been proposed for the solitary tumor-like nodule that occurs, rarely, on other parts of the body.[681,682]

Histopathology[683]

The large spherical sporangia (100–400 μm in diameter), containing from hundreds to thousands of endospores, each measuring up to 7 μm in diameter, are characteristic (Fig. 25.22). There is also a mixed inflammatory cell infiltrate, with the formation of some granulomas.

ALGAL INFECTIONS

PROTOTHECOSIS

Protothecosis s a rare infection caused by achlorophyllic alga-like organisms of the genus *Prototheca*.[684] There are several species, but *P. wickerhamii* is most often found in humans.[685] It can be cultured on Sabouraud's medium, which is the usual medium used for the culture of fungi.[686]

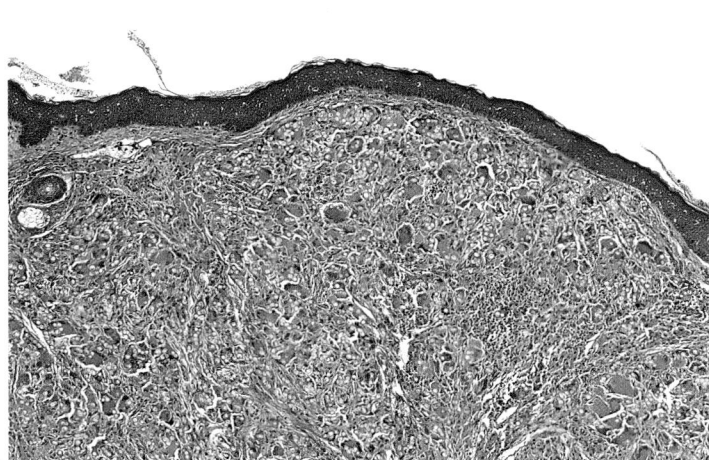

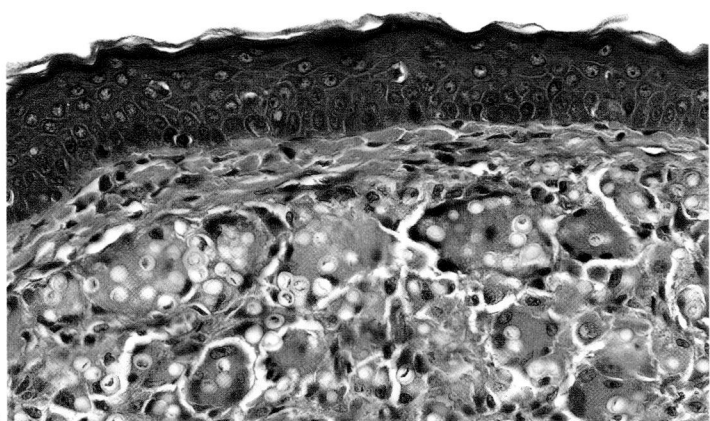

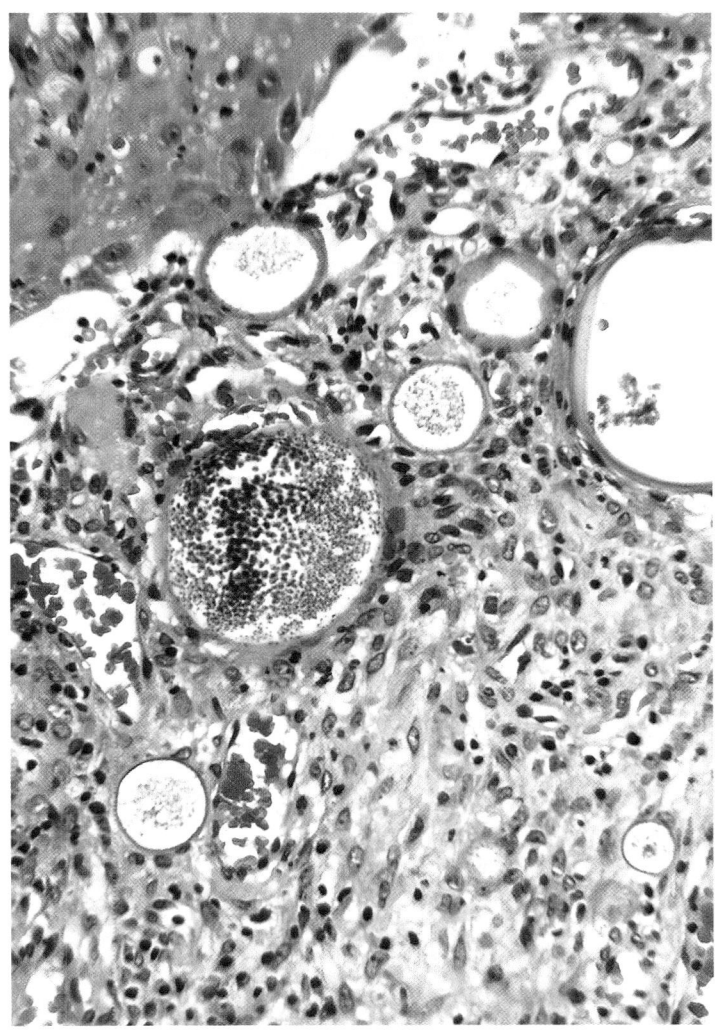

Fig. 25.21 **(A) Keloidal blastomycosis. (B)** Numerous fungi with slightly refractile cell walls are present in the cytoplasm of macrophages and giant cells. (H & E)

Fig. 25.22 **Rhinosporidiosis.** Large spherical sporangia contain numerous endospores. (H & E)

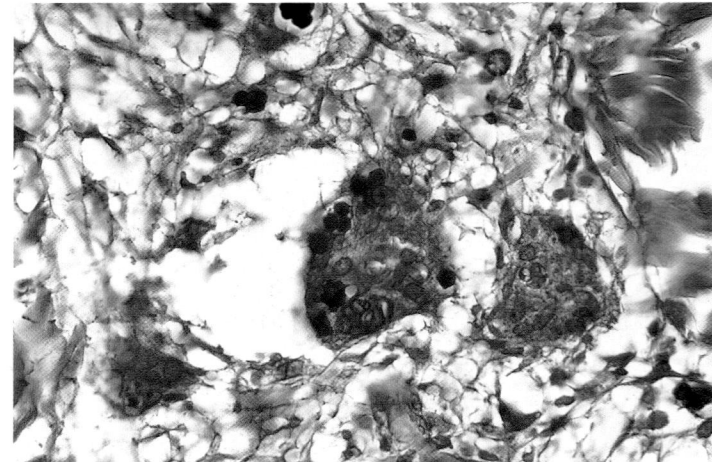

Fig. 25.23 **Protothecosis.** Sporangia are present in the cytoplasm of multinucleate giant cells. (PAS stain)

Infection usually results from traumatic inoculation in an immuno-compromised host.[687–691] It may involve the skin and subcutaneous tissue.[692,693] Infection of an olecranon bursa has been recorded.[688] Rarely there is visceral dissemination. Cutaneous lesions are eczematous,[694] herpetiform,[695] or papules[696] and papulonodules which may coalesce, resulting in the formation of slowly progressive plaques.[688,697,698]

Histopathology[685]

The usual picture is a chronic granulomatous reaction throughout the dermis, with a variable admixture of lymphocytes, plasma cells and occasionally eosinophils and even neutrophils.[699] In early lesions there are fewer multi-nucleate giant cells and the infiltrate shows greater localization to a peri-vascular and periappendageal position. There is focal necrosis in some lesions, particularly those with subcutaneous involvement. Epidermal changes are variable.[687]

Organisms (sporangia) are found in the cytoplasm of macrophages and multinucleate giant cells as thick-walled spherical bodies, often with a clear halo around them (Fig. 25.23). They may also be free in the dermis, but are difficult to see in hematoxylin and eosin-stained preparations. *Prototheca wickerhamii*, the species usually responsible for the infection in humans, measures from 3 to 11 μm in diameter. Many show internal septation, with endospore formation. Prototheca sporangia are much smaller than those of *Coccidioides immitis*.[693] They stain with the PAS and silver methenamine stains. Specific identification can be made with a fluorescein-labeled monoclonal antibody.

REFERENCES

Introduction

1 McGinnis MR. Dematiaceous fungi. In: Lennette EH, Balows A, Hausler WJ Jr, Shadomy HJ, eds. Manual of clinical microbiology, 4th ed. Washington DC: American Society for Microbiology, 1985; 561–574.

2 Kimura M, McGinnis MR. Nomenclature for fungus infections. Int J Dermatol 1998; 37: 825–826.

3 Elewski BE, Hazen PG. The superficial mycoses and the dermatophytes. J Am Acad Dermatol 1989; 21: 655–673.

4 Mann JL. Autofluorescence of fungi: an aid to detection in tissue sections. Am J Clin Pathol 1983; 79: 587–590.

5 Monheit JE, Cowan DF, Moore DG. Rapid detection of fungi in tissues using calcofluor white and fluorescence microscopy. Arch Pathol Lab Med 1984; 108: 616–618.

6 Anthony PP. A guide to the histological identification of fungi in tissues. J Clin Pathol 1973; 26: 828–831.

7 Graham AR. Fungal autofluorescence with ultraviolet illumination. Am J Clin Pathol 1983; 79: 231–234.

8 Byrd J, Mehregan DR, Mehregan DA. Use of anti-bacillus Calmette–Guérin antibodies as a screen for organisms in sporotrichoid infections. J Am Acad Dermatol 2001; 44: 261–264.

9 Moskowitz LB, Ganjei P, Ziegels-Weissman J et al. Immunohistologic identification of fungi in systemic and cutaneous mycoses. Arch Pathol Lab Med 1986; 110: 433–436.

10 Liu D, Coloe S, Baird R, Pedersen J. Molecular determination of dermatophyte fungi using the arbitrarily primed polymerase chain reaction. Br J Dermatol 1997; 137: 351–355.

11 Gräser Y, El Fari M, Presber W et al. Identification of common dermatophytes (*Trichophyton, Microsporum, Epidermophyton*) using polymerase chain reactions. Br J Dermatol 1998; 138: 576–582.

12 El Fari M, Tietz H-J, Presber W et al. Development of an oligonucleotide probe specific for *Trichophyton rubrum*. Br J Dermatol 1999; 141: 240–245.

13 Kac G, Bougnoux ME, Feuilhade de Chauvin M et al. Genetic diversity among *Trichophyton mentagrophytes* isolates using random amplified polymorphic DNA method. Br J Dermatol 1999; 140: 839–844.

Superficial filamentous infections

14 Matsumoto T, Ajello L. Current taxonomic concepts pertaining to the dermatophytes and related fungi. Int J Dermatol 1987; 26: 491–499.

15 McGinnis MR, Ajello L, Schell WA. Mycotic diseases. A proposed nomenclature. Int J Dermatol 1985; 24: 9–15.

16 Macura AB. Dermatophyte infections. Int J Dermatol 1993; 32: 313–323.

17 Svejgaard E. Epidemiology and clinical features of dermatomycoses and dermatophytoses. Acta Derm Venereol (Suppl) 1986; 121: 19–26.

18 Rinaldi MG. Dermatophytosis: Epidemiological and microbiological update. J Am Acad Dermatol 2000; 43: S120–S124.

19 Marks R. Tinea incognito. Int J Dermatol 1978; 17: 301–302.

20 Grossman ME, Pappert AS, Garzon MC, Silvers DN. Invasive *Trichophyton rubrum* infection in the immunocompromised host: report of three cases. J Am Acad Dermatol 1995; 33: 315–318.

21 Svejgaard E. Immunologic investigations of dermatophytoses and dermatophytosis. Semin Dermatol 1985; 4: 201–221.

22 Mayou SC, Calderon RA, Goodfellow A, Hay RJ. Deep (subcutaneous) dermatophyte infection presenting with unilateral lymphoedema. Clin Exp Dermatol 1987; 12: 385–388.

23 Sommer S, Barton RC, Wilkinson SM et al. Microbiological and molecular diagnosis of deep localized cutaneous infection with *Trichophyton mentagrophytes*. Br J Dermatol 1999; 141: 323–325.

24 Voisard JJ, Weill FX, Beylot-Barry M et al. Dermatophytic granuloma caused by *Microsporum canis* in a heart-lung recipient. Dermatology 1999; 198: 317–319.

25 Margolis DJ, Weinberg JM, Tangoren IA et al. Trichophytic granuloma of the vulva. Dermatology 1998; 197: 69–70.

26 Swart E, Smit FJA. *Trichophyton violaceum* abscesses. Br J Dermatol 1979; 101: 177–184.

27 Faergemann J, Gisslen H, Dahlberg E et al. *Trichophyton rubrum* abscesses in immunocompromised patients. Acta Derm Venereol 1989; 69: 244–247.

28 Elewski BE, Sullivan J. Dermatophytes as opportunistic pathogens. J Am Acad Dermatol 1994; 30: 1021–1022.

29 Muñoz-Pèrez MA, Rodriguez-Pichardo A, Camacho F, Rios JJ. Extensive and deep dermatophytosis caused by *Trichophyton mentagrophytes* var. *interdigitalis* in an HIV-1 positive patient. J Eur Acad Dermatol Venereol 2000; 14: 61–63.

30 Squeo RF, Beer R, Silvers D et al. Invasive *Trichophyton rubrum* resembling blastomycosis infection in the immunocompromised host. J Am Acad Dermatol 1998; 39: 379–380.

31 Hironaga M, Okazaki N, Saito K, Watanabe S. *Trichophyton mentagrophytes* granulomas. Arch Dermatol 1983; 119: 482–490.

32 Tsang P, Hopkins T, Jimenez-Lucho V. Deep dermatophytosis caused by *Trichophyton rubrum* in a patient with AIDS. J Am Acad Dermatol 1996; 34: 1090–1091.

33 Özdemir F, Erboz S, Ünal İ et al. Generalized *Trichophyton rubrum* infection in a subject with pemphigus vulgaris. J Eur Acad Dermatol Venereol 2000; 14: 228–230.

34 Stephens CJM, Hay RJ, Black MM. Fungal kerion – total scalp involvement due to *Microsporum canis* infection. Clin Exp Dermatol 1989; 14: 442–444.

35 Feder HM Jr. Tinea incognito misdiagnosed as erythema migrans. N Engl J Med 2000; 343: 69.

36 Romano C, Asta F, Massai L. Tinea incognito due to *Microsporum gypseum* in three children. Pediatr Dermatol 2000; 17: 41–44.

37 Gamborg Nielsen P. The prevalence of dermatophyte infections in hereditary palmo-plantar keratoderma. Acta Derm Venereol 1983; 63: 439–441.

38 De Vroey C. Epidemiology of ringworm (dermatophytosis). Semin Dermatol 1985; 4: 185–200.

39 Svejgaard EL. Epidemiology of dermatophytes in Europe. Int J Dermatol 1995; 34: 525–528.

40 Sinski JT, Flouras K. A survey of dermatophytes isolated from human patients in the United States from 1979 to 1981 with chronological listings of worldwide incidence of five dermatophytes often isolated in the United States. Mycopathologia 1984; 85: 97–120.

41 Bhakhtaviziam C, Shafi M, Mehta MC et al. Tinea capitis in Tripoli. Clin Exp Dermatol 1984; 9: 84–88.

42 Maslen MM, Andrew PJ. Tinea due to *Trichophyton violaceum* in Victoria, Australia. Australas J Dermatol 1997; 38: 124–128.

43 Onsberg P. Human infections with *Microsporum gypseum* in Denmark. Br J Dermatol 1978; 99: 527–536.

44 Muir DB, Pritchard RC, Gregory JD. Dermatophytes identified at the Australian National Reference Laboratory in Medical Mycology 1966–1982. Pathology 1984; 16: 179–183.

45 McLean T, Levy H, Lue YA. Ecology of dermatophyte infections in South Bronx, New York, 1969 to 1981. J Am Acad Dermatol 1987; 16: 336–340.

46 Aly R. Ecology and epidemiology of dermatophyte infection. J Am Acad Dermatol 1994; 31: S21–S25.

47 Maslen MM. Human cases of cattle ringworm due to *Trichophyton verrucosum* in Victoria, Australia. Australas J Dermatol 2000; 41: 90–94.

48 Harari Z, Sommer B, Feinstein A. *Trichophyton soudanense* infection in two white families. Br J Dermatol 1973; 88: 243–244.

49 Hay RJ, Reid S, Talwat E, Macnamara K. Immune responses of patients with tinea imbricata. Br J Dermatol 1983; 108: 581–586.

50 Hay RJ. Tinea imbricata. The factors affecting persistent dermatophytosis. Int J Dermatol 1985; 24: 562–564.

51 Simpson JR. Tinea barbae caused by *Trichophyton erinacei*. Br J Dermatol 1974; 90: 697–698.

52 Roller JA, Westblom TU. *Microsporum nanum* infection in hog farmers. J Am Acad Dermatol 1986; 15: 935–939.

53 Barsky S, Knapp D, McMillen S. *Trichophyton simii* infection in the United States not traceable to India. Arch Dermatol 1978; 114: 118.

54 O'Grady KJ, English MP, Warin RP. *Microsporum equinum* infection of the scalp in an adult. Br J Dermatol 1972; 86: 175–176.

55 Shwayder T, Andreae M, Babel D. *Trichophyton equinum* from riding bareback: first reported US case. J Am Acad Dermatol 1994; 30: 785–787.

56 Svejgaard E, Christiansen AH, Stahl D, Thomsen K. Clinical and immunological studies in chronic dermatophytosis caused by *Trichophyton rubrum*. Acta Derm Venereol 1984; 64: 493–500.

57 Hay RJ. Chronic dermatophyte infections. I. Clinical and mycological features. Br J Dermatol 1982; 106: 1–7.

58 Ahmed AR. Immunology of human dermatophyte infections. Arch Dermatol 1982; 118: 521–525.

59 Hay RJ, Shennan G. Chronic dermatophyte infections. II. Antibody and cell-mediated immune responses. Br J Dermatol 1982; 106: 191–198.

60 Sherwin WK, Ross TH, Rosenthal CM, Petrozzi JW. An immunosuppressive serum factor in widespread cutaneous dermatophytosis. Arch Dermatol 1979; 115: 600–604.

61 Svejgaard E, Jakobsen B, Svejgaard A. HLA studies in chronic dermatophytosis caused by *Trichophyton rubrum*. Acta Derm Venereol 1983; 63: 254–255.

62 Zaias N, Rebell G. Chronic dermatophytosis syndrome due to *Trichophyton rubrum*. Int J Dermatol 1996; 35: 614–617.

63 Pigué E, Copado R, Cabrera A et al. An outbreak of tinea gladiatorum in Lanzarote. Clin Exp Dermatol 1999; 24: 7–9.

64 Adams BB. Tinea corporis gladiatorum: A cross-sectional study. J Am Acad Dermatol 2000; 43: 1039–1041.

65 Koumantaki E, Georgala S, Rallis E, Papadavid E. *Microsporum canis* tinea capitis in an 8-month-old infant successfully treated with 2 weekly pulses of oral itraconazole. Pediatr Dermatol 2001; 18: 60–62.

66 Hebert AA. Tinea capitis. Current concepts. Arch Dermatol 1988; 124: 1554–1557.

67 Bronson DM, Desai DR, Barsky S, Foley SMc. An epidemic of infection with *Trichophyton tonsurans* revealed in a 20-year survey of fungal infections in Chicago. J Am Acad Dermatol 1983; 8: 322–330.

68 Lee JY-Y, Hsu M-L. Pathogenesis of hair infection and black dots in tinea capitis caused by *Trichophyton violaceum*: a histopathological study. J Cutan Pathol 1992; 19: 54–58.

69 Frieden IJ, Howard R. Tinea capitis: epidemiology, diagnosis, treatment, and control. J Am Acad Dermatol 1994; 31: S42–S46.

70 Elewski BE. Tinea capitis: itraconazole in *Trichophyton tonsurans* infection. J Am Acad Dermatol 1994; 31: 65–67.

71 Korstanje MJ, Staats CCG. Tinea capitis in northwestern Europe 1963–1993: etiologic agents and their changing prevalence. Int J Dermatol 1994; 33: 548–549.

72 Leeming JG, Elliott TSJ. The emergence of *Trichophyton tonsurans* tinea capitis in Birmingham, UK. Br J Dermatol 1995; 133: 929–931.

73 Weitzman I, Chin N-X, Kunjukunju N, Della-Latta P. A survey of dermatophytes isolated from human patients in the United States from 1993 to 1995. J Am Acad Dermatol 1998; 39: 255–261.

74 Jahangir M, Hussain I, Khurshid K, Haroon TS. A clinico-etiologic correlation in tinea capitis. Int J Dermatol 1999; 38: 275–278.

75 Elewski BE. Tinea capitis: A current perspective. J Am Acad Dermatol 2000; 42: 1–20.

76 Cuétara MS, Del Palacio A, Pereiro M, Noriega AR. Prevalence of undetected tinea capitis in a prospective school survey in Madrid: emergence of new causative fungi. Br J Dermatol 1998; 138: 658–660.

77 Gupta AK, Hofstader SLR, Adam P, Summerbell RC. Tinea capitis: an overview with emphasis on management. Pediatr Dermatol 1999; 16: 171–189.

78 Ravenscroft J, Goodfield MJD, Evans EGV. *Trichophyton tonsurans* tinea capitis and tinea corporis: treatment and follow-up of four affected family members. Pediatr Dermatol 2000; 17: 407–409.

79 Shelley WB, Shelley ES. The infected hairs of tinea capitis due to *Microsporum canis*: demonstration of uniqueness of the hair cuticle by scanning electron microscopy. J Am Acad Dermatol 1987; 16: 354–361.

80 Anstey A, Lucke TW, Philpot C. Tinea capitis caused by *Trichophyton rubrum*. Br J Dermatol 1996; 135: 113–115.

81 Suite M, Moore MK, Hay RJ. Leucocyte chemotaxis to antigens of dermatophytes causing scalp ringworm. Clin Exp Dermatol 1987; 12: 171–174.

82 Hebert AA, Head ES, Macdonald EM. Tinea capitis caused by *Trichophyton tonsurans*. Pediatr Dermatol 1985; 2: 219–223.

83 Bournerias I, Feuilhade De Chauvin M, Datry A et al. Unusual *Microsporum canis* infections in adult HIV patients. J Am Acad Dermatol 1996; 35: 808–810.

84 Lateur N, André J, De Maubeuge J et al. Tinea capitis in two black African adults with HIV infection. Br J Dermatol 1999; 140: 722–724.

85 Takwale A, Agarwal S, Holmes SC, Berth-Jones J. Tinea capitis in two elderly women: transmission at the hairdresser. Br J Dermatol 2001; 144: 898–900.

86 Rudolph AH. The diagnosis and treatment of tinea capitis due to *Trichophyton tonsurans*. Int J Dermatol 1985; 24: 426–431.

87 Urbanek M, Neill SM, Miller JA. Kerion – a case report. Clin Exp Dermatol 1995; 20: 413–414.

88 Jahan V, LeBoit PE, Frieden AJ. Inflammatory nodule on the scalp. Pediatr Dermatol 1990; 7: 153–155.

89 Aste N, Pau M, Biggio P. *Trichophyton mentagrophytes* kerion in a woman. Br J Dermatol 1996; 135: 1010–1011.

90 Powell FC, Muller SA. Kerion in the glabrous skin. J Am Acad Dermatol 1982; 7: 490–494.

91 Beswick SJ, Das S, Lawrence CM, Tan BB. Kerion formation due to *Trichophyton rubrum*. Br J Dermatol 1999; 141: 953–954.

92 Gupta G, Burden AD, Roberts DT. Acute suppurative ringworm (kerion) caused by *Trichophyton rubrum*. Br J Dermatol 1999; 140: 369–370.

93 Ive FA. Kerion formation caused by *Trichophyton rubrum*. Br J Dermatol 2000; 142: 1065–1066.

94 Jury CS, Lucke TW, Bilsland D. *Trichophyton erinacei*: an unusual cause of kerion. Br J Dermatol 1999; 141: 606–607.

95 Dvoretzky I, Fisher BK, Movshovitz M, Schewach-Millet M. Favus. Int J Dermatol 1980; 19: 89–93.

96 Gargoom AM, Elyazachi MB, Al-Ani SM, Duweb GA. Tinea capitis in Benghazi, Libya. Int J Dermatol 2000; 39: 263–265.

97 Garcia-Sánchez MS, Pereiro M Jr, Pereiro MM, Toribio J. Favus due to *Trichophyton mentagrophytes* var. quinckeanum. Dermatology 1997; 194: 177–179.

98 Pravda DJ, Pugliese MM. Tinea faciei. Arch Dermatol 1978; 114: 250–252.

99 Bardazzi F, Raone B, Neri I, Patrizi A. Tinea faciei in a newborn: a new case. Pediatr Dermatol 2000; 17: 494–495.

100 Cirillo-Hyland V, Humphreys T, Elenitsas R. Tinea faciei. J Am Acad Dermatol 1993; 29: 119–120.

101 Raimer SS, Beightler EL, Hebert AA et al. Tinea faciei in infants caused by *Trichophyton tonsurans*. Pediatr Dermatol 1986; 3: 452–454.

102 Frankel DH, Soltani K, Medenica MM, Rippon JW. Tinea of the face caused by *Trichophyton rubrum* with histologic changes of granuloma faciale. J Am Acad Dermatol 1988; 18: 403–406.

103 Patel GK, Mills CM. Tinea faciei due to *Microsporum canis* abscess formation. Clin Exp Dermatol 2000; 25: 608–610.

104 Beller M, Gessner BD. An outbreak of tinea corporis gladiatorum on a high school wrestling team. J Am Acad Dermatol 1994; 31: 197–201.

105 Kemna ME, Elewski BE. A U.S. epidemiologic survey of superficial fungal diseases. J Am Acad Dermatol 1996; 35: 539–542.

106 Kawada A, Aragane Y, Maeda A et al. Tinea barbae due to *Trichophyton rubrum* with possible involvement of autoinoculation. Br J Dermatol 2000; 142: 1064–1065.

107 Bakos L, Bonamigo RR, Pisani AC et al. Scutular favus-like tinea cruris et pedis in a patient with AIDS. J Am Acad Dermatol 1996; 34: 1086–1087.

108 Pielop J, Rosen T. Penile dermatophytosis. J Am Acad Dermatol 2001; 44: 864–867.

109 Baudraz-Rosselet F, Ruffieux Ph, Mancarella A et al. Diaper dermatitis due to *Trichophyton verrucosum*. Pediatr Dermatol 1993; 10: 368–369.

110 Logan RA, Kobza-Black A. Tinea imbricata in a British nurse. Clin Exp Dermatol 1988; 13: 232–233.

111 Cohen PR, Maor MH. Tinea corporis confined to irradiated skin. Cancer 1992; 70: 1634–1637.

112 Jang K-A, Chi D-H, Choi J-H et al. Tinea pedis in Korean children. Int J Dermatol 2000; 9: 25–27.

113 Merlin K, Kilkenny M, Plunkett A, Marks R. The prevalence of common skin conditions in Australian school students: 4 Tinea pedis. Br J Dermatol 1999; 140: 897–901.

114 Hirschmann JV, Raugi GJ. Pustular tinea pedis. J Am Acad Dermatol 2000; 42: 132–133.

115 Raboobee N, Aboobaker J, Peer AK. Tinea pedis et unguium in the Muslim community of Durban, South Africa. Int J Dermatol 1998; 37: 759–765.

116 Geary RJ, Lucky AW. Tinea pedis in children presenting as unilateral inflammatory lesions of the sole. Pediatr Dermatol 1999; 16: 255–258.

117 Barson WJ. Granuloma and pseudogranuloma of the skin due to *Microsporum canis*. Arch Dermatol 1985; 121: 895–897.

118 Smith KJ, Neafie RC, Skelton HG III et al. Majocchi's granuloma. J Cutan Pathol 1991; 18: 28–35.

119 Mikhail GR. *Trichophyton rubrum* granuloma. Int J Dermatol 1970; 9: 41–46.

120 Liao Y-H, Chu S-H, Hsiao G-H et al. Majocchi's granuloma caused by *Trichophyton tonsurans* in a cardiac transplant recipient. Br J Dermatol 1999; 140: 1194–1196.

121 Sequeira M, Burdick AE, Elgart GW, Berman B. New-onset Majocchi's granuloma in two kidney transplant recipients under tacrolimus treatment. J Am Acad Dermatol 1998; 38: 486–488.

122 Gupta S, Kumar B, Radotra BD, Rai R. Majocchi's granuloma trichophyticum in an immunocompromised patient. Int J Dermatol 2000; 39: 140–141.

123 Haneke E, Roseeuw D. The scope of onychomycosis: epidemiology and clinical features. Int J Dermatol 1999; 38 (Suppl 2): 7–12.

124 Elewski BE. Onychomycosis caused by *Scytalidium dimidiatum*. J Am Acad Dermatol 1996; 35: 336–338.

125 Tosti A, Piraccini BM, Lorenzi S. Onychomycosis caused by nondermatophytic molds: Clinical features and response to treatment of 59 cases. J Am Acad Dermatol 2000; 42: 217–224.

126 Sehgal VN, Jain S. Onychomycosis: clinical perspective. Int J Dermatol 2000; 39: 241–249.

127 Jain S, Sehgal VN. Onychomycosis: an epidemio-etiologic perspective. Int J Dermatol 2000; 39: 100–103.

128 Arrese JE, Piérard-Franchimont C, Piérard GE. Onychomycosis and keratomycosis caused by *Alternaria* sp. Am J Dermatopathol 1996; 18: 611–613.

129 Tosti A, Piraccini BM. Proximal subungual onychomycosis due to *Aspergillus niger*: report of two cases. Br J Dermatol 1998; 139: 156–157.

130 Kam KM, Au WF, Wong PY, Cheung MM. Onychomycosis in Hong Kong. Int J Dermatol 1997; 36: 757–761.

131 Scher RK. Onychomycosis: A significant medical disorder. J Am Acad Dermatol 1996; 35: S2–S5.

132 Ghannoum MA, Hajjeh RA, Scher R et al. A large-scale North American study of fungal isolates from nails: The frequency of onychomycosis, fungal distribution, and antifungal susceptibility patterns. J Am Acad Dermatol 2000; 43: 641–648.

133 Weismann K, Knudsen EA, Pedersen C. White nails in AIDS/ARC due to *Trichophyton rubrum* infection. Clin Exp Dermatol 1988; 13: 24–25.

134 Hay RJ, Baran R, Moore MK, Wilkinson JD. Candida onychomycosis – an evaluation of the role of *Candida* species in nail disease. Br J Dermatol 1988; 118: 47–58.

135 Ploysangam T, Lucky AW. Childhood white superficial onychomycosis caused by *Trichophyton rubrum*: Report of seven cases and review of the literature. J Am Acad Dermatol 1997; 36: 29–32.

136 Baran R, Hay RJ, Tosti A, Haneke E. A new classification of onychomycosis. Br J Dermatol 1998; 139: 567–571.

137 Lee S, Bang D. Hyphae on the ventral nailplate as a clue to onychomycosis. Am J Dermatopathol 1987; 9: 445–446.

138 Scher RK, Ackerman AB. Histologic differential diagnosis of onychomycosis and psoriasis of the nail unit from cornified cells of the nail bed alone. Am J Dermatopathol 1980; 2: 255–257.

139 Roberts DT, Evans EGV. Subungual dermatophytoma complicating dermatophyte onychomycosis. Br J Dermatol 1998; 138: 189–190.

140 Lawry MA, Haneke E, Strobeck K et al. Methods for diagnosing onychomycosis. A comparative study and review of the literature. Arch Dermatol 2000; 136: 1112–1116.

141 Graham JH. Superficial fungus infections. In: Graham JH, Johnson WC, Helwig EB, eds. Dermal pathology. Hagerstown, MD: Harper & Row, 1972; 137–253.

142 Ackerman AB. Neutrophils within the cornified layer as clues to infection by superficial fungi. Am J Dermatopathol 1979; 1: 69–75.

143 Ollague J, Ackerman AB. Compact orthokeratosis as a clue to chronic dermatophytosis and candidiasis. Am J Dermatopathol 1982; 4: 359–363.

144 Gottlieb GJ, Ackerman AB. The 'sandwich sign' of dermatophytosis. Am J Dermatopathol 1986; 8: 347–350.

145 Carter RL. Majocchi's granuloma. J Am Acad Dermatol 1980; 2: 75.

146 Kuo T-T, Chen S-Y, Chan H-L. Tinea infection histologically simulating eosinophilic pustular folliculitis. J Cutan Pathol 1986; 13: 118–122.

147 Tsang P, Hopkins T, Jimenez-Lucho V. Deep dermatophytosis caused by *Trichophyton rubrum* in a patient with AIDS. J Am Acad Dermatol 1996; 34: 1090–1091.

148 Graham JH, Johnson WC, Burgoon CF Jr, Helwig EB. Tinea capitis. A histopathological and histochemical study. Arch Dermatol 1964; 89: 528–543.

149 Greer DL, Gutierrez MM. Tinea pedis caused by *Hendersonula toruloidea*. A new problem in dermatology. J Am Acad Dermatol 1987; 16: 1111–1115.

150 Little MG, Hammond ML. *Scytalidium dimidiatum* in Australia. Australas J Dermatol 1995; 36: 204–205.

151 Peiris S, Moore MK, Marten RH. *Scytalidium hyalinum* infection of skin and nails. Br J Dermatol 1979; 100: 579–584.

152 Elewski BE, Greer DL. *Hendersonula toruloidea* and *Scytalidium hyalinum*. Review and update. Arch Dermatol 1991; 127: 1041–1044.

153 Hay RJ, Moore MK. Clinical features of superficial fungal infections caused by *Hendersonula toruloidea* and *Scytalidium hyalinum*. Br J Dermatol 1984; 110: 677–683.

154 Creus L, Umbert P, Torres-Rodríguez JM, López-Gil F. Ulcerous granulomatous cheilitis with lymphatic invasion caused by *Scopulariopsis brevicaulis* infection. J Am Acad Dermatol 1994; 31: 881–883.

155 Bruynzeel I, Starink TM. Granulomatous skin infection caused by *Scopulariopsis brevicaulis*. J Am Acad Dermatol 1998; 39: 365–367.

Yeast infections

156 Cooper BH, Silva-Hutner M. Yeasts of medical importance. In: Lennette EH, Balows A, Hausler WJ Jr, Shadomy HJ, eds. Manual of clinical microbiology, 4th ed. Washington DC: American Society for Microbiology, 1985; 526–541.

157 Stenderup A. Ecology of yeast and epidemiology of yeast infections. Acta Derm Venereol (Suppl) 1986; 121: 27–37.

158 Groisser D, Bottone EJ, Lebwohl M. Association of *Pityrosporum orbiculare (Malassezia furfur)* with seborrheic dermatitis in patients with acquired immunodeficiency syndrome (AIDS). J Am Acad Dermatol 1989; 20: 770–773.

159 Faergemann J, Maibach HI. The Pityrosporon yeasts. Their role as pathogens. Int J Dermatol 1984; 23: 463–465.

160 Bergman AG, Kauffman CA. Dermatitis due to *Sporobolomyces* infection. Arch Dermatol 1984; 120: 1059–1060.

161 DeCastro P, Jorizzo JL. Cutaneous aspects of candidosis. Semin Dermatol 1985; 4: 165–172.

162 Ro BI. Chronic mucocutaneous candidosis. Int J Dermatol 1988; 27: 457–462.

163 Thomas I. Superficial and deep candidosis. Int J Dermatol 1993; 32: 778–783.

164 Winton GB. Skin diseases aggravated by pregnancy. J Am Acad Dermatol 1989; 20: 1–13.

165 Odds FC. Pathogenesis of *Candida* infections. J Am Acad Dermatol 1994; 31: S2–S5.

166 Dekio S, Imaoka C, Jidoi J. Candida folliculitis associated with hypothyroidism. Br J Dermatol 1987; 117: 663–664.

167 Giandoni MB, Grabski WJ. Cutaneous candidiasis as a cause of delayed surgical wound healing. J Am Acad Dermatol 1994; 30: 981–984.

168 Kapdağli H, Öztürk G, Dereli T et al. *Candida* folliculitis mimicking tinea barbae. Int J Dermatol 1997; 36: 295–297.

169 Kurita M, Kishimoto S, Kibe Y et al. Candida folliculitis mimicking tinea barbae. Acta Derm Venereol 2000; 80: 153–154.

170 Trizna Z, Chen S-H, Lockhart S et al. *Candida parapsilosis* chondritis successfully treated with oral fluconazole. Arch Dermatol 2000; 136: 804.

171 Scherwitz C. Ultrastructure of human cutaneous candidosis. J Invest Dermatol 1982; 78: 200–205.

172 Montes LF, Wilborn WH. Fungus-host relationship in candidiasis. A brief review. Arch Dermatol 1985; 121: 119–124.

173 Kirkpatrick CH, Montes LF. Chronic mucocutaneous candidiasis. J Cutan Pathol 1974; 1: 211–229.

174 Jorizzo JL. Chronic mucocutaneous candidosis. An update. Arch Dermatol 1982; 118: 963–965.

175 Kirkpatrick CH. Chronic mucocutaneous candidiasis. J Am Acad Dermatol 1994; 31: S14–S17.

176 Helm TN, Calabrese LH, Longworth DL et al. Vascular nodules and plaques resembling chronic mucocutaneous candidiasis in a patient with a low interleukin 2 level. J Am Acad Dermatol 1993; 29: 473–477.

177 Lilic D, Gravenor I. Immunology of chronic mucocutaneous candidiasis. J Clin Pathol 2001; 54: 81–83.

178 Shama SK, Kirkpatrick CH. Dermatophytosis in patients with chronic mucocutaneous candidiasis. J Am Acad Dermatol 1980; 2: 285–294.

179 Steensma DP, Tefferi A, Weiler CR. Autoimmune hemolytic anemia in a patient with 75: 853–855.

180 Coleman R, Hay RJ. Chronic mucocutaneous candidosis associated with hypothyroidism: a distinct syndrome? Br J Dermatol 1997; 136: 24–29.

181 Palestine RF, Su WPD, Liesegang TJ. Late-onset chronic mucocutaneous and ocular candidiasis and malignant thymoma. Arch Dermatol 1983; 119: 580–586.

182 Anstey A, Spickett GP, Beechey-Newman N et al. A case of candidal umbilical granuloma. Br J Dermatol 1991; 124: 475–478.

183 Ollague J, Ackerman AB. Compact orthokeratosis as a clue to chronic dermatophytosis and candidiasis. Am J Dermatopathol 1982; 4: 359–363.

184 Radentz WH. Opportunistic fungal infections in immunocompromised hosts. J Am Acad Dermatol 1989; 20: 989–1003.

185 Jacobs MI, Magid MS, Jarowski CI. Disseminated candidiasis. Newer approaches to early recognition and treatment. Arch Dermatol 1980; 116: 1277–1279.

186 Marcus J, Grossman ME, Yunakow MJ, Rappaport F. Disseminated candidiasis, Candida arthritis, and unilateral skin lesions. J Am Acad Dermatol 1992; 26: 295–297.

187 Grossman ME, Silvers DN, Walther RR. Cutaneous manifestations of disseminated candidiasis. J Am Acad Dermatol 1980; 2: 111–116.

188 File TM Jr, Marina OA, Flowers FP. Necrotic skin lesions associated with disseminated candidiasis. Arch Dermatol 1979; 115: 214–215.

189 Fine JD, Miller JA, Harrist TJ, Haynes HA. Cutaneous lesions in disseminated candidiasis mimicking ecthyma gangrenosum. Am J Med 1981; 70: 1133–1135.

190 Dupont B, Drouhet E. Cutaneous, ocular, and osteoarticular candidiasis in heroin addicts: new clinical and therapeutic aspects in 38 patients. J Infect Dis 1985; 152: 577–591.

191 Podzamczer D, Ribera M, Gudiol F. Skin abscesses caused by Candida albicans in heroin abusers. J Am Acad Dermatol 1987; 16: 386–387.

192 Kam LA, Giacoia GP. Congenital cutaneous candidiasis. Am J Dis Child 1975; 129: 1215–1218.

193 Cosgrove BF, Reeves K, Mullins D et al. Congenital cutaneous candidiasis associated with respiratory distress and elevation of liver function tests: A case report and review of the literature. J Am Acad Dermatol 1997; 37: 817–823.

194 Chapel TA, Gagliardi C, Nichols W. Congenital cutaneous candidiasis. J Am Acad Dermatol 1982; 6: 926–928.

195 Raval DS, Barton LL, Hansen RC, Kling PJ. Congenital cutaneous candidiasis: case report and review. Pediatr Dermatol 1995; 12: 355–358.

196 Bonifazi E, Garofalo L, Lospalluti M et al. Granuloma gluteale infantum with atrophic scars: clinical and histological observations in eleven cases. Clin Exp Dermatol 1981; 6: 23–29.

197 Concannon P, Gisoldi E, Phillips S, Grossman R. Diaper dermatitis: a therapeutic dilemma. Results of a double-blind placebo controlled trial of metronidazole nitrate 0.25%. Pediatr Dermatol 2001; 18: 149–155.

198 Montes LF. The histopathology of diaper dermatitis. Historical review. J Cutan Pathol 1978; 5: 1–4.

199 Lovell CR, Atherton DJ. Infantile gluteal granulomata – case report. Clin Exp Dermatol 1984; 9: 522–525.

200 Maekawa Y, Sakazaki Y, Hayashibara T. Diaper area granuloma of the aged. Arch Dermatol 1978; 114: 382–383.

201 Mooney MA, Thomas I, Sirois D. Oral candidosis. Int J Dermatol 1995; 34: 759–765.

202 Jolly M. White lesions of the mouth. Int J Dermatol 1977; 16: 713–725.

203 Klein RS, Harris CA, Small CB et al. Oral candidiasis in high-risk patients as the initial manifestation of the acquired immunodeficiency syndrome. N Engl J Med 1984; 311: 354–358.

204 Cooke BED. Median rhomboid glossitis. Candidiasis and not a developmental anomaly. Br J Dermatol 1975; 93: 399–405.

205 Brandrup F, Wantzin GL, Thomsen K. Perioral pustular eruption caused by Candida albicans. Br J Dermatol 1981; 105: 327–329.

206 Odds FC. Genital candidosis. Clin Exp Dermatol 1982; 7: 345–354.

207 Ganor S, Pumpianski R. Chronic Candida albicans paronychia in adult Israeli women. Sources and spread. Br J Dermatol 1974; 90: 77–83.

208 Hay RJ. Cryptococcus neoformans and cutaneous cryptococcosis. Semin Dermatol 1985; 4: 252–259.

209 Goonetilleke AKE, Krause K, Slater DN et al. Primary cutaneous cryptococcosis in an immunocompromised pigeon keeper. Br J Dermatol 1995; 133: 650–652.

210 Sampaio RN, Medeiros B, Milfort M et al. Systemic cryptococcosis with solitary cutaneous lesion in an immunocompetent patient. Int J Dermatol 1999; 38: 773–775.

211 Micalizzi C, Persi A, Parodi A. Primary cutaneous cryptococcosis in an immunocompetent pigeon keeper. Clin Exp Dermatol 1997; 22: 195–197.

212 Barfield L, Iacobelli D, Hashimoto K. Secondary cutaneous cryptococcosis: case report and review of 22 cases. J Cutan Pathol 1988; 15: 385–392.

213 Gordon LA, Gordon DL. Cryptococcal infection simulating varicella. Australas J Dermatol 1987; 28: 24–26.

214 Sussman EJ, McMahon F, Wright D, Friedman HM. Cutaneous cryptococcosis without evidence of systemic involvement. J Am Acad Dermatol 1984; 11: 371–374.

215 Webling DD'A, Mahajani A. Localized dermal cryptococcosis following a scorpion sting. Australas J Dermatol 1981; 22: 127–128.

216 Gordon PM, Ormerod AD, Harvey G et al. Cutaneous cryptococcal infection without immunodeficiency. Clin Exp Dermatol 1994; 19: 181–184.

217 Ng WF, Loo KT. Cutaneous cryptococcosis – primary versus secondary disease: report of two cases with review of literature. Am J Dermatopathol 1993; 15: 372–377.

218 Patel P, Ramanathan J, Kayser M, Baran J Jr. Primary cutaneous cryptococcosis of the nose in an immunocompetent woman. J Am Acad Dermatol 2000; 43: 344–345.

219 Granier F, Kanitakis J, Hermier C et al. Localized cutaneous cryptococcosis successfully treated with ketoconazole. J Am Acad Dermatol 1987; 16: 243–249.

220 Gloster HM Jr, Swerlick RA, Solomon AR. Cryptococcal cellulitis in a diabetic, kidney transplant patient. J Am Acad Dermatol 1994; 30: 1025–1026.

221 Lauerma AI, Jeskanen L, Rantanen T et al. Cryptococcosis during systemic glucocorticosteroid treatment. Dermatology 1999; 199: 180–182.

222 Hunger RE, Paredes BE, Quattroppani C et al. Primary cutaneous cryptococcosis in a patient with systemic immunosuppression after liver transplantation. Dermatology 2000; 200: 352–355.

223 Borton LK, Wintroub BU. Disseminated cryptococcosis presenting as herpetiform lesions in a homosexual man with acquired immunodeficiency syndrome. J Am Acad Dermatol 1984; 10: 387–390.

224 Piérard GE, Piérard-Franchimont C, Estrada JE et al. Cutaneous mixed infections in AIDS. Am J Dermatopathol 1990; 12: 63–66.

225 Rico MJ, Penneys NS. Cutaneous cryptococcosis resembling molluscum contagiosum in a patient with AIDS. Arch Dermatol 1985; 121: 901–902.

226 Picon L, Vaillant L, Duong T et al. Cutaneous cryptococcosis resembling molluscum contagiosum: a first manifestation of AIDS. Acta Derm Venereol 1989; 69: 365–367.

227 Dimino-Emme L, Gurevitch AW. Cutaneous manifestations of disseminated cryptococcosis. J Am Acad Dermatol 1995; 32: 844–850.

228 Durden FM, Elewski B. Cutaneous involvement with Cryptococcus neoformans in AIDS. J Am Acad Dermatol 1994; 30: 844–848.

229 Myers SA, Kamino H. Cutaneous cryptococcosis and histoplasmosis coinfection in a patient with AIDS. J Am Acad Dermatol 1996; 34: 898–900.

230 Murakawa GJ, Kerschmann R, Berger T. Cutaneous cryptococcal infection and AIDS. Report of 12 cases and review of the literature. Arch Dermatol 1996; 132: 545–548.

231 Tomasini C, Caliendo V, Puiatti P, Grazia Bernengo M. Granulomatous-ulcerative vulvar cryptococcosis in a patient with advanced HIV disease. J Am Acad Dermatol 1997; 37: 116–117.

232 Hall JC, Brewer JH, Crouch TT, Watson KR. Cryptococcal cellulitis with multiple sites of involvement. J Am Acad Dermatol 1987; 17: 329–332.

233 Carlson KC, Mehlmauer M, Evans S, Chandrasoma P. Cryptococcal cellulitis in renal transplant recipients. J Am Acad Dermatol 1987; 17: 469–472.

234 Hamann ID, Gillespie RJ, Ferguson JK. Primary cryptococcal cellulitis caused by Cryptococcus neoformans var. gattii in an immunocompetent host. Australas J Dermatol 1997; 38: 29–32.

235 Sanchez-Albisua B, Rodriguez-Peralto JL, Romero G et al. Cryptococcal cellulitis in an immunocompetent host. J Am Acad Dermatol 1997; 36: 109–112.

236 Massa MC, Doyle JA. Cutaneous cryptococcosis simulating pyoderma gangrenosum. J Am Acad Dermatol 1981; 5: 32–36.

237 Manrique P, Mayo J, Alvarez JA et al. Polymorphous cutaneous cryptococcosis: nodular, herpes-like, and molluscum-like lesions in a patient with the acquired immunodeficiency syndrome. J Am Acad Dermatol 1992; 26: 122–124.

238 Hecker MS, Weinberg JM. Cutaneous cryptococcosis mimicking keloid. Dermatology 2001; 202: 78–79.

239 Muñoz-Pérez MA, Colmenero MA, Rodriguez-Pichardo A et al. Disseminated cryptococcosis presenting as molluscum-like lesions as the first manifestation of AIDS. Int J Dermatol 1996; 35: 646–648.

240 Kamalam A, Yesudian P, Thambiah AS. Cutaneous infection by Cryptococcus laurentii. Br J Dermatol 1977; 97: 221–223.

241 Narayan S, Batta K, Colloby P, Tan CY. Cutaneous Cryptococcus infection due to C. albidus associated with Sézary syndrome. Br J Dermatol 2000; 143: 632–634.

242 Chu AC, Hay RJ, MacDonald DM. Cutaneous cryptococcosis. Br J Dermatol 1980; 103: 95–100.

243 Leidel GD, Metcalf JS. Formation of palisading granulomas in a patient with chronic cutaneous cryptococcosis. Am J Dermatopathol 1989; 11: 560–562.

244 Gutierrez F, Fu YS, Lurie HI. Cryptococcosis histologically resembling histoplasmos s. A light and electron microscopical study. Arch Pathol 1975; 99: 347–352.

245 Naka W, Masuda M, Konohana A et al. Primary cutaneous cryptococcosis and *Cryptococcus neoformans* serotype D. Clin Exp Dermatol 1995; 20: 221–225.

246 Noble RC, Fajardo LF. Primary cutaneous cryptococcosis: review and morphologic study. Am J Clin Pathol 1972; 57: 13–22.

247 Faergemann J. Lipophilic yeasts in skin disease. Semin Dermatol 1985; 4: 173–184.

248 Borelli D, Jacobs PH, Nall L. Tinea versicolor: epidemiologic, clinical, and therapeutic aspects. J Am Acad Dermatol 1991; 25: 300–305.

249 El-Gothamy Z, Ghozzi M. Tinea versicolor of the scalp. Int J Dermatol 1995; 34: 533–534.

250 Rapelanoro R, Mortureux P, Couprie B et al. Neonatal *Malassezia furfur* pustulosis. Arch Dermatol 1996; 132: 190–193.

251 Kim TY, Jang IG, Park YM et al. Head and neck dermatitis: the role of *Malassezia furfur*, topical steroid use and environmental factors in its causation. Clin Exp Dermatol 1999; 24: 226–231.

252 Mayser P, Gross A. IgE antibodies to *Malassezia furfur, M. sympodialis* and *Pityrosporum orbiculare* in patients with atopic dermatitis, seborrheic eczema or pityriasis versicolor, and identification of respective allergens. Acta Derm Venereol 2000; 80: 357–361.

253 Saadatzadeh MR, Ashbee HR, Cunliffe WJ, Ingham E. Cell-mediated immunity to the mycelial phase of *Malassezia* spp. in patients with pityriasis versicolor and controls. Br J Dermatol 2001; 144: 77–84.

254 Borgers M, Cauwenbergh G, Van de Ven M-A et al. Pityriasis versicolor and *Pityrosporum ovale*. Morphogenetic and ultrastructural considerations. Int J Dermatol 1987; 26: 586–589.

255 Silva-Lizama E. Tinea versicolor. Int J Dermatol 1995; 34: 611–617.

256 Faergemann J. *Pityrosporum* infections. J Am Acad Dermatol 1994; 31: S18–S20.

257 Sunenshine PJ, Schwartz RA, Janniger CK. Tinea versicolor. Int J Dermatol 1998; 37: 648–655.

258 Crespo Erchiga V, Ojeda Martos A, Vera Casaño A et al. *Malassezia globosa* as the causative agent of pityriasis versicolor. Br J Dermatol 2000; 143: 799–803.

259 Faergemann J, Fredriksson T. Tinea versicolor: some new aspects on etiology, pathogenesis, and treatment. Int J Dermatol 1982; 21: 8–11.

260 Galadari I, Elkomy M, Mousa A et al. Tinea versicolor: histologic and ultrastructural investigation of pigmentary changes. Int J Dermatol 1992; 31: 253–256.

261 Allen HB, Charles CR, Johnson BL. Hyperpigmented tinea versicolor. Arch Dermatol 1976; 112: 1110–1112.

262 Karaoui R, Bou-Resli M, Al-Zaid NS, Mousa A. Tinea versicolor: ultrastructural studies on hypopigmented and hyperpigmented skin. Dermatologica 1981; 162: 69–85.

263 Dotz WI, Henrikson DM, Yu GSM, Galey CI. Tinea versicolor: a light and electron microscopic study of hyperpigmented skin. J Am Acad Dermatol 1985; 12: 37–44.

264 Scheynius A, Faergemann J, Forsum U, Sjöberg O. Phenotypic characterization *in situ* of inflammatory cells in pityriasis (tinea) versicolor. Acta Derm Venereol 1984: 64: 473–479.

265 Marinaro RE, Gershenbaum MR, Roisen FJ, Papa CM. Tinea versicolor: a scanning electron microscopic view. J Cutan Pathol 1978; 5: 15–22.

266 Back O, Faergemann J, Hornqvist R. *Pityrosporum* folliculitis: a common disease of the young and middle-aged. J Am Acad Dermatol 1985; 12: 56–61.

267 Abdel-Razek M, Fadaly G, Abdel-Raheim M, Al-Morsy F. Pityrosporum (*Malassezia*) folliculitis in Saudi Arabia – diagnosis and therapeutic trials. Clin Exp Dermatol 1995; 20: 406–409.

268 Berretty PJM, Neumann HAM, Hulsebosch HJ. Pityrosporum folliculitis: is it a real entity? Br J Dermatol 1980; 103: 565.

269 Ford GP, Ive FA, Midgley G. *Pityrosporum* folliculitis and ketoconazole. Br J Dermatol 1982; 107: 691–695.

270 Faergemann J, Johansson S, Back O, Scheynius A. An immunologic and cultured study of *Pityrosporum* folliculitis. J Am Acad Dermatol 1986; 14: 429–433.

271 Kavanagh GM, Leeming JP, Marshman GM et al. Folliculitis in Down's syndrome. Br J Dermatol 1993; 129: 696–699.

272 Heymann WR, Wolf DJ. *Malassezia (Pityrosporon)* folliculitis occurring during pregnancy. Int J Dermatol 1986; 25: 49–51.

273 Bufill JA, Lum LG, Caya JG et al. Pityrosporum folliculitis after bone marrow transplantation. Clinical observations in five patients. Ann Intern Med 1988; 108: 560–563.

274 Helm KF, Lookingbill DP. *Pityrosporum* folliculitis and severe pruritus in two patients with Hodgkin's disease. Arch Dermatol 1993; 129: 380–381.

275 Klotz SA, Drutz DJ, Huppert M, Johnson JE. *Pityrosporum* folliculitis. Its potential for confusion with skin lesions of systemic candidiasis. Arch Intern Med 1982; 142: 2126–2129.

276 Archer-Dubon C, Icaza-Chivez ME, Orozco-Topete R et al. An epidemic outbreak of *Malassezia* folliculitis in three adult patients in an intensive care unit: a previously unrecognized nosocomial infection. Int J Dermatol 1999; 38: 453–456.

277 Hill MK, Goodfield MJD, Rodgers FG et al. Skin surface electron microscopy in Pityrosporum folliculitis. Arch Dermatol 1990; 126: 181–184.

278 Potter BS, Burgoon CF, Johnson WC. Pityrosporum folliculitis. Arch Dermatol 1973; 107: 388–391.

279 Sina B, Kauffman L, Samorodin CS. Intrafollicular mucin deposits in *Pityrosporum* folliculitis. J Am Acad Dermatol 1995; 32: 807–809.

280 Hanna JM, Johnson WT, Wyre HW. *Malassezia (Pityrosporum)* folliculitis occurring with granuloma annulare and alopecia areata. Arch Dermatol 1983; 119: 869–871.

281 Clemmensen OJ, Hagdrup H. Splendore–Hoeppli phenomenon in *Pityrosporum* folliculitis (pseudoactinomycosis of the skin). J Cutan Pathol 1991; 18: 293–297.

282 Nahass GT, Rosenberg SP, Leonardi CL, Penneys NS. Disseminated infection with *Trichosporon beigelii*. Arch Dermatol 1993; 129: 1020–1023.

283 Walsh TJ, Newman KR, Moody M et al. Trichosporonosis in patients with neoplastic disease. Medicine (Baltimore) 1986; 65: 268–279.

284 Piérard GE, Read D, Piérard-Franchimont C et al. Cutaneous manifestions in systemic trichosporonosis. Clin Exp Dermatol 1992; 17: 79–82.

285 Otsuka F, Seki Y, Takizawa K et al. Facial granuloma associated with *Trichosporon cutaneum* infection. Arch Dermatol 1986; 122: 1176–1179.

286 Nakagawa T, Nakashima K, Takaiwa T, Negayama K. *Trichosporon cutaneum (Trichosporon asabii)* infection mimicking hand eczema in a patient with leukemia. J Am Acad Dermatol 2000; 42: 929–931.

287 Han M-H, Choi J-H, Sung K-J et al. Onychomycosis and *Trichosporon beigelii* in Korea. Int J Dermatol 2000; 39: 266–269.

288 Steinman HK, Pappenfort RB. White piedra – a case report and review of the literature. Clin Exp Dermatol 1984; 9: 591–598.

289 Mostafa WZ, Al Jabre SH. White piedra in Saudi Arabia. Int J Dermatol 1992; 31: 501–502.

290 Benson PM, Lapins NA, Odom RB. White piedra. Arch Dermatol 1983; 119: 602–604.

291 Manzella JP, Berman IJ, Kukrika MD. *Trichosporon beigelii* fungemia and cutaneous dissemination. Arch Dermatol 1982; 118: 343–345.

292 Lassus A, Kanerva L, Stubb S. White piedra. Report of a case evaluated by scanning electron microscopy. Arch Dermatol 1982; 118: 208–211.

Systemic mycoses

293 Harrell ER, Curtis AC. North American blastomycosis. Am J Med 1959; 27: 750–766.

294 Malak JA, Farah FS. Blastomycosis in the Middle East. Report of a suspected case of North American blastomycosis. Br J Dermatol 1971; 84: 161–166.

295 Verma KK, Lakhanpal S, Sirka CS et al. Disseminated mucocutaneous blastomycosis in an immunocompetent Indian patient. J Eur Acad Dermatol Venereol 2000; 14: 332–333.

296 Yen A, Knipe RC, Tyring SK. Primary cutaneous blastomycosis: report of a case acquired by direct inoculation of a bullous pemphigoid lesion. J Am Acad Dermatol 1994; 31: 277–278.

297 Hay RJ. Blastomycosis: what's new? J Eur Acad Dermatol Venereol 2000; 14: 249–250.

298 Witorsch P, Utz JP. North American blastomycosis: a study of 40 patients. Medicine (Baltimore) 1968; 47: 169–200.

299 Hashimoto K, Kaplan RJ, Daman LA et al. Pustular blastomycosis. Int J Dermatol 1977; 16: 277–280.

300 Basler RSW, Lagomarsino SL. Coccidioidomycosis: clinical review and treatment update. Int J Dermatol 1979; 18: 104–110.

301 Stevens DA. Coccidioidomycosis. N Engl J Med 1995; 332: 1077–1082.

302 Deresinski SC, Stevens DA. Coccidioidomycosis in compromised hosts. Medicine (Baltimore) 1975; 54: 377–395.

303 Schwartz RA, Lamberts RJ. Isolated nodular cutaneous coccidioidomycosis. The initial manifestation of disseminated disease. J Am Acad Dermatol 1981; 4: 38–46.

304 Hamner RW, Baum EW, Pritchett PS. Coccidioidal meningitis diagnosed by skin biopsy. Cutis 1982; 29: 603–610.

305 Quimby SR, Connolly SM, Winkelmann RK, Smilack JD. Clinicopathologic spectrum of specific cutaneous lesions of disseminated coccidioidomycosis. J Am Acad Dermatol 1992; 26: 79–85.

306 Bayer AS, Yoshikawa TT, Galpin JE, Guze LB. Unusual syndromes of coccidioidomycosis: diagnostic and therapeutic considerations. A report of 10 cases and review of the English literature. Medicine (Baltimore) 1976; 55: 131–152.

307 Hobbs ER, Hempstead RW. Cutaneous coccidioidomycosis simulating lepromatous leprosy. Int J Dermatol 1984; 23: 334–336.

308 Choon SE, Khoo JJ. Coccidioidomycosis in Malaysia. Br J Dermatol 1999; 140: 557–558.

309 Bonifaz A, Saúl A, Galindo J, Andrade R. Primary cutaneous coccidioidomycosis treated with itraconazole. Int J Dermatol 1994; 33: 720–722.

310 Carroll GF, Haley LD, Brown JM. Primary cutaneous coccidioidomycosis. A review of the literature and a report of a new case. Arch Dermatol 1977; 113: 933–936.

311 Levan NE, Huntington RW. Primary cutaneous coccidioidomycosis in agricultural workers. Arch Dermatol 1965; 92: 215–220.

312 Westphal SA. Disseminated coccidioidomycosis associated with hypercalcemia. Mayo Clin Proc 1998; 73: 893–894.

313 Beard JS, Benson PM, Skillman L. Rapid diagnosis of coccidioidomycosis with a DNA probe to ribosomal RNA. Arch Dermatol 1993; 129: 1589–1593.

314 Waldman JS, Barr RJ, Espinoza FP, Simmons GE. Subcutaneous myospherulosis. J Am Acad Dermatol 1989; 21: 400–403.

315 Negroni R. Paracoccidioidomycosis (South American blastomycosis, Lutz's mycosis). Int J Dermatol 1993; 32: 847–859.

316 Dias MFRG, Pereira AC Jr, Pereira A Jr, Alves MSR. The role of HLA antigens in the development of paracoccidioidomycosis. J Eur Acad Dermatol Venereol 2000; 14: 166–171.

317 Murray HW, Littman ML, Roberts RB. Disseminated paracoccidioidomycosis (South American blastomycosis) in the United States. Am J Med 1974; 56: 209–220.

318 Bakos L, Kronfeld M, Hampse S et al. Disseminated paracoccidioidomycosis with skin lesions in a patient with acquired immunodeficiency syndrome. J Am Acad Dermatol 1989; 20: 854–855.

319 Gimenez MF, Tausk F, Gimenez MM, Gigli I. Langerhans' cells in paracoccidioidomycosis. Arch Dermatol 1987; 123: 479–481.

320 Bustinduy MG, Guimerá FJ, Arévalo P et al. Cutaneous primary paracoccidioidomycosis. J Eur Acad Dermatol Venereol 2000; 14: 113–117.

321 Kroll JJ, Walzer RA. Paracoccidioidomycosis in the United States. Arch Pathol 1972; 106: 543–546.

322 Ollague JM, de Zurita AM, Calero G. Paracoccidioidomycosis (South American blastomycosis) successfully treated with terbinafine: first case report. Br J Dermatol 2000; 143: 188–191.

323 Hernández-Pérez E, Orellana-Diaz O. Paracoccidioidomycosis. Report of the first autochthonous case in El Salvador. Int J Dermatol 1984; 23: 617–618.

324 Salfelder K, Doehnert G, Doehnert H-R. Paracoccidioidomycosis. Anatomic study with complete autopsies. Virchows Arch (Pathol Anat) 1969; 348: 51–76.

325 Goodwin RA, Shapiro JL, Thurman GH et al. Disseminated histoplasmosis: clinical and pathologic correlations. Medicine (Baltimore) 1980; 59: 1–33.

326 Peterson PK, Dahl MV, Howard RJ et al. Mucormycosis and cutaneous histoplasmosis in a renal transplant recipient. Arch Dermatol 1982; 118: 275–277.

327 Mayoral F, Penneys NS. Disseminated histoplasmosis presenting as a transepidermal elimination disorder in an AIDS victim. J Am Acad Dermatol 1985; 13: 842–844.

328 Hazelhurst JA, Vismer HF. Histoplasmosis presenting with unusual skin lesions in acquired immunodeficiency syndrome (AIDS). Br J Dermatol 1985; 113: 345–348.

329 Krunic AL, Calonje E, Jeftovic D et al. Primary localized cutaneous histoplasmosis in a patient with acquired immunodeficiency syndrome. Int J Dermatol 1995; 34: 558–562.

330 Chaker MB, Cockerell CJ. Concomitant psoriasis, seborrheic dermatitis, and disseminated cutaneous histoplasmosis in a patient infected with human immunodeficiency virus. J Am Acad Dermatol 1993; 29: 311–313.

331 Souza Filho FJ, Lopes M, Almeida OP, Scully C. Mucocutaneous histoplasmosis in AIDS. Br J Dermatol 1995; 133: 472–474.

332 Eidbo J, Sanchez RL, Tschen JA, Ellner KM. Cutaneous manifestations of histoplasmosis in the acquired immune deficiency syndrome. Am J Surg Pathol 1993; 17: 110–116.

333 Cohen PR, Bank DE, Silvers DN, Grossman ME. Cutaneous lesions of disseminated histoplasmosis in human immunodeficiency virus-infected patients. J Am Acad Dermatol 1990; 23: 422–428.

334 Bellman B, Berman B, Sasken H, Kirsner RS. Cutaneous disseminated histoplasmosis in AIDS patients in south Florida. Int J Dermatol 1997; 36: 599–603.

335 Bonifaz A, Cansela R, Novales J et al. Cutaneous histoplasmosis associated with acquired immunodeficiency syndrome (AIDS). Int J Dermatol 2000; 39: 35–38.

336 Paya CV, Roberts GD, Cockerill FR. Laboratory methods for the diagnosis of disseminated histoplasmosis: clinical importance of the lysis-centrifugation blood culture technique. Mayo Clin Proc 1987; 62: 480–485.

337 Sathapatayavongs B, Batteiger BE, Wheat J et al. Clinical and laboratory features of disseminated histoplasmosis during two large urban outbreaks. Medicine (Baltimore) 1983; 62: 263–270.

338 Witty LA, Steiner F, Curfman M et al. Disseminated histoplasmosis in patients receiving low-dose methotrexate therapy for psoriasis. Arch Dermatol 1992; 128: 91–93.

339 Yilmaz GG, Yilmaz E, Coskun M et al. Cutaneous histoplasmosis in a child with hyper-IgM. Pediatr Dermatol 1995; 12: 235–238.

340 Studdard J, Sneed WF, Taylor MR et al. Cutaneous histoplasmosis. Am Rev Respir Dis 1976; 113: 689–693.

341 Samovitz M, Dillon TK. Disseminated histoplasmosis presenting as exfoliative erythroderma. Arch Dermatol 1970; 101: 216–219.

342 Ozols II, Wheat LJ. Erythema nodosum in an epidemic of histoplasmosis in Indianapolis. Arch Dermatol 1981; 117: 709–712.

343 Soo-Hoo TS, Adam BA, Yusof D. Disseminated primary cutaneous histoplasmosis. Australas J Dermatol 1980; 21: 105–107.

344 Chanda JJ, Callen JP. Isolated nodular cutaneous histoplasmosis. Arch Dermatol 1978; 114: 1197–1198.

345 Nethercott JR, Schachter RK, Givan KF, Ryder DE. Histoplasmosis due to *Histoplasma capsulatum* var *duboisii* in a Canadian immigrant. Arch Dermatol 1978; 114: 595–598.

346 Williams AO, Lawson EA, Lucas AO. African histoplasmosis due to *Histoplasma duboisii*. Arch Pathol 1971; 92: 306–318.

347 Abildgaard WH, Hargrove RH, Kalivas J. *Histoplasma* panniculitis. Arch Dermatol 1985; 121: 914–916.

348 Johnston CA, Tang C-K, Jiji RM. Histoplasmosis of skin and lymph nodes and chronic lymphocytic leukemia. Arch Dermatol 1979; 115: 336–337.

349 Rodríguez G, Ordóñez N, Motta A. *Histoplasma capsulatum* var. *capsulatum* within cutaneous nerves in patients with disseminated histoplasmosis and AIDS. Br J Dermatol 2001; 144: 205–207.

350 Dumont A, Piche C. Electron microscopic study of human histoplasmosis. Arch Pathol 1969; 87: 168–178.

Infections by dematiaceous fungi

351 McGinnis MR, Hilger AE. Infections caused by black fungi. Arch Dermatol 1987; 123: 1300–1302.

352 Vollum DI. Chromomycosis: a review. Br J Dermatol 1977; 96: 454–458.

353 Wood C, Russel-Bell B. Characterization of pigmented fungi by melanin staining. Am J Dermatopathol 1983; 5: 77–81.

354 Fukushiro R. Chromomycosis in Japan. Int J Dermatol 1983; 22: 221–229.

355 Sindhuphak W, MacDonald E, Head E, Hudson RD. *Exophiala jeanselmei* infection in a postrenal transplant patient. J Am Acad Dermatol 1985; 13: 877–881.

356 McGinnis MR. Chromoblastomycosis and phaeohyphomycosis: New concepts, diagnosis, and mycology. J Am Acad Dermatol 1983; 8: 1–16.

357 Barba-Gómez JF, Mayorga J, McGinnis MR, González-Mendoza A. Chromoblastomycosis caused by *Exophiala spinifera*. J Am Acad Dermatol 1992; 26: 367–370.

358 Turiansky GW, Benson PM, Sperling LC et al. *Phialophora verrucosa*: a new cause of mycetoma. J Am Acad Dermatol 1995; 32: 311–315.

359 Matsumoto T, Matsuda T. Chromoblastomycosis and phaeohyphomycosis. Semin Dermatol 1985; 4: 240–251.

360 Ajello L, Georg LK, Steibgel RT, Wang CJK. A case of phaeohyphomycosis caused by a new species of *Phialophora*. Mycologia 1974; 66: 490–498.

361 Zaias N. Chromomycosis. J Cutan Pathol 1978; 5: 155–164.

362 Leslie DF, Beardmore GL. Chromoblastomycosis in Queensland: a retrospective study of 13 cases at the Royal Brisbane Hospital. Australas J Dermatol 1979; 20: 23–30.

363 Wortman PD. Concurrent chromoblastomycosis caused by *Fonsecaea pedrosoi* and actinomycetoma caused by *Nocardia brasiliensis*. J Am Acad Dermatol 1995; 32: 390–392.

364 Tomecki KJ, Steck WD, Hall GS, Dijkstra JWE. Subcutaneous mycoses. J Am Acad Dermatol 1989; 21: 785–790.

365 Santos LD, Arianayagam S, Dwyer B et al. Chromoblastomycosis: a retrospective study of six cases at the Royal Darwin Hospital from 1989 to 1994. Pathology 1996; 28: 182–187.

366 Iwatsu T, Takano M, Okamoto S. Auricular chromomycosis. Arch Dermatol 1983; 119: 88–89.

367 Bayles MAH. Chromomycosis. Treatment with thiabendazole. Arch Dermatol 1971; 104: 476–485.

368 Hiruma M, Ohnishi Y, Ohata H et al. Chromomycosis of the breast. Int J Dermatol 1992; 31: 184–185.

369 Rajendran C, Ramesh V, Misra RS et al. Chromoblastomycosis in India. Int J Dermatol 1997; 36: 29–33.

370 Sharma NL, Sharma RC, Grover PS et al. Chromoblastomycosis in India. Int J Dermatol 1999; 38: 846–851.

371 Mahaisavariya P, Chaiprasert A, Sivayathorn A, Khemngern S. Deep fungal and higher bacterial skin infections in Thailand: clinical manifestations and treatment regimens. Int J Dermatol 1999; 38: 279–284.

372 Redondo-Bellón P, Idoate M, Rubio M, Ignacio-Herrero J. Chromoblastomycosis produced by *Aureobasidium pullulans* in an immunosuppressed patient. Arch Dermatol 1997; 133: 663–664.

373 Ajello L. Phaeohyphomycosis: definition and etiology. In: Mycoses. Pan American Health Organization Scientific Publication No. 304. Washington DC: Pan American Health Organization, 1975; 126–130.

374 Rosen T, Overholt M. Persistent viability of the Medlar body. Int J Dermatol 1996; 35: 96–98.

375 Walter P, Garin Y, Richard-Lenoble D. Chromoblastomycosis. A morphological investigation of the host-parasite interaction. Virchows Arch (Pathol Anat) 1982; 397: 203–214.

376 Rosen T, Gyorkey F, Joseph LM, Batres E. Ultrastructural features of chromoblastomycosis. Int J Dermatol 1980; 19: 461–468.

377 Blakely FA, Rao BK, Wiley EL et al. Chromoblastomycosis with unusual histological features. J Cutan Pathol 1988; 15: 298 (abstract).

378 Lee M-WC, Hsu S, Rosen T. Spores and mycelia in cutaneous chromomycosis. J Am Acad Dermatol 1998; 39: 850–852.

379 Goette DK, Robertson D. Transepithelial elimination in chromomycosis. Arch Dermatol 1984; 120: 400–401.

380 Uitto J, Santa-Cruz DJ, Eisen AZ, Kobayashi GS. Chromomycosis. Successful treatment with 5-fluorocytosine. J Cutan Pathol 1979; 6: 77–84.

381 Caplan RM. Epidermoid carcinoma arising in extensive chromoblastomycosis. Arch Dermatol 1968; 97: 38–41.

382 Minotto R, Bernardi CDV, Mallmann LF et al. Chromoblastomycosis: A review of 100 cases in the state of Rio Grande do Sul, Brazil. J Am Acad Dermatol 2001; 44: 585–592.

383 Chuan M-T, Wu M-C. Subcutaneous phaeohyphomycosis caused by *Exophiala jeanselmei*: successful treatment with itraconazole. Int J Dermatol 1995; 34: 563–566.

384 Kim HU, Kang SH, Matsumoto T. Subcutaneous phaeohyphomycosis caused by *Exophiala jeanselmei* in a patient with advanced tuberculosis. Br J Dermatol 1998; 138: 351–353.

385 McCown HF, Sahn EE. Subcutaneous phaeohyphomycosis and nocardiosis in a kidney transplant patient. J Am Acad Dermatol 1997; 36: 863–866.

386 Kotylo PK, Israel KS, Cohen JS, Bartlett MS. Subcutaneous phaeohyphomycosis of the finger caused by *Exophiala spinifera*. Am J Clin Pathol 1989; 91: 624–627.

387 Woollons A, Darley CR, Pandian S et al. Phaeohyphomycosis caused by *Exophiala dermatitidis* following intra-articular steroid injection. Br J Dermatol 1996; 135: 475–477.

388 Berg D, Garcia JA, Schell WA et al. Cutaneous infection caused by *Curvularia pallescens*: a case report and review of the spectrum of disease. J Am Acad Dermatol 1995; 32: 375–378.

389 Coldiron BM, Wiley EL, Rinaldi MG. Cutaneous phaeohyphomycosis caused by a rare fungal pathogen, *Hormonema dematioides*: successful treatment with ketoconazole. J Am Acad Dermatol 1990; 23: 363–367.

390 Adam RD, Paquin ML, Petersen EA et al. Phaeohyphomycosis caused by the fungal genera *Bipolaris* and *Exserohilum*. A report of 9 cases and review of the literature. Medicine (Baltimore) 1986; 65: 203–217.

391 Straka BF, Cooper PH, Body BA. Cutaneous *Bipolaris spicifera* infection. Arch Dermatol 1989; 125: 1383–1386.

392 Hirsh AH, Schiff TA. Subcutaneous phaeohyphomycosis caused by an unusual pathogen: *Phoma* species. J Am Acad Dermatol 1996; 34: 679–680.

393 Oh C-K, Kwon K-S, Lee J-B et al. Subcutaneous pheohyphomycosis caused by *Phoma* species. Int J Dermatol 1998; 38: 874–876.

394 Suzuki Y, Udagawa S, Wakita H et al. Subcutaneous phaeohyphomycosis caused by *Geniculosporium* species: a new fungal pathogen. Br J Dermatol 1998; 138: 346–350.

395 Jacyk WK, Du Bruyn JH, Holm N et al. Cutaneous infection due to *Cladophialophora bantiana* in a patient receiving immunosuppressive therapy. Br J Dermatol 1997; 136: 428–430.

396 Patterson JW, Warren NG, Kelly LW. Cutaneous phaeohyphomycosis due to *Cladophialophora bantiana*. J Am Acad Dermatol 1999; 40: 364–366.

397 Pereiro M Jr, Jo-Chu J, Toribio J. Phaeohyphomycotic cyst due to *Cladosporium cladosporioides*. Dermatology 1998; 197: 90–92.

398 Ikai K, Tomono H, Watanabe S. Phaeohyphomycosis caused by *Phialophora richardsiae*. J Am Acad Dermatol 1988; 19: 478–481.

399 Burges GE, Walls CT, Maize JC. Subcutaneous phaeohyphomycosis caused by *Exserohilum rostratum* in an immunocompetent host. Arch Dermatol 1987; 123: 1346–1350.

400 Tieman JM, Furner BB. Phaeohyphomycosis caused by *Exserohilum rostratum* mimicking hemorrhagic herpes zoster. J Am Acad Dermatol 1991; 25: 852–854.

401 Hsu MM-L, Lee JY-Y. Cutaneous and subcutaneous phaeohyphomycosis caused by *Exserohilum rostratum*. J Am Acad Dermatol 1993; 28: 340–344.

402 Ronan SG, Uzoaru I, Nadimpalli V et al. Primary cutaneous phaeohyphomycosis: report of seven cases. J Cutan Pathol 1993; 20: 223–228.

403 Fathizadeh A, Rippon JW, Rosenfeld SI et al. Pheomycotic cyst in an immunosuppressed host. J Am Acad Dermatol 1981; 5: 423–427.

404 Hachisuka H, Matsumoto T, Kusuhara M et al. Cutaneous phaeohyphomycosis caused by *Exophiala jeanselmei* after renal transplantation. Int J Dermatol 1990; 29: 198–200.

405 Faulk CT, Lesher JL Jr. Phaeohyphomycosis and *Mycobacterium fortuitum* abscesses in a patient receiving corticosteroids for sarcoidosis. J Am Acad Dermatol 1995; 33: 309–311.

406 Weedon D, Ritchie G. Cystic chromomycosis of the skin. Pathology 1979; 11: 389–392.

407 Kempson RL, Sternberg WH. Chronic subcutaneous abscesses caused by pigmented fungi, a lesion distinguishable from cutaneous chromoblastomycosis. Am J Clin Pathol 1963; 39: 598–606.

408 Noel SB, Greer DL, Abadie SM et al. Primary cutaneous phaeohyphomycosis. Report of three cases. J Am Acad Dermatol 1988; 18: 1023–1030.

409 Schwartz IS, Emmons CW. Subcutaneous cystic granuloma caused by a fungus of wood pulp (*Phialophora richardsiae*). Am J Clin Pathol 1968; 49: 500–505.

410 Zackheim HS, Halde C, Goodman RS et al. Phaeohyphomycotic cyst of the skin caused by *Exophiala jeanselmei*. J Am Acad Dermatol 1985; 12: 207–212.

411 Tschen JA, Knox JM, McGavran MH, Duncan WC. Chromomycosis. The association of fungal elements and wood splinters. Arch Dermatol 1984; 120: 107–108.

412 Iwatsu T, Miyaji M. Phaeomycotic cyst. A case with a lesion containing a wood splinter. Arch Dermatol 1984; 120: 1209–1211.

413 Estes SA, Merz WG, Maxwell LG. Primary cutaneous phaeohyphomycosis caused by *Drechslera spicifera*. Arch Dermatol 1977; 113: 813–815.

414 Werner AH, Werner BE. Sporotrichosis in man and animal. Int J Dermatol 1994; 33: 692–700.

415 Grotte M, Younger B. Sporotrichosis associated with sphagnum moss exposure. Arch Pathol Lab Med 1981; 105: 50–51.

416 Auld JC, Beardmore GL. Sporotrichosis in Queensland: a review of 37 cases at the Royal Brisbane Hospital. Australas J Dermatol 1979; 20: 14–22.

417 Conias S, Wilson P. Epidemic cutaneous sporotrichosis: report of 16 cases in Queensland due to mouldy hay. Australas J Dermatol 1998; 39: 34–37.

418 Nusbaum BP, Gulbas N, Horwitz SN. Sporotrichosis acquired from a cat. J Am Acad Dermatol 1983; 8: 386–391.

419 Dunstan RW, Langham RF, Reimann KA, Wakenell PS. Feline sporotrichosis: A report of five cases with transmission to humans. J Am Acad Dermatol 1986; 15: 37–45.

420 Lurie HI. Histopathology of sporotrichosis. Notes on the nature of the asteroid body. Arch Pathol 1963; 75: 421–437.

421 Whitfield MJ, Faust HB. Lymphocutaneous sporotrichosis. Australas J Dermatol 1995; 36: 161–163.

422 Nakagawa T, Sasaki M, Ishihama Y, Takaiwa T. Reinfection with lymphocutaneous sporotrichosis. Br J Dermatol 1997; 137: 834–835.

423 Dolezal JF. Blastomycoid sporotrichosis. Response to low-dose amphotericin B. J Am Acad Dermatol 1981; 4: 523–527.

424 Shiraishi H, Gomi H, Kawada A et al. Solitary sporotrichosis lasting for 10 years. Dermatology 1999; 198: 100–101.

425 Prose NS, Milburn PB, Papayanopulos DM. Facial sporotrichosis in children. Pediatr Dermatol 1986; 3: 311–314.

426 Rudolph RI. Facial sporotrichosis in an infant. Cutis 1984; 33: 171–176.

427 Rafal ES, Rasmussen JE. An unusual presentation of fixed cutaneous sporotrichosis: a case report and review of the literature. J Am Acad Dermatol 1991; 25: 928–932.

428 Kwon K-S, Yim C-S, Jang H-S et al. Verrucous sporotrichosis in an infant treated with itraconazole. J Am Acad Dermatol 1998; 38: 112–114.

429 Dellatorre DL, Lattanand A, Buckley HR, Urbach F. Fixed cutaneous sporotrichosis of the face. J Am Acad Dermatol 1982; 6: 97–100.

430 Bonifaz A, Saúl A, Montes-de-Oca G, Mercadillo P. Superficial cutaneous sporotrichosis in specific anergic patient. Int J Dermatol 1999; 38: 700–703.

431 Kwon-Chung KJ. Comparison of isolates of *Sporothrix schenckii* obtained from fixed cutaneous lesions with isolates from other types of lesions. J Infect Dis 1979; 139: 424–431.

432 Bargman H. Sporotrichosis of the skin with spontaneous cure – report of a second case. J Am Acad Dermatol 1983; 8: 261–262.

433 Grekin RH. Sporotrichosis. Two cases of exogenous second infection. J Am Acad Dermatol 1984; 10: 233–234.

434 Kim S, Rusk MH, James WD. Erysipeloid sporotrichosis in a woman with Cushing's disease. J Am Acad Dermatol 1999; 40: 272–274.

435 Schamroth JM, Grieve TP, Kellen P. Disseminated sporotrichosis. Int J Dermatol 1988; 27: 28–30.

436 Smith PW, Loomis GW, Luckasen JL, Osterholm RK. Disseminated cutaneous sporotrichosis. Three illustrative cases. Arch Dermatol 1981; 117: 143–144.

437 Campos P, Arenas R, Coronado H. Primary cutaneous sporotrichosis. Int J Dermatol 1994; 33: 38–41.

438 Spiers EM, Hendrick SJ, Jorizzo JL, Solomon AR. Sporotrichosis masquerading as pyoderma gangrenosum. Arch Dermatol 1986; 122: 691–694.

439 Wilson DE, Mann JJ, Bennett JE, Utz JP. Clinical features of extracutaneous sporotrichosis. Medicine (Baltimore) 1967; 46: 265–279.

440 Ewing GE, Bosl GJ, Peterson PK. *Sporothrix schenckii* meningitis in a farmer with Hodgkin's disease. Am J Med 1980; 68: 455–457.

441 Purvis RS, Diven DG, Drechsel RD et al. Sporotrichosis presenting as arthritis and subcutaneous nodules. J Am Acad Dermatol 1993; 28: 879–884.

442 Shaw JC, Levinson W, Montanaro A. Sporotrichosis in the acquired immunodeficiency syndrome. J Am Acad Dermatol 1989; 21: 1145–1147.

443 Ware AJ, Cockerell CJ, Skiest DJ, Kussman HM. Disseminated sporotrichosis with extensive cutaneous involvement in a patient with AIDS. J Am Acad Dermatol 1999; 40: 350–355.

444 Lynch PJ, Voorhees JJ, Harrell ER. Sporotrichosis and sarcoidosis. Arch Dermatol 1971; 103: 298–303.

445 Plouffe JF, Silva J, Fekety R et al. Cell-mediated immune responses in sporotrichosis. J Infect Dis 1979; 139: 152–157.

446 del Pilar Agudelo S, Restrepo S, Darío Vélez I. Cutaneous New World leishmaniasis-sporotrichosis coinfection: Report of 3 cases. J Am Acad Dermatol 1999; 40: 1002–1004.

447 Bullpitt P, Weedon D. Sporotrichosis: a review of 39 cases. Pathology 1978; 10: 249–256.

448 Maberry JD, Mullins JF, Stone OJ. Sporotrichosis with demonstration of hyphae in human tissue. Arch Dermatol 1966; 93: 65–67.

449 Shelley WB, Sica PA. Disseminate sporotrichosis of skin and bone cured with 5-fluorocytosine: photosensitivity as a complication. J Am Acad Dermatol 1983; 8: 229–235.

450 Rodríguez G, Sarmiento L. The asteroid bodies of sporotrichosis. Am J Dermatopathol 1998; 20: 246–249.

451 Fetter BF, Tindall JP. Cutaneous sporotrichosis. Arch Dermatol 1964; 78: 613–617.

452 Hachisuka H, Sasai Y. A peculiar case of sporotrichosis. Dermatologica 1980; 160: 37–40.

453 Bickley LK, Berman IJ, Hood AF. Fixed cutaneous sporotrichosis: unusual histopathology following intralesional corticosteroid administration. J Am Acad Dermatol 1985; 12: 1007–1012.

454 Reid BJ. Exophiala werneckii causing tinea nigra in Scotland. Br J Dermatol 1998; 139: 157–158.

455 Gupta G, Burden AD, Shankland GS et al. Tinea nigra secondary to Exophiala werneckii responding to itraconazole. Br J Dermatol 1997; 137: 483–484.

456 Chadfield HW, Campbell CK. A case of tinea nigra in Britain. Br J Dermatol 1972; 87: 505–508.

457 Hughes JR, Moore MK, Pembroke AC. Tinea nigra palmaris. Clin Exp Dermatol 1993; 18: 481–482.

458 Tay Y-K, Koh M-T. Pigmented palmar patch in a child. Pediatr Dermatol 1998; 15: 233–234.

459 Miles WJ, Branom WT, Frank SB. Tinea nigra. Arch Dermatol 1966; 94: 203–204.

460 Isaacs F, Reiss-Levy E. Tinea nigra plantaris: a case report. Australas J Dermatol 1980; 21: 13–15.

461 Dummer R, Meyer J. A growing brownish macule on the sole of a doctor's spouse. Dermatology 2000; 200: 368–369.

462 Babel DE, Pelachyk JM, Hurley JP. Tinea nigra masquerading as acral lentiginous melanoma. J Dermatol Surg Oncol 1986; 12: 502–504.

463 Mitchell AJ, Solomon AR, Beneke ES, Anderson TF. Subcutaneous alternariosis. J Am Acad Dermatol 1983; 8: 673–676.

464 Saenz-Santamaria MC, Gilaberte Y, Garcia-Latasa FJ, Carapeto FJ. Cutaneous alternariosis in a nonimmunocompromised patient. Int J Dermatol 1995; 34: 556–557.

465 del Palacio A, Gómez-Hernando C, Revenga F. Cutaneous Alternaria alternata infection successfully treated with itraconazole. Clin Exp Dermatol 1996; 21: 241–243.

466 Altomare GF, Capella GL, Boneschi V, Viviani MA. Effectiveness of terbinafine in cutaneous alternariosis. Br J Dermatol 2000; 142: 840–841.

467 Baykal C, Kazancioğlu R, Büyükbabani N et al. Simultaneous cutaneous and ungual alternariosis in a renal transplant recipient. Br J Dermatol 2000; 143: 910–912.

468 Gilmour TK, Rytina E, O'Connell PB, Sterling JC. Cutaneous alternariosis in a cardiac transplant recipient. Australas J Dermatol 2001; 42: 46–49.

469 Pedersen NB, Mardh P-A, Hallberg T, Jonsson N. Cutaneous alternariosis. Br J Dermatol 1976; 94: 201–209.

470 Iwatsu T. Cutaneous alternariosis. Arch Dermatol 1988; 124: 1822–1825.

471 Duffill MB, Coley KE. Cutaneous phaeohyphomycosis due to Alternaria alternata responding to itraconazole. Clin Exp Dermatol 1993; 18: 156–158.

472 Palencarova E, Jesenska Z, Plank L et al. Phaeohyphomycosis caused by Alternaria species and Phaeosclera dematioides Sigler, Tsuneda and Carmichael. Clin Exp Dermatol 1995; 20: 419–422.

473 Lerner LH, Lerner EA, Bello YM. Co-existence of cutaneous and presumptive pulmonary alternariosis. Int J Dermatol 1997; 36: 285–288.

474 Acland KM, Hay RJ, Groves R. Cutaneous infection with Alternaria alternata complicating immunosuppression: successful treatment with itraconazole. Br J Dermatol 1998; 138: 354–356.

475 Ioannidou DJ, Stefanidou MP, Maraki SG et al. Cutaneous alternariosis in a patient with idiopathic pulmonary fibrosis. Int J Dermatol 2000; 39: 293–295.

476 Magina S, Lisboa C, Santos P et al. Cutaneous alternariosis by Alternaria chartarum in a renal transplanted patient. Br J Dermatol 2000; 142: 1261–1262.

477 Bartolome B, Valks R, Fraga J et al. Cutaneous alternariosis due to Alternaria chlamydospora after bone marrow transplantation. Acta Derm Venereol 1999; 79: 244.

478 Bourlond A, Alexandre G. Dermal alterniasis in a kidney transplant recipient. Dermatologica 1984; 168: 152–156.

479 Farmer SG, Komorowski RA. Cutaneous microabscess formation from Alternaria alternata. Am J Clin Pathol 1976; 66: 565–569.

480 Higashi N, Asada Y. Cutaneous alternariosis with mixed infection of Candida albicans. Arch Dermatol 1973; 108: 558–560.

481 Bourlond A. Alternariasis: ultrastructure of skin granuloma. J Cutan Pathol 1983; 10: 123–132.

Mycetoma and morphologically similar conditions

482 Zaias N, Taplin D, Rebell G. Mycetoma. Arch Dermatol 1969; 99: 215–225.

483 Palestine RF, Rogers RS III. Diagnosis and treatment of mycetoma. J Am Acad Dermatol 1982; 6: 107–111.

484 Fahal AH, Hassan MA. Mycetoma. Br J Surg 1992; 79: 1138–1141.

485 Welsh O. Mycetoma. Current concepts in treatment. Int J Dermatol 1991; 30: 387–396.

486 Barnetson RStC, Milne LJR. Mycetoma. Br J Dermatol 1978; 99: 227–231.

487 Mahgoub ES. Mycetoma. Semin Dermatol 1985; 4: 230–239.

488 Degavre B, Joujoux JM, Dandurand M, Guillot B. First report of mycetoma caused by Arthrographis kalrae: Successful treatment with itraconazole. J Am Acad Dermatol 1997; 37: 318–320.

489 Satta R, Sanna S, Cottoni F. Madurella infection in an immunocompromised host. Int J Dermatol 2000; 39: 939–941.

490 Welsh O, Sauceda E, Gonzalez J, Ocampo J. Amikacin alone and in combination with trimethoprim-sulfamethoxazole in the treatment of actinomycotic mycetoma. J Am Acad Dermatol 1987; 17: 443–448.

491 West BC, Kwon-Chung KJ. Mycetoma caused by Microsporum audouinii. Am J Clin Pathol 1980; 73: 447–454.

492 Chen AWJ, Kuo JWL, Chen J-S et al. Dermatophyte pseudomycetoma: a case report. Br J Dermatol 1993; 129: 729–732.

493 Magana M. Mycetoma. Int J Dermatol 1984; 23: 221–236.

494 Butz WC, Ajello L. Black grain mycetoma. A case due to Madurella grisea. Arch Dermatol 1971; 104: 197–201.

495 Hay RJ, Mackenzie DWR. Mycetoma (madura foot) in the United Kingdom – a survey of forty-four cases. Clin Exp Dermatol 1983; 8: 553–562.

496 Muir DB, Pritchard RC. Eumycotic mycetoma due to Madurella grisea. Australas J Dermatol 1986; 27: 33–34.

497 Sindhuphak W, Macdonald E, Head E. Actinomycetoma caused by Nocardiopsis dassonvillei. Arch Dermatol 1985; 121: 1332–1334.

498 Kandhari KC, Mohapatra LN, Sehgal VN, Gugnani HC. Black grain mycetoma of foot. Arch Dermatol 1964; 89: 867–870.

499 Findlay GH, Vismer HF. Black grain mycetoma. Br J Dermatol 1974; 91: 297–303.

500 Hay RJ, Mackenzie DWR. The histopathological features of pale grain eumycetoma. Trans R Soc Trop Med Hyg 1982; 76: 839–844.

501 Venugopal PV, Venugopal TV. Pale grain eumycetomas in Madras. Australas J Dermatol 1995; 36: 149–151.

502 Hood SV, Moore CB, Cheesbrough JS et al. Atypical eumycetoma caused by Phialophora parasitica successfully treated with itraconazole and flucytosine. Br J Dermatol 1997; 136: 953–956.

503 Moeller CA, Burton CS III. Primary lymphocutaneous Nocardia brasiliensis infection. Arch Dermatol 1987; 122: 1180–1182.

504 Satterwhite TK, Wallace RJ Jr. Primary cutaneous nocardiosis. JAMA 1979; 242: 333–336.

505 Callen JP, Kingman J. Disseminated cutaneous Nocardia brasiliensis infection. Pediatr Dermatol 1984; 2: 49–51.

506 Naka W, Miyakawa S, Niizeki H et al. Unusually located lymphocutaneous nocardiosis caused by Nocardia brasiliensis. Br J Dermatol 1995; 132: 609–613.

507 Saul A, Bonifaz A, Messina M, Andrade R. Mycetoma due to Nocardia caviae. Int J Dermatol 1987; 26: 174–177.

508 Yang L-J, Chan H-L, Chen W-J, Kuo T-T. Lymphocutaneous nocardiosis caused by Nocardia caviae: the first case report from Asia. J Am Acad Dermatol 1993; 29: 639–641.

509 Shimizu T, Furumoto H, Asagami C et al. Disseminated subcutaneous Nocardia farcinica abscesses in a nephrotic syndrome patient. J Am Acad Dermatol 1998; 38: 874–876.

510 Schiff TA, Goldman R, Sanchez M et al. Primary lymphocutaneous nocardiosis caused by an unusual species of Nocardia: Nocardia transvalensis. J Am Acad Dermatol 1993; 28: 336–340.

511 Saarinen KA, Lestringant GG, Czechowski J, Frossard PM. Cutaneous nocardiosis of the chest wall and pleura – 10-year consequences of a hand actinomycetoma. Dermatology 2001; 202: 131–133.

512 Curry WA. Human nocardiosis. A clinical review with selected case reports. Arch Intern Med 1980; 140: 818–826.

513 Frazier AR, Rosenow EC III, Roberts GD. Nocardiosis. A review of 25 cases occurring during 24 months. Mayo Clin Proc 1975; 50: 657–663.

514 Shapiro PE, Grossman MC. Disseminated Nocardia asteroides with pustules. J Am Acad Dermatol 1989; 20: 889–892.

515 Kalb RE, Kaplan MH, Grossman ME. Cutaneous nocardiosis. Case reports and review. J Am Acad Dermatol 1985; 13: 125–133.

516 Boixeda P, España A, Suarez J et al. Cutaneous nocardiosis and human immunodeficiency virus infection. Int J Dermatol 1991; 30: 804–805.

517 Karakayali G, Karaarslan A, Artüz F et al. Primary cutaneous Nocardia asteroides. Br J Dermatol 1998; 139: 919–920.

518 Merigou D, Beylot-Barry M, Ly S et al. Primary cutaneous Nocardia asteroides infection after heart transplantation. Dermatology 1998; 196: 246–247.

519 Hornef MW, Gandorfer A, Heesemann J, Roggenkamp A. Humoral response in a patient with cutaneous nocardiosis. Dermatology 2000; 200: 78–80.

520 Chung YL, Park J-C, Takatori K, Lee KH. Primary cutaneous nocardiosis mimicking lupus erythematosus. Br J Dermatol 2001; 144: 639–641.

521 Moore M, Conrad AH. Sporotrichoid nocardiosis caused by Nocardia brasiliensis. Arch Dermatol 1967; 95: 390–393.

522 Rapaport J. Primary chancriform syndrome caused by Nocardia brasiliensis. Arch Dermatol 1966; 93: 62–64.

523 Lampe RM, Baker CJ, Septimus EJ, Wallace RJ Jr. Cervicofacial nocardiosis in children. J Pediatr 1981; 99: 593–595.

524 Wlodaver CG, Tolomeo T, Benear JB. Primary cutaneous nocardiosis mimicking sporotrichosis. Arch Dermatol 1988; 124: 659–660.

525 Paredes BE, Hunger RE, Braathen LR, Brand CU. Cutaneous nocardiosis caused by Nocardia brasiliensis after an insect bite. Dermatology 1999; 198: 159–161.

526 Hironaga M, Mochizuki T, Watanabe S. Acute primary cutaneous nocardiosis. J Am Acad Dermatol 1990; 23: 399–400.

527 Harth Y, Friedman-Birnbaum R, Lefler E, Bergman R. Two patients with simultaneous, unusually located primary cutaneous nocardiosis. J Am Acad Dermatol 1992; 26: 132–133.

528 Angelika J, Hans-Jürgen G, Uwe-Frithjof H. Primary cutaneous nocardiosis in a husband and wife. J Am Acad Dermatol 1999; 41: 338–340.

529 Zecler E, Gilboa Y, Elkina L et al. Lymphocutaneous nocardiosis due to Nocardia brasiliensis. Arch Dermatol 1977; 113: 642–643.

530 Aydingöz İE, Candan İ, Dervent B, Hitit G. Primary cutaneous nocardiosis associated with intra-articular corticosteroid injection. Int J Dermatol 2001; 40: 196–198.

531 Tsuboi R, Takamori K, Ogawa H et al. Lymphocutaneous nocardiosis caused by Nocardia asteroides. Case report and literature review. Arch Dermatol 1986; 122: 1183–1185.

532 Schreiner DT, de Castro P, Jorizzo JL et al. Disseminated Nocardia brasiliensis infection following cryptococcal disease. Arch Dermatol 1986; 122: 1186–1190.

533 Lee M-S, Sippe JR. Primary cutaneous nocardiosis. Australas J Dermatol 1999; 40: 103–105.

534 Kannon GA, Kuechle MK, Garrett AB. Superficial cutaneous Nocardia asteroides infection in an immunocompetent pregnant woman. J Am Acad Dermatol 1996; 35: 1000–1002.

535 Ng CS, Hellinger WC. Superficial cutaneous abscess and multiple brain abscesses from Nocardia asteroides in an immunocompetent patient. J Am Acad Dermatol 1998; 39: 793–794.

536 Soto-Mendoza N, Bonifaz A. Head actinomycetoma with a double aetiology, caused by Nocardia brasiliensis and N. asteroides. Br J Dermatol 2000; 143: 192–194.

537 Pelzer K, Tietz HJ, Sterry W, Haas N. Isolation of both Sporothrix schenckii and Nocardia asteroides from a mycetoma of the forefoot. Br J Dermatol 2000; 143: 1311–1315.

538 Nishimoto K, Ohno M. Subcutaneous abscesses caused by Nocardia brasiliensis complicated by malignant lymphoma. Int J Dermatol 1985; 24: 437–440.

539 Boudoulas O, Camisa C. Nocardia asteroides infection with dissemination to skin and joints. Arch Dermatol 1985; 121: 898–900.

540 Curley RK, Hayward T, Holden CA. Cutaneous abscesses due to systemic nocardiosis – a case report. Clin Exp Dermatol 1990; 15: 459–461.

541 Brown JR. Human actinomycosis. A study of 181 subjects. Hum Pathol 1973; 4: 319–330.

542 Verma KK, Lakhanpal S, Sirka CS et al. Primary cutaneous actinomycosis. Acta Derm Venereol 1999; 79: 327.

543 Chang SN, Wee SH, Shim JY et al. Primary cutaneous actinomycosis on the thigh. J Cutan Pathol 2000; 27: 552–553 (abstract).

544 Ramam M, Garg T, D'Souza P et al. A two-step schedule for the treatment of actinomycotic mycetomas. Acta Derm Venereol 2000; 80: 378–380.

545 Cirillo-Hyland V, Herzberg A, Jaworsky C. Cervicofacial actinomycosis resembling a ruptured cyst. J Am Acad Dermatol 1993; 29: 308–311.

546 Varkey B, Landis FB, Tang TT, Rose HD. Thoracic actinomycosis. Dissemination to skin, subcutaneous tissue, and muscle. Arch Intern Med 1974; 134: 689–693.

547 Rigopoulos D, Mavridou M, Nicolaidou E et al. Mycetoma due to actinomycetes: a rare entity in Europe. Int J Dermatol 2000; 39: 557–558.

548 Elgart GW, Rotman DA. Localized cutaneous actinomycetoma due to Streptomyces infection: histologic features and clinical course. J Cutan Pathol 2000; 27: 555 (abstract).

549 Robboy SJ, Vickery AL Jr. Tinctorial and morphologic properties distinguishing actinomycosis and nocardiosis. N Engl J Med 1970; 282: 593–596.

550 Hacker P. Botryomycosis. Int J Dermatol 1983; 22: 455–458.

551 Mehregan DA, Su WPD, Anhalt JP. Cutaneous botryomycosis. J Am Acad Dermatol 1991; 24: 393–396.

552 Bonifaz A, Carrasco E. Botryomycosis. Int J Dermatol 1996; 35: 381–388.

553 Picou K, Batres E, Jarratt M. Botryomycosis. A bacterial cause of mycetoma. Arch Dermatol 1979; 115: 609–610.

554 Waisman M. Staphylococcic actinophytosis (botryomycosis). Arch Dermatol 1962; 86: 525–529.

555 Simantov A, Chosidow O, Fraitag S et al. Disseminated cutaneous botryomycosis – an unexpected diagnosis after 20 years' duration. Clin Exp Dermatol 1994; 19: 259–261.

556 Calegari L, Gezuele E, Torres E, Carmona C. Botryomycosis caused by Pseudomonas vesicularis. Int J Dermatol 1996; 35: 817–818.

557 Brunken RC, Lichon-Chao N, van den Broek H. Immunologic abnormalities in botryomycosis. J Am Acad Dermatol 1983; 9: 428–434.

558 Defraigne JO, Demoulin JC, Piérard GE et al. Fatal mural endocarditis and cutaneous botryomycosis after heart transplantation. Am J Dermatopathol 1997; 19: 602–605.

559 Patterson JW, Kitces EN, Neafie RC. Cutaneous botryomycosis in a patient with acquired immunodeficiency syndrome. J Am Acad Dermatol 1987; 16: 238–242.

560 Leibowitz MR, Asvat MS, Kalla AA, Wing G. Extensive botryomycosis in a patient with diabetes and chronic active hepatitis. Arch Dermatol 1981; 117: 739–742.

561 Toth IR, Kazal HL. Botryomycosis in acquired immunodeficiency syndrome. Arch Pathol Lab Med 1987; 111: 246–249.

562 Harman RRM, English MP, Halford M et al. Botryomycosis: a complication of extensive follicular mucinosis. Br J Dermatol 1980; 102: 215–222.

563 Olmstead PM, Finn M. Botryomycosis in pierced ears. Arch Dermatol 1982; 118: 925–927.

564 Bishop GF, Greer KE, Horwitz DA. Pseudomonas botryomycosis. Arch Dermatol 1976; 112: 1568–1570.

565 Hoffman TE, Russell B, Jacobs PH. Mycetoma-like infection caused by previously undescribed bacterium. Arch Dermatol 1978; 114: 1199–1202.

566 Goette DK. Transepithelial elimination in botryomycosis. Int J Dermatol 1981; 20: 198–200.

567 Martin-Pascual A, Perez AG. Botryomycosis. Dermatologica 1975; 151: 302–308.

Zygomycoses

568 Parker C, Kaminski G, Hill D. Zygomycosis in a tattoo, caused by Saksenaea vasiformis. Australas J Dermatol 1986; 27: 107–111.

569 Bateman CP, Umland ET, Becker LE. Cutaneous zygomycosis in a patient with lymphoma. J Am Acad Dermatol 1983; 8: 890–894.

570 Kerr PG, Turner H, Davidson A et al. Zygomycosis requiring amputation of the hand: an isolated case in a patient receiving haemodialysis. Med J Aust 1988; 148: 258–259.

571 du Plessis PJ, Wentzel LF, Delport SD, van Damme E. Zygomycotic necrotizing cellulitis in a premature infant. Dermatology 1997; 195: 179–181.

572 Marchevsky AM, Bottone EJ, Geller SA, Giger DK. The changing spectrum of disease, etiology, and diagnosis of mucormycosis. Hum Pathol 1980; 11: 457–464.

573 Howard DH. Classification of the Mucorales. In: Lehrer RI, Moderator. Mucormycosis. Ann Intern Med 1980; 93: 93–94.

574 Edwards JE. Clinical aspects of mucormycosis. In: Lehrer RI, Moderator. Mucormycosis. Ann Intern Med 1980; 93: 96–99.

575 Clark R, Greer DL, Carlisle T, Carroll B. Cutaneous zygomycosis in a diabetic HTLV-1-seropositive man. J Am Acad Dermatol 1990; 22: 956–959.

576 Woods SG, Elewski BE. Zosteriform zygomycosis. J Am Acad Dermatol 1995; 32: 357–361.

577 Weinberg JM, Baxt RD, Egan CL et al. Mucormycosis in a patient with acquired immunodeficiency syndrome. Arch Dermatol 1997; 133: 249–251.

578 Gartenberg G, Bottone EJ, Keusch GT, Weitzman I. Hospital-acquired mucormycosis (Rhizopus rhizopodiformis) of skin and subcutaneous tissue. N Engl J Med 1978; 299: 1115–1118.

579 Hammond DE, Winkelmann RK. Cutaneous phycomycosis. Report of three cases with identification of Rhizopus. Arch Dermatol 1979; 115: 990–992.

580 Veliath AJ, Rao R, Prabhu MR, Aurora AL. Cutaneous phycomycosis (mucormycosis) with fatal pulmonary dissemination. Arch Dermatol 1976; 112: 509–512.

581 Maliwan N, Reyes CV, Rippon JW. Osteomyelitis secondary to cutaneous mucormycosis. Am J Dermatopathol 1984; 6: 479–481.

582 Myskowski PL, Brown AE, Dinsmore R et al. Mucormycosis following bone marrow transplantation. J Am Acad Dermatol 1983; 9: 111–115.

583 Wirth F, Perry R, Eskenazi A et al. Cutaneous mucormycosis with subsequent visceral dissemination in a child with neutropenia: A case report and review of the pediatric literature. J Am Acad Dermatol 1996; 35: 336–341.

584 Meyer RD, Kaplan MH, Ong M, Armstrong D. Cutaneous lesions in disseminated mucormycosis. JAMA 1973; 225: 737–738.

585 Sanchez MR, Ponge-Wilson I, Moy JA, Rosenthal S. Zygomycosis and HIV infection. J Am Acad Dermatol 1994; 30: 904–908.

586 Craig NM, Lueder FL, Pensler JM et al. Disseminated *Rhizopus* infection in a premature infant. Pediatr Dermatol 1994; 11: 346–350.

587 Stoebner PE, Gaspard C, Mourad G et al. Fulminant mucormycosis in a renal transplant recipient. Acta Derm Venereol 2000; 80: 305.

588 Kramer BS, Hernandez AD, Reddick RL, Levine AS. Cutaneous infarction. Manifestation of disseminated mucormycosis. Arch Dermatol 1977; 113: 1075–1076.

589 Khardori N, Hayat S, Rolston K, Bodey GP. Cutaneous *Rhizopus* and *Aspergillus* infections in five patients with cancer. Arch Dermatol 1989; 125: 952–956.

590 Prevoo RLMA, Starink TM, de Haan P. Primary cutaneous mucormycosis in a healthy young girl. J Am Acad Dermatol 1991; 24: 882–885.

591 Umbert IJ, Su WPD. Cutaneous mucormycosis. J Am Acad Dermatol 1989; 21: 1232–1234.

592 Geller JD, Peters MS, Su WPD. Cutaneous mucormycosis resembling superficial granulomatous pyoderma in an immunocompetent host. J Am Acad Dermatol 1993; 29: 462–465.

593 Tio TH, Djojopranoto M, Eng N-IT. Subcutaneous phycomycosis. Arch Dermatol 1966; 93: 550–553.

594 Harman RRM, Jackson H, Willis AJP. Subcutaneous phycomycosis in Nigeria. Br J Dermatol 1964; 76: 408–420.

595 Bittencourt AL, Arruda SM, Freire de Andrade JA, Carvalho EM. Basidiobolomycosis: a case report. Pediatr Dermatol 1991; 8: 325–328.

596 Sivaraman, Thappa DM, Karthikeyan, Hemanthkumar. Subcutaneous phycomycosis mimicking synovial sarcoma. Int J Dermatol 1999; 38: 920–923.

597 Mugerwa JW. Subcutaneous phycomycosis in Uganda. Br J Dermatol 1976; 94: 539–544.

598 Miller RI, Campbell RSF. The comparative pathology of equine cutaneous phycomycosis. Vet Pathol 1984; 21: 325–332.

599 Miller RI, Olcott BM, Archer M. Cutaneous pythiosis in beef calves. JAVMA 1985; 186: 984–985.

600 Triscott JA, Weedon D, Cabana E. Human subcutaneous pythiosis. J Cutan Pathol 1993; 20: 267–271.

601 Symmers W St C. Histopathologic aspects of the pathogenesis of some opportunistic fungal infections, as exemplified in the pathology of aspergillosis and the phycomycetoses. Lab Invest 1962; 11: 1073–1090.

602 Herstoff JK, Bogaars H, McDonald CJ. *Rhinophycomycosis entomophthorae*. Arch Dermatol 1978; 114: 1674–1678.

603 Towersey L, Wanke B, Ribeiro Estrella R et al. *Conidiobolus coronatus* infection treated with ketoconazole. Arch Dermatol 1988; 124: 1392–1396.

604 Williams AO. Pathology of phycomycosis due to *Entomophthora* and *Basidiobolus* species. Arch Pathol 1969; 87: 13–20.

605 Williams AO, von Lichtenberg F, Smith JH, Martinson FD. Ultrastructure of phycomycosis due to *Entomophthora, Basidiobolus*, and associated 'Splendore–Hoeppli' phenomenon. Arch Pathol 1969; 87: 459–468.

606 de León-Bojorge B, Ruiz-Maldonado R, López-Martinez R. Subcutaneous phycomycosis caused by *Basidiobolus haptosporus*: a clinicopathologic and mycologic study in a child. Pediatr Dermatol 1988; 5: 33–36.

607 Scholtens RE, Harrison SM. Subcutaneous phycomycosis. Trop Geogr Med 1994; 46: 371–373.

Hyalohyphomycoses

608 Griffin TD, McFarland JP, Johnson WC. Hyalohyphomycosis masquerading as squamous cell carcinoma. J Cutan Pathol 1991; 18: 116–119.

609 Vasiloudes P, Morelli JG, Weston WL. Painful skin papules caused by concomitant *Acremonium* and *Fusarium* infection in a neutropenic child. J Am Acad Dermatol 1997; 37: 1006–1008.

610 Bernstein EF, Schuster MG, Stieritz DD et al. Disseminated cutaneous *Pseudallescheria boydii*. Br J Dermatol 1995; 132: 456–460.

611 Leigheb G, Mossini A, Boggio P et al. Sporotrichosis-like lesions caused by a *Paecilomyces* genus fungus. Int J Dermatol 1994; 33: 275–276.

612 Itin PH, Frei R, Lautenschlager S et al. Cutaneous manifestations of *Paecilomyces lilacinus* infection induced by a contaminated skin lotion in patients who are severely immunosuppressed. J Am Acad Dermatol 1998; 39: 401–409.

613 Hecker MS, Weinberg JM, Bagheri B et al. Cutaneous *Paecilomyces lilacinus* infection: Report of two novel cases. J Am Acad Dermatol 1997; 37: 270–271.

614 Marchese SM, Smoller BR. Cutaneous *Paecilomyces lilacinus* infection in a hospitalized patient taking corticosteroids. Int J Dermatol 1998; 37: 438–441.

615 Diven DG, Newton RC, Sang JL et al. Cutaneous hyalohyphomycosis caused by *Paecilomyces lilacinus* in a patient with lymphoma. J Am Acad Dermatol 1996; 35: 779–781.

616 Naldi L, Lovati S, Farina C et al. *Paecilomyces marquandii* cellulitis in a kidney transplant patient. Br J Dermatol 2000; 143: 647–649.

617 Blackwell V, Ahmed K, O'Docherty C, Hay RJ. Cutaneous hyalohyphomycosis caused by *Paecilomyces lilacinus* in a renal transplant patient. Br J Dermatol 2000; 143: 873–875.

618 English MP. Invasion of the skin by filamentous non-dermatophyte fungi. Br J Dermatol 1968; 80: 282–286.

619 Alvarez-Franco M, Reyes-Mugica M, Paller AS. Cutaneous *Fusarium* infection in an adolescent with acute leukemia. Pediatr Dermatol 1992; 9: 62–65.

620 Prins C, Chavaz P, Tamm K, Hauser C. Ecthyma gangrenosum-like lesions: a sign of disseminated *Fusarium* infection in the neutropenic patient. Clin Exp Dermatol 1995; 20: 428–430.

621 Arrese JE, Piérard-Franchimont C, Piérard GE. Fatal hyalohyphomycosis following *Fusarium* onychomycosis in an immunocompromised patient. Am J Dermatopathol 1996; 18: 196–198.

622 Repiso T, García-Patos V, Martin N et al. Disseminated fusariosis. Pediatr Dermatol 1996; 13: 118–121.

623 Pereiro M Jr, Labandeira J, Toribio J. Plantar hyperkeratosis due to *Fusarium verticillioides* in a patient with malignancy. Clin Exp Dermatol 1999; 24: 175–178.

624 Antony SJ. Disseminated *Fusarium* infection in an immunocompromised host. Int J Dermatol 1996; 35: 815–816.

625 Costa AR, Valente NYS, Criado PR et al. Invasive hyalohyphomycosis due to *Fusarium solani* in a patient with acute lymphocytic leukemia. Int J Dermatol 2000; 39: 717–718.

626 Pereiro M Jr, Abalde MT, Zulaica A et al. Chronic infection due to *Fusarium oxysporum* mimicking lupus vulgaris: case report and review of cutaneous involvement in fusariosis. Acta Derm Venereol 2001; 81: 51–53.

627 Borradori L, Schmit J-C, Stetzkowski M et al. *Penicilliosis marneffei* infection in AIDS. J Am Acad Dermatol 1994; 31: 843–846.

628 Liu M-T, Wong C-K, Fung C-P. Disseminated *Penicillium marneffei* infection with cutaneous lesions in an HIV-positive patient. Br J Dermatol 1994; 131: 280–283.

629 Wortman PD. Infection with *Penicillium marneffei*. Int J Dermatol 1996; 35: 393–399.

630 Nelson KE, Sirisanthana T. Disseminated *Penicillium marneffei* infection in a patient with AIDS. N Engl J Med 2001; 344: 1763.

631 Gillum PS, Gurswami A, Taira JW. Localized cutaneous infection by *Scedosporium prolificans (inflatum)*. Int J Dermatol 1997; 36: 297–299.

632 Kim HU, Kim SC, Lee HS. Localized skin infection due to *Scedosporium apiospermum*: report of two cases. Br J Dermatol 1999; 141: 605–606.

633 Miyamoto T, Sasaoka R, Kawaguchi M et al. *Scedosporium apiospermum* skin infection: A case report and review of the literature. J Am Acad Dermatol 1998; 39: 498–500.

634 Kusuhara M, Hachisuka H. Lymphocutaneous infection due to *Scedosporium apiospermum*. Int J Dermatol 1997; 36: 684–688.

635 Liu YF, Zhao XD, Ma CL et al. Cutaneous infection by *Scedosporium apiospermum* and its successful treatment with itraconazole. Clin Exp Dermatol 1997; 22: 198–200.

636 Lavigne C, Maillot F, de Muret A et al. Cutaneous infection with *Scedosporium apiospermum* in a patient treated with corticosteroids. Acta Derm Venereol 1999; 79: 402–403.

637 Veglia KS, Marks VJ. Fusarium as a pathogen. A case report of *Fusarium* sepsis and review of the literature. J Am Acad Dermatol 1987; 16: 260–263.

638 Bushelman SJ, Callen JP, Roth DN, Cohen LM. Disseminated *Fusarium solani* infection. J Am Acad Dermatol 1995; 32: 346–351.

639 Helm TN, Longworth DL, Hall GS et al. Case report and review of resolved fusariosis. J Am Acad Dermatol 1990; 23: 393–398.

640 Benjamin RP, Callaway JL, Conant NF. Facial granuloma associated with *Fusarium* infection. Arch Dermatol 1970; 101: 598–600.

641 Young RC, Bennett JE, Vogel CL et al. Aspergillosis. The spectrum of the disease in 98 patients. Medicine (Baltimore) 1970; 49: 147–173.

642 Caro I, Dogliotti M. Aspergillosis of the skin. Report of a case. Dermatologica 1973; 146: 244–248.

643 Khatri ML, Stefanato CM, Benghazeil M et al. Cutaneous and paranasal aspergillosis in an immunocompetent patient. Int J Dermatol 2000; 39: 853–856.

644 Cahill KM, El Mofty AM, Kawaguchi TP. Primary cutaneous aspergillosis. Arch Dermatol 1967; 96: 545–547.

645 Diamond HJ, Phelps RG, Gordon ML et al. Combined *Aspergillus* and zygomycotic *(Rhizopus)* infection in a patient with acquired immunodeficiency syndrome. Presentation as inflammatory tinea capitis. J Am Acad Dermatol 1992; 26: 1017–1018.

646 Böhler K, Metze D, Poitschek Ch, Jurecka W. Cutaneous aspergillosis. Clin Exp Dermatol 1990; 15: 446–450.

647 Thakur BK, Bernardi DM, Murali MR et al. Invasive cutaneous aspergillosis complicating immunosuppressive therapy for recalcitrant pemphigus vulgaris. J Am Acad Dermatol 1998; 38: 488–490.

648 Munn S, Keane F, Child F et al. Primary cutaneous aspergillosis. Br J Dermatol 1999; 141: 378–380.

649 Galimberti R, Kowalczuk A, Hidalgo Parra I et al. Cutaneous aspergillosis: a report of six cases. Br J Dermatol 1998; 139: 522–526.

650 Roilides E, Farmaki E. Human immunodeficiency virus infection and cutaneous aspergillosis. Arch Dermatol 2000; 136: 412–414.

651 Murakawa GJ, Harvell JD, Lubitz P et al. Cutaneous aspergillosis and acquired immunodeficiency syndrome. Arch Dermatol 2000; 136: 365–369.

652 Stanford D, Boyle M, Gillespie R. Human immunodeficiency virus-related primary cutaneous aspergillosis. Australas J Dermatol 2000; 41: 112–116.

653 Estes SA, Hendricks AA, Merz WG, Prystowsky SD. Primary cutaneous aspergillos s. J Am Acad Dermatol 1980; 3: 397–400.

654 Grossman ME, Fithian EC, Behrens C et al. Primary cutaneous aspergillosis in six leukemic children. J Am Acad Dermatol 1985; 12: 313–318.

655 Carlile JR, Millet RE, Cho CT, Vats TS. Primary cutaneous aspergillosis in a leukemic child. Arch Dermatol 1978; 114: 78–80.

656 Romero LS, Hunt SJ. Hickman catheter-associated primary cutaneous aspergillosis in a patient with the acquired immunodeficiency syndrome. Int J Dermatol 1995; 34: 551–553.

657 Hunt SJ, Nagi C, Gross KG et al. Primary cutaneous aspergillosis near central venous catheters in patients with the acquired immunodeficiency syndrome. Arch Dermatol 1992; 128: 1229–1232.

658 Mowad CM, Nguyen TV, Jaworsky C, Honig PJ. Primary cutaneous aspergillosis in an immunocompetent child. J Am Acad Dermatol 1995; 32: 136–137.

659 Googe PB, DeCoste SD, Herold WH, Mihm MC Jr. Primary cutaneous aspergillosis mimicking dermatophytosis. Arch Pathol Lab Med 1989; 113: 1284–1286.

660 Watsky KL, Eisen RN, Bolognia JL. Unilateral cutaneous emboli of Aspergillus. Arch Dermatol 1990; 126: 1214–1217.

661 Granstein RD, First LR, Sober AJ. Primary cutaneous aspergillosis in a premature neonate. Br J Dermatol 1980; 103: 681–684.

662 Ricci RM, Evans JS, Meffert JJ et al. Primary cutaneous Aspergillus ustus infection: Second reported case. J Am Acad Dermatol 1998; 38: 797–798.

663 Stiller MJ, Teperman L, Rosenthal SA et al. Primary cutaneous infection by Aspergillus ustus in a 62-year-old liver transplant recipient. J Am Acad Dermatol 1994; 31: 344–347.

664 Panke TW, McManus AT, Spebar MJ. Infection of a burn wound by Aspergillus niger. Gross appearance simulating ecthyma gangrenosa. Am J Clin Pathol 1979; 72: 230–232.

665 Harmon CB, Su WPD, Peters MS. Cutaneous aspergillosis complicating pyoderma gangrenosum. J Am Acad Dermatol 1993; 29: 656–658.

666 Goel R, Wallace ML. Pseudoepitheliomatous hyperplasia secondary to cutaneous Aspergillus. Am J Dermatopathol 2001; 23: 224–226.

Miscellaneous mycoses

667 Tapia A, Torres-Calcindo A, Arosemena R. Keloidal blastomycosis (Lobo's disease) in Panama. Int J Dermatol 1978; 17: 572–574.

668 Rodríguez-Toro G. Lobomycosis. Int J Dermatol 1993; 32: 324–332.

669 Azulay RD, Carneiro JA, Da Graca M et al. Keloidal blastomycosis (Lobo's disease) with lymphatic involvement. A case report. Int J Dermatol 1976; 15: 40–44.

670 Bhawan J, Bain RW, Purtilo DT et al. Lobomycosis. An electronmicroscopic, histochemical and immunologic study. J Cutan Pathol 1976; 3: 5–16.

671 Brun AM. Lobomycosis in three Venezuelan patients. Int J Dermatol 1999; 38: 302–305.

672 Baruzzi RG, Rodriques DA, Michalany NS, Salomão R. Squamous-cell carcinoma and lobomycosis (Jorge Lobo's disease). Int J Dermatol 1989; 28: 183–185.

673 Jaramillo D, Cortés A, Restrepo A et al. Lobomycosis. Report of the eighth Colombian case and review of the literature. J Cutan Pathol 1976; 3: 180–189.

674 Mikat DM. Unusual fungal conditions of the skin. Int J Dermatol 1980; 19: 18–22.

675 Sahoo S, Das S. Rhinosporidiosis of subcutaneous tissue. J Indian Med Assoc 1982; 78: 114–116.

676 Friedman I. Ulcerative/necrotizing diseases of the nose and paranasal sinuses. Curr Diagn Pathol 1995; 2: 236–255.

677 Ramanan C, Ghorpade A. Giant cutaneous rhinosporidiosis. Int J Dermatol 1996; 35: 441–442.

678 Gaines JJ, Clay JR, Chandler FW et al. Rhinosporidiosis: three domestic cases. South Med J 1996; 89: 65–67.

679 Mahakrisnan A, Rajasekaram V, Pandian PI. Disseminated cutaneous rhinosporidiosis treated with dapsone. Trop Geogr Med 1981; 33: 189–192.

680 Agrawal S, Sharma KD, Shrivastava JB. Generalized rhinosporidiosis with visceral involvement. Report of a case. Arch Dermatol 1959; 80: 22–26.

681 Date A, Ramakrishna B, Lee VN, Sundararaj GD. Tumoral rhinosporidiosis. Histopathology 1995; 27: 288–290.

682 Angunawela P, De Tissera A, Dissanaike AS. Rhinosporidiosis presenting with two soft tissue tumors followed by dissemination. Pathology 1999; 31: 57–58.

683 Yesudian P. Cutaneous rhinosporidiosis mimicking verruca vulgaris. Int J Dermatol 1988; 27: 47–48.

Algal infections

684 Boyd AS, Langley M, King LE Jr. Cutaneous manifestations of Prototheca infections. J Am Acad Dermatol 1995; 32: 758–764.

685 Venezio FR, Lavoo E, Williams JE et al. Progressive cutaneous protothecosis. Am J Clin Pathol 1982; 77: 485–493.

686 Sudman MS. Protothecosis. A critical review. Am J Clin Pathol 1974; 61: 10–19.

687 Tindall JP, Fetter BF. Infections caused by achloric algae (protothecosis). Arch Dermatol 1971; 104: 490–500.

688 McAnally T, Parry EL. Cutaneous protothecosis presenting as recurrent chromomycosis. Arch Dermatol 1985; 121: 1066–1069.

689 Woolrich A, Koestenblatt E, Don P, Szaniawski W. Cutaneous protothecosis and AIDS. J Am Acad Dermatol 1994; 31: 920–924.

690 Monopoli A, Accetturi MP, Lombardo GA. Cutaneous protothecosis. Int J Dermatol 1995; 34: 766–767.

691 Laeng RH, Egger C, Schaffner T et al. Protothecosis in an HIV-positive patient. Am J Surg Pathol 1994; 18: 1261–1264.

692 Mars PW, Rabson AR, Rippey JJ, Ajello L. Cutaneous protothecosis. Br J Dermatol (Suppl) 1971; 7: 76–84.

693 Walsh SV, Johnson RA, Tahan SR. Prototheosis: an unusual cause of chronic subcutaneous and soft tissue infection. Am J Dermatopathol 1998; 20: 379–382.

694 Kuo T-t, Hsueh S, Wu J-L, Wang A-M. Cutaneous prototheosis. A clinicopathologic study. Arch Pathol Lab Med 1987; 111: 737–740.

695 Goldstein GD, Bhatia P, Kalivas J. Herpetiform prototheosis. Int J Dermatol 1986; 25: 54–55.

696 Tyring SK, Lee PC, Walsh P et al. Papular prototheosis of the chest. Arch Dermatol 1989; 125: 1249–1252.

697 Mayhall CG, Miller CW, Eisen AZ et al. Cutaneous prototheosis. Successful treatment with amphotericin B. Arch Dermatol 1976; 112: 1749–1752.

698 Mendez CM, Silva-Lizama E, Logemann H. Human cutaneous prototheosis. Int J Dermatol 1995; 34: 554–555.

699 Tang WYM, Lo KK, Lam WY et al. Cutaneous prototheosis: report of a case in Hong Kong. Br J Dermatol 1995; 133: 479–482.

Viral diseases

INTRODUCTION

Viral infections of the skin are of increasing clinical importance, particularly in patients who are immunocompromised. Viruses may reach the skin by direct inoculation, as in warts, milker's nodule and orf, or by spread from other locations, as in herpes zoster. Many viral exanthems result from a generalized infection, with localization of the virus in the epidermis or dermis or in the endothelium of blood vessels.[1] The usual clinical appearance of this group is an erythematous maculopapular rash, but sometimes macular, vesicular, petechial, purpuric or urticarial reactions may be seen. Some of the varied manifestations of viral diseases may result from an immune reaction to the virus. This is the probable explanation for the erythema multiforme and erythema nodosum that occasionally follow viral infections. Other dermatoses appear to be in this category of a post-viral dermatosis (see below).

Viruses are separated into families on the basis of the type and form of the nucleic acid genome, of the morphological features of the virus particle, and of the mode of replication. There are four important families involved in cutaneous diseases: the DNA families of Poxviridae, Herpesviridae and Papovaviridae, and the RNA family Picornaviridae. In addition to these four families, exanthems can occur in the course of infections with the following families: Adenoviridae, Reoviridae,[2] Togaviridae, Paramyxoviridae, Arenaviridae, and an unclassified group which includes hepatitis B and C viruses and Marburg virus.[1] The three major DNA families produce lesions that are histologically diagnostic for a disease or group of diseases, whereas the other viruses produce lesions that are often histologically non-specific. These non-specific features include a superficial perivascular infiltrate of lymphocytes, mild epidermal spongiosis, occasional Civatte bodies and, sometimes, urticarial edema or mild hemorrhage. Inclusion bodies, which represent sites of virus replication, are uncommon in skin lesions produced by viruses outside the four major families.

Various laboratory techniques can be used to assist in the specific diagnosis of a suspected viral disease.[3] These include light and electron microscopy of a biopsy or smear, serology, viral culture and immunomorphological methods. Although viral isolation in tissue culture remains the paramount diagnostic method, the development of monoclonal antibodies to various viruses, for use with fluorescent, immunoperoxidase and ELISA (enzyme-linked immunosorbent assay) techniques, has made possible the rapid diagnosis of many viral infections with a high degree of specificity.[4] Techniques using the polymerase chain reaction (PCR) are now being used routinely in some laboratories for the diagnosis of certain viral diseases. Serology is still the preferred method of diagnosis for certain viral infections, such as rubella and infectious mononucleosis. Brief mention must be made of the Tzanck smear, which was traditionally used by clinicians, especially dermatologists, in the diagnosis of certain vesicular lesions, especially those caused by the herpes simplex and varicella-zoster viruses. A smear is made by scraping the lesion. This is then stained by the Giemsa or Papanicolaou methods and examined for the presence of viral inclusion bodies. This use is declining with the advent of the more specific immunomorphological techniques.

The various virus families, and the cutaneous diseases they produce, will be considered in turn, after a brief discussion of the concept of the post-viral dermatoses.

Post-viral dermatoses

Dermatoses are seen, occasionally, which appear to be a reaction to an earlier viral infection. As mentioned above, erythema multiforme and erythema nodosum sometimes follow a viral infection. At other times the viral etiology is presumptive, such as the appearance of skin lesions some days after an upper respiratory tract or gastrointestinal infection of possible viral etiology. Serological evidence of a viral illness, such as IgM antibodies to a particular virus, is sometimes present. Although the dermatoses are thought to result from an immunological reaction to a virus, it does not necessarily persist in the body. There are circumstances in which viral persistence has been demonstrated. Such is the case with the herpes simplex virus and erythema multiforme (see p. 43).

The histological pattern seen in these various post-viral dermatoses is similar – a lichenoid lymphocytic vasculitis. This pattern is characterized by a lymphocytic vasculitis, usually mild and without the presence of fibrin in vessel walls, accompanied by a lichenoid (interface) reaction in which there are variable numbers of apoptotic keratinocytes. Variations on this theme may allow a specific diagnosis to be attached to the process. For example, some cases of pityriasis lichenoides appear to follow a viral illness. On histological examination, there is parakeratosis in addition to a lichenoid lymphocytic vasculitis. In erythema multiforme, associated with herpes simplex, there is a prominent lichenoid (interface) dermatitis with cell death at all layers of the epidermis. In Gianotti–Crosti syndrome (see p. 706), associated with many different viruses, spongiosis is an additional modification to the usual pattern of lichenoid lymphocytic vasculitis.

This concept may need to be modified as additional information becomes available. In the meantime, it provides a plausible explanation of observed cases.

POXVIRIDAE

Poxvirus infections of humans include cowpox, vaccinia, variola (smallpox), molluscum contagiosum, milker's nodule (paravaccinia) and orf (ecthyma contagiosum). Rarely, human infection with *Parapoxvirus* has been acquired after exposure to wildlife.[5] Other poxviruses (including monkeypox and tanapox) have been reported as causing human disease in Africa.[6,7] They will not be considered further. The causative viruses are large, with a DNA core and a surrounding capsid. There are two subgroups, based on the morphological features of the virus. The viruses of molluscum contagiosum and orf are oval or cylindrical in shape and measure approximately 150 × 300 nm. The remaining viruses are brick-shaped and range in size from 250 to 300 nm × 200 to 250 nm. Clusters of these poxviruses can be identified in hematoxylin and eosin-stained sections as intracytoplasmic eosinophilic inclusions.

COWPOX

Cowpox is a viral disease of cattle. It may be contracted by milkers, who develop a pustular eruption on the hands, forearms or face, accompanied by slight fever and lymphadenitis. Crusted lesions resembling anthrax[8] and sporotrichoid spread[9] have also been reported. A generalized eruption due to cowpox infection may develop, rarely, in patients with atopic dermatitis.[10,11] This variant, known as Kaposi's varicelliform eruption, resembles eczema herpeticum (see p. 698). The disease is of historical interest, because it was the immunity to smallpox of those who had had cowpox that led Jenner to substitute inoculation with cowpox for the more dangerous procedure of variolation. Doubt has been cast recently on the role of cattle as a reservoir of infection in cowpox.[8,12] It appears that the domestic cat and rodents have an important role in the transmission of cowpox virus.[8,11–13] Rare cases continue to be reported from Europe[14] and other parts of the world.[15]

Buffalopox is a similar condition, reported in persons who milk infected buffaloes.[16]

VACCINIA

Vaccination against smallpox was carried out with the vaccinia virus, a laboratory-developed member of the poxvirus group. In previously unvaccinated individuals, a papule developed on about the fifth day at the site of inoculation. This quickly became vesicular and gradually dried up, producing a crust which fell away, leaving a scar.

With the eradication of smallpox, vaccination is no longer given. As a result, generalized vaccinia infection (eczema vaccinatum), a serious complication of vaccination, is now of historical interest only. Eczema vaccinatum has many similarities to eczema herpeticum, an infection by the herpes simplex virus seen also in predisposed patients, such as those with an atopic diathesis.

Histopathology

The appearances are similar to those of herpes simplex, zoster and varicella, except that intracytoplasmic rather than intranuclear inclusion bodies are seen in vaccinia.

Complications of vaccination

Many cutaneous and systemic complications of smallpox vaccination have been reported.[17,18] They are now of historical interest only, except for late complications, which may continue to be seen.

Late sequelae have included keloid formation, basal and squamous cell carcinoma,[19] malignant melanoma, dermatofibrosarcoma protuberans, and malignant fibrous histiocytoma.[20] Dermatoses have also developed, including discoid lupus erythematosus,[21] lichen sclerosus et atrophicus,[22] contact dermatitis and 'localized eczema'.[18] It is possible that some of the late complications represent the chance localization of a particular lesion at the site of previous vaccination.

VARIOLA (SMALLPOX)

Variola has now been eradicated.[23] The last known case occurred in Somalia in 1977. Two types were encountered: variola major, a severe form with a significant fatality rate, and variola minor (alastrim), a mild form with a fatality rate of less than 1%. Umbilicated papules were seen. They became crusted and healed with scarring.

Variola remains a potential threat in biological warfare as laboratory cultures of the virus still exist.[24]

Histopathology

Variola resulted in vesicular lesions that resembled those of herpes simplex, zoster and varicella, except (usually) for the absence of multinucleate epidermal cells and for the intracytoplasmic localization of the inclusion bodies.[25]

MOLLUSCUM CONTAGIOSUM

Molluscum contagiosum occurs as solitary or multiple dome-shaped, umbilicated, waxy papules with a predilection for the head and neck, flexural areas or the genitalia of children and adolescents.[26–30] Sexual and fomite transmission may occur.[31,32] Papules range from 2 to 8 mm in diameter, although solitary lesions may be slightly larger.[33] Spontaneous regression often occurs within a year, although more persistent lesions are encountered. Pitted scarring is a rare complication in atopic individuals.[34] Antibodies to the virus have been found in nearly 60% of patients with skin lesions, but they are less frequent in patients with AIDS.[35] Extensive lesions can occur in immuno-

compromised patients, particularly those with AIDS.[36–44] Cidofovir, a drug with broad-spectrum anti-DNA virus activity, has been successfully used in the treatment of recalcitrant lesions in patients with HIV.[45]

The disease is caused by a large brick-shaped DNA poxvirus with an ultrastructural resemblance to vaccinia virus.[46] A well-defined sac encloses the virion colony of each infected keratinocyte.[47] The sequencing of the viral genome is known.[45]

Histopathology

A lesion consists of several inverted lobules of hyperplastic squamous epithelium which expand into the underlying dermis (Fig. 26.1).[46] The lobules are separated by fine septa of compressed dermis. Eosinophilic inclusion bodies form in the cytoplasm of keratinocytes just above the basal layer, and progressively enlarge. At the level of the granular layer, the bodies become increasingly hematoxyphile and occupy the entire cell (Fig. 26.2). These molluscum bodies are eventually extruded with keratinous debris into dilated ostia, which lead to the surface.[48,49] Areas of hair bulb differentiation, or epithelial proliferation mimicking a basal cell carcinoma, may occur at the margins of a lesion.[48] Molluscum contagiosum has been reported in epidermal cysts,[46,50,51] but some of these cases may simply represent pilar infundibula dilated by cornified cells and molluscum bodies.[52]

Secondary infection and ulceration may occur.[53] Molluscum folliculitis is an uncommon pattern seen mainly in immunocompromised persons.[54] A variable chronic inflammatory cell infiltrate is seen in regressing lesions, and is thought to represent a cell-mediated immune reaction.[48,55] However, in the early eruptive phase there is no inflammatory response.[56] Inflammation and a foreign-body reaction may also be related to extrusion of molluscum bodies into the dermis. Rarely, an atypical lymphocytic infiltrate ('pseudoleukemia cutis', 'pseudolymphoma') may be found.[57,58] In one case, the atypical cells were CD8+ T lymphocytes with scattered CD30+ cells.[59]

Molluscum contagiosum has also been reported in association with a nevocellular nevus, a halo nevus,[60,61] with the Meyerson phenomenon (see p. 808),[62] with cutaneous lupus erythematosus[63] and with human papilloma-virus (HPV).[64] In one patient with systemic lupus erythematosus, metaplastic bone was present in the dermis adjacent to each lesion of molluscum contagiosum.[65]

MILKER'S NODULE

Milker's nodule results from infection with the paravaccinia virus, transmitted from the udders of infected cows. Indirect transmission from contaminated

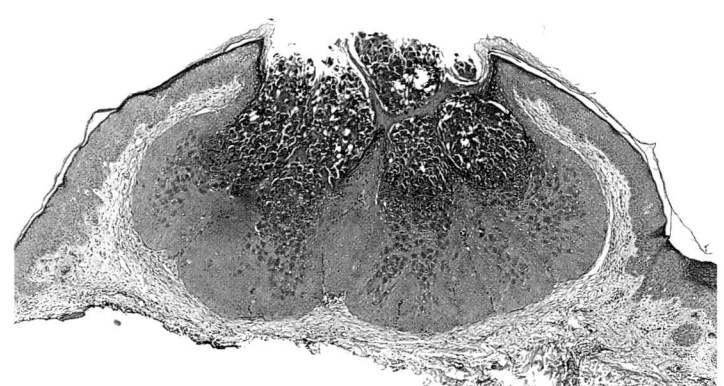

Fig. 26.1 **Molluscum contagiosum** showing inverted lobules of squamous epithelium with molluscum bodies maturing toward the surface. (H & E)

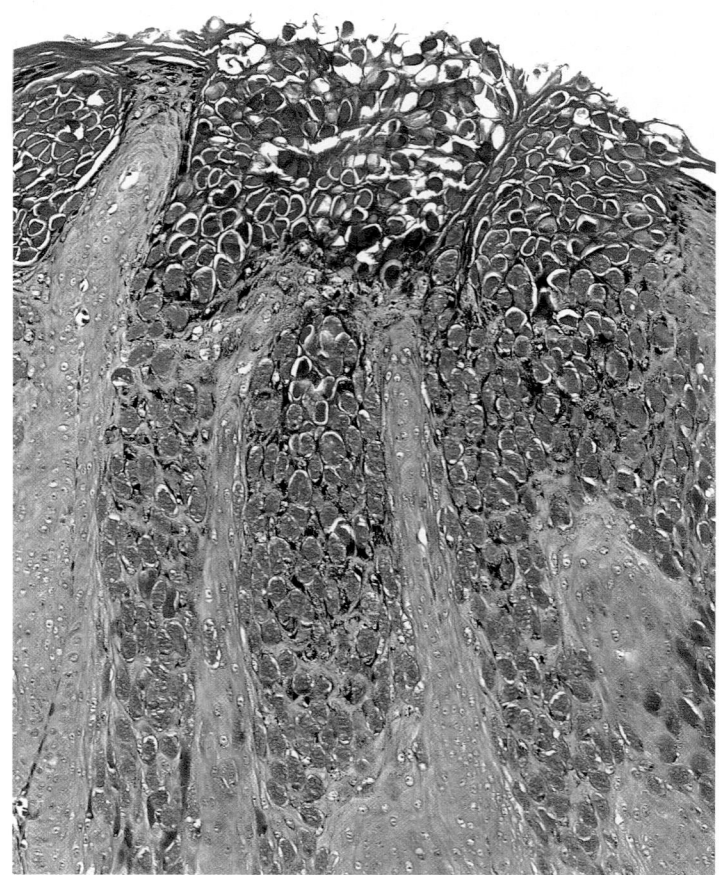

Fig. 26.2 Molluscum contagiosum. The large molluscum bodies occupy almost the whole of each infected cell. (H & E)

objects has also been reported in several patients with recent burns.[66] Lesions are usually solitary, and on the hands. Multiple nodules and involvement of other sites have been described. Lesions heal, with scarring, in 6–8 weeks. Six clinical stages have been delineated, but the usual lesion, when the patient presents, is a red-violaceous, sometimes erosive or crusted nodule measuring 0.5–2 cm in diameter.[67] Erythema multiforme, erythema nodosum or urticarial lesions may develop in a small number of cases.[68]

The clinical and histopathological similarities between milker's nodule and human orf have led to the collective term 'farmyard-pox' being proposed for these two conditions.[69]

Histopathology

The appearances vary with the stage of the lesion.[67] An early milker's nodule shows vacuolization and ballooning of the cells in the upper third of the epidermis, leading sometimes to multilocular vesicles.[70] Intracytoplasmic and, rarely, intranuclear inclusions may be seen.[71] Focal epidermal necrosis sometimes occurs, and this may lead to ulceration and secondary scale crust formation. Neutrophils are found in the epidermis and superficial papillary dermis when epidermal necrosis occurs. Mature lesions will show acanthosis of the epidermis, with the formation of finger-like downward projections of

the epidermis (Fig. 26.3). There is prominent edema of the papillary dermis, with an inflammatory infiltrate comprised of lymphocytes, histiocytes, plasma cells and occasional eosinophils. There are numerous small blood vessels, many of which are ectatic, in the papillary dermis (Fig. 26.4). In regressing lesions there is progressive diminution of the acanthosis, and eventually of the inflammatory infiltrate.[67]

Electron microscopy

Electron microscopy may show a large oval viral particle with a central electron-dense core surrounded by a less dense homogeneous coat and two narrow electron-dense layers. Rapid diagnosis may be made by electron microscopy of the crust from an early lesion.[72]

ORF

Orf (ecthyma contagiosum) is primarily a disease of young sheep and goats, involving the lips and perioral area.[69,73–79] It is caused by a poxvirus of the paravaccinia subgroup. Orf can be transmitted to humans by contact with infected animals; rarely, lesions have developed at sites of trauma produced by an inanimate object.[78] Lesions, which measure approximately 1–3 cm or more[75,76] in diameter, develop most commonly on the hands and forearms. Other sites of involvement have included the face,[80] scalp, temple[81] and perianal region.[77] Several lesions may be present in the one area. Spontaneous regression is usual after about 7 weeks. Recurrent lesions have been reported in immunocompromised persons.[82] A mature lesion is nodular with central umbilication and an erythematous halo. Regional adenitis, superinfection, toxic erythema, erythema multiforme, widespread lesions or a generalized varicelliform eruption may complicate the infection.[83] Bullous pemphigoid may also develop following orf.[84,85]

Histopathology

The appearances vary with the stage of the disease (Fig. 26.5).[73,74] Early lesions of orf show moderate acanthosis and pale vacuolated cytoplasm, involving particularly the upper epidermis.[86] Cytoplasmic inclusion bodies are usually present (Fig. 26.6).[69] An unusual change, which has been called 'spongiform degeneration', can be seen, particularly in follicular structures.[69] This is characterized by vacuolated cells having wispy strands of eosinophilic

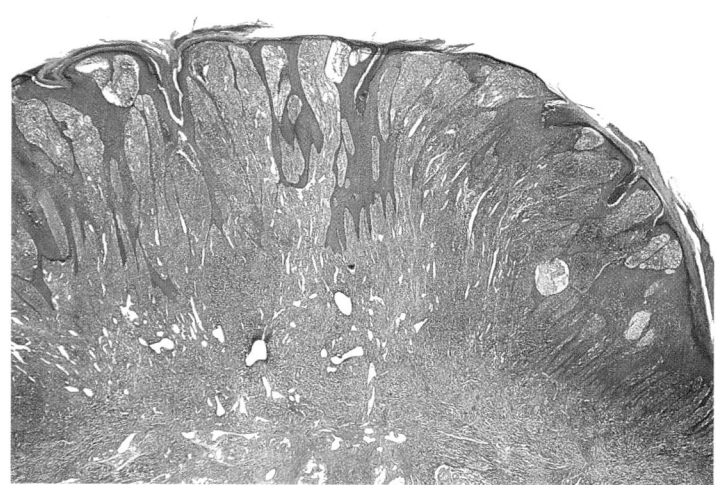

Fig. 26.3 Milker's nodule. The elongated thin rete pegs with intervening heavy inflammation of the upper dermis are characteristic features of mature lesions. (H & E)

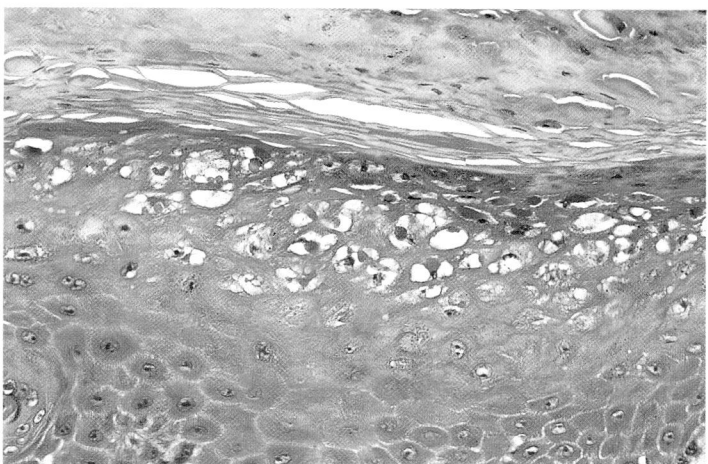

Fig. 26.6 **Orf.** Inclusion bodies are present in the cytoplasm of the keratinocytes in the upper epidermis. (H & E)

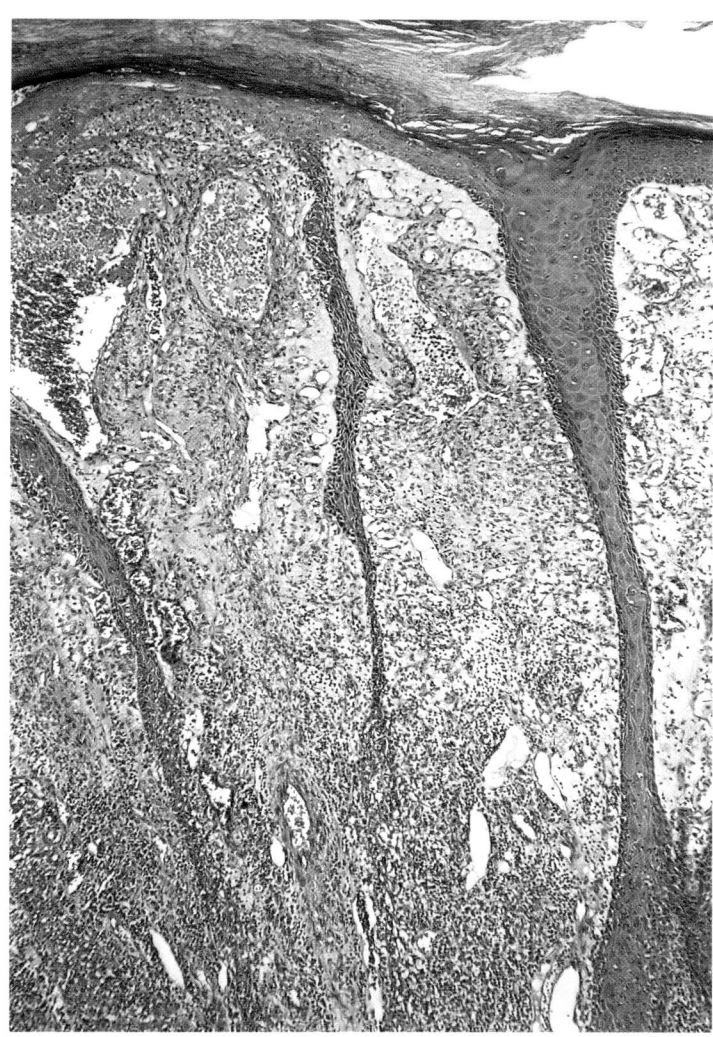

Fig. 26.4 **Milker's nodule.** The dermis between the thin rete pegs is vascular and inflamed. (H & E)

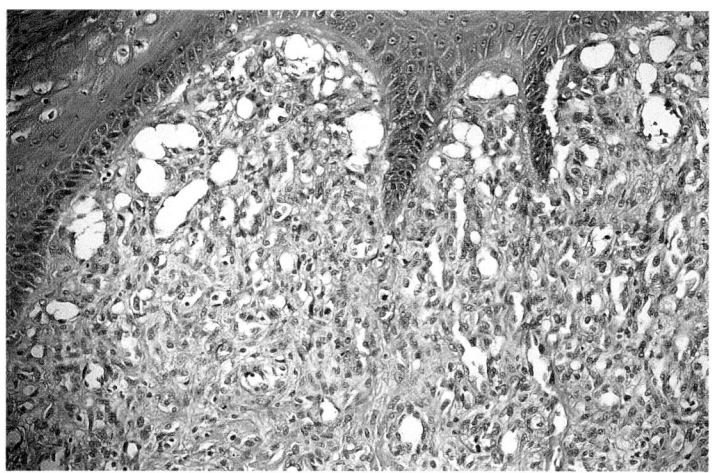

Fig. 26.7 **Orf.** The papillary dermis may be so vascular that a vascular tumor is suspected. (H & E)

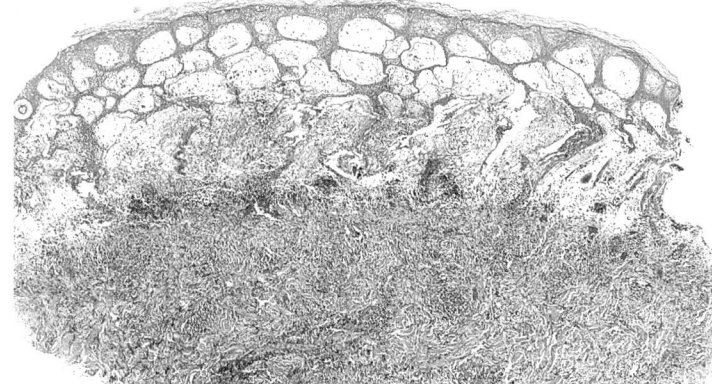

Fig. 26.5 **Orf.** There is epidermal necrosis, acanthosis and subepidermal edema. (H & E)

cytoplasm. Intraepidermal vesicles or bullae may form. The dermis contains dilated thin-walled vessels and an infiltrate of lymphocytes, macrophages and occasional eosinophils and plasma cells.[74] Cells expressing CD30 are sometimes present in this infiltrate.[87] Later lesions often show epidermal necrosis, particularly in the center. Neutrophils are often found within and adjacent to the necrotic epidermis. Other biopsies may show elongated rete pegs with dilated vessels in the intervening dermal papillae. Sometimes there is an unusual proliferation of endothelial cells in the dermal papillae which may even simulate a vascular tumor (Fig. 26.7).[81] Eventually the inflammatory infiltrate and epithelial hyperplasia resolve. The lesions of orf are generally regarded as indistinguishable from milker's nodules,[69] although full-thickness epidermal necrosis seems to be more common in orf. Immunoperoxidase techniques using orf-specific monoclonal antibodies can be used to confirm the diagnosis, if necessary.

Electron microscopy

Electron microscopy shows an oval virus with an electron-dense core, surrounded by a laminated capsule similar to the virus of milker's nodule (Fig. 26.8).[83] Rapid diagnosis may be made by electron microscopy of negatively stained suspensions from the lesion. The number of virus-containing cells is greatest in the first 2 weeks of the disease; they may be absent by the fourth week.[89]

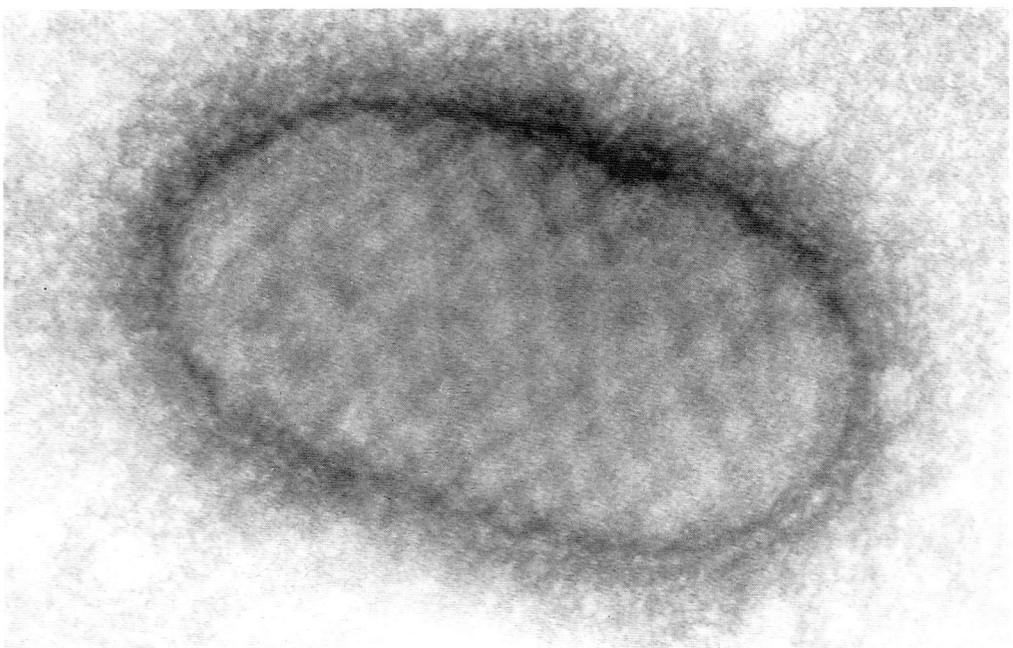

Fig. 26.8 **Orf.** Ultrastructural features of the orf virus with its laminated capsule and internal cross-hatched appearance. Electron micrograph × 20 000

HERPESVIRIDAE

There are three major subgroups within the family Herpesviridae. The α-herpesviruses are neurotropic and include herpes simplex virus (types 1 and 2) and the varicella-zoster virus.[90,91] The γ-herpesviruses are lymphotropic and include Epstein–Barr virus, human herpesvirus-8 (HHV-8) and herpesvirus saimiri. The predominant sites of latency of the β-herpesviruses – cytomegalovirus and human herpesviruses 6 and 7 (HHV-6 and HHV-7) – are not known.[91] Concurrent infection by two viruses of this family is a rare occurrence, seen in immunocompromised patients.[92,93]

Type-specific identification of the two main types of herpes simplex virus can be made in paraffin sections using immunoperoxidase techniques; furthermore, varicella-zoster virus can be distinguished from them.[94,95] Techniques using the polymerase chain reaction (PCR) can also be used.[92,96,97]

HERPES SIMPLEX

There are two main types of herpes simplex virus, type 1 (HSV-1) and type 2 (HSV-2).[98] Primary infection with HSV-1 usually occurs in childhood and is mild. Recurrent lesions occur most commonly around the lips (herpes labialis – 'cold sores'). Other sites of infection include the oral cavity, pharynx, esophagus, eye, lung and brain.[99–101]

Infection with HSV-2 generally involves the genitalia and surrounding areas after puberty; it is usually sexually transmitted.[102–104] The incubation period for genital lesions averages 5 days. HSV-2 may also result in generalized or cutaneous lesions of the newborn.[105,106] The relationship between the site of infection and HSV type is not absolute.

Once infected, a person will usually harbor the virus for life. The virus can travel along sensory nerves to infect the neurons in the sensory ganglia. Recurrent disease follows this latency in the sensory ganglia and can be stimulated by ultraviolet light,[107] trauma, fever, HIV infection,[108] menstruation and stress, to name the most common factors.[109] Prostaglandins and

diminished production of IFN-γ may play a role in the reactivation of infections.[110,111] A recent study found that reactivation of genital HSV-2 infection in asymptomatic seropositive persons is quite frequent.[112] Asymptomatic perianal shedding of HSV is common in patients with AIDS.[113]

The usual lesions of herpes simplex consist of a group of clear vesicles which heal without scarring, except in cases where secondary bacterial infection supervenes. Special clinical variants[114] include herpes folliculitis of the beard or scalp, herpetic whitlow[115] (usually in medical or nursing personnel), necrotizing balanitis[116] (a very rare HSV-2 complication), a varicella-like eruption,[117] infection localized to sites of atopic dermatitis[118] or photoexposure,[119] vegetating plaques,[120] flaccid intracorneal blisters,[121] acquired lymphedema of the hand[122] and eczema herpeticum (see p. 698).[123] Severe primary or secondary infection with systemic involvement may occur in immunocompromised patients.[124,125] Disseminated herpes simplex infection is a rare complication of pregnancy.[126] Herpes simplex virus DNA is present in lesional skin in a significant number of patients with erythema multiforme (see p. 43).[127,128]

HSV-1 and HSV-2 are biologically and serologically distinct. They are usually isolated using human embryonic fibroblast cell cultures.[129] Characteristic cytopathic changes can be seen after 1 or 2 days. Rapid diagnosis of cutaneous infections of herpes simplex can be made using smears of lesions and monoclonal antibodies, with an immunofluorescence technique.[130] Reliable and convenient serologic tests for antibodies against both HSV-1 and HSV-2 are now available commercially.[131] These methods indicate that viral culture has significantly underestimated the number of infected individuals.[131] PCR-based methods are now being used routinely in some laboratories for diagnosis.

Histopathology

The histological appearances of herpes simplex, varicella and herpes zoster are very similar. The earliest changes involve the epidermal cell nuclei, which develop peripheral clumping of chromatin and a homogeneous ground-glass appearance, combined with ballooning of the nucleus.[132] Vacuolization is the earliest cytoplasmic alteration. These changes begin focally along the basal layer, but soon involve the entire epidermis.[132] By the time lesions are biopsied there is usually an established intraepidermal vesicle (Fig. 26.9). This results from two types of degenerative change, ballooning degeneration and reticular degeneration. *Ballooning degeneration* is peculiar to viral vesicles. The affected cells swell and lose their attachment to adjacent cells, thus separating from them (secondary acantholysis). The cytoplasm of these cells becomes homogeneous and intensely eosinophilic, and some are also multinucleate (Tzanck cells). At times the basal layer of the epidermis is also destroyed in this way, leading to the formation of a subepidermal vesicle. The change known as *reticular degeneration* is characterized by progressive hydropic swelling of epidermal cells, which become large and clear with only fine cytoplasmic strands remaining at the edge of the cells. These eventually rupture, contributing further to the formation of a vesicle. This change is not specific for viral infection and can be seen also in allergic contact dermatitis. Whereas ballooning degeneration is found mainly at the base of the vesicle, reticular degeneration is seen on its superficial aspect and margin.

Eosinophilic intranuclear inclusion bodies are found, particularly in ballooned cells (Fig. 26.10). They are more common in multinucleate cells of lesions that have been present for several days. Neutrophils are present within established vesicles. There are also moderate numbers in the underlying dermis, as well as lymphocytes. Neutrophils are prominent in the lesions of herpetic whitlow. Marked inflammation and even vasculitis have been noted in some lesions.[133] As a rule, the dermal inflammation is more severe in herpes simplex than in zoster. Atypical lymphoid cells may be present in the infiltrate where herpes simplex complicates an underlying hematological malignancy.[134] Atypical lymphocytes have been noted in 32 of 45 routine cases of herpes simplex submitted for microscopy.[135]

Uncommonly, erythema multiforme-like changes may be seen in the adjacent skin, concurrent with a vesicle of herpes simplex. A related reaction pattern is so-called 'lichenoid lymphocytic vasculitis', a term coined for the changes seen in presumptive cases of herpes simplex with an immunological response (see p. 692).[136] There is an upper dermal infiltrate of lymphocytes and histiocytes, with lichenoid changes in the epidermis and a dermal lymphocytic vasculitis.

Focal involvement of pilosebaceous units is not uncommon in recurrent lesions.[132] In the variant known as herpes folliculitis,[137] pilosebaceous involvement is the dominant lesion (Fig. 26.11). Rarely, the eccrine ducts and glands are involved (herpetic syringitis).[138] Ballooning degeneration may involve cells of the outer root sheath of the deep portion of the follicle. A dermal inflammatory infiltrate is often present in these cases; it is heaviest in the deep reticular dermis – a so-called 'bottom-heavy' infiltrate.

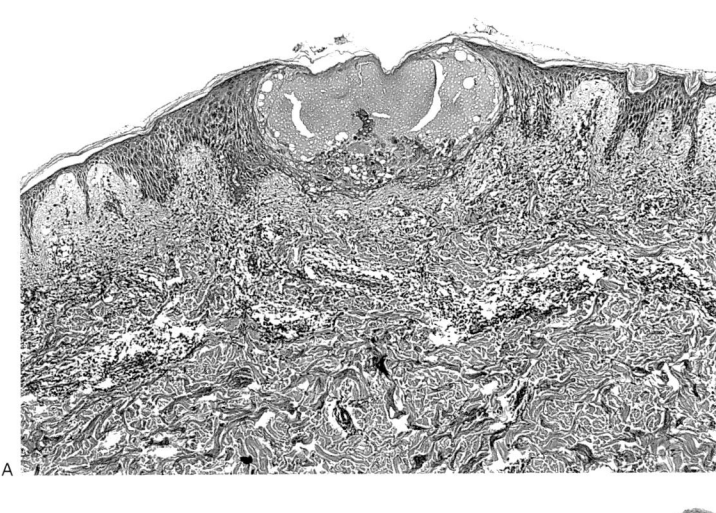

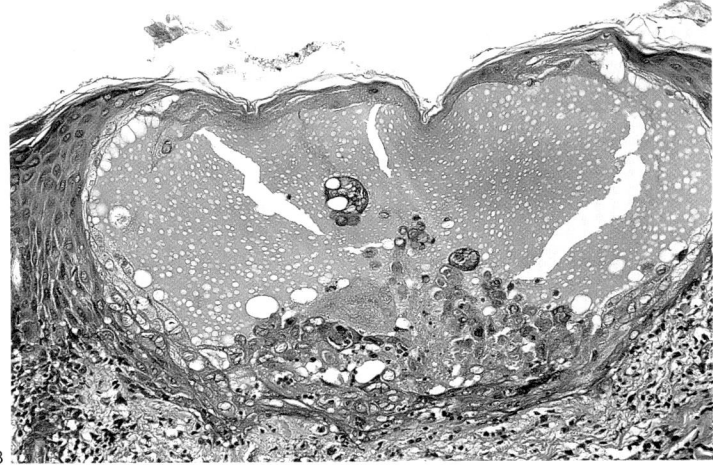

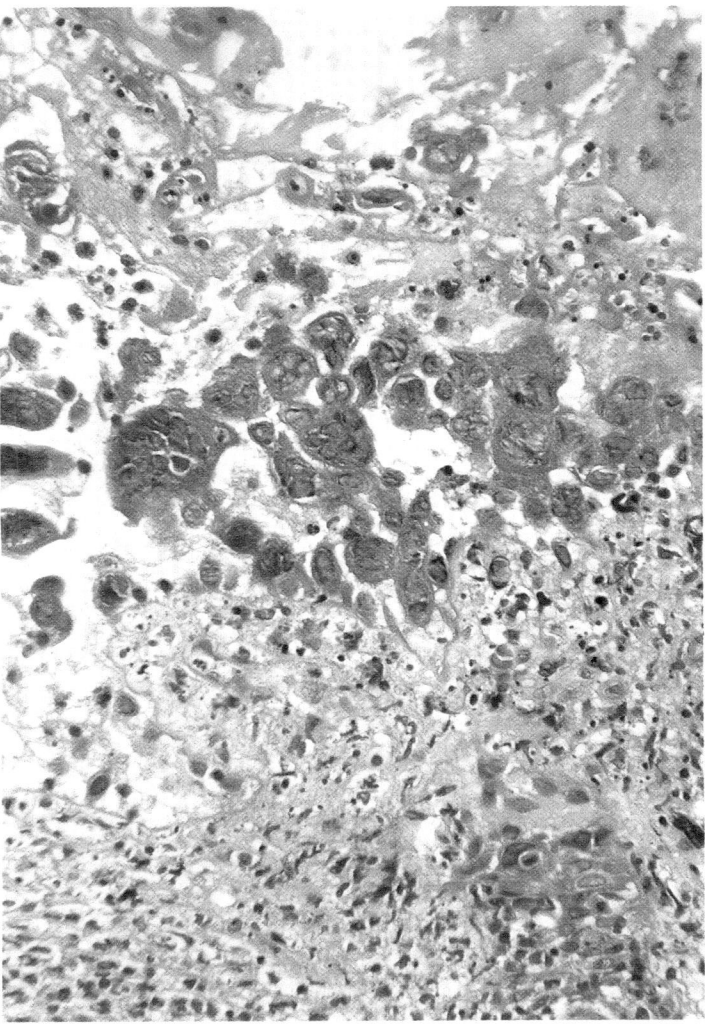

Fig. 26.9 **(A) Herpes simplex. (B)** There is an intraepidermal vesicle containing ballooned, acantholytic keratinocytes in which there are intranuclear inclusion bodies. (H & E)

Fig. 26.10 **Herpes simplex.** The multinucleate keratinocytes have intranuclear inclusion bodies. (H & E)

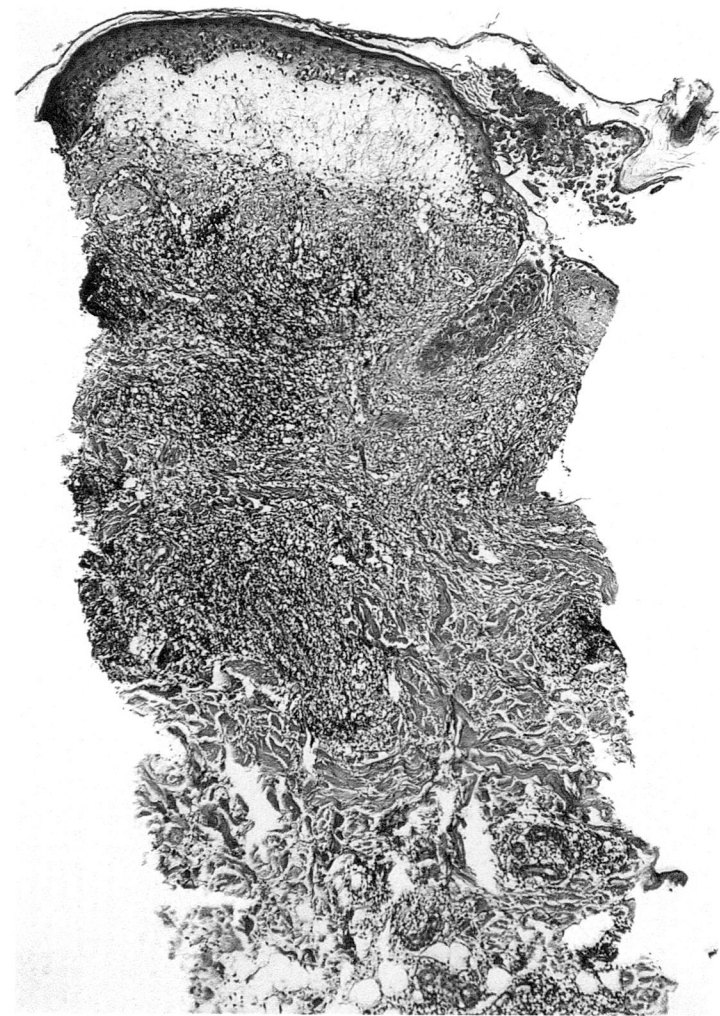

Fig. 26.11 **Herpes folliculitis.** There is a heavy superficial and deep dermal infiltrate of lymphocytes. A necrotic follicle is present in the upper third of the dermis. (H & E)

Dermal nerves in lesional skin in both herpes simplex and herpes zoster show perineural and some intraneural inflammation. Viral antigen can be detected in these inflamed nerve twigs, indicating that they are not just passive conduits for viral spread.[139] Schwann cell hypertrophy and neuronal necrosis with cytopathic changes may also be present.[139] Sometimes the perineural infiltration is out of proportion to the overlying dermal inflammation.

In late lesions of herpes simplex, ulceration is often present. Ghosts of acantholytic, multinucleate epithelial cells with slate-gray nuclei on routine staining may still be seen in the overlying crust.

Recently, attention has been drawn to the histological appearance of the lesions that recur at the site of previous surgery. These vesicles are sub-epidermal, with an inflammatory response, complete with multinucleate giant cells,[140] in the uppermost dermis.

A rapid cytological diagnosis of a vesicular lesion can be made by making a smear from the base of a freshly opened vesicle and staining it with the Giemsa stain. Ballooned cells, some of which are multinucleate, will be seen in herpes simplex, varicella and zoster.

Electron microscopy

Virus particles of *Herpesvirus hominis*, measuring between 90 and 130 nm, can be seen in the nuclei of the basal cells. Cells in the malpighian layer often contain other virus-related material, such as nuclear granules and capsules. Viral capsids have also been seen within the nuclei of monocytes, young histiocytes and lymphocytes in the epidermal vesicles.[141] Large lymphocytes are sometimes seen adjacent to keratinocytes exhibiting lytic changes, suggesting that cell-mediated immunity may be partly responsible for the epidermal damage that occurs.[142]

Eczema herpeticum

Eczema herpeticum is a generalized infection of the skin with the herpes simplex virus.[143–145] A similar condition (eczema vaccinatum) occurred, in the past, with the vaccinia virus.[146] Both lesions have been grouped together as Kaposi's varicelliform eruption. This condition occurs most commonly in association with atopic dermatitis, but it has also been reported in Darier's disease,[147,148] Hailey–Hailey disease,[149] pityriasis rubra pilaris,[150] pemphigus foliaceus, seborrheic dermatitis, ichthyosiform erythroderma, multiple myeloma,[151] the Sézary syndrome and mycosis fungoides,[152] and following thermal injury.[153] It has been suggested that interleukin-4, which may be increased in atopic dermatitis, may downregulate the response against herpes simplex virus and contribute to generalized infection.[154] Reduced numbers of natural killer (NK) cells and a decrease in interleukin-2 receptors probably also contribute.[155]

Histopathology

Although eczema herpeticum is characterized by the presence of multinucleate epidermal cells and intranuclear inclusions, rather than the intracytoplasmic inclusions seen in the past with eczema vaccinatum, these features are often obscured by the heavy inflammatory cell infiltrate of neutrophils and early breakdown of the vesicles. Recently formed lesions usually show the typical features of a vesicle of herpes simplex.

VARICELLA

Varicella (chickenpox) is characterized by an acute vesicular eruption. It is predominantly a disease of childhood. The lesions develop in successive crops, so that the rash typically consists of pocks at different stages of development. Thus, papules, vesicles, pustules, crusted lesions and healing lesions may all be present. Varicella pneumonia may be seen in adults as a primary infection. In immunocompromised hosts dissemination may occur, or large ulcerated and necrotic lesions (varicella gangrenosa) may develop; chronic verrucous lesions have also been described.[156–158] An interesting observation is the finding of marked intensification of the varicella eruption in areas of skin which are normally covered but which become sunburnt just before the eruption commences.[159] Photodistributed varicella, mimicking polymorphous light eruption, has been reported.[160] Varicella has also been reported largely restricted to an area covered by a plaster cast,[161] and in a patient with Kawasaki disease.[162] Viral exanthems, particularly varicella, may localize early and preferentially to areas of prior inflammation.[163]

Cutaneous lesions, usually scars, can be seen in neonates with the congenital varicella syndrome. The incidence of an embryopathy after infection in the first 20 weeks of gestation is estimated at 1–2%.[164]

Histopathology

The appearances are virtually indistinguishable from those of herpes simplex, although the degree of inflammation is said to be greater in herpes simplex than in varicella-zoster lesions.[165] Direct immunofluorescence and immunoperoxidase methods,[94] using a monoclonal antibody specific for varicella-zoster virus,[166] and the Tzanck smear are superior to viral culture in the diagnosis of varicella zoster;[167] monoclonal antibody techniques have the advantage of specificity over the Tzanck smear.[166]

The chronic verrucous lesions reported in immunocompromised patients show pseudoepitheliomatous hyperplasia and massive hyperkeratosis.[156] Herpetic cytopathic changes are also present in keratinocytes.

Electron microscopy

The ultrastructural features of *Herpesvirus varicellae* are similar to those of *Herpesvirus hominis*. However, colloidal gold immunoelectron microscopy using monoclonal antibodies can distinguish between the two.[168]

HERPES ZOSTER

Herpes zoster is caused by the same virus as varicella.[169–171] It occurs in individuals with partial immunity resulting from a prior varicella infection. With few exceptions, zoster appears to represent reactivation of latent virus in sensory ganglia, often in an immunocompromised host. The virus travels through the sensory nerves to reach the skin, where it replicates in the epidermal keratinocytes. Now that a varicella vaccine is available, it is hoped that this may lessen the incidence of herpes zoster in the future.[172] Nevertheless, herpes zoster has been reported in a child following immunization for varicella using the Oka strain of live, attenuated varicella. This strain was recovered from lesional skin.[173]

Zoster is not highly infectious. When children are infected by adults suffering from zoster they develop varicella and not zoster. An attack of either disease leaves the patient with some measure of immunity against both. Recurrent attacks of zoster can occur,[169] although many cases diagnosed as recurrent herpes zoster are probably recurrent herpes simplex.[174,175] Herpes simplex virus has been detected by PCR in two cases with a persistent, painful papular eruption in a zosteriform pattern.[176] Conversely, there is also evidence from PCR studies that initial herpes zoster is sometimes misdiagnosed as herpes simplex.[177] Disseminated herpes zoster is a rare complication of AIDS.[171,178] It has also been reported in idiopathic CD4+ lymphocytopenia.[179]

Clinically, herpes zoster (shingles) is an acute disease that occurs almost exclusively in adults. The illness is febrile and begins with pain in the area innervated by the affected sensory ganglia. The skin in this area becomes red, and papules soon develop.[180] These quickly transform into vesicles and then pustules. There is one report of bullous lesions.[181] Crusts then form and, later, healing takes place. Chronic hyperkeratotic and verrucous lesions may occur in immunocompromised patients.[182–184] Chronicity appears to be associated with a particular pattern of viral gene expression with reduced or undetectable levels of the viral envelope glycoproteins gE and gB.[183] Sometimes there is residual scarring, particularly if there has been secondary bacterial infection of the vesicles. There is one report of herpes zoster localizing to recent surgical scars.[185] Granuloma annulare has been reported at sites of healing herpes zoster.[186] Other lesions reported in herpes zoster scars include a keloid, comedones, lichen planus, giant cell lichenoid dermatitis, urticaria, granulomatous vasculitis, granulomatous folliculitis, sarcoidosis, lichen sclerosus et atrophicus, morphea, an eosinophilic dermatosis, fungal infections, pseudolymphoma, lymphoma, leukemia cutis, Rosai–Dorfman disease, Kaposi's sarcoma, various skin cancers and metastases.[187–195] Necrotizing fasciitis is another rare complication of disseminated cutaneous herpes zoster.[196]

The ganglia most commonly involved are those of the lumbar and thoracic nerves. Post-herpetic neuralgia is a serious complication.[197] Severe ocular damage may result when the ophthalmic division of a trigeminal nerve is involved. If multiple dermatomes are involved, they are usually contiguous.

There is one report of an immunocompromised patient in whom seven disparate dermatomes were involved (zoster multiplex).[198]

Histopathology

The appearances resemble those described for herpes simplex. Despite the comment made earlier that lesions of herpes simplex are usually more inflammatory than those due to varicella-zoster infection,[165] dermal inflammation may be prominent in some cases of herpes zoster, and there may occasionally be a vasculitis.[199] If the vasculitis is severe, necrotizing lesions will be present.[200] A granulomatous vasculitis and lesions resembling granuloma annulare may be seen in healing or healed lesions.[186,201,202] These factors, as well as secondary infection, contribute to the scarring which sometimes ensues. Eccrine duct involvement has been reported, but it is quite uncommon.[203]

The chronic verrucous lesions show hyperkeratosis, verruciform acanthosis and virus-induced cytopathic changes.[183]

CYTOMEGALOVIRUS

Cytomegalovirus belongs to the subgroup of β-herpesviruses. Like other members of the family Herpesviridae, this virus produces primary infection, latent infection and reinfection;[204] however, its site of latency is not known.

There are few reports of cutaneous involvement with cytomegalovirus.[205–207] A maculopapular eruption is the most common clinical presentation, and is seen most often in patients with cytomegalovirus infection who are treated with ampicillin. This is analogous to the situation in infectious mononucleosis.[206] Urticaria,[208] vesiculobullous lesions,[209] ulceration,[210,211] keratotic lesions,[212] diaper dermatitis[213] and even epidermolysis have been reported. Often the clinical picture is quite non-specific.[214,215] The patients are usually immunocompromised,[209,216] a clinical setting in which mixed infections with other agents may occur.[204,217–221]

Infants with congenital infection with cytomegalovirus may present with petechiae and blue-red macular or plaque-like (so-called 'blueberry muffin') lesions, in addition to neurological abnormalities.[222]

Histopathology

There is usually a non-specific dermal infiltrate. The characteristic changes are enlarged endothelial cells in small dermal vessels (Fig. 26.12).[206] The nuclei of these cells contain large eosinophilic inclusions, surrounded by a clear halo. Cytomegalic changes in the absence of nuclear inclusions have been reported.[223] There may also be prominent neutrophilic infiltration of the involved vessel walls, although an unequivocal leukocytoclastic vasculitis is quite rare.[224] Other cells that may harbor viral inclusions include fibrocytes and macrophages. Ductal epithelial cells are rarely involved.[225] The 'blueberry muffin' lesions associated with congenital infections are the result of dermal erythropoiesis.[222] They may also be seen in congenital rubella infections.[222]

Monoclonal antibodies are available for use with immunoperoxidase methods, should it be necessary to confirm the diagnosis in cases with unusual histopathological changes.[226,227] PCR-based methods are also available.[211]

EPSTEIN–BARR VIRUS

A cutaneous rash is seen in approximately 10% of patients with infectious mononucleosis, but this incidence increases dramatically if ampicillin is administered to the patient. The rash is usually erythematous, macular or maculopapular. Erythema multiforme and urticaria may occur.[1] Rare cutaneous manifestations of Epstein–Barr virus infection include a granuloma

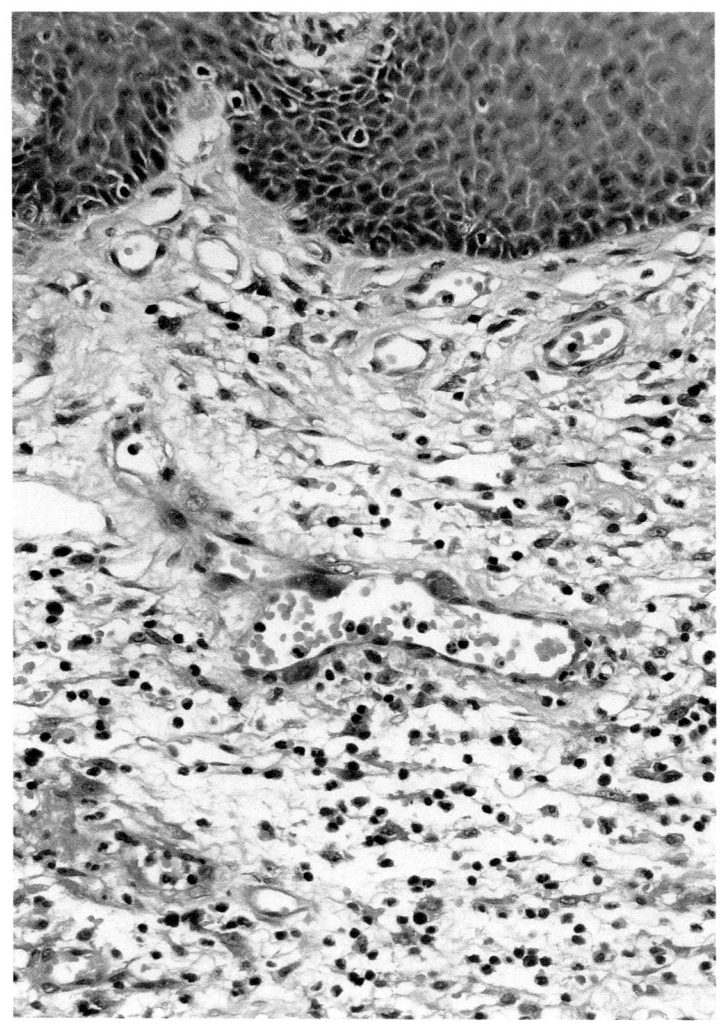

Fig. 26.12 **Cytomegalovirus infection.** A blood vessel in the dermis contains several enlarged endothelial cells, each containing an inclusion body. (H & E) (Photomicrograph kindly supplied by Dr G Strutton)

annulare-like eruption,[228] the Gianotti–Crosti syndrome,[229] oral hairy leukoplakia and lymphoproliferative lesions in immunocompromised patients, particularly following transplantation.[230] Although the lesions may histologically mimic malignant lymphoma, the lesions disappear completely in some patients after the degree of immunosuppression is lowered.[230–232] Epstein–Barr virus has also been implicated in the etiology of Kikuchi's disease.[233,234]

Histopathology
There is usually a mild perivascular infiltrate of inflammatory cells. The changes are non-specific.

HUMAN HERPESVIRUS-6

Human herpesvirus-6 (HHV-6) is the sixth member of the family Herpesviridae to be identified. It shows closest homology with cytomegalovirus and HHV-7.[235] Most of the reports of this recently described infection are in the pediatric literature. The virus produces a cutaneous eruption (exanthem subitum) resembling measles or rubella in infants.[236] The illness may be accompanied by fever.

HHV-6 infection in infants is said to be the commonest cause of fever-induced seizures.[235,237] In adults, infection is seen primarily in immuno-compromised individuals. Although it may play a role in multiple sclerosis and a demyelinating disease in patients with HIV infection, it plays no role in the etiology of lymphomatoid papulosis.[237] Although parvovirus B19 is usually implicated in the etiology of papular-purpuric 'gloves and socks' syndrome (see p. 706), a case has been reported in association with HHV-6 infection.[238]

There are now several reports of a drug hypersensitivity syndrome occurring in association with reactivation of HHV-6.[239–241] In one case a fulminant hemophagocytic syndrome developed.[242] HHV-7 may also act in concert with HHV-6 in producing a drug hypersensitivity syndrome.[240] The drugs implicated were sulfasalazine,[239] allopurinol[240] and phenobarbital.[242] There is some controversy regarding the role of HHV-6 and HHV-7 in the etiology of pityriasis rosea (see p. 112).[243] It is possible that viral reactivation is the explanation for its detection in a number of circumstances.[244]

Histopathology
The cutaneous lesions of exanthem subitum are characterized by spongiosis, small spongiotic vesicles and exocytosis of lymphocytes, sometimes producing Pautrier-like lesions. There is often edema of the papillary dermis and a superficial perivascular infiltrate of mononuclear cells.[236] Cytopathic changes, resembling those seen in herpes simplex and varicella-zoster infections, are absent.

HUMAN HERPESVIRUS-7

Human herpesvirus-7 (HHV-7) was first isolated from a peripheral blood T cell in 1990, and isolated again in 1992 from a patient with chronic fatigue syndrome.[237] HHV-7 can provide a transactivating function for HHV-6. HHV-7 is ubiquitous and infects more than 80% of children in infancy.[237] It has been implicated in the etiology of pityriasis rosea (see p. 112), but reactivation of the virus is a possible explanation for its occurrence in some cases. There is no clear link between HHV-7 and any specific disease at this time.[245]

HUMAN HERPESVIRUS-8

Unlike the other recently described herpesviruses (HHV-6 and HHV-7), this virus (HHV-8) does not appear to be ubiquitous.[246] Its role in the etiology of Kaposi's sarcoma in HIV-positive individuals was confirmed in 1994 when unique DNA sequences were isolated from biopsies of Kaposi's sarcoma. The virus, initially called Kaposi's sarcoma-associated herpesvirus (KSHV), was subsequently renamed HHV-8. Sequence analysis confirms that it is related to *Herpes saimiri* virus, which induces lymphoid malignancies in some primates, and to Epstein–Barr virus (EBV).[247]

The role of HHV-8 in the etiology of Kaposi's sarcoma in patients infected with HIV is now beyond doubt.[248–250] It has also been found in a variable but significant number of HIV-negative cases.[251] The viral load of HHV-8 is relatively low in both HIV-positive and HIV-negative cases.[252] HHV-8 infects the endothelial-derived spindle cells of Kaposi's sarcoma as well as CD19+ B cells. This latter event may be etiologically significant in the causation of some cases of Castleman's disease (see p. 1064) and primary effusion lymphoma. Its presence in a surprising number of skin cancers and in lesions of pemphigus has not been satisfactorily explained, although tropism for lesional skin has been postulated.[253–255] Other studies have failed to confirm these findings.[256,257]

Most studies suggest that the mode of spread is by sexual transmission, but other modes of spread are also likely.[258]

PAPOVAVIRIDAE

Papovaviruses are DNA viruses which replicate in the nucleus. The only important virus in this group in dermatopathology is the human papillomavirus (HPV), which produces various types of warts on different parts of the skin.[259–263] The use of new techniques, such as DNA hybridization, has allowed the separation of over 80 antigenically distinct strains of HPV.[264,265] Further genotypes have been identified, but not fully characterized.[266] In recent years attempts have been made to relate specific antigenic strains of HPV to particular clinicopathological groups of verrucae.[267,268] Some strains have oncogenic potential, and the theoretical mechanisms by which HPV may cause cancer have been reviewed,[269] as has the role of the various immune defense mechanisms to these oncogenic strains of HPV.[270] The following correlations have been recorded: HPV-1 – plantar warts,[271,272] but also common warts and anogenital warts; HPV-2 – common warts, but also plantar,[271] oral[273] and anogenital lesions; HPV-3 – plane warts and epidermodysplasia verruciformis; HPV-3 (variant) – common warts;[274] HPV-4 – plantar and common warts; HPV-5 – epidermodysplasia, which in cases associated with this strain of HPV is usually complicated by carcinoma; HPV-6 – anogenital warts and also epidermodysplasia; HPV-7 – warts in meat and fish handlers;[275–279] HPV-8, 9, 10, 12, 14, 17, 19, 22, 24, and many others – epidermodysplasia; HPV-11 – anogenital lesions;[280] HPV-13 and 32 – focal epithelial hyperplasia (Heck's disease);[281,282] HPV-57 – plantar epidermoid cysts and nail dystrophy;[283,284] HPV-60 – plantar warts and epidermal cysts;[285] HPV-63, 65 and 66 – plantar warts; and HPV-75, 76 and 77 – common warts in immunosuppressed patients.[266] There is now great interest in the role of HPV-16 and 18 in the etiology of uterine cervical intraepithelial neoplasia (CIN) and invasive carcinoma of the cervix. HPV-16 is also the strain most frequently implicated in the etiology of bowenoid papulosis, a disease which sometimes progresses to invasive carcinoma. HPV-16 has also been detected in anogenital warts[286] and in a squamous cell carcinoma of the finger.[287] Various HPV strains may be present in immunosuppressed patients[288] and in skin tumors removed from them.[289–292] Individuals whose immunosuppression results from HIV infection have an increased prevalence of HPV infections, a more rapid progression of the disease, and a higher number of invasive carcinomas.[293] Recent studies have detected HPV strains usually associated with epidermodysplasia verruciformis in some of the malignant and pre-malignant skin lesions of renal transplant recipients.[294,295] This was not found in an earlier study.[296] Furthermore, HPV-5 has recently been found in psoriatic skin lesions, but it is not known if it has any etiological role (see below).

The traditional classification of verrucae will be used here:

- verruca vulgaris or common wart
- palmoplantar warts, including superficial and deep types
- verruca plana
- epidermodysplasia verruciformis
- condyloma acuminatum.

It should be noted that there is some clinical and histological overlap between these groups.[297] Focal epithelial hyperplasia and bowenoid papulosis will also be discussed.

VERRUCA VULGARIS

The common wart (verruca vulgaris) occurs predominantly in children and adolescents, although adults are also frequently infected.[298] Warts have been found in approximately 20% of school students.[299] The lesions may be solitary or multiple, and they are usually found on exposed parts, most frequently on the fingers.[300] They are hard, rough-surfaced papules that range in diameter from about 0.2 cm to as much as 2 cm. New warts may form at sites of trauma (Koebner phenomenon), though not so frequently as in cases of plane warts. They are preferentially associated with HPV-2, but may be induced by HPV-1, HPV-4 and HPV-7.[281] In children, HPV-6 and/or 11 are rarely found in common warts,[301] while HPV-75, 76 and 77 have been identified in lesions from immunosuppressed patients of all ages.[266] Extensive verrucae have been reported in immunodeficiency syndromes.[302–304] They may clear following the use of highly active antiretroviral therapy (HAART).[305]

Histopathology[306]

Common warts show marked hyperkeratosis and acanthosis. There is often some inward turning of the elongated rete ridges at the edge of the lesion (Fig. 26.13). There is some papillomatosis, but this is particularly prominent in filiform variants (Fig. 26.14). Columns of parakeratosis overlie the papillomatous projections. Sometimes there is a small amount of hemorrhage within these columns. The granular layer is lacking in these areas, but elsewhere it is thickened, the cells containing coarse clumps of keratohyaline granules (hypergranulosis). A characteristic feature is the presence of large vacuolated cells in the more superficial parts of the malpighian layer and in the granular layer. These cells (koilocytes) have a small pyknotic nucleus surrounded by clear cytoplasm. There may be small amounts of keratohyaline material in the cytoplasm. These vacuolated cells are not seen in older lesions.

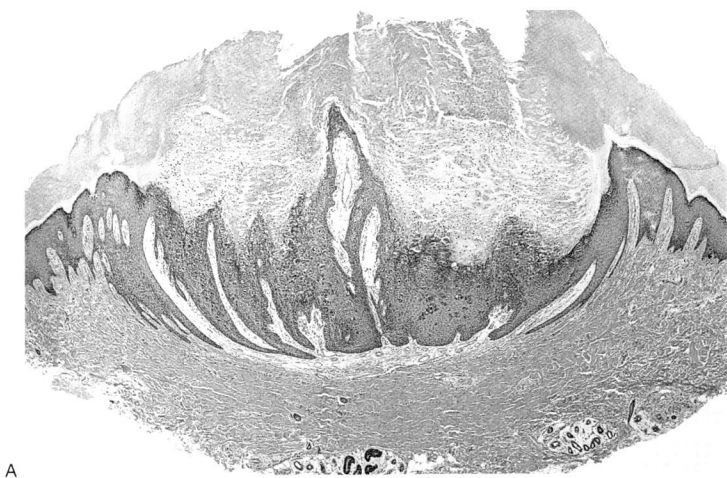

A

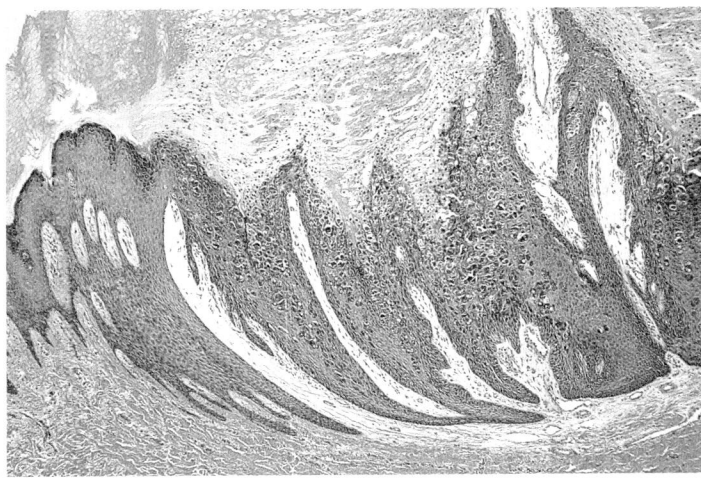

B

Fig. 26.13 **(A) Verruca vulgaris. (B)** Note the papillomatosis, large keratohyaline granules and the characteristic inturning of the rete pegs. (H & E)

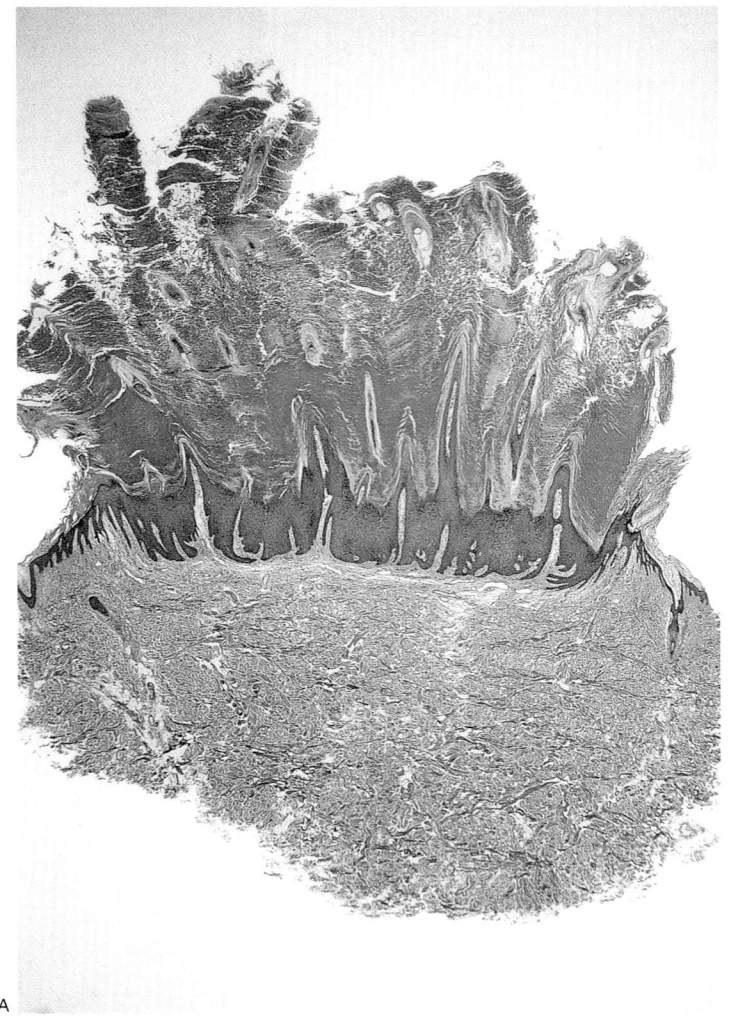

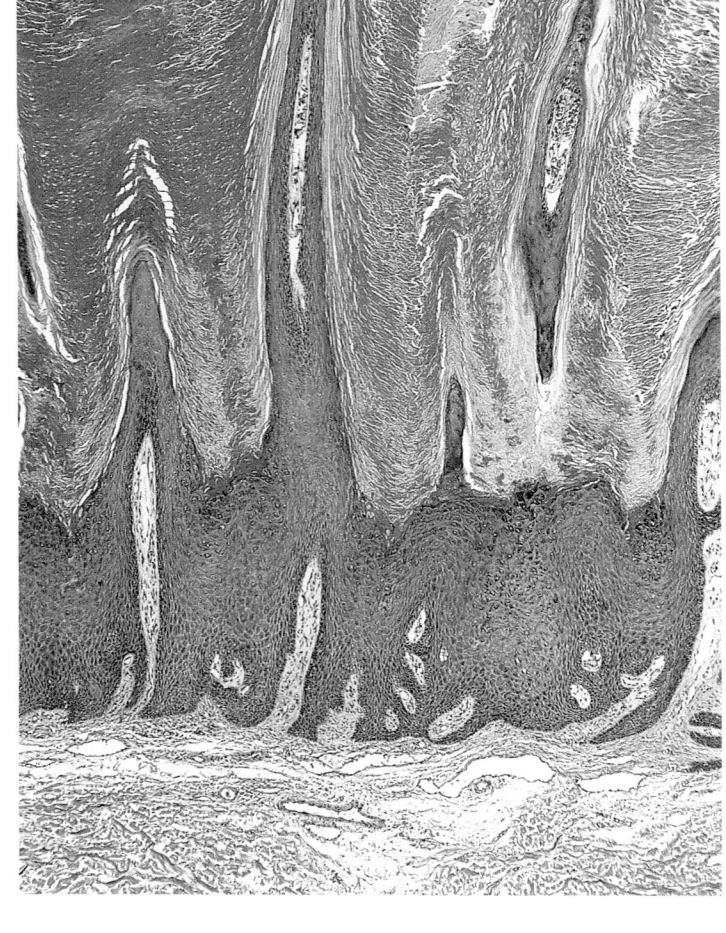

Fig. 26.14 **(A) Verruca vulgaris of filiform type. (B)** There is marked papillomatosis. (H & E)

Cells with pale cytoplasm, representing tricholemmal differentiation, may be seen in the lower epidermis and follicular infundibula of old warts. This has led to controversy regarding the specificity of the appendageal tumor known as tricholemmoma (see p. 867).[307] It seems likely that trichoemmoma is a specific entity, but that local areas of similar appearance can be seen in old warts, particularly if they involve the follicular infundibulum.[308] A similar controversy surrounds the presence of squamous eddies in old warts, and the relationship of these lesions to inverted follicular keratosis (see p. 867).[307] Sebaceous differentiation may rarely be seen. Acantholytic dyskeratosis has been reported in the viral warts that developed in a boy with Darier's disease.[309]

The nuclei of some of the cells in verruca vulgaris may also be vacuolated. They may contain basophilic inclusions representing viral inclusion bodies, or eosinophilic material which is possibly nuclear debris. Papillomavirus antigen can be detected by immunoperoxidase methods.[310]

Most warts show few changes in the dermis, although dilated vessels often extend into the core of the papillomatous projections. A review of 500 verrucae at the Mayo Clinic showed that 8% had a lymphocytic dermal infiltrate, with lichenoid features.[311] The patients were usually elderly. The authors suggested that this might represent an immunological response, although there was no clinical evidence of regression. Earlier observations suggested that the regression of common warts followed the lesions turning

black, a result of thromboses in the capillaries and venules in the upper dermis, accompanied by hemorrhage. However, another study found that in all but one instance, regression took place without the lesions turning black.[312] These verrucae had a heavy mononuclear cell infiltrate in the dermis, with features of a lichenoid tissue reaction. Civatte bodies were not confined to the basal layer. The findings suggest that cell-mediated regression may occur in common warts, similar to that described in plane warts. Warts treated with injections of bleomycin show confluent epidermal necrosis, single apoptotic keratinocytes and diffuse neutrophil infiltration of the epidermis, with abscess formation in the granular layer.[313]

Carcinoma in situ[314,315] and squamous cell carcinoma have developed only very rarely in common warts.[303,307,316] Some of the squamous cell carcinomas that develop in renal transplant patients arise in warts.

Electron microscopy
Wart virus particles range from 45 to 55 nm in diameter. They are initially seen in the nucleus.

PALMOPLANTAR WARTS

Palmoplantar warts are found on the palm of the hand or sole of the foot, and are of clinical importance because they are often painful. They usually occur beneath pressure points, where they may be confused with callosities. They are preferentially associated with HPV-1 or HPV-4 infection,[281] although other subtypes, including HPV-45, 57, 60, 63, 65 and 66, have recently been incriminated (see below).[317] Warts on the palms and soles have traditionally been divided into superficial (mosaic) warts, which are ordinary verrucae, and a deep variety (myrmecia – so named for its supposed resemblance to an anthill). Several other variants[285] have recently been described:

1. A nodular form with retention of the surface ridge pattern ('ridged wart') associated with HPV-60;[318] this HPV type has also been associated with epidermal cysts on the soles,[319] as has HPV-57.[283] HPV-60-induced warts are often pigmented.[320,321]
2. A pigmented verrucous variant associated with HPV-65.
3. A whitish punctate keratotic wart, usually multiple, showing endophytic growth and associated with HPV-63.[322] Cyst formation is sometimes present.[266]
4. A large plantar wart caused by HPV-66.[323]

Histopathology

There are many similarities between the usual variant caused by HPV-1 and the common wart, except that the greater part of the lesion lies deep to the plane of the skin surface and intrudes well into the dermis.[306] There is prominent hyperkeratosis. The HPV-60-associated lesions show acanthosis, but only mild papillomatosis.[324]

It is now accepted that there are correlations between certain HPV types and specific cytopathic changes:[285,322]

- HPV-1 – vacuolated cells in the upper epidermis with large eosinophilic keratohyaline granules (granular inclusions)
- HPV-2 – condensed heterogeneous keratohyaline granules
- HPV-4 – large vacuolated keratinocytes with almost no keratohyaline granules and small peripherally located nuclei
- HPV-60 and 65 – eosinophilic, homogeneous and solitary inclusions, sometimes seen also with HPV-4 (homogeneous inclusions)
- HPV-63 – intracytoplasmic, heavily stained keratohyaline material with filamentous structures that may encase the vacuolated nucleus (filamentous inclusions). Similar inclusions have recently been reported with an HPV genotype that could not be characterized, but which was not HPV-63.[325]

Regression of plantar warts is usually associated with thrombosis of superficial vessels, hemorrhage and necrosis of the epidermis. There is often a mixed inflammatory cell infiltrate.[326]

Pigmented warts are associated with one of the related types of HPV (HPV-4, 60 and 65). The pigmentation is due to the presence of 'melanin blockade melanocytes', resulting from a failure of the transfer of melanosomes to keratinocytes.[327] As a consequence melanocytes become highly dendritic and engorged with melanin pigment.[327]

VERRUCA PLANA

Plane warts (verrucae planae) are flesh-colored or brownish, flat-topped papules, a few millimeters in diameter. They occur most frequently on the back of the hands and on the face. The warts are preferentially associated with HPV-3 and HPV-10;[281] HPV-5 is rarely involved in patients with HIV infection.[328,329] They may develop at sites of trauma (the Koebner phenomenon). Plane warts may disappear suddenly after a few weeks or months, or they may persist for years. Involution is usually preceded by an erythematous change in the warts,[330] but other presentations have included the development of depigmented haloes,[331] and the sudden eruption of large numbers of tiny plane warts.[332] The regression is probably the result of cell-mediated immune mechanisms.[333,334] The epidermodysplasia verruciformis induced by HPV-3 and HPV-10 is characterized by widely disseminated plane warts or large brownish plaques (see below). In these circumstances the warts persist as a result of impaired cell-mediated immunity.[281]

Histopathology

There is hyperkeratosis and acanthosis, with vacuolation of the cells of the granular and upper malpighian layers. The stratum corneum has a 'basket-weave' appearance (Fig. 26.15). The dermis is usually normal. In spontaneously regressing warts there is a superficial lymphocytic infiltrate in the dermis with exocytosis of these cells into the epidermis.[330] This is accompanied by the death of single epidermal cells by the process of apoptosis.[335] Often more than one lymphocyte is in contact with a degenerating epidermal cell. These latter cells are shrunken, with eosinophilic cytoplasm and pyknotic nuclear remnants. Regressing plane warts lose their histological features.

EPIDERMODYSPLASIA VERRUCIFORMIS

Epidermodysplasia verruciformis (EV) usually begins in infancy or childhood.[336] More than 20 different human papillomavirus types have been incriminated, including HPV-3, 5, 8, 9, 10, 12, 14, 15, 17, 19–25, 28, 29, 36–38, 46, 47, 49, 51 and 59.[266] Two forms of the disease are currently recognized.[337] One form is induced by HPV-3, and sometimes HPV-10; these virus types are also responsible for plane warts.[281] Not surprisingly, this form is characterized by multiple plane warts, but the disease is distinguished by the persistence of the lesions, their wider distribution and the presence of plaques. The distinction between this type of EV and multiple plane warts is not always clear cut. Some of the cases are familial. There may be disturbed cellular immune function.[338–341] There is no tendency to malignant transformation in this form. Regression of the lesions has been reported.[337]

The second form of EV is related to HPV-5, and sometimes HPV-8, 9, 14, 20, 24, 38, 47 and others.[342–345] There is often a familial history with an autosomal recessive inheritance, or a history of parental consanguinity. Two susceptibility loci have been mapped to chromosome regions 2p21–p24 and 17q25.[346] This latter region also contains a locus for psoriasis, which is of interest in view of the finding of some EV-related strains of HPV in patients

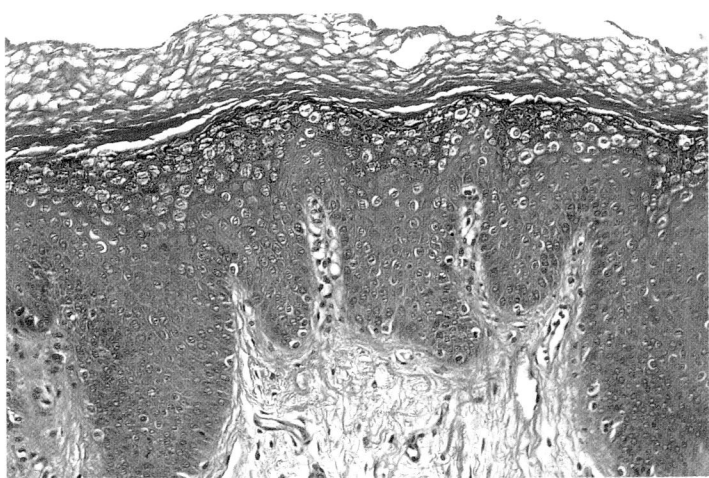

Fig. 26.15 **Verruca plana.** There are vacuolated cells in the upper epidermis and a basket-weave pattern in the overlying stratum corneum. (H & E)

with psoriasis (see below).[347] X-linked recessive inheritance and vertical transmission have also been reported.[348,349] In addition to the plane warts, reddish-brown patches and lesions resembling scaling pityriasis versicolor and seborrheic keratosis develop,[350] with the eventual complication of Bowen's disease[351] or invasive squamous cell carcinoma. Malignant transformation, which occurs in about 25% of patients with EV, depends on the oncogenic potential of the infecting virus.[281] This is highest for HPV-5, followed by HPV-8. Carcinomas develop mainly in light-exposed lesions. Such tumors have a very low rate of metastasis,[342] although patients with advanced squamous cell carcinomas have a much higher rate.[352] Patients with this oncogenic form of EV have an altered natural killer-cell cytotoxic response.[342] p53 protein expression is common in lesional skin.[353]

An epidermodysplasia verruciformis-like eruption, caused by HPV, may complicate HIV infection.[354]

Some of the HPV types involved in epidermodysplasia verruciformis have been implicated in other conditions. For example, HPV-8 has been found in actinic keratoses in patients without epidermodysplasia verruciformis.[355] HPV-5 has been found on the skin of both normal and immunocompromised individuals and also in lesional skin of psoriasis.[347,356–359]

Finally, neurological manifestations and isolated IgM deficiency have been reported in patients with epidermodysplasia verruciformis.[360,361]

Histopathology[362]

The cases induced by HPV-3 resemble plane warts. In the other form there is some variability in the changes seen. Some lesions may resemble plane warts, whereas others consist of thickened epidermis with swollen cells in the upper epidermis (Figs 26.16, 26.17). This latter change is a specific cytopathic effect seen in the various HPV types associated with epidermodysplasia verruciformis. Its full expression is characterized by large cells, sometimes in nests, in the granular and spinous layers. There is a conspicuous perinuclear halo.[362] The nucleoplasm is clear and the cytoplasm, which has a blue-gray pallor, contains keratohyaline granules of various sizes and shapes.[363] The horny layer is loose and has a basket-weave-like appearance.[363] Dysplastic epidermal cells may be seen. Changes of Bowen's disease or squamous cell carcinoma may ultimately supervene.

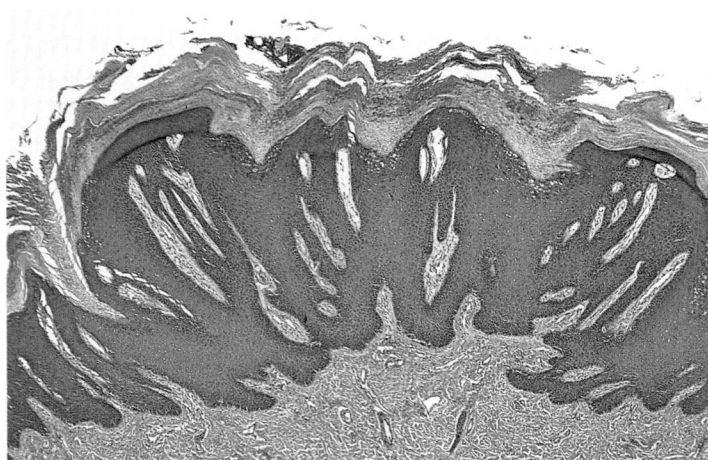

Fig. 26.16 **Epidermodysplasia verruciformis.** The epidermal changes resemble, somewhat, a condyloma acuminatum. Squamous cell carcinoma was present in a neighboring area. (H & E)

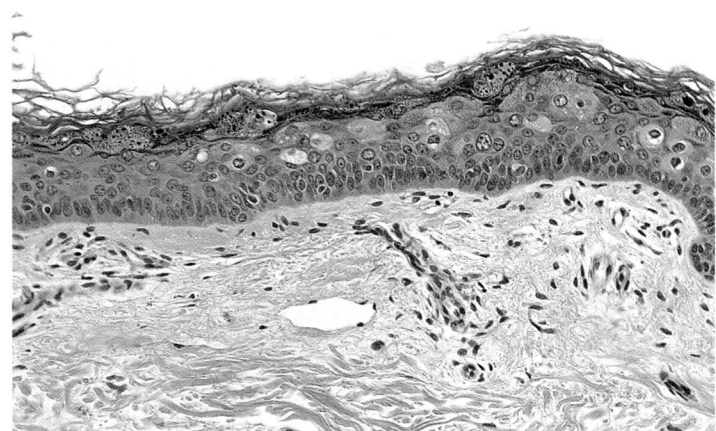

Fig. 26.17 **Epidermodysplasia verruciformis** in a patient with HIV infection. Large pale keratinocytes are present. (H & E)

CONDYLOMA ACUMINATUM

Although condyloma acuminatum is traditionally defined as a fleshy exophytic lesion of the anogenital region,[364,365] it is now known that small inconspicuous lesions may occur on the penis,[366–368] vulva and cervix.[369–371] They are usually sexually transmitted and spread rapidly.[280] Extensive lesions may occur in immunosuppressed persons.[372] The incubation period is variable, but averages 2–3 months.[373] Lesions resembling condyloma acuminatum have been reported as an unusual complication of intertrigo,[374] and of healed herpes progenitalis.[375] A giant-sized condyloma, related to HPV-6 and 11, has been reported on the breast.[376] Children occasionally develop lesions, raising the issue of sexual abuse.[377–381] Condylomas in children regress spontaneously in more than 50% of cases.[382] Condylomas in all age groups are recurrent in up to one-third of cases.[383] This may be related to the persistence of HPV DNA in the dermis.[384] Although malignant transformation of condylomas of the anogenital region is rare, it is more common than in other types of warts, with the exception of epidermodysplasia verruciformis.[385] Giant condyloma acuminatum of Buschke–Lowenstein is now regarded as a variant of verrucous carcinoma,[386–388] although this is still disputed by some.[389] Regression of a deeply infiltrating variant has been reported following long-term intralesional interferon alfa therapy.[390]

As only small amounts of virus are present, characterization of the etiological subtype of HPV involved in the causation of condylomas was made only in the last decade. HPV-6 and 11 are most commonly identified, but other types have been implicated, including HPV-2, 6, 11, 16, 18, 31, 33, 35, 39, 41–45, 51, 56 and 59.[265,281,364,391–393] More than one HPV type may be present.[394] In one study, 83% of cases were positive for HPV-6 and/or 11, whereas 6% were positive for type 16.[265] HPV-16 has oncogenic properties and is sometimes isolated from condylomas, although more usually HPV-16 is seen in association with bowenoid papulosis.[395] The concurrence of condyloma acuminatum and bowenoid papulosis has been reported.[396]

Histopathology[280]

There is marked acanthosis, with some papillomatosis and hyperkeratosis. Vacuolization of granular cells is not as prominent as in other varieties of warts, although there are usually some vacuolated koilocytes in the upper malpighian layer. Lesions resembling seborrheic keratoses may be seen; they usually contain human papillomavirus.[397] Small penile lesions may only show a slightly thickened granular layer.[398] Coarse keratohyaline granules may also be present. Langerhans cells are sometimes prominent.[399] Acantholysis has been reported in one case.[376]

If the lesions are treated with podophyllum resin (podophyllin) 48 hours or so prior to removal, there are striking histological changes. These include pallor of the epidermis, numerous degenerate keratinocytes in the lower half of the epidermis, and a marked increase in this region in the number of mitotic figures.[400] Persistent lesions, resistant to treatment with the immune-response modifier imiquimod, have only rare factor XIIIa-positive dendrocytes in the upper dermis.[401] This feature may be responsible for low cytokine production and explain the resistance to treatment.

Papillomavirus common antigen can be detected in about 60% of lesions by immunoperoxidase techniques.[402] Its presence correlates with that of coarse keratohyaline granules and koilocytes.[402] More sophisticated techniques increase this detection to almost 100%. The presence of MIB-1 immunostaining in the nuclei of the upper two-thirds of the epidermis correlates with the presence of HPV in lesions in which the morphology is suggestive, but not diagnostic, of condyloma.[403]

FOCAL EPITHELIAL HYPERPLASIA

Also known as Heck's disease, focal epithelial hyperplasia is characterized by multiple soft pink or white papules and confluent plaques, particularly on the mucosa of the lips and cheeks.[404] There is a high incidence among Inuits (Eskimos) and American Indians, but there are isolated reports of involvement in other races.[405] HPV-13 and 32 have been implicated in the etiology of this condition.[282,406–408]

Histopathology

The involved mucosa is hyperplastic, with acanthosis and some clubbing of rete pegs. There is a characteristic pallor of epidermal cells, particularly in the upper layers.[409] There are often binucleate cells, but inclusion bodies are not found.

BOWENOID PAPULOSIS

Bowenoid papulosis is the presence, usually on the genitalia, of solitary or multiple verruca-like papules or plaques having a close histological resemblance to Bowen's disease.[410,411] It has a predilection for sexually active young adults. If children develop lesions, the possibility of child sexual abuse should be considered.[412] In males it tends to involve the glans penis and also the foreskin, whereas in females the vulval lesions are often bilateral and pigmented.[413] This condition was first described as multicentric pigmented Bowen's disease,[414] and several other terms were used before acceptance of the term 'bowenoid papulosis'.[415] Although increasing in incidence, it is still a relatively uncommon condition. Cases localized to extragenital sites such as the neck,[416,417] face[418] and fingers[419] have been reported.

Lesions are often resistant to treatment and may have a protracted course, particularly in those with depressed immunity.[420] Spontaneous regression is uncommon. Sometimes there is a history of a previous condyloma. In a small number of cases invasive carcinoma develops. This risk is greatest in women over the age of 40,[413,421] but men are not immune.[422,423] It has been suggested that a cocarcinogenic factor, as yet undetected, may be implicated in this malignant transformation.[424] Most cases of bowenoid papulosis are due to HPV-16, but in a small number HPV-18, 35 and 39, or mixed infections, have been present.[422,425–428] The HPV-16 strain has also been implicated in the pathogenesis of vulval carcinomas and cervical intraepithelial neoplasia.[429,430] The latter condition is occasionally present in the sexual partner of patients with bowenoid papulosis of the penis.[413]

Anogenital cancers have been associated, not only with the HPV types already mentioned, but also with some of the more recently identified types such as HPV-30, 31, 33, 45, 51, 52, 56, 58, 66 and 69.[266]

Histopathology

The histological differentiation of bowenoid papulosis and Bowen's disease is difficult, and may be impossible. Bowenoid papulosis is characterized by full-thickness epidermal atypia and loss of architecture. The basement membrane is intact. Mitoses are frequent, sometimes with abnormal forms. They are often in metaphase. Dyskeratotic cells are also present. True koilocytes are uncommon,[431] although partly vacuolated cells with a 'koilocytotic aura' are sometimes present (Fig. 26.18). The stratum corneum and granular cell layer often contain small inclusion-like bodies which are deeply basophilic, rounded and sometimes surrounded by a halo. These bodies, together with the numerous metaphase mitoses, are the features that suggest a diagnosis of bowenoid papulosis rather than Bowen's disease itself.

Bowenoid papulosis is commonly classified by gynecological pathologists as vulvar intraepithelial neoplasia (VIN) III.[421]

PICORNAVIRIDAE

The picornaviridae are an important family of RNA viruses which includes the coxsackievirus and ECHOvirus. They are now the most common cause of exanthems in children.[1] Most of the cutaneous manifestations are transient macular or maculopapular lesions in the course of an obvious viral illness, and biopsies are rarely taken. As a result, very little is known of the histology. Urticarial and vesicular lesions have also been reported.[432] The most important of the vesicular group is so-called 'hand, foot and mouth disease', caused mostly by coxsackievirus A16. This virus has also been associated with an eruption resembling that of the Gianotti–Crosti syndrome,[433] although this condition is more usually associated with hepatitis B infection (see below).[434]

HAND, FOOT AND MOUTH DISEASE

Most cases are caused by coxsackievirus A16, although other types have also been implicated. The disease is a febrile illness characterized by vesicles in the

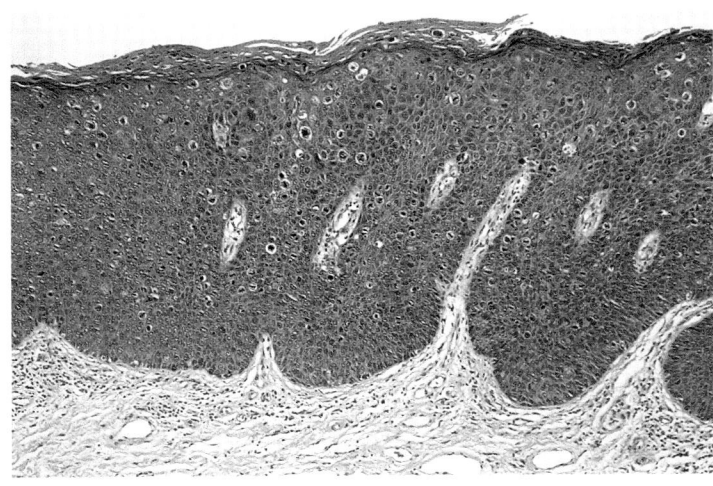

Fig. 26.18 **Bowenoid papulosis.** There are atypical keratinocytes throughout the full thickness of the epidermis with several mitoses in metaphase. Small basophilic inclusions are present in the granular layer. (H & E)

anterior parts of the mouth and on the hands and feet.[435] The vesicles are usually small and they may be sparse.

Histopathology

There are intraepidermal vesicles with prominent reticular degeneration, and sometimes a few ballooned cells in the base. There are no multinucleate cells or inclusion bodies. Similar changes, usually without ballooning, are seen in the vesicular lesions of other viruses in this family. There is sometimes the additional feature of papillary dermal edema and a mild perivascular inflammatory infiltrate.

OTHER VIRAL DISEASES

PARVOVIRUS

Human parvovirus is a member of the family Parvoviridae, a group of single-stranded DNA viruses. Parvovirus B19 is the type most often implicated in human disease. It can produce an influenza-like illness, miscarriages, fetal hydrops, neonatal angioedema,[436] polyarthritis, aplastic crises, purpura, vasculitis, erythema multiforme, dermatomyositis,[437] a Sweet's syndrome-like eruption,[437] lupus erythematosus-like syndromes,[437] an asymptomatic papular eruption, livedo reticularis,[438] acral pruritus,[439] the papular-purpuric (petechial) 'gloves-and-socks' syndrome[440] and erythema infectiosum (fifth disease).[441–445]

The *papular-purpuric 'gloves-and-socks' syndrome* is a self-limited infection characterized by pruritic, erythematous papules with petechiae and edema involving predominantly the hands and feet.[446] Fever, arthralgias and oral lesions may be present. This exanthem usually occurs in adults. Although parvovirus B19 has been implicated most often, there are reports of a similar illness following measles virus, Epstein–Barr virus, human herpesvirus-6, human herpesvirus-7, coxsackievirus B6 and cytomegalovirus.[447,448] In immunocompromised patients, persistent skin lesions and anemia often develop.[449] Serological confirmation can be used to confirm the diagnosis.[450] Approximately 50% of the adult population is immune.[451]

Erythema infectiosum (fifth disease) is an exanthem which may be difficult to distinguish from rubella. A distinctive well-marginated rash often appears on the cheeks a few days after the onset of prodromal symptoms. The rash usually becomes more generalized after a few days.

Parvovirus B19 is spread by a respiratory droplet and has an incubation period of 5–14 days.[451] The receptor for the virus is the erythrocyte P antigen which is also expressed on endothelial cells. The virus has been demonstrated in endothelial cells in lesional skin by several methods, including PCR.[452,453] It has also been identified in keratinocytes.[454] Parvovirus B19 has been reported as producing four distinct clinical presentations in the one family.[451] This suggests that the immunological response to the virus may play a role in determining the clinical presentation.[455]

Histopathology[452,453,455]

The changes resemble other viral infections with a mild, usually tight perivascular infiltrate of lymphocytes, mild exocytosis of lymphocytes and mild basal vacuolar change with rare apoptotic keratinocytes. Extravasation of red cells is often present. At times, the appearances are those of a lichenoid lymphocytic vasculitis (see p. 243) but fibrin is rarely present. Eosinophils and occasional neutrophils may be present. Interstitial lymphocytes and histiocytes have been described, resembling incomplete granuloma annulare,[437] but this may be a late manifestation of a previous lymphocytic vasculitis in which a hypercellular interstitium ('busy' dermis) and mucin may be present.

MEASLES

A biopsy from the rash of measles shows epidermal spongiosis and mild vesiculation, with scattered shrunken and degenerate keratinocytes.[456,457] This latter feature may be prominent in patients with AIDS.[457] Occasional multinucleate epithelial giant cells may be seen in the upper epidermis and in hair follicles and acrosyringial cells.[458]

TOGAVIRUSES

The togavirus group includes the viruses that cause rubella and dengue,[459] as well as the Sindbis, Ross River, West Nile, Chikungunya and O'nyong-nyong viruses.[1,460] West Nile virus has been reported in countries outside Africa.[461] Very little is known about the host response to arboviruses such as West Nile. Experimentally, Langerhans cells migrate from the skin to local lymph nodes following cutaneous infection.[462] This migration appears to be important in the development of an immune response to the virus. The rashes are usually maculopapular, but petechial or purpuric lesions are not uncommon. There is a light perivascular infiltrate of lymphocytes with mild endothelial swelling. Red cell extravasation is present in the purpuric lesions.[463,464] Large, atypical lymphoid cells have been reported in a heavy perifollicular lymphohistiocytic infiltrate in a papular eruption in a patient with Sindbis infection.[465]

HEPATITIS A VIRUS

Skin manifestations associated with infection by hepatitis A virus have been rarely reported. They include a photo-accentuated eruption, accompanied by the deposition of IgA in endothelial cells of the upper dermis.[466] The Gianotti–Crosti syndrome (see below) and a vasculitis are other rare manifestations.

HEPATITIS B VIRUS

The dermatological manifestations of the hepatitis B virus include:

1. a serum sickness-like prodrome with urticarial or vasculitic lesions and, rarely, an erythema multiforme or lichenoid picture[467]
2. a rare, photolocalized pustular eruption[468]
3. polyarteritis nodosa[469,470]
4. essential mixed cryoglobulinemia
5. papular acrodermatitis of childhood (Gianotti–Crosti syndrome).[434,471,472]

Gianotti–Crosti syndrome

Gianotti–Crosti syndrome is characterized by a non-relapsing erythematopapular rash, lasting about 3 weeks and localized to the face and limbs, with the addition sometimes of lymphadenopathy and acute hepatitis, usually anicteric.[473,474] It has also been associated with many other viruses, including hepatitis A,[475] cytomegalovirus,[476] Epstein–Barr virus,[477,478] adenovirus,[476] rotavirus,[479] parainfluenza virus[480] and coxsackievirus.[481,482] It has also been reported following various immunizations.[483,484] The histology can show a characteristic mixture of three tissue reactions: spongiotic, lichenoid and lymphocytic vasculitis. Usually the lichenoid features consist of mild basal vacuolar change; rarely, this is a dominant feature.[485] Red cell extravasation and papillary dermal edema are other features.

A recurrent erythematous asymptomatic papular rash on the trunk and proximal extremities has been reported in hepatitis B carriers.[486] Histopathological study showed a superficial and deep perivascular mononuclear infiltrate in the dermis.[486]

HEPATITIS C VIRUS

Since its discovery in 1989, the hepatitis C virus has assumed great clinical importance as a cause of chronic hepatitis. Other organs may be involved, usually through immunological mechanisms.[487–489] Skin disorders have been reported in up to 15% of patients afflicted with this virus. Most of these conditions are discussed in more detail elsewhere. They include:

- vasculitis (mainly cryoglobulin-associated vasculitis or polyarteritis nodosa)[490]
- pigmented purpuric dermatosis (see p. 247)[491]
- sporadic porphyria cutanea tarda (see p. 559)[492–494]
- lichen planus (see p. 33)
- erythema nodosum (see p. 522)
- urticaria (see p. 227)[495]
- erythema multiforme (see p. 43)
- Behçet's syndrome (see p. 241)
- necrolytic acral erythema (see p. 554)
- symmetric polyarthritis with livedo reticularis[496]
- pruritus.[490]

There appears to be a high incidence of cutaneous reactions in patients with chronic hepatitis C viral infection treated with the combination of interferon alfa and ribavirin.[497] The eruptions may be eczematous, lichenoid or non-specific.

KIKUCHI'S DISEASE

Kikuchi's disease (histiocytic necrotizing lymphadenitis) is of presumptive viral origin, based on its clinical features and course. Most cases have been reported from Japan. Viruses implicated have included HHV-6, HHV-8,[498] HTLV-1,[499] EBV[233 234] and cytomegalovirus. Cutaneous involvement occurs in about 30% of patients. The eruption may be morbilliform, urticarial, maculopular or disseminated erythema.[500,501] Lymphadenopathy is an important clinical feature. Kikuchi's disease has been reported in association with cutaneous lupus erythematosus[502] and Still's disease.[503]

Histopathology[500,504,505]

The histological changes may show some resemblance to lupus erythematosus, with a lichenoid (interface) reaction with basal vacuolar change and some apoptotic keratinocytes. There is a variable superficial and deep perivascular infiltrate of lymphocytes and histiocytes in the dermis. Extension into the subcutis is not uncommon.

Subepidermal edema is often present and histiocytes containing nuclear debris are often seen in the base of the edema.[505] A CD68 stain confirms that many of the cells that initially seem to be lymphocytes are of histiocytic lineage.[503] Cells with a cleaved or deformed nucleus, sometimes resembling Reed–Sternberg cells, have been reported. There is a conspicuous absence of neutrophils and a paucity of plasma cells.[505]

ASYMMETRIC PERIFLEXURAL EXANTHEM

Also known as unilateral laterothoracic exanthem, asymmetric periflexural exanthem is of presumptive viral etiology, although no virus has yet been detected by various methods.[506] It begins as a unilateral eruption close to the axilla with centrifugal spread.[507] There is spontaneous resolution after several weeks. This disorder is rare after childhood.[508,509]

Histopathology

There is a superficial perivascular infiltrate of lymphocytes which often forms a tight cuff around the vessels. Some authors have described a lymphocytic infiltrate around eccrine ducts with mild miliarial spongiosis and exocytosis of lymphocytes into the acrosyringium.[507,510] Mild lichenoid changes may be present in late lesions.

ACQUIRED IMMUNODEFICIENCY SYNDROME (AIDS)

AIDS is one manifestation of a variety of disorders caused by infection with the human T-cell lymphotropic virus type III (HTLV III), now known as human immunodeficiency virus (HIV). It is a retrovirus that infects and destroys helper T lymphocytes, with resulting disturbances in cellular immune function.[511,512] It also infects cells of the central nervous system, producing dementia and motor disturbances. Lymphadenopathy is another manifestation of HIV infection. AIDS is found most commonly in male homosexuals, in hemophiliacs who have received infected blood, in intravenous drug users and in parts of Africa, where heterosexual transmission is important. Viremia is lifelong.

Kaposi's sarcoma was the first cutaneous manifestation of AIDS to be reported (see p. 1021). It is found in up to one-third of patients, and is an adverse prognostic factor. Its incidence is lower in some non-Western countries, such as India.[513] The role of human herpesvirus-8 in its etiology is discussed elsewhere (see p. 700). Many other cutaneous effects have been described in recent years. These fall into three broad categories: infections, usually of an opportunistic nature, neoplasms[514,515] and non-infectious dermatoses.[516–527] These are detailed in Table 26.1. Detailed references can be found in a number of reviews of this subject.[528–534]

Table 26.1 Cutaneous manifestations of AIDS

Infections

Viral: molluscum contagiosum, herpes simplex, herpes zoster, verruca vulgaris, condylomas, cytomegalovirus, oral hairy leukoplakia, Kaposi's sarcoma

Bacterial: mycobacterial infections, more usual bacterial infections, bacillary angiomatosis

Spirochetal: syphilis

Fungal: candidosis, dermatophytosis, histoplasmosis, cryptococcosis, tinea versicolor, phaeonyphomycosis, nocardiosis, mucormycosis, *Penicillium marneffei* infection

Protozoa: acanthamebiasis, pneumocytosis

Arthropod: scabies, demodicosis

Neoplasms

Kaposi's sarcoma, cutaneous lymphomas, Bowen's disease, squamous and basal cell carcinomas, cutaneous melanomas

Dermatoses

Psoriasis, seborrheic dermatitis, pityriasis rubra pilaris, acquired ichthyosis, asteatosis, porokeratosis, vasculitis, folliculitis, contact dermatitis, photosensitivity, vitiligo, yellow nail syndrome, papular eruption, idiopathic pruritus, a chronic diffuse dermatitis, severe drug reactions, alopecia, palmoplantar keratoderma, porphyria cutanea tarda, acrodermatitis enteropathica and neutrophilic eccrine hidradenitis

Opportunistic infections have decreased in patients with HIV since the introduction in 1997 of so-called 'highly active antiretroviral therapy' (HAART). Viral titers fall with this therapy and there is a progressive increase in CD4[+] cells. Over time, reappearance of the complete T-cell repertoire occurs.[535] Restoration of immunity can result in the appearance of quiescent or latent infections such as herpes zoster and *M. avium-intracellulare* infection.

Other skin conditions that seem to improve or decline in incidence with HAART include Kaposi's sarcoma, eosinophilic folliculitis, Norwegian scabies and verrucous lesions of herpes zoster.[535] Complications of HAART, using protease inhibitors, include a lipodystrophy (see p. 531) and paronychia.[536]

Early signs of HIV infection may be a roseola-like rash associated with recent infection and seroconversion,[537-540] or the development of psoriasis/seborrheic dermatitis,[541] pruritic lesions,[542,543] herpes simplex and zoster, a chronic acneiform folliculitis, oral candidosis, tinea, or impetigo of the neck and beard region.[544,545] Infections in immunocompromised patients may differ in severity and other clinical features from those in normal hosts.[546-548]

A unique manifestation of HIV infection is *oral 'hairy' leukoplakic*, which is characterized by raised, poorly demarcated projections on the lateral borders of the tongue, resulting in a corrugated or 'hairy' surface.[549,550] It has been observed in nearly 25% of patients with HIV-associated skin disorders.[532,551] It is induced by Epstein–Barr virus but human papillomavirus has also been identified in some biopsy specimens.[552] *Candida* is frequently present. The development of oral 'hairy' leukoplakia in patients with HIV infection indicates advanced immunosuppression.[551] In other clinical settings of immunosuppression, however, oral 'hairy' leukoplakia is quite rare.

Pruritic papular eruption is the most common cutaneous manifestation in HIV-infected patients.[553,554] It consists of chronic, pruritic, discrete papules on the trunk, extremities and face. Excoriation is often present. This eruption is distinct from the rare widespread, pruritic disorder, often with pigment changes, seen in late stage HIV infection and characterized by atypical lymphocytes in the skin, which are CD8[+]. This pseudo-Sézary syndrome rarely progresses to frank lymphoma.[555]

Changes in the immune system, including T-cell function, antigen response and shifting cytokine expression, as well as a propensity for autoimmune reactions, appear to underlie the skin changes occurring in AIDS.[556,557] Their occurrence correlates with low CD4 lymphocyte counts.[558-561] Cutaneous infections and a pruritic eruption have been reported in association with a 'syndrome' characterized by idiopathic CD4[+] lymphocytopenia but no evidence of HIV infection.[562-564]

Histopathology[557]

Various inflammatory dermatoses occur in patients infected with the human immunodeficiency virus type I (HIV-1). Subtle differences have been found in the expression of the diseases in these patients compared to patients without HIV infection. The number of neutrophils and eosinophils in inflammatory infiltrates may increase during the course of the disease. Plasma cells are sometimes present in diseases in which they are not usually found. Spotty parakeratosis is also more common. Apoptotic keratinocytes, often with an adjacent lymphocyte, are sometimes seen. At times the appearances resemble those seen in graft-versus-host disease (see p. 46). T cells, negative for CD7, are increased in cutaneous infiltrates.[565] This class of lymphocyte is epidermotropic. Increased numbers of CD30[+] cells appear in the infiltrates of inflammatory dermatoses in later stages of AIDS.[566]

The *pruritic papular eruption* of HIV infection shows variable features. There is a superficial perivascular infiltrate of lymphocytes, often with some eosinophils. Neutrophils and plasma cells are less common.[567,568] Extension of the infiltrate around the deep plexus and appendages also occurs. Factor XIIIa-positive cells are usually increased. Dermal fibrosis and changes suggestive of early 'necrobiosis' are often present.

In the *acute exanthem* of HIV infection (seroconversion) there is a tight perivascular infiltrate of lymphocytes. Epidermal changes are usually mild, but may include spongiosis, vacuolar alteration, scattered apoptotic keratinocytes or epidermal necrosis.[569-572] Folliculitis is uncommon. In many cases the changes resemble those seen in other viral exanthems.

In *oral 'hairy' leukoplakia* there is some acanthosis and parakeratosis. Large pale-staining cells resembling koilocytes are present in the upper stratum malpighii. *Candida* is frequently present in the keratin projections on the surface.

HUMAN T-LYMPHOTROPHIC VIRUS TYPE I (HTLV-1)

The human retrovirus HTLV-1 was first isolated in 1980. It is found in parts of Japan, the Caribbean and central Africa. Immigration has led to its dissemination to other countries, although its seroprevalence in the USA is very low.[573] This virus was originally found to be the cause of adult T-cell leukemia/lymphoma (see p. 1116), but recently it has been associated with infective dermatitis of children, a condition with close clinical and histopathological similarities to atopic dermatitis. Both diseases are a chronic dermatitis with a propensity for colonization with *Staphylococcus aureus* and β-hemolytic streptococci.[574] Infective dermatitis presents as an eczema of the scalp, axillae and groins, external ear and retroauricular region. Dermatopathic lymphadenopathy is common.[573,574]

HTLV-1 infection can also produce tropical spastic paraparesis and a myelopathy.[573,575]

REFERENCES

Introduction

1 Cherry JD. Viral exanthems. Dis Mon 1982; 28 (8): 1–56.
2 Ruzicka T, Rosendahl C, Braun-Falco O. A probable case of rotavirus exanthem. Arch Dermatol 1985; 121: 253–254.
3 Drew WL. Laboratory diagnosis of viral skin disease. Semin Dermatol 1984; 3: 146–153.
4 Solomon AR. New diagnostic tests for herpes simplex and varicella zoster infections. J Am Acad Dermatol 1988; 18: 218–221.

Poxviridae

5 Smith KJ, Skelton HG III, James WD, Lupton GP. *Parapoxvirus* infections acquired after exposure to wildlife. Arch Dermatol 1991; 127: 79–82.
6 Birge MB, Rudikoff D, Tan MH et al. Orthopoxvirus from Sierra Leone. J Cutan Pathol 2000; 27: 549 (abstract).
7 Diven DG. An overview of poxviruses. J Am Acad Dermatol 2001; 44: 1–14.
8 Lewis-Jones MS, Baxby D, Cefai C, Hart CA. Cowpox can mimic anthrax. Br J Dermatol 1993; 129: 625–627.
9 Motley RJ, Holt PJA. Cowpox presenting with sporotrichoid spread: a case report. Br J Dermatol 1990; 122: 705–708.
10 Blackford S, Roberts DL, Thomas PD. Cowpox infection causing a generalized eruption in a patient with atopic dermatitis. Br J Dermatol 1993; 129: 628–629.
11 Baxby D, Bennett M, Getty B. Human cowpox 1969–93: a review based on 54 cases. Br J Dermatol 1994; 131: 598–607.
12 Casemore DP, Emslie ES, Whyler DK et al. Cowpox in a child, acquired from a cat. Clin Exp Dermatol 1987; 12: 286–287.
13 Vestey JP, Yirrell DL, Norval M. What is human catpox/cowpox infection? Int J Dermatol 1991; 30: 696–698.
14 Wienecke R, Wolff H, Schaller M et al. Cowpox virus infection in an 11-year-old girl. J Am Acad Dermatol 2000; 42: 892–894.

15 Amer M, El-Gharib I, Rashed A et al. Human cowpox infection in Sharkia Governorate, Egypt. Int J Dermatol 2001; 40: 14–17.

16 Ramanan C, Ghorpade A, Kalra SK, Mann S. Buffalopox. Int J Dermatol 1996; 35: 128–130.

17 Lane JM, Ruben FL, Neff JM, Millar JD. Complications of smallpox vaccination, 1968; national surveillance in the United States. N Engl J Med 1968; 281: 1201–1208.

18 Sarkany I, Caron GA. Cutaneous complications of smallpox vaccination. Trans St Johns Hosp Dermatol Soc 1962; 48: 163–170.

19 Marmelzat WL. Malignant tumors in smallpox vaccination scars. A report of 24 cases. Arch Dermatol 1968; 97: 400–406.

20 Slater DN, Parsons MA, Fussey IV. Malignant fibrous histiocytoma arising in a smallpox vaccination scar. Br J Dermatol 1981; 105: 215–217.

21 Lupton GP. Discoid lupus erythematosus occurring in a smallpox vaccination scar. J Am Acad Dermatol 1987; 17: 688–690.

22 Anderton RL, Abele DC. Lichen sclerosus et atrophicus in a vaccination site. Arch Dermatol 1976; 112: 1787.

23 Breman JG, Arita I. The confirmation and maintenance of smallpox eradication. N Engl J Med 1980; 303: 1263–1273.

24 McGovern TW, Christopher GW, Eitzen EM. Cutaneous manifestations of biological warfare and related threat agents. Arch Dermatol 1999; 135: 311–322.

25 Michelson HE, Ikeda K. Microscopic changes in variola. Arch Dermatol Syph 1927; 15: 138–164.

26 Epstein WL. Molluscum contagiosum. Semin Dermatol 1992; 11: 184–189.

27 Gottlieb SL, Myskowski PL. Molluscum contagiosum. Int J Dermatol 1994; 33: 453–461.

28 Smith KJ, Yeager J, Skelton H. Molluscum contagiosum: its clinical, histopathologic, and immunohistochemical spectrum. Int J Dermatol 1999; 38: 664–672.

29 Silverberg NB, Sidbury R, Mancini AJ. Childhood molluscum contagiosum: Experience with cantharidin therapy in 300 patients. J Am Acad Dermatol 2000; 43: 503–507.

30 Cribier B, Scrivener Y, Grosshans E. Molluscum contagiosum: histologic patterns and associated lesions. A study of 578 cases. Am J Dermatopathol 2001; 23: 99–103.

31 Myskowski PL. Molluscum contagiosum. New insights, new directions. Arch Dermatol 1997; 133: 1039–1041.

32 Choong KY, Roberts LJ. Molluscum contagiosum, swimming and bathing: a clinical analysis. Australas J Dermatol 1999; 40: 89–92.

33 Ha S-J, Park Y-M, Cho S-H et al. Solitary giant molluscum contagiosum of the sole. Pediatr Dermatol 1998; 15: 222–224.

34 Ghura HS, Camp RDR. Scarring molluscum contagiosum in patients with severe atopic dermatitis: report of two cases. Br J Dermatol 2001; 144: 1094–1095.

35 Watanabe T, Nakamura K, Wakugawa M et al. Antibodies to molluscum contagiosum virus in the general population and susceptible patients. Arch Dermatol 2000; 136: 1518–1522.

36 Cotton DWK, Cooper C, Barrett DF, Leppard BJ. Severe atypical molluscum contagiosum infection in an immunocompromised host. Br J Dermatol 1987; 116: 871–876.

37 Katzman M, Carey JT, Elmets CA et al. Molluscum contagiosum and the acquired immunodeficiency syndrome: clinical and immunological details of two cases. Br J Dermatol 1987; 116: 131–138.

38 Smith KJ, Skelton HG III, Yeager J et al. Molluscum contagiosum. Ultrastructural evidence for its presence in skin adjacent to clinical lesions in patients infected with human immunodeficiency virus type 1. Arch Dermatol 1992; 128: 223–227.

39 Izu R, Manzano D, Gardeazabal J, Diaz-Perez JL. Giant molluscum contagiosum presenting as a tumor in an HIV-infected patient. Int J Dermatol 1994; 33: 266–267.

40 Schwartz JJ, Myskowski PL. Molluscum contagiosum in patients with human immunodeficiency virus infection. A review of twenty-seven patients. J Am Acad Dermatol 1992; 27: 583–588.

41 Vozmediano JM, Manrique A, Petraglia S et al. Giant molluscum contagiosum in AIDS. Int J Dermatol 1996; 35: 45–47.

42 Cronin TA Jr, Resnik BI, Elgart G, Kerdel FA. Recalcitrant giant molluscum contagiosum in a patient with AIDS. J Am Acad Dermatol 1996; 35: 266–267.

43 Mastrolorenzo A, Urbano FG, Salimbeni L et al. Atypical molluscum contagiosum infection in an HIV-infected patient. Int J Dermatol 1998; 37: 378–380.

44 Au WY, Lie AKW, Shek TW. Fulminant molluscum contagiosum infection and concomitant leukaemia cutis after bone marrow transplantation for chronic myeloid leukaemia. Br J Dermatol 2000; 143: 1097–1098.

45 Meadows KP, Tyring SK, Pavia AT, Rallis TM. Resolution of recalcitrant molluscum contagiosum virus lesions in human immunodeficiency virus-infected patients treated with cidofovir. Arch Dermatol 1997; 133: 987–990.

46 Kwittken J. Molluscum contagiosum: some new histologic observations. Mt Sinai J Med 1980; 47: 583–588.

47 Shelley WB, Burmeister V. Demonstration of a unique viral structure: the molluscum viral colony sac. Br J Dermatol 1986; 115: 557–562.

48 Reed RJ, Parkinson RP. The histogenesis of molluscum contagiosum. Am J Surg Pathol 1977; 1: 161–166.

49 Uehara M, Danno K. Central pitting of molluscum contagiosum. J Cutan Pathol 1980; 7: 149–153.

50 Aloi FG, Pippione M. *Molluscum contagiosum* occurring in an epidermoid cyst. J Cutan Pathol 1985; 12: 163–165.

51 Egawa K, Honda Y, Ono T. Multiple giant molluscum contagiosa with cyst formation. Am J Dermatopathol 1995; 17: 414–416.

52 Ackerman AB. Epidermal inclusion cysts. Arch Dermatol 1974; 109: 736.

53 Brandrup F, Asschenfeldt P. Molluscum contagiosum-induced comedo and secondary abscess formation. Pediatr Dermatol 1989; 6: 118–121.

54 Jang KA, Choi J-H, Sung K-J et al. Molluscum folliculitis in the absence of HIV infection. Br J Dermatol 1999; 140: 171–172.

55 Steffen C, Markman J-A. Spontaneous disappearance of molluscum contagiosum. Report of a case. Arch Dermatol 1980; 116: 923–924.

56 Heng MCY, Steuer ME, Levy A et al. Lack of host cellular immune response in eruptive molluscum contagiosum. Am J Dermatopathol 1989; 11: 248–254.

57 Ackerman AB, Tanski EV. Pseudoleukemia cutis. Report of a case in association with molluscum contagiosum. Cancer 1977; 40: 813–817.

58 de Diego J, Berridi D, Saracibar N, Requena L. Cutaneous pseudolymphoma in association with molluscum contagiosum. Am J Dermatopathol 1998; 20: 518–521.

59 Guitart J, Hurt MA. Pleomorphic T-cell infiltrate associated with molluscum contagiosum. Am J Dermatopathol 1999; 21: 178–180.

60 Marks JG Jr, White JW Jr. Molluscum contagiosum in a halo nevus. Int J Dermatol 1980; 19: 258–259.

61 Hanau D, Grosshans E. Response to molluscum contagiosum in a halo nevus. Int J Dermatol 1981; 20: 218–220.

62 Crovato F, Nazzari G. Halo dermatitis around molluscum contagiosum: Meyerson's phenomenon? Br J Dermatol 1994; 131: 452.

63 Charley MR, Sontheimer RD. Clearing of subacute cutaneous lupus erythematosus around molluscum contagiosum lesions. J Am Acad Dermatol 1982; 6: 529–533.

64 Payne D, Yen A, Tyring S. Coinfection of molluscum contagiosum with human papillomavirus. J Am Acad Dermatol 1997; 36: 641–644.

65 Naert F, Lachapelle JM. Multiple lesions of molluscum contagiosum with metaplastic ossification. Am J Dermatopathol 1989; 11: 238–241.

66 Schuler G, Honigsmann H, Wolff K. The syndrome of milker's nodules in burn injury. Evidence for indirect viral transmission. J Am Acad Dermatol 1982; 6: 334–339.

67 Leavell UW Jr, Phillips IA. Milker's nodules. Pathogenesis, tissue culture, electron microscopy, and calf inoculation. Arch Dermatol 1975; 111: 1307–1311.

68 Kuokkanen K, Launis J, Morttinen A. Erythema nodosum and erythema multiforme associated with milker's nodules. Acta Derm Venereol 1976; 56: 69–72.

69 Groves RW, Wilson-Jones E, MacDonald DM. Human orf and milkers' nodule: a clinicopathologic study. J Am Acad Dermatol 1991; 25: 706–711.

70 Labeille B, Duverlie G, Daniel P, Denoeux J-P. Bullous eruption complicating a milker's nodule. Int J Dermatol 1988; 27: 115–116.

71 Evins S, Leavell UW Jr, Phillips IA. Intranuclear inclusions in milker's nodules. Arch Dermatol 1971; 103: 91–93.

72 Davis CM, Musil G. Milker's nodule. A clinical and electron microscopic report. Arch Dermatol 1970; 101: 305–311.

73 Leavell UW Jr, McNamara MJ, Muelling R et al. Orf, report of 19 human cases with clinical and pathological observations. JAMA 1968; 204: 657–664.

74 Johannessen JV, Krogh H-K, Solberg I et al. Human orf. J Cutan Pathol 1975; 2: 265–283.

75 Hunskaar S. Giant orf in a patient with chronic lymphocytic leukaemia. Br J Dermatol 1986; 114: 631–634.

76 Pether JVS, Guerrier CJW, Jones SM et al. Giant orf in a normal individual. Br J Dermatol 1986; 115: 497–499.

77 Kennedy CTC, Lyell A. Perianal orf. J Am Acad Dermatol 1984; 11: 72–74.

78 Rees J, Marks JM. Two unusual cases of orf following trauma to the scalp. Br J Dermatol 1988; 118: 445–447.

79 Yirrell DL, Vestey JP, Norval M. Immune responses of patients to orf virus infection. Br J Dermatol 1994; 130: 438–443.

80 Bodnar MG, Miller F III, Tyler WB. Facial orf. J Am Acad Dermatol 1999; 40: 815–817.

81 Mayet A, Sommer B, Heenan P. Rapidly growing cutaneous tumour of the right temple: Orf. Australas J Dermatol 1997; 38: 217–219.

82 Degraeve C, De Coninck A, Senneseael J, Roseeuw D. Recurrent contagious ecthyma (orf) in an immunocompromised host successfully treated with cryotherapy. Dermatology 1999; 198: 162–163.

83 Kahn D, Hutchinson EA. Generalized bullous orf. Int J Dermatol 1980; 19: 340–341.

84 Murphy JK, Ralfs IG. Bullous pemphigoid complicating human orf. Br J Dermatol 1996; 134: 929–930.

85 Macfarlane AW. Human orf complicated by bullous pemphigoid. Br J Dermatol 1997; 137: 656–657.

86 Sanchez RL, Hebert A, Lucia H, Swedo J. Orf. A case report with histologic, electron microscopic, and immunoperoxidase studies. Arch Pathol Lab Med 1985; 109: 166–170.

87 Rose C, Starostik P, Bröcker E-B. Infection with parapoxvirus induces CD30-positive cutaneous infiltrates in humans. J Cutan Pathol 1999; 26: 520–522.

88 Gill MJ, Arlette J, Buchan KA, Barber K. Human orf. A diagnostic consideration? Arch Dermatol 1990; 126: 356–358.

89 Taieb A, Guillot M, Carlotti D, Maleville J. Orf and pregnancy. Int J Dermatol 1988; 27: 31–33.

Herpesviridae

90 Rockley PF, Tyring SK. Pathophysiology and clinical manifestations of varicella zoster virus infections. Int J Dermatol 1994; 33: 227–232.

91 Nicholas J. Evolutionary aspects of oncogenic herpesviruses. J Clin Pathol: Mol Pathol 2000; 53: 222–237.

92 Gibney MD, Leonardi CL, Glaser DA. Concurrent herpes simplex and varicella-zoster infection in an immunocompromised patient. J Am Acad Dermatol 1995; 33: 126–129.

93 Smith KJ, Skelton HG III, James WD et al. Concurrent epidermal involvement of cytomegalovirus and herpes simplex virus in two HIV-infected patients. J Am Acad Dermatol 1991; 25: 500–506.

94 Martin JR, Holt RK, Langston C et al. Type-specific identification of herpes simplex and varicella-zoster virus antigen in autopsy tissues. Hum Pathol 1991; 22: 75–80.

95 Zirn JR, Tompkins SD, Huie C, Shea CR. Rapid detection and distinction of cutaneous herpesvirus infections by direct immunofluorescence. J Am Acad Dermatol 1995; 33: 724–728.

96 Nahass GT, Mandel MJ, Cook S et al. Detection of herpes simplex and varicella-zoster infection from cutaneous lesions in different clinical stages with the polymerase chain reaction. J Am Acad Dermatol 1995; 32: 730–733.

97 Thomas CA, Smith SE, Morgan TM et al. Clinical application of polymerase chain reaction amplification to diagnosis of herpes virus infection. Am J Dermatopathol 1994; 16: 268–274.

98 Rawls WE, Hammerberg O. Epidemiology of the herpes simplex viruses. Clin Dermatol 1984; 2 (2): 29–45.

99 Vestey JP, Norval M. Mucocutaneous infections with herpes simplex virus and their management. Clin Exp Dermatol 1992; 17: 221–237.

100 Spruance SL. The natural history of recurrent oral-facial herpes simplex virus infection. Semin Dermatol 1992; 11: 200–206.

101 Whitley RJ, Roizman B. Herpex simplex virus infections. Lancet 2001; 357: 1513–1518.

102 Corey L, Vontver LA, Brown ZA. Genital herpes simplex virus infections: clinical manifestations, course, and complications. Semin Dermatol 1984; 3: 89–101.

103 Vanderhooft S, Kirby P. Genital herpes simplex virus infection: natural history. Semin Dermatol 1992; 11: 190–199.

104 Petersen CS, Larsen FG, Zachariae C, Heidenheim M. Herpes simplex virus-type 2 seropositivity in a Dutch adult population denying previous episodes of genital herpes. Acta Derm Venereol 2000; 80: 158.

105 Cliff S, Ostlere LS, Hague K, Harland CC. Segmental scarring following intrauterine herpes simplex virus infection. Clin Exp Dermatol 1997; 22: 96–98.

106 Tang WYM, Lo JYC, Yuen MK, Lam WY. Herpes simplex virus type 2 infection in a 5-year-old boy presenting with recurrent chest wall vesicles and a possible history of herpes encephalitis. Br J Dermatol 1997; 137: 440–444.

107 Perna JJ, Mannix ML, Rooney JF et al. Reactivation of latent herpes simplex virus infection by ultraviolet light: a human model. J Am Acad Dermatol 1987; 17: 473–478.

108 Severson JL, Tyring SK. Relation between herpes simplex viruses and human immunodeficiency virus infections. Arch Dermatol 1999; 135: 1393–1397.

109 Pereira FA. Herpes simplex: Evolving concepts. J Am Acad Dermatol 1996; 35: 503–520.

110 Hill TJ, Altman DM, Blyth WA et al. Herpes simplex virus latency. Clin Dermatol 1984; 2: 46–55.

111 McKenna DB, Neill WA, Norval M. Herpes simplex virus-specific immune responses in subjects with frequent and infrequent orofacial recrudescences. Br J Dermatol 2001; 144: 459–464.

112 Liu V, Bigby M. Reactivation of genital herpes simplex virus 2 infection in asymptomatic seropositive persons is frequent. Arch Dermatol 2000; 136: 1141–1142.

113 Pannuti CS, Finck MCDS, Grimbaun RS et al. Asymptomatic perianal shedding of herpes simplex virus in patients with acquired immunodeficiency syndrome. Arch Dermatol 1997; 133: 180–183.

114 Snavely SR, Liu C. Clinical spectrum of herpes simplex virus infections. Clin Dermatol 1984; 2: 8–22.

115 Giacobetti R. Herpetic whitlow. Int J Dermatol 1979; 18: 55–58.

116 Peutherer JF, Smith IW, Robertson DH. Necrotising balanitis due to a generalised primary infection with herpes simplex virus type 2. Br J Vener Dis 1979; 55: 48–51.

117 Long JC, Wheeler CE Jr, Briggaman RA. Varicella-like infection due to herpes simplex. Arch Dermatol 1978; 114: 406–409.

118 Leyden JJ, Baker DA. Localized herpes simplex infections in atopic dermatitis. Arch Dermatol 1979; 115: 311–312.

119 Boyd AS, Neldner KH, Zemtsov A, Shihada B. Photolocalized varicella. J Am Acad Dermatol 1992; 26: 772–774.

120 Beasley KL, Cooley GE, Kao GF et al. Herpes simplex vegetans: Atypical genital herpes infection in a patient with common variable immunodeficiency. J Am Acad Dermatol 1997; 37: 860–863.

121 Das S, Leonard N, Reynolds NJ. Herpes simplex virus type 1 as a cause of widespread intracorneal blistering of the lower limbs. Clin Exp Dermatol 2000; 25: 119–121.

122 Butler DF, Malouf PJ, Batz RC, Stetson CL. Acquired lymphedema of the hand due to herpes simplex virus type 2. Arch Dermatol 1999; 135: 1125–1126.

123 Toole JWP, Hofstader SL, Ramsay CA. Darier's disease and Kaposi's varicelliform eruption. J Am Acad Dermatol 1979; 1: 321–324.

124 Langtry JAA, Ostlere LS, Hawkins DA, Staughton RCD. The difficulty in diagnosis of cutaneous herpes simplex virus infection in patients with AIDS. Clin Exp Dermatol 1994; 19: 224–226.

125 Saijo M, Suzutani T, Murono K et al. Recurrent aciclovir-resistant herpes simplex in a child with Wiskott–Aldrich syndrome. Br J Dermatol 1998; 139: 311–314.

126 Hillard P, Seeds J, Cefalo R. Disseminated herpes simplex in pregnancy: two cases and a review. Obstet Gynecol Surv 1982; 37: 449–453.

127 Darragh TM, Egbert BM, Berger TG, Yen TSB. Identification of herpes simplex virus DNA in lesions of erythema multiforme by the polymerase chain reaction. J Am Acad Dermatol 1991; 24: 23–26.

128 Huff JC. Erythema multiforme and latent herpes simplex infection. Semin Dermatol 1992; 11: 207–210.

129 Hsiung GD, Landry ML, Mayo DR, Fong CKY. Laboratory diagnosis of herpes simplex virus type 1 and type 2 infections. Clin Dermatol 1984; 2: 67–82.

130 Goodyear HM, Wilson P, Cropper L et al. Rapid diagnosis of cutaneous herpes simplex infections using specific monoclonal antibodies. Clin Exp Dermatol 1994; 19: 294–297.

131 Goldman BD. Herpes serology for dermatologists. Arch Dermatol 2000; 136: 1158–1161.

132 Huff JC, Krueger GG, Overall JC Jr et al. The histopathologic evolution of recurrent herpes simplex labialis. J Am Acad Dermatol 1981; 5: 550–557.

133 Cohen C, Trapuckd S. Leukocytoclastic vasculitis associated with cutaneous infection by herpesvirus. Am J Dermatopathol 1984; 6: 561–565.

134 Hassel MH, Lesher JL Jr. Herpes simplex mimicking leukemia cutis. J Am Acad Dermatol 1989; 21: 367–371.

135 Resnik KS, DiLeonardo M. Herpes incognito. Am J Dermatopathol 2000; 22: 144–150.

136 Ferguson DL, Hawk RJ, Covington NM, Reed RJ. Lichenoid lymphocytic vasculitis with a high component of histiocytes. Histogenetic implications in a specified clinical setting. Am J Dermatopathol 1989; 11: 259–269.

137 Jang K-A, Kim S-H, Choi J-H et al. Viral folliculitis on the face. Br J Dermatol 2000; 142: 555–559.

138 Sangueza OP, Gordon MD, White CR Jr. Subtle clues to the diagnosis of the herpesvirus by light microscopy. Herpetic syringitis. Am J Dermatopathol 1995; 17: 163–168.

139 Worrell JT, Cockerell CJ. Histopathology of peripheral nerves in cutaneous herpesvirus infection. Am J Dermatopathol 1997; 19: 133–137.

140 Shelley WB, Wood MG. Surgical conversion of herpes simplex from an epidermal to a dermal disease. Br J Dermatol 1979; 100: 649–655.

141 Boddingius J, Dijkman H, Hendriksen E et al. HSV-2 replication sites, monocyte and lymphocytic cell infection and virion phagocytosis by neutrophils, in vesicular lesions on penile skin. J Cutan Pathol 1987; 14: 165–175.

142 Heng MCY, Allen SG, Heng SY et al. An electron microscopic study of the epidermal infiltrate in recurrent herpes simplex. Clin Exp Dermatol 1989; 14: 199–202.

143 Vestey JP, Howie SEM, Norval M et al. Immune responses to herpes simplex virus in patients with facial herpes simplex and those with eczema herpeticum. Br J Dermatol 1988; 118: 775–782.

144 Fukuda M, Kono T, Ishii M, Hamada T. Detection of herpes simplex viral DNA in Kaposi's varicelliform eruption using in situ hybridization method. Clin Exp Dermatol 1991; 16: 407–410.

145 Amatsu A, Yoshida M. Detection of herpes simplex virus DNA in non-herpetic areas of patients with eczema herpeticum. Dermatology 2000; 200: 104–107.

146 Keane JT, James K, Blankenship ML, Pearson RW. Progressive vaccinia associated with combined variable immunodeficiency. Arch Dermatol 1983; 119: 404–408.

147 Parslew R, Verbov JL. Kaposi's varicelliform eruption due to herpes simplex in Darier's disease. Clin Exp Dermatol 1994; 19: 428–429.

148 Pantazi V, Potouridou I, Katsarou A et al. Darier's disease complicated by Kaposi's varicelliform eruption due to herpes simplex virus. J Eur Acad Dermatol Venereol 2000; 14: 209–211.

149 Flint ID, Spencer DM, Wilkin JK. Eczema herpeticum in association with familial benign chronic pemphigus. J Am Acad Dermatol 1993; 28: 257–259.

150 Ng SK, Ang CB, Tham A. Kaposi's varicelliform eruption in a patient with pityriasis rubra pilaris. J Am Acad Dermatol 1992; 27: 263.

151 Fukuzawa M, Oguchi S, Saida T. Kaposi's varicelliform eruption of an elderly patient with multiple myeloma. J Am Acad Dermatol 2000; 42: 921–922.

152 Hayashi S, Yamada Y, Dekio S, Jidoi J. Kaposi's varicelliform eruption in a patient with mycosis fungoides. Clin Exp Dermatol 1997; 22: 41–43.

153 Nishimura M, Maekawa M, Hino Y et al. Kaposi's varicelliform eruption. Development in a patient with a healing second-degree burn. Arch Dermatol 1984; 120: 799–800.

154 Raychaudhuri SP, Raychaudhuri SK. Revisit to Kaposi's varicelliform eruption: role of IL-4. Int J Dermatol 1995; 34: 854–856.

155 Goodyear HM, McLeish P, Randall S et al. Immunological studies of herpes simplex virus infection in children with atopic eczema. Br J Dermatol 1996; 134: 85–93.

156 LeBoit PE, Limová M, Yen TSB et al. Chronic verrucous varicella-zoster virus infection in patients with the acquired immunodeficiency syndrome (AIDS). Am J Dermatopathol 1992; 14: 1–7.

157 Vaughan Jones SA, McGibbon DH, Bradbeer CS. Chronic verrucous varicella-zoster infection in a patient with AIDS. Clin Exp Dermatol 1994; 19: 327–329.

158 Zampogna JC, Flowers FP. Persistent verrucous varicella as the initial manifestation of HIV infection. J Am Acad Dermatol 2001; 44: 391–394.

159 Findlay GH, Forman L, Hull PR. Actinic chickenpox. Light-distributed varicella eruption. S Afr Med J 1979; 55: 989–991.

160 Osborne GEN, Hawk JLM. Photodistributed chickenpox mimicking polymorphic light eruption. Br J Dermatol 2000; 142: 584–585.

161 Wilkin JK, Ribble JC, Wilkin OC. Vascular factors and the localization of varicella lesions. J Am Acad Dermatol 1981; 4: 665–666.

162 Ogboli MI, Parslew R, Verbov J, Smyth R. Kawasaki disease associated with varicella: a rare association. Br J Dermatol 1999; 141: 1145–1146.

163 Messner J, Miller JJ, James WD, Honig PJ. Accentuated viral exanthems in areas of inflammation. J Am Acad Dermatol 1999; 40: 345–346.

164 Liang CD, Yu TJ, Ko SF. Ipsilateral renal dysplasia with hypertensive heart disease in an infant with cutaneous varicella lesions: An unusual presentation of congenital varicella syndrome. J Am Acad Dermatol 2000; 43: 864–866.

165 McSorley J, Shapiro L, Brownstein MH, Hsu KC. Herpes simplex and varicella-zoster: comparative histopathology of 77 cases. Int J Dermatol 1974; 13: 69–75.

166 Sadick NS, Swenson PD, Kaufman RL, Kaplan MH. Comparison of detection of varicella-zoster virus by the Tzanck smear, direct immunofluorescence with a monoclonal antibody, and virus isolation. J Am Acad Dermatol 1987; 17: 64–69.

167 Solomon AR, Rasmussen JE, Weiss JS. A comparison of the Tzanck smear and viral isolation in varicella and herpes zoster. Arch Dermatol 1986; 122: 282–285.

168 Folkers E, Vreeswijk J, Oranje AP, Duivenvoorden JN. Rapid diagnosis in varicella and herpes zoster: re-evaluation of direct smear (Tzanck test) and electron microscopy including colloidal gold immuno-electron microscopy in comparison with virus isolation. Br J Dermatol 1989; 121: 287–296.

169 Liesegang TJ. The varicella-zoster virus: systemic and ocular features. J Am Acad Dermatol 1984; 11: 165–191.

170 Tyring SK. Natural history of varicella zoster virus. Semin Dermatol 1992; 11: 211–217.

171 McCrary ML, Severson J, Tyring SK. Varicella zoster virus. J Am Acad Dermatol 1999; 41: 1–14.

172 Liesegang TJ. Varicella zoster viral disease. Mayo Clin Proc 1999; 74: 983–998.

173 Liang MG, Heidelberg KA, Jacobson RM, McEvoy MT. Herpes zoster after varicella immunization. J Am Acad Dermatol 1998; 38: 761–763.

174 Heskel NS, Hanifin JM. "Recurrent herpes zoster": An unproved entity? J Am Acad Dermatol 1984; 10: 486–490.

175 Kakourou T, Theodoridou M, Mostrou G. Herpes zoster in children. J Am Acad Dermatol 1998; 39: 207–210.

176 Snow JL, el-Azhary RA, Gibson LE et al. Granulomatous vasculitis associated with herpes virus: a persistent, painful, postherpetic papular eruption. Mayo Clin Proc 1997; 72: 851–853.

177 Rübben A, Baron JM, Grussendorf-Conen E-I. Routine detection of herpes simplex virus and varicella zoster virus by polymerase chain reaction reveals that initial herpes zoster is frequently misdiagnosed as herpes simplex. Br J Dermatol 1997; 137: 259–261.

178 Cohen PR, Grossman ME. Clinical features of human immunodeficiency virus-associated disseminated herpes zoster virus infection – a review of the literature. Clin Exp Dermatol 1989; 14: 273–276.

179 Manchado Lopez P, Ruiz de Morales JMG, Ruiz González I, Rodriguez Prieto MA. Cutaneous infections by papillomavirus, herpes zoster and *Candida albicans* as the only manifestation of idiopathic CD4+ T lymphocytopenia. Int J Dermatol 1999; 38: 119–121.

180 Sehgal VN, Kumar S, Jain S, Bhattacharya SN. Typical varicella zoster (ophthalmicus) in an HIV-infected person. J Eur Acad Dermatol Venereol 2000; 14: 59–60.

181 Veraldi S, Carrera C, Gianotti R, Caputo R. Bullous herpes zoster. Acta Derm Venereol 2000; 80: 55.

182 Grossman MC, Grossman ME. Chronic hyperkeratotic herpes zoster and human immunodeficiency virus infection. J Am Acad Dermatol 1993; 28: 306–308.

183 Nikkels AF, Snoeck R, Rentier B, Piérard GE. Chronic verrucous varicella zoster virus skin lesions: clinical, histological, molecular and therapeutic aspects. Clin Exp Dermatol 1999; 24: 346–353.

184 Tsao H, Tahan SR, Johnson RA. Chronic varicella zoster infection mimicking a basal cell carcinoma in an AIDS patient. J Am Acad Dermatol 1997; 36: 831–833.

185 Nikkels AF, Piérard GE. Shingles developing within recent surgical scars. J Am Acad Dermatol 1999; 41: 309–311.

186 Davis Gibney M, Nahass GT, Leonardi CL. Cutaneous reactions following herpes zoster infections: report of three cases and a review of the literature. Br J Dermatol 1996; 134: 504–509.

187 Requena L, Kutzner H, Escalonilla P et al. Cutaneous reactions at sites of herpes zoster scars: an expanded spectrum. Br J Dermatol 1998; 138: 161–168.

188 del Rio E, Allegue F, Fachal C et al. Comedones appearing after herpes zoster infection: a report of 7 cases. Arch Dermatol 1997; 133: 1316–1317.

189 Bahadoran P, Lacour J-P, Ortonne J-P. Leukaemia cutis at the site of prior herpes zoster. Br J Dermatol 1997; 136: 465.

190 Turner RJ, Sviland L, Lawrence CM. Acute infiltration by non-Hodgkin's B-cell lymphoma of lesions of disseminated herpes zoster. Br J Dermatol 1998; 139: 295–298.

191 Bahadoran P, Lacour J-P, Ortonne J-P. Leukaemia cutis at the site of prior herpes zoster. Br J Dermatol 1997; 136: 465.

192 Córdoba S, Fraga J, Bartolomé B et al. Giant cell lichenoid dermatitis within herpes zoster scars in a bone marrow recipient. J Cutan Pathol 2000; 27: 255–257.

193 Corazza M, Bacilieri S, Strumia R. Post-herpes zoster scar sarcoidosis. Acta Derm Venereol 1999; 79: 95.

194 Lee H-J, Ahn W-K, Chae K-S et al. Localized chronic urticaria at the site of healed herpes zoster. Acta Derm Venereol 1999; 79: 168.

195 Braun RP, Barua D, Masouyé I. Zosteriform lichen planus after herpes zoster. Dermatology 1998; 197: 87–88.

196 Jarrett P, Ha T, Oliver F. Necrotizing fasciitis complicating disseminated cutaneous herpes zoster. Clin Exp Dermatol 1998; 23: 87–88.

197 Goh C-L, Khoo L. A retrospective study of the clinical presentation and outcome of herpes zoster in a tertiary dermatology outpatient referral clinic. Int J Dermatol 1997; 36: 667–672.

198 Vu AQ, Radonich MA, Heald PW. Herpes zoster in seven disparate dermatomes (zoster multiplex): Report of a case and review of the literature. J Am Acad Dermatol 1999; 40: 868–869.

199 Erhard H, Rünger TM, Kreienkamp M et al. Atypical varicella-zoster virus infection in an immunocompromised patient: result of a virus-induced vasculitis. J Am Acad Dermatol 1995; 32: 908–911.

200 Böni R, Dummer R, Dommann-Scherrer C et al. Necrotizing herpes zoster mimicking relapse of vasculitis in angioimmunoblastic lymphadenopathy with dysproteinaemia. Br J Dermatol 1995; 133: 978–982.

201 Guill MA, Goette DK. Granuloma annulare at sites of healing herpes zoster. Arch Dermatol 1978; 114: 1383.

202 Serfling U, Penneys NS, Zhu W-Y et al. Varicella-zoster virus DNA in granulomatous skin lesions following herpes zoster. J Cutan Pathol 1993; 20: 28–33.

203 Rinder HM, Murphy GF. Eccrine duct involvement by herpes zoster. Arch Dermatol 1984; 120: 261–262.

204 Drago F, Aragone MG, Lugani C, Rebora A. Cytomegalovirus infection in normal and immunocompromised humans. Dermatology 2000; 200: 189–195.

205 Lesher JL Jr. Cytomegalovirus infections and the skin. J Am Acad Dermatol 1988; 18: 1333–1338.

206 Walker JD, Chesney TMcC. Cytomegalovirus infection of the skin. Am J Dermatopathol 1982; 4: 263–265.

207 Feldman PS, Walker AN, Baker R. Cutaneous lesions heralding disseminated cytomegalovirus infection. J Am Acad Dermatol 1982; 7: 545–548.

208 Doeglas HMG, Rijnten WJ, Schroder FP, Schirm J. Cold urticaria and virus infections: a clinical and serological study in 39 patients. Br J Dermatol 1986; 114: 311–318.

209 Bhawan J, Gellis S, Ucci A, Chang T-W. Vesiculobullous lesions caused by cytomegalovirus infection in an immunocompromised adult. J Am Acad Dermatol 1984; 11: 743–747.

210 Aloi F, Solaroli C, Papotti M. Perianal cytomegalovirus ulcer in an HIV-infected patient. Dermatology 1996; 192: 81–83.

211 Colsky AS, Jegasothy SM, Leonardi C et al. Diagnosis and treatment of a case of cutaneous cytomegalovirus infection with a dramatic clinical presentation. J Am Acad Dermatol 1998; 38: 349–351.

212 Bournerias I, Boisnic S, Patey O et al. Unusual cutaneous cytomegalovirus involvement in patients with acquired immunodeficiency syndrome. Arch Dermatol 1989; 125: 1243–1246.

213 Thiboutot DM, Beckford A, Mart CR et al. Cytomegalovirus diaper dermatitis. Arch Dermatol 1991; 127: 396–398.

214 Horn TD, Hood AF. Clinically occult cytomegalovirus present in skin biopsy specimens in immunosuppressed hosts. J Am Acad Dermatol 1989; 21: 781–784.

215 Sugiura H, Sawai T, Miyauchi H et al. Successful treatment of disseminated cutaneous cytomegalic inclusion disease associated with Hodgkin's disease. J Am Acad Dermatol 1991; 24: 346–352.

216 Minars N, Silverman JF, Escobar MR, Martinez AJ. Fatal cytomegalic inclusion disease. Associated skin manifestations in a renal transplant patient. Arch Dermatol 1977; 113: 1569–1571.

217 Lee JY-Y, Peel R. Concurrent cytomegalovirus and herpes simplex virus infections in skin biopsy specimens from two AIDS patients with fatal CMV infection. Am J Dermatopathol 1989; 11: 136–143.

218 Boudreau S, Hines HC, Hood AF. Dermal abscesses with *Staphylococcus aureus*, cytomegalovirus and acid-fast bacilli in a patient with acquired immunodeficiency syndrome (AIDS). J Cutan Pathol 1988; 15: 53–57.

219 Abel EA. Cutaneous manifestations of immunosuppression in organ transplant recipients. J Am Acad Dermatol 1989; 21: 167–179.

220 Wong J, McCracken G, Ronan S, Aronson I. Coexistent cutaneous Aspergillus and cytomegalovirus infection in a liver transplant recipient. J Am Acad Dermatol 2001; 44: 370–372.

221 Daudén E, Fernández-Buezo G, Fraga J et al. Mucocutaneous presence of cytomegalovirus associated with human immunodeficiency virus infection. Arch Dermatol 2001; 137: 443–448.

222 Fine J-D, Arndt KA. The TORCH syndrome: a clinical review. J Am Acad Dermatol 1985; 12: 697–706.

223 Pariser RJ. Histologically specific skin lesions in disseminated cytomegalovirus infection. J Am Acad Dermatol 1983; 9: 937–946.

224 Curtis JL, Egbert BM. Cutaneous cytomegalovirus vasculitis: an unusual clinical presentation of a common opportunistic pathogen. Hum Pathol 1982; 13: 1138–1141.

225 Resnik KS, DiLeonardo M, Maillet M. Histopathologic findings in cutaneous cytomegalovirus infection. Am J Dermatopathol 2000; 22: 397–407.

226 Patterson JW, Broecker AH, Kornstein MJ, Mills AS. Cutaneous cytomegalovirus infection in a liver transplant patient. Diagnosis by in situ DNA hybridization. Am J Dermatopathol 1988; 10: 524–530.

227 Toome BK, Bowers KE, Scott GA. Diagnosis of cutaneous cytomegalovirus infection: a review and report of a case. J Am Acad Dermatol 1991; 24: 857–863.

228 Spencer SA. Fenske NA, Espinoza CG et al. Granuloma annulare-like eruption due to chronic Epstein–Barr virus infection. Arch Dermatol 1988; 124: 250–255.

229 Lowe L, Hebert AA, Duvic M. Gianotti–Crosti syndrome associated with Epstein–Barr virus infection. J Am Acad Dermatol 1989; 20: 336–338.

230 Chai C, White WL, Shea CR, Prieto VG. Epstein Barr virus-associated lymphoproliferative-disorders primarily involving the skin. J Cutan Pathol 1999; 26: 242–247.

231 Salama S. Epstein–Barr virus (EBV) associated cutaneous lympho-proliferative disorders (LPDs). J Cutan Pathol 2000; 27: 571 (abstract).

232 Sangueza OP. Epstein–Barr virus. A serial killer or an innocent bystander? Arch Dermatol 1997; 133: 1156–1157.

233 Hudnall SD. Kikuchi–Fujimoto disease. Is Epstein–Barr virus the culprit? Am J Clin Pathol 2000; 113: 761–764.

234 Yen A, Fearneyhough P, Raimer SS, Hudnall SD. EBV-associated Kikuchi's histiocytic necrotizing lymphadenitis with cutaneous manifestations. J Am Acad Dermatol 1997; 36: 342–346.

235 Dockrell DH, Smith TF, Paya CV. Human herpesvirus 6. Mayo Clin Proc 1999; 74: 163–170.

236 Yoshida M, Fukui K, Orita T et al. Exanthem subitum (roseola infantum) with vesicular lesions. Br J Dermatol 1995; 132: 614–616.

237 Drago F, Rebora A. The new herpesviruses. Emerging pathogens of dermatological interest. Arch Dermatol 1999; 135: 71–75.

238 Ruzicka T, Kalka K, Diercks K, Schuppe H-C. Papular-purpuric 'gloves and socks' syndrome associated with human herpesvirus 6 infection. Arch Dermatol 1998; 134: 242–244.

239 Tohyama M, Yahata Y, Yasukawa M et al. Severe hypersensitivity syndrome due to sulfasalazine associated with reactivation of human herpesvirus 6. Arch Dermatol 1998; 134: 1113–1117.

240 Suzuki Y, Inagi R, Aono T et al. Human herpesvirus 6 infection as a risk factor for the development of severe drug-induced hypersensitivity syndrome. Arch Dermatol 1998; 134: 1108–1112.

241 Descamps V, Valance A, Edlinger C et al. Association of human herpesvirus 6 infection with drug reaction with eosinophilia and systemic symptoms. Arch Dermatol 2001; 137: 301–304.

242 Descamps V, Bouscarat F, Laglenne S et al. Human herpesvirus 6 infection associated with anticonvulsant hypersensitivity syndrome and reactive haemophagocytic syndrome. Br J Dermatol 1997; 137: 605–608.

243 Kosuge H, Tanaka-Taya K, Miyoshi H et al. Epidemiological study of human herpesvirus-6 and human herpesvirus-7 in pityriasis rosea. Br J Dermatol 2000; 143: 795–798.

244 Le Cleach L, Fillet AM, Agut H, Chosidow O. Human herpesviruses 6 and 7. New roles yet to be discovered? Arch Dermatol 1998; 134: 1155–1157.

245 Drago F, Rebora A. Pityriasis rosea: one virus, two viruses, more viruses? Br J Dermatol 2001; 144: 1090.

246 Lebbé C. Human herpesvirus 8 as the infectious cause of Kaposi sarcoma. Evidence and involvement of cofactors. Arch Dermatol 1998; 134: 736–738.

247 Gill J, Powles T, Bower M. The molecular genetics of human herpesvirus 8. Hosp Med 2000; 61: 306–309.

248 Herman PS, Shogreen MR, White WL. The evaluation of human herpesvirus 8 (Kaposi's sarcoma-associated herpesvirus) in cutaneous lesions of Kaposi's sarcoma. Am J Dermatopathol 1998; 20: 7–11.

249 Kemény L, Gyulai R, Kiss M et al. Kaposi's sarcoma-associated herpesvirus/human herpesvirus-8: A new virus in human pathology. J Am Acad Dermatol 1997; 37: 107–113.

250 Sachsenberg-Studer EM, Dobrynski N, Sheldon J et al. Human herpes-virus 8 seropositive patient with skin and graft Kaposi's sarcoma after lung transplantation. J Am Acad Dermatol 1999; 40: 308–311.

251 Cattani, P, Capuano M, Lesnoni La Parola I et al. Human herpesvirus 8 in Italian HIV-seronegative patients with Kaposi sarcoma. Arch Dermatol 1998; 134: 695–699.

252 Bezold G, Messer G, Peter RU et al. Quantitation of human herpes virus 8 DNA in paraffin-embedded biopsies of HIV-associated and classical Kaposi's sarcoma by PCR. J Cutan Pathol 2001; 28: 127–130.

253 Nishimoto S, Inagi R, Yamanishi K et al. Prevalence of human herpesvirus-8 in skin lesions. Br J Dermatol 1997; 137: 179–184.

254 Dupin N, Marcelin A-G, Gorin I et al. Prevalence of human herpesvirus 8 infection measured by antibodies to a latent nuclear antigen in patients with various dermatologic diseases. Arch Dermatol 1998; 134: 700–702.

255 Memar OM, Rady PL, Goldblum RM et al. Human herpesvirus 8 DNA sequences in blistering skin from patients with pemphigus. Arch Dermatol 1997; 133: 1247–1251.

256 Cohen SS, Weinstein MD, Herndier BG et al. No evidence of human herpesvirus 8 infection in patients with paraneoplastic pemphigus, pemphigus vulgaris, or pemphigus foliaceus. J Invest Dermatol 1998; 111: 781–783.

257 Kohler S, Kamel OW, Chang PP, Smoller BR. Absence of human herpesvirus 8 and Epstein–Barr virus genome sequences in cutaneous epithelial neoplasms arising in immunosuppressed organ-transplant patients. J Cutan Pathol 1997; 24: 559–563.

258 Masini C, Abeni DD, Cattaruzza MS et al. Antibodies against human herpesvirus 8 in subjects with non-venereal dermatological conditions. Br J Dermatol 2000; 143: 484–490.

Papovaviridae

259 Orth G, Favre M. Human papillomaviruses. Biochemical and biologic properties. Clin Dermatol 1985; 3: 27–42.

260 Androphy EJ. Human papillomavirus. Current concepts. Arch Dermatol 1989; 125: 683–685.

261 Highet AS. Viral warts. Semin Dermatol 1988; 7: 53–57.

262 Cobb MW. Human papillomavirus infection. J Am Acad Dermatol 1990; 22: 547–566.

263 Bosch FX, Rohan T, Schneider A et al. Papillomavirus research update: highlights of the Barcelona HPV 2000 international papillomavirus conference. J Clin Pathol 2001; 54: 163–175.

264 Vogel LN. Epidemiology of human papilloma virus infection. Semin Dermatol 1992; 11: 226–228.

265 Brown TJ, Yen-Moore A, Tyring SK. An overview of sexually transmitted diseases. Part II. J Am Acad Dermatol 1999; 41: 661–677.

266 Majewski S, Jablonska S. Human papillomavirus-associated tumors of the skin and mucosa. J Am Acad Dermatol 1997; 36: 659–685.

267 Gross G, Pfister H, Hagedorn M, Gissmann L. Correlation between human papillomavirus (HPV) type and histology of warts. J Invest Dermatol 1982; 78: 160–164.

268 Jablonska S, Orth G, Obalek S, Croissant O. Cutaneous warts. Clinical, histologic, and virologic correlations. Clin Dermatol 1985; 3: 71–82.

269 Androphy EJ. Molecular biology of human papillomavirus infection and oncogenesis. J Invest Dermatol 1994; 103: 248–256.

270 Majewski S, Jablonska S. Immunology of HPV infection and HPV-associated tumors. Int J Dermatol 1998; 37: 81–95.

271 Laurent R, Kienzler JL, Croissant O, Orth G. Two anatomoclinical types of warts with plantar localization: specific cytopathogenic effects of papillomavirus. Type 1 (HPV-1) and type 2 (HPV-2). Arch Dermatol Res 1982; 274: 101–111.

272 Jenson AB, Lim LY, Singer E. Comparison of human papillomavirus type 1 serotyping by monoclonal antibodies with genotyping by in situ hybridization of plantar warts. J Cutan Pathol 1989; 16: 54–59.

273 Eversole LR, Laipis PJ, Green TL. Human papillomavirus type 2 DNA in oral and labial verruca vulgaris. J Cutan Pathol 1987; 14: 319–325.

274 Ostrow R, Zachow K, Watts S et al. Characterization of two HPV-3 related papillomaviruses from common warts that are distinct clinically from flat warts or epidermodysplasia verruciformis. J Invest Dermatol 1983; 80: 436–440.

275 Finkel ML, Finkel DJ. Warts among meat handlers. Arch Dermatol 1984; 120: 1314–1317.

276 de Villiers E-M, Neumann C, Olsterdorf T et al. Butcher's wart virus (HPV 7) infections in non-butchers. J Invest Dermatol 1986; 87: 236–238.

277 Rudlinger R, Bunney MH, Grob R, Hunter JAA. Warts in fish handlers. Br J Dermatol 1989; 120: 375–381.

278 Keefe M, Al-Ghamdi A, Coggon D et al. Cutaneous warts in butchers. Br J Dermatol 1994; 130: 9–14.

279 Keefe M, Al-Ghamdi A, Coggon D et al. Butchers' warts: no evidence for person to person transmission of HPV7. Br J Dermatol 1994; 130: 15–17.

280 von Krogh G. Condyloma acuminata 1983: an up-dated review. Semin Dermatol 1983; 2: 109–129.

281 Jablonska S. Wart viruses: human papillomaviruses. Semin Dermatol 1984; 3: 120–129.

282 Beaudenon S, Praetorius F, Kremsdorf D et al. A new type of human papillomavirus associated with oral focal epithelial hyperplasia. J Invest Dermatol 1987; 88: 130–135.

283 Egawa K, Kitasato H, Honda Y et al. Human papillomavirus 57 identified in a plantar epidermoid cyst. Br J Dermatol 1998; 138: 510–514.

284 McCown H, Thiers B, Cook J, Acker S. Global nail dystrophy associated with human papillomavirus type 57 infection. Br J Dermatol 1999; 141: 731–735.

285 Bender ME. The protean manifestations of human papillomavirus infection. Arch Dermatol 1994; 130: 1429–1430.

286 von Krogh G, Syrjanen SM, Syrjanen KJ. Advantage of human papillomavirus typing in the clinical evaluation of genitoanal warts. J Am Acad Dermatol 1988; 18: 495–503.

287 Ostrow RS, Shaver MK, Turnquist S et al. Human papillomavirus-16 DNA in a cutaneous invasive cancer. Arch Dermatol 1989; 125: 666–669.

288 van der Leest RJ, Zachow KR, Ostrow RS et al. Human papillomavirus heterogeneity in 36 renal transplant recipients. Arch Dermatol 1987; 123: 354–357.

289 Obalek S, Favre M, Jablonska S et al. Human papillomavirus type 2-associated basal cell carcinoma in two immunosuppressed patients. Arch Dermatol 1988; 124: 930–934.

290 Quan MB, Moy RL. The role of human papillomavirus in carcinoma. J Am Acad Dermatol 1991; 25: 698–705.

291 Liranzo MO, Golitz L, Shroyer KR. Detection of human papillomavirus DNA in squamous cell carcinomas of a patient with mycosis fungoides: report of a case. J Cutan Pathol 1997; 24: 47–50.

292 Bishop JW, Emanuel JM, Sims KL. Disseminated mucosal papilloma/condyloma secondary to human papillomavirus. Am J Surg Pathol 1998; 22: 1291–1295.

293 Chopra KF, Tyring SK. The impact of the human immunodeficiency virus on the human papillomavirus epidemic. Arch Dermatol 1997; 133: 629–633.

294 Tieben LM, Berkhout RJM, Smits HL et al. Detection of epidermodysplasia verruciformis-like human papillomavirus types in malignant and premalignant skin lesions of renal transplant recipients. Br J Dermatol 1994; 131: 226–230.

295 Stark S, Petridis AK, Ghim SJ et al. Prevalence of antibodies against virus-like particles of epidermodysplasia verruciformis-associated HPV8 in patients at risk of skin cancer. J Invest Dermatol 1998; 111: 696–701.

296 Dyall-Smith D, Trowell H, Dyall-Smith ML. Benign human papillomavirus infection in renal transplant recipients. Int J Dermatol 1991; 30: 785–789.

297 Guillet GY, del Grande P, Thivolet J. Cutaneous and mucosal warts. Clinical and histopathological criteria for classification. Int J Dermatol 1982; 21: 89–93.

298 Laurent R, Kienzler J-L. Epidemiology of HPV infections. Clin Dermatol 1985; 3: 64–70.

299 Kilkenny M, Merlin K, Young R, Marks R. The prevalence of common skin conditions in Australian school students: 1. Common, plane and plantar viral warts. Br J Dermatol 1998; 138: 840–845.

300 Young R, Jolley D, Marks R. Comparison of the use of standardized diagnostic criteria and intuitive clinical diagnosis in the diagnosis of common viral warts (verrucae vulgaris). Arch Dermatol 1998; 134: 1586–1589.

301 Payne DA, Sanchez R, Tyring SK. Cutaneous verruca with genital human papillomavirus in a 2-year-old girl. Am J Dermatopathol 1997; 19: 258–260.

302 Barnett N, Mak H, Winkelstein JA. Extensive verrucosis in primary immunodeficiency diseases. Arch Dermatol 1983; 119: 5–7.

303 Milburn PB, Brandsma JL, Goldsman CI et al. Disseminated warts and evolving squamous cell carcinoma in a patient with acquired immunodeficiency syndrome. J Am Acad Dermatol 1988; 19: 401–405.

304 Kang S, Fitzpatrick TB. Debilitating verruca vulgaris in a patient infected with the human immunodeficiency virus. Arch Dermatol 1994; 130: 294–296.

305 Spach DH, Colven R. Resolution of recalcitrant hand warts in an HIV-infected patient treated with potent antiretroviral therapy. J Am Acad Dermatol 1999; 40: 818–821.

306 Steigleder G-K. Histology of benign virus induced tumors of the skin. J Cutan Pathol 1978; 5: 45–52.

307 Phillips ME, Ackerman AB. "Benign" and "malignant" neoplasms associated with verrucae vulgares. Am J Dermatopathol 1982; 4: 61–84.

308 Kimura S, Komatsu T, Ohyama K. Common and plantar warts with trichilemmal keratinization-like keratinizing process: a possible existence of pseudo-trichilemmal keratinization. J Cutan Pathol 1982; 9: 391–395.

309 Jacyk WK, du Plessis PJ. Viral warts in a patient with Darier's disease show acantholytic dyskeratosis. Am J Dermatopathol 1997; 19: 87–88.

310 Eng AM, Jin Y-T, Matsuoka LY et al. Correlative studies of verruca vulgaris by H&E, PAP immunostaining, and electronmicroscopy. J Cutan Pathol 1985; 12: 46–54.

311 Kossard S, Xenias SJ, Palestine RF et al. Inflammatory changes in verruca vulgaris. J Cutan Pathol 1980; 7: 217–221.

312 Berman A, Winkelmann RK. Involuting common warts. Clinical and histopathologic findings. J Am Acad Dermatol 1980; 3: 356–362.

313 James MP, Collier PM, Aherne W et al. Histologic, pharmacologic, and immunocytochemical effects of injection of bleomycin into viral warts. J Am Acad Dermatol 1993; 28: 933–937.

314 Goette DK. Carcinoma in situ in verruca vulgaris. Int J Dermatol 1980; 19: 98–101.

315 Inaba Y, Egawa K, Yoshimura K, Ono T. Demonstration of human papillomavirus type 1 DNA in a wart with bowenoid histologic changes. Am J Dermatopathol 1993; 15: 172–175.

316 Shelley WB, Wood MG. Transformation of the common wart into squamous cell carcinoma in a patient with primary lymphedema. Cancer 1981; 48: 820–824.

317 Ratoosh SL, Glombicki AP, Lockhart SG et al. Mastication of verruca vulgaris associated with esophageal papilloma: HPV-45 sequences detected in oral and cutaneous tissues. J Am Acad Dermatol 1997; 36: 853–857.

318 Honda A, Iwasaki T, Sata T et al. Human papillomavirus type 60-associated plantar wart. Ridged wart. Arch Dermatol 1994; 130: 1413–1417.

319 Egawa K, Hayashibara T, Ono T. Inverted plantar wart. Arch Dermatol 1993; 129: 385–386.

320 Kashima M, Tanabe Y, Kaminishi K et al. Human papillomavirus type 60 plantar warts are predominately pigmented when discovered after early adulthood. Br J Dermatol 1999; 141: 601–603.

321 Egawa K, Kasai S, Hattori N et al. A case of a human-papillomavirus-60-induced wart with clinical appearance of both pigmented and ridged warts. Dermatology 1998; 197: 268–270.

322 Egawa K. New types of human papillomaviruses and intracytoplasmic inclusion bodies: a classification of inclusion warts according to clinical features, histology and associated HPV types. Br J Dermatol 1994; 130: 158–166.

323 Davis MDP, Gostout BS, McGovern RM et al. Large plantar wart caused by human papillomavirus-66 and resolution by topical cidofovir therapy. J Am Acad Dermatol 2000; 43: 340–343.

324 Kashima M, Adachi M, Honda M et al. A case of peculiar plantar warts. Human papillomavirus type 60 infection. Arch Dermatol 1994; 130: 1418–1420.

325 Egawa K, Honda Y, Ono T, Kitasato H. A case of viral warts with particular fibrillar intracytoplasmic inclusion bodies. Dermatology 2000; 200: 275–278.

326 Berman A, Domnitz JM, Winkelmann RK. Plantar warts recently turned black. Clinical and histopathologic findings. Arch Dermatol 1982; 118: 47–51.

327 Egawa K, Honda Y, Inaba Y, Ono T. Pigmented viral warts: a clinical and histopathological study including human papillomavirus typing. Br J Dermatol 1998; 138: 381–389.

328 Prose NS, von Knebel-Doeberitz C, Miller S et al. Widespread flat warts associated with human papillomavirus type 5: a cutaneous manifestation of human immunodeficiency virus infection. J Am Acad Dermatol 1990; 23: 978–981.

329 Berger TG, Sawchuk WS, Leonardi C et al. Epidermodysplasia verruciformis-associated papillomavirus infection complicating human immunodeficiency virus disease. Br J Dermatol 1991; 124: 79–83.

330 Tagami H, Takigawa M, Ogino A et al. Spontaneous regression of plane warts after inflammation: clinical and histologic studies in 25 cases. Arch Dermatol 1977; 113: 1209–1213.

331 Berman A. Depigmented haloes associated with the involution of flat warts. Br J Dermatol 1977; 97: 263–265.

332 Berman A, Berman JE. Efflorescence of new warts: a sign of onset of involution in flat warts. Br J Dermatol 1978; 99: 179–182.

333 Iwatsuki K, Tagami H, Takigawa M, Yamada M. Plane warts under spontaneous regression. Arch Dermatol 1986; 122: 655–659.

334 Bender ME. Concepts of wart regression. Arch Dermatol 1986; 122: 645–647.

335 Weedon D, Robertson I. Regressing plane warts – an ultrastructural study. Australas J Dermatol 1978; 19: 65–68.

336 Jablonska S, Orth G. Epidermodysplasia verruciformis. Clin Dermatol 1985; 3: 83–96.

337 Jablonska S, Obalek S, Orth G et al. Regression of the lesions of epidermodysplasia verruciformis. Br J Dermatol 1982; 107: 109–115.

338 Majewski S, Skcpinska-Rozewska E, Jablonska S et al. Partial defects of cell-mediated immunity in patients with epidermodysplasia verruciformis. J Am Acad Dermatol 1986; 15: 966–973.

339 Ostrow RS, Manias D, Mitchell AJ et al. Epidermodysplasia verruciformis. A case associated with primary lymphatic dysplasia, depressed cell-mediated immunity, and Bowen's disease containing human papillomavirus 16 DNA. Arch Dermatol 1987; 123: 1511–1516.

340 Majewski S, Malejczyk J, Jablonska S et al. Natural cell-mediated cytotoxicity against various target cells in patients with epidermodysplasia verruciformis. J Am Acad Dermatol 1990; 22: 423–427.

341 Aizawa H, Abo T, Aiba S et al. Epidermodysplasia verruciformis accompanied by large granular lymphocytosis. Report of a case and immunological studies. Arch Dermatol 1989; 125: 660–665.

342 Kaminski M, Pawinska M, Jablonska S et al. Increased natural killer cell activity in patients with epidermodysplasia verruciformis. Arch Dermatol 1985; 121: 84–86.

343 van Voorst Vader PC, Orth G, Dutronquay V et al. Epidermodysplasia verruciformis. Acta Derm Venereol 1986; 66: 231–236.

344 Harris AJ, Purdie K, Leigh IM et al. A novel human papillomavirus identified in epidermodysplasia verruciformis. Br J Dermatol 1997; 136: 587–591.

345 Ishiji T, Kawase M, Honda M et al. Distinctive distribution of human papillomavirus type 16 and type 20 DNA in the tonsillar and the skin carcinomas of a patient with epidermodysplasia verruciformis. Br J Dermatol 2000; 143: 1005–1010.

346 Ramoz N, Taïeb A, Rueda L-A et al. Evidence for a nonallelic heterogeneity of epidermodysplasia verruciformis with two susceptibility loci mapped to chromosome regions 2p21-p24 and 17q25. J Invest Dermatol 2000; 114: 1148–1153.

347 Ramoz N, Rueda L-A, Bouadjar B et al. A susceptibility locus for epidermodysplasia verruciformis, an abnormal predisposition to infection with the oncogenic human papillomavirus type 5, maps to chromosome 17qter in a region containing a psoriasis locus. J Invest Dermatol 1999; 112: 259–263.

348 Androphy EJ, Dvoretzky I, Lowy DR. X-linked inheritance of epidermodysplasia verruciformis. Genetic and virologic studies of a kindred. Arch Dermatol 1985; 121: 864–868.

349 Favre M, Majewski S, De Jesus N et al. A possible vertical transmission of human papillomavirus genotypes associated with epidermodysplasia verruciformis. J Invest Dermatol 1998; 111: 333–336.

350 Jacyk WK, De Villiers EM. Epidermodysplasia verruciformis in Africans. Int J Dermatol 1993; 32: 806–810.

351 Cortés-Franco R, Tyring SK, Vega E et al. Divergent clinical course of epidermodysplasia verruciformis in siblings. Int J Dermatol 1997; 36: 442–445.

352 Kaspar TA, Wagner RF Jr, Jablonska S et al. Prognosis and treatment of advanced squamous cell carcinoma secondary to epidermodysplasia verruciformis: a worldwide analysis of 11 patients. J Dermatol Surg Oncol 1991; 17: 237–240.

353 Pizarro A, Gamallo C, Castresana JS et al. p53 protein expression in viral warts from patients with epidermodysplasia verruciformis. Br J Dermatol 1995; 132: 513–519.

354 Barzegar C, Paul C, Saiag P et al. Epidermodysplasia verruciformis-like eruption complicating human immunodeficiency virus infection. Br J Dermatol 1998; 139: 122–127.

355 Bouwes Bavinck JN, Stark S, Petridis AK et al. The presence of antibodies against virus-like particles of epidermodysplasia verruciformis-associated human papillomavirus type 8 in patients with actinic keratoses. Br J Dermatol 2000; 142: 103–109.

356 Boxman ILA, Mulder LHC, Russell A et al. Human papillomavirus type 5 is commonly present in immunosuppressed and immunocompetent individuals. Br J Dermatol 1999; 141: 246–249.

357 Favre M, Orth G, Majewski S et al. Psoriasis: a possible reservoir for human papillomavirus type 5, the virus associated with skin carcinomas of epidermodysplasia verruciformis. J Invest Dermatol 1998; 110: 311–317.

358 Weissenborn SJ, Höpfl R, Weber F et al. High prevalence of a variety of epidermodysplasia verruciformis-associated human papillomaviruses in psoriatic skin of patients treated or not treated with PUVA. J Invest Dermatol 1999; 113: 122–126.

359 Astori G, Lavergne D, Benton C et al. Human papillomaviruses are commonly found in normal skin of immunocompetent hosts. J Invest Dermatol 1998; 110: 752–755.

360 Iraji F, Faghihi G. Epidermodysplasia verruciformis: association with isolated IgM deficiency and response to treatment with acitretin. Clin Exp Dermatol 2000; 25: 41–43.

361 Al Rubaie S, Breuer J, Inshasi J et al. Epidermodysplasia verruciformis with neurological manifestations. Int J Dermatol 1998; 37: 766–771.

362 Nuovo GJ, Ishag M. The histologic spectrum of epidermodysplasia verruciformis. Am J Surg Pathol 2000; 24: 1400–1406.

363 Majewski S, Jablonska S. Epidermodysplasia verruciformis as a model of human papillomavirus-induced genetic cancer of the skin. Arch Dermatol 1995; 131: 1312–1318.

364 Rock B, Shah KV, Farmer ER. A morphologic, pathologic, and virologic study of anogenital warts in men. Arch Dermatol 1992; 127: 495–500.

365 Sykes NL Jr. Condyloma acuminatum. Int J Dermatol 1995; 34: 297–302.

366 Comite SL, Castadot M-J. Colposcopic evaluation of men with genital warts. J Am Acad Dermatol 1988; 18: 1274–1278.

367 von Krogh G. Clinical relevance and evaluation of genitoanal papilloma virus infection in the male. Semin Dermatol 1992; 11: 229–240.

368 Mazzatenta C, Andreassi L, Biagioli M et al. Detection and typing of genital papillomaviruses in men with a single polymerase chain reaction and type-specific DNA probes. J Am Acad Dermatol 1993; 28: 704–710.

369 Chuang T-Y. Condylomata acuminata (genital warts). An epidemiologic view. J Am Acad Dermatol 1987; 16: 376–384.

370 Oriel JD. Genital papillomavirus infection. Semin Dermatol 1989; 8: 48–53.

371 Sehgal VN, Koranne RV, Srivastava SB. Genital warts. Current status. Int J Dermatol 1989; 28: 75–85.

372 Euvrard S, Kanitakis J, Chardonnet Y et al. External anogenital lesions in organ transplant recipients. Arch Dermatol 1997; 133: 175–178.

373 Grussendorf-Conen E-I. Condylomata acuminata. Clin Dermatol 1985; 3: 97–103.

374 Yell JA, Sinclair R, Mann S et al. Human papillomavirus type 6-induced condylomata: an unusual complication of intertrigo. Br J Dermatol 1993; 128: 575–577.

375 Ruocco E. Genital warts at the site of healed herpes progenitalis: the isotopic response. Int J Dermatol 2000; 39: 705–706.

376 Googe PB, Chung SJ, Simmons J, King R. Giant-sized condyloma of the breast with focal acantholytic changes. J Cutan Pathol 2000; 27: 319–322.

377 Rock B, Naghashfar Z, Barnett N et al. Genital tract papillomavirus infection in children. Arch Dermatol 1986; 122: 1129–1132.

378 Bender ME. New concepts of condyloma acuminata in children. Arch Dermatol 1986; 122: 1121–1124.

379 Handley JM, Maw RD, Bingham EA et al. Anogenital warts in children. Clin Exp Dermatol 1993; 18: 241–247.

380 Yun K, Joblin L. Presence of human papillomavirus DNA in condylomata acuminata in children and adolescents. Pathology 1993; 25: 1–3.

381 Sagerman PM, Kadish AS, Niedt GW. Condyloma acuminatum with superficial spirochetosis simulating condyloma latum. Am J Dermatopathol 1993; 15: 176–179.

382 Allen AL, Siegfried EC. The natural history of condyloma in children. J Am Acad Dermatol 1998; 39: 951–955.

383 Chuang T-Y, Perry HO, Kurland LT, Ilstrup DM. Condyloma acuminatum in Rochester, Minn, 1950–1978. I. Epidemiology and clinical features. Arch Dermatol 1984; 120: 469–475.

384 Zhu W-Y, Leonardi C, Blauvelt A et al. Human papillomavirus DNA in the dermis of condyloma acuminatum. J Cutan Pathol 1993; 20: 447–450.

385 Lee SH, McGregor DH, Kuziez MN. Malignant transformation of perianal condyloma acuminatum: a case report with review of the literature. Dis Colon Rectum 1981; 24: 462–467.

386 Bogomoletz WV, Potet F, Molas G. Condylomata acuminata, giant condyloma acuminatum (Buschke–Loewenstein tumour) and verrucous squamous carcinoma of the perianal and anorectal region: a continuous precancerous spectrum? Histopathology 1985; 9: 1155–1169.

387 Norris CS. Giant condyloma acuminatum (Buschke–Lowenstein tumor) involving a pilonidal sinus: a case report and review of the literature. J Surg Oncol 1983; 22: 47–50.

388 Grassegger A, Höpfl R, Hussl H et al. Buschke–Loewenstein tumour infiltrating pelvic organs. Br J Dermatol 1994; 130: 221–225.

389 Anadolu R, Boyvat A, Çalikoğlu E, Gürler A. Buschke–Lowenstein tumour is not a low-grade carcinoma but a giant verruca. Acta Derm Venereol 1999; 79: 253–254.

390 Geusau A, Heinz-Peer G, Volc-Platzer B et al. Regression of deeply infiltrating giant condyloma (Buscke–Löwenstein tumor) following long-term intralesional interferon alfa therapy. Arch Dermatol 2000; 136: 707–710.

391 Gross G, Ikenberg H, Gissmann L, Hagedorn M. Papillomavirus infection of the anogenital region: correlation between histology, clinical picture, and virus type. Proposal of a new nomenclature. J Invest Dermatol 1985; 85: 147–152.

392 Obalek S, Misiewicz J, Jablonska S et al. Childhood condyloma acuminatum: association with genital and cutaneous human papillomaviruses. Pediatr Dermatol 1993; 10: 101–106.

393 Obalek S, Jablonska S, Favre M et al. Condylomata acuminata in children: frequent association with human papillomaviruses responsible for cutaneous warts. J Am Acad Dermatol 1990; 23: 205–213.

394 Langenberg A, Cone RW, McDougall J et al. Dual infection with human papillomavirus in a population with overt genital condylomas. J Am Acad Dermatol 1993; 28: 434–442.

395 Bradshaw BR, Nuovo GJ, DiCostanzo D, Cohen SR. Human papillomavirus type 16 in a homosexual man. Arch Dermatol 1992; 128: 949–952.

396 Steffen C. Concurrence of condylomata acuminata and bowenoid papulosis. Am J Dermatopathol 1982; 4: 5–8.

397 Li J, Ackerman AB. "Seborrheic keratoses" that contain human papillomavirus are condylomata acuminata. Am J Dermatopathol 1994; 16: 398–405.

398 Nuovo GJ, Becker J, Margiotta M et al. Histological distribution of polymerase chain reaction-amplified human papillomavirus 6 and 11 DNA in penile lesions. Am J Surg Pathol 1992; 16: 269–275.

399 Bhawan J, Dayal Y, Bhan AK. Langerhans' cells in molluscum contagiosum, verruca vulgaris, plantar wart, and condyloma acuminatum. J Am Acad Dermatol 1986; 15: 645–649.

400 Wade TR, Ackerman AB. The effects of resin of podophyllin on condyloma acuminatum. Am J Dermatopathol 1984; 6: 109–122.

401 Arrese JE, Paquet P, Claessens N et al. Dermal dendritic cells in anogenital warty lesions unresponsive to an immune-response modifier. J Cutan Pathol 2001; 28: 131–134.

402 Kimura S, Masuda M. A comparative immunoperoxidase and histopathologic study of condylomata acuminata. J Cutan Pathol 1985; 12: 142–146.

403 Pirog EC, Chen Y-T, Isacson C. MIB-1 immunostaining is a beneficial adjunct test for accurate diagnosis of vulvar condyloma acuminatum. Am J Surg Pathol 2000; 24: 1393–1399.

404 Cohen PR, Hebert AA, Adler-Storthz K. Focal epithelial hyperplasia: Heck disease. Pediatr Dermatol 1993; 10: 245–251.

405 Vilmer C, Cavelier-Balloy B, Pinquier L et al. Focal epithelial hyperplasia and multifocal human papillomavirus infection in an HIV-seropositive man. J Am Acad Dermatol 1994; 30: 497–498.

406 Lutzner M, Kuffer R, Blanchet-Bardon C, Croissant O. Different papillomaviruses as the causes of oral warts. Arch Dermatol 1982; 118: 393–399.

407 Obalek S, Janniger C, Jablonska S et al. Sporadic cases of Heck disease in two Polish girls: association with human papillomavirus type 13. Pediatr Dermatol 1993; 10: 240–244.

408 Steinhoff M, Metze D, Stockfleth E, Luger TA. Successful topical treatment of focal epithelial hyperplasia (Heck's disease) with interferon-β. Br J Dermatol 2001; 144: 1067–1069.

409 Stiefler RE, Solomon MP, Shalita AR. Heck's disease (focal epithelial hyperplasia). J Am Acad Dermatol 1979; 1: 499–502.

410 Kimura S. Bowenoid papulosis of the genitalia. Int J Dermatol 1982; 21: 432–436.

411 Schwartz RA, Janniger CK. Bowenoid papulosis. J Am Acad Dermatol 1991; 24: 261–264.

412 Halasz C, Silvers D, Crum CP. Bowenoid papulosis in three-year-old girl. J Am Acad Dermatol 1986; 14: 326–330.

413 Obalek S, Jablonska S, Baudenon S et al. Bowenoid papulosis of the male and female genitalia: risk of cervical neoplasia. J Am Acad Dermatol 1986; 14: 433–444.

414 Lloyd KM. Multicentric pigmented Bowen's disease of the groin. Arch Dermatol 1970; 101: 48–51.

415 Wade TR, Kopf AW, Ackerman AB. Bowenoid papulosis of the genitalia. Arch Dermatol 1979; 115: 306–308.

416 Johnson TM, Saluja A, Fader D et al. Isolated extragenital bowenoid papulosis of the neck. J Am Acad Dermatol 1999; 41: 867–870.

417 Baron JM, Rübben A, Grussendorf-Conen E-I. HPV 18-induced pigmented bowenoid papulosis of the neck. J Am Acad Dermatol 1999; 40: 633–634.

418 Olhoffer IH, Davidson M, Longley J et al. Facial bowenoid papulosis secondary to human papillomavirus type 16. Br J Dermatol 1999; 140: 761–762.

419 Purnell D, Ilchyshyn A, Jenkins D et al. Isolated human papillomavirus 18-positive extragenital bowenoid papulosis and idiopathic CD4+ lymphocytopenia. Br J Dermatol 2001; 144: 619–621.

420 Feldman SB, Sexton FM, Glenn JD, Lookingbill DP. Immunosuppression in men with bowenoid papulosis. Arch Dermatol 1989; 125: 651–654.

421 Crum CP, Liskow A, Petras P et al. Vulvar intraepithelial neoplasia (severe atypia and carcinoma in situ). A clinicopathologic analysis of 41 cases. Cancer 1984; 54: 1429–1434.

422 Jablonska S, Majewski S. Bowenoid papulosis transforming into squamous cell carcinoma of the genitalia. Br J Dermatol 1999; 141: 576–577.

423 Park K-C, Kim K-H, Youn S-W et al. Heterogeneity of human papillomavirus DNA in a patient with Bowenoid papulosis that progressed to squamous cell carcinoma. Br J Dermatol 1998; 139: 1087–1091.

424 Guillet GY, Braun L, Masse R et al. Bowenoid papulosis. Demonstration of human papillomavirus (HPV) with anti-HPV immune serum. Arch Dermatol 1984; 120: 514–516.

425 Penneys NS, Mogollon RJ, Nadji M, Gould E. Papillomavirus common antigens. Arch Dermatol 1984; 120: 859–861.

426 Lookingbill DP, Kreider JW, Howett MK et al. Human papillomavirus type 16 in bowenoid papulosis, intraoral papillomas, and squamous cell carcinoma of the tongue. Arch Dermatol 1987; 123: 363–368.

427 Abdennader S, Lessana-Leibowitch M, Pelisse M. An atypical case of penile carcinoma in situ associated with human papillomavirus DNA type 18. J Am Acad Dermatol 1989; 20: 887–889.

428 Rudlinger R, Grob R, Yu YX, Schnyder UW. Human papillomavirus-35-positive bowenoid papulosis of the anogenital area and concurrent human papillomavirus-35-positive verruca with bowenoid dysplasia of the periungual area. Arch Dermatol 1989; 125: 655–659.

429 Gupta J, Pilotti S, Shah KV et al. Human papillomavirus-associated early vulvar neoplasia investigated by in situ hybridization. Am J Surg Pathol 1987; 11: 430–434.

430 Ochiai T, Honda A, Morishima T et al. Human papillomavirus types 16 and 39 in a vulval carcinoma occurring in a woman with Hailey–Hailey disease. Br J Dermatol 1999; 140: 509–513.

431 Gross G, Hagedorn M, Ikenberg H et al. Bowenoid papulosis. Presence of human papillomavirus (HPV) structural antigens and of HPV 16-related DNA sequences. Arch Dermatol 1985; 121: 858–863.

Picornaviridae

432 Deseda-Tous J, Byatt PH, Cherry JD. Vesicular lesions in adults due to echovirus 11 infections. Arch Dermatol 1977; 113: 1705–1706.

433 James WD, Odom RB, Hatch MH. Gianotti–Crosti-like eruption associated with Coxsackievirus A-16 infection. J Am Acad Dermatol 1982; 6: 862–866.

434 McElgunn PSJ. Dermatologic manifestations of hepatitis B virus infection. J Am Acad Dermatol 1983; 8: 539–548.

435 Fields JP, Mihm MC Jr, Hellreich PD, Danoff SS. Hand, foot and mouth disease. Arch Dermatol 1969; 99: 243–246.

Other viral diseases

436 Miyagawa S, Takahashi Y, Nagai A et al. Angio-oedema in a neonate with IgG antibodies to parvovirus B19 following intrauterine parvovirus B19 infection. Br J Dermatol 2000; 143: 428–430.

437 Magro CM, Dawood MR, Crowson AN. The cutaneous manifestations of human parvovirus B19 infection. Hum Pathol 2000; 31: 488–497.

438 Dereure O, Montes B, Guilhou JJ. Acute generalized livedo reticularis with myasthenialike syndrome revealing parvovirus B19 primary infection. Arch Dermatol 1995; 131: 744–745.

439 Lyon CC. Severe acral pruritus associated with parvovirus B19 infection. Br J Dermatol 1998; 139: 153–154.

440 Halasz CLG, Cormier D, Den M. Petechial glove and sock syndrome caused by parvovirus B19. J Am Acad Dermatol 1992; 27: 835–838.

441 Lefrere J-J, Courouce A-M, Muller J-Y et al. Human parvovirus and purpura. Lancet 1985; ii: 730–731.

442 Bialecki C, Feder HM Jr, Grant-Kels JM. The six classic childhood exanthems: a review and update. J Am Acad Dermatol 1989; 21: 891–903.

443 Berry PJ, Gray ES, Porter HJ, Burton PA. Parvovirus infection of the human fetus and newborn. Semin Diagn Pathol 1992; 9: 4–12.

444 Evans LM, Grossman ME, Gregory N. Koplik spots and a purpuric eruption associated with parvovirus B19 infection. J Am Acad Dermatol 1992; 27: 466–467.

445 Shishiba T, Matsunaga Y. An outbreak of erythema infectiosum among hospital staff members including a patient with pleural fluid and pericardial effusion. J Am Acad Dermatol 1993; 29: 265–267.

446 Saulsbury FT. Petechial gloves and socks syndrome caused by parvovirus B19. Pediatr Dermatol 1998; 15: 35–37.

447 Ongradi J, Becker K, Horvath A et al. Simultaneous infection by human herpesvirus 7 and human parvovirus B19 in papular-purpuric gloves-and-socks syndrome. Arch Dermatol 2000; 136: 672.

448 Segui N, Zayas A, Fuertes A, Marquina A. Papular-purpuric 'gloves-and-socks' syndrome related to rubella virus infection. Dermatology 2000; 200: 89.

449 Ghigliotti G, Mazzarello G, Nigro A et al. Papular-purpuric gloves and socks syndrome in HIV-positive patients. J Am Acad Dermatol 2000; 43: 916–917.

450 Jones MF, Wold AD, Espy MJ, Smith TF. Serologic diagnosis of parvovirus B19 infections. Mayo Clin Proc 1993; 68: 1107–1108.

451 Leahy ST, Marshman G. Variable presentation of parvovirus B19 in a family. Australas J Dermatol 1998; 39: 112–115.

452 Takahashi M, Ito M, Sakamoto F et al. Human parvovirus B19 infection: immunohistochemical and electron microscopic studies of skin lesions. J Cutan Pathol 1995; 22: 168–172.

453 Grilli R, Izquierdo MJ, Fariña MC et al. Papular-purpuric "gloves and socks" syndrome: Polymerase chain reaction demonstration of parvovirus B19 DNA in cutaneous lesions and sera. J Am Acad Dermatol 1999; 41: 793–796.

454 Aractingi S, Bakhos D, Flageul B et al. Immunohistochemical and virological study of skin in the papular-purpuric gloves and socks syndrome. Br J Dermatol 1996; 135: 599–602.

455 Vargas-Diez E, Buezo GF, Aragües M et al. Papular-purpuric gloves-and-socks syndrome. Int J Dermatol 1996; 35: 626–632.

456 Ackerman AB, Suringa DWR. Multinucleate epidermal cells in measles. A histologic study. Arch Dermatol 1971; 103: 180–184.

457 McNutt NS, Kindel S, Lugo J. Cutaneous manifestations of measles in AIDS. J Cutan Pathol 1992; 19: 315–324.

458 Yanagihara M, Fujii T, Mochizuki T et al. Measles virus was present in the inner cell of the acrosyringium in the skin rash. Pediatr Dermatol 1998; 15: 456–458.

459 de Andino RM, Vazquez Botet M, Gubler DJ et al. The absence of dengue virus in the skin lesions of dengue fever. Int J Dermatol 1985; 24: 48–51.

450 Hart CA. Viral redskins. Semin Dermatol 1988; 7: 48–52.

461 Cernescu C, Nedelcu N-I, Tardei G et al. Continued transmission of West Nile virus to humans in Southeastern Romania, 1997–1998. J Infect Dis 2000; 181: 710–712.

462 Johnston LJ, Halliday GM, King NJC. Langerhans cells migrate to local lymph nodes following cutaneous infection with an arbovirus. J Invest Dermatol 2000; 114: 560–568.

463 Fraser JRE. Epidemic polyarthritis and Ross River virus disease. Clin Rheum Dis 1986; 12: 369–388.

464 Fraser JRE, Ratnamohan VM, Dowling JPG et al. The exanthem of Ross River virus infection: histology, location of virus antigen and nature of inflammatory infiltrate. J Clin Pathol 1983; 36: 1256–1263.

465 Autio P, Niemi KM, Kariniemi A-L. An eruption associated with alphavirus infection. Br J Dermatol 1996; 135: 320–323.

466 Kano Y, Kokaji T, Shiohara T. Photo-accentuated eruption and vascular deposits of immunoglobulin A associated with hepatitis A virus infection. Dermatology 2000; 200: 266–269.

467 Rosen LB, Rywlin AM, Resnick L. Hepatitis B surface antigen positive skin lesions. Two case reports with an immunoperoxidase study. Am J Dermatopathol 1985; 7: 507–514.

468 Hayakawa K, Shiohara T. Photolocalized eruption associated with acute hepatitis B virus infection. Br J Dermatol 1996; 134: 167–169.

469 Whittaker SJ, Dover JS, Greaves MW. Cutaneous polyarteritis nodosa associated with hepatitis B surface antigen. J Am Acad Dermatol 1986; 15: 1142–1145.

470 van de Pette JEW, Jarvis JM, Wilton JMA, MacDonald DM. Cutaneous periarteritis nodosa. Arch Dermatol 1984; 120: 109–111.

471 Lee S, Kim KY, Hahn CS et al. Gianotti–Crosti syndrome associated with hepatitis B surface antigen (subtype adr). J Am Acad Dermatol 1985; 12: 629–633.

472 Magyarlaki M, Drobnitsch I, Schneider I. Papular acrodermatitis of childhood (Gianotti–Crosti disease). Pediatr Dermatol 1991; 8: 224–227.

473 Gianotti F. Papular acrodermatitis of childhood and other papulo-vesicular acro-located syndromes. Br J Dermatol 1979; 100: 49–59.

474 Gibbs S, Burrows NP. Gianotti–Crosti syndrome in two unrelated adults. Clin Exp Dermatol 2000; 25: 594–596.

475 Sagi EF, Linder N, Shouval D. Papular acrodermatitis of childhood associated with hepatitis A virus infection. Pediatr Dermatol 1985; 3: 31–33.

476 Patrizi A, Di Lernia V, Ricci G et al. Papular and papulovesicular acrolocated eruptions and viral infections. Pediatr Dermatol 1990; 7: 22–26.

477 Hofmann B, Schuppe H-C, Adams O et al. Gianotti–Crosti syndrome associated with Epstein–Barr virus infection. Pediatr Dermatol 1997; 14: 273–277.

478 Smith KJ, Skelton H. Histopathologic features seen in Gianotti–Crosti syndrome secondary to Epstein–Barr virus. J Am Acad Dermatol 2000; 43: 1076–1079.

479 Di Lernia V. Gianotti–Crosti syndrome related to rotavirus infection. Pediatr Dermatol 1998; 15: 485–486.

480 Harangi F, Várszegi D, Szücs G. Asymmetric periflexural exanthem of childhood and viral examinations. Pediatr Dermatol 1995; 12: 112–115.

481 Taieb A, Plantin P, Du Pasquier P et al. Gianotti–Crosti syndrome: a study of 26 cases. Br J Dermatol 1986; 115: 49–59.

482 Spear KL, Winkelmann RK. Gianotti–Crosti syndrome. A review of ten cases not associated with hepatitis B. Arch Dermatol 1984; 120: 891–896.

483 Velangi SS, Tidman MJ. Gianotti–Crosti syndrome after measles, mumps and rubella vaccination. Br J Dermatol 1998; 139: 1122–1123.

484 Murphy L-A, Buckley C. Gianotti–Crosti syndrome in an infant following immunization. Pediatr Dermatol 2000; 17: 225–226.

485 Stefanato CM, Goldberg LJ, Andersen WK, Bhawan J. Gianotti–Crosti syndrome presenting as lichenoid dermatitis. Am J Dermatopathol 2000; 22: 162–165.

486 Martinez MI, Sanchez JL, Lopez-Malpica F. Peculiar papular skin lesions occurring in hepatitis B carriers. J Am Acad Dermatol 1987; 16: 31–34.

487 Pawlotsky J-M, Dhumeaux D, Bagot M. Hepatitis C virus in dermatology. A review. Arch Dermatol 1995; 131: 1185–1193.

488 Doutre M-S. Hepatitis C virus-related skin diseases. Arch Dermatol 1999; 135: 1401–1403.

489 Bonkovsky HL, Mehta S. Hepatitis C: A review and update. J Am Acad Dermatol 2001; 44: 159–179.

490 Schwaber MJ, Zlotogorski A. Dermatologic manifestations of hepatitis C infection. Int J Dermatol 1997; 36: 251–254.

491 Rao BK, Igwegbe I, Wiederkehr M et al. Gougerot–Blum disease as a manifestation of hepatitis C infection. J Cutan Pathol 2000; 27: 569 (abstract).

492 Hussain I, Hepburn NC, Jones A et al. The association of hepatitis C viral infection with porphyria cutanea tarda in the Lothian region of Scotland. Clin Exp Dermatol 1996; 21: 283–285.

493 Jackson JM, Callen JP. Scarring alopecia and sclerodermatous changes of the scalp in a patient with hepatitis C infection. J Am Acad Dermatol 1998; 39: 824–826.

494 O'Connor WJ, Badley AD, Dicken CH, Murphy GM. Porphyria cutanea tarda and human immunodeficiency virus: two cases associated with hepatitis C. Mayo Clin Proc 1998; 73: 895–897.

495 Llanos F, Raison-Peyron N, Meunier L et al. Hepatitis C virus infection in patients with urticaria. J Am Acad Dermatol 1998; 38: 646.

496 Shearer CM, Jackson JM, Callen JP. Symmetric polyarthritis with livedo reticularis: A newly recognized manifestation of hepatitis C virus infection. J Am Acad Dermatol 1997; 37: 659–661.

497 Sookoian S, Neglia V, Castaño G et al. High prevalence of cutaneous reactions to interferon alfa plus ribavirin combination therapy in patients with chronic hepatitis C virus. Arch Dermatol 1999; 135: 1000–1001.

498 Huh J, Kang GH, Gong G et al. Kaposi's sarcoma-associated herpesvirus in Kikuchi's disease. Hum Pathol 1998; 29: 1091–1096.

499 Bataille V, Harland CC, Behrens J et al. Kikuchi disease (histiocytic necrotizing lymphadenitis) in association with HTLV1. Br J Dermatol 1997; 136: 610–612.

500 Seno A, Torigoe R, Shimoe K et al. Kikuchi's disease (histiocytic necrotizing lymphadenitis) with cutaneous involvement. J Am Acad Dermatol 1994; 30: 504–506.

501 Yasukawa K, Matsumura T, Sato-Matsumura KC et al. Kikuchi's disease and the skin: case report and review of the literature. Br J Dermatol 2001; 144: 885–889.

502 Lopez C, Oliver M, Olavarria R et al. Kikuchi–Fujimoto necrotizing lymphadenitis associated with cutaneous lupus erythematosus. A case report. Am J Dermatopathol 2000; 22: 328–333.

503 Cousin F, Grézard P, Roth B et al. Kikuchi disease associated with Still disease. Int J Dermatol 1999; 38: 464–473.

504 Kuo T-t. Cutaneous manifestations of Kikuchi's histiocytic necrotizing lymphadenitis. Am J Surg Pathol 1990; 14: 872–876.

505 Spies J, Foucar K, Thompson CT, LeBoit PE. The histopathology of cutaneous lesions of Kikuchi's disease (necrotizing lymphadenitis). A report of five cases. Am J Surg Pathol 1999; 23: 1040–1047.

506 Coustou D, Masquelier B, Lafon ME et al. Asymmetric periflexural exanthem of childhood: microbiologic case-control study. Pediatr Dermatol 2000; 17: 169–173.

507 McCuaig CC, Russo P, Powell J et al. Unilateral laterothoracic exanthem. A clinicopathologic study of forty-eight patients. J Am Acad Dermatol 1996; 34: 979–984.

508 Bauzá A, Redondo P, Fernández J. Asymmetric periflexural exanthem in adults. Br J Dermatol 2000; 143: 224–226.

509 Gutzmer R, Herbst RA, Kiehl P et al. Unilateral laterothoracic exanthem (asymmetrical periflexural exanthem of childhood): Report of an adult patient. J Am Acad Dermatol 1997; 37: 484–485.

510 Coustou D, Léauté-Labrèze C, Bioulac-Sage P et al. Asymmetric periflexural exanthem of childhood. A clinical, pathologic, and epidemiologic prospective study. Arch Dermatol 1999; 135: 799–803.

511 Nutting WB, Beerman H, Parish LC, Witkowski JA. Retrovirus (HIV). Transfer, potential vectors, and biomedical concerns. Int J Dermatol 1987; 26: 426–433.

512 Lisby G, Lisby S, Wantzin GL. Retroviruses in dermatology. Int J Dermatol 1988; 27: 463–467.

513 Kumarasamy N, Solomon S, Madhivanan P et al. Dermatologic manifestations among human immunodeficiency virus patients in south India. Int J Dermatol 2000; 39: 192–195.

514 Cockerell CJ. Mucocutaneous neoplasms in patients with human immunodeficiency virus infection. Semin Diagn Pathol 1996; 13: 19–39.

515 Whittaker SJ, Ng YL, Rustin M et al. HTLV-1-associated cutaneous disease: a clinicopathological and molecular study of patients from the UK. Br J Dermatol 1993; 128: 483–492.

516 Smith KJ, Skelton HG, Yeager J et al. Cutaneous findings in HIV-1-positive patients: a 42-month prospective study. J Am Acad Dermatol 1994; 31: 746–754.

517 Farthing CF, Staughton RCD, Rowland Payne CME. Skin disease in homosexual patients with acquired immune deficiency syndrome (AIDS) and lesser forms of human T cell leukaemia virus (HTLV III) disease. Clin Exp Dermatol 1985; 10: 3–12.

518 Barlow RJ, Schulz EJ. Necrotizing folliculitis in AIDS-related complex. Br J Dermatol 1987; 116: 581–584.

519 Gregory N, DeLeo VA. Clinical manifestations of photosensitivity in patients with human immunodeficiency virus infection. Arch Dermatol 1994; 130: 630–633.

520 Duvic M, Rapini R, Hoots WK, Mansell PW. Human immunodeficiency virus-associated vitiligo: expression of autoimmunity with immunodeficiency? J Am Acad Dermatol 1987; 17: 656–662.

521 James WD, Redfield RR, Lupton GP et al. A papular eruption associated with human T cell lymphotropic virus type III disease. J Am Acad Dermatol 1985; 13: 563–566.

522 Shapiro RS, Samorodin C, Hood AF. Pruritis as a presenting sign of acquired immunodeficiency syndrome. J Am Acad Dermatol 1987; 16: 1115–1117.

523 Coopman SA, Stern RS. Cutaneous drug reactions in human immunodeficiency virus infection. Arch Dermatol 1991; 127: 714–717.

524 Smith KJ, Skelton HG, DeRusso D et al. Clinical and histopathologic features of hair loss in patients with HIV-1 infection. J Am Acad Dermatol 1996; 34: 63–68.

525 Sadick NS, McNutt NS, Kaplan MH. Papulosquamous dermatoses of AIDS. J Am Acad Dermatol 1990; 22: 1270–1277.

526 O'Connor WJ, Murphy GM, Darby C et al. Porphyrin abnormalities in acquired immunodeficiency syndrome. Arch Dermatol 1996; 132: 1443–1447.

527 Lim HW, Pereira A, Sassa S et al. Early-stage HIV infection and hepatitis C virus infection are associated with elevated serum porphyrin levels. J Am Acad Dermatol 1998; 39: 956–959.

528 Smith KJ, Skelton HG, Yeager J et al. Clinical features of inflammatory dermatoses in human immunodeficiency virus type 1 disease and their correlation with Walter Reed stage. J Am Acad Dermatol 1993; 28: 167–173.

529 Smith KJ, Skelton HG, Wagner KF. Pathogenesis of HIV-1 disease. Int J Dermatol 1995; 34: 308–318.

530 Francis N. Non-neoplastic, cutaneous and mucocutaneous manifestations of HIV infection. Histopathology 1993; 23: 297–305.

531 Myers SA, Prose NS, Bartlett JA. Progress in the understanding of HIV infection: an overview. J Am Acad Dermatol 1993; 29: 1–21.

532 Samet JH, Muz P, Cabral P et al. Dermatologic manifestations in HIV-infected patients: a primary care perspective. Mayo Clin Proc 1999; 74: 658–660.

533 Spira R, Mignard M, Doutre M-S et al. Prevalence of cutaneous disorders in a population of HIV-infected patients. Southwestern France, 1996. Arch Dermatol 1998; 134: 1208–1212.

534 Ramdial PK. Selected topics in HIV-associated skin pathology. Curr Diagn Pathol 2000; 6: 113–124.

535 Costner M, Cockerell CJ. The changing spectrum of the cutaneous manifestations of HIV disease. Arch Dermatol 1998; 134: 1290–1292.

536 Tosti A, Piraccini BM, D'Antuono A et al. Paronychia associated with antiretroviral therapy. Br J Dermatol 1999; 140: 1165–1168.

537 Wantzin GRL, Lindhardt BO, Weismann K, Ulrich K. Acute HTLV III infection associated with exanthema, diagnosed by seroconversion. Br J Dermatol 1986; 115: 601–606.

538 Hulsebosch HJ, Claessen FAP, van Ginkel CJW et al. Human immunodeficiency virus exanthem. J Am Acad Dermatol 1990; 23: 483–486.

539 Alessi E, Cusini M. The exanthem of HIV-1 seroconversion syndrome. Int J Dermatol 1995; 34: 238–239.

540 Hamann ID, Barnetson RStC. Non-infective mucocutaneous presentations of human immunodeficiency virus infection. Australas J Dermatol 1997; 38: 105–114.

541 Berger RS, Stoner MF, Hobbs ER et al. Cutaneous manifestations of early human immunodeficiency virus exposure. J Am Acad Dermatol 1988; 19: 298–303.

542 Liautaud B, Pape JW, DeHovitz JA et al. Pruritic skin lesions. A common initial presentation of acquired immunodeficiency syndrome. Arch Dermatol 1989; 125: 629–632.

543 Berk MA, Medenica M, Laumann A. Tubuloreticular structures in a papular eruption associated with human immunodeficiency virus disease. J Am Acad Dermatol 1988; 18: 452–456.

544 Muhlemann MF, Anderson MG, Paradinas FJ et al. Early warning skin signs in AIDS and persistent generalized lymphadenopathy. Br J Dermatol 1986; 114: 419–424.

545 Jensen BL, Weismann K, Sindrup JH et al. Incidence and prognostic significance of skin disease in patients with HIV/AIDS: a 5-year observational study. Acta Derm Venereol 2000; 80: 140–143.

546 Leyden JL. Infection in the immunocompromised host. Arch Dermatol 1985; 121: 855–857.

547 Czelusta A, Yen-Moore A, Van der Straten M et al. An overview of sexually transmitted diseases. Part III. Sexually transmitted diseases in HIV-infected patients. J Am Acad Dermatol 2000; 43: 409–432.

548 Wananukul S, Thisyakorn U. Mucocutaneous manifestations of HIV infection in 91 children born to HIV-seropositive women. Pediatr Dermatol 1999; 16: 359–363.

549 Winzer M, Gilliar U, Ackerman AB. Hairy lesions of the oral cavity. Clinical and histopathologic differentiation of hairy leukoplakia from hairy tongue. Am J Dermatopathol 1988; 10: 155–159.

550 Southam JC, Felix DH, Wray D, Cubie HA. Hairy leukoplakia – a histological study. Histopathology 1991; 19: 63–67.

551 Husak R, Garbe C, Orfanos CE. Oral hairy leukoplakia in 71 HIV-seropositive patients: Clinical symptoms, relation to immunologic status, and prognostic significance. J Am Acad Dermatol 1996; 35: 928–934.

552 Lupton GP, James WD, Redfield RR et al. Oral hairy leukoplakia. Arch Dermatol 1987; 123: 624–628.

553 Boonchai W, Laohasrisakul R, Manonukul J, Kulthanan K. Pruritic papular eruption in HIV seropositive patients: a cutaneous marker for immunosuppression. Int J Dermatol 1999; 38: 348–350.

554 Aires JM, Rosatelli JB, de Castro Figueiredo JF, Roselino AMF. Cytokines in the pruritic papular eruption of HIV. Int J Dermatol 2000; 39: 903–906.

555 Friedler S, Parisi MT, Waldo E et al. Atypical cutaneous lymphoproliferative disorder in patients with HIV infection. Int J Dermatol 1999; 38: 111–118.

556 Duvic M. Human immunodeficiency virus and the skin: selected controversies. J Invest Dermatol 1995; 105: 117S–121S.

557 Smith KJ, Skelton HG, Yeager J et al. Histopathologic and immunohistochemical findings associated with inflammatory dermatoses in human immunodeficiency virus type 1 disease and their correlation with Walter Reed stage. J Am Acad Dermatol 1993; 28: 174–184.

558 Goldstein B, Berman B, Sukenik E. Correlation of skin disorders with CD4 lymphocyte counts in patients with HIV/AIDS. J Am Acad Dermatol 1997; 36: 262–264.

559 Uthayakumar S, Nandwani R, Drinkwater T et al. The prevalence of skin disease in HIV infection and its relationship to the degree of immunosuppression. Br J Dermatol 1997; 137: 595–598.

560 Muñoz-Pérez MA, Rodriquez-Pichardo A, Camacho F, Colmenero MA. Dermatological findings correlated with CD4 lymphocyte counts in a prospective 3 year study of 1161 patients with human immunodeficiency virus disease predominantly acquired through intravenous drug abuse. Br J Dermatol 1998; 139: 33–39.

561 El Hachem M, Bernardi S, Pianosi G et al. Mucocutaneous manifestations in children with HIV infection and AIDS. Pediatr Dermatol 1998; 15: 429–434.

562 Wakeel RAP, Urbaniak SJ, Armstrong SS et al. Idiopathic CD4+ lymphocytopenia associated with chronic pruritic papules. Br J Dermatol 1994; 131: 371–375.

563 Kurwa HA, Marks R. Protracted cutaneous disorders in association with low CD4+ lymphocyte counts. Br J Dermatol 1995; 133: 625–629.

564 Stetson CL, Rapini RP, Tyring SK. Disseminated human papillomavirus infection with idiopathic CD4+ T-cell lymphocytopenia. J Cutan Pathol 2000; 27: 574 (abstract).

565 Smith KJ, Skelton HG, Chu WS et al. Decreased CD7 expression in cutaneous infiltrates of HIV-1+ patients. Am J Dermatopathol 1995; 17: 564–569.

566 Smith KJ, Barrett TL, Neafie R et al. Is CD30 (Ki-1) immunostaining in cutaneous eruptions useful as a marker of Th1 to Th2 cytokine switching and/or as a marker of advanced HIV-1 disease? Br J Dermatol 1998; 138: 774–779.

567 Smith KJ, Skelton HG III, James WD et al. Papular eruption of human immunodeficiency virus disease. A review of the clinical, histologic, and immunohistochemical findings in 48 cases. Am J Dermatopathol 1991; 13: 445–451.

568 Hevia O, Jimenez-Acosta F, Ceballos PI et al. Pruritic papular eruption of the acquired immunodeficiency syndrome: a clinicopathologic study. J Am Acad Dermatol 1991; 24: 231–235.

569 Goldman GD, Milstone LM, Shapiro PE. Histologic findings in acute HIV exanthem. J Cutan Pathol 1995; 22: 371–373.

570 Lapins J, Lindbäck S, Lidbrink P et al. Mucocutaneous manifestations in 22 consecutive cases of primary HIV-1 infection. Br J Dermatol 1996; 134: 257–261.

571 Barnadas MA, Alegre M, Baselga E et al. Histopathological changes of primary HIV infection. Description of three cases and review of the literature. J Cutan Pathol 1997; 24: 507–510.

572 Sapacin AN, Gelfand JM, Gumprecht J et al. Eruption of human immunodeficiency virus seroconversion. Int J Dermatol 1998; 37: 436–438.

573 Tschachler E, Franchini G. Infective dermatitis. A pabulum for human T-lymphotrophic virus type I leukemogenesis? Arch Dermatol 1998; 134: 487–488.

574 La Grenade L, Manns A, Fletcher V et al. Clinical, pathologic, and immunologic features of human T-lymphotrophic virus type I-associated infective dermatitis in children. Arch Dermatol 1998; 134: 439–444.

575 Sharata HH, Colvin JH, Fujiwara K et al. Cutaneous and neurologic disease associated with HTLV-1 infection. J Am Acad Dermatol 1997; 36: 869–871.

Protozoal infections

INTRODUCTION

The protozoa are single-celled organisms of great medical importance. There are six categories, covering several phyla; not all are of dermatopathological interest.

- Amebae
- Flagellates
- Coccidia
- Microsporidia
- Ciliates
- Sporozoa.

The amebae include the organisms that cause amebiasis and acanthamebiasis. The flagellates constitute an important group that includes the organisms for trypanosomiasis, leishmaniasis, trichomoniasis and giardiasis. The coccidia include *Toxoplasma gondii* and *Cryptosporidium parvum*; only toxoplasmosis will be considered further. The microsporidia and ciliates include a range of ntestinal parasites but no organisms of dermatopathological interest. Finally, the sporozoa include *Plasmodium* spp. and *Babesia* spp., responsible for malaria and babesiosis respectively.[1] *Pneumocystis carinii* has recently been reclassified as a fungus, but it lacks many of their features. It is considered here by tradition.

AMEBAE

Amebae are single-celled organisms with trophozoite and cyst stages in the life cycle. Their motility results from pseudopods.

AMEBIASIS

Cutaneous infection with *Entamoeba histolytica* is quite rare, occurring chiefly in the tropics.[2] It usually develops as a complication of amebic colitis, producing irregular areas of ulceration with verrucous borders around the anus, sometimes spreading to the thighs and genitalia.[3–5] Cutaneous lesions may also arise by fistulous extension from a gastrointestinal or hepatic abscess, around a colostomy or abdominal wound, or as a consequence of venereal transmission.[6] Penile lesions are being seen with increasing frequency in male homosexuals.

The ulcers are covered by gray slough and have a peculiarly unpleasant smell. Large exophytic lesions resembling squamous cell carcinoma may develop, particularly in genital areas.[7] These lesions may lead to an erroneous diagnosis of carcinoma, with unnecessary surgery being carried out.

Histopathology

Sections usually show an ulcerated lesion with extensive necrosis in the base, pseudoepitheliomatous hyperplasia at the margins, and a non-specific inflammatory infiltrate extending into the deep dermis and subcutaneous tissues beneath the ulcer base.[8] Sometimes there is extensive pseudo-epitheliomatous hyperplasia involving much of the lesion, with only small punctate areas of ulceration (Fig. 27.1). This may resemble a verrucous carcinoma. *E. histolytica* may be found, singly and in clusters, in the overlying exudate (Fig. 27.2). They differ from histiocytes by the presence of a single eccentric nucleus with a prominent central karyosome and occasional phagocytosed red blood cells in the cytoplasm.[4] In sections of fixed tissue their diameters are usually within the range 12–20 μm.

ACANTHAMEBIASIS

The free-living amebae of soil and water, *Acanthamoeba* and *Naegleria*, are facultative parasites of man.[9,10] Although meningoencephalitis is the major clinical feature, there have been a number of reports of pustular, chronic ulcerating or nodular lesions in the skin,[11,12] particularly in patients with the acquired immunodeficiency syndrome (AIDS).[13–18]

Histopathology

Sections have shown tuberculoid granulomatous lesions in the deep dermis and subcutaneous tissue, often with accompanying vasculitis.[11,14] In patients with AIDS, granulomas are not always present. There may be a diffuse neutrophilic infiltrate with numerous organisms, and abscess formation. A suppurative panniculitis has also been described.[15,16,18] Amebae, 15–40 μm in width, can often be seen lying free in the tissues;[19] they may take the form of trophozoites or cysts.[16] Organisms are not invariably present in immuno-competent individuals with granulomas.

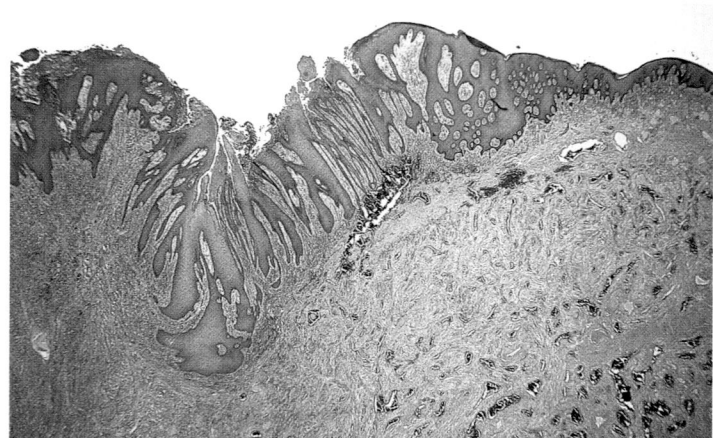

Fig. 27.1 **Amebiasis of the penis.** This case was misdiagnosed on biopsy as a squamous cell carcinoma because of the marked pseudoepitheliomatous hyperplasia. (H & E)

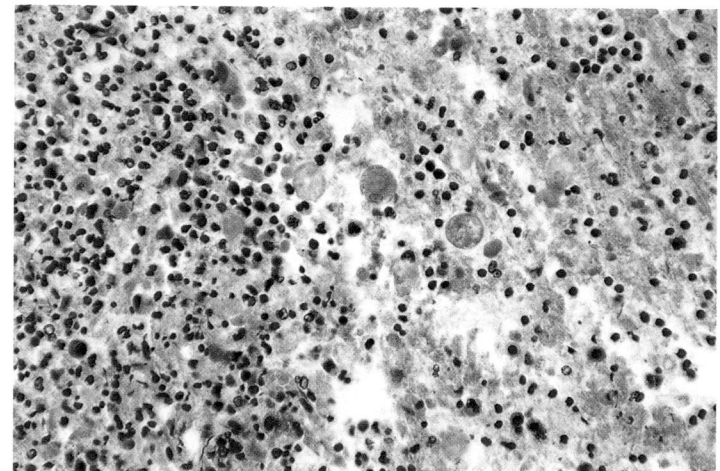

Fig. 27.2 **Amebiasis.** Organisms are present in the ulcer base. (H & E)

FLAGELLATES

The flagellates are a group of protozoa that move by means of a flagella. They are of considerable medical importance. The following diseases will be considered:

- trypanosomiasis
- leishmaniasis
- trichomoniasis
- giardiasis.

TRYPANOSOMIASIS

African trypanosomiasis is caused by the protozoa *Trypanosoma brucei gambiense* and *Trypanosoma brucei rhodesiense*, which are transmitted by the bite of the tsetse fly (*Glossina* species).[20,21] The Gambian variant has increased in incidence in Central Africa, with nearly 100 000 new infections each year.[21] Although the major clinical manifestations are fever and neurological signs, cutaneous lesions develop in about half of the patients.[22] These consist of an indurated erythematous 'chancre' at the site of the bite, followed several weeks later by a fleeting erythematous maculopapular rash, often with circinate lesions.[23] The lesions in this latter secondary stage are known as trypanids.[24] The diagnosis is made by finding hemoflagellates in thick peripheral blood smears.[25]

There are usually no significant skin lesions in American trypanosomiasis (Chagas' disease), caused by *T. cruzi*, although a macular and ulcerative eruption due to parasitosis of the skin by amastigotes of this organism has been reported in an immunosuppressed patient. Visceral lesions include a cardiomyopathy and gastrointestinal involvement.[26]

Histopathology

Sections of the chancre show a superficial and deep, predominantly perivascular infiltrate with lymphocytes and prominent plasma cells, with some resemblance to the lesions of secondary syphilis.[22] Organisms can be seen in Giemsa-stained smears taken from the exudate of a chancre, but they are not usually seen in tissue sections.[22] In the secondary stage the trypanids show mild spongiosis with exocytosis of lymphocytes, a superficial perivascular infiltrate of lymphocytes, and a mild diffuse infiltrate of neutrophils with some leukocytoclasis.[24] Amastigotes of *T. cruzi* were present in the walls of blood vessels, in arrector pili muscles and in the cytoplasm of inflammatory cells in the immunosuppressed patient referred to above.

LEISHMANIASIS

Leishmaniasis is an important protozoal infection, with an estimated 400 000 new cases occurring worldwide each year.[27–29] Its incidence is increasing.[30] Leishmaniasis can be classified into three types, each caused by a different species of *Leishmania*:

1. cutaneous (oriental) leishmaniasis caused by *L. tropica* in Asia and Africa, and by *L. mexicana* in Central and South America[31]
2. mucocutaneous (American) leishmaniasis caused by *L. brasiliensis*
3. visceral leishmaniasis (kala-azar) caused by *L. donovani*.

This classification is an oversimplification, as a great deal of clinical overlap exists between the various forms.[32,33] For example, visceral infection, caused by *L. tropica*, was reported in American soldiers infected in Saudi Arabia during the operation known as 'Desert Storm'.[34,35] The diagnosis can be made by identifying parasites on histological section,[36] or in smears,[37] by culture on specialized media, by the leishmanin intradermal skin test (Montenegro test), by fluorescent antibody tests using the patient's serum,[38] or by polymerase chain reaction (PCR) using species-specific primers. Results of PCR can be falsely positive.[39] The leishmanin test is usually negative in the forms with cell-mediated hyporeactivity, such as the diffuse cutaneous forms and the visceral form (kala-azar).[34]

Various subspecies of *Leishmania* have been documented in recent years (see below).[34]

Cutaneous leishmaniasis

Cutaneous leishmaniasis, a chronic self-limited granulomatous disease of the skin, is usually caused by *L. tropica*. It is endemic in the Middle East, around the eastern Mediterranean, in North Africa and in parts of Asia.[35,40–45] The term 'Old World' leishmaniasis has been used for such cases. Subspecies of *L. tropica* include *L. major*, *L. minor* and *L. aethiopica*.[34,46] Sandflies of the genus *Phlebotomus* are the usual vectors. The incubation period following the sandfly bite is weeks to months and depends on the size of the inoculum.[47] In Central and South America, and in parts of Texas ('New World'), *L. mexicana* is the species involved.[48] Subspecies include *L. amazonensis*, *L. pifanoi* and *L. venezuelensis*.[34,49] Other species of *Leishmania* involved in 'New World' disease include *L. guyanensis* and *L. panamensis*[50] as well as *L. brasiliensis* (once considered an exclusive cause of mucocutaneous disease). A recent series of cases caused by this species found mucosal disease in only 12.7% of cases.[51] *L. infantum*, long considered an exclusive cause of visceral leishmaniasis (see below), has now been identified in cutaneous leishmaniasis.[52,53] These two examples highlight the artificiality of 'matching' organisms to each of the three categories (cutaneous, mucocutaneous and visceral) in the traditional classification.

Acute, chronic, recidivous and disseminated forms are recognized.[47] The acute lesions are usually single papules, which become nodules, ulcerate and heal, leaving a scar.[40,54–56] Unusual presentations include paronychial, chancriform, annular, palmoplantar, zosteriform and erysipeloid forms.[57] Chronic lesions, which persist for 1–2 years, are single, or occasionally multiple, raised non-ulcerated plaques. The recidivous (lupoid) form consists of erythematous papules, often circinate, near the scars of previously healed lesions.[36,58–63] The recidivous form is mostly seen with so-called 'Old World' leishmaniasis caused by *L. tropica*. Several cases have now been reported from South America ('New World').[64] The disseminated form (primary diffuse cutaneous leishmaniasis) develops in anergic individuals as widespread nodules and macules, without ulceration or visceral involvement.[65] It is quite rare in *L. tropica* infections, but less so with *L. mexicana*.[49,66] Sporotrichoid[67,68] and satellite lesions[69] are very uncommon clinical manifestations of cutaneous leishmaniasis. A tardive form, in which a lesion developed at the site of recent cutaneous surgery, has been reported.[70] The likely source of infection was encountered over 50 years previously.[70]

Histopathology

In acute lesions there is a massive dermal infiltrate of lymphocytes, parasitized macrophages, epithelioid cells and occasional giant cells, plasma cells and sometimes a few eosinophils (Fig. 27.3).[71] Both CD4+ and CD8+ lymphocytes are present.[50] Variable numbers of neutrophils are present in the upper dermis. Granulated calcific Michaelis–Gutmann bodies have been reported in the cytoplasm of macrophages in two cases.[72] Rarely, the inflammatory infiltrate extends around small nerves in the deep dermis in a manner similar to leprosy.[73] The parasites are round to oval basophilic structures, 2–4 μm in

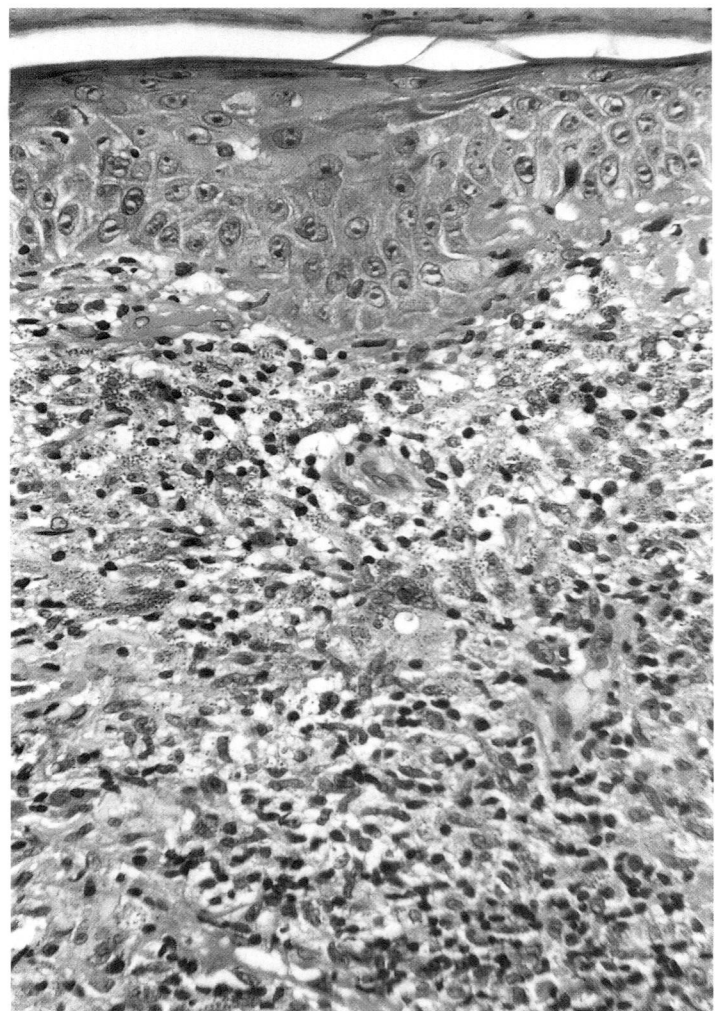

Fig. 27.3 **Leishmaniasis.** The dermal infiltrate is composed of lymphocytes, some plasma cells and parasitized macrophages. (H & E)

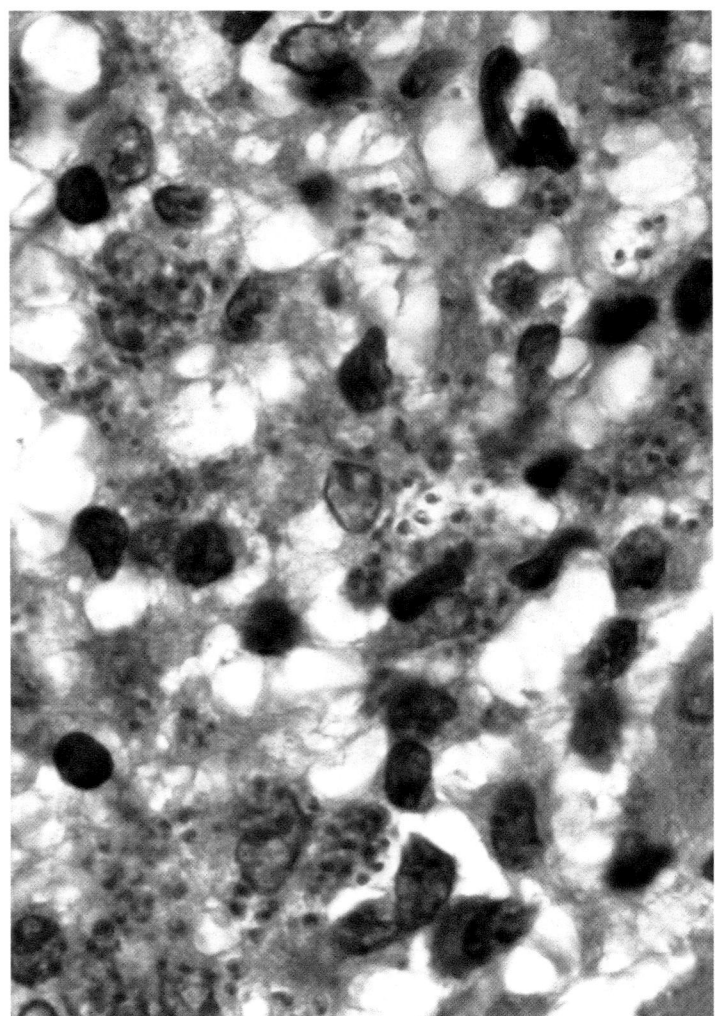

Fig. 27.4 **Leishmaniasis.** Numerous organisms are present in the cytoplasm of macrophages. (H & E)

size. They have an eccentrically located kinetoplast. Their lack of a capsule is helpful in distinguishing them from *Histoplasma capsulatum*. Although organisms can be seen in macrophages in hematoxylin and eosin-stained sections (Fig. 27.4), the morphological details are better seen on a Giemsa stain, preferably of a slit-skin smear.[74] Organisms tend to localize at the periphery of the macrophages, the so-called 'marquee' sign. The epidermis shows hyperkeratosis and acanthosis, but sometimes atrophy, ulceration or intraepidermal abscesses.[67,75] Pseudoepitheliomatous hyperplasia is present in some long-standing lesions.

With increasing chronicity there is a reduction in the number of parasitized macrophages, and the appearance of small tuberculoid granulomas which consist predominantly of epithelioid cells and histiocytes with occasional giant cells.[75] Central necrosis is rare.[76] There is an intervening mild to moderate mononuclear cell infiltrate.

In the recidivous form the appearances resemble those seen in lupus vulgaris, with tubercles surrounded by lymphocytes and histiocytes with some giant cells.[36,75] However, there is no necrosis and only sparse plasma cells. Occasional organisms may be found on careful search. The polymerase chain reaction can be used to demonstrate the presence of DNA of *Leishmania* amastigotes in tissue sections.[36] An immunohistochemical method using a

monoclonal anti-*Leishmania* (G2D10) antibody has been developed.[77] It has only marginally greater sensitivity and specificity than the routine H & E stain.

In the disseminated anergic lesions the infiltrate is almost entirely composed of parasitized macrophages, with scant lymphocytes.[78] Eosinophils were abundant in one reported case.[79]

Mucocutaneous leishmaniasis

The initial lesions of mucocutaneous (American) leishmaniasis, caused by *L. brasiliensis*, resemble those seen in the cutaneous form.[80] In an increasing number of cases, only cutaneous lesions are being seen with this organism (see above). Vegetating, verrucous and sporotrichoid[81] lesions may also occur. In up to 20% of cases destructive ulcerative lesions of mucous membranes develop, particularly in the tongue, nasopharynx and at body orifices.[82,83] This complication, known as espundia, may develop up to 25 years after the apparent clinical cure of the primary lesion.[30,80] Mucocutaneous leishmaniasis is found in Central and South America, or in travelers from those areas.[84,85] The disseminated anergic form is a rare complication;[78] it may occur in patients with AIDS.[86]

Histopathology

The appearances resemble those seen in the acute cutaneous form, although the number of organisms is considerably smaller and occasional tuberculoid granulomas may be seen. Suppurative granulomas have been described.[80] The mucosal lesions show non-specific chronic inflammation, with only a few parasitized macrophages. Pseudoepitheliomatous hyperplasia may be prominent in some lesions, particularly at the periphery.[84] There may be fibrosis in the dermis in cicatricial lesions.[84] A favorable prognostic feature is the presence of necrosis with a reactive response.[87]

Visceral leishmaniasis

Visceral leishmaniasis (kala-azar), caused by *L. donovani*, results in fever, anemia and hepatosplenomegaly.[78] It is endemic in many tropical countries. Cutaneous involvement (post-kala-azar dermal leishmaniasis) develops in about 5% of cases, some 1–5 years after the original infection.[88] This figure was much higher in a recent series.[89] This cutaneous form is most frequent in countries of the Indian subcontinent.[90,91] The lesions comprise areas of erythema (usually on the face), macules which may be hyper- or hypo-pigmented (usually on the trunk), and nodules (usually on the face, but not infrequently on the limbs).[88,92,93] Lesions may clinically resemble leprosy, but differ by having normal sensation.[89] Cutaneous lesions have recently been reported during the course of visceral leishmaniasis in patients with AIDS.[94–99] Rare variants of AIDS-associated cases have included the occurrence of leishmaniasis in lesions of herpes zoster,[100] parasitization of cells in a dermatofibroma[101] and the development of dermatomyositis-like lesions.[102]

Subspecies within the *L. donovani* complex include *L. donovani*, *L. infantum*, *L. chagasi* and *L. nilotica*.[34]

Histopathology

There is usually a dense infiltrate of inflammatory cells in the upper dermis beneath an atrophic epidermis.[91] The infiltrate is composed of a variable admixture of macrophages, lymphocytes, plasma cells and epithelioid cells.[103] Occasional eosinophils can usually be found. Neutrophils are present in a few cases.[92] There may be an occasional tuberculoid granuloma. In nodular lesions the infiltrate may occupy the entire thickness of the dermis.[92] In patients with a neuropathy, the inflammatory cell infiltrate shows perineural accentuation.[104] Follicular plugging is often present, particularly in lesions from the face.[91] Organisms (Leishman–Donovan bodies) are nearly always present, but their number varies from case to case and from lesion to lesion. They may be visualized better in sections stained with Weigert iron hematoxylin than in those stained with hematoxylin and eosin or the Giemsa stain.[92]

TRICHOMONIASIS

Although genital infections with *Trichomonas vaginalis* are common, cutaneous infections with this organism are exceedingly rare and usually confined to the median raphe of the penis.[105] An underlying cyst or tract is usually present. Trichomonads may be demonstrated by microscopy of the pus, drained from the abscess that forms.

GIARDIASIS

The cutaneous manifestations most commonly associated with gastrointestinal infection by *Giardia lamblia* are urticaria and angioedema. Other associations have included atopic dermatitis and a papulovesicular eruption that cleared on treatment of the parasite.[106] The protozoan has not been found in skin lesions.

COCCIDIA

Coccidia have both asexual and sexual cycles. They are usually acquired from contaminated food or water. They are particularly important in immuno-compromised patients. They include the genera *Cryptosporidium*, *Sarcocystis* and *Toxoplasma*. The cat family are the only known definite hosts for the sexual stages of *Toxoplasma gondii*. They are an important reservoir of infection. Congenital infection is the other important route of transmission.

TOXOPLASMOSIS

There are two clinical forms of toxoplasmosis, congenital and acquired.[107,108] The acquired form is seen most often in immunocompromised patients.[109] Skin changes in both are rare and not clinically distinctive. Macular, hemorrhagic and even exfoliative lesions have been reported in congenital toxoplasmosis,[110] whereas in the acquired form the lesions have been described as maculopapular, hemorrhagic, lichenoid,[111] nodular and erythema multiforme-like.[110,112] There have been several reports of a dermatomyositis-like syndrome.[113,114] The recent report of acute toxoplasmosis presenting as erythroderma[115] has subsequently been challenged.[116]

Histopathology

There is a superficial and mid-dermal perivascular lymphohistiocytic infiltrate. In about half the cases parasites can be seen in the cytoplasm of macrophages, in the form of pseudocysts, or lying free in the dermis,[112] or rarely the epidermis,[109] in the form of trophozoites. Pseudoepitheliomatous hyperplasia may develop in a few cases.[112] The histology has resembled dermatomyositis in those cases presenting with a dermatomyositis-like syndrome. Some of the rare histological expressions of the disease have recently been reviewed.[117]

MISCELLANEOUS

Although traditionally classified as a protozoan, *Pneumocystis carinii* has recently been reclassified as a fungus on the basis of several morphological features. Pneumocystosis is considered here by tradition.

PNEUMOCYSTOSIS

Cutaneous pneumocystosis is a rare infection in patients with AIDS.[118,119] There may be polypoid lesions in the external auditory canals, or necrotic papules and nodules elsewhere on the skin.[119]

Histopathology

Sections show perivascular mantles of amphophilic, foamy to finely stippled material similar to that seen in pulmonary pneumocystosis.[118] The methenamine silver stain may show large numbers of small cysts typical of *Pneumocystis carinii*. The other two structural forms of *P. carinii*, the intracystic sporozoite and the trophozoite (the encysted form), may be seen with polychrome stains such as the Giemsa or Wright stain.[119]

REFERENCES

Introduction
1 Javed MZ, Srivastava M, Zhang S, Kandathil M. Concurrent babesiosis and ehrlichiosis in an elderly host. Mayo Clin Proc 2001; 76: 563–565.

Amebae

2 El-Zawahry M, El-Komy M. Amoebiasis cutis. Int J Dermatol 1973; 12: 305–307.

3 Binford CH, Connor DH. Amebiasis. In: Pathology of tropical and extraordinary diseases. Vol 1. Washington DC: Armed Forces Institute of Pathology, 1976; 308–316.

4 Fujita WH, Barr RJ, Gottschalk HR. Cutaneous amebiasis. Arch Dermatol 1981; 117: 309–310.

5 Magaña-García M. Arista-Viveros A. Cutaneous amebiasis in children. Pediatr Dermatol 1993; 10: 352–355.

6 Elsahy NI. Cutaneous amoebiasis. Br J Plast Surg 1978; 31: 48–49.

7 Majmudar B, Chaiken ML, Lee KU. Amebiasis of clitoris mimicking carcinoma. JAMA 1976; 236: 1145–1146.

8 Loschiavo F, Guarneri B, Ventura-Spagnolo T et al. Cutaneous amebiasis in an Iranian immunodeficient alcoholic: immunohistochemical and histological study. Dermatology 1997; 194: 370–371.

9 Beaver PC, Jung RC, Cupp EW. Clinical parasitology, 9th ed. Philadelphia: Lea & Febiger, 1984.

10 Wortman PD. Acanthamoeba infection. Int J Dermatol 1996; 35: 48–51.

11 Bhagwandeen SB, Carter RF, Naik KG, Levitt D. A case of Hartmannellid amebic meningoencephalitis in Zambia. Am J Clin Pathol 1975; 63: 483–492.

12 Gullett J, Mills J, Hadley K et al. Disseminated granulomatous acanthamoeba infection presenting as an unusual skin lesion. Am J Med 1979; 67: 891–896.

13 May LP, Sidhu GS, Buchness MR. Diagnosis of *Acanthamoeba* infection by cutaneous manifestations in a man seropositive to HIV. J Am Acad Dermatol 1992; 26: 352–355.

14 Helton J, Loveless M, White CR Jr. Cutaneous *Acanthamoeba* infection associated with leukocytoclastic vasculitis in an AIDS patient. Am J Dermatopathol 1993; 15: 146–149.

15 Murakawa GJ, McCalmont T, Altman J et al. Disseminated acanthamebiasis in patients with AIDS. Arch Dermatol 1995; 131: 1291–1296.

16 Tan B, Weldon–Linne M, Rhone DP et al. *Acanthamoeba* infection presenting as skin lesions in patients with the acquired immunodeficiency syndrome. Arch Pathol Lab Med 1993; 117: 1043–1046.

17 Torno MS Jr, Babapour R, Gurevitch A, Witt MD. Cutaneous acanthamoebiasis in AIDS. J Am Acad Dermatol 2000; 42: 351–354.

18 Rosenberg AS, Morgan MB. Disseminated acanthamoebiasis presenting as lobular panniculitis with necrotizing vasculitis in a patient with AIDS. J Cutan Pathol 2001; 28: 307–313.

19 Ringsted J, Jager BV, Suk D, Visvesvara GS. Probable acanthamoeba meningoencephalitis in a Korean child. Am J Clin Pathol 1976; 66: 723–730.

Flagellates

20 Robinson B, Clark RM, King JF et al. Chronic Gambian trypanosomiasis. South Med J 1980; 73: 516–518.

21 Murray HW, Pépin J, Nutman TB et al. Tropical medicine. BMJ 2000; 320: 490–494.

22 Cochran R, Rosen T. African trypanosomiasis in the United States. Arch Dermatol 1983; 119: 670–674.

23 Spencer HC Jr, Gibson JJ Jr, Brodsky RE, Schultz MG. Imported African trypanosomiasis in the United States. Ann Intern Med 1975; 82: 633–638.

24 McGovern TW, Williams W, Fitzpatrick JE et al. Cutaneous manifestations of African trypanosomiasis. Arch Dermatol 1995; 131: 1178–1182.

25 Maddocks S, O'Brien R. African trypanosomiasis in Australia. N Engl J Med 2000; 342: 1254.

26 Tomimori-Yamashita J, Deps PD, Almeida DR et al. Cutaneous manifestation of Chagas' disease after heart transplantation: successful treatment with allopurinol. Br J Dermatol 1997; 137: 626–630.

27 Koff AB, Rosen T. Treatment of cutaneous leishmaniasis. J Am Acad Dermatol 1994; 31: 693–708.

28 Marsella R, Ruiz de Gopegui R. Leishmaniasis: a re-emerging zoonosis. Int J Dermatol 1998; 37: 801–814.

29 Herwaldt BL. Leishmaniasis. Lancet 1999; 354: 1191–1199.

30 Hepburn NC. Cutaneous leishmaniasis. Clin Exp Dermatol 2000; 25: 363–370.

31 Nelson DA, Gustafson TL, Spielvogel RL. Clinical aspects of cutaneous leishmaniasis acquired in Texas. J Am Acad Dermatol 1985; 12: 985–992.

32 Dowlati Y. Cutaneous leishmaniasis. Int J Dermatol 1979; 18: 362–368.

33 Grevelink SA, Lerner EA. Leishmaniasis. J Am Acad Dermatol 1996; 34: 257–272.

34 Azulay RD, Azulay DR Jr. Immune–clinical–pathologic spectrum of leishmaniasis. Int J Dermatol 1995; 34: 303–307.

35 Samady JA, Schwartz RA. Old World cutaneous leishmaniasis. Int J Dermatol 1997; 36: 161–166.

36 Momeni AZ, Yotsumoto S, Mehregan DR et al. Chronic lupoid leishmaniasis. Arch Dermatol 1996; 132: 198–202.

37 Berger RS, Perez-Figaredo RA, Spielvogel RL. Leishmaniasis: the touch preparation as a rapid means of diagnosis. J Am Acad Dermatol 1987; 16: 1096–1105.

38 Moriearty PL, Pereira C. Diagnosis and prognosis of new world leishmaniasis. Arch Dermatol 1978; 114: 962–963.

39 Palmer RA, Tran D, Hepburn NC, Ashton RE. The management of cutaneous leishmaniasis from Belize. Clin Exp Dermatol 2001; 26: 16–20.

40 Azab AS, Kamal MS, El Haggar MS et al. Early surgical treatment of cutaneous leishmaniasis. J Dermatol Surg Oncol 1983; 9: 1007–1012.

41 Marsden PD. Current concepts in parasitology: leishmaniasis. N Engl J Med 1979; 300: 350–352.

42 Farah FS, Malak JA. Cutaneous leishmaniasis. Arch Dermatol 1971; 103: 467–474.

43 Norton SA, Frankenburg S, Klaus SN. Cutaneous leishmaniasis acquired during military service in the Middle East. Arch Dermatol 1992; 128: 83–87.

44 Momeni AZ, Jalayer T, Emamjomeh M et al. Treatment of cutaneous leishmaniasis with itraconazole. Randomized double-blind study. Arch Dermatol 1996; 132: 784–786.

45 Mujtaba G, Khalid M. Cutaneous leishmaniasis in Multan, Pakistan. Int J Dermatol 1998; 37: 843–845.

46 Vardy DA, Frankenburg S, Goldenhersh M et al. Unusually extensive disease caused by *Leishmania major* parasites. Clin Exp Dermatol 1993; 18: 36–40.

47 Barsky S, Storino W, Salgea K, Knapp DP. Cutaneous leishmaniasis. Arch Dermatol 1978; 114: 1354–1355.

48 Furner BB. Cutaneous leishmaniasis in Texas: report of a case and review of the literature. J Am Acad Dermatol 1990; 23: 368–371.

49 Bonfante-Garrido R, Barroeta S, Mejía De Alejos MA et al. Disseminated American cutaneous leishmaniasis. Int J Dermatol 1996; 35: 561–565.

50 Palma GI, Saravia NG. In situ characterization of the human host response to *Leishmania panamensis*. Am J Dermatopathol 1997; 19: 585–590.

51 de Oliveira-Neto MP, Mattos MS, Perez MA et al. American tegumentary leishmaniasis (ATL) in Rio de Janeiro State, Brazil: main clinical and epidemiologic characteristics. Int J Dermatol 2000; 39: 506–514.

52 del Giudice P, Marty P, Lacour JP et al. Cutaneous leishmaniasis due to *Leishmania infantum*. Arch Dermatol 1998; 134: 193–198.

53 Gállego M, Pratlong F, Riera C et al. Cutaneous leishmaniasis due to Leishmania infantum in the northeast of Spain: the isoenzymatic analysis of parasites. Arch Dermatol 2001; 137: 667–668.

54 Kubba R, Al-Gindan Y, El-Hassan AM, Omer AHS. Clinical diagnosis of cutaneous leishmaniasis (oriental sore). J Am Acad Dermatol 1987; 16: 1183–1189.

55 Albanese G, Giorgetti P, Santagostino L et al. Cutaneous leishmaniasis. Treatment with itraconazole. Arch Dermatol 1989; 125: 1540–1542.

56 Uzun S, Uslular C, Yücel A et al. Cutaneous leishmaniasis: evaluation of 3074 cases in the Çukurova region of Turkey. Br J Dermatol 1999; 140: 347–350.

57 Raja KM, Khan AA, Hameed A, Rahman SB. Unusual clinical variants of cutaneous leishmaniasis in Pakistan. Br J Dermatol 1998; 139: 111–113.

58 Stratigos J, Tosca A, Nicolis G et al. Epidemiology of cutaneous leishmaniasis in Greece. Int J Dermatol 1980; 19: 86–88.

59 Kanj LF, Kibbi A-G, Zaynoun S. Cutaneous leishmaniasis: an unusual case with atypical recurrence. J Am Acad Dermatol 1993; 28: 495–496.

60 Bittencourt AL, Costa JML, Carvalho EM, Barral A. Leishmaniasis recidiva cutis in American cutaneous leishmaniasis. Int J Dermatol 1993; 32: 802–805.

61 Landau M, Srebrnik A, Brenner S. Leishmaniasis recidivans mimicking lupus vulgaris. Int J Dermatol 1996; 35: 572–573.

62 Gündüz K, Afsar S, Ayhan S et al. Recidivans cutaneous leishmaniasis unresponsive to liposomal amphotericin B (AmBisome®). J Eur Acad Dermatol Venereol 2000; 14: 11–13.

63 Cannavò SP, Vaccaro M, Guarneri F. Leishmaniasis recidiva cutis. Int J Dermatol 2000; 39: 205–206.

64 Oliveira-Neto MP, Mattos M, Souza CS et al. Leishmaniasis recidiva cutis in New World cutaneous leishmaniasis. Int J Dermatol 1998; 37: 846–849.

65 Al-Qurashi AR, Ghandour AM, Osman M, Al-Juma M. Dissemination in cutaneous leishmaniasis due to *Leishmania major* in different ethnic groups in Saudi Arabia. Int J Dermatol 2000; 39: 832–836.

66 Barral A, Costa JML, Bittencourt AL et al. Polar and subpolar diffuse cutaneous leishmaniasis in Brazil: clinical and immunopathologic aspects. Int J Dermatol 1995; 34: 474–479.

67 Kibbi A-G, Karam PG, Kurban AK. Sporotrichoid leishmaniasis in patients from Saudi Arabia: clinical and histologic features. J Am Acad Dermatol 1987; 17: 759–764.

68 Walsh DS, Balagon MV, Abalos RM et al. Multiple lesions of sporotrichoid leishmaniasis in a Filipino expatriate. J Am Acad Dermatol 1997; 36: 847–849.

69 Kubba R, Al-Gindan Y, El-Hassan AM et al. Dissemination in cutaneous leishmaniasis. II. Satellite papules and subcutaneous induration. Int J Dermatol 1988; 27: 702–706.

70 Czechowicz RT, Millard TP, Smith HR et al. Reactivation of cutaneous leishmaniasis after surgery. Br J Dermatol 1999; 141: 1113–1116.

71 Kurban AK, Malak JA, Farah FS, Chaglassian HT. Histopathology of cutaneous leishmaniasis. Arch Dermatol 1966; 93: 396–401.

72 Sandbank M. Michaelis–Gutmann bodies in macrophages of cutaneous leishmaniasis. J Cutan Pathol 1976; 3: 263–268.

73 Satti MB, El-Hassan AM, Al-Gindan Y et al. Peripheral neural involvement in cutaneous leishmaniasis. Int J Dermatol 1989; 28: 243–247.

74 Bryceson A. Tropical dermatology. Cutaneous leishmaniasis. Br J Dermatol 1976; 94: 223–226.

75 Nicolis GD, Tosca AD, Stratigos JD, Capetanakis JA. A clinical and histological study of cutaneous leishmaniasis. Acta Derm Venereol 1978; 58: 521–525.

76 Peltier E, Wolkenstein P, Deniau M et al. Caseous necrosis in cutaneous leishmaniasis. J Clin Pathol 1996; 49: 517–519.

77 Kenner JR, Aronson NE, Bratthauer GL et al. Immunohistochemistry to identify *Leishmania* parasites in fixed tissues. J Cutan Pathol 1999; 26: 130–136.

78 Rau RC, Dubin HV, Taylor WB. *Leishmania tropica* infections in travellers. Arch Dermatol 1976; 112: 197–201.

79 Bittencourt AL, Barral A, Costa JML et al. Diffuse cutaneous leishmaniasis with atypical aspects. Int J Dermatol 1992; 31: 568–570.

80 Price SM, Silvers DN. New world leishmaniasis. Serologic aids to diagnosis. Arch Dermatol 1977; 113: 1415–1416.

81 Spier S, Medenica M, McMillan S, Virtue C. Sporotrichoid leishmaniasis. Arch Dermatol 1977; 113: 1104–1105.

82 Farge D, Frances C, Vouldoukis I et al. Chronic destructive ulcerative lesion of the midface and nasal cavity due to leishmaniasis contracted in Djibouti. Clin Exp Dermatol 1987; 12: 211–213.

83 Iborra C, Caumes E, Carrière J et al. Mucosal leishmaniasis in a heart transplant recipient. Br J Dermatol 1998; 138: 190–192.

84 Sangueza OP, Sangueza JM, Stiller MJ, Sangueza P. Mucocutaneous leishmaniasis: a clinicopathologic classification. J Am Acad Dermatol 1993; 28: 927–932.

85 Rosbotham JL, Corbett EL, Grant HR et al. Imported mucocutaneous leishmaniasis. Clin Exp Dermatol 1996; 21: 288–290.

86 Nogueira-Castañon MCM, Pereira CAC, Furtado T. Unusual association of American cutaneous leishmaniasis and acquired immunodeficiency syndrome. Int J Dermatol 1996; 35: 295–297.

87 Ridley DS, Marsden PD, Cuba CC, Barreto AC. A histological classification of mucocutaneous leishmaniasis in Brazil and its clinical evaluation. Trans R Soc Trop Med Hyg 1980; 74: 508–514.

88 Girgla HS, Marsden RA, Singh GM, Ryan TJ. Post-kala-azar dermal leishmaniasis. Br J Dermatol 1977; 97: 307–311.

89 Zijlstra EE, Khalil EAG, Kager PA, El-Hassan AM. Post-kala-azar dermal leishmaniasis in the Sudan: clinical presentation and differential diagnosis. Br J Dermatol 2000; 143: 136–143.

90 Ramesh V, Mukherjee A. Post-kala-azar dermal leishmaniasis. Int J Dermatol 1995; 34: 85–91.

91 Singh N, Ramesh V, Arora VK et al. Nodular post-kala-azar dermal leishmaniasis: a distinct histopathological entity. J Cutan Pathol 1998; 25: 95–99.

92 Mukherjee A, Ramesh V, Misra RS. Post-kala-azar dermal leishmaniasis: a light and electron microscopic study of 18 cases. J Cutan Pathol 1993; 20: 320–325.

93 Ramesh V, Misra RS, Saxena U, Mukherjee A. Post-kala-azar dermal leishmaniasis: a clinical and therapeutic study. Int J Dermatol 1993; 32: 272–275.

94 Perrin C, Taillan B, Hofman P et al. Atypical cutaneous histological features of visceral leishmaniasis in acquired immunodeficiency syndrome. Am J Dermatopathol 1995; 17: 145–150.

95 Ara M, Maillo C, Peón G et al. Visceral leishmaniasis with cutaneous lesions in a patient infected with human immunodeficiency virus. Br J Dermatol 1998; 139: 114–117.

96 Colebunders R, Depraetere K, Verstraetan T et al. Unusual cutaneous lesions in two patients with visceral leishmaniasis and HIV infection. J Am Acad Dermatol 1999; 41: 847–850.

97 Abajo P, Buezo GF, Fraga J et al. Leishmaniasis and Kaposi's sarcoma in an HIV-infected patient. Am J Dermatopathol 1997; 19: 101–102.

98 Hofman V, Marty P, Perrin C et al. The histological spectrum of visceral leishmaniasis caused by *Leishmania infantum* MON-1 in acquired immune deficiency syndrome. Hum Pathol 2000; 31: 75–84.

99 González-Beato MJ, Moyano B, Sánchez C et al. Kaposi's sarcoma-like lesions and other nodules as cutaneous involvement in AIDS-related visceral leishmaniasis. Br J Dermatol 2000; 143: 1316–1318.

100 del Giudice P. *Leishmania* infection occurring in herpes zoster lesions in an HIV positive patient. Br J Dermatol 1996; 135: 1005–1006.

101 Castellano VM, Rodriquez-Peralto JL, Alonso S et al. Dermatofibroma parasitized by Leishmania in HIV infection: a new morphologic expression of dermal Kala Azar in an immunodepressed patient. J Cutan Pathol 1999; 26: 516–519.

102 Daudén E, Peñas PF, Rios L et al. Leishmaniasis presenting as a dermatomyositis-like eruption in AIDS. J Am Acad Dermatol 1996; 35: 316–319.

103 Yesudian P, Thambiah AS. Amphotericin B therapy in dermal leishmaniasis. Arch Dermatol 1974; 109: 720–722.

104 Elhassan AM, Ali MS, Zijlstra E et al. Post-kala-azar dermal leishmaniasis in the Sudan: peripheral neural involvement. Int J Dermatol 1992; 31: 400–403.

105 Pavithran K. Trichomonal abscess of the median raphe of the penis. Int J Dermatol 1993; 32: 820–821.

106 Sánchez-Carpintero I, Vázquez-Doval FJ. Cutaneous lesions in giardiasis. Report of two cases. Br J Dermatol 1998; 139: 152–153.

Coccidia

107 Justus J. Cutaneous manifestations of toxoplasmosis. Curr Probl Dermatol 1971; 4: 24–47.

108 Mawhorter SD, Effron D, Blinkhorn R, Spagnuolo PJ. Cutaneous manifestations of toxoplasmosis. Clin Infect Dis 1992; 14: 1084–1088.

109 Leyva WH, Santa Cruz DJ. Cutaneous toxoplasmosis. J Am Acad Dermatol 1986; 14: 600–605.

110 Andreev VC, Angelov N, Zlatkov NB. Skin manifestations in toxoplasmosis. Arch Dermatol 1969; 100: 196–199.

111 Menter MA, Morrison JGL. Lichen verrucosus et reticularis of Kaposi (porokeratosis striata of Nekam): a manifestation of acquired adult toxoplasmosis. Br J Dermatol 1976; 94: 645–654.

112 Binazzi M, Papini M. Cutaneous toxoplasmosis. Int J Dermatol 1980; 19: 332–335.

113 Tobi GC, D'Alessandro L, Catricala C, Zardi O. Dermatomyositis-like syndrome due to toxoplasma. Br J Dermatol 1979; 101: 589–591.

114 Pollock JL. Toxoplasmosis appearing to be dermatomyositis. Arch Dermatol 1979; 115: 736–737.

115 Fernandez DF, Wolff AH, Bagley MP. Acute cutaneous toxoplasmosis presenting as erythroderma. Int J Dermatol 1994; 33: 129–130.

116 Delaporte E, Alfandari S, Piette F, Fortier B. Cutaneous manifestations of toxoplasmosis. Int J Dermatol 1995; 34: 443.

117 Binazzi M. Profile of cutaneous toxoplasmosis. Int J Dermatol 1986; 25: 357–363.

Miscellaneous

118 Coulman CU, Greene I, Archibald RWR. Cutaneous pneumocystosis. Ann Intern Med 1987; 106: 396–398.

119 Sandler B, Potter TS, Hashimoto K. Cutaneous *Pneumocystis carinii* and *Cryptococcus neoformans* in AIDS. Br J Dermatol 1996; 134: 159–163.

Marine injuries

INTRODUCTION

Cutaneous injuries from various forms of marine life are uncommon recreational and occupational hazards. In most instances a localized urticarial and inflammatory lesion results at the point of injury, but this may be accompanied by a laceration if a sharp dorsal spine is involved. Severe systemic reactions and even fatality may result from the toxins of some marine organisms.

There have been several reviews of the cutaneous manifestations of marine animal injuries,[1–4] including Fisher's *Atlas of Aquatic Dermatology*.[5] Although of great dermatological and medical interest, these cutaneous lesions are of little dermatopathological importance. Biopsies are rarely taken, and, if they are, the findings, with several exceptions, are not diagnostically or etiologically specific.

In the brief account that follows, various categories of marine organisms will be considered.

CNIDARIANS

Although the phylum Cnidaria, formerly Coelenterata, has over 9 000 species, fewer than 80 are of clinical significance.[2–5] The toxic effects of cnidarians (coelenterates) result from contact with the nematocyst, a coiled thread-like tube, found particularly on the tentacles, which pierces the skin on contact. The toxin contained in the nematocysts of some species is capable of producing such diverse reactions as erythema, urticaria, a burning sensation or, rarely, fatal anaphylaxis and cardiorespiratory arrest.[6] The cnidarians of dermatological or medical importance include the Portuguese man-of-war[7] (*Physalia physalis*) in the class Hydrozoa, the box jellyfish[8] (*Chironex fleckeri*) in the order Scyphozoa, and the corals in the order Anthozoa.

More than 70 deaths have resulted from the sting of the box jellyfish.[8] In the areas of contact with the tentacles, linear erythematous and urticarial lesions are produced. These may persist for several days or longer, and be followed by postinflammatory pigmentation or keloid formation.[9]

Attention has also been given to the development of delayed and recurrent eruptions, not necessarily at the previous site of contact, which may follow solitary episodes of envenomation by different species of cnidarians.[9–13] An immunological mechanism has been postulated for these delayed or recurrent reactions.[12,14]

In the case of corals the nematocysts are relatively innocuous, but some coral cuts are slow to heal. Localized persistent inflammatory reactions have been reported at the site of contact with coral.[15]

Seabather's eruption is a highly pruritic maculopapular eruption, under swimwear, that occurs after bathing in the ocean.[16] It appears to result from the nematocyst of a cnidarian larva;[16] *Edwardsiella lineata* and *Linuche unguiculata* have been implicated.[17–19] It should be distinguished from 'swimmer's itch', which occurs primarily in fresh water and is caused by schistosomal cercariae (see p. 732).[20] Paresthesias and pruritus, particularly in the axillae, groins and genital region, can result from contact with *Liriope tetraphylla* medusa, from the class Hydrozoa. It forms a bloom in the shallow waters of the South American Atlantic coast.[21]

Histopathology

A biopsy from the site of contact with the tentacles of jellyfish (Fig. 28.1) will show nematocyst capsules in the swollen stratum corneum.[22] There is some thinning of the malpighian layer, with focal pyknosis of nuclei. With reduced

light, fine refractile threads, sometimes continuous with the nematocysts, can be seen penetrating for variable distances into the dermis (Fig. 28.2).[22–24] The threads are further highlighted with a reticulin stain.

In some of the recurrent eruptions produced by cnidarians a heavy dermal lymphocytic infiltrate may be present.[11,12] Spongiosis of the overlying epidermis is sometimes present.[25] Rare reactions include granulomas, papular urticaria, local necrosis[26] and subcutaneous atrophy.[10] Rarely, corals can produce an inflammatory reaction which on biopsy shows the pattern of a persistent arthropod reaction or papular urticaria.[15]

In seabather's eruption there is a superficial and deep perivascular and interstitial infiltrate of lymphocytes, neutrophils and eosinophils.

MOLLUSCS

The phylum Mollusca includes such well-known delicacies as scallops and oysters, as well as slugs, squid, cone shells and several types of octopus.[5] Cone shell snails of the genus *Conus* produce a painful puncture wound if handled carelessly, followed by systemic toxic symptoms which are sometimes fatal.

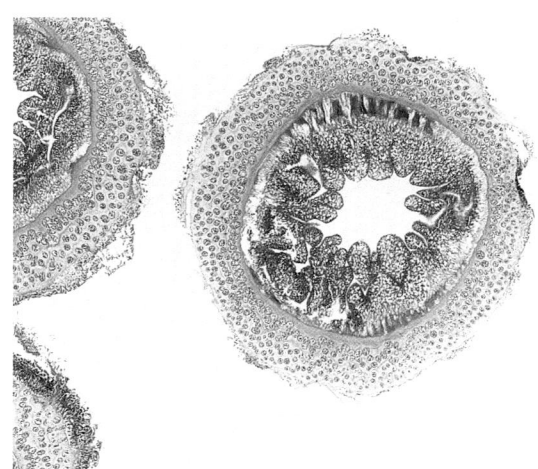

Fig. 28.1 **A box jellyfish tentacle in cross-section.** (H & E)

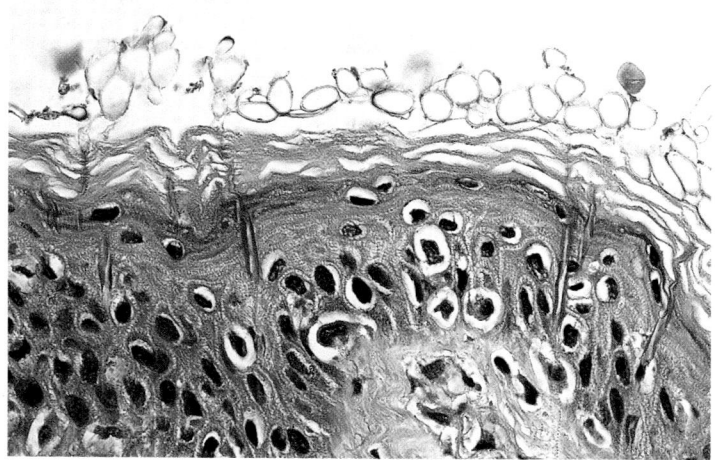

Fig. 28.2 **The site of a box jellyfish sting.** Nematocysts are present above the stratum corneum. Several fine thread-like tubules penetrate the epidermis. (H & E) (Photograph kindly provided by Dr G Strutton)

Another highly venomous mollusc is the blue-ringed octopus (*Hapalochlaena maculosa*), which can produce neuromuscular paralysis leading to respiratory failure.[27] The puncture wounds on the skin will have surrounding erythema and edema.[5] An urticarial reaction has also been recorded.[28]

ECHINODERMS

There are approximately 80 venomous species among the 6 000 that comprise the phylum Echinodermata.[5] This phylum includes sea urchins, starfish and sea cucumbers, all of which possess an array of sharp or toxic spines.

Sea urchins are widely distributed in several tropical and subtropical oceans. Their brittle spines break off in the skin, where they may produce several different lesions. A neurotoxin is present in the spines of some species. There is an immediate reaction with burning pain, followed by edema and erythema. Small nodules may develop several months after the injury. The resulting dermal reaction has been reported as sarcoidal granulomas,[29] although the illustrations suggest non-caseating tuberculoid granulomas.[29,30] A recent study found granulomas of sarcoidal, tuberculoid, suppurative, necrobiotic and foreign-body types in 39 biopsies with granulomas.[31] A foreign-body granulomatous reaction, probably to the debris of a spine, has been observed.[32] Implantation cysts may also form.[29]

A contact dermatitis can result from contact with certain starfish and sea cucumbers.[4]

SPONGES

Several species of sponge can produce a contact dermatitis, and the spicules from some may produce a foreign-body reaction if implanted in the skin.[5] A severe vesicular dermatitis can occur in some people who come in contact with the 'fire sponge', *Tedania ignis*.[33] It has been suggested that the reaction may be a primary irritant one, and not a contact allergic reaction.[33] An erythema multiforme-like reaction has also been reported which developed 10 days after the contact.[33]

SEAWEED

The marine alga *Lyngba* can produce an acute dermatitis characterized by intraepidermal vesiculation.[34] An allergic contact dermatitis can be produced by a completely different species, *Alcyonidium hirsutum*, which produces a seaweed-like animal colony known as the sea chervil or Dogger bank moss.[5,35] These sea 'mosses' are found on the Dogger bank and give rise to a pruritic vesiculobullous dermatitis ('Dogger bank itch') in fishermen who come into contact with them.[5]

VENOMOUS FISH

Contact with the venomous spines of several marine vertebrates can produce severe systemic reactions that may be fatal. Excruciating pain is usual at the site of the injury. This group includes the stingray, stonefish, weever fish and catfish.[36] The stonefish possesses a potent neurotoxin and is the most dangerous in this group.[5,37] Both the stonefish and stingray can produce local tissue necrosis, sometimes extensive, in the region of the injury.[38–40] TIA+

lymphocytes are found in the infiltrate adjacent to the zone of necrosis; these cells may contribute to the delayed healing that is frequently encountered.[41]

Scales from certain species may produce an irritant dermatitis in workers cleaning fish.[42] The lesions are 0.5–1 cm in diameter, raised and non-scaling.

An erythematous eruption, accompanied by systemic symptoms, may follow the eating of spoiled fish of the families *Scomberesocidae* and *Scombridae* (tuna, mackerel, skipjack and bonito). Bacterial proliferation allows the conversion of histidine in the fish into histamine, which is thought to be responsible for the symptoms.[43]

REFERENCES

Introduction
1 Cleland JB, Southcott RV. Injuries to man from marine invertebrates in the Australian region. Special Report Series No.12. Canberra: National Health and Medical Research Council, 1965.
2 Manowitz NR, Rosenthal RR. Cutaneous–systemic reactions to toxins and venoms of common marine organisms. Cutis 1979; 23: 450–454.
3 Mitchell JC. Biochemical basis of geographic ecology: Part 1. Int J Dermatol 1975; 14: 239–250.
4 Rosco MD. Cutaneous manifestations of marine animal injuries including diagnosis and treatment. Cutis 1977; 19: 507–510.
5 Fisher AA. Atlas of aquatic dermatology. New York: Grune & Stratton, 1978.

Cnidarians
6 Tong DW. Skin hazards of the marine aquarium industry. Int J Dermatol 1996; 35: 153–158.
7 Ioannides G, Davis JH. Portuguese man-of-war stinging. Arch Dermatol 1965; 91: 448–451.
8 Williamson JA, Le Ray LE, Wohlfahrt M, Fenner PJ. Acute management of serious envenomation by box-jellyfish (*Chironex fleckeri*). Med J Aust 1984; 141: 851–853.
9 Mansson T, Randle HW, Mandojana RM et al. Recurrent cutaneous jellyfish eruptions without envenomation. Acta Derm Venereol 1985; 65: 72–75.
10 Burnett JW, Calton GJ, Burnett HW. Jellyfish envenomation syndromes. J Am Acad Dermatol 1986; 14: 100–106.
11 Reed KM, Bronstein BR, Baden HP. Delayed and persistent cutaneous reactions to coelenterates. J Am Acad Dermatol 1984; 10: 462–466.
12 Burnett JW, Hepper KP, Aurelian L et al. Recurrent eruptions following unusual solitary coelenterate envenomations. J Am Acad Dermatol 1987; 17: 86–92.
13 Veraldi S, Carrera C. Delayed cutaneous reaction to jellyfish. Int J Dermatol 2000; 39: 28–29.
14 Kokelj F, Stinco G, Avian M et al. Cell-mediated sensitization to jellyfish antigens confirmed by positive patch test to *Olindias sambaquiensis* preparations. J Am Acad Dermatol 1995; 33: 307–309.
15 Weedon D, Hart V, Beardmore G, Dickson P. Coral dermatitis. Australas J Dermatol 1981; 22: 104–105.
16 Wong DE, Meinking TL, Rosen LB et al. Seabather's eruption. Clinical, histologic, and immunologic features. J Am Acad Dermatol 1994; 30: 399–406.
17 Basler RSW, Basler GC, Palmer AH, Garcia MA. Special skin symptoms seen in swimmers. J Am Acad Dermatol 2000; 43: 299–305.
18 Segura Puertas L, Burnett JW, Heimer de la Cotera E. The medusa stage of the coronate scyphomedusa *Linuche unguiculata* ('thimble jellyfish') can cause seabather's eruption. Dermatology 1999; 198: 171–172.
19 Segura-Puertas L, Ramos ME, Aramburo C et al. One *Linuche* mystery solved: All 3 stages of the coronate scyphomedusa *Linuche unguiculata* cause seabather's eruption. J Am Acad Dermatol 2001; 44: 624–628.
20 Bastert J, Sing A, Wollenberg A, Korting HC. Aquarium dermatitis: cercarial dermatitis in an aquarist. Dermatology 1998; 197: 84–86.
21 Mianzan H, Sorarrain D, Burnett JW, Lutz LL. Mucocutaneous junctional and flexural paresthesias caused by the holoplanktonic trachymedusa *Liriope tetraphylla*. Dermatology 2000; 201: 46–48.
22 Kingston CW, Southcott RV. Skin histopathology in fatal jellyfish stinging. Trans R Soc Trop Med Hyg 1960; 54: 373–384.
23 Yaffee HS. A delayed cutaneous reaction following contact with jellyfish. Derm Int 1968; 7: 75–77.
24 Strutton G, Lumley J. Cutaneous light microscopic and ultrastructural changes in a fatal case of jellyfish envenomation. J Cutan Pathol 1988; 15: 249–255.
25 Piérard GE, Letot B, Piérard-Franchimont C. Histologic study of delayed reactions to coelenterates. J Am Acad Dermatol 1990; 22: 599–601.

26 Drury JK, Noonan JD, Pollock JG, Reid WH. Jelly fish sting with serious hand complications. Injury 1980; 12: 66–68.

Molluscs

27 Sutherland SK, Lane WR. Toxins and mode of envenomation of the common ringed or blue-banded octopus. Med J Aust 1969; 1: 893–898.
28 Edmonds C. A non-fatal case of blue-ringed octopus bite. Med J Aust 1969; 2: 601.

Echinoderms

29 Kinmont PDC. Sea-urchin sarcoidal granuloma. Br J Dermatol 1965; 77: 335–343.
30 Rocha G, Fraga S. Sea urchin granuloma of the skin. Arch Dermatol 1962; 85: 406–408.
31 De la Torre C, Toribio J. Sea-urchin granuloma: histologic profile. A pathologic study of 50 biopsies. J Cutan Pathol 2001; 28: 223–228.
32 Strauss MB, MacDonald RI. Hand injuries from sea urchin spines. Clin Orthop 1976; 114: 216–218.

Sponges

33 Yaffee HS, Stargardter F. Erythema multiforme from *Tedania ignis*. Arch Dermatol 1963; 87: 601–604.

Seaweed

34 Grauer FH, Arnold HL Jr. Seaweed dermatitis. Arch Dermatol 1961; 84: 720–730.
35 Seville RH. Dogger Bank itch. Br J Dermatol 1957; 69: 92–93.

Venomous fish

36 Carducci M, Mussi A, Leone G, Catricalà C. Raynaud's phenomenon secondary to weever fish stings. Arch Dermatol 1996; 132: 838–839.
37 Wiener S. A case of stone-fish sting treated with antivenene. Med J Aust 1965; 1: 191.
38 Russell FE. Stingray injuries: a review and discussion of their treatment. Am J Med Sci 1953; 226: 611–622.
39 Russell FE, Panos TC, Kang LW et al. Studies on the mechanism of death from stingray venoms. A report of two fatal cases. Am J Med Sci 1958; 235: 566–583.
40 Barss P. Wound necrosis caused by the venom of stingrays. Pathological findings and surgical management. Med J Aust 1984; 141: 854–855.
41 Germain M, Smith KJ, Skelton H. The cutaneous cellular infiltrate to stingray envenomization contains increased TIA+ cells. Br J Dermatol 2000; 143: 1074–1077.
42 Chiou FY, Tschen JA. Fish scale-induced dermatitis. J Am Acad Dermatol 1993; 29: 962–965.
43 Sabroe RA, Kobza Black A. Scombrotoxic fish poisoning. Clin Exp Dermatol 1998; 23: 258–259.

Helminth infestations

INTRODUCTION

Helminthic parasites are responsible for a number of important diseases of tropical countries. These include schistosomiasis, caused by the trematode flukes; cysticercosis and sparganosis, resulting from the larvae of certain tapeworms (cestodes); and onchocerciasis, dirofilariasis and larva migrans occurring as a consequence of nematode infestations.[1]

TREMATODE INFESTATIONS

SCHISTOSOMIASIS

It has been estimated that 200 million people are infested with one or other of the three major species of schistosome fluke.[2] *Schistosoma haematobium* (found in most of Africa and in the near East) has a predilection for the bladder, *S. japonicum* (common in parts of the orient) for the gut, and *S. mansoni* (found in Africa and parts of the Caribbean region and the northeast part of South America) for the portal circulation.[3] Four types of skin lesions have been described:[4–13]

1. a pruritic, erythematous and urticarial papular rash (cercarial dermatitis, 'swimmer's itch') associated with the penetration of the cercariae through the skin en route to the various venous plexuses to mature
2. urticarial lesions associated with the dissemination of the cercariae or the laying of eggs by the adult flukes
3. papular, granulomatous and even warty vegetating lesions of the genital and perineal skin secondary to the deposition of ova in dermal vessels[11,14]
4. extragenital cutaneous lesions secondary to lodgement of ova and, rarely, worms.[12,15]

Urticarial lesions are more common with *S. japonicum*,[6] and perineal lesions with *S. haematobium*,[7,16] whereas extragenital cutaneous manifestations are usually a complication of *S. japonicum* and *S. haematobium*, but are quite rare with *S. mansoni*.[17] The term 'bilharziasis' is used for the ectopic deposition of ova within the dermis. The late development of squamous cell carcinoma has been reported in the verrucous genital lesions.[8]

Cercarial dermatitis may also be seen, rarely, as a result of penetration of the skin by cercariae of species of schistosome that are unable to develop further in humans, being destroyed before they reach the venous plexus.[8,18]

Histopathology

The cercarial dermatitis shows intraepidermal spongiosis with exocytosis of eosinophils and neutrophils, sometimes forming microabscesses.[6] Cercariae are not usually seen. The dermal reaction is mild, with edema, vascular dilatation and a mild perivascular inflammatory cell infiltrate and some interstitial eosinophils.

Genital and perineal lesions show hyperkeratosis and acanthosis. There may be prominent pseudoepitheliomatous hyperplasia, and at times focal ulceration or draining sinuses with accompanying acute inflammation.[5,11] The dermis contains numerous ova, some associated with a granulomatous reaction, including foreign-body giant cells. Other eggs are in microabscesses, often containing numerous eosinophils. Flukes may be seen in cutaneous vessels.

Extragenital lesions show numerous ova in the superficial dermis associated with necrobiosis and palisading granulomas.[9,10,13] Eosinophils, neutrophils and foreign-body giant cells are found in most lesions, whereas in later lesions

there may be degenerating or calcified ova, plasma cells and fibroblasts, with variable fibrosis (Fig. 29.1). Identification of ova in late fibrous lesions may be difficult.[17]

The ova of the three major species have characteristic features. The ova of *S. haematobium* have an apical spine, those of *S. mansoni* a lateral spine, and those of *S. japonicum* have no spine.[6] The ova of *S. mansoni* and *S. japonicum* may be acid fast.

OTHER TREMATODES

A larval trematode, identified as a mesocercaria of an undescribed species belonging to the subfamily Alariinae, has been removed from an intradermal swelling.[19] The lung fluke *Paragonimus westermani* can also produce a cutaneous inflammatory lesion, which includes eosinophils and plasma cells.[20]

CESTODE INFESTATIONS

CYSTICERCOSIS

The larval phase of *Taenia solium*, the pork tapeworm, may infect man as an accidental intermediate host, with the formation of one or more asymptomatic subcutaneous nodules 1–3 cm in diameter.[21–28] The larvae have a predilection for the chest wall, upper arms and thighs.[29] The nodules are composed of a white cystic structure with an outer membrane containing clear fluid and a cysticercus larva attached to one edge. Surrounding the gelatinous cyst is a host response of fibrous tissue.

Histopathology

The diagnosis is made by the characteristic appearance of the scolex of the cysticercus larva (Fig. 29.2). The fibrous tissue reaction in the subcutaneous tissue contains a moderate chronic inflammatory cell infiltrate which includes variable numbers of eosinophils. A few scattered giant cells are sometimes present.

SPARGANOSIS

Sparganosis is a rare infestation caused by the larval form of a tapeworm of the genus Spirometra.[30,31] It occurs in many parts of the world, mainly in the

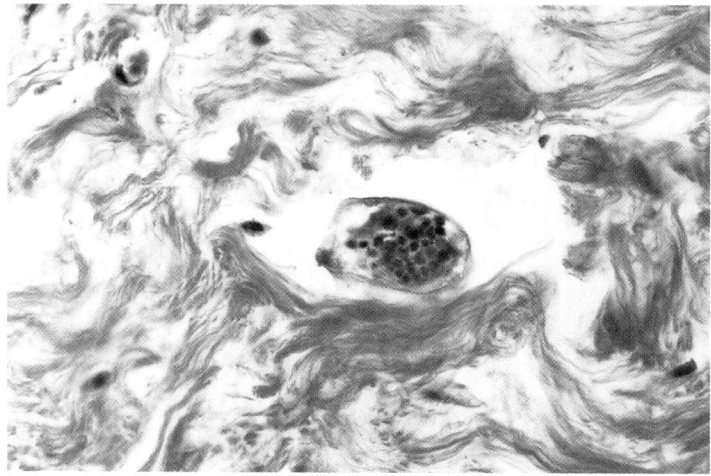

Fig. 29.1 **An ovum of *Schistosoma*** in an area of fibrosis. No reaction is present. (H & E)

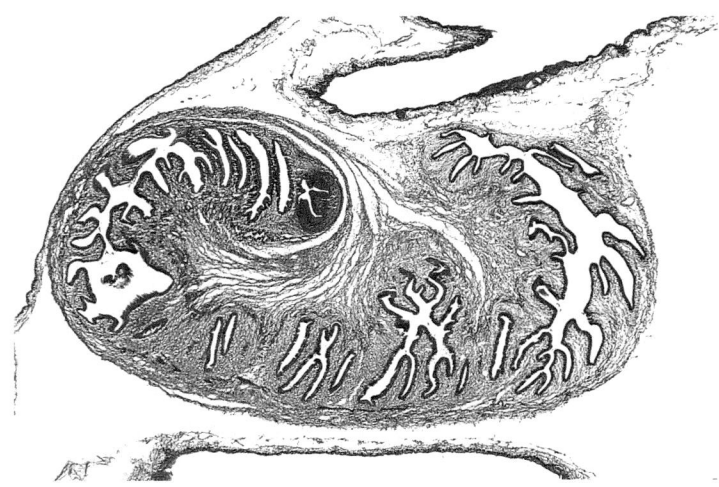

Fig. 29.2 **Cysticercus larva** removed from a subcutaneous 'cyst' of the skin.

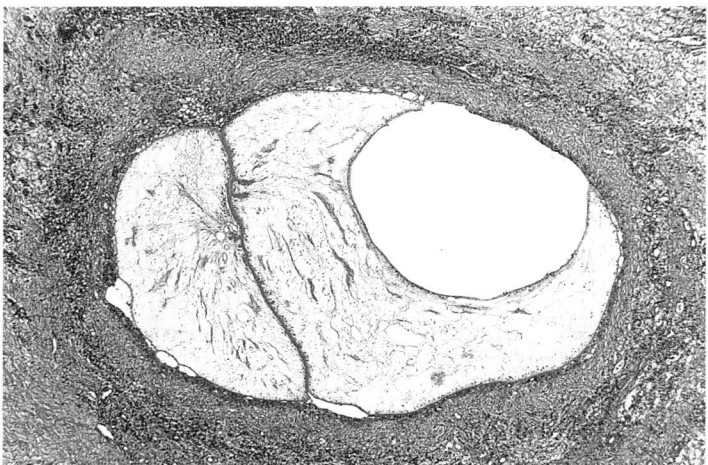

Fig. 29.3 **Sparganosis.** Portions of worm are present in a subcutaneous cavity. There is an inflammatory reaction in the surrounding tissue and some fibrosis. (H & E) (Photograph kindly supplied by Professor Robin Cooke)

tropics. Humans are a second intermediate host. Infestation may result in a subcutaneous nodule which slowly migrates. Bisection of the nodule after excision will reveal a white thread-like worm about 1 mm in width and from a few centimeters to 50 cm in length.[32]

Histopathology

There is a subcutaneous, partly granulomatous, inflammatory mass composed of lymphocytes, plasma cells, neutrophils and variable numbers of eosinophils.[33] Portions of worm are usually seen within the mass,[30] or there may be a cavity where the larva has been (Fig. 29.3). The larva has a flattened structure with both longitudinal and horizontal muscle bundles, giving a 'checkerboard' appearance. A longitudinal excretory canal is also present, and basophilic calcareous corpuscles, a characteristic feature of cestodes, may also be seen scattered in varying numbers throughout the matrix.[31]

ECHINOCOCCOSIS

Cutaneous lesions have been reported on the abdomen in two patients with alveolar echinococcosis, an uncommon parasitic disease of the liver caused by the larvae of *Echinococcus multilocularis*.[34] This cestode is closely related to *E. granulosus*, which causes hydatid disease of the liver and other sites.

Histopathology

The lesions were characterized by a dense granulomatous infiltrate within the dermis, surrounding larval elements.[34]

NEMATODE INFESTATIONS

ONCHOCERCIASIS

Onchocerciasis, which is common in tropical Africa, the Yemen, and Central and South America, is caused by the nematode *Onchocerca volvulus*.[35–38] The larvae are transmitted by several species of flies of the genus *Simulium*. Onchocerciasis mainly affects people living close to fast-flowing rivers, where the flies breed.[38] The larvae mature into adult worms in the subcutaneous tissue, where they form non-tender subcutaneous nodules 2.5–10 cm in diameter. The nodules, which may occur anywhere on the body, are either

isolated or grouped in large conglomerations. They may contain one or several tightly coiled worms, which may live for many years.

The adult worms produce microfilariae, which are found in the neighboring lymphatics. The microfilariae may migrate to the dermis and eye. Visual impairment and blindness (river blindness) is an important complication of onchocerciasis.[39] Onchocercal dermatitis, which results from infiltration of the skin by these microfilariae, is a pruritic papular rash with altered pigmentation.[36] The dermatitis is typically generalized, but an eruption localized to one limb, usually a leg, is found in the northern Sudan and also in the Yemen, where it is known as sowda.[40] Pruritic urticarial plaques may also form.[41]

Histopathology[42–44]

The subcutaneous nodules have an outer wall of dense fibrous tissue which usually extends between the worms (Fig. 29.4). Centrally, there is granulation tissue and a mixed inflammatory cell infiltrate in early lesions, although in long-standing lesions in which the worms are dead there is only dense fibrous tissue, with some calcification and foreign-body giant cells and a chronic inflammatory cell infiltrate. Eosinophils are usually present at all stages. Microfilariae may be seen in lymphatics in this region.

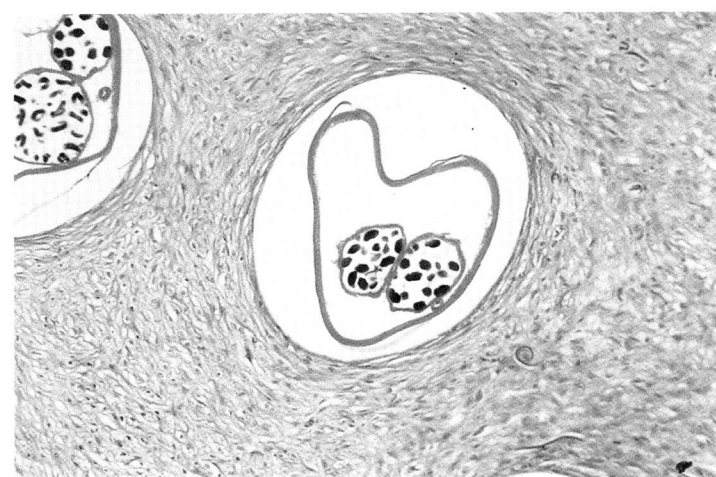

Fig. 29.4 **Onchocerciasis.** Several fine coiled microfilariae are present in the fibrous tissue that surrounds the worm. (H&E)

In onchocercal dermatitis there is a light superficial and deep infiltrate of chronic inflammatory cells and eosinophils in the dermis. Microfilariae may be seen in slits between collagen bundles in the upper dermis.[43,45] Eosinophils and eosinophil major basic protein are usually present around degenerating microfilariae.[40,42] There is progressive fibrosis of the dermis. The epidermis shows acanthosis and hyperkeratosis.

DIROFILARIASIS

Human infection with *Dirofilaria* spp. is uncommon except in endemic areas, notably the Mediterranean region.[46–51] The usual species found in this region is *Dirofilaria repens*, which may cause subcutaneous nodules.[52] In the case of *Dirofilaria immitis* (the dog heartworm) pulmonary lesions, which are usually asymptomatic, can also occur.[53] Skin lesions are usually solitary, erythematous and tender subcutaneous nodules. Sometimes there is a sensation of 'movement' under the skin.[54]

Histopathology

The center of the nodule contains a degenerating filaria with a thick laminated cuticle, distinct longitudinal ridges and large lateral chords, as well as typical musculature.[55] There is an intense surrounding inflammatory reaction of lymphocytes, plasma cells, histiocytes, eosinophils and sometimes giant cells. There is usually central suppuration, and neutrophils may extend out into the adjacent inflammatory zone.[55] The diagnostic histological features of various zoonotic filariae in tissue sections have been reviewed by Gutierrez.[48]

LARVA MIGRANS

Cutaneous larva migrans is caused by the intracutaneous wanderings of hookworm and certain other nematode larvae.[56–59] The creeping eruption caused by fly larvae is usually considered separately. In larva migrans there are pruritic papules that form serpiginous tunnels, which are at first erythematous but soon become elevated and vesicular. Bullae may rarely form.[60] The lesion may extend several millimeters per day. Older parts of the track may become crusted. Epiluminescence microscopy has been used, with mixed success, in the attempted clinical diagnosis of this condition.[61]

Larva migrans is most commonly caused by larvae of *Ancylostoma braziliense*, a hookworm of dogs and cats, but *Necator americanus* may give a creeping eruption of shorter duration.[1] Other hookworms that may produce cutaneous larva migrans include *Ancylostoma caninum*, *Uncinaria stenocephala* and *Bunostomum phlebotomum*.

A deep subcutaneous form of larva migrans may be seen with *Gnathostoma spinigerum*.[62–64] Infection with *Toxocara* sp. may cause visceral and ocular larva migrans, but not the cutaneous form. Urticaria and prurigo are cutaneous manifestations associated with toxocariasis.[65]

The larvae of *Strongyloides stercoralis* usually provoke little reaction as they migrate through the skin to reach vessels for their passage to the lung. In some individuals with strongyloidiasis, a variant of larva migrans is found with a rapidly progressing linear urticarial lesion, which may extend at up to 10 cm per hour.[66,67] The term larva currens (racing larva) has been used for these cases.[67–70] There is still a high incidence of *Strongyloides stercoralis* infestation in former prisoners of war interned many years ago in southeast Asia.[71–73] In one series, almost one-third had suffered episodes of larva currens.[74] Another cutaneous manifestation of strongyloidiasis is the presence of widespread petechiae and purpura. These features are seen in immunosuppressed patients with disseminated infections.[67,75–79] Prurigo nodularis and lichen simplex chronicus are further manifestations of infection with this parasite.[80,81]

Recently, a creeping eruption caused by larvae of the suborder *Spirurina* has been reported from Japan.[82,83] The eating of raw squid has been implicated in these patients.

Histopathology

In larva migrans there are small cavities in the epidermis corresponding to the track of the larva, although the parasite itself is uncommonly seen in section. There may be a diffuse spongiotic dermatitis, with intraepidermal vesicles containing some eosinophils.[84] There is usually no inflammatory reaction around the larva (when it can be found), whereas there is a mixed inflammatory reaction behind the migrating larva with a superficial dermal infiltrate of neutrophils, lymphocytes, plasma cells and usually abundant eosinophils.[84] An eosinophilic folliculitis has been recorded.[85,86]

Reports of larva currens have mentioned a perivascular round-cell infiltrate with interstitial eosinophils, a picture common to many parasitic infestations.[87] In disseminated strongyloidiasis there are numerous larvae, 9–15 µm in diameter, in the dermal collagen and rarely in the lumina of small blood vessels.[67,75]

OTHER NEMATODES

Various other nematodes are sometimes of dermatopathological interest.[1] *Mansonella streptocerca* is found in West Africa. The adult worm lives in the dermis, and microfilariae may also be seen. It usually presents with hypopigmented macules and itching. The adult worms of *Loa loa*, which is endemic in the rain forests of West and Central Africa, live in the subcutaneous tissue and migrate, producing fugitive swellings and temporary inflammation.[88] The elevated outline of the subcutaneous worms may be visible on the skin surface.[89] There is high eosinophilia. Liberation of the microfilariae may produce urticarial lesions. *Wuchereria bancrofti* (Fig. 29.5) and *Brugia malayi* produce lymphangitis and lymphadenopathy, with the later development of elephantiasis.[90] Further discussion is beyond the scope of this chapter.

Dracunculus medinensis may produce a blistering lesion due to the migration of the worm, which will eventually be extruded through rupture of the bleb. The female worm measures 70–120 cm in length and is coiled through the subcutaneous tissues. The anterior end is surrounded by granulation tissue containing a mixed inflammatory infiltrate, and there is fibrosis and some inflammation in the deeper parts.

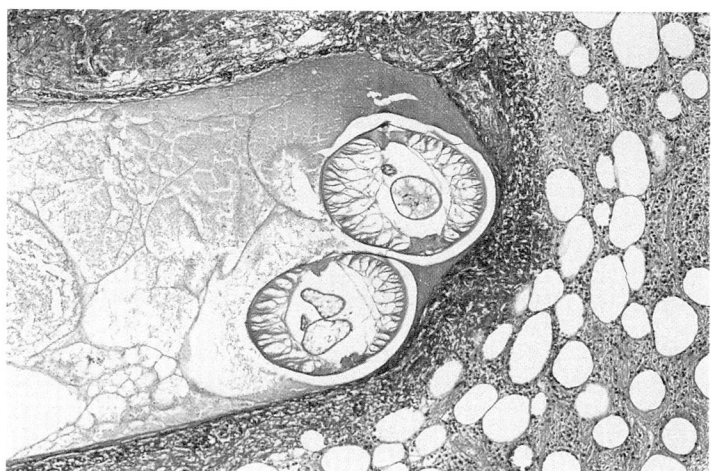

Fig. 29.5 **Sections of the nematode *Wuchereria bancrofti*** are present in a cavity in the subcutaneous fat. There are numerous eosinophils in the adjacent fat. (H & E)

Trichinella spiralis may produce variable clinical lesions ranging from urticaria to maculopapular lesions following its development in striated muscle.[91] The changes are not diagnostic.

Gnathostoma spinigerum is endemic in southeast Asia and Japan. It is rare in other countries, including the Americas.[92] Other species of *Gnathostoma* are rarely implicated.[93–95] Human infestation results from eating uncooked infested meat from the second intermediate host, such as pigs, chickens, and fresh-water fish of the genus *Ophicephalus*.[64] It may produce migratory cutaneous swellings with localized erythema, or a true creeping eruption.[62,64,96,97] Excoriation of a pruritic patch may reveal the worm, which measures up to 3 cm in length.

There are rare reports of larvae of the soil nematode *Pelodera (Rhabditis) strongyloides* producing nodular lesions associated with a heavy mixed dermal inflammatory infiltrate and the presence of larvae in tissue sections.[98,99] There are five pathogenic species of *Lagochilascaris*, found in Central and South America. It produces abscesses and fistulas in the skin, particularly in the neck region.[100]

Larvae of *Dioctophyme renale*, the giant kidney worm, which occurs naturally in several fish-eating mammals throughout the world, have been recovered from the subcutaneous tissues of humans on several occasions.[101]

REFERENCES

Introduction

1 Beaver PC, Jung RC, Cupp EW. Clinical parasitology, 9th ed. Philadelphia: Lea & Febiger, 1984.

Trematode infestations

2 Mahmoud AA. Schistosomiasis. N Engl J Med 1977; 297: 1329–1331.

3 Scrimgeour EM, Daar AS. Schistosomiasis: clinical relevance to surgeons in Australasia and diagnostic update. Aust NZ J Surg 2000; 70: 157–161.

4 Obasi OE. Cutaneous schistosomiasis in Nigeria. An update. Br J Dermatol 1986; 114: 597–602.

5 Amer M. Cutaneous schistosomiasis. Int J Dermatol 1982; 21: 44–46.

6 Wood MG, Srolovitz H, Schetman D. Schistosomiasis. Paraplegia and ectopic skin lesions as admission symptoms. Arch Dermatol 1976; 112: 690–695.

7 Torres VM. Dermatologic manifestations of schistosomiasis mansoni. Arch Dermatol 1976; 112: 1539–1542.

8 Walther RR. Chronic papular dermatitis of the scrotum due to *Schistosoma mansoni*. Arch Dermatol 1979; 115: 869–870.

9 Jacyk WK, Lawande RV, Tulpule SS. Unusual presentation of extragenital cutaneous schistosomiasis mansoni. Br J Dermatol 1980; 103: 205–208.

10 Findlay GH, Whiting DA. Disseminated and zosteriform cutaneous schistosomiasis. Br J Dermatol (Suppl) 1971; 7: 98–101.

11 McKee PH, Wright E, Hutt MSR. Vulval schistosomiasis. Clin Exp Dermatol 1983; 8: 189–194.

12 Mulligan A, Burns DA. Ectopic cutaneous schistosomiasis and schistosomal ocular inflammatory disease. Br J Dermatol 1988; 119: 793–798.

13 Eulderink F, Gryseels B, van Kampen WJ, de Regt J. Haematobium schistosomiasis presenting in the Netherlands as a skin disease. Am J Dermatopathol 1994; 16: 434–438.

14 Davis-Reed L, Theis JH. Cutaneous schistosomiasis: Report of a case and review of the literature. J Am Acad Dermatol 2000; 42: 678–680.

15 Farrell AM, Woodrow D, Bryceson ADB et al. Ectopic cutaneous schistosomiasis: extragenital involvement with progressive upward spread. Br J Dermatol 1996; 135: 110–112.

16 Leman JA, Small G, Wilks D, Tidman MJ. Localized papular cutaneous schistosomiasis: two cases in travellers. Clin Exp Dermatol 2001; 26: 50–52.

17 Kick G, Schaller M, Korting HC. Late cutaneous schistosomiasis representing an isolated skin manifestation of *Schistosoma mansoni* infection. Dermatology 2000; 200: 144–146.

18 Kullavanijaya P, Wongwaisayawan H. Outbreak of cercarial dermatitis in Thailand. Int J Dermatol 1993; 32: 113–115.

19 Beaver PC, Little MD, Tucker CF, Reed RJ. Mesocercaria in the skin of man in Louisiana. Am J Trop Med Hyg 1977; 26: 422–426.

20 Brenes RR, Little MD, Raudales O et al. Cutaneous paragonimiasis in man in Honduras. Am J Trop Med Hyg 1983; 32: 376–378.

Cestode infestations

21 King DT, Gilbert DJ, Gurevitch AW et al. Subcutaneous cysticercosis. Arch Dermatol 1979; 115: 236.

22 Tschen EH, Tschen EA, Smith EB. Cutaneous cysticercosis treated with metrifonate. Arch Dermatol 1981; 117: 507–509.

23 Falanga V, Kapoor W. Cerebral cysticercosis: diagnostic value of subcutaneous nodules. J Am Acad Dermatol 1985; 12: 304–307.

24 Wortman PD. Subcutaneous cysticercosis. J Am Acad Dermatol 1991; 25: 409–414.

25 Schmidt DKT, Jordaan HF, Schneider JW, Cilliers J. Cerebral and subcutaneous cysticercosis treated with albendazole. Int J Dermatol 1995; 34: 574–579.

26 O'Grady TC, Robbins BA, Barrett TL, Higginbottom PA. Subcutaneous cysticercosis simulating metastatic breast carcinoma. Int J Dermatol 1993; 32: 62–64.

27 Amatya BM, Kimula Y. Cysticercosis in Nepal. A histopathologic study of sixty-two cases. Am J Surg Pathol 1999; 23: 1276–1279.

28 Miura H, Itoh Y, Kozuka T. A case of subcutaneous cysticercosis (*Cysticercus cellulosae* cutis). J Am Acad Dermatol 2000; 43: 538–540.

29 Raimer S, Wolf JE Jr. Subcutaneous cysticercosis. Arch Dermatol 1978; 114: 107–108.

30 Taylor RL. Sparganosis in the United States: report of a case. Am J Clin Pathol 1976; 66: 560–564.

31 Norman SH, Kreutner A Jr. Sparganosis: clinical and pathologic observations in ten cases. South Med J 1980; 73: 297–300.

32 Sarma DP, Weilbaecher TG. Human sparganosis. J Am Acad Dermatol 1986; 15: 1145–1148.

33 Griffin MP, Tompkins KJ, Ryan MT. Cutaneous sparganosis. Am J Dermatopathol 1996; 18: 70–72.

34 Bresson-Hadni S, Humbert P, Paintaud G et al. Skin localization of alveolar echinococcosis of the liver. J Am Acad Dermatol 1996; 34: 873–877.

Nematode infestations

35 Somorin AO. Onchocerciasis. Int J Dermatol 1983; 22: 182–188.

36 Hay RJ, Mackenzie CD, Guderian R et al. Onchodermatitis – correlation between skin disease and parasitic load in an endemic focus in Ecuador. Br J Dermatol 1989; 121: 187–198.

37 Yarzabal L. The immunology of onchocerciasis. Int J Dermatol 1985; 24: 349–358.

38 Murdoch ME, Hay RJ, MacKenzie CD et al. A clinical classification and grading system of the cutaneous changes in onchocerciasis. Br J Dermatol 1993; 129: 260–269.

39 Richards F, Hopkins D, Cupp E. Programmatic goals and approaches to onchocerciasis. Lancet 2000; 355: 1663–1664.

40 Connor DH, Gibson DW, Neafie RC et al. Sowda-onchocerciasis in North Yemen: a clinicopathologic study of 18 patients. Am J Trop Med Hyg 1983; 32: 123–137.

41 Weilepp A, O'Grady T. An unusual presentation of filariasis in a world traveler. J Cutan Pathol 1997; 24: 132.

42 Connor DH, George GH, Gibson DW. Pathologic changes of human onchocerciasis: implications for future research. Rev Inf Dis 1985; 7: 809–819.

43 Connor DH, Williams PH, Helwig EB, Winslow DJ. Dermal changes in onchocerciasis. Arch Pathol 1969; 87: 193–200.

44 Stingl P. Onchocerciasis: clinical presentation and host parasite interactions in patients of Southen Sudan. Int J Dermatol 1997; 36: 23–28.

45 Rozenman D, Kremer M, Zuckerman F. Onchocerciasis in Israel. Arch Dermatol 1984; 120: 505–507.

46 Payan HM. Human infection with *Dirofilaria*. Arch Dermatol 1978; 114: 593–594.

47 Santamaría B, Di Sacco B, Muro A et al. Serological diagnosis of subcutaneous dirofilariosis. Clin Exp Dermatol 1995; 20: 19–21.

48 Gutierrez Y. Diagnostic features of zoonotic filariae in tissue sections. Hum Pathol 1984; 15: 514–525.

49 Van den Ende J, Kumar V, Van Gompel A et al. Subcutaneous dirofilariasis caused by *Dirofilaria (Nochtiella) repens* in a Belgian patient. Int J Dermatol 1995; 34: 274–277.

50 Herzberg AJ, Boyd PR, Gutierrez Y. Subcutaneous dirofilariasis in Collier County, Florida, USA. Am J Surg Pathol 1995; 19: 934–939.

51 Jelinek T, Schulte-Hillen J, Löscher T. Human dirofilariasis. Int J Dermatol 1996; 35: 872–875.

52 Pampiglione S, Rivasi F, Angeli G et al. Dirofilariasis due to *Dirofilaria repens* in Italy, an emergent zoonosis: report of 60 new cases. Histopathology 2001; 38: 344–354.

53 Billups J, Schenken JR, Beaver PC. Subcutaneous dirofilariasis in Nebraska. Arch Pathol Lab Med 1980; 104: 11–13.

54 Shenefelt PD, Esperanza L, Lynn A. Elusive migratory subcutaneous dirofilariasis. J Am Acad Dermatol 1996; 35: 260–262.

55 Fisher BK, Homayouni M, Orihel TC. Subcutaneous infection with *Dirofilaria*. Arch Dermatol 1964; 89: 837–840.

56 Williams HC, Monk B. Creeping eruption stopped in its tracks by albendazole. Clin Exp Dermatol 1989; 14: 355–356.

57 Davies HD, Sakuls P, Keystone JS. Creeping eruption. A review of clinical presentation and management of 60 cases presenting to a tropical disease unit. Arch Dermatol 1993; 129: 588–591.

58 Albanese G, Di Cintio R, Beneggi M et al. Larva migrans in Italy. Int J Dermatol 1995; 34: 464–465.

59 Grassi A, Angelo C, Grosso MG, Paradisi M. Perianal cutaneous larva migrans in a child. Pediatr Dermatol 1998; 15: 367–369.

60 Wong-Waldamez A, Silva-Lizama E. Bullous larva migrans accompanied by Loeffler's syndrome. Int J Dermatol 1995; 34: 570–571.

61 Veraldi S, Schianchi R, Carrera C. Epiluminescence microscopy in cutaneous larva migrans. Acta Derm Venereol 2000; 80: 233.

62 Pinkus H, Fan J, De Giusti D. Creeping eruption due to *Gnathostoma spinigerum* in a Taiwanese patient. Int J Dermatol 1981; 20: 46–49.

63 Feinstein RJ, Rodriguez-Valdes J. Gnathostomiasis, or larva migrans profundus. J Am Acad Dermatol 1984; 11: 738–740.

64 Kagen CN, Vance JC, Simpson M. Gnathostomiasis. Infestation in an Asian immigrant. Arch Dermatol 1984; 120: 508–510.

65 Humbert P, Niezborala M, Salembier R et al. Skin manifestations associated with toxocariasis: a case-control study. Dermatology 2000; 201: 230–234.

66 Stone OJ, Newell GB, Mullins JF. Cutaneous strongyloidiasis: larva currens. Arch Dermatol 1972; 106: 734–736.

67 von Kuster LC, Genta RM. Cutaneous manifestations of strongyloidiasis. Arch Dermatol 1988; 124: 1826–1830.

68 Arthur RP, Shelley WB. Larva currens. Arch Dermatol 1958; 78: 186–190.

69 Amer M, Attia M, Ramadan AS, Matout K. Larva currens and systemic disease. Int J Dermatol 1984; 23: 402–403.

70 Iwamoto T, Kitoh M, Kayashima K, Ono T. Larva currens: the usefulness of the agar plate method. Dermatology 1998; 196: 343–345.

71 Gill GV, Bell DR. Longstanding tropical infections amongst former war prisoners of the Japanese. Lancet 1982; 1: 958–959.

72 Speight EL, Myers B, Davies JM. Strongyloidiasis, angio-oedema and natural killer cell lymphocytosis. Br J Dermatol 1999; 140: 1179–1180.

73 del Giudice P. Strongyloidiasis and natural killer cell lymphocytosis. Br J Dermatol 2000; 142: 1066.

74 Grove DI. Strongyloidiasis in allied ex-prisoners of war in south-east Asia. Br Med J 1980; 280: 598–601.

75 Ronan SG, Reddy RL, Manaligod JR et al. Disseminated strongyloidiasis presenting as purpura. J Am Acad Dermatol 1989; 21: 1123–1125.

76 Gordon SM, Gal AA, Solomon AR, Bryan JA. Disseminated strongyloidiasis with cutaneous manifestations in an immunocompromised host. J Am Acad Dermatol 1994; 31: 255–259.

77 Purvis RS, Beightler EL, Diven DG et al. *Strongyloides stercoralis* hyperinfection. Int J Dermatol 1992; 31: 160–164.

78 Purvis RS, Beightler EL, Diven DG et al. *Strongyloides* hyperinfection presenting with petechiae and purpura. Int J Dermatol 1992; 31: 169–171.

79 Kao D, Murakawa GJ, Kerschmann R, Berger T. Disseminated strongyloidiasis in a patient with acquired immunodeficiency syndrome. Arch Dermatol 1996; 132: 977–978.

80 Jacob CI, Patten SF. *Strongyloides stercoralis* infection presenting as generalized prurigo nodularis and lichen simplex chronicus. J Am Acad Dermatol 1999; 41: 357–361.

81 Albanese G, Venturi C, Galbiati G. Prurigo in a patient with intestinal strongyloidiasis. Int J Dermatol 2001; 40: 52–54.

82 Taniguchi Y, Ando K, Shimizu M et al. Creeping eruption due to larvae of the suborder *Spirurina* – a newly recognized causative parasite. Int J Dermatol 1994; 33: 279–281.

83 Goto Y, Tamura A, Ishikawa O et al. Creeping eruption caused by a larva of the suborder Spirurina type X. Br J Dermatol 1998; 139: 315–318.

84 Sulica VI, Berberian B, Kao GF. Histopathologic findings of cutaneous larva migrans. J Cutan Pathol 1988; 15: 346 (abstract).

85 Czarnetzki BM, Springorum M. Larva migrans with eosinophilic papular folliculitis. Dermatologica 1982; 164: 36–40.

86 Miller AC, Walker J, Jaworski R et al. Hookworm folliculitis. Arch Dermatol 1991; 127: 547–549.

87 Smith JD, Goette DK, Odom RB. Larva currens. Cutaneous strongyloidiasis. Arch Dermatol 1976; 112: 1161–1163.

88 de Viragh PA, Guggisberg D, Derighetti M et al. Monosymptomatic *Loa loa* infection. Dermatology 1998; 197: 303–305.

89 Marriott WRV. Loiasis in a young child in Oregon. Int J Dermatol 1986; 25: 252–254.

90 Routh HB. Elephantiasis. Int J Dermatol 1992; 31: 845–852.

91 Pun KK. Rose spots and trichinosis – report of a case. Clin Exp Dermatol 1985; 10: 587–589.

92 Vargas-Ocampo F, Alarcón-Rivera E, Alvarado-Alemán FJ. Human gnathostomiasis in Mexico. Int J Dermatol 1998; 37: 441–444.

93 Taniguchi Y, Ando K, Isoda K-I et al. Human gnathostomiasis: successful removal of *Gnathostoma hispidum*. Int J Dermatol 1992; 31: 175–177.

94 Taniguchi Y, Hashimoto K, Ichikawa S et al. Human gnathostomiasis. J Cutan Pathol 1991; 18: 112–115.

95 Taniguchi Y, Ando K, Sugimoto K, Yamanaka K. Creeping eruption due to *Gnathostoma hispidum* – one way to find the causative parasite with artificial digestion method. Int J Dermatol 1999; 38: 873–874.

96 Crowley JJ, Kim YH. Cutaneous gnathostomiasis. J Am Acad Dermatol 1995; 33: 825–828.

97 Elgart ML. Creeping eruption. Arch Dermatol 1998; 134: 619–620.

98 Ginsburg B, Beaver PC, Wilson ER, Whitley RJ. Dermatitis due to larvae of a soil nematode, *Pelodera strongyloides*. Pediatr Dermatol 1984; 2: 33–37.

99 Pasyk K. Dermatitis rhabditidosa in an 11-year-old girl. Br J Dermatol 1978; 98: 107–112.

100 Vargas-Ocampo F, Alvarado-Aleman FJ. Infestation from *Lagochilascaris minor* in Mexico. Int J Dermatol 1997; 36: 56–58.

101 Gutierrez Y, Cohen M, Machicao CN. *Dioctophyme* larva in the subcutaneous tissues of a woman in Ohio. Am J Surg Pathol 1989; 13: 800–802.

Arthropod-induced diseases

INTRODUCTION

The phylum Arthropoda, which accounts for approximately 75% of animal species, is one of the most important sources of human pathogens. As well as acting as vectors of bacteria, viruses, rickettsiae, chlamydiae, spirochetes, protozoa and helminths, arthropods may also produce lesions at their portal of entry into the skin. Furthermore, immunological reactions to the parasite or its parts may result in more widely disseminated cutaneous lesions.

There are five major classes of arthropods.[1,2] The class Insecta is the largest group, although the class Arachnida, which includes ticks, spiders and mites, is probably of greater dermatopathological interest. The class Crustacea, which includes lobsters, crabs and shrimps, and the classes Diplopoda and Chilopoda, which include millipedes and centipedes respectively, are not of major dermatopathological importance and will not be considered in detail. They may produce local reactions at the site of contact. These include erythema, urticaria and purpura in the case of millipedes and centipedes. A brief classification of the arthropods is given in Table 30.1. Mention should also be made of the comprehensive monograph on arthropods and the skin by Alexander[3] and the review on venomous arthropods by Vetter and Visscher.[4]

ARACHNIDS

SCORPION AND SPIDER BITES

Scorpion venom may produce throbbing indurated lesions at the site of attack, usually on acral parts. Erythema, purpura, bullae, necrosis, ulcers, lymphadenitis and systemic symptoms may develop.[1]

Local necrosis may be produced at the site of spider bites; in some cases, e.g. following the bite of a black widow spider (usually *Latrodectus mactans*), severe systemic symptoms and even death may result. The genus *Loxosceles* (which includes the brown recluse spider *Loxosceles reclusa*) may produce

Table 30.1 **A general classification of arthropods**

Class crustacea
Lobsters, crabs, shrimps

Class diplopoda
Millipedes

Class chilopoda
Centipedes

Class arachnida
Scorpions
Spiders
Ticks
Demodex
Sarcoptes
Cheyletiella
Miscellaneous mites

Class insecta
Sucking lice (Anoplura)
Bugs (Hemiptera)
Flies, mosquitoes, sandflies (Diptera)
Fleas (Siphonaptera)
Beetles (Coleoptera)
Moths and butterflies (Lepidoptera)
Bees, wasps, hornets (Hymenoptera)

a local lesion with quite extensive necrosis, hemorrhage, blistering and ulceration.[5–10] A chronic pyoderma gangrenosum-like reaction has also been reported.[11,12] Less severe reactions, such as erythema and edema, are more usual with other species of spiders.[13] An excellent review of spider bites has been published by Wong and colleagues.[14]

Histopathology

The appearances change from a neutrophilic vasculitis with hemorrhage, through a phase with arterial wall necrosis, to eschar-covered ulceration and subcutaneous necrosis.[5] There are usually eosinophils in the accompanying inflammatory infiltrate. The term 'necrotizing arachnidism' is given to the necrotic lesions produced by some spider bites (Fig. 30.1).[15–17]

TICK BITES

Ticks are important as hosts and transmitters of a wide range of diseases.[18] Their salivary secretions may produce systemic toxemia and their embedded mouthparts may produce a local erythematous lesion or a more persistent granulomatous or nodular response.[19] Unusual reactions include panniculitis,[20] papular urticaria, bullae and hemorrhage. There are two major families of ticks, soft ticks (Argasidae) and hard ticks (Ixodidae). Soft ticks (*Ornithodoros*

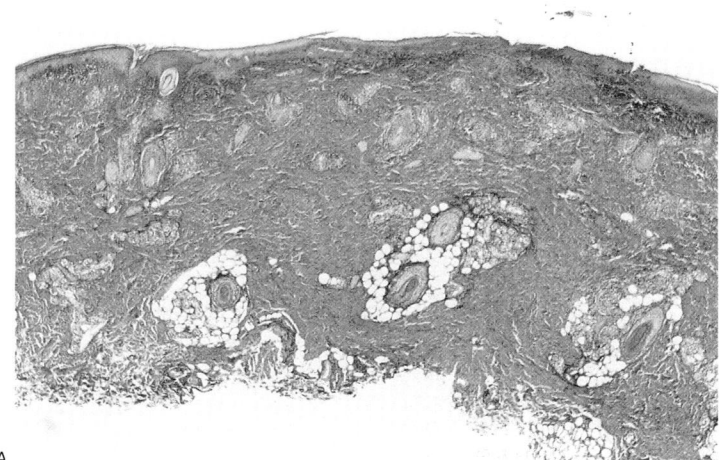

A

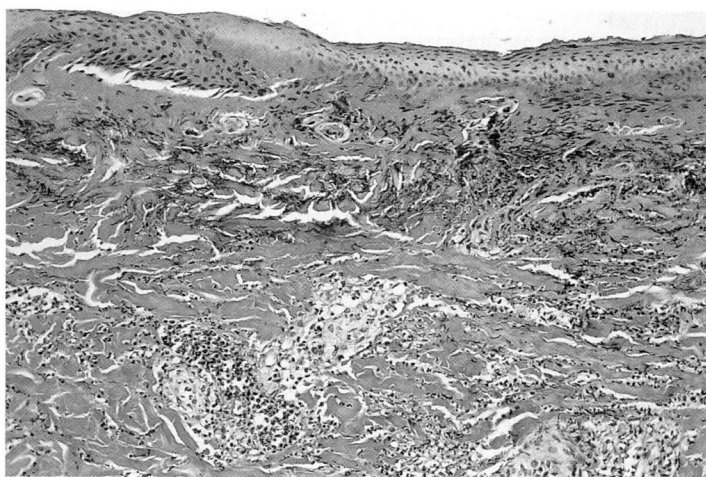

B

Fig. 30.1 **(A) Necrotizing arachnidism. (B)** There is epidermal and superficial dermal necrosis. (H & E)

species)[21] are generally not perceived by the victim, although hard ticks — of which there are several genera, including *Ixodes* and *Dermacentor* — are eventually noticed because they remain attached for days and slowly engorge with blood. Attempts to remove the tick may cause the embedded mouthparts to separate and remain in the tissue.

Histopathology

In acute lesions there is an intradermal cavity, below which the mouthparts may be seen (Fig. 30.2). There is often a tract of 'necrosis' on either side, and in the first few days intense extravasation of fibrin may be seen in relation to vessels.[19] Fibrin thrombi are sometimes present in dermal capillaries.[22] A moderately dense, predominantly perivascular infiltrate of neutrophils, lymphocytes, plasma cells and histiocytes is present, with a variable admixture of eosinophils.[23] Neutrophils are sometimes prominent in recent bites. The diagnosis may be difficult if tick mouthparts are not seen (Fig. 30.3). A panniculitis, with a preponderance of neutrophils in the infiltrate, may occur.[20]

In chronic persistent lesions there is a diffuse superficial and deep infiltrate which includes all the cells found in acute lesions, but usually with many fewer neutrophils and more lymphocytes. There may be occasional giant cells, dermal fibrosis and even granuloma formation.[24] The epidermis may show acanthosis or pseudoepitheliomatous hyperplasia.

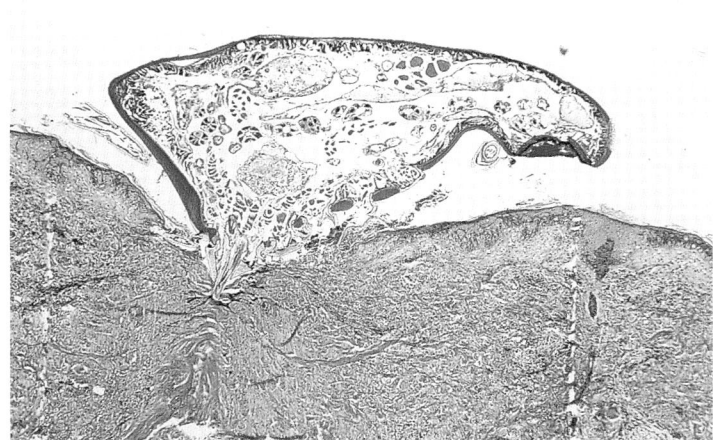

Fig. 30.2 **A tick in situ.** (H & E)

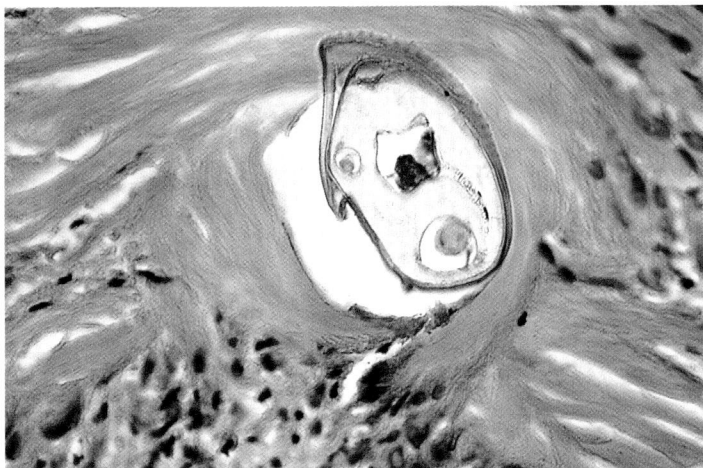

Fig. 30.3 **A tick-bite reaction.** Mouthparts are present in the dermis. (H & E)

Erythema chronicum migrans (Lyme disease), which follows the bite of *Ixodes*, has been shown to be caused by a spirochete transmitted by the tick.[25] It is considered with other spirochetal diseases in Chapter 24 (p. 654).

DEMODICOSIS

Two species of follicle mites are found as normal inhabitants of human skin:[26–37] *Demodex folliculorum* lives mainly in the hair follicles and *Demodex brevis* in the sebaceous glands. The larger of the two, *Demodex folliculorum*, measures about 0.4 mm in length. Mites of this species are often aggregated in a follicle, whereas *D. brevis* is usually solitary.[28] The mites have been found in 10% of routine skin biopsies (from all sites), and in 12% of all follicles examined in these same biopsies.[29] They are not increased in pregnancy.[38] The face is most often involved, although *D. brevis* has a wider distribution.[35] Although increased numbers of mites are found in sections of rosacea and in subclinical forms of folliculitis, this does not prove a causal relationship.[39–41] It is generally accepted that demodex mites are not etiologically involved in the usual form of rosacea, although they may possibly play a role in the granulomatous form, in which extrafollicular mites are sometimes seen. *Demodex* may produce a blepharitis[30] and so-called 'rosacea-like' demodicosis.[34,42–45] It has been incriminated as a cause of localized pustular folliculitis of the face,[31,44,46] and of a more widespread eruption in patients with an immunosuppressed state.[47–51] However, mite density is not always increased in immunosuppressed patients.[52] Facial erythema with follicular plugging (pityriasis folliculorum) is another manifestation of *Demodex* infestation.[53] Genital lesions are rare.[54]

Histopathology

The effects of *Demodex* infestation include follicular dilatation, the presence of dense homogeneous eosinophilic material surrounding the mites, folliculitis, and perifollicular chronic inflammation (Figs 30.4, 30.5). Tiny follicular spicules resulting from the combination of follicular hyperkeratosis and protruding mites have been reported.[55] There are several reports of a granulomatous reaction to extrafollicular *Demodex*, usually in granulomatous or pustular rosacea.[32,33]

In rosacea-like demodicosis, up to 10–15 *D. folliculorum* may be found in individual follicles.[34] Telangiectasia of superficial vessels, perifollicular granulomas and mild perivascular chronic inflammation may also be seen in this condition.

SCABIES

Scabies is a contagious disease caused by the mite *Sarcoptes scabiei* var. *hominis*. It is acquired particularly under conditions of overcrowding and poor personal hygiene, or during sexual contact. Patients with both minimal disease and only a few mites[56] and exaggerated atypical lesions complicating AIDS[57–62] are now being seen. The disease tends to appear in epidemics, which have a cyclical character, recurring at intervals of about 30 years and lasting for about 15 years.[63] The reasons for these cyclic fluctuations are not understood. A new cycle probably commenced in 1993, although there are conflicting reports on the date of commencement of this most recent cycle.[64]

Three clinical forms are found: papulovesicular lesions, persistent nodules and Norwegian (crusted) scabies. The usual lesions are papules and papulovesicles which are intensely pruritic. The vesicles are usually found at the end of very fine wavy dark lines, best seen with the help of a hand lens or by applying a small amount of ink to the surface and removing the excess.[65] These lines represent the excreta-soiled burrows in the horny layer in which

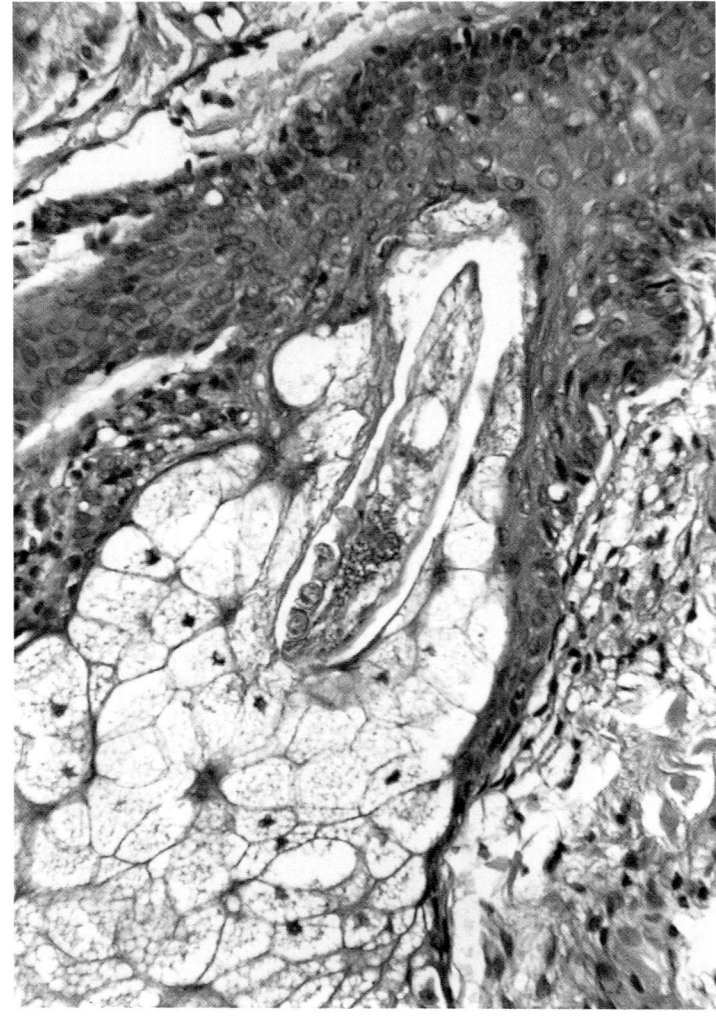

Fig. 30.4 **A demodex mite** in the lower sebaceous duct. (H & E)

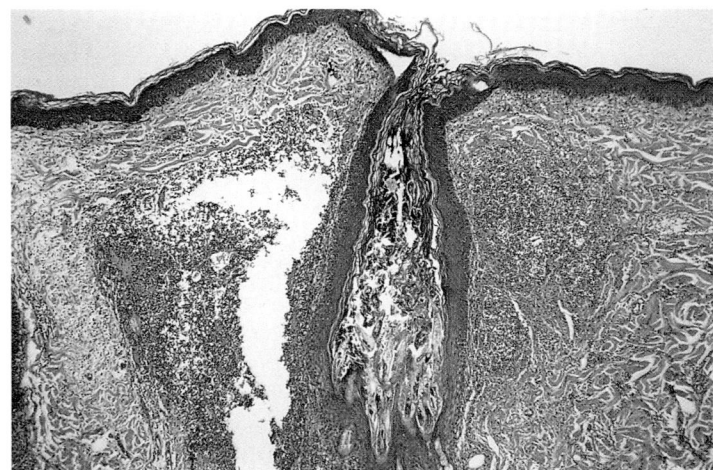

Fig. 30.5 ***Demodex* perifolliculitis.** There are numerous mites in the follicle. (H & E)

the female travels to deposit her eggs. Epiluminescence microscopy enhances the diagnosis of scabies; it gives a low number of false-negative results.[66] Amplification of *Sarcoptes* DNA in the cutaneous scale, using PCR, has been used to confirm inapparent infection.[67]

The female mite measures up to 0.4 mm in length and rather less in breadth, whereas the adult male, which dies after copulation, is much smaller (Fig. 30.6). The sites most commonly affected are the interdigital skin folds, the palmar surfaces of the hands and fingers, the wrists, the nipples, the inframammary regions and the male genitals. A more generalized eruption is sometimes seen in infants and young children.[68] In addition to the burrows, there is nearly always a secondary rash of small urticarial papules with no mites, which may result from autosensitization.[69,70] Bullae, resembling bullous pemphigoid, are rarely seen.[71–74] The presence of circulating antibodies against BP180 and/or BP230 suggests that scabies may induce true bullous pemphigoid.[75]

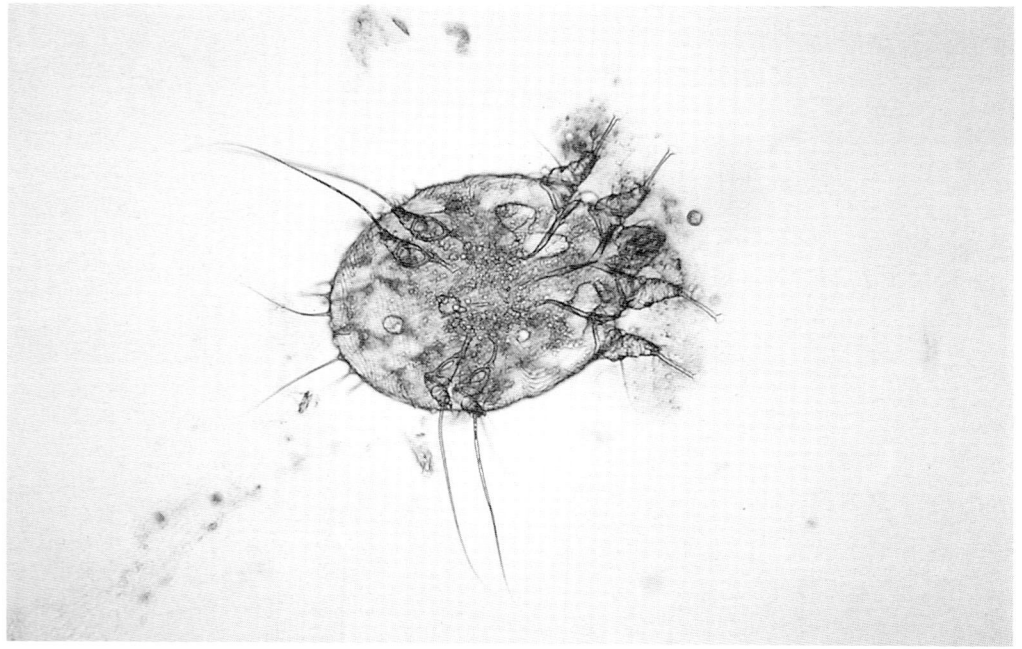

Fig. 30.6 ***Sarcoptes* mite.** (×100)

In about 7% of patients, particularly children and young adults, reddish-brown pruritic nodules develop with a predilection for the lower trunk, scrotum and thighs.[63] These lesions may persist for a year, despite treatment. Mites are rarely found, and this form (persistent nodular scabies) is thought to represent a delayed hypersensitivity reaction similar to that found following some other arthropod bites.

Norwegian (crusted) scabies is a rare contagious form consisting of widespread crusted and secondarily infected hyperkeratotic lesions, found in the mentally and physically debilitated[76-78] as well as in immunosuppressed patients.[62,79-88] This form has also been reported in an otherwise healthy pregnant woman[89] and in patients with epidermolysis bullosa.[90,91] There is an extremely heavy infestation with mites.

Human infestation with varieties of *Sarcoptes scabiei* of animal origin is not uncommon.[92] They produce a self-limiting disease without the presence of burrows.[93,94] These animal variants are morphologically indistinguishable from the human variant of *Sarcoptes scabiei*.

The conventional antiscabetics have poor compliance; however, ivermectin, an oral scabicide, is proving a useful substitute.[95,96]

Immunological features

There is some evidence that immunological phenomena are involved in scabies.[97-99] Immediate hypersensitivity may result in the primary lesions, and delayed hypersensitivity in the persistent nodular lesions. Elevated levels of IgE have been found in the serum of some patients with scabies, but the serum IgA is reduced in many with the Norwegian form.[100,101] IgE has been demonstrated by immunofluorescence in vessel walls in the dermis,[102] IgA and C3 in the stratum corneum, and IgM and/or C3 along the basement membrane in some cases.[103] IgE-containing plasma cells have been found in nodular lesions.[104]

Histopathology

The histological changes are sufficiently distinctive at least to suggest the diagnosis.[105] There is a superficial and deep infiltrate of lymphocytes, histiocytes, mast cells[106] and eosinophils, together with some interstitial eosinophils. These features are common to many arthropod reactions. Flame figures and a vasculitis are found, rarely.[107,108] In addition there are spongiotic foci and spongiotic vesicles within the epidermis, with exocytosis of variable numbers of eosinophils and sometimes neutrophils (Fig. 30.7). Subepidermal

bullae, resembling bullous pemphigoid, have been reported.[71-73] Eggs, larvae, mites and excreta may be seen in the stratum corneum if an obvious burrow is excised (Fig. 30.8).[109,110] If the secondary (autosensitization) lesions are biopsied, the picture may not be diagnostic: no mites will be seen, and there is a report which suggests that even eosinophils may be absent.[69] Older lesions may simply show excoriation and overlying scale crusts.[105]

The lesions of persistent nodular scabies resemble those of other persistent bite reactions, with a more dense superficial and deep inflammatory cell infiltrate which includes lymphocytes, macrophages, plasma cells, eosinophils, Langerhans cells and sometimes atypical mononuclear cells (Fig. 30.9).[109,111] Lymphoid follicles are sometimes present, and the infiltrate may even extend into the subcutaneous fat. Pseudoepitheliomatous hyperplasia is not a feature. Cases have been published that purportedly resembled cutaneous lymphoma, but the descriptions provided in those instances are not those of lymphoma.[112] Mites are rarely found in routine sections, but if serial sections are studied mite parts can be seen in about 20% of cases.[113]

In Norwegian scabies there is a massive orthokeratosis and parakeratosis containing mites in all stages of development (Fig. 30.10). The underlying epidermis shows psoriasiform hyperplasia with focal spongiosis and exocytosis of eosinophils and neutrophils, sometimes producing intraepidermal microabscesses. The dermis contains a superficial and deep infiltrate of chronic inflammatory cells, and usually some interstitial eosinophils.

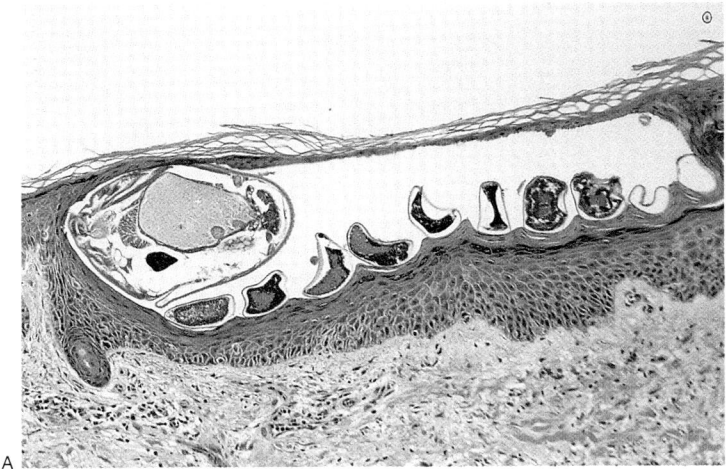

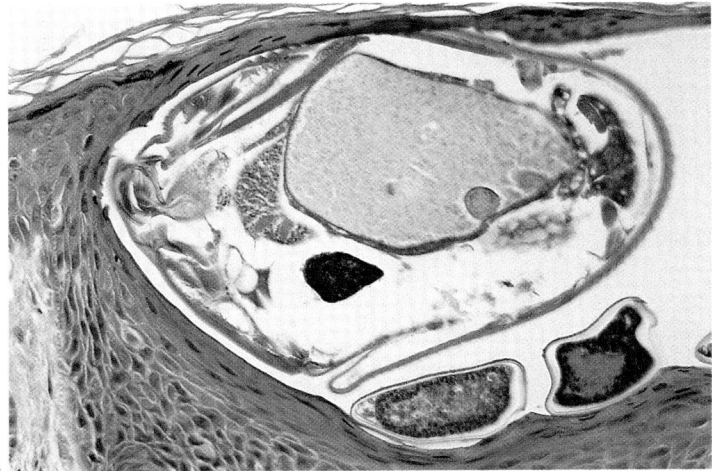

Fig. 30.8 **Scabies. (A)** A burrow is present in the stratum corneum. A mite is present at one end with a trail of debris. **(B)** A higher-power view of the mite. (H & E)

Fig. 30.7 **Scabies.** There are spongiotic vesicles containing many eosinophils. (H & E)

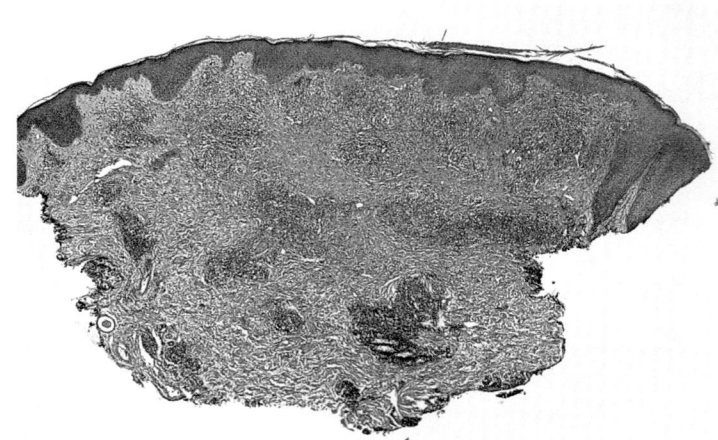

Fig. 30.9 **Persistent nodular scabies.** There is a superficial and deep infiltrate within the dermis. The interstitial eosinophils are not obvious at this magnification. (H & E)

CHEYLETIELLA DERMATITIS

Several species of *Cheyletiella*, a mite found on dogs, rabbits and cats, can produce an intensely pruritic dermatitis in humans.[114–116] In animals it produces so-called 'walking dandruff'. There are erythematous papules and papulovesicles, sometimes grouped, with a predilection for the chest, abdomen and proximal extremities.[117] Involved areas usually correspond to the sites of close physical contact with the infested pet.[118] The mite is almost never found on humans, and the diagnosis may be confirmed by examining fur brushings of the patient's pet for the mite.[119,120] This condition is no longer thought to be synonymous with so-called 'itchy red bump' disease (papular dermatitis), a papular pruritic disorder of uncertain histogenesis which was originally reported from Florida, USA (see p. 111).[114,121] Delayed hypersensitivity mechanisms are thought to play a role in the pathogenesis of the eruption.[122]

Histopathology

Sections show focal epidermal spongiosis at the site of the bite. There is a superficial and mid-dermal predominantly perivascular infiltrate composed of lymphocytes, macrophages and some eosinophils. There are usually some interstitial eosinophils, suggesting an arthropod bite; however, the reaction is more superficial and less inflammatory than the usual arthropod reaction.

OTHER MITE LESIONS

Four other families of mites have been incriminated in the production of cutaneous lesions: Tyroglyphoidea (food mites), Pyemotidae (predacious or grain itch mites), Dermanyssidae (parasitoid or rat mites) and Trombiculidae (trombiculid or harvest mites, chiggers).[1,2,115]

Food mites and predacious mites produce erythematous papules, papulovesicles or urticaria in workers handling certain foods and grain. The lesions may be mistaken for scabies, but there are no burrows.[19] The genera involved include *Glycophagus* (grocery mite), *Acarus* (cheese mite), *Tyrophagus* (copra mite), *Pyemotes* (grain itch mite) and *Tyroglyphus*.[19,93,123] The house dust mite *Dermatophagoides pteronyssinus* and related species are widely distributed in bedding and clothing, and may play a role in producing or exacerbating chronic dermatitis.[124,125] Paper mites may also produce a mild pruritic rash in persons handling stored paper or old books.

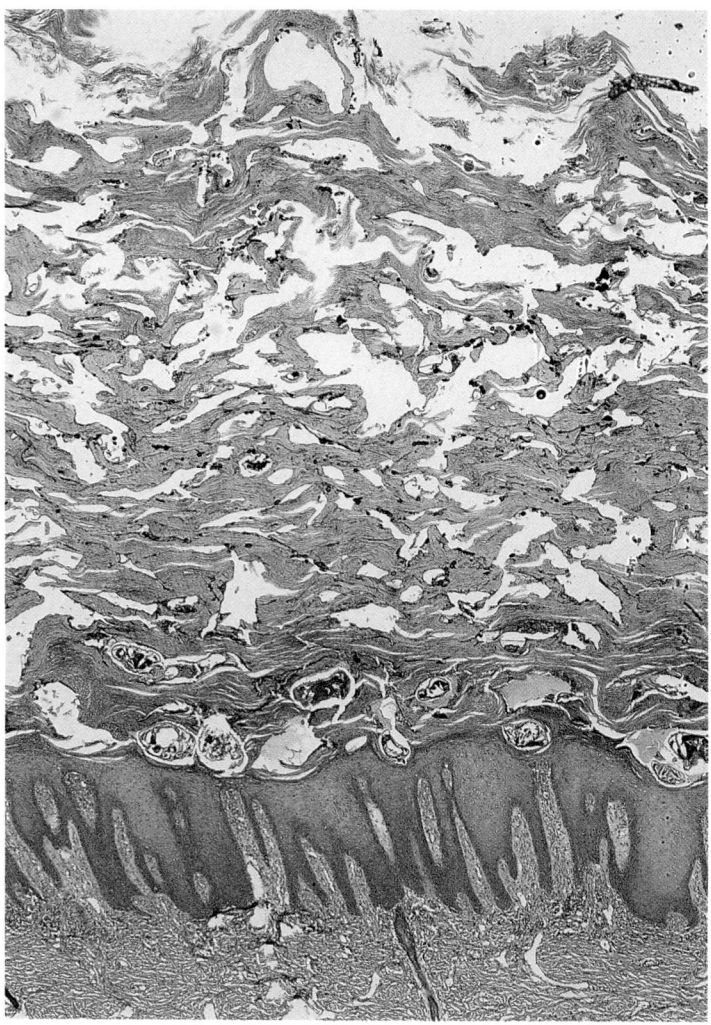

Fig. 30.10 **Norwegian scabies.** The thick keratin layer overlying the psoriasiform epidermis contains many mites. (H & E)

The parasitoid mites may produce papular urticaria in people employed in grain stores or living in places harboring rats.[126,127] Pet rabbits may be infected by the mite *Listrophorus gibbus*, which can produce a papular urticaria in the handler.[128] Various birds, including pet gerbils, may harbor mites from the family Dermanyssidae.[129–132] The term 'gamasoidosis' has been used to describe the human skin disease caused by mites from birds and other animals.[129]

The trombiculid mites may produce a severe dermatitis with minute, intensely pruritic red elevations.[133] They have a predilection for the lower legs, groin and waistline.

Histopathology

The lesions produced by mites other than chiggers resemble those generally seen in mild arthropod reactions, with a superficial and mid-dermal perivascular infiltrate, some interstitial eosinophils and mild epidermal spongiosis. The mite is almost never found. Some neutrophils are usually present in lesions produced by *Pyemotes* species.[19]

Bites by chiggers (*Trombicula* species) may be centered on hair follicles or in skin having a thin horny layer. A tissue canal or 'stylostome' surrounded by a mass of hyaline tissue runs into the malpighian layer. There is usually epidermal spongiosis, dermal edema with some neutrophils, and later a more mixed dermal inflammatory infiltrate, as in other arthropod lesions. A chronic granulomatous response has been described.[19]

INSECTS

HUMAN LICE (PEDICULOSIS)

Pediculosis, which has been known for over 10 000 years, is caused by three types of lice, each having a separate microenvironment. The head louse (*Pediculus humanus capitis*) infests the hairs of the scalp. It is an increasing problem in many urban communities, with outbreaks particularly in schools.[134–137]

The pubic louse (*Phthirus pubis*) infests pubic and axillary hair in particular, although there may be colonization of any heavy growth of hair on the trunk and limbs.[138] Occasionally the eyebrows are infested, and very rarely the scalp.[139,140] The HIV status of the patient does not appear to influence the severity of the infestation. Both the pubic louse and the head louse cement their eggs to hair, forming the minute gritty projection that is known as a nit. Multiple bluish spots (maculae ceruleae) may be found, particularly on the trunk, in persons infested with the pubic louse.[141]

The body louse (*Pediculus humanus corporis*) divides its existence between the host and the host's clothing, in the seams of which it deposits its eggs.

The lice are blood-suckers and the injected saliva produces an allergic reaction. The resulting itching may lead to excoriation or secondary bacterial infection.

Histopathology
A louse may be removed from the body and examined microscopically for confirmation (Fig. 30.11). Nits may also be identified by examining involved hairs (Fig. 30.12).

Scanning electron microscopy of the egg of the pubic louse has found that the egg is totally encased by a proteinaceous sheath, except for the operculum, through which oxygen exchange occurs.[142] The operculum is the target of topical insecticides for ovicidal kill.[142]

BEDBUGS

Bedbugs (*Cimicidae*) are found usually in dirty and dilapidated housing, associated with unwashed bedlinen.[143] They may also infest wooden seating in public transport. They are notoriously difficult to eliminate.[144]

The common bedbug (*Cimex lectularius*) can produce urticarial, vesicular and even bullous lesions. Anaphylactic reactions and persistent nodular lesions are rare. The distribution of the lesions is influenced by the method of infestation and the wearing of bedclothes.[144]

Histopathology
Urticarial lesions show variable edema of the upper dermis with perivascular lymphocytes, eosinophils and mast cells. A few interstitial eosinophils are also present. Vesiculobullous lesions show both intraepidermal and subepidermal edema. Hemorrhage may be present in the dermis in bullous lesions.[144]

MYIASIS

Myiasis is the infestation of live human tissues by the larvae of flies in the order Diptera.[145–147] In Central and South America dermal myiasis is usually caused by the 'human botfly', *Dermatobia hominis*.[148–155] In West and Central

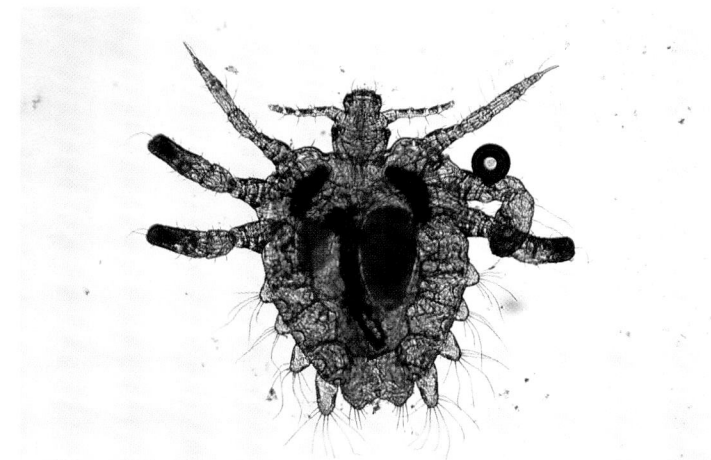

Fig. 30.11 **Crab louse (*Phthirus pubis*).** (×27)

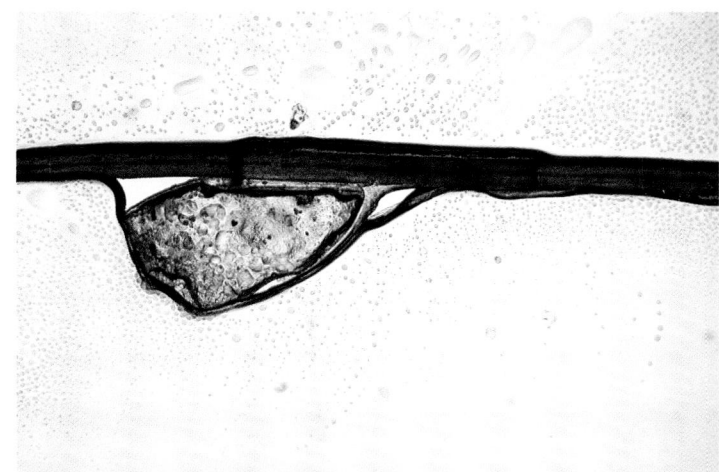

Fig. 30.12 **Pediculosis.** Hair shaft with an attached egg (nit) of the head louse. (×40)

Africa the tumbu fly (*Cordylobia anthropophaga*) is involved.[156–162] Other flies, some of them of restricted geographical distribution, can produce myiasis, including species of *Parasarcophaga*,[163] *Gasterophilus*, *Hypoderma*,[164,165] *Cuterebra*,[166–168] *Cochliomyia*,[169,170] *Chrysomya*[171] and *Wohlfahrtia*.[1,172] The larvae of the common housefly *Musca domestica* may rarely infest the skin of debilitated and extremely neglected patients.[173,174] The eggs may be transmitted to humans by another insect, such as the mosquito in the case of *Dermatobia hominis*, or the larvae may burrow into the skin of a suitable host after hatching on the ground or on clothing, as with the tumbu fly.

The larva completes its molts in from about 2 weeks to 3 months or longer, depending on the species. It then works its way out of the skin and falls to the ground, where pupation occurs. This may be noted by the patient.

The lesions have a predilection for exposed surfaces such as the feet and forearms.[175] The scalp is uncommonly involved, while penile involvement is very rare.[161] Lesions have a furuncle-like presentation which culminates in ulceration.[176,177] Sometimes there are plaques with draining sinuses.[178] There may be throbbing pain as the lesion enlarges.

Histopathology
There is usually a small cavity, in the dermis and sometimes in the subcutaneous tissue, containing the developing larva (Fig. 30.13). Surrounding

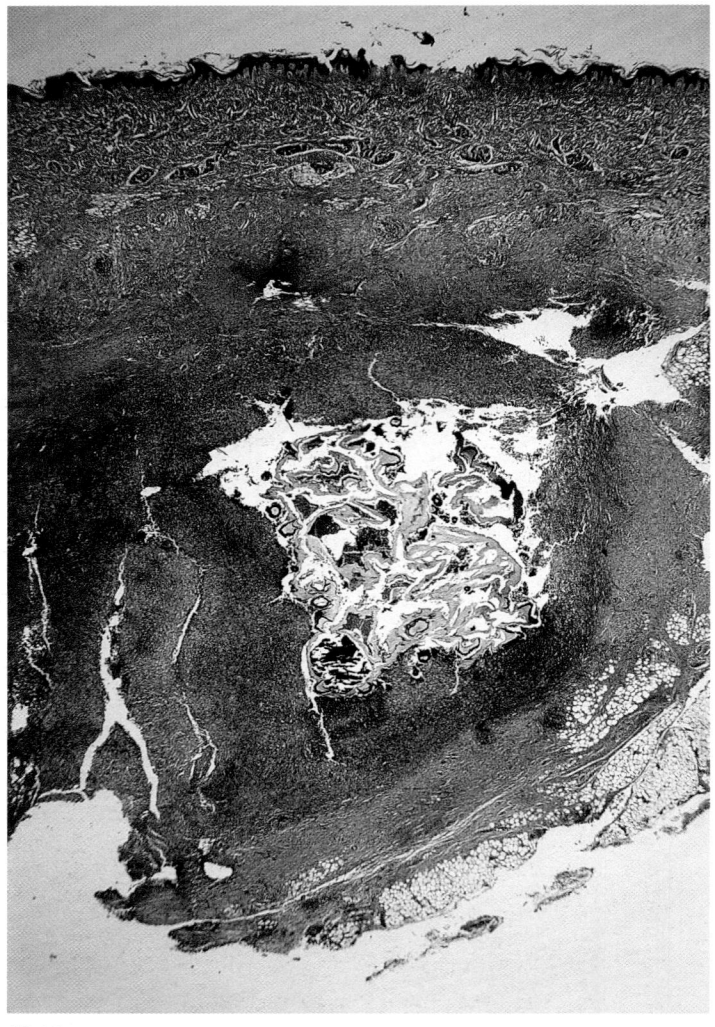

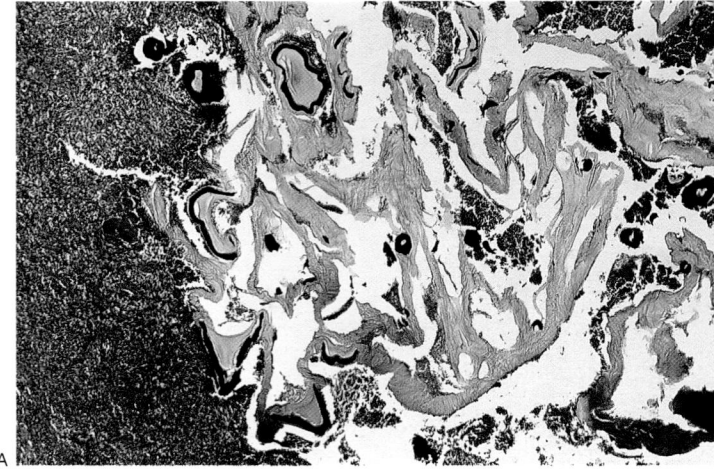

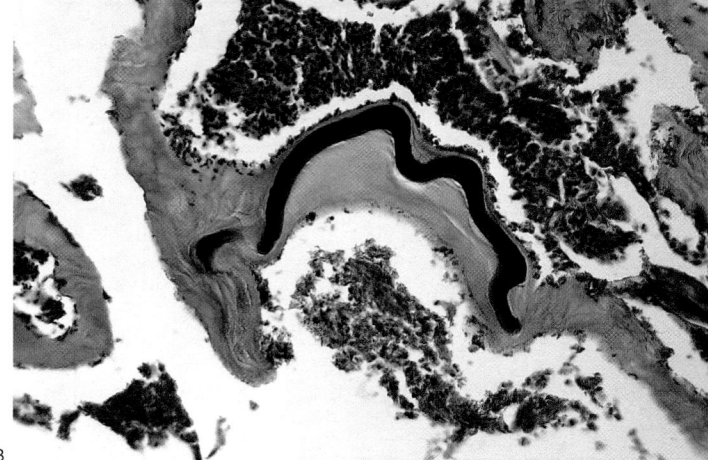

Fig. 30.14 **(A) Myiasis. (B)** Higher magnification of the case in Fig. 30.13 showing fragments of the larval wall. (H & E)

Fig. 30.13 **Myiasis.** Larval parts are present within a subcutaneous cavity, the wall of which contains a heavy inflammatory cell infiltrate. (H & E)

this is a heavy mixed inflammatory cell infiltrate which includes lymphocytes, histiocytes, occasional foreign-body giant cells and plasma cells, as well as eosinophils; neutrophils are also present near the cavity.[145] There are abundant activated fibroblasts elaborating collagen, which may relate to larval containment.[145] A sinus tract may lead to the surface, with ulceration. Fragments of larva are usually seen within the cavity (Fig. 30.14). It s encased by a thick chitinous cuticle with widely spaced spines on the surface. Beneath the cuticle, layers of striated muscle and internal organs may be seen.[179]

Immunohistochemical studies have shown that 30% of the cells in the inflammatory infiltrate are cytotoxic CD4 positive T cells that produce a Th2 cytokine pattern.[180]

TUNGIASIS

Tungiasis is produced by infestation of the skin by the pregnant female sandflea *Tunga penetrans*.[181] It occurs in Central and South America, tropical Africa and Pakistan.[182–185] International travel has resulted in its occurrence in many countries.[186–189] As the flea is a poor jumper, lesions are usually found on the feet. Penetration into the dermis by the flea produces characteristic single or multiple white papules, and eventually nodules about 1 cm in diameter.[190] Lesions have a central black dot and erythematous margins. On

entering the skin the female tunga is about 0.1 cm in diameter, but this increases to 0.6 cm or more as the 150–200 eggs within the abdomen of the gravid female mature. Once the ova have been shed through an opening in the skin and the tunga has died, the nodule usually becomes frankly ulcerated.

Histopathology

The diagnosis is made by finding the tunga in the epidermis or dermis, with its characteristic exoskeleton and internal parts, including ova (Fig. 30.15).[190,191] There is a surrounding mixed inflammatory cell infiltrate of lymphocytes, plasma cells and eosinophils. A mass of eggs may be seen within the stratum corneum, with underlying epidermal necrosis; in later lesions there is ulceration.[190]

OTHER INSECT BITES

Species within the order Diptera may be responsible for cutaneous lesions other than myiasis. These insects include mosquitoes, gnats and midges. Mosquitoes may cause urticarial and even bullous lesions in occasional sensitized hosts. In some cases of severe hypersensitivity to mosquito bites, a lymphocytosis with many natural killer cells has been present.[192] The biting gnats and midges may give urticarial wheals or pruritic papules.[193] Papular urticaria is a common reaction to fleas. Large persistent lesions may develop

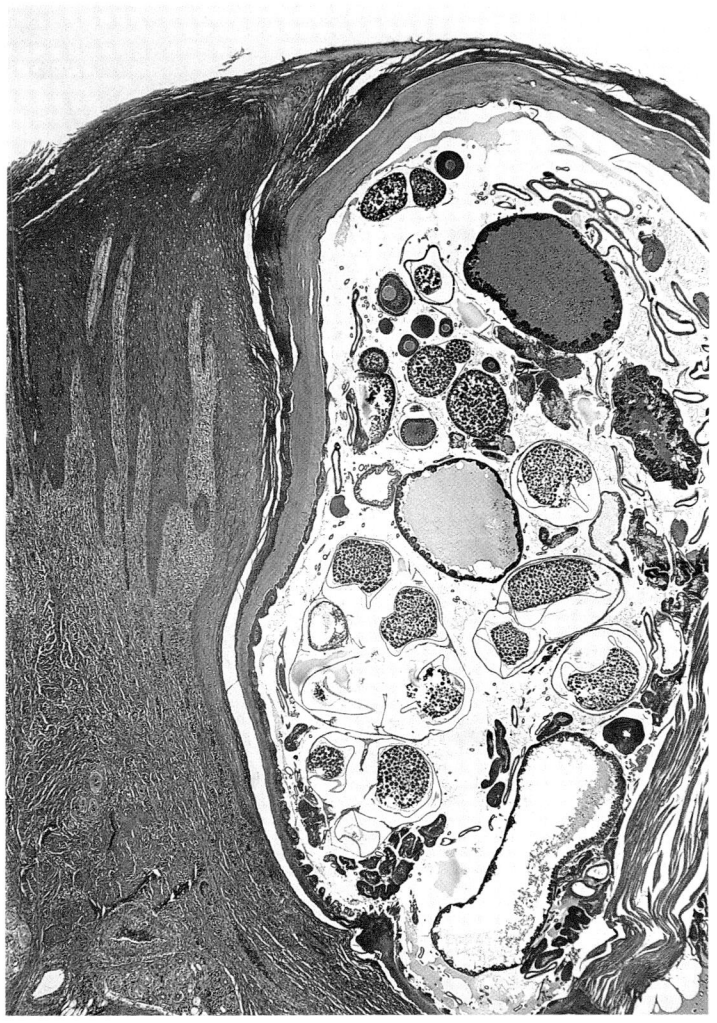

Fig. 30.15 **Tungiasis.** The parasite has penetrated the epidermis and occupies much of the dermis. (H & E)

in patients infected with the human immunodeficiency virus.[194] A related phenomenon is the development of exuberant lesions in patients with hematological disorders, particularly chronic lymphocytic leukemia (see below).

Beetles (order Coleoptera) can produce slowly forming blisters, necrotizing lesions or papular urticaria.[195–197] The best known blister beetle is *Lytta vesicatoria* (the Spanish fly), an insect endemic to Southern Europe.[198] The blisters are produced by cantharidin, a substance found in certain beetles.[199] Other families of beetle have a different vesicating toxin in their coelomic fluid, known as pederin, which is released when the beetle is accidentally crushed on the skin.[200] Recently, an outbreak of over 250 cases of a vesicular dermatitis was reported from Australia.[198] It was caused by the genus *Paederus* (whiplash rove beetles).[198] An earlier outbreak was reported from Sri Lanka.[201]

Some species of moths and butterflies (order Lepidoptera) have larvae (caterpillars) with surface hairs that may produce urtication on entering the skin. Erythematous macules and papules and urticarial wheals may be seen.[202–204]

Moths of the genus *Hylesia* (found particularly in South America) may produce an intensely pruritic urticarial rash within a few minutes to several hours after contact with the abdominal hairs of the adult female moth.[205]

Severe urticarial edema and even anaphylaxis may follow the stings of species within the order Hymenoptera (bees, wasps and hornets) in some susceptible individuals.[206]

There was a recent review on the cutaneous side effects of insect repellents.[207] Despite the widespread use of repellents, complications, such as an irritant contact dermatitis, are quite uncommon.[207]

Histopathology

The appearances will depend on many factors, such as the nature of the arthropod, the duration of the lesion, the immunological reaction (immediate or delayed hypersensitivity), the presence of arthropod parts and the discharge of toxins.

Lesions of papular urticaria show prominent papillary dermal edema and a superficial and deep inflammatory infiltrate, with perivascular accentuation and usually some interstitial eosinophils. Papular and papulovesicular lesions resemble those produced by other arthropods.

Some neutrophils are often present in lesions biopsied in the first day or so, particularly with certain insects. Flea bites usually have some neutrophils in the exudate, as do the necrotizing lesions produced by beetles.

Plasma cells may be prominent, particularly in the deep dermis, in some persistent insect bites; rarely the appearances may simulate a plasmacytoma.

Focal epidermal necrosis is seen with some gnat and beetle bites.[193,197,208] The vesicular dermatitis associated with the whiplash rove beetle (*Paederus*), see page 99, is characterized by intraepidermal and suprabasal vesicles and pustules with reticular and confluent necrosis of the epidermis and the superficial zones of the appendages (Fig. 30.16).[198] There are occasional eosinophils in the dermal infiltrate.

Bullous lesions seen in some hosts susceptible to mosquitoes have large intraepidermal vesicles with thin strands of epidermis between the vesicles and prominent edema of the papillary dermis. Intraepidermal vesicles containing eosinophils may be seen in caterpillar dermatitis and in some other bite reactions, particularly at the point of entry of any mouthparts. Moths of the genus *Hylesia* produce a spongiotic epidermal reaction related to a fine hair shaft implanted by the moth; there is some exocytosis of neutrophils and lymphocytes.

Other findings that may be seen in persistent insect bite reactions include pseudoepitheliomatous hyperplasia, sometimes quite severe (Fig. 30.17), and atypical dermal infiltrates which may be mistaken for malignant lymphoma.[209,210] The presence of a heterogeneous cell population with interstitial eosinophils is a reassuring sign in these rare atypical lesions.

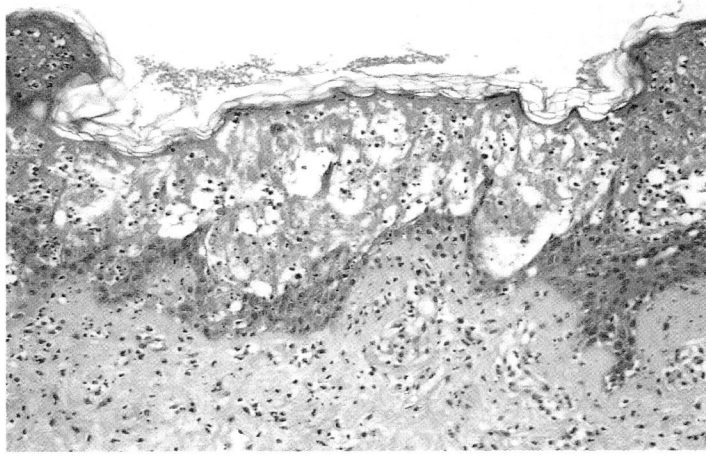

Fig. 30.16 *Paederus* **bite reaction.** A neutrophilic spongiosis with focal necrosis is present. (H & E) (Photograph kindly provided by Dr Dominic Wood)

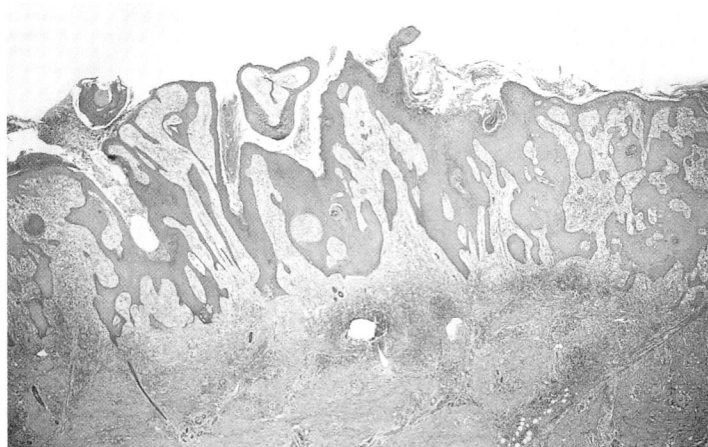

Fig. 30.17 **Arthropod bite reaction.** There is pronounced pseudoepitheliomatous hyperplasia, an uncommon pattern of reaction. (H & E)

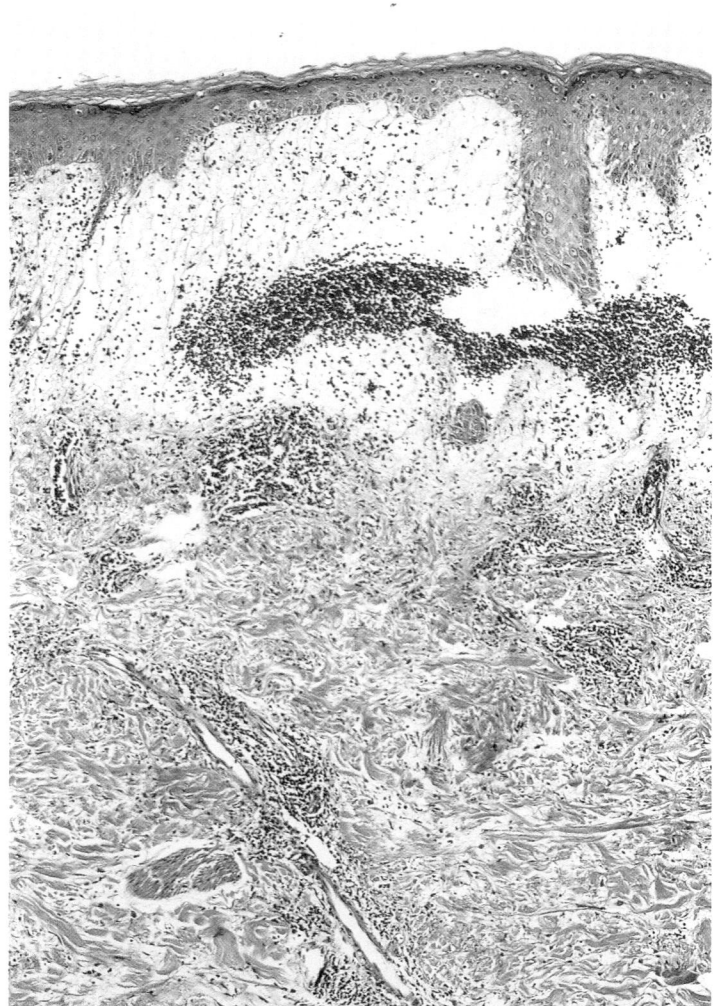

Fig. 30.18 **Exaggerated bite reaction** in a patient with chronic lymphocytic leukemia. (H & E)

It should be noted that the cnidarians (coelenterates) can produce lesions which mimic both clinically and histologically those produced by arthropods (see p. 728), including the development of persistent nodular lesions.

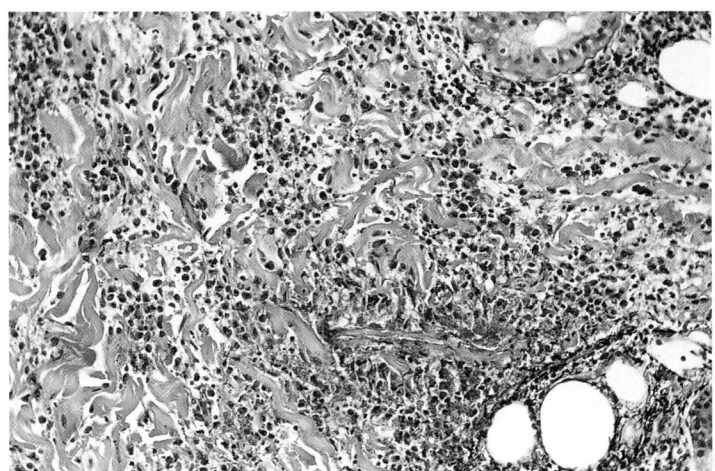

Fig. 30.19 **Exaggerated bite reaction.** There are numerous eosinophils and flame figures. (H & E)

EXAGGERATED BITE REACTIONS

Exuberant papular and vesiculobullous lesions may develop in patients with leukemia, particularly chronic lymphocytic leukemia, apparently as an exaggerated response to arthropod bites.[211,212] Patients usually do not recall being bitten. The reaction may precede the diagnosis of the hematological disorder. Lesions may persist for many years.[212] Immunodeficiency may play a role in their pathogenesis, as similar lesions have been reported in HIV infection (see above). Further studies are required to determine the exact nature of these lesions.[212]

Histopathology[211]
The epidermal changes include eosinophilic spongiosis, vesiculation and full-thickness necrosis. Both intraepidermal and subepidermal vesicles may be present (Fig. 30.18). There is a superficial and deep perivascular and interstitial infiltrate of lymphocytes and eosinophils of variable density. Flame figures and lymphoid nodules are sometimes seen (Fig. 30.19). A vasculitis, usually of lymphocytic type, may be present.

REFERENCES

Introduction
1   Beaver PC, Jung RC, Cupp EW. Clinical parasitology, 9th ed. Philadelphia: Lea & Febiger, 1984.
2   Southcott RV. Some harmful Australian arthropods. Med J Aust 1986; 145: 590–595.
3   Alexander JO'D. Arthropods and human skin. Berlin: Springer Verlag, 1984.
4   Vetter RS, Visscher PK. Bites and stings of medically important venomous arthropods. Int J Dermatol 1998; 37: 481–496.

Arachnids
5   Pucevich MV, Chesney TMcC. Histopathologic analysis of human bites by the brown recluse spider. Arch Dermatol 1983; 119: 851 (abstract).
6   Hillis TJ, Grant-Kels JM, Jacoby LM. Presumed arachnidism. Int J Dermatol 1986; 25: 44–48.
7   Ingber A, Trattner A, Cleper R, Sandbank M. Morbidity of brown recluse spider bites. Clinical picture, treatment and prognosis. Acta Derm Venereol 1991; 71: 337–340.
8   Elston DM, Eggers JS, Schmidt WE et al. Histological findings after brown recluse spider envenomation. Am J Dermatopathol 2000; 22: 242–246.
9   Lung JM, Mallory SB. A child with spider bite and glomerulonephritis: a diagnostic challenge. Int J Dermatol 2000; 39: 287–289.
10 Sams HH, Hearth SB, Long LL et al. Nineteen documented cases of *Loxosceles reclusa* envenomation. J Am Acad Dermatol 2001; 44: 603–608.
11 King LE. Spider bites. Arch Dermatol 1987; 123: 41–43.

12 Rees RS, Fields JP, King LE Jr. Do brown recluse spider bites induce pyoderma gangrenosum? South Med J 1985; 78: 283–287.

13 White J, Hirst D, Hender E. 36 cases of bites by spiders, including the white-tailed spider, *Lampona cylindrata*. Med J Aust 1989; 150: 401–403.

14 Wong RC, Hughes SE, Voorhees JJ. Spider bites. Arch Dermatol 1987; 123: 98–104.

15 White J. Necrotising arachnidism. Does the white-tailed spider deserve its bad name? Med J Aust 1999; 171: 98.

16 Pincus SJ, Winkel KD, Hawdon GM, Sutherland SK. Acute and recurrent skin ulceration after spider bite. Med J Aust 1999; 171: 99–102.

17 Sams HH, Dunnick CA, Smith ML, King LE Jr. Necrotic arachnidism. J Am Acad Dermatol 2001; 44: 561–573.

18 Marshall J. Ticks and the human skin. Dermatologica 1967; 135: 60–65.

19 Krinsky WL. Dermatoses associated with the bites of mites and ticks (Arthropoda: Acari). Int J Dermatol 1983; 22: 75–91.

20 Cho BK, Kang H, Bang D et al. Tick bites in Korea. Int J Dermatol 1994; 33: 552–555.

21 Leker RR, Felsenstein I, Raveh D et al. *Ornithodoros tholozani* bites: a unique clinical picture. J Am Acad Dermatol 1992; 27: 1025–1026.

22 Shim H, Phelps RG. Intravascular fibrin thrombi and suppuration as a clue to tick bite reaction. J Cutan Pathol 1997; 24: 124 (abstract).

23 Patterson JW, Fitzwater JE, Connell J. Localized tick bite reaction. Cutis 1979; 24: 168–172.

24 Russell FE. Dermatitis due to imbedded tick parts. JAMA 1974; 228: 1581.

25 Berger BW. Erythema chronicum migrans of Lyme disease. Arch Dermatol 1984; 120: 1017–1021.

26 Nutting WB. Hair follicle mites (Acari: Demodicidae) of man. Int J Dermatol 1976; 15: 79–98.

27 Nutting WB, Beerman H. Demodicosis and symbiophobia: status, terminology and treatments. Int J Dermatol 1983; 22: 13–17.

28 Nutting WB, Green AC. Pathogenesis associated with hair follicle mites (*Demodex spp.*) in Australian Aborigines. Br J Dermatol 1976; 94: 307–312.

29 Aylesworth R, Vance JC. *Demodex folliculorum* and *Demodex brevis* in cutaneous biopsies. J Am Acad Dermatol 1982; 7: 583–589.

30 English FP, Nutting WB, Cohn D. Demodectic oviposition in the eyelid. Aust NZ J Ophthalmol 1985; 13: 71–73.

31 Purcell SM, Hayes TJ, Dixon SL. Pustular folliculitis associated with *Demodex folliculorum*. J Am Acad Dermatol 1986; 15: 1159–1162.

32 Ecker RI, Winkelmann RK. *Demodex* granuloma. Arch Dermatol 1979; 115: 343–344.

33 Grosshans EM, Kremer M, Maleville J. *Demodex folliculorum* und die Histogenese der granulomatosen Rosacea. Hautarzt 1974; 25: 166–177.

34 Ayres S Jr, Mihan R. *Demodex* granuloma. Arch Dermatol 1979; 115: 1285–1286.

35 Crosti C, Menni S, Sala F, Piccinno RJ. Demodectic infestation of the pilosebaceous follicle. J Cutan Pathol 1983; 10: 257–261.

36 Burns DA. Follicle mites and their role in disease. Clin Exp Dermatol 1992; 17: 152–155.

37 Kanitakis J, Al-Rifai I, Faure M, Claudy A. Demodex mites of human skin express Tn but not T (Thomsen–Friedenreich) antigen immunoreactivity. J Cutan Pathol 1997; 24: 454–455.

38 Aydıngöz İE, Dervent B, Güney O. *Demodex folliculorum* in pregnancy. Int J Dermatol 2000; 39: 743–745.

39 Bonnar E, Eustace P, Powell FC. The *Demodex* mite population in rosacea. J Am Acad Dermatol 1993; 28: 443–448.

40 Forton F. Demodex-associated folliculitis. Am J Dermatopathol 1998; 20: 536–537.

41 Vollmer RT. Demodex-associated folliculitis. Am J Dermatopathol 1996; 18: 589–591.

42 Shelley WB, Shelley ED, Burmeister V. Unilateral demodectic rosacea. J Am Acad Dermatol 1989; 20: 915–917.

43 Hoekzema R, Hulsebosch HJ, Bos JD. Demodicidosis or rosacea: what did we treat? Br J Dermatol 1995; 133: 294–299.

44 Patrizi A, Neri I, Chieregato C, Misciali M. Demodicidosis in immunocompetent young children: report of eight cases. Dermatology 1997; 195: 239–242.

45 Forstinger C, Kittler H, Binder M. Treatment of rosacea-like demodicidosis with oral ivermectin and topical permethrin cream. J Am Acad Dermatol 1999; 41: 775–777.

46 Sahn EE, Sheridan DM. Demodicidosis in a child with leukemia. J Am Acad Dermatol 1992; 27: 799–801.

47 Ashack RJ, Frost ML, Norins AL. Papular pruritic eruption of *Demodex* folliculitis in patients with acquired immunodeficiency syndrome. J Am Acad Dermatol 1989; 21: 306–307.

48 Nakagawa T, Sasaki M, Fujita K et al. Demodex folliculitis on the trunk of a patient with mycosis fungoides. Clin Exp Dermatol 1996; 21: 148–150.

49 Sarro RA, Hong JJ, Elgart ML. An unusual demodicidosis manifestation in a patient with AIDS. J Am Acad Dermatol 1998; 38: 120–121.

50 Castanet J, Monpoux F, Mariani R et al. Demodicidosis in an immunodeficient child. Pediatr Dermatol 1997; 14: 219–220.

51 Jansen T, Kastner U, Kreuter A, Altmeyer P. Rosacea-like demodicidosis associated with acquired immunodeficiency syndrome. Br J Dermatol 2001; 144: 139–142.

52 Aydıngöz IE, Mansur T, Dervent B. *Demodex folliculorum* in renal transplant patients. Dermatology 1997; 195: 232–234.

53 Dominey A, Tschen J, Rosen T et al. Pityriasis folliculorum revisited. J Am Acad Dermatol 1989; 21: 81–84.

54 Hwang SM, Yoo MS, Ahn SK, Choi EH. Demodecidosis manifested on the external genitalia. Int J Dermatol 1998; 37: 634–636.

55 Fariña MC, Requena L, Sarasa JL et al. Spinulosis of the face as a manifestation of demodicidosis. Br J Dermatol 1998; 138: 901–903.

56 Orkin M, Maibach HI. Current concepts in parasitology: this scabies pandemic. N Engl J Med 1978; 298: 496–498.

57 Sadick N, Kaplan MH, Pahwra SG, Sarngadharan MG. Unusual features of scabies complicating human T-lymphotropic virus type III infection. J Am Acad Dermatol 1986; 15: 482–486.

58 Jucowics P, Ramon ME, Don PC et al. Norwegian scabies in an infant with acquired immunodeficiency syndrome. Arch Dermatol 1989; 125: 1670–1671.

59 Orkin M. Scabies in AIDS. Semin Dermatol 1993; 12: 9–14.

60 Chosidow O. Scabies and pediculosis. Lancet 2000; 355: 819–826.

61 Czelusta A, Yen-Moore A, Van der Straten M et al. An overview of sexually transmitted diseases. Part III. Sexually transmitted diseases in HIV-infected patients. J Am Acad Dermatol 2000; 43: 409–432.

62 Guggisberg D, de Viragh PA, Constantin Ch, Panizzon RG. Norwegian scabies in a patient with acquired immunodeficiency syndrome. Dermatology 1998; 197: 306–308.

63 Orkin M. Today's scabies. Arch Dermatol 1975; 111: 1431–1432.

64 Mimouni D, Gdalevich M, Mimouni FB et al. The epidemiologic trends of scabies among israeli soldiers: a 28-year follow-up. Int J Dermatol 1998; 37: 586–587.

65 Woodley D, Saurat JH. The Burrow Ink Test and the scabies mites. J Am Acad Dermatol 1981; 4: 715–722.

66 Argenziano G, Fabbrocini G, Delfino M. Epiluminescence microscopy. A new approach to in vivo detection of *Sarcoptes scabiei*. Arch Dermatol 1997; 133: 751–753.

67 Bezold G, Lange M, Schiener R et al. Hidden scabies: diagnosis by polymerase chain reaction. Br J Dermatol 2001; 144: 614–618.

68 Paller AS. Scabies in infants and small children. Semin Dermatol 1993; 12: 3–8.

69 Falk ES, Eide TJ. Histologic and clinical findings in human scabies. Int J Dermatol 1981; 20: 600–605.

70 Brenner S, Wolf R, Landau M. Scabid: an unusual id reaction to scabies. Int J Dermatol 1993; 32: 128–129.

71 Bhawan J, Milstone E, Malhotra R et al. Scabies presenting as bullous pemphigoid-like eruption. J Am Acad Dermatol 1991; 24: 179–181.

72 Sard S, Jay S, Kang J et al. Localized bullous scabies. Am J Dermatopathol 1993; 15: 590–593.

73 Ostlere LS, Harris D, Rustin MHA. Scabies associated with a bullous pemphigoid-like eruption. Br J Dermatol 1993; 128: 217–219.

74 Slawsky LD, Maroon M, Tyler WB, Miller OF III. Association of scabies with a bullous pemphigoid-like eruption. J Am Acad Dermatol 1996; 34: 878–879.

75 Konishi N, Suzuki K, Tokura Y et al. Bullous eruption associated with scabies: evidence for scabetic induction of true bullous pemphigoid. Acta Derm Venereol 2000; 80: 281–283.

76 Wolf R, Krakowski A. Atypical crusted scabies. J Am Acad Dermatol 1987; 17: 434–436.

77 Gach JE, Heagerty A. Crusted scabies looking like psoriasis. Lancet 2000; 356: 650.

78 Almond DS, Green CJ, Geurin DM, Evans S. Norwegian scabies misdiagnosed as an adverse drug reaction. BMJ 2000; 320: 35–36.

79 Hubler WR Jr, Clabaugh W. Epidemic Norwegian scabies. Arch Dermatol 1976; 112: 179–181.

80 Dick GF, Burgdorf WHC, Gentry WC Jr. Norwegian scabies in Bloom's syndrome. Arch Dermatol 1979; 115: 212–213.

81 Espy PD, Jolly HW Jr. Norwegian scabies. Occurrence in a patient undergoing immunosuppression. Arch Dermatol 1976; 112: 193–196.

82 Anolik MA, Rudolph RI. Scabies simulating Darier disease in an immunosuppressed host. Arch Dermatol 1976; 112: 73–74.

83 Barnes L, McCallister RE, Lucky AW. Crusted (Norwegian) scabies. Occurrence in a child undergoing a bone marrow transplant. Arch Dermatol 1987; 123: 95–97.

84 Magee KL, Hebert AA, Rapini RP. Crusted scabies in a patient with chronic graft-versus-host disease. J Am Acad Dermatol 1991; 25: 889–891.

85 Aricò M, Noto G, La Rocca E et al. Localized crusted scabies in the acquired immunodeficiency syndrome. Clin Exp Dermatol 1992; 17: 339–341.

86 Portu JJ, Santamaria JM, Zubero Z et al. Atypical scabies in HIV-positive patients. J Am Acad Dermatol 1996; 34: 915–917.

87 Farrell AM, Ross JS, Bunker CB, Staughton RCD. Crusted scabies with scalp involvement in HIV-1 infection. Br J Dermatol 1998; 138: 192–193.

88 Cestari SCP, Petri V, Rotta O, Alchorne MMA. Oral treatment of crusted scabies with ivermectin: report of two cases. Pediatr Dermatol 2000; 17: 410–414.

89 Judge MR, Kobza-Black A. Crusted scabies in pregnancy. Br J Dermatol 1995; 132: 116–119.

90 Van Der Wal VB, Van Voorst Vader PC, Mandema JM, Jonkman MF. Crusted (Norwegian) scabies in a patient with dystrophic epidermolysis bullosa. Br J Dermatol 1999; 141: 918–921.

91 Torrelo A, Zambrano A. Crusted scabies in a girl with epidermolysis bullosa simplex. Br J Dermatol 2000; 142: 197–198.

92 Estes SA, Estes J. Scabies research: another dimension. Semin Dermatol 1993; 12: 34–38.

93 Fain A. Epidemiological problems of scabies. Int J Dermatol 1978; 17: 20–30.

94 Arlian LG, Runyan RA, Estes SA. Cross infestivity of *Sarcoptes scabiei*. J Am Acad Dermatol 1984; 10: 979–986.

95 Dourmishev AL, Serafimova DK, Dourmishev LA et al. Crusted scabies of the scalp in dermatomyositis patients: three cases treated with oral ivermectin. Int J Dermatol 1998; 37: 231–234.

96 Usha V, Nair TVG. A comparative study of oral ivermectin and topical permethrin cream in the treatment of scabies. J Am Acad Dermatol 2000; 42: 236–240.

97 van Neste D, Lachapelle JM. Host–parasite relationships in hyperkeratotic (Norwegian) scabies: pathological and immunological findings. Br J Dermatol 1981; 105: 667–678.

98 Falk ES, Bolle R. *In vitro* demonstration of specific immunological hypersensitivity to scabies mite. Br J Dermatol 1980; 103: 367–373.

99 Cabrera R, Agar A, Dahl MV. The immunology of scabies. Semin Dermatol 1993; 12: 15–21.

100 Van Neste DJJ. Human scabies in perspective. Int J Dermatol 1988; 27: 10–15.

101 Shindo K, Kono T, Kitajima J-I, Hamada T. Crusted scabies in acquired selective IgA deficiency. Acta Derm Venereol 1991; 71: 250–251.

102 Frentz G, Keien NK, Eriksen K. Immunofluorescence studies in scabies. J Cutan Pathol 1977; 4: 191–193.

103 Hoefling KK, Schroeter AL. Dermatoimmunopathology of scabies. J Am Acad Dermatol 1980; 3: 237–240.

104 Reunala T, Ranki A, Rantanen T, Salo OP. Inflammatory cells in skin lesions of scabies. Clin Exp Dermatol 1984; 9: 70–77.

105 Hejazi N, Mehregan AH. Scabies. Histological study of inflammatory lesions. Arch Dermatol 1975; 111: 37–39.

106 Amer M, Mostafa FF, Nasr AN, El-Harras M. The role of mast cells in treatment of scabies. Int J Dermatol 1995; 34: 186–189.

107 Seraly MP, Shockman J, Jacoby RA. Flame figures in scabies: a case report. Arch Dermatol 1991; 127: 1850–1851.

108 Jarrett P, Snow J. Scabies presenting as a necrotizing vasculitis in the presence of lupus anticoagulant. Br J Dermatol 1998; 139: 701–703.

109 Fernandez N, Torres A, Ackerman AB. Pathologic findings in human scabies. Arch Dermatol 1977; 113: 320–324.

110 Head ES, Macdonald EM, Ewert A, Apisarnthanarax P. *Sarcoptes scabiei* in histopathologic sections of skin in human scabies. Arch Dermatol 1990; 126: 1475–1477.

111 Walton S, Bottomley WW, Wyatt EH, Bury HPR. Pseudo T-cell lymphoma due to scabies in a patient with Hodgkin's disease. Br J Dermatol 1991; 124: 277–278.

112 Thomson J, Cochrane T, Cochran R, McQueen A. Histology simulating reticulosis in persistent nodular scabies. Br J Dermatol 1974; 90: 421–429.

113 Liu H-N, Sheu W-J, Chu T-L. Scabietic nodules: a dermatopathologic and immunofluorescent study. J Cutan Pathol 1992; 19: 124–127.

114 Lee BW. *Cheyletiella* dermatitis. Arch Dermatol 1981; 117: 677–678.

115 Millikan LE. Mite infestations other than scabies. Semin Dermatol 1993; 12: 46–52.

116 Paradis M. Mite dermatitis caused by *Cheyletiella blakei*. J Am Acad Dermatol 1998; 38: 1014–1015.

117 Cohen SR. *Cheyletiella* dermatitis. A mite infestation of rabbit, cat, dog, and man. Arch Dermatol 1980; 116: 435–437.

118 Wagner R, Stallmeister N. *Cheyletiella* dermatitis in humans, dogs and cats. Br J Dermatol 2000; 143: 1110–1112.

119 Powell RF, Palmer SM, Palmer CH, Smith EB. Cheyletiella dermatitis. Int J Dermatol 1977; 16: 679–682.

120 Rivers JK, Martin J, Pukay B. Walking dandruff and *Cheyletiella* dermatitis. J Am Acad Dermatol 1986; 15: 1130–1133.

121 Ackerman AB. Histologic diagnosis of inflammatory skin diseases. Philadelphia: Lea & Febiger, 1978; 184.

122 Maurice PDL, Schofield O, Griffiths WAD. Cheyletiella dermatitis: a case report and the role of specific immunological hypersensitivity in its pathogenesis. Clin Exp Dermatol 1987; 12: 381–384.

123 Uenotsuchi T, Satoh E, Kiryu H, Yano Y. *Pyemotes* dermatitis caused by indirect contact with husk rice. Br J Dermatol 2000; 143: 680–682.

124 Hewitt M, Barrow GI, Miller DC et al. Mites in the personal environment and their role in skin disorders. Br J Dermatol 1973; 89: 401–409.

125 Aylesworth R. Feather pillow dermatitis caused by an unusual mite, *Dermatophagoides scheremetewskyi*. J Am Acad Dermatol 1985; 13: 680–681.

126 Theis J, Lavoipierre MM, La Perriere R, Kroese H. Tropical rat mite dermatitis. Arch Dermatol 1981; 117: 341–343.

127 Chung SL, Hwang SJ, Kwon SB et al. Outbreak of rat mite dermatitis in medical students. Int J Dermatol 1998; 37: 591–594.

128 Burns DA. Papular urticaria produced by the mite *Listrophorus gibbus*. Clin Exp Dermatol 1987; 12: 200–201.

129 Schulze KE, Cohen PR. Dove-associated gamasoidosis: a case of avian mite dermatitis. J Am Acad Dermatol 1994; 30: 278–280.

130 Uesugi Y, Aiba S, Suetake T, Tagami H. Multiple infestations with avian mites within a family. Int J Dermatol 1994; 33: 566–567.

131 Orton DI, Warren LJ, Wilkinson JD. Avian mite dermatitis. Clin Exp Dermatol 2000; 25: 129–131.

132 Lucky AW, Sayers CP, Argus JD, Lucky A. Avian mite bites acquired from a new source – pet gerbils. Arch Dermatol 2001; 137: 167–170.

133 Yates VM. Harvest mites – a present from the Lake District. Clin Exp Dermatol 1991; 16: 277–278.

Insects

134 Gillis D, Slepon R, Karsenty E, Green M. Seasonality and long-term trends of pediculosis capitis and pubis in a young adult population. Arch Dermatol 1990; 126: 638–641.

135 Mumcuoglu KY, Klaus S, Kafka D et al. Clinical observations related to head lice infestation. J Am Acad Dermatol 1991; 25: 248–251.

136 Chouela E, Abeldaño A, Cirigliano M et al. Head louse infestations: epidemiologic survey and treatment evaluation in Argentinian schoolchildren. Int J Dermatol 1997; 36: 819–825.

137 de Berker D, Sinclair R. Getting ahead of head lice. Australas J Dermatol 2000; 41: 209–212.

138 Burns DA, Sims TA. A closer look at *Pthirus pubis*. Br J Dermatol 1988; 118: 497–503.

139 Gartmann H, Dickmans-Burmeister D. Phthiri im Bereich der Kopfhaare. Hautarzt 1970; 21: 279–281.

140 Parish LC, Witkowski JA. The saga of ectoparasitoses: scabies and pediculosis. Int J Dermatol 1999; 38: 432–433.

141 Miller RAW. Maculae ceruleae. Int J Dermatol 1986; 25: 383–384.

142 Burkhart CN, Gunning W, Burkhart CG. Scanning electron microscopic examination of the egg of the pubic louse (Anoplura: *Pthirus pubis*). Int J Dermatol 2000; 39: 201–202.

143 Crissey JT. Bedbugs. An old problem with a new dimension. Int J Dermatol 1981; 20: 411–414.

144 Tharakaram S. Bullous eruption due to *Cimex lecticularis*. Clin Exp Dermatol 1999; 24: 241–242.

145 Grogan TM, Payne CM, Payne TB et al. Cutaneous myiasis. Am J Dermatopathol 1987; 9: 232–239.

146 Lane RP, Lovell CR, Griffiths WAD, Sonnex TS. Human cutaneous myiasis – a review and report of three cases due to *Dermatobia hominis*. Clin Exp Dermatol 1987; 12: 40–45.

147 Lukin LG. Human cutaneous myiasis in Brisbane: a prospective study. Med J Aust 1989; 150: 237–240.

148 Dondero TJ Jr, Schaffner W, Athanasiou R, Maguire W. Cutaneous myiasis in visitors to Central America. South Med J 1979; 72: 1508–1511.

149 Sauder DN, Hall RP, Wurster CF. Dermal myiasis: the porcine lipid cure. Arch Dermatol 1981; 117: 681–682.

150 Poindexter HA. Cutaneous myiasis. Arch Dermatol 1979; 115: 235.

151 Rubel DM, Walder BK, Jopp-McKay A, Rosen R. Dermal myiasis in an Australian traveller. Australas J Dermatol 1993; 34: 45–47.

152 Arosemena R, Booth SA, Su WPD. Cutaneous myiasis. J Am Acad Dermatol 1993; 28: 254–256.

153 Gordon PM, Hepburn NC, Williams AE, Bunney MH. Cutaneous myiasis due to *Dermatobia hominis*: a report of six cases. Br J Dermatol 1995; 132: 811–814.

154 Tsuda S, Nagaji J, Kurose K et al. Furuncular cutaneous myiasis caused by *Dermatobia hominis* larvae following travel to Brazil. Int J Dermatol 1996; 35: 121–123.

155 Veraldi S, Gorani A, Süss L, Tadini G. Cutaneous myiasis caused by *Dermatobia hominis*. Pediatr Dermatol 1998; 15: 116–118.

156 Gunther S. Furuncular Tumbu fly myiasis of man in Gabon, Equatorial Africa. J Trop Med Hyg 1967; 70: 169–174.

157 Ockenhouse CF, Samlaska CP, Benson PM et al. Cutaneous myiasis caused by the African tumbu fly (*Cordylobia anthropophaga*). Arch Dermatol 1990; 126: 199–202.

158 Lodi A, Bruscagin C, Gianni C et al. Myiasis due to *Cordylobia anthropophaga* (Tumbu-fly). Int J Dermatol 1994; 33: 127–128.

159 Ng SOC, Yates M. Cutaneous myiasis in a traveller returning from Africa. Australas J Dermatol 1997; 38: 38–39.

160 Geary MJ, Hudson BJ, Russell RC, Hardy A. Exotic myiasis with Lund's fly (*Cordylobia rodhaini*). Med J Aust 1999; 171: 654–655.

161 Petersen CS, Zachariae C. Acute balanoposthitis caused by infestation with *Cordylobia anthropophaga*. Acta Derm Venereol 1999; 79: 170.

162 Hasegawa M, Harada T, Kojima Y et al. An important case of furuncular myiasis due to *Cordylobia anthropophaga* which emerged in Japan. Br J Dermatol 2000; 143: 912–914.

163 Burgess I, Spraggs PDR. Myiasis due to *Parasarcophaga argyrostoma* – first recorded case in Britain. Clin Exp Dermatol 1992; 17: 261–263.

164 Jelinek T, Nothdurft HD, Rieder N, Loscher T. Cutaneous myiasis: review of 13 cases in travelers returning from tropical countries. Int J Dermatol 1995; 34: 624–626.

165 Starr J, Pruett JH, Yunginger JW, Gleich GJ. Myiasis due to *Hypoderma lineatum* infection mimicking the hypereosinophilic syndrome. Mayo Clin Proc 2000; 75: 755–759.

166 Newell GB. Dermal myiasis caused by the rabbit botfly (*Cuterebra* sp). Arch Dermatol 1979; 115: 101.

167 Baird JK, Baird CR, Sabrosky CW. North American cuterebrid myiasis. Report of seventeen new infections of human beings and review of the disease. J Am Acad Dermatol 1989; 21: 763–772.

168 Schiff TA. Furuncular cutaneous myiasis caused by *Cuterebra* larva. J Am Acad Dermatol 1993; 28: 261–263.

169 Kron MA. Human infestation with *Cochliomyia hominivorax*, the New World screwworm. J Am Acad Dermatol 1992; 27: 264–265.

170 Victoria J, Trujillo R, Barreto M. Myiasis: a successful treatment with topical ivermectin. Int J Dermatol 1999; 38: 142–144.

171 Kumarasinghe SPW, Karunaweera ND, Ihalamulla RL. A study of cutaneous myiasis in Sri Lanka. Int J Dermatol 2000; 39: 689–694.

172 Delir S, Handjani F, Emad M, Ardehali S. Vulvar myiasis due to *Wohlfahrtia magnifica*. Clin Exp Dermatol 1999; 24: 279–280.

173 Logan JCP, Walkey M. A case of endemic cutaneous myiasis. Br J Dermatol 1964; 76: 218–222.

174 Burgess I, Davies EA. Cutaneous myiasis caused by the housefly, *Musca domestica*. Br J Dermatol 1991; 125: 377–379.

175 García-Doval I, de la Torre C, Losada A et al. Subungual myiasis. Acta Derm Venereol 2000; 80: 236.

176 Guillozet N. Erosive myiasis. Arch Dermatol 1981; 117: 59–60.

177 File TM, Thomson RB, Tan JS. *Dermatobia hominis* dermal myiasis. Arch Dermatol 1985; 121: 1195–1196.

178 Swetter SM, Stewart MI, Smoller BR. Cutaneous myiasis following travel to Belize. Int J Dermatol 1996; 35: 118–120.

179 Baker DJ, Kantor GR, Stierstorfer MB, Brady G. Furuncular myiasis from *Dermatobia hominis* infestation. Diagnosis by light microscopy. Am J Dermatopathol 1995; 17: 389–394.

180 Norwood C, Smith KJ, Neafie R, Skelton H. Are cutaneous reactions to fly larvae mediated by CD1-restricted T cells? J Cutan Pathol 2000; 27: 567 (abstract).

181 Goldman L. Tungiasis in travelers from tropical Africa. JAMA 1976; 236: 1386.

182 Sanusi ID, Brown EB, Shepard TG, Grafton WD. Tungiasis: Report of one case and review of the 14 reported cases in the United States. J Am Acad Dermatol 1989; 20: 941–944.

183 Burke WA, Jones BE, Park HK, Finley JL. Imported tungiasis. Int J Dermatol 1991; 30: 881–883.

184 De Carvalho Bezerra SM. Tungiasis – an unusual case of severe infestation. Int J Dermatol 1994; 33: 725.

185 Campos Macías P, Méndez Sashida P. Cutaneous infestation by *Tunga penetrans*. Int J Dermatol 2000; 39: 296–298.

186 Mashek H, Licznerski B, Pincus S. Tungiasis in New York. Int J Dermatol 1997; 36: 276–278.

187 Gelmetti C, Carrera C, Veraldi S. Tungiasis in a 3-year-old child. Pediatr Dermatol 2000; 17: 293–295.

188 Grunwald MH, Shai A, Mosovich B, Avinoach I. Tungiasis. Australas J Dermatol 2000; 41: 46–47.

189 Veraldi S, Carrera C, Schianchi R. Tungiasis has reached Europe. Dermatology 2000; 201: 382.

190 Zalar GL, Walther RR. Infestation by *Tunga penetrans*. Arch Dermatol 1980; 116: 80–81.

191 Wentzell JM, Schwartz BK, Pesce JR. Tungiasis. J Am Acad Dermatol 1986; 15: 117–119.

192 Tokura Y, Tamura Y, Takigawa M et al. Severe hypersensitivity to mosquito bites associated with natural killer cell lymphocytosis. Arch Dermatol 1990; 126: 362–368.

193 Steffen C. Clinical and histopathologic correlation of midge bites. Arch Dermatol 1981; 117: 785–787.

194 Smith KJ, Skelton HG III, Vogel P et al. Exaggerated insect bite reactions in patients positive for HIV. J Am Acad Dermatol 1993; 29: 269–272.

195 Rustin MHA, Munro DD. Papular urticaria caused by *Dermestes maculatus Degeer*. Clin Exp Dermatol 1984; 9: 317–321.

196 Kerdel-Vegas F, Goihman-Yahr M. *Paederus* dermatitis. Arch Dermatol 1966; 94: 175–185.

197 Borroni G, Brazzelli V, Rosso R, Pavan M. *Paederus fuscipes* dermatitis. A histopathological study. Am J Dermatopathol 1991; 13: 467–474.

198 Banney LA, Wood DJ, Francis GD. Whiplash rove beetle dermatitis in central Queensland. Australas J Dermatol 2000; 41: 162–167.

199 Samlaska CP, Samuelson GA, Faran ME, Shparago NI. Blister beetle dermatosis in Hawaii caused by *Thelyphassa apicata* (Fairmaire). Pediatr Dermatol 1992; 9: 246–250.

200 Veraldi S, Süss L. Dermatitis caused by *Paederus fuscipes Curt.* Int J Dermatol 1994; 33: 277–278.

201 Kamaladasa SD, Perera WDH, Weeratunge L. An outbreak of paederus dermatitis in a suburban hospital in Sri Lanka. Int J Dermatol 1997; 36: 34–36.

202 Henwood BP, MacDonald DM. Caterpillar dermatitis. Clin Exp Dermatol 1983; 8: 77–93.

203 Garty BZ, Danon YL. Processionary caterpillar dermatitis. Pediatr Dermatol 1985; 2: 194–196.

204 Allen VT, Miller OF III, Tyler WB. Gypsy moth caterpillar dermatitis – revisited. J Am Acad Dermatol 1991; 24: 979–981.

205 Dinehart SM, Archer ME, Wolf JE et al. Caripito itch: dermatitis from contact with *Hyselia* moths. J Am Acad Dermatol 1985; 13: 743–747.

206 O'Hehir RE, Douglass JA. Stinging insect allergy. Safe, effective immunotherapy is available. Med J Aust 1999; 171: 649–650.

207 Brown M, Hebert AA. Insect repellents: An overview. J Am Acad Dermatol 1997; 36: 243–249.

208 Altchek DD, Kurtin SB. An unusual histopathologic response to an insect bite. Cutis 1980; 25: 169–170.

209 Allen AC. Persistent "insect bites" (dermal eosinophilic granulomas) simulating lymphoblastomas, histiocytoses, and squamous cell carcinomas. Am J Pathol 1948; 24: 367–387.

210 Kolbusz RV, Micetich K, Armin A-R, Massa MC. Exaggerated response to insect bites. An unusual cutaneous manifestation of chronic lymphocytic leukemia. Int J Dermatol 1989; 28: 186–187.

211 Davis MDP, Perniciaro C, Dahl PR et al. Exaggerated arthropod-bite lesions in patients with chronic lymphocytic leukemia: A clinical, histopathologic, and immunopathologic study of eight patients. J Am Acad Dermatol 1998; 39: 27–35.

212 Barzilai A, Shpiro D, Goldberg I et al. Insect bite-like reaction in patients with hematologic malignant neoplasms. Arch Dermatol 1999; 135: 1503–1507.

Tumors

Tumors of the epidermis

INTRODUCTION

Tumors of the epidermis are a histopathologically diverse group of entities which have in common a localized proliferation of keratinocytes resulting in a clinically discrete lesion. They may be divided into a number of categories, reflecting their different biological behaviors. These include hamartomas (epidermal nevi), reactive hyperplasias (pseudoepitheliomatous hyperplasia), and benign tumors (acanthomas), as well as premalignant, in situ and invasive carcinomas. There is a tendency in some countries to regard the epidermal dysplasias as squamous cell carcinoma in situ and to include keratoacanthoma as a variant of squamous cell carcinoma despite its different biological potential.

EPIDERMAL AND OTHER NEVI

Some authors use the term 'epithelial nevus' or 'epidermal nevus' as a group generic term to cover malformations of adnexal epithelium, as well as those involving the epidermis alone.[1,2] The term 'epidermal nevus' is used here in a restricted sense and does not include organoid, sebaceous, eccrine and pilar nevi. These are considered with the appendageal tumors in Chapter 33. An exception has been made for nevus comedonicus, an abnormality of the infundibulum of the hair follicle. It is considered here because its histological appearance suggests an abnormality of the epidermis, rather than of appendages. Furthermore, the report of the coexistence of nevus comedonicus and an epidermal nevus suggests that the two entities are closely related.[3]

EPIDERMAL NEVUS

An epidermal nevus is a developmental malformation of the epidermis in which an excess of keratinocytes, sometimes showing abnormal maturation, results in a visible lesion with a variety of clinical and histological patterns.[4] Such lesions are of early onset, with a predilection for the neck, trunk and extremities.[5,6] There may be one only, or a few small warty brown or pale plaques may be present. At other times the nevus takes the form of a linear or zosteriform lesion, or just a slightly scaly area of discoloration.[4,7,8] Various terms have been applied, not always in a consistent manner, to the different clinical patterns.[8] The term 'nevus verrucosus' has been used for localized wart-like variants,[9] and 'nevus unius lateris' for long, linear, usually unilateral lesions on the extremities. 'Ichthyosis hystrix' refers to large, often disfiguring nevi with a bilateral distribution on the trunk.[10,11]

Various tumors have been reported arising in epidermal nevi, as a rare complication. These include basal cell[12] and squamous cell carcinomas[13–15] as well as a keratoacanthoma.[16] Verrucous epidermal nevus (nevus verrucosus) has been reported in association with an organoid nevus (nevus sebaceus).[17]

The term 'epidermal nevus syndrome' refers to the association of epidermal nevi with neurological, ocular and skeletal abnormalities, such as epilepsy, mental retardation, cataracts, kyphoscoliosis and limb hypertrophy; there may also be cutaneous hemangiomas.[2,18–26] There are potentially many different epidermal nevus syndromes based on variable genetic mosaicism.[6,27,28] Systemic cancers of various types may arise at a young age in those with the syndrome.[29,30] The epidermal nevi, which are often particularly extensive in patients with the syndrome, may be of any histological type.[31–33] Epidermal nevi have also been reported in association with polyostotic fibrous dysplasia[34] and the Proteus syndrome, a very rare disorder with various mesodermal malformations.[35–39]

Histopathology

At least 10 different histological patterns have been found in epidermal nevi (Figs 31.1, 31.2).[4,8] More than one such pattern may be present in a given example. In over 60% of cases the pattern is that of hyperkeratosis, with papillomatosis of relatively flat and broad type, together with acanthosis. There is thickening of the granular layer and often a slight increase in basal melanin pigment. This is the so-called 'common type' of epidermal nevus.

Less frequently the histological pattern resembles acrokeratosis verruciformis, epidermolytic hyperkeratosis or seborrheic keratosis.[4,8] Epidermal nevi with a seborrheic keratosis-like pattern often have thin, elongated rete ridges with 'flat bottoms', a feature not usually seen in seborrheic keratoses. Rare patterns include the verrucoid, porokeratotic, focal acantholytic dyskeratotic,[40–43] acanthosis nigricans-like,[44] Hailey–Hailey disease-like[45] and the incontinentia pigmenti-like (verrucous phase) variants.[46] A lichenoid inflammatory infiltrate has also been reported in an epidermal nevus, although usually the dermis is devoid of inflammatory cells.[47] Inflammatory linear verrucous epidermal nevus and nevus comedonicus are regarded as distinct entities, although they are sometimes included as histological patterns of epidermal nevus.

The epidermis overlying an organoid nevus (see p. 899) frequently will show the histological picture of an epidermal nevus. In such cases this is usually of the common type.

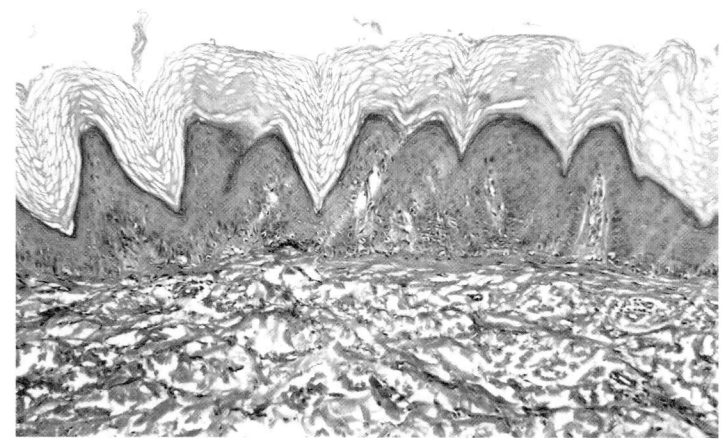

Fig. 31.1 **Epidermal nevus.** There is papillomatosis and acanthosis with overlying laminated hyperkeratosis. (H & E)

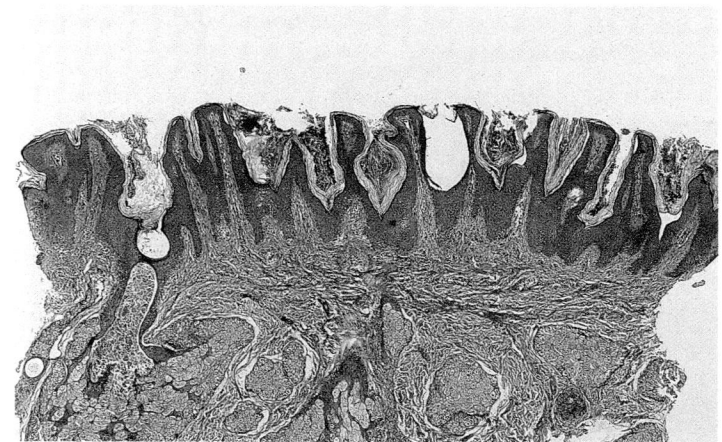

Fig. 31.2 **Epidermal nevus.** This variant resembles acanthosis nigricans. (H & E)

INFLAMMATORY LINEAR VERRUCOUS EPIDERMAL NEVUS

Also known by the acronym of ILVEN, inflammatory linear verrucous epidermal nevus is a specific clinicopathological subgroup of epidermal nevi which most often presents as a pruritic linear eruption on the lower extremities.[2,48–52] The lesions are usually arranged along the lines of Blaschko.[53] The condition is of early onset. Asymptomatic variants and widespread bilateral distribution have been reported.[54,55] ILVEN has been described in association with the epidermal nevus syndrome (see above)[56] and in a burn scar.[57]

The lesions resemble linear psoriasis both clinically and histologically; in this context it must be noted that the existence of a linear form of psoriasis has been questioned.[58] Interestingly, the epidermal fibrous protein isolated from the scale in ILVEN is different from that found in psoriasis.[59,60]

Histopathology

There is psoriasiform epidermal hyperplasia with overlying areas of parakeratosis, alternating with orthokeratosis. Beneath the orthokeratotic areas of hyperkeratosis there is hypergranulosis, often with a depressed cup-like appearance; the parakeratosis overlies areas of agranulosis of the upper epidermis.[61] The zones of parakeratosis are usually much broader than in psoriasis. Focal mild spongiosis with some exocytosis and even vesiculation may be seen in some lesions.[62] There is also a mild perivascular lymphocytic infiltrate in the upper dermis. A dense lichenoid infiltrate was present in one case, perhaps representing the attempted immunological regression of the lesion.[63]

The immunohistochemical features of this lesion differ from those found in epidermal nevi.[64] This may simply be a reflection of the inflammatory component of ILVEN.

NEVUS COMEDONICUS

Nevus comedonicus (comedo nevus) is a rare abnormality of the infundibulum of the hair follicle in which grouped or linear comedonal papules develop at any time from birth to middle age.[65–67] They are usually restricted to one side of the body, particularly the face, trunk and neck.[68–70] Rare clinical presentations have included penile,[71] palmar,[72–74] bilateral[75] and verrucous lesions.[72] Rarely, abnormalities of other systems are present, indicating that a nevus comedonicus syndrome, akin to the epidermal nevus syndrome, may occur.[76–79] Inflammation of the lesions is an important complication, resulting in scarring.[75,80,81]

Histopathology[82]

There are dilated keratin-filled invaginations of the epidermis. An atrophic sebaceous or pilar structure sometimes opens into the lower pole of the invagination.[82] A small lanugo hair is occasionally present in the keratinous material.

Inflammation and subsequent dermal scarring are a feature in some cases. A tricholemmal cyst has also been reported arising in a comedo nevus.[83]

The epithelial invagination in some cases of palmar involvement has opened into a recognizable eccrine duct.[73,84] Cornoid lamellae have also been present.[85–87] It has been suggested that these are cases of eccrine hamartomas, akin to nevus comedonicus and unrelated to porokeratosis.[88]

Rare histological patterns associated with comedo nevus-like lesions have included a basal cell nevus,[89] a linear variant with underlying tumors of sweat gland origin,[90] and a variant with epidermolytic hyperkeratosis in the wall of the invaginations.[91] Epithelial proliferation, resembling that seen in the dilated pore of Winer, has been noted.[92] A form with dyskeratosis, accompanied often by acantholysis in the wall, is regarded as a distinct entity – familial dyskeratotic comedones (see below).

FAMILIAL DYSKERATOTIC COMEDONES

Familial dyskeratotic comedones is a rare autosomal dominant condition in which multiple comedones develop in childhood or adolescence, sometimes in association with acne.[93–96] Sites of involvement include the trunk and extremities and, uncommonly, the palms and soles, the scrotum and the penis.[93,97] This entity appears to be distinct from nevus comedonicus, and also from the rare condition of familial comedones.[98,99]

Histopathology[94,97]

A follicle-like invagination in the epidermis is filled with laminated keratinous material. Dyskeratotic cells are present in the wall of the invagination, particularly in the base. This is associated with acantholysis, which may, however, be mild or inapparent.[94]

PSEUDOEPITHELIOMATOUS HYPERPLASIA

Pseudoepitheliomatous (pseudocarcinomatous) hyperplasia is a histopathological reaction pattern rather than a disease sui generis.[100–102] It is characterized by irregular hyperplasia of the epidermis which also involves follicular infundibula and acrosyringia.[100,103] This proliferation occurs in response to a wide range of stimuli comprising chronic irritation, including around urostomy and colostomy sites,[104] trauma, cryotherapy, chronic lymphedema, and various dermal inflammatory processes such as chromomycosis, sporotrichosis, aspergillosis, pyodermas and actinomycosis.[101,102,105,106] Pseudoepitheliomatous hyperplasia has recently been reported in the chronic verrucous lesions that develop in immunocompromised patients who develop herpes zoster/varicella infection (see p. 699). It may also develop in the halogenodermas and in association with chondrodermatitis nodularis helicis,[107] Spitz nevi, malignant melanomas, overlying granular cell tumors and cutaneous T-cell lymphomas.[108] The term 'pseudorecidivism' has been used for the pseudoepitheliomatous hyperplasia that sometimes develops a few weeks after treatment, by various methods,[109] of a cutaneous tumor.

On microscopic examination there are prominent, somewhat bulbous, acanthotic downgrowths which in many instances represent expanded follicular infundibula.[100] The hyperplasia is not as regular as that seen in psoriasiform hyperplasia. The cells have abundant cytoplasm, which is sometimes pale staining. Unlike squamous cell carcinoma there are few mitoses and only minimal cytological atypia. Aneuploidy is present in a small number of cases.[110] Where the process overlies dermal inflammation, transepidermal elimination of the inflammatory debris may occur, resulting in intraepidermal microabscesses.

In addition to those conditions already mentioned, pseudoepitheliomatous hyperplasia occurs in granuloma fissuratum and prurigo nodularis: these conditions are discussed below.

GRANULOMA FISSURATUM

Granuloma fissuratum[111] (acanthoma fissuratum,[112] spectacle-frame acanthoma[113]) is a firm, flesh-colored or pink nodule with a grooved central depression which develops at the site of focal pressure and friction from poorly fitting prostheses such as spectacles.[112,114] Accordingly, such lesions are found on the lateral aspect of the bridge of the nose near the inner canthus,[115] in the retroauricular region[111] and, rarely, on the cheeks.

A similar lesion develops in the mouth as a result of poorly fitting dentures. The lesions are painful or tender and they may ulcerate. Clinically they resemble basal cell carcinomas, although the central groove corresponding to the point of contact with the spectacle frame usually allows a correct diagnosis to be made.[116] Lesions heal within weeks of correction of the ill-fitting prosthesis.

Histopathology[111,113]

The lesion is characterized by marked acanthosis of the epidermis with broad and elongated rete pegs (Fig. 31.3). There is a central depression, corresponding with the groove noted macroscopically, and here the epidermis is attenuated and sometimes ulcerated. There is mild hyperkeratosis and often a prominent granular layer overlying the acanthotic epidermis; there may be parakeratosis and mild spongiosis in the region of the groove or adjacent to it.

The dermis shows telangiectasia of the small blood vessels with an accompanying chronic inflammatory cell infiltrate, which is usually mild and patchy. The infiltrate includes plasma cells, lymphocytes and some histiocytes. There is focal fibroblastic activity and focal dermal fibrosis, with mild hyalinization of collagen beneath the groove. There may be mild edema of the superficial dermis.

PRURIGO NODULARIS

Prurigo nodularis is an uncommon disorder in which there are usually numerous persistent, intensely pruritic nodules. They involve predominantly the extensor aspects of the limbs, often symmetrically, but they may also develop on the trunk, face, scalp and neck.[117–120] The nodules are firm, pink, and sometimes verrucous or focally excoriated. They are approximately 5–12 mm in diameter and range from few in number to over 100.[117] Solitary lesions also occur. The intervening skin may be normal or xerotic; sometimes there is a lichenified eczema.[117] There may be an underlying cause for the pruritus, such as a metabolic disorder, bites, folliculitis, the pruritic eruption of HIV infection[121,122] or atopic state.[117,123] Mycobacteria have been cultured from, or demonstrated in, tissue sections in nearly one-quarter of cases in one study.[124] The significance of this finding is uncertain; it has not been

confirmed. The tretinoin derivative etretinate, used in the treatment of a range of skin conditions, has been incriminated in several cases.[125] Stress is sometimes a factor. Prurigo nodularis is regarded by some authors as an exaggerated form of lichen simplex chronicus (see p. 86).

Capsaicin, an alkaloid which interferes with the perception of pruritus and pain by depletion of neuropeptides in small sensory nerves in the skin, has been used successfully in the treatment of prurigo nodularis.[126]

Histopathology[117,127]

There is prominent hyperkeratosis, often focal parakeratosis, and marked irregular acanthosis that often is of pseudoepitheliomatous proportions (Fig. 31.4). Sometimes the hyperplasia is more regular and vaguely psoriasiform in type. There may be pinpoint ulceration from excoriation. Mitoses are usually increased among the keratinocytes. A hair follicle is often present in the center of each acanthotic downgrowth (Fig. 31.5).[128]

The upper dermis shows an increase in small blood vessels, and there is often an increase in the numbers of dermal fibroblasts, some of which may be stellate. There are usually fine collagen bundles in a vertical orientation in the papillary dermis. The arrectores pilorum muscles may be prominent. A syringomatous proliferation of eccrine sweat ducts is a rare finding.[129] The inflammatory cell infiltrate in the dermis is usually only mild and includes lymphocytes, mast cells, histiocytes, and sometimes eosinophils. Extracellular deposition of eosinophil granule protein is usually present.[130] Epidermal mast cells and Merkel cells may be seen.[127,131] The mast cells are increased in size and become more dendritic.[132] They are seen in close vicinity to nerves which functionally express increased amounts of nerve growth factor receptor (NGFr).[132]

Hypertrophy and proliferation of dermal nerve fibers has been emphasized by most,[133–136] but it was not a prominent feature in two large series of cases.[127,137] Small neuroid nodules with numerous Schwann cells have been reported in the dermis.[138,139] Immunohistochemistry has revealed that calcitonin gene-related peptide (CGRP) is expressed in increased amounts in nerve fibers in prurigo nodularis; this may be of significance in the recruitment of eosinophils and mast cells into lesional tissue.[140]

Electron microscopy

There is an increase in cutaneous nerves in some cases[138] and vacuolization of the cytoplasm of Schwann cells.[127,141] Myelinated nerves may show various degrees of demyelination.[141]

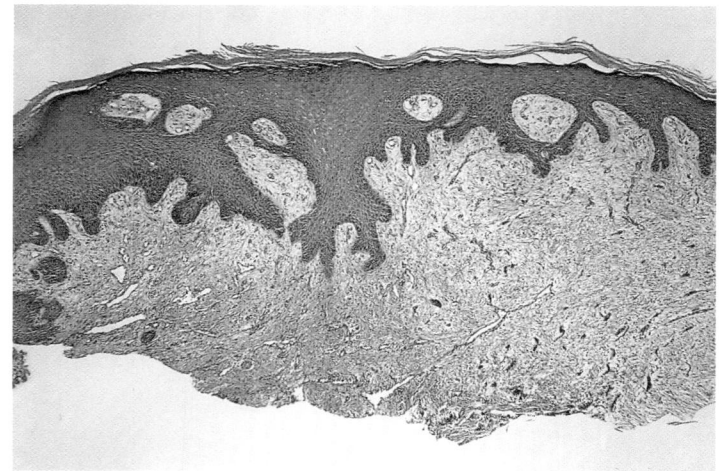

Fig. 31.3 **Granuloma fissuratum.** There is focal pseudoepitheliomatous hyperplasia. (H & E)

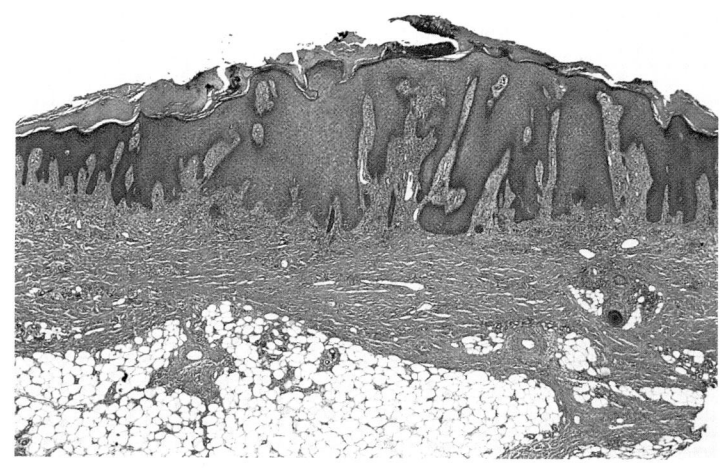

Fig. 31.4 **Prurigo nodularis.** There is marked pseudoepitheliomatous hyperplasia. (H & E)

EPIDERMOLYTIC ACANTHOMA

Epidermolytic acanthoma is an uncommon lesion which may be solitary, resembling a wart, or multiple. It shows the histopathological changes of epidermolytic hyperkeratosis and is therefore considered in Chapter 9 with other lesions showing this disorder of epidermal maturation and keratinization (see p. 294).

WARTY DYSKERATOMA

Warty dyskeratomas are rare, usually solitary, papulonodular lesions with a predilection for the head and neck of middle-aged and elderly individuals (see p. 299). They show suprabasilar clefting, with numerous acantholytic and dyskeratotic cells within the cleft and an overlying keratinous plug.

ACANTHOLYTIC ACANTHOMA

Acantholytic acanthoma is a solitary tumor with a predilection for the trunk of older individuals.[143,144] It usually presents as an asymptomatic keratotic papule or nodule. Multiple lesions have been reported in a renal transplant recipient.[145]

Histopathology[143]

The features include variable hyperkeratosis, papillomatosis and acanthosis, together with prominent acantholysis, most often involving multiple levels of the epidermis (Fig. 31.6). There is sometimes suprabasilar or subcorneal cleft formation, but there is no dyskeratosis. The pattern resembles that seen in pemphigus or Hailey–Hailey disease, but there has been no evidence of these diseases in the cases reported.

SEBORRHEIC KERATOSIS

Seborrheic keratoses (senile warts, basal cell papillomas) are common, often multiple, benign tumors which usually first appear in middle life.[146,147] They may occur on any part of the body except the palms and soles, although there is a predilection for the chest, interscapular region, waistline and forehead. Seborrheic keratoses are sharply demarcated gray-brown to black lesions, which are slightly raised. They may be covered with greasy scales. Most

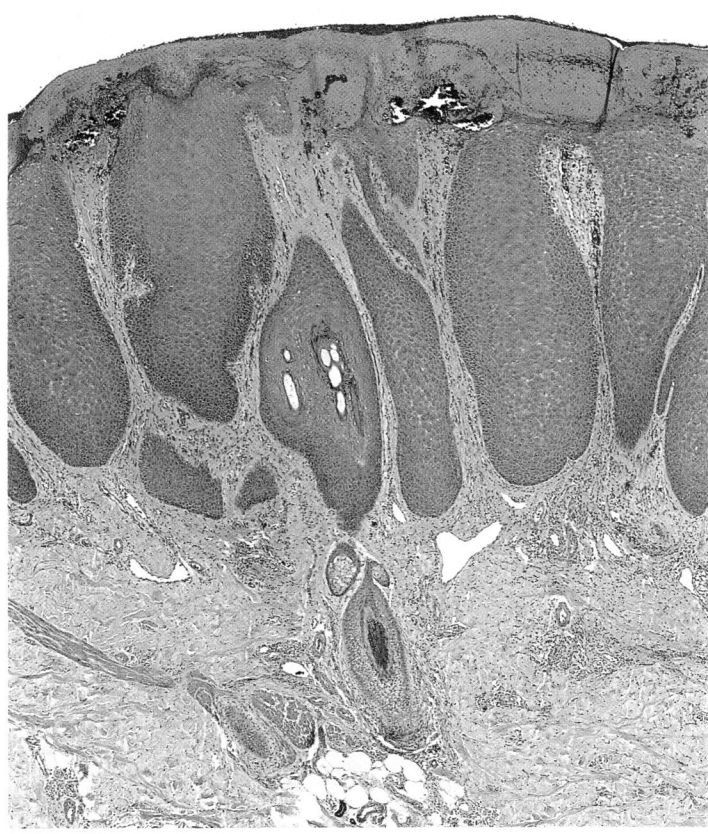

Fig. 31.5 **Prurigo nodularis.** There is focal excoriation and bulbous rete pegs. (H & E)

ACANTHOMAS

Acanthomas are benign tumors of epidermal keratinocytes.[142] The proliferating cells may show normal epidermoid keratinization or a wide range of aberrant keratinization, including epidermolytic hyperkeratosis (epidermolytic acanthoma), dyskeratosis with acantholysis (warty dyskeratoma) or acantholysis alone (acantholytic acanthoma).[142] These abnormal forms of keratinization occur in a much broader context and have already been discussed in Chapter 9 (pp. 294–299). Brief mention of these forms of acanthoma is made again for completeness. Keratoacanthomas (see p. 778) are not usually considered in this category, although there is no logical reason for their exclusion. The following acanthomas are discussed below:

- epidermolytic acanthoma
- warty dyskeratoma
- acantholytic acanthoma
- seborrheic keratosis
- dermatosis papulosa nigra
- melanoacanthoma
- clear cell acanthoma
- clear cell papulosis
- large cell acanthoma.

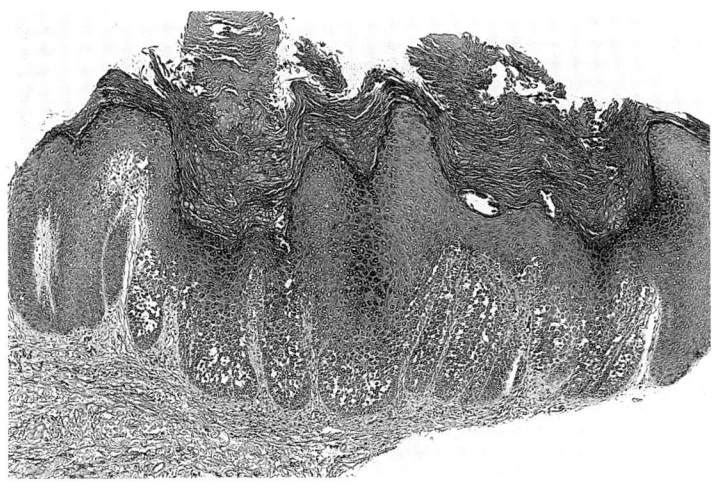

Fig. 31.6 **Acantholytic acanthoma.** Acantholysis involves the lower layers of the hyperplastic epidermis. There is a thick, orthokeratotic stratum corneum. (H & E)

lesions are no more than a centimeter or so in diameter, but larger variants, sometimes even pedunculated, have been reported.[148-150] A flat plaque-like form is sometimes found on the buttocks or thighs. This should not be confused with the lightly pigmented plaques of unwashed skin which have variously been called keratoderma simplex,[151] dermatitis artefacta and 'terra firma-forme' dermatosis (see p. 334).

Rare clinical variants include a familial form, which may be of early or late onset,[152,153] and a halo variant with a depigmented halo around each lesion.[154] Multiple seborrheic keratoses may sometimes assume a patterned arrangement along lines of cleavage[155] or a linear ('raindrop') pattern.[156] The eruptive form associated with internal cancer (sign of Leser and Trélat) is discussed below.

The nature of seborrheic keratoses is still disputed. A follicular origin has been proposed. They have also been regarded as a late-onset nevoid disturbance, or the result of a local arrest of maturation of keratinocytes.[157] Human papillomavirus (HPV) has been detected in a small number of cases,[158] particularly from the genital region.[159] It has also been found in the seborrheic keratoses of patients who have epidermodysplasia verruciformis.[160,161] Several cases of necrotizing herpesvirus infection complicating a seborrheic keratosis have been reported.[162] Endothelin-1, a keratinocyte-derived cytokine with a stimulatory effect on melanocytes, is thought to be involved in the melanization of seborrheic keratoses.[163] The basosquamous cell acanthoma of Lund, the inverted follicular keratosis and the stucco keratosis have all been regarded, at some time, as variants of seborrheic keratosis.[142,164]

A case can be made for submitting all suspected seborrheic keratoses for histological examination as clinical misdiagnosis can occur.[165,166]

Histopathology[142,167]

Seborrheic keratoses are sharply defined tumors which may be endophytic or exophytic.[167] They are composed of basaloid cells with a varying admixture of squamoid cells. Keratin-filled invaginations and small cysts (horn cysts) are a characteristic feature. Nests of squamous cells (squamous eddies) may be present, particularly in the irritated type. Approximately one-third of seborrheic keratoses appear hyperpigmented in hematoxylin and eosin-stained sections.[149]

At least five distinct histological patterns have been recognized: acanthotic (solid), reticulated (adenoid), hyperkeratotic (papillomatous), clonal and irritated.[167] Overlapping features are quite common. The acanthotic type is composed of broad columns or sheets of basaloid cells with intervening horn cysts. The reticulated type has interlacing thin strands of basaloid cells, often pigmented, enclosing small horn cysts. This variant often evolves from a solar lentigo.[167] The hyperkeratotic type is exophytic, with varying degrees of hyperkeratosis, papillomatosis and acanthosis (Fig. 31.7). There are both basaloid and squamous cells. Clonal seborrheic keratoses (Fig. 31.8) have intraepidermal nests of basaloid cells resembling the Borst–Jadassohn phenomenon (see p. 765).[168] In the irritated variant there is a heavy inflammatory cell infiltrate, with lichenoid features, in the upper dermis (Fig. 31.9). Apoptotic cells are present in the base of the lesion and in areas of squamous differentiation.[169] This represents the attempted immunological regression of a seborrheic keratosis.[170,171] Sometimes there is a heavy inflammatory cell infiltrate without lichenoid qualities;[172] rarely neutrophils are abundant in the infiltrate.[149] This may be regarded as a true inflammatory variant, although often lesions with features overlapping with those of the irritated type are found.[172]

Tricholemmal differentiation with glycogen-rich cells is an uncommon, usually focal, change.[173,174] So too is sebaceous differentiation.[175] Acantholysis is another uncommon histological feature.[176,177] Trichostasis spinulosa with multiple retained hair shafts has also been reported.[178] Amyloid in the underlying dermis is another incidental finding.[167]

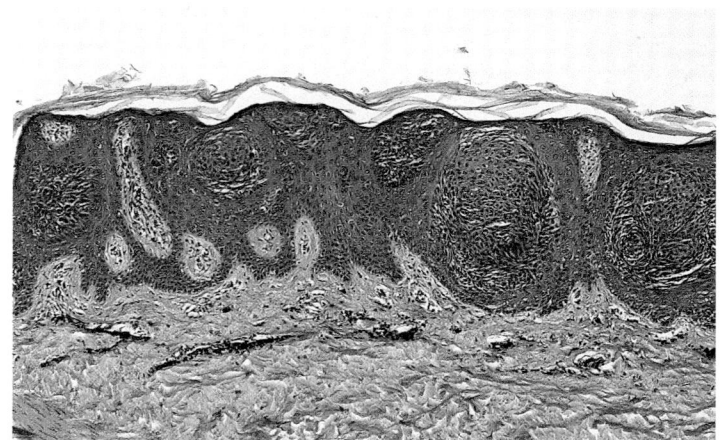

Fig. 31.8 **Clonal seborrheic keratosis.** Nests of keratinocytes show the Borst–Jadassohn phenomenon. (H & E)

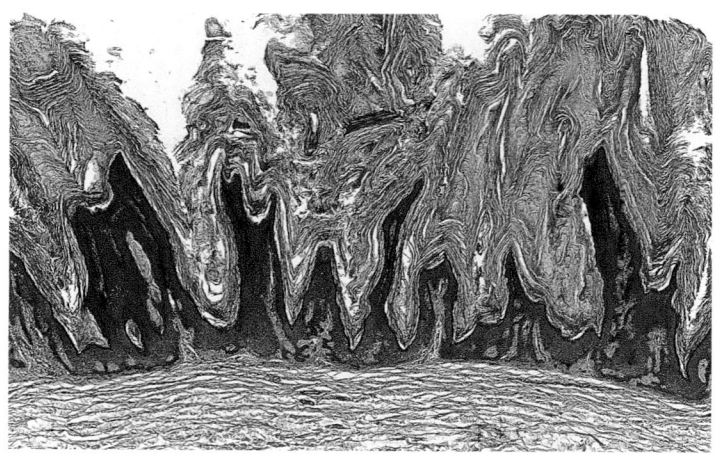

Fig. 31.7 **Seborrheic keratosis of hyperkeratotic type** with marked papillomatosis and hyperkeratosis. (H & E)

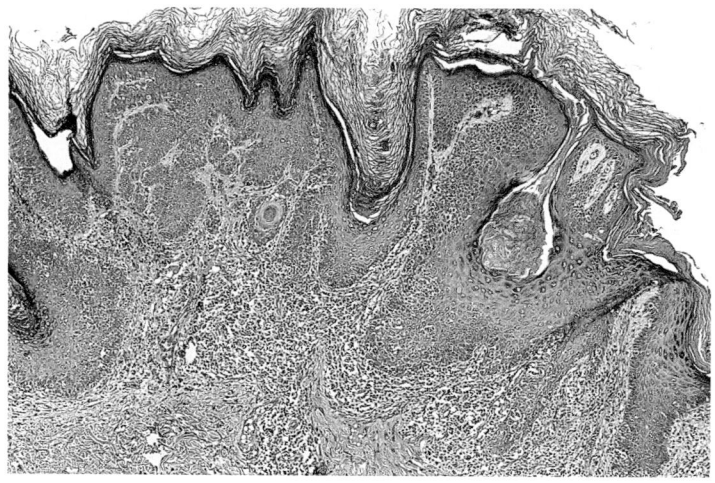

Fig. 31.9 **Irritated seborrheic keratosis.** There is a lichenoid inflammatory infiltrate. (H & E)

The development of a basal cell or squamous cell carcinoma or a keratoacanthoma in a seborrheic keratosis is an exceedingly rare event.[179–185] More common is the juxtaposition or 'collision' of these lesions.[186] Another finding is epidermal atypia of varying severity in the cells of a seborrheic keratosis; a progressive transformation to in situ squamous cell carcinoma (bowenoid transformation) may occur.[187–193] Rarely, a malignant melanoma may develop in a seborrheic keratosis.[194]

Electron microscopy
Ultrastructural studies have shown that the small basaloid cells are related to cells of the epidermal basal cell layer. Clusters of melanosomes, which are often membrane bound, may be found within the cells.[195] Langerhans cells are probably not increased,[196] as originally reported.[197]

Leser–Trélat sign
The sign of Leser and Trélat is defined as the sudden increase in the number and size of seborrheic keratoses associated with an internal cancer.[198–200] Approximately 100 such cases have been reported,[201–204] although some of them are poorly documented as genuine examples of the sign.[205,206] Other cutaneous paraneoplastic conditions, such as acanthosis nigricans, hypertrichosis lanuginosa and acquired ichthyosis, are sometimes present as well.[207–210] Pruritus is also common.[201] A gastrointestinal tract adenocarcinoma is the most frequent accompanying cancer,[211,212] followed by lymphoproliferative disorders.[213–216] The various cancers reported with this sign are analyzed in several reviews.[202,208,209] Metastases are frequently present and most patients have a poor prognosis.[207,209]

The seborrheic keratoses may precede,[217] follow, or develop concurrently with the onset of symptoms of the cancer.[209] Cases purporting to represent chemotherapy-induced lesions have been reported.[218] Involution of the seborrheic keratoses has followed treatment of the cancer. The lesions are most frequent on the trunk. A variant in which they were linear in distribution has been reported.[219]

The mechanism responsible for the appearance of these keratoses is not known. Epidermal growth factor does not appear to be increased,[212] although the structurally related α-transforming growth factor was increased in one report.[202]

Eruptive seborrheic keratoses have rarely been reported during the course of an erythrodermic condition.[220,221] They have also been reported in a patient with acromegaly.[222]

Histopathology[209]
Histological examination of the skin lesions has only been made in isolated cases.[223] In some reports typical seborrheic keratoses have been present. In other instances non-specific hyperkeratosis and papillomatosis without acanthosis have been noted.[209] Florid cutaneous papillomatosis with hyperkeratosis and acanthosis has also been described.[224] The regression of lesions following treatment of the underlying cancer appears to be associated with a mononuclear cell infiltrate in the upper dermis and lower epidermis.[221]

DERMATOSIS PAPULOSA NIGRA
Although regarded by some as a variant of seborrheic keratosis,[149] dermatosis papulosa nigra is a clinically distinctive entity, found almost exclusively in black adults, with a female preponderance.[225] There are multiple small pigmented papules, with a predilection for the malar area of the face. The neck and upper part of the trunk may also be involved. Lesions have been found in from 10% to 35% of the black population in the USA.[226]

Histopathology[226]
Dermatosis papulosa nigra is characterized by hyperkeratosis, elongated and interconnected rete ridges, and hyperpigmentation of the basal layer (Fig. 31.10). There are often keratin-filled invaginations of the epidermis. The picture is similar to that of the reticulate type of seborrheic keratosis. In contrast to seborrheic keratoses, the epithelial proliferation in dermatosis papulosa nigra is not usually composed of basaloid cells.

MELANOACANTHOMA
The term 'melanoacanthoma' was introduced in 1960 for a rare benign pigmented lesion which is composed of both melanocytes and keratinocytes.[227] The lesion is a slowly growing, usually solitary, tumor of the head and neck, or trunk, of older people.[228,229] Clinically, a melanoacanthoma resembles a seborrheic keratosis or a melanoma, and may grow to 3 cm or more in diameter.[230] Melanoacanthoma has been recorded as arising from mucous membranes (see p. 804): the nature of the lesion in such cases appears to be distinct from that of cutaneous melanoacanthoma.[231,232]

Histopathology[228,230,233]
There is some resemblance to a seborrheic keratosis, with an acanthotic, slightly verrucous epidermis composed of both basaloid and spinous cells.[233] The basaloid cells sometimes form islands, whereas the spinous cells form foci with central keratinization and horn pearl formation (endokeratinization). Numerous dendritic melanocytes are scattered throughout the lesion.[228] The melanocytes contain mature melanosomes and are heavily pigmented. The neighboring keratinocytes are only sparsely pigmented.[234] There is usually pigment in macrophages in the upper dermis.

CLEAR CELL ACANTHOMA
Clear cell acanthoma (pale cell acanthoma) is an uncommon firm brown-red dome-shaped nodule or papule, 5–10 mm or more in diameter, with a predilection for the lower part of the legs of middle-aged and elderly individuals.[235–239] Giant forms have been described.[240,241] Rarely, other sites have been involved;[242,243] onset in younger patients has also been recorded.[244] Although usually solitary, multiple tumors have been described and a few patients with multiple clear cell acanthomas have also had varicose veins

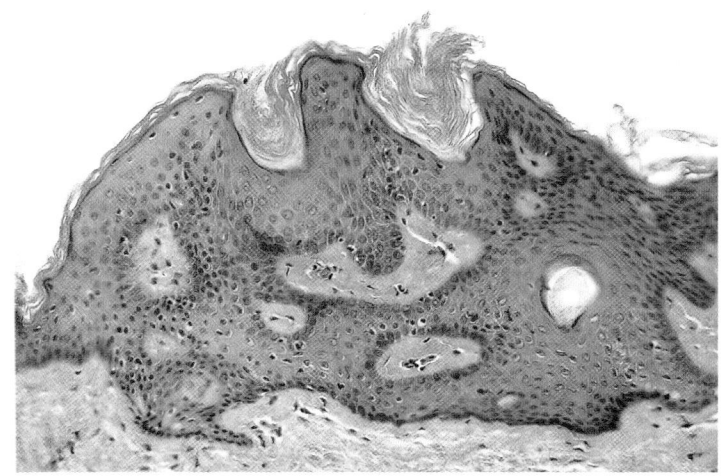

Fig. 31.10 **Dermatosis papulosa nigra.** There are interconnected rete pegs and hyperpigmentation of the basal layer. (H & E)

and/or ichthyosis.[245–249] In one case, the lesion developed over a melanocytic nevus.[250] The lesions may have a crusted surface and may bleed with minor trauma. A scaly collarette and vascular puncta on the surface of the lesion are common.[235,251,252] Growth is slow and the tumor may persist for many years. Spontaneous involution has been reported.[253]

The exact nosological position of this lesion is uncertain, but it has generally been considered to be a benign epidermal neoplasm (as originally proposed by Degos) rather than a reactive hyperplasia of inflammatory origin.[242,254] However, the expression of cytokeratins is similar to that seen in some inflammatory dermatoses.[255] Furthermore, clear cell acanthoma has developed in a psoriatic plaque.[256]

Histopathology[238,242,257]

Histological examination shows a well-demarcated area of psoriasiform epidermal hyperplasia in which the keratinocytes have pale-staining cytoplasm. The epithelium of the adnexa is spared. There are intermittent broad and slender rete pegs, and a tendency for the acanthosis to be more prominent centrally. There may be fusion of the acanthotic downgrowths. Usually there is slight acanthosis of the epidermis, involving one or two rete ridges bordering the area of pale acanthosis (Fig. 31.11).[257]

Other epidermal changes include mild spongiosis, exocytosis of neutrophils which may form tiny intraepidermal microabscesses, and thinning of the suprapapillary plates. The epidermal surface shows parakeratotic scale and sometimes focal pustulation. The cytoplasm of the basal cells may not be as pale as that of the other keratinocytes: it is often devoid of melanin pigment, although melanocytes are present.[258] A pigmented variant with dendritic melanocytes has been reported.[259] Cellular atypia is a rare occurrence.[260]

The dermal papillae are edematous, with increased vascularity and a mixed inflammatory cell infiltrate which includes a variable proportion of lymphocytes, plasma cells and neutrophils. In several cases the sweat ducts have been dilated, and rarely they may be hyperplastic.

A PAS stain, with and without diastase, will confirm the presence of abundant glycogen in the pale cells. Electron microscopy has also confirmed that the keratinocytes contain glycogen.[261,262] Langerhans cells are also abundant.[247,263] Immunohistochemistry shows that the cells contain keratin and involucrin, but not carcinoembryonic antigen.[264]

It has been suggested that there is a distinct tissue reaction, pale cell acanthosis (clear cell acanthosis), characterized by the presence of pale cells in an acanthotic epidermis.[265] This histological pattern can be seen not only in clear cell acanthoma but also in some seborrheic keratoses, usually the clonal subtype, and rarely in verruca vulgaris. The lesion reported as a cystic clear cell acanthoma may represent this tissue reaction occurring in an epidermal cyst or dilated follicle.[266]

CLEAR CELL PAPULOSIS

Clear cell papulosis is an exceedingly rare condition characterized by multiple white papules on the face, chest, abdomen or lumbar region of young women.[267–271] Some lesions may develop along the 'milk lines'. The lesions measure 2–10 mm in size. The number of lesions has ranged from 5 to more than 100. It has been suggested that there may be some histogenetic relationship with Toker's clear cells of the nipple and that cases reported away from the 'milk lines' may be a different entity.[272]

Histopathology

The epidermis is mildly acanthotic with a slightly disorganized arrangement of the epidermal cells. The characteristic feature is the presence of clear cells scattered mainly among the basal cells, with a few cells in the malpighian layer. The cells are larger than the adjacent keratinocytes. The clear cells are variably stained by the PAS, mucicarmine, alcian blue and colloidal iron methods. A characteristic feature is the positive immunostaining for gross cystic disease fluid protein-15 (GCDFP).[267]

The clear cells in pagetoid dyskeratosis, an incidental histological finding in a variety of lesions, are found at a higher level in the epidermis (see p. 300). They do not stain with the PAS or mucicarmine methods.

LARGE CELL ACANTHOMA

Large cell acanthoma occurs as a sharply demarcated, scaly, often lightly pigmented patch, approximately 3–10 mm in diameter, on the sun-exposed skin of middle-aged and elderly individuals.[273–275] It is usually solitary. Clinically, it resembles a seborrheic or actinic keratosis. Large cell acanthoma is thought to comprise sunlight-induced clones of abnormal cells, without a tendency to malignancy.[273,276] As such it is a distinctive condition[277–279] and not a variant of solar lentigo, as proposed by Roewert and Ackerman.[280]

Histopathology[273,274]

There is epidermal thickening caused by the enlargement of keratinocytes to about twice their normal size (Fig. 31.12). There is also a proportional

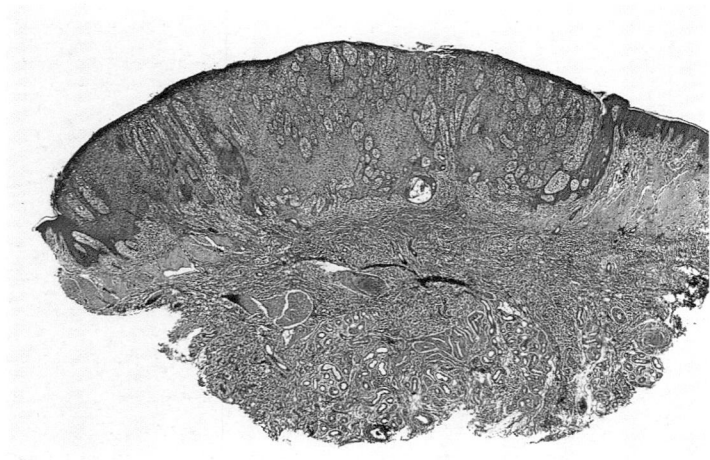

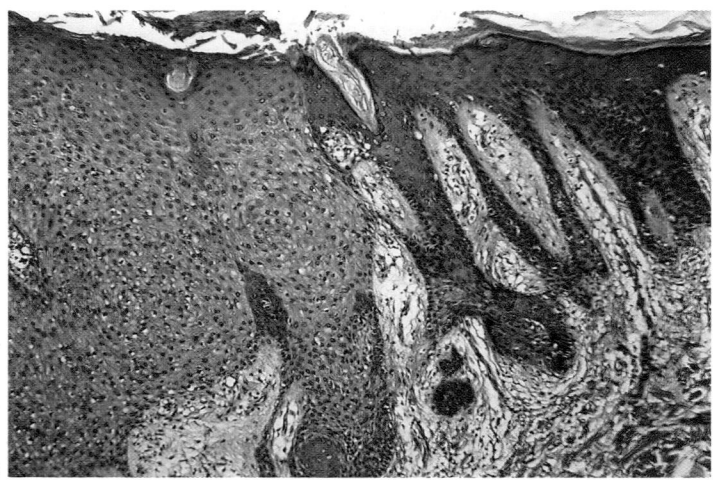

Fig. 31.11 **(A) Clear cell acanthoma. (B)** The lesion is acanthotic, with pale-staining keratinocytes, except at the periphery of the lesion where they appear normal. (H & E)

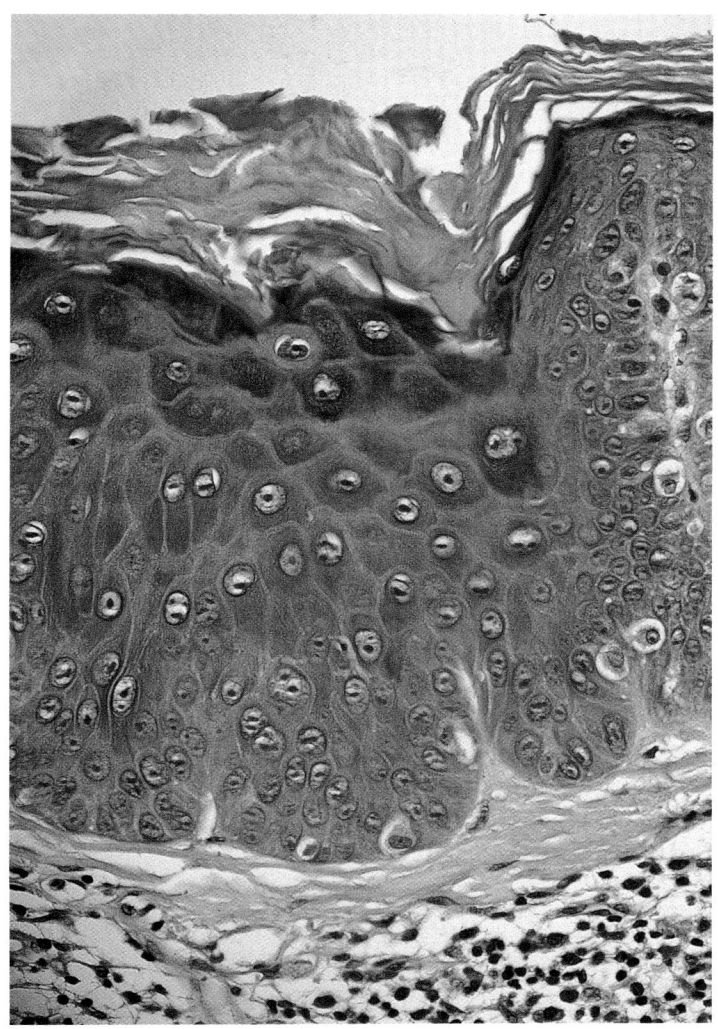

Fig. 31.12 **Large cell acanthoma.** The keratinocytes are larger than usual and the granular layer is thickened. Normal epidermis is present at the edge of the photograph. (H & E)

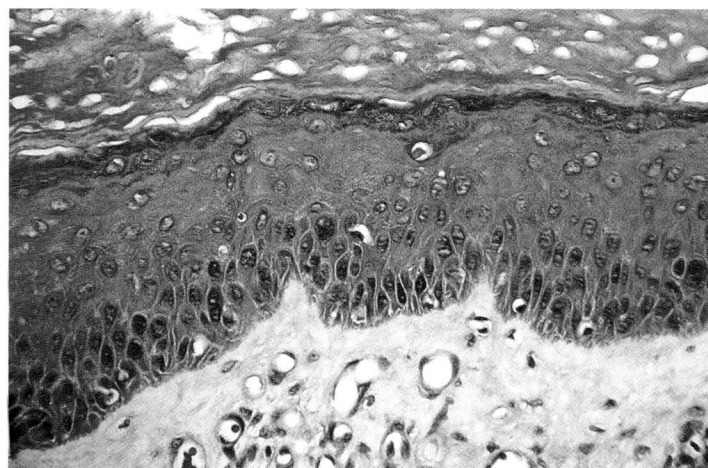

Fig. 31.13 **Large cell acanthoma.** There is mild basal cell atypia. There would be parakeratosis overlying a solar keratosis. There is orthokeratosis here. (H & E)

increase in nuclear size. The lesions are sharply demarcated from the adjacent normal keratinocytes; the adnexal epithelium within a lesion is usually spared. Other features include orthokeratosis, a prominent granular layer, mild papillomatosis, mild basal pigmentation, and some downward budding of the rete ridges.[279] Occasionally there is a focal lichenoid inflammatory cell infiltrate. Atypia may develop in large cell acanthoma; only rarely is this bowenoid (Fig. 31.13).

EPIDERMAL DYSPLASIAS

The epidermal dysplasias have the potential for malignant transformation. This group includes actinic (solar) keratosis, actinic cheilitis, arsenical keratoses and PUVA keratosis.

ACTINIC KERATOSIS

Actinic (solar) keratoses present clinically as circumscribed scaly erythematous lesions, usually less than I cm in diameter, on the sun-exposed skin of older individuals.[281–283] The face, ears, scalp, hands and forearms are sites of predilection. In Australia, actinic keratoses are found in 40–60% of people aged 40 years and over.[284,285] They develop most often in those with a fair complexion, who do not tan readily.[286] They may also develop in lesions of vitiligo.[287]

Actinic keratoses may remit, or remain unchanged for many years.[288–291] It has been stated that 8–20% gradually transform into squamous cell carcinoma if left untreated.[281,292,293] The hyperplastic variant appears to have a relatively high rate of malignant transformation.[294] In one study the annual incidence rate of malignant transformation of a solar keratosis was less than 0.25% for each keratosis,[295] but this study has been criticized on several grounds.[296,297]

Ackerman has proposed that actinic keratoses are morphological expressions of squamous cell carcinoma (see p. 773)[298,299] while Cockerell has suggested that actinic (solar) keratoses be renamed 'keratinocytic intra-epidermal neoplasia' or 'solar keratotic intraepidermal SCC'.[300] It is difficult to envisage clinicians embracing this latter terminology.

Several clinical variants of actinic keratosis have been described. In the hyperplastic (hypertrophic) form, found almost exclusively on the dorsum of the hands and the forearms, individual lesions are quite thick.[301,302] The changes probably result in part from the superadded changes caused by rubbing and scratching. They may be overdiagnosed clinically as squamous cell carcinoma.[301] The spreading pigmented actinic keratosis is a brown patch or plaque, usually greater than I cm in diameter, that tends to spread centrifugally.[303,304] Some cases appear to represent the collision of a solar keratosis and solar lentigo.[305] The cheeks and forehead are sites of predilection. The lichenoid actinic keratosis (not to be confused with the lichen planus-like keratosis) is not usually distinctive, although sometimes local irritation is noted.[306]

Cumulative exposure to sunlight appears to be important in the etiology. Intermittent, intense UV exposure in childhood, manifest as sunburn, is also strongly associated with the prevalence of actinic keratoses.[307] Despite educational programs, a significant number of individuals still experience sunburns.[308] Abnormalities in DNA synthesis in keratinocytes in the skin around the lesion suggest that there is a gradual stepwise progression from sun-damaged epidermis to clinically obvious keratoses, and eventually to squamous cell carcinoma.[309] The keratinocytes in solar keratoses, like those in squamous cell carcinomas, lose various surface carbohydrates.[310] Approximately 50% of actinic keratoses and squamous cell carcinomas show overexpression of cyclin D protein as well as p53 positivity.[311–316] Activated *ras* genes are found in a small percentage of cases.[317] However, no genetic susceptibility to actinic keratoses has been found.[315]

Histopathology[318]

Diagnostic biopsy is undertaken in only a small percentage of actinic keratoses diagnosed clinically.[284] The usual actinic keratosis is characterized by focal parakeratosis, with loss of the underlying granular layer and a slightly thickened epidermis with some irregular downward buds. Uncommonly, the epidermis is thinner than normal. In all cases there is variable loss of the normal orderly stratified arrangement of the epidermis; this is associated with cytological atypia of keratinocytes, which varies from slight to extreme. The term 'bowenoid keratosis' may be used when the atypia is close to full thickness.[303] Sometimes the dysplastic epithelium shows suprabasal cleft formation.[281,319,320] There is often a sharp slanting border between the normal epidermis of the acrotrichia and acrosyringia and the parakeratotic atypical epithelium of the keratosis.[321] However, dysplastic epithelium may involve the infundibular portion of the hair follicle.[321–323] The parakeratotic scale may sometimes pile up to form a cutaneous horn.[281]

Actinic keratoses must be distinguished from the **epidermal dysmaturation** that may be seen following chemotherapy. It is a histological diagnosis characterized by disruption of keratinocyte maturation, loss of polarity, widened intercellular spaces, irregular large nuclei, mid-epidermal mitotic figures, and apoptosis.[324]

The dermal changes include actinic elastosis, which is usually quite severe, and a variable, but usually mild, chronic inflammatory cell infiltrate.[281] Histological studies have not been reported on the inflammatory keratoses that may develop during chemotherapy of malignant disease with fluorouracil,[325,326] but in the one case the author has studied there was vascular telangiectasia and a moderately heavy mixed inflammatory cell infiltrate in the upper dermis.

In the hyperplastic (hypertrophic) form there is prominent orthokeratosis with alternating parakeratosis.[301] The epidermis usually shows irregular psoriasiform hyperplasia, and sometimes there is mild papillomatosis. Dysplastic changes are sometimes minimal and confined to the basal layer.[302] The presence of vertical collagen bundles and some dilated vessels in the papillary dermis is evidence that these lesions represent actinic keratoses, with superimposed changes due to rubbing or scratching (lichen simplex chronicus).[301]

In the pigmented variant there is excess melanin in the lower epidermis, usually in both keratinocytes and melanocytes, but sometimes only in one or the other.[303] Melanophages are usually found in the papillary dermis.[303]

In lichenoid actinic keratoses there is a superficial, often band-like, chronic inflammatory cell infiltrate, with occasional apoptotic keratinocytes in the basal layer and some basal vacuolar change.[306] The acral keratotic lesions with a lichenoid infiltrate, reported as a possible manifestation of graft-versus-host disease, may have been a manifestation of HPV infection, as wart-virus features sometimes remit in the presence of a lichenoid infiltrate.[327]

In all types of actinic keratoses in immunosuppressed patients there is usually marked atypia of the keratinocytes;[328] multinucleate forms may be present.[328] Confluent parakeratosis and verruciform changes may also occur.[329]

It is sometimes a matter of personal judgment whether a lesion is considered to show early squamous cell carcinomatous change or not.[330] The protrusion of atypical cells into the reticular dermis and the detachment of individual nests of keratinocytes from the lower layers of the epidermis are criteria used to diagnose invasive transformation.[330] Step sections are important in small biopsies initially regarded as solar keratosis. More significant pathology may emerge in the deeper sections.[331,332]

Confocal laser microscopic imaging of actinic keratoses has been used. Its widespread use will probably await further technological advances.[333]

Electron microscopy
Ultrastructural studies suggest that the hyperpigmentation in the pigmented variant is due to enhanced melanosome formation and distribution, and not to a block in the transfer of melanosomes to keratinocytes.[304]

ACTINIC CHEILITIS

Actinic cheilitis (solar cheilosis, actinic keratosis of the lip) is a premalignant condition seen predominantly on the vermilion part of the lower lip. It results from chronic exposure to sunlight,[334] although smoking and chronic irritation may also contribute.[335] There are dry, whitish-gray scaly plaques in which areas of erythema, erosions and ulceration may develop.[334] The whitish areas were known in the past as leukoplakia.[336] Large areas of the lower lip may be affected. Squamous cell carcinoma may develop after a latent period of 20–30 years,[337,338] although the incidence of this transformation is difficult to quantify.[335]

An acute form of actinic cheilitis, characterized by edema, erythema and erosions, has been recognized.[336] It is an uncommon response to prolonged exposure to sunlight.

Histopathology[336,339]

The lesions show alternating areas of orthokeratosis and parakeratosis. The epidermis may be hyperplastic or atrophic. Other features are disordered maturation of epidermal cells, increased mitotic activity and variable cytological atypia.[337] Squamous cell carcinoma may develop in areas of marked atypia.

There is prominent solar elastosis of the submucosal connective tissue, some vascular telangiectasia, and a mild to moderate infiltrate of chronic inflammatory cells. Plasma cells are usually prominent, particularly beneath areas of ulceration.[339]

ARSENICAL KERATOSES

For more than a century inorganic arsenic was used in the treatment of many diverse conditions.[340] The recognition of its adverse effects, and its replacement by more effective therapeutic agents, has led to a marked reduction in the incidence of arsenic-related conditions.[341] However, there is a high arsenic content in some drinking waters and naturopathic medicines.[342–348]

The best-known effect of chronic arsenicism is cutaneous pigmentation, which may be diffuse or of 'raindrop' type.[349] More than 40% of affected individuals develop keratoses on the palms and soles, and sometimes this is associated with a mild diffuse keratoderma.[349] There is an increased incidence of multiple skin cancers, which include Bowen's disease, basal cell carcinomas and squamous cell carcinomas.[346,350] The lesions are sometimes quite exophytic in appearance. Visceral cancers, particularly involving the lung and genitourinary system, may also be found.[351]

Many arsenical skin cancers express p53, although arsenic-related basal cell carcinomas express it less intensely than sporadic ones.[352] It is also found in perilesional skin.[353,354] The expression of p53 is reduced after UV-B therapy.[355]

Histopathology[342,343]

Arsenical keratoses are of the hyperkeratotic type. Sometimes there is prominent hyperkeratosis and papillomatosis, but no atypia. These lesions have a superficial resemblance to the hyperkeratotic type of seborrheic keratosis. Similar lesions follow exposure to tar (Fig. 31.14).[356] In other cases there is mild atypia resembling the hyperkeratotic variant of actinic keratosis.

In some lesions of Bowen's disease related to exposure to arsenic there may be areas resembling seborrheic keratosis, superficial basal cell carcinoma or intraepidermal epithelioma of Jadassohn. Invasive carcinomas arising in Bowen's disease show the non-keratinizing pattern of squamous cell carcinoma, sometimes with areas of appendageal differentiation (see below).

The basal cell carcinomas that develop may be of solid or multifocal superficial type.

PUVA KERATOSIS

A PUVA keratosis is a distinctive form of keratosis, often found on non-sun-exposed skin of patients who have received long-term treatment with psoralens and ultraviolet-A radiation (PUVA).[357] It is a raised papule with a broad base and a scaly surface, often with a warty appearance. There is an increased risk of developing non-melanoma skin cancer, particularly with long-term, high-dose exposure.[358–360] Punctate keratoses on the hands and feet are a rare complication of PUVA therapy.[361]

Histopathology

There is a variable degree of acanthosis, orthokeratosis and parakeratosis. Papillomatosis is present in one-half of the lesions. PUVA keratoses differ from actinic keratoses by their paucity of atypical cells and an absence of solar elastosis.[357] The lesions reported as disseminated hypopigmented keratoses developed in young patients who had previously received PUVA therapy.[362] They had some histological resemblance to stucco keratoses (see p. 778).[362]

INTRAEPIDERMAL CARCINOMAS

Although the term 'intraepidermal carcinoma' is often used synonymously with Bowen's disease, it is used here in a broader sense to include not only carcinoma in situ of the skin (Bowen's disease) and penis (erythroplasia of Queyrat), but also intraepidermal epithelioma of Jadassohn, a controversial entity of disputed histogenesis. Paget's disease is sometimes included in this category because of the presence of cytologically malignant cells within

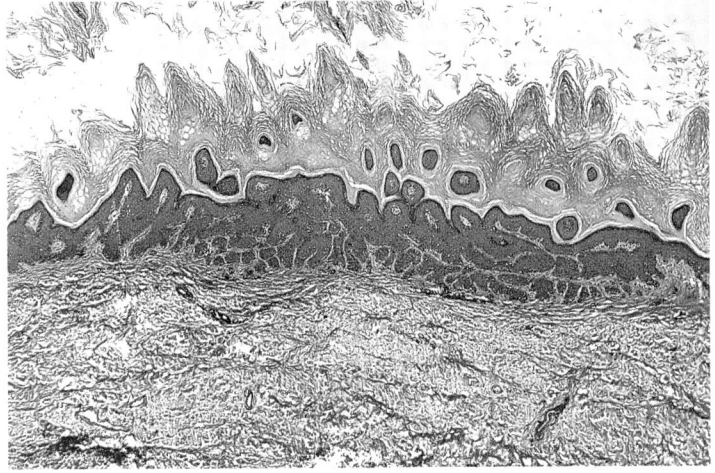

Fig. 31.14 Tar keratosis. There is pronounced hyperkeratosis, papillomatosis and acanthosis. (H & E)

the epidermis. Paget's disease is discussed with the appendageal tumors on page 883.

BOWEN'S DISEASE

Bowen's disease is a clinical expression of squamous cell carcinoma in situ of the skin.[363] It presents as an asymptomatic well-defined erythematous scaly plaque, which expands centrifugally. Verrucous, nodular, eroded and pigmented[364–367] variants occur. Many of the pigmented lesions reported in the anogenital area as Bowen's disease[368–370] would now be regarded as examples of bowenoid papulosis[371] (see p. 705).

Bowen's disease has a predilection for the sun-exposed areas (particularly the face and legs) of fair-skinned older individuals.[372–374] It is uncommon in black people,[375] in whom it is found more often on areas of the skin that are not exposed to the sun.[376] Lesions may also develop on the trunk and the vulva, and rarely on the nail bed,[377–381] lip,[382] nipple,[383] palm,[384–386] sole,[387] and the margin of an eyelid.[388] Bowen's disease has been reported in the wall of an epidermoid cyst,[389] in a lesion of porokeratosis of Mibelli,[390] above a scar,[391] in erythema ab igne[392] and in seborrheic keratoses (see p. 757).

Several investigators have proposed that Bowen's disease should be considered to be a skin marker for internal malignant disease,[393–395] although more recent studies have shown no evidence for this association.[397–399] However, patients with Bowen's disease have the same increased risk of developing a subsequent skin cancer as do those with invasive squamous cell carcinoma.[400]

Invasive carcinoma develops in up to 8% of untreated cases.[401,402] This complication, which is not well recognized, is characterized by the development of a rapidly growing tumor, 1–15 cm in diameter, in a pre-existing scaly lesion.[402] It appears to be more common in older people. The invasive tumor has metastatic potential, which has been stated to be as high as 13%,[402] although this would appear to be an overestimation of the risk.[401,403,404] Spontaneous complete regression of Bowen's disease has also been reported.[405]

Several factors have been implicated in the etiology of Bowen's disease. They include prolonged exposure to solar radiation, the ingestion of arsenic,[349,393] and infection with the human papillomavirus (HPV).[406] Whereas HPV type 16 (HPV-16) and HPV-18, and to a lesser extent HPV-18, 31, 33, 39, 52 and 67, have been detected in Bowen's disease of the genital region and its precursors,[407,408] there are now several reports of non-genital Bowen's disease related to infections with HPV-2,[409] HPV-16,[410–413] HPV-34,[414] HPV-56[415] and HPV-58.[416] Bowen's disease is a rare complication of the treatment of psoriasis with psoralens and ultraviolet-A radiation (PUVA).[417–419]

Various modalities have been used to treat Bowen's disease including curettage and cautery, cryotherapy, imiquimod cream, and photodynamic therapy.[420–425]

Bowenoid papulosis (see p. 705) consists of one or more indolent, verrucous papules on the genitalia with a clinical resemblance to condyloma acuminatum and a histological resemblance to Bowen's disease. It usually responds to local therapies, but recurrences and the development of invasive carcinoma have been reported.[408]

Histopathology[281,426]

Bowen's disease is a form of carcinoma in situ, and accordingly shows full-thickness involvement of the epidermis, and sometimes the pilosebaceous epithelium, by atypical keratinocytes.[427,428] This is associated with disorderly maturation of the epidermis, mitoses at different levels, multinucleate keratinocytes and dyskeratotic cells. Usually there is loss of the granular layer, with overlying parakeratosis and sometimes hyperkeratosis.

Several histological variants have been described, and more than one of these patterns may be present in different areas of the same lesion.[426] In the psoriasiform pattern there is regular acanthosis with thickening of the rete ridges and overlying parakeratosis (Fig. 31.15).[426] In the atrophic form there is thinning of the epidermis, which shows full-thickness atypia and disorganization.[426] There is usually overlying hyperkeratosis and parakeratosis. The verrucous-hyperkeratotic type is characterized by hyperkeratosis, papillomatosis, and sometimes intervening pit-like invaginations.[426] The irregular variant shows irregular acanthosis, and often extensive chronic inflammation in the underlying dermis.[426] In the pigmented type there is melanin in individual tumor cells and melanophages in the underlying dermis.[371] The pagetoid variant has nests of cells with pale cytoplasm and thin strands of relatively normal keratinocytes intervening; the basal layer may also be spared (Fig. 31.16). Sometimes this is associated with psoriasiform hyperplasia of the epidermis. Mucinous and sebaceous metaplasia characterize two other rare histological patterns.[429]

As already mentioned, the atypical epithelium may also involve the pilosebaceous units. This may lead to treatment failure when superficial methods of destruction are used.[430,431] Involvement of the eccrine ducts is uncommon,[432,433] and in the author's experience it has usually been confined to cases of Bowen's disease of the temple region.[434]

Changes in the underlying dermis include increased vascularity and a variable inflammatory response, which is usually composed of lymphocytes. Occasionally this has lichenoid features. Partial regression may ensue.[435] Small deposits of amyloid may be found in the papillary dermis, particularly in lesions of long standing.[426]

The pagetoid variant of Bowen's disease is sometimes difficult to distinguish from Paget's disease and from in situ superficial spreading melanoma, particularly if only a small biopsy is available. In these instances immunoperoxidase markers may be of assistance. Melanoma cells are positive for S100 protein, whereas Paget cells usually demonstrate carcinoembryonic antigen (CEA).[436] Melanoma cells do not contain cytokeratins, although Paget cells are positive for cytokeratins with a molecular weight of 54 kilodaltons (kd) and negative for those of 66 kd; the reverse applies with the cells in Bowen's disease.[437] Although cytokeratin 7 (CK7) has been regarded as a specific marker of Paget's disease, it has also been reported in pagetoid Bowen's disease, but not in the other types.[438] In Bowen's disease there is a diffuse pattern of staining of the keratinocyte nuclei for PCNA (proliferating cell nuclear antigen).[439–441] CD1a+ cells are significantly decreased.[442]

In the invasive form there are large islands of non-keratinizing squamoid cells throughout the dermis.[402] The cells usually have pale cytoplasm. Basaloid and adnexal differentiation are common patterns.[402,443,444] The invasive tumor that supervenes is best regarded as a variant of squamous cell carcinoma. Invasion may be facilitated by the production of metalloproteinases which are involved in the destruction of basement membrane.[445]

The term 'Bowen's disease' is no longer used in gynecological pathology, having been replaced by the concept of vulvar intraepithelial neoplasia (VIN).[446–448] Progressive atypia of the epithelium is semiquantified, VIN I representing atypia confined to the basal third of the epidermis, and VIN II corresponding to involvement of from one-third to two-thirds of the epithelium. In VIN III, the atypical cells involve more than two-thirds of the thickness of the epidermis. Bowen's disease therefore corresponds to severe VIN III. There has been an attempt to apply this concept, in part, to other areas of the skin.[449] The term 'squamous intraepidermal neoplasia, Bowen's type' has been suggested for full-thickness atypia of the epidermis, and 'squamous intraepidermal neoplasia, non-Bowen's type' when the atypia is limited to the lower two-thirds of the epidermis.[449] This categorization has not received wide acceptance. As the criteria used for grading cervical intraepithelial neoplasia (CIN) are not strictly applicable to VIN, it has been suggested that only two categories of VIN should be recognized: classic (bowenoid) VIN corresponding to Bowen's disease, and simplex (differentiated) VIN. Simplex VIN is often seen adjacent to invasive squamous cell carcinoma. The epidermis is thickened by a proliferation of enlarged and abnormal keratinocytes showing less maturation than the adjacent normal epidermis. Full-thickness atypia may not be present. This topic has been the subject of a recent review.[450]

Vulvar intraepithelial neoplasia should be distinguished from the recently described entity **multinucleated atypia of the vulva**, in which cells with 2–10 nuclei are found in the cells of the lower layers of the epithelium of the vulva.[451] The cells lack hyperchromasia or variation in nuclear size. HPV has not been detected. The nature of this process is uncertain. Parenthetically, the author has seen multinucleate cells in the epidermis of patients who have applied retinoic acid for a long time (unpublished observation).

Bowen's disease differs from actinic (solar) keratosis in the full-thickness atypia of the epithelium and in usually sparing the acrosyringium. Both lesions may show aneuploidy of the constituent cells,[452] and both may express mutant p53 protein and p21.[453–455] In solar keratoses the keratin and involucrin distribution is similar to normal epidermis, whereas in Bowen's

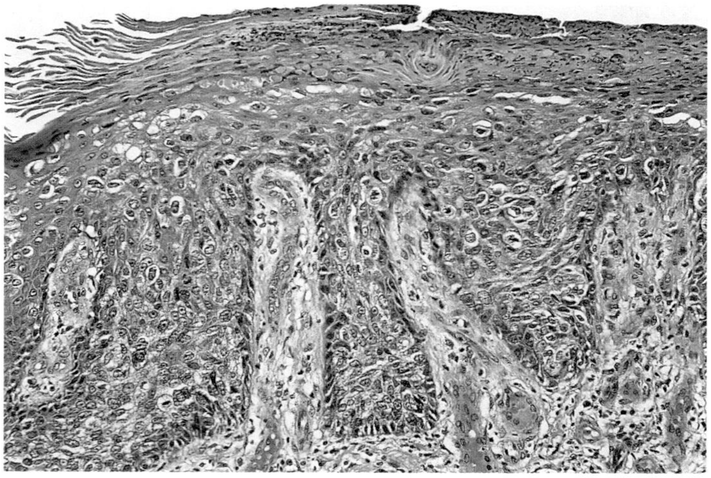

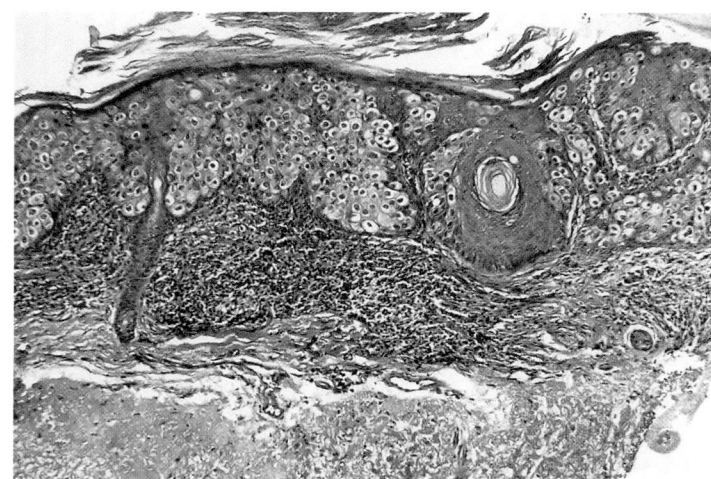

Fig. 31.15 **Bowen's disease.** There is full-thickness atypia of the epidermis, which also shows psoriasiform hyperplasia. (H & E)

Fig. 31.16 **Bowen's disease.** The atypical keratinocytes are pale, with a pagetoid appearance. (H & E)

disease the keratin distribution is variable.[456] In arsenical keratoses, in situ carcinoma indistinguishable from Bowen's disease may develop.

Bowenoid papulosis of the genitalia is regarded by some as a variant of Bowen's disease of the genitalia; although the two conditions may be histologically indistinguishable, features that favor a diagnosis of bowenoid papulosis include numerous mitoses in metaphase, small basophilic inclusions in the cytoplasm of the granular layer, and the presence sometimes of cells with a resemblance to koilocytes (Fig. 31.17).

Electron microscopy[457]

The keratinocytes have large nuclei and nucleoli, and a reduced number of desmosomal attachments.[458] The dyskeratotic cells show an aggregation of cytoplasmic tonofilaments. Occasional apoptotic bodies are present in the intercellular spaces, whereas others have been phagocytosed by neighboring keratinocytes.[459,460] Cytoplasmic projections of keratinocytes may extend through gaps in the basement membrane.[457]

ERYTHROPLASIA OF QUEYRAT

Erythroplasia of Queyrat is a clinical expression of carcinoma in situ of the penis.[46–466] It is found most commonly on the glans penis of uncircumcised males as a sharply circumscribed, asymptomatic, bright red shiny plaque.[463] It may also arise on the coronal sulcus or the inner surface of the prepuce. As in Bowen's disease, invasive carcinoma may develop in up to 10% of cases of erythroplasia of Queyrat, and such tumors have metastatic potential.[461]

The etiology of this condition has been regarded as multifactorial: chronic irritation, poor hygiene, genital herpes simplex, and infection with human papillomavirus (HPV) have all been incriminated.[467] Recently, the rare epidermodysplasia verruciformis-associated subtype, HPV-8, was detected in all cases studied.[468] A coinfection with other HPV types, particularly HPV-16, HPV-39 and HPV-51, was usually present.[468]

Histopathology[461,462]

The changes are those of a carcinoma in situ, as in Bowen's disease.[469] There are said to be fewer multinucleate and dyskeratotic cells than in Bowen's disease.[461] The accompanying inflammatory cell infiltrate in the dermis is often rich in plasma cells.[461]

INTRAEPIDERMAL EPITHELIOMA (JADASSOHN)

The intraepidermal epithelioma (Jadassohn) has been regarded by some as a distinct clinicopathological entity, characterized by the presence of nests of atypical keratinocytes within the epidermis and having the potential to progress to invasive squamous cell carcinoma in a small number of cases.[470–472] As defined, it presents as a scaly plaque, usually on the lower part of the trunk, the buttocks or the thighs, measuring from 0.5 to 10 cm in diameter.[471]

Most authors do not recognize the existence of such an entity, which they believe is simply an expression of the Borst–Jadassohn phenomenon, a term used to describe the presence of sharply defined nests of morphologically different cells within the epidermis.[473,474] This phenomenon may be seen in seborrheic keratoses (clonal variant), hidroacanthoma simplex and some cases of Bowen's disease, actinic keratosis and, rarely, epidermal nevi.[475,476] It has also been seen in a tumor in which the nests of cells exhibited markers for hair follicle cells by immunoperoxidase: accordingly, the lesion was called an **intraepidermal pilar epithelioma**.[477]

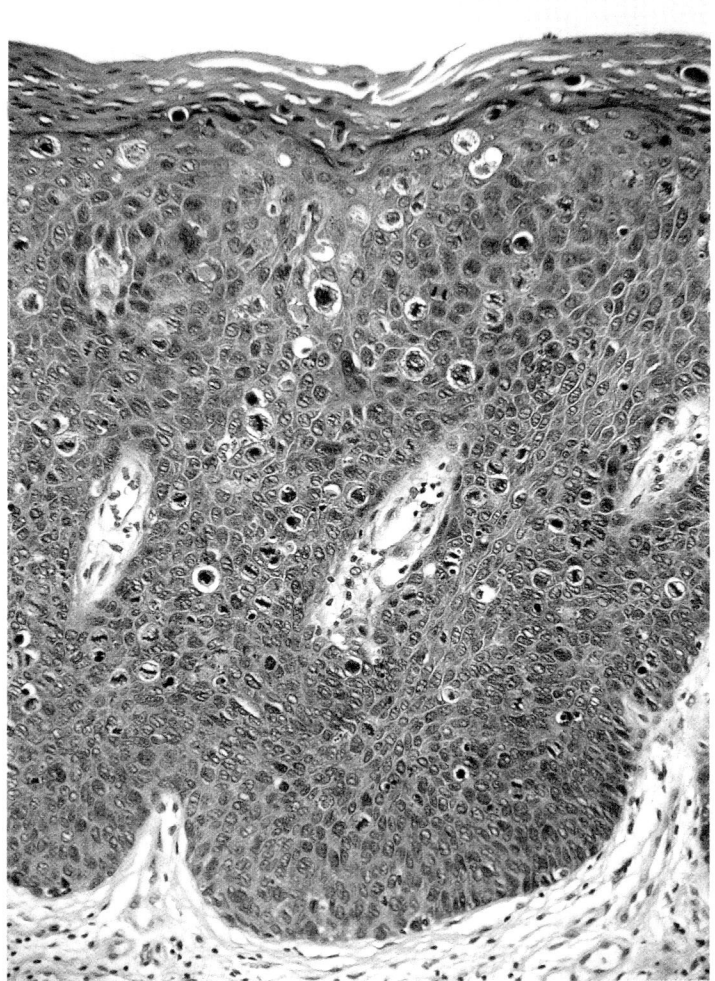

Fig. 31.17 **Bowenoid papulosis.** There is full-thickness atypia, scattered mitoses in metaphase, basophilic inclusions in the granular layer and koilocytes. (H & E)

MALIGNANT TUMORS

This group, which includes basal cell and squamous cell carcinomas, accounts for approximately 90% or more of all skin malignancies. These tumors constitute an important public health problem,[478] despite their comparatively low mortality rate.[479,480] The lifetime risk for the development of skin cancer in the USA is now 1 in 5.[481] In most instances the histopathological diagnosis is straightforward, but very occasionally tumors are encountered which are difficult to classify because of some apparent morphological overlap with various appendageal tumors, or because the tumor exhibits both basaloid and squamous differentiation. In these circumstances immunohistochemistry may be of assistance.[482]

BASAL CELL CARCINOMA

Basal cell carcinomas are the most common cutaneous tumors, accounting for approximately 70% of all malignant diseases of the skin.[483] They exceed squamous cell carcinomas in frequency by a factor of approximately 5:1, although this ratio varies from 3:1 to 7:1 in different latitudes.[484–486] Of course, if solar keratoses are regarded as squamous cell carcinomas (see

p. 773) then squamous cell carcinoma becomes more common than basal cell carcinoma.[487,488] The incidence of basal cell carcinomas appears to be increasing.[489]

Clinical aspects

Basal cell carcinomas are found predominantly on areas of skin exposed to the sun, particularly in fair-skinned individuals.[490–492] They are rare in black people.[493–496] Up to 80% of all lesions are found on the head and neck,[484,497] whereas approximately 15% develop on the shoulders, back or chest.[498] There are isolated reports documenting involvement of the breast,[499] nipple,[500] axilla,[501] perianal region,[502–504] vulva,[505,506] penis,[507–509] scrotum,[510–512] inguinal region,[513] subungual skin,[514–516] lower part of the legs,[517] and the palms[513,518] and soles.[519,520] Other unusual sites of involvement include pilonidal sinuses,[521] venous ulcers,[522] sternotomy scars,[523] the skin overlying arteriovenous malformations,[524,525] the nose affected by rhinophyma,[526,527] and the scars that follow thermal burns,[528] radiation,[529–531] chickenpox,[532] leishmaniasis,[533] smallpox[534] and BCG vaccination.[535] Basal cell carcinomas develop in approximately 20% of organoid nevi,[536,537] and, rarely, in epidermal nevi,[538,539] fibroepithelial polyps,[540] 'port wine' stains[541,542] and solar lentiges.[543] Multiple basal cell carcinomas may develop in the basal cell nevus syndrome (see p. 771) and in the rare Bazex's syndrome, in which there is also follicular atrophoderma and hypohidrosis.[544–547] Furthermore, any patient who has had one basal cell carcinoma has a high probability of subsequently developing a further lesion.[548,549] Patients with truncal lesions represent a high susceptibility group for the development of further lesions.[550,551] Tumors in this site are commonly of the multifocal superficial type with a male predominance.[552] There appears to be no risk for the development of non-cutaneous cancers.[553]

Basal cell carcinomas are more common in males, presumably related to occupational and recreational exposure to ultraviolet light. They tend to occur in older people, although they have also been documented in children[554–556] and young adults.[557] In children there is often a clinical association with the basal cell nevus syndrome, Bazex's syndrome, xeroderma pigmentosum or an organoid nevus.[554]

The clinical presentation of a basal cell carcinoma can be quite variable. It may be a papulonodular lesion with a pearly translucent edge, an ulcerated destructive lesion ('rodent ulcer'), a pale plaque with variable induration, an erythematous plaque with visible telangiectasia, or a partly cystic nodule.[558,559] Giant lesions up to 20 cm in diameter,[560–562] and variants with mutilation of the face have also been documented.[563,564] Rare linear and polypoid forms have been reported.[565,566] Approximately 2–5% of lesions are pigmented; basal cell carcinomas in black people and in the Japanese are often pigmented.[495,567,568] Rarely, these pigmented variants mimic a malignant melanoma[569] or develop a depigmented halo.[570] The surface microscopy of pigmented basal cell carcinomas is distinctive.[571] Despite the marked variability of their appearance, the accuracy rate in the clinical diagnosis of basal cell carcinomas is still 60–70%.[572,573]

Although most basal cell carcinomas are slow-growing, relatively non-aggressive tumors that are cured by most methods of treatment, a minority have an aggressive behavior with local tissue destruction and, rarely, metastasis.[574] These aspects will be considered in further detail after the histopathology has been discussed.

Etiology

Although the prime etiological factor in the development of basal cell carcinoma is exposure to ultraviolet light, particularly the UV-B wavelengths, solar dosimetry studies show a poor correlation between tumor density and ultraviolet dose.[575–577] Indeed, susceptibility to UV-B induced inhibition of

contact hypersensitivity appears to be a better indicator of cancer risk than cumulative sun exposure, suggesting an important role for immune surveillance in protecting against the development of basal cell carcinoma.[578] Tumor necrosis factor (TNF) may be an important mediator of the immuno-suppression produced by UV-B.[578] Various mediators of UV-B induced damage are now being reported.[579,580] Sunlight exposure in adolescence and childhood appears to be a risk factor for the development of basal cell carcinoma.[581–583] UV-B radiation produces DNA damage at mutation hot spots on the p53 tumor suppressor gene. Approximately 50% of all basal cell carcinomas studied have mutations of this gene.[584,585] Whereas squamous cell carcinomas tend to develop at the sites of direct exposure to sunlight (dorsum of hands, ears, bald scalp and lower lip), basal cell carcinomas are more common in sites slightly removed from this, such as the paranasal region and inner canthus. Other predisposing factors include exposure to X-rays,[529,586–588] arsenical intoxication,[348,589] adjuvant treatment of melanoma with isolated limb perfusion,[590] HPV infection,[591] welding[592] and stasis dermatitis of the legs.[593–595] In females, the risk of developing a basal cell carcinoma increases with the increasing number of nevocellular nevi.[596] Tumors have also developed following PUVA therapy in patients with psoriasis.[597]

Basal cell carcinomas have occurred in renal transplant recipients[598–600] and in other circumstances of immunosuppression, such as malignant lymphoma or leukemia[601–604] and the AIDS-related complex.[605–608] Tumors are more aggressive in these circumstances. They are also aggressive in albinos.[609] Basal cell carcinomas are now being seen after prolonged hydroxyurea therapy used in the treatment of myeloproliferative disorders.[610]

Genetic aspects

There is increasing evidence that genetic factors play a role in the susceptibility of some individuals to basal cell carcinoma.[577] Mutations in the PATCHED gene (ptc, PTCH), which is known to be responsible for the nevoid basal cell carcinoma syndrome (see below), have also been reported in sporadic cases of basal cell carcinoma.[611–614] There is also an association with HLA-DR7 and HLA-DR4 in some populations.[615,616] Mutations in the ptc gene have downstream effects leading to the accumulation of the transcription factor Gli-1, which may play a role in the development of basal cell carcinomas.[617,618] Frameshift mutations in the BAX gene (bcl-2 associated X protein) have also been found in sporadic cases.[619]

Cell of origin

Basal cell carcinomas usually arise from the lowermost layers of the epidermis, although a small percentage may originate from the outer root sheath of the pilosebaceous unit.[575,620] Whatever their origin – lower epidermis or follicle – the cells in the basal cell carcinoma have many features in common with follicular epithelium, particularly follicular matrix cells, rather than follicular bulge cells as once thought.[621] There is a virtually identical cytokeratin pattern in basal cell carcinomas, trichoblastomas and developing fetal hair follicles, compelling evidence for a common histogenetic pathway.[622,623] Ackerman now classifies basal cell carcinomas as trichoblastic carcinomas. Further circumstantial evidence of this shared antigenicity is the finding of T lymphocytes in the upper portion of hair follicles, adjacent to a regressing basal cell carcinoma.[624] In contrast to squamous cell carcinomas, basal cell carcinomas are difficult to produce experimentally in animals, although they have been produced in rats using chemical carcinogens.[625] Human lesions can, however, be transplanted to nude mice, but only if the animals are athymic and lacking in natural killer-cell activity.[605] Basal cell carcinomas are stroma dependent, and autotransplantation is unsuccessful if the stroma is not included.[626] This stromal dependency is the most likely reason for the low incidence of metastasis of these tumors.[575] The cells can be cultured.[627]

Therapy

Various studies have been published recently relating to the treatment of basal cell carcinoma.[628–639] They are beyond the scope of this book but are referenced in case they are of interest to readers.

Histopathology[640]

There is considerable variability in the morphology of basal cell carcinomas, and as a consequence a number of histopathological subtypes have been defined. Certain features are shared by more than one of these subtypes, and these will be considered first.

Basal cell carcinomas are composed of islands or nests of basaloid cells, with palisading of the cells at the periphery and a haphazard arrangement of those in the centers of the islands. The tumor cells have a hyperchromatic nucleus with relatively little, poorly defined cytoplasm. The intercellular bridges are invisible on routine light microscopy. There are numerous mitotic figures, sometimes atypical,[641] and a correspondingly high number of apoptotic tumor cells. This high rate of cell death accounts for the paradoxically slow growth of basal cell carcinomas which possess numerous mitoses.[642]

The vast majority of cases show some attachment to the undersurface of the epidermis. Ulceration is not infrequent in larger lesions. Lesions of long standing and aggressive tumors usually extend into the lower dermis. Deep extension occurs either diffusely or within the paths of the cutaneous adnexae.[643] Involvement of the subcutis or of the underlying cartilage in lesions of the nose and ear is quite uncommon.[644] Perineural invasion is present in nearly 1% of cases, although the incidence is higher in aggressive variants.[645–647]

Islands of tumor cells are surrounded by a stroma, which is newly formed and different from the adjacent dermis. This stroma contains variable amounts of acid mucopolysaccharides. Laminin and types IV, V and VII collagen are present in the basement membrane, which separates the tumor cells from the stroma.[648,649] However, there is decreased expression of some other basement membrane components, which may facilitate their ability to invade.[650] Aggressive basal cell carcinomas show discontinuous staining for laminin and type IV collagen, but a marked stromal myofibroblastic response with an increase in stromal fibronectin.[651] They are also more likely to express p53 protein.[652] Amyloid, which is formed by the tumor cells, is present in the stroma in up to 50% of cases.[653–655] It is less common in aggressive variants.[654] The adjacent dermis shows solar elastosis in over 90% of cases, although its degree is sometimes mild.[656] The overlying epidermis may show the changes of a solar keratosis, although this is only rarely the precursor of a basal cell carcinoma.[657]

A variable inflammatory cell infiltrate is usually present, although there is a paucity of cells in some recurrences. The presence of plasma cells in the infiltrate correlates with ulceration. The infiltrate is usually composed mainly of T cells, the majority of which are CD4+.[658–660] Natural killer cells, mast cells and Langerhans cells are also present.[658,661–663] Cell-mediated immunity appears to play a role in the focal regression seen in up to 20% of tumors.[659,664] The expression of interleukin-2 receptor is increased in regressing lesions.[659] Active regression is characterized by the presence of a lymphocytic infiltrate which surrounds and penetrates tumor nests, with disruption of the normal palisaded outline and the formation of numerous apoptotic tumor cells.[661,664] Both C4+ and CD8+ cells are present in regressing lesions.[665] Past regression can be recognized by finding areas of eosinophilic new collagen within a tumor, associated with absence of tumor nests, an increase in small blood vessels, loss of appendages and a variable inflammatory cell infiltrate.[664] Prominent central regression with the formation of scar tissue is a feature of the so-called 'field fire' type of basal cell carcinoma.

Calcification may be present in the center of the keratin cysts that form in several of the histological subtypes. Ossification is an exceedingly rare event.[656–669] Another rare finding is the presence of transepidermal elimination of tumor nests.[670] Also rare is the development of pseudoepitheliomatous hyperplasia or keratoacanthoma-like changes in the epidermis following irradiation or excision of a basal cell carcinoma;[671] this is known as pseudorecidivism.[672]

Basal cell carcinomas or closely related changes may overlie a dermatofibroma.[673] This has been discussed on page 932. Basal cell carcinomas have also been reported in association with seborrheic keratoses (see p. 759), intradermal nevi, porokeratosis, Darier's disease, lupus vulgaris, keratoacanthoma, desmoplastic tricholemmoma,[674] neurofibromas and, as already mentioned, organoid nevi.[675]

Sometimes no tumor can be found in a biopsy specimen despite a strong clinical suspicion that basal cell carcinoma is present. This is particularly so with the multifocal superficial basal cell carcinoma where nests can be widely spaced or undergo regression. It is good practice to order, routinely, three levels of all punch and shave biopsies to prevent sampling errors. Clues in an initial non-diagnostic slide that suggest that deeper sections may yield basal cell carcinoma include focal basal atypia, stromal or superficial fibrosis, empty dermal spaces, equivocal adnexae and microcalcifications.[676]

The tumor cells in basal cell carcinoma resemble epidermal basal cells, both in their glycoconjugate pattern, their keratin expression[677,678] and the presence of *bcl-2*.[679–684] Clinically aggressive basal cell carcinomas have low labeling with *bcl-2*.[685] However, the cells also express cytokeratins, which are found only in follicular epithelium.[677,686] Tumor cells stain with the murine monoclonal antibody VM-1;[687] they usually do not stain for involucrin, epithelial membrane antigen or CD44, as occurs in squamous cell carcinomas,[688–692] although CD44 has been found in infiltrative tumor strands.[693] However, they do stain diffusely for Ber EP4, unlike squamous cell carcinomas, which are always negative;[694–696] basaloid carcinoma of the anus is also negative.[504] A band-like peritumorous reaction with peanut agglutinin has been reported in most basal cell carcinomas,[697] but not in trichoepitheliomas.[698] Other features that can be used to distinguish these two tumors are the staining pattern for *bcl-2* (expressed in virtually all cells in most basal cell carcinomas, but only weakly in some aggressive variants, and only in the basal layer of trichoepitheliomas) and CD34 (found in the peritumoral fibroblasts around trichoepitheliomas but not in those around sclerosing basal cell carcinomas).[698–700] In contrast, stromelysin-3 is expressed by the fibroblastic cells of nearly 70% of morpheic basal cell carcinomas, but not by fibroblasts in desmoplastic trichoepithelioma.[701,702] Light microscopy is still the most reliable method of distinguishing these two tumors, although the diffuse staining of basal cell carcinomas with *bcl-2* is of some value.[695,703]

Various morphological subtypes have been defined. These include solid (nodular), micronodular, cystic, multifocal superficial (superficial multifocal), pigmented, adenoid, infiltrating, sclerosing, keratotic, infundibulocystic, metatypical, basosquamous and fibroepitheliomatous.[704] Mixed patterns are quite common (Fig. 31.18).[705] Several other rare variants have also been described. It should be remembered that punch and shave biopsy techniques provide approximately 80% accuracy in the diagnosis of the various subtypes of basal cell carcinoma.[706]

Solid (nodular) type

The solid variant, also known as the large nest type, accounts for approximately 70% of all cases. It is composed of islands of cells with peripheral palisading and a haphazard arrangement of the more central cells. Retraction spaces sometimes form between the tumor islands and the surrounding stroma. Ulceration may be present in larger lesions.

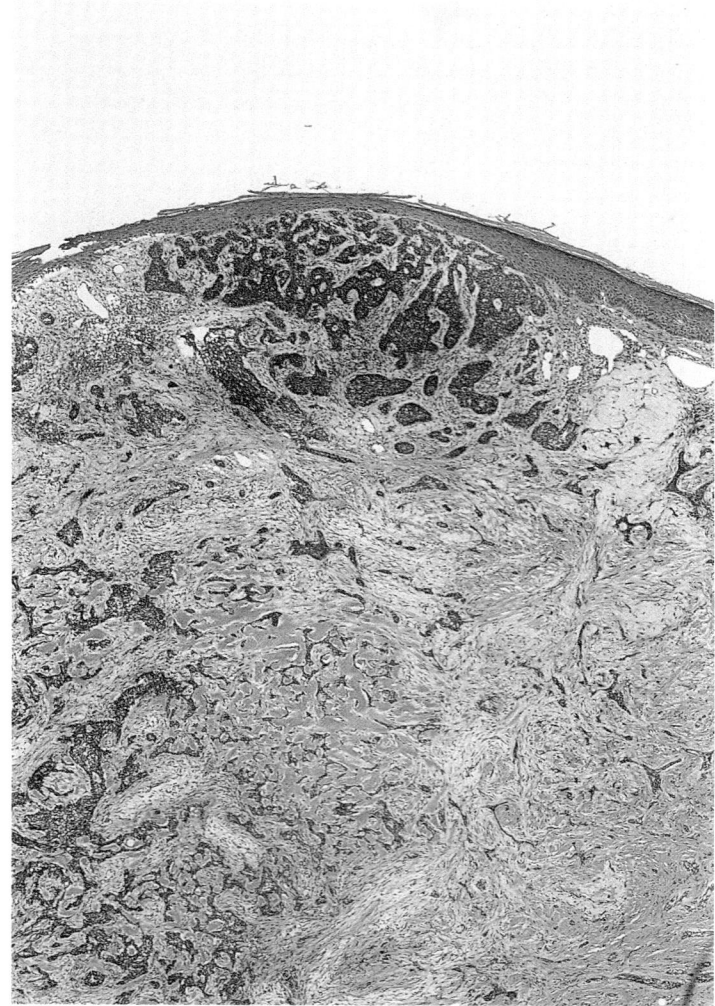

Fig. 31.18 **Basal cell carcinoma of mixed type** with a superficial solid and micronodular component and a deep sclerosing/morpheic area. This lesion had not been treated previously, supporting the view that aggressive lesions may develop *de novo*, without previous treatment. (H & E)

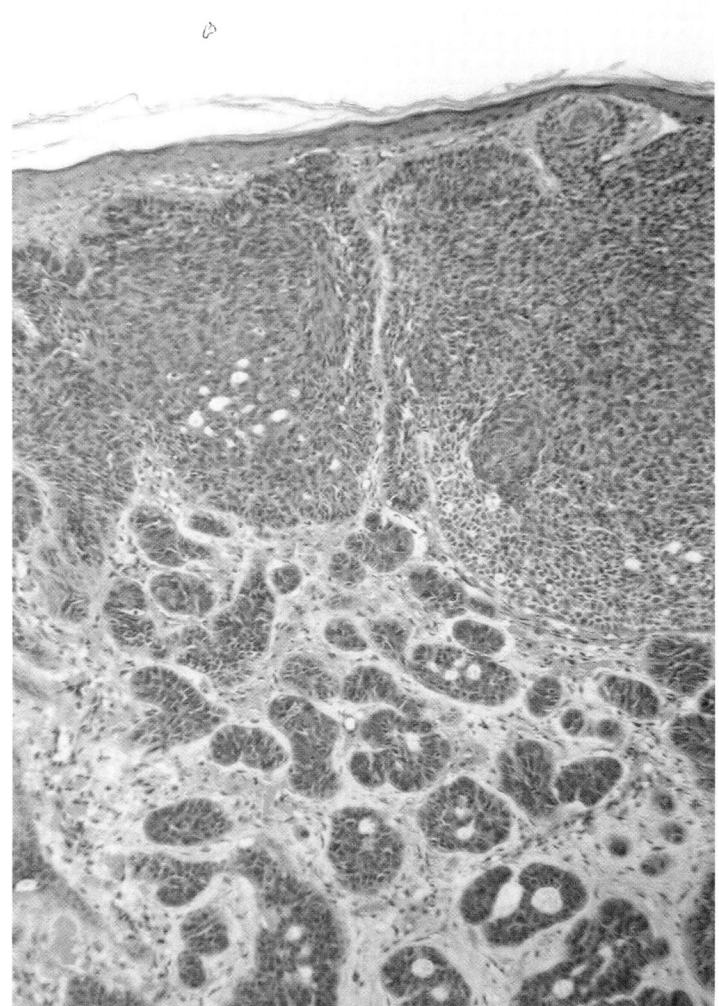

Fig. 31.19 **Basal cell carcinoma.** The superficial part is of solid type and the deeper nests are of micronodular type. (H & E)

Micronodular type

The micronodular variant resembles the solid type, but the nests are much smaller and the peripheral palisading is not always as well developed (Fig. 31.19). The micronodular type has a much greater propensity for local recurrence than the solid type.[707] Sometimes it infiltrates quite widely through the dermis and extends into the subcutis. The micronodular type is often included incorrectly with the infiltrating or solid types.

Cystic type

One or more cystic spaces are present toward the center of some or all of the tumor islands.[558] This results from the degeneration of tumor cells centrally, and it may be associated with increased mucin between the tumor cells adjacent to the cyst.

Multifocal superficial (superficial multifocal) type

Although a three-dimensional reconstruction study has shown that the apparently discrete nests of tumor cells are interconnected, suggesting a unicentric origin,[708] inclusion of the word 'multifocal' in the title is still recommended for the full characterization of this variant (Fig. 31.20). The author has difficulty in accepting the concept of a unicentric origin for all such

cases, given the wide separation of nests that is sometimes found. The multifocal superficial basal cell carcinoma is composed of multiple small islands of basaloid cells attached to the undersurface of the epidermis, and usually confined to the papillary dermis. Acantholysis has been reported in a few cases.[709] A narrow zone of fibrous stroma may surround the nests. There is usually a patchy band-like lymphocytic infiltrate and an increase in thin-walled vessels.[710] This pattern accounts for 10–15% of all tumors, and is the usual pattern seen in lesions removed from the shoulder region.[510] The age of patients with this subtype is lower than for other types.[711]

Pigmented type

Melanin pigment is usually formed in solid, micronodular, multifocal super-ficial, or follicular variants.[712] Functional melanocytes are scattered through the tumor islands and there are numerous melanophages in the stroma.[713] There are few melanosomes within the tumor cells. Melanosome complexes form in tumor cells as a consequence of repeated cycles of phagocytosis of melanosome-containing tumor cells that have undergone apoptosis.[714] Basal cell carcinomas of the usual type are also populated by some melanocytes.[715] Other pigmented phenomena in basal cell carcinomas are the colonization of one by a melanoma in situ, the metastasis of a melanoma to one, and the presence of a combined melanoma and basal cell carcinoma.[716–718]

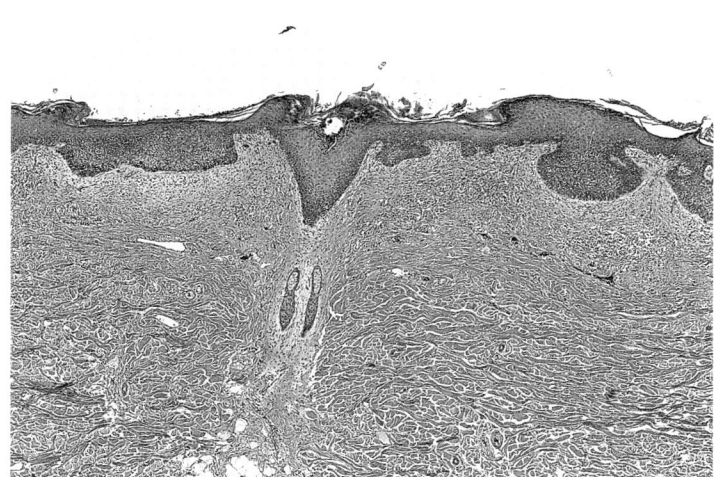

Fig. 31.20 **Basal cell carcinoma of multifocal superficial type.** (H & E)

Adenoid type

The adenoid variant consists of thin strands of basaloid cells in a reticulate pattern. Stromal mucin is often quite prominent. The adenoid type is quite uncommon in a pure form. It may occur in association with the solid type.

Infiltrating type

This non-sclerosing variant has an infiltrative rather than an expansile pattern of growth.[719] It accounts for approximately 5% of all tumors, although this figure is higher in some patient groups.[720] The histological features are distinctive, with elongated strands of basaloid cells, 4–8 cells thick, infiltrating between collagen bundles (Fig. 31.21).[719] Sometimes, even narrower strands are present, with spiking projections.[719] There may be a slight increase in fibroblasts, but there is no significant fibrosis. Often there is a solid pattern superficially with the infiltrating nests at the periphery or base of the lesion. Sometimes a focal infiltrative pattern is seen in the re-excision specimen of a biopsy proven solid (nodular) basal cell carcinoma.[721] These changes are limited to the region of the biopsy scar and appear to represent a scar-induced phenomenon without any sinister connotations. Like the sclerosing variant, it has a clinically indistinct border, but it differs from that variant in its opaque, yellow-white color.[719] Metallothionein, a presumptive marker of aggressive clinical behavior, is increased in the infiltrative variant.[722]

Sclerosing type

The sclerosing category includes lesions which have also been referred to as fibrosing, scirrhous, desmoplastic and morpheic.[723,724] The uncommon 'field fire' type with central fibrosis resulting from regression should not be included in this category. Up to 5% of all basal cell carcinomas are of the sclerosing type.[723] The tumor presents as an indurated, pale plaque with a slightly shiny surface and clinically indistinct margins.[723] There are narrow elongated strands and small islands of tumor cells embedded in a dense fibrous stroma.[724] If the stroma has dense, eosinophilic areas resembling a keloid, then the term 'morpheic' has traditionally been used, although at other times this term has been used interchangeably with 'sclerosing'. The term 'keloidal' has been applied to basal cell carcinomas with thick sclerotic keloidal collagen bundles in the stroma.[725,726] A selectively enhanced procollagen gene expression has been found in the sclerosing variant.[727] Also, large defects have been found in the basal lamina that surrounds the tumor nests.[728] Smooth muscle α-actin and myosin are often present in the stroma.

Keratotic type

The keratotic variant is similar to the solid type, with nests and islands of basaloid cells with peripheral palisading.[729] It differs in the presence of squamous differentiation and keratinization in the centers of the islands.[730] There is usually very little stroma, and no lobular arrangement or follicular differentiation.[729]

Infundibulocystic type

The uncommon infundibulocystic variant, found most often on the face, is often confused with the keratotic type.[731–735] It is small, well circumscribed, and composed of nests of cells arranged in an anastomosing fashion with little stroma (Fig. 31.22). There are numerous small infundibular cyst-like structures containing keratinous material and sometimes melanin.[731] The stroma may contain amyloid and/or melanin.[731] Multiple lesions are sometimes present.[736]

Metatypical type

Although the term 'metatypical' is sometimes applied to tumors with mixed basaloid and squamous features, it should be reserved for the rare basal cell carcinoma composed of nests and strands of cells maturing into larger and paler cells (Fig. 31.23).[640,730] Peripheral palisading is often lost. The cells express much less keratin 17 and keratin 8 than do the cells in the more usual types of basal cell carcinoma.[737] Peripheral palisading is less obvious than usual, and

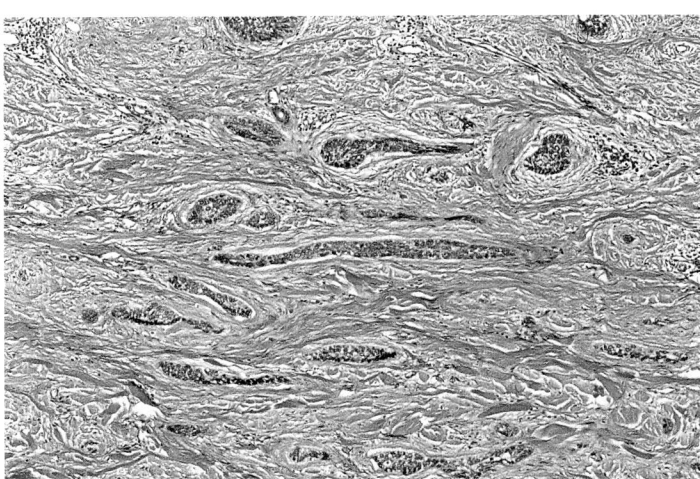

Fig. 31.21 **Basal cell carcinoma of infiltrating type,** with elongated nests of basaloid cells infiltrating between the collagen bundles of the dermis. (H & E)

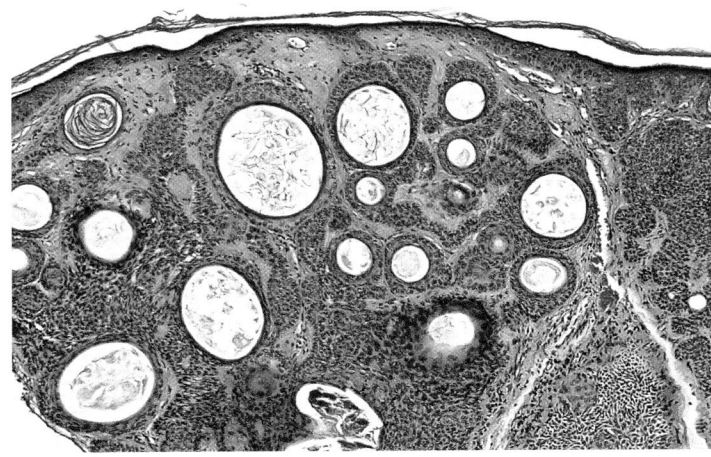

Fig. 31.22 **Basal cell carcinoma of infundibulocystic type.** (H & E)

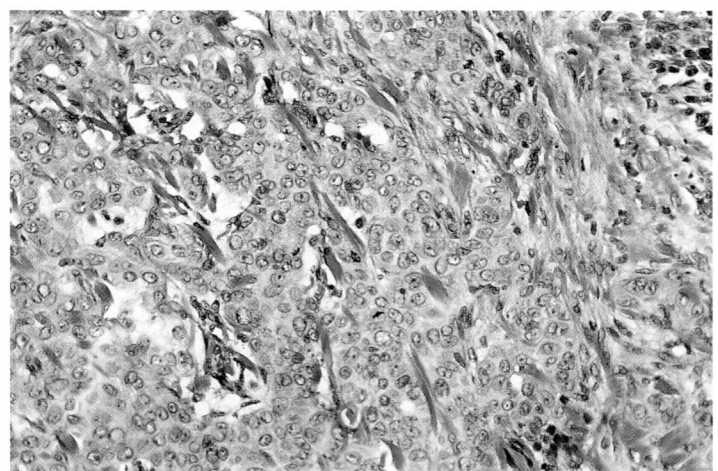

Fig. 31.23 **Basal cell carcinoma of metatypical type.** There are larger cells with loss of palisading. (H & E)

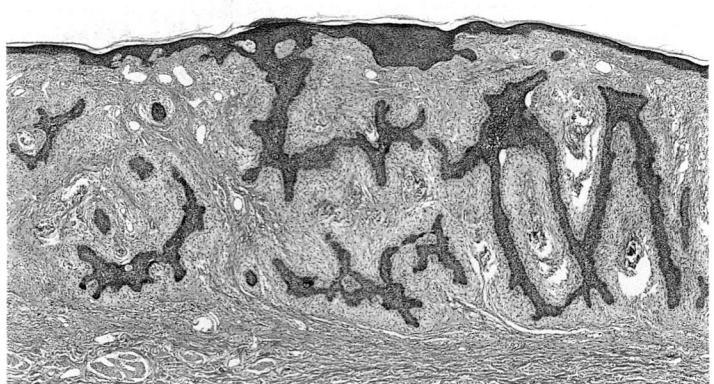

Fig. 31.24 **Fibroepithelioma variant of basal cell carcinoma,** with thin cords of cells set in a fibrous stroma. (H & E)

the stroma is often prominent. This variant is regarded by some as having metastatic potential.[738]

Basosquamous carcinoma

Basosquamous carcinoma is a controversial entity which can be defined as a basal cell carcinoma differentiating into a squamous cell carcinoma.[730,739–741] It is composed of three types of cell: basaloid cells, which are slightly larger, paler and more rounded than the cells of a solid basal cell carcinoma; squamoid cells with copious eosinophilic cytoplasm; and an intermediate cell which resembles that seen in metatypical tumors.[730,741] Accordingly, the basosquamous carcinoma is sometimes confused with metatypical and keratotic basal cell carcinomas. It is an aggressive lesion with metastatic potential.[742] This tumor shows some areas of Ber EP4 positivity, in contrast to squamous cell carcinoma which is always negative.[696]

Fibroepithelioma

Fibroepithelioma presents as a soft nodular lesion resembling a fibroma or papilloma, often on the lower part of the back.[743,744] It is composed of thin anastomosing strands of basaloid cells set in a prominent loose stroma (Fig. 31.24).[745] The stroma has no elastic tissue.[743] Merkel cells are quite prominent.[746] It has been suggested, and subsequently disputed, that this variant derives its histological pattern from the spread of basal cell carcinoma down eccrine ducts, eventually replacing them with solid strands of tumor.[519,747,748] A rare cystic variant of fibroepithelioma has been reported.[749]

Miscellaneous variants

Appendageal differentiation is sometimes present in basal cell carcinomas. Follicular (pilar) variants have already been mentioned (see above). Matrical and tricholemmal differentiation may also occur:[750–752] basal cell carcinomas that show this feature require differentiation from matrical carcinomas (see p. 869). Sebaceous differentiation is sometimes seen in areas of an otherwise typical basal cell carcinoma: such lesions require differentiation from other sebaceous tumors (see p. 872). A rare variant with histochemical and ultra-structural features of apocrine differentiation has been reported.[753] Tumors with eccrine differentiation also occur, and these shade into lesions best classifed with eccrine carcinomas[754,755] (see p. 895).

Other variants include the exceedingly rare granular cell,[756,757] clear cell (Fig. 31.25)[758–762] and 'signet-ring' cell (hyaline inclusion) types.[763–767] Lesions with giant tumor cells and large nuclei have been variously reported as 'basal

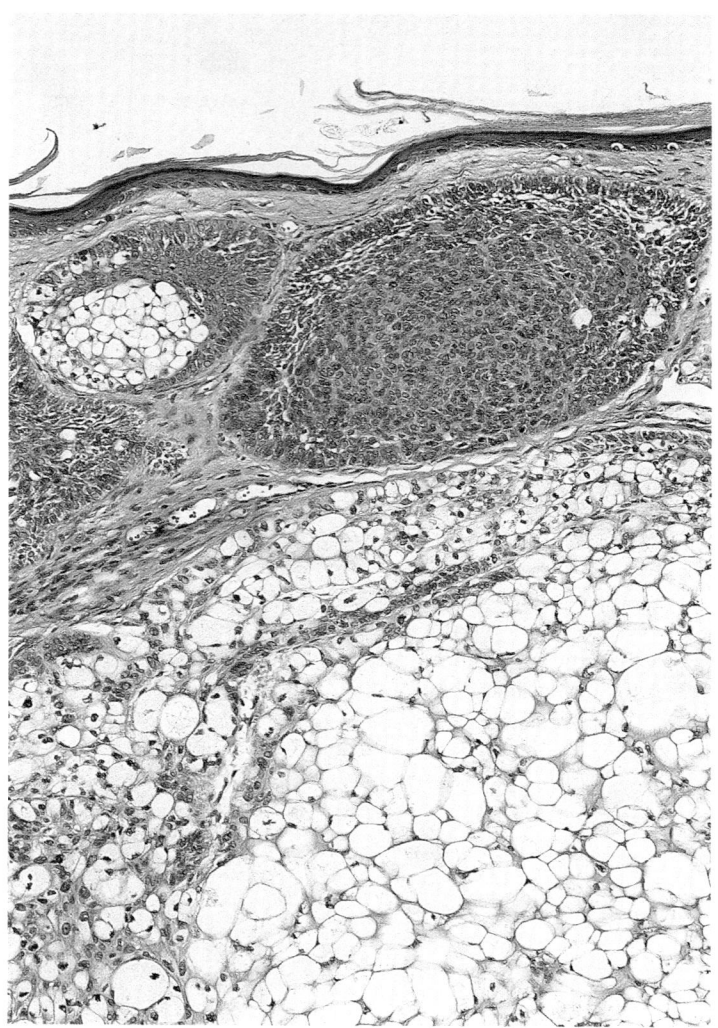

Fig. 31.25 **Basal cell carcinoma with solid and clear cell areas.** (H & E)

cell epithelioma with giant tumor cells', 'basal cell carcinoma with monster cells' and 'pleomorphic basal cell carcinoma'.[768–770] The giant cells are cycling and they do not appear to represent a senescent change.[771] There is one report of this variant in which there were stromal giant cells as well.[772] Adamantinoid,[773] schwannoid[774,775] and neuroendocrine differentiation[776–779] are further variants. It has been suggested that the tumor reported as a basal cell carcinoma with thickened basement membrane was really a trichilemmal carcinoma.[780,781] The rare lesion showing myoepithelial differentiation needs to be distinguished from a carcinosarcoma (see p 776).[782]

Electron microscopy

The tumor cells have a large nucleus and cytoplasm containing a few tonofilaments. There are a small number of desmosomes and some thin processes on the cell surface.[783] The appearances resemble those of the primary epithelial germ.[784] Stromal amyloid is sometimes present, and this appears to be formed in the cytoplasm of tumor cells. Myofibroblasts have been found in the stroma.[785]

Cytology

The cytological diagnosis of basal cell carcinoma is made by finding large clusters of cells with crowded nuclei.[786,787] Peripheral palisading can seldom be appreciated in cytological preparations.[786]

Recurrences

The 5-year recurrence rate for basal cell carcinomas is approximately 5%, although this varies with the type of treatment.[788–790] The figure rises to 9% with long-term follow-up.[791] Although one study found almost no difference in the recurrence rate of completely excised tumors and those with tumor at one excision margin,[792] this is contrary to most reports,[793,794] which have found that the distance to the closest resection margin is an important predictor of recurrence.[795] In another report the recurrence rate was noted to be 1.2% in cases of adequately excised lesions, 12% if tumor was present within 1 high-power field of a margin, and 33% if tumor was present at the excision margin.[796] Residual tumor is found in only 60% of re-excision specimens following a report of tumor at an excision margin.[797] Failure to find tumor in all such re-excisions may result from an insufficient amount of tumor surviving to be detected, or because the residual cells spontaneously die or are destroyed by a local inflammatory reaction. Another possibility is that the incompleteness of the initial excision was more apparent than real. Failure to detect tumor in re-excision specimens, combined with a recurrence rate thought to be 30–50%, has resulted in a view that additional resection is not always necessary when margins are positive. However, if recurrence does occur, subsequent recurrences are sometimes difficult to control.[798,799] Patients with small primary basal cell carcinomas that appear to have been completely removed after a biopsy procedure are at risk for recurrence without further treatment.[800]

Recurrences are more common in lesions on the nose and nasolabial fold, but this may in part be related to a difficulty in achieving adequate margins in these sites.[793,801] Infiltrative, micronodular[793] and multifocal types of basal cell carcinoma are more likely to recur than nodular types.[705,795,802–804] Metatypical and sclerosing variants may also be associated with more aggressive behavior.[805–807] Recurrences are also more likely in patients who have multiple skin cancers.[808,809] It is now generally accepted that the majority of recurrent basal cell carcinomas are aggressive from the onset, and that in many cases this can be predicted from the histological appearances of the original tumor.[810,811] Notwithstanding these studies, tumors recurring after previous radiotherapy are usually aggressive and infiltrative.[812] It is unlikely that all such lesions were of an aggressive type initially. It should be noted that some studies have shown no correlation between the histological type and the recurrence rate, although a lack of uniformity in the histological classification of basal cell carcinomas makes the comparison of some series almost meaningless.[792,805] Basal cell carcinomas in young adults are not more aggressive than those occurring in older patients, as once thought.[813]

Numerous reports document changes in the cells and stroma of basal cell carcinoma, some of which appear to provide explanations for the aggressiveness or otherwise of particular variants of basal cell carcinoma.[814–821] Tumors showing aneuploidy and hyperexpression of cyclin D1 are more likely to have an unfavorable outcome.[822] Angiogenesis may be an important step in the acquisition of an aggressive phenotype.[823,824] Acquisition of trisomy 6 by tumor cells may lead to the emergence of metastatic potential.[825]

Metastases

The usual criteria used for the acceptance of metastatic basal cell carcinoma are a previous or present primary lesion in the skin and a metastatic lesion that has a histological picture similar to that of the primary, and which could not have arisen by direct extension from the primary lesion.[826] Metastases are rare, occurring in approximately 0.05% of cases.[826–828] This low incidence is probably related to the stromal dependence of basal cell carcinomas, which presupposes that only large tumor emboli with attached stroma are successful in implanting.[829] Accordingly, it is not surprising that lesions that give origin to metastases are large, ulcerated and neglected.[830] Metatypical features and/or squamous differentiation have also been regarded as important,[738,742] although these changes were present in only 15% of the primary lesions in one review of metastasizing basal cell carcinomas.[826]

Metastases occur most commonly in the regional lymph nodes;[831,832] bones, lungs[833] and liver are less frequent sites of involvement.[834] Other organs and the subcutis are rarely affected.[738] Aspiration metastasis to the lung has been recorded.[835] The median interval between the diagnosis of the primary lesion and signs of metastasis is approximately 9 years, whereas the interval between the appearance of the metastases and the death of the patient is approximately 1 year.[826] Long survivals have occasionally been reported.[336] Systemic amyloidosis[837,838] and a myelophthisic anemia secondary to marrow infiltration[839] have been documented in patients with metastatic basal cell carcinomas.

NEVOID BASAL CELL CARCINOMA SYNDROME

The nevoid basal cell carcinoma syndrome is a multisystem disorder characterized by multiple basal cell carcinomas with an early age of onset, odontogenic keratocysts, pits on the palms and/or soles, cutaneous cysts,[840] skeletal and neurological anomalies and ectopic calcifications.[841–843] Often there is a characteristic facies, with hypertelorism and an enlarged calvaria.[844] Less common manifestations include lipomas and fibromas of various organs,[845] fetal rhabdomyoma,[846] ovarian cysts and medulloblastomas.[841,847] The inheritance is autosomal dominant with high gene penetrance and variable expressivity.[848] The responsible gene, the *PATCHED* gene (*ptc*), is on chromosome 9q22.3–q31.[849–851] Sporadic cases of basal cell carcinoma with this gene mutation have been found (see above).[611]

Only 15% of affected individuals have basal cell carcinomas before puberty, and these may take the form of pigmented macules resembling nevi.[841] The development of acrochordon-like basal cell carcinomas may be the first manifestation of the syndrome.[852] Tumors are usually harmless before puberty and only a small percentage become aggressive in later life.[844,853] The tumors may develop anywhere, including within the palmar pits,[854] but there is a predilection for sun-exposed areas, such as the face, neck and upper part of the trunk.[855] They may vary in number from few to hundreds of lesions. A defective in vitro cellular response to X-irradiation has been found in the syndrome,[856] and this may help explain the development of skin tumors in these patients at sites of X-irradiation.[854,857]

The unilateral linear basal cell nevus is an unrelated condition which may be associated with comedones and, rarely, osteoma cutis[858] (see p. 865).

Multiple basal cell carcinomas can occur in a familial setting without other manifestations of a systemic syndrome. In one such family, segmental distribution of the tumors occurred representing mosaicism.[859] Multiple hereditary infundibulocystic basal cell carcinomas have also been reported. Genetic studies have mapped the defect to chromosome 9q22.3, flanking the *ptc* gene.[860] Multiple infundibulocystic basal cell carcinomas have also been reported in a patient with HIV infection.[736]

Histopathology[861]

The whole spectrum of histological variants of basal cell carcinoma is found in the nevoid basal cell carcinoma syndrome.[862] Calcification, keratinizing cysts, pigmentation and osteoid tissue have all been said to occur more frequently in basal cell carcinomas occurring in the syndrome than in sporadic cases, although some studies have failed to confirm this.[862]

The cutaneous cysts usually take the form of epidermal cysts.[840] Occasionally they may have a festooned lining of squamous cells that form keratin without the presence of a granular layer, thus resembling the keratocysts of the jaws.[863]

The palmar and plantar pits show marked thinning of the stratum corneum, with a thin parakeratotic or orthokeratotic layer in the base overlying a mildly acanthotic epidermis.[864] Basal cell hyperplasia, and rarely basal cell carcinomas, may be found in the base of the pits.[865,866]

SQUAMOUS CELL CARCINOMA

Squamous cell carcinoma is the second most common form of skin cancer in Caucasians.[867] Its incidence in an Australian study was 166 cases per 100 000 of the population, the highest in the world.[868] There is a predisposition for it to arise in the sun-damaged skin of fair-skinned people who tan poorly.[868–870] It is relatively uncommon in black people, in whom the tumors often arise in association with scarring processes.[871]

Clinical aspects

Most squamous cell carcinomas arise in areas of direct exposure to the sun, such as the forehead, face, neck, and dorsum of the hands.[872–875] The ears, scalp and vermilion part of the lower lip are also involved, particularly in males.[872] Non-exposed areas such as the buttocks, genitalia[876,877] and subungual regions[878–881] are occasionally affected. Uncommonly, squamous cell carcinomas may develop at sites of chronic ulceration,[882] trauma, burns, frostbite,[883] vaccination scars,[884] a pyoderma gangrenosum scar,[884a] skin grafts,[885] fistula tracts,[886] pilonidal sinuses of long standing,[887,888] hidradenitis suppurativa and acne conglobata.[889,890] The term 'Marjolin's ulcer' has been used for cancers arising in sites of chronic injury or irritation such as scars, ulcers and sinuses,[891–893] although Marjolin did not describe the condition with which he is eponymously credited.[894] Tumors arising in these circumstances are sometimes aggressive, and local recurrences are common.[392]

There are isolated reports of the occurrence of squamous cell carcinomas in various conditions such as dystrophic epidermolysis bullosa,[895] Hailey–Hailey disease,[896] porokeratosis,[897,898] discoid lupus erythematosus,[899] lichen planus,[900,901] erythema ab igne, leprosy,[902] lupus vulgaris,[903] lichen sclerosus et atrophicus,[904,905] balanitis xerotica obliterans, acrodermatitis chronica atrophicans, chronic lymphedema,[906] organoid and epidermal nevi,[907] granuloma inguinale, lymphogranuloma venereum, poikiloderma,[908] epidermodysplasia verruciformis, acrokeratosis verruciformis, and the Jadassohn phenomenon. Squamous cell carcinomas are also increased in frequency among patients with xeroderma pigmentosum, vitiligo and albinism.[909,910] Several cases have been associated with hypercalcemia.[911–913]

Squamous cell carcinomas are found predominantly in older people; they are rare in adolescence and childhood.[914] Clinically, they present as shallow ulcers, often with a keratinous crust and elevated, indurated surrounds. The adjacent skin usually shows features of actinic damage. The acantholytic variant is usually a nodular tumor on the head or neck, and is almost invariably misdiagnosed clinically as a basal cell carcinoma. It tends to be more aggressive than the conventional squamous cell carcinoma.[915] The metastatic potential of this tumor will be considered after discussion of the histopathology.

Occurrence in organ transplant recipients

Patients whose immune status is deficient,[916] particularly organ transplant recipients,[917–924] are also predisposed to develop these tumors. It has been estimated that renal transplant recipients have a risk of developing squamous cell carcinoma of the skin which is 18 times that of the general population. The incidence of carcinoma of the lip is also increased in these patients.[925] They also develop warts with varying dysplasia, and verrucous keratoses with a putative viral contribution.[599] In a significant number of these tumors HPV-5 or HPV-8 is found, suggesting a role for the virus in the etiology of the skin cancers that result.[599] In genital lesions HPV-16 and/or HPV-18 have been detected.[926,927] HPV-16 appears to be a risk factor for squamous cell carcinoma of the head and neck.[928] Human papillomavirus has been specifically excluded in some series of post-transplant skin cancers;[929,930] however, the frequency and spectrum of HPV types detected depend on the HPV detection system used, indicating a need for standardization of techniques.[931] There may be a synergistic interaction of HPV and HIV in the carcinogenic process leading to the development of some penile carcinomas.[932] It appears that background levels of *p53* mutations may be increased in the normal skin of post-transplant and HIV patients and this may contribute to the increased incidence of skin cancers in these patients.[933–935] It should be remembered that the immunohistochemical overexpression of p53 does not necessarily reflect the degree of *p53* gene mutations as short gene deletions will not be reflected in increased p53 immunoreactivity.[936] The tumors often infiltrate widely, indicating their aggressive nature. They have a diminished cellular immune response in the stroma.[937,938] Low-dose acitretin produces a reduction in the number of skin cancers in these post-transplant patients.[939] Most of the fatal cases have been reported from Australia, suggesting that sunlight, which has a profound effect on the cutaneous immune system,[282] plays a role in the formation of these aggressive lesions.[919,940] Exposure to sunlight before the age of 30 appears to be a risk factor for the development of skin cancers in renal transplant recipients,[941] although not necessarily for aggressive ones. Information is now being published which indicates that recipients of cardio-thoracic transplants have a greater risk of developing aggressive cutaneous malignancies than recipients of renal transplants.[942] Cardiac transplant patients generally receive quantitatively more immunosuppression than their renal counterparts and this is the presumed explanation for the significant incidence of cutaneous malignancies in this group.[942–944] Cessation of immunosuppressants appears to result in deceleration of cutaneous carcinogenesis.[945]

Etiology

Ultraviolet-B radiation appears to be the most important etiological factor; ultraviolet-A plays a minor role.[358,946–949] Ultraviolet radiation is known to damage the DNA of epidermal cells, but there appear to be other complex mechanisms involved in UV-induced carcinogenesis. Squamous cell carcinomas can be produced in various animals with ultraviolet radiation, almost to the exclusion of other types of tumors.[947,950] Less important etiological agents include radiation therapy,[529] arsenic, coal tar and various hydrocarbons.[951]

Human papillomavirus may play a role in immunosuppressed patients (see above);[599,926] it has a significant role in genital lesions and, rarely, in squamous cell carcinomas on the finger.[930,952–956] HPV is now being detected in squamous cell carcinomas of immunocompetent patients.[957–960]

Genetic aspects

The role of gene mutations in the development of this skin cancer is now being studied. Chromosomal instability at 13q14 adjacent to the retinoblastoma tumor suppressor gene (*Rb*) has been detected in some cases.[961] Inactivation of the *Rb* gene can result from interaction with some HPV types.[961]

It should be kept in mind that, in simple terms, carcinogenesis is a three-step process that consists of initiation, promotion and progression.[962]

Unitarian theory of squamous cell carcinoma

Ackerman has proposed that solar keratoses should be regarded as squamous cell carcinomas *de novo* and that they should not be regarded as premalignancies or precancers that may convert into squamous cell carcinoma.[298,963] Others have agreed with this approach.[964,965]

According to this 'unitarian' viewpoint the following conditions are morphological expressions of squamous cell carcinoma:

- solar keratosis and its analogs, arsenical and radiation keratoses
- Bowen's disease and bowenoid papulosis
- giant condyloma and verrucous carcinoma
- keratoacanthoma
- proliferating tricholemmal cysts.

However, this approach assumes the inevitable progression of solar keratoses to squamous cell carcinomas, which is not proved. It is also likely to alarm patients who have one of these lesions. This approach also has a significant impact on reimbursement schedules in some jurisdictions.

Histopathology

The usual squamous cell carcinoma consists of nests of squamous epithelial cells which arise from the epidermis and extend into the dermis for a variable distance. The cells have abundant eosinophilic cytoplasm and a large, often vesicular, nucleus. There is variable central keratinization and horn pearl formation, depending on the differentiation of the tumor. Individual cell keratinization is often present. The degree of anaplasia in the tumor nests has been used to grade squamous cell carcinomas. Usually, a rather subjective assessment of differentiation is made using the categories of 'well', 'moderately' and 'poorly' differentiated, rather than Broder's classic grading of 1–4, where grade 4 applies to the most poorly differentiated lesions (Fig. 31.26).

Most squamous cell carcinomas arise in solar keratoses or sun-damaged skin.[640,966,967] The borderline between a thick solar keratosis and a superficial squamous cell carcinoma is somewhat arbitrary (see p. 762). Squamous cell carcinomas sometimes arise in Bowen's disease, and in these cases the cells are usually non-keratinizing; they may show variable tricholemmal or even sebaceous-like differentiation.[402] These tumors should not be confused with the rare clear cell[762,968–970] and 'signet-ring'[971,972] variants of squamous cell carcinoma, both of which have cells with pale cytoplasm; in the case of the 'signet-ring' variant the nucleus is eccentric. Tumors developing in renal transplant recipients cannot be reliably distinguished from those arising in immunocompetent people.[973]

Squamous cell carcinomas occasionally infiltrate along nerve sheaths, the adventitia of blood vessels, lymphatics, fascial planes and embryological fusion planes.[974,975] The presence of perineural lymphocytes is an important clue to the likely presence of perineural invasion in deeper sections.[976] There is often

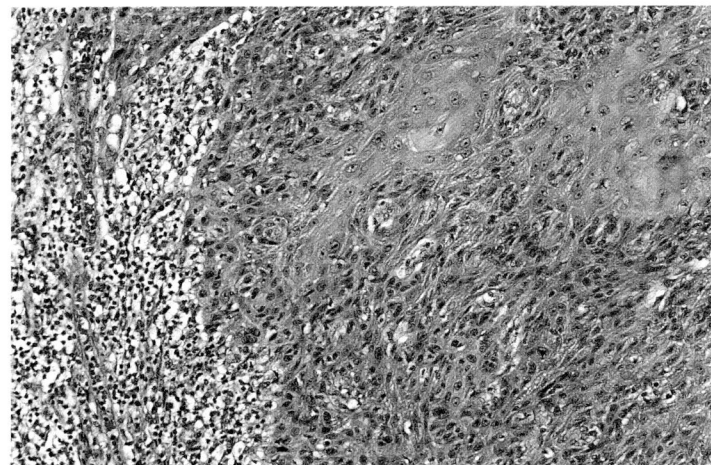

Fig. 31.26 **Moderately well differentiated squamous cell carcinoma.** (H & E)

a mild to moderate chronic inflammatory cell infiltrate at the periphery of the tumor.[977] A subpopulation of these cells express the TCR-αβ heterodimer.[978] Eosinophils are occasionally prominent in the infiltrate and sometimes extend into the tumor islands.[979] Erythrophagocytosis by tumor cells has been reported in one case.[980] The tumor cells may evoke a stromal desmoplastic response.[981]

Immunoperoxidase studies are sometimes helpful if the tumor is poorly differentiated or of spindle-cell type.[982] The cells are positive for epithelial membrane antigen[696,983] and cytokeratin.[984,985] Squamous cell carcinomas contain keratins of higher molecular weight than those in basal cell carcinomas.[986] Involucrin is present in larger keratinized cells.[688] Stains for lysozyme, S100 protein and desmin are negative. Vimentin may be expressed in poorly differentiated and spindle-cell variants (see below). The expression of Ki-67 and MIB-1 is higher in squamous cell carcinoma than in basal cell carcinoma.[987] However, the level of expression is not a predictor of prognosis.[983]

Spindle-cell squamous carcinoma

Spindle-cell squamous carcinoma is an uncommon variant that usually arises in sun-damaged or irradiated skin. It may be composed entirely of spindle cells, or have a variable component of more conventional squamous cell carcinoma.[989–992] The spindle cells have a large vesicular nucleus and scanty eosinophilic cytoplasm, often with indistinct cell borders. There is variable pleomorphism, usually with many mitoses. The presence of squamous differentiation, dyskeratotic cells and continuity with the epidermis may assist in making the diagnosis. Electron microscopy and immunoperoxidase markers may be necessary in some circumstances to differentiate this variant from malignant melanoma and atypical fibroxanthoma.[993–995] Some spindle-cell squamous carcinomas may coexpress cytokeratin and vimentin, suggesting metaplastic change of a squamous cell carcinoma to a neoplasm with mesenchymal characteristics.[996,997] Vimentin is sometimes found in squamous cell carcinomas arising in Marjolin's ulcers.[998] As the spindle cells are often negative with Cam 5.2, it is necessary to use a pankeratin marker or 'cocktail'. MNF116 is suitable for this purpose.

Adenoid squamous cell carcinoma

The adenoid (acantholytic, pseudoglandular) variant, which is found most often on the head and neck, accounts for 2–4% of all squamous cell carcinomas.[999–1002] It consists of nests of squamous cells with central acantholysis leading to an impression of gland formation,[999] although the peripheral cells are cohesive (Fig. 31.27). Acantholysis is sometimes minimal. Mucin has been reported in some,[1001] but these tumors may have been variants of adenosquamous carcinoma (see p. 776). Adenoid variants often arise from an acantholytic solar keratosis. Sometimes this is in the vicinity of the pilosebaceous follicle.[1001]

Pseudovascular squamous cell carcinoma

Pseudovascular squamous cell carcinoma is a rare variant of adenoid squamous cell carcinoma which may be mistaken for an angiosarcoma.[1003] The terms 'pseudovascular adenoid squamous cell carcinoma'[1004] and 'pseudoangiosarcomatous carcinoma'[1005] have also been used for this tumor. It presents as an ulcer or crusted nodule on sun-exposed skin. The tumor usually has an aggressive behavior, with a high mortality rate.[1006] Microscopically, the lesion is composed of pseudovascular structures lined by cords of polygonal or flattened tumor cells.[1004] The cells express cytokeratin, epithelial membrane antigen and, sometimes, vimentin. They are negative for CD31, CD34 and factor VIII-related antigen.[1004]

Other variants of squamous cell carcinoma

There are several other histological variants of squamous cell carcinoma, a knowledge of which may prevent misdiagnosis. The *clear cell* and 'signet-ring' types have already been mentioned (see above). The cells express keratin markers.[972] A *pigmented* variant also occurs. Melanin is found in epithelial tumor cells as well as in macrophages and dendritic melanocytes. The dendritic cells express S100 protein and HMB-45.[1007–1012] This variant must be distinguished from the squamomelanocytic tumor, in which both a squamous cell carcinoma and melanoma component develop (see p. 835). The *inflammatory* squamous cell carcinoma has a dense lymphocytic stromal infiltrate surrounding poorly differentiated squamous nests (Fig. 31.28). Focal regression is sometimes present. This variant appears to have a high metastatic potential. The *basaloid* squamous cell carcinoma is a distinctive variant of squamous cell carcinoma found in the oropharynx[1013] and anogenital region.[1014] In this latter region it has a high association with HPV infection. It is composed of small basaloid cells with a high mitotic rate.[1014] Central comedonecrosis is sometimes present in the tumor cell islands. It has a higher histological grade, deeper extension and higher mortality rate than conventional tumors. Other rare variants are the *infiltrative* type (Fig. 31.29)

with small nests and strands or single cells infiltrating a dermis which is fibrous and/or mucinous,[1015] and a *desmoplastic* variant analogous to morpheic basal cell carcinoma.[1016] Finally, there has been one report of *rhabdoid* differentiation in a squamous cell carcinoma.[1017]

Electron microscopy

The tumor cells in conventional lesions have tonofilaments and well-developed desmosomes and some interdigitating microvilli. In some studies of spindle-cell lesions, the cells have shown the features of squamous epithelium with well-developed desmosomes and tonofilaments.[1018,1019] In other cases there have been cells resembling fibroblasts, as well as cells exhibiting both mesenchymal and epithelial features.[1020] This mixed pattern of differentiation may result from cell fusion rather than metaplasia.[1020]

Recurrences and metastases

Recurrences are more likely in those tumors with aggressive histological features such as deep invasion,[1021] poor differentiation, perineural invasion and acantholytic features.[807,1022–1025] Aneuploidy does not appear to correlate with the risk of metastasis.[1026] Narrow surgical margins also contribute to local recurrence.[1027] Squamous cell carcinomas developing in patients who

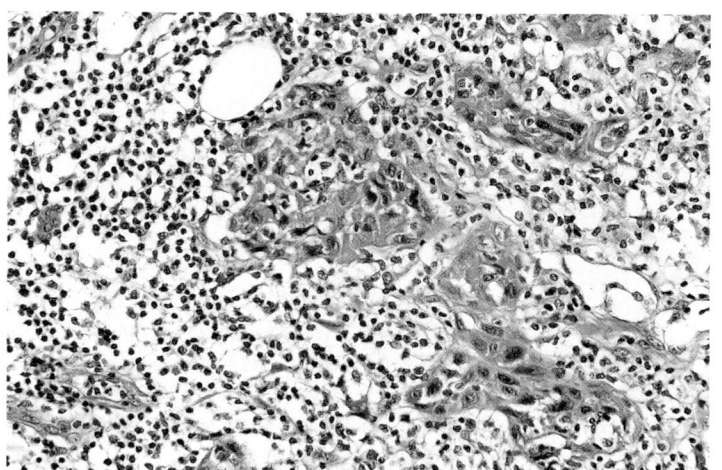

Fig. 31.28 **Squamous cell carcinoma of inflammatory type.** There is usually a heavy infiltrate throughout the entire tumor. (H & E)

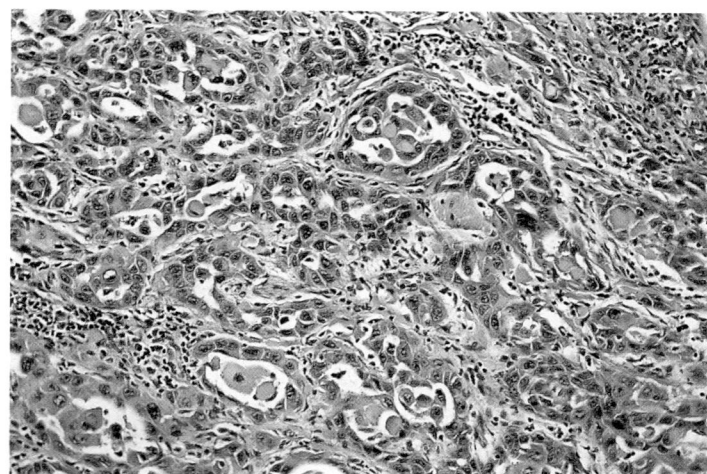

Fig. 31.27 **Squamous cell carcinoma of acantholytic type.** The cells at the periphery of the tumor nests are still cohesive. (H & E)

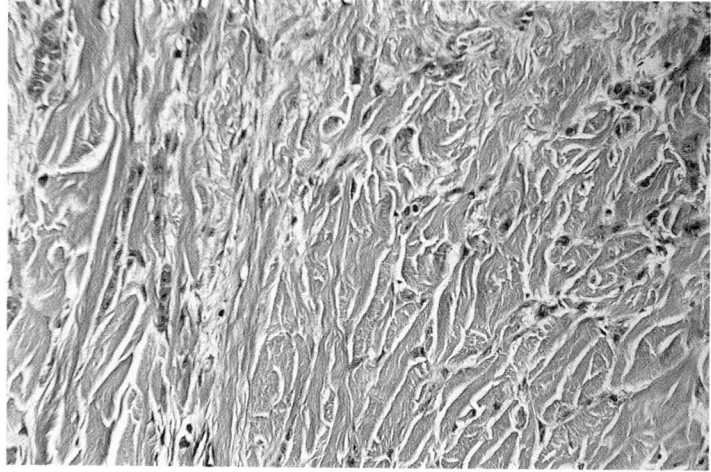

Fig. 31.29 **Squamous cell carcinoma of infiltrating type.** There are strands and small clusters of cells infiltrating between collagenous bundles. (H & E)

are immunosuppressed or who have an underlying malignant lymphoma or leukemia are often more aggressive.[1028–1030] The majority of squamous cell carcinomas are only locally aggressive and are cured by several different methods of treatment. The recurrence rate is approximately double that for basal cell carcinomas.[1031]

The risk of metastasis varies with the clinical setting in which the lesion arises.[1032] The lowest risk is for tumors arising in sun-damaged skin.[1033,1034] The usually quoted figure of 0.5%[1033] has been challenged as being too low on the basis of several hospital series, which might be expected to be weighted in favor of more aggressive and deeply invasive lesions.[947] In this regard it appears that vertical tumor thickness is a prognostic variable, just as it is for melanomas,[1021,1035] although further studies are required to ascertain the critical tumor thickness required for metastasis. Acantholytic variants arising in sun-damaged skin have a slightly greater risk of metastasis, of the order of 2%,[1032] although in one study it was as high as 19%.[1002] Invasive lesions arising in Bowen's disease metastasize in 2–5% of cases.[402] They have been regarded as high-risk squamous cell carcinomas.[1036]

For lesions arising in skin not exposed to the sun, the incidence of metastases is approximately 2–3%.[1037,1038] There is a further increase in this risk for lesions of the lip, although the quoted range (2–16%) is quite wide.[1035,1038–1040] Tumors of the lip are more likely to metastasize if there is perineural invasion, if the tumor is of high grade with a dispersed pattern, and if the tumor thickness exceeds 2 mm.[1035,1041] Metastasis is almost invariable for tumors thicker than 6 mm.[1041] Muscle invasion is not useful in predicting the development of lymph node metastases, as was once thought. Tumor vascularity is not a risk factor.[1042] A strong dendritic cell response appears to be favorable.[1043] In a recent retrospective review of 323 patients with squamous cell carcinoma of the lip, the cause-specific survival at 10 years was 98%.[1044] For squamous cell carcinomas arising in Marjolin's ulcers the incidence of metastasis is thought to be 10–30%,[1038] whereas for vulval, perineal and penile tumors it may be as high as 30–80%.[1032,1045–1047]

Metastases usually occur in the regional lymph nodes in the first instance. For this reason, sentinel lymph node biopsy has been advocated for some high-risk lesions.[1048] Uncommonly the lung is involved, and then it is usually a terminal phenomenon associated with metastases to other organs. Cutaneous metastases are exceedingly rare.[1049] In one case they produced a bowenoid (epidermotropic) pattern.[1050] A zosteriform pattern of cutaneous metastasis has also been recorded.[1051] A circulating tumor antigen, thought to be specific for squamous cell carcinoma, has been detected in patients with metastatic disease;[1052] however, this antigen has been reported recently in patients with inflammatory dermatoses.[1053]

It has been suggested that tumor spread may be facilitated by a loss of skin-derived antileukoproteinase (SKALP), an inhibitor of elastase and proteinase 3. This enzyme is found in well-differentiated tumors but is absent in poorly differentiated tumor cells.[1054] Other factors undoubtedly contribute, such as reduced expression of the adherens junction protein vinculin[1055] and the surface proteoglycan syndecan-1.[1056,1057] There is increased expression of the matrix metalloproteinases (which degrade extracellular matrix),[1058] of cathepsin B and D,[1059,1060] of carcinoembryonic antigen[1061] and of ornithine decarboxylase.[1062] Several cases of burn scar-related squamous cell carcinoma, an aggressive variant, have had mutations in the *Fas* gene, involved in cell death signaling.[1063] Apoptosis is increased in squamous cell carcinomas.[1064]

A not uncommon problem is the finding of a predominantly cystic squamous cell carcinoma in the soft tissues of the neck. Often, no primary tumor can be found although there may be a history of past skin cancers. A recent study has shown that, in the majority of cases, the primary lesion will be in the faucial or lingual tonsillar crypt epithelium.[1065]

VERRUCOUS CARCINOMA

Verrucous carcinoma is a distinctive clinicopathological variant of squamous cell carcinoma which may involve the oral cavity,[1066] larynx, esophagus and skin.[1067–1069] It is a slow-growing, often large, warty tumor which invades contiguous structures but rarely metastasizes.[1070] Cutaneous lesions are usually in the genitocrural area[1071–1074] or on the plantar surface of the foot (epithelioma cuniculatum), although exceptionally it can arise in any part of the skin surface.[1075–1080]

Plantar lesions are the most common form of verrucous carcinoma.[1081–1085] They are usually exophytic, pale lesions, sometimes with draining sinuses,[1086] and are often painful and tender. Similar lesions have rarely been reported on the palm or thumb.[1087,1088] Occasionally, explosive growth occurs after a prolonged period of slow progression. The mean duration of lesions at the time of diagnosis is 13–16 years.[1089]

Various factors have been implicated in the etiology of verrucous carcinomas. The chewing of tobacco or betel may predispose to oral lesions, whereas human papillomavirus has been implicated in the etiology of genitocrural lesions[1075] and, rarely, of tumors at other sites.[1090] HPV-6, 11, 16 and 18 have been implicated in various cases.[1069,1091–1093] However, if the concept of **warty carcinoma** is adopted (see below) then the incidence of HPV in verrucous carcinomas will considerably decrease. A case of plantar verrucous carcinoma has been reported contiguous with a plantar wart, and this may have been of etiological significance.[1094] Trauma and chronic irritation have also been implicated in the etiology.[1095]

Histopathology[1075,1081,1085,1096]

Multiple biopsies are often required for the diagnosis of verrucous carcinoma. Lesions are both exophytic, with papillomatosis and a covering of hyperkeratosis and parakeratosis, and endophytic (Fig. 31.30).[1085] The rete pegs have a bulbous appearance and are composed of large well-differentiated squamous epithelial cells with a deceptively benign appearance.[1096] These acanthotic downgrowths sometimes extend into the deep reticular dermis and even the subcutis.[1097] They are blunted projections, in contrast to the uneven, sharply pointed and jagged downgrowths seen in pseudoepitheliomatous hyperplasia.[1096] There is usually only very low mitotic activity and this is confined to the basal layer.[1098] The downgrowths are mostly contained by an intact basement membrane, although frankly invasive features are sometimes present. A more aggressive, cytologically malignant squamous

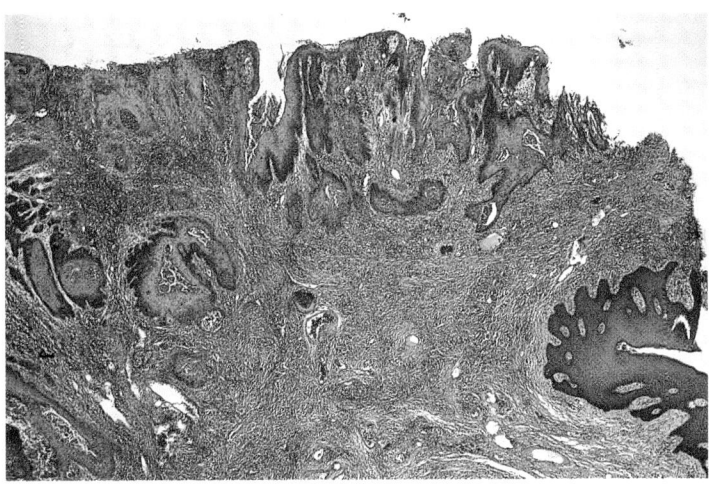

Fig. 31.30 **Verrucous carcinoma.** Well-differentiated nests of squamous epithelium extend into the dermis. (H & E)

cell carcinoma may sometimes arise in a verrucous carcinoma, either *de novo* or following X-irradiation of the lesion.[1099] The combination of verrucous and conventional squamous cell carcinoma is called hybrid verrucous-squamous carcinoma.[1100]

Other features include the presence of burrows in the surface filled with parakeratotic horn, as well as draining sinuses containing inflammatory and keratinous debris. Keratin-filled cysts may develop within the tumor mass.[1096] The fibrous stroma surrounding the epithelial downgrowths contains ectatic vessels and a variable inflammatory infiltrate, in which eosinophils and neutrophils are sometimes prominent.[1081,1101] The presence of neutrophils is an important diagnostic clue. Intraepidermal abscesses are often present in lesions of long standing.

A rare entity affecting the glans penis and known as **pseudo-epitheliomatous, keratotic and micaceous balanitis** may present with the histological features of a verrucous carcinoma; in other instances it has features of a hyperplastic dystrophy akin to vulval dystrophy.[1102-1104] A true verrucous carcinoma may arise within it.[1105] Its etiology is unknown; HPV infection was excluded in one case.[1106]

Verrucous carcinoma should be distinguished from the exceedingly rare papillary variant of squamous cell carcinoma, which is a purely exophytic lesion, in contrast to the mixed endophytic and exophytic character of verrucous carcinoma.[1107]

Recently, the concept of **warty (condylomatous) squamous cell carcinoma** has been proposed for an exophytic warty tumor of the penis (a similar lesion occurs on the vulva) usually related to HPV-16 infection.[1108,1109] This tumor is distinguished from verrucous carcinoma on the basis of long and undulating, condylomatous papillae, with prominent fibrovascular cores and a base which is rounded or irregular and jagged. Furthermore, koilocytotic atypia is prominent and diffuse, while it is absent in the 'pure' verrucous carcinoma.[1108] Warty carcinoma of the penis appears to have a better prognosis than typical squamous cell carcinoma of the penis.[1110]

Proliferating cell nuclear antigen (PCNA) is expressed at the periphery of squamous nests (similar to keratoacanthomas), in contrast to the more widespread distribution in the usual type of squamous cell carcinoma.[1111]

ADENOSQUAMOUS CARCINOMA

Primary adenosquamous carcinoma of the skin is a rare, usually aggressive, tumor with a potential for local recurrence and metastasis.[1112-1114] The penis is a favored site.[1115] Most cases in the literature have been reported as mucoepidermoid carcinomas,[1116,1117] but this term is best reserved for morphologically related tumors arising in the salivary gland and lung.[1112,1118,1119]

Histopathology[1112,1113]
Adenosquamous carcinomas are usually deeply invasive tumors composed of islands and strands of squamous cell carcinoma admixed with glandular structures containing mucin (Fig. 31.31). The mucin, which is of epithelial type (sialomucin), is present in the lumen and the cytoplasm of the lining cells. It stains with mucicarmine, alcian blue at pH 2.5, and the PAS method, and it is digested by sialidase. The cells are positive for epithelial membrane antigen and cytokeratin, whereas those lining the glandular spaces stain for carcinoembryonic antigen.

Adenosquamous carcinoma has been confused with adenoid (acantholytic) squamous cell carcinoma, but in the latter there is no mucin and the glandular spaces contain acantholytic squamous cells.[1120] Adenosquamous carcinoma also differs from the case reported as 'squamous cell carcinoma with mucinous metaplasia', which was composed of mucin-containing vacuolated cells resembling 'signet-ring' cells; there were no gland spaces.[1112]

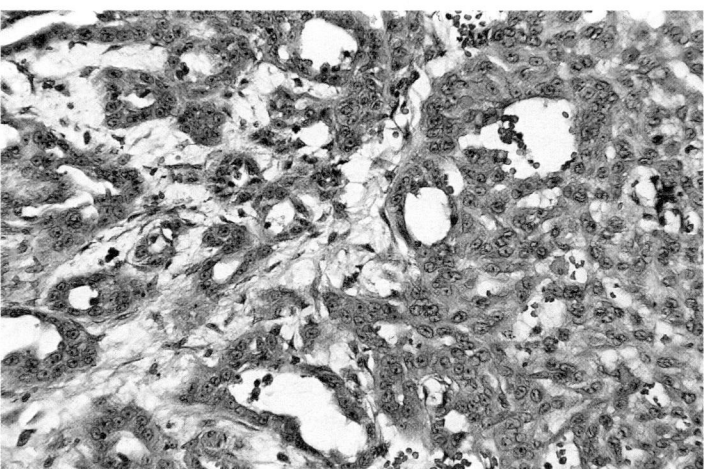

Fig. 31.31 **Adenosquamous carcinoma.** There are glandular spaces containing a small amount of mucin. There are no acantholytic cells, distinguishing this lesion from an acantholytic type of squamous cell carcinoma. (H & E)

CARCINOSARCOMA (METAPLASTIC CARCINOMA)

Carcinosarcoma of the skin is an exceedingly rare biphasic tumor with fewer than 20 cases reported to date.[1121-1126] This tumor has metastatic potential.[1127]

Histopathology
For this diagnosis the tumor must contain an intimate admixture of epithelial and mesenchymal elements, both of which are malignant (Fig. 31.32).[1122] In most cases reported, the epithelial component has been a basal or squamous cell carcinoma,[1121,1128] whereas the mesenchymal component has included fibrosarcoma, chondrosarcoma and osteogenic sarcoma, and sometimes other elements such as leiomyosarcoma and rhabdomyosarcoma.[1126] Rare epithelial components have included eccrine porocarcinoma and spiradenocarcinoma.[1126]

LYMPHOEPITHELIOMA-LIKE CARCINOMA

Lymphoepithelioma-like carcinoma of the skin is a rare tumor which resembles histologically the nasopharyngeal tumor of the same name.[1129-1132] It presents clinically as a papulonodular lesion, usually on the face or scalp.[1133] The shoulder and vulva are rare sites of involvement.[1134] Metastasis is uncommon. Epstein–Barr virus has not been detected in tumor cells.[1133,1135-1137] Wick's group believes that this lesion is a morphological manifestation of squamous cell carcinoma.[1138]

Histopathology[1129]
The tumor may arise in the dermis or subcutis. It is composed of islands of large epithelial cells surrounded by a dense infiltrate of lymphocytes and some plasmacytoid cells (Fig. 31.33). The epithelial cells have a vesicular nucleus and a large nucleolus. There is no evidence of overt squamous differentiation such as the formation of keratin 'pearls', intercellular bridges or dyskeratotic cells.[1138] Adnexal differentiation has been reported in the epithelial nests in several cases.[1136,1139] The overlying epidermis has been reported as normal in many cases, but as dysplastic in a few.[1140]

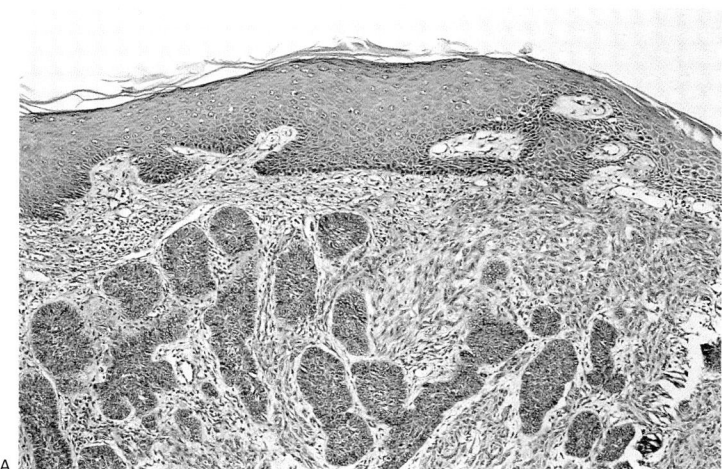

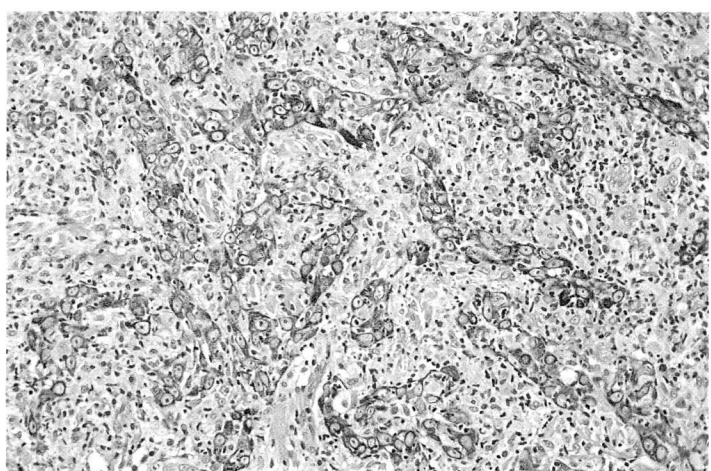

Fig. 31.34 **Lymphoepithelioma-like carcinoma.** This is the same case as Fig. 31.33. There are more epithelial cells than might be expected from the H & E preparation. (Broad keratin immunoperoxidase)

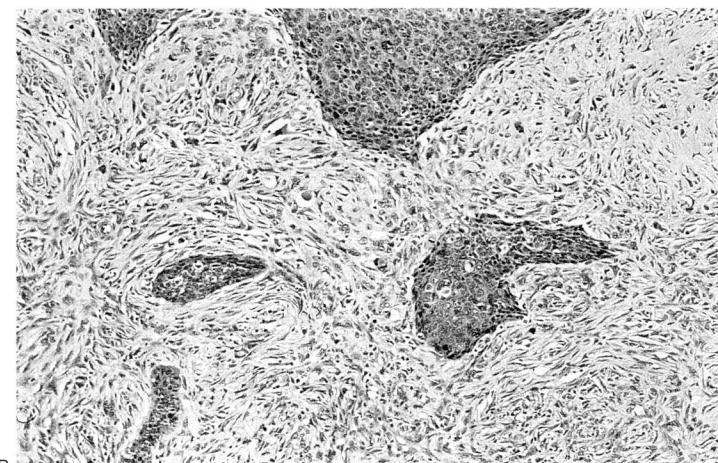

Fig. 31.32 **(A) Carcinosarcoma. (B)** There is a pleomorphic sarcomatous component surrounding basisquamous epithelial nests. (H & E)

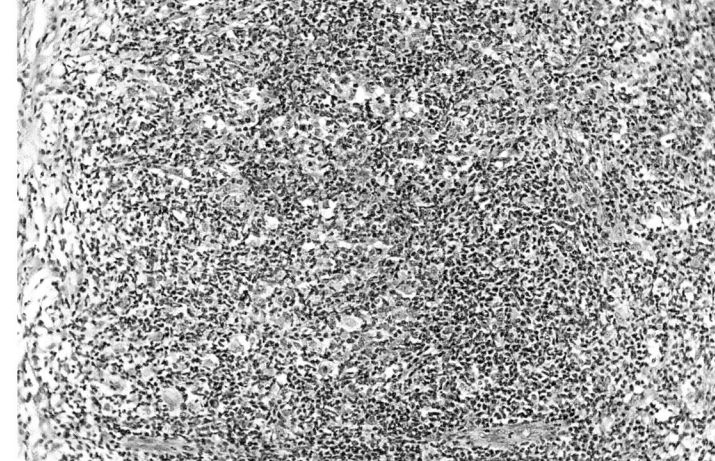

Fig. 31.33 **Lymphoepithelioma-like carcinoma.** Tumor cells are difficult to distinguish from the surrounding lymphoid cells. (H & E)

The epithelial cells contain cytokeratin (Fig. 31.34) and express epithelial membrane antigen but not S100 protein, whereas the stromal lymphocytes express CD45 (leukocyte common antigen). Some cases have numerous factor XIIIa-positive dendritic cells in the stroma.[1133]

Lymphoepithelioma-like carcinoma must be distinguished from cutaneous lymphadenoma, a variant of trichoblastoma peppered by lymphocytes (see p. 863).

MISCELLANEOUS 'TUMORS'

CUTANEOUS HORN

A cutaneous horn is a hard, yellowish-brown keratotic excrescence: to earn the designation of 'horn' its height conventionally must exceed at least one-half its greatest diameter.[1141] It may be straight or curved, and up to several centimeters in length.[1142] Cutaneous horns are usually solitary. They have a predilection for the face, the ears, and the dorsum of the hands of older individuals.[1143] A rare site is the penis.[1144,1145] It is a clinical entity which may be associated with many different pathological lesions. Most commonly a horn overlies an actinic keratosis, seborrheic keratosis, inverted follicular keratosis,[1143] tricholemmoma, verruca vulgaris or squamous cell carcinoma.[1141,1146,1147] Rarely, there may be an underlying keratoacanthoma, epidermal nevus, lichen simplex chronicus, epidermal cyst, angiokeratoma or basal cell carcinoma.[1148,1149] The pathology in the base of the horn is more likely to be premalignant or malignant in lesions with a wide base or a low height-to-base ratio and in lesions occurring on the nose, scalp, forearms and back of the hands.[1147] There is one report of underlying Kaposi's sarcoma,[1150] and one of psoriasis.[1151]

Histopathology

Horns are composed of keratotic material which may be amorphous or lamellated. Any of the lesions mentioned above may be present in the base. Occasionally, there is underlying epidermal hyperplasia without cellular atypia, and in these circumstances a 'descriptive' diagnosis of cutaneous horn is appropriate.

The pattern of keratinization is usually epidermal, but a special variant of horn with tricholemmal keratinization has been reported.[1152–1154] Human papillomaviruses have been suggested as being causally related to these tricholemmal horns, on the basis of intranuclear inclusions demonstrated on electron microscopy.[1155] The tricholemmal horns must be distinguished from the so-called 'tricholemmomal horn',[1156] which represents the usual type of horn, with epidermal keratinization, overlying a tricholemmoma. The term 'onycholemmal horn' has been used for a tricholemmal horn on the nail groove.[1157] Nail horns showing epidermal keratinization may also occur, particularly on the big toe.[1142] Filiform parakeratotic horns have also been reported.[1158]

STUCCO KERATOSIS

The stucco keratosis (keratoelastoidosis verrucosa) has received little attention in the literature, despite its reported incidence in the elderly of approximately 5%.[1159–1161] Lesions are usually multiple and distributed symmetrically on the distal parts of the extremities, particularly the legs.[1159,1160] Individual lesions are small (1–4 mm), grayish-white keratotic papules. The surface scale may be scratched off with the finger to reveal a non-bleeding, slightly scaly surface. The lesions have some morphological resemblance to the hyperkeratotic variant of seborrheic keratosis and to tar keratoses, and their continued separation as a distinct entity is of doubtful validity. Several HPV types were detected in one case reported recently.[1162]

Histopathology[1159,1160,1163]

Stucco keratoses have prominent orthokeratosis and papillomatosis. There is some acanthosis, often associated with fusion of the rete ridges. There is little or no inflammatory infiltrate in the underlying dermis, which may show some solar elastotic changes. There is no increase in basaloid cells in the lesions and there are no horn cysts.

CLAVUS (CORN)

A clavus (corn) is a localized callosity which develops a small horny plug, pressure on which is usually painful. It results from pressure or friction, usually from footwear, on the skin overlying a bony prominence.

Histopathology

A clavus is composed of a thick parakeratotic plug set in a cup-shaped depression of the epidermis (Fig. 31.35). There is usually loss of the granular layer beneath the plug and thinning of the epidermis. A few telangiectatic vessels may be present in the upper dermis.

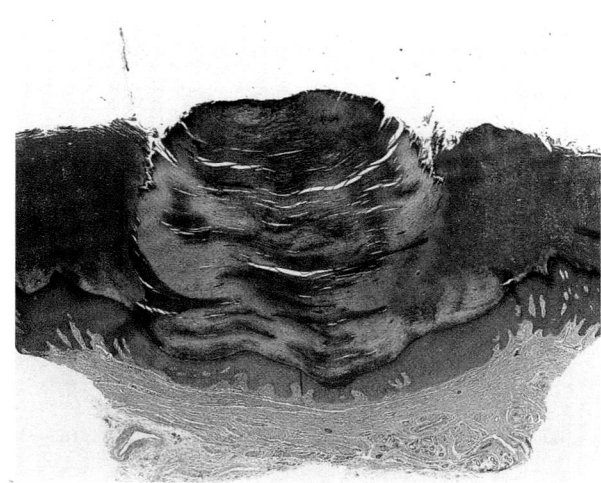

Fig. 31.35 **Clavus.** A thick parakeratotic plug is set in a cup-shaped depression of the epidermis. (H & E)

CALLUS

A callus is a circumscribed area of hyperkeratosis resulting from chronic friction or pressure. Callosities develop most frequently on the soles, overlying the metatarsal heads, but they may also arise on the hands in manual workers. Other sites may be affected in individuals involved in certain occupations and recreational pursuits.

Histopathology

The stratum corneum is thickened and compact, resulting in a slight cup-shaped depression of the underlying epidermis. The granular layer may be thickened, in contrast to a clavus (corn) in which it is usually lost (see above). There is usually some parakeratosis overlying the dermal papillae, but much less than in a clavus.

ONYCHOMATRIXOMA

Onychomatrixoma, a benign entity described comparatively recently, presents as a yellow discoloration of the nail plate, with transverse overcurvature of the affected nail.[1164] It may rarely present as longitudinal melanonychia or with nail bleeding.[1165,1166] This tumor appears to originate from the nail matrix cells.[1167]

Histopathology

The tumor is composed of epithelial cell strands originating from the nail matrix and penetrating vertically into the dermis. Some of the strands anastomose. In the central parts of the strands the keratinocytes evolve into parakeratotic cells, orientated along the axis of the strands.[1164,1168] The fibrous stroma is sharply delineated from the tumor cells.[1169]

KERATOACANTHOMA

Keratoacanthoma was first described in 1889 by Sir Jonathan Hutchinson, as 'crateriform ulcer of the face'.[1170] Several other terms, including 'molluscum sebaceum' and 'self-healing squamous cell carcinoma', have been applied since that time; the term 'keratoacanthoma' is now universally accepted.[1171,1172] Notwithstanding this comment, there is a growing trend in some countries to regard keratoacanthoma as a variant of squamous cell carcinoma.[1173] This cannot be justified on morphological or biological grounds.

A keratoacanthoma is most often a solitary, pink or flesh-colored dome-shaped nodule with a central keratin plug. It grows rapidly to a size of 1–2 cm over a period of 1–2 months, and has a tendency to involute spontaneously after 3–6 months. The duration of the lesion is more variable than is generally recognized, and lesions may persist for over a year without involuting. A keratoacanthoma may cause extensive local destruction, particularly if on the nose or eyelids, before regression occurs, and for this reason active treatment is usually advocated.

Keratoacanthomas develop most often in the older age groups, particularly in the sixth and seventh decades, and there is a male preponderance.[1174] It is estimated that one keratoacanthoma is diagnosed for every four squamous cell carcinomas of the skin, although keratoacanthomas are proportionately more frequent in subtropical areas.[1175] Whereas 70% of lesions develop on the face in temperate climates, there is a much greater tendency for lesions to arise on the arms, dorsum of the hands and the lower extremity in patients in subtropical areas.[1176] In a recent series of 40 consecutive cases studied by the author (in subtropical Brisbane, Australia), 85% were on the extremities.[1177] Nearly all lesions develop on hair-bearing areas (follicular keratoacanthomas), although there are some exceptions, to be mentioned below. Rare sites of involvement include the eyelids,[1178] conjunctiva,[1179] lip,[1180,1181] mouth,[1182] glans penis,[1183] perianal region and male nipple.[1184]

Nearly all keratoacanthomas are solitary lesions, less than 2 cm in diameter, arising on skin exposed to the sun. They may arise on areas not exposed to the sun.[1185] However, there are a number of rare clinical variants that are worthy of mention.[1171,1186,1187]

Giant keratoacanthoma

The term 'giant keratoacanthoma' is applied to a tumor greater than 2–3 cm in diameter. Such lesions have a predilection for the nose and the dorsum of the hands.[1188–1190] It has been reported on the lip.[1191]

Keratoacanthoma centrifugum marginatum (multinodular keratoacanthoma)

Keratoacanthoma centrifugum marginatum is a rare variant characterized by progressive peripheral growth with coincident central healing.[1192–1195] Such lesions may be 20 cm or more in diameter. The plaque-like variant reported as keratoacanthoma dyskeratoticum et segregans[1196] is probably related.

Subungual keratoacanthoma

Subungual keratoacanthoma may be solitary or it may be associated with multiple keratoacanthomas of the common type: in the latter case more than one subungual lesion may be present. Subungual keratoacanthomas grow rapidly, often fail to regress spontaneously,[1197–1199] and usually cause pressure erosion of the distal phalanx.[1200] Paradoxically, they are more destructive than squamous cell carcinomas in this site.[1201] They appear to be identical to the subungual keratotic tumors found in incontinentia pigmenti.[1202] Subungual keratoacanthomas can be grouped with lesions derived from mucous membranes as non-follicular keratoacanthomas.[1173]

Multiple keratoacanthomas[1203–1212]

There are several distinct clinical types of multiple keratoacanthomas. These include the Ferguson Smith type,[1204] the Grzybowski (eruptive) type,[1205,1213–1219] a mixed group with overlap or unusual features,[1206] a limited type in which the keratoacanthomas are restricted to one side or area of the body,[1207,1220,1221] and a secondary type in which the lesions develop at sites of trauma,[1186] treatment or an underlying dermatosis.[1222] Multiple keratoacanthomas may be associated with internal cancer,[1223–1225] as in Torre's syndrome (Muir–Torre syndrome), in which multiple keratoacanthomas accompany the presence of a primary visceral cancer, particularly of the gastrointestinal tract.[1208,1226,1227]

The Ferguson Smith type is characterized by the development of a succession of lesions, one or a few at a time, on covered as well as exposed areas of the body, and beginning usually in adolescence.[1186,1209,1228] These heal, leaving an atrophic and sometimes disfiguring scar. It seems that the variant found in Scottish kindreds is a more aggressive form with an autosomal dominant inheritance and histological appearances which may resemble those found in a squamous cell carcinoma.[1210] The term 'multiple self-healing squamous carcinomas' is still applied to this variant.[1210,1211] The locus implicated in this condition is on chromosome 9q22–q31.[1229]

In the eruptive type there are multiple (often several hundred) papules and nodules of varying size, with an onset in the fifth and sixth decades.[1212] Lesions may develop on the palms and soles and mucous membranes, as well as in the more usual sites. They may exemplify the Koebner phenomenon. The lesions may be intensely pruritic.[1212] The Witten and Zak type of multiple keratoacanthomas is a rare familial syndrome that combines features of the Grzybowski and Ferguson Smith types.[1230]

Etiology

Although viruses have long been suggested as an etiological agent, there are only isolated examples of their discovery in keratoacanthomas in immunocompetent individuals.[1231] However, DNA sequences of HPV of both genital and cutaneous types have been detected in 20% of keratoacanthomas in immunosuppressed patients.[1232,1233] In animals, chemical carcinogens can produce lesions resembling keratoacanthomas; such tumors develop from the hair follicles.[1234] Exposure to tars, either industrial or therapeutic, will induce lesions in humans.[356] Exposure to excessive sunlight is the most frequently incriminated factor in the etiology of keratoacanthomas.[1235] Other factors include trauma,[1186] immunosuppressed states (in which the keratoacanthomas are prone to aggressive growth, early recurrence, and even transformation into squamous cell carcinoma)[917] and xeroderma pigmentosum.[1180] They have rarely followed bites, vaccinations,[1236] arterial puncture,[1237] burns,[1238] the smoking of 'Goza' and 'Shisha' in the Middle East[1181] and PUVA therapy.[1239] They have been known to develop in linear epidermal nevi,[1240] in organoid nevi,[1241] in prurigo nodularis treated with cryotherapy,[1242] within an in situ malignant melanoma,[1243] at the site of treated psoriatic lesions[1244] and in association with several dermatoses, particularly hypertrophic lichen planus.[1245,1246]

Histopathology

As there is no single consistent histological feature that characterizes a keratoacanthoma,[1247] the diagnosis may cause difficulty for the inexperienced pathologist, particularly if only a snippet biopsy is submitted. However, there should be no difficulty in making a correct diagnosis on excision or shave specimens and in fusiform biopsies, which extend across the central diameter of the lesion for its full width or at least well into its center. A constellation of histological features needs to be assessed.

Keratoacanthomas are exoendophytic lesions with an invaginating mass of keratinizing, well-differentiated squamous epithelium at the sides and bottom of the lesion. There is a central keratin-filled crater which enlarges with the maturation and evolution of the lesion. Another key feature is the lipping (also known as buttressing) of the edges of the lesion which overlap the central crater, giving it a symmetrical appearance (Fig. 31.36). In some lesions a keratotic plug overlies discrete infundibula, and a central horn-filled crater is not formed.

The component cells have a distinctive eosinophilic hue to their cytoplasm and, as they mature, toward the center of the islands of squamous epithelium,

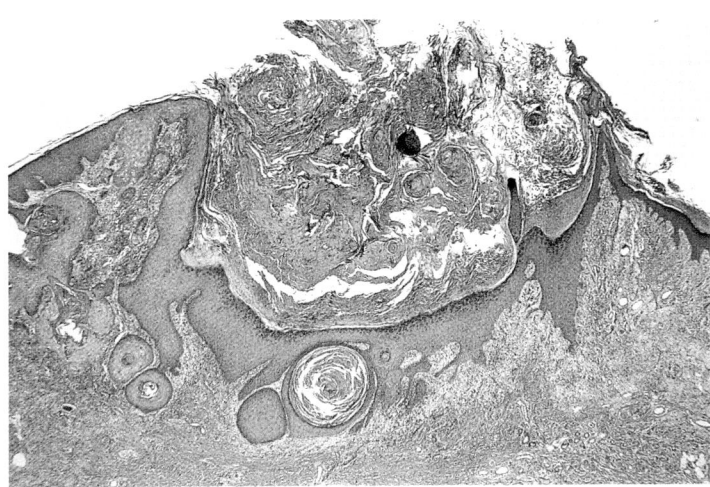

Fig. 31.36 **Keratoacanthoma.** This regressing lesion has a large keratin plug. (H & E)

they can become quite large (Fig. 31.37). Epithelial atypia and mitoses are not a usual feature. There is a mixed infiltrate of inflammatory cells in the adjacent dermis, and this is sometimes moderately heavy. Eosinophils and neutrophils may be prominent, and these may extend into the epithelial nests to form

small microabscesses. There is no stromal desmoplasia except in late involuting lesions.[1248] Extension below the level of the sweat glands is unusual;[1249] if it is present, particularly careful assessment of the other histological features is required. Atypical hyperplasia of the sweat duct epithelium may be present in some cases.[1250] Perineural invasion is an incidental and infrequent finding which does not usually affect the prognosis or behavior of the lesion,[1251,1252] although local recurrence has been reported in two perioral keratoacanthomas with extensive perineural invasion and intravenous growth (Fig. 31.38).[1253] Of the 40 cases reported from the author's institution, 27 were from the head or neck region. We found no metastasis in the 35 cases for which follow-up information was available. Local recurrence occurred in only one case, and this was not considered to be directly attributable to the presence of perineural invasion.[1177] Intravenous growth has also been recorded in a keratoacanthoma of the scalp.[1254] No recurrence occurred, although wider excision was carried out. The author has now seen five such cases that have had no untoward consequences (Fig. 31.39).

In *keratoacanthoma centrifugum marginatum* there is progressive involution and fibrosis toward the center of the lesion, although the advancing edge will show the typical overhanging lip with nests of squamous epithelium in the underlying dermis.

Subungual keratoacanthomas contain more dyskeratotic cells (Fig. 31.40) and fewer neutrophils and eosinophils than the usual keratoacanthoma, and

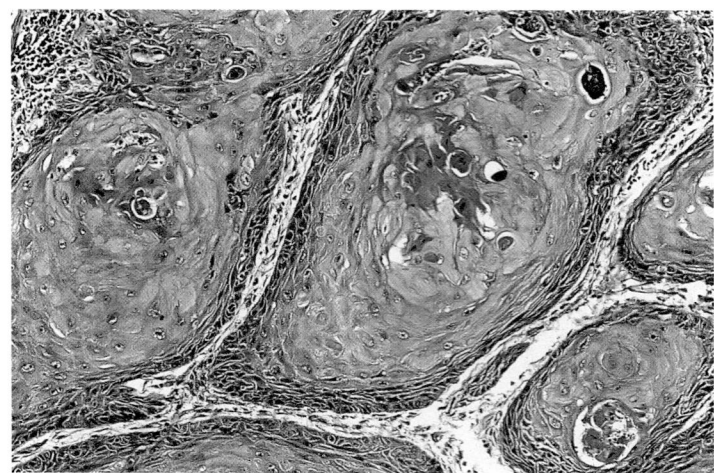

Fig. 31.37 **Keratoacanthoma.** The keratinocytes are large, particularly toward the center of the tumor cell nests. (H & E)

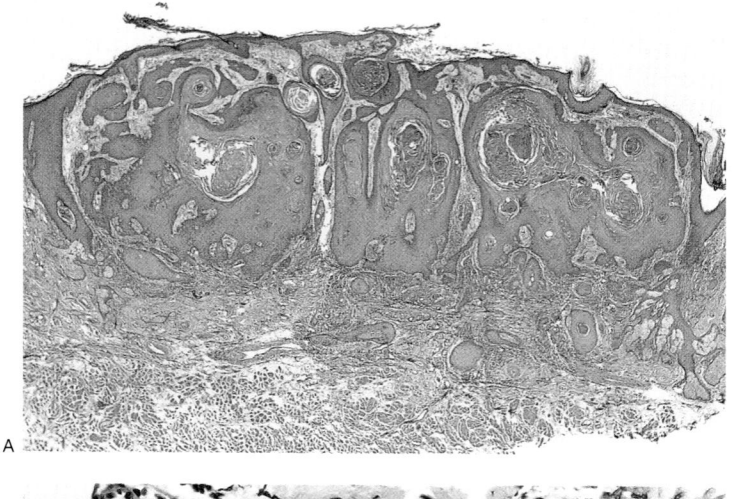

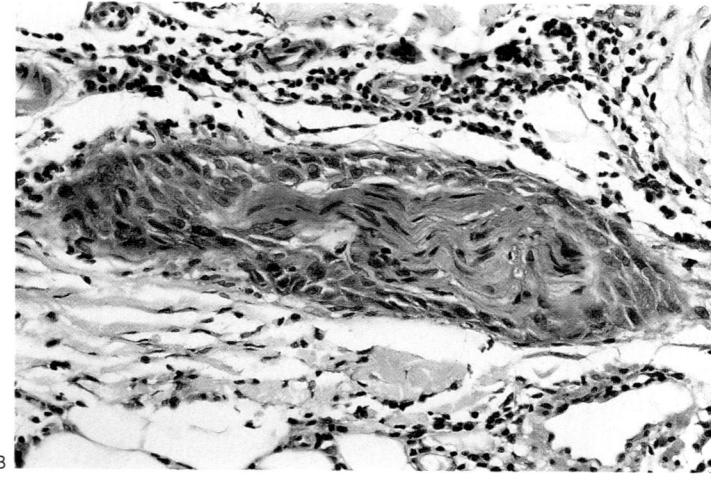

Fig. 31.38 **(A) Keratoacanthoma with perineural invasion. (B)** There has been no recurrence after five years. (H & E)

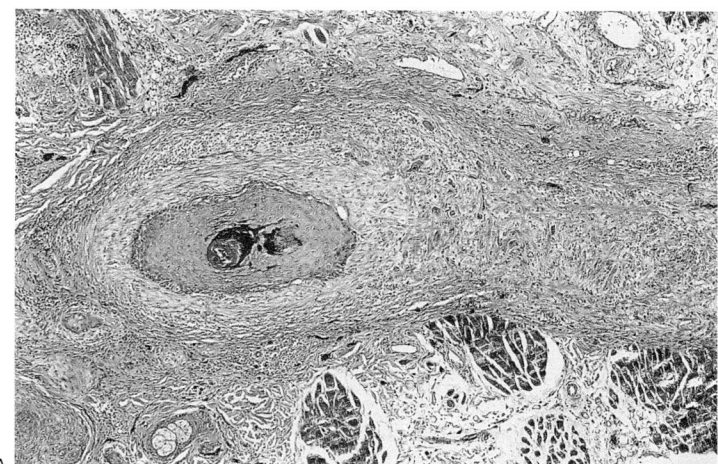

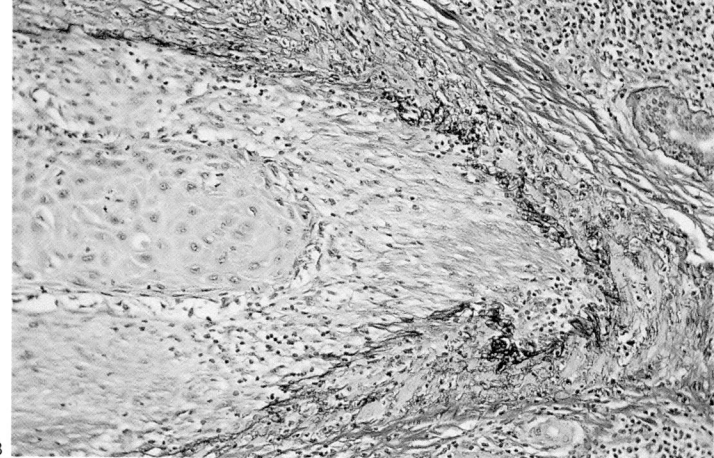

Fig. 31.39 **Keratoacanthoma in a vein. (A)** There has been no recurrence (H & E). **(B)** The elastic tissue stain confirms this is a vein with intimal thickening. (Verhoeff van Gieson)

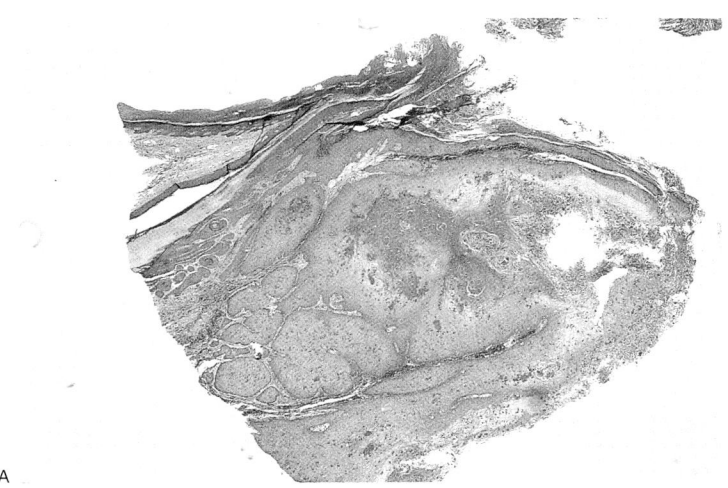

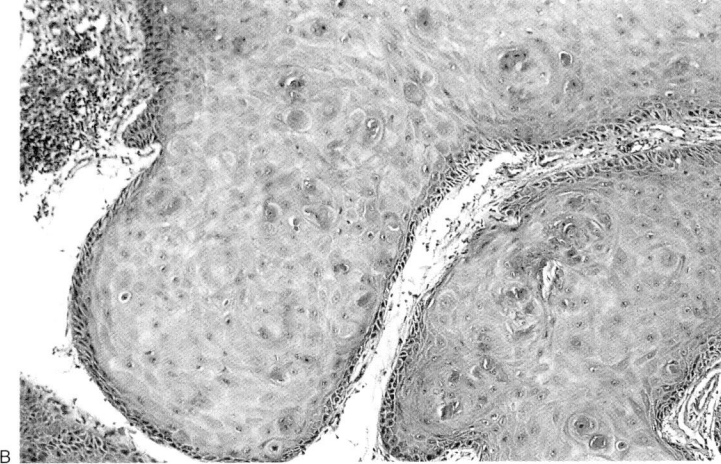

Fig. 31.40 **(A) Subungual keratoacanthoma. (B)** There are numerous dyskeratotic cells. (H & E)

their orientation is more vertical.[1197,1200] The dyskeratotic cells may show focal calcification. Some of the smaller lesions in the various syndromes of multiple keratoacanthomas may show a dilated follicle or cup-shaped depression filled with keratin and showing only limited proliferation of squamous epithelium in the base. Keratoacanthomas developing in the Muir–Torre syndrome may have an accompanying sebaceous proliferation.[1255]

Some authorities believe that the *Ferguson Smith type* of lesion should be separated from keratoacanthoma.[1211] There is histological support for this view. The Ferguson Smith tumor may have an indefinite edge, some pleomorphism of cells, and the production of only a small amount of keratin. The infiltrate is usually lymphocytic rather than composed of polymorphs.[1211]

Electron microscopy

The cells in a keratoacanthoma resemble keratinocytes with abundant tonofibrils and numerous desmosomes.[1247] Intracytoplasmic desmosomes are sometimes observed.[1247]

Distinction of keratoacanthoma from squamous cell carcinoma

Histological features that favor a diagnosis of keratoacanthoma over squamous cell carcinoma include the characteristic low-power architecture with a flask-like configuration and central keratin plug, as well as the pattern of cell keratinization with large central cells that have slightly paler eosinophilic cytoplasm.[1247,1249,1256] Not every craterifom lesion is a

keratoacanthoma: this architecture can occur in squamous cell carcinomas arising over cartilage, such as on the ear and the base of the nose. In keratoacanthomas, the crater is usually multiloculated and the lips are perforated.[1185] Other features favoring keratoacanthoma include lack of anaplasia, a sharp outline between tumor nests and stroma,[1257] and absence of stromal desmoplasia. The presence of intraepithelial elastic fibers and intracytoplasmic glycogen has also been said to favor the diagnosis of keratoacanthoma.[1258,1259] Involucrin, a marker for preterminal squamous differentiation, has been demonstrated by immunoperoxidase methods to be present in all but the basal cells of a keratoacanthoma and in a homogeneous pattern, whereas the staining in squamous cell carcinomas was of variable intensity from cell to cell.[1260,1261] The volume-weighted mean nuclear volume is higher in keratoacanthomas than in squamous cell carcinomas.[1262] Peanut lectin has been demonstrated in the cell membranes of keratinocytes, in a uniform pattern, in keratoacanthomas but not in most squamous cell carcinomas.[1263] The expression of stromelysin-3, collagenase-3, p21 and the oncoprotein C-*erb*B-2/*neu*/HER-2 are all higher in squamous cell carcinomas than in keratoacanthomas.[1264–1267] Both proliferating cell nuclear antigen (PCNA) and MIB 1 (raised against recombinant Ki-67 antigen) are found in the periphery of the squamous nests in keratoacanthoma, in contrast to a more diffuse staining pattern throughout the nests in squamous cell carcinomas, although some overlap occurs.[1268–1271] Expression of the p53 oncoprotein is found in both entities.[1269,1272–1276] Analysis of loss of heterozygosity reveals only low loss in keratoacanthomas, contrasting with the high loss in squamous cell carcinomas.[1229]

Behavior of keratoacanthomas

The literature contains many examples of lesions which on clinical, and sometimes even pathological, grounds were regarded as keratoacanthomas, but which on the basis of their subsequent course were reclassified as squamous cell carcinomas.[1249,1277] There are four possible explanations for this occurrence.[1277] First, the initial diagnosis of keratoacanthoma could have been wrong; this is the usually accepted and most likely explanation.[1256] Second, the initial lesion may have combined a keratoacanthoma and a squamous cell carcinoma. Third, a keratoacanthoma may have transformed into a squamous cell carcinoma, either as a result of therapy or at some point in its evolution (see below).[1278,1279] Fourth, keratoacanthoma may actually be a variant of squamous cell carcinoma, as proposed recently by Ackerman.[1280,1281] The author believes with strong conviction that the biological potential and histopathology of keratoacanthomas and squamous cell carcinomas are so different that their continued separation is essential, if mistreatment of keratoacanthomas with perineural and/or venous invasion is to be avoided.

The author has seen many examples in which part of the lesion was an undoubted keratoacanthoma, but in which, usually toward the base or at one edge, there were areas of typical squamous cell carcinoma. Support for the concept of malignant transformation of keratoacanthoma comes from animal experiments, in which ultraviolet irradiation of hairless mice produced some squamous cell carcinomas that appeared to arise in keratoacanthomas.[1282] This transformation also occurs in immunocompromised patients.[1256] Recently, Sánchez Yus and colleagues have reported focal squamous cell carcinoma change in at least a quarter of all cases.[1185] This is considerably higher than the author's anecdotal experience of about 1%. One explanation might be that keratoacanthoma in subtropical countries is not the same as in temperate lands.

It should be remembered that keratoacanthomas can recur in up to 3% of cases.[1283] Recurrence is more likely with lesions on the fingers, hands, lips and pinnae.[1278] Lesions on the nose and eyelids can be very destructive.[1178, 284]

Metastasis

The published photomicrographs accompanying a report of a giant metastasizing keratoacanthoma show a pattern of keratinization more in keeping with a squamous cell carcinoma than a keratoacanthoma.[1285] Ackerman and colleagues have reported three cases purporting to be keratoacanthomas in which metastasis occurred.[1280] On this basis, they concluded that keratoacanthoma is a squamous cell carcinoma.[1280]

Regression

The mechanism responsible for the regression of keratoacanthomas is still poorly understood. There is only limited evidence that regression is immunologically mediated. Activated CD4-positive T lymphocytes expressing the interleukin-2 receptor (IL-2R) are present in the infiltrate.[1286] Langerhans cells are also increased.[1287] Deletion of many of the cells results from their maturation and keratinization, with subsequent extrusion as a keratin plug. Other cells show dyskeratotic changes (filamentous degeneration), and these tonofilament-rich masses are extruded into the stroma where they become incorporated into the dermal collagen. Still other cells undergo cell death at an earlier stage by the process of apoptosis. It is worth recalling that many keratoacanthomas appear to arise from hair follicle epithelium: in the normal follicle the cells have a programmed ability to be deleted by apoptosis, resulting in catagen involution of the follicle. Expression of *bcl-2*, a proto-oncogene which inhibits apoptosis, is lost in regressing keratoacanthomas.[1288] It has recently been found that expression of the cyclin-dependent kinase inhibitor p27 is elevated significantly in regressing keratoacanthomas when compared with growing lesions.[1289] This protein induces a G1 block in the cell cycle. Another study has found sialyl-Tn, a tumor-associated carbohydrate expressed on the cell surface, more often in keratoacanthomas than in squamous cell carcinomas. It may be linked to the regression of keratoacanthomas.[1290]

REFERENCES

Epidermal and other nevi

1 Solomon LM, Esterly NB. Epidermal and other congenital organoid nevi. Curr Probl Dermatol 1975; 6: 3–56.
2 Rogers M, McCrossin I, Commens C. Epidermal nevi and the epidermal nevus syndrome. A review of 131 cases. J Am Acad Dermatol 1989; 20: 476–488.
3 Kim SC, Kang WH. Nevus comedonicus associated with epidermal nevus. J Am Acad Dermatol 1989; 21: 1085–1088.
4 Su WPD. Histopathologic varieties of epidermal nevus. A study of 160 cases. Am J Dermatopathol 1982; 4: 161–170.
5 Hayashi N, Soma Y. A case of epidermal nevi showing a divided form on the fingers. J Am Acad Dermatol 1993; 29: 281–282.
6 Rogers M. Epidermal nevi and the epidermal nevus syndromes: a review of 233 cases. Pediatr Dermatol 1992; 9: 342–344.
7 Mehregan AH, Rahbari H. Benign epithelial tumors of the skin. Part 1: epidermal tumors. Cutis 1977; 19: 43–48.
8 Submoke S, Piamphongsant T. Clinico-histopathological study of epidermal naevi. Australas J Dermatol 1983; 24: 130–136.
9 Adams BB, Mutasim DF. Adult onset verrucous epidermal nevus. J Am Acad Dermatol 1999; 41: 824–826.
10 Basler RSW, Jacobs SI, Taylor WB. Ichthyosis hystrix. Arch Dermatol 1978; 114: 1059–1060.
11 Adam JE, Richards R. Ichthyosis hystrix. Arch Dermatol 1973; 107: 278–282.
12 Horn MS, Sausker WF, Pierson DL. Basal cell epithelioma arising in a linear epidermal nevus. Arch Dermatol 1981; 117: 247.
13 Levin A, Amazon K, Rywlin AM. A squamous cell carcinoma that developed in an epidermal nevus. Am J Dermatopathol 1984; 6: 51–55.
14 Dogliotti M, Frenkel A. Malignant change in a verrucous nevus. Int J Dermatol 1978; 17: 225–227.
15 Cramer SF, Mandel MA, Hauler R et al. Squamous cell carcinoma arising in a linear epidermal nevus. Arch Dermatol 1981; 117: 222–224.
16 Braunstein BL, Mackel SE, Cooper PH. Keratoacanthoma arising in a linear epidermal nevus. Arch Dermatol 1982; 118: 362–363.
17 Waltz KM, Helm KF, Billingsley EM. The spectrum of epidermal nevi: a case of verrucous epidermal nevus contiguous with nevus sebaceus. Pediatr Dermatol 1999; 16: 211–213.
18 Solomon LM, Fretzin DF, Dewald RL. The epidermal nevus syndrome. Arch Dermatol 1968; 97: 273–285.
19 Eichler C, Flowers FP, Ross J. Epidermal nevus syndrome: case report and review of clinical manifestations. Pediatr Dermatol 1989; 6: 316–320.
20 Goldberg LH, Collins SAB, Siegel DM. The epidermal nevus syndrome: case report and review. Pediatr Dermatol 1987; 4: 27–33.
21 Mahakrishnan A. Megalopinna in naevus uniuslateris: a case report. Acta Derm Venereol 1981; 61: 365–367.
22 Happle R. How many epidermal nevus syndromes exist? A clinicogenetic classification. J Am Acad Dermatol 1991; 25: 550–556.
23 Hodge JA, Ray MC, Flynn KJ. The epidermal nevus syndrome. Int J Dermatol 1991; 30: 91–98.
24 Mostafa WZ, Satti MB. Epidermal nevus syndrome: a clinicopathologic study with six-year follow-up. Pediatr Dermatol 1991; 8: 228–230.
25 Ivker R, Resnick SD, Skidmore RA. Hypophosphatemic vitamin D-resistant rickets, precocious puberty, and the epidermal nevus syndrome Arch Dermatol 1997; 133: 1557–1561.
26 Tay Y-K, Weston WL, Ganong CA, Klingensmith GJ. Epidermal nevus syndrome: Association with central precocious puberty and woolly hair nevus. J Am Acad Dermatol 1996; 35: 839–842.
27 Stosiek N, Ulmer R, von den Driesch P et al. Chromosomal mosaicism in two patients with epidermal verrucous nevus. J Am Acad Dermatol 1994; 30: 622–625.
28 Inglesias Zamora ME, Vázquez-Doval FJ. Epidermal naevi associated with trichilemmal cysts and chromosomal mosaicism. Br J Dermatol 1997; 137: 821–824.
29 Dimond RL, Amon RB. Epidermal nevus and rhabdomyosarcoma. Arch Dermatol 1976; 112: 1424–1426.
30 Rosenthal D, Fretzin DF. Epidermal nevus syndrome: report of association with transitional cell carcinoma of the bladder. Pediatr Dermatol 1986; 3: 455–458.
31 Obasi OE, Isitor GN. Extensive congenital bilateral epidermal naevus syndrome – a case report from Nigeria with ultrastructural observations. Clin Exp Dermatol 1987; 12: 132–135.
32 Attia MK, Abdel-Aziz AM. Epidermal naevus syndrome. Br J Dermatol 1976; 95: 647–648.
33 Gobello T, Mazzanti C, Zambruno G et al. New type of epidermal nevus syndrome. Dermatology 2000; 201: 51–53.
34 Rustin MHA, Bunker CB, Gilkes JJH et al. Polyostotic fibrous dysplasia associated with extensive linear epidermal naevi. Clin Exp Dermatol 1989; 14: 371–375.
35 Samlaska CP, Levin SW, James WD et al. Proteus syndrome. Arch Dermatol 1989; 125: 1109–1114.
36 Nazzaro V, Cambiaghi S, Montagnani A et al. Proteus syndrome. Ultrastructural study of linear verrucous and depigmented nevi. J Am Acad Dermatol 1991; 25: 377–383.
37 Child FJ, Werring DJ, Du Vivier AWP. Proteus syndrome: diagnosis in adulthood. Br J Dermatol 1998; 139: 132–136.
38 Cavero JA, Castro EG, Junco L. Proteus syndrome. Int J Dermatol 2000; 39: 707–709.
39 Barona-Mazuera MdR, Hidalgo-Galván LR, Orozco-Covarrubias MdL et al. Proteus syndrome: new findings in seven patients. Pediatr Dermatol 1997; 14: 1–5.
40 Demetree JW, Lang PG, St Clair JT. Unilateral, linear, zosteriform epidermal nevus with acantholytic dyskeratosis. Arch Dermatol 1979; 115: 875–877.
41 Delacretaz J, Christeler A. Dyskeratose acantholytique regionale. Dermatologica 1981; 163: 113–116.
42 Starink TM, Woerdeman MJ. Unilateral systematized keratosis follicularis. A variant of Darier's disease or an epidermal naevus (acantholytic dyskeratotic epidermal naevus)? Br J Dermatol 1981; 105: 207–214.
43 van der Wegen-Keijser MH, Prevoo RLMH, Bruynzeel DP. Acantholytic dyskeratotic epidermal naevus in a patient with guttate psoriasis on PUVA therapy. Br J Dermatol 1991; 124: 603–605.
44 Curth HO. Unilateral epidermal naevus resembling acanthosis nigricans. Br J Dermatol 1976; 95: 433–436.
45 Vakilzadeh F, Kolde G. Relapsing linear acantholytic dermatosis. Br J Dermatol 1985; 112: 349–355.
46 Fletcher V, Williams ML, Lane AT. Histologic changes resembling the verrucous phase of incontinentia pigmenti within epidermal nevi: report of two cases. Pediatr Dermatol 1985; 3: 69–74.
47 Brownstein MH, Silverstein L, Lefing W. Lichenoid epidermal nevus: 'linear lichen planus'. J Am Acad Dermatol 1989; 20: 913–915.

48 Altman J, Mehregan AH. Inflammatory linear verrucose epidermal nevus. Arch Dermatol 1971; 104: 385–389.

49 Morag C, Metzker A. Inflammatory linear verrucous epidermal nevus: report of seven new cases and review of the literature. Pediatr Dermatol 1985; 3: 15–18.

50 De Jong EMGJ, Rulo HFC, Van De Kerkhof PCM. Inflammatory linear verrucous epidermal naevus (ILVEN) versus linear psoriasis. Acta Derm Venereol 1991; 71: 343–346.

51 Zvulunov A, Grunwald MH, Halvy S. Topical calcipotriol for treatment of inflammatory linear verrucous epidermal nevus. Arch Dermatol 1997; 133: 567–568.

52 Kim JJ, Chang MW, Shwayder T. Topical tretinoin and 5-fluorouracil in the treatment of linear verrucous epidermal nevus. J Am Acad Dermatol 2000; 43: 129–132.

53 Alsaleh QA, Nanda A, Hassab-El-Naby HMM, Sakr MF. Familial inflammatory linear verrucous epidermal nevus (ILVEN). Int J Dermatol 1994; 33: 52–54.

54 Landwehr AJ, Starink TM. Inflammatory linear verrucous epidermal naevus. Report of a case with bilateral distribution and nail involvement. Dermatologica 1983; 166: 107–109.

55 Cheesbrough MJ, Kilby PE. The inflammatory linear verrucous epidermal naevus – a case report. Clin Exp Dermatol 1978; 3: 293–298.

56 Golitz LE, Weston WL. Inflammatory linear verrucous epidermal nevus. Association with epidermal nevus syndrome. Arch Dermatol 1979; 115: 1208–1209.

57 Lee IW, Ahn SK, Choi EH. Inflammatory linear verrucous epidermal naevus arising on a burn scar. Acta Derm Venereol 1999; 79: 164–165.

58 Goujon C, Pierini A-M, Thivolet J. Le psoriasis linéaire; existe-t-il? Ann Dermatol Venereol 1981; 108: 643–650.

59 Adrian RM, Baden HP. Analysis of epidermal fibrous proteins in inflammatory linear verrucous epidermal nevus. Arch Dermatol 1980; 116: 1179–1180.

60 Bernhard JD, Owen WR, Steinman HK et al. Inflammatory linear verrucous epidermal nevus. Epidermal protein analysis in four patients. Arch Dermatol 1984; 120: 214–215.

61 Dupre A, Christol B. Inflammatory linear verrucose epidermal nevus. A pathologic study. Arch Dermatol 1977; 113: 767–769.

62 Hodge SJ, Barr JM, Owen LG. Inflammatory linear verrucose epidermal nevus. Arch Dermatol 1978; 114: 436–438.

63 Ahrens EM, Hodge SJ. Lichen planus arising in an inflammatory linear verrucous epidermal nevus. Int J Dermatol 1986; 25: 527–528.

64 Welch ML, Smith KJ, Skelton HG et al. Immunohistochemical features in inflammatory linear verrucous epidermal nevi suggest a distinctive pattern of clonal dysregulation of growth. J Am Acad Dermatol 1993; 29: 242–248.

65 Grimalt R, Caputo R. Posttraumatic nevus comedonicus. J Am Acad Dermatol 1993; 28: 273–274.

66 Inoue Y, Miyamoto Y, Ono T. Two cases of nevus comedonicus: Successful treatment of keratin plugs with a pore strip. J Am Acad Dermatol 2000; 43: 927–929.

67 Lefkowitz A, Schwartz RA, Lambert WC. Nevus comedonicus. Dermatology 1999; 199: 204–207.

68 Beck MH, Dave VK. Extensive nevus comedonicus. Arch Dermatol 1980; 116: 1048–1050.

69 Cestari TF, Rubim M, Valentini BC. Nevus comedonicus: case report and brief review of the literature. Pediatr Dermatol 1991; 8: 300–305.

70 Fletcher CL, Acland KM, Powles AV. Unusual giant comedo naevus. Clin Exp Dermatol 1999; 24: 186–188.

71 Abdel-Aal H, Abdel-Aziz AHM. Nevus comedonicus. Report of three cases localized on the glans penis. Acta Derm Venereol 1975; 55: 78–80.

72 Cripps DJ, Bertram JR. Nevus comedonicus bilateralis et verruciformis. J Cutan Pathol 1976; 3: 273–281.

73 Wood MG, Thew MA. Nevus comedonicus. A case with palmar involvement and review of the literature. Arch Dermatol 1968; 98: 111–116.

74 Harper KE, Spielvogel RL. Nevus comedonicus of the palm and wrist. J Am Acad Dermatol 1985; 12: 185–188.

75 Paige TN, Mendelson CG. Bilateral nevus comedonicus. Arch Dermatol 1967; 96: 172–175.

76 Engber PB. The nevus comedonicus syndrome: a case report with emphasis on associated internal manifestations. Int J Dermatol 1978; 17: 745–749.

77 Whyte HJ. Unilateral comedo nevus and cataract. Arch Dermatol 1968; 97: 533–535.

78 Woods KA, Larcher VF, Harper JI. Extensive naevus comedonicus in a child with Alagille syndrome. Clin Exp Dermatol 1994; 19: 163–164.

79 Patrizi A, Neri I, Fiorentini C, Marzaduri S. Nevus comedonicus syndrome: a new pediatric case. Pediatr Dermatol 1998; 15: 304–306.

80 Rodriguez JM. Nevus comedonicus. Arch Dermatol 1975; 111: 1363–1364.

81 Vasiloudes PE, Morelli JG, Weston WL. Inflammatory nevus comedonicus in children. J Am Acad Dermatol 1998; 38: 834–836.

82 Nabai H, Mehregan AH. Nevus comedonicus. A review of the literature and report of twelve cases. Acta Derm Venereol 1973; 53: 71–74.

83 Leppard BJ. Trichilemmal cysts arising in an extensive comedo naevus. Br J Dermatol 1977; 96: 545–548.

84 Marsden RA, Fleming K, Dawber RPR. Comedo naevus of the palm – a sweat duct naevus? Br J Dermatol 1979; 101: 717–722.

85 Abell E, Read SI. Porokeratotic eccrine ostial and dermal duct naevus. Br J Dermatol 1980; 103: 435–441.

86 Coskey RJ, Mehregan AH. Porokeratotic eccrine duct and hair follicle nevus. J Am Acad Dermatol 1982; 6: 940–943.

87 Aloi FG, Pippione M. Porokeratotic eccrine ostial and dermal duct nevus. Arch Dermatol 1986; 122: 892–895.

88 Moreno A, Pujol RM, Salvatella N et al. Porokeratotic eccrine ostial and dermal duct nevus. J Cutan Pathol 1988; 15: 43–48.

89 Horio T, Komura J. Linear unilateral basal cell nevus with comedo-like lesions. Arch Dermatol 1978; 114: 95–97.

90 Blanchard L, Hodge SJ, Owen LG. Linear eccrine nevus with comedones. Arch Dermatol 1981; 117: 357–359.

91 Plewig G, Christophers E. Nevoid follicular epidermolytic hyperkeratosis. Arch Dermatol 1975; 111: 223–226.

92 Resnik KS, Kantor GR, Howe NR, Ditre CM. Dilated pore nevus. A histologic variant of nevus comedonicus. Am J Dermatopathol 1993; 15: 169–171.

93 Price M, Russell Jones R. Familial dyskeratotic comedones. Clin Exp Dermatol 1985; 10: 147–153.

94 Hall JR, Holder W, Knox JM et al. Familial dyskeratotic comedones. J Am Acad Dermatol 1987; 17: 808–814.

95 Carneiro SJC, Dickson JE, Knox JM. Familial dyskeratotic comedones. Arch Dermatol 1972; 105: 249–251.

96 Van Geel NAC, Kockaert M, Neumann HAM. Familial dyskeratotic comedones. Br J Dermatol 1999; 140: 956–959.

97 Leppard BJ. Familial dyskeratotic comedones. Clin Exp Dermatol 1982; 7: 329–332.

98 Cantú JM, Gómez-Bustamente MO, González-Mendoza A, Sánchez-Corona J. Familial comedones. Evidence for autosomal dominant inheritance. Arch Dermatol 1978; 114: 1807–1809.

99 Rodin HH, Blankenship ML, Bernstein G. Diffuse familial comedones. Arch Dermatol 1967; 95: 145–146.

Pseudoepitheliomatous hyperplasia

100 Grumwald MH, Lee JY-Y, Ackerman AB. Pseudocarcinomatous hyperplasia. Am J Dermatopathol 1988; 10: 95–103.

101 Civatte J. Pseudo-carcinomatous hyperplasia. J Cutan Pathol 1985; 12: 214–223.

102 Ju DMC. Pseudoepitheliomatous hyperplasia of the skin. Dermatol Int 1967; 6: 82–92.

103 Freeman RG. On the pathogenesis of pseudoepitheliomatous hyperplasia. J Cutan Pathol 1974; 1: 231–237.

104 Goldberg NS, Esterly NB, Rothman KF et al. Perianal pseudoverrucous papules and nodules in children. Arch Dermatol 1992; 128: 240–242.

105 Vaccaro M, Borgia F, Guarneri F, Cannavò SP. Elephantiasis nostras verrucosa. Int J Dermatol 2000; 39: 764–766.

106 Goel R, Wallace ML. Pseudoepitheliomatous hyperplasia secondary to cutaneous Aspergillus. Am J Dermatopathol 2001; 23: 224–226.

107 Hurwitz RM. Pseudocarcinomatous or infundibular hyperplasia. Am J Dermatopathol 1989; 11: 189–191.

108 Courville P, Wechsler J, Thomine E et al. Pseudoepitheliomatous hyperplasia in cutaneous T-cell lymphoma. A clinical, histopathological and immunohistochemical study with particular interest in epithelial growth factor expression. Br J Dermatol 1999; 140: 421–426.

109 Weber PJ, Johnson BL, Dzubow LM. Pseudoepitheliomatous hyperplasia following Mohs micrographic surgery. J Dermatol Surg Oncol 1989; 15: 557–560.

110 Gattuso P, Candel AG, Castelli MJ et al. Pseudoepitheliomatous hyperplasia in chronic cutaneous wounds. A flow cytometric study. J Cutan Pathol 1994; 21: 312–315.

111 Epstein E. Granuloma fissuratum of the ears. Arch Dermatol 1965; 91: 621–622.

112 Cerroni L, Soyer HP, Chimenti S. Acanthoma fissuratum. J Dermatol Surg Oncol 1988; 14: 1003–1005.

113 MacDonald DM, Martin SJ. Acanthoma fissuratum – spectacle frame acanthoma. Acta Derm Venereol 1975; 55: 485–487.

114 Betti R, Inselvini E, Pozzi G, Crosti C. Bilateral spectacle frame acanthoma. Clin Exp Dermatol 1994; 19: 503–504.

115 Farrell WJ, Wilson JW. Granuloma fissuratum of the nose. Arch Dermatol 1968; 97: 34–37.

116 Delaney TJ, Stewart TW. Granuloma fissuratum. Br J Dermatol 1971; 84: 373–375.

117 Rowland Payne CME, Wilkinson JD, McKee PH. Nodular prurigo – a clinicopathological study of 46 patients. Br J Dermatol 1985; 113: 431–439.

118 Berth-Jones J, Smith SG, Graham-Brown RAC. Nodular prurigo responds to cyclosporin. Br J Dermatol 1995; 132: 795–799.

119 Woo P-N, Finch TM, Hindson C, Foulds IS. Nodular prurigo successfully treated with the pulsed dye laser. Br J Dermatol 2000; 143: 215–216.

120 Accioly-Filho JW, Nogueira A, Ramos-e-Silva M. Prurigo nodularis of Hyde: an update. J Eur Acad Dermatol Venereol 2000; 14: 75–82.

121 Matthews SN, Cockerell CJ. Prurigo nodularis in HIV-infected individuals. Int J Dermatol 1998; 37: 401–409.

122 Herranz P, Pizarro A, de Lucas R et al. Treatment of AIDS-associated prurigo nodularis with thalidomide. Clin Exp Dermatol 1998; 23: 233–235.

123 Tanaka M, Aiba S, Matsumura N et al. Prurigo nodularis consists of two distinct forms: early-onset atopic and late-onset non-atopic. Dermatology 1995; 190: 269–276.

124 Mattila JO, Vornanen M, Vaara J, Katila M-L. Mycobacteria in prurigo nodularis: the cause or a consequence? J Am Acad Dermatol 1996; 34: 224–228.

125 Boer J, Smeenk G. Nodular prurigo-like eruptions induced by etretinate. Br J Dermatol 1987; 116: 271–274.

126 Ständer S, Luger T, Metze D. Treatment of prurigo nodularis with topical capsaicin. J Am Acad Dermatol 2001; 44: 471–478.

127 Doyle JA, Connolly SM, Hunziker N, Winkelmann RK. Prurigo nodularis: a reappraisal of the clinical and histologic features. J Cutan Pathol 1979; 6: 392–403.

128 Miyauchi H, Uehara M. Follicular occurrence of prurigo nodularis. J Cutan Pathol 1988; 15: 208–211.

129 Corredor F, Cohen PR, Tschen JA. Syringomatous changes of eccrine sweat ducts associated with prurigo nodularis. Am J Dermatopathol 1998; 20: 296–301.

130 Perez GL, Peters MS, Reda AM et al. Mast cells, neutrophils, and eosinophils in prurigo nodularis. Arch Dermatol 1993; 129: 861–865.

131 Nahass GT, Penneys NS. Merkel cells and prurigo nodularis. J Am Acad Dermatol 1994; 31: 86–88.

132 Liang Y, Marcusson JA, Jacobi HH et al. Histamine-containing mast cells and their relationship to NGFr-immunoreactive nerves in prurigo nodularis: a reappraisal. J Cutan Pathol 1998; 25: 189–198.

133 Cowan MA. Neurohistological changes in prurigo nodularis. Arch Dermatol 1964; 89: 754–758.

134 Abadia Molina F, Burrows NP, Russell Jones R et al. Increased sensory neuropeptides in nodular prurigo: a quantitative immunohistochemical analysis. Br J Dermatol 1992; 127: 344–351.

135 Hirschel-Scholz S, Salomon D, Merot Y, Saurat J-H. Anetodermic prurigo nodularis (with Pautrier's neuroma) responsive to arotinoid acid. J Am Acad Dermatol 1991; 25: 437–442.

136 Harris B, Harris K, Penneys NS. Demonstration by S-100 protein staining of increased numbers of nerves in the papillary dermis of patients with prurigo nodularis. J Am Acad Dermatol 1992; 26: 56–58.

137 Lindley RP, Rowland Payne CME. Neural hyperplasia is not a diagnostic prerequisite in nodular prurigo. J Cutan Pathol 1989; 16: 14–18.

138 Feuerman EJ, Sandbank M. Prurigo nodularis. Histological and electron microscopical study. Arch Dermatol 1975; 111: 1472–1477.

139 Runne U, Orfanos CE. Cutaneous neural proliferation in highly pruritic lesions of chronic prurigo. Arch Dermatol 1977; 113: 787–791.

140 Liang Y, Jacobi HH, Reimert CM et al. CGRP-immunoreactive nerves in prurigo nodularis – an exploration of neurogenic inflammation. J Cutan Pathol 2000; 27: 359–366.

141 Sandbank M. Cutaneous nerve lesions in prurigo nodularis. Electron microscopic study of two patients. J Cutan Pathol 1976; 3: 125–132.

Acanthomas

142 Brownstein MH. The benign acanthomas. J Cutan Pathol 1985; 12: 172–188.

143 Brownstein MH. Acantholytic acanthoma. J Am Acad Dermatol 1988; 19: 783–786.

144 Megahed M, Scharffetter-Kochanek K. Acantholytic acanthoma. Am J Dermatopathol 1993; 15: 283–285.

145 Ramos-Caro FA, Sexton FM, Browder JF, Flowers FP. Acantholytic acanthomas in an immunosuppressed patient. J Am Acad Dermatol 1992; 27: 452–453.

146 Yeatman JM, Kilkenny M, Marks R. The prevalence of seborrhoeic keratoses in an Australian population: does exposure to sunlight play a part in their frequency? Br J Dermatol 1997; 137: 411–414.

147 Gill D, Dorevitch A, Marks R. The prevalence of seborrheic keratoses in people aged 15 to 30 years. Is the term senile keratosis redundant? Arch Dermatol 2000; 136: 759–762.

148 Baer RL. Giant pedunculated seborrheic keratosis. Arch Dermatol 1979; 115: 627.

149 Becker SW. Seborrheic keratosis and verruca, with special reference to the melanotic variety. Arch Dermatol 1951; 63: 358–372.

150 Satterfield PA, Haas AF. Postoperative localized eruption of seborrheic keratoses. J Am Acad Dermatol 1998; 38: 267–268.

151 Shelley WB, Shelley ED. Keratoderma simplex: a novel entity simulating seborrhoeic keratosis. Br J Dermatol 1997; 136: 792.

152 Bedi TR. Familial congenital multiple seborrheic verrucae. Arch Dermatol 1977; 113: 1441–1442.

153 Reiches AJ. Seborrheic keratoses. Are they delayed hereditary nevi? Arch Dermatol 1952; 65: 596–600.

154 Migally M, Migally N. Halo seborrheic keratosis. Int J Dermatol 1983; 22: 307–309.

155 Kaminsky CA, De Kaminsky AR, Sanguinetti O, Shaw M. Acquired pigmentation of skin folds with the histological picture of seborrhoeic wart. Br J Dermatol 1975; 93: 713–716.

156 Heffernan MP, Khavari PA. Raindrop seborrheic keratoses: a distinctive pattern on the backs of elderly patients. Arch Dermatol 1998; 134: 382–383.

157 Sanderson KV. The structure of seborrhoeic keratoses. Br J Dermatol 1968; 80: 588–593.

158 Zhao Y, Lin Y, Luo R et al. Human papillomavirus (HPV) infection in seborrheic keratosis. Am J Dermatopathol 1989; 11: 209–212.

159 Leonardi CL, Zhu W-Y, Kinsey WH, Penneys NS. Seborrheic keratoses from the genital region may contain human papillomavirus DNA. Arch Dermatol 1991; 127: 1203–1206.

160 Jacyk WK, Dreyer L, de Villiers EM. Seborrheic keratoses of black patients with epidermodysplasia verruciformis contain human papillomavirus DNA. Am J Dermatopathol 1993; 15: 1–6.

161 Tomasini C, Aloi F, Pippione M. Seborrheic keratosis-like lesions in epidermodysplasia verruciformis. J Cutan Pathol 1993; 20: 237–241.

162 Googe PB, King K. Herpesvirus infection of seborrheic keratoses. Am J Dermatopathol 2001; 23: 146–148.

163 Teraki E, Tajima S, Manaka I et al. Role of endothelin-1 in hyperpigmentation in seborrhoeic keratosis. Br J Dermatol 1996; 135: 918–923.

164 Morales A, Hu F. Seborrheic verruca and intraepidermal basal cell epithelioma of Jadassohn. Arch Dermatol 1965; 91: 342–344.

165 Eads TJ, Hood AF, Chuang T-Y et al. The diagnostic yield of histologic examination of seborrheic keratoses. Arch Dermatol 1997; 133: 1417–1420.

166 Murphy M, Watson R, Sweeney EC, Barnes L. Accuracy of diagnosis of seborrheic keratoses in a dermatology clinic. Arch Dermatol 2000; 136: 800–801.

167 Wade TR, Ackerman AB. The many faces of seborrheic keratoses. J Dermatol Surg Oncol 1979; 5: 378–382.

168 Trotter MJ, Donn WB. Pagetoid seborrheic keratosis. J Cutan Pathol 1997; 24: 130 (abstract).

169 Pesce C, Scalora S. Apoptosis in the areas of squamous differentiation of irritated seborrheic keratosis. J Cutan Pathol 2000; 27: 121–123.

170 Berman A, Winkelmann RK. Seborrheic keratoses. Appearance in course of exfoliative erythroderma and regression associated with histologic mononuclear cell inflammation. Arch Dermatol 1982; 118: 615–618.

171 Berman A, Winkelmann RK. Histologic changes in seborrheic keratoses after rubbing. J Cutan Pathol 1980; 7: 32–38.

172 Berman A, Winkelmann RK. Inflammatory seborrheic keratoses with mononuclear cell infiltration. J Cutan Pathol 1978; 5: 353–360.

173 Nakayasu K, Nishimura A, Maruo M, Wakabayashi S. Trichilemmal differentiation in seborrheic keratosis. J Cutan Pathol 1981; 8: 256–262.

174 Masuda M, Kimura S. Trichilemmal keratinization in seborrheic keratoses. J Cutan Pathol 1984; 11: 12–17.

175 Requena L, Kuztner H, Fariña MC. Pigmented and nested sebomatricoma or seborrheic keratosis with sebaceous differentiation? Am J Dermatopathol 1998; 20: 383–388.

176 Tagami H, Yamada M. Seborrheic keratosis: an acantholytic variant. J Cutan Pathol 1978; 5: 145–149.

177 Chen M, Shinmori H, Takemiya M, Miki Y. Acantholytic variant of seborrheic keratosis. J Cutan Pathol 1990; 17: 27–31.

178 Kossard S, Berman A, Winkelmann RK. Seborrheic keratoses and trichostasis spinulosa. J Cutan Pathol 1979; 6: 492–495.

179 Kwittken J. Squamous cell carcinoma arising in seborrheic keratosis. Mt Sinai J Med 1981; 48: 61–62.

180 Kwittken J. Keratoacanthoma arising in seborrheic keratosis. Cutis 1974; 14: 546–547.

181 Mikhail GR, Mehregan AH. Basal cell carcinoma in seborrheic keratosis. J Am Acad Dermatol 1982; 6: 500–506.

182 Suvarna SK, Bagary M, Glazer G. Radiation-induced squamous carcinoma arising within a seborrhoeic keratosis. Br J Dermatol 1993; 128: 443–447.

183 Maize JC, Snider RL. Nonmelanoma skin cancers in association with seborrheic keratoses. Dermatol Surg 1995; 21: 960–962.

184 Helm TN, Helm F, Marsico R et al. Seborrheic keratoses with occult underlying basal cell carcinoma. J Am Acad Dermatol 1993; 29: 791–793.

185 Díaz Cascajo C, Reichel M, Sánchez JL. Malignant neoplasms associated with seborrheic keratoses. An analysis of 54 cases. Am J Dermatopathol 1996; 18: 278–282.

186 Boyd AS, Rapini RP. Cutaneous collision tumors. An analysis of 69 cases and review of the literature. Am J Dermatopathol 1994; 16: 253–257.

187 Baer RL, Garcia RL, Partsalidou V, Ackerman AB. Papillated squamous cell carcinoma in situ arising in a seborrheic keratosis. J Am Acad Dermatol 1981; 5: 561–565.

188 Bloch PH. Transformation of seborrheic keratosis into Bowen's disease. J Cutan Pathol 1978; 5: 361–367.

189 Monteagudo JC, Jorda E, Terencio C, Llombart-Bosch A. Squamous cell carcinoma in situ (Bowen's disease) arising in seborrheic keratosis: three lesions in two patients. J Cutan Pathol 1989; 16: 348–352.

190 Kwittken J. Malignant changes in seborrheic keratoses. Mt Sinai J Med (NY) 1974; 41: 792–801.

191 Gallimore AP. Malignant transformation of a clonal seborrhoeic keratosis. Br J Dermatol 1991; 124: 287–290.

192 Marschall SF, Ronan SG, Massa MC. Pigmented Bowen's disease arising from pigmented seborrheic keratosis. J Am Acad Dermatol 1990; 23: 440–444.

193 Yen A, Austin P, Sanchez R. Is Bowenoid seborrheic keratosis a form of squamous cell carcinoma in-situ? J Cutan Pathol 1997; 24: 133 (abstract).

194 Zabel RJ, Vinson RP, McCollough ML. Malignant melanoma arising in a seborrheic keratosis. J Am Acad Dermatol 2000; 42: 831–833.

195 Shelley WB, Shelley ED, Burmeister V. Melanosome macrocomplex: an ultrastructural component of patterned and nonpatterned seborrheic keratoses. J Am Acad Dermatol 1987; 16: 124–128.

196 Nyfors A, Kruger PG. Langerhans' cells in seborrheic keratosis. A clinical and ultrastructural study. Acta Derm Venereol 1985; 65: 333–335.

197 Wilborn WH, Dismukes DE, Montes LF. Ultrastructural identification of Langerhans cells in seborrheic keratosis. J Cutan Pathol 1978; 5: 368–372.

198 Dantzig PI. Sign of Leser–Trélat. Arch Dermatol 1973; 108: 700–701.

199 Barron LA, Prendiville JS. The sign of Leser–Trélat in a young woman with osteogenic sarcoma. J Am Acad Dermatol 1992; 26: 344–347.

200 Heaphy MR Jr, Millns JL, Schroeter AL. The sign of Leser–Trélat in a case of adenocarcinoma of the lung. J Am Acad Dermatol 2000; 43: 386–390.

201 Holdiness MR. The sign of Leser–Trélat. Int J Dermatol 1986; 25: 564–572.

202 Holdiness MR. On the classification of the sign of Leser–Trélat. J Am Acad Dermatol 1988; 19: 754–757.

203 Yaniv R, Servadio Y, Feinstein A, Trau H. The sign of Leser–Trélat associated with transitional cell carcinoma of the urinary-bladder – a case report and short review. Clin Exp Dermatol 1994; 19: 142–145.

204 Schwartz RA. Sign of Leser–Trélat. J Am Acad Dermatol 1996; 35: 88–95.

205 Rampen FHJ, Schwengle LEM. The sign of Leser–Trélat: does it exist? J Am Acad Dermatol 1989; 21: 50–55.

206 Lindelöf B, Sigurgeirsson B, Melander S. Seborrheic keratoses and cancer. J Am Acad Dermatol 1992; 26: 947–950.

207 Czarnecki DB, Rotstein H, O'Brien TJ et al. The sign of Leser–Trélat. Australas J Dermatol 1983; 24: 93–99.

208 Venencie PY, Perry HO. Sign of Leser–Trélat: Report of two cases and review of the literature. J Am Acad Dermatol 1984; 10: 83–88.

209 Elewski BE, Gilgor RS. Eruptive lesions and malignancy. Int J Dermatol 1985; 24: 617–629.

210 Yeh JSM, Munn SE, Plunkett TA et al. Coexistence of acanthosis nigricans and the sign of Leser–Trélat in a patient with gastric adenocarcinoma: A case report and literature review. J Am Acad Dermatol 2000; 42: 357–362.

211 Sperry K, Wall J. Adenocarcinoma of the stomach with eruptive seborrheic keratoses. The sign of Leser–Trélat. Cancer 1980; 45: 2434–2437.

212 Curry SS, King LE. The sign of Leser–Trélat. Report of a case with adenocarcinoma of the duodenum. Arch Dermatol 1980; 116: 1059–1060.

213 Wagner RF Jr, Wagner KD. Malignant neoplasms and the Leser–Trélat sign. Arch Dermatol 1981; 117: 598–599.

214 Safai B, Grant JM, Good RA. Cutaneous manifestations of internal malignancies (II): the sign of Leser–Trélat. Int J Dermatol 1978; 17: 494–495.

215 Wieselthier JS, Bhawan J, Koh HK. Transformation of Sézary syndrome and the sign of Leser–Trélat: A histopathologic study. J Am Acad Dermatol 1990; 23: 520–522.

216 McCrary ML, Davis LS. Sign of Leser–Trélat and mycosis fungoides. J Am Acad Dermatol 1998; 38: 644.

217 Liddell D, White JE, Caldwell IW. Seborrhoeic keratoses and carcinoma of the large bowel. Br J Dermatol 1975; 92: 449–452.

218 Williams JV, Helm KF, Long D. Chemotherapy-induced inflammation in seborrheic keratoses mimicking disseminated herpes zoster. J Am Acad Dermatol 1999; 40: 643–644.

219 Heng MCY, Soo-Hoo K, Levine S, Petresek D. Linear seborrheic keratoses associated with underlying malignancy. J Am Acad Dermatol 1988; 18: 1316–1321.

220 Schwengle LEM, Rampen FHJ. Eruptive seborrheic keratoses associated with erythrodermic pityriasis rubra pilaris. Acta Derm Venereol 1988; 68: 443–445.

221 Berman A, Winkelmann RK. Seborrheic keratoses. Appearances in course of exfoliative erythroderma and regression associated with histologic mononuclear cell inflammation. Arch Dermatol 1982; 118: 615–618.

222 Kilmer SL, Berman B, Morhenn VB. Eruptive seborrheic keratoses in a young woman with acromegaly. J Am Acad Dermatol 1990; 23: 991–994.

223 Halevy S, Feuerman EJ. The sign of Leser–Trélat. A cutaneous marker for internal malignancy. Int J Dermatol 1985; 24: 359–361.

224 Schwartz RA, Burgess GH. Florid cutaneous papillomatosis. Arch Dermatol 1978; 114: 1803–1806.

225 Babapour R, Leach J, Levy H. Dermatosis papulosa nigra in a young child. Pediatr Dermatol 1993; 10: 356–358.

226 Hairston MA, Reed RJ, Derbes VJ. Dermatosis papulosa nigra. Arch Dermatol 1964; 89: 655–658.

227 Mishima Y, Pinkus H. Benign mixed tumor of melanocytes and malpighian cells. Melanoacanthoma: its relationship to Bloch's benign non-nevoid melanoepithelioma. Arch Dermatol 1960; 81: 539–550.

228 Sexton FM, Maize JC. Melanotic macules and melanoacanthomas of the lip. Am J Dermatopathol 1987; 9: 438–444.

229 Delacretaz J. Mélano-acanthome. Dermatologica 1975; 151: 236–240.

230 Prince C, Mehregan AH, Hashimoto K, Plotnick H. Large melanoacanthomas: a report of five cases. J Cutan Pathol 1984; 11: 309–317.

231 Matsuoka LY, Glasser S, Barsky S. Melanoacanthoma of the lip. Arch Dermatol 1979; 115: 1116–1117.

232 Matsuoka LY, Barsky S, Glasser S. Melanoacanthoma of the lip. Arch Dermatol 1982; 118: 290.

233 Schlappner OLA, Rowden G, Phillips TM, Rahim Z. Melanoacanthoma. Ultrastructural and immunological studies. J Cutan Pathol 1978; 5: 127–141.

234 Spott DA, Wood MG, Heaton CL. Melanoacanthoma of the eyelid. Arch Dermatol 1972; 105: 898–899.

235 Zak FG, Martinez M, Statsinger AL. Pale cell acanthoma. Arch Dermatol 1966; 93: 674–678.

236 Wells GC, Wilson Jones E. Degos' acanthoma (acanthome à cellules claires). Br J Dermatol 1967; 79: 249–258.

237 Petzelbauer P, Konrad K. Polypous clear cell acanthoma. Am J Dermatopathol 1990; 12: 393–395.

238 Degos R, Civatte J. Clear-cell acanthoma. Experience of 8 years. Br J Dermatol 1970; 83: 248–254.

239 Inalöz HS, Patel G, Knight AG. Polypoid clear cell acanthoma: case report. J Eur Acad Dermatol Venereol 2000; 14: 511–512.

240 Murphy R, Kesseler ME, Slater DN. Giant clear cell acanthoma. Br J Dermatol 2000; 143: 1114–1115.

241 Nijssen A, Laeijendecker R, Heinbuis RJ, Dekker SK. Polypoid clear cell acanthoma of unusual size. J Am Acad Dermatol 2001; 44: 314–316.

242 Wilson Jones E, Wells GC. Degos' acanthoma (acanthome à cellules claires). Arch Dermatol 1966; 94: 286–294.

243 Langtry JAA, Torras H, Palou J et al. Giant clear cell acanthoma in an atypical location. J Am Acad Dermatol 1989; 21: 313–315.

244 Witkowski JA, Parish LC. Clear cell acanthoma. Int J Dermatol 1979; 18: 162–163.

245 Trau H, Fisher BK, Schewach-Millet M. Multiple clear cell acanthomas. Arch Dermatol 1980; 116: 433–434.

246 Goette DK, Diakon NC. Multiple clear cell acanthomas. Arch Dermatol 1983; 119: 359–361.

247 Landry M, Winkelmann RK. Multiple clear-cell acanthoma and ichthyosis. Arch Dermatol 1972; 105: 371–383.

248 Baden TJ, Woodley DT, Wheeler CE. Multiple clear cell acanthomas. Case report and delineation of basement membrane zone antigens. J Am Acad Dermatol 1987; 16: 1075–1078.

249 Burg G, Würsch Th, Fäh J, Elsner P. Eruptive hamartomatous clear-cell acanthomas. Dermatology 1994; 189: 437–439.

250 Yang SG, Moon SH, Lim JG et al. Clear cell acanthoma presenting as polypoid papule combined with melanocytic nevus. Am J Dermatopathol 1999; 21: 63–65.

251 Fine RM, Chernosky ME. Clinical recognition of clear-cell acanthoma (Degos'). Arch Dermatol 1969; 100: 559–562.

252 Kim D-H, Kim C-W, Kang S-J, Kim T-Y. A case of clear cell acanthoma presenting as nipple eczema. Br J Dermatol 1999; 141: 950–951.

253 Bonnetblanc JM, Delrous JL, Catanzano G et al. Multiple clear cell acanthoma. Arch Dermatol 1981; 117: 1.

254 Cotton DWK, Mills PM, Stephenson TJ, Underwood JCE. On the nature of clear cell acanthomas. Br J Dermatol 1987; 117: 569–574.

255 Ohnishi T, Watanabe S. Immunohistochemical characterization of keratin expression in clear cell acanthoma. Br J Dermatol 1995; 133: 186–193.

256 Finch TM, Tan CY. Clear cell acanthoma developing on a psoriatic plaque: further evidence of an inflammatory aetiology? Br J Dermatol 2000; 142: 842–844.

257 Brownstein MH, Fernando S, Shapiro L. Clear cell acanthoma. Clinicopathologic analysis of 37 new cases. Am J Clin Pathol 1973; 59: 306–311.

258 Fanti PA, Passarini B, Varotti C. Melanocytes in clear cell acanthoma. Am J Dermatopathol 1990; 12: 373–376.

259 Langer K, Wuketich S, Konrad K. Pigmented clear cell acanthoma. Am J Dermatopathol 1994; 16: 134–139.

260 Grunwald MH, Rothem A, Halevy S. Atypical clear cell acanthoma. Int J Dermatol 1991; 30: 848–850.

261 Hu F, Sisson JK. The ultrastructure of the pale cell acanthoma. J Invest Dermatol 1969; 52: 185–188.

262 Kerl H. Das Klarzellakanthom. Hautarzt 1977; 28: 456–462.

263 Desmons F, Breuillard F, Thomas P et al. Multiple clear-cell acanthoma (Degos): histochemical and ultrastructural study of two cases. Int J Dermatol 1977; 16: 203–213.

264 Hashimoto T, Inamoto N, Nakamura K. Two cases of clear cell acanthoma: an immunohistological study. J Cutan Pathol 1988; 15: 27–30.

265 Fukushiro S, Takei Y, Ackerman AB. Pale cell acanthosis. A distinctive histologic pattern of epidermal epithelium. Am J Dermatopathol 1985; 7: 515–527.

266 Hamaguchi T, Penneys N. Cystic clear cell acanthoma. J Cutan Pathol 1995; 22: 188–190.

267 Kuo T-t, Huang C-L, Chan H-L et al. Clear cell papulosis: report of three cases of a newly recognized disease. J Am Acad Dermatol 1995; 33: 230–233.

268 Kuo T-t, Chan H-L, Hsueh S. Clear cell papulosis of the skin. Am J Surg Pathol 1987; 11: 827–834.

269 Lee JY-Y, Chao S-C. Clear cell papulosis of the skin. Br J Dermatol 1998; 138: 678–683.

270 Moulonguet I, Cavelier-Balloy B, Broissin M et al. Clear cell papulosis – report of a case. Am J Dermatopathol 2000; 22: 348 (abstract).

271 Kim Y-C, Bang D, Cinn Y-W. Clear cell papulosis: case report and literature review. Pediatr Dermatol 1997; 14: 380–382.

272 Lee JY-Y. Clear cell papulosis: a unique disorder in early childhood characterized by white macules in milk-line distribution. Pediatr Dermatol 1998; 15: 328.

273 Rahbari H, Pinkus H. Large cell acanthoma. One of the actinic keratoses. Arch Dermatol 1978; 114: 49–52.

274 Rabinowitz AD. Multiple large cell acanthomas. J Am Acad Dermatol 1983 8: 840–845.

275 Sánchez Yus E, de Diego V, Urrutia S. Large cell acanthoma. A cytologic variant of Bowen's disease? Am J Dermatopathol 1988; 10: 197–208.

276 Argenyi ZB, Huston BM, Argenyi EE et al. Large-cell acanthoma of the skin. A study by image analysis cytometry and immunohistochemistry. Am J Dermatopathol 1994; 16: 140–144.

277 Weinstock MA. Large-cell acanthoma. Am J Dermatopathol 1992; 14: 133–134.

278 Rabinowitz AD, Inghirami G. Large-cell acanthoma. A distinctive keratosis. Am J Dermatopathol 1992; 14: 136–138.

279 Sánchez Yus E, del Rio E, Requena L. Large-cell acanthoma is a distinctive entity. Am J Dermatopathol 1992; 14: 140–147.

280 Roewert HJ, Ackerman AB. Large-cell acanthoma is a solar lentigo. Am J Dermatopathol 1992; 14: 122–132.

Epidermal dysplasias

281 Pinkus H, Mehregan AH. Premalignant skin lesions. Clin Plast Surg 1980; 7: 289–300.

282 Sander CA, Pfeiffer C, Kligman AM, Plewig G. Chemotherapy for disseminated actinic keratoses with 5-fluorouracil and isotretinoin. J Am Acad Dermatol 1997; 36: 236–238.

283 Feldman SR, Fleischer AB Jr, Williford PM, Jorizzo JL. Destructive procedures are the standard of care for treatment of actinic keratoses. J Am Acad Dermatol 1999; 40: 43–47.

284 Marks R. Nonmelanotic skin cancer and solar keratoses. The quiet 20th century epidemic. Int J Dermatol 1987; 26: 201–205.

285 Frost CA, Green AC. Epidemiology of solar keratoses. Br J Dermatol 1994; 131: 455–464.

286 Memon AA, Tomenson JA, Bothwell J, Friedmann PS. Prevalence of solar damage and actinic keratosis in a Merseyside population. Br J Dermatol 2000; 142: 1154–1159.

287 Yashiro K, Nakagawa T, Takaiwa T, Inai M. Actinic keratoses arising only on sun-exposed vitiligo skin. Clin Exp Dermatol 1999; 24: 199–201.

288 Salasche SJ. Epidemiology of actinic keratoses and squamous cell carcinoma. J Am Acad Dermatol 2000; 42: S4–S7.

289 Moy RL. Clinical presentation of actinic keratoses and squamous cell carcinoma. J Am Acad Dermatol 2000; 42: S8–S10.

290 Frost C, Williams G, Green A. High incidence and regression rates of solar keratoses in a Queensland community. J Invest Dermatol 2000; 115: 273–277.

291 Merino MJG-B, Ackerman AB. Solar keratoses have not been proven to regress! Dermatopathology: Practical & Conceptual 2000; 6: 5–9.

292 Glogau RG. The risk of progression to invasive disease. J Am Acad Dermatol 2000; 42: S23–S24.

293 Callen JP, Bickers DR, Moy RL. Actinic keratoses. J Am Acad Dermatol 1997; 36: 650–653.

294 Suchniak JM, Baer S, Goldberg LH. High rate of malignant transformation in hyperkeratotic actinic keratoses. J Am Acad Dermatol 1997; 37: 392–394.

295 Marks R, Foley P, Goodman G et al. Spontaneous remission of solar keratoses: the case for conservative management. Br J Dermatol 1986; 115: 649–655.

296 Commens C. Solar keratosis: fallacies in measuring remission rate and conversion rate to squamous cell carcinoma. Br J Dermatol 1987; 117: 261.

297 Dodson JM, DeSpain J, Hewett JE, Clark DP. Malignant potential of actinic keratoses and the controversy over treatment. Arch Dermatol 1991; 127: 1029–1031.

298 Heaphy MR Jr, Ackerman AB. The nature of solar keratosis: A critical review in historical perspective. J Am Acad Dermatol 2000; 43: 138–150.

299 Ackerman AB. Respect at last for solar keratosis. Dermatopathology: Practical & Conceptual 1997; 3: 101–103.

300 Cockerell CJ. Histopathology of incipient intraepidermal squamous cell carcinoma ("actinic keratosis"). J Am Acad Dermatol 2000; 42: S11–S17.

301 Billano RA, Little WP. Hypertrophic actinic keratosis. J Am Acad Dermatol 1982; 7: 484–489.

302 Rabkin MS, Weems WS. Hyperplastic acral keratoses – association with invasive squamous cell carcinoma. J Dermatol Surg Oncol 1987; 13: 1223–1228.

303 James MP, Wells GC, Whimster IW. Spreading pigmented actinic keratoses. Br J Dermatol 1978; 98: 373–379.

304 Dinehart SM, Sanchez RL. Spreading pigmented actinic keratosis. An electron microscopic study. Arch Dermatol 1988; 124: 680–683.

305 Subrt P, Jorizzo JL, Apisarnthanarax P et al. Spreading pigmented actinic keratosis. J Am Acad Dermatol 1983; 8: 63–67.

306 Tan CY, Marks R. Lichenoid solar keratosis – prevalence and immunologic findings. J Invest Dermatol 1982; 79: 365–367.

307 Frost CA, Green AC, Williams GM. The prevalence and determinants of solar keratoses at a subtropical latitude (Queensland, Australia). Br J Dermatol 1998; 139: 1033–1039.

308 Robinson JK, Rigel DS, Amonette RA. Summertime sun protection used by adults for their children. J Am Acad Dermatol 2000; 42: 746–753.

309 Pearse AD, Marks R. Actinic keratoses and the epidermis on which they arise. Br J Dermatol 1977; 96: 45–51.

310 Schaumburg-Lever G, Alroy J, Ucci A, Lever WF. Cell surface carbohydrates in proliferative epidermal lesions. J Cutan Pathol 1986; 13: 163–171.

311 Bito T, Ueda M, Ahmed NU et al. Cyclin D and retinoblastoma gene product expression in actinic keratosis and cutaneous squamous cell carcinoma in relation to p53 expression. J Cutan Pathol 1995; 22: 427–434.

312 McNutt NS, Saenz-Santamaría C, Volkenandt M et al. Abnormalities of p53 protein expression in cutaneous disorders. Arch Dermatol 1994; 130: 225–232.

313 Onodera H, Nakamura S, Sugai T. Cell proliferation and p53 protein expression in cutaneous epithelial neoplasms. Am J Dermatopathol 1996; 18: 580–588.

314 Park W-S, Lee H-K, Lee J-Y et al. *p53* mutations in solar keratoses. Hum Pathol 1996; 27: 1180–1184.

315 Lea RA, Selvey S, Ashton KJ. The null allele of GSTM1 does not affect susceptibility to solar keratoses in the Australian white population. J Am Acad Dermatol 1998; 38: 631–633.

316 McCarron K, Ormsby A, Bergfeld W. p53 mutation immunoexpression in cutaneous squamous neoplasia: an adjunct to histomorphology. J Cutan Pathol 2000; 27: 564–565 (abstract).

317 Spencer JM, Kahn SM, Jiang W et al. Activated *ras* genes occur in human actinic keratoses, premalignant precursors to squamous cell carcinomas. Arch Dermatol 1995; 31: 796–800.

318 Bhawan J. Histology of epidermal dysplasia. J Cutan Aging Cosm Dermatol 1988; 1: 95–103.

319 Lever L, Marks R. The significance of the Darier-like solar keratosis and acantholytic changes in preneoplastic lesions of the epidermis. Br J Dermatol 1989; 120: 383–389.

320 Javier BJ, Ackerman AB. Solar keratosis with "Darier-like features" is "pseudoglandular" squamous-cell carcinoma. Dermatopathology: Practical & Conceptual 2000; 6: 114–121.

321 Pinkus H. Keratosis senilis. Am J Clin Pathol 1958; 29: 193–207.

322 Goldberg LH, Joseph AK, Tschen JA. Proliferative actinic keratosis. Int J Dermatol 1994; 33: 341–345.

323 Kaufman D, Ackerman AB. Acrosyringia and acrotrichia in solar keratosis are "spared", but affected nonetheless by the process! Dermatopathology: Practical & Conceptual 2000; 6: 383–386.

324 Chun Y-S, Chang SN, Oh D, Park WH. A case of cutaneous reaction to chemotherapeutic agents showing epidermal dysmaturation. J Am Acad Dermatol 2000; 43: 358–360.

325 Johnson TM, Rapini RP, Duvic M. Inflammation of actinic keratoses from systemic chemotherapy. J Am Acad Dermatol 1987; 17: 192–197.

326 Bataille V, Cunningham D, Mansi J, Mortimer P. Inflammation of solar keratoses following systemic 5-fluorouracil. Br J Dermatol 1996; 135: 478–480.

327 Kossard S, Ma DDF. Acral keratotic graft versus host disease simulating warts. Australas J Dermatol 1999; 40: 161–163.

328 Price ML, Tidman MJ, Fagg NLK et al. Distinctive epidermal atypia in immunosuppression-associated cutaneous malignancy. Histopathology 1988; 13: 89–94.

329 Boyd AS, Stasko TH, Cameron G et al. Histopathologic features of actinic keratoses in solid organ transplant recipients and healthy controls. J Cutan Pathol 2000; 27: 549–550.

330 Jones RE Jr, ed. What is the boundary that separates a thick solar keratosis and a thin squamous cell carcinoma? Am J Dermatopathol 1984; 6: 301–306.

331 Guillén DR, Cockerell CJ. Accurate diagnosis of cutaneous keratinocytic neoplasms. The importance of histological step sections (and other factors). Arch Dermatol 2000; 136: 535–537.

332 Carag HR, Prieto VG, Yballe LS, Shea CR. Utility of step sections. Demonstration of additional pathological findings in biopsy samples initially diagnosed as actinic keratosis. Arch Dermatol 2000; 136: 471–475.

333 Aghassi D, Anderson RR, González S. Confocal laser microscopic imaging of actinic keratoses in vivo: A preliminary report. J Am Acad Dermatol 2000; 43: 42–48.

334 Ficascia DD, Robinson JK. Actinic cheilitis: a review of the etiology, differential diagnosis and treatment. J Am Acad Dermatol 1987; 17: 255–264.

335 Cataldo E, Doku HC. Solar cheilitis. J Dermatol Surg Oncol 1981; 7: 989–995.

336 Gibson LE, Perry HO. Skin lesions from sun exposure: a treatment guide. Geriatrics 1985; 40: 87–92.

337 Stanley RJ. Actinic cheilitis: treatment with the carbon dioxide laser. Mayo Clin Proc 1988; 63: 230–235.

338 Nicolau SG, Balus L. Chronic actinic cheilitis and cancer of the lower lip. Br J Dermatol 1964; 76: 278–289.

339 Koten JW, Verhagen ARHB, Frank GL. Histopathology of actinic cheilitis. Dermatologica 1967; 135: 465–471.

340 Gerdsen R, Stockfleth E, Uerlich M et al. Papular palmoplantar hyperkeratosis following chronic medical exposure to arsenic: human papillomavirus as a co-factor in the pathogenesis of arsenical keratosis? Acta Derm Venereol 2000; 80: 292–293.

341 Schwartz RA. Arsenic and the skin. Int J Dermatol 1997; 36: 241–250.

342 Yeh S, How SW, Lin CS. Arsenical cancer of skin. Histologic study with special reference to Bowen's disease. Cancer 1968; 21: 312–339.

343 Yeh S. Skin cancer in chronic arsenicism. Hum Pathol 1973; 4: 469–485.

344 Alain G, Tousignant J, Rozenfarb E. Chronic arsenic toxicity. Int J Dermatol 1993; 32: 899–901.

345 Schwartz RA. Premalignant keratinocytic neoplasms. J Am Acad Dermatol 1996; 35: 223–242.

346 Wong SS, Tan KC, Goh CL. Cutaneous manifestations of chronic arsenicism: Review of seventeen cases. J Am Acad Dermatol 1998; 38: 179–185.

347 Piamphongsant T. Chronic environmental arsenic poisoning. Int J Dermatol 1999; 38: 401–410.

348 Boorchai W, Green A, Ng J et al. Basal cell carcinoma in chronic arsenicism occurring in Queensland, Australia, after ingestion of an asthma medication. J Am Acad Dermatol 2000; 43: 664–669.

349 Jackson R, Grainge JW. Arsenic and cancer. Can Med Assoc J 1975; 113: 396–399.

350 Graham JH, Helwig EB. Bowen's disease and its relationship to systemic cancer. Arch Dermatol 1961; 83: 738–758.

351 Sommers SC, McManus RG. Multiple arsenical cancers of skin and internal organs. Cancer 1953; 6: 347–359.

352 Boonchai W, Walsh M, Cummings M, Chenevix-Trench G. Expression of p53 in arsenic-related and sporadic basal cell carcinoma. Arch Dermatol 2000; 136: 195–198.

353 Chang C-H, Tsai R-K, Chen G-S et al. Expression of bcl-2, p53 and Ki-67 in arsenical skin cancers. J Cutan Pathol 1998; 25: 457–462.

354 Kuo T-T, Hu S, Lo S-K, Chan H-L. p53 expression and proliferative activity in Bowen's disease with or without chronic arsenic exposure. Hum Pathol 1997; 28: 786–790.

355 Chai C-Y, Yu H-S, Yen H-T et al. The inhibitory effect of UVB irradiation on the expression of p53 and Ki-67 proteins in arsenic-induced Bowen's disease. J Cutan Pathol 1997; 24: 8–13.

356 Letzel S, Drexler H. Occupationally related tumors in tar refinery workers. J Am Acad Dermatol 1998; 39: 712–720.

357 van Praag MCG, Bavinck JNB, Bergman W et al. PUVA keratosis. A clinical and histopathologic entity associated with an increased risk of nonmelanoma skin cancer. J Am Acad Dermatol 1993; 28: 412–417.

358 Stern RS, Lunder EJ. Risk of squamous cell carcinoma and methoxsalen (psoralen) and UV-A radiation (PUVA). Arch Dermatol 1998; 134: 1582–1585.

359 Buckley DA, Rogers S. Multiple keratoses and squamous carcinoma after PUVA treatment of vitiligo. Clin Exp Dermatol 1996; 21: 43–45.

360 McKenna KE, Patterson CC, Handley J et al. Cutaneous neoplasia following PUVA therapy for psoriasis. Br J Dermatol 1996; 134: 639–642.

361 Turner RJ, Sviland L, Charlton F, Farr PM. PUVA-related punctate keratoses on the hands and feet. J Am Acad Dermatol 2000; 42: 476–479.

362 Morison WL, Kerker BJ, Tunnessen WW, Farmer ER. Disseminated hypopigmented keratoses. Arch Dermatol 1991; 127: 848–850.

Intraepidermal carcinomas

363 Callen JP. Bowen's disease and internal malignant disease. Arch Dermatol 1988; 124: 675–676.

364 Scarborough DA, Bisaccia EP, Yoder FW. Solitary pigmented Bowen's disease. Arch Dermatol 1982; 118: 954–955.

365 Fisher GB Jr, Greer KE, Walker AN. Bowen's disease mimicking melanoma. Arch Dermatol 1982; 118: 444–445.

366 Burns DA. Bilateral pigmented Bowen's disease of the web-spaces of the feet. Clin Exp Dermatol 1981; 6: 435–437.

367 Papageorgiou PP, Koumarianou AA, Chu AC. Pigmented Bowen's disease. Br J Dermatol 1998; 138: 515–518.

368 Katz HI, Posalaky Z, McGinley D. Pigmented penile papules with carcinoma in situ changes. Br J Dermatol 1978; 99: 155–162.

369 Kimura S, Hirai A, Harada R, Nagashima M. So-called multicentric pigmented Bowen's disease. Dermatologica 1978; 157: 229–237.

370 Lloyd KM. Multicentric pigmented Bowen's disease of the groin. Arch Dermatol 1970; 101: 48–51.

371 Ragi G, Turner MS, Klein LE, Stoll HL Jr. Pigmented Bowen's disease and review of 420 Bowen's disease lesions. J Dermatol Surg Oncol 1988; 14: 765–769.

372 Thestrup-Pedersen K, Ravnborg L, Reymann F. Morbus Bowen. A description of the disease in 617 patients. Acta Derm Venereol 1988; 68: 236–239.

373 Cox NH. Body site distribution of Bowen's disease. Br J Dermatol 1994; 130: 714–716.

374 Kossard S, Rosen R. Cutaneous Bowen's disease. An analysis of 1001 cases according to age, sex, and site. J Am Acad Dermatol 1992; 27: 406–410.

375 Rosen T, Tucker SB, Tschen J. Bowen's disease in blacks. J Am Acad Dermatol 1982; 7: 364–368.

376 Mora RG, Perniciaro C, Lee B. Cancer of the skin in blacks. III. A review of nineteen black patients with Bowen's disease. J Am Acad Dermatol 1984; 11: 557–562.

377 Coskey RJ, Mehregan A, Fosnaugh R. Bowen's disease of the nail bed. Arch Dermatol 1972; 106: 79–80.

378 Mikhail GR. Bowen disease and squamous cell carcinoma of the nail bed. Arch Dermatol 1974; 110: 267–270.

379 Baran RL, Gormley DE. Polydactylous Bowen's disease of the nail. J Am Acad Dermatol 1987; 17: 201–204.

380 Sau P, McMarlin SL, Sperling LC, Katz R. Bowen's disease of the nail bed and periungual area. Arch Dermatol 1994; 130: 204–209.

381 Baran R, Perrin C. Longitudinal erythronychia with distal subungual keratosis: onychopapilloma of the nail bed and Bowen's disease. Br J Dermatol 2000; 143: 132–135.

382 Biediger TL, Grabski WJ, McCollough ML. Bilateral pigmented Bowen's disease of the lower lip. Int J Dermatol 1995; 34: 116–118.

383 Venkataseshan VS, Budd DC, Kim DU, Hutter RVP. Intraepidermal squamous carcinoma (Bowen's disease) of the nipple. Hum Pathol 1994; 25: 1371–1374.

384 Wagers LT, Shapiro L, Kroll JJ. Bowen disease of the hand. Arch Dermatol 1973; 107: 745–746.

385 Starke WR. Bowen's disease of the palm associated with Hodgkin's lymphoma. Cancer 1972; 30: 1315–1318.

386 Jacyk WK. Bowen's disease of the palm. Report of a case in an African. Dermatologica 1980; 161: 285–287.

387 Grekin RC, Swanson NA. Verrucous Bowen's disease of the plantar foot. J Dermatol Surg Oncol 1984; 10: 734–736.

388 McCallum DI, Kinmont PDC, Williams DW et al. Intra-epidermal carcinoma of the eyelid margin. Br J Dermatol 1975; 93: 239–252.

389 Shelley WB, Wood MG. Occult Bowen's disease in keratinous cysts. Br J Dermatol 1981; 105: 105–108.

390 Coskey RJ, Mehregan A. Bowen disease associated with porokeratosis of Mibelli. Arch Dermatol 1975; 111: 1480–1481.

391 Keefe M, Smith GD. Bowen's disease arising in a scar – a case report and review of the relationship between trauma and malignancy. Clin Exp Dermatol 1991; 16: 478–480.

392 Arrington JH III, Lockman DS. Thermal keratoses and squamous cell carcinoma in situ associated with erythema ab igne. Arch Dermatol 1979; 115: 1226–1228.

393 Miki Y, Kawatsu T, Matsuda K et al. Cutaneous and pulmonary cancers associated with Bowen's disease. J Am Acad Dermatol 1982; 6: 26–31.

394 Graham JH, Helwig EB. Bowen's disease and its relationship to systemic cancer. Arch Dermatol 1959; 80: 133–159.

395 Epstein E. Association of Bowen's disease with visceral cancer. Arch Dermatol 1960; 80: 349–351.

396 Peterka ES, Lynch FW, Goltz RW. An association between Bowen's disease and internal cancer. Arch Dermatol 1961; 84: 623–629.

397 Chuang T-Y, Reizner GT. Bowen's disease and internal malignancy. A matched case-control study. J Am Acad Dermatol 1988; 19: 47–51.

398 Arbesman H, Ransohoff DF. Is Bowen's disease a predictor for the development of internal malignancy? A methodological critique of the literature. JAMA 1987; 257: 516–518.

399 Reymann F, Ravnborg L, Schou G et al. Bowen's disease and internal malignant diseases. A study of 581 patients. Arch Dermatol 1988; 124: 677–679.

400 Hemminki K, Dong C. Subsequent cancers after in situ and invasive squamous cell carcinoma of the skin. Arch Dermatol 2000; 136: 647–651.

401 McGovern VJ. Bowen's disease. Australas J Dermatol 1965; 8: 48–50.

402 Kao GF. Carcinoma arising in Bowen's disease. Arch Dermatol 1986; 122: 1124–1126.

403 Brownstein MH, Rabinowitz AD. The precursors of cutaneous squamous cell carcinoma. Int J Dermatol 1979; 18: 1–16.

404 González-Pérez R, Gardeazábal J, Eizaguirre X, Diaz-Pérez JL. Metastatic squamous cell carcinoma arising in Bowen's disease of the palm. J Am Acad Dermatol 1997; 36: 635–636.

405 Chisiki M, Kawada A, Akiyama M et al. Bowen's disease showing spontaneous complete regression associated with apoptosis. Br J Dermatol 1999; 140: 939–944.

406 Collina G, Rossi E, Bettelli S et al. Detection of human papillomavirus in extragenital Bowen's disease using in situ hybridization and polymerase chain reaction. Am J Dermatopathol 1995; 17: 236–241.

407 Ikenberg H, Gissmann L, Gross G et al. Human papillomavirus type-16-related DNA in genital Bowen's disease and in Bowenoid papulosis. Int J Cancer 1983; 32: 563–565.

408 Yoneta A, Yamashita T, Jin H-Y et al. Development of squamous cell carcinoma by two high-risk human papillomaviruses (HPVs), a novel HPV-67 and HPV-31 from bowenoid papulosis. Br J Dermatol 2000; 143: 604–608.

409 Pfister H, Haneke E. Demonstration of human papilloma virus type 2 DNA in Bowen's disease. Arch Dermatol Res 1984; 276: 123–125.

410 Stone MS, Noonan CA, Tschen J, Bruce S. Bowen's disease of the feet. Presence of human papillomavirus 16 DNA in tumor tissue. Arch Dermatol 1987; 123: 1517–1520.

411 McGrae JD Jr, Greer CE, Manos MM. Multiple Bowen's disease of the fingers associated with human papilloma virus type 16. Int J Dermatol 1993; 32: 104–107

412 Forslund O, Nordin P, Andersson K et al. DNA analysis indicates patient-specific human papillomavirus type 16 strains in Bowen's disease on fingers and in archival samples from genital dysplasia. Br J Dermatol 1997; 136: 678–682.

413 Clavel CE, Huu VP, Durlach AP et al. Mucosal oncogenic human papillomaviruses and extragenital Bowen disease. Cancer 1999; 86: 282–287.

414 Kawashima M, Jablonska S, Favre M et al. Characterization of a new type of human papillomavirus found in a lesion of Bowen's disease of the skin. J Virol 1986; 57: 688–692.

415 Uezato H, Hagiwara K, Ramuzi ST et al. Detection of human papilloma virus type 56 in extragenital Bowen's disease. Acta Derm Venereol 1999; 79: 311–313.

416 Mitsuishi T, Kawashima M, Matsukura T, Sata T. Human papillomavirus type 58 in Bowen's disease of the elbow. Br J Dermatol 2001; 144: 384–386.

417 Hofmann C, Plewig G, Braun-Falco O. Bowenoid lesions, Bowen's disease and keratoacanthomas in long-term PUVA-treated patients. Br J Dermatol 1979; 101: 685–692.

418 Tam DW, Van Scott EJ, Urbach F. Bowen's disease and squamous cell carcinoma. Occurrence in a patient with psoriasis after topical, systemic, and PUVA therapy. Arch Dermatol 1979; 115: 203–204.

419 Takeda H, Mitsuhashi Y, Kondo S. Multiple squamous cell carcinomas in situ in vitiligo lesions after long-term PUVA therapy. J Am Acad Dermatol 1998; 38: 268–270.

420 Cox NH, Eedy DJ, Morton CA. Guidelines for management of Bowen's disease. Br J Dermatol 1999; 141: 633–641.

421 Bell HK, Rhodes LE. Bowen's disease – a retrospective review of clinical management. Clin Exp Dermatol 1999; 24: 338–339.

422 Cox NH. Bowen's disease: where now with therapeutic trials? Br J Dermatol 2000; 143: 699–700.

423 Ahmed I, Berth-Jones J, Charles-Holmes S et al. Comparison of cryotherapy with curettage in the treatment of Bowen's disease: a prospective study. Br J Dermatol 2000; 143: 759–766.

424 Morton CA, Whitehurst C, Moore JV, MacKie RM. Comparison of red and green light in the treatment of Bowen's disease by photodynamic therapy. Br J Dermatol 2000; 143: 767–772.

425 Mackenzie-Wood A, Kossard S, de Launey J et al. Imiquimod 5% cream in the treatment of Bowen's disease. J Am Acad Dermatol 2001; 44: 462–470.

426 Strayer DS, Santa Cruz DJ. Carcinoma in situ of the skin: a review of histopathology. J Cutan Pathol 1980; 7: 244–259.

427 Ackerman AB. Carcinoma in situ. Another view. Am J Dermatopathol 1979; 1: 147–149.

428 Jones RE Jr, ed. Questions to the Editorial Board and other authorities. Am J Dermatopathol 1982; 4: 91–95.

429 Fulling KH, Strayer DS, Santa Cruz DJ. Adnexal metaplasia in carcinoma in situ of the skin. J Cutan Pathol 1981; 8: 79–88.

430 Hunter GA, Donald GF, Burry JN. Bowen's disease: A clinical and histological re-evaluation. Australas J Dermatol 1967; 9: 132–135.

431 Hunter GA. Follicular Bowen's disease. Br J Dermatol (Suppl) 1977; 15: 20.

432 Peralta OC, Barr RJ, Romansky SG. Mixed carcinoma in situ: an immunohistochemical study. J Cutan Pathol 1983; 10: 350–358.

433 Argenyi ZB, Hughes AM, Balogh K, Vo T-L. Cancerization of eccrine sweat ducts in Bowen's disease as studied by light microscopy, DNA spectrophotometry and immunohistochemistry. Am J Dermatopathol 1990; 12: 433–440.

434 Weedon D. Unpublished observations.

435 Murata Y, Kumano K, Sashikata T. Partial spontaneous regression of Bowen's disease. Arch Dermatol 1996; 132: 429–432.

436 Guldhammer B, Nrgaard T. The differential diagnosis of intraepidermal malignant lesions using immunohistochemistry. Am J Dermatopathol 1986; 8: 295–301.

437 Shah KD, Tabibzadeh SS, Gerber MA. Immunohistochemical distinction of Paget's disease from Bowen's disease and superficial spreading melanoma with the use of monoclonal cytokeratin antibodies. Am J Clin Pathol 1987; 88: 689–695.

438 Williamson JD, Colome MI, Sahin A et al. Pagetoid Bowen disease. A report of 2 cases that express cytokeratin 7. Arch Pathol Lab Med 2000; 124: 427–430.

439 Geary WA, Cooper PH. Proliferating cell nuclear antigen (PCNA) in common epidermal lesions. J Cutan Pathol 1992; 19: 458–468.

440 Baum H-P, Meurer I, Unteregger G. Expression of proliferation-associated proteins (proliferating cell nuclear antigen and Ki-67 antigen) in Bowen's disease. Br J Dermatol 1994; 131: 231–236.

441 Tsuji T, Kitajima S, Koashi Y. Expression of proliferating cell nuclear antigen (PCNA) and apoptosis related antigen (Le^Y) in epithelial skin tumors. Am J Dermatopathol 1998; 20: 164–169.

442 Duan H, Koga T, Masuda T et al. CD1a+, CD3+, CD4+, CD8+, CD68+ and cutaneous lymphocyte-associated antigen positive cells in Bowen's disease. Br J Dermatol 2000; 143: 1211–1216.

443 Jacobs DM, Sandles LG, LeBoit PE. Sebaceous carcinoma arising from Bowen's disease of the vulva. Arch Dermatol 1986; 122: 1191–1193.

444 Saida T, Okabe Y, Uhara H. Bowen's disease with invasive carcinoma showing sweat gland differentiation. J Cutan Pathol 1989; 16: 222–226.

445 Verdolini R, Amerio P, Goteri G et al. Cutaneous carcinomas and preinvasive neoplastic lesions. Role of MMP-2 and MMP-9 metalloproteinases in neoplastic invasion and their relationship with proliferative activity and p53 expression. J Cutan Pathol 2001; 28: 120–126.

446 Mene A, Buckley CH. Involvement of the vulval skin appendages by intraepithelial neoplasia. Br J Obstet Gynaecol 1985; 92: 634–638.

447 Voet RL. Classification of vulvar dystrophies and premalignant squamous lesions. J Cutan Pathol 1994; 21: 86–90.

448 Yang B, Hart WR. Vulvar intraepithelial neoplasia of the simplex (differentiated) type. A clinicopathologic study including analysis of HPV and p53 expression. Am J Surg Pathol 2000; 24: 429–441.

449 Callen JP, Headington J. Bowen's and non-Bowen's squamous intraepidermal neoplasia of the skin. Relationship to internal malignancy. Arch Dermatol 1980; 116: 422–426.

450 Hart WR. Vulvar intraepithelial neoplasia: historical aspects and current status. Int J Gynecol Pathol 2001; 20: 16–30.

451 McLachlin CM, Mutter GL, Crum CP. Multinucleated atypia of the vulva. Report of a distinct entity not associated with human papillomavirus. Am J Surg Pathol 1994; 18: 1233–1239.

452 Biesterfeld S, Pennings K, Grussendorf-Conen E-I, Böcking A. Aneuploidy in actinic keratosis and Bowen's disease – increased risk for invasive squamous cell carcinoma? Br J Dermatol 1995; 133: 557–560.

453 Sim CS, Slater S, McKee PH. Mutant p53 expression in solar keratosis: an immunohistochemical study. J Cutan Pathol 1992; 19: 302–308.

454 Sim CS, Slater SD, McKee PH. Mutant p53 is expressed in Bowen's disease. Am J Dermatopathol 1992; 14: 195–199.

455 Kawakami T, Saito R, Takahashi K. Overexpression of p21$^{WAf1/Cip1}$ immunohistochemical staining in Bowen's disease, but not in disseminated superficial porokeratosis. Br J Dermatol 1999; 141: 647–651.

456 Ichikawa E, Watanabe S, Otsuka F. Immunohistochemical localization of keratins and involucrin in solar keratosis and Bowen's disease. Am J Dermatopathol 1995; 17: 151–157.

457 Olson RL, Nordquist RE, Everett MA. Dyskeratosis in Bowen's disease. Br J Dermatol 1969; 81: 676–680.

458 Lupulescu A, Mehregan AH. Bowen's disease of genital areas. An ultrastructural study. J Cutan Pathol 1977; 4: 266–274.

459 Seiji M, Mizuno F. Electron microscopic study of Bowen's disease. Arch Dermatol 1969; 99: 3–16.

460 Kuligowski M, Dabrowski JH, Jablonska S. Apoptosis in Bowen's disease. An ultrastructural study. Am J Dermatopathol 1989; 11: 13–21.

461 Graham JH, Helwig EB. Erythroplasia of Queyrat. A clinicopathologic and histochemical study. Cancer 1973; 32: 1396–1414.

462 Mikhail GR. Cancers, precancers, and pseudocancers on the male genitalia. A review of clinical appearances, histopathology, and management. J Dermatol Surg Oncol 1980; 6: 1027–1035.

463 Goette DK. Erythroplasia of Queyrat. Arch Dermatol 1974; 110: 271–273.

464 English JC III, Laws RA, Keough GC et al. Dermatoses of the glans penis and prepuce. J Am Acad Dermatol 1997; 37: 1–24.

465 Varma S, Holt PJA, Anstey AV. Erythroplasia of Queyrat treated by topical aminolaevulinic acid photodynamic therapy: a cautionary tale. Br J Dermatol 2000; 142: 825–826.

466 Stables GI, Stringer MR, Robinson DJ, Ash DV. Erythroplasia of Queyrat treated by topical aminolaevulinic acid photodynamic therapy. Br J Dermatol 1999; 140: 514–517.

467 Mitsuishi T, Sata T, Iwasaki T et al. The detection of human papillomavirus 16 DNA in erythroplasia of Queyrat invading the urethra. Br J Dermatol 1998; 138: 188–189.

468 Wieland U, Jurk S, Weißenborn S et al. Erythroplasia of Queyrat: coinfection with cutaneous carcinogenic human papillomavirus type 8 and genital papillomaviruses in a carcinoma in situ. J Invest Dermatol 2000; 115: 396–401.

469 Sonnex TS, Ralfs IG, Plaza de Lanza M, Dawber RPR. Treatment of erythroplasia of Queyrat with liquid nitrogen cryosurgery. Br J Dermatol 1982; 106: 581–584.

470 Berger P, Baughman R. Intra-epidermal epithelioma. Report of case with invasion after many years. Br J Dermatol 1974; 90: 343–349.

471 Cook MG, Ridgway HA. The intra-epidermal epithelioma of Jadassohn: a distinct entity. Br J Dermatol 1979; 101: 659–667.

472 Larsson A, Hammarstrom L, Nethander G, Sjogren S. Multiple lesions of the lip exhibiting the 'Jadassohn phenomenon'. Br J Dermatol 1977; 96: 307–312.

473 Steffen C, Ackerman AB. Intraepidermal epithelioma of Borst–Jadassohn. Am J Dermatopathol 1985; 7: 5–24.

474 Helm KF, Helm TN, Helm F. Borst–Jadassohn phenomenon associated with an undifferentiated spindle cell neoplasm. Int J Dermatol 1994; 33: 563–565.

475 Mehregan AH, Pinkus H. Intraepidermal epithelioma: a critical study. Cancer 1964; 17: 609–636.

476 Hodge SJ, Turner JE. Histopathologic concepts of intraepithelial epithelioma. Int J Dermatol 1986; 25: 372–375.

477 Ito M, Tazawa T, Shimizu N et al. Intraepidermal pilar epithelioma: A new dermatopathologic interpretation of a skin tumor. J Am Acad Dermatol 1988; 18: 123–132.

Malignant tumors

478 Miller DL, Weinstock MA. Nonmelanoma skin cancer in the United States: Incidence. J Am Acad Dermatol 1994; 30: 774–778.

479 Weinstock MA, Bogaars HA, Ashley M et al. Nonmelanoma skin cancer mortality. Arch Dermatol 1991; 127: 1194–1197.

480 Weinstock MA. Death from skin cancer among the elderly. Epidemiological patterns. Arch Dermatol 1997; 133: 1207–1209.

481 Rigel DS, Friedman RJ, Kopf AW. Lifetime risk for development of skin cancer in the U.S. population: Current estimate is now 1 in 5. J Am Acad Dermatol 1996; 35: 1012–1013.

482 Wallace ML, Smoller BR. Immunohistochemistry in diagnostic dermatopathology. J Am Acad Dermatol 1996; 34: 163–183.

483 Casson P. Basal cell carcinoma. Clin Plast Surg 1980; 7: 301–311.

484 Scotto J, Kopf AW, Urbach F. Non-melanoma skin cancer among Caucasians in four areas of the United States. Cancer 1974; 34: 1333–1338.

485 Marks R, Jolley D, Dorevitch AP, Selwood TS. The incidence of non-melanocytic skin cancers in an Australian population: results of a five-year prospective study. Med J Aust 1989; 150: 475–478.

486 Yiannias JA, Goldberg LH, Carter-Campbell S et al. The ratio of basal cell carcinoma to squamous cell carcinoma in Houston, Texas. J Dermatol Surg Oncol 1988; 14: 886–889.

487 Cohn BA. Squamous cell carcinoma: Could it be the most common skin cancer? J Am Acad Dermatol 1998; 39: 134–135.

488 Brand D, Ackerman AB. Squamous cell carcinoma, not basal cell carcinoma, is the most common cancer in humans. J Am Acad Dermatol 2000; 42: 523–526.

489 Dahl E, Åberg M, Rausing A, Rausing E-L. Basal cell carcinoma. An epidemiologic study in a defined population. Cancer 1992; 70: 104–108.

490 Robinson JK. Risk of developing another basal cell carcinoma. A 5-year prospective study. Cancer 1987; 60: 118–120.

491 Hogan DJ, To T, Gran L et al. Risk factors for basal cell carcinoma. Int J Dermatol 1989; 28: 591–594.

492 Long CC, Marks R. Increased risk of skin cancer: another Celtic myth? J Am Acad Dermatol 1995; 33: 658–661.

493 Mora RG, Burris R. Cancer of the skin in blacks. A review of 128 patients with basal-cell carcinoma. Cancer 1981; 47: 1436–1438.

494 Abreo F, Sanusi ID. Basal cell carcinoma in North American blacks. Clinical and histopathologic study of 26 patients. J Am Acad Dermatol 1991; 25: 1005–1011.

495 Altman A, Rosen T, Tschen JA et al. Basal cell epithelioma in black patients. J Am Acad Dermatol 1987; 17: 741–745.

496 Bhat L, Goldberg LH, Rosen T. Basal cell carcinoma in a black woman with syringomas. J Am Acad Dermatol 1998; 39: 1033–1034.

497 Lober CW, Fenske NA. Basal cell, squamous cell, and sebaceous gland carcinomas of the periorbital region. J Am Acad Dermatol 1991; 25: 685–690.

498 Maafs E, De la Barreda F, Delgado R et al. Basal cell carcinoma of trunk and extremities. Int J Dermatol 1997; 36: 622–628.

499 Wong SW, Smith JG Jr, Thomas WO. Bilateral basal cell carcinoma of the breasts. J Am Acad Dermatol 1993; 28: 777.

500 Cain RJ, Sau P, Benson PM. Basal cell carcinoma of the nipple. Report of two cases. J Am Acad Dermatol 1990; 22: 207–210.

501 Betti R, Bruscagin C, Inselvini E, Crosti C. Basal cell carcinomas of covered and unusual sites of the body. Int J Dermatol 1997; 36: 503–505.

502 España A, Redondo P, Idoate MA et al. Perianal basal cell carcinoma. Clin Exp Dermatol 1992; 17: 360–362.

503 Kort R, Fazaa B, Bouden S et al. Perianal basal cell carcinoma. Int J Dermatol 1995; 34: 427–428.

504 Alvarez-Cañas MC, Fernández FA, Rodilla IG, Val-Bernal JF. Perianal basal cell carcinoma: a comparative histologic, immunohistochemical, and flow cytometric study with basaloid carcinoma of the anus. Am J Dermatopathol 1996; 18: 371–379.

505 Cruz-Jimenez PR, Abell MR. Cutaneous basal cell carcinoma of vulva. Cancer 1975; 36: 1860–1868.

506 Stiller M, Klein W, Dorman R, Albom M. Bilateral vulvar basal cell carcinomata. J Am Acad Dermatol 1993; 28: 836–838.

507 Greenbaum SS, Krull EA, Simmons EB Jr. Basal cell carcinoma at the base of the penis in a black patient. J Am Acad Dermatol 1989; 20: 317–319.

508 Goldminz D, Scott G, Klaus S. Penile basal cell carcinoma. Report of a case and review of the literature. J Am Acad Dermatol 1989; 20: 1094–1097.

509 Smith HR, Black MM. Basal cell carcinoma of the penis. Br J Dermatol 1999; 140: 361–362.

510 Rahbari H, Mehregan AH. Basal cell epitheliomas in usual and unusual sites. J Cutan Pathol 1979; 6: 425–431.

511 Nahass GT, Blauvelt A, Leonardi CL, Penneys NS. Basal cell carcinoma of the scrotum. Report of three cases and review of the literature. J Am Acad Dermatol 1992; 26: 574–578.

512 Esquivias Gómez JI, González-López A, Velasco E et al. Basal cell carcinoma of the scrotum. Australas J Dermatol 1999; 40: 141–143.

513 Robins P, Rabinovitz HS, Rigel D. Basal-cell carcinomas on covered or unusual sites of the body. J Dermatol Surg Oncol 1981; 7: 803–806.

514 Rudolph RI. Subungual basal cell carcinoma presenting as longitudinal melanonychia. J Am Acad Dermatol 1987; 16: 229–233.

515 Kim H-J, Kim Y-S, Suhr K-B et al. Basal cell carcinoma of the nail bed in a Korean woman. Int J Dermatol 2000; 39: 397–398.

516 Grine RC, Parlette HL III, Wilson BB. Nail unit basal cell carcinoma: A case report and literature review. J Am Acad Dermatol 1997; 37: 790–793.

517 Pearson G, King LE Jr, Boyd AS. Basal cell carcinoma of the lower extremities. Int J Dermatol 1999; 38: 852–854.

518 Piro GF, Collier DU. Basal cell carcinoma of the palm. J Am Acad Dermatol 1995; 33: 823–824.

519 Roth MJ, Stern JB, Haupt HM et al. Basal cell carcinoma of the sole. J Cutan Pathol 1995; 22: 349–353.

520 Alcalay J, Goldberg LH. Pedal basal cell carcinoma. Int J Dermatol 1991; 30: 727–729.

521 Pilipshen SJ, Gray G, Goldsmith E, Dineen P. Carcinoma arising in pilonidal sinuses. Ann Surg 1981; 193: 506–512.

522 Lutz ME, Davis MDP, Otley CC. Infiltrating basal cell carcinoma in the setting of a venous ulcer. Int J Dermatol 2000; 39: 519–520.

523 Dolan OM, Lowe L, Orringer MB et al. Basal cell carcinoma arising in a sternotomy scar: A report of three cases. J Am Acad Dermatol 1998; 38: 491–493.

524 Sagi E, Aram H, Peled IJ. Basal cell carcinoma developing in a nevus flammeus. Cutis 1984; 33: 311–318.

525 Feinmesser M, Taube E, Badani E, Kristt D. Basal cell carcinoma arising over arteriovenous malformations. Some speculations on the theme. Am J Dermatopathol 1997; 19: 575–579.

526 Keefe M, Wakeel RA, McBride DI. Basal cell carcinoma mimicking rhinophyma. Arch Dermatol 1988; 124: 1077–1079.

527 Silvis NG, Zachary CB. Occult basal-cell carcinoma within rhinophyma. Clin Exp Dermatol 1990; 15: 282–284.

528 Margolis MH. Superficial multicentric basal cell epithelioma arising in thermal burn scar. Arch Dermatol 1970; 102: 474–476.

529 Martin H, Strong E, Spiro RH. Radiation-induced skin cancer of the head and neck. Cancer 1970; 25: 61–71.

530 Frentz G. Grenz ray-induced nonmelanoma skin cancer. J Am Acad Dermatol 1989; 21: 475–478.

531 Beswick SJ, Garrido MC, Fryer AA et al. Multiple basal cell carcinomas and malignant melanoma following radiotherapy for ankylosing spondylitis. Clin Exp Dermatol 2000; 25: 381–383.

532 Hendricks WM. Basal cell carcinoma arising in a chickenpox scar. Arch Dermatol 1980; 116: 1304–1305.

533 Suster S, Ronnen M. Basal cell carcinoma arising in a leishmania scar. Int J Dermatol 1988; 27: 175–176.

534 Riley KA. Basal cell epithelioma in smallpox vaccination scar. Arch Dermatol 1970; 101: 416–417.

535 Nielsen T. Basal cell epithelioma in a BCG vaccination scar. Arch Dermatol 1979; 115: 678.

536 Goldstein GD, Whitaker DC, Argenyi ZB, Bardach J. Basal cell carcinoma arising in a sebaceous nevus during childhood. J Am Acad Dermatol 1988; 18: 429–430.

537 Piansay-Soriano EF, Pineda VB, Jimenez RI, Mungcal VC. Basal cell carcinoma and infundibuloma arising in separate sebaceous nevi during childhood. J Dermatol Surg Oncol 1989; 15: 1283–1286.

538 Horn MS, Sausker WF, Pierson DL. Basal cell epithelioma arising in a linear epidermal nevus. Arch Dermatol 1981; 117: 247.

539 Joshi A, Sah SP, Agarwalla A et al. Basal cell carcinoma arising in a localized linear verrucous epidermal naevus. Acta Derm Venereol 2000; 80: 227–228.

540 Hayes AG, Berry AD III. Basal cell carcinoma arising in a fibroepithelial polyp. J Am Acad Dermatol 1993; 28: 493–495.

541 Magaña-García M, Magaña-Lozana M. Multiple basal cell carcinomas arising in port-wine haemangiomas. Br J Dermatol 1988; 119: 393–396.

542 Duhra P, Foulds IS. Basal-cell carcinoma complicating a port-wine stain. Clin Exp Dermatol 1991; 16: 63–65.

543 Padilha-Goncalves A, Basilio de Oliveira CA. Basal cell carcinoma arising from solar lentigo. J Cutan Pathol 1989; 16: 319 (abstract).

544 Mehta VR, Potdar R. Bazex syndrome. Follicular atrophoderma and basal cell epitheliomas. Int J Dermatol 1985; 24: 444–446.

545 Plosila M, Kiistala R, Niemi K-M. The Bazex syndrome: follicular atrophoderma with multiple basal cell carcinomas, hypotrichosis and hypohidrosis. Clin Exp Dermatol 1981; 6: 31–41.

546 Vabres P, Lacombe D, Rabinowitz LG et al. The gene for Bazex–Dupré–Christol syndrome maps to chromosome Xq. J Invest Dermatol 1995; 105: 87–91.

547 Goeteyn M, Geerts M-L, Kint A, De Weert J. The Bazex–Dupré–Christol syndrome. Arch Dermatol 1994; 130: 337–342.

548 Marghoob A, Kopf AW, Bart RS et al. Risk of another basal cell carcinoma developing after treatment of a basal cell carcinoma. J Am Acad Dermatol 1993; 28: 22–28.

549 Marcil I, Stern RS. Risk of developing a subsequent nonmelanoma skin cancer in patients with a history of nonmelanoma skin cancer. A critical review of the literature and meta-analysis. Arch Dermatol 2000; 136: 1524–1530.

550 Lear JT, Smith AG, Strange RC, Fryer AA. Patients with truncal basal cell carcinoma represent a high-risk group. Arch Dermatol 1998; 134: 373.

551 Levi F, La Vecchia C, Te V-C et al. Incidence of invasive cancers following basal cell skin cancer. Am J Epidemiol 1998; 147: 722–726.

552 Bastiaens MT, Hoefnagel JJ, Bruijn JA et al. Differences in age, site distribution, and sex between nodular and superficial basal cell carcinomas indicate different types of tumors. J Invest Dermatol 1998; 110: 880–884.

553 Bower CPR, Lear JT, Bygrave S et al. Basal cell carcinoma and risk of subsequent malignancies: A cancer registry-based study in southwest England. J Am Acad Dermatol 2000; 42: 988–991.

554 Rahbari H, Mehregan AH. Basal cell epithelioma (carcinoma) in children and teenagers. Cancer 1982; 49: 350–353.

555 Orozco-Covarrubias ML, Tamayo-Sanchez L, Duran-McKinster C et al. Malignant cutaneous tumors in children. Twenty years of experience at a large pediatric hospital. J Am Acad Dermatol 1994; 30: 243–249.

556 Ledwig PA, Paller AS. Congenital basal cell carcinoma. Arch Dermatol 1991; 127: 1066–1067.

557 Cox NH. Basal cell carcinoma in young adults. Br J Dermatol 1992; 127: 26–29.

558 Schwartz RA, Hansen RC, Maize JC. The blue-gray cystic basal cell epithelioma. J Am Acad Dermatol 1980; 2: 155–160.

559 Bruce AJ, Brodland DG. Overview of skin cancer detection and prevention for the primary care physician. Mayo Clin Proc 2000; 75: 491–500.

560 Curry MC, Montgomery H, Winkelmann RK. Giant basal cell carcinoma. Arch Dermatol 1977; 113: 316–319.

561 Randle HW, Roenigk RK, Brodland DG. Giant basal cell carcinoma (T3). Cancer 1993; 72: 1624–1630.

562 Sahl WJ Jr, Snow SN, Levine NS. Giant basal cell carcinoma. Report of two cases and review of the literature. J Am Acad Dermatol 1994; 30: 856–859.

563 Jackson R, Adams RH. Horrifying basal cell carcinoma: a study of 33 cases and a comparison with 435 non-horror cases and a report on four metastatic cases. J Surg Oncol 1973; 5: 431–463.

564 Ko CB, Walton S, Keczkes K. Extensive and fatal basal cell carcinoma: a report of three cases. Br J Dermatol 1992; 127: 164–167.

565 Oliveira da Silva M, Dadalt P, da Rosa Santos OL et al. Linear basal cell carcinoma. Int J Dermatol 1995; 34: 488.

566 Megahed M. Polypoid basal cell carcinoma: a new clinicopathological variant. Br J Dermatol 1999; 140: 701–703.

567 Kikuchi A, Shimizu H, Nishikawa T. Clinical and histopathological characteristics of basal cell carcinoma in Japanese patients. Arch Dermatol 1996; 132: 320–324.

568 Shoji T, Lee J, Hong SH et al. Multiple pigmented basal cell carcinomas. Am J Dermatopathol 1998; 20: 199–202.

569 Fellner MJ, Katz JM. Pigmented basal cell cancer masquerading as superficial spreading malignant melanoma. Arch Dermatol 1977; 113: 946–947.

570 Johnson DB Jr, Ceilley RI. Basal cell carcinoma with annular leukoderma mimicking leukoderma acquisitum centrifugum. Arch Dermatol 1980; 116: 352–353.

571 Menzies SW, Westerhoff K, Rabinovitz H et al. Surface microscopy of pigmented basal cell carcinoma. Arch Dermatol 2000; 136: 1012–1016.

572 Presser SE, Taylor JR. Clinical diagnostic accuracy of basal cell carcinoma. J Am Acad Dermatol 1987; 16: 988–990.

573 Green A, Leslie D, Weedon D. Diagnosis of skin cancer in the general population: clinical accuracy in the Nambour survey. Med J Aust 1988; 148: 447–450.

574 Miller SJ. Biology of basal cell carcinoma (Part 1). J Am Acad Dermatol 1991; 24: 1–13.

575 Pollack SV, Goslen JB, Sherertz EF, Jegasothy BV. The biology of basal cell carcinoma: a review. J Am Acad Dermatol 1982; 7: 569–577.

576 Armstrong BK, Kricker A, English DR. Sun exposure and skin cancer. Australas J Dermatol 1997; 38 (Suppl): S1–S6.

577 Naldi L, DiLandro A, D'Avanzo B et al. Host-related and environmental risk factors for cutaneous basal cell carcinoma: Evidence from an Italian case-control study. J Am Acad Dermatol 2000; 42: 446–452.

578 Hajeer AH, Lear JT, Ollier WER et al. Preliminary evidence of an association of tumour necrosis factor microsatellites with increased risk of multiple basal cell carcinomas. Br J Dermatol 2000; 142: 441–445.

579 Slominski A, Heasley D, Mazurkiewicz JE et al. Expression of proopiomelanocortin (POMC)-derived melanocyte-stimulating hormone (MSH) and adrenocorticotropic hormone (ACTH) peptides in skin of basal cell carcinoma patients. Hum Pathol 1999; 30: 208–215.

580 Grimbaldeston MA, Skov L, Baadsgaard O et al. High dermal mast cell prevalence is a predisposing factor for basal cell carcinoma in humans. J Invest Dermatol 2000; 115: 317–320.

581 Gallagher RP, Hill GB, Bajdik CD et al. Sunlight exposure, pigmentary factors and risk of nonmelanocytic skin cancer. I. Basal cell carcinoma. Arch Dermatol 1995; 131: 157–163.

582 Stern RS. The mysteries of geographic variability in nonmelanoma skin cancer incidence. Arch Dermatol 1999; 135: 843–844.

583 Melia J, Pendry L, Eiser JR et al. Evaluation of primary prevention initiatives for skin cancer: a review from a U.K. perspective. Br J Dermatol 2000; 143: 701–708.

584 Barrett TL, Smith KJ, Hodge JJ et al. Immunohistochemical nuclear staining for p53, PCNA, and Ki-67 in different histologic variants of basal cell carcinoma. J Am Acad Dermatol 1997; 37: 430–437.

585 Wikonkal NM, Berg RJW, van Haselen CW et al. bcl-2 vs p53 protein expression and apoptotic rate in human nonmelanoma skin cancers. Arch Dermatol 1997; 133: 599–602.

586 van Dijk TJA, Mali WJH. Multiple basal cell carcinoma 58 years after X-ray therapy. Arch Dermatol 1979; 115: 1287.

587 Davis MM, Hanke CW, Zollinger TW et al. Skin cancer in patients with chronic radiation dermatitis. J Am Acad Dermatol 1989; 20: 608–616.

588 Lichter MD, Karagas MR, Mott LA et al. Therapeutic ionizing radiation and the incidence of basal cell carcinoma and squamous cell carcinoma. Arch Dermatol 2000; 136: 1007–1011.

589 Wagner SL, Maliner JS, Morton WE, Braman RS. Skin cancer and arsenical intoxication from well water. Arch Dermatol 1979; 115: 1205–1207.

590 Lamb PM, Menaker GM, Moy RL. Multiple basal cell carcinomas of the limb after adjuvant treatment of melanoma with isolated limb perfusion. J Am Acad Dermatol 1998; 38: 767–768.

591 Sass U, Theunis A, Noël JC, Song M. Multiple HPV-positive basal cell carcinoma (BCC) on the abdomen in a young pregnant woman. Am J Dermatopathol 2000; 22: 344 (abstract).

592 Currie CLA, Monk BE. Welding and non-melanoma skin cancer. Clin Exp Dermatol 2000; 25: 28–29.

593 Lanehart WH, Sanusi ID, Misra RP, O'Neal B. Metastasizing basal cell carcinoma originating in a stasis ulcer in a black woman. Arch Dermatol 1983; 119: 587–591.

594 Ryan JF. Basal cell carcinoma and chronic venous stasis. Histopathology 1989; 14: 657–659.

595 Black MM, Walkden VM. Basal cell carcinomatous changes on the lower leg: a possible association with chronic venous stasis. Histopathology 1983; 7: 219–227.

596 Lock-Andersen J, Drzewiecki KT, Wulf HC. Naevi as a risk factor for basal cell carcinoma in Caucasians: Danish case-control study. Acta Derm Venereol 1999; 79: 314–319.

597 Brown FS, Burnett JW, Robinson HM Jr. Cutaneous carcinoma following psoralen and long-wave ultraviolet radiation (PUVA) therapy for psoriasis. J Am Acad Dermatol 1980; 2: 393–395.

598 Cohen EB, Komorowski RA, Clowry LJ. Cutaneous complications in renal transplant recipients. Am J Clin Pathol 1987; 88: 32–37.

599 Blessing K, McLaren KM, Benton EC et al. Histopathology of skin lesions in renal allograft recipients – an assessment of viral features and dysplasia. Histopathology 1989; 14: 129–139.

600 Ferrándiz C, Fuente MJ, Ribera M et al. Epidermal dysplasia and neoplasia in kidney transplant recipients. J Am Acad Dermatol 1995; 33: 590–596.

601 Parnes R, Safai B, Myskowski PL. Basal cell carcinomas and lymphoma: biologic behavior and associated factors in sixty-three patients. J Am Acad Dermatol 1988; 19: 1017–1023.

602 Schön MP, Reifenberger J, Von Schmiedeberg S et al. Multiple basal cell carcinomas associated with hairy cell leukaemia. Br J Dermatol 1999; 140: 150–153.

603 Ramsay HM, Fryer A, Strange RC, Smith AG. Multiple basal cell carcinomas in a patient with acute myeloid leukaemia and chronic lymphocytic leukaemia. Clin Exp Dermatol 1999; 24: 281–282.

604 Cliff S, Mortimer PS. Skin cancer and non-Hodgkin's lymphoproliferative diseases: is sunlight to blame? Clin Exp Dermatol 1999; 24: 40–41.

605 Myskowski PL, Safai B. The immunology of basal cell carcinoma. Int J Dermatol 1988; 27: 601–607.

606 Sitz KV, Keppen M, Johnson DF. Metastatic basal cell carcinoma in acquired immunodeficiency syndrome-related complex. JAMA 1987; 257: 340–343.

607 Hruza GJ, Snow SN. Basal cell carcinoma in a patient with acquired immunodeficiency syndrome: treatment with Mohs micrographic surgery fixed-tissue technique. J Dermatol Surg Oncol 1989; 15: 545–551.

608 Wang C-Y, Brodland DG, Su WPD. Skin cancers associated with acquired immunodeficiency syndrome. Mayo Clin Proc 1995; 70: 766–772.

609 Itayemi SO, Abioye AA, Ogan O et al. Aggressive basal cell carcinoma in Nigerians. Br J Dermatol 1979; 101: 465–468.

610 Best PJM, Petitt RM. Multiple skin cancers associated with hydroxyurea therapy. Mayo Clin Proc 1998; 73: 961–963.

611 Shen T, Park W-S, Böni R et al. Detection of loss of heterozygosity on chromosome 9q22.3 in microdissected sporadic basal cell carcinoma. Hum Pathol 1999; 30: 284–287.

612 Nagano T, Bito T, Kallassy M et al. Overexpression of the human homologue of *Drosophila patched* (PTCH) in skin tumours: specificity for basal cell carcinoma. Br J Dermatol 1999; 140: 287–290.

613 Saridaki Z, Koumantaki E, Liloglou T et al. High frequency of loss of heterozygosity on chromosome region 9p21–p22 but lack of p16^{INK4a}/p19^{ARF} mutations in Greek patients with basal cell carcinoma of the skin. J Invest Dermatol 2000; 115: 719–725.

614 Ratner D, Peacocke M, Zhang H et al. UV-specific p53 and PTCH mutations in sporadic basal cell carcinoma of sun-exposed skin. J Am Acad Dermatol 2001; 44: 293–297.

615 Bouwes Bavinck JN, Bastiaens MT, Marugg ME et al. Further evidence for an association of HLA-DR7 with basal cell carcinoma on the tropical island of Saba. Arch Dermatol 2000; 136: 1019–1022.

616 Long CC, Darke C, Marks R. Celtic ancestry, HLA phenotype and increased risk of skin cancer. Br J Dermatol 1998; 138: 627–630.

617 Green J, Leigh IM, Poulsom R, Quinn AG. Basal cell carcinoma development is associated with induction of the expression of the transcription factor Gli-1. Br J Dermatol 1998; 139: 911–915.

618 Ghali L, Wong ST, Green J et al. Gli 1 protein is expressed in basal cell carcinomas, outer root sheath keratinocytes and a subpopulation of mesenchymal cells in normal human skin. J Invest Dermatol 1999; 113: 595–599.

619 Cho S, Hahm J-H, Hong Y-S. Analysis of p53 and BAX mutations, loss of heterozygosity, p53 and BCL2 expression and apoptosis in basal cell carcinoma in Korean patients. Br J Dermatol 2001; 144: 841–848.

620 Miller SJ. Biology of basal cell carcinoma (Part II). J Am Acad Dermatol 1991; 24: 161–175.

621 Kore-eda S, Horiguchi Y, Ueda M et al. Basal cell carcinoma cells resemble follicular matrix cells rather than follicular bulge cells: immunohistochemical and ultrastructural comparative studies. Am J Dermatopathol 1998; 20: 362–369.

622 Schirren CG, Rütten A, Kaudewitz P et al. Trichoblastoma and basal cell carcinoma are neoplasms with follicular differentiation sharing the same profile of cytokeratin intermediate filaments. Am J Dermatopathol 1997; 19: 341–350.

623 Bowman P, Abdelsayed R, Sangueza O. Immunohistochemical evaluation of morpheaform and infundibulocystic variants of basal cell carcinoma, desmoplastic trichoepithelioma, trichoblastoma, and basaloid follicular hamartoma using Bcl-2, Ki67 and PCNA. J Cutan Pathol 2000; 27: 544 (abstract).

624 Lespi PJ, Gregorini SD. Folliculotropic T cells in regressive basal cell carcinoma of skin. Am J Dermatopathol 2000; 22: 30–33.

625 Zackheim HS. The origin of experimental basal cell epitheliomas in the rat. J Invest Dermatol 1962; 38: 57–64.

626 Hales SA, Stamp G, Evans M, Fleming KA. Identification of the origin of cells in human basal cell carcinoma xenografts in mice using *in situ* hybridization. Br J Dermatol 1989; 120: 351–357.

627 Grando SA, Schofield OMV, Skubitz APN et al. Nodular basal cell carcinoma in vivo vs in vitro. Arch Dermatol 1996; 132: 1185–1193.

628 Fleischer AB Jr, Feldman SR, Barlow JO et al. The specialty of the treating physician affects the likelihood of tumor-free resection margins for basal cell carcinoma: Results from a multi-institutional retrospective study. J Am Acad Dermatol 2001; 44: 224–230.

629 Lawrence CM. Mohs' micrographic surgery for basal cell carcinoma. Clin Exp Dermatol 1999; 24: 130–133.

630 Nordin P. Curettage-cryosurgery for non-melanoma skin cancer of the external ear: excellent 5-year results. Br J Dermatol 1999; 140: 291–293.

631 Eedy DJ. Non-melanoma skin cancer and the 'new National Health Service': implications for U.K. Dermatology? Br J Dermatol 2000; 142: 397–399.

632 Chiller K, Passaro D, McCalmont T, Vin-Christian K. Efficacy of curettage before excision in clearing surgical margins of nonmelanoma skin cancer. J Am Acad Dermatol 2000; 136: 1327–1332.

633 Thissen MRTM, Neumann MHA, Schouten LJ. A systematic review of treatment modalities for primary basal cell carcinomas. Arch Dermatol 1999; 135: 1177–1183.

634 Gordon PM, Cox NH, Paterson WD, Lawrence CM. Basal cell carcinoma: are early appointments justifiable? Br J Dermatol 2000; 142: 446–448.

635 Kirkup ME, De Berker DAR. Clinical measurement of dimensions of basal cell carcinoma: effect of waiting for elective surgery. Br J Dermatol 1999; 141: 876–879.

636 Telfer NR, Colver GB, Bowers PW. Guidelines for the management of basal cell carcinoma. Br J Dermatol 1999; 141: 415–423.

637 Kuflik EG, Gage AA. Recurrent basal cell carcinoma treated with cryosurgery. J Am Acad Dermatol 1997; 37: 82–84.

638 Lindgren G, Larkö O. Long-term follow-up of cryosurgery of the eyelid. J Am Acad Dermatol 1997; 36: 742–746.

639 Fink-Puches R, Soyer HP, Hofer A et al. Long-term follow-up and histological changes of superficial nonmelanoma skin cancers treated with topical δ-aminolevulinic acid photodynamic therapy. Arch Dermatol 1998; 134: 821–826.

640 McGibbon DH. Malignant epidermal tumours. J Cutan Pathol 1985; 12: 224–238.

641 Pritchard BN, Youngberg GA. Atypical mitotic figures in basal cell carcinoma. A review of 208 cases. Am J Dermatopathol 1993; 15: 549–552.

642 Kerr JFR, Searle J. A suggested explanation for the paradoxically slow growth rate of basal cell carcinomas that contain numerous mitotic figures. J Pathol 1972; 107: 41–44.

643 Mehregan AH. Aggressive basal cell epithelioma on sunlight-protected skin. Report of eight cases, one with pulmonary and bone metastases. Am J Dermatopathol 1983; 5: 221–229.

644 Robinson JK, Pollack SV, Robins P. Invasion of cartilage by basal cell carcinoma. J Am Acad Dermatol 1980; 2: 499–505.

645 Mark GJ. Basal cell carcinoma with intraneural invasion. Cancer 1977; 40: 2181–2187.

646 Ratner D, Lowe L, Johnson TM, Fader DJ. Perineural spread of basal cell carcinomas treated with Mohs micrographic surgery. Cancer 2000; 88: 1605–1613.

647 Brown CI, Perry AE. Incidence of perineural invasion in histologically aggressive types of basal cell carcinoma. Am J Dermatopathol 2000; 22: 123–125.

648 Van Cawenberge D, Pierard GE, Foidart JM, Lapiere CM. Immunohistochemical localization of laminin, type IV and type V collagen in basal cell carcinoma. Br J Dermatol 1983; 108: 163–170.

649 Jones JCR, Steinman HK, Goldsmith BA. Hemidesmosomes, collagen VII, and intermediate filaments in basal cell carcinoma. J Invest Dermatol 1989; 93: 662–671.

650 Chopra A, Maitra B, Korman NJ. Decreased mRNA expression of several basement membrane components in basal cell carcinoma. J Invest Dermatol 1998; 110: 52–56.

651 DeRosa G, Barra E, Guarino M et al. Fibronectin, laminin, type IV collagen distribution, and myofibroblastic stromal reaction in aggressive and nonaggressive basal cell carcinoma. Am J Dermatopathol 1994; 16: 258–267.

652 De Rosa G, Staibano S, Barra E et al. p53 protein in aggressive and non-aggressive basal cell carcinoma. J Cutan Pathol 1993; 20: 429–434.

653 Looi LM. Localized amyloidosis in basal cell carcinoma. A pathologic study. Cancer 1983; 52: 1833–1836.

654 Weedon D, Shand E. Amyloid in basal cell carcinoma. Br J Dermatol 1979; 101: 141–146.

655 Satti MB, Azzopardi JG. Amyloid deposits in basal cell carcinoma of the skin. A pathologic study of 199 cases. J Am Acad Dermatol 1990; 22: 1082–1087.

656 Zaynoun S, Ali LA, Shaib J, Kurban A. The relationship of sun exposure and solar elastosis to basal cell carcinoma. J Am Acad Dermatol 1985; 12: 522–525.

657 Lambert WC, Schwartz RA. Evidence for origin of basal cell carcinomas in solar (actinic) keratoses. J Cutan Pathol 1988; 15: 322 (abstract).

658 Habets JMW, Tank B, Vuzevski VD et al. Characterization of the mononuclear cell infiltrate in basal cell carcinoma: a predominantly T cell-mediated immune response with minor participation of Leu-7+ (natural killer) cells and Leu-14+(B) cells. J Invest Dermatol 1988; 90: 289–292.

659 Hunt MJ, Halliday GM, Weedon D et al. Regression of basal cell carcinoma: an immunohistochemical analysis. Br J Dermatol 1994; 130: 1–8.

660 Wong DA, Bishop GA, Lowes MA et al. Cytokine profiles in spontaneously regressing basal cell carcinomas. Br J Dermatol 2000; 143: 91–98.

661 Murphy GF, Krusinski PA, Myzak LA, Ershler WB. Local immune response in basal cell carcinoma: characterization by transmission electron microscopy and monoclonal anti-T6 antibody. J Am Acad Dermatol 1983; 8: 477–485.

662 Azizi E, Bucana C, Goldberg L, Kripke ML. Perturbation of epidermal Langerhans cells in basal cell carcinomas. Am J Dermatopathol 1987; 9: 465–473.

663 Deng JS, Brod BA, Saito R, Tharp MD. Immune-associated cells in basal cell carcinomas of skin. J Cutan Pathol 1996; 23: 140–146.

664 Curson C, Weedon D. Spontaneous regression in basal cell carcinoma. J Cutan Pathol 1979; 6: 432–437.

665 Deng J-S, Falo LD Jr, Kim B, Abell E. Cytotoxic T cells in basal cell carcinomas of skin. Am J Dermatopathol 1998; 20: 143–146.

666 Buselmeier TJ, Uecker JH. Invasive basal cell carcinoma with metaplastic bone formation associated with a long-standing dermatofibroma. J Cutan Pathol 1979; 6: 496–500.

667 Tomsick RS, Menn H. Ossifying basal cell epithelioma. Int J Dermatol 1982; 21: 218–219.

668 Shoji T, Burlage AM, Bhawan J. Basal cell carcinoma with massive ossification. Am J Dermatopathol 1999; 21: 34–36.

669 Boyd AS, King LE Jr. Basal cell carcinoma with ossification. J Am Acad Dermatol 1998; 38: 906–910.

670 Goette DK. Transepithelial elimination of benign and malignant tumors. J Dermatol Surg Oncol 1987; 13: 68–73.

671 Poyzer KG, de Launey WE. Pseudorecidivism of irradiated basal cell carcinoma. Australas J Dermatol 1974; 15: 77–83.

672 Frank SB, Cohen HJ, Minkin W. Pseudorecidive following excision of a basal cell epithelioma. Arch Dermatol 1970; 101: 578–579.

673 Goette DK, Helwig EB. Basal cell carcinomas and basal cell carcinoma-like changes overlying dermatofibromas. Arch Dermatol 1975; 111: 589–592.

674 Crowson AN, Magro CM. Basal cell carcinoma arising in association with desmoplastic trichilemmoma. Am J Dermatopathol 1996; 18: 43–48.

675 Coskey RJ, Mehregan AH. The association of basal cell carcinomas with other tumors. J Dermatol Surg Oncol 1987; 13: 553–555.

676 Haupt HM, Stern JB, Dilaimy MS. Basal cell carcinoma. Clues to its presence in histologic sections when the initial slide is nondiagnostic. Am J Surg Pathol 2000; 24: 1291–1294.

677 Kariniemi A-L, Holthofer H, Vartio T, Virtanen I. Cellular differentiation of basal cell carcinoma studied with fluorescent lectins and cytokeratin antibodies. J Cutan Pathol 1984; 11: 541–548.

678 Markey AC, Lane EB, MacDonald DM, Leigh IM. Keratin expression in basal cell carcinomas. Br J Dermatol 1992; 126: 154–160.

679 Morales-Ducret CRJ, van de Rijn M, LeBrun DP, Smoller BR. bcl-2 expression in primary malignancies of the skin. Arch Dermatol 1995; 131: 909–912.

680 Nakagawa K, Yamamura K, Maeda S, Ichihashi M. bcl-2 expression in epidermal keratinocytic diseases. Cancer 1994; 74: 1720–1724.

681 Verhaegh MEJM, Sanders CJG, Arends JW, Neumann HAM. Expression of the apoptosis-suppressing protein Bcl-2 in non-melanoma skin cancer. Br J Dermatol 1995; 132: 740–744.

682 Cerroni L, Kerl H. Aberrant bcl-2 protein expression provides a possible mechanism of neoplastic cell growth in cutaneous basal cell carcinoma. J Cutan Pathol 1994; 21: 398–403.

683 Mills AE. Solar keratosis can be distinguished from superficial basal cell carcinoma by expression of bcl-2. Am J Dermatopathol 1997; 19: 443–445.

684 Nakagawa K, Yamamura K, Maeda S, Ichihashi M. bcl-2 expression in epidermal keratinocytic diseases. Cancer 1994; 74: 1720–1724.

685 Ramdial PK, Madaree A, Reddy R, Chetty R. bcl-2 protein expression in aggressive and non-aggressive basal cell carcinomas. J Cutan Pathol 2000; 27: 283–291.

686 Shimizu N, Ito M, Tazawa T, Sato Y. Immunohistochemical study on keratin expression in certain cutaneous epithelial neoplasms. Basal cell carcinoma, pilomatricoma, and seborrheic keratosis. Am J Dermatopathol 1989; 11: 534–540.

687 Oseroff AR, Roth R, Lipman S, Morhenn VB. Use of a murine monoclonal antibody which binds to malignant keratinocytes to detect tumor cells in microscopically controlled surgery. J Am Acad Dermatol 1983; 8: 616–619.

688 Said JW, Sassoon AF, Shintaku IP, Banks-Schlegel S. Involucrin in squamous and basal cell carcinomas of the skin: an immunohistochemical study. J Invest Dermatol 1984; 82: 449–452.

689 Prieto VG, Reed JA, McNutt S et al. Differential expression of CD44 in malignant cutaneous epithelial neoplasms. Am J Dermatopathol 1995; 17: 447–451.

690 Hale LP, Patel DD, Clark RE, Haynes BF. Distribution of CD44 variant isoforms in human skin: differential expression in components of benign and malignant epithelia. J Cutan Pathol 1995; 22: 536–545.

691 Kooy AJW, Tank B, de Jong AAW et al. Expression of E-cadherin, α- and β-catenin, and CD44V$_6$ and the subcellular localization of E-cadherin and CD44V$_6$ in normal epidermis and basal cell carcinoma. Hum Pathol 1999; 30: 1328–1335.

692 Ichikawa T, Masumoto J, Kaneko M et al. Expression of moesin and its associated molecule CD44 in epithelial skin tumors. J Cutan Pathol 1998; 25: 237–243.

693 Dingemans KP, Ramkema MD, Koopman G et al. The expression of CD44 glycoprotein adhesion molecules in basal cell carcinomas is related to growth pattern and invasiveness. Br J Dermatol 1999; 140: 17–25.

694 Tellechea O, Reis JP, Domingues JC, Baptista AP. Monoclonal antibody Ber EP4 distinguishes basal-cell carcinoma from squamous-cell carcinoma of the skin. Am J Dermatopathol 1993; 15: 452–455.

695 Swanson PE, Fitzpatrick MM, Ritter JH et al. Immunohistologic differential diagnosis of basal cell carcinoma, squamous cell carcinoma, and trichoepithelioma in small cutaneous biopsy specimens. J Cutan Pathol 1998; 25: 153–159.

696 Beer TW, Shepherd P, Theaker JM. Ber EP4 and epithelial membrane antigen aid distinction of basal cell, squamous cell and basosquamous carcinomas of the skin. Histopathology 2000; 37: 218–223.

697 Vigneswaran N, Haneke E, Peters KP. Peanut agglutinin immunohistochemistry of basal cell carcinoma. J Cutan Pathol 1987; 14: 147–153.

698 Haneke E. Differentiation of basal cell carcinoma from trichoepithelioma by lectin histochemistry. Br J Dermatol 1995; 132: 1024–1025.

699 Smoller BR, van de Rijn M, Lebrun D, Warnke RA. bcl-2 expression reliably distinguishes trichoepitheliomas from basal cell carcinomas. Br J Dermatol 1994; 131: 28–31.

700 Crowson AN, Magro CM, Kadin ME, Stranc M. Differential expression of the bcl-2 oncogene in human basal cell carcinoma. Hum Pathol 1996; 27: 355–359.

701 Thewes M, Worret WI, Engst R, Ring J. Stromelysin-3. A potent marker for histopathologic differentiation between desmoplastic trichoepithelioma and morphealike basal cell carcinoma. Am J Dermatopathol 1998; 20: 140–142.

702 Thewes M, Worret WI, Engst R, Ring J. Stromelysin-3 (ST-3): immunohistochemical characterization of the matrix metalloproteinase (MMP)-11 in benign and malignant skin tumours and other skin disorders. Clin Exp Dermatol 1999; 24: 122–126.

703 Poniecka AW, Alexis JB. An immunohistochemical study of basal cell carcinoma and trichoepithelioma. Am J Dermatopathol 1999; 21: 332–336.

704 Strutton GM. Pathological variants of basal cell carcinoma. Australas J Dermatol 1997; 38 (Suppl): S31–S35.

705 Sexton M, Jones DB, Maloney ME. Histologic pattern analysis of basal cell carcinoma. Study of a series of 1039 consecutive neoplasms. J Am Acad Dermatol 1990; 23: 1118–1126.

706 Russell EB, Carrington PR, Smoller BR. Basal cell carcinoma: A comparison of shave biopsy versus punch biopsy techniques in subtype diagnosis. J Am Acad Dermatol 1999; 41: 69–71.

707 Hendrix JD Jr, Parlette HL. Micronodular basal cell carcinoma. Arch Dermatol 1996; 132: 295–298.

708 Lang PG Jr, McKelvey AC, Nicholson JH. Three-dimensional reconstruction of the superficial multicentric basal cell carcinoma using serial sections and a computer. Am J Dermatopathol 1987; 9: 198–203.

709 Mehregan AH. Acantholysis in basal cell epithelioma. J Cutan Pathol 1979; 6: 280–283.

710 LeBoit PE. Stroma, interrupted. Am J Dermatopathol 2001; 23: 67–68.

711 McCormack CJ, Kelly JW, Dorevitch AP. Differences in age and body site distribution of the histological subtypes of basal cell carcinoma. A possible indicator of differing causes. Arch Dermatol 1997; 133: 593–596.

712 Maloney ME, Jones DB, Sexton FM. Pigmented basal cell carcinoma: investigation of 70 cases. J Am Acad Dermatol 1992; 27: 74–78.

713 Bleehen SS. Pigmented basal cell epithelioma. Br J Dermatol 1975; 93: 361–370.

714 Lao L-M, Kumakiri M, Kiyohara T et al. Sub-populations of melanocytes in pigmented basal cell carcinoma: a quantitative, ultrastructural investigation. J Cutan Pathol 2001; 28: 34–43.

715 Florell SR, Zone JJ, Gerwels JW. Basal cell carcinomas are populated by melanocytes and Langerhan's cells. Am J Dermatopathol 2001; 23: 24–28.

716 Burkhalter A, White WL. Malignant melanoma in situ colonizing basal cell carcinoma. A simulator of invasive melanoma. Am J Dermatopathol 1997; 19: 303–307.

717 Cowley GP, Gallimore A. Malignant melanoma metastasising to a basal cell carcinoma. Histopathology 1996; 29: 469–470.

718 Barbosa AdeA Jr, Guimaraes NS, de Lourdes Lopes M et al. Malignant melanoma and basal cell carcinoma in a combined tumour. Br J Dermatol 1999; 140: 360–361.

719 Siegle RJ, MacMillan J, Pollack SV. Infiltrative basal cell carcinoma: a nonsclerosing subtype. J Dermatol Surg Oncol 1986; 12: 830–836.

720 Wrone DA, Swetter SM, Egbert BM et al. Increased proportion of aggressive-growth basal cell carcinoma in the Veterans Affairs population of Palo Alto, California. J Am Acad Dermatol 1996; 35: 907–910.

721 Swetter SM, Yaghmai D, Egbert BM. Infiltrative basal cell carcinoma occurring in sites of biopsy-proven nodular basal cell carcinoma. J Cutan Pathol 1998; 25: 420–425.

722 Rossen K, Haerslev T, Hou-Jensen K, Krag Jacobsen G. Metallothionein expression in basaloid proliferations overlying dermatofibromas and in basal cell carcinomas. Br J Dermatol 1997; 136: 30–34.

723 Salasche SJ, Amonette RA. Morpheaform basal-cell epitheliomas. A study of subclinical extensions in a series of 51 cases. J Dermatol Surg Oncol 1981; 7: 387–394.

724 Richman T, Penneys NS. Analysis of morpheaform basal cell carcinoma. J Cutan Pathol 1988; 15: 359–362.

725 Requena L, Martin L, Farina MC. Keloidal basal cell carcinoma. A new clinicopathological variant of basal cell carcinoma. Br J Dermatol 1996; 134: 953–957.

726 Murphy B, Camacho A, Lewis J, Cockerell C. Keloidal basal cell carcinoma: an underreported variant? J Cutan Pathol 2000; 27: 566 (abstract).

727 Moy RL, Moy LS, Matsuoka LY et al. Selectively enhanced procollagen gene expression in sclerosing (morphea-like) basal cell carcinoma as reflected by elevated proα1 (I) and proα1 (III) procollagen messenger RNA steady-state levels. J Invest Dermatol 1988; 90: 634–638.

728 Barsky SH, Grossman DA, Bhuta S. Desmoplastic basal cell carcinomas possess unique basement membrane-degrading properties. J Invest Dermatol 1987; 88: 324–329.

729 Ackerman AB. Basal cell carcinoma with follicular differentiation. Reply. Am J Dermatopathol 1988; 10: 458–466.

730 Lopes de Faria J. Basal cell carcinoma of the skin with areas of squamous cell carcinoma: a basosquamous cell carcinoma? J Clin Pathol 1985; 38: 1273–1277.

731 Tozawa T, Ackerman AB. Basal cell carcinoma with follicular differentiation. Am J Dermatopathol 1987; 9: 474–482.

732 Rosai J. Basal cell carcinoma with follicular differentiation. Am J Dermatopathol 1988; 10: 457–458.

733 Ackerman AB. Basal cell carcinoma with follicular differentiation. Reply. Am J Dermatopathol 1989; 11: 481–497.

734 Kato N, Ueno H. Infundibulocystic basal cell carcinoma. Am J Dermatopathol 1993; 15: 265–267.

735 de Eusebio E, Sánchez Yus E, López Bran E et al. Infundibulocystic basaloid neoplasm. J Cutan Pathol 1996; 23: 147–150.

736 Kagen MH, Hirsch RJ, Chu P et al. Multiple infundibulocystic basal cell carcinomas in association with human immunodeficiency virus. J Cutan Pathol 2000; 27: 316–318.

737 Kazantseva IA, Khlebnikova AN, Babaev VR. Immunohistochemical study of primary and recurrent basal cell and metatypical carcinomas of the skin. Am J Dermatopathol 1996; 18: 35–42.

738 Farmer ER, Helwig EB. Metastatic basal cell carcinoma: a clinicopathologic study of seventeen cases. Cancer 1980; 46: 748–757.

739 Borel DM. Cutaneous basosquamous carcinoma. Arch Pathol 1973; 95: 293–297.

740 Pena YM, Bason MM, Grant-Kels JM. Basosquamous cell carcinoma with leptomeningeal carcinomatosis. Arch Dermatol 1990; 126: 195–198.

741 Lopes de Faria J, Nunes PHF. Basosquamous cell carcinoma of the skin with metastases. Histopathology 1988; 12: 85–94.

742 Martin RCG II, Edwards MJ, Cawte TG et al. Basosquamous carcinoma. Analysis of prognostic factors influencing recurrence. Cancer 2000; 88: 1365–1369.

743 Pinkus H. Premalignant fibroepithelial tumors of skin. Arch Dermatol 1953; 67: 598–615.

744 Betti R, Inselvini E, Carducci M, Crosti C. Age and site prevalence of histologic subtypes of basal cell carcinoma. Int J Dermatol 1995; 34: 174–176.

745 Gellin GA, Bender B. Giant premalignant fibroepithelioma. Arch Dermatol 1966; 94: 70–73.

746 Hartschuh W, Schulz T. Merkel cell hyperplasia in chronic radiation-damaged skin: its possible relationship to fibroepithelioma of Pinkus. J Cutan Pathol 1997; 24: 477–483.

747 Stern JB, Haupt HM, Smith RRL. Fibroepithelioma of Pinkus. Eccrine duct spread of basal cell carcinoma. Am J Dermatopathol 1994; 16: 585–587.

748 Sina B, Kauffman CL. Fibroepithelioma of Pinkus: eccrine duct spread of basal cell carcinoma. Am J Dermatopathol 1995; 17: 634–635.

749 Jones CC, Ansari SJ, Tschen JA. Cystic fibroepithelioma of Pinkus. J Cutan Pathol 1991; 18: 220–222.

750 Aloi FG, Molinero A, Pippione M. Basal cell carcinoma with matrical differentiation. Matrical carcinoma. Am J Dermatopathol 1988; 10: 509–513.

751 Ambrojo P, Aguilar A, Simón P et al. Basal cell carcinoma with matrical differentiation. Am J Dermatopathol 1992; 14: 293–297.

752 Misago N, Ackerman AB. Trichoblastic (basal-cell) carcinoma with tricholemmal (at the bulb) differentiation. Dermatopathology: Practical & Conceptual 1999; 5: 200–204.

753 Sakamoto F, Ito M, Sato S, Sato Y. Basal cell tumor with apocrine differentiation: apocrine epithelioma. J Am Acad Dermatol 1985; 13: 355–363.

754 Sanchez NP, Winkelmann RK. Basal cell tumor with eccrine differentiation (eccrine epithelioma). J Am Acad Dermatol 1982; 6: 514–518.

755 Heenan PJ, Bogle MS. Eccrine differentiation in basal cell carcinoma. J Invest Dermatol 1993; 100: 295S–299S.

756 Barr RJ, Graham JH. Granular basal cell carcinoma. Arch Dermatol 1979; 115: 1064–1067.

757 Mrak RE, Baker GF. Granular basal cell carcinoma. J Cutan Pathol 1987; 14: 37–42.

758 Oliver GF, Winkelmann RK. Clear-cell basal cell carcinoma: histopathological, histochemical, and electron microscopic findings. J Cutan Pathol 1988; 15: 404–408.

759 Barnadas MA, Freeman RG. Clear cell basal cell epithelioma: light and electron microscopic study of an unusual variant. J Cutan Pathol 1988; 15: 1–7.

760 Starink TM, Blomjous CEM, Stoof TJ, van der Linden JC. Clear cell basal cell carcinoma. Histopathology 1990; 17: 401–405.

761 Barr RJ, Alpern KS, Santa Cruz DJ, Fretzin DF. Clear cell basal cell carcinoma: an unusual degenerative variant. J Cutan Pathol 1993; 20: 308–316.

762 Suster S. Clear cell tumors of the skin. Semin Diagn Pathol 1996; 13: 40–59.

763 Cohen RE, Zaim MT. Signet-ring clear-cell basal cell carcinoma. J Cutan Pathol 1988; 15: 183–187.

764 Sahin AA, Ro JY, Grignon DJ, Ordonez NG. Basal cell carcinoma with hyaline inclusions. Arch Pathol Lab Med 1989; 113: 1015–1018.

765 Seo IS, Warner TFCS, Priest JB. Basal cell carcinoma – signet ring type. J Cutan Pathol 1979; 6: 101–107.

766 James CL. Basal cell carcinoma with hyaline inclusions. Pathology 1995; 27: 97–100.

767 White GM, Barr RJ, Liao S-Y. Signet ring basal cell carcinoma. Am J Dermatopathol 1991; 13: 288–292.

768 Ochiai T, Suzuki H, Morioka S. Basal cell epithelioma with giant tumor cells: light and electron microscopic study. J Cutan Pathol 1987; 14: 242–247.

769 Elston DM, Bergfeld WF, Petroff N. Basal cell carcinoma with monster cells. J Cutan Pathol 1993; 20: 70–73.

770 Garcia JA, Cohen PR, Herzberg AJ et al. Pleomorphic basal cell carcinoma. J Am Acad Dermatol 1995; 32: 740–746.

771 Cutlan RT, Maluf HM. Immunohistochemical characterization of pleomorphic giant cells in basal cell carcinoma. J Cutan Pathol 1999; 26: 353–356.

772 Meehan SA, Egbert BM, Rouse RV. Basal cell carcinoma with tumor epithelial and stromal giant cells. Am J Dermatopathol 1999; 21: 473–478.

773 Lerchin E, Rahbari H. Adamantinoid basal cell epithelioma. Arch Dermatol 1975; 111: 586–588.

774 Kadono T, Okada H, Okuno T, Ohara K. Basal cell carcinoma with neuroid type nuclear palisading: a report of three cases. Br J Dermatol 1998; 138: 1064–1066.

775 San Juan J, Monteagudo C, Navarro P, Terrádez JJ. Basal cell carcinoma with prominent central palisading of epithelial cells mimicking schwannoma. J Cutan Pathol 1999; 26: 528–532.

776 Visser R, Bosman FT. Neuroendocrine differentiation in basal cell carcinomas: a retrospective immunohistochemical and ultrastructural study. J Cutan Pathol 1985; 12: 117–124.

777 Dardi LE, Memoli VA, Gould VE. Neuroendocrine differentiation in basal cell carcinomas. J Cutan Pathol 1981; 8: 335–341.

778 George E, Swanson PE, Wick MR. Neuroendocrine differentiation in basal cell carcinoma. An immunohistochemical study. Am J Dermatopathol 1989; 11: 131–135.

779 Tawfik O, Casparian JM, Garrigues N et al. Neuroendocrine differentiation of a metastatic basal cell carcinoma in a patient with basal cell nevus syndrome. J Cutan Pathol 1999; 26: 306–310.

780 El-Shabrawi L, LeBoit PE. Basal cell carcinoma with thickened basement membrane. Am J Dermatopathol 1997; 19: 568–574.

781 Khan ZM. Basal cell carcinoma with thickened basement membrane. Am J Dermatopathol 1999; 21: 111.

782 Suster S, Ramon y Cajal S. Myoepithelial differentiation in basal cell carcinoma. Am J Dermatopathol 1991; 13: 350–357.

783 Cutler B, Posalaky Z, Katz HI. Cell processes in basal cell carcinoma. J Cutan Pathol 1980; 7: 310–314.

784 Kumakiri M, Hashimoto K. Ultrastructural resemblance of basal cell epithelioma to primary epithelial germ. J Cutan Pathol 1978; 5: 53–67.

785 Nagao S, Nemoto H, Suzuki M et al. Myofibroblasts in basal cell epithelioma: with special reference to the phagocytic function of myofibroblasts. J Cutan Pathol 1986; 13: 261–267.

786 Youngberg GA, Laucirica R, Leicht SS. Frequency of occurrence of diagnostic cytologic parameters in basal cell carcinoma. Am J Clin Pathol 1989; 91: 24–30.

787 Vega-Memije E, Martinez-de Larios N, Waxtein LM, Dominguez-Soto L. Cytodiagnosis of cutaneous basal and squamous cell carcinoma. Int J Dermatol 2000; 39: 116–120.

788 Rigel DS, Robins P, Friedman RJ. Predicting recurrence of basal-cell carcinomas treated by microscopically controlled excision. J Dermatol Surg Oncol 1981; 7: 807–810.

789 Silverman MK, Kopf AW, Grin CM et al. Recurrence rates of treated basal cell carcinomas. Part 1: overview. J Dermatol Surg Oncol 1991; 17: 713–718.

790 Silverman MK, Kopf AW, Grin CM et al. Recurrence rates of treated basal cell carcinomas. Part 2: Curettage-electrodesiccation. J Dermatol Surg Oncol 1991; 17: 720–726.

791 Rowe DE, Carroll RJ, Day CL Jr. Long-term recurrence rates in previously untreated (primary) basal cell carcinoma: implications for patient follow-up. J Dermatol Surg Oncol 1989; 15: 315–328.

792 Hauben DJ, Zirkin H, Mahler D, Sacks M. The biologic behavior of basal cell carcinoma: analysis of recurrence in excised basal cell carcinoma: Part II. Plast Reconstr Surg 1982; 69: 110–116.

793 Dixon AY, Lee SH, McGregor DH. Factors predictive of recurrence of basal cell carcinoma. Am J Dermatopathol 1989; 11: 222–232.

794 Wolf DJ, Zitelli JA. Surgical margins for basal cell carcinoma. Arch Dermatol 1987; 123: 340–344.

795 Dixon AY, Lee SH, McGregor DH. Histologic features predictive of basal cell carcinoma recurrence: results of a multivariate analysis. J Cutan Pathol 1993; 20: 137–142.

796 Pascal RR, Hobby LW, Lattes R, Crikelair GF. Prognosis of 'incompletely excised' versus 'completely excised' basal cell carcinoma. Plast Reconstr Surg 1968; 41: 328–332.

797 Koplin L, Zarem HA. Recurrent basal cell carcinoma. Plast Reconstr Surg 1980; 65: 656–664.

798 Robinson JK, Fisher SG. Recurrent basal cell carcinoma after incomplete resection. J Am Acad Dermatol 2000; 136: 1318–1324.

799 Rippey JJ, Rippey E. Characteristics of incompletely excised basal cell carcinomas of the skin. Med J Aust 1997; 166: 581–583.

800 Holmkvist KA, Rogers GS, Dahl PR. Incidence of residual basal cell carcinoma in patients who appear tumor free after biopsy. J Am Acad Dermatol 1999; 41: 600–605.

801 Dubin N, Kopf AW. Multivariate risk score for recurrence of cutaneous basal cell carcinomas. Arch Dermatol 1983; 119: 373–377.

802 Sloane JP. The value of typing basal cell carcinomas in predicting recurrence after surgical excision. Br J Dermatol 1977; 96: 127–132.

803 Emmett AJJ. Surgical analysis and biological behaviour of 2277 basal cell carcinomas. Aust NZ J Surg 1990; 60: 855–863.

804 Orengo IF, Salasche SJ, Fewkes J et al. Correlation of histologic subtypes of primary basal cell carcinoma and number of Mohs stages required to achieve a tumor-free plane. J Am Acad Dermatol 1997; 37: 395–397.

805 Lang PG Jr, Maize JC. Histologic evolution of recurrent basal cell carcinoma and treatment implications. J Am Acad Dermatol 1986; 14: 186–196.

806 Metcalf JS, Maize JC. Histopathologic considerations in the management of basal cell carcinoma. Semin Dermatol 1989; 8: 259–265.

807 Freeman RG, Duncan WC. Recurrent skin cancer. Arch Dermatol 1973; 107: 395–399.

808 Czarnecki D. The prognosis of patients with basal and squamous cell carcinoma of the skin. Int J Dermatol 1998; 37: 656–658.

809 Ramachandran S, Fryer AA, Smith AG et al. Basal cell carcinoma. Tumor clustering is associated with increased accrual in high risk subgroups. Cancer 2000; 89: 1012–1018.

810 Jacobs GH, Rippey JJ, Altini M. Prediction of aggressive behavior in basal cell carcinoma. Cancer 1982; 49: 533–537.

811 Dixon AY, Lee SH, McGregor DH. Histologic evolution of basal cell carcinoma recurrence. Am J Dermatopathol 1991; 13: 241–247.

812 Smith SP, Grande DJ. Basal cell carcinoma recurring after radiotherapy: a unique, difficult treatment subclass of recurrent basal cell carcinoma. J Dermatol Surg Oncol 1991; 17: 26–30.

813 Roudier-Pujol C, Auperin A, Nguyen T et al. Basal cell carcinoma in young adults: not more aggressive than in older patients. Dermatology 1999; 199: 119–123.

814 Bayer-Garner IB, Dilday B, Sanderson RD, Smoller BR. Syndecan-1 expression is decreased with increasing aggressiveness of basal cell carcinoma. Am J Dermatopathol 2000; 22: 119–122.

815 Tada H, Hatoko M, Tanaka A et al. Expression of desmoglein I and plakoglobin in skin carcinomas. J Cutan Pathol 2000; 27: 24–29.

816 Bahadoran Ph, Perrin Ch, Aberdam D et al. Altered expression of the hemidesmosome-anchoring filament complex proteins in basal cell carcinoma: possible role in the origin of peritumoral lacunae. Br J Dermatol 1997; 136: 35–42.

817 Bernemann T-M, Podda M, Wolter M, Boehncke W-H. Expression of the basal cell adhesion molecule (B-CAM) in normal and diseased human skin. J Cutan Pathol 2000; 27: 108–111.

818 Cousin F, Baldassini S, Bourchany D et al. Expression of the pro-apoptotic caspase 3/CPP32 in cutaneous basal and squamous cell carcinomas. J Cutan Pathol 2000; 27: 235–241.

819 Reynolds NJ, Todd C, Angus B. Overexpression of protein kinase C-α and -β isozymes by stromal dendritic cells in basal and squamous cell carcinoma. Br J Dermatol 1997; 136: 666–673.

820 Wu A, Ichihashi M, Ueda M. Correlation of the expression of human telomerase subunits with telomerase activity in normal skin and skin tumors. Cancer 1999; 86: 2038–2044.

821 Kanitakis J, Euvrard S, Bourchany D et al. Expression of the nm23 metastasis-suppressor gene product in skin tumors. J Cutan Pathol 1997; 24: 151–156.

822 Staibano S, Muzio LL, Pannone G et al. DNA ploidy and cyclin D1 expression in basal cell carcinoma of the head and neck. Am J Clin Pathol 2001; 115: 805–813.

823 Staibano S, Boscaino A, Salvatore G et al. The prognostic significance of tumor angiogenesis in nonaggressive and aggressive basal cell carcinoma of the human skin. Hum Pathol 1996; 27: 695–700.

824 Weninger W, Rendl M, Pammer J et al. Differences in tumor microvessel density between squamous cell carcinomas and basal cell carcinomas may relate to their different biologic behavior. J Cutan Pathol 1997; 24: 364–369.

825 Nangia R, Sait SNJ, Block AW, Zhang PJ. Trisomy 6 in basal cell carcinomas correlates with metastatic potential. Cancer 2001; 91: 1927–1932.

826 Domarus H, Stevens PJ. Metastatic basal cell carcinoma. Report of five cases and review of 170 cases in the literature. J Am Acad Dermatol 1984; 10: 1043–1060.

827 Weedon D, Wall D. Metastatic basal cell carcinoma. Med J Aust 1975; 2: 177–179.

828 Oram Y, Orengo I, Alford E et al. Basal cell carcinoma of the scalp resulting in spine metastasis in a black patient. J Am Acad Dermatol 1994; 31: 916–920.

829 Blewitt RW. Why does basal cell carcinoma metastasize so rarely? Int J Dermatol 1980; 19: 144–146.

830 Snow SN, Sahl W, Lo JS et al. Metastatic basal cell carcinoma. Report of five cases. Cancer 1994; 73: 328–335.

831 Lo JS, Snow SN, Reizner GT. Metastatic basal cell carcinoma: report of twelve cases with a review of the literature. J Am Acad Dermatol 1991; 24: 715–719.

832 Peck GL, Krisnan J, Dugan E et al. Late occult nodal metastasis of basal cell carcinoma. J Cutan Pathol 2000; 27: 568 (abstract).

833 Keenan R, Hopkinson JM. Pulmonary metastases from a basal cell carcinoma. J Cutan Pathol 1981; 8: 235–240.

834 Mikhail GR, Nims LP, Kelly AP Jr et al. Metastatic basal cell carcinoma. Review, pathogenesis, and report of two cases. Arch Dermatol 1977; 113: 1261–1269.

835 Guillan RA, Johnson RP. Aspiration metastases from basal cell carcinoma. The 92nd known case. Arch Dermatol 1978; 114: 589–590.

836 Hartman R, Hartman S, Green N. Long-term survival following bony metastases from basal cell carcinoma. Arch Dermatol 1986; 122: 912–914.

837 Lichtenstein HL, Lee JCK. Amyloidosis associated with metastasizing basal cell carcinoma. Cancer 1980; 46: 2693–2696.

838 Beck H-I, Andersen JA, Birkler NE, Ottosen PD. Giant basal cell carcinoma with metastasis and secondary amyloidosis: report of case. Acta Derm Venereol 1983; 63: 564–567.

839 Kleinberg C, Penetrante RB, Milgrom H, Pickren JW. Metastatic basal cell carcinoma of the skin. J Am Acad Dermatol 1982; 7: 655–659.

840 Leppard BJ. Skin cysts in the basal cell naevus syndrome. Clin Exp Dermatol 1983; 8: 603–612.

841 Gorlin RJ. Nevoid basal-cell carcinoma syndrome. Medicine (Baltimore) 1987; 66: 98–113.

842 Hall J, Johnston KA, McPhillips JP et al. Nevoid basal cell carcinoma syndrome in a black child. J Am Acad Dermatol 1998; 38: 363–365.

843 Tsao H. Update on familial cancer syndromes and the skin. J Am Acad Dermatol 2000; 42: 939–969.

844 Southwick GJ, Schwartz RA. The basal cell nevus syndrome. Disasters occurring among a series of 36 patients. Cancer 1979; 44: 2294–2305.

845 Johnson AD, Hebert AA, Esterly NB. Nevoid basal cell carcinoma syndrome: bilateral ovarian fibromas in a 3?-year-old girl. J Am Acad Dermatol 1986; 14: 371–374.

846 Hardisson D, Jimenez-Heffernan JA, Nistal M et al. Neural variant of fetal rhabdomyoma and naevoid basal cell carcinoma syndrome. Histopathology 1996; 29: 247–252.

847 Vortmeyer AO, Stavrou T, Selby D et al. Deletion analysis of the adenomatous polyposis coli and *PTCH* gene loci in patients with sporadic and nevoid basal cell carcinoma syndrome-associated medulloblastoma. Cancer 1999; 85: 2662–2667.

848 Howell JB. The roots of the naevoid basal cell carcinoma syndrome. Clin Exp Dermatol 1980; 5: 339–348.

849 Compton JG, Goldstein AM, Turner M et al. Fine mapping of the locus for nevoid basal cell carcinoma syndrome on chromosome 9q. J Invest Dermatol 1994; 103: 178–181.

850 Rees J. Genetic alterations in non-melanoma skin cancer. J Invest Dermatol 1994; 103: 747–750.

851 Harada H, Hashimoto K, Toi Y et al. Basal cell carcinoma occurring in multiple familial trichoepithelioma: detection of loss of heterozygosity in chromosome 9q. Arch Dermatol 1997; 133: 666–667.

852 Chiritescu E, Maloney ME. Acrochordons as a presenting sign of nevoid basal cell carcinoma syndrome. J Am Acad Dermatol 2001; 44: 789–794.

853 Pratt MD, Jackson R. Nevoid basal cell carcinoma syndrome. A 15-year follow-up of cases in Ottawa and the Ottawa Valley. J Am Acad Dermatol 1987; 16: 964–970.

854 Golitz LE, Norris DA, Luekens CA Jr, Charles DM. Nevoid basal cell carcinoma syndrome. Multiple basal cell carcinomas of the palm after radiation therapy. Arch Dermatol 1980; 116: 1159–1163.

855 Goldstein AM, Bale SJ, Peck GL, DiGiovanna JJ. Sun exposure and basal cell carcinomas in the nevoid basal cell carcinoma syndrome. J Am Acad Dermatol 1993; 29: 34–41.

856 Frentz G, Munch-Petersen B, Wulf HC et al. The nevoid basal cell carcinoma syndrome: sensitivity to ultraviolet and X-ray irradiation. J Am Acad Dermatol 1987; 17: 637–643.

857 Howell JB. Nevoid basal cell carcinoma syndrome. Profile of genetic and environmental factors in oncogenesis. J Am Acad Dermatol 1984; 11: 98–104.

858 Aloi FG, Tomasini CF, Isaia G, Bernengo MG. Unilateral linear basal cell nevus associated with diffuse osteoma cutis, unilateral anodontia, and abnormal bone mineralization. J Am Acad Dermatol 1989; 20: 973–978.

859 Guarneri B, Borgia F, Cannavò SP et al. Multiple familial basal cell carcinomas including a case of segmental manifestation. Dermatology 2000; 200: 299–302.

860 Requena L, del Carmen Fariña M, Robledo M et al. Multiple hereditary infundibulocystic basal cell carcinomas. A genodermatosis different from nevoid basal cell carcinoma syndrome. Arch Dermatol 1999; 135: 1227–1235.

861 Mason JK, Helwig EB, Graham JH. Pathology of the nevoid basal cell carcinoma syndrome. Arch Pathol 1965; 79: 401–408.

862 Lindberg H, Jepsen FL. The nevoid basal cell carcinoma syndrome. Histopathology of the basal cell tumors. J Cutan Pathol 1983; 10: 68–73.

863 Barr RJ, Headley JL, Jensen JL, Howell JB. Cutaneous keratocysts of nevoid basal cell carcinoma syndrome. J Am Acad Dermatol 1986; 14: 572–576.

864 Zackheim HS, Howell JB, Loud AV. Nevoid basal cell carcinoma syndrome. Arch Dermatol 1966; 93: 317–323.

865 Holubar K, Matras H, Smalik AV. Multiple palmar basal cell epitheliomas in basal cell nevus syndrome. Arch Dermatol 1970; 101: 679–682.

866 Howell JB, Mehregan AH. Pursuit of the pits in the nevoid basal cell carcinoma syndrome. Arch Dermatol 1970; 102: 586–597.

867 Gray DT, Suman VJ, Su WPD et al. Trends in the population-based incidence of squamous cell carcinoma of the skin first diagnosed between 1984 and 1992. Arch Dermatol 1997; 133: 735–740.

868 Giles GG, Marks R, Foley P. Incidence of non-melanocytic skin cancer treated in Australia. Br Med J 1988; 296: 13–17.

869 Gallagher RP, Hill GB, Bajdik CD et al. Sunlight exposure, pigmentation factors, and risk of nonmelanocytic skin cancer. II. Squamous cell carcinoma. Arch Dermatol 1995; 131: 164–169.

870 Alam M, Ratner D. Cutaneous squamous-cell carcinoma. N Engl J Med 2001; 344: 975–983.

871 Mora RG, Perniciaro C. Cancer of the skin in blacks. I. A review of 163 black patients with cutaneous squamous cell carcinoma. J Am Acad Dermatol 1981; 5: 535–543.

872 Epstein JH. Photocarcinogenesis, skin cancer, and aging. J Am Acad Dermatol 1983; 9: 487–502.

873 Johnson TM, Rowe DE, Nelson BR, Swanson NA. Squamous cell carcinoma of the skin (excluding lip and oral mucosa). J Am Acad Dermatol 1992; 26: 467–484.

874 Strom SS, Yamamura Y. Epidemiology of nonmelanoma skin cancer. Clin Plast Surg 1997; 24: 627–636.

875 Lohmann CM, Solomon AR. Clinicopathologic variants of cutaneous squamous cell carcinoma. Adv Anat Pathol 2001; 8: 27–36.

876 Hubbell CR, Rabin VR, Mora RG. Cancer of the skin in blacks. V. A review of 175 black patients with squamous cell carcinoma of the penis. J Am Acad Dermatol 1988; 18: 292–298.

877 Micali G, Innocenzi D, Nasca MR et al. Squamous cell carcinoma of the penis. J Am Acad Dermatol 1996; 35: 432–451.

878 Lumpkin LR III, Rosen T, Tschen JA. Subungual squamous cell carcinoma. J Am Acad Dermatol 1984; 11: 735–738.

879 Mikhail GR. Subungual epidermoid carcinoma. J Am Acad Dermatol 1984; 11: 291–298.

880 Guitart J, Bergfeld WF, Tuthill RJ et al. Squamous cell carcinoma of the nail bed: a clinicopathological study of 12 cases. Br J Dermatol 1990; 123: 215–222.

881 Hale LR, Dawber RPR. Subungual squamous cell carcinoma presenting with minimal nail changes: a factor in delayed diagnosis? Australas J Dermatol 1998; 39: 86–88.

882 Baldursson B, Sigurgeirsson B, Lindelöf B. Venous leg ulcers and squamous cell carcinoma: a large-scale epidemiological study. Br J Dermatol 1995; 133: 571–574.

883 Rossis CG, Yiacoumettis AM, Elemenoglou J. Squamous cell carcinoma of the heel developing at site of previous frostbite. J R Soc Med 1982; 75: 715–718.

884 Marmelzat WL. Malignant tumors in smallpox vaccination scars. A report of 24 cases. Arch Dermatol 1968; 97: 400–406.

884a Sánchez-Díez A, Díaz-Ramón L, Agesta N et al. Squamous cell carcinoma on a pyoderma gangrenosum scar. Am J Dermatopathol 2000; 22: 351 (abstract).

885 Kavouni A, Shibu M, Carver N. Squamous cell carcinoma arising in transplanted skin. Clin Exp Dermatol 2000; 25: 302–304.

886 Bowers RF, Young JM. Carcinoma arising in scars, osteomyelitis, and fistulae. Arch Surg 1960; 80: 564–570.

887 Sagi A, Rosenberg L, Greiff M, Mahler D. Squamous-cell carcinoma arising in a pilonidal sinus: a case report and review of the literature. J Dermatol Surg Oncol 1984; 10: 210–212.

888 Anscombe AM, Isaacson P. An unusual variant of squamous cell carcinoma (inverted verrucous carcinoma) arising in a pilonidal sinus. Histopathology 1983; 7: 123–127.

889 Quintal D, Jackson R. Aggressive squamous cell carcinoma arising in familial acne conglobata. J Am Acad Dermatol 1986; 14: 207–214.

890 Whipp MJ, Harrington CI, Dundas S. Fatal squamous cell carcinoma associated with acne conglobata in a father and daughter. Br J Dermatol 1987; 117: 389–392.

891 Cruickshank AH, McConnell EM, Miller DG. Malignancy in scars, chronic ulcers, and sinuses. J Clin Pathol 1963; 16: 573–580.

892 Barr LH, Menard JW. Marjolin's ulcer. The LSU experience. Cancer 1983; 52: 173–175.

893 Goldberg DJ, Arbesfeld D. Squamous cell carcinoma arising in a site of chronic osteomyelitis. J Dermatol Surg Oncol 1991; 17: 788–790.

894 Steffen C. Marjolin's ulcer. Am J Dermatopathol 1984; 6: 187–193.

895 Yoshioka K, Kono T, Kitajima J et al. Squamous cell carcinoma developing in epidermolysis bullosa dystrophica. Int J Dermatol 1991; 30: 718–721.

896 Chun SI, Whang KC, Su WPD. Squamous cell carcinoma arising in Hailey–Hailey disease. J Cutan Pathol 1988; 15: 234–237.

897 Leache A, Soto de Delás J, Vázquez-Doval J et al. Squamous cell carcinoma arising from a lesion of disseminated superficial actinic porokeratosis. Clin Exp Dermatol 1991; 16: 460–462.

898 Chang S-E, Lim Y-S, Lee H-J et al. Expression of p53, pRb, p16 and proliferating cell nuclear antigen in squamous cell carcinoma arising on a giant porokeratosis. Br J Dermatol 1999; 141: 575–576.

899 Martin S, Rosen T, Locker E. Metastatic squamous cell carcinoma of the lip. Occurrence in blacks with discoid lupus erythematosus. Arch Dermatol 1979; 115: 1214.

900 Bam L, Geronemus R. The association of lichen planus of the penis with squamous cell carcinoma in situ and with verrucous squamous carcinoma. J Dermatol Surg Oncol 1989; 15: 413–417.

901 Mayron R, Grimwood RE, Siegle RJ, Camisa C. Verrucous carcinoma arising in ulcerative lichen planus of the soles. J Dermatol Surg Oncol 1988; 14: 547–551.

902 Kontochristopoulos G, Kyriakis K, Symeonidou S et al. Squamous cell carcinoma in chronic trophic ulcers of leprosy patients. J Eur Acad Dermatol Venereol 2000; 14: 230–231.

903 Gooptu C, Marks N, Thomas J, James MP. Squamous cell carcinoma associated with lupus vulgaris. Clin Exp Dermatol 1998; 23: 99–102.

904 Scurry JP, Vanin K. Vulvar squamous cell carcinoma and lichen sclerosus. Australas J Dermatol 1997; 38 (Suppl): S20–S25.

905 Derrick EK, Ridley CM, Kobza-Black A et al. A clinical study of 23 cases of female anogenital carcinoma. Br J Dermatol 2000; 143: 1217–1223.

906 Lister RK, Black MM, Calonje E, Burnand KG. Squamous cell carcinoma arising in chronic lymphoedema. Br J Dermatol 1997; 136: 384–387.

907 Levin A, Amazon K, Rywlin AM. A squamous cell carcinoma that developed in an epidermal nevus. Am J Dermatopathol 1984; 6: 51–55.

908 Colver G, Mortimer P, Dawber R. Premycotic poikiloderma, mycosis fungoides and cutaneous squamous cell carcinoma. Int J Dermatol 1986; 25: 376–378.

909 Cohn BA. From sunlight to actinic keratosis to squamous cell carcinoma. J Am Acad Dermatol 2000; 42: 143–144.

910 Akimoto S, Suzuki Y, Ishikawa O. Multiple actinic keratoses and squamous cell carcinomas on the sun-exposed areas of widespread vitiligo. Br J Dermatol 2000; 142: 824–825.

911 Picascia DD, Caro WA. Cutaneous squamous cell carcinoma and hypercalcemia. J Am Acad Dermatol 1987; 17: 347–351.

912 Sparks MM, Kuhlman DS, Prieto A, Callen JP. Hypercalcemia in association with cutaneous squamous cell carcinoma. Occurrence as a late complication of hidradenitis suppurativa. Arch Dermatol 1985; 121: 243–246.

913 Loche F, Bennet A, Bazex J, Thouvenin MD. Hypercalcaemia of malignancy associated with invasive cutaneous squamous cell carcinoma. Br J Dermatol 1999; 141: 577–579.

914 Harvey RA, Chaglassian T, Knapper W, Goulian D. Squamous cell carcinoma of the skin in adolescence. Report of a case. JAMA 1977; 238: 513.

915 Watanabe K, Mukawa A, Miyazaki K, Tsukahara K. Adenoid squamous cell carcinoma of the penis. Acta Pathol Jpn 1983; 33: 1243–1250.

916 Howe NR, Lang PG. Squamous cell carcinoma of the sole in a patient with chronic graft-vs-host disease. Arch Dermatol 1988; 124: 1244–1245.

917 Walder BK, Robertson MR, Jeremy D. Skin cancer and immunosuppression. Lancet 1971; 2: 1282–1283.

918 Gupta AK, Cardella CJ, Haberman HF. Cutaneous malignant neoplasms in patients with renal transplants. Arch Dermatol 1986; 122: 1288–1293.

919 Cohen EB, Kormorowski RA, Clowry LJ. Cutaneous complications in renal transplant recipients. Am J Clin Pathol 1987; 88: 32–37.

920 España A, Redondo P, Fernández AL et al. Skin cancer in heart transplant recipients. J Am Acad Dermatol 1995; 32: 458–465.

921 Euvrard S, Kanitakis J, Pouteil-Noble C et al. Comparative epidemiologic study of premalignant and malignant epithelial cutaneous lesions developing after kidney and heart transplantation. J Am Acad Dermatol 1995; 33: 222–229.

922 Cowen EW, Billingsley EM. Awareness of skin cancer by kidney transplant patients. J Am Acad Dermatol 1999; 40: 697–701.

923 Penn I. Skin disorders in organ transplant recipients. Arch Dermatol 1997; 133: 221–223.

924 Lindelöf B, Sigurgeirsson B, Gäbel H, Stern RS. Incidence of skin cancer in 5356 patients following organ transplantation. Br J Dermatol 2000; 143: 513–519.

925 van Zuuren EJ, de Visscher JGAM, Bouwes Bavinck JN. Carcinoma of the lip in kidney transplant recipients. J Am Acad Dermatol 1998; 38: 497–499.

926 Blessing K, McLaren KM, Morris R et al. Detection of human papillomavirus in skin and genital lesions of renal allograft recipients by *in situ* hybridization. Histopathology 1990; 16: 181–185.

927 Harwood CA, McGregor JM, Proby CM, Breuer J. Human papillomavirus and the development of non-melanoma skin cancer. J Clin Pathol 1999; 52: 249–253.

928 Mork J, Lie AK, Glattre E et al. Human papillomavirus infection as a risk factor for squamous-cell carcinoma of the head and neck. N Engl J Med 2001; 344: 1125–1131.

929 McGregor JM, Farthing A, Crook T et al. Posttransplant skin cancer: A possible role for p53 gene mutation but not for oncogenic human papillomaviruses. J Am Acad Dermatol 1994; 30: 701–706.

930 Smith SE, Davis IC, Leshin B et al. Absence of human papillomavirus in squamous cell carcinomas of nongenital skin from immunocompromised renal transplant patients. Arch Dermatol 1993; 129: 1585–1588.

931 Meyer T, Arndt R, Christophers E, Stockfleth E. Frequency and spectrum of HPV types detected in cutaneous squamous-cell carcinomas depend on the HPV detection system: a comparison of four PCR assays. Dermatology 2000; 201: 204–211.

932 Poblet E, Alfaro L, Fernander-Segoviano P et al. Human papillomavirus-associated penile squamous cell carcinoma in HIV-positive patients. Am J Surg Pathol 1999; 23: 1119–1123.

933 Gasparro FP. *p53* in dermatology. Arch Dermatol 1998; 134: 1029–1032.

934 Maurer TA, Vin Christian K, Kerschmann RL et al. Cutaneous squamous cell carcinoma in human immunodeficiency virus-infected patients. A study of epidemiologic risk factors, human papillomavirus, and p53 expression. Arch Dermatol 1997; 133: 577–583.

935 Hudson AR, Antley CM, Kohler S, Smoller BR. Increased p53 staining in normal skin of posttransplant, immunocompromised patients and implications for carcinogenesis. Am J Dermatopathol 1999; 21: 442–445.

936 Sakatani S, Kusakabe H, Kiyokane K, Suzuki K. p53 gene mutations in squamous cell

937 Hoyo E, Kanitakis J, Euvrard S, Thivolet J. Proliferation characteristics of cutaneous squamous cell carcinomas developing in organ graft recipients. Arch Dermatol 1993; 129: 324–327.

938 Galvão MM, Sotto MN, Kihara SM et al. Lymphocyte subsets and Langerhans cells in sun-protected and sun-exposed skin of immunosuppressed renal allograft recipients. J Am Acad Dermatol 1998; 38: 38–44.

939 McKenna DB, Murphy GM. Skin cancer chemoprophylaxis in renal transplant recipients: 5 years of experience using low-dose acitretin. Br J Dermatol 1999; 140: 656–660.

940 Rosenblatt L, Marks R. Deaths due to squamous cell carcinoma in Australia: Is there a case for a public health intervention? Australas J Dermatol 1996; 37: 26–29.

941 Bouwes Bavinck JN, De Boer A, Vermeer BJ et al. Sunlight, keratotic skin lesions and skin cancer in renal transplant recipients. Br J Dermatol 1993; 129: 242–249.

942 Veness MJ, Quinn DI, Ong CS et al. Aggressive cutaneous malignancies following cardiothoracic transplantation. The Australian experience. Cancer 1999; 85: 1758–1764.

943 Ong CS, Keogh AM, Kossard S et al. Skin cancer in Australian heart transplant recipients. J Am Acad Dermatol 1999; 40: 27–34.

944 Jensen P, Hansen S, Møller B et al. Skin cancer in kidney and heart transplant recipients and different long-term immunosuppressive therapy regimens. J Am Acad Dermatol 1999; 40: 177–186.

945 Otley CC, Coldiron BM, Stasko T, Goldman GD. Decreased skin cancer after cessation of therapy with transplant-associated immunosuppressants. Arch Dermatol 2001; 137: 459–463.

946 Honigsmann H, Wolff K, Gschnait F et al. Keratoses and nonmelanoma skin tumors in long-term photochemotherapy (PUVA). J Am Acad Dermatol 1980; 3: 406–414.

947 Epstein E. Malignant sun-induced squamous-cell carcinoma of the skin. J Dermatol Surg Oncol 1983; 9: 505–506.

948 Altman JS, Adler SS. Development of multiple cutaneous squamous cell carcinomas during PUVA treatment for chronic graft-versus-host disease. J Am Acad Dermatol 1994; 31: 505–507.

949 Kwa RE, Campana K, Moy RL. Biology of cutaneous squamous cell carcinoma. J Am Acad Dermatol 1992; 26: 1–26.

950 Canfield PJ, Greenoak GE, Mascasaet EN et al. The characterization of squamous cell carcinoma induced by ultraviolet irradiation in hairless mice. Pathology 1988; 20: 109–117.

951 Swanbeck G. Aetiological factors in squamous cell skin cancer. Br J Dermatol 1971; 85: 394–396.

952 Moy R, Eliezri YD. Significance of human papillomavirus-induced squamous cell carcinoma to dermatologists. Arch Dermatol 1994; 130: 235–238.

953 Eliezri YD, Silverstein SJ, Nuovo GJ. Occurrence of human papillomavirus type 16 DNA in cutaneous squamous and basal cell neoplasms. J Am Acad Dermatol 1990; 23: 836–842.

954 Kao GF, Kao WH. Malignant transformation of keratinocytes by human papillomaviruses. J Cutan Pathol 1994; 21: 193–199.

955 Ashinoff R, Li JJ, Jacobson M et al. Detection of human papillomavirus DNA in squamous cell carcinoma of the nail bed and finger determined by polymerase chain reaction. Arch Dermatol 1991; 127: 1813–1818.

956 Theunis A, André J, Noël J-Ch. Evaluation of the role of genital human papillomavirus in the pathogenesis of ungual squamous cell carcinoma. Dermatology 1999; 198: 206–208.

957 Amerio P, Offidani A, Cellini A, Bossi G. Well-differentiated squamous cell carcinoma of the penis associated with HPV type 33. Int J Dermatol 1998; 37: 128–130.

958 McHugh RW, Hazen P, Eliezri YD, Nuovo GJ. Metastatic periungual squamous cell carcinoma: Detection of human papillomavirus type 35 RNA in the digital tumor and axillary lymph node metastases. J Am Acad Dermatol 1996; 34: 1080–1082.

959 Forslund O, Nordin P, Hansson BG. Mucosal human papillomavirus types in squamous cell carcinomas of the uterine cervix and subsequently on fingers. Br J Dermatol 2000; 142: 1148–1153.

960 Rust A, McGovern RM, Gostout BS et al. Human papillomavirus in cutaneous squamous cell carcinoma and cervix of a patient with psoriasis and extensive ultraviolet radiation exposure. J Am Acad Dermatol 2001; 44: 681–686.

961 O'Connor DP, Kay EW, Leader M et al. A high degree of chromosomal instability at 13q14 in cutaneous squamous cell carcinomas: indication for a role of a tumour suppressor gene other than Rb. J Clin Pathol: Mol Pathol 2001; 54: 165–169.

962 Brodland DG. The life of a skin cancer. Mayo Clin Proc 1997; 72: 475–478.

963 Ng P, Ackerman AB. The major types of squamous-cell carcinoma. Dermatopathology: Practical & Conceptual 1999; 5: 250–252.

964 Lober BA, Lober CW, Accola J. Actinic keratosis is squamous cell carcinoma. J Am Acad Dermatol 2000; 43: 881–882.

965 DiLeonardo M. Solar keratosis vs. Bowen's disease vs. bowenoid papulosis. Dermatopathology: Practical & Conceptual 1997; 3: 130–131.

966 Mittelbronn MA, Mullins DL, Ramos-Caro FA, Flowers FP. Frequency of pre-existing actinic keratosis in cutaneous squamous cell carcinoma. Int J Dermatol 1998; 37: 677–681.

967 Guenthner ST, Hurwitz RM, Buckel LJ, Gray HR. Cutaneous squamous cell carcinomas consistently show histologic evidence of in situ changes: A clinicopathologic correlation. J Am Acad Dermatol 1999; 41: 443–448.

968 Kuo T. Clear cell carcinoma of the skin. A variant of the squamous cell carcinoma that simulates sebaceous carcinoma. Am J Surg Pathol 1980; 4: 573–583.

969 Requena L, Sánchez M, Requena I et al. Clear cell squamous cell carcinoma. J Dermatol Surg Oncol 1991; 17: 656–660.

970 Cruces M, Losada A, de la Torre C. Clear cell squamous cell carcinoma. Am J Dermatopathol 1996; 18: 438 (abstract).

971 Cramer SF, Heggeness LM. Signet-ring squamous cell carcinoma. Am J Clin Pathol 1989; 91: 488–491.

972 McKinley E, Valles R, Bang R, Bocklage T. Signet-ring squamous cell carcinoma: a case report. J Cutan Pathol 1998; 25: 176–181.

973 Glover M, Cerio R, Corbett M et al. Cutaneous squamoproliferative lesions in renal transplant recipients. Am J Dermatopathol 1995; 17: 551–554.

974 Mohs FE, Lathrop TG. Modes of spread of cancer of skin. Arch Dermatol 1952; 66: 427–439.

975 Bernstein SC, Lim KK, Brodland DG, Heidelberg KA. The many faces of squamous cell carcinoma. Dermatol Surg 1996; 22: 243–254.

976 Subtil A, LeBoit PE. Lymphocytes + nerves = ? Am J Dermatopathol 2000; 22: 362–364.

977 Smolle J, Wolf P. Is favorable prognosis of squamous cell carcinoma of the skin due to efficient immune surveillance? Arch Dermatol 1997; 133: 645–646.

978 Haeffner AC, Zepter K, Elmets CA, Wood GS. Analysis of tumor-infiltrating lymphocytes in cutaneous squamous cell carcinoma. Arch Dermatol 1997; 133: 585–590.

979 Lowe D, Fletcher CDM, Shaw MP, McKee PH. Eosinophil infiltration in keratoacanthoma and squamous cell carcinoma of the skin. Histopathology 1984; 8: 619–625.

980 Monteagudo C, Jordá E, Carda C et al. Erythrophagocytic tumour cells in melanoma and squamous cell carcinoma of the skin. Histopathology 1997; 31: 367–373.

981 Stenbäck F, Mäkinen MJ, Jussila T et al. The extracellular matrix in skin tumor development – a morphological study. J Cutan Pathol 1999; 26: 327–338.

982 Wick MR, Swanson PE, Ritter JH, Fitzgibbon JF. The immunohistology of cutaneous neoplasia: a practical perspective. J Cutan Pathol 1993; 20: 481–497.

983 Pinkus GS, Kurtin PJ. Epithelial membrane antigen – a diagnostic discriminant in surgical pathology. Hum Pathol 1985; 16: 929–940.

984 Wick MR, Kaye VN. The role of diagnostic immunohistochemistry in dermatology. Semin Dermatol 1986; 5: 346–358.

985 Silvis GN, Swanson PE, Manivel JC et al. Spindle-cell and pleomorphic neoplasms of the skin. Am J Dermatopathol 1988; 10: 9–19.

986 Nadji M. Immunoperoxidase techniques. II. Application to cutaneous neoplasms. Am J Dermatopathol 1986; 8: 124–129.

987 Al-Sader MH, Doyle E, Kay EW et al. Proliferation indexes – a comparison between cutaneous basal and squamous cell carcinomas. J Clin Pathol 1996; 49: 549–551.

988 Mansoor A, McKee PH, Simpson JA et al. Prognostic significance of Ki-67 and p53 immunoreactivity in cutaneous squamous cell carcinomas. Am J Dermatopathol 1996; 18: 351–357.

989 Evans HL, Smith JL. Spindle cell squamous carcinomas and sarcoma-like tumors of the skin. A comparative study of 38 cases. Cancer 1980; 45: 2687–2697.

990 Harwood CA, Proby CM, Leigh IM, Cerio R. Aggressive spindle cell squamous cell carcinoma in renal transplant recipients. Br J Dermatol (Suppl) 1996; 47: 23 (abstract).

991 Kanitakis J, Narvaez D, Euvrard S et al. Proliferation markers Ki67 and PCNA in cutaneous squamous cell carcinomas: lack of prognostic value. Br J Dermatol 1997; 136: 643–644.

992 Cockayne SE, Shah M, Slater DN, Harrington CI. Spindle and pseudoglandular squamous cell carcinoma arising in lichen sclerosus of the vulva. Br J Dermatol 1998; 138: 695–697.

993 Penneys NS, Nadji M, Ziegels-Weissman J, Morales AR. Prekeratin in spindle cell tumors of the skin. Arch Dermatol 1983; 119: 476–479.

994 Argenyi ZB. Spindle cell neoplasms of the skin: a comprehensive diagnostic approach. Semin Dermatol 1989; 8: 283–297.

995 Eusebi V, Ceccarelli C, Piscioli F et al. Spindle cell tumours of the skin of debatable origin. An immunocytochemical study. J Pathol 1984; 144: 189–199.

996 Smith KJ, Skelton HG III, Morgan AM et al. Spindle cell neoplasms coexpressing cytokeratin and vimentin (metaplastic squamous cell carcinoma). J Cutan Pathol 1992; 19: 286–293.

997 Iyer PV, Leong AS-Y. Poorly differentiated squamous cell carcinomas of the skin can express vimentin. J Cutan Pathol 1992; 19: 34–39.

998 Kim JM, Su WPD, Kurtin PJ, Ziesmer S. Marjolin's ulcer: immunohistochemical study of 17 cases and comparison with common squamous cell carcinoma and basal cell carcinoma. J Cutan Pathol 1992; 19: 278–285.

999 Wooldridge WE, Frerichs JB. Multiple adenoid squamous cell carcinoma. Arch Dermatol 1971; 104: 202–206.

1000 Ikegawa S, Saida T, Takizawa Y et al. Vimentin-positive squamous cell carcinoma arising in a burn scar. A highly malignant neoplasm composed of acantholytic round keratinocytes. Arch Dermatol 1989; 125: 1672–1676.

1001 Johnson WC, Helwig EB. Adenoid squamous cell carcinoma (adenoacanthoma). A clinicopathologic study of 155 patients. Cancer 1966; 19: 1639–1650.

1002 Nappi O, Pettinato G, Wick MR. Adenoid (acantholytic) squamous cell carcinoma of the skin. J Cutan Pathol 1989; 16: 114–121.

1003 Ritter JH, Mills SE, Nappi O, Wick MR. Angiosarcoma-like neoplasms of epithelial organs: true endothelial tumors or variants of carcinoma? Semin Diagn Pathol 1995; 12: 270–282.

1004 Nappi O, Wick MR, Pettinato G et al. Pseudovascular adenoid squamous cell carcinoma of the skin. A neoplasm that may be mistaken for angiosarcoma. Am J Surg Pathol 1992; 16: 429–438.

1005 Banerjee SS, Eyden BP, Wells S et al. Pseudoangiosarcomatous carcinoma: a clinicopathological study of seven cases. Histopathology 1992; 21: 13–23.

1006 Nagore E, Sánchez-Motilla JM, Pérez-Vallés A et al. Pseudovascular squamous cell carcinoma of the skin. Clin Exp Dermatol 2000; 25: 206–208.

1007 Kossard S, Cook D. Pigmented squamous cell carcinoma with dendritic melanocytes. Australas J Dermatol 1997; 38: 145–147.

1008 Matsumoto M, Sonobe H, Takeuchi T et al. Pigmented squamous cell carcinoma of the scrotum associated with a lentigo. Br J Dermatol 1999; 141: 132–136.

1009 Jurado I, Saez A, Luelmo J et al. Pigmented squamous cell carcinoma of the skin. Report of two cases and review of the literature. Am J Dermatopathol 1998; 20: 578–581.

1010 Chapman MS, Quitadamo MJ, Perry AE. Pigmented squamous cell carcinoma. J Cutan Pathol 2000; 27: 93–95.

1011 Morgan MB, Lima-Maribona J, Miller RA et al. Pigmented squamous cell carcinoma of the skin: morphologic and immunohistochemical study of five cases. J Cutan Pathol 2000; 27: 381–386.

1012 Diaz-Cano SJ. Melanocytes in squamous cell carcinoma of the skin. Br J Dermatol 2000; 142: 184.

1013 Morice WG, Ferreiro JA. Distinction of basaloid squamous cell carcinoma from adenoid cystic and small cell undifferentiated carcinoma by immunohistochemistry. Hum Pathol 1998; 29: 609–612.

1014 Cubilla AL, Reuter VE, Gregoire L et al. Basaloid squamous cell carcinoma: a distinctive human papilloma virus-related penile neoplasm. A report of 20 cases. Am J Surg Pathol 1998; 22: 755–761.

1015 Lee PK, Olbricht SM, Gonzalez-Serva A, Harrist TH. Infiltrative squamous cell carcinoma: histopathologic and clinical characterization of a newly described skin cancer. J Cutan Pathol 1997; 24: 108 (abstract).

1016 McCalmont TH, Salmon PJM, Geisse JK, Grekin RG. Desmoplastic squamous and adenosquamous carcinoma: 60 examples of an overlooked pattern of epithelial malignancy. J Cutan Pathol 1997; 24: 111 (abstract).

1017 Mathers ME, O'Donnell M. Squamous cell carcinoma of skin with a rhabdoid phenotype: a case report. J Clin Pathol 2000; 53: 868–870.

1018 Feldman PS, Barr RJ. Ultrastructure of spindle cell squamous carcinoma. J Cutan Pathol 1976; 3: 17–24.

1019 Harris M. Differential diagnosis of spindle cell tumours by electron microscopy – personal experience and a review. Histopathology 1981; 5: 81–105.

1020 Harris M. Spindle cell squamous carcinoma: ultrastructural observations. Histopathology 1982; 6: 197–210.

1021 Friedman HI, Cooper PH, Wanebo HJ. Prognostic and therapeutic use of microstaging of cutaneous squamous cell carcinoma of the trunk and extremities. Cancer 1985; 56: 1099–1105.

1022 Immerman SC, Scanlon EF, Christ M, Knox KL. Recurrent squamous cell carcinoma of the skin. Cancer 1983; 51: 1537–1540.

1023 Rowe DE, Carroll RJ, Day CL Jr. Prognostic factors for local recurrence, metastasis, and survival rates in squamous cell carcinoma of the skin, ear, and lip. J Am Acad Dermatol 1993; 26: 976–990.

1024 Lawrence N, Cottel WI. Squamous cell carcinoma of skin with perineural invasion. J Am Acad Dermatol 1994; 31: 30–33.

1025 Veness MJ. Perineural spread in head and neck skin cancer. Australas J Dermatol 2000; 41: 117–119.

1026 Tamura A, Ohnishi K, Ishikawa O, Miyachi Y. Flow cytometric DNA content analysis on squamous cell carcinomas according to the preceding lesions. Br J Dermatol 1996; 134: 40–43.

1027 Turner RJ, Leonard N, Malcolm AJ et al. A retrospective study of outcome of Mohs' micrographic surgery for cutaneous squamous cell carcinoma using formalin fixed sections. Br J Dermatol 2000; 142: 752–757.

1028 Turner JE, Callen JP. Aggressive behavior of squamous cell carcinoma in a patient with preceding lymphocytic lymphoma. J Am Acad Dermatol 1981; 4: 446–450.

1029 Frierson HF Jr, Deutsch BD, Levine PA. Clinicopathologic features of cutaneous squamous cell carcinomas of the head and neck in patients with chronic lymphocytic leukemia/small cell lymphocytic lymphoma. Hum Pathol 1988; 19: 1397–1402.

1030 Mora RG. Metastatic squamous cell carcinoma of the skin occurring in a lymphomatous lymph node. J Am Acad Dermatol 1985; 12: 571–575.

1031 Riefkohl R, Pollack S, Georgiade GS. A rationale for the treatment of difficult basal cell and squamous cell carcinomas of the skin. Ann Plast Surg 1985; 15: 101–104.

1032 Wilkinson JD. Current treatment of epitheliomas of the skin. Clin Exp Dermatol 1982; 7: 75–88.

1033 Lund HZ. How often does squamous cell carcinoma of the skin metastasize? Arch Dermatol 1965; 92: 635–637.

1034 Lund HZ. Metastasis from sun-induced squamous-cell carcinoma of the skin: an uncommon event. J Dermatol Surg Oncol 1984; 10: 169–170.

1035 Frierson HF Jr, Cooper PH. Prognostic factors in squamous cell carcinoma of the lower lip. Hum Pathol 1986; 17: 346–354.

1036 Graham BS, Del Rosario RN, Barr RJ. Classification of cutaneous squamous cell carcinoma. J Cutan Pathol 2000; 27: 558 (abstract).

1037 Chuang T-Y, Popescu NA, Su WPD, Chute CG. Squamous cell carcinoma. A population-based incidence study in Rochester, Minn. Arch Dermatol 1990; 126: 185–188.

1038 Moller R, Raymann F, Hou-Jensen K. Metastases in dermatological patients with squamous cell carcinoma. Arch Dermatol 1979; 115: 703–705.

1039 Dinehart SM, Pollack SV. Metastases from squamous cell carcinoma of the skin and lip. An analysis of twenty-seven cases. J Am Acad Dermatol 1989; 21: 241–248.

1040 Hendricks JL, Mendelson BC, Woods JE. Invasive carcinoma of the lower lip. Surg Clin North Am 1977; 57: 837–844.

1041 Stein AL, Tahan SR. Histologic correlates of metastasis in primary invasive squamous cell carcinoma of the lip. J Cutan Pathol 1994; 21: 16–21.

1042 Tahan SR, Stein AL. Angiogenesis in invasive squamous cell carcinoma of the lip: tumor vascularity is not an indicator of metastatic risk. J Cutan Pathol 1995; 22: 236–240.

1043 Wei N, Tahan SR. S100+ cell response to squamous cell carcinoma of the lip: inverse correlation with metastasis. J Cutan Pathol 1998; 25: 463–468.

1044 McCombe D, MacGill K, Ainslie J et al. Squamous cell carcinoma of the lip: a retrospective review of the Peter MacCallum Cancer Institute experience 1979–88. Aust NZ J Surg 2000; 70: 358–361.

1045 Cubilla AL, Barreto J, Caballero C et al. Pathologic features of epidermoid carcinoma of the penis. A prospective study of 66 cases. Am J Surg Pathol 1993; 17: 753–763.

1046 Maggino T, Landoni F, Sartori E et al. Patterns of recurrence in patients with squamous cell carcinoma of the vulva. A multicenter CTF study. Cancer 2000; 89: 116–122.

1047 Preti M, Ronco G, Ghiringhello B, Micheletti L. Recurrent squamous cell carcinoma of the vulva. Clinicopathologic determinants identifying low risk patients. Cancer 2000; 88: 1869–1876.

1048 Weisberg NK, Bertagnolli MM, Becker DS. Combined sentinel lymphadenectomy and Mohs micrographic surgery for high-risk cutaneous squamous cell carcinoma. J Am Acad Dermatol 2000; 43: 483–488.

1049 Buecker JW, Ratz JL. Cutaneous metastatic squamous-cell carcinoma in zosteriform distribution. J Dermatol Surg Oncol 1984; 10: 718–720.

1050 Ihm C-W, Park S-L, Sung S-Y, Lee I-S. Bowenoid epidermotropic metastatic squamous cell carcinoma. J Cutan Pathol 1996; 23: 479–484.

1051 Kato N, Aoyagi S, Sugawara H, Mayuzumi M. Zosteriform and epidermotropic metastatic primary cutaneous squamous cell carcinoma. Am J Dermatopathol 2001; 23: 216–220.

1052 Yagi H, Danno K, Maruguchi Y et al. Significance of squamous cell carcinoma (SCC)-related antigens in cutaneous SCC. Arch Dermatol 1987; 123: 902–906.

1053 Campbell B, De'Ambrosis B. Squamous cell carcinoma antigen in patients with cutaneous disorders. J Am Acad Dermatol 1990; 22: 639–642.

1054 Alkemade HAC, van Vlijmen-Willems IMJJ, van Haelst UJGM et al. Demonstration of skin-derived antileukoproteinase (SKALP) and its target enzyme human leukocyte elastase in squamous cell carcinoma. J Pathol 1994; 174: 121–129.

1055 Lifschitz-Mercer B, Czernobilsky B, Feldberg E, Geiger B. Expression of the adherens junction protein vinculin in human basal and squamous cell tumors: relationship to invasiveness and metastatic potential. Hum Pathol 1997; 28: 1230–1236.

1056 Bayer-Garner IB, Sanderson RD, Smoller BR. Syndecan-1 expression is diminished in acantholytic cutaneous squamous cell carcinoma. J Cutan Pathol 1999; 26: 386–390.

1057 Bayer-Garner IB, Smoller BR. The expression of syndecan-1 is preferentially reduced compared with that of E-cadherin in acantholytic squamous cell carcinoma. J Cutan Pathol 2001; 28: 83–89.

1058 Imanishi Y, Fujii M, Tokumaru Y et al. Clinical significance of expression of membrane type

1 matrix metalloproteinase and matrix metalloproteinase-2 in human head and neck squamous cell carcinoma. Hum Pathol 2000; 31: 895–904.

1059 Kawada A, Hara K, Kominami E et al. Cathepsin B and D expression in squamous cell carcinoma. Br J Dermatol 1996; 135: 905–910.

1060 Kawada A, Hara K, Kominami E et al. Expression of cathepsin D and B in invasion and metastasis of squamous cell carcinoma. Br J Dermatol 1997; 137: 361–366.

1061 Egawa K, Honda Y, Ono T, Kuroki M. Immunohistochemical demonstration of carcinoembryonic antigen and related antigens in various cutaneous keratinous neoplasms and verruca vulgaris. Br J Dermatol 1998; 139: 178–185.

1062 Kagoura M, Toyoda M, Matsui C, Morohashi M. Immunohistochemical localization of ornithine decarboxylase in skin tumors. J Cutan Pathol 2000; 27: 338–343.

1063 Lee SH, Shin MS, Kim HS et al. Somatic mutations of Fas (Apo-1/CD95) gene in cutaneous squamous cell carcinoma arising from a burn scar. J Invest Dermatol 1999; 114: 122–126.

1064 Makino T, Tatebe S, Goto A et al. Apoptosis and cellular proliferation in human epidermal squamous cell neoplasia. J Cutan Pathol 1998; 25: 136–142.

1065 Thompson LDR, Heffner DK. The clinical importance of cystic squamous cell carcinoma in the neck. A study of 136 cases. Cancer 1998; 82: 944–956.

1066 Grinspan D, Abulafia J. Oral florid papillomatosis (verrucous carcinoma). Int J Dermatol 1979; 18: 608–622.

1067 Kraus FT, Perez-Mesa C. Verrucous carcinoma. Clinical and pathologic study of 105 cases involving oral cavity, larynx and genitalia. Cancer 1966; 19: 26–38.

1068 Klima M, Kurtis B, Jordan PH Jr. Verrucous carcinoma of skin. J Cutan Pathol 1980; 7: 88–98.

1069 Schwartz RA. Verrucous carcinoma of the skin and mucosa. J Am Acad Dermatol 1995; 32: 1–21.

1070 McKee PH, Wilkinson JD, Corbett MF et al. Carcinoma cuniculatum: a case metastasizing to skin and lymph nodes. Clin Exp Dermatol 1981; 6: 613–618.

1071 Carson TE. Verrucous carcinoma of the penis. Arch Dermatol 1978; 114: 1546–1547.

1072 Schwartz RA. Buschke–Loewenstein tumor: Verrucous carcinoma of the penis. J Am Acad Dermatol 1990; 23: 723–727.

1073 Kanik AB, Lee J, Wax F, Bhawan J. Penile verrucous carcinoma in a 37-year-old circumcised man. J Am Acad Dermatol 1997; 37: 329–331.

1074 Mehta RK, Rytina E, Sterling JC. Treatment of verrucous carcinoma of vulva with acitretin. Br J Dermatol 2000; 142: 1195–1198.

1075 Sánchez-Yus E, Velasco E, Robledo A. Verrucous carcinoma of the back. J Am Acad Dermatol 1986; 14: 947–950.

1076 Nguyen KQ, McMarlin SL. Verrucous carcinoma of the face. Arch Dermatol 1984; 120: 383–385.

1077 Baruchin AM, Lupo L, Goldstein J. Carcinoma cuniculatum capitis. A variant of squamous cell carcinoma of the skin. Int J Dermatol 1984; 23: 67–69.

1078 Ruppe JP Jr. Verrucous carcinoma. Papillomatosis cutis carcinoides. Arch Dermatol 1981; 117: 184–185.

1079 Dogan G, Oram Y, Hazneci E et al. Three cases of verrucous carcinoma. Australas J Dermatol 1998; 39: 251–254.

1080 D'Aniello C, Grimaldi L, Meschino N et al. Verrucous 'cuniculatum' carcinoma of the sacral region. Br J Dermatol 2000; 143: 459–460.

1081 McKee PH, Wilkinson JD, Black MM, Whimster IW. Carcinoma (epithelioma) cuniculatum: a clinico-pathological study of nineteen cases and review of the literature. Histopathology 1981; 5: 425–436.

1082 Seehafer JR, Muller SA, Dicken CH, Masson JK. Bilateral verrucous carcinoma of the feet. Arch Dermatol 1979; 115: 1222–1223.

1083 Swanson NA, Taylor WB. Plantar verrucous carcinoma. Literature review and treatment by the Mohs' chemosurgery technique. Arch Dermatol 1980; 116: 794–797.

1084 Kathuria S, Rieker J, Jablokow VR, Van Den Broek H. Plantar verrucous carcinoma (epithelioma cuniculatum): case report with review of the literature. J Surg Oncol 1986; 31: 71–75.

1085 Kao GF, Graham JH, Helwig EB. Carcinoma cuniculatum (verrucous carcinoma of the skin). A clinicopathologic study of 46 cases with ultrastructural observations. Cancer 1982; 49: 2395–2403.

1086 Reingold IM, Smith BR, Graham JH. Epithelioma cuniculatum pedis, a variant of squamous cell carcinoma. Am J Clin Pathol 1978; 69: 561–565.

1087 Coldiron BM, Brown FC, Freeman RG. Epithelioma cuniculatum (carcinoma cuniculatum) of the thumb: a case report and literature review. J Dermatol Surg Oncol 1986; 12: 1150–1155.

1088 Cowen P. Epithelioma cuniculatum. Australas J Dermatol 1983; 24: 83–85.

1089 Brownstein MH, Shapiro L. Verrucous carcinoma of skin. Epithelioma cuniculatum plantare. Cancer 1976; 38: 1710–1716.

1090 Garven TC, Thelmo WL, Victor J, Pertschuk L. Verrucous carcinoma of the leg positive for human papillomavirus DNA 11 and 18: a case report. Hum Pathol 1991; 22: 1170–1173.

1091 Cuesta KH, Palazzo JP, Mittal KR. Detection of human papillomavirus in verrucous carcinoma from HIV-seropositive patients. J Cutan Pathol 1998; 25: 165–170.

1092 Miyamoto T, Sasaoka R, Hagari Y, Mihara M. Association of cutaneous verrucous carcinoma with human papillomavirus type 16. Br J Dermatol 1999; 140: 168–169.

1093 Lu S, Bodemer W, Ostwald C et al. Anal verrucous carcinoma and penile condylomata acuminata. Dermatology 2000; 200: 320–323.

1094 Wilkinson JD, McKee PH, Black MM et al. A case of carcinoma cuniculatum with coexistant viral plantar wart. Clin Exp Dermatol 1981; 6: 619–623.

1095 Aton JK, Kinstrey TE. Verrucous carcinoma arising from a burn scar. Int J Dermatol 1981; 20: 359–361.

1096 Headington JT. Verrucous carcinoma. Cutis 1978; 21: 207–211.

1097 Yip KMH, Lin-Yip J, Kumta S, Leung PC. Subcutaneous ("inverted") verrucous carcinoma with bone invasion. Am J Dermatopathol 1997; 19: 83–86.

1098 Prioleau PG, Santa Cruz DJ, Meyer JS, Bauer WC. Verrucous carcinoma. A light and electron microscopic, autoradiographic, and immunofluorescence study. Cancer 1980; 45: 2849–2857.

1099 Youngberg GA, Thornthwaite JT, Inoshita T, Franzus D. Cytologically malignant squamous-cell carcinoma arising in a verrucous carcinoma of the penis. J Dermatol Surg Oncol 1983; 9: 474–479.

1100 Kato N, Onozuka T, Yasukawa K et al. Penile hybrid verrucous-squamous carcinoma associated with a superficial inguinal lymph node metastasis. Am J Dermatopathol 2000; 22: 339–343.

1101 Takematsu H, Watanabe M, Matsunaga J et al. Verrucous carcinoma of the face with a massive neutrophil infiltrate. Analysis of leucocyte chemotactic activity in the tumour extract. Clin Exp Dermatol 1994; 19: 26–30.

1102 Read SI, Abell E. Pseudoepitheliomatous, keratotic, and micaceous balanitis. Arch Dermatol 1981; 117: 435–437.

1103 Jenkins D Jr, Jakubovic HR. Pseudoepitheliomatous, keratotic, micaceous balanitis. A clinical lesion with two histologic subsets: hyperplastic dystrophy and verrucous carcinoma. J Am Acad Dermatol 1988; 18: 419–422.

1104 Beljaards RC, Van Dijk E, Hausman R. Is pseudoepitheliomatous, micaceous and keratotic balanitis synonymous with verrucous carcinoma? Br J Dermatol 1987; 117: 641–646.

1105 Child FJ, Kim BK, Ganesan R et al. Verrucous carcinoma arising in pseudoepitheliomatous keratotic and micaceous balanitis, without evidence of human papillomavirus. Br J Dermatol 2000; 143: 183–187.

1106 Kim BK, Ganesan R, Herrington CS, Colonje E. Absence of human papillomavirus in verrucous carcinoma arising in pseudoepitheliomatous, keratotic, micaceous balanitis: a case report. J Cutan Pathol 1997; 24: 107 (abstract).

1107 Masouyé I, Kapanci Y. A third case of cutaneous papillary squamous cell carcinoma. J Cutan Pathol 1991; 18: 142–143.

1108 Cubilla AL, Velazques EF, Reuter VE et al. Warty (condylomatous) squamous cell carcinoma of the penis. A report of 11 cases and proposed classification of 'verruciform' penile tumors. Am J Surg Pathol 2000; 24: 505–512.

1109 Aroni K, Lazaris AC, Ioakim-Liossi A et al. Histological diagnosis of cutaneous "warty" carcinoma on a pre-existing HPV lesion. Acta Derm Venereol 2000; 80: 294–296.

1110 Bezerra ALR, Lopes A, Landman G et al. Clinicopathologic features and human papillomavirus DNA prevalence of warty and squamous cell carcinoma of the penis. Am J Surg Pathol 2001; 25: 673–678.

1111 Noel JC, Heenen M, Peny MO et al. Proliferating cell nuclear antigen distribution in verrucous carcinoma of the skin. Br J Dermatol 1995; 133: 868–873.

1112 Friedman KJ, Hood AF, Farmer ER. Cutaneous squamous cell carcinoma with mucinous metaplasia. J Cutan Pathol 1988; 15: 176–182.

1113 Weidner N, Foucar E. Adenosquamous carcinoma of the skin. Arch Dermatol 1985; 121: 775–779.

1114 Banks ER, Cooper PH. Adenosquamous carcinoma of the skin: a report of 10 cases. J Cutan Pathol 1991; 18: 227–234.

1115 Cubilla AL, Ayala MT, Barreto JE et al. Surface adenosquamous carcinoma of the penis. A report of three cases. Am J Surg Pathol 1996; 20: 156–160.

1116 Revercomb CH, Reitmeyer WJ, Pulitzer DR. Clear cell variant of mucoepidermoid carcinoma of the skin. J Am Acad Dermatol 1993; 29: 642–644.

1117 Landman G, Farmer ER. Primary cutaneous mucoepidermoid carcinoma: report of a case. J Cutan Pathol 1991; 18: 56–59.

1118 Yen A, Sanchez RL, Fearneyhough P et al. Mucoepidermoid carcinoma with cutaneous presentation. J Am Acad Dermatol 1997; 37: 340–342.

1119 Fernández-Figueras M-T, Fuente M-J, Bielsa I, Ferrándiz C. Low-grade mucoepidermoid carcinoma on the vermilion border of the lip. Am J Dermatopathol 1997; 19: 197–201.

1120 Underwood JW, Adcock LL, Okagaki T. Adenosquamous carcinoma of skin appendages (adenoid squamous cell carcinoma, pseudoglandular squamous cell carcinoma, adenoacanthoma of sweat gland of Lever) of the vulva. Cancer 1978; 42: 1851–1858.

1121 Dawson EK. Carcinosarcoma of the skin. J Roy Coll Surg Edinb 1972; 17: 242–246.

1122 Quay SC, Harrist TJ, Mihm MC Jr. Carcinosarcoma of the skin. Case report and review. J Cutan Pathol 1981; 8: 241–246.

1123 Tschen JA, Goldberg LH, McGavran MH. Carcinosarcoma of the skin. J Cutan Pathol 1988; 15: 31–35.

1124 Izaki S, Hirai A, Yoshizawa Y et al. Carcinosarcoma of the skin: immunohistochemical and electron microscopic observations. J Cutan Pathol 1993; 20: 272–278.

1125 Leen EJ, Saunders MP, Vollum DI, Keen CE. Carcinosarcoma of skin. Histopathology 1995; 26: 367–371.

1126 Patel NK, McKee PH, Smith NP, Fletcher CDM. Primary metaplastic carcinoma (carcinosarcoma) of the skin. Am J Dermatopathol 1997; 19: 363–372.

1127 Harrist TJ, Hassell LA, Bronstein BR, Mihm MC Jr. Follow-up of a previously reported carcinosarcoma of the skin. J Cutan Pathol 1983; 10: 359–360.

1128 Biernat W, Kordek R, Liberski PP, Woźniak L. Carcinosarcoma of the skin. Case report and literature review. Am J Dermatopathol 1996; 18: 614–619.

1129 Swanson SA, Cooper PH, Mills SE, Wick JR. Lymphoepithelioma-like carcinoma of the skin. Mod Pathol 1988; 1: 359–365.

1130 Walker AN, Kent D, Mitchell AR. Lymphoepithelioma-like carcinoma in the skin. J Am Acad Dermatol 1990; 22: 691–693.

1131 Ortiz-Frutos FJ, Zarco C, Gil R et al. Lymphoepithelioma-like carcinoma of the skin. Clin Exp Dermatol 1993; 18: 83–86.

1132 Jimenez F, Clark RE, Buchanan MD, Kamino H. Lymphoepithelioma-like carcinoma of the skin treated with Mohs micrographic surgery in combination with immune staining for cytokeratins. J Am Acad Dermatol 1995; 32: 878–881.

1133 Ferlicot S, Plantier F, Rethers L et al. Lymphoepithelioma-like carcinoma of the skin: a report of 3 Epstein–Barr virus (EBV)-negative additional cases. Immunohistochemical study of the stroma reaction. J Cutan Pathol 2000; 27: 306–311.

1134 Axelsen SM, Stamp IM. Lymphoepithelioma-like carcinoma of the vulvar region. Histopathology 1995; 27: 281–283.

1135 Carr KA, Bulengo-Ransby SM, Weiss LM, Nickoloff BJ. Lymphoepitheliomalike carcinoma of the skin. A case report with immunophenotypic analysis and in situ hybridization for Epstein–Barr viral genome. Am J Surg Pathol 1992; 16: 909–913.

1136 Requena L, Sánchez Yus E, Jiménez E, Roo E. Lymphoepithelioma-like carcinoma of the skin: a light-microscopic and immunohistochemical study. J Cutan Pathol 1994; 21: 541–548.

1137 Gillum PS, Morgan MB, Naylor MF, Everett MA. Absence of Epstein–Barr virus in lymphoepitheliomalike carcinoma of the skin. Polymerase chain reaction evidence and review of five cases. Am J Dermatopathol 1996; 18: 478–482.

1138 Lind AC, Breer WA, Wick MR. Lymphoepithelioma-like carcinoma of the skin with apparent origin in the epidermis – a pattern or an entity? A case report. Cancer 1999; 85: 884–890.

1139 Wick MR, Swanson PE, LeBoit PE et al. Lymphoepithelioma-like carcinoma of the skin with adnexal differentiation. J Cutan Pathol 1991; 18: 93–102.

1140 Shek TWH, Leung EYF, Luk ISC et al. Lymphoepithelioma-like carcinoma of the skin. Am J Dermatopathol 1996; 18: 637–644.

Miscellaneous 'tumors'

1141 Bart RS, Andrade R, Kopf AW. Cutaneous horns. A clinical and histopathologic study. Acta Derm Venereol 1968; 48: 507–515.

1142 Ingram NP. Cutaneous horns: a review and case history. Ann Roy Coll Surg Engl 1978; 60: 128–129.

1143 Mehregan AH. Cutaneous horn: a clinicopathologic study. Dermatol Digest 1965; 4: 45–54.

1144 Lowe FC, McCullough AR. Cutaneous horns of the penis: an approach to management. J Am Acad Dermatol 1985; 13: 369–373.

1145 Solivan GA, Smith KJ, James WD. Cutaneous horn of the penis: its association with squamous cell carcinoma and HPV-16 infection. J Am Acad Dermatol 1990; 23: 969–972.

1146 Hubler WR. Horrendous cutaneous horns. Cutis 1978; 22: 592–593.

1147 Yu RCH, Pryce DW, Macfarlane AW, Stewart TW. A histopathological study of 643 cutaneous horns. Br J Dermatol 1991; 124: 449–452.

1148 Sandbank M. Basal cell carcinoma at the base of cutaneous horn (cornu cutaneum). Arch Dermatol 1971; 104: 97–98.

1149 Khaitan BK, Sood A, Singh MK. Lichen simplex chronicus with a cutaneous horn. Acta Derm Venereol 1999; 79: 243.

1150 Gibbs RC, Hyman AB. Kaposi's sarcoma at the base of cutaneous horn. Arch Dermatol 1968; 98: 37–40.

1151 Lucky PA, Carter DM. Psoriasis presenting as cutaneous horns. J Am Acad Dermatol 1981; 5: 681–683.

1152 Brownstein MH. Trichilemmal horn: cutaneous horn showing trichilemmal keratinization. Br J Dermatol 1979; 100: 303–309.

1153 Nakamura K. Two cases of trichilemmal-like horn. Arch Dermatol 1984; 120: 386–387.

1154 Peteiro MC, Toribio J, Caeiro JL. Trichilemmal horn. J Cutan Pathol 1984; 11: 326–328.

1155 Kimura S. Trichilemmal keratosis (horn): a light and electron microscopic study. J Cutan Pathol 1983; 10: 59–68.

1156 Brownstein MH, Shapiro EE. Trichilemmomal horn: cutaneous horn overlying trichilemmoma. Clin Exp Dermatol 1979; 4: 59–63.

1157 Haneke E. 'Onycholemmal' horn. Dermatologica 1983; 167: 155–158.

1158 Kuokkanen K, Niemi K-M, Reunala T. Parakeratotic horns in a patient with myeloma. J Cutan Pathol 1987; 14: 54–58.

1159 Kocsard E, Ofner F. Keratoelastoidosis verrucosa of the extremities (stucco keratoses of the extremities). Dermatologica 1966; 133: 225–235.

1160 Kocsard E, Carter JJ. The papillomatous keratoses. The nature and differential diagnosis of stucco keratosis. Aust J Dermatol 1971; 12: 80–88.

1161 Shall L, Marks R. Stucco keratoses. A clinico-pathological study. Acta Derm Venereol 1991; 71: 258–261.

1162 Stockfleth E, Röwert J, Arndt R et al. Detection of human papillomavirus and response to topical 5% imiquimod in a case of stucco keratosis. Br J Dermatol 2000; 143: 846–850.

1163 Willoughby C, Soter NA. Stucco keratosis. Arch Dermatol 1972; 105: 859–861.

1164 Baran R, Kint A. Onychomatrixoma. Filamentous tufted tumour in the matrix of a funnel-shaped nail: a new entity (report of three cases). Br J Dermatol 1992; 126: 510–515.

1165 Fayol J, Baran R, Perrin C, Labrousse F. Onychomatricoma with misleading features. Acta Derm Venereol 2000; 80: 370–372.

1166 Raison-Peyron N, Alirezai M, Meunier L et al. Onychomatricoma: an unusual cause of nail bleeding. Clin Exp Dermatol 1998; 23: 138.

1167 Kint A, Baran R, Geerts ML. The onychomatricoma: an electron microscopic study. J Cutan Pathol 1997; 24: 183–188.

1168 Fraga GR, Patterson JW, McHargue CA. Onychomatricoma. Report of a case and its comparison with fibrokeratoma of the nailbed. Am J Dermatopathol 2001; 23: 36–40.

1169 Perrin Ch, Goettmann S, Baran R. Onychomatricoma: Clinical and histopathologic findings in 12 cases. J Am Acad Dermatol 1998; 39: 560–564.

1170 Hutchinson J. The crateriform ulcer of the face: a form of epithelial cancer. Trans Pathol Soc London 1889; 40: 275–281.

1171 Schwartz RA. Keratoacanthoma. J Am Acad Dermatol 1994; 30: 1–19.

1172 Sullivan JJ. Keratoacanthoma: the Australian experience. Australas J Dermatol 1997; 38 (Suppl): S36–S39.

1173 Choonhakarn C, Ackerman AB. Keratoacanthomas: a new classification based on morphologic findings and on anatomic site. Dermatopathology: Practical & Conceptual 2001; 7: 7–16.

1174 Chuang T-Y, Reizner GT, Elpern DJ et al. Keratoacanthoma in Kauai, Hawaii. The first documented incidence in a defined population. Arch Dermatol 1993; 129: 317–319.

1175 Cohen N, Plaschkes Y, Pevzner S, Loewenthal M. Review of 57 cases of keratoacanthoma. Plast Reconstr Surg 1972; 49: 138–142.

1176 Sullivan JJ, Colditz GA. Keratoacanthoma in a sub-tropical climate. Australas J Dermatol 1979; 20: 34–40.

1177 Godbolt AM, Sullivan JJ, Weedon D. Keratoacanthoma with perineural invasion: a report of 40 cases. Australas J Dermatol 2001; 42: 168–171.

1178 Rank BK, Dixon PL. Another look at keratoacanthoma. Aust NZ J Surg 1979; 49: 654–658.

1179 Friedman RP, Morales A, Burnham TK. Multiple cutaneous and conjunctival keratoacanthomata. Arch Dermatol 1965; 92: 162–165.

1180 Azaz B, Lustmann J. Keratoacanthoma of the lower lip. Oral Surg 1974; 38: 918–927.

1181 El-Hakim IE, Uthman MAE. Squamous cell carcinoma and keratoacanthoma of the lower lip associated with "Goza" and "Shisha" smoking. Int J Dermatol 1999; 38: 108–110.

1182 Svirsky JA, Freedman PD, Lumerman H. Solitary intraoral keratoacanthoma. Oral Surg 1977; 43: 116–119.

1183 Tkach JR, Thorne EG. Keratoacanthoma of the glans penis. Cutis 1979; 24: 615–616.

1184 Drut R. Solitary keratoacanthoma of the nipple in a male. Case report. J Cutan Pathol 1976; 3: 195–198.

1185 Sánchez Yus E, Simón P, Requena L et al. Solitary keratoacanthoma. A self-healing proliferation that frequently becomes malignant. Am J Dermatopathol 2000; 22: 305–310.

1186 Sullivan JJ, Donoghue MF, Kynaston B, McCaffrey JF. Multiple keratoacanthomas: report of four cases. Australas J Dermatol 1980; 21: 16–24.

1187 Schwartz RA. The keratoacanthoma: a review. J Surg Oncol 1979; 12: 305–317.

1188 Rapaport J. Giant keratoacanthoma of the nose. Arch Dermatol 1975; 111: 73–75.

1189 Wolinsky S, Silvers DN, Kohn SR. Spontaneous regression of a giant keratoacanthoma. J Dermatol Surg Oncol 1981; 7: 897–900.

1190 Grob JJ, Suzini F, Richard MA et al. Large keratoacanthomas treated with intralesional interferon alfa-2a. J Am Acad Dermatol 1993; 29: 237–241.

1191 Spieth K, Gille J, Kaufmann R. Intralesional methotrexate as effective treatment in solitary giant keratoacanthoma of the lower lip. Dermatology 2000; 200: 317–319.

1192 Weedon D, Barnett L. Keratoacanthoma centrifugum marginatum. Arch Dermatol 1975; 111: 1024–1026.

1193 Eliezri YD, Libow L. Multinodular keratoacanthoma. J Am Acad Dermatol 1988; 19: 826–830.

1194 Benest L, Kaplan RP, Salit R, Moy R. Keratoacanthoma centrifugum marginatum of the lower extremity treated with Mohs micrographic surgery. J Am Acad Dermatol 1994; 31: 501–502.

1195 de la Torre C, Losada A, Cruces MJ. Keratoacanthoma centrifugum marginatum: Treatment with intralesional bleomycin. J Am Acad Dermatol 1997; 37: 1010–1011.

1196 Stevanovic DV. Keratoacanthoma dyskeratoticum and segregans. Arch Dermatol 1965; 92: 666–669.

1197 Oliwiecki S, Peachey RDG, Bradfield JWB et al. Subungual keratoacanthoma — a report of four cases and review of the literature. Clin Exp Dermatol 1994; 19: 230–235.

1198 Keeney GL, Banks PM, Linscheid RL. Subungual keratoacanthoma. Report of a case and review of the literature. Arch Dermatol 1988; 124: 1074–1076.

1199 Allen CA, Stephens M, Steel WM. Subungual keratoacanthoma. Histopathology 1994; 25: 181–183.

1200 Stoll DM, Ackerman AB. Subungual keratoacanthoma. Am J Dermatopathol 1980; 2: 265–271.

1201 Shapiro L, Baraf CS. Subungual epidermoid carcinoma and keratoacanthoma. Cancer 1970; 25: 141–152.

1202 Baran R, Goettmann S. Distal digital keratoacanthoma: a report of 12 cases and a review of the literature. Br J Dermatol 1998; 139: 512–515.

1203 Ahmed AR. Multiple keratoacanthoma. Int J Dermatol 1980; 19: 496–499.

1204 Ferguson Smith J. A case of multiple primary squamous-celled carcinomata of the skin in a young man, with spontaneous healing. Br J Dermatol 1934; 46: 267–272.

1205 Grzybowski M. A case of peculiar generalized epithelial tumours of the skin. Br J Dermatol 1950; 62: 310–313.

1206 Sohn D, Chin TCM, Fellner MJ. Multiple keratoacanthomas associated with steatocystoma multiplex and rheumatoid arthritis. A case report. Arch Dermatol 1980; 116: 913–914.

1207 Rook A, Moffatt JL. Multiple self-healing epithelioma of Ferguson Smith type. Report of a case of unilateral distribution. Arch Dermatol 1956; 74: 525–532.

1208 Schwartz RA, Flieger DN, Saied NK. The Torre syndrome with gastrointestinal polyposis. Arch Dermatol 1980; 116: 312–314.

1209 Benoldi D, Alinovi A. Multiple persistent keratoacanthomas: treatment with oral etretinate. J Am Acad Dermatol 1984; 10: 1035–1038.

1210 Alexander JO'D, Lyell A. Multiple keratoacanthomas. J Am Acad Dermatol 1985; 12: 376.

1211 Jackson IT, Alexander JO'D, Verheyden CN. Self-healing squamous epithelioma: a family affair. Br J Plast Surg 1983; 36: 22–28.

1212 Winkelmann RK, Brown J. Generalized eruptive keratoacanthoma. Arch Dermatol 1968; 97: 615–623.

1213 Lloyd KM, Madsen DK, Lin PY. Grzybowski's eruptive keratoacanthoma. J Am Acad Dermatol 1989; 21: 1023–1024.

1214 Jaber PW, Cooper PH, Greer KE. Generalized eruptive keratoacanthoma of Grzybowski. J Am Acad Dermatol 1993; 29: 299–304.

1215 Kavanagh GM, Marshman G, Hanna MM. A case of Grzybowski's generalized eruptive keratoacanthomas. Australas J Dermatol 1995; 36: 83–85.

1216 Dessoukey MW, Omar MF, Abdel-Dayem H. Eruptive keratoacanthomas associated with immunosuppressive therapy in a patient with systemic lupus erythematosus. J Am Acad Dermatol 1997; 37: 478–480.

1217 Czubak A, Kalbarczyk K, Maciejowska E et al. [Keratoacanthoma eruptivum varietas Grzybowski: coexistence with keratoacanthoma marginatum-centrifugum and typical solitary tumor]. Przegl Dermatol 1995; 82: 413–419.

1218 Consigli JE, González ME, Morsino R et al. Generalized eruptive keratoacanthoma (Grzybowski variant). Br J Dermatol 2000; 142: 800–803.

1219 Grine RC, Hendrix JD, Greer KE. Generalized eruptive keratoacanthoma of Grzybowski: Response to cyclophosphamide. J Am Acad Dermatol 1997; 36: 786–787.

1220 Higuchi M, Tanikawa E, Nomura H et al. Multiple keratoacanthomas with peculiar manifestations and course. J Am Acad Dermatol 1990; 23: 389–392.

1221 Frank TL, Maguire HC Jr, Greenbaum SS. Multiple painful keratoacanthomas. Int J Dermatol 1996; 35: 648–650.

1222 Guitart J, Gordon K. Keratoacanthomas and lymphomatoid papulosis. Am J Dermatopathol 1998; 20: 430–432.

1223 Fathizadeh A, Medenica MM, Soltani K et al. Aggressive keratoacanthoma and internal malignant neoplasm. Arch Dermatol 1982; 118: 112–114.

1224 Inoshita T, Youngberg GA. Keratoacanthomas associated with cervical squamous cell carcinoma. Arch Dermatol 1984; 120: 123–124.

1225 Snider BL, Benjamin DR. Eruptive keratoacanthoma and internal malignant neoplasm. Arch Dermatol 1981; 117: 788–790.

1226 Housholder MS, Zeligman I. Sebaceous neoplasms associated with visceral carcinomas. Arch Dermatol 1980; 116: 61–64.

1227 Halleng KC, Honchel R, Pittelkow MR, Thibodeau SN. Microsatellite instability in keratoacanthoma. Cancer 1995; 76: 1765–1771.

1228 Kumar V, Kumar H, Thappa DM, Ratnakar C. Multiple keratoacanthoma with neonatal onset in a girl. Pediatr Dermatol 1999; 16: 411–412.

1229 Waring AJ, Takata M, Rehman I, Rees JL. Loss of heterozygosity analysis of keratoacanthoma reveals multiple differences from cutaneous squamous cell carcinoma. Br J Cancer 1996; 73: 649–653.

1230 Agarwal M, Chander R, Karmakar S, Walia R. Multiple familial keratoacanthoma of Witten and Zak — a report of three siblings. Dermatology 1999; 198: 396–399.

1231 Hsi ED, Svoboda-Newman SM, Stern RA et al. Detection of human papillomavirus DNA in keratoacanthomas by polymerase chain reaction. Am J Dermatopathol 1997; 19: 10–15.

1232 Payne D, Newman C, Tyring S. Human papillomavirus DNA in nonanogenital keratoacanthoma and squamous cell carcinoma of patients with HIV infection. J Am Acad Dermatol 1995; 33: 1047–1049.

1233 Stockfleth E, Meinke B, Arndt R et al. Identification of DNA sequences of both genital and cutaneous HPV types in a small number of keratoacanthomas of nonimmunosuppressed patients. Dermatology 1999; 198: 122–125.

1234 Ghadially FN, Barton BW, Kerridge DF. The etiology of keratoacanthoma. Cancer 1963; 16: 603–610.

1235 Dufresne RG, Marrero GM, Robinson-Bostom L. Seasonal presentation of keratoacanthomas in Rhode Island. Br J Dermatol 1997; 136: 227–229.

1236 Bart RS, Lagin S. Keratoacanthoma following pneumococcal vaccination: a case report. J Dermatol Surg Oncol 1983; 9: 381–382.

1237 Shellito JE, Samet JM. Keratoacanthoma as a complication of arterial puncture for blood gases. Int J Dermatol 1982; 21: 349.

1238 Tamir G, Morgenstern S, Ben-Amitay D et al. Synchronous appearance of keratoacanthomas in burn scar and skin graft donor site shortly after injury. J Am Acad Dermatol 1999; 40: 870–871.

1239 Sina B, Adrian RM. Multiple keratoacanthomas possibly induced by psoralens and ultraviolet A photochemotherapy. J Am Acad Dermatol 1983; 9: 686–688.

1240 Rosen T. Keratoacanthoma arising within a linear epidermal nevus. J Dermatol Surg Oncol 1982; 8: 878–880.

1241 Wilkinson SM, Tan CY, Smith AG. Keratoacanthoma arising within organoid naevi. Clin Exp Dermatol 1991; 16: 58–60.

1242 Okuyama R, Takahashi K, Ohi T, Tagami H. Keratoacanthoma developing in prurigo nodularis treated with cryotherapy. Dermatology 1997; 194: 290–292.

1243 Sánchez Yus E, Requena L. Keratoacanthoma within a superficial spreading malignant melanoma in situ. J Cutan Pathol 1991; 18: 288–292.

1244 Maddin WS, Wood WS. Multiple keratoacanthomas and squamous cell carcinomas occurring at psoriatic treatment sites. J Cutan Pathol 1979; 6: 96–100.

1245 Allen JV, Callen JP. Keratoacanthomas arising in hypertrophic lichen planus. Arch Dermatol 1981; 117: 519–521.

1246 Sakai H, Minami M, Satoh E et al. Keratoacanthoma developing on a pigmented patch in incontinentia pigmenti. Dermatology 2000; 200: 258–261.

1247 Fisher ER, McCoy MM, Wechsler HL. Analysis of histopathologic and electron microscopic determinants of keratoacanthoma and squamous cell carcinoma. Cancer 1972; 29: 1387–1397.

1248 Blessing K, Al Nafussi A, Gordon PM. The regressing keratoacanthoma. Histopathology 1994; 24: 381–384.

1249 Mikhail GR. Squamous cell carcinoma diagnosed as keratoacanthoma. Cutis 1974; 13: 378–382.

1250 Santa Cruz DJ, Clausen K. Atypical sweat duct hyperplasia accompanying keratoacanthoma. Dermatologica 1977; 154: 156–160.

1251 Lapins NA, Helwig EB. Perineural invasion by keratoacanthoma. Arch Dermatol 1980; 116: 791–793.

1252 Janecka IP, Wolff M, Crikelair GF, Cosman B. Aggressive histological features of keratoacanthoma. J Cutan Pathol 1977; 4: 342–348.

1253 Cooper PH, Wolfe JT III. Perioral keratoacanthomas with extensive perineural invasion and intravenous growth. Arch Dermatol 1988; 124: 1397–1401.

1254 Calonje E, Wilson Jones E. Intravascular spread of keratoacanthoma. An alarming but benign phenomenon. Am J Dermatopathol 1992; 14: 414–417.

1255 Burgdorf WHC, Pitha J, Fahmy A. Muir–Torre syndrome. Histologic spectrums of sebaceous proliferations. Am J Dermatopathol 1986; 8: 202–208.

1256 Kern WH. McCray MK. The histopathologic differentiation of keratoacanthoma and squamous cell carcinoma of the skin. J Cutan Pathol 1980; 7: 318–325.

1257 Cribier B, Asch P-H, Grosshans E. Differentiating squamous cell carcinoma from keratoacanthoma using histopathological criteria. Is it possible? A study of 296 cases. Dermatology 1999; 199: 208–212.

1258 King DF, Barr RJ. Intraepithelial elastic fibers and intracytoplasmic glycogen: diagnostic aids in differentiating keratoacanthoma from squamous cell carcinoma. J Cutan Pathol 1980; 7: 140–148.

1259 Jordan RCK, Kahn HJ, From L, Jambrosic J. Immunohistochemical demonstration of actinically damaged elastic fibers in keratoacanthomas: an aid in diagnosis. J Cutan Pathol 1991; 18: 81–86.

1260 Smoller BR, Kwan TH, Said JW, Banks-Schlegel S. Keratoacanthoma and squamous cell carcinoma of the skin. Immunohistochemical localization of involucrin and keratin proteins. J Am Acad Dermatol 1986; 14: 226–234.

1261 Suo Z, Holm R, Nesland JM. Squamous cell carcinomas. An immunohistochemical study of cytokeratins and involucrin in primary and metastatic tumours. Histopathology 1993; 23: 45–54.

1262 Binder M, Steiner A, Mossbacher U et al. Estimation of the volume-weighted mean nuclear volume discriminates keratoacanthoma from squamous cell carcinoma. Am J Dermatopathol 1998; 20: 453–458.

1263 Kannon G, Park HK. Utility of peanut agglutinin (PNA) in the diagnosis of squamous cell carcinoma and keratoacanthoma. Am J Dermatopathol 1990; 12: 31–36.

1264 Ahmed NU, Ueda M, Ichihashi M. Increased levels of c-erbB-2/neu/HER-2 protein in cutaneous squamous cell carcinoma. Br J Dermatol 1997; 136: 908–912.

1265 Airola K, Johansson N, Kariniemi A-L et al. Human collagenase-3 is expressed in malignant squamous epithelium of the skin. J Invest Dermatol 1997; 109: 225–231.

1266 Asch P-H, Basset P, Roos M et al. Expression of stromelysin 3 in keratoacanthoma and squamous cell carcinoma. Am J Dermatopathol 1999; 21: 146–150.

1267 Ahmed NU, Ueda M, Ichihashi M. p21$^{WAF1/CIP1}$ expression in non-melanoma skin tumors. J Cutan Pathol 1997; 24: 223–227.

1268 Phillips P, Helm KF. Proliferating cell nuclear antigen distribution in keratoacanthoma and squamous cell carcinoma. J Cutan Pathol 1993; 20: 424–428.

1269 Cain CT, Niemann TH, Argenyi ZB. Keratoacanthoma versus squamous cell carcinoma. An immunohistochemical reappraisal of p53 protein and proliferating cell nuclear antigen expression in keratoacanthoma-like tumors. Am J Dermatopathol 1995; 17: 324–331.

1270 Skálová A, Michal M. Patterns of cell proliferation in actinic keratoacanthomas and squamous cell carcinomas of the skin. Am J Dermatopathol 1995; 17: 332–334.

1271 Tsuji T. Keratoacanthoma and squamous cell carcinoma: study of PCNA and Le^Y expression. J Cutan Pathol 1997; 24: 409–415.

1272 Kerschmann RL, McCalmont TH, LeBoit PE. p53 oncoprotein expression and proliferation index in keratoacanthoma and squamous cell carcinoma. Arch Dermatol 1994; 130: 181–186.

1273 Borkowski A, Bennett WP, Jones RT et al. Quantitative image analysis of p53 protein accumulation in keratoacanthomas. Am J Dermatopathol 1995; 17: 335–338.

1274 Pilch H, Weiss J, Heubner C, Heine M. Differential diagnosis of keratoacanthomas and squamous cell carcinomas: diagnostic value of DNA image cytometry and p53 expression. J Cutan Pathol 1994; 21: 507–513.

1275 Lee Y-S, Teh M. p53 expression in pseudoepitheliomatous hyperplasia, keratoacanthoma, and squamous cell carcinoma of skin. Cancer 1994; 73: 2317–2323.

1276 Perez MI, Robins P, Biria S et al. p53 oncoprotein expression and gene mutations in some keratoacanthomas. Arch Dermatol 1997; 133: 189–193.

1277 Goldenhersh MA, Olsen TG. Invasive squamous cell carcinoma initially diagnosed as a giant keratoacanthoma. J Am Acad Dermatol 1984; 10: 372–378.

1278 Rook A, Whimster I. Keratoacanthoma — a thirty year retrospect. Br J Dermatol 1979; 100: 41–47.

1279 Requena L, Romero E, Sanchez M et al. Aggressive keratoacanthoma of the eyelid: 'malignant' keratoacanthoma or squamous cell carcinoma? J Dermatol Surg Oncol 1990; 16: 564–568.

1280 Hodak E, Jones RE, Ackerman AB. Solitary keratoacanthoma is a squamous-cell carcinoma: three examples with metastases. Am J Dermatopathol 1993; 15: 332–342.

1281 Cheville JC, Bromley C, Argenyi ZB. Trisomy 7 in keratoacanthoma and squamous cell carcinoma detected by fluorescence in-situ hybridization. J Cutan Pathol 1995; 22: 546–550.

1282 Kligman LH, Kligman AM. Histogenesis and progression of ultraviolet light-induced tumors in hairless mice. J Natl Cancer Inst 1981; 67: 1289–1293.

1283 Kingman J, Callen JP. Keratoacanthoma. A clinical study. Arch Dermatol 1984; 120: 736–740.

1284 Grossniklaus HE, Wojno TH, Yanoff M, Font RL. Invasive keratoacanthoma of the eyelid and ocular adnexa. Ophthalmology 1996; 103: 937–941.

1285 Piscioli F, Zumiani G, Boi S, Christofolini M. A gigantic, metastasizing keratoacanthoma. Report of a case and discussion on classification. Am J Dermatopathol 1984; 6: 123–129.

1286 Patel A, Halliday GM, Cooke BE, Barnetson RStC. Evidence that regression in keratoacanthoma is immunologically mediated: a comparison with squamous cell carcinoma. Br J Dermatol 1994; 131: 789–798.

1287 Korenberg R, Penneys NS, Kowalczyk A, Nadji M. Quantitation of S100 protein-positive cells in inflamed and non-inflamed keratoacanthoma and squamous cell carcinoma. J Cutan Pathol 1988; 15: 104–108.

1288 Sleater JP, Beers BB, Stephens CA, Hendricks JB. Keratoacanthoma: a deficient squamous cell carcinoma? Study of *bcl-2* expression. J Cutan Pathol 1994; 21: 514–519.

1289 Hu W, Cook T, Oh CW, Penneys NS. Expression of the cyclin-dependent kinase inhibitor p27 in keratoacanthoma. J Am Acad Dermatol 2000; 42: 473–475.

1290 Jensen P, Clausen OPF, Bryne M. Differences in sialyl-Tn antigen expression between keratoacanthomas and cutaneous squamous cell carcinomas. J Cutan Pathol 1999; 26: 183–189.

Lentigines, nevi and melanomas

INTRODUCTION

The histopathological diagnosis of pigmented skin tumors is an important area of dermatopathology. It should be noted that melanin pigment may also be present in skin tumors other than nevocellular nevi and malignant melanomas. For instance, seborrheic keratoses, basal cell carcinomas and, rarely, squamous cell carcinomas, schwannomas and dermatofibrosarcoma protuberans may contain melanin. Furthermore, there is a group of dermatoses characterized by variable patterns of hyperpigmentation covering, at times, significant areas of the body.[1] This chapter is devoted to proliferative disturbances of the melanocyte–nevus-cell system. Other disorders of pigmentation are considered in Chapter 10 (pp. 321–334).

LESIONS WITH BASAL MELANOCYTE PROLIFERATION

Lesions with basal melanocyte proliferation are characterized by basal hyperpigmentation and an increase in melanocytes in the basal layer. The melanocytes are usually single and cytologically normal. Small junctional nests are sometimes seen. Epidermal acanthosis and the presence of melanophages in the papillary dermis are additional histological features that are usually seen in entities within this group.

LENTIGO SIMPLEX (SIMPLE LENTIGO)

The simple lentigo is a brown to black, sharply circumscribed and usually uniformly pigmented macule, measuring a few millimeters in diameter. It may be found anywhere on the body surface.[2]

The term 'labial melanotic macule' is now used for a clinically similar lesion on the lip that was previously referred to as a lentigo (see below).

Histopathology

There is variable basal hyperpigmentation with an increased number of single melanocytes in the basal layer. There is usually acanthosis, with regular elongation of the rete ridges. The papillary dermis may contain a sparse lymphohistiocytic infiltrate, including scattered melanophages. Some lesions evolve with the formation of nests of melanocytes in the junctional zone,[3] but it is best to designate these lesions with mixed features of a lentigo and a junctional or compound nevus as lentiginous nevi.

MULTIPLE LENTIGINES

Various syndromes characterized by the presence of numerous lentigines developing in childhood or adolescence have been described.[1,2] The pigmented macules may be unilateral in distribution,[4-7] or generalized,[8-10] the latter form sometimes being a marker of an underlying developmental defect (see below).[11] The terms 'lentiginous mosaicism' and 'partial lentiginosis' have been used for cases with regional or segmental lesions,[1] but the older term 'lentiginosis profusa' is still used sometimes for cases of multiple lentigines with or without associated abnormalities. Partial (segmental) lentiginosis differs from speckled lentiginous nevus (nevus spilus) by occurring on normal skin, in contrast to the background of macular pigmentation seen in speckled lentiginous nevus.[12-15] Multiple lentigines are associated with internal manifestations in several rare syndromes: the LEOPARD syndrome, the NAME and LAMB syndromes, and centrofacial lentiginosis. In the Peutz–Jeghers

syndrome (see p. 331) there are conflicting views as to whether the lesions are lentiginous (with an increased number of melanocytes) on histological examination.

The LEOPARD syndrome is inherited as an autosomal dominant trait.[16,17] It is characterized by lentigines (L), electrocardiographic conduction defects (E), ocular hypertelorism (O), pulmonary stenosis (P), gonadal hypoplasia (A), retarded growth (R) and nerve deafness (D). Hyperplastic skin may be present.[18] These features are not all present in every case. Sporadic cases also occur.[19]

The NAME syndrome is another rare cardiocutaneous syndrome.[20] Its features include nevi (N) as well as lentigines, ephelides and blue nevi, atrial myxoma (A), myxoid tumors of the skin (M) and endocrine abnormalities (E). A similar syndrome has been reported as the LAMB syndrome: mucocutaneous lentigines (L), atrial myxoma (A), mucocutaneous myxomas (M) and blue nevi (B).[21] The NAME and LAMB syndromes are now referred to collectively as Carney's syndrome,[22,23] although this properly refers to multiple lentigines and blue nevi, melanotic schwannoma, myxomas and endocrine overactivity.[24] Lentigines have been reported in association with an atrial myxoma,[11] with blue nevi[24] and with segmental achromic nevi.[6,25]

LABIAL AND GENITAL MELANOTIC MACULES

The *labial melanotic macule* is a recently delineated pigmented lesion of the lip that may occur in up to 3% of the population.[26] Previously, lesions of this type were classified as lentigos. It presents as a tan-brown to brown-black macule, 2–15 mm in diameter, on the vermilion border of the lip, particularly the lower.[27-29] Multiple lesions may be present.[26] They tend to remain stable and unchanged when followed over a long period. Oral and labial melanotic macules appear to be more common in patients infected with the human immunodeficiency virus.[30]

The term '*genital melanotic macule (genital lentiginosis)*' has been suggested for similar lesions, up to 2 cm in diameter, that develop uncommonly on the penis and vulva.[31-33] These are sometimes referred to as 'penile melanosis' and 'melanosis of the vulva', respectively.[34,35] The oral melanoacanthoma (mucosal melanotic macule – reactive type, oral melanoacanthosis) is sometimes included in this group of lesions.[36-39]

Histopathology

There is prominent hyperpigmentation of the basal layer which is accentuated at the tip of the rete ridges (Fig. 32.1). There is only mild acanthosis, in contrast to the regular elongation of the rete ridges found in the lentigo simplex. Melanocytes are said to be normal in number; in some cases they have prominent dendritic processes containing melanin pigment, which can be seen between the keratinocytes of the lower epidermis. These melanocytes are HMB-45 negative.[29] Melanophages are present in the papillary dermis in about half of the cases.

Genital lesions are histologically similar, although melanophages are almost invariably present.[40] The oral melanoacanthoma is characterized by dendritic melanocytes of benign morphology at all levels of the acanthotic epithelium, in contrast to their basal location in lentigos and labial melanotic macules.

The lesions reported as volar melanotic macules appear to be heterogeneous with some resembling post-inflammatory pigmentation. They were reported as the volar counterpart of mucosal melanotic macules.[41]

SOLAR (SENILE) LENTIGO

Solar lentigos are dark-brown to black macules, 3–12 mm or more in diameter, which develop on the sun-exposed skin of middle-aged to elderly patients.

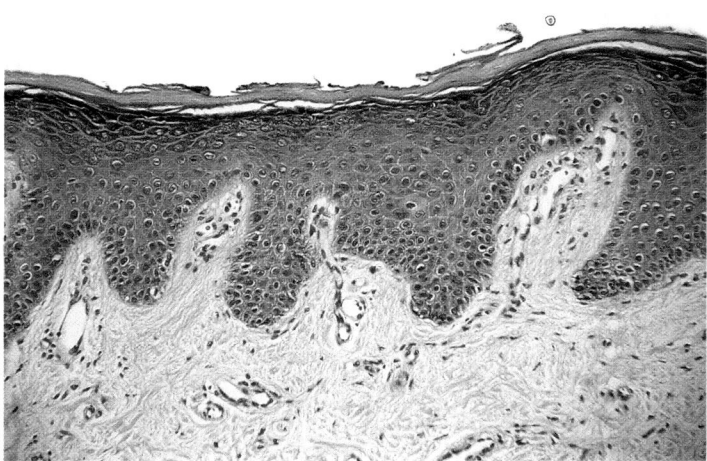

Fig. 32.1 **Labial melanotic macule.** There is basal pigmentation limited to the tips of the rete pegs. Melanocytes appear normal. This entity is considered here because it was regarded in the past as a variant of lentigo. (H & E)

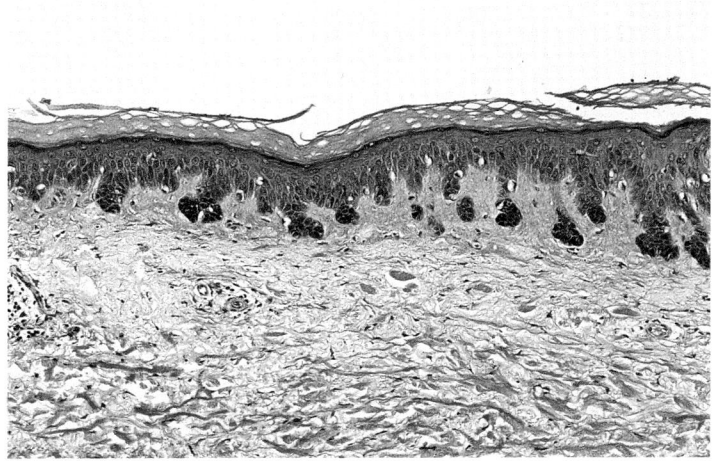

Fig. 32.2 **Solar lentigo.** There is hyperpigmentation of the bulbous rete ridges. Lesions on the face do not have bulbous downgrowths. (H & E)

They are often multiple. The term 'ink-spot' lentigo is sometimes used for a clinical variant characterized by its black color and a markedly irregular outline, resembling a spot of ink on the skin.[42] Lesions may increase slowly in size over many years. Solar lentigos may evolve into the reticulate form of seborrheic keratosis, such lesions developing a slightly verrucose surface.[43]

Solar lentigos increase with age. They are related to freckling during adolescence and frequent sunburns during adulthood.[44,45] They appear to be a common precursor lesion of malignant melanoma in patients with xeroderma pigmentosum.[46]

Histopathology

The solar lentigo is characterized by elongation of the rete ridges, which are usually short and bulb-like (Fig. 32.2). As they extend more deeply into the dermis, finger-like projections form and connect with adjacent rete ridges to form a reticulate pattern resembling that seen in the reticulate type of seborrheic keratosis.[43,47] Rete ridge hyperplasia is less conspicuous, and may be absent, in lesions from the face.[48] In addition, there is basal hyperpigmentation which is sometimes quite heavy. There is an increased number of melanocytes, particularly at the bases of the clubbed and budding rete ridges;[47] sometimes the increase is not appreciated on casual examination. Variable numbers of melanophages are present in the papillary dermis. When solar lentigos undergo regression they develop a heavy lichenoid inflammatory cell infiltrate in the papillary dermis. These features are referred to as a lichen planus-like keratosis (see p. 40).

The author has seen a number of cases of lentigo maligna (Hutchinson's melanotic freckle) developing in solar lentigos. The presence of transitional features suggests that this is not a 'collision phenomenon'. Others have also documented this transformation.[46,49]

Electron microscopy

The melanosome complexes are much larger than those found in non-involved skin.[47]

LENTIGINOUS NEVUS

The lentiginous nevus is a neglected entity which appears to represent the evolution of a lentigo simplex into a junctional and sometimes a compound nevus.[3] It has also been called nevoid lentigo and nevus incipiens.[50] They are

well-circumscribed, sometimes deeply pigmented, often quite small lesions, found most frequently on the trunk of adults between the ages of 20 and 40 years.

Histopathology

At the advancing edge there is a lentiginous proliferation of melanocytes resembling that seen in a simple lentigo, whereas in the more central areas there is junctional nest formation and sometimes a small number of mature intradermal nevus cell nests as well. Elongation of the rete pegs and some melanophages in the papillary dermis are usually present.

The **hypermelanotic nevus** appears to be a closely related entity characterized by dark brown to black macules or papules, often on the back, and prominent melanin pigmentation histologically.[51] The pigment is present in the stratum corneum, in keratinocytes and nevomelanocytes in the basal layer, and in melanophages in the upper dermis.[51]

SPECKLED LENTIGINOUS NEVUS (NEVUS SPILUS)

Speckled lentiginous nevus is the preferred term for a lesion composed of small dark hyperpigmented speckles, superimposed on a tan-brown macular background.[50,52] Lesions are present at birth or appear in childhood.[53] As such, they have been regarded as a variant of congenital nevus.[54] They may have a zosteriform or regional distribution. Rarely, lesions are widespread.[55] Similar cases have been reported as nevus spilus,[56] but this does not accord with the original use of this term. The term 'zosteriform lentiginous nevus' has also been used synonymously, but it is sometimes used for speckled lesions without the background macular pigmentation.[57,58] These latter lesions are best regarded as variants of partial lentiginosis. However, the occurrence of cases of speckled pigmentation in which only part of the lesion has a background of macular pigmentation suggests that overlap cases between speckled lentiginous nevus (nevus spilus) and partial (segmental) lentiginosis occur.[59] Finally, the term 'spotted grouped pigmented nevus' has been used for a closely related lesion.[60] Malignant melanoma has been reported as a very rare complication.[61–68]

Speckled lentiginous nevus (nevus spilus) is one of the components of at least two of the subtypes of phakomatosis pigmentovascularis, which combines vascular and pigmentary malformations (see p. 819).[69]

Histopathology

Whereas the background pigmented area resembles lentigo simplex, the speckled areas usually show the features of a lentiginous nevus with lentigo-like areas progressing to junctional and even small compound nevi.[50,70] An associated old neurotized nevus was present in one case,[71] while in another the dermal component resembled a congenital and a blue nevus.[72]

Atypia of the intraepidermal melanocytes is an uncommon change in speckled lentiginous nevi; it may be a predisposing factor for the development of a malignant melanoma, a rare complication.[61]

PUVA LENTIGO

Freckles,[73] lentigines[74,75] and nevus spilus-like pigmentation[75] have been reported in patients treated with psoralens and ultraviolet-A radiation (PUVA), particularly in sun-protected sites such as the buttock.[77] Palmoplantar involvement has also been recorded.[78] There is confusion in terminology in the literature concerning PUVA-induced pigmentary changes.[79] Clinically similar lesions have resulted from exposure to ultraviolet-A radiation, without concomitant psoralen administration, in tanning parlors.[80,81] Similar lesions have developed following accidental exposure to ionizing radiation.[82]

Histopathology

Many of the lentigines have relatively large, even cytologically atypical, melanocytes in the basal layer (Fig. 32.3).[83] Melanoma in situ change and malignant melanoma have also been reported.[84,85] Atypical melanocytes may develop in pre-existing nevi exposed to ultraviolet light in an experimental situation.[86] PUVA-exposed skin that is without clinically evident lesions may also show melanocytic atypia.[87] Many of the lesions are simply freckles without any increase in melanocytes.

SCAR LENTIGO

The development of a pigmented lesion in the surgical scar of a previously excised pigmented lesion can give rise to clinical concern.[88,89] Similar lesions have also been reported in surgical scars, unrelated to previous nevomelanocytic lesions.[90] In a recent study, three types of clinical pigmentation were observed: lentigo-like lesions, pigmented streaks, and diffuse pigmentation in grafts.[91] It has been suggested that the scar tissue is responsible for the induction of melanocytic hyperplasia and/or hyperfunction.[91]

Histopathology

Two different patterns can be seen. In one there is lentiginous epidermal hyperplasia, hyperpigmentation, and a normal or moderately increased number of melanocytes. In the other there is melanocytic hyperplasia without accompanying epidermal hyperplasia.[91]

MELANOCYTIC NEVI

Melanocytic nevi are occasionally present at birth (congenital melanocytic nevi), but the majority appear in childhood or adolescence (acquired melanocytic nevi).[92,93] Congenital nevi show some distinct morphological features and are therefore considered separately (see p. 815). Various studies have been undertaken in recent years to ascertain the prevalence of nevi in certain population groups and the role of environmental factors in their etiology. All of these studies have concluded that sun exposure in childhood predisposes to the development of more nevi, some of which may be larger

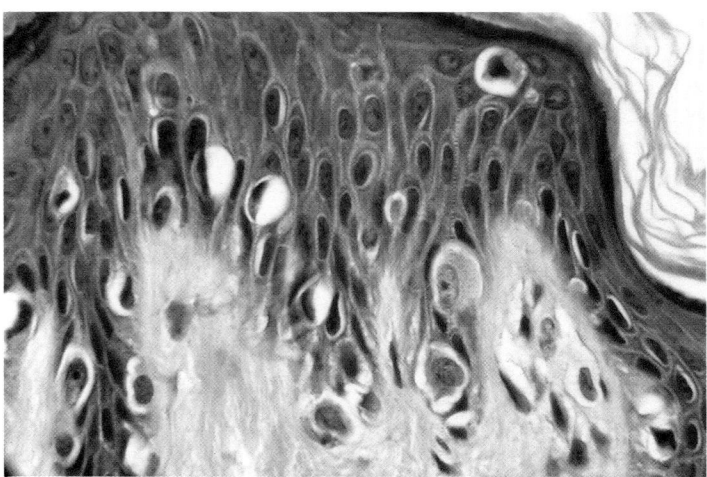

Fig. 32.3 **PUVA lentigo** showing an increase in basal melanocytes, some of which are large and mildly atypical. (H & E)

than usual or have atypical features.[94–98] Nevi are more prevalent in boys than girls, in white children than in other ethnic groups,[94] and in children with fair skin and blond or red hair.[99] Whereas both immunosuppression and solar radiation are associated with increased numbers of nevi in children, this may not be the case in adults.[100–107] Experimentally, ultraviolet radiation produces transient melanocytic activation.[108]

Acquired melanocytic nevi undergo progressive maturation with increasing age of the lesion. Initially, the acquired melanocytic nevus is a flat macular lesion (junctional nevus) in which nests of proliferating melanocytes are confined to the dermoepidermal junction. The lesion becomes progressively more elevated as nests of nevus cells extend ('drop off') into the underlying dermis (compound nevus). Unna's concept of *Abtropfung* ('dropping off') has been challenged in recent times,[109,110] although the higher reactivity of proliferating cell nuclear antigen (PCNA) in junctional and compound nevi than in intradermal nevi supports the epidermal origin of acquired melanocytic nevi.[111] The MDP (melanocyte differentiation pathway) hypothesis is an attempt to explain the origin of melanocytes and their subsequent upward migration into the epidermis, the reverse of *Abtropfung*.[112,113] With further maturation junctional activity ceases and the lesion is composed only of dermal nevus cells (intradermal nevus). Intradermal nevi usually become progressively less pigmented over the ensuing years. This process of maturation is somewhat variable in duration, but most nevi are intradermal in type by early adult life. However, nevi on the palms of the hands, soles of the feet and the genital region are often slow to mature, and remain as junctional nevi for some time. This feature gave rise in the past to the erroneous belief that nevi in these sites were prone to malignant change. Some nevi may increase in size during pregnancy and adolescence.[114–117] They do not appear to change as a consequence of growth hormone therapy.[118,119] However, nevi may change in their dermatoscopic appearance (and histology) following ultraviolet radiation.[120]

It has been customary to refer to the cells comprising a melanocytic nevus as 'nevus cells' or 'nevomelanocytes'. Nevus cells are melanocytes which have lost their long dendritic processes, probably as an adaptive response associated with the formation of nests of cells. As this change cannot usually be appreciated in hematoxylin and eosin-stained preparations, it has been suggested that all cells in melanocytic nevi (epidermal and dermal) should be referred to as melanocytes.[121] Many nevi appear to be clonal.[122] Interestingly, the 'maturation' of melanocytes is accompanied by an alteration in the antigens they express. Cells in the junctional layer contain S100 protein and sometimes one or more of the melanoma-associated antigens (including NK1/C-3 and HMB-45), but usually only S100 protein is expressed by dermal nevus cells.[123]

With advancing age there is a progressive decrease in the number of nevi. Whereas the number of nevi in young adults varies from approximately 15 to 40, this decreases markedly over the age of 50 years.[124–126] It has been proposed that this comes about by progressive fibrosis of nevi, and in some cases by transformation into skin tags which may self-amputate, but others have not confirmed this theory.[127] The presence of large numbers of nevi is a risk factor for the development of malignant melanoma.[128]

Rarely, multiple nevi may develop in a patient over the course of several months. An underlying bullous disease, including hereditary epidermolysis bullosa, has sometimes been present in these cases of eruptive nevi.[129–131] Eruptive nevi have also followed exposure to sulfur mustard gas used in warfare.[132]

It is generally accepted that all nevi be submitted for histological examination for medicolegal reasons. In a recent study, 2.3% of clinically diagnosed benign nevi were microscopically diagnosed as malignant tumors, either melanomas or basal or squamous cell carcinomas.[133]

JUNCTIONAL NEVUS

The junctional melanocytic nevus is a well-circumscribed brown to black macule, which may clinically resemble a lentigo. It may develop anywhere on the body surface. Usually it appears during childhood or early adolescence, and matures with time into a compound nevus and later into an intradermal nevus. The small 'active junctional nevus' reported by Eng in adolescents has some resemblance to the lesion described earlier as a lentiginous nevus.[134]

Histopathology

The junctional nevus is composed of discrete nests of melanocytes/nevus cells at the dermoepidermal junction, usually located on the rete ridges, which often show some accentuation. The cells are oval to cuboidal in shape, with clear cytoplasm containing a variable amount of melanin pigment. Mitoses are rare or absent. Nests of nevus cells sometimes bulge into the underlying dermis, which may contain a few melanophages and a sparse lymphohistiocytic infiltrate.[135]

Junctional nevi of the nail matrix are one cause of **longitudinal melanonychia**, a characteristic pattern of pigmentation of nail. This pattern of pigmentation can be produced by lesions that resemble lentigos, ephelides, acanthomas, seborrheic keratoses and even malignant melanomas.[136,137]

COMPOUND NEVUS

Compound melanocytic nevi are most common in children and adolescents. They vary from minimally elevated lesions to dome-shaped or polypoid configurations. They may be tan or dark brown in color.

Histopathology

Compound nevi have both junctional nests and an intradermal component of nevus cells (Fig. 32.4). Whereas the cells in the upper dermis are usually cuboidal, with melanin pigment in the cytoplasm, deeper cells are often smaller and contain less melanin. Apoptosis is sometimes seen in the deeper cells.[138] The nevus cells are arranged in orderly nests or cords. The overlying epidermis may be flat, show some acanthosis, or have a seborrheic keratosis-like appearance, even with horn cysts. These nevi have been called 'keratotic melanocytic nevi'.[139] These papillomatous nevi are more common in females;

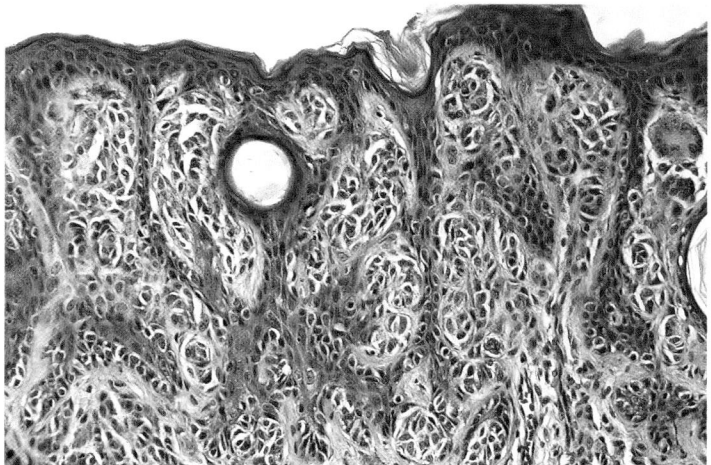

Fig. 32.4 **Benign compound nevus** with both junctional and dermal nests of nevus cells. (H & E)

the nevus cells in this variant often express estrogen-inducible pS2 protein.[140] Ackerman has suggested the designation of Unna's nevus for these exophytic papillomatous nevi, and Miescher's nevus for the dome-shaped exoendophytic nevi that extend far into the reticular dermis.[141]

Site-specific variations

Benign melanocytic nevi in certain anatomical sites may show unusual histopathological features.[142] The best known of these are nevi of the vulva and acral region. Nevi in other sites such as the ear, breast and flexural locations may show similar features.[143] The author has received, for a second opinion, the histology slides of many atypical nevi from the ears of adolescent males.

Some *vulval* nevi in premenopausal women show atypical histological features characterized by enlargement of junctional melanocytic nests, with variability in the size, shape and position of the nests.[144–146] Pagetoid spread of melanocytes is often present.[147] Nevi in pregnant women may also show some 'activation', with an increase in basal melanocytes and an increase in mitotic activity in these cells.[148] The changes are usually mild and never of sufficient degree to result in diagnostic confusion.[148]

Flexural nevi may show a nested and dyshesive pattern with some variability in nest size and arrangement.[149] *Conjunctival* nevi are another example of nevi at special sites that may present with worrisome features.[150]

Melanocytic lesions of the *palms and soles* may also cause diagnostic difficulties. This appears to be related, in part, to the presence of skin markings (dermatoglyphics) in these sites.[151] If sections are cut perpendicular, rather than parallel to the dermatoglyphics, symmetry and circumscription are seen more often.[151] Transepidermal elimination of well-circumscribed nests of nevus cells is sometimes seen in benign nevi, but pagetoid infiltration of the epidermis by single atypical cells, or small groups of atypical cells with pale cytoplasm, should be viewed with suspicion.[147,152,153] A lymphocytic infiltrate in the dermis is suspicious but not diagnostic of melanoma.[152] There is a unique variant of nevus on plantar skin – acral lentiginous nevus.[154] The appearances in this lesion have some resemblance to a dysplastic (atypical) nevus, although they lack cytological atypia and lamellar fibroplasia.[154]

Another special group of nevi are the *nail matrix* nevi.[155] Most are junctional in type, but when compound there is usually little maturation of cells in the dermis. The distribution of melanocytes in the basal layer may not be symmetrical. Pagetoid spread of melanocytes is confined to the suprabasal layer. The lesions present clinically as longitudinal melanonychia.[155]

INTRADERMAL NEVUS

Intradermal nevi are the most common type of melanocytic nevi. The vast majority are found in adults. They are usually dome-shaped, nodular or polypoid lesions which are flesh-colored or only lightly pigmented. Coarse hairs may protrude from the surface. Rare clinical variants have had a lobulated[156] or cerebriform appearance.[157]

Histopathology

Nevus cells are confined to the dermis, where they are arranged in nests and cords. Multinucleate nevus cells may be present. In the deeper parts of the lesion the nevus cells may assume a neuroid appearance ('neural nevus', neurotized melanocytic nevus), with spindle-shaped cells and structures resembling Meissner's tactile body (Fig. 32.5). These various patterns may represent different expressions of peripheral nerve sheath differentiation.[158]

These neuroid cells are quite distinct with electron microscopy and immunohistochemistry from those seen in a neurofibroma.[159,160] The cells in a neurofibroma show focal staining for Leu 7, glial fibrillary acid protein (GFAP) and myelin basic protein (MBP), antigens not expressed in neurotized melanocytic nevi.[159] Neither cell expresses peripherin, an intermediate filament found in neurons and some melanomas.[161,162] However, nerve growth factor receptor expression is increased in neural nevi[163] and S100A6 stains the Schwann cell-like type C cells.[164] With increasing age of the lesion

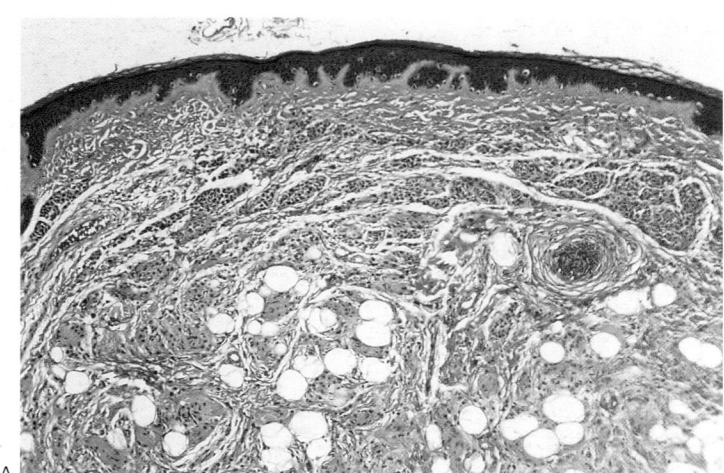

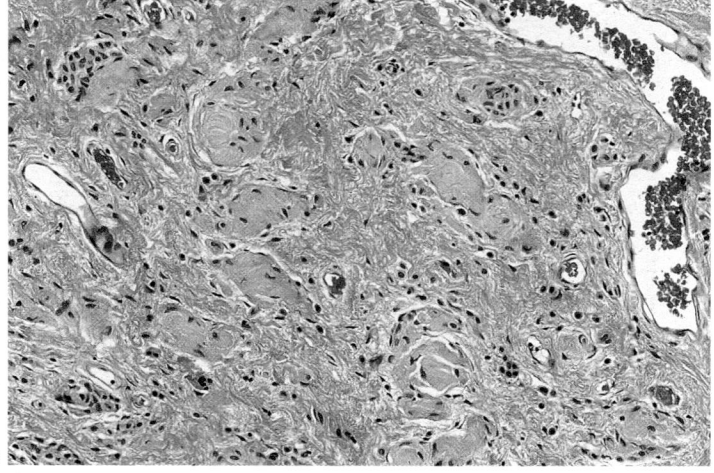

Fig. 32.5 **(A) Intradermal nevus** with stromal fat. **(B)** Some nevus cell nests have a neuroid appearance. (H &E)

there may also be replacement of nevus cells within the dermis by collagen, fat,[165] elastin and ground substance.[127]

Electron microscopy

The ultrastructural features of nevus cells are similar to those of melanocytes, although they lack the long dendritic processes of the melanocyte. Instead they have microvillous processes. The cells contain abundant cytoplasmic organelles, including melanosomes.[166]

Secondary changes in nevi

Many interesting changes may be found in nevi.[157] They include the incidental finding of amyloid[168] or of bone (osteonevus of Nanta);[169] epidermal spongiosis producing a clinical eczematous halo – Meyerson's nevus (see below);[170–174] the concurrence of psoriasis;[175] increased amounts of elastic tissue;[176] nodular myxoid change;[177] cystic dilatation of related hair follicles,[178] folliculitis,[179] epidermal, dermoid or tricholemmal cyst formation,[180,181] sometimes with rupture, producing sudden clinical enlargement; psammoma body formation;[182] sebocyte-like melanocytes;[183] paramyxovirus-like inclusions;[184] perinevoid alopecia;[185] focal epidermal necrosis;[186] an incidental molluscum contagiosum;[187] and an associated trichoepithelioma,[188] basal cell carcinoma,[189] syringoma[190] or sweat duct proliferation.[167,191] Artifacts may be caused by paraffin processing or by the injection of local anesthetic.[192] In the latter instance there is separation of nevus cells into parallel rows. Changes associated with tissue processing include the formation of clefts and spaces resembling vascular or lymphatic channels. The cells lining these pseudo-vascular spaces have been identified as nevus cells by immunoperoxidase studies using various markers.[193]

Tiny foci of hyperpigmentation ('small dark dots') may develop in nevi. The increased pigment may be in epidermal melanocytes, melanophages or dermal nevus cells. The heavily pigmented foci sometimes correspond to circumscribed nodules of atypical epithelioid cells – **clonal nevi**.[194,195] The cells possess fine dusty melanin pigment and often have an irregular nuclear contour. There are stromal melanophages. The appearances differ slightly from an epithelioid Spitz nevus. Rarely, the 'small dark dots' represent melanoma change.[196] Perifollicular hypopigmentation results from a variety of histological changes, including reduced numbers of nevomelanocytes and decreased pigmentation of keratinocytes, in the follicular region.[197] It may lead to variegate pigmentation and an irregular border to the nevus.

MEYERSON'S NEVUS

The Meyerson's nevus is a junctional, compound or intradermal nevus surrounded by an eczematous halo which may be pruritic.[170–173] The change may involve one or more nevi simultaneously. It occurs more often in young adults than in children.[174] Unlike the halo nevus, Meyerson's nevus does not undergo regression as a consequence of this change; however, the evolution of a Meyerson's nevus into a halo nevus has been reported recently.[198] The nature of the process is uncertain, but resolution of the eczematous halo has followed the excision of the central nevus alone. Multiple Meyerson's nevi appeared in a patient with Behçet's syndrome and the dysplastic nevus syndrome when the dosage of interferon alfa-2b was increased.[199]

An eczematous halo (the Meyerson phenomenon) has also been reported around dysplastic (atypical) nevi,[200] and also around a lesion of molluscum contagiosum.

Histopathology

There is a subacute spongiotic dermatitis associated with a nevocellular nevus (Fig. 32.6). Eosinophils are usually present in the cellular infiltrate, and

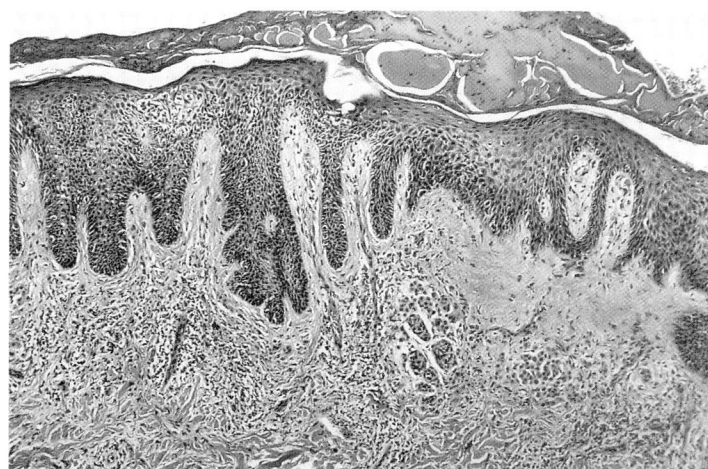

Fig. 32.6 **Meyerson's nevus.** Spongiotic (eczematous) changes superimposed on a benign compound nevus. Clinically, the lesion had recently developed an 'eczematous halo'. (H & E)

they may show exocytosis into the epidermis. There is no regression of the nevus.

ANCIENT NEVUS

Some nevi, particularly from the face of older individuals, can show a degree of cytological atypia that may lead to the erroneous diagnosis of malignant melanoma.[201,202] Clinically, the lesion is usually a dome-shaped, skin-colored or reddish brown papule or nodule.

Histopathology

Most lesions are intradermal in type although there is sometimes a junctional component. One population of dermal nevomelanocytes has large pleomorphic nuclei while the other has small monomorphous ones (Fig. 32.7).[201] The large melanocytes may resemble those of the epithelioid variant of Spitz nevus. Occasional mitotic figures may be present. Degenerative changes such as thrombi, hemorrhage, sclerosis around dilated venules, stromal fibrosis and mucin are usually present.[201]

DEEP PENETRATING NEVUS

The deep penetrating nevus (plexiform spindle cell nevus) is a variant of melanocytic nevus found on the face, the upper part of the trunk, and the proximal part of the limbs of young adults.[203] It is often deeply pigmented, with some variegation in color, leading to a mistaken clinical diagnosis of blue nevus or malignant melanoma. There are also histological features that overlap with these two entities and with the Spitz nevus. Deep penetrating nevi have been regarded as a variant of congenital nevus.

Histopathology[203]

The deep penetrating nevus is usually of compound type but the junctional nests are only small in most cases. It may have a wedge shape on low power, with the apex of the wedge directed toward the deep dermis.[204,205] The lesion is composed of loosely arranged nests and fascicles of pigmented nevus cells, interspersed with melanophages. Spindle cells are the predominant cell type, but varying numbers of epithelioid cells are also present.[204] The nests extend into the deep reticular dermis and often into the subcutaneous fat (Fig. 32.8). They surround hair follicles, sweat glands and nerves. Pilar muscles are sometimes infiltrated.

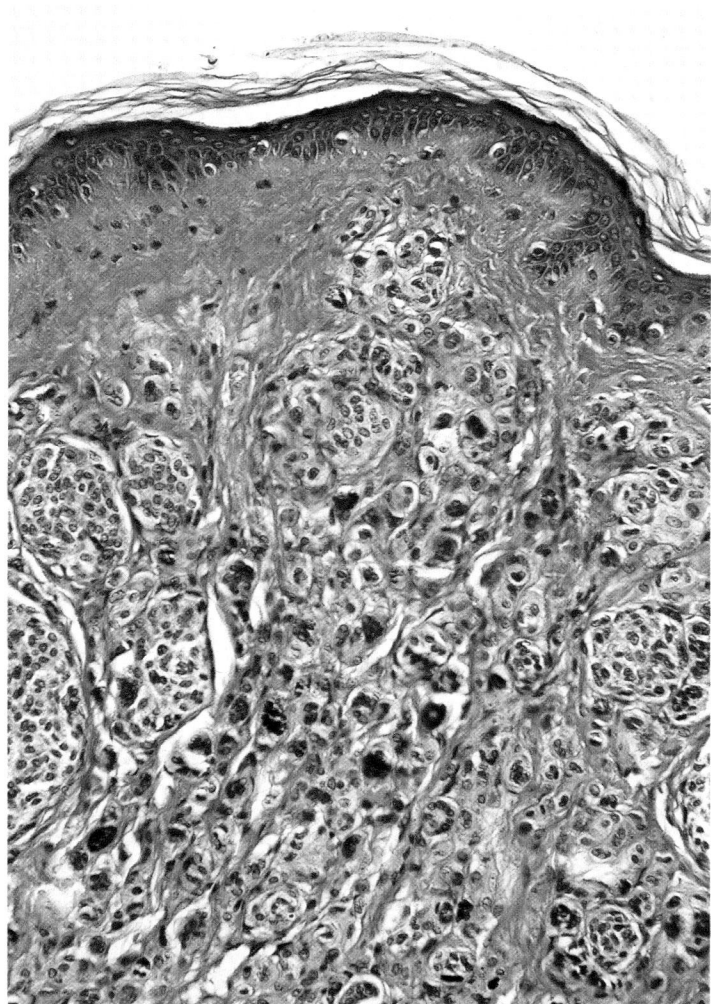

Fig. 32.7 **Ancient nevus.** One population of cells is large with hyperchromatic nuclei. (H & E)

Although there is some pleomorphism of the nuclei of the nevus cells, nucleoli are generally inconspicuous and mitoses are rare. Nuclear vacuoles and smudging of the chromatin pattern are additional features. A superficial variant of deep penetrating nevus has been recognized. It shows overlap features with the epithelioid blue nevus (see p. 818).[206]

Immunohistochemical studies have shown that the cells express S100 protein and HMB-45.[204,205,207] Proliferating cell nuclear antigen (PCNA) is present in only scattered melanocytes (<5%) in the deep penetrating nevus, whereas 25–75% of the cells in a melanoma will usually stain.[208]

BALLOON CELL NEVUS

The balloon cell nevus is a rare lesion which is clinically indistinguishable from an ordinary melanocytic nevus. A depigmented halo has rarely been described.[209]

Histopathology

The balloon cell nevus is composed of somewhat swollen nevus cells, with clear cytoplasm and a central nucleus which appears comparatively hyperchromatic (Fig. 32.9). Multinucleate balloon cells are often present. The diagnosis should be restricted to lesions containing a preponderance of

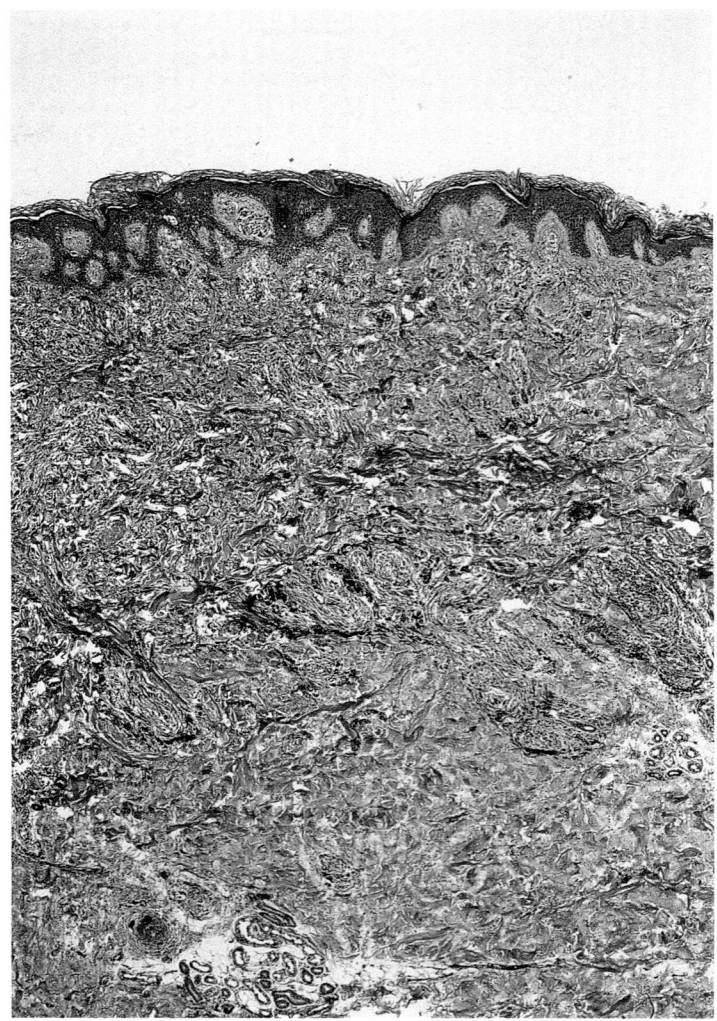

Fig. 32.8 **Deep penetrating nevus.** Nests of nevus cells extend into the deep reticular dermis. (H & E)

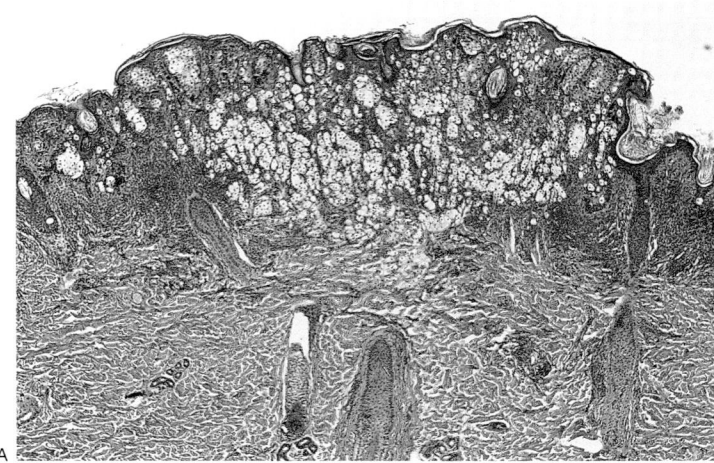

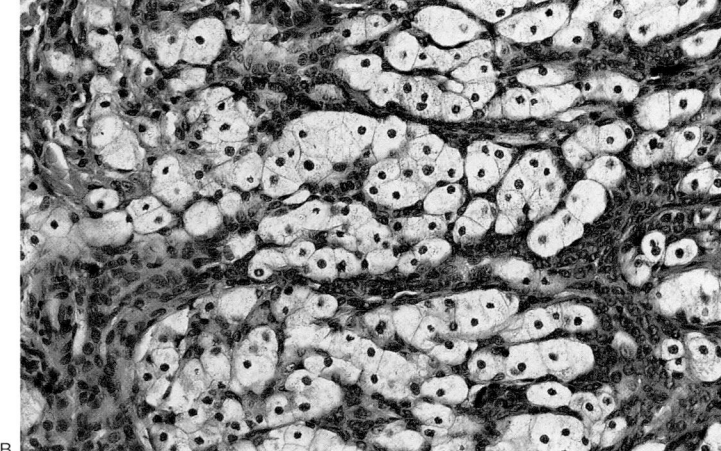

Fig. 32.9 **(A) Balloon cell nevus. (B)** Many of the cells have clear cytoplasm. (H & E)

balloon cells (over 50%), and not applied to nevi showing only a few foci of balloon cell change.[210] Balloon cell change has also been reported in dysplastic (atypical) nevi.[211] Balloon cell melanomas have also been described (see p. 828). The cells have larger nuclei than those in the balloon cell nevus, and mitoses can usually be found in the dermis.

Electron microscopy
The balloon cells appear to form by the progressive vacuolization of nevus cells resulting from the enlargement and eventual destruction of melanosomes.[212]

HALO NEVUS

A halo nevus is characterized by the presence of a depigmented halo up to several millimeters in width around a melanocytic nevus. This change is most often an idiopathic phenomenon which precedes the lymphocytic destruction of the nevus cells and the clinical regression of the lesion.[213,2 4] It should be noted that the lymphocyte-mediated regression of a nevus can take place without the development of a clinical halo. Halo change may involve one or several nevi. Very rarely a halo may develop around a congenital melanocytic nevus or a nodular melanoma.[215,216] Another rare phenomenon is the development of a targetoid halo.[217] Familial cases have been reported.[218]

Circulating antibodies that react against melanoma cells have been found in a high proportion of individuals with halo nevi, as have circulating lymphocytes with an activated phenotype,[219] suggesting that both humoral and cell-mediated immunity are involved in the rejection of nevus cells and the formation of the halo (see below).[216]

The halo nevus must be distinguished from the Meyerson's nevus (see p. 808), in which there is an eczematous halo surrounding a nevus.

Histopathology
There is usually a dense lymphocytic infiltrate within the dermis, with nevus cells surviving in nests or singly among the lymphocytes. The number of nevus cells will, of course, depend on the stage at which the biopsy is taken. Surviving nevus cells may appear slightly swollen, with some variation in size, and these changes may be worrisome. In one study 51% of lesions showed cells with some degree of atypia, ranging from minimal to moderate severity.[214] However, a heavy diffuse infiltrate of lymphocytes of the type seen in halo nevi is most unusual in a malignant melanoma. Macrophages are also present in the infiltrate. Rarely, a halo nevus is devoid of inflammatory cells.[220] Regression would not occur in such cases. Immunohistochemical staining for the presence of S100 protein may assist in the identification of residual nevus cells in cases in which a dense inflammatory infiltrate tends to obscure the

nature of the lesion.[221] Immunohistochemistry has also been used to characterize the nature of the lymphocytes present in the dermis. They are mostly CD8-positive T lymphocytes that express the activation molecule CD69 as well as tumor necrosis factor-α (TNF-α).[222,223] Macrophages and factor XIIIa-positive dendrocytes are also found in the infiltrate.[224]

The depigmented halo shows an absence of melanin pigment and melanocytes in the basal layer. Lymphocytes are sometimes noted in close proximity to residual melanocytes in the halo zone of newly forming lesions, but they are not usually present in the basal layer of established lesions. In one case, the adjacent epidermis showed interface changes resembling erythema multiforme with keratinocytes targeted by lymphocytes.[225]

Electron microscopy

Ultrastructural studies have shown non-specific injury changes in some nevus cells and destruction of others.[226,227] It seems likely that the nevus cells die by the process of apoptosis, but this requires confirmation.

COCKARDE NEVUS

The term 'cockarde nevus' (cocarde nevus, cockade nevus) refers to nevi which develop a peripheral pigmented halo with an intervening zone that is non-pigmented.[228,229] Several cases have been reported in association with spinal dysraphism.[230]

Histopathology

The central nevus is of junctional or compound type, whereas the peripheral halo is usually composed of junctional nests. The intervening non-pigmented zone is usually devoid of nevus cells.

ECCRINE-CENTERED NEVUS

The eccrine-centered nevus is a rare variety of nevocellular nevus in which the nevus cell proliferation is closely related to eccrine sweat ducts.[231]

RECURRENT NEVUS

Nevi may recur following shave biopsy of the lesion, with or without electrodesiccation. As the histological features of these recurrent nevi may be worrisome, Kornberg and Ackerman coined the term 'pseudomelanoma' for them.[232] However, as only a minority of such lesions mimic melanoma histologically, it has been suggested that this term be dropped.[233] Their appearances on dermoscopy may cause difficulties in diagnosis.[234] Recurrent nevi are not uncommon following inadequate excision of dysplastic (atypical) nevi.[235] This phenomenon can also be seen after non-biopsy trauma such as chronic irritation[236] and laser therapy.[237]

Histopathology

These recurrent nevi show a lentiginous and junctional epidermal component. Although there may be some upward epidermal spread of the tumor cells, the lesion is sharply circumscribed and there is no lateral extension of melanocytes. There is usually dermal fibrosis resulting from the previous procedure, and nests of mature nevus cells may be found in the dermis deep to, or at the edge of, the scar tissue.[232] Within the scar tissue are scattered nevus cells which resemble fibroblasts on light microscopy.[238]

Immunohistochemistry shows that the junctional melanocytes in the recurrent lesion express greater amounts of HMB-45 than the melanocytes in the original lesion.[239]

SPITZ NEVUS

The eponymous designation 'Spitz nevus' is the preferred term for the variant of nevocellular nevus that has also been known in the past by the terms 'spindle cell nevus', 'epithelioid cell nevus', 'nevus of large spindle and/or epithelioid cells' and 'benign juvenile melanoma'.[186,240,241] This title recognizes the important contribution of Sophie Spitz, who for the first time, in 1948, published criteria for the diagnosis of a specific lesion of childhood which, despite some histological resemblance to malignant melanoma, was known to behave in a benign fashion.[242–244]

The typical Spitz nevus is a pink or flesh-colored papule or nodule arising on the face, trunk or extremities,[245,246] particularly the lower limbs, of children or young adults. They are uncommon in black children.[247] Pigmented variants and lesions in other sites or in older individuals are not uncommon.[248] Pigmented lesions accounted for 71.7% of cases in one study.[249] The halo phenomenon has been observed in several cases.[250] Most lesions are less than 1 cm in diameter and solitary, but multiple Spitz nevi have been described in a clustered (agminate) or disseminated pattern.[251–260] Rare clinical variants include congenital onset,[261] the presence of multiple lesions with intervening (background) hyperpigmentation,[262,263] development within a speckled lentiginous nevus,[264,265] and the development of a large nodule following attempted removal.[266] Clinical diagnostic accuracy can be increased by the use of epiluminescence microscopy, but there are still many diagnostic pitfalls.[267,268]

Spitz nevi account for approximately 0.5–1% of surgically excised nevi in children and adolescents.[241] There is a low recurrence rate, even after incomplete excision.[269–271] Rarely, satellite lesions may occur in recurrent lesions.[272] Comparative genomic hybridization studies of recurrent lesions suggest that Spitz nevi with an 11p gain may be more apt to recur.[271]

Cramer has applied the MDP hypothesis (melanocyte differentiation pathway) to Spitz nevi. He has suggested that relatively impaired melanocyte–keratinocyte interactions in Spitz nevi may contribute to lack of dark pigmentation and to relatively accelerated accumulation of dermal nevus cells.[113]

Histopathology

The majority of Spitz nevi are compound in type, although 5–10% are junctional and 20% are intradermal lesions. The diagnosis depends on the assessment of a constellation of histological features (Table 32.1), some of which are more important than others.[241,273–277] The major diagnostic criteria include the cell type, the symmetrical appearance of the lesion, maturation of nevus cells, the lack of pagetoid spread of single melanocytes, and the presence of coalescent eosinophilic globules (Kamino bodies). These features are discussed in further detail below.

Table 32.1 **Diagnostic criteria for Spitz nevi**

Major criteria	Minor criteria
Symmetry	Junctional cleavage
Cell type – epithelioid and/or spindle cells	Superficial multinucleate nevus cells
Maturation of cells	Perivascular inflammation
Absent pagetoid spread of single melanocytes	Absence of nuclear pleomorphism
Coalescent, pale pink Kamino bodies	No deep atypical mitoses
	Deep outlying, solitary nevus cells
	Superficial edema, telangiectasia
	Low AgNOR score
	Stratification of HMB-45 staining
	Low PCNA staining
	Low chromosomal aberrations

A Spitz nevus may be composed of either epithelioid or spindle cells, the latter type being much more common. In one large study, spindle cells only were found in 45% of lesions, spindle and epithelioid cells in 34%, and epithelioid cells only in 21%.[278] Sometimes the spindle cells are quite plump (Fig. 32.10). On low-power magnification, Spitz nevi are usually quite symmetrical in appearance, with no lateral extension of junctional activity beyond the limits of the dermal component (Fig. 32.11). A recent paper has suggested that this is an 'unsupportable criterion' for distinguishing a Spitz nevus from a melanoma,[279] although subsequent correspondence has disputed this assertion.[280] There is usually 'maturation' of nevus cells in depth; this refers to the presence of cells in the deeper parts of the lesion which are smaller and resemble ordinary nevus cells. It has been suggested, on the basis of ultrastructural studies, that the process of 'maturation' of nevus cells is really one of atrophy.[281] Confusion may be caused by a rare subset of malignant melanomas which show paradoxical maturation in depth.[282] Single melanocytes extending upward within the epidermis are quite uncommon in Spitz nevi,[147,283] although clusters of three or more cells may be found within the epidermis, in places appearing to be undergoing transepidermal elimination (Fig. 32.12). Recently, prominent pagetoid spread of epithelioid melanocytes was reported in a series of small, uniformly pigmented macules, which often occurred on the lower legs of young female patients.[284] The melanocytes were purely intraepidermal. There was a perception of ordered growth and minimal atypia. The term *'pagetoid Spitz nevus'* has been used for these lesions, which show little, if any, junctional nesting (Fig. 32.13).[285,286]

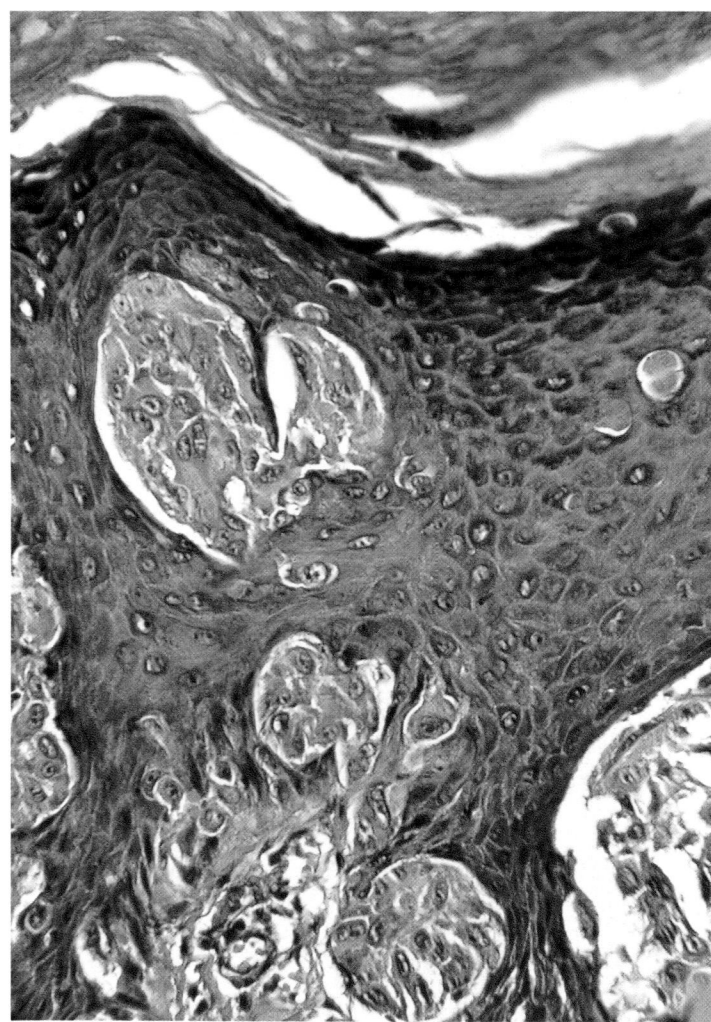

Fig. 32.12 **Spitz nevus.** There is some upward spread of melanocytes within the epidermis, but most of the cells are in small nests and not single cells. (H & E)

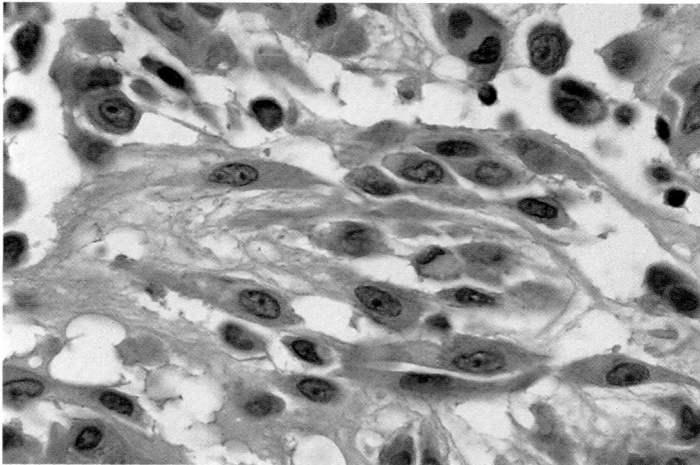

Fig. 32.10 **Spitz nevus** composed of plump, spindle-shaped cells. (H & E)

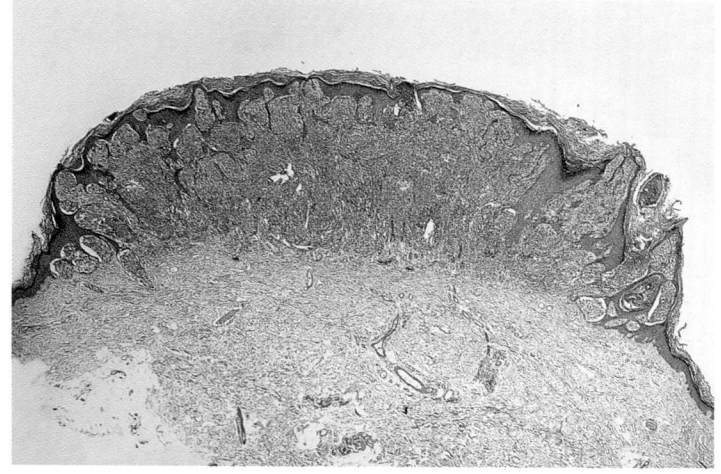

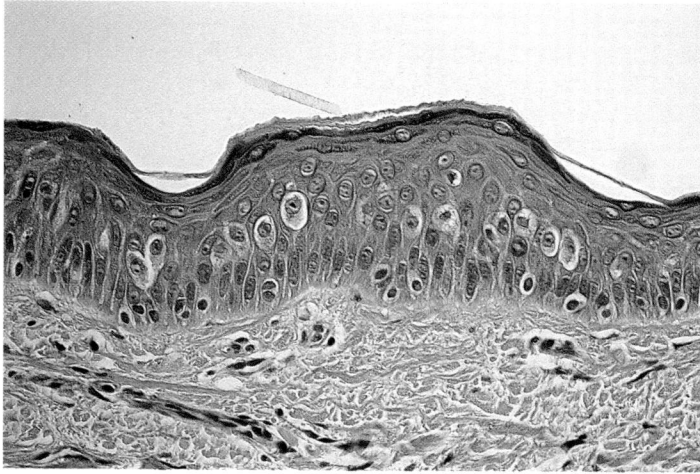

Fig. 32.11 **Spitz nevus.** Although this lesion is large, it shows symmetry. (H & E)

Fig. 32.13 **Pagetoid Spitz nevus.** The cells are large and pagetoid but there is no nesting or significant atypia. A Spitz nevus was present adjacent to this change. (H & E)

Solitary or coalescent eosinophilic globules (Kamino bodies) may be found at the dermoepidermal junction.[287,288] The presence of coalescent globules is an important diagnostic sign, but multiple step sections may be needed to demonstrate them (Fig. 32.14). They are usually PAS positive and trichrome positive.[241] On immunohistochemistry they contain various components of the basement membrane, including laminin and type IV and VII collagen[289] but no keratin or S100 protein.[290] They are not an apoptotic product of keratinocytes or melanocytes.[291] Electron microscopy shows them to be composed of bundles of filaments situated extracellularly.[287,288]

Minor diagnostic criteria include the presence of junctional cleavage (separation of the epidermis from nests of nevus cells at the junctional zone; Fig. 32.15), pseudoepitheliomatous hyperplasia,[292] superficial dermal edema and telangiectasia, giant nevus cells (both multinucleate and uninucleate), and an absence of nuclear pleomorphism.[241] Mitoses may be quite frequent in some actively growing lesions, but extreme caution should be adopted in making a diagnosis of Spitz nevus if mitoses, particularly atypical ones, are present in the deeper portion of a lesion. There may be an inflammatory infiltrate which shows perivascular localization.[248] The infiltrate is more intense in the halo variant (see below). The vascularity of Spitz nevi is usually higher than that of melanomas, despite an earlier study which reached the opposite conclusion.[293,294] Not infrequently, individual nevus cells may be found at a depth of up to 1 high-power field or more below the deep aspect of the tumor. In some Spitz nevi of epithelioid cell type a distinct component

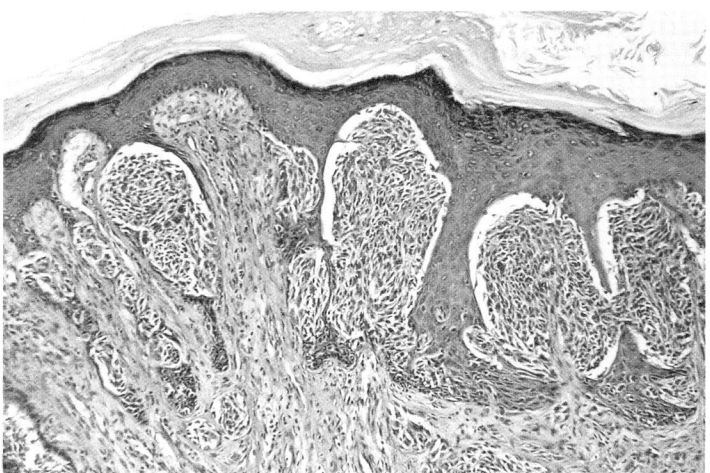

Fig. 32.15 **Spitz nevus.** There is conspicuous 'cleavage' at the junctional zone resulting from the artifactual separation of nevus cells from the basal layer of the epidermis. (H & E)

of smaller nevus cells is present, usually at the periphery of the lesion. The term 'combined nevus' has been used for this association of an intradermal nevus with a Spitz nevus, but it is also used for the combination of any two histological patterns of nevi, congenital or acquired, found in the same lesion.[295–298] Other histological changes that occur, rarely, are stromal fibrosis and hyalinization of the stroma.[299] The presence of tubules and microcystic structures may represent an artifact of fixation rather than a distinctive variant (tubular Spitz nevus), as originally thought.[300–302]

Distinction from malignant melanoma

In a histological review of Spitz nevi and melanomas in teenagers, McCarthy and colleagues found that features favoring malignancy were fine dusty cytoplasmic pigment, marginal or abnormal mitoses, epithelioid intraepidermal melanocytes below parakeratosis, dermal nests larger than junctional nests, and the mitotic rate in the papillary dermis.[303] In a similar study, Peters and Goellner found that pagetoid spread, cellular pleomorphism, nuclear hyperchromatism and mitotic activity were greater in melanomas than in Spitz nevi.[304] These nuclear differences can be quantified using image analysis cytometry.[305] One study showed that multivariate DNA cytometry could be used with high accuracy to discriminate between Spitz nevi and malignant melanoma.[306] Microfluorimetric analysis, computer-assisted image analysis and flow cytometry have also been used.[307–309] DNA in situ hybridization is another recently described diagnostic tool with excellent discriminatory value.[310] Molecular cytogenetic analysis of Spitz nevi shows clear differences to melanoma.[311] Whereas melanomas show frequent chromosomal deletions, as well as some gains, the majority of Spitz nevi have a normal chromosomal complement with the technique used.[311] Another recently introduced technique that shows some promise in the distinction of Spitz nevi and malignant melanoma is the measurement of telomerase activity, which is much lower in Spitz nevi than malignant melanoma.[312]

Although the misdiagnosis of malignant melanoma as a Spitz nevus is a well-recognized error, the reverse phenomenon, diagnosing a Spitz nevus as a melanoma, also occurs.[313] Even so-called 'experts' can occasionally disagree as to the correct diagnosis.[314]

Other techniques which may be applied in the diagnosis of Spitz nevi are immunohistochemistry[315] and the measurement of nucleolar organizer regions (loops of DNA that transcribe ribosomal RNA and which are easily identified in paraffin-embedded sections using a silver stain).[316] Unfortunately, neither method gives unequivocal results in borderline lesions.[317] With

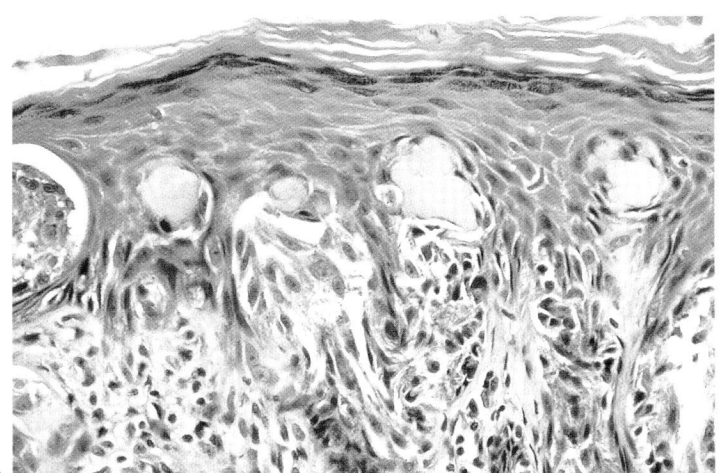

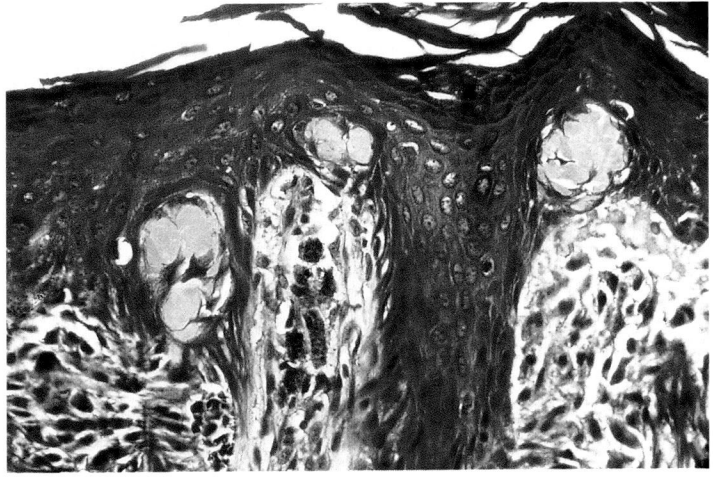

Fig. 32.14 **Spitz nevus. (A)** Coalescent eosinophilic globules ('Kamino bodies') are present in the junctional zone (H & E). **(B)** They are well seen in the trichrome stain. (Masson trichrome)

immunohistochemistry the cells express NK1/C-3, melan-A (MART-1) and S100 protein; the results are inconsistent with HMB-45. This latter marker is usually expressed weakly in the superficial cells, but sometimes there is staining throughout the tumor in a pattern near to that seen in malignant melanoma.[315] Nevertheless, even in these cases it is often possible to discern less intense staining in the deeper cells than in the more superficial cells. This pattern, known as stratification, is not seen in melanomas.[317,318] Stratification also occurs with cyclin D1, positive cells in Spitz nevi being restricted to the upper dermis.[319] No stratification is seen with melan-A (MART-1), which stains some cells in a high proportion of Spitz nevi as well as melanomas.[320] Proliferating cell nuclear antigen (PCNA) is expressed, usually weakly, in a variable number of nevus cells in a Spitz nevus; in melanomas the expression of this antigen is usually stronger and more diffuse.[321,322] Only 2–3% of cells express Ki-67, in contrast to malignant melanoma in which approximately 15% or more of the cells are positive.[319,323] p53 protein is detected in only occasional Spitz nevi by immunohistochemistry.[324] The number of silver-positive nucleolar organizer regions (AgNOR score) is lower in Spitz nevi (mean 1.2 per cell) than in malignant melanoma (mean 2.0 per cell), but overlap occurs.[316] Immunohistochemistry using S100 protein, melan-A (MART-1) and CD68 can be used to distinguish epithelioid Spitz nevi from epithelioid histiocytomas; the latter entity is positive for CD68.[325] C-fos protein expression does not distinguish Spitz nevi, common melanocytic nevi and malignant melanomas.[326]

Atypical Spitz nevus

'Atypical Spitz nevus' is the term used for a lesion in which a number of histological features deviate from the 'stylized depiction' of the Spitz nevus.[202,273] The connotation of this diagnosis is that the malignant potential is uncertain, although untoward events have proved to be rare in retrospective series and in the pathologist's experience.[273] It has been suggested that a diagnosis of 'probable Spitz nevus' is a more appropriate designation.[327] It seems likely that a histological continuum exists encompassing Spitz nevi at one end and Spitzoid melanoma at the other, with varying degrees of 'atypia' along this path.[314] The degree of deviation from the 'norm' is sometimes semiquantified as mild/moderate/severe or low/intermediate/high.[328,329] This latter scoring system has been used to indicate risk of metastasis (Spitzoid melanoma); it is an extension of the concept of atypical Spitz tumors.[329] Factors contributing to a high risk of likely metastasis (that is, the lesion was a melanoma and not a Spitz nevus) were age greater than 10 years, diameter of the lesion greater than 10 mm, the presence of ulceration, involvement of the subcutis (Clark level V), and a mitotic rate of at least 6/mm^2.[329] Spitzoid melanomas developing in teenagers do not have a better prognosis than that of other forms of melanoma.[330] Some of the cases now reported as atypical Spitz nevi (tumors) have been reported in the past as minimal deviation melanoma of Spitz nevus-like type.[331] The author believes that this diagnosis should not be used indiscriminately as an 'insurance policy' against misdiagnosis. Atypical Spitz nevus is not the same as dysplastic Spitz nevus, a recently recognized variant of dysplastic nevus.

Halo Spitz nevus

The term 'halo Spitz nevus' is used here for nevi with a depigmented rim, corresponding to that seen in the usual halo nevus, and for nevi with a heavy lymphocytic response resembling that seen in halo nevi, but with sparing of adjacent basal melanocytes.[250,332,333] This latter group, which does not develop a depigmented halo clinically, may also be designated *nevus with halo reaction*.[332] This phenomenon represents an early stage of nevus involution. It is often seen in combined nevi in which one component is an epithelioid Spitz nevus and the other a more traditional nevocellular nevus.[333]

The inflammatory response may induce reactive cytological atypia. Mitoses, if present, are superficial in location.

Desmoplastic nevus

Desmoplastic nevus, which may be mistaken clinically for a fibrohistiocytic lesion such as a dermatofibroma or epithelioid histiocytoma,[334,335] is probably a variant of Spitz nevus with stromal desmoplasia, although desmoplastic variants of common melanocytic nevi probably develop. MacKie and Doherty believe that it is a discrete entity.[336]

Angiomatoid Spitz nevus is a distinct variant of desmoplastic nevus with prominent vasculature and some plump endothelial cells.[337]

Histopathology

The desmoplastic nevus is characterized by a sclerotic dermis, sparse pigmentation, and little or no junctional activity and nest formation.[334] Well-defined intranuclear invaginations of cytoplasm are present in most cases. The cells express S100 protein.[336] Superficial dermal cells may also express HMB-45.[335]

A related variant is the hyalinizing Spitz nevus, in which there is extensive stromal hyalinization.[299]

Plexiform Spitz nevus

The exceedingly rare plexiform variant of Spitz nevus has no distinguishing clinical features. It is characterized by a plexiform arrangement of bundles and lobules of enlarged spindle to epithelioid melanocytes throughout the dermis.[338] Some lobules are surrounded by a thin rim of compressed stroma. A myxoid stroma was present in the two cases initially reported.[338]

Malignant Spitz tumor

The term 'malignant Spitz tumor' has been used for a very rare lesion with a close histological resemblance to a Spitz nevus but larger (with a diameter greater than 1 cm), and which extends into the subcutaneous fat.[273] It may metastasize to regional lymph nodes, but not beyond.[241,339,340] Barnhill's review of his cases of childhood melanomas gives some support to the notion that there is a Spitz-like tumor in childhood that may metastasize to regional nodes without further aggressive disease.[341] The diagnosis should not be used for all diagnostically difficult tumors or for melanomas that have been misdiagnosed as Spitz nevi and which are reviewed after metastases have developed.

Histopathology

The malignant Spitz tumor is characterized by a relatively high mitotic rate and mitoses deep within the lesion. There is more cellular pleomorphism, less maturation in depth and less cohesion of cells than in the usual Spitz nevus. In the few cases examined by immunohistochemistry the cells contained S100 protein.[339] HMB-45 was expressed either focally or diffusely.

PIGMENTED SPINDLE CELL NEVUS

Pigmented spindle cell nevus is now regarded as a distinct entity and not as a variant of the spindle cell type of Spitz nevus.[342,343] It is an uncommon lesion, with a distinctive clinical presentation: a well-circumscribed deeply pigmented papule, usually of recent onset, frequently located on the thighs of young adults.[342] Pigmented spindle cell nevus is more common in females. Clinical follow-up has not so far suggested any aggressive behavior.[342]

Histopathology

The histological appearances are sometimes quite worrisome because of the presence of some pagetoid spread of cells and also some cytological atypia.[147,344,345] The tumor is composed of spindle-shaped cells in nests, with the formation of interconnected fascicles (Fig. 32.16).[343] It is usually heavily pigmented, and many melanophages may also be present. Eosinophilic globules (Kamino bodies), resembling those seen in a Spitz nevus (see above), can be demonstrated in most cases if 'step sections' are examined.[346] They are present in about half the cases if only one section is examined.[347] They sometimes contain melanin granules. Junctional clefting, similar to that seen in the Spitz nevus, is often present.[347] Features distinguishing the pigmented spindle cell nevus from malignant melanoma include a symmetrical and orderly growth pattern, maturation of nevus cells in the deeper aspects of the lesion, and limitation of any pagetoid spread of melanocytes to the lower half of the epidermis.[344]

A pigmented epithelioid cell nevus also occurs; this is best regarded as a variant of Spitz nevus.[348]

CONGENITAL NEVUS

Congenital nevi are found in approximately 1% of newborn infants.[349,350] They are usually solitary,[351] with a predilection for the trunk, although other sites such as the lower extremities and scalp may also be involved.[241] In one series, 29% of congenital nevi were 1–9 mm in diameter, 63% were 10–40 mm, and the remainder were larger.[351] The majority of nevi that appear subsequent

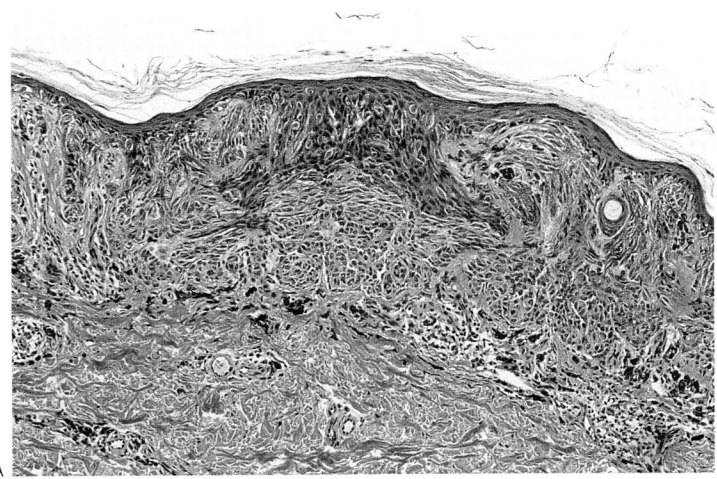

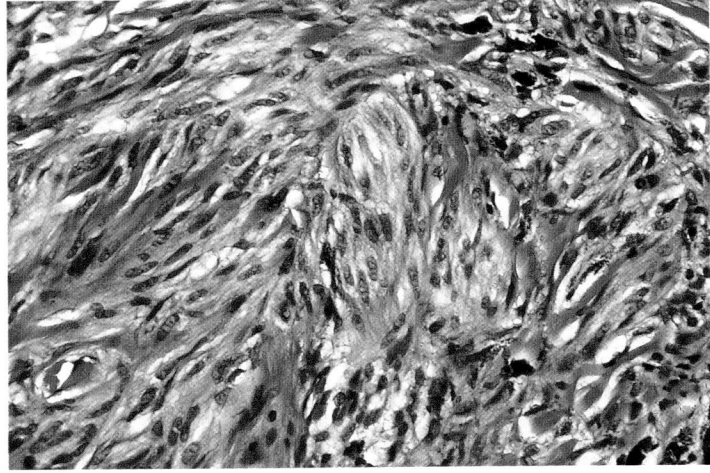

Fig. 32.16 **Pigmented spindle cell nevus. (A)** The fascicles of spindle-shaped cells are confined, as is usual with this lesion, to the epidermis and the papillary dermis. There is some melanin incontinence at the base of the lesion. **(B)** The cells are nested. (H & E)

to birth are less than 10 mm in diameter. Giant congenital nevi, i.e. those measuring more than 20 cm in greatest diameter, often have a garment (e.g. a bathing trunk) distribution.[352,353] They may be associated with leptomeningeal melanocytosis (neurocutaneous melanosis).[354–360] The receptor for hepatocyte growth factor/scatter factor (HGF/SF), a multifunctional cytokine, has been detected in a congenital nevus in a patient with neurocutaneous melanosis. Transgenic mice overexpressing this factor develop similar lesions, support for the pathogenetic role of this proto-oncogene in neurocutaneous melanosis.[361]

Studies have been undertaken to ascertain whether the size of congenital nevi remains static during overall body growth. In infants less than 6 months of age, more than half of the small congenital nevi followed in one study enlarged disproportionately to the growth of the anatomical region, whereas beyond 6 months of age such growth was very uncommon.[362] Erosions and ulcerations are sometimes noted in giant congenital nevi in the neonatal period. Such changes are not necessarily an indication of malignancy.[363] In adults, congenital nevi remain static in appearance in the absence of malignancy, trauma, infection or stretching of the skin.[362]

Congenital nevi can be associated with several syndromes: these include Carney's syndrome (including LAMB and NAME syndromes – see p. 804), the epidermal nevus syndrome, neurocutaneous melanosis (see above), neurofibromatosis type I, the premature aging syndrome, and occult spinal dysraphism.[364] A retroperitoneal malignant schwannoma has been reported in an infant with a giant congenital nevus.[365] This may represent a further 'syndrome', previously unreported. Other clinical presentations include a halo variant,[366,367] an exceedingly rare linear form[368] and an equally rare segmental agminate form.[369]

There is a significant risk of melanoma, both cutaneous and extracutaneous, developing in a giant congenital nevus.[370,371] This risk has been placed at between 2% and 31%, although a figure of approximately 5% or less would seem more realistic.[241] A more recent paper, based on a prospective study of 46 patients, reported a cumulative 5-year risk of melanoma of 5.7%.[372] Axial lesions appear to be more at risk for developing melanomas than lesions on the extremities.[373] The risk with small and medium-sized congenital nevi is more controversial.[370,374–377] Some have claimed that it is quite small,[352,370,377–379] or non-existent,[380,381] whereas others have estimated the cumulative risk as 3–20 times the usual risk.[382] Evidence of a pre-existing congenital nevus has been found in 1.1%[352] and 8.1%[383] of melanomas in two studies. One of the problems in assessing this risk is that the histological features of congenital nevi are not always distinguishable from those of acquired nevi. Accordingly, Rhodes and colleagues[384] have subsequently cautioned that their earlier work suggesting the presence of a pre-existing congenital nevus in 8.1% of melanomas[383] may be giving a falsely high figure. Another study found that 44% of melanomas developing in patients under 30 years of age developed in a small nevus present either from birth or from early childhood. This study suggests that small early-onset nevi may have a higher potential for postpubertal malignant change than has been previously recognized.[385] The author's anecdotal experience is that congenital nevi on the scalp have a slightly higher risk of developing a melanoma than those in other sites, in which the risk is very small. Melanoma change has not been reported so far in lesions treated with laser therapy.[386,387]

A **congenital melanoma** arising in a giant congenital nevus is an exceedingly rare event.[388] It has also been recorded in the absence of an underlying congenital nevus.[389] Prenatal metastases have also been recorded,[388] although many of the reported cases have done well, with no evidence of metastasis.[390] Nevus cells may be found in the placenta in association with giant congenital pigmented nevi. They should not be overdiagnosed as indicating malignancy.[390–392]

Finally, a rare form of congenital nevus is the divided (kissing) nevus that occurs on adjacent parts, such as the upper and lower eyelids, and may appear as one lesion when the eyelids are closed. A divided nevus has also been reported on the penis.[393,394]

Histopathology

Congenital nevi may be junctional, compound or intradermal in type, depending on the age at which they are removed. In neonates they are often junctional,[395] and if biopsied in the first week of life the melanocytic hyperplasia may be quite prominent in the epidermis and adnexal epithelium.[396] Two types of cells have been reported in congenital nevi removed in the first year of life. There are small nevus cells in the reticular dermis, usually separated by a space from overlying larger cells in the epidermis or close under it.[397] Features that have traditionally been regarded as characteristic of congenital nevi removed after the neonatal period are the presence of nevus cells in the lower two-thirds of the dermis, extension of nevus cells between collagen bundles singly or in Indian file, and extension of cells around nerves, vessels and adnexae (Fig. 32.17).[398,399] Although one study showed extension of nevus cells into the deep dermis in only 37% of congenital nevi,[400] a more recent immunohistological investigation using S100 protein staining found nevus cell involvement of adnexae in all cases.[401] Another study has found a poor correlation between the histology and the clinical history of the lesion – congenital or acquired.[402] Involvement of eccrine glands and septa are said to be the most specific features of a true congenital nevus.[402] Full-thickness dermal involvement, which is clearly visible in routine hematoxylin and eosin-stained sections, seems to be a feature of the larger congenital nevi, but not the smaller ones,[403] which may have a patchy distribution of nevus cells in the dermis.[284] According to some, small congenital nevi do not differ appreciably from acquired nevi.[404,405] The contrary view is that use of the traditional histological criteria (see above) makes it possible to differentiate the majority of small congenital melanocytic nevi from acquired melanocytic nevi.[406] Underlying hypoplasia of the subcutaneous fat and loss of elastic tissue from the papillary dermis producing anetoderma-like changes have both been reported in congenital nevi.[407,408]

The melanomas that develop in small congenital nevi have been said to have less aggressive growth than other melanomas,[383] but this remains to be confirmed. In giant congenital nevi the melanomas are often non-epidermal in origin.[409] Their metastatic potential is well recognized.[410] Patterns described include spindle and round cell differentiation, malignant

blue nevus and heterologous malignant mesenchymal differentiation, including neurosarcoma,[411] rhabdomyosarcoma, liposarcoma and undifferentiated spindle cell carcinoma.[412]

Sometimes, a cellular 'nodule' of large epithelioid cells is present at birth or develops in a congenital nevus;[413] it should not be misdiagnosed as a melanoma. It is usually less than 5 mm in diameter.[414] Features that favor a diagnosis of malignancy include the presence of atypical mitoses or focal necrosis within the 'nodule', or a lack of circumscription, with nests of cells infiltrating into the adjacent nevus. The 'melanoma simulant cells', as they have been called,[415] often blend imperceptibly with the more banal nevus cells surrounding the nodule.[390,416,417] Similar cellular nodules may develop in acquired nevi ('clonal nevi'), although they do not usually have the nuclear variability seen in the cellular nodules of congenital nevi. Atypical features, resembling those seen in dysplastic nevi, are occasionally seen in congenital nevi.[418]

DERMAL MELANOCYTIC LESIONS

In this group, dendritic melanocytes are present in the dermis.[419] These melanocytes may be derived from precursor cells which did not complete their migration from the neural crest to the epidermis during embryogenesis.

MONGOLIAN SPOT

Mongolian spots are slate-colored patches of discoloration with a predilection for the sacral region of certain races, particularly orientals.[420] They are present at birth or soon afterwards, but tend to disappear with increasing age, except in the Japanese, among whom persistent lesions may be found in approximately 3% of middle-aged adults.[421] Rare clinical variants include the presence of a depigmented halo,[422] adult onset,[423] and occurrence on the scalp, temple, and in cleft lips.[424–426] Mongolian spots have been reported in patients with mucopolysaccharidoses.[427,428] The pigmentation associated with minocycline therapy may rarely simulate a Mongolian spot.[429]

Histopathology

There are widely scattered, melanin-containing melanocytes in the lower half of the dermis. The cells are elongated and slender. Occasional melanophages are also present.

NEVUS OF OTA AND NEVUS OF ITO

The nevus of Ota is a diffuse, although sometimes slightly speckled, macular area of blue to dark-brown pigmentation of skin in the region of the ophthalmic and maxillary divisions of the trigeminal nerve.[430] There is often conjunctival involvement as well. Lesions are bilateral in a small number of cases.[431] There is a predilection for certain races and for females. The nevus of Ito is a similar condition located in the supraclavicular and deltoid regions, and sometimes in the scapular area.[432] Both lesions are occasionally present in the same patient.[431] Pigmentation is often present at birth, but it may not become apparent until early childhood. Malignant change is exceptionally rare.[433,434] There is one report of a nevus of Ota which locally invaded bone and dura over a period of 50 years. It was histologically benign in appearance.[435]

Histopathology

There are often nodular collections of melanocytes which resemble those of blue nevi (see below). The intervening macular areas are composed of a more diffuse infiltrate of elongated melanocytes situated in the upper dermis.[436]

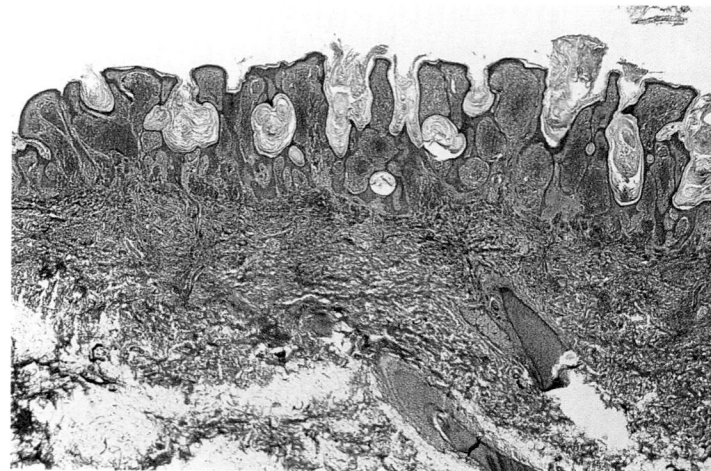

Fig. 32.17 **Congenital nevus.** Nests of nevus cells extend deeply in the dermis. (H & E)

BLUE NEVUS

The common or classic blue nevus is a small slate-blue to blue-black macule or papule found most commonly on the extremities. It is almost invariably acquired after infancy,[437] but a giant congenital lesion has been reported.[438] The cellular variant is a much larger nodular lesion, often found on the buttocks but sometimes on the scalp[439] or the extremities.[440–443] Eruptive,[444–446] plaque,[447–449] target,[450] linear,[451] satellite,[452] disseminated[453–455] and familial[456,457] forms have been described. The term 'agminate blue nevus' has sometimes been used for the eruptive and plaque variants.[458]

The epithelioid blue nevus is a recently described variant which clinically resembles the common blue nevus, except for its distinct histological appearance, its tendency to be multiple, and its association with the Carney complex (see p. 804).[459–461] However, it is not always associated with the Carney complex.[462,463]

Histopathology

The *common blue nevus* is composed of elongated, sometimes finely branching, melanocytes in the interstices of the dermal collagen of the mid and upper dermis (Fig. 32.18). There are some melanophages. Some lesions show dermal fibrosis (sclerosing blue nevus). In about 3% of cases, there is minimal pigment present. Such cases have been called 'amelanotic' or 'hypopigmented' blue nevi.[464–466] Occasionally, an overlying intradermal nevus is present: such lesions are called combined[295,467,468] or 'true and blue' nevi. A rare finding is an overlying lentigo or junctional lentiginous nevus,[469–473] a junctional Spitz nevus[474] or a dendritic component.[475] Melanoma in situ has also developed over a combined blue nevus.[476]

The *cellular blue nevus* is composed of dendritic melanocytes, as in the common type, together with islands of epithelioid and plump spindle cells with abundant pale cytoplasm and usually little pigment (Fig. 32.19). Heavily pigmented variants do occur. Melanophages are found between the cellular islands. The tumor often bulges into the subcutaneous fat as a nodular downgrowth which has a rather characteristic appearance. There are solitary reports of a lesion with subcutaneous cellular nodules[448] and one of bony infiltration by a scalp lesion.[477] Stromal desmoplasia (desmoplastic cellular blue nevus) and balloon cell change are rare occurrences.[478,479]

Mihm and colleagues have proposed the concept of *atypical cellular blue nevus* for a lesion that has clinicopathological features intermediate between typical cellular blue nevus and the rare malignant blue nevus.[480] No metastases were recorded. The lesions were characterized by architectural and/or cytological atypia including necrosis.[480] No atypical mitoses were present, indicating the importance of this finding in the distinction from malignant blue nevus.[480]

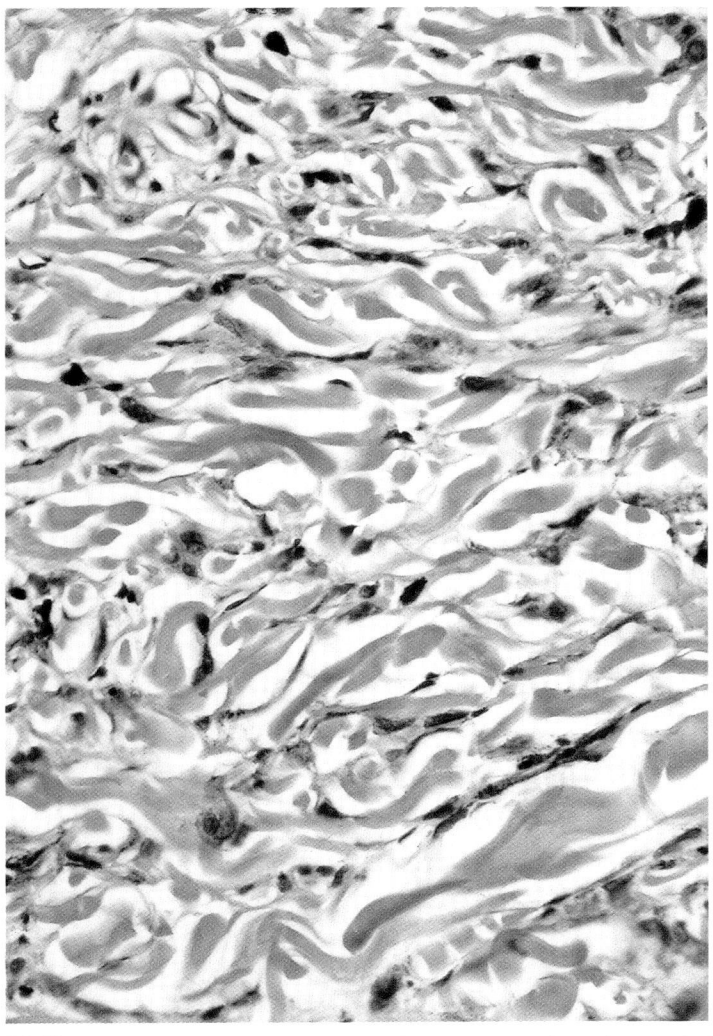

Fig. 32.18 **Blue nevus.** Melanocytes with long dendritic processes and cytoplasmic melanin are present between the collagen bundles in the dermis. (H & E)

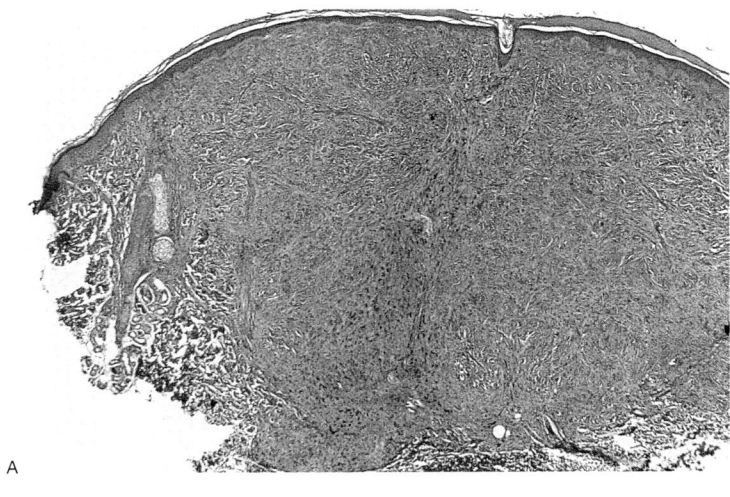

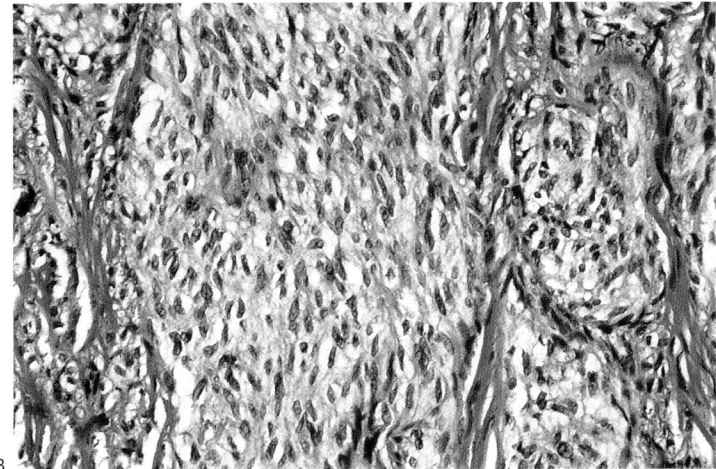

Fig. 32.19 **Cellular blue nevus. (A)** The lesion fills the dermis and bulges into the subcutaneous fat. **(B)** There are nests and fascicles of melanocytes, some with a spindle shape. The cytoplasm of the cells is pale staining. (H & E)

The *epithelioid blue nevus* is composed of intensely pigmented globular and fusiform cells admixed with lightly pigmented polygonal and spindle cells. The melanocytes are usually dispersed as single cells among the collagen bundles, although occasional fascicles exist. This pattern distinguishes this entity from the deep penetrating nevus, although some cases of epithelioid blue nevus resemble what has been called the superficial variant of deep penetrating nevus. The epithelioid blue nevus is often part of a combined nevus that may include Spitz nevus, desmoplastic nevus or congenital nevus. The combination of epithelioid blue and Spitz features in the one lesion has been called a **blitz nevus**.[481] Some consolidation of the nomenclature is clearly needed in this area.

Rare variants include the association of a blue nevus with osteoma cutis,[482] and with a trichoepithelioma,[483] and a bizarre blue nevus with striking cytological atypia, but without any other features of malignancy.[484] Perifollicular pigment-laden spindle cells, similar to those seen in a pilar neurocristic hamartoma are rarely present.[485] Central myxoid change is another rare histological finding.[486]

The melanocytes in blue nevi of all types express S100 protein, melan-A (MART-1) and HMB-45.[487,488] They do not stain for CEA.[489] CD34 expression has been reported in a rare congenital form of cellular blue nevus with spindle-shaped cells, suggesting some overlap with neurocristic cutaneous hamartoma (see below).[490]

Electron microscopy

Melanosomes are present in both the dendritic melanocytes and the paler cells of the cellular blue nevus. Some authors have highlighted schwannian features in this variant of blue nevus.[491]

BLUE NEVUS-LIKE METASTATIC MELANOMA

One of the most difficult diagnostic problems in dermatopathology is the recognition of the rare form of metastatic melanoma that closely simulates a blue nevus.[492,493] The lesions usually occur in the same anatomic region as the primary tumor, but if no clinical history of a previous melanoma is provided, it is virtually impossible to make the diagnosis.

Histopathology

The lesions are composed of pigmented melanocytes and melanophages in a blue nevus-like growth pattern.[493] Atypical epithelioid melanocytes and mitotic figures are often present. In the author's experience, the presence of an associated inflammatory reaction at the periphery of the lesion is sometimes the only clue to the diagnosis (Fig. 32.20).

MALIGNANT BLUE NEVUS

Malignant blue nevus is an exceedingly rare, aggressive tumor found on the scalp, face, buttocks and chest.[494] It affects middle-aged to elderly patients, with a slight male predominance.[495] Rare cases in childhood have been reported.[496] The term is sometimes restricted to tumors arising in blue nevi with no concurrent junctional component, but it may be used for tumors that arise in a nevus of Ota,[497] or *de novo*.[498] It usually arises in a cellular blue nevus. Nodal metastases and distant metastases, particularly to the lungs, have been reported in malignant blue nevi.[499–501] In one series of 12 cases (8 of which were on the scalp) metastases developed in 10, and 8 died of their metastases.[495] Metastases may not develop for many years.[502]

Histopathology

There is usually an underlying blue nevus, in which a poorly circumscribed cellular nodule occupies a variable proportion of the lesion. The diagnosis is made by finding cytological features of malignancy, such as nuclear pleomorphism and atypical mitoses, combined with subcutaneous invasion and often some necrosis. The presence of atypical mitoses appears to be a more specific feature of malignancy than necrosis. Cytoplasmic vacuolization is often present in malignant lesions. A cellular blue nevus will often extend into the subcutaneous fat, but on low magnification it has a rounded, non-infiltrating pattern which is quite distinct from that seen in the malignant blue nevus (Fig. 32.19). Furthermore, recurrence is a rare phenomenon in blue nevi. Cytological atypia and frequent mitoses may be seen but necrosis and atypical mitoses are usually absent, distinguishing such cases from malignant blue nevus.[503] The distinction from other types of melanoma, particularly metastatic melanoma, is aided by the absence of junctional activity and the presence of dendritic melanocytes.

AgNOR counts (see p. 813) and immunostaining for proliferating cell nuclear antigen (PCNA) and Ki-67 (MIB-1) are useful additional parameters for the diagnosis. Both are significantly different from that seen in benign nevomelanocytic lesions.[504,505]

Cells resembling those found in a blue nevus may be found in the capsule of lymph nodes, either as an isolated phenomenon[506,507] or in association with

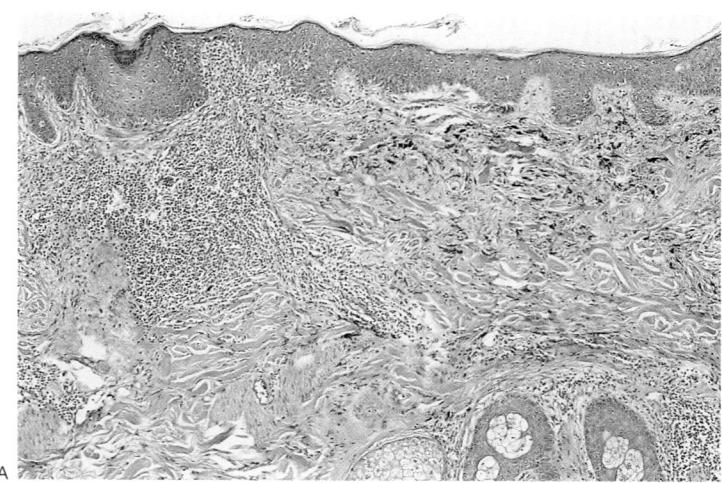
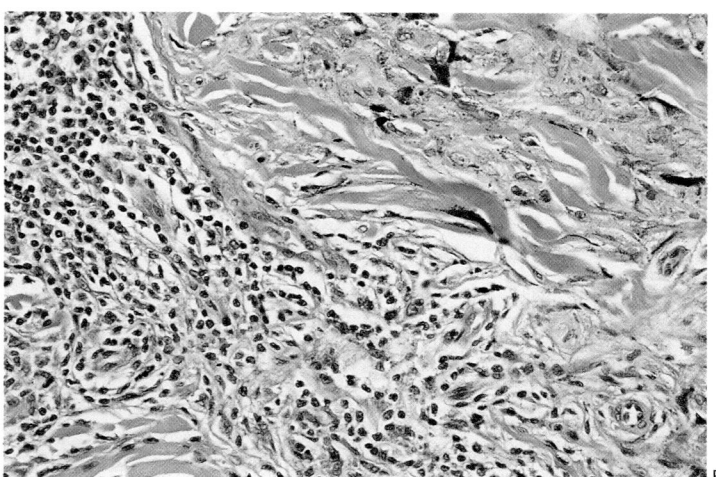

Fig. 32.20 **(A) Blue nevus-like melanoma. (B)** There is a lymphocytic infiltrate at the edge of a lesion that closely resembles a blue nevus. (H & E)

a cellular blue nevus.[508] Migration arrest during embryogenesis has been favored over 'benign metastasis' in explanation of this lesion.[509] Metastases from a malignant blue nevus will usually involve much of the node.

DERMAL MELANOCYTE HAMARTOMA

Dermal melanocyte hamartoma is a very rare condition characterized by large areas of diffuse gray-blue pigmentation or coalescing macular lesions, present at birth, and with similarities to the nevi of Ota and Ito (see above).[510] A segmental distribution of the pigmentation has been reported.[511] Related entities are the pilar neurocristic hamartoma,[512,513] and phakomatosis pigmentovascularis, in which there is a disorder of pigmentation associated with vascular abnormalities (see below). A rare acquired variant of dermal melanocytosis **(acquired dermal melanocytosis)** has been reported.[514,515] In one report the cases had symmetrical spotted pigmentation on the face and extremities,[516] and in others localized lesions have developed.[517]

Histopathology

In both dermal melanocyte hamartoma and phakomatosis pigmentovascularis there are moderate numbers of dendritic melanocytes scattered throughout the upper and mid dermis, similar to the macular areas of the nevus of Ota.[518] In the pilar neurocristic hamartoma the pigment-laden spindle cells have a perifollicular arrangement similar to that of equine melanotic disease.[485,512] In **acquired dermal melanocytosis** the melanocytes are usually more dispersed in the dermis than in the blue nevus.[517] Numerous melanophages are often present.[519]

PHAKOMATOSIS PIGMENTOVASCULARIS

Phakomatosis pigmentovascularis is a rare congenital syndrome with the combination of vascular anomalies, usually a large nevus flammeus, combined with cutaneous pigmentary abnormalities.[518,520–530] Four subtypes have been recognized on the basis of the accompanying pigmented lesion and the presence of systemic or localized disease. Most cases have been reported from Japan. The pigmented lesions described include nevus spilus, Mongolian spots, nevus depigmentosus, blue nevus and nevus of Ota.[531,532]

CUTANEOUS NEUROCRISTIC HAMARTOMA

Cutaneous neurocristic hamartoma is a recently delineated entity composed of nevomelanocytes, pigmented spindle and dendritic cells, and Schwann cells.[533] These hamartomas are often present at birth, but may develop in childhood or adolescence. The lesions, which resemble blue nevi or congenital nevi clinically, average 3–7 cm in diameter. The pilar neurocristic hamartoma can also be included in this concept (see above). They are of presumed neural crest origin.

There is a high incidence of malignant transformation, but the melanomas that develop run a more indolent course than common melanoma, or melanoma arising in a blue nevus.[533]

Histopathology

Cutaneous neurocristic hamartoma most resembles a congenital nevus with neuroid features. There is a variable admixture of nevomelanocytes, Schwann cells and dendritic blue nevus cells. The hamartomas involve the dermis and can extend into the subcutis and skeletal muscle.

The melanomas that may develop are subepidermal, often multinodular tumors, composed of small, round to spindle cells displaying a trabecular or nested growth pattern. Nuclear palisading and perivascular pseudorosettes are sometimes present.[533] The cells express S100 protein and vimentin; in a majority of cases they also stain for HMB-45 and neuron-specific enolase.[533]

ATYPICAL NEVOMELANOCYTIC LESIONS

DYSPLASTIC (ATYPICAL, CLARK'S) NEVUS

Dysplastic (atypical, Clark's) nevi are clinically distinctive nevi with characteristic histology and an increased risk of melanoma change.[141,296,534–536] One or more dysplastic nevi can be found in from 2% to 18% of the population.[537,538] They are uncommon in the Japanese.[539] They constitute approximately 10% of the nevomelanocytic lesions received by a pathology laboratory.[540]

The term 'dysplastic (atypical) nevus syndrome' refers to the familial or sporadic occurrence of multiple dysplastic (atypical) nevi in an individual.[541] Familial cases of this syndrome were originally called the B-K mole syndrome[542] (based on the surnames of two of the probands) and the FAMMM syndrome[543] (familial atypical mole/malignant melanoma syndrome). Controversy surrounding the use of the term 'dysplastic' in the title has led to the suggestion that the term 'atypical mole syndrome' is more appropriate.[544–546]

Despite repeated calls for the diagnosis of dysplastic nevus to be dropped,[547] the diagnosis survives because proponents for its continued use can still be found[548–550] and because alternative designations and definitions lack general support. The use of the term 'Clark's nevus' as a synonymous term ignores its origin; the term was used by Ackerman for a nevus with architectural atypia in the form of a junctional shoulder extending beyond the dermal one.[551] Lentiginous nevi are 'captured' by this definition. The suggestion of the second NIH Consensus Conference – 'nevus with architectural disorder' – had no chance of acceptance because it lacked brevity.

Clinically, dysplastic (atypical, Clark's) nevi are usually larger than ordinary nevi and often show a mixture of tan, dark brown and pink areas.[552] Non-pigmented variants are rare.[553] There is often persistence of a somewhat indistinct peripheral macular area in a lesion which, by its size, would be expected to be solely papular.[554] The surface texture is often 'pebbly'. Not all nevi with these clinical characteristics have the histological features of dysplastic (atypical) nevi (see below).

In patients with the dysplastic (atypical) nevus syndrome the number of nevi is large – up to 80 or more. In childhood, nevi usually appear normal, the abnormal lesions appearing in adolescence and adult life.[555] The incidence of dysplastic nevi in the pediatric population is extremely low,[556] although a significant number of cases on the scalp and forehead were reported in one study of children under 18 years of age.[557] Atypical nevi may continue to appear in up to 20% of patients over the age of 50.[558] However, many of those in adults with the syndrome are not of dysplastic (atypical) type: there are many junctional lentiginous nevi and compound melanocytic nevi.[559] Persistence of junctional activity is a feature of most nevi in this condition, even in late adult life.[560] Dysplastic (atypical) nevi predominate on the trunk. In females there may be considerable numbers on the legs as well.[561] There is some evidence that sunlight induces the formation and enlargement of nevi in patients with the dysplastic (atypical) nevus syndrome,[562–567] although this has been disputed.[568]

In familial cases the melanoma trait is inherited as an autosomal dominant with incomplete penetrance. The dysplastic (atypical) nevus trait has a more complicated inheritance, occurring more commonly than is usual for dominant inheritance. Mutations in a gene on chromosome 9p21 *(CDKN2A)* have been found in patients with familial melanoma,[569] but mutations in the *CDKN2A* gene are uncommon in dysplastic nevi.[570] Interestingly, the dysplastic (atypical) nevus syndrome has also been associated with partial deletion of chromosome 11[571] and with deletion of 17p13 (p53).[572] Intraocular melanomas,[573] oral melanoma in situ,[574] other tumors (particularly pancreatic)[575] and endocrine abnormalities[576] have been reported in families with the dysplastic (atypical) nevus syndrome, but a recent study showed no increase in cancers other than malignant melanoma.[577]

It has been calculated that for a Caucasian resident in the USA the lifetime risk of developing a melanoma is 0.6%, whereas in patients with dysplastic (atypical) nevi, this risk is 10% or more.[578–582] The risk exceeds 50% in melanoma-prone families with the dysplastic (atypical) nevus syndrome.[583] Blood relatives of patients who have had a melanoma or dysplastic (atypical) nevus removed also have an increased risk of developing a dysplastic (atypical) nevus[584,585] or melanoma.[586]

A rare clinical presentation of dysplastic (atypical) nevi is an eruptive form; it has been reported in a patient with the acquired immunodeficiency syndrome,[587] and in one with chronic myelocytic leukemia[588] and following renal transplantation.[589] Dysplastic (atypical) nevi localized to one area of the body have also been reported.[590]

Histopathology[554,591,592]

Dysplastic (atypical) nevi, as originally defined, have three characteristic histological features: intraepidermal lentiginous hyperplasia of melanocytes, random cytological atypia of these cells, and a stromal response.[541,554,593] A fourth feature, architectural atypia, is generally regarded as a diagnostic requirement.[594] *Lentiginous hyperplasia* refers here to a proliferation of melanocytes singly, but also in nests along the basal layer. The nests may involve the sides of the elongated rete ridges as well as the tips (Fig. 32.21); bridging nests also form. The term 'junctional nest disarray' has been applied to the uneven distribution and pattern of the junctional component.[595,596] The cells commonly show shrinkage artifact, with scant cytoplasm and a spindle-shaped pattern, but in some lesions there are larger cuboidal (epithelioid) cells with dusty pigment.

Random cytological atypia refers to the presence of occasional cells with enlarged hyperchromatic nuclei, sometimes with prominent nucleoli. The nuclei equal the nucleus of the overlying keratinocytes in size, or are larger.[597] The atypia is usually graded into low-grade and severe, although there are no universally acceptable criteria for this.[534] There is often a progression of cytological atypia with increasing age of the patient.[598] Furthermore, increasing atypia has been found to correlate with increasing darkness and confluence of pigmentation clinically.[599] Several reports have implied that severe atypia is associated with an increased risk of melanoma change, but this was not confirmed in one study.[600–602] Atypia may also be present in nevi that do not otherwise fulfil the criteria for the diagnosis of a dysplastic (atypical) nevus.[603,604]

The *stromal response* consists of lamellar and concentric fibroplasia of the papillary dermis, associated with a proliferation of dermal dendrocytes. Sometimes there is fibrosis in the upper reticular dermis, resulting in more widely spaced nests, often larger than usual. Such cases can be worrisome; they are often received in consultation (Fig. 32.22). There is also a patchy superficial lymphocytic infiltrate[554] and, sometimes, new vessel formation.

Ackerman and others have placed emphasis on *architectural atypia* rather than cytological atypia in defining a dysplastic (atypical, Clark's) nevus. They stress the importance of the 'shoulder phenomenon' (peripheral extension of the junctional component beyond the dermal component) in making the diagnosis.[601,605,606]

A dermal nevus-cell component is usually present in the central part of the lesion, consisting of small cells or epithelioid cells but showing only slight evidence of maturation and with impairment of pigment synthesis. In other

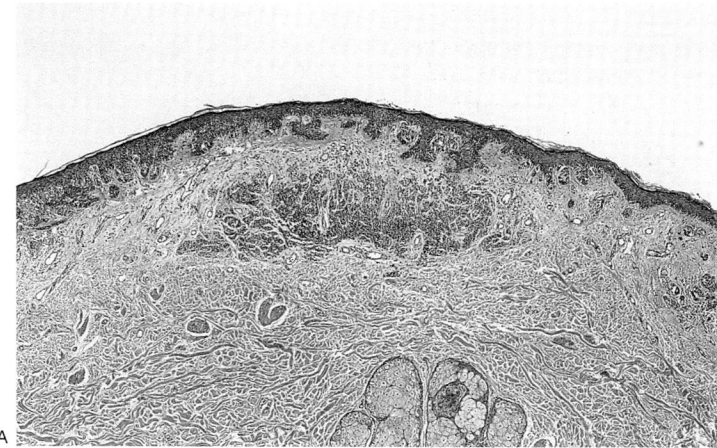

A

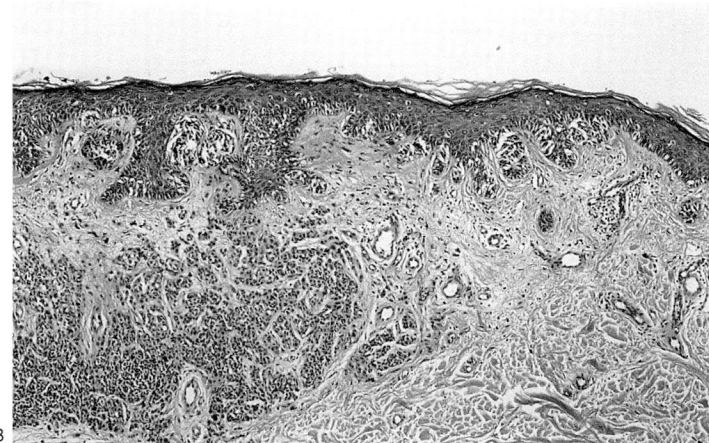

B

Fig. 32.21 **Dysplastic nevus. (A)** There is a lentiginous proliferation of melanocytes in the basal layer, with some nests of nevomelanocytes in the junctional zone and in the dermis. Only mild cytological atypia is present. **(B)** There is mild fibroplasia involving the papillary dermis. (H & E)

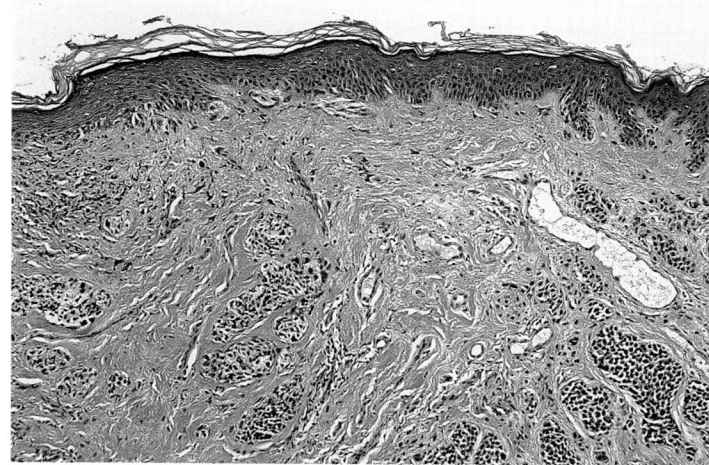

Fig. 32.22 **Dysplastic nevus of compound type.** There is fibrosis of the superficial dermis and an absence of nevomelanocytes in the overlying junctional zone, suggesting focal regression. Focal scarring of this type is not uncommon in dysplastic nevi. (H & E)

words, dysplastic (atypical) nevi are usually compound nevi with peripheral lentiginous and junctional activity and random cytological atypia in the epidermal component.

Toussaint and Kamino have examined a large series of dysplastic nevi and found that the dermal component of some cases may show features of other varieties of nevi, such as a congenital nevus, Spitz nevus, blue nevus, halo nevus or dermal neuronevus.[607]

Several studies have assessed the interobserver and intraobserver concordance in the diagnosis of dysplastic (atypical) nevi and the histological grading of their atypia. Although some centers have reported good reproducibility of results for both diagnosis and grading (into mild, moderate and severe),[608–611] others have reported limited or 'only fair' concordance for one or both of these features, particularly at the mild to moderate (low-grade) end of the spectrum.[612–614] Although there is usually agreement on the presence of architectural atypia, problems can arise in the assessment of cytological atypia (Fig. 32.23).[615,616] Sometimes, lesions that display clinical features thought to indicate a dysplastic (atypical) nevus do not do so on histology.[617,618] Conversely, some common nevi may show the histological features of a dysplastic nevus, leading to a suggestion that a continuum of cases exists.[619] Color variegation often correlates with atypia, whereas the absence of a macular component clinically usually indicates a lack of atypia histologically.[620,621] Another study found that nevus size and irregular borders corresponded with the greatest number of individual histological parameters of a dysplastic (atypical) nevus.[622]

Dysplastic (atypical) nevi have been reported in contiguity with up to one-third or more of superficial spreading melanomas.[623–627] In determining whether a dysplastic (atypical) nevus is present it has been proposed that the atypical lentiginous melanocytic hyperplasia should extend three or more rete pegs beyond the most lateral margin of the in situ or invasive melanoma.[624] Critics of this definition would argue that the diagnosis of dysplastic (atypical) nevus is being applied indiscriminately in this and other situations.[628–630] Dysplastic (atypical) melanocytes in an evolving melanoma in situ should not be regarded as indicative of a precursor dysplastic (atypical) nevus.

The AgNOR rating (see p. 813) of dysplastic (atypical) nevi is not significantly different from that of common nevi.[631–634] Nuclei are usually diploid in type.[635] With immunoperoxidase techniques, S100 protein can be detected in the cells. However, the expression of HMB-45 is limited to epidermal melanocytes and cells in the papillary dermis.[636–638]

Electron microscopy

The melanosomes in epidermal melanocytes in dysplastic (atypical) nevi are abnormal, with incompletely developed lamellae and uneven melanization.[639,640]

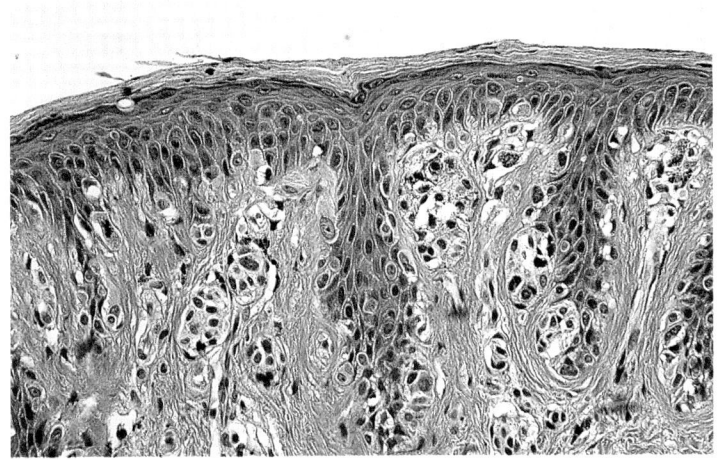

Fig. 32.23 **Dysplastic nevus.** There is mild cytological atypia of the cells and mild fibroplasia of the papillary dermis. (H & E)

The melanosomes are spherical. These abnormal melanosomes are transferred to keratinocytes before being completely melanized, and they reveal marked degradation.[639]

LENTIGINOUS DYSPLASTIC NEVUS OF THE ELDERLY

This variant of dysplastic (atypical) nevus was described by Kossard and colleagues some years ago.[641] The term 'pigmented lentiginous nevus with atypia' is favored by Blessing.[642] It is an important precursor of melanoma and melanoma in situ in the elderly. The melanomas that develop are usually of superficial spreading type, but sometimes they are of indeterminate type, having overlapping features with lentigo maligna. This distinctive clinico-pathological entity has been ignored. Similar lesions have been categorized in the past (and presumably still are in most centers) as dysplastic nevus, atypical junctional nevus, melanoma in situ (early or evolving) and premalignant melanosis.

Clinically, the nevi occur sporadically in individuals over the age of 60. There is a predilection for the back in males and the legs in females. There is usually solar damage.

Histopathology[641]

Lentiginous dysplastic nevus of the elderly is characterized by elongated rete ridges of uneven size and pattern in which there is extensive junctional nesting as well as single melanocytes. The nests are of irregular size and distribution. There is confluence of melanocytes over occasional single suprapapillary plates. The cells have hyperchromatic nuclei with focal atypia. In some lesions, progression to melanoma in situ has occurred.

The dermis shows prominent lamellar fibrosis around the dermal papillae. There is a variable lymphocytic infiltrate and pigment incontinence. A small dermal component of nevus cells is quite uncommon.

MALIGNANT MELANOCYTIC LESIONS

This section discusses malignant melanoma. The malignant blue nevus has been discussed with its benign counterpart (see p. 818). The malignant lesion that may arise in a cutaneous neurocristic hamartoma is discussed on page 819.

MALIGNANT MELANOMA

The incidence of malignant melanoma has increased significantly over the last two decades in the white populations of various industrialized countries,[643] although there is some evidence to suggest that incidence rates have now begun to stabilize or even decline.[644–646] Furthermore, the prognosis has continued to improve because patients are presenting at an earlier stage with smaller and therefore potentially curable lesions.[647–650] The incidence of melanoma is highest in the subtropical state of Queensland in northern Australia: 42.89 new cases in women and 55.8 in men, annually, per 100 000 of the population.[651] The incidence in Sweden is 8.7/100 000 for men and 10.2/100 000 for women,[652] in white South Africans it is 24.4/100 000,[653] and in Scotland it is 4.9/100 000. In the USA, the lifetime risk of developing a melanoma in 1987 was estimated to be 1 in 120; in 2000 it was estimated to be 1 in 75.[645 654]

The increased incidence rates noted in the last decade appear not to have been caused solely by the increased early detection of clinically insignificant melanomas, but may also have represented a true increase in melanoma incidence.[655–657] It has been suggested that the recent decline in the incidence of melanoma in some countries may be due, in part, to the influx of immigrants at low risk for the development of malignant melanoma.[658] Melanoma in the elderly appears to be the new public health problem for this decade.[659]

Risk factors

The incidence data (see above) suggest a role for sun in the etiology of malignant melanoma. Many studies have examined the sun-exposure habits of patients with melanoma, and have found increased sun sensitivity which is associated with pale skin, blond or red hair, the presence of numerous freckles, and a tendency to burn and to tan poorly.[660–663] There is sometimes a history of painful or blistering sunburns during childhood or adolescence.[664] Two or more such episodes before the age of 15 appear to be important as a risk factor.[45] Recent studies suggest that childhood, per se, may not be a critical period for sunburn and that melanoma risk is increased regardless of the timing in life of the sunburns.[665]

The use of sunscreens has not always been followed by a reduction in the incidence of melanoma. It has even been suggested that their use might increase the risk. However, it appears that the use of sunscreens modifies sun-exposure behavior, leading to sun exposures of greater duration.[666] This finding has important public health implications.[667,668]

The role of chronic sun exposure is more controversial.[669,670] Whereas some studies have suggested that total accumulated exposure to sunlight is an important risk factor, others have found that long-term occupational exposure to sunlight may even be protective against melanoma.[671] Although the role of chronic exposure remains unresolved, there is general acceptance that intermittent intense exposure to sunlight in individuals who are untanned (and who tan poorly) is one of the most important risk factors.[662,672] Experimentally, melanocytes appear to have a protective effect on epidermal basal cells, although they do not seem to prevent DNA damage.[673]

Patients who have received multiple PUVA exposures in the treatment of psoriasis appear to have an increased risk of melanoma about 15 years after the first treatment.[674–676]

The presence of certain types of nevi is also a risk factor. Large congenital nevi and dysplastic (atypical) nevi have been recognized as precursor lesions for some time.[677,678] The dysplastic (atypical) nevus syndrome phenotype is present in 15% or more of patients with melanoma.[678,679] It is only comparatively recently that the etiological significance of large numbers of common (banal, typical), acquired nevi has been appreciated.[680–684] This risk appears to be significant when the number of nevi exceeds 50.[685] The presence of nevi greater than 6 mm in diameter appears to be an independent risk factor.[686] Proneness to develop nevi correlates not only with sun exposure, including blistering episodes, but also with skin complexion, hair color and tanning ability.[45]

Various other associations have been reported. Some of these may represent the chance occurrence of two conditions, but others appear to be a definite although, in some cases, small risk factor. Malignant melanomas have been reported in association with xeroderma pigmentosum (particularly complementation groups C and D),[46,687] Cowden's disease (see p. 868), neurofibromatosis,[688,689] retinoblastoma,[690,691] stasis dermatitis,[692] Turner's syndrome,[693,694] soft tissue sarcomas,[695] subsequent carcinoma of the pancreas,[696] lymphoproliferative disorders,[341,697–702] systemic mastocytosis,[703] the 'cancer family syndrome of Lynch'[704] and infection with the human papilloma virus-16 or human immunodeficiency virus.[705–708]

Other uncommon risk factors include frequent use of tanning salons (although the risk may be limited to use before age 25),[709–712] exposure to polyvinyl chloride, insecticides[713] and solvents, ingestion of arsenic-polluted water, burn scars[714] and Marjolin's ulcers.[715,716] There is no evidence that trauma or the use of oral contraceptives is a risk factor.[717,718] Melanomas have also been recorded after electron beam radiation for cutaneous T-cell lymphoma,[719] in immunosuppressed patients after renal transplantation,[720] following the use of levodopa,[721,722] and in a tattoo.[723]

These various risk factors are listed in Table 32.2.

Genetic factors

The fact that 8–12% of melanomas occur in a familial setting[724] has led to attempts to find a candidate gene or genes for this familial basis. A gene for melanomas associated with the dysplastic (atypical) nevus syndrome was originally localized to the short arm of chromosome 1,[725–727] but subsequent studies, involving other kindreds, failed to confirm this locus. It is now known that mutations of the gene *CDKN2A* (cyclin-dependent kinase inhibitor 2A), encoding the tumor-suppressor protein p16^{INK4a} (p16) and linked to chromosome 9p21, confer susceptibility to familial melanoma.[728–735] Nearly half of the families predisposed to melanoma are linked to this abnormality. In Queensland, Australia, mutations were found in 10% of the most 'melanoma-dense families', but were estimated to occur in only 0.2% of all melanomas.[736] Recently, germline mutations within the exon 2 of the *CDK4* gene on chromosome 12q15 have been reported in families with familial melanoma.[737] However, there is only a low prevalence of germline *CDKN2A* and *CDK4* mutations in patients with early - onset melanoma.[738]

Partial or complete loss of p16 expression is also prevalent in sporadic melanomas.[729,739,740] In one study, loss of chromosome 9 was found in 81% of melanomas studied by comparative genomic hybridization.[741] Other chromosomal losses (and gains) have also been demonstrated.[742–747] One such gain may involve the *C-myc* gene,[748] but there may also be additions to chromosome 7.[749] Karyotypic abnormalities on chromosomes 1, 2, 3, 6, 7, 9, 10, 11, 19 and 22 have been described as melanoma-associated genomic changes.[748] Increased chromosome 1 copy numbers occur with progression of melanoma.[749] Somatic mutations in the Peutz–Jeghers gene (*LKB1/STK11*) have been found in sporadic melanomas.[750]

Increased expression of p16^{INK4a} has been found in cultured human melanocytes after UVB radiation.[728] This substance may have a protective effect against the propagation of melanocytes harboring potentially carcinogenic DNA damage.

Finally, a gene for mole density, another risk factor for melanoma, is linked to the familial melanoma gene *CDKN2A*.[736]

Classification of melanoma

The clinicopathological classification of malignant melanoma has evolved into six groups, based on proposals by Clark[751] and McGovern[752] around 30 years ago. The relative incidence of each type of melanoma varies considerably in

Table 32.2 **Risk factors for the development of melanoma**

Skin and hair color
Numerous freckles
Tendency to burn and tan poorly
Blistering sunburns (? any age)
PUVA therapy
Tanning salons
Presence of nevi (numerous, large, atypical)
Genetic factors (*CDKN2A* and *CDK4* mutations)
Xeroderma pigmentosum
Immunosuppression
Exposure to chemicals
Miscellaneous rare associations

different areas – for example, there is a higher proportion of lentigo maligna melanomas in Caucasians living in subtropical and tropical areas[753] and of acral lentiginous melanomas in Japanese.[754] The figures quoted in parentheses are therefore only a guide to the relative incidence of each type:

- lentigo maligna melanoma (5–15%)
- superficial spreading melanoma (50–75%)
- nodular melanoma (15–35%)
- acral lentiginous melanoma (5–10%)
- desmoplastic (and neurotropic) melanoma (rare)
- miscellaneous group (rare).

Included in the miscellaneous group are melanomas arising in blue nevi, and minimal deviation melanoma, the latter diagnosis not being universally accepted as a distinct entity (see p. 826). The rare examples of a melanoma developing within an intradermal nevus without junctional activity are also included in this category.[755] Amelanotic melanoma is best regarded as a poorly differentiated melanoma, usually of nodular type, rather than as a special type.[756,757] Rare histological variants such as the signet-ring cell melanoma, the balloon cell melanoma, the small cell melanoma, the nevoid melanoma and the myxoid melanoma can be included in the miscellaneous group. These histological variants are considered further on page 827.

Ackerman has continued to question the validity of this traditional classification of melanomas.[758] He states in support of his 'unifying concept' of melanoma that no list of repeatable and reliable criteria for differentiation of the reputed types of melanoma has been published.[758] This statement has been supported by some but questioned by others.[759,760]

Clinical features[761]

Although there is some validity in Ackerman's contention that a clinical distinction cannot always be made between the various types of melanoma that have traditionally been recognized,[761] a clinical description of each of these generally accepted types will be given below.[762] First, however, there are several unrelated clinical aspects of melanoma that should be mentioned. These include the rarity of melanomas in childhood,[763–765] the very rare occurrence of congenital melanomas,[388,389,766] and the development in some patients of a paraneoplastic syndrome.[767] Some of the melanomas in children and in adolescents arise in small congenital nevi;[764,768] others arise *de novo*. The natural history of melanomas in children appears to be similar to that in adults,[769] although the survival advantage for adult females is not seen in children.[770] Diagnosis is sometimes difficult, both clinically and histopathologically,[303,771] sometimes leading to delayed diagnosis and the removal of thicker lesions.[772–774]

Attempts have been made to characterize the clinical features of melanoma in an easily remembered mnemonic. The ABCD rule highlights the clinical characteristics: asymmetry, border irregularity, color variegation, and diameter greater than 6 mm.[775–777] Many exceptions to this rule occur,[778–780] leading to clinical misdiagnoses.[781–785]

Lentigo maligna melanoma occurs most frequently on the face and sun-exposed upper extremities of elderly people.[786] Its precursor lesion, the lentigo maligna (Hutchinson's melanotic freckle), is an irregularly pigmented macule which expands slowly. There is great variation in color, with tan-brown, black and even pink areas present. An amelanotic variant has been reported;[787–793] rarely, this takes the form of an inflammatory plaque[794] or follows cryosurgery for lentigo maligna.[795] Invasive malignancy (vertical growth phase) is characterized by thickening of the lesion with the development of elevated plaques or discrete nodules. The proportion of lentigo malignas that progress to lentigo maligna melanoma is said to be quite small, with a lifetime risk of only about 5%.[796] Rapid progression to a deeply invasive tumor has

been reported[790,797] Cryotherapy, superficial radiotherapy, surgical excision with mapping[798] or peripheral vertical sections for margin control,[799,800] and a modified Mohs' micrographic technique, using immunoperoxidase staining with HMB-45, have all been proposed as suitable methods of treatment for lentigo maligna.[801–806] Unfortunately, cryotherapy may be followed by lentiginous hyperpigmentation in the scar, which requires differentiation from a recurrence.[807]

The **superficial spreading melanoma** may develop on any part of the body, and at any age.[808] It is particularly common on the trunk in males and the lower extremities in females. It has a shorter radial growth phase than lentigo maligna melanoma and is usually at least superficially invasive at the time of presentation. It also has a variegated color with an irregular expanding margin. An amelanotic variant has also been reported;[809] rarely, it may clinically simulate a patch of vitiligo.[810] Areas of regression are not uncommon in both this type of melanoma and the lentigo maligna form.

Nodular melanomas have no antecedent radial growth phase. They are therefore nodular, polypoid[811,812] or occasionally pedunculated,[813] dark brown or blue-black lesions occurring anywhere on the body. Occasionally flesh-colored amelanotic variants are found.[814,815] Ulceration may be present.

Acral lentiginous melanomas[816] develop on palmar, plantar and sub-ungual skin.[817–825] They are particularly common in black people and the Japanese[826-830] and Taiwanese,[831] and are found predominantly in elderly patients, with a male preponderance. They present as pigmented plaques or nodules which are often ulcerated. Subungual melanomas may present as longitudinal melanonychia.[832] Atypical presentations such as intertriginous ulcerated areas and amelanotic variants have been reported.[186,833,834] Not all melanomas on volar and subungual skin are of acral lentiginous type, some being of superficial spreading, nodular or unclassifiable type.[835–839] In one series of subungual melanomas, only half were of acral lentiginous type.[840] Melanomas of the oral cavity and other mucous surfaces, such as the vagina, have been included in this group by some, but excluded by others.[336,841,842] There are some clinical and histological similarities between mucosal melanomas and those of volar skin.[843] The term 'mucosal (lentiginous) melanomas' is sometimes used.

In a large Swedish series of 219 cases of melanoma of the vulva, the vast majority were of the mucosal (acral) lentiginous type.[844] The prognosis of vulval melanomas (37–47% 5-year survival) is poorer than for other cutaneous melanomas.[845,846] They tend to be thicker lesions and to occur in older women.[847]

Desmoplastic melanoma is usually found on the head and neck region as a spreading indurated plaque or bulky, firm tumefaction.[848–855] Atypical presentations occur.[856,857] The lesions are often non-pigmented, although areas of lentigo maligna may overlie part of the lesion or be found at the periphery.[858] Sometimes the desmoplastic pattern is found only in the recurrence, or in the metastases of a more usual type of melanoma. Desmoplastic melanomas are often stubbornly recurrent;[848] in many instances this is a reflection of inadequate surgical excision of a lesion which is often, locally, quite advanced in its growth.[851,859] In one series the 5-year disease-free survival rate was 68%, better than is seen for other categories of melanoma of comparable thickness.[860] In another, desmoplastic melanomas with neurotropism had a significant decrease in survival.[861] In a large series reported from the Sydney Melanoma Unit, the 5-year survival was 75%, which was similar to that for patients with other cutaneous melanomas of similar thickness.[862]

Histopathology

Before considering the histopathological features of each subtype of melanoma, there are two related aspects that require consideration. These are:

- the concept of radial and vertical growth phase
- the nomenclature for precursor lesions, including the radial growth phase.

Clark and colleagues introduced the concept of radial and vertical growth phases in the evolution of a malignant melanoma.[863] The radial growth phase refers to the progressive centrifugal spread of a flat pigmented area, which is characterized by intraepidermal proliferation of atypical melanocytes with features that differ in lentigo maligna, superficial spreading melanoma and acral lentiginous melanoma. It is generally agreed that multiple melanocytes (a 'field'), rather than a single melanocyte, are responsible for the beginning of a melanoma.[864,865] The radial growth phase precedes the development of the vertical growth phase, although nodular melanomas have no radial growth. Invasion of the papillary dermis may not have the same prognostic connotations as penetration of the reticular dermis; the concept of radial growth has therefore been redefined to include lesions with invasion of the papillary dermis by cells, either single or in small nests, resembling those in the epidermis.[863,866] This stage has been called the invasive radial growth phase. The presence of dermal mitoses excludes this diagnosis. Melanomas in this phase are probably incapable of metastasis.[867] Angiogenesis and expression of vascular endothelial growth factor are associated with the development of the vertical growth phase and tumor progression.[868,869] Other mechanisms are also involved, but they are complex and poorly understood.[870–876] Destruction or loss of the basement membrane is not mandatory for melanoma invasion.[877]

There is considerable controversy regarding the nomenclature to be used for presumed precursor lesions of malignant melanoma.[878–885] Terms such as 'atypical melanocytic hyperplasia', 'pagetoid melanocytic proliferation', 'pagetoid melanocytosis', 'precancerous melanosis', 'severe melanocytic dysplasia' and, more recently, 'dysplastic (atypical) nevus' have been used for these precursor lesions, and not always consistently.[886–888] Some have used the term 'melanoma in situ' for evolving melanocytic atypias,[887,889] whereas others have avoided the term because of the connotation for insurance purposes of the word 'melanoma' in this title. This latter practice has been criticized.[890,891] The Consensus Conference on the early diagnosis and treatment of melanomas, convened by the National Institutes of Health (USA), agreed that 'melanoma in situ' was a distinct entity.[892] Their report has been criticised by Ackerman.[893] To overcome this controversy, it has been suggested that the term 'melanocytic intraepidermal neoplasia (MIN)' be applied to these lesions in the same way that cervical intraepithelial neoplasia (CIN) is used for the cervix.[894,895] This term is little used outside the United Kingdom.

Despite the above, the epidermal component (radial growth phase) of melanomas of the lentigo maligna, superficial spreading and acral lentiginous types is usually histologically distinctive.[896,897] It may be difficult to assign a classification in about 5% of melanomas, because of overlap features.

There is a disappointing degree of disagreement between experts in the diagnosis of melanocytic neoplasms.[327,898–902] Errors in diagnosis, leading to litigation, are not uncommon.[903] Nevertheless, it is generally agreed that in a very small number of cases the diagnosis is elusive and that expressing diagnostic uncertainty is acceptable.[904]

Criteria for the diagnosis of malignant melanoma[905] are listed in Table 32.3.

Lentigo maligna melanoma is characterized by an epidermal component of atypical melanocytes, singly and in nests, usually confined to the basal layer and with little pagetoid invasion of the epidermis (Fig. 32.24).[786,906,907] It is controversial whether the precursor lentigo maligna should be regarded as a melanocytic dysplasia or as an in situ melanoma.[786,908] No consistent criteria have been proposed for distinguishing these evolutionary stages, although the presence of junctional nesting, deep adnexal involvement, melanocyte crowding with confluence, atypia, and the presence of melanocytes above the

Table 32.3 **Histological criteria for the diagnosis of malignant melanoma (after Ackerman)**[905]

Architectural criteria
Asymmetry
Poor circumscription
Epidermal nests of melanocytes showing:
- confluence
- variability in size and shape
- haphazard interval and array

Solitary epidermal melanocytes showing:
- predominance over nests
- pagetoid spread
- haphazard arrangement

Dermal nests showing:
- variability in size and shape
- confluence
- lack of maturation in depth
- variability in melanin distribution

Melanocytes within lymphovascular spaces

Cytological criteria
Nuclear pleomorphism
Nucleolar variability
Mitoses:
- even deep
- sometimes atypical

Apoptosis increased

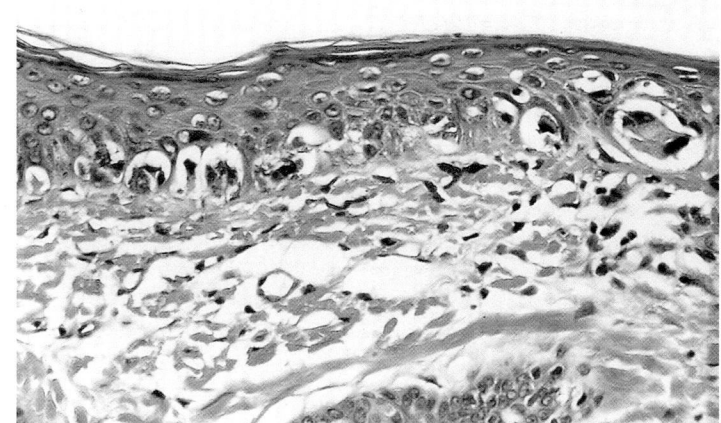

Fig. 32.24 **Lentigo maligna.** There are atypical melanocytes in the basal layer of the epidermis. Elastotic changes are present in the dermis. (H & E)

basal layer have been used as markers of melanoma in situ.[909,910] There is often some epidermal atrophy. Multinucleate melanocytes with prominent dendritic processes (the 'starburst giant cell') are often present in the basal layer.[911,912] The invasive component may be composed of spindle or epithelioid melanocytes. There is variable cytological atypia. In some cases there are plentiful mitoses, with considerable nuclear pleomorphism and even tumor giant cells. The upper dermis usually shows moderate to severe solar elastosis and the presence of pigment-containing macrophages and small collections of lymphocytes. However, solar elastosis is not a prerequisite for the diagnosis.[760] Microinvasive foci, which may be difficult to see in hematoxylin and eosin-stained sections, can be highlighted by the demonstration of S100 protein and HMB-45 in invasive melanocytes by immunoperoxidase techniques.[913]

It is a well-recognized phenomenon that a subsequent excision may show more pronounced (atypical) features than a previous biopsy specimen. This is particularly so for lesions on actinically damaged skin, in which up to 40% of excisions may show more pronounced changes.[914,915]

On electron microscopy, the melanosomes in the atypical melanocytes are usually ellipsoidal and resemble those of normal melanocytes, unlike the spheroidal and abnormal appearance of the melanosomes in superficial spreading and nodular melanomas.[916]

Superficial spreading melanoma is characterized by a proliferation of atypical melanocytes, singly and in nests, at all levels within the epidermis. This pagetoid spread within the epidermis is sometimes known as 'buckshot scatter' (Fig. 32.25). Superficial adnexal epithelium may also be involved. The infiltrative component may be arranged in solid masses or may have a fascicular arrangement. The cells may be epithelioid, nevus cell-like, or even spindle-shaped without evidence of maturation during their descent into the dermis. Again the degree of cytological atypia varies from case to case.[917]

A rare variant of melanoma, usually of the superficial spreading type, is the **verrucous melanoma**.[918] This occurs most often on the back and limbs of middle-aged to older males.[919] It is characterized by marked epidermal hyperplasia, elongation of the rete ridges and overlying hyperkeratosis.[920,921] This variant is often misdiagnosed clinically as a seborrheic keratosis.[918]

Nodular melanoma has no adjacent intraepidermal component of atypical melanocytes, although there is usually epidermal invasion by malignant cells directly overlying the dermal mass. The dermal component is usually composed of oval to round epithelioid cells but, as in other types of melanoma, this can be quite variable (Fig. 32.26). Mast cells are increased in this and other types of melanoma.[922] Erythrophagocytosis by tumor cells is an exceedingly rare phenomenon.[923]

Acral lentiginous melanomas have a radial growth phase which is characterized by a lentiginous pattern of atypical melanocytes, with some nesting (Fig. 32.27).[816] There may be some 'buckshot scatter' of melanocytes, but this is never as marked as in superficial spreading melanoma (see above). The melanocytes may be plump with a surrounding clear halo, giving a lacunar appearance, or they may have heavily pigmented dendritic processes. The epidermal component may look misleadingly benign. Against this background, the recent report of three patients from Japan with 'atypical melanosis of the foot' must be viewed with some reservations.[924] It is possible that regression resulted in the bland histological appearances seen in these cases, which clinically resembled acral lentiginous melanoma, in which the epidermis is usually hyperplastic; focal ulceration may occur. The invasive component may consist of epithelioid cells or spindle cells, or resemble nevus cells. There may be a desmoplastic stromal response. Osteosarcomatous change has been reported in the stroma. It is not uncommon for tumor cells to have infiltrated the deep dermis or subcutaneous tissue by the time of diagnosis.[925]

Ahmed has reviewed the histological spectrum of acral melanomas and proposed that this term be used for all melanomas in acral locations, not just those traditionally called acral lentiginous melanoma.[926] In a significant number of these cases, the dermal component shows an unusual morphology including the presence of giant, nevoid and clear cells.[926]

Desmoplastic/spindle-cell melanomas are composed of strands of elongated spindle-shaped cells surrounded by mature collagen bundles (Fig. 32.28). The stromal component varies considerably in different tumors. Sometimes there are scattered spindle cells and abundant collagen, whereas in others there is little stroma. This latter group is usually referred to as spindle-cell melanomas, although it should be noted that desmoplastic melanoma and spindle-cell melanoma form a continuum without a discrete separation.[927] The desmoplastic features are usually more prominent in the local recurrences, in contrast to lymph node and visceral metastases, which often resemble conventional melanomas.[928] The cells resemble fibroblasts, but there are scattered cells with hyperchromatic and even bizarre nuclei.[929]

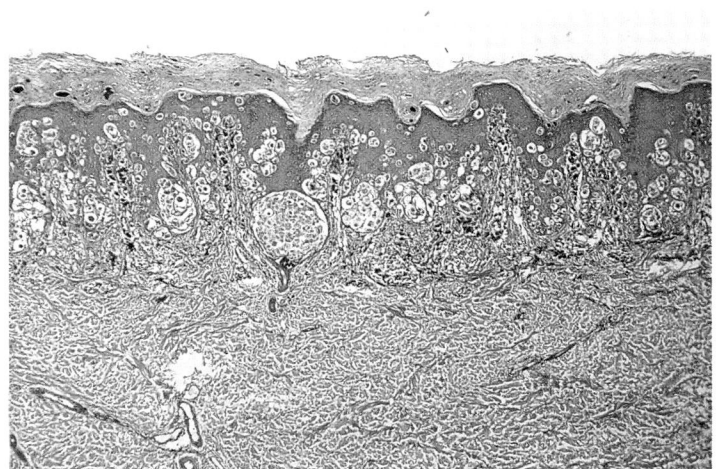

Fig. 32.25 **Superficial spreading melanoma.** This lesion is level I (in situ). Atypical melanocytes show 'buckshot scatter' within the epidermis. (H & E)

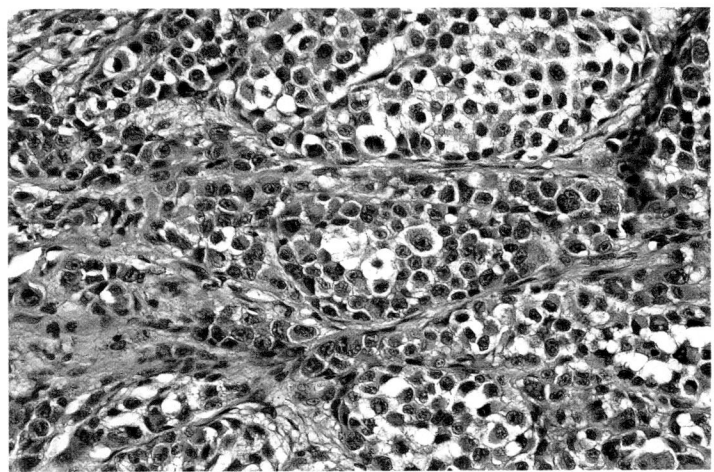

Fig. 32.26 **Nodular melanoma.** The tumor cells in the dermis have large, hyperchromatic nuclei. There is no melanin present in the cells. They were positive for S100 protein. (H & E)

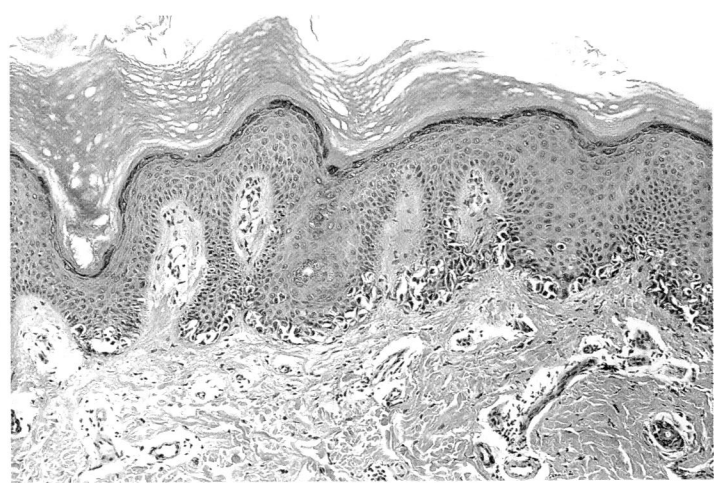

Fig. 32.27 **Acral lentiginous melanoma** (radial growth phase). There are atypical melanocytes within the basal layer that show only slight upward spread. (H & E)

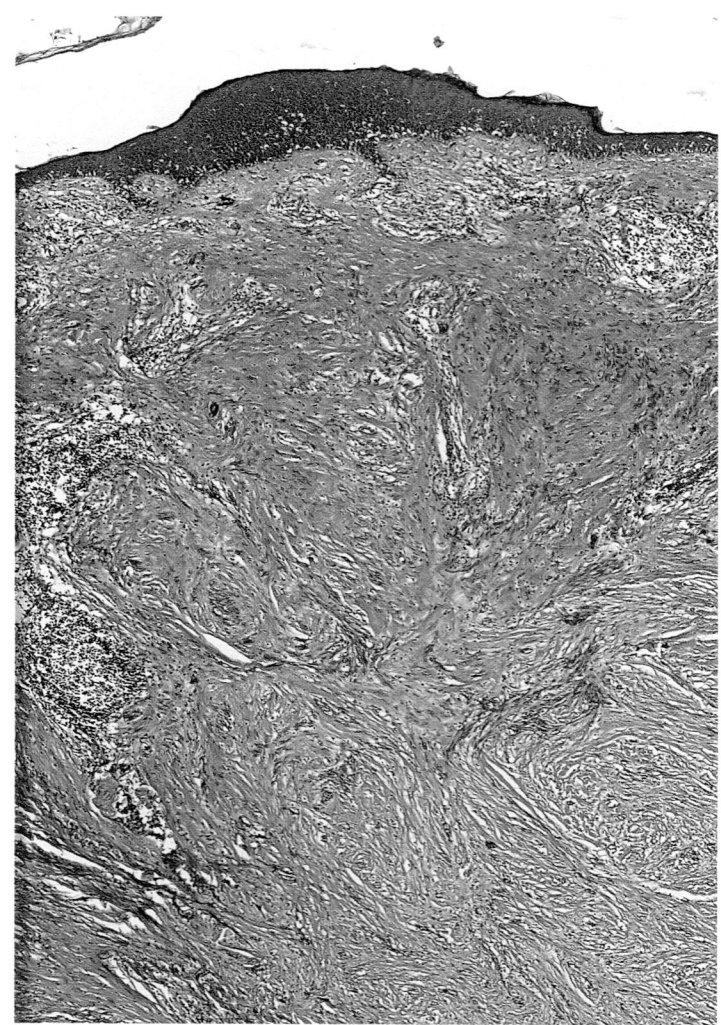

Fig. 32.28 **Desmoplastic melanoma.** Bundles of spindle-shaped cells are present in the dermis admixed with collagen and blood vessels. Note the characteristic lymphoid collections. This case was initially misdiagnosed as 'scar tissue'. (H & E)

into two groups, pure desmoplastic melanomas are negative for HMB-45.[940,941] Nearly 50% of spindle-cell melanomas show some staining for HMB-45, and this subset of tumors appears to have a more aggressive biologic potential than negative lesions.[940] Sensitivity is increased if antigen retrieval methods are used.[942] Melan-A (MART-1) gives mostly negative results with desmoplastic melanoma and is of little use with this morphologic type.[943] NK1/C-3 is expressed in approximately one-quarter of cases.[938] In one study, microphthalmia transcription factor (MiTF) had a sensitivity for desmoplastic/spindle-cell melanomas that equalled or exceeded that of HMB-45 or melan-A.[944] In another series, it stained only one case of desmoplastic melanoma.[945] Overall, this new marker lacks sufficient sensitivity and specificity for widespread diagnostic use.[946,947] Smooth muscle actin is present in a patchy distribution in nearly half the cases.[860,948] Basic fibroblast growth factor (bFGF), an established growth factor for melanocytes, and other fibrogenic cytokines are expressed in the nuclei of the tumor cells in most desmoplastic melanomas.[547] They presumably play a role in mediating the desmoplastic phenotype.[949] p75 nerve growth factor receptor stains the cells in desmoplastic and neurotropic tumors, but it also stains other tumors of putative neural crest origin.[939,950] Basement membrane antigens such as laminin and type IV collagen are often expressed in spindle-cell melanomas.[951] CD34 expression has been reported in a metastatic desmoplastic melanoma.[952] The cells in a desmoplastic melanoma have abundant rough endoplasmic reticulum, and sometimes intracytoplasmic collagen and macular desmosomes. Non-membrane-bound melanin granules and premelanosomes have been noted in some cases,[953] although they have been specifically excluded in others.[937] The most widely accepted view is that the desmoplastic component is derived from melanocytes that have undergone adaptive fibroplasia,[929] although contrary views favor a fibroblastic stromal response[858] or neurosarcomatous differentiation.[954] Although mature scars are easily differentiated from desmoplastic melanoma on light microscopy, immature scars share many features including lymphoid infiltrates, myxoid change, hypercellularity and atypia.[955] Kaneishi and Cockerell found that an epidermal proliferation of melanocytes, neurotropism and S100 and/or HMB-45 positivity were the only distinguishing features.[955] Parallelism of fibrocyte nuclei may be present in scar tissue. Nuclei in desmoplastic melanoma have a haphazard array.

In the **neurotropic** variant (Fig. 32.29) there are spindle-shaped cells with neuroma-like patterns (neural transformation) and a tendency to adopt a circumferential arrangement around small nerves in the deep dermis and subcutaneous tissue (neurotropism).[852,956,957] Interlacing bundles of cells are seen. Desmoplastic and neurotropic patterns often occur together in the same neoplasm.[958] The cells vary in size and nuclear staining. The cells usually lack melanin pigment, although a case with prominent melanization of the cells has been reported.[959] The absence of S100 protein using immunoperoxidase techniques does not exclude the diagnosis, as this antigen may be absent in up to 20% of cases;[960] this figure seems unusually high in the author's experience. There is a significant risk of local recurrence in the presence of neurotropism.[862]

'Minimal deviation melanoma' is the term applied to melanomas in which the vertical growth phase is composed of a uniform population of cells whose cytological features deviate only minimally from those of nevus cells.[961–965] Epithelioid or spindle-cell features may be present. Included in this group by some pathologists is the melanoma composed of cells resembling small nevus cells (see p. 828). The concept of minimal deviation melanoma has not gained universal acceptance, largely because of an absence of standardized histological criteria.[966–969] There is some evidence that this diagnosis has been applied indiscriminately to difficult and borderline lesions.

Multinucleate cells are often present. Small foci of neural transformation and neurotropism may be seen.[860,930] The tumor infiltrates deeply. The full extent of the tumor is sometimes difficult to discern with accuracy. The use of S100 staining is a valuable adjunct in determining the extent of some lesions.[931] There may be scattered collections of lymphocytes and plasma cells within the tumor. In paucicellular tumors these small foci of inflammatory cells can provide a clue to the diagnosis on scanning magnification. This paucicellular variant is easy to misdiagnose on a small punch biopsy or superficial shave. There may even be a resemblance to dermatofibroma with a storiform appearance. Another variant is the superficial or early lesion characterized by cytological atypia, stromal myxoid change, aggregates of lymphocytes and poor circumscription.[932] Heterotopic bone and cartilage and sweat duct proliferation may form.[933–936] There is often a lentigo maligna epidermal component overlying or towards one edge of the lesion.[859] The tumor cells are nearly always amelanotic, but they are positive for vimentin in all cases and for S100 protein and neuron-specific enolase in approximately 95% of cases.[929,937,938] Sometimes only a minority of the malignant cells (10–20%) express S100 protein. HMB-45, which detects premelanosomes, is detected in from 0 to 20% of cases, but only small clusters of cells are stained in the positive cases.[860,938,939] If desmoplastic/spindle-cell melanomas are separated

Level and thickness

In any report on a malignant melanoma the anatomical level of invasion

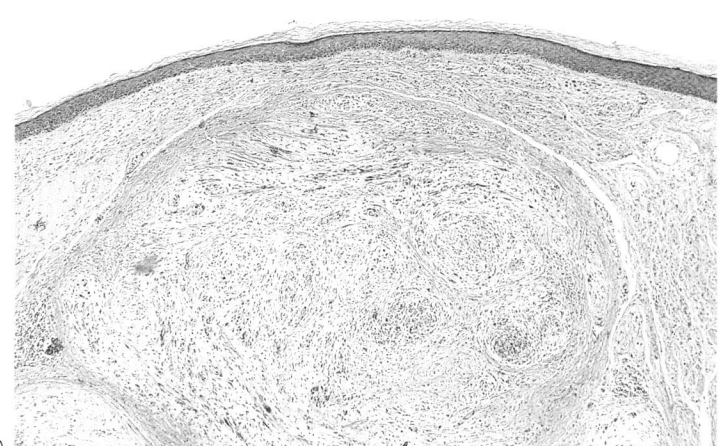

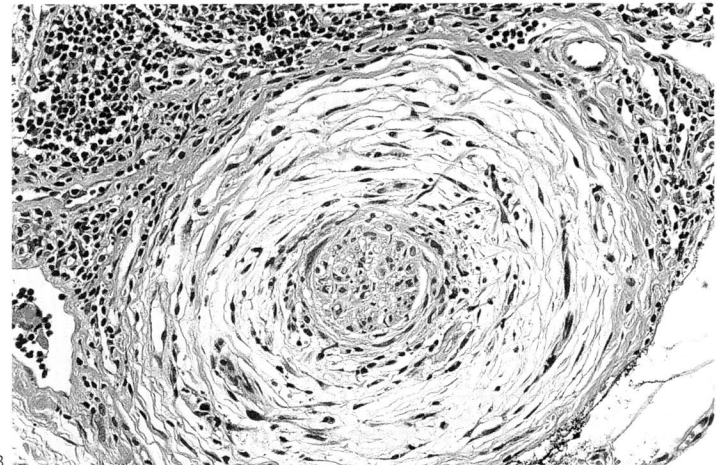

Fig. 32.29 **(A) Neurotropic melanoma. (B)** Tumor cells are loosely arranged in a concentric fashion around a small nerve in the subcutis. Lymphocytes are present in the surrounding tissue. (H & E)

(Clark's level) and the thickness of the tumor (Breslow thickness)[970] should be stated. Five anatomical levels are recognized:[752]

1. confined to the epidermis (in situ melanoma)
2. invasion of the papillary dermis
3. invasion to the papillary/reticular dermal interface
4. invasion into the reticular dermis
5. invasion into subcutaneous fat.

The thickness of a melanoma is measured from the top of the granular layer (undersurface of the stratum corneum) to the deepest tumor cell. The Breslow thickness is a reproducible measurement, although some interobserver variation occurs.[971] Melanomas less than 0.76 mm in thickness are regarded as being 'thin melanomas' and generally have an excellent prognosis. It has been suggested that either 0.85 mm or 1 mm is a better breakpoint than 0.76 mm for defining a prognostically favorable group of melanomas.[972,973] Numerous clinical and histological features are related to tumor thickness.[974]

Associated nevi

A contiguous nevus, either dysplastic or common (banal) type, is found in approximately one-third of all melanomas.[652,975–977] The nevus is more often of acquired than congenital type, although in some instances a distinction cannot be made. The great majority of the acquired nevi found in association with melanomas are of the dysplastic (atypical) type.[978] Melanomas develop only rarely from intradermal nevi.[979]

Regression

Partial regression may be found in up to one-third of melanomas;[980,981] the figure is higher in thin melanomas.[982–985] Active regression is recognized by the presence of a heavy lymphocytic infiltrate in the dermis, with loss or degeneration of tumor cells.[986] It seems likely that tumor cells are removed by lymphocyte-mediated apoptosis. Previous (old) regression is characterized by the presence of vascular fibrous tissue with or without melanophages, and a variable lymphocytic infiltrate.[986] If numerous melanophages are present, the term **'nodular melanosis'** is sometimes used. This pattern is not exclusive to regressed melanomas; it can be produced by the regression of solar lentigos and epithelial lesions, such as a pigmented basal cell carcinoma.[987] It has been suggested that as the different stages of regression often coexist in the one specimen, 'subdividing the process is impractical and unrealistic'.[988] The prognostic significance of partial regression will be considered later (see p. 832).

Approximately 2% of patients with melanoma present with metastatic disease in the absence of a recognized primary tumor.[989] In many of these cases of so-called 'occult primary melanoma' it is probable that the primary lesion underwent spontaneous regression.[990] Sometimes the patient can recall an earlier pigmented lesion that enlarged, darkened, then flattened and depigmented.[991] Other possibilities include origin of the tumor in lymph nodes or in visceral organs, or a primary cutaneous lesion which is initially undetectable.[992] A related phenomenon is the occurrence of a single focus of melanoma, of presumed metastatic origin, confined to the dermis and/or subcutis, but without evidence of an overlying epidermal component or inflammation. Such tumors may be the result of previous partial regression of which no evidence remains or local recurrence following previous complete regression. Such cases have a better prognosis than other examples of stage IV disease, suggesting that they are not true metastases.[993]

Electron microscopy

Stage II melanosomes are considered the hallmark of malignant melanoma and melanin synthesis. They are found rarely in other tumors.[994] Care must be taken to avoid mistaking myelin figures for aberrant melanosomes. In some desmoplastic melanomas it may not be possible to find melanosomes.[994] Ultrastructural features of the various histological subtypes have already been mentioned (see above).

Special variants of malignant melanoma

In recent years a number of histologically distinct variants of malignant melanoma have been described.[995] Some of these have already been referred to, as they represent unusual histological changes in one of the major categories of melanoma. Smooth muscle differentiation has been reported in one case of a metastatic sarcomatoid melanoma in an axillary lymph node.[996] This finding does not warrant a special diagnostic category.

Myxoid melanoma[997–1003]

The myxoid variant was first described in a metastatic deposit, but it has since been described in primary lesions as well.[1004] Spindle and stellate-shaped cells are embedded in a myxoid stroma. The stroma stains with alcian blue, and the tumor cells express S100 protein and neuron-specific enolase. HMB-45 may not be expressed, despite the presence of premelanosomes in one case examined ultrastructurally.[1000] However, HMB-45 was present in nine of 10 cases in one recent study.[1005]

Balloon cell melanoma

Balloon cell change may occur in primary or secondary melanomas.[860,1006,1007] The presence of nuclear pleomorphism, mitoses and cytological atypia help to distinguish this lesion from balloon cell nevus (see p. 809). The cells express the usual immunohistochemical markers of a malignant melanoma. The prognosis correlates with tumor thickness.[1008] The nature of the clear cell change is uncertain; it is not a degenerative change, as was once thought.[1009]

Signet-ring cell melanoma

The presence of signet-ring cells has been reported in several metastatic and recurrent melanomas, and in one primary lesion (Fig. 32.30).[1010–013] These cells are quite different from the scattered sebocyte-like cells occasionally seen in nevi and metastatic melanoma.[1014]

Rhabdoid melanoma

The presence of cells resembling those seen in rhabdoid tumors (see p. 972) is a rare change described in metastatic melanomas.[1015,1016] It has since been reported in primary melanomas.[1017] Large pleomorphic multinucleated cells can be seen in a rare variant that masquerades as malignant fibrous histiocytoma.[1018]

Osteogenic melanoma

Osteocartilaginous metaplasia is an exceedingly rare finding in malignant melanomas.[1019,1020] The change usually occurs in acral lentiginous melanomas, particularly subungual lesions.[1021] There is a high-grade sarcomatoid component, with osteoid matrix and sometimes chondroblastic differentiation. Junctional activity assists in making the diagnosis. The cells are positive for S100 protein and vimentin. HMB-45 staining is variable. Osteocartilaginous differentiation has been described in two cases of primary mucosal melanoma.[1022] A melanoma with osteoclast-like giant cells has also been reported.[1023]

Small cell melanoma

Small cell carcinoma refers to the presence of cells resembling those seen in a Merkel cell carcinoma (see p. 989). It is not the same as the nevoid melanoma (see below). In one reported case the cells were focally positive for S100 protein and strongly positive for HMB-45. The cells contained premelanosomes and melanosomes on electron microscopy.[1024] Spatz and Barnhill have proposed the use of the term 'small cell melanoma' for a variant of nevoid melanoma in which more than 50% of the melanoma cell population have nuclei smaller than keratinocytic nuclei.[1025]

Nevoid melanoma

The existence of a melanoma composed of nevus-like cells has been known for a long time, but it is only comparatively recently that it has been separated from nodular melanoma.[1026–1029] It sometimes causes problems in diagnosis.[902,1030] Two histological variants of nevoid melanoma are now recognized: one composed of small nevus-like cells (Fig. 32.31), and the other composed of larger cells resembling those seen in a Spitz nevus.[1026,1031,1032] Mixed variants are rare. The term 'small cell melanoma' (see above) is often used for the small cell variant of nevoid melanoma. It is the author's practice to restrict the use of the term 'nevoid melanoma' to lesions that resemble a benign nevus and that do not possess an intraepidermal component resembling the radial growth phase of one of the more usual types of melanoma (Fig. 32.32). Kossard and Wilkinson have included as nevoid melanomas cases composed of small cells in the dermis, all but one of which had a lentiginous intraepidermal component.[1033]

Nevoid melanomas superficially resemble a nevus by their cell type, symmetry and lack of a prominent intraepidermal component. They may even show maturation of cells in depth, although this is often impaired.[1034] The diagnosis can be made by the presence of dermal mitoses, often deep, and cells in the base with prominent nucleoli. The cells often form sheets or cords in part of the lesion, with the loss of an orderly arrangement of nests. Subtle pleomorphism is often present.[1034] An epidermal verrucous pattern with prominent acanthosis is sometimes seen in the 'Spitzoid' variant.[1028,1034] The continuous pattern of melanocytes along the basal layer helps distinguish this lesion from a Spitz nevus. The increased number of AgNORs (see p. 813) may assist in making a diagnosis of nevoid melanoma.[1035]

McNutt and colleagues have studied the immunohistochemical features of nevoid melanomas. They express S100 protein, HMB-45, proliferating cell nuclear antigen (PCNA) and Ki-67 (using the antibody MIB-1). In contrast, a Spitz nevus usually shows stratification of staining (not always with PCNA), with less intense staining of cells in the base of the lesion.[1026,1036] The author has seen two cases (the subject of litigation) in which metastasis occurred but which were negative for HMB-45.

Although one study has shown a better than expected prognosis for nevoid melanomas,[1028] this has not been confirmed.[1026,1027] In fact, a recent study showed a significant local recurrence and mortality rate in those cases with sufficient follow-up information.[1034]

Small-diameter melanoma

Approximately 5% of melanomas are less than 6 mm in diameter.[1037–1040] These tend to occur in patients younger than the usual average age for melanoma. Initially they were thought to have a better prognosis than melanomas of the same thickness, but this does not appear to be the case.

Ganglioneuroblastic melanoma

A case of metastatic melanoma showing ganglioneuroblastic differentiation has been reported. It combined large ganglion cells with abundant cytoplasm separated by pale pink fibrillar material.[1041] Other areas resembled an epithelioid melanoma. The ganglioneuroblastic component stained for S100 protein, melan-A, neurofilament, GFAP, synaptophysin and chromogranin.[1041]

Angiomatoid melanoma

The term 'angiomatoid melanoma' has been used for metastatic lesions in which the tumor cells show features suggesting vascular differentiation.[1042,1043] It should not be confused with angiotropic melanoma (see p. 830) in which there is periendothelial cuffing of microvessels by melanoma cells.

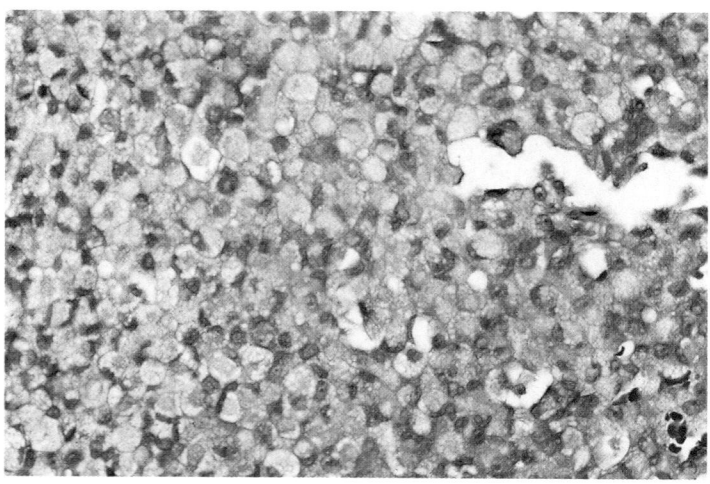

Fig. 32.30 **Signet-ring cell melanoma.** The cells have an eccentric nucleus and foamy cytoplasm. (H & E)

Metastatic melanoma resembling MPNST

Recently, 16 cases of metastatic malignant melanoma resembling malignant peripheral nerve sheath tumor (MPNST) were reported.[1044] Histologically, the tumors were composed of an atypical spindle-cell proliferation arranged in fascicles, often accompanied by a peritheliomatous growth pattern.[1044] Foci of necrosis and numerous mitoses were often seen. Strong, diffuse staining for S100 protein was usually present.[1044] A subsequent report has shown that this pattern may also be found in primary malignant melanomas.[1045]

Animal type (equine) melanoma

The rare animal type variant of melanoma, also known as malignant melanoma with prominent pigment synthesis, is jet black in color and composed of heavily pigmented epithelioid and dendritic cells with numerous melanophages. It may occur at any site but several personally studied cases have been on the scalp.[766] It resembles the tumor seen in many gray horses, which is a slow-growing, progressive lesion; it is usually benign in horses. In humans its behavior has been unpredictable, with metastasis recorded in several cases.[1046,1047]

Bullous melanoma

The presence of suprabasal clefting in a melanoma has been regarded as a possible localized manifestation of paraneoplastic pemphigus.[1048] The author has seen two cases in which the clefting was subepidermal and quite extensive (Fig. 32.33).

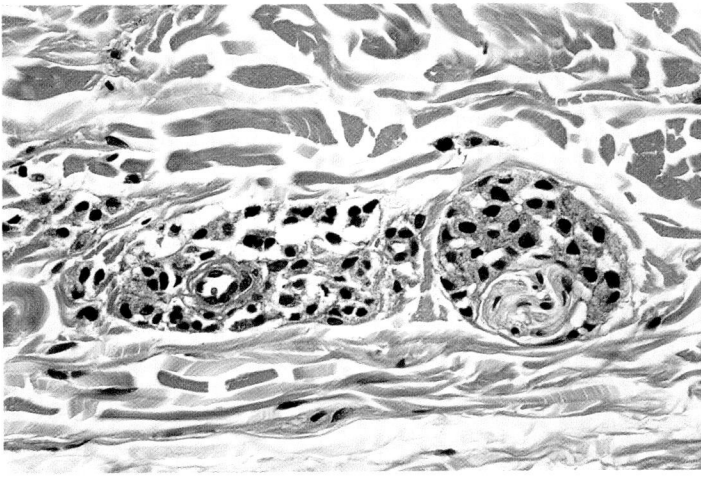

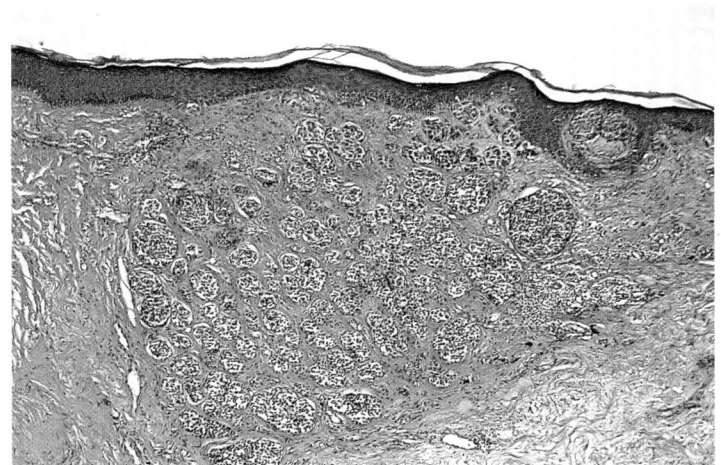

Fig. 32.32 **Nevoid melanoma.** This case was initially diagnosed as benign, but it metastasizec. There is variability in nest size and arrangement. (H & E)

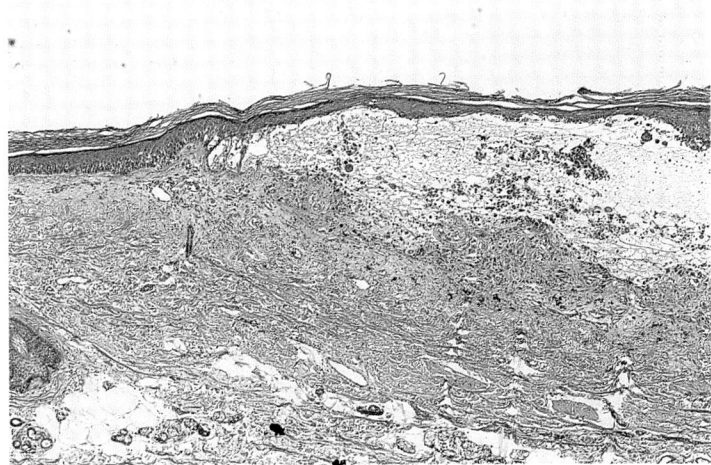

Fig. 32.31 **(A) Melanoma composed of small nevus-like cells. (B)** Tumor cells surround a small nerve in the deep dermis. The patient developed metastases 1 year after the removal of this lesion. (H & E)

Fig. 32.33 **Bullous melanoma.** The lesion presented as a pigmented blister. Acantholytic melanoma cells are in the subepidermal space. (H & E)

Melanoma of soft parts (clear cell sarcoma)[496,1049]

Melanoma of soft parts is mentioned here for completeness because it may involve the skin secondarily. Rarely, a dermal nodule of the tumor may be a major component. It arises mainly in adolescents and young adults, but there is a wide age range. The extremities, particularly the lower, are commonly involved. Its course is marked by frequent local recurrences, with eventual metastasis in many.[1050] The tumor is composed of nests and strands of relatively bland oval or elongated cells separated by thin collagenous septa.[1049] Large amounts of pale or granular amphophilic cytoplasm are present.[1049] Melanin and glycogen can be demonstrated in about two-thirds of cases. Multinucleate tumor cells are often present, but mitoses may be scarce. The cells express S100 protein and/or HMB-45. Keratin markers, such as CAM5.2, are expressed in up to one-third of cases. A specific chromosomal translocation involving chromosomes 22 and 12 characterizes 60% of cases. The translocation is t(12;22)(q13;q12). Other abnormalities involving chromosome 22 are observed in most of the remaining tumors.[1051]

Metastases

Metastases in cases of malignant melanoma are usually to regional lymph nodes in the first instance. The probability of nodal metastases is related to the Clark level[1052] and the Breslow tumor thickness (see above).[1053] Nodal metastases are quite uncommon in lesions less than 1 mm in thickness; their frequency exceeds 50% among lesions greater than 4 mm in thickness.[1052,1053] It has been suggested that the propensity for spindle-cell melanomas to metastasize to lymph nodes is relatively low, despite their thickness.[927] Metastases also take place to the skin and subcutaneous tissue,[1054,1055] skin graft donor sites,[1056] lungs, brain and dura,[1057] gastrointestinal tract, heart,[1058] liver and adrenal glands.[1059] Nodal and pulmonary granulomatosis, usually of sarcoidal type, is a rare finding in patients with malignant melanoma.[1060] Its presence may lead to a clinical misdiagnosis of metastatic disease. Fine needle aspiration (FNA) can be used as a reliable technique to diagnose metastatic melanoma.[1061] Rarely, dermal lymphatic invasion associated with cutaneous metastatic disease may give a picture resembling that of so-called 'inflammatory' carcinoma of the breast.[1062–1066] Lymphatic permeation in primary cutaneous melanoma is rarely seen;[1067] however, it is the likely cause of in-transit metastases.[1068] Such metastases are clonal in type.[1069] Rare cases of blood vessel wall invasion (*angiotropic melanoma*) have been reported.[1043,1070–1072] This usually takes the form of periendothelial cuffing of microvessels by melanoma cells, although extension of cells throughout the vessel wall may occur.[1073] Other tropic phenomena (neurotropism and eccrine duct tropism) may accompany the vascular lesions.[1073]

When cutaneous metastases of malignant melanoma extend into the epidermis (epidermotropic metastases), differentiating them from a primary melanoma can be particularly difficult.[1074] The epidermotropic component can extend beyond the dermal component, a finding which used to be regarded as specific for a primary lesion.[1074] Even an epidermis-only pattern of epidermotropic metastasis can occur. The pattern seen in local recurrences can be identical.[1075,1076]

The development of *generalized melanosis* in patients with malignant melanoma has been attributed by some to an unlimited spread of single melanoma cells throughout the dermis,[1077–1079] but others have specifically excluded the presence of tumor cells and have found numerous perivascular melanophages in the dermis.[1080–1083] Pigment may also be present in endothelial cells.[1082] A recent study has attributed the pigmentation to activation of the pigment system by melanocyte peptide growth factors and not to widely dispersed melanoma cells.[1084] Exceptions appear to occur.

There is one rare complication of treatment of metastatic disease that warrants mention – the tumor lysis syndrome. This complication, seen mostly with hematologic malignancies, results from the rapid death of numerous malignant cells releasing intracellular products that overwhelm the renal tubules, producing metabolic derangements that may end in death. It has been reported in a patient with metastatic melanoma. [085]

Multiple primary lesions

Additional primary lesions may develop in approximately 2% of patients with malignant melanoma.[1086–1088] Up to a third are diagnosed concurrently with the initial melanoma.[1089] Sometimes it is difficult to distinguish between a new primary lesion and an epidermotropic metastasis.[1090,1091] The usually accepted criteria for diagnosing an additional primary lesion, as opposed to a cutaneous secondary – that is, junctional activity extending beyond the dermal component, lack of central epidermal attenuation and of lymphatic permeation – may not always be reliable (see above).[1091] The second primary melanoma is usually thinner than the first, probably the result of increased clinical surveillance.[1092] Furthermore, some overdiagnosis appears more likely to occur with second lesions.[1093]

Patients with multiple primary lesions will show the *CDKN2A* and *CDK4* mutations more often than patients with solitary lesions, a reflection of the familial setting of an underlying risk factor for multiple lesions, the dysplastic nevus syndrome.[1093,1094]

Special techniques to aid diagnosis

In suspected cases of melanoma which are amelanotic or oligomelanotic, a number of special stains and techniques may be used to establish a diagnosis.[757,1095] These include the Masson–Fontana, Schmorl's and modified Warthin–Starry stains for melanin,[1096] the identification of premelanosomes on electron microscopy, and the demonstration of S100 protein, HMB-45, melan-A (MART-1) and NKI/C-3 using immunoperoxidase techniques.[1097–1100] In one study of 144 melanomas, all stained for S100 protein, 95% stained for NKI/C-3 and 92% for HMB-45. Negative staining was experienced in lesions with little pigment and/or a spindle-cell growth pattern.[1101] Melanomas that are S100 negative are found from time to time. Such lesions may be positive for HMB-45, or retest as positive using monoclonal and polyclonal antibodies against S100 protein.[1102] S100 protein is also found in nevi and Langerhans cells, as well as cutaneous neural tumors. S100 protein is not a single protein but a family of acidic calcium-binding proteins that are important in intracellular calcium metabolism.[1103] False-positive staining of melanophages will occur if the section used for the immunoperoxidase technique has been subjected to prolonged prior melanin bleaching.[1104]

HMB-45, a monoclonal antibody with putative specificity for melanoma cells, stains stimulated melanocytes such as junctional melanocytes in nevi, dermal nevus cells in pigmented lesions removed from some patients with HIV infection,[1105] the cells in deep penetrating nevi,[207] some cells in the papillary dermis in dysplastic (atypical) nevi, melanocytes in blue nevi, and some cells in Spitz nevi (see p. 814). It is a highly sensitive marker for melanoma cells, although it does not stain the cells of desmoplastic melanomas.[207,1098–1100,1106–1108] Some nevoid melanomas (with proven metastasis) fail to stain. Rapid HMB-45 staining has been used to aid in the interpretation of frozen sections during Mohs surgery in the treatment of melanoma.[1109] Both HMB-45 and NKI/C-3 are expressed in a small number of breast carcinomas.[1110] HMB-45 appears to stain melanosomes early in their formation, but not late (stage IV) melanosomes.[1111] Neuron-specific enolase[1112] and vimentin[1113] have also been found in melanomas, but myelin basic protein has not. Cytokeratin staining has been noted in some metastatic melanomas.[1114] Such lesions may be negative for HMB-45, even though the initial primary lesion was positive for HMB-45 and negative for cytokeratin.

That is, a change in immunophenotype appears to take place in some tumors that metastasize.[1115] The immunohistochemical profile of desmoplastic and spindle-cell melanomas has been discussed on page 826.

Melan-A and MART-1 (melanoma antigen recognized by T cells) are the names given independently to the same gene which encodes a melanocytic differentiation antigen with expression in skin, retina and melanocyte cell lines, but not in other normal tissues.[943] A monoclonal antibody to this protein has been called A103. Melan-A is broadly expressed in benign and malignant melanocytic lesions but not in most desmoplastic melanomas.[1116] It is more sensitive than HMB-45[1117,1118] and more specific than stains for S100 protein.[943,1119,1120] A recent study using alcohol-fixed tissue found only faint staining with nevi and strong staining for melanomas, although one-third of the congenital nevi examined were stained.[1121] Another recently introduced marker, microphthalmia transcription factor, is expressed in most benign nevi and melanomas, with the exception of desmoplastic melanomas.[1122]

Melanoma cells and some nevi will show positive fluorescence when unstained sections from formalin-fixed paraffin-embedded tissue are examined.[1123] To date, this method has not been used in routine diagnosis.

A technique which is of some value in the assessment of borderline lesions is the measurement of silver-positive nucleolar organizer regions (AgNOR count) in a representative number of tumor cells.[1124] The mean AgNOR count for melanoma cells is significantly higher than for benign neval cells, although some overlap occurs, particularly with Spitz nevi and dysplastic (atypical) nevi.[1125,1126] However, an AgNOR count of more than 2.5 per cell is very suggestive of a malignant melanoma.[631–634,1125,1127] The AgNOR count appears to have no value in prognostication,[1128,1129] although a contrary view has been expressed, particularly for thin melanomas.[1130,1131]

Various other markers and techniques have been tested in recent years to ascertain their potential as a diagnostic tool in the assessment of borderline lesions. The *bcl-2* oncoprotein is expressed in the cells of melanomas and nevi, and is therefore of no diagnostic value.[1132–1136] Variable results have been obtained with CD44.[1137–1143] The tumor-suppressor protein p53 is expressed in up to 50% of melanomas, but not in benign nevi, although occasional foci of weak nuclear immunoreactivity can be seen in some dysplastic (atypical) nevi and in rare Spitz nevi.[1144–1146] It was strongly expressed in melanomas with a poor prognosis in one study,[1144] but associated with improved survival in another.[1147] Telomerase activity is significantly increased in primary melanomas and metastases.[1148] Cyclin expression is also elevated during tumor progression.[1149–1151] The apoptosis inhibitor, survivin, is expressed in metastatic melanoma; its pathogenetic role in the spread of melanomas remains to be determined.[1152] The tumor-associated antigen TA90 can be detected in the sera of patients with melanoma recurrence an average of 19 months sooner than clinical evaluation.[1153,1154]

Proliferating cell nuclear antigen (PCNA) is expressed in nearly all melanomas, although the intensity of staining in a few cases is weak, with only 20–30% of the cells stained.[322,1155] In the great majority of melanomas more than 40% of the cells stain strongly for PCNA.[322] A significant number of Spitz nevi express PCNA, but staining is weak, with only 10–40% of the cells staining.[322] Expression of PCNA has little role in predicting the prognostic outcome of patients with melanoma.[1156–1158] The Ki-67 antigen, a marker of cellular proliferation, is expressed variably in melanomas, but not nevi.[1133,1145,1159,1160] It can be identified in paraffin sections using the monoclonal antibody MIB-1. Thick melanomas (>4 mm) with high MIB-1 reactivity have a poor prognosis.[1161–1163] Ki-67 does not appear to have independent prognostic significance for most melanomas;[1164–1167] it may have diagnostic value in the borderline lesion, particularly in distinguishing melanoma from a Spitz nevus.[323,1168,1169]

Assessment of nuclear characteristics by various techniques shows differ-ences between benign and malignant nevomelanocytic lesions.[1170–1172] These techniques are now being used in some borderline lesions, such as atypical Spitz nevi.

Frozen sections are now used infrequently in the surgical management of melanoma. The technique is reliable in experienced hands.[1173–1175]

Attempts have been made to identify melanoma/melanocyte autoantigens in melanomas because of their possible use as a target in immunotherapy.[1176,1177] Other studies are focused on identifying specific subsets of lymphocytes with natural killer cell activity.[1178]

Surface microscopy using the dermatoscope (epiluminescence microscopy) is the most recent method to have been suggested in the assessment of pigmented lesions. It is becoming a useful clinical tool for the discrimination of benign and malignant nevomelanocytic lesions.[1179–1192] The ABCD rule for the clinical assessment of melanoma (see p. 823) has been adapted for epiluminescence microscopy to produce a score.[1193–1196] It is derived from a multivariate analysis of four criteria (*a*symmetry, abrupt cutoff of the pigment pattern at the *b*order, *c*olor variegation and *d*ermatoscopic structure).[1197] The rule has not received universal acceptance.[1198,1199]

Prognostic factors in melanoma

The introduction of sophisticated statistical techniques, such as multivariate analysis, has led to the delineation of histological criteria with independent predictive value with respect to prognosis.[1200–1202]

Survival rates for malignant melanoma continue to improve because patients are now presenting earlier with thinner (and therefore low-risk) melanomas.[1203–1206] However, this trend for presentation with thinner lesions appears to be declining.[1207] Five-year survival rates of 85% or better for females and 75% for males are being reported.[1208,1209] Survival rates approaching 100% are seen with superficial melanomas in the invasive radial growth phase (see p. 824). The various prognostic features, with their significance, are listed in Table 32.4.

Table 32.4 **Prognostic features of malignant melanoma**

Morphological
Increasing Breslow thickness (A)
Ulceration (A)
Mitotic rate/mitotic index (A)
Increased nuclear volume (A)
Satellite deposits (A)
Hemangiolymphatic invasion (A)
Advanced clinical stage (A)
'Occult' metastasis (A)
Local recurrence (A)
Clark level (C)
Site (C)
Histological subtype (C)
Coexisting nevus (C)
Lymphocytic infiltrate (C/F)
Absence of regression (C/F)

Clinical
Female (F)
Vitiligo (F)
Increasing age (A)
Pregnancy (C)

Immunohistochemical
Metallothionein (A)
Osteonectin (A)
Integrins (A)
Serum S100 (A)

A = adverse; F = favorable; C = conflicting reports or limited value.

Tumor thickness

It is now accepted that the maximum tumor thickness (Breslow thickness) is the most important single predictor of survival in clinical stage I melanomas.[1210–1214] A possible caveat applies for thin melanomas, where the level may be a more reliable predictor of low-risk status,[1208] and for thin melanomas with regression, where several reports[1215–1217] (but not the majority[982,1218–1221]) have suggested that the presence of regression may carry a significant risk of metastasis. Put another way, the 5-year survival rate for thin melanomas in some series has been 100%,[1203] although some studies have recorded a small number of deaths, particularly in patients whose tumors were more than level 2, or for those with regression.[985,1222–1226] Thicker lesions are associated with a far more ominous prognosis; the 10-year mortality for lesions thicker than 3.5 mm is 65%.[1227] Thicker tumors may, in some instances, be a consequence of an inherently more aggressive tumor rather than a reflection of delay in diagnosis.[1228,1229] This has medicolegal implications. It is accepted that tumor thickness alone can only be used in a general statistical sense to prognosticate on any individual lesion.[1230] Thickness is not an infallible predictor of prognosis. Better prognostic information can be obtained by using more cut points in the Breslow thickness. Initially, 0.76 mm and multiples of it, were used as cut points in various prognostic studies. Subsequently, 1.7 mm was used as a cut point. Prognosis appears to be related to a continuum of thickness.[1231] There is a correlation between tumor thickness and increasing age.[1232] The volume of a melanoma may be superior to thickness as a prognostic indicator.[1233] The cross-sectional area is another measurement that may be helpful in assessing prognosis.[1234]

Attempts have been made to look at melanomas of different thickness that behave in a manner not in keeping with the expected outcome.[1235] One such study looked at thick melanomas (>3 mm) with a good clinical outcome. Such cases were characterized by a 'pushing' as opposed to an infiltrative deep margin, absence of vascular invasion, and location on the head and neck and arm.[1235] Another study of patients with thick melanomas (>5 mm) and survival beyond 10 years found that low mitotic rate, desmoplasia, lack of vascular invasion and the presence of spindle-cell and Spitz-like cell populations correlated with long-term survival.[1236] A study looking at thin melanomas (<1.5 mm) with a poor prognosis found that the Clark level, the presence of regression and the depth of the uninvolved dermis influenced prognosis.[1237]

Clark level

Most authors now agree that the prognostic significance of the Clark level is derived from its secondary correlation with tumor thickness.[1238] The level of invasion may have independent prognostic significance in certain circumstances, particularly as a predictor of outcome in thin melanomas,[1208,1239–1241] although this has been questioned.[1242]

Ulceration

Ulceration, particularly where its width is greater than 3 mm, has adverse prognostic significance.[1243–1246] Ulcerated melanomas also have significantly more mitoses.[1247] Despite its prognostic significance, only 28% of reports in one study commented on the presence or absence of ulceration.[1248]

Site

In some studies the anatomical site has been shown to be a prognostic predictive variable.[1249–1251] High-risk sites include the so-called 'BANS areas' of the body – B (back), A (posterior upper arm), N (posterior neck), S (scalp) – and the feet and genitalia.[983,1249] The thorax (including the back) has been identified in one study as being a prognostically adverse region.[1251] Other studies have been unable to confirm a site-dependent difference in mortality

for the BANS area,[1239,1252] except for melanomas of intermediate thickness (0.76–1.69 mm)[1253] and stage II melanomas.[1254] As a rule, tumors in less visible body areas are significantly thicker at the time of diagnosis than those occurring in more visible areas.[1255] Melanomas in hair-bearing regions of the scalp have a considerably worse prognosis than tumors in other areas of the scalp. One study has shown that the survival of patients with melanoma of the lower extremity decreased with distance from the trunk.[1256]

Mitotic rate

The mitotic rate, particularly if greater than $6/mm^2$, has prognostic significance.[1257] The product of the thickness in millimeters and the number of mitoses per square millimeter (the prognostic index) may give prognostic information.[1258,1259]

Satellite deposits

The presence of microscopic satellite deposits separated from the main body of the tumor has an adverse influence.[1260–1263] The presence of satellites has been shown to be a better indicator of occult regional lymph node metastases in clinical stage I melanoma than the tumor thickness.[1264]

Lymphocytic infiltration

Although some investigators have found no association between prognosis and lymphocytic infiltration of the lesion,[1265] Clark's group found that tumor-infiltrating lymphocytes, particularly when 'brisk', were a favorable feature.[866] A study since that time has found that a high ratio, when comparing the width of the lymphocytic infiltrate to the tumor width, correlated with improved survival.[1266] Interobserver agreement in assessing this feature is good.[1267]

Histological subtype

It is generally agreed that there is no survival difference between superficial spreading, nodular and acral lentiginous melanomas[1268] when these are corrected for thickness.[827,981,1208,1269] Although McGovern and colleagues presented evidence that lentigo maligna melanoma, particularly in women, has a more favorable prognosis, independent of thickness,[1270,1271] this finding has usually not been confirmed in studies from other centers.[1272,1273] A study from Germany has found that the prognosis for nodular melanomas is slightly worse than for non-nodular melanomas, independent of thickness.[1274] Desmoplasia is not associated with a worse prognosis but neurotropism is, particularly when it is associated with desmoplasia.[861] Melanoma with Spitzoid features, occurring in teenagers, does not have a better prognosis than other types of melanoma if the follow-up is sufficiently prolonged.[330]

Nuclear characteristics

Increased nuclear volume and deviation from diploidy are two further parameters that have an adverse prognostic significance.[1275–1278]

Stage

The clinical[1279,1280] and pathological stages[1281] of the disease obviously have a bearing on the survival of the patient. The 5-year survival rate for clinical stage II melanoma is between 35% and 50%.[1282] Among patients with regional lymph node metastasis, an advantage for survival is seen in those with a single involved lymph node and a thin primary tumor, especially if located on an extremity.[1283] The probability of lymph nodal metastases is directly related to the Clark level[1052] and the thickness of the tumor.[1053,1284] The presence of plasma cells in the primary lesion is a recently delineated criterion for the occurrence of lymph node metastases.[1285,1286] Hemangiolymphatic invasion, regarded by some as indicative of metastasis, is an adverse feature.[1287–1289] The sentinel nodes in the lymphatic basins are the first nodes to be involved in metastatic disease.[1290] Their involvement, including the presence of so-called 'occult metastases', is of adverse prognostic significance.[1291] This aspect will be considered further below. The detection of circulating melanocytes, by polymerase chain reaction (PCR) techniques, is also an adverse prognostic finding.[1292]

There is a subset of patients in whom local recurrence is the first event. The prognosis of this group is only slightly better than for a group presenting with lymph node metastasis.[1293] Histopathological features in the cutaneous metastases that are associated with an adverse prognosis include invasion between collagen bundles of the reticular dermis and between fat cells in the subcutis, with preservation of these structures, and a lack of any inflammatory reaction or fibroblastic stromal response.[1294]

In patients with stage IV melanoma, the main prognostic factors are the number of metastatic lesions and their site; visceral involvement portends a poor outcome.[1295]

Coexisting nevus

The prognostic significance of a coexisting intradermal nevus has been controversial.[186,1296] Nevi have been found in approximately one-third of all melanomas, depending on the diligence with which a search is made and the criteria used for accepting a nevus. It has been suggested that this feature may be associated with a more favorable prognosis,[383,1297] but this has not been confirmed when tumor thickness is controlled.[385]

Immunohistochemical findings

Various immunohistochemical markers with prognostic significance have not been found to improve upon a prognostic model that included tumor thickness, localization and mitotic rate.[1298] Expression of metallothionein appears to be associated with adverse prognosis.[1299,1300] The monoclonal antibody KP1, which recognizes the CD68 antigen on macrophages and myeloid precursors, often stains variable numbers of cells in primary and metastatic melanomas. This should be kept in mind when secondary tumors of unknown type are being assessed. The mRNA levels of the proteases cathepsin B and L are increased in melanomas.[1301] Cathepsin D is also increased.[1302] So too is the expression of topoisomerase IIα,[1303,1304] transforming growth factor-β1,[1305] CD95 ligand,[1306,1307] laminin-containing periendothelial matrix,[1308,1309] histidine decarboxylase,[1310] matrix metalloproteinases,[1310,1311] p21[1312] and XMEL.[313] Expression of osteonectin, a multifunctional glycoprotein involved in tissue mineralization, correlates with risk of progression and distant metastases.[1314] Expression of β3 integrin and the cytoplasmic accumulation of peanut agglutinin-binding glycoconjugates[1315] are also associated with adverse prognosis.[1316] α3 integrin is increased in melanomas compared to normal skin;[1317] however, expression of β3 integrin in Spitz nevi is likely to limit its application.[1318] Tumor–stroma interactions appear to be an important facet of melanoma growth and require further study.[1319]

The serum S100 protein level has been found to have some prognostic significance as an indicator of disease progression.[1320–1323] The S100β level also has prognostic value in patients with metastatic disease. High levels are of adverse significance.[1324]

Clinical features with prognostic significance

Various clinical aspects have been studied for prognostic significance. It is well established that *females* with clinical stage I and stage II melanoma have superior survival rates to males.[1325–1328] This may result from the occurrence of lesions in prognostically more favorable sites than in males (lower extremities rather than the trunk) and the presence of thinner tumors at the time of removal.[1208,1329] However, other factors may lead to a more favorable prognosis in premenopausal[1247,1330] and, in some circumstances, postmeno-

pausal women.[1331] This enhanced survival does not appear to apply to stage IV disease.[1332]

There are conflicting results regarding the influence of *pregnancy* on survival rates.[1333,1334] An intercurrent melanoma arising during pregnancy may[1335] or may not[1336,1337] lead to a worse prognosis than in control groups. One study found that melanomas arising during pregnancy are thicker, on average, than in a control group, but this may be balanced in part by a possible pregnancy-associated prognostic advantage.[1338] However, pregnancy seems to have no effect on patients who have had a melanoma diagnosed and treated prior to the pregnancy.[1334,1335]

Another clinical parameter with prognostic significance is *age*. Elderly patients tend to have lesions with adverse prognostic features, such as increased thickness and ulceration.[1246,1339,1340] This increased thickness may be the consequence of inherently more aggressive tumors in the elderly.

The presence of *vitiligo*, usually commencing after the diagnosis of melanoma, appears to be prognostically favorable in patients with secondary melanoma.[1341–1343] Antimelanoma autoantibodies have been detected in the sera of these patients.[1344]

Retention of the novel melanocyte-specific gene melastatin is associated with a good prognosis.[1345]

Features with no prognostic implications

The following factors have not been shown to have independent prognostic significance, according to various studies:[1265] tumor vascularity,[1346,1347] regression[980] (except possibly in thin melanomas), size and shape of the lesion,[1038,1039,1348] cell type,[1349] pigmentation[1350] and incisional biopsy prior to excision,[1351] although in the latter circumstance one group has found an adverse effect.[1352]

Management of malignant melanoma

The treatment of malignant melanoma is beyond the scope of this book. However, three related aspects impinge upon the dermatopathologist:

- resection margins
- handling the re-excision specimens
- sentinel lymph node biopsy.

They will be discussed in turn.

Resection margins

Controlled studies suggest that arbitrary wide margins of excision are not justified.[1262,1353–1357] Local recurrence rates for thick melanomas are increased when the surgical margin is less than 3 cm, although the overall survival rates do not appear to be affected.[1358] In the light of available information from these various studies, the current recommendations for the excision margins for melanomas of various Breslow thicknesses are as follows:[1359–1363]

- melanoma in situ – 0.5 cm margins
- <1 mm – 1 cm margins
- 1–2 mm – 1–2 cm margins (2 cm if primary closure can be achieved)
- 2–4 mm – 2 cm margins (1.5–2.5 cm also suggested)[1364]
- >4 mm – 3 cm margins.

Despite these recommendations, Piepkorn and Barnhill have stated that 'the choice of a resection margin materially more than 1 cm has no basis in scientifically observable fact'.[1365–1367] These margins are usually reduced for facial lesions for cosmetic reasons.[1368]

With subungual melanomas the survival rate is reasonably good provided a radical surgical approach is adopted initially.[1369,1370] Parenthetically, immune therapy is now being used with some success in advanced disease.[1371–1374]

Re-excision specimens

This is the appropriate place to consider the laboratory's approach to the handling of re-excision specimens. Studies have shown that, in the absence of a macroscopic abnormality, the detection of a residual lesion in the re-excision specimen of a completely excised lesion is unusual.[1375] Accordingly, small block numbers have been recommended in these circumstances with sampling restricted to the center of the previous excision biopsy scar.[1375,1376]

Sentinel lymph node biopsy

Lymphatic mapping and sentinel lymph node (SLN) biopsy have had a significant impact on the management and prognostication of patients with melanoma.[1377–1379] The status of the regional lymph node is a powerful predictor of recurrence rates and survival for most solid tumors, including melanoma.[1380] The SLN is defined as the first node in the lymphatic basin that drains the lesion in question. It is at the greatest risk for the development of a metastasis.[1381] The histology of the SLN has been shown to be representative of the entire lymph node basin, although the use of a tyrosinase PCR has shown that micrometastasis may occur in non-sentinel lymph nodes and be undetectable using standard techniques.[1382] This technique enhances the yield of positive SLNs and has prognostic importance.[1383]

If histological examination reveals melanoma metastasis in the SLN, completion lymphadenopathy is performed and adjuvant therapy considered.[1384] The survival advantage of this process remains to be confirmed by a trial currently under way, leading to a view that SLN biopsy should currently be limited to patients in trials.[1385–1387]

The handling of the SLN by the laboratory should be done in accordance with any trial protocol. The cutting of deeper sections and the use of immunohistochemical stains for S100, HMB-45 and melan-A (MART-1) are routine. This procedure increases the yield of positive cases.[1384,1388–1391] Micrometastases should not be confused with nodal nevi, which appear to be increased in patients with a melanoma.[1392] Frozen section assessment of the SLN is not warranted, in view of the low sensitivity of this procedure.[1393]

Micrometastases have been found in the SLN in approximately 20% of melanomas greater than 0.76 mm in thickness, although some institutions restrict the procedure to melanomas more than 1 mm in thickness.[1394] The presence of one or more high-risk histological features in the primary lesion significantly increases the incidence of microscopic nodal involvement.[1395] Those patients in whom the SLN is free of disease have a low rate of nodal recurrence.[1394] It has even been suggested that SLN biopsy be used as an adjunct to the management of lesions over 1 mm in thickness that are histologically difficult to diagnose.[1396]

Although thick melanomas (>3–4 mm) have been excluded from many protocols on the basis that the risk of hematogenous dissemination is considered to be significant, a recent study of SLN status in thick melanomas indicated that it was also predictive of disease-free survival in this group of patients.[1381]

The SLN from patients with desmoplastic/spindle-cell melanoma only rarely harbors a micrometastasis, despite the relative thickness of such lesions.[927]

Imaging techniques are of little value in detecting micrometastases.[1397–1399]

Survival data

A pooled study of 15 798 stage I and 2116 stage II melanomas recorded a 5-year survival of 79% for stage I and 34% for stage II.[1400] The pooled 5-year survival for thin melanomas was 96%. Multifactorial analyses using the data from eight centers found that the most significant prognostic variables (in descending order of significance) were tumor thickness, the presence of ulceration, the anatomical site, the patient's sex, and the tumor growth pattern.[1400] This compares with a study by Clark's group which found that the

favorable prognostic features in a stage I melanoma were low mitotic rate, tumor-infiltrating lymphocytes, a thin lesion, location on the extremities, female sex, and absence of regression.[866] Adverse factors in a Swedish study were increasing age, ulceration, tumor thickness, and male gender.[1401]

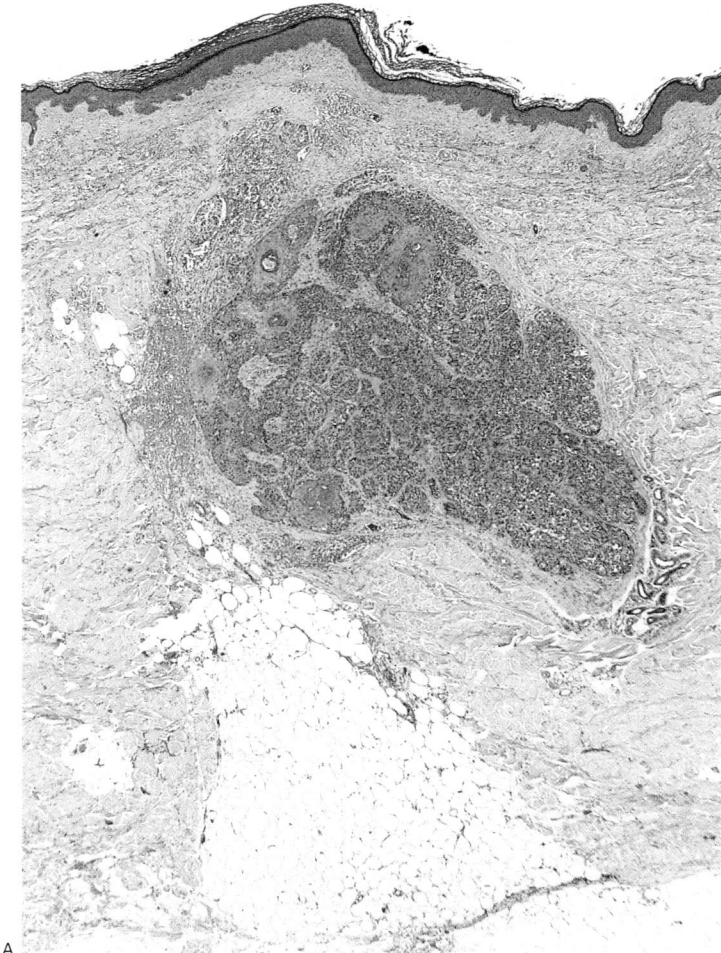

A

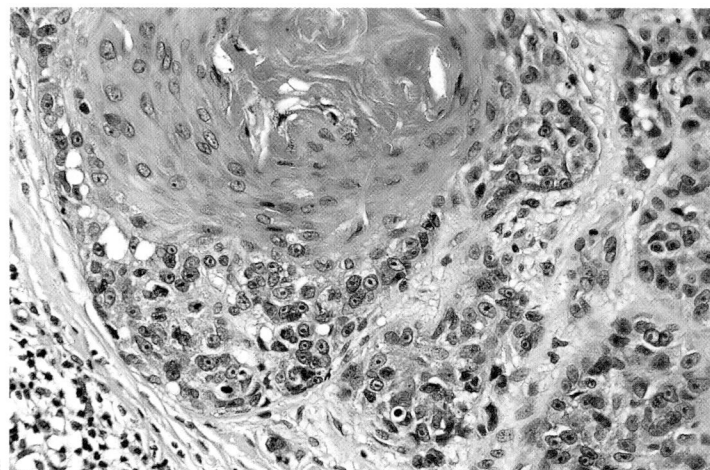

B

Fig. 32.34 **Squamo-melanocytic tumor. (A)** This lesion is not connected with the surface. **(B)** There is an intimate admixture of squamous cells and cytologically malignant melanocytes that stained with HMB-45. (H & E)

The discussion so far has considered risk categories that do not allow accurate prognostication on an individual patient basis.[1402] An individualized prognosis can be provided using a two-step approach and five prognostic variables.[1403] It is little used in clinical practice.

Finally, hazard-rate analyses suggest that the peak hazard rate for death in clinical stage I cutaneous melanoma is the 48th month of follow-up, and that after 120 months' survival the risk of dying from melanoma is virtually zero.[1404] With respect to recurrences, patients with thick melanomas have a marked reduction in future risk (of recurrence) with time.[1405] Put another way, their greatest risk is in the first few years after removal of their thick lesion. With melanomas 0.76–1.5 mm thick there is a relatively constant risk of recurrent disease and death. Overall, 80% of recurrences occur within the first three years.[1406] Although rare, late recurrences (beyond 10 years) are recorded.[1407–1413] Low tumor vascularity and low but comparable rates of proliferation and apoptosis may account for the long period of dormancy of micrometastases, the ultimate source of macrometastases.[1414,1415]

SQUAMO-MELANOCYTIC TUMOR

Four cases of squamo-melanocytic tumor were described in 1999, although a similar case had been described much earlier.[1416] The four cases developed on

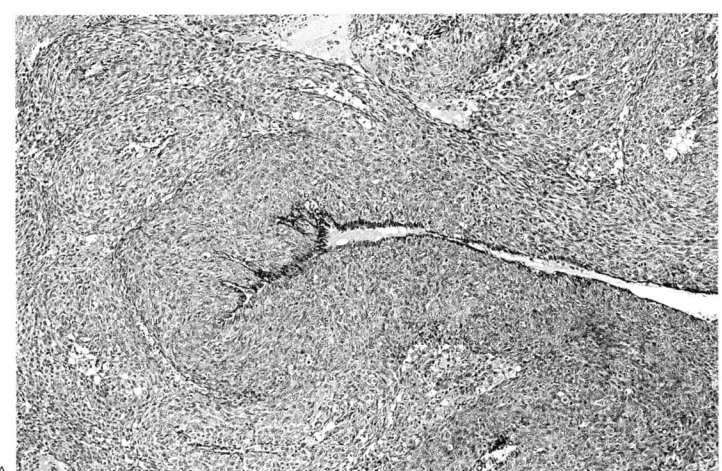

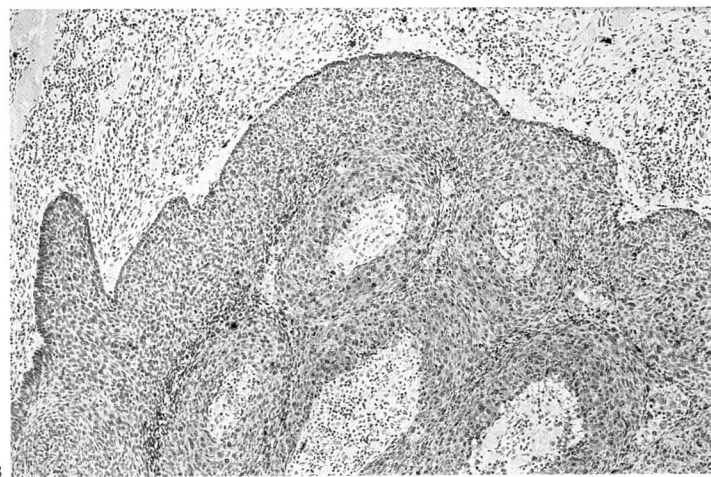

Fig. 32.35 **Basi-melanocytic tumor. (A)** This appears to be the basaloid equivalent of squamo-melanocytic tumor (H & E). **(B)** The intimate admixture of basaloid cells and melanocytes (or biphenotypic differentiation) can be seen on this S100 preparation. (Immunohistochemistry for S100 protein)

the face of middle-aged and older individuals as a purple-black nodule, ranging in size from 3 to 10 mm. Neither recurrence nor metastasis has developed following complete excision and a mean follow-up period of 3.25 years.

This tumor appears to represent a biphasic neoplasm with features of malignancy and uncertain biological behavior.[1416] The author has seen three such cases, but their fate is unknown.

Histopathology

The lesion usually presents as a discrete dermal nodule surrounded by a fibroblastic stroma. In most instances there is no connection with the overlying epidermis and no epidermal component. However, in one of the reported cases and in two personally studied cases there was connection to an overlying lentigo maligna component.

The tumor is composed of two cell types that are diffusely admixed or clustered in small groups within the nodule.[1416] The squamoid component comprises atypical epithelial cells with focal formation of squamous pearls. The other component consists of small, atypical epithelioid cells with nuclear atypia and cytoplasmic melanin (Fig. 32.34). The pigment-containing cells express S100 protein, with fewer cells expressing HMB-45, while the squamoid cells stain for cytokeratin.[1416]

The intimate admixture of the two components distinguishes this lesion from the more common collision tumor which may involve malignant melanoma as one component and basal cell carcinoma[1417] or squamous cell carcinoma as the other.[1418,1419] Biphenotypic tumors with dedifferentiated cells, yet two components on immunohistochemistry, have also been reported (Fig. 32.35).[1420] A squamous cell carcinoma in situ of the skin with melanocyte colonization is another variation on this biphasic theme.[1421]

REFERENCES

Introduction
1   Fulk CS. Primary disorders of hyperpigmentation. J Am Acad Dermatol 1984; 10: 1–16.

Lesions with basal melanocyte proliferation
2   Rahman SB, Bhawan J. Lentigo. Int J Dermatol 1996; 35: 229–239.
3   Ackerman AB, Ragaz A. The lives of lesions. Chronology in dermatology. New York: Masson Publishing USA, 1984: 203–209.
4   Thompson GW, Diehl AK. Partial unilateral lentiginosis. Arch Dermatol 1980; 116: 356.
5   Marchesi L, Naldi L, Di Landro A et al. Segmental lentiginosis with 'jentigo' histologic pattern. Am J Dermatopathol 1992; 14: 323–327.
6   Alkemade H, Juhlin L. Unilateral lentiginosis with nevus depigmentosus on the other side. J Am Acad Dermatol 2000; 43: 361–363.
7   Schafer JV, Lazova R, Bolognia JL. Partial unilateral lentiginosis with ocular involvement. J Am Acad Dermatol 2001; 44: 387–390.
8   O'Neill JF, James WD. Inherited patterned lentiginosis in blacks. Arch Dermatol 1989; 125: 1231–1235.
9   Uhle P, Norvell SS Jr. Generalized lentiginosis. J Am Acad Dermatol 1988; 18: 444–447.
10 Arnsmeier SL, Paller AS. Pigmentary anomalies in the multiple lentigines syndrome: is it distinct from LEOPARD syndrome? Pediatr Dermatol 1996; 13: 100–104.
11 Peterson LL, Serrill WS. Lentiginosis associated with left atrial myxoma. J Am Acad Dermatol 1984; 10: 337–340.
12 Parslew R, Verbov JL. Partial lentiginosis. Clin Exp Dermatol 1995; 20: 141–142.
13 Micali G, Nasca MR, Innocenzi D, Lembo D. Agminated lentiginosis: case report and review of the literature. Pediatr Dermatol 1994; 11: 241–245.
14 Piqué E, Aguiar A, Fariña MC et al. Partial unilateral lentiginosis: report of seven cases and review of the literature. Clin Exp Dermatol 1995; 20: 319–322.
15 Trattner A, Metzker A. Partial unilateral lentiginosis. J Am Acad Dermatol 1993; 29: 693–695.
16 Jóźwiak S, Schwartz RA, Janniger CK, Zaremba J. Familial occurrence of the LEOPARD syndrome. Int J Dermatol 1998; 37: 48–51.
17 Schepis C, Greco D, Siragusa M et al. An intriguing case of LEOPARD syndrome. Pediatr Dermatol 1998; 15: 125–128.

18 Ohkura T, Ohnishi Y, Kawada A et al. Leopard syndrome associated with hyperelastic skin: analysis of collagen metabolism in cultured skin fibroblasts. Dermatology 1999; 198: 385–387.

19 Shamsadini S, Abazardi H, Shamsadini F. Leopard syndrome. Lancet 1999; 354: 1530.

20 Atherton DJ, Pitcher DW, Wells RS, MacDonald DM. A syndrome of various cutaneous pigmented lesions, myxoid neurofibromata and atrial myxoma: the NAME syndrome. Br J Dermatol 1980; 103: 421–429.

21 Rhodes AR, Silverman RA, Harrist TJ, Perez-Atayde AR. Mucocutaneous lentigines, cardiocutaneous myxomas, and multiple blue nevi: the 'LAMB' syndrome. J Am Acad Dermatol 1984; 10: 72–82.

22 Carney JA, Gordon H, Carpenter PG et al. The complex of myxomas, spotty pigmentation, and endocrine overactivity. Medicine (Baltimore) 1985; 64: 270–283.

23 Egan CA, Stratakis CA, Turner ML. Multiple lentigines associated with cutaneous myxomas. J Am Acad Dermatol 2001; 44: 282–284.

24 Holder JE, Graham-Brown RAC, Camp RDR. Partial unilateral lentiginosis associated with blue naevi. Br J Dermatol 1994; 130: 390–393.

25 Bolognia JL, Lazova R, Watsky K. The development of lentigines within segmental achromic nevi. J Am Acad Dermatol 1998; 39: 330–333.

26 Gupta G, Williams REA, MacKie RM. The labial melanotic macule: a review of 79 cases. Br J Dermatol 1997; 136: 772–775.

27 Sexton FM, Maize JC. Melanotic macules and melanoacanthomas of the lip Am J Dermatopathol 1987; 9: 438–444.

28 Spann CR, Owen LG, Hodge SJ. The labial melanotic macule. Arch Dermatol 1987; 123: 1029–1031.

29 Ho KK-L, Dervan P, O'Loughlin S, Powell FC. Labial melanotic macule: a clinical, histopathologic, and ultrastructural study. J Am Acad Dermatol 1993; 28: 33–39.

30 Cohen LM, Callen JP. Oral and labial melanotic macules in a patient infected with human immunodeficiency virus. J Am Acad Dermatol 1992; 26: 653–654.

31 Barnhill RL, Albert LS, Shama SK et al. Genital lentiginosis: a clinical and histopathologic study. J Am Acad Dermatol 1990; 22: 453–460.

32 Leicht S, Youngberg G, Diaz-Miranda C. Atypical pigmented penile macules. Arch Dermatol 1988; 124: 1267–1270.

33 Revuz J, Clerici T. Penile melanosis. J Am Acad Dermatol 1989; 20: 567–570.

34 Rudolph RI. Vulvar melanosis. J Am Acad Dermatol 1990; 23: 982–984.

35 Jih DM, Elder DE, Elenitsas R. A histopathologic evaluation of vulvar melanosis. Arch Dermatol 1999; 135: 857–858.

36 Lambert WC, Lambert MW, Mesa ML et al. Melanoacanthoma and related disorders. Simulants of acral-lentiginous (P-P-S-M) melanoma. Int J Dermatol 1987; 26: 508–510.

37 Tomich CE, Zunt SL. Melanoacanthosis (melanoacanthoma) of the oral mucosa. J Dermatol Surg Oncol 1990; 16: 231–236.

38 Horlick HP, Walther RR, Zegarelli DJ et al. Mucosal melanotic macule, reactive type: a simulation of melanoma. J Am Acad Dermatol 1988; 19: 786–791.

39 Zemtsov A, Bergfeld WF. Oral melanoacanthoma with prominent spongiotic intraepithelial vesicles. J Cutan Pathol 1989; 16: 365–369.

40 Lenane P, Keane CO, Connell BO et al. Genital melanotic macules: Clinical, histologic, immunohistochemical, and ultrastructural features. J Am Acad Dermatol 2000; 42: 640–644.

41 Kiyohara T, Kumakiri M, Kouraba S et al. Volar melanotic macules in a Japanese man with histopathological postinflammatory pigmentation: the volar counterpart of mucosal melanotic macules. J Cutan Pathol 2001; 28: 303–306.

42 Bolognia JL. Reticulated black solar lentigo ('ink spot' lentigo). Arch Dermatol 1992; 128: 934–940.

43 Mehregan AH. Lentigo senilis and its evolutions. J Invest Dermatol 1975; 65: 429–433.

44 Skender-Kalnenas TM, English DR, Heenan PJ. Benign melanocytic lesions: risk markers or precursors of cutaneous melanoma? J Am Acad Dermatol 1995; 33: 1000–1007.

45 Garbe C, Büttner P, Weiss J et al. Associated factors in the prevalence of more than 50 common melanocytic nevi, atypical melanocytic nevi, and actinic lentigines: multicenter case-control study of the Central Malignant Melanoma Registry of the German Dermatological Society. J Invest Dermatol 1994; 102: 700–705.

46 Stern JB, Peck GL, Haupt HM et al. Malignant melanoma in xeroderma pigmentosum: search for a precursor lesion. J Am Acad Dermatol 1993; 28: 591–594.

47 Montagna W, Hu F, Carlisle K. A reinvestigation of solar lentigines. Arch Dermatol 1980; 116: 1151–1154.

48 Andersen WK, Labadie RR, Bhawan J. Histopathology of solar lentigines of the face: A quantitative study. J Am Acad Dermatol 1997; 36: 444–447.

49 Walton RG. Recognition and importance of precursor lesions in the diagnosis of early cutaneous malignant melanoma. Int J Dermatol 1994; 33: 302–307.

50 Stewart DM, Altman J, Mehregan AH. Speckled lentiginous nevus. Arch Dermatol 1978; 114: 895–896.

51 Cohen LM, Bennion SD, Johnson TW, Golitz LE. Hypermelanotic nevus: clinical, histopathologic, and ultrastructural features in 316 cases. Am J Dermatopathol 1997; 19: 23–30.

52 Welch ML, James WD. Widespread nevus spilus. Int J Dermatol 1993; 32: 120–122.

53 Crosti C, Betti R. Inherited extensive speckled lentiginous nevus with ichthyosis: report of a previously undescribed association. Arch Dermatol 1994; 130: 393–395.

54 Schaffer JV, Orlow SJ, Lazova R, Bolognia JL. Speckled lentiginous nevus. Within the spectrum of congenital melanocytic nevi. Arch Dermatol 2001; 137: 172–178.

55 Roma P, Sanjeev H, Bhusan K. Generalized naevus spilus: a rare entity? J Eur Acad Dermatol Venereol 2000; 14: 430.

56 Cohen HJ, Munkin W, Frank SB. Nevus spilus. Arch Dermatol 1970; 102: 433–437.

57 Ruth WK, Shelburne JD, Jegasothy BV. Zosteriform lentiginous nevus. Arch Dermatol 1980; 116: 478.

58 Carmichael AJ, Tan CY. Speckled compound naevus. Clin Exp Dermatol 1990; 15: 137–138.

59 Betti R, Inselvini E, Crosti C. Extensive unilateral speckled lentiginous nevus. Am J Dermatopathol 1994; 16: 554–556.

60 Morishima T, Endo M, Imagawa I, Morioka S. Clinical and histopathological studies on spotted grouped pigmented nevi with special reference to eccrine-centered nevus. Acta Derm Venereol 1976; 56: 345–351.

61 Rhodes AR, Mihm MC Jr. Origin of cutaneous melanoma in a congenital dysplastic nevus spilus. Arch Dermatol 1990; 126: 500–505.

62 Wagner RF Jr, Cottel WI. In situ malignant melanoma arising in a speckled lentiginous nevus. J Am Acad Dermatol 1989; 20: 125–126.

63 Kurban RS, Preffer FI, Sober AJ et al. Occurrence of melanoma in 'dysplastic' nevus spilus: report of case and analysis by flow cytometry. J Cutan Pathol 1992; 19: 423–428.

64 Borrego L, Hernandez Santana J, Baez O, Hernandez Hernandez B. Naevus spilus as a precursor of cutaneous melanoma: report of a case and literature review. Clin Exp Dermatol 1994; 19: 515–517.

65 Vázquel-Doval J, Sola MA, Contreras-Mejuto F et al. Malignant melanoma developing in a speckled lentiginous nevus. Int J Dermatol 1995; 34: 637–638.

66 Bolognia JL. Fatal melanoma arising in a zosteriform speckled lentiginous nevus. Arch Dermatol 1991; 127: 1240–1241.

67 Stern JB, Haupt HM, Aaronson CM. Malignant melanoma in a speckled zosteriform lentiginous nevus. Int J Dermatol 1990; 29: 583–584.

68 Grinspan D, Casala A, Abulafia J et al. Melanoma on dysplastic nevus spilus. Int J Dermatol 1997; 36: 499–502.

69 Bielsa I, Paradelo C, Ribera M, Ferrándiz C. Generalized nevus spilus and nevus anemicus in a patient with a primary lymphedema: a new type of phakomatosis pigmentovascularis? Pediatr Dermatol 1998; 15: 293–295.

70 Altman DA, Banse L. Zosteriform speckled lentiginous nevus. J Am Acad Dermatol 1992; 27: 106–108.

71 Hwang SM, Choi EH, Lee WS et al. Nevus spilus (speckled lentiginous nevus) associated with a nodular neurotized nevus. Am J Dermatopathol 1997; 19: 308–311.

72 Stefanato CM, Kurban A, Bhawan J. Nevus spilus with features of congenital nevus and blue nevus: case report. J Cutan Pathol 2000; 27: 573 (abstract).

73 Bleehen SS. Freckles induced by PUVA treatment. Br J Dermatol (Suppl) 1978; 16: 20.

74 Farber EM, Abel EA, Cox AJ. Long-term risks of psoralen and UV-A therapy for psoriasis. Arch Dermatol 1983; 119: 426–431.

75 Rhodes AR, Stern RS, Melski JW. The PUVA lentigo: an analysis of predisposing factors. J Invest Dermatol 1983; 81: 459–463.

76 Burrows NP, Handfield-Jones S, Monk BE et al. Multiple lentigines confined to psoriatic plaques. Clin Exp Dermatol 1994; 19: 380–382.

77 Basarab T, Millard TP, McGregor JM, Barker JNWN. Atypical pigmented lesions following extensive PUVA therapy. Clin Exp Dermatol 2000; 25: 135–137.

78 Bruce DR, Berger TG. PUVA-induced pigmented macules: a case involving palmoplantar skin. J Am Acad Dermatol 1987; 16: 1087–1090.

79 Swart R, Kenter I, Suurmond D. The incidence of PUVA-induced freckles. Dermatologica 1984; 168: 304–305.

80 Salisbury JR, Williams H, du Vivier AWP. Tanning-bed lentigines: ultrastructural and histopathologic features. J Am Acad Dermatol 1989; 21: 689–693.

81 Kadunce DP, Piepkorn MW, Zone JJ. Persistent melanocytic lesions associated with cosmetic tanning bed use: 'sunbed lentigines'. J Am Acad Dermatol 1990; 23: 1029–1031.

82 Peter RU, Gottlöber P, Nadeshina N et al. Radiation lentigo. A distinct cutaneous lesion after accidental radiation exposure. Arch Dermatol 1997; 133: 209–211.

83 Rhodes AR, Harrist TJ, Momtaz TK. The PUVA-induced pigmented macule: a lentiginous proliferation of large, sometimes cytologically atypical, melanocytes. J Am Acad Dermatol 1984; 9: 47–58.

84 Marx JL, Auerbach R, Possick P et al. Malignant melanoma in situ in two patients treated with psoralens and ultraviolet A. J Am Acad Dermatol 1983; 9: 904–911.

85 Gupta AK, Stern RS, Swanson NA et al. Cutaneous melanomas in patients treated with psoralens plus ultraviolet A. J Am Acad Dermatol 1988; 19: 67–76.

86 Tronnier M, Wolff HH. U-V irradiated melanocytic nevi simulating melanoma in situ. Am J Dermatopathol 1995; 17: 1–6.

87 Abel EA, Reid H, Wood C, Hu C-H. PUVA-induced melanocytic atypia: is it confined to PUVA lentigines? J Am Acad Dermatol 1985; 13: 761–768.

88 Ho VC, Sober AJ. Pigmented streaks in melanoma scars. J Dermatol Surg Oncol 1990; 16: 663–666.

89 Dwyer CM, Kerr RE, Knight SL, Walker E. Pseudomelanoma after dermabrasion. J Am Acad Dermatol 1993; 28: 263–264.

90 Duve S, Schmoeckel C, Burgdorf WHC. Melanocytic hyperplasia in scars. A histopathological investigation of 722 cases. Am J Dermatopathol 1996; 18: 236–240.

91 Botella-Estrada R, Sanmartín O, Sevila A et al. Melanotic pigmentation in excision scars of melanocytic and non-melanocytic skin tumors. J Cutan Pathol 1999; 26: 137–144.

Melanocytic nevi

92 Hurwitz S. Pigmented nevi. Semin Dermatol 1988; 7: 17–25.

93 Cochran AJ, Bailly C, Paul E, Dolbeau D. Nevi, other than dysplastic and Spitz nevi. Semin Diagn Pathol 1993; 10: 3–17.

94 Pope DJ, Sorahan T, Marsden JR et al. Benign pigmented nevi in children. Arch Dermatol 1992; 128: 1201–1206.

95 Richard MA, Grob J-J, Gouvernet J et al. Role of sun exposure on nevus. Arch Dermatol 1993; 129: 1280–1285.

96 Fritsche L, McHenry P, Green A et al. Naevi in schoolchildren in Scotland and Australia. Br J Dermatol 1994; 130: 599–603.

97 Rivers JK, MacLennan R, Kelly JW et al. The Eastern Australian childhood nevus study: prevalence of atypical nevi, congenital nevus-like nevi, and other pigmented lesions. J Am Acad Dermatol 1995; 32: 957–963.

98 Kelly JW, Rivers JK, MacLennan R et al. Sunlight: a major factor associated with the development of melanocytic nevi in Australian schoolchildren. J Am Acad Dermatol 1994; 30: 40–48.

99 Brogelli L, De Giorgi V, Bini F, Giannotti B. Melanocytic naevi: clinical features and correlation with the phenotype in healthy young males in Italy. Br J Dermatol 1991; 125: 349–352.

100 McGregor JM, Barker JNWN, MacDonald DM. The development of excess numbers of melanocytic naevi in an immunosuppressed identical twin. Clin Exp Dermatol 1991; 16: 131–132.

101 Smith CH, McGregor JM, Barker JNWN et al. Excess melanocytic nevi in children with renal allografts. J Am Acad Dermatol 1993; 28: 51–55.

102 Harth Y, Friedman-Birnbaum R, Linn S. Influence of cumulative sun exposure on the prevalence of common acquired nevi. J Am Acad Dermatol 1992; 27: 21–24.

103 Bouwes Bavinck JN, Crijns M, Vermeer BJ et al. Chronic sun exposure and age are inversely associated with nevi in adult renal transplant recipients. J Invest Dermatol 1996; 106: 1036–1041.

104 Luther H, Altmeyer P, Garbe C et al. Increase of melanocytic nevus counts in children during 5 years of follow-up and analysis of associated factors. Arch Dermatol 1996; 132: 1473–1478.

105 Harrison SL, Buettner PG, MacLennan R. Body-site distribution of melanocytic nevi in young Australian children. Arch Dermatol 1999; 135: 47–52.

106 Nguyen TD, Siskind V, Green L et al. Ultraviolet radiation, melanocytic naevi and their dose-response relationship. Br J Dermatol 1997; 137: 91–95.

107 Fariñas-Álvarez C, Ródenas JM, Herranz MT, Delgado-Rodríguez M. The naevus count on the arms as a predictor of the number of melanocytic naevi on the whole body. Br J Dermatol 1999; 140: 457–462.

108 Tronnier M, Smolle J, Wolff HH. Ultraviolet irradiation induces acute changes in melanocytic nevi. J Invest Dermatol 1995; 104: 475–478.

109 Cramer SF. The origin of epidermal melanocytes. Arch Pathol Lab Med 1991; 115: 115–119.

110 Schmoeckel C. Classification of melanocytic nevi: do nodular and flat nevi develop differently? Am J Dermatopathol 1997; 19: 31–34.

111 Tokuda Y, Saida T, Mukai K, Takasaki Y. Growth dynamics of acquired melanocytic nevi. J Am Acad Dermatol 1994; 31: 220–224.

112 Worret W-I, Burgdorf WHC. Which direction do nevus cells move? *Abtropfung* reexamined. Am J Dermatopathol 1998; 20: 135–139.

113 Cramer SF. The melanocytic differentiation pathway in Spitz nevi. Am J Dermatopathol 1998; 20: 555–570.

114 Pennoyer JW, Grin CM, Driscoll MS et al. Changes in size of melanocytic nevi during pregnancy. J Am Acad Dermatol 1997; 36: 378–382.

115 Kittler H, Seltenheim M, Dawid M et al. Frequency and characteristics of enlarging common melanocytic naevi. Arch Dermatol 2000; 136: 316–320.

116 Lee H-J, Ha S-J, Lee S-J, Kim J-W. Melanocytic nevus with pregnancy-related changes in size accompanied by apoptosis of nevus cells. A case report. J Am Acad Dermatol 2000; 42: 936–938.

117 Rhodes AR. Common acquired nevomelanocytic nevi and the fourth dimension. Arch Dermatol 2000; 136: 400–405.

118 Zvulunov A, Wyatt DT, Laud PW, Esterly NB. Lack of effect of growth hormone therapy on the count and density of melanocytic naevi in children. Br J Dermatol 1997; 137: 545–548.

119 McLean DI, Gallagher RP. Hormones, immunology, nevi, and melanoma. Arch Dermatol 1997; 133: 783–784.

120 Böni R, Matt D, Burg G et al. Ultraviolet-induced acute histological changes in irradiated nevi are not associated with allelic loss. Arch Dermatol 1998; 134: 853–856.

121 Magana-Garcia M, Ackerman AB. What are nevus cells? Am J Dermatopathol 1990; 12: 93–102.

122 Hui P, Perkins AS, Glusac EJ. Assessment of clonality in melanocytic nevi. J Cutan Pathol 2001; 28: 140–144.

123 Paul E, Cochran AJ, Wen D-R. Immunohistochemical demonstration of S-100 protein and melanoma-associated antigens in melanocytic nevi. J Cutan Pathol 1988; 15: 161–165.

124 MacKie RM, English J, Aitchison TC et al. The number and distribution of benign pigmented moles (melanocytic naevi) in a healthy British population. Br J Dermatol 1985; 113: 167–174.

125 Green A, Siskind V, Hansen M-E et al. Melanocytic nevi in schoolchildren in Queensland. J Am Acad Dermatol 1989; 20: 1054–1060.

126 English JSC, Swerdlow AJ, Mackie RM et al. Site-specific melanocytic naevus counts as predictors of whole body naevi. Br J Dermatol 1988; 118: 641–644.

127 Maize JC, Foster G. Age-related changes in melanocytic naevi. Clin Exp Dermatol 1979; 4: 49–58.

128 Swerdlow AJ, Green A. Melanocytic naevi and melanoma: an epidemiological perspective. Br J Dermatol 1987; 117: 137–146.

129 Soltani K, Pepper MC, Simjee S, Apatoff BR. Large acquired nevocytic nevi induced by the Koebner phenomenon. J Cutan Pathol 1984; 11: 296–299.

130 Shoji T, Cockerell CJ, Koff AB, Bhawan J. Eruptive melanocytic nevi after Stevens–Johnson syndrome. J Am Acad Dermatol 1997; 37: 337–339.

131 Bauer JW, Schaeppi H, Kaserer C et al. Large melanocytic nevi in hereditary epidermolysis bullosa. J Am Acad Dermatol 2001; 44: 577–584.

132 Firooz A, Komeili A, Dowlati Y. Eruptive melanocytic nevi and cherry angiomas secondary to exposure to sulfur mustard gas. J Am Acad Dermatol 1999; 40: 646–647.

133 Reeck MC, Chuang T-Y, Eads TJ et al. The diagnostic yield in submitting nevi for histologic examination. J Am Acad Dermatol 1999; 40: 567–571.

134 Eng AM. Solitary small active junctional nevi in juvenile patients. Arch Dermatol 1983; 119: 35–38.

135 Benz G, Hölzel D, Schmoeckel C. Inflammatory cellular infiltrates in melanocytic nevi. Am J Dermatopathol 1991; 13: 538–542.

136 Goettmann-Bonvallot S, André J, Belaich S. Longitudinal melanonychia in children: A clinical and histopathologic study of 40 cases. J Am Acad Dermatol 1999; 41: 17–22.

137 Baran R, Perrin C. Linear melanonychia due to subungual keratosis of the nail bed: a report of two cases. Br J Dermatol 1999; 140: 730–733.

138 Sprecher E, Bergman R, Meilick A et al. Apoptosis, Fas and Fas-ligand expression in melanocytic tumors. J Cutan Pathol 1999; 26: 72–77.

139 Horenstein MG, Prieto VG, Burchette JL Jr, Shea CR. Keratotic melanocytic nevus: a clinicopathologic and immunohistochemical study. J Cutan Pathol 2000; 27: 344–350.

140 Morgan MB, Raley BA, Vannarath RL et al. Papillomatous melanocytic nevi: an estrogen related phenomenon. J Cutan Pathol 1995; 22: 446–449.

141 Ackerman AB, Milde P. Naming acquired melanocytic nevi. Common and dysplastic, normal and atypical, or Unna, Miescher, Spitz and Clark? Am J Dermatopathol 1992; 14: 447–453.

142 LeBoit PE. A diagnosis for maniacs. Am J Dermatopathol 2000; 22: 556–558.

143 Murphy B, Guillen D, Cockerell C. Unusual features of melanocytic nevi at specific anatomical sites. J Cutan Pathol 2000; 27: 566 (abstract).

144 Rock B, Hood AF, Rock JA. Prospective study of vulvar nevi. J Am Acad Dermatol 1990; 22: 104–106.

145 Christensen WN, Friedman KJ, Woodruff JD, Hood AF. Histologic characteristics of vulvar nevocellular nevi. J Cutan Pathol 1987; 14: 87–91.

146 Clark WH Jr, Hood AF, Tucker MA, Jampel RM. Atypical melanocytic nevi of the genital type with a discussion of reciprocal parenchymal–stromal interactions in the biology of neoplasia Hum Pathol 1998; 29 (Suppl 1): S1–S24.

147 Haupt HM, Stern JB. Pagetoid melanocytosis. Histologic features in benign and malignant lesions. Am J Surg Pathol 1995; 19: 792–797.

148 Foucar E, Bentley TJ, Laube DW, Rosai J. A histopathologic evaluation of nevocellular nevi in pregnancy. Arch Dermatol 1985; 121: 350–354.

149 Rongioletti F, Ball RA, Marcus R, Barnhill RL. Histopathological features of flexural melanocytic nevi: a study of 40 cases. J Cutan Pathol 2000; 27: 215–217.

150 Kabukçuoğlu S, McNutt NS. Conjunctival melanocytic nevi of childhood. J Cutan Pathol 1999; 26: 248–252.

151 Signoretti S, Annessi G, Puddu P, Faraggiana T. Melanocytic nevi of palms and soles. A histological study according to the plane of section. Am J Surg Pathol 1999; 23: 283–287.

152 Fallowfield ME, Collina G, Cook MG. Melanocytic lesions of the palm and sole. Histopathology 1994; 24: 463–467.

153 Boyd AS, Rapini RP. Acral melanocytic neoplasms: a histologic analysis of 158 lesions. J Am Acad Dermatol 1994; 31: 740–745.

154 Clemente C, Zurrida S, Bartoli C et al. Acral-lentiginous naevus of plantar skin. Histopathology 1995; 27: 549–555.

155 Tosti A, Baran R, Piraccini BM et al. Nail matrix nevi: a clinical and histopathologic study of twenty-two patients. J Am Acad Dermatol 1996; 34: 765–771.

156 Cho KH, Lee AY, Suh DH et al. Lobulated intradermal nevus. J Am Acad Dermatol 1991; 24: 74–77.

157 Tabata H, Yamakage A, Yamazaki S. Cerebriform intradermal nevus. Int J Dermatol 1995; 34: 634.

158 Misago N. The relationship between melanocytes and peripheral nerve sheath cells (Part I): melanocytic nevus (excluding so-called "blue nevus") with peripheral nerve sheath differentiation. Am J Dermatopathol 2000; 22: 217–229.

159 Gray MH, Smoller BR, McNutt NS, Hsu A. Neurofibromas and neurotized melanocytic nevi are immunohistochemically distinct neoplasms. Am J Dermatopathol 1990; 12: 234–241.

160 Van Paesschen M-A, Goovaerts G, Buyssens N. A study of the so-called neurotization of nevi. Am J Dermatopathol 1990; 12: 242–248.

161 Prieto VG, McNutt NS, Lugo J, Reed JA. The intermediate filament peripherin is expressed in cutaneous melanocytic lesions. J Cutan Pathol 1997; 24: 145–150.

162 Prieto VG, McNutt NS, Lugo J, Reed JA. Differential expression of the intermediate filament peripherin in cutaneous neural lesions and neurotized melanocytic nevi. Am J Surg Pathol 1997; 21: 1450–1454.

163 Argenyi ZB, Rodgers J, Wick M. Expression of nerve growth factor and epidermal growth factor receptors in neural nevi with nevic corpuscles. Am J Dermatopathol 1996; 18: 460–464.

164 Fullen D, Reed J, Finnerty B, McNutt NS. S100A6 preferentially labels type C nevus cells and nevic corpuscles: additional support for schwannian differentiation of dermal nevi. J Cutan Pathol 2000; 27: 556 (abstract).

165 Eng W, Cohen PR. Nevus with fat: Clinical characteristics of 100 nevi containing mature adipose cells. J Am Acad Dermatol 1998; 39: 704–711.

166 Gottlieb B, Brown AL Jr, Winkelmann RK. Fine structure of the nevus cell. Arch Dermatol 1965; 92: 81–87.

167 Weedon D. Unusual features of nevocellular nevi. J Cutan Pathol 1982; 9: 284–292.

168 MacDonald DM, Black MM. Secondary localized cutaneous amyloidosis in melanocytic naevi. Br J Dermatol 1980; 103: 553–556.

169 Culver W, Burgdorf WHC. Malignant melanoma arising in a nevus of Nanta. J Cutan Pathol 1993; 20: 375–377.

170 Weedon D, Farnsworth J. Spongiotic changes in melanocytic nevi. Am J Dermatopathol (Suppl) 1984; 1: 257–259.

171 Crovato F, Nazzari G, Gambini C, Massone L. Meyerson's naevi in pityriasis rosea. Br J Dermatol 1989; 120: 318–319.

172 Nicholls DSH, Mason GH. Halo dermatitis around a melanocytic naevus: Meyerson's naevus. Br J Dermatol 1988; 118: 125–129.

173 Fernandez Herrera JM, Argues Montanes M, Fraga Fernandez J, Garcia Diez A. Halo eczema in melanocytic nevi. Acta Derm Venereol 1988; 68: 161–163.

174 Shifer O, Tchetchik R, Glazer O, Metzker A. Halo dermatitis in children. Pediatr Dermatol 1992; 9: 275–277.

175 Fabrizi G, Massi G. Histological changes in naevi with superimposed psoriasis. Br J Dermatol 2000; 143: 688–690.

176 Mehregan AH, Staricco RG. Elastic fibers in pigmented nevi. J Invest Dermatol 1962; 38: 271–276.

177 Mehregan DR, Mehregan DA, Mehregan AH. Nodular myxoid change in melanocytic nevi. A report of two cases. Am J Dermatopathol 1996; 18: 400–402.

178 Haber H. Some observations on common moles. Br J Dermatol 1962; 74: 224–228.

179 Sánchez Yus E, Requena L. Nevus with cyst and nevus with folliculitis. Am J Dermatopathol 1994; 16: 574–575.

180 Requena L, Ambrojo P, Sánchez Yus E. Trichilemmal cyst under a compound melanocytic nevus. J Cutan Pathol 1990; 17: 185–188.

181 Cohen PR, Rapini RP. Nevus with cyst. A report of 93 cases. Am J Dermatopathol 1993; 15: 229–234.

182 Weitzner S. Intradermal nevus with psammoma body formation. Arch Dermatol 1968; 98: 287–289.

183 Eftychiadis AS, Iozzo RV, Ackerman AB. Sebocyte-like melanocytes in melanocytic nevi. Dermatopathology: Practical & Conceptual 1996; 2: 49–50.

184 Tschen JA, Tyring SK, Font RL. Paramyxovirus-like inclusions in an intradermal nevus from a healthy woman. Am J Dermatopathol 1994; 16: 422–425.

185 Yesudian P, Thambiah AS. Perinevoid alopecia. An unusual variant of alopecia areata. Arch Dermatol 1976; 112: 1432–1434.

186 Weedon D. Melanoma and other melanocytic skin lesions. Curr Top Pathol 1985; 74: 1–55.

187 Marks JG, White JW. Molluscum contagiosum in a halo nevus. Int J Dermatol 1980; 19: 258–259.

188 Rahbari H, Mehregan AH. Trichoepithelioma and pigmented nevus. A combined malformation. J Cutan Pathol 1975; 2: 225–231.

189 Sigal C, Saunders TS. Basal cell epithelioma and nevus pigmentosus, their simultaneous occurrence. Arch Dermatol 1967; 96: 520–523.

190 Schellander F, Mark R, Wilson Jones E. Basal cell hamartoma and cellular naevus. An unusual combined malformation. Br J Dermatol 1974; 90: 413–419.

191 Stefanato CM, Simkin DA, Bhawan J. An unusual melanocytic lesion associated with eccrine duct fibroadenomatosis and syringoid features. Am J Dermatopathol 2001; 23: 139–142.

192 Sagebiel RW. Histologic artifacts of benign pigmented nevi. Arch Dermatol 1972; 106: 691–693.

193 Collina G, Eusebi V. Naevocytic naevi with vascular-like spaces. Br J Dermatol 1991; 124: 591–595.

194 Ball NJ, Golitz LE. Melanocytic nevi with focal atypical epithelioid cell components: a review of seventy-three cases. J Am Acad Dermatol 1994; 30: 724–729.

195 Collina G, Deen S, Cliff S et al. Atypical dermal nodules in benign melanocytic naevi. Histopathology 1997; 31: 97–101.

196 Bolognia JL, Lin A, Shapiro PE. The significance of eccentric foci of hyperpigmentation ('small dark dots') within melanocytic nevi. Analysis of 59 cases. Arch Dermatol 1994; 130: 1013–1017.

197 Bolognia JL, Shapiro PE. Perifollicular hypopigmentation. A cause of variegate pigmentation and irregular border in melanocytic nevi. Arch Dermatol 1992; 128: 514–517.

198 Ramón R, Silvestre JF, Betlloch I et al. Progression of Meyerson's naevus to Sutton's naevus. Dermatology 2000; 200: 337–338.

199 Krischer J, Pechère M, Salomon D et al. Interferon alfa-2b-induced Meyerson's nevi in a patient with dysplastic nevus syndrome. J Am Acad Dermatol 1999; 40: 105–106.

200 Elenitsas R, Halpern AC. Eczematous halo reaction in atypical nevi. J Am Acad Dermatol 1996; 34: 357–361.

201 Kerl H, Soyer HP, Cerroni L et al. Ancient melanocytic nevus. Semin Diagn Pathol 1998; 15: 210–215.

202 Edwards SL, Blessing K. Problematic pigmented lesions: approach to diagnosis. J Clin Pathol 2000; 53: 409–418.

203 Seab JA Jr, Graham JH, Helwig EB. Deep penetrating nevus. Am J Surg Pathol 1989; 13: 39–44.

204 Barnhill RL, Mihm MC Jr, Magro CM. Plexiform spindle cell naevus: a distinctive variant of plexiform melanocytic naevus. Histopathology 1991; 18: 243–247.

205 Mehregan DA, Mehregan AH. Deep penetrating nevus. Arch Dermatol 1993; 129: 328–331.

206 Alanen KW, Golitz LE. Is melanocytic nevus with focal atypical epithelioid components a superficial variant of deep penetrating nevus? a study of 227 cases. J Cutan Pathol 2000; 27: 547–548 (abstract).

207 Skelton HG III, Smith KJ, Barrett TL et al. HMB-45 staining in benign and malignant melanocytic lesions. A reflection of cellular activation. Am J Dermatopathol 1991; 13: 543–550.

208 Mehregan DR, Mehregan DA, Mehregan AH. Proliferating cell nuclear antigen staining in deep-penetrating nevi. J Am Acad Dermatol 1995; 33: 685–687.

209 Cote J, Watters AK, O'Brien EA. Halo balloon cell nevus. J Cutan Pathol 1986; 13: 123–127.

210 Schrader WA, Helwig EB. Balloon cell nevi. Cancer 1967; 20: 1502–1514.

211 Smoller BR, Kindel S, McNutt NS et al. Balloon cell transformation in multiple dysplastic nevi. J Am Acad Dermatol 1991; 24: 290–292.

212 Okun MR, Donellan B, Edelstein L. An ultrastructural study of balloon cell nevus. Cancer 1974; 34: 615–625.

213 Berman A, Herszenson S. Vascular response in halo of recent halo nevus. J Am Acad Dermatol 1981; 4: 537–540.

214 Mooney MA, Barr RJ, Buxton MG. Halo nevus or halo phenomenon? A study of 142 cases. J Cutan Pathol 1995; 22: 342–348.

215 Langer K, Konrad K. Congenital melanocytic nevi with halo phenomenon: report of two cases and a review of the literature. J Dermatol Surg Oncol 1990; 16: 377–380.

216 Berman B, Shaieb AM, France DS, Altechek DD. Halo giant congenital melanocytic nevus: in vitro immunologic studies. J Am Acad Dermatol 1988; 19: 954–960.

217 del-Rio E, Aguilar A, Gallego MA et al. Targetoid halo nevus. J Am Acad Dermatol 1993; 29: 267–268.

218 Herd RM, Hunter JAA. Familial halo naevi. Clin Exp Dermatol 1998; 23: 68–69.

219 Baranda L, Torres-Alvarez B, Moncada B et al. Presence of activated lymphocytes in the peripheral blood of patients with halo nevi. J Am Acad Dermatol 1999; 41: 567–572.

220 Gauthier Y, Surleve-Bazeille JE, Texier L. Halo nevi without dermal infiltrate. Arch Dermatol 1978; 114: 1718.

221 Penneys NS, Mayoral F, Barnhill R et al. Delineation of nevus cell nests in inflammatory infiltrates by immunohistochemical staining for the presence of S100 protein. J Cutan Pathol 1985; 12: 28–32.

222 Fernández-Herrera J, Fernández-Ruiz E, López-Cabrera M et al. CD69 expression and tumour necrosis factor-α immunoreactivity in the inflammatory cell infiltrate of halo naevi. Br J Dermatol 1996; 134: 388–393.

223 Zeff RA, Freitag A, Grin CM, Grant-Kels JM. The immune response in halo nevi. J Am Acad Dermatol 1997; 37: 620–624.

224 Akasu R, From L, Kahn HJ. Characterization of the mononuclear infiltrate involved in regression of halo nevi. J Cutan Pathol 1994; 21: 302–311.

225 Fabrizi G, Massi G. Halo naevus with histological changes resembling epidermal erythema multiforme. Br J Dermatol 1999; 141: 369–370.

226 Hashimoto K. Ultrastructural studies of halo nevus. Cancer 1974; 34: 1653–1666.

227 Gauthier Y, Surleve-Bazeille JE, Gauthier O, Texier L. Ultrastructure of halo nevi. J Cutan Pathol 1975; 2: 71–81.

228 James MP, Wells RS. Cockade naevus: an unusual variant of the benign cellular naevus. Acta Derm Venereol 1980; 60: 360–363.

229 Guzzo C, Johnson B, Honig P. Cockarde nevus: a case report and review of the literature. Pediatr Dermatol 1988; 5: 250–253.

230 Capella GL, Altomare G. Cockade nevi and spinal dysraphism. Int J Dermatol 2000; 39: 318–320.

231 Mishima Y. Eccrine-centered nevus. Arch Dermatol 1973; 107: 59–61.

232 Kornberg R, Ackerman AB. Pseudomelanoma. Recurrent melanocytic nevus following partial surgical removal. Arch Dermatol 1975; 111: 1588–1590.

233 Park HK, Leonard DD, Arrington JH, Lund HZ. Recurrent melanocytic nevi: clinical and histologic review of 175 cases. J Am Acad Dermatol 1987; 17: 285–292.

234 Marghoob AA, Kopf AW. Persistent nevus: An exception to the ABCD rule of dermoscopy. J Am Acad Dermatol 1997; 36: 474–475.

235 Cochran AJ. The role of the histopathologist in the diagnosis of dysplastic naevi. Histopathology 1994; 24: 589–590.

236 Langel DJ, White WL. Pseudomelanoma after non-biopsy trauma – expanding the spectrum of persistent nevi. J Cutan Pathol 2000; 27: 562 (abstract).

237 Dummer R, Kempf W, Burg G. Pseudo-melanoma after laser therapy. Dermatology 1998; 197: 71–73.

238 Estrada JA, Piérard-Franchimont C, Piérard GE. Histogenesis of recurrent nevus. Am J Dermatopathol 1990; 12: 370–372.

239 Sexton M, Sexton CW. Recurrent pigmented melanocytic nevus. Arch Pathol Lab Med 1991; 115: 122–126.

240 Weedon D, Little JH. Spindle and epithelioid cell nevi in children and adults. A review of 211 cases of the Spitz nevus. Cancer 1977; 40: 217–225.

241 Weedon D. The Spitz naevus. Clin Oncol 1984; 3: 493–507.

242 Spitz S. Melanomas of childhood. Am J Pathol 1948; 24: 591–609.

243 Shimek CM, Golitz LE. The golden anniversary of the Spitz nevus. Arch Dermatol 1999; 135: 333–335.

244 Spatz A, Barnhill RL. The Spitz tumor 50 years later: Revisiting a landmark contribution and unresolved controversy. J Am Acad Dermatol 1999; 40: 223–228.

245 Nogita T, Nagayama M, Kawashima M et al. Spitz naevus of the toe. Br J Dermatol 1992; 126: 520–522.

246 Fabrizi G, Massi G. Polypoid Spitz naevus: the benign counterpart of polypoid malignant melanoma. Br J Dermatol 2000; 142: 128–132.

247 Carr EM, Heilman E, Prose NS. Spitz nevi in black children. J Am Acad Dermatol 1990; 23: 842–845.

248 Paniago-Pereira C, Maize JC, Ackerman AB. Nevus of large spindle and/or epithelioid cells (Spitz's nevus). Arch Dermatol 1978; 114: 1811–1823.

249 Dal Pozzo V, Benelli C, Restano L et al. Clinical review of 247 case records of Spitz nevus (epithelioid cell and/or spindle cell nevus). Dermatology 1997; 194: 20–25.

250 Yasaka N, Furue M, Tamaki K. Histopathological evaluation of halo phenomenon in Spitz nevus. Am J Dermatopathol 1995; 17: 484–486.

251 Lancer HA, Muhlbauer JE, Sober AJ. Multiple agminated spindle cell nevi. Unique clinical presentation and review. J Am Acad Dermatol 1983; 8: 707–711.

252 Smith SA, Day CL. Eruptive widespread Spitz nevi. J Am Acad Dermatol 1986; 15: 1155–1159.

253 Paties CT, Borroni G, Rosso R, Vassalo G. Relapsing eruptive multiple Spitz nevi or metastatic Spitzoid malignant melanoma? Am J Dermatopathol 1987; 9: 520–527.

254 Hamm H, Happle R, Brocker E-B. Multiple agminate Spitz naevi: review of the literature and report of a case with distinctive immunohistological features. Br J Dermatol 1987; 117: 511–522.

255 Bullen R, Snow SN, Larson PO et al. Multiple agminated Spitz nevi: report of two cases and review of the literature. Pediatr Dermatol 1995; 12: 156–158.

256 Abramovits W, Gonzalez-Serva A. Multiple agminated pigmented Spitz nevi (mimicking acral lentiginous malignant melanoma and dysplastic nevus) in an African-American girl. Int J Dermatol 1993; 32: 280–285.

257 Onsun N, Saraçoğlu Ş, Demirkesen C et al. Eruptive widespread Spitz nevi: Can pregnancy be a stimulating factor? J Am Acad Dermatol 1999; 40: 866–867.

258 Dawe RS, Wainwright NJ, Evans AT, Lowe JG. Multiple widespread eruptive Spitz naevi. Br J Dermatol 1998; 138: 872–874.

259 Sabroe RA, Vaingankar NV, Rigby HS, Peachey RDG. Agminate Spitz naevi occurring in an adult after the excision of a solitary Spitz naevus – report of a case and review of the literature. Clin Exp Dermatol 1996; 21: 197–200.

260 Menni S, Betti R, Boccardi D, Gualandri L. Both unilateral naevus achromicus and congenital agminated Spitz naevi in a checkerboard mosaic pattern. Br J Dermatol 2001; 144: 187–188.

261 Palazzo JP, Duray PH. Congenital agminated Spitz nevi: immunoreactivity with a melanoma-associated monoclonal antibody. J Cutan Pathol 1988; 15: 166–170.

262 Renfro L, Grant-Kels JM, Brown SA. Multiple agminate Spitz nevi. Pediatr Dermatol 1989; 6: 114–117.

263 Herd RM, Allan SM, Biddlestone L et al. Agminate Spitz naevi arising on hyperpigmented patches. Clin Exp Dermatol 1994; 19: 483–486.

264 Aloi F, Tomasini C, Pippione M. Agminated Spitz nevi occurring within a congenital speckled lentiginous nevus. Am J Dermatopathol 1995; 17: 594–598.

265 Betti R, Inselvini E, Palvarini M, Crosti C. Agminated intradermal Spitz nevi arising on an unusual speckled lentiginous nevus with localized lentiginosis. A continuum? Am J Dermatopathol 1997; 19: 524–527.

266 Krasovec M, Gianadda B, Hohl D. Giant recurrence of a multiple agminated Spitz nevus. J Am Acad Dermatol 1995; 33: 386–388.

267 Argenziano G, Scalvenzi M, Staibano S et al. Dermatoscopic pitfalls in differentiating pigmented Spitz naevi from cutaneous melanomas. Br J Dermatol 1999; 141: 788–793.

268 Pellacani G, Cesinaro AM, Seidenari S. Morphological features of Spitz naevus as observed by digital videomicroscopy. Acta Derm Venereol 2000; 80: 117–121.

269 Kaye VN, Dehner LP. Spindle and epithelioid cell nevus (Spitz nevus). Natural history following biopsy. Arch Dermatol 1990; 126: 1581–1583.

270 Ko CB, Walton S, Wyatt EH, Bury HP. Spitz nevus. Int J Dermatol 1993; 32: 354–357.

271 Harvell JD, Bastian BC, LeBoit PE. Persistent and recurrent Spitz nevi: a series of 21 cases. J Cutan Pathol 2000; 27: 559 (abstract).

272 Gambini C, Rongioletti F. Recurrent Spitz nevus. Case report and review of the literature. Am J Dermatopathol 1994; 16: 409–413.

273 Piepkorn M. On the nature of histologic observations: the case of the Spitz nevus. J Am Acad Dermatol 1995; 32: 248–254.

274 Casso EM, Grin-Jorgensen CM, Grant-Kels JM. Spitz nevi. J Am Acad Dermatol 1992; 27: 901–913.

275 Binder SW, Asnong C, Paul E, Cochran AJ. The histology and differential diagnosis of Spitz nevus. Semin Diagn Pathol 1993; 10: 36–46.

276 Crotty KA. Spitz naevus: Histological features and distinction from malignant melanoma. Australas J Dermatol 1997; 38 (Suppl): S49–S53.

277 Ackerman AB, Miyauchi Y, Takeuchi A, Ohata C. Melanomas that simulate Spitz's nevi histopathologically (and vice versa): an exercise in differentiation based on dependable criteria. Dermatopathology: Practical & Conceptual 1999; 5: 9–13.

278 Gartmann H, Ganser M. Der Spitz-Naevus. Z Hautkr 1985; 60: 22–28.

279 Okun MR. Histological demarcation of lateral borders: an unsupportable criterion for distinguishing malignant melanoma from Spitz naevus and compound naevus. Histopathology 1998; 33: 158–162.

280 Slater DN. Histological demarcation of lateral borders: an unsupportable criterion for distinguishing malignant melanoma from Spitz naevus and compound naevus. Histopathology 1998; 33: 576.

281 Goovaerts G, Buyssens N. Nevus cell maturation or atrophy? Am J Dermatopathol 1988; 10: 20–27.

282 Ruhoy SM, Prieto VG, Eliason SL et al. Malignant melanoma with paradoxical maturation. Am J Surg Pathol 2000; 24: 1600–1614.

283 Mérot Y, Frenk E. Spitz nevus (large spindle cell and/or epithelioid cell nevus). Virchows Arch [A] 1989; 415: 97–101.

284 Barnhill RL, Fleischli M. Histologic features of congenital melanocytic nevi in infants 1 year of age or younger. J Am Acad Dermatol 1995; 33: 780–785.

285 Busam KJ, Barnhill RL. Pagetoid Spitz nevus. Intraepidermal Spitz tumor with prominent pagetoid spread. Am J Surg Pathol 1995; 19: 1061–1067.

286 Han M-H, Koh K-J, Choi J-H et al. Pagetoid Spitz nevus: a variant of Spitz nevus. Int J Dermatol 2000; 39: 555–557.

287 Kamino H, Flotte TJ, Misheloff E. Eosinophilic globules in Spitz's nevi. New findings and a diagnostic sign. Am J Dermatopathol 1979; 1: 319–324.

288 Arbuckle S, Weedon D. Eosinophilic globules in the Spitz nevus. J Am Acad Dermatol 1982; 7: 324–327.

289 Schmoeckel C, Stolz W, Burgeson R, Krieg T. Identification of basement membrane components in eosinophilic globules in a case of Spitz's nevus. Am J Dermatopathol 1990; 12: 272–274.

290 Skelton HG, Miller ML, Lupton GP, Smith KJ. Eosinophilic globules in spindle cell and epithelioid cell nevi. Composition and possible origin. Am J Dermatopathol 1998; 20: 547–550.

291 Wesselmann U, Becker LR, Bröcker EB et al. Eosinophilic globules in Spitz nevi: no evidence for apoptosis. Am J Dermatopathol 1998; 20: 551–554.

292 Scott G, Chen KTK, Rosai J. Pseudoepitheliomatous hyperplasia in Spitz nevi. A possible source of confusion with squamous cell carcinoma. Arch Pathol Lab Med 1989; 113: 61–63.

293 Cockerell CJ, Sonnier G, Kelly L, Patel S. Comparative analysis of neovascularization in primary cutaneous melanoma and Spitz nevus. Am J Dermatopathol 1994; 16: 9–13.

294 Binder M, Steiner A, Mossbacher U et al. Quantification of vascularity in nodular melanoma and Spitz's nevus. J Cutan Pathol 1997; 24: 272–277.

295 Pulitzer DR, Martin PC, Cohen AP, Reed RJ. Histologic classification of the combined nevus. Analysis of the variable expression of melanocytic nevi. Am J Surg Pathol 1991; 15: 1111–1122.

296 Marchesi L, Naldi L, Locati F et al. Combined Clark's nevus. Am J Dermatopathol 1994; 16: 364–371.

297 Nakagawa S, Kumasaka K, Kato T et al. Spitz naevus arising on congenital compound nevus pigmentosus. Int J Dermatol 1995; 34: 863–864.

298 McCalmont TH. Brace yourself and tread cautiously: surprises and pitfalls in the diagnosis of melanocytic neoplasms. Pathology Case Reviews 1999; 4: 63–76.

299 Suster S. Hyalinizing spindle and epithelioid cell nevus. A study of five cases of a distinctive histologic variant of Spitz's nevus. Am J Dermatopathol 1994; 16: 593–598.

300 Burg G, Kempf W, Höchli M et al. 'Tubular' epithelioid cell nevus: a new variant of Spitz's nevus. J Cutan Pathol 1998; 25: 475–478.

301 Soyer HP, Breier F, Cerroni L, Kerl H. 'Tubular' structures within melanocytic proliferations: a distinctive morphologic finding not restricted to Spitz nevi. J Cutan Pathol 1999; 26: 315–316.

302 Ziemer M, Diaz-Cascajo C, Köhler G, Weyers W. "Tubular Spitz's nevus" – an artifact of fixation? J Cutan Pathol 2000; 27: 500–504.

303 McCarthy SW, Crotty KA, Palmer AA et al. Cutaneous malignant melanoma in teenagers. Histopathology 1994; 24: 453–461.

304 Peters MS, Goellner JR. Spitz naevi and malignant melanomas of childhood and adolescence. Histopathology 1986; 10: 1289–1302.

305 LeBoit PE, van Fletcher H. A comparative study of Spitz nevus and nodular malignant melanoma using image analysis cytometry. J Invest Dermatol 1987; 88: 753–757.

306 Vogt T, Stolz W, Glässl A et al. Multivariate DNA cytometry discriminates between Spitz nevi and malignant melanomas because large polymorphic nuclei in Spitz nevi are not aneuploid. Am J Dermatopathol 1996; 18: 142–150.

307 Otsuka F, Chi H-I, Umebayashi Y. Successful differentiation of Spitz naevus from malignant melanoma by microfluorometric analysis of cellular DNA content. Clin Exp Dermatol 1993; 18: 421–424.

308 Winokur TS, Palazzo JP, Johnson WC, Duray PH. Evaluation of DNA ploidy in dysplastic and Spitz nevi by flow cytometry. J Cutan Pathol 1990; 17: 342–347.

309 Bergman R, Sabo E, Schafer I. Measurement of the maturation parameter by using computer-assisted interactive image analysis may be helpful in the differential diagnosis between compound Spitz nevus and malignant melanoma. Am J Dermatopathol 1996; 18: 567–570.

310 de Wit PEJ, Kerstens HMJ, Poddighe PJ et al. DNA in situ hybridization as a diagnostic tool in the discrimination of melanoma and Spitz naevus. J Pathol 1994; 173; 227–233.

311 Bastian BC, Wesselmann U, Pinkel D, LeBoit PE. Molecular cytogenetic analysis of Spitz nevi shows clear differences to melanoma. J Invest Dermatol 1999; 13: 1065–1069.

312 Tosi P, Miracco C, Santopietro R et al. Possible diagnostic role of telomerase activity evaluation in the differential diagnosis between Spitz naevi and cutaneous malignant melanoma. Br J Dermatol 2000; 142: 1060–1061.

313 Orchard DC, Dowling JP, Kelly JW. Spitz naevi misdiagnosed histologically as melanoma: prevalence and clinical profile. Australas J Dermatol 1997; 38: 12–14.

314 Barnhill RL, Argenyi ZB, From L et al. Atypical Spitz nevi/tumors: lack of consensus for diagnosis, discrimination from melanoma, and prediction of outcome. Hum Pathol 1999; 30: 513–520.

315 Palazzo J, Duray PH. Typical, dysplastic, congenital, and Spitz nevi: a comparative histochemical study. Hum Pathol 1989; 20: 341–346.

316 Howat AJ, Giri DD, Cotton DWK, Slater DN. Nucleolar organizer regions in Spitz nevi and malignant melanomas. Cancer 1989; 63: 474–478.

317 Lazzaro B, Elder DE, Rebers A et al. Immunophenotyping of compound and Spitz nevi and vertical-growth phase melanoma using a panel of monoclonal antibodies reactive in paraffin sections. J Invest Dermatol 1993; 100: 313S–317S.

318 Bergman R, Dromi R, Trau H et al. The pattern of HMB-45 antibody staining in compound Spitz nevi. Am J Dermatopathol 1995; 17: 542–546.

319 Nagasaka T, Lai R, Medeiros LJ et al. Cyclin D1 overexpression in Spitz nevi: an immunohistochemical study. Am J Dermatopathol 1999; 21: 115–120.

320 Bergman R, Azzam H, Sprecher E et al. A comparative immunohistochemical study of MART-1 expression in Spitz nevi, ordinary melanocytic nevi, and malignant melanomas. J Am Acad Dermatol 2000; 42: 496–500.

321 Penneys N, Seigfried E, Nahass G, Vogler C. Expression of proliferating cell nuclear antigen in Spitz nevus. J Am Acad Dermatol 1995; 32: 964–967.

322 Niemann TH, Argenyi ZB. Immunohistochemical study of Spitz nevi and malignant melanoma with use of antibody to proliferating cell nuclear antigen. Am J Dermatopathol 1993; 15: 441–445.

323 Bergman R, Malkin L, Sabo E, Kerner H. MIB-1 monoclonal antibody to determine proliferative activity of Ki-67 antigen as an adjunct to the histopathologic differential diagnosis of Spitz nevi. J Am Acad Dermatol 2001; 44: 500–504.

324 Bergman R, Shemer A, Levy R et al. Immunohistochemical study of p53 protein expression in Spitz nevus as compared with other melanocytic lesions. Am J Dermatopathol 1995; 17: 547–550.

325 Busam KJ, Granter SR, Iversen K, Jungbluth AA. Immunohistochemical distinction of epithelioid histiocytic proliferations from epithelioid melanocytic nevi. Am J Dermatopathol 2000; 22: 237–241.

326 Bergman R, Kerner H, Manov L, Friedman-Birnbaum R. C-fos protein expression in Spitz nevi, common melanocytic nevi, and malignant melanomas. Am J Dermatopathol 1998; 20: 262–265.

327 Weyers W. The 21st Colloquium of the International Society of Dermatopathology. Am J Dermatopathol 2001; 23: 232–236.

328 Kohler S. Spitz (spindle and epithelioid) nevi. Pathology Case Reviews 1999; 4: 87–91.

329 Spatz A, Calonje E, Handfield-Jones S, Barnhill RL. Spitz tumors in children. A grading system for risk stratification. Arch Dermatol 1999; 135: 282–285.

330 Fabrizi G, Massi G. Spitzoid malignant melanoma in teenagers: an entity with no better prognosis than that of other forms of melanoma. Histopathology 2001; 38: 448–453.

331 Reed RJ. Atypical Spitz nevus/tumor. Hum Pathol 1999; 30: 1523–1525.

332 Harvell JD, Meehan SA, LeBoit PE. Halo Spitz nevi. Pathology Case Reviews 1999; 4: 92–96.

333 Harvell JD, Meehan SA, LeBoit PE. Spitz's nevi with halo reaction: a histopathologic study of 17 cases. J Cutan Pathol 1997; 24: 611–619.

334 Barr RJ, Morales RV, Graham JH. Desmoplastic nevus. A distinct histologic variant of mixed spindle cell and epithelioid cell nevus. Cancer 1980; 46: 557–564.

335 Harris GR, Shea CR, Horenstein MG et al. Desmoplastic (sclerotic) nevus. Am J Surg Pathol 1999; 23: 786–794.

336 MacKie RM, Doherty VR. The desmoplastic melanocytic naevus: a distinct histological entity. Histopathology 1992; 20: 207–211.

337 Diaz-Cascajo C, Borghi S, Weyers W. Angiomatoid Spitz nevus. A distinct variant of desmoplastic Spitz nevus with prominent vasculature. Am J Dermatopathol 2000; 22: 135–139.

338 Spatz A, Peterse S, Fletcher CDM, Barnhill RL. Plexiform Spitz nevus. Am J Dermatopathol 1999; 21: 542–546.

339 Smith KJ, Barrett TL, Skelton HG III et al. Spindle cell and epithelioid cell nevi with atypia and metastasis (malignant Spitz nevus). Am J Surg Pathol 1989; 13: 931–939.

340 Skelton HG III, Smith KJ, Holland TT et al. Malignant Spitz nevus. Int J Dermatol 1992; 31: 639–641.

341 Barnhill RL. Childhood melanoma. Semin Diagn Pathol 1998; 15: 189–194.

342 Barnhill RL, Barnhill MA, Berwick M, Mihm MC. The histologic spectrum of pigmented spindle cell nevus. Hum Pathol 1991; 22: 52–58.

343 Smith NP. The pigmented spindle cell tumor of Reed: an underdiagnosed lesion. Semin Diagn Pathol 1987; 4: 75–87.

344 Barnhill RL, Mihm MC Jr. Pigmented spindle cell naevus and its variants: distinction from melanoma. Br J Dermatol 1989; 121: 717–726.

345 Requena L, Sánchez Yus E. Pigmented spindle cell naevus. Br J Dermatol 1990; 123: 757–763.

346 Wistuba I, Gonzalez S. Eosinophilic globules in pigmented spindle cell nevus. Am J Dermatopathol 1990; 12: 268–271.

347 Sau P, Graham JH, Helwig EB. Pigmented spindle cell nevus: a clinicopathologic analysis of ninety-five cases. J Am Acad Dermatol 1993; 28: 565–571.

348 Choi JH, Sung KJ, Koh JK. Pigmented epithelioid cell nevus: a variant of Spitz nevus? J Am Acad Dermatol 1993; 28: 497–498.

349 Kroon S, Clemmensen OJ. Incidence of congenital melanocytic nevi in newborn babies in Denmark. J Am Acad Dermatol 1987; 17: 422–426.

350 Schleicher SM, Lim SJM. Congenital nevi. Int J Dermatol 1995; 34: 825–829.

351 Castilla EE, Dutra MDG, Orioli-Parreiras IM. Epidemiology of congenital pigmented naevi: 1. Incidence rates and relative frequencies. Br J Dermatol 1981; 104: 307–315.

352 Kopf AW, Bart RS, Hennessey P. Congenital nevocytic nevi and malignant melanoma. J Am Acad Dermatol 1979; 1: 123–130.

353 Dawson HA, Atherton DJ, Mayou B. A prospective study of congenital melanocytic naevi: progress report and evaluation after 6 years. Br J Dermatol 1996; 134: 617–623.

354 Frieden IJ, Williams ML, Barkovich AJ. Giant congenital melanocytic nevi: brain magnetic resonance findings in neurologically asymptomatic children. J Am Acad Dermatol 1994; 31: 423–429.

355 Kadonaga JN, Barkovich AJ, Edwards MSB, Frieden IJ. Neurocutaneous melanosis in association with the Dandy–Walker complex. Pediatr Dermatol 1992; 9: 37–43.

356 Kadonaga JN, Frieden IJ. Neurocutaneous melanosis: definition and review of the literature. J Am Acad Dermatol 1991; 24: 747–755.

357 DeDavid M, Orlow SJ, Provost N et al. Neurocutaneous melanosis: Clinical features of large congenital melanocytic nevi in patients with manifest central nervous system melanosis. J Am Acad Dermatol 1996; 35: 529–538.

358 Green LJ, Nanda VS, Roth GM, Barr RJ. Neurocutaneous melanosis and Dandy–Walker syndrome in an infant. Int J Dermatol 1997; 36: 356–358.

359 Ruiz-Maldonado R, del Rosario Barona-Mazuera M, Hidalgo-Galván LR et al. Giant congenital melanocytic nevi, neurocutaneous melanosis and neurological alterations. Dermatology 1997; 195: 125–128.

360 Holmes G, Wines N, Ryman W. Giant congenital melanocytic naevus and symptomatic thoracic arachnoid cyst. Australas J Dermatol 2001; 42: 124–128.

361 Takayama H, Nagashima Y, Hara M et al. Immunohistochemical detection of the *c-met* proto-oncogene product in the congenital melanocytic nevus of an infant with neurocutaneous melanosis. J Am Acad Dermatol 2001; 44: 538–540.

362 Rhodes AR, Albert LS, Weinstock MA. Congenital nevomelanocytic nevi: proportionate area expansion during infancy and early childhood. J Am Acad Dermatol 1996; 34: 51–62.

363 Giam Y-C, Williams ML, LeBoit PE et al. Neonatal erosions and ulcerations in giant congenital melanocytic nevi. Pediatr Dermatol 1999; 16: 354–358.

364 Marghoob AA, Orlow SJ, Kopf AW. Syndromes associated with melanocytic nevi. J Am Acad Dermatol 1993; 29: 373–388.

365 Roth MJ, Medeiros LJ, Kapur S et al. Malignant schwannoma with melanocytic and neuroepithelial differentiation in an infant with congenital giant melanocytic nevus: a complex neurocristopathy. Hum Pathol 1993; 24: 1371–1375.

366 Tokura Y, Yamanaka K, Wakita H et al. Halo congenital nevus undergoing spontaneous regression. Arch Dermatol 1994; 130: 1036–1041.

367 Goulden V, Highet AS. Halo congenital naevus. Br J Dermatol 1994; 131: 295–296.

368 Effendy I, Happle R. Linear arrangement of multiple congenital melanocytic nevi. J Am Acad Dermatol 1992; 27: 853–854.

369 Brunner M, Vardarman E, Megahed M, Ruzicka T. Congenital agminated segmental naevi. Br J Dermatol 1995; 133: 315–316.

370 Swerdlow AJ, English JSC, Qiao Z. The risk of melanoma in patients with congenital nevi: a cohort study. J Am Acad Dermatol 1995; 32: 595–599.

371 Marghoob AA, Schoenbach SP, Kopf AW et al. Large congenital melanocytic nevi and the risk for the development of malignant melanoma. Arch Dermatol 1996; 132: 170–175.

372 Egan CL, Oliveria SA, Elenitsas R et al. Cutaneous melanoma risk and phenotypic changes in large congenital nevi: A follow-up study of 46 patients. J Am Acad Dermatol 1998; 39: 923–932.

373 DeDavid M, Orlow SJ, Provost N et al. A study of large congenital melanocytic nevi and associated malignant melanomas: Review of cases in the New York University Registry and the world literature. J Am Acad Dermatol 1997; 36: 409–416.

374 Alper JC. Congenital nevi. The controversy rages on. Arch Dermatol 1985; 121: 734–735.

375 Illig L, Weidner F, Hundeiker M et al. Congenital nevi ≦ 10 cm as precursors to melanoma. 52 cases, a review, and a new conception. Arch Dermatol 1985; 121: 1274–1281.

376 Elder DE. The blind men and the elephant. Different views of small congenital nevi. Arch Dermatol 1985; 121: 1263–1265.

377 Shpall S, Frieden I, Chesney M, Newman T. Risk of malignant transformation of congenital melanocytic nevi in blacks. Pediatr Dermatol 1994; 11: 204–208.

378 Clemmensen O, Ackerman AB. All small congenital nevi need not be removed. Am J Dermatopathol (Suppl) 1984; 1: 189–194.

379 Keipert JA. Giant pigmented naevus: the frequency of malignant change and indications for treatment in prepubertal children. Australas J Dermatol 1985; 26: 81–85.

380 Sahin S, Levin L, Kopf AW et al. Risk of melanoma in medium-sized congenital melanocytic nevi: A follow-up study. J Am Acad Dermatol 1998; 39: 428–433.

381 Otley CC. Risk of melanoma in medium-sized congenital melanocytic nevi. J Am Acad Dermatol 1999; 41: 131.

382 Rhodes AR, Melski JW. Small congenital nevocellular nevi and the risk of cutaneous melanoma. J Pediatr 1982; 100: 219–224.

383 Rhodes AR, Sober AJ, Day CL et al. The malignant potential of small congenital nevocellular nevi. An estimate of association based on a histologic study of 234 primary cutaneous melanomas. J Am Acad Dermatol 1982; 6: 230–241.

384 Rhodes AR, Silverman RA, Harrist TJ, Melski JW. A histologic comparison of congenital and acquired nevomelanocytic nevi. Arch Dermatol 1985; 121: 1266–1273.

385 MacKie RM, Watt D, Doherty V, Aitchison T. Malignant melanoma occurring in those aged under 30 in the west of Scotland 1979–1986: a study of incidence, clinical features, pathological features and survival. Br J Dermatol 1991; 124: 560–564.

386 Grevelink JM, van Leeuwen RL, Anderson RR, Byers HR. Clinical and histological responses of congenital melanocytic nevi after single treatment with Q-switched lasers. Arch Dermatol 1997; 133: 349–353.

387 Imayama S, Ueda S. Long- and short-term histological observations of congenital nevi treated with the normal-mode ruby laser. Arch Dermatol 1999; 135: 1211–1218.

388 Schneiderman H, Wu AY-Y, Campbell WA et al. Congenital melanoma with multiple prenatal metastases. Cancer 1987; 60: 1371–1377.

389 Ishii N, Ichiyama S, Saito S et al. Congenital malignant melanoma. Br J Dermatol 1991; 124: 492–494.

390 Carroll CB, Ceballos P, Perry AE et al. Severely atypical medium-sized congenital nevus with widespread satellitosis and placental deposits in a neonate: the problem of congenital melanoma and its simulants. J Am Acad Dermatol 1994; 30: 825–828.

391 Antaya RJ, Keller RA, Wilkerson JA. Placental nevus cells associated with giant congenital pigmented nevi. Pediatr Dermatol 1995; 12: 260–262.

392 Ball RA, Genest D, Sander M et al. Congenital melanocytic nevi with placental infiltration by melanocytes. A benign condition that mimics metastatic melanoma. Arch Dermatol 1998; 134: 711–714.

393 Desruelles F, Lacour J-P, Mantoux F, Ortonne J-P. Divided nevus of the penis: an unusual location. Arch Dermatol 1998; 134: 879–880.

394 Choi G-S, Won D-H, Lee S-J et al. Divided naevus on the penis. Br J Dermatol 2000; 143: 1126–1127.

395 Walton RG, Jacobs AH, Cox AJ. Pigmented lesions in newborn infants. Br J Dermatol 1976; 95: 389–396.

396 Silvers DN, Helwig EB. Melanocytic nevi in neonates. J Am Acad Dermatol 1981; 4: 166–175.

397 Kuehnl-Petzoldt C, Volk B, Kunze J et al. Histology of congenital nevi during the first year of life. Am J Dermatopathol (Suppl) 1984; 1: 81–88.

398 Mark GJ, Mihm MC, Liteplo MG et al. Congenital melanocytic nevi of the small and garment type. Clinical, histologic, and ultrastructural studies. Hum Pathol 1973; 4: 395–418.

399 Rhodes AR. Congenital nevomelanocytic nevi. Histologic patterns in the first year of life and evolution during childhood. Arch Dermatol 1986; 122: 1257–1262.

400 Stenn KS, Arons M, Hurwitz S. Patterns of congenital nevocellular nevi. A histologic study of thirty-eight cases. J Am Acad Dermatol 1983; 9: 388–393.

401 Nickoloff BJ, Walton R, Pregerson-Rodan K et al. Immunohistologic patterns of congenital nevocellular nevi. Arch Dermatol 1986; 122: 1263–1268.

402 Cribier BJ, Santinelli F, Grosshans E. Lack of clinical-pathological correlation in the diagnosis of congenital naevi. Br J Dermatol 1999; 141: 1004–1009.

403 Zitelli JA, Grant MG, Abell E, Boyd JB. Histologic patterns of congenital nevocytic nevi and implications for treatment. J Am Acad Dermatol 1984; 11: 402–409.

404 Everett MA. Histopathology of congenital pigmented nevi. Am J Dermatopathol 1989; 11 11–12.

405 Clemmensen OJ, Kroon S. The histology of 'congenital features' in early acquired melanocytic nevi. J Am Acad Dermatol 1988; 19: 742–746.

406 Walsh MY, Mackie RM. Histological features of value in differentiating small congenital melanocytic naevi from acquired naevi. Histopathology 1988; 12: 145–154.

407 Cardona SA, Skidmore R, Gupta A et al. Giant congenital melanocytic nevus with underlying hypoplasia of the subcutaneous fat. Pediatr Dermatol 2000; 17: 387–390.

408 Cockayne SE, Gawkrodger DJ. Hamartomatous congenital melanocytic nevi showing secondary anetoderma-like changes. J Am Acad Dermatol 1998; 39: 843–845.

409 Padilla RS, McConnell TS, Gribble JT, Smoot C. Malignant melanoma arising in a giant congenital melanocytic nevus. A case report with cytogenetic and histopathologic analyses. Cancer 1988; 62: 2589–2594.

4 0 Cutlan RT, Wesche WA, Jenkins JJ III. Malignant melanoma arising in giant congenital nevi: a clinical and histopathological study of 3 cases. J Cutan Pathol 2000; 27: 554 (abstract).

411 Weidner N, Flanders DJ, Jochimsen PR, Stamler FW. Neurosarcomatous malignant melanoma arising in a neuroid giant congenital melanocytic nevus. Arch Dermatol 1985; 121: 1302–1306.

412 Hendrickson MR, Ross JC. Neoplasms arising in congenital giant nevi. Morphologic study of seven cases and a review of the literature. Am J Surg Pathol 1981; 5: 109–135.

413 Lowes MA, Norris D, Whitfeld M. Benign melanocytic proliferative nodule within a congenital naevus. Australas J Dermatol 2000; 41: 109–111.

414 Borbujo J, Jara M, Cortes L, Sanchez de Leon L. A newborn with nodular ulcerated lesion on a giant congenital nevus. Pediatr Dermatol 2000; 17: 299–301.

415 Mancianti ML, Clark WH, Hayes FA et al. Malignant melanoma simulants arising in congenital melanocytic nevi do not show experimental evidence for a malignant phenotype. Am J Pathol 1990; 136: 817–829.

416 Angelucci D, Natali PG, Amerio PL et al. Rapid perinatal growth mimicking malignant transformation in a giant congenital melanocytic nevus. Hum Pathol 1991; 22: 297–301.

417 Reed RJ. Giant congenital nevi: a conceptualization of patterns. J Invest Dermatol 1993; 100: 300S–312S.

418 Thomas JE, Selim MA, Allee J et al. Comparative histomorphology of congenital versus atypical nevi, with an emphasis on overlapping and distinguishing features. J Cutan Pathol 2000; 27: 574–575 (abstract).

Dermal melanocytic lesions

419 Stanford DG, Georgouras KE. Dermal melanocytosis: a clinical spectrum. Australas J Dermatol 1996; 37: 19–25.

420 Leung AKC. Mongolian spots in Chinese children. Int J Dermatol 1988; 27: 106–108.

421 Kikuchi I, Inoue S. Natural history of the Mongolian spot. J Dermatol 1980; 7: 449–450.

422 Bart BJ, Olson CL. Congenital halo Mongolian spot. J Am Acad Dermatol 1991; 25: 1082–1083.

423 Carmichael AJ, Tan CY, Abraham SM. Adult onset Mongolian spot. Clin Exp Dermatol 1993; 18: 72–74.

424 Igawa HH, Ohura T, Sugihara T et al. Cleft lip Mongolian spot: Mongolian spot associated with cleft lip. J Am Acad Dermatol 1994; 30: 566–569.

425 Leung AKC, Kao CP. Extensive Mongolian spots with involvement of the scalp. Pediatr Dermatol 1999; 16: 371–372.

426 Leung AKC, Kao CP, Lee TKM. Mongolian spots with involvement of the temporal area. Int J Dermatol 2001; 40: 288–289.

427 Sapadin AN, Friedman IS. Extensive Mongolian spots associated with Hunter syndrome. J Am Acad Dermatol 1998; 39: 1013–1015.

428 Grant BP, Beard JS, de Castro F et al. Extensive Mongolian spots in an infant with Hurler syndrome. Arch Dermatol 1998; 134: 108–109.

429 Ridgway HB, Reizner GT. Acquired pseudo-Mongolian spot associated with minocycline therapy. Arch Dermatol 1992; 128: 565–566.

430 Suh DH, Hwang JH, Lee HS et al. Clinical features of Ota's naevus in Koreans and its treatment with Q-switched alexandrite laser. Clin Exp Dermatol 2000; 25: 269–273.

431 Hidano A, Kajima H, Endo Y. Bilateral nevus Ota associated with nevus Ito. A case of pigmentation on the lips. Arch Dermatol 1965; 91: 357–359.

432 Mishima Y, Mevorah B. Nevus Ota and nevus Ito in American negroes. J Invest Dermatol 1961; 36: 133–154.

433 van Krieken JHJM, Boom BW, Scheffer E. Malignant transformation in a naevus of Ito. A case report. Histopathology 1988; 12: 100–102.

434 Patel BCK, Egan CA, Lucius RW et al. Cutaneous malignant melanoma and oculodermal melanocytosis (nevus of Ota): Report of a case and review of the literature. J Am Acad Dermatol 1998; 38: 862–865.

435 Juhasz ES, Rees MJW, Miller MV. Invasive naevus of Ota. Pathology 1993; 25: 95–97.

436 Cowan TH, Balistocky M. The nevus of Ota or oculodermal melanocytosis: the ocular changes. Arch Ophthalmol 1977; 95: 1820–1824.

437 Radentz WH. Congenital common blue nevus. Arch Dermatol 1990; 126: 124–125.

438 Kawasaki T, Tsuboi R, Ueki R et al. Congenital giant common blue nevus. J Am Acad Dermatol 1993; 28: 653–654.

439 McDonagh AJG, Laing RW, Harrington CI, Griffiths RW. Giant alopecic nodule of the scalp: unusual presentation of a cellular blue naevus in an adult. Br J Dermatol 1992; 126: 375–377.

440 Rodriguez HA, Ackerman LV. Cellular blue nevus. Clinicopathologic study of forty-five cases. Cancer 1968; 21: 393–405.

441 Temple-Camp CRE, Saxe N, King H. Benign and malignant cellular blue nevus. A clinicopathological study of 30 cases. Am J Dermatopathol 1988; 10: 289–296.

442 Suchniak JM, Griego RD, Rudolph AH, Waidhofer W. Acquired multiple blue nevi on an extremity. J Am Acad Dermatol 1995; 33: 1051–1052.

443 Vidal S, Sanz A, Hernández B et al. Subungual blue naevus. Br J Dermatol 1997; 137: 1023–1025.

444 Hendricks WM. Eruptive blue nevi. J Am Acad Dermatol 1981; 4: 50–53.

445 Walsh MY. Eruptive disseminated blue naevi of the scalp. Br J Dermatol 1999; 141: 581–582.

446 Nardini P, De Giorgi V, Massi D, Carli P. Eruptive disseminated blue naevi of the scalp. Br J Dermatol 1999; 140: 178–180.

447 Hsiao G-H, Hsiao C-W. Plaque-type blue nevus on the face: a variant of Ota's nevus? J Am Acad Dermatol 1994; 30: 849–851.

448 Busam KJ, Woodruff JM, Erlandson RA, Brady MS. Large plaque-type blue nevus with subcutaneous cellular nodules. Am J Surg Pathol 2000; 24: 92–99.

449 Park YM, Kang H, Cho BK. Plaque-type blue nevus combined with nevus spilus and smooth muscle hyperplasia. Int J Dermatol 1999; 38: 775–777.

450 Bondi EE, Elder D, Guerry D, Clark WH. Target blue nevus. Arch Dermatol 1983; 119: 919–920.

451 Bart BJ. Acquired linear blue nevi. J Am Acad Dermatol 1997; 36: 268–269.

452 Kang DS, Chung K-Y. Common blue naevus with satellite lesions: possible perivascular dissemination resulting in a clinical resemblance to malignant melanoma. Br J Dermatol 1999; 141: 922–925.

453 Balloy BC, Mallet V, Bassile G et al. Disseminated blue nevus: abnormal nevoblast migration or proliferation? Arch Dermatol 1998; 134: 245–246.

454 Krause MH, Bonnekoh B, Weisshaar E, Gollnick H. Coincidence of multiple, disseminated, tardive-eruptive blue nevi with cutis marmorata teleangiectatica congenita. Dermatology 2000; 200: 134–138.

455 Kasahara N, Kazama T, Sakamoto F, Ito M. Acquired multiple blue naevi scattered over the whole body. Br J Dermatol 2001; 144: 440–442.

456 Blackford S, Roberts DL. Familial multiple blue naevi. Clin Exp Dermatol 1991; 16: 308–309.

457 Knoell KA, Nelson KC, Patterson JW. Familial multiple blue nevi. J Am Acad Dermatol 1998; 39: 322–325.

458 Marchesi L, Naldi L, Parma A et al. Agminate blue nevus combined with lentigo: a variant of speckled lentiginous nevus? Am J Dermatopathol 1993; 15: 162–165.

459 Carney JA, Ferreiro JA. The epithelioid blue nevus. A multicentric familial tumor with important associations, including cardiac myxoma and psammomatous melanotic schwannoma. Am J Surg Pathol 1996; 20: 259–272.

460 Bleasel NR, Stapleton KM. Carney complex: in a patient with multiple blue naevi and lentigines, suspect cardiac myxoma. Australas J Dermatol 1999; 40: 158–160.

461 Carney JA, Stratakis CA. Epithelioid blue nevus and psammomatous melanotic schwannoma: the unusual pigmented skin tumors of the Carney complex. Semin Diagn Pathol 1998; 15: 216–224.

462 O'Grady TC, Barr RJ, Billman G, Cunningham BB. Epithelioid blue nevus occurring in children with no evidence of Carney complex. Am J Dermatopathol 1999; 21: 483–486.

463 Moreno C, Requena L, Kutzner H et al. Epithelioid blue nevus: a rare variant of blue nevus not always associated with the Carney complex. J Cutan Pathol 2000; 27: 218–223.

464 Carr S, See J, Wilkinson B, Kossard S. Hypopigmented common blue nevus. J Cutan Pathol 1997; 24: 494–498.

465 Bhawan J, Cao S-L. Amelanotic blue nevus: a variant of blue nevus. Am J Dermatopathol 1999; 21: 225–228.

466 Bolognia JL, Glusac EJ. Hypopigmented common blue nevi. Arch Dermatol 1998; 134: 754–756.

467 Leopold JG, Richards DB. The interrelationship of blue and common naevi. J Pathol 1968; 95: 37–46.

468 Gartmann H, Muller HD. Über das gemeinsame Vorkommen von blauem Naevus und Naevuszellnaevus in em und derselbem Geschwulst ('combined nevus'). Z Hautkr 1977; 52: 389–398.

469 Pock L, Trnka J, Vosmík F, Záruba F. Systematized progradient multiple combined melanocytic and blue nevus. Am J Dermatopathol 1991; 13: 282–287.

470 Ishibashi A, Kimura K, Kukita A. Plaque-type blue nevus combined with lentigo (nevus spilus). J Cutan Pathol 1990; 17: 241–245.

471 Hofmann UB, Ogilvie P, Müllges W et al. Congenital unilateral speckled lentiginous blue nevi with asymmetric spinal muscular atrophy. J Am Acad Dermatol 1998; 39: 326–329.

472 Betti R, Inselvini E, Crosti E. Blue nevi and basal cell carcinoma within a speckled lentiginous nevus. J Am Acad Dermatol 1999; 41: 1039–1041.

473 Betti R, Inselvini E, Palvarini M, Crosti C. Agminate and plaque-type blue nevus combined with lentigo, associated with follicular cyst and eccrine changes: a variant of speckled lentiginous nevus. Dermatology 1997; 195: 387–390.

474 van Leeuwen RL, Vink J, Bergman W et al. Agminate-type combined nevus consisting of a common blue nevus with a junctional Spitz nevus. Arch Dermatol 1994; 130: 1074–1075.

475 Kamino H, Tam ST. Compound blue nevus: a variant of blue nevus with an additional junctional dendritic component. Arch Dermatol 1990; 126: 1330–1333.

476 Requena L, Barat A, Hasson A et al. Malignant combined nevus. Am J Dermatopathol 1991; 13: 169–173.

477 Micali G, Innocenzi D, Nasca MR. Cellular blue nevus of the scalp infiltrating the underlying bone: case report and review. Pediatr Dermatol 1997; 14: 199–203.

478 Michal M, Kerekes Z, Kinkor Z et al. Desmoplastic cellular blue nevi. Am J Dermatopathol 1995; 17: 230–235.

479 Perez MT, Suster S. Balloon cell change in cellular blue nevus. Am J Dermatopathol 1999; 21: 181–184.

480 Tran TA, Carlson JA, Basaca PC, Mihm MC. Cellular blue nevus with atypia (atypical cellular blue nevus): a clinicopathologic study of nine cases. J Cutan Pathol 1998; 25: 252–258.

481 Groben PA, Harvell JD, White WL. Epithelioid blue nevus. Neoplasm *sui generis* or variation on a theme? Am J Dermatopathol 2000; 22: 473–488.

482 Collina G, Annessi G, Di Gregorio C. Cellular blue naevus associated with osteoma cutis. Histopathology 1991; 19: 473–475.

483 Newton JA, McGibbon DH. Blue naevus associated with trichoepithelioma: a report of two cases. J Cutan Pathol 1984; 11: 549–552.

484 Youngberg GA, Rasch EM, Douglas HL. Bizarre blue nevus: a case report with deoxyribonucleic acid content analysis. J Am Acad Dermatol 1986; 15: 336–341.

485 Pathy AL, Helm TN, Elston D et al. Malignant melanoma arising in a blue nevus with features of pilar neurocristic hamartoma. J Cutan Pathol 1993; 20: 459–464.

486 Michal M, Baumruk L, Skálová A. Myxoid change within cellular blue naevi: a diagnostic pitfall. Histopathology 1992; 20: 527–530.

487 Sun J, Morton TH Jr, Gown AM. Antibody HMB-45 identifies the cells of blue nevi. Am J Surg Pathol 1990; 14: 748–751.

488 Wood WS, Tron VA. Analysis of HMB-45 immunoreactivity in common and cellular blue nevi. J Cutan Pathol 1991; 18: 261–263.

489 Egawa K, Honda Y, Kuroki M, Ono T. The carcinoembryonic antigen (CEA) family (CD66) expressed in melanocytic naevi is not expressed in blue naevuscell naevi in dendritic type. J Cutan Pathol 2000; 27: 351–358.

490 Smith KJ, Germain M, Williams J, Skelton HG. CD34-positive cellular blue nevi. J Cutan Pathol 2001; 28: 145–150.

491 Bhawan J, Chang WH, Edelstein LM. Cellular blue nevus. An ultrastructural study. J Cutan Pathol 1980; 7: 109–122.

492 White WL, Hitchcock MG. Blue-nevus like metastatic melanoma. Pathology Case Reviews 1999; 4: 97–102.

493 Busam KJ. Metastatic melanoma to the skin simulating blue nevus. Am J Surg Pathol 1999; 23: 276–282.

494 Granter SR, McKee PH, Calonje E et al. Melanoma associated with blue nevus and melanoma mimicking cellular blue nevus. A clinicopathologic study of 10 cases on the spectrum of so-called 'malignant blue nevus.' Am J Surg Pathol 2001; 25: 316–323.

495 Connelly J, Smith JL Jr. Malignant blue nevus. Cancer 1991; 67: 2653–2657.

496 Scott GA, Trepeta R. Clear cell sarcoma of tendons and aponeuroses and malignant blue nevus arising in prepubescent children: report of two cases and review of the literature. Am J Dermatopathol 1993; 15: 139–145.

497 Kopf AW, Bart RS. Malignant Blue (Ota's?) nevus. J Dermatol Surg Oncol 1982; 8: 442–445.

498 Gartmann H, Lischka G. Maligner blauer naevus (Malignes dermales Melanozytom). Hautarzt 1972; 23: 175–178.

499 Kwittken J, Negri L. Malignant blue nevus. Case report of a negro woman. Arch Dermatol 1966; 94: 64–69.

500 Kuhn A, Groth W, Gartmann H, Steigleder GK. Malignant blue nevus with metastases to the lung. Am J Dermatopathol 1988; 10: 436–441.

501 Calista D, Schianchi S, Landi C. Malignant blue nevus of the scalp. Int J Dermatol 1998; 37: 126–127.

502 Spatz A, Zimmermann U, Bachollet B et al. Malignant blue nevus of the vulva with late ovarian metastasis. Am J Dermatopathol 1998; 20: 408–412.

503 Harvell JD, White WL. Persistent and recurrent blue nevi. Am J Dermatopathol 1999; 21: 506–517.

504 Pich A, Chiusa L, Margaria E, Aloi F. Proliferative activity in the malignant cellular blue nevus. Hum Pathol 1993; 24: 1323–1329.

505 Böni R, Panizzon R, Huch Böni RA et al. Malignant blue naevus with distant subcutaneous metastasis. Clin Exp Dermatol 1996; 21: 427–430.

506 Bautista NC, Cohen S, Anders KH. Benign melanocytic nevus cells in axillary lymph nodes. Am J Clin Pathol 1994; 102: 102–108.

507 Carson KF, Wen D-R, Li P-X et al. Nodal nevi and cutaneous melanomas. Am J Surg Pathol 1996; 20: 834–840.

508 Lambert WC, Brodkin RH. Nodal and subcutaneous cellular blue nevi. A pseudometastasizing pseudomelanoma. Arch Dermatol 1984; 120: 367–370.

509 Lamovec J. Blue nevus of the lymph node capsule. Report of a new case with review of the literature. Am J Clin Pathol 1984; 81: 367–372.

510 Levene A. Disseminated dermal melanocytosis terminating in melanoma. Br J Dermatol 1979; 101: 197–205.

511 Vélez A, Fuente C, Belinchón I et al. Congenital segmental dermal melanocytosis in an adult. Arch Dermatol 1992; 128: 521–525.

512 Tuthill RJ, Clark WH Jr, Levene A. Pilar neurocristic hamartoma. Its relationship to blue nevus and equine melanotic disease. Arch Dermatol 1982; 118: 592–596.

513 Misago N. The relationship between melanocytes and peripheral nerve sheath cells (Part II): blue nevus with peripheral nerve sheath differentiation. Am J Dermatopathol 2000; 22: 230–236.

514 Mizushima J, Nogita T, Higaki Y et al. Dormant melanocytes in the dermis: do dermal melanocytes of acquired dermal melanocytosis exist from birth? Br J Dermatol 1998; 139: 349–350.

515 Buka R, Mauch J, Phelps R, Rudikoff D. Acquired dermal melanocytosis in an African-American: a case report. J Am Acad Dermatol 2000; 43: 934–936.

516 Hidano A, Kaneko K. Acquired dermal melanocytosis of the face and extremities. Br J Dermatol 1991; 124: 96–99.

517 Jimenez E, Valle P, Villegas C et al. Unusual acquired dermal melanocytosis. J Am Acad Dermatol 1994; 30: 277–278.

518 Hasegawa Y, Yasuhara M. Phakomatosis pigmentovascularis type IVa. Arch Dermatol 1985; 121: 651–655.

519 Murakami F, Baba T, Mizoguchi M. Ultraviolet-induced generalized acquired dermal melanocytosis with numerous melanophages. Br J Dermatol 2000; 142: 184–186.

520 Ruiz-Maldonado R, Tamayo L, Laterza AM. Phacomatis pigmentovascularis: a new syndrome? Report of four cases. Pediatr Dermatol 1987; 4: 189–196.

521 Libow LF. Phakomatosis pigmentovascularis type IIIb. J Am Acad Dermatol 1993; 29: 305–307.

522 Larralde de Luna M, Barquin MA, Casas JG, Sidelsky S. Phacomatosis pigmentovascularis with a selective IgA deficiency. Pediatr Dermatol 1995; 12: 159–163.

523 Gilliam AC, Ragge NK, Perez MI, Bolognia JL. Phakomatosis pigmentovascularis type IIb with iris mammillations. Arch Dermatol 1993; 129: 340–342.

524 Mahroughan M, Mehregan AH, Mehregan DA. Phakomatosis pigmentovascularis: report of a case. Pediatr Dermatol 1996; 13: 36–38.

525 Huang C-Y, Lee P-Y. Phakomatosis pigmentovascularis IIb with renal anomaly. Clin Exp Dermatol 2000; 25: 51–54.

526 Hermes B, Cremer B, Happle R, Henz BM. Phacomatosis pigmentokeratotica: a patient with the rare melanocytic-epidermal twin nevus syndrome. Dermatology 1997; 194: 77–79.

527 Tsuruta D, Fukai K, Seto M et al. Phakomatosis pigmentovascularis type IIIb associated with Moyamoya disease. Pediatr Dermatol 1999; 16: 35–38.

528 Langenbach N, Hohenleutner U, Landthaler M. Phacomatosis pigmentokeratotica: speckled-lentiginous nevus in association with nevus sebaceus. Dermatology 1998; 197: 377–380.

529 Tadini G, Restano L, Gonzáles-Pérez R et al. Phacomatosis pigmentokeratotica. Report of new cases and further delineation of the syndrome. Arch Dermatol 1998; 134: 333–337.

530 Mandt N, Blume-Peytavi U, Pfrommer C et al. Phakomatosis pigmentovascularis type IIa. J Am Acad Dermatol 1999; 40: 318–321.

531 Ono I, Tateshita T. Phacomatosis pigmentovascularis type IIa successfully treated with two types of laser therapy. Br J Dermatol 2000; 142: 358–361.

532 Di Landro A, Tadini GL, Marchesi L, Cainelli T. Phacomatosis pigmentovascularis: a new case with renal angiomas and some considerations about the classification. Pediatr Dermatol 1999; 16: 25–30.

533 Pearson JP, Weiss SW, Headington JT. Cutaneous malignant melanotic neurocristic tumors arising in neurocristic hamartomas. Am J Surg Pathol 1996; 20: 665–677.

Atypical nevomelanocytic lesions

534 Sagebiel RW. The dysplastic melanocytic nevus. J Am Acad Dermatol 1989; 20: 496–501.

535 Rigel DS, Rivers JK, Kopf AW et al. Dysplastic nevi. Markers for increased risk for melanoma. Cancer 1989; 63: 386–389.

536 Barnhill RL. Current status of the dysplastic melanocytic nevus. J Cutan Pathol 1991; 18: 147–159.

537 Cooke KR, Spears GFS, Elder DE, Greene MH. Dysplastic nevi in a population-based survey. Cancer 1989; 63: 1240–1244.

538 Augustsson A, Stierner U, Suurkülla M, Rosdahl I. Prevalence of common and dysplastic naevi in a Swedish population. Br J Dermatol 1991; 124: 152–156.

539 Hara K, Nitta Y, Ikeya T. Dysplastic nevus syndrome among Japanese. Am J Dermatopathol 1992; 14: 24–31.

540 Barnhill RL, Kiryu H, Sober AJ, Mihm MC Jr. Frequency of dysplastic nevi among nevomelanocytic lesions submitted for histopathologic examination. Time trends over a 37-year period. Arch Dermatol 1990; 126: 463–465.

541 Elder DE, Goldman LI, Goldman SC et al. Dysplastic nevus syndrome. A phenotypic association of sporadic cutaneous melanoma. Cancer 1980; 46: 1787–1794.

542 Clark WH, Reimer RR, Greene M et al. Origin of familial malignant melanomas from heritable melanocytic lesions. 'The B-K mole syndrome'. Arch Dermatol 1978; 114: 732–738.

543 Lynch HT, Frichot BC, Lynch JF. Familial atypical multiple mole-melanoma syndrome. J Med Genet 1978; 15: 352–356.

544 Kopf AW, Friedman RJ, Rigel DS. Atypical mole syndrome. J Am Acad Dermatol 1990; 22: 117–118.

545 Newton JA. Familial melanoma. Clin Exp Dermatol 1993; 18: 5–11.

546 Slade J, Marghoob AA, Salopek TG et al. Atypical mole syndrome: risk factor for cutaneous malignant melanoma and implications for management. J Am Acad Dermatol 1995; 32: 479–494.

547 Kubo M, Kikuchi K, Nashiro K et al. Expression of fibrogenic cytokines in desmoplastic malignant melanoma. Br J Dermatol 1998; 139: 192–197.

548 Murphy GF, Mihm MC Jr. Recognition and evaluation of cytological dysplasia in acquired melanocytic nevi. Hum Pathol 1999; 30: 506–512.

549 Mooi WJ. The dysplastic naevus. J Clin Pathol 1997; 50: 711–715.

550 Cramer SF. To the Editor. Am J Dermatopathol 2001; 23: 160.

551 Ackerman AB. Enough mysticism about dysplastic nevi! Dermatopathology: Practical & Conceptual 2001; 7: 86–88.

552 Greene MH, Clark WH Jr, Tucker MA et al. Acquired precursors of cutaneous malignant melanoma. The familial dysplastic nevus syndrome. N Engl J Med 1985; 312: 91–97.

553 Knoell KA, Hendrix JD Jr, Patterson JW et al. Nonpigmented dysplastic melanocytic nevi. Arch Dermatol 1997; 133: 992–994.

554 Elder DE, Kraemer KH, Greene MH et al. The dysplastic nevus syndrome. Our definition. Am J Dermatopathol 1982; 4: 455–460.

555 Barnes LM, Nordlund JJ. The natural history of dysplastic nevi. A case history illustrating their evolution. Arch Dermatol 1987; 123: 1059–1061.

556 Haley JC, Hood AF, Chuang T-Y, Rasmussen J. The frequency of histologically dysplastic nevi in 199 pediatric patients. Pediatr Dermatol 2000; 17: 266–269.

557 Fernandez M, Raimer SS, Sánchez RL. Dysplastic nevi of the scalp and forehead in children. Pediatr Dermatol 2001; 18: 5–8.

558 Halpern AC, Guerry DP IV, Elder DE et al. Natural history of dysplastic nevi. J Am Acad Dermatol 1993; 29: 51–57.

559 Clark WH Jr. The dysplastic nevus syndrome. Arch Dermatol 1988; 124: 1207–1210.

560 Mehregan AH. Dysplastic nevi: a histopathological investigation. J Cutan Pathol 1988; 15: 276–281.

561 Crijns MB, Bergman W, Berger MJ et al. On naevi and melanomas in dysplastic naevus syndrome patients. Clin Exp Dermatol 1993; 18: 248–252.

562 Kopf AW, Lindsay AC, Rogers GS et al. Relationship of nevocytic nevi to sun exposure in dysplastic nevus syndrome. J Am Acad Dermatol 1985; 12: 656–662.

563 Kopf AW, Gold RS, Rogers GS et al. Relationship of lumbosacral nevocytic nevi to sun exposure in dysplastic nevus syndrome. Arch Dermatol 1986; 122: 1003–1006.

564 Crijns MB, Vink J, Van Hees CLM et al. Dysplastic nevi. Occurrence in first- and second-degree relatives of patients with 'sporadic' dysplastic nevus syndrome. Arch Dermatol 1991; 127: 1346–1351.

565 Weinstock MA, Stryker WS, Stampfer MJ et al. Sunlight and dysplastic nevus risk. Results of a clinic-based case-control study. Cancer 1991; 67: 1701–1706.

566 Abadir MC, Marghoob AA, Slade J et al. Case-control study of melanocytic nevi on the buttocks in atypical mole syndrome: role of solar radiation in the pathogenesis of atypical moles. J Am Acad Dermatol 1995; 33: 31–36.

567 Carli P, Biggeri A, Nardini P et al. Sun exposure and large numbers of common and atypical melanocytic naevi: an analytical study in a southern European population. Br J Dermatol 1998; 138: 422–425.

568 Rampen FHJ, Fleuren BAM, de Boo TM, Lemmens WAJG. Prevalence of common "acquired" nevocytic nevi and dysplastic nevi is not related to ultraviolet exposure. J Am Acad Dermatol 1988; 18: 679–683.

569 Piepkorn MW. Genetic basis of susceptibility to melanoma. J Am Acad Dermatol 1994; 31: 1022–1039.

570 Piepkorn M. Whither the atypical (dysplastic) nevus? Am J Clin Pathol 2001; 115: 177–179.

571 McDonagh AJG, Wright AL, Messenger AG. Dysplastic naevi in association with partial deletion of chromosome 11. Clin Exp Dermatol 1990; 15: 44–45.

572 Park W-S, Vortmeyer AO, Pack S et al. Allelic deletion at chromosome 9p21(p16) and 17p13(p53) in microdissected sporadic dysplastic nevus. Hum Pathol 1998; 29: 127–130.

573 Bataille V, Pinney E, Hungerford JL et al. Five cases of coexistent primary ocular and cutaneous melanoma. Arch Dermatol 1993; 129: 198–201.

574 Tremblay J-F, O'Brien EA, Chauvin PJ. Melanoma in situ of the oral mucosa in an adolescent with dysplastic nevus syndrome. J Am Acad Dermatol 2000; 42: 844–846.

575 Hille ETM, van Duijn E, Gruis NA et al. Excess cancer mortality in six Dutch pedigrees with the familial atypical multiple mole-melanoma syndrome from 1830 to 1994. J Invest Dermatol 1998; 110: 788–792.

576 Adams SJ, Rustin MHA, Robinson TWE, Munro DD. The dysplastic naevus syndrome and endocrine disease. Br Med J 1984; 288: 1790–1791.

577 Greene MH, Tucker MA, Clark WH et al. Hereditary melanoma and the dysplastic nevus syndrome: The risk of cancers other than melanoma. J Am Acad Dermatol 1987; 16: 792–797.

578 National Institutes of Health Consensus Development Conference. Precursors to malignant melanoma, 1983; volume 4, number 9.

579 Marghoob AA, Kopf AW, Rigel DS et al. Risk of cutaneous malignant melanoma in patients with 'classic' atypical-mole syndrome. Arch Dermatol 1994; 130: 993–998.

580 Kang S, Barnhill RL, Mihm MC Jr et al. Melanoma risk in individuals with clinically atypical nevi. Arch Dermatol 1994; 130: 999–1001.

581 Marghoob AA, Slade J, Kopf AW et al. Risk of developing multiple primary cutaneous melanomas in patients with the classic atypical-mole syndome: a case-control study. Br J Dermatol 1996; 135: 704–711.

582 Snels DGCTM, Hille ETM, Gruis NA, Bergman W. Risk of cutaneous malignant melanoma in patients with nonfamilial atypical nevi from a pigmented lesions clinic. J Am Acad Dermatol 1999; 40: 686–693.

583 Carey WP Jr, Thompson CJ, Synnestvedt M et al. Dysplastic nevi as a melanoma risk factor in patients with familial melanoma. Cancer 1994; 74: 3118–3125.

584 Tucker MA, Crutcher WA, Hartge P, Sagebiel RW. Familial and cutaneous features of dysplastic nevi: a case-control study. J Am Acad Dermatol 1993; 28: 558–564.

585 Novakovic B, Clark WH Jr, Fears TR et al. Melanocytic nevi, dysplastic nevi, and malignant melanoma in children from melanoma-prone families. J Am Acad Dermatol 1995; 33: 631–636.

586 Albert LS, Rhodes AR, Sober AJ. Dysplastic melanocytic nevi and cutaneous melanoma: Markers of increased melanoma risk for affected persons and blood relatives. J Am Acad Dermatol 1990; 22: 69–75.

587 Duvic M, Lowe L, Rapini RP et al. Eruptive dysplastic nevi associated with human immunodeficiency virus infection. Arch Dermatol 1989; 125: 397–401.

588 Richert S, Bloom EJ, Flynn K, Seraly MP. Widespread eruptive dermal and atypical melanocytic nevi in association with chronic myelocytic leukemia: case report and review of the literature. J Am Acad Dermatol 1996; 35: 326–329.

589 Barker JNWN, MacDonald DM. Eruptive dysplastic naevi following renal transplantation. Clin Exp Dermatol 1988; 13: 123–125.

590 Sterry W, Christophers E. Quadrant distribution of dysplastic nevus syndrome. Arch Dermatol 1988; 124: 926–929.

591 Cook MG, Fallowfield ME. Dysplastic naevi – an alternative view. Histopathology 1990; 16: 29–35.

592 Elder DE, Clark WH Jr, Elenitsas R et al. The early and intermediate precursor lesions of tumor progression in the melanocytic system: common acquired nevi and atypical (dysplastic) nevi. Semin Diagn Pathol 1993; 10: 18–35.

593 Clemente C, Cochran AJ, Elder DE et al. Histopathologic diagnosis of dysplastic nevi: concordance among pathologists convened by the World Health Organization Melanoma Programme. Hum Pathol 1991; 22: 313–319.

594 Shea CR, Vollmer RT, Prieto VG. Correlating architectural disorder and cytologic atypia in Clark (dysplastic) melanocytic nevi. Hum Pathol 1999; 30: 500–505.

595 Rivers JK, Cockerell CJ, McBride A, Kopf AW. Quantification of histologic features of dysplastic nevi. Am J Dermatopathol 1990; 12: 42–50.

596 Barnhill RL, Roush GC, Duray PH. Correlation of histologic architectural and cytoplasmic features with nuclear atypia in atypical (dysplastic) nevomelanocytic nevi. Hum Pathol 1990; 21: 51–58.

597 Steijlen PM, Bergman W, Hermans J et al. The efficacy of histopathological criteria required for diagnosing dysplastic naevi. Histopathology 1988; 12: 289–300.

598 Sagebiel RW, Banda PW, Schneider JS, Crutcher WA. Age distribution and histologic patterns of dysplastic nevi. J Am Acad Dermatol 1985; 13: 975–982.

599 Kelly JW, Crutcher WA, Sagebiel RW. Clinical diagnosis of dysplastic melanocytic nevi. A clinicopathologic correlation. J Am Acad Dermatol 1986; 14: 1044–1052.

600 Bergman W, Ruiter DJ, Scheffer E, van Vloten WA. Melanocytic atypia in dysplastic nevi. Immunohistochemical and cytophotometrical analysis. Cancer 1988; 61: 1660–1666.

601 Murphy GF, Halpern A. Dysplastic melanocytic nevi. Normal variants or melanoma precursors? Arch Dermatol 1990; 126: 519–522.

602 Ahmed I, Piepkorn MW, Rabkin MS et al. Histopathologic characteristics of dysplastic nevi. Limited association of conventional histologic criteria with melanoma risk group. J Am Acad Dermatol 1990; 22: 727–733.

603 Klein LJ, Barr RJ. Histologic atypia in clinically benign nevi. A prospective study. J Am Acad Dermatol 1990; 22: 275–282.

604 Piepkorn M, Meyer LJ, Goldgar D et al. The dysplastic melanocytic nevus: a prevalent lesion that correlates poorly with clinical phenotype. J Am Acad Dermatol 1989; 20: 407–415.

605 Ackerman AB. What naevus is dysplastic, a syndrome and the commonest precursor of malignant melanoma? A riddle and an answer. Histopathology 1988; 13: 241–256.

606 Clark WH Jr, Ackerman AB. An exchange of views regarding the dysplastic nevus controversy. Semin Dermatol 1989; 8: 229–250.

607 Toussaint S, Kamino H. Dysplastic changes in different types of melanocytic nevi. A unifying concept. J Cutan Pathol 1999; 26: 84–90.

608 Smoller BR, Egbert BM. Dysplastic nevi can be diagnosed and graded reproducibly: a longitudinal study. J Am Acad Dermatol 1992; 27: 399–402.

609 Weinstock MA. Dysplastic nevi revisited. J Am Acad Dermatol 1994; 30: 807–810.

610 Duncan LM, Berwick M, Bruijn JA et al. Histopathologic recognition and grading of dysplastic melanocytic nevi: an interobserver agreement study. J Invest Dermatol 1993; 100: 318S–321S.

611 Weinstock MA, Barnhill RL, Rhodes AR et al. Reliability of the histopathologic diagnosis of melanocytic dysplasia. Arch Dermatol 1997; 133: 953–958.

612 Piepkorn MW, Barnhill RL, Cannon-Albright LA et al. A multiobserver, population-based analysis of histologic dysplasia in melanocytic nevi. J Am Acad Dermatol 1994; 30: 707–714.

613 Duray PH, DerSimonian R, Barnhill R et al. An analysis of interobserver recognition of the histopathologic features of dysplastic nevi from a mixed group of nevomelanocytic lesions. J Am Acad Dermatol 1992; 27: 741–749.

614 Pozo L, Naase M, Cerio R et al. Critical analysis of histologic criteria for grading atypical (dysplastic) melanocytic nevi. Am J Clin Pathol 2001; 115: 194–204.

615 Hastrup N, Clemmensen OJ, Spaun E, Søndergaard K. Dysplastic naevus: histological criteria and their inter-observer reproducibility. Histopathology 1994; 24: 503–509.

616 Roth ME, Grant-Kels JM, Ackerman AB et al. The histopathology of dysplastic nevi. Continued controversy. Am J Dermatopathol 1991; 13: 38–51.

617 Grob JJ, Andrac L, Romano MH et al. Dysplastic naevus in non-familial melanoma. A clinicopathological study of 101 cases. Br J Dermatol 1988; 118: 745–752.

618 Black WC, Hunt WC. Histologic correlations with the clinical diagnosis of dysplastic nevus. Am J Surg Pathol 1990; 14: 44–52.

619 Urso C. Atypical histologic features in melanocytic nevi. Am J Dermatopathol 2000; 22: 391–396.

620 Meyer LJ, Piepkorn M, Goldgar DE et al. Interobserver concordance in discriminating clinical atypia of melanocytic nevi, and correlations with histologic atypia. J Am Acad Dermatol 1996; 34: 618–625.

621 Roush GC, Dubin N, Barnhill RL. Prediction of histologic melanocytic dysplasia from clinical observation. J Am Acad Dermatol 1993; 29: 555–562.

622 Barnhill RL, Roush GC. Correlation of clinical and histopathologic features in clinically atypical melanocytic nevi. Cancer 1991; 67: 3157–3164.

623 McGovern VJ, Shaw HM, Milton GW. Histogenesis of malignant melanoma with an adjacent component of superficial spreading type. Pathology 1985; 17: 251–254.

624 Rhodes AR, Harrist TJ, Day CL et al. Dysplastic melanocytic nevi in 234 primary cutaneous melanomas. J Am Acad Dermatol 1983; 9: 563–574.

625 Duray PH, Ernstoff MS. Dysplastic nevus in histologic contiguity with acquired nonfamilial melanoma. Clinicopathologic experience in a 100-bed hospital. Arch Dermatol 1987; 123: 80–84.

626 Black WC. Residual dysplastic and other nevi in superficial spreading melanoma. Clinical correlations and association with sun damage. Cancer 1988; 62: 163–173.

627 Hastrup N, Østerlind A, Drzewiecki KT, Hou-Jensen K. The presence of dysplastic nevus remnants in malignant melanomas. Am J Dermatopathol 1991; 13: 378–385.

628 Maize JC. Dysplastic melanocytic nevi in histologic association with primary cutaneous melanomas. J Am Acad Dermatol 1984; 10: 831–835.

629 Ackerman AB. Critical commentary on statements in "Precursors to Malignant Melanoma". Am J Dermatopathol (Suppl) 1984; 1: 181–183.

630 Ackerman AB, Ng P. What are the differences between the way melanoma evolves *de novo* and the manner in which it develops in association with a Clark's ("dysplastic") nevus? Dermatopathology: Practical & Conceptual 1999; 5: 256–257.

631 Fallowfield ME, Dodson AR, Cook MG. Nucleolar organizer regions in melanocytic dysplasia and melanoma. Histopathology 1988; 13: 95–99.

632 Fallowfield ME, Cook MG. The value of nucleolar organizer region staining in the differential diagnosis of borderline melanocytic lesions. Histopathology 1989; 14: 299–304.

633 Mackie RM, White SI, Seywright MM, Young H. An assessment of the value of Ag NOR staining in the identification of dysplastic and other borderline melanocytic naevi. Br J Dermatol 1989; 120: 511–516.

634 Howat AJ, Wright AL, Cotton DWK et al. AgNORs in benign, dysplastic, and malignant melanocytic skin lesions. Am J Dermatopathol 1990; 12: 156–161.

635 Sanguenza OP, Hyder DM, Bakke AC, White CR Jr. DNA determination in dysplastic nevi. A comparative study between flow cytometry and image analysis. Am J Dermatopathol 1993; 15: 99–105.

636 Smoller BR, McNutt NS, Hsu A. HMB-45 recognizes stimulated melanocytes. J Cutan Pathol 1989; 16: 49–53.

637 Smoller BR, McNutt NS, Hsu A. HMB-45 staining of dysplastic nevi. Support for a spectrum of progression toward melanoma. Am J Surg Pathol 1989; 13: 680–684.

638 Ahmed I, Piepkorn M, Goldgar DE et al. HMB-45 staining of dysplastic melanocytic nevi in melanoma risk groups. J Cutan Pathol 1991; 18: 257–260.

639 Takahashi H, Yamana K, Maeda K et al. Dysplastic melanocytic nevus. Electron-microscopic observation as a diagnostic tool. Am J Dermatopathol 1987; 9: 189–197.

640 Rhodes AR, Seki Y, Fitzpatrick TB, Stern RS. Melanosomal alterations in dysplastic melanocytic nevi. A quantitative, ultrastructural investigation. Cancer 1988; 61: 358–369.

641 Kossard S, Commens C, Symons M, Doyle J. Lentiginous dysplastic naevi in the elderly: a potential precursor for malignant melanoma. Australas J Dermatol 1991; 32: 27–37.

642 Blessing K. Benign atypical naevi: diagnostic difficulties and continued controversy. Histopathology 1999; 34: 189–198.

Malignant melanocytic lesions

643 Rigel DS. Malignant melanoma: incidence issues and their effect on diagnosis and treatment in the 1990s. Mayo Clin Proc 1997; 72: 367–371.

644 Chuang T-Y, Charles J, Reizner GT et al. Melanoma in Kauai, Hawaii, 1981–1990: the significance of *in situ* melanoma and the incidence trend. Int J Dermatol 1999; 38: 101–107.

645 Hall HI, Miller DR, Rogers JD, Bewerse B. Update on the incidence and mortality from melanoma in the United States. J Am Acad Dermatol 1999; 40: 35–42.

646 van der Rhee HJ, van der Spek-Keijser LMT, van Westering R, Coebergh JWW. Increase in and stabilization of incidence and mortality of primary cutaneous malignant melanoma in western Netherlands, 1980–95. Br J Dermatol 1999; 140: 463–467.

647 Shafir R, Hiss J, Tsur H, Bubis JJ. The thin malignant melanoma: changing patterns of epidemiology and treatment. Cancer 1982; 50: 817–819.

648 van der Spek-Keijser LMT, van der Rhee HJ, Tóth G et al. Site, histological type, and thickness of primary cutaneous malignant melanoma in western Netherlands since 1980. Br J Dermatol 1997; 136: 565–571.

649 MacKie RM. Melanoma and the dermatologist in the third millennium. Arch Dermatol 2000; 136: 71–73.

650 Richert SM, D'Amico F, Rhodes AR. Cutaneous melanoma: Patient surveillance and tumor progression. J Am Acad Dermatol 1998; 39: 571–577.

651 MacLennan R, Green AC, McLeod GRC, Martin NG. Increasing incidence of cutaneous melanoma in Queensland, Australia. J Natl Cancer Inst 1992; 84: 1427–1432.

652 Måsbäck A, Westerdahl J, Ingvar C et al. Cutaneous malignant melanoma in South Sweden 1965, 1975, and 1985. A histopathologic review. Cancer 1994; 73: 1625–1630.

653 Saxe N, Hoffman M, Krige JE et al. Malignant melanoma in Cape Town, South Africa. Br J Dermatol 1998; 138: 998–1002.

654 Rigel DS, Friedman RJ, Kopf AW. The incidence of malignant melanoma in the United States: issues as we approach the 21st century. J Am Acad Dermatol 1996; 34: 839–847.

655 Dennis LK. Analysis of the melanoma epidemic, both apparent and real. Data from the 1973 through 1994 Surveillance, Epidemiology, and End Results Program Registry. Arch Dermatol 1999; 135: 275–280.

656 Swerlick RA, Chen S. The melanoma epidemic. Is increased surveillance the solution or the problem? Arch Dermatol 1996; 132: 881–884.

657 Swerlick RA, Chen S. The melanoma epidemic: more apparent than real? Mayo Clin Proc 1997; 72: 559–564.

658 Czarnecki D, Meehan CJ. Is the incidence of malignant melanoma decreasing in young Australians? J Am Acad Dermatol 2000; 42: 672–674.

659 Kelly JW. Melanoma in the elderly – a neglected public health challenge. Med J Aust 1998; 169: 403–404.

660 Beitner H, Ringborg U, Wennersten G, Lagerlof B. Further evidence for increased light sensitivity in patients with malignant melanoma. Br J Dermatol 1981; 104: 289–294.

661 Beral V, Evans S, Shaw H, Milton G. Cutaneous factors related to the risk of melanoma. Br J Dermatol 1983; 109: 165–172.

662 Katsambas A, Nicolaidou E. Cutaneous malignant melanoma and sun exposure. Recent developments in epidemiology. Arch Dermatol 1996; 132: 444–450.

663 Whiteman DC, Green AC. Melanoma and sun exposure: where are we now? Int J Dermatol 1999; 38: 481–489.

664 Lew RA, Sober AJ, Cook N et al. Sun exposure habits in patients with cutaneous melanoma: a case control study. J Dermatol Surg Oncol 1983; 9: 981–986.

665 Pfahlberg A, Kölmel K-F, Gefeller O. Timing of excessive ultraviolet radiation and melanoma: epidemiology does not support the existence of a critical period of high susceptibility to solar ultraviolet radiation-induced melanoma. Br J Dermatol 2001; 144: 471–475.

666 Autier P. Sunscreen and melanoma revisited. Arch Dermatol 2000; 136: 423.

667 Rogers RS III. Malignant melanoma in the 21st century. Int J Dermatol 2000; 39: 178–179.

668 Marks R. Epidemiology of melanoma. Clin Exp Dermatol 2000; 25: 459–463.

669 Schreiber MM, Moon TE, Bozzo PD. Chronic solar ultraviolet damage associated with malignant melanoma of the skin. J Am Acad Dermatol 1984; 10: 755–759.

670 Kopf AW, Kripke ML, Stern RS. Sun and malignant melanoma. J Am Acad Dermatol 1984; 11: 674–684.

671 Green A, MacLennan R, Youl P, Martin N. Site distribution of cutaneous melanoma in Queensland. Int J Cancer 1993; 53: 232–236.

672 Armstrong BK. Epidemiology of malignant melanoma: intermittent or total accumulated exposure to the sun? J Dermatol Surg Oncol 1988; 14: 835–849.

673 Cario-André M, Pain C, Gall Y et al. Studies on epidermis reconstructed with and without melanocytes: melanocytes prevent sunburn cell formation but not appearance of DNA damaged cells in fair-skinned Caucasians. J Invest Dermatol 2000; 115: 193–199.

674 Wolf P, Schöllnast R, Hofer A et al. Malignant melanoma after psoralen and ultraviolet A (PUVA) therapy. Br J Dermatol 1998; 138: 1100–1101.

675 Stern RS and the PUVA Follow up Study. The risk of melanoma in association with long-term exposure to PUVA. J Am Acad Dermatol 2001; 44: 755–761.

676 Wang SQ, Setlow R, Berwick M et al. Ultraviolet A and melanoma: A review. J Am Acad Dermatol 2001; 44: 837–846.

677 Schneider JS, Moore DH, Sagebiel RW. Risk factors for melanoma incidence in prospective follow-up. The importance of atypical (dysplastic) nevi. Arch Dermatol 1994; 130: 1002–1007.

678 Newton JA, Bataille V, Griffiths K et al. How common is the atypical mole syndrome phenotype in apparently sporadic melanoma? J Am Acad Dermatol 1993; 29: 989–996.

679 Halpern AC, Guerry D, Elder DE et al. Dysplastic nevi as risk markers of sporadic (nonfamilial) melanoma. Arch Dermatol 1991; 127: 995–999.

680 English JSC, Swerdlow AJ, MacKie RM et al. Relation between phenotype and banal melanocytic naevi. Br Med J 1987; 294: 152–154.

681 Rampen FHJ, van der Meeren HLM, Boezeman JBM. Frequency of moles as a key to melanoma incidence? J Am Acad Dermatol 1986; 15: 1200–1203.

682 Evans RD, Kopf AW, Lew RA et al. Risk factors for the development of malignant melanoma – I: Review of case-control studies. J Dermatol Surg Oncol 1988; 14: 393–408.

683 Beitner H, Norell SE, Ringborg U et al. Malignant melanoma: aetiological importance of individual pigmentation and sun exposure. Br J Dermatol 1990; 122: 43–51.

684 Carli P, Massi D, Santucci M et al. Cutaneous melanoma histologically associated with a nevus and melanoma de novo have a different profile of risk: Results from a case-control study. J Am Acad Dermatol 1999; 40: 549–557.

685 Mikkilineni R, Weinstock MA. Is the self-counting of moles a valid method of assessing melanoma risk? Arch Dermatol 2000; 136: 1550–1551.

686 Naldi L, Imberti GL, Parazzini F et al. Pigmentary traits, modalities of sun reaction, history of sunburns, and melanocytic nevi as risk factors for cutaneous malignant melanoma in the Italian population. Cancer 2000; 88: 2703–2710.

687 Greene SL, Thomas JR, Doyle JA. Cowden's disease with associated malignant melanoma. Int J Dermatol 1984; 23: 466–467.

688 Duve S, Rakoski J. Cutaneous melanoma in a patient with neurofibromatosis: a case report and review of the literature. Br J Dermatol 1994; 131: 290–294

689 Stokkel MPM, Kroon BBR, van der Sande JJ, Neering H. Malignant cutaneous melanoma associated with neurofibromatosis in two sisters from a family with familial atypical multiple mole melanoma syndrome. Cancer 1993; 72: 2370–2375.

690 Bataille V, Hiles R, Newton Bishop JA. Retinoblastoma, melanoma and the atypical mole syndrome. Br J Dermatol 1995; 132: 134–138.

691 Albert LS, Sober AJ, Rhodes AR. Cutaneous melanoma and bilateral retinoblastoma. J Am Acad Dermatol 1990; 23: 1001–1004.

692 Blessing K. Malignant melanoma in stasis dermatitis. Histopathology 1997; 30: 135–139.

693 Zvulunov A, Wyatt DT, Laud PW, Esterly NB. Influence of genetic and environmental factors on melanocytic naevi: a lesson from Turner's syndrome. Br J Dermatol 1998; 138: 993–997.

694 Gibbs P, Brady BMR, Gonzalez R, Robinson WA. Nevi and melanoma: lessons from Turner's syndrome. Dermatology 2001; 202: 1–3.

695 Berking C, Brady MS. Cutaneous melanoma in patients with sarcoma. Cancer 1997; 79: 843–848.

696 Schenk M, Severson RK, Pawlish KS. The risk of subsequent primary carcinoma of the pancreas in patients with cutaneous malignant melanoma. Cancer 1998; 82: 1672–1676.

697 Koeppel M-C, Grego F, Andrac L, Berbis P. Primary cutaneous large B-cell lymphoma of the legs and malignant melanoma: coincidence or association? Br J Dermatol 1998; 139: 751–752.

698 Milton GW, Shaw HM, Thompson JF, McCarthy WH. Cutaneous melanoma in childhood: incidence and prognosis. Australas J Dermatol 1997; 38 (Suppl.): S44–S48.

699 Ruiz-Maldonado R, de la Luz Orozsco-Covarrubias M. Malignant melanoma in children. A review. Arch Dermatol 1997; 133: 363–371.

700 McKenna DB, Doherty VR, McLaren KM, Hunter JAA. Malignant melanoma and lymphoproliferative malignancy: is there a shared aetiology? Br J Dermatol 2000; 143: 171–173.

701 Wu SJ, Lambert DR. Melanoma in children and adolescents. Pediatr Dermatol 1997; 14: 87–92.

702 Goggins WB, Finkelstein DM, Tsao H. Evidence for an association between cutaneous melanoma and non-Hodgkin lymphoma. Cancer 2001; 91: 874–880.

703 Todd P, Garioch J, Seywright M et al. Malignant melanoma and systemic mastocytosis – a possible association? Clin Exp Dermatol 1991; 16: 455–457.

704 Buckley C, Thomas V, Crow J et al. Cancer family syndrome associated with multiple malignant melanomas and a malignant fibrous histiocytoma. Br J Dermatol 1992; 126: 83–85.

705 Tindall B, Finlayson R, Mutimer K et al. Malignant melanoma associated with human immunodeficiency virus infection in three homosexual men. J Am Acad Dermatol 1989; 20: 587–591.

706 Rockley PF, Trieff N, Wagner RF Jr, Tyring SK. Nonsunlight risk factors for malignant melanoma Part II: immunity, genetics, and workplace prevention. Int J Dermatol 1994; 33: 462–467.

707 van Ginkel CJW, Sang RTL, Blaauwgeers JLG et al. Multiple primary malignant melanomas in an HIV-positive man. J Am Acad Dermatol 1991; 24: 284–285.

708 Takamiyagi A, Asato T, Nakashima Y, Nonaka S. Association of human papillomavirus type 16 with malignant melanoma. Am J Dermatopathol 1998; 20: 69–73.

709 Higgins EM, Du Vivier AWP. Possible induction of malignant melanoma by sunbed use. Clin Exp Dermatol 1992; 17: 357–359.

710 Setlow RB. Spectral regions contributing to melanoma: a personal view. J Invest Dermatol (Symposium Proceedings) 1999; 4: 46–49.

711 Swerdlow AJ, Weinstock MA. Do tanning lamps cause melanoma? An epidemiologic assessment. J Am Acad Dermatol 1998; 38: 89–98.

712 Cattaruzza MS. Does sunlamp use increase the risk of cutaneous malignant melanoma? Arch Dermatol 2000; 136: 389–390.

713 Burkhart CG, Burkhart CN. Melanoma and insecticides: Is there a connection? J Am Acad Dermatol 2000; 42: 302–303.

714 Lee JY-Y, Kapadia SB, Musgrave RH, Futrell WJ. Neurotropic malignant melanoma occurring in a stable burn scar. J Cutan Pathol 1992; 19: 145–150.

715 Rockley PF, Trieff N, Wagner RF Jr, Tyring SK. Nonsunlight risk factors for malignant melanoma Part I: chemical agents, physical conditions, and occupation. Int J Dermatol 1994; 33: 398–406.

716 Gan BS, Colcleugh RG, Scilley CG, Craig ID. Melanoma arising in a chronic (Marjolin's) ulcer. J Am Acad Dermatol 1995; 32: 1058–1059.

717 Kaskel P, Kind P, Sander S et al. Trauma and melanoma formation: a true association? Br J Dermatol 2000; 143: 749–753.

718 Gefeller O, Hassan K, Wille L. Cutaneous malignant melanoma in women and the role of oral contraceptives. Br J Dermatol 1998; 138: 122–124.

719 Licata AG, Wilson LD, Braverman IM et al. Malignant melanoma and other second cutaneous malignancies in cutaneous T-cell lymphoma. Arch Dermatol 1995; 131: 432–435.

720 Merkle T, Landthaler M, Eckert F, Braun-Falco O. Acral verrucous malignant melanoma in an immunosuppressed patient after kidney transplantation. J Am Acad Dermatol 1991; 24: 505–506.

721 Rampen F. Melanoma and levodopa. J Am Acad Dermatol 1998; 38: 782–783.

722 Pfützner W, Przybilla B. Malignant melanoma and levodopa: Is there a relationship? Two new cases and a review of the literature. J Am Acad Dermatol 1997; 37: 332–336.

723 Kircik L, Armus S, Van den Broek H. Malignant melanoma in a tattoo. Int J Dermatol 1993; 32: 297–298.

724 Grange F, Chompret A, Guilloud-Bataille M et al. Comparison between familial and nonfamilial melanoma in France. Arch Dermatol 1995; 131: 1154–1159.

725 Greene MH, Goldin LR, Clark WH et al. Familial cutaneous malignant melanoma: autosomal dominant trait possibly linked to the Rh locus. Proc Natl Acad Sci USA 1983; 80: 6071–6075.

726 Bale SJ, Dracopoli NC, Tucker MA et al. Mapping the gene for hereditary cutaneous malignant melanoma-dysplastic nevus to chromosome 1p. N Engl J Med 1989; 320: 1367–1372.

727 Greene MH. Genetics of cutaneous melanoma and nevi. Mayo Clin Proc 1997; 72: 467–474.

728 Piepkorn M. The expression of p16^{INK4a}, the product of a tumor suppressor gene for melanoma, is upregulated in human melanocytes by UVB irradiation. J Am Acad Dermatol 2000; 42: 741–745.

729 Funk JO, Schiller PI, Barrett MT et al. p16^{INK4a} expression is frequently decreased and associated with 9p21 loss of heterozygosity in sporadic melanoma. J Cutan Pathol 1998; 25: 291–296.

730 Rees JL, Healy E. Molecular genetic approaches to non-melanoma and melanoma skin cancer. Clin Exp Dermatol 1996; 21: 253–262.

731 Gruis NA, van der Velden PA, Bergman W, Frants RR. Familial melanoma; CDKN2A and beyond. J Invest Dermatol (Symposium Proceedings) 1999; 4: 50–54.

732 MacKie RM, Andrew N, Lanyon WG, Connor JM. *CDKN2A* germline mutations in U.K. patients with familial melanoma and multiple primary melanomas. J Invest Dermatol 1998; 111: 269–272.

733 Piepkorn M. Melanoma genetics: An update with focus on the CDKN2A (p16)/ARF tumor suppressors. J Am Acad Dermatol 2000; 42: 705–722.

734 Newton Bishop JA, Harland M, Bishop DT. The genetics of melanoma: the U.K. experience. Clin Exp Dermatol 1998; 23: 158–161.

735 Bataille V. Genetics of familial and sporadic melanoma. Clin Exp Dermatol 2000; 25: 464–470.

736 Zhu G, Duffy DL, Eldridge A et al. A major quantitative-trait locus for mole density is linked to the familial melanoma gene *CDKN2A*: a maximum-likelihood combined linkage and association analysis in twins and their sibs. Am J Hum Genet 1999; 65: 483–492.

737 Nagore E, Climent J, Planelles MD et al. Analysis of the CDKN2A and CDK4 genes and HLA-DR and HLA-DQ alleles in two Spanish familial melanoma kindreds. Acta Derm Venereol 2000; 80: 440–442.

738 Tsao H, Zhang X, Kwitkiwski K et al. Low prevalence of germline *CDKN2A* and CDK4 mutations in patients with early-onset melanoma. Arch Dermatol 2000; 136: 1118–1122.

739 Wagner SN, Wagner C, Briedigkeit L, Goos M. Homozygous deletion of the p16[INK4a] and the p15[INK4b] tumour suppressor genes in a subset of human sporadic cutaneous malignant melanoma. Br J Dermatol 1998; 138: 13–21.

740 Burden AD, Newell J, Andrew N et al. Genetic and environmental influences in the development of multiple primary melanoma. Arch Dermatol 1999; 135: 261–265.

741 Bastian BC, LeBoit PE, Hamm H et al. Chromosomal gains and losses in primary cutaneous melanomas detected by comparative genomic hybridization. Cancer Research 1998; 58: 2170–2175.

742 Lee CS, Pirdas A, Lee MWK. Immunohistochemical demonstration of the nm23-H1 gene product in human malignant melanoma and Spitz nevi. Pathology 1996; 28: 220–224.

743 Birck A, Ahrenkiel V, Zuethen J et al. Mutation and allelic loss of the *PTEN/MMAC1* gene in primary and metastatic melanoma biopsies. J Invest Dermatol 2000; 114: 277–280.

744 Matsuta M, Imamura Y, Matsuta M et al. Detection of numerical chromosomal aberrations in malignant melanomas using fluorescence in situ hybridization. J Cutan Pathol 1997; 24: 201–205.

745 Wolfe KQ, Southern SA, Herrington CS. Interphase cytogenetic demonstration of chromosome 9 loss in thick melanomas. J Cutan Pathol 1997; 24: 398–402.

746 Basarab T, Picard JK, Simpson E, Russell-Jones R. Melanoma antigen-encoding gene expression in melanocytic naevi and cutaneous malignant melanomas. Br J Dermatol 1998; 140: 106–108.

747 D'Alessandro I, Zitzelsberger H, Hutzler P et al. Numerical aberrations of chromosome 7 detected in 15Φm paraffin-embedded tissue sections of primary cutaneous melanomas by fluorescence in situ hybridization and confocal laser scanning microscopy. J Cutan Pathol 1997; 24: 70–75.

748 Greulich KM, Utikal J, Peter R-U, Krähn G. c-MYC and nodular malignant melanoma. A case report. Cancer 2000; 89: 97–103.

749 Lee JD, Unger ER, Gittenger C et al. Interphase cytogenetic analysis of 1q12 satellite III DNA in melanocytic lesions. Increased aneuploidy with malignant histology. Am J Dermatopathol 2001; 23: 176–180.

750 Rowan A, Bataille V, MacKie R et al. Somatic mutations in the Peutz–Jeghers *(LKB1/STKII)* gene in sporadic malignant melanomas. J Invest Dermatol 1999; 112: 509–511.

751 Clark WH, From L, Bernadino EA, Mihm MC. The histogenesis and biologic behavior of primary human malignant melanomas of the skin. Cancer Res 1969; 29: 705–727.

752 McGovern VJ, Mihm MC, Bailly C et al. The classification of malignant melanoma and its histologic reporting. Cancer 1973; 32: 1446–1457.

753 Green A, MacLennan R, Siskind V. Common acquired naevi and the risk of malignant melanoma. Int J Cancer 1985; 35: 297–300.

754 Kukita A, Ishihara K. Clinical features and distribution of malignant melanoma and pigmented nevi on the soles of the feet in Japan. J Invest Dermatol 1989; 92: 210s–213s.

755 Tajima Y, Nakajima T, Sugano I et al. Malignant melanoma within an intradermal nevus. Am J Dermatopathol 1994; 16: 301–306.

756 Bhawan J. Amelanotic melanoma or poorly differentiated melanoma? J Cutan Pathol 1980; 7: 55–56.

757 Gibson LE, Goellner JR. Amelanotic melanoma: cases studied by Fontana stain, S-100 immunostain, and ultrastructural examination. Mayo Clin Proc 1988; 63: 777–782.

758 Ackerman AB, David KM. A unifying concept of malignant melanoma: biologic aspects. Hum Pathol 1986; 17: 438–440.

759 Flotte TJ, Mihm MC. Melanoma: the art versus the science of dermatopathology. Hum Pathol 1986; 17: 441–442.

760 Weyers W, Euler M, Diaz-Cascajo C et al. Classification of cutaneous malignant melanoma. A reassessment of histopathologic criteria for the distinction of different types. Cancer 1999; 86: 288–299.

761 Sober AJ, Fitzpatrick TB, Mihm MC. Primary melanoma of the skin: recognition and management. J Am Acad Dermatol 1980; 2: 179–197.

762 Su WPD. Malignant melanoma: basic approach to clinicopathologic correlation. Mayo Clin Proc 1997; 72: 267–272.

763 Roth ME, Grant-Kels JM, Kuhn K et al. Melanoma in children. J Am Acad Dermatol 1990; 22: 265–274.

764 Chun K, Vázquez M, Sánchez JL. Malignant melanoma in children. Int J Dermatol 1993; 32: 41–43.

765 Mehregan AH, Mehregan DA. Malignant melanoma in childhood. Cancer 1993; 71: 4096–4103.

766 Richardson SK, Mihm MC, Tannous ZS. Congenital and infantile melanoma: review of the literature and report of an uncommon variant, "equine-type" melanoma. J Cutan Pathol 2000; 27: 570 (abstract).

767 Wagner RF, Nathanson L. Paraneoplastic syndromes, tumor markers, and other unusual features of malignant melanoma. J Am Acad Dermatol 1986; 14: 249–256.

768 Öztürkcan S, Göze F, Atakan N, İçli F. Malignant melanoma in a child. J Am Acad Dermatol 1994; 30: 493–494.

769 Temple WJ, Mulloy RH, Alexander F et al. Childhood melanoma. J Pediatr Surg 1991; 26: 135–137.

770 Saenz NC, Saenz-Badillos J, Busam K et al. Childhood melanoma survival. Cancer 1999; 85: 750–754.

771 Handfield-Jones SE, Smith NP. Malignant melanoma in childhood. Br J Dermatol 1996; 134: 607–616.

772 Eedy DJ. Malignant melanoma in childhood. Br J Dermatol 1997; 136: 137–138.

773 Berg P, Lindelöf B. Differences in malignant melanoma between children and adolescents. A 35-year epidemiological study. Arch Dermatol 1997; 133: 295–297.

774 Egan CA, Bradley RR, Logsdon VK et al. Vulvar melanoma in childhood. Arch Dermatol 1997; 133: 345–348.

775 Polk HC Jr. Surgical progress and understanding in the treatment of the melanoma epidemic. Am J Surg 1999; 178: 443–448.

776 Guibert P, Mollat F, Ligen M, Dreno B. Melanoma screening. Report of a survey in occupational medicine. Arch Dermatol 2000; 136: 199–202.

777 Baade PD, Balanda KP, Stanton WR et al. Community perceptions about the important signs of early melanoma. J Am Acad Dermatol 1997; 36: 33–39.

778 Koch SE, Henneberry JM. Clinically subtle primary cutaneous melanoma. J Am Acad Dermatol 1999; 40: 252–254.

779 Piepkorn M, Odland PB. Quality of care in the diagnosis of melanoma and related melanocytic lesions. Arch Dermatol 1997; 133: 1393–1396.

780 Green J, Ackerman AB. 6mm for diameter in the ABCDs of melanoma? Dermatopathology: Practical & Conceptual 2000; 6: 379–382.

781 Osborne JE, Bourke JF, Graham-Brown RAC, Hutchinson PE. False negative clinical diagnoses of malignant melanoma. Br J Dermatol 1999; 140: 902–908.

782 MacKenzie-Wood AR, Milton GW, de Launey JW. Melanoma: accuracy of clinical diagnosis. Australas J Dermatol 1998; 39: 31–33.

783 Grant-Kels JM, Bason ET, Grin CM. The misdiagnosis of malignant melanoma. J Am Acad Dermatol 1999; 40: 539–548.

784 Morton CA, MacKie RM. Clinical accuracy of the diagnosis of cutaneous malignant melanoma. Br J Dermatol 1998; 138: 283–287.

785 Khorshid SM, Pinney E, Newton Bishop JA. Melanoma excision by general practitioners in North-East Thames region, England. Br J Dermatol 1998; 138: 412–417.

786 Cohen LM. Lentigo maligna and lentigo maligna melanoma. J Am Acad Dermatol 1995; 33: 923–936.

787 Borkovic SP, Schwartz RA. Amelanotic lentigo maligna melanoma manifesting as a dermatitislike plaque. Arch Dermatol 1983; 119: 423–425.

788 Kaufmann R, Nikelski K, Weber L, Sterry W. Amelanotic lentigo maligna melanoma. J Am Acad Dermatol 1995; 32: 339–342.

789 Kelly RI, Cook MG, Mortimer PS. Aggressive amelanotic lentigo maligna. Br J Dermatol 1994; 131: 562–565.

790 Kelly JW. Following lentigo maligna may not prevent the development of life-threatening melanoma. Arch Dermatol 1992; 128: 657–660.

791 Rahbari H, Nabai H, Mehregan AH et al. Amelanotic lentigo maligna melanoma. Diagnostic conundrum – presentation of four new cases. Cancer 1996; 77: 2052–2057.

792 Cliff S, Otter M, Holden CA. Amelanotic lentigo maligna melanoma of the face: a case report and review of the literature. Clin Exp Dermatol 1997; 22: 177–179.

793 Kiene P, Christophers E. From melanotic to amelanotic lentigo maligna: an aggressive variant presenting as an inflammatory lesion. Int J Dermatol 1997; 36: 123–125.

794 Tschen JA, Fordice DB, Reddick M, Stehlin J. Amelanotic melanoma presenting as inflammatory plaques. J Am Acad Dermatol 1992; 27: 464–465.

795 McKenna DB, Cooper EJ, Kavanagh GM et al. Amelanotic malignant melanoma following cryosurgery for atypical lentigo maligna. Clin Exp Dermatol 2000; 25: 600–604.

796 Weinstock MA, Sober AJ. The risk of progression of lentigo maligna to lentigo maligna melanoma. Br J Dermatol 1987; 116: 303–310.

797 Michalik EE, Fitzpatrick TB, Sober AJ. Rapid progression of lentigo maligna to deeply invasive lentigo maligna melanoma. Report of two cases. Arch Dermatol 1983; 119: 831–835.

798 Hill DC, Gramp AA. Surgical treatment of lentigo maligna and lentigo maligna melanoma. Australas J Dermatol 1999; 40: 25–30.

799 Johnson TM, Headington JT, Baker SR, Lowe L. Usefulness of the staged excision for lentigo maligna and lentigo maligna melanoma: The "square" procedure. J Am Acad Dermatol 1997; 37: 758–764.

800 Breuninger H, Schlagenhauff B, Stroebel W et al. Patterns of local horizontal spread of melanomas. Consequences for surgery and histopathologic investigation. Am J Surg Pathol 1999; 23: 1493–1498.

801 Stonecipher MR, Leshin B, Patrick J, White WL. Management of lentigo maligna and lentigo maligna melanoma with paraffin-embedded tangential sections: utility of immunoperoxidase staining and supplemental vertical sections. J Am Acad Dermatol 1993; 29: 589–594.

802 Kuflik EG, Gage AA. Cryosurgery for lentigo maligna. J Am Acad Dermatol 1994; 31: 75–78.

803 Robinson JK. Margin control for lentigo maligna. J Am Acad Dermatol 1994; 31: 79–85.

804 Tsang RW, Liu F-F, Wells W, Payne DG. Lentigo maligna of the head and neck. Results of treatment by radiotherapy. Arch Dermatol 1994; 130: 1008–1012.

805 Mahendran R, Newton-Bishop JA. Survey of U.K. current practice in the treatment of lentigo maligna. Br J Dermatol 2001; 144: 71–76.

806 Schmid-Wendtner MH, Brunner B, Konz B et al. Fractionated radiotherapy of lentigo maligna and lentigo maligna melanoma in 64 patients. J Am Acad Dermatol 2000; 43: 477–482.

807 Böhler-Sommeregger K, Schuller-Petrovic S, Knobler R, Neumann PR. Reactive lentiginous hyperpigmentation after cryosurgery for lentigo maligna. J Am Acad Dermatol 1992; 27: 523–526.

808 Demitsu T, Nagato H, Nishimaki K et al. Melanoma in situ of the penis. J Am Acad Dermatol 2000; 42: 386–388.

809 Holder JE, Colloby PS, Fletcher A, Camp RDR. Amelanotic superficial spreading malignant melanoma mimicking Bowen's disease. Br J Dermatol 1996; 134: 519–521.

810 Kossard S, Commens C. Hypopigmented malignant melanoma simulating vitiligo. J Am Acad Dermatol 1990; 22: 840–842.

811 McGovern VJ, Shaw HM, Milton GW. Prognostic significance of a polypoid configuration in malignant melanoma. Histopathology 1983; 7: 663–672.

812 Plotnick H, Rachmaninoff N, VandenBerg HJ Jr. Polypoid melanoma: a virulent variant of nodular melanoma. J Am Acad Dermatol 1990; 23: 880–884.

813 Kiene P, Petres-Dunsche C, Fölster-Holst R. Pigmented pedunculated malignant melanoma. A rare variant of nodular melanoma. Br J Dermatol 1995; 133: 300–302.

814 Zellman GL. Amelanotic melanoma in a black man. J Am Acad Dermatol 1997; 37: 665–666.

815 Koch SE, Lange JR. Amelanotic melanoma: The great masquerader. J Am Acad Dermatol 2000; 42: 731–734.

816 Arrington JH, Reed RJ, Ichinose H, Krementz ET. Plantar lentiginous melanoma: a distinctive variant of human cutaneous malignant melanoma. Am J Surg Pathol 1977; 1: 131–143.

817 Vazquez M, Ramos FA, Sanchez JL. Melanomas of volar and subungual skin in Puerto Ricans. A clinicopathologic study. J Am Acad Dermatol 1984; 10: 39–45.

818 Patterson RH, Helwig EB. Subungual malignant melanoma: a clinical-pathologic study. Cancer 1980; 46: 2074–2087.

819 Lin C-S, Wang W-J, Wong C-K. Acral melanoma. A clinicopathologic study of 28 patients. Int J Dermatol 1990; 29: 107–112.

820 O'Toole EA, Stephens R, Young MM et al. Subungual melanoma: a relation to direct injury? J Am Acad Dermatol 1995; 33: 525–528.

821 Ishihara Y, Matsumoto K, Kawachi S, Saida T. Detection of early lesions of "ungual" malignant melanoma. Int J Dermatol 1993; 32: 44–47.

822 Levit EK, Kagen MH, Scher RK et al. The ABC rule for clinical detection of subungual melanoma. J Am Acad Dermatol 2000; 42: 269–274.

823 Banfield CC, Redburn JC, Dawber RPR. The incidence and prognosis of nail apparatus melanoma. A retrospective study of 105 patients in four English regions. Br J Dermatol 1998; 139: 276–279.

824 Banfield CC, Dawber RPR. Nail melanoma: a review of the literature with recommendations to improve patient management. Br J Dermatol 1999; 141: 628–632.

825 Thai K-E, Young R, Sinclair RD. Nail apparatus melanoma. Australas J Dermatol 2001; 42: 71–83.

826 Coleman WP, Loria PR, Reed RJ, Krementz ET. Acral lentiginous melanoma. Arch Dermatol 1980; 116: 773–776.

827 Jimbow K, Ikeda S, Takahashi H et al. Biological behavior and natural course of acral malignant melanoma. Am J Dermatopathol (Suppl) 1984; 1: 43–53.

828 Saida T. Malignant melanoma in situ on the sole of the foot. Its clinical and histopathologic characteristics. Am J Dermatopathol 1989; 11: 124–130.

829 Saida T, Yoshida N, Ikegawa S et al. Clinical guidelines for the early detection of plantar malignant melanoma. J Am Acad Dermatol 1990; 23: 37–40.

830 Kato T, Suetake T, Tabata N et al. Epidemiology and prognosis of plantar melanoma in 62 Japanese patients over a 28-year period. Int J Dermatol 1999; 38: 515–519.

831 Chen Y-J, Wu C-Y, Chen J-T et al. Clinicopathologic analysis of malignant melanoma in Taiwan. J Am Acad Dermatol 1999; 41: 945–949.

832 Tomizawa K. Early malignant melanoma manifested as longitudinal melanonychia: subungual melanoma may arise from suprabasal melanocytes. Br J Dermatol 2000; 143: 431–434.

833 Yasuoka N, Ueda M, Ohgami Y et al. Amelanotic acral lentiginous malignant melanoma. Br J Dermatol 1999; 141: 370–372.

834 Kato T, Tabata N, Suetake T, Tagami H. Non-pigmented nodular plantar melanoma in 12 Japanese patients. Br J Dermatol 1997; 136: 207–211.

835 Krementz ET, Reed RJ, Coleman WP et al. Acral lentiginous melanoma. A clinicopathologic entity. Ann Surg 1982; 195: 632–645.

836 Paladugu RR, Winberg CD, Yonemoto RH. Acral lentiginous melanoma. A clinicopathologic study of 36 patients. Cancer 1983; 52: 161–168.

837 Scrivner D, Oxenhandler RW, Lopez M, Perez-Mesa C. Plantar lentiginous melanoma. A clinicopathologic study. Cancer 1987; 60: 2502–2509.

838 Dwyer PK, MacKie RM, Watt DC, Aitchison TC. Plantar malignant melanoma in a white Caucasian population. Br J Dermatol 1993; 128: 115–120.

839 Kuchelmeister C, Schaumburg-Lever G, Garbe C. Acral cutaneous melanoma in caucasians: clinical features, histopathology and prognosis in 112 patients. Br J Dermatol 2000; 143: 275–280.

840 Blessing K, Kernohan NM, Park KGM. Subungual malignant melanoma: clinicopathological features of 100 cases. Histopathology 1991; 19: 425–429.

841 Ronan SG, Eng AM, Briele HA et al. Malignant melanoma of the female genitalia. J Am Acad Dermatol 1990; 22: 428–435.

842 Batsakis JG, Suarez P. Mucosal melanomas: a review. Adv Anat Pathol 2000; 7: 167–180.

843 Kato T, Takematsu H, Tomita Y et al. Malignant melanoma of mucous membranes. A clinicopathologic study of 13 cases in Japanese patients. Arch Dermatol 1987; 123: 216–220.

844 Ragnarsson-Olding BK, Nilsson BR, Kanter-Lewensohn LR et al. Malignant melanoma of the vulva in a nationwide, 25-year study of 219 Swedish females. Predictors of survival. Cancer 1999; 86: 1285–1293.

845 Dunton CJ, Berd D. Vulvar melanoma, biologically different from other cutaneous melanomas. Lancet 1999; 354: 2013–2014.

846 Räber G, Mempel V, Jackisch C et al. Malignant melanoma of the vulva. Report of 89 patients. Cancer 1996; 78: 2353–2358.

847 Rogers RS III, Gibson LE. Mucosal, genital, and unusual clinical variants of melanoma. Mayo Clin Proc 1997; 72: 362–366.

848 Conley J, Lattes R, Orr W. Desmoplastic malignant melanoma. Cancer 1971; 28: 914–936.

849 Reiman HM, Goellner JR, Woods JE, Mixter RC. Desmoplastic melanoma of the head and neck. Cancer 1987; 60: 2269–2274.

850 Jain S, Allen PW. Desmoplastic malignant melanoma and its variants. A study of 45 cases. Am J Dermatopathol 1989; 13: 358–373.

851 Smithers BM, McLeod GR, Little JH. Desmoplastic melanoma: patterns of recurrence. World J Surg 1992; 16: 186–190.

852 Smithers BM, McLeod GR, Little JH. Desmoplastic, neural transforming and neurotropic melanoma: a review of 45 cases. Aust NZ J Surg 1990; 60: 967–972.

853 Sagebiel RW. Who needs zebras? Comments on desmoplastic melanoma. J Am Acad Dermatol 1995; 32: 800–802.

854 Anstey A, McKee P, Wilson Jones E. Desmoplastic malignant melanoma: a clinicopathological study of 25 cases. Br J Dermatol 1993; 129: 359–371.

855 Whitaker DC, Argenyi Z, Smith AC. Desmoplastic malignant melanoma: rare and difficult to diagnose. J Am Acad Dermatol 1992; 26: 704–709.

856 Chan GSW, Choy C, Ng WK, Chan KW. Desmoplastic malignant melanoma on the buttock of an 18-year-old girl. Differentiation from desmoplastic nevus. Am J Dermatopathol 1999; 21: 170–173.

857 Jennings TA, Okby NT, Schroer KR et al. Parotid involvement by desmoplastic melanoma. Histopathology 1996; 29: 165–170.

858 Man D, Weiner LJ, Reiman HM. Desmoplastic malignant melanoma: a case report. Br J Plast Surg 1981; 34: 79–82.

859 Egbert B, Kempson R, Sagebiel R. Desmoplastic malignant melanoma. A clinicohistopathologic study of 25 cases. Cancer 1988; 62: 2033–2041.

860 Skelton HG, Smith KJ, Laskin WB et al. Desmoplastic malignant melanoma. J Am Acad Dermatol 1995; 32: 717–725.

861 Baer SC, Schultz D, Synnesvedt M, Elder DE. Desmoplasia and neurotropism. Prognostic variables in patients with stage I melanoma. Cancer 1995; 76: 2242–2247.

862 Quinn MJ, Crotty KA, Thompson JF et al. Desmoplastic and desmoplastic neurotropic melanoma. Experience with 280 patients. Cancer 1998; 83: 1128–1135.

863 Clark WH, Elder DE, van Horn M. The biologic forms of malignant melanoma. Hum Pathol 1986; 17: 443–450.

864 Ackerman AB. How does primary cutaneous melanoma begin? A point of view. Dermatopathology: Practical & Conceptual 1999; 5: 177.

865 Hunter C, Bernert R, Maillet M. Another point of view. Dermatopathology: Practical & Conceptual 1999; 5: 178–179.

866 Clark WH, Elder DE, Guerry D IV et al. Model for predicting survival in stage I melanoma based on tumor progression. J Natl Cancer Inst 1989; 81: 1893–1904.

867 Guerry DP IV, Synnestvedt M, Elder DE, Schultz D. Lessons from tumor progression: the invasive radial growth phase of melanoma is common, incapable of metastasis, and indolent. J Invest Dermatol 1993; 100: 342S–345S.

868 Marcoval J, Moreno A, Graells J et al. Angiogenesis and malignant melanoma. Angiogenesis is related to the development of vertical (tumorigenic) growth phase. J Cutan Pathol 1997; 24: 212–218.

869 Tóth T, Tóth-Jakatics R, Jimi S et al. Cutaneous malignant melanoma: correlation between neovascularisation and peritumor accumulation of mast cells overexpressing vascular endothelial growth factor. Hum Pathol 2000; 31: 955–960.

870 Nagahama M, Funasaka Y, Fernandez-Frez ML et al. Immunoreactivity of α-melanocyte-stimulating hormone, adrenocorticotrophic hormone and β-endorphin in cutaneous malignant melanoma and benign melanocytic naevi. Br J Dermatol 1998; 138: 981–985.

871 van den Oord JJ. Expression of CD26/dipeptidyl-peptidase IV in benign and malignant pigment-cell lesions of the skin. Br J Dermatol 1998; 138: 615–621.

872 Reed JA, McNutt NS, Bogdany JK, Albino AP. Expression of the mast cell growth factor interleukin-3 in melanocytic lesions correlates with an increased number of mast cells in the perilesional stroma: implications for melanoma progression. J Cutan Pathol 1996; 23: 495–505.

873 Sparrow LE, Eldon MJ, English DR, Heenan PJ. p16 and p21 WAF1 protein expression in melanocytic tumors by immunohistochemistry. Am J Dermatopathol 1998; 20: 255–261.

874 Böni R, Wellmann A, Man Y-G et al. Expression of the proliferation and apoptosis-associated CAS protein in benign and malignant cutaneous melanocytic lesions. Am J Dermatopathol 1999; 21: 125–128.

875 Geertsen RC, Hofbauer GFL, Yue F-Y et al. Higher frequency of selective losses of HLA-A and -B allospecificities in metastasis than in primary melanoma lesions. J Invest Dermatol 1998; 111: 497–502.

876 Kurschat P, Mauch C. Mechanisms of metastasis. Clin Exp Dermatol 2000; 25: 482–489.

877 Schaumburg-Lever G, Lever I, Fehrenbacher B et al. Melanocytes in nevi and melanomas synthesize basement membrane and basement membrane-like material. An immunohistochemical and electron microscopic study including immunoelectron microscopy. J Cutan Pathol 2000; 27: 67–75.

878 Urso C, Giannini A, Bartolini M, Bondi R. Histologic analysis of intraepidermal proliferations of atypical melanocytes. Am J Dermatopathol 1990; 12: 150–155.

879 Flotte TJ. Malignant melanoma in situ. Hum Pathol 1990; 21: 1199–1201.

880 Tron VA, Barnhill RL, Mihm MC Jr. Malignant melanoma in situ: functional considerations of cancer. Hum Pathol 1990; 21: 1202–1205.

881 Clark WH Jr. Malignant melanoma in situ. Hum Pathol 1990; 21: 1197–1198.

882 Kopf AW. What is early melanoma? Am J Dermatopathol 1993; 15: 44–45.

883 Reed RJ. Melanoma *in situ*: images, segments, appellations, and implications. Hum Pathol 1998; 29: 1–3.

884 Ackerman AB. Melanoma *in situ*. Hum Pathol 1998; 29: 1328–1329.

885 Ackerman AB. Melanoma *in situ* and matters that transcend it. Hum Pathol 1998; 29: 4–5.

886 Schmoeckel C. How consistent are dermatopathologists in reading early malignant melanomas and lesions "precursor" to them? An international survey. Am J Dermatopathol (Suppl) 1984; 1: 13–24.

887 Ackerman AB, Borghi S. "Pagetoid melanocytic proliferation" is the latest evasion from a diagnosis of "melanoma in situ". Am J Dermatopathol 1991; 13: 583–604.

888 Stern JB, Haupt HM. Pagetoid melanocytosis: tease or tocsin? Semin Diagn Pathol 1998; 15: 225–229.

889 Ackerman AB. Histopathologists can diagnose malignant melanoma *in situ* correctly and consistently. Am J Dermatopathol (Suppl) 1984; 1: 103–107.

890 Weedon D. A reappraisal of melanoma in situ. J Dermatol Surg Oncol 1982; 8: 774–775.

891 Mihm MC Jr, Murphy GF. Malignant melanoma *in situ*: an oxymoron whose time has come. Hum Pathol 1998; 29: 6–7.

892 National Institutes of Health Consensus Development Conference Statement on Diagnosis and Treatment of Early Melanoma, January 27–29, 1992. Am J Dermatopathol 1993; 15: 34–43.

893 Ackerman AB. A critique of an NIH Consensus Development Conference about "early" melanoma. Am J Dermatopathol 1993; 15: 52–58.

894 Cook MG, Clarke TJ, Humphreys S et al. The evaluation of diagnostic and prognostic criteria and the terminology of thin cutaneous malignant melanoma by the CRC Melanoma Pathology Panel. Histopathology 1996; 28: 497–512.

895 CRC Melanoma Pathology Panel. A nationwide survey of observer variation in the diagnosis of thin cutaneous malignant melanoma including the MIN terminology. J Clin Pathol 1997; 50: 202–205.

896 Perniciaro C. Dermatopathologic variants of malignant melanoma. Mayo Clin Proc 1997; 72: 273–279.

897 MacKie RM. Malignant melanoma: clinical variants and prognostic indicators. Clin Exp Dermatol 2000; 25: 471–475.

898 Ackerman AB. Discordance among expert pathologists in diagnosis of melanocytic neoplasms. Hum Pathol 1996; 27: 1115–1116.

899 Farmer ER, Gonin R, Hanna MP. Discordance in the histopathologic diagnosis of melanoma and melanocytic nevi between expert pathologists. Hum Pathol 1996; 27: 528–531.

900 Cramer SF. Interobserver variability in dermatopathology. Arch Dermatol 1997; 133: 1033–1036.

901 LeBoit PE. The 21st Colloquium of The International Society of Dermatopathology. Symposium on Melanocytic Lesions. Am J Dermatopathol 2001; 23: 244–245.

902 Cerroni L, Kerl H. Tutorial on melanocytic lesions. Am J Dermatopathol 2001; 23: 237–241.

903 Ming ME. The histopathologic misdiagnosis of melanoma: Sources and consequences of "false positives" and "false negatives". J Am Acad Dermatol 2000; 43: 704–706.

904 Okun MR, Edelstein LM, Kasznica J. What criteria reliably distinguish melanoma from benign melanocytic lesions? Histopathology 2000; 37: 464–472.

905 Tan MAL, Ackerman AB. Criteria for histopathologic diagnosis of melanoma, 1947–2000: a critique in historical perspective. Dermatopathology: Practical & Conceptual 2001; 7: 39–53.

906 Clark WH, Mihm MC. Lentigo maligna and lentigo-maligna melanoma. Am J Pathol 1969; 53: 39–67.

907 Acker SM, Nicholson JH, Rust PF, Maize JC. Morphometric discrimination of melanoma in situ of sun-damaged skin from chronically sun-damaged skin. J Am Acad Dermatol 1998; 39: 239–245.

908 Trotter MJ, Tron VA. Dermal vascularity in lentigo maligna. J Pathol 1994; 173: 341–345.

909 Weyers W, Bonczkowitz M, Weyers I et al. Melanoma in situ versus melanocytic hyperplasia in sun-damaged skin. Assessment of the significance of histopathologic criteria for differential diagnosis. Am J Dermatopathol 1996; 18: 560–566.

910 Flotte TJ, Mihm MC Jr. Lentigo maligna and malignant melanoma in situ, lentigo maligna type. Hum Pathol 1999; 30: 533–536.

911 Cohen LM. The starburst giant cell is useful for distinguishing lentigo maligna from photodamaged skin. J Am Acad Dermatol 1996; 35: 962–968.

912 Katz SK, Guitart J. Starburst giant cells in benign nevomelanocytic lesions. J Am Acad Dermatol 1998; 38: 283.

913 Penneys NS. Microinvasive lentigo maligna melanoma. J Am Acad Dermatol 1987; 17: 675–680.

914 Somach SC, Taira JW, Pitha JV, Everett MA. Pigmented lesions in actinically damaged skin. Arch Dermatol 1996; 132: 1297–1302.

915 Stevens G, Cockerell CJ. Avoiding sampling error in the biopsy of pigmented lesions. Arch Dermatol 1996; 132: 1380–1382.

916 Hunter JAA, Zaynoun S, Paterson WD et al. Cellular fine structure in the invasive nodules of different histogenetic types of malignant melanoma. Br J Dermatol 1978; 98: 255–272.

917 Stolz W, Schmoeckel C, Welkovich B, Braun-Falco O. Semiquantitative analysis of histologic criteria in thin malignant melanomas. J Am Acad Dermatol 1989; 20: 1115–1120.

918 Steiner A, Konrad K, Pehamberger H, Wolff K. Verrucous malignant melanoma. Arch Dermatol 1988; 124: 1534–1537.

919 Blessing K, Evans AT, Al-Nafussi A. Verrucous naevoid and keratotic malignant melanoma: a clinico-pathological study of 20 cases. Histopathology 1993; 23: 453–458.

920 Kamino H, Tam ST, Alvarez L. Malignant melanoma with pseudocarcinomatous hyperplasia – an entity that can simulate squamous cell carcinoma. Am J Dermatopathol 1990; 12: 446–451.

921 Hanly AJ, Jorda M, Elgart GW. Cutaneous malignant melanoma associated with extensive pseudoepitheliomatous hyperplasia. Report of a case and discussion of the origin of pseudoepitheliomatous hyperplasia. J Cutan Pathol 2000; 27: 153–156.

922 Duncan LM, Richards LA, Mihm MC Jr. Increased mast cell density in invasive melanoma. J Cutan Pathol 1998; 25: 11–15.

923 Monteagudo C, Jordá E, Carda C et al. Erythrophagocytic tumour cells in melanoma and squamous cell carcinoma of the skin. Histopathology 1997; 31: 367–373.

924 Nogita T, Wong T-Y, Ohara K et al. Atypical melanosis of the foot. Arch Dermatol 1994; 130: 1042–1045.

925 Feibleman CE, Stoll H, Maize JC. Melanomas of the palm, sole, and nailbed: a clinicopathologic study. Cancer 1980; 46: 2492–2504.

926 Ahmed I. The histological spectrum of acral melanomas. J Cutan Pathol 2000: 27: 547 (abstract).

927 Thelmo MC, Sagebiel RW, Treseler PA et al. Evaluation of sentinel lymph node status in spindle cell melanomas. J Am Acad Dermatol 2001; 44: 451–455.

928 Bruijn JA, Mihm MC Jr, Barnhill RL. Desmoplastic melanoma. Histopathology 1992; 20: 197–205.

929 From L, Hanna W, Kahn HJ et al. Origin of the desmoplasia in desmoplastic malignant melanoma. Hum Pathol 1983; 14: 1072–1080.

930 Walsh NMG, Roberts JT, Orr W, Simon GT. Desmoplastic malignant melanoma. A clinicopathologic study of 14 cases. Arch Pathol Lab Med 1988; 112: 922–927.

931 Eng W, Tschen JA. Comparison of S-100 versus hematoxylin and eosin staining for evaluating dermal invasion and peripheral margins by desmoplastic malignant melanoma. Am J Dermatopathol 2000; 22: 26–29.

932 Wharton JM, Carlson JA, Mihm MC Jr. Desmoplastic malignant melanoma: diagnosis of early clinical lesions. Hum Pathol 1999; 30: 537–542.

933 Moreno A, Lamarca J, Martinez R, Guix M. Osteoid and bone formation in desmoplastic malignant melanoma. J Cutan Pathol 1986; 13: 128–134.

934 Grunwald MH, Rothem A. Desmoplastic cartilaginous formation in malignant melanoma. J Cutan Pathol 1987; 14: 255.

935 Vadmal MS, Usmani A, Chang S, Pellegrini AE. Desmoplastic malignant melanoma with bone formation. Am J Dermatopathol 2000; 22: 348 (abstract).

936 Langman G, Mehregan DA, Bhawan J. Proliferation of sweat ducts in a melanocytic neoplasm. Am J Dermatopathol 2001; 23: 268–270.

937 Tuthill RJ, Weinzweig N, Yetman RJ. Desmoplastic melanoma: a clinicopathologic study of ten cases with electron microscopy and immunohistology. J Cutan Pathol 1988; 15: 348.

938 Anstey A, Cerio R, Ramnarain N et al. Desmoplastic malignant melanoma. An immunocytochemical study of 25 cases. Am J Dermatopathol 1994; 16: 4–22.

939 Kanik AB, Yaar M, Bhawan J. p75 nerve growth factor receptor staining helps identify desmoplastic and neurotropic melanoma. J Cutan Pathol 1996; 23: 205–210

940 Skelton HG, Maceira J, Smith KJ et al. HMB45 negative spindle cell malignant melanoma. Am J Dermatopathol 1997; 19: 580–584.

941 Longacre TA, Egbert BM, Rouse RV. Desmoplastic and spindle-cell malignant melanoma. An immunohistochemical study. Am J Surg Pathol 1996; 20: 1489–1500.

942 Prieto VG, Woodruff JM. Expression of HMB45 antigen in spindle cell melanoma. J Cutan Pathol 1997; 24: 580–581.

943 Orosz Z. Melan-A/Mart-1 expression in various melanocytic lesions and in non-melanocytic soft tissue tumours. Histopathology 1999; 34: 517–525.

944 Koch MB, Shih I-M, Weiss SW, Folpe AL. Microphthalmia transcription factor and melanoma cell adhesion molecule expression distinguish desmoplastic/spindle cell melanoma from morphologic mimics. Am J Surg Pathol 2001; 25: 58–64.

945 Miettinen M, Fernandez M, Franssila K et al. Microphthalmia transcription factor in the immunohistochemical diagnosis of metastatic melanoma. Comparison with four other melanoma markers. Am J Surg Pathol 2001; 25: 205–211.

946 Busam KJ, Iversen K, Coplan KC, Jungbluth AA. Analysis of microphthalmia transcription factor expression in normal tissues and tumors, and comparison of its expression with S-100 protein, gp100, and tyrosinase in desmoplastic malignant melanoma. Am J Surg Pathol 2001; 25: 197–204.

947 Granter SR, Weilbaecher KN, Quigley C et al. Microphthalmia transcription factor. Not a sensitive or specific marker for the diagnosis of desmoplastic melanoma and spindle cell (non-desmoplastic) melanoma. Am J Dermatopathol 2001; 23: 185–189.

948 Riccioni L, Di Tommaso L, Collina G. Actin-rich desmoplastic malignant melanoma. Report of three cases. Am J Dermatopathol 1999; 21: 537–541.

949 Al-Alousi S, Carlson JA, Blessing K et al. Expression of basic fibroblast growth factor in desmoplastic melanoma. J Cutan Pathol 1996; 23: 118–125.

950 Iwamoto S, Odland PB, Piepkorn M, Bothwell M. Evidence that the p75 neurotrophin receptor mediates perineural spread of desmoplastic melanoma. J Am Acad Dermatol 1996; 35: 725–731.

951 Prieto VG, Woodruff JM. Expression of basement membrane antigens in spindle cell melanoma. J Cutan Pathol 1998; 25: 297–300.

952 Hoang MP, Bentley R, Selim MA et al. CD34 expression in desmoplastic melanoma. J Cutan Pathol 2000; 27: 560 (abstract).

953 Berry RB, Subbuswamy SG, Hackett MEJ. Desmoplastic malignant melanoma: the first British report. Br J Plast Surg 1982; 35: 324–327.

954 Di Maio SM, Mackay B, Smith JL, Dickersin GR. Neurosarcomatous transformation in malignant melanoma. An ultrastructural study. Cancer 1982; 50: 2345–2354.

955 Kaneishi NK, Cockerell CJ. Histologic differentiation of desmoplastic melanoma from cicatrices. Am J Dermatopathol 1998; 20: 128–134.

956 Reed RJ, Leonard DD. Neurotropic melanoma. A variant of desmoplastic melanoma. Am J Surg Pathol 1979; 3: 301–311.

957 Schadendorf D, Haas N, Worm M et al. Amelanotic malignant melanoma presenting as malignant schwannoma. Br J Dermatol 1993; 129: 609–614.

958 Ackerman AB, Godomski J. Neurotropic malignant melanoma and other neurotropic neoplasms in the skin. Am J Dermatopathol (Suppl) 1984; 1: 63–80.

959 Barnhill RL, Bolognia JL. Neurotropic melanoma with prominent melanization. J Cutan Pathol 1995; 22: 450–459.

960 Kossard S, Doherty E, Murray E. Neurotropic melanoma. A variant of desmoplastic melanoma. Arch Dermatol 1987; 123: 907–912.

961 Reed RJ. Consultation case. Am J Surg Pathol 1978; 2: 215–220.

962 Muhlbauer JE, Margolis RJ, Mihm MC, Reed RJ. Minimal deviation melanoma: a histologic variant of cutaneous malignant melanoma in its vertical growth phase. J Invest Dermatol 1983; 80: 63s–65s.

963 Phillips ME, Margolis RJ, Merot Y et al. The spectrum of minimal deviation melanoma: a clinicopathologic study of 21 cases. Hum Pathol 1986; 17: 796–806.

964 Reed RJ, Webb SV, Clark WH Jr. Minimal deviation melanoma (halo nevus variant). Am J Surg Pathol 1990; 14: 53–68.

965 Reed RJ. Minimal deviation melanoma. Hum Pathol 1990; 21: 1206–1211.

966 Vollmer RT. Minimal deviation melanoma. Hum Pathol 1987; 18: 869–870.

967 Jones RE Jr (Ed). Questions to the Editorial Board and other authorities. Am J Dermatopathol 1988; 10: 163–175.

968 Barnhill RL, Mihm MC Jr. The histopathology of cutaneous malignant melanoma. Semin Diagn Pathol 1993; 10: 47–75.

969 Reed RJ. Dimensionalities: borderline and intermediate melanocytic neoplasia. Hum Pathol 1999; 30: 521–524.

970 Breslow A. Thickness, cross-sectional area and depth of invasion in the prognosis of cutaneous melanoma. Ann Surg 1970; 172: 902–908.

971 Colloby PS, West KP, Fletcher A. Observer variation in the measurement of Breslow depth and Clark's level in thin cutaneous malignant melanoma. J Pathol 1991; 163: 245–250.

972 Day CL, Lew RA, Mihm MC et al. The natural break points for primary tumor thickness in clinical stage I melanoma. N Engl J Med 1981; 305: 1155.

973 Büttner P, Garbe C, Bertz J et al. Primary cutaneous melanoma. Optimized cutoff points of tumor thickness and importance of Clark's level for prognostic classification. Cancer 1995; 75: 2499–2506.

974 Kopf AW, Welkovich B, Frankel RE et al. Thickness of malignant melanoma: global analysis of related factors. J Dermatol Surg Oncol 1987; 13: 345–420.

975 Gruber SB, Barnhill RL, Stenn KS, Roush GC. Nevomelanocytic proliferations in association with cutaneous malignant melanoma: a multivariate analysis. J Am Acad Dermatol 1989; 21: 773–780.

976 Stolz W, Schmoeckel C, Landthaler M, Braun-Falco O. Association of early malignant melanoma with nevocytic nevi. Cancer 1989; 63: 550–555.

977 Sagebiel RW. Melanocytic nevi in histologic association with primary cutaneous melanoma of superficial spreading and nodular types: effect of tumor thickness. J Invest Dermatol 1993; 100: 322S–325S.

978 Harley S, Walsh N. A new look at nevus-associated melanomas. Am J Dermatopathol 1996; 18: 137–141.

979 Hashiro M, Miyamoto T, Sonoda S, Okumura M. Malignant melanoma developing from an intradermal nevus. Dermatology 1998; 196: 425–426.

980 Trau H, Kopf AW, Rigel DS et al. Regression in malignant melanoma. J Am Acad Dermatol 1983; 8: 363–368.

981 McGovern VJ, Shaw HM, Milton GW, Farago GA. Prognostic significance of the histological features of malignant melanoma. Histopathology 1979; 3: 385–393.

982 McGovern VJ, Shaw HM, Milton GW. Prognosis in patients with thin malignant melanoma: influence of regression. Histopathology 1983; 7: 673–680.

983 Day CL, Mihm MC, Sober AJ et al. Prognostic factors for melanoma patients with lesions 0.76–1.69 mm in thickness. An appraisal of 'thin' level IV lesions. Ann Surg 1982; 195: 30–34.

984 Trau H, Rigel DS, Harris MN et al. Metastases of thin melanomas. Cancer 1983; 51: 553–556.

985 Blessing K, McLaren KM. Histological regression in primary cutaneous melanoma: recognition, prevalence and significance. Histopathology 1992; 20: 315–322.

986 McGovern VJ. Spontaneous regression of melanoma. Pathology 1975; 7: 91–99.

987 Flax SH, Skelton HG, Smith KJ, Lupton GP. Nodular melanosis due to epithelial neoplasms. A finding not restricted to regressed melanomas. Am J Dermatopathol 1998; 20: 118–122.

988 Kang S, Barnhill RL, Mihm MC Jr, Sober AJ. Histologic regression in malignant melanoma: an interobserver concordance study. J Cutan Pathol 1993; 20: 126–129.

989 Velez A, Walsh D, Karakousis CP. Treatment of unknown primary melanoma. Cancer 1991; 68: 2579–2581.

990 Chang P, Knapper WH. Metastatic melanoma of unknown primary. Cancer 1982; 49: 1106–1111.

991 Avril MF, Charpentier P, Margulis A, Guillaume JC. Regression of primary melanoma with metastases. Cancer 1992; 69: 1377–1381.

992 Shenoy BV, Ford L III, Benjamin SP. Malignant melanoma primary in lymph node. The case of the missing link. Am J Surg Pathol 1987; 11: 140–146.

993 Bowen GM, Chang AE, Lowe L et al. Solitary melanoma confined to the dermal and/or subcutaneous tissue. Evidence for revisiting the staging classification. J Am Acad Dermatol 2000; 136: 1397–1399.

994 Bhuta S. Electron microscopy in the evaluation of melanocytic tumors. Semin Diagn Pathol 1993; 10: 92–101.

995 Banerjee SS, Harris M. Morphological and immunophenotypic variations in malignant melanoma. Histopathology 2000; 36: 387–402.

996 Banerjee SS, Bishop PW, Nicholson CM, Eyden BP. Malignant melanoma showing smooth muscle differentiation. J Clin Pathol 1996; 49: 950–951.

997 Prieto VG, Kanik A, Salob S, McNutt NS. Primary cutaneous myxoid melanoma: immunohistologic clues to a difficult diagnosis. J Am Acad Dermatol 1994; 30: 335–339.

998 Sarode VR, Joshi K, Ravichandran P, Das R. Myxoid variant of primary cutaneous malignant melanoma. Histopathology 1992; 20: 186–187.

999 Garcia-Caballero T, Fraga M, Antunez JR et al. Myxoid metastatic melanoma. Histopathology 1991; 18: 371–373.

1000 McCluggage WG, Shah V, Toner PG. Primary cutaneous myxoid melanoma. Histopathology 1996; 28: 179–182.

1001 Urso C, Giannotti B, Bondi R. Myxoid melanoma of the skin. Arch Pathol Lab Med 1990; 114: 527–528.

1002 Nottingham JF, Slater DN. Malignant melanoma: a new mimic of colloid adenocarcinoma. Histopathology 1988; 13: 576–578.

1003 Hitchcock MG, White WL. Malicious masquerade: myxoid melanoma. Semin Diagn Pathol 1998; 15: 195–202.

1004 Collina G, Losi L, Taccagni GL, Maiorana A. Myxoid metastases of melanoma: report of three cases and review of the literature. Am J Dermatopathol 1997; 19: 52–57.

1005 Hitchcock MG, McCalmont TH, White WL. Cutaneous melanoma with myxoid features. Twelve cases with differential diagnosis. Am J Surg Pathol 1999; 23: 1506–1513.

1006 Peters MS, Su WPD. Balloon cell malignant melanoma. J Am Acad Dermatol 1985; 13: 351–354.

1007 Aloi FG, Coverlizza S, Pippione M. Balloon cell melanoma: a report of two cases. J Cutan Pathol 1988; 15: 230–233.

1008 Kao GF, Helwig EB, Graham JH. Balloon cell malignant melanoma of the skin. A clinicopathologic study of 34 cases with histochemical, immunohistochemical, and ultrastructural observations. Cancer 1992; 69: 2942–2952.

1009 Macák J, Krc I, Elleder M, Lukás Z. Clear cell melanoma of the skin with regressive changes. Histopathology 1991; 18: 276–277.

1010 Sheibani K, Battifora H. Signet-ring cell melanoma. A rare morphologic variant of malignant melanoma. Am J Surg Pathol 1988; 12: 28–34.

1011 Bonetti F, Colombari R, Zamboni G et al. Signet ring melanoma, S-100 negative. Am J Surg Pathol 1989; 13: 522–526.

1012 Al-Talib RK, Theaker JM. Signet-ring cell melanoma: light microscopic, immunohistochemical and ultrastructural features. Histopathology 1991; 18: 572–575.

1013 Breier F, Feldmann R, Fellenz C et al. Primary invasive signet-ring cell melanoma. J Cutan Pathol 1999; 26: 533–536.

1014 Reichel M, Ackerman AB. Sebocyte-like melanocytes in metastatic melanoma. Dermatopathology: Practical & Conceptual 1996; 2: 51–52.

1015 Bittesini L, Dei Tos AP, Fletcher CDM. Metastatic malignant melanoma showing a rhabdoid phenotype: further evidence of a non-specific histological pattern. Histopathology 1992; 20: 167–170.

1016 Chang ES, Wick MR, Swanson PE, Dehner LP. Metastatic malignant melanoma with "rhabdoid" features. Am J Clin Pathol 1994; 102: 426–431.

1017 Borek BT, McKee PH, Freeman JA et al. Primary malignant melanoma with rhabdoid features: a histologic and immunocytochemical study of three cases. Am J Dermatopathol 1998; 20: 123–127.

1018 Helm KF. Malignant melanoma masquerading as malignant fibrous histiocytoma. Am J Dermatopathol 1997; 19: 473–476.

1019 Lucas DR, Tazelaar HD, Unni KK et al. Osteogenic melanoma: a rare variant of malignant melanoma. Am J Surg Pathol 1993; 17: 400–409.

1020 Pellegrini AE, Scalamogna PA. Malignant melanoma with osteoid formation. Am J Dermatopathol 1990; 12: 607–611.

1021 Cachia AR, Kedziora AM. Subungual malignant melanoma with cartilaginous differentiation. Am J Dermatopathol 1999; 21: 165–169.

1022 Banerjee SS, Coyne JD, Menasce LP et al. Diagnostic lessons of mucosal melanoma with osteocartilaginous differentiation. Histopathology 1998; 33: 255–260.

1023 Denton KJ, Stretch J, Athanasou N. Osteoclast-like giant cells in malignant melanoma. Histopathology 1992; 20: 179–181.

1024 House NS, Fedok F, Maloney ME, Helm KF. Malignant melanoma with clinical and histologic features of Merkel cell carcinoma. J Am Acad Dermatol 1994; 31: 839–842.

1025 Spatz A, Barnhill RL. Small cell melanoma in childhood. Pathology Case Reviews 1999; 4: 103–106.

1026 McNutt NS, Urmacher C, Hakimian J et al. Nevoid malignant melanoma: morphologic patterns and immunohistochemical reactivity. J Cutan Pathol 1995; 22: 502–517.

1027 Schmoeckel C, Castro CE, Braun-Falco O. Nevoid malignant melanoma. Arch Dermatol Res 1985; 277: 362–369.

1028 Wong T-Y, Suster S, Duncan LM, Mihm MC Jr. Nevoid melanoma: a clinicopathological study of seven cases of malignant melanoma mimicking spindle and epithelioid cell nevus and verrucous dermal nevus. Hum Pathol 1995; 26: 171–179.

1029 Wong T-Y, Duncan LM, Mihm MC Jr. Melanoma mimicking dermal and Spitz's nevus ("nevoid" melanoma). Semin Surg Oncol 1993; 9: 188–193.

1030 LeBoit PE, Ming ME. Litigious melanocytic proliferations and how to avoid them. Pathology Case Reviews 1999; 4: 77–86.

1031 Walsh N, Crotty K, Palmer A, McCarthy S. Spitz nevus versus spitzoid malignant melanoma: an evaluation of the current distinguishing histopathologic criteria. Hum Pathol 1998; 29: 1105–1112.

1032 Miyauchi Y, Ackerman AB. Melanomas that simulate Spitz's nevi histopathologically (and vice versa): an exercise in differentiation based on dependable criteria. Dermatopathology: Practical & Conceptual 1999; 5: 113–117.

1033 Kossard S, Wilkinson B. Small cell (naevoid) melanoma: A clinicopathologic study of 131 cases. Australas J Dermatol 1997; 38 (Suppl.): S54–S58.

1034 Zembowicz A, McCusker M, Chiarelli C et al. Morphological analysis of nevoid melanoma. A study of 20 cases with a review of the literature. Am J Dermatopathol 2001; 23: 167–175.

1035 Kossard S, Wilkinson B. Nucleolar organizer regions and image analysis nuclear morphometry of small cell (nevoid) melanoma. J Cutan Pathol 1995; 22: 132–136.

1036 McNutt NS, "Triggered trap": nevoid malignant melanoma. Semin Diagn Pathol 1998; 15: 203–209.

1037 Gonzalez A, West AJ, Pitha JV, Taira JW. Small-diameter invasive melanomas: clinical and pathologic characteristics. J Cutan Pathol 1996; 23: 126–132.

1038 Shaw HM, McCarthy WH. Small-diameter malignant melanoma: a common diagnosis in New South Wales, Australia. J Am Acad Dermatol 1992; 27: 679–682.

1039 Bergman R, Katz I, Lichtig C et al. Malignant melanomas with histologic diameters less than 6 mm. J Am Acad Dermatol 1992; 26: 462–466.

1040 Shaw HM, McCarthy WH. Concerning small-diameter invasive melanoma. J Cutan Pathol 1997; 24: 261.

1041 Banerjee SS, Menasce LP, Eyden BP, Brain AN. Malignant melanoma showing ganglioneuroblastic differentiation. Am J Surg Pathol 1999; 23: 582–588.

1042 Adler MJ, Beckstead J, White CR Jr. Angiomatoid melanoma: a case of metastatic melanoma mimicking a vascular malignancy. Am J Dermatopathol 1997; 19: 606–609.

1043 Baron JA, Monzon F, Galaria N, Murphy GF. Angiomatoid melanoma: a novel pattern of differentiation in invasive periocular desmoplastic malignant melanoma. Hum Pathol 2000; 31: 1520–1522.

1044 King R, Busam K, Rosai J. Metastatic malignant melanoma resembling malignant peripheral nerve sheath tumor. Report of 16 cases. Am J Surg Pathol 1999; 23: 1499–1505.

1045 Diaz-Cascajo C, Hoos A. Histopathologic features of malignant peripheral nerve sheath tumor are not restricted to metastatic malignant melanoma and can be found in primary malignant melanoma also. Am J Surg Pathol 2000; 24: 1438–1439.

1046 Elder DE, Murphy GF. Melanocytic tumors of the skin. Washington: Armed Forces Institute of Pathology, 1991; 184–185.

1047 Crowson AN, Magro CM, Mihm MC Jr. Malignant melanoma with prominent pigment synthesis: "Animal type" melanoma – a clinical and histological study of six cases with a consideration of other melanocytic neoplasms with prominent pigment synthesis. Hum Pathol 1999; 30: 543–550.

1048 Schaeppi H, Hametner R, Metze D et al. Focal suprabasal acantholysis in malignant melanoma – a localized variant of paraneoplastic pemphigus? Am J Dermatopathol 2000; 22: 359 (abstract).

1049 Mooi WJ, Deenik W, Peterse JL, Hogendoorn PCW. Keratin immunoreactivity in melanoma of soft parts (clear cell sarcoma). Histopathology 1995; 27: 61–65.

1050 Deenik W, Mooi WJ, Rutgers EJ et al. Clear cell sarcoma (malignant melanoma) of soft parts. A clinicopathologic study of 30 cases. Cancer 1999; 86: 969–975.

1051 d'Amore ESG, Ninfo V. Clear cell tumors of the somatic soft tissues. Semin Diagn Pathol 1997; 14: 270–280.

1052 Wanebo HJ, Woodruff J, Fortner JG. Malignant melanoma of the extremities a clinicopathologic study using levels of invasion (microstage). Cancer 1975; 35: 666–676.

1053 Balch CM, Murad TM, Soong SJ et al. Tumor thickness as a guide to surgical management of clinical stage I melanoma patients. Cancer 1979; 43: 883–888.

1054 Assmann A, Farthmann B, Burkhardt O et al. Cerebriform nodular amelanotic metastases of malignant melanoma: a challenge in differential diagnosis of a rare variant. Br J Dermatol 2000; 142: 533–536.

1055 Cagnoni ML, Graziani MP, Ghersetich I et al. Multiple cutaneous melanoma metastases. Int J Dermatol 1997; 36: 136–138.

1056 Trefzer U, Schwürzer-Voit M, Audring H et al. Multiple melanoma metastases in split-thickness skin graft donor sites. J Am Acad Dermatol 1998; 38: 997–998.

1057 Wong A, Koszyca B, Blumbergs PC et al. Malignant melanoma metastatic to a meningioma. Pathology 1999; 31: 162–165.

1058 Gibbs P, Cebon JS, Calafiore P, Robinson WA. Cardiac metastases from malignant melanoma. Cancer 1999; 85: 78–84.

1059 Amer MH, Al-Sarraf M, Baker LH, Vaitkevicius VK. Malignant melanoma and central nervous system metastases. Incidence, diagnosis, treatment and survival. Cancer 1978; 42: 660–668.

1060 Robert C, Schoenlaub P, Avril M-F et al. Malignant melanoma and granulomatosis. Br J Dermatol 1997; 137: 787–792.

1061 Rodrigues LKE, Leong SPL, Ljung B-M et al. Fine needle aspiration in the diagnosis of metastatic melanoma. J Am Acad Dermatol 2000; 42: 735–740.

1062 Haupt HM, Hood AF, Cohen MH. Inflammatory melanoma. J Am Acad Dermatol 1984; 10: 52–55.

1063 Böni R, Meuli C, Dummer R. Erysipelas melanomatosum. Br J Dermatol 1997; 137: 833–834.

1064 Botev IN. Malignant melanoma in association with inflammatory skin metastasis. J Am Acad Dermatol 1997; 36: 280.

1065 Flórez A, Sánchez-Aguilar D, Peteiro C et al. Inflammatory metastatic melanoma. J Cutan Pathol 1999; 26: 105–108.

1066 Hillen U, Willers C, Goos M. Melanoma erysipeloides: successful treatment by chemoimmunotherapy. Br J Dermatol 2000; 143: 904–906.

1067 Fallowfield ME, Cook MG. Lymphatics in primary cutaneous melanoma. Am J Surg Pathol 1990; 14: 370–374.

1068 Cotton J, Armstrong DJ, Wedig R, Hood AF. Melanoma-in-transit presenting as panniculitis. J Am Acad Dermatol 1998; 39: 876–878.

1069 Nakayama T, Taback B, Turner R et al. Molecular clonality of in-transit melanoma metastasis. Am J Pathol 2001; 158: 1371–1378.

1070 Moreno A, Español I, Romagosa V. Angiotropic malignant melanoma. J Cutan Pathol 1992; 19: 325–329.

1071 Saluja A, Money N, Zivony DI, Solomon AR. Angiotropic malignant melanoma: A rare pattern of local metastases. J Am Acad Dermatol 2001; 44: 829–832.

1072 Siegel DM, McClain SA. Angiotropic malignant melanoma: More common than we think? J Am Acad Dermatol 2001; 44: 870–871.

1073 Barnhill RL, Sagebiel RW, Lugassy C. Angiotropic melanoma: report of seven additional cases. J Cutan Pathol 2000; 27: 548 (abstract).

1074 White WL, Hitchcock MG. Dying dogma: the pathological diagnosis of epidermotropic metastatic malignant melanoma. Semin Diagn Pathol 1998; 15: 176–188.

1075 Yu LL, Heenan PJ. The morphological features of locally recurrent melanoma and cutaneous metastases of melanoma. Hum Pathol 1999; 30: 551–555.

1076 Heenan PJ. Local recurrence of melanoma. Australas J Dermatol 1997; 38 (Suppl): S59–S62.

1077 Schuler G, Honigsmann H, Wolff K. Diffuse melanosis in metastatic melanoma. Further evidence for disseminated single cell metastases. J Am Acad Dermatol 1980; 3: 363–369.

1078 Péc J, Plank L, Mináriková E et al. Generalized melanosis with malignant melanoma metastasizing to skin – a pathological study with S-100 protein and HMB-45. Clin Exp Dermatol 1993; 18: 454–457.

1079 Tsukamoto K, Furue M, Sato Y et al. Generalized melanosis in metastatic malignant melanoma: the possible role of DOPAquinone metabolites. Dermatology 1998; 197: 338–342.

1080 Eide J. Pathogenesis of generalized melanosis with melanuria and melanoptysis secondary to malignant melanoma. Histopathology 1981; 5: 285–294.

1081 Adrian RM, Murphy GF, Sato S et al. Diffuse melanosis secondary to metastatic malignant melanoma. Light and electron microscopic findings. J Am Acad Dermatol 1981; 5: 308–318.

1082 Steiner A, Rappersberger K, Groh V, Pehamberger H. Diffuse melanosis in metastatic malignant melanoma. J Am Acad Dermatol 1991; 24: 625–628.

1083 Murray C, D'Intino Y, MacCormick R et al. Melanosis in association with metastatic malignant melanoma. Report of a case and a unifying concept of pathogenesis. Am J Dermatopathol 1999; 21: 28–30.

1084 Böhm M, Schiller M, Nashan D et al. Diffuse melanosis arising from metastatic melanoma: Pathogenetic function of elevated melanocyte peptide growth factors. J Am Acad Dermatol 2001; 44: 747–754.

1085 Castro MP, VanAuken J, Spencer-Cisek P et al. Acute tumor lysis syndrome associated with concurrent biochemotherapy of metastatic melanoma. A case report and review of the literature. Cancer 1999; 85: 1055–1059.

1086 Kang S, Barnhill RL, Mihm MC Jr, Sober AJ. Multiple primary cutaneous melanomas. Cancer 1992; 70: 1911–1916.

1087 Gupta BK, Piedmonte MR, Karakousis CP. Attributes and survival patterns of multiple primary cutaneous malignant melanoma. Cancer 1991; 67: 1984–1989.

1088 Bhatia S, Estrada-Batres L, Maryon T et al. Second primary tumors in patients with cutaneous malignant melanoma. Cancer 1999; 86: 2014–2020.

1089 Johnson TM, Hamilton T, Lowe L. Multiple primary melanomas. J Am Acad Dermatol 1998; 39: 422–427.

1090 Unger SW, Wanebo HJ, Cooper PH. Multiple cutaneous malignant melanomas with features of primary melanoma. Ann Surg 1981; 193: 245–250.

1091 Bengoechea-Beeby MP, Velasco-Osés A, Mouriño Fernández F et al. Epidermotropic metastatic melanoma. Are the current histologic criteria adequate to differentiate primary from metastatic melanoma? Cancer 1993; 72: 1909–1913.

1092 DiFronzo LA, Wanek LA, Morton DL. Earlier diagnosis of second primary melanoma confirms the benefits of patient education and routine postoperative follow-up. Cancer 2001; 91: 1520–1524.

1093 Grob J-J. Multiple primary melanoma is not a distinct biological entity. Arch Dermatol 1999; 135: 325–327.

1094 Stam-Posthuma JJ, van Duinen C, Scheffer E et al. Multiple primary melanomas. J Am Acad Dermatol 2001; 44: 22–27.

1095 van Duinen SG, Ruiter DJ, Hageman P et al. Immunohistochemical and histochemical tools in the diagnosis of amelanotic melanoma. Cancer 1984; 53: 1566–1573.

1096 van Duinen SG, Ruiter DJ, Scheffer E. A staining procedure for melanin in semithin and ultrathin epoxy sections. Histopathology 1983; 7: 35–48.

1097 Hagen EC, Vennegoor C, Schlingemann RO et al. Correlation of histopathological characteristics with staining patterns in human melanoma assessed by (monoclonal) antibodies reactive on paraffin sections. Histopathology 1986; 10: 689–700.

1098 Thomson W, Mackie RM. Comparison of five antimelanoma antibodies for identification of melanocytic cells on tissue sections in routine dermatopathology. J Am Acad Dermatol 1989; 21: 1280–1284.

1099 Wick MR, Swanson PE, Rocamora A. Recognition of malignant melanoma by monoclonal antibody HMB-45. An immunohistochemical study of 200 paraffin-embedded cutaneous tumors. J Cutan Pathol 1988; 15: 201–207.

1100 Walts AE, Said JW, Shintaku IP. Cytodiagnosis of malignant melanoma. Immunoperoxidase staining with HMB-45 antibody as an aid to diagnosis. Am J Clin Pathol 1988; 90: 77–80.

1101 Fernando SSE, Johnson S, Bate J. Immunohistochemical analysis of cutaneous malignant melanoma: comparison of S-100 protein, HMB-45 monoclonal antibody and NKI/C3 monoclonal antibody. Pathology 1994; 26: 16–19.

1102 Argenyi ZB, Cain C, Bromley C et al. S-100 protein-negative malignant melanoma: fact or fiction? Light-microscopic and immunohistochemical study. Am J Dermatopathol 1994; 16: 233–240.

1103 McNutt NS. The S100 family of multipurpose calcium-binding proteins. J Cutan Pathol 1998; 25: 521–529.

1104 Orchard GE, Calonje E. The effect of melanin bleaching on immunohistochemical staining in heavily pigmented melanocytic neoplasms. Am J Dermatopathol 1998; 20: 357–361.

1105 Smith KJ, Skelton HG, Heimer W et al. Melanocytic activation in HIV-1 disease: HMB-45 staining in common acquired nevi. J Am Acad Dermatol 1993; 29: 539–544.

1106 Lane H, O'Loughlin S, Powell F et al. A quantitative immunohistochemical evaluation of lentigo maligna and pigmented solar keratosis. Am J Clin Pathol 1993; 100: 681–685.

1107 Yates AJ, Banerjee SS, Bishop PW, Graham KE. HMB-45 in non-melanocytic tumours. Histopathology 1993; 23: 477–478.

1108 Ruiter DJ, Bröcker E-B. Immunohistochemistry in the evaluation of melanocytic tumors. Semin Diagn Pathol 1993; 10: 76–91.

1109 Menaker GM, Chiang JK, Tabila B, Moy RL. Rapid HMB-45 staining in Mohs micrographic surgery for melanoma in situ and invasive melanoma. J Am Acad Dermatol 2001; 44: 833–836.

1110 Biesterfeld S, Kusche M, Viereck E, Füzesi L. Limited value of the NK1/C3-antibody for the differential diagnosis of Paget's disease of the nipple and intra-epidermal malignant melanoma. Histopathology 1996; 28: 269–270.

1111 Schaumburg-Lever G, Metzler G, Kaiserling E. Ultrastructural localization of HMB-45 binding sites. J Cutan Pathol 1991; 18: 432–435.

1112 Dhillon AP, Rode J. Patterns of staining of neurone specific enolase in benign and malignant melanocytic lesions of the skin. Diagn Histopathol 1982; 5: 169–174.

1113 Puches R, Smolle J, Rieger E et al. Expression of cytoskeletal components in melanocytic skin lesions. Am J Dermatopathol 1991; 13: 137–144.

1114 Ben-Izhak O, Stark P, Levy R et al. Epithelial markers in malignant melanoma. Am J Dermatopathol 1994; 16: 241–246.

1115 Bishop PW, Menasce LP, Yates AJ et al. An immunophenotypic survey of malignant melanomas. Histopathology 1993; 23: 159–166.

1116 Busam KJ, Chen Y-T, Old LJ et al. Expression of Melan-A (MART1) in benign melanocytic nevi and primary cutaneous malignant melanoma. Am J Surg Pathol 1998; 22: 976–982.

1117 Blessing K, Sanders DSA, Grant JJH. Comparison of immunohistochemical staining of the novel antibody melan-A with S100 protein and HMB-45 in malignant melanoma and melanoma variants. Histopathology 1998; 32: 139–146.

1118 Clarkson KS, Sturdgess IC, Molyneux AJ. The usefulness of tyrosinase in the immunohistochemical assessment of melanocytic lesions: a comparison of the novel T311 antibody (anti-tyrosinase) with S-100, HMB45, and A103 (anti-melan-A). J Clin Pathol 2001; 54: 196–200.

1119 Jungbluth AA, Busam KJ, Gerald WL et al. A103. An anti- Melan-A monoclonal antibody for the detection of malignant melanoma in paraffin-embedded tissues. Am J Surg Pathol 1998; 22: 595–602.

1120 Fetsch PA, Marincola FM, Abati A. The new melanoma markers: MART-1 and Melan-A (the NIH experience). Am J Surg Pathol 1999; 23: 607–613.

1121 Mehregan DR, Hamzavi I. Staining of melanocytic neoplasms by melanoma antigen recognized by T cells. Am J Dermatopathol 2000; 22: 247–250.

1122 King R, Googe PB, Weilbaecher KN et al. Microphthalmia transcription factor expression in cutaneous benign, malignant melanocytic, and nonmelanocytic tumors. Am J Surg Pathol 2001; 25: 51–57.

1123 Temple-Camp CRE, Hainsworth M. The fluorescence of melanocytic lesions. Am J Dermatopathol 1986; 8: 290–294.

1124 Orrell JM, Evans AT, Grant A. A critical evaluation of AgNOR counting in benign naevi and malignant melanoma. J Pathol 1991; 163: 239–244.

1125 Gonzalez AP, Kumar D, Sánchez RL. AgNOR area measurements differentiate benign and malignant melanocytic lesions more accurately than simple counting. Am J Dermatopathol 1994; 16: 372–376.

1126 Di Gregorio C, Losi L, Annessi G, Botticelli A. Nucleolar organizer regions in malignant melanoma and melanocytic nevi. Comparison of two counting methods. Am J Dermatopathol 1991; 13: 329–333.

1127 Leong A S-Y, Gilham P. Silver staining of nucleolar organizer regions in malignant melanoma and melanotic nevi. Hum Pathol 1989; 20: 257–262.

1128 Evans AT, Blessing K, Orrell JM, Grant A. Mitotic indices, anti-PCNA immunostaining, and AgNORS in thick cutaneous melanomas displaying paradoxical behaviour. J Pathol 1992; 168: 15–22.

1129 Ronan SG, Farolan MJ, McDonald A et al. Prognostic significance of nucleolar organizer regions (NORS) in malignant melanoma. J Cutan Pathol 1994; 21: 494–499.

1130 Gambini C, Casazza S, Borgiani L et al. Counting the nucleolar organizer region-associated proteins is a prognostic clue of malignant melanoma. Arch Dermatol 1992; 128: 487–490.

1131 Barzilai A, Goldberg I, Yulash M et al. Silver-stained nucleolar organizer regions (AgNORs) as a prognostic value in malignant melanoma. Am J Dermatopathol 1998; 20: 473–477.

1132 Morales-Ducret CRJ, van de Rijn M, Smoller BR. bcl-2 expression in melanocytic nevi. Arch Dermatol 1995; 131: 915–918.

1133 Saenz-Santamaria MC, Reed JA, McNutt NS, Shea CR. Immunohistochemical expression of BCL-2 in melanomas and intradermal nevi. J Cutan Pathol 1994; 21: 393–397.

1134 Cerroni L, Soyer HP, Kerl H. bcl-2 protein expression in cutaneous malignant melanoma and benign melanocytic nevi. Am J Dermatopathol 1995; 17: 7–11.

1135 Collins KA, White WL. Intercellular adhesion molecule 1 (ICAM-1) and bcl-2 are differentially expressed in early evolving malignant melanoma. Am J Dermatopathol 1995; 17: 429–438.

1136 Miracco C, Santopietro R, Biagioli M et al. Different patterns of cell proliferation and death and oncogene expression in cutaneous malignant melanoma. J Cutan Pathol 1998; 25: 244–251.

1137 Fernández-Figueras M-T, Ariza A, Calatrava A et al. CD44 and melanocytic tumors: a possible role for standard CD44 in the epidermotropic spread of melanoma. J Cutan Pathol 1996; 23: 133–139.

1138 Schaider H, Soyer HP, Heider K-H et al. CD44 and variants in melanocytic skin neoplasms. J Cutan Pathol 1998; 25: 199–203.

1139 Schaider H, Rech-Weichselbraun I, Richtig E et al. Circulating adhesion molecules as prognostic factors for cutaneous melanoma. J Am Acad Dermatol 1997; 36: 209–213.

1140 Harwood CA, Green MA, Cook MG. CD44 expression in melanocytic lesions: a marker of malignant progression? Br J Dermatol 1996; 135: 876–882.

1141 Seelentag WKF, Böni R, Günthert U et al. Expression of CD44 isoforms and β1, 6-branched oligosaccharides in human malignant melanoma is correlated with tumour progression but not with metastatic potential. J Cutan Pathol 1997; 24: 206–211.

1142 Ichikawa T, Masumoto J, Kaneko M et al. Moesin and CD44 expression in cutaneous melanocytic tumours. Br J Dermatol 1998; 138: 763–768.

1143 Leigh CJ, Palechek PL, Knutson JR et al. CD44 expression in benign and malignant nevomelanocytic lesions. Hum Pathol 1996; 27: 1288–1294.

1144 McGregor JM, Yu CC-W, Dublin EA et al. p53 immunoreactivity in human malignant melanoma and dysplastic naevi. Br J Dermatol 1993; 128: 606–611.

1145 Saenz-Santamaria MC, McNutt NS, Bogdany JK, Shea CR. p53 expression is rare in cutaneous melanomas. Am J Dermatopathol 1995; 17: 344–349.

1146 Lee CS, Pirdas A, Lee MWK. p53 in cutaneous melanoma: immunoreactivity and correlation with prognosis. Australas J Dermatol 1995; 36: 192–195.

1147 Essner R, Kuo CT, Wang H et al. Prognostic implications of p53 overexpression in cutaneous melanoma from sun-exposed and nonexposed sites. Cancer 1998; 82: 309–316.

1148 Miracco C, Pacenti L, Santopietro R et al. Evaluation of telomerase activity in cutaneous melanocytic proliferations. Hum Pathol 2000; 31: 1018–1021.

1149 Tran T-A, Ross JS, Carlson JA, Mihm MC Jr. Mitotic cyclins and cyclin-dependent kinases in melanocytic lesions. Hum Pathol 1998; 29: 1085–1090.

1150 Bales ES, Dietrich C, Bandyopadhyay D et al. High levels of expression of $p27^{KIP1}$ and cyclin E in invasive primary malignant melanomas. J Invest Dermatol 1999; 113: 1039–1046.

1151 Georgieva J, Sinha P, Schadendorf D. Expression of cyclins and cyclin dependent kinases in human benign and malignant melanocytic lesions. J Clin Pathol 2001; 54: 229–235.

1152 Grossman D, McNiff JM, Li F, Altieri DC. Expression and targeting of the apoptosis inhibitor, survivin, in human melanoma. J Invest Dermatol 1999; 113: 1076–1081.

1153 Kelley MC, Jones RC, Gupta RK et al. Tumor-associated antigen TA-90 immune complex assay predicts subclinical metastasis and survival for patients with early stage melanoma. Cancer 1998; 83: 1355–1361.

1154 Kelley MC, Gupta RK, Hsueh EC et al. Tumor-associated antigen TA90 immune complex assay predicts recurrence and survival after surgical treatment of stage I–III melanoma. J Clin Oncol 2001; 19: 1176–1182.

1155 Björnhagen V, Bonfoco E, Brahme EM et al. Morphometric, DNA, and proliferating cell nuclear antigen measurements in benign melanocytic lesions and cutaneous malignant melanoma. Am J Dermatopathol 1994; 16: 615–623.

1156 Woosley JT, Dietrich DR. Prognostic significance of PCNA grade in malignant melanoma. J Cutan Pathol 1993; 20: 498–503.

1157 Rieger E, Hofmann-Wellenhof R, Soyer HP et al. Comparison of proliferative activity as assessed by proliferating cell nuclear antigen (PCNA) and Ki-67 monoclonal antibodies in melanocytic skin lesions. A quantitative immunohistochemical study. J Cutan Pathol 1993; 20: 229–236.

1158 Reddy VB, Gattuso P, Aranha G, Carson HJ. Cell proliferation markers in predicting metastases in malignant melanoma. J Cutan Pathol 1995; 22: 248–251.

1159 Soyer HP. Ki 67 immunostaining in melanocytic skin tumors. Correlation with histologic parameters. J Cutan Pathol 1991; 18: 264–272.

1160 Fogt F, Vortmeyer AO, Tahan SR. Nucleolar organizer regions (AgNOR) and Ki-67 immunoreactivity in cutaneous melanocytic lesions. Am J Dermatopathol 1995; 17: 12–17.

1161 Ramsay JA, From L, Iscoe NA, Kahn HJ. MIB-1 proliferative activity is a significant prognostic factor in primary thick cutaneous melanomas. J Invest Dermatol 1995; 105: 22–26.

1162 Vogt T, Zipperer K-H, Vogt A et al. p53-protein and Ki-67-antigen expression are both reliable biomarkers of prognosis in thick stage I nodular melanomas of the skin. Histopathology 1997; 30: 57–63.

1163 Böni R, Doguoglu A, Burg G et al. MIB-1 immunoreactivity correlates with metastatic dissemination in primary thick cutaneous melanoma. J Am Acad Dermatol 1996; 35: 416–418.

1164 Sparrow LE, English DR, Taran JM, Heenan PJ. Prognostic significance of MIB-1 proliferative activity in thin melanomas and immunohistochemical analysis of MIB-1 proliferative activity in melanocytic tumors. Am J Dermatopathol 1998; 20: 12–16.

1165 Talve LAI, Collan YUI, Ekfors TO. Nuclear morphometry, immunohistochemical staining with Ki-67 antibody and mitotic index in the assessment of proliferative activity and prognosis of primary malignant melanomas of the skin. J Cutan Pathol 1996; 23: 335–343.

1166 Moretti S, Spallanzani A, Chiarugi A et al. Correlation of Ki-67 expression in cutaneous primary melanoma with prognosis in a prospective study: Different correlation according to thickness. J Am Acad Dermatol 2001; 44: 188–192.

1167 Henrique R, Azevedo R, Bento MJ et al. Prognostic value of Ki-67 expression in localized cutaneous malignant melanoma. J Am Acad Dermatol 2000; 43: 991–1000.

1168 Rudolph P, Schubert C, Schubert B, Parwaresch R. Proliferation marker Ki-S5 as a diagnostic tool in melanocytic lesions. J Am Acad Dermatol 1997; 37: 169–178.

1169 Li L-XL, Crotty KA, McCarthy SW et al. A zonal comparison of MIB1-Ki67 immunoreactivity in benign and malignant melanocytic lesions. Am J Dermatopathol 2000; 22: 489–495.

1170 Bruijn JA, Berwick M, Mihm MC Jr, Barnhill RL. Common acquired melanocytic nevi, dysplastic melanocytic nevi and malignant melanomas: an image analysis cytometric study. J Cutan Pathol 1993; 20: 121–125.

1171 Stolz W, Vogt T, Landthaler M et al. Differentiation between malignant melanomas and benign melanocytic nevi by computerized DNA cytometry of imprint specimens. J Cutan Pathol 1994; 21: 7–15.

1172 Pilch H, Günzel S, Schäffer U et al. Evaluation of DNA ploidy and degree of DNA abnormality in benign and malignant melanocytic lesions of the skin using video imaging. Cancer 2000; 88: 1370–1377.

1173 Shafir R, Hiss J, Tsur H, Bubis JJ. Pitfalls in frozen section diagnosis of malignant melanoma. Cancer 1983; 51: 1168–1170.

1174 Zitelli JA, Moy RL, Abell E. The reliability of frozen sections in the evaluation of surgical margins for melanoma. J Am Acad Dermatol 1991; 24: 102–106.

1175 Kiehl P, Matthies B, Ehrich K et al. Accuracy of frozen section measurements for the determination of Breslow tumour thickness in primary malignant melanoma. Histopathology 1999; 34: 257–261.

1176 Hofbauer GFL, Kamarashev J, Geertsen R et al. Tyrosinase immunoreactivity in formalin-fixed, paraffin-embedded primary and metastatic melanoma: frequency and distribution. J Cutan Pathol 1998; 25: 204–209.

1177 Huang SKS, Okamoto T, Morton DL, Hoon DSB. Antibody responses to melanoma/melanocyte autoantigens in melanoma patients. J Invest Dermatol 1998; 111: 662–667.

1178 Vetter CS, Straten PT, Terheyden P et al. Expression of CD94/NKG2 subtypes on tumor-infiltrating lymphocytes in primary and metastatic melanoma. J Invest Dermatol 2000; 114: 941–947.

1179 Bono A, Tomatis S, Bartoli C et al. The ABCD system of melanoma detection. A spectrophotometric analysis of the asymmetry, border, color, and dimension. Cancer 1999; 85: 72–77.

1180 Ascierto PA, Palmieri G, Celentano E et al. Sensitivity and specificity of epiluminescence microscopy: evaluation on a sample of 2731 excised cutaneous pigmented lesions. Br J Dermatol 2000; 142: 893–898.

1181 Andreassi L, Perotti R, Rubegni P et al. Digital dermoscopy analysis for the differentiation of atypical nevi and early melanoma. Arch Dermatol 1999; 135: 1459–1465.

1182 Argenziano G, Fabbrocini G, Carli P et al. Clinical and dermatoscopic criteria for the preoperative evaluation of cutaneous melanoma thickness. J Am Acad Dermatol 1999; 40: 61–68.

1183 Menzies SW. Surface microscopy of pigmented skin tumours. Australas J Dermatol 1997; 38 (Suppl): S40–S43.

1184 Argenziano G, Fabbrocini G, Carli P et al. Epiluminesence microscopy: Criteria of cutaneous melanoma progression. J Am Acad Dermatol 1997; 37: 68–74.

1185 Schiffner R, Schiffner-Rohe J, Vogt T et al. Improvement of early recognition of lentigo maligna using dermatoscopy. J Am Acad Dermatol 2000; 42: 25–32.

1186 Braun RP, Meier M-L, Pelloni F et al. Teledermatoscopy in Switzerland: A preliminary evaluation. J Am Acad Dermatol 2000; 42: 770–775.

1187 Binder M, Puespoeck-Schwarz M, Steiner A et al. Epiluminescence microscopy of small pigmented skin lesions: Short-term formal training improves the diagnostic performance of dermatologists. J Am Acad Dermatol 1997; 36: 197–202.

1188 Menzies SW, Ingvar C, Crotty KA, McCarthy WH. Frequency and morphologic characteristics of invasive melanomas lacking specific surface microscopic features. Arch Dermatol 1996; 132: 1178–1182.

1189 Kittler H, Pehamberger H, Wolff K, Binder M. Follow-up of melanocytic skin lesions with digital epiluminescence microscopy: Patterns of modifications observed in early melanoma, atypical nevi, and common nevi. J Am Acad Dermatol 2000; 43: 467–476.

1190 Carli P, de Giorgi V, Massi D, Giannotti B. The role of pattern analysis and the ABCD rule of dermoscopy in the detection of histological atypia in melanocytic naevi. Br J Dermatol 2000; 143: 290–297.

1191 Westerhoff K, McCarthy WH, Menzies SW. Increase in the sensitivity for melanoma diagnosis by primary care physicians using skin surface microscopy. Br J Dermatol 2000; 143: 1016–1020.

1192 Elbaum M, Kopf AW, Rabinovitz HS et al. Automatic differentiation of melanoma from melanocytic nevi with multispectral digital dermoscopy: A feasibility study. J Am Acad Dermatol 2001; 44: 207–218.

1193 Binder M, Kittler H, Steiner A et al. Reevaluation of the ABCD rule for epiluminescence microscopy. J Am Acad Dermatol 1999; 40: 171–176.

1194 Oguchi S, Saida T, Koganehira Y et al. Characteristic epiluminescent microscopic features of early malignant melanoma on glabrous skin. Arch Dermatol 1998; 134: 563–568.

1195 Lorentzen H, Weismann K, Kenet RO et al. Comparison of dermatoscopic ABCD rule and risk stratification in the diagnosis of malignant melanoma. Acta Derm Venereol 2000; 80: 122–126.

1196 Carli P, de Giorgi V, Palli D et al. Preoperative assessment of melanoma thickness by ABCD score of dermatoscopy. J Am Acad Dermatol 2000; 43: 459–466.

1197 Kittler H, Seltenheim M, Dawid M et al. Morphologic changes of pigmented skin lesions: A useful extension of the ABCD rule for dermatoscopy. J Am Acad Dermatol 1999; 40: 558–562.

1198 Lorentzen H, Weismann K, Secher L et al. The dermatoscopic ABCD rule does not improve diagnostic accuracy of malignant melanoma. Acta Derm Venereol 1999; 79: 469–472.

1199 Argenziano G, Fabbrocini G, Carli P et al. Epiluminescence microscopy for the diagnosis of doubtful melanocytic skin lesions. Comparison of the ABCD rule of dermatoscopy and a new 7-point checklist based on pattern analysis. Arch Dermatol 1998; 134: 1563–1570.

1200 Rivers JK, Ho VC. Malignant melanoma. Who shall live and who shall die? Arch Dermatol 1992; 128: 537–542.

1201 Smolle J, Hofmann-Wellenhof R, Kofler R et al. Computer simulations of histologic patterns in melanoma using a cellular automaton provide correlations with prognosis. J Invest Dermatol 1995; 105: 797–801.

1202 Rigel DS, Friedman RJ, Kopf AW, Silverman MK. Factors influencing survival in melanoma. Dermatol Clin 1991; 9: 631–642.

1203 Lemish WM, Heenan PJ, Holman CDJ, Armstrong BK. Survival from preinvasive and invasive malignant melanoma in Western Australia. Cancer 1983; 52: 580–585.

1204 Krige JEJ, Isaacs S, Hudson DA et al. Delay in the diagnosis of cutaneous malignant melanoma. A prospective study in 250 patients. Cancer 1991; 68: 2064–2068.

1205 Herd RM, Cooper EJ, Hunter JAA et al. Cutaneous malignant melanoma. Publicity, screening clinics and survival – the Edinburgh experience 1982–90. Br J Dermatol 1995; 132: 563–570.

1206 Lipsker DM, Hedelin G, Heid E et al. Striking increase of thin melanomas contrasts with stable incidence of thick melanomas. Arch Dermatol 1999; 135: 1451–1456.

1207 Johnson TM, Dolan OM, Hamilton TA et al. Clinical and histologic trends of melanoma. J Am Acad Dermatol 1998; 38: 681–686.

1208 Blois MS, Sagebiel RW, Abarbanel RM et al. Malignant melanoma of the skin. I. The association of tumor depth and type, and patient sex, age, and site with survival. Cancer 1983; 52: 1330–1341.

1209 Heenan PJ, English DR, Holman CDJ, Armstrong BK. Survival among patients with clinical Stage I cutaneous malignant melanoma diagnosed in Western Australia in 1975/1976 and 1980/1981. Cancer 1991; 68: 2079–2087.

1210 van der Esch EP, Cascinelli N, Preda F et al. Stage I melanoma of the skin: evaluation of prognosis according to histologic characteristics. Cancer 1981; 48: 1668–1673.

1211 Prade M, Bognel C, Charpentier P et al. Malignant melanoma of the skin: prognostic factors derived from a multifactorial analysis of 239 cases. Am J Dermatopathol 1982; 4: 411–412.

1212 Smolle J. Biologic significance of tumor thickness. Am J Dermatopathol 1995; 17: 281–286.

1213 Barnhill RL, Fine JA, Roush GC, Berwick M. Predicting five-year outcome for patients with cutaneous melanoma in a population-based study. Cancer 1996; 78: 427–432.

1214 Margolis DJ, Halpern AC, Rebbeck T et al. Validation of a melanoma prognostic model. Arch Dermatol 1998; 134: 1597–1601.

1215 Ronan SG, Eng AM, Briele HA et al. Thin malignant melanomas with regression and metastases. Arch Dermatol 1987; 123: 1326–1330.

1216 Slingluff CL Jr, Seigler HF. "Thin" malignant melanoma: risk factors and clinical management. Ann Plast Surg 1992; 28: 89–94.

1217 Massi D, Franchi A, Borgognoni L et al. Thin cutaneous malignant melanomas (≤1.5 mm). Identification of risk factors indicative of progression. Cancer 1999; 85: 1067–1076.

1218 Kelly JW, Sagebiel RW, Blois MS. Regression in malignant melanoma. A histologic feature without independent prognostic significance. Cancer 1985; 56: 2287–2291.

1219 Cooper PH, Wanebo HJ, Hagar RW. Regression in thin malignant melanoma. Microscopic diagnosis and prognostic importance. Arch Dermatol 1985; 121: 1127–1131.

1220 Wanebo HJ, Cooper PH, Hagar RW. Thin (less than or equal to 1mm) melanomas of the extremities are biologically favourable lesions not influenced by regression. Ann Surg 1985; 201: 499–504.

1221 Shaw HM, McCarthy SW, McCarthy WH et al. Thin regressing malignant melanoma: significance of concurrent regional lymph node metastases. Histopathology 1989; 15: 257–265.

1222 Woods JE, Soule EH, Creagan ET. Metastasis and death in patients with thin melanomas (less than 0.76 mm). Ann Surg 1983; 198: 63–64.

1223 Kelly JW, Sagebiel RW, Clyman S, Blois MS. Thin level IV malignant melanoma. A subset in which level is the major prognostic indicator. Ann Surg 1985; 202: 98–103.

1224 Salman SM, Rogers GS. Prognostic factors in thin cutaneous malignant melanoma. J Dermatol Surg Oncol 1990; 16: 413–418.

1225 Sim FH, Nelson TE, Pritchard DJ. Malignant melanoma: Mayo Clinic experience. Mayo Clin Proc 1997; 72: 565–569.

1226 Taran JM, Heenan PJ. Clinical and histologic features of level 2 cutaneous malignant melanoma associated with metastasis. Cancer 2001; 91: 1822–1825.

1227 Creagan ET. Malignant melanoma: an emerging and preventable medical catastrophe. Mayo Clin Proc 1997; 72: 570–574.

1228 Richard MA, Grob JJ, Avril MF et al. Melanoma and tumor thickness. Challenges of early diagnosis. Arch Dermatol 1999; 135: 269–274.

1229 MacKie RM. Thickness and delay in diagnosis of melanoma. How far can we go? Arch Dermatol 1999; 135: 339–340.

1230 Green MS, Ackerman AB. Thickness is not an accurate gauge of prognosis of primary cutaneous melanoma. Am J Dermatopathol 1993; 15: 461–473.

1231 Vollmer RT, Seigler HF. Using a continuous transformation of the Breslow thickness for prognosis in cutaneous melanoma. Am J Clin Pathol 2001; 115: 205–212.

1232 Osborne JE, Hutchinson PE. Clinical correlates of Breslow thickness of malignant melanoma. Br J Dermatol 2001; 144: 476–483.

1233 Friedman RJ, Rigel DS, Kopf AW et al. Volume of malignant melanoma is superior to thickness as a prognostic indicator. Preliminary observation. Dermatol Clin 1991; 9: 643–648.

1234 Smolle J, Okcu A, Hofmann-Wellenhof R et al. Automated measurement of melanoma cross-sectional area. Am J Dermatopathol 1998; 20: 155–159.

1235 Blessing K, McLaren KM, McLean A, Davidson P. Thick malignant melanomas (>3 mm Breslow) with good clinical outcome: a histological study and survival analysis. Histopathology 1991; 18: 143–148.

1236 Spatz A, Shaw HM, Crotty KA et al. Analysis of histopathological factors associated with prolonged survival of 10 years or more for patients with thick melanomas (>5mm). Histopathology 1998; 33: 406–413.

1237 Park KGM, Blessing K, McLaren KM, Watson ACH. A study of thin (<1.5 mm) malignant melanomas with poor prognosis. Br J Plast Surg 1993; 46: 607–610.

1238 Maize JC. Primary cutaneous malignant melanoma. An analysis of the prognostic value of histologic characteristics. J Am Acad Dermatol 1983; 8: 857–863.

1239 Blois MS, Sagebiel RW, Tuttle MS et al. Judging prognosis in malignant melanoma of the skin. A problem of inference over small data sets. Ann Surg 1983; 198: 200–206.

1240 Vilmer C, Bailly C, Le Doussal V et al. Thin melanomas with unusual aggressive behavior: a report of nine cases. J Am Acad Dermatol 1996; 34: 439–444.

1241 Marghoob AA, Koenig K, Bittencourt FV et al. Breslow thickness and Clark level in melanoma. Support for including level in pathology reports and in American Joint Committee on Cancer Staging. Cancer 2000; 88: 589–595.

1242 Owen SA, Sanders LL, Edwards LJ et al. Identification of higher risk thin melanomas should be based on Breslow depth not Clark level IV. Cancer 2001; 91: 983–991.

1243 Day CL, Lew RA, Harrist TJ. Malignant melanoma prognostic factors 4: Ulceration width. J Dermatol Surg Oncol 1984; 10: 23–24.

1244 McGovern VJ, Shaw HM, Milton GW, McCarthy WH. Ulceration and prognosis in cutaneous malignant melanoma. Histopathology 1982; 6: 399–407.

1245 Kuehnl-Petzoldt C, Wiebelt H, Berger H. Prognostic groups of patients with stage I melanoma. Arch Dermatol 1983; 119: 816–819.

1246 Andersson AP, Gottlieb J, Drzewiecki KT et al. Skin melanoma of the head and neck. Prognostic factors and recurrence-free survival in 512 patients. Cancer 1992; 69: 1153–1156.

1247 Mascaro JM, Castro J, Castel T et al. Why do melanomas ulcerate? J Cutan Pathol 1984; 11: 269–273.

1248 Busam KJ. Lack of relevant information for tumor staging in pathology reports of primary cutaneous melanoma. Am J Clin Pathol 2001; 115: 743–746.

1249 Rogers GS, Kopf AW, Rigel DS et al. Effect of anatomical location on prognosis in patients with clinical stage I melanoma. Arch Dermatol 1983; 119: 644–649.

1250 Ringborg U, Afzelius L-E, Lagerlöf B et al. Cutaneous malignant melanoma of the head and neck. Analysis of treatment results and prognostic factors in 581 patients: a report from the Swedish Melanoma Study Group. Cancer 1993; 71: 751–758.

1251 Garbe C, Büttner P, Bertz J et al. Primary cutaneous melanoma. Prognostic classification of anatomic site. Cancer 1995; 75: 2492–2498.

1252 Rogers GS, Kopf AW, Rigel DS et al. Influence of anatomic location on prognosis of malignant melanoma: attempt to verify the BANS model. J Am Acad Dermatol 1986; 15: 231–237.

1253 Weinstock MA, Morris BT, Lederman JS et al. Effect of BANS location on the prognosis of clinical stage I melanoma: new data and meta-analysis. Br J Dermatol 1988; 119: 559–565.

1254 Wong JH, Wanek L, Chang L-JC et al. The importance of anatomic site in prognosis in patients with cutaneous melanoma. Arch Surg 1991; 126: 486–489.

1255 Hemo Y, Gutman M, Klausner JM. Anatomic site of primary melanoma is associated with depth of invasion. Arch Surg 1999; 134: 148–150.

1256 Hsueh EC, Lucci A, Qi K, Morton DL. Survival of patients with melanoma of the lower extremity decreases with distance from the trunk. Cancer 1999; 85: 383–388.

1257 Day CL, Sober AJ, Kopf AW et al. A prognostic model for clinical stage I melanoma of the trunk. Location near the midline is not an independent risk factor for recurrent disease. Am J Surg 1981; 142: 247–251.

1258 Schmoeckel C, Bockelbrink A, Bockelbrink H, Braun-Falco O. Low- and high-risk malignant melanoma – II. Multivariate analyses for a prognostic classification. Eur J Cancer Clin Oncol 1983; 19: 237–243.

1259 Kopf AW, Gross DF, Rogers GS et al. Prognostic index for malignant melanoma. Cancer 1987; 59: 1236–1241.

1260 Sober AJ, Day CL, Fitzpatrick TB et al. Early death from clinical stage I melanoma. J Invest Dermatol 1983; 80: 50s–52s.

1261 Day CL, Mihm MC, Lew RA et al. Prognostic factors for patients with clinical stage I melanoma of intermediate thickness (1.51–3.39 mm). A conceptual model for tumor growth and metastasis. Ann Surg 1982; 195: 35–43.

1262 Kelly JW, Sagebiel RW, Calderon W et al. The frequency of local recurrence and microsatellites as a guide to reexcision margins for cutaneous malignant melanoma. Ann Surg 1984; 200: 759–763.

1263 León P, Daly JM, Synnestvedt M et al. The prognostic implications of microscopic satellites in patients with clinical stage I melanoma. Arch Surg 1991; 126: 1461–1468.

1264 Harrist TJ, Rigel DS, Day CL et al. "Microscopic satellites" are more highly associated with lymph node metastases than is primary melanoma thickness. Cancer 1984; 53: 2183–2187.

1265 Hacene K, Le Doussal V, Brunet M et al. Prognostic index for clinical stage I cutaneous malignant melanoma. Cancer Res 1983; 43: 2991–2996.

1266 Pastorfide GC, Kibbi A-G, de Roa AL et al. Image analysis of stage I melanoma (1.00–2.50 mm): lymphocytic infiltrates related to metastasis and survival. J Cutan Pathol 1992; 19: 390–397.

1267 Busam KJ, Antonescu CR, Marghoob AA et al. Histologic classification of tumor-infiltrating lymphocytes in primary cutaneous malignant melanoma. A study of interobserver agreement. Am J Clin Pathol 2001; 115: 856–860.

1268 Ridgeway CA, Hieken TJ, Ronan SG et al. Acral lentiginous melanoma. Arch Surg 1995; 130: 88–92.

1269 Sondergaard K. Histological type and biological behavior of primary cutaneous malignant melanoma. 2. An analysis of 86 cases located on so-called acral region as plantar, palmar and sub-/parungual areas. Virchows Arch [A] 1983; 401: 333–343.

1270 McGovern VJ, Shaw HM, Milton GW, Farago GA. Is malignant melanoma arising in a Hutchinson's melanotic freckle a separate disease entity? Histopathology 1980; 4: 235–242.

1271 O'Brien CJ, Coates AS, Petersen-Schaefer K et al. Experience with 998 cutaneous melanomas of the head and neck over 30 years. Am J Surg 1991; 162: 310–314.

1272 Koh HK, Michalik E, Sober AJ et al. Lentigo maligna melanoma has no better prognosis than other types of melanoma. J Clin Oncol 1984; 2: 994–1001.

1273 Popescu NA, Beard CM, Treacy PJ et al. Cutaneous malignant melanoma in Rochester, Minnesota: trends in incidence and survivorship, 1950 through 1985. Mayo Clin Proc 1990; 65: 1293–1302.

1274 Garbe C, Büttner P, Bertz J et al. Primary cutaneous melanoma. Identification of prognostic groups and estimation of individual prognosis for 5093 patients. Cancer 1995; 75: 2484–2491.

1275 Heenan PJ, Jarvis LR, Armstrong BK. Nuclear indices and survival in cutaneous melanoma. Am J Dermatopathol 1989; 11: 308–312.

1276 Sørensen FB, Kristensen IB, Grymer F, Jakobsen A. DNA level, tumor thickness, and stereological estimates of nuclear volume in stage I cutaneous malignant melanomas. Am J Dermatopathol 1991; 13: 11–19.

1277 Mossbacher U, Knollmayer S, Binder M et al. Increased nuclear volume in metastasizing "thick" melanomas. J Invest Dermatol 1996; 106: 437–440.

1278 Binder M, Dolezal I, Wolff K, Pehamberger H. Stereologic examination of volume-weighted mean nuclear volume as a predictor of prognosis in "thin" malignant melanoma. J Invest Dermatol 1992; 99: 180–183.

1279 Karakousis CP, Temple DF, Moore R, Ambrus JL. Prognostic parameters in recurrent malignant melanoma. Cancer 1983; 52: 575–579.

1280 Day CL, Lew RA. Malignant melanoma prognostic factors 5: Clinical staging. J Dermatol Surg Oncol 1984; 10: 351–353.

1281 Balch CM, Murad TM, Soong S-J et al. A multifactorial analysis of melanoma: prognostic histopathological features comparing Clark's and Breslow's staging methods. Ann Surg 1978; 188: 732–742.

1282 Robert ME, Wen D-R, Cochran AJ. Pathological evaluation of the regional lymph nodes in malignant melanoma. Semin Diagn Pathol 1993; 10: 102–115.

1283 Buzzell RA, Zitelli JA. Favorable prognostic factors in recurrent and metastatic melanoma. J Am Acad Dermatol 1996; 34: 798–803.

1284 Lee YTN. Diagnosis, treatment and prognosis of early melanoma. The importance of depth of microinvasion. Ann Surg 1980; 191: 87–97.

1285 Weissmann A, Harris M, Roses D, Dibin N. Prediction of lymph node metastases from the histologic features of primary cutaneous malignant melanomas. Am J Dermatopathol (Suppl) 1984; 1: 35–41.

1286 Mascaro JM, Molgo M, Castel T, Castro J. Plasma cells within the infiltrate of primary cutaneous malignant melanoma of the skin. A confirmation of its histoprognostic value. Am J Dermatopathol 1987; 9: 497–499.

1287 Straume O, Akslen LA. Independent prognostic importance of vascular invasion in nodular melanomas. Cancer 1996; 78: 1211–1219.

1288 Paichitrojjana A. Hemangiolymphatic invasion at the site of a primary cutaneous melanoma is virtually equivalent to metastasis. Dermatopathology: Practical & Conceptual 2001; 7: 21–27.

1289 Emberger M. Implication for prognosis of "vascular invasion" by neoplastic cells of a primary melanoma. Dermatopathology: Practical & Conceptual 2000; 6: 243–244.

1290 Reintgen D, Cruse CW, Wells K et al. The orderly progression of melanoma nodal metastases. Ann Surg 1994; 220: 759–767.

1291 Cochran AJ, Wen D-R, Morton DL. Occult tumor cells in the lymph nodes of patients with pathological stage I malignant melanoma. An immunohistological study. Am J Surg Pathol 1988; 12: 612–618.

292 Battayani Z, Grob JJ, Xerri L et al. Polymerase chain reaction detection of circulating melanocytes as a prognostic marker in patients with melanoma. Arch Dermatol 1995; 131: 443–447.

1293 Dong XD, Tyler D, Johnson JL et al. Analysis of prognosis and disease progression after local recurrence of melanoma. Cancer 2000; 88: 1063–1071.

1294 Hofmann-Wellenhof R, Woltsche-Kahr I, Smolle J, Kerl H. Clinical and histological features of poor prognosis in cutaneous metastatic melanomas. J Cutan Pathol 1996; 23: 199–204.

1295 Ahmed I. Malignant melanoma: prognostic indicators. Mayo Clin Proc 1997; 72: 356–361.

1296 Schmoeckel C, Bockelbrink A, Bockelbrink H et al. Low- and high-risk malignant melanoma – I. Evaluation of clinical and histological prognosticators in 585 cases. Eur J Cancer Clin Oncol 1983; 19: 227–235.

1297 Friedman RJ, Rigel DS, Kopf AW et al. Favorable prognosis for malignant melanomas associated with acquired melanocytic nevi. Arch Dermatol 1983; 119: 455–462.

1298 Ostmeier H, Fuchs B, Otto F et al. Can immunohistochemical markers and mitotic rate improve prognostic precision in patients with primary melanoma? Cancer 1999; 85: 2391–2399.

1299 Zelger B, Hittmair A, Schir M et al. Immunohistochemically demonstrated metallothionein expression in malignant melanoma. Histopathology 1993; 23: 257–264.

1300 Sugita K, Yamamoto O, Asahi M. Immunohistochemical analysis of metallothionein expression in malignant melanoma in Japanese patients. Am J Dermatopathol 2001; 23: 29–35.

1301 Fröhlich E, Schlagenhauff B, Möhrle M et al. Activity, expression, and transcription rate of the cathepsins B, D, H, and L in cutaneous malignant melanoma. Cancer 2001; 91: 972–982.

1302 Bartenjev I, Rudolf Z, Štabuc B et al. Cathepsin D expression in early cutaneous malignant melanoma. Int J Dermatol 2000; 39: 599–602.

1303 Mu XC, Tran TA, Ross JS, Carlson JA. Topoisomerase II-alpha expression in melanocytic nevi and malignant melanoma. J Cutan Pathol 2000; 27: 242–248.

1304 Lynch BJ, Komaromy-Hiller G, Bronstein IB, Holden JA. Expression of DNA topoisomerase I, DNA topoisomerase II-alpha, and p53 in metastatic malignant melanoma. Hum Pathol 1998; 29: 1240–1245.

1305 Golomb C, Wilkel C, Falanga V et al. Distribution of transforming growth factor-β1 in benign and malignant melanocytic neoplasms. J Cutan Pathol 2000; 27: 557 (abstract).

1306 Soubrane C, Mouawad R, Antoine EC et al. A comparative study of Fas and Fas-ligand expression during melanoma progression. Br J Dermatol 2000; 143: 307–312.

1307 Maeda A, Aragane Y, Tezuka T. Expression of CD95 ligand in melanocytic lesions as a diagnostic marker. Br J Dermatol 1998; 139: 198–206.

1308 Lugassy C, Dickersin GR, Christensen L et al. Ultrastructural and immunohistochemical studies of the periendothelial matrix in human melanoma: evidence for an amorphous matrix containing laminin. J Cutan Pathol 1999; 26: 78–83.

1309 Lugassy C, Shahsafaei A, Bonitz P et al. Tumor microvessels in melanoma express the beta-2 chain of laminin. Implications for melanoma metastasis. J Cutan Pathol 1999; 26: 222–226.

1310 Haak-Frendscho M, Darvas Z, Hegyesi H et al. Histidine decarboxylase expression in human melanoma. J Invest Dermatol 2000; 115: 345–352.

1311 Hofmann UB, Westphal JR, van Muijen GNP, Ruiter DJ. Matrix metalloproteinases in human melanoma. J Invest Dermatol 2000; 115: 337–344.

1312 Trotter MJ, Tang L, Tron VA. Overexpression of the cyclin-dependent kinase inhibitor p21 WAF1/CIP1 in human cutaneous malignant melanoma. J Cutan Pathol 1997; 24: 265–271.

1313 Vielkind JR, Huhn K, Tron VA. The Xiphophorus-derived antibody, XMEL, shows sensitivity and specificity for human cutaneous melanoma but is not a prognostic marker. J Cutan Pathol 1997; 24: 620–627.

1314 Massi D, Franchi A, Borgognoni L et al. Osteonectin expression correlates with clinical outcome in thin cutaneous malignant melanomas. Hum Pathol 1999; 30: 339–344.

1315 Cochran AJ, Wen D-R, Berthier-Vergnes O et al. Cytoplasmic accumulation of peanut agglutinin-binding glycoconjugates in the cells of primary melanoma correlates with clinical outcome. Hum Pathol 1999; 30: 556–561.

1316 Hieken TJ, Ronan SG, Farolan M et al. Molecular prognostic markers in intermediate-thickness cutaneous malignant melanoma. Cancer 1999; 85: 375–382.

1317 Schumacher D, Schaumburg-Lever G. Ultrastructural localization of alpha-3 integrin subunit in malignant melanoma and adjacent epidermis. J Cutan Pathol 1999; 26: 321–326.

1318 Van Belle PA, Elenitsas R, Satyamoorthy K et al. Progression-related expression of β3 integrin in melanomas and nevi. Hum Pathol 1999; 33: 562–567.

1319 Fink-Puches R, Smolle J, Hofmann-Wellenhof R, Kerl H. Expression of two morphologic parameters concerning tumor–stroma interaction in benign and malignant melanocytic skin lesions. Am J Dermatopathol 1998; 20: 468–472.

1320 Abraha HD, Fuller LC, Du Vivier AWP et al. Serum S-100 protein: a potentially useful prognostic marker in cutaneous melanoma. Br J Dermatol 1997; 137: 381–385.

1321 Kaskel P, Berking C, Sander S et al. S-100 protein in peripheral blood: A marker for melanoma metastases. A prospective 2-center study of 570 patients with melanoma. J Am Acad Dermatol 1999; 41: 962–969.

1322 Brochez L, Naeyaert J-M. Serological markers for melanoma. Br J Dermatol 2000; 143: 256–268.

1323 Jury CS, McAllister EJ, MacKie RM. Rising levels of serum S100 protein precede other evidence of disease progression in patients with malignant melanoma. Br J Dermatol 2000; 143: 269–274.

1324 Schulz ES, Diepgen TL, von den Driesch P. Clinical and prognostic relevance of serum S-100β protein in malignant melanoma. Br J Dermatol 1998; 138: 426–430.

1325 Shaw HM, McGovern VJ, Milton GW et al. The female superiority in survival in clinical stage II cutaneous malignant melanoma. Cancer 1982; 49: 1941–1944.

1326 Karjalainen S, Hakulinen T. Survival and prognostic factors of patients with skin melanoma. A regression-model analysis based on nationwide cancer registry data. Cancer 1988; 62: 2274–2280.

1327 Stidham KR, Johnson JL, Seigler HF. Survival superiority of females with melanoma. Arch Surg 1994; 129: 316–324.

1328 Miller JG, MacNeil S. Gender and cutaneous melanoma. Br J Dermatol 1997; 136: 657–665.

1329 Vossaert KA, Silverman MK, Kopf AW et al. Influence of gender on survival in patients with stage I malignant melanoma. J Am Acad Dermatol 1992; 26: 429–440.

1330 Shaw HM, McGovern VJ, Milton GW et al. Malignant melanoma: influence of site of lesion and age of patient in the female superiority in survival. Cancer 1980; 46: 2731–2735.

1331 O'Doherty CJ, Prescott RJ, White H et al. Sex differences in presentation of cutaneous malignant melanoma and in survival from Stage I disease. Cancer 1986; 58: 788–792.

1332 Unger JM, Flaherty LE, Liu PY et al. Gender and other survival predictors in patients with metastatic melanoma on Southwest Oncology Group trials. Cancer 2001; 91: 1148–1155.

1333 Schwartz BK, Zashin SJ, Spencer SK et al. Pregnancy and hormonal influences on malignant melanoma. J Dermatol Surg Oncol 1987; 13: 276–281.

1334 Driscoll MS, Grin-Jorgensen CM, Grant-Kels JM. Does pregnancy influence the prognosis of malignant melanoma? J Am Acad Dermatol 1993; 29: 619–630.

1335 Reintgen DS, McCarty KS, Vollmer R et al. Malignant melanoma and pregnancy. Cancer 1985; 55: 1340–1344.

1336 Houghton AN, Flannery J, Viola MV. Malignant melanoma of the skin occurring during pregnancy. Cancer 1981; 48: 407–410.

1337 Martins Ferreira CM, Pineiro Maceira JM, de Oliveira Coelho JMC. Melanoma and pregnancy with placental metastases. Report of a case. Am J Dermatopathol 1998; 20: 403–407.

1338 Travers RL, Sober AJ, Berwick M et al. Increased thickness of pregnancy-associated melanoma. Br J Dermatol 1995; 132: 876–883.

1339 Loggie B, Ronan SG, Bean J, Das Gupta TK. Invasive cutaneous melanoma in elderly patients. Arch Dermatol 1991; 127: 1188–1193.

1340 Helfenstein U, Schüler G, Morf S, Schüler D. Action profiles of predictors of death and survival time in stage I malignant melanoma. Dermatology 1996; 192: 1–7.

1341 Koh HK, Sober AJ, Nakagawa H et al. Malignant melanoma and vitiligo-like leukoderma. An electron microscopic study. J Am Acad Dermatol 1983; 9: 696–708.

1342 Bystryn J-C, Rigel D, Friedman RJ, Kopf A. Prognostic significance of hypopigmentation in malignant melanoma. Arch Dermatol 1987; 123: 1053–1055.

1343 Duhra P, Ilchyshyn A. Prolonged survival in metastatic malignant melanoma associated with vitiligo. Clin Exp Dermatol 1991; 16: 303–305.

1344 Fishman P, Azizi E, Shoenfeld Y et al. Vitiligo autoantibodies are effective against melanoma. Cancer 1993; 72: 2365–2369.

1345 Duncan LM, Deeds J, Cronin FE et al. Melastatin expression and prognosis in cutaneous malignant melanoma. J Clin Oncol 2001; 19: 568–576.

1346 Guffey JM, Chaney JV, Stevens GL et al. Immunohistochemical assessment of tumor vascularity in recurrent Clark II melanomas using antibody to type IV collagen. J Cutan Pathol 1995; 22: 122–127.

1347 Rongioletti F, Miracco C, Gambini C et al. Tumor vascularity as a prognostic indicator in intermediate-thickness (0.76–4 mm) cutaneous melanoma. A quantitative assay. Am J Dermatopathol 1996; 18: 474–477.

1348 Kamino H, Kiryu H, Ratech H. Small malignant melanomas: clinicopathologic correlation and DNA ploidy analysis. J Am Acad Dermatol 1990; 22: 1032–1038.

1349 Drzewiecki KT, Christensen HE, Ladefoged C, Poulsen H. Clinical course of cutaneous malignant melanoma related to histopathological criteria of primary tumour. Scand J Plast Reconstr Surg 1980; 14: 229–234.

1350 McGovern VJ. The classification of melanoma and its relationship with prognosis. Pathology 1970; 2: 85–98.

1351 Lederman JS, Sober AJ. Does biopsy type influence survival in clinical stage I cutaneous melanoma? J Am Acad Dermatol 1985; 13: 983–987.

1352 Rampen FHJ, van der Esch EP. Biopsy and survival of malignant melanoma. J Am Acad Dermatol 1985; 12: 385–388.

1353 Ackerman AB, Scheiner AM. A critique of surgical practice in excisions of primary cutaneous malignant melanoma. Am J Dermatopathol (Suppl) 1984; 1: 109–111.

1354 Urist MM, Balch CM, Soong S-J et al. The influence of surgical margins and prognostic factors predicting the risk of local recurrence in 3445 patients with primary cutaneous melanoma. Cancer 1985; 55: 1398–1402.

1355 Fallowfield ME, Cook MG. Re-excisions of scar in primary cutaneous melanoma: a histopathological study. Br J Dermatol 1992; 126: 47–51.

1356 Heenan PJ, English DR, Holman CDJ, Armstrong BK. The effects of surgical treatment on survival and local recurrence of cutaneous malignant melanoma. Cancer 1992; 69: 421–426.

1357 Månsson-Brahme E, Carstensen J, Erhardt K et al. Prognostic factors in thin cutaneous malignant melanoma. Cancer 1994; 73: 2324–2332.

1358 Day CL, Lew RA. Malignant melanoma prognostic factors 3: Surgical margins. J Dermatol Surg Oncol 1983; 9: 797–801.

1359 Johnson TM, Smith JW II, Nelson BR, Chang A. Current therapy for cutaneous melanoma. J Am Acad Dermatol 1995; 32: 689–707.

1360 Green MS. The changing controversy over surgical resection margins for stage I cutaneous melanoma. Mt Sinai Med J 1991; 58: 341–346.

1361 O'Rourke MGE, Altmann CR. Melanoma recurrence after excision. Is a wide margin justified? Ann Surg 1993; 217: 2–5.

1362 Balch CM, Unst MM, Karakousis CP et al. Efficacy of 2-cm surgical margins for intermediate-thickness melanomas (1 to 4 mm). Ann Surg 1993; 218: 262–269.

1363 Ringborg U, Andersson R, Eldh J et al. Resection margins of 2 versus 5 cm for cutaneous malignant melanoma with a tumor thickness of 0.8 to 2.0 mm. Cancer 1996; 77: 1809–1814.

1364 Zitelli JA, Brown CD, Hanusa BH. Surgical margins for excision of primary cutaneous melanoma. J Am Acad Dermatol 1997; 37: 422–429.

1365 Piepkorn M, Barnhill RL. A factual, not arbitrary, basis for choice of resection margins in melanoma. Arch Dermatol 1996; 132: 811–814.

1366 Weinstock MA. Resection margins in primary cutaneous melanoma. Arch Dermatol 1997; 133: 103.

1367 Piepkorn M. Melanoma resection margin recommendations, unconventionally based on available facts. Semin Diagn Pathol 1998; 15: 230–234.

1368 Zitelli JA, Brown C, Hanusa BH. Mohs micrographic surgery for the treatment of primary cutaneous melanoma. J Am Acad Dermatol 1997; 37: 236–245.

1369 Milton GW, Shaw HM, McCarthy WH. Subungual malignant melanoma: a disease entity separate from other forms of cutaneous melanoma. Australas J Dermatol 1985; 26: 61–64.

1370 Heaton KM, El-Naggar A, Ensign LG et al. Surgical management and prognostic factors in patients with subungual melanoma. Ann Surg 1994; 219: 197–204.

1371 Demierre M-F, Koh HK. Adjuvant therapy for cutaneous malignant melanoma. J Am Acad Dermatol 1997; 36: 747–764.

1372 Hsueh EC, Nathanson L, Foshag LJ et al. Active specific immunotherapy with polyvalent melanoma cell vaccine for patients with in-transit melanoma metastases. Cancer 1999; 85: 2160–2169.

1373 Curiel-Lewandrowski C, Demierre M-F. Advances in specific immunotherapy of malignant melanoma. J Am Acad Dermatol 2000; 43: 167–185.

1374 Schneeberger A, Goos M, Stingl G, Wagner SN. Management of malignant melanoma: new developments in immune and gene therapy. Clin Exp Dermatol 2000; 25: 509–519.

1375 Martin HM, Birkin AJ, Theaker JM. Malignant melanoma re-excision specimens – how many blocks? Histopathology 1998; 32: 362–367.

1376 Kirham N. What is there to find in malignant melanoma re-excision specimens? Histopathology 1998; 32: 566–567.

1377 Walsh P, Gibbs P, Gonzalez R. Newer strategies for effective evaluation of primary melanoma and treatment of stage III and IV disease. J Am Acad Dermatol 2000; 42: 480–489.

1378 Brady MS, Coit DG. Sentinel lymph node evaluation in melanoma. Arch Dermatol 1997; 133: 1014–1020.

1379 Piepkorn M, Weinstock MA, Barnhill RL. Theoretical and empirical arguments in relation to elective lymph node dissection for melanoma. Arch Dermatol 1997; 133: 995–1002.

1380 Reintgen D, Shivers S. Sentinel lymph node micrometastasis from melanoma. Proven methodology and evolving significance. Cancer 1999; 86: 551–552.

1381 Cherpelis BS, Haddad F, Messina J et al. Sentinel lymph node micrometastasis and other histologic factors that predict outcome in patients with thicker melanomas. J Am Acad Dermatol 2001; 44: 762–766.

1382 Lukowsky A, Bellmann B, Ringk A et al. Detection of melanoma micrometastases in the sentinel lymph node and in nonsentinel nodes by tyrosinase polymerase chain reaction. J Invest Dermatol 1999; 113: 554–559.

1383 Blaheta H-J, Ellwanger U, Schittek B et al. Examination of regional lymph nodes by sentinel node biopsy and molecular analysis provides new staging facilities in primary cutaneous melanoma. J Invest Dermatol 2000; 114: 637–642.

1384 Yu LL, Flotte TJ, Tanabe KK et al. Detection of microscopic melanoma metastases in sentinel lymph nodes. Cancer 1999; 86: 617–627.

1385 Thomas JM, Patocskai EJ. The argument against sentinel node biopsy for malignant melanoma. Its use should be confined to patients in clinical trials. BMJ 2000; 321: 3–4.

1386 Glass FL, Cottam JA, Reintgen DS, Fenske NA. Lymphatic mapping and sentinel node biopsy in the management of high-risk melanoma. J Am Acad Dermatol 1998; 39: 603–610.

1387 McCarthy WH. Evidence-based management of melanoma. Med J Aust 2000; 173: 286–288.

1388 Messina JL, Glass LF, Cruse CW et al. Pathologic examination of the sentinel lymph node in malignant melanoma. Am J Surg Pathol 1999; 23: 686–690.

1389 Baisden BL, Askin FB, Lange JR, Westra WH. HMB-45 immunohistochemical staining of sentinel lymph nodes. A specific method for enhancing detection of micrometastases in patients with melanoma. Am J Surg Pathol 2000; 24: 1140–1146.

1390 Hatta N, Takata M, Takehara K, Ohara K. Polymerase chain reaction and immunohistochemistry frequently detect occult melanoma cells in regional lymph nodes of melanoma patients. J Clin Pathol 1998; 51: 597–601.

1391 Cochran AJ. Surgical pathology remains pivotal in the evaluation of 'sentinel' lymph nodes. Am J Surg Pathol 1999; 23: 1169–1172.

1392 Carson KF, Wen D-R, Li P-X et al. Nodal nevi and cutaneous melanomas. Am J Surg Pathol 1996; 20: 834–840.

1393 Koopal SA, Tiebosch ATMG, Piers DA et al. Frozen section analysis of sentinel lymph nodes in melanoma patients. Cancer 2000; 89: 1720–1725.

1394 Landi G, Polverelli M, Moscatelli G et al. Sentinel lymph node biopsy in patients with primary cutaneous melanoma: study of 455 cases. J Eur Acad Dermatol Venereol 2000; 14: 35–45.

1395 Mraz-Gernhard S, Sagebiel RW, Kashani-Sabet M et al. Prediction of sentinel lymph node micrometastasis by histological features in primary cutaneous malignant melanoma. Arch Dermatol 1998; 134: 983–987.

1396 Kelley SW, Cockerell CJ. Sentinel lymph node biopsy as an adjunct to management of histologically difficult to diagnose melanocytic lesions: A proposal. J Am Acad Dermatol 2000; 42: 527–530.

1397 Böni R, Huch-Böni RA, Steinert H et al. Early detection of melanoma metastasis using fludeoxyglucose F18 positron emission tomography. Arch Dermatol 1996; 132: 875–876.

1398 Moehrle M, Blum A, Rassner G, Juenger M. Lymph node metastases of cutaneous melanoma: Diagnosis by B-scan and color Doppler sonography. J Am Acad Dermatol 1999; 41: 703–709.

1399 Tyler DS, Onaitis M, Kherani A et al. Positron emission tomography scanning in malignant melanoma. Clinical utility in patients with Stage III disease. Cancer 2000; 89: 1019–1025.

1400 Balch CM, Soong S-J, Shaw HM. A comparison of worldwide melanoma data. In: Balch CM, Milton GW, eds. Cutaneous melanoma. Clinical management and treatment results worldwide. Philadelphia: JB Lippincott, 1985; 507–518.

1401 Måsbäck A, Westerdahl J, Ingvar C et al. Cutaneous malignant melanoma in southern Sweden 1965, 1975, and 1985. Prognostic factors and histologic correlations. Cancer 1997; 79: 275–283.

1402 Ackerman AB. Mythology and numerology in the sphere of melanoma. Cancer 2000; 88: 491–496.

1403 Cochran AJ, Elashoff D, Morton DL, Elashoff R. Individualized prognosis for melanoma patients. Hum Pathol 2000; 31: 327–331.

1404 Rogers GS, Kopf AW, Rigel DS et al. Hazard-rate analysis in stage I malignant melanoma. Arch Dermatol 1986; 122: 999–1002.

1405 Slingluff CL Jr, Dodge RK, Stanley WE, Seigler HF. The annual risk of melanoma progression. Implications for the concept of cure. Cancer 1992; 70: 1917–1927.

1406 Dicker TJ, Kavanagh GM, Herd RM et al. A rational approach to melanoma follow-up in patients with primary cutaneous melanoma. Br J Dermatol 1999; 140: 249–254.

1407 Steiner A, Wolf C, Pehamberger H, Wolff K. Late metastases of cutaneous malignant melanoma. Br J Dermatol 1986; 114: 737–740.

1408 Raderman D, Giler S, Rothem A, Ben-Bassat M. Late metastases (beyond ten years) of cutaneous malignant melanoma. Literature review and case report. J Am Acad Dermatol 1986; 15: 374–378.

1409 Boi S, Amichetti M. Late metastases of cutaneous melanoma: case report and literature review. J Am Acad Dermatol 1991; 24: 335–338.

1410 Vignale R, Brugnini S, Martinez M et al. Regional ganglionar metastasis 24 years after surgical resection of a malignant melanoma. Int J Dermatol 1998; 37: 44–45.

1411 Filizel F, Demirkesen C, Yildu N, Oruç N. Late metastasis of malignant melanoma. Int J Dermatol 1997; 36: 955–957.

1412 Googe P, Griffin W, Rash P, King R. Late metastasis from regressed cutaneous melanoma. J Cutan Pathol 2000; 27: 557–558 (abstract).

1413 Schmid-Wendtner M-H, Baumert J, Schmidt M et al. Late metastases of cutaneous melanoma: An analysis of 31 patients. J Am Acad Dermatol 2000; 43: 605–609.

1414 Barnhill RL, Piepkorn MW, Cochran AJ et al. Tumor vascularity, proliferation, and apoptosis in human melanoma micrometastases and macrometastases. Arch Dermatol 1998; 134: 991–994.

1415 Arbiser JL. Melanoma. Lessons from metastases. Arch Dermatol 1998; 134: 1027–1028.

1416 Pool SE, Manieei F, Clark WH Jr, Harrist TJ. Dermal squamo-melanocytic tumor: A unique biphenotypic neoplasm of uncertain biological potential. Hum Pathol 1999; 30: 525–529.

1417 Piérard GE, Fazaa B, Henry F et al. Collision of primary malignant neoplasms of the skin: the connection between malignant melanoma and basal cell carcinoma. Dermatology 1997; 194: 378–379.

1418 Akiyama M, Inamoto N, Nakamura K. Malignant melanoma and squamous cell carcinoma forming one tumour on a burn scar. Dermatology 1997; 194: 157–161.

1419 Bridges AG, Mutasim DF. Malignant melanoma arising in association with squamous cell carcinoma. J Cutan Pathol 2000; 27: 551 (abstract).

1420 Cutlan RT, Wesche WA, Chesney TM. A cutaneous neoplasm with histopathological and immunohistochemical features of both malignant melanoma and squamous cell carcinoma. J Cutan Pathol 2000; 27: 554 (abstract).

1421 Umlas J, Liteplo M, Ucci A. Squamous carcinoma in situ of the skin containing premelanosomes, with melanocytic colonization of the tumor. Hum Pathol 1999; 30: 530–532.

Tumors of cutaneous appendages

33

INTRODUCTION

The cutaneous appendages give rise to a bewildering number of neoplasms – more than 80 at a recent count. Various classifications have been proposed in the past, which have required modification from time to time in the light of the most recent ultrastructural and histochemical findings and the reporting of new morphological entities. Ackerman and colleagues have been systematically reclassifying many of the traditional 'eccrine' tumors into apocrine categories, based largely on their morphology rather than their histochemical chacteristics. The classification used here is based, in part, on Ackerman's recent writings.

Appendageal tumors will be considered under the traditional headings:

- hair follicle tumors
- sebaceous tumors
- apocrine tumors
- eccrine tumors
- complex adnexal tumors.

A case could be made on embryological grounds to have only two categories – folliculosebaceous-apocrine, and eccrine.[1] More and more tumors are being recognized in the first of these two categories with divergent differentiation, although monophasic differentiation is the usual characteristic.

Occasional tumors defy classification such as the extraparotid Warthin's tumor and the ocular adnexal oncocytoma.[2–4]

Hair follicle tumors

There is as yet no universally acceptable classification of hair follicle tumors. Headington, in his comprehensive review in 1976, proposed a detailed histogenetic classification,[5] whereas Mehregan in 1985 used a much simpler classification[6] with three subgroups: hyperplasias (nevi), adenomas and epitheliomas. Rosen has published a classification in which the benign tumors are divided into seven categories, depending on which part or parts of the hair follicle the lesion differentiates towards or most closely resembles.[7]

In their book on follicular neoplasms, Ackerman, Reddy and Soyer have published, with a critique, the classifications used in eight textbooks of dermatopathology.[8] No two classifications are the same, although there is some unanimity as to the entities that ought to be regarded as follicular tumors. The new classification of Ackerman and colleagues differs in categorization and nomenclature from the one used here.[8] For example, they now classify trichoepitheliomas as trichoblastomas while conceding that what is known as desmoplastic trichoepithelioma is clinically distinctive. Tricholemmomas and inverted follicular keratoses are warts (still), and basal cell carcinomas have been renamed trichoblastic carcinoma. It is not proposed to modify substantially the classification previously used for follicular tumors.

HAMARTOMAS AND TUMORS OF HAIR GERM

The hamartomas and tumors of hair germ constitute the largest group of pilar tumors. They have in common the formation of nests, strands and cords of basaloid cells with varying degrees of differentiation towards a hair follicle. At one end of the spectrum there are highly structured and differentiated tumors, such as the hair follicle nevus and trichofolliculoma, whereas at the other end the epithelial proliferations show only limited follicular differentiation and may resemble basal cell carcinomas. Included in this group are the rare trichogenic tumors, which are somewhat analogous to odontogenic tumors in having variants that may contain both epithelial and mesenchymal components. The better differentiated variants will be considered first.

HAIR FOLLICLE NEVUS

These hamartomas are exceedingly rare lesions of the head and neck, presenting as a small nodule or area of hypertrichosis.[6,9,10] A linear variant has been reported.[11] They are composed of closely arranged mature vellus follicles.[12] Headington has suggested the term 'congenital vellus hamartoma' for these lesions.[5] They must be distinguished from accessory tragi, in which many vellus follicles can also be seen.[13] The hair follicle nevus has been confused with the trichofolliculoma, but they are histologically distinct.[14]

Also included in this group is the entity known as 'faun-tail', a patch of hairs over the lower sacral area.[6] It is relevant to mention here the rare occurrence of hair follicles on the palms and soles.[15] Becker's nevus (see p. 331) is sometimes included in the general category of hair follicle hamartomas.[5]

TRICHOFOLLICULOMA

Trichofolliculoma is a rare pilar tumor, intermediate in differentiation between a hair follicle nevus and a trichoepithelioma (see below). It usually presents as a solitary tumor, approximately 0.5 cm in diameter, on the head and neck, usually the face.[16] A tuft of fine hairs may protrude from a central umbilication.

Recently, Schulz and Hartschuh have published their detailed observations on the evolution of a trichofolliculoma.[17] They suggest that the trichofolliculoma undergoes changes corresponding to the regressing hair follicle in its well-known cycle.[17]

Histopathology[5,6,16]

There are one or several dilated follicles from which radiate numerous small follicles of varying degrees of maturity (Fig. 33.1). The central follicle, which opens on to the surface, usually contains keratinous material and sometimes vellus hairs. The follicles that branch off the central follicle may in turn give rise to secondary or even tertiary follicles. Sometimes only rudimentary pilar structures or epithelial cords are formed. In older lesions, catagen and telogen follicles are present.[17] Trichofolliculomas have a relatively cellular connective tissue stroma. This complex pattern is quite different from the hair follicle nevus (see above), which is composed of mature vellus follicles. Merkel cells are found in the outer sheath of the small follicles.[18]

Scattered vacuolated cells representing sebaceous differentiation may be present within the follicles or the rudimentary structures. Sebocytes are seen more often in late stage lesions. Epidermolytic hyperkeratosis has been found as an incidental change.[19] A variant of trichofolliculoma in which large sebaceous follicles connect to a central cavity or sinus has been reported as a **sebaceous trichofolliculoma**.[20] It has some similarities to the folliculosebaceous cystic hamartoma (see p. 873), which appears to be a trichofolliculoma at a late stage in its evolution.[17,21,22]

TRICHOADENOMA

Trichoadenoma (of Nikolowski)[23] is a rare tumor with hair follicle-like differentiation; it is found as a nodular lesion, particularly on the face and buttocks.[24,25]

Histopathology[24]

Trichoadenoma is a well-defined dermal tumor composed of epithelial islands, most of which have a central cystic cavity containing keratinous material. The multilayered squamous epithelium shows epidermoid keratinization toward the central cavity. The appearances resemble multiple cross-sections of the infundibular portion of hair follicles (Fig. 33.2). There are no hair shafts present. Collagen fibers are present between the follicular structures.

Verrucous trichoadenoma is a variant of trichoadenoma which clinically resembles a seborrheic keratosis.[26] It is composed of small epidermoid cysts, some of which contain vellus hairs. There is abundant keratin on the epidermal surface.[26]

TRICHOEPITHELIOMA

Trichoepitheliomas (trichoblastomas in the classification of Ackerman et al) are regarded as poorly differentiated hamartomas of hair germ.[5,8] There are three variants of trichoepithelioma: solitary, multiple and desmoplastic. The histological features of the solitary and multiple types are identical and they will be considered together. Desmoplastic trichoepithelioma is a distinct clinicopathological entity and it will be discussed separately below.

Solitary trichoepitheliomas are found as skin-colored papules, with a predilection for the nose, upper lip and cheeks. They measure up to 0.5 cm in diameter. Most of the lesions reported as giant solitary trichoepitheliomas are trichoblastomas.[27–30] Rare presentations include a linear form and as a large, hemifacial plaque.[31,32]

Multiple trichoepitheliomas (epithelioma adenoides cysticum) have an autosomal dominant mode of inheritance, with lessened expressivity and

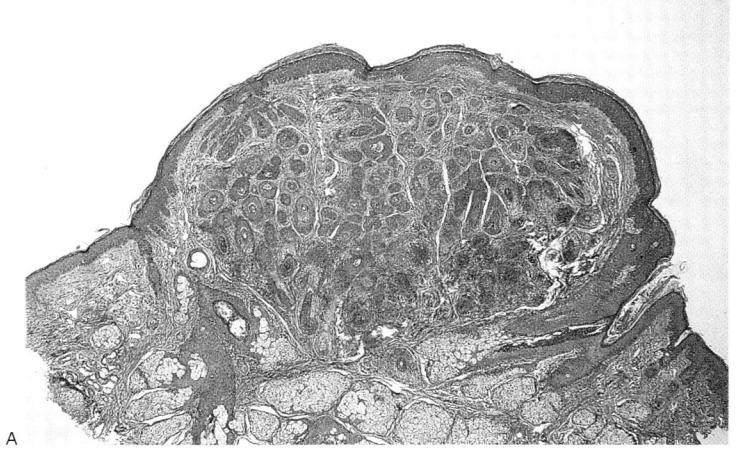

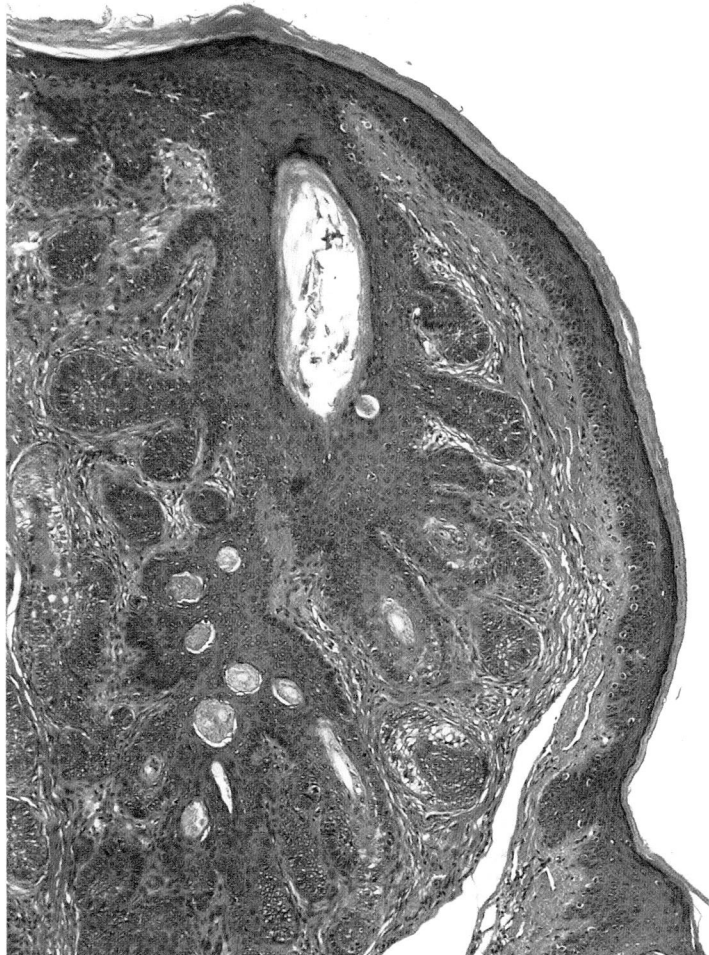

Fig. 33.1 **(A) Trichofolliculoma. (B)** Small follicles with variable maturity radiate from a larger central follicle. (H & E)

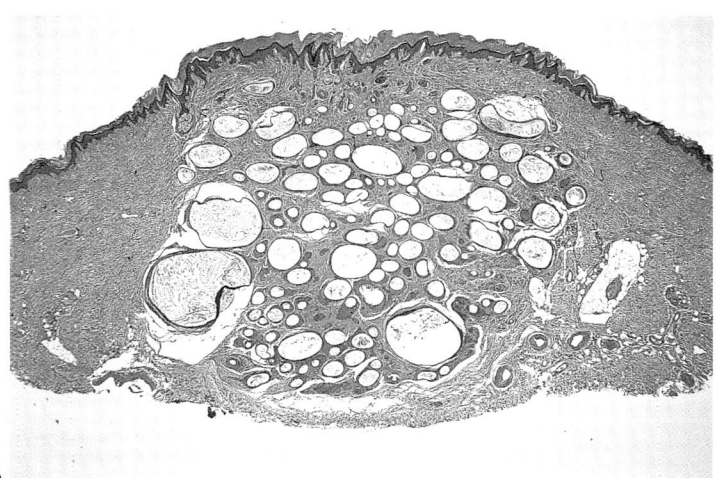

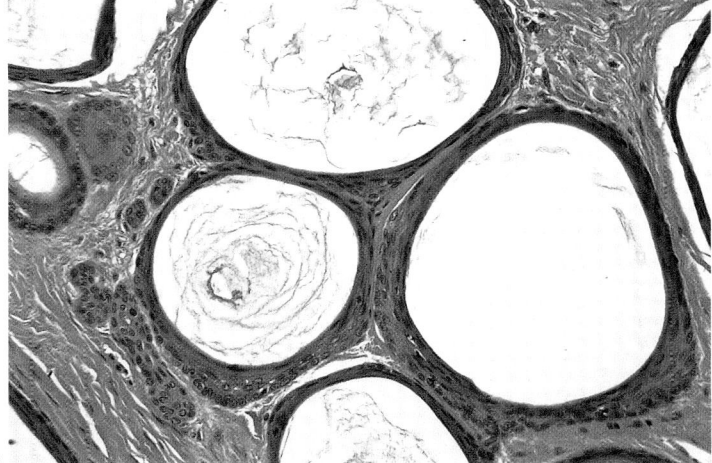

Fig. 33.2 **(A) Trichoadenoma. (B)** There are multiple 'cystic structures' resembling cross-sections of the infundibular portion of hair follicles. (H & E)

penetrance in the male. Sporadic cases of this condition also occur.[5] Multiple trichoepitheliomas present as small papules with a strong predilection for the central part of the face. The trunk, neck and scalp are sometimes involved. The papules may coalesce to give plaques.[33–35] The onset of lesions is usually in childhood or at the time of puberty.[36] Rare presentations include a linear and dermatomal distribution,[37] development in an epidermal nevus,[38] an association with cylindromas[34,39] and sometimes also with spiradenomas,[40] and an association with ungual fibromas,[41] dystrophia unguis congenita[42] and the ROMBO syndrome (vermiculate atrophoderma, milia, hypotrichosis, trichoepithelioma, basal cell carcinomas and peripheral vasodilatation).[43–45] The simultaneous appearance of trichoepitheliomas and carcinoma of the breast has also been reported.[46]

Trichoepitheliomas are benign lesions. Many of the cases of malignant transformation reported in the older literature represent cases of the nevoid basal cell carcinoma syndrome and not trichoepitheliomas.[5] Nevertheless, there are several documented cases of basal cell carcinoma developing in trichoepithelioma,[47–49] and one case of a malignant tumor, with pilar (including matrical) differentiation, arising in a trichoepithelioma.[50]

One study has shown deletions at 9q22.3 (the location of the *patched* (*PATCH*) gene of the basal cell nevus syndrome) in sporadic trichoepitheliomas.[51] In the Brooke–Spiegler syndrome (multiple trichoepitheliomas and cylindromas) the locus has been assigned to 16q12–q13.[52]

Histopathology

Trichoepitheliomas are dermal tumors with focal continuity with the epidermis in up to one-third of cases. They are composed of islands of uniform basaloid cells, sometimes showing peripheral palisading. This may lead to a mistaken diagnosis of basal cell carcinoma if features of pilar differentiation are not noted. In addition, there are usually branching nests of basaloid cells. Epithelial structures resembling hair papillae or abortive hair follicles may be seen (Fig. 33.3). Small keratinous cysts lined by stratified squamous epithelium are quite common. Rupture of these cysts with liberation of the keratinous debris results in a small foreign-body granuloma in the stroma. Foci of calcification are often present; amyloid is generally considered to be uncommon although it was present in 33% of cases in one study.[53,54] The stroma is prominent and loosely arranged. Aggregations of fibroblasts, representing abortive attempts to form papillary mesenchyme, are characteristic of trichoepithelioma.[55]

Immunohistochemical staining of trichoepitheliomas resembles that seen in the outer root sheath, with strong reactions for keratins (K) 5/6 and K8. Some K17 is present in cells surrounding horn cysts.[56] Conflicting views have been expressed on the specificity of cytokeratin types in the distinction between trichoepithelioma and trichoblastoma. Although one study concluded that there were no differences,[57] another study found K7 in trichoblastomas but not trichoepithelioma.[58] Trichoepitheliomas express K15, whereas only a subset of basal cell carcinomas do this.[59] Basal cell carcinomas differ from trichoepitheliomas by having stronger and more diffuse expression of PCNA and Ki-67.[60]

Electron microscopy

In trichoepitheliomas there is a proliferation of basaloid cells similar to basal cell carcinoma.[61] Abortive hair papillae and keratinous cysts may be seen. The cells sometimes contain paranuclear glycogen, a feature not seen in basal cell carcinomas.[61]

DESMOPLASTIC TRICHOEPITHELIOMA

Desmoplastic trichoepithelioma is a histological variant of trichoepithelioma that occurs almost exclusively on the face.[62–69] There is a predilection for females and relatively young adults. Solitary familial desmoplastic trichoepithelioma[62] and multiple familial and non-familial tumors[63,70] have been reported. Desmoplastic trichoepitheliomas usually present as asymptomatic solitary hard annular lesions with a raised border and a depressed center. They vary from 3 to 8 mm in diameter. Atypical clinical presentations have been reported.[71]

The finding of Merkel cells as an integral constituent of this tumor raises the possibility of a bulge-derived origin because of the high number of Merkel cells known to reside in this area of the follicle.[72]

Histopathology[73]

Desmoplastic trichoepitheliomas are reasonably well circumscribed tumors in the upper and mid dermis, with an overlying central depression. They are composed of cords and small nests of basaloid cells with scanty cytoplasm (Fig. 33.4). Tumor strands may be attached to the epidermis. There are usually many keratinous (horn) cysts, with a peripheral basaloid layer and several layers of stratified squamous epithelium with central loosely laminated

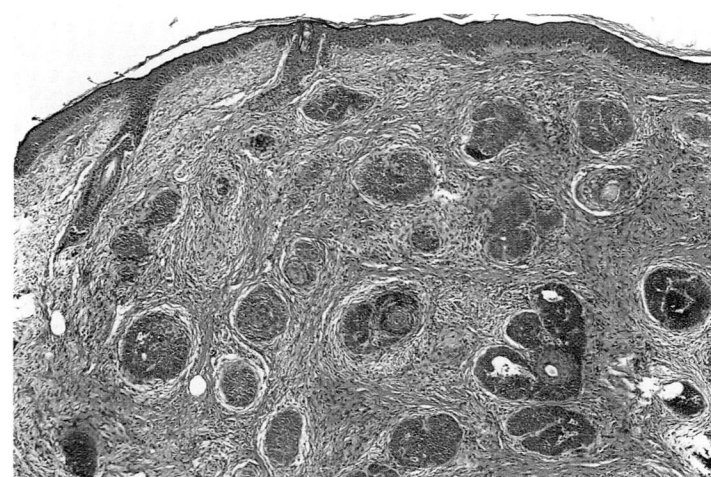

Fig. 33.3 Trichoepithelioma. There are multiple nests of basaloid cells, some showing abortive hair follicle differentiation. (H & E)

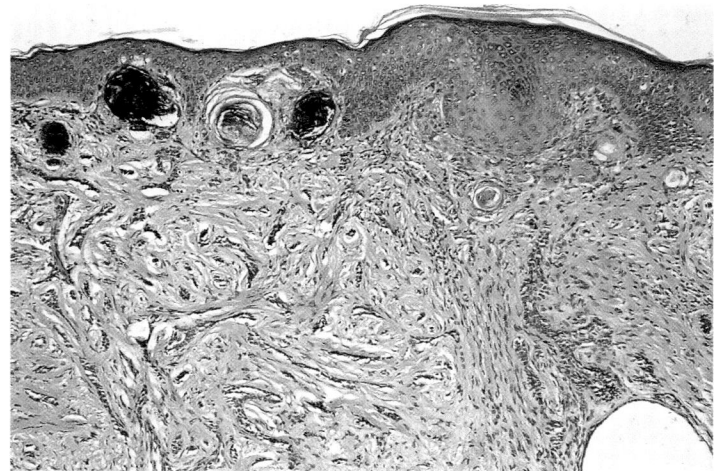

Fig. 33.4 Desmoplastic trichoepithelioma. It is composed of small cords and islands of basaloid cells set in a fibrous stroma. Small keratinous cysts are also present. (H & E)

horn.[74] Sometimes this epithelial lining is attenuated and one cell thick. Tadpole or comma-shaped epithelial projections extend from the peripheral layer of some of the keratinous cysts. Sometimes, structures resembling eccrine ducts are present.

The desmoplastic stroma is dense and hypocellular, with fewer elastic fibers and more acid mucopolysaccharides than in the normal dermis. Other features which are frequently present include foreign-body granulomas, usually related to ruptured cysts, and calcification. Stromal ossification is rare. Occasionally foci of sebaceous cells or shadow cells are present. Rarely, a nevocellular nevus is also present.[64]

The tumor cells do not contain carcinoembryonic antigen, unlike the cells in a syringoma, which are usually positive.[65] In contrast, involucrin is expressed in desmoplastic trichoepitheliomas but not in syringomas.[66] The spindle-shaped cells surrounding the cellular islands in desmoplastic trichoepithelioma are focally strongly positive for CD34, whereas the stromal cells around basal cell carcinomas and microcystic adnexal carcinomas are usually negative.[75–77] Whereas bcl-2 is expressed in most basal cell carcinomas, it is found only in the basal layer of trichoepitheliomas. Unfortunately these markers do not always differentiate reliably between basal cell carcinoma and desmoplastic trichoepithelioma.[78] Merkel cells are present in desmoplastic trichoepitheliomas but uncommon in basal cell carcinoma.[79]

The differential diagnosis includes syringoma and morphea-like basal cell carcinoma.[68,73,80] Syringomas rarely have horn cysts, foreign-body granulomas or calcification.[73] Narrow strands of tumor cells are also unusual in syringomas. Furthermore, syringomas are usually periorbital and multiple. Basal cell carcinomas of morpheic type may form clefts between the nests and the stroma.[68] There is often coexisting nodular basal cell carcinoma. Mitoses and apoptotic bodies are also quite common in basal cell carcinomas, whereas foreign-body granulomas and ruptured keratinous cysts are uncommon.[68] The staining pattern for CD34 and bcl-2 (see above) is also of use in the differentiation of these two tumors.

Electron microscopy
Ultrastructural studies[62,67] have shown basaloid cells surrounded by a basal lamina. Individual cells contain tonofilaments and are connected to adjacent cells by desmosomes.

TRICHOBLASTOMA

Trichoblastomas are extremely rare benign tumors of the hair germ in which follicle development may be partly or completely recapitulated.[29,81–84] They are constituted largely of follicular germinative cells.[85] They have been likened to the odontogenic tumors, which may also be epithelial and/or mesenchymal.[5] As initially reported by Headington, the trichogenic tumors were further classified on the basis of the relative proportions of epithelial and mesenchymal components: the predominantly epithelial trichogenic tumor was called a trichoblastoma and the predominantly mesenchymal variant was labeled trichogenic fibroma.[86] Other categories were included.[5] Other terms have also been used for tumors in this group, including solitary, giant and immature trichoepithelioma,[29,87,88] and trichogerminoma.[89] The cutaneous lymphadenoma is a distinctive variant of trichoblastoma which will be considered separately. The tumor reported as a 'rippled-pattern trichomatricoma' is also a trichoblastoma.[90]

Trichoblastomas are usually greater than 1 cm in diameter and involve the deep dermis and subcutis. Lesions confined to the subcutis are seen occasionally.[91] The head, particularly the scalp, is a common site.[92] Multiple lesions have been reported.[93] Trichoblastomas are not aggressive, unless they have been misdiagnosed or contain an element of basal cell carcinoma.[8,94]

Histopathology[5,83]
The low-power view is usually quite striking: a large, circumscribed basaloid tumor with no epidermal connection. It is usually situated in the mid and lower dermis, with extension into the subcutis. The tumor shows irregular nests of basaloid cells resembling a basal cell carcinoma, but with variable stromal condensation and pilar differentiation (Fig. 33.5). The variant reported as trichogerminoma was composed of closely packed lobules of basaloid cells resembling hair bulbs, with little intervening stroma.[89] At the other end of the spectrum is the *trichoblastic fibroma*, with an intimate relationship between basaloid nests and strands, and a fibrocellular stroma.[95–97] A desmoplastic stroma has been reported.[98] So-called 'stromal induction', with the formation of primitive hair bulbs, is present. Keratinous cysts may be present in this group of trichoblastomas but they are not seen in the cellular, basaloid variants that may resemble basal cell carcinoma.

Ackerman and colleagues have used 'trichoblastoma' as a generic term for all neoplasms of the skin and subcutaneous fat that are composed mostly of follicular germinative cells. Trichoepitheliomas are included in this definition.[8] They have reported nodular, retiform, cribriform, racemiform and columnar patterns of trichoblastoma.[8]

Stromal amyloid and Merkel cells are quite common in trichoblastomas.[29,99] Rare variants include clear cell, pigmented (pigmented trichoblastoma)[100,101] and adamantinoid lesions (Fig. 33.6).[85] Focal sebaceous differentiation is also rare.[102] It is generally agreed that the cutaneous lymphadenoma is an adamantinoid variant of trichoblastoma with lymphocytic infiltration of the basaloid nests (see below). The cells in a trichoblastoma express K8 and K19.[103] K7 is also expressed, in contrast to trichoepithelioma.[58]

The *rippled-pattern trichoblastoma* has a palisaded arrangement of epithelial ribbons with areas of nuclear palisading resembling Verocay bodies. Focal sebaceous differentiation may occur. The expression of cytokeratins is similar to the more usual trichoblastoma.[104]

CUTANEOUS LYMPHADENOMA (TRICHOBLASTOMA VARIANT)

Cutaneous lymphadenoma is a rare adnexal tumor with a prominent lymphocytic infiltrate in the tumor nests.[105–113] It is a distinctive variant of trichoblastoma.[106]

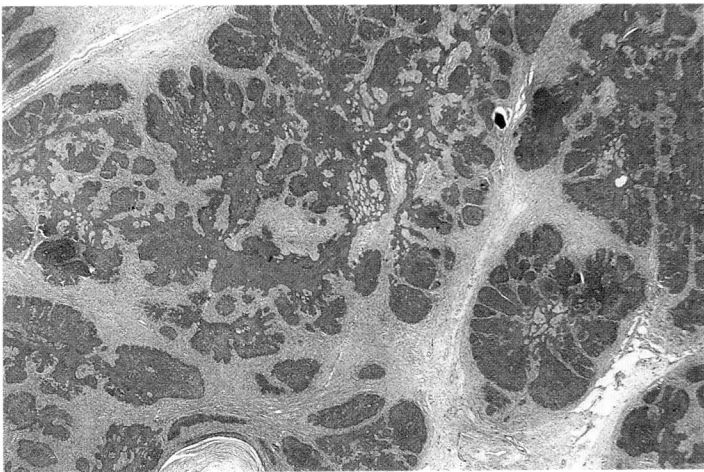

Fig. 33.5 **Trichoblastoma.** This basaloid tumor resembles basal cell carcinoma. There is some trichogenic differentiation and stromal induction. (H & E)

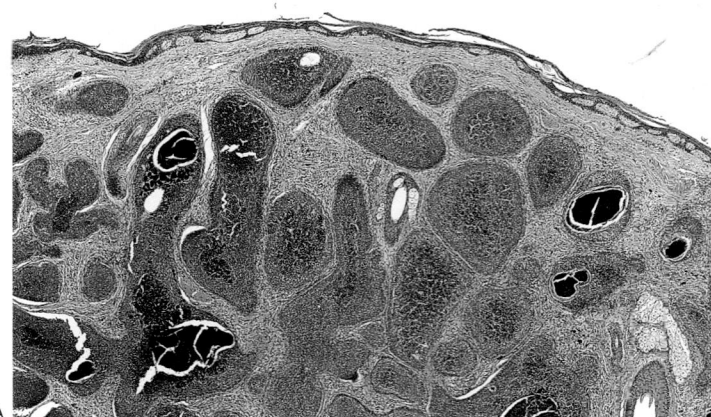

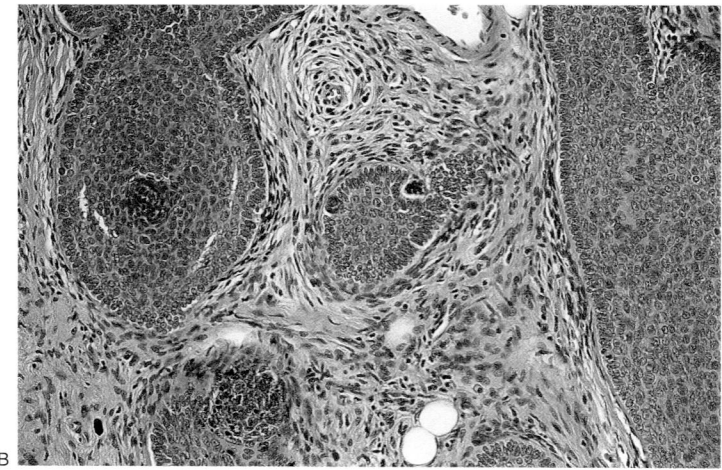

Fig. 33.6 **(A) Pigmented trichoblastoma. (B)** There is focal stromal induction with the formation of primitive follicular structures. (H & E)

The tumor presents as a small nodule on the face or legs. The lesion has usually been present for many months or years. Local excision is curative.

Histopathology

Cutaneous lymphadenoma is composed of multiple rounded lobules of basaloid cells with some degree of peripheral palisading, embedded in a fibrous stroma of variable density (Fig. 33.7). The stroma may rarely be desmoplastic.[114] There is an intense infiltrate of small mature lymphocytes within the lobules, with some spillage into the stroma.[109] A hint of follicular differentiation and focal sebaceous differentiation is sometimes present.[110] Some nests may show adamantinoid features, but this does not appear to be a universal change, a strong point against cutaneous lymphadenoma being synonymous with adamantinoid trichoblastoma.[115] Focal stromal mucinosis is an uncommon finding.[112]

Both T and B lymphocytes are found within the lobules, as well as some S100-positive dendritic cells.[107] The pattern of staining with CD34 and *bcl-2* is similar to that seen in trichoblastomas and trichoepitheliomas.[116] There are scattered CD30-positive cells within the tumor nests.[116,117]

PANFOLLICULOMA

Panfolliculoma is an exceedingly rare, but distinctive tumor, with advanced follicular differentiation. It was described by Ackerman and colleagues.[8] It has

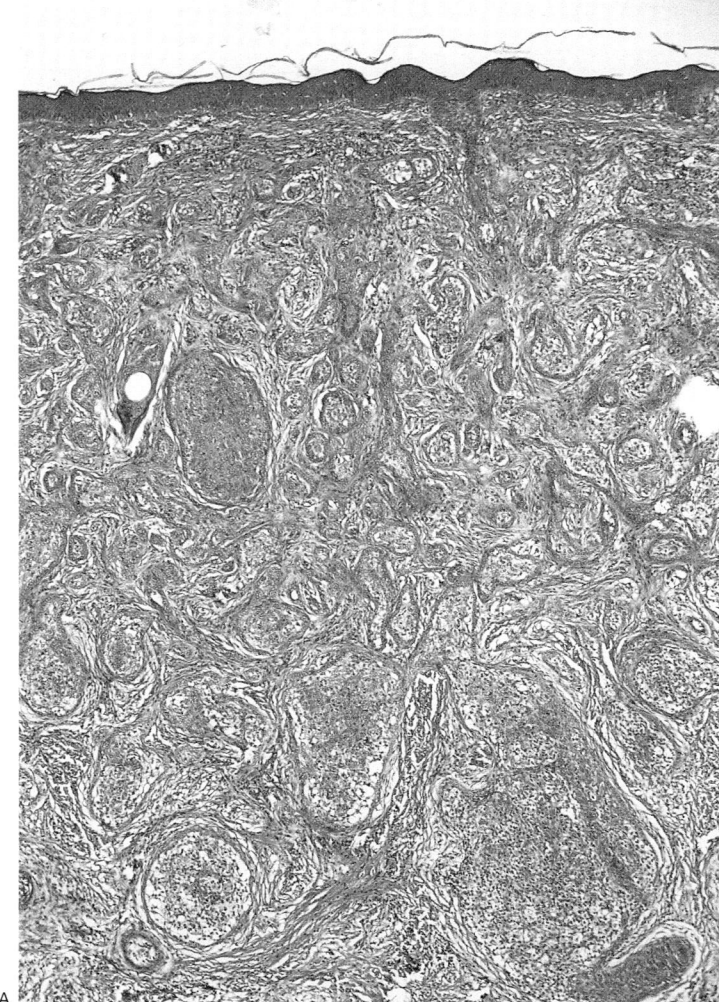

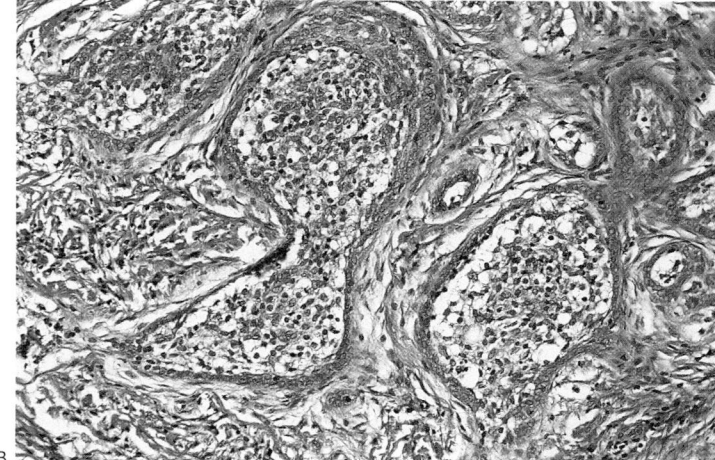

Fig. 33.7 **(A) Cutaneous lymphadenoma. (B)** Lymphocytes extend into the basaloid nests. (H & E)

overlap features between a trichoblastoma (see above) and a matricoma (see p. 870), but it differs from the former by the presence of differentiation towards all elements of the follicle, including cystic structures containing corneocytes. Matrical differentiation is less conspicuous than it is in matricoma.

FOLLICULAR HAMARTOMA SYNDROMES

Several extremely rare syndromes are characterized by the development of localized, zosteriform or linear tumors with overlapping histological features. Cases have been both familial and sporadic, and the associated clinical features have been varied. Ackerman has challenged the validity of these syndromes, believing them to be different expressions of infundibulocystic basal cell carcinomas occurring in variants of the basal cell nevus syndrome, although this has been disputed.[118] Some of the cases to be mentioned here have only a vague resemblance to infundibulocystic basal cell carcinomas. It is acknowledged that they may not all be discrete entities.

Generalized hair follicle hamartoma

Generalized hair follicle hamartoma has been applied to patients with papules and plaques on the face, progressive alopecia and myasthenia gravis.[119,120] Cystic fibrosis is a further association of this follicular hamartoma.[121] Involved skin shows a spectrum of changes, with some lesions resembling trichoepithelioma and others 'basaloid follicular hamartoma', whereas uninvolved skin may show small islands of basaloid cells.[120] A case with diffuse sclerosis of the face has been reported.[122]

Basaloid follicular hamartoma

The term 'basaloid follicular hamartoma' was coined by Mehregan and Baker for three patients with localized or systematized lesions in which individual hair follicles were replaced or were associated with solid strands and branching cords of undifferentiated basaloid cells with some intervening fibrous stroma.[123] Although they regarded the condition as a localized variant of generalized hair follicle hamartoma, in their cases there was less resemblance to trichoepithelioma and more to a premalignant fibroepithelial tumor of Pinkus.[123] A linear variant has also been reported.[124]

Similar cases, both solitary and multiple familial cases, have been reported by Brownstein and others.[125,126] The lesions were 1–2 mm smooth facial papules composed of anastomosing strands of basaloid and squamoid cells in a loose stroma. Horn cysts and pigmentation were common.

The family reported recently by Wheeler and colleagues as dominantly inherited *generalized basaloid follicular hamartoma syndrome* had clinical and histological differences to Brownstein's cases.[127] The lesions were composed of nests of bland basaloid cells surrounded by scant fibrous stroma. They were usually associated with hair follicles. There were infundibular cysts and comedone-like lesions but they had no resemblance to the infundibulocystic basal cell carcinoma.[127]

Linear unilateral basal cell nevus with comedones

Linear unilateral basal cell nevus with comedones refers to linear or zosteriform lesions, some with comedone plugs, that are present at birth or soon after.[128] Although there is some clinical resemblance to nevus comedonicus (see p. 755), the histology resembles a basal cell carcinoma. Some cases have had a lattice-like growth of basaloid cells attached to the undersurface of the epidermis and vague follicular differentiation. These features were also present in the case reported as **localized follicular hamartoma**.[129]

INFUNDIBULAR AND ISTHMIC TUMORS

Two tumors arise from the infundibulum, the uppermost portion of the hair follicle above the opening of the sebaceous duct, and a further two arise from the segment below, the isthmus, which extends from the origin of the sebaceous duct to the level of the bulge. The infundibular tumors are the dilated pore of Winer and the inverted follicular keratosis, while the isthmic tumors are the tumor of the follicular infundibulum (better renamed the tumor of the follicular isthmus) and the pilar sheath acanthoma.[8]

All are characterized by a superficial location, connection with the epidermis and pilar structures, and infundibular (epidermoid) keratinization. The epidermal cyst could be included here, but for convenience it has been considered with other cysts (see Ch. 16, p. 504).

TUMOR OF THE FOLLICULAR INFUNDIBULUM

Despite its name, the tumor of the follicular infundibulum is really of isthmic origin.[130] It usually occurs as a solitary, asymptomatic, smooth or slightly keratotic papule on the head and neck or upper chest.[131] Multiple lesions, including a mantle distribution on the upper trunk (infundibulomatosis, eruptive infundibulomas),[132,133] have been reported.[134] The tumor of the follicular infundibulum may also occur in Cowden's disease, the Schöpf–Schu tz–Passarge syndrome and in an organoid nevus.[135]

Histopathology[131]

The growth pattern resembles that of a superficial basal cell carcinoma. There is a plate-like fenestrated subepidermal tumor composed of pale or pink-staining glycogen-containing cells, with a peripheral palisade of basal cells (Fig. 33.8). Some of the cords are basaloid without pale-staining cytoplasm. The tumor connects at intervals with the undersurface of the epidermis by slender pedicles. Hair follicles entering the tumor from below lose their identity and merge with it. Small follicular bulbs and papillary mesenchymal bodies may be found. Focal sebaceous differentiation is rare.[136] Ductal structures, resembling eccrine ducts, have been reported in the tumor strands.[137] The surrounding loose connective tissue stroma contains a network of elastic fibers.[131,132] The histological features sometimes overlap those of tricholemmoma, but the low-power architecture is quite different.

The tumor of the follicular infundibulum appears to be the same as that reported as a basal cell hamartoma with follicular differentiation.[138] However, it is histologically dissimilar to the cases reported as **multiple infundibular tumors of the head and neck**.[139] In these latter cases clusters of enlarged follicular infundibula comprised each lesion, somewhat similar to the

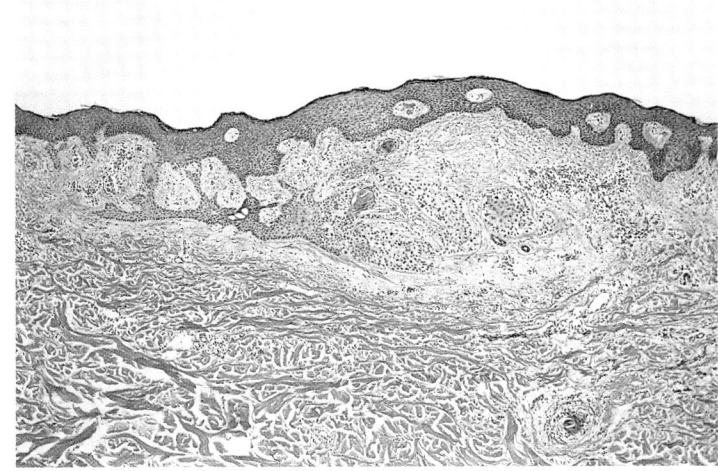

Fig. 33.8 **Tumor of the follicular infundibulum.** Anastomosing cords of basaloid cells are present on the undersurface of the epidermis. (H & E)

appearances of prurigo nodularis. The illustrations in the report of a tumor called an **infundibular keratosis** showed some features of the multiple infundibular tumor referred to above, and others of an inverted follicular keratosis (see below) but without squamous eddies.[140]

DILATED PORE OF WINER

The dilated pore of Winer[141] is a relatively common adnexal lesion which occurs predominantly on the head and neck, but also on the upper trunk of elderly individuals.[142] Clinically and histologically it is a comedo-like structure. Dilated pores may be acquired as a sequel of inflammatory cystic acne, or of actinic damage.[5]

Histopathology[131]

There is a markedly dilated follicular pore, which may extend to the mid or lower dermis. The follicle is lined by outer root sheath epithelium in which there is infundibular keratinization with the formation of keratohyaline granules. The epithelium shows acanthosis and finger-like projections that radiate into the surrounding dermis (Fig. 33.9). There is sometimes heavy melanin pigmentation of the follicular wall; pigmentation may also involve the central horny plug. The pilary unit of the involved follicle and the sebaceous gland are absent or rudimentary.

PILAR SHEATH ACANTHOMA

Pilar sheath acanthoma is a rare, benign follicular tumor found almost exclusively on the upper lip of older individuals.[143–145] The tumors, which measure 5–10 mm in diameter, have a central pore-like opening plugged with keratin.

Histopathology[143–145]

There is a central, cystically dilated follicle containing keratinous material which opens on to the surface (Fig. 33.10). Tumor lobules composed of outer root sheath epithelium extend from the wall of the cystic cavity into the adjacent dermis. Lobules sometimes reach the subcutis. Occasional abortive hair follicles may be present. The tumor epithelium shows infundibular keratinization, although it is of isthmic origin. There may be abundant glycogen in some of the tumor cells.

The condition may be distinguished from the dilated pore of Winer, in which there is a patulous follicle with only small projections of epithelium

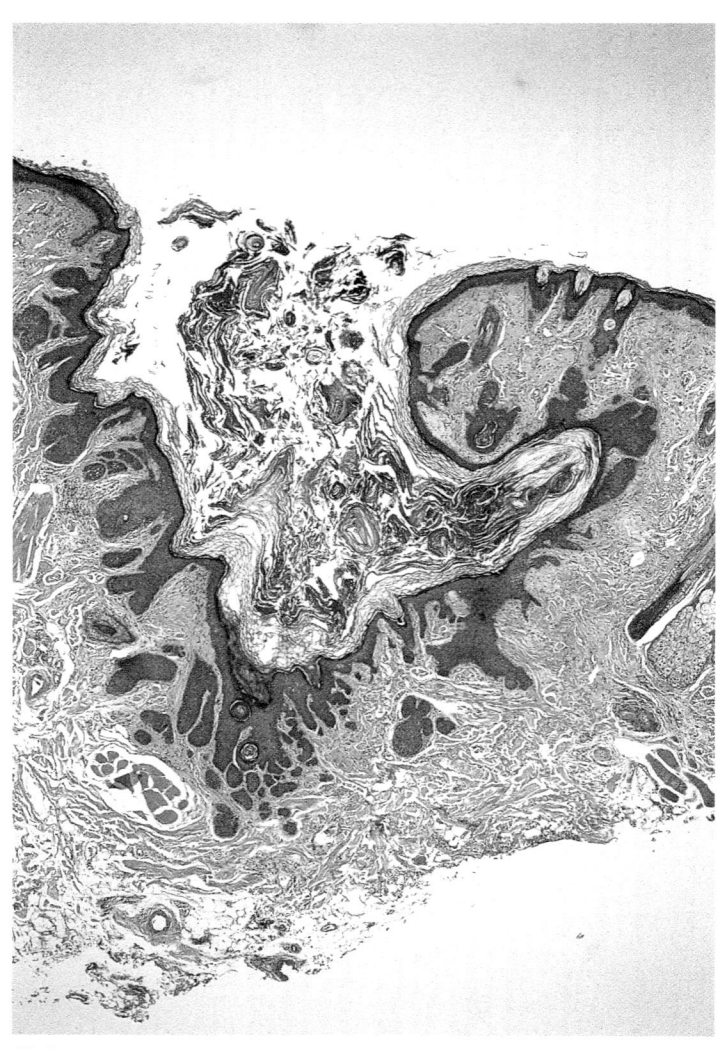

Fig. 33.9 **Dilated pore of Winer.** Acanthotic projections extend from the base of a dilated follicular pore. (H & E)

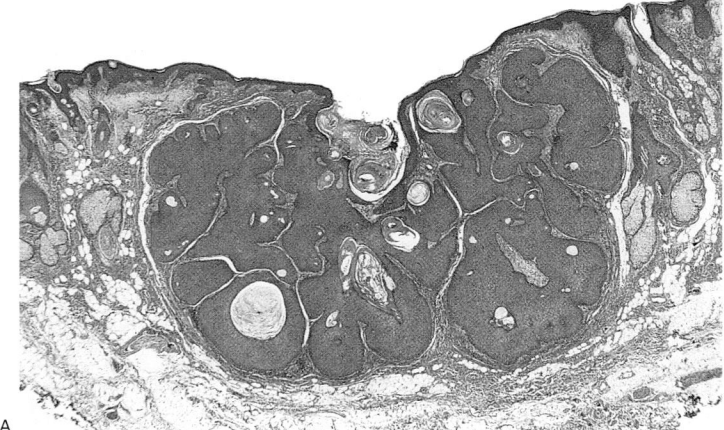

A

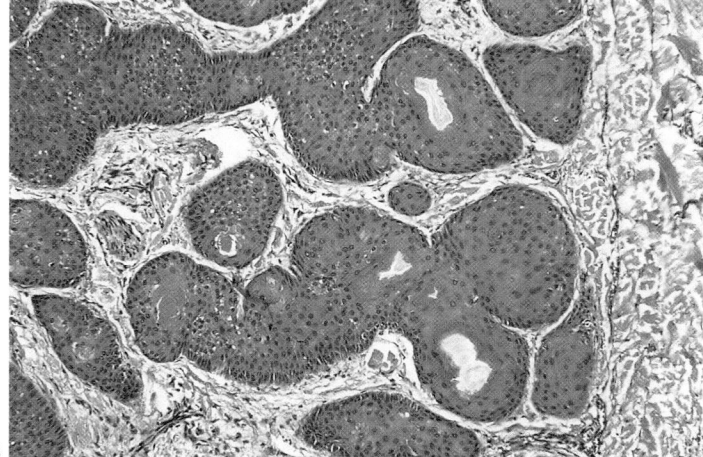

B

Fig. 33.10 **Pilar sheath acanthoma. (A)** Tumor lobules, composed of outer root sheath epithelium, radiate from a central depression. **(B)** The tumor lobules are composed of outer root sheath epithelium. (H & E)

extending into the surrounding connective tissue. In trichofolliculoma, well-formed follicles radiate from the central keratin-filled sinus and there is a well-formed stroma, which is absent in pilar sheath acanthoma.

INVERTED FOLLICULAR KERATOSIS

Inverted follicular keratosis is a benign tumor of the follicular infundibulum that was first described by Helwig in 1954. It is a somewhat controversial entity, having been regarded by some as a variant of seborrheic keratosis or verruca vulgaris.[146,147] It occurs as a solitary flesh-colored nodular or filiform lesion which measures from 0.3 to 1 cm in diameter.[131] In about 90% of cases the tumor occurs on the head and neck, the cheeks and upper lip being the sites of predilection.[147] The eyelids may be involved.[148] It is more common in males and older individuals. Human papillomavirus has not been detected in most cases, suggesting that the inverted follicular keratosis is not a variant of verruca vulgaris, as has been claimed.[149,150] However, some cases of verruca vulgaris do develop areas with features of inverted follicular keratosis and/or tricholemmoma.

Histopathology[131]

Inverted follicular keratoses are predominantly endophytic tumors with large lobules or finger-like projections of tumor cells extending into the dermis. An exophytic growth pattern is present in some lesions, and it is occasionally the dominant feature. Mehregan has described four growth patterns:

1. a papillomatous wart-like variant, which is largely exophytic with overlying hyperkeratosis and parakeratosis
2. a keratoacanthoma-like pattern with marginal buttress formation and a central exo-endophytic mass of solid epithelium
3. a solid nodular form, which is largely endophytic with solid, lobulated masses of epithelium
4. an uncommon cystic type, with irregular clefts within the tumor and the formation of small cysts.[131]

Each tumor lobule is composed of basaloid and squamous cells, with the basaloid cells at the periphery and larger keratinizing cells toward the center. Mitoses are not uncommon in the basaloid cells.

A characteristic feature is the presence of squamous eddies, which are formed by concentric layers of squamous cells in a whorled pattern and which may become keratinized with the formation of keratohyalin and sometimes keratin at the center of these islands (Fig. 33.11). There is sometimes clefting at the periphery of the squamous eddies, and even focal acantholysis. Melanin pigment is usually inconspicuous. The surrounding dermis sometimes contains a mild inflammatory cell infiltrate which is predominantly lymphohistiocytic. Telangiectatic vessels may be found in the dermal papillae in the filiform lesions.

Overlying the tumor there is variable hyperkeratosis and parakeratosis. Funnel-shaped keratinous plugs may form. Occasionally a prominent cutaneous horn is present.

TRICHOLEMMAL (EXTERNAL SHEATH) TUMORS

This group of tumors is characterized by cells which differentiate toward those of the outer sheath of the hair follicle.[5] As such, they show a variable extent of clear cell change resulting from cytoplasmic accumulation of glycogen. There are also cells that are intermediate between those of the outer sheath

and infundibular keratinocytes. These cells may have anisotropic tonofibrils, a characteristic feature of tricholemmal keratinization and one that is also seen in both tricholemmal cysts and proliferating tricholemmal cysts.

OUTER ROOT SHEATH ACANTHOMA

The term 'outer root sheath acanthoma' has been used for a distinctive tumor that developed on the cheek of an 80-year-old male.[151] On lower power, it has some features of the tumor of the follicular infundibulum with anastomosing columns of cells on the undersurface of the epidermis. With progressive descent into the dermis, the tumor cells show outer root sheath differentiation characteristic of the infundibulum, isthmus, stem and anagen bulb.[151]

TRICHOLEMMOMA

Tricholemmomas (trichilemmomas) are small solitary asymptomatic papular lesions found almost exclusively on the face.[5,81,131,152] Multiple tricholemmomas are a cutaneous marker of Cowden's disease (see below).

Although they appear to arise from the follicular infundibulum, they differentiate toward the outer root sheath. Ackerman regards tricholemmomas as old viral warts,[8,153] a view not supported by most dermatopathologists[154,155] or by immunoperoxidase studies to detect viral antigens.[156]

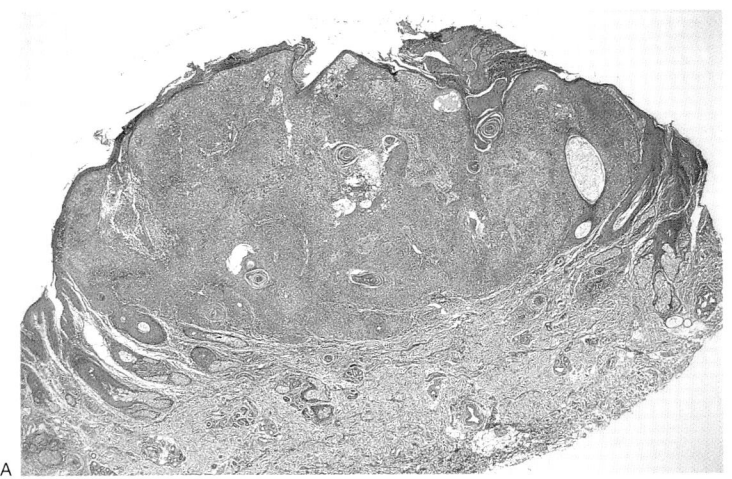

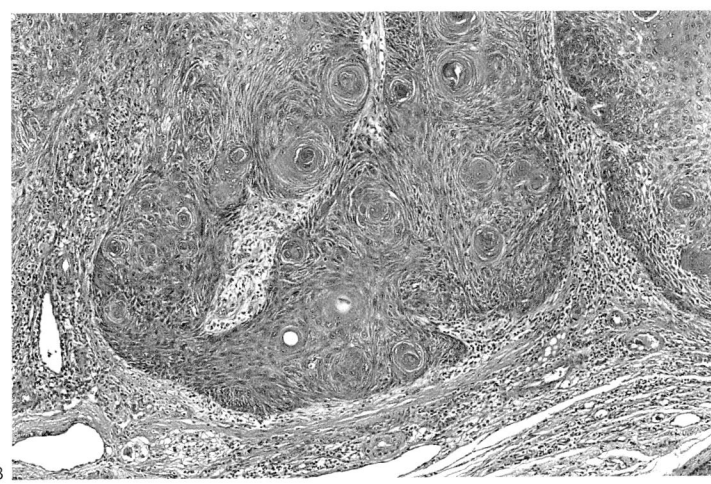

Fig. 33.11 **(A) Inverted follicular keratosis. (B)** Squamous eddies are seen toward the base of the tumor. (H & E)

Histopathology[157]

Tricholemmomas are sharply circumscribed tumors composed of one or more lobules which extend into the upper dermis and are in continuity with the epidermis or follicular epithelium at several points. In small lesions follicular concentricity is apparent.[158] The tumor is composed of squamoid cells showing variable glycogen vacuolation, this change being most marked deeply (Fig. 33.12). Centrally, there may be foci of epidermal keratinization and occasionally small squamous eddies. Keratinous microcysts may form in large lesions. There is a peripheral layer of columnar cells with nuclear palisading resembling the outer root sheath of hair follicles. A thickened glassy basement membrane surrounds the tumor in part. This is PAS positive, and diastase resistant. The stroma is occasionally hyalinized or desmoplastic.[152,159] The term 'desmoplastic tricholemmoma' is used for this histological variant. A case of desmoplastic tricholemmoma arising in an organoid nevus has been reported.[160]

The overlying epidermis shows hyperkeratosis, mild acanthosis and sometimes a prominent granular layer. Uncommonly, a cutaneous horn will form (tricholemmomal horn).[161] This differs from the tricholemmal horn, in which a horn showing tricholemmal keratinization overlies a depression in the epidermis which usually has a prominent basement membrane.[162] Warts, basal and squamous cell carcinomas, and inverted follicular keratoses and seborrheic keratoses sometimes contain areas of tricholemmal differentiation.[153,163]

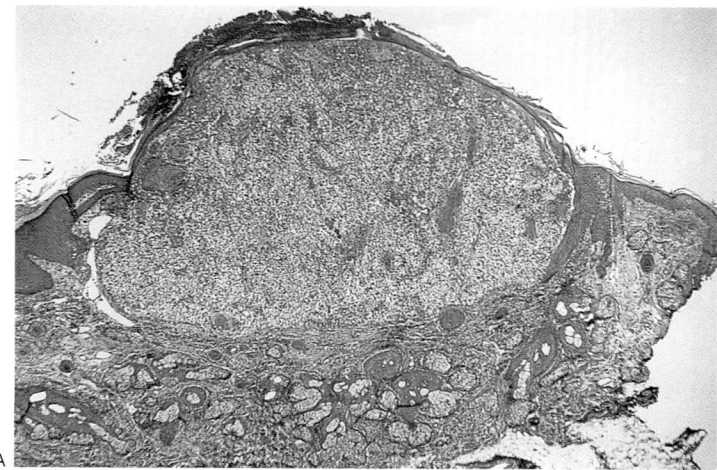

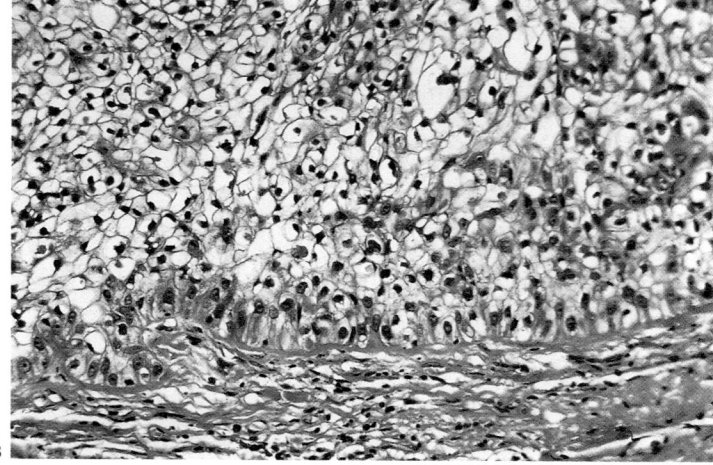

Fig. 33.12 **(A) Tricholemmoma. (B)** Vacuolation of the tumor cells near the base of the lesion is marked. (H & E)

CD34 has been reported in tricholemmomas and also in the external root sheath of normal hair follicles.[164] Its presence in desmoplastic tricholemmoma may be of diagnostic value; it is not present in basal cell carcinoma.[165]

COWDEN'S DISEASE

Cowden's disease (Cowden's syndrome, multiple hamartoma and neoplasia syndrome) is a rare multisystem condition with autosomal dominant inheritance.[166–169] The eponym is the surname of the propositus of the report by Lloyd and Dennis in 1963.[170] The mucocutaneous features are the most constant findings. These include multiple tricholemmomas,[171] which are usually on the face, acral keratoses, palmar pits and oral fibromas.[167] They usually appear in late adolescence. The tumor of the follicular infundibulum may also arise in Cowden's disease.[135] There is also a high incidence of visceral hamartomas and tumors, including fibrocystic disease of the breast,[172] thyroid adenomas, ovarian cysts, subcutaneous lipomas and neuromas, gastrointestinal polyps,[173] and carcinomas of the breast and thyroid.[169] Also documented are eye changes,[174] skeletal abnormalities,[175] acromelanosis,[174] non-Hodgkin's lymphoma,[171] and carcinomas of the skin, tongue[176] and cervix. Impaired T-cell function has been reported in this syndrome.[175]

Cowden's disease involves a mutation in the *PTEN* gene on chromosome 10q23, a tumor suppressor gene with tyrosine phosphatase and tensin homology.[177,178] A similar genetic abnormality occurs in the Bannayan–Zonana syndrome, suggesting that they are different phenotypic expressions of the one disease.[179] The Bannayan–Zonana syndrome has also been reported as the Bannayan–Riley–Ruvalcaba syndrome[180,181] and the Ruvalcaba–Myre syndrome.[179] Macrocephaly is the hallmark of the Bannayan–Zonana syndrome. It may present with tricholemmomas and lipomas. No increased risk of malignancy has been documented. An association of Cowden's disease and Lhermitte–Duclos disease (cerebellar gangliocytoma) has been reported.[182]

Histopathology[183–186]

Most of the facial lesions are tricholemmomas or tumors of the follicular infundibulum. The tricholemmomas are cylindrical or lobular in configuration.[183] Sometimes the lesions keratinize with squamous eddies, resembling an inverted follicular keratosis. Non-specific verrucous acanthomas and lesions resembling digitate warts may also be present.[183]

The extrafacial lesions are mostly hyperkeratotic papillomas that resemble either verruca vulgaris, acrokeratosis verruciformis or a non-descript hyperkeratotic acanthoma.[184] This latter change may take the form of hyperplasia of the follicular infundibulum.[184] No evidence of a viral etiology has been found on electron microscopy,[175,187] or with immunoperoxidase studies.

Distinctive dermal fibromas (sclerotic fibromas) with interwoven fascicles of coarse collagen, sometimes showing marked hyalinization, are not uncommon in Cowden's disease.[184,188] They may have a plywood-like appearance histologically (see p. 922).

TRICHOLEMMAL CARCINOMA

Headington has defined tricholemmal carcinoma (tricholemmocarcinoma)[189] as a 'histologically invasive, cytologically atypical clear cell neoplasm of adnexal keratinocytes which is in continuity with the epidermis and/or follicular epithelium'.[5,190] Only a small number of cases purporting to be this entity have been reported.[5,189,191–197] The illustrations in some of the reported cases resemble invasive intraepidermal carcinoma, a tumor which often shows adnexal differentiation in its dermal component.[189,198] Ackerman believes that true tricholemmal carcinoma is a rare expression of basal cell carcinoma (tricholemmal carcinoma) and that what 'conventionally is called tricholemmal carcinoma is a clear-cell variant of squamous-cell carcinoma'.[199]

The tumors reported as tricholemmal carcinoma have usually arisen in the sun-exposed skin of the face and extremities of elderly patients. They are usually diagnosed clinically as a basal cell carcinoma. Their development in Cowden's disease is surprisingly rare.[200]

The hypercalcemia of malignancy was present in one extensive lesion that arose in a burn scar.[201]

Histopathology

The tumors are multilobulate, infiltrative growths connected to the epidermis and pilosebaceous structures and showing features reminiscent of the outer root sheath.[193] The lobules often show peripheral palisading, hyaline basement membranes and tricholemmal keratinization (Fig. 33.13).[193] A high mitotic rate is often present.[192,194]

The tumor reported as '**clear cell pilar sheath tumor of scalp**' had some histological similarities to the tricholemmal carcinoma. The reported case was composed of small nests of glycogen-containing clear cells infiltrating the dermis and subcutis.[202] There was no underlying cyst or evidence of tricholemmal keratinization.[202]

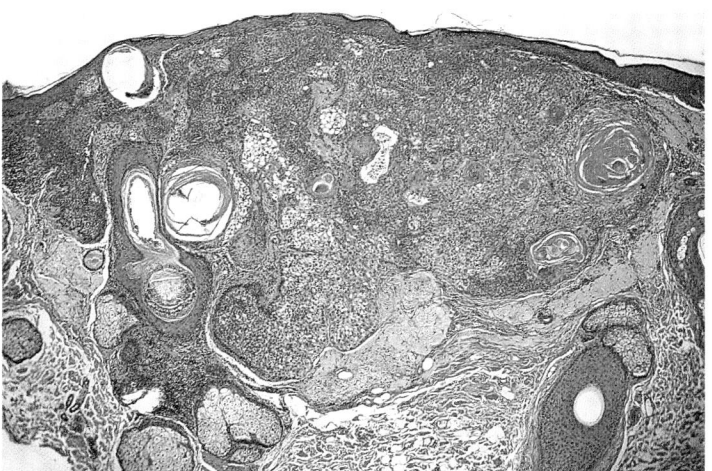

Fig. 33.13 **Tricholemmal carcinoma.** This tumor is focally infiltrative. Some clear cells are present near the base of the tumor. (H & E)

TUMORS WITH MATRICAL DIFFERENTIATION

In this group there is differentiation toward cells of the hair matrix and hair cortex and cells of the inner sheath. The prototype tumor is the pilomatrixoma. A rare malignant variant, the pilomatrix carcinoma, has also been described. Matrical differentiation can also be seen in other tumors:

- melanocytic matricoma (see below)
- epidermal cyst
- trichoblastoma[203]
- trichoepithelioma
- panfolliculoma
- basal cell carcinoma
- apocrine mixed tumor
- complex adnexal tumors.

PILOMATRIXOMA AND PILOMATRIX CARCINOMA

Pilomatrixoma (pilomatricoma, calcifying epithelioma of Malherbe), which accounts for almost 20% of pilar tumors, is a benign lesion with differentiation toward the matrix of the hair follicle.[204] It is found particularly on the head and neck and upper extremities.[6,205] About 60% develop in the first two decades of life.[206,207] They are mostly solitary, but multiple lesions – usually less than five in all – are sometimes found.[208–211] Some patients with multiple lesions have myotonic dystrophy.[6,212–214] They have also been reported in Turner's syndrome and with other abnormalities.[215,216] A familial occurrence is rarely noted.[217] A pilomatrixoma-like change is not uncommon in the epidermal cysts found in Gardner's syndrome.[218] This syndrome has also been described in a patient with multiple pilomatrixomas.[219]

Pilomatrixomas are firm nodules, approximately 0.5–3.0 cm in diameter. Giant forms have been recorded.[220] Overlying striae and anetodermic changes have been reported in a few cases.[221] Pilomatrixomas are usually slow growing, but rapid enlargement due to hemorrhage has been reported.[222] Rarely, there is sufficient melanin pigment in the lesion to be visible clinically.[223] These tumors have a variegated appearance macroscopically, with gray, white and brown areas on the cut surface. Small spicules of bone and minute thorny fragments may be discernible.[224] The consistency of the nodules depends on the amount of calcification and ossification.

Activating mutations in β-catenin, a constituent of the adherens junctions, have been found in sporadic pilomatrixomas.[225] A similar defect is also found in colonic carcinomas.[225]

Most tumors, even if inadequately excised, will not recur. However, local recurrence and aggressive forms have been documented.[226,227] More than 40 examples of a malignant variant, **pilomatrix carcinoma**, have been reported.[228–239] In one case the patient was only 8 years old,[240] while another had multiple pilomatrixomas.[241] In a further case, a pilomatrixoma had been treated at the same site.[242] A diagnosis of malignancy is usually based on cytological atypia and local aggressive behavior. In only some of these cases have metastases developed.[229,243–246] Wide local excision is the preferred treatment.[247]

Histopathology

The appearances vary according to the age of the lesion. Established lesions are sharply demarcated tumors in the lower dermis, extending quite often into the subcutis. There are masses of epithelial cells of various shapes, with an intervening connective tissue stroma containing blood vessels, a mixed inflammatory cell infiltrate, foreign-body giant cells, and sometimes hemosiderin, melanin, bone, and rarely amyloid.[5,248]

There are two basic cell types, basophilic cells and eosinophilic shadow cells (Fig. 33.14). The basophilic cells tend to be at the periphery of the cell islands and have little cytoplasm, indistinct cell borders, hyperchromatic nuclei and plentiful mitoses. They resemble the cells of a basal cell carcinoma. They are sometimes the predominant cell in lesions removed from elderly patients. The term 'proliferating pilomatricoma' has been proposed for this variant (Fig. 33.15).[249] The eosinophilic shadow cells are found toward the central areas of the cell masses. They have more cytoplasm and distinct cell borders, but no nuclear staining. These shadow (mummified) cells form from the basophilic cells, and the transition may be relatively abrupt or take place over several layers of cells (transitional cells). The intermediary cells develop progressively more eosinophilic cytoplasm and the nucleus becomes pyknotic. The mode of cell death has been reported as apoptotic[250,251] but it is more likely that the shadow cells represent terminal differentiation rather than apoptosis.[252,253]

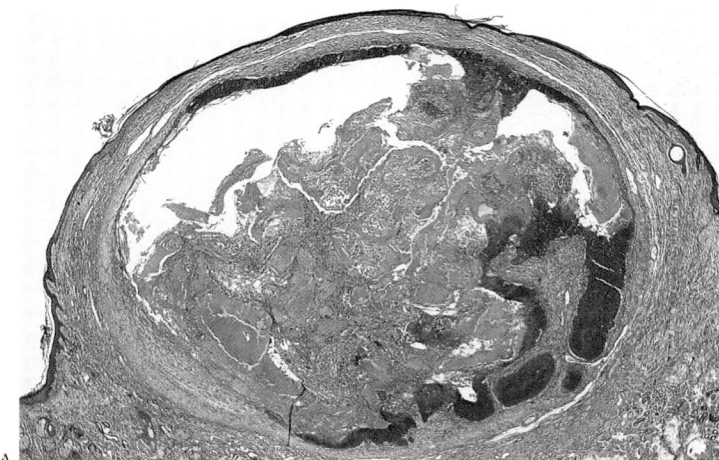

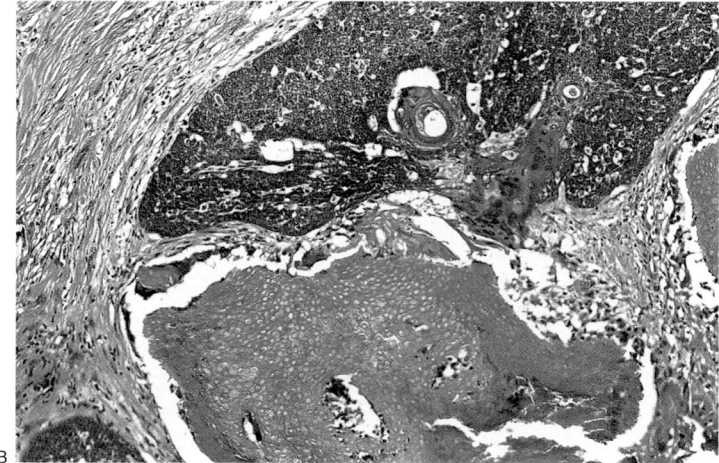

Fig. 33.14 **(A) Pilomatrixoma. (B)** There are two cell types present – nests of basaloid cells and shadow cells. The lesion is partly cystic. (H & E)

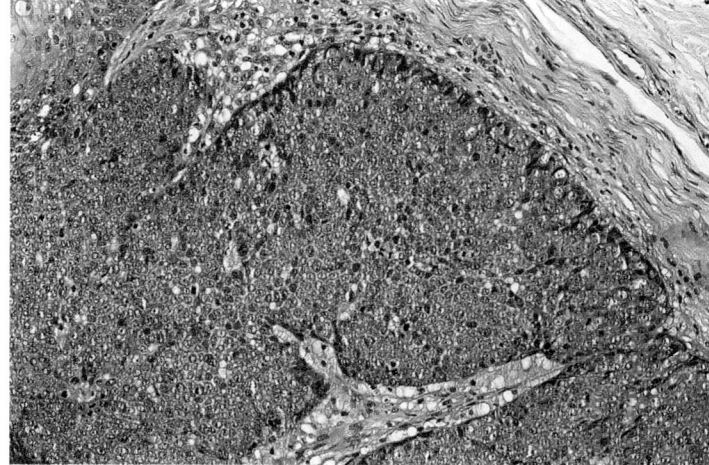

Fig. 33.15 **Pilomatrixoma of proliferating type.** Mitotic figures can be seen. (H & E)

Hyalinization of the cells, squamous change or disruption into amorphous debris may result.

Calcification occurs in more than two-thirds of the tumors and is usually in the shadow cells. Ossification of the stroma occurs in about 13%;[254]

hemosiderin is found in about 25% of cases;[255] melanin is present in nearly 20% of lesions and may be in the shadow cells as well as in the stroma.[255,256] Extramedullary hematopoiesis may occur adjacent to the spicules of bone.[257] Bone morphogenetic protein (BMP)-2, which plays an important role in ectopic bone formation, has been found in the shadow cells, suggesting that it may play a role in generating bone formation in pilomatrixomas.[258] Dendritic cells are sometimes seen among the basophilic cells in the cases with pigmentation.

In early lesions there is often a small cyst with basophilic cells in the wall.[259] Rarely, a pilomatrixoma appears to arise in an established epidermal cyst[260] or hair follicle.[261] Pilomatrixoma-like changes can also develop in the epidermal cysts in Gardner's syndrome (see above). As the lesion ages, the number of basophilic cells decreases as the process of mummification outstrips the proliferation of the basophilic cells. About 20% of lesions are fully keratinized (mummified) at the time of removal and have no basophilic cells remaining.[255,259] Transepidermal elimination of the tumor is a rare outcome.[206,262–266]

The immunohistochemical pattern indicates a tumor differentiating into both the hair cortex and outer root sheath.[267] The hard keratins hHa1, a2 and a5 are expressed in pilomatrixomas but not in other tumors of follicular origin.[268] Maturation to shadow cells is associated with a gradual loss of differentiation-specific hair keratins.[269] K15, found in trichoepitheliomas, some basal cell carcinomas and proliferating tricholemmal cysts, inter alia, is not found in pilomatrixomas.[59] The transitional cells show strong staining for involucrin[267] and *bcl-2*.[270]

Pilomatrix dysplasia was the term used for a histologically distinctive pattern seen in a patient with facial dysmorphism and follicular papules who was receiving four immunosuppressive drugs.[271] Hair follicles were dilated and contained hyperkeratotic and parakeratotic debris in place of hair shafts. There were hyperplastic areas of differentiation into hair matrix with cellular disorganization and loss of nuclear polarity.[271] A similar lesion has been reported as trichodysplasia spinulosa (see p. 462). The authors proposed a viral origin for their case.

Matricoma is the designation used by Ackerman and colleagues for a tumor with the same constituent cells as a pilomatrixoma but with a different silhouette.[8] The lesions are well circumscribed, not fundamentally cystic (although cystic areas can be present in some lobules), and composed of discrete aggregations. Some of these cases have probably been included with the 'proliferating pilomatrixoma' (see above).

Pilomatrix carcinoma (pilomatrical carcinoma, malignant pilomatrixoma) is a somewhat subjective diagnosis. The usual criteria are high mitotic activity, cytological atypia, locally aggressive behavior and, rarely, vascular or lymphatic invasion.[228,232] Sometimes, pilomatrixomas that are not malignant show a locally aggressive pattern of growth.[206] Some of the cases reported in the past as pilomatrix carcinoma may well have been 'proliferating pilomatricomas'.

Electron microscopy

The cells differentiate and keratinize in a manner analogous to the cells that form the cortex of the hair.[272] The fully developed shadow cells contain interlacing sworls of keratin that form a mantle around the nuclear remnants.[272]

MELANOCYTIC MATRICOMA

Melanocytic matricoma is a recently described entity that presents as a small circumscribed papule.[273] Despite some histological atypia, the two lesions did not recur after limited follow-up. A case seen by the author has not recurred either.

Histopathology

Melanocytic matricoma is a well-circumscribed dermal nodule composed of variably melanized, pleomorphic and mitotically active matrical and supramatrical cells with islands of shadow cells (Fig. 33.16).[273] The shadow cells are not always plentiful. Admixed with these cells are numerous dendritic melanocytes containing melanin pigment. There has been no discernible connection with the overlying epidermis or a hair follicle. Pigmented matrical cells are sometimes seen in normal hair follicles (Fig. 33.17).

TUMORS WITH PROMINENT PERIFOLLICULAR MESENCHYME

The two tumors in this category are characterized by a prominent component of perifollicular mesenchyme, but follicular elements are also present. The fibrofolliculoma and trichodiscoma, previously regarded as separate tumors, will be considered together, for the reasons listed below. The second tumor in this category, the neurofollicular hamartoma, has many features in common with the folliculosebaceous cystic hamartoma, regarded as an end-stage variant of trichofolliculoma, but the presence of a unique mesenchymal component justifies its continued existence as a discrete entity.

The *perifollicular fibroma* is a controversial entity of doubtful existence. This term has been used for angiofibromas[274,275] and fibrofolliculomas.[276,277] It should no longer be used.

FIBROFOLLICULOMA/TRICHODISCOMA

Although fibrofolliculomas and trichodiscomas are quite different at first glance, Ackerman and colleagues have presented evidence that they are different stages in the development of a single entity.[8] For this reason the composite designation fibrofolliculoma/trichodiscoma will be used here.

Both variants are found as asymptomatic skin-colored papules 1–3 mm in diameter, usually on the face. Other sites include the arms, trunk and thighs. A hair follicle may be present within the lesion. The lesions may be solitary or multiple with up to several hundred lesions present. Most cases develop in the third decade of life and persist thereafter.[8] A linear and a congenital annular variant have been described.[278,279] Multiple lesions may be found in pure form, sometimes with early onset and autosomal dominant inheritance,[280,281] or they may be associated with acrochordons — the Birt–Hogg–Dubé syndrome.[282–289] The Hornstein–Knickenberg syndrome appears to be the same syndrome, but confirmation of this will require genetic studies.[275,290] Both are autosomal dominant. On the basis of a histological study that showed that the acrochordons were also fibrofolliculoma/trichodiscoma, the existence of the Birt–Hogg–Dubé syndrome has been called in to question.[291] Colonic polyps and renal tumors have been associated with this syndrome.[292]

The origin of these tumors is uncertain. Ackerman and colleagues regard these tumors as hamartomas, but not one related to the hair disk (Haarscheibe), as was originally proposed for trichodiscoma.[8] The hair disk, a specialized component of the perifollicular mesenchyme, is a richly vascular dermal pad which serves as a slowly adapting mechanoreceptor.[280,293,294]

Histopathology

The *fibrofolliculoma* end of the spectrum consists of cords and strands of epithelial cells, 2–4 cells thick, radiating from a follicular structure with infundibular features. This may be dilated and contain keratin. The strands may anastomose or rejoin the infundibulum at several points. One or more sebocytes may be seen within the epithelial cords. They may form tiny

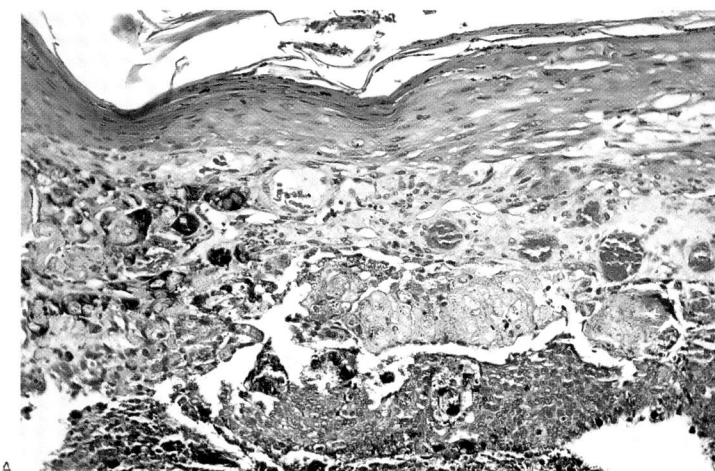
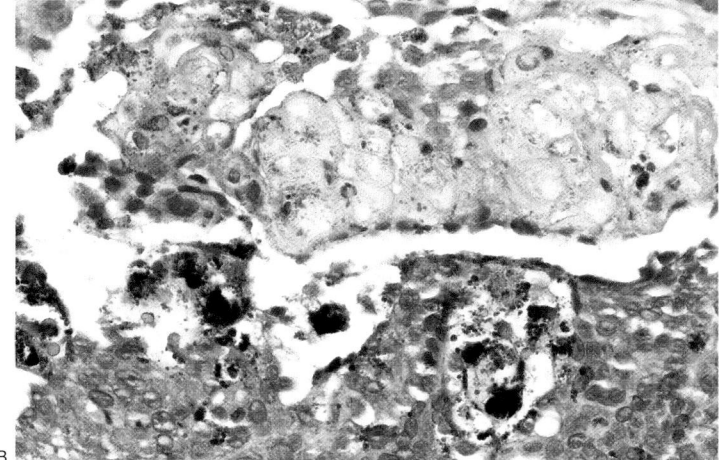

Fig. 33.16 **(A) Melanocytic matricoma. (B)** Matrical cells and atypical melanocytic cells are present. (H & E)

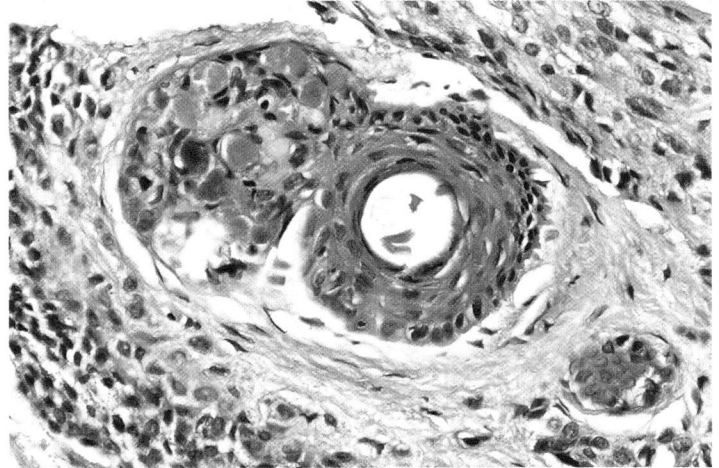

Fig. 33.17 **Pigmented matrical cells in a normal hair follicle.** (H & E)

lobules. Sebaceous ducts may also be present. The term '*mantleoma*' has also been used for these tumors. Around the epithelial cords there is a well-circumscribed proliferation of loose connective tissue composed of fine fibers with some intervening mucin. Elastic fibers are scant or absent.

The *trichodiscoma* component is usually a well-demarcated and non-encapsulated tumor, which often has a folliculosebaceous collarette of variable maturity. Areas resembling fibrofolliculoma may be seen, particularly at the periphery. Trichodiscomas are composed of fascicles of loose, finely fibrillar connective tissue with intervening mucinous ground substance (Fig. 33.18). There is a moderate increase in fibroblasts, with occasional stellate forms. Elastic fibers are sparse or absent. There are prominent small vessels, some of which are telangiectatic. Sometimes, blood vessels with a concentric arrangement of PAS-positive collagen, forming a thickened wall, have been present toward the lower edge of the tumor. The term 'perivascular fibroma' has been used for these changes.[295] Nerve fibers have been described at the periphery of the lesions, and also extending into the base.

Multiple giant tumors with the appearances of a trichodiscoma have been reported as '**giant fibromyxoid tumors of the adventitial dermis**'.

Electron microscopy

Trichodiscomas have shown deposits of fibrillar–amorphous material between the collagen bundles.[293] The significance of this material is uncertain. Banded structures and a Merkel cell–neurite complex in the basal layer of the epidermis have also been noted, although Merkel cells are not seen in the dermis.[293]

NEUROFOLLICULAR HAMARTOMA

The neurofollicular hamartoma is a rare tumor found on the face, usually near the nose. It presents as a pale papule, usually solitary, that measures 3–7 mm in diameter.[296–299]

Histopathology

The lesion consists of hyperplastic pilosebaceous units with an intervening stroma of spindle cells arranged in broad, haphazard fascicles. The stroma has features of both an angiofibroma and a neurofibroma. It also resembles a trichodiscoma.

It has been suggested that the neurofollicular hamartoma, trichodiscoma and fibrofolliculoma are part of the same spectrum of hamartomas.[296] The folliculosebaceous cystic hamartoma is closely related (see p. 873).[300]

Immunohistochemistry shows scattered cells that are positive for S100 and factor XIIIa. Diffuse staining for S100 has also been reported.[299] Most of the connective tissue cells are positive for vimentin.[296]

Sebaceous tumors

Sebaceous tumors are relatively uncommon tumors of the skin. They are derived from the sebaceous gland, which begins its development as a bulge or collar at the junction of the infundibulum and isthmus of the hair follicle. Early in life, small cords of basaloid cells extend downward on either side of the follicle, forming the so-called 'mantle'. Maturation of the mantle occurs slowly in childhood with the accumulation of lipid in some of the cells, forming sebocytes at the base of the mantle. Sebocytes increase in number and size such that a fully developed sebaceous lobule is present by puberty. Mantles are best seen around vellus follicles on the face, but they also develop in association with terminal follicles. Later in life, the sebaceous glands undergo progressive involution so that mantles are again seen, this time as vestiges. Initially, Steffen and Ackerman suggested that sebaceous glands had several cycles of growth, involution and rest, independent of the cycle of the hair follicle.[301] Ackerman has since modfied this view by suggesting that the cycle occurs 'but twice in a lifetime (involution early in infancy, evolution at puberty, and involution again at menopause)'.[302] The latest theory may not be absolute as one occasionally sees a mantle in mid-adult life.

The following categories of sebaceous tumors will be considered:

- ectopic sebaceous glands
- hamartomas and hyperplasias of sebaceous glands
- benign sebaceous tumors
- malignant sebaceous tumors
- tumors with focal sebaceous differentiation.

ECTOPIC SEBACEOUS GLANDS

FORDYCE'S SPOTS AND RELATED ECTOPIAS

Sebaceous glands are usually found in association with hair follicles, the so-called 'pilosebaceous unit'. Ectopic sebaceous glands without attached follicles (Fig. 33.19) may be found as tiny yellow papules near mucocutaneous junctions, particularly the upper lip, and in the buccal mucosa (*Fordyce's spots*).[204] They may also be found in the areolae of the breasts, where they are known as *Montgomery's tubercles*. They are said to be restricted to the

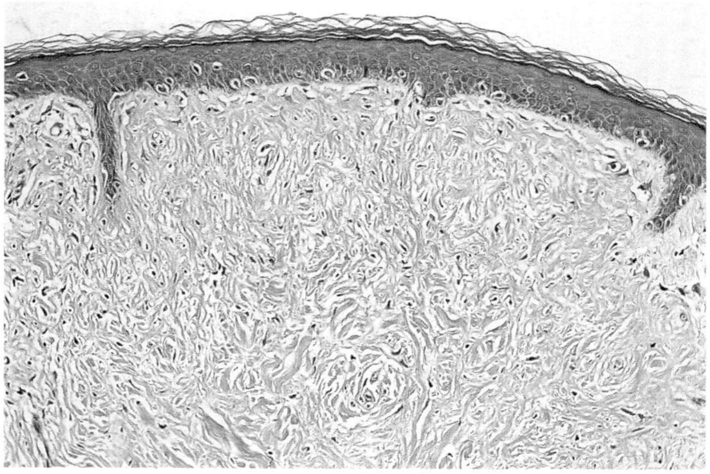

Fig. 33.18 **Trichodiscoma.** A poorly defined angiofibroma-like proliferation is present in the upper dermis. (H & E)

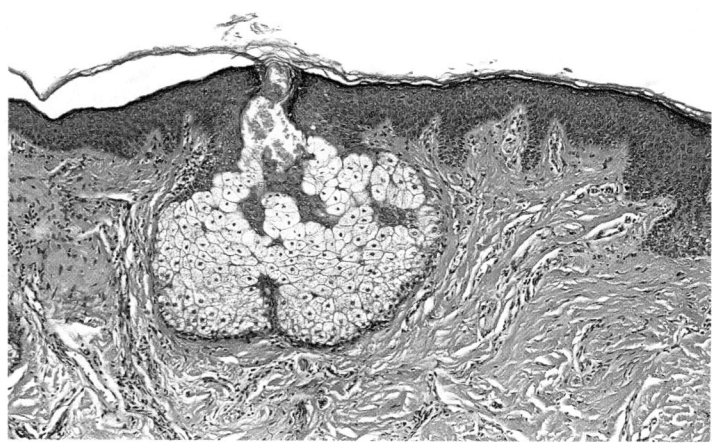

Fig. 33.19 **Montgomery's tubercle.** An ectopic sebaceous gland opens directly onto the surface. (H & E)

female breast, but the author has seen a case from a male breast. Like Fordyce's spots, the sebaceous gland in a Montgomery's tubercle opens directly onto the surface.

Ectopic sebaceous glands can also be found on the penis,[303,304] labia minora and, very rarely, in the esophagus and vagina.[305]

HAMARTOMAS AND HYPERPLASIAS

By far the most common abnormality of the sebaceous gland is sebaceous hyperplasia. The hamartomas are quite uncommon and include folliculosebaceous cystic hamartoma and steatocystoma. Organoid nevus (nevus sebaceus) involves other appendageal components and is considered with the complex adnexal tumors (see p. 899).

FOLLICULOSEBACEOUS CYSTIC HAMARTOMA

The folliculosebaceous cystic hamartoma is a distinctive hamartoma composed of folliculosebaceous structures surrounded by a stroma consisting of various mesenchymal components.[300,306–309] It presents as a solitary papule or nodule 0.5–2 cm or more in diameter, usually on the face.[310] Lesions are usually removed in adulthood, although they have often been present for many years. Schulz and Hartschuh have presented convincing evidence that this lesion is a trichofolliculoma at its very late stage with the follicular structures in a state of involution, corresponding to the normal hair cycle.[21] Others agree with this concept but suggest the designation sebofolliculomas as a pole of the spectrum of tricho-sebo-folliculoma.[22] This entity is discussed here because the sebaceous elements are usually the most prominent feature.

Histopathology

The lesion is composed of infundibular structures, sometimes cystic, with numerous radiating sebaceous lobules. Occasional rudimentary hair structures and even apocrine glands may be present. The pilosebaceous units are embedded in a mesenchymal stroma composed of variable proportions of fibrous, adipose, vascular and neural tissue. There are usually spindle-shaped cells in the stroma, and some of these stain for CD34 or factor XIIIa.[309]

The case reported with a prominent neural component in the stroma has some features in common with the neurofollicular hamartoma (see p. 872), although this latter entity lacks the haphazard cystic infundibular structures.[300] The morphologically related sebaceous trichofolliculoma (see p. 860) lacks a mesenchymal stromal component.

SEBACEOUS HYPERPLASIA

Sebaceous hyperplasia occurs as asymptomatic, solitary or multiple yellowish papules, often umbilicated, on the forehead and cheeks of elderly, and sometimes younger, individuals.[311–314] Clinically it may mimic basal cell carcinoma. Rare variants include a 'giant' form,[315,316] a linear or zosteriform arrangement,[317] a diffuse form,[318] a familial occurrence[319,320] and involvement of the areola[321,322] or the vulva.[323] Sebaceous hyperplasia is seen in heart transplant recipients. It is thought to be related to the process of dysplastic epithelial proliferation in transplant recipients and not to the effects of cyclosporine.[324] It has also been seen in a bone marrow recipient; cyclosporine was implicated in this case.[325]

Juxtaclavicular beaded lines – tiny papules arranged in closely placed parallel rows, resembling 'strands of beads' – are a variant of sebaceous gland hyperplasia.[326–328] They are said to be arranged along skin tension lines and they may be seen at other sites, such as the face[329] and penis.[330]

The etiopathogenesis of sebaceous hyperplasia is unknown. Interestingly, sebaceous hyperplasia can be produced in rats by the topical application of Citrol (3,7-dimethyl-2,6-octadienol), a chemical used in foods as a flavoring agent.[331]

Histopathology

Large, mature sebaceous lobules are grouped around a central dilated duct, which is usually filled with debris, bacteria and occasionally a vellus hair. The lobules usually lack the indentations by fibrous septa that characterize the normal gland (Fig. 33.20). The sebocytes are smaller than usual and there are more basal cells per unit basement membrane length than in normal glands. Autoradiographic studies have shown a lower labeling index.[332] Sebaceous hyperplasia may be a clue to an underlying dermatofibroma. In shallow shave biopsies, sebaceous glands may be the most conspicuous feature.[333]

In **juxtaclavicular beaded lines** there may be isolated sebaceous lobules in the upper dermis, not obviously connected with hair follicles.[326]

Although sebaceous glands are prominent in rhinophyma, the sebaceous lobules are not as well defined and grouped as in sebaceous hyperplasia.

STEATOCYSTOMA

The steatocystoma is a cystic structure lined by epithelium resembling the sebaceous duct (Fig. 33.21). Sebaceous lobules and individual sebaceous cells are present within the lining epithelium. Steatocystoma has been considered in detail with other cysts (see p. 508).

BENIGN SEBACEOUS TUMORS

The four tumors in this category are sebaceous adenoma, sebaceoma, mantleoma and superficial epithelioma with sebaceous differentiation, although the latter entity is of doubtful validity. As sebaceous tumors are an important component of the Muir–Torre syndrome, it is considered here also.

SEBACEOUS ADENOMA

The sebaceous adenoma is an uncommon benign tumor which usually presents as a slowly growing, pink or flesh-colored solitary nodule, predominantly on

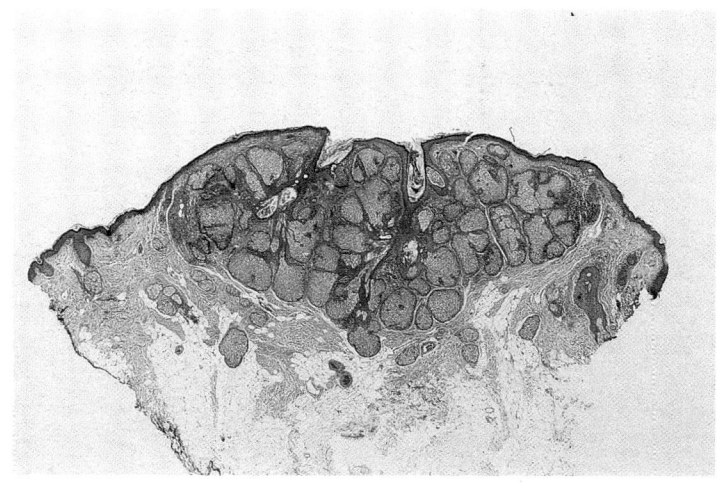

Fig. 33.20 **Sebaceous gland hyperplasia.** Lobules of enlarged, mature sebaceous glands are attached to a central hair follicle. (H & E)

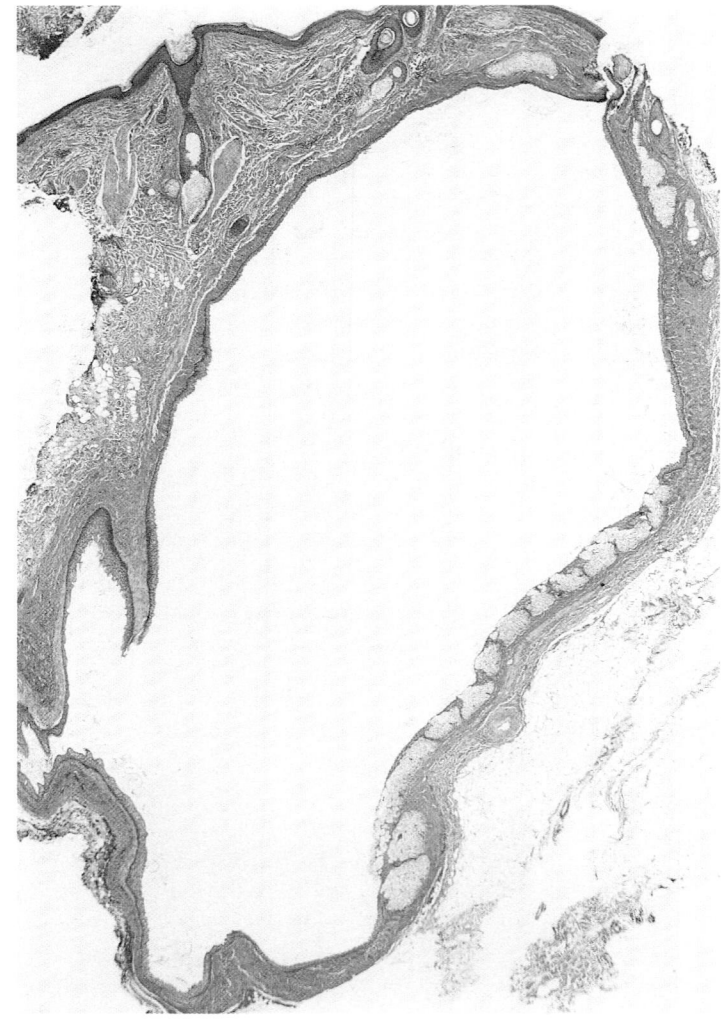

Fig. 33.21 **Steatocystoma.** There are mature sebaceous glands in the wall of a cyst. (H & E)

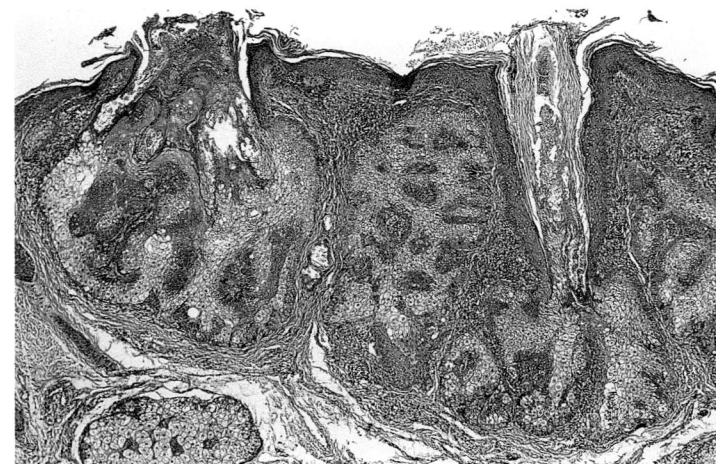

Fig. 33.22 **Sebaceous adenoma.** The sebaceous lobules have a peripheral layer of smaller basaloid cells. (H & E)

the head and neck of older individuals.[334] Rarely, it may involve the buccal mucosa.[335] Sebaceous adenomas are usually about 0.5 cm in diameter but larger variants, up to 9 cm in diameter, can develop. Occasionally they ulcerate and bleed or become tender. Sebaceous adenomas, either solitary or multiple, may be associated with visceral cancer, usually of the gastrointestinal tract – the Muir–Torre syndrome (see below).

Ackerman has been suggesting for the last few years that sebaceous adenoma is really a carcinoma.[336] However, the evidence for this is not convincing.

Histopathology[334]

The tumor is composed of multiple sharply circumscribed sebaceous lobules separated by compressed connective tissue septa. It is usually centered on the mid dermis, but may adjoin the epidermis or exhibit multiple openings on to the skin surface, with partial replacement of the epidermis by basaloid epithelium showing sebaceous differentiation (Fig. 33.22). The sebaceous lobules have a peripheral germinative layer of small cells, with mature sebaceous cells centrally and transitional forms in between. This maturation is not as orderly or as well developed as in normal sebaceous glands. Nevertheless, mature cells still outnumber the darker germinative cells.[204] There is variable central holocrine degeneration, with granular debris scattered in the area of cystic change. Cystic sebaceous tumors are now regarded as a marker for the mismatch repair-deficient subtype of the Muir–Torre syndrome. The connective tissue stroma may contain a patchy chronic inflammatory cell infiltrate.

An overlying cutaneous horn is a rare occurrence.[337]

MUIR–TORRE SYNDROME

Muir–Torre syndrome, the first examples of which were reported in 1967,[338] is characterized by the development of sebaceous tumors, often multiple, in association with visceral neoplasms, usually gastrointestinal carcinomas.[339–347] Keratoacanthomas, epidermal cysts and colonic polyps may also be present. The sebaceous tumors are sometimes difficult to classify,[348] but they most resemble either sebaceous adenoma or sebaceoma, and occasionally sebaceous carcinomas.[349] The cutaneous tumors may precede or follow the first direct manifestation of the visceral cancer, and they may occur sporadically in other family members. The visceral tumor is usually of the gastrointestinal tract, particularly adenocarcinoma or polyps of the large bowel, but other sites, such as the larynx, the genitourinary system in men,[350] and the ovary and uterus may be involved.[351] Lymphoma has been reported. The visceral tumors may behave in a less aggressive fashion than would be expected from the histology.[339,352,353] This is particularly so for tumors displaying widespread microsatellite instability (MSI).[353] Detection of MSI in cutaneous tumors of various types may form the basis of a non-invasive screening technique for hereditary non-polyposis colon syndrome, of which the Muir–Torre syndrome is regarded as a variant.[354,355]

The Muir–Torre syndrome is inherited as an autosomal dominant trait. Mutations in one of the DNA mismatch repair genes *hMLH1* and *hMSH2* have been found in some patients.[356,357] Their sebaceous tumors may show widespread microsatellite instability.[357] It has been suggested that treatment with isotretinoin and interferon-α2A can prevent tumor development.[347]

Histopathology[339,348]

The sebaceous tumors resemble to varying degrees those already described. Often they appear 'unique' and difficult to classify.[348] There may be solid sheets of basaloid cells in some lobules, or an intermingling of these cells and sebaceous cells without any orderly maturation. It has been suggested that these atypical features are predictive of malignant transformation, if not completely removed.[358] Sometimes the tumors resemble a basal cell carcinoma, but with focal sebaceous differentiation. Mucinous and cystic areas may be present (Fig. 33.23). Cystic lesions are an important component of this syndrome (see above).[359] Other tumors may connect with the surface and have a central debris-filled crater resembling, in part, a keratoacanthoma.

The cells express epithelial membrane antigen and nuclear androgen receptor.[360]

SEBACEOMA

The term 'sebaceoma' was coined by Ackerman for a distinctive sebaceous tumor,[361] examples of which have been reported in the past as basal cell carcinoma with sebaceous differentiation[334] or sebaceous epithelioma.[204,362] These tumors are usually solitary, yellowish papulonodules on the face or scalp, but they are sometimes multiple, particularly in the Muir–Torre syndrome (see above), or associated with organoid nevi.[334] They grow slowly and do not usually recur after treatment.

Histopathology[334,361]
There are multiple nests of basaloid cells with a random admixture of sebaceous cells, either solitary or in clusters (Fig. 33.24). The tumor is centered on the upper and mid dermis, but some nests may be continuous with the basal layer of the epidermis. The small basaloid cells of the tumor

outnumber the mature sebaceous component. Cysts and duct-like structures containing the debris of holocrine degeneration may be present.[362] There are scattered mitoses, but the tumor lacks the atypia of sebaceous carcinoma.

The sebaceoma can exhibit an amazing diversity of patterns.[301] Sebocytes and sebaceous ducts may be plentiful or scarce, and the sebocytes may show variable vacuolation. Adenoid, reticulated, cribriform, cystic and cornified areas may be present.[363,364] Sometimes, areas resembling a seborrheic keratosis with sebaceous differentiation may be present.[365] Furthermore, a sebaceoma has been reported arising in association with a seborrheic keratosis.[366] It has been suggested that some of the cystic cases of sebaceoma pictured in Steffen and Ackerman's book[301] are really sebocrine adenomas (see p. 901).[367]

There exist tumors with close morphological resemblance to basal cell carcinoma which may show focal sebaceous differentiation. Such tumors are best classified as basal cell carcinomas with sebaceous differentiation. It is acknowledged that there is some overlap of this tumor with what has been designated sebaceoma.[361]

Rare variants have been reported with sweat gland differentiation in part of the lesion.[368]

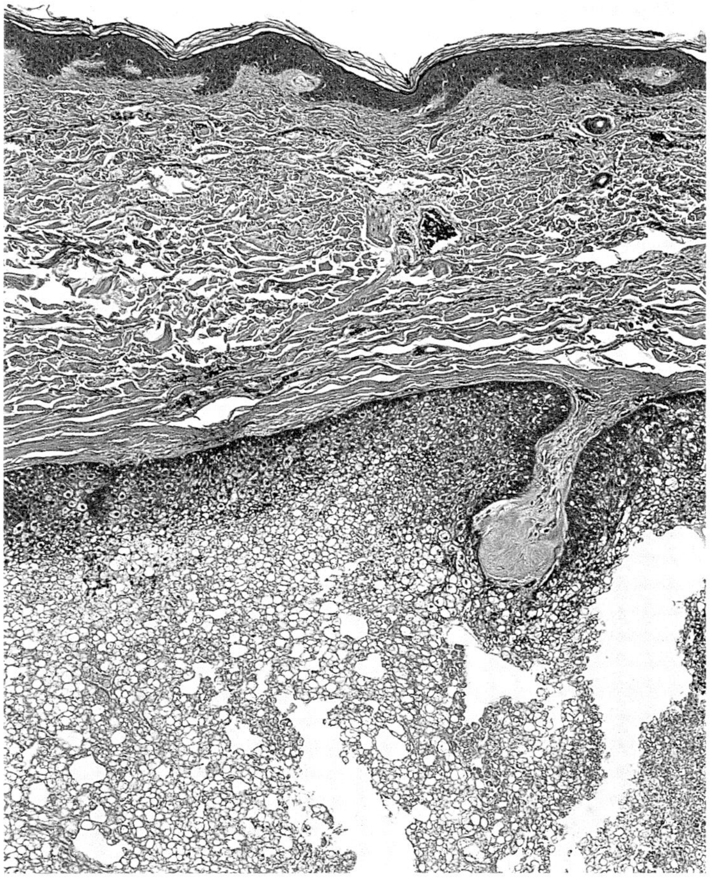

SUPERFICIAL EPITHELIOMA WITH SEBACEOUS DIFFERENTIATION

The term 'superficial epithelioma with sebaceous differentiation' has been applied to a rare tumor with a predilection for the face of elderly individuals. It is usually solitary,[369] but multiple papules have been recorded.[370] It behaves in a benign fashion.

Only one further case with features similar to earlier descriptions has been reported in recent times.[371] It had areas showing features of a sebaceous adenoma, prompting Sánchez Yus and colleagues to reinforce their view that the term 'sebomatricoma' should be adopted for all benign sebaceous neoplasms, which they believe form a continuum.[372,373] Similar cases have been reported by Steffen and Ackerman as a **reticulated acanthoma with sebaceous differentiation**.[301]

Histopathology
The tumor is characterized by a superficial plate-like proliferation of basaloid to squamoid cells with broad attachments to the overlying epidermis.[369]

Fig. 33.23 **Cystic sebaceous adenoma** in a patient with Muir–Torre syndrome. (H & E)

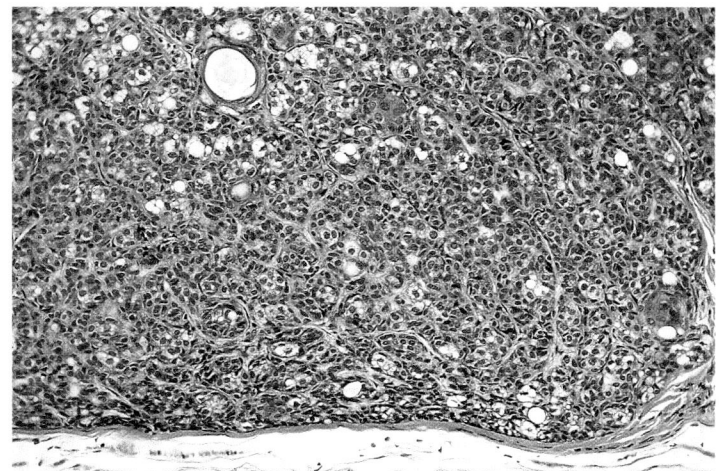

Fig. 33.24 **Sebaceoma.** Sheets of basaloid cells are randomly admixed with small sebocytes and sebaceous ducts. (H & E)

Clusters of mature sebaceous cells are present within the tumor. The low-power pattern is somewhat analogous to that seen in basaloid follicular hamartoma, an entity that lacks sebaceous differentiation.[374]

MANTLEOMA

The mantleoma is a tumor of the sebaceous mantle, a neglected structure which gives rise to sebaceous glands. The mantle is composed of cords of basaloid cells that hang downwards from the side of the follicular infundibulum like a skirt. Unfortunately, the term 'mantleoma' has been used for two different lesions. It has been applied by Steffen to a small, incidental tumor on the face, and described below.[375] It was also used in the book by Steffen and Ackerman for what is often called a fibrofolliculoma.[301]

Histopathology

The mantleoma consists of cords and columns of undifferentiated cells that radiate from the infundibulum of a hair follicle. The cords may interweave into a retiform pattern. Varying degrees of vacuolization of the cells, representing sebocyte formation, can be seen. Some sebaceous ductal structures may be present.[375]

The **folliculocentric basaloid proliferation** of Leshin and White is a hyperplasia of mantle epithelium that may become so pronounced that the term 'mantleoma' would be appropriate (Fig. 33.25). It would probably be best to regard the two as variants of the same lesion. It may be confused with basal cell carcinomas, particularly on frozen section.

MALIGNANT SEBACEOUS TUMORS

Although some tumors, particularly basal cell carcinomas, may show focal sebaceous differentiation, the sebaceous carcinoma is the only 'pure' tumor in this category.

SEBACEOUS CARCINOMA

Sebaceous carcinomas have traditionally been considered in two groups: those arising in the ocular adnexa, particularly the meibomian glands and glands of Zeiss, and tumors arising in extraocular sites.[376,377] The latter are uncommon and are usually found as yellow-tan firm nodules, often ulcerated, measuring 1–4 cm or more in diameter. They are found particularly on the head and neck of elderly patients. Rare sites include the foot,[378] labia[334,379] and penis.[380]

Those arising in the ocular adnexa are more common and comprise 1% of all eyelid neoplasms. They have a slight female preponderance and tend to involve the upper eyelid more than the lower.[381,382] They often masquerade clinically as a chalazion, delaying effective treatment. Mohs micrographic surgery has been used with excellent results.[383] Rarely, there is a history of radiation to the area.[382] Up to one-third develop lymph node metastases, usually to the preauricular and cervical nodes, and there is a 20% 5-year mortality. Recently, extraocular cases with nodal and even visceral metastases have been reported, leading the authors to question the notion that extraocular tumors are less aggressive than sebaceous carcinomas of the eyelid.[380,384]

Rarely, sebaceous carcinomas are associated with the Muir–Torre syndrome (see above),[376] organ transplant recipients,[385] or a rhinophyma.[386]

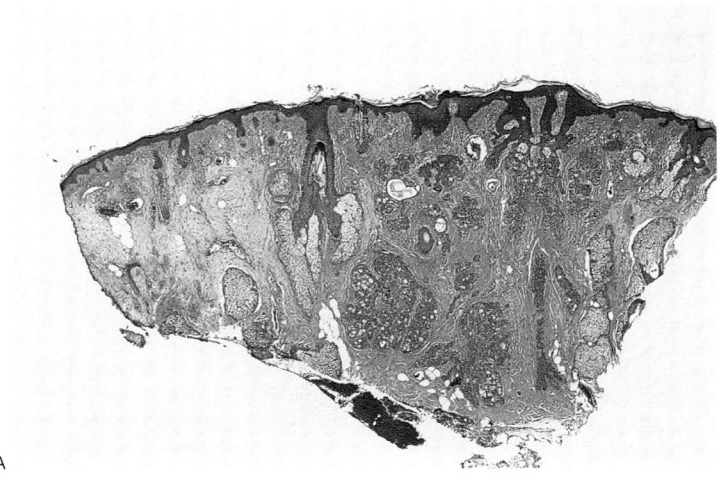

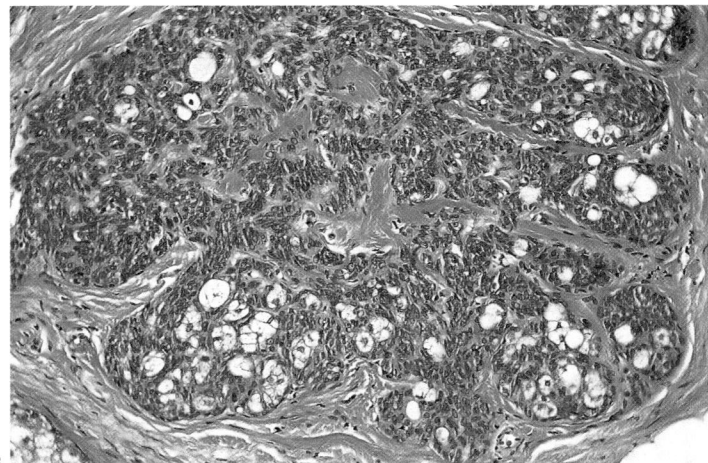

Fig. 33.25 **(A) Mantleoma** (folliculocentric basaloid proliferation). **(B)** This is a very large lesion found incidentally in the re-excision specimen of a previously removed melanoma. Basaloid cells, sebocytes and ducts are present. (H & E)

Histopathology[334,382]

The tumor is composed of lobules or sheets of cells separated by a fibrovascular stroma. The cells extend deeply and often involve the subcutaneous tissue and even the underlying muscle. There is infiltration at the edges. The cells show variable sebaceous differentiation, manifest as finely vacuolated or foamy rather than clear cytoplasm (Fig. 33.26). There is usually more differentiation at the center of the nests. The nuclei are large, with large nucleoli. There are scattered mitoses. Smaller basaloid cells and cells resembling those in a squamous cell carcinoma may be present; even focal keratinization does not negate the diagnosis. Focal necrosis is not uncommon and this may have a 'comedo-like' pattern. Sometimes pseudoglandular formation occurs. The vacuolated cells show abundant lipid if a frozen section is stained with oil red O or Sudan black. There may be a very small amount of PAS-positive diastase-resistant material in some cells. Focal apocrine differentiation is sometimes present.[387] This is not surprising in view of the common embryological origin of the folliculosebaceous–apocrine unit.

The periocular lesions often show a pagetoid or, less commonly, a carcinoma-in-situ change in the overlying conjunctiva or epidermis of the eyelid (Fig. 33.27).[381,382] Such changes are not usually seen in extraocular cases. The presence of such a change above extraocular tumors should prompt reassessment of the lesion in case it is invasive Bowen's disease, which may rarely mimic sebaceous carcinoma.[388]

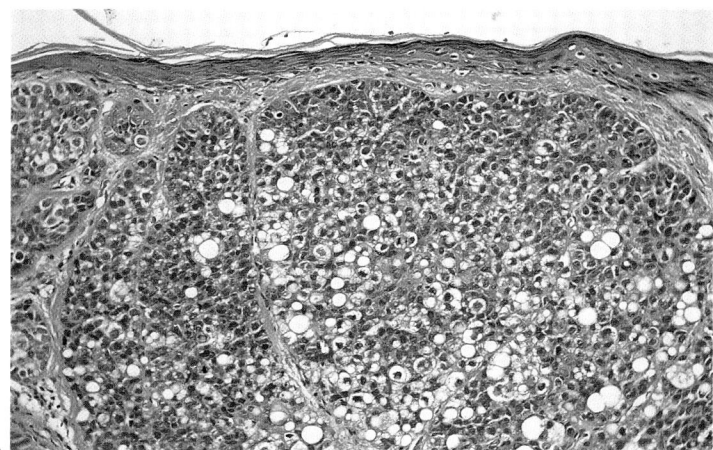

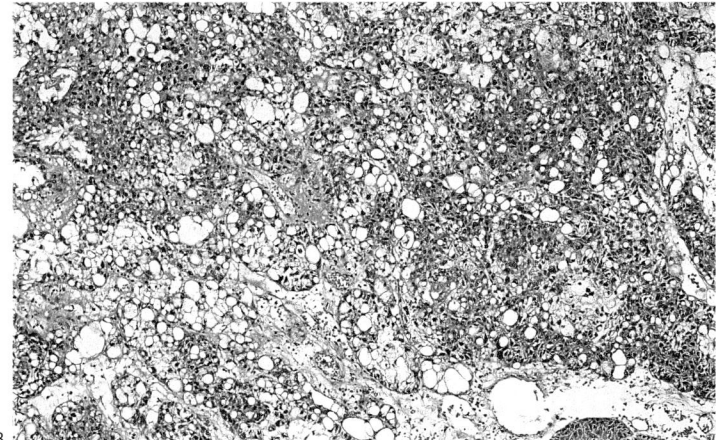

Fig. 33.26 (A) Sebaceous carcinoma. (B) Vacuolated sebaceous cells are present. (H & E)

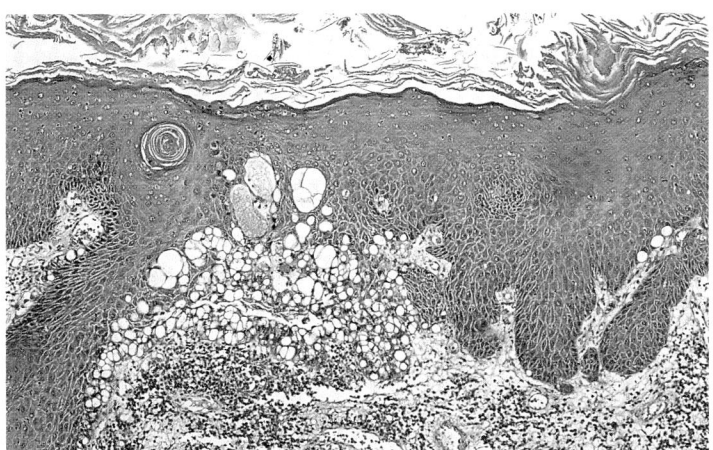

Fig. 33.27 Sebaceous carcinoma. There is early epidermotropism. (H & E)

Adverse prognostic features for tumors of the ocular adnexa include vascular and lymphatic invasion, orbital extension, poor differentiation, an infiltrative growth pattern and large tumor size.[382]

Immunohistochemically, the tumor cells show positive reactions for epithelial membrane antigen (EMA) and androgen receptor (AR), but not for carcinoembryonic antigen (CEA), S100 protein or gross cystic disease fluid protein-15 (GCDFP).[389] In one report, two cases reacted with CD36.[390] It

should be noted that EMA staining is often absent in poorly differentiated tumors but nuclear staining for AR is present, making it the more reliable marker.[360] Approximately 60% of basal cell carcinomas show focal positivity for AR.[360] Ocular sebaceous carcinomas contain cytokeratin 7 (CK7) but ocular basal cell carcinomas and squamous cell carcinomas do not.[391,392]

Electron microscopy
The tumor cells contain cytoplasmic lipid droplets and tonofilaments that insert into well-formed desmosomes.[380,381]

TUMORS WITH FOCAL SEBACEOUS DIFFERENTIATION

This category is included for completeness so that tumors considered in other sections of this book can be grouped together. Sebaceous differentiation or sebaceous glands can be seen in:

- basal cell carcinoma
- squamous cell carcinoma
- seborrheic keratosis
- verruca vulgaris
- inverted follicular keratosis
- dermatofibroma
- reticulated acanthoma
- sebocrine adenoma.

The occurrence of basal cell carcinomas with sebaceous differentiation is mentioned above. Sebaceous differentiation is very rare in squamous cell carcinomas, and such cases must be distinguished from sebaceous carcinomas and from invasive Bowen's disease.

The *seborrheic keratosis with sebaceous differentiation* usually has recognizable areas of seborrheic keratosis with admixed sebocytes occurring in clusters or as single cells. Microcysts with variable resemblance to sebaceous ducts are usually present.[301] They are much smaller than the horn cysts of a seborrheic keratosis. There is some overlap with apocrine poroma with sebaceous differentiation.[393]

The *verruca vulgaris with sebaceous differentiation* is a rare entity. Sometimes, focal apocrine differentiation is also present. Several of the cases pictured in the excellent book by Steffen and Ackerman (and currently under revision)[301] would be regarded by many as examples of *inverted follicular keratosis*. The induction of folliculosebaceous units by *dermatofibromas* is mentioned elsewhere (see p. 932). The *reticulated acanthoma with sebaceous differentiation* is the term used by Steffen and Ackerman for what others have called superficial epithelioma with sebaceous differentiation (see p. 875). Sebocrine adenoma is discussed with the complex adnexal tumors (see p. 901).

Apocrine tumors

Normal apocrine glands
Apocrine glands, which are derived from the folliculosebaceous–apocrine germ, are restricted to the axillae, anogenital and inguinal regions, the periumbilical and periareolar regions and, rarely, the face and scalp. Specialized apocrine glands are found on the eyelids (the glands of Moll) and

in the auditory canal (ceruminous glands). The breast is sometimes regarded as a modified apocrine gland.

Apocrine glands are composed of a secretory coil in the lower dermis and subcutis, a straight ductal component which is indistinguishable from the eccrine duct, and a terminal intra-infundibular duct which opens into the follicular infundibulum. A conspicuous feature of apocrine secretory cells is their 'decapitation' mode of secretion whereby an apical cap, formed at the luminal border of the apocrine cells, separates off from the cell and is discharged into the lumen. Apocrine secretions produce a characteristic odor.[394]

Alternate classification

Despite the relative paucity of apocrine glands in comparison with the ubiquitous eccrine gland, found everywhere in the skin, it would seem that many tumors arising in non-apocrine areas, and formerly regarded as being of eccrine origin, are probably apocrine in type. This reclassification of some tumors has taken place as a consequence of the identification of decapitation secretion, either as a regular or occasional feature, and the presence of, or association with, cells or other tumors showing follicular and/or sebaceous differentiation. The rationale is their common embryological origin from the folliculo-sebaceous apocrine germ.

Using these and other criteria, Requena, Kiryu and Ackerman, in a superbly illustrated book, have reclassified as apocrine the following tumors which were previously regarded as being of eccrine type:[395]

- eccrine hidrocystoma
- papillary eccrine adenoma
- hidradenoma (nodular, cystic)
- cylindroma
- spiradenoma
- syringoma
- poromas (some)
- malignant variants of the above
- microcystic adnexal carcinoma
- mucinous carcinoma
- signet-ring cell carcinoma
- adenoid cystic carcinoma.

This classification is likely to be regarded in some centers as controversial. Cynics will argue (a) does it matter whether they are called eccrine or apocrine, particularly when the ducts of either gland are indistinguishable, and (b) can the folliculosebaceous–apocrine germ be so unstable that it produces apocrine tumors at sites not normally frequented by apocrine glands? Immunohistochemical markers such as lysozyme, Leu M1 and gross cystic disease fluid protein-15 (GCDFP-15, AP-15, Brst-2)[396] are no longer regarded as being of much assistance in this debate.[397]

Of interest are the results obtained using a novel monoclonal antibody, IKH-4, which stains the eccrine secretory coil, but not the apocrine secretory segment.[398] Unfortunately, specific markers have a habit in dermatopathology of becoming less specific with time, and subsequent studies do not invariably confirm the initial ones. Notwithstanding these reservations, the study mentioned found staining that would support an eccrine origin for hidradenoma, poroma, spiradenoma, cylindroma, syringoma and eccrine carcinoma and the occurrence of an eccrine variant of hidrocystoma, papillary adenoma and syringocystadenoma papilliferum.[398] These tumors have also stained with the eccrine gland-associated monoclonal antibodies EKH-5 and EKH-6.[398]

In the light of these studies, it is not proposed to make major changes from the traditional subdivision of eccrine and apocrine tumors.

CYSTS AND HAMARTOMAS

Three entities will be considered in this category:

- apocrine nevus
- apocrine hidrocystoma (apocrine gland cyst)
- syringocystadenoma papilliferum.

APOCRINE NEVUS

The apocrine nevus is a rare tumor composed of increased numbers of mature apocrine glands.[399–402] It has been reported on the upper chest and in the axilla; more often, it is an element of an organoid nevus (nevus sebaceus). The lesion reported as congenital apocrine hamartoma was thought to represent a form of organoid nevus with pure apocrine differentiation on the basis of a deformed follicular structure present in the lesion.[403]

APOCRINE HIDROCYSTOMA (APOCRINE GLAND CYST)

Apocrine hidrocystoma has been regarded by some as an adenomatous cystic proliferation of apocrine glands, and by others as a simple retention cyst. For this reason, the term 'apocrine cystadenoma' is sometimes used for these cases. The tumor has a predilection for the head and neck, and is uncommon in the sites in which apocrine glands are usually found. Clinically, it may have a bluish colour. Apocrine hidrocystoma is considered further with other cutaneous cysts (see p. 509).

Histopathology

The cysts are lined by two layers of cells: an inner lining of large columnar cells with eosinophilic cytoplasm often showing luminal decapitation secretion, and an outer flattened layer of myoepithelial cells. Papillary projections of epithelium into the lumen are found in about one-half of cases. The term '*papillary apocrine gland cyst*' has been used for these cases.[395] The cytokeratin expression suggests that it is a complex tumor, differentiating into each portion of the apocrine gland.[404] There is a suggestion from immunohistochemistry that lesions with a proliferative component (apocrine cystadenoma) are different from the pure cystic form.[405]

SYRINGOCYSTADENOMA PAPILLIFERUM

Syringocystadenoma papilliferum is an uncommon benign tumor of disputed histogenesis,[406] with a predilection for the scalp and forehead.[407,408] Less common sites of involvement are the chest,[409] upper arms,[410] male breast,[411] eyelids,[412] scrotum[413] and thighs. There is an associated organoid nevus in approximately one-third of cases,[407] and for this reason it is not always possible to be certain at what age the syringocystadenoma (syringoadenoma) papilliferum component developed.[414] Probably half are present at birth or develop in childhood. A coexisting basal cell carcinoma is noted in 10% of cases,[407] and there are two reports of an associated condyloma acuminatum[413,415] and another of a verrucous carcinoma.[416] Other congenital lesions have been associated with the presence of the tumor.

The tumor has a varied clinical appearance, most often presenting as a raised warty plaque or as an irregular, flat, gray or reddened area.[417] Linear papules and nodules are occasionally present.[410] The lesions measure from 1 to 3 cm in diameter and are usually solitary. Alopecia accompanies those on the scalp.

There is increasing evidence for an apocrine histogenesis,[418,419] but the possibility of an eccrine origin for a few cases seems likely. Another theory suggests the apoeccrine glands as the origin of this tumor.[420] Allelic deletions have been reported at 9p21 (p16) and 9q22 (the patched gene).[421]

Several examples of a malignant variant, **syringadenocarcinoma papilliferum**, have been reported.[422–425] Some have been present for many years, suggesting the possibility of malignant transformation of a benign lesion.

Histopathology[407]

The tumor is composed of duct-like structures that extend as invaginations from the surface epithelium into the underlying dermis (Fig. 33.28). These may be lined by squamous epithelium near the epidermal surface, with a transition to double-layered cuboidal and columnar epithelium below. Sometimes this latter epithelium partly replaces the overlying epidermis. At other times the surface is composed of irregular papillary projections covered by stratified squamous epithelium. An unusual keratotic lesion, thought to be derived from the apocrine acrosyringium, has been reported in association with syringocystadenoma papilliferum.[426] It showed hyperkeratotic columns surrounded by acanthotic epidermis with features of trichilemmal keratinization. The term '**apocrine acrosyringeal keratosis**' was used for this associated proliferation.[426]

The dilated and contorted ducts may lead into cystic spaces, into which villous projections of diverse size and shape protrude. The ducts and papillary projections are usually covered by an inner layer of columnar epithelium and an outer layer of cuboidal or flattened cells. Goblet cells may be present.[427]

The stroma of the papillary processes contains connective tissue, dilated vessels and, characteristically, numerous plasma cells admixed with a few lymphocytes. The underlying dermis also contains a few inflammatory cells.

There may be underlying dilated sweat glands and, occasionally, dilated apocrine glands. In those cases associated with an organoid nevus, apocrine glands are said to be always present.[428]

Carcinoembryonic antigen is usually present in the epithelial cells.[429,430] Gross cystic disease fluid protein-15 (GCDFP-15) is variably positive in the tumor cells.[431] IgA and secretory component have also been demonstrated in these cells, and it has been suggested that the cells attract plasma cells by a similar mechanism to that utilized by glands of the secretory immune system.[419]

Further evidence for the existence of an eccrine variant comes from a study of the eccrine-specific marker IKH-4 which has labeled one case.[398]

Although Hashimoto has found evidence ultrastructurally for an eccrine origin,[432] Niizuma has suggested that the tumor differentiates toward the intrafollicular and intradermal duct of the embryonic apocrine gland.[418]

Syringadenocarcinoma papilliferum lacks precise morphological definition, but some have a close but cytologically malignant similarity to their benign counterpart.[424] Solid areas of tumor may be present, in addition to the cystic and papillary areas.[423,425] In one instance a ductal sweat gland carcinoma was reported arising in syringocystadenoma papilliferum.[433]

BENIGN APOCRINE TUMORS

This group is expanding as tumors previously regarded as being of eccrine origin are reclassified as apocrine tumors. The following tumors will be considered here:

- hidradenoma papilliferum
- apocrine adenoma (tubular adenoma)
- apocrine hidradenoma
- apocrine mixed tumor
- myoepithelioma (often apocrine associated)
- apocrine poroma.

Their association with follicular tumors and the occasional presence of sebocytes and other structures indicate that the cylindroma and its frequent associate the spiradenoma are probably also of apocrine origin, as stated by Ackerman and colleagues. There is less convincing evidence that syringomas are of apocrine origin. At this stage, they will be considered with the eccrine tumors.

HIDRADENOMA PAPILLIFERUM

Hidradenoma papilliferum is a variant of apocrine adenoma with specific morphology. It is almost always found in the vulval and perianal regions.[434,435] There are reports of ectopic lesions developing on the face, scalp, eyelid,[436] auditory canal[437] and arm. It presents usually as a solitary nodule, usually less than 1 cm in diameter and usually in middle-aged women.

Histopathology[438]

The tumor is usually partly cystic and has both papillary and glandular areas (Fig. 33.29). The papillae often have an arborizing trabecular pattern; the glandular structures vary in size. Two types of epithelium are noted in both the papillary and glandular areas. Usually, the cells are tall and columnar with pale eosinophilic cytoplasm and nipple-like cytoplasmic projections on the surface. An underlying thin myoepithelial layer is often present. In about one-third of lesions, cuboidal cells with eosinophilic cytoplasm and small round nuclei, resembling apocrine metaplasia as seen in the breast, are present in some areas of the tumor.

PAS-positive diastase-resistant granules are present in the apices of the large cells, and material in the glandular spaces stains with the colloidal iron method for acid mucopolysaccharides.

Electron microscopy

Electron microscopy has shown characteristic secretory granules and 'decapitation' secretion.[439]

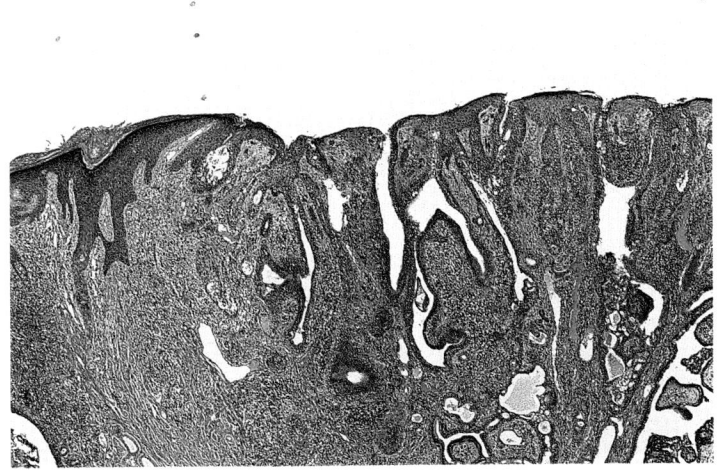

Fig. 33.28 **Syringocystadenoma papilliferum.** Irregular papillary projections protrude into the invaginations of the surface epithelium. The stroma contains numerous plasma cells. (H & E)

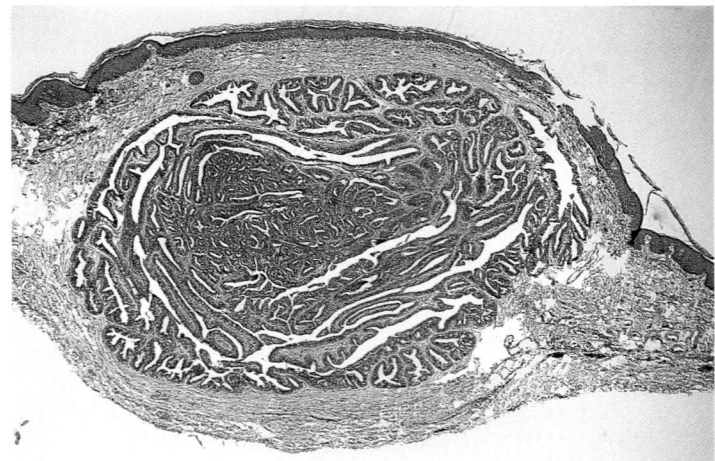

Fig. 33.29 **Hidradenoma papilliferum** with papillary and glandular areas. (H & E)

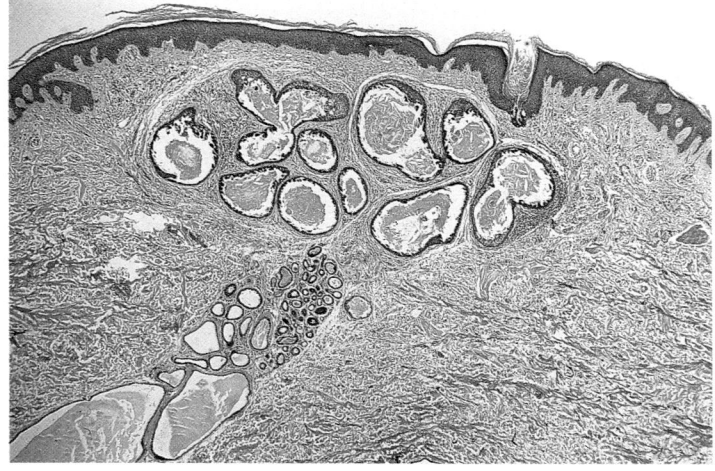

Fig. 33.30 **Tubular apocrine adenoma.** There are multiple tubular structures lined by apocrine-type epithelium. (H & E)

APOCRINE ADENOMA (TUBULAR ADENOMA)

Apocrine adenoma is a very rare tumor which may be found in the axilla,[440] cheek[441] and breast,[442] or in association with an organoid nevus.[443,444] Lesions of the vulval and perianal area reported as apocrine adenoma[445] and apocrine fibroadenoma probably represent variants of what are now called **'adenomas of anogenital mammary-like glands'** (see p. 837).

The *tubular apocrine adenoma*, first described by Landry and Winkelmann in 1972, is part of this spectrum. It has a predilection for the scalp. Furthermore, tumors reported by Rulon and Helwig as papillary eccrine adenomas have been regarded by some authors as examples of apocrine adenomas, whereas others have regarded them as separate entities on the basis of different sites of origin and their microscopic and immunohistochemical characteristics.[446,447] They will be considered separately here. An origin from apoeccrine glands has also been suggested to explain their dual differentiation.[448]

Requena, Kiryu and Ackerman use the term '*tubular adenoma*' for this spectrum of cases, and include tumors known as papillary eccrine adenoma.[395]

Apocrine adenomas are slowly growing, circumscribed nodules situated in the dermis or subcutaneous tissue.

Histopathology[449–451]

The tumor is composed of circumscribed lobules of well-differentiated tubular structures situated in the dermis but sometimes extending into the subcutis (Fig. 33.30). A transition to normal apocrine glands may be present. The tubules have apocrine features with an inner layer of cylindrical cells, often showing 'decapitation' secretion. Papillae devoid of stroma project into the lumina of some tubules. There is often an outer layer of flattened cuboidal cells. Occasional comedo-like conduits extend into the epidermis and form a communication with some of the tubules of the tumor.[452] The epidermis may be hyperplastic. The stroma consists of fibrous tissue with only a paucity of inflammatory cells, in contrast to syringocystadenoma papilliferum, in which inflammatory cells, particularly plasma cells, are prominent. However, cases of tubular apocrine adenoma have been reported with features of syringocystadenoma papilliferum in the upper part of the lesion.[446,453–455]

These tumors differ from apocrine adenocarcinomas by lack of infiltration of surrounding tissues, and by less marked cytological atypia. Myoepithelial cells are usually present in adenomas, whereas they are absent in adenocarcinomas.[441]

Immunoperoxidase studies have shown that the tumor cells contain cytokeratin; human milk protein and CEA are localized to the apical region of the cells.[454]

Electron microscopy

Ultrastructural features confirm the apocrine nature of apocrine adenoma; luminal cells show vacuolar change, lipid granules and multiple microvilli projecting into the lumen.[450] Most of the cells are rich in organelles such as mitochondria and endoplasmic reticulum, and have a prominent Golgi apparatus. Cases with some eccrine features have been reported.[448]

APOCRINE HIDRADENOMA

Most of the cases reported previously as eccrine hidradenoma and eccrine acrospiroma have been reclassified as apocrine hidradenoma on the basis of their presumed apocrine histogenesis. They usually present as solitary nodules 2–3 cm in diameter, but larger variants occur. There is no site predilection. They can occur at all ages. Local recurrence can occur, particularly if the lesion is incompletely excised. The malignant variant, hidradenocarcinoma, is exceedingly rare. It may arise ab initio or by transformation of a benign lesion.

Histopathology[456]

Hidradenomas are usually circumscribed non-encapsulated multilobular tumors, centered on the dermis but sometimes extending into the subcutis. Epidermal connections are present in up to one-quarter of cases.[457] Mucinous syringometaplasia has been described in one case, overlying a clear cell variant of hidradenoma.[458] Hidradenomas may be solid or cystic in varying proportions. Sometimes, large cystic spaces are present and may contain sialomucin attached to the surface of the lining cells. The closely arranged tumor cells, which may be round, fusiform or polygonal in shape, are biphasic in cytoplasmic architecture, with one type having clear and the other eosinophilic cytoplasm (Fig. 33.31). There are variable proportions of each cell type in different tumors, but clear cells predominate in less than one-third.[457] Sometimes, only a few clear cells can be seen. They contain glycogen and some PAS-positive diastase-resistant material, but no lipid. The nuclei of the clear cells tend to be smaller than those in the eosinophilic cells. Focal goblet-cell metaplasia is sometimes seen.[459] Mitoses are variable in number;

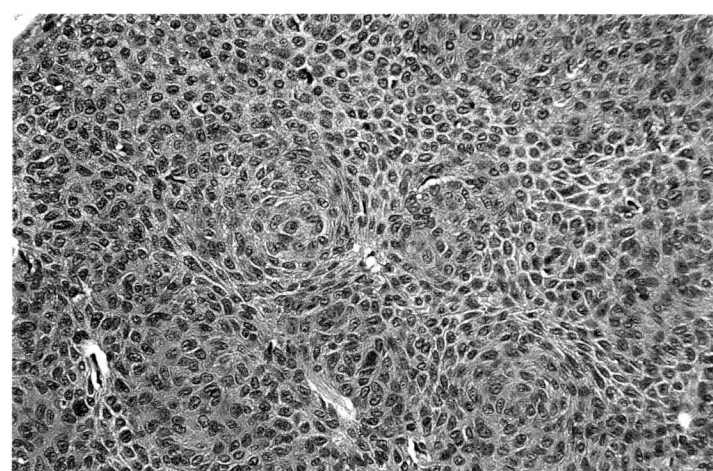

Fig. 33.31 **Apocrine hidradenoma.** This lesion was previously classified as an eccrine hidradenoma. (H & E)

their presence does not necessarily indicate malignancy.[460] However, in one study mitoses and atypical nuclear changes were associated with an increased local recurrence rate, and even subsequent malignant transformation.[461] Other cellular variations include an oncocytic variant,[462] an epidermoid variant[463,464] with large polyhedral cells having a squamous appearance, and a pigmented variant with some melanocytes and melanin pigment in cells and macrophages.[465,466] A racemiform and reticulated pattern of growth has been recorded.[467]

Duct-like structures are often present in the tumor. Some resemble eccrine or apocrine ducts, whereas others consist of several layers of concentric squamous cells with slit-like lumina. The stroma between the lobules varies from thin, delicate, vascularized cords of fibrous tissue to abundant focally hyalinized collagen. A myxoid or chondroid stroma is rarely present.

Immunohistochemistry demonstrates low molecular weight cytokeratin (CAM 5.2) in most tumors. Some also express CEA and epithelial membrane antigen.[468] There is some variability in the expression of the various keratin subtypes in different parts of the tumor.[469,470]

The malignant variant has an infiltrative growth pattern, frequent mitoses (although some overlap exists in the mitotic rate between benign and malignant variants),[460,471] and sometimes angiolymphatic invasion.

Electron microscopy[472]

The cells composing the tumor are connected by desmosomes. The clear cells have abundant glycogen and few tonofilaments, whereas the other cell type has abundant tonofilaments and small amounts of glycogen.

APOCRINE MIXED TUMOR

More than 30 years ago it was suggested that chondroid syringomas (cutaneous mixed tumors), as they were called, had eccrine and apocrine variants.[473] In 1989, Ackerman's group supported this contention.[474] This view is now generally accepted.

Apocrine mixed tumor (chondroid syringoma, apocrine type) is an uncommon tumor, usually occurring as a solitary, slowly growing nodule on the head or neck of the middle-aged and elderly.[475] There is a male predilection. Most tumors are well circumscribed and measure 0.5–3 cm in diameter.

Malignant variants are rare.

Histopathology

Apocrine mixed tumors are circumscribed dermal tumors with an epithelial component distributed through a myxoid, chondroid and fibrous stroma (Fig. 33.32). The epithelial component includes clusters and solid cords of cells as well as ductal structures, sometimes branching, lined by two layers of

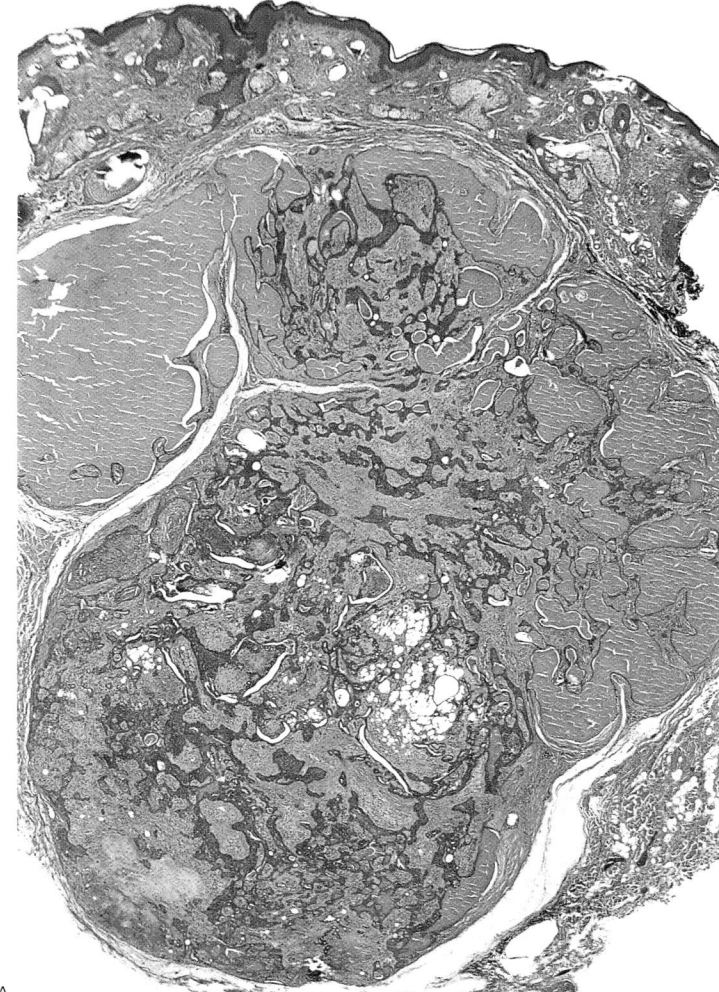

A

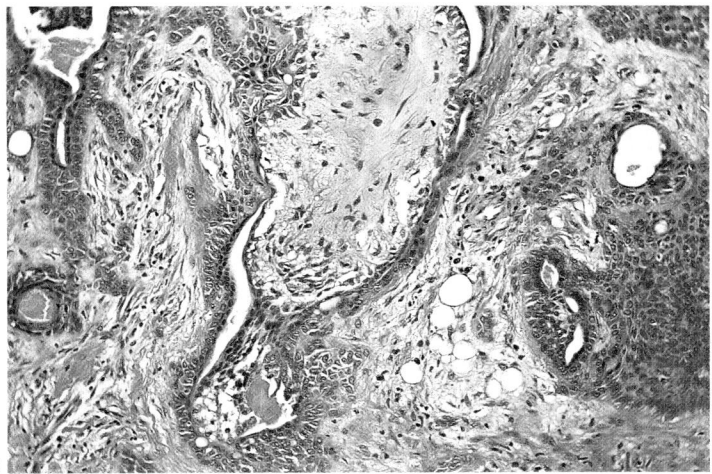

B

Fig. 33.32 **(A) Apocrine mixed tumor. (B)** It is composed of ductal structures set in a myxoid and chondroid matrix. (H & E)

cuboidal cells.[476] Some of the ducts are variably dilated, and keratinous cysts may form.[477] The finding of an apocrine duct in continuity with this tumor is further support for an apocrine origin.[478] Eosinophilic globules composed of collagen (collagenous spherulosis) may be found in the lumina of the glandular elements.[479] This change was present in the stroma in one case.[480] Solid islands of squamous epithelium may be present. Focal calcification and sebaceous and matrical differentiation are sometimes present.[481,482] Hyaline epithelial cells are uncommon.[483,484] Rare cases are composed almost exclusively of these hyaline cells, which have a 'plasmacytoid' appearance because of the peripheral displacement of the nucleus.[485,486] Such cases have been called hyaline-cell rich chondroid syringomas, but hyaline-cell rich apocrine mixed tumor would now be more appropriate (Fig. 33.33).

It has been suggested that the stromal components are derived from the outer cells of the tubuloglandular elements, some of which are myoepithelial in type.[487,488]

The term '**atypical mixed tumor**' has been suggested for tumors with borderline features of malignancy such as an infiltrative edge, but which do not develop metastasis after follow-up.[489]

The cells express CEA and cytokeratin, whereas cells in the outer layer of the tubular structures contain vimentin and S100 protein.[474,437,490,491] This coexpression of CEA and cytokeratins suggests that the keratin cysts may contain cells differentiating toward the intrafollicular portion of the apocrine duct.[492] Extracellular matrix components, such as type IV collagen, laminin, fibronectin and tenascin, are prominently expressed in the chondromyxoid matrix.[493] Type II collagen, which is expressed almost exclusively in cartilage, has been found not only in the stroma but also in epithelial portions of the tumor.[494] The chondroid matrix expresses BM-1.[495]

Electron microscopy

Ultrastructural studies have shown tubuloalveolar spaces lined by ductal epithelium.[477,496] There are myoepithelial cells, which appear to be responsible for producing the chondroid material.[497] The epithelial cells in the solid nests of cells show intracytoplasmic luminal formation.[497]

MYOEPITHELIOMA

Myoepitheliomas are exceedingly rare cutaneous tumors that present as dome-shaped, exophytic nodules on the face, extremities or trunk.[498,499] They may occur at any age. Myoepitheliomas also occur in salivary glands, deep soft tissues[500] and other organs. They are derived from myoepithelial cells which are found in the skin as a discontinuous peripheral layer around eccrine and apocrine glands.[499] Their contraction aids in the delivery of their secretory products. Focal myoepithelial proliferation is not uncommon in apocrine mixed tumors. Some of the mixed tumors and myoepitheliomas of soft tissue reported by Fletcher and colleagues were probably apocrine mixed tumors with areas of myoepitheliomatous change.[500]

The lesions are almost invariably benign; no local recurrence has been recorded. However, a malignant variant has been reported on the vulva.[501]

Histopathology

Myoepitheliomas are circumscribed, non-encapsulated tumors situated in the dermis or subcutis. They are composed of spindle-shaped, epithelioid and plasmacytoid (hyaline) cells.[502] The cells usually have pale eosinophilic cytoplasm and relatively monomorphous ovoid nuclei.

Immunohistochemistry shows that the cells express vimentin, S100 protein, epithelial membrane antigen, smooth muscle actin and muscle specific actin (HHF35).[499] Keratin staining is quite variable.[503]

The rare **adenomyoepithelioma** combines glandular sweat gland elements with myoepithelial cells.[504]

APOCRINE POROMA

Undoubted examples of a poroid neoplasm with apocrine features occur.[505] Often there is follicular and/or sebaceous differentiation as well, reflecting the common origin of the folliculosebaceous–apocrine unit.[506] Such tumors could also be regarded as complex adnexal tumors, examples of which have been reported in the past as poroma-like adnexal adenoma and sebocrine adenoma (see p. 901). Apocrine poromas appear to originate from follicular infundibula.

Histopathology

Anastomosing lobules of small uniform basaloid cells form small ductular structures lined by eosinophilic cuticles.[505] Focal hair follicle and/or sebaceous differentiation are common. One case resembled hidroacanthoma simplex with underlying sebaceous glands.[393] Similar cases were regarded by Steffen and Ackerman as seborrheic keratoses with sebaceous differentiation.[301]

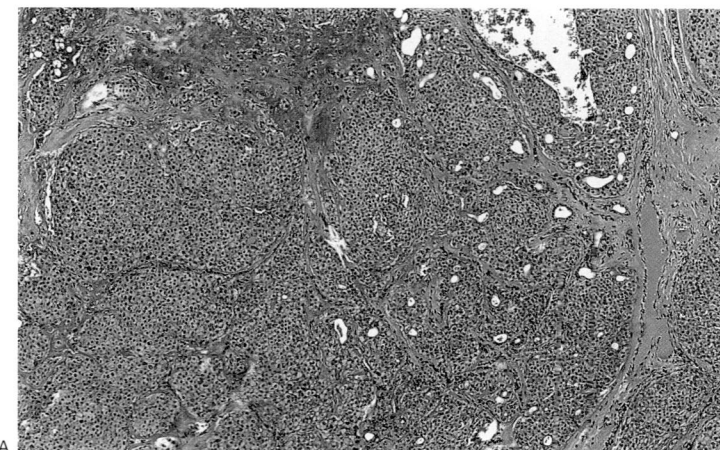
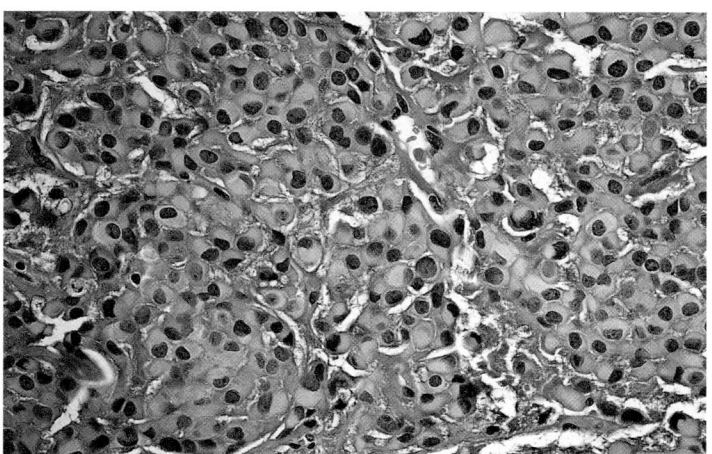

Fig. 33.33 **(A) Hyaline-cell rich apocrine mixed tumor (chondroid syringoma). (B)** The hyaline cells have a plasmacytoid appearance. (H & E)

Cytokeratin expression has not assisted in the differentiation of apocrine and eccrine poromas.[507]

MALIGNANT APOCRINE TUMORS

This group of tumors is expanding with the reclassification of some eccrine tumors. The following tumors will be considered:

- apocrine adenocarcinoma
- extramammary Paget's disease
- adenoid cystic carcinoma
- mucinous carcinoma
- endocrine mucin-producing sweat gland carcinoma
- malignant mixed tumor
- hidradenocarcinoma.

It is possible that the malignant variants of cylindroma and spiradenoma are apocrine. There is also some evidence that the microcystic adnexal carcinoma belongs to this group. They have been considered in their traditional eccrine category here.

APOCRINE ADENOCARCINOMA

Apocrine adenocarcinoma is a very rare tumor with no distinctive clinical features.[406,440,508] It usually presents as a single or multinodular mass in the axilla[440,509,510] or anogenital region, and rarely in other sites such as the chest, nipple, finger[511] and the scalp in association with organoid nevi.[443] A case arising in apocrine hyperplasia (nevus) of the axilla has been reported.[512] Those in the anogenital region may be associated with extramammary Paget's disease.[513,514] The tumors vary from 2 to 8 cm in diameter.

Metastasis is to regional lymph nodes in the first instance, but death, usually from visceral metastases, has been reported in 40% of the reported cases.[406] This may be an underestimation of the eventual mortality, as the follow-up period of some reported cases has been short. There is some correlation between survival and the differentiation of the tumor.[508]

Histopathology[406,440]
There is great variability between tumors, and even in different areas of the same tumor. Apocrine adenocarcinomas are non-encapsulated and centered on the lower dermis and subcutaneous tissue. There is a complex glandular arrangement which includes papillary, tubular, solid and cord-like areas. Small lumina may be present in some of the solid areas. The cells have abundant eosinophilic cytoplasm, which may be granular and sometimes partly vacuolated. A case with signet-ring cells has been reported.[515] Some cells may show decapitation secretion, but this may be absent. There is variable nuclear pleomorphism and mitotic activity. The latter features, together with the degree of invasion, have been used to distinguish these tumors from apocrine adenomas.[441] Normal or hyperplastic apocrine glands may be seen in the vicinity; the lumen of these glands may contain foamy macrophages.[516]

Tumor cells have PAS-positive diastase-resistant granules in the cytoplasm; in contrast to eccrine tumors, glycogen is virtually absent. Cytoplasmic granules of hemosiderin are present in about one-third of cases.[440] The tumor cells express cytokeratin and gross cystic disease fluid protein-15, but, not usually, carcinoembryonic antigen.[508,516] S100 protein has been reported in some cases,[508] but not others.[510]

A tumor resembling a basal cell carcinoma but with histochemical and ultrastructural features of apocrine cells has been reported.[517] It is best regarded as a variant of basal cell carcinoma.

EXTRAMAMMARY PAGET'S DISEASE

Extramammary Paget's disease usually affects sites with a high density of apocrine glands, such as the anogenital region,[518,519] and less commonly the axilla.[520,521] It has also been reported in areas with modified apocrine glands, such as the external auditory canal in association with ceruminous carcinoma,[522] and possibly in the eyelid accompanying carcinoma of Moll's glands. Rare sites of involvement include the buttock,[520] thigh, knee,[523] umbilicus,[524] abdomen[525] and lower anterior chest.[526,527] Rare presentations have included the concurrence of mammary and vulval Paget's disease,[528] the concurrence of genital Paget's disease with clear cells in the epidermis of the axilla,[529] its association with metastatic breast carcinoma in the arm,[530] and the concurrent involvement of both axillae and the genital region in an elderly male.[531,532] Paget's disease has been reported in a supernumerary nipple[533] and overlying a hidradenoma papilliferum.[534]

Extramammary Paget's disease presents as an erythematous, eczematoid, slowly spreading plaque. A rare pattern of erythema, localized to the underpants area, is associated with lymphatic permeation and a bad prognosis.[535] Rarely, the lesions may be focally pigmented or depigmented.[535,537] The size of the lesion usually correlates with its duration. There is a predilection for older individuals. It has been reported in elderly sibs.[538,539] There is an overall female preponderance because the vulva is a common site of involvement.[540,541] Intractable pruritus is a common presenting symptom. In one study, nearly 50% of the patients had an elevated serum carcinoembryonic antigen (CEA).[542]

Pathogenesis
Although it is generally accepted that mammary Paget's disease results from the direct extension into the epidermis of an underlying intraductal adenocarcinoma in the breast,[543] the histogenesis of the extramammary type remains controversial.[544,545] The evidence would seem to indicate that extramammary Paget's disease does not have a uniform histogenesis.[546] About 25% of all cases have an underlying cutaneous adnexal carcinoma, mostly of apocrine type,[547] but sometimes derived from eccrine,[548–550] periurethral, perianal or Bartholin's glands.[551] The underlying appendageal component may include mucinous carcinoma or porocarcinoma. A further 10–15% of patients have an internal carcinoma involving the rectum,[520] prostate,[518,552,553] bladder,[540,554] cervix[520,540,555] or urethra, which appears to be of etiological significance.[551] In the case of perianal Paget's disease, an underlying adnexal or visceral carcinoma is present in nearly 80% of cases.[556] Several explanations have been proposed for the pathogenesis of those cases in which no underlying carcinoma is found. These have included the presence of an underlying in-situ adnexal carcinoma which for technical (sampling) reasons has not been discovered, or an origin from the dermal or coral portion of sweat glands.[540] Alternatively, such cases could be derived from apocrine or eccrine cells or other pluripotential cells in the epidermis.[520,557] In the latter category are the pagetoid clear cells of the nipple, first described by Toker and thought to give rise to clear cell papulosis (see p. 760).[558] These cells may give rise to a primary form of Paget's disease, while epidermal spread of an underlying malignancy may constitute a secondary form.[559]

Local recurrence of extramammary Paget's disease is quite common because of histological extension beyond the clinically abnormal area.[560–562] The prognosis is generally good, except in those cases with an underlying adnexal or visceral carcinoma, in which the mortality is 50% or higher. Spontaneous regression has been reported after partial surgical excision.[563]

Histopathology[520,564]
The tumor cells in Paget's disease have abundant pale cytoplasm and large

pleomorphic nuclei, sometimes with a prominent nucleolus (Fig. 33.34). Occasional cells have an eccentric nucleus and the appearance of a signet ring.[564] Mitoses are usually present. In early lesions the cells are arranged singly or in small groups, sometimes with glandular formation, in the basal and parabasal regions of the epidermis. Later, the entire thickness of the epidermis

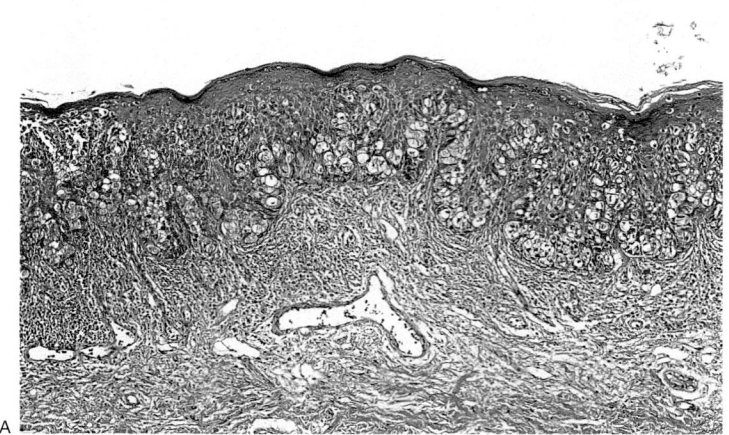

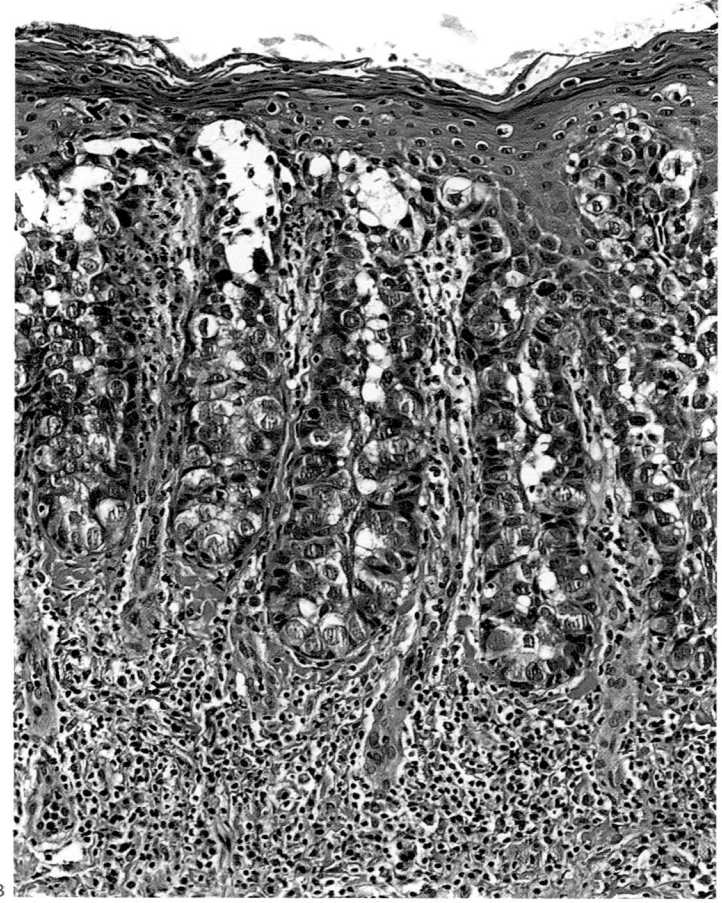

Fig. 33.34 **(A) Extramammary Paget's disease. (B)** Note the pale tumor cells at all levels of the epidermis. (H & E)

may be involved, although the greatest concentration of tumor cells is in the lower epidermis.[564] They usually spread into the contiguous epithelium of hair follicles and eccrine ducts. Uncommonly, Paget cells may invade the dermis.[520] Rarely, an invasive microacinar adenocarcinoma may develop.[565,566] The epidermis is usually hyperplastic and there is often overlying hyperkeratosis and parakeratosis. The epidermal hyperplasia has been categorized into three types – squamous hyperplasia, fibroepithelioma-like hyperplasia and papillomatous hyperplasia.[567] The rare pigmented form has melanocytic colonization. The dendritic cells stain for both S100 protein and HMB-45.[537] A chronic inflammatory cell infiltrate is found in the upper dermis. An underlying in situ or invasive adnexal carcinoma may be present. This may show apocrine differentiation, but in other cases it is not possible to determine the cell of origin. An unusual variant of anogenital Paget's disease has the concurrence of a dermal mucinous carcinoma and fibroepithelioma (of Pinkus)-like changes. This latter phenomenon may represent an unusual form of eccrine duct spread of the Paget's cells.[549] Another case mimicked pemphigus vulgaris with prominent acantholysis due to scant desmosomes in the tumor cells.[568]

Unlike the great majority of cases of mammary Paget's disease, the tumor cells in extramammary Paget's disease contain abundant mucin, which may be confirmed by positive staining with mucicarmine, alcian blue at pH 2.5, Hale's colloidal iron and the PAS method.[564,569–571] However, small 'skip areas', devoid of mucin, have been described.[572] Such areas may resemble Bowen's disease.[557] The cells of clear cell papulosis (see p. 760) do not contain mucin or show cytological atypia.[573] With immunoperoxidase techniques the Paget cells stain for carcinoembryonic antigen (CEA),[557,571,574–576] CA15.3 and KA-93,[577] low molecular weight cytokeratins[571,572,576,578–580] and epithelial membrane antigen.[557,560,576,581] In a recent study, all 15 cases of primary extramammary Paget's disease had the cytokeratin immunophenotype CK7+/CK20−, while only some cases secondary to underlying carcinomas were CK7+; furthermore, some were CK20+.[582] Interestingly, CK7 is also found in Toker cells and Merkel cells.[583] Others have confirmed these findings.[541,567,584,585] The Paget cells also contain apocrine epithelial antigen[574] and gross cystic disease fluid protein (GCDFP), which was thought to be specific for apocrine cells.[431,523,556] However, GCDFP sometimes localizes in eccrine cells.[397,564] Variable staining of cells has been reported for human milk fat globulin.[586] There is a consistent lack of estrogen and progesterone receptors but, in about half the cases, androgen receptors are expressed. However, they involve from only 1% of cells to more than 75% of them.[587] Prostate-specific antigen is expressed in the pagetoid cells of many cases associated with an underlying adenocarcinoma of the prostate (Fig. 33.35).[552] The cells do not contain CD44 or S100 protein.[569,576,577,580] The various immunoperoxidase markers can be used to distinguish Paget's disease from Bowen's disease and superficial spreading melanoma in situ, should any difficulty be experienced on examining hematoxylin and eosin-stained sections.[588]

Electron microscopy
There are secretory and non-secretory cells, the former having a prominent Golgi complex, numerous free ribosomes and clusters of mucinous secretory granules.[589] Some cells have a few surface microvilli, and a few may border a small lumen. Adjacent Paget cells are joined by small desmosomes, and these may also exist between Paget cells and keratinocytes.[564]

ADENOID CYSTIC CARCINOMA

Over 40 cases have now been reported with the designation 'adenoid cystic carcinoma',[422,590–594] excluding purported cases in the external auditory canal.[595]

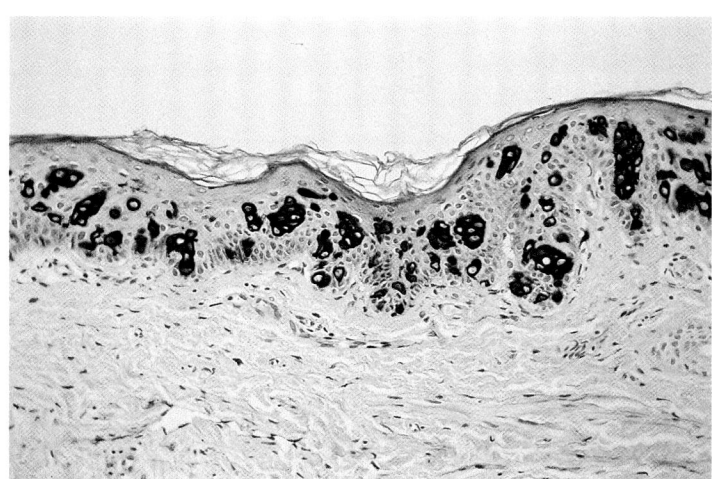

Fig. 33.35 **Extramammary Paget's disease.** The intraepidermal tumor cells stain for prostate-specific antigen. The patient had advanced cancer of the prostate. (Immunoperoxidase stain for PSA)

Santa Cruz, in his major review,[424] appears to have accepted as adenoid cystic carcinomas all cases reported with this title. However, Cooper[596] has pointed out that some of these cases[595,597] belong to a category of eccrine tumor, which has been reported as eccrine carcinoma (eccrine epithelioma) and basal cell carcinoma with eccrine differentiation.[598,599] There are rare cutaneous tumors that do have a striking resemblance to adenoid cystic carcinoma of the salivary gland, and therefore it seems appropriate to accept the existence of adenoid cystic carcinoma of the skin.[592]

The scalp and chest have been the sites of predilection.[600,601] Although local recurrence is common, only a few cases with distant metastases have been reported.[592,600,601] The histogenesis of these tumors has been disputed. They have been regarded in the past as eccrine tumors, although it has been acknowledged that many arise from ceruminous glands, which are modified apocrine glands. It seems best to regard these tumors as apocrine in origin.[601]

Histopathology

The tumor is composed of islands and cords of basaloid cells showing cribriform and some tubular areas. There is abundant basophilic mucin (hyaluronic acid) in the small cysts and between cells. Mitoses are uncommon. Perineural invasion is almost invariably present.[602] The histological features closely resemble those of the corresponding tumor in salivary glands.[603] The tumor cells express epithelial membrane antigen and, sometimes, CEA.[590,603] There is focal staining for cytokeratin, vimentin and S100 protein.[601,604]

MUCINOUS CARCINOMA

Over 80 cases of primary mucinous carcinoma of the skin have been reported.[424,605–609] This is a slowly growing tumor arising on the face (particularly the eyelids),[610,611] scalp,[422,612–614] axilla and trunk of middle-aged and older individuals. The tumor nodules are often reddish and painless, measuring 0.5–7 cm in diameter. Larger variants have been recorded.[615] Late recurrences are common. Metastases to regional nodes and widespread dissemination occur in about 15% of cases.[605]

Histopathology

Mucinous carcinomas are dermal tumors that sometimes extend into the subcutis and deeper tissues. There are large pools of basophilic mucin

separated by thin fibrovascular septa. Small islands of epithelial cells appear to float in these mucinous pools (Fig. 33.36). The epithelial component is denser at the periphery of the lesion. The tumor cells are small and cuboidal, and some have vacuolated cytoplasm. The cell nests in some areas have a cribriform appearance, whereas other cells form small glandular or tubular spaces containing mucin. Focal neuroendocrine differentiation was present in a lesion removed from the vulva,[616] suggesting that it may have been an endocrine mucin-producing sweat gland carcinoma (see below). Another rare component may mimic infiltrating mammary carcinoma.[617] Epidermotropism, resembling Paget's disease, has been reported.[549]

The mucin is PAS positive and stains with mucicarmine and colloidal iron. It is hyaluronidase resistant and sialidase labile, indicating that it is a sialomucin. This feature assists in differentiating this tumor from a metastatic mucinous carcinoma, which it may closely mimic on histological examination.[618] Some mucinous carcinomas express apocrine markers.[397,619] They also express low molecular weight cytokeratins, CEA, epithelial membrane antigen and, sometimes, S100 protein.[614,619,620] There is strong nuclear expression of estrogen receptors, but a more variable pattern for progesterone receptors.[621]

Electron microscopy

The tumor is composed of peripheral dark cells, some of which contain mucin-like material, and inner pale cells which are less well differentiated.[622]

ENDOCRINE MUCIN-PRODUCING SWEAT GLAND CARCINOMA

Endocrine mucin-producing sweat gland carcinoma is an exceedingly rare but distinctive tumor reported on the eyelids; it is analogous to a similar tumor reported recently in the breast.[623,624] There are solid and cystic dermal nodules, some containing mucin pools with adjacent areas resembling mucinous carcinoma. The cells express estrogen and progesterone receptors as well as chromogranin and synaptophysin.[623]

Its origin may be the apocrine glands of Moll.[624] However, the cases of mucinous carcinoma reported by Hanby et al appeared to include both mucinous carcinomas and the lesion reported here. These authors listed tumors on the eyelids and other sites but it is not possible from their paper to correlate site with histological pattern.[621]

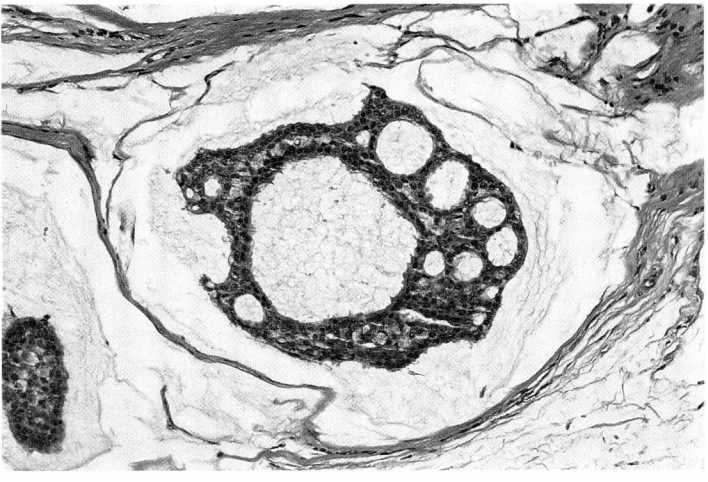

Fig. 33.36 **Mucinous carcinoma.** A cystic and somewhat cribriform nest is present in a pool of mucin. (H & E)

MALIGNANT MIXED TUMOR

Malignant mixed tumor (malignant chondroid syringoma, malignant apocrine mixed tumor) is most often found on the trunk and extremities, which are not the usual sites of the benign variant.[424,625–629] Sometimes, juxtaposed areas of benign and malignant tumor are found, evidence for malignant transformation of an apocrine mixed tumor, at least in some cases.[424] Local or distant metastases are common, although there is usually a prolonged course.[630]

Histopathology

The tumors have a lobulated appearance. They are composed of an epithelial and a mesenchyme-like component, the latter consisting of myxomatous and cartilaginous areas.[625,627] The epithelial component predominates at the periphery of the tumor, where there are cords and nests of cuboidal or polygonal cells with some glandular structures. There is variable pleomorphism (Fig. 33.37). Scattered mitoses are present. Mesenchymal elements are progressively more abundant toward the center.[626] They may also be present in lymph node metastases (Fig. 33.38). Ossification is occasionally present.[625] The histological appearance may be a poor indicator of the biological behavior of a particular tumor in this category.[424,631]

The epithelial cells express cytokeratins. The luminal epithelial cells show binding to the lectin *Ulex europaeus*; intraluminal cells are CEA positive.[632]

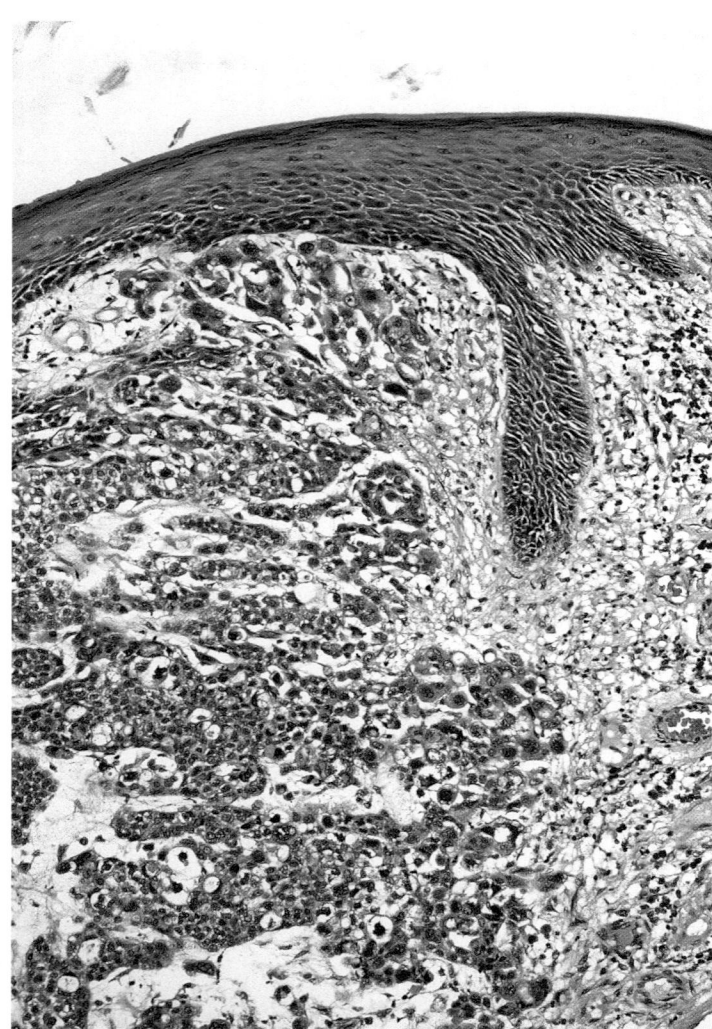

Fig. 33.37 **Malignant mixed tumor.** This obviously malignant tumor shows no obvious mixed differentiation. (H & E)

Androgen receptors have not been detected.[633] The chondroid areas express S100 protein.[632]

HIDRADENOCARCINOMA

Although the term 'malignant acrospiroma' is sometimes used for hidradenocarcinoma,[634,635] it has also been applied to a heterogeneous group of eccrine carcinomas. Because of the likely apocrine origin of most of these lesions the terms 'hidradenocarcinoma' or 'malignant hidradenoma' are preferred. This is a rare tumor with a predilection for the face and extremities.[636] It usually presents as an ulcerated reddish nodule in older individuals, but cases have been recorded in children[637,638] and at birth.[639] The tumors have an aggressive course, with eventual distant metastasis to lymph nodes, bones and lungs.[635,636,640]

Histopathology[636,639]

The tumor is composed of sheets of cells with glycogen-containing pale cytoplasm and distinct cell membranes.[641] The term 'clear cell eccrine carcinoma' has been used in the past for those with a prominent clear cell component.[642] In some cases there is little clear cell change and the cells have a basaloid or even squamoid appearance. Sometimes, squamous differentiation is widespread.[643] Cytoplasmic vacuoles, representing intracellular lumina formation, are an important feature.[424] Peripheral lobules of the tumors are often irregular and appear invasive.[644] Focal necrosis is sometimes present.[645] An occasional malignant tumor is deceptively bland in appearance[639] whereas others have numerous mitoses.[424] Melanocytes are sometimes present in the tumor lobules.[424]

Electron microscopy

The tumor cells contain cytoplasmic glycogen and form intracellular lumina,[424] around which tonofilaments are arranged in a circumferential pattern. Desmosomes are usually well developed.

TUMORS OF MODIFIED APOCRINE GLANDS

The glands of Moll on the eyelid, and the ceruminous glands of the external ear are examples of modified apocrine glands. The breast can also be regarded as a modified apocrine gland. Ectopic mammary glands do occur (see below).

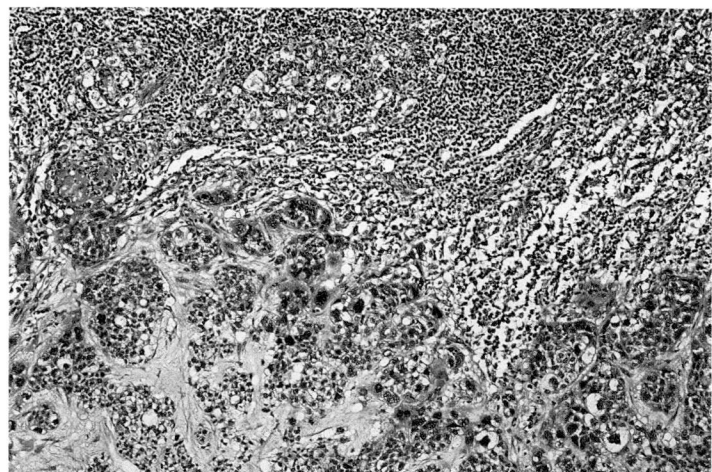

Fig. 33.38 **Malignant mixed tumor.** This deposit in a lymph node shows stromal myxoid and chondroid differentiation. (H & E)

ADENOCARCINOMA OF MOLL'S GLANDS

The glands of Moll are modified apocrine glands in the eyelids. Retention cysts (resembling apocrine cystadenoma), hidradenoma papilliferum[436] and malignant tumors resembling apocrine adenocarcinoma have been reported.[406,646] There are too few cases of adenocarcinoma in the literature for significant clinical comment.

Histopathology

The tumors resemble apocrine adenocarcinoma with architectural and cytological features of malignancy. There may be iron granules in the cytoplasm of the tumor cells. Cases reported in the past with pagetoid epidermal involvement have been regarded as possibly sebaceous rather than apocrine tumors.[647]

EROSIVE ADENOMATOSIS OF THE NIPPLE

Erosive adenomatosis (florid papillomatosis, papillary adenoma) is a benign tumor involving the nipple which may clinically mimic Paget's disease.[648,649] It is thought to arise from the ducts of the nipple. It may rarely occur in males and in children.[650]

Histopathology[651]

This dermal tumor is a well-circumscribed non-encapsulated lesion with an adenomatous configuration (Fig. 33.39). Some of the ducts have papillary projections into the lumen, and a few show cystic dilatation. The lining epithelium is of apocrine secretory type and there is usually a backing of myoepithelial cells. Some ducts connect with the surface epithelium; squamous epithelium may extend into them.

The fibrous stroma sometimes contains a mild inflammatory infiltrate, which may be rich in plasma cells.

CERUMINOUS ADENOMA AND ADENOCARCINOMA

The ceruminous glands are modified apocrine glands in the external auditory canal. They give rise to rare tumors in which the distinction between adenoma and adenocarcinoma may be difficult on histological grounds.[652–654] The term

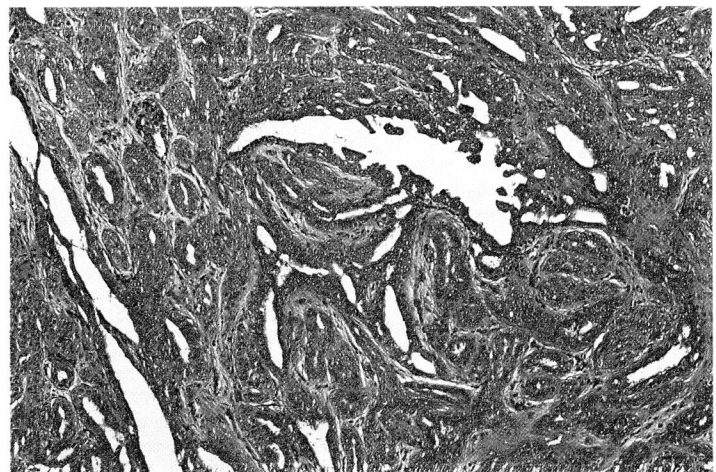

Fig. 33.39 **Erosive adenomatosis of the nipple** composed of duct-like structures of varying size. (H & E)

'ceruminoma' has been used in the past, not only for the ceruminous adenoma and adenocarcinoma, but also for adenoid cystic carcinomas and mixed tumors of the auditory canal. The term is best abandoned.

TUMORS OF ANOGENITAL MAMMARY-LIKE GLANDS

Mammary-like glands are a newly recognized variant of cutaneous adnexal gland found in the anogenital region.[655] They resemble mammary glands, although they have variously been regarded in the past as modified eccrine or apocrine glands. Both adenomas[655,656] and adenocarcinomas[657] may arise in these glands. Decapitation secretion is sometimes present. These glands possess receptors for estrogen and progesterone proteins which help to distinguish them from classical eccrine and apocrine glands. Mammary-like sweat glands can occur in other parts of the body, outside the milk line. Three cases of breast-like lesions arising in the skin of the thigh, scalp and umbilicus have recently been reported.[658] They presumably arose in ectopic mammary-like sweat glands.

Eccrine tumors

In the past there has been some debate as to the eccrine or apocrine origin and differentiation of certain adnexal tumors. Histochemistry and electron microscopy sometimes gave conflicting results, with features suggestive of both apocrine and eccrine differentiation in some tumors. The recent development of various monoclonal antibodies, for use with immunoperoxidase techniques, has assisted marginally in the classification of the various adnexal tumors.[429–431,659] The various markers have not lived up to initial expectations. The first of these markers to have diagnostic value was the finding of carcinoembryonic antigen (CEA) in sweat gland tumors.[660] This does not represent a single oncofetal antigen, but comprises a family of homologous glycoproteins that include classic CEA-180, biliary glycoprotein (BGP), and non-specific cross-reacting antigens (NCA). If these monospecific antibodies are used, a rather consistent profile emerges: staining for both CEA-180 and NCA indicates ductal differentiation of both apocrine and eccrine type; co-expression of all three is consistent with differentiation toward the secretory portion of eccrine glands or the transitional portion of proximal ducts.[661]

Other monoclonal antibodies have been developed with variable specificity and sensitivity for eccrine-related antigens. They include:

1. SKH1, which reacts with the secretory portion and coiled duct of the eccrine gland and the secretory portion of apocrine glands[662]
2. ferritin antibody, which demonstrates ferritin in the outermost layer of the eccrine and apocrine duct[663]
3. antibodies to IgA and secretory component, which detect antigen in the lumen and on the surface of the epithelium of sweat glands[654]
4. IKH-4, EKH-5 and EKH-6, which stain the eccrine secretory coil[398]
5. Dako-CK1 and Cam 5.2 (both commercially available), which react with two cytokeratins of different molecular weight.[665]

Whereas Dako-CK1 detects a cytokeratin in the intraepidermal eccrine duct and the inner layer of the intradermal portion of the duct but not other structures, Cam 5.2 reacts with the apocrine gland and supposedly the duct, and the eccrine secretory coils but not the eccrine duct.[665] Numerous other monoclonal antibodies have been prepared to various cytokeratins.

The monoclonal antibody MNF116, which detects the low and intermediate molecular weight keratins (5, 6, 8, 17 and 19), stains the basal cells of the epidermis and adnexae. It is found in all epithelial tumors, including adnexal ones.[666] Antibodies to individual keratins have not been of much assistance in routine diagnosis, but they have given a valuable insight into the possible derivation and/or differentiation of various eccrine tumors.[56,667,668] For example, syringomas exhibit a pattern similar to normal dermal eccrine ducts (EMA in peripheral cells, CK10 in intermediate cells and CK6, CK19 and CEA in luminal cells), and eccrine poromas exhibit a widespread reaction for CK5/6 and EMA, analogous to peripheral dermal duct cells.[56] Cylindromas and eccrine spiradenomas have a more complex pattern.[56]

Although CD44 is strongly expressed in the eccrine coil secretory cells, it has not proved a useful marker of sweat gland differentiation in tumors.[669] It is expressed not only in syringomas and eccrine poromas but in tumors of undoubted apocrine origin such as hidradenoma papilliferum.[669]

Some eccrine tumors contain estrogen receptor protein, a feature of some breast carcinomas.[670] Myoepithelial cells (as determined by the expression of vimentin and α-smooth muscle actin) are seen in most sweat gland tumors considered to differentiate toward the secretory coil of sweat glands, such as cylindroma, eccrine spiradenoma, papillary eccrine adenoma and most of the traditional apocrine tumors.[671-673] The myoepithelioma has been considered with the apocrine tumors (see p. 882). Another feature of some sweat gland carcinomas is the presence of p53 protein; it is rarely present in benign tumors.[674] The mitotic rate is also an important indicator of malignancy.[675]

It has been mentioned already that some of the tumors traditionally regarded as being of eccrine origin are apocrine in type, while the evidence for the histogenesis of a further group of these tumors is still being evaluated. The results obtained with the antibody IKH-4 (see above) suggest that it is premature to embark on a wholesale reclassification of the 'eccrine' tumors.

The eccrine hamartomas will be considered first, followed by a discussion of the benign eccrine tumors and the eccrine carcinomas. Hyperplastic and metaplastic lesions of the eccrine glands are discussed in Chapter 15 (pp. 486–487).

HAMARTOMAS AND BENIGN TUMORS

ECCRINE HAMARTOMAS

The term 'eccrine hamartomas' is used to cover the diverse group of nevoid conditions involving the eccrine sweat glands. The simplest lesion is an **eccrine nevus**,[676-679] a rare abnormality in which there is an increased number of normal-appearing eccrine coils or an increase in the size of the coils (Fig. 33.40). **Eccrine duct hyperplasia** usually occurs as a reactive process (see eccrine syringofibroadenomatosis – page 894), but it has been reported in association with a nasal glioma, a hamartomatous lesion.[680]

In **eccrine angiomatous hamartoma**[681-691] there is an increase in the number of small blood vessels, and sometimes of nerve fibers, mucin or fat, in addition to the increase in eccrine glands.[692] Hair follicles are sometimes associated with this lesion. Overlying verrucous features have been recorded.[693] Gross cystic disease fluid protein-15 was present in the eccrine glands in one case.[694] The lesion reported as a **palmar cutaneous hamartoma** had neurovascular glomic bodies in addition to fat, angiomatous vessels and eccrine glands.[695]

The **acrosyringeal nevus** consists of a proliferation of PAS-positive acrosyringeal keratinocytes, which extend down into the dermis as thin anastomosing cords from the undersurface of the epidermis (Fig. 33.41).[696] Some of these structures are recognizable as eccrine ducts. Stromal plasma cells may be prominent. Lesions may be linear,[697] plaque-like or multiple.[696] Diffuse lesions have been observed in ectodermal dysplasia.[698] Although

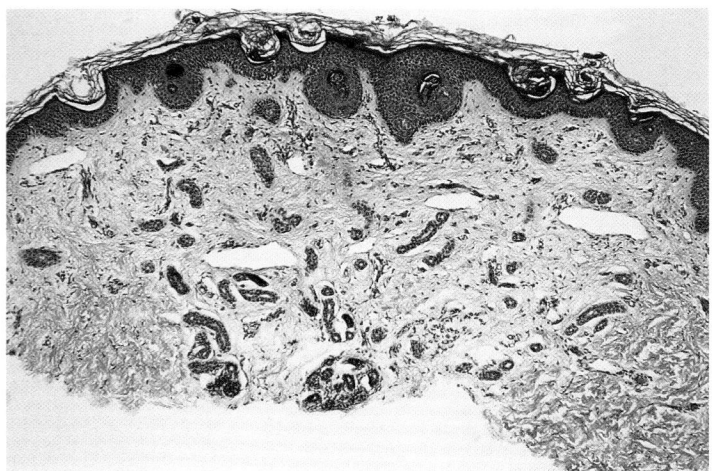
Fig. 33.40 **Eccrine nevus.** There is an increase in eccrine glands and ducts. (H & E)

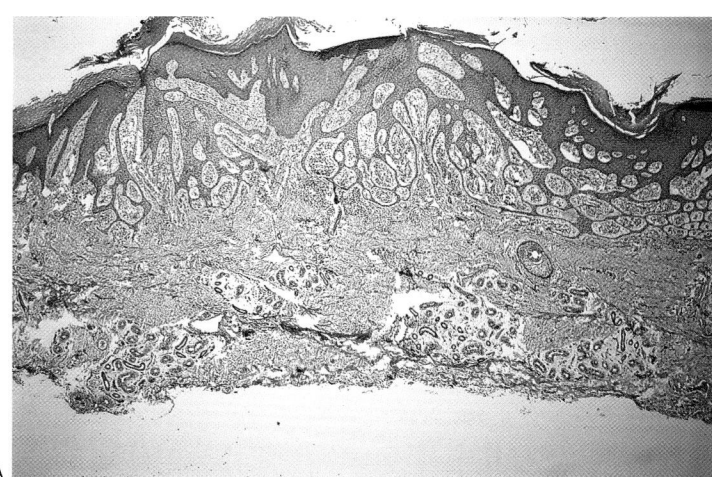
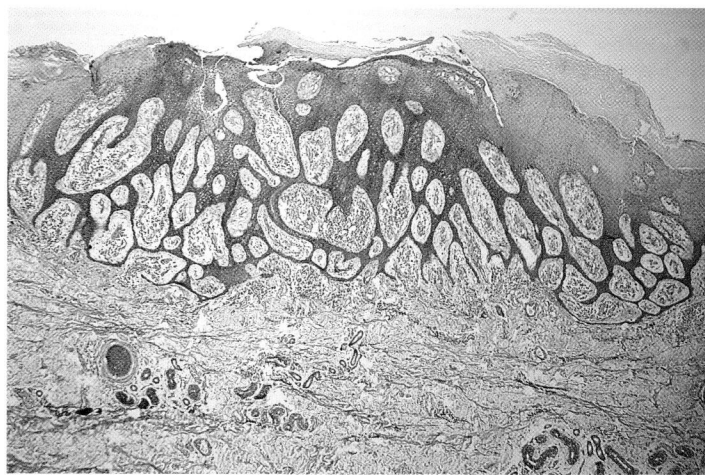
Fig. 33.41 **(A) Acrosyringeal nevus** (H & E). **(B)** Thin anastomosing cords of cells extend from the undersurface of the epidermis. The cells are PAS positive. (Periodic acid–Schiff)

usually regarded as an identical lesion,[699,700] the solitary tumor reported as a syringofibroadenoma[701] does have clinicopathological differences; it will be considered with the benign tumors (see p. 894).[702,703] Incidentally, the term 'acrosyringeal nevus' was suggested to the author by the late Dr Hermann

Pinkus, who agreed that the lesion had clinical and pathological features that distinguished it from the lesion reported earlier by Mascaro.

The **phakomatous choristoma** is a benign congenital lesion of the eyelid consisting of lens tissue in an ectopic location.[704] It is mentioned here because the irregularly branched ducts and cords, some cystically dilated, can mimic an adnexal tumor. Furthermore, there is no other suitable place for its inclusion. There is a densely fibrotic stroma, psammoma body-like calcifications and intraluminal degenerated ghost cells. There is strong staining for vimentin and weak focal staining for S100 protein.[704]

There are three somewhat related lesions characterized by comedonal dilatation of eccrine ostia, with or without cornoid lamellae. These lesions are comedo nevus of the palm, linear eccrine nevus with comedones, and porokeratotic eccrine ostial nevus. In **comedo nevus of the palm**[705] there are keratotic pits formed by parakeratotic plugs within dilated eccrine ostia. The lesion reported as **linear eccrine nevus with comedones**[706] resembles nevus comedonicus, with the addition of basaloid nests in the dermis resembling eccrine spiradenoma in some areas and eccrine acrospiroma in others. In **porokeratotic eccrine ostial nevus** there are cornoid lamellae associated with eccrine ducts.[707-711]

In **eccrine-centered nevus** there are nevus cells intimately associated with eccrine sweat ducts.[712,713]

ECCRINE HIDROCYSTOMA

Eccrine hidrocystoma is usually solitary, but multiple lesions may occur.[714,715] There is a predilection for the periorbital area. It is discussed further with the other cystic lesions in Chapter 16 (p. 508).

The existence of this entity has been challenged; many, if not all of these lesions are now regarded as being of apocrine type.[395,716]

Histopathology

The cysts are unilocular and lined by two layers of cuboidal epithelium. Cytokeratins 7, 8 and 19 were present in some cases. On this basis they were regarded as being of eccrine origin.[717]

PAPILLARY ECCRINE ADENOMA

The benign papillary eccrine adenoma was first described by Rulon and Helwig in 1977.[718] It presents as a slowly growing firm nodule with a predilection for the extremities of black people.[718-725] Ackerman and colleagues include this group with their tubular adenomas of apocrine origin.[395]

Histopathology[718,719]

Papillary eccrine adenoma is a circumscribed dermal tumor composed of multiple variably dilated duct-like structures lined by two or more layers of cells.[720] The inner layer often forms intraluminal papillations of variable complexity (Fig. 33.42).[719] This latter feature is not always prominent in all areas of the tumor. There is no decapitation secretion. The epithelial cells may show focal clear-cell change and even focal squamous differentiation. Some of the lumina contain an amorphous eosinophilic material.[725] Immunoperoxidase studies have demonstrated the presence of CEA, cytokeratins, particularly CK8 and CK14, and S100 protein.[720,722,723,726,727] The unique pattern of some cases, which are devoid of apocrine features, together with the positive staining with the eccrine-specific antibody IKH-4 are reasons for the retention of an eccrine variant of tubular adenoma. It is acknowledged that apocrine variants are far more common. The stromal connective tissue may show hyalinized collagen and a focal increase in fibroblasts. Inflammatory cells are usually sparse.

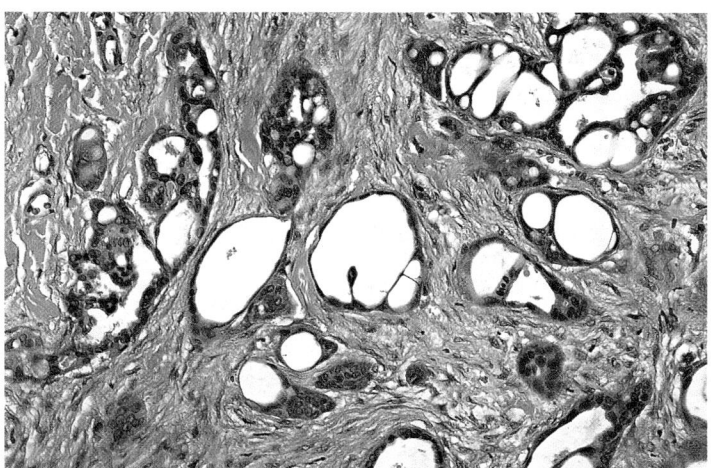

Fig. 33.42 **Papillary eccrine adenoma.** A few intraluminal papillations arise from the wall of the duct-like structures in the dermis. (H & E)

Electron microscopy

The duct-like structures are composed of basal and luminal cells, the latter containing intracytoplasmic cavities but not secretory granules.[721]

SYRINGOMA

Syringomas are usually found as multiple small papules on the lower eyelids and cheeks of adolescent females.[728] Other variants include solitary and giant[729] lesions, a plaque form, milia-like lesions,[730] tumors limited to the vulva,[729] penis,[731-733] buttocks[734] or scalp,[735] and acral,[736] linear[737,738] or bathing-trunk distributions.[739] Eruptive[740-743] and disseminated forms,[744] some of which may be familial,[745] have also been described. The clear-cell variant of syringoma has been associated clinically with diabetes mellitus in many instances.[746,747] Syringomas appear to be more common in patients with Down syndrome.[740,748]

They are regarded as probable apocrine tumors by Ackerman and colleagues.[395]

Histopathology[728]

Syringomas are dermal tumors composed of multiple small ducts lined usually by two layers of cuboidal epithelium (Fig. 33.43). Sometimes, the ducts have a comma-like tail resembling those seen in desmoplastic trichoepithelioma. Solid nests and strands of cells, sometimes having a basaloid appearance, may be present. Some ducts are dilated and contain eosinophilic material. There is usually a dense fibrous stroma.

In the clear-cell variant the ducts are lined by larger epithelial cells with pale or clear cytoplasm (Fig. 33.44).[746,749] This clear-cell change may involve only part of the tumor or be limited to the cells adjacent to the duct lumina. The clear cells contain abundant glycogen. It is regarded as a 'metabolic' variant of the conventional syringoma.[750]

Rare variants include the presence of numerous mast cells in the stroma[751] or of nevus cells admixed with the syringomatous elements.[728,752] Syringoma-like sweat duct proliferation is found as an incidental finding in scalp biopsies taken for the histological evaluation of alopecia.[753,754] It has also been found in prurigo nodularis.[755] Malignant degeneration is very rare, and the tumors designated as malignant syringoma (syringoid eccrine carcinoma) are probably malignant ab initio. Syringomas differ from microcystic adnexal carcinoma by

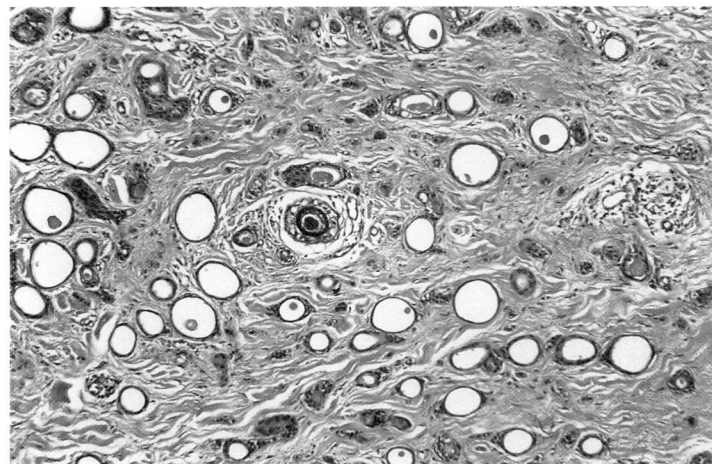

Fig. 33.43 **Syringoma.** Multiple small ductal structures, lined by two layers of cuboidal epithelium, are present in a fibrous stroma. (H & E)

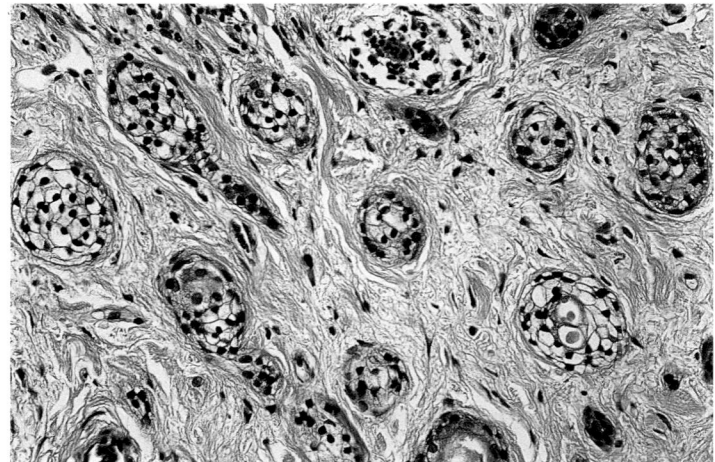

Fig. 33.44 **Syringoma** (clear cell variant). The ductal structures are lined by epithelium having pale cytoplasm. (H & E)

their lack of deep extension and of perineural infiltration.[756] They are easily distinguished from the exceedingly rare change known as sclerosing adenosis of sweat ducts.[757]

Staining with monoclonal anti-eccrine gland antibodies has shown positivity for EKH-6 (eccrine secretory and ductal structures), but the tumor cells are negative for EKH-5 and SKH1, which label eccrine secretory elements.[662,758] The cytokeratin pattern has been further characterized: the cells express CK1/5/10/11/19, and CK14 variably.[750,759] Syringomas usually contain CEA, whereas desmoplastic trichoepitheliomas do not.[65] Ferritin is present in the outermost layer of cells in the epithelial elements of the syringoma, in a similar pattern to that seen in normal eccrine ducts.[663] Progesterone receptors are expressed in most syringomas, supporting the view that they are under hormonal control.[760]

Electron microscopy

There are numerous microvilli on the cells bordering the lumina and a band of periluminal tonofilaments.[758,761] Intracytoplasmic lumen formation and keratohyaline granules in luminal cells have also been reported.[761]

ECCRINE MIXED TUMOR

Eccrine mixed tumor (chondroid syringoma, eccrine type) is a rare tumor which was formerly included with the apocrine variant of mixed tumor as a chondroid syringoma. It is found as a solitary, slowly growing nodule on the head or extremities of the middle-aged and elderly. Local recurrence occurs only if the tumor is incompletely excised.

Histopathology

The eccrine mixed tumor has small, non-branching ducts resembling a syringoma, set in a myxoid and cartilaginous stroma (Fig. 33.45). The tumor is well circumscribed and may extend into the subcutis. The cells express CEA and cytokeratin.

CYLINDROMA

Cylindromas are usually found as small solitary lesions on the head and neck. There is a strong predilection for middle-aged and elderly females. Large variants, usually with multiple coalescing tumors (turban tumors), may arise on the scalp and forehead. A rare variant with multiple lesions in linear array has been reported.[762] The multiple type is often inherited as an autosomal dominant trait.[763,764] Cylindromas have also been associated with the multiple, inherited form of trichoepitheliomas,[764–766] with monomorphic adenomas of the parotid gland[767] and with eccrine spiradenoma.[768–771] Local aggressive behavior and malignant transformation are uncommon and usually associated with long-standing turban tumors of the scalp.[772–775] However, metastasis is very rare.[776]

The origin of this tumor has been controversial: some immunohisto-chemical studies suggest that cylindroma is linked to the secretory coil of the apocrine gland, rather than the coiled duct region of the eccrine gland as previously thought.[777–779] A more recent study using the monoclonal antibody IKH-4, thought to be eccrine specific, showed positive staining, again putting the histogenesis of cylindroma into dispute.[398]

Histopathology

Cylindromas are poorly circumscribed dermal tumors composed of irregularly shaped islands and cords of basaloid cells surrounded by conspicuous eosinophilic hyaline bands which are PAS positive and diastase resistant (Fig. 33.46). Droplets of similar hyaline material may be present in the cell nests. The hyaline basement membrane contains type IV and type VII collagen.[780,781] There is usually a thin band of uninvolved connective tissue beneath the epidermis; however, the large turban tumors will ulcerate. Subcutaneous extension may also occur.

Most of the tumor islands have two cell types: a peripheral cell with a dark-staining nucleus and a tendency for palisading, and a larger cell with a vesicular nucleus more centrally located. Small duct-like structures are some-times present.

The stroma is composed of loosely arranged collagen containing an increased number of fibroblasts. A more compact stroma is occasionally present.

Areas resembling spiradenoma (see below) will sometimes be present, and there may also be tumor lobules with overlap features between these two entities.[770,782,783]

Aggressive or malignant behavior is characterized by loss of the hyaline sheath and expanded cellular islands composed predominantly of larger cells, devoid of peripheral palisading.[775]

Although the expression of cytokeratins could be interpreted as indicating an eccrine origin, the presence of lysozyme, human milk factor globulin 1, α-smooth muscle actin and α_1-antichymotrypsin favors an apocrine origin. CEA

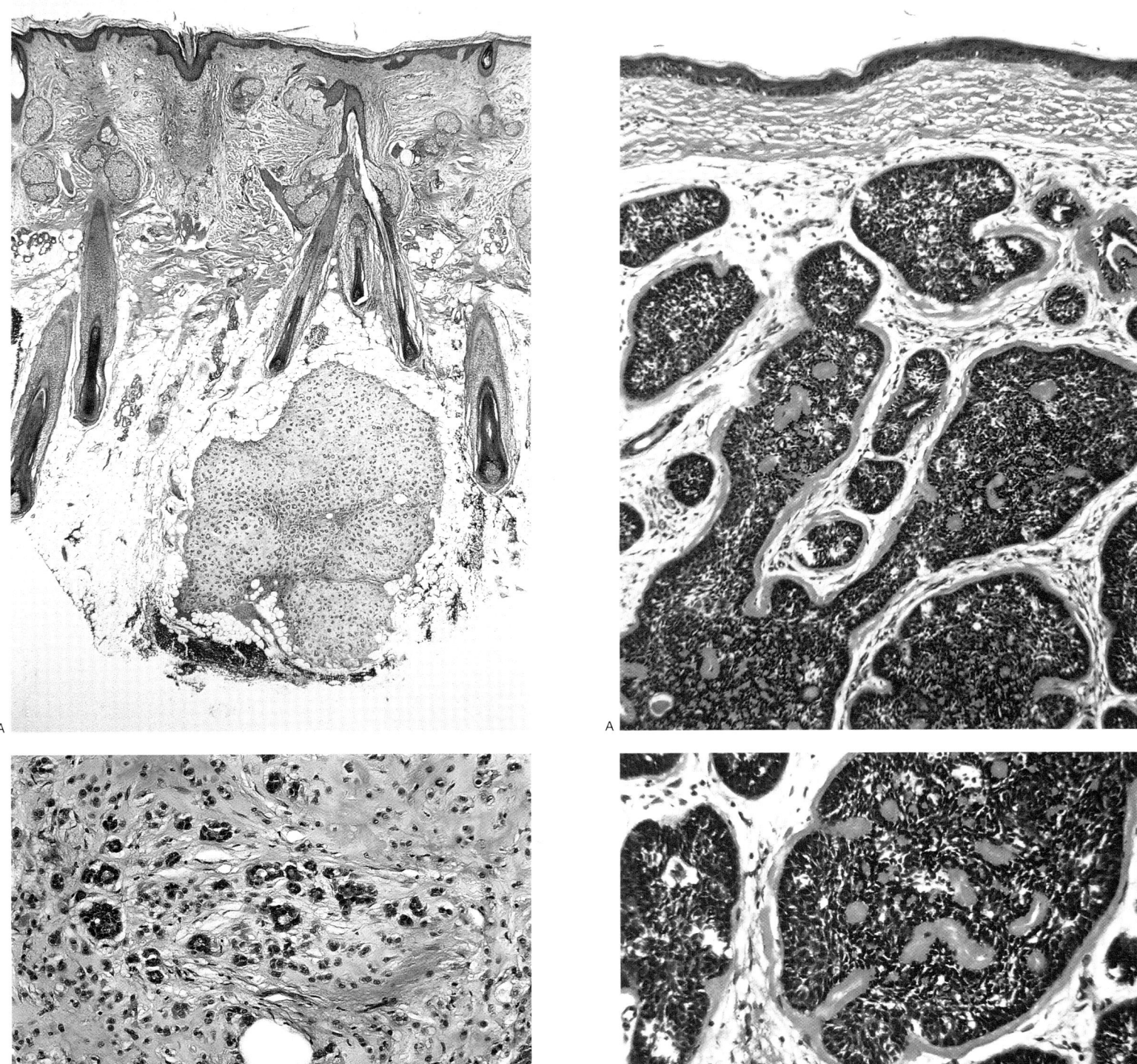

Fig. 33.45 **(A) Eccrine mixed tumor** (chondroid syringoma of eccrine type). **(B)** This variant is composed of small, non-branching ducts set in a myxoid and chondroid stroma. (H & E)

Fig. 33.46 **(A) Cylindroma. (B)** The basaloid cells are arranged in irregularly shaped islands surrounded by a thin band of hyaline material. (H & E)

and epithelial membrane antigen are also expressed.[778] Both cylindroma and spiradenoma express cytokeratins 7, 8 and 18.[783]

Electron microscopy[761,784]

Electron microscopy shows small dense basal cells, large light indeterminate

cells, ductal cells, secretory cells containing secretory granules, and some Langerhans cells. Ductal structures are also present. The thick hyaline band is composed of thickened amorphous basal lamina and a fibrous component consisting of anchoring fibrils.[761] Collagen fibrils of varying width are also present.

SPIRADENOMA

Spiradenoma is usually a solitary gray-pink nodule, less than 1 cm in diameter, arising on the head and neck, trunk or, less commonly, the extremities of adults.[785] Satellite tumors, multiple lesions,[728,786–788] giant variants,[789] a linear[790–792] or zosteriform[793] distribution and occurrence at birth[794] and in infancy[795] have also been described. Pain and/or tenderness are frequently present, but one recent study has suggested that these features may have been overstressed in the past.[785]

Spiradenoma has been associated with cylindromas in the same patient (see above),[769,787,796] and tumors with overlap features between these two types have also been described.[770] Ackerman and colleagues regard both tumors as apocrine in type. Malignant transformation is a very rare event.[770,775,785,797–801] It appears to be accompanied by increased expression of p53 protein.[802]

Histopathology[785,803]

The tumor is composed of one or more large, sharply delineated basophilic nodules in the dermis, unattached to the epidermis and sometimes extending into the subcutis. Small satellite lobules may be present. The tumor nodules are composed of aggregates of cells in sheets, cords or islands, or with a trabecular arrangement (Fig. 33.47). Two cell types are present: small dark basaloid cells with hyperchromatic nuclei, and a more frequent larger cell with a pale nucleus which tends to be near the center of the clusters. The cells are PAS negative, but droplets of PAS-positive hyalin may be present in some areas of the tumor. A few duct-like structures are often present (Fig. 33.48). Other findings include squamous eddies, small cysts, and lymphocytes infiltrating the tumor nests. Irregular, thin bands of fibrous tissue containing blood vessels are present within the tumor lobules. Perivascular spaces, containing some lymphocytes, sometimes form between the blood vessels and the tumor cells.[804] The stroma between lobules may be edematous and sometimes there are prominent vessels with telangiectasia and even hemorrhage.[789,805] Dilated vessels rimmed by sclerosis have been called 'ancient' changes.[806] Cylindromatous areas are sometimes present.[770,782,783]

The strands of cells are cytokeratin positive and the lumina are CEA positive.[789] The pattern of cytokeratin expression mirrors that seen in the transitional portion between the secretory segments and the coiled ducts of eccrine glands.[807] Abundant T lymphocytes and Langerhans cells are found within the tumor lobules.[808]

Electron microscopy

There is some variability in the ultrastructural findings.[789,803,809] The tumor is composed of sheets of cells separated into lobules by strands of amorphous and fibrillar material.[803] The most common cell is a clear polygonal or

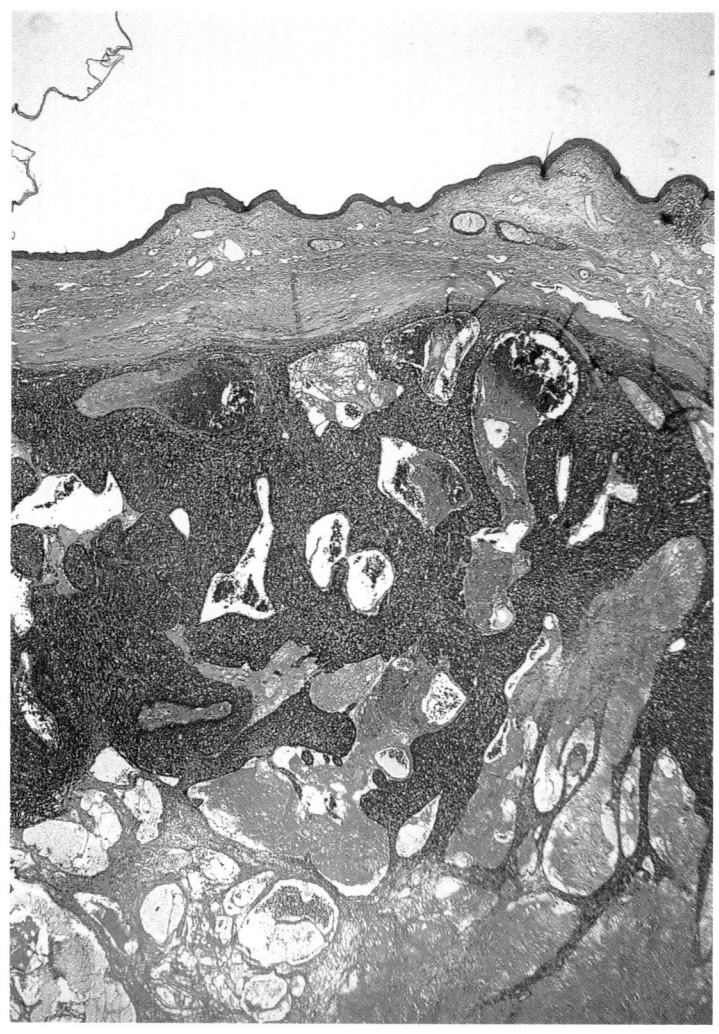

Fig. 33.47 **Spiradenoma.** This large lesion is partly cystic and hemorrhagic (H & E)

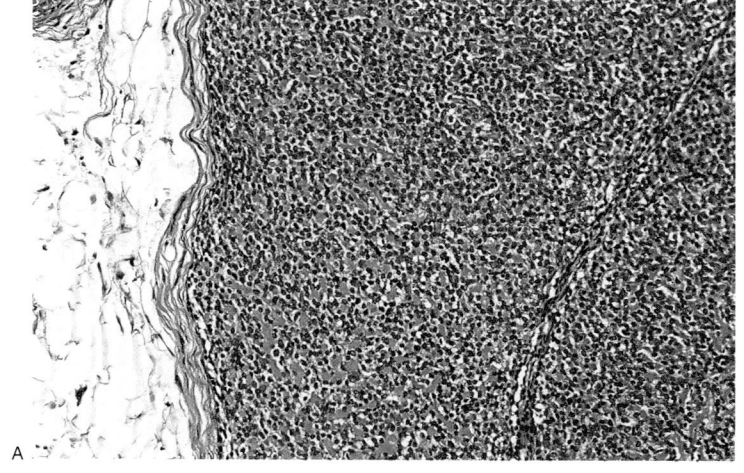

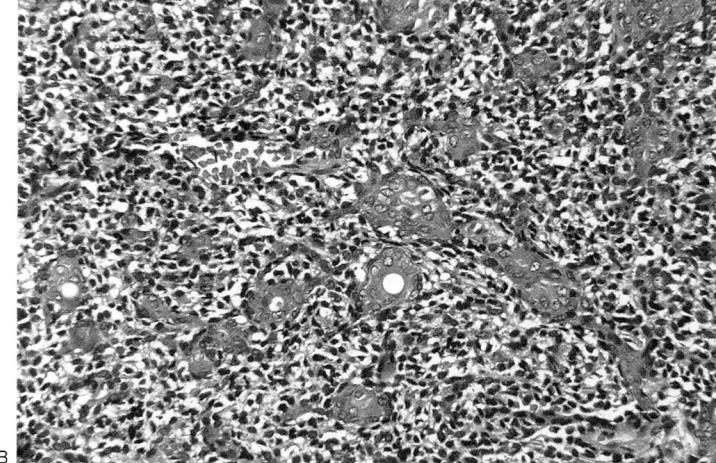

Fig. 33.48 **Spiradenoma. (A)** The tumor lobule has a thin fibrous capsule. There are small basaloid cells admixed with some larger cells. **(B)** Small duct-like structures are present within a tumor lobule. (H & E)

round cell with mitochondria, small vesicles, and sometimes glycogen in the cytoplasm.[789] A rare dark cell is present. Although lumina have not always been seen,[803] they have been reported, with microvilli on the lining cells. Intracytoplasmic lumina have also been seen within the epithelial cells.[809]

POROMA GROUP

The subclassification of the poroma group and the hidradenomas is a confusing area of dermatopathology. Not only does an overlap in histological features occur between the various entities within each of these two groups, but also between the two. For example, it is not uncommon for a tumor to resemble poroma superficially and to have a deeper dermal component of solid–cystic hidradenoma. Some authors have used the terms 'solid–cystic hidradenoma' and 'acrospiroma' to encompass both the poroma and hidradenoma group, whereas others have used the terms for an individual tumor in the hidradenoma group.[456] The term 'poroid hidradenoma' has been applied to a dermal tumor with solid and cystic components resembling the hidradenoma but composed of poroid-type cells.[395,810] It is regarded as the eccrine equivalent of apocrine hidradenoma (see below).

Here the poroma group will be subdivided into eccrine poroma, dermal duct tumor (dermal eccrine poroma), hidroacanthoma simplex (intra-epidermal poroma), syringoacanthoma and syringofibroadenoma. A lesion has been described which contained three histologically distinct components: hidroacanthoma simplex, eccrine poroma and dermal duct tumor.[811]

Ackerman believes that some poromas are of apocrine origin, but they can only be inferred to be apocrine on the basis of a connection of one or more elongated tubules to infundibula.[395]

ECCRINE POROMA

Eccrine poroma, a tumor derived from the acrosyringium, presents as a solitary, pink or red exophytic nodule, usually on plantar or palmar skin.[812,813] It may also be found elsewhere on the lower extremities and hands, and at times on any other area of the body with sweat glands. Some of the lesions on the head and neck may be of apocrine origin.[814] Multiple lesions (eccrine poromatosis) are very rare and some purported cases appear to be examples of acrosyringeal nevus.[696,815] Origin in an area of chronic radiation dermatitis has been reported once.[816]

Histopathology[817]

Eccrine poroma is a circumscribed tumor composed of cords and broad columns of uniform basaloid cells extending into the dermis from the undersurface of the epidermis (Fig. 33.49). The cells are smaller than, and well delineated from, the epidermal cells with which they are in contact. They are PAS positive and much of the PAS-positive material is diastase sensitive. Melanin pigment is sometimes present and is sometimes visible clinically.[818] Ducts and, less commonly, small cysts may also be seen within the tumor columns. The stroma is usually richly vascular with some telangiectatic vessels, contributing to the clinical appearance.

Uncommonly, divergent adnexal differentiation is seen in eccrine poromas, with focal sebaceous, pilar and possibly apocrine secretory differentiation.[819] On the basis of the common embryological origin of follicular, sebaceous and apocrine structures, it has been suggested that some 'eccrine' poromas might be of apocrine origin (see above).[814,819] Keratins 1 and 10 are expressed in the tumor nests.[820]

Electron microscopy

The tumor cells have numerous connecting desmosomes, cytoplasmic tonofilaments, glycogen granules and intracytoplasmic lumina. The latter appear to coalesce to form larger intercellular duct-like structures resembling embryonic intraepidermal sweat ducts.[821]

DERMAL DUCT TUMOR

The term 'dermal duct tumor' was coined by Winkelmann and McLeod in 1966 for a tumor composed of basaloid cells, like an eccrine poroma, but located in the dermis.[822] Relatively few cases have been reported since, and this may simply reflect the hesitation of some dermatopathologists to make the diagnosis, particularly when multiple sections through a presumed dermal duct tumor often show a connection with the undersurface of the epidermis or areas resembling solid–cystic hidradenoma (poroid hidradenoma). Clinically, dermal duct tumor presents as a firm nodule, particularly on the lower limbs or head and neck region.[823]

Histopathology

The tumor is composed of islands of basaloid tumor cells within the dermis. Duct-like structures are prominent in many of the nests, and the tumor may

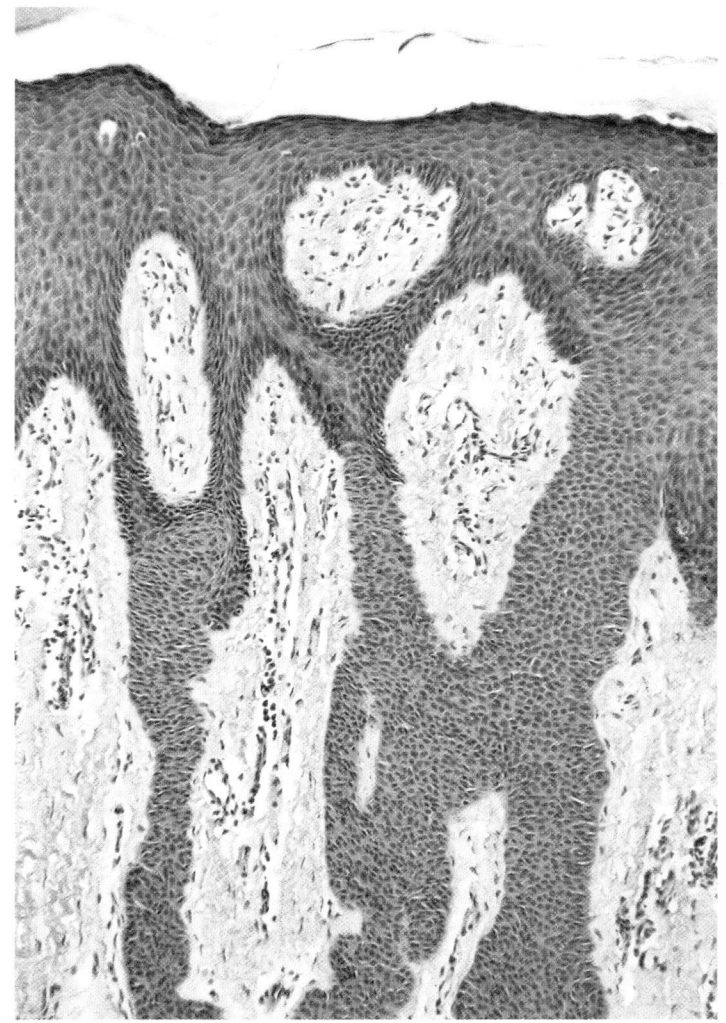

Fig. 33.49 **Poroma.** Cords of basaloid cells extend into the dermis. (H & E)

tself connect with a normal-appearing eccrine duct. An epidermal connection s often found if multiple sections are examined.[824] The cells are PAS positive, but this is usually not as striking as in eccrine poroma. Melanin pigment is sometimes present.

Electron microscopy
The tumor is composed of clear, dark and luminal cells, the clear cell being predominant.[823] There are microvilli on the luminal side of the cells lining the ducts within the cell nests.

HIDROACANTHOMA SIMPLEX

Hidroacanthoma simplex (intraepidermal eccrine poroma) is a solitary plaque or nodular lesion found particularly on the extremities and the trunk.[825–827] It arises throughout adult life and there is an equal sex incidence. Clinically, it resembles a seborrheic keratosis or basal cell carcinoma. Many of the cases reported in the literature as hidroacanthoma simplex are probably examples of the clonal variant of seborrheic keratosis;[828] two cases purporting to be hidroacanthoma simplex with porocarcinomatous transformation[829,830] are possibly other entities.[831]

Histopathology
Hidroacanthoma simplex is composed of well-circumscribed nests of cuboidal to oval basaloid cells within the epidermis, resembling those seen in eccrine poroma (Fig. 33.50). The cells are smaller than neighboring epidermal keratinocytes and they contain some glycogen. Rarely, melanin pigment is present.[832] Reports that mention squamous and spindle-cell variants[826] probably included seborrheic keratoses.[831]

A few ductal structures may sometimes be seen within the islands. The epidermis is usually acanthotic with some overlying hyperkeratosis. A dermal component resembling solid–cystic hidradenoma is sometimes present.

One immunohistochemical study has shown that the tumor cells stain intensely with antikeratin antibodies (using an AE1/AE3 cytokeratin 'cocktail'), but not with CEA, which did stain adjacent normal acrosyringium.[833] On the basis of these findings and the electron microscopy (see below) the authors concluded that the case studied 'did not appear to arise from or differentiate toward the luminal cells of the acrosyringium'.[833] Hidroacanthoma simplex may arise from the outer cells of the intraepidermal eccrine duct.

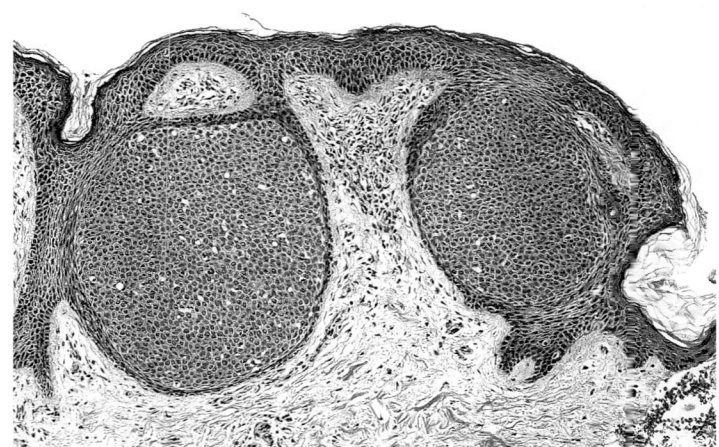

Fig. 33.50 **Hidroacanthoma simplex.** Well-circumscribed nests of basaloid cells are present within the epidermis. (H & E)

Seborrheic keratoses of the clonal type may have islands of cells within the epidermis, the so-called 'Jadassohn phenomenon'. However, the cells in seborrheic keratoses are not as small and basaloid and do not contain glycogen. Another tumor that shows the Jadassohn phenomenon of intra-epidermal nesting is the so-called 'intraepidermal epithelioma of Jadassohn'.[834] This is perhaps the most controversial entity in dermatopathology.[835] It is assumed to be derived from acrosyringeal keratinocytes (as are hidroacanthoma simplex, acrosyringeal nevus and syringofibroadenoma). Many believe that this entity is heterogeneous and includes seborrheic keratoses with atypia or bowenoid transformation, and variants of intraepidermal carcinoma.[831,836] It has not been mentioned in the recent literature.

Electron microscopy
The tumor cells contain few desmosomes, decreased numbers of tonofilaments, and abundant cytoplasmic glycogen.[833]

SYRINGOACANTHOMA

Syringoacanthoma was described by Rahbari in 1984 as a tumor derived from the acrosyringium.[837] It is said to differ from hidroacanthoma simplex by the presence of prominent acanthosis and papillomatosis, and less orderly intraepidermal nests. Steffen and Ackerman believe that it is not a distinct entity.[831]

SYRINGOFIBROADENOMA

It has been suggested[699] that eccrine syringofibroadenoma, as described by Mascaro in 1963,[701] is identical to the acrosyringeal nevus of Weedon and Lewis[696] (see eccrine hamartomas, p. 888), but there do appear to be some clinicopathological differences.[703] The eccrine syringofibroadenoma presents as a solitary, often large, hyperkeratotic nodular lesion with a predilection for the extremities.[699,702,838,839] Rare sites of involvement include the nail apparatus[840] and an organoid nevus.[841] This term has also been applied to diffuse, zosteriform and multiple lesions resembling the case reported as an acrosyringeal nevus.[842] The terms 'acrosyringeal adenomatosis' and 'eccrine syringofibroadenomatosis (Mascaro)' have been suggested as appropriate designations for the more diffuse cases.[843–845] Eccrine syringofibroadenomatosis can occur in association with hidrotic ectodermal dysplasia.[846,847] It has been said that the lesions are somewhat different in the two variants, Clouston's syndrome and the Schöpf syndrome. HPV-10 has been detected in the lesions occurring in Clouston's syndrome.[848] Eccrine syringofibroadenomatosis has also been reported in a familial setting in association with ophthalmological abnormalities.[849]

The occurrence of this phenomenon next to inflammatory dermatoses and tumors, often in an acral location, has been called reactive eccrine syringofibroadenomatosis. As stromal changes are minimal in some instances, 'eccrine duct hyperplasia' would be a better term. This reactive change has been seen next to palmoplantar erosive lichen planus,[850] bullous pemphigoid,[851] a burn scar,[852] pincer nail,[853] squamous cell carcinoma[854] and a chronic diabetic foot ulcer.[855]

It has also presented as a 'mossy' leg, resembling lymphedematous keratoderma.[856]

Histopathology[699,702,857]
There are thin anastomosing epithelial cords and strands forming a lattice and connected to the undersurface of the epidermis (Fig. 33.51). The cells are smaller and more basophilic than the epidermal keratinocytes. Nests of clear

to 6 cm or more in diameter have been recorded.[471,872] The behavior of the eccrine variant is probably no different to that of the apocrine variant (see p. 880).

Histopathology

Despite their identical clinical appearances, the eccrine variant of hidradenoma differs histologically from the apocrine hidradenoma. Eccrine hidradenoma (poroid hidradenoma) is a circumscribed, non-encapsulated dermal tumor composed of poroid and cuticular cells. Ductal structures may form, particularly within the zones of cuticular cells. It has the architectural features of the apocrine hidradenoma but with the cytological characteristics of a poroma.[810] It lacks the polygonal, clear and mucinous cells of the apocrine variant.[395]

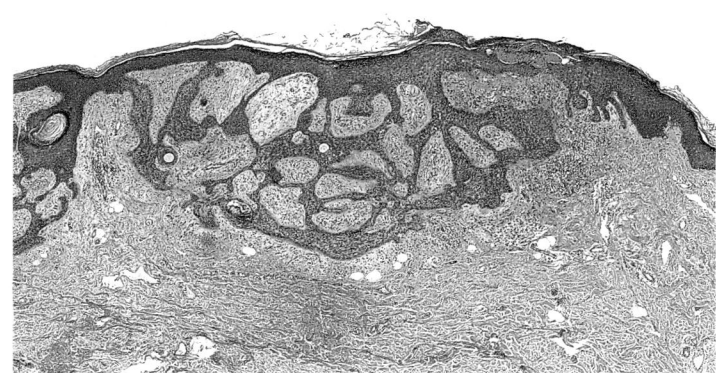

Fig. 33.51 **Syringofibroadenoma.** A lattice of thin epithelial cords is connected to the under-surface of the epidermis. The cells are smaller and more basaloid than the overlying epidermal keratinocytes. (H & E)

cells have been reported.[858,859] Ducts are present within the tumor. Between the strands there is a rich fibrovascular stroma. The tumor does not have the strong PAS positivity or the abundant stromal plasma cells noted in the case reported as an acrosyringeal nevus.[696] However, plasma cells have not been a feature in many of the other multiple/diffuse cases.

The term '**syringofibrocarcinoma**' has been suggested for a single case in which a net-like arrangement of cytologically malignant cells showing ductal differentiation impinged on a benign component.[860]

Immunohistochemical studies have not shown consistent results with respect to cytokeratin expression, but they seem to indicate differentiation toward the acrosyringium and dermal duct.[838,861–865]

Electron microscopy

Intracellular duct formation, characteristic of developing acrosyringia, has been observed. Abundant glycogen is also present.[861,866]

HIDRADENOMA

Considerable confusion exists in the literature concerning the most appropriate designation for this tumor. Wilson Jones has called it a 'nosological jungle'.[465] Terms used have included 'solid–cystic hidradenoma',[457] 'eccrine acrospiroma',[456] 'clear cell hidradenoma',[644] 'eccrine sweat gland adenoma'[867] and 'clear cell myoepithelioma'.[868] This topic is further confused by the recent separation of apocrine hidradenomas from a less common eccrine group, which has also been called poroid hidradenoma. The apocrine group (apocrine hidradenoma) are composed of clear, polygonal and mucinous cells while the eccrine lesion (hidradenoma, poroid hidradenoma) consists of poroid and cuticular cells.[467,869]

HIDRADENOMA (POROID HIDRADENOMA)

Hidradenoma refers to a tumor that includes both an eccrine and apocrine variant. The two are clinically indistinguishable. Both usually present as a solitary, solid or partially cystic nodule with a slight preponderance in females of middle age,[644] but with no site predilection. Cases occurring in children are rare.[870,87] Hidradenoma averages 1–2 cm in diameter, but larger variants up

MALIGNANT ECCRINE TUMORS

The classification of malignant eccrine tumors is one of the most confusing areas of dermatopathology, with identical tumors reported in the literature under three or more designations. Furthermore, tumors with heterogeneous histological features that defy classification are common. Some earlier reports give scant histological details, precluding reassessment.[873] It is tempting to suggest that the term 'eccrine carcinoma' be applied to all malignant eccrine tumors, in much the same way that the term 'basal cell carcinoma' has proved adequate for a histologically diverse group of tumors.

In his major review of sweat gland carcinomas, Santa Cruz lists the synonyms and related terms used for each of the tumors he describes.[424] He also suggests a classification based on the malignant potential as currently understood. For the most part, the eccrine tumors with the highest malignant potential are the malignant counterparts of the benign eccrine tumors (malignant spiradenoma and malignant cylindroma), and some of the ductal adenocarcinomas. The malignant eccrine poroma is of intermediate malignancy. The low-malignancy group includes microcystic adnexal carcinoma and eccrine epithelioma.[424] If there is any doubt about the potential malignancy of a sweat gland tumor, aneuploidy detected by DNA image cytometry is a clear and specific indicator of prospective malignancy.[874]

Rarely, a pleomorphic or mixed sarcoma may arise in a sweat gland adenoma, or *de novo*, that is assumed to be derived from the myoepithelial elements of eccrine tumors. Recognition of an underlying benign tumor is usually necessary to make the diagnosis.[875]

There has been much interest in assessing the various immunohistochemical markers of the eccrine carcinomas. In a study of 32 cases, epithelial membrane antigen and cytokeratin were present in all cases, CEA was detected in 25, and S100 in 19 cases.[876] Diffuse staining for ferritin is another marker of eccrine carcinomas.[663] These studies need reassessing in the light of the suggested reclassification of many eccrine tumors as apocrine in type.

A recent study of genetic and other markers in a mixed group of 21 sweat gland carcinomas found loss of heterozygosity (LOH), confined mostly to chromosome arm 17p, in 4 cases.[877] There was only a low frequency of p53 alterations.

MICROCYSTIC ADNEXAL CARCINOMA

Microcystic adnexal carcinoma was first reported in 1982 by Goldstein and colleagues.[878] It has also been referred to as malignant syringoma,[879] sweat gland carcinoma with syringomatous features[880] and sclerosing sweat duct carcinoma.[881] **Syringomatous adenoma of the nipple** is a closely related entity.[882]

Microcystic adnexal carcinoma is a slowly growing, locally aggressive tumor which presents as an indurated plaque or nodule, usually on the upper lip or elsewhere on the face.[883–886] It has a predilection for the left side of the face.[887] It may also be found in the axilla,[888] the extremities,[889] genital skin[890] and on the trunk and scalp.[891,892] It affects adults of all ages. In several cases the patient has previously received radiotherapy for adolescent acne or cancers.[881,893–896] Other associations have included an underlying 'systematized compound epithelial nevus'[897] and a primary immunodeficiency syndrome.[898]

Local recurrence occurs in nearly 50% of cases,[881] but this is less likely if the excision margins are free of tumor in the initial excision.[896] The recurrence rate has recently been calculated as 1.98% per patient-year.[887] Only one case has had histological evidence of lymph node involvement, and this was almost certainly due to in-continuity extension.[881] Microcystic adnexal carcinoma is included within the spectrum of *locally aggressive adnexal carcinomas*.[899] It has been regarded recently as an apocrine tumor.[395]

Histopathology[424,881]

The tumor usually involves the subcutis as well as the dermis, and it may extend into the underlying muscle. There is some stratification of the various histological changes.[424] The superficial part is composed of numerous keratinous cysts and small islands and strands of basaloid and squamous epithelium showing variable ductal differentiation. Focal clear cell change may be present in some of the cells. Rarely, this is a prominent feature.[900] Sebaceous differentiation has also been reported.[899,901]

The deeper component has smaller nests and strands of cells in a dense, hyalinized stroma, giving a scirrhous appearance (Fig. 33.52). Perineural invasion is frequently present.[902,903] The aggressive growth and perineural spread allow a distinction to be made from syringoma and desmoplastic trichoepithelioma.

The microcystic adnexal carcinoma has become an expanding 'entity' with the inclusion of tumors that bear no relationship to those originally described. Cases of eccrine (syringoid) carcinoma are sometimes included.

The **solid carcinoma**, previously included with either the eccrine (syringoid) carcinoma or the microcystic adnexal carcinoma, has now been regarded as a discrete entity by Requena, Kiryu and Ackerman.[395] It consists of numerous small nests and strands of cells having a predominantly solid pattern. There is stromal desmoplasia and perineural spread.

In some of the reported cases the luminal cells have been CEA positive.[884,904] The cells stain for epithelial membrane antigen and various keratins, particularly CK7.[905–907] Some S100-positive cells are also present.[908] The low level of Ki-67 supports a low proliferative rate.[907] It has been suggested, on the basis of the electron microscopy and the immunophenotype, that microcystic adnexal carcinoma expresses both eccrine and pilar differentiation, but this is at variance with other views that it is of apocrine type.

ECCRINE CARCINOMA (SYRINGOID CARCINOMA)

Eccrine carcinoma (syringoid carcinoma) is a rare tumor which usually presents as a slowly growing infiltrating plaque on the scalp,[909] or as a plaque or nodule on the extremities or trunk.[424,598,599,910–912] It has a propensity for local recurrence, but metastases are quite rare.[424,913]

These tumors were originally reported as basal cell tumors with eccrine differentiation (eccrine epitheliomas).[598] Subsequently, they have been reported as syringoid eccrine carcinomas[914,915] and also as eccrine

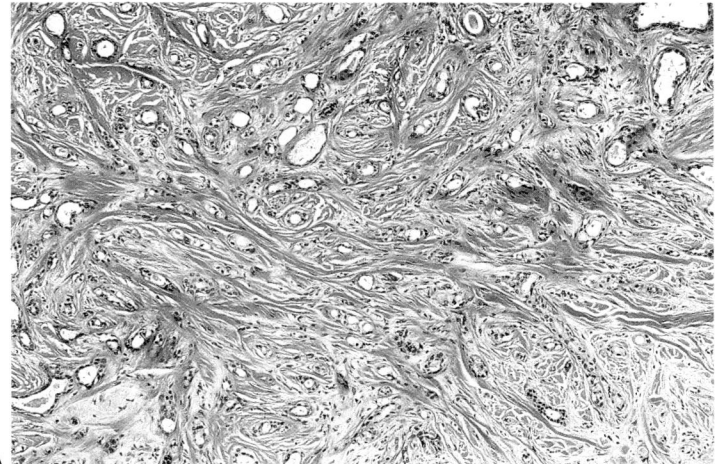

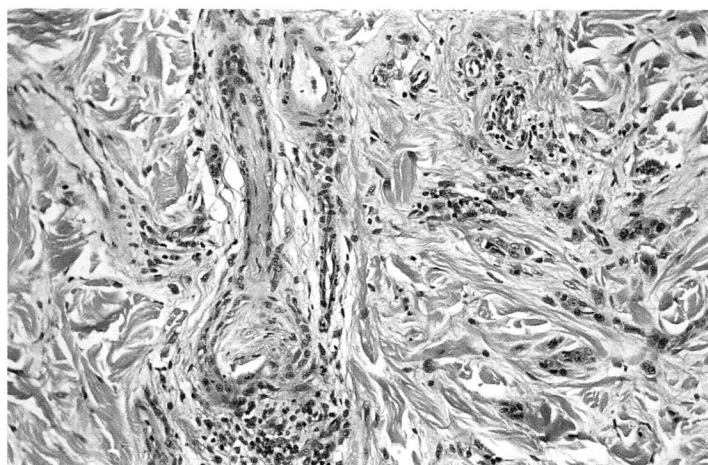

Fig. 33.52 **Microcystic adnexal carcinoma. (A)** Ductal structures and small cords of cells are set in a fibrous stroma. **(B)** Perineural invasion is present. (H & E)

syringomatous carcinoma.[916] It has been the author's practice to use this term for a group of malignant eccrine tumors composed of varying numbers of tubular structures which may be basaloid at one end of the spectrum and syringoma-like at the other end. Other components may be present (see below). Excluded from this category are tumors with morphologically specific features, such as the microcystic adnexal carcinoma (see above), the adenoid cystic carcinoma, the mucinous carcinoma and the polymorphous sweat gland carcinoma.

Histopathology

The tumor is composed of numerous tubular structures lined by one or several layers of atypical basaloid cells (Fig. 33.53).[598,599,917] Thin strands and solid nests of similar cells also occur.[918] Foci with syringomatous features are often present.[919] A clear cell variant and one with possible acrosyringeal differentiation have been reported.[920,921] PAS-positive diastase-resistant material is present in the lumina of the tubular structures.

The tumor is centered on the dermis, but often extends into the subcutis or deeper.[919] Perineural invasion is common.

Eccrine carcinoma differs from microcystic adnexal carcinoma by having areas with a basaloid cell pattern, in contrast to the squamoid features of the other.[596] However, some eccrine carcinomas may have syringoma-like ducts (syringoid carcinoma), but these are often larger and better formed than those seen in microcystic adnexal carcinoma. Unlike the latter tumor, a

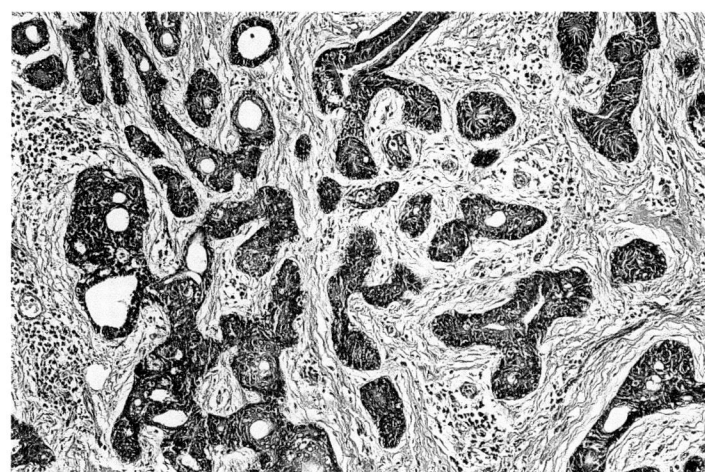

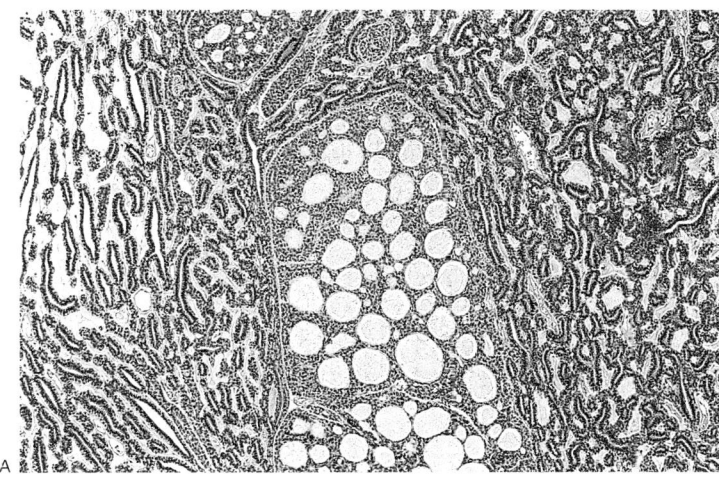

Fig. 33.53 **Eccrine carcinoma.** It is composed of tubular structures lined by atypical basaloid cells. A few ducts have features resembling those seen in a syringoma. (H & E)

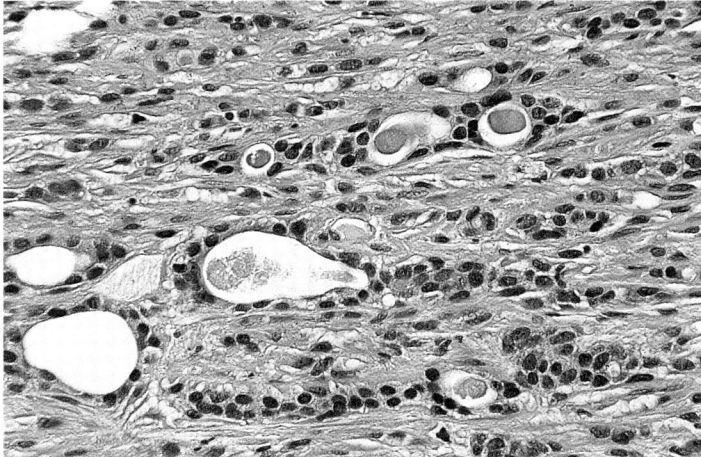

desmoplastic stroma is minimal or absent in eccrine carcinoma. Despite the above, it must be acknowledged that cases with overlap features arise (Fig. 33.54).[920] There is a growing tendency to regard this tumor as a variant of microcystic adnexal carcinoma.

POLYMORPHOUS SWEAT GLAND CARCINOMA

Polymorphous sweat gland carcinoma is a recently described adnexal tumor characterized by a variegated histological appearance and low-grade malignant behavior.[922] The lesions present as large, slow-growing dermal nodules with a marked predilection for the extremities. Local recurrence can occur, but metastasis is uncommon.

Histopathology
The lesions are characterized by a highly cellular proliferation with a variety of growth patterns, including solid, trabecular, tubular, pseudopapillary and cylindromatous (Fig. 33.55). Focal small tubules resembling eccrine ducts are often present. The stroma may show hemorrhage and some hyalinization.[922]

Fig. 33.55 **(A) Polymorphous sweat gland carcinoma. (B)** An area with syringoid features is also present. (H & E)

DIGITAL PAPILLARY ADENOCARCINOMA

Digital papillary adenocarcinoma occurs as a solitary painless mass, almost exclusively on the fingers, toes and adjacent parts of the palms and soles.[923,924] Most tumors are nodular growths, less than 2 cm in diameter. Over 90% are grossly cystic.

On the basis of a review of 67 cases of this entity at the Armed Forces Institute of Pathology, the original suggestion that both a benign and malignant form of this tumor existed was modified.[925] Since none of the histological or clinical parameters studied was predictive of recurrence or metastasis, all lesions were regarded as adenocarcinomas. Metastases occurred in 14% of cases that were available for follow-up. Ackerman and colleagues call it papillary carcinoma and regard it as being of apocrine origin.[395] Now that all tumors are regarded as being malignant, it seems pointless to retain the term 'aggressive' in the title, as originally used.

Histopathology[728,923]
The tumor involves the dermis and subcutis; it is usually poorly circumscribed. There are tubuloalveolar and ductal structures with areas of papillary projections protruding into cystic lumina (Fig. 33.56). The ductal structures are usually larger and more dilated than those in the papillary eccrine adenoma. A cribriform pattern without obvious epithelial papillations is seen in about 20% of cases. The glandular lumina may contain eosinophilic secretory

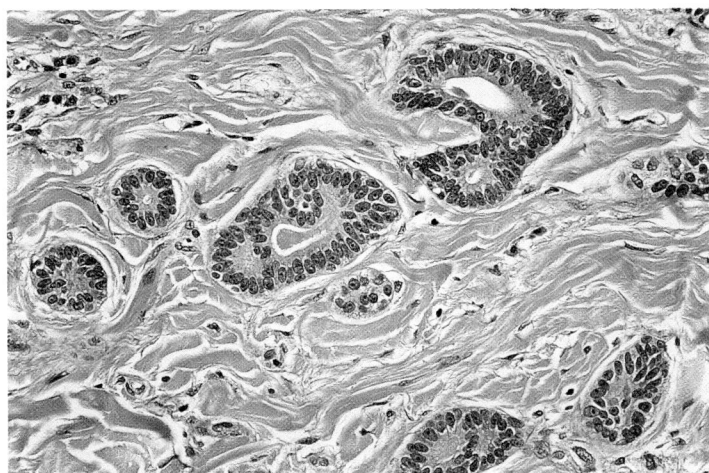

Fig. 33.54 **Eccrine carcinoma.** This tumor has ductal structures with syringoid features. (H & E)

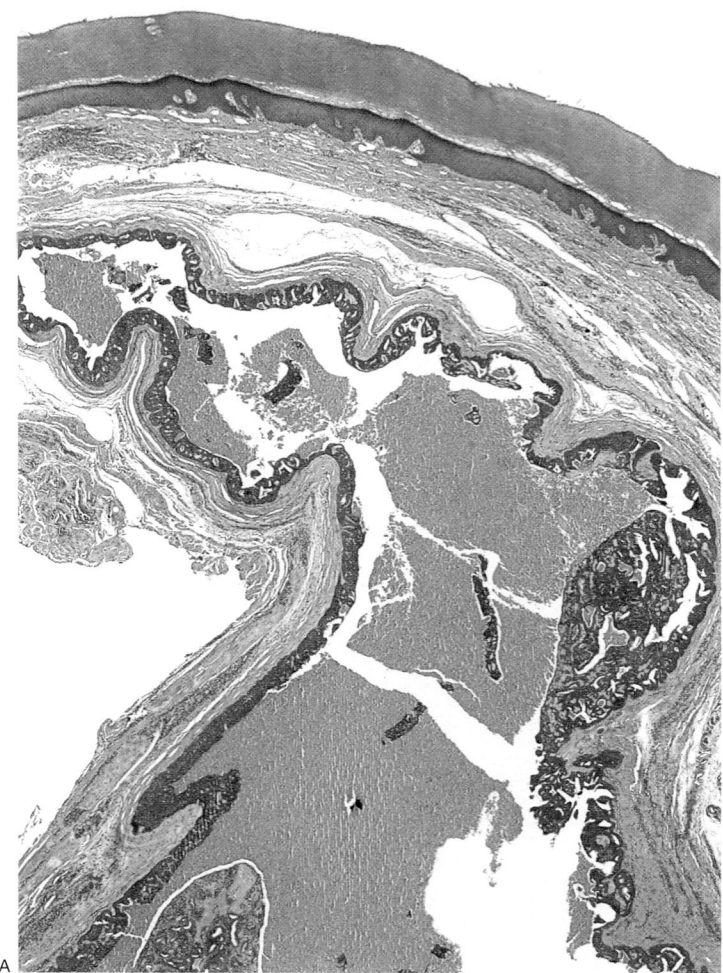

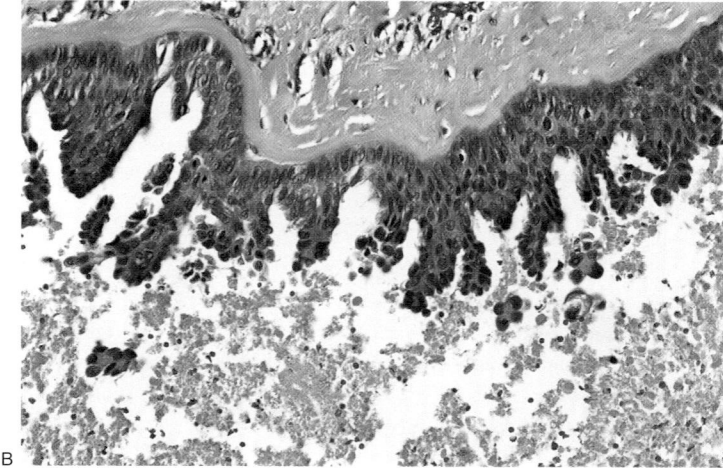

Fig. 33.56 **(A) Digital papillary adenocarcinoma. (B)** The cells lining the cystic space show papillary infolding and some atypia of cells. (H & E)

material. Scattered mitoses are present. The stroma varies from thin fibrous septa to areas of dense hyalinized collagen.

In some cases there is poor glandular differentiation, focal necrosis, cellular atypia and pleomorphism, and invasion of soft tissues, blood vessels and sometimes the underlying bone.[923,925,926]

Immunoperoxidase studies have shown positivity for S100 protein, CEA and cytokeratins.[923] This staining is not eccrine specific. Electron microscopy has shown eccrine glandular differentiation.

MALIGNANT CYLINDROMA

Malignant cylindroma is a very rare tumor that usually arises in a long-standing cylindroma of the scalp.[772,774,775,927] It develops more often in patients with multiple cylindromas.[928,929] Ab initio variants probably also occur.[424] Multiple malignant cylindromas have been reported in a patient who also had a basal cell adenocarcinoma of minor salivary gland.[930] The tumors are aggressive, although subsequent metastasis is rare.[776]

This tumor may be of apocrine type.

Histopathology

The tumor is composed of nests and cords of basaloid cells showing frequent mitoses, focal necrosis and loss of the PAS-positive hyaline membrane. It has been suggested that the rare variants that have partially preserved hyaline membranes have a good prognosis.[931] Foci of squamous differentiation occur. A contiguous benign cylindroma is usually present.[932]

MALIGNANT SPIRADENOMA (SPIRADENOCARCINOMA)

The malignant transformation of spiradenoma is a rare event, heralded by the rapid enlargement of a cutaneous nodule of long standing.[799,800,933,934] Many different sites have been involved, several of these tumors occurring around the elbow and on the digits.[424,935] The trunk is the favored site.[936] The tumors are quite aggressive, with fatal metastasis developing in at least 20% of cases.[424]

A case has been reported of a mixed eccrine spiradenoma and cylindroma in which malignant transformation of both components occurred.[937]

Histopathology

There are solid islands of tumor cells, which may show either a squamous or a basaloid pattern. Glandular and sarcomatous areas have also been reported.[424,798,938] The diagnosis depends on finding a contiguous spiradenoma, as the malignant component usually lacks any distinguishing features. Sometimes, an abrupt transition between the benign and malignant components is present.[936]

The tumor cells express cytokeratins, epithelial membrane antigen[935] and p53.[939]

POROCARCINOMA

Porocarcinoma (malignant poroma) was first described by Pinkus and Mehregan as 'epidermotropic eccrine carcinoma'.[940] Since that time over 200 cases have been reported; there have been three large series.[914,941,942] The tumor occurs at all ages, although there is a predilection for older individuals. Acral locations are favored.[943,944] Porocarcinomas present as verrucous plaques or polypoid growths which sometimes bleed with minor trauma.[941,945] Pigmented variants, due to melanocyte colonization, are uncommon.[946,947]

Some are of long duration, suggesting malignant transformation of an eccrine or apocrine poroma or hidroacanthoma simplex.[948,949] Rarely, a porocarcinoma arises in an organoid nevus.[950] Local recurrences and metastasis, particularly to regional nodes, occur.[942,951] Distant metastases are less common than in some of the other malignant counterparts of benign sweat gland tumors.[952–955] An unusual pattern of metastasis is the development of multiple cutaneous deposits with a lymphangitic pattern and microscopic epidermotropic deposits.

In the light of the distinction between apocrine and eccrine poromas, it is likely that many porocarcinomas are of apocrine origin, but further studies are needed before wholesale reclassification is done.

Histopathology[424,914,941]

The intraepidermal component is composed of nests and islands of small basaloid cells, sharply demarcated from the adjacent keratinocytes.[914] Broad anastomosing cords and solid columns and nests of large cells extend into the dermis to varying levels. Clear cell areas, squamous differentiation, melanin pigment and focal necrosis may be present in the dermal nests.[947,956,957] Clear cell change has been found in a diabetic patient.[958] Ductal structures are also found (Fig. 33.57). A similar lesion, but with only an intraepidermal component, has been reported as an in situ porocarcinoma.[959] This pattern must be distinguished from epidermotropic porocarcinoma, a pattern that can be seen adjacent to porocarcinomas and in cutaneous metastases.[960] A benign component of poroma or hidroacanthoma simplex may be present.[775,829,830] An acrosyringeal and ductal proliferation resembling syringofibroadenomatosis has been reported adjacent to a porocarcinoma of the heel.[944]

The cells contain variable amounts of PAS-positive material, much of which is diastase labile. They stain positively for CEA, cytokeratin and epithelial membrane antigen.[876] Porocarcinomas have a significantly higher proportion of cells expressing proliferating cell nuclear antigen (PCNA) than do benign poromas.[961]

Electron microscopy

The tumor cells contain a variable amount of glycogen, rare tonofilaments and intracellular lumina. The cell membranes have complex interdigitating microvilli-like cell processes.[424] Crystalline membrane-bound granules have also been reported.[962]

SQUAMOID ECCRINE DUCTAL CARCINOMA

Squamoid eccrine ductal carcinoma is an exceedingly rare tumor that shows eccrine ductal differentiation combined with a squamoid component characterized by prominent squamous proliferation with atypia, keratinous cyst formation and squamous eddies (Fig. 33.58).[963] Tumors present as nodules on the head and neck or extremities.[963,964] Multiple local recurrences have been recorded in one case.[963]

MISCELLANEOUS SWEAT GLAND CARCINOMAS

Very rare tumors include the mucoepidermoid carcinoma of the skin (see p. 776),[422,965,966] the signet-ring cell carcinoma of the eyelids[424,967] and the small-cell sweat gland carcinoma in childhood.[968] The tumor reported as a trabecular carcinoma of the skin was regarded as adnexal in origin, but no evidence was presented to support this contention.[969] It was composed of long, irregularly branching serpiginous trabeculae.

Complex adnexal tumors

The term 'complex adnexal tumors' is proposed for those tumors, including hamartomas, in which differentiation toward more than one adnexal structure

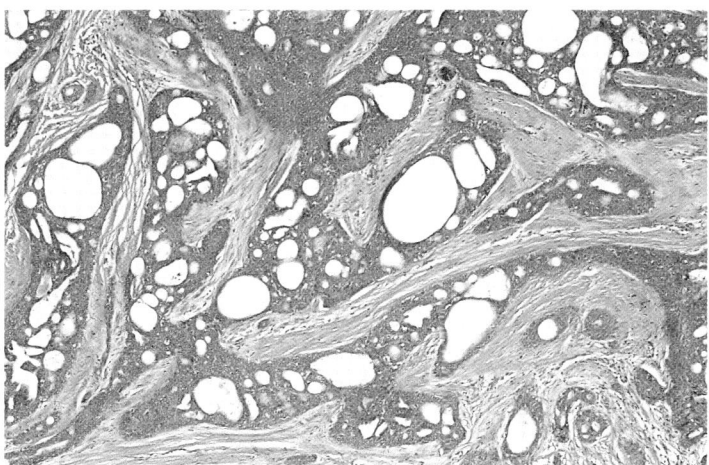

Fig. 33.57 **Porocarcinoma.** There are columns of cells with cystic change. Nests infiltrate the stroma. (H & E)

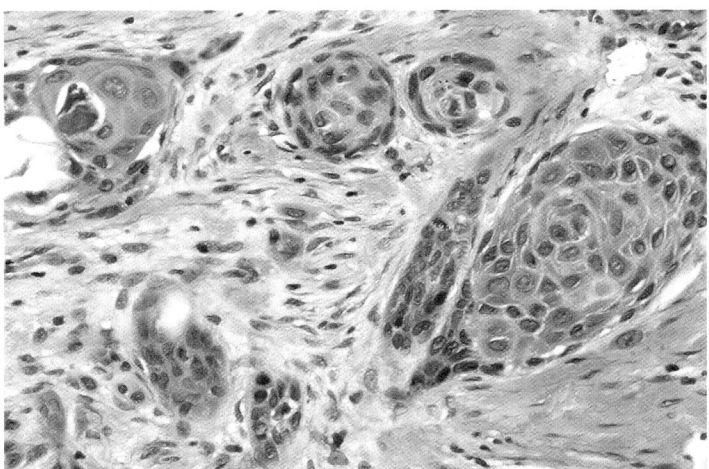

Fig. 33.58 **Squamoid eccrine ductal adenocarcinoma.** There are squamoid nests with focal duct formation. (H & E)

is present. The most important lesion in this group is the organoid nevus (nevus sebaceus of Jadassohn), in which abnormalities of all adnexal structures as well as of the epidermis may be present. Other tumors in this group include the adnexal polyp of neonatal skin,[970] combined adnexal tumor,[971] poroma-like adnexal adenoma,[972,973] sebaceous epithelioma with sweat gland differentiation[368] and hemifacial mixed appendage tumor.[974] The linear eccrine nevus with comedones (see eccrine hamartomas, p. 889) could also have been included.

ORGANOID NEVUS

Organoid nevus (nevus sebaceus of Jadassohn) is a complex hamartoma involving not only the pilosebaceous follicle, but also the epidermis, and often other adnexal structures.[975,976] It evolves through different stages. Nearly all lesions are on the scalp, forehead or face. It is present at birth or develops in early childhood. Familial cases have been recorded.[977,978] Most lesions are plaques 1–6 cm in diameter. A lesion 9.5 cm in diameter, with a cerebriform surface, has been reported on the scalp.[979] Linear or zosteriform patterns are uncommon. The tumor is usually hairless, yellow or waxy in color, with a smooth, warty or mamillated surface. There are some reports of patients with large organoid nevi of the scalp with associated neuroectodermal and other defects,[980–982] but these associations were not present in the large series of Mehregan and Pinkus[976] and of Wilson Jones and Heyl.[983] Other associated abnormalities have included segmental neurofibromatosis,[984] retinoblastoma with associated lipomata and a meningioma,[985] and tuberous sclerosis.[986] The term 'nevus sebaceus syndrome' is applied to cases with associated ectodermal or mesodermal defects.[987] Tumors such as basal cell carcinoma, trichoblastomas, syringocystadenoma papilliferum and hidracenomas may develop in organoid nevi in adults.[988] Recent studies have confirmed that the vast majority of basaloid neoplasms arising in organoid nevi are trichoblastomas and not basal cell carcinomas as once thought.[989–991] Other rare associations include leiomyoma,[992] syringoma, spiradenoma,[993] squamous cell carcinoma, nevoid growths of melanocytes,[994] keratoacanthoma, porocarcinoma[950] and various sebaceous and apocrine tumors.[983,995,996] Many of the associated tumors do not correspond precisely with described entities.[975]

Histopathology[976,983,997]

In infants and young children the dominant feature is the presence of immature and abnormally formed pilosebaceous units, which may also be reduced in number (Fig. 33.59). The epidermal changes are usually mild, with some acanthosis and mild papillomatosis. Around puberty there is enlargement of the sebaceous glands, which are often located abnormally high in the dermis, with an increased number of closely set lobules and malformed ducts. Some lobules may be incompletely lipidized. Sebaceous glands are sometimes reduced or even absent at this age. Hair follicles are usually vellus rather than terminal, and are often reduced in number. The follicular dysgenesis and hair follicle numbers are easier to assess in lesions from the scalp than from other sites. The epidermis is now more papillomatous and acanthotic. At other times the epidermal pattern may resemble a seborrheic keratosis, an epidermal nevus or acanthosis nigricans (Fig. 33.60); rarely, there is pseudo-epitheliomatous hyperplasia, a keratoacanthoma-like proliferation[993] or epidermal downgrowths showing both apocrine and sebaceous differentiation.[999] Apocrine glands are present in up to half of the cases and sometimes the duct or secretory unit is dilated. Calcification within the apocrine glands has been reported in one case.[1000] Eccrine glands may be reduced in number, or show focal dilatation of the duct or secretory gland. In approximately 20% of cases 'apoeccrine' glands are present, but they have been said to represent eccrine glands with variable apocrine metaplasia rather than the separate category of sweat glands usually included under this designation.[1001] This explanation does not fit well with the embryological derivatives of the primary epithelial germ – follicular, sebaceous and apocrine.

The dermis is often thickened, particularly the adventitial dermis. There may be a slight increase in vascularity and a reduction in elastic fibers. Immature adipose tissue and extramedullary hematopoiesis have been reported.[1002] A mild chronic inflammatory cell infiltrate of lymphocytes and plasma cells is often present. Merkel cells are increased in those cases with follicular germ structures or with a superimposed trichoblastoma.[1003]

In older patients, other tumors may develop, as mentioned above. These may include syringocystadenoma papilliferum, which sometimes occupies only a small area of the entire nevus.

ADNEXAL POLYP OF NEONATAL SKIN

The adnexal polyp of neonatal skin is a small, usually solitary lesion, occurring mostly on the areola of the nipple of the neonate.[970] It was present in 4% of 3257 newborn infants in the one Japanese study of this entity, but it has

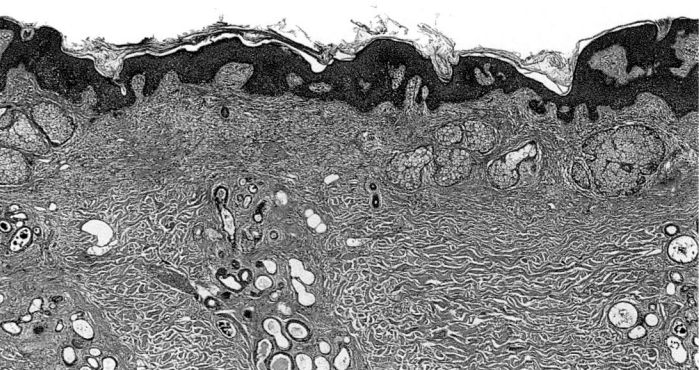

Fig. 33.59 **Organoid nevus.** The pilosebaceous follicles are small and abnormally formed. A few apocrine glands are present in the lower dermis. (H & E)

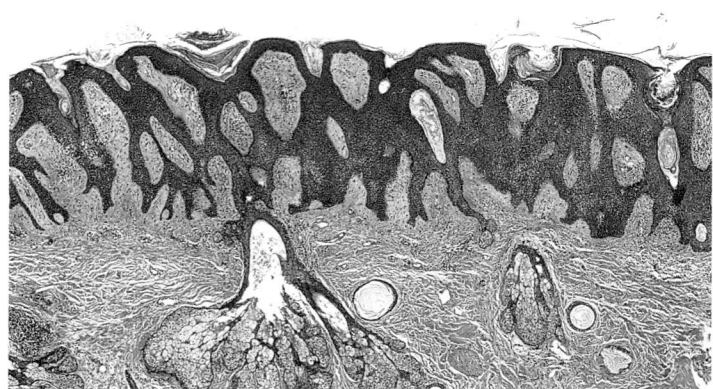

Fig. 33.60 **Organoid nevus.** The epidermis shows features of an epidermal nevus while the dermal changes are not striking in this area. (H & E)

received little attention in the literature. It drops off in the first week of life. Histologically, it contains hair follicles, eccrine glands and vestigial sebaceous glands.

COMBINED ADNEXAL TUMOR

The term 'combined adnexal tumor' has been used for a tumor with differentiation toward the formation of sebaceous glands and pilar and sweat duct structures.[971] It has also been applied to a tumor showing only pilar and sweat duct structures, but the case was probably a microcystic adnexal carcinoma.[904] Apocrine, sebaceous and pilar differentiation has been reported in apocrine mixed tumors of the skin. Embryologically, this combination of structures is explicable, as all three are derivatives of the primary epithelial germ.[1004] Notwithstanding this explanation, tumors with all four patterns of differentiation (pilar, sebaceous, apocrine and eccrine) have been described.[1005] It should also be noted that divergent differentiation is sometimes seen in various eccrine carcinomas. The term 'cutaneous adnexal carcinoma with divergent differentiation' has been used in these circumstances.[1006] All of these tumors would now fit into a category of apocrine or sebaceous tumors.

Requena and Ackerman have described a distinctive adnexal lesion with retiform and racemiform patterns.[1007] It showed both follicular and apocrine differentiation but differed from the sebocrine adenoma (see below).

SEBOCRINE ADENOMA

The sebocrine adenoma at first glance resembles an eccrine poroma, but the epithelial proliferations show apocrine and sebaceous, rather than eccrine, differentiation.[972,1008] The term 'poroma-like adnexal adenoma' has also been proposed for such cases.[973] It is likely that all these lesions will be recategorized as apocrine poromas. A similar case, but with prominent cystic degeneration, has been reported.[367]

HEMIFACIAL MIXED APPENDAGEAL TUMOR

The condition to which the name hemifacial mixed appendageal tumor was given was an erythematous papulonodular eruption confined to one side of the face of an infant.[974] It had a linear array on the cheek. The lesion was composed of islands of cells with eccrine, apocrine and basaloid features. Similar cases in the literature, usually with comedones, have been classed as linear basal cell nevi.

REFERENCES

Introduction

1 McCalmont TH. A call for logic in the classification of adnexal neoplasms [guest editorial]. Am J Dermatopathol 1996; 18(2).
2 Somach SC, Morgan MB. Benign keratosis with a spectrum of follicular differentiation: a case series and investigation of a potential role of human papilloma virus. J Cutan Pathol 2001; 28: 156–159.
3 Patterson JW, Wright ED, Camden S. Extraparotid Warthin's tumor. J Am Acad Dermatol 1999; 40: 468–470.
4 Morgan MB, Truitt CA, Romer C et al. Ocular adnexal oncocytoma. A case series and clinicopathologic review of the literature. Am J Dermatopathol 1998; 20: 487–490.

Hair follicle tumors

5 Headington JT. Tumors of the hair follicle. A review. Am J Pathol 1976; 85: 480–505.
6 Mehregan AH. Hair follicle tumors of the skin. J Cutan Pathol 1985; 12: 189–195.
7 Rosen LB. A review and proposed new classification of benign acquired neoplasms with hair follicle differentiation. Am J Dermatopathol 1990; 12: 496–516.
8 Ackerman AB, Reddy VB, Soyer HP. Neoplasms with follicular differentiation. New York: Ardor Scribendi, 2000.

Hamartomas and tumors of hair germ

9 Choi EH, Ahn SK, Lee SH, Bang D. Hair follicle nevus. Int J Dermatol 1992; 31: 578–581.
10 Davis DA, Cohen PR. Hair follicle nevus: case report and review of the literature. Pediatr Dermatol 1996; 13: 135–138.
11 Bass J, Pomeranz JR. Linear hair follicle nevus. Presentation American Society of Dermatopathology Meeting, San Antonio; 1987.
12 Pippione M, Aloi F, Depaoli MA. Hair-follicle nevus. Am J Dermatopathol 1984; 6: 245–247.
13 Weir TW. Hair-follicle nevus. Am J Dermatopathol 1985; 7: 304.
14 Labandeira J, Peteiro C, Toribio J. Hair follicle nevus. Case report and review. Am J Dermatopathol 1996; 18: 90–93.
15 Jackson CE, Callies QC, Krull EA, Mehregan A. Hairy cutaneous malformations of palms and soles. Arch Dermatol 1975; 111: 1146–1149.
16 Gray HR, Helwig EB. Trichofolliculoma. Arch Dermatol 1962; 86: 619–625.
17 Schulz T, Hartschuh W. The trichofolliculoma undergoes changes corresponding to the regressing normal hair follicle in its cycle. J Cutan Pathol 1998; 25: 341–353.
18 Hartschuh W, Schulz T. Immunohistochemical investigation of the different developmental stages of trichofolliculoma with special reference to the Merkel cell. Am J Dermatopathol 1999; 21: 8–15.
19 Stefanato CM, Simkin D, Bhawan J. Epidermolytic hyperkeratosis in trichofolliculoma: apropos of a case. J Cutan Pathol 2000; 27: 573 (abstract).
20 Plewig G. Sebaceous trichofolliculoma. J Cutan Pathol 1980; 7: 394–403.
21 Schulz T, Hartschuh W. Folliculo-sebaceous cystic hamartoma is a trichofolliculoma at its very late stage. J Cutan Pathol 1998; 25: 354–364.
22 Simón RS, de Eusebio E, Alvarez-Viéitez A, Sánchez Yus E. Folliculo-sebaceous cystic hamartoma is but the sebaceous end of the tricho-sebo-folliculoma spectrum. J Cutan Pathol 1999; 26: 109.

23 Nikolowski W. Tricho-Adenom (Organoides Follikel-Hamartoma). Arch Klin Exp Dermatol 1958; 207: 34–45.
24 Rahbari H, Mehregan A, Pinkus H. Trichoadenoma of Nikolowski. J Cutan Pathol 1977; 4: 90–98.
25 Bañuls J, Silvestre JF, Sevila A et al. Trichoadenoma of Nikolowski. Int J Dermatol 1995; 34: 711–712.
26 Jaqueti G, Requena L, Sánchez Yus E. Verrucous trichoadenoma. J Cutan Pathol 1989; 16: 145–148.
27 Filho GB, Toppa NH, Miranda D et al. Giant solitary trichoepithelioma. Arch Dermatol 1984; 120: 797–798.
28 Beck S, Cotton DWK. Recurrent solitary giant trichoepithelioma located in the perianal area; a case report. Br J Dermatol 1988; 118: 563–566.
29 Tatnall FM, Wilson Jones E. Giant solitary trichoepitheliomas located in the perianal area: a report of three cases. Br J Dermatol 1986; 115: 91–99.
30 Lorenzo MJ, Yebra-Pimentel MT, Peteiro C, Toribio J. Cystic giant solitary trichoepithelioma. Am J Dermatopathol 1992; 14: 155–160.
31 Singh A, Thappa DM, Ratnakar C. Unilateral linear trichoepitheliomas. Int J Dermatol 1999; 38: 236–237.
32 Oh DH, Lane AT, Turk AE, Kohler S. A young boy with a large hemifacial plaque with histopathologic features of trichoepithelioma. J Am Acad Dermatol 1997; 37: 881–883.
33 Gray HR, Helwig EB. Epithelioma adenoides cysticum and solitary trichoepithelioma. Arch Dermatol 1963; 87: 102–114.
34 Schirren CG, Wörle B, Kind P, Plewig G. A nevoid plaque with histological changes of trichoepithelioma and cylindroma in Brooke–Spiegler syndrome. J Cutan Pathol 1995; 22: 563–569.
35 Alessi E, Azzolini A. Localized hair follicle hamartoma. J Cutan Pathol 1993; 20: 364–367.
36 Marrogi AJ, Wick MR, Dehner LP. Benign cutaneous adnexal tumors in childhood and young adults, excluding pilomatrixoma: review of 28 cases and literature. J Cutan Pathol 1991; 18: 20–27.
37 Geffner RE, Goslen JB, Santa Cruz DJ. Linear and dermatomal trichoepitheliomas. J Am Acad Dermatol 1986; 14: 927–930.
38 Lambert WC, Bilinski DL, Khan MY, Brodkin RH. Trichoepithelioma in a systematized epidermal nevus with acantholytic dyskeratosis. Arch Dermatol 1984; 120: 227–230.
39 Burrows NP, Russell Jones R, Smith NP. The clinicopathological features of familial cylindromas and trichoepitheliomas (Brooke–Spiegler syndrome): a report of two families. Clin Exp Dermatol 1992; 17: 332–336.
40 Puig L, Nadal C, Fernández-Figueras MT et al. Brooke–Spiegler syndrome variant: segregation of tumor types with mixed differentiation in two generations. Am J Dermatopathol 1998; 20: 56–60.
41 Parhizgar B, Leppard BJ. Epithelioma adenoides cysticum. A condition mimicking tuberose sclerosis. Clin Exp Dermatol 1977; 2: 145–152.
42 Cramers M. Trichoepithelioma multiplex and dystrophia unguis congenita: a new syndrome? Acta Derm Venereol 1981; 61: 364–365.
43 Michaelsson G, Olsson E, Westermark P. The ROMBO syndrome: a familial disorder with vermiculate atrophoderma, milia, hypotrichosis, trichoepitheliomas, basal cell carcinomas and peripheral vasodilation with cyanosis. Acta Derm Venereol 1981; 61: 497–503.
44 Ashinoff R, Jacobson M, Belsito DV. Rombo syndrome: a second case report and review. J Am Acad Dermatol 1993; 28: 1011–1014.
45 Pujol RM, Nadal C, Matias-Guiu X et al. Multiple follicular hamartomas with sweat gland and sebaceous differentiation, vermiculate atrophoderma, milia, hypotrichosis, and late development of multiple basal cell carcinomas. J Am Acad Dermatol 1998; 39: 853–857.
46 Sandbank M, Bashan D. Multiple trichoepithelioma and breast carcinoma. Arch Dermatol 1978; 114: 1230.
47 Pariser RJ. Multiple hereditary trichoepitheliomas and basal cell carcinomas. J Cutan Pathol 1986; 13: 111–117.
48 Johnson SC, Bennett RG. Occurrence of basal cell carcinoma among multiple trichoepitheliomas. J Am Acad Dermatol 1993; 28: 322–326.
49 Wallace ML, Smoller BR. Trichoepithelioma with an adjacent basal cell carcinoma, transformation or collision? J Am Acad Dermatol 1997; 37: 343–345.
50 Hunt SJ, Abell E. Malignant hair matrix tumor ('malignant trichoepithelioma') arising in the setting of multiple hereditary trichoepithelioma. Am J Dermatopathol 1991; 13: 275–281.
51 Matt D, Xin H, Vortmeyer AO et al. Sporadic trichoepithelioma demonstrates deletions at 9q22.3. Arch Dermatol 2000; 136: 657–660.
52 Fenske C, Banerjee P, Holden C, Carter N. Brooke–Spiegler syndrome locus assigned to 16q12–q13. J Invest Dermatol 2000; 114: 1057–1058.
53 Lee Y-S, Fong P-H. Secondary localized amyloidosis in trichoepithelioma. A light microscopic and ultrastructural study. Am J Dermatopathol 1990; 12: 469–478.
54 Bettencourt MS, Prieto VG, Shea CR. Trichoepithelioma: a 19-year clinicopathologic re-evaluation. J Cutan Pathol 1999; 26: 398–404.

55 Brooke JD, Fitzpatrick JE, Golitz LE. Papillary mesenchymal bodies: a histologic finding useful in differentiating trichoepitheliomas from basal cell carcinomas. J Am Acad Dermatol 1989; 21: 523–528.

56 Demirkesen G, Hoede N, Moll R. Epithelial markers and differentiation in adnexal neoplasms of the skin: an immunohistochemical study including individual cytokeratins. J Cutan Pathol 1995; 22: 518–535.

57 Ohnishi T, Watanabe S. Immunohistochemical analysis of cytokeratin expression in various trichogenic tumors. Am J Dermatopathol 1999; 21: 337–343.

58 Yamamoto O, Asahi M. Cytokeratin expression in trichoblastic fibroma (small nodular type trichoblastoma), trichoepithelioma and basal cell carcinoma. Br J Dermatol 1999; 140: 8–16.

59 Jih DM, Lyle S, Elenitsas R et al. Cytokeratin 15 expression in trichoepitheliomas and a subset of basal cell carcinomas suggests they originate from hair follicle stem cells. J Cutan Pathol 1999; 26: 113–118.

60 Abdelsayed RA, Guijarro-Rojas M, Ibrahim NA, Sangueza OP. Immunohistochemical evaluation of basal cell carcinoma and trichoepithelioma using Bcl-2, Ki67, PCNA and P53. J Cutan Pathol 2000; 27: 169–175.

61 Ueda K, Komori Y, Maruo M, Kusaba K. Ultrastructure of trichoepithelioma papulosum multiplex. J Cutan Pathol 1981; 8: 188–198.

62 Dervan PA, O'Loughlin S, O'Hegarty M, Corrigan T. Solitary familial desmoplastic trichoepithelioma. Am J Dermatopathol 1985; 7: 277–282.

63 Lazorik FC, Wood MG. Multiple desmoplastic trichoepitheliomas. Arch Dermatol 1982; 118: 361–362.

64 Brownstein MH, Starink TM. Desmoplastic trichoepithelioma and intradermal nevus: a combined malformation. J Am Acad Dermatol 1987; 17: 489–492.

65 Landau-Price D, Barnhill RL, Kowalcyzk AP et al. The value of carcinoembryonic antigen in differentiating sclerosing epithelial hamartoma from syringoma. J Cutan Pathol 1985; 12: 8–12.

66 Hashimoto T, Inamoto N, Nakamura K, Harada R. Involucrin expression in skin appendage tumors. Br J Dermatol 1987; 117: 325–332.

67 Bondi R, Donati E, Santucci M et al. An ultrastructural study of a sclerosing epithelial hamartoma. Am J Dermatopathol 1985; 7: 223–229.

68 Takei Y, Fukushiro S, Ackerman AB. Criteria for histologic differentiation of desmoplastic trichoepithelioma (sclerosing epithelial hamartoma) from morphea-like basal-cell carcinoma. Am J Dermatopathol 1985; 7: 207–221.

69 Zuccati G, Massi D, Mastrolorenzo A et al. Desmoplastic trichoepithelioma. Australas J Dermatol 1998; 39: 273–274.

70 Shapiro PE, Kopf AW. Familial multiple desmoplastic trichoepitheliomas. Arch Dermatol 1991; 127: 83–87.

71 Orozco-Covarrubias M de la L, Uribe-Rea C, Tamayo-Sánchez L et al. Trichoepitheliomatous infiltration of the skin simulating leprosy. Pediatr Dermatol 1993; 10: 252–255.

72 Hartschuh W, Schulz T. Merkel cells are integral constituents of desmoplastic trichoepithelioma: an immunohistochemical and electron microscopic study. J Cutan Pathol 1995; 22: 413–421.

73 Brownstein MH, Shapiro L. Desmoplastic trichoepithelioma. Cancer 1977; 40: 2979–2986.

74 Sumithra S, Jayaraman M, Yesudian P. Desmoplastic trichoepithelioma and multiple epidermal cysts. Int J Dermatol 1993; 32: 747–748.

75 Kirchmann TTT, Prieto VG, Smoller BR. Use of CD34 in assessing the relationship between stroma and tumor in desmoplastic keratinocytic neoplasms. J Cutan Pathol 1995; 22: 422–426.

76 Kirchmann TTT, Prieto VG, Smoller BR. CD34 staining pattern distinguishes basal cell carcinoma from trichoepithelioma. Arch Dermatol 1994; 130: 589–592.

77 Bryant D, Penneys NS. Immunostaining for CD34 to determine trichoepithelioma. Arch Dermatol 1995; 131: 616–617.

78 Basarab T, Orchard G, Russell-Jones R. The use of immunostaining for bcl-2 and CD34 and the lectin peanut agglutinin in differentiating between basal cell carcinomas and trichoepitheliomas. Am J Dermatopathol 1998; 20: 448–452.

79 Abesamis-Cubillan E, El-Shabrawi-Caelen L, LeBoit PE. Merkel cells and sclerosing epithelial neoplasms. Am J Dermatopathol 2000; 22: 311–315.

80 San Juan EB, Guana AL, Goldberg LH et al. Aggressive trichoepithelioma versus keratotic basal cell carcinoma. Int J Dermatol 1993; 32: 728–730.

81 Headington JT, French AJ. Primary neoplasms of the hair follicle. Histogenesis and classification. Arch Dermatol 1962; 86: 430–441.

82 Grouls V, Hey A. Trichoblastic fibroma. Pathol Res Pract 1988; 183: 462–468.

83 Slater DN. Trichoblastic fibroma: hair germ (trichogenic) tumors revisited. Histopathology 1987; 11: 327–331.

84 Wong T-Y, Reed JA, Suster S et al. Benign trichogenic tumors: a report of two cases supporting a simplified nomenclature. Histopathology 1993; 22: 575–580.

85 Ackerman AB, de Viragh PA, Chongchitnant N. Neoplasms with follicular differentiation. Philadelphia: Lea & Febiger, 1993.

86 Escalonilla P, Requena L. Plaque variant of trichoblastic fibroma. Arch Dermatol 1996; 132: 1388–1390.

87 Long SA, Hurt MA, Santa Cruz DJ. Immature trichoepithelioma: report of six cases. J Cutan Pathol 1988; 15: 353–358.

88 Zaim MT. 'Immature' trichoepithelioma. J Cutan Pathol 1989; 16: 287–289.

89 Sau P, Lupton GP, Graham JH. Trichogerminoma. Report of 14 cases. J Cutan Pathol 1992; 19: 357–365.

90 Hashimoto K, Prince C, Kato I et al. Rippled-pattern trichomatricoma. J Cutan Pathol 1989; 16: 19–30.

91 Kaddu S, Schaeppi H, Kerl H, Soyer HP. Subcutaneous trichoblastoma. J Cutan Pathol 1999; 26: 490–496.

92 Requena L, Barat A. Giant trichoblastoma on the scalp. Am J Dermatopathol 1993; 15: 497–502.

93 Cohen C, Davis TS. Multiple trichogenic adnexal tumors. Am J Dermatopathol 1986; 8: 241–246.

94 Helm KF, Cowen EW, Billingsley EM, Ackerman AB. Trichoblastoma or trichoblastic carcinoma? J Am Acad Dermatol 2001; 44: 547.

95 Gilks CB, Clement PB, Wood WS. Trichoblastic fibroma. A clinicopathologic study of three cases. Am J Dermatopathol 1989; 11: 397–402.

96 Requena L, Renedo G, Sarasa J et al. Trichoblastic fibroma. J Cutan Pathol 1990; 17: 381–384.

97 Watanabe S, Torii H, Matsuyama T, Harada S. Trichoblastic fibroma. A case report and an immunohistochemical study of cytokeratin expression. Am J Dermatopathol 1996; 18: 308–313.

98 Altman DA, Mikhail GR, Johnson TM, Lowe L. Trichoblastic fibroma. A series of 10 cases with report of a new plaque variant. Arch Dermatol 1995; 131: 198–201.

99 Schulz T, Hartschuh W. Merkel cells are absent in basal cell carcinomas but frequently found in trichoblastomas. An immunohistochemical study. J Cutan Pathol 1997; 24: 14–24.

100 Aloi F, Tomasini C, Pippione M. Pigmented trichoblastoma. Am J Dermatopathol 1992; 14: 345–349.

101 Ackerman AB. Pigmented trichoblastoma. Am J Dermatopathol 1997; 19: 619.

102 Graham BS, Barr RJ. Rippled-pattern sebaceous trichoblastoma. J Cutan Pathol 2000; 27: 455–459.

103 Torii H, Ohnishi T, Matsuyama T et al. Trichogenic trichoblastoma arising on the supraclavicular fossa with an immunohistochemical study of cytokeratin expression. Clin Exp Dermatol 1997; 22: 183–188.

104 Yamamoto O, Hisaoka M, Yasuda H et al. A rippled-pattern trichoblastoma: an immunohistochemical study. J Cutan Pathol 2000; 27: 460–465.

105 Betti R, Alessi E. Nodular trichoblastoma with adamantinoid features. Am J Dermatopathol 1996; 18: 192–195.

106 Diaz-Cascajo C, Borghi S, Rey-Lopez A, Carretero-Hernandez G. Cutaneous lymphadenoma. A peculiar variant of nodular trichoblastoma. Am J Dermatopathol 1996; 18: 186–191.

107 Aloi F, Tomasini C, Pippione M. Cutaneous lymphadenoma: a basal cell carcinoma with unusual inflammatory reaction pattern? Am J Dermatopathol 1993; 15: 353–357.

108 Tsang WYW, Chan JKC. So-called cutaneous lymphadenoma: a lymphotropic solid syringoma? Histopathology 1991; 19: 382–385.

109 Santa Cruz DJ, Barr RJ, Headington JT. Cutaneous lymphadenoma. Am J Surg Pathol 1991; 15: 101–110.

110 Requena L, Sánchez Yus E. Cutaneous lymphadenoma with ductal differentiation. J Cutan Pathol 1992; 19: 429–433.

111 Pardal-de-Oliveira F, Sanches A. Cutaneous lymphadenoma. Histopathology 1994; 25: 384–387.

112 Wechsler J, Fromont G, André J-M, Zafrani ES. Cutaneous lymphadenoma with focal mucinosis. J Cutan Pathol 1992; 19: 142–144.

113 Botella R, MacKie RM. Cutaneous lymphadenoma: a case report and review of the literature. Br J Dermatol 1993; 128: 339–341.

114 Schroh RG. Cutaneous lymphadenoma with desmoplastic trichoepitheliomatoid features. J Cutan Pathol 1997; 24: 123.

115 Soyer HP, Kutzner H, Jacobson M et al. Cutaneous lymphadenoma is adamantinoid trichoblastoma. Dermatopathology: Practical and Conceptual 1996; 2: 32–38.

116 McNiff JM, Eisen RN, Glusac EJ. Immunohistochemical comparison of cutaneous lymphadenoma, trichoblastoma, and basal cell carcinoma: support for classification of lymphadenoma as a variant of trichoblastoma. J Cutan Pathol 1999; 26: 119–124.

117 Rodríguez-Diaz E, Román C, Yuste M et al. Cutaneous lymphadenoma. An adnexal neoplasm with intralobular activated lymphoid cells. Am J Dermatopathol 1998; 20: 74–78.

118 Walsh N, Ackerman AB. Basaloid follicular hamartoma: solitary and multiple types. J Am Acad Dermatol 1993; 29: 125–127.

119 Starink TM, Lane EB, Meijer CJLM. Generalized trichoepitheliomas with alopecia and myasthenia gravis: clinicopathologic and immunohistochemical study and comparison with classic and desmoplastic trichoepithelioma. J Am Acad Dermatol 1986; 15: 1104–1112.

120 Weltfriend S, David M, Ginzburg A, Sandbank M. Generalized hair follicle hamartoma: the third case reported in association with myasthenia gravis. Am J Dermatopathol 1987; 9: 428–432.

121 Mascaró JM, Ferrando J, Bombi JA et al. Congenital generalized follicular hamartoma associated with alopecia and cystic fibrosis in three siblings. Arch Dermatol 1995; 131: 454–458.

122 Shimizu H, Takai T, Ichihashi M, Ueda M. A case of generalized hair follicle hamartoma associated with diffuse sclerosis of the face. Br J Dermatol 2000; 143: 1103–1105.

123 Mehregan AH, Baker S. Basaloid follicular hamartoma: three cases with localized and systematized unilateral lesions. J Cutan Pathol 1985; 12: 55–65.

124 Jiménez-Acosta FJ, Redondo E, Baez O, Hernandez B. Linear unilateral basaloid follicular hamartoma. J Am Acad Dermatol 1992; 27: 316–319.

125 Brownstein MH. Basaloid follicular hamartoma: solitary and multiple types. J Am Acad Dermatol 1992; 27: 237–240.

126 Girardi M, Federman GL, McNiff JM. Familial multiple basaloid follicular hamartomas: a report of two affected sisters. Pediatr Dermatol 1999; 16: 281–284.

127 Wheeler CE Jr, Carroll MA, Groben PA et al. Autosomal dominantly inherited generalized basaloid follicular hamartoma syndrome: Report of a new disease in a North Carolina family. J Am Acad Dermatol 2000; 43: 189–206.

128 Horio T, Komura J. Linear unilateral basal cell nevus with comedo-like lesions. Arch Dermatol 1978; 114: 95–97.

129 Morohashi M, Sakamoto F, Takenouchi T et al. A case of localized follicular hamartoma: an ultrastructural and immunohistochemical study. J Cutan Pathol 2000; 27: 191–198.

Infundibular and isthmic tumors

130 Hurt MA. Pilar sheath acanthoma (lobular infundibuloisthmicoma). Am J Dermatopathol 1996; 18: 435 (abstract).

131 Mehregan AH. Infundibular tumors of the skin. J Cutan Pathol 1984; 11: 387–395.

132 Kossard S, Kocsard E, Poyzer KG. Infundibulomatosis. Arch Dermatol 1983; 119: 267–268.

133 Kossard S, Finley AG, Poyzer K, Kocsard E. Eruptive infundibulomas. A distinctive presentation of the tumor of follicular infundibulum. J Am Acad Dermatol 1989; 21: 361–366.

134 Kolenik SA III, Bolognia JL, Castiglione FM Jr, Longley BJ. Multiple tumors of the follicular infundibulum. Int J Dermatol 1996; 25: 282–284.

135 Cribier B, Grosshans E. Tumor of the follicular infundibulum: a clinicopathologic study. J Am Acad Dermatol 1995; 33: 979–984.

136 Mahalingam M, Bhawan J, Finn R, Stefanato CM. Tumor of the follicular infundibulum with sebaceous differentiation. J Cutan Pathol 2001; 28: 314–317.

137 Horn TD, Vennos EM, Bernstein BD, Cooper PH. Multiple tumors of follicular infundibulum with sweat duct differentiation. J Cutan Pathol 1995; 22: 281–287.

138 Johnson WC, Hookerman BJ. Basal cell hamartoma with follicular differentiation. Arch Dermatol 1972; 105: 105–106.

139 Findlay GH. Multiple infundibular tumors of the head and neck. Br J Dermatol 1989; 120: 633–638.

140 Ishida-Yamamoto A, Iizuka H. Infundibular keratosis – a prototype of benign infundibular tumors. Clin Exp Dermatol 1989; 14: 145–149.

141 Winer LH. The dilated pore, a trichoepithelioma. J Invest Dermatol 1954; 23: 181–188.

142 Steffen C. Winer's dilated pore. The infundibuloma. Am J Dermatopathol 2001; 23: 246–253.

143 Smolle J, Kerl H. Das Pilar Sheath Acanthoma – ein gutartiges follikuläres Hamartom. Dermatologica 1983; 167: 335–338.

144 Mehregan AH, Brownstein MH. Pilar sheath acanthoma. Arch Dermatol 1978; 114: 1495–1497.

145 Bhawan J. Pilar sheath acanthoma. A new benign follicular tumor. J Cutan Pathol 1979; 6: 438–440.

146 Spielvogel RL, Austin C, Ackerman AB. Inverted follicular keratosis is not a specific keratosis but a verruca vulgaris (or seborrheic keratosis) with squamous eddies. Am J Dermatopathol 1983; 5: 427–445.

147 Mehregan AH. Inverted follicular keratosis is a distinct follicular tumor. Am J Dermatopathol 1983; 5: 467–470.

148 Sassani JW, Yanoff M. Inverted follicular keratosis. Am J Ophthalmol 1979; 87: 810–813.

149 Mehregan AH, Nadji M. Inverted follicular keratosis and *Verruca vulgaris*. An investigation for the papillomavirus common antigen. J Cutan Pathol 1984; 11: 99–102.

150 Hori K. Inverted follicular keratosis and papillomavirus infection. Am J Dermatopathol 1991; 13: 145–151.

Tricholemmal (external sheath) tumors

151 Reichel M, Heilman ER. Outer root sheath acanthoma. J Cutan Pathol 1999; 26: 441–443.

152 Hunt SJ, Kilzer B, Santa Cruz DJ. Desmoplastic trichilemmoma: histologic variant resembling invasive carcinoma. J Cutan Pathol 1990; 17: 45–52.

153 Ackerman AB, Wade TR. Tricholemmoma. Am J Dermatopathol 1980; 2: 207–224.

154 Headington JT. Tricholemmoma. To be or not to be? Am J Dermatopathol 1980; 2: 225–228.

155 Brownstein MH. Trichilemmoma. Benign follicular tumor or viral wart? Am J Dermatopathol 1980; 2: 229–231.

156 Leonardi CL, Zhu WY, Kinsey WH, Penneys NS. Trichilemmomas are not associated with human papillomavirus DNA. J Cutan Pathol 1991; 18: 193–197.

157 Brownstein MH, Shapiro L. Trichilemmoma. Analysis of 40 new cases. Arch Dermatol 1973; 107: 866–869.

158 Reed RJ. Tricholemmoma. A cutaneous hamartoma. Am J Dermatopathol 1980; 2: 227–228.

159 Tellechea O, Reis JP, Poiares Baptista A. Desmoplastic trichilemmoma. Am J Dermatopathol 1992; 14: 107–114.

160 Rosón E, Gómez-Centeno P, Sánchez-Aguilar D et al. Desmoplastic trichilemmoma arising within a nevus sebaceus. Am J Dermatopathol 1998; 20: 495–497.

161 Brownstein MH, Shapiro EE. Trichilemmomal horn: cutaneous horn overlying trichilemmoma. Clin Exp Dermatol 1979; 4: 59–63.

162 DiMaio DJM, Cohen PR. Trichilemmal horn: Case presentation and literature review. J Am Acad Dermatol 1998; 39: 368–371.

163 Richfield DF. Tricholemmoma. True and false types. Am J Dermatopathol 1980; 2: 233–234.

164 Poblet E, Jimenez-Acosta F, Rocamora A. QBEND/10 (anti-CD34 antibody) in external root sheath cells and follicular tumors. J Cutan Pathol 1994; 21: 224–228.

165 Illueca C, Monteagudo C, Revert A, Llombart-Bosch A. Diagnostic value of CD34 immunostaining in desmoplastic trichilemmoma. J Cutan Pathol 1998; 25: 435–439.

166 Gentry WC Jr. Autosomal dominant genodermatoses associated with internal malignant disease. Semin Dermatol 1984; 3: 273–281.

167 Salem OS, Steck WD. Cowden's disease (multiple hamartoma and neoplasia syndrome). A case report and review of the English literature. J Am Acad Dermatol 1983; 8: 686–696.

168 Shapiro SD, Lambert WC, Schwartz RA. Cowden's disease. A marker for malignancy. Int J Dermatol 1988; 27: 232–237.

169 Starink TM. Cowden's disease: analysis of fourteen new cases. J Am Acad Dermatol 1984; 11: 1127–1141.

170 Lloyd KM, Dennis M. Cowden's disease. A possible new symptom complex with multiple system involvement. Ann Intern Med 1963; 58: 136–142.

171 Elston DM, James WD, Rodman OG, Graham GF. Multiple hamartoma syndrome (Cowden's disease) associated with non-Hodgkin's lymphoma. Arch Dermatol 1986; 122: 572–575.

172 Grattan CEH, Hamburger J. Cowden's disease in two sisters, one showing partial expression. Clin Exp Dermatol 1987; 12: 360–363.

173 Ortonne JP, Lambert R, Daudet J et al. Involvement of the digestive tract in Cowden's disease. Int J Dermatol 1980; 19: 570–576.

174 Aram H, Zidenbaum M. Multiple hamartoma syndrome (Cowden's disease). J Am Acad Dermatol 1983; 9: 774–776.

175 Halevy S, Sandbank M, Pick AI, Feuerman EJ. Cowden's disease in three siblings: electron-microscope and immunological studies. Acta Derm Venereol 1985; 65: 126–131.

176 Camisa C, Bikowski JB, McDonald SG. Cowden's disease. Association with squamous cell carcinoma of the tongue and perianal basal cell carcinoma. Arch Dermatol 1984; 120: 677–678.

177 Raizis AM, Ferguson MM, Nicholls DT et al. A novel 5' (40'41insA) mutation in a patient with numerous manifestations of Cowden disease. J Invest Dermatol 2000; 114: 597–598.

178 Kubo Y, Urano Y, Hida Y et al. A novel *PTEN* mutation in a Japanese patient with Cowden disease. Br J Dermatol 2000; 142: 1100–1105.

179 Wanner M, Çelebi JT, Peacocke M. Identification of a *PTEN* mutation in a family with Cowden syndrome and Bannayan–Zonana syndrome. J Am Acad Dermatol 2001; 44: 183–187.

180 Fargnoli MC, Orlow SJ, Semel-Concepcion J, Bolognia JL. Clinicopathologic findings in the Bannayan–Riley–Ruvalcaba syndrome. Arch Dermatol 1996; 132: 1214–1218.

181 Perriard J, Saurat J-H, Harms M. An overlap of Cowden's disease and Bannayan–Riley–Ruvalcaba syndrome in the same family. J Am Acad Dermatol 2000; 42: 348–350.

182 Chapman MS, Perry AE, Baughman RD. Cowden's syndrome, Lhermitte–Duclos disease, and sclerotic fibroma. Am J Dermatopathol 1998; 20: 413–416.

183 Starink TM, Hausman R. The cutaneous pathology of facial lesions in Cowden's disease. J Cutan Pathol 1984; 11: 331–337.

184 Starink TM, Hausman R. The cutaneous pathology of extrafacial lesions in Cowden's disease. J Cutan Pathol 1984; 11: 338–344.

185 Starink TM, Meijer CJLM, Brownstein MH. The cutaneous pathology of Cowden's disease: new findings. J Cutan Pathol 1985; 12: 83–93.

186 Brownstein MH, Mehregan AH, Bikowski JB et al. The dermatopathology of Cowden's syndrome. Br J Dermatol 1979; 100: 667–673.

187 Johnson BL, Kramer EM, Lavker RM. The keratotic tumors of Cowden's disease: an electronmicroscopic study. J Cutan Pathol 1987; 14: 291–298.

188 Barax CN, Lebwohl M, Phelps RG. Multiple hamartoma syndrome. J Am Acad Dermatol 1987; 17: 342–346.

189 Ten Seldam REJ. Tricholemmocarcinoma. Australas J Dermatol 1977; 18: 62–72.

190 Headington JT. Tricholemmal carcinoma. J Cutan Pathol 1992; 19: 83–84.

19 Lee JY, Tank CK, Leung YS. Clear cell carcinoma of the skin: a tricholemmal carcinoma. J Cutan Pathol 1989; 16: 31–39.

192 Wong T-Y, Suster S. Tricholemmal carcinoma. A clinicopathologic study of 13 cases. Am J Dermatopathol 1994; 16: 463–473.

193 Reis JP, Tellechea O, Cunha MF, Poiares Baptista A. Trichilemmal carcinoma: review of 8 cases. J Cutan Pathol 1993; 20: 44–49.

194 Boscaino A, Terracciano LM, Donofrio V et al. Tricholemmal carcinoma: a study of seven cases. J Cutan Pathol 1992; 19: 94–99.

195 Swanson PE, Marrogi AJ, Williams DJ et al. Tricholemmal carcinoma; clinicopathologic study of 10 cases. J Cutan Pathol 1992; 19: 100–109.

196 Takata M, Rehman I, Rees JL. A trichilemmal carcinoma arising from a proliferating trichilemmal cyst: the loss of the wild-type p53 is a critical event in malignant transformation. Hum Pathol 1998; 29: 193–195.

197 Monteagudo C. A trichilemmal carcinoma arising from a proliferating trichilemmal cyst: a response. Hum Pathol 1999; 30: 247–248.

98 Billingsley EM, Davidowski TA, Maloney ME. Trichilemmal carcinoma. J Am Acad Dermatol 1997; 36: 107–109.

199 Misago N, Ackerman AB. Tricholemmal carcinoma? Dermatopathology: Practical & Conceptual 1999; 5: 205–206.

200 O'Hare AM, Cooper PH, Parlette HL III. Trichilemmomal carcinoma in a patient with Cowden's disease (multiple hamartoma syndrome). J Am Acad Dermatol 1997; 36: 1021–1023.

201 Ikeda T, Tsuru K, Hayashi K et al. Hypercalcemia of malignancy associated with trichilemmal carcinoma in burn scar. Acta Derm Venereol 2000; 80: 396–397.

202 Mehregan AH, Medenica M, Whitney D, Kato I. A clear cell pilar sheath tumor of scalp: case report. J Cutan Pathol 1988; 15: 380–384.

Tumors with matrical differentiation

203 Jacobson M, Ackerman AB. 'Shadow' cells as clues to follicular differentiation. Am J Dermatopathol 1987; 9: 51–57.

204 Brownstein MH, Shapiro L. The pilosebaceous tumors. Int J Dermatol 1977, 16: 340–352.

205 Julian CG, Bowers PW. A clinical review of 209 pilomatricomas. J Am Acad Dermatol 1998; 39: 191–195.

206 Marrogi AJ, Wick MR, Dehner LP. Pilomatrical neoplasms in children and young adults. Am J Dermatopathol 1992; 14: 87–94.

207 Behnke N, Schulte K, Ruzicka T, Megahed M. Pilomatricoma in elderly individuals. Dermatology 1998; 197: 391–393.

208 Schlechter R, Hartsough NA, Guttman FM. Multiple pilomatricomas (calcifying epitheliomas of Malherbe). Pediatr Dermatol 1984; 2: 23–25.

209 Taaffe A, Wyatt EH, Bury HPR. Pilomatricoma (Malherbe). A clinical and histopathologic survey of 78 cases. Int J Dermatol 1988; 27: 477–480.

210 Hernández-Pérez E, Cestoni-Parducci RF. Pilomatricoma (calcifying epithelioma). A study of 100 cases in El Salvador. Int J Dermatol 1981; 20: 491–494.

211 White GM. Multiple pilomatricomas of the scalp. Int J Dermatol 1992; 31: 348–350.

212 Schwartz BK, Peraza JE. Pilomatricomas associated with myotonic dystrophy. J Am Acad Dermatol 1987; 16: 887–888.

213 Farrell AM, Ross JS, Barton SE, Bunker CB. Multiple pilomatricomas and myotonic dystrophy in a patient with AIDS. Clin Exp Dermatol 1995; 20: 423–424.

214 Berberian BJ, Colonna TM, Battaglia M, Sulica VI. Multiple pilomatricomas in association with myotonic dystrophy and a family history of melanoma. J Am Acad Dermatol 1997; 37: 268–269.

215 Noguchi H, Kayashima K, Nishiyama S, Ono T. Two cases of pilomatrixoma in Turner's syndrome. Dermatology 1999; 199: 338–340.

216 Strumia R, Sansone D, Voghenzi A. Multiple pilomatricomas, sternal cleft and mild coagulative defect. Acta Derm Venereol 2000; 80: 77.

217 Demircan M, Balik E. Pilomatricoma in children: a prospective study. Pediatr Dermatol 1997; 14: 430–432.

218 Cooper PH, Fechner RE. Pilomatricoma-like changes in the epidermal cysts of Gardner's syndrome. J Am Acad Dermatol 1983; 8: 639–644.

219 Pujol RM, Casanova JM, Egido R et al. Multiple familial pilomatricomas: a cutaneous marker for Gardner syndrome? Pediatr Dermatol 1995; 12: 331–335.

220 Kawakami M, Akiyama M, Kimoto M et al. Extraordinarily large calcifying epithelioma without aggressive behavior. Dermatology 2001; 202: 74–75.

221 Jones CC, Tschen JA. Anetodermic cutaneous changes overlying pilomatricomas. J Am Acad Dermatol 1991; 25: 1072–1076.

222 Swerlick RA, Cooper PH, Mackel SE. Rapid enlargement of pilomatricoma. J Am Acad Dermatol 1982; 7: 54–56.

223 Spitz D, Fisher D, Friedman RJ, Kopf AW. Pigmented pilomatricoma. A clinical simulator of malignant melanoma. J Dermatol Surg Oncol 1981; 7: 903–906.

224 Zina AM, Bundino S, Torre C. Gross pathology and scanning electron microscopy of pilomatricoma. J Cutan Pathol 1985; 12: 33–36.

225 Chan EF. Pilomatricomas contain activating mutations in β-catenin. J Am Acad Dermatol 2000; 43: 701–702.

226 Wickremaratchi T, Collins CMP. Pilomatrixoma or calcifying epithelioma of Malherbe invading bone. Histopathology 1992; 21: 79–81.

227 Kaddu S, Soyer HP, Cerroni L et al. Clinical and histopathologic spectrum of pilomatricomas in adults. Int J Dermatol 1994; 33: 705–708.

228 Manivel C, Wick MR, Mukai K. Pilomatrix carcinoma: an immunohistochemical comparison with benign pilomatrixoma and other benign cutaneous lesions of pilar origin. J Cutan Pathol 1986; 13: 22–29.

229 Gould E, Kurzon R, Kowalczyk AP, Saldana M. Pilomatrix carcinoma with pulmonary metastasis. Report of a case. Cancer 1984; 54: 370–372.

230 Wood MG, Parhizgar B, Beerman H. Malignant pilomatricoma. Arch Dermatol 1984; 120: 770–773.

231 Rabkin M, Wittwer CT, Soong VY. Flow cytometric DNA content analysis of a case of pilomatrix carcinoma showing multiple recurrences and invasion of the cranial vault. J Am Acad Dermatol 1990; 23: 104–108.

232 van der Walt JD, Rohlova B. Carcinomatous transformation in a pilomatrixoma. Am J Dermatopathol 1984; 6: 63–69.

233 Green DE, Sanusi ID, Fowler MR. Pilomatrix carcinoma. J Am Acad Dermatol 1987; 17: 264–270.

234 Bridger L, Koh HK, Smiddy M et al. Giant pilomatrix carcinoma: report and review of the literature. J Am Acad Dermatol 1990; 23: 985–988.

235 Zagarella SS, Kneale KL, Stern HS. Pilomatrix carcinoma of the scalp. Australas J Dermatol 1992; 33: 39–42.

236 Tateyama H, Eimoto T, Tada T, Niwa T. Malignant pilomatricoma. An immunohistochemical study with antihair keratin antibody. Cancer 1992; 69: 127–132.

237 Waxtein L, Vega E, Alvarez L et al. Malignant pilomatricoma: a case report. Int J Dermatol 1998; 37: 538–540.

238 Dutta R, Boadle R, Ng T. Pilomatrix carcinoma: case report and review of literature. Pathology 2001; 33: 248–251.

239 Khammash MR, Todd DJ, Abalkhail A. Concurrent pilomatrix carcinoma and giant pilomatrixoma. Australas J Dermatol 2001; 42: 120–123.

240 Joshi A, Sah SP, Agrawal CS et al. Pilomatrix carcinoma in a child. Acta Derm Venereol 1999; 79: 476–477.

241 McCulloch TA, Singh S, Cotton DWK. Pilomatrix carcinoma and multiple pilomatrixomas. Br J Dermatol 1996; 134: 368–371.

242 Sassmannshausen J, Chaffins M. Pilomatrix carcinoma: A report of a case arising from a previously excised pilomatrixoma and a review of the literature. J Am Acad Dermatol 2001; 44: 358–361.

243 Hanly MG, Allsbrook WC, Pantazis CG et al. Pilomatrical carcinosarcoma of the cheek with subsequent pulmonary metastases. A case report. Am J Dermatopathol 1994; 16: 196–200.

244 Monchy D, McCarthy SW, Dubourdieu D. Malignant pilomatrixoma of the scalp. Pathology 1995; 27: 201–203.

245 O'Donovan DG, Freemont AJ, Adams JE, Markham DE. Malignant pilomatrixoma with bone metastasis. Histopathology 1993; 23: 385–386.

246 Cross P, Richmond I, Wells S, Coyne J. Malignant pilomatrixoma with bone metastasis. Histopathology 1994; 24: 499–500.

247 Sau P, Lupton GP, Graham JH. Pilomatrix carcinoma. Cancer 1993; 71: 2491–2498.

248 Sano Y, Mihara M, Miyamoto T, Shimao S. Simultaneous occurrence of calcification and amyloid deposit in pilomatricoma. Acta Derm Venereol 1990; 70: 256–259.

249 Kaddu S, Soyer HP, Wolf IH, Kerl H. Proliferating pilomatricoma. A histopathologic simulator of matrical carcinoma. J Cutan Pathol 1997; 24: 228–234.

250 Fayyazi A, Soruri A, Radzun HJ et al. Cell renewal, cell differentiation and programmed cell death (apoptosis) in pilomatrixoma. Br J Dermatol 1997; 137: 714–720.

251 Kishimoto S, Nagata M, Takenaka H, Yasuno H. Detection of apoptosis by in situ labeling in pilomatricoma. Am J Dermatopathol 1996; 18: 339–343.

252 Nakamura T. A reappraisal on the modes of cell death in pilomatricoma. J Cutan Pathol 1999; 26: 125–129.

253 Zámečnik M, Michal M, Mukensnabl P. Cell death in pilomatricoma. J Cutan Pathol 2000; 27: 100.

254 Kumasa S, Mori H, Tsujimura T, Mori M. Calcifying epithelioma of Malherbe with ossification. Special reference to lectin binding and immunohistochemistry of ossified sites. J Cutan Pathol 1987; 14: 181–187.

255 Moehlenbeck FW. Pilomatrixoma (calcifying epithelioma). A statistical study. Arch Dermatol 1973; 108: 532–534.

256 Sloan JB, Sueki H, Jaworsky C. Pigmented malignant pilomatrixoma: report of a case and review of the literature. J Cutan Pathol 1992; 19: 240–246.

257 Kaddu S, Beham-Schmid C, Soyer HP et al. Extramedullary hematopoiesis in pilomatricomas. Am J Dermatopathol 1995; 17: 126–130.

258 Kurokawa I, Kusumoto K, Bessho K et al. Immunohistochemical expression of bone morphogenetic protein-2 in pilomatricoma. Br J Dermatol 2000; 143: 754–758.

259 Kaddu S, Soyer HP, Hödl S, Kerl H. Morphological stages of pilomatricoma. Am J Dermatopathol 1996; 18: 333–338.

260 Benharroch D, Sacks MI. Pilomatricoma associated with epidermoid cyst. J Cutan Pathol 1989; 16: 40–43.

261 Noguchi H, Kayashima K, Ono T. Pilomatricoma associated with several hair follicles. Am J Dermatopathol 1999; 21: 458–461.

262 Uchiyama N, Shindo Y, Saida T. Perforating pilomatricoma. J Cutan Pathol 1986; 13: 312–318.

263 Zulaica A, Peteiro C, Quintas C et al. Perforating pilomatricoma. J Cutan Pathol 1988; 15: 409–411.

264 Tsoitis G, Mandinaos C, Kanitakis JC. Perforating calcifying epithelioma of Malherbe with a rapid evolution. Dermatologica 1984; 168: 233–237.

265 Arnold M, McGuire LJ. Perforating pilomatricoma – difficulty in diagnosis. J Am Acad Dermatol 1988; 18: 754–755.

266 Alli N, Güngör E, Artüz F. Perforating pilomatricoma. J Am Acad Dermatol 1996; 35: 116–118.

267 Watanabe S, Wagatsuma K, Takahashi H. Immunohistochemical localization of cytokeratins and involucrin in calcifying epithelioma: comparative studies with normal skin. Br J Dermatol 1994; 131: 506–513.

268 Cribier B, Asch P-H, Regnier C et al. Expression of human hair keratin basic 1 in pilomatrixoma. A study of 128 cases. Br J Dermatol 1999; 140: 600–604.

269 Cribier B, Peltre B, Langbein L et al. Expression of type I hair keratins in follicular tumours. Br J Dermatol 2001; 144: 977–982.

270 Farrier S, Morgan M. bcl-2 expression in pilomatricoma. Am J Dermatopathol 1997; 19: 254–257.

271 Chastain MA, Millikan LE. Pilomatrix dysplasia in an immunosuppressed patient. J Am Acad Dermatol 2000; 43: 118–122.

272 McGavran MH. Ultrastructure of pilomatrixoma (calcifying epithelioma). Cancer 1965; 18: 1445–1456.

273 Carlson JA, Healy K, Slominski A, Mihm MC Jr. Melanocytic matricoma: a report of two cases of a new entity. Am J Dermatopathol 1999; 21: 344–349.

Tumors of perifollicular mesenchyme

274 Meigel WN, Ackerman AB. Fibrous papule of the face. Am J Dermatopathol 1979; 1: 329–340.

275 Schulz T, Hartschuh W. Birt–Hogg–Dubé-syndrome and the Hornstein–Knickenberg-syndrome are the same. Different sectioning technique as the cause of different histology. J Cutan Pathol 1999; 26: 55–61.

276 Junkins-Hopkins JM, Cooper PH. Multiple perifollicular fibromas: report of a case and analysis of the literature. J Cutan Pathol 1994; 21: 467–471.

277 Sasai S, Takahashi K, Tagami H. Coexistence of multiple perifollicular fibromas and colonic polyp and cancer. Dermatology 1996; 192: 262–263.

278 Park YM, Ham SH, Cho SH et al. Congenital annular multiple fibrofolliculomas occurring with deformity of the ear and ventricular septal defect. Br J Dermatol 1999; 141: 332–334.

279 Aroni K, Aivaliotis M, Tsagroni E, Davaris P. Fibrofolliculomas with acne scar-like appearance. Int J Dermatol 1999; 38: 857–859.

280 Camarasa JG, Calderon P, Moreno A. Familial multiple trichodiscomas. Acta Derm Venereol 1988; 68: 163–165.

281 Starink TM, Kisch LS, Meijer CJLM. Familial multiple trichodiscomas. A clinicopathologic study. Arch Dermatol 1985; 121: 888–891.

282 Birt AR, Hogg GR, Dubé WJ. Hereditary multiple fibrofolliculomas with trichodiscomas and acrochordons. Arch Dermatol 1977; 113: 1674–1677.

283 Ubogy-Rainey Z, James WD, Lupton GP, Rodman OG. Fibrofolliculomas, trichodiscomas, and acrochordons: the Birt–Hogg–Dubé syndrome. J Am Acad Dermatol 1987; 16: 452–457.

284 Rongioletti F, Hazini R, Gianotti G, Rebora A. Fibrofolliculomas, tricodiscomas and acrochordons (Birt–Hogg–Dubé) associated with intestinal polyposis. Clin Exp Dermatol 1989; 14: 72–74.

285 Fujita WH, Barr RJ, Headley JL. Multiple fibrofolliculomas with trichodiscomas and acrochordons. Arch Dermatol 1981; 117: 32–35.

286 Burgdorf WHC, Koester G. Multiple cutaneous tumors: what do they mean? J Cutan Pathol 1992; 19: 449–457.

287 Jacob CI, Dover JS. Birt–Hogg–Dubé syndrome: treatment of cutaneous manifestations with laser skin resurfacing. Arch Dermatol 2001; 137: 98–99.

288 Liu V, Kwan T, Page EH. Parotid oncocytoma in the Birt–Hogg–Dubé syndrome. J Am Acad Dermatol 2000; 43: 1120–1122.

289 Gambichler T, Wolter M, Altmeyer P, Hoffman K. Treatment of Birt–Hogg–Dubé syndrome with erbium: YAG laser. J Am Acad Dermatol 2000; 43: 856–858.

290 Schulz T, Hartschuh W. Characteristics of the Birt–Hogg–Dubé/Hornstein–Knickenberg syndrome. Am J Dermatopathol 2000; 22: 293.

291 De La Torre C, Ocampo C, Doval IG et al. Acrochordons are not a component of the Birt–Hogg–Dubé syndrome. Does this syndrome exist? Case reports and review of the literature. Am J Dermatopathol 1999; 21: 369–374.

292 Toro JR, Glenn G, Duray P et al. Birt–Hogg–Dubé syndrome. A novel marker of kidney neoplasia. Arch Dermatol 1999; 135: 1195–1202.

293 Balus L, Crovato F, Breathnach AS. Familial multiple trichodiscomas. J Am Acad Dermatol 1986; 15: 603–607.

294 Pinkus H, Coskey R, Burgess GH. Trichodiscoma. A benign tumor related to Haarscheibe (hair disk). J Invest Dermatol 1974; 63: 212–218.

295 Schulz T, Ebschner U, Hartschuh W. Localized Birt–Hogg–Dubé syndrome with prominent perivascular fibromas. Am J Dermatopathol 2001; 23: 149–153.

296 Sanguez OP, Requena L. Neurofollicular hamartoma. A new histogenetic interpretation. Am J Dermatopathol 1994; 16: 150–154.

297 Barr RJ, Goodman MM. Neurofollicular hamartoma: a light microscopic and immunohistochemical study. J Cutan Pathol 1989; 16: 336–341.

298 Nova MP, Zung M, Halperin A. Neurofollicular hamartoma. A clinicopathological study. Am J Dermatopathol 1991; 13: 459–462.

299 Xie D, Nielsen TA, Pellegrini AE, Hessel AB. Neurofollicular hamartoma with strong diffuse S-100 positivity. A case report. Am J Dermatopathol 1999; 21: 253–255.

300 Donati P, Balus L. Folliculosebaceous cystic hamartoma. Reported case with a neural component. Am J Dermatopathol 1993; 15: 277–279.

Sebaceous tumors

301 Steffen C, Ackerman AB. Neoplasms with sebaceous differentiation. Philadelphia: Lea & Febiger, 1994.

302 Sanguez M, Radonich MA, Ackerman AB. Uncloaking the mantle. Dermatopathology: Practical and Conceptual 1996; 2: 3–16.

Ectopic sebaceous glands

303 Massmanian A, Valls GS, Sempere VFJ. Fordyce spots on the glans penis. Br J Dermatol 1995; 133: 498–500.

304 Piccinno R, Carrel C-F, Menni S, Brancaleon W. Preputial ectopic sebaceous glands mimicking molluscum contagiosum. Acta Derm Venereol 1990; 70: 344–345.

305 Zak FG, Lawson W. Sebaceous glands in the esophagus. Arch Dermatol 1976; 112: 1153–1154.

Hamartomas and hyperplasias

306 Fogt F, Tahan SR. Cutaneous hamartoma of adnexa and mesenchyme. A variant of folliculosebaceous cystic hamartoma with vascular-mesenchymal overgrowth. Am J Dermatopathol 1993; 15: 73–76.

307 Yamamoto O, Suenaga Y, Bhawan J. Giant folliculosebaceous cystic hamartoma. J Cutan Pathol 1994; 21: 170–172.

308 Kimura T, Miyazawa H, Aoyagi T, Ackerman AB. Folliculosebaceous cystic hamartoma. A distinctive malformation of the skin. Am J Dermatopathol 1991; 13: 213–220.

309 Templeton SF. Folliculosebaceous cystic hamartoma: a clinical pathologic study. J Am Acad Dermatol 1996; 34: 77–81.

310 Bolognia JL, Longley BJ. Genital variant of folliculosebaceous cystic hamartoma. Dermatology 1998; 197: 258–260.

311 Prioleau PG, Santa Cruz DJ. Sebaceous gland neoplasia. J Cutan Pathol 1984; 11: 396–414.

312 Burton CS, Sawchuk WS. Premature sebaceous gland hyperplasia. Successful treatment with isotretinoin. J Am Acad Dermatol 1985; 12: 182–184.

313 De Villez RL, Roberts LC. Premature sebaceous gland hyperplasia. J Am Acad Dermatol 1982; 6: 933–935.

314 Grimalt R, Ferrando J, Mascaro JM. Premature familial sebaceous hyperplasia: Successful response to oral isotretinoin in three patients. J Am Acad Dermatol 1997; 37: 996–998.

315 Kudoh K, Hosokawa M, Miyazawa T, Tagami H. Giant solitary sebaceous gland hyperplasia clinically simulating epidermoid cyst. J Cutan Pathol 1988; 15: 396–398.

316 Czarnecki DB, Dorevitch AP. Giant senile sebaceous hyperplasia. Arch Dermatol 1986; 122: 1101.

317 Fernandez N, Torres A. Hyperplasia of sebaceous glands in a linear pattern of papules. Report of four cases. Am J Dermatopathol 1984; 6: 237–243.

318 Schirren CG, Jansen T, Lindner A et al. Diffuse sebaceous gland hyperplasia. Am J Dermatopathol 1996; 18: 296–301.

319 Dupre A, Bonafe JL, Lamon R. Functional familial sebaceous hyperplasia of the face. Clin Exp Dermatol 1980; 5: 203–207.

320 Boonchai W, Leenutaphong V. Familial presenile sebaceous gland hyperplasia. J Am Acad Dermatol 1997; 36: 120–122.

321 Catalano PM, Ioannides G. Areolar sebaceous hyperplasia. J Am Acad Dermatol 1985; 13: 867–868.

322 Sánchez Yus E, Montull C, Valcayo A, Robledo A. Areolar sebaceous hyperplasia: a new entity? J Cutan Pathol 1988; 15: 62–63.

323 Rocamora A, Santonja C, Vives R, Varona C. Sebaceous gland hyperplasia of the vulva: a case report. Obstet Gynecol (Suppl) 1986; 68: 63s–65s.

324 de Berker DAR, Taylor AE, Quinn AG, Simpson NB. Sebaceous hyperplasia in organ transplant recipients: Shared aspects of hyperplastic and dysplastic processes? J Am Acad Dermatol 1996; 35: 696–699.

325 Marini M, Saponaro A, Remorino L et al. Eruptive lesions in a patient with bone marrow transplantation. Int J Dermatol 2001; 40: 133–135.

326 Finan MC, Apgar JT. Juxta-clavicular beaded lines: a subepidermal proliferation of sebaceous gland elements. J Cutan Pathol 1991; 18: 464–468.

327 Sanchez JL. Juxta-clavicular beaded lines. Am J Dermatopathol 1996; 18: 434 (abstract).

328 Donati P, Muscardin LM, Maini A. Juxtaclavicular beaded lines: a malformative condition affecting sebaceous glands. Dermatology 2000; 200: 283.

329 del Rio E. Juxtaclavicular beaded lines are a universal condition arranged along tension lines. Dermatology 1998; 197: 94–95.

330 Kumar A, Kossard S. Band-like sebaceous hyperplasia over the penis. Australas J Dermatol 1999; 40: 47–48.

331 Sandbank M, Abramovici A, Wolf R, David EB. Sebaceous gland hyperplasia following topical application of citral. An ultrastructural study. Am J Dermatopathol 1983; 10: 415–418.

332 Kumar P, Barton SP, Marks R. Tissue measurements in senile sebaceous gland hyperplasia. Br J Dermatol 1988; 118: 397–402.

333 Fuciarelli K, Cohen PR. Sebaceous hyperplasia: A clue to the diagnosis of dermatofibroma. J Am Acad Dermatol 2001; 44: 94–95.

Benign sebaceous tumors

334 Rulon DB, Helwig EB. Cutaneous sebaceous neoplasms. Cancer 1974; 33 82–102.

335 Ferguson JW, Geary CP, MacAlister AD. Sebaceous cell adenoma. Rare intra-oral occurrence of a tumor which is a frequent marker of Torre's syndrome. Pathology 1987; 19: 204–208.

336 Nussen S, Ackerman AB. Sebaceous "adenoma" is sebaceous carcinoma. Dermatopathology: Practical and Conceptual 1998; 4: 5–14.

337 Thornton CM, Hunt SJ. Sebaceous adenoma with a cutaneous horn. J Cutan Pathol 1995; 22: 185–187.

338 Torre D. Society transactions: New York Dermatological Society, Oct 24, 1967 (multiple sebaceous tumors). Arch Dermatol 1968; 98: 549–551.

339 Banse-Kupin L, Morales A, Barlow M. Torre's syndrome: report of two cases and review of the literature. J Am Acad Dermatol 1984; 10: 803–817.

340 Ródenas JM, Herranz MT, Tercedor J et al. Muir–Torre syndrome associated with a family history of hyperlipidemia. J Am Acad Dermatol 1993; 28: 285–288.

341 Schwartz RA, Torre DP. The Muir–Torre syndrome: a 25-year retrospect. J Am Acad Dermatol 1995; 33: 90–104.

342 Weitzer M, Pokos V, Jeevaratnam P et al. Isolated expression of the Muir–Torre phenotype in a member of a family with hereditary non-polyposis colorectal cancer. Histopathology 1995; 27: 573–575.

343 Gregory B, Ho VC. Cutaneous manifestations of gastrointestinal disorders. Part I. J Am Acad Dermatol 1992; 26: 153–166.

344 Rothenberg J, Lambert WC, Vail JT Jr et al. The Muir–Torre (Torre's) syndrome: the significance of a solitary sebaceous tumor. J Am Acad Dermatol 1990; 23: 638–640.

345 Guitart J, McGillis ST, Bergfeld WF et al. Muir–Torre syndrome associated with α1-antitrypsin deficiency and cutaneous vasculitis. J Am Acad Dermatol 1991; 24: 875–877.

346 Akhtar S, Oza KK, Khan SA, Wright J. Muir–Torre syndrome: Case report of a patient with concurrent jejunal and ureteral cancer and a review of the literature. J Am Acad Dermatol 1999; 41: 681–686.

347 Graefe T, Wollina U, Schulz H-J, Burgdorf W. Muir–Torre syndrome – treatment with isotretinoin and interferon alpha-2a can prevent tumour development. Dermatology 2000; 200: 331–333.

348 Burgdorf WHC, Pitha J, Fahmy A. Muir–Torre syndrome. Histologic spectrum of sebaceous proliferations. Am J Dermatopathol 1986; 8: 202–208.

349 Graham R, McKee P, McGibbon D, Heyderman E. Torre–Muir syndrome. An association with isolated sebaceous carcinoma. Cancer 1985; 55: 2868–2873.

350 Davis DA, Cohen PR. Genitourinary tumors in men with the Muir–Torre syndrome. J Am Acad Dermatol 1995; 33: 909–912.

351 Finan MC, Connolly SM. Sebaceous gland tumors and systemic disease: a clinicopathologic analysis. Medicine (Baltimore) 1984; 63: 232–242.

352 Kanitakis J, Petiot-Roland A, Souillet A-L et al. Sebaceous adenomas with atypical immunohistochemical features in the Muir–Torre syndrome. Br J Dermatol 1999; 140: 749–750.

353 Warschaw KE, Eble JN, Hood AF et al. The Muir–Torre syndrome in a black patient with AIDS: histopathology and molecular genetic studies. J Cutan Pathol 1997; 24: 511–518.

354 Lynch HT, Fusaro RM. The Muir–Torre syndrome in kindreds with hereditary nonpolyposis colorectal cancer (Lynch syndrome): A classic obligation in preventive medicine. J Am Acad Dermatol 1999; 41: 797–799.

355 Swale VJ, Quinn AG, Wheeler JM et al. Microsatellite instability in benign skin lesions in hereditary non-polyposis colorectal cancer syndrome. J Invest Dermatol 1999; 113: 901–905.

356 Esche C, Kruse R, Lamberti C et al. Muir–Torre syndrome: clinical features and molecular genetic analysis. Br J Dermatol 1997; 136: 913–917.

357 Peris K, Onorati MT, Keller G et al. Widespread microsatellite instability in sebaceous tumours of patients with the Muir–Torre syndrome. Br J Dermatol 1997; 137: 356–360.

358 Misago N, Narisawa Y. Sebaceous neoplasms in Muir–Torre syndrome. Am J Dermatopathol 2000; 22: 155–161.

359 Rütten A, Burgdorf W, Hügel H et al. Cystic sebaceous tumors as marker lesions for the Muir–Torre syndrome. Am J Dermatopathol 1999; 21: 405–413.

360 Bayer-Garner IB, Givens V, Smoller B. Immunohistochemical staining for androgen receptors. A sensitive marker of sebaceous differentiation. Am J Dermatopathol 1999; 21: 426–431.

361 Troy JL, Ackerman AB. Sebaceoma. A distinctive benign neoplasm of adnexal epithelium differentiating toward sebaceous cells. Am J Dermatopathol 1984; 6: 7–13.

362 Dinneen AM, Mehregan DR. Sebaceous epithelioma: a review of twenty-one cases. J Am Acad Dermatol 1996; 34: 47–50.

363 Nielsen TA, Maia-Cohen S, Hessel AB et al. Sebaceous neoplasm with reticulated and cribriform features: a rare variant of sebaceoma. J Cutan Pathol 1998; 25: 233–235.

364 Di Leonardo M. Sebaceous adenoma vs. sebaceoma vs. sebaceous carcinoma. Dermatopathology: Practical & Conceptual 1997; 3: 11.

365 Requena L, Kutzner H, Fariña MC. Pigmented and nested sebaceous keratosis with sebaceous differentiation? Am J Dermatopathol 1998; 20: 383–388.

366 Betti R, Inselvini E, Vergani R et al. Sebaceoma arising in association with seborrheic keratosis. Am J Dermatopathol 2001; 23: 58–61.

367 Mahalingam M, Byers HR. Intra-epidermal and intra-dermal sebocrine adenoma with cystic degeneration and hemorrhage. J Cutan Pathol 2000; 27: 472–475.

368 Okuda C, Ito M, Fujiwara H, Takenouchi T. Sebaceous epithelioma with sweat gland differentiation. Am J Dermatopathol 1995; 17: 523–528.

369 Friedman KJ, Boudreau S, Farmer ER. Superficial epithelioma with sebaceous differentiation. J Cutan Pathol 1987; 14: 193–197.

370 Rothko K, Farmer ER, Zeligman I. Superficial epithelioma with sebaceous differentiation. Arch Dermatol 1980; 116: 329–331.

371 Toyoda M, Shoji T, Morohashi M, Bhawan J. Benign sebaceous neoplasm with prominent epidermal component. Am J Dermatopathol 1998; 20: 194–198.

372 Sánchez Yus E, Requena L, Simón P, de Rio E. Sebomatricoma: a unifying term that encompasses all benign neoplasms with sebaceous differentiation. Am J Dermatopathol 1995; 17: 213–221.

373 Sánchez Yus E, Simón P. About benign neoplasms with sebaceous differentiation. Am J Dermatopathol 1999; 21: 298–299.

374 Vaughan TK, Sau P. Superficial epithelioma with sebaceous differentiation. J Am Acad Dermatol 1990; 23: 760–762.

375 Steffen C. Mantleoma: a benign neoplasm with mantle differentiation. Am J Dermatopathol 1993; 15: 306–310.

Malignant sebaceous tumors

376 Graham RM, McKee PH, McGibbon D. Sebaceous carcinoma. Clin Exp Dermatol 1984; 9: 466–471.

377 Nelson BR, Hamlet KR, Gillard M et al. Sebaceous carcinoma. J Am Acad Dermatol 1995; 33: 1–15.

378 Pricolo VE, Rodil JV, Vezeridis MP. Extraorbital sebaceous carcinoma. Arch Surg 1985; 120: 853–855.

379 Jacobs DM, Sandles LG, LeBoit PE. Sebaceous carcinoma arising from Bowen's disease of the vulva. Arch Dermatol 1986; 122: 1191–1193.

380 Wick MR, Goellner JR, Wolfe JT, Su WPD. Adnexal carcinomas of the skin. II. Extraocular sebaceous carcinomas. Cancer 1985; 56: 1163–1172.

381 Wolfe JT, Campbell RJ, Yeatts RP et al. Sebaceous carcinoma of the eyelid. Errors in clinical and pathologic diagnosis. Am J Surg Pathol 1984; 8: 597–606.

382 Rao NA, Hidayat A, McLean IW, Zimmerman LE. Sebaceous carcinomas of the ocular adnexa: a clinicopathologic study of 104 cases with five-year follow-up data. Hum Pathol 1982; 13: 113–122.

383 Spencer JM, Nossa R, Tse DT, Sequeira M. Sebaceous carcinoma of the eyelid treated with Mohs micrographic surgery. J Am Acad Dermatol 2001; 44: 1004–1009.

384 Jensen ML. Extraocular sebaceous carcinoma of the skin with visceral metastases: case report. J Cutan Pathol 1990; 17: 117–121.

385 Harwood CA, Swale VJ, Bataille VA et al. An association between sebaceous carcinoma and microsatellite instability in immunosuppressed organ transplant recipients. J Invest Dermatol 2001; 116: 246–253.

386 Motley RJ, Douglas-Jones AF, Holt PJA. Sebaceous carcinoma: an unusual cause of a rapidly enlarging rhinophyma. Br J Dermatol 1991; 124: 283–284.

387 Misago N, Narisawa Y. Sebaceous carcinoma with apocrine differentiation. Am J Dermatopathol 2001; 23: 50–57.

388 Escalonilla P, Grilli R, Cañamero M et al. Sebaceous carcinoma of the vulva. Am J Dermatopathol 1999; 21: 468–472.

389 Ansai S, Hashimoto H, Aoki T et al. A histochemical and immunohistochemical study of extra-ocular sebaceous carcinoma. Histopathology 1993; 22: 127–133.

390 Zhao Y, Chen H, He C. Reactivity of monoclonal antibody OKM5 with sebaceous carcinoma. J Cutan Pathol 1991; 18: 323–327.

391 Schirren CG, Stefani F, Sander CA, Kind P. Ocular sebaceous carcinoma and basal cell carcinoma show different profiles of cytokeratin intermediate filaments. J Cutan Pathol 1997; 24: 123 (abstract).

392 Martinka M, Trotter M, White V. Cytokeratin 7: aid to differential diagnosis of ocular sebaceous carcinomas, squamous cell and basal cell carcinomas. J Cutan Pathol 2000; 27: 564 (abstract).

Tumors with focal sebaceous differentiation

393 Lee NH, Lee SH, Ahn SK. Apocrine poroma with sebaceous differentiation. Am J Dermatopathol 2000; 22: 261–263.

Apocrine tumors

394 Spielman AI, Sunavala G, Harmony JAK et al. Identification and immunohistochemical localization of protein precursors to human axillary odors in apocrine glands and secretions. Arch Dermatol 1998; 134: 813–818.

395 Requena L, Kiryu H, Ackerman AB. Neoplasms with apocrine differentiation. Philadelphia: Lippincott-Raven and Ardor Scribendi, 1997.

396 Perrone T. Signet-ring cell formation in cutaneous neoplasms. J Am Acad Dermatol 2001; 44: 549–550.

397 Ansai S, Koseki S, Hozumi Y, Kondo S. An immunohistochemical study of lysozyme, CD-15 (Leu M1), and gross cystic disease fluid protein-15 in various skin tumors. Am J Dermatopathol 1995; 17: 249–255.

398 Ishihara M, Mehregan DR, Hashimoto K et al. Staining of eccrine and apocrine neoplasms and metastatic adenocarcinoma with IKH-4, a monoclonal antibody specific for the eccrine gland. J Cutan Pathol 1998; 25: 100–105.

Cysts and hamartomas

399 Kim JH, Hur H, Lee CW, Kim YT. Apocrine nevus. J Am Acad Dermatol 1988; 18: 579–581.

400 Mori O, Hachisuka H, Sasai Y. Apocrine nevus. Int J Dermatol 1993; 32: 448–449.

401 Neill JSA, Park HK. Apocrine nevus: light microscopic, immunohistochemical and ultrastructural studies of a case. J Cutan Pathol 1993; 20: 79–83.

402 Ando K, Hashikawa Y, Nakashima M et al. Pure apocrine nevus. A study of light-microscopic and immunohistochemical features of a rare tumor. Am J Dermatopathol 1991; 13: 71–76.

403 Herrmann JJ, Eramo LR. Congenital apocrine hamartoma: an unusual clinical variant of organoid nevus with apocrine differentiation. Pediatr Dermatol 1995; 12: 248–251.

404 Ohnishi T, Watanabe S. Immunohistochemical analysis of cytokeratin expression in apocrine cystadenoma or hidrocystoma. J Cutan Pathol 1999; 26: 295–300.

405 de Viragh PA, Szeimies RM, Eckert F. Apocrine cystadenoma, apocrine hidrocystoma, and eccrine hidrocystoma: three distinct tumors defined by expression of keratins and human milk fat globulin 1. J Cutan Pathol 1997; 24: 249–255.

406 Warkel RL. Selected apocrine neoplasms. J Cutan Pathol 1984; 11: 437–449.

407 Helwig EB, Hackney VC. Syringadenoma papilliferum. Arch Dermatol 1955; 71: 361–372.

408 Larralde M, Brunet A, Corbella MC. Congenital alopecic plaque. Pediatr Dermatol 1999; 16: 473–474.

409 Premalatha S, Rao NR, Yesudian P et al. Segmental syringocystadenoma papilliferum. Int J Dermatol 1985; 24: 520–521.

410 Rostan SE, Waller JD. Syringocystadenoma papilliferum in an unusual location. Report of a case. Arch Dermatol 1976; 112: 835–836.

411 Nowak M, Pathan A, Fatteh S et al. Syringocystadenoma papilliferum of the male breast. Am J Dermatopathol 1998; 20: 422–424.

412 Abanmi A, Joshi RK, Atukorala D, Okla R. Syringocystadenoma papilliferum mimicking basal cell carcinoma. J Am Acad Dermatol 1994; 30: 127–128.

413 Coyne JD, Fitzgibbon JF. Mixed syringocystadenoma papilliferum and papillary eccrine adenoma occurring in a scrotal condyloma. J Cutan Pathol 2000; 27: 199–201.

414 Koga T, Kubota Y, Nakayama J. Syringocystadenoma papilliferum without an antecedent naevus sebaceous. Acta Derm Venereol 1999; 79: 237.

415 Skelton HG III, Smith KJ, Young D, Lupton GP. Condyloma acuminatum associated with syringocystadenoma papilliferum. Am J Dermatopathol 1994; 16: 628–630.

416 Contreras F, Rodriguez-Peralto JL, Palacios J et al. Verrucous carcinoma of the skin associated with syringadenoma papilliferum: a case report. J Cutan Pathol 1987; 14: 238–241.

417 Wen SY. Syringocystadenoma papilliferum presenting as a cutaneous horn. Br J Dermatol 2000; 142: 1242–1244.

418 Niizuma K. Syringocystadenoma papilliferum: light and electron microscopic studies. Acta Derm Venereol 1976; 56: 327–336.

419 Vanatta PR, Bangert JL, Freeman RG. Syringocystadenoma papilliferum. A plasmacytotropic tumor. Am J Surg Pathol 1985; 9: 678–683.

420 Mammino JJ, Vidmar DA. Syringocystadenoma papilliferum. Int J Dermatol 1991; 30: 763–766.

421 Böni R, Xin H, Hohl D et al. Syringocystadenoma papilliferum. A study of potential tumor suppressor genes. Am J Dermatopathol 2001; 23: 87–89.

422 Dissanayake RVP, Salm R. Sweat-gland carcinomas: prognosis related to histological type. Histopathology 1980; 4: 445–466.

423 Numata M, Hosoe S, Itoh N et al. Syringadenocarcinoma papilliferum. J Cutan Pathol 1985; 12: 3–7.

424 Santa Cruz DJ. Sweat gland carcinomas: a comprehensive review. Semin Diagn Pathol 1987; 4: 38–74.

425 Bondi R, Urso C. Syringocystadenocarcinoma papilliferum. Histopathology 1996; 28: 475–477.

426 Kishimoto S, Wakabayashi S, Yamamoto M et al. Apocrine acrosyringeal keratosis in association with syringocystadenoma papilliferum. Br J Dermatol 2000; 142: 543–547.

427 Donati P, Requena L. Syringocystadenoma papilliferum with goblet cells at the margin of an eyelid. Dermatopathology: Practical & Conceptual 1999; 5: 14–15.

428 Mehregan AH. The origin of the adnexal tumors of the skin: a viewpoint. J Cutan Pathol 1985; 12: 459–467.

429 Penneys NS, Nadji M, Morales A. Carcinoembryonic antigen in benign sweat gland tumors. Arch Dermatol 1982; 118: 225–227.

430 Maiorana A, Nigrisoli E, Papotti M. Immunohistochemical markers of sweat gland tumors. J Cutan Pathol 1986; 13: 187–196.

431 Mazoujian G, Margolis R. Immunohistochemistry of gross cystic disease fluid protein (GCDFP-15) in 65 benign sweat gland tumors of the skin. Am J Dermatopathol 1988; 10: 28–35.

432 Hashimoto K. Syringocystadenoma papilliferum. An electron microscopic study. Arch Dermatol Forsch 1972; 245: 353–369.

433 Ansai S, Koseki S, Hashimoto H et al. A case of ductal sweat gland carcinoma connected to syringocystadenoma papilliferum arising in nevus sebaceus. J Cutan Pathol 1994; 21: 557–563.

Benign apocrine tumors

434 Woodworth H, Dockerty MB, Wilson RB, Pratt JH. Papillary hidradenoma of the vulva: a clinicopathologic study of 69 cases. Am J Obstet Gynecol 1971; 110: 501–508.

435 Vang R, Cohen PR. Ectopic hidradenoma papilliferum: A case report and review of the literature. J Am Acad Dermatol 1999; 41: 115–118.

436 Santa Cruz DJ, Prioleau PG, Smith ME. Hidradenoma papilliferum of the eyelid. Arch Dermatol 1981; 117: 55–56.

437 Nissim F, Czernobilsky B, Ostfeld E. Hidradenoma papilliferum of the external auditory canal. J Laryngol Otol 1981; 95: 843–848.

438 Meeker JH, Neubecker RD, Helwig EB. Hidradenoma papilliferum. Am J Clin Pathol 1962; 37: 182–195.

439 Hashimoto K. Hidradenoma papilliferum. An electron microscopic study. Acta Derm Venereol 1973; 53: 22–30.

440 Warkel RL, Helwig EB. Apocrine gland adenoma and adenocarcinoma of the axilla. Arch Dermatol 1978; 114: 198–203.

441 Okun MR, Finn R, Blumental G. Apocrine adenoma versus apocrine carcinoma. J Am Acad Dermatol 1980; 2: 322–326.

442 De Potter CR, Cuvelier CA, Roels HJ. Apocrine adenoma presenting as gynaecomastia in a 14-year-old boy. Histopathology 1988; 13: 697–699.

443 Domingo J, Helwig EB. Malignant neoplasms associated with nevus sebaceus of Jadassohn. J Am Acad Dermatol 1979; 1: 545–556.

444 Jacyk WK, Requena L, Sánchez Yus E, Judd MJ. Tubular apocrine carcinoma arising in a nevus sebaceus of Jadassohn. Am J Dermatopathol 1998; 20: 389–392.

445 Weigand DA, Burgdorf WHC. Perianal apocrine gland adenoma. Arch Dermatol 1980; 116: 1051–1053.

446 Toribio J, Zulaica A, Peteiro C. Tubular apocrine adenoma. J Cutan Pathol 1987; 14: 114–117.

447 Burket JM, Zelickson AS. Tubular apocrine adenoma with perineural invasion. J Am Acad Dermatol 1984; 11: 639–642.

448 Fox SB, Cotton DWK. Tubular apocrine adenoma and papillary eccrine adenoma. Entities or unity? Am J Dermatopathol 1992; 14: 149–154.

449 Landry M, Winkelmann RK. An unusual tubular apocrine adenoma. Histochemical and ultrastructural study. Arch Dermatol 1972; 105: 869–879.

450 Umbert P, Winkelmann RK. Tubular apocrine adenoma. J Cutan Pathol 1976; 3: 75–87.

451 Kanitakis J, Hermier C, Thivolet J. Adénome tubulaire apocrine: à propos d'un cas. Dermatologica 1984; 169: 23–28.

452 Tellechea O, Reis JP, Marques C, Baptista AP. Tubular apocrine adenoma with eccrine and apocrine immunophenotypes or papillary tubular adenoma? Am J Dermatopathol 1995; 17: 499–505.

453 Epstein BA, Argenyi ZB, Goldstein G, Whitaker D. An unusual presentation of a congenital benign apocrine hamartoma. J Cutan Pathol 1990; 17: 53–58.

454 Ansai S, Watanabe S, Aso K. A case of tubular apocrine adenoma with syringocystadenoma papilliferum. J Cutan Pathol 1989; 16: 230–236.

455 Ishiko A, Shimizu H, Inamoto N, Nakmura K. Is tubular apocrine adenoma a distinct clinical entity? Am J Dermatopathol 1993; 15: 482–487.

456 Johnson BL, Helwig EB. Eccrine acrospiroma. A clinicopathologic study. Cancer 1969; 23: 641–657.

457 Winkelmann RK, Wolff K. Solid-cystic hidradenoma of the skin. Clinical and histopathologic study. Arch Dermatol 1968; 97: 651–661.

458 Hunt SJ, Abell E. Mucinous syringometaplasia mimicked by a clear cell hidradenoma with mucinous change. J Cutan Pathol 1991; 18: 339–343.

459 Fitzgibbon JF, Googe PB. Mucinous differentiation in adnexal sweat gland tumors. J Cutan Pathol 1996; 23: 259–263.

460 Cooper PH. Mitotic figures in sweat gland adenomas. J Cutan Pathol 1987; 14: 10–14.

461 Mambo NC. The significance of atypical nuclear changes in benign eccrine acrospiromas: a clinical and pathological study of 18 cases. J Cutan Pathol 1984; 11: 35–44.

462 Roth MJ, Stern JB, Hijazi Y et al. Oncocytic nodular hidradenoma. Am J Dermatopathol 1996; 18: 314–316.

463 Stanley RJ, Sanchez NP, Massa MC et al. Epidermoid hidradenoma. A clinicopathologic study. J Cutan Pathol 1982; 9: 293–302.

464 Satoh T, Katsumata M, Tokura Y et al. Clear cell hidradenoma with whorl formation of squamoid cells: immunohistochemical and electron microscopic studies. J Am Acad Dermatol 1989; 21: 271–277.

465 Wilson-Jones E. Pigmented nodular hidradenoma. Arch Dermatol 1971; 104: 117–123.

466 Fathizadeh A, Miller-Catchpole R, Medenica MM, Lorincz AL. Pigmented eccrine acrospiroma. Report of a case. Arch Dermatol 1981; 117: 599–600.

467 Biernat W, Pytel J. Retiform/racemiform neoplasm with features of clear cell hidradenoma. Am J Dermatopathol 1999; 21: 479–482.

468 Haupt HM, Stern JB, Berlin SJ. Immunohistochemistry in the differential diagnosis of nodular hidradenoma and glomus tumor. Am J Dermatopathol 1992; 14: 310–314.

469 Ohnishi T, Watanabe S. Histogenesis of clear cell hidradenoma: immunohistochemical study of keratin expression. J Cutan Pathol 1997; 24: 30–36.

470 Biernat W, Kordek R, Woźniak L. Phenotypic heterogeneiety of nodular hidradenoma. Immunohistochemical analysis with emphasis on cytokeratin expression. Am J Dermatopathol 1996; 18: 592–596.

471 Hunt SJ, Santa Cruz DJ, Kerl H. Giant eccrine acrospiroma. J Am Acad Dermatol 1990; 23: 663–668.

472 Hashimoto K, DiBella RJ, Lever WF. Clear cell hidradenoma. Histological, histochemical, and electron microscopic studies. Arch Dermatol 1967; 96: 18–38.

473 Requena L, Sánchez Yus E, Santa Cruz DJ. Apocrine type of cutaneous mixed tumor with follicular and sebaceous differentiation. Am J Dermatopathol 1992; 14: 186–194.

474 Hassab-El-Naby HM, Tam S, White WL, Ackerman AB. Mixed tumors of the skin. A histological and immunohistochemical study. Am J Dermatopathol 1989; 11: 413–428.

475 Hirsch P, Helwig EB. Chondroid syringoma: mixed tumor of skin, salivary gland type. Arch Dermatol 1961; 84: 835–847.

476 Sheikh SS, Pennanen M, Montgomery E. Benign chondroid syringoma: report of a case clinically mimicking a malignant neoplasm. J Surg Oncol 2000; 73: 228–230.

477 Hernandez FJ. Mixed tumors of the skin of the salivary gland type: a light and electron microscopic study. J Invest Dermatol 1976; 66: 49–52.

478 Gianotti R, Coggi A, Alessi E. Cutaneous apocrine mixed tumor: derived from the apocrine duct of the folliculo-sebaceous-apocrine unit? Am J Dermatopathol 1998; 20: 323–325.

479 Argenyi ZB, Balogh K. Collagenous spherulosis in chondroid syringoma. J Cutan Pathol 1989; 16: 293 (abstract).

480 Argenyi ZB, Balogh K. Collagenous spherulosis in chondroid syringomas. Am J Dermatopathol 1991; 13: 115–121.

481 Rapini RP, Kennedy LJ, Golitz LE. Hair matrix differentiation in chondroid syringoma. J Cutan Pathol 1984; 11: 318–321.

482 Triguero M, Schroh R. Apocrine type of cutaneous mixed tumor with follicular and sebaceous differentiation. J Cutan Pathol 1997; 24: 129 (abstract).

483 Argenyi ZB, Goeken JA, Balogh K. Hyaline cells in chondroid syringomas. A light-microscopic, immunohistochemical, and ultrastructural study. Am J Dermatopathol 1989; 11: 403–412.

484 Mambo NC. Hyaline cells in a benign chondroid syringoma. Am J Dermatopathol 1984; 6: 265–272.

485 Ferreiro JA, Nascimento AG. Hyaline-cell rich chondroid syringoma. A tumor mimicking malignancy. Am J Surg Pathol 1995; 19: 912–917.

486 Banerjee SS, Harris M, Eyden BP et al. Chondroid syringoma with hyaline cell change. Histopathology 1993; 22: 235–245.

487 Argenyi ZB, Balogh K, Goeken JA. Immunohistochemical characterization of chondroid syringomas. Am J Clin Pathol 1988; 90: 662–669.

488 Dominguez Iglesias F, Fresno Forcelledo F, Soler Sanchez T et al. Chondroid syringoma: a histological and immunohistochemical study of 15 cases. Histopathology 1990; 17: 311–317.

489 Bates AW, Baithun SI. Atypical mixed tumor of the skin. Histologic, immunohistochemical, and ultrastructural features in three cases and a review of the criteria for malignancy. Am J Dermatopathol 1998; 20: 35–40.

490 Terui T, Obata M, Tagami H. Immunohistochemical studies on epithelial cells in mixed tumor of the skin. J Cutan Pathol 1986; 13: 197–206.

491 Yamamoto O, Yasuda H. An immunohistochemical study of the apocrine type of cutaneous mixed tumors with special reference to their follicular and sebaceous differentiation. J Cutan Pathol 1999; 26: 232–241.

492 Ohnishi T, Watanabe S. Histogenesis of mixed tumor of the skin, apocrine type. Immunohistochemical study of keratin expression. Am J Dermatopathol 1997; 19: 456–461.

493 Franchi A, Dini M, Paglierani M, Bondi R. Immunolocalization of extracellular matrix components in mixed tumors of the skin. Am J Dermatopathol 1995; 17: 36–41.

494 Phelps RG, Klauer J, Wolfe D, Cernainu G. Type II collagen in mixed tumors of the skin. Am J Dermatopathol 1995; 17: 42–47.

495 Tsuji T. Chondroid syringoma: an immunohistochemical study using antibodies to Ca 15-3, KA-93, Ca 19-9, CD44 and BM-1. J Cutan Pathol 1996; 23: 530–536.

496 Mihara M. Chondroid syringoma associated with hidrocystoma-like changes. Possible differentiation into eccrine gland. A histologic, immunohistochemical and electron microscopic study. J Cutan Pathol 1989; 16: 281–286.

497 Varela-Duran J, Diaz-Flores L, Varela-Nunez R. Ultrastructure of chondroid syringoma. Role of the myoepithelial cell in the development of the mixed tumor of the skin and soft tissues. Cancer 1979; 44: 148–156.

498 Mangini J, Farber JN, Palko MJ. Cytokeratin negative cutaneous myoepithelioma. J Cutan Pathol 2000; 27: 564 (abstract).

499 Kutzner H, Mentzel T, Kaddu S et al. Cutaneous myoepithelioma. An under-recognized cutaneous neoplasm composed of myoepithelial cells. Am J Surg Pathol 2001; 25: 348–355.

500 Kilpatrick SE, Hitchcock MG, Kraus MD et al. Mixed tumors and myoepitheliomas of soft tissue. A clinicopathologic study of 19 cases with a unifying concept. Am J Surg Pathol 1997; 21: 13–22.

501 Hinze P, Feyler S, Berndt J et al. Malignant myoepithelioma of the vulva resembling a rhabdoid tumour. Histopathology 1999; 35: 50–54.

502 Fernández-Figueras M-T, Puig L, Trias I et al. Benign myoepithelioma of the skin. Am J Dermatopathol 1998; 20: 208–212.

503 Requena L. Cutaneous myoepithelioma? Am J Dermatopathol 2000; 22: 360–361.

504 Wallis NT, Banerjee SS, Eyden BP, Armstrong GR. Adenomyoepithelioma of the skin: a case report with immunohistochemical and ultrastructural observations. Histopathology 1997; 31: 374–377.

505 Groben PA, Hitchcock MG, Leshin B, White WL. Apocrine poroma: a distinctive case in a patient with nevoid basal cell carcinoma syndrome. Am J Dermatopathol 1999; 21: 31–33.

506 Kamiya H, Oyama Z, Kitajima Y. "Apocrine" poroma: review of the literature and case report. J Cutan Pathol 2001; 28: 101–104.

507 Yamamoto O, Hisaoka M, Yasuda H et al. Cytokeratin expression of apocrine and eccrine poromas with special reference to its expression in cuticular cells. J Cutan Pathol 2000; 27: 367–373.

Malignant apocrine tumors

508 Paties C, Taccagni GL, Papotti M et al. Apocrine carcinoma of the skin. A clinicopathologic, immunocytochemical, and ultrastructural study. Cancer 1993; 71: 375–381.

509 Yoshida A, Kodama Y, Hatanaka S et al. Apocrine adenocarcinoma of the bilateral axillae. Acta Pathol Jpn 1991; 41: 927–932.

510 Katagiri Y, Ansai S. Two cases of cutaneous apocrine ductal carcinoma of the axilla. Case report and review of the literature. Dermatology 1999; 199: 332–337.

511 Dhawan SS, Nanda VS, Grekin S, Ranbinovitz HS. Apocrine adenocarcinoma: case report and review of the literature. J Dermatol Surg Oncol 1990; 16: 468–470.

512 Nishikawa Y, Tokusashi Y, Saito Y et al. A case of apocrine adenocarcinoma associated with hamartomatous apocrine gland hyperplasia of both axillae. Am J Surg Pathol 1994; 18: 832–836.

513 Helwig EB, Graham JH. Anogenital (extramammary) Paget's disease. A clinicopathological study. Cancer 1963; 16: 387–403.

514 Yamamoto O, Haratake J, Hisaoka M et al. A unique case of apocrine carcinoma on the male pubic skin: histopathologic and ultrastructural observations. J Cutan Pathol 1993; 20: 378–383.

515 Kuno Y, Numata T, Kanzaki T. Adenocarcinoma with signet ring cells of the axilla showing apocrine features: a case report. Am J Dermatopathol 1999; 21: 37–41.

516 Nishimura M, Urabe A, Hori Y. Nature of so-called 'metaplasia of the apocrine epithelium'. Macrophages attack apocrine epithelium. Am J Dermatopathol 1989; 11: 563–569.

517 Sakamoto F, Ito M, Sato S, Sato Y. Basal cell tumor with apocrine differentiation: apocrine cell epithelioma. J Am Acad Dermatol 1985; 13: 355–363.

518 Koh KBH, Nazarina AR. Paget's disease of the scrotum: report of a case with underlying carcinoma of the prostate. Br J Dermatol 1995; 133: 306–307.

519 Kageyama N, Izumi AK. Bilateral scrotal extramammary Paget's disease in a Chinese man. Int J Dermatol 1997; 36: 695–696.

520 Jones RE, Austin C, Ackerman AB. Extramammary Paget's disease. A critical reexamination. Am J Dermatopathol 1979; 1: 101–132.

521 Mazoujian G, Pinkus GS, Haagensen DE. Extramammary Paget's disease – evidence for an apocrine origin. Am J Surg Pathol 1984; 8: 43–50.

522 Gonzalez-Castro J, Iranzo P, Palou J, Mascaró JM. Extramammary Paget's disease involving the external ear. Br J Dermatol 1998; 138: 914–915.

523 de Blois GG, Patterson JW, Hunter SB. Extramammary Paget's disease. Arising in knee region in association with sweat gland carcinoma. Arch Pathol Lab Med 1984; 108: 713–716.

524 Remond B, Aractingi S, Blanc F et al. Umbilical Paget's disease and prostatic carcinoma. Br J Dermatol 1993; 128: 448–450.

525 Onishi Y, Ohara K. Ectopic extramammary Paget's disease affecting the upper abdomen. Br J Dermatol 1996; 134: 958–961.

526 Saida T, Iwata M. 'Ectopic' extramammary Paget's disease affecting the lower anterior aspect of the chest. J Am Acad Dermatol 1987; 17: 910–913.

527 Kao GF, Graham JH, Helwig EB. Paget's disease of the ectopic breast with an underlying intraductal carcinoma: report of a case. J Cutan Pathol 1986; 13: 59–66.

528 Tsukada Y, Lopez RG, Pickren JW. Paget's disease of the vulva. A clinicopathologic study of eight cases. Obstet Gynecol 1975; 45: 73–78.

529 Makino T, Nakamura S, Nakayama H, Mihara M. Genital Paget's disease with clear cells in the epidermis of the axilla. J Cutan Pathol 1998; 25: 568–571.

530 Greenwood SM, Minkowitz S. Paget's disease in metastatic breast carcinoma. Arch Dermatol 1971; 104: 312–315.

531 Kawatsu T, Miki Y. Triple extramammary Paget's disease. Arch Dermatol 1971; 104: 316–319.

532 Imakado S, Abe M, Okuno T et al. Two cases of genital Paget's disease with bilateral axillary involvement: mutability of axillary lesions. Arch Dermatol 1991; 127: 1243.

533 Martin VG, Pellettiere EV, Gress D, Miller AW. Paget's disease in an adolescent arising in a supernumerary nipple. J Cutan Pathol 1994; 21: 283–286.

534 Stefanato CM, Finn R, Bhawan J. Extramammary Paget disease and underlying hidradenoma papilliferum. Guilt by association? Am J Dermatopathol 2000; 22: 439–442.

535 Murata Y, Kumano K, Tani M. Underpants-pattern erythema: A previously unrecognized cutaneous manifestation of extramammary Paget's disease of the genitalia with advanced metastatic spread. J Am Acad Dermatol 1999; 40: 949–956.

536 Kakinuma H, Iwasawa U, Kurakata N, Suzuki H. A case of extramammary Paget's disease with depigmented macules as the sole manifestation. Br J Dermatol 1994; 130: 102–105.

537 Chiba H, Kazama T, Takenouchi T et al. Two cases of vulval pigmented extramammary Paget's disease: histochemical and immunohistochemical studies. Br J Dermatol 2000; 142: 1190–1194.

538 Demitsu T, Gonda K, Tanita M et al. Extramammary Paget's disease in two siblings. Br J Dermatol 1999; 141: 951–952.

539 Inoue S, Aki T, Mihara M. Extramammary Paget's disease in siblings. Dermatology 2000; 201: 178.

540 Lee SC, Roth LM, Ehrlich C, Hall JA. Extramammary Paget's disease of the vulva. A clinicopathologic study of 13 cases. Cancer 1977; 39: 2540–2549.

541 Goldblum JR, Hart WR. Vulvar Paget's disease: a clinicopathologic and immunohistochemical study of 19 cases. Am J Surg Pathol 1997; 21: 1178–1187.

542 Furukawa F, Kashihara M, Miyauchi H et al. Evaluation of carcinoembryonic antigen in extramammary Paget's disease. J Cutan Pathol 1984; 11: 558–561.

543 Bodnar M, Miller OF III, Tyler W. Paget's disease of the male breast associated with intraductal carcinoma. J Am Acad Dermatol 1999; 40: 829–831.

544 Wood WS, Hegedus C. Mammary Paget's disease and intraductal carcinoma. Histologic, histochemical, and immunocytochemical comparison. Am J Dermatopathol 1988; 10: 183–188.

545 Whitaker-Worth DL, Carlone V, Susser WS et al. Dermatologic diseases of the breast and nipple. J Am Acad Dermatol 2000; 43: 733–751.

546 Hamm H, Vroom TM, Czarnetzki BM. Extramammary Paget's cells: further evidence of sweat gland derivation. J Acad Dermatol 1986; 15: 1275–1281.

547 Piura B, Zirkin HJ. Vulvar Paget's disease with an underlying sweat gland adenocarcinoma. J Dermatol Surg Oncol 1988; 14: 533–537.

548 Misago N, Toda S, Hikichi Y et al. A unique case of extramammary Paget's disease: derivation from eccrine porocarcinoma? Am J Dermatopathol 1992; 14: 553–559.

549 Hurt MA, Hardarson S, Stadecker MJ, Santa Cruz DJ. Fibroepithelioma-like changes associated with anogenital epidermotropic mucinous carcinoma. J Cutan Pathol 1992; 19: 134–141.

550 Farrell AM, Charnock FM, Millard PR, Wojnarowska F. Paget's disease of the vulva associated with local adenocarcinoma and previous breast adenocarcinoma: report of two cases. Br J Dermatol 1999; 141: 146–149.

551 Chanda JJ. Extramammary Paget's disease: prognosis and relationship to internal malignancy. J Am Acad Dermatol 1985; 13: 1009–1014.

552 Perez MA, LaRossa DD, Tomaszewski JE. Paget's disease primarily involving the scrotum. Cancer 1989; 63: 970–975.

553 Allan SJR, McLaren K, Aldridge RD. Paget's disease of the scrotum: a case exhibiting positive prostate-specific antigen staining and associated prostatic adenocarcinoma. Br J Dermatol 1998; 138: 689–691.

554 Ojeda VJ, Heenan PJ, Watson SH. Paget's disease of the groin associated with adenocarcinoma of the urinary bladder. J Cutan Pathol 1987; 14: 227–231.

555 McKee PH, Hertogs KT. Endocervical adenocarcinoma and vulval Paget's disease: a significant association. Br J Dermatol 1980; 103: 443–448.

556 Merot Y, Mazoujian G, Pinkus G et al. Extramammary Paget's disease of the perianal and perineal regions. Evidence of apocrine derivation. Arch Dermatol 1985; 121: 750–752.

557 Yamamura T, Honda T, Matsui Y et al. Ultrastructural study of extramammary Paget's disease – histologically showing transition from bowenoid pattern to Paget's disease pattern. Br J Dermatol 1993; 128: 189–193.

558 Chen Y-H, Wong T-W, Lee JY-Y. Depigmented genital extramammary Paget's disease: a possible histogenetic link to Toker's clear cells and clear cell papulosis. J Cutan Pathol 2001; 28: 105–108.

559 Lloyd J, Flanagan AM. Mammary and extramammary Paget's disease. J Clin Pathol 2000; 53: 742–749.

560 Anthony PP, Freeman K, Warin AP. Extramammary Paget's disease. Clin Exp Dermatol 1986; 11: 387–395.

561 Zollo JD, Zeitouni NC. The Roswell Park Cancer Institute experience with extramammary Paget's disease. Br J Dermatol 2000; 142: 59–65.

562 Lloyd J, Evans DJ, Flanagan AM. Extension of extramammary Paget disease of the vulva to the cervix. J Clin Pathol 1999; 52: 538–540.

563 Archer CB, Louback JB, MacDonald DM. Spontaneous regression of perianal extramammary Paget's disease after partial surgical excision. Arch Dermatol 1987; 123: 379–382.

564 Ordonez NG, Awalt H, Mackay B. Mammary and extramammary Paget's disease. An immunocytochemical and ultrastructural study. Cancer 1987; 59: 1173–1183.

565 Evans AT, Neven P. Invasive adenocarcinoma arising in extramammary Paget's disease of the vulva. Histopathology 1991; 18: 355–360.

566 Hawley IC, Husain F, Pryse-Davies J. Extramammary Paget's disease of the vulva with dermal invasion and vulval intra-epithelial neoplasia. Histopathology 1991; 18: 374–376.

567 Brainard JA, Hart WR. Proliferative epidermal lesions associated with anogenital Paget's disease. Am J Surg Pathol 2000; 24: 543–552.

568 Kohler S, Smoller BR. A case of extramammary Paget's disease mimicking pemphigus vulgaris on histologic examination. Dermatology 1997; 195: 54–56.

569 Glasgow BJ, Wen DR, Al-Jitawi S, Cochran AJ. Antibody to S-100 protein aids the separation of pagetoid melanoma from mammary and extramammary Paget's disease. J Cutan Pathol 1987; 14: 223–226.

570 Sitakalin C, Ackerman AB. Mammary and extramammary Paget's disease. Am J Dermatopathol 1985; 7: 335–340.

571 Helm KF, Goellner JR, Peters MS. Immunohistochemical stains in extramammary Paget's disease. Am J Dermatopathol 1992; 14: 402–407.

572 Alguacil-Garcia A, O'Connor R. Mucin-negative biopsy in extra-mammary Paget's disease. A diagnostic problem. Histopathology 1989; 15: 429–431.

573 Piérard-Franchimont C, Dosal FL, Arrese Estrada J, Piérard GE. Cutaneous hamartoma with pagetoid cells. Am J Dermatopathol 1991; 13: 158–161.

574 Kariniemi A-L, Forsman L, Wahlstrom T et al. Expression of differentiation antigens in mammary and extramammary Paget's disease. Br J Dermatol 1984; 110: 203–210.

575 Vanstapel M-J, Gatter KC, de Wolf-Peeters C et al. Immunohistochemical study of mammary and extra-mammary Paget's disease. Histopathology 1984; 8: 1013–1023.

576 Guarner J, Cohen C, DeRose PB. Histogenesis of extramammary and mammary Paget cells. An immunohistochemical study. Am J Dermatopathol 1989; 11: 313–318.

577 Tsuji T. Mammary and extramammary Paget's disease: expression of Ca 15-3, Ka-93, Ca 19-9 and CD44 in Paget cells and adjacent normal skin. Br J Dermatol 1995; 132: 7–14.

578 Kariniemi A-L, Ramaekers F, Lehto V-P, Virtanen I. Paget cells express cytokeratins typical of glandular epithelia. Br J Dermatol 1985; 112: 179–183.

579 Tazawa T, Ito M, Fujiwara H et al. Immunologic characteristics of keratins in extramammary Paget's disease. Arch Dermatol 1988; 124: 1063–1068.

580 Miller LR, McCunniff AJ, Randall ME. An immunohistochemical study of perianal Paget's disease. Possible origins and clinical implications. Cancer 1992; 69: 2166–2171.

581 Russell Jones R, Spaull J, Gusterson B. The histogenesis of mammary and extramammary Paget's disease. Histopathology 1989; 14: 409–416.

582 Ohnishi T, Watanabe S. The use of cytokeratins 7 and 20 in the diagnosis of primary and secondary extramammary Paget's disease. Br J Dermatol 2000; 142: 243–247.

583 Lundquist K, Kohler S, Rouse RV. Intraepidermal cytokeratin 7 expression is not restricted to Paget cells but is also seen in Toker cells and Merkel cells. Am J Surg Pathol 1999; 23: 212–219.

584 Wu ML-C, Guitart J. Low specificity of cytokeratin 20 in the diagnosis of extramammary Paget's disease. Br J Dermatol 2000; 142: 569.

585 Goldblum JR, Hart WR. Perianal Paget's disease. A histologic and immunohistochemical study of 11 cases with and without associated rectal adenocarcinoma. Am J Surg Pathol 1998; 22: 170–179.

586 Ohnishi T, Watanabe S. Immunohistochemical analysis of human milk fat globulin expression in extramammary Paget's disease. Clin Exp Dermatol 2001; 26: 192–195.

587 Diaz de Leon E, Carcangiu ML, Prieto VG et al. Extramammary Paget disease is characterized by the consistent lack of estrogen and progesterone receptors but frequently expresses androgen receptor. Am J Clin Pathol 2000; 113: 572–575.

588 Reed W, Oppedal BR, Eeg Larsen T. Immunohistology is valuable in distinguishing between Paget's disease, Bowen's disease and superficial spreading malignant melanoma. Histopathology 1990; 16: 583–588.

589 Belcher RW. Extramammary Paget's disease. Enzyme histochemical and electron microscopic study. Arch Pathol 1972; 94: 59–64.

590 Van der Kwast TH, Vuzevski VD, Ramaekers F et al. Primary cutaneous adenoid cystic carcinoma: case report, immunohistochemistry, and review of the literature. Br J Dermatol 1988; 118: 567–578.

591 Kuramoto Y, Tagami H. Primary adenoid cystic carcinoma masquerading as syringoma of the scalp. Am J Dermatopathol 1990; 12: 169–174.

592 Seab JA, Graham JH. Primary cutaneous adenoid cystic carcinoma. J Am Acad Dermatol 1987; 17: 113–118.

593 Chesser RS, Bertler DE, Fitzpatrick JE, Mellette JR. Primary cutaneous adenoid cystic carcinoma treated with Mohs micrographic surgery toluidine blue technique. J Dermatol Surg Oncol 1992; 18: 175–176.

594 Urso C. Primary cutaneous adenoid cystic carcinoma. Am J Dermatopathol 1999; 21: 400.

595 Perzin KH, Gullane P, Conley J. Adenoid cystic carcinoma involving the external auditory canal. A clinicopathologic study of 16 cases. Cancer 1982; 50: 2873–2883.

596 Cooper PH. Sclerosing carcinomas of sweat ducts (microcystic adnexal carcinoma). Arch Dermatol 1986; 122: 261–264.

597 Cooper PH, Adelson GL, Holthaus WH. Primary cutaneous adenoid cystic carcinoma. Arch Dermatol 1984; 120: 774–777.

598 Freeman RG, Winkelmann RK. Basal cell tumor with eccrine differentiation (eccrine epithelioma). Arch Dermatol 1969; 100: 234–242.

599 Sanchez NP, Winkelmann RK. Basal cell tumor with eccrine differentiation (eccrine epithelioma). J Am Acad Dermatol 1982; 6: 514–518.

600 Chang S-E, Ahn S-J, Choi J-H et al. Primary adenoid cystic carcinoma of skin with lung metastasis. J Am Acad Dermatol 1999; 40: 640–642.

601 Kato N, Yasukawa K, Onozuka T. Primary cutaneous adenoid cystic carcinoma with lymph node metastasis. Am J Dermatopathol 1998; 20: 571–577.

602 Fukai K, Ishii M, Kobayashi H et al. Primary cutaneous adenoid cystic carcinoma: ultrastructural study and immunolocalization of types I, III, IV, V collagens and laminin. J Cutan Pathol 1990; 17: 374–380.

603 Wick MR, Swanson PE. Primary adenoid cystic carcinoma of the skin. Am J Dermatopathol 1986; 8: 2–13.

604 Bergman R, Lichtig C, Moscona RA, Friedman-Birnbaum R. A comparative immunohistochemical study of adenoid cystic carcinoma of the skin and salivary glands. Am J Dermatopathol 1991; 13: 162–168.

605 Pilgrim JP, Wolfish PS, Kloss SG, Heng MCY. Primary mucinous carcinoma of the skin with metastases to the lymph nodes. Am J Dermatopathol 1985; 7: 461–469.

606 Balin AK, Fine RM, Golitz LE. Mucinous carcinoma. J Dermatol Surg Oncol 1988; 14: 521–524.

607 Wick MR, Goellner JR, Wolfe JT, Su WPD. Adnexal carcinomas of the skin. I. Eccrine carcinomas. Cancer 1985; 56: 1147–1162.

608 Weber PJ, Hevia O, Gretzula JC, Rabinovitz HC. Primary mucinous carcinoma. J Dermatol Surg Oncol 1988; 14: 170–172.

609 Prasad RRA, Ratnakar C, Veliath AJ, Srinivasan K. Eccrine carcinoma of the forearm. Int J Dermatol 1995; 34: 859–860.

610 Snow SN, Reizner GT. Mucinous eccrine carcinoma of the eyelid. Cancer 1992; 70: 2099–2104.

611 Tanaka A, Hatoko M, Kuwahara M et al. Recurrent mucinous carcinoma of the skin invading to the frontal skull base. Br J Dermatol 2000; 143: 458–459.

612 Karimipour DJ, Johnson TM, Kang S et al. Mucinous carcinoma of the skin. J Am Acad Dermatol 1996; 34: 323–326.

613 Breier F, Clabian M, Pokieser W et al. Primary mucinous carcinoma of the scalp. Dermatology 2000; 200: 250–253.

614 Bellezza G, Sidoni A, Bucciarelli E. Primary mucinous carcinoma of the skin. Am J Dermatopathol 2000; 22: 166–170.

615 Kavanagh GM, Rigby HS, Archer CB. Giant primary mucinous sweat gland carcinoma of the scalp. Clin Exp Dermatol 1993; 18: 375–377.

616 Rahilly MA, Beattie GJ, Lessells AM. Mucinous eccrine carcinoma of the vulva with neuroendocrine differentiation. Histopathology 1995; 27: 82–86.

617 Yamamoto O, Nakayama K, Asahi M. Sweat gland carcinoma with mucinous and infiltrating duct-like patterns. J Cutan Pathol 1992; 19: 334–339.

618 Baandrup U, Sogaard H. Mucinous (adenocystic) carcinoma of the skin. Dermatologica 1982; 164: 338–342.

619 Carson HJ, Gattuso P, Raslan WF, Reddy V. Mucinous carcinoma of the eyelid. An immunohistochemical study. Am J Dermatopathol 1995; 17: 494–498.

620 Eckert F, Schmid U, Hardmeier T, Altmannsberger M. Cytokeratin expression in mucinous sweat gland carcinomas: an immunohistochemical analysis of four cases. Histopathology 1992; 21: 161–165.

621 Hanby AM, McKee P, Jeffrey M et al. Primary mucinous carcinomas of the skin express TFF1, TFF3, estrogen receptor, and progesterone receptors. Am J Surg Pathol 1998; 22: 1125–1131.

622 Headington JT. Primary mucinous carcinoma of skin. Histochemistry and electron microscopy. Cancer 1977; 39: 1055–1063.

623 Flieder A, Koerner FC, Pilch BZ, Maluf HM. Endocrine mucin-producing sweat gland carcinoma. A cutaneous neoplasm analogous to solid papillary carcinoma of breast. Am J Surg Pathol 1997; 21: 1501–1506.

624 Allan A, Barnhill R, Wladis WP et al. A unique mucin-producing adnexal carcinoma of the eyelid. J Cutan Pathol 2000; 27: 548 (abstract).

625 Harrist TJ, Aretz TH, Mihm MC Jr. Cutaneous malignant mixed tumor. Arch Dermatol 1981; 117: 719–724.

626 Redono C, Rocamora A, Villoria F, Garcia M. Malignant mixed tumor of the skin. Malignant chondroid syringoma. Cancer 1982; 49: 1690–1696.

627 Shvili D, Rothem A. Fulminant metastasizing chondroid syringoma of the skin. Am J Dermatopathol 1986; 8: 321–325.

628 Trown K, Heenan PJ. Malignant mixed tumor of the skin (malignant chondroid syringoma). Pathology 1994; 26: 237–243.

629 Tsoitis G, Papadimitriou C, Kanitakis J et al. Malignant cutaneous mixed tumor. Am J Dermatopathol 2000; 22: 347 (abstract).

630 Watson JAS, Walker MM, Smith NP, Hunt DM. Malignant chondroid syringoma – a rare cause of secondary bone tumor. Clin Exp Dermatol 1991; 16: 306–307.

631 Ishimura E, Iwamoto H, Kobashi Y et al. Malignant chondroid syringoma. Report of a case with widespread metastasis and review of pertinent literature. Cancer 1983; 52: 1966–1973.

632 Metzler G, Schaumburg-Lever G, Hornstein O, Rassner G. Malignant chondroid syringoma. Immunohistopathology. Am J Dermatopathol 1996; 18: 83–89.

633 Bayer-Garner IB, Smoller BR. Chondroid syringioma versus salivary ductal carcinoma: is immunohistochemistry an aid in distinguishing these two entities? J Cutan Pathol 2000; 27: 549 (abstract).

634 Cyrlak D, Barr RJ, Wile AG. Malignant eccrine acrospiroma of the breast. Int J Dermatol 1995; 34: 271–273.

635 Junkins-Hopkins JM. Polypoid malignant acrospiroma: a clinical variant with aggressive behavior. J Cutan Pathol 2000; 27: 561 (abstract).

636 Berg JW, McDivitt RW. Pathology of sweat gland carcinoma. Pathol Annu 1968; 3: 123–144.

637 Chow CW, Campbell PE, Burry AF. Sweat gland carcinomas in children. Cancer 1984; 53: 1222–1227.

638 Biddlestone LR, McLaren KM, Tidman MJ. Malignant hidradenoma – a case report demonstrating insidious histological and clinical progression. Clin Exp Dermatol 1991; 16: 474–477.

639 Hernández-Pérez E, Cestoni-Parducci R. Nodular hidradenoma and hidradenocarcinoma. J Am Acad Dermatol 1985; 12: 15–20.

640 Waxtein L, Vega E, Cortes R et al. Malignant nodular hidradenoma. Int J Dermatol 1998; 37: 225–228.

641 Czarnecki DB, Aarons I, Dowling JP et al. Malignant clear cell hidradenoma: a case report. Acta Derm Venereol 1982; 62: 173–176.

642 Wong T-Y, Suster S, Nogita T et al. Clear cell eccrine carcinomas of the skin. Cancer 1994; 73: 1631–1643.

643 Park HJ, Kim YC, Cinn YW. Nodular hidradenocarcinoma with prominent squamous differentiation: case report and immunohistochemical study. J Cutan Pathol 2000; 27: 423–427.

644 Kersting DW. Clear cell hidradenoma and hidradenocarcinoma. Arch Dermatol 1963; 87: 323–333.

645 Wick MR, Goellner JR, Wolfe JT, Su WPD. Vulvar sweat gland carcinomas. Arch Pathol Lab Med 1985; 109: 43–47.

Tumors of modified apocrine glands

646 Futrell JW, Krueger GR, Chretien PB, Ketcham AS. Multiple primary sweat gland carcinomas. Cancer 1971; 28: 686–691.

647 Aurora AL, Luxenberg MN. Case report of adenocarcinoma of glands of Moll. Am J Ophthalmol 1970; 70: 984–990.

648 Montemarano AD, Sau P, James WD. Superficial papillary adenomatosis of the nipple: a case report and review of the literature. J Am Acad Dermatol 1995; 33: 871–875.

649 Kuflik EG. Erosive adenomatosis of the nipple treated with cryosurgery. J Am Acad Dermatol 1998; 38: 270–271.

650 Albers SE, Barnard M, Thorner P, Krafchik BR. Erosive adenomatosis of the nipple in an eight-year-old girl. J Am Acad Dermatol 1999; 40: 834–837.

651 Smith NP, Wilson Jones E. Erosive adenomatosis of the nipple. Clin Exp Dermatol 1977; 2: 79–84.

652 Michel RG, Woodard BH, Shelburne JD, Bossen EH. Ceruminous gland adenocarcinoma. A light and electron microscopic study. Cancer 1978; 41: 545–553.

653 Lynde CW, McLean DI, Wood WS. Tumors of ceruminous glands. J Am Acad Dermatol 1984; 11: 841–847.

654 Wassef M, Kanavaros P, Polivka M et al. Middle ear adenoma. A tumor displaying mucinous and neuroendocrine differentiation. Am J Surg Pathol 1989; 13: 838–847.

655 Donati P, Amantea A. Adenoma of anogenital mammary-like glands. Am J Dermatopathol 1996; 18: 73–76.

656 Higgins CM, Strutton GM. Papillary apocrine fibroadenoma of the vulva. J Cutan Pathol 1997; 24: 256–260.

657 van der Putte SCJ, Van Gorp LHM. Adenocarcinoma of the mammary-like glands of the vulva. J Cutan Pathol 1994; 21: 157–163.

658 Pfeifer JD, Barr RJ, Wick MR. Ectopic breast tissue and breast-like sweat gland metaplasias: an overlapping spectrum of lesions. J Cutan Pathol 1999; 26: 190–196.

Eccrine tumors

659 Kanitakis J, Schmitt D, Bernard A et al. Anti-D47: a monoclonal antibody reacting with the secretory cells of human eccrine sweat glands. Br J Dermatol 1983; 109: 509–513.

660 Metze D, Soyer H-P, Zelger B et al. Expression of a glycoprotein of the carcinoembryonic antigen family in normal and neoplastic sebaceous glands. J Am Acad Dermatol 1996; 34: 735–744.

661 Metze D, Grunert F, Neumaier M et al. Neoplasms with sweat gland differentiation express various glycoproteins of the carcinoembryonic antigen (CEA) family. J Cutan Pathol 1996; 23: 1–11.

662 Suzuki Y, Hashimoto K, Kato I et al. A monoclonal antibody, SKHI, reacts with 40Kd sweat gland-associated antigen. J Cutan Pathol 1989; 16: 66–71.

663 Penneys NS, Zlatkiss I. Immunohistochemical demonstration of ferritin in sweat gland and sweat gland neoplasms. J Cutan Pathol 1990; 17: 32–36.

664 Metze D, Jurecka W, Gebhart W, Schuller-Petrovic S. Secretory immunoglobulin A in sweat gland tumors. J Cutan Pathol 1989; 16: 126–132.

665 Zuk JA, West KP, Fletcher A. Immunohistochemical staining patterns of sweat glands and their neoplasms using two monoclonal antibodies to keratins. J Cutan Pathol 1988; 15: 8–17.

666 Prieto VG, Lugo J, McNutt NS. Intermediate- and low-molecular-weight keratin detection with the monoclonal antibody MNF116. An immunohistochemical study on 232 paraffin-embedded cutaneous lesions. J Cutan Pathol 1996; 23: 234–241.

667 Watanabe S, Ichikawa E, Takanashi S, Takahashi H. Immunohistochemical localization of cytokeratins in normal eccrine glands, with monoclonal antibodies in routinely processed, formalin-fixed, paraffin-embedded sections. J Am Acad Dermatol 1993; 28: 203–212.

668 Tazawa T, Ito M, Fujiwara H et al. Monoclonal antibody analysis of keratin expression in carcinomas of sweat glands. J Cutan Pathol 1992; 19: 407–414.

669 Fernández-Figueras M-T, Puig L, Ariza A et al. CD44 distribution in sweat gland tumors suggests it has different functional roles in the various cell types. Am J Dermatopathol 1996; 18: 483–489.

670 Swanson PE, Mazoujian G, Mills SE et al. Immunoreactivity for estrogen receptor protein in sweat gland tumors. Am J Surg Pathol 1991; 15: 835–841.

671 Wiley EL, Milchgrub S, Freeman RG, Kim ES. Sweat gland adenomas: immunohistochemical study with emphasis on myoepithelial differentiation. J Cutan Pathol 1993; 20: 337–343.

672 Eckert F, Betke M, Schmoeckel C et al. Myoepithelial differentiation in benign sweat gland tumors. J Cutan Pathol 1992; 19: 294–301.

673 Eckert F, de Viragh PA, Schmid U. Coexpression of cytokeratin and vimentin intermediate filaments in benign and malignant sweat gland tumors. J Cutan Pathol 1994; 21: 140–150.

674 Wienecke R, Eckert F, Kaudewitz P et al. p53 protein in benign and malignant sweat gland tumors. Am J Dermatopathol 1994; 16: 126–129.

675 Pozo L, Camacho F, Rios-Martin JJ, Diaz-Cano SJ. Cell proliferation in skin tumors with ductal differentiation: patterns and diagnostic applications. J Cutan Pathol 2000; 27: 292–297.

Hamartomas and benign tumors

676 Mayou SC, Black MM, Russell Jones R. Sudoriferous hamartoma. Clin Exp Dermatol 1988; 13: 107–108.

677 Ruiz de Erenchun F, Vázquez-Doval FJ, Contreras Mejuto F, Quintanilla E. Localized unilateral hyperhidrosis: eccrine nevus. J Am Acad Dermatol 1992; 27: 115–116.

678 Parslew R, Lewis-Jones MS. Localized unilateral hyperhidrosis secondary to an eccrine naevus. Clin Exp Dermatol 1997; 22: 246–247.

679 Nightingale KJ, Newman P, Davies MG. A functioning eccrine hamartoma associated with Down's syndrome (46, xx, -21, +t(21q21q). Clin Exp Dermatol 1998; 23: 264–266.

680 Gambini C, Rongioletti F, Rebora A. Proliferation of eccrine sweat ducts associated with heterotopic neural tissue (nasal glioma). Am J Dermatopathol 2000; 22: 179–182.

681 Donati P, Amantea A, Balus L. Eccrine angiomatous hamartoma: a lipomatous variant. J Cutan Pathol 1989; 16: 227–229.

682 Nair LV, Kurien AM. Eccrine angiomatous hamartoma. Int J Dermatol 1994; 33: 650–651.

683 Calderone DC, Glass LF, Seleznick M, Fenske NA. Eccrine angiomatous hamartoma. J Dermatol Surg Oncol 1994; 20: 837–838.

684 Sulica RL, Kao GF, Sulica VI, Penneys NS. Eccrine angiomatous hamartoma (nevus): immunohistochemical findings and review of the literature. J Cutan Pathol 1994; 21: 71–75.

685 Seraly MP, Magee K, Abell E et al. Eccrine angiomatous nevus, a new variant. J Am Acad Dermatol 1993; 29: 274–275.

686 Sanmartin O, Botella R, Alegre V et al. Congenital eccrine angiomatous hamartoma. Am J Dermatopathol 1992; 14: 161–164.

687 Gabrielsen T-Ø, Elgjo K, Sommerschild H. Eccrine angiomatous hamartoma of the finger leading to amputation. Clin Exp Dermatol 1991; 16: 44–45.

688 Smith VC, Montesinos E, Revert A et al. Eccrine angiomatous hamartoma: report of three patients. Pediatr Dermatol 1996; 13: 139–142.

689 Kwon O-C, Oh S-T, Kim S-W et al. Eccrine angiomatous hamartoma. Int J Dermatol 1998; 37: 787–789.

690 Nakatsui TC, Schloss E, Krol A, Lin AN. Eccrine angiomatous hamartoma: Report of a case and literature review. J Am Acad Dermatol 1999; 41: 109–111.

691 Morrell DS, Ghali FE, Stahr BJ, McCauliffe DP. Eccrine angiomatous hamartoma: a report of symmetric and painful lesions of the wrists. Pediatr Dermatol 2001; 18: 117–119.

692 Cebreiro C, Sánchez-Aguilar D, Goméz Centeno P et al. Eccrine angiomatous hamartoma: report of seven cases. Clin Exp Dermatol 1998; 23: 267–270.

693 Tsuji T, Sawada H. Eccrine angiomatous hamartoma with verrucous features. Br J Dermatol 1999; 141: 167–169.

694 Tanaka M, Shimizu S, Miyakawa S. Hypertrophic eccrine glands in eccrine angiomatous hamartoma produce gross cystic disease fluid protein 15. Dermatology 2000; 200: 336–337.

695 Damiani S, Riccioni L. Palmar cutaneous hamartoma. Am J Dermatopathol 1998; 20: 65–68.

696 Weedon D, Lewis J. Acrosyringeal nevus. J Cutan Pathol 1977; 4: 166–168.

697 Ogino A. Linear eccrine poroma. Arch Dermatol 1976; 112: 841–844.

698 Aloi FG, Torre C. Hidrotic ectodermal dysplasia with diffuse eccrine syringofibroadenomatosis. Arch Dermatol 1989; 125: 1715.

699 Mehregan AH, Marufi M, Medenica M. Eccrine syringofibroadenoma (Mascaro) Report of two cases. J Am Acad Dermatol 1985; 13: 433–436.

700 Civatte J, Jeanmougin M, Barrandon Y, Jimenez de Franch A. Syringofibroadenoma ecrino de Mascaro. Med Cutan Iber Lat Am 1981; 9: 193–196.

701 Mascaro JM. Considérations sur les tumeurs fibro-épithéliales: le syringofibroadénome eccrine. Ann Dermatol Syphil 1963; 90: 146–153.

702 Kanitakis J, Zambruno G, Euvrard S et al. Eccrine syringofibroadenoma. Immunohistological study of a new case. Am J Dermatopathol 1987; 9: 37–40.

703 Weedon D. Eccrine syringofibroadenoma versus acrosyringeal nevus. J Am Acad Dermatol 1987; 16: 622.

704 Blenc AM, Gómez JA, Lee MW et al. Phakomatous choristoma. A case report and review of the literature. Am J Dermatopathol 2000; 22: 55–59.

705 Marsden RA, Fleming K, Dauber RPR. Comedo nevus of the palm – a sweat duct nevus? Br J Dermatol 1979; 101: 717–722.

706 Blanchard L, Hodge SJ, Owen LG. Linear eccrine nevus with comedones. Arch Dermatol 1981; 117: 357–359.

707 Abell E, Read SI. Porokeratotic eccrine ostial and dermal duct nevus. Br J Dermatol 1980; 103: 435–441.

708 Driban NE, Cavicchia JC. Porokeratotic eccrine ostial and dermal duct nevus. J Cutan Pathol 1987; 14: 118–121.

709 Fernandez-Redondo V, Toribio J. Porokeratotic eccrine ostial and dermal duct nevus. J Cutan Pathol 1988; 15: 393–395.

710 Stoof TJ, Starink TM, Nieboer C. Porokeratotic eccrine ostial and dermal duct nevus. Report of a case of adult onset. J Am Acad Dermatol 1989; 20: 924–927.

711 Beer K, Medenica M. Solitary truncal porokeratotic eccrine ostial and dermal duct nevus in a sixty-year-old man. Int J Dermatol 1996; 35: 124–125.

712 Mishima Y. Eccrine-centered nevus. Arch Dermatol 1973; 107: 59–61.

713 Hollander A. Eccrine-centered nevus. Arch Dermatol 1973; 108: 177.

714 Ohnishi T, Watanabe S. Immunohistochemical analysis of cytokeratin expression in multiple eccrine hidrocystoma. J Cutan Pathol 1999; 26: 91–94.

715 Armstrong DKB, Walsh MY, Corbett JR. Multiple facial eccrine hidrocystomas: effective topical therapy with atropine. Br J Dermatol 1998; 139: 558–559.

716 Simón RS, Sánchez Yus E. Does eccrine hidrocystoma exist? J Cutan Pathol 1998; 25: 182–183.

717 Kamishima T, Igarashi S, Takeuchi Y et al. Pigmented hidrocystoma of the eccrine secretory coil in the vulva: clinicopathologic, immunohistochemical and ultrastructural studies. J Cutan Pathol 1999; 26: 145–149.

718 Rulon DB, Helwig EB. Papillary eccrine adenoma. Arch Dermatol 1977; 113: 596–598.

719 Cooper PH, Frierson HF. Papillary eccrine adenoma. Arch Pathol Lab Med 1984; 108: 55–57.

720 Sexton M, Maize JC. Papillary eccrine adenoma. A light microscopic and immunohistochemical study. J Am Acad Dermatol 1988; 18: 1114–1120.

721 Jerasutus S, Suvanprakorn P, Wongchinchai M. Papillary eccrine adenoma: an electron microscopic study. J Am Acad Dermatol 1989; 20: 1111–1114.

722 Urmacher C, Lieberman PH. Papillary eccrine adenoma. Light-microscopic, histochemical, and immunohistochemical studies. Am J Dermatopathol 1987; 9: 243–249.

723 Megahed M, Hölzle E. Papillary eccrine adenoma. A case report with immunohistochemical examination. Am J Dermatopathol 1993; 15: 150–155.

724 Requena L, Peña M, Sánchez M, Sánchez Yus E. Papillary eccrine adenoma – a light-microscopic and immunohistochemical study. Clin Exp Dermatol 1990; 15: 425–428.

725 Falck VG, Jordaan HF. Papillary eccrine adenoma. A tubulopapillary hidradenoma with eccrine differentiation. Am J Dermatopathol 1986; 8: 64–72.

726 Mizuoka H, Senzaki H, Shikata N et al. Papillary eccrine adenoma: immunohistochemical study and literature review. J Cutan Pathol 1998; 25: 59–64.

727 Ichikawa E, Okabe S, Umebayashi Y et al. Papillary eccrine adenoma: immunohistochemical studies of keratin expression. J Cutan Pathol 1997; 24: 564–570.

728 Weedon D. Eccrine tumors: a selective review. J Cutan Pathol 1984; 11: 421–436.

729 Blasdale C, McLelland J. Solitary giant vulval syringoma. Br J Dermatol 1999; 141: 374–375.

730 Friedman SJ, Butler DF. Syringoma presenting as milia. J Am Acad Dermatol 1987; 16: 310–314.

731 Lo JS, Dijkstra JW, Bergfeld WF. Syringomas on the penis. Int J Dermatol 1990; 29: 309–310.

732 Sola Casas MA, Soto de Delás J, Redondo Bellón P, Quintanilla Gutierrez E. Syringomas localized to the penis (case report). Clin Exp Dermatol 1993; 18: 384–385.

733 Rongioletti F, Semino MT, Rebora A. Unilateral multiple plaque-like syringomas. Br J Dermatol 1996; 135: 623–625.

734 Paquette DL, Massa MC. An unusual presentation of syringomas on the buttocks. J Am Acad Dermatol 1998; 39: 1032–1033.

735 Shelley WB, Wood MG. Occult syringomas of scalp associated with progressive hair loss. Arch Dermatol 1980; 116: 843–844.

736 Port M, Farmer ER. Syringoma of the ankle. J Am Acad Dermatol 1984; 10: 291–293.

737 Yung CW, Soltani K, Bernstein JE, Lorincz AL. Unilateral linear nevoidal syringoma. J Am Acad Dermatol 1981; 4: 412–416.

738 Creamer D, Macdonald A, Griffiths WAD. Unilateral linear syringomata. A case report. Clin Exp Dermatol 1999; 24: 428–430.

739 Holden CA, MacDonald DM. Syringomata: a bathing trunk distribution. Clin Exp Dermatol 1981; 6: 555–559.

740 Urban CD, Cannon JR, Cole RD. Eruptive syringomas in Down's syndrome. Arch Dermatol 1981; 117: 374–375.

741 Weiss E, Paez E, Greenberg AS et al. Eruptive syringomas associated with milia. Int J Dermatol 1995; 34: 193–195.

742 Lee AY, Kawashima M, Nakagawa H, Ishibashi Y. Generalized eruptive syringoma. J Am Acad Dermatol 1991; 25: 570–571.

743 Sánchez TS, Daudén E, Peréz Casas A, García-Diez A. Eruptive pruritic syringomas: Treatment with topical atropine. J Am Acad Dermatol 2001; 44: 148–149.

744 Haneke E, Gutschmidt E. Generalisierte Syringome. Hautarzt 1978; 29: 222–223.

745 Hashimoto K, Blum D, Fukaya T, Eto H. Familial syringoma. Case history and application of monoclonal anti-eccrine gland antibodies. Arch Dermatol 1985; 121: 756–760.

746 Furue M, Hori Y, Nakabayashi Y. Clear-cell syringoma. Association with diabetes mellitus. Am J Dermatopathol 1984; 6: 131–138.

747 Saitoh A, Ohtake N, Fukuda S, Tamaki K. Clear cells of eccrine glands in a patient with clear cell syringoma associated with diabetes mellitus. Am J Dermatopathol 1993; 15: 166–168.

748 Rhodes LE, Verbov JL. Widespread syringomata in Down's syndrome. Clin Exp Dermatol 1993; 18: 333–334.

749 Feibelman CE, Maize JC. Clear-cell syringoma. A study by conventional and electron microscopy. Am J Dermatopathol 1984; 6: 139–150.

750 Ohnishi T, Watanabe S. Immunohistochemical analysis of keratin expression in clear cell syringoma. A comparative study with conventional syringoma. J Cutan Pathol 1997; 24: 370–376.

751 Seifert HW. Multiple Syringome mit Vermehrung von Mastzellen unter dem klinischen Bild einer Urticaria pigmentosa. Z Hautkr 1981; 56: 303–306.

752 Schellander F, Marks R, Wilson Jones E. Basal cell hamartoma and cellular nevus: an unusual combined malformation. Br J Dermatol 1974; 90: 413–419.

753 Helm TN, Guitart J, Bergfeld WF, Benedetto E. Occult syringoma associated with alopecia. Int J Dermatol 1992; 31: 437–438.

754 Mehregan AH, Mehregan DA. Syringoma-like sweat duct proliferation in scalp alopecias. J Cutan Pathol 1990; 17: 355–357.

755 Corredor F, Cohen PR, Tschen JA. Syringomatous changes of eccrine sweat ducts associated with prurigo nodularis. Am J Dermatopathol 1998; 20: 296–301.

756 Henner MS, Shapiro PE, Ritter JH et al. Solitary syringoma. Report of five cases and clinicopathologic comparison with microcystic adnexal carcinoma of the skin. Am J Dermatopathol 1995; 17: 465–470.

757 Urso C, Anichini C. Sclerosing adenosis-like lesion of sweat glands. Am J Dermatopathol 2000; 22: 561–562.

758 Hashimoto K, Gross BG, Lever WF. Syringoma. Histochemical and electron microscopic studies. J Invest Dermatol 1966; 46: 150–166.

759 Eckert F, Nilles M, Schmid U, Altmannsberger M. Distribution of cytokeratin polypeptides in syringomas. Am J Dermatopathol 1992; 14: 115–121.

760 Wallace ML, Smoller BR. Progesterone receptor positivity supports hormonal control of syringomas. J Cutan Pathol 1995; 22: 442–445.

761 Hashimoto K, Lever WF. Histogenesis of skin appendage tumors. Arch Dermatol 1969; 100: 356–369.

762 Martinez W, Yebra MT, Arnal F et al. Multiple linear cylindromas. J Am Acad Dermatol 1992; 26: 821–824.

763 Vernon HJ, Olsen EA, Vollmer RT. Autosomal dominant multiple cylindromas associated with solitary lung cylindroma. J Am Acad Dermatol 1988; 19: 397–400.

764 Gerretsen AL, Beemer FA, Deenstra W et al. Familial cutaneous cylindromas: investigations in five generations of a family. J Am Acad Dermatol 1995; 33: 199–206.

765 Rockerbie N, Solomon AR, Woo TY et al. Malignant dermal cylindroma in a patient with multiple dermal cylindromas, trichoepitheliomas, and bilateral dermal analogue tumors of the parotid gland. Am J Dermatopathol 1989; 11: 353–359.

766 van der Putte SCJ. The pathogenesis of familial multiple cylindromas, trichoepitheliomas, milia, and spiradenomas. Am J Dermatopathol 1995; 17: 271–280.

767 Schmidt KT, Ma A, Goldberg R, Medenica M. Multiple adnexal tumors and a parotid basal cell adenoma. J Am Acad Dermatol 1991; 25: 960–964.

768 Gottschalk HR, Graham JH, Aston EE. Dermal eccrine cylindroma, epithelioma adenoides cysticum of Brooke, and eccrine spiradenoma. Arch Dermatol 1974; 110: 473–474.

769 Ferrandiz C, Campo E, Baumann E. Dermal cylindromas (Turban tumor) and eccrine spiradenomas in a patient with membranous basal cell adenoma of the parotid gland. J Cutan Pathol 1985; 12: 72–79.

770 Goette DK, McConnell MA, Fowler VR. Cylindroma and eccrine spiradenoma coexistent in the same lesion. Arch Dermatol 1982; 118: 273–274.

771 Lee MW, Kelly JW. Dermal cylindroma and eccrine spiradenoma. Australas J Dermatol 1996; 37: 48–49.

772 Urbanski SJ, From L, Abramowicz A et al. Metamorphosis of dermal cylindroma: possible relation to malignant transformation. J Am Acad Dermatol 1985; 12: 188–195.

773 Lin PY, Fatteh SM, Lloyd KM. Malignant transformation in a solitary dermal cylindroma. Arch Pathol Lab Med 1987; 111: 765–767.

774 Tsambaos D, Greither A, Orfanos CE. Brachydactyly and racket-nails. Light and electron microscopic study. J Cutan Pathol 1979; 6: 31–41.

775 Galadari E, Mehregan AH, Lee KC. Malignant transformation of eccrine tumors. J Cutan Pathol 1987; 14: 15–22.

776 Iyer PV, Leong A S-Y. Malignant dermal cylindromas. Do they exist? A morphological and immunohistochemical study and review of the literature. Pathology 1989; 21: 269–274.

777 Cotton DWK, Braye SG. Dermal cylindromas originate from the eccrine sweat gland. Br J Dermatol 1984; 111: 53–61.

778 Tellechea O, Reis JP, Ilheu O, Baptista AP. Dermal cylindroma. An immunohistochemical study of thirteen cases. Am J Dermatopathol 1995; 17: 260–265.

779 Penneys NS, Kaiser M. Cylindroma expresses immunohistochemical markers linking it to eccrine coil. J Cutan Pathol 1993; 20: 40–43.

780 Pfaltz M, Bruckner-Tuderman L, Schnyder UW. Type VII collagen is a component of cylindroma basement membrane zone. J Cutan Pathol 1989; 16: 388–395.

781 Bruckner-Tuderman L, Pfaltz M, Schnyder UW. Cylindroma overexpresses collagen VII, the major anchoring fibril protein. J Invest Dermatol 1991; 96: 729–734.

782 Soyer HP, Kerl H, Ott A. Spiradenocylindroma – more than a coincidence? Am J Dermatopathol 1998; 20: 315–317.

783 Meybehm M, Fischer H-P. Spiradenoma and dermal cylindroma: comparative immunohistochemical analysis and histogenetic considerations. Am J Dermatopathol 1997; 19: 154–161.

784 Munger BL, Graham JH, Helwig EB. Ultrastructure and histochemical characteristics of dermal eccrine cylindroma (turban tumor). J Invest Dermatol 1962; 39: 577–595.

785 Mambo NC. Eccrine spiradenoma: clinical and pathologic study of 49 tumors. J Cutan Pathol 1983; 10: 312–320.

786 Revis P, Chyu J, Medenica M. Multiple eccrine spiradenoma: case report and review. J Cutan Pathol 1988; 15: 226–229.

787 Wright S, Ryan J. Multiple familial eccrine spiradenoma with cylindroma. Acta Derm Venereol 1990; 70: 79–82.

788 Bedlow AJ, Cook MG, Kurwa A. Extensive naevoid eccrine spiradenoma. Br J Dermatol 1999; 140: 154–157.

789 Cotton DWK, Slater DN, Rooney N et al. Giant vascular eccrine spiradenomas: a report of two cases with histology, immunohistology and electron microscopy. Histopathology 1986; 10: 1093–1099.

790 Tsur H, Lipskier E, Fisher BK. Multiple linear spiradenomas. Plast Reconstr Surg 1981; 68: 100–102.

791 Noto G, Bongiorno MR, Pravatà G, Aricò M. Multiple nevoid spiradenomas. Am J Dermatopathol 1994; 16: 280–284.

792 Gupta S, Radotra BD, Kaur I et al. Multiple linear eccrine spiradenomas with eyelid involvement. J Eur Acad Dermatol Venereol 2001; 15: 163–166.

793 Shelley WB, Wood MG. A zosteriform network of spiradenomas. J Am Acad Dermatol 1980; 2: 59–61.

794 Schmoeckel C, Burg G. Congenital spiradenoma. Am J Dermatopathol 1988; 10: 541–545.

795 Kao GF, Laskin WB, Weiss SW. Eccrine spiradenoma occurring in infancy mimicking mesenchymal tumor. J Cutan Pathol 1990; 17: 214–219.

796 Weyers W, Nilles M, Eckert F, Schill W-B. Spiradenomas in Brooke–Spiegler syndrome. Am J Dermatopathol 1993; 15: 156–161.

797 Evans HL, Su WPD, Smith JL, Winkelmann RK. Carcinoma arising in eccrine spiradenoma. Cancer 1979; 43: 1881–1884.

798 McKee PH, Fletcher CDM, Stavrinos P, Pambakian H. Carcinosarcoma arising in eccrine spiradenoma. Am J Dermatopathol 1990; 12: 335–343.

799 Cooper PH, Frierson HF, Morrison AG. Malignant transformation of eccrine spiradenoma. Arch Dermatol 1985; 121: 1445–1448.

800 Wick MR, Swanson PE, Kaye VN, Pittelkow MR. Sweat gland carcinoma ex eccrine spiradenoma. Am J Dermatopathol 1987; 9: 90–98.

801 Dijkhuizen T, van den Berg E, Nikkels PGJ et al. Cytogenetics of a case of eccrine spiradenoma. Hum Pathol 1992; 23: 1085–1087.

802 Biernat W, Kordek R, Wozniak L. Over-expression of p53 protein as an indicator of the malignant transformation in spiradenoma. Histopathology 1995; 26: 439–443.

803 Castro C, Winkelmann RK. Spiradenoma. Histochemical and electron microscopic study. Arch Dermatol 1974; 109: 40–48.

804 van den Oord JJ, Dé Wolf-Peeters C. Perivascular spaces in eccrine spiradenoma. Am J Dermatopathol 1995; 17: 266–270.

805 Senol M, Ozcan A, Sasmaz S et al. Giant vascular eccrine spiradenoma. Int J Dermatol 1998; 37: 221–223.

806 Soyer HP, El Shabrawi-Caelen L. A spiradenoma with "ancient" stromal features. Dermatopathology: Practical & Conceptual 2000; 6: 29–32.

807 Watanabe S, Hirose M, Sato S, Takahashi H. Immunohistochemical analysis of cytokeratin expression in eccrine spiradenoma: similarities to the transitional portions between secretory segments and coiled ducts of eccrine glands. Br J Dermatol 1994; 131: 799–807.

808 Al-Nafussi A, Blessing K, Rahilly M. Non-epithelial cellular components in eccrine spiradenoma: a histological and immunohistochemical study of 20 cases. Histopathology 1991; 18: 155–160.

809 Jitsukawa K, Sueki H, Sato S, Anzai T. Eccrine spiradenoma. An electron microscopic study. Am J Dermatopathol 1987; 9: 99–108.

Poroma group

810 Cho S, Kim J-S, Shin J-H et al. Poroid hidradenoma. Int J Dermatol 2001; 40: 62–64.

811 Kakinuma H, Miyamoto R, Iwasawa U et al. Three subtypes of poroid neoplasia in a single lesion: eccrine poroma, hidroacanthoma simplex, and dermal duct tumor. Am J Dermatopathol 1994; 16: 66–72.

812 Pinkus H, Rogin JR, Goldman P. Eccrine poroma. Tumors exhibiting features of the epidermal sweat duct unit. Arch Dermatol 1956; 74: 511–521.

813 Lemont H, Snyder H. Eccrine poroma of the heel. Int J Dermatol 2000; 39: 453–454.

814 Moore TO, Orman HL, Orman SK, Helm KF. Poromas of the head and neck. J Am Acad Dermatol 2001; 44: 48–52.

815 Wilkinson RD, Schopflocher P, Rozenfeld M. Hidrotic ectodermal dysplasia with diffuse eccrine poromatosis. Arch Dermatol 1977; 113: 472–476.

816 Penneys NS, Ackerman AB, Indgin SN, Mandy SH. Eccrine poroma: two unusual variants. Br J Dermatol 1970; 82: 613–615.

817 Hyman AB, Brownstein MH. Eccrine poroma. An analysis of forty-five new cases. Dermatologica 1969; 138: 29–38.

818 Mousawi A, Kibbi A-G. Pigmented eccrine poroma: a simulant of nodular melanoma. Int J Dermatol 1995; 34: 857–858.

819 Harvell JD, Kerschmann RL, LeBoit PE. Eccrine or apocrine poroma? Six poromas with divergent adnexal differentiation. Am J Dermatopathol 1996; 18: 1–9.

820 Ban M, Yoneda K, Kitajima Y. Differentiation of eccrine poroma cells to cytokeratin 1- and 10-expressing cells, the intermediate layer cells of eccrine sweat duct, in the tumor cell nests. J Cutan Pathol 1997; 24: 246–248.

821 Hashimoto K, Lever WF. Eccrine poroma. Histochemical and electron microscopic studies. J Invest Dermatol 1964; 43: 237–247.

822 Winkelmann RK, McLeod WA. The dermal duct tumor. Arch Dermatol 1966; 94: 50–55.

823 Hu C-H, Marques AS, Winkelmann RK. Dermal duct tumor. A histochemical and electron microscopic study. Arch Dermatol 1978; 114: 1659–1664.

824 Faure M, Colomb D. Dermal duct tumor. J Cutan Pathol 1979; 6: 317–322.

825 Smith JLS, Coburn JG. Hidroacanthoma simplex. Br J Dermatol 1956; 68: 400–418.

826 Rahbari H. Hidroacanthoma simplex – a review of 15 cases. Br J Dermatol 1983 109: 219–225.

827 Nakagawa T, Inai M, Yamamoto S, Takaiwa T. Hidroacanthoma simplex showing variation in the appearance of tumor cells in different nests. J Cutan Pathol 1988; 15: 238–244.

828 Warner TFCS, Goell WS, Cripps DJJ. Hidroacanthoma simplex: an ultrastructural study. J Cutan Pathol 1982; 9: 189–195.

829 Zina AM, Bundino S, Pippione MG. Pigmented hidroacanthoma simplex with porocarcinoma. Light and electron microscopic study of a case. J Cutan Pathol 1982; 9: 104–112.

830 Bardach H. Hidroacanthoma simplex with in situ porocarcinoma. A case suggesting malignant transformation. J Cutan Pathol 1978; 5: 236–248.

831 Steffen C, Ackerman AB. Intraepidermal epithelioma of Borst–Jadassohn. Am J Dermatopathol 1985; 7: 5–24.

832 Kennedy C, Bhogal B, Moss R, Sanderson KV. Pigmented intraepidermal eccrine poroma. Br J Dermatol (Suppl) 1979; 17: 76–78.

833 Perniciaro C, Muller SA, Zelickson BD, Snow JL. Hidroacanthoma simplex: an ultrastructural and immunohistochemical study. J Cutan Pathol 1994; 21: 274–279.

834 Cook MG, Ridgway HA. The intra-epidermal epithelioma of Jadassohn: a distinct entity. Br J Dermatol 1979; 101: 659–667.

835 Freeman RG. Questions to the Editorial Board and other authorities. Am J Dermatopathol 1985; 7: 37–38.

836 Mehregan AH, Pinkus H. Intraepidermal epithelioma: a critical study. Cancer 1969; 17: 609–636.

837 Rahbari H. Syringoacanthoma. Acanthotic lesion of the acrosyringium. Arch Dermatol 1984; 120: 751–756.

838 Takeda H, Mitsuhashi Y, Yoshikawa K et al. Eccrine syringofibroadenoma: report of a case and analysis of cytokeratin expression. Dermatology 1998; 196: 242–245.

839 Takeda H, Mitsuhashi Y, Hayashi M, Kondo S. Eccrine syringofibroadenoma: case report and review of the literature. J Eur Acad Dermatol Venereol 2001; 15: 147–149.

840 Fouilloux B, Perrin C, Dutoit M, Cambazard F. Clear cell syringofibroadenoma (of Mascaro) of the nail. Br J Dermatol 2001; 144: 625–627.

841 Noguchi M, Akiyama M, Kawakami M et al. Eccrine syringofibroadenoma developing in a sebaceous naevus. Br J Dermatol 2000; 142: 1050–1051.

842 Billson VR, Dyall-Smith DJ. Eccrine syringofibroadenoma: a report of 2 cases. Pathology 1991; 23: 259–262.

843 Hara K, Mizuno E, Nitta Y, Ikeya T. Acrosyringeal adenomatosis (eccrine syringofibroadenoma of Mascaro). A case report and review of the literature. Am J Dermatopathol 1992; 14: 328–339.

844 Lui H, Stewart WD, English JC, Wood WS. Eccrine syringofibroadenomatosis: a clinical and histologic study and review of the literature. J Am Acad Dermatol 1992; 26: 805–813.

845 Ochonisky S, Wechsler J, Marinho E, Revuz J. Eccrine syringofibroadenomatosis (Mascaro) with mucous involvement. Arch Dermatol 1994; 130: 933–934.

846 Simpson EL, Styles AR, Cockerell CJ. Eccrine syringofibroadenomatosis associated with hidrotic ectodermal dysplasia. Br J Dermatol 1998; 138: 879–884.

847 Starink TM. Eccrine syringofibroadenoma: Multiple lesions representing a new cutaneous marker of the Schöpf syndrome, and solitary nonhereditary tumors. J Am Acad Dermatol 1997; 36: 569–576.

848 Carlson JA, Rohwedder A, Daulat S et al. Detection of human papillomavirus type 10 DNA in eccrine syringofibroadenomatosis occurring in Clouston's syndrome. J Am Acad Dermatol 1999; 40: 259–262.

849 Chen S, Palay D, Templeton SF. Familial eccrine syringofibroadenomatosis with associated ophthalmologic abnormalities. J Am Acad Dermatol 1998; 39: 356–358.

850 French LE, Masgrau E, Chavaz P, Saurat J-H. Eccrine syringofibroadenoma in a patient with erosive palmoplantar lichen planus. Dermatology 1997; 195: 399–401.

851 Nomura K, Hashimoto I. Eccrine syringofibroadenomatosis in two patients with bullous pemphigoid. Dermatology 1997; 195: 395–398.

852 Ichikawa E, Fujisawa Y, Tateishi Y et al. Eccrine syringofibroadenoma in a patient with a burn scar ulcer. Br J Dermatol 2000; 143: 591–594.

853 Theunis A, Andre J, Forton F et al. Reactive eccrine syringofibroadenoma: report of a subungual case. Am J Dermatopathol 2000; 22: 354 (abstract).

854 Lele SM, Gloster ES, Heilman ER et al. Eccrine syringofibroadenoma surrounding a squamous cell carcinoma: A case report. J Cutan Pathol 1997; 24: 193–196.

855 Utani A, Yabunami H, Kakuta T et al. Reactive eccrine syringofibroadenoma: An association with chronic foot ulcer in a patient with diabetes mellitus. J Am Acad Dermatol 1999; 41: 650–651.

856 Rongioletti F, Gambini C, Parodi A et al. Mossy leg with eccrine syringofibroadenomatous hyperplasia resembling multiple eccrine syringofibroadenoma. Clin Exp Dermatol 1996; 21: 454–456.

857 Sanusi ID, Byrd LN. Eccrine syringofibroadenoma. Int J Dermatol 1988; 27: 523–525.

858 Fretzin DF, Sloan JB, Beer K, Fretzin SA. Eccrine syringofibroadenoma. A clear-cell variant. Am J Dermatopathol 1995; 17: 591–593.

859 van Leeuwen RL, Lavrijsen APM, Starink TM. Eccrine syringofibroadenoma: the simultaneous occurrence of two histopathological variants (conventional and clear-cell type) in one patient. Br J Dermatol 1999; 141: 947–949.

860 González-Serva A, Pró-Risquez MA, Oliver M, Caruso MG. Syringofibrocarcinoma versus squamous cell carcinoma involving syringofibroadenoma: is there a malignant counterpart of Mascaró's syringofibroadenoma? Am J Dermatopathol 1997; 19: 58–65.

861 Ishida-Yamamoto A, Iizuka H. Eccrine syringofibroadenoma (Mascaro). An ultrastructural and immunohistochemical study. Am J Dermatopathol 1996; 18: 207–211.

862 Ohnishi T, Suzuki T, Watanabe S. Eccrine syringofibroadenoma. Report of a case and immunohistochemical study of keratin expression. Br J Dermatol 1995; 134: 449–454.

863 Eckert F, Nilles M, Altmannsberger M. Eccrine syringofibroadenoma: a case report with analysis of cytokeratin expression. Br J Dermatol 1992; 126: 257–261.

864 Komine M, Hattori N, Tamaki K. Eccrine syringofibroadenoma (Mascaro). An immunohistochemical study. Am J Dermatopathol 2000; 22: 171–175.

865 Ohnishi T, Watanabe S, Nomura K. Immunohistochemical analysis of cytokeratin expression in reactive eccrine syringofibroadenoma-like lesion: a comparative study with eccrine syringofibroadenoma. J Cutan Pathol 2000; 27: 164–168.

866 Sueki H, Miller SJ, Dzubow LM, Murphy GF. Eccrine syringofibroadenoma (Mascaro): an ultrastructural study. J Cutan Pathol 1992; 19: 232–239.

Hidradenoma

867 O'Hara JM, Bensch K, Ioannides G, Klaus SN. Eccrine sweat gland adenoma, clear cell type. A histochemical study. Cancer 1966; 19: 1438–1450.

868 Lever WF, Castleman B. Clear cell myo-epithelioma of the skin. Report of ten cases. Am J Pathol 1952; 28: 691–699.

869 Gianotti R, Alessi E. Clear cell hidradenoma associated with the folliculo-sebaceous-apocrine unit. Histologic study of five cases. Am J Dermatopathol 1997; 19: 351–357.

870 Yashar SS, Newbury RO, Cunningham BB. Tender blue mass in an 8 year old. Pediatr Dermatol 2000; 17: 235–237.

871 Faulhaber D, Wörle B, Trautner B, Sander CA. Clear cell hidradenoma in a young girl. J Am Acad Dermatol 2000; 42: 693–695.

872 Morain WD. Large eccrine acrospiroma of the nose. Br J Plast Surg 1979; 32: 43–45.

Malignant eccrine tumors

873 El-Domeiri AA, Brasfield RD, Huvos AG, Strong EW. Sweat gland carcinoma: a clinico-pathologic study of 83 patients. Ann Surg 1971; 173: 270–274.

874 Vogelbruch M, Böcking A, Rütten A et al. DNA image cytometry in malignant and benign sweat gland tumours. Br J Dermatol 2000; 142: 688–693.

875 Coscia Porrazzi L, Sapere P. Cutaneous mixed sarcoma probably arising in a sweat gland adenoma. Histopathology 1995; 26: 471–472.

876 Swanson PE, Cherwitz DL, Neumann MP, Wick MR. Eccrine sweat gland carcinoma: an histologic and immunohistochemical study of 32 cases. J Cutan Pathol 1987; 14: 65–86.

877 Takata M, Hashimoto K, Mehregan P et al. Genetic changes in sweat gland carcinomas. J Cutan Pathol 2000; 27: 30–35.

878 Goldstein DJ, Barr RJ, Santa Cruz DJ. Microcystic adnexal carcinoma. A distinct clinicopathologic entity. Cancer 1982; 50: 566–572.

879 Glatt HJ, Proia AD, Tsoy EA et al. Malignant syringoma of the eyelid. Ophthalmology 1984; 91: 987–990.

880 Lipper S, Peiper SC. Sweat gland carcinoma with syringomatous features. A light microscopic and ultrastructural study. Cancer 1979; 44: 157–163.

881 Cooper PH, Headington JT, Mills SE et al. Sclerosing sweat duct (syringomatous) carcinoma. Am J Surg Pathol 1985; 9: 422–433.

882 Jones MW, Norris HJ, Snyder RC. Infiltrating syringomatous adenoma of the nipple. A clinical and pathological study of 11 cases. Am J Surg Pathol 1989; 13: 197–201.

883 Lupton GP, McMarlin SL. Microcystic adnexal carcinoma. Report of a case with 30-year follow-up. Arch Dermatol 1986; 122: 286–289.

884 LeBoit PE, Sexton M. Microcystic adnexal carcinoma of the skin. J Am Acad Dermatol 1993; 29: 609–618.

885 Moy RL, Tahery DP, Howe K. Microcystic adnexal carcinoma: in vitro growth characteristics and effect of stromal collagen production. Int J Dermatol 1993; 32: 341–344.

886 Rackett SC, Jones RM, Perry AE. Multifocal microcystic adnexal carcinoma. J Cutan Pathol 1997; 24: 118.

887 Chiller K, Passaro D, Scheuller M et al. Microcystic adnexal carcinoma. Forty-eight cases, their treatment, and their outcome. J Am Acad Dermatol 2000; 136: 1355–1359.

888 Ceballos PI, Penneys NS, Cohen BH. Microcystic adnexal carcinoma: a case showing eccrine duct differentiation. J Dermatol Surg Oncol 1988; 14: 1236–1239.

889 Sabhikhi AK, Rao CR, Kumar RV, Hazarika D. Microcystic adnexal carcinoma. Int J Dermatol 1997; 36: 134–136.

890 Landow S, Santoso P, Heilman E. Microcystic adnexal carcinoma in genital skin. J Cutan Pathol 2000; 27: 545 (abstract).

891 Chow WC, Cockerell CJ, Geronemus RG. Microcystic adnexal carcinoma of the scalp. J Dermatol Surg Oncol 1989; 15: 768–771.

892 Peterdy GA, Lind AC, Ackerman LV. Microcystic adnexal carcinoma: 5 cases presenting in unusual anatomic sites. J Cutan Pathol 2000; 27: 568 (abstract).

893 Cooper PH, Mills SE. Microcystic adnexal carcinoma. J Am Acad Dermatol 1984; 10: 908–914.

894 Schwarze HP, Loche F, Lamant L et al. Microcystic adnexal carcinoma induced by multiple radiation therapy. Int J Dermatol 2000; 39: 369–372.

895 Antley CA, Carney M, Smoller BR. Microcystic adnexal carcinoma arising in the setting of previous radiation therapy. J Cutan Pathol 1999; 26: 48–50.

896 Friedman PM, Friedman RH, Jiang SB et al. Microcystic adnexal carcinoma: Collaborative series review and update. J Am Acad Dermatol 1999; 41: 225–231.

897 Martin PC, Smith JL, Pulitzer DR, Reed RJ. Compound (primordial) adnexal carcinoma arising in a systematized compound epithelial nevus. Am J Surg Pathol 1992; 16: 417–425.

898 Lei J-Y, Wang Y, Jaffe ES et al. Microcystic adnexal carcinoma associated with primary immunodeficiency, recurrent diffuse herpes simplex virus infection, and cutaneous T-cell lymphoma. Am J Dermatopathol 2000; 22: 524–529.

899 Pujol RM, LeBoit PE, Su WPD. Microcystic adnexal carcinoma with extensive sebaceous differentiation. Am J Dermatopathol 1997; 19: 358–362.

900 Cooper PH, Robinson CR, Greer KE. Low-grade clear cell eccrine carcinoma. Arch Dermatol 1984; 120: 1076–1078.

901 Heenan PJ. Sebaceous differentiation in microcystic adnexal carcinoma. Am J Dermatopathol 1998; 20: 537.

902 Birkby CS, Argenyi ZB, Whitaker DC. Microcystic adnexal carcinoma with mandibular invasion and bone marrow replacement. J Dermatol Surg Oncol 1989; 15: 308–312.

903 Sebastien TS, Nelson BR, Lowe L et al. Microcystic adnexal carcinoma. J Am Acad Dermatol 1993; 29: 840–845.

904 Nickoloff BJ, Fleischmann HE, Carmel J et al. Microcystic adnexal carcinoma. Immunohistologic observations suggesting dual (pilar and eccrine) differentiation. Arch Dermatol 1986; 122: 290–294.

905 Wick MR, Cooper PH, Swanson PE et al. Microcystic adnexal carcinoma. An immunohistochemical comparison with other cutaneous appendage tumors. Arch Dermatol 1990; 126: 189–194.

906 Rongioletti F, Grosshans E, Rebora A. Microcystic adnexal carcinoma. Br J Dermatol 1986; 115: 101–104.

907 Smith KJ, Williams J, Corbett D. Skelton H. Microcystic adnexal carcinoma. An immunohistochemical study including markers of proliferation and apoptosis. Am J Surg Pathol 2001; 25: 464–471.

908 Requena L, Marquina A, Alegre V et al. Sclerosing-sweat-duct (microcystic adnexal) carcinoma – a tumor from a single eccrine origin. Clin Exp Dermatol 1990; 15: 222–224.

909 Alessi E, Caputo R. Syringomatous carcinoma of the scalp presenting as a slowly enlarging patch of alopecia. Am J Dermatopathol 1993; 15: 503–505.

910 Sequeira J, Wright S, Baker H. Basal cell tumor with eccrine differentiation (eccrine epithelioma) – a histochemical and immunocytochemical analysis of a case. Clin Exp Dermatol 1987; 12: 58–60.

911 Goto M, Sonoda T, Shibuya H et al. Digital syringomatous carcinoma mimicking basal cell carcinoma. Br J Dermatol 2001; 144: 438–439.

912 Gregurek-Novak T, Talan-Hranilović J, Troskot N et al. Syringoid eccrine carcinoma. J Eur Acad Dermatol Venereol 2001; 15: 143–146.

913 Evans AT, Parham DM, Van Niekerk LJA. Metastasising eccrine syringomatous carcinoma. Histopathology 1995; 26: 185–187.

914 Mehregan AH, Hashimoto K, Rahbari H. Eccrine adenocarcinoma. A clinicopathologic study of 35 cases. Arch Dermatol 1983; 119: 104–114.

915 Moy RL, Rivkin JE, Lee H et al. Syringoid eccrine carcinoma. J Am Acad Dermatol 1991; 24: 864–867.

916 McKee PH, Fletcher CDM, Rasbridge SA. The enigmatic eccrine epithelioma (eccrine syringomatous carcinoma). Am J Dermatopathol 1990; 12: 552–561.

917 Urso C, Paglierani M, Bondi R. Histologic spectrum of carcinomas with eccrine ductal differentiation (sweat-gland ductal carcinomas). Am J Dermatopathol 1993; 15: 435–440.

918 Hanke CW, Temofeew RK. Basal cell carcinoma with eccrine differentiation (eccrine epithelioma). J Dermatol Surg Oncol 1986; 12: 820–824.

919 Serrano G, Aliaga A, Bonillo J et al. Basal cell tumor with eccrine differentiation (eccrine epithelioma). J Cutan Pathol 1984; 11: 553–557.

920 Sánchez Yus E, Caballero LR, Salazar IG, Menchero SC. Clear cell syringoid eccrine carcinoma. Am J Dermatopathol 1987; 9: 225–231.

921 Gianotti R, Grimalt R, Alessi E, Caputo R. Spiralled variant of syringomatous carcinoma. Am J Dermatopathol 1993; 15: 568–571.

922 Suster S, Wong T-Y. Polymorphous sweat gland carcinoma. Histopathology 1994; 25: 31–39.

923 Kao GF, Helwig EB, Graham JH. Aggressive digital papillary adenoma and adenocarcinoma. A clinicopathological study of 57 patients, with histochemical, immunopathological, and ultrastructural observations. J Cutan Pathol 1987; 14: 129–146.

924 Jih DM, Elenitsas R, Vittorio CC et al. Aggressive digital papillary adenocarcinoma. A case report and review of the literature. Am J Dermatopathol 2001; 23: 154–157.

925 Duke WH, Sherrod TT, Lupton GP. Aggressive digital papillary adenocarcinoma (aggressive digital papillary adenoma and adenocarcinoma revisited). Am J Surg Pathol 2000; 24: 775–784.

926 Ceballos PI, Penneys NS, Acosta R. Aggressive digital papillary adenocarcinoma. J Am Acad Dermatol 1990; 23: 331–334.

927 Lo JS, Peschen M, Snow SN et al. Malignant cylindroma of the scalp. J Dermatol Surg Oncol 1991; 17: 897–901.

928 Gerretsen AL, van der Putte SCJ, Deenstra W, van Vloten WA. Cutaneous cylindroma with malignant transformation. Cancer 1993; 72: 1618–1623.

929 Pizinger K, Michal M. Malignant cylindroma in Brooke–Spiegler syndrome. Dermatology 2000; 201: 255–257.

930 Antonescu CR, Terzakis JA. Multiple malignant cylindromas of skin in association with basal cell adenocarcinoma with adenoid cystic features of minor salivary gland. J Cutan Pathol 1997; 24: 449–453.

931 Donner LR, Ruff T, Diaz JA. Well-differentiated malignant cylindroma with partially preserved hyaline sheaths. A locally invasive neoplasm? Am J Dermatopathol 1995; 17: 169–173.

932 Lotem M, Trattner A, Kahanovich S et al. Multiple dermal cylindroma undergoing a malignant transformation. Int J Dermatol 1992; 31: 642–644.

933 Argenyi ZB, Nguyen AV, Balogh K et al. Malignant eccrine spiradenoma. A clinicopathologic study. Am J Dermatopathol 1992; 14: 381–390.

934 Fernández-Aceñero MJ, Manzarbeitia F, Mestre de Juan MJ, Requena L. Malignant spiradenoma: Report of two cases and literature review. J Am Acad Dermatol 2001; 44: 395–398.

935 Biernat W, Wozniak L. Spiradenocarcinoma: a clinicopathologic and immunohistochemical study of three cases. Am J Dermatopathol 1994; 16: 377–382.

936 Granter SR, Seeger K, Calonje E et al. Malignant eccrine spiradenoma (spiradenocarcinoma). A clinicopathologic study of 12 cases. Am J Dermatopathol 2000; 22: 97–103.

937 Biernat W, Biernat S. Cutaneous adnexal carcinoma arising within a solitary cylindroma-spiradenoma. Am J Dermatopathol 1996; 18: 77–82.

938 McCluggage WG, Fon LJ, O'Rourke D et al. Malignant eccrine spiradenoma with carcinomatous and sarcomatous features. J Clin Pathol 1997; 50: 871–873.

939 Fernández-Aceñero MJ, Manzarbeitia F, Mestre MJ, Requena L. p53 expression in two cases of spiradenocarcinomas. Am J Dermatopathol 2000; 22: 104–107.

940 Pinkus H, Mehregan AH. Epidermotropic eccrine carcinoma. A case combining features of eccrine poroma and Paget's dermatosis. Arch Dermatol 1963; 88: 597–606.

941 Shaw M, McKee PH, Lowe D, Black MM. Malignant eccrine poroma: a study of twenty-seven cases. Br J Dermatol 1982; 107: 675–680.

942 Robson A, Greene J, Ansari N et al. Eccrine porocarcinoma (malignant eccrine poroma). A clinicopathologic study of 69 cases. Am J Surg Pathol 2001; 25: 710–720.

943 Snow SN, Reizner GT. Eccrine porocarcinoma of the face. J Am Acad Dermatol 1992; 27: 306–311.

944 D'Amato MS, Patterson RH, Guccion JG et al. Porocarcinoma of the heel. A case report with unusual histologic features. Cancer 1996; 78: 751–757.

945 Pylyser K, De Wolf-Peeters C, Marien K. The histology of eccrine poromas: a study of 14 cases. Dermatologica 1983; 167: 243–249.

946 Lee H-J, Jeong S-H, Seo E-J et al. Melanocyte colonization associated with malignant transformation of eccrine poroma. Br J Dermatol 1999; 141: 582–583.

947 Nakanishi Y, Matsuno Y, Shimoda T et al. Eccrine porocarcinoma with melanocyte colonization. Br J Dermatol 1998; 138: 519–521.

948 Ishikawa K. Malignant hidroacanthoma simplex. Arch Dermatol 1971; 104: 529–532.

949 Puttick L, Ince P, Comaish JS. Three cases of eccrine porocarcinoma. Br J Dermatol 1986; 115: 111–116.

950 Tarkhan II, Domingo J. Metastasizing eccrine porocarcinoma developing in a sebaceous nevus of Jadassohn. Report of a case. Arch Dermatol 1985; 121: 413–415.

951 Ryan JF, Darley CR, Pollock DJ. Malignant eccrine poroma: report of three cases. J Clin Pathol 1986; 39: 1099–1104.

952 Huet P, Dandurand M, Pignodel C, Guillot B. Metastasizing eccrine porocarcinoma: report of a case and review of the literature. J Am Acad Dermatol 1996; 35: 860–864.

953 Maeda T, Mori H, Matsuo T et al. Malignant eccrine poroma with multiple visceral metastases: report of a case with autopsy findings. J Cutan Pathol 1996; 23: 566–570.

954 Grimme H, Petres A, Bergen E et al. Metastasizing porocarcinoma of the head with lethal outcome. Dermatology 1999; 198: 298–300.

955 Goel R, Wallace ML. Widespread metastatic eccrine porocarcinoma: a case report. J Cutan Pathol 2000; 27: 557 (abstract).

956 Gschnait F, Horn F, Lindlbauer R, Sponer D. Eccrine porocarcinoma. J Cutan Pathol 1980; 7: 349–353.

957 Hara K, Kamiya S. Pigmented eccrine porocarcinoma: a mimic of malignant melanoma. Histopathology 1995; 27: 86–88.

958 Requena L, Sarasa JL, Piqué E et al. Cell-cell porocarcinoma. Another cutaneous marker of diabetes mellitus. Am J Dermatopathol 1997; 19: 540–544.

959 Miyashita M, Suzuki H. In situ porocarcinoma: a case with malignant expression in clear tumor cells. Int J Dermatol 1993; 32: 749–750.

960 Landa NG, Winkelmann RK. Epidermotropic eccrine porocarcinoma. J Am Acad Dermatol 1991; 24: 27–31.

961 Tateyama H, Eimoto T, Tada T et al. p53 protein and proliferating cell nuclear antigen in eccrine poroma and porocarcinoma. An immunohistochemical study. Am J Dermatopathol 1995; 17: 457–464.

962 Bottles K, Sagebiel RW, McNutt NS et al. Malignant eccrine poroma. Case report and review of the literature. Cancer 1984; 53: 1579–1585.

963 Wong T-Y, Suster S, Mihm MC. Squamoid eccrine ductal carcinoma. Histopathology 1997; 30: 288–293.

964 Herrero J, Monteagudo C, Jordá E, Llombart-Bosch A. Squamoid eccrine ductal carcinoma. Histopathology 1998; 32: 478–480.

965 Friedman KJ. Low-grade primary cutaneous adenosquamous (mucoepidermoid) carcinoma. Report of a case and review of the literature. Am J Dermatopathol 1989; 11: 43–50.

966 Santa Cruz DJ, Prioleau PG. Adnexal carcinomas of the skin. J Cutan Pathol 1984; 11: 450–456.

967 Rosen Y, Kim B, Yermakov VA. Eccrine sweat gland tumor of clear cell origin involving the eyelids. Cancer 1975; 36: 1034–1041.

968 Busam KJ, Gellis S, Shimamura A et al. Small cell sweat gland carcinoma in childhood. Am J Surg Pathol 1998; 22: 215–220.

969 Collina G, Quarto F, Eusebi V. Trabecular carcinoid of the skin with cellular stroma. Am J Dermatopathol 1988; 10: 430–435.

Complex adnexal tumors

970 Hidano A, Kobayashi T. Adnexal polyp of neonatal skin. Br J Dermatol 1975; 92: 659–662.

971 Apisarnthanarax P, Bovenmyer DA, Mehregan AH. Combined adnexal tumor of the skin. Arch Dermatol 1984; 120: 231–233.

972 Hanau D, Grosshans E, Laplanche G. A complex poroma-like adnexal adenoma. Am J Dermatopathol 1984; 6: 567–572.

973 Zaim MT. Sebocrine adenoma. An adnexal adenoma with sebaceous and apocrine poroma-like differentiation. Am J Dermatopathol 1988; 10: 311–318.

974 Robinson HN, Barnett NK. Hemifacial mixed appendageal tumor in an infant. Pediatr Dermatol 1986; 3: 406–409.

975 Alessi E, Wong SN, Advani HH, Ackerman AB. Nevus sebaceus is associated with unusual neoplasms. An atlas. Am J Dermatopathol 1988; 10: 116–127.

976 Mehregan AH, Pinkus H. Life history of organoid nevi. Arch Dermatol 1965; 91: 574–588.

977 Fearfield LA, Bunker CB. Familial naevus sebaceus of Jadassohn. Br J Dermatol 1998; 139: 1119–1120.

978 Happle R, König A. Familial naevus sebaceus may be explained by paradominant transmission. Br J Dermatol 1999; 141: 377.

979 Ramesh A, Murugusundaram S, Kumar KVS et al. Cerebriform sebaceous nevus. Int J Dermatol 1998; 37: 220.

980 Moskowitz R, Honig PJ. Nevus sebaceus in association with an intracranial mass. J Am Acad Dermatol 1982; 6: 1078–1080.

981 Kang WH, Koh YJ, Chun SI. Nevus sebaceus syndrome associated with intracranial arteriovenous malformation. Int J Dermatol 1987; 26: 382–384.

982 Diven DG, Solomon AR, McNeely MC, Font RL. Nevus sebaceus associated with major ophthalmologic abnormalities. Arch Dermatol 1987; 123: 383–386.

983 Wilson Jones E, Heyl T. Naevus sebaceus. A report of 140 cases with special regard to the development of secondary malignant tumors. Br J Dermatol 1970; 82: 99–117.

984 Lupton JR, Elgart ML, Sulica VI. Segmental neurofibromatosis in association with nevus sebaceus of Jadassohn. J Am Acad Dermatol 2000; 43: 895–897.

985 Morris SD, Onadim Z, Yu RO. A case of naevus sebaceous associated with familial retinoblastoma, multiple lipomata and meningioma. Br J Dermatol 2000; 143: 211–214.

986 Hwang SM, Choi EH, Ahn SK, Lee WS. Tuberous sclerosis with naevus sebaceus. Clin Exp Dermatol 1998; 23: 44–45.

987 Jang IG, Choi JM, Park KW, Kim S-Y. Nevus sebaceus syndrome. Int J Dermatol 1999; 38: 531–533.

988 Chun K, Vázquez M, Sánchez JL. Nevus sebaceus: clinical outcome and considerations for prophylactic excision. Int J Dermatol 1995; 34: 538–541.

989 Kaddu S, Schaeppi H, Kerl H, Soyer HP. Basaloid neoplasms in nevus sebaceus. J Cutan Pathol 2000; 27: 327–337.

990 Jaqueti G, Requena L, Sánchez Yus E. Trichoblastoma is the most common neoplasm developed in nevus sebaceus of Jadassohn. A clinicopathologic study of a series of 155 cases. Am J Dermatopathol 2000; 22: 108–118.

991 Cribier B, Scrivener Y, Grosshans E. Tumors arising in nevus sebaceus: A study of 596 cases. J Am Acad Dermatol 2000; 42: 263–268.

992 Burden PA, Gentry RH, Fitzpatrick JE. Piloleiomyoma arising in an organoid nevus: a case report and review of the literature. J Dermatol Surg Oncol 1987; 13: 1213–1218.

993 Shapiro M, Johnson B Jr, Witmer W, Elenitsas R. Spiradenoma arising in a nevus sebaceus of Jadassohn. Case report and literature review. Am J Dermatopathol 1999; 21: 462–467.

994 Misago N, Narisawa Y, Nishi T, Kohda H. Association of nevus sebaceus with an unusual type of "combined nevus". J Cutan Pathol 1994; 21: 76–81.

995 Kaddu S, Schäppi H, Kerl H, Soyer HP. Trichoblastoma and sebaceoma in nevus sebaceus. Am J Dermatopathol 1999; 21: 552–556.

996 Stavrianeas NG, Katoulis AC, Stratigeas NP et al. Development of multiple tumors in a sebaceous nevus of Jadassohn. Dermatology 1997; 195: 155–158.

997 Alessi E, Sala F. Nevus sebaceus. A clinicopathologic study of its evolution. Am J Dermatopathol 1986; 8: 27–31.

998 Morioka S. The natural history of nevus sebaceus. J Cutan Pathol 1985; 12: 200–213.

999 Ng WK. Nevus sebaceus with apocrine and sebaceous differentiation. Am J Dermatopathol 1996; 18: 420–423.

1000 Choi SW, Woo HJ, Rho K-Y et al. Calcification in the apocrine glands of naevus sebaceus. Br J Dermatol 2000; 142: 1241–1242.

1001 van der Putte SCJ. Apoeccrine glands in nevus sebaceus. Am J Dermatopathol 1994; 16: 23–30.

1002 Massa LR, Stone MS. An unusual hematopoietic proliferation seen in a nevus sebaceous. J Am Acad Dermatol 2000; 42: 881–882.

1003 Schulz T, Hartschuh W. Merkel cells in nevus sebaceus. An immunohistochemical study. Am J Dermatopathol 1995; 17: 570–579.

1004 Sánchez Yus E, Requena L, Simón P, Sánchez M. Complex adnexal tumor of the primary epithelial germ with distinct patterns of superficial epithelioma with sebaceous differentiation, immature trichoepithelioma, and apocrine adenocarcinoma. Am J Dermatopathol 1992; 14: 245–252.

1005 Wong T-Y, Suster S, Cheek RF, Mihm MC Jr. Benign cutaneous adnexal tumors with combined folliculosebaceous, apocrine, and eccrine differentiation. Am J Dermatopathol 1996; 18: 124–136.

1006 Nakhleh RE, Swanson PE, Wick MR. Cutaneous adnexal carcinomas with divergent differentiation. Am J Dermatopathol 1990; 12: 325–334.

1007 Requena L, Ackerman AB. A distinctive cutaneous benign adnexal neoplasm with retiform and racemiform patterns. Dermatopathology: Practical & Conceptual 1997; 3: 104–109.

1008 Gianotti R, Coggi A, Alessi E. Poral neoplasm with combined sebaceous and apocrine differentiation. Am J Dermatopathol 1998; 20: 491–494.

Tumors and tumor-like proliferations of fibrous and related tissues

34

INTRODUCTION

Recent immunohistochemical findings have assisted in the histogenetic classification of many of the soft tissue tumors.[1] However the 'fibrohistiocytic' tumors are still largely enigmatic with respect to their histogenesis, and the diagnosis is largely dependent on H&E inspection.[2] In addition to the 'fibrohistiocytic' tumors, this chapter includes those entities that have traditionally been grouped together on the basis of collagen production and/or the presence of fibroblasts or fibroblast-like cells forming an integral component of the tumor. It also includes tumors of presumptive origin from dermal dendrocytes and myofibroblasts.

Dermal dendrocytes

Dermal dendrocytes are bone marrow-derived cells found in different parts of the dermis.[3–6] They are closely related to mast cells in the perivascular space.[6] They express factor XIIIa and von Willebrand factor receptor, suggesting a possible role in tissue repair and hemostasis. An antigen-processing function has also been proposed.[7–9] The subset of dendrocytes expressing factor XIIIa is found in some of the acral angiofibromas and in dermatofibromas. They are also increased in many other situations. Another subset of dendrocytes, comprising 10–30% of all interstitial cells in the reticular dermis, expresses CD34.[10] This antigen is expressed in vascular endothelial cells, some perivascular and interstitial dendritic cells in the dermis, as mentioned above, and spindle cells in the basement membrane zone of eccrine ducts and the bulge area of the hair follicle. The two subsets of dendrocytes appear to interact in many situations.[11] A hamartoma composed of CD34-positive cells has been reported as a **'dermal dendrocyte hamartoma'**.[12] A granular cell variant of CD34-positive cells, presenting as multiple papules and plaques in a baby has been called **'granular cell dendrocytosis'**,[13] while a post-traumatic myxoid tumor of the thumb composed of both CD34[+] and factor XIIIa[+] cells has been called a **'myxoid dermatofibrohistiocytoma'**.[14] Yet another term, **'CD34-positive eruptive fibroma'**, has been used for the multiple papules composed of CD34[+] spindle cells reported on the neck and upper chest of a female teenager.[15]

Myofibroblasts

Tumors of myofibroblasts are also considered in this chapter. They often coexist with ordinary fibroblasts in many of the lesions. There is still a lack of consensus regarding their exact role in the formation of the soft tissue tumors usually attributed to them.[2] It has even been suggested that myofibroblasts are merely a functional stage of fibroblasts, smooth muscle cells or pericytes, and that their identification requires the ultrastructural recognition of the so-called 'fibronexus' (microtendons).[16,17] Neoplastic myofibroblasts express vimentin, muscle actin, α-smooth muscle actin, and/or desmin, although the specificity of desmin has been questioned.

Various attempts have been made to simplify this difficult subject including an algorithmic approach based on colors,[18,19] and the application of molecular genetics.[20]

ACRAL ANGIOFIBROMAS

Acral angiofibromas are a clinically diverse group of entities that share distinctive histological features.[21,22] They are thought by some to represent hyperplasias of the papillary and/or periadnexal dermis (the adventitial dermis).[23] Immunohistochemical studies have shown that the large stellate fibroblast-like cells that characterize these tumors express factor XIIIa.[24,25] They are not mesenchymally derived fibroblasts.[26] Factor XIIIa appears to be important in the promulgation of fibroplasia.[27]

Tumors derived from the perifollicular mesenchyme – the perifollicular fibroma, trichodiscoma and fibrofolliculoma – are usually considered separately from the acral angiofibromas.[28] They are discussed with the tumors of the hair follicle (see p. 871).

The following clinical conditions will be discussed:

- adenoma sebaceum (tuberous sclerosis)
- angiofibromas in other syndromes
- fibrous papule of the face
- pearly penile papules
- acral fibrokeratoma
- familial myxovascular fibromas.

The entity reported as linear papular ectodermal–mesodermal hamartoma has some features of this group.[29]

ADENOMA SEBACEUM

'Adenoma sebaceum' is the misnomer (there is no adenomatous proliferation of sebaceous glands as the name implies) used for the angiofibromatous lesions found in most patients with tuberous sclerosis, an autosomal dominant neurocutaneous syndrome in which mental retardation and epilepsy are often present.[30,31] Other organ systems are often involved.[32,33] Other cutaneous angiofibromatous lesions may accompany adenoma sebaceum, and these include plaque-like lesions of the forehead and scalp and ungual fibromas (see acral fibrokeratomas on p. 920).[34,35] 'Shagreen patches', with the histology of connective tissue nevi, are commonly found in tuberous sclerosis.[36] They are usually present by puberty.[37] Hypopigmented macules are a common finding.[38] Genetic linkage studies indicate that about half of all families with tuberous sclerosis show linkage to chromosome 9q34 (*TSC1*), and the remainder to chromosome 16p13 (*TSC2*).[39,40] Hamartin is encoded by *TSC1* and tuberin, a tumor suppressor, by *TSC2*. Approximately two-thirds of all cases are sporadic and assumed to result from new mutations, many of which are in *TSC2*.[41] Other cases are inherited as an autosomal dominant trait. Mutation screening in tuberous sclerosis is labor intensive and expensive.[42]

Adenoma sebaceum consists of several or multiple papules and nodules, sometimes grouped, with a predilection for the butterfly area of the face, particularly the nasolabial groove.[32,34] They appear in early childhood as pink-red to yellow-brown lesions and their growth is usually progressive until adult life. A giant angiofibromatous plaque and a cluster growth of large nodules[43] have been reported. Unilateral facial involvement is another clinical variant.[44] It probably represents mosaicism.[45–47]

Histopathology[22,48]

The lesions vary from rounded elevations to raised pedunculated growths (Fig. 34.1).[48] The epidermis shows some flattening of rete ridges with patchy melanocytic hyperplasia, and mild overlying hyperkeratosis. The dermal component consists of a network of collagen fibers, often oriented perpendicular to the surface in the subepidermal zone, and having an onion-skin arrangement around follicles and sometimes blood vessels (Fig. 34.2). There is an increase in fibroblastic cells, which are plump, spindle shaped, stellate or even multinucleate. There is often a sparse inflammatory infiltrate which includes mast cells. The blood vessels are increased in number, and some are dilated with an irregular outline. Follicles may show epithelial proliferation and there

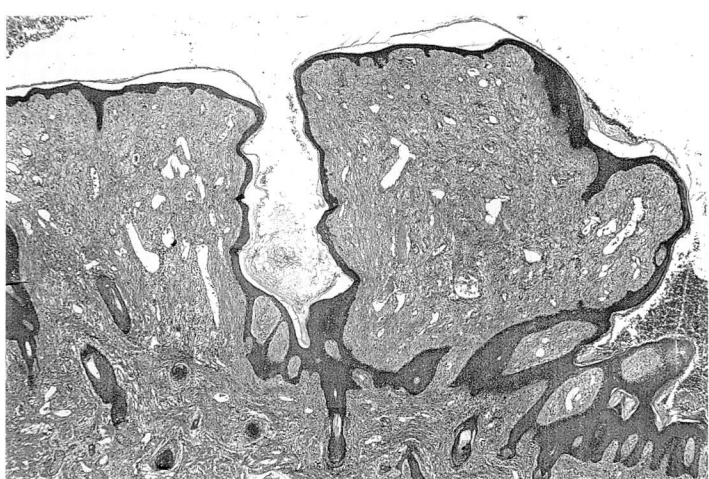

Fig. 34.1 **Adenoma sebaceum.** There are pedunculated outgrowths with an angiofibromatous stroma. (H & E)

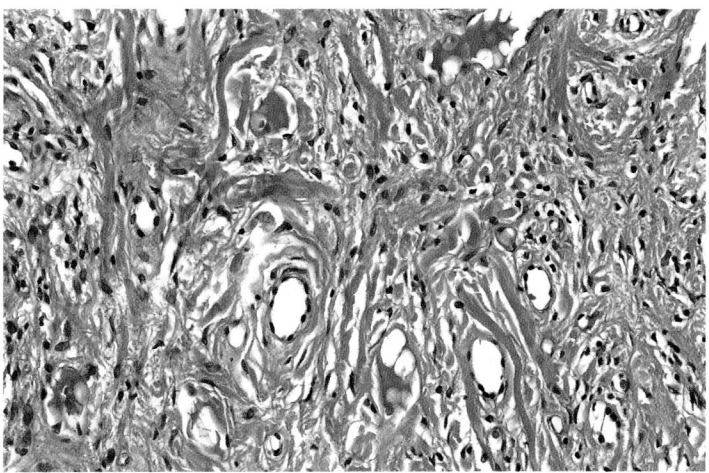

Fig. 34.2 **Adenoma sebaceum.** Collagen is arranged around the small blood vessels in the upper dermis. Fibroblasts are increased in number, but they are not as stellate as usual. (H & E)

may be primitive small follicles.[49] Elastic tissue is absent from the stromal fibrous tissue. The extracellular glycoproteins fibronectin and tenascin are increased in the stroma.[50]

Staining for CD31 confirms the increased vascularity of these lesions.

Electron microscopy

Ultrastructural examination[51] has shown large numbers of microvilli on the luminal surface of the endothelial cells of the vessels. The stroma contains many banded structures. No myofibroblasts have been seen.

ANGIOFIBROMAS IN OTHER SYNDROMES

Facial angiofibromas, both unilateral and bilateral, have already been mentioned as an important manifestation of *tuberous sclerosis* (see above). They have also been described in a patient with *neurofibromatosis 2* (NF-2) as a cluster of small papules on the ear.[52] Multiple facial angiofibromas are seen quite often in patients with *multiple endocrine neoplasia* (MEN) type I. They tend to present in adult life.[53] Other cutaneous tumors in this syndrome include collagenomas and lipomas.[54] There may also be café-au-lait macules and confetti-like hypopigmented macules.[55] The tumors show allelic deletion of the *MEN1* gene. It encodes a protein called menin, which is presumed to act as a tumor suppressor. Basic fibroblast growth factor (BFGF) is elevated in many patients and may be responsible for the formation of the cutaneous tumors.[53]

Angiofibromas (often reported as perifollicular fibromas) have been reported in the *Hornstein–Knickenberg syndrome*, which appears to be a slightly different phenotypic expression of the Birt–Hogg–Dubé syndrome (see p. 871).

FIBROUS PAPULE OF THE FACE

Fibrous papules of the face are usually solitary, dome-shaped papules, measuring 3–5 mm in diameter, found particularly on the nose of middle-aged adults.[22,56,57] They are flesh colored and usually asymptomatic, although some may bleed after minor trauma. They were originally regarded as fibrosed dermal nevi,[56–58] a proposition which has been disproved by electron microscopy[59,60] and immunohistochemistry.[61–63] The presence of factor XIIIa

in the spindle cells and in some stellate cells suggests that fibrous papule is a proliferative reactive process consisting mainly of dermal dendritic cells.[62,63]

Histopathology[22,48,56,57]

The changes are similar to those described for adenoma sebaceum. However, the vessels are sometimes more ectatic and less likely to show concentric fibrosis than in adenoma sebaceum (Fig. 34.3). Furthermore, the bizarre cells in the dermis are usually more numerous and the basal melanocytic hyperplasia more prominent in fibrous papule of the face. Rarely, the stromal cells may contain coarse cytoplasmic granules leading to a granular-cell appearance.[64] Another rare pattern involves the presence of numerous fibroblasts/histiocytes/dendrocytes with clear vacuolated cytoplasm embedded in a dense sclerotic and hyalinized stroma. A few multinucleate 'floret'-like cells may be present. Only a few cells stain for factor XIIIa and CD68. This lesion, *clear cell fibrous papule*, may eventually prove to be unrelated to fibrous papule, although the cases reported were all on the face, predominantly the nose (Fig. 34.4).[65]

The spindle and stellate cells in fibrous papule of the face contain vimentin and factor XIIIa (see above), but not S100 protein.[62,66,67] α_1-Antitrypsin and lysozyme were detected in one study, although this has not been confirmed subsequently.[68] A case with CD34$^+$ cells has been reported.[69]

Electron microscopy

Ultrastructural studies have suggested that the stellate cells are fibroblastic or fibrohistiocytic.[59,60]

PEARLY PENILE PAPULES

Pearly penile papules are persistent asymptomatic pearly-white papules, 1–3 mm in diameter, occurring in groups or rows on the coronal margin and sulcus of the penis.[21,70–73] Rarely they may be found on the penile shaft[74] or glans.[75] They are found in about 10% of young adult males, and are more common in the uncircumcised.[71] They may be misdiagnosed as warts.[72]

Histopathology[21]

There is a rich vascular network, surrounded by dense connective tissue containing an increased number of plump and stellate fibroblasts. They

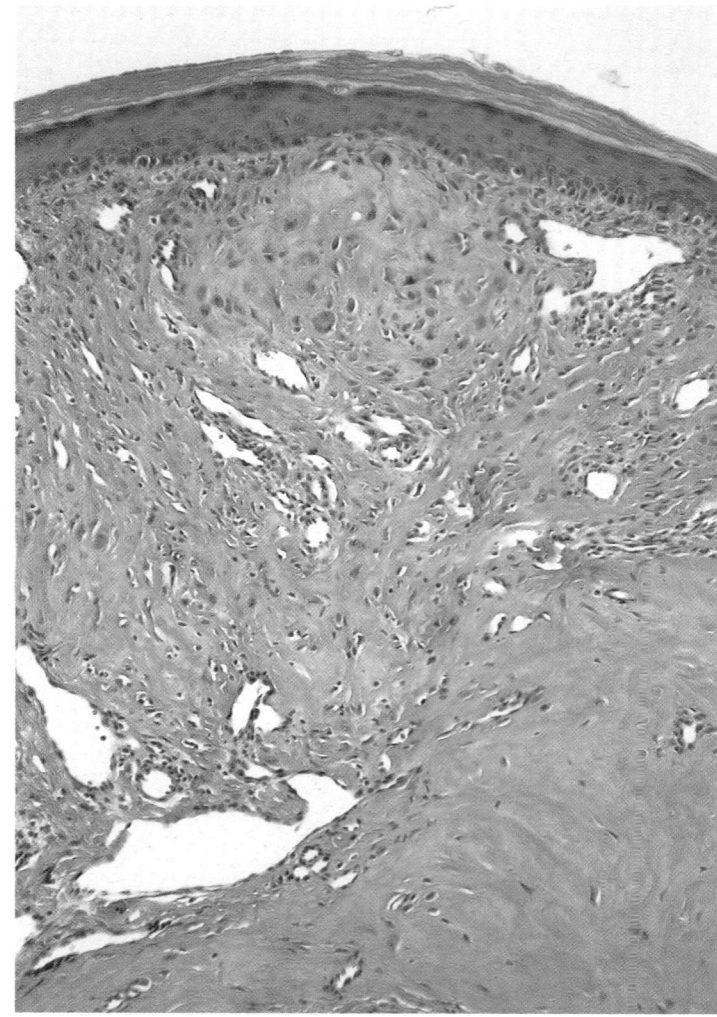

Fig. 34.3 **Fibrous papule of the nose.** Note the bizarre stellate cells in the upper dermis. (H & E)

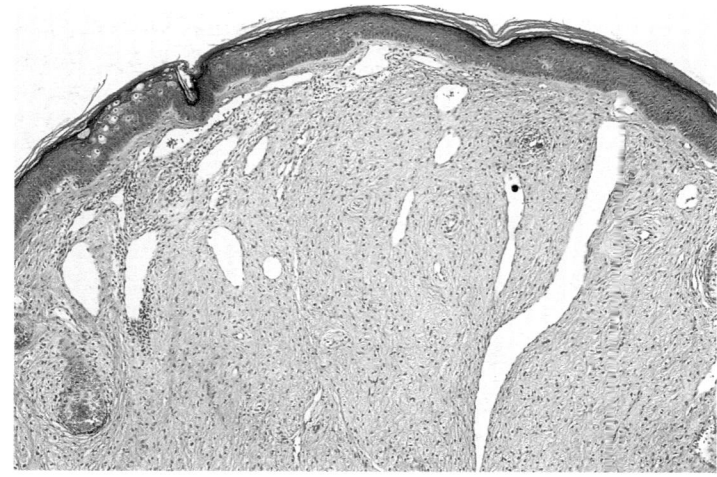

Fig. 34.4 **Clear-cell fibrous papule.** This lesion from the nasal ala contains telangiectatic vessels and sheets of clear cells. (H & E)

resemble other lesions in this group, except for the absence of pilosebaceous follicles.

ACRAL FIBROKERATOMA

Included in the acral fibrokeratoma group[76] are lesions reported as acquired digital fibrokeratoma,[77–80] acquired periungual fibrokeratoma, 'garlic clove fibroma',[81] and the subungual and periungual fibromas of tuberous sclerosis.[34] This unifying concept is an attempt to overcome the needless proliferation of terms, and it gives recognition not only to the common histopathological features, but also to the fact that occasional lesions have been reported in sites other than digits.[82]

The lesions are usually solitary, dome-shaped or elongated thin horns, 1–3 mm in diameter and up to 15 mm in height. There is sometimes a history of trauma.[78] The ungual fibromas of tuberous sclerosis are often multiple, sometimes in clusters, and develop at about puberty.[83] They are found in about half the patients with tuberous sclerosis.[31,34]

Some fibrokeratomas originate from the dermal connective tissue, whereas others appear to originate from the proximal nail fold.[84] An invaginated variant has been reported in relation to the nail apparatus.[85] This difference in the site of origin may account for the heterogeneous features observed in this entity.

Multiple acral fibromas with a myxoid but poorly vascularized stroma have been reported in a patient with familial retinoblastoma, leading to the suggestion that multiple acral benign tumors with a fibrous component might be a cutaneous marker of tumor-suppressor gene germline mutation.[86] Lesions reported as **familial multiple acral mucinous fibrokeratomas**[87] and familial myxovascular fibroma (see below) are probably further examples of this hypothesis.

Histopathology

The epidermal covering usually shows hyperkeratosis, and sometimes acanthosis. There is a core of thick collagen bundles which are oriented predominantly in the vertical axis (Fig. 34.5). Stellate fibroblasts are often present. There is sometimes prominent cellularity,[84] and a rich vascular supply. These latter two features have not been prominent,[79] or have been specifically excluded[88] in some of the reports, suggesting that some of the lesions might best be regarded as fibromas[76,86] rather than angiofibromas. The rare invaginated variant is characterized by a deep epithelial invagination proximal to the normal matrix.[85] A pseudo-nail plate is produced.

There are usually sparse elastic fibers, few inflammatory cells, and no hair follicles. Neural tissue is not present, unlike the clinically similar entity of supernumerary (rudimentary) digits.[79,89]

FAMILIAL MYXOVASCULAR FIBROMA

Three kindreds have been reported in which multiple verrucous papules developed on the fingers and hands.[87,90,91] On histological examination the papules showed a fibrovascular proliferation of the papillary dermis, with variable myxoid change and overlying epidermal acanthosis and hyperkeratosis. There is some overlap with the lesions included within the concept of cutaneous myxomas (see p. 942).

FIBROUS OVERGROWTHS, FIBROMATOSES, MYOFIBROBLASTIC PROLIFERATIONS AND FIBROSARCOMA

This heterogeneous group of lesions forms a histological spectrum, at one end of which is the fibroma and at the other end the fibrosarcoma. In

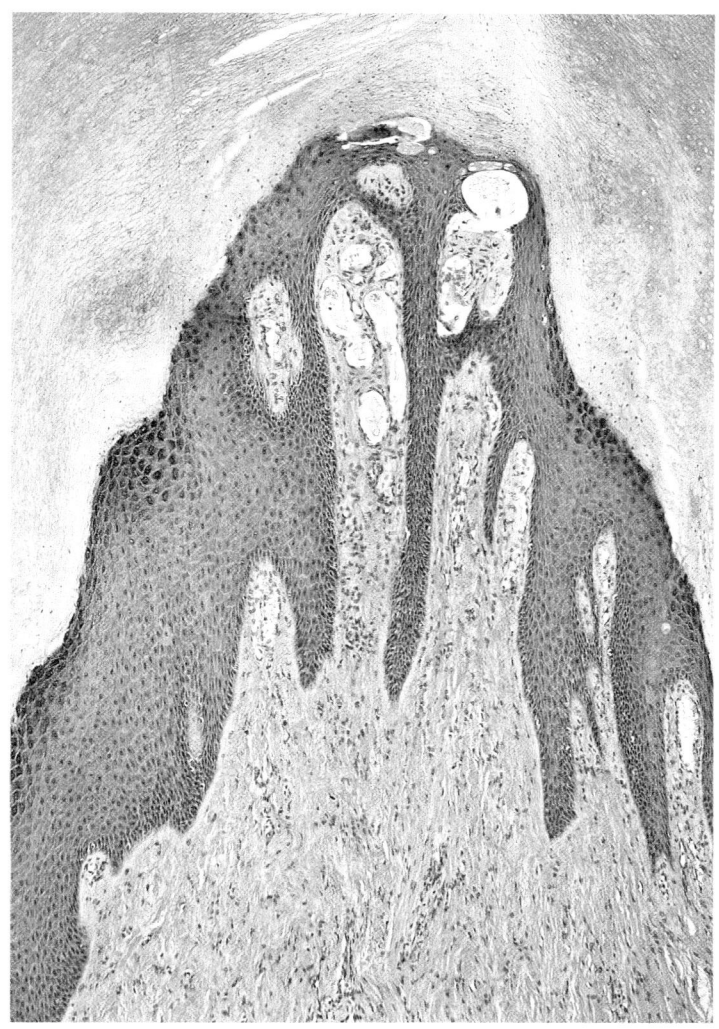

Fig. 34.5 **Acral fibrokeratoma.** This lesion, which was clinically horn-like, has a core of fibrous tissue and an epidermal covering with overlying orthokeratosis. Dilated vessels are present at the tip. (H & E)

between are the 'fibromatoses', which have been defined as a 'group of non-metastasizing fibrous tumors which tend to invade locally and recur after surgical excision'.[92]

The 'fibromatoses' include entities such as palmar and plantar fibromatosis,[93] extra-abdominal desmoid,[94,95] knuckle pads, pachydermodactyly, Peyronie's disease of the penis, and various 'juvenile fibromatoses' such as juvenile aponeurotic fibroma, fibrous hamartoma of infancy, digital fibromatosis of childhood, and infantile myofibromatosis. The tumors in this latter category usually contain an admixture of fibroblasts and myofibroblasts. This is the explanation for their inclusion also as tumors of myofibroblasts (see below).

Plantar fibromatosis is a benign, but sometimes locally aggressive, proliferation of fibrous tissue involving the deep subcutis and fascia of the plantar surface of the foot. A variant with distinct nodules occurs.[93] *Peyronie's disease* of the penis and *Dupuytren's disease* of the palmar fascia are similar fibromatoses.[96] The *desmoid tumor* (a clonal process) and *extra-abdominal desmoid tumor* are usually regarded as belonging to the domain of soft tissue tumors.[97-100] They will not be considered further. The nuchal fibroma (see p. 359)[101] and the nuchal fibrocartilaginous tumor (see p. 428)[102] are considered elsewhere. The nuchal-type fibromas that arise in Gardner's syndrome may be multiple and occur in unusual locations.[103]

Tumors of myofibroblasts include nodular fasciitis, fibrous hamartoma of infancy, digital fibromatosis of childhood, dermatomyofibroma, infantile myofibromatosis, inflammatory myofibroblastic tumor, plexiform fibrohistiocytic tumor and myofibroblastic sarcoma. Partial myofibroblastic differentiation is seen in low-grade fibromyxoid sarcoma and angiomyofibroblastoma of the vulva. Plexiform fibrohistiocytic tumor is considered with the fibrohistiocytic tumors (see p. 933) because of the dual population of cells. Congenital-infantile fibrosarcoma is sometimes included as a myofibroblastic lesion in some classifications.[16] The case with myofibroblastic proliferation confined to the skin of the neck defies classification.[104]

SKIN TAGS

Skin tags (soft fibromas, acrochordons, fibrolipomas) are common cutaneous lesions that have received little attention in the dermatological literature, because hitherto they have been regarded as being of little consequence. However, there have been several reports suggesting an association between the presence of skin tags and underlying diabetes,[105-108] abnormal lipid profile,[109] colonic polyps[110-113] or acromegaly.[114] The association with colonic polyps is controversial, and several studies have failed to confirm its existence.[115-117] HPV types 6/11 were detected in a significant number of cases in one study.[118] This finding remains to be confirmed.

Skin tags have a predilection for the axilla, neck, groin, eyelids and beneath pendulous breasts. They are more common in obese females, and they may develop in pregnancy.[119] In one autopsy study they were present in 64% of individuals over the age of 50,[115] whereas in a more recent study they were present in 46% of 750 individuals examined.[120] There are three clinical types:[115] furrowed papules approximately 2 mm in width and height; filiform lesions, approximately 2 mm in width and 5 mm in height; and large bag-like protuberances, usually on the lower trunk.[121,122] These larger lesions are very occasionally multiple.[105,123]

Vestibular papillae of the vulva are skin tag-like smooth projections of the vestibular mucosa that appear to be normal anatomical variants.[124] They are not related to human papillomavirus infection, as previously suggested.[124]

Fibroepithelial polyps of the anus are relatively common lesions, some of which are thought to arise from enlargement of anal papillae.[125] They should be distinguished from the much smaller **infantile perianal pyramidal protrusion** which occurs predominantly in young girls in the midline, anterior to the anus.[126]

Histopathology

The histological features vary with the clinical type. The furrowed papules show epidermal hyperplasia and sometimes horn cyst formation. These lesions, with seborrheic keratosis-like surface changes, are most common on the neck and eyelids.[127] The filiform lesions are covered by an epidermis which shows only mild acanthosis. The connective tissue stalk is usually composed of well-vascularized, loosely arranged collagen. Elastic fibers are present in normal amounts.[128] A few fat cells and, sometimes, nevus cells may be present. The larger, bag-like lesions (fibroepithelial polyps, fibrolipomas) usually have a stroma composed of loosely arranged collagen and a central core of adipose tissue. It has been suggested, and subsequently challenged, that there is little utility in submitting these lesions for histological examination.[129,130]

Vestibular papillae of the vulva consist of connective tissue projections covered by normal stratified squamous epithelium.[124]

An unusual cutaneous polyp with bizarre stromal cells, thought to represent a degenerative phenomenon, has been reported as a **'pseudosarcomatous polyp'**.[131] Subsequent correspondence raised the possibility that the lesion may have been a dermal spindle-cell lipoma or 'ancient' (degenerative) change in a polyp.[132]

The **fibroepithelial polyp of the anus** has a myxoid and/or collagenous stroma covered by stratified squamous epithelium which may show some swollen cells with vacuolation near the surface.[133] The stroma sometimes contains atypical cells showing fibroblastic and myofibroblastic differentiation.[125] The **infantile perianal pyramidal protrusion** reveals epidermal acanthosis, marked edema in the upper dermis and a mild inflammatory cell infiltrate.[126]

PLEOMORPHIC FIBROMA

Pleomorphic fibroma of the skin was described by Kamino et al in 1989.[134] It presents as a slow-growing lesion, clinically indistinguishable from a polypoid skin tag.[135] A subungual lesion has been reported.

Histopathology

The lesion is usually a dome-shaped nodule with variable cellularity. The spindle-shaped cells show striking nuclear pleomorphism with rare mitotic figures. A variant with myxoid stroma occurs.[136,137] The cells express vimentin and CD34, but not desmin, Ki-M1p[138] or S100 protein, suggesting a possible origin from dendrocytes, rather than myofibroblasts as originally thought.[134,138] Staining for factor XIIIa has been moderate in some studies, but negative or patchy in others.[137–139] The nuclear atypia is similar to the 'degenerative' changes seen in a number of benign mesenchymal tumors.[140]

SCLEROTIC FIBROMA

Sclerotic ('plywood') fibroma is an uncommon fibrocytic neoplasm that occurs sporadically as a solitary lesion, and in a multifocal form in patients with Cowden's disease.[141–145] The terms 'hypocellular fibroma' and 'circumscribed, storiform collagenoma'[146] have also been used for this entity. The lesions are flesh-colored papules or nodules measuring 0.5–3 cm in diameter.

Although it was initially regarded as an involutional lesion, one study has demonstrated ongoing type I collagen synthesis and deposition, suggesting that the lesion is a proliferating neoplasm.[143,147] Local recurrence has been reported.[148]

Histopathology

The lesions are circumscribed, unencapsulated dermal nodules, often with an attenuated overlying epidermis.[143] They are composed of thickened and homogenized eosinophilic collagen bundles arranged in a laminated fashion with intervening prominent clefts.[149] Vaguely storiform or whorled patterns of collagen may be present (Fig. 34.6). The lesions are of low cellularity. The nuclei are tapered to stellate. Elastic fibers are absent from the lesion, but there is often some stromal mucin. Similar collagenous changes have been seen as a focal phenomenon in the vicinity of inflammatory lesions, such as folliculitis,[150] and in dermatofibromas, where the sclerosis may be more extensive.[151] This has led to the view that sclerotic fibromas may not have a common origin.

The spindle cells stain for vimentin and factor XIIIa.[147,152] CD34 positivity occurs focally, with no consistent localization.[147,153] Both PCNA and Ki-67 immunoreactivity have been detected, as would be expected in a growing neoplasm.[143]

The lesion reported as a **pacinian collagenoma** is probably a variant.[154] It was composed of paucicellular collagen fibers arranged in concentric lamellations giving an 'onion-skin' appearance. The cells stained for CD34. It had some resemblance to the perineurioma (see p. 981).

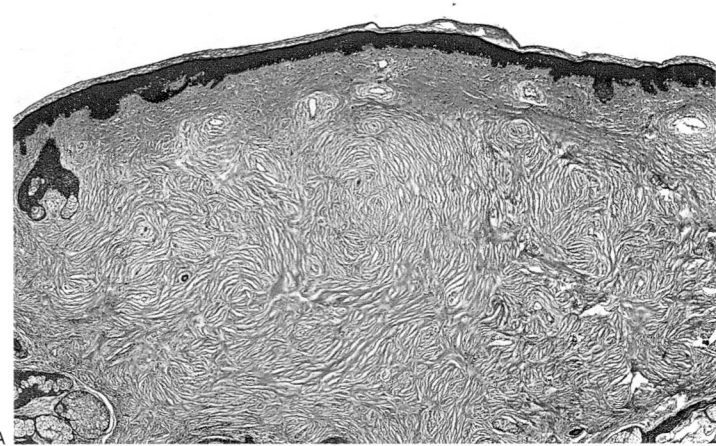
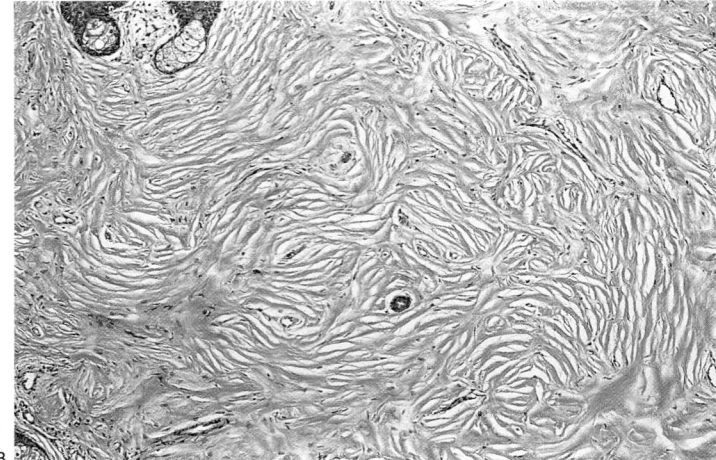

Fig. 34.6 **(A) Sclerotic fibroma. (B)** There is a storiform and whorled pattern. (H & E)

Cases resembling sclerotic fibroma but with variable numbers of bizarre, multinucleated cells, often with a foamy cytoplasm, have been reported as **pleomorphic sclerotic fibroma** and **giant cell collagenoma**.[155,156]

Electron microscopy

The widened collagen bundles contain tightly packed collagen fibrils, only 50 nm in diameter.[149]

COLLAGENOUS FIBROMA (DESMOPLASTIC FIBROBLASTOMA)

Collagenous fibroma, a recently described tumor, may arise in the subcutaneous tissue or muscle.[157,158] Dermal involvement is rare.[159] The tumors are firm and non-tender. Most measure 2–3 cm in diameter but larger lesions have been reported.[160] There is a predilection for adult males.[161] Any part of the body may be involved.[161]

Histopathology

Collagenous fibroma is usually a well-demarcated tumor in the subcutis, although some infiltration is often present at the periphery. It is hypocellular and composed of large, stellate or spindle cells set in a densely collagenous or fibromyxoid stroma. There are usually no mitoses. There are inconspicuous small vessels. The cells express vimentin. Factor XIIIa was present in one case. Scattered cells may show a myofibroblastic immunophenotype.[162]

KNUCKLE PADS

Knuckle pads (discrete keratodermas over the knuckle and finger articulations) are well-formed skin-colored nodules overlying the interphalangeal and metacarpophalangeal joints of the hands.[163-165] They are usually multiple. There are several clinical variants, including a familial group, an occupational or recreational-related group, and an acquired idiopathic group. An association with knuckle cracking and with pseudoxanthoma elasticum has been reported.[166,167] Of historical interest is the prominent knuckle pad on the right thumb of Michelangelo's statue of David.[168]

Histopathology[168]

There appear to be at least three histological types. The usual lesions show prominent hyperkeratosis and epidermal acanthosis. There is minimal thickening of the papillary dermis. Another type has macronodules of swollen collagen fibers surrounded by thickened elastic fibers.[169] A third variant with prominent subcutaneous fibrosis, belonging to the fibromatoses, has been documented.[168]

PACHYDERMODACTYLY

Pachydermodactyly is characterized by fibrous thickening of the lateral aspects of the proximal interphalangeal joints of the fingers, usually in males.[170-175] The thumbs and fifth fingers are usually not involved. More extensive lesions have been reported.[173,176,177]

Pachydermodactyly is regarded as a localized form of superficial fibromatosis. Trauma, such as finger rubbing, has been implicated in the etiology.[178]

Histopathology

There is thickening of the dermis, with coarse collagen bundles and a mild proliferation of fibroblasts. Small deposits of mucin are sometimes present in the interstitium.[173] Elastic fibers are reduced. There is no inflammation.

The overlying epidermis shows mild hyperplasia and compact orthokeratosis.

NODULAR FASCIITIS

Nodular fasciitis is a reactive proliferation of fibroblast-like cells with a predilection for the subcutaneous tissues of the forearm, upper arm and thigh of young and middle-aged adults.[179,180] Dermal and intravascular variants have been reported.[181-185] It usually grows quite quickly to reach a median diameter of 1.5 cm. Multiple lesions have been reported.[186] Recurrences are rare, even after incomplete surgical removal, and their occurrence should lead to a reappraisal of the original histological diagnosis.[187,188] Regression may occur after the use of intralesional corticosteroids.[189] Despite having high activity for proliferating cell nuclear antigen (PCNA), the cells do not express p53 or show aneuploidy.[190,191]

Cranial fasciitis of childhood is a distinct clinical variant arising in the deep soft tissues of the scalp, with involvement of the underlying cranium.[192,193]

Histopathology[179,194,195]

Nodular fasciitis is composed of a proliferation of spindle-shaped to plump fibroblasts which may be arranged in haphazard array ('tissue culture appearance'), or in bundles that form S-shaped curves (Fig. 34.7).[195] A vague storiform pattern is sometimes present focally. Mitoses are frequent, but atypical forms are rare. Cleft-like spaces may be seen between the fibroblasts. There is a variable amount of myxoid stroma and extravasated erythrocytes. Collagen is usually sparse. Capillaries with plump endothelial cells are common. Scattered lymphocytes are dispersed throughout the lesion.

Intravascular fasciitis, in which the proliferation occurs within small and medium-sized arteries and veins, appears to represent an origin from myofibroblasts within vessel walls rather than extension from the extravascular component which is often present.[183,196] It is not associated with aggressive growth or metastasis.[181] Vascular involvement results in a plexiform appearance.

Less common findings include the presence of bone and cartilage;[195,197,198] osteoid is not uncommon in the variant known as cranial fasciitis.[192] Scattered multinucleate fibroblasts and osteoclast-like giant cells are often present and, rarely, the latter cells are quite common.[187,195] The term **'ossifying fasciitis'** has been used if there is a significant component of osteoid or bone.[199] A variant with numerous cells resembling ganglion cells, akin to those seen in proliferative myositis,[200,201] may be separated off as a distinct entity – **proliferative fasciitis** (Fig. 34.8).[202-204]

Various histological subtypes of nodular fasciitis have been proposed, based on the cellularity, the amount of myxoid stroma, and the presence of collagen or other histological features such as osteoclast-like cells, ganglion-like cells or bone. Some of the proposed subtypes merely reflect changes in the histological composition during the evolution of the lesion.[179]

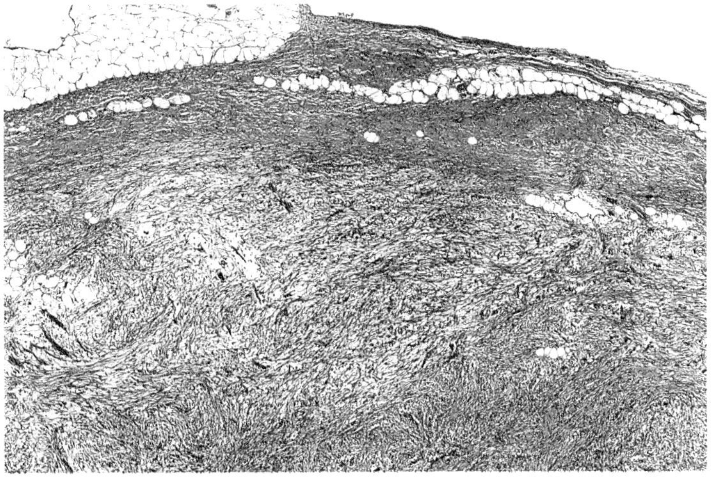

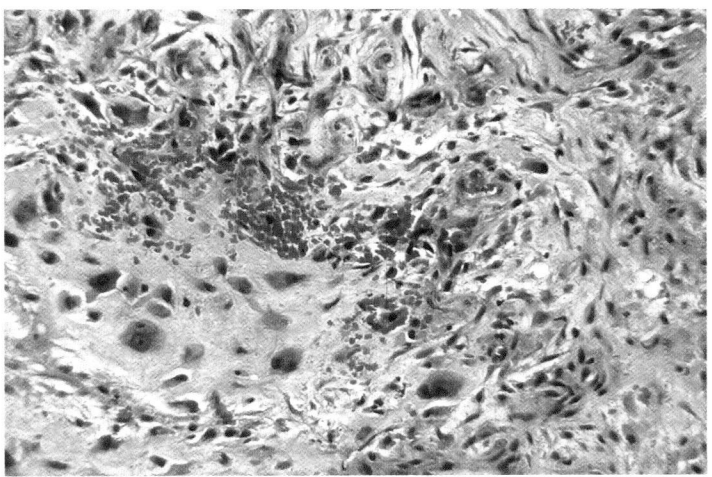

Fig. 34.7 **Nodular fasciitis.** A condensed fibrous capsule surrounds a tumor which is composed of swirling bundles of spindle-shaped cells set in a myxoid stroma. (H & E)

Fig. 34.8 **Proliferative fasciitis.** Ganglion-like cells are present within a spindle-cell tumor. (H & E)

Immunoperoxidase studies demonstrate smooth muscle actin, muscle-specific actin, vimentin and KP1, but not desmin or S100 protein.[82,205,206] A similar staining pattern is seen in proliferative fasciitis, although the ganglion cells express only vimentin.[204]

Electron microscopy

Few ultrastructural studies have been carried out but, in one study of eight cases, myofibroblasts were the predominant cell present.[207] Cells with features of fibroblasts or histiocytes are also seen.[206] Myofibroblasts and fibroblasts are also present in cranial fasciitis.[193]

ATYPICAL DECUBITAL FIBROPLASIA

Atypical decubital fibroplasia (ischemic fasciitis) is a pseudosarcomatous proliferation, found in immobilized or debilitated patients, which is different to decubitus ulcers.[208] There is involvement of the deep dermis, subcutis and deep fascia with fibrinoid necrosis, reactive fibrosis, neovascularization, fat necrosis and ectatic vessels.[208] Atypical fibroblasts are usually present.

POSTOPERATIVE SPINDLE-CELL NODULE

Postoperative spindle-cell nodule is a rare lesion that develops soon after a surgical procedure in genital skin or the genitourinary system.[209] Lesions have now been reported at other sites.[210] It is composed of spindle-shaped cells in a pattern of interlacing fascicles. There are occasional mitotic cells. The cells express vimentin; desmin and muscle-specific actin have been present in some cases.[209] They do not express keratin.[210]

SOLITARY FIBROUS TUMOR

Solitary fibrous tumor is a rare mesenchymal tumor that most commonly involves the pleura. It has been reported in many other sites, including the skin.[211–213] It presents as a circumscribed nodule, often mistaken for a cyst. Most cases have been on the head and neck.[214] Cases have also been reported in the vagina.[215,216] Although 10–20% of lesions in other organs have been malignant,[217,218] all cutaneous tumors reported so far have behaved in a benign fashion.[211]

The tumor cells are predominantly fibroblastic although focal myo-fibroblastic differentiation is often seen.[211]

Histopathology

Cutaneous tumors are circumscribed with alternating hypercellular and less cellular areas. There are short spindle and ovoid cells with scant cytoplasm in a fascicular, haphazard or storiform arrangement (Fig. 34.9). Areas with a hemangiopericytoma-like appearance are quite common. There is a variable collagenous stroma and some ectatic vessels. Lesions need to be distinguished from spindle-cell lipoma.[213,219]

Immunohistochemistry shows generalized staining for CD34 and vimentin.[213] The cells are negative for smooth muscle and epithelial markers. The mesothelial markers calretinin and HBME-1 have not been detected in five dermal cases.[214]

The **giant cell angiofibroma**, originally described in the orbit, and subsequently in other locations, including the skin, appears to be a giant cell-rich variant of solitary fibrous tumor.[220,221]

FIBROUS HAMARTOMA OF INFANCY

Fibrous hamartoma of infancy is an uncommon fibroproliferative lesion of the subcutaneous tissue that is present at birth or develops in the first 2 years of life.[222–226] It most commonly occurs around the shoulder, axilla and upper arms, but cases involving the scalp,[227] inguinal region, scrotum,[228] perianal area[229] and lower extremities[230] have been reported. There is a male predominance of 3:1.[223] The clinical course is benign, despite its infiltrative appearance and tendency to local recurrence.[224]

The subcutaneous tissue of excised lesions has a glistening gray-white appearance interspersed with fatty tissue. The involved area measures 2–8 cm in maximum diameter.

Histopathology[223,231]

Fibrous hamartoma of infancy has poorly defined margins. It is centered on the subcutis. There are three different tissue components:[223,232] interlacing trabeculae of fibrocollagenous tissue, small nests of loosely arranged mesenchymal cells, and interspersed mature fat (Fig. 34.10). The fibrous trabeculae vary in thickness and arrangement and contain spindle-shaped cells; they express vimentin but not S100 protein.[224] Desmin and smooth muscle actin are found in the fascicular-fibroblastic regions.[233] The myxoid areas are more cellular, with immature oval or stellate cells, sometimes having a whorled pattern. Sparse lymphocytes may be present in the stroma.

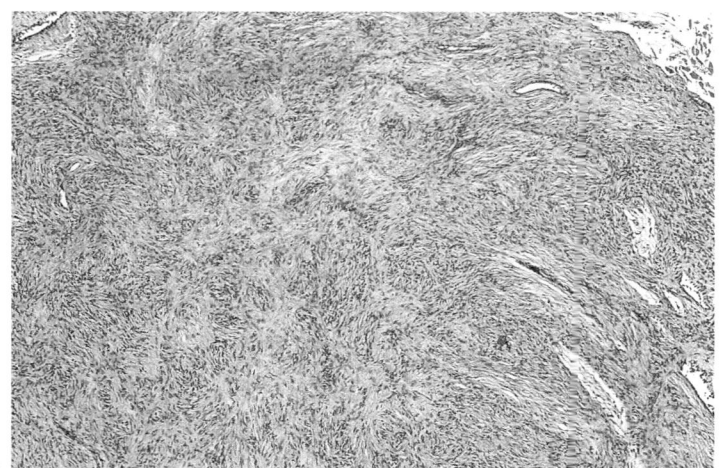
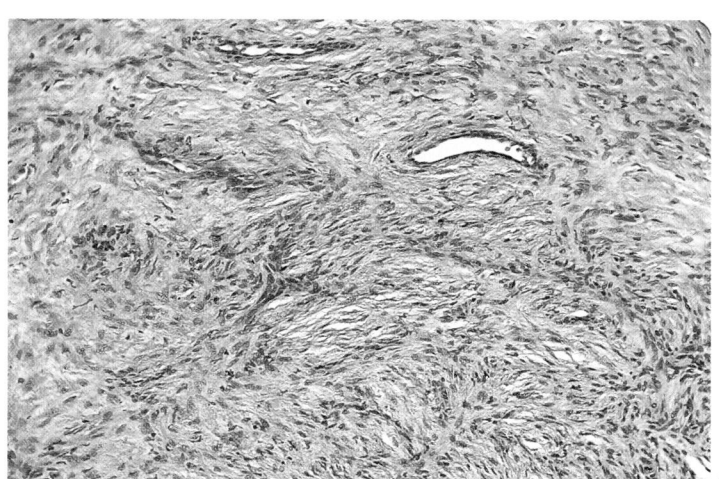

Fig. 34.9 **Solitary fibrous tumor. (A)** There is variable cellularity. **(B)** The tumor is composed of spindle cells. (H & E)

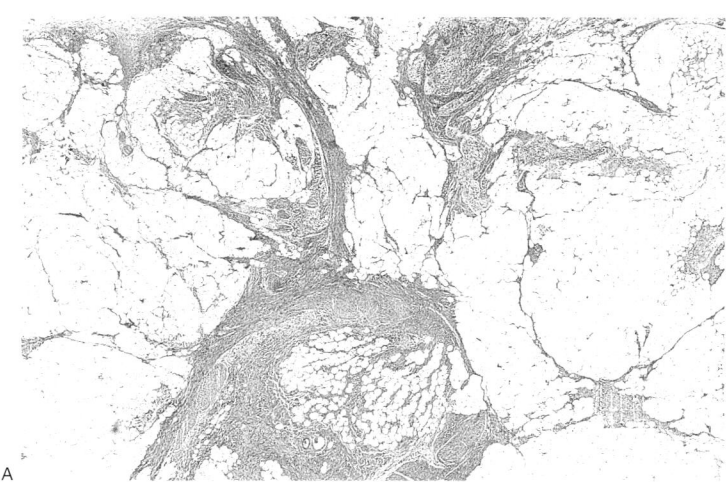
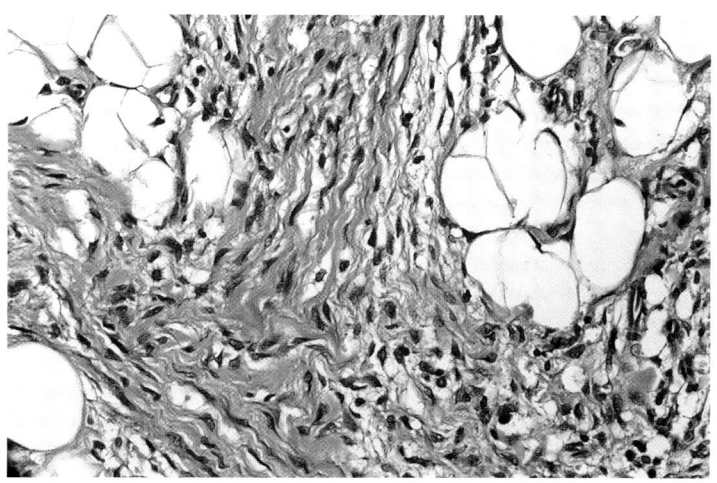

Fig. 34.10 **(A) Fibrous hamartoma of infancy. (B)** There are bundles of fibrous tissue, some mesenchymal cells, and interspersed mature fat. (H & E)

Electron microscopy

The constituent cells have the features of myofibroblasts, although some fibroblasts are also present.[227,234] Fibroblasts alone were present in one reported case.[235] Primitive mesenchymal cells are present in the immature-appearing areas.[233]

DIGITAL FIBROMATOSIS OF CHILDHOOD

Digital fibromatosis of childhood (infantile digital fibromatosis,[236] recurring digital fibrous tumor of childhood,[237] inclusion body fibromatosis[238]) is a rare benign tumor of myofibroblasts with characteristic cytoplasmic inclusion bodies.[225] It presents as a dome-shaped firm nodule, up to 1 cm in diameter, usually on the digits.[239,240] The thumbs and great toes are spared.[241] Lesions are usually solitary, but a second tumor is sometimes noted at the time of presentation, or develops subsequently.[239] The tumors may be present at birth, or appear in the first year of life. Onset in late childhood or adult life is rare.[238,242,243] A history of preceding trauma has been reported.[244] The tumor often recurs after local excision; very occasionally it may regress spontaneously.[245,246]

There is a rare syndrome consisting of recurrent digital fibroma, focal dermal hypoplasia and limb malformations.[247]

A viral etiology was originally suspected because of the characteristic inclusion bodies, but all cultures have been negative, excluding this hypothesis.[248–250] The inclusions are now known to be filamentous aggregations composed largely of actin.[251,252]

Histopathology[239,241,253]

The tumor is non-encapsulated and extends from beneath the epidermis, through the dermis and usually into the subcutis. It is composed of interlacing bundles of spindle-shaped cells and collagen bundles. There may be some vertical orientation of the cells and fibers superficially (Fig. 34.11). The appendages become incorporated within the tumor. The nuclei of the cells are oval or spindle shaped, and some stellate forms may be present. There are only occasional mitoses. The cytoplasm of the cells merges imperceptibly with the collagen. There are characteristic small eosinophilic inclusion bodies within the cytoplasm of the tumor cells, often in a paranuclear position (Fig. 34.12). A clear halo is sometimes discernible in well-stained sections. These bodies measure 2–10 µm in diameter, and may be mistaken for red blood cells.

The cells stain red with the Masson trichrome stain, and deep purple with the PTAH method. They are PAS negative but actin positive.[254]

There are small capillaries and a few scattered elastic fibers in the stroma. The overlying epidermis usually shows flattening of the rete ridges. Ulceration is rare.

The immunocytochemical localization of vimentin and muscle-specific actin in the proliferating cells confirms their myofibroblastic nature.[238] The cells also express desmin.[251]

Electron microscopy

The spindle cells are myofibroblasts[244,255] and the inclusion bodies are compact masses of amorphous and granular material with some discernible microfilaments, but with no limiting membrane. Actin has been demonstrated within the myofibroblasts, and it has been suggested that the inclusions are masses of actin[236] or, more likely, degradation products of it.[256] This viewpoint has subsequently been challenged.[257] Cultured tumor cells also develop inclusion bodies.[236]

ANGIOFIBROBLASTOMA

Only two cases of angiofibroblastoma have been described.[258] It consists of stellate and spindle-shaped cells, with the phenotype of fibroblasts, embedded in a fibromyxoid to dense fibrous stroma. Numerous capillary-sized vessels, often in small groups, are scattered throughout the stroma.

ANGIOMYOFIBROBLASTOMA OF THE VULVA

Angiomyofibroblastoma is a rare tumor of the vulva that may be confused with aggressive angiomyxoma of the pelvic soft tissues and vulval region, which appears to be a related tumor.[259–264] It now appears that a similar lesion occurs in the male genital tract.[265] These latter cases have some similarity to spindle-cell lipoma.[265] Angiomyofibroblastoma is often misdiagnosed clinically as a Bartholin's cyst.[266] The tumors are well circumscribed, measuring 0.5–12 cm in diameter. They do not recur if completely excised. Sarcomatous transformation has been reported.[267]

Histopathology[266,268]

The lesion is composed of an edematous stroma in which abundant blood vessels (predominantly of the capillary type) are irregularly distributed. Spindle

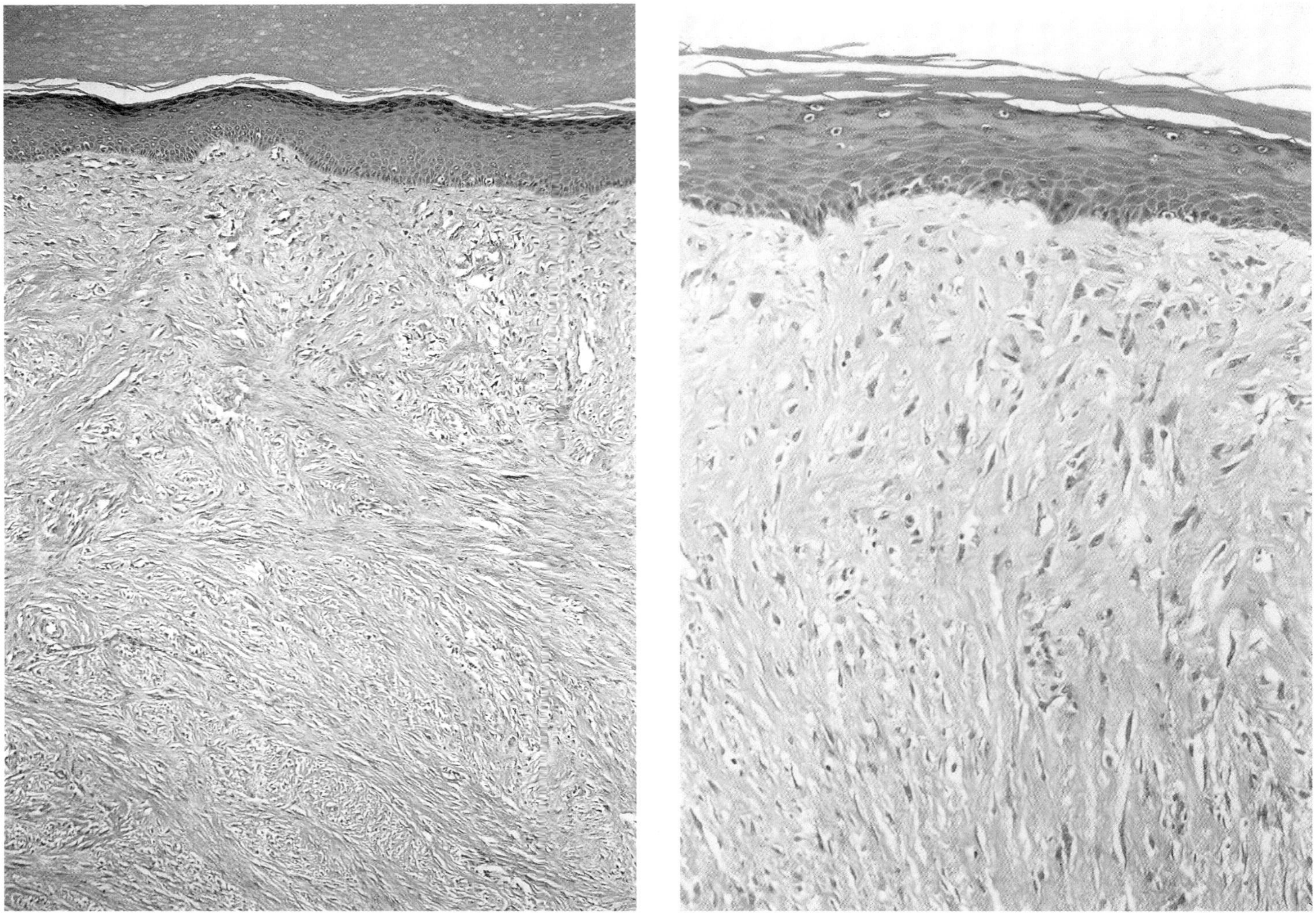

Fig. 34.11 **(A) Digital fibromatosis of childhood. (B)** The spindle-shaped cells and some collagen bundles have a vertical orientation within the dermis. (H & E)

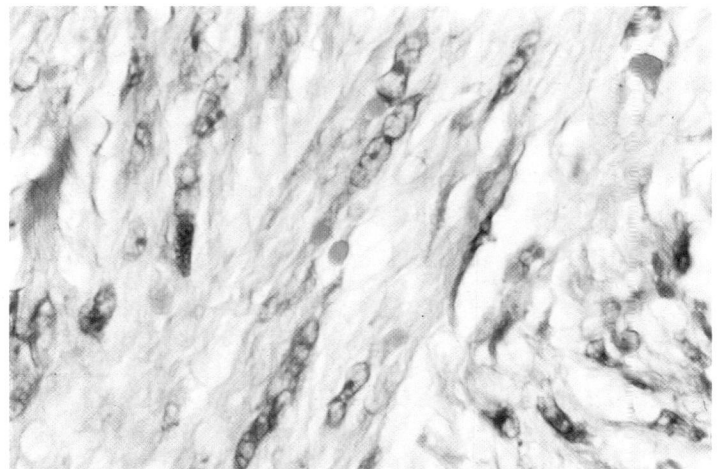

Fig. 34.12 **Digital fibromatosis.** Pale pink inclusion bodies, composed of actin, are present in the cytoplasm of the spindle-shaped cells. (H & E)

cells, some of which are plump, are present in the stroma, often aggregated around the vessels. Some cells may have abundant hyaline cytoplasm. Hyper-

cellular areas may be present. Wavy collagen bundles are scattered through the stroma. Intralesional fat is often present. A lipomatous variant with abundant fat has been reported.[269]

The stromal cells express vimentin and desmin but not S100 protein, smooth muscle actin or muscle-specific actin.[266]

The recently described **cellular angiofibroma** is a benign neoplasm with a propensity for the vulva[270,271] which is distinct from angiomyofibroblastoma and spindle-cell lipoma. It is composed of uniform spindled stromal cells, numerous thick-walled and often hyalinized vessels, and a small component of mature adipocytes.[270] Immunohistochemical markers are all negative, except for vimentin.

DERMATOMYOFIBROMA

Dermatomyofibroma is a benign tumor of fibroblasts and myofibroblasts first reported by Hügel in 1991.[271a] It has a predilection for the shoulder girdle, axilla and abdomen of young adults.[272,273] There is a female predominance. Cases in young males have a predilection for the posterior neck.[274] The lesions present as firm red-brown plaques or nodules, 1–2 cm in diameter; they may resemble a keloid.[275] A linear variant occurs.[276] A similar lesion has been reported under the term 'myoid fibroma'.[277,278]

Histopathology

The tumor is a non-encapsulated plaque-like lesion composed of fascicles of monomorphic spindle cells predominantly orientated parallel to the skin surface; some intersecting bundles are present (Fig. 34.13).[279] The cells have faintly eosinophilic cytoplasm and elongated vesicular tapering nuclei. The lesion fills the reticular dermis and sometimes extends into the upper subcutis. It spares adnexal structures. The stroma contains collagen bundles with an increase in small blood vessels. Elastic fibers are preserved and some are thicker than usual. There is usually a sparse chronic inflammatory cell infiltrate around the vessels.

Most of the tumor cells express vimentin and non-specific muscle actin.[279,280] They are negative for smooth muscle-specific actin, desmin, S100, CD34 and factor XIIIa.[279,280]

Electron microscopy

There is a mixture of fibroblasts, myofibroblasts and mesenchymal cells.[272,281]

INFANTILE MYOFIBROMATOSIS

The entity of infantile myofibromatosis, which is regarded as a proliferative disorder of myofibroblasts, was established by Chung and Enzinger in 1981, with their report of 61 cases.[282] Previous reports had appeared under several designations including congenital fibrosarcoma,[283] congenital generalized fibromatosis,[231,284,285] and congenital mesenchymal hamartoma.[286] Fletcher and colleagues have suggested that the spindle-cell component shows true smooth muscle differentiation rather than being of a myofibroblastic nature.[287] Requena et al have suggested an origin from myopericytes.[288] More recently, Fletcher and colleagues have described a spectrum of tumors showing perivascular myoid differentiation, which included adult cases of myofibromatosis (myofibroma).[289]

The lesions are solitary in approximately 70% of cases.[282,290] Almost half of these are situated in the deep soft tissues, and the remainder are located in the skin and/or subcutaneous tissue.[225,291] The head, neck and trunk are the usual sites of involvement.[282,290] There is a male predominance. Most lesions are present at birth, or appear in the first 2 years of life; onset in adult life has been recorded.[292,293] The term 'solitary cutaneous myofibroma' would seem to be an appropriate designation for the solitary lesions occurring in adults.[294–296] The prognosis is excellent, with recurrence unlikely after excision; aggressive variants are rare.[297]

In approximately 30% of cases the lesions are multicentric and involve the skin, soft tissues, bones and, uncommonly, the viscera.[282,298] They are usually present at birth, and there is a female predominance. Spontaneous regression of soft tissue and osseous lesions sometimes occurs,[282,299,300] but cases with visceral involvement are usually fatal.[282,290,301] The various clinical types of myofibromatosis are shown in Table 34.1. Recurrence after a long period of quiescence has been documented.[302] Central nervous system abnormalities were present in one case.[303] Both autosomal recessive[304] and dominant inheritance with reduced penetrance have been proposed.[302]

Macroscopically, the tumors measure 0.5–7 cm or more in diameter. They are grayish-white in color, and fibrous in consistency.

Histopathology[282,287]

The nodules are reasonably well circumscribed, although there may be an infiltrative border in the subcutis. There are plump to elongated spindle cells with features of myofibroblasts. They are grouped in short fascicles. Delicate bundles of collagen separate or enclose the cellular aggregates (Fig. 34.14). Mitoses are variable in number, but they are not atypical.

Vascular spaces resembling those of hemangiopericytoma are often found in the center of the tumor.[282,305] This gives most lesions a biphasic appearance, with a central hemangiopericytoma-like area and a peripheral leiomyoma-like region. A monophasic variant with a prominence of tiny capillaries has been reported.[306] Sometimes there is an intravascular pattern of growth. Necrosis, hyalinization, calcification and focal hemorrhage may be present centrally.[287]

Immunoperoxidase studies have shown that the tumor cells are positive for vimentin and α-smooth muscle actin but negative for S100 protein, myoglobin and cytokeratin.[287,292,305] Conflicting results have been reported for desmin,[287,292] although it has been negative in recently reported cases.[296,307]

Electron microscopy

The cells have the ultrastructural features of myofibroblasts.[286] Primitive vascular formations, with a pattern of irregular clefts between adjoining cells, were noted by Requena and colleagues.[288] Regressing lesions show vacuoation of the cytoplasm of spindle cells with their eventual disruption.[301]

PERIVASCULAR MYOMAS

'Perivascular myoma' is the suggested designation by Granter, Badizadegan and Fletcher for a histological continuum of three lesional groups of tumor – myofibromatosis in adults, glomangiopericytoma and myopericytoma – showing perivascular myoid differentiation.[289] Such lesions were reported in patients of all ages, with a predilection for the subcutis and superficial soft tissues of the extremities.[289] Some lesions were multifocal. Further studies are needed to confirm the exact nature of these lesions.

INFLAMMATORY MYOFIBROBLASTIC TUMOR

Inflammatory myofibroblastic tumor, also known as inflammatory fibrosarcoma, occurs predominantly in the lungs and mesentery, although the soft tissues of the head and neck, or the extremities, may be involved.[308] Systemic

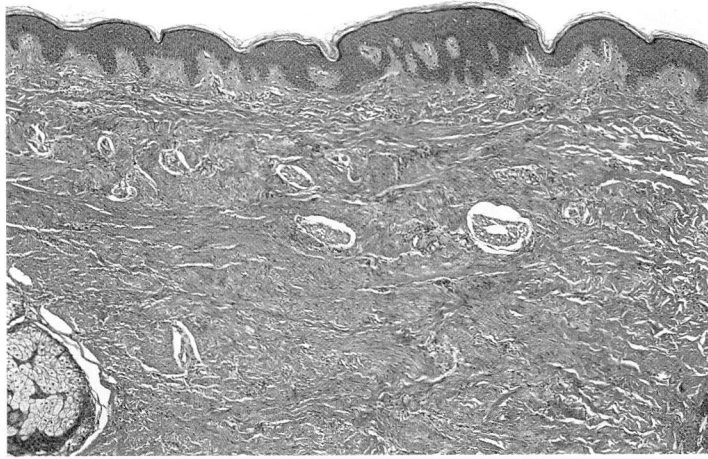

Fig. 34.13 **Dermatomyofibroma.** This scar-like lesion has cells orientated parallel to the epidermis. (H & E)

Table 34.1 **Types of myofibromatosis**

- Solitary, infantile
- Congenital, multiple without visceral involvement
- Congenital, generalized with cutaneous and visceral involvement
- Solitary cutaneous myofibroma of adulthood

symptoms are often present. It appears to represent a spectrum of myofibroblastic proliferations, some of which have been included in the past as inflammatory pseudotumor, a heterogeneous 'entity'.[16,309]

This tumor has a potential for recurrence and persistent local growth.[310] Metastases have been recorded but no reliable morphological parameters

have been identified that predict prognosis.[308,311] It has been suggested that inflammatory myofibroblastic tumor and inflammatory fibrosarcoma are synonymous or closely related entities.[312] They have been regarded as synonymous here.

Histopathology

The lesions are characterized by an admixture of myofibroblasts and fibroblasts, usually arranged in short interwoven fascicles (Fig. 34.15).[313] In addition there is a polymorphic inflammatory cell component, consisting principally of lymphocytes and plasma cells.[313] Xanthoma cells are sometimes prominent. Myxoid areas and focal stromal hyalinization are usually present.

Immunoperoxidase stains for vimentin, muscle-specific actin, smooth muscle actin and cytokeratin are usually positive, indicative of a myofibroblastic tumor with admixed inflammatory cells.[310,314]

JUVENILE HYALINE FIBROMATOSIS

Juvenile hyaline fibromatosis, an exceedingly rare autosomal recessive condition, is characterized by large tumors, especially on the scalp, whitish cutaneous nodules, hypertrophy of the gingiva, flexural contractures, and often focal bone erosion.[225,315-323] Onset is in infancy and childhood. A localized form,

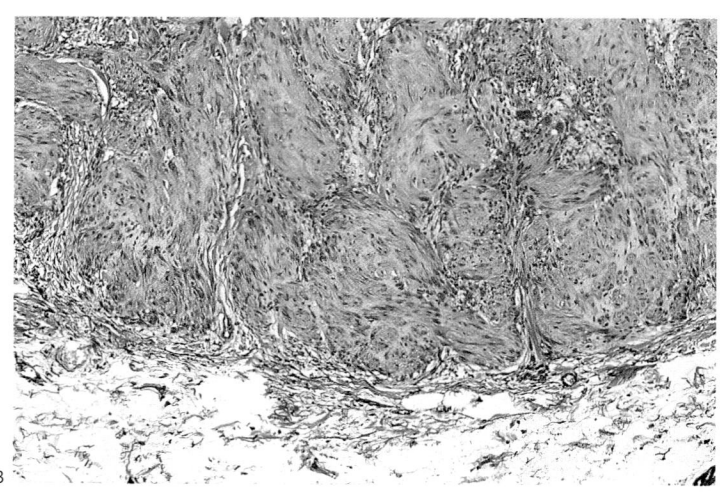

Fig. 34.14 **(A) Infantile myofibroma. (B)** Short fascicles of plump, spindle-shaped cells are separated by thin bundles of collagen. (H & E)

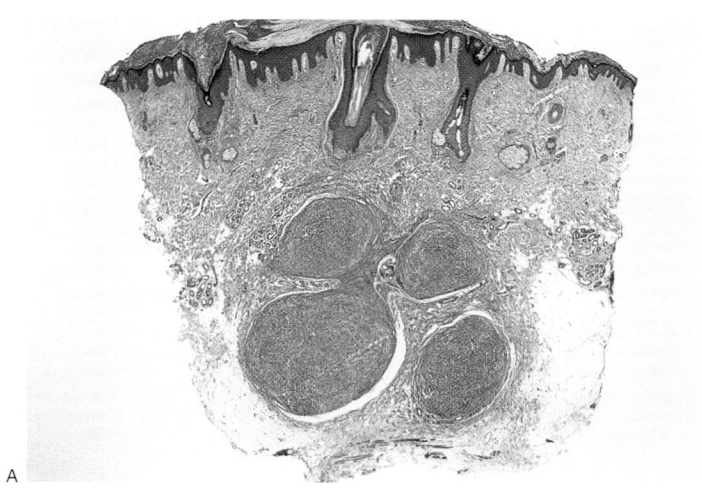
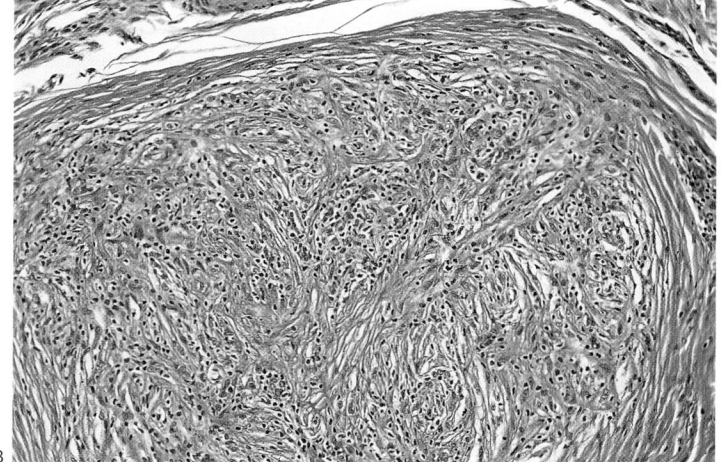

Fig. 34.15 **(A) Inflammatory myofibroblastic tumor. (B)** There is an intimate admixture of inflammatory cells and spindle-shaped cells. (H & E)

with slow progression and no visceral involvement, has been reported.[324] Spontaneous regression of tumors sometimes occurs. Recurrent infections may lead to death. Some overlap features exist with the condition reported as infantile systemic hyalinosis (see p. 438). This condition has stiff skin but it lacks the large cutaneous nodules of juvenile hyaline fibromatosis.[322,325] Both conditions are probably part of the same disease spectrum.

Histopathology[315–319]

The tumor nodules are composed of a markedly thickened dermis with a vaguely chondroid appearance. They are composed of fibroblast-like cells, with abundant granular cytoplasm, embedded in an amorphous eosinophilic ground substance that is PAS positive and diastase resistant. It does not stain with alcian blue.[320] The ground substance is abundant in older lesions and presumably represents a collagen precursor produced by the fibroblast-like tumor cells.

Electron microscopy[326]

The spindle-shaped cells are fibroblasts with dilated rough endoplasmic reticulum and vacuoles in their cytoplasm filled with fine granular or filamentous material.[320] There are plentiful collagen fibrils in the stroma, as well as abundant granular material.[320]

CUTANEOUS MYXOID FIBROBLASTOMA

There has been one report of a benign fibroblastic tumor, with a myxoid matrix, that does not fit into one of the recognized entities.[327] The well-circumscribed tumor was confined to the dermis and composed of stellate and spindle-shaped cells arranged loosely in a fascicular pattern resembling 'tissue cultures of fibroblasts'. There was abundant stromal mucin. The cells expressed vimentin only and had the ultrastructural characteristics of fibroblasts.[327]

FIBROMYXOID SARCOMA (LOW GRADE)

Low-grade fibromyxoid sarcoma is a rare tumor characterized by bland histological features and a paradoxically aggressive clinical course.[328–332] The **hyalinizing spindle-cell tumor with giant rosettes** (low-grade fibrosarcoma with palisaded granuloma-like bodies) is a closely related entity (see below).[332,333] Low-grade fibromyxoid sarcoma has a tendency to develop in the deep soft tissues of young adults. Local recurrence is common; distant metastasis, particularly to the lungs, occurs in up to 50% of cases.

The immunophenotype and ultrastructure suggest a fibroblastic tumor with focal myofibroblastic differentiation.

Histopathology[328,329]

The tumor consists of bland spindle cells, showing a mainly whorled or focally linear arrangement, set in areas with an alternating fibrous or myxoid stroma.[329] Cellularity is low to moderate, and mitotic figures uncommon.[328] The tumor cells are small, spindle to stellate, with pale, poorly defined cytoplasm.

Most tumor cells express vimentin, but occasional cells stain positively for actin, desmin and cytokeratin.[329]

FIBROSARCOMA

Enzinger and Weiss have defined a fibrosarcoma as a malignant tumor of fibroblasts that shows no evidence of other cellular differentiation.[334] There has been a marked decline in the diagnosis of fibrosarcoma in the last 15–20

years as a result of the delineation of the fibromatoses as a diagnostic entity and the recognition of the malignant fibrous histiocytoma. Furthermore, other spindle-cell tumors, which in the past were sometimes misdiagnosed as fibrosarcoma, such as spindle-cell melanoma and spindle-cell squamous carcinoma, as well as malignant peripheral nerve sheath tumors, can now be more confidently diagnosed with the assistance of various monoclonal antibodies and immunoperoxidase techniques.

Very little has been written on fibrosarcoma in recent years.[335] However, as it is primarily a tumor of the deep soft tissues which only rarely develops in the skin and superficial subcutis, only brief mention will be made of it. Cutaneous fibrosarcomas may follow thermal burns and radiation therapy, or result from extension of a tumor arising in deeper tissues. The tumor affects predominantly middle-aged adults, although there is an uncommon clinical subset involving neonates and young children (congenital-infantile fibrosarcoma).[336–339]

Congenital-infantile fibrosarcoma is much less aggressive than adult-type fibrosarcoma despite a similar histological appearance. Recently, a novel chromosomal translocation t(12;15)(p13;q25) has been identified in the congenital-infantile group.[340] This translocation gives rise to an *ETV6–NTRK3* gene fusion.[340] It can be detected in paraffin-embedded tissue.[341]

Histopathology[334,342]

Typically, fibrosarcomas are composed of interlacing fascicles of spindle cells forming a so-called 'herringbone' pattern. Mitoses are common. There is a variable meshwork of collagen and reticulin between the individual cells, the amount depending on the differentiation of the tumor.

The *sclerosing epithelioid fibrosarcoma* is composed of small to medium-sized cells with a clear or pale cytoplasm and arranged in cords and strands.[343,344] The cells are surrounded by a prominent collagenous stroma.

The low-grade *fibrosarcoma with palisaded granuloma-like bodies (giant rosettes)* is another exceedingly rare variant characterized by a collagenized fibroma-like component, cellular patches of hyperchromatic spindle cells, and hyalinized bodies ringed by nuclei giving the appearance of a rosette or palisaded granuloma.[345] It has also been reported as *hyalinizing spindle cell tumor with giant rosettes*.[332] As mentioned above, it appears to be related to the low-grade fibromyxoid sarcoma.

The *inflammatory* fibrosarcoma appears to be synonymous with the inflammatory myofibroblastic tumor (see above).

The *congenital infantile* variant is usually more cellular and composed of smaller cells with prominent mitotic activity.

The tumor cells express vimentin but not desmin, S100 protein or smooth muscle actin.[339]

MYOFIBROBLASTIC SARCOMA (LOW GRADE)

A low-grade, spindle-cell sarcoma showing myofibroblastic differentiation was reported by Fletcher and colleagues in 1998.[346] Of the 18 cases, only two involved the subcutis. Recurrence and metastases were recorded for some of the cases, but there was no follow-up for the subcutaneous cases.

FIBROHISTIOCYTIC TUMORS

The term 'fibrous histiocytoma' was introduced for a group of tumors that share certain morphological features, such as the presence of fibroblast-like spindle cells and presumptive histiocytes, cells that were assumed to arise from a tissue histiocyte that could function as, or transform into, a fibroblast.

Although these tumors appear to be histogenetically heterogeneous, it is still convenient to retain the term 'fibrohistiocytic' in a morphologically descriptive sense for tumors which show features of fibroblastic and histiocytic differentiation. Some of these tumors appear to be derived from the dermal dendrocyte.

DERMATOFIBROMA (FIBROUS HISTIOCYTOMA)

The large number of terms that have been used for dermatofibroma (histiocytoma,[347,348] fibrous histiocytoma,[349–351] sclerosing hemangioma,[352] nodular subepidermal fibrosis[353,354]) reflects the remarkable variation in its histological features, and continuing controversy regarding its histogenesis.[355] However, the presence of transitional patterns and different morphological components in the same lesion is strong evidence in favor of its basically common nature and histogenesis.[349] There has been a tendency to use the term 'dermatofibroma' for the usual fibrocollagenous and storiform variant and 'fibrous histiocytoma' for some of the unusual variants.

Dermatofibromas are common, accounting for almost 3% of specimens received by one dermatopathology laboratory.[356] There is a predilection for the extremities, particularly the lower, of young adults.[347,356] There is a female preponderance.[356] Rare sites of involvement have included the fingers,[353,357] palms and soles,[358] the scalp,[353] the face[359] and a vaccination scar.[360]

Dermatofibromas are round or ovoid, firm dermal nodules, usually less than 1 cm in diameter. A 'giant' variant has been recorded.[361–363] Polypoid, flat, atrophic and depressed configurations occur.[364,365] Lesions with a preponderance of histiocytes are often larger, and the aneurysmal (angiomatoid) variants may measure up to 10 cm in diameter.[366,367] Dermatofibromas are usually a dusky brown in color but aneurysmal variants may be red, and tumors with abundant lipid can be cream/yellow, particularly on the cut surface of the excised lesion. They often show a characteristic central white, scar-like patch on dermatoscopic examination.[368] Dermatofibromas are most often solitary, but 2–5 lesions are present in 10% or so of individuals.[347] Multiple lesions have been reported,[369,370] usually as a rare complication of immunosuppressive therapy[358,371–373] or the acquired immunodeficiency syndrome.[374–378] Eruptive lesions have appeared after the commencement of highly active antiretroviral therapy (HAART).[379] There are only a few reports of patients with large numbers of tumors;[351,380–384] one such case was reported as 'disseminated dermal dendrocytomas'. This case may have been a different entity – progressive nodular histiocytosis (see p. 1070). Clinical variants include the aneurysmal type, already referred to,[366] and the rare annular hemosiderotic histiocytoma in which multiple brown papules in annular configurations were present on the buttocks.[385] Spreading satellitosis has been reported in one case.[386]

Although regarded as a benign tumor or reactive inflammatory process that may uncommonly recur locally (see below), several cases of metastasizing cellular dermatofibroma have been recorded.[387,388] Clonality has since been found in some cases of dermatofibroma but no consistent karyotypic aberration has been found.[389,390]

Fibroblasts, non-lysozyme containing histiocytes,[354] and endothelial cells have all been regarded at some time as the cell of origin.[347] Dermatofibromas have been regarded by some authors as a benign tumor, and by others as a fibrosing inflammatory or reactive process.[391,392] In support of the latter concept is the history of trauma, blunt or piercing, recorded in up to 20% of cases.[353] An insect bite has preceded the development of a dermatofibroma.[347] HHV-8 has not been detected.[393] On the basis of the immunoreactivity of 30–70% of the constituent cells with factor XIIIa, an origin from the 'dermal dendrocyte' has been proposed.[394–396] The dendritic cells appear to be derived from blood monocytes or a stem cell common to both.[397]

Histopathology[347,349,350]

Dermatofibromas are poorly demarcated tumors centered on the dermis. There is sometimes extension into the superficial subcutis which may take the form of septal extension or a well-demarcated bulge.[398,399] A 'pure' subcutaneous form is exceedingly rare.[400] A grenz zone of variable thickness is present in about 70% of cases.[347] Sometimes this contains dilated vessels.[347] Dermatofibromas are composed of a variable admixture of fibroblast-like cells, histiocytes, some of which may be xanthomatous or multinucleate, and blood vessels. The terms 'nodular subepidermal fibrosis', 'histiocytoma' and 'sclerosing hemangioma' were used in the past for variants where one of these three components predominated. Nowadays it is usual practice to refer to fibrocollagenous, histiocytic and angiomatous variants to reflect these differences in composition.[349,401] Storiform, aneurysmal (angiomatoid) and fibrous histiocytoma variants are also recognized (see below). Numerous other variants have been described in recent years. Many are histological curiosities. They are listed in Table 34.2.

The *fibrocollagenous type* has a predominance of collagen and fibroblast-like cells in an irregular or whorled arrangement (Fig. 34.16).[349] Sometimes there is striking cellularity of the lesion beneath the epidermis, with less cellular areas deeply.[349] The *lichenoid* dermatofibroma has a dense cellular infiltrate impinging on the undersurface of the epidermis producing basal cell damage that often leads to clefting.[402] Mitoses are rare. Histiocytes are usually imperceptible, but there is a variable vascular component. Hemosiderin is sometimes present in the cellular areas, but is uncommon elsewhere. Bone[403] and calcification[353] are rare constituents of the stroma. Another variant of the fibrocollagenous type has nuclear *palisading* and prominent Verocay-like bodies in part of the lesion, usually the center.[401] This palisading variant is positive for vimentin and factor XIIIa.[404]

Those cases with a prominent *storiform* pattern are sometimes termed 'fibrous histiocytoma' to distinguish them from the more usual fibrocollagenous type.[349,405] Included within this group is the so-called '*cellular benign fibrous histiocytoma*'.[406,407] These tumors often extend into the subcutis; they sometimes recur locally after incomplete surgical removal.[408] Normal mitotic figures are common in the cellular variant, and 12% of cases show central necrosis. Up to 60% of cases show focal positivity for smooth muscle actin in a minority of the cells. The cellular variant differs from dermatofibrosarcoma protuberans by its smaller size, fewer mitoses and less extensive involvement of the subcutis.[405] It is negative for CD34, in contrast to dermatofibrosarcoma protuberans.[406] Another variant of fibrous histiocytoma occurs in the subcutis and deep soft tissues.[409]

The histiocytic variant ('*histiocytoma*') has nests and sheets of histiocytes in a poorly cellular collagenous stroma (Fig. 34.17).[347,349] There are often many foam cells and giant cells, which may be of foreign body or Touton type.[347]

Table 34.2 **Histological variants of dermatofibroma**

• Fibrocollagenous	• 'Monster' cell
• Storiform	• Osteoclastic
• Cellular	• Myofibroblastic
• Histiocytoma	• Myxoid
• Lipidized	• Keloidal
• Angiomatous	• Palisading
• Aneurysmal	• Atrophic
• Clear cell	• Subcutaneous
• Granular cell	• Combined
• Halo	

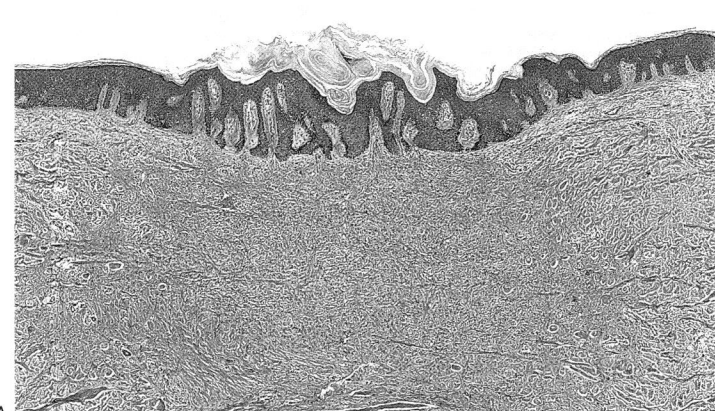

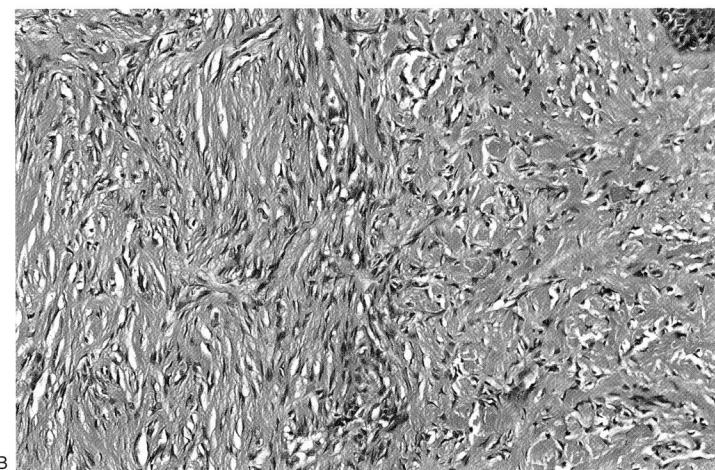

Fig. 34.16 **Dermatofibroma. (A)** The epidermis overlying the dermal tumor is acanthotic and papillomatous. There is a central 'dell'. **(B)** The cells have a storiform arrangement. (H & E)

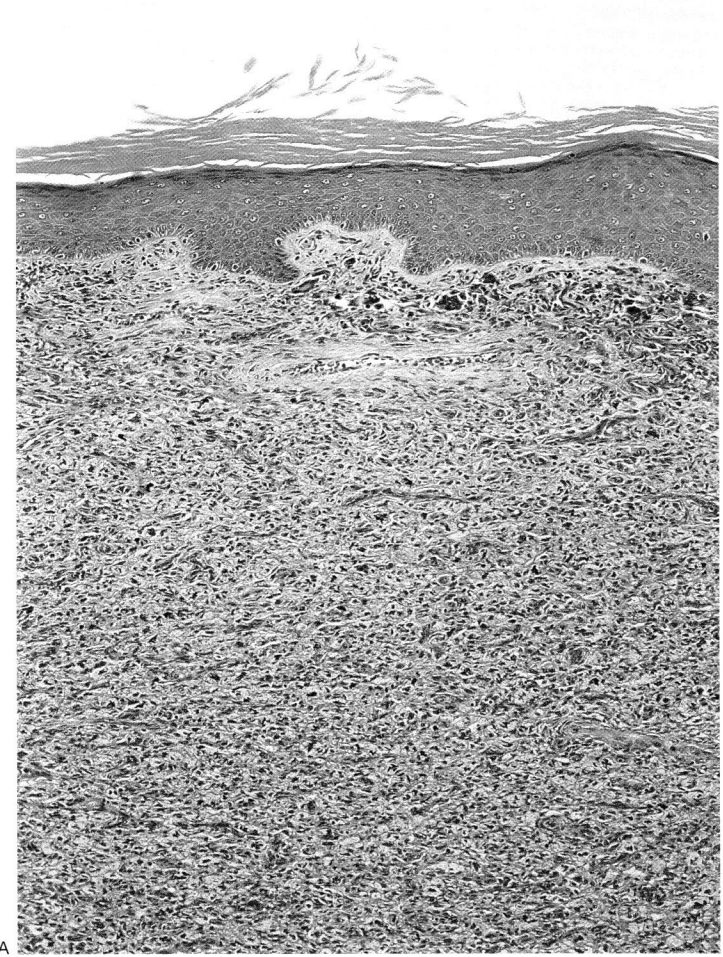

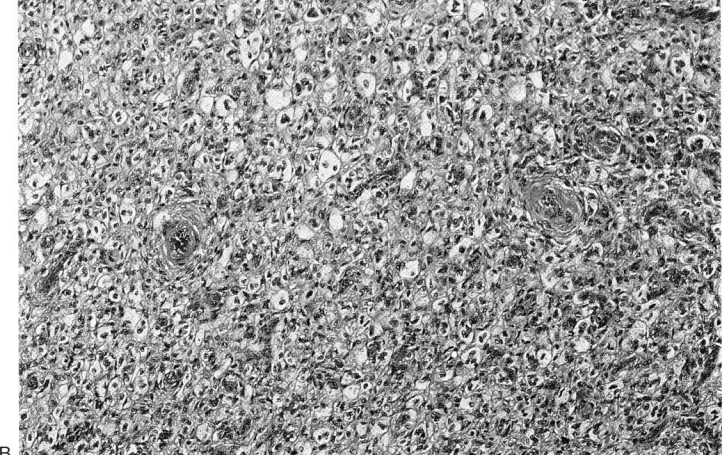

Fig. 34.17 **(A) Dermatofibroma (histiocytic variant). (B)** Sheets of 'histiocytes', some with vacuolated cytoplasm, are admixed with spindle-shaped cells. (H & E)

Hemosiderin and lipid are commonly present.[353] Foam cells and cholesterol clefts may be prominent in dermatofibromas if there is underlying hyperlipoproteinemia.[410] These foam cells are different from the clear cells seen in the rare *clear cell* dermatofibroma (Fig. 34.18), in which the intrinsic spindle cells have pale cytoplasm.[411–414] The *granular cell* dermatofibroma has epithelioid cells with a granular cytoplasm (Fig. 34.19).[415–419] More traditional-appearing areas are usually present.

The *lipidized* variant, which tends to be large and situated around the ankle region, is composed of numerous foam cells, smaller numbers of siderophages, and stromal hyalinization, which is typically 'wiry', keloid-like or osteoid-like.[420] These stromal changes set it apart from the more usual histiocytoma variant.

In the *angiomatous* (vascular) variant there are numerous small branching vessels in a variable collagenous stroma. Focal hypercellularity resembling that seen in the fibrocollagenous type is often present. Hemosiderin is present in about half the cases.

The *aneurysmal* (angiomatoid) variant is distinct, with blood-filled spaces occupying up to one-half of the lesion.[366,421–424] These vary from narrow clefts to large cavernous cysts (Fig. 34.20). The vascular channels are surrounded by histiocytes which contain hemosiderin, and by foam cells and fibroblasts.[366] Solid areas with the more usual appearance of a dermatofibroma are almost invariably present. This feature, together with the presence of foam cells, allows a distinction to be made from Kaposi's sarcoma.[421] The aneurysmal

variant of malignant fibrous histiocytoma is much more pleomorphic and is usually centered on the deeper soft tissues.

Large, bizarre cells with abundant foamy cytoplasm and hyperchromatic nuclei have been reported in some dermatofibromas.[391,406,425–427] These '*monster cells*' are sometimes binucleate or multinucleate.[391,428] Numerous

931

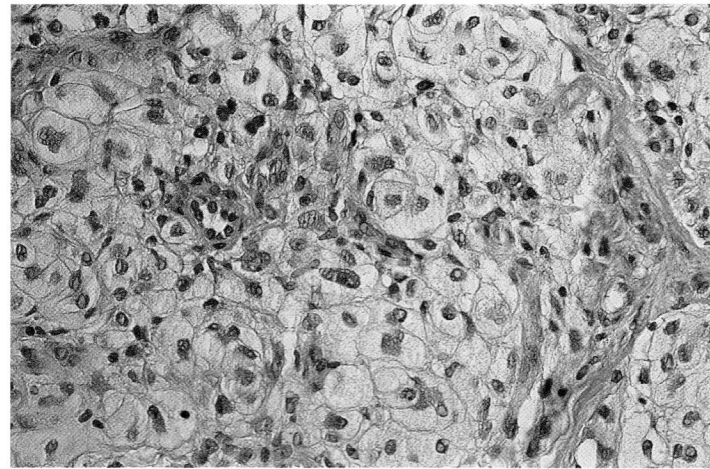

Fig. 34.18 **Dermatofibroma of clear cell type.** (H & E)

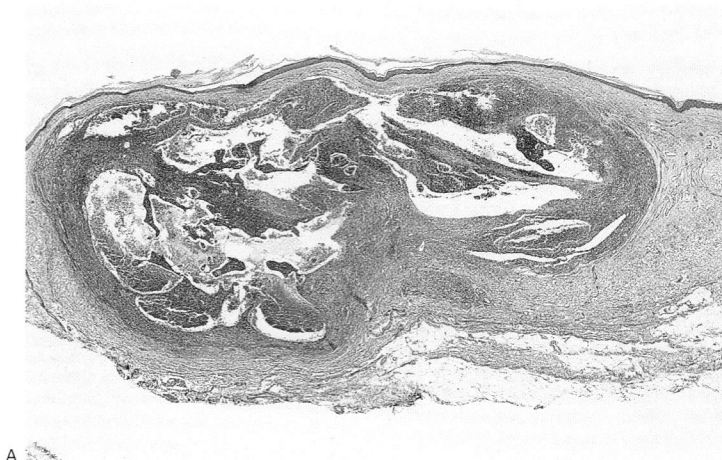

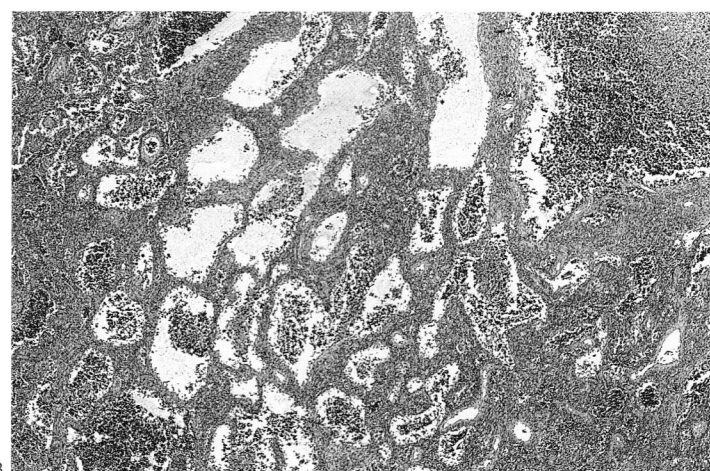

Fig. 34.20 **(A) Dermatofibroma (aneurysmal variant). (B)** There are large vascular spaces and abundant hemosiderin in the surrounding stroma. (H & E)

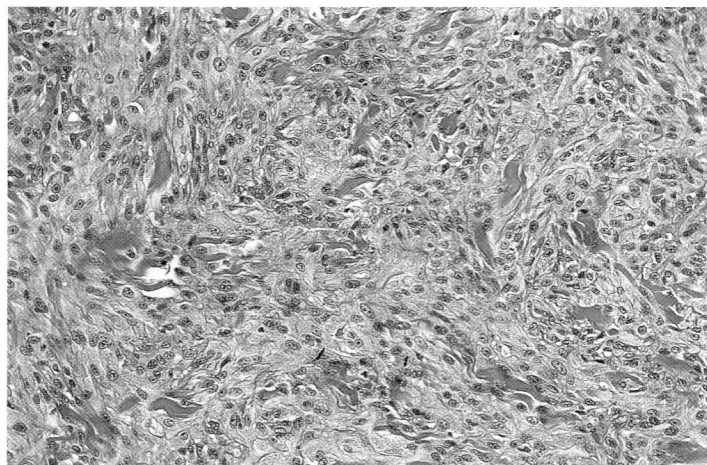

Fig. 34.19 **Dermatofibroma of granular cell type.** (H & E)

cells express Ki-M1p.[138] The term 'atypical (pseudosarcomatous) fibrous histiocytoma' has also been used for this variant. A variant with osteoclast-like giant cells (*osteoclastic*) has also been reported.[429,430] In the *combined* dermatofibroma two or more variant patterns coexist in a single lesion.[431]

Two other rare variants are the *myxoid* dermatofibroma with abundant stromal mucin mimicking a cutaneous myxoma[432] and the *keloidal* dermatofibroma with areas of thick eosinophilic collagen.[433] There is marked thinning of the dermis in the *atrophic* variant. The proliferating cells in this variant appear to phagocytose the elastic fibers within the lesion.[434] Ulcerated and erosive variants have also been described.[402]

Other histological changes that can be seen in dermatofibromas include the presence of lymphoid nodules.[347,435] They are an uncommon finding. The lymphoid tissue is usually in the subjacent fat, or at the periphery of the lesion.[435] Germinal center formation is faint but definite in many instances.[435] Mast cells and a sparse infiltrate of chronic inflammatory cells are sometimes present. A diffuse stromal infiltrate of eosinophils was present in one case.[436] Another uncommon finding is the presence of smooth muscle bundles in the adjacent dermis.[437] *Myofibroblastic* differentiation may occur within the tumor cells.[438] Rarely it is a prominent feature.[439,440] The cells express smooth muscle actin and HHF35.[439]

A morphologically related entity is the epithelioid cell histiocytoma (see below), which is composed of large angulated epithelioid cells that have some resemblance to the cells of a Spitz nevus.[441] It is considered separately because of its distinctive appearance.

Various changes may be present in the overlying epidermis in dermatofibromas.[442] Acanthosis, sometimes with basal hyperpigmentation, is present in approximately 70% of lesions.[443,444] Other changes include a seborrheic keratosis-like pattern,[444] epidermal atrophy[444] or, rarely, intraepidermal carcinoma[445] or pseudoepitheliomatous hyperplasia and focal acantholytic dyskeratosis.[446] In 5–8% of cases there is a spectrum of distinctive epidermal changes ranging from basaloid hyperplasia, often with rudimentary pilar structures, to undoubted basal cell carcinoma.[348,442,447–449] Sebaceous structures are uncommonly present (Fig. 34.21).[348,450] Unequivocal basal cell carcinoma is uncommon,[403,451] and some of the cases reported as this are examples of exuberant basaloid hyperplasia;[452] the distinction is not always easy. It has been suggested that the hair follicle-like structures represent regressive changes in pre-existing follicles and not the induction of new pilar units.[356] Epidermal growth factor or some other factor produced by the underlying tumor cells may be responsible for these proliferative changes.[453,454] Loss of heterozygosity in the *patch* gene is often present in the basal cell carcinoma-like changes in the epidermis.[455]

A small percentage of cells, usually at the periphery, are S100 positive.[401] α_1-Antitrypsin and macrophage markers such as CD68 and HAM-56 have been reported in some of the tumor cells.[456,457] Vimentin and α-smooth

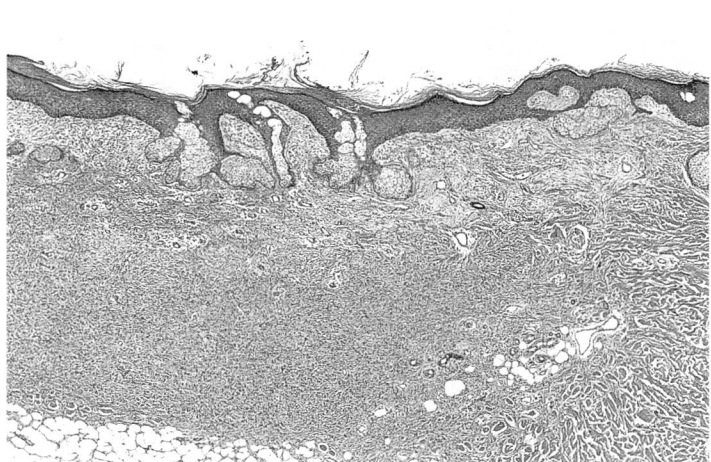

Fig. 34.21 **Dermatofibroma with overlying sebaceous glands.** (H & E)

muscle actin are often present in the spindle-shaped cells.[458,459] The finding of factor XIIIa in many dermatofibromas provides a marker for this tumor,[394] although it is also present in acral angiofibromas, scars, keloids and some atypical fibroxanthomas, but not in dermatofibrosarcoma protuberans (DFSP).[395] The staining in dermatofibromas is often restricted to the periphery of the lesions, leading some authorities to question its specificity for dermatofibromas.[458] It is usually absent in the aneurysmal variant.[424] It was initially thought that the use of CD34 and factor XIIIa staining would differentiate dermatofibroma from DFSP. Unfortunately some overlap occurs,[460] including the occurrence of indeterminate fibrohistiocytic lesions with a dual population of CD34 and factor XIIIa-positive cells (see below). In a recent study of the immunohistochemical properties of dermatofibroma and DFSP, CD34 was strongly expressed in 25% of dermatofibromas and 80% of DFSP, whereas factor XIIIa was strongly expressed in 95% of dermatofibromas and 15% of DFSP.[461] This same study demonstrated the strong expression of tenascin (an extracellular matrix glycoprotein) at the dermal–epidermal junction in all cases of dermatofibroma but not in any DFSP.[461] Staining within the lesion was of no help in differentiating these two lesions. Similar results were recorded in an earlier study.[462] The expression of metallothionein has been reported in dermatofibromas but not DFSP.[399]

Electron microscopy

Ultrastructural studies have given conflicting results, with the cells variously reported as resembling fibroblasts, histiocytes and even myofibroblasts.[463,464] Endothelial cells with Weibel–Palade bodies were the prominent cell noted in one study.[352] Vessels are conspicuous in the angiomatoid variant.[422] There is a need for a reappraisal of the ultrastructural findings in the light of the immunoperoxidase studies implicating the dermal dendrocyte as the cell of origin (see above).

EPITHELIOID CELL HISTIOCYTOMA

Epithelioid cell histiocytoma is regarded as a variant of fibrous histiocytoma (dermatofibroma).[441] It is considered separately from dermatofibroma because of its distinctive histological appearance, which resembles to some extent the intradermal variant of Spitz nevus.[465] The lesion usually presents as an elevated nodule on the extremities of adults, although other sites have been recorded.[466] Although a dendrocyte origin is usually favored, an endothelial cell origin has also been proposed on the basis of the ultrastructural findings in one case.[467]

Histopathology

The polypoid lesions often have an epidermal collarette.[466] There is relatively sharp circumscription.[468] All lesions are characterized by sheets of angulated epithelioid cells with abundant eosinophilic cytoplasm. Scattered mitoses are usually present. There are many small blood vessels, and there is often a perivascular mosaic pattern of epithelioid and plump spindle cells. Xanthoma and/or giant cells are often present in small numbers.[469] The stroma contains a light mononuclear inflammatory cell infiltrate.[466] A cellular variant, with one or more dermal nodules composed of large epithelioid cells, has been reported.[470] It usually extends into the deep dermis. Rare cases occur with combined features of dermatofibroma and epithelioid cell histiocytoma (Fig. 34.22).

Factor XIIIa is expressed by 50–70% of the cells, whereas S100 and HAM-56 may be expressed by up to 5% of cells. HMB-45 is negative.[470] The vascularity is confirmed by a CD31 preparation.[471] Vimentin positivity was recorded in one study.[472]

PLEXIFORM FIBROHISTIOCYTIC TUMOR

Plexiform fibrohistiocytic tumor is a rare tumor that involves predominantly the upper limb of infants and children. It has an immunophenotype suggestive of myofibroblastic differentiation.[473,474] It involves the superficial soft tissue,

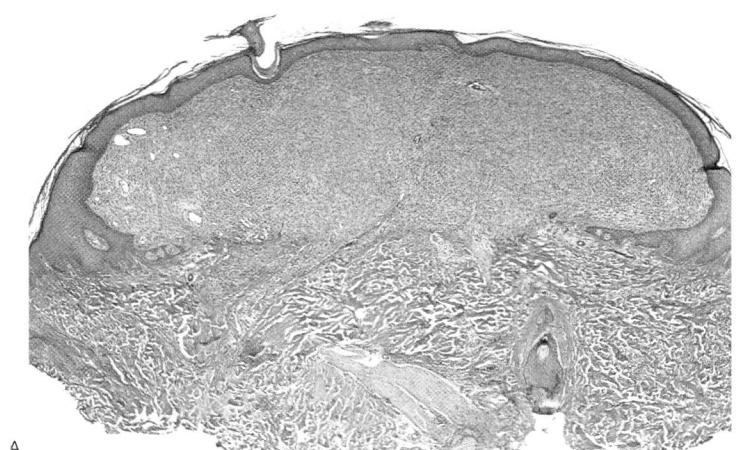

A

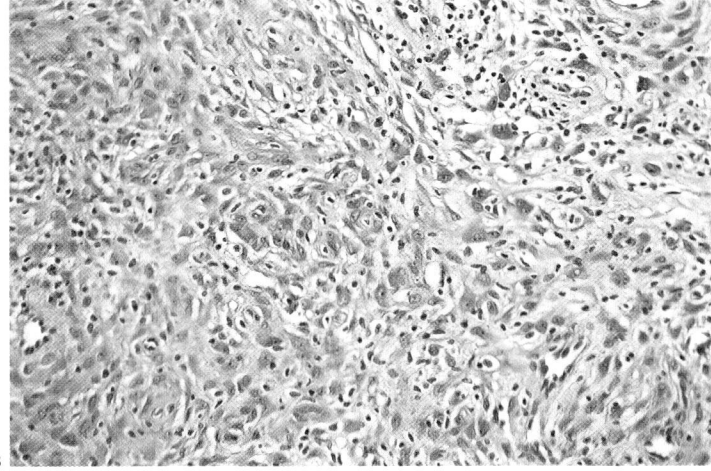

B

Fig. 34.22 **(A) Epithelioid cell histiocytoma. (B)** This case has both epithelioid cells and overlap features with dermatofibroma. (H & E)

often arising at the dermal–subcutaneous junction.[475] Dermal variants have been described.[476] Local recurrence is common, usually because of incomplete removal. Metastasis has been recorded.[477] It is included here with the fibrohistiocytic lesions, rather than the myofibroblastic tumors, because of the dual cell population.

Histopathology[475]

The appearances vary, depending on the relative proportion of the two major components – fascicles of fibroblastic cells, and aggregates or discrete nodules of histiocyte-like cells. The fascicles often ramify, giving a plexiform appearance. The 'histiocytic' nodules are composed of eosinophilic epithelioid cells. Osteoclast-like giant cells with 3–10 nuclei are often present. Granular cell change is a rare finding.[478] The cases reported as **plexiform xanthomatous tumor** had some areas resembling this lesion with the addition of numerous xanthoma cells.[479]

The tumor cells express smooth muscle actin but not factor XIIIa. They are positive with HHF35.[476] A minority of the cells in the histiocytic nodules stain for CD68 but not CD45 or Mac387.[475,477] The osteoclast-like giant cells are positive with KP1.[476]

GIANT CELL FIBROBLASTOMA

Giant cell fibroblastoma is a rare soft tissue tumor occurring predominantly in childhood.[480] The back, thigh and chest are the favored sites. There is a male predominance. Macroscopically, the tumor appears gray-pink with a partly gelatinous consistency.[481] Local recurrence is common, following incomplete surgical removal.[482] Cases recurring as, or transforming to, dermatofibrosarcoma protuberans (DFSP) have been reported.[483–486] Foci resembling giant cell fibroblastoma have also been seen within a DFSP,[487] as has the phenomenon of a DFSP recurring as a giant cell fibroblastoma.[488,489] Furthermore, both possess a similar cytogenetic abnormality (see below). These findings have led to the suggestion that giant cell fibroblastoma is a juvenile variant of DFSP.

Histopathology[480,481,490–493]

The dermis and subcutis are involved by an infiltrating spindle-cell tumor in which the tumor cells are embedded in a loose connective tissue matrix showing areas of mucinous change. Scattered through the tumor are uninucleate and multinucleate giant cells. A characteristic feature is the presence of branching sinusoidal spaces lined by cytoplasmic extensions of the spindle and giant cells.[490,494] These cells are negative for S100 protein, desmin, muscle-specific actin and factor VIII, but show scattered positivity for α_1-antitrypsin.[490,491,495] Both the spindle cells and the giant cells stain consistently for vimentin.[493] Although earlier reports gave conflicting results on the expression of CD34 by this tumor,[496] recent reports have found positivity in a significant number of cases.[497] The giant cells are almost invariably positive.[496,498]

Electron microscopy

Ultrastructural examination of this tumor has shown the cells to be fibroblasts, some of which have cytoplasmic extensions.[481] Cross-striated fibrils have been demonstrated in the cytoplasm of the cells.[499]

DERMATOFIBROSARCOMA PROTUBERANS

Dermatofibrosarcoma protuberans (DFSP) is a slow-growing, locally aggressive tumor of disputed histogenesis, with a marked tendency to local recurrence, but which rarely metastasizes.[500–502] It has a predilection for the

trunk and proximal extremities of young and middle-aged adults,[500,503,504] but other sites are rarely involved.[498,505–507] Congenital and familial cases and onset in childhood are all rare.[508–513] The lesions are solitary or multiple polypoid nodules, often arising in an indurated plaque of tumor.[514–517] Atrophic variants are uncommon; they may be difficult to diagnose clinically.[508,518,519] The involved area of skin measures from 0.5 to 10 cm or more in greatest diameter. A violaceous or red color is sometimes present, but at other times the nodules are flesh colored.[515] A history of previous trauma at the site is sometimes given.[500,505,520] Accelerated growth has been reported during pregnancy.[521] Previous arsenic exposure was present in one case.[522]

Local recurrence occurs in up to one-third of all cases.[500,515,523] Lower recurrence rates have been reported using Mohs micrographic surgery.[524,525] Hematogenous metastases, although rare,[526] are more common than those to regional lymph nodes.[527–530] Progression of a recurrent DFSP to a malignant fibrous histiocytoma[531] and the development of fibrosarcomatous and myxofibrosarcomatous areas in a DFSP have been reported.[532,533] The fibrosarcomatous variant of DFSP is said to be a much more aggressive lesion with metastatic potential;[534,535] however, a recent study of 17 cases showed that only four cases recurred and none developed metastasis within the 5-year follow-up period.[536] The lesions were treated initially with wide local excision with negative margins.[536] Giant cell fibroblastoma has a close relationship with DFSP; either tumor may recur with features of the other (see above).

The pigmented storiform neurofibroma of Bednar (Bednar tumor) is now regarded as a pigmented variant of DFSP.[537–544] It is an exceedingly rare tumor which accounts for only 1–5% of all cases of DFSP.[542] It occurs in a similar clinical setting to DFSP but, as yet, no metastases have been recorded. It is thought to represent the colonization of a DFSP by melanocytes.[545] A case has been reported that arose at the site of a previous immunization.[546]

Although DFSP is traditionally regarded as a fibrohistiocytic tumor, several ultrastructural and immunohistochemical studies have questioned this viewpoint;[547] a neuroectodermal origin has also been suggested, but the immunophenotype (see below) does not support this concept. Fletcher and colleagues have commented that 'the most pragmatic solution at this time may be to regard these tumours as a heterogeneous group, in line with the pluripotentiality of mesenchyme'.[548] A fibroblastic origin seems most likely on the basis of the immunophenotype and ultrastructure of the cells.[549] Platelet-derived growth factor has been identified in DFSP and other fibrohistiocytic lesions.[550]

Cytogenetically, DFSP is characterized by a reciprocal translocation, t(17;22)(q22;q13), and a supernumerary ring chromosome derived from the translocation r(17;22).[551] Other rare abnormalities have been found. Cloning studies reveal that the translocations result in the fusion of two genes, COLIAI and PDGFB, related respectively to the formation of type I collagen and platelet-derived growth factor.[551]

Macroscopically, the cut surface of the tumor nodules appears firm, and gray-white in color. Recurrent lesions with abundant mucin may have a more glistening appearance. The pigmented variant may appear slate gray or black if sufficient melanin is present within the tumor.[542]

Histopathology[500]

Dermatofibrosarcoma protuberans is a dermal tumor which almost invariably extends into the subcutis, where it infiltrates around small groups of fat cells in a characteristic manner (Figs 34.23 and 34.24).[514] A variant localized to the subcutis has been reported.[552] Deeper extension to underlying muscle is rare.[553] A superficial grenz zone is often present, but extension to the epidermis, with ulceration, is sometimes seen.[548] Dermal appendages are surrounded but not invaded.

DFSP is a spindle-cell tumor composed of interwoven bundles of rather uniform, small spindle cells with plump nuclei. There are small amounts of intermingled collagen. At points of intersection of the fascicles there may be

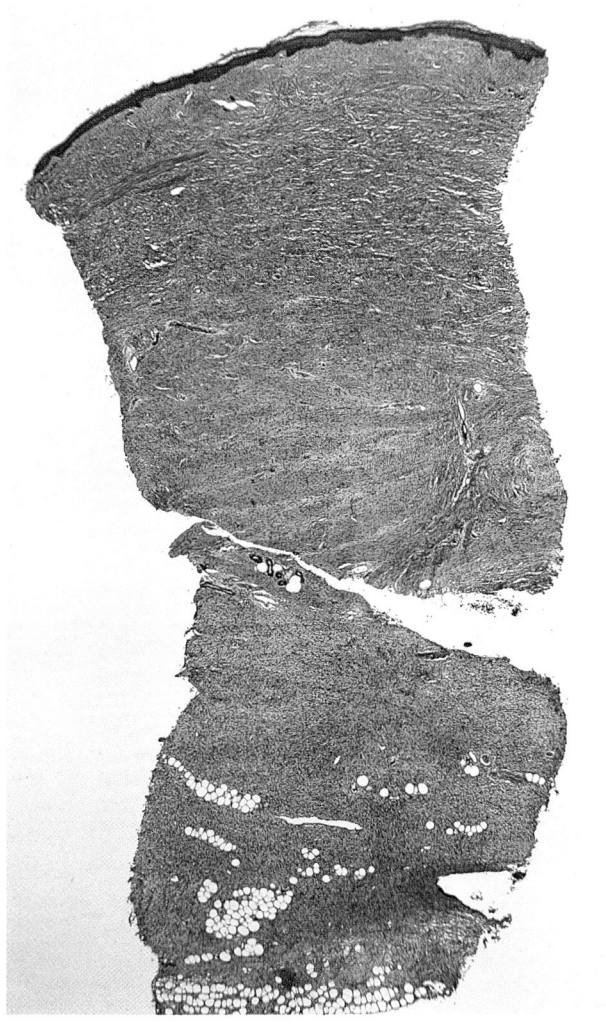

Fig. 34.23 **Dermatofibrosarcoma protuberans.** This deep biopsy shows a tumor involving dermis and subcutis. (H & E)

an acellular collagenous focus from which the fascicles appear to radiate (Fig. 34.25).[526] This is referred to as a storiform or cartwheel pattern. Scattered mitoses are present, but atypical forms are rare. Increased cellularity of the tumor, and more than eight mitoses per 10 high-power fields, appear to be associated with a predisposition to metastasis.[526] Other histological features include an occasional histiocyte and multinucleate giant cell.[547] Thin-walled capillaries are randomly distributed. *Fibrosarcomatous* change, seen particularly in recurrences represents a form of tumor progression.[500,554] The proportion of this element varies markedly from case to case.[497] The fibrosarcomatous areas may show focal myxoid change,[533] keloid-like hyalinization, giant rosettes,[555] pigmented melanocytes,[556] and myoid nodules and bundles.[557–560] The leiomyomatous nodules appear to be, at least in part, of vascular origin and reactive in nature.[561] The fibrosarcomatous areas express CD34 in less than 50% of cases.[556] The expression of fusion transcripts in both conventional and fibrosarcomatous areas supports a common histogenesis of the two components.[551]

Myxoid DFSP is a distinct variant, often found for the first time in recurrent lesions. There are large myxoid areas which are paucicellular, surrounded by more typical areas with storiform features.[562] *Atrophic* and *granular cell* variants of DFSP have also been proposed.[563–565] Some cases of DFSP have areas resembling *giant cell fibroblastoma* (see above).[497] Furthermore, either tumor may, rarely, recur as the other.[483–485,487,488,496] The related giant cell angiofibroma may also occur within a DFSP.[221]

The *pigmented* variant has melanin-containing dendritic cells (melanocytes) scattered throughout the tumor.[542] The amount of melanin pigment is quite variable (Fig. 34.26). Although Bednar reported three cases in which this pigmented variant was present in the core of a nevocellular nevus,[538] no further examples of this phenomenon have been reported. There is one report of a recurrent DFSP transforming into the pigmented form.[566] The various types are listed in Table 34.3.

Although usually inconspicuous, the stromal collagen in a DFSP will stain with the trichrome method, but unlike the collagen in a dermatofibroma it is not polarizable.[567] Unlike dermatofibromas, hemosiderin is rarely present in a DFSP.[500] Furthermore, a dermatofibroma is usually smaller and less cellular, with fewer mitoses than DFSP.

Lesions with overlap features between dermatofibroma and DFSP have been reported as **indeterminate fibrohistiocytic lesions**.[568] The tumors all had keloidal collagen, infiltration of the subcutis in a honeycomb pattern, low mitotic counts, and a dual population of CD34+ and factor XIIIa

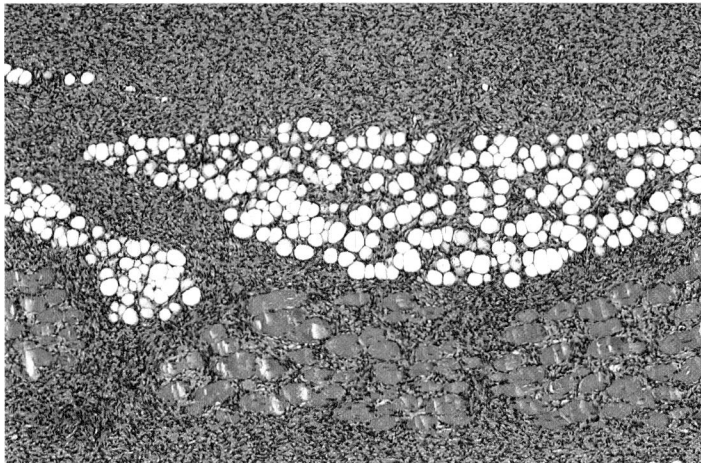

Fig. 34.24 **Dermatofibrosarcoma protuberans.** Tumor cells insinuate between fat cells in the subcutis and extend into the underlying muscle. (H & E)

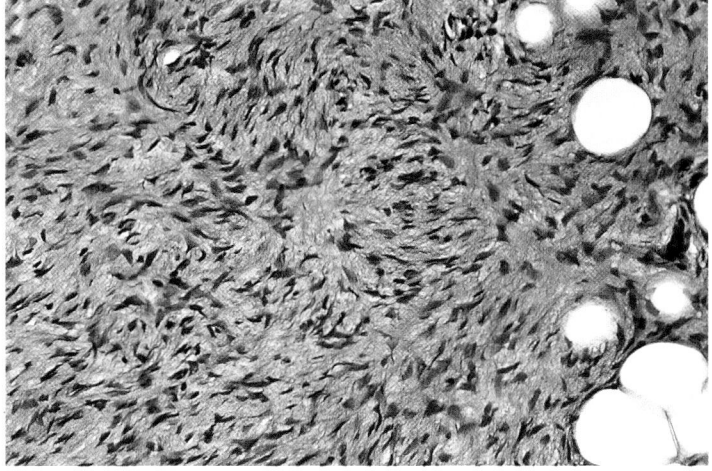

Fig. 34.25 **Dermatofibrosarcoma protuberans.** The spindle-shaped cells have a storiform or cartwheel arrangement. (H & E)

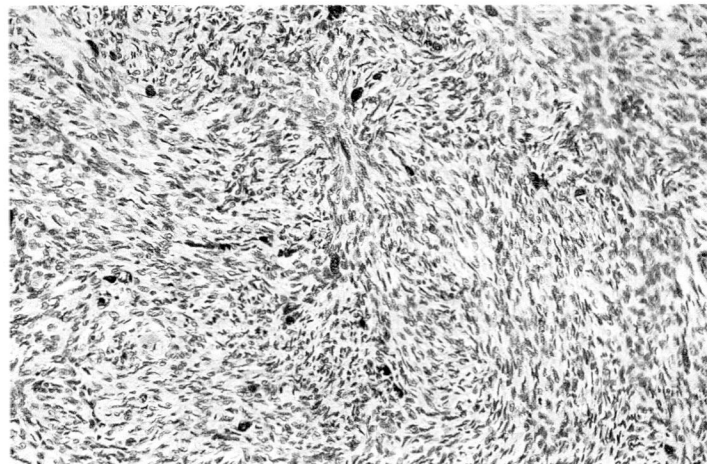

Fig. 34.26 **Dermatofibrosarcoma protuberans** with melanin pigment. This variant is known as a Bednar tumor. (H & E)

cells in varying proportions from tumor to tumor. A single recurrence was noted.[568]

Immunohistochemical studies have shown that the tumor cells in DFSP contain vimentin,[549,569] but they are negative for S100 protein. A few scattered cells may stain for lysozyme and α_1-antichymotrypsin.[548] The most diagnostic marker is the human progenitor cell antigen, CD34, which stains 50–100% of the cells in DFSP.[570–575] Conflicting results have been reported in the giant cell fibroblastoma component that is sometimes present.[487,496] In contrast, CD34 stains only focal areas, in a small percentage of cases, in dermatofibroma[576] and some neural tumors.[577] Factor XIIIa, which stains most dermatofibromas, is only focally positive in a small number of cases of DFSP. MIB-1 is not a useful marker in distinguishing DFSP from dermatofibroma.[578] The pigment-laden cells in the Bednar tumor are positive for S100 protein and vimentin, whereas the non-pigmented cells are usually positive only for vimentin.[545] The expression of CD34 is not present in all cases of pigmented DFSP.[544,546,579]

Electron microscopy

The spindle-shaped cells usually have an indented or deeply lobulated nucleus. In some studies, including one concerning the Bednar tumor,[542] a basal lamina suggesting a perineurial origin was present.[580,581] In other studies the predominant cell has been interpreted as a modified fibroblast[582,583] or histiocyte.[584] Of interest are the rare reports in which the metastases of a DFSP have assumed a histiocytic appearance.[530] The primary lesion in such cases may have been a malignant fibrous histiocytoma incorrectly diagnosed as a DFSP.[548]

ATYPICAL FIBROXANTHOMA

'Atypical fibroxanthoma' is the term coined by Helwig for a cutaneous tumor with marked cellular pleomorphism, yet with a course that is usually benign.[585] As such it has been regarded as one of the so-called 'pseudomalignancies' of the skin.[586] This view must be modified somewhat in the light of rare reports of metastasis (see below). Similar cases were reported about the same time as those of Helwig, under several different names.[587,588] The tumors usually occur as a solitary, gray to pink or red nodule, often dome-shaped, on the head or neck of the elderly.[589,590] There is a rare plaque form. In some series there has been a predominance in males.[591] They may develop quickly, but they are usually less than 2 cm in diameter. Another clinical variant occurs in younger patients, and these lesions may be larger, more slowly growing, and

Table 34.3 **Histological variants of DFSP**

- Fibrosarcomatous
- Fibrosarcomatous with myoid/myofibroblastic change
- Myxoid
- Granular cell
- Atrophic
- Sclerosing
- Palisaded
- Giant cell fibroblastoma
- Combined
- Indeterminate

with a predilection for the trunk and extremities.[590,592] Atypical fibroxanthoma has been reported in children with xeroderma pigmentosum.[593,594] In both groups, the lesions may be ulcerated and bleed.

The nature of atypical fibroxanthoma is speculative. It has been regarded as a proliferative mesenchymal, possibly fibrohistiocytic, response to a variety of cutaneous injuries.[595] The diversity of immunoperoxidase markers raises the possibility of heterogeneous, bimodal 'fibrohistiocytic' and 'myofibroblastic' phenotypes.[596] In older patients there is often a history of prolonged actinic exposure, but lesions may also develop at sites of irradiation and even trauma.[597] This tumor may also develop in renal transplant recipients.[598,599] It has been suggested that there is a close relationship to malignant fibrous histiocytoma (see below), and that it is merely the small size and dermal location of most cases of atypical fibroxanthoma that lead to its benign behavior.[600,601] Although the large atypical cells in atypical fibroxanthoma are aneuploid, as they are in malignant fibrous histiocytoma, the smaller spindle-shaped cells in atypical fibroxanthoma are diploid.[602,603]

Recurrences develop in approximately 5% of cases, but in most instances this is due to incomplete removal. Lesions may even regress spontaneously or after incomplete removal. The diagnosis of atypical fibroxanthoma has been questioned in those cases that have behaved aggressively.[604] There is no doubt that atypical fibroxanthoma, as reported in the past, was a hetero-geneous entity that included cases of malignant melanoma and the spindle-cell variant of squamous cell carcinoma.[605,606] The advent of immunoperoxidase markers, and the wider use of electron microscopy, should allow more accurate assessment and diagnosis of these tumors in the future. More than 10 cases of atypical fibroxanthoma with metastases have now been reported, and several of these have been studied with immunoperoxidase or electron microscopy to exclude melanoma and squamous cell carcinoma.[595,607] The cases reported have tended to metastasize to regional lymph nodes,[595] but more widespread systemic spread has been reported.[608]

The author's personal (anecdotal) experience with over 300 cases may be of interest. The tumor is usually histologically distinctive with its bizarre cells, numerous mitoses, level 4 extension (except for the rare plaque form), frequent 'collarette', and usual occurrence on the ear, forehead or bald scalp. Experience has shown that it is prudent to perform immunohistochemistry for S100 protein and keratin, as melanoma and squamous cell carcinoma can produce morphological simulants. The author is not aware of any metastasis in these cases but at least 10 have recurred. All these recurrent lesions were excised with positive or narrow margins and there was usually subcutaneous extension. It should be noted that most lesions were completely excised, as shave excisions have not been used widely in Australia until recently. It has been suggested recently that atypical fibroxanthoma is a 'myth', and yet another variant of squamous cell carcinoma.[609] This is not my experience.

Histopathology[590]

Atypical fibroxanthoma is usually a well-circumscribed, non-encapsulated, highly cellular tumor centered on the dermis (Fig. 34.27). It is contiguous with the epidermis, or separated from it by a thin zone of collagen. Sometimes cells appear to stream out from the basal layer, and in these areas the dermo-epidermal junction is not always distinct.[604] In one series, nearly half the tumors extended into the subcutaneous fat,[605] but most observers would regard subcutaneous extension as uncommon, and an indicator of possible recurrence. The epidermis is often thin or even ulcerated, but there may be peripheral acanthosis and, occasionally, a peripheral 'collarette'.

There is florid pleomorphism and polymorphism, with many atypical and often bizarre cells. There are usually admixtures of three cell types, although a *spindle-cell* variant without the other two cell types has been recorded.[406,610] The predominant cell is a plump, spindle-shaped cell in poorly arranged fascicles. Although it may occur in an atypical fibroxanthoma,[589] a storiform arrangement should raise the possibility that the correct diagnosis is in fact a malignant fibrous histiocytoma or dermatofibrosarcoma protuberans. The spindle cells have a prominent nucleus, which is often vesicular. There is also a haphazard arrangement of large polyhedral cells in the tumor. Some have vacuolated, lipid-containing cytoplasm. A *clear cell* variant has been described (Fig. 34.28).[611–613] They do not contain glycogen.[614] True xanthoma cells are uncommon. The third cell type is a giant cell, which may be mononucleate or multinucleate. These cells have hyperchromatic nuclei, and mitoses, including bizarre forms, are common. The cytoplasm of these cells is often partly vacuolated. Lipid stains on frozen sections will show variable amounts of lipid, usually in the polyhedral and giant cells, with only sparse amounts in the spindle cells. Hemosiderin may also be present.

Necrosis is uncommon and is usually limited to the ulcerated surface. Large areas of necrosis should raise doubts about the diagnosis of atypical fibroxanthoma. The adnexae may be distorted by the growth of the tumor, but they are not usually destroyed.

There is usually only a very small amount of interspersed collagen, although variants with prominent fibrosis have been reported.[590] Foci of stromal *osteoid*[615] or *chondroid*[616] differentiation and the presence of numerous *osteoclast-like* giant cells[616–620] are rare findings. *Pigmented* and *granular cell* variants have also been reported.[621,622] The various forms are listed in Table 34.4. Some tumors are richly vascular. The adjacent uninvolved dermis may show solar elastosis. Any inflammatory infiltrate is usually sparse

Table 34.4 **Histological variants of atypical fibroxanthoma**

- Spindle cell
- Clear cell
- Osteoid
- Osteoclastic
- Chondroid
- Pigmented
- Granular cell

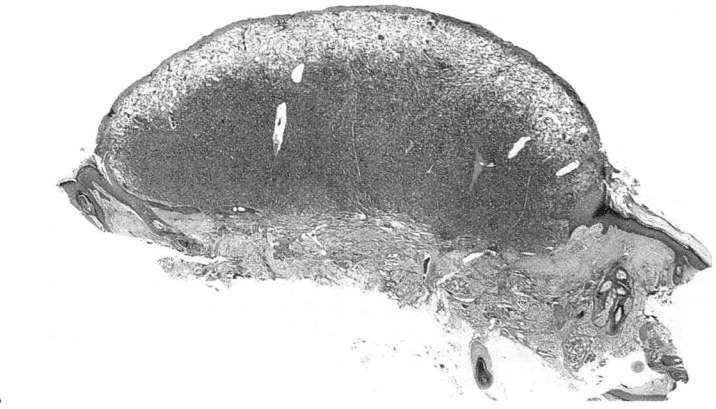
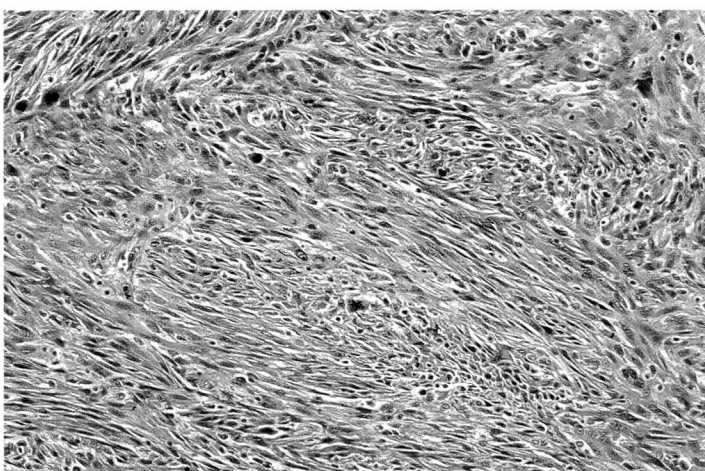

Fig. 34.27 **(A) Atypical fibroxanthoma. (B)** This cellular tumor is composed of spindle-shaped cells and some bizarre cells with hyperchromatic nuclei. Several mitotic figures are present. (H & E)

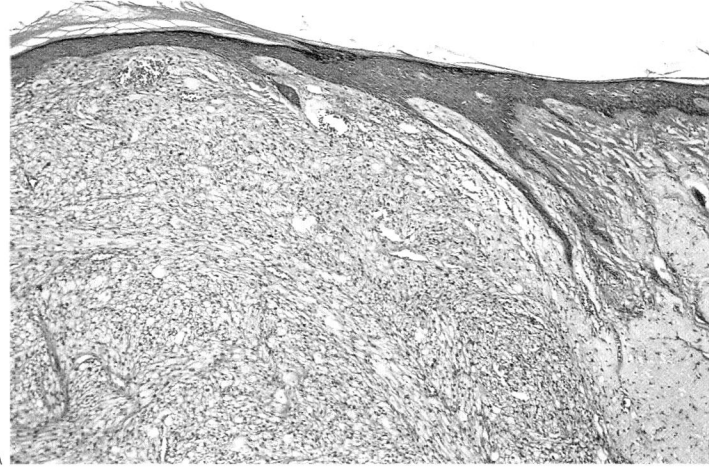
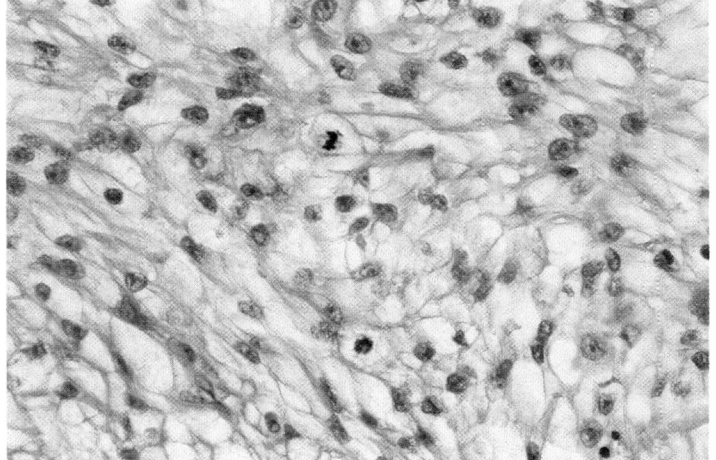

Fig. 34.28 **(A) Atypical fibroxanthoma of clear cell type. (B)** A mitotic figure is present. (H & E)

and peripheral, although neutrophils may be abundant near an ulcerated surface.

Features that may portend a more aggressive behavior include vascular invasion (the most reliable feature), deep tissue invasion, tumor necrosis,[595] and possibly impaired host immunity.[607]

Immunoperoxidase studies for α_1-antitrypsin and α_1-antichymotrypsin are positive in more than half of the cases.[592,623] Although some S100-positive cells may be found, these constitute only a small percentage of the cells present.[596,624,625] However, S100A6 is expressed in many cases.[626] These cells may represent part of the inflammatory response. The tumor cells are reactive for vimentin and, in a few cases, scattered cells stain for factor XIIIa[395,627] but not for cytokeratin or epithelial membrane antigen.[628] In one study, 41% of cases stained for muscle-specific actin or smooth muscle actin, 57% expressed CD68 (a monocyte–macrophage marker), but no case expressed CD34 (other than stromal blood vessels).[596] Recently, weak positivity with CD74 has been reported in atypical fibroxanthoma, in contrast to the strong staining for this marker in malignant fibrous histiocytoma.[629] Positivity for CD99 has been reported in two-thirds of the cases tested.[630]

Electron microscopy

The spindle cells have abundant rough endoplasmic reticulum, small vesicles and cytoplasmic filaments, and surface indentations in the nuclei.[631] These features suggest a fibroblastic or myofibroblastic origin. The large cells have a histiocytic appearance with lipid vacuoles.[632] Transition forms between these two cell types have been noted, as have histiocytic cells with Langerhans granules.[624,633]

MALIGNANT FIBROUS HISTIOCYTOMA

Malignant fibrous histiocytoma is the most common soft tissue sarcoma of late adult life.[547] It usually involves the deep soft tissues and striated muscles of the proximal part of the extremities, particularly the lower.[634] The retroperitoneum is another favored site.[547,635] Up to 25% of cases may arise in the subcutaneous tissues, although less than 10% are confined to the subcutis without underlying fascial involvement.[635–638] Cutaneous tumors are even rarer.[639,640] Adults between the ages of 50 and 70 years are most often affected, although the angiomatoid variant involves primarily children and adolescents.[641–643] There are usually no predisposing factors but, rarely, cases have followed radiotherapy,[636,644] or developed at the site of a chronic ulcer,[645] vaccination scar[646] or burn scar.[647]

The tumors are multilobulated, often circumscribed, gray-white fleshy masses.[636] The majority are 5 cm or more in diameter. Focal areas of hemorrhage and necrosis are quite common. The myxoid variant has a somewhat gelatinous appearance and the inflammatory variant may be yellow in color.

The prognosis is generally poor, with 5-year survivals ranging from 15% to 30%.[648] Tumors that are small and superficially located have a better prognosis than large, deep ones.[635,649,650] Proliferative activity (MIB-1 index) is not an independent prognostic parameter, despite being so in other soft tissue sarcomas.[651] Proximal deep tumors and those in the retroperitoneum have a poor prognosis. The angiomatoid variant (see below) has a better prognosis than the other histological subtypes.[652] Local recurrence and metastases are common, with the lungs and regional lymph nodes most often affected.[635]

The histogenesis of this tumor has been controversial. The tumor cells show partial fibroblastic and histiocytic differentiation, as reflected by collagen production and the presence of cells which may be immunoreactive for the histiocytic markers, as well as showing occasional phagocytosis.[653] The angiomatoid variant has some myoid features.[642] It is now believed that the

progenitor cell is not the mononuclear phagocyte but rather a poorly defined mesenchymal cell, which may differentiate along histiocytic and fibroblastic lines.[654–656]

Multiple structural and numerical aberrations in many chromosomes have been found in this tumor.[657] It appears that genes involved in the RB1- and TP53-associated cell-cycle regulatory pathways may play a prominent role in the development of malignant fibrous histiocytoma.[658]

Histopathology

Five histological subtypes of malignant fibrous histiocytoma have been recognized: pleomorphic, angiomatoid, myxoid, giant cell and inflammatory.[547,636] The presence of myofibroblastic differentiation may constitute a sixth type (pleomorphic myofibrosarcoma) but this is not yet a well-delineated entity.[659] Overlap features occur between the various types.[648] All tumors usually have an infiltrative margin. They may show areas of hemorrhage and necrosis, particularly the larger tumors. Chronic inflammatory cells are usually present throughout the tumor, particularly at the periphery. The various types will be considered in further detail.

Pleomorphic

The pleomorphic variant is the most common.[635,636,660] It is composed of an admixture of plump spindle-shaped cells, clusters or sheets of histiocytes, and scattered pleomorphic multinucleate giant cells (Fig. 34.29). Mitoses are common. The spindle cells may be arranged in whorls or have a storiform appearance. There is usually a delicate collagenous stroma, which in some areas may be more prominent. Focal myxoid change is quite common. Rarely, metaplastic osteoid or chondroid material is formed.[661] Xanthoma cells and siderophages are sometimes present. Similar appearances can be seen in pleomorphic sarcomas presumed to be of other cell lineage:[656] that is, pleomorphic malignant fibrous histiocytoma, as currently reported, is probably a heterogeneous entity.

Angiomatoid

The angiomatoid variant tends to involve the subcutis.[641] There are large blood-filled cystic spaces and areas of hemorrhage in addition to the solid nests of fibroblast-like and histiocyte-like cells.[641,662] A lymphoplasmacytic infiltrate is present to some degree in about 80% of cases.[642] Xanthoma cells, siderophages and giant cells are often present. The cells show strong staining

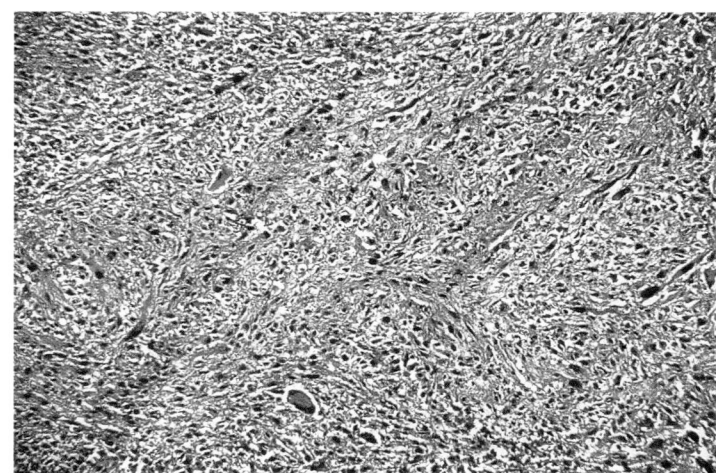

Fig. 34.29 **Malignant fibrous histiocytoma** composed of spindle-shaped and polygonal cells and scattered pleomorphic giant cells, some of which are multinucleate. (H & E)

for vimentin and intermediate staining for CD34.[663,664] Approximately 50% of the cases show positivity for desmin and CD99.[642] In a recent study, fusion of the *FUS* and *ATF-1* genes, resulting from a chromosomal translocation involving bands 12q13 and 16p11, was demonstrated.[665]

The lesion reported as a **pleomorphic hyalinizing angiectatic tumor of soft parts** appears to be a low-grade malignancy that shares some histological features with malignant fibrous histiocytoma and neurilemmoma.[666] The cells have prominent intranuclear cytoplasmic inclusions and focal CD34 expression.[666,667]

Myxoid

Approximately 10% of all malignant fibrous histiocytomas are of the myxoid type.[668,669] They are also known as myxofibrosarcoma. It has a better prognosis than most other types. Prominent myxoid foci comprise nearly 50% of the tumor.[668,670] Other areas resemble the pleomorphic variant.

The recently described acral **myxoinflammatory fibroblastic sarcoma** has some histological similarities, but with the addition of numerous inflammatory cells.[671] It is a low-grade sarcoma of the hands and feet, possibly of synovial origin.

Giant cell

Formerly known as giant cell tumor of soft parts, this variant has numerous osteoclast-like giant cells in addition to the spindle and histiocytic cells (Fig. 34.30).[672]

Inflammatory

The rare inflammatory variant, which is most frequently retroperitoneal, has a grave prognosis. A diffuse and at times intense neutrophilic infiltrate, unassociated with tissue necrosis, is present not only in the primary tumor, but also in recurrences and metastases.[673-675] Xanthoma cells, both bland and anaplastic, are also present. A storiform fibrous pattern is usually seen in some areas of the tumor.[673]

The tumor cells contain vimentin;[676,677] cytokeratin has also been present in a few tumors.[678] Strong staining for CD74 has been reported.[629] Various histiocyte markers can be demonstrated, using immunoperoxidase techniques, in from 60% to 80% of malignant fibrous histiocytomas. Those used have included α_1-antitrypsin and α_1-antichymotrypsin.[456] CD68 is frequently positive, whereas CD34 is negative.[679-681]

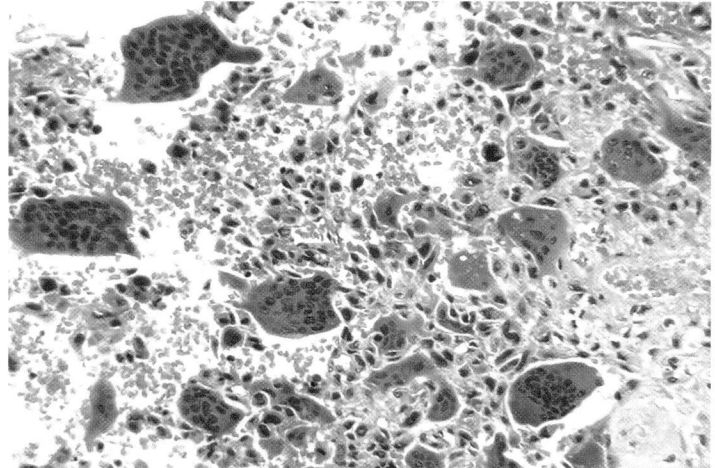

Fig. 34.30 **Malignant fibrous histiocytoma** composed of numerous osteoclast-like giant cells. (H & E)

Electron microscopy

Studies have consistently shown cells with fibroblastic and histiocytic morphology, as well as undifferentiated mesenchymal cells with a narrow rim of cytoplasm and scattered ribosomes.[654,682] Myofibroblasts were said to be the predominant cell in one case.[683]

PRESUMPTIVE SYNOVIAL AND TENDON SHEATH TUMORS

FIBROMA OF TENDON SHEATH

Chung and Enzinger formally documented fibroma of tendon sheath in 1979, with a report of 138 cases.[684] It is a solitary, slow-growing subcutaneous tumor with a predilection for the fingers, hands and wrists of middle-aged adults, particularly males.[685,686] Recurrences occur in approximately 20% of cases.

The fibromas are well-circumscribed, often lobulated, gray to white tumors that measure 1–2 cm in diameter. They are usually attached to a tendon sheath.

A (2;11) translocation has been found in some of the tumor cells in one case, suggesting that this lesion is neoplastic and not a reactive process.[687]

Histopathology[684,688]

These tumors are situated in the subcutaneous tissue, sometimes with dermal extension. There are relatively sparse spindle or stellate cells embedded in a dense fibrocollagenous stroma. Cellular areas are present, sometimes toward the periphery. The stroma shows variable hyalinization and sometimes has a whorled pattern with associated artifactual clefting. Myxoid degeneration and, rarely, focal calcification of the stroma may be present. A characteristic feature is the presence of dilated or slit-like vascular channels. A sparse mononuclear cell infiltrate is sometimes present at the periphery.

A rare pleomorphic variant (**pleomorphic fibroma of tendon sheath**) has been reported. There are scattered large cells with pleomorphic, hyperchromatic nuclei, but no mitoses.[689] A further variant of pleomorphic fibroma exists: it has overlap features with the giant cell tumor of tendon sheath (see below). This has given rise to the suggestion that fibroma of tendon sheath is the end and sclerosing stage of giant cell tumor,[690] although this has been strongly disputed.[691]

Electron microscopy

Ultrastructural examination has shown the spindle cells to be myofibroblasts[692] with some fibroblasts.[686,693]

GIANT CELL TUMOR OF TENDON SHEATH

Giant cell tumor of tendon sheath is a not uncommon benign tumor with a predilection for the dorsal surface of the fingers, in the vicinity of the distal interphalangeal joint.[694,695] Periungual lesions are rare.[696] It occurs particularly in young and middle-aged adults. It is a slow-growing, usually asymptomatic lesion, which may measure up to 3 cm in diameter at the time of removal. Local recurrence, usually a result of incomplete removal, occurs in 15% of cases.[694]

Giant cell tumors are lobulated and gray-brown in color, with yellowish areas. They are usually attached to a tendon sheath or joint capsule, but cutaneous involvement can occur.[697,698] The histogenesis of giant cell tumors has been controversial. They have been regarded as a variant of fibrous histiocytoma, and as a tumor derived from mesenchymal cells.[699] One study concluded that the cells are of monocyte–macrophage lineage, closely resembling osteoclasts.[700] The immunophenotype (see below) is more suggestive of a synovial cell origin.[691] It appears to be a polyclonal proliferation.[701]

This tumor must be distinguished from the **giant cell tumor of soft tissue**, a rare tumor resembling the lesion of bone. There is a benign variant and a malignant one, the latter usually being designated as a variant of malignant fibrous histiocytoma. It is beyond the scope of this book.[702,703]

Histopathology[694,704]

The lesion has an eosinophilic collagenous stroma with variable cellularity. In the sparsely cellular areas the cells are plump and spindle shaped, set in a partly hyalinized stroma, whereas in the more cellular areas the cells are usually polygonal. Small clusters of lipid-laden histiocytes are often present. Multinucleate giant cells with up to 60 or more nuclei are a characteristic feature. They are variable in number and haphazardly distributed. Hemosiderin is invariably present, and sometimes there are cholesterol clefts.

The proliferating mononuclear cells stain positively for CD68, HAM-56 and vimentin, but not for S100, cytokeratins, EMA, CD45, CD34, desmin or smooth muscle actin.[691] The giant cells stain for CD68, vimentin and CD45.[691]

Electron microscopy

Ultrastructural studies have usually supported a synovial or fibrohistiocytic origin,[705] although another report documented a pleomorphic cell population in which the giant cells had some similarity to osteoclasts and the stromal cells similarities to primitive mesenchymal cells, osteoblasts, fibroblasts and histiocytes.[699]

EPITHELIOID SARCOMA

Epithelioid sarcoma, first delineated by Enzinger,[706] is a rare malignant tumor that usually involves the deep subcutis and underlying soft tissues. Infrequently, it arises in the dermis and superficial subcutis, where it may be confused both clinically[707] and histologically with various benign cutaneous diseases, including granuloma annulare.[708] It has a predilection for the extremities, particularly the hands, of young adult males.[709,710] Childhood cases occur.[711] Lesions of the face,[712] vulva[713] and penis[714] have also been described. A history of trauma is sometimes given.[709] A case has been reported in a patient with neurofibromatosis type 2.[715]

It presents as one or more slow-growing tan-white nodules with an indistinct infiltrating margin. Ulceration develops late, if at all. Local recurrence occurs in nearly 80% of cases, and metastases in 30–45%.[709,716–7 8] The regional lymph nodes and lungs are the most common initial sites of metastases. The skin of the scalp represents another site of distant metastasis.[719] Adverse prognostic features are a proximal or axial location, tumor size greater than 5 cm, deep extension, vascular invasion, metastases, and numerous mitotic figures.[709,720]

Epithelioid sarcoma is of disputed histogenesis, with a synovial origin most favored.[721,722] A histiocytic, fibroblastic,[723] myofibroblastic[724] and mesenchymal reserve cell[725] origin have all been suggested. One tumor produced granulocyte colony-stimulating factor, but it is difficult to draw any histogenetic conclusions.[726] An N-*ras* oncogene mutation has been demonstrated in the tumor cells in one study.[717] In another, allelic loss on chromosome 22q was present in 60% of cases.[727]

Fletcher and colleagues have drawn attention to an aggressive tumor with epithelioid and rhabdoid features, which they have called 'proximal-type' epithelioid sarcoma.[728] Most of the cases involved the deep soft tissues but several, in the region of the vulva, involved the subcutis.

Histopathology[708,709]

The low-power appearance often resembles a necrobiotic or granulomatous process, or an epithelial tumor. Epithelioid sarcoma is an ill-defined cellular lesion forming vague nodules in the dermis and subcutis. There is subtle extension into the contiguous fascial and tendinous structures. Perineural invasion is present in approximately 20% of cases.[720] The tumor is composed of oval to polygonal cells with abundant, often eosinophilic, cytoplasm, and a gradual transition to plump spindle cells (Fig. 34.31).[729,730] Rarely, a spindle-cell pattern predominates.[731] Nuclear pleomorphism and scattered mitoses are present. Multinucleate giant cells are rare or absent. Sometimes the pattern can look deceptively bland.[732]

A characteristic feature is the presence of central necrosis or fibrosis. Collagen also extends between the cells. Calcification is present in approximately 20% of cases, and osseous metaplasia in 10%.[709] Hemosiderin is often present. A perinodular inflammatory cell infiltrate of lymphocytes and histiocytes is a usual feature.[733]

The 'proximal-type' variant grows in a multinodular pattern and shows prominent epithelioid and rhabdoid features. There is marked cytological atypia. The cells are positive for vimentin, cytokeratin and EMA. Some tumors express desmin and CD34.[728]

Immunoperoxidase studies of the usual type show that many tumor cells contain cytokeratin, epithelial membrane antigen (EMA) and vimentin, but not

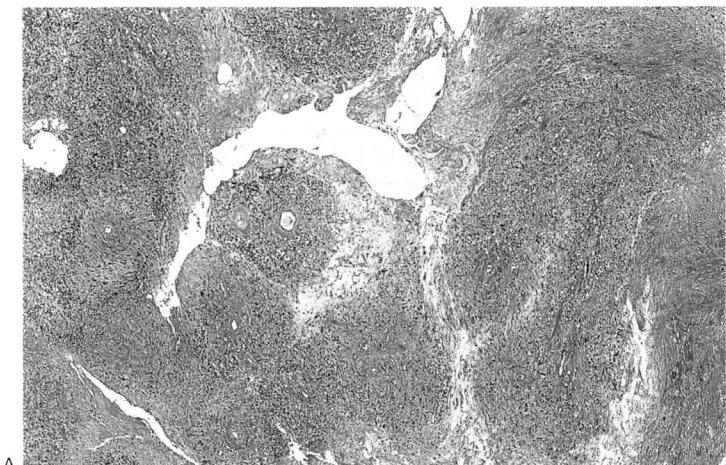

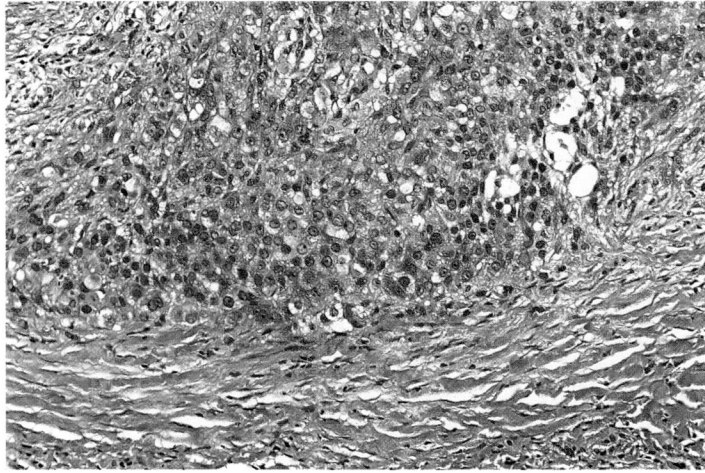

Fig. 34.31 **(A) Epithelioid cell sarcoma. (B)** There are sheets of epithelioid and polygonal cells. (H & E)

CD45 or S100 protein.[734–737] The combination of keratin, EMA and vimentin positivity is a characteristic feature of this tumor, although exceptions occur.[738] Nearly all epithelioid sarcomas express keratin 8 (K8), whereas about 75% express K19.[739] Patchy membrane staining for CD34 and more diffuse staining for muscle-specific actin[739] occur in more than half of the cases.[738] Most cells express vascular-endothelial cadherin.[740] Histiocytic markers have usually been negative.[736]

Electron microscopy

Light and dark cells are present within the tumor cell population. There are many filopodia-like surface extensions of cytoplasm[721] and there are bundles of intermediate filaments in the cytoplasm.[736] Occasional pseudoglandular spaces have been present in some tumors.[722]

SYNOVIAL SARCOMA

Only brief mention will be made of this soft tissue sarcoma, which has a predilection for the extremities of young and middle-aged adults. It exhibits a wide spectrum of biological behavior. The high-risk group includes older patients, tumor size greater than 5 cm, and poor differentiation.[741,742]

Only one case of superficial synovial sarcoma involving the dermis has been reported.[743] It involved the skin overlying the knee in a young woman. It recurred six times over a 24-year period.[743]

The chromosomal translocation t(X;18) has been described in 90% of synovial sarcomas, and the presence of SYT–SSX fusion products is quite characteristic.[744]

Histopathology

Synovial sarcoma occurs in two predominant patterns: a monophasic form composed of spindle cells, sometimes in a fascicular pattern, and a biphasic form with spindle cells admixed with glandular structures of varying size. The biphasic lesions usually stain for cytokeratin and EMA while about 70% of the monophasic form stain for at least one of the cytokeratins or EMA.[741] Focal staining for S100 protein is seen in about 10% of cases.

The cutaneous lesion (see above) was composed predominantly of spindle cells with scattered epithelial nests. Focal myxoid and hemangiopericytoma areas were present.[743] The spindle cells stained for vimentin, Cam 5.2 and EMA.[743]

MISCELLANEOUS ENTITIES

The miscellaneous group of disorders includes several very rare entities in which fibrous tissue forms a significant component, and another group with a myxoid stroma.

FIBRO-OSSEOUS PSEUDOTUMOR OF THE DIGITS

Fibro-osseous pseudotumor is a rare tumor of the subcutaneous and soft tissues of the digits, usually in young adults.[745,746] There is a close histological resemblance to myositis ossificans, with osteoid formation and a background stroma of fibroblasts, collagen and myxoid material.[745,747] Unlike myositis ossificans, the lesion usually involves the subcutis and has an irregular multinodular growth pattern.[745]

OSSIFYING FIBROMYXOID TUMOR

Ossifying fibromyxoid tumor is a rare tumor of soft tissues that sometimes involves the subcutaneous tissue.[748–750] It occurs preferentially on the upper and lower extremities, but many sites can be involved. The tumor is benign, but local recurrences are common unless an adequate clearance is obtained. The lesion appears to be of neural origin.

Histopathology

The tumor is circumscribed, with a characteristic fibrous capsule and an incomplete peripheral shell of new bone.[749] There are cords, nests and sheets of oval to round and spindle-shaped cells with a well-vascularized stroma.[748] The stroma may be mucoid, fibromyxoid or fibrous. Tumor cells stain for vimentin and show strong focal staining for S100 protein. Some cases have shown staining for desmin, glial fibrillary acidic protein and neuron-specific enolase.

FIBROADENOMA

Fibroadenomas resembling those seen in the breast may arise along the embryonic milk line and elsewhere.[751]

NODULAR FIBROSIS IN ELEPHANTIASIS

Multiple nodules, sometimes large, are a common complication of non-filarial elephantiasis of the lower legs.[752] This idiopathic condition is endemic in Ethiopia.[752] Microscopy shows bundles of collagen in the dermis. in irregular whorls, with a variable number of fibroblasts depending on the age of the lesion.[752] A few small blood vessels, some with a surrounding cuff of lymphocytes, are also present. The overlying epidermis shows pseudoepitheliomatous hyperplasia.[753]

Discrete fibroma-like nodules have been recorded in a patient with Kaposi's sarcoma and lymphedema.[754]

MULTIFOCAL FIBROSCLEROSIS

Subcutaneous fibrosis is an uncommon complication of multifocal fibrosclerosis, a condition in which progressive fibrosis of several discrete regions of the body, particularly the retroperitoneum and mediastinum, occurs.[755] Ulceration and vasculitic lesions may also develop in the skin.

MESENCHYMAL HAMARTOMA

The designation mesenchymal hamartoma is preferred to the alternative suggestion of benign polymorphous mesenchymal tumor of soft parts. Only two cases have been reported of this benign tumor of uncertain histogenesis.[756] It is characterized by a prominent lobular configuration with distinctive garland-shaped structures composed of cells expressing glial fibrillary acidic protein (GFAP) encased in concentric loops of fine collagen fibers. The clusters of cells are surrounded by a copious myxoid matrix. The reported lesions were located in the subcutis with no dermal extension.

COLLAGENOUS PAPULES OF THE EAR

There have been several reports of patients with papules, 1–4 mm in size, on the inner surfaces of the aural conchae and characterized histologically by sclerotic, hyalinized and focally clefted masses of collagen in the upper dermis.[757] The material abutted against the epidermis and contained scattered spirdle, stellate and binucleated fibroblasts. Superficial telangiectatic vessels were present. Earlier reports of the same entity have been included with lichen amyloidosus on the basis of positive histochemical staining for amyloid.[758] However, a recent publication has confirmed the presence of amyloid by electron microscopy and the use of the monoclonal antikeratin antibody EKH-4.[759]

CUTANEOUS MYXOMA

Cutaneous myxomas are rare tumors that may be associated with a systemic syndrome – Carney's complex – which includes cardiac myxomas, spotty cutaneous pigmentation and endocrine overactivity as its usual manifestations.[760] At other times, myxomas are solitary tumors, usually on the digits, and unassociated with any systemic abnormalities.[761,762] Cutaneous myxomas are discussed in further detail with the mucinoses (see Ch. 13, p. 413) because of their close resemblance to digital mucous cysts.

Histopathology[761,762]

Cutaneous myxomas are composed of stellate and spindle-shaped cells set in a loose myxoid stroma.

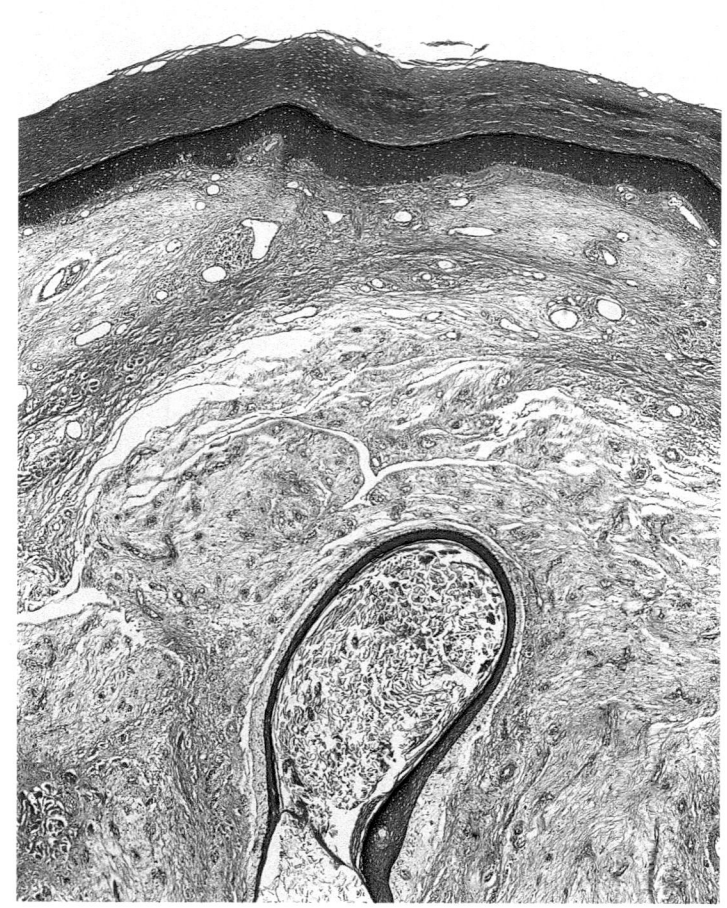

Fig. 34.32 **Superficial angiomyxoma.** There is a keratinous cyst in the center of the tumor, which has a vascular and myxoid stroma. (H & E)

SUPERFICIAL ANGIOMYXOMA

Angiomyxomas are a distinct variant of myxoma which may also contain epithelial elements (see p. 413).[763,764] They present as slow-growing, painless nodules that may involve the dermis and subcutis of any part of the body. One case was present at birth.[765] They usually measure 1–5 cm in diameter, but larger variants have been recorded.[763] Local recurrence may occur after surgical removal, but not metastasis.[766]

Histopathology[763]

Angiomyxomas are usually centered on the subcutis, but extension into the dermis is almost invariable. They are composed of spindle-shaped and stellate cells set in a copious, well-vascularized basophilic matrix (Fig. 34.32). Another distinguishing feature of these lesions is the presence, in more than half, of an epithelial component, which takes the form of epithelial strands or a keratin-filled cyst.[763]

The stromal cells are positive for vimentin and focally positive for smooth muscle actin, but negative for desmin, S100 and factor XIIIa.[767]

REFERENCES

Introduction

1 Schach CP, Smoller BR, Hudson AR, Horn TD. Immunohistochemical stains in dermatopathology. J Am Acad Dermatol 2000; 43: 1094–1100.

2 Suster S. Recent advances in the application of immunohistochemical markers for the diagnosis of soft tissue tumors. Semin Diagn Pathol 2000; 17: 225–235.

3 Steinman R, Hoffman L, Pope M. Maturation and migration of cutaneous dendritic cells. J Invest Dermatol 1995; 105: 2s–7s.

4 Nestle FO, Nickoloff BJ. A fresh morphological and functional look at dermal dendritic cells. J Cutan Pathol 1995; 22: 385–393.

5 Derrick EK, Barker JNWN, Khan A et al. The tissue distribution of factor XIIIa positive cells. Histopathology 1993; 22: 157–162.

6 Monteiro MR, Murphy EE, Galaria NA et al. Cytological alterations in dermal dendrocytes in vitro: evidence for transformation to a non-dendritic phenotype. Br J Dermatol 2000; 143: 84–90.

7 Wright-Browne V, McClain KL, Talpaz M et al. Physiology and pathophysiology of dendritic cells. Hum Pathol 1997; 28: 563–579.

8 Nestle FO, Burg G. Dendritic cells: role in skin diseases and therapeutic applications. Clin Exp Dermatol 1999; 24: 204–207.

9 Nestle FO, Filgueira L, Nickoloff BJ, Burg G. Human dermal dendritic cells process and present soluble protein antigens. J Invest Dermatol 1998; 110: 762–766.

10 Narvaez D, Kanitakis J, Faure M, Claudy A. Immunohistochemical study of CD34-positive dendritic cells of human dermis. Am J Dermatopathol 1996; 18: 283–288.

11 Silverman JS, Tamsen A. CD34 and factor XIIIa-positive microvascular dendritic cells and the family of fibrohistiocytic mesenchymal tumors. Am J Dermatopathol 1998; 20: 533–536.

12 Koizumi H, Kumakiri M, Yamanaka K et al. Dermal dendrocyte hamartoma with stubby white hair: a novel connective tissue hamartoma of infancy. J Am Acad Dermatol 1995; 32: 318–321.

13 Chang SE, Choi JH, Sung KJ et al. Congenital CD34-positive granular cell dendrocytosis. J Cutan Pathol 1999; 26: 253–258.

14 Silverman JS, Brustein S. Myxoid dermatofibrohistiocytoma: an indolent post-traumatic tumor composed of CD34+ epithelioid and dendritic cells and factor XIIIa+ dendrophages. J Cutan Pathol 1996; 23: 551–557.

15 Pursley HG, Williford PM, Groben PA, White WL. CD34-positive eruptive fibromas. J Cutan Pathol 1998; 25: 122–125.

16 Mentzel T. Myofibroblastic sarcomas: a brief review of sarcomas showing a myofibroblastic line of differentiation and discussion of the differential diagnosis. Curr Diagn Pathol 2001; 7: 17–24.

17 Schürch W, Seemayer TA, Gabbiani G. The myofibroblast. A quarter century after its discovery. Am J Surg Pathol 1998; 22: 141–147.

18 Diaz-Cascajo C. Histopathologic diagnosis of superficial soft tissue tumors, related lesions, and simulators. An algorithmic approach based on colors. Am J Dermatopathol 1999; 21: 193–199.

19 Diaz-Cascajo C. Histopathologic diagnosis of superficial soft tissue tumors, related lesions, and simulators: an algorithmic approach based on colors. Tumors with predominance of pink. Am J Dermatopathol 2000; 22: 191–196.

20 Pfeifer JD, Hill DA, O'Sullivan MJ, Dehner LP. Diagnostic gold standard for soft tissue tumours: morphology or molecular genetics? Histopathology 2000; 37: 485–500.

Acral angiofibromas

21 Ackerman AB, Kornberg R. Pearly penile papules. Acral angiofibromas. Arch Dermatol 1973; 108: 673–675.

22 Meigel WN, Ackerman AB. Fibrous papule of the face. Am J Dermatopathol 1979; 1: 329–340.

23 Reed RJ, Ackerman AB. Pathology of the adventitial dermis. Anatomic observations and biologic speculations. Hum Pathol 1973; 4: 207–217.

24 Nemeth AJ, Penneys NS. Factor XIIIa is expressed by fibroblasts in fibrovascular tumors. J Cutan Pathol 1989; 16: 266–271.

25 Cerio R, Griffiths CEM, Cooper KD et al. Characterization of factor XIIIa positive dermal dendritic cells in normal and inflamed skin. Br J Dermatol 1989; 121: 421–431.

26 Schaumburg-Lever G, Gehring B, Kaiserling E. Ultrastructural localization of factor XIIIa. J Cutan Pathol 1994; 21: 129–134.

27 Penneys NS. Factor XIII expression in the skin: observations and a hypothesis. J Am Acad Dermatol 1990; 22: 484–488.

28 Pinkus H. Perifollicular fibromas. Pure periadnexal adventitial tumors. Am J Dermatopathol 1979; 1: 341–342.

29 Butterworth T, Graham JH. Linear papular ectodermal-mesodermal hamartoma (hamartoma moniliformis). Arch Dermatol 1970; 101: 191–204.

30 Reed RJ. Cutaneous manifestations of neural crest disorders (neurocristopathies). Int J Dermatol 1977; 16: 807–826.

31 Schnur RE. Tuberous sclerosis. The persistent challenge of clinical diagnosis. Arch Dermatol 1995; 131: 1460–1462.

32 Sanchez NP, Wick MR, Perry HO. Adenoma sebaceum of Pringle: a clinicopathologic review, with a discussion of related pathologic entities. J Cutan Pathol 1981; 8: 395–403.

33 Sahoo B, Handa S, Kumar B. Tuberous sclerosis with macrodactyly. Pediatr Dermatol 2000; 17: 463–465.

34 Nickel WR, Reed WB. Tuberous sclerosis; special reference to the microscopic alterations in the cutaneous hamartomas. Arch Dermatol 1962; 85: 209–224.

35 Finch TM, Hindson C, Cotterill JA. Successful treatment of adenoma sebaceum with the potassium titanyl phosphate laser. Clin Exp Dermatol 1998; 23: 201–203.

36 Webb DW, Clarke A, Fryer A, Osborne JP. The cutaneous features of tuberous sclerosis. Br J Dermatol 1996; 135: 1–5.

37 Verhoef S, Vrtel R, van Essen T et al. Somatic mosaicism and clinical variation in tuberous sclerosis complex. Lancet 1995; 345: 202.

38 Jóźwiak S, Schwartz RA, Janniger CK et al. Skin lesions in children with tuberous sclerosis complex: their prevalence, natural course, and diagnostic significance. Int J Dermatol 1998; 37: 911–917.

39 Kwiatkowski DJ, Short MP. Tuberous sclerosis. Arch Dermatol 1994; 130: 348–354.

40 Wienecke R, Maize JC Jr, Lowy DR, DeClue JE. The tuberous sclerosis gene TSC2 is a tumor suppressor gene whose protein product co-localizes with its putative substrate RAP1 in the cis/medial golgi. J Invest Dermatol 1996; 106: 811 (abstract).

41 Yamashita Y, Ono J, Okada S et al. Analysis of all exons of TSC1 and TSC2 genes for germline mutations in Japanese patients with tuberous sclerosis: report of 10 mutations. Am J Med Genet 2000; 90: 123–126.

42 Osborne JP, Jones AC, Burley MW et al. Non-penetrance in tuberous sclerosis. Lancet 2000; 355: 1698.

43 Park Y-K, Hann SK. Cluster growths in adenoma sebaceum associated with tuberous sclerosis. J Am Acad Dermatol 1989; 20: 918–920.

44 McGrae JD Jr, Hashimoto K. Unilateral facial angiofibromas – a segmental form of tuberous sclerosis. Br J Dermatol 1996; 134: 727–730.

45 Silvestre JF, Bañuls J, Ramón R et al. Unilateral multiple facial angiofibromas: A mosaic form of tuberous sclerosis. J Am Acad Dermatol 2000; 43: 127–129.

46 Iitoyo M. Unilateral facial angiofibromas. Am J Dermatopathol 2000; 22: 353 (abstract).

47 Anliker MD, Dummer R, Burg G. Unilateral agminated angiofibromas: a segmental expression of tuberous sclerosis? Dermatology 1997; 195: 176–178.

48 Reed RJ, Hairston MA, Palomeque FE. The histologic identity of adenoma sebaceum and solitary melanocytic angiofibroma. Dermatol Int 1966; 5: 3–11.

49 Reed RJ. Fibrous papule of the face. Melanocytic angiofibroma. Am J Dermatopathol 1979; 1: 343–344.

50 Uysal H, Hemming FW. Changes in the expression and distribution of fibronectin, laminin and tenascin by cultured fibroblasts from skin lesions of patients with tuberous sclerosis. Br J Dermatol 1999; 141: 658–666.

51 Bhawan J, Edelstein L. Angiofibromas in tuberous sclerosis: a light and electron microscopic study. J Cutan Pathol 1977; 4: 300–307.

52 Jaffe AT, Heymann W, Schnur RE. Clustered angiofibromas on the ear of a patient with neurofibromatosis type 2. Arch Dermatol 1998; 134: 760–761.

53 Hoang-Xuan T, Steger JW. Adult-onset angiofibroma and multiple endocrine neoplasia type 1. J Am Acad Dermatol 1999; 41: 890–892.

54 Pack S, Turner ML, Zhuang Z et al. Cutaneous tumors in patients with multiple endocrine neoplasia type 1 show allelic deletion of the MEN1 gene. J Invest Dermatol 1998; 110: 438–440.

55 Darling TN, Skarulis MC, Steinberg SM et al. Multiple facial angiofibromas and collagenomas in patients with multiple endocrine neoplasia type 1. Arch Dermatol 1997; 133: 853–857.

56 Graham JH, Sanders JB, Johnson WC, Helwig EB. Fibrous papule of the nose; a clinicopathological study. J Invest Dermatol 1965; 45: 194–203.

57 Saylan T, Marks R, Wilson Jones E. Fibrous papule of the nose. Br J Dermatol 1971; 85: 111–118.

58 McGibbon DH, Wilson Jones E. Fibrous papule of the face (nose). Fibrosing nevocytic nevus. Am J Dermatopathol 1979; 1: 345–348.

59 Santa Cruz DJ, Prioleau PG. Fibrous papule of the face. An electron-microscopic study of two cases. Am J Dermatopathol 1979; 1: 349–352.

60 Ragaz A, Berezowsky V. Fibrous papule of the face. A study of five cases by electron microscopy. Am J Dermatopathol 1979; 1: 353–355.

61 Nemeth AJ, Penneys NS, Bernstein HB. Fibrous papule: a tumour of fibrohistiocytic cells that contain factor XIIIa. J Am Acad Dermatol 1988; 19: 1102–1106.

62 Cerio R, Rao BK, Spaull J, Wilson Jones E. An immunohistochemical study of fibrous papule of the nose: 25 cases. J Cutan Pathol 1989; 16: 194–198.

63 Cerio R, Wilson Jones E. Factor XIIIa positivity in fibrous papule. J Am Acad Dermatol 1990; 22: 138–139.

64 Guitart J, Bergfeld WF, Tuthill RJ. Fibrous papule of the nose with granular cells: two cases. J Cutan Pathol 1991; 18: 284–287.

65 Soyer HP, Kutzner H, Metze D et al. Clear-cell fibrous papule. J Cutan Pathol 1996; 23: 62 (abstract).

66 Spiegel J, Nadji M, Penneys NS. Fibrous papule: an immunohistochemical study with antibody to S-100 protein. J Am Acad Dermatol 1983; 9: 360–362.

67 Rosen LB, Suster S. Fibrous papule. A light microscopic and immunohistochemical study. Am J Dermatopathol 1988; 10: 109–115.

68 Kwan TH, Smoller BR, Schneider DR. α1-antitrypsin and lysozyme in fibrous papules and angiofibromas. J Am Acad Dermatol 1985; 12: 99–101.

69 Shea CR, Salob S, Reed JA et al. CD34-reactive fibrous papule of the nose. J Am Acad Dermatol 1996; 35: 342–345.

70 Johnson BL, Baxter DL. Pearly penile papules. Arch Dermatol 1964; 90: 166–167.

71 Glicksman JM, Freeman RG. Pearly penile papules. A statistical study of incidence. Arch Dermatol 1966; 93: 56–59.

72 Hyman AB, Brownstein MH. Tyson's "glands". Ectopic sebaceous glands and papillomatosis penis. Arch Dermatol 1969; 99: 31–36.

73 Porter WM, Bunker CB. Treatment of pearly penile papules with cryotherapy. Br J Dermatol 2000; 142: 847–848.

74 O'Neil CA, Hansen RC. Pearly penile papules on the shaft. Arch Dermatol 1995; 131: 491–492.

75 Vesper JL, Messina J, Glass LF, Fenske NA. Profound proliferating pearly penile papules. Int J Dermatol 1995; 34: 425–426.

76 Reed RJ, Elmer LC. Multiple acral fibrokeratomas (a variant of prurigo nodularis). Arch Dermatol 1971; 103: 286–297.

77 Kint A, Baran R, De Keyser H. Acquired (digital) fibrokeratoma. J Am Acad Dermatol 1985; 12: 816–821.

78 Herman PS, Datnow B. Acquired (digital) fibrokeratomas. Acta Derm Venereol 1974; 54: 73–76.

79 Bart RS, Andrade R, Kopf AW, Leider M. Acquired digital fibrokeratomas. Arch Dermatol 1968; 97: 120–129.

80 Hare PJ, Smith PAJ. Acquired (digital) fibrokeratoma. Br J Dermatol 1969; 81: 667–670.

81 Steel HH. Garlic-clove fibroma. JAMA 1965; 191: 1082–1083.

82 Cooper PH, Mackel SE. Acquired fibrokeratoma of the heel. Arch Dermatol 1985; 121: 386–388.

83 Zeller J, Friedman D, Clerici T, Revuz J. The significance of a single periungual fibroma: report of seven cases. Arch Dermatol 1995; 131: 1465–1466.

84 Kint A, Baran R. Histopathologic study of Koenen tumors. Are they different from acquired digital fibrokeratoma? J Am Acad Dermatol 1988; 18: 369–372.

85 Perrin C, Baran R. Invaginated fibrokeratoma with matrix differentiation: a new histological variant of acquired fibrokeratoma. Br J Dermatol 1994; 130: 654–657.

86 Dereure O, Savoy D, Doz F et al. Multiple acral fibromas in a patient with familial retinoblastoma: a cutaneous marker of tumour-suppressor gene germline mutation? Br J Dermatol 2000; 143: 856–859.

87 Moulin G, Balme B, Thomas L. Familial multiple acral mucinous fibrokeratomas. J Am Acad Dermatol 1998; 38: 999–1001.

88 Cahn RL. Acquired periungual fibrokeratoma. Arch Dermatol 1977; 113: 1564–1568.

89 Verallo VVM. Acquired digital fibrokeratomas. Br J Dermatol 1968; 80: 730–736.

90 Coskey RJ, Mehregan AH, Lupulescu AP. Multiple vascular fibromas and myxoid fibromas of the fingers. A histologic and ultrastructural study. J Am Acad Dermatol 1980; 2: 425–431.

91 Peterson JL, Read SI, Rodman OG. Familial myxovascular fibromas. J Am Acad Dermatol 1982; 6: 470–472.

Fibrous overgrowths, fibromatoses, myofibroblastic proliferations and fibrosarcoma

92 Allen PW. The fibromatoses: a clinicopathologic classification based on 140 cases. Part 1. Am J Surg Pathol 1977; 1: 255–270.

93 Jacob CI, Kumm RC. Benign anteromedial plantar nodules of childhood: a distinct form of plantar fibromatosis. Pediatr Dermatol 2000; 17: 472–474.

94 Pereyo NG, Heimer WL II. Extraabdominal desmoid tumor. J Am Acad Dermatol 1996; 34: 352–356.

95 Keltz M, DiCostanzo D, Desai P, Cohen SR. Infantile (desmoid-type) fibromatosis. Pediatr Dermatol 1995; 12: 149–151.

96 Connelly TJ. Development of Peyronie's and Dupuytren's diseases in an individual after single episodes of trauma: A case report and review of the literature. J Am Acad Dermatol 1999; 41: 106–108.

97 Lucas DR, Shroyer KR, McCarthy PJ et al. Desmoid tumor is a clonal cellular proliferation: PCR amplification of HUMARA for analysis of patterns of X-chromosome inactivation. Am J Surg Pathol 1997; 21: 306–311.

98 Merchant NB, Lewis JJ, Woodruff JM et al. Extremity and trunk desmoid tumors. A multifactorial analysis of outcome. Cancer 1999; 86: 2045–2052.

99 Li M, Cordon-Cardo C, Gerald WL, Rosai J. Desmoid fibromatosis is a clonal process. Hum Pathol 1996; 27: 939–943.

100 Simpson JL, Petropolis AA, Styles AR et al. Extra-abdominal desmoid tumor: an unusual subcutaneous lesion presenting as shoulder pain. Int J Dermatol 1998; 37: 780–784.

101 Michal M, Fetsch JF, Hes O, Miettinen M. Nuchal-type fibroma. A clinicopathologic study of 52 cases. Cancer 1999; 85: 156–163.

102 O'Connell JX, Janzen DL, Hughes TR. Nuchal fibrocartilaginous pseudotumor: a distinctive soft-tissue lesion associated with prior neck injury. Am J Surg Pathol 1997; 21: 836–840.

103 Wehrli BM, Weiss SW, Yandow S, Coffin CM. Gardner-associated fibromas (GAF) in young patients. A distinct fibrous lesion that identifies unsuspected Gardner syndrome and risk for fibromatosis. Am J Surg Pathol 2001; 25: 645–651.

104 Reissenweber N, Panuncio AL, De Anda G. Localized myofibroblastic proliferation in the neck of a patient with an IgG myeloma. Am J Dermatopathol 1997; 19: 265–270.

105 Huntley AC. Eruptive lipofibromata. Arch Dermatol 1983; 119: 612–614.

106 Margolis J, Margolis LS. Skin tags: a frequent sign of diabetes mellitus. N Engl J Med 1976; 294: 1184.

107 Kahana M, Grossman E, Feinstein A et al. Skin tags: a cutaneous marker for diabetes mellitus. Acta Derm Venereol 1987; 67: 175–177.

108 Agarwal JK, Nigam PK. Acrochordon: a cutaneous sign of carbohydrate intolerance. Australas J Dermatol 1987; 28: 132–133.

109 Crook MA. Skin tags and the atherogenic lipid profile. J Clin Pathol 2000; 53: 873–874.

110 Chobanian SJ, Van Ness MM, Winters C, Cattau EL. Skin tags as a marker for adenomatous polyps of the colon. Am Intern Med 1985; 103: 892–893.

111 Beitler M, Eng A, Kilgour H, Lebwohl M. Association between acrochordons and colonic polyps. J Am Acad Dermatol 1986; 14: 1042–1044.

112 Chobanian SJ, Van Ness MM, Winters C et al. Skin tags as a screening marker for colonic neoplasia. Gastrointest Endosc 1986; 32: 162.

113 Chobanian SJ. Skin tags and colonic polyps – a gastroenterologist's perspective. J Am Acad Dermatol 1987; 16: 407–409.

114 Lawrence JH, Tobias CA, Linfoot JA et al. Successful treatment of acromegaly: metabolic and clinical studies in 145 patients. J Clin Endocrinol Metabol 1970; 31: 180–198.

115 Dalton ADA, Coghill SB. No association between skin tags and colorectal adenomas. Lancet 1985; 1: 1332–1333.

116 Luk GD. Colonic polyps and acrochordons (skin tags) do not correlate in familial colonic polyposis kindreds. Ann Intern Med 1986; 104: 209–210.

117 Graffeo M, Cesari P, Buffoli F et al. Skin tags: markers for colonic polyps? J Am Acad Dermatol 1989; 21: 1029–1030.

118 Dianzani C, Calvieri S, Pierangeli A et al. The detection of human papillomavirus DNA in skin tags. Br J Dermatol 1998; 138: 649–651.

119 Wong RC, Ellis CN. Physiologic skin changes in pregnancy. J Am Acad Dermatol 1984; 10: 929–940.

120 Banik R, Lubach D. Skin tags: localization and frequencies according to sex and age. Dermatologica 1987; 174: 180–183.

121 Field LM. A giant pendulous fibrolipoma. J Dermatol Surg Oncol 1982; 8: 54–55.

122 Kitajima T, Okuwa T, Imamura S. Giant pendulous fibroma with unusual clinical appearance arising on the scrotum. Clin Exp Dermatol 1994; 19: 278–279.

123 Worm M, Skarabis W, Audring H et al. Nevoid bag-like soft fibromas. Dermatology 1999; 199: 167–168.

124 Moyal-Barracco M, Leibowitch M, Orth G. Vestibular papillae of the vulva. Lack of evidence for human papillomavirus etiology. Arch Dermatol 1990; 126: 1594–1598.

125 Groisman GM, Polak-Charcon S. Fibroepithelial polyps of the anus. Am J Surg Pathol 1998; 22: 70–76.

126 Kayashima K, Kitoh M, Ono T. Infantile perianal pyramidal protrusion. Arch Dermatol 1996; 132: 1481–1484.

127 Waisman M. Cutaneous papillomas of the neck. Papillomatous seborrheic keratoses. South Med J 1957; 50: 725–731.

128 Adams BB, Mutasim DF. Elastic tissue in fibroepithelial polyps. Am J Dermatopathol 1999; 21: 446–448.

129 Eads TJ, Chuang T-Y, Fabré VC et al. The utility of submitting fibroepithelial polyps for histological examination. Arch Dermatol 1996; 132: 1459–1462.

130 Brodell RT, Pokorney DR. Fibroepithelial polyps and pathologic evaluation. Arch Dermatol 1997; 133: 915.

131 Williams BT, Barr RJ, Barrett TL et al. Cutaneous pseudosarcomatous polyp: a histological and immunohistochemical study. J Cutan Pathol 1996; 23: 189–193.

132 Zelger BG, Zelger B. Cutaneous pseudosarcomatous polyp – another variant of dermal lipoma or only an "ancient" skin tag? J Cutan Pathol 1997; 24: 390–391.

133 Beer TW, Carr NJ. Fibroepithelial polyps of the anus with epithelial vacuolation. Am J Surg Pathol 1999; 23: 488–489.

134 Kamino H, Lee JY-Y, Berke A. Pleomorphic fibroma of the skin: a benign neoplasm with cytologic atypia. A clinicopathologic study of eight cases. Am J Surg Pathol 1989; 13: 107–113.

135 Garcia-Doval I, Casas L, Toribio J. Pleomorphic fibroma of the skin, a form of sclerotic fibroma: an immunohistochemical study. Clin Exp Dermatol 1998; 23: 22–24.

136 Miliauskas JR. Myxoid cutaneous pleomorphic fibroma. Histopathology 1994; 24: 179–181.

137 Hassanein A, Telang G, Benedetto E, Spielvogel R. Subungual myxoid pleomorphic fibroma. Am J Dermatopathol 1998; 20: 502–505.

138 Rudolph P, Schubert C, Zelger BG et al. Differential expression of CD34 and Ki-M1p in pleomorphic fibroma and dermatofibroma with monster cells. Am J Dermatopathol 1999; 21: 414–419.

139 Ioffreda MD, Kantor GR, Abrams BJ et al. Cutaneous pleomorphic fibroma. J Cutan Pathol 1997; 24: 104 (abstract).

140 Layfield LJ, Fain JS. Pleomorphic fibroma of skin. Arch Pathol Lab Med 1991; 115: 1046–1049.

141 Rapini RP, Golitz LE. Sclerotic fibromas of the skin. J Am Acad Dermatol 1989; 20: 266–271.

142 Starink TM, Meijer CJLM, Brownstein MH. The cutaneous pathology of Cowden's disease: new findings. J Cutan Pathol 1985; 12: 83–93.

143 McCalmont TH. Sclerotic fibroma: a fossil no longer. J Cutan Pathol 1994; 21: 82–85.

144 Requena L, Gutiérrez J, Sánchez Yus E. Multiple sclerotic fibromas of the skin. A cutaneous marker of Cowden's disease. J Cutan Pathol 1992; 19: 346–351.

145 Herrera Sánchez M, Suárez-Fernández R, del Cerro Heredero M et al. Sclerotic fibroma. Dermatology 1998; 196: 429–430.

146 Metcalf JS, Maize JC, LeBoit PE. Circumscribed storiform collagenoma (sclerosing fibroma). Am J Dermatopathol 1991; 13: 122–129.

147 Shitabata PK, Crouch EC, Fitzgibbon JF et al. Cutaneous sclerotic fibroma. Immunohistochemical evidence of a fibroblastic neoplasm with ongoing type I collagen synthesis. Am J Dermatopathol 1995; 17: 339–343.

148 Cohen PR, Tschen JA, Abaya-Blas R, Cochran RJ. Recurrent sclerotic fibroma of the skin. Am J Dermatopathol 1999; 21: 571–574.

149 Lo WL, Wong CK. Solitary sclerotic fibroma. J Cutan Pathol 1990; 17: 269–273.

150 Chang S-N, Chun SI, Moon TK, Park W-H. Solitary sclerotic fibroma of the skin. Degenerated sclerotic change of inflammatory conditions, especially folliculitis. Am J Dermatopathol 2000; 22: 22–25.

151 Pujol RM, de Castro F, Schroeter AL, Su WPD. Solitary sclerotic fibroma of the skin: a sclerotic dermatofibroma? Am J Dermatopathol 1996; 18: 620–624.

152 Satoh T, Katsumata M, Asaka Y et al. Solitary sclerotic fibroma of the skin. Int J Dermatol 1991; 30: 505–506.

153 Hanft VN, Shea CR, McNutt NS et al. Expression of CD34 in sclerotic ("plywood") fibromas. Am J Dermatopathol 2000; 22: 17–21.

154 Pillay P, Essa AS, Chetty R. Pacinian collagenoma. Br J Dermatol 1999; 141: 119–122.

155 Martin-López R, Feal-Cortizas C, Fraga J. Pleomorphic sclerotic fibroma. Dermatology 1999; 198: 69–72.

156 Rudolph P, Schubert C, Harms D, Parwaresch R. Giant cell collagenoma. A benign dermal tumor with distinctive multinucleate cells. Am J Surg Pathol 1998; 22: 557–563.

157 Jang J-G, Jung H-H, Suh K-S, Kim S-T. Desmoplastic fibroblastoma (collagenous fibroma). Am J Dermatopathol 1999; 21: 256–258.

158 Weisberg NK, DiCaudo DJ, Meland NB. Collagenous fibroma (desmoplastic fibroblastoma). J Am Acad Dermatol 1999; 41: 292–294.

159 Junkins-Hopkins JM, Johnson WC. Desmoplastic fibroblastoma. J Cutan Pathol 1998; 25: 450–454.

160 Wesche WA, Cutlan RT. Collagenous fibroma: case report of a recently described benign soft tissue tumor. J Cutan Pathol 2000; 27: 576 (abstract).

161 Miettinen M, Fetsch JF. Collagenous fibroma (desmoplastic fibroblastoma): a clinicopathologic analysis of 63 cases of a distinctive soft tissue lesion with stellate-shaped fibroblasts. Hum Pathol 1998; 29: 676–682.

162 Nielsen GP, O'Connell JX, Dickersin GR, Rosenberg AE. Collagenous fibroma (desmoplastic fibroblastoma): a report of seven cases. Mod Pathol 1996; 9: 781–785.

163 Morginson WJ. Discrete keratodermas over the knuckle and finger articulations. Arch Dermatol 1955; 71: 349–353.

164 Sehgal VN, Singh M, Saxena HMK, Nayar M. Primary knuckle pads. Clin Exp Dermatol 1979; 4: 337–339.

165 Köse O, Baloğlu H. Knuckle pads, leukonychia and deafness. Int J Dermatol 1996; 35: 728–729.

166 Stankler L. Pseudoxanthoma elasticum with a knuckle pad on the thumb. Acta Derm Venereol 1967; 47: 263–266.

167 Peterson CM, Barnes CJ, Davis LS. Knuckle pads: does knuckle cracking play an etiologic role? Pediatr Dermatol 2000; 17: 450–452.

168 Allison JR Jr, Allison JR Sr. Knuckle pads. Arch Dermatol 1966; 93: 311–316.

169 Abulafia J, Vignale RA. Degenerative collagenous plaques of the hands and acrokeratoelastoidosis: pathogenesis and relationship with knuckle pads. Int J Dermatol 2000; 39: 424–432.

170 Curley RK, Hudson PM, Marsden RA. Pachydermodactyly: a rare form of digital fibromatosis – report of four cases. Clin Exp Dermatol 1991; 16: 121–123.

171 Kopera D, Soyer HP, Kerl H. An update on pachydermodactyly and a report of three additional cases. Br J Dermatol 1995; 133: 433–437.

172 Draluck JC, Kopf AW, Hodak E. Pachydermodactyly: first report in a woman. J Am Acad Dermatol 1992; 27: 303–305.

173 Sola A, Vazquez-Doval J, Sola J, Quintanilla E. Pachydermodactyly transgrediens. Int J Dermatol 1992; 31: 796–797.

174 Iraci S, Bianchi L, Innocenzi D et al. Pachydermodactyly: a case of an unusual type of reactive digital fibromatosis. Arch Dermatol 1993; 129: 247–248.

175 Kang BD, Hong SH, Kim IH et al. Two cases of pachydermodactyly. Int J Dermatol 1997; 36: 768–772.

176 Tompkins SD, McNutt NS, Shea CR. Distal pachydermodactyly. J Am Acad Dermatol 1998; 38: 359–362.

177 Kopera D, Soyer HP, Kerl H. Pachydermodactyly. Int J Dermatol 1999; 38: 237.

178 Meunier L, Pailler C, Barneon G, Meynadier J. Pachydermodactyly or acquired digital fibromatosis. Br J Dermatol 1994; 131: 744–746.

179 Shimizu S, Hashimoto H, Enjoji M. Nodular fasciitis: an analysis of 250 patients. Pathology 1984; 16: 161–166.

180 Krasovec M, Burg G. Nodular fasciitis (pseudotumor of the skin). Dermatology 1999; 198: 431–433.

181 Price SK, Kahn LB, Saxe N. Dermal and intravascular fasciitis: unusual variants of nodular fasciitis. Am J Dermatopathol 1993; 15: 539–543.

182 Goodlad JR, Fletcher CDM. Intradermal variant of nodular 'fasciitis'. Histopathology 1990; 17: 569–571.

183 Samaratunga H, Searle J, O'Loughlin B. Intravascular fasciitis: a case report and review of the literature. Pathology 1996; 28: 8–11.

184 Lai FM-M, Lam WY. Nodular fasciitis of the dermis. J Cutan Pathol 1993; 20: 66–69.

185 Meffert JJ, Kennard CD, Davis TL, Quinn BD. Intradermal nodular fasciitis presenting as an eyelid mass. Int J Dermatol 1996; 35: 548–552.

186 Mehregan AH. Nodular fasciitis. Arch Dermatol 1966; 93: 204–210.

187 Bernstein KE, Lattes R. Nodular (pseudosarcomatous) fasciitis, a nonrecurrent lesion: clinicopathologic study of 134 cases. Cancer 1982; 49: 1668–1678.

188 Tay Y-K, Tan S-H. A subcutaneous nodule on the face. Pediatr Dermatol 2000; 17: 487–489.

89 Graham BS, Barrett TL, Goltz RW. Nodular fasciitis: Response to intralesional corticosteroids. J Am Acad Dermatol 1999; 40: 490–492.

190 Oshiro Y, Fukuda T, Tsuneyoshi M. Fibrosarcoma versus fibromatoses and cellular nodular fasciitis. Am J Surg Pathol 1994; 18: 712–719.

191 El-Jabbour JN, Wilson GD, Bennett MH et al. Flow cytometric study of nodular fasciitis, proliferative fasciitis, and proliferative myositis. Hum Pathol 1991; 22: 1146–1149.

192 Lauer DH, Enzinger FM. Cranial fasciitis of childhood. Cancer 1980; 45: 401–406.

193 Patterson JW, Moran SL, Konerding H. Cranial fasciitis. Arch Dermatol 1989; 125: 674–678.

194 Price EB Jr, Silliphant WM, Shuman R. Nodular fasciitis: a clinicopathologic analysis of 65 cases. Am J Clin Pathol 1961; 35: 122–136.

195 Allen PW. Nodular fasciitis. Pathology 1972; 4: 9–26.

196 Beer K, Katz S, Medenica M. Intravascular fasciitis. Int J Dermatol 1996; 35: 147–148.

197 Kwittken J, Branche M. Fasciitis ossificans. Am J Clin Pathol 1969; 51: 251–255.

198 Daroca PJ Jr, Pulitzer DR, LoCicero J III. Ossifying fasciitis. Arch Pathol Lab Med 1982; 106: 682–685.

199 Innocenzi D, Giustini S, Barduagni F et al. Ossifying fasciitis of the nose. J Am Acad Dermatol 1997; 37: 357–361.

200 El-Jabbour JN, Bennett MH, Burke MM et al. Proliferative myositis. An immunohistochemical and ultrastructural study. Am J Surg Pathol 1991; 15: 654–659.

201 Turner R, Robson A, Motley R. Proliferative myositis: an unusual cause of multiple subcutaneous nodules. Clin Exp Dermatol 1997; 22: 101–103.

202 Chung EB, Enzinger FM. Proliferative fasciitis. Cancer 1975; 36: 1450–1485.

203 Diaz-Flores L, Martin Herrera AI, Garcia Montelongo R, Gutierrez Garcia R. Proliferative fasciitis: ultrastructure and histogenesis. J Cutan Pathol 1989; 16: 85–92.

204 Kiryu H, Takeshita H, Hori Y. Proliferative fasciitis. Report of a case with histopathologic and immunohistochemical studies. Am J Dermatopathol 1997; 19: 396–399.

205 Montgomery EA, Meis JM. Nodular fasciitis. Its morphologic spectrum and immunohistochemical profile. Am J Surg Pathol 1991; 15: 942–948.

206 Meis JM, Enzinger FM. Proliferative fasciitis and myositis of childhood. Am J Surg Pathol 1992; 16: 364–372.

207 Wirman JA. Nodular fasciitis, a lesion of myofibroblasts. An ultrastructural study. Cancer 1976; 38: 2378–2389.

208 Baldassano MF, Rosenberg AE, Flotte TJ. Atypical decubital fibroplasia: a series of three cases. J Cutan Pathol 1998; 25: 149–152.

209 Manson CM, Hirsch PJ, Coyne JD. Post-operative spindle cell nodule of the vulva. Histopathology 1995; 26: 571–574.

210 Wick MR, Mills SE, Ritter JH, Lind AC. Postoperative/posttraumatic spindle cell nodule of the skin. The dermal analogue of nodular fasciitis. Am J Dermatopathol 1999; 21: 220–224.

21 Chan JKC. Solitary fibrous tumour – everywhere, and a diagnosis in vogue. Histopathology 1997; 31: 568–576.

212 Okamura JM, Barr RJ, Battifora H. Solitary fibrous tumor of the skin. Am J Dermatopathol 1997; 19: 515–518.

213 Cowper SE, Kilpatrick T, Proper S, Morgan MB. Solitary fibrous tumor of the skin. Am J Dermatopathol 1999; 21: 213–219.

214 Morgan MB, Smoller BR. Solitary fibrous tumors are immunophenotypically distinct from mesothelioma(s). J Cutan Pathol 2000; 27: 451–454.

215 Vadmal MS, Pellegrini AE. Solitary fibrous tumor of the vagina. Am J Dermatopathol 2000; 22: 83–86.

216 Smith KJ, Skelton HG. Solitary fibrous tumor. Am J Dermatopathol 2001; 23: 81–82.

217 Yokoi T, Tsuzuki T, Yatabe Y et al. Solitary fibrous tumour: significance of p53 and CD34 immunoreactivity in its malignant transformation. Histopathology 1998; 32: 423–432.

218 Guillou L, Fletcher CDM. Newer entities in soft tissue tumours. Curr Diagn Pathol 1997; 4: 210–221.

219 Sigel JE, Goldblum JR. Solitary fibrous tumor of the skin. Am J Dermatopathol 2001; 23: 275–276.

220 Guillou L, Gebhard S, Coindre J-M. Orbital and extraorbital giant cell angiofibroma: a giant cell-rich variant of solitary fibrous tumor? Am J Surg Pathol 2000; 24: 971–979.

221 Silverman JS, Tamsen A. A cutaneous case of giant cell angiofibroma occurring with dermatofibrosarcoma protuberans and showing bimodal CD34+ fibroblastic and FXIIIa+ histiocytic immunophenotype. J Cutan Pathol 1998; 25: 265–270.

222 Reye RDK. A consideration of certain "fibromatous tumours" of infancy. J Pathol Bacteriol 1956; 72: 149–154.

223 Enzinger FM. Fibrous hamartoma of infancy. Cancer 1965; 18: 241–248.

224 Maung R, Lindsay R, Trevenen C, Hwang WS. Fibrous hamartoma of infancy. Hum Pathol 1987; 18: 652–653.

225 Cooper PH. Fibrous proliferations of infancy and childhood. J Cutan Pathol 1992; 19: 257–267.

226 Scott DM, Peña JR, Omura EF. Fibrous hamartoma of infancy. J Am Acad Dermatol 1999; 41: 857–859.

227 Mitchell ML, di Sant'Agnese PA, Gerber JE. Fibrous hamartoma of infancy. Hum Pathol 1982; 13: 586–588.

228 Harris CJ, Das S, Vogt PJ. Fibrous hamartoma of infancy in the scrotum. J Urol 1982; 127: 781–782.

229 Alburkerk J, Wexler H, Dana M, Silverman J. A case of fibrous hamartoma of infancy. J Pediatr Surg 1979; 14: 80–82.

230 Robbins LB, Hoffman S, Kahn S. Fibrous hamartoma of infancy. Case report. Plast Reconstr Surg 1970; 46: 197–200.

231 Allen PW. The fibromatoses: a clinicopathologic classification based on 140 cases. Part 2. Am J Surg Pathol 1977; 1: 305–321.

232 King DF, Barr RJ, Hirose FM. Fibrous hamartoma of infancy. J Dermatol Surg Oncol 1979; 5: 482–483.

233 Groisman G, Lichtig C. Fibrous hamartoma of infancy: an immunohistochemical and ultrastructural study. Hum Pathol 1991; 22: 914–918.

234 Greco MA, Schinella RA, Vuletin JC. Fibrous hamartoma of infancy: an ultrastructural study. Hum Pathol 1984; 15: 717–723.

235 Paller AS, Gonzalez-Crussi F, Sherman JO. Fibrous hamartoma of infancy. Eight additional cases and a review of the literature. Arch Dermatol 1989; 125: 88–91.

236 Iwasaki H, Kikuchi M, Ohtsuki I et al. Infantile digital fibromatosis. Identification of actin filaments in cytoplasmic inclusions by heavy meromyosin binding. Cancer 1933; 52: 1653–1661.

237 Reye RDK. Recurring digital fibrous tumors of childhood. Arch Pathol 1965; 80: 228–231.

238 Viale G, Doglioni C, Iuzzolino P et al. Infantile digital fibromatosis-like tumour (inclusion body fibromatosis) of adulthood: report of two cases with ultrastructural and immunocytochemical findings. Histopathology 1988; 12: 415–424.

239 Allen PW. Recurring digital fibrous tumours of childhood. Pathology 1972; 4: 215–223.

240 Azam SH, Nicholas JL. Recurring infantile digital fibromatosis: report of two cases. J Pediatr Surg 1995; 30: 89–90.

241 Santa Cruz DJ, Reiner CB. Recurrent digital fibroma of childhood. J Cutan Pathol 1978; 5: 339–346.

242 Sarma DP, Hoffman EO. Infantile digital fibroma-like tumor in an adult. Arch Dermatol 1980; 116: 578–579.

243 Plusjé LGJM, Bastiaens M, Chang A, Hogendoorn PCW. Infantile-type digital fibromatosis tumour in an adult. Br J Dermatol 2000; 143: 1107–1108.

244 Miyamoto T, Mihara M, Hagari Y et al. Posttraumatic occurrence of infantile digital fibromatosis. A histologic and electron microscopic study. Arch Dermatol 1986; 122: 915–918.

245 Ishii N, Matsui K, Ichiyama S et al. A case of infantile digital fibromatosis showing spontaneous regression. Br J Dermatol 1989; 121: 129–133.

246 Rimareix F, Bardot J, Andrac L et al. Infantile digital fibroma: Report on eleven cases. Eur J Pediatr Surg 1997; 7: 345–348.

247 Breuning MH, Oranje AP, Langemeijer RAThM et al. Recurrent digital fibroma, focal dermal hypoplasia, and limb malformations. Am J Med Genet 2000; 94: 91–101.

248 Burry AF, Kerr JFR, Pope JH. Recurring digital fibrous tumour of childhood: an electron microscopic and virological study. Pathology 1970; 2: 287–291.

249 Mehregan AH, Nabai H, Matthews JE. Recurring digital fibrous tumor of childhood. Arch Dermatol 1972; 106: 375–378.

250 Zhu WY, Xia MY, Huang YF et al. Infantile digital fibromatosis: ultrastructural human papillomavirus and herpes simplex virus DNA observation. Pediatr Dermatol 1991; 8: 137–139.

251 Choi KC, Hashimoto K, Setoyama M et al. Infantile digital fibromatosis. Immunohistochemical and immunoelectron microscopic studies. J Cutan Pathol 1990; 17: 225–232.

252 Mukai M, Torikata C, Iri H et al. Immunohistochemical identification of aggregated actin filaments in formalin-fixed, paraffin-embedded sections. 1. A study of infantile digital fibromatosis by a new pretreatment. Am J Surg Pathol 1992; 16: 110–115.

253 Mehregan AH. Superficial fibrous tumors in childhood. J Cutan Pathol 1981; 8: 321–324.

254 Shapiro L. Infantile digital fibromatosis and aponeurotic fibroma. Arch Dermatol 1969; 99: 37–42.

255 Bhawan J, Bacchetta C, Joris I, Majno G. A myofibroblastic tumor. Infantile digital fibroma (recurrent digital fibrous tumor of childhood). Am J Pathol 1979; 94: 19–36.

256 Zina AM, Rampini E, Fulcheri E et al. Recurrent digital fibromatosis of childhood. An ultrastructural and immunohistochemical study of two cases. Am J Dermatopathol 1986; 8: 22–26.

257 Yun K. Infantile digital fibromatosis. Immunohistochemical and ultrastructural observations of cytoplasmic inclusions. Cancer 1988; 61: 500–507.

258 Diaz-Cascajo C, Metze D. Angiofibroblastoma of the skin: a histological, immunohistochemical and ultrastructural report of two cases of an undescribed fibrous tumour. Histopathology 1999; 35: 109–113.

259 Skálová A, Michal M, Husek K et al. Aggressive angiomyxoma of the pelvioperineal region: immunohistological and ultrastructural study of seven cases. Am J Dermatopathol 1993; 15: 446–451.

260 Tsang WYW, Chan JKC, Lee KC et al. Aggressive angiomyxoma. A report of four cases occurring in men. Am J Surg Pathol 1992; 16: 1059–1065.

261 Fetsch JF, Laskin WB, Lefkowitz M et al. Aggressive angiomyxoma. A clinicopathologic study of 29 female patients. Cancer 1996; 78: 79–90.

262 Granter SR, Nucci MR, Fletcher CDM. Aggressive angiomyxoma: reappraisal of its relationship to angiomyofibroblastoma in a series of 16 cases. Histopathology 1997; 30: 3–10.

263 Zamecnik M, Skalova A, Michal M, Gomolcak P. Aggressive angiomyxoma with multinucleated giant cells. A lesion mimicking liposarcoma. Am J Dermatopathol 2000; 22: 368–371.

264 Heymans O, Médot M, Hermanns-Lê T et al. Recurrent pleomorphic solitary angiomyxoma of the face. Dermatology 1999; 198: 195–197.

265 Laskin WB, Fetsch JF, Mostofi FK. Angiomyofibroblastomalike tumor of the male genital tract. Am J Surg Pathol 1998; 22: 6–16.

266 Fletcher CDM, Tsang WYW, Fisher C et al. Angiomyofibroblastoma of the vulva. A benign neoplasm distinct from aggressive angiomyxoma. Am J Surg Pathol 1992; 16: 373–382.

267 Nielsen GP, Young RH, Dickersin GR, Rosenberg AE. Angiomyofibroblastoma of the vulva with sarcomatous transformation ("angiomyofibrosarcoma"). Am J Surg Pathol 1997; 21: 1104–1108.

268 Goodlad JR, Fletcher CDM. Recent developments in soft tissue tumours. Histopathology 1995; 27: 103–120.

269 Laskin WB, Fetsch JF, Tavassoli FA. Angiomyofibroblastoma of the female genital tract. Analysis of 17 cases including a lipomatous variant. Hum Pathol 1997; 28: 1046–1055.

270 Nucci MR, Granter SR, Fletcher CDM. Cellular angiofibroma: a benign neoplasm distinct from angiomyofibroblastoma and spindle cell lipoma. Am J Surg Pathol 1997; 21: 636–644.

271 Garijo MF, Val-Bernal JF. Extravulvar subcutaneous cellular angiofibroma. J Cutan Pathol 1998; 25: 327–332.

271a Hügel H. Die plaqueförmige dermale fibromatose. Hautarzt 1991; 42: 223–226.

272 Kamino H, Reddy VB, Gero M, Greco MA. Dermatomyofibroma. A benign cutaneous, plaque-like proliferation of fibroblasts and myofibroblasts in young adults. J Cutan Pathol 1992; 19: 85–93.

273 Rose C, Bröcker E-B. Dermatomyofibroma: case report and review. Pediatr Dermatol 1999; 16: 456–459.

274 Mortimore RJ, Whitehead KJ. Dermatomyofibroma: a report of two cases, one occurring in a child. Australas J Dermatol 2001; 42: 22–25.

275 Cooper PH. Dermatomyofibroma: a case of fibromatosis revisited. J Cutan Pathol 1992; 19: 81–82.

276 Trotter MJ, McGregor GI, O'Connell JX. Linear dermatomyofibroma. Clin Exp Dermatol 1996; 21: 307–309.

277 Poomeechaiwong S, Bonelli JE, DeSpain JD et al. Myoid fibroma: piloleiomyoma-like fibroma of the skin. J Cutan Pathol 1989; 16: 320 (abstract).

278 Hügel H. Plaque-like dermal fibromatosis/dermatomyofibroma. J Cutan Pathol 1993; 20: 94.

279 Mentzel T, Calonje E, Fletcher CDM. Dermatomyofibroma: additional observations on a distinctive cutaneous myofibroblastic tumour with emphasis on differential diagnosis. Br J Dermatol 1993; 129: 69–73.

280 Colomé MI, Sánchez RL. Dermatomyofibroma: report of two cases. J Cutan Pathol 1994; 21: 371–376.

281 Ng WK, Cheung MF, Ma L. Dermatomyofibroma: further support of its myofibroblastic nature by electronmicroscopy. Histopathology 1996; 29: 181–183.

282 Chung EB, Enzinger FM. Infantile myofibromatosis. Cancer 1981; 48: 1807–1818.

283 Williams JO, Schrum D. Congenital fibrosarcoma: report of a case in a newborn infant. Arch Pathol 1951; 51: 548–552.

284 Stout AP. Juvenile fibromatoses. Cancer 1954; 7: 953–978.

285 Kauffman SL, Stout AP. Congenital mesenchymal tumors. Cancer 1965; 18: 460–476.

286 Benjamin SP, Mercer RD, Hawk WA. Myofibroblastic contraction in spontaneous regression of multiple congenital mesenchymal hamartomas. Cancer 1977; 40: 2343–2352.

287 Fletcher CDM, Achu P, Van Noorden S, McKee PH. Infantile myofibromatosis: a light microscopic, histochemical and immunohistochemical study suggesting true smooth muscle differentiation. Histopathology 1987; 11: 245–258.

288 Requena L, Kutzner H, Hügel H et al. Cutaneous adult myofibroma: a vascular neoplasm. J Cutan Pathol 1996; 23: 445–457.

289 Granter SR, Badizadegan K, Fletcher CDM. Myofibromatosis in adults, glomangiopericytoma, and myopericytoma. A spectrum of tumors showing perivascular myoid differentiation. Am J Surg Pathol 1998; 22: 513–525.

290 Stanford D, Rogers M. Dermatological presentations of infantile myofibromatosis: a review of 27 cases. Australas J Dermatol 2000; 41: 156–161.

291 Parker RK, Mallory SB, Baker GF. Infantile myofibromatosis. Pediatr Dermatol 1991; 8: 129–132.

292 Daimaru Y, Hashimoto H, Enjoji M. Myofibromatosis in adults (adult counterpart of infantile myofibromatosis). Am J Surg Pathol 1989; 13: 859–865.

293 Wolfe JT III, Cooper PH. Solitary cutaneous "infantile" myofibroma in a 49-year-old woman. Hum Pathol 1990; 21: 562–564.

294 Guitart J, Ritter JH, Wick MR. Solitary cutaneous myofibroma(tosis) in adults. J Cutan Pathol 1996; 23: 51 (abstract).

295 Val-Bernal JF, Garijo MF. Solitary cutaneous myofibroma of the glans penis. Am J Dermatopathol 1996; 18: 317–321.

296 Guitart J, Ritter JH, Wick MR. Solitary cutaneous myofibromas in adults: report of six cases and discussion of differential diagnosis. J Cutan Pathol 1996; 23: 437–444.

297 Goldberg NS, Bauer BS, Kraus H et al. Infantile myofibromatosis: a review of clinicopathology with perspectives on new treatment choices. Pediatr Dermatol 1988; 5: 37–46.

298 Dimson OG, Drolet BA, Southern JF et al. Congenital generalized myofibromatosis in a neonate. Arch Dermatol 2000; 136: 597–600.

299 Dimmick JE, Wood WS. Congenital multiple fibromatosis. Am J Dermatopathol 1983; 5: 289–295.

300 Bellman B, Wooming G, Landsman L et al. Infantile myofibromatosis: a case report. Pediatr Dermatol 1991; 8: 306–309.

301 Iijima S, Suzuki R, Otsuka F. Solitary form of infantile myofibromatosis: a histologic, immunohistochemical, and electronmicroscopic study of a regressing tumor over a 20-month period. Am J Dermatopathol 1999; 21: 375–380.

302 Jennings TA, Sabetta J, Duray PH et al. Infantile myofibromatosis. Evidence for an autosomal-dominant disorder. Am J Surg Pathol 1984; 8: 529–538.

303 Spraker MK, Stack C, Esterly NB. Congenital generalized fibromatosis: a review of the literature and report of a case associated with porencephaly, hemiatrophy, and cutis marmorata telangiectatica congenita. J Am Acad Dermatol 1984; 10: 365–371.

304 Venencie PY, Bigel P, Desgruelles C et al. Infantile myofibromatosis. Report of two cases in one family. Br J Dermatol 1987; 117: 255–259.

305 Variend S, Bax NMA, Van Gorp J. Are infantile myofibromatosis, congenital fibrosarcoma and congenital haemangiopericytoma histogenetically related? Histopathology 1995; 26: 57–62.

306 Zelger BWH, Calonje E, Sepp N et al. Monophasic cellular variant of infantile myofibromatosis. An unusual histopathologic pattern in two siblings. Am J Dermatopathol 1995; 17: 131–138.

307 Bracko M, Cindro L, Golouh R. Familial occurrence of infantile myofibromatosis. Cancer 1992; 69: 1294–1299.

308 Meis-Kindblom JM, Kjellström C, Kindblom L-G. Inflammatory fibrosarcoma: update, reappraisal, and perspective on its place in the spectrum of inflammatory myofibroblastic tumors. Semin Diagn Pathol 1998; 15: 133–143.

309 Carlson JA, Ackerman AB, Fletcher CDM, Zelger B. A cutaneous spindle-cell lesion. Am J Dermatopathol 2001; 23: 62–66.

310 Coffin CM, Watterson J, Priest JR, Dehner LP. Extrapulmonary inflammatory myofibroblastic tumor (inflammatory pseudotumor). Am J Surg Pathol 1995; 19: 859–872.

311 Donner LR, Trompler RA, White RR IV. Progression of inflammatory myofibroblastic tumor (inflammatory pseudotumor) of soft tissue into sarcoma after several recurrences. Hum Pathol 1996; 27: 1095–1098.

312 Coffin CM, Dehner LP, Meis-Kindblom JM. Inflammatory myofibroblastic tumor, inflammatory fibrosarcoma, and related lesions: an historical review with differential diagnostic considerations. Semin Diagn Pathol 1998; 15: 102–110.

313 Ramachandra S, Hollowood K, Bisceglia M, Fletcher CDM. Inflammatory pseudotumour of soft tissues: a clinicopathological and immunohistochemical analysis of 18 cases. Histopathology 1995; 27: 313–323.

314 Vadmal MS, Pellegrini AE. Inflammatory myofibroblastic tumor of the skin. Am J Dermatopathol 1999; 21: 449–453.

315 Puretic S, Puretic B, Fiser-Herman M, Adamcic M. A unique form of mesenchymal dysplasia. Br J Dermatol 1962; 74: 8–19.

316 Kitano Y. Juvenile hyalin fibromatosis. Arch Dermatol 1976; 112: 86–88.

317 Kitano Y, Horiki M, Aoki T, Sagami S. Two cases of juvenile hyalin fibromatosis. Arch Dermatol 1972; 106: 877–883.

318 Mayer-da-Silva A, Poiares-Baptista A, Guerra Rodrigo F, Teresa-Lopes M. Juvenile hyaline fibromatosis. A histologic and histochemical study. Arch Pathol Lab Med 1988; 112: 928–931.

319 Kan AE, Rogers M. Juvenile hyaline fibromatosis: an expanded clinicopathologic spectrum. Pediatr Dermatol 1989; 6: 68–75.

320 Miyake I, Tokumaru H, Sugino H et al. Juvenile hyaline fibromatosis. Case report with five years' follow-up. Am J Dermatopathol 1995; 17: 584–590.

321 Jacyk WK, Wentzel LF. Juvenile hyaline fibromatosis in two South African black children. Int J Dermatol 1996; 35: 740–742.

322 Mancini GMS, Stojanov L, Willemsen R et al. Juvenile hyaline fibromatosis: clinical heterogeneity in three patients. Dermatology 1999; 198: 18–25.

323 Allen PW. Selected case from the Arkadi M. Rywlin International Pathology Slide Seminar: hyaline fibromatosis. Adv Anat Pathol 2001; 8: 173–178.

324 De Rosa G, Tornillo L, Orabona P et al. Juvenile hyaline fibromatosis. A case report of a localized form? Am J Dermatopathol 1994; 16: 624–627.

325 Glover MT, Lake BD, Atherton DJ. Clinical, histologic, and ultrastructural findings in two cases of infantile systemic hyalinosis. Pediatr Dermatol 1992; 9: 255–258.

326 Winik BC, Boente MC, Asial R. Juvenile hyaline fibromatosis: ultrastructural study. Am J Dermatopathol 1998; 20: 373–378.

327 Rieger E, Soyer HP, Auboeck L, Kerl H. Cutaneous myxoid fibroblastoma: a histological, immunohistochemical, and ultrastructural study. Am J Dermatopathol 1992; 14: 536–541.

328 Evans HL. Low-grade fibromyxoid sarcoma. A report of 12 cases. Am J Surg Pathol 1993; 17: 595–600.

329 Goodlad JR, Mentzel T, Fletcher CDM. Low grade fibromyxoid sarcoma: clinicopathological analysis of eleven new cases in support of a distinct entity. Histopathology 1995; 26: 229–237.

330 Dvornik G, Barbareschi M, Gallotta P, Dalla Palma P. Low grade fibromyxoid sarcoma. Histopathology 1997; 30: 274–276.

331 Graadt van Roggen JF, Hogendoorn PCW, Fletcher CDM. Myxoid tumours of soft tissue. Histopathology 1999; 35: 291–312.

332 Folpe AL, Lane KL, Paull G, Weiss SW. Low-grade fibromyxoid sarcoma and hyalinizing spindle cell tumor with giant rosettes. Am J Surg Pathol 2000; 24: 1353–1360.

333 Nielsen GP, Selig MK, O'Connell JX et al. Hyalinizing spindle cell tumor with giant rosettes. A report of three cases with ultrastructural analysis. Am J Surg Pathol 1999; 23: 1227–1232.

334 Enzinger FM, Weiss SW. Soft tissue tumours. St. Louis: CV Mosby, 1983: 103–124.

335 Hajdu SI. Fibrosarcoma. A historic commentary. Cancer 1998; 82: 2081–2089.

336 Gonzalez-Crussi F, Wiederhold MD, Sotelo-Avila C. Congenital fibrosarcoma. Presence of a histiocytic component. Cancer 1980; 46: 77–86.

337 Soule EH, Pritchard DJ. Fibrosarcoma in infants and children. A review of 110 cases. Cancer 1977; 40: 1711–1721.

338 Chung EB, Enzinger FM. Infantile fibrosarcoma. Cancer 1976; 38: 729–739.

339 Schofield DE, Fletcher JA, Grier HE, Yunis EJ. Fibrosarcoma in infants and children. Application of new techniques. Am J Surg Pathol 1994; 18: 14–24.

340 Bourgeois JM, Knezevich SR, Mathers JA, Sorensen PHB. Molecular detection of the *ETV6–NTRK3* gene fusion differentiates congenital fibrosarcoma from other childhood spindle cell tumors. Am J Surg Pathol 2000; 24: 937–946.

341 Sheng W-Q, Hisaoka M, Okamoto S et al. Congenital-infantile fibrosarcoma. Am J Clin Pathol 2001; 115: 348–355.

342 Pritchard DJ, Soule EH, Taylor WF, Ivins JC. Fibrosarcoma – a clinicopathologic and statistical study of 199 tumors of the soft tissues of the extremities and trunk. Cancer 1974; 33: 888–897.

343 Eyden BP, Manson C, Banerjee SS et al. Sclerosing epithelioid fibrosarcoma: a study of five cases emphasizing diagnostic criteria. Histopathology 1998; 33: 354–360.

344 Antonescu CR, Rosenblum MR, Pereira P et al. Sclerosing epithelioid fibrosarcoma. A study of 16 cases and confirmation of a clinicopathologically distinct tumor. Am J Surg Pathol 2001; 25: 699–709.

345 Woodruff JM, Antonescu CR, Erlandson RA, Boland PJ. Low-grade fibrosarcoma with palisaded granulomalike bodies (giant rosettes). Am J Surg Pathol 1999; 23: 1423–1428.

346 Mentzel T, Dry S, Katenkamp D, Fletcher CDM. Low-grade myofibroblastic sarcoma. Analysis of 18 cases in the spectrum of myofibroblastic tumors. Am J Surg Pathol 1998; 22: 1228–1238.

Fibrohistiocytic tumors

347 Niemi KM. The benign fibrohistiocytic tumours of the skin. Acta Derm Venereol (Suppl) 1970; 63: 1–60.

348 Dalziel K, Marks R. Hair follicle-like change over histiocytomas. Am J Dermatopathol 1986; 8: 462–466.

349 Vilanova JR, Flint A. The morphological variations of fibrous histiocytomas. J Cutan Pathol 1974; 1: 155–164.

350 Gonzalez S, Duarte I. Benign fibrous histiocytoma of the skin. A morphologic study of 290 cases. Pathol Res Pract 1982; 174: 379–391.

351 Baraf CS, Shapiro L. Multiple histiocytomas. Report of a case. Arch Dermatol 1970; 101: 588–590.

352 Carstens PHB, Schrodt GR. Ultrastructure of sclerosing hemangioma. Am J Pathol 1974; 77: 377–386.

353 Rentiers PL, Montgomery H. Nodular subepidermal fibrosis (dermatofibroma versus histiocytoma). Arch Dermatol 1949; 59: 568–583.

354 Burgdorf W, Moreland A, Wasik R. Negative immunoperoxidase staining for lysozyme in nodular subepidermal fibrosis. Arch Dermatol 1982; 118: 241–243.

355 Sanchez RL. The elusive dermatofibromas. Arch Dermatol 1990; 126: 522–523.

356 Rahbari H, Mehregan AH. Adnexal displacement and regression in association with histiocytoma (dermatofibroma). J Cutan Pathol 1985; 12: 94–102.

357 Baran R, Perrin Ch, Baudet J, Requena L. Clinical and histological patterns of dermatofibromas of the nail apparatus. Clin Exp Dermatol 1994; 19: 31–35.

358 Bargman HB, Fefferman I. Multiple dermatofibromas in a patient with myasthenia gravis treated with prednisone and cyclophosphamide. J Am Acad Dermatol 1986; 14: 351–352.

359 Gray MH, Smoller BR, McNutt NS et al. Giant dermal dendrocytoma of the face: a distinct clinicopathologic entity. Arch Dermatol 1990; 126: 689–690.

360 Hendricks WM. Dermatofibroma occurring in a smallpox vaccination scar. J Am Acad Dermatol 1987; 16: 146–147.

361 Requena L, Fariña C, Fuente C et al. Giant dermatofibroma. A little-known clinical variant of dermatofibroma. J Am Acad Dermatol 1994; 30: 714–718.

362 Kim BK, Smith MA, McKee PH, Calonje E. Giant multinodular fibrous histiocytoma clinically mimicking dermatofibrosarcoma protuberans: report of two cases. J Cutan Pathol 1997; 24: 107 (abstract).

363 Numajiri T, Kishimoto S, Shibagaki R et al. Giant combined dermatofibroma. Br J Dermatol 2000; 143: 655–657.

364 Puig L, Esquius J, Fernández-Figueras MT et al. Atypical polypoid dermatofibroma: report of two cases. J Am Acad Dermatol 1991; 24: 561–565.

365 Beer M, Eckert F. The atrophic dermatofibroma. J Am Acad Dermatol 1991 25: 1081–1082.

366 Santa Cruz DJ, Kyriakos M. Aneurysmal ("angiomatoid") fibrous histiocytoma of the skin. Cancer 1981; 47: 2053–2061.

367 Hairston MA Jr, Reed RJ. Aneurysmal sclerosing hemangioma of skin. Arch Dermatol 1966; 93: 439–442.

368 Ferrari A, Soyer HP, Peris K et al. Central white scarlike patch: A dermatoscopic clue for the diagnosis of dermatofibroma. J Am Acad Dermatol 2000; 43: 1123–1125.

369 Stainforth J, Goodfield MJD. Multiple dermatofibromata developing during pregnancy. Clin Exp Dermatol 1994; 19: 59–60.

370 Veraldi S, Bocor M, Gianotti R, Gasparini G. Multiple eruptive dermatofibromas localized exclusively to the buttock. Int J Dermatol 1991; 30: 507–508.

371 Newman DM, Walter JB. Multiple dermatofibromas in patients with systemic lupus erythematosus on immunosuppressive therapy. N Engl J Med 1973; 289: 842–843.

372 Cohen PR. Multiple dermatofibromas in patients with autoimmune disorders receiving immunosuppressive therapy. Int J Dermatol 1991; 30: 266–270.

373 Chang S-E, Choi J-H, Sung K-J et al. Multiple eruptive dermatofibromas occurring in a patient with acute myeloid leukaemia. Br J Dermatol 2000; 142: 1062–1063.

374 Pechère M, Chavaz P, Saurat J-H. Multiple eruptive dermatofibromas in an AIDS patient: a new differential diagnosis of Kaposi's sarcoma. Dermatology 1995; 190: 319.

375 Lu I, Cohen PR, Grossman ME. Multiple dermatofibromas in a woman with HIV infection and systemic lupus erythematosus. J Am Acad Dermatol 1995; 32: 901–903.

376 Kanitakis J, Carbonnel E, Delmonte S et al. Multiple eruptive dermatofibromas in a patient with HIV infection: case report and literature review. J Cutan Pathol 2000; 27: 54–56.

377 Ammirati CT, Mann C, Hornstra IK. Multiple eruptive dermatofibromas in three men with HIV infection. Dermatology 1997; 195: 344–348.

378 Silvestre JF, Betlloch I, Jiménez MJ. Eruptive dermatofibromas in AIDS patients: a form of mycobacteriosis? Dermatology 1997; 194: 197.

379 Bachmeyer C, Cordier F, Blum L et al. Multiple eruptive dermatofibromas after highly active antiretroviral therapy. Br J Dermatol 2000; 143: 1336–1337.

380 Gelfarb M, Hyman AB. Multiple noduli cutanei. Arch Dermatol 1962; 85: 89–94.

381 Bedi TR, Pandhi RK, Bhutani LK. Multiple palmoplantar histiocytomas. Arch Dermatol 1976; 112: 1001–1003.

382 Ashworth J, Archard L, Woodrow D, Cream JJ. Multiple eruptive histiocytoma cutis in an atopic. Clin Exp Dermatol 1990; 15: 454–456.

383 Zheng P, Hanke CW, Faust HB et al. Progressing dermatofibromas following surgery. Int J Dermatol 1997; 36: 697–699.

384 de Unamuno P, Carames Y, Fernandez-Lopez E et al. Congenital multiple clustered dermatofibroma. Br J Dermatol 2000; 142: 1040–1043.

385 Saga K. Annular hemosiderotic histiocytoma. J Cutan Pathol 1981; 8: 251–255.

386 Curcó N, Jucglà A, Bordas X, Moreno A. Dermatofibroma with spreading satellitosis. J Am Acad Dermatol 1992; 27: 1017–1019.

387 Colome-Grimmer MI, Evans HL. Metastasizing cellular dermatofibroma. A report of two cases. Am J Surg Pathol 1996; 20: 1361–1367.

388 Colby TV. Metastasizing dermatofibroma. Am J Surg Pathol 1997; 21: 976.

389 Calonje E. Is cutaneous benign fibrous histiocytoma (dermatofibroma) a reactive inflammatory process or a neoplasm? Histopathology 2000; 37: 278–280.

390 Chen T-C, Kuo T-t, Chan H-L. Dermatofibroma is a clonal proliferative disease. J Cutan Pathol 2000; 27: 36–39.

391 Tamada S, Ackerman AB. Dermatofibroma with monster cells. Am J Dermatopathol 1987; 9: 380–387.

392 Zelger BG, Zelger B. Dermatofibroma (fibrous histiocytoma): an inflammatory or neoplastic disorder? Histopathology 2001; 38: 379–381.

393 Foreman K, Bonish B, Nickoloff B. Absence of human herpesvirus 8 DNA sequences in patients with immunosuppression-associated dermatofibromas. Arch Dermatol 1997; 133: 108–109.

394 Cerio R, Spaull J, Wilson Jones E. Histiocytoma cutis: a tumour of dermal dendrocytes (dermal dendrocytoma). Br J Dermatol 1989; 120: 197–206.

395 Cerio R, Spaull J, Oliver GF, Wilson Jones E. A study of factor XIIIa and MAC 387 immunolabeling in normal and pathological skin. Am J Dermatopathol 1990; 12: 221–233.

396 Nestle FO, Nickoloff BJ, Burg G. Dermatofibroma: an abortive immunoreactive process mediated by dermal dendritic cells? Dermatology 1995; 190: 265–268.

397 Aiba S, Tagami H. Phorbol 12-myristate 13-acetate can transform monocyte-derived dendritic cells to different cell types similar to those found in dermatofibroma. J Cutan Pathol 1998; 25: 65–71.

398 Kamino H, Jacobson M. Dermatofibroma extending into the subcutaneous tissue. Differential diagnosis from dermatofibrosarcoma protuberans. Am J Surg Pathol 1990; 14: 1156–1164.

399 Zelger B, Sidoroff A, Stanzl U et al. Deep penetrating dermatofibroma versus dermatofibrosarcoma protuberans. A clinicopathologic comparison. Am J Surg Pathol 1994; 18: 677–686.

400 Chang S-E, Choi J-H, Sung K-J et al. Subcutaneous dermatofibroma showing a depressed surface. Int J Dermatol 2001; 40: 77–78.

401 Schwob VS, Santa Cruz DJ. Palisading cutaneous fibrous histiocytoma. J Cutan Pathol 1986; 13: 403–407.

402 Sánchez Yus E, Soria L, de Eusebio E, Requena L. Lichenoid, erosive and ulcerated dermatofibromas. Three additional clinico-pathologic variants. J Cutan Pathol 2000; 27: 112–117.

403 Buselmeier TJ, Uecker JH. Invasive basal cell carcinoma with metaplastic bone formation associated with a long-standing dermatofibroma. J Cutan Pathol 1979; 6: 496–500.

404 Helm KF, Helm T, Helm F. Palisading cutaneous fibrous histiocytoma. An immunohistochemical study demonstrating differentiation from dermal dendrocytes. Am J Dermatopathol 1993; 15: 559–561.

405 Franquemont DW, Cooper PH, Shmookler BM, Wick MR. Benign fibrous histiocytoma of the skin with potential for recurrence. J Cutan Pathol 1989; 16: 303 (abstract).

406 Calonje E, Fletcher CDM. Cutaneous fibrohistiocytic tumors: an update. Adv Anat Pathol 1994; 1: 2–15.

407 Calonje E, Mentzel T, Fletcher CDM. Cellular benign fibrous histiocytoma. Am J Surg Pathol 1994; 18: 668–676.

408 Fraga G, Patterson J. Mitotic activity in dermatofibromas. J Cutan Pathol 2000; 27: 556 (abstract).

409 Fletcher CDM. Benign fibrous histiocytoma of subcutaneous and deep soft tissue: a clinicopathologic analysis of 21 cases. Am J Surg Pathol 1990; 14: 801–809.

410 Hunt SJ, Santa Cruz DJ, Miller CW. Cholesterotic fibrous histiocytoma. Its association with hyperlipoproteinemia. Arch Dermatol 1990; 126: 506–508.

411 Zelger BW, Steiner H, Kutzner H. Clear cell dermatofibroma. Case report of an unusual fibrohistiocytic lesion. Am J Surg Pathol 1996; 20: 483–491.

412 Wambacher-Gasser B, Zelger B, Zelger BG, Steiner H. Clear cell dermatofibroma. Histopathology 1997; 30: 64–69.

413 Zelger B. Clear cell dermatofibroma. Am J Surg Pathol 1997; 21: 737.

414 Paties C, Vassallo G, Taccagni GL. Clear cell dermatofibroma. Am J Surg Pathol 1997; 21: 250–252.

415 Zelger BG, Steiner H, Kutzner H et al. Granular cell dermatofibroma. Histopathology 1997; 31: 258–262.

416 Soyer HP, Metze D, Kerl H. Granular cell dermatofibroma. Am J Dermatopathol 1997; 19: 168–173.

417 Val-Bernal JF, Mira C. Dermatofibroma with granular cells. J Cutan Pathol 1996; 23: 562–565.

418 Sanz-Trelles A, Weil-Lara B, Acedo-Rodriguez C. Dermatofibroma with granular cells. Histopathology 1997; 30: 495–497.

419 Aloi F, Albertazzi D, Pippione M. Dermatofibroma with granular cells: a report of two cases. Dermatology 1999; 199: 54–56.

420 Iwata J, Fletcher CDM. Lipidized fibrous histiocytoma. Clinicopathologic analysis of 22 cases. Am J Dermatopathol 2000; 22: 126–134.

421 Sood U, Mehregan AH. Aneurysmal (angiomatoid) fibrous histiocytoma. J Cutan Pathol 1985; 12: 157–162.

422 Sun C-CJ, Toker C, Breitenecker R. An ultrastructural study of angiomatoid fibrous histiocytoma. Cancer 1982; 49: 2103–2111.

423 Cerio R, McGibbon D, Wilson Jones E. Angiomatoid fibrous histiocytoma. J Cutan Pathol 1989; 16: 298 (abstract).

424 Calonje E, Fletcher CDM. Aneurysmal benign fibrous histiocytoma: clinicopathological analysis of 40 cases of a tumour frequently misdiagnosed as a vascular neoplasm. Histopathology 1995; 26: 323–331.

425 Leyva WH, Santa Cruz DJ. Atypical cutaneous fibrous histiocytoma. Am J Dermatopathol 1986; 8: 467–471.

426 Fukamizu H, Oku T, Inoue K et al. Atypical ("pseudosarcomatous") cutaneous histiocytoma. J Cutan Pathol 1983; 10: 327–333.

427 Marrogi AJ, Dehner LP, Coffin CM, Wick MR. Atypical fibrous histiocytoma of the skin and subcutis in childhood and adolescence. J Cutan Pathol 1992; 19: 268–277.

428 Setoyama M, Fukumaru S, Kanzaki T. Case of dermatofibroma with monster cells: a review and an immunohistochemical study. Am J Dermatopathol 1997; 19: 312–315.

429 Kutchemeshgi M, Barr RJ, Henderson CD. Dermatofibroma with osteoclast-like giant cells. Am J Dermatopathol 1992; 14: 397–401.

430 Kuo T-t, Chan H-L. Ossifying dermatofibroma with osteoclast-like giant cells. Am J Dermatopathol 1994; 16: 193–195.

431 Zelger BG, Sidoroff A, Zelger B. Combined dermatofibroma: co-existence of two or more variant patterns in a single lesion. Histopathology 2000; 36: 529–539.

432 Zelger BG, Calonje E, Zelger B. Myxoid dermatofibroma. Histopathology 1999; 34: 357–364.

433 Kuo T-t, Hu S, Chan H-L. Keloidal dermatofibroma. Am J Surg Pathol 1998; 22: 564–568.

434 Kiyohara T, Kumakiri M, Kobayashi H et al. Atrophic dermatofibroma. Elastophagocytosis by the tumor cells. J Cutan Pathol 2000; 27: 312–315.

435 Barker SM, Winkelmann RK. Inflammatory lymphadenoid reactions with dermatofibroma/histiocytoma. J Cutan Pathol 1986; 13: 222–226.

436 Aiba S, Terui T, Tagami H. Dermatofibroma with diffuse eosinophilic infiltrate. Am J Dermatopathol 2000; 22: 281–284.

437 LeBoit PE, Barr RJ. Smooth-muscle proliferation in dermatofibromas. Am J Dermatopathol 1994; 16: 155–160.

438 Usmani A, Lal P, Li H et al. Myofibroblastic differentiation in dermatofibromas. J Cutan Pathol 2000; 27: 576 (abstract).

439 Zelger BWH, Zelger BG, Rappersberger K. Prominent myofibroblastic differentiation. A pitfall in the diagnosis of dermatofibroma. Am J Dermatopathol 1997; 19: 138–146.

440 Zelger B. Author's reply. Am J Dermatopathol 1998; 20: 321–322.

441 Wilson Jones E, Cerio R, Smith NP. Epithelioid cell histiocytoma: a new entity. Br J Dermatol 1989; 120: 185–195.

442 Goette DK, Helwig EB. Basal cell carcinomas and basal cell carcinoma-like changes overlying dermatofibromas. Arch Dermatol 1975; 111: 589–592.

443 Schoenfeld RJ. Epidermal proliferations overlying histiocytomas. Arch Dermatol 1964; 90: 266–270.

444 Halpryn HJ, Allen AC. Epidermal changes associated with sclerosing hemangiomas. Arch Dermatol 1959; 80: 160–166.

445 Herman KL, Kantor GR, Katz SM. Squamous cell carcinoma in situ overlying dermatofibroma. J Cutan Pathol 1990; 17: 385–387.

446 Ackerman AB, Capland L, Rywlin AM. Focal keratosis follicularis overlying dermatofibroma. Br J Dermatol 1971; 84: 167–168.

447 Caron GA, Clink HM. Clinical association of basal cell epithelioma with histiocytoma. Arch Dermatol 1964; 90: 271–273.

448 Fujisawa H, Matsushima Y, Hoshino M et al. Differentiation of the basal cell epithelioma-like changes overlying dermatofibroma. Acta Derm Venereol 1991; 71: 354–356.

449 Cheng L, Amini SB, Zaim MT. Follicular basal cell hyperplasia overlying dermatofibroma. Am J Surg Pathol 1997; 21: 711–718.

450 Requena L, Roó E, Sánchez Yus E. Plate-like sebaceous hyperplasia overlying dermatofibroma. J Cutan Pathol 1992; 19: 253–255.

451 Rotteleur G, Chevallier JM, Piette F, Bergoend H. Basal cell carcinoma overlying histiocytofibroma. Acta Derm Venereol 1983; 63: 567–569.

452 Bryant J. Basal cell carcinoma overlying long-standing dermatofibromas. Arch Dermatol 1977; 113: 1445–1446.

453 Morgan MB, Howard HG, Everett MA. Epithelial induction in dermatofibroma: a role for the epidermal growth factor (EGF) receptor. Am J Dermatopathol 1997; 19: 35–40.

454 Han K-H, Huh C-H, Cho K-H. Proliferation and differentiation of the keratinocytes in hyperplastic epidermis overlying dermatofibroma. Immunohistochemical characterization. Am J Dermatopathol 2001; 23: 90–98.

455 Leong PM, Kauffman CL, Moresi JM et al. Basal cell carcinoma-like epidermal changes overlying dermatofibromas often reveal loss of heterozygosity in the PTCH gene. J Invest Dermatol 1999; 113: 279–280.

456 du Boulay CEH. Demonstration of alpha-1-antitrypsin and alpha-1-antichymotrypsin in fibrous histiocytomas using the immunoperoxidase technique. Am J Surg Pathol 1982; 6: 559–564.

457 Soini Y. Cell differentiation in benign cutaneous fibrous histiocytomas. An immunohistochemical study with antibodies to histiomonocytic cells and intermediate filament proteins. Am J Dermatopathol 1990; 12: 134–140.

458 Li D-F, Iwasaki H, Kikuchi M et al. Dermatofibroma: superficial fibrous proliferation with reactive histiocytes. Cancer 1994; 74: 66–73.

459 Prieto VG, Reed JA, Shea CR. Immunohistochemistry of dermatofibromas and benign fibrous histiocytomas. J Cutan Pathol 1995; 22: 336–341.

460 Goldblum JR, Tuthill RJ. CD34 and factor-XIIIa immunoreactivity in dermatofibrosarcoma protuberans and dermatofibroma. Am J Dermatopathol 1997; 19: 147–153.

461 Kahn HJ, Fekete E, From L. Tenascin differentiates dermatofibroma from dermatofibrosarcoma protuberans: comparison with CD34 and factor XIIIa. Hum Pathol 2001; 32: 50–56.

462 Franchi A, Santucci M. Tenascin expression in cutaneous fibrohistiocytic tumors. Immunohistochemical investigation of 24 cases. Am J Dermatopathol 1996; 18: 454–459.

463 Carrington SG, Winkelmann RK. Electron microscopy of the histiocytic diseases of the skin. Acta Derm Venereol 1972; 52: 161–178.

464 Katenkamp D, Stiller D. Cellular composition of the so-called dermatofibroma (histiocytoma cutis). Virchows Arch [A] 1975; 367: 325–336.

465 Zelger BG, Wambacher B, Steiner H, Zelger B. Cutaneous epithelioid hemangioendothelioma, epithelioid cell histiocytoma and Spitz nevus. Three separate epithelioid tumors in one patient. J Cutan Pathol 1997; 24: 641–647.

466 Singh Gomez C, Calonje E, Fletcher CDM. Epithelioid benign fibrous histiocytoma of skin: clinico-pathological analysis of 20 cases of a poorly known variant. Histopathology 1994; 24: 123–129.

467 Manente L, Schmitt I, Onetti AM et al. Cutaneous epithelioid cell histiocytoma. Immunohistochemical and ultrastructural findings suggesting endothelial origin. Am J Dermatopathol 1997; 19: 519–523.

468 Diaz-Cascajo C. What is your diagnosis and why? (epithelioid-cell dermatofibroma). Dermatopathology: Practical & Conceptual 2000; 6: 133–137.

469 McCarron K, Oriba H, Bergfeld W, Goldblum J. The epithelioid variant of benign fibrous histiocytoma (BFH): a clinicopathologic & immunohistochemical analysis of 19 cases. J Cutan Pathol 2000; 27: 564 (abstract).

470 Glusac EJ, Barr RJ, Everett MA et al. Epithelioid cell histiocytoma. A report of 10 cases including a new cellular variant. Am J Surg Pathol 1994; 18: 583–590.

471 Glusac EJ, McNiff JM. Epithelioid cell histiocytoma: a simulant of vascular and melanocytic neoplasms. Am J Dermatopathol 1999; 21: 1–7.

472 Mehregan AH, Mehregan DR, Broecker A. Epithelioid cell histiocytoma. A clinicopathologic and immunohistochemical study of eight cases. J Am Acad Dermatol 1992; 26: 243–246.

473 Enzinger FM, Zhang R. Plexiform fibrohistiocytic tumor presenting in children and young adults. An analysis of 65 cases. Am J Surg Pathol 1988; 12: 818–826.

474 Fisher C. Atypical plexiform fibrohistiocytic tumour. Histopathology 1997; 30: 271–273.

475 Hollowood K, Holley MP, Fletcher CDM. Plexiform fibrohistiocytic tumour: clinicopathological, immunohistochemical and ultrastructural analysis in favour of a myofibroblastic lesion. Histopathology 1991; 19: 503–513.

476 Zelger B, Weinlich G, Steiner H et al. Dermal and subcutaneous variants of plexiform fibrohistiocytic tumor. Am J Surg Pathol 1997; 21: 235–241.

477 Remstein ED, Arndt CAS, Nascimento AG. Plexiform fibrohistiocytic tumor: clinicopathologic analysis of 22 cases. Am J Surg Pathol 1999; 23: 662–670.

478 Sigel JE, Bergfeld WF, Goldblum JR. Plexiform fibrous histiocytoma with granular cell change: an unusual morphologic variant of a rare neoplasm. J Cutan Pathol 2000; 27: 572 (abstract).

479 Michal M. Plexiform xanthomatous tumor. A report of three cases. Am J Dermatopathol 1994; 16: 532–536.

480 Shmookler BM, Enzinger FM. Giant cell fibroblastoma: a peculiar childhood tumor. Lab Invest 1982; 46: 76A (abstract).

481 Abdul-Karim FW, Evans HL, Silva EG. Giant cell fibroblastoma: a report of three cases. Am J Clin Pathol 1985; 83: 165–170.

482 Dymock RB, Allen PW, Stirling JW et al. Giant cell fibroblastoma. A distinctive, recurrent tumor of childhood. Am J Surg Pathol 1987; 11: 263–272.

483 Allen PW, Zwi J. Giant cell fibroblastoma transforming into dermatofibrosarcoma protuberans. Am J Surg Pathol 1992; 16: 1127–1128.

484 Perry DA, Schultz LR, Dehner LP. Giant cell fibroblastoma with dermatofibrosarcoma protuberans-like transformation. J Cutan Pathol 1993; 20: 451–454.

485 Alguacil-Garcia A. Giant cell fibroblastoma recurring as dermatofibrosarcoma protuberans. Am J Surg Pathol 1991; 15: 798–801.

486 Michal M, Zamecnik M. Giant cell fibroblastoma with a dermatofibrosarcoma protuberans component. Am J Dermatopathol 1992; 14: 549–552.

487 Heller P, McDonough D, Burchette JL et al. Dermatofibrosarcoma protuberans with a giant cell fibroblastomatous component. J Cutan Pathol 1996; 23: 51 (abstract).

488 Coyne J, Kaftan SM, Craig RDP. Dermatofibrosarcoma protuberans recurring as a giant cell fibroblastoma. Histopathology 1992; 21: 184–187.

489 Harvell JD, Kilpatrick SE, White WL. Histogenetic relations between giant cell fibroblastoma and dermatofibrosarcoma protuberans. CD34 staining showing the spectrum and a simulator. Am J Dermatopathol 1998; 20: 339–345.

490 Barr RJ, Young EM Jr, Liao S-Y. Giant cell fibroblastoma: an immunohistochemical study. J Cutan Pathol 1986; 13: 301–307.

491 Chou P, Gonzalez-Crussi F, Mangkornkanok M. Giant cell fibroblastoma. Cancer 1989; 63: 756–762.

492 Rosen LB, Amazon K, Weitzner J, Resnick L. Giant cell fibroblastoma. A report of a case and review of the literature. Am J Dermatopathol 1989; 11: 242–247.

493 Fletcher CDM. Giant cell fibroblastoma of soft tissue: a clinicopathological and immunohistochemical study. Histopathology 1988; 13: 499–508.

494 Díaz-Cascajo C, Borrego L, Bastida-Iñarrea J, Borghi S. Giant cell fibroblastoma. New histological observations. Am J Dermatopathol 1996; 18: 403–408.

495 Kanai Y, Mukai M, Sugiura H et al. Giant cell fibroblastoma. Acta Pathol Jpn 1991; 41: 552–560.

496 Harvell J, Kilpatrick S, White W. The giant cell patterns in giant cell fibroblastoma with dermatofibrosarcoma protuberans: CD34 staining showing the spectrum and a simulator. J Cutan Pathol 1996; 23: 51 (abstract).

497 Sigel JE, Bergfeld WF, Goldblum JR. A morphologic study of dermatofibrosarcoma protuberans: expansion of a histologic profile. J Cutan Pathol 2000; 27: 159–163.

498 Rockley PF, Robinson JK, Magid M, Goldblatt D. Dermatofibrosarcoma protuberans of the scalp: a series of cases. J Am Acad Dermatol 1989; 21: 278–283.

499 Yang AH, Chen BF. Intracytoplasmic giant cross-striated fibrils in giant cell fibroblastoma. Histopathology 1995; 27: 383–385.

500 Taylor HB, Helwig EB. Dermatofibrosarcoma protuberans. A study of 115 cases. Cancer 1962; 15: 717–725.

501 Garcia C, Clark RE, Buchanan M. Dermatofibrosarcoma protuberans. Int J Dermatol 1996; 35: 867–871.

502 Gloster HM Jr. Dermatofibrosarcoma protuberans. J Am Acad Dermatol 1996; 35: 355–374.

503 McKee PH, Fletcher CDM. Dermatofibrosarcoma protuberans presenting in infancy and childhood. J Cutan Pathol 1991; 18: 241–246.

504 Annessi G, Cimitan A, Girolomoni G, Giannetti A. Congenital dermatofibrosarcoma protuberans. Pediatr Dermatol 1993; 10: 40–42.

505 McLelland J, Chu T. Dermatofibrosarcoma protuberans arising in a BCG vaccination scar. Arch Dermatol 1988; 124: 496–497.

506 Hacker SM, Ford MJ. Dermatofibrosarcoma protuberans of the face. Int J Dermatol 1994; 33: 568–569.

507 Meehan SA, Napoli JA, Perry AE. Dermatofibrosarcoma protuberans of the oral cavity. J Am Acad Dermatol 1999; 41: 863–866.

508 Martin L, Combemale P, Dupin M et al. The atrophic variant of dermatofibrosarcoma protuberans in childhood: a report of six cases. Br J Dermatol 1998; 139: 719–725.

509 Gardner TL, Elston DM, Wotowic PJ. A familial dermatofibrosarcoma protuberans. J Am Acad Dermatol 1998; 39: 504–505.

510 Mooney E, Sigurgeirsson B, Johannsson JH, Hood AF. Dermatofibrosarcoma protuberans on the neck of a young child. J Cutan Pathol 2000; 27: 565 (abstract).

511 Patrizi A, Vespignani F, Fraternali GO, Neri I. A pediatric case of dermatofibrosarcoma protuberans: an immunohistochemical study. Pediatr Dermatol 2000; 17: 29–33.

512 Checketts SR, Hamilton TK, Baughman RD. Congenital and childhood dermatofibrosarcoma protuberans: A case report and review of the literature. J Am Acad Dermatol 2000; 42: 907–913.

513 Bouyssou-Gauthier M-L, Labrousse F, Longis B et al. Dermatofibrosarcoma protuberans in childhood. Pediatr Dermatol 1997; 14: 463–465.

514 Hawk JLM. Dermatofibrosarcoma protuberans. Clin Exp Dermatol 1977; 2: 85–89.

515 Burkhardt BR, Soule EH, Winkelmann RK, Ivins JC. Dermatofibrosarcoma protuberans. Study of fifty-six cases. Am J Surg 1966; 111: 638–644.

516 Weber PJ, Gretzula JC, Hevia O et al. Dermatofibrosarcoma protuberans. J Dermatol Surg Oncol 1988; 14: 555–558.

517 Lauritz BV, Mason GH. Dermatofibrosarcoma protuberans: an early non-protuberant phase of the tumour. Australas J Dermatol 1999; 40: 35–36.

518 Davis DA, Sánchez RL. Atrophic and plaquelike dermatofibrosarcoma protuberans. Am J Dermatopathol 1998; 20: 498–501.

519 Fujimoto M, Kikuchi K, Okochi H, Furue M. Atrophic dermatofibrosarcoma protuberans: a case report and review of the literature. Dermatology 1998; 196: 422–424.

520 Morman MR, Lin R-Y, Petrozzi JW. Dermatofibrosarcoma protuberans arising in a site of multiple immunizations. Arch Dermatol 1979; 115: 1453.

521 Parlette E, Smith KJ, Germain M et al. Accelerated growth of dermatofibrosarcoma protuberans during pregnancy. J Am Acad Dermatol 1999; 41: 778–783.

522 Shneidman D, Belizaire R. Arsenic exposure followed by the development of dermatofibrosarcoma protuberans. Cancer 1986; 58: 1585–1587.

523 Koh CK, Ko CB, Bury HPR, Wyatt EH. Dermatofibrosarcoma protuberans. Int J Dermatol 1995; 34: 256–260.

524 Ratner D, Thomas CO, Johnson TM et al. Mohs micrographic surgery for the treatment of dermatofibrosarcoma protuberans. J Am Acad Dermatol 1997; 37: 600–613.

525 Gloster HM Jr, Harris KR, Roenigk RK. A comparison between Mohs micrographic surgery and wide surgical excision for the treatment of dermatofibrosarcoma protuberans. J Am Acad Dermatol 1996; 35: 82–87.

526 McPeak CJ, Cruz T, Nicastri AD. Dermatofibrosarcoma protuberans: an analysis of 86 cases – five with metastasis. Ann Surg 1967; 166: 803–816.

527 Kahn LB, Saxe N, Gordon W. Dermatofibrosarcoma protuberans with lymph node and pulmonary metastases. Arch Dermatol 1978; 114: 599–601.

528 Hausner RJ, Vargas-Cortes F, Alexander RW. Dermatofibrosarcoma protuberans with lymph node involvement. A case report of simultaneous occurrence with an atypical fibroxanthoma of the skin. Arch Dermatol 1978; 114: 88–91.

529 Brenner W, Schaefler K, Chhabra H, Postel A. Dermatofibrosarcoma protuberans metastatic to a regional lymph node. Report of a case and review. Cancer 1975; 36: 1897–1902.

530 Volpe R, Carbone A. Dermatofibrosarcoma protuberans metastatic to lymph nodes and showing a dominant histiocytic component. Am J Dermatopathol 1983; 5: 327–334.

531 O'Dowd J, Laidler P. Progression of dermatofibrosarcoma protuberans to malignant fibrous histiocytoma: Report of a case with implications for tumor histogenesis. Hum Pathol 1988; 19: 368–370.

532 Wrotnowski U, Cooper PH, Shmookler BM. Fibrosarcomatous change in dermatofibrosarcoma protuberans. Am J Surg Pathol 1988; 12: 287–293.

533 Zámečník M, Michal M, Mukenšnábl P. Composite tumor consisting of dermatofibrosarcoma protuberans and myxofibrosarcoma. J Cutan Pathol 1998; 25: 445–449.

534 Díaz-Cascajo C, Weyers W, Borrego L et al. Dermatofibrosarcoma protuberans with fibrosarcomatous areas: a clinico-pathologic and immunohistochemic study in four cases. Am J Dermatopathol 1997; 19: 562–567.

535 Bowne WB, Antonescu CR, Leung DHY et al. Dermatofibrosarcoma protuberans. A clinicopathologic analysis of patients treated and followed at a single institution. Cancer 2000; 88: 2711–2720.

536 Goldblum JR, Reith JD, Weiss SW. Sarcomas arising in dermatofibrosarcoma protuberans. A reappraisal of biologic behavior in eighteen cases treated by wide local excision with extended clinical follow up. Am J Surg Pathol 2000; 24: 1125–1130.

537 Bednar B. Storiform neurofibromas of the skin, pigmented and nonpigmented. Cancer 1957; 10: 368–376.

538 Bednar B. Storiform neurofibroma in the core of naevocellular naevi. J Pathol 1970; 101: 199–201.

539 Santa Cruz DJ, Yates AJ. Pigmented storiform neurofibroma. J Cutan Pathol 1977; 4: 9–13.

540 Nakamura T, Ogata H, Katsuyama T. Pigmented dermatofibrosarcoma protuberans. Am J Dermatopathol 1987; 9: 18–25.

541 Miyamoto Y, Morimatsu M, Nakashima T. Pigmented storiform neurofibroma. Acta Pathol Jpn 1984; 34: 821–826.

542 Dupree WB, Langloss JM, Weiss SW. Pigmented dermatofibrosarcoma protuberans (Bednar tumor). A pathologic, ultrastructural, and immunohistochemical study. Am J Surg Pathol 1985; 9: 630–639.

543 Chuan M-T, Tsai T-F, Wu M-C, Wong T-H. Atrophic pigmented dermatofibrosarcoma presenting an infraorbital hyperpigmentation. Dermatology 1997; 194: 65–67.

544 Kaburagi Y, Hatta N, Kawara S, Takehara K. Pigmented dermatofibrosarcoma protuberans (Bednář tumor) occurring in a Japanese infant. Dermatology 1998; 197: 48–51.

545 Fletcher CDM, Theaker JM, Flanagan A, Krausz T. Pigmented dermatofibrosarcoma protuberans (Bednar tumour): melanocytic colonization or neuroectodermal differentiation? A clinicopathological and immunohistochemical study. Histopathology 1988; 13: 631–643.

546 Elgart GW, Hanly A, Busso M, Spencer JM. Bednar tumor (pigmented dermatofibrosarcoma protuberans) occurring in a site of prior immunization: Immunochemical findings and therapy. J Am Acad Dermatol 1999; 40: 315–317.

547 Fletcher CDM, McKee PH. Sarcomas – a clinicopathological guide with particular reference to cutaneous manifestation I. Dermatofibrosarcoma protuberans, malignant fibrous histiocytoma and the epithelioid sarcoma of Enzinger. Clin Exp Dermatol 1984; 9: 451–465.

548 Fletcher CDM, Evans BJ, Macartney JC et al. Dermatofibrosarcoma protuberans: a clinicopathological and immunohistochemical study with a review of the literature. Histopathology 1985; 9: 921–938.

549 Calonje E, Fletcher CDM. Myoid differentiation in dermatofibrosarcoma protuberans and its fibrosarcomatous variant: clinicopathologic analysis of 5 cases. J Cutan Pathol 1996; 23: 30–36.

550 Taniuchi K, Yamada Y, Nonomura A, Takehara K. Immunohistochemical analysis of platelet-derived growth factor and its receptors in fibrohistiocytic tumors. J Cutan Pathol 1997; 24: 393–397.

551 Wang J, Morimitsu Y, Okamoto S et al. COL1A1–PDGFB fusion transcripts in fibrosarcomatous areas of six dermatofibrosarcomas protuberans. J Mol Diagn 2000; 2: 47–52.

552 Diaz-Cascajo C, Weyers W, Rey-Lopez A, Borghi S. Deep dermatofibrosarcoma protuberans: a subcutaneous variant. Histopathology 1998; 32: 552–555.

553 Sauter LS, DeFeo CP. Dermatofibrosarcoma protuberans of the face. Arch Dermatol 1971; 104: 671–673.

554 Connelly JH, Evans HL. Dermatofibrosarcoma protuberans. A clinicopathologic review with emphasis on fibrosarcomatous areas. Am J Surg Pathol 1992; 16: 921–925.

555 Zamecnik M. Fibrosarcomatous dermatofibrosarcoma protuberans with giant rosettes. Am J Dermatopathol 2001; 23: 41–45.

556 Mentzel T, Beham A, Katenkamp D et al. Fibrosarcomatous ("high grade") dermatofibrosarcoma protuberans. Clinicopathologic and immunohistochemical study of a series of 41 cases with emphasis on prognostic significance. Am J Surg Pathol 1998; 22: 576–587.

557 Zámecnik M. Myoid cells in the fibrosarcomatous variant of dermatofibrosarcoma protuberans. Histopathology 2000; 36: 186.

558 Morimitsu Y, Hisaoka M, Okamoto S et al. Dermatofibrosarcoma protuberans and its fibrosarcomatous variant with areas of myoid differentiation: a report of three cases. Histopathology 1998; 32: 547–551.

559 Sanz-Trelles A. Myoid cells in the fibrosarcomatous variant of dermatofibrosarcoma protuberans. Are they neoplastic? Histopathology 1999; 34: 179–180.

560 Diaz-Cascajo C. Myoid differentiation in dermatofibrosarcoma protuberans and its fibrosarcomatous variant. J Cutan Pathol 1997; 24: 197–198.

561 Sanz-Trelles A, Ayala-Carbonero A, Rodrigo-Fernández I, Weil-Lara B. Leiomyomatous nodules and bundles of vascular origin in the fibrosarcomatous variant of dermatofibrosarcoma protuberans. J Cutan Pathol 1998; 25: 44–49.

562 Orlandi A, Bianchi L, Spagnoli LG. Myxoid dermatofibrosarcoma protuberans: morphological, ultrastructural and immunohistochemical features. J Cutan Pathol 1998; 25: 386–393.

563 Frierson HF, Cooper PH. Myxoid variant of dermatofibrosarcoma protuberans. Am J Surg Pathol 1983; 7: 445–450.

564 Zelger BW, Öfner D, Zelger BG. Atrophic variants of dermatofibroma and dermatofibrosarcoma protuberans. Histopathology 1995; 26: 519–527.

565 Banerjee SS, Harris M, Eyden BP, Hamid BNA. Granular cell variant of dermatofibrosarcoma protuberans. Histopathology 1990; 17: 375–378.

566 Rytina ERC, Ball RY. Transformation of recurrent dermatofibrosarcoma protuberans to its pigmented variant (Bednar tumour). Histopathology 1998; 32: 384–385.

567 Barr RJ, Young EM Jr, King DF. Non-polarizable collagen in dermatofibrosarcoma protuberans: a useful diagnostic aid. J Cutan Pathol 1986; 13: 339–346.

568 Horenstein MG, Prieto VG, Nuckols JD et al. Indeterminate fibrohistiocytic lesions of the skin. Is there a spectrum between dermatofibroma and dermatofibrosarcoma protuberans? Am J Surg Pathol 2000; 24: 996–1003.

569 Lautier R, Wolff HH, Jones RE. An immunohistochemical study of dermatofibrosarcoma protuberans supports its fibroblastic character and contradicts neuroectodermal or histiocytic components. Am J Dermatopathol 1990; 12: 25–30.

570 Aiba S, Tabata N, Ishii H et al. Dermatofibrosarcoma protuberans is a unique fibrohistiocytic tumour expressing CD34. Br J Dermatol 1992; 127: 79–84.

571 Kutzner H. Expression of the human progenitor cell antigen CD34 (HPCA-1) distinguishes dermatofibrosarcoma protuberans from fibrous histiocytoma in formalin-fixed, paraffin-embedded tissue. J Am Acad Dermatol 1993; 28: 613–617.

572 Cohen PR, Rapini RP, Farhood AI. Expression of the human hematopoietic progenitor cell antigen CD34 in vascular and spindle cell tumors. J Cutan Pathol 1993; 20: 15–20.

573 Prieto VG, Reed JA, Shea CR. CD34 immunoreactivity distinguishes between scar tissue and residual tumor in re-excisional specimens of dermatofibrosarcoma protuberans. J Cutan Pathol 1994; 21: 324–329.

574 Cohen PR, Rapini RP, Farhood AI. Dermatofibroma and dermatofibrosarcoma protuberans: differential expression of CD34 and factor XIIIa. Am J Dermatopathol 1994; 16: 573–574.

575 Haycox CL, Odland PB, Olbricht SM, Piepkorn M. Immunohistochemical characterization of dermatofibrosarcoma protuberans with practical applications for diagnosis and treatment. J Am Acad Dermatol 1997; 37: 438–444.

576 Abenoza P, Lillemoe T. CD34 and factor XIIIa in the differential diagnosis of dermatofibroma and dermatofibrosarcoma protuberans. Am J Dermatopathol 1993; 15: 429–434.

577 Cohen PR, Rapini RP, Farhood AI. Expression of the human hematopoietic progenitor cell antigen CD34 in dermatofibrosarcoma protuberans, other spindle cell tumors, and vascular lesions. J Am Acad Dermatol 1994; 30: 147–148.

578 Diaz-Cascajo C, Bastida-Iñarrea J, Borrego L, Carretero-Hernández G. Comparison of p53 expression in dermatofibrosarcoma protuberans and dermatofibroma: lack of correlation with proliferation rate. J Cutan Pathol 1995; 22: 304–309.

579 Kobayashi T, Hasegawa Y, Konohana A, Nakamura N. A case of Bednar tumor. Immunohistochemical positivity for CD34. Dermatology 1997; 195: 57–59.

580 Hashimoto K, Brownstein MH, Jakobiec FA. Dermatofibrosarcoma protuberans. A tumor with perineural and endoneural cell features. Arch Dermatol 1974; 110: 874–885.

581 Alguacil-Garcia A, Unni KK, Goellner RJ. Histogenesis of dermatofibrosarcoma protuberans. An ultrastructural study. Am J Clin Pathol 1978; 69: 427–434.

582 Escalona-Zapata J, Fernandez EA, Escuin FL. The fibroblastic nature of dermatofibrosarcoma protuberans. A tissue culture and ultrastructural study. Virchows Arch [A] 1981; 391: 165–175.

583 Zina AM, Bundino S. Dermatofibrosarcoma protuberans. An ultrastructural study of five cases. J Cutan Pathol 1979; 6: 265–271.

584 Ozzello L, Hamels J. The histiocytic nature of dermatofibrosarcoma protuberans. Tissue culture and electron microscopic study. Am J Clin Pathol 1976; 65: 136–148.

585 Helwig EB. Atypical fibroxanthoma. Texas J Med 1963; 59: 664–667.

586 Connors RC, Ackerman AB. Histologic pseudomalignancies of the skin. Arch Dermatol 1976; 112: 1767–1780.

587 Finlay-Jones LR, Nicoll P, Ten Seldam REJ. Pseudosarcoma of the skin. Pathology 1971; 3: 215–222.

588 Bourne RG. Paradoxical fibrosarcoma of skin (pseudosarcoma): a review of 13 cases. Med J Aust 1963; 1: 504–510.

589 Vargas-Cortes F, Winkelmann RK, Soule EH. Atypical fibroxanthomas of the skin. Further observations with 19 additional cases. Mayo Clin Proc 1973; 48: 211–218.

590 Fretzin DF, Helwig EB. Atypical fibroxanthoma of the skin. A clinicopathologic study of 140 cases. Cancer 1973; 31: 1541–1552.

591 Kempson RL, McGavran MH. Atypical fibroxanthomas of the skin. Cancer 1964; 17: 1463–1471.

592 Leong AS-Y, Milios J. Atypical fibroxanthoma of the skin: a clinicopathological and immunohistochemical study and a discussion of its histogenesis. Histopathology 1987; 11: 463–475.

593 Patterson JW, Jordan WP Jr. Atypical fibroxanthoma in a patient with xeroderma pigmentosum. Arch Dermatol 1987; 123: 1066–1070.

594 Dilek FH, Akpolat N, Metin A, Ugras S. Atypical fibroxanthoma of the skin and the lower lip in xeroderma pigmentosum. Br J Dermatol 2000; 143: 618–620.

595 Helwig EB, May D. Atypical fibroxanthoma of the skin with metastases. Cancer 1986; 57: 368–376.

596 Longacre TA, Smoller BR, Rouse RV. Atypical fibroxanthoma. Multiple immunohistologic profiles. Am J Surg Pathol 1993; 17: 1199–1209.

597 Kemmett D, Gawkrodger DJ, Mclaren KM, Hunter JAA. Two atypical fibroxanthomas arising separately in X-irradiated skin. Clin Exp Dermatol 1988; 13: 382–384.

598 Kanitakis J, Euvrard S, Montazeri A et al. Atypical fibroxanthoma in a renal graft recipient. J Am Acad Dermatol 1996; 35: 262–264.

599 Hafner J, Künzi W, Weinreich T. Malignant fibrous histiocytoma and atypical fibroxanthoma in renal transplant recipients. Dermatology 1999; 198: 29–32.

600 Enzinger FM. Questions to the Editorial Board and other authorities. Am J Dermatopathol 1979; 1: 185.

601 Westermann FN, Langlois NEI, Simpson JG. Apoptosis in atypical fibroxanthoma and pleomorphic malignant fibrous histiocytoma. Am J Dermatopathol 1997; 19: 228–231.

602 Michie BA, Reid RP, Fallowfield ME. Aneuploidy in atypical fibroxanthoma: DNA content quantification of 10 cases by image analysis. J Cutan Pathol 1994; 21: 404–407.

603 Worrell JT, Ansari MQ, Ansari SJ, Cockerell CJ. Atypical fibroxanthoma: DNA ploidy analysis of 14 cases with possible histogenetic implications. J Cutan Pathol 1993; 20: 211–215.

604 Starink TM, Hausman R, Van Delden L, Neering H. Atypical fibroxanthoma of the skin. Presentation of 5 cases and a review of the literature. Br J Dermatol 1977; 97: 167–177.

605 Dahl I. Atypical fibroxanthoma of the skin. A clinico-pathological study of 57 cases. Acta Pathol Microbiol Immunol Scand (A) 1976; 84: 183–197.

606 Hudson AW, Winkelmann RK. Atypical fibroxanthoma of the skin: a reappraisal of 19 cases in which the original diagnosis was spindle-cell squamous carcinoma. Cancer 1972; 29: 413–422.

607 Kemp JD, Stenn KS, Arons M, Fischer J. Metastasizing atypical fibroxanthoma. Coexistence with chronic lymphocytic leukemia. Arch Dermatol 1978; 114: 1533–1535.

608 Glavin FL, Cornwell ML. Atypical fibroxanthoma of the skin metastatic to a lung. Am J Dermatopathol 1985; 7: 57–63.

609 Zelger B, Soyer HP. Between Scylla and Charybdis: mythology in dermatopathology. Dermatopathology: Practical & Conceptual 2000; 6: 348–355.

610 Calonje E, Wadden C, Wilson-Jones E, Fletcher CDM. Spindle-cell non-pleomorphic atypical fibroxanthoma: analysis of a series and delineation of a distinctive variant. Histopathology 1993; 22: 247–254.

611 Patterson JW, Konerding H, Kramer WM. "Clear cell" atypical fibroxanthoma. J Dermatol Surg Oncol 1987; 13: 1109–1114.

612 Requena L, Sánchez Yus E. Clear-cell atypical fibroxanthoma: a new histopathologic variant of atypical fibroxanthoma. J Cutan Pathol 1996; 23: 59 (abstract).

613 Lázaro-Santander R, Andrés-Gozalbo C, Rodríguez-Pereira C, Vera-Román JM. Clear cell atypical fibroxanthoma. Histopathology 1999; 35: 484–485.

614 Requena L, Sangueza OP, Sánchez Yus E, Furio V. Clear-cell atypical fibroxanthoma: an uncommon histopathologic variant of atypical fibroxanthoma. J Cutan Pathol 1997; 24: 176–182.

615 Chen KTK. Atypical fibroxanthoma of the skin with osteoid production. Arch Dermatol 1980; 116: 113–114.

616 Wilson PR, Strutton GM, Stewart MR. Atypical fibroxanthoma: two unusual variants. J Cutan Pathol 1989; 16: 93–98.

617 Tomaszewski M-M, Lupton GP. Atypical fibroxanthoma. An unusual variant with osteoclast-like giant cells. Am J Surg Pathol 1997; 21: 213–218.

618 Khan ZM, Cockerell CJ. Atypical fibroxanthoma with osteoclast-like multinucleated giant cells. Am J Dermatopathol 1997; 19: 174–179.

619 Zelger BG, Soyer HP, Zelger B. Giant cell atypical fibroxanthoma: does it really exist? Am J Dermatopathol 1999; 21: 108–109.

620 Val-Bernal JF, Fernández FA. Atypical fibroxanthoma with osteoclastlike giant cells. Am J Surg Pathol 1997; 21: 1393.

621 Diaz-Cascajo C, Borghi S, Bonczkowitz M. Pigmented atypical fibroxanthoma. Histopathology 1998; 33: 537–541.

622 Orosz Z. Atypical fibroxanthoma with granular cells. Histopathology 1998; 33: 88–89.

623 Kuwano H, Hashimoto H, Enjoji M. Atypical fibroxanthoma distinguishable from spindle cell carcinoma in sarcoma-like skin lesions. A clinicopathologic and immunohistochemical study of 21 cases. Cancer 1985; 55: 172–180.

624 Winkelmann RK, Peters MS. Atypical fibroxanthoma. A study with antibody to S-100 protein. Arch Dermatol 1985; 121: 753–755.

625 Ricci A Jr, Cartun RW, Zakowski MF. Atypical fibroxanthoma. A study of 14 cases emphasizing the presence of Langerhans' histiocytes with implications for differential diagnosis by antibody panels. Am J Surg Pathol 1988; 12: 591–598.

626 Fullen DR, Reed JA, Finnerty B, McNutt NS. S100A6 expression in fibrohistiocytic lesions. J Cutan Pathol 2001; 28: 229–234.

627 Altman DA, Nicholoff BJ, Fivenson DP. Differential expression of factor XIIIa and CD34 in cutaneous mesenchymal tumors. J Cutan Pathol 1993; 20: 154–158.

628 Silvis NG, Swanson PE, Manivel JC et al. Spindle-cell and pleomorphic neoplasms of the skin. A clinicopathologic and immunohistochemical study of 30 cases, with emphasis on "atypical fibroxanthomas". Am J Dermatopathol 1988; 10: 9–19.

629 Lazova R, Moynes R, Scott G. CD-74: a useful marker to distinguish atypical fibroxanthoma from malignant fibrous histiocytoma. J Cutan Pathol 1996; 23: 54 (abstract).

630 Monteagudo C, Calduch L, Navarro S et al. Immunodetection of CD99 in atypical fibroxanthoma: a helpful diagnostic marker. Am J Dermatopathol 2000; 22: 351 (abstract).

631 Weedon D, Kerr JFR. Atypical fibroxanthoma of skin: an electron microscope study. Pathology 1975; 7: 173–177.

632 Barr RJ, Wuerker RB, Graham JH. Ultrastructure of atypical fibroxanthoma. Cancer 1977; 40: 736–743.

633 Carson JW, Schwartz RA, McCandless CM, French SW. Atypical fibroxanthoma of the skin. Report of a case with Langerhans-like granules. Arch Dermatol 1984; 120: 234–239.

634 Salo JC, Lewis JJ, Woodruff JM et al. Malignant fibrous histiocytoma of the extremity. Cancer 1999; 85: 1765–1772.

635 Weiss SW, Enzinger FM. Malignant fibrous histiocytoma. An analysis of 200 cases. Cancer 1978; 41: 2250–2266.

636 Weiss SW. Malignant fibrous histiocytoma. Am J Surg Pathol 1982; 6: 773–784.

637 Rothman AE, Lowitt MH, Pfau RG. Pediatric cutaneous malignant fibrous histiocytoma. J Am Acad Dermatol 2000; 42: 371–373.

638 Lim S-C, Kim D-C, Jeong Y-K, Suh C-H. Malignant fibrous histiocytoma in a child's hand. Histopathology 1998; 33: 191–192.

639 Headington JT, Niederhuber JE, Repola DA. Primary malignant fibrous histiocytoma of skin. J Cutan Pathol 1978; 5: 329–338.

640 Moran CA, Kaneko M. Malignant fibrous histiocytoma of the glans penis. Am J Dermatopathol 1990; 12: 182–187.

641 Enzinger FM. Angiomatoid malignant fibrous histiocytoma. A distinct fibrohistiocytic tumor of children and young adults simulating a vascular neoplasm. Cancer 1979; 44: 2147–2157.

642 Fanburg-Smith JC, Miettinen M. Angiomatoid "malignant" fibrous histiocytoma: a clinicopathologic study of 158 cases and further exploration of the myoid phenotype. Hum Pathol 1999; 30: 1336–1343.

643 Gambini C, Haupt R, Rongioletti F. Angiomatoid (malignant) fibrous histiocytoma as a second tumour in a child with neuroblastoma. Br J Dermatol 2000; 142: 537–539.

644 Seo IS, Warner TFCS, Warren JS, Bennett JE. Cutaneous postirradiation sarcoma. Ultrastructural evidence of pluripotential mesenchymal cell derivation. Cancer 1985; 56: 761–767.

645 Routh A, Hickman BT, Johnson WW. Malignant fibrous histiocytoma arising from chronic ulcer. Arch Dermatol 1985; 121: 529–531.

646 Slater DN, Parsons MA, Fussey IV. Malignant fibrous histiocytoma arising in a smallpox vaccination scar. Br J Dermatol 1981; 105: 215–217.

647 Yamamura T, Aozasa K, Honda T et al. Malignant fibrous histiocytoma developing in a burn scar. Br J Dermatol 1984; 110: 725–730.

648 Kearney MM, Soule EH, Ivins JC. Malignant fibrous histiocytoma. A retrospective study of 167 cases. Cancer 1980; 45: 167–178.

649 Bertoni F, Capanna R, Biagini R et al. Malignant fibrous histiocytoma of soft tissue. An analysis of 78 cases located and deeply seated in the extremities. Cancer 1985; 56: 356–367.

650 Pezzi CM, Rawlings MS Jr, Esgro JJ et al. Prognostic factors in 227 patients with malignant fibrous histiocytoma. Cancer 1992; 69: 2098–2103.

651 Jensen V, Brandt Sørensen F, Bentzen SM et al. Proliferative activity (MIB-1 index) is an independent prognostic parameter in patients with high-grade soft tissue sarcomas of subtypes other than malignant fibrous histiocytomas: a retrospective immunohistological study including 216 soft tissue sarcomas. Histopathology 1998; 32: 536–546.

652 Costa MJ, Weiss SW. Angiomatoid malignant fibrous histiocytoma. A follow-up study of 108 cases with evaluation of possible histologic predictors of outcome. Am J Surg Pathol 1990; 14: 1126–1132.

653 Oku T, Takigawa M, Fukamizu H, Yamada M. Tissue cultures of benign and malignant fibrous histiocytomas: SEM observations. J Cutan Pathol 1984; 11: 534–540.

654 Lattes R. Malignant fibrous histiocytoma. A review article. Am J Surg Pathol 1982; 6: 761–771.

655 Dehner LP. Malignant fibrous histiocytoma. Nonspecific morphologic pattern, specific pathologic entity, or both? Arch Pathol Lab Med 1988; 112: 236–237.

656 Hollowood K, Fletcher CDM. Malignant fibrous histiocytoma: morphologic pattern or pathologic entity? Semin Diagn Pathol 1995; 12: 210–220.

657 Derré J, Lagacé R, Nicolas A et al. Leiomyosarcomas and most malignant fibrous histiocytomas share very similar comparative genomic hybridization imbalances: an analysis of a series of 27 leiomyosarcomas. Lab Invest 2001; 81: 211–215.

658 Simons A, Schepens M, Jeuken J et al. Frequent loss of 9p21 [p16 INK4A] and other genomic imbalances in human malignant fibrous histiocytoma. Cancer Genet Cytogenet 2000; 118: 89–98.

659 Montgomery E, Fisher C. Myofibroblastic differentiation in malignant fibrous histiocytoma (pleomorphic myofibrosarcoma): a clinicopathological study. Histopathology 2001; 38: 499–509.

660 Fletcher CDM. Pleomorphic malignant fibrous histiocytoma: fact or fiction? A critical reappraisal based on 159 tumors diagnosed as pleomorphic sarcoma. Am J Surg Pathol 1992; 16: 213–228.

661 Bhagavan BS, Dorfman HD. The significance of bone and cartilage formation in malignant fibrous histiocytoma of soft tissue. Cancer 1982; 49: 480–488.

662 Argenyi ZB, Van Rybroek JJ, Kemp JD, Soper RT. Congenital angiomatoid malignant fibrous histiocytoma. A light-microscopic, immunopathologic, and electron-microscopic study. Am J Dermatopathol 1988; 10: 59–67.

663 Morgan MB, Pitha J, Johnson S et al. Angiomatoid malignant fibrous histiocytoma revisited. An immunohistochemical and DNA ploidy analysis. Am J Dermatopathol 1997; 19: 223–227.

664 Silverman JS, Tamsen A. Interactive CD34-positive fibroblasts and factor XIII-a positive histiocytes in cutaneous mesenchymal tumors. Am J Dermatopathol 1998; 20: 317–320.

665 Waters BL, Panagopoulos I, Allen EF. Genetic characterization of angiomatoid fibrous histiocytoma identifies fusion of the FUS and ATF-1 genes induced by a chromosomal translocation involving bands 12q13 and 16p11. Cancer Genet Cytogenet 2000; 121: 109–116.

666 Smith MEF, Fisher C, Weiss SW. Pleomorphic hyalinizing angiectatic tumor of soft parts. A low-grade neoplasm resembling neurilemmoma. Am J Surg Pathol 1996; 20: 21–29.

667 Silverman JS, Dana MM. Pleomorphic hyalinizing angiectatic tumor of soft parts: immunohistochemical case study shows cellular composition by CD34+ fibroblasts and factor XIIIa+ dendrophages. J Cutan Pathol 1997; 24: 377–383.

668 Weiss SW, Enzinger FM. Myxoid variant of malignant fibrous histiocytoma. Cancer 1977; 39: 1672–1685.

669 Lillemoe T, Steeper T, Manivel JC, Wick MR. Myxoid malignant fibrous histiocytoma (MMFH) of the skin. J Cutan Pathol 1988; 15: 324 (abstract).

670 Stephen MR, Morton R. Myxoid malignant fibrous histiocytoma mimicking papular mucinosis. Am J Dermatopathol 1998; 20: 290–295.

671 Meis-Kindblom JM, Kindblom L-G. Acral myxoinflammatory fibroblastic sarcoma. A low-grade tumor of the hands and feet. Am J Surg Pathol 1998; 22: 911–924.

672 Angervall L, Hagmar B, Kindblom L-G, Merck C. Malignant giant cell tumor of soft tissues; a clinicopathologic, cytologic, ultrastructural, angiographic, and microangiographic study. Cancer 1981; 47: 736–747.

673 Kyriakos M, Kempson RL. Inflammatory fibrous histiocytoma. An aggressive and lethal lesion. Cancer 1976; 37: 1584–1606.

674 Miller R, Kreutner A Jr, Kurtz SM. Malignant inflammatory histiocytoma (inflammatory fibrous histiocytoma). Report of a patient with four lesions. Cancer 1980; 45: 179–187.

675 Ritter JH, Humphrey PA, Wick MR. Malignant neoplasms capable of simulating inflammatory (myofibroblastic) pseudotumors and tumefactive fibroinflammatory lesions: pseudopseudotumors. Semin Diagn Pathol 1998; 15: 111–132.

676 Iwasaki H, Yoshitake K, Ohjimi Y et al. Malignant fibrous histiocytoma. Proliferative compartment and heterogeneity of "histiocytic" cells. Am J Surg Pathol 1992; 16: 735–745.

677 Wick MR, Fitzgibbon J, Swanson PE. Cutaneous sarcomas and sarcomatoid neoplasms of the skin. Semin Diagn Pathol 1993; 10: 148–158.

678 Miettin M, Soini Y. Malignant fibrous histiocytoma. Heterogeneous patterns of intermediate filament proteins by immunohistochemistry. Arch Pathol Lab Med 1989; 113: 1363–1366.

679 Costa MJ, McGlothlen L, Pierce M et al. Angiomatoid features in fibrohistiocytic sarcomas. Arch Pathol Lab Med 1995; 119: 1065–1071.

680 Smith MEF, Costa MJ, Weiss SW. Evaluation of CD68 and other histiocytic antigens in angiomatoid malignant fibrous histiocytoma. Am J Surg Pathol 1991; 15: 757–763.

681 Brooks JSJ. The spectrum of fibrohistiocytic tumours with special emphasis on malignant fibrous histiocytoma. Curr Diagn Pathol 1994; 1: 3–12.

682 Alguacil-Garcia A, Unni KK, Goellner JR. Malignant fibrous histiocytoma. An ultrastructural study of six cases. Am J Clin Pathol 1978; 69: 121–129.

683 Hayashi Y, Kikuchi-Tada A, Jitsukawa K et al. Myofibroblasts in malignant fibrous histiocytoma – histochemical, immunohistochemical, ultrastructural and tissue culture studies. Clin Exp Dermatol 1988; 13: 402–405.

Presumptive synovial and tendon sheath tumors

684 Chung EB, Enzinger FM. Fibroma of tendon sheath. Cancer 1979; 44: 1945–1954.

685 Humphreys S, McKee PH, Fletcher CDM. Fibroma of tendon sheath: a clinicopathologic study. J Cutan Pathol 1986; 13: 331–338.

686 Pulitzer DR, Martin PC, Reed RJ. Fibroma of tendon sheath. A clinicopathologic study of 32 cases. Am J Surg Pathol 1989; 13: 472–479.

687 Dal Cin P, Sciot R, De Smet L, Van den Berghe H. Translocation 2;11 in a fibroma of tendon sheath. Histopathology 1998; 32: 433–435.

688 Azzopardi JG, Tanda F, Salm R. Tenosynovial fibroma. Diagn Histopathol 1983; 6: 69–76.

689 Lamovec J, Bracko M, Voncina D. Pleomorphic fibroma of tendon sheath. Am J Surg Pathol 1991; 15: 1202–1205.

690 Satti MB. Tendon sheath tumours: a pathological study of the relationship between giant cell tumour and fibroma of tendon sheath. Histopathology 1992; 20: 213–220.

691 O'Connell JX, Fanburg JC, Rosenberg AE. Giant cell tumor of tendon sheath and pigmented villonodular synovitis: immunophenotype suggests a synovial cell origin. Hum Pathol 1995; 26: 771–775.

692 Hashimoto H, Tsuneyoshi M, Daimaru Y et al. Fibroma of tendon sheath: a tumor of myofibroblasts. A clinicopathologic study of 18 cases. Acta Pathol Jpn 1985; 35: 1099–1107.

693 Lundgren LG, Kindblom L-G. Fibroma of tendon sheath. A light and electron-microscopic study of 6 cases. Acta Pathol Microbiol Immunol Scand (A) 1984; 92: 401–409.

694 Jones FE, Soule EH, Coventry MB. Fibrous xanthoma of synovium (giant-cell tumor of tendon sheath, pigmented nodular synovitis). J Bone Joint Surg 1969; 51-A: 76–86.

695 Sapra S, Prokopetz R, Murray AH. Giant cell tumor of tendon sheath. Int J Dermatol 1989; 28: 587–590.

696 Richert B, André J. Laterosubungual giant cell tumor of the tendon sheath: An unusual location. J Am Acad Dermatol 1999; 41: 347–348.

697 King DT, Millman AJ, Gurevitch AW, Hirose FM. Giant cell tumor of the tendon sheath involving skin. Arch Dermatol 1978; 114: 944–946.

698 Rustin MHA, Robinson TWE. Giant-cell tumour of the tendon sheath – an uncommon tumour presenting to dermatologists. Clin Exp Dermatol 1989; 14: 466–468.

699 Carstens PHB. Giant cell tumors of tendon sheath. An electron microscopical study of 11 cases. Arch Pathol Lab Med 1978; 102: 99–103.

700 Wood GS, Beckstead JH, Medeiros LJ et al. The cells of giant cell tumor of tendon sheath resemble osteoclasts. Am J Surg Pathol 1988; 12: 444–452.

701 Vogrincic GS, O'Connell JX, Gilks CB. Giant cell tumor of tendon sheath is a polyclonal cellular proliferation. Hum Pathol 1997; 28: 815–819.

702 O'Connell JX, Wehrli BM, Nielsen GP, Rosenberg AE. Giant cell tumors of soft tissue. A clinicopathologic study of 18 benign and malignant tumors. Am J Surg Pathol 2000; 24: 386–395.

703 Oliveira AM, Dei Tos AP, Fletcher CDM, Nascimento AG. Primary giant cell tumor of soft tissues. A study of 22 cases. Am J Surg Pathol 2000; 24: 248–256.

704 Phalen GS, McCormack LJ, Gazale WJ. Giant-cell tumor of tendon sheath (benign synovioma) in the hand. Evaluation of 56 cases. Clin Orthop 1959; 15: 140–151.

705 Wolff HH, Braun-Falco O. Das benigne riesenzell synovialom. Zur klinik, histologie und elektronenmikroskopie. Hautarzt 1972; 23: 499–508.

706 Enzinger FM. Epithelioid sarcoma. A sarcoma simulating a granuloma or a carcinoma. Cancer 1970; 26: 1029–1041.

707 Ratnam AV, Naik KG. Epithelioid sarcoma – a case report. Br J Dermatol 1978; 99: 451–453.

708 Shmookler BM, Gunther SF. Superficial epithelioid sarcoma: a clinical and histologic simulant of benign cutaneous disease. J Am Acad Dermatol 1986; 14: 893–898.

709 Chase DR, Enzinger FM. Epithelioid sarcoma. Diagnosis, prognostic indicators, and treatment. Am J Surg Pathol 1985; 9: 241–263.

710 Zanolli MD, Wilmoth G, Shaw J et al. Epithelioid sarcoma: clinical and histologic characteristics. J Am Acad Dermatol 1992; 26: 302–305.

711 Theunis A, André J, Larsimont D, Song M. Epithelioid sarcoma: a puzzling soft tissue neoplasm in a child. Dermatology 2000; 200: 179–180.

712 Billings SD, Hood AF. Epithelioid sarcoma arising on the nose of a child: a case report and review of the literature. J Cutan Pathol 2000; 27: 186–190.

713 Ulbright TM, Brokaw SA, Stehman FB, Roth LM. Epithelioid sarcoma of the vulva. Evidence suggesting a more aggressive behavior than extra-genital epithelioid sarcoma. Cancer 1983; 52: 1462–1469.

714 Moore SW, Wheeler JE, Hefter LG. Epithelioid sarcoma masquerading as Peyronie's disease. Cancer 1975; 35: 1706–1710.

715 Rose DSC, Fisher C, Smith MEF. Epithelioid sarcoma arising in a patient with neurofibromatosis type 2. Histopathology 1994; 25: 379–380.

716 Prat J, Woodruff JM, Marcove RC. Epithelioid sarcoma. An analysis of 22 cases indicating the prognostic significance of vascular invasion and regional lymph node metastasis. Cancer 1978; 41: 1472–1487.

717 Kusakabe H, Yonebayashi K, Sakatani S et al. Metastic epithelioid sarcoma with an N-*ras* oncogene mutation. Am J Dermatopathol 1994; 16: 294–300.

718 Halling AC, Wollan PC, Pritchard DJ et al. Epithelioid sarcoma: a clinicopathologic review of 55 cases. Mayo Clin Proc 1996; 71: 636–642.

719 Sugarbaker PH, Auda S, Webber BL et al. Early distant metastases from epithelioid sarcoma of the hand. Cancer 1981; 48: 852–855.

720 Evans HL, Baer SC. Epithelioid sarcoma: a clinicopathologic and prognostic study of 26 cases. Semin Diagn Pathol 1993; 10: 286–291.

721 Miettinen M, Lehto V-P, Vartio T, Virtanen I. Epithelioid sarcoma. Ultrastructural and immunohistologic features suggesting a synovial origin. Arch Pathol Lab Med 1982; 106: 620–623.

722 Cooney TP, Hwang WS, Robertson DI, Hoogstraten J. Monophasic synovial sarcoma, epithelioid sarcoma and chordoid sarcoma: ultrastructural evidence for a common histogenesis, despite light microscopic diversity. Histopathology 1982; 6: 163–190.

723 Fisher ER, Horvat B. The fibrocytic origin of the so-called epithelioid sarcoma. Cancer 1972; 30: 1074–1081.

724 Blewitt RW, Aparicio SGR, Bird CC. Epithelioid sarcoma: a tumour of myofibroblasts. Histopathology 1983; 7: 573–584.

725 Bloustein PA, Silverberg SG, Waddell WR. Epithelioid sarcoma. Case report with ultrastructural review, histogenetic discussion, and chemotherapeutic data. Cancer 1976; 38: 2390–2400.

726 Sonobe H, Ohtsuki Y, Ido E et al. Epithelioid sarcoma producing granulocyte colony-stimulating factor. Hum Pathol 1997; 28: 1433–1435.

727 Quezado MM, Middleton LP, Bryant B et al. Allelic loss on chromosome 22Q in epithelioid sarcomas. Hum Pathol 1998; 29: 604–608.

728 Guillou L, Wadden C, Coindre J-M et al. "Proximal-typ" epithelioid sarcoma, a distinctive aggressive neoplasm showing rhabdoid features. Am J Surg Pathol 1997; 21: 130–146.

729 Santiago H, Feinerman LK, Lattes R. Epithelioid sarcoma. A clinical and pathologic study of nine cases. Hum Pathol 1972; 3: 133–147.

730 Tan SH, Ong BH. Spindle cell variant of epithelioid sarcoma – a case mimicking squamous cell carcinoma. Am J Dermatopathol 2000; 22: 346 (abstract).

731 Tan SH, Ong BH. Spindle cell variant of epithelioid sarcoma: an easily misdiagnosed tumour. Australas J Dermatol 2001; 42: 139–141.

732 Mirra JM, Kessler S, Bhuta S, Eckardt J. The fibroma-like variant of epithelioid sarcoma. Cancer 1992; 69: 1382–1395.

733 Medenica M, Casas C, Lorincz AL, Van Dam DP. Epithelioid sarcoma: ultrastructural observation of lymphoid cell-induced lysis of tumor cells. Acta Derm Venereol 1979; 59: 333–339.

734 Chase DR, Weiss SW, Enzinger FM, Langloss JM. Keratin in epithelioid sarcoma. An immunohistochemical study. Am J Surg Pathol 1984; 8: 435–441.

735 Wick MR, Manivel JC. Epithelioid sarcoma and isolated necrobiotic granuloma: a comparative immunocytochemical study. J Cutan Pathol 1986; 13: 253–260.

736 Heenan PJ, Quirk CJ, Papadimitriou JM. Epithelioid sarcoma. A diagnostic problem. Am J Dermatopathol 1986; 8: 95–104.

737 Fisher C. Epithelioid sarcoma: the spectrum of ultrastructural differentiation in seven immunohistochemically defined cases. Hum Pathol 1988; 19: 265–275.

738 Arber DA, Kandalaft PL, Mehta P, Battifora H. Vimentin-negative epithelioid sarcoma. The value of an immunohistochemical panel that includes CD34. Am J Surg Pathol 1993; 17: 302–307.

739 Miettinen M, Fanburg-Smith JC, Virolainen M et al. Epithelioid sarcoma: an immunohistochemical analysis of 112 classical and variant cases and a discussion of the differential diagnosis. Hum Pathol 1999; 30: 934–942.

740 Smith MEF, Brown JI, Fisher C. Epithelioid sarcoma: presence of vascular-endothelial cadherin and lack of epithelial cadherin. Histopathology 1998; 33: 425–431.

741 Bergh P, Meis-Kindblom JM, Gherlinzoni F et al. Synovial sarcoma. Identification of low and high risk groups. Cancer 1999; 85: 2596–2607.

742 Hasegawa T, Yokoyama R, Matsuno Y et al. Prognostic significance of histologic grade and nuclear expression of β-catenin in synovial sarcoma. Hum Pathol 2001; 32: 257–263.

743 Flieder DB, Moran CA. Primary cutaneous synovial sarcoma. A case report. Am J Dermatopathol 1998; 20: 509–512.

744 van de Rijn M, Barr FG, Collins MH et al. Absence of SYT-SSX fusion products in soft tissue tumors other than synovial sarcoma. Am J Clin Pathol 1999; 112: 43–49.

Miscellaneous entities

745 Dupree WB, Enzinger FM. Fibro-osseous pseudotumor of the digits. Cancer 1986; 58: 2103–2109.

746 Takahashi A, Tamura A, Ishikawa O. A case of fibro-osseous pseudotumour of the digits. Br J Dermatol 2001; 144: 1274–1275.

747 Chan KW, Khoo US, Ho CM. Fibro-osseous pseudotumor of the digits: report of a case with immunohistochemical and ultrastructural studies. Pathology 1993; 25: 193–196.

748 Barrett TL, Skelton HG, Smith KJ et al. Ossifying fibromyxoid tumor of soft parts: a case report and review. J Cutan Pathol 1996; 23: 378–380.

749 Velasco-Pastor AM, Martínez-Escribano J, del Pino Gil-Mateo M et al. Ossifying fibromyxoid tumor of soft parts. J Cutan Pathol 1996; 23: 381–384.

750 Nakayama F, Kuwahara T. Ossifying fibromyxoid tumor of soft parts of the back. J Cutan Pathol 1996; 23: 385–388.

751 Amazon K, Glick H. Subcutaneous fibroadenoma on an arm. Am J Dermatopathol 1985; 7: 127–130.

752 Price EW. Nodular subepidermal fibrosis in non-filarial endemic elephantiasis of the legs. Br J Dermatol 1973; 89: 451–456.

753 Zouboulis ChC, Biczó S, Gollnick H et al. Elephantiasis nostras verrucosa: beneficial effect of oral etretinate therapy. Br J Dermatol 1992; 127: 411–416.

754 Caputo R, Gianotti R, Grimalt R et al. Soft fibroma-like lesions on the legs of a patient with Kaposi's sarcoma and lymphedema. Am J Dermatopathol 1991; 13: 493–496.

755 Fischer GO, de Launey WE. Multifocal fibrosclerosis: cutaneous associations. Case report and review of the literature. Australas J Dermatol 1986; 27: 19–26.

756 Michal M, Sokol L. Benign polymorphous mesenchymal tumor (mesenchymal hamartoma) of soft parts. Report of two cases. Am J Dermatopathol 1997; 19: 271–275.

757 Sanchez JL. Collagenous papules on the conchae. Am J Dermatopathol 1983; 5: 231–233.

758 Iranzo P, Mascaro JM. Comments on previously reported cases of collagenous papules on the aural conchae. Am J Dermatopathol 1985; 7: 502–503.

759 Hicks BC, Weber PJ, Hashimoto K et al. Primary cutaneous amyloidosis of the auricular concha. J Am Acad Dermatol 1988; 18: 19–25.

760 Handley J, Carson D, Sloan J et al. Multiple lentigines, myxoid tumours and endocrine overactivity: four cases of Carney's complex. Br J Dermatol 1992; 126: 367–371.

761 Sanusi ID. Subungual myxoma. Arch Dermatol 1982; 118: 612–614.

762 Hill TL, Jones BE, Park KH. Myxoma of the skin of a finger. J Am Acad Dermatol 1990; 22: 343–345.

763 Allen PW, Dymock RB, MacCormac LB. Superficial angiomyxomas with and without epithelial components. Report of 30 tumors in 28 patients. Am J Surg Pathol 1988; 12: 519–530.

764 Guerin D, Calonje E, McCormick D, Fletcher CDM. Superficial angiomyxoma: clinicopathological analysis of 26 cases of a distinctive cutaneous tumour with tendency for recurrence. J Pathol (Suppl) 1995; 176: 51A (abstract).

765 Bedlow AJ, Sampson SA, Holden CA. Congenital superficial angiomyxoma. Clin Exp Dermatol 1997; 22: 237–239.

766 Calonje E, Guerin D, McCormick D, Fletcher CDM. Superficial angiomyxoma. Clinicopathologic analysis of a series of distinctive but poorly recognized cutaneous tumors with tendency for recurrence. Am J Surg Pathol 1999; 23: 910–917.

767 Wilk M, Schmoeckel C, Kaiser HW et al. Cutaneous angiomyxoma: a benign neoplasm distinct from cutaneous focal mucinosis. J Am Acad Dermatol 1995; 33: 352–355.

Tumors of fat

INTRODUCTION

The tumors of fat are a histologically diverse group. Fortunately, most have well-established diagnostic criteria and present no difficulty in diagnosis. However, there are three comparatively recently delineated fatty tumors – spindle-cell lipoma, sclerotic lipoma and pleomorphic lipoma – which may cause diagnostic problems, sometimes leading to a mistaken diagnosis of liposarcoma.

Lipomatous tumors of different types appear to harbor CD34[+] interstitial dendritic cells. Clonal expansion of the CD34[+] cells may account for the development of spindle-cell lipomas and the spindle-cell component in some dedifferentiated liposarcomas.[1,2]

Most tumors of fat, excluding angiolipomas, have specific aberrations of their karyotype. On this basis, it has been suggested that angiolipomas (see below) are not true lipomas, but a hamartoma of blood vessels and fat.[3]

NEVUS LIPOMATOSUS

Nevus lipomatosus, also known by the complicated term 'nevus lipomatosus cutaneus superficialis (Hoffmann–Zurhelle)[4,5] is a rare type of connective tissue nevus characterized by the presence of mature adipose tissue in the dermis. It is found as plaques or solitary lesions, or in an extremely rare generalized form.

The plaque type has aggregations of flesh-colored or yellow papules and nodules which are present at birth, or which develop in the first two decades of life. There is a predilection for the pelvic girdle, particularly the gluteal region. Other sites may be involved.[6] Lesions are usually unilateral, and sometimes in a linear or zosteriform arrangement. The surface of most lesions is smooth, although it may be verrucous or dimpled. Surface comedones have been noted occasionally. Lesions usually develop insidiously, but later become reasonably stable.

The solitary form consists of isolated papules or nodules, anywhere on the body, but with a predilection for the trunk.[7] They may not appear until the fifth decade. They usually have a broader base than the common skin tag (acrochordon), but there are some who doubt the existence of the solitary form, preferring to regard them as skin tags or 'pedunculated lipofibromas'.[4,8]

There are reports of more generalized body involvement with a markedly folded skin surface ('Michelin man' appearance).[9,10]

Histopathology[4,11]

The basic abnormality is the presence of varying amounts of mature adipose tissue in the dermis, often not connecting with the fat of the underlying subcutis. The fat can constitute from less than 10%, to 70% of the lesion. When there is only a small amount of fat, it is usually localized around the subpapillary blood vessels. Some authors have indicated a requirement for fat to be present in the papillary dermis in solitary cases to distinguish them from skin tags,[11] but this feature is not always present, even in the plaque variant (Fig. 35.1).

There are also abnormalities in the other connective tissue components of the dermis,[4] including some thickening of the collagen bundles.[12] In about half of the cases the deeper elastic tissue is increased, although there may be a reduction in elastic fibers superficially. There is an increase in the number of fibroblasts in the papillary dermis, and also of mononuclear cells, including mast cells, elsewhere in the dermis. Blood vessels are increased in the papillary dermis, and subjacent to this there may be some ectatic vessels. Vessels are also increased in the ectopic dermal fat. Pilosebaceous follicles are often reduced.

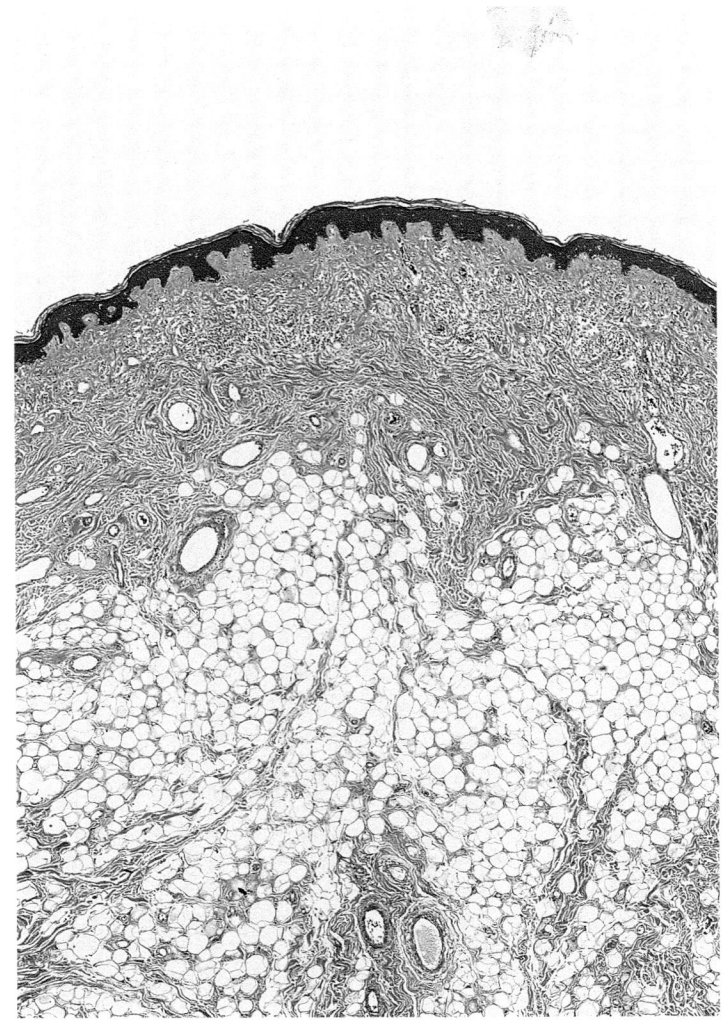

Fig. 35.1 **Nevus lipomatosus.** Mature fat cells replace much of the dermis. Sometimes they extend to the undersurface of the epidermis. (H & E)

The epidermal changes are variable. There is often some undulation with acanthosis and even mild papillomatosis,[13] and there may be mild hyperpigmentation of the basal layer. The changes may resemble those of an epidermal nevus. Dilated follicular ostia will be present, if there are comedones clinically.

Nevus lipomatosus should be distinguished from old nevocellular nevi, in which there may be large amounts of fat and sometimes only small areas of nevus cells. Focal dermal hypoplasia also has fat in the dermis, but in this condition there is extreme attenuation of collagen as well as vast clinical differences. The dermal variant of spindle-cell lipoma has more spindle-shaped cells present as well as a fibromucinous stroma.

Electron microscopy

Electron microscopy has shown mature lipocytes in the perivascular region,[14] and, in one study, a vascular origin for the fat cells was suggested.[15]

PIEZOGENIC PEDAL PAPULES

In piezogenic pedal papules there are usually multiple small papulonodules on the heels[16–21] which have a tendency to disappear when pressure is relieved from the heels.[21] Although most are painless and small,[22] there are a few reports of a painful variant.[17–19,23] This entity has recently been reported in one-third of a group of patients with Ehlers–Danlos syndrome.[20]

Piezogenic pedal papules are thought to represent pressure-induced herniations of the subcutaneous fat through acquired or inherited defects in the connective tissue of the heel.[20,24,25]

Similar lesions (piezogenic wrist papules) have been reported on the wrist.[26]

Histopathology[18,19]

There is thickening of the dermis in the painful variant, with loss of the normal small fat compartments in the lower dermis and subcutis. These appear to coalesce as a result of degeneration of the thin fibrous septa.[18,20,21] There may also be protrusion of these enlarged fat lobules into the dermis.[19] Such cases need to be distinguished from the rare condition of **bilateral congenital adipose plantar nodules**, in which there are well-defined lobules of mature fat in the mid and deep dermis, mostly in a periadnexal distribution;[27] **congenital fibrolipomatous hamartoma** appears to be the same condition.[28]

LIPOBLASTOMA

Lipoblastoma is a rare, benign tumor of infants and young children, thought to be related to fetal white fat.[29–32] Some earlier reports of liposarcoma in infants probably included examples of this entity.[33] Chung and Enzinger delineated a circumscribed, usually superficial type, and a less common diffuse form, often in the deeper soft tissues, analogous to diffuse lipomatosis.[31] In one study of 14 cases, 6 were of the circumscribed type and 8 were diffuse and ill defined (lipoblastomatosis),[34] while in another study of 25 cases, 11 were circumscribed (discrete) and 14 were diffuse.[35] Lipoblastoma/lipoblastomatosis behaves in a benign fashion, although local recurrence sometimes occurs.[35]

Cytogenetic studies have consistently shown alterations in chromosome 8, band q11–13, in contrast to the translocation t(12;16)(q13;p11) found in myxoid liposarcoma.[36]

Lipoblastomas are light yellow to tan-yellow tumors, averaging 5 cm in greatest diameter, with focal myxoid areas on the cut surface. They are usually thinly encapsulated.

Histopathology[31]

The tumor is lobulated, with thin, well-vascularized connective tissue septa. The lobules contain mature fat cells, intermingled with spindle-shaped mesenchymal cells and various types of lipoblasts. These cells may be univacuolated, resembling signet-ring cells, multivacuolated, or granular resembling hibernoma cells (Fig. 35.2). In contrast to liposarcoma, there are no mitoses or nuclear atypia in the lipoblasts. There is often a plexiform capillary pattern in the lobules, and patchy myxoid stroma containing mucopolysaccharides. The cytogenetic abnormality differs from liposarcoma (see above).

Electron microscopy

Ultrastructural examination has confirmed the presence of lipocytes, lipoblasts and mesenchymal cells.[37] The lipid vacuoles may or may not be membrane bound.[38]

LIPOFIBROMATOSIS

Lipofibromatosis is a rare pediatric neoplasm, with a propensity for the hands and feet, which occurs in the subcutis and deep soft tissues.[39] It may be

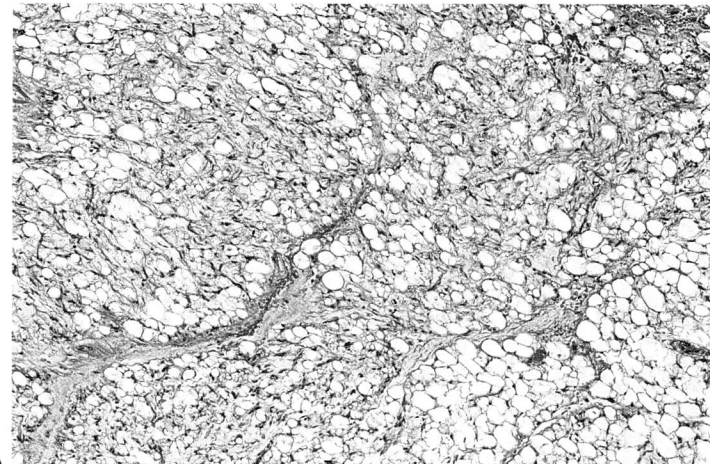
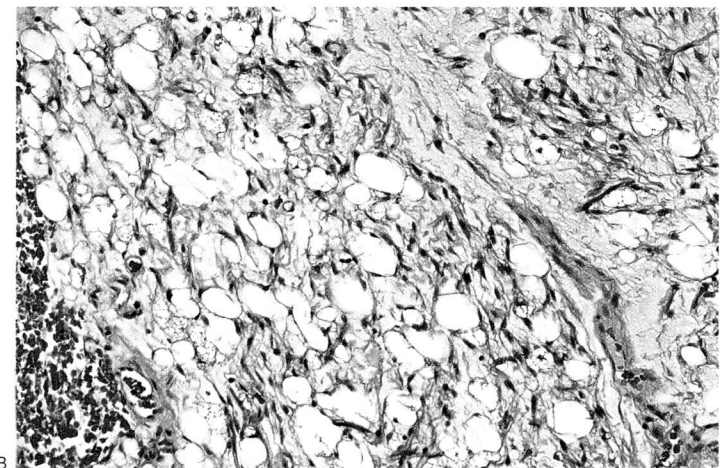

Fig. 35.2 **Lipoblastoma. (A)** The tumor is composed of mature fat cells, spindle-shaped mesenchymal cells, and a few cells with granular cytoplasm. **(B)** A higher power view of the same lesion. (H & E)

present at birth. Similar cases have been diagnosed in the past as infantile fibromatosis, fibrous hamartoma of infancy, and fibrosing lipoblastoma. Regrowth or persistence of the tumor is common following incomplete excision.[39]

Histopathology

There is abundant adipose tissue, typically comprising more than 50% of the specimen, dissected by thickened septa containing a spindled fibroblastic element.[39] These cells sometimes show a fascicular growth pattern and limited mitotic activity. Small collections of univacuolated cells are often present at the interface between the fat and the fibroblastic element. Rare pigmented cells have been described.[39]

PSEUDOLIPOMATOSIS CUTIS

The term 'pseudolipomatosis cutis' was coined by Trotter and Crawford for the incidental finding of grouped and coalescent spaces in the dermis resembling fatty infiltration.[40] Similar changes have been reported in acrodermatitis chronica atrophicans (see p. 654) and in a case of psoriasis (see p. 80).[41] Although Trotter and Crawford regarded these spaces as artifactual, subsequent correspondence refuted this suggestion in favor of a prelymphatic origin.[41]

LIPOMA AND LIPOMATOSIS

Lipomas are relatively common, usually asymptomatic, subcutaneous tumors with a predilection for the upper trunk, upper extremities, thighs and neck of individuals in the fifth and sixth decades.[42] A deep variant arising on the forehead has recently been described.[43] Lipomas account for 90% or more of tumors of fat seen in most laboratories. They are soft, often mobile, encapsulated tumors of varying size, but averaging 3–5 cm in diameter. 'Giant' variants have been recorded.[44]

There are several distinct clinical syndromes in which disfiguring masses of mature adipose tissue develop in the subcutaneous tissues. These are discussed in some detail by Allen.[45] In **benign symmetric lipomatosis** (multiple symmetric lipomatosis/Madelung's disease), the tumors develop on the neck, back and upper trunk, with a predilection for middle-aged men.[46–51] Variants involving the hands,[52] the thighs[53] or the feet[54] have been reported. The distinction between obesity and localized (zonal) variants of the buttocks and thighs is often problematic in females.[55] Familial cases have also been recorded, but no pattern of inheritance has been delineated. Some cases have been associated with the mitochondrial DNA syndromes.[56] Various metabolic abnormalities may occur in this condition,[57,58] and there is sometimes alcohol-related liver disease.[55,59–61] In **familial multiple lipomatosis**,[59,62–64] multiple discrete, usually asymptomatic, lipomas develop on the forearms, trunk and thighs in the third decade. Non-symmetrical lesions may be present.[65] An autosomal dominant inheritance has been proposed, despite the predominance in males. The masses are encapsulated and vary from a few millimeters to 5 cm or more in diameter. In **adiposis dolorosa (Dercum's disease)** there are painful, circumscribed or diffuse fatty deposits with a predilection for the lower legs, abdomen and buttocks.[66,67] There may be obesity, weakness and mental disturbances. Familial cases related to an autosomal dominant gene with variable expressivity have been reported.[58,69] Juxta-articular fatty deposits, resembling those seen in adiposis dolorosa, have been reported in a patient receiving long-term treatment with high doses of corticosteroids.[70] **Diffuse lipomatosis**[33,71–73] consists of infiltrating masses of mature adipose tissue, extensively involving part of a limb or the trunk, with onset before 2 years of age. It has been associated with tuberous sclerosis.[71] In **encephalocraniocutaneous lipomatosis**[74–76] there are subcutaneous lipomas on the scalp with overlying alopecia, as well as cranial and ocular abnormalities. The cutaneous component has been called 'nevus psiloliparus'.[77] **Infiltrating lipoma of the face**[78] is another variant of this hamartomatous condition. Other variants of infiltrating lipoma occur.[79] **Lipedematous scalp** refers to a thickening of the subcutaneous fat of the scalp, leading to a clinically thickened and soft scalp.[80] It may present as an alopecia (see p. 481).

The use of protease inhibitors in the treatment of human immunodeficiency virus type 1 (HIV-1) may be associated with several abnormalities of fat including subcutaneous lipomas,[81] angiolipomas,[82] peripheral lipodystrophy (see p. 530) and benign symmetrical lipomatosis.[81]

Cytogenetically, approximately 30% of lipomas are characterized by aberrations of 12q13–15. Others probably have subtle abnormalities that are undetectable by standard cytogenetic methods.[3]

Histopathology

Lipomas are composed of sheets of mature fat dissected by thin, incomplete fibrous septa containing a few blood vessels. A fibrous capsule is present. Variants with increased stromal fibrous tissue (fibrolipomas) are found. If blood vessels constitute more than 5% of the mass, the lesion is best regarded as an angiolipoma (see below). Eccrine sweat ducts are rarely present. Such variants have been termed 'adenolipomas'.[83] The admixture of smooth muscle and fat constitutes a myolipoma. Rarely, the lipomatous component is mildly atypical.[84] A unique case with myxoid change and synovial metaplasia has been reported.[85] Membranous fat necrosis is another rare secondary change.[86]

The histological appearances of the various lipomatosis syndromes are similar, except for the absence of a capsule and increased fibrous tissue in multiple symmetrical lipomatosis, and the 'infiltrative' properties of the fat in diffuse lipomatosis. Granulomatous panniculitis has been found in a painful mass in Dercum's disease, although most reports have shown normal fat.[66]

ANGIOLIPOMA

Angiolipomas are subcutaneous tumors of the extremities and trunk; they comprise approximately 10% of tumors of fat.[87–89] They are often multiple, with the first tumors appearing just after puberty.[87] A family history is found in about 10% of cases, but no pattern of inheritance has been proposed. A history of previous trauma to the site or the therapeutic use of protease inhibitors is rarely elicited.[82,90] Mild pain or discomfort is often noted when pressure is applied or the lesions are moved;[91] the pain appears to be related to the vascularity of the lesions.

Subcutaneous angiolipomas have a normal karyotype, setting them apart from most other tumors of fat, including lipomas.[92] For this reason, they have been regarded as a hamartoma of blood vessels and fat, rather than a true tumor of fat.[3]

Macroscopically, they are yellow, firm, circumscribed tumors, from 1 to 4 cm in diameter. They may have a yellow-red appearance on the cut surface, reflecting the degree of vascularity.

Subcutaneous angiolipomas must be distinguished from the infiltrating angiolipoma, which is a solitary lesion of the deep soft tissues.[93,94] It will not be discussed further.

Histopathology[87,88,95]

Angiolipomas have a thin fibrous capsule with incomplete fibrous septa extending into the lesion, dividing it into lobules of different size. They are composed of variable proportions of fatty tissue and blood vessels (Fig. 35.3). The fat cells are mature, with a single vacuole and an eccentric nucleus. The vascular component, which comprises 5–50% or more of the tumor, consists of groups of capillaries and occasional vessels of larger caliber.[95] Only sparse fat cells were present in the lesion reported as a cellular angiolipoma,[96] which was composed almost entirely of small vessels. In the usual type of angiolipoma there are prominent pericytes around the vessels.[88] Erythrocytes are present within the lumen, and scattered fibrin thrombi are easily found. In one report, hemorrhagic infarction of the fat was present in association with numerous fibrin thrombi and disseminated intravascular coagulation.[97] Two cases with a myxoid stroma have been reported (angiomyxolipoma).[98] This tumor shares cytogenetic changes with lipoma, spindle-cell/pleomorphic lipoma and myxoma, setting it apart from the angiolipoma, which has a normal karyotype.[99]

There are numerous mast cells throughout the tumor.[100] Bodian stains for small nerves have been consistently negative, but large myelinated nerves have been found in the surrounding connective tissue.[95]

Electron microscopy

Ultrastructural examination has shown mature fat cells interspersed with blood vessels lined by one or more endothelial cells.[88] Interestingly, Weibel–Palade bodies, characteristic of endothelial cells, were exceedingly sparse in the endothelium.[88] The significance of this finding is uncertain.

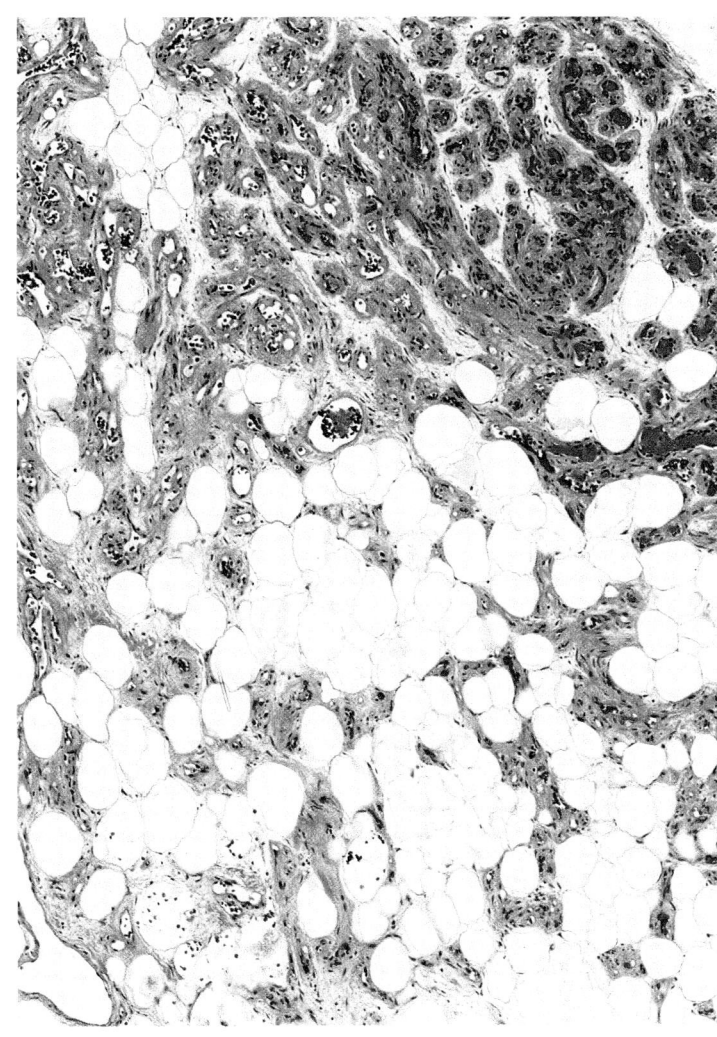

Fig. 35.3 **Angiolipoma.** Mature fat cells are admixed with small blood vessels. (H & E)

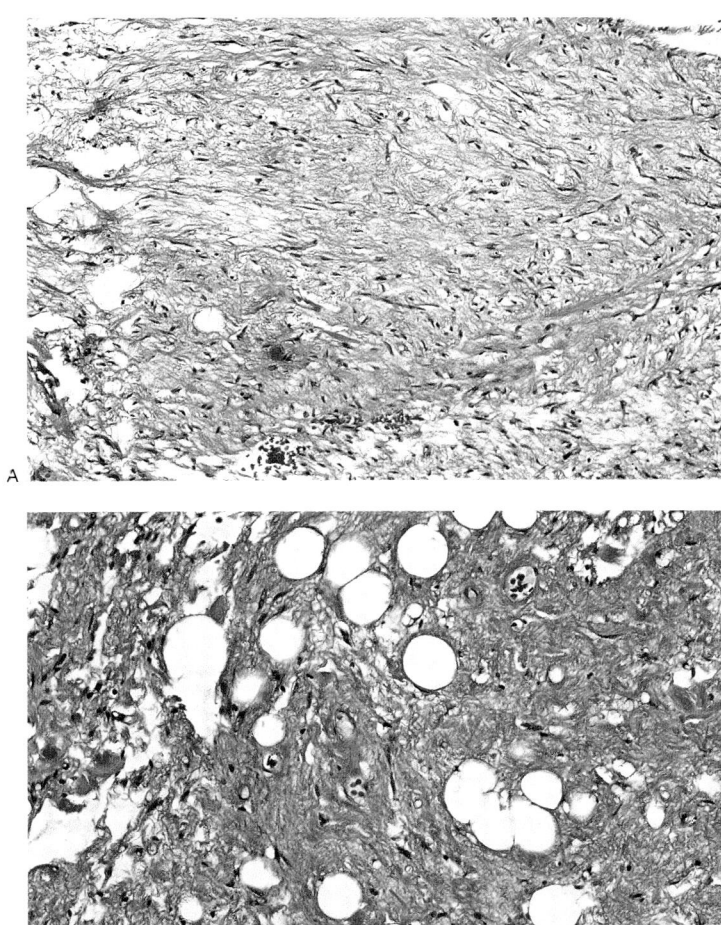

Fig. 35.4 **(A) Spindle-cell lipoma. (B)** The tumor is composed of fat cells, fibrous tissue and scattered spindle-shaped cells. (H & E)

SPINDLE-CELL LIPOMA

Spindle-cell lipoma is a slow-growing benign tumor of the subcutis. It primarily affects the shoulders, upper back, and back of the neck of men in the fifth to seventh decades.[101,102] Uncommonly, the tumors arise on the extremities,[101] lower trunk[103] and the head.[104,105] They are generally painless. Multiple lesions are rare; the clinical presentation of such cases may mimic symmetrical lipomatosis (see above).[106] Some cases are familial.[106] Cytogenetic studies generally show monosomy 16 or partial loss of 16q, a finding distinct from liposarcoma.[3] Anomalies of chromosome 13 have also been reported.[107]

Macroscopically, the tumors are soft, oval, lobular masses with an average diameter of 5 cm. They are yellow or gray-yellow in color, and sometimes have a glistening or mucoid appearance on the cut surface.

Histopathology[101,103,108]

Spindle-cell lipomas are usually circumscribed unencapsulated tumors of the subcutis, although occasionally they are poorly delimited and extend into the dermis or underlying tissues. A variant confined to the dermis (dermal spindle-cell lipoma) has been reported.[109,110] They are composed of a variable mixture of spindle cells and adipose tissue (Fig. 35.4). Sometimes the proliferation of spindle cells is localized. The spindle cells are usually small and elongated and arranged haphazardly. Occasionally they may show a palisaded or fascicular pattern in some areas. A few spindle cells may show small cytoplasmic vacuoles. There is no increase in mitoses, although there may be some nuclear variability. The spindle cells are separated by variable amounts of collagen. Sometimes this stroma shows focal myxomatous change, which stains positively for acid mucopolysaccharides.

The intervening fat cells are mature and univacuolated, resembling normal fat. There are no lipoblasts present. A few tumors have a prominent vascular pattern,[111] and this may resemble a lymphangioma or hemangiopericytoma in some areas.[101] At other times there are irregular and branching spaces with villiform connective tissue projections, giving a striking angiomatoid appearance.[112] This is the so-called *'pseudoangiomatous variant'* (Fig. 35.5). A few inflammatory cells may be found in the walls of these vessels. Mast cells are usually present throughout the stroma. The cytoplasm of the spindle cells stains for vimentin[102] and CD34.[2,113,114] Some factor XIIIa-positive stromal cells are also present.[1]

In the past, spindle-cell lipoma was sometimes confused histologically with liposarcoma and other spindle-cell sarcomas. The absence of multivacuolated lipoblasts and lack of significant nuclear atypia excludes liposarcoma.

Electron microscopy

Ultrastructurally, the spindle cells resemble fibroblasts. A few contain cytoplasmic lipid droplets.[101,102]

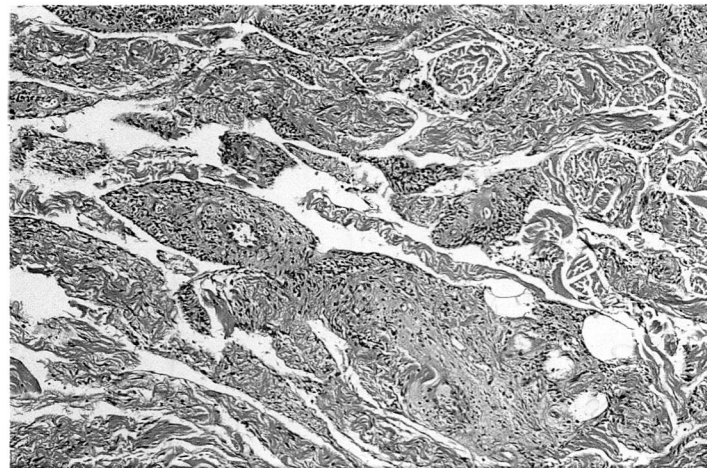

Fig. 35.5 **Spindle-cell lipoma.** This is the pseudoangiomatous variant with vascular-like spaces of irregular shape. (H & E)

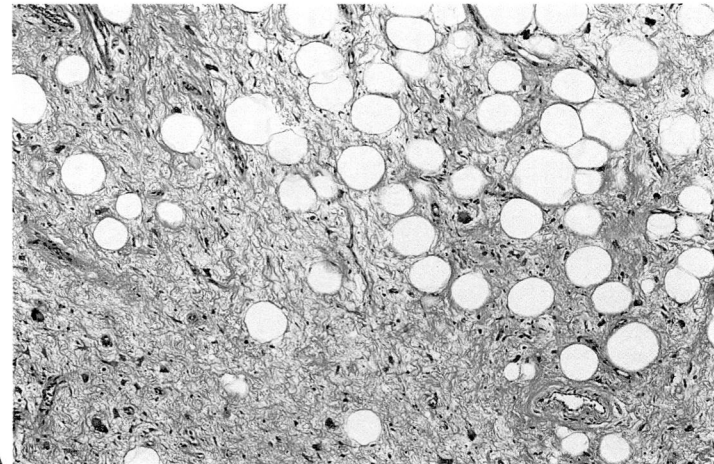

A

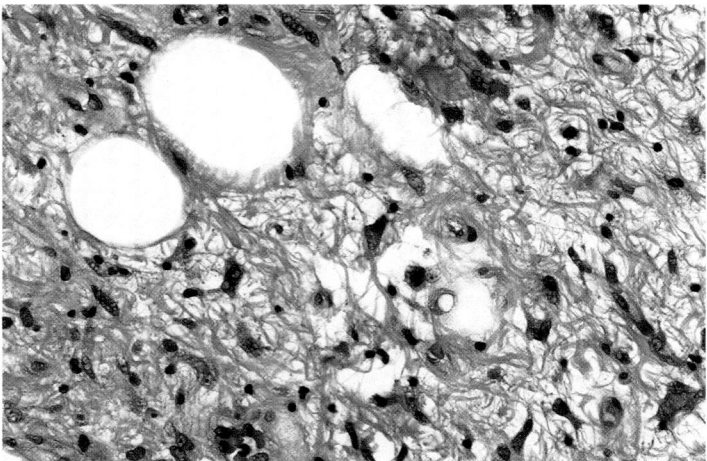

B

Fig. 35.6 **(A) Pleomorphic lipoma. (B)** Some fat cells have hyperchromatic nuclei with a smudgy appearance. There are no mitoses. (H & E)

SCLEROTIC LIPOMA

Sclerotic lipoma is a recently delineated subtype of lipoma with prominent stromal sclerosis. The reported cases have all been in young adult males.[115] Three lesions were on the scalp and two on the hands.

Histopathology

Sclerotic fibromas are circumscribed nodules in the subcutis with a prominent sclerotic stroma in a storiform arrangement. There is a resemblance to fibrolipoma or sclerotic fibroma (circumscribed storiform collagenoma), depending on the amount of admixed fat. The number of adipocytes varies from case to case and in different parts of the same tumor. Small foci containing numerous spindle-shaped to stellate cells may be found. The *fibrous spindle-cell lipoma* has abundant fibrous stroma; sclerosis is not a feature.[116]

Immunohistochemistry shows staining for vimentin and also for S100 protein at the margins of the adipocytes.[115]

PLEOMORPHIC LIPOMA

Pleomorphic (giant-cell) lipoma is a benign tumor of adipose tissue with atypical histological features that may lead to a misdiagnosis of liposarcoma.[117,118] It presents as a soft subcutaneous mass, averaging 5 cm in diameter. A case confined to the dermis has been reported.[119] Pleomorphic lipoma has a predilection for the shoulders, back of the neck, back[117,120] and, less frequently, the face and thighs[121] of middle-aged to elderly males.[117] Pleomorphic lipomas resemble spindle-cell lipomas cytogenetically with a consistent loss of chromosome 16q material.[3] Macroscopically, the tumor resembles a lipoma, although gelatinous gray areas may be present on the cut surface. Some of the reported cases of atypical lipoma are examples of this entity.[122,123]

Histopathology[117,121]

These circumscribed tumors have an intricate mixture of mature adipose tissue, collagen, and myxoid areas interspersed with cellular foci of varying amounts. In addition to lipoblast-like cells, the tumor includes spindle and giant cells, the latter being both uninucleate and multinucleate in type (Fig. 35.6). There are variable numbers of giant cells with marginally placed and often overlapping nuclei, the so-called 'floret giant cells'. Sometimes the nuclei of some giant cells are smudgy, with indistinct chromatin. Mitoses are rare. Focal collections of lymphocytes and plasma cells are often found within the tumor. A variant with pseudopapillary structures resembling those seen in pseudoangiomatous spindle-cell lipoma (see above) has been described.[124]

At times the pleomorphic lipoma is a circumscribed nodule within an otherwise typical lipoma. Areas resembling spindle-cell lipoma may sometimes be present within pleomorphic lipomas. As in spindle-cell lipoma, there are CD34+ and factor XIIIa+ stromal cells.[1]

Pleomorphic lipoma may be distinguished from liposarcoma by the floret giant cells, the pyknotic or smudgy nuclear features, and the absence of mitoses.[125]

CHONDROID LIPOMA

The chondroid variant of lipogenic tumor was described by Meis and Enzinger in 1993.[126] The lesion is usually deep seated, although subcutaneous variants occur. It has a predilection for females. The lower extremity is the most common location. Its histogenesis is disputed. One view is that the lesion is composed only of white adipocytes, but the other view suggests that the cells have features of embryonal fat and, to a lesser extent, embryonal cartilage.[127] A recent cytogenetic study showed a three-way translocation between chromosomes 1, 2, and 5 together with an 11;16 translocation with a breakpoint in 11q13.[128]

Chondroid lipomas are firm yellow tumors averaging 3–5 cm in diameter.

Histopathology

The tumors are lobulated, with a thin capsule.[126,127,129] There are multi-vacuolated tumor cells within a chondromyxoid matrix. In addition, there are clusters of mature adipocytes with a single vacuole that occupies most of the cytoplasm. The cells contain glycogen and fat. The stroma is strongly metachromatic with toluidine blue at pH 4.0.

Immunoperoxidase methods demonstrate vimentin and S100 protein in the tumor cells.[127–129]

Electron microscopy[129]

The tumor cells have numerous lipid vacuoles of varying size in the cytoplasm. There are glycogen granules, mitochondria and pinocytotic vesicles. The cells are set in a flocculent stroma, with cartilage demonstrable in some areas.[127]

HIBERNOMA

Hibernoma is a rare benign tumor of the subcutaneous[130] and deeper soft tissues,[131] generally considered to arise from brown fat. It is found in the scapular area, axilla,[132] lower neck[130] and, less commonly, in the thigh,[133,134] abdominal wall[135] and retroperitoneum.[136] It grows slowly. There may be increased warmth over the area.[137] Cytogenetic studies have shown re-arrangements in both homologs of chromosome 11, frequently including deletions in the region between *PLCB3* and *PPP1A*, leading to loss of the *MEN1* gene.[128,138] In addition, abnormalities involving chromosome 10q22 have been reported.[3]

Grossly, hibernomas are tan-brown lobulated tumors, averaging 10 cm in diameter. Several possible malignant variants have been reported, but these have been disputed by others.[130,139]

Histopathology[130,135]

The tumors are thinly encapsulated, and divided into lobules by thin septa. There are usually prominent blood vessels in the septa and lobules; in one case with possible endocrine activity[133] they assumed a prominent sinusoidal pattern.

There are three cell types with transitional forms.[136] These include large, coarsely vacuolated cells with multiple vacuoles, univacuolated cells, and smaller cells with granular cytoplasm (Fig. 35.7). Vacuoles stain with oil red O in frozen sections. Lipofuscin pigment is also present.[140] There is often a prominent nucleolus, but there are no mitoses.

Electron microscopy

Electron microscopy shows abundant lipid droplets, numerous pleomorphic mitochondria with transverse cristae, and a well-formed basal lamina.[135,136,140,141]

ATYPICAL SUBCUTANEOUS FATTY TUMORS

This category of fatty tumors is not a distinct entity, but the name given by Allen and colleagues to borderline lesions seen in a consultation practice.[142] It comprises a histological spectrum ranging from atypical fibrolipomas, through various mixed spindle-cell and pleomorphic lipoma patterns, to tumors indistinguishable from dedifferentiated liposarcomas.[142,143] Of interest is the extremely good prognosis of atypical lesions confined to the subcutaneous fat, despite sometimes alarming histological features, including the presence of lipoblasts.[142] Local recurrence can occur.

LIPOSARCOMA

Liposarcomas are uncommon tumors of the deep soft tissues and retroperitoneum that only rarely arise in the subcutis, although they may eventually extend into it from below.[144–146] Accordingly, they will be considered only briefly. They have a predilection for the thighs and buttocks, but may sometimes involve the head and neck[147,148] or upper extremities. They arise in older adults, and are exceedingly rare in children.[33,149] Although a few cases have developed in patients with multiple lipomas, liposarcomas are not thought to arise from pre-existing lipomas.[144,150] They are often large and non-encapsulated, varying in color from yellow to gray, to gray-white. There may be some firmer areas and gelatinous foci in the generally soft tissue.

Recently, primary liposarcoma of the skin (dermis) has been described.[151] Four of the seven cases arose on the scalp. The median age of the patients was 72 years. Local recurrence occurred in two patients, but no metastases or disease-related deaths were recorded.[151]

Cytogenetic studies have shown clonal karyotypic abnormalities, which often correlate with the histological subtype.[152] For example, the myxoid liposarcoma often demonstrates a balanced translocation t(12;16)(q13;p11).[36,152,153] A similar chromosomal abnormality has been found in the round cell liposarcoma, suggesting that this variant may be a poorly differentiated form of myxoid liposarcoma.[154] The well-differentiated liposarcoma (including sclerosing, inflammatory and dedifferentiated variants) is characterized by ring

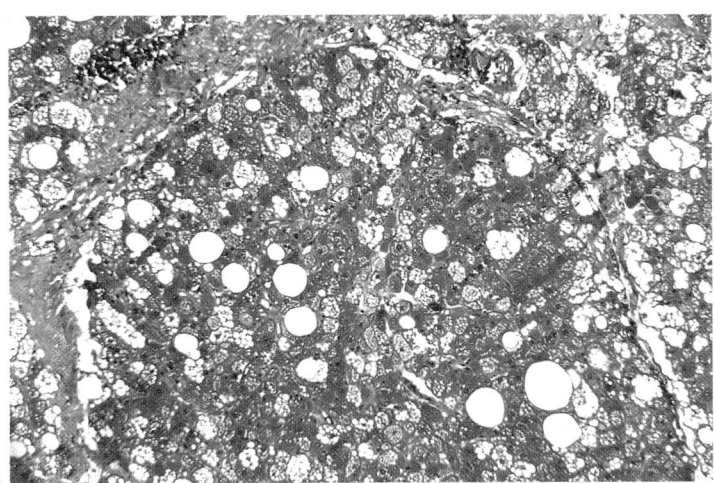
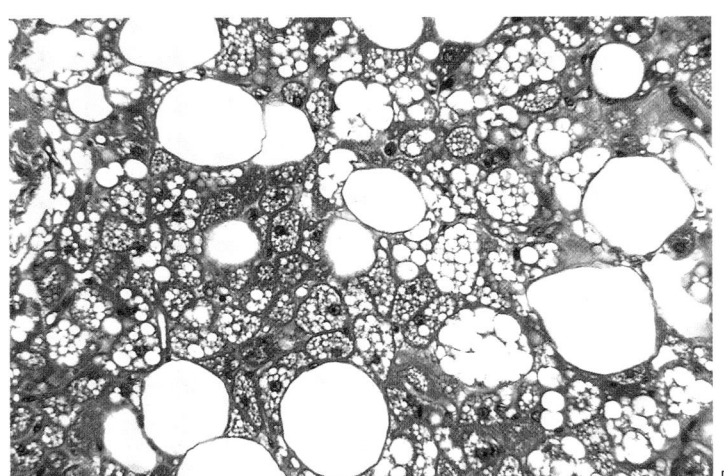

Fig. 35.7 **(A) Hibernoma. (B)** Some cells are coarsely vacuolated while others have a 'granular' cytoplasm. (H & E)

or long marker chromosomes derived from chromosome 12, while the pleomorphic liposarcoma has complex karyotypes.[155]

Histopathology[145,156,157]

There are four histological variants, although mixed forms occur. The *well-differentiated (lipoma-like) liposarcoma* (atypical lipomatous tumor) resembles normal fat.[158] There is some nuclear pleomorphism and hyperchromatism and scattered multivacuolated lipoblasts. The diagnosis is often made in retrospect, after the first recurrence. A sclerosing variant with abundant fibrous tissue is also recognized.[159] The spindle-cell liposarcoma is a further variant: a relatively bland spindle-cell proliferation is arranged in fascicles and whorls and set in a variably myxoid stroma.[160,161] Numerous lymphocytes are sometimes present, but this feature is usually associated with the pleomorphic variant (see below).[162,163] Well-differentiated liposarcomas have a good prognosis. The *myxoid liposarcoma* consists of fusiform or stellate cells, with abundant mucoid stroma, a delicate plexiform network of small capillaries, and a variable number of multivacuolated lipoblasts.[149] Tumor cells stain for vimentin and S100 protein. There is often focal expression of desmin and smooth muscle actin.[152] This variant often metastasizes to extrapulmonary sites.[164] The *round cell liposarcoma*, which is a poorly differentiated form of myxoid liposarcoma,[165,166] has diffuse sheets of closely arranged round or oval cells, frequently with a single small cytoplasmic vacuole. Lipoblasts are present but may be difficult to find. Mitoses are abundant in some areas. Fibrosarcoma-like areas are sometimes present. The *pleomorphic liposarcoma* (Fig. 35.8) is a highly cellular tumor with numerous mitoses and some bizarre and extremely pleomorphic multivacuolated lipoblasts with one or more hyperchromatic nuclei.[167] Fibrous areas with bizarre tumor cells are also present. Sometimes the cytoplasmic vacuolation is insignificant, making it difficult to differentiate from other pleomorphic sarcomas. A lipid stain sometimes helps in these cases. Inflammatory cells are sometimes prominent in the stroma of pleomorphic liposarcoma (*inflammatory liposarcoma*). Rarely, an extensive lymphoplasmacytic infiltrate may be seen in the other variants of liposarcoma.[163] Another variant of pleomorphic liposarcoma is the so-called '*dedifferentiated liposarcoma*', which includes a well-differentiated (lipoma-like) component and dedifferentiated areas resembling malignant fibrous histiocytoma or myxofibrosarcoma.[168–170] A variant of dedifferentiated liposarcoma with meningothelial-like whorls has been reported. The whorls represent a mesenchymal proliferation that may undergo myofibroblastic or osteoblastic differentiation.[171,172] The whorls do not represent meningothelial differentiation.[171] Dedifferentiation can also occur in myxoid liposarcomas.[173] Dedifferentiated liposarcomas have a variable course.[168,170] In one series, nearly half of all liposarcomas showed p53 immunostaining.[174] Tumor size, grade and histological subtype are predictors of metastasis in soft tissue liposarcomas.[175]

The dermal liposarcoma may have unusually high-grade features resembling the pleomorphic liposarcoma. Myxoid, round cell and well-differentiated variants have also been described. Despite these cytological features, metastases have not been recorded with dermal liposarcomas, analogous to other dermal sarcomas.[151]

Liposarcomas must be distinguished from the changes seen in **massive localized lymphedema** of the morbidly obese, which is characterized by a large, ill-defined mass composed of mature fat interrupted by expanded connective tissue septa showing edema and neovascularization at the interface between fat and septa.[176]

Electron microscopy

Liposarcomas are composed of cells showing lipoblastic differentiation with lipid droplets, micropinocytotic vesicles, glycogen, external lamina and intermediate filaments.[177] Most tumors contain lipid-free, poorly differentiated mesenchymal cells and cells resembling early lipoblasts with non-membrane bound lipid vacuoles.[177]

REFERENCES

1 Silverman JS, Tamsen A. Fibrohistiocytic differentiation in subcutaneous fatty tumors. J Cutan Pathol 1997; 24: 484–493.

2 Suster S, Fisher C. Immunoreactivity for the human hematopoietic progenitor cell antigen (CD34) in lipomatous tumors. Am J Surg Pathol 1997; 21: 195–200.

3 Rubin BP, Fletcher CDM. The cytogenetics of lipomatous tumours. Histopathology 1997; 30: 507–511.

4 Mehregan A, Tavafoghi V, Ghandchi A. Nevus lipomatosus superficialis cutaneus (Hoffmann–Zurhelle). J Cutan Pathol 1975; 2: 307–313.

5 Finley AG, Musso LA. Naevus lipomatosus cutaneus superficialis (Hoffmann–Zurhelle). Br J Dermatol 1972; 87: 557–564.

6 Park HJ, Park CJ, Yi JY et al. Nevus lipomatosus superficialis on the face. Int J Dermatol 1997; 36: 435–437.

7 Weitzner S. Solitary nevus lipomatosus cutaneus superficialis of scalp. Arch Dermatol 1968; 97: 540–542.

8 Nogita T, Wong T-Y, Hidano A et al. Pedunculated lipofibroma. A clinicopathologic study of thirty-two cases supporting a simplified nomenclature. J Am Acad Dermatol 1994; 31: 235–240.

9 Gardner EW, Miller HM, Lowney ED. Folded skin associated with underlying nevus lipomatosus. Arch Dermatol 1979; 115: 978–979.

10 Ross CM. Generalized folded skin with an underlying lipomatous nevus. "The Michelin tire baby". Arch Dermatol 1969; 100: 320–323.

11 Wilson Jones E, Marks R, Pongsehirun D. Naevus superficialis lipomatosus. A clinicopathological report of twenty cases. Br J Dermatol 1975; 93: 121–133.

12 Ioannidou DJ, Stefanidou MP, Panayiotides JG, Tosca AD. Nevus lipomatosus cutaneous superficialis (Hoffmann–Zurhelle) with localized scleroderma like appearance. Int J Dermatol 2001; 40: 54–57.

13 Fergin PE, MacDonald DM. Naevus superficialis lipomatosus. Clin Exp Dermatol 1980; 5: 365–367.

14 Dotz W, Prioleau PG. Nevus lipomatosus cutaneus superficialis. Arch Dermatol 1984; 120: 376–379.

15 Reymond JL, Stoebner P, Amblard P. Nevus lipomatosus cutaneous superficialis. An electron microscopic study of four cases. J Cutan Pathol 1980; 7: 295–301.

16 Shelley WB, Rawnsley HM. Painful feet due to herniation of fat. JAMA 1968; 205: 308–309.

17 Woerdeman MJ, van Dijk E. Piezogenic papules of the feet. Acta Derm Venereol 1972; 52: 411–414.

18 Schlappner OLA, Wood MG, Gerstein W, Gross PR. Painful and nonpainful piezogenic pedal papules. Arch Dermatol 1972; 106: 729–733.

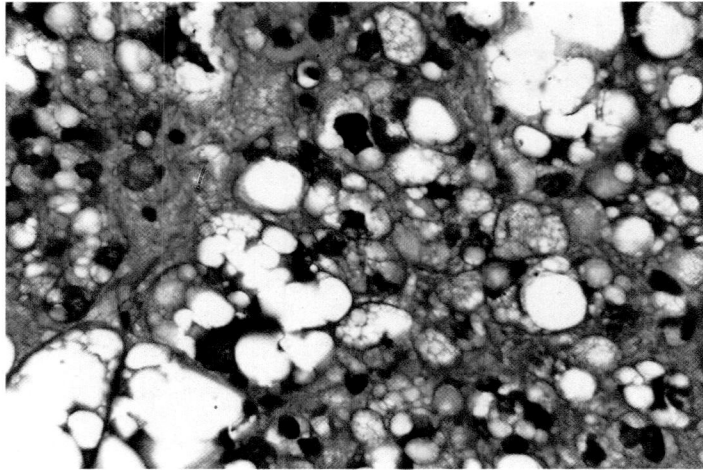
Fig. 35.8 **Pleomorphic liposarcoma.** Many vacuolated lipoblasts are present. (H & E)

19 Harman RRM, Matthews CNA. Painful piezogenic pedal papules. Br J Dermatol 1974; 90: 573–574.

20 Kahana M, Feinstein A, Tabachnic E et al. Painful piezogenic pedal papules in patients with Ehlers–Danlos syndrome. J Am Acad Dermatol 1987; 17: 205–209.

21 Ronnen M, Suster S, Huszar M, Schewach-Millet M. Solitary painful piezogenic pedal papule in a patient with rheumatoid arthritis. Int J Dermatol 1987; 26: 240–241.

22 van Straaten EA, van Langen IM, Oorthuys JWE, Oosting J. Piezogenic papules of the feet in healthy children and their possible relation with connective tissue disorders. Pediatr Dermatol 1991; 8: 277–279.

23 Graham BS, Barrett TL. Solitary painful piezogenic pedal papule. J Am Acad Dermatol 1997; 36: 780–781.

24 Böni R, Dummer R. Compression therapy in painful piezogenic pedal papules. Arch Dermatol 1996; 132: 127–128.

25 Woodrow SL, Brereton-Smith G, Handfield-Jones S. Painful piezogenic pedal papules: response to local electro-acupuncture. Br J Dermatol 1997; 136: 628–630.

26 Laing VB, Fleischer AB Jr. Piezogenic wrist papules: a common and asymptomatic finding. J Am Acad Dermatol 1991; 24: 415–417.

27 España A, Pujol RM, Idoate MA et al. Bilateral congenital adipose plantar nodules. Br J Dermatol 2000; 142: 1262–1264.

28 Ortega-Monzó C, Molina-Gallardo I, Monteagudo-Castro C et al. Precalcaneal congenital fibrolipomatous hamartoma: a report of four cases. Pediatr Dermatol 2000; 17: 429–431.

29 Vellios F, Baez J, Shumacker HB. Lipoblastomatosis: a tumor of fetal fat different from hibernoma. Am J Pathol 1958; 34: 1149–1159.

30 Enghardt MH, Warren RC. Congenital palpebral lipoblastoma. First report of a case. Am J Dermatopathol 1990; 12: 408–411.

31 Chung EB, Enzinger FM. Benign lipoblastomatosis. An analysis of 35 cases. Cancer 1973; 32: 482–492.

32 Calobrisi SD, Garland JS, Esterly NB. Congenital lipoblastomatosis of the lower extremity in a neonate. Pediatr Dermatol 1998; 15: 210–213.

33 Kauffman SL, Stout AP. Lipoblastic tumors of children. Cancer 1959; 12: 912–925.

34 Mentzel T, Calonje E, Fletcher CDM. Lipoblastoma and lipoblastomatosis: a clinicopathological study of 14 cases. Histopathology 1993; 23: 527–533.

35 Collins MH, Chatten J. Lipoblastoma/lipoblastomatosis: a clinicopathologic study of 25 tumors. Am J Surg Pathol 1997; 21: 1131–1137.

36 Tallini G, Akerman M, Dal Cin P et al. Combined morphologic and karyotypic study of 28 myxoid liposarcomas. Am J Surg Pathol 1996; 20: 1047–1055.

37 Chaudhuri B, Ronan SG, Ghosh L. Benign lipoblastoma. Report of a case. Cancer 1980; 46: 611–614.

38 Greco MA, Garcia RL, Vuletin JC. Benign lipoblastomatosis. Ultrastructure and histogenesis. Cancer 1980; 45: 511–515.

39 Fetsch JF, Miettinen M, Laskin WB et al. A clinicopathologic study of 45 pediatric soft tissue tumors with an admixture of adipose tissue and fibroblastic elements, and a proposal for classification as lipofibromatosis. Am J Surg Pathol 2000; 24: 1491–1500.

40 Trotter MJ, Crawford RI. Pseudolipomatosis cutis: superficial dermal vacuoles resembling fatty infiltration of the skin. Am J Dermatopathol 1998; 20: 443–447.

41 Brehmer-Andersson E, Hovmark A, Åsbrink E. Pseudolipomatosis cutis. Am J Dermatopathol 1999; 21: 398–399.

42 Adair FE, Pack GT, Farrior JH. Lipomas. Am J Cancer 1932; 16: 1104–1120.

43 Salasche SJ, McCollough ML, Angeloni VL, Grabski WJ. Frontalis-associated lipoma of the forehead. J Am Acad Dermatol 1989; 20: 462–468.

44 Sanchez MR, Golomb FM, Moy JA, Potozkin JR. Giant lipoma: case report and review of the literature. J Am Acad Dermatol 1993; 28: 266–268.

45 Allen PW. Tumors and proliferations of adipose tissue. A clinicopathologic approach. New York: Masson Publishing USA, 1981.

46 Enzi G. Multiple symmetric lipomatosis: an updated clinical report. Medicine (Baltimore) 1984; 63: 56–64.

47 Uhlin SR. Benign symmetric lipomatosis. Arch Dermatol 1979; 115: 94–95.

48 Ruzicka T, Vieluf D, Landthaler M, Braun-Falco O. Benign symmetric lipomatosis Launois–Bensaude. Report of ten cases and review of the literature. J Am Acad Dermatol 1987; 17: 663–674.

49 Carlin MC, Ratz JL. Multiple symmetric lipomatosis: treatment with liposuction. J Am Acad Dermatol 1988; 18: 359–362.

50 Ross M, Goodman MM. Multiple symmetric lipomatosis (Launois–Bensaude syndrome). Int J Dermatol 1992; 31: 80–82.

51 Ho MH, Lo KK. Benign symmetric lipomatosis in a Chinese man with bullous pemphigoid. Int J Dermatol 1999; 38: 131–133.

52 Findlay GH, Duvenage M. Acquired symmetrical lipomatosis of the hands – a distal form of the Madelung–Launois–Bensaude syndrome. Clin Exp Dermatol 1989; 14: 58–59.

53 Hacker SM, Ramos-Caro FA. An uncommon presentation of multiple symmetric lipomatosis. Int J Dermatol 1993; 32: 594–597.

54 Requena L, Hasson A, Arias D et al. Acquired symmetric lipomatosis of the soles. J Am Acad Dermatol 1992; 26: 860–862.

55 Stavropoulos PG, Zouboulis ChC, Trautmann Ch, Orfanos CE. Symmetric lipomatoses in female patients. Dermatology 1997; 194: 26–31.

56 Flynn MK, Wee SA, Lane AT. Skin manifestations of mitochondrial DNA syndromes: Case report and review. J Am Acad Dermatol 1998; 39: 819–823.

57 Greene ML, Glueck CJ, Fujimoto WY, Seegmiller JE. Benign symmetric lipomatosis (Launois–Bensaude adenolipomatosis) with gout and hyperlipoproteinemia. Am J Med 1970; 48: 239–246.

58 Springer HA, Whitehouse JS. Launois–Bensaude adenolipomatosis. Case report. Plast Reconstr Surg 1972; 50: 291–294.

59 Leffell DJ, Braverman IM. Familial multiple lipomatosis. Report of a case and a review of the literature. J Am Acad Dermatol 1986; 15: 275–279.

60 Paredes BE, Braathen LR, Brand CU. Benign symmetrical lipomatosis – one cutaneous manifestation of alcoholism. Dermatology 1999; 198: 436–438.

61 Saiz Hervás E, Martín Llorens M, López Alvarez J. Peripheral neuropathy as the first manifestation of Madelung's disease. Br J Dermatol 2000; 143: 684–686.

62 Rabbiosi G, Borroni G, Scuderi N. Familial multiple lipomatosis. Acta Derm Venereol 1977; 57: 265–267.

63 Mohar N. Familial multiple lipomatosis. Acta Derm Venereol 1980; 60: 509–513.

64 Tsao H, Sober AJ. Multiple lipomatosis in a patient with familial atypical mole syndrome. Br J Dermatol 1998; 139: 1118–1119.

65 Rubinstein A, Goor Y, Gazit E, Cabili S. Non-symmetric subcutaneous lipomatosis associated with familial combined hyperlipidaemia. Br J Dermatol 1989; 120: 689–694.

66 Blomstrand R, Juhlin L, Nordenstam H et al. Adiposis dolorosa associated with defects of lipid metabolism. Acta Derm Venereol 1971; 51: 243–250.

67 Held JL, Andrew JA, Kohn SR. Surgical amelioration of Dercum's disease: a report and review. J Dermatol Surg Oncol 1989; 15: 1294–1296.

68 Lynch HT, Harlan WL. Hereditary factors in adiposis dolorosa (Dercum's disease). Am J Hum Genet 1963; 15: 184–190.

69 Campen R, Mankin H, Louis DN et al. Familial occurrence of adiposis dolorosa. J Am Acad Dermatol 2001; 44: 132–136.

70 Greenbaum SS, Varga J. Corticosteroid-induced juxta-articular adiposis dolorosa. Arch Dermatol 1991; 127: 231–233.

71 Klein JA, Barr RJ. Diffuse lipomatosis and tuberous sclerosis. Arch Dermatol 1986; 122: 1298–1302.

72 Nixon HH, Scobie WG. Congenital lipomatosis: a report of four cases. J Pediatr Surg 1971; 6: 742–745.

73 Schlicht D. Recurrent lipomatosis in a child. Med J Aust 1965; 2: 959–962.

74 Grimalt R, Ermacora E, Mistura L et al. Encephalocraniocutaneous lipomatosis: case report and review of the literature. Pediatr Dermatol 1993; 10: 164–168.

75 Nosti-Martínez D, del Castillo V, Durán-Mckinster C et al. Encephalocraniocutaneous lipomatosis: an uncommon neurocutaneous syndrome. J Am Acad Dermatol 1995; 32: 387–389.

76 Ciatti S, Del Monaco M, Hyde P, Bernstein EF. Encephalocraniocutaneous lipomatosis: A rare neurocutaneous syndrome. J Am Acad Dermatol 1998; 38: 102–104.

77 Happle R, Küster W. Nevus psiloliparus: a distinct fatty tissue nevus. Dermatology 1998; 197: 6–10.

78 Slavin SA, Baker DC, McCarthy JG, Mufarrij A. Congenital infiltrating lipomatosis of the face: clinicopathologic evaluation and treatment. Plast Reconstr Surg 1983; 72: 158–164.

79 Lasso JM, España A, Zudaire MI et al. Congenital infiltrating lipoma of the upper limb in a patient with von Willebrand disease. Br J Dermatol 2000; 143: 180–182.

80 Lee JH, Sung YH, Yoon JS, Park JK. Lipedematous scalp. Arch Dermatol 1994; 130: 802–803.

81 Bornhövd E, Sakrauski AK, Brühl H et al. Multiple circumscribed subcutaneous lipomas associated with use of human immunodeficiency virus protease inhibitors? Br J Dermatol 2000; 143: 1113–1114.

82 Dank JP, Colven R. Protease-inhibitor associated angiolipomatosis. J Am Acad Dermatol 2000; 42: 129–131.

83 Hitchcock MG, Hurt MA, Santa Cruz DJ. Adenolipoma of the skin: a report of nine cases. J Am Acad Dermatol 1993; 29: 82–85.

84 Záměčník M, Michal M, Šulc M. Atypical lipomatous tumors with smooth muscle differentiation: report of two cases. Pathology 1999; 31: 425–427.

85 Michal M, Záměčník M. Synovial metaplasia in lipoma. Am J Dermatopathol 1998; 20: 285–289.

86 Ramdial PK, Madaree A, Singh B. Membranous fat necrosis in lipomas. Am J Surg Pathol 1997; 21: 841–846.

87 Howard WR, Helwig EB. Angiolipoma. Arch Dermatol 1960; 82: 924–931.

88 Dixon AY, McGregor DH, Lee SH. Angiolipomas: an ultrastructural and clinicopathological study. Hum Pathol 1981; 12: 739–747.

89 Goodfield MJD, Rowell NR. The clinical presentation of cutaneous angiolipomata and the response to β-blockade. Clin Exp Dermatol 1988; 13: 190–192.

90 Rasanen O, Nohteri H, Dammert K. Angiolipoma and lipoma. Acta Chir Scand 1967; 133: 461–465.

91 Sahl WJ Jr. Mobile encapsulated lipomas. Formerly called encapsulated angiolipomas. Arch Dermatol 1978; 114: 1684–1686.

92 Sciot R, Akerman M, Dal Cin P et al. Cytogenetic analysis of subcutaneous angiolipoma: further evidence supporting its difference from ordinary pure lipomas. Am J Surg Pathol 1997; 21: 441–444.

93 Dionne GP, Seemayer TA. Infiltrating lipomas and angiolipomas revisited. Cancer 1974; 33: 732–738.

94 Lin JJ, Lin F. Two entities in angiolipoma. Cancer 1974; 34: 720–727.

95 Belcher RW, Czarnetzki BM, Carney JF, Gardner E. Multiple (subcutaneous) angiolipomas. Arch Dermatol 1974; 110: 583–585.

96 Kanik AB, Oh CH, Bhawan J. Cellular angiolipoma. Am J Dermatopathol 1995; 17: 312–315.

97 Rustin GJS. Diffuse intravascular coagulation in association with myocardial infarction and multiple angiolipomata. Postgrad Med J 1977; 53: 228–229.

98 Zámečník M. Vascular myxolipoma (angiomyxolipoma) of subcutaneous tissue. Histopathology 1999; 34: 180–181.

99 Sciot R, Debiec-Rychter M, De Wever I, Hagemeijer A. Angiomyxolipoma shares cytogenetic changes with lipoma, spindle cell/pleomorphic lipoma and myxoma. Virchows Arch 2001; 438: 66–69.

100 Shea CR, Prieto VG. Mast cells in angiolipomas and hemangiomas of human skin: are they important for angiogenesis? J Cutan Pathol 1994; 21: 247–251.

101 Enzinger FM, Harvey DA. Spindle cell lipoma. Cancer 1975; 36: 1852–1859.

102 Duve S, Müller-Höcker J, Worret WI. Spindle-cell lipoma of the skin. Am J Dermatopathol 1995; 17: 529–533.

103 Angervall L, Dahl I, Kindblom L-G, Save-Soderbergh J. Spindle cell lipoma. Acta Pathol Microbiol Scand (A) 1976; 84: 477–487.

104 Brody HJ, Meltzer HD, Someren A. Spindle cell lipoma. An unusual dermatologic presentation. Arch Dermatol 1978; 114: 1065–1066.

105 Meister P. Spindle cell lipoma (report of 2 cases and differential diagnosis). Beitr Path 1977; 161: 376–384.

106 Fanburg-Smith JC, Devaney KO, Miettinen M, Weiss, SW. Multiple spindle cell lipomas. A report of 7 familial and 11 nonfamilial cases. Am J Surg Pathol 1998; 22: 40–48.

107 Dal Cin P, Sciot R, Polito P et al. Lesions of 13q may occur independently of deletion of 16q in spindle cell/pleomorphic lipomas. Histopathology 1997; 31: 222–225.

108 Fletcher CDM, Martin-Bates E. Spindle cell lipoma: a clinicopathological study with some original observations. Histopathology 1987; 11: 803–817.

109 Zelger BWH, Zelger BG, Plörer A et al. Dermal spindle cell lipoma: plexiform and nodular variants. Histopathology 1995; 27: 533–540.

110 French CA, Mentzel T, Kutzner H, Fletcher CDM. Intradermal spindle cell/pleomorphic lipoma. A distinct subset. Am J Dermatopathol 2000; 22: 496–502.

111 Warkel RL, Rehme CG, Thompson WH. Vascular spindle cell lipoma. J Cutan Pathol 1982; 9: 113–118.

112 Hawley IC, Krausz T, Evans DJ, Fletcher CDM. Spindle cell lipoma – a pseudoangiomatous variant. Histopathology 1994; 24: 565–569.

113 Templeton SF, Solomon AR. Spindle cell lipoma is CD34 positive, an immunohistochemical study. J Cutan Pathol 1996; 23: 62 (abstract).

114 Templeton SF, Solomon AR Jr. Spindle cell lipoma is strongly CD34 positive. An immunohistochemical study. J Cutan Pathol 1996; 23: 546–550.

115 Zelger BG, Zelger B, Steiner H, Rütten A. Sclerotic lipoma: lipomas simulating sclerotic fibroma. Histopathology 1997; 31: 174–181.

116 Diaz-Cascajo C, Borghi S, Weyers W. Fibrous spindle cell lipoma. Report of a new variant. Am J Dermatopathol 2001; 23: 112–115.

117 Shmookler BM, Enzinger FM. Pleomorphic lipoma: a benign tumor simulating liposarcoma. A clinicopathologic analysis of 48 cases. Cancer 1981; 47: 126–133.

118 Digregorio F, Barr RJ, Fretzin DF. Pleomorphic lipoma. Case reports and review of the literature. J Dermatol Surg Oncol 1992; 18: 197–202.

119 Nigro MA. Chieregato GC, Querci della Rovere G. Pleomorphic lipoma of the dermis. Br J Dermatol 1987; 116: 713–717.

120 Griffin TD, Goldstein J, Johnson WC. Pleomorphic lipoma. Case report and discussion of "atypical" lipomatous tumors. J Cutan Pathol 1992; 19: 330–333.

121 Azzopardi JG, Iocco J, Salm R. Pleomorphic lipoma: a tumour simulating liposarcoma. Histopathology 1983; 7: 511–523.

122 Evans HL, Soule EH, Winkelmann RK. Atypical lipoma, atypical intramuscular lipoma, and well differentiated retroperitoneal liposarcoma. Cancer 1979; 43: 574–584.

123 Kindblom LG, Angervall L, Fassina AS. Atypical lipoma. Acta Pathol Microbiol Immunol Scand (A) 1982; 90: 27–36.

124 Diaz-Cascajo C, Borghi S, Weyers W. Pleomorphic lipoma with pseudopapillary structures: a pleomorphic counterpart of pseudoangiomatous spindle cell lipoma. Histopathology 2000; 36: 475–476.

125 Bryant J. A pleomorphic lipoma in the scalp. J Dermatol Surg Oncol 1981; 7: 323–325.

126 Meis JM, Enzinger FM. Chondroid lipoma. A unique tumor simulating liposarcoma and myxoid chondrosarcoma. Am J Surg Pathol 1993; 17: 1103–1112.

127 Kindblom L-G, Meis-Kindblom JM. Chondroid lipoma: an ultrastructural and immunohistochemical analysis with further observations regarding its differentiation. Hum Pathol 1995; 26: 706–715.

128 Gisselsson D, Domanski HA, Höglund M et al. Unique cytological features and chromosome aberrations in chondroid lipoma. Am J Surg Pathol 1999; 23: 1300–1304.

129 Nielsen GP, O'Connell JX, Dickersin GR, Rosenberg AE. Chondroid lipoma, a tumor of white fat cells. Am J Surg Pathol 1995; 19: 1272–1276.

130 Novy FG Jr, Wilson JW. Hibernomas, brown fat tumors. Arch Dermatol 1956; 73: 149–157.

131 Kindblom L-G, Angervall L, Stener B, Wickbom I. Intermuscular and intramuscular lipomas and hibernomas. Cancer 1974; 33: 754–762.

132 Lay K, Velasco C, Akin H, Mancini M. Axillary hibernoma: an unusual soft tissue tumor. Am Surg 2000; 66: 787–788.

133 Allegra SR, Gmuer C, O'Leary GP Jr. Endocrine activity in a large hibernoma. Hum Pathol 1983; 14: 1044–1052.

134 Angervall L, Nilsson L, Stener B. Microangiographic and histological studies in 2 cases of hibernoma. Cancer 1964; 17: 685–692.

135 Dardick I. Hibernoma: a possible model of brown fat histogenesis. Hum Pathol 1978; 9: 321–329.

136 Rigor VU, Goldstone SE, Jones J et al. Hibernoma. A case report and discussion of a rare tumor. Cancer 1986; 57: 2207–2211.

137 Brines OA, Johnson MH. Hibernoma, a special fatty tumor. Report of a case. Am J Pathol 1949; 25: 467–479.

138 Gisselsson D, Höglund M, Mertens F et al. Hibernomas are characterized by homozygous deletions in the *MEN1* region. Metaphase fluorescence in situ hybridization reveals complex rearrangements not detected by conventional cytogenetics. Am J Pathol 1999; 155: 61–66.

139 Enterline HT, Lowry LD, Richman AV. Does malignant hibernoma exist? Am J Surg Pathol 1979; 3: 265–271.

140 Levine GD. Hibernoma. An electron microscopic study. Hum Pathol 1972; 3: 351–359.

141 Seemayer TA, Knaack J, Wang N-S, Ahmed MN. On the ultrastructure of hibernoma. Cancer 1975; 36: 1785–1793.

142 Allen PW, Strungs I, MacCormac LB. Atypical subcutaneous fatty tumors: a review of 37 referred cases. Pathology 1998; 30: 123–135.

143 Challis D. Atypical subcutaneous fatty tumors. Adv Anat Pathol 2000; 7: 94–99.

144 Spittle MF, Newton KA, Mackenzie DH. Liposarcoma. A review of 60 cases. Br J Cancer 1970; 24: 696–704.

145 Kindblom L-G, Angervall L, Svendsen P. Liposarcoma. A clinicopathologic, radiographic and prognostic study. Acta Pathol Microbiol Scand (A) 1975; Suppl 253: 1–71

146 Azumi N, Curtis J, Kempson RL, Hendrickson MR. Atypical and malignant neoplasms showing lipomatous differentiation. A study of 111 cases. Am J Surg Pathol 1987; 11: 161–183.

147 Saunders JR, Jaques DA, Casterline PF et al. Liposarcoma of the head and neck. A review of the literature and addition of four cases. Cancer 1979; 43: 162–168.

148 Golledge J, Fisher C, Rhys-Evans PH. Head and neck liposarcoma. Cancer 1995; 76: 1051–1058.

149 Vocks E, Worret W-I, Burgdorf WHC. Myxoid liposarcoma in a 12-year-old girl. Pediatr Dermatol 2000; 17: 129–132.

150 Kindblom L-G, Angervall L, Jarlstedt J. Liposarcoma of the neck. A clinicopathologic study of 4 cases. Cancer 1978; 42: 774–780.

151 Dei Tos AP, Mentzel T, Fletcher CDM. Primary liposarcoma of the skin: a rare neoplasm with unusual high grade features. Am J Dermatopathol 1998; 20: 332–338.

152 Gibas Z, Miettinen M, Limon J et al. Cytogenetic and immunohistochemical profile of myxoid liposarcoma. Am J Clin Pathol 1995; 103: 20–26.

153 Sreekantaiah C, Karakousis CP, Leong SPL, Sandberg AA. Cytogenetic findings in liposarcoma correlate with histopathologic subtypes. Cancer 1992; 69: 2484–2495.

154 Mrózek K, Szumigala J, Brooks JSJ et al. Round cell liposarcoma with the insertion (12; 16) (q13; p11.2p13). Am J Clin Pathol 1997; 108: 35–39.

155 Dei Tos AP. Lipomatous tumours. Curr Diagn Pathol 2001; 7: 8–16.

156 Enterline HT, Culberson JD, Rochlin DB, Brady LW. Liposarcoma. A clinical and pathological study of 53 cases. Cancer 1960; 13: 932–950.

157 Enzinger FM, Winslow DJ. Liposarcoma. A study of 103 cases. Virchows Arch Pathol Anat 1962; 335: 367–388.

158 Rosai J, Akerman M, Dal Cin P et al. Combined morphologic and karyotypic study of 59 atypical lipomatous tumors. Am J Surg Pathol 1996; 20: 1182–1189.

159 Lucas DR, Nascimento AG, Sanjay BKS, Rock MG. Well-differentiated liposarcoma. The Mayo Clinic experience with 58 cases. Am J Clin Pathol 1994; 102: 677–683.

160 Nascimento AG. Spindle cell liposarcoma. Adv Anat Pathol 1995; 2: 320–325.

161 Dei Tos AP, Mentzel T, Newman PL, Fletcher CDM. Spindle cell liposarcoma, a hitherto unrecognized variant of liposarcoma. Analysis of six cases. Am J Surg Pathol 1994; 18: 913–921.

162 Argani P, Facchetti F, Inghirami G, Rosai J. Lymphocyte-rich well-differentiated liposarcoma: report of nine cases. Am J Surg Pathol 1997; 21: 884–895.

163 Kraus MD, Guillou L, Fletcher CDM. Well-differentiated inflammatory liposarcoma: an uncommon and easily overlooked variant of a common sarcoma. Am J Surg Pathol 1997; 21: 518–527.

164 Pearlstone DB, Pisters PWT, Bold RJ et al. Patterns of recurrence in extremity liposarcoma. Implications for staging and follow-up. Cancer 1999; 85: 85–92.

165 Smith TA, Easley KA, Goldblum JR. Myxoid/round cell liposarcoma of the extremities. A clinicopathologic study of 29 cases with particular attention to extent of round cell liposarcoma. Am J Surg Pathol 1996; 20: 171–180.

166 Kilpatrick SE, Doyon J, Choong PFM et al. The clinicopathologic spectrum of myxoid and round cell liposarcoma. A study of 95 cases. Cancer 1996; 77: 1450–1458.

167 Schwimer CJ, Bergfeld WF, Goldblum JR. Primary cutaneous pleomorphic liposarcoma: a rare high-grade sarcoma demonstrating site-dependent clinical behavior. J Cutan Pathol 2000; 27: 571 (abstract).

158 McCormick D, Mentzel T, Beham A, Fletcher CDM. Dedifferentiated liposarcoma. Clinicopathologic analysis of 32 cases suggesting a better prognostic subgroup among pleomorphic sarcomas. Am J Surg Pathol 1994; 18: 1213–1223.

169 Yoshikawa H, Ueda T, Mori S et al. Differentiated liposarcoma of the subcutis. Am J Surg Pathol 1996; 20: 1525–1530.

170 Henricks WH, Chu YC, Goldblum JR, Weiss SW. Dedifferentiated liposarcoma. A clinicopathological analysis of 155 cases with a proposal for an expanded definition of dedifferentiation. Am J Surg Pathol 1997; 21: 271–281.

171 Fanburg-Smith JC, Miettinen M. Liposarcoma with meningothelial-like whorls: a study of 17 cases of a distinctive histological pattern associated with dedifferentiated liposarcoma. Histopathology 1998; 33: 414–424.

172 Nascimento AG, Kurtin PJ, Guillou L, Fletcher CDM. Dedifferentiated liposarcoma. A report of nine cases with a peculiar neurallike whorling pattern associated with metaplastic bone formation. Am J Surg Pathol 1998; 22: 945–955.

173 Mentzel T, Fletcher CDM. Dedifferentiated myxoid liposarcoma: a clinicopathological study suggesting a closer relationship between myxoid and well-differentiated liposarcoma. Histopathology 1997; 30: 457–463.

174 Taubert H, Würl P, Meye A et al. Molecular and immunohistochemical p53 status in liposarcoma and malignant fibrous histiocytoma. Cancer 1995; 76: 1187–1196.

175 Coindre J-M, Terrier P, Guillou L et al. Predictive value of grade for metastasis development in the main histologic types of adult soft tissue sarcomas. Cancer 2001; 91: 1914–1926.

176 Farshid G, Weiss SW. Massive localized lymphedema in the morbidly obese. A histologically distinct reactive lesion simulating liposarcoma. Am J Surg Pathol 1998; 22: 1277–1283.

177 Rossouw DJ, Cinti S, Dickersin GR. Liposarcoma. An ultrastructural study of 15 cases. Am J Clin Pathol 1986; 85: 649–667.

Tumors of muscle, cartilage and bone

TUMORS OF SMOOTH MUSCLE

Smooth muscle is found in the skin in three distinct settings: the arrector pili muscles, the walls of blood vessels, and the specialized muscle of genital skin, which includes the scrotum (dartos muscle), vulva and nipple (areolar smooth muscle). Each of these sources of smooth muscle can give rise to benign tumors, resulting in three categories of cutaneous leiomyoma: piloleiomyoma, leiomyoma of genital skin, and angioleiomyoma.[1,2] The rare leiomyoma of deep soft tissue, and the case reported as 'leiomyomatosis' on the basis of numerous large and widespread tumoral masses of smooth muscle, are additional categories.[3,4] Leiomyomas of the scrotum and vulva show some histopathological differences from piloleiomyomas and leiomyomas of the nipple. These differences will be highlighted below.

For completeness, it should be noted that smooth muscle has also been reported, rarely, in organoid[5] and blue nevi.[6]

LEIOMYOMA

Leiomyomas derived from the arrector pili muscle (*piloleiomyomas*) are more often multiple than solitary. Multiple lesions usually have their onset in the late second or third decade of life. They present as multiple, firm, reddish-brown papulonodules with a predilection for the face,[7] back, and extensor surfaces of the extremities.[8] Several hundred lesions may be present. They may cluster to form plaques,[9–11] which usually involve more than one area of the body.[12,13] Rarely, tumors are zosteriform or symmetrically distributed,[14,15] suggesting a nevoid condition, and these cases have been designated 'nevus leiomyomatosus systematicus'.[16] Some of the multiple cases are familial, with an autosomal dominant inheritance.[17,18] There is a report of identical twins being involved.[19] Multiple leiomyomas have been associated with uterine leiomyomas in some females.[20–22] Erythropoietic activity of the tumors is a rare finding.[21] Minor trauma or exposure to cold temperatures may lead to severe pain in the tumors.[9,23,24]

Solitary piloleiomyomas,[25,26] which are infrequently painful, are usually slightly larger than those found in patients with the multiple form, sometimes reaching 2 cm or more in diameter. Rarely they are present at birth.[27] There has been a female preponderance.

There are only sparse reports of *leiomyoma of the nipple*[12,28] in the dermatopathological literature. Leiomyomas of genital skin are quite uncommon, with only small numbers of scrotal and vulval lesions reported.[12,28–31] *Scrotal leiomyomas* present as firm, solitary asymptomatic nodules, measuring 1–14 cm in diameter.[32] *Vulval leiomyomas* usually arise in the labia majora.[28,31] They usually measure 1–5 cm in diameter. Most are asymptomatic.

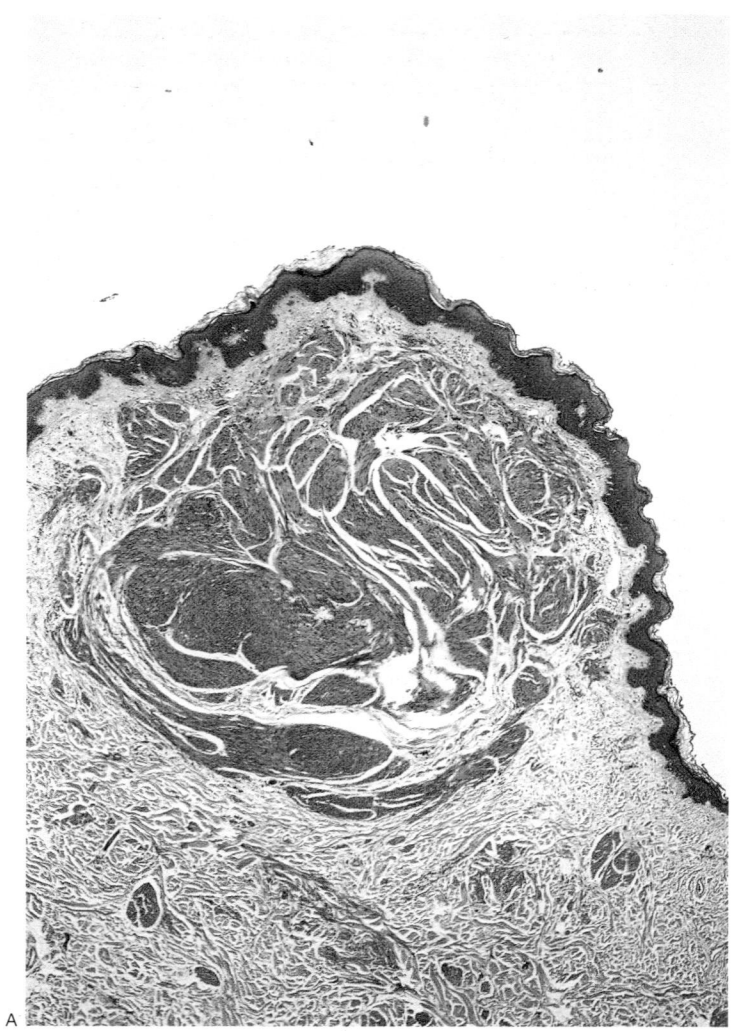
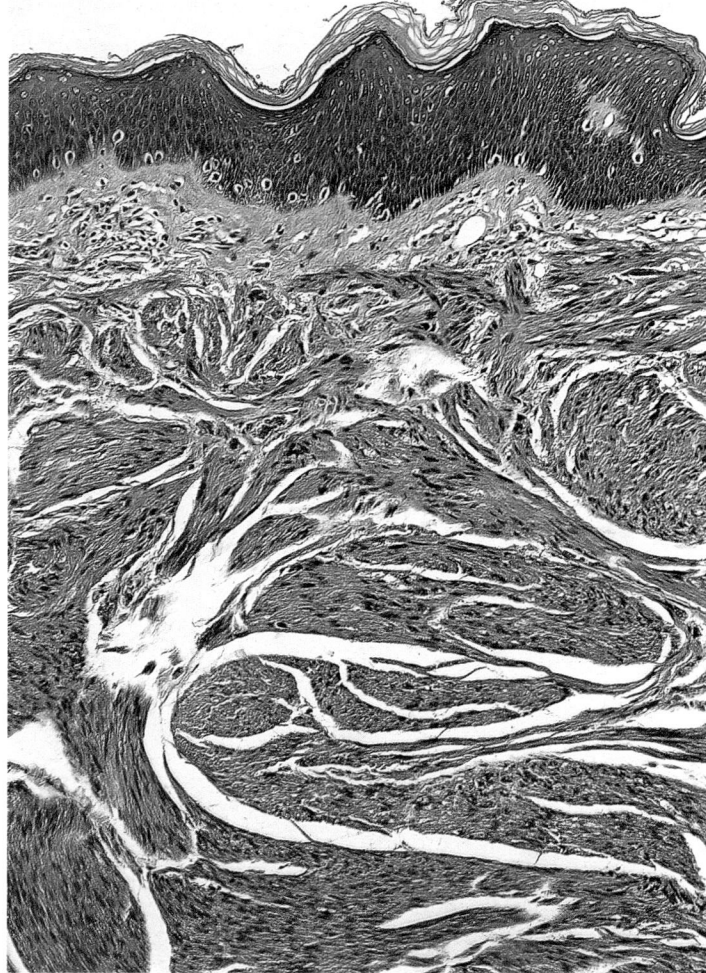

Fig. 36.1 **(A)** Leiomyoma. **(B)** The reticular dermis is replaced by interlacing bundles of smooth muscle cells. (H & E)

Histopathology

Piloleiomyomas are circumscribed non-encapsulated tumors, centered on the dermis.[12,13] An overlying zone of uninvolved subepidermal tissue (so-called 'grenz zone') is usually present, and there may be some flattening of the epidermis. Epidermal hyperplasia was present in over 50% of cases in one series.[2] The tumor is composed of bundles of smooth muscle arranged in an interlacing and sometimes a whorled pattern (Fig. 36.1). The cells have abundant eosinophilic cytoplasm and elongated nuclei with blunt ends. Nuclear palisading and the formation of Verocay bodies was reported in one case.[33] Granular cell change is a rare variant.[34] There are usually no mitoses in the pilar variant. Tumors of long standing may have fibrous tissue in the stroma, and occasionally this shows focal hyalinization.[28] Focal stromal myxoid change and small lymphoid collections have been noted. Hair follicles are sometimes found surviving within the tumor.[12] The smooth muscle nature of the cells can be confirmed with the Masson trichrome stain or the use of immunoperoxidase markers for smooth muscle. A Bodian stain has shown increased numbers of nerve fibers interlacing with the muscle fibers, and also in the surrounding tissue.[13]

Scrotal leiomyomas often have ill-defined or focally infiltrative margins, differing from the circumscribed tumors of pilar origin. Scrotal lesions are often more cellular with occasional mitoses. Symplastic features have been reported in all types.[28,35] Clear cell and granular cell variants are rare.[36] Lymphoid aggregates are sometimes present. Dartoic muscle is seen adjacent to the tumor.

Vulval leiomyomas are usually of spindle-cell type, although rare epithelioid and myxoid variants occur.[28,37] Sparse mitoses may be present. Stromal hyalinization is found in nearly one-half of the cases. Small fascicles of spindle cells may be trapped in these hyaline areas producing a plexiform appearance.[28] The majority of cases express estrogen and progesterone receptors,[37] a feature not found in pilar lesions.[38]

Smooth muscle hamartoma differs from leiomyoma by having discrete bundles of smooth muscle fibers set in dermal collagen (see below). The multiple papular variant of pilar leiomyoma not infrequently exhibits small bundles of collagen between the smooth muscle bundles, but usually the collagen is not as plentiful as it is in smooth muscle hamartoma.[39]

ANGIOLEIOMYOMA

Angioleiomyoma usually presents as a solitary, slow-growing nodule on the extremities, particularly the lower leg, of middle-aged individuals.[40,41] There is a female preponderance.[42,43] More than half the lesions are painful or tender, but this feature is usually absent in those found on the face and upper trunk.[40,44]

The tumors are firm, gray-white round to oval nodules in the lower dermis and subcutis.[45] They are usually less than 2 cm in diameter. Most authors assume that they arise from veins, although some may be hamartomas.[43] A rare intravascular variant has been reported.[46]

Histopathology

The tumor is usually well circumscribed with a fibrous capsule of variable thickness and completeness (Fig. 36.2). The main component is smooth muscle, which is present as interlacing bundles between the numerous vascular channels.[40,43,45] Most of the vessels have several layers of smooth muscle in the walls which often merges peripherally with the intervascular fascicles (Fig. 36.3). Sometimes there are large sinusoidal vessels with little smooth muscle in their walls. Small slit-like channels are sometimes present. Most vessels have only scant and scattered elastic fibers in their walls.

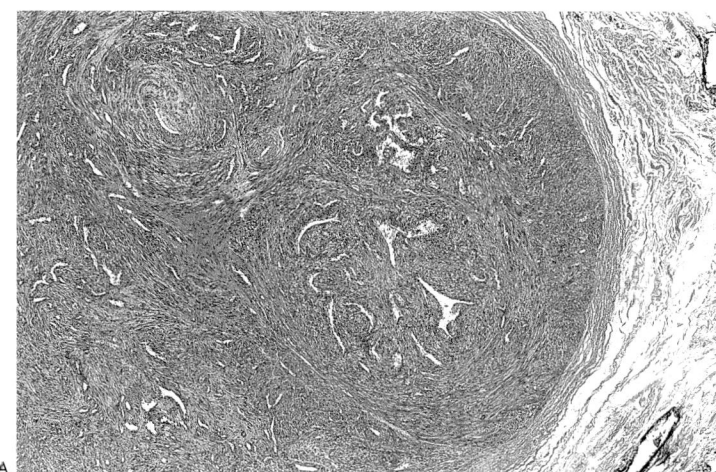

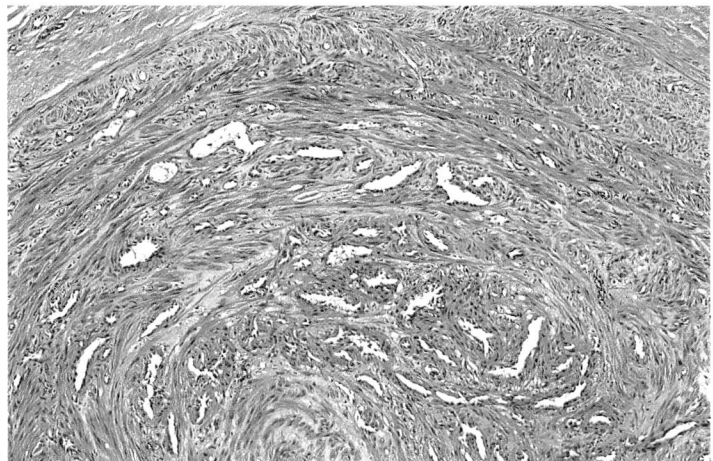

Fig. 36.2 **(A) Angioleiomyoma. (B)** The smooth muscle bundles are admixed with small blood vessels. (H & E)

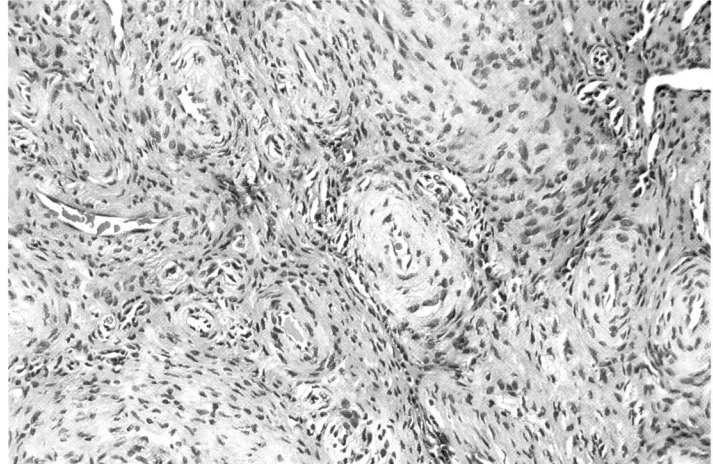

Fig. 36.3 **Angioleiomyoma.** In this case the individual vessels are thick walled; their outer layers of smooth muscle merge with the intervascular muscle fascicles. (H & E)

The stroma contains varying amounts of fibrous tissue, and in about a third of cases there is a sparse lymphocytic infiltrate. Myxoid change is quite common in the stroma, particularly in the larger tumors.[42] The presence of fat in a few cases has led to suggestions of a hamartomatous origin;[43] a designation of 'angiomyolipoma' can be used for these cases which also contain fat (Fig. 36.4).[47–52] The HMB-45 is negative in cutaneous tumors, in contrast to the finding in renal lesions.[53,54] The term 'myolipoma' is used for the rare tumors containing smooth muscle and adipose tissue, but no vascular component.[55] Uncommon changes include thrombosis of vascular channels, focal calcification, stromal hemosiderin, and hyalinization of vessel walls. Nuclear palisading, producing Verocay-like bodies, is a rare occurrence.[56] Nerve fibers are only seen occasionally.[1] An angioleiomyoma arising in a histiocytoma has been reported.[57]

In a review of 562 cases, three histological variants were described: a *solid type*, in which smooth muscle bundles surround numerous small slit-like channels; a *cavernous type*, with dilated vascular channels, the walls of which are difficult to distinguish from the intervascular smooth muscle; and a *venous type*, with thick-walled vessels which are easily distinguished from the intervascular smooth muscle.[43] Two further variants have since been reported: an *epithelioid type* composed of cells with round to oval nuclei and a moderate amount of finely granular eosinophilic cytoplasm with occasional vacuoles;[58] and a *pleomorphic type* with marked nuclear pleomorphism but only rare or absent mitoses. There is some resemblance to the symplastic change seen in uterine leiomyomas.[59–61]

The smooth muscle cells express vimentin, desmin and smooth muscle actin.

SMOOTH MUSCLE HAMARTOMA

The smooth muscle hamartoma is a rare, usually congenital, hyperplasia of dermal smooth muscle fibers which presents as a flesh-colored or lightly pigmented plaque up to 10 cm in diameter on the extremities or trunk.[62–69] The scrotum is rarely involved.[70] Within the plaques small gooseflesh-like papules may be discernible, and these may transiently elevate when rubbed (pseudo-Darier's sign).[71,72] A rare linear variant with perifollicular papules has been reported.[73] Hairs are usually more prominent in the skin of the affected site, being slightly longer and thicker than in the adjoining skin.[74] A more generalized variant with prominent skin folds has been reported as a 'Michelin tire baby'.[75–78] Multiple lesions have been described in three members of the same family.[79]

Smooth muscle bundles, indistinguishable from those seen in this condition, may also occur in Becker's nevus,[80,81] and this has led to some controversy about the relationship of these two entities.[71,74] Becker's nevus has its onset in adolescence, with invariable hyperpigmentation and hypertrichosis. Recent reports of patients with the clinical features of smooth muscle hamartoma which developed in late childhood[82] or early adulthood[83,84] suggest that Becker's nevus and smooth muscle hamartoma belong at different poles of the same developmental spectrum, involving hamartomatous change to the pilar unit and arrectores pilorum.[68,85,86]

Histopathology

There are well-defined smooth muscle bundles in the dermis, oriented in various directions. Some are attached to, or surround, hair follicles.[68,71] Often there is a thin retraction space around the bundles, separating them from the adjacent dermal collagen (Fig. 36.5). The smooth muscle bundles are clearly seen with the Masson trichrome stain. Bundles of nerve fibers may also be present.[67] These findings can be confirmed with appropriate immunohistochemical stains. Interestingly, large numbers of CD34-positive cells are present in the stroma surrounding the smooth muscle bundles.[87] There is often slight elongation of the rete ridges of the overlying epidermis, and mild basal hypermelanosis.[85]

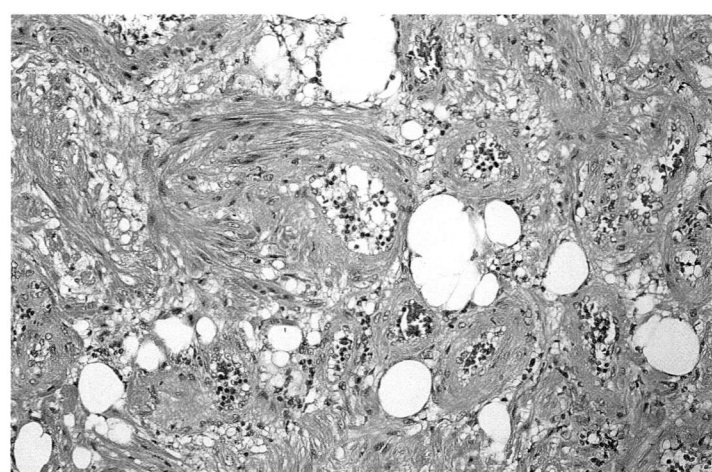

Fig. 36.4 **Angiomyolipoma.** There is an admixture of blood vessels, smooth muscle and adipocytes. (H & E)

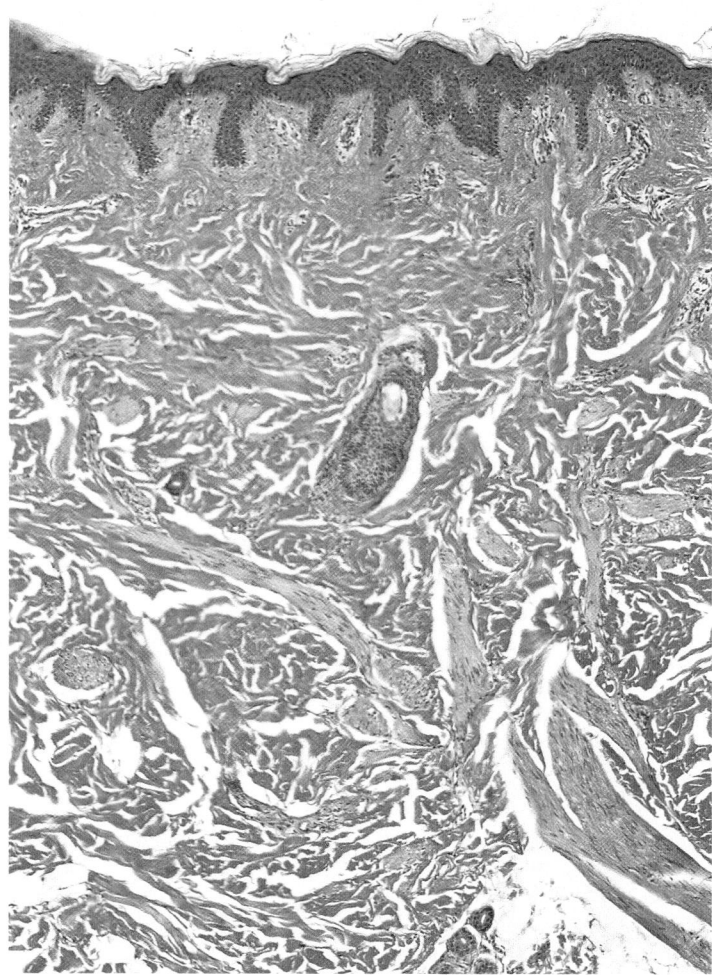

Fig. 36.5 **Smooth muscle hamartoma.** There are scattered smooth muscle bundles in the dermis. (H & E)

Electron microscopy

Ultrastructural examination confirms the presence of normal smooth muscle cells in this lesion.[74,86]

LEIOMYOSARCOMA

According to their different biological behavior, leiomyosarcomas of the skin can be divided into three categories: dermal, subcutaneous and secondary tumors.[88,89]

Over 100 acceptable cases of *dermal leiomyosarcoma* have now been recorded.[88,90] These tumors have a predilection for the extensor surfaces of the extremities,[88,89] and to a lesser extent the scalp[91] and trunk.[92–95] Rare sites include the upper lip,[96] nipple,[97,98] scrotum,[99,100] a chronic venous stasis ulcer,[101] and the face.[25] There is a male predominance, and the average age of presentation is in the sixth decade. Childhood presentation is rare.[102,103] The tumors vary in size from 0.5 to 3 cm or more in maximum diameter. Subcutaneous extension is present in two-thirds of cases.[88] Pain or tenderness is present in some.[89] Occasionally there is a history of previous injury to the site.[89,92] These tumors presumably arise from the arrector pili muscles, except for scrotal lesions, which derive from the dartos muscle.[88,99] A case apparently arising in an angioleiomyoma has been reported.[104] Dermal leiomyosarcomas may recur locally in up to 30% of cases (5% in the author's experience), but metastases of confirmed cases are unknown.[88]

Subcutaneous leiomyosarcomas tend to be slightly larger at presentation and more circumscribed in outline.[89] They may also be tender or painful. They presumably arise from the smooth muscle in vessel walls.[105] They have a greater tendency for local recurrence (50–70%), and metastases to lung, liver, bone and other sites occur in about one-third of cases.[89,106,107] Assessment of the DNA content of the tumor cells by flow cytometry may be used to predict those with metastatic potential.[108–110] The most frequent genomic alterations in leiomyosarcomas involve losses in the 13q4–21 region, but other chromosomal losses occur.[111] Malignant fibrous histiocytoma shares many of these genomic imbalances.[111]

Secondary leiomyosarcomas are rare in the skin and arise from retroperitoneal and uterine primary lesions.[112] There are usually several dermal or subcutaneous nodules. There has been a predilection for the scalp and back.

Histopathology

Dermal leiomyosarcomas are irregular in outline, with tumor cells blending into the collagenous stroma at the periphery.[113] By definition, the major portion of the tumor is in the dermis, although subcutaneous extension occurs in two-thirds.[88] A superficial grenz zone is present in many. Ulceration and pseudoepithelial hyperplasia are rare. There is usually some flattening of the rete ridges of the overlying epidermis.

Leiomyosarcomas are composed of interlacing fascicles of elongated spindle-shaped cells with eosinophilic cytoplasm and eccentric, blunt-ended (cigar-shaped) nuclei (Fig. 36.6). Rare variants with intracytoplasmic eosinophilic granules (*granular cell leiomyosarcoma*)[34,114,115] or with epithelioid cells (*epithelioid leiomyosarcoma*)[116] have been reported. Sometimes there is a suggestion of nuclear palisading. There is variable nuclear pleomorphism, with at least one mitosis per 10 high-power fields in cellular areas. Pockets of greater mitotic activity (mitotic 'hot spots')[117] are found. Tumor giant cells are usually present in the less well differentiated variants. Perinuclear halos are rare. Small lymphoid aggregates are sometimes present within the tumor,[88] but a dense infiltrate (*inflammatory leiomyosarcoma*) is quite rare.[102] Stromal sclerosis (*desmoplastic leiomyosarcoma*) is a rare phenomenon.[118,119] The resemblance of this tumor to other desmoplastic tumors of the skin is striking

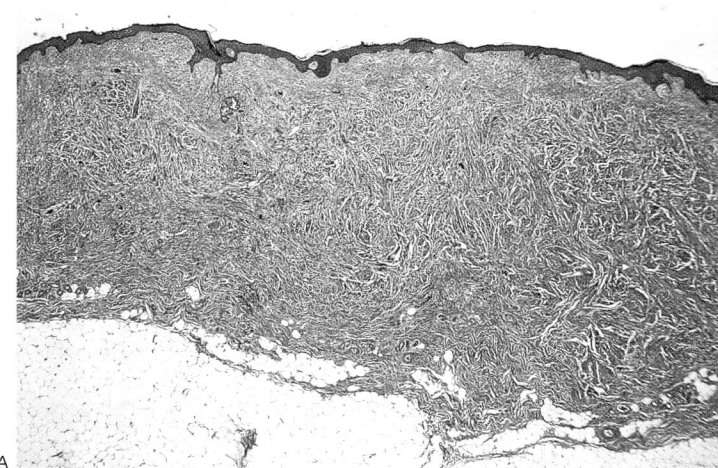
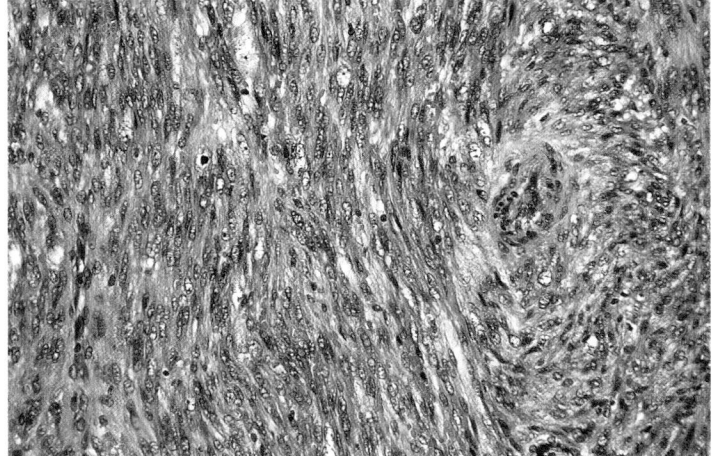

Fig. 36.6 **Leiomyosarcoma. (A)** The tumor is composed of plump spindle-shaped cells. **(B)** Scattered mitoses are present. (H & E)

and immunohistochemistry is necessary for its diagnosis.[119] Arrector pili muscles are often prominent or hyperplastic, and in some cases transitions from normal to hyperplastic, to benign neoplastic, and to a frankly sarcomatous pattern occur.[88,99]

In one large series, two predominant growth patterns were observed: nodular and diffuse.[90] Nodular tumors were usually quite cellular with nuclear atypia and many mitoses. Sometimes there were small foci of necrosis. Diffuse tumors were less cellular with well-differentiated smooth muscle cells and inconspicuous mitoses.[90]

Subcutaneous leiomyosarcomas often extend into the lower dermis (Fig. 36.7). They frequently have a prominent vascular pattern;[89] vascular invasion is an adverse prognostic feature.[109] Small areas of necrosis are sometimes present. Deep variants with either a heavy inflammatory cell component[120] or osteoclast-like giant cells[121] have been reported. A *myxoid* variant has been reported in the deeper soft tissues.[122]

Secondary leiomyosarcomas are often multiple, spheroidal in outline, and sometimes present in vascular lumina.[88]

Leiomyosarcomas of all three types will have myofilaments, demonstrated by the Masson trichrome stain. Reticulin stains show a fine reticulin network interspersed between adjacent fibers. A small amount of glycogen is usually present.[123] Immunoperoxidase preparations show the presence of vimentin and smooth muscle actin in the cytoplasm.[124] Desmin is present in about 70% of cases but is less common in the higher-grade tumors.[90,110] Pan-muscle

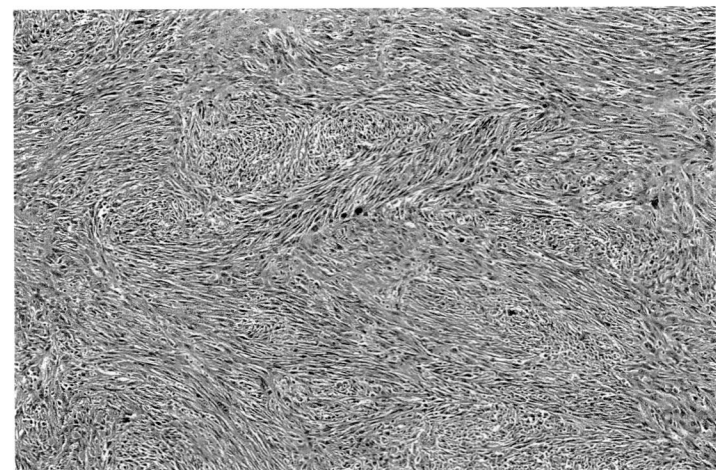

Fig. 36.7 **Subcutaneous leiomyosarcoma.** The lesion is quite cellular. (H & E)

actin (HHF-35) is usually present. Cytokeratin and S100 protein have been demonstrated in a small number of cases.[90,125]

Reliable criteria for malignancy remain to be established.[117] Usually accepted features include high cellularity, significant nuclear atypia, tumor giant cells, and at least one mitosis per 10 high-power fields. Tumor size of 5 cm or more is an adverse feature in subcutaneous tumors.[126]

Electron microscopy

Electron microscopy confirms the smooth muscle origin of the tumor cells, with numerous fine myofilaments in the cytoplasm, some marginal plaques, pinocytotic vesicles, glycogen, and a basal lamina surrounding individual cells.[99,117] Junctional complexes are uncommon.[117] Some myofibroblasts may also be present.[100]

TUMORS OF STRIATED MUSCLE

There is an exceedingly rare group of cutaneous tumors that contain either mature striated muscle, or cells differentiating toward striated muscle, as a major component of the lesion. Mature striated muscle is found in some parts of the face as a normal constituent,[127] in the striated muscle hamartoma (see below), the accessory tragus (see p. 572), and in the first arch abnormality reported as dermatorynchus geneae (see p. 572). Rarely, a few striated muscle fibers may be present adjacent to developmental cysts of the head and neck. Rhabdomyomas are usually found in the vicinity of the aerodigestive tract.[128] Rarely, they occur elsewhere (see below). Malignant cells showing ultrastructural, immunohistochemical and sometimes light microscopic differentiation toward striated muscle are a feature of rhabdomyosarcomas. Brief mention will also be made of the malignant rhabdoid tumor, which has some histopathological similarities to a rhabdomyosarcoma, but which is of uncertain histogenesis.

STRIATED MUSCLE HAMARTOMA

The term 'striated muscle hamartoma' has been proposed for an exceedingly rare entity of neonates in which there is a polypoid (skin tag-like) lesion of the head and neck region which contains striated muscle bundles.[129,130] A lesion in the perianal region has been reported.[131] Similar tumors have been reported as rhabdomyomatous mesenchymal hamartoma[132–135] and congenital midline hamartoma.[136] Striated muscle hamartomas have a midline location, whereas accessory tragi, which may also contain striated muscle, are usually found in the preauricular region or in the upper, lateral neck.

Histopathology

The polypoid tumors contain multiple bundles of normal-appearing striated muscle surrounded by fibrofatty tissue containing a few telangiectatic vessels.[129,132] Numerous vellus hair follicles or folliculosebaceous structures are usually present.[130]

The subcutaneous tumor with desmin-positive spindle cells, reported as **pleomorphic hamartoma of the subcutis**, is of uncertain histogenesis.[137]

RHABDOMYOMA (ADULT TYPE)

The adult rhabdomyoma is a rare, benign neoplasm that usually occurs in the head and neck region.[138] Rarely, they may arise elsewhere.[139] Rhabdomyomas are well circumscribed, soft tumors with a reddish-brown appearance. They may recur locally if incompletely excised.

Histopathology

Adult rhabdomyomas are composed of sheets of large polygonal cells with granular, eosinophilic cytoplasm. The cells are partly vacuolated due to their glycogen content. 'Spider-web' cells, with residual strands of cytoplasm between the vacuoles, and cells with cross-striations may both be present.[138] The tumor cells stain strongly for desmin and myoglobin; some may stain weakly for S100 protein.[139]

RHABDOMYOSARCOMA

Rhabdomyosarcoma, a tumor composed of malignant cells showing some differentiation toward striated muscle, has a predilection for the head and neck region,[140,141] the genitourinary tract, the retroperitoneum and the soft tissues of the extremities. It is the most common soft tissue sarcoma of childhood. Rarely, rhabdomyosarcoma may present as a dermal nodule, particularly on the head or neck, usually as a result of the dermal extension of a lesion arising in the underlying soft tissues.[142] Lesions of dermal origin are rare.[143,144]

Rhabdomyosarcomas have been reported in patients with neurofibromatosis, in the basal cell nevus syndrome, and many years after radiotherapy.[145]

Histopathology

There are three major histological subtypes of rhabdomyosarcoma: embryonal (including the botryoid variant), alveolar[146] and pleomorphic.[147,148] They may be composed of small round cells, spindle or polygonal cells, or large pleomorphic cells. Cross-striations are sometimes seen using the phosphotungstic–acid-hematoxylin stain.

Immunoperoxidase techniques using monoclonal antibodies to vimentin, desmin, myoglobin and muscle actin may be used to confirm the diagnosis.[142,144]

MALIGNANT RHABDOID TUMOR

Malignant rhabdoid tumors were initially regarded as a subset of Wilms' tumor of the kidney showing rhabdomyosarcomatous differentiation.[149] Subsequent studies have not confirmed this, and their histogenesis is currently uncertain. Tumors of similar morphology to the renal lesions have been reported in the skin.[150–156] Cutaneous lesions are highly aggressive neoplasms, often present at birth. The average survival following diagnosis is less than 6 weeks.[157] Genetic studies show a consistent pattern of abnormalities of chromosome 22q11, involving deletions and/or translocations.[157]

There is a report of two children with papulonodular skin lesions, present at birth, who subsequently developed malignant rhabdoid tumors, in one case in contiguity. The term 'neurovascular hamartoma' was used for these lesions composed of bland spindle cells in a vascular stroma.[158] Another case developed adjacent to a 'benign myofibromatous proliferation'.[159]

Histopathology

The tumor is composed of sheets of polygonal cells with abundant hyaline eosinophilic cytoplasm and a peripherally displaced vesicular nucleus. Mitotic activity is prominent, and there are usually areas of tumor necrosis.[150]

The cells invariably express vimentin and cytokeratins AE1/AE3 and/or CAM5.2. They often show strong focal to diffuse membranous staining for epithelial membrane antigen.[157,160] Focal positivity for muscle-specific actin and desmin may occur.[157] Malignant rhabdoid tumor has some morphological and immunohistochemical features in common with epithelioid sarcoma (see p. 940), although the cells in epithelioid sarcoma do not contain rhabdoid filamentous masses.[150,151] Rhabdoid differentiation has been reported in some malignant nerve sheath tumors.[161]

TUMORS OF CARTILAGE

Cartilage can be found in the skin in hamartomas (see p. 428), in certain tumors (such as chondroid syringomas), and in chondromas and osteochondromas. The latter two entities will be discussed here, together with the morphologically similar tumor known as parachordoma. The extraskeletal myxoid chondrosarcoma is a deep soft tissue tumor and beyond the scope of this book.[162]

CHONDROMA

True cutaneous chondromas, without bony connection, are exceedingly rare.[163,164] They occur most commonly on the fingers, but have been recorded at other sites, such as the ear[165] and nose.[165] Multiple lesions were present in one patient, who had a suggested autosomal dominant mode of inheritance.[165]

Histopathology

Chondroma is a well-circumscribed expansile tumor composed of single and grouped chondrocytes embedded in a cartilaginous matrix. It usually produces effacement of the epidermal rete ridge pattern.[165] The cells exhibit reactivity for S100 protein.

SUBUNGUAL OSTEOCHONDROMA

Subungual osteochondroma (exostosis) is a fairly common, often painful, tumor occurring on the distal phalanx of a digit, usually the great toe.[166–171]

Histopathology

The lesion consists of a base of mature trabecular bone with a proliferating cap of mature cartilage.[170] Osteogenesis occurs by endochondral ossification.

PARACHORDOMA

Parachordoma is an exceedingly rare soft tissue neoplasm with a superficial resemblance to a chordoma. It develops on the extremities adjacent to a tendon, synovium or bone, unlike chordoma which is axial in location.[172,173] Parachordomas are slow-growing tumors with occasional late recurrence. Cases with reported metastasis have not been convincing.[174]

Chordomas may develop in the skin by direct extension from an underlying sacrococcygeal tumor, or by distant metastasis (see p. 1052).

Histopathology

As in chordomas, there are strands and cords of vacuolated (physaliperous) cells set in a myxoid stroma (Fig. 36.8).[172] The cells stain for S100 protein, vimentin and epithelial membrane antigen.[173,174] Parachordomas are strongly positive for cytokeratin 8/18, but not for CK1/10, 7, and 20.[174] Extraskeletal myxoid chondrosarcoma is negative for all cytokeratins.[174,175]

TUMORS OF BONE

Mature bone may be found in the skin in the various forms of osteoma cutis (see p. 425). True neoplasms with differentiation toward bone (osteosarcoma) are exceedingly rare in the skin.[176–178] A case purporting to be a cutaneous osteoblastoma has been reported.[179]

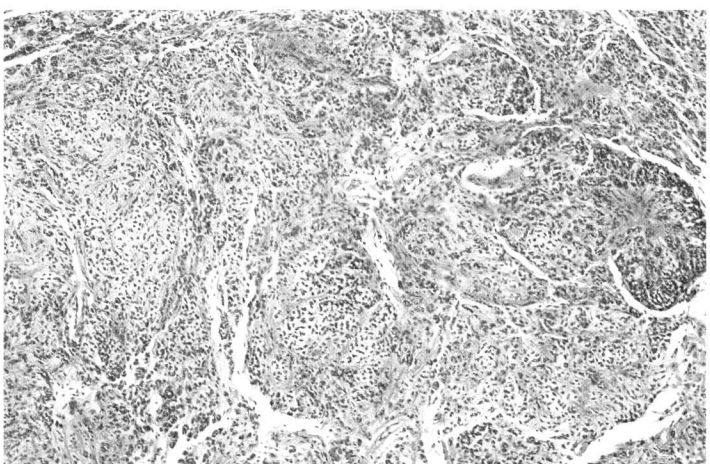
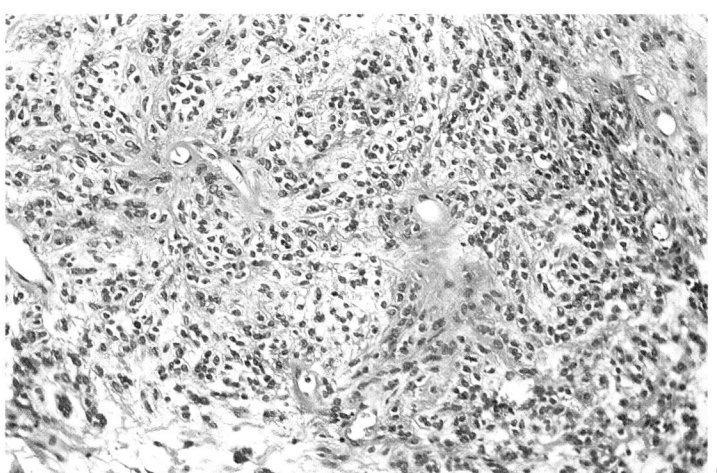

Fig. 36.8 **(A) Parachordoma. (B)** Nests of vacuolated cells are set in a fibromyxoid stroma. (H & E)

OSTEOSARCOMA

Osteosarcoma (osteogenic sarcoma) of the skin may arise *de novo* or within heterotopic bone.[176] An origin from underlying bone or metastasis from a primary lesion elsewhere must be excluded. Primary osteosarcoma of the skin can recur locally[178] and/or spread to the lungs and other organs.[176,177,180]

Histopathology

The tumor may be found in the dermis and/or the subcutis.[181] Ulceration often occurs. Highly cellular areas composed of spindle cells with scant eosinophilic cytoplasm and elongated hyperchromatic nuclei are usually present, in addition to foci of chondroid and osteoid differentiation. The tumor cells are positive for vimentin but negative for S100 protein and cytokeratins.

REFERENCES

Tumors of smooth muscle

1 Montgomery H, Winkelmann RK. Smooth-muscle tumors of the skin. Arch Dermatol 1959; 79: 32–39.

2 Raj S, Calonje E, Kraus M et al. Cutaneous pilar leiomyoma: clinicopathologic analysis of 53 lesions in 45 patients. Am J Dermatopathol 1997; 19: 2–9.

3 Kilpatrick SE, Mentzel T, Fletcher CDM. Leiomyoma of deep soft tissue. Am J Surg Pathol 1994; 18: 576–582.

4 Díaz-Pérez JL, Sánchez Díez A, Díaz-Ramón L et al. Leiomyomatosis. Am J Dermatopathol 2000; 22: 350 (abstract).

5 Burden PA, Gentry RH, Fitzpatrick JE. Piloleiomyoma arising in an organoid nevus: a case report and review of the literature. J Dermatol Surg Oncol 1987; 13: 1213–1218.

6 Pinkus H. Discussion. Arch Dermatol 1959; 79: 40.

7 Gökdemir G, Altunay IK, Köslü A, Ince Ü. A case of multiple facial painless leiomyomata. J Eur Acad Dermatol Venereol 2000; 14: 144–145.

8 Kanitakis J, Carbonnel E, Chouvet B et al. Cutaneous leiomyomas (piloleiomyomas) in adult patients with human immunodeficiency virus infection. Br J Dermatol 2000; 143: 1338–1340.

9 Abraham Z, Cohen A, Haim S. Muscle relaxing agent in cutaneous leiomyoma. Dermatologica 1983; 166: 255–256.

10 Thompson JA Jr. Therapy for painful cutaneous leiomyomas. J Am Acad Dermato 1985; 13: 865–867.

11 Henderson CA, Ruban E, Porter DI. Multiple leiomyomata presenting in a child. Pediatr Dermatol 1997; 14: 287–289.

12 Fisher WC, Helwig EB. Leiomyomas of the skin. Arch Dermatol 1963; 88: 510–520.

13 Thyresson HN, Su WPD. Familial cutaneous leiomyomatosis. J Am Acad Dermatol 1981; 4: 430–434.

14 Smith CG, Glaser DA, Leonardi C. Zosteriform multiple leiomyomas. J Am Acad Dermatol 1998; 38: 272–273.

15 Agarwalla A, Thakur A, Jacob M et al. Zosteriform and disseminated lesions in cutaneous leiomyoma. Acta Derm Venereol 2000; 80: 446.

16 Peters CW, Hanke CW, Reed JC. Nevus leiomyomatosus systematicus. Cutis 1981; 27: 484–486.

17 Kloepfer HW, Krafchuk J, Derbes V, Burks J. Hereditary multiple leiomyoma of the skin. Am J Hum Genet 1958; 10: 48–52.

18 Fernández-Pugnaire MA, Delgado-Florencio V. Familial multiple cutaneous leiomyomas. Dermatology 1995; 191: 295–298.

19 Rudner EJ, Schwartz OD, Grekin JN. Multiple cutaneous leiomyomata in identical twins. Arch Dermatol 1964; 90: 81–82.

20 Jolliffe DS. Multiple cutaneous leiomyomata. Clin Exp Dermatol 1978; 3: 89–92.

21 Venencie PY, Puissant A, Boffa GA et al. Multiple cutaneous leiomyomata and erythrocytosis with demonstration of erythropoietic activity in the cutaneous leiomyomata. Br J Dermatol 1982; 107: 483–486.

22 Engelke H, Christophers E. Leiomyomatosis cutis et uteri. Acta Derm Venereol (Suppl) 1979; 85: 51–54.

23 Spencer JM, Amonette RA. Tumors with smooth muscle differentiation. Dermatol Surg 1996; 22: 761–768.

24 Vergani R, Betti R, Uziel L et al. Eruptive multiple sporadic cutaneous piloleiomyomas in a patient with chronic lymphocytic leukaemia. Br J Dermatol 2000; 143: 907–909.

25 Orellana-Diaz O, Hernandez-Perez E. Leiomyoma cutis and leiomyosarcoma: a 10-year study and a short review. J Dermatol Surg Oncol 1983; 9: 283–287.

26 Stout AP. Solitary cutaneous and subcutaneous leiomyoma. Am J Cancer 1937; 29: 435–469.

27 Lupton GP, Naik DG, Rodman OG. An unusual congenital leiomyoma. Pediatr Dermatol 1986; 3: 158–160.

28 Newman PL, Fletcher CDM. Smooth muscle tumours of the external genitalia: clinicopathological analysis of a series. Histopathology 1991; 18: 523–529.

29 Livne PM, Nobel M, Savir A et al. Leiomyoma of the scrotum. Arch Dermatol 1983; 119: 358–359.

30 Siegal GP, Gaffey TA. Solitary leiomyomas arising from the tunica dartos scroti. J Urol 1976; 116: 69–71.

31 Jansen LH. Leiomyoma cutis. Acta Derm Venereol 1952; 32: 40–50.

32 Ohtake N, Maeda S, Kanzaki T, Shimoinaba K. Leiomyoma of the scrotum. Dermatology 1997; 194: 299–301.

33 Lespi PJ, Smit R. Verocay-body prominent cutaneous leiomyoma. Am J Dermatopathol 1999; 21: 110–111.

34 Mentzel T, Wadden C, Fletcher CDM. Granular cell change in smooth muscle tumours of skin and soft tissue. Histopathology 1994; 24: 223–231.

35 Mahalingam M, Goldberg LJ. Atypical pilar leiomyoma — the cutaneous counterpart of uterine symplastic leiomyoma. J Cutan Pathol 2000; 27: 563 (abstract).

36 Dobashi Y, Iwabuchi K, Nakahata J et al. Combined clear and granular cell leiomyoma of soft tissue: evidence of transformation to a histiocytic phenotype. Histopathology 1999; 34: 526–531.

37 Nielsen GP, Rosenberg AE, Koerner FC et al. Smooth-muscle tumors of the vulva. A clinicopathological study of 25 cases and review of the literature. Am J Surg Pathol 1996; 20: 779–793.

38 McGinley KM, Bryant S, Kattine AA et al. Cutaneous leiomyomas lack estrogen and progesterone receptor immunoreactivity. J Cutan Pathol 1997; 24: 241–245.

39 Lun KR, Spelman LJ. Multiple piloleiomyomas. Australas J Dermatol 2000; 41: 185–186.

40 Duhig JT, Ayer JP. Vascular leiomyoma. A study of sixty-one cases. Arch Pathol 1959; 68: 424–430.

41 Requena L, Baran R. Digital angioleiomyoma: an uncommon neoplasm. J Am Acad Dermatol 1993; 29: 1043–1044.

42 MacDonald DM, Sanderson KV. Angioleiomyoma of the skin. Br J Dermatol 1974; 91: 161–168.

43 Hachisuga T, Hashimoto H, Enjoji M. Angioleiomyoma. A clinicopathologic reappraisal of 562 cases. Cancer 1984; 54: 126–130.

44 Fox SB, Heryet A, Khong TY. Angioleiomyomas: an immunohistological study. Histopathology 1990; 16: 495–496.

45 Magner D, Hill DP. Encapsulated angiomyoma of the skin and subcutaneous tissues. Am J Clin Pathol 1961; 35: 137–141.

46 Sajben FP, Barnette DJ, Barrett TL. Intravascular angioleiomyoma. J Cutan Pathol 1999; 26: 165–167.

47 Argenyi ZB, Piette WW, Goeken J. Cutaneous angiomyolipoma: a light microscopic, immunohistochemical, and electronmicroscopic study. J Cutan Pathol 1986; 13: 434.

48 Fitzpatrick JE, Mellette JR Jr, Zaim MT et al. Cutaneous angiolipoleiomyoma (angiomyolipoma). J Cutan Pathol 1988; 15: 305 (abstract).

49 Mehregan DA, Mehregan DR, Mehregan AH. Angiomyolipoma. J Am Acad Dermatol 1992; 27: 331–333.

50 Rodriguez-Fernández A, Caro-Mancilla A. Cutaneous angiomyolipoma with pleomorphic changes. J Am Acad Dermatol 1993; 29: 115–116.

51 Argenyi ZB, Piette WW, Goeken JA. Cutaneous angiomyolipoma. Am J Dermatopathol 1991; 13: 497–502.

52 Fitzpatrick JE, Mellette JR Jr, Hwang RJ et al. Cutaneous angiolipoleiomyoma. J Am Acad Dermatol 1990; 23: 1093–1098.

53 Val-Bernal JF, Mira C. Cutaneous angiomyolipoma. J Cutan Pathol 1996; 23: 364–368.

54 Nonomura A, Minato H, Kurumaya H. Angiomyolipoma predominantly composed of smooth muscle cells: problems in histological diagnosis. Histopathology 1998; 33: 20–27.

55 Meis JM, Enzinger FM. Myolipoma of soft tissue. Am J Surg Pathol 1991; 15: 121–125.

56 Baugh W, Quigley MM, Barrett TL. Palisaded angioleiomyoma. J Cutan Pathol 2000; 27: 526–528.

57 Requena L, Ortiz S, Sánchez M, Sánchez Yus E. Angioleiomyoma within a histiocytoma. J Cutan Pathol 1990; 17: 278–280.

58 Heffernan MP, Smoller BR, Kohler S. Cutaneous epithelioid angioleiomyoma. Am J Dermatopathol 1998; 20: 213–217.

59 Martínez JA, Quecedo E, Fortea JM et al. Pleomorphic angioleiomyoma. Am J Dermatopathol 1996; 18: 409–412.

60 Rosai J. Pleomorphic angioleiomyoma. Am J Dermatopathol 1997; 19: 419.

61 Kawagishi N, Kashiwagi T, Ibe M et al. Pleomorphic angioleiomyoma. Report of two cases with immunohistochemical studies. Am J Dermatopathol 2000; 22: 268–271.

62 Tsambaos D, Orfanos CE. Cutaneous smooth muscle hamartoma. J Cutan Pathol 1982; 9: 33–42.

63 Bronson DM, Fretzin DF, Farrell LN. Congenital pilar and smooth muscle nevus. J Am Acad Dermatol 1983; 8: 111–114.

64 Karo KR, Gange RW. Smooth-muscle hamartoma. Possible congenital Becker's nevus. Arch Dermatol 1981; 117: 678–679.

65 Metzker A, Amir J, Rotem A, Merlob P. Congenital smooth muscle hamartoma of the skin. Pediatr Dermatol 1984; 2: 45–48.

66 Plewig G, Schmoeckel C. Naevus musculi arrector pili. Hautarzt 1979; 30: 503–505.

67 Goldman MP, Kaplan RP, Heng MCY. Congenital smooth-muscle hamartoma. Int J Dermatol 1987; 26: 448–452.

68 Johnson MD, Jacobs AH. Congenital smooth muscle hamartoma. A report of six cases and a review of the literature. Arch Dermatol 1989; 125: 820–822.

69 Gerdsen R, Lagarde C, Steen A et al. Congenital smooth muscle hamartoma of the skin: clinical classification. Acta Derm Venereol 1999; 79: 408–409.

70 Quinn TR, Young RH. Smooth-muscle hamartoma of the tunica dartos of the scrotum: report of a case. J Cutan Pathol 1997; 24: 322–326.

71 Berberian BJ, Burnett JW. Congenital smooth muscle hamartoma: a case report. Br J Dermatol 1986; 115: 711–714.

72 Gagné EJ, Su WPD. Congenital smooth muscle hamartoma of the skin. Pediatr Dermatol 1993; 10: 142–145.

73 Jang H-S, Kim MB, Oh C-K et al. Linear congenital smooth muscle hamartoma with follicular spotted appearance. Br J Dermatol 2000; 142: 138–142.

74 Berger TG, Levin MW. Congenital smooth muscle hamartoma. J Am Acad Dermatol 1984; 11: 709–712.

75 Wallach D, Sorin M, Saurat JH. Naevus musculaire généralisé avec aspect clinique de "bébé Michelin". Ann Dermatol Venereol 1980; 107: 923–927.

76 Glover MT, Malone M, Atherton DJ. Michelin-tire baby syndrome resulting from diffuse smooth muscle hamartoma. Pediatr Dermatol 1989; 6: 329–331.

77 Oku T, Iwasaki K, Fujita H. Folded skin with an underlying cutaneous smooth muscle hamartoma. Br J Dermatol 1993; 129: 606–608.

78 Schnur RE, Herzberg AJ, Spinner N et al. Variability in the Michelin tire syndrome. J Am Acad Dermatol 1993; 28: 364–370.

79 Gualandri L, Cambiaghi S, Ermacora E et al. Multiple familial smooth muscle hamartomas. Pediatr Dermatol 2001; 18: 17–20.

80 Haneke E. The dermal component in melanosis naeviformis Becker. J Cutan Pathol 1979; 6: 53–58.

81 Urbanek RW, Johnson WC. Smooth muscle hamartoma associated with Becker's nevus. Arch Dermatol 1978; 114: 104–106.

82 Wong RC, Solomon AR. Acquired dermal smooth-muscle hamartoma. Cutis 1985; 35: 369–370.

83 Hsiao G-H, Chen J-S. Acquired genital smooth-muscle hamartoma. A case report. Am J Dermatopathol 1995; 17: 67–70.

84 Darling TN, Kamino H, Murray JC. Acquired cutaneous smooth muscle hamartoma. J Am Acad Dermatol 1993; 28: 844–845.

85 Slifman NR, Harrist TJ, Rhodes AR. Congenital arrector pili hamartoma. Arch Dermatol 1985; 121: 1034–1037.

86 Fishman SJ, Phelps RG, Lebwohl M, Lieber C. Immunofluorescence and electron microscopic findings in a congenital arrector pili hamartoma. Am J Dermatopathol 1989; 11: 369–374.

87 Koizumi H, Kodama K, Tsuji Y et al. CD34-positive dendritic cells are an intrinsic part of smooth muscle hamartoma. Br J Dermatol 1999; 140: 172–174.

88 Wolff M, Rothenberg J. Dermal leiomyosarcoma: a misnomer? Prog Surg Pathol 1986; 6: 147–159.

89 Fields JP, Helwig EB. Leiomyosarcoma of the skin and subcutaneous tissue. Cancer 1981; 47: 156–169.

90 Kaddu S, Beham A, Cerroni L et al. Cutaneous leiomyosarcoma. Am J Surg Pathol 1997; 21: 979–987.

91 Montes LF, Ocampo JC, Garcia NJ et al. Response of leiomyosarcoma to cryosurgery: clinicopathological and ultrastructural study. Clin Exp Dermatol 1995; 20: 22–26.

92 Chow J, Sabet LM, Clark BL, Coire CI. Cutaneous leiomyosarcoma: case reports and review of the literature. Ann Plast Surg 1987; 18: 319–322.

93 Davidson LL, Frost ML, Hanke W, Epinette WW. Primary leiomyosarcoma of the skin. Case report and review of the literature. J Am Acad Dermatol 1989; 21: 1156–1160.

94 Landry MM, Sarma DP, Boucree JB Jr. Leiomyosarcoma of the buttock. J Am Acad Dermatol 1991; 24: 618–620.

95 Wargon O. Primary leiomyosarcoma of the skin. Australas J Dermatol 1997; 38: 26–28.

96 Bañuls J, Botella R, Sevila A et al. Leiomyosarcoma of the upper lip. Int J Dermatol 1994; 33: 48–49.

97 Lonsdale RN, Widdison A. Leiomyosarcoma of the nipple. Histopathology 1992; 20: 537–539.

98 Alessi E, Sala F. Leiomyosarcoma in ectopic areola. Am J Dermatopathol 1992; 14: 165–169.

99 Flotte TJ, Bell DA, Sidhu GS, Plair CM. Leiomyosarcoma of the dartos muscle. J Cutan Pathol 1981; 8: 69–74.

100 Johnson S, Rundell M, Platt W. Leiomyosarcoma of the scrotum. A case report with electron microscopy. Cancer 1978; 41: 1830–1835.

101 Nunnery EW, Lipper S, Reddick R, Kahn LB. Leiomyosarcoma arising in a chronic venous stasis ulcer. Hum Pathol 1981; 12: 951–953.

102 Aubain Somerhausen N de S, Fletcher CDM. Leiomyosarcoma of soft tissue in children. Clinicopathologic analysis of 20 cases. Am J Surg Pathol 1999; 23: 755–763.

103 Yanguas I, Goday J, González-Güemes M et al. Cutaneous leiomyosarcoma in a child. Pediatr Dermatol 1997; 14: 281–283.

104 White IR, MacDonald DM. Cutaneous leiomyosarcoma with coexistent superficial angioleiomyoma. Clin Exp Dermatol 1981; 6: 333–337.

105 Del-Río R, Vilalta A, Palou J, Mascaró JM. Giant vascular leiomyosarcoma. Int J Dermatol 1994; 33: 856–857.

106 Stout AP, Hill WT. Leiomyosarcoma of the superficial soft tissues. Cancer 1958; 11: 844–854.

107 Wascher RA, Lee MYT. Recurrent cutaneous leiomyosarcoma. Cancer 1992; 70: 490–492.

108 Oliver GF, Reiman HM, Gonchoroff NJ, Muller SA, Umbert I. Cutaneous and subcutaneous leiomyosarcoma: a clinicopathologic review of 14 cases with reference to anti-desmin staining and nuclear DNA patterns studied by flow cytometry. J Cutan Pathol 1988; 15: 332 (abstract).

109 Gustafson P, Willén H, Baldetorp B et al. Soft tissue leiomyosarcoma. Cancer 1992; 70: 114–119.

110 Oliver GF, Reiman HM, Gonchoroff NJ et al. Cutaneous and subcutaneous leiomyosarcoma: a clinicopathological review of 14 cases with reference to antidesmin staining and nuclear DNA patterns studied by flow cytometry. Br J Dermatol 1991; 124: 252–257.

111 Derré J, Lagacé R, Nicolas A et al. Leiomyosarcomas and most malignant fibrous histiocytomas share very similar comparative genomic hybridization imbalances: an analysis of a series of 27 leiomyosarcomas. Lab Invest 2001; 81: 211–215.

112 Alessi E, Innocenti M, Sala F. Leiomyosarcoma metastatic to the back and scalp from a primary neoplasm in the uterus. Am J Dermatopathol 1985; 7: 471–476.

113 Jegasothy BV, Gilgor RS, Hull DM. Leiomyosarcoma of the skin and subcutaneous tissue. Arch Dermatol 1981; 117: 478–481.

114 Suster S, Rosen LB, Sanchez JL. Granular cell leiomyosarcoma of the skin. Am J Dermatopathol 1988; 10: 234–239.

115 Sironi M, Assi A, Pasquinelli G, Cenacchi G. Not all granular cell tumors show Schwann cell differentiation: a granular cell leiomyosarcoma of the thumb, a case report. Am J Dermatopathol 1999; 21: 307–309.

116 Suster S. Epithelioid leiomyosarcoma of the skin and subcutaneous tissue. Am J Surg Pathol 1994; 18: 232–240.

117 Headington JT, Beals TF, Niederhuber JE. Primary leiomyosarcoma of skin: a report and critical appraisal. J Cutan Pathol 1977; 4: 308–317.

118 Karroum JE, Zappi EG, Cockerell CJ. Sclerotic primary cutaneous leiomyosarcoma. Am J Dermatopathol 1995; 17: 292–296.

119 Diaz-Cascajo C, Borghi S, Weyers W. Desmoplastic leiomyosarcoma of the skin. Am J Dermatopathol 2000; 22: 251–255.

120 Merchant W, Calonje E, Fletcher CDM. Inflammatory leiomyosarcoma: a morphological subgroup within the heterogeneous family of so-called inflammatory malignant fibrous histiocytoma. Histopathology 1995; 27: 525–532.

121 Mentzel T, Calonje E, Fletcher CDM. Leiomyosarcoma with prominent osteoclast-like giant cells. Am J Surg Pathol 1994; 18: 258–265.

122 Rubin BP, Fletcher CDM. Myxoid leiomyosarcoma of soft tissue, an underrecognized variant. Am J Surg Pathol 2000; 24: 927–936.

123 Fletcher CDM, McKee PH. Sarcomas – a clinicopathological guide with particular reference to cutaneous manifestation II. Malignant nerve sheath tumour, leiomyosarcoma and rhabdomyosarcoma. Clin Exp Dermatol 1985; 10: 201–216.

124 Miettinen M, Lehto V-P, Virtanen I. Antibodies to intermediate filament proteins. The differential diagnosis of cutaneous tumors. Arch Dermatol 1985; 121: 736–741.

125 Swanson PE, Stanley MW, Scheithauer BW, Wick MR. Primary cutaneous leiomyosarcoma. A histological and immunohistochemical study of 9 cases, with ultrastructural correlation. J Cutan Pathol 1988; 15: 129–141.

126 Lidang Jensen M, Myhre Jensen O, Michalski W et al. Intradermal and subcutaneous leiomyosarcoma: a clinicopathological and immunohistochemical study of 41 cases. J Cutan Pathol 1996; 23: 458–463.

Tumors of striated muscle

127 Sánchez Yus E, Simón P. Striated muscle. A normal component of the dermis and subcutis in many areas of the face. Am J Dermatopathol 2000; 22: 503–509.

128 Kapadia SB, Meis JM, Frisman DM et al. Adult rhabdomyoma of the head and neck: a clinicopathologic and immunophenotypic study. Hum Pathol 1993; 24: 608–617.

129 Hendrick SJ, Sanchez RL, Blackwell SJ, Raimer SS. Striated muscle hamartoma: description of two cases. Pediatr Dermatol 1986; 3: 153–157.

130 Sánchez RL, Raimer SS. Clinical and histologic features of striated muscle hamartoma: possible relationship to Delleman's syndrome. J Cutan Pathol 1994; 21: 40–46.

13 Scrivener Y, Petiau P, Rodier-Bruant C et al. Perianal striated muscle hamartoma associated with hemangioma. Pediatr Dermatol 1998; 15: 274–276.

132 Mills AE. Rhabdomyomatous mesenchymal hamartoma. Am J Dermatopathol 1989; 11: 58–63.

133 Sahn EE, Garen PD, Pai GS et al. Multiple rhabdomyomatous mesenchymal hamartomas of skin. Am J Dermatopathol 1990; 12: 485–491.

134 Farris PE, Manning S, Vuitch F. Rhabdomyomatous mesenchymal hamartoma. Am J Dermatopathol 1994; 16: 73–75.

135 Hayes M, van der Westhuizen N. Congenital rhabdomyomatous mesenchymal hamartoma. Am J Dermatopathol 1992; 14: 64–65.

136 Elgart GW, Patterson JW. Congenital midline hamartoma: case report with histochemical and immunohistochemical findings. Pediatr Dermatol 1990; 7: 199–201.

137 Shitabata PK, Ritter JH, Fitzgibbon JF et al. Pleomorphic hamartoma of the subcutis: a lesion with possible myogenous and neural lineages. J Cutan Pathol 1995; 22: 269–275.

138 Verdolini R, Goteri G, Brancorsini D et al. Adult rhabdomyoma: report of two cases of rhabdomyoma of the lip and of the eyelid. Am J Dermatopathol 2000; 22: 264–267.

139 Cronin CT, Keel SB, Grabbe J, Schuler JG. Adult rhabdomyoma of the extremity: a case report and review of the literature. Hum Pathol 2000; 31: 1074–1080.

140 Lyos AT, Goepfert H, Luna MA et al. Soft tissue sarcoma of the head and neck in children and adolescents. Cancer 1996; 77: 193–200.

141 Ansai S, Takeda H, Koseki S et al. A patient with rhabdomyosarcoma and clear cell sarcoma of the skin. J Am Acad Dermatol 1994; 31: 871–876.

142 Wiss K, Solomon AR, Raimer SS et al. Rhabdomyosarcoma presenting as a cutaneous nodule. Arch Dermatol 1988; 124: 1687–1690.

143 Chang Y, Dehner LP, Egbert B. Primary cutaneous rhabdomyosarcoma. Am J Surg Pathol 1990; 14: 977–982.

144 Wong T-Y, Suster S. Primary cutaneous sarcomas showing rhabdomyoblastic differentiation. Histopathology 1995; 26: 25–32.

145 Miracco C, Materno M, Margherita De Santi M et al. Unusual second malignancies following radiation therapy: subcutaneous pleomorphic rhabdomyosarcoma and cutaneous melanoma. Two case reports. J Cutan Pathol 2000; 27: 419–422.

146 Bianchi L, Orlandi A, Iraci S et al. Solid alveolar rhabdomyosarcoma of the hand in adolescence: a clinical, histologic, immunologic, and ultrastructural study. Pediatr Dermatol 1995; 12: 343–347.

147 Gaffney EF, Dervan PA, Fletcher CDM. Pleomorphic rhabdomyosarcoma in adulthood. Analysis of 11 cases with definition of diagnostic criteria. Am J Surg Pathol 1993; 17: 601–609.

148 Kodet R, Newton WA Jr, Hamoudi AB et al. Childhood rhabdomyosarcoma with anaplastic (pleomorphic) features. Am J Surg Pathol 1993; 17: 443–453.

149 Wick MR, Ritter JH, Dehner LP. Malignant rhabdoid tumors: a clinicopathologic review and conceptual discussion. Semin Diagn Pathol 1995; 12: 233–248.

150 Dabbs DJ, Park HK. Malignant rhabdoid skin tumor: an uncommon primary skin neoplasm. Ultrastructural and immunohistochemical analysis. J Cutan Pathol 1988; 15: 109–115.

51 Perrone T, Swanson PE, Twiggs L et al. Malignant rhabdoid tumor of the vulva: is distinction from epithelioid sarcoma possible? A pathologic and immunohistochemical study. Am J Surg Pathol 1989; 13: 848–858.

152 Dominey A, Paller AS, Gonzalez-Crussi F. Congenital rhabdoid sarcoma with cutaneous metastases. J Am Acad Dermatol 1990; 22: 969–974.

153 Sangueza OP, Meshul CK, Sangueza P, Mendoza R. Rhabdoid tumor of the skin. Int J Dermatol 1992; 31: 484–487.

154 Matias C, Nunes JFM, Vicente LF, Almeida MO. Primary malignant rhabdoid tumour of the vulva. Histopathology 1990; 17: 576–578.

155 Davies MRQ, Mogilner JG. Congenital malignant rhabdoid tumour of the skin. Pediatr Surg Int 1991; 6: 230–232.

156 Boscaino A, Donofrio V, Tornillo L et al. Primary rhabdoid tumour of the skin in a 14-month-old child. Dermatology 1994; 188: 322–325.

157 White FV, Dehner LP, Belchis DA et al. Congenital disseminated malignant rhabdoid tumor. A distinct clinicopathologic entity demonstrating abnormalities of chromosome 22q11. Am J Surg Pathol 1999; 23: 249–256.

158 Perez-Atayde AR, Newburg R, Fletcher JA et al. Congenital "neurovascular hamartoma" of the skin. A possible marker of malignant rhabdoid tumour. Am J Surg Pathol 1994; 18: 1030–1038.

159 García-Bustinduy M, Álvarez-Arguelles H, Guimerá F et al. Malignant rhabdoid tumor beside benign skin mesenchymal neoplasm with myofibromatous features. J Cutan Pathol 1999; 26: 509–515.

160 Kodet R, Newton WA Jr, Sachs N et al. Rhabdoid tumors of soft tissues: a clinicopathologic study of 26 cases enrolled on the intergroup rhabdomyosarcoma study. Hum Pathol 1991; 22: 674–684.

161 Morgan M, Stevens L, Tannenbaum M. Cutaneous epithelioid malignant nerve sheath tumor with rhabdoid features. J Cutan Pathol 2000; 27: 565 (abstract).

Tumors of cartilage

162 Cummings TJ, Shea CR, Reed JA et al. Expression of the intermediate filament peripherin in extraskeletal myxoid chondrosarcoma. J Cutan Pathol 2000; 27: 141–146.

163 Holmes HS, Bovenmeyer DA. Cutaneous cartilaginous tumor. Arch Dermatol 1976; 112: 839–840.

164 Ayala F, Lembo G, Montesano M. A rare tumor: subungual chondroma. Dermatologica 1983; 167: 339–340.

165 Humphreys TR, Herzberg AJ, Elenitsas R et al. Familial occurrence of multiple cutaneous chondromas. Am J Dermatopathol 1994; 16: 56–59.

166 Landon GC, Johnson KA, Dahlin DC. Subungual exostoses. J Bone Joint Surg 1979; 61A: 256–259.

167 Miller-Breslow A, Dorman HD. Dupuytren's (subungual) exostosis. Am J Surg Pathol 1988; 12: 368–378.

168 Matthewson MH. Subungual exostoses of the fingers. Are they really uncommon? Br J Dermatol 1978; 98: 187–189.

169 Cohen HJ, Frank SB, Minkin W, Gibbs RC. Subungual exostoses. Arch Dermatol 1973; 107: 431–432.

170 Kato H, Nakagawa K, Tsuji T, Hamada T. Subungual exostoses – clinicopathological and ultrastructural studies of three cases. Clin Exp Dermatol 1990; 15: 429–432.

171 Schulze KE, Hebert AA. Diagnostic features, differential diagnosis, and treatment of subungual osteochondroma. Pediatr Dermatol 1994; 11: 39–41.

172 Sangueza OP, White CR Jr. Parachordoma. Am J Dermatopathol 1994; 16: 185–188.

173 Imlay SP, Argenyi ZB, Stone MS et al. Cutaneous parachordoma. A light microscopic and immunohistochemical report of two cases and review of the literature. J Cutan Pathol 1998; 25: 279–284.

174 Fisher C. Parachordoma exists – but what is it? Adv Anat Pathol 2000; 7: 141–148.

175 Folpe AL, Agoff SN, Willis J, Weiss SW. Parachordoma is immunohistochemically and cytogenetically distinct from axial chordoma and extraskeletal myxoid chondrosarcoma. Am J Surg Pathol 1999; 23: 1059–1067.

Tumors of bone

176 Sacker AR, Oyama KK, Kessler S. Primary osteosarcoma of the penis. Am J Dermatopathol 1994; 16: 285–287.

177 Kircik L, Mohs FE, Snow SN. Osteogenic sarcoma of the scalp. Int J Dermatol 1995; 34: 861–862.

178 Kobos JW, Yu GH, Varadarajan S, Brooks JSJ. Primary cutaneous osteosarcoma. Am J Dermatopathol 1995; 17: 53–57.

179 Cannavo SP, Marafioti T. Cutaneous aggressive osteoblastoma. Int J Dermatol 1996; 35: 504–505.

180 Pillay P, Simango S, Govender D. Extraskeletal osteosarcoma of the scalp. Pathology 2000; 32: 154–157.

181 Kuo T-t. Primary osteosarcoma of the skin. J Cutan Pathol 1992; 19: 151–155.

Neural and neuroendocrine tumors

INTRODUCTION

Neural tumors are an important category of cutaneous tumors. Although the vast majority of them can be diagnosed without difficulty, there are cases which require distinction from other spindle-cell tumors, including melanoma. Markers are still being sought that will allow a reliable distinction between neural tumors and spindle-cell melanomas.

Cutaneous neural tumors arise from, or differentiate toward, one or more elements of the nervous system. Most of the tumors found in the skin and subcutaneous tissue are derived from peripheral nerves or their neuro-cutaneous end organs. There are three principal cells comprising the sheath of peripheral nerves: the perineurial cell, the Schwann cell and the fibroblast. Perineurial cells, which differ from Schwann cells by having no basement membrane, give rise to the perineurioma. Schwann cells give rise to the three main types of cutaneous neural tumors: neuromas, schwannomas (neurilemmomas) and neurofibromas. The tumors differ from one another by having a different proportion and arrangement of the various constituents of a peripheral nerve – Schwann cells, axons, fibroblasts and supporting stroma. Although Schwann cells are generally viewed as neuroectodermal cells derived from the neural crest, it has been suggested that they may be of mesenchymal origin.[1] The perineurial cell may also be of neural crest derivation.[2]

The other categories to be considered in this chapter are the herniations and heterotopias of glial and meningeal cells, giving rise to nasal gliomas, cutaneous meningiomas and related heterotopias, and the neuroendocrine carcinoma (Merkel cell tumor), which may be derived from another neural crest derivative, the Merkel cell. This cell subserves a neurosensory function in the skin. Merkel cell hyperplasia has been found in many settings, including sun- and radiation-damaged skin, as well as in some tumors of follicular origin.[3]

NERVE SHEATH TUMORS

The principal tumors in the nerve sheath category are neuromas, schwannomas (neurilemmomas), neurofibromas and their variants. As malignant peripheral nerve sheath tumors are rare, and often deep-seated, only a brief account will be given. The granular cell tumor (myoblastoma) is possibly of Schwann cell origin and is also included. Nerve sheath tumors express both S100 protein and myelin basic protein.[4] The reaction for these substances is less intense in the malignant peripheral nerve sheath tumors.[4] Epithelial membrane antigen is present in the perineurial cell, the capsule of some nerve sheath tumors (see below), and in the nerve sheath myxoma.[5] Perineurial cells also express vascular endothelial cadherin.[6] The human progenitor cell antigen CD34 is present in a dendritic cell within the endoneurium of normal nerves,[7] as well as in neurofibromas, Antoni B areas of neurilemmomas, and dermatofibrosarcomas.[8,9]

NEUROMAS

Neuromas are nerve sheath tumors in which the ratio of axons to Schwann cell fascicles approaches 1:1.[10] There are four distinct clinicopathological groups: traumatic neuromas, rudimentary polydactyly, solitary neuromas and neuromas associated with the multiple endocrine neoplasia syndrome (type 2b). Ganglioneuromas will also be considered here.

Traumatic neuroma

Traumatic neuromas result when a nerve is sectioned or traumatized in some way, and continuity cannot be re-established.[11] They are therefore found at sites of trauma, in scars, and in amputation stumps.[12] Traumatic neuromas are usually firm, oval, pea-sized nodules in the subcutis or deeper soft tissues.[11] They may be painful.

Histopathology[12]

Traumatic neuromas are composed of an irregular arrangement of nerve fascicles embedded in fibrous scar tissue. There may be concentric condensations of fibrous tissue around individual fascicles, giving the appearance of multiple separate nerves (Fig. 37.1). Perineurial cells, which contain epithelial membrane antigen, surround each fascicle, in contrast to solitary circumscribed neuromas, in which only the peripheral capsule contains these cells.[13] A Bodian stain will confirm the presence of numerous axons (Fig. 37.2). As in most neural tumors, mast cells are scattered throughout.

Electron microscopy

Studies have shown that each fascicle is ensheathed by multiple laminae of perineurial cells.[14] Furthermore, there is wide variation in the size of the axons.[14]

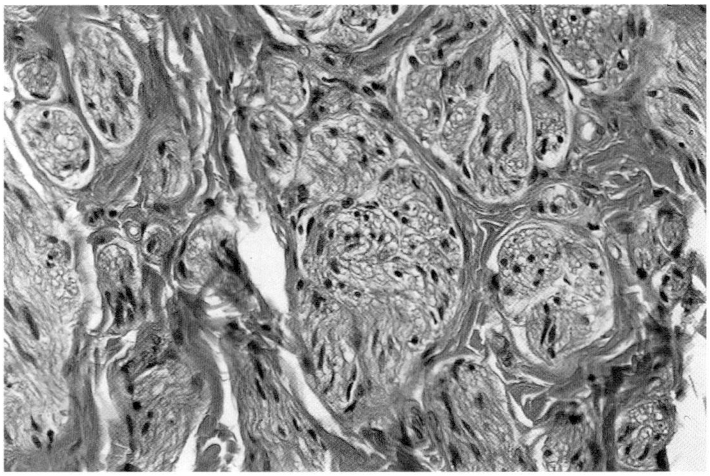

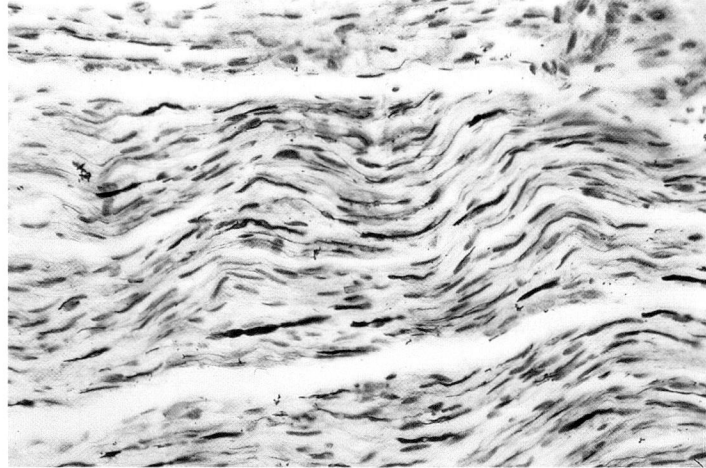

Fig. 37.1 **Traumatic neuroma** composed of nerve fascicles separated by thin septa of fibrous tissue. (H & E)

Fig. 37.2 **Traumatic neuroma.** Numerous axons are present. (Bodian preparation)

Rudimentary polydactyly

The term 'rudimentary polydactyly' is applied to a small nodular tumor which is found rarely near the base of the fifth finger, along its ulnar border.[15-17] The traditional view, that it is a variant of amputation neuroma at the site of a supernumerary sixth digit, presumed to have undergone spontaneous auto-amputation, has been challenged.[18] It has been suggested that such lesions are neural malformations unrelated to a supernumerary digit.[18] A lesion with similar histology has been reported on the penis.[18]

Histopathology

There are numerous bundles of nerve fibers embedded in connective tissue in the upper dermis, and in dermal papillae (Fig. 37.3). Many oval corpuscles, resembling small Meissner corpuscles, are also present. This latter feature, together with the indefinite outline and the position in the upper dermis, all differ from the usual traumatic neuroma.[16,19] This supports the view that the traditional explanation for these lesions is incorrect.[18]

Electron microscopy

There are normal Merkel cells along the basal layer of the epidermis, in addition to the nerve fibers and encapsulated corpuscles.[16]

Solitary circumscribed neuroma

Solitary circumscribed neuromas, also described as 'palisaded and encapsulated neuromas',[10] are uncommon, slow-growing painless nodules found usually on the face of middle-aged individuals.[20,21] An extremely rare site of involvement is the glans penis.[22] They average 0.5 cm in diameter. A patient with multiple cutaneous neuromas, but no other abnormality, has been reported.[23] Their morphological resemblance of solitary neuromas to traumatic neuromas has led to the suggestion that they represent a regenerative lesion in response to minor trauma to the site.[13,24]

Histopathology[10]

Solitary circumscribed neuroma usually presents as a single nodule confined to the dermis (Fig. 37.4). A multinodular or plexiform growth pattern is uncommon.[25] The neuroma is composed of well-developed fascicles separated by a loose matrix resembling the endoneurium of normal nerve (Fig. 37.5). Rarely, cells with an epithelioid appearance are present.[26] A thin perineural connective tissue capsule often surrounds the tumor, but there is no fibrous tissue sheath around fascicles, as seen in a traumatic neuroma.[12] The perineurial cells in the capsule contain epithelial membrane antigen.[20] The fascicles contain axons, and many are also myelinated;[27] they stain for S100 protein.[28,29] Kossard and colleagues have presented evidence challenging the concept that these tumors always contain axons.[30] They found that some tumors lacked a significant axonal content, thus merging with the features of a schwannoma.[30]

The superficial part of a solitary neuroma is sometimes more loosely arranged, with a myxomatoid stroma, resembling a neurofibroma.[10] Prominent stromal vascularity has been reported.[31] Occasionally a nerve can be traced into the lesion from below.

The overlying epidermis is usually normal or attenuated, but there is one report of overlying pseudoepitheliomatous hyperplasia.[32]

Neuromas and the multiple endocrine neoplasia syndrome

Multiple mucosal neuromas may be the first manifestation[33,34] of the multiple endocrine neoplasia syndrome (type 2b), a rare autosomal dominant condition which also includes medullary carcinoma of the thyroid, pheochromocytoma

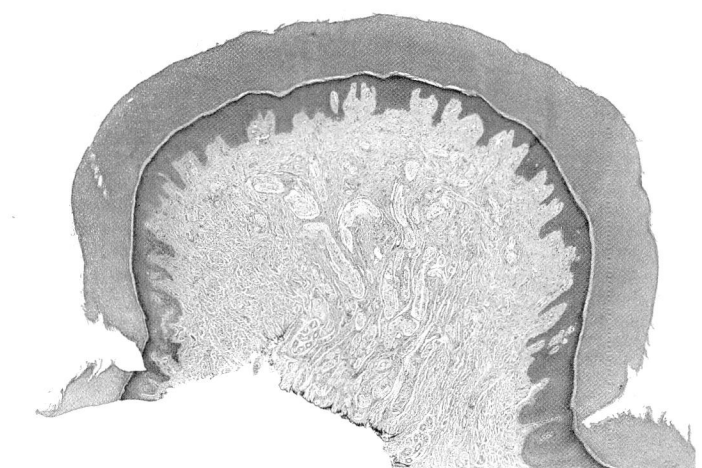

A

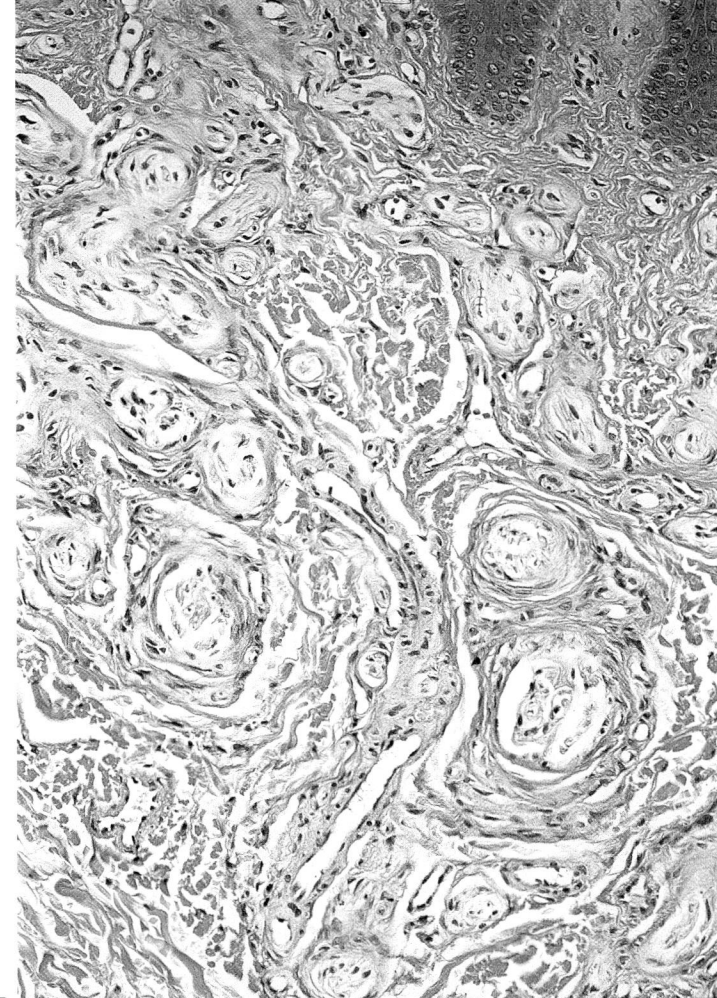

B

Fig. 37.3 **(A) Rudimentary polydactyly. (B)** There are many small nerves and some Meissner corpuscles in the upper dermis. (H & E)

and somatic abnormalities.[35-39] Mucosal neuromas have been reported without any other systemic features of the syndrome.[40]

Histopathology

Two different patterns may be seen.[10] The usual mucosal neuromas resemble solitary neuromas with haphazardly arranged bundles of Schwann cell fascicles.

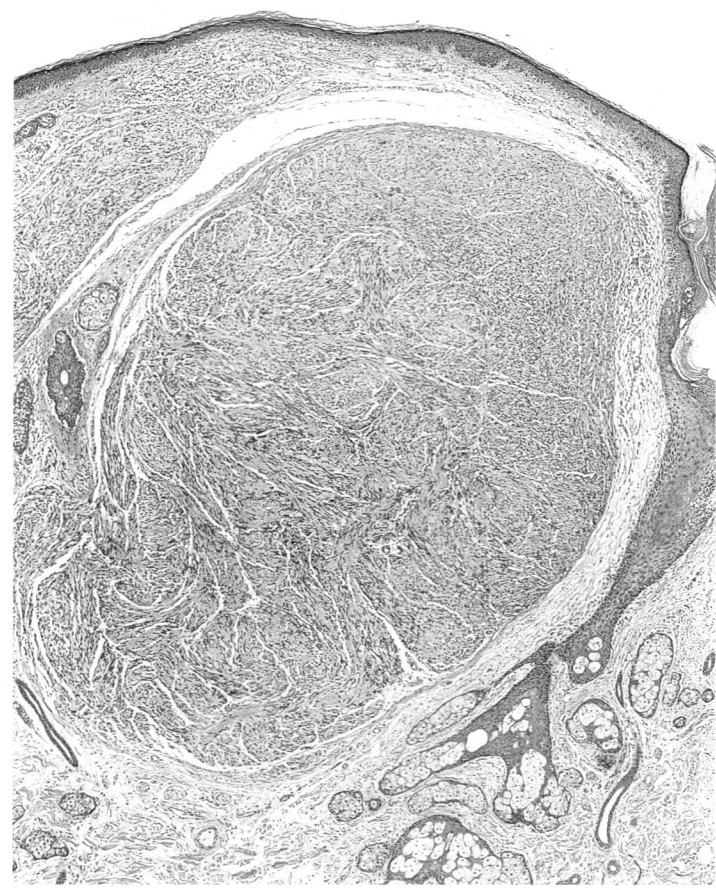

Fig. 37.4 **Solitary neuroma.** A circumscribed dermal tumor is present. (H & E)

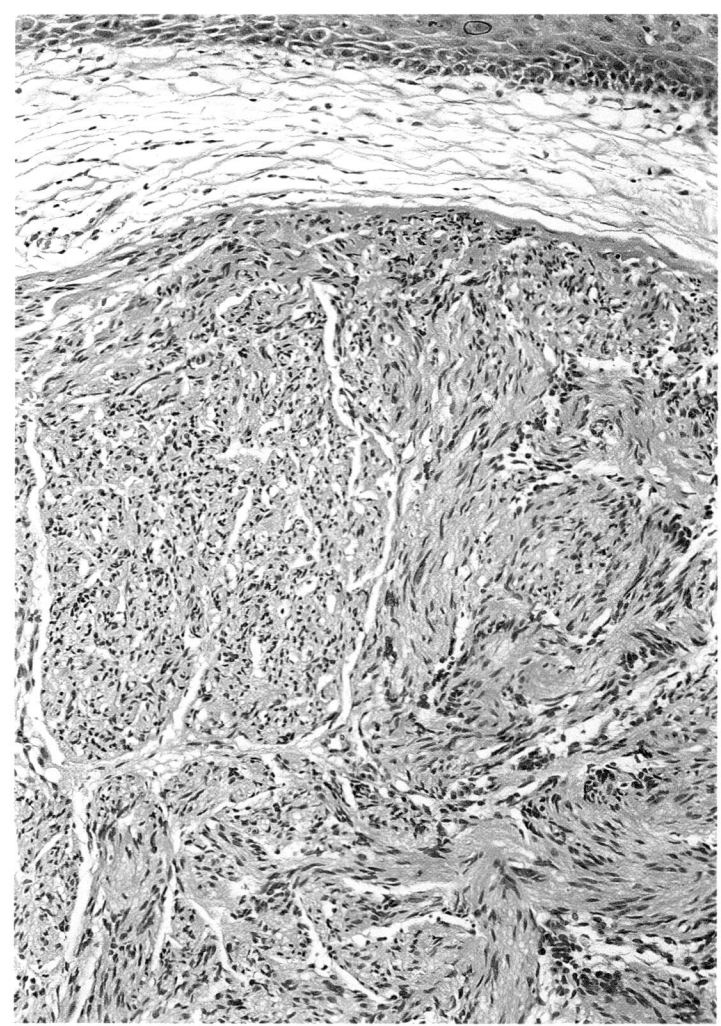

Fig. 37.5 **Solitary neuroma** composed of nerve fascicles with no intervening collagen. (H & E)

In the other pattern there are tortuous hyperplastic nerves with a thickened perineurium.[10]

Hypertrophy of small nerves in the dermis ('**dermal hyperneury**') has also been noted in the clinically normal skin of patients with this syndrome.[41] Nerve hypertrophy has been reported in a patient with striated pigmentation and a marfanoid habitus, a possible forme fruste of this syndrome, but without the endocrine tumors.[42] Rarely, it may follow chronic irritation or rubbing of the skin (Fig. 37.6).[43]

Ganglioneuroma

Ganglioneuromas may be found in the skin in patients with neuroblastomas and mature cutaneous secondary deposits, and in von Recklinghausen's disease where ganglion cells have been entrapped by a neurofibroma.[44] Primary cutaneous ganglioneuromas are exceedingly rare.[45–47] Most cases develop after birth, but a congenital lesion has been reported.[48]

Histopathology

Ganglioneuromas consist of mature ganglion cells, which are usually inter-mixed with fascicles of spindle cells.[46] In one reported case the ganglion cells were separate from the neuromatous elements.[49] The term 'ganglion cell choristoma' has been used for rare cases with ganglion cells and no stromal

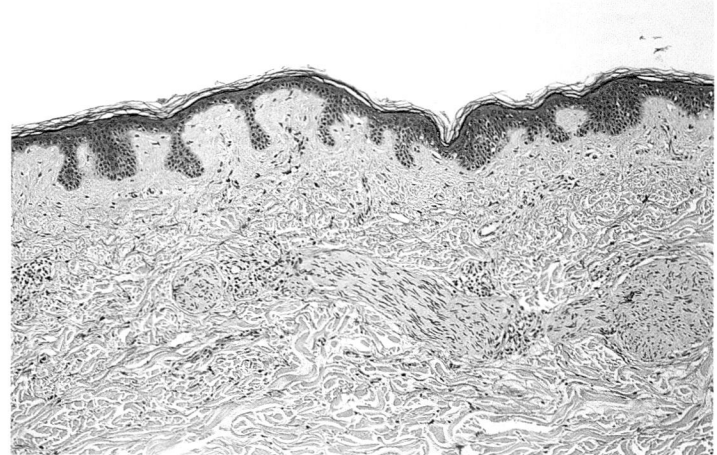

Fig. 37.6 **Dermal hyperneury.** A large nerve fiber is present just above the mid dermis. (H & E)

component.[50,51] At the other end of the spectrum is a case with abundant collagenous stroma containing scattered spindle and ganglion cells – a desmoplastic ganglioneuroma.[52]

The fusiform cells are strongly positive for S100 protein, but not the ganglion cells.[53]

EPITHELIAL SHEATH NEUROMA

Four cases of an unusual tumor, characterized by a proliferation of enlarged nerve fibers in the upper dermis ensheathed by squamous epithelium, have recently been reported.[54] The nerve fibers were much larger than normal for the dermis, and the perineural squamous epithelium was mature with focal cornification.[55] These structures were surrounded by delicate fibroplasia and a mild inflammatory cell infiltrate of lymphocytes with a few plasma cells.[56]

As expected, the nerves stained for a variety of neural markers, including S100 protein, and the epithelial sheaths for cytokeratins.[54] This entity differs from perineural invasion by the increased number and size of nerve fibers and by the lack of cytological atypia of the ensheathing cells.[57]

Reexcision perineural invasion refers to the presence of mature squamous epithelium in the perineural spaces of normal cutaneous nerves in reexcision specimens. It was originally described in the reexcision specimens of melanocytic lesions, but it has also been noted in reexcision specimens of other cutaneous tumors, when its distinction from perineural invasion can be more difficult. The perineural epithelium, however, is mature. The origin of the epithelium is uncertain as no connection can be demonstrated with surface or adnexal epithelium.[58] It may result from implantation during the initial procedure.

PERINEURIOMA

Perineurioma (storiform perineurial fibroma) is a rare tumor composed exclusively of perineurial cells which develops in the dermis, subcutis or deep soft tissue.[53] Unfortunately, this term was used in the past for localized hypertrophic neuropathy ('dermal hyperneury', see above), with which it has no relationship at all.[59,60]

The *sclerosing perineurioma* is a distinctive variant with a predilection for the fingers and palms of young adults.[61,62] This variant has been associated with a cryptic deletion of the *NF2* gene on chromosome 22.[62] This supports other evidence linking other types of perineurioma to this chromosome.[63]

Histopathology

The neoplasms are circumscribed non-encapsulated lesions composed of spindle cells with elongated, bipolar cytoplasmic processes.[59] On low power they usually resemble neurofibromas, with fascicles or individual cells oriented either parallel to each other or forming small concentric collections (Fig. 37.7).[53] These concentric whorls ('onion bulbs') are an important clue to the diagnosis.[64] Variants with granular cells and others with a plexiform or reticular pattern have been reported.[65–67] The stroma is fibromyxoid in type; rarely, it contains calcospherites.[60] Uncommonly, there is a fibrous or sclerotic stroma.[68]

The cases described by Mentzel and colleagues were more cellular lesions with a mixed lamellar and whorled pattern, sometimes with a marked storiform pattern. Focal stromal hyalinization and small aggregates of foam cells were present in some of their cases.[59] Such cases can be misdiagnosed as epithelioid histiocytomas.[69]

Most of the tumor cells stain for EMA and vimentin. Focal positivity for factor XIIIa is often present.[69] They do not stain for S100 protein, CD34, chromogranin or neuron-specific enolase.[59,60] In the variant with granular cells (see above), however, these cells expressed S100 protein but not epithelial membrane antigen (EMA), supporting their Schwann cell origin.[65]

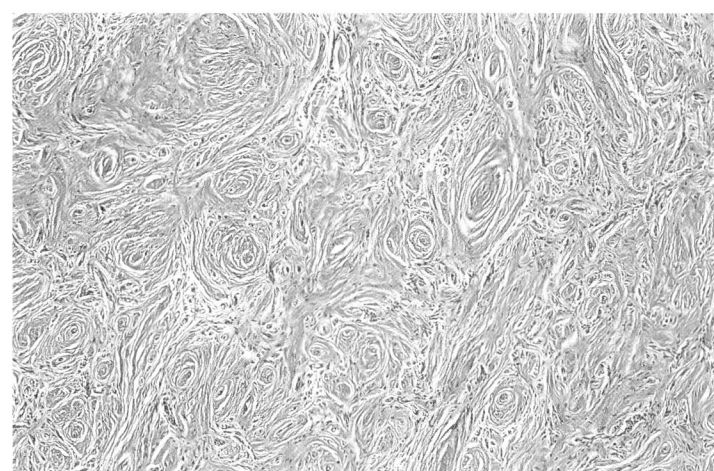

Fig. 37.7 **Perineurioma.** This is a paucicellular fibrous variant. Typical 'onion bulb' structures can be seen. (H & E)

The *sclerosing perineurioma* is composed of abundant dense collagen and variable numbers of small, epithelioid and spindled cells exhibiting corded, trabecular and whorled (onion skin) patterns.[61] This tumor may be confused with the fibroma of tendon sheath, the sclerotic fibroma of Cowden's disease (see p. 922) and the recently described pacinian collagenoma (see p. 922).[70] The cells stain for EMA and vimentin and often muscle-specific actin as well.[61] The *fibrous perineurioma* is probably a less dense, more cellular and better vascularized variant of the sclerosing perineurioma.[68]

SCHWANNOMA (NEURILEMMOMA)

Cutaneous schwannomas (neurilemmomas) are uncommon, slow-growing, usually solitary tumors with a propensity for the limbs of adults.[12] Pain, tenderness and paresthesiae may be present in up to one-third of lesions.[71–74] They measure 2–4 cm in diameter.[12] Multiple tumors are uncommon and can occur in several clinical settings: as multiple, localized (agminate) tumors;[75] in association with neurofibromas in von Recklinghausen's disease;[76] or as the syndrome of schwannomatosis (neurilemmomatosis), in which widespread subcutaneous and intradermal tumors are often associated with tumors of internal organs.[77–80] This latter syndrome is non-hereditary and not associated with café-au-lait spots or neurofibromas. It has been reported mainly from Japan.[77,81] A study suggesting that the genes for neurilemmomatosis and neurofibromatosis 2 (NF-2) are identical[82] and part of the same clinical disease has been disputed.[80,83]

Schwannomas also occur in the deep soft tissues, retroperitoneum, mediastinum and tongue,[84] and on the vestibulocochlear nerve. Local recurrence and malignant transformation are exceedingly rare.[85,86] The tumors are of Schwann cell origin.[2,87]

The tumor is gray-white in color, encapsulated, with a smooth, glistening appearance.[88] Cystic change is sometimes present, particularly in the larger, deeper tumors.

Histopathology[87]

Schwannomas are circumscribed encapsulated tumors, usually confined to the subcutis. The nerve of origin may sometimes be seen along one border (Fig. 37.8). The agminate tumors and some of those in schwannomatosis are often situated in the dermis.[75] Multiple small tumor nodules may be present in these forms, as well as hypertrophied peripheral nerves.[75,77] The term 'plexiform schwannoma' has been applied to this type (Fig. 37.9).[89–91]

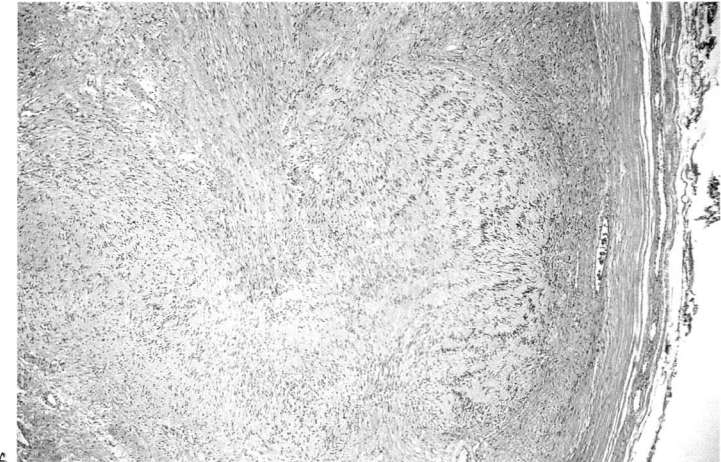

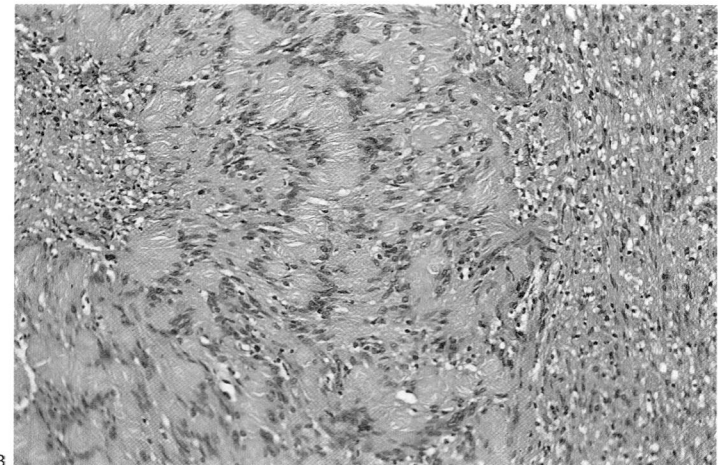

Fig. 37.8 **(A) Schwannoma. (B)** There are Verocay bodies in the interlacing bundles of spindle-shaped cells (Antoni A tissue). (H & E)

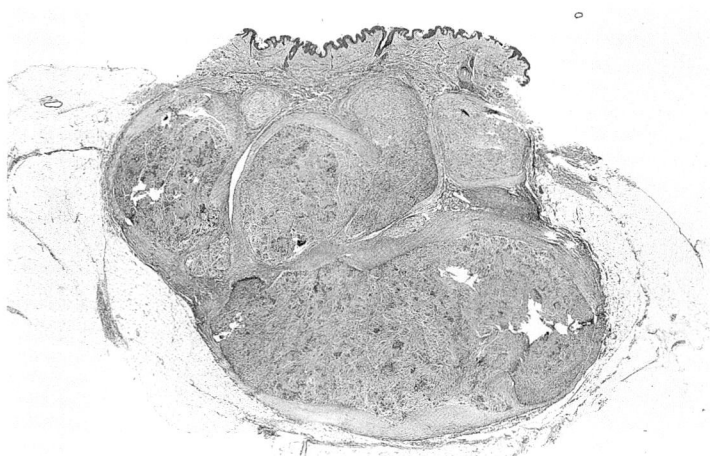

Fig. 37.9 **Plexiform schwannoma.** The tumor bulges into the subcutis. There are multiple nodules. (H & E)

Schwannomas are characteristically composed of two tissue types.[87] In the so-called 'Antoni A' areas there are spindle-shaped Schwann cells arranged in interlacing fascicles. The cells have indistinct cytoplasmic borders. The nuclei may be aligned in rows or palisades, between which the cell processes are fused into eosinophilic masses forming Verocay bodies. A variant in which the Verocay bodies form 75–100% of the tumor has been described.[52] No axons are present.[10] Antoni B tissue consists of a loose meshwork of gelatinous and microcystic tissue with widely separated Schwann cells. Lipid-laden macrophages, dilated blood vessels with thick hyaline walls, old and recent hemorrhage, lipofuscin and sometimes calcified hyaline areas may also be present in Antoni B areas.[2,87,93] 'Collagenous spherulosis' (radiating eosinophilic collagen fibers) has been reported in one case.[94] Mast cells and non-specific cholinesterase may be demonstrated.[12] Merkel cells are increased in the epidermis overlying schwannomas.[95]

Immunoperoxidase methods demonstrate S100 protein,[75] vimentin[96] and myelin basic protein[97] in the tumor cells. Glial fibrillary acidic protein (GFAP) is present in a small number of cases.[96,98] Epithelial membrane antigen is found in the perineurial cells in the capsule of schwannomas, as in that of solitary neuromas (see above).[92,99]

A cellular variant *(cellular schwannoma)*, mostly found in the deeper tissues, has been described.[100,101] There are compact spindle-shaped cells with mitoses and some storiform areas, and a near absence of Verocay bodies and Antoni B tissue.[100] Rare variants with multiple glandular elements,[102] with pseudoglandular structures,[103] and with sweat duct differentiation[104] have been reported.

A *neuroblastoma-like variant*, with large rosette-like structures and fibrillary collagenous centers, has been noted.[105] The presence of intervening Antoni B areas and an absence of necrosis or mitoses assist in making a diagnosis. The cells express S100 protein.

The *epithelioid schwannoma* is an extremely rare variant composed largely of epithelioid cells, in which there is a lack of mitotic activity.[106–108] Features of classic schwannoma are usually present in some areas of the tumor.[107] There is a thin capsule containing EMA-positive cells. Type IV collagen encircles individual cells within the tumor.[106] The cells stain for S100 protein but not HMB-45.

Another type of schwannoma is the *psammomatous melanotic schwannoma*, which contains melanin and scattered psammoma bodies (see below).

The term *'congenital neural hamartoma (fascicular schwannoma)'* has been used for an unencapsulated dermal tumor composed of fascicles of Schwann cells with frequent Verocay body-like structures.[109] Unlike cutaneous neuromas, there are no axons present.

Electron microscopy

There are aggregates of mature Schwann cells with thin, complexly entangled cytoplasmic processes, but only rare cell junctions.[2,110] One report suggested that the Antoni B areas showed features of degeneration,[111] but this finding has not been confirmed by others.[14]

PSAMMOMATOUS MELANOTIC SCHWANNOMA

The rare psammomatous melanotic schwannoma is an unusual component of Carney's complex (myxomas, spotty pigmentation and endocrinopathy).[112,113] The most common locations are the posterior spinal nerve roots, gastrointestinal tract, bone and soft tissue;[114] the skin is an uncommon site.[115] Multiple lesions may be present.[112]

Histopathology

This tumor is usually well circumscribed but only partly encapsulated. There is a mixture of polygonal and fusiform cells, many of which are heavily pigmented melanocytes.[53] Psammoma bodies are present in varying numbers.

Sometimes they coalesce to form larger, irregular masses. Adipocytes are often present.

The tumor cells stain positively for S100 protein, HMB-45, MART-1, synaptophysin and vimentin.[116]

A **malignant melanotic schwannoma** has been reported.[117] It did not occur in the setting of Carney's complex, nor were there psammoma bodies. Epithelioid cells with melanin were seen in the primary lesion, whereas spindle cells dominated in the recurrence.[117]

NEUROFIBROMA AND NEUROFIBROMATOSIS

Neurofibromas may occur as a solitary tumor or as multiple lesions in a segmental or widespread distribution, referred to as neurofibromatosis. The histopathology of the neurofibromas in these different clinical settings is similar and will be considered together.

Solitary neurofibromas are papular, nodular or pedunculated tumors with a predilection for the upper trunk.[12] They are soft and tend to invaginate on pressure (the 'buttonhole' sign). A subungual lesion has been reported.[118]

Neurofibromatosis, described by von Recklinghausen in 1882, is a clinically heterogeneous disorder with varied manifestations affecting the skin, soft tissues, blood vessels, and the peripheral and central nervous systems.[119,120] It is said to affect 80 000 individuals in the USA.[121] Riccardi has proposed eight clinical subtypes of neurofibromatosis (NF-1 to NF-8).[122] NF-1 is classic von Recklinghausen's disease, which accounts for 85–90% of all cases. NF-2 is associated with acoustic neuromas and sometimes other intracranial tumors. Cutaneous tumors, particularly schwannomas, are found in more than 50% of cases.[123] The inheritance of NF-2 is autosomal dominant, the gene being located on chromosome 22q12.2. NF-3 is a mixed form combining features of NF-1 and NF-2. NF-4 is a variant form with diffuse neurofibromas and café-au-lait pigmentation, but without many of the other clinical features that typify NF-1. NF-5 is the segmental form. NF-6 has prominent café-au-lait pigmentation as the sole manifestation. NF-7 is a late-onset type, and NF-8 is a miscellaneous group not categorized into the other subtypes.[122,124] Prenatal diagnosis of neurofibromatosis is not routinely available because of the large size of the gene. Furthermore, the high rate of new mutations (approximately 50% of all cases) means that the index of suspicion that a fetus may be affected is consequently lowered.[125]

Classic neurofibromatosis (NF-1)

Classic neurofibromatosis (NF-1) is the usual form of the disease. It is inherited as an autosomal dominant trait, although spontaneous mutations account for up to 50% of all NF-1 probands.[125] It is linked to the *NF1* gene located on the long arm of chromosome 17 (17q11.2).[126] Neurofibromin is the protein encoded by the gene, which appears to have a tumor-suppressor function. Café-au-lait pigmentation, which varies from small macular areas to large patches of pigmentation, is present in 99% of cases.[121] The pigmentation is present at birth or appears early in childhood before other stigmata of the disease. It may be found in other conditions, but the presence of six or more patches is said to be diagnostic of neurofibromatosis.[127] Axillary freckling is present in about 20% of patients.

The neurofibromas are multiple and sometimes disfiguring. They appear at about puberty, although late onset has been recorded.[128] Neurofibromas may develop for the first time in pregnancy; women who already have tumors may experience an increase in the size and number of the lesions during pregnancy.[129] Plexiform neurofibromas,[12] which were thought to be pathognomonic of neurofibromatosis, may rarely present as solitary lesions

without any features of neurofibromatosis.[130] They may present as large deep tumors or localized areas of deformity.[131] They are found in about 25% of cases.[127,132] Schwannomas are sometimes present as well.

Other clinical features of the classic form are pigmented hamartomas of the iris (Lisch nodules),[133,134] macrocephaly, mental retardation, kyphoscoliosis, bone hypertrophy, pseudoarthrosis and vascular lesions.[133,135–138] Somatic mutations may explain the variable expressivity of the *NF1* phenotype.[139] The classic form has been reported in a patient with tuberous sclerosis,[140] and in one with the McCune–Albright syndrome.[141] Elephantiasis neuromatosa, with localized gigantism or thick redundant folds of skin, is rare.[135] Neurofibromas, each with a halo of depigmentation, have been reported in one patient with presumptive mild neurofibromatosis.[142]

Malignant degeneration of neurofibromas occurs in 2–3% of patients,[127] although higher figures have been reported in some series.[132] In addition, various other sarcomas,[143] melanomas[132,144,145] and visceral carcinomas[132] have been reported, although the latter may not be increased in incidence.[146]

Segmental neurofibromatosis (NF-5)

The segmental variant (NF-5) is a heterogeneous group.[147–154] Café-au-lait pigmentation is present in some cases;[131,155–158] there are usually no other stigmata of neurofibromatosis (other than neurofibromas) and no family history.[159–162] This localized form may be due to mosaicism.[163] Variants of the segmental form include a localized,[164] a unilateral[147,160] and a bilateral[147,165,166] segmental form, a form associated with deep neural tumors,[167] and a rare hereditary form.[168] Over 100 cases of NF-5 have been reported.

Neurofibromatosis localized to the vulva can be classified with this group.[169]

Histopathology

Cutaneous neurofibromas are non-encapsulated, loosely textured tumors centered on the dermis.[12,170] There is often extension into the subcutis, sometimes in a diffuse infiltrative pattern.[170] An overlying grenz zone separates the lesion from the undersurface of the epidermis. The lesion is composed of delicate fascicles, usually only a single cell thick.[10] The cells have an oval or spindle-shaped nucleus and scant, indefinite cytoplasm (Fig. 37.10). There is sometimes nuclear pleomorphism, but mitoses are rare. The matrix is pale

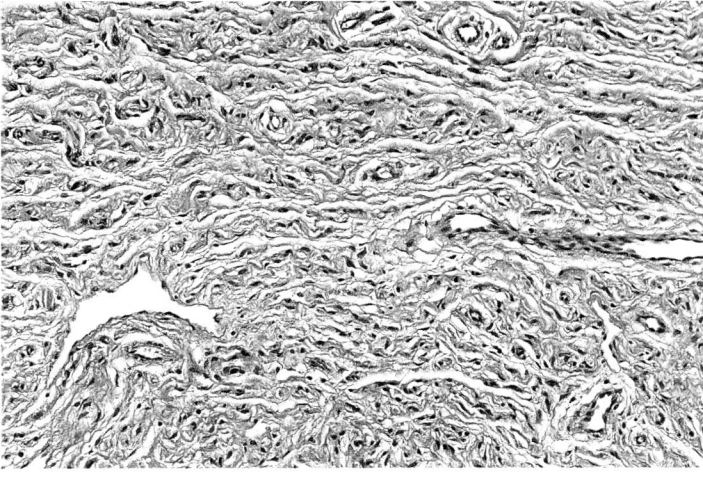

Fig. 37.10 **Neurofibroma** composed of thin fascicles of cells, each with a 'wavy', spindle-shaped nucleus. (H & E)

staining with delicate wavy collagen; rarely, the matrix is rich in mucin or is sclerosing or hyalinized.[170,171] Solitary neurofibromas are sometimes more compact than those in neurofibromatosis.[87] Blood vessels are increased in number in the stroma.[172] A Bodian stain will demonstrate some axonal material, but not in the 1:1 ratio with Schwann cells, as occurs in neuromas.[10] Mast cells,[173] non-specific cholinesterase,[162] S100 protein, myelin basic protein[97] and factor XIIIa[174,175] can be demonstrated by the appropriate techniques.

Various growth factors and their receptors are also present.[176] Neural cell adhesion molecule (NCAM – CD56) was present in one recent study in 100% of schwannomas and MPNSTs, in 86% of neurofibromas, 76% of neurotized nevi, but only 50% of desmoplastic/spindle cell melanomas.[177] The staining was less intense in the melanomas than in the neural tumors.[177]

Plexiform neurofibromas are a distinct variant in which there is irregular cylindrical or fusiform enlargement of a subcutaneous or deep nerve;[12] rarely, they arise in the dermis.[178] Numerous large nerve fascicles are embedded in a cellular matrix containing abundant mucin as well as collagen, fibroblasts and Schwann cells.[10] Initially, this proliferation of nerve fibers is confined within the epineurium of the involved nerve.[10] The massive soft tissue neurofibroma is highly specific for NF-1. It is worrisome because its size may mask the development of a malignant peripheral nerve sheath tumor.[179]

Other findings in neurofibromatosis are schwannomas (neurilemmomas), tumors with features of both neurofibroma and schwannoma (hybrid lesions),[180,181] and neurofibromas containing scattered, possibly entrapped, ganglion cells. Pilar dysplasia and folliculosebaceous proliferations have been reported overlying neurofibromas.[182,183] Vascular changes are rarely found. They include smooth muscle islands in the intima of vessels.[136] If random biopsies are taken from apparently normal skin in patients with NF-1, microscopic (occult) neurofibromas are sometimes found. Abundant S100-positive cells may also be found within the perifollicular fibrous tissue.[184,185] In elephantiasis neuromatosa there is a diffuse proliferation of Schwann cells and axons in the subcutis.[87] Islands of cartilage are present, rarely, in this tissue.[87] Glandular epithelial structures *(epithelioid neurofibroma)* have been reported in the stroma.[151,186]

In a recent review of the histopathological variants of neurofibroma, Megahed listed 10 variants:[170] classic, cellular, myxoid, hyalinized, epithelioid, plexiform, diffuse, pigmented, granular cell and pacinian. Some of these variants are regarded by others as discrete entities, whereas others represent morphological curiosities. An additional variant is the recently described *dendritic cell neurofibroma* with pseudorosettes.[187]

The rare *pigmented neurofibroma*, six cases of which were described by Bird and Willis in 1969,[188] had received scant attention until the recent report of 19 cases.[189] It is composed of whorled fibrillar ovoid structures resembling Wagner–Meissner bodies.[189,190] Melanin is present in macrophages and in some of the tumor cells, which stain for S100 protein, HMB-45 and melan-A. In the few cases tested, the cells also expressed CD34.[189]

The *cellular neurofibroma* can be difficult to distinguish from a malignant peripheral nerve sheath tumor (MPNST), particularly if atypia and low-grade mitotic activity are present. It has been suggested that ancillary studies (p53 expression, Ki-67 immunostaining and flow cytometry to assess DNA content) may be useful in confirming a benign diagnosis in these cases.[191] Further studies are needed to confirm these findings.[192]

Giant pigment granules (macromelanosomes) are often present in melanocytes and basal keratinocytes in the *café-au-lait spots* of neurofibromatosis.[193] The granules can just be seen with the light microscope. They are probably increased in older individuals.[194] Macromelanosomes are not present in all cases of neurofibromatosis; their presence is not pathognomonic, as they can also be found in several other conditions.[193,195]

Electron microscopy

Neurofibromas are composed of fusiform or stellate cells which are widely separated by individual collagen bundles and matrix.[14,110] They have usually been interpreted as Schwann cells,[14] but one report has claimed that the principal cell is the perineurial cell, although scattered Schwann cell–axon complexes are also present.[2]

PACINIOMA AND PACINIAN NEUROFIBROMA

The term 'pacinioma' has been applied to the rare finding of a hamartomatous overgrowth of mature Vater–Pacini corpuscles (Fig. 37.11).[196,197] Another term used is 'hyperplasia and hypertrophy of pacinian corpuscles'.[198] Bale has reported two such lesions in the sacral region associated with spina bifida occulta.[196] Pain and local tenderness are often present. Sometimes a history of prior trauma to the site can be elicited.[198]

Pacinian neurofibroma (pacinian neuroma) is a rare tumor of the digits, hands and feet. It is composed of round or ovoid corpuscles with multiple concentric lamellae.[199–201] They do not have the perfect structure of a Vater–Pacini corpuscle, but the resemblance is close. The report of a case with multiple hairy lesions on the buttock composed of rudimentary Vater–Pacini corpuscles suggests that the distinction between the hamartomatous pacinioma and the pacinian neurofibroma is artificial.[202] In another case, multiple tiny lesions were present on the ring finger in one patient, associated with marked vascular changes of the glomus type of arteriovenous anastomoses.[203] Some of the cases reported in the literature as pacinian neurofibromas would now be reclassified as nerve sheath myxomas.[204] These latter tumors have less resemblance to Vater–Pacini corpuscles and they contain more stromal mucin than true pacinian neurofibromas.

NEUROTHEKEOMA AND NERVE SHEATH MYXOMA

The terms 'neurothekeoma' and 'nerve sheath myxoma' refer to neural tumors at either end of a spectrum of histological appearances.[205–209] The term 'nerve sheath myxoma' was at one stage applied to all variants along the spectrum, but in recent years the term 'neurothekeoma' has been used for this spectrum. This has led to considerable confusion. Three variants of neurothekeoma are now recognized:[210]

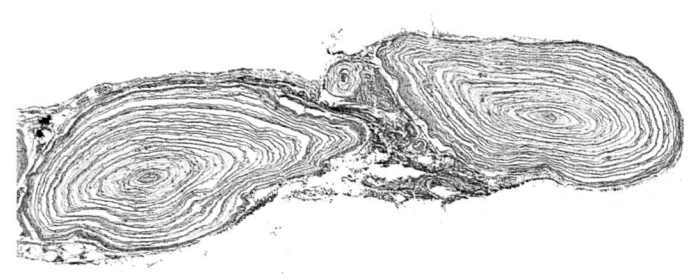

Fig. 37.11 **Pacinioma** composed of two enlarged Vater–Pacini corpuscles. (H & E)

- myxoid (formerly nerve sheath myxoma)
- intermediate (also called 'mixed')
- cellular.

In some reports, the term 'cellular' has been applied to a specific variant of neurothekeoma which has a more cellular apearance than the more usual neurothekeoma.

Neurothekeomas are found mostly on the face and upper extremities.[211,212] They are not associated with neurofibromatosis. There is a predilection for females. The cellular variant often occurs at a younger age than the myxoid type.[213] They present as asymptomatic, dome-shaped nodules that measure 0.5–3 cm or more in diameter.[214,215] The cellular variants are usually larger and firmer than the myxoid lesions. Rarely, they recur if inadequately excised.

The histogenesis is in doubt but there are features of schwannian, perineurial, fibroblastic and smooth muscle differentiation.[5,216–218]

Histopathology[207,211]

The *myxoid variant (nerve sheath myxoma)* is multilobulated and non-encapsulated (Fig. 37.12). It is centered on the reticular dermis but often extends into the superficial subcutis.[219] The lobules are composed of spindle-shaped, stellate and sometimes epithelioid cells arranged in a swirling, lamellar and often concentric pattern. The cellular elements are embedded in a myxoid stroma, which is usually abundant in those tumors in which stellate and bipolar cells predominate, but scanty in those with a predominantly epithelioid pattern.[211] Chondroitin-4 or chondroitin-6 sulfate is the principal heteroglycan present.[205,216] There is variable nuclear hyperchromatism and sometimes nuclear atypia. Mitoses are also variable. In one case, melanin was present in some tumor cells.[220]

The *cellular (neurothekeoma)* variant is composed of nests and fascicles, giving a multilobular appearance (Fig. 37.13). The intervening stroma may be hyalinized; less often there are myxoid foci. The nests of spindle cells sometimes have a concentric or whorling arrangement. There may be a poorly differentiated interface between the fascicles and the dermal collagen.[207,221] Some of the cells may have large hyperchromatic nuclei and some mitoses are common.[222] These atypical (worrisome) features do not appear to influence prognosis: surgical excision has been curative.[214] Extensive dystrophic calcification[223] and ossification have been reported.[224] A variant of neurothekeoma, with epithelioid as well as spindle-shaped cells and a cellular morphology, has been reported as a 'cellular neurothekeoma' (Fig. 37.14).[225] The authors speculated that it was an epithelioid variant of pilar leiomyoma, although only three were positive for smooth muscle actin.[225] More recently, Zelger and colleagues have speculated on the relationship of this tumor to dermatofibroma.[226] Although this is usually a dermal tumor, subcutaneous extension or localization may occur.[227]

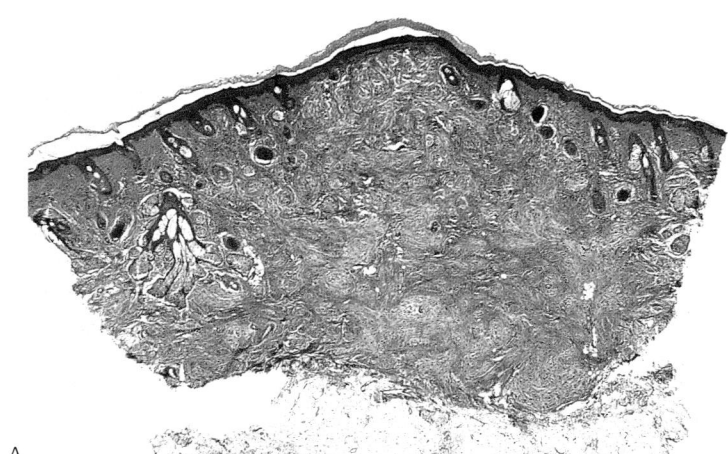

A

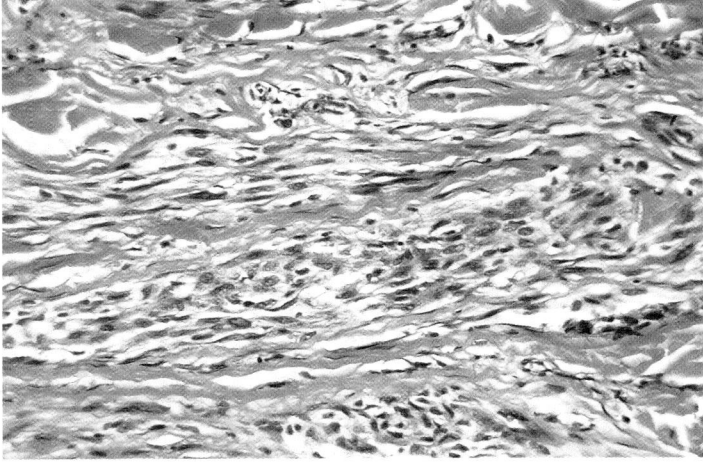

B

Fig. 37.12 **Nerve sheath myxoma.** Spindle-shaped cells are arranged in a swirling and concentric fashion. The stroma is myxoid. (H & E)

Fig. 37.13 **(A) Neurothekeoma. (B)** Tumor fascicles merge with the intervening dermal collagen. (H & E)

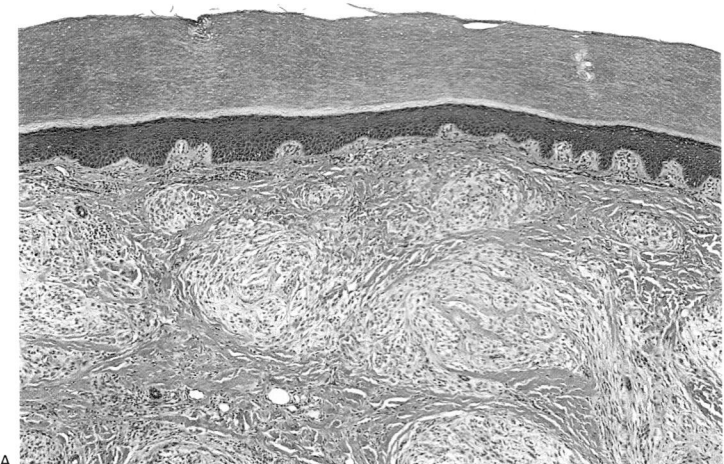

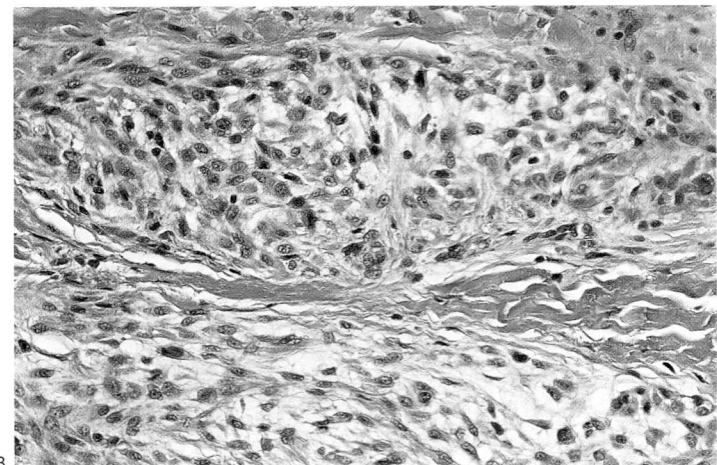

Fig. 37.14 (A) Neurothekeoma. (B) This is a further case with both epithelioid and spindle cells and some nuclear atypia. (H & E)

The immunohistochemical findings are variable.[228] In the myxoid type of neurothekeoma, the cells stain for vimentin and S100 protein and, sometimes, epithelial membrane antigen.[220,228–230] The cellular variant is negative for S100 protein and desmin, but sometimes positive for smooth muscle-specific actin and neuron-specific enolase.[228] It is frequently positive for vimentin and the melanoma-specific antigen NKI/C-3.[231] Focal positivity for factor XIIIa has also been noted.[232,233] A recently introduced marker, protein gene product 9.5 (PGP9.5), has been positive in 100% of cases, but only if the antigen retrieval method is used.[210]

Electron microscopy

There have been conflicting reports of the ultrastructural changes.[234–236] It appears that the myxoid type is composed mainly of Schwann cells, whereas the cellular (neurothekeoma) variant is composed of undifferentiated cells with partial features of Schwann cells, smooth muscle cells, myofibroblasts and fibroblasts, suggesting a divergent differentiation.[236]

PIGMENTED STORIFORM NEUROFIBROMA

The pigmented storiform neurofibroma, also known as the Bednar tumor, is now regarded as a variant of dermatofibrosarcoma protuberans that shows some neural differentiation. It is discussed further in Chapter 34, page 934.

GRANULAR CELL TUMOR

The granular cell tumor, previously known as granular cell myoblastoma, is an uncommon, benign tumor of disputed histogenesis. It may develop in many anatomical sites:[237–240] most are found in the oral cavity, especially the tongue, and in the skin and subcutaneous tissue.[237,241,242] There is a female predominance and a predilection for black races. Familial cases are rare.[243] The average age of presentation is 40–50 years, but the tumors may arise in children.[244,245] Most lesions are asymptomatic solitary skin-colored nodules, less than 2 cm in diameter. They are multiple in about 10% of cases.[244,246–252] Sometimes there are associated visceral granular cell tumors,[253] or defects in other organs.[250,251,254] Multiple granular cell tumors have been associated with neurofibromatosis.[255]

Morphologically similar tumors are found on the anterior alveolar ridge of neonates, almost exclusively in females.[256] Occasionally they are multiple,[256] or they may involve other areas of the oral cavity.[257] These gingival giant cell tumors (congenital epulis) may regress spontaneously, or following inadequate removal. They are about one-tenth as common as the acquired variant.

Malignant granular cell tumors are exceedingly rare, accounting for only 1–3% of all acquired granular cell tumors.[237,258] Very few have been reported in the skin.[259–266] They may metastasize to regional lymph nodes, or more widely.[243,261] Of interest is the report of a patient with neurofibromatosis in whom a malignant granular cell tumor developed.[267]

Some immunohistochemical studies have been interpreted as indicating an origin from a 'neural crest-derived peripheral nerve-related cell',[268] but most investigators still favor a Schwann cell origin.[240,269] Ultrastructural studies of gingival giant cell tumors of the newborn have suggested an origin from undifferentiated mesenchymal cells;[257,270] by analogy, a similar origin has been proposed for the acquired variant.[257] These theories are not mutually exclusive.[268,271]

Histopathology[237,238,272]

The tumors are non-encapsulated and composed of irregularly arranged sheets of large polyhedral cells with a small central hyperchromatic nucleus and abundant fine to coarsely granular eosinophilic cytoplasm (Fig. 37.15). Dermal tumors often extend into the upper subcutis. Cells infiltrate between collagen bundles and may displace them. They surround appendages, but may extend into the arrector pili muscle. Rarely, a plexiform or dermatofibroma-like pattern is present.[273–275] Cytoplasmic borders are not always distinct. The cytoplasmic granules are PAS positive and diastase resistant. They are also well seen with Movat's pentachrome technique.[272] The nuclei contain one or two nucleoli. Elastosis is common in the stroma of granular cell tumors.[276]

The overlying epithelium often shows prominent pseudoepitheliomatous hyperplasia, which may be misdiagnosed as squamous cell carcinoma if only a superficial biopsy is available for examination.[237] This epithelial response is usually not present in congenital gingival tumors,[257] and is absent in some cutaneous tumors, especially if multiple.[247]

Congenital gingival tumors have a more prominent vascular stroma, often with perivascular collections of lymphocytes and histiocytes.[270] The amount of stromal collagen increases as the lesion ages. Small nerve fibers are sometimes found in and around acquired granular cell tumors.[247]

The *polypoid granular cell tumors* of the skin described by LeBoit et al are thought to be from a different cell lineage from the usual granular cell tumor (Fig. 37.16).[277] The cells showed cytological atypia, numerous mitoses and a 'primitive' immunophenotype.[277]

Immunohistological studies have given conflicting results. Granular cell tumors usually contain S100 protein,[266,278–280] neuron-specific enolase,[268] PGP9.5[281] and the melanoma-associated antigen NKI/C-3.[268] Myelin basic

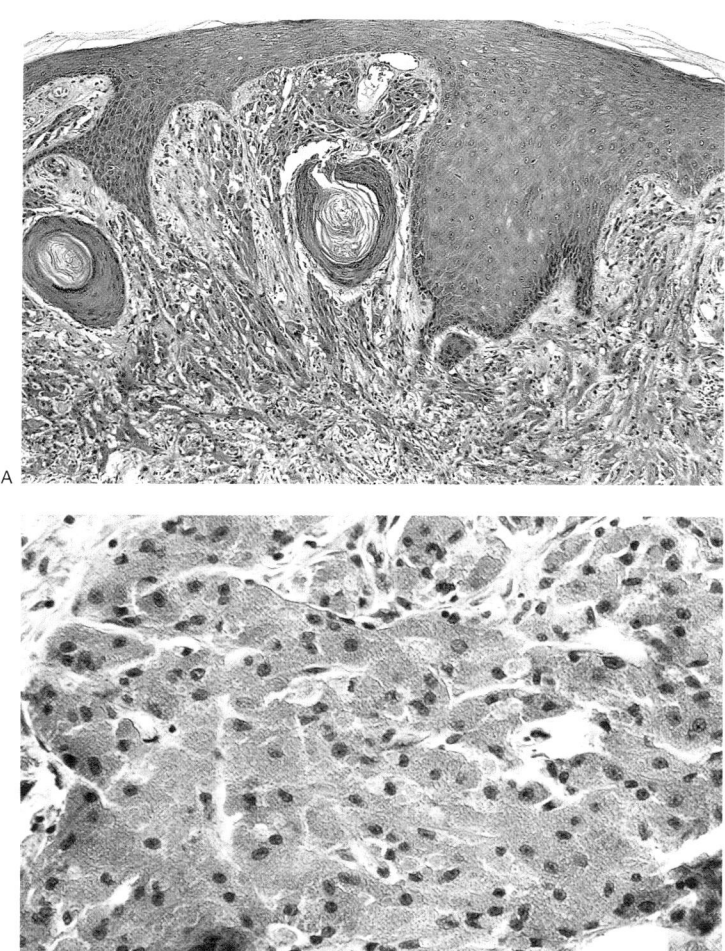

Fig. 37.15 **Granular cell tumor. (A)** The epidermal hyperplasia may overshadow the dermal granular cells. **(B)** The eosinophilic granular cytoplasm is characteristic. (H & E)

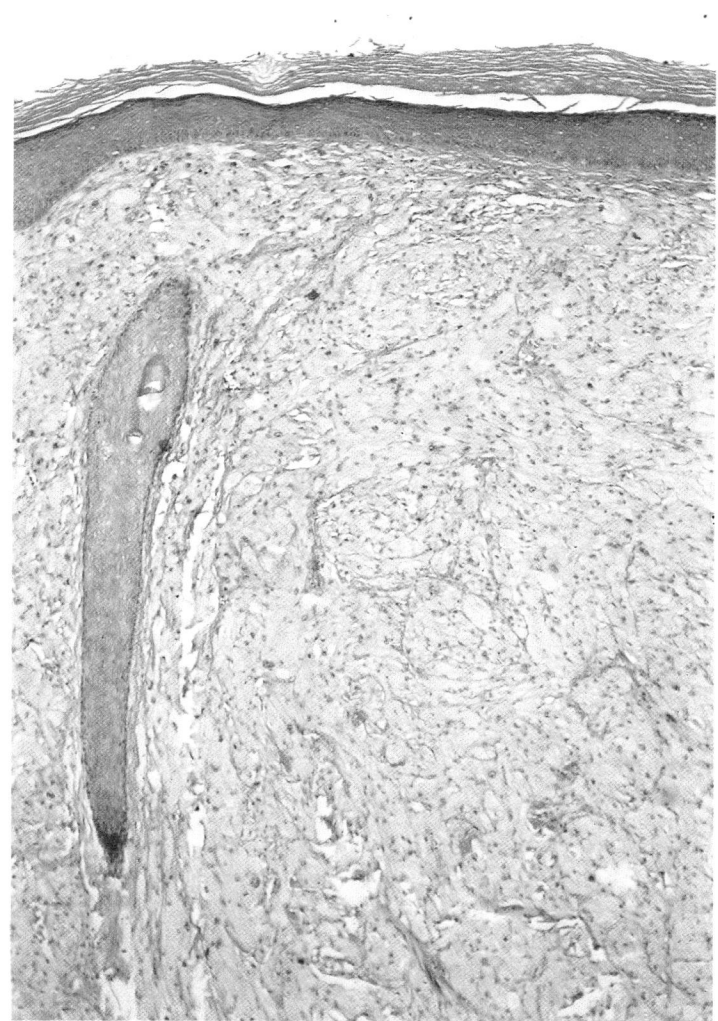

Fig. 37.16 **Polypoid granular cell tumor.** There is some cytological atypia and mitoses. (H & E)

protein has been present in some cases;[282] it was absent in all 25 cases in one series.[268] The cells are negative for myoglobin[280,283] and glial fibrillary acidic protein.[98] Some reports have suggested the presence of carcinoembryonic antigen (CEA),[283] but this appears to be a false positive result, due to a related antigen in the tumor cells.[284,285] The cells are also positive for esterase and acid phosphatase.[272]

There are no well-defined criteria for malignancy. Tumor size greater than 5 cm, vascular invasion, necrosis and rapid growth are important indicators of malignant behavior.[253,264] Mitoses, apoptotic cells and pleomorphic nuclei may also be present, but not necessarily so; they are invariably absent in benign variants.[265] Cell spindling and angiogenesis have been reported in malignant lesions.

The exact nosological position of the congenital lesion reported as **CD34-positive granular cell dendrocytosis** is currently unknown.[286] The patient had numerous papules and plaques on the face and extremities. The lesions were composed of S100-negative, CD34-positive dermal dendrocytes, with a granular morphology due to an abundance of phagolysosomes and an appearance resembling a granular cell tumor.[286]

Electron microscopy
The tumor cells are surrounded by a basal lamina.[253] The cytoplasm contains numerous granules of various sizes and shapes; the majority of these are

phagolysosomes.[240,283,287] Microfilaments and microtubules have been reported.[287] Angulate bodies may also be found in acquired tumors,[283] and sometimes these are also found in satellite fibroblasts.[288] Congenital tumors have immature mesenchymal cells as well as forms transitional between these and the granular cells.[257]

MALIGNANT PERIPHERAL NERVE SHEATH TUMOR

Malignant peripheral nerve sheath tumor (MPNST)[2] is the preferred designation for a tumor which has in the past been called neurosarcoma, neurogenic sarcoma, neurofibrosarcoma[289,290] and malignant schwannoma.[291–293] This latter tumor is not always included under this 'umbrella' term.[294] MPNST is a rare tumor, accounting for approximately 2% of all nerve sheath tumors.[295] Most cases are thought to arise by malignant transformation of a neurofibroma.[179] Only two forms of neurofibroma – the plexiform and massive soft tissue variant – are significant precursors of MPNST.[179] Although tumor is sometimes present in the dermis,[296,297] this usually represents extension of a growth that originated in the deeper soft tissues.[298]

A recently described variant is the perineurial malignant peripheral nerve sheath tumor derived from perineurial rather than Schwann cells. Only 4% of MPNSTs show perineurial cell differentiation.[299]

Neurofibromatosis is present in more than 50% of cases of malignant peripheral nerve sheath tumor.[300,301] There is a predilection for the deep soft tissues of the proximal extremities of young and middle-aged adults. The mean survival for patients with these tumors is 2–3 years.[302]

Histopathology

There is usually a spindle-cell growth pattern with cells arranged in tight wavy or interlacing bundles (Fig. 37.17).[303] There are sometimes densely cellular areas alternating with more loosely textured areas.[304] A rare plexiform variant has been reported.[305] The cellularity and number of mitoses determine the grading of the tumor.

Purely epithelioid variants have been reported (malignant epithelioid schwannoma).[306–311] There appears to be a tendency for MPNSTs arising in a benign schwannoma to show epithelioid morphology.[312]

Focal divergent differentiation, with the formation of foci of osteogenic sarcoma, chondrosarcoma, angiosarcoma,[313] rhabdomyosarcoma or an epithelial element, is present in about 15% of tumors.[314,315] The epithelial element is usually glandular in type.[186] The presence of rhabdomyosarcomatous elements can be confirmed by immunoperoxidase stains for myoglobin.[316] This variant is known as a 'triton tumor'.[311,316,317] It should not be confused with the rare neuromuscular hamartoma of infancy composed of nerve fibers admixed with well-differentiated skeletal muscle.[318]

In the past, the diagnosis of a malignant nerve sheath tumor was difficult, particularly in the absence of a clinical history of neurofibromatosis, and in those tumors in which no anatomical relationship to a nerve trunk could be demonstrated. The development of immunoperoxidase techniques has assisted considerably in making a specific diagnosis.[319] These tumors contain S100 protein, neuron-specific enolase, neurofilament protein and myelin basic protein, although sometimes this staining is weak.[4,290,293] Vimentin, AE1/AE3, and EMA may also be present.[98,320] Whereas the majority of monophasic synovial sarcomas stain for one or both of cytokeratins 7 and 19, most MPNSTs do not express these cytokeratin subsets.[320]

The *perineurial variant* is composed of spindle cells with long processes disposed in whorls or storiform patterns. Necrosis is sometimes present. Their characteristic immunohistochemical profile is EMA positive, S100 negative.[299]

Electron microscopy

Electron microscopy shows undifferentiated cells with some features of Schwann and perineurial cells.[2] Fibroblastic cells have also been identified.[2,321]

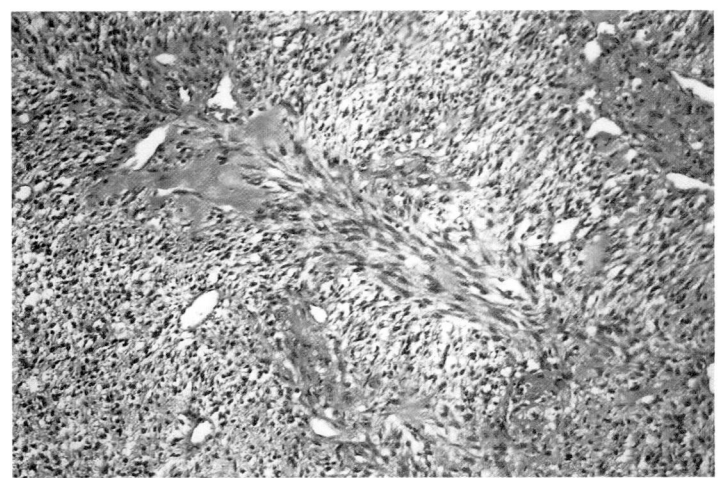

Fig. 37.17 **Malignant nerve sheath tumor.** This cellular tumor is composed of interlacing bundles of spindle-shaped cells. Several mitoses are present. (H & E)

HERNIATIONS AND ECTOPIAS

NASAL GLIOMA AND NEURAL HETEROTOPIAS

The unsatisfactory term 'nasal glioma' refers to the presence of heterotopic neural tissue, predominantly glial in nature, at or near the root of the nose. Approximately 60% of these lesions are confined to the subcutaneous tissue, whereas 30% are intranasal in location.[322–324] The remainder have both external and intranasal components. In approximately 20% of cases intracranial connections are present, sometimes with an associated bony defect in the nasofrontal region,[325,326] but there is no fluid-filled space connecting with the ventricular system, as in an encephalocele.[322,327] Nasal gliomas present at birth, or in early infancy, as a red to blue, firm smooth tumor near the bridge of the nose. Those confined to the intranasal region may present later with nasal obstruction or epistaxis, or as a nasal polyp.

Rarely, similar tissue has been reported in the scalp,[328] either as a midline parietal nodule[329] or as multiple subcutaneous nodules in the scalp.[330] A ring of dark long hair encircling a congenital scalp lesion (the 'hair collar sign') is sometimes present as a marker of an associated encephalocele or heterotopic brain tissue. Hair anomalies may also overlie sequestrated meningoceles.[331] Heterotopic glial tissue has been reported in the subcutaneous tissues overlying T12. There was no associated spinal defect.[332] The term 'heterotopic neural tissue' is the preferred collective term for these lesions, and for nasal gliomas.[329] They are hamartomas, resulting from sequestration of neural tissue early in embryogenesis.[333]

The meningeal–cutaneous relationships in anencephaly have recently been reviewed.[334] This study is mentioned for completeness.

Histopathology[333,335]

There are islands of neural and fibrovascular tissue in the subcutis. The neural tissue is composed of astrocytes enmeshed in a neurofibrillary stroma (Fig. 37.18). Multinucleate astrocytes are not uncommon, but neurons are usually inconspicuous and few in number. They were the predominant element in one case.[336] The nodules are interlaced with vascular fibrous septa. A markedly sclerosed stroma may be seen in older lesions.[337] Calcification and sweat duct hyperplasia are two other rare associations.[338]

Heterotopic neural islands occurring on the scalp may be surrounded by a capsule that structurally resembles the leptomeninges.[329,339] Clusters of ependymal cells with central vascular channels and myxoid stroma (myxopapillary ependymal rests) are found rarely in the sacrococcygeal region.[340]

Immunoperoxidase staining demonstrates glial fibrillary acid protein (GFAP) and S100 protein in the glial tissue.[337]

CUTANEOUS MENINGIOMA

Meningiomas (cutaneous meningothelial tumors, cutaneous heterotopic meningeal nodules) are found only rarely in extracranial sites, including the skin.[341–346] The scalp, forehead and paravertebral areas are most commonly involved. Three distinct clinicopathological groups have been recognized.[344] Type I lesions arise in the subcutaneous tissue of the scalp, forehead and paravertebral region. They are usually present at birth, and are thought to be derived from ectopic arachnoid cells misplaced during embryogenesis. A familial occurrence has been reported.[347] This group includes lesions with only scattered meningothelial cells in a collagenous nodule (acellic meningeal hamartoma), lesions with a rudimentary cystic channel (rudimentary

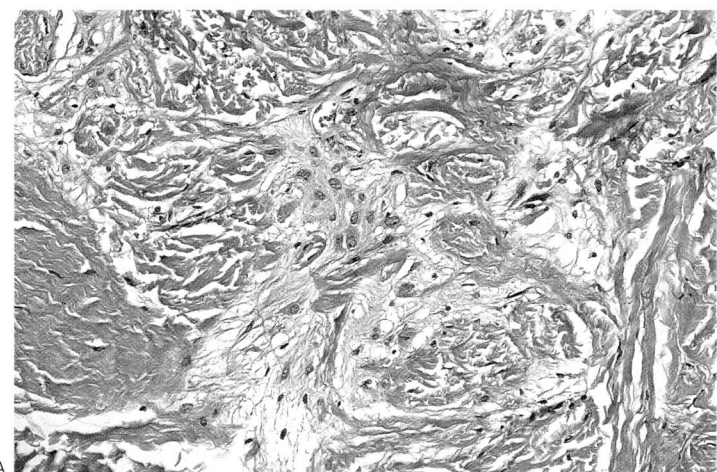

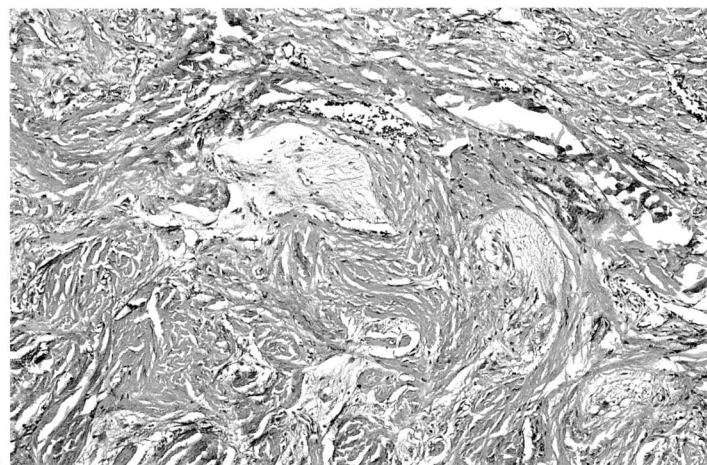

Fig. 37.18 **Heterotopic glial tissue** admixed with collagen bundles. **(A)** This lesion was removed from the occipital region (H & E). **(B)** The pale pink glial fibers contrast with the green stromal collagen. (Masson trichrome)

meningocele variant) and those with well-circumscribed nodules resembling intracranial meningiomas.[327,331,348–353] Type II lesions are found in adults around sensory organs of the head (periorbital, aural and paranasal) and along the course of cranial and spinal nerves. They are thought to be derived from nests of arachnoid cells which are found along the course of these nerves after they penetrate the dura. Type III lesions represent the direct cutaneous extension or distant metastasis of an intracranial tumor.[344,354,355]

Primary cutaneous meningioma has been reported in association with von Recklinghausen's disease.[356] Another rare presentation is as an aural polyp.[357]

Histopathology[344]

Whereas type I lesions are usually confined to the subcutis, type II and III tumors may also involve the dermis. Some type I lesions consist merely of irregular strands of meningothelial cells set in a collagenous stroma,[358] whereas others resemble type II and III tumors in being circumscribed and more cellular, akin to intracranial meningiomas and including spindle-cell areas and meningothelial whorls. Psammoma bodies are variable in number. Inflammatory cells may be present in type II and III lesions.

When meningoceles and related malformations are studied a range of tissue types can be identified, including dura-like tissue, blood vessels, lipoma formation, hypertrophy of the arrector pili muscle, nerve fibers, meningothelial cells and neural tissue.[327]

Immunoperoxidase studies for S100, vimentin and epithelial membrane antigen have been positive.[341,342,359] Ultrastructural studies have shown a similar appearance to intracranial meningiomas.[343,344]

Barr and colleagues have described three cases of an unusual cutaneous tumor with a superficial resemblance to a meningioma or the canine hemangiopericytoma.[360] The tumors had a whorled configuration of spindle cells, some concentrically arranged around blood vessels. Only vimentin positivity was present.

NEUROENDOCRINE CARCINOMAS

MERKEL CELL (NEUROENDOCRINE) CARCINOMA

In 1972, Toker reported five cases of this tumor as trabecular carcinoma.[361] Some years later, on the basis of the electron microscopic findings of neurosecretory granules, Tang and Toker suggested that the tumor had a Merkel cell origin.[362] Because a Merkel cell origin is not established beyond doubt,[363] and because a trabecular pattern is not usually a dominant feature, the designation 'neuroendocrine carcinoma' is favored by some.[364,365] Another term used is 'primary small-cell carcinoma of the skin'.[366] Most reports in the literature still use the term 'Merkel cell carcinoma'.

This tumor usually arises on the sun-exposed skin of elderly patients, particularly on the head and neck and extremities.[367,368] Perianal involvement has been recorded.[369] It occurs, rarely, in children.[370] Rare associations include chronic lymphocytic leukemia,[371,372] chronic arsenicism,[373,374] therapeutic immunosuppression[375–377] and ectodermal dysplasia.[378,379] There is a relatively high incidence of second neoplasms in patients with Merkel cell carcinoma.[380] There was a slight female preponderance in one series and a predilection for males in others.[381,382] The tumors are often indistinguishable from other skin cancers. They may have a reddish, nodular appearance which sometimes resembles an angiosarcoma or granulation tissue.[383,384] They average 2 cm in diameter, although 'giant' and small variants have been recorded.[385,386]

Local recurrences occur in about one-third of cases. The tumor spreads to the regional lymph nodes in up to 75% of cases,[367,387,388] and distant metastasis with eventual death occurs in one-third or more.[389] Spontaneous regression of the tumor has been reported.[390–394] In a large series reported from the Memorial Sloan Kettering Cancer Center, the overall 5-year disease-specific survival rate was 75%.[395] It is generally agreed that the primary tumor should be treated aggressively.[396,397] Chemotherapy is usually restricted to those with metastatic or locally advanced disease.[398] A high incidence of toxic death due to chemotherapy has been reported in the literature.[399] Merkel cell carcinoma involving lymph nodes and lacking an identifiable primary site may result from regression of a cutaneous primary, although an origin in lymph nodes may be the explanation in other cases.[400]

Ectopic peptide production is not uncommon (see below),[401] but the levels are not high enough to produce a clinical endocrinopathy.[402] Paraneoplastic syndromes are rare.[403]

Now that tumor cell lines have been established in the laboratory, it is hoped that further studies may give some insight into the origin of this enigmatic tumor.[404]

Histopathology[367,405]

The tumor is composed of small, round to oval cells of uniform size with a vesicular nucleus and multiple small nucleoli (Fig. 37.19). Mitoses and apoptotic bodies are usually numerous.[406] The cytoplasm is scanty and amphophilic and

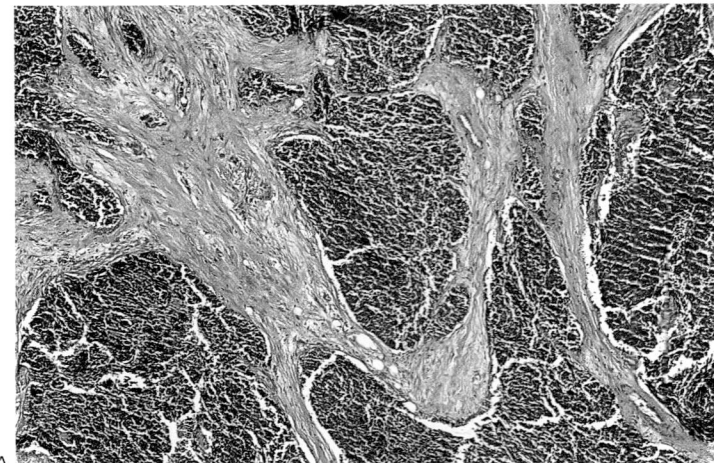

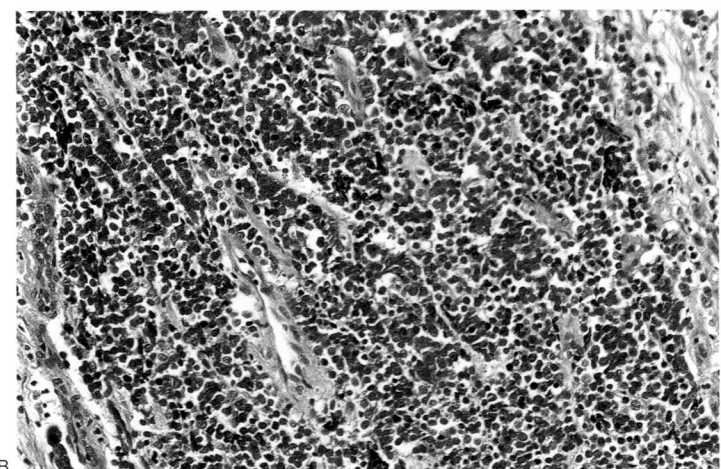

Fig. 37.19 **(A)** Merkel cell carcinoma. **(B)** The cells are small, with indistinct cytoplasmic borders and a hyperchromatic nucleus. (H & E)

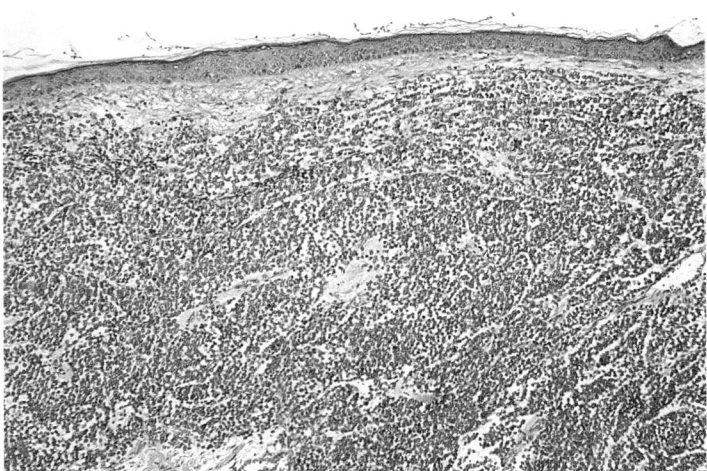

Fig. 37.20 **Merkel cell carcinoma.** Sheets of small cells with hyperchromatic nuclei extend throughout the dermis. (H & E)

the cell borders are vaguely defined. A few tumors have scattered areas with spindle-shaped nuclei. The cells are present as sheets and solid nests, infiltrating the entire dermis and sometimes extending into the subcutis (Fig. 37.20). Some authors have attempted to define three distinct patterns of histological differentiation: trabecular, small cell, and intermediate. Overlap features are common and the trabecular pattern may be limited to the peripheral areas of the tumor.[407] Pseudorosettes are quite uncommon.[408] There is a dissociation of tumor cells in poorly fixed areas. Other features include focal necrosis, particularly in large tumors, frequent involvement of dermal lymphatics,[407] and a scattered infiltrate of lymphocytes and sometimes plasma cells. Stromal desmoplasia is a rare finding.[409] Tumor cells may be larger in recurrences after radiotherapy.[410] Amyloid has been demonstrated in a few tumors.[411,412] Focal argyrophilia is sometimes present, and this is enhanced by fixation in Bouin's solution.[406]

The overlying epidermis is ulcerated in about 20% of cases. Sometimes there is epidermal hyperplasia. Epidermotropism of tumor cells is uncommon.[363,413–415] Epidermal involvement was present in 11 of 132 cases in one series.[416] Two cases have been reported in which the tumor cells were confined exclusively to the epidermis.[417] Cases with prominent epidermal involvement have been used as evidence of a Merkel cell origin of these tumors.[414] Overlying and contiguous Bowen's disease has also been reported,[367,418,419] as has the admixture of a Merkel and squamous cell carcinoma.[420–422] No transition was seen between the two cell types.[421]

Another rarity is the finding of a tumor composed of Merkel, squamous and basal cell carcinoma.[423] Patients with Merkel cell carcinoma have often had numerous skin cancers in the past.[421] Small swirls of squamoid differentiation[424] and even sweat duct differentiation[416,418,425,426] are occasionally seen within the tumor itself. Tripartite differentiation (squamous, glandular and melanocytic) has been recorded.[427] This has led to the suggestion that the tumor arises from a primitive cell that can differentiate in either a neuroendocrine or a sudoriferous direction.[418] Other exceedingly rare patterns of differentiation include skeletal muscle, leiomyosarcomatous, lymphoepithelioma-like and atypical fibroxanthoma-like.[428–433] Well-differentiated follicular structures were present in one of these cases.[430] One case was purported to have arisen in an epidermal cyst[434] and another has been associated with a trichilemmal cyst.[435]

Examination of the sites of a regressed lesion shows perivascular lymphocytes, some lymphoid nodules, variable numbers of foamy histiocytes, and some fibrosis. No tumor cells remain.[394] In partial regression, there is usually a heavy lymphocytic infiltrate with prominent apoptosis of tumor cells and some fibrosis.[436]

Histological features associated with a worse survival include small cell size and a high mitotic rate.[437] The expression of *bcl-2*, *bax* and p53 did not correlate with survival in one study,[438] although in another small series, the presence of p53 did correlate with increased recurrence/death.[439] Large tumor size, location on the buttocks/thigh region or trunk, and advanced clinical stage are other adverse prognostic features.[395,437]

Merkel cell carcinomas need to be differentiated histologically from anaplastic primary and secondary tumors; therefore there have been numerous immunoperoxidase studies assessing the specificity of various markers.[440,441] The variability in the reported results for the same marker probably reflects the different sensitivity of the techniques used and the level of specificity of the monoclonal antibodies. Most tumors are positive for neuron-specific enolase[424,442] and epithelial membrane antigen.[440] Cytokeratin is usually present as paranuclear globules (Fig. 37.21),[443–446] which are present in mitotic as well as interphase cells.[447] Cytokeratin 20 (CK20) was initially regarded as a sensitive and specific marker for Merkel cell carcinoma, which allowed distinction from other small cell carcinomas.[448–450] However, a recent study has shown that one-third of small cell carcinomas of the lung are positive for CK20.[451] In this same study, 28 of 33 of the lung tumors stained for thyroid transcription factor-1 but none of the 21 Merkel cell carcinomas stained.[451] CK20 can also be used for the detection of micrometastases in

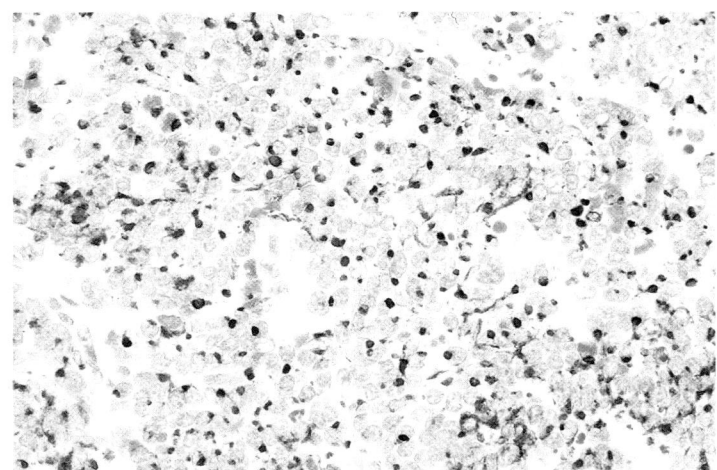

Fig. 37.21 **Merkel cell carcinoma.** Paranuclear filaments are seen as small globules ('dots'). (Immunoperoxidase preparation for cytokeratin)

lymph nodes.[452] Tumor cells may also stain with Ber-EP4, an antibody directed against an epithelium-specific membrane antigen.[416] Neurofilaments,[453] chromogranin,[454,455] guanine nucleotide-binding proteins,[456] and polypeptides such as calcitonin,[457] gastrin,[458] somatostatin and corticotropin are sometimes present.[364] Expression of CD44 may indicate a metastatic potential.[459] The tumor cells are negative for S100 protein, laminin, CD45 (leukocyte common antigen)[440] and metenkephalin,[402,444] the latter being a marker for normal Merkel cells. Tumor cells often contain high levels of *bcl-2* protein.[460,461] The cells of secondary 'oat-cell' carcinomas and carcinoids, some of which are spindle shaped, usually have more cytoplasm; they may be immunoperoxidase positive for bombesin, leucine, enkephalin and β-endorphin, markers which are absent in Merkel cell carcinomas.[441]

Nearly 50% of Merkel cell carcinomas exhibit trisomy 6.[462] A distal deletion involving chromosome 1p35–36 is also quite common, a feature shared with other neoplasms of neural crest derivation.[463] Other chromosomes implicated include 18q and 20.[464]

Electron microscopy

The tumor cells contain dense core neurosecretory granules in the cytoplasm,[465] but these tend to be lost in formalin-fixed material.[466] A characteristic feature is the presence of paranuclear aggregates of intermediate-sized filaments.[467,468] Complex intercellular junctions and cytoplasmic spinous processes are also present.[367,469,470]

MALIGNANT PRIMITIVE NEUROECTODERMAL TUMOR

The term 'malignant primitive (peripheral) neuroectodermal tumor' (MPNET) is the preferred designation for a rare small-cell malignancy of the skin that differs from Merkel cell carcinoma on immunohistochemical and ultrastructural features.[471–474] Other terms used for this tumor include 'malignant neuroepithelioma'[475] and 'peripheral neuroepithelioma'.

Extraskeletal Ewing's sarcoma and MPNET are generally regarded as two ends of a morphological spectrum of the same biological entity.[476,477] They both contain the cell surface product of the *MIC2* gene, CD99, and both have a consistent chromosomal translocation t(11;22)(q24;q12), found in up to 90% of all cases.[478,479] Variant translocations, all of which involve the *EWS* gene on chromosome 22q12, have been reported.[478] The overall 5-year

survival rate for lesions designated as extraskeletal Ewing's sarcoma was 61% in one series.[480] A younger age and wide initial surgical excision correlated with improved overall survival.[480]

Most MPNETs are situated in the deep soft tissues.[475] The subcutis and dermis are involved quite uncommonly.[481,482] They are highly aggressive tumors that eventually metastasize widely.

Histopathology

Malignant primitive neuroectodermal tumors are composed of sheets of hyperchromatic cells with small amounts of cytoplasm. Homer Wright rosettes are frequently present, and central neurofibrillary material may be seen in them.[482] Glycogen may be present, a feature once thought to be restricted to Ewing's sarcoma (see below).[483] The tumor cells contain neurosecretory granules and are usually positive for neuron-specific enolase, CD99, and PGP9.5.[483] They show restricted expression of S100 protein and the various neuropeptides.

Extraskeletal Ewing's sarcoma has cells that often contain glycogen, but there are no neurosecretory granules or well-developed desmosomes.[484] The cells express CD99 in a characteristic membranous pattern,[478,485] but are negative for S100 protein and desmin.[486] Merkel cell carcinomas are frequently positive for epithelial membrane antigen and cytokeratin 20 (CK20), features not seen usually in MPNETs. Neuroblastomas are usually negative for CD99.[487]

A final diagnosis can usually be made only after the electron microscopic findings and immunohistochemistry results have been correlated.

REFERENCES

Introduction

1 Feigin I. Skin tumors of neural origin. Am J Dermatopathol 1983; 5: 397–399.
2 Erlandson RA, Woodruff JM. Peripheral nerve sheath tumors: an electron microscopic study of 43 cases. Cancer 1982; 49: 273–287.
3 Hartschuh W, Schulz T. Merkel cell hyperplasia in chronic radiation-damaged skin: its possible relationship to fibroepithelioma of Pinkus. J Cutan Pathol 1997; 24: 477–483.

Nerve sheath tumors

4 Nadji M. Immunoperoxidase techniques II. Application to cutaneous neoplasms. Am J Dermatopathol 1986; 8: 124–129.
5 Theaker JM, Fletcher CDM. Epithelial membrane antigen expression by the perineurial cell: further studies of peripheral nerve lesions. Histopathology 1989; 14: 581–592.
6 Smith MEF, Jones TA, Hilton D. Vascular endothelial cadherin is expressed by perineurial cells of peripheral nerves. Histopathology 1998; 32: 411–413.
7 Jimenez FJ, Grichnik JM, Clark RE. CD34-positive spindle cells in nerves. J Cutan Pathol 1994; 21: 189–190.
8 Weiss SW, Nickoloff BJ. CD-34 is expressed by a distinctive cell population in peripheral nerve, nerve sheath tumors, and related lesions. Am J Surg Pathol 1993; 17: 1039–1045.
9 Khalifa MA, Montgomery EA, Ismiil N, Azumi N. What are the CD34+ cells in benign peripheral nerve sheath tumors? Am J Clin Pathol 2000; 114: 123–126.
10 Reed RJ, Fine RM, Meltzer HD. Palisaded, encapsulated neuromas of the skin. Arch Dermatol 1972; 106: 865–870.
11 Mathews GJ, Osterholm JL. Painful traumatic neuromas. Surg Clin North Am 1972; 51: 1313–1324.
12 Reed ML, Jacoby RA. Cutaneous neuroanatomy and neuropathology. Am J Dermatopathol 1983; 5: 335–362.
13 Argenyi ZB, Santa Cruz D, Bromley C. Comparative light-microscopic and immunohistochemical study of traumatic and palisaded encapsulated neuromas of the skin. Am J Dermatopathol 1992; 14: 504–510.
14 Waggener JD. Ultrastructure of benign peripheral nerve sheath tumors. Cancer 1966; 19: 699–709.
15 Hare PJ. Rudimentary polydactyly. Br J Dermatol 1954; 66: 402–408.
16 Suzuki H, Matsuoka S. Rudimentary polydactyly (cutaneous neuroma) case report with ultrastructural study. J Cutan Pathol 1981; 8: 299–307
17 Shapiro L, Juhlin EA, Brownstein MH. "Rudimentary polydactyly". An amputation neuroma. Arch Dermatol 1973; 108: 223–225.

18 Brehmer-Andersson EE. Penile neuromas with multiple Meissner's corpuscles. Histopathology 1999; 34: 555–556.

19 Ban M, Kitajima Y. The number and distribution of Merkel cells in rudimentary polydactyly. Dermatology 2001; 202: 31–34.

20 Fletcher CDM. Solitary circumscribed neuroma of the skin (so-called palisaded, encapsulated neuroma). A clinicopathologic and immunohistochemical study. Am J Surg Pathol 1989; 13: 574–580.

21 Dakin MC, Leppard B, Theaker JM. The palisaded, encapsulated neuroma (solitary circumscribed neuroma). Histopathology 1992; 20: 405–410.

22 Navarro M, Vilata J, Requena C, Aliaga A. Palisaded encapsulated neuroma (solitary circumscribed neuroma) of the glans penis. Br J Dermatol 2000; 142: 1061–1062.

23 Holm TW, Prawer SE, Sahl WJ, Bart BJ. Multiple cutaneous neuromas. Arch Dermatol 1973; 107: 608–610.

24 Dover JS, From L, Lewis A. Palisaded encapsulated neuromas. A clinicopathologic study. Arch Dermatol 1989; 125: 386–389.

25 Argenyi ZB, Cooper PH, Santa Cruz D. Plexiform and other unusual variants of palisaded encapsulated neuroma. J Cutan Pathol 1993; 20: 34–39.

26 Tsang WYW, Chan JKC. Epithelioid variant of solitary circumscribed neuroma of the skin. Histopathology 1992; 20: 439–441.

27 Argenyi ZB. Immunohistochemical characterization of palisading, encapsulated neuroma. J Cutan Pathol 1989; 16: 293 (abstract).

28 Megahed M. Palisaded encapsulated neuroma (solitary circumscribed neuroma). A clinicopathologic and immunohistochemical study. Am J Dermatopathol 1994; 16: 120–125.

29 Argenyi ZB. Immunohistochemical characterization of palisaded, encapsulated neuroma. J Cutan Pathol 1990; 17: 329–335.

30 Kossard S, Kumar A, Wilkinson B. Neural spectrum: palisaded encapsulated neuroma and verocay body poor dermal schwannoma. J Cutan Pathol 1999; 26: 31–36.

31 Argenyi ZB, Penick GD. Vascular variant of palisaded encapsulated neuroma. J Cutan Pathol 1993; 20: 92–93.

32 Alexander J, Theaker JM. An unusual solitary circumscribed neuroma (palisaded encapsulated neuroma) of the skin – with observations on the nature of pseudo-epitheliomatous hyperplasia. Histopathology 1991; 18: 175–177.

33 Walker DM. Oral mucosal neuroma–medullary thyroid carcinoma syndrome. Br J Dermatol 1973; 88: 599–603.

34 Brown RS, Colle E, Tashjian AH. The syndrome of multiple mucosal neuromas and medullary thyroid carcinoma in childhood. J Pediatr 1975; 86: 77–83.

35 Williams ED, Pollock DJ. Multiple mucosal neuromata with endocrine tumours: a syndrome allied to Von Recklinghausen's disease. J Pathol Bacteriol 1966; 91: 71–80.

36 Ayala F, De Rosa G, Scippa L, Vecchio P. Multiple endocrine neoplasia, type IIb. Report of a case. Dermatologica 1981; 162: 292–299.

37 Gorlin RJ, Sedano HO, Vickers RA, Cervenka J. Multiple mucosal neuromas pheochromocytoma and medullary carcinoma of the thyroid – a syndrome. Cancer 1968; 22: 293–299.

38 Khairi MRA, Dexter RN, Burzynski NJ, Johnston CC. Mucosal neuroma, pheochromocytoma and medullary thyroid carcinoma: multiple endocrine neoplasia type 3. Medicine (Baltimore) 1975; 54: 89–112.

39 Lashgari AR, Friedlander SF. The importance of early diagnosis in multiple endocrine neoplasia III: Report of a case with thyroid C-cell hyperplasia. J Am Acad Dermatol 1997; 36: 296–300.

40 Pujol RM, Matias-Guiu X, Miralles J et al. Multiple idiopathic mucosal neuromas: A minor form of multiple endocrine neoplasia type 2B or a new entity? J Am Acad Dermatol 1997; 37: 349–352.

41 Winkelmann RK, Carney JA. Cutaneous neuropathology in multiple endocrine neoplasia, type 2b. J Invest Dermatol 1982; 79: 307–312.

42 Guillet G, Gauthier Y, Tamisier JM et al. Linear cutaneous neuromas (dermatoneurie en stries): a limited phakomatosis with striated pigmentation corresponding to cutaneous hypernneury (featuring multiple endocrine neoplasia syndrome?). J Cutan Pathol 1987; 14: 43–48.

43 Mason GH, Pitt TE, Tay E. Cutaneous nerve hypertrophy. Pathology 1998; 30: 422–424.

44 Bolande RP, Towler WF. A possible relationship of neuroblastoma to von Recklinghausen's disease. Cancer 1970; 26: 162–175.

45 Collins J-P, Johnson WC, Burgoon CF. Ganglioneuroma of the skin. Arch Dermatol 1972; 105: 256–258.

46 Geffner RE, Hassell CM. Ganglioneuroma of the skin. Arch Dermatol 1986; 122: 377–378.

47 Hammond RR, Walton JC. Cutaneous ganglioneuromas: a case report and review of the literature. Hum Pathol 1996; 27: 735–738.

48 Gambini C, Rongioletti F. Primary congenital cutaneous ganglioneuroma. J Am Acad Dermatol 1996; 35: 353–354.

49 Lee JY, Martinez AJ, Abell E. Ganglioneuromatous tumor of the skin: a combined

heterotopia of ganglion cells and hamartomatous neuroma: report of a case. J Cutan Pathol 1988; 15: 58–61.

50 Radice F, Gianotti R. Cutaneous ganglion cell tumor of the skin. Case report and review of the literature. Am J Dermatopathol 1993; 15: 488–491.

51 Rios JJ, Diaz-Cano SJ, Rivera-Hueto F, Villar JL. Cutaneous ganglion cell choristoma. Report of a case. J Cutan Pathol 1991; 18: 469–473.

52 Franchi A, Massi D, Santucci M. Desmoplastic cutaneous ganglioneuroma. Histopathology 1999; 34: 82–84.

53 Requena L, Sangüeza OP. Benign neoplasms with neural differentiation. A review. Am J Dermatopathol 1995; 17: 75–96.

54 Requena L, Grosshans E, Kutzner H et al. Epithelial sheath neuroma: a new entity. Am J Surg Pathol 2000; 24: 190–196.

55 Zelger BG, Zelger B. Epithelial sheath neuroma: a benign neoplasm? Am J Surg Pathol 2001; 25: 696–698.

56 Grosshans EM, Kutzner HH, Resnik K. Of epithelium and nerve. Am J Dermatopathol 2000; 22: 38–39.

57 Wu ML, Guitart J. Unusual neurotropism. Am J Dermatopathol 2000; 22: 468–469.

58 Wu ML, Caro WA, Richards KA, Guitart J. Atypical reexcision perineural invasion. Am J Surg Pathol 2000; 24: 895–896.

59 Mentzel T, Dei Tos AP, Fletcher CDM. Perineurioma (storiform perineurial fibroma): clinico-pathological analysis of four cases. Histopathology 1994; 25: 261–267.

60 Tsang WYW, Chan JKC, Chow LTC, Tse CCH. Perineurioma: an uncommon soft tissue neoplasm distinct from localized hypertrophic neuropathy and neurofibroma. Am J Surg Pathol 1992; 16: 756–763.

61 Fetsch JF, Miettinen M. Sclerosing perineurioma. A clinicopathologic study of 19 cases of a distinctive soft tissue lesion with a predilection for the fingers and palms of young adults. Am J Surg Pathol 1997; 21: 1433–1442.

62 Sciot R, Dal Cin P, Hagemeijer A et al. Cutaneous sclerosing perineurioma with cryptic *NF2* gene deletion. Am J Surg Pathol 1999; 23: 849–853.

63 Giannini C, Scheithauer BW, Jenkins RB et al. Soft-tissue perineurioma. Evidence for an abnormality of chromosome 22, criteria for diagnosis, and review of the literature. Am J Surg Pathol 1997; 21: 164–173.

64 Zelger B. Clue to diagnosis. Dermatopathology: Practical & Conceptual 2000; 6: 80–85.

65 Díaz-Flores L, Alvarez-Argüelles H, Madrid JF et al. Perineural cell tumor (perineurioma) with granular cells. J Cutan Pathol 1997; 24: 575–579.

66 Zelger BG, Weinlich G, Zelger B. Perineurioma. A frequently unrecognized entity with emphasis on a plexiform variant. Adv Clin Pathol 2000; 4: 25–33.

67 Graadt van Roggen JF, McMenamin ME, Belchis DA et al. Reticular perineurioma. A distinctive variant of soft tissue perineurioma. Am J Surg Pathol 2001; 25: 485–493.

68 Skelton HG, Williams J, Smith KJ. The clinical and histologic spectrum of fibrous perineuriomas. Am J Dermatopathol 2001; 23: 190–196.

69 Robson AM, Calonje E. Cutaneous perineurioma: a poorly recognized tumour often misdiagnosed as epithelioid histiocytoma. Histopathology 2000; 37: 332–339.

70 Pillay P, Essa AS, Chetty R. Pacinian collagenoma. Br J Dermatol 1999; 141: 119–122.

71 Whitaker WG, Droulias C. Benign encapsulated neurilemmoma: a report of 76 cases. Am Surg 1976; 42: 675–678.

72 White NB. Neurilemomas of the extremities. J Bone Joint Surg 1967; 49–A: 1605–1610.

73 Jacobs RL, Barmada R. Neurilemoma. A review of the literature with six case reports. Arch Surg 1971; 102: 181–186.

74 Buscher CA, Izumi AK. A painful subcutaneous neurilemmoma attached to a peripheral nerve. J Am Acad Dermatol 1998; 38: 122–124.

75 Berger TG, Lapins NA, Engel ML. Agminated neurilemomas. J Am Acad Dermatol 1987; 17: 891–894.

76 Izumi AK, Rosato FE, Wood MG. Von Recklinghausen's disease associated with multiple neurolemomas. Arch Dermatol 1971; 104: 172–176.

77 Shishiba T, Niimura M, Ohtsuka F, Tsuru N. Multiple cutaneous neurilemmomas as a skin manifestation of neurilemmomatosis. J Am Acad Dermatol 1984; 10: 744–754.

78 Murata Y, Kumano K, Ugai K et al. Neurilemmomatosis. Br J Dermatol 1991; 125: 466–468.

79 Sasaki T, Nakajima H. Congenital neurilemmomatosis. J Am Acad Dermatol 1992; 26: 786–787.

80 Wolkenstein P, Benchikhi H, Zeller J et al. Schwannomatosis: a clinical entity distinct from neurofibromatosis type 2. Dermatology 1997; 195: 228–231.

81 Purcell SM, Dixon SL. Schwannomatosis. An unusual variant of neurofibromatosis or a distinct clinical entity? Arch Dermatol 1989; 125: 390–393.

82 Honda M, Arai E, Sawada S et al. Neurofibromatosis 2 and neurilemmomatosis gene are identical. J Invest Dermatol 1995; 104: 74–77.

83 Iyengar V, Golomb CA, Schachner L. Neurilemmomatosis, NF2, and juvenile xanthogranuloma. J Am Acad Dermatol 1998; 39: 831–834.

84 Mercantini ES, Mopper C. Neurilemmoma of the tongue. Arch Dermatol 1959; 79: 542–544.

85 Woodruff JM, Selig AM, Crowley K, Allen PW. Schwannoma (neurilemmoma) with malignant transformation. Am J Surg Pathol 1994; 18: 882–895.

86 Nayler SJ, Leiman G, Omar T, Cooper K. Malignant transformation in a schwannoma. Histopathology 1996; 29: 189–192.

87 Abell MR, Hart WR, Olson JR. Tumors of the peripheral nervous system. Hum Pathol 1970; 1: 503–551.

88 Phalen GS. Neurilemmomas of the forearm and hand. Clin Orthop 1976; 114: 219–222.

89 Kao GF, Laskin WB, Olson TG. Solitary cutaneous plexiform neurilemmoma (Schwannoma). J Cutan Pathol 1988; 15: 318 (abstract).

90 Megahed M. Plexiform schwannoma. Am J Dermatopathol 1994; 16: 288–293.

91 Val-Bernal JF, Figols J, Vázquez-Barquero A. Cutaneous plexiform schwannoma associated with neurofibromatosis type 2. Cancer 1995; 76: 1181–1186.

92 Zelger BG, Steiner H, Kutzner H et al. Verocay body-prominent cutaneous schwannoma. Am J Dermatopathol 1997; 19: 242–249.

93 Argenyi ZB, Balogh K, Abraham AA. Degenerative ("ancient") changes in benign cutaneous schwannoma. A light microscopic, histochemical and immunohistochemical study. J Cutan Pathol 1993; 20: 148–153.

94 Skelton HG III, Smith KJ, Lupton GP. Collagenous spherulosis in a Schwannoma. Am J Dermatopathol 1994; 16: 549–553.

95 Nahass GT, Penneys NS. Merkel cells in neurofibromas and neurilemmomas. Br J Dermatol 1994; 131: 664–666.

96 Kawahara E, Oda Y, Ooi A et al. Expression of glial fibrillary acidic protein (GFAP) in peripheral nerve sheath tumors. Am J Surg Pathol 1988; 12: 115–120.

97 Penneys NS, Mogollon R, Kowalczyk A et al. A survey of cutaneous neural lesions for the presence of myelin basic protein. An immunohistochemical study. Arch Dermatol 1984; 120: 210–213.

98 Gray MH, Rosenberg AE, Dickersin GR, Bhan AK. Glial fibrillary acid protein and keratin expression by benign and malignant nerve sheath tumors. Hum Pathol 1989; 20: 1089–1096.

99 Theaker JM, Gatter KC, Puddle J. Epithelial membrane antigen expression by the perineurium of peripheral nerve and in peripheral nerve tumours. Histopathology 1988; 13: 171–179.

100 Woodruff JM, Susin M, Godwin TA et al. Cellular schwannoma. A variety of schwannoma sometimes mistaken for a malignant tumor. Am J Surg Pathol 1981; 5: 733–744.

101 Megahed M, Ruzicka T. Cellular schwannoma. Am J Dermatopathol 1994; 16: 418–421.

102 Fletcher CDM, Madziwa D, Heyderman E, McKee PH. Benign dermal Schwannoma with glandular elements – true heterology or a local 'organizer' effect? Clin Exp Dermatol 1986; 11: 475–485.

103 Chan JKC, Fok KO. Pseudoglandular schwannoma. Histopathology 1996; 29: 481–483.

104 Elston DM, Bergfeld WF, Biscotti CV, McMahon JT. Schwannoma with sweat duct differentiation. J Cutan Pathol 1993; 20: 254–258.

105 Fisher C, Chappell ME, Weiss SW. Neuroblastoma-like epithelioid schwannoma. Histopathology 1995; 26: 193–194.

106 Smith K, Mezebish D, Williams JP et al. Cutaneous epithelioid schwannomas: a rare variant of a benign peripheral nerve sheath tumor. J Cutan Pathol 1998; 25: 50–55.

107 Kindblom L-G, Meis-Kindblom JM, Havel G, Busch C. Benign epithelioid schwannoma. Am J Surg Pathol 1998; 22: 762–770.

108 Orosz Z. Cutaneous epithelioid schwannoma: an unusual benign neurogenic tumor. J Cutan Pathol 1999; 26: 213–214.

109 Argenyi ZB, Goodenberger ME, Strauss JS. Congenital neural hamartoma ("fascicular schwannoma"). Am J Dermatopathol 1990; 12: 283–293.

110 Lassmann H, Jurecka W, Lassmann G et al. Different types of benign nerve sheath tumors. Virchows Arch [A] 1977; 375: 197–210.

111 Sian CS, Ryan SF. The ultrastructure of neurilemoma with emphasis on Antoni B tissue. Hum Pathol 1981; 12: 145–160.

112 Carney JA. Psammomatous melanotic schwannoma. A distinctive, heritable tumor with special associations, including cardiac myxoma and the Cushing syndrome. Am J Surg Pathol 1990; 14: 206–222.

113 Killeen RM, Davy CL, Bauserman SC. Melanocytic schwannoma. Cancer 1988; 62: 174–183.

114 Utiger CA, Headington JT. Psammomatous melanotic schwannoma. A new cutaneous marker for Carney's complex. Arch Dermatol 1993; 129: 202–204.

115 Thornton CM, Handley J, Bingham EA et al. Psammomatous melanotic schwannoma arising in the dermis in a patient with Carney's complex. Histopathology 1992; 20: 71–73.

116 Foad MS, Kleiner DE, Dugan EM. A case of psammomatous melanotic schwannoma in the setting of the Carney complex. J Cutan Pathol 2000; 27: 556 (abstract).

117 Murakami T, Kiyosawa T, Murata S et al. Malignant schwannoma with melanocytic differentiation arising in a patient with neurofibromatosis. Br J Dermatol 2000; 143: 1078–1082.

118 Bhushan M, Telfer NR, Chalmers RJG. Subungual neurofibroma: an unusual cause of nail dystrophy. Br J Dermatol 1999; 140: 777–778.

119 Riccardi VM. Neurofibromatosis. The importance of localized or otherwise atypical forms. Arch Dermatol 1987; 123: 882–883.

120 Zvulunov A, Esterly NB. Neurocutaneous syndromes associated with pigmentary skin lesions. J Am Acad Dermatol 1995; 32: 915–935.

121 Riccardi VM. Von Recklinghausen neurofibromatosis. N Engl J Med 1981; 305: 1617–1627.

122 Riccardi VM. Neurofibromatosis: clinical heterogeneity. Curr Probl Cancer 1982; 7: 1–35.

123 Mautner VF, Lindenau M, Baser ME et al. Skin abnormalities in neurofibromatosis 2. Arch Dermatol 1997; 133: 1539–1543.

124 Bousema MT, Vuzevski VD, Oranje AP et al. Non-von Recklinghausen's neurofibromatosis resembling a giant pigmented nevus. J Am Acad Dermatol 1989; 20: 358–362.

125 Friedman JM. Epidemiology of neurofibromatosis type 1. Am J Med Genet (Semin Med Genet) 1999; 89: 1–6.

126 Koivunen J, Ylä-Outinen H, Korkiamäki T et al. New function for NF1 tumor suppressor. J Invest Dermatol 2000; 114: 473–479.

127 Person JR, Perry HO. Recent advances in the phakomatoses. Int J Dermatol 1978; 17: 1–13.

128 Miller MB, Tonsgard JH, Soltani K. Late-onset neurofibromatosis in a liver transplant recipient. Int J Dermatol 2000; 39: 376–379.

129 Swapp GH, Main RA. Neurofibromatosis in pregnancy. Br J Dermatol 1973; 80: 431–435.

130 Fisher DA, Chu P, McCalmont T. Solitary plexiform neurofibroma is not pathognomonic of von Recklinghausen's neurofibromatosis: a report of a case. Int J Dermatol 1997; 36: 439–442.

131 Wasserteil V, Bruce S, Riccardi VM. Non von Recklinghausen's neurofibromatosis presenting as hemifacial neurofibromas and contralateral café au lait spots. J Am Acad Dermatol 1987; 16: 1090–1096.

132 Brasfield RD, Das Gupta TK. Von Recklinghausen's disease: a clinicopathological study. Ann Surg 1972; 175: 86–104.

133 Riccardi VM. Pathophysiology of neurofibromatosis IV. Dermatologic insights into heterogeneity and pathogenesis. J Am Acad Dermatol 1980; 3: 157–166.

134 Otsuka F, Kawashima T, Imakado S et al. Lisch nodules and skin manifestation in neurofibromatosis type 1. Arch Dermatol 2001; 137: 232–233.

135 McCarroll HR. Soft-tissue neoplasms associated with congenital neurofibromatosis. J Bone Joint Surg 1956; 38-A: 717–731.

136 Greene JF Jr, Fitzwater JE, Burgess J. Arterial lesions associated with neurofibromatosis. Am J Clin Pathol 1974; 62: 481–487.

137 Karnes PS. Neurofibromatosis: a common neurocutaneous disorder. Mayo Clin Proc 1998; 73: 1071–1076.

138 Wolkenstein P, Frèche B, Zeller J, Revuz J. Usefulness of screening investigations in neurofibromatosis type 1. A study of 152 patients. Arch Dermatol 1996; 132: 1333–1336.

139 Eisenbarth I, Beyer K, Krone W, Assum G. Toward a survey of somatic mutation of the *NF1* gene in benign neurofibromas of patients with neurofibromatosis type 1. Am J Hum Genet 2000; 66: 393–401.

140 Phillips CM, Rye B. Neurofibromatosis type 1 and tuberous sclerosis: a case of a double phakomatosis. J Am Acad Dermatol 1994; 31: 799–800.

141 Gonzalez-Martin J, Glover S, Dixon S et al. Neurofibromatosis type 1 and McCune–Albright syndrome occurring in the same patient. Br J Dermatol 2000; 143: 1288–1291.

142 Smith WE, Moseley JC. Multiple halo neurofibromas. Arch Dermatol 1976; 112: 987–990.

143 Chaudhuri B, Ronan SG, Manaligod JR. Angiosarcoma arising in a plexiform neurofibroma. A case report. Cancer 1980; 46: 605–610.

144 Knight WA III, Murphy WK, Gottlieb JA. Neurofibromatosis associated with malignant neurofibromas. Arch Dermatol 1973; 107: 747–750.

145 Mastrangelo MJ, Goepp CE, Patel YA, Clark WH Jr. Cutaneous melanoma in a patient with neurofibromatosis. Arch Dermatol 1979; 115: 864–865.

146 Sorensen SA, Mulvihill JJ, Nielsen A. Long-term follow-up of von Recklinghausen neurofibromatosis. Survival and malignant neoplasms. N Engl J Med 1986; 314: 1010–1015.

147 Roth RR, Martines R, James WD. Segmental neurofibromatosis. Arch Dermatol 1987; 123: 917–920.

148 McFadden JP, Logan R, Griffiths WAD. Segmental neurofibromatosis and pruritus. Clin Exp Dermatol 1988; 13: 265–268.

149 Allegue F, España A, Fernandez-Garcia JM, Ledo A. Segmental neurofibromatosis with contralateral lentiginosis. Clin Exp Dermatol 1989; 14: 448–450.

150 Sloan JB, Fretzin DF, Boyenmyer DA. Genetic counseling in segmental neurofibromatosis. J Am Acad Dermatol 1990; 22: 461–467.

151 Jaakkola S, Muona P, James WD et al. Segmental neurofibromatosis: immunocytochemical analysis of cutaneous lesions. J Am Acad Dermatol 1990; 22: 617–621.

152 Moss C, Green SH. What is segmental neurofibromatosis? Br J Dermatol 1994; 130: 106–110.

153 Trattner A, David M, Hodak E et al. Segmental neurofibromatosis. J Am Acad Dermatol 1990; 23: 866–869.

154 Hager CM, Cohen PR, Tschen JA. Segmental neurofibromatosis: Case reports and review. J Am Acad Dermatol 1997; 37: 864–869.

155 Miller RM, Sparkes RS. Segmental neurofibromatosis. Arch Dermatol 1977; 113: 837–838.

156 Goldberg NS. What is segmental neurofibromatosis? J Am Acad Dermatol 1992; 26: 638–640.

157 Micali G, Lembo D, Giustini S, Calvieri S. Segmental neurofibromatosis with only macular lesions. Pediatr Dermatol 1993; 10: 43–45.

158 Finley EM, Kolbusz RV. Segmental neurofibromatosis clinically appearing as a nevus spilus. Int J Dermatol 1993; 32: 358–360.

159 Oranje AP, Vuzevski VD, Kalis TJ et al. Segmental neurofibromatosis. Br J Dermatol 1985; 112: 107–112.

160 Pullara TJ, Greeson JD, Stoker GL, Fenske NA. Cutaneous segmental neurofibromatosis. J Am Acad Dermatol 1985; 13: 999–1003.

161 Garcia RL. Multiple localized neurofibromas. JAMA 1971; 215: 1670.

162 Winkelmann RK, Johnson LA. Cholinesterases in neurofibromas. Arch Dermatol 1962; 85: 106–114.

163 Carey JC, Viskochil DH. Neurofibromatosis type 1: a model condition for the study of the molecular basis of variable expressivity in human disorders. Am J Med Genet (Semin Med Genet) 1999; 89: 7–13.

164 Mohri S, Atsusaka K, Sasaki T. Localized multiple neurofibromas. Clin Exp Dermatol 1992; 17: 195–196.

165 Takiguchi PS, Ratz JL. Bilateral dermatomal neurofibromatosis. J Am Acad Dermatol 1984; 10: 451–453.

166 Wong SS. Bilateral segmental neurofibromatosis with partial unilateral lentiginosis. Br J Dermatol 1997; 136: 380–383.

167 Nicholls EM. Somatic variation and multiple neurofibromatosis. Hum Hered 1969; 19: 473–479.

168 Rubenstein AE, Bader JL, Aron AA et al. Familial transmission of segmental neurofibromatosis. Neurology 1983; 33 (Suppl 2): 76.

169 Lewis FM, Lewis-Jones MS, Toon PG, Rollason TP. Neurofibromatosis of the vulva. Br J Dermatol 1992; 127: 540–541.

170 Megahed M. Histopathological variants of neurofibroma. A study of 114 lesions. Am J Dermatopathol 1994; 16: 486–495.

171 Shek TWH. Sclerosing neurofibroma. Histopathology 2000; 36: 377–378.

172 Arbiser JL, Flynn E, Barnhill RL. Analysis of vascularity of human neurofibromas. J Am Acad Dermatol 1998; 39: 950–954.

173 Johnson MD, Kamso-Pratt J, Federspiel CF, Whetsell WO Jr. Mast cell and lymphoreticular infiltrates in neurofibromas. Comparison with nerve sheath tumors. Arch Pathol Lab Med 1989; 113: 1263–1270.

174 Gray MH, Smoller BR, McNutt NS, Hsu A. Immunohistochemical demonstration of factor XIIIa expression in neurofibromas. Arch Dermatol 1990; 126: 472–476.

175 Takata M, Imai T, Hirone T. Factor-XIIIa-positive cells in normal peripheral nerves and cutaneous neurofibromas of type-I neurofibromatosis. Am J Dermatopathol 1994; 16: 37–43.

176 Kadono T, Kikuchi K, Nakagawa H, Tamaki K. Expression of various growth factors and their receptors in tissues from neurofibroma. Dermatology 2000; 201: 10–14.

177 Jukic DM, Busam KJ. Neural cell adhesion molecule (NCAM-CD56) and HU staining in the differential diagnosis of cutaneous spindle cell neoplasms. J Cutan Pathol 2000; 27: 560–561 (abstract).

178 Jurecka W. Plexiforme neurofibroma of the skin. Am J Dermatopathol 1988; 10: 209–217.

179 Woodruff JM. Pathology of tumors of the peripheral nerve sheath in type I neurofibromatosis. Am J Med Genet (Semin Med Genet) 1999; 89: 23–30.

180 Feany MB, Anthony DC, Fletcher CDM. Nerve sheath tumours with hybrid features of neurofibroma and schwannoma: a conceptual challenge. Histopathology 1998 32: 405–410.

181 Zamecnik M. Hybrid neurofibroma/schwannoma versus schwannoma with Antoni B areas. Histopathology 2000; 36: 473.

182 Henkes J, Ferrandiz C, Peyri J, Fontarnau R. Pilar dysplasia overlying two neurofibromas of the scalp. J Cutan Pathol 1984; 11: 65–70.

183 del Rio E, Sánchez Yus E, Simón P, Vázquez Veiga HA. Stimulation of folliculo-sebaceous proliferations by neurofibromas: a report of two cases. J Cutan Pathol 1998; 25: 228–232.

184 Karvonen S-L, Kallioinen M, Ylä-Outinen H et al. Occult neurofibroma and increased S100 protein in the skin of patients with neurofibromatosis type 1. Arch Dermatol 2000; 136: 1207–1209.

185 Riccardi VM. Of mass and men. Neurofibromas and histogenesis. Arch Dermatol 2000; 136: 1257–1258.

186 Woodruff JM, Christensen WN. Glandular peripheral nerve sheath tumors. Cancer 1993; 72: 3618–3628.

187 Michal M, Fanburg-Smith JC, Mentzel T et al. Dendritic cell neurofibroma with pseudorosettes. A report of 18 cases of a distinct and hitherto unrecognized neurofibroma variant. Am J Surg Pathol 2001; 25: 587–594.

188 Bird CC, Willis RA. The histogenesis of pigmented neurofibromas. J Pathol 1969; 97: 631–637.

189 Fetsch JF, Michal M, Miettinen M. Pigmented (melanotic) neurofibroma. A clinicopathologic and immunohistochemical analysis of 19 lesions from 17 patients. Am J Surg Pathol 2000; 24: 331–343.

190 Williamson DM, Suggit RIC. Pigmented neurofibroma. Br J Dermatol 1977; 97: 685–688.

191 Lin BT-Y, Weiss LM, Medeiros LJ. Neurofibroma and cellular neurofibroma with atypia. A report of 14 tumors. Am J Surg Pathol 1997; 21: 1443–1449.

192 Liapis H, Dehner LP, Gutmann DH. Neurofibroma and cellular neurofibroma with atypia: a report of 14 tumors. Am J Surg Pathol 1999; 23: 1156–1157.

193 Slater C, Hayes M, Saxe N et al. Macromelanosomes in the early diagnosis of neurofibromatosis. Am J Dermatopathol 1986; 8: 284–289.

194 Silvers DN, Greenwood RS, Helwig EB. Café au lait spots without giant pigment granules. Occurrence in suspected neurofibromatosis. Arch Dermatol 1974; 110: 87–88.

195 Jimbow K, Horikoshi T. The nature and significance of macromelanosomes in pigmented skin lesions. Am J Dermatopathol 1982; 4: 413–420.

196 Bale PM. Sacrococcygeal paciniomas. Pathology 1980; 12: 231–235.

197 Fraitag S, Gherardi R, Wechsler J. Hyperplastic pacinian corpuscles: an uncommonly encountered lesion of the hand. J Cutan Pathol 1994; 21: 457–460.

198 Reznik M, Thiry A, Fridman V. Painful hyperplasia and hypertrophy of pacinian corpuscles in the hand. Am J Dermatopathol 1998; 20: 203–207.

199 Prose PH, Gherardi GJ, Coblenz A. Pacinian neurofibroma. Arch Dermatol 1957; 76: 65–69.

200 Fletcher CDM, Theaker JM. Digital pacinian neuroma: a distinctive hyperplastic lesion. Histopathology 1989; 15: 249–256.

201 Bennin B, Barsky S, Salgia K. Pacinian neurofibroma. Arch Dermatol 1976; 112: 1558.

202 McCormack K, Kaplan D, Murray JC, Fetter BF. Multiple hairy pacinian neurofibromas (nerve-sheath myxomas). J Am Acad Dermatol 1988; 18: 416–419.

203 Levi L, Curri SB. Multiple pacinian neurofibroma and relationship with the finger-tip arterio-venous anastomoses. Br J Dermatol 1980; 102: 345–349.

204 MacDonald DM, Wilson Jones E. Pacinian neurofibroma. Histopathology 1977; 1: 247–255.

205 Angervall L, Kindblom L-G, Haglid K. Dermal nerve sheath myxoma. A light and electron microscopic, histochemical and immunohistochemical study. Cancer 1984; 53: 1752–1759.

206 King DT, Barr RJ. Bizarre cutaneous neurofibromas. J Cutan Pathol 1980; 7: 21–31.

207 Gallagher RL, Helwig EB. Neurothekeoma – a benign cutaneous tumor of neural origin. Am J Clin Pathol 1980; 74: 759–764.

208 Holden CA, Wilson-Jones E, MacDonald DM. Cutaneous lobular neuromyxoma. Br J Dermatol 1982; 106: 211–215.

209 Argenyi ZB. Recent developments in cutaneous neural neoplasms. J Cutan Pathol 1993; 20: 97–108.

210 Wang AR, May D, Bourne P, Scott G. PGP9.5. A marker for cellular neurothekeoma. Am J Surg Pathol 1999; 23: 1401–1407.

211 Pulitzer DR, Reed RJ. Nerve-sheath myxoma (perineurial myxoma). Am J Dermatopathol 1985; 7: 409–421.

212 Cecchi A, Giomi A, Rapicano V, Apicella P. Cellular neurothekeoma on the left auricle. J Eur Acad Dermatol Venereol 2000; 14: 314–315.

213 Pepine M, Flowers F, Ramos-Caro FA. Neurothekeoma in a 15-year-old boy: case report. Pediatr Dermatol 1992; 9: 272–274.

214 Busam KJ, Mentzel T, Colpaert C et al. Atypical or worrisome features in cellular neurothekeoma. A study of 10 cases. Am J Surg Pathol 1998; 22: 1067–1072.

215 Strumia R, Lombardi AR, Cavazzini L. Cellular neurothekeoma. Acta Derm Venereol 1999; 79: 162–163.

216 Fletcher CDM, Chan J K-C, McKee PH. Dermal nerve sheath myxoma: a study of three cases. Histopathology 1986; 10: 135–145.

217 Tuthill RJ. Nerve-sheath myxoma: a case report with immunohistologic evidence of its perineurial cell origin. J Cutan Pathol 1988; 15: 348 (abstract).

218 Salama S, Chorneyko K. Neurothekeoma (N.T.), a clinicopathologic study of 13 new cases with emphasis on immunohistochemical and ultrastructural features. J Cutan Pathol 2000; 27: 571 (abstract).

219 Goldstein L, Lifshitz T. Myxoma of the nerve sheath. Am J Dermatopathol 1985; 7: 423–429.

220 Barnhill RL, Dickersin GR, Nickeleit V et al. Studies on the cellular origin of neurothekeoma: clinical, light microscopic, immunohistochemical, and ultrastructural observations. J Am Acad Dermatol 1991; 25: 80–88.

221 Aronson PJ, Fretzin DF, Potter BS. Neurothekeoma of Gallager and Helwig (dermal nerve sheath myxoma variant): report of a case with electron microscopic and immunohistochemical studies. J Cutan Pathol 1985; 12: 506–519.

222 Barnhill RL, Mihm MC Jr. Cellular neurothekeoma. A distinctive variant of neurothekeoma mimicking nevomelanocytic tumors. Am J Surg Pathol 1990; 14: 113–120.

223 Goette DK. Calcifying neurothekeoma. J Dermatol Surg Oncol 1986; 12: 958–960.

224 Rooney MT, Nascimento AG, Tung RLK. Ossifying plexiform tumor. Report of a cutaneous ossifying lesion with histologic features of neurothekeoma. Am J Dermatopathol 1994; 16: 189–192.

225 Calonje E, Wilson-Jones E, Smith NP, Fletcher CDM. Cellular 'neurothekeoma': an epithelioid variant of pilar leiomyoma? Morphological and immunohistochemical analysis of a series. Histopathology 1992; 20: 397–404.

226 Zelger BG, Steiner H, Kutzner H et al. Cellular 'neurothekeoma': an epithelioid variant of dermatofibroma? Histopathology 1998; 32: 414–422.

227 Watanabe K, Kusakabe T, Hoshi N, Suzuki T. Subcutaneous cellular neurothekeoma: a pseudosarcomatous tumour. Br J Dermatol 2001; 144: 1273–1274.

228 Argenyi ZB, LeBoit PE, Santa Cruz D et al. Nerve sheath myxoma (neurothekeoma) of the skin: light microscopic and immunohistochemical reappraisal of the cellular variant. J Cutan Pathol 1993; 20: 294–303.

229 Husain S, Silvers DN, Halperin AJ, McNutt NS. Histologic spectrum of neurothekeoma and the value of immunoperoxidase staining for S-100 protein in distinguishing it from melanoma. Am J Dermatopathol 1994; 16: 496–503.

230 Strumia R, Lombardi AR, Cavazzini L. S-100 negative myxoid neurothekeoma. Am J Dermatopathol 2001; 23: 82–83.

231 Barnhill RL. Nerve sheath myxoma (neurothekeoma). J Cutan Pathol 1994; 21: 91–93.

232 Tomasini C, Aloi F, Pippione M. Cellular neurothekeoma. Dermatology 1996; 192: 160–163.

233 Laskin WB, Fetsch JF, Miettinen M. The "neurothekeoma": immunohistochemical analysis distinguishes the true nerve sheath myxoma from its mimics. Hum Pathol 2000; 31: 1230–1241.

234 Weiser G. An electron microscope study of "pacinian neurofibroma". Virchows Arch [A] 1975; 366: 331–340.

235 Webb JN. The histogenesis of nerve sheath myxoma: report of a case with electron microscopy. J Pathol 1979; 127: 35–37.

236 Argenyi ZB, Kutzner H, Seaba MM. Ultrastructural spectrum of cutaneous nerve sheath myxoma/cellular neurothekeoma. J Cutan Pathol 1995; 22: 137–145.

237 Apisarnthanarax P. Granular cell tumor. An analysis of 16 cases and review of the literature. J Am Acad Dermatol 1981; 5: 171–182.

238 Lack EE, Worsham GF, Callihan MD et al. Granular cell tumor: a clinicopathologic study of 110 patients. J Surg Oncol 1980; 13: 301–316.

239 Enghardt MH, Jordan SE. Granular cell tumor of a digital nerve. Cancer 1991; 68: 1764–1769.

240 Ordóñez NG. Granular cell tumor: a review and update. Adv Anat Pathol 1999; 6: 186–203.

241 Peterson LJ. Granular-cell tumor. Review of the literature and report of a case. Oral Surg 1974; 37: 728–735.

242 Ortiz-Hidalgo C, de la Vega G, Moreno-Collado C. Granular cell tumor (Abrikossoff tumor) of the clitoris. Int J Dermatol 1997; 36: 935–937.

243 Khansur T, Balducci L, Tavassoli M. Granular cell tumor. Clinical spectrum of the benign and malignant entity. Cancer 1987; 60: 220–222.

244 Apted JH. Multiple granular-cell myoblastoma (schwannoma) in a child. Br J Dermatol 1968; 80: 257–260.

245 Guenther L, Shum D. Granular cell tumor of the vulva. Pediatr Dermatol 1993; 10: 153–155.

246 Price ML, MacDonald DM. Multiple granular cell tumour. Clin Exp Dermatol 1984; 9: 375–378.

247 Papageorgiou S, Litt JZ, Pomeranz JR. Multiple granular cell myoblastomas in children. Arch Dermatol 1967; 96: 168–171.

248 Goette DK, Olson EG. Multiple cutaneous granular cell tumors. Int J Dermatol 1982; 21: 271–272.

249 Noppakun N, Apisarnthanarax P. Multiple cutaneous granular cell tumors simulating prurigo nodularis. Int J Dermatol 1981; 20: 126–129.

250 Guiglia MC, Prendiville JS. Multiple granular cell tumors associated with giant speckled lentiginous nevus and nevus flammeus in a child. J Am Acad Dermatol 1991; 24: 359–363.

251 Seiter S, Ugurel S, Tilgen W, Reinhold U. Multiple granular cell tumors and growth hormone deficiency in a child. Pediatr Dermatol 1999; 16: 308–310.

252 Dorta S, Sánchez R, García-Bustinduy M et al. Multiple granular cell tumour in a teenager. Br J Dermatol 2000; 143: 906–907.

253 Seo IS, Azzarelli B, Warner TF et al. Multiple visceral and cutaneous granular cell tumors. Ultrastructural and immunocytochemical evidence of Schwann cell origin. Cancer 1984; 53: 2104–2110.

254 Bakos L. Multiple cutaneous granular cell tumors with systemic defects: a distinct entity? Int J Dermatol 1993; 32: 432–435.

255 Sahn EE, Dunlavey ES, Parsons JL. Multiple cutaneous granular cell tumors in a child with possible neurofibromatosis. J Am Acad Dermatol 1996; 34: 327–330.

256 Lack EE, Crawford BE, Worsham GF et al. Gingival granular cell tumors of the newborn (congenital "epulis"). Am J Surg Pathol 1981; 5: 37–46.

257 de la Monte SM, Radowsky M, Hood AF. Congenital granular-cell neoplasms. An unusual case report with ultrastructural findings and a review of the literature. Am J Dermatopathol 1986; 8: 57–63.

258 Simsir A, Osborne BM, Greenebaum E. Malignant granular cell tumor: a case report and review of the recent literature. Hum Pathol 1996; 27: 853–858.

259 Gamboa LG. Malignant granular-cell myoblastoma. Arch Pathol 1955; 60: 663–668.

260 Cadotte M. Malignant granular-cell myoblastoma. Cancer 1974; 33: 1417–1422.

261 Robertson AJ, McIntosh W, Lamont P, Guthrie W. Malignant granular cell tumour (myoblastoma) of the vulva: report of a case and review of the literature. Histopathology 1981; 5: 69–79.

262 Klima M, Peters J. Malignant granular cell tumor. Arch Pathol Lab Med 1987; 111: 1070–1073.

263 Thunold S, von Eyben FE, Maehle B. Malignant granular cell tumour of the neck: immunohistochemical and ultrastructural studies of a case. Histopathology 1989; 14: 655–657.

264 Gokaslan ST, Terzakis JA, Santagada EA. Malignant granular cell tumor. J Cutan Pathol 1994; 21: 263–270.

265 Miracco C, Andreassi A, Laurini L et al. Granular cell tumour with histological signs of malignancy: report of a case and comparison with 10 benign and 4 atypical cases. Br J Dermatol 1999; 41: 573–575.

266 Schoedel KE, Bastacky S, Silverman A. An S100 negative granular cell tumor with malignant potential: Report of a case. J Am Acad Dermatol 1998; 39: 894–898.

267 Finkel G, Lane B. Granular cell variant of neurofibromatosis: ultrastructure of benign and malignant tumors. Hum Pathol 1982; 13: 959–963.

268 Buley ID, Gatter KC, Kelly PMA et al. Granular cell tumours revisited. An immunohistological and ultrastructural study. Histopathology 1988; 12: 263–274.

269 Penneys NS, Adachi K, Ziegels-Weissman J, Nadji M. Granular cell tumors of the skin contain myelin basic protein. Arch Pathol Lab Med 1983; 107: 302–303.

270 Lack EE, Perez-Atayde AR, McGill TJ, Vawter GF. Gingival granuloma cell tumor of the newborn (congenital "epulis"): ultrastructural observations relating to histogenesis. Hum Pathol 1982; 13: 686–689.

271 Sobel HJ, Marquet E, Schwarz R. Is schwannoma related to granular cell myoblastoma? Arch Pathol 1973; 95: 396–401.

272 Alkek DS, Johnson WC, Graham JH. Granular cell myoblastoma. A histological and enzymatic study. Arch Dermatol 1968; 98: 543–547.

273 Lee J, Bhawan J, Wax F, Farber J. Plexiform granular cell tumor. A report of two cases. Am J Dermatopathol 1994; 16: 537–541.

274 Usmani AS, Pellegrini AE, Hessel AB et al. Plexiform granular cell tumor. Am J Dermatopathol 2000; 22: 344 (abstract).

275 Cheng SD, Usmani AS, DeYoung BR et al. Dermatofibroma-like granular cell tumor. J Cutan Pathol 2001; 28: 49–52.

276 McMahon JN, Rigby HS, Davies JD. Elastosis in granular cell tumours: prevalence and distribution. Histopathology 1990; 16: 37–41.

277 LeBoit PE, Barr RJ, Burall S et al. Primitive polypoid granular-cell tumor and other cutaneous granular-cell neoplasms of apparent nonneural origin. Am J Surg Pathol 1991; 15: 48–58.

278 Stefansson K, Wollmann RL. S-100 protein in granular cell tumors (granular cell myoblastomas). Cancer 1982; 49: 1834–1838.

279 Armin A, Connelly EM, Rowden G. An immunoperoxidase investigation of S-100 protein in granular cell myoblastomas: evidence for schwann cell derivation. Am J Clin Pathol 1983; 79: 37–44.

280 Raju GC, O'Reilly AP. Immunohistochemical study of granular cell tumour. Pathology 1987; 19: 402–406.

281 Mahalingam M, LoPiccolo D, Byers HR. Expression of PGP 9.5 in granular cell nerve sheath tumors: an immunohistochemical study of six cases. J Cutan Pathol 2001; 28: 282–286.

282 Kanitakis J, Mauduit G, Viac J, Thivolet J. [Granular cell tumour (Abrikosoff). Immunohistological study of four cases with review of the literature]. Ann Dermatol Venereol 1985; 112: 871–876.

283 Ingram DL, Mossler JA, Snowhite J et al. Granular cell tumors of the breast. Arch Pathol Lab Med 1984; 108: 897–901.

284 Matthews JB, Mason GI. Granular cell myoblastoma: an immunoperoxidase study using a variety of antisera to human carcinoembryonic antigen. Histopathology 1983; 7: 77–82.

285 Kanitakis J, Zambruno G, Viac J, Thivolet J. Granular-cell tumours of the skin do not express carcino-embryonic antigen. J Cutan Pathol 1986; 13: 370–374.

286 Chang SE, Choi JH, Sung KJ et al. Congenital CD34-positive granular cell dendrocytosis. J Cutan Pathol 1999; 26: 253–258.

287 Manara GC, De Panfilis G, Bottazzi Bacchi A et al. Fine structure of granular cell tumor of Abrikossoff. J Cutan Pathol 1981; 8: 277–282.

288 Christian MA, Gambarelli D, Hassoun J et al. Granular cell myoblastoma. J Cutan Pathol 1977; 4: 80–89.

289 Storm FK, Eilber FR, Mirra J, Morton DL. Neurofibrosarcoma. Cancer 1980; 45: 126–129.

290 Dabski C, Reiman HM Jr, Muller SA. Neurofibrosarcoma of skin and subcutaneous tissues. Mayo Clin Proc 1990; 65: 164–172.

291 Das Gupta TK, Brasfield RD. Solitary malignant schwannoma. Ann Surg 1970; 171: 419–428.

292 Robson DK, Ironside JW. Malignant peripheral nerve sheath tumour arising in a schwannoma. Histopathology 1990; 16: 295–308.

293 Kikuchi A, Akiyama M, Han-yaku H et al. Solitary cutaneous malignant schwannoma: immunohistochemical and ultrastructural studies. Am J Dermatopathol 1993; 15: 15–19.

294 Ogata H, Sawada Y, Narita T et al. Solitary malignant schwannoma of the lower extremity – a case report. Clin Exp Dermatol 1996; 21: 383–387.

295 Trojanowski JQ, Kleinman GM, Proppe KH. Malignant tumors of nerve sheath origin. Cancer 1980; 46: 1202–1212.

296 George E, Swanson PE, Wick MR. Malignant peripheral nerve sheath tumors of the skin. Am J Dermatopathol 1989; 11: 213–221.

297 Misago N, Ishii Y, Kohda H. Malignant peripheral nerve sheath tumor of the skin: a superficial form of this tumor. J Cutan Pathol 1996; 23: 182–188.

298 Mogollon R, Penneys N, Albores-Saavedra J, Nadji M. Malignant schwannoma presenting as a skin mass. Cancer 1984; 53: 1190–1193.

299 Hirose T, Scheithauer BW, Sano T. Perineurial malignant peripheral nerve sheath tumor (MPNST). A clinicopathologic, immunohistochemical, and ultrastructural study of seven cases. Am J Surg Pathol 1998; 22: 1368–1378.

300 Sordillo PP, Helson L, Hadju SI et al. Malignant schwannoma – clinical characteristics, survival, and response to therapy. Cancer 1981; 47: 2503–2509.

301 Wanebo JE, Malik JM, VandenBerg SR et al. Malignant peripheral nerve sheath tumors. A clinicopathologic study of 28 cases. Cancer 1993; 71: 1247–1253.

302 Hajdu SI. Peripheral nerve sheath tumors. Histogenesis, classification, and prognosis. Cancer 1993; 72: 3549–3552.

303 Ghosh BC, Ghosh L, Huvos AG, Fortner JG. Malignant schwannoma. A clinicopathologic study. Cancer 1973; 31: 184–190.

304 Taxy JB, Battifora H, Trujillo Y, Dorfman HD. Electron microscopy in the diagnosis of malignant schwannoma. Cancer 1981; 48: 1381–1391.

305 Meis-Kindblom JM, Enzinger FM. Plexiform malignant peripheral nerve sheath tumor of infancy and childhood. Am J Surg Pathol 1994; 18: 479–485.

306 Di Carlo EF, Woodruff JM, Bansal M, Erlandson RA. The purely epithelioid malignant peripheral nerve sheath tumor. Am J Surg Pathol 1986; 10: 478–490.

307 Suster S, Amazon K, Rosen LB, Ollague JM. Malignant epithelioid schwannoma of the skin. A low-grade neurotropic malignant melanoma? Am J Dermatopathol 1989; 11: 338–344.

308 Laskin WB, Weiss SW, Bratthauer GL. Epithelioid variant of malignant peripheral nerve sheath tumor (malignant epithelioid schwannoma). Am J Surg Pathol 1991; 15: 1136–1145.

309 Shimizu S, Teraki Y, Ishiko A et al. Malignant epithelioid schwannoma of the skin showing partial HMB-45 positivity. Am J Dermatopathol 1993; 15: 378–384.

310 Meis JM, Enzinger FM, Martz KL, Neal JA. Malignant peripheral nerve sheath tumors (malignant schwannomas) in children. Am J Surg Pathol 1992; 16: 694–707.

311 Sangüeza OP, Requena L. Neoplasms with neural differentiation: a review. Part II: malignant neoplasms. Am J Dermatopathol 1998; 20: 89–102.

312 McMenamin ME, Fletcher CDM. Expanding the spectrum of malignant change in schwannomas. Epithelioid malignant change, epithelioid malignant nerve sheath tumor, and epithelioid angiosarcoma: a study of 17 cases. Am J Surg Pathol 2001; 25: 13–25.

313 Morphopoulos GD, Banerjee SS, Ali HH et al. Malignant peripheral nerve sheath tumour with vascular differentiation: a report of four cases. Histopathology 1996; 28: 401–410.

314 Ducatman BS, Scheithauer BW. Malignant peripheral nerve sheath tumors with divergent differentiation. Cancer 1984; 54: 1049–1057.

315 Morgan MB, Stevens L, Patterson J, Tannenbaum M. Cutaneous epithelioid malignant nerve sheath tumor with rhabdoid features: a histologic, immunohistochemical, and ultrastructural study of three cases. J Cutan Pathol 2000; 27: 529–534.

316 Daimaru Y, Hashimoto H, Enjoji M. Malignant "triton" tumors: a clinicopathologic and immunohistochemical study of nine cases. Hum Pathol 1984; 15: 768–778.

317 Kiryu H, Urabe H. Malignant triton tumor. A case with protean histopathological patterns. Am J Dermatopathol 1992; 14: 255–262.

318 Markel SF, Enzinger FM. Neuromuscular hamartoma: a benign "triton tumor" composed of mature neural and striated muscle elements. Cancer 1982; 49: 140–144.

319 Wick MR. Immunohistology of neuroendocrine and neuroectodermal tumors. Semin Diagn Pathol 2000; 17: 194–203.

320 Smith TA, Machen SK, Fisher C, Goldblum JR. Usefulness of cytokeratin subsets for distinguishing monophasic synovial sarcoma from malignant peripheral nerve sheath tumor. Am J Clin Pathol 1999; 112: 641–648.

321 Hirose T, Hasegawa T, Kudo E et al. Malignant peripheral nerve sheath tumors: an immunohistochemical study in relation to ultrastructural features. Hum Pathol 1992; 23: 865–870.

Herniations and ectopias

322 Fletcher CDM, Carpenter G, McKee PH. Nasal glioma. A rarity. Am J Dermatopathol 1986; 8: 341–346.

323 Paller AS, Pensler JM, Tomita T. Nasal midline masses in infants and children. Dermoids, encephaloceles, and gliomas. Arch Dermatol 1991; 127: 362–366.

324 Yashar SS, Newbury RO, Cunningham BB. Congenital midline nasal mass in a toddler. Pediatr Dermatol 2000; 17: 62–64.

325 Kopf AW, Bart RS. Nasal glioma. J Dermatol Surg Oncol 1978; 4: 128–130.

326 Lowe RS, Robinson DW, Ketchum LD, Masters FW. Nasal gliomata. Plast Reconstr Surg 1971; 47: 1–5.

327 Berry AD III, Patterson JW. Meningoceles, meningomyeloceles, and encephaloceles: a neuro-dermatopathologic study of 132 cases. J Cutan Pathol 1990; 18: 164–177.

328 Commens C, Rogers M, Kan A. Heterotopic brain tissue presenting as bald cysts with a collar of hypertrophic hair. The 'hair collar' sign. Arch Dermatol 1989; 125: 1253–1256.

329 Orkin M, Fisher I. Heterotopic brain tissue (heterotopic neural rest). Arch Dermatol 1966; 94: 699–708.

330 Musser AW, Campbell R. Nasal glioma. Arch Otolaryngol 1961; 73: 732–736.

331 Khallouf R, Fétissof F, Machet MC et al. Sequestrated meningocele of the scalp: diagnostic value of hair anomalies. Pediatr Dermatol 1994; 11: 315–318.

332 Skelton HG, Smith KJ. Glial heterotopia in the subcutaneous tissue overlying T-12. J Cutan Pathol 1999; 26: 523–527.

333 Gebhart W, Hohlbrugger H, Lassmann H, Ramadan W. Nasal glioma. Int J Dermatol 1982; 21: 212–215.

334 Kashani AH, Hutchins GM. Meningeal-cutaneous relationships in anencephaly: evidence for a primary mesenchymal abnormality. Hum Pathol 2001; 32: 553–558.

335 Christianson HB. Nasal glioma. Arch Dermatol 1966; 93: 68–70.

336 Mirra SS, Pearl GS, Hoffman JC, Campbell WG. Nasal 'glioma' with prominent neuronal component. Arch Pathol Lab Med 1981; 105: 540–541.

337 Theaker JM, Fletcher CDM. Heterotopic glial nodules: a light microscopic and immunohistochemical study. Histopathology 1991; 18: 255–260.

338 Gambini C, Rongioletti F, Rebora A. Proliferation of eccrine sweat ducts associated with heterotopic neural tissue (nasal glioma). Am J Dermatopathol 2000; 22: 179–182.

339 Lee CM, McLaurin RL. Heterotopic brain tissue as an isolated embryonic rest. J Neurosurg 1955; 12: 190–195.

340 Argenyi ZB. Cutaneous neural heterotopias and related tumors relevant for the dermatopathologist. Semin Diagn Pathol 1996; 13: 60–71.

341 Theaker JM, Fleming KA. Meningioma of the scalp: a case report with immunohistological features. J Cutan Pathol 1987; 14: 49–53.

342 Theaker JM, Fletcher CDM, Tudway AJ. Cutaneous heterotopic meningeal nodules. Histopathology 1990; 16: 475–479.

343 Nochomovitz LE, Jannotta F, Orenstein JM. Meningioma of the scalp. Light and electron microscopic observations. Arch Pathol Lab Med 1985; 109: 92–95.

344 Lopez DA, Silvers DN, Helwig EB. Cutaneous meningiomas – a clinicopathologic study. Cancer 1974; 34: 728–744.

345 Peñas PF, Jones-Caballero M, Amigo A et al. Cutaneous meningioma underlying congenital localized hypertrichosis. J Am Acad Dermatol 1994; 30: 363–366.

346 Peñas PF, Jones-Cabellero M, Garcia-Diez A. Cutaneous heterotopic meningeal nodules. Arch Dermatol 1995; 131: 731.

347 Tron V, Bellamy C, Wood W. Familial cutaneous heterotopic meningeal nodules. J Am Acad Dermatol 1993; 28: 1015–1017.

348 Sibley DA, Cooper PH. Rudimentary meningocele: a variant of "primary cutaneous meningioma". J Cutan Pathol 1989; 16: 72–80.

349 Stone MS, Walker PS, Kennard CD. Rudimentary meningocele presenting with a scalp hair tuft. Arch Dermatol 1994; 130: 775–777.

350 Marrogi AJ, Swanson PE, Kyriakos M, Wick MR. Rudimentary meningocele of the skin. Clinicopathologic features and differential diagnosis. J Cutan Pathol 1991; 18: 178–188.

351 El Shabrawi-Caelen L, White WL, Soyer HP et al. Rudimentary meningocele – remnant of a neural tube defect? Am J Dermatopathol 2000; 22: 357 (abstract).

352 Chan HHL, Fung JWK, Lam WM, Choi P. The clinical spectrum of rudimentary meningocele. Pediatr Dermatol 1998; 15: 388–389.

353 El Shabrawi-Caelen L, White WL, Soyer HP et al. Rudimentary meningocele: remnant of a neural tube defect? Arch Dermatol 2001; 137: 45–50.

354 Umbert I, Nasarre J, Rovira E, Umbert P. Cutaneous meningioma: report of a case with immunohistochemical study. J Cutan Pathol 1989; 16: 328 (abstract).

355 Iglesias ME, Vázquez-Doval FJ, Idoate MA et al. Intracranial osteolytic meningioma affecting the scalp. J Am Acad Dermatol 1996; 35: 641–642.

356 Argenyi ZB, Thieberg MD, Hayes CM, Whitaker DC. Primary cutaneous meningioma associated with von Recklinghausen's disease. J Cutan Pathol 1994; 21: 549–556.

357 Brugler G. Tumors presenting as aural polyps: a report of four cases. Pathology 1992; 24: 315–319.

358 Suster S, Rosai J. Hamartoma of the scalp with ectopic meningothelial elements. A distinctive benign soft tissue lesion that may simulate angiosarcoma. Am J Surg Pathol 1990; 14: 1–11.

359 Gelli MC, Pasquinelli G, Martinelli G, Gardini G. Cutaneous meningioma: histochemical, immunohistochemical and ultrastructural investigation. Histopathology 1993; 23: 576–578.

360 Barr RJ, Yi ES, Jensen JL et al. Meningioma-like tumor of the skin. An ultrastructural and immunohistochemical study. Am J Surg Pathol 1993; 17: 779–787.

Neuroendocrine carcinomas

361 Toker C. Trabecular carcinoma of the skin. Arch Dermatol 1972; 105: 107–110.

362 Tang C-K, Toker C. Trabecular carcinoma of the skin. An ultrastructural study. Cancer 1978; 42: 2311–2321.

363 Rocamora A, Badia N, Vives R et al. Epidermotropic primary neuroendocrine (Merkel cell) carcinoma of the skin with Pautrier-like microabscesses. Report of three cases and review of the literature. J Am Acad Dermatol 1987; 16: 1163–1168.

364 Hoefler H, Rauch H-J, Kerl H, Denk H. New immunocytochemical observations with diagnostic significance in cutaneous neuroendocrine carcinoma. Am J Dermatopathol 1984; 6: 525–530.

365 Wick MR, Scheithauer BW. In: Wick MR. Pathology of unusual malignant cutaneous tumors. New York: Marcel Dekker, 1985: 107–180.

366 Foschini MP, Eusebi V. The spectrum of endocrine tumours of skin. Curr Diagn Pathol 1995; 2: 2–9.

367 Sibley RK, Dehner LP, Rosai J. Primary neuroendocrine (Merkel cell?) carcinoma of the skin. I. A clinicopathologic and ultrastructural study of 43 cases. Am J Surg Pathol 1985; 9: 95–108.

368 Jemec B, Chana J, Grover R, Grobbelaar AO. The Merkel cell carcinoma: survival and oncogene markers. J Eur Acad Dermatol Venereol 2000; 14: 400–404.

369 Micali G, Ferraú F, Innocenzi D. Primary Merkel cell tumor: a clinical analysis of eight cases. Int J Dermatol 1993; 32: 345–349.

370 Schmid Ch, Beham A, Feichtinger J et al. Recurrent and subsequently metastasizing Merkel cell carcinoma in a 7-year-old girl. Histopathology 1992; 20: 437–439.

371 Ziprin P, Smith S, Salerno G, Rosin RD. Two cases of Merkel cell tumour arising in patients with chronic lymphocytic leukaemia. Br J Dermatol 2000; 142: 525–528.

372 Warakaulle DR, Rytina E, Burrows NP. Merkel cell tumour associated with chronic lymphocytic leukaemia. Br J Dermatol 2001; 144: 216–217.

373 Lien H-C, Tsai T-F, Lee YY, Hsiao C-H. Merkel cell carcinoma and chronic arsenicism. J Am Acad Dermatol 1999; 41: 641–643.

374 Tsuruta D, Hamada T, Mochida K et al. Merkel cell carcinoma, Bowen's disease and chronic occupational arsenic poisoning. Br J Dermatol 1998; 139: 291–294.

375 Gooptu C, Woollons A, Ross J et al. Merkel cell carcinoma arising after therapeutic immunosuppression. Br J Dermatol 1997; 137: 637–641.

376 Urbatsch A, Sams WM Jr, Urist MM, Sturdivant R. Merkel cell carcinoma occurring in renal transplant patients. J Am Acad Dermatol 1999; 41: 289–291.

377 Gilaberte M, Pujol RM, Sierra J et al. Merkel cell carcinoma developing after bone marrow transplantation. Dermatology 2000; 201: 80–82.

378 Wick MR, Thomas JR, Scheithauer BW, Jackson IT. Multifocal Merkel's cell tumors associated with a cutaneous dysplasia syndrome. Arch Dermatol 1983; 119: 409–414.

379 Moya CE, Guarda LA, Dyer GA et al. Neuroendocrine carcinoma of the skin in a young adult. Am J Clin Pathol 1982; 78: 783–785.

380 Brenner B, Sulkes A, Rakowsky E et al. Second neoplasms in patients with Merkel cell carcinoma. Cancer 2001; 91: 1358–1362.

381 Pilotti S, Rilke F, Lombardi L. Neuroendocrine (Merkel cell) carcinoma of the skin. Am J Dermatopathol 1982; 6: 243–254.

382 Akhtar S, Oza KK, Wright J. Merkel cell carcinoma: Report of 10 cases and review of the literature. J Am Acad Dermatol 2000; 43: 755–767.

383 Tyring SK, Lee PC, Omura EF et al. Recurrent and metastatic cutaneous neuroendocrine (Merkel cell) carcinoma mimicking angiosarcoma. Arch Dermatol 1987; 123: 1368–1370.

384 Goldenhersh MA, Prus D, Ron N, Rosenmann E. Merkel cell tumor masquerading as granulation tissue on a teenager's toe. Am J Dermatopathol 1992; 14: 560–563.

385 Tada J, Toi Y, Yamada T et al. Giant neuroendocrine (Merkel cell) carcinoma of the skin. J Am Acad Dermatol 1991; 24: 827–831.

386 Chiarelli TG, Grant-Kels JM, Sporn JR et al. Unusual presentation of a Merkel cell carcinoma. J Am Acad Dermatol 2000; 42: 366–370.

387 Raaf JH, Urmacher C, Knapper WK et al. Trabecular (Merkel cell) carcinoma of the skin. Treatment of primary, recurrent, and metastatic disease. Cancer 1986; 57: 178–182.

388 Haag ML, Glass LF, Fenske NA. Merkel cell carcinoma. Diagnosis and treatment. Dermatol Surg 1995; 21: 669–683.

389 Hanke CW, Conner AC, Temofeew RK, Lingeman RE. Merkel cell carcinoma. Arch Dermatol 1989; 125: 1096–1100.

390 O'Rourke MGE, Bell JR. Merkel cell tumor with spontaneous regression. J Dermatol Surg Oncol 1986; 12: 994–997.

391 Duncan WC, Tschen JA. Spontaneous regression of Merkel cell (neuroendocrine) carcinoma of the skin. J Am Acad Dermatol 1993; 29: 653–654.

392 Kayashima K, Ono T, Johno M et al. Spontaneous regression in Merkel cell (neuroendocrine) carcinoma of the skin. Arch Dermatol 1991; 127: 550–553.

393 Yanguas I, Goday JJ, González-Güemes M et al. Spontaneous regression of Merkel cell carcinoma of the skin. Br J Dermatol 1997; 137: 296–298.

394 Maruo K, Kayashima K-I, Ono T. Regressing Merkel cell carcinoma – a case showing replacement of tumour cells by foamy cells. Br J Dermatol 2000; 142: 1184–1189.

395 Allen PJ, Zhang Z-F, Coit DG. Surgical management of Merkel cell carcinoma. Ann Surg 1999; 229: 97–105.

396 Krasagakis K, Almond-Roesler B, Zouboulis CC et al. Merkel cell carcinoma: Report of ten cases with emphasis on clinical course, treatment, and in vitro drug sensitivity. J Am Acad Dermatol 1997; 36: 727–732.

397 Gollard R, Weber R, Kosty MP et al. Merkel cell carcinoma. Review of 22 cases with surgical, pathologic, and therapeutic considerations. Cancer 2000; 88: 1842–1851.

398 Waldmann V, Goldschmidt H, Jäckel A et al. Transient complete remission of metastasized Merkel cell carcinoma by high-dose polychemotherapy and autologous peripheral blood stem cell transplantation. Br J Dermatol 2000; 143: 837–839.

399 Voog E, Biron P, Martin J-P, Blay J-Y. Chemotherapy for patients with locally advanced or metastatic Merkel cell carcinoma. Cancer 1999; 85: 2589–2595.

400 Eusebi V, Capella C, Cossu A, Rosai J. Neuroendocrine carcinoma within lymph nodes in the absence of a primary tumor, with special reference to merkel cell carcinoma. Am J Surg Pathol 1992; 16: 658–666.

401 Rustin MHA, Chambers TJ, Levison DA, Munro DD. Merkel cell tumour: report of a case. Br J Dermatol 1983; 108: 711–715.

402 Silva EG, Ordonez NG, Lechago J. Immunohistochemical studies in endocrine carcinoma of the skin. Am J Clin Pathol 1984; 81: 558–562.

403 Eggers SDZ, Salomao DR, Dinapoli RP, Vernino S. Paraneoplastic and metastatic neurologic complications of Merkel cell carcinoma. Mayo Clin Proc 2001; 76: 327–330.

404 Leonard JH, Bell JR. Insights into the Merkel cell phenotype from Merkel cell carcinoma cell lines. Australas J Dermatol 1997; 38 (Suppl): S91–S98.

405 Ratner D, Nelson BR, Brown MD, Johnson TM. Merkel cell carcinoma. J Am Acad Dermatol 1993; 29: 143–156.

406 Frigerio B, Capella C, Eusebi V et al. Merkel cell carcinoma of the skin: the structure and origin of normal Merkel cells. Histopathology 1983; 7: 229–249.

407 Leong A S-Y, Phillips GE, Pieterse AS, Milios J. Criteria for the diagnosis of primary endocrine carcinoma of the skin (Merkel cell carcinoma). A histological, immunohistochemical and ultrastructural study of 13 cases. Pathology 1986; 18: 393–399.

408 Warner TFCS, Uno H, Hafez GR et al. Merkel cells and Merkel cell tumors. Ultrastructure, immunocytochemistry and review of the literature. Cancer 1983; 52: 238–245.

409 Kossard S, Wittal R, Killingsworth M. Merkel cell carcinoma with a desmoplastic portion. Am J Dermatopathol 1995; 17: 517–522.

410 Schnitt SJ, Wang H, Dvorak AM. Morphologic changes in primary neuroendocrine carcinoma of the skin following radiation therapy. Hum Pathol 1986; 17: 198–201.

411 Zak FG, Lawson W, Statsinger AL et al. Intracellular amyloid in trabecular (Merkel cell) carcinoma of the skin: ultrastructural study. Mt Sinai J Med 1982; 49: 46–54.

412 Abaci IF, Zac FG. Multicentric amyloid containing cutaneous trabecular carcinoma. Case report with ultrastructural study. J Cutan Pathol 1979; 6: 292–303.

413 Gillham SL, Morrison RG, Hurt MA. Epidermotrophic neuroendocrine carcinoma. Immunohistochemical differentiation from simulators, including malignant melanoma. J Cutan Pathol 1991; 18: 120–127.

414 Hashimoto K, Lee MW, D'Annunzio DR et al. Pagetoid Merkel cell carcinoma: epidermal origin of the tumor. J Cutan Pathol 1998; 25: 572–579.

415 Traest K, De Vos R, van den Oord JJ. Pagetoid Merkel cell carcinoma: speculations on its origin and the mechanism of epidermal spread. J Cutan Pathol 1999; 26: 362–365.

416 Smith KJ, Skelton HG III, Holland TT et al. Neuroendocrine (Merkel cell) carcinoma with an intraepidermal component. Am J Dermatopathol 1993; 15: 528–533.

417 Brown HA, Sawyer DM, Woo T. Intraepidermal Merkel cell carcinoma with no dermal involvement. Am J Dermatopathol 2000; 22: 65–69.

418 Kroll MH, Toker C. Trabecular carcinoma of the skin. Arch Pathol Lab Med 1982; 106: 404–408.

419 LeBoit PE, Crutcher WA, Shapiro PE. Pagetoid intraepidermal spread in Merkel cell (primary neuroendocrine) carcinoma of the skin. Am J Surg Pathol 1992; 16: 584–592.

420 Tang C-K, Nedwich A, Toker C, Zaman ANF. Unusual cutaneous carcinoma with features of small cell (oat cell-like) and squamous cell carcinomas. A variant of malignant Merkel cell neoplasm. Am J Dermatopathol 1982; 4: 537–548.

421 Gomez LG, Silva EG, Di Maio S, Mackay B. Association between neuroendocrine (Merkel cell) carcinoma and squamous carcinoma of the skin. Am J Surg Pathol 1983; 7: 171–177.

422 Iacocca MV, Abernethy JL, Stefanato CM et al. Mixed Merkel cell carcinoma and squamous cell carcinoma of the skin. J Am Acad Dermatol 1998; 39: 882–887.

423 Cerroni L, Kerl H. Primary cutaneous neuroendocrine (Merkel cell) carcinoma in association with squamous- and basal-cell carcinoma. Am J Dermatopathol 1997; 19: 610–613.

424 Layfield L, Ulich T, Liao S et al. Neuroendocrine carcinoma of the skin: an immunohistochemical study of tumor markers and neuroendocrine products. J Cutan Pathol 1986; 13: 268–273.

425 Gould E, Albores-Saavedra J, Dubner B et al. Eccrine and squamous differentiation in Merkel cell carcinoma. An immunohistochemical study. Am J Surg Pathol 1988; 12: 768–772.

426 Yamamoto O, Tanimoto A, Yasuda H et al. A combined occurrence of neuroendocrine carcinoma of the skin and a benign appendageal neoplasm. J Cutan Pathol 1993; 20: 173–176.

427 Isimbaldi G, Sironi M, Taccagni G et al. Tripartite differentiation (squamous, glandular, and melanocytic) of a primary cutaneous neuroendocrine carcinoma. Am J Dermatopathol 1993; 15: 260–264.

428 Rosso R, Paulli M, Carnevali L. Neuroendocrine carcinoma of the skin with lymphoepithelioma-like features. Am J Dermatopathol 1998; 20: 483–486.

429 Eusebi V, Damiani S, Pasquinelli G et al. Small cell neuroendocrine carcinoma with skeletal muscle differentiation. Report of three cases. Am J Surg Pathol 2000; 24: 223–230.

430 Bastian BC, Kreipe HH, Bröcker EB. Primary neuroendocrine carcinoma of the skin with an unusual follicular lymphocytic infiltrate of the dermis. Am J Dermatopathol 1996; 18: 625–628.

431 Rios-Martin JJ, Solorzano-Amoreti A, González-Cámpora R, Galera-Davidson H. Neuroendocrine carcinoma of the skin with a lymphoepithelioma-like histological pattern. Br J Dermatol 2000; 143: 460–462.

432 Foschini MP, Eusebi V. Divergent differentiation in endocrine and nonendocrine tumors of the skin. Semin Diagn Pathol 2000; 17: 162–168.

433 Cooper L, DeBono R, Alsanjari N, Al-Nafussi A. Merkel cell tumour with leiomyosarcomatous differentiation. Histopathology 2000; 36: 540–543.

434 Perse RM, Klappenbach S, Ragsdale BD. Trabecular (Merkel cell) carcinoma arising in the wall of an epidermal cyst. Am J Dermatopathol 1987; 9: 423–427.

435 Collina G, Bagni A, Fano RA. Combined neuroendocrine carcinoma of the skin (Merkel cell tumor) and trichilemmal cyst. Am J Dermatopathol 1997; 19: 545–548.

436 Takenaka H, Kishimoto S, Shibagaki R et al. Merkel cell carcinoma with partial spontaneous regression. An immunohistochemical, ultrastructural, and TUNEL labeling study. Am J Dermatopathol 1997; 19: 614–618.

437 Skelton HG, Smith KJ, Hitchcock CL et al. Merkel cell carcinoma: Analysis of clinical, histologic, and immunohistologic features of 132 cases with relation to survival. J Am Acad Dermatol 1997; 37: 734–739.

438 Feinmesser M, Halpern M, Fenig E et al. Expression of the apoptosis-related oncogenes bcl-2, bax, and p53 in Merkel cell carcinoma: can they predict treatment response and clinical outcome? Hum Pathol 1999; 30: 1367–1372.

439 Carson HJ, Reddy V, Taxy JB. Proliferation markers and prognosis in Merkel cell carcinoma. J Cutan Pathol 1998; 25: 16–19.

440 Wick MR, Kaye VN, Sibley RK et al. Primary neuroendocrine carcinoma and small-cell malignant lymphoma of the skin. A discriminant immunohistochemical comparison. J Cutan Pathol 1986; 13: 347–358.

441 Wick MR, Millns JL, Sibley RK et al. Secondary neuroendocrine carcinomas of the skin. J Am Acad Dermatol 1985; 13: 134–142.

442 Hall PA, D'Ardenne AJ, Butler MG et al. Cytokeratin and laminin immunostaining in the diagnosis of cutaneous neuro-endocrine (Merkel cell) tumours. Histopathology 1986; 10: 1179–1190.

443 Dreno B, Mousset S, Stalder JF et al. A study of intermediate filaments (cytokeratin, vimentin, neurofilament) in two cases of Merkel cell tumor. J Cutan Pathol 1985; 12: 37–45.

444 Tazawa T, Ito M, Okuda C, Sato Y. Immunohistochemical demonstration of simple epithelia-type keratin intermediate filament in a case of Merkel cell carcinoma. Arch Dermatol 1987; 123: 489–492.

445 Heenan PJ, Cole JM, Spagnolo DV. Primary cutaneous neuroendocrine carcinoma (Merkel cell tumor). An adnexal epithelial neoplasm. Am J Dermatopathol 1990; 12: 7–16.

446 Mount SL, Taatjes DJ. Neuroendocrine carcinoma of the skin (Merkel cell carcinoma). An immunoelectron-microscopic case study. Am J Dermatopathol 1994; 16: 60–65.

447 Alvarez-Gago T, Bullón MM, Rivera F et al. Intermediate filament aggregates in mitoses of primary cutaneous neuroendocrine (Merkel cell) carcinoma. Histopathology 1996; 28: 349–355.

448 Scott MP, Helm KF. Cytokeratin 20: a marker for diagnosing Merkel cell carcinoma. Am J Dermatopathol 1999; 21: 16–20.

449 Chan JKC, Suster S, Wenig BM et al. Cytokeratin 20 immunoreactivity distinguishes Merkel cell (primary cutaneous neuroendocrine) carcinomas and salivary gland small cell carcinomas from small cell carcinomas of various sites. Am J Surg Pathol 1997; 21: 226–234.

450 Schmidt U, Müller U, Metz KA, Leder L-D. Cytokeratin and neurofilament protein staining in Merkel cell carcinoma of the small cell type and small cell carcinoma of the lung. Am J Dermatopathol 1998; 20: 346–351.

451 Hanly AJ, Elgart GW, Jorda M et al. Analysis of thyroid transcription factor-1 and cytokeratin 20 separates merkel cell carcinoma from small cell carcinoma of lung. J Cutan Pathol 2000; 27: 118–120.

452 Herman CM, Reed JA, Shea CR, Prieto VG. Use of anti-CK20 for detection of lymph node micrometastases in Merkel cell carcinoma. J Cutan Pathol 2000; 27: 559–560 (abstract).

453 Sibley RK, Dahl D. Primary neuroendocrine (Merkel cell?) carcinoma of the skin. II. An immunocytochemical study of 21 cases. Am J Surg Pathol 1985; 9: 109–116.

454 Battifora H, Silva EG. The use of antikeratin antibodies in the immunohistochemical distinction between neuroendocrine (Merkel cell) carcinoma of the skin, lymphoma, and oat cell carcinoma. Cancer 1986; 58: 1040–1046.

455 Haneke E, Schulze H-J, Mahrle G. Immunohistochemical and immunoelectron microscopic demonstration of chromogranin A in formalin-fixed tissue of Merkel cell carcinoma. J Am Acad Dermatol 1993; 28: 222–226.

456 Uhara H, Wang Y-L, Matsumoto S et al. Expression of α subunit of guanine nucleotide-binding protein Go in merkel cell carcinoma. J Cutan Pathol 1995; 22: 146–148.

457 Johannessen JV, Gould VE. Neuroendocrine skin carcinoma associated with calcitonin production: a Merkel cell carcinoma? Hum Pathol 1980; 11: 586–589.

458 Drijkoningen M, De Wolf-Peeters C, van Limbergen E, Desmet V. Merkel cell tumor of the skin. An immunohistochemical study. Hum Pathol 1986; 17: 301–307.

459 Penneys NS, Shapiro S. CD44 expression in Merkel cell carcinoma may correlate with risk of metastasis. J Cutan Pathol 1994; 21: 22–26.

460 Kennedy MM, Blessing K, King G, Kerr KM. Expression of bcl-2 and p53 in Merkel cell carcinoma. An immunohistochemical study. Am J Dermatopathol 1996; 18: 273–277.

461 Moll I, Gillardon F, Waltering S et al. Differences of bcl-2 protein expression between Merkel cells and Merkel cell carcinomas. J Cutan Pathol 1996; 23: 109–117.

462 Gancberg D, Feoli F, Hamels J et al. Trisomy 6 in Merkel cell carcinoma: a recurrent chromosomal aberration. Histopathology 2000; 37: 445–451.

463 Vortmeyer AO, Merino MJ, Böni R et al. Genetic changes associated with primary Merkel cell carcinoma. Am J Clin Pathol 1998; 109: 565–570.

464 Härle M, Arens N, Moll I et al. Comparative genomic hybridization (CGH) discloses chromosomal and subchromosomal copy number changes in Merkel cell carcinomas. J Cutan Pathol 1996; 23: 391–397.

465 Sibley RK, Rosai J, Foucar E et al. Neuroendocrine (Merkel cell) carcinoma of the skin. A histologic and ultrastructural study of two cases. Am J Surg Pathol 1980; 4: 211–221.

466 Haneke E. Electron microscopy of Merkel cell carcinoma from formalin-fixed tissue. J Am Acad Dermatol 1985; 12: 487–492.

467 Kirkham N, Isaacson P. Merkel cell carcinoma: a report of three cases with neurone-specific enolase activity. Histopathology 1983; 7: 251–259.

468 Bayrou O, Avril MF, Charpentier P et al. Primary neuroendocrine carcinoma of the skin. Clinicopathologic study of 18 cases. J Am Acad Dermatol 1991; 24: 198–207.

469 Muijen GNP, Ruiter DJ, Warnaar SO. Intermediate filaments in Merkel cell tumors. Hum Pathol 1985; 16: 590–595.

470 Sidhu GS, Mullins JD, Feiner H et al. Merkel cell neoplasms. Histology, electron microscopy, biology, and histogenesis. Am J Dermatopathol 1980; 2: 101–119.

471 Nesland JM, Sobrinko-Simões MA, Holm R, Johannessen JV. Primitive neuroectodermal tumor (peripheral neuroblastoma). Ultrastruct Pathol 1985; 9: 59–64.

472 Dehner LP. Peripheral and central primitive neuroectodermal tumors. Arch Pathol Lab Med 1986; 110: 997–1005.

473 Seemayer TA, Thelmo WL, Bolande RP, Wiglesworth FW. Peripheral neuroectodermal tumors. Perspect Pediatr Pathol 1975; 2: 151–172.

474 Jurgens H, Bier V, Harms D et al. Malignant peripheral neuroectodermal tumors. A retrospective analysis of 42 patients. Cancer 1988; 61: 349–357.

475 Hashimoto H, Kiryu H, Enjoji M et al. Malignant neuroepithelioma (peripheral neuroblastoma). Am J Surg Pathol 1983; 7: 309–318.

476 Mierau GW. Extraskeletal Ewing's sarcoma (peripheral neuroepithelioma). Ultrastruct Pathol 1985; 9: 91–98.

477 Stefanko J, Turnbull AD, Helson L et al. Primitive neuroectodermal tumors of the chest wall. J Surg Oncol 1988; 37: 33–37.

478 Hasegawa SL, Davison JM, Rutten A et al. Primary cutaneous Ewing's sarcoma. Immunophenotypic and molecular cytogenetic evaluation of five cases. Am J Surg Pathol 1998; 22: 310–318.

479 Morris R, Sequeira J, Folpe A, Solomon A. Extraosseous Ewing's sarcoma (primitive neuroectodermal tumor) presenting in the skin. J Cutan Pathol 2000; 27: 566 (abstract).

480 Ahmad R, Mayol BR, Davis M, Rougraff BT. Extraskeletal Ewing's sarcoma. Cancer 1999; 85: 725–731.

481 Argenyi ZB, Bergfeld WF, McMahon JT et al. Primitive neuroectodermal tumor in the skin with features of neuroblastoma in an adult patient. J Cutan Pathol 1986; 13: 420–430.

432 Sangüeza OP, Sangüeza P, Valda LR et al. Multiple primitive neuroectodermal tumors. J Am Acad Dermatol 1994; 31: 356–361.

483 Banerjee SS, Agbamu DA, Eyden BP, Harris M. Clinicopathological characteristics of peripheral primitive neuroectodermal tumour of skin and subcutaneous tissue. Histopathology 1997; 31: 355–366.

484 Peters MS, Reiman HM, Muller SA. Cutaneous extraskeletal Ewing's sarcoma. J Cutan Pathol 1985; 12: 476–485.

485 Sexton CW, White WL. Primary cutaneous Ewing's family sarcoma. Report of a case with immunostaining for glycoprotein p30/32 *mic 2*. Am J Dermatopathol 1996; 18: 601–605.

486 Patterson JW, Maygarden SJ. Extraskeletal Ewing's sarcoma with cutaneous involvement. J Cutan Pathol 1986; 13: 46–58.

487 Sur M, Cooper K. PNETs everywhere. Histopathology 1999; 35: 279–280.

Vascular tumors

INTRODUCTION

This chapter is based on the one written for the last edition by Geoffrey Strutton. His contribution is gratefully acknowledged.

A renewed interest in vascular tumors was provoked by the emergence of AIDS-related Kaposi's sarcoma in the 1980s, and since then a number of new entities have been described.[1] Although many of these are rare, they may produce diagnostic dilemmas, several having many features in common with Kaposi's sarcoma.

The classification of the vascular tumors and ectasias is far from straightforward. First, there is difficulty in separating true neoplasms from reactive proliferations or developmental abnormalities. Secondly, some vascular lesions represent a dilatation of pre-existing vessels rather than a proliferation of new vessels. Finally, it may be difficult to distinguish between a lesion showing blood vessel differentiation and one with lymphatic features as, for example, in the case of Kaposi's sarcoma. Immunohistochemical, ultrastructural and morphometric studies are helping to resolve some of these difficulties.

Vascular abnormalities of the skin are common. Approximately 50% of all neonates have some type of congenital vascular lesion.[2] The classification adopted here is based on recently delineated clinical classifications.[3] The distinction between malformations and vascular proliferations (tumors) has important clinical consequences. The distinction is more clear cut clinically than it is on a shave or punch biopsy of skin. This is a dilemma that remains to be resolved (Fig. 38.1). Furthermore, some overlap does occur between vascular tumors and malformations.[4,5] The following categories will be considered:

- hamartomas and malformations
- vascular dilatations (telangiectases)
- vascular proliferations
- tumors with variable or uncertain behavior
- malignant tumors
- tumors with a significant vascular component.

HAMARTOMAS AND MALFORMATIONS

Hamartomas result from an error in embryological development and are present at birth. In the case of vascular hamartomas and malformations, they may become more obvious clinically some time after birth as a consequence of progressive ectasia. The constituent vessels may be capillaries, veins, arteries, lymphatics or a combination of these vessels. Vascular malformations are associated with a range of dysmorphic syndromes such as the Sturge–Weber syndrome and 'blue rubber bleb' nevus syndrome (see below).

ECCRINE ANGIOMATOUS HAMARTOMA

Eccrine angiomatous hamartoma is a rare malformation characterized by an increased number of small blood vessels, admixed with or adjacent to an increased number of eccrine glands (see p. 888). There may also be an increase in mucin, fat or nerve fibers.

PHAKOMATOSIS PIGMENTOVASCULARIS

The term 'phakomatosis pigmentovascularis' refers to the coexistence of a vascular hamartoma, in the form of nevus flammeus, with a melanocytic

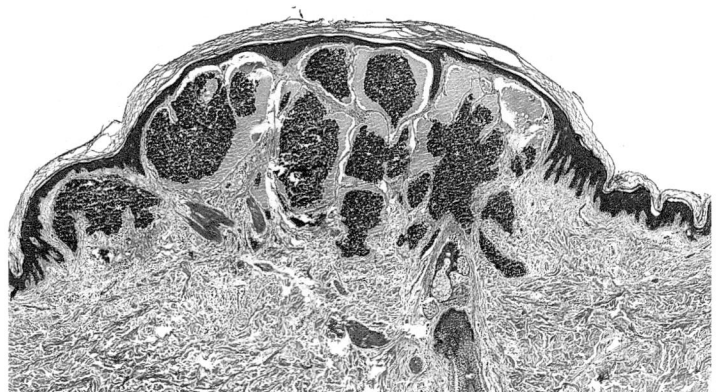

Fig. 38.1 This lesion illustrates some of the problems with nomenclature. It would have been called cavernous hemangioma in the past. It does not fit neatly into the venous malformations or other entities. (H & E)

lesion – usually a mongolian spot or nevus spilus. Nevus anemicus, a functional abnormality of blood vessels (see p. 328) is often present. Four types of phakomatosis pigmentovascularis have been recognized based on the nature of the constituent abnormalities.[6] The condition is thought to result from an abnormality of neural crest development. The nevus flammeus is similar to the 'port wine' stain (see below) although there may also be an increase in perivascular nerve fibers.[6]

NEVUS FLAMMEUS

'Nevus flammeus' is a generic term for a group of congenital vascular malformations that commonly involve the forehead, face and neck of newborns. The term includes the 'port wine' stain, the 'salmon' patch and the 'stork bite', the latter representing the combination of glabellar lesions with lesions on the nape of the neck. The lesions generally grow proportionately with the child's development and there is usually no tendency for spontaneous involution, although the small 'salmon' patch usually fades early in life (see below).[7]

The *'port wine' stain* is present at birth in 0.3% of children.[8,9] Familial occurrence is rare.[10] An acquired variant, which follows antecedent trauma, is said to occur very rarely.[11] Although any area may be affected, the lesion occurs most frequently on the face and neck. Single or multiple lesions may be present, and they are often sharply unilateral or segmental. Small or extensive areas of skin may be involved. At birth the lesions are flat and light pink in color. Lesions may become darker and thickened with time.[12] This change is most common in facial lesions in the area of the second and third branches of the facial nerve.[13]

The *'salmon' patch* is a pink macular area present at birth in approximately 40% of the population. The nape of the neck, the eyelids or the skin over the glabella may be involved.[14] In the majority of cases the lesions fade in the first year of life.[14] There are usually no associated congenital abnormalities.[15] In a small number of cases the condition persists for life, particularly a lesion in the nuchal region.

Clinical syndromes associated with nevus flammeus include:

- Sturge–Weber syndrome
- Klippel–Trenaunay–Weber syndrome
- Cobb's syndrome.

Histopathology

Initially, there is a barely detectable dilatation of the thin-walled vessels of the superficial vascular plexus. Progressive ectasia occurs and there is obvious erythrocyte stasis.[16] There is no significant increase in thickness or number of vessels with age in typical superficial lesions. In some cases there is an underlying cavernous hemangioma, which may blend with the superficial lesion. Localized exaggeration of the vascular ectasia produces the roughened surface of the older lesions.[13,17] Secondary angiomatous lesions and pyogenic granulomas may occur within the main lesion.[18]

One study has shown that the lesions are produced by dilatations of postcapillary venules of the superficial horizontal plexus, with no evidence of new vessel formation. The walls of the venules are thickened by basement membrane-like material and reticulin fibers.[19] Progressive dilatation does not appear to be related to decreased fibronectin or type IV collagen in the vessel walls.[20] A decreased nerve density has been demonstrated within affected areas, and it has been proposed that abnormal neural control of blood flow may be important in the pathogenesis of this lesion.[21] One immunohistochemical study showed that vessels were typical of capillaries, postcapillary venules and small veins.[22]

Sturge–Weber syndrome

The essential components of Sturge–Weber syndrome, also known as encephalotrigeminal angiomatosis, are:

- a unilateral facial port wine stain which includes that area of skin supplied by the ophthalmic branch of the trigeminal nerve (forehead and upper eyelid)
- an ipsilateral vascular abnormality of the leptomeninges
- an ipsilateral vascular abnormality of the choroid of the eye.[23]

The 'port wine' stain may be associated with only one or other of the other components of the syndrome.

Klippel–Trenaunay–Weber syndrome

The literature on Klippel–Trenaunay–Weber syndrome, also known as angioosteohypertrophy, is somewhat confusing. However, the major elements are a 'port wine' stain, usually on a limb, associated with varicose veins and limb overgrowth. Since the original description, a number of other abnormalities have been described in conjunction with this syndrome. The majority of cases are sporadic, but familial cases have also been described.[24,25] In some cases there is a hemodynamically significant arteriovenous fistula.[26] Capillary hemangiomas and venous malformations may be present.[27] There are many incomplete forms of this syndrome, and in one large series a 'port wine' stain was present in only 32% of cases.[28]

Cobb's syndrome

In Cobb's syndrome there is a 'port wine' stain (or another vascular lesion) on the trunk or limb in a dermatomal distribution, corresponding to a segment of the spinal cord in which there is an arteriovenous or venous hemangioma.[29]

VENOUS MALFORMATIONS

The term 'venous malformation' refers to a congenital vascular malformation that has been known in the past as *cavernous hemangioma*. Superficial venous malformations are blue or purple papules or nodules, which may have a grouped configuration. Deeper lesions may impart little color to the skin.[30]

Multiple lesions are present in the 'blue rubber bleb' nevus syndrome and Maffucci's syndrome (see below). Occasionally venous malformations have a unilateral dermatomal (zosteriform) distribution.[31] This may represent a form of mosaicism of a more generalized process.[32] Unlike (capillary) hemangiomas, venous malformations lack a proliferative phase with thymidine incorporation and have little tendency to regress with time. Venous malformations are generally at a deeper level in the skin than hemangiomas.

The distinction between venous malformations and hemangiomas is not quite as clear cut as the classification system of Mulliken et al would suggest.[7,33] Dysmorphic syndromes occur with hemangiomas as well as with venous malformations and in some, such as Maffucci's syndrome, overlap lesions may occur.

There are several, somewhat overlapping syndromes in which multiple venous malformations form the major part. These include:

- the 'blue rubber bleb' nevus syndrome
- Maffucci's syndrome.

Histopathology

The malformations may be found at any level of the skin, but there is a tendency for them to occur in the deep dermis and subcutis. They consist of large dilated vascular channels lined by flat endothelium (Fig. 38.2). The walls of the vessels vary in thickness, but they are generally thin and fibrous. Some vessels may have smooth muscle in their walls and resemble dilated veins. Thrombosis may complicate these lesions. Calcification of the walls and phlebolith-like calcific bodies in the lumina may be found.

Electron microscopy

The endothelium is flattened and the basal lamina duplicated, with interspersed collagen fibrils.[34]

'Blue rubber bleb' nevus syndrome

The 'blue rubber bleb' nevus syndrome was first named by Bean.[35] It is characterized by multiple compressible blue rubbery cavernous hemangiomas of the skin and of the gastrointestinal tract, and occasionally other organs.[36–40] The skin lesions may be present at birth or develop in childhood. They do not regress. Some, but not all, are characteristically painful or tender on palpation. There may be associated hyperhidrosis in the region of the tumors.[41] Iron-deficiency anemia sometimes results from gastrointestinal hemorrhage.[42]

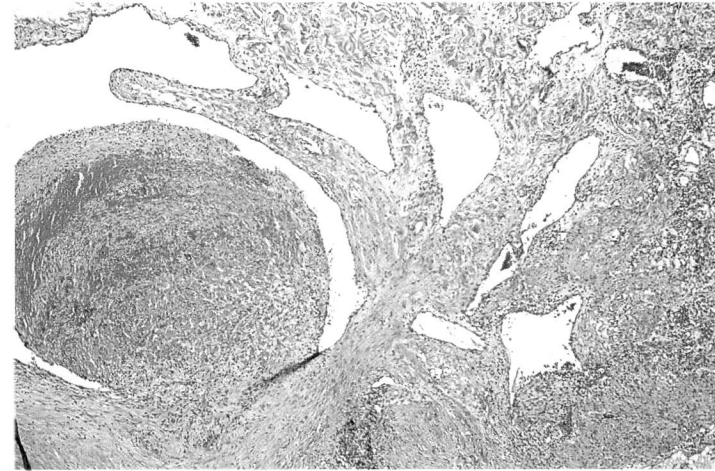

Fig. 38.2 **Venous malformation.** There are dilated vascular channels in the deep dermis and subcutis. One of the channels contains a thrombus. (H & E)

Most cases are sporadic, but there is evidence for an autosomal dominant mode of inheritance.[42] In one family males only were affected.[43]

The cutaneous lesions are composed of irregular cavernous channels in the deep dermis and subcutis. There is smooth muscle in the vessel walls. In some cases vessels may be intimately related to dermal sweat glands.[41]

Maffucci's syndrome

Maffucci's syndrome is characterized by multiple vascular tumors of the skin and subcutis associated with multiple enchondromas of bone, particularly the long bones. The vascular tumors are usually cavernous hemangiomas, but capillary hemangiomas, phlebectasias (dilated venules and veins) and lymphangiomas also occur. Spindle-cell hemangioendothelioma is associated with this syndrome. Phlebolith-like bodies may develop in vascular channels. In one case, only lymphangiomas were present.[44] The vascular tumors are present at birth or appear during childhood; they do not regress.[45,46] Mucous membrane and visceral hemangiomas have also been reported.[46]

Enchondromatosis results in variable shortening and deformity of the extremities. Skeletal lesions are predominantly unilateral in approximately half the reported cases.[46] There is no anatomical relationship between the osseous and vascular components.

There is probably an equal sex incidence and no familial grouping of cases.[46] Chondrosarcomas develop in approximately 15–30% of cases, and other cancers have also been reported.[46,47] The condition appears to be a generalized disorder of mesenchymal tissues.[48]

CUTIS MARMORATA TELANGIECTATICA CONGENITA

Cutis marmorata telangiectatica congenita, also known as congenital generalized phlebectasia, is a rare sporadic condition. It is characterized by a persistent patterning of the skin by a reticulate network of dark violet-blue vessels (cutis marmorata), spider nevus-like telangiectases, and venous abnormalities variously described as phlebectasia, venous lakes or venous hemangiomas.[49–54] Lesions are usually located on the trunk or extremities where they may be localized or generalized. They are often unilateral.[55,56] The skin changes appear in the neonatal period, and in many cases have a tendency to improve with time.[57] In addition to cutaneous atrophy and ulceration or hypertrophy of the involved tissues, a range of other associated vascular and skeletal abnormalities has been described.[51,58–63] There is no involvement of internal organs by the vascular abnormalities.[49]

The etiology is uncertain. The condition may be a genodermatosis with autosomal dominant inheritance and reduced penetrance of the gene. It has been suggested recently that it may represent a functional disturbance resulting from reduced α-adrenergic innervation of cutaneous terminal vessels.[64]

Histopathology

Various changes, including dilated capillaries and veins in the dermis and subcutis, have been described in this condition.[49,65]

LYMPHANGIOMA (CYSTIC LYMPHATIC MALFORMATION)

The term 'cystic lymphatic malformation' has been suggested as a more appropriate designation than lymphangioma for localized malformations of lymphatics.[66] Most are present at birth or arise in infancy or early childhood.[67,68] It has been suggested that lymphangiomas represent sequestrated lymphatic vessels that have failed to link up with the rest of the lymphatic

system or with the venous system during embryological development.[69,70] Histologically identical lesions arising because of acquired obstruction of lymphatics, often in association with lymphedema, are classified as lymphangiectases (see p. 1009). There have been several attempts to classify lymphangiomas: the classification of Flanagan and Helwig[67] divided them into superficial and deep types. Lymphangiomatosis is an additional category. Mulliken and colleagues,[33] who prefer the term 'cystic lymphatic malformation', have subdivided them into microcystic (lymphangiomas, verrucous hemangiomas and angiokeratoma circumscriptum) and macrocystic (cystic hygromas and cavernous lymphangiomas). Combined macrocystic and microcystic lesions may occur.

Superficial lymphangioma

The superficial lymphangioma is also known as superficial microcystic lymphatic malformation and lymphangioma circumscriptum. Although these lesions may occur on almost any part of the body, they are most common on the proximal parts of the limbs and in the limb girdle regions.[68,71] There are typically multiple scattered or grouped translucent vesicles and papulovesicles in an area of skin; single small lesions composed of a group of vessels also occur.[68] The lesions have been likened to frogspawn. Secondary hemorrhage and thrombus formation in vesicles may produce red or purple coloration in the lesions. Some lesions have a warty appearance owing to epidermal hyperplasia and hyperkeratosis.[72] There may be an underlying deep lymphangioma or other abnormality of lymphatic drainage, resulting in lymphedema and enlargement of the limb.[73,74] Most of the lesions are present at birth or develop in early infancy or childhood. Occasionally the lesions appear first in adult life: this is most common in the small localized form.[68] In the typical extensive lesion the superficial vessels communicate through deep vessels with large closed lymphatic cisterns in the subcutaneous or deeper tissues;[75] the superficial ectatic lymphatic vessels appear to result from raised pressure in these cisterns.[69] Magnetic resonance imaging has been used to demonstrate the full extent of these lesions.[76] This underlying abnormality may explain the tendency of the lesions to recur after superficial excision. Lesions may enlarge and spread with time, and they may persist indefinitely. The development of lymphangiosarcoma has been reported in an area of superficial lymphangioma treated with radiotherapy.[77] Squamous cell carcinoma may also develop in these lesions.[78]

Histopathology

The epidermis is elevated above the general level of the skin by solitary or grouped ectatic lymphatics located in the papillary dermis (Fig. 38.3). This accounts for the raised vesicles seen clinically. These channels abut closely on the overlying epidermis and are thin walled, consisting predominantly of an endothelial lining. The vessels may contain eosinophilic proteinaceous lymph or blood or thrombus, and occasionally foamy histiocytes or multinucleate giant cells.[69] Scattered lymphoid cells are sometimes seen in the dermis. There is atrophy of the epidermis directly over the vessels, with elongation of the rete ridges such that the vessels may appear to be intraepidermal, the picture resembling that of angiokeratoma. Deep irregular lymphatics are sometimes seen beneath the surface vessels in the dermis and subcutis, particularly in the extensive lesions.[69]

Deep lymphangioma

Deep lymphangioma (macrocystic lymphatic malformation) includes the lesions known as lymphangioma cavernosum (cavernous lymphangioma) and cystic hygroma.[67] The term *'cystic hygroma'* has generally been used for large deep lymphangiomas in the neck or axilla which consist of single or

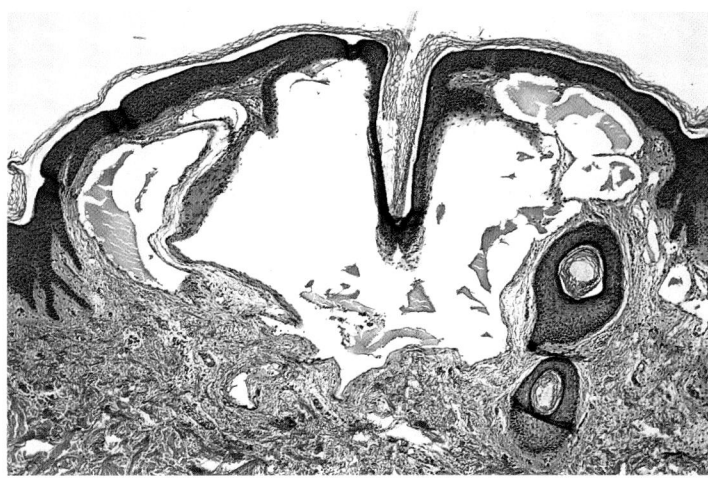

Fig. 38.3 **Superficial lymphangioma.** There are dilated lymphatic channels in the upper dermis. (H & E)

multiloculate fluid-filled cavities. Cystic hygromas of the posterior triangle of the neck are associated with hydrops fetalis and fetal death.[79] There is an association with the 45,XO karyotype (Turner's syndrome), other congenital malformation syndromes and several varieties of chromosomal aneuploidy.[79] A coexisting nevus flammeus has been reported overlying a cystic hygroma.[80] It is thought that these lesions represent failed connection between the jugular lymph sac and the internal jugular vein.[70,79] There is no clear-cut distinction between other deep lymphangiomas and classic cystic hygromas,[67] and it has been suggested that the appearance of the tumor is determined by the site and nature of the tissues in which it arises.[81] Deep lymphangiomas present as soft swellings in the skin and subcutaneous tissues. Progressive extension into deeper structures, such as muscle, is said to be an unfavorable sign.[67] The overlying epidermis is normal except in those cases in which there is an associated superficial lymphangioma. When cut across, these tumors vary from a spongy mass of small vascular spaces to large and 'multicystic'. Most are present at birth or arise in the first few years of life.[67,81]

Histopathology

The histological picture of these tumors is inconstant. There are irregular dilated lymphatic channels of variable size in the dermis, subcutis and deeper tissues. These vary from an endothelium-lined channel with no obvious supporting stroma to vessels with thick fibromuscular walls. The intervening dermis or subcutis may be unaltered, or there may be loose or compact fibrous stroma.[67] Blood may be present in some channels. In larger lesions collections of lymphocytes are sometimes present in the stroma and cause the endothelium to bulge into the vascular lumen.

Lymphangiomatosis

Lymphangiomatosis, a rare disorder occurring mainly in children, may have skin lesions, although it primarily involves bones, parenchymal organs and soft tissue.[82–84] The prognosis in this form is related to the extent of the disease. A variant limited to bone, soft tissue and skin, and with a good prognosis, has been described.[82]

Histopathology

In lymphangiomatosis involving skin, the dermis and subcutis are infiltrated by dilated lymphatic channels which dissect dermal collagen and surround pre-existing structures, a pattern seen in well-differentiated angiosarcoma. Vessels are lined by a single layer of flat endothelium which stains positively for factor

VIII-related antigen, *Ulex europaeus*-1 antigen and, variably, with CD31 and CD34.[82] Thrombomodulin is a more recent marker, which is said to be specific for lymphatic endothelium.[85]

VERRUCOUS HEMANGIOMA

Verrucous hemangioma is a vascular malformation which appears to arise at birth or in childhood, and enlarges and spreads in later life.[86–88] Lesions occur predominantly on the legs, and consist of bluish-red soft papules, plaques and nodules which become wart-like as the patient ages, or following trauma. Satellite nodules may develop. Recurrence is frequent after removal of the lesions because of involvement of the deeper tissues. An eruptive form with multiple disseminated cutaneous lesions and a linear variant have also been described.[89,90]

Histopathology

Fully evolved lesions consist of dermal and subcutaneous foci of small and large vessels, with overlying verrucous hyperplasia of the epidermis (Fig. 38.4). There is irregular papillomatosis with acanthosis and hyperkeratosis. Angiokeratomatous areas may be present; however, unlike angiokeratomas,

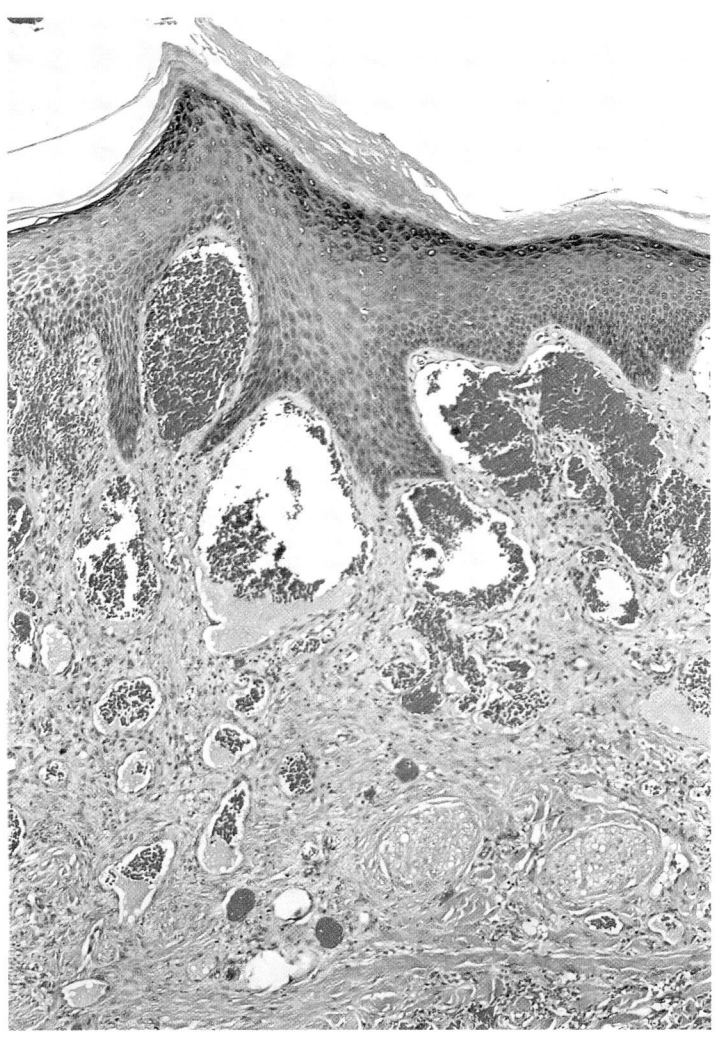

Fig. 38.4 **Early verrucous hemangioma** with much less epidermal response than usual. Unlike angiokeratoma, in which the vessels are limited to the papillary dermis, this entity has vessels extending deeply in the dermis. (H & E)

which are ectasias of superficial vessels (see p. 1007), verrucous hemangiomas involve deeper levels.[86,87] Verrucous hemangiomas have been included in some classifications with the microcystic lymphatic malformations.[66]

CALIBER-PERSISTENT ARTERY

Chronic ulceration of the vermilion border of the lips is sometimes associated with the presence of an artery of abnormally large caliber running in a very superficial location beneath the squamous epithelium. These vessels have been called 'caliber-persistent arteries' because of the failure of normal narrowing of the lumen as the vessel approaches the mucosal surface.[91,92] Some cases have been misdiagnosed clinically as squamous cell carcinoma.[93] The vessel may show fibroelastotic intimal thickening.[94] Multiple sections may be necessary to demonstrate the vessels.[91]

VASCULAR DILATATIONS (TELANGIECTASES)

In this group, the vascular channels of which the lesion is composed are predominantly pre-existing blood vessels which have undergone dilatation.

HEREDITARY HEMORRHAGIC TELANGIECTASIA

In hereditary hemorrhagic telangiectasia, also known as Osler–Rendu–Weber disease, multiple punctate telangiectases occur in the skin and mucous membranes. The respiratory tract, gastrointestinal tract and urinary tract may be involved.[95] The nasal mucosa, lips, mouth and face are frequently affected, and epistaxis is the most common presenting symptom. Although lesions may be present in childhood, they do not usually appear until puberty. The number and size of the lesions increase with advancing age, and with pregnancy. Fibrovascular abnormalities of the liver, cerebral arteriovenous fistulae and pulmonary arteriovenous fistulae are associated abnormalities.[96–98] Cerebral abscesses are occasionally a complication.[99] Inheritance is by an autosomal dominant trait. Linkage studies have identified at least three loci, on chromosomes 9, 12, and elsewhere. The mutated genes on chromosomes 9 and 12 encode respectively for endoglin and activin receptor-like kinase 1, both transmembrane proteins expressed on endothelial cells.[7,100]

Histopathology
Within the dermal papillae, dilated thin-walled vessels are lined by a single layer of endothelium. Ultrastructural studies have shown these to be venules.[101] Abnormalities in the endothelial lining have also been reported.[102]

GENERALIZED ESSENTIAL TELANGIECTASIA

Telangiectatic macules and diffuse erythematous areas likewise composed of a fine meshwork of ectatic vessels are seen in this condition, which occurs most frequently in women, appearing in early childhood. Lesions appear first on the lower extremities and spread gradually to involve the trunk and arms.[103] Gastrointestinal bleeding from an associated 'watermelon' stomach has been reported.[104]

Histopathology
Thin-walled vascular channels are found in the upper dermis. They are produced by dilatation of postcapillary venules of the upper horizontal plexus (Fig. 38.5).[19]

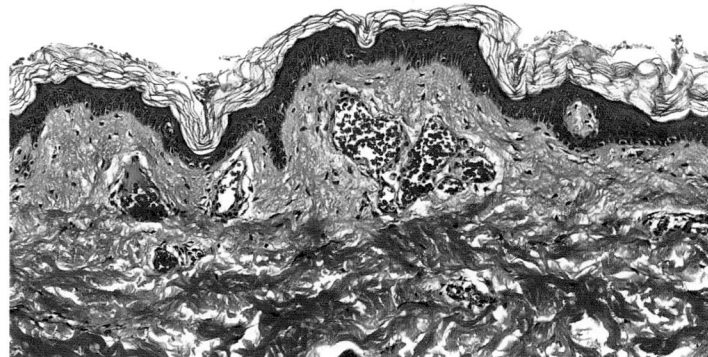

Fig. 38.5 **Generalized essential telangiectasia.** The upper dermis contains congested and dilated vessels. (H & E)

HEREDITARY BENIGN TELANGIECTASIA

Hereditary benign telangiectasia is inherited as an autosomal dominant trait. It is characterized by widespread cutaneous telangiectases, which commonly appear in childhood. Many lesions resemble spider nevi. There are no systemic vascular lesions associated with this form of telangiectasia.[105,106]

UNILATERAL NEVOID TELANGIECTASIA

Unilateral nevoid telangiectasia is also known as unilateral dermatomal superficial telangiectasia. The telangiectases have a dermatomal distribution and particularly involve the trigeminal and the third and fourth cervical and adjacent dermatomes.[107] The lesions may be present at birth or they may be acquired at times of physiological or pathological estrogen excess, including puberty and pregnancy in females, and chronic liver disease.[108,109] The condition has been reported in association with metastatic carcinoid tumor[110] and also in two males with hepatitis C but without evidence of cirrhosis or abnormal hormone levels.[111] Increased numbers of receptors for estrogen and progesterone have been reported in the lesional area compared to normal skin.[112]

ATAXIA–TELANGIECTASIA

Telangiectases are a constant but clinically unimportant part of this syndrome, which is also known as Louis–Bar syndrome.[113,114] Telangiectases appear in childhood in the bulbar conjunctiva and in the skin of the face, pinnae, neck and limbs. They arise from the superficial vascular plexus. These changes are followed by progressive cerebellar ataxia from cerebellar cortical atrophy. Other skin changes have been described including granulomas, segmental pigmentation, progeric changes and seborrheic dermatitis.[115–119] Profound dysfunction of both cell-mediated and humoral immunity results in decreased resistance to viruses and recurrent sinus and pulmonary infections. Thymic aplasia or hypoplasia and a decrease in the lymphoid tissue in lymph nodes, spleen and elsewhere are associated with deficiency of IgA, IgE and IgG, and abnormal function of T lymphocytes. An increased sensitivity to ionizing radiation and a markedly increased risk of developing cancers, particularly lymphomas and leukemias, are other facets of this syndrome.

Inheritance is autosomal recessive with variable penetrance. Mutations occur on chromosome band 11q22. 'Homozygotes' (strictly speaking, many are compound heterozygotes because each of their chromosomes 11 carries a different mutation) express the full syndrome. Heterozygotes have an elevated risk of cancer, especially female breast cancer, of ischemic heart disease and early mortality.[120]

'SPIDER' ANGIOMA

One or more 'spider' angiomas (nevi) are present in 10–15% of normal adults.[121] The face, neck, upper part of the trunk and arms are the regions usually involved; it is very uncommon for lesions to occur below the level of the umbilicus. There is a higher incidence in pregnant women and in patients with chronic liver disease. Lesions may regress following the pregnancy. In children, 'spider' nevi tend to arise on the hands and fingers.[122]

'Spider' angiomas consist of a central punctum within a generally circular area of erythema. Fine branching vessels or 'legs' radiate from the punctum.

Histopathology

These lesions are rarely biopsied or excised. They consist of a central ascending spiral thick-walled arteriole which ends in a thin-walled ampulla just beneath the epidermis (Fig. 38.6). From the ampulla, thin-walled branching channels radiate peripherally in the papillary dermis. Glomus cells have been described in the wall of the central arteriole.[121]

VENOUS LAKE

Venous lakes are dark-blue, often multiple, papules a few millimeters in diameter, which occur on the ears, face, lips or neck of the elderly.[123,124] Minor trauma to the lesions may produce persistent bleeding.

The lesions reported as *capillary aneurysms* probably represent venous lakes.[125] The clinical similarity of these lesions to malignant melanomas has been highlighted, particularly if thrombosis of the vascular lumen occurs.

Histopathology

Usually only a single large dilated vascular channel is present, in the upper dermis (Fig. 38.7). It has a very thin fibrous wall and a flat endothelial lining. A thrombus is sometimes present in the lumen or part thereof. These lesions appear to represent a dilated segment of a vein or venule.[123]

ANGIOKERATOMA

The angiokeratoma is characterized by ectasia of superficial dermal blood vessels, with associated epidermal changes. Five clinical variants have been recognized: all have similar histopathological features.[126] The variants are discussed below:

1. The *Mibelli type* develops in childhood and adolescence, with warty lesions over the bony prominences of the hands, feet, elbows and knees.[126,127] It is more common in females and it may be associated with pernio.

2. The *Fordyce (scrotal) type* arises as early as the second and third decades, but is seen most commonly in elderly men.[128,129] The penis, upper part of the thighs and lower part of the abdomen may also be involved.[130] The lesions are single or multiple, red to black papules, occurring along the course of the superficial scrotal vessels. Scrotal angiokeratomas may be associated with varicoceles, inguinal hernias and thrombophlebitis.[128] Spontaneous regression has been reported following the surgical treatment of an associated varicocele.[131] An equivalent lesion occurs on the vulva in young adult females. Increased venous pressure associated with pregnancy, vulval varicosities and hemorrhoids has been implicated in the pathogenesis of the vulval lesions.[132] An association with the contraceptive pill has also been suggested.[133]

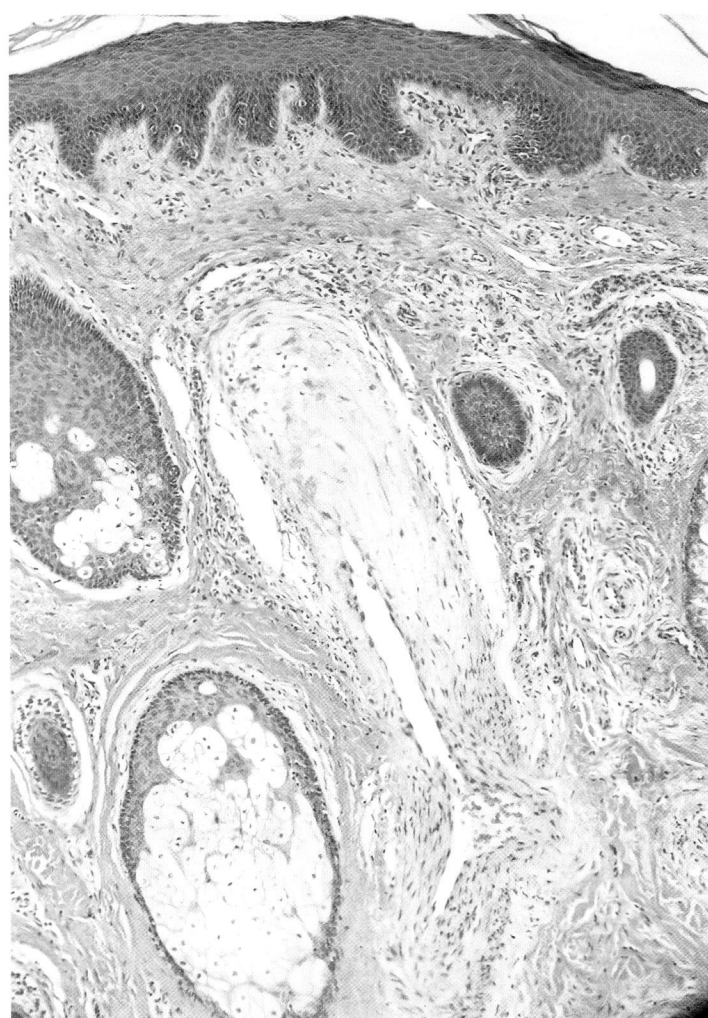

Fig. 38.6 **'Spider' angioma (nevus).** A deep dermal vessel has given rise to a vertically oriented vessel leading into a superficial ampulla. There are thin-walled vessels in the upper dermis. (H & E)

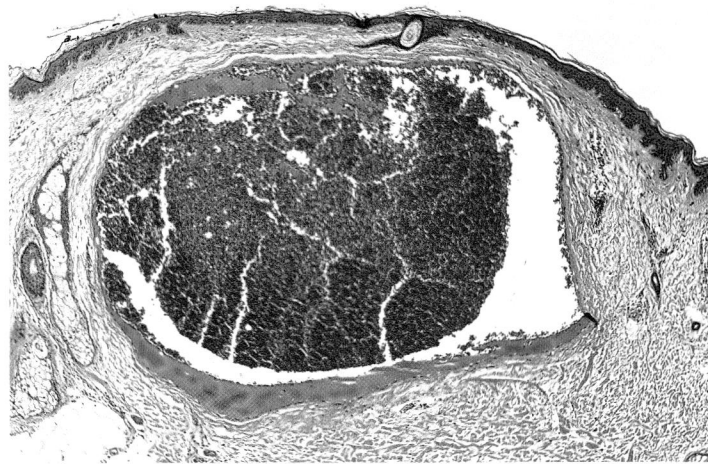

Fig. 38.7 **Venous lake.** There is a solitary large vascular channel in the upper dermis. (H & E)

3. *Solitary and multiple types* occur on any part of the body, but the lower extremities are most commonly affected. In one series the lesions were solitary in 83% of cases and multiple in 17%.[126] A zosteriform distribution has been described.[134] Angiokeratomas have been reported in a patient with juvenile dermatomyositis.[135] It was postulated that the lesions developed as a compensatory response to the obliterative angiopathy of the dermatomyositis.

4. *Angiokeratoma circumscriptum* is the least common variant. It consists either of a plaque composed of small discrete papules, or of variable hyperkeratotic papules and nodules with a tendency to confluence.[136] Lesions are almost always unilateral, and they occur predominantly on the leg, trunk or arm. They develop in infancy or childhood, predominantly in females.

5. *Angiokeratoma corporis diffusum* consists of multiple papules, frequently in clusters, and usually in a bathing-trunk distribution. Originally thought to be synonymous with Anderson–Fabry disease, it is now evident that this vascular lesion may occur in association with other enzyme disorders and also in people with normal enzyme activity (see p. 548).[137–139] Anderson–Fabry disease is an X-linked recessive disorder characterized by a deficiency of the lysosomal enzyme α-galactosidase A and the accumulation of the neutral glycolipid ceramide trihexidose in lysosomes in many types of cell.[140] Homozygous male patients generally, but not always, develop the lesions of the disease.[141] The skin lesions are usually present by adult life; the changes are often absent or slight in childhood.[142] An eruptive form is exceedingly rare.[143] Females with the genetic abnormality may also develop the lesion, but this occurs in less than 25% of cases.[142] Other enzyme deficiencies associated with angiokeratoma corporis diffusum include α-L-fucosidase deficiency (fucosidosis), β-galactosidase deficiency, α-N-acetylgalactosaminidase deficiency,[144,145] β-mannosidase deficiency[146] and neuraminidase deficiency.[147–149] A dominantly inherited form, associated with arteriovenous fistulae but no metabolic disorder, has been reported.[150]

Histopathology

In angiokeratomas there is marked dilatation of papillary dermal vessels to form large cavernous channels. There is associated irregular acanthosis of the epidermis with elongation of the rete ridges which partially or completely enclose the vascular channels (Fig. 38.8). A collarette may be formed at the margins of the lesions and there may be thrombosis of the vessels. The surface epidermis may show varying degrees of hyperkeratosis. The occurrence of a deep dermal hemangioma has been reported in association with angiokeratoma circumscriptum.[136,151] This combination may represent a verrucous hemangioma. In patients with Anderson–Fabry disease there is vacuolation of smooth muscle in arterioles and arteries and in the arrectores pilorum. Frozen sections of lesions may show PAS-positive and Sudan black-positive granules in endothelial cells, pericytes, arrectores pilorum and eccrine sweat glands. The vessels do not usually express CD34.[151]

Electron microscopy

Examination of lesions or of normal skin from patients with Anderson–Fabry disease shows electron-dense lipid bodies in the cytoplasm; they are either membrane bound or free in the endothelial cells, pericytes, smooth muscle cells and fibroblasts. These bodies may show a characteristic lamellar pattern. They are not seen in the other types of angiokeratoma or in the lesions in cases of angiokeratoma corporis diffusum with normal enzyme activities.[137]

The ultrastructure of the vessels in scrotal angiokeratomas and in Anderson–Fabry disease is similar to that of the small valve-containing collecting veins at the junction of the dermis and subcutaneous fat.[19] The possible role of raised intravenous pressure in the formation of scrotal and vulval angiokeratomas has been mentioned. It has been suggested that the lesions in Anderson–Fabry disease may follow weakening of vessel walls and subsequent dilatation, the result of lysosomal storage of lipid and consequent cellular damage.[152]

MISCELLANEOUS TELANGIECTASES

Numerous skin disorders are associated with telangiectases. These include such disparate conditions as collagen vascular disease, cutaneous mastocytosis and chronic graft-versus-host disease. Telangiectases may appear following trauma, including repetitive injury from the use of a keyboard ('computer palms'),[153] or be associated with skin damage due to solar and other forms of radiation (Fig. 38.9).

Several syndromes are associated with cutaneous telangiectases, such as Cockayne's syndrome, Bloom's syndrome (congenital telangiectatic erythema) and Rothmund–Thomson syndrome (poikiloderma congenitale).[113] Bloom's syndrome is a rare autosomal recessive genodermatosis consisting of photo-

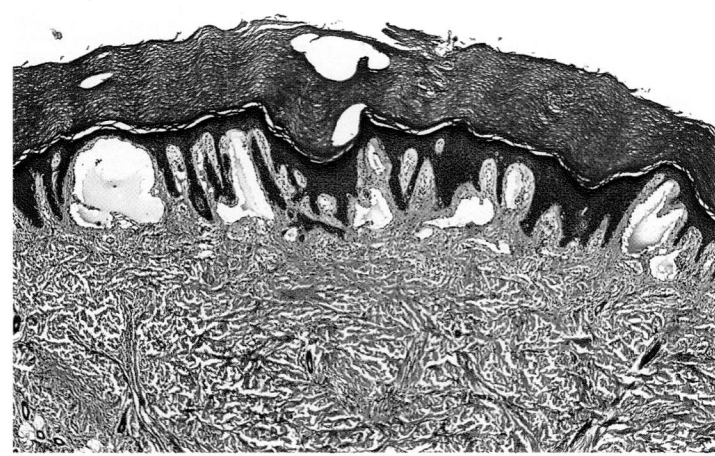

Fig 38.8 **Angiokeratoma.** The elongated rete ridges partly surround the vascular channels in the papillary dermis. (H & E)

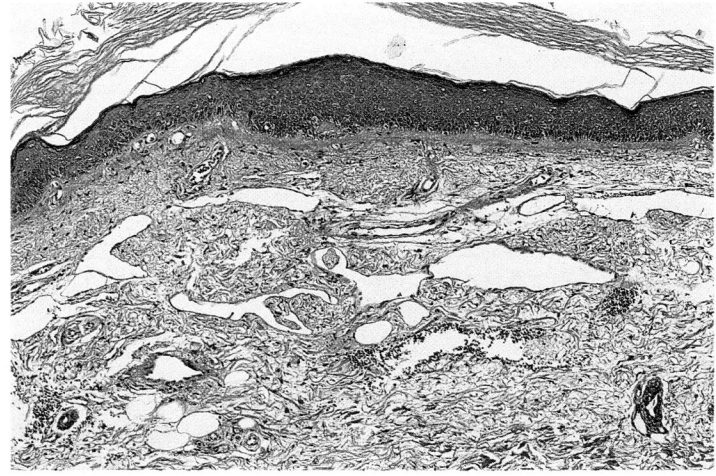

Fig. 38.9 **Secondary telangiectasia** occurring in sun-damaged skin. (H & E)

sensitivity, telangiectases, growth retardation and an increased incidence of malignancies.[154] The defect has been mapped to chromosome 15q26.1.

A unique case, characterized by telangiectasia with marked collagen deposition around the basal lamina of the vessels resembling amyloid, has been reported as **cutaneous collagenous vasculopathy**.[155]

DRUG-INDUCED TELANGIECTASIA

Iatrogenic telangiectases have been produced by lithium, isotretinoin and interferon-alfa. Photo-distributed telangiectases have been reported following the use of cefotaxime (a cephalosporin) and the calcium channel blockers nifedipine, felodipine and amlodipine.[156–159]

COSTAL FRINGE

Costal fringe is an acquired lesion in elderly men and, less frequently, elderly women. It consists of a band-like pattern of telangiectases across the anterior aspect of the thorax, usually near the costal margin. It is uncommon in young adults.[160] The telangiectases represent dilated postcapillary venules of the superficial vascular plexus.[161]

LYMPHANGIECTASES

Lesions that are clinically and histologically similar to superficial lymphangiomas (cystic lymphatic malformations) may develop in areas of skin affected by obstruction or destruction of the lymphatic drainage.[72,162] The interference with the lymphatics may result from radiotherapy or surgery,[163,164] and has been described in the chest and arm following radical mastectomy and radiotherapy,[165–167] in the penis and scrotum following surgery for a sacrococcygeal tumor,[168] and on the vulva and on the thigh following surgery and radiotherapy for carcinoma of the cervix.[169–173]

Cutaneous lymphangiectases have also been reported in association with severe photoaging and topical corticosteroid application.[174] Facial lymphangiectases are a rare complication of porphyria.[175]

VASCULAR PROLIFERATIONS (HYPERPLASIAS AND BENIGN NEOPLASMS)

This group of vascular tumors includes a variety of lesions in which there is a hyperplasia or a benign neoplastic proliferation of blood vessels of different types.[176]

HEMANGIOMA OF INFANCY

Hemangioma of infancy, a benign proliferation of blood vessels, has also been called 'strawberry' nevus, infantile capillary hemangioma and benign infantile hemangioendothelioma. They are the most common tumors of infancy, with an incidence in the newborn population of approximately 2%. They are especially common among infants born prematurely.[177]

In most series there is a female preponderance of cases.[178,179] Familial cases are rare.[180] One or more lesions may be present on any part of the body, but the head, neck and trunk are the most commonly affected sites.[181] The parotid gland and overlying skin may be involved, this being the most common tumor of the parotid gland in children.[182] Lesions are often not visible at birth but appear in the first few weeks of life. Rarely, a faint

erythematous macule or an area of pallor with telangiectasia is present at birth.[183] The lesions evolve and enlarge over a period of months to become raised and bright red in color, with a smooth or irregular surface. Most lesions have reached maximum size by the age of 3–6 months.[181,183] Total or partial regression then occurs in the majority of lesions and is usually maximal by 5–7 years of age.[179,181] This regression appears to be mediated by apoptosis accompanied by reduced proliferation of cells.[184] Most cases therefore require no surgical intervention,[183,185] although newer laser techniques and even cryosurgery are being used with success.[183,185,186] Periorbital lesions may warrant active therapy because of the association of visual complications.[183,187] Complete involution is less likely to occur where there is a deep cavernous component or more complex vascular malformation.[188–190]

A locus for an autosomal dominant predisposition to hemangiomas has recently been identified on chromosome 5q. A similar locus may be involved in the formation of sporadic hemangiomas.[191,192] It has been suggested that the incidence of infantile hemangiomas is increased following chorionic villus sampling during pregnancy.[193] Interestingly, these hemangiomas share a phenotype with the placental microvasculature.[194]

Multiple disseminated cutaneous hemangiomas are sometimes associated with multiple visceral hemangiomas (diffuse neonatal hemangiomatosis). This is usually a fatal disorder (see below).

Recent work has shown that the endothelial cells of these hemangiomas have the cell morphology and protein expression of embryonic endothelial cells, indicating a dysfunction in maturation of the endothelial cells in these lesions.[195] Another study has shown that the endothelial cells of these hemangiomas have high levels of erythrocyte-type glucose transporter protein (GLUT1), but this is not found in vascular malformations.[196] Cellular adhesion molecules are also involved in the formation and maturation of hemangiomas. ICAM-3 appears to play a role in the early stages of vessel formation.[197]

A recent finding[198] that the endothelial cells in this tumor are clonal has major implications for our understanding of this lesion. It supports their separation from venous malformations.[199] This finding is consistent with the possibility that these tumors are caused by somatic mutations in one or more genes regulating endothelial cell proliferation.[198]

Histopathology

Early lesions are highly cellular and involve the dermis, but extension into the subcutis may occur. Vascular lumina are small, often slit-like and unapparent, and lined by plump endothelial cells (Fig. 38.10). Moderate numbers of normal mitotic figures are present, and mast cells and dermal dendrocytes are frequent in the intervening stroma.[200] It has been suggested that the mast cells may play a role in angiogenesis and therefore in the formation of these lesions.[201] The vascular proliferation often has a marked lobular configuration; this is often more obvious in the subcutis. Here fat lobules are partly or completely replaced and the appearance may resemble that of angiolipomas.[181] Perineural infiltration can be present.[202] Lesions with vessel proliferation, in and around sweat glands, have also been described.[203] As the lesions evolve, vascular lumina become larger and more obvious. A central draining lumen may become evident in each lobule. The endothelium lining the vessels becomes flatter. With regression of lesions there is disappearance of vessels, interstitial fibrosis, and fat replacement of vascular tissue in the lobules of the subcutis.[181] Immunohistochemical studies have demonstrated endothelial and pericytic differentiation in cells.[204]

Electron microscopy

Ultrastructural studies of capillary hemangiomas have shown plump endothelial cells surrounded by a basement membrane and pericytes.[34] Intracytoplasmic vacuoles are present in endothelial cells, and are thought to represent an early

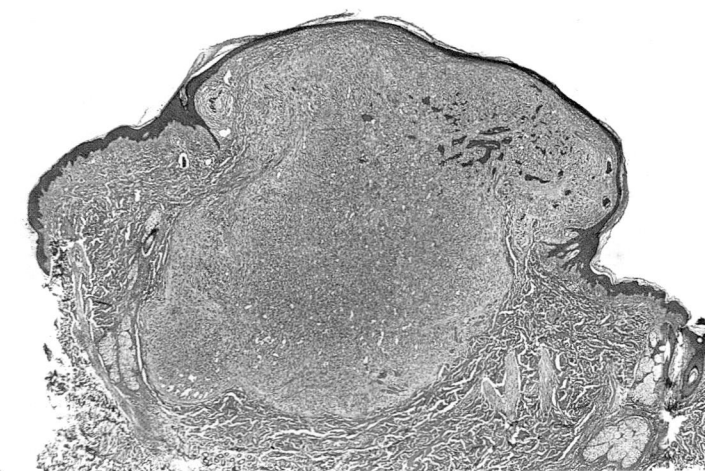

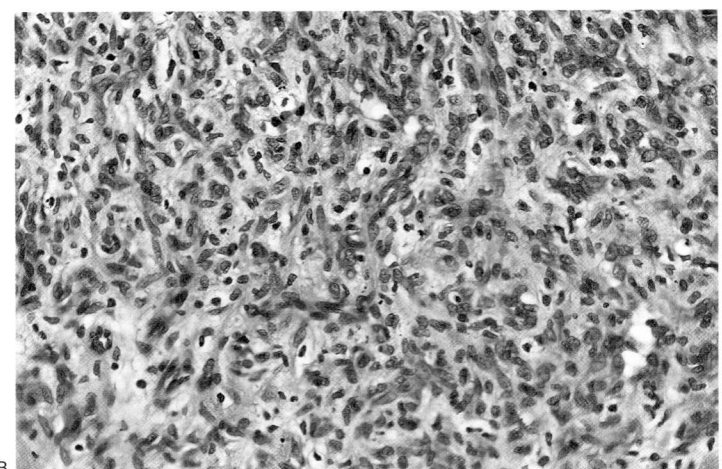

Fig. 38.10 **(A) Hemangioma of infancy. (B)** The lumina are slit-like and unapparent. (H & E)

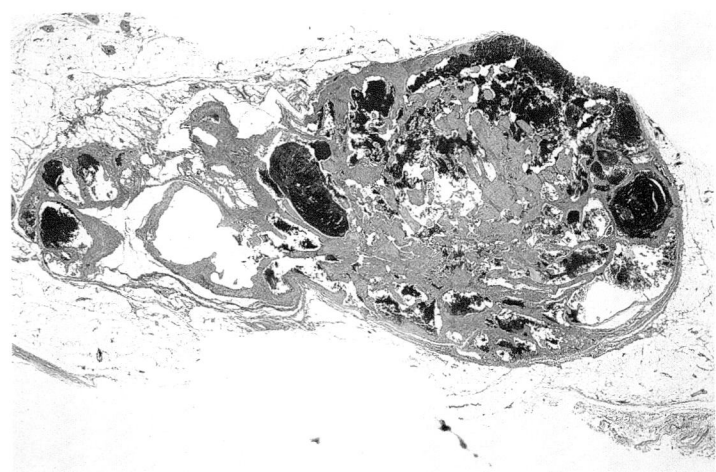

Fig. 38.11 **Sinusoidal hemangioma.** There is a lobular pattern, with interconnecting vascular channels. (H & E)

The prognosis in this group is good. In these patients, and in some survivors of those with visceral hemangiomas, spontaneous regression of lesions occurs.[215–217]

SINUSOIDAL HEMANGIOMA

Sinusoidal hemangioma is an uncommon benign vascular tumor with some similarities to a venous malformation ('cavernous' hemangioma). However, it occurs as an acquired lesion in adults, rather than in children.[218] This variant is most common in females, the trunk (including the breast) and limbs being the most common sites. The tumor involves the subcutis and deep dermis.

It is an acquired lesion and has therefore not been included with the 'Hamartomas and Malformations'.

Histopathology[218]
A lobular architecture is characteristic of sinusoidal hemangioma (Fig. 38.11). Lobules are composed of thin-walled interconnecting vascular channels forming a sinusoidal pattern. Vessels are closely approximated, with little intervening stroma. Tangential sectioning of vessel walls produces a pseudo-papillary pattern. Unlike typical 'cavernous' hemangiomas, lining cells may appear focally atypical with nuclear hyperchromatism. Mitotic figures are not seen. Calcification is a rare complication.[219]

'CHERRY' ANGIOMA

'Cherry' angiomas (senile angioma, Campbell de Morgan spots) are very common single or multiple bright red papules, up to a few millimeters in diameter, which occur predominantly on the trunk and proximal parts of the limbs. There is typically a pallid halo surrounding the lesions. Rare before puberty, the incidence rises sharply in the fourth decade, such that they are almost universal in old age.[220]

Histopathology
In small early lesions, one or more dilated interconnecting thin-walled vascular channels are present in the dermal papillae. In older lesions there is loss of rete ridges and atrophy of the superficial epidermis, with formation of a polypoid lesion composed of a network of dilated communicating channels with scant intervening connective tissue (Fig. 38.12). A collarette may be present at the periphery of the lesions.

stage in lumen formation.[205] Crystalloid inclusions have been identified in endothelial cells in early cellular lesions.[206] Vessels within a hemangioma may have features of capillaries, venules or arterioles.[34]

Diffuse neonatal hemangiomatosis
Multiple cutaneous hemangiomas may occur with or without disseminated visceral hemangiomas.[207] The cutaneous lesions are capillary hemangiomas, which are present at birth or appear in infancy. In those cases with visceral involvement, any organ may be affected. Visceral involvement is a poor prognostic sign, death occurring in the majority of cases, usually within a few months of birth.[208] Common causes of death include high-output congestive cardiac failure associated with arteriovenous shunts (particularly in the liver), central nervous system complications, and bleeding associated with the Kasabach–Merritt syndrome.[208–212] Other developmental abnormalities have been reported in association with this condition.[213]

Hemangiomas of the head and neck region are sometimes associated with anomalies of the major blood vessels, including aortic coarctation.[214] Another associated syndrome is PHACES (posterior fossa malformations, hemangiomas – especially large, plaque-like, facial lesions – arterial anomalies, cardiac anomalies, eye abnormalities and sternal cleft and/or supraumbilical raphe).[177]

A purely cutaneous form of diffuse neonatal hemangiomatosis has also been reported, and has been called 'benign neonatal hemangiomatosis'.[215,216]

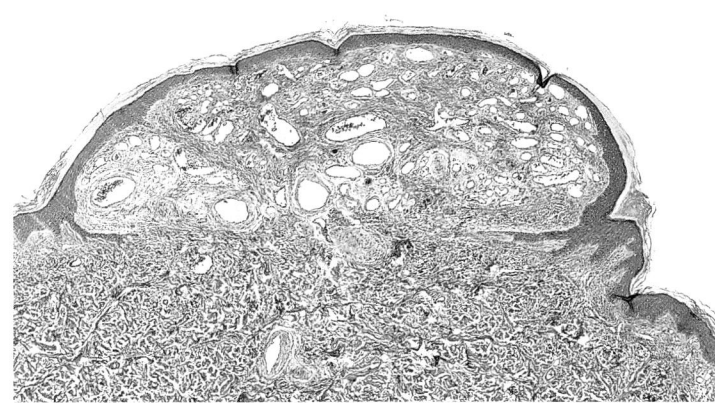

Fig. 38.12 **'Cherry angioma'.** This polypoid lesion is composed of dilated vascular channels and scant intervening stroma. A collarette is present at the periphery. (H & E)

These lesions appear to be the dilated and interconnected segments of venous capillaries and postcapillary venules in the dermal papillae. The vessels of the upper horizontal plexus are not involved. The non-replicating nature of the endothelial cells comprising these lesions indicates that they are probably not true neoplasms.[221] The high incidence of these lesions in old age suggests that their occurrence is an age-related degenerative phenomenon.

Laser-treated lesions undergo inflammation, necrosis and eventual healing by four weeks.[222]

GLOMERULOID HEMANGIOMA

Chan and colleagues coined the term 'glomeruloid hemangioma' for a characteristic benign vascular tumor which they considered a cutaneous marker for POEMS syndrome.[223,224] POEMS syndrome is a multisystem disorder characterized by polyneuropathy (peripheral sensorimotor neuropathy, papilledema), organomegaly (hepatosplenomegaly, lymphadenopathy), endocrinopathy (impotence, gynecomastia, amenorrhea, glucose intolerance, hypothyroidism, adrenal insufficiency), M-protein (paraproteinemia, osteosclerotic myeloma, marrow plasmacytosis) and skin changes (hyperpigmentation, hypertrichosis, sclerodermoid features and hemangiomas).[225,226] Multicentric Castleman's disease and POEMS syndrome are overlapping conditions.[227,228]

Vascular tumors in POEMS syndrome are eruptive, multiple, red or purple in color, and distributed on the trunk and limbs. Lesions are usually small papules from pinhead in size to a few millimeters, although larger, bluish subcutaneous compressible tumors have also been described.[229] The tumors have variously been described as showing features of cherry angioma, capillary hemangioma, cavernous hemangioma, lobular hemangioma (pyogenic granuloma and tufted angioma) and targetoid hemangioma.[230] Lesions may show overlap features.[229,231–233]

Glomeruloid hemangiomas appear to be more common in the Japanese than in other races or ethnic groups.

Histopathology[223]

In the characteristic glomeruloid hemangiomas described by Chan et al there are dilated (sinusoidal) dermal vascular spaces filled by grape-like aggregates of small capillary vessels, resulting in structures resembling renal glomeruli. Between these small vessels are plump cells which appear to be endothelial cells, being positive for factor VIII-related antigen. These cells and endothelial cells lining vessels contain PAS-positive eosinophilic globules, which stain for immunoglobulins at their periphery.

A recent study has shown endothelial cells with two different immunophenotypes.[224] The capillary-type endothelium had a CD31$^+$/CD34$^+$/UEA I$^+$/CD68$^-$ phenotype, while the sinusoidal endothelium had a CD31$^+$/CD34$^-$/UEA I$^-$/CD68$^+$ phenotype.[224]

ARTERIOVENOUS HEMANGIOMA

Arteriovenous hemangioma (acral arteriovenous tumor) presents as a solitary, red or purple papule with a predilection for the lips, the perioral skin, the nose and the eyelids of middle-aged to elderly men.[234–236] It is usually asymptomatic. It appears to have an association with chronic liver disease.[237]

Histopathology[234,235]

There is a well-circumscribed non-encapsulated collection of large, thick-walled vessels in the upper and mid dermis (Fig. 38.13). These vessels are lined by endothelium and have a fibromuscular wall which contains elastic fibers but no definite elastic laminae. Most vessels have the characteristics of veins.[238] In approximately one-third of cases there are thin-walled dilated angiomatous capillaries superficial to the large tumor vessels. The stroma is often myxoid.

Acquired digital arteriovenous malformations are a distinct entity thought to result from shunts between an artery and a vein in a fingertip.[239,240] They are composed of thick- and thin-walled vessels, some of the former having small amounts of smooth muscle in their walls. The lesions lack the tumor-like qualities of the arteriovenous hemangioma. Shunts are visible between the two classes of vessels.[239]

MICROVENULAR HEMANGIOMA

Microvenular hemangioma, a benign vascular tumor, occurs predominantly in young and middle-aged adults as a single, slow-growing lesion on the trunk or limbs. Lesions are purple to red papules or nodules, usually less than 1 cm in diameter.[241,242] Larger plaque forms have been reported.[243]

Histopathology[241]

The main characteristic of this tumor is a proliferation of thin uniform branching collapsed-looking vessels with inconspicuous lumina. The vessels involve the dermis and occasionally the superficial subcutis. The intervening stroma is collagenous, sometimes with a desmoplastic appearance. Endothelial cells are sometimes plumper than normal, but not atypical; they stain for factor VIII-related antigen, CD34 and *Ulex europaeus*-1 lectin. A peripheral layer of pericytes stains for smooth muscle actin.[243,244] Eosinophilic globules, commonly seen in Kaposi's sarcoma, are not seen in this tumor.

TARGETOID HEMOSIDEROTIC HEMANGIOMA

Targetoid hemosiderotic hemangiomas are single lesions occurring in young or middle-aged persons, with a male predominance. They involve the trunk or limbs.[176,245–250] Characteristically the lesion has a 'targetoid' appearance with a violaceous central papule surrounded by an area of pallor and an ecchymotic or brown ring,[251] which expands and subsequently disappears. The central papule persists. It has been reported in pregnancy,[246,247] and in a father and son.[252]

It has been suggested that targetoid hemosiderotic hemangioma is a larger variant of solitary angiokeratoma resulting from trauma.[250] Trauma to other lesions may produce a simulant of this tumor.[253] Others have suggested lymphatic differentiation.[249]

The term **'hobnail hemangioma'** has been used for a group of vascular lesions related to targetoid hemosiderotic hemangioma, but encompassing tumors with morphological features of retiform hemangioendothelioma, progressive lymphangioma and Dabska's tumor.[254,255]

Histopathology[251]

Initially there are ectatic vascular channels lined by plump (hobnail) endothelial cells in the upper dermis. The vessels have intraluminal papillary projections. In the deep dermis and subcutis the channels dissect collagen bundles and surround sweat glands. There is a variable mild inflammatory infiltrate about vessels and considerable extravasation of erythrocytes and hemosiderin (Fig. 38.14). Fibrin thrombi may be seen in the superficial vessels, a feature not present in the early lesions of Kaposi's sarcoma. Plasma cells are also uncommon; eosinophilic globules have not been reported. Old lesions are composed of collapsed thin-walled anastomosing vascular channels with hemosiderin.

In one series, the tumor cells stained for CD31 in all cases tested, whereas only 3 of the 28 cases stained completely for CD34. In addition, 4 out of 8 cases stained positively for vascular endothelial growth factor receptor-3 (VEGFR-3), suggesting lymphatic differentiation.[249] Another series showed variable reactivity of endothelial cells for CD31, CD34, factor VIII-related antigen and *Ulex europaeus*-1 lectin in all cases.[255]

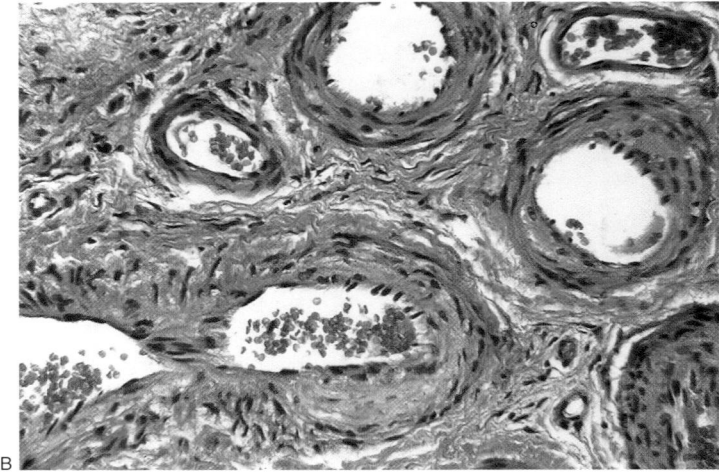

Fig. 38.13 **(A) Arteriovenous hemangioma. (B)** It is composed of thick-walled vascular channels. (H & E)

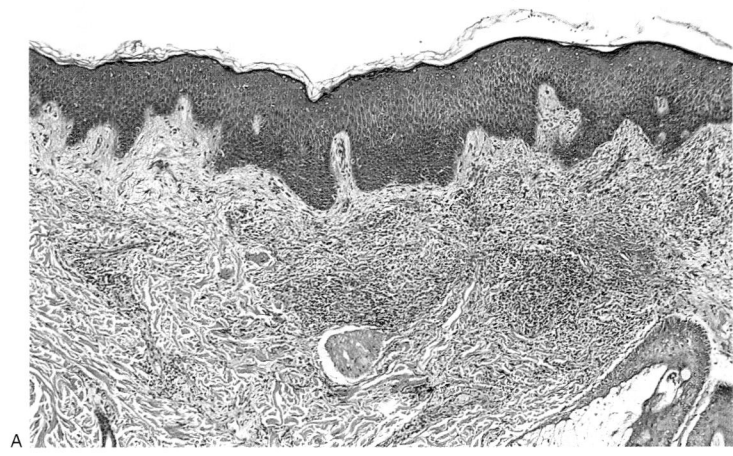

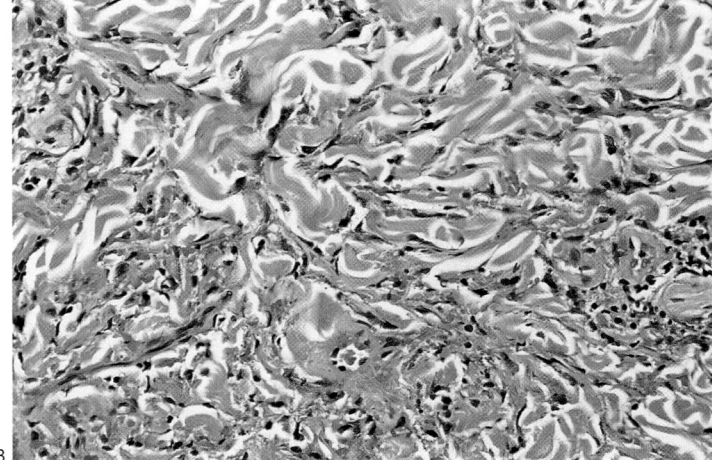

Fig. 38.14 **Targetoid hemosiderotic hemangioma. (A)** There is no superficial vascular dilatation in this case. **(B)** There are small vessels and abundant hemosiderin. The lesion was clinically typical. (H & E)

SPINDLE-CELL HEMANGIOENDOTHELIOMA (HEMANGIOMA)

Although spindle-cell hemangioendothelioma was originally believed to be a vascular tumor of low-grade malignancy,[256] there is convincing evidence that this entity may in fact represent a non-neoplastic process.[257–265] Accordingly, Requena and Ackerman believe it should be renamed 'spindle-cell hemangioma'.[264] Fletcher et al have suggested that these lesions represent a reactive vascular process arising in association with a local abnormality of blood flow, because the lesions are often associated with local malformation of blood vessels, have an integral smooth muscle component, occasionally regress spontaneously, and do not metastasize.[257] A similar view has been expressed by Perkins and Weiss.[261] This tumor has been reported in Maffucci's syndrome and in association with venous malformations and the Klippel–Trenaunay syndrome.[256,258,261,266,267]

Although tumors may occur at any age from birth to adulthood, approximately 50% of cases arise before the age of 25. Lesions may be single or multiple; multiple lesions tend to occur in a single area. Occasionally lesions are widespread. The hands and feet are the most common sites, but lesions also occur on the trunk.[256,268] Tumors are circumscribed, hemorrhagic nodules. They may increase in size and number with time, often over a long period. Local recurrence of lesions is common after removal. In one study 'recurrences' were noted to arise in adjacent, previously unaffected tissue, suggesting a new lesion. Such recurrences may arise from contiguous spread along, or multifocal involvement of a vessel.[261] There is only one documented case of metastasis by this tumor and that followed multiple recurrences, radiotherapy and transformation to a conventional angiosarcoma.[256]

Histopathology[256,257]

Tumors are situated in the dermis and subcutis; rarely, they occur in the lumen of a vein. There are three main components. The first is a vascular component of thin-walled cavernous channels which may contain thrombi or phleboliths. The second is a solid area of spindle cells with slit-like vascular spaces; these areas may resemble Kaposi's sarcoma (Fig. 38.15). The third component is plump endothelial cells, either in groups or lining vascular channels. Some of these cells have intracytoplasmic vacuoles. Fletcher et al have also noted the frequent presence of large, malformed, thick- or thin-walled vessels adjacent to the tumor, as well as bundles of smooth muscle

cells near cavernous vessels or in solid areas.[257] Nuclear atypia is minimal; mitoses are rarely seen. Lymphocytes and siderophages may be associated with the lesions, but eosinophilic globules, as seen in Kaposi's sarcoma, have not been reported. The spindle cells in this tumor are generally more bland-looking and regular in appearance than those in Kaposi's sarcoma. Furthermore, the spindle-cell fascicles are not as well-formed as those in Kaposi's sarcoma.[269]

Immunohistochemical studies have confirmed the endothelial nature of the cells lining cavernous channels which stain for CD31, factor VIII-related antigen and *Ulex europaeus*-1 lectin. Solid epithelioid and spindle-cell areas are negative for these antigens.[257] DNA flow cytometric and immunohistochemical studies have shown that this tumor has low proliferative activity and is diploid, consistent with a reactive lesion.[258]

Electron microscopy

Ultrastructural studies have shown a heterogeneous cell population in solid areas; however, occasional cells contain Weibel–Palade bodies, confirming that some cells are showing endothelial differentiation.

ANGIOMA SERPIGINOSUM

Angioma serpiginosum is a rare condition in which multiple pin-sized vascular puncta occur either singly or in clusters on any part of the body except mucous membranes and the palms and soles.[270,271] The legs are the most common site. Lesions appear before puberty and progress by the development of further puncta at the periphery of the involved area. The lesions do not regress. Females are more commonly affected, and a familial grouping of cases has been reported.[272]

Histopathology

Microscopic examination shows single or grouped ectatic, congested, thin-walled capillaries in the papillary dermis. Thick-walled capillaries and downgrowth of the rete ridges between groups of vessels have also been described.[273,274] The latter lesions resemble angiokeratomas. Although previously regarded as a telangiectatic process, an element of vascular proliferation appears to be present.[273]

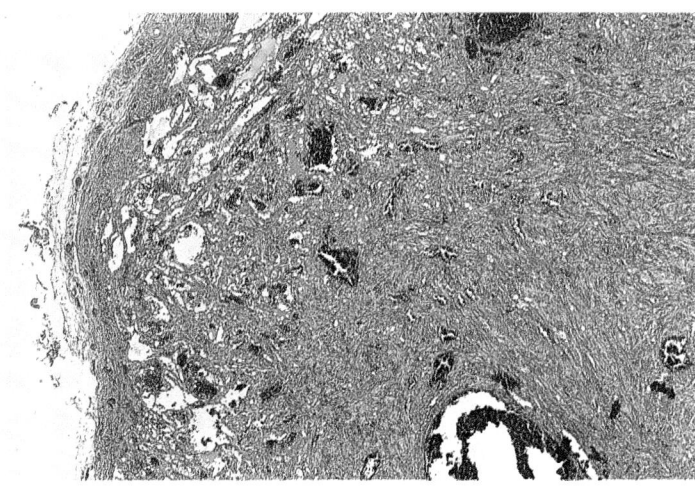
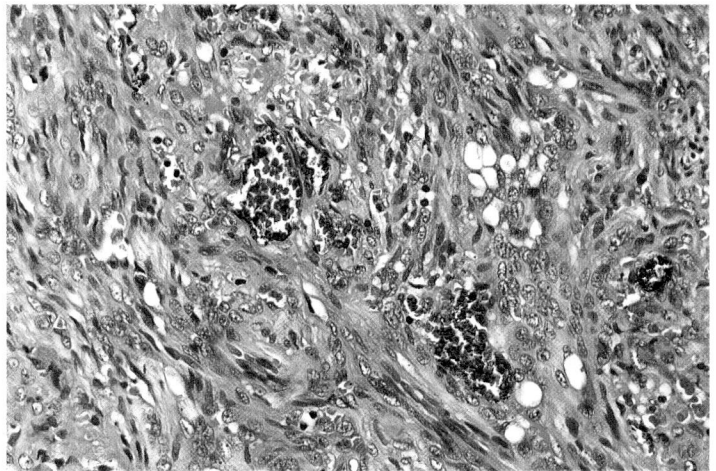

Fig. 38.15 **(A) Spindle-cell hemangioendothelioma. (B)** There are thin bundles of spindle cells between the vascular channels. (H & E)

GIANT CELL ANGIOBLASTOMA

Only four cases of giant cell angioblastoma, an exceedingly rare tumor of skin and soft tissues, have been reported.[275] The tumor is present at birth or noted soon after. It is locally infiltrative, but grows slowly. The morphology suggests an unusual form of neoplastic angiogenesis.[275] Metastases have not been recorded.

Histopathology[275]

There are concentric arrays of oval-to-spindle cells around small endothelium-lined channels. These primitive cells arranged around the vessels tend to differentiate toward pericytes and express smooth muscle actin while the endothelial cells express CD31 and factor VIII-related antigen. Large mononuclear and multinucleate giant cells are also present. Perineural and intraneural involvement by small vessels is common. A stromal infiltrate of lymphocytes and plasma cells is another feature.

ANGIOLYMPHOID HYPERPLASIA WITH EOSINOPHILIA

Angiolymphoid hyperplasia with eosinophilia is a tumor of skin and subcutaneous tissues composed of vessels, a proliferation of a distinctive type of endothelial cell, and a variable component of inflammatory cells.[276] Whether it is a true neoplasm or a reactive process is at present undecided. It appears to be identical to the lesions known as pseudopyogenic granuloma, atypical pyogenic granuloma, epithelioid hemangioma, histiocytoid hemangioma, intravenous atypical vascular proliferation, and nodular angioblastic hyperplasia with eosinophilia and lymphofolliculosis.[277–282]

Kimura's disease (eosinophilic lymphogranuloma),[283–287] although previously included by some in this group of conditions, is a separate entity.[288–290] It is clinically different, typically presenting as large subcutaneous masses in young Asian men. The majority of lesions are located around the ears or in the parotid gland.[291] Its etiology is unknown but it may be an aberrant immune reaction to an as yet unknown stimulus. Epstein–Barr virus DNA has been detected in lesional tissue in one case.[292]

In angiolymphoid hyperplasia, lesions involve the subcutaneous tissue or the dermis or both. Single or multiple pink to red-brown papules or nodules occur, predominantly on the face, scalp and ears; they are uncommon on the limbs and trunk. Widespread lesions and multiple lesions limited to one limb have been reported.[293,294] Cases have been reported in a port wine stain[295] and on the vulva,[280,296] lip[297] and oral mucosa.[298] It has been reported in association with HIV infection.[299] Symptomatic lesions may be painful, pruritic or pulsatile.[300] In some series there is a female predominance.[301] Young to middle-aged people are most commonly affected. Some cases are associated with a blood eosinophilia. Lesions may remain for years without evidence of involution, and they may recur after excision.[281] They have been treated successfully with the pulsed dye laser,[302] intralesional interferon alfa-2a[303] and oral isotretinoin.[304]

The true nature of this lesion is uncertain. A few examples appear to be associated with trauma, oral contraceptives,[300,305] HIV infection[299] or pregnancy, but not HHV-8.[294] It has been suggested that the lesions are a reactive hyperplastic process secondary to an underlying arteriovenous malformation or traumatic pseudoaneurysm.[176,306,307] The interleukin-5 levels are increased, which may explain the eosinophilia.[307] Recently, clonal populations of T cells were detected in several of the cases tested.[308]

Histopathology

The lesions consist of circumscribed collections of vessels and inflammatory cells. The vascular component comprises thick- and thin-walled vessels lined by plump endothelial cells (Fig. 38.16). These cells also occur in clumps that appear solid or sometimes contain small lumina. They are 'epithelioid' in appearance, with a large nucleus and abundant eosinophilic cytoplasm, and are characteristic of this condition. Prominent cytoplasmic vacuoles are seen in some cells. Normal mitotic figures are sometimes present. Intravascular proliferations of these cells may be seen in the lumina of larger vessels.[280] There is one report of multinucleated cells, some of which were endothelial sprouts and others fibrohistiocytic cells.[309] Associated with the vascular and endothelial proliferations is a stromal cellular infiltrate which varies in intensity and consists of lymphocytes (sometimes with lymphoid follicle formation), eosinophils and mast cells. The stroma may be fibrous or myxoid in character.

Although these epithelioid cells share some enzymes with histiocytes[310] they do not contain lysozyme; they have ultrastructural features of endothelial cells, including Weibel–Palade bodies.[300] The epithelioid cells stain for factor VIII-related antigen and *Ulex europaeus*-1 lectin, but not for cytokeratins or epithelial membrane antigen.[311,312] The vacuoles in their cytoplasm possibly represent primitive vascular lumina.

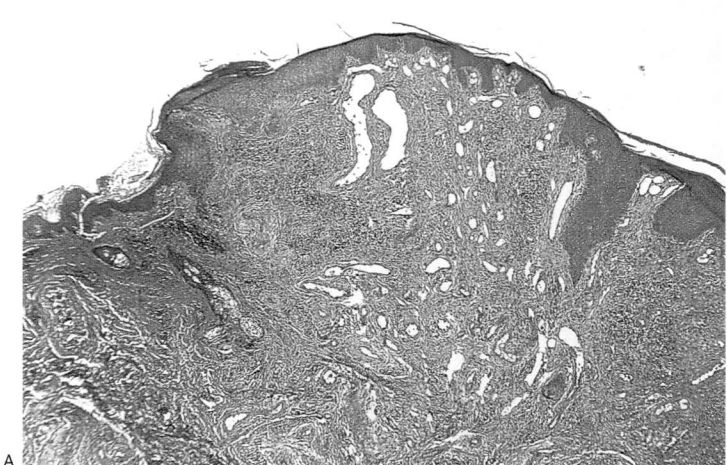
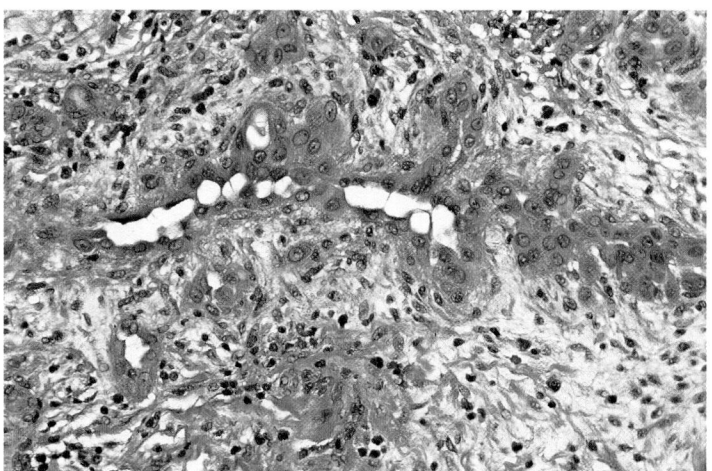

Fig. 38.16 **(A) Angiolymphoid hyperplasia with eosinophils. (B)** The vascular channels are lined by plump, partly vacuolated endothelial cells. There are scattered eosinophils in the stroma. (H & E)

Kimura's disease is composed of reactive lymphoid follicles with a dense infiltration of eosinophils, sometimes forming eosinophilic abscesses.[313–315] Mast cells are increased.[315,316] Vessels are increased in number, but their endothelial cells are usually flat. Vascular cords are unusual.[293]

'Angiolymphoid hyperplasia with high endothelial venules' is the term suggested recently for a cutaneous lesion with a characteristic admixture of lymphoid hyperplasia (without eosinophils) and a vascular proliferation previously called APACHE – *acral pseudolymphomatous angiokeratoma of children* (see p. 1124).[317]

LOBULAR CAPILLARY HEMANGIOMAS

The term 'lobular capillary hemangiomas' refers to a group of vascular tumors characterized by the presence of capillary-sized vessels arranged in lobules.[318,319] Included in this category are pyogenic granuloma and its variants, acquired tufted angioma (angioblastoma, progressive capillary hemangioma),[318] and glomeruloid hemangioma. The infection-related angiomatoses (bacillary epithelioid angiomatosis and verruga peruana) may also have a lobular pattern.

Pyogenic granuloma and variants

Pyogenic granuloma is a common benign vascular tumor of mucous membranes and skin. Studies suggest that it represents a hemangioma and not simply a florid proliferation of granulation tissue.[320,321] Common sites include the gingiva, lips, fingers and face.[322] Less common sites include the trunk, arms, legs and conjunctiva.[323] These tumors are commonly polypoid and pedunculated, but they may be sessile. Most are red or red-brown in color. Some darker lesions may clinically mimic nodular malignant melanoma. The lesions typically evolve rapidly to maximum size over a period of weeks. In one series this varied from 0.5 to 4 cm, with a mean diameter of 1.1 cm.[324] The surface is often ulcerated and bleeds easily.

Spontaneous involution of lesions is uncommon but has been reported in cases of disseminated pyogenic granuloma[325] and post partum in women who develop lesions during pregnancy (epulis gravidarum).[326] The lesions may develop at any age, and both sexes are affected. There is a female predominance in some reports,[327] but not in others.[328] In one series of oral and nasal mucosal lesions there was a marked male predominance in the first two decades and a female predominance during the childbearing years.[320] Children most commonly develop this tumor after the age of 1 year; rarely, congenital lesions occur.[323] Occasionally, the tumors may be multiple or disseminated.[325,329–333] Multiple satellite recurrences sometimes occur after treatment of the primary lesion, particularly when the latter was on the trunk, an uncommon site for pyogenic granuloma.[334–336] Satellite vascular lesions resembling a vascular malformation have been reported following removal of a nevocellular nevus.[337] Pyogenic granulomas have been reported in a pre-existing nevus flammeus,[338] a portwine stain[323,339,340] and a 'spider' angioma.[341]

In the majority of cases there is no apparent cause for these lesions; a minority follow trauma,[320,323,324] retinoid therapy,[342,343] insect bite,[323] burn,[311,333] scald[344] or cryotherapy.[345] The higher incidence in women during the child-bearing years, the occurrence in pregnancy, an association with use of the oral contraceptive pill, and the spontaneous regression of lesions following parturition suggest that a hormonal factor is involved in their genesis.[326] This theory has been disputed for cutaneous pyogenic granulomas, but not for mucosal ones.[328] It has also been suggested that pyogenic granulomas represent small acquired arteriovenous fistulae.[322] Immunohistochemical and ultrastructural studies have confirmed that pyogenic granulomas are tumors of vessels and endothelial cells.[346,347]

Histopathology

Pyogenic granulomas are lobular capillary hemangiomas (Fig. 38.17).[320] The lobular arrangement of the lesions is distinct from the pattern of capillaries in granulation tissue and, unlike granulation tissue, the capillaries do not usually involute with time. The underlying morphology is often obscured by secondary ulceration, edema, hemorrhage and inflammatory changes. In uncomplicated lesions there is a lobulated proliferation of capillary-sized vessels. The deep lobules are compact and cellular, with small indistinct lumina. Occasional mitotic figures may be seen within the cellular lobules. The apoptotic rate is low, possibly a reflection of its rapid growth.[348] Toward the surface, the lobules are larger and less tightly packed, and have distinct capillaries with larger branching lumina. The lobules are separated by myxoid or fibrous connective tissue septa.[349] The rare presence of spindle cells may mimic Kaposi's sarcoma.[350] Extramedullary hematopoiesis has been reported in the stroma in one case.[351]

The surface epithelium is attenuated, and at the margins of the lesion there is often an epidermal collarette formed by elongated rete ridges or sweat ducts. Surface ulceration and inflammation are secondary events, and some-times lead to the formation of true granulation tissue near the surface of the lesions. Mast cells are not increased in pyogenic granuloma, unlike proliferative-phase hemangiomas.[201,323]

Lesions with the same lobular hemangiomatous pattern have also been described within veins[352] and in subcutaneous tissues.[353] *Intravenous pyogenic granuloma* occurs predominantly on the neck, arms and hands.[352,354] The lesions are composed of a lobular proliferation of capillaries set in a fibro-myxoid stroma. A fibrovascular stalk usually connects the lesion to the intima of the involved vein.[355] *Subcutaneous pyogenic granuloma* occurs predominantly on the upper extremities.[353]

Acquired tufted angioma

Wilson Jones first gave the name acquired tufted angioma to an unusual acquired vascular proliferation[356,357] that had previously been reported as progressive capillary hemangioma,[358] and 'angioblastoma (Nakagawa)' in the Japanese literature.[359,360] The Japanese cases have some clinical differences and may not be identical to acquired tufted angioma. The condition is characterized by slowly spreading erythematous macules and plaques; rarely, there are multiple lesions.[177] Raised papules resembling pyogenic granulomas are sometimes seen within the lesion.[318] This vascular tumor occurs

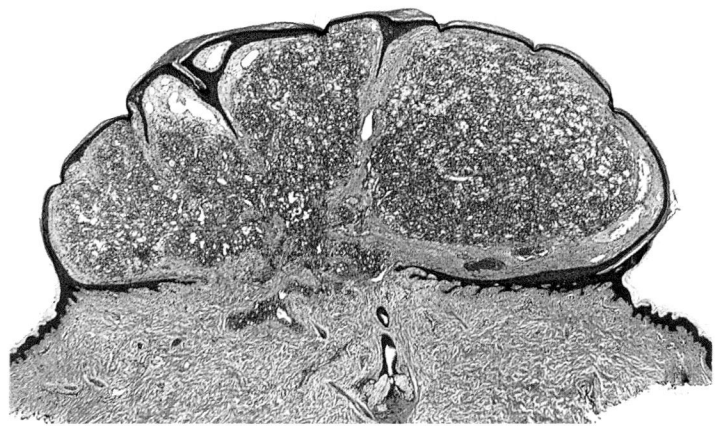

Fig. 38.17 **Pyogenic granuloma.** There is a well-developed collarette at the margins of this lobular vascular proliferation. (H & E)

predominantly in children and young adults, but has also been reported in older individuals.[361–363] Lesions arise most commonly on the neck and upper trunk, but also at other sites;[364,365] they are sometimes painful.[364,366] Platelet trapping in the lesions, producing the Kasabach–Merritt syndrome, is an uncommon complication.[367–371] There are rare associations with pregnancy,[372] liver transplantation[366] and nevus flammeus.[373,374] Familial cases have also been described. Most cases do not regress, as do 'strawberry nevi' of infancy and childhood, but there are reports of partial or complete regression and the recurrence of lesions.[362,372,375–378] Familial lesions have been described.[379]

Histopathology

There are multiple separated cellular lobules within the dermis and subcutis. Some lobules bulge the walls of dilated thin-walled vascular channels which are within the lobules or at their periphery. This sometimes gives the vessels a semilunar profile.[318] These larger vessels have a distinct endothelial lining.

Each lobule is composed of cells with spindle-shaped and oval nuclei (Fig. 38.18). Mitotic figures may be seen but there is no cellular atypia. Small capillary-sized vascular lumina are present in these areas. The morphology of the lobules resembles those seen in pyogenic granulomas. Hemosiderin may be present in the lesions; inflammation and edema are not usually seen. Some authors have noted proliferation of eccrine sweat glands near the vascular lobules.[372,380]

The pattern of cellular nodules with a peripheral dilated channel superficially resembles Kaposi's sarcoma, but the lobules lack the characteristic interlacing bundles of spindle cells and slit-like vessels, and usually lack an inflammatory infiltrate with plasma cells. In endovascular papillary angioendothelioma of childhood, papillary processes lined by atypical endothelial cells protrude into vascular lumina. In Masson's 'vegetant intravascular hemangioendothelioma', papular processes, composed of hyperplastic endothelium supported by fibrous stalks, are confined within vascular lumina.

Tumor cells are positive for CD34, but stain only weakly or not at all for factor VIII-related antigen.[381]

Electron microscopy

Ultrastructural studies have confirmed cell-marker studies, which have shown that these lesions consist of endothelial cells and pericytes with small lumina.[357] In one study of 'angioblastoma (Nakagawa)' crystalloid inclusions were seen in endothelial cells.[359]

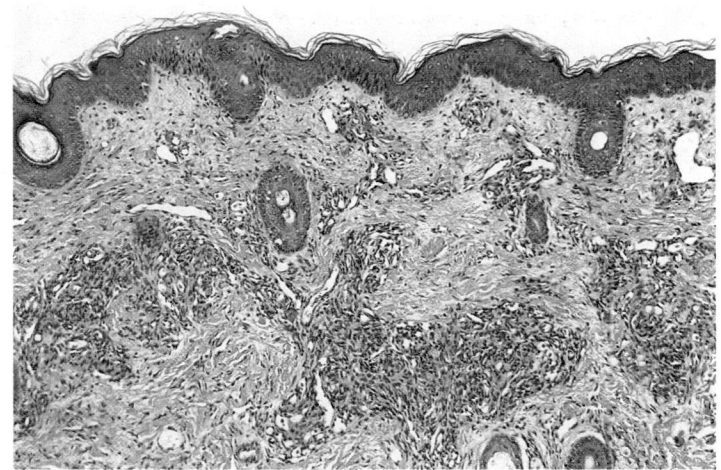

Fig. 38.18 **Acquired tufted angioma.** The multiple vascular lobules are composed of spindle-shaped and polygonal cells. (H & E)

GLOMUS TUMOR

Glomus tumors are variably regarded as hamartomas or neoplasms which resemble elements of the glomus apparatus in the skin. The glomus apparatus contains a central coiled canal, the Sucquet–Hoyer canal, which is lined by endothelium and several layers of glomus cells. Glomus tumors combine cells resembling glomus cells and vascular structures. Although they almost always occur in the skin, rare lesions have been reported at other sites, including the deep soft tissues,[382] bone,[383,384] vagina,[385] trachea,[386] lung,[387] gastrointestinal tract,[388,389] oral cavity,[390] nasal cavity,[391,392] within veins[374,393] and in cutaneous nerves.[394,395] The intravenous lesions tend to involve the forearm. There is no evidence of aggressive clinical behavior.[396] Glomus tumors may be solitary or multiple; multiple forms may be disseminated or regional.[397–401] Variants of the regional form are the congenital plaque-like[399,402–404] and patch-like types.[405] The plaque-like variant may have the histological features of a glomangioma or glomangiomyoma (see below).[402,403,406] Rare glomangiosarcomas, a malignant form, have been reported; they may arise *de novo* or in association with a benign glomus tumor.[407–410] Benign lesions are occasionally locally infiltrative;[411] they may recur after removal.[408] Atypical glomus tumors are discussed further below.

The *glomus tumor proper* is almost always a solitary, purple dermal nodule on the extremities, particularly the fingers and toes. It may have a subungual location and lie within a slight depression in the underlying phalanx. This variant usually presents in adults and occurs with an equal sex incidence. The tumors are almost always painful. The pain varies in intensity but may be severe and paroxysmal, and occur spontaneously or be induced by pressure or cold. Rarely, a small cluster of tumors may occur.[412]

The *glomangioma* is most often solitary, but multiple lesions may also occur. Familial instances of multiple lesions have been reported and there may be an autosomal dominant mode of inheritance, linked to a locus on chromosome 1p21–p22.[397,413,414] Glomangiomas are usually painless and vary in size from small to moderately large protuberant hemangioma-like lesions. Glomangiomas may occur on the extremities or trunk, and rarely have a subungual location.[415] They may have a segmental distribution reflecting mosaicism. They usually exhibit so-called 'type 2 mosaicism', which reflects loss of heterozygosity and is characterized by severe/prominent lesions locally superimposed on 'milder' disseminated lesions.[416,417] Glomangiomas present at an earlier age (usually in adolescence), and are less common than the glomus tumor proper.

Histopathology

The *glomus tumor proper* is a well-circumscribed or encapsulated dermal tumor which may extend into the subcutis. It is composed of solid aggregates of glomus cells surrounding inconspicuous vessels. Glomus cells are rounded, regular cells with eosinophilic cytoplasm and darkly staining round to oval nuclei (Fig. 38.19). Tumor cells and vessels are embedded in a fibrous stroma. Some tumors contain large amounts of myxoid stroma (Fig. 38.20).[418] The tumor matrix contains small unmyelinated nerve fibers and mast cells. The uniformity of the cells and their lack of pleomorphism are features of these tumors. Oncocytic and epithelioid variants have been described.[419,420] The latter are composed of large polygonal to spindle-shaped cells with abundant eosinophilic cytoplasm and large irregular nuclei. The cytological atypia is thought to represent cellular senescence.[420] The term 'symplastic glomus tumor' has been used for these lesions, which have a high nuclear grade in the absence of any other malignant features.[421] Another variant is the *infiltrative glomus tumor*, characterized by an infiltrative growth pattern at the periphery of the lesion.[422] Some of these lesions have been regarded in the past as malignant glomus tumors. This category of infiltrative glomus tumor is not

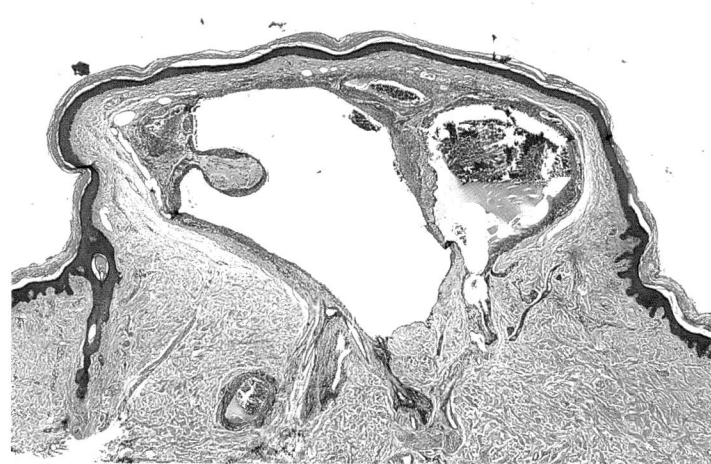

Fig. 38.21 **Glomangioma.** Only several layers of glomus cells surround the large vascular channels. (H & E)

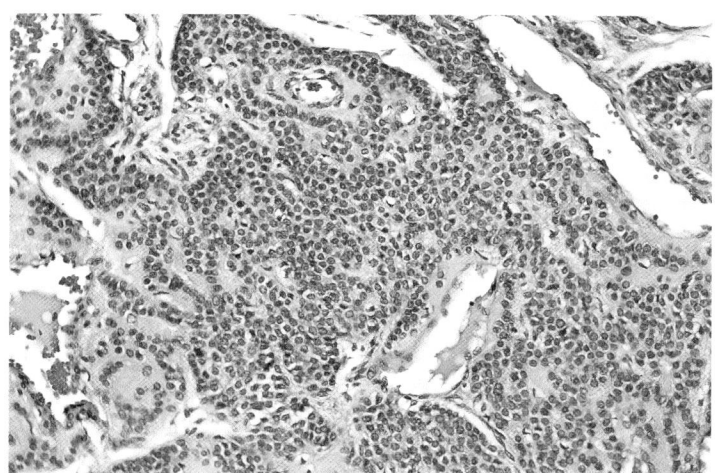

Fig. 38.19 **Glomus tumor.** There are sheets of glomus cells and a few blood vessels. (H & E)

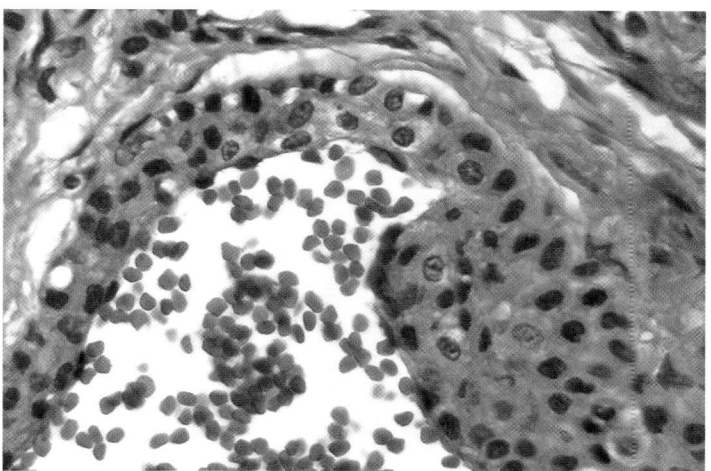

Fig. 38.22 **Glomangioma.** A few layers of glomus cells surround a vascular channel. (H & E)

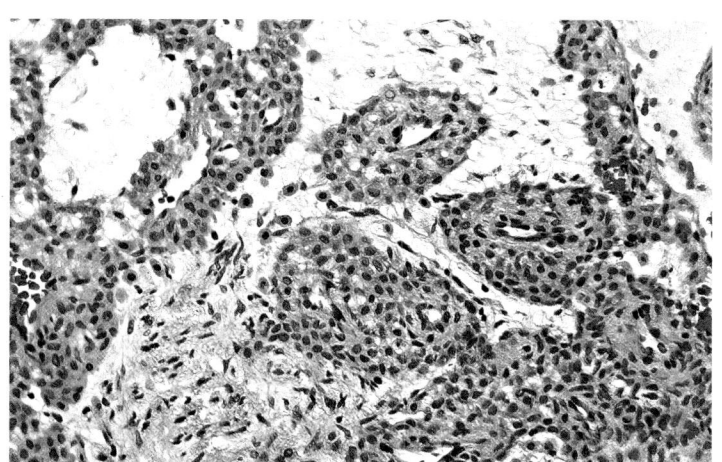

Fig. 38.20 **Glomus tumor.** The stroma between some of the nests of glomus cells contains mucin. (H & E)

included in the recent classification proposed by Folpe et al.[421] Extensive *glomus cell hyperplasia* has been reported in the vicinity of a cluster of multiple glomus tumors.[412]

Glomangiomas have more prominent vessels and less conspicuous glomus cells than the glomus tumor proper (Fig. 38.21). Glomangiomas are poorly circumscribed and unencapsulated and consist of irregular ectatic vascular channels irregularly surrounded by small numbers of glomus cells (Fig. 38.22). Glomus cells may be so sparse that the lesions can be difficult to distinguish from conventional hemangiomas. *Glomangiomatosis* refers to diffuse angiomatosis with a histological excess of glomus cells.[421]

Some glomus tumors of both types show an apparent transition from glomus cells to smooth muscle cells. They have been called *glomangiomyomas*.[403]

Immunohistochemical techniques have demonstrated vimentin, muscle-specific actin and α-smooth muscle actin in the cytoplasm; laminin and type IV collagen are present in the basal lamina-like material.[399,423,424] The cells lack the cell markers of endothelial cells. The absence of desmin from the tumor cells is a feature shared with some cells of vascular smooth muscle.[399,424]

Multiple nerve fibers containing substance P have been identified within solitary glomus tumors.[425] Substance P is known to be a sensory afferent neurotransmitter for mediating painful stimuli.

Electron microscopy

The tumor cells show similar ultrastructural features to smooth muscle cells. Each cell is surrounded by a basal lamina and contains cytoplasmic intermediate filaments, microfilaments, pinocytotic vesicles, and dense bodies in the cytoplasm and adjacent to the plasma membrane.[399,424]

ERUPTIVE PSEUDOANGIOMATOSIS

Prose and colleagues reported three children who, during an apparent viral illness, developed angiomatous papules that resolved spontaneously. The lesions were composed of dilated dermal blood vessels with plump, 'hobnail' endothelial cells.[426] Subsequent cases have not always been associated with an obvious viral illness, suggesting multiple etiologies.[427] Furthermore, the endothelial cells have not always been enlarged.[427] A mild perivascular infiltrate of lymphocytes has been present in some cases.[428]

PAPULAR ANGIOPLASIA

The two recorded cases of papular angioplasia were in elderly patients who presented with vascular papules of the face and scalp in which the dermal vascular proliferation contained atypical bizarre endothelial cells.[429] The lesions, which were termed 'papular angioplasia', were thought of as a 'pseudo-malignancy'. Their relationship to pyogenic granuloma and angiolymphoid hyperplasia is uncertain.

MULTINUCLEATE CELL ANGIOHISTIOCYTOMA

Multinucleate cell angiohistiocytoma was first described by Smith and Wilson Jones. It is characterized by grouped, red to violet papules that may resemble Kaposi's sarcoma;[430,431] almost all reported cases have been in females over 40.[431–434] The legs, particularly the calves and thighs, are most commonly involved; the hands are the second most common site.[431,433] Occasional cases have occurred on the chest[431] and face.[431,435,436] Papules develop over several months and then growth ceases.

The etiology is not known; HHV-8 has not been detected.[437]

Histopathology[431]

It is not clear whether multinucleate cell angiohistiocytoma is primarily a vascular or stromal cell tumor. The two main components are increased numbers of ectatic or narrow vessels in the upper and mid dermis, and large angulated multinucleate cells (Fig. 38.23). The vessels are small venules and capillaries, lined by endothelial cells with prominent nuclei. Angulated multinucleate cells have 3–10 nuclei arranged in a ring or clumped together; they are basophilic. These large cells stain with vimentin but not with macrophage markers (Mac387, CD68, lysozyme), CD31, CD34, S100 or factor XIIIa.[437] Varying numbers of mononuclear interstitial cells are present; they appear to be dermal dendrocytes (factor XIIIa positive), indeterminate or Langerhans' cells (CD1a positive) or macrophages (lysozyme, CD68 and Mac387 positive).[431,435] Discrete foci of inflammatory cells are also present. The ultrastructural features have also been described.[432]

REACTIVE ANGIOENDOTHELIOMATOSIS

Reactive angioendotheliomatosis is a cutaneous vascular proliferation that presents as infiltrated, red-to-blue patches and plaques, often with purpura. Necrosis and ulceration may sometimes develop.[438] The lesions may occur at any body site. They measure from 1 to 3 cm or more in diameter. This vascular proliferation may be associated with a variety of conditions, many of which have in common luminal obstruction by thrombi or abnormal proteins. It may occur in association with chronic disseminated intravascular coagulation (DIC),[439] cryoglobulinemia,[440] infections, paraproteinemia with myelomatosis, intravascular immunoglobulin deposits associated with a monoclonal gammopathy, the lupus anticoagulant, hepatopathy and arteriovenous fistulae used for hemodialysis.[438,441–443] A similar lesion has been reported overlying an implanted nickel nail for delayed union of a fracture and as an idiopathic phenomenon in a child.[444,445] The lesions usually resolve after the withdrawal or the cure of the initiating process. It must be distinguished from malignant angioendotheliomatosis, an angiotropic lymphoma, and from the intravascular simulant seen in patients with rheumatoid arthritis and variously called reactive angioendotheliomatosis, cutaneous histiocytic lymphangitis and intravascular histiocytosis (see p. 208).[446]

Diffuse dermal angiomatosis is a variant of reactive angio-endotheliomatosis associated with severe atherosclerosis causing vascular narrowing.[447,448] Lesions resolve completely with revascularization. Interestingly, two cases of vascular proliferation have been reported in the skin distal to an arteriovenous fistula made for hemodialysis: one case resembled reactive angioendotheliomatosis and the other diffuse dermal angiomatosis, indicating the close relationship between these two entities.[442]

Histopathology

Reactive angioendotheliomatosis is characterized by a benign intraluminal proliferation of endothelial cells which may occlude the vascular lumina. The vessels are dilated. Sometimes the proliferated endothelial cells produce a glomeruloid appearance. The cells may be large and mildly atypical but they are not malignant. Thrombi and protein deposits are sometimes found. There is usually only minimal inflammation, if any. The cells express CD31, CD34 and factor VIII-related antigen.

In **diffuse dermal angiomatosis** the hyperplastic endothelial cells diffusely infiltrate the reticular dermis, sometimes forming small lumina.[447,448] This contrasts with the intravascular proliferation seen in reactive angio-endotheliomatosis.

MISCELLANEOUS LESIONS

Rarely, patients with chronic disseminated intravascular coagulation (DIC) develop plaques of purplish discoloration which on biopsy show an apparent increase in small vessels arranged in leashes in the dermis and subcutaneous fat (Fig. 38.24). The vessel proliferation represents organization of thrombosed vessels.[439] A similar 'angiomatosis' has been reported in cryoproteinemia.[440] So-called 'reactive angioendotheliomatosis' is poorly defined.[449]

INTRAVASCULAR PAPILLARY ENDOTHELIAL HYPERPLASIA

Pierre Masson first described this vascular proliferation in hemorrhoidal veins; he regarded it as a neoplastic process. He named it 'hémangioendothéliome végétant intravasculaire'.[450] Its importance lies in its histological resemblance to angiosarcoma: the name 'Masson's pseudoangiosarcoma' has also been proposed.[451–455] The condition is now generally regarded as an unusual pattern of organization of a thrombus within a vein,[176,452,454,456] or within one or more of the component vessels of various vascular abnormalities. These include cavernous hemangiomas,[451,453] pyogenic granulomas[451,457] and lymphangiomas.[458] Organizing hematomas of soft tissues may also show this pattern.[459] In most cases there is a single lesion, but multiple lesions have also been described.[460] They usually present clinically as firm, sometimes painful

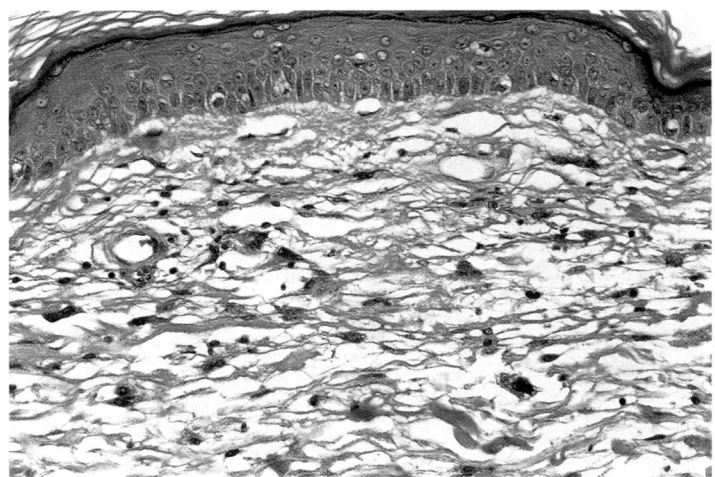

Fig. 38.23 **Multinucleate cell angiohistiocytoma.** There are atypical cells and an increase in small vessels in the papillary dermis. (H & E)

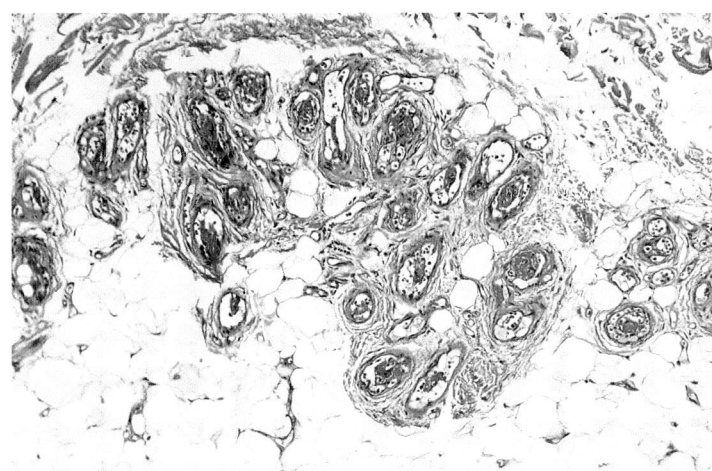

Fig. 38.24 **Vascular proliferation in a patient with chronic disseminated intravascular coagulation (DIC).** Thrombi are present in some of the vessels. (H & E)

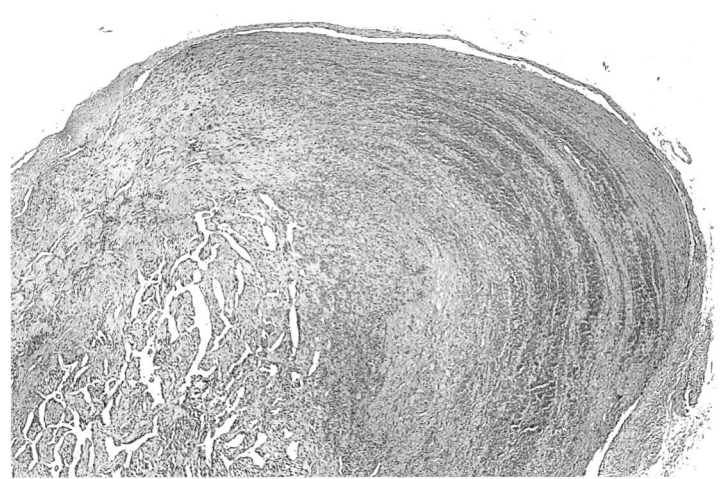

Fig. 38.25 **Intravascular papillary endothelial hyperplasia.** Vascular channels are present within the lumen of a dilated vein. (H & E)

nodules which appear blue or purple through the overlying skin.[454] On section, typical lesions appear encapsulated and cystic; they contain variable amounts of thrombus. Although lesions can occur at any site, including the tongue,[455] they are most commonly found on the fingers, head and neck, and trunk.[451,454,461] There is a female predominance in most series.[451,454] Local excision is curative.

Histopathology

In most examples the proliferation is limited to the lumen of an identifiable vein or vessel in a vascular abnormality (Fig. 38.25). Occasionally there is only a fibrous capsule lacking definite features of a vessel wall. Rarely, the proliferation extends outside the lumen, possibly due to rupture of the wall of the vessel. Masses of papillary processes are present within the lumen and they are almost always associated with some thrombus. Each papillary frond is covered by a single layer of plump endothelial cells. Mitotic figures may be present but they are never frequent. There is no multilayering of the cells, and solid cellular areas, cellular tufts, atypia and necrosis are not usually evident; however, Renshaw and Rosai have described severe cytological atypia in lesions from the lip.[462] The core of the papillae consists of fibrin or collagenous connective tissue, depending on the stage of organization.

Electron microscopy

Electron microscopy confirms the endothelial nature of the cells and demonstrates that they lie on a basement membrane, outside of which are pericytes.[463]

ACRO-ANGIODERMATITIS

The vasoproliferative disorder acro-angiodermatitis resembles Kaposi's sarcoma both clinically and histologically, and has been termed 'pseudo-Kaposi sarcoma'.[176,464,465] The lesions arise in a background of increased venous pressure due to chronic venous insufficiency,[466–468] paralysis of a limb,[469] congenital arteriovenous malformation,[470,471] Klippel–Trenaunay–Weber syndrome[472] or acquired arteriovenous fistula.[473,474] Acro-angiodermatitis has also been reported in an above-knee amputation stump.[475,476] The majority occur on the lower part of the legs and on the feet; in cases associated with arteriovenous malformations they are found over the site of the malformation. In most cases affecting the legs there is also stasis dermatitis. The lesions consist of purple papules and nodules with variable surface scale.[477]

Those cases associated with venous insufficiency or paralysis of the legs have a characteristic distribution, occupying a triangular region on the extensor surface of the foot and toes, with the most prominent lesions on the first and second toes.[466] Lesions may be unilateral or bilateral, depending on the cause. There is a male preponderance.[478]

Histopathology[479,480]

The papules and nodules consist of a proliferation of small dilated vessels in an edematous dermis (Fig. 38.26). The vessels have fairly regular profiles and lack the jagged outline and 'promontory' sign seen in early lesions of Kaposi's sarcoma.[479] Plump endothelial cells, without atypia, line the vessels. The cells are positive for CD34.[481] A slight perivascular fibroblastic proliferation is also seen but is not marked. Some lesions show nodular collections of vessels with narrow lumina.[480] Extravasated red blood cells, hemosiderin and a variable round-cell infiltrate are seen around the vascular proliferation. Plasma cells are usually not present. The overlying epidermis may show hyperkeratosis.

BACILLARY ANGIOMATOSIS

The condition now known as bacillary angiomatosis[482] was first described by Stoler et al in 1983.[483] It is a systemic disorder but was first identified because of cutaneous lesions resembling Kaposi's sarcoma. Unlike Kaposi's sarcoma, this condition responds readily to antibiotic therapy. Bacillary angiomatosis is caused by two closely related Gram-negative coccobacilli, *Bartonella (Rochalimaea) henselae* and *Bartonella (Rochalimaea) quintana*.[484–488] *Bartonella henselae* is also a common cause of cat-scratch disease; it has also been associated with a bacteremic syndrome and peliosis hepatis.[484] *Bartonella quintana* is the causative agent of trench fever.

Bacillary angiomatosis occurs primarily in those with HIV infection,[482,489–491] but has also been reported in organ transplant recipients,[484] in patients with leukemia,[492,493] in patients on systemic steroid therapy[494] and even immunocompetent individuals, including children.[495–499] Up to two-thirds of cases are associated with exposure to cats; lesions sometimes follow a bite or scratch.[500] Cutaneous tumors are usually multiple and take the form of pyogenic granuloma-like lesions, subcutaneous nodules or, uncommonly, hyperpigmented indurated plaques, the last form occurring particularly in black people.[501] Pyogenic granuloma-like lesions are dusky-red in color, often pedunculated, frequently bleed and may be mildly tender. They resemble the lesions of verruga peruana. Spontaneous regression sometimes occurs. The lesions of bacillary angiomatosis also occur on respiratory and gastrointestinal tract mucosa, and in the heart, liver, spleen, bone marrow, muscle, soft tissue and brain. Patients often have constitutional symptoms, particularly when extracutaneous lesions are present.[484]

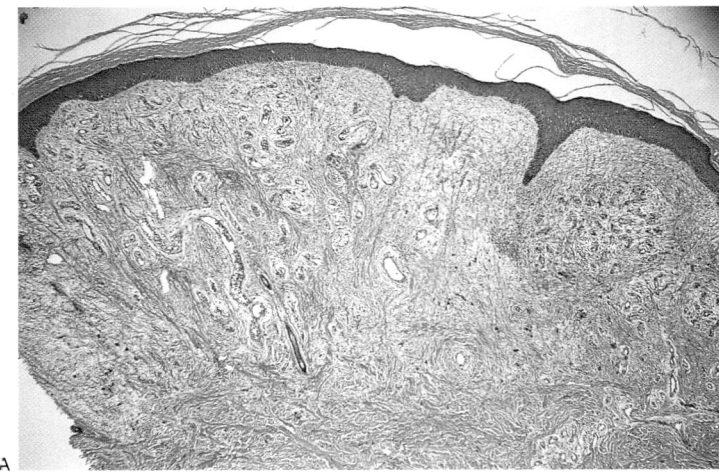

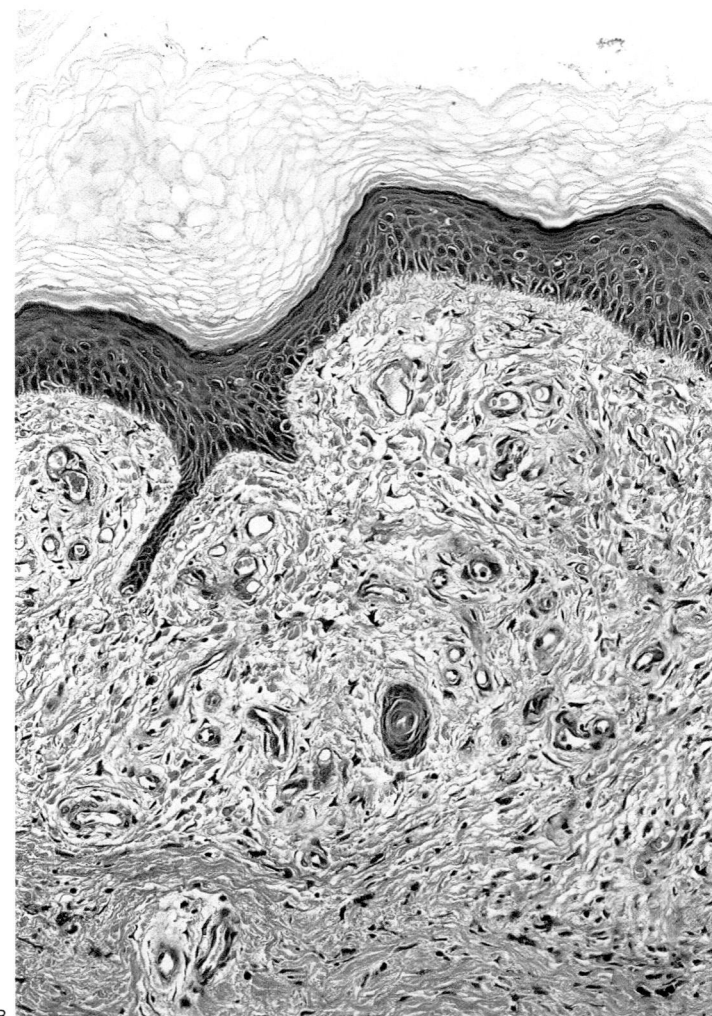

Fig. 38.26 **Acro-angiodermatitis.** There is a proliferation of small vessels in an edematous dermis. Fibroblasts are also increased. (H & E)

Histopathology[489,501]

Superficial lesions are characterized by small round blood vessels in an edematous stroma. Deeper lesions are more cellular and compact. In both forms blood vessels are lined by plump, epithelioid endothelial cells. A background inflammatory cell infiltrate of lymphocytes, histiocytes and neutrophils is also present. Neutrophils are plentiful in deeper lesions. A peripheral collarette and ulceration are seen in superficial lesions (Fig. 38.27). Organisms are seen as clumps of amphophilic granular material, particularly near neutrophils; they are readily demonstrated by a Warthin–Starry or Grocott–methenamine silver stain.[489,502] Immunohistochemical techniques and PCR-based methods have also been used to identify organisms.[487,503] Ultrastructurally, organisms are seen in the interstitium of lesions and are pleomorphic structures with a trilaminar wall and coarsely granular cytoplasm.[504]

Differential diagnosis

Bacillary angiomatosis is usually easy to differentiate from Kaposi's sarcoma because of the presence of epithelioid endothelial cells, neutrophils and organisms in the former, and spindle cells and slit-like vessels in the latter. The two conditions may occur concurrently,[505] but bacillary angiomatosis is much less common than Kaposi's sarcoma in patients with AIDS. Neutrophils are

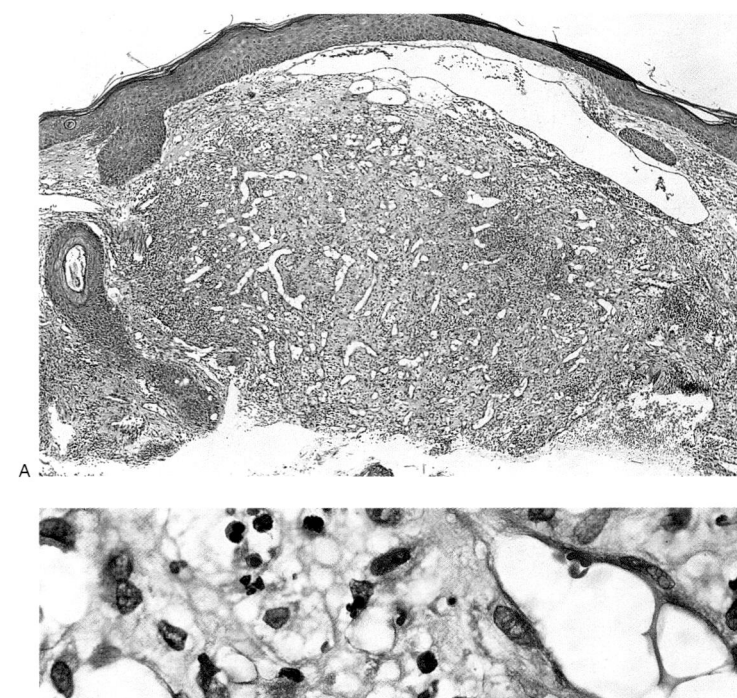

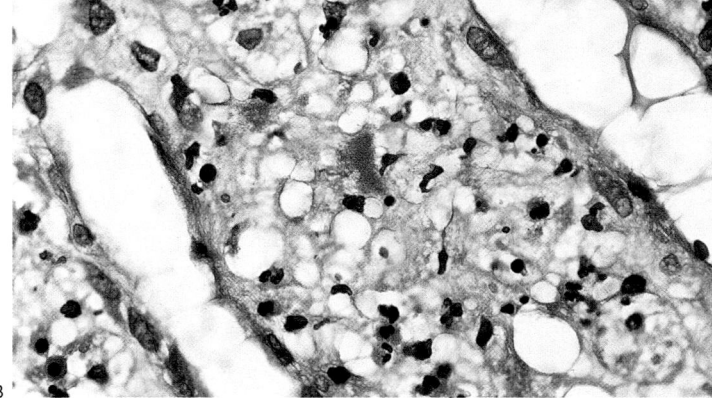

Fig. 38.27 **(A) Bacillary angiomatosis in a patient with AIDS. (B)** Neutrophils, nuclear dust and a clump of granular material (representing bacteria) are present in the stroma between the small vascular channels. (H & E) (Microscopic slide kindly provided by Dr Philip LeBoit, Department of Pathology and Dermatology, University of California, San Francisco, USA)

confined to the surface of ulcerated lesions of pyogenic granuloma; this lesion is usually more obviously lobulated. Organisms are not seen in pyogenic granuloma.

VERRUGA PERUANA

The skin lesion of the eruptive phase of Carrión's disease (bartonellosis), caused by *Bartonella bacilliformis*, is known as verruga peruana (Peruvian wart).[506,507] Carrión's disease is endemic at altitudes between 800 and 2500 meters in parts of Peru, Ecuador and Colombia. Multiple, miliary superficial hemangioma-like lesions or larger, deeper, sometimes ulcerated lesions occur in this condition. They resolve spontaneously over weeks to months.[506,507]

Histopathology

Superficial lesions consist of a proliferation of capillary-like vessels in the papillary dermis, with the formation of a collarette. There is an associated inflammatory infiltrate composed of lymphocytes and plasma cells. In nodular lesions there is a multilobular proliferation or more solid aggregation of cells in the dermis, and sometimes also in the subcutis. Vascular lumina are fewer and smaller. The 'tumor cells' are large and epithelioid; groups of them are surrounded by a reticulin network. Mitotic figures are frequent. A spindle-cell element is occasionally seen and may make distinction from Kaposi's sarcoma extremely difficult. Immunohistochemical studies have identified these cells as endothelial in nature, as they are positive for both factor VIII-associated antigen and *Ulex europaeus*-1 lectin.[506] In regressing lesions there is involution and necrosis of the vascular elements, associated with a heavy infiltrate of lymphocytes, histiocytes and neutrophils. There is subsequent fibrosis.

The causative organism is not seen by light microscopy but may be found on ultrastructural examination, predominantly in an extracellular location but occasionally in phagosomes.[506] Rocha Lima inclusions, consisting of conglomerates of apparently intracellular cytoplasmic granules that are colored red by Romanowsky–Giemsa stains, may be seen within the endothelial cells. Ultrastructurally these appear to consist of phagosomes containing organisms and interstitial matrix-like material as well as a labyrinth of cisternal channels with similar contents.[506]

ACQUIRED PROGRESSIVE LYMPHANGIOMA

Acquired progressive lymphangioma[508] is a rare vascular proliferative lesion which has also been called benign lymphangioendothelioma.[509] Although it was initially presumed to be of lymphatic origin, immunohistochemical and ultrastructural studies have been conflicting: some studies suggest a possible blood vessel derivation, but others suggest overlap features.[510] There are histological similarities to cutaneous angiosarcoma, but the course of the reported cases has been benign. The lesion presents as an erythematous patch or plaque which gradually enlarges, often over many years.[511] There is no site predilection, cases having been reported on the abdomen, leg, arm and head.[511] Most tumors reported have been in adults[512] but this lesion may also arise in children;[508,510,511] rarely, it is congenital.[513] It has been associated with previous femoral arteriography,[514] trauma to a 'vascular birthmark', a tick bite and radiotherapy.[515–517] One case resolved spontaneously.[518] The lesions reported as **benign lymphangiomatous papules of the skin (BLAP)** are related lesions occurring at sites of radiotherapy.[519] The lesions present as solitary or multiple papules or vesicles.

Histopathology[512]

The main feature is the presence of thin-walled interconnecting vascular channels at various levels of the dermis or subcutis. These vessels tend to be arranged horizontally, particularly in the upper dermis. Vessels are smaller, more irregular, angular and cleft-like at deeper levels, and 'dissect' the dermal collagen bundles. The vessels are lined by flat to plump endothelial cells with some focal nuclear hyperchromasia and crowding. No frank atypia or mitotic figures have been reported. No intraluminal cell clumps are seen. Vessels contain proteinaceous material, a few red blood cells, or are empty. The vessels are usually surrounded by chronic inflammatory cells, often including a few plasma cells.[520]

Immunohistochemical studies are conflicting: endothelial cells have been reported as staining positively or negatively for factor VIII-related antigen and *Ulex europaeus*-1 lectin, and positively for CD34 and CD31.[516,521] Basement membrane has been shown to be present by positive staining for type IV collagen and laminin. It has been absent by electron microscopy. A smooth muscle component has also been demonstrated focally, around the vascular spaces.[510,512–515,518]

Histologically, this lesion may mimic angiosarcoma and patch-stage Kaposi's sarcoma. The distinction from well-differentiated angiosarcoma can be very difficult; usually there is more cellular atypia or cellular tufts in angiosarcoma. The long clinical history and the site of the lesion may be helpful. The face and scalp are the usual sites for cutaneous angiosarcoma. Early Kaposi's sarcoma may be impossible to distinguish from acquired progressive lymphangioma, but in the former there may be red blood cells, hemosiderin and an inflammatory cell infiltrate which includes plasma cells. Inflammation is minimal in acquired progressive lymphangioma.[512] The patch stage of Kaposi's sarcoma is usually seen in AIDS-related cases, and lesions are often multiple.

Benign lymphangiomatous papules of the skin (BLAP) consist of markedly dilated vascular spaces in the upper dermis exhibiting atypical features which include endothelial cells with plump or flattened nuclei, and numerous small papillary projections. As the lesions descend into the deeper dermis, the spaces become smaller and their lumina irregular, focally dissecting the collagen.[519] The endothelial cells are positive for *Ulex europaeus*-1 lectin and weakly positive for CD31, CD34 and factor VIII-related antigen.

TUMORS WITH VARIABLE OR UNCERTAIN BEHAVIOR

This category of vascular tumors has evoked considerable controversy, particularly the use of the term 'borderline' malignancy to describe the behavior of some tumors in this group.[522] The term 'hemangioendothelioma' has also attracted criticism because it has been applied to both benign and malignant vascular tumors.[264] While acknowledging the validity of this comment, the designations originally reported will be used here to avoid confusion.

The following tumors have a variable behavior and outcome:

- Kaposi's sarcoma
- hemangiopericytoma
- Kaposiform hemangioendothelioma.

KAPOSI'S SARCOMA

Kaposi's sarcoma, composed of vessels and spindle-shaped cells, was first described by Kaposi in 1872 as 'idiopathic multiple pigment-sarcoma of the skin'.[523] The epidemic type of Kaposi's sarcoma, first reported in the United States in 1981, has provoked considerable interest in this previously uncommon condition.[524] There are four clinicopathological types: classic, African (endemic type), a variant associated with immunosuppressive therapy, and an HIV-associated (epidemic) type. Human herpesvirus type 8 is the etiological agent in all types.[525]

Classic type

The classic type affects predominantly men in the fifth to seventh decades. It is exceedingly rare in children.[526] There is an increased incidence in Jews and Eastern Europeans and in people of Mediterranean origin.[527,528] In most cases the lesions are limited to the skin of the extremities, particularly the lower part of the legs and feet; occasionally lymph nodes and other organs are involved. The incidence of visceral involvement varies in different parts of the world, possibly reflecting the incidence of the different serotypes of the HHV-8 virus.[529] Edema sometimes precedes or follows the appearance of the lesions.[530] This type of Kaposi's sarcoma has a chronic course, with the development of more lesions; death is usually due to other causes. There is an increased risk of developing other tumors, particularly malignant lymphomas.[531-536] Spontaneous regression of the lesions may occur.

African (endemic) type

The African type of Kaposi's sarcoma is endemic in parts of tropical Africa, with the highest prevalence in eastern Zaire and western Uganda.[537] There are three main subtypes,[538] the most common being nodular disease, similar to classic Kaposi's sarcoma with a benign clinical course. A more aggressive subtype is characterized by extensive florid and infiltrative skin lesions, which may involve soft tissues and underlying bone. A lymphadenopathic subtype occurs predominantly in children: in this variety there is involvement of lymph nodes, often without cutaneous lesions, and the prognosis is poor.[539] There is a marked male predominance in endemic African Kaposi's sarcoma.[540] Epstein–Barr virus (EBV), as well as HHV-8, is frequently present in African cases.[541]

Kaposi's sarcoma associated with immunosuppressive therapy

Kaposi's sarcoma is a rare complication of organ transplantation, chemotherapy for tumors and long-term corticosteroid treatment for a variety of dermatological and other conditions.[532,542-547] It has been reported in renal transplant recipients, but only rarely in cardiac transplant recipients. In two recent studies the prevalence in renal transplant patients was 0.3% and 1.6%.[548,549] In cardiac transplant recipients the prevalence has been reported as 0.41%.[550] The male preponderance of cases is less marked than in the other forms of the disease; younger age groups are also affected. Tumors may appear within a short time of commencement of immunosuppressive therapy and may regress spontaneously following cessation of therapy.[543] There may be a more aggressive clinical course than in classic Kaposi's sarcoma. Death may follow widespread disease, particularly from gastrointestinal hemorrhage.

Epidemic (HIV-associated) type

The epidemic type of Kaposi's sarcoma is associated with AIDS, caused predominantly by the retrovirus human immunodeficiency virus type-1 (HIV-1).[551-553] In West Africa, AIDS is also associated with a second retrovirus, HIV-2; Kaposi's sarcoma is also reported in this group.[554] In Europe, the USA and Australia, this form of Kaposi's sarcoma is most common in homosexual and bisexual men. HIV-associated Kaposi's sarcoma also occurs in women, children, hemophiliacs and intravenous drug users. The prevalence of the tumor in risk groups other than homosexual and bisexual men varies. It is uncommon in hemophiliacs and in recipients of blood transfusions who develop HIV infection.[555,556] There is an intermediate risk in intravenous drug users.[557] In women who have contracted HIV infection by sexual contact, the

prevalence of Kaposi's sarcoma is highest in those who have had a bisexual partner.[556] Kaposi's sarcoma in HIV infection is rare before the age of 15.[556] Children of parents in high-risk groups for Kaposi's sarcoma and those children who acquire HIV infection by blood transfusion have the highest risk of developing Kaposi's sarcoma.[558] The proportion of patients with AIDS who develop Kaposi's sarcoma has fallen from 33% in 1981 to about 10% in 2000.[559]

The distribution of lesions in this form differs from that in classic Kaposi's sarcoma. The trunk, arms, head and neck are frequently involved. Lesions are usually multiple. There is frequent involvement of mucosal surfaces and internal organs. In one autopsy study the lungs were involved in 37% of cases, the gastrointestinal tract in 50%, and lymph nodes in 50%; 29% had evidence of visceral lesions without skin lesions.[560] The extent of cutaneous involvement does not correlate well with the extent of visceral disease.[561] The clinical course ranges from chronic to rapidly progressive. Most patients die from opportunistic infections or other complications of AIDS, rather than from Kaposi's sarcoma. In one large series of AIDS patients, survival was best in those whose only manifestation was Kaposi's sarcoma.[562] The lesions may regress spontaneously.[563]

Skin lesions are similar in all groups, but in the epidemic form they tend to occur earlier and to be smaller and more subtle. Early lesions are brown to red macules or patches which may resemble a bruise. Papules, nodules and plaques may be bluish or purple in color and may ulcerate. Unusual presentations include occurrence in a lymphedematous penis,[564] and localization to an area of previous radiation.[565]

Etiology and pathogenesis

In 1994, Chang et al identified DNA belonging to a novel virus in tissue affected by Kaposi's sarcoma. This virus, human herpesvirus type-8 (HHV-8) was originally known as Kaposi's sarcoma-associated herpesvirus (KSHV).[566] It has now been detected in all epidemiological forms of Kaposi's sarcoma.[567-571] The occasional negative case may be related to technical difficulties with the identification.[572] HHV-8 has also been implicated in the pathogenesis of multicentric Castleman's disease and primary effusion lymphomas.[573-575] The virus is not ubiquitous in the community and seropositivity is limited to a small percentage of the population.[576] However, there are small geographical areas in Italy with a high incidence of the classic type of Kaposi's sarcoma; they appear to be 'hot-spots' for HHV-8 infection.[577]

The mode of transmission of the virus has attracted considerable attention. HHV-8 is not shed in appreciable amounts in seminal fluid or from the rectum.[577,578] The virus is found in oral secretions. It appears that penile–oral contact is a high-risk activity, but this is obviously not the entire 'story'.[577] The virus was found in 44% of the heterosexual partners of patients with classic Kaposi's sarcoma, but this study did not categorize the sexual contact/ practices involved.[579,580] Transmission through needle sharing in drug use is another documented method of spread.[581]

As with other cell-transforming DNA viruses, infection with HHV-8 alone is probably not sufficient for the development of Kaposi's sarcoma; additional cofactors are probably required.[528] Isolated cases have been reported in which HHV-8 has been associated with other viruses, such as EBV[582] and HPV (in the case of penile lesions of Kaposi's sarcoma).[583,584] Furthermore, the explosive incidence of HIV-associated Kaposi's sarcoma in the early 1980s (later in some countries) resulted from colliding epidemics of HIV and HHV-8 infections in the homosexual and bisexual communities.[577,585] Kaposi's sarcoma is said to be 20 000 times more common in patients with HIV infection/AIDS than in the general population.[559] In most cases, no cofactors have been identified.[586] The tumor-suppressor gene p53 is an inconstant finding and appears not to have a significant role as a cofactor.[587–589] Studies of HLA subtype in patients with HIV-associated and the classic form of the condition have suggested a significant association with HLA-A2, B5, B8, B18 and DR5.[548,590,591]

HHV-8 infects CD19[+] B cells as well as T cells, monocytes, endothelial-derived spindle cells,[577] and CD34[+] cells in the peripheral blood of patients with Kaposi's sarcoma.[592] Three subtypes of HHV-8 (A, B and C) have been recognized. Type C infection tends not to be asociated with extracutaneous disease compared with subtypes A and B.[525]

It has been considered that disseminated Kaposi's sarcoma represents a multifocal reactive process, rather than a true sarcoma with the potential to metastasize.[593–595] In one study the cell population was found to be polyclonal, but another has shown a monoclonal population in multifocal lesions.[596] The controversy can be partly resolved by regarding Kaposi's sarcoma as binomial (hyperplastic/neoplastic), beginning as a reactive proliferation but behaving as a multifocal neoplasm in advanced stages.[530,597–599] Abnormalities have been detected in various angiogenic cytokines and cellular control systems.[597,600–605] The spindle cells are thought to be the proliferating component, while the endothelial cell population is thought to undergo a reactive hyperplasia. Other evidence suggests that the spindle-cell elements show endothelial differentiation.[606–613] Chronic stimulation of endothelial cells (possibly by viral infection) can produce transdifferentiation to a spindle-shaped cell.[614] Derivation from lymphatic endothelium has also been suggested.[615]

The response of a disease to various treatments may provide a valuable insight into its etiology and pathogenesis. Treatment with interferon alfa-2a has been associated with regression of the lesions although HHV-8 DNA persists in lesional skin.[616,617] However, with highly active antiretroviral therapy (HAART) there has not only been regression of the lesions but also undetectable levels of HHV-8 DNA.[618–620] The advent of HAART has led to a declining incidence of Kaposi's sarcoma.[621] Remission of lesions in renal transplant recipients may follow a reduction in the immunosuppressive therapy.[525]

Histopathology

The microscopic appearance of the lesions is identical in the different types of Kaposi's sarcoma.[622,623] They evolve through patch, plaque and nodular stages.[624] The earliest lesions, corresponding to the flat macule or patch stage, are predominantly vascular in nature. Within the dermis there is a proliferation of irregular, often jagged, vascular channels which partly surround pre-existing blood vessels in some areas. This characteristic appearance has been termed the 'promontory sign' (Fig. 38.28).[479] The vascular proliferation is also present about appendages and between collagen bundles. The vessels are thin walled and lined by plump or inconspicuous endothelial cells. Scattered groups of perivascular lymphocytes and plasma cells may also be present (Fig. 38.29). Extravasated erythrocytes and deposits of hemosiderin are also found in the dermis.

The papules, nodules and plaques consist of a dermal proliferation of interlacing bundles of spindle cells and intimately related, poorly defined slit-like vessels (Fig. 38.30). The proportion of vessels and spindle cells varies. There is an associated inflammatory cell infiltrate consisting predominantly of lymphocytes and plasma cells. Dilated thin-walled vessels are found at the periphery of the tumor. The spindle-cell component shows variable nuclear pleomorphism. Mitotic figures are present, but not usually frequent. Erythrocytes can be seen within vascular lumina and extravasated in and around the lesion. In one study, the spindle cells labeled for CD34 but not for CD31 or *Ulex europaeus*-1 lectin.[625] Other studies have demonstrated labeling for CD31 and factor VIII-related antigen.[626]

Clusters of eosinophilic hyaline globules, varying in size from just visible with the light microscope to larger than an erythrocyte, may be seen within spindle cells and macrophages or in an extracellular location. These were first

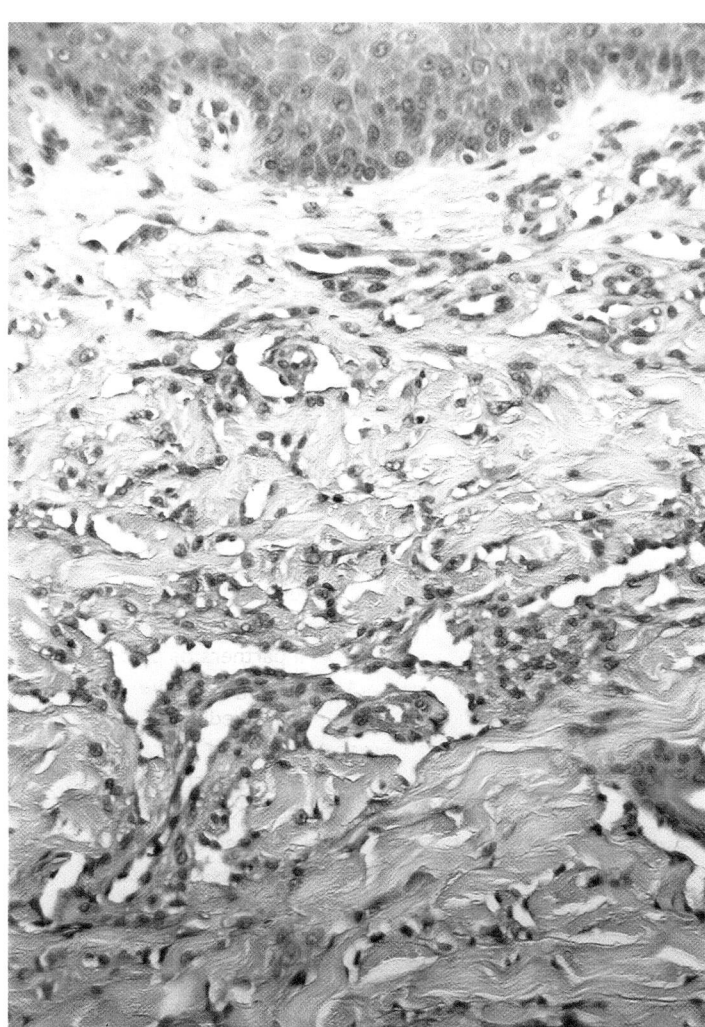

Fig. 38.28 **Kaposi's sarcoma.** Dilated irregular vascular channels surround a pre-existing vessel ('promontory sign'). (H & E)

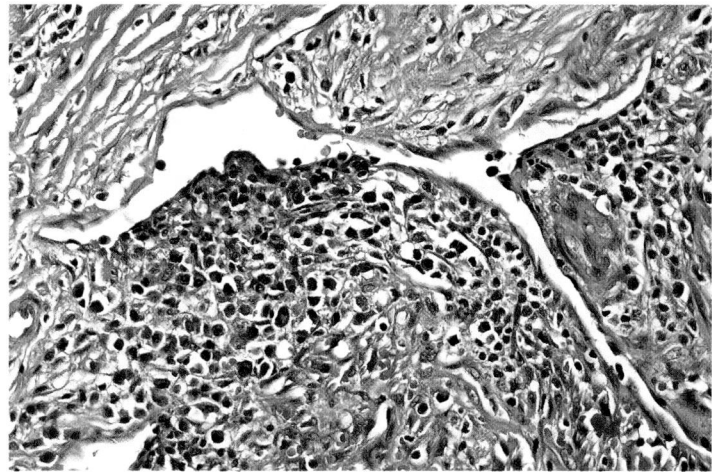

Fig. 38.29 **Kaposi's sarcoma.** Lymphocytes and plasma cells are present in the stroma adjacent to an irregularly shaped vascular channel. (H & E)

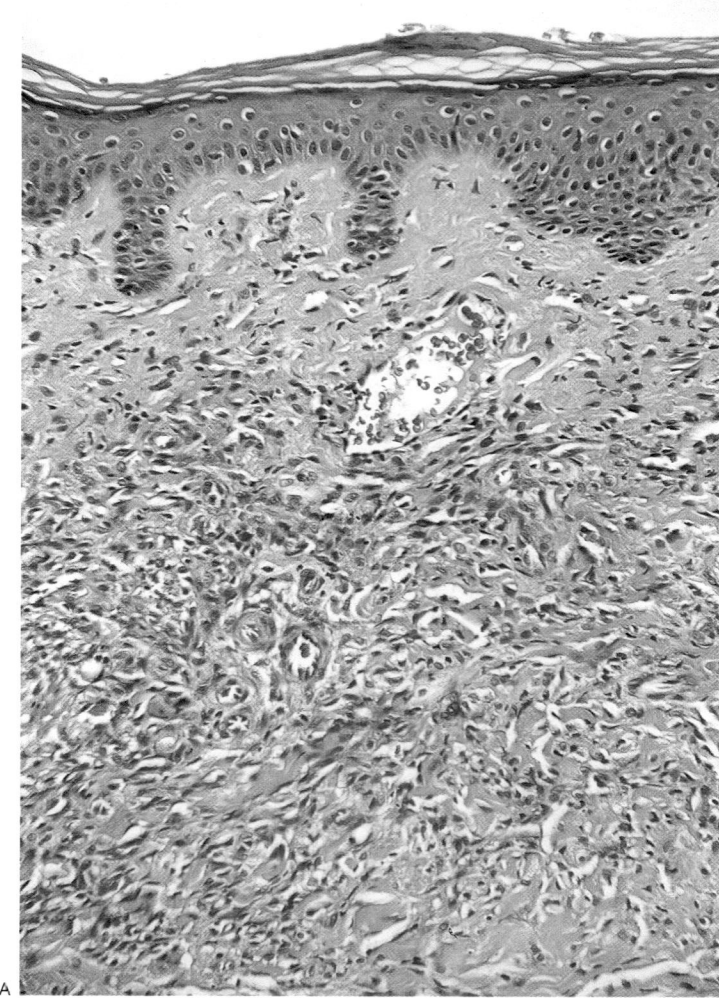

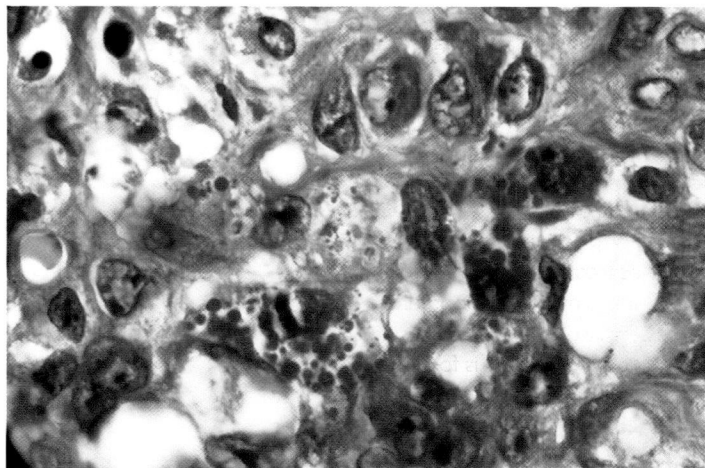

Fig. 38.31 **Kaposi's sarcoma.** Small hyaline globules are present in the cytoplasm of some macrophages and spindle-shaped cells. (Mallory's trichrome ×1500)

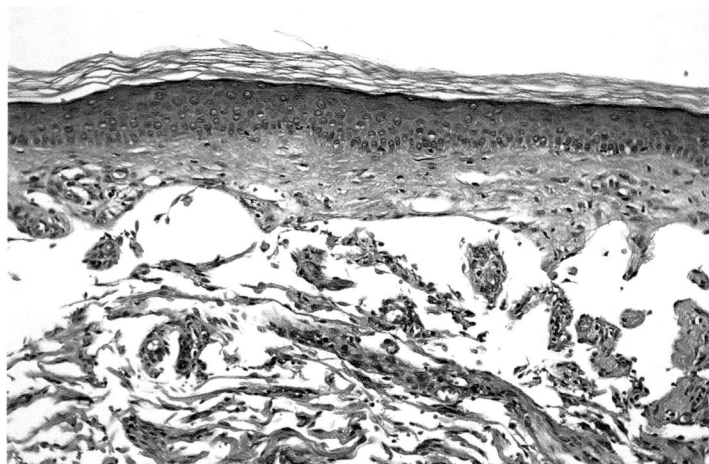

Fig. 38.32 **Lymphangioma-like area in a Kaposi's sarcoma.** Deeper areas resembled the more usual tumor. (H & E)

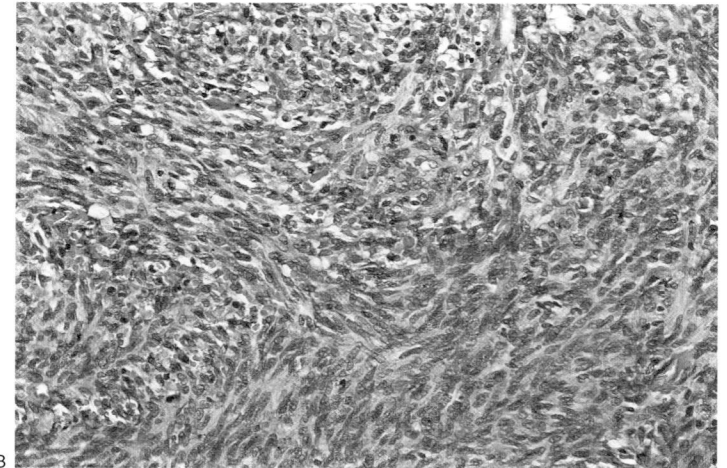

Fig. 38.30 **Kaposi's sarcoma. (A)** This variant is composed of vascular spaces and spindle-shaped cells. **(B)** Parts of another lesion show atypical spindle cells and less obvious vessels. (H & E)

described in African cases, but are also seen in classic Kaposi's sarcoma and in the epidemic form.[593,627] They resemble Russell bodies and are PAS positive, stain bright red with Mallory's trichrome stain (Fig. 38.31) and are auto-fluorescent.[628] They are seen in early patch lesions in some cases.[593] They appear to represent effete red blood cell fragments that have been

phagocytosed.[629] Erythrophagocytosis by tumor cells has been described in all stages of Kaposi's sarcoma.[630] Apoptosis of endothelial cells is seen quite often in plaques and nodules; it is seen less often in patch-stage lesions.[631] Lesions regressing as a consequence of HAART become surrounded by a dense fibrous stroma which eventually obliterates the lesion.[621]

Lymphangioma-like Kaposi's sarcoma is an uncommon variant accounting for less than 5% of all cases.[632] It consists of grossly dilated channels lined by flattened endothelial cells with a bland appearance (Fig. 38.32).[633] There are irregular, anastomosing channels, closely applied to the dermal collagen, with slender papillary projections into the lumen. Most of the spaces are devoid of erythrocytes, further enhancing the lymphangioma-like features. Clinically, the lesions may have a bulla-like appearance.[634] There is usually an admixture of more typical lesions.

An anaplastic form has been reported in African and sporadic cases.[538,635] The anaplastic lesions exhibit greater cellularity, nuclear pleomorphism and more frequent mitotic figures, and may have areas resembling angiosarcoma or fibrosarcoma.[530,635] Epidermal changes vary with the lesion and include atrophy and ulceration over raised lesions. A peripheral epidermal collarette is sometimes present about papules and nodules. Lesions with prominent hyperkeratosis sometimes occur.[636]

HHV-8 can be detected by PCR in paraffin-embedded tissue, although the viral load is low.[637,638] The molecular demonstration of HHV-8 DNA may be a useful adjunct in the diagnosis of Kaposi's sarcoma by fine needle aspiration[639] and when difficult lesions are encountered.[640]

Differential diagnosis

The early vascular lesions are subtle and must be differentiated from telangiectases, pigmented purpuric dermatosis, acroangiodermatitis and low-grade angiosarcoma. The vessels in Kaposi's sarcoma are usually more irregular than in most developmental or acquired telangiectases, pigmented purpuric dermatosis or acroangiodermatitis.[480] An inflammatory infiltrate which includes plasma cells is found in some early lesions of Kaposi's sarcoma. In low-grade angiosarcoma there is usually some evidence of cellular atypia. Small intravascular endothelial buds are sometimes seen. Irregular jagged vessels, dissection of collagen bundles by vascular structures, and an inflammatory cell infiltrate may all be seen in low-grade angiosarcoma.

Lesions with a spindle-cell component must be differentiated from cutaneous smooth muscle tumors, some forms of dermatofibroma (fibrous histiocytoma)[641] and spindle-cell hemangioendothelioma.[256] Smooth muscle tumors lack the intimate mingling of spindle cells, slit-like vessels and eosinophilic globules, and are usually positive for desmin intermediate filaments on immunoperoxidase staining. Aneurysmal fibrous histiocytoma can usually be differentiated from Kaposi's sarcoma because of the presence of foamy macrophages, multinucleate giant cells and the overlying epidermal changes, which range from epidermal hyperplasia to basal budding resembling hair differentiation.

The lesions of spindle-cell hemangioendothelioma closely mimic Kaposi's sarcoma, but the component vessels are usually more cavernous and, focally, the endothelial cells are epithelioid and vacuolated. Eosinophilic globules have not been reported in these tumors.

HEMANGIOPERICYTOMA

Hemangiopericytoma is a tumor first delineated by Stout and Murray in 1942.[642] Enzinger and Smith have divided this uncommon tumor into two groups.[643] The usual form of hemangiopericytoma (adult type) occurs in adults and rarely in children. It arises in deep soft tissues, particularly the lower extremities, pelvis and retroperitoneum, and occasionally other organs.[643,644] It rarely arises in the subcutis.[643–645] A second form (congenital or infantile hemangiopericytoma) is present at birth or arises in the first year of life; it is more common in boys.[646–648] The tumors in this group are multilobulate and arise almost exclusively in the subcutis of the head and neck, extremities or trunk; occasionally they arise in the dermis.[643,649] Most are solitary, but multiple lesions also occur.[646,650] Conventional hemangiopericytomas have an unpredictable course and may recur after treatment; they may metastasize, predominantly to the lungs and bone.[643] Fewer than 25% of cases behave as malignant tumors.[651] Congenital and infantile tumors have a benign clinical course, although they may grow rapidly during infancy or be complicated by hemorrhage.[643,652,653] Hemangiopericytoma in children older than 1 year does not differ in behavior from the adult type.[654]

The concept of hemangiopericytoma has been questioned.[651] Many soft tissue sarcomas may have a 'hemangiopericytoma-like pattern'.[655] Fletcher questions the existence of this entity, because tumor cells have only a limited morphological similarity to pericytes. Furthermore, a diagnosis is made without positive criteria.[651] Nappi et al have concluded that 'hemangiopericytoma represents both a pattern and a pathologic entity…and should be considered to represent an exclusionary interpretation'.[655a] Infantile hemangiopericytoma

is now considered by some to be the same entity as infantile myofibromatosis, or one end of a spectrum of infantile myofibroblastic lesions.[651,656]

Histopathology[643]

The *adult type* exhibits the characteristic pattern of tightly packed cellular areas surrounding endothelium-lined ramifying vessels. The cell boundaries are poorly defined; the nuclei are round or oval. Tumor cells are separated from the endothelial cells by a basement membrane and are themselves surrounded by a meshwork of reticulin fibers. Histological variations include myxoid areas, fibrotic areas and, rarely, osseous and cartilaginous metaplasia.[643] The deep variant with mature fat reported as a *lipomatous hemangiopericytoma*[657] has been regarded by others as a fat-containing variant of solitary fibrous tumor.[658] Epithelioid histiocytomas may exhibit hemangiopericytoma-like areas.[659,660] Tumor cells express vimentin only; they are negative for α-smooth muscle actin and α-sarcomeric actin.[424] Normal vascular pericytes are uniformly reactive for vimentin and α-isoforms of actin, and sometimes stain for desmin and HLA-DR. Tumor cells also stain for factor XIIIa, CD34, CD57 and HLA-DR[661] but these are not specific markers. Pericytes express 3G5 ganglioside.[662] Further studies are needed to see if this marker leads to the retention of hemangiopericytoma as a diagnostic entity. Several studies have stressed the difficulty in predicting the behavior of these tumors from their histological appearance, but frequent mitotic figures, necrosis, hemorrhage and increased cellularity are features that indicate a poor prognosis.[644] DNA flow cytometry and immunohistochemical stains for PCNA are not helpful in predicting outcome in these tumors.[663]

Congenital and infantile hemangiopericytomas have the typical pattern of cells and vessels as described above, but they are multilobulate, with perivascular and intravascular tumor outside the main tumor mass.[643,650] Endothelial proliferation within vascular lumina has been described.[643] Mitotic figures and necrosis may be seen but do not indicate a bad prognosis as these tumors have a benign course.[646] Hemangiopericytoma-like areas are sometimes seen in infantile myofibromatosis (see p. 927), which affects infants and children and may involve skin and subcutis.[664] Conversely, foci of cells having a spindled, myoid appearance typical of myofibroblasts can be seen in typical cases of infantile hemangiopericytoma. These cases show focal staining for actin.

Electron microscopy

Ultrastructural studies of adult cases have shown that the tumor cells are partially or completely surrounded by well-formed basement membranes. Pinocytotic vesicles and cytoplasmic filaments, sometimes with dense-body formation, are seen within the cells.[665] More than half the cases do not show pericytic features.[666]

KAPOSIFORM HEMANGIOENDOTHELIOMA

Kaposiform hemangioendothelioma is a locally aggressive vascular proliferation in children that usually presents in the skin as a single lesion, although a multifocal congenital case has been reported.[667,668] Requena and Ackerman believe it should be renamed Kaposiform hemangioma because there are no reports of unequivocal metastasis.[264]

In the largest series of this rare tumor published to date, a variety of sites were involved, including deep soft tissues of the upper extremities, retroperitoneum, chest wall, scalp and neck.[669] Earlier reports had emphasized peritoneal and retroperitoneal sites.[670] It is often associated with Kasabach–Merritt syndrome or lymphangiomatosis.[177,667] HHV-8 has not been detected in several cases.[667] The outcome depends on the site and the extent of the disease. Deaths have been reported from the associated Kasabach–Merritt syndrome and lymphangiomatosis.

Histopathology[669]

As with Kaposi's sarcoma, there are interconnecting sheets or nodules of spindled endothelial cells lining slit-like or crescent-shaped vessels. The spindle-cell fascicles are generally shorter and narrower than those found in Kaposi's sarcoma.[269] Small rounded vessels may also be seen. Unlike Kaposi's sarcoma, there may be nests of epithelioid-like endothelial cells with eosinophilic cytoplasm containing hemosiderin and cytoplasmic vacuoles. Cellular atypia is minimal and mitoses infrequent. Hemosiderin may also be present in the spindle cells. Hyaline eosinophilic globules similar to those in Kaposi's sarcoma are also seen. An occasional finding is microthrombi in vessel lumina. In the skin and subcutis there is surrounding dense hyaline fibrosis. Spindle cells stain for CD34 and focally for CD31.[669,671] The tumor has some similarities to spindle-cell hemangioendothelioma, but the latter occurs predominantly in adults, is superficial, and may have cavernous vessels and phleboliths. Kaposi's sarcoma is usually multifocal; it is very rare in children, except as the endemic form.

MALIGNANT TUMORS

Several of the rare vascular tumors previously categorized as being of variable or uncertain behavior have been reclassified as malignant tumors, although it is acknowledged that they are usually associated with an excellent prognosis. The following tumors will be considered in this category:

- angiosarcoma and lymphangiosarcoma
- endovascular papillary angioendothelioma of childhood
- epithelioid hemangioendothelioma
- retiform hemangioendothelioma
- composite hemangioendothelioma
- malignant and atypical glomus tumors.

ANGIOSARCOMA AND LYMPHANGIOSARCOMA

As the distinction between malignant tumors showing blood vessel differentiation (angiosarcoma) and those showing lymphatic differentiation (lymphangiosarcoma) is often unclear or controversial, it is proposed to discuss both types together. However, a new marker, vascular endothelial cell growth factor receptor type 3, has recently been shown to have high specificity for lymphatic endothelium and it may aid in the distinction of these two tumor types.[672]

There are three main clinicopathological subtypes: idiopathic cutaneous angiosarcoma of the head and neck, angiosarcoma complicating lymphedema, and postirradiation angiosarcoma.[594] A miscellaneous category is sometimes added.

Idiopathic cutaneous angiosarcoma of the head and neck[673–676]

Idiopathic cutaneous angiosarcoma of the head and neck most commonly involves the upper part of the face or the scalp of elderly people.[677] Men are affected more frequently than women.[678] The lesions are single or multifocal, bluish or violaceous nodules, plaques or flat infiltrating areas; they may occasionally bleed or ulcerate. Rare clinical presentations include recurrent angioedema of the face,[679] an inflammatory process,[680] a rosacea-like eruption[681]

and involvement of an area of radiodermatitis.[682] Thrombocytopenia may develop as a consequence of enlargement of the primary lesion or the development of metastatic deposits.[683] Extensive local growth is common and margins are difficult to define surgically. Metastasis to regional lymph nodes and to the lungs occurs, often after repeated surgical excision of the primary growth. A reduction in adhesion molecules, such as cadherin, has been implicated in the local invasiveness and metastasis of angiosarcoma.[684] The prognosis is poor. In one series, only 15% of patients survived for 5 years or more after diagnosis.[678] This may reflect the fact that clinical diagnosis is often delayed until the lesions are advanced. Complete spontaneous regression of the tumor has been reported.[685]

Various treatments have been used for angiosarcoma with limited success. They include surgery, paclitaxel (a taxane with antiangiogenic and apoptotic effects),[686] doxorubicin, combination interferon alfa-2a and 13-cis-retinoic acid,[687] interferon alfa-2b with interleukin-2 and surface radiotherapy,[688] and combined chemotherapy and radiotherapy in various schedules.[689]

Lymphangiosarcoma arising in chronic lymphedematous limbs

Since 1948, when Stewart and Treves recognized the syndrome of post-mastectomy lymphangiosarcoma, the association of such tumors with chronic lymphedema has become well known.[690] In their original series they described the appearance of purplish-red raised macular or polypoid tumors in the chronically edematous arm of women who had undergone radical mastectomy on that side. The tumors appeared on average 12.5 years after surgery. Similar tumors have been reported in men after mastectomy. They have also occurred in cases without lymph node dissection and without preceding edema. Much less commonly, similar tumors arise in the limbs of patients with chronic lymphedema due to other causes.[691] These include congenital lymphedema (Milroy's disease), lymphedema following other types of surgery, and chronic venous stasis.[692–698] Lymphangiosarcoma has also been reported in association with chronic filarial lymphedema, but appears to be a rare complication of this condition.[699] Rarely, cutaneous angiosarcoma has been reported in lymphedematous extremities which have developed as a complication of malignancies other than breast carcinoma, such as Hodgkin's disease.[700,701]

Postirradiation angiosarcoma

Postirradiation angiosarcomas are rare and have been documented after radiotherapy for a variety of benign and malignant conditions.[702,703] At least 10 cases of angiosarcoma have been reported following irradiation of benign hemangiomas; the median latent period from irradiation to diagnosis of angiosarcoma was 21.8 years.[704,705] Angiosarcomas have also been reported following treatment of eczema,[706] tinea capitis and sinusitis.[707] This form of angiosarcoma is more common following therapy of a variety of malignant tumors,[704] including carcinoma of the breast[708] and cervix.[709] The latent period between treatment and diagnosis is reported to be shorter than for benign conditions – an average of 12 years in one report[702] – but it may be much shorter.[708]

Miscellaneous angiosarcoma

Angiosarcomas have been reported to arise in pre-existing benign vascular tumors, including lymphangioma[710] and 'port wine' stains[711] and in benign and malignant peripheral nerve sheath tumors.[712] They have also occurred as a complication of varicose ulceration,[713] arteriovenous fistulae,[714] renal transplantation,[715] hereditary epidermolysis bullosa,[716] xeroderma pigmentosum,[717] a gouty tophus,[718] retained foreign materials such as shrapnel, surgical sponges and adjacent to a Dacron vascular prosthesis.[719] HHV-8 has been detected in several cases, but specifically excluded in others.[714,720,721] Intravascular dissemination of an angiosarcoma, mimicking angioendotheliomatosis, has been reported.[722]

Histopathology

The appearances are similar in the three groups.[673–675,690] The lesions are poorly circumscribed dermal tumors which infiltrate subcutaneous fat and other tissues and often have a multifocal distribution. Angiomatous and solid patterns may be seen. In the angiomatous areas a meshwork of anastomosing dilated vessels extends between pre-existing dermal collagen bundles and around skin appendages. The vessels are irregular and lined by crowded endothelial cells, which range in appearance from virtually normal-looking to plump atypical protuberant cells with enlarged hyperchromatic nuclei (Fig. 38.33). Papillary processes may extend into the lumen of the vessel. In the solid areas of the poorly differentiated tumors the cells vary from spindle-shaped to polygonal. Some areas may resemble Kaposi's sarcoma. Cytoplasmic vacuoles resembling primitive vascular lumina may be seen in some cells. Reticulin stains show that the cellular proliferation is on the luminal side of the reticulin fibers in the angiomatous areas. Generally, as architectural differentiation decreases, cytological atypia and cell size tend to increase.[674] Lymphocytic infiltrates are commonly seen and may obscure the underlying lesion, particularly in well-differentiated tumors with minimal cellular atypia.[674] Mast cells appear to be increased.[717,723] Distinguishing the well-differentiated angiomatous areas from benign vascular proliferations depends on the recognition of cellular atypia, the presence of crowding of lining cells and of solid papillary clusters of cells, and an irregular interconnecting pattern of vessels. The use of antibodies specific for signal transduction pathways is a feasible method for distinguishing benign from malignant endothelial processes in paraffin-embedded tissue. There is strong expression of mitogen-activated protein kinase (MAPK) in benign endothelial tumors and a greatly decreased expression in angiosarcoma.[724] Infectious endothelial lesions (Kaposi's sarcoma and verruga peruana) stain strongly.[724] Caveolin, a scaffolding cell membrane protein, has a higher level of expression in benign vascular tumor than in angiosarcomas, including the well-differentiated variants.[725] It has been suggested that caveolin expression might be useful in separating benign and malignant vascular tumors.[725] The differentiation of early lesions from early lesions of Kaposi's sarcoma may be dependent on clinicopathological correlation.

Poorly differentiated tumors with polygonal and epithelioid cells can resemble carcinomas and even amelanotic melanoma. Immunohistochemical markers for keratins and S100 protein will help to distinguish between these tumors. *Epithelioid*, *spindle* and *granular* cell variants of angiosarcoma have also been described.[269] The epithelioid variant sometimes expresses keratin (see below).[691,726–728] Another histological variant is the verrucous angiosarcoma, in which there are striking verrucous changes in the overlying epidermis.[729]

Many immunohistochemical markers for endothelial cell differentiation have been used, including factor VIII-related antigen, *Ulex europaeus*-I lectin,[730,731] PAL-E[732] and, more recently, CD34[673] and CD31.[625] Epithelioid angiosarcomas often express K8 and K18 (approximately 50%), whereas the non-epithelioid types express K7, K8, and K18 in about 20% of cases. Epithelial membrane antigen (EMA) is expressed in about a third of non-epithelioid angiosarcomas.[728] Thus caution is needed in interpreting EMA positivity as evidence for an epithelial tumor. The monoclonal antibody AE1, which does not react with keratins 7, 8 and 18, is advantageous in the differential diagnosis of angiosarcoma and carcinoma.[728,733]

Poorly differentiated tumors are, unfortunately, less likely to stain with immunohistochemical markers than well-differentiated tumors, in which the vascular differentiation is already more obvious. In some cases, the use of frozen instead of paraffin sections, and special fixation techniques may

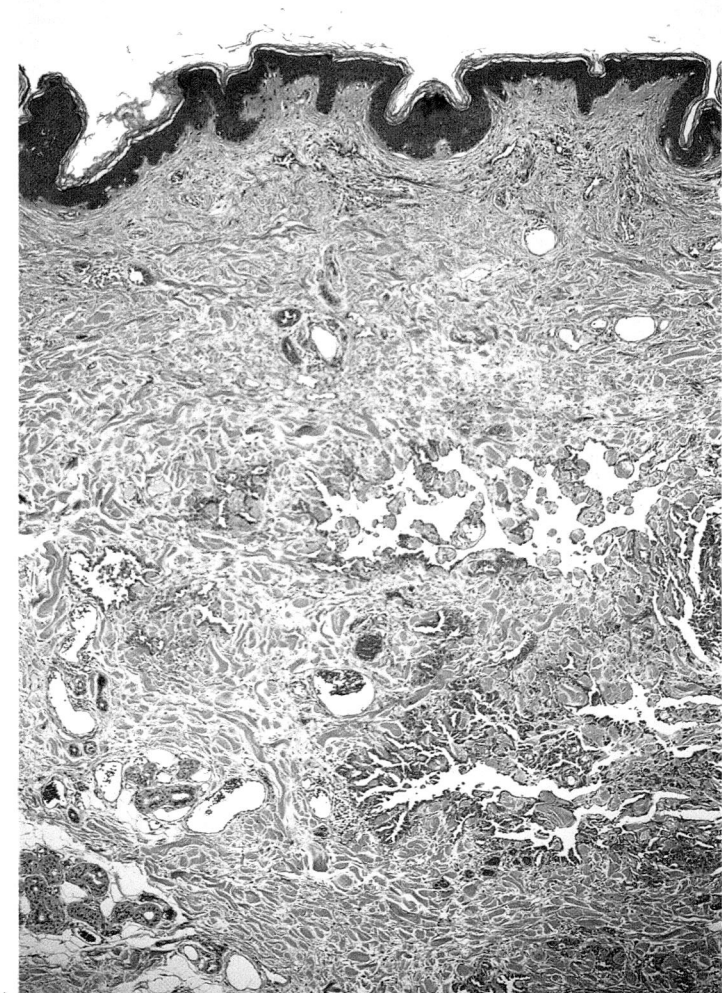

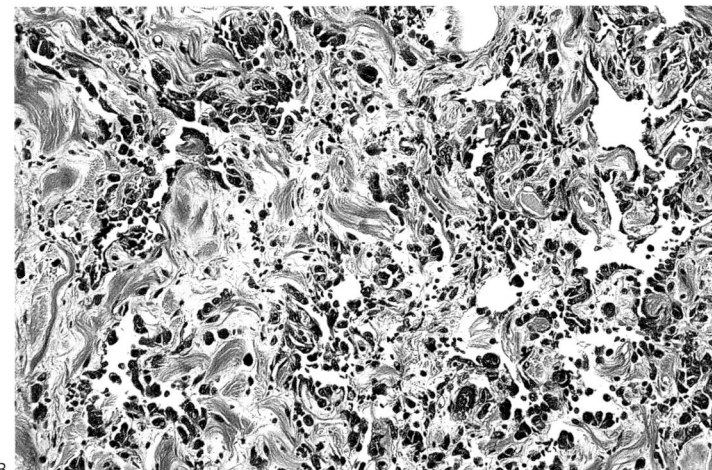

Fig. 38.33 **(A) Angiosarcoma. (B)** The vascular channels are lined by atypical endothelial cells. (H & E)

produce positive reactions. At present CD31 appears to be the most useful marker for endothelial differentiation, being both relatively sensitive and specific compared to other markers.[625,734] *Ulex europaeus*-I lectin labels some non-vascular neoplasms, as does CD34.[625] Factor VIII-related antigen was positive in only 29% of non- or poorly vasoformative areas of angiosarcoma in one study.[734] CD31, CD34 and *Ulex europaeus*-1 lectin label blood vessel as well as lymphatic endothelium.[625] The presence of factor VIII-related antigen in the endothelium of blood vessels and its absence in that of lymphatics has been reported by some[735] but not by others.[736] PAL-E monoclonal antibody is reported to be more specific for blood vessel endothelium.[732] Further studies are needed to confirm the specificity of vascular endothelial cell growth factor receptor type 3 for lymphatic endothelium. Initia studies appear promising.[672]

Ultrastructural and immunohistochemical studies have confirmed that postmastectomy lymphangiosarcomas are of endothelial origin[735,737,738] and not secondary breast carcinoma as has been suggested.[739] As alluded to in the introduction, the distinction between angiosarcoma and lymphangiosarcoma has, in some cases, become blurred with the use of modern investigative techniques. Immunohistochemical studies have suggested that tumors arising in edematous extremities are angiosarcomas rather than lymphangiosarcomas.[735,740] One study of angiosarcoma of the face and scalp suggested that these tumors are more akin to lymphangiosarcomas than angiosarcomas.[741] As noted above, poorly differentiated tumors tend to lose the characteristic cell markers that would indicate their nature.

Electron microscopy

Ultrastructural features of blood vessel endothelium include well-formed junctional complexes of the zonula adherens type, a well-developed basal lamina, and Weibel–Palade bodies.[742] Lymphatic endothelial cells are said to lack Weibel–Palade bodies, to have cell junctions that are inconspicuous, and to have incomplete, if any, basal laminae.

ENDOVASCULAR PAPILLARY ANGIOENDOTHELIOMA OF CHILDHOOD

Endovascular papillary angioendothelioma of childhood has had a confusing taxonomic evolution. Dabska, in the first report of this very rare vascular tumor, described it as malignant endovascular papillary angioendothelioma because it was locally invasive and appeared to have the potential to metastasize.[743] Subsequently, others suggested that this lesion should be classified as of borderline malignancy because of its good long-term prognosis, minimal cellular atypia and controversial metastatic potential.[744,745] It was next regarded as a low-grade angiosarcoma[746,747] and, now, on the basis of its staining pattern, it has been renamed papillary intralymphatic angio-endothelioma (PILA),[672] reflecting its presumed lymphatic origin.

The majority of reported cases have been in children; rarely, adults are affected.[748] There is a recent report of this lesion developing in a pre-existing vascular malformation in an adult.[748] A tumor showing some similarities to this entity has also been reported in a background of lymphedema.[749] In the majority of cases the lesions are present at birth. They occur in a variety of sites, either as a diffuse swelling of the skin or as an intradermal tumor. The tumors enlarge and may eventually invade deeper soft tissues and bone. Metastasis to regional lymph nodes and lungs has been reported.[743] One of the original cases reported by Dabska subsequently died of widespread pulmonary metastases, putting beyond doubt the malignant nature of this tumor.[747]

Histopathology

There is some variability.[743,750] Irregular vascular channels are present in the dermis and subcutis. They are lined by endothelial cells ranging from flattened to columnar in shape. Some cells have a 'hobnail' appearance. Within the lumina of these vessels are papillary structures covered by similar cells. The cores of the papillae are avascular and consist of fibrous tissue or peculiar eosinophilic hyaline globules, some with central clearing.

Some of these vascular structures have a glomeruloid appearance. Lymphocytes are seen both within the lumina of the vascular channels, in intimate association with the endothelial cells, and also in the extravascular stroma. There is nuclear hyperchromatism and mitotic figures are present.[743]

Immunohistochemical and ultrastructural studies have confirmed the endothelial nature of the tumor cells and identified the hyaline globules as basal lamina-like material.[744,745] Tumor cells are positive for vimentin, factor VIII-related antigen, CD31 and focally for CD34. They are negative for keratins, EMA, S100 protein and desmin.[672] Vascular endothelial growth factor receptor type 3, a recently introduced marker for lymphatic endothelia, was positive in all cases studied – hence the latest redesignation of this tumor.[672]

EPITHELIOID HEMANGIOENDOTHELIOMA

Epithelioid hemangioendothelioma is a rare tumor with a clinical course intermediate between hemangioma and angiosarcoma.[751] Although most cases occur in soft tissues and other organs, including bone and liver, these tumors have also been reported in the skin.[752–760] Skin lesions have been reported with underlying bone lesions.[761] These tumors have low-grade or borderline malignant potential and may metastasize. They are less aggressive than conventional angiosarcomas.

A 1;3 translocation has been identified in two cases of this tumor.[762] Its full characterization is t(1;3)(p36.3;q25).

Histopathology

There is a proliferation of nests and cords of plump, epithelioid to spindle-shaped endothelial cells in a fibromyxoid stroma. Many of the cells contain cytoplasmic vacuoles. Well-formed vascular channels are not a feature of this tumor.[752] Slight cellular pleomorphism and occasional mitotic figures are sometimes present. A spindle-cell element may rarely be present.[763] Lamellar bone has been reported in one case.[764] These tumors may be difficult to distinguish from secondary adenocarcinoma, but the cells stain for *Ulex europaeus*-1 lectin, factor VIII-related antigen, CD31 and CD34. Cases are always positive for at least one vascular endothelial marker, but not usually all.[760] About half the cases express smooth muscle actin.[757] Occasional cases express cytokeratin.[751,765] Using specific keratin markers, the cells of epithelioid hemangioendothelioma express K7 and K18 in the majority of cases.[728] An epithelioid variant of angiosarcoma has also been described (see above), but in this tumor there are largely confluent sheets of tumor cells with greater cellular atypia and areas of necrosis.[766,767]

Electron microscopy

Features include immature cell junctions, abundant intermediate filaments, Weibel–Palade bodies and intracytoplasmic lumen formation; lumina may contain red blood cells.[751]

RETIFORM HEMANGIOENDOTHELIOMA

In 1994, Calonje et al described 15 cases of retiform hemangioendothelioma, which they regarded as a low-grade angiosarcoma.[767] Lesions are slow-growing, exophytic or plaque-like tumors of the dermis and subcutis. They occur predominantly on the limbs and trunk of young and middle-aged adults. Occasionally, lesions have been associated with radiotherapy or chronic lymphedema. DNA sequences of HHV-8 have recently been detected in one case.[768] Local recurrence is common, but metastasis to local lymph nodes has occurred in only one case. In another case, multiple lesions developed in non-contiguous sites over a 10-year period.[769] The relationship of this tumor to endovascular papillary angioendothelioma of childhood (Dabska's tumor) is unclear.

Histopathology[767]

The distinctive feature of this tumor is the pattern of arborizing vessels which resembles the rete testis. Vessels are lined by 'hobnail', monomorphous endothelial cells which have scant cytoplasm and minimal or no atypia. Mitoses are not seen. The tumor involves the dermis, subcutis and, rarely, underlying muscle. A further characteristic is the presence of a prominent lymphocytic infiltrate, which may be so heavy as to almost obscure the vessels. As well as surrounding vessels, lymphocytes are also present in the lumina of vessels, closely applied to the endothelial cells. This feature, as well as the presence of occasional intraluminal papillae with collagenous cores, resembles Dabska's tumor. Conspicuous papillary structures are rarely present.[770] Some tumors also have solid areas with spindle cells arranged in closely packed cords with narrow vascular lumina. Endothelial cells express CD34, *Ulex europaeus*-1 lectin, and are weakly positive for CD31 and factor VIII-associated antigen. Lymphocytes about the vessels are a mixture of B and T cells (CD20+, CD3+); those within the vessel are predominantly T cells (CD3+).

COMPOSITE HEMANGIOENDOTHELIOMA

The term 'composite hemangioendothelioma' has been applied recently to a low-grade malignant vascular tumor showing varying combinations of benign, low-grade malignant, and malignant vascular components.[771] The predominant components were epithelioid hemangioendothelioma, retiform hemangioendothelioma and spindle-cell hemangioendothelioma. Angiosarcoma-like elements were present in most cases. Local recurrence was common while only one of the six cases followed has metastasized.[771]

MALIGNANT AND ATYPICAL GLOMUS TUMORS

A group of tumors with glomus cell differentiation and aberrant behavior on histological appearance has been described by Gould et al.[408] They divided this group into three categories:

1. a locally infiltrative glomus tumor
2. a cytologically malignant tumor arising and merging with an otherwise typical glomus tumor (glomangiosarcoma arising in a benign glomus tumor)[409,772,773]
3. *de novo* glomangiosarcoma.[773,774]

Recently, Folpe et al reported their findings on 52 unusual glomus tumors.[421] They ranged in size from 0.2 to 12 cm and occurred predominantly on the extremities, in both the superficial and deep soft tissues. Most cases had a benign-appearing component. Eight of their cases had histologically confirmed metastases. Local recurrence occurred in a further seven cases. Based on their cases, they proposed a new classification of atypical glomus tumors (see Table 38.1).[421]

Histopathology

Based on the findings of Gould et al,[408] locally aggressive tumors have the appearance of a glomus tumor or glomangioma and infiltrate the adjacent tissue.[408] Intraneural spread is sometimes seen. In the second group there is a component of conventional glomus tumor and an adjacent component with increased cellularity, nuclear atypia and mitotic figures (Fig. 38.34).[407,408,410,775] The cells form solid sheets with intervening vascular spaces. Enzinger and Weiss describe similar tumors, the atypical component consisting of 'short spindle cells having features somewhat intermediate between a fibrosarcoma and leiomyosarcoma'.[774,776] *De novo* glomangiosarcoma is a more controversial entity, but it would seem to occur. Table 38.1 lists the distinguishing features of the various tumors described by Folpe et al.[421] The tumor cells in malignant glomus tumors stain positively for vimentin, muscle-specific actin and smooth muscle actin.[775]

Table 38.1 **Classification of atypical glomus tumors** (after Folpe et al)[421]

Malignant glomus tumor	Deep location; size >2 cm; atypical mitotic figures; moderate to high nuclear grade
Symplastic glomus tumor	High nuclear grade without other malignant features
Glomus tumors of uncertain malignant potential	Lack criteria of above 2 categories; high mitotic activity and superficial location only, or large size only, or deep location only
G omangiomatosis	Diffuse angiomatosis and excess glomus cells

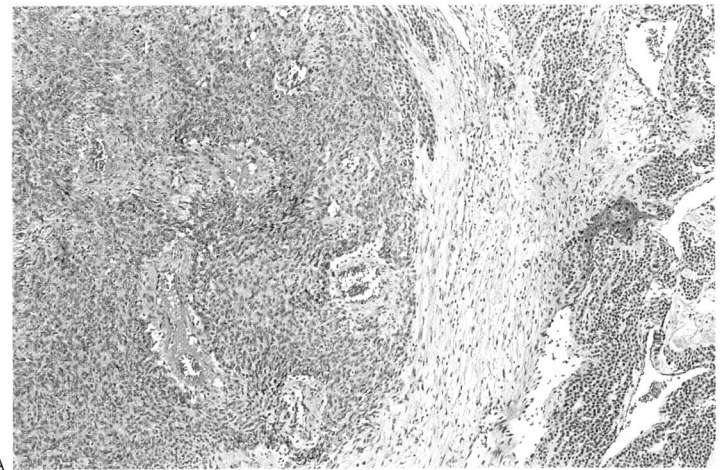
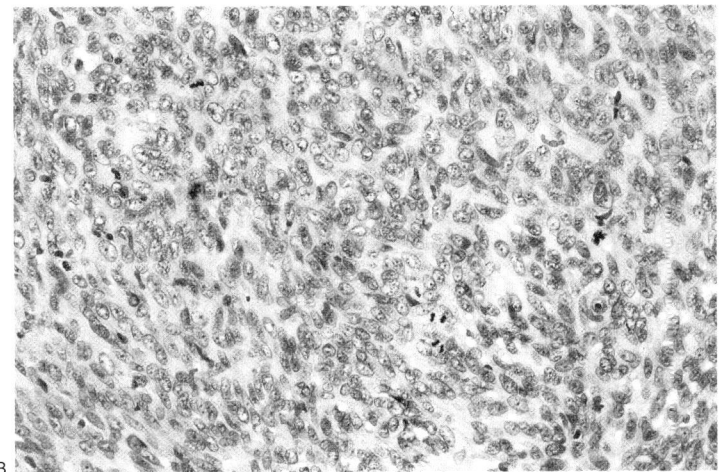

Fig. 38.34 **Malignant glomus tumor. (A)** Normal glomus tumor is present along one edge. **(B)** The malignant component is quite cellular with mitotic figures. (H & E)

The risk of metastasis increases significantly for tumors with a deep location, with a size of more than 2 cm, and with atypical mitotic figures.[421] High cellularity and mitotic rate, the presence of necrosis, and moderate to high nuclear grade are of lesser importance.[421]

TUMORS WITH A SIGNIFICANT VASCULAR COMPONENT

Some tumors of mesenchymal derivation may have two or more components, one of which may be of vascular type. These tumors are considered in detail elsewhere, but they are mentioned here briefly for completeness:

- angiofibromas
- angioleiomyoma
- angiolipoma
- spindle-cell lipoma (angiomatoid variant)
- angiomyolipoma
- angiomyxoma
- angiomyofibroblastoma
- dermatofibroma – aneurysmal variant
- angioplasmocellular hyperplasia.

The multinucleate cell angiohistiocytoma has been included in this category in some classifications. It has been considered here with the vascular proliferations (see p. 1018).

ANGIOFIBROMAS

The angiofibromas are a clinically diverse group of entities that share similar histological features, namely the presence of small vessels of capillary type with a collagenous stroma containing some spindle cells. Multinucleate cells are sometimes present. Examples include fibrous papule of the face, adenoma sebaceum, pearly penile papules, acral fibrokeratomas (the vessels are often not prominent), and familial myxovascular fibromas (see p. 918).

ANGIOLEIOMYOMA

The angioleiomyoma usually presents as a solitary nodule on the extremities, particularly the lower legs (see p. 969). They are well-circumscribed lesions composed of interlacing bundles of smooth muscle arranged around and between vascular channels. The vessels vary in size from large sinusoidal vessels to small slit-like channels.

ANGIOLIPOMA

Angiolipomas are subcutaneous tumors with a predilection for the extremities, particularly the forearm (see p. 958). Mild pain or discomfort is sometimes present. They are composed of lobules of mature fat, admixed with capillaries which may comprise from 5% to 50% or more of the lesion.

SPINDLE-CELL LIPOMA (ANGIOMATOID VARIANT)

Some spindle-cell lipomas have areas resembling a lymphangioma or hemangiopericytoma. Another variant has irregular and branching spaces with villiform connective tissue projections giving a striking angiomatoid appear-ance. This is the so-called 'angiomatoid' or 'pseudoangiomatous variant' (see p. 959).

ANGIOMYOLIPOMA

The angiomyolipoma is a rare tumor resembles an angioleiomyoma with the admixture of foci of mature fat cells of varying size between the muscle bundles (see p. 970). The blood vessels resemble those seen in angioleiomyomas.

ANGIOMYXOMA

The superficial angiomyxoma usually involves the dermis and subcutis. It is composed of spindle-shaped and stellate cells set in a basophilic myxoid matrix containing numerous small blood vessels. Epithelial strands or keratin-filled cysts are present in more than half (see p. 942).

ANGIOMYOFIBROBLASTOMA

Angiomyofibroblastoma is a rare tumor of the vulva composed of an edematous stroma containing abundant blood vessels, predominantly of the capillary type (see p. 925). Spindle cells are present in the stroma, often aggregated around the vessels.

DERMATOFIBROMA (ANEURYSMAL VARIANT)

Rarely, a dermatofibroma is composed of such large vascular spaces that it can be confused at first glance with a vascular tumor. The stroma, which is composed of spindle cells, often in a storiform arrangement, contains abundant hemosiderin (see p. 931).

ANGIOPLASMOCELLULAR HYPERPLASIA

Angioplasmocellular hyperplasia is an exceedingly rare condition characterized by a proliferation of small blood vessels, some with vacuolated endothelium, and a mixed inflammatory cell infiltrate with a predominance of polyclonal plasma cells (see p. 1064).

REFERENCES

Introduction

1 Tsang WYW, Chan JKC, Fletcher CDM. Recently characterized vascular tumours of skin and soft tissues. Histopathology 1991; 19: 489–501.
2 Metzker A. Cutaneous vascular lesions. Semin Dermatol 1988; 7: 9–16.
3 Enjolras O, Mulliken JB. Vascular tumors and vascular malformations (new issues). Adv Dermatol 1998; 13: 375–422.
4 Garzon MC, Enjolras O, Frieden IJ. Vascular tumors and vascular malformations: Evidence for an association. J Am Acad Dermatol 2000; 42: 275–279.
5 Enjolras O. Vascular tumors and vascular malformations: are we at the dawn of a better knowledge? Pediatr Dermatol 1999; 16: 238–241.

Hamartomas and malformations

6 Tsuruta D, Fukai K, Seto M et al. Phakomatosis pigmentovascularis type IIIb associated with moyamoya disease. Pediatr Dermatol 1999; 16: 35–38.
7 Eichenfield LF. Evolving knowledge of hemangiomas and vascular malformations. Beyond strawberries and port wine. Arch Dermatol 1998; 134: 740–742.
8 Jacobs AH, Walton RG. The incidence of birthmarks in the neonate. Pediatrics 1976; 58: 218–222.

9 Nguyen CM, Yohn JJ, Huff C et al. Facial port wine stains in childhood: prediction of the rate of improvement as a function of the age of the patient, size and location of the port wine stain and the number of treatments with the pulsed dye (585 nm) laser. Br J Dermatol 1998; 138: 821–825.

10 Redondo P, Vázquez-Doval FJ. Familial multiple nevi flammei. J Am Acad Dermatol 1996; 35: 769–770.

11 Adams BB, Lucky AW. Acquired port-wine stains and antecedent trauma. Arch Dermatol 2000; 136: 897–899.

12 Woodrow SL, Handfield-Jones SE. Enlarging congenital haemangioma in an adult – a new entity? Clin Exp Dermatol 1997; 22: 283–286.

13 Klapman MH, Yao JF. Thickening and nodules in port-wine stains. J Am Acad Dermatol 2001; 44: 300–302.

14 Smith MA, Manfield PA. The natural history of salmon patches in the first year of life. Br J Dermatol 1962; 74: 31–33.

15 Tan KL. Nevus flammeus of the nape, glabella and eyelids. Clin Pediatrics 1972; 11: 112–118.

16 Barsky SH, Rosen S, Geer DE, Noe JM. The nature and evolution of port wine stains: a computer-assisted study. J Invest Dermatol 1980; 74: 154–157.

17 Finley JL, Noe JM, Arndt KA, Rosen S. Port-wine stains. Morphologic variations and developmental lesions. Arch Dermatol 1984; 120: 1453–1455.

18 Holloway KB, Ramos-Caro FA, Brownlee RE Jr, Flowers FP. Giant proliferative hemangiomas arising in a port-wine stain. J Am Acad Dermatol 1994; 31: 675–676.

19 Braverman IM, Keh-Yen A. Ultrastructure and three-dimensional reconstruction of several macular and papular telangiectases. J Invest Dermatol 1983; 81: 489–497.

20 Finley JL, Clark RAF, Colvin RB et al. Immunofluorescence staining with antibodies to factor VIII, fibronectin, and collagenous basement membrane protein in normal human skin and port wine stains. Arch Dermatol 1982; 118: 971–975.

21 Smoller BR, Rosen S. Port-wine stains. A disease of altered neural modulation of blood vessels? Arch Dermatol 1986; 122: 177–179.

22 Neumann R, Leonhartsberger H, Knobler R, Honigsmann H. Immunohistochemistry of port-wine stains and normal skin with endothelium-specific antibodies PAL-E, anti-ICAM-1, anti-ELAM-1, and anti-factor VIIIrAg. Arch Dermatol 1994; 130: 879–883.

23 Enjolras O, Riche MC, Merland JJ. Facial port-wine stains and Sturge–Weber syndrome. Pediatrics 1985; 76: 48–51.

24 Craven N, Wright AL. Familial Klippel–Trenaunay syndrome: a case report. Clin Exp Dermatol 1995; 20: 76–79.

25 Aelvoet GE, Jorens PG, Roelen LM. Genetic aspects of the Klippel–Trenaunay syndrome. Br J Dermatol 1992; 126: 603–607.

26 Baskerville PA, Ackroyd JS, Browse NL. The etiology of the Klippel–Trenaunay syndrome. Ann Surg 1985; 202: 624–627.

27 Viljoen D, Saxe N, Pearn J, Beighton P. The cutaneous manifestations of the Klippel–Trenaunay–Weber syndrome. Clin Exp Dermatol 1987; 12: 12–17.

28 Servelle M. Klippel and Trenaunay's syndrome. 768 operated cases. Ann Surg 1985; 201: 365–373.

29 Jessen RT, Thompson S, Smith EB. Cobb syndrome. Arch Dermatol 1977; 113: 1587–1590.

30 Enjolras O, Ciabrini D, Mazoyer E et al. Extensive pure venous malformations in the upper or lower limb: A review of 27 cases. J Am Acad Dermatol 1997; 36: 219–225.

31 Steinway DM, Fretzin DF. Acquired zosteriform cavernous hemangiomas: brief clinical observation. Arch Dermatol 1977; 113: 848–849.

32 Watabe H, Kashima M, Baba T, Mizoguchi M. A case of unilateral dermatomal cavernous haemangiomatosis. Br J Dermatol 2000; 143: 888–891.

33 Mulliken JB, Young A. Vascular birthmarks, hemangiomas and vascular malformations. Philadelphia: WB Saunders, 1988.

34 Waldo ED, Vuletin JC, Kaye GI. The ultrastructure of vascular tumors: additional observations and a review of the literature. Pathol Annu 1977; 12 (part 2): 279–308.

35 Bean WB. Vascular spiders and related lesions of the skin. Oxford: Blackwell Scientific Publications, 1958; 178.

36 Rice JS, Fischer DS. Blue rubber-bleb nevus syndrome. Arch Dermatol 1962; 86: 503–511.

37 Ishii T, Asuwa N, Suzuki S et al. Blue rubber bleb naevus syndrome. Virchows Archiv A (Pathol Anat) 1988; 413: 485–490.

38 Morris L, Lynch PM, Gleason WA Jr et al. Blue rubber bleb nevus syndrome: laser photocoagulation of colonic hemangiomas in a child with microcytic anemia. Pediatr Dermatol 1992; 9: 91–94.

39 Wilson JR, Weston MJ, Singh P, Eardley I. Blue rubber bleb naevus syndrome: an unusual cause of urethral bleeding. Br J Dermatol 2000; 143: 677–678.

40 Boente MdC, Cordisco MR, Frontini MdV, Asial RA. Blue rubber bleb nevus (Bean syndrome): evolution of four cases and clinical response to pharmacologic agents. Pediatr Dermatol 1999; 16: 222–227.

41 Fine RM, Derbes VJ, Clark WH Jr. Blue rubber bleb nevus. Arch Dermatol 1961; 84: 802–805.

42 Berlyne GM, Berlyne N. Anaemia due to "blue rubber-bleb" naevus disease. Lancet 1960; 2: 1275–1277.

43 Talbot S, Wyatt EH. Blue rubber bleb naevi. (Report of a family in which only males were affected). Br J Dermatol 1970; 82: 37–39.

44 Suringa DWR, Ackerman AB. Cutaneous lymphangiomas with dyschondroplasia (Maffucci's syndrome). A unique variant of an unusual syndrome. Arch Dermatol 1970; 101: 472–474.

45 Bean WB. Dyschondroplasia and hemangiomata (Maffucci's syndrome). Arch Intern Med 1955; 95: 767–778.

46 Lewis RJ, Ketcham AS. Maffucci's syndrome: functional and neoplastic significance. J Bone Joint Surg (A) 1973; 55: 1465–1479.

47 Kaplan RP, Wang JT, Amron DM, Kaplan L. Maffucci's syndrome: two case reports with a literature review. J Am Acad Dermatol 1993; 29: 894–899.

48 Loewinger RJ, Lichtenstein JR, Dodson WE, Eisen AZ. Maffucci's syndrome: a mesenchymal dysplasia and multiple tumour syndrome. Br J Dermatol 1977; 96: 317–322.

49 Way BH, Hermann J, Gilbert EF et al. Cutis marmorata telangiectatica congenita. J Cutan Pathol 1974; 1: 10–25.

50 Rogers M, Poyzer KG. Cutis marmorata telangiectatica congenita. Arch Dermatol 1982; 118: 895–899.

51 South DA, Jacobs AH. Cutis marmorata telangiectatica congenita (congenital generalized phlebectasia). J Pediatr 1978; 93: 944–947.

52 Suarez SM, Grossman ME. Localized cutis marmorata telangiectatica congenita. Pediatr Dermatol 1991; 8: 329–331.

53 Kennedy C, Oranje AP, Keizer K et al. Cutis marmorata telangiectatica congenita. Int J Dermatol 1992; 31: 249–252.

54 Pehr K, Moroz B. Cutis marmorata telangiectatica congenita: long-term follow-up, review of the literature, and report of a case in conjunction with congenital hypothyroidism. Pediatr Dermatol 1993; 10: 6–11.

55 Yi G, Oh M. Cutis marmorata telangiectasia congenita: early detection in two premature infants. Pediatr Dermatol 2000; 17: 240–241.

56 Amitai DB, Fichman S, Merlob P et al. Cutis marmorata telangiectatica congenita: clinical findings in 85 patients. Pediatr Dermatol 2000; 17: 100–104.

57 Devillers ACA, de Waard-van der Spek FB, Oranje AP. Cutis marmorata telangiectatica congenita. Clinical features in 35 cases. Arch Dermatol 1999; 135: 34–38.

58 Picascia DD, Esterly NB. Cutis marmorata telangiectatica congenita: report of 22 cases. J Am Acad Dermatol 1989; 20: 1098–1104.

59 Nicholls DSH, Harper JI. Cutis marmorata telangiectatica congenita with soft-tissue herniations on the lower legs. Clin Exp Dermatol 1989; 14: 369–370.

60 Lewis-Jones MS, Evans S, Graham-Brown RAC. Cutis marmorata telangiectatica congenita – a report of two cases occurring in male children. Clin Exp Dermatol 1988; 13: 97–99.

61 Gerritsen MJP, Steijlen PM, Brunner HG, Rieu P. Cutis marmorata telangiectatica congenita: report of 18 cases. Br J Dermatol 2000; 142: 366–369.

62 Chen C-P, Chen H-C, Liu F-F et al. Cutis marmorata telangiectatica congenita associated with an elevated maternal serum human chorionic gonadotrophin level and transitory isolated fetal ascites. Br J Dermatol 1997; 136: 267–271.

63 Morgan JM, Naisby GP, Carmichael AJ. Cutis marmorata telangiectatica congenita with hypoplasia of the right iliac and femoral veins. Br J Dermatol 1997; 137: 119–122.

64 Bormann G, Wohlrab J, Fischer M, Marsch WCh. Cutis marmorata telangiectatica congenita: laser Doppler fluxmetry evidence for a functional nervous defect. Pediatr Dermatol 2001; 18: 110–113.

65 Lynch PJ, Zelickson AS. Congenital phlebectasia. A histopathologic study. Arch Dermatol 1967; 95: 98–101.

66 Davies D, Rogers M, Lam A, Cooke-Yarborough C. Localized microcystic lymphatic malformations – ultrasound diagnosis. Pediatr Dermatol 1999; 16: 423–429.

67 Flanagan BP, Helwig EB. Cutaneous lymphangioma. Arch Dermatol 1977; 113: 24–30.

68 Peachey RDG, Lim C-C, Whimster IW. Lymphangioma of skin. A review of 65 cases. Br J Dermatol 1970; 83: 519–527.

69 Whimster IW. The pathology of lymphangioma circumscriptum. Br J Dermatol 1976; 94: 473–486.

70 Singh RP, Carr DH. The anatomy and histology of XO human embryos and fetuses. Anat Rec 1966; 155: 369–383.

71 Egan CA, Rallis TM, Zone JJ. Multiple scrotal lymphangiomas (lymphangiectases) treated by carbon dioxide laser ablation. Br J Dermatol 1998; 139: 561–562.

72 Mu XC, Tran T-AN, Dupree M, Carlson JA. Acquired vulvar lymphangioma mimicking genital warts. A case report and review of the literature. J Cutan Pathol 1999; 26: 150–154.

73 Burstein JH. Lymphangioma circumscriptum with congenital unilateral lymphedema. Arch Dermatol 1956; 74: 689.

74 Palmer LC, Strauch WG, Welton WA. Lymphangioma circumscriptum. A case with deep lymphatic involvement. Arch Dermatol 1978; 114: 394–396.

75 Irvine AD, Sweeney L, Corbett JR. Lymphangioma circumscriptum associated with paravesical cystic retroperitoneal lymphangioma. Br J Dermatol 1996; 134: 1135–1137.

76 McAlvany JP, Jorizzo JL, Zanolli D et al. Magnetic resonance imaging in the evaluation of lymphangioma circumscriptum. Arch Dermatol 1993; 129: 194–197.

77 King DT, Duffy DM, Hirose FM, Gurevitch AW. Lymphangiosarcoma arising from lymphangioma circumscriptum. Arch Dermatol 1979; 115: 969–972.

78 Wilson GR, Cox NH, McLean NR, Scott D. Squamous cell carcinoma arising within congenital lymphangioma circumscriptum. Br J Dermatol 1993; 129: 337–339.

79 Chervenak FA, Isaacson G, Blakemore KJ et al. Fetal cystic hygroma. Cause and natural history. N Engl J Med 1983; 309: 822–825.

80 Chen C-P, Chen H-C, Liu F-F et al. Progressive fetal axillary cystic lymphangioma with coexistent naevus flammeus. Br J Dermatol 1997; 136: 102–104.

81 Bill AH Jr, Sumner DS. A unified concept of lymphangioma and cystic hygroma. Surg Gynecol Obstet 1965; 120: 79–86.

82 Gomez CS, Calonje E, Ferrar DW et al. Lymphangiomatosis of the limbs. Clinicopathologic analysis of a series with a good prognosis. Am J Surg Pathol 1995; 19: 125–133.

33 Ramani P, Shah A. Lymphangiomatosis: histologic and immunohistochemical analysis of four cases. Am J Surg Pathol 1993; 17: 329–335.

84 Dutheil P, Leraillez J, Guillemette J, Wallach D. Generalized lymphangiomatosis with chylothorax and skin lymphangiomas in a neonate. Pediatr Dermatol 1998; 15: 296–298.

85 Appleton MAC, Attanoos RL, Jasani B. Thrombomodulin as a marker of vascular and lymphatic tumours. Histopathology 1996; 29: 153–157.

86 Imperial R, Helwig EB. Verrucous hemangioma. A clinicopathologic study of 21 cases. Arch Dermatol 1967; 96: 247–253.

87 Rossi A, Bozzi M, Barra E. Verrucous hemangioma and angiokeratoma circumscriptum: clinical and histologic differential characteristics. J Dermatol Surg Oncol 1989; 15: 88–91.

88 Calduch L, Ortega C, Navarro V et al. Verrucous hemangioma: report of two cases and review of the literature. Pediatr Dermatol 2000; 17: 213–217.

89 Cruces MJ, De la Torre C. Multiple eruptive verrucous hemangiomas: a variant of multiple hemangiomatosis. Dermatologica 1985; 171: 106–111.

90 Wentscher U, Happle R. Linear verrucous hemangioma. J Am Acad Dermatol 2000; 42: 516–518.

91 Miko T, Adler P, Endes P. Simulated cancer of the lower lip attributed to a 'caliber persistent' artery. J Oral Pathol 1980; 9: 137–144.

92 Kua H, Blessing K, Holmes J, Burrell M. Calibre persistent artery of the lip: an underdiagnosed entity? J Clin Pathol 2000; 53: 885.

93 Miko TL, Molnar P, Vereckei L. Interrelationships of calibre persistent artery, chronic ulcer and squamous cancer of the lower lip. Histopathology 1983; 7: 595–599.

94 Marshall RJ, Leppard BJ. Ulceration of the lip associated with a 'calibre-persistent artery'. Br J Dermatol 1985; 113: 757–760.

Vascular dilatations (telangiectases)

95 Bean WB. Vascular spiders and related lesions of the skin. Oxford: Blackwell Scientific Publications, 1958; 132.

96 Daly JJ, Schiller AL. The liver in hereditary hemorrhagic telangiectasia (Osler–Weber–Rendu disease). Am J Med 1976; 60: 723–726.

97 Chandler D. Pulmonary and cerebral arteriovenous fistula with Osler's disease. Arch Intern Med 1965; 116: 277–282.

98 Dines DE, Arms RA, Bernatz PE, Gomes MR. Pulmonary arteriovenous fistulas. Mayo Clin Proc 1974; 49: 460–465.

99 Swanson DL, Dahl MV. Embolic abscesses in hereditary hemorrhagic telangiectasia. J Am Acad Dermatol 1991; 24: 580–583.

100 Mager JJ, Westermann CJJ. Value of capillary microscopy in the diagnosis of hereditary hemorrhagic telangiectasia. Arch Dermatol 2000; 136: 732–734.

101 Hashimoto K, Pritzker MS. Hereditary hemorrhagic telangiectasia. An electron microscopic study. Oral Surg 1972; 34: 751–758.

102 Menefee MG, Flessa HC, Glueck HI, Hogg SP. Hereditary hemorrhagic telangiectasia (Osler–Weber–Rendu disease). An electron microscopic study of the vascular lesions before and after therapy with hormones. Arch Otolaryngol 1975; 101: 246–251.

103 McGrae JD Jr, Winkelmann RK. Generalized essential telangiectasia. Report of a clinical and histochemical study of 13 patients with acquired cutaneous lesions. JAMA 1963; 185: 909–913.

104 Checketts SR, Burton PS, Bjorkman DJ, Kadunce DP. Generalized essential telangiectasia in the presence of gastrointestinal bleeding. J Am Acad Dermatol 1997 37: 321–325.

105 Ryan TJ, Wells RS. Hereditary benign telangiectasia. Trans St John's Hosp Dermatol Soc 1971; 57: 148–156.

106 Gold MH, Eramo L, Prendiville JS. Hereditary benign telangiectasia. Pediatr Dermatol 1989; 6: 194–197.

107 Wagner RF Jr, Grande DJ, Bhawan J et al. Unilateral dermatomal superficial telangiectasia overlapping Becker's melanosis. Int J Dermatol 1989; 28: 595–596.

108 Wilkin JK, Smith JG Jr, Cullison DA et al. Unilateral dermatomal superficial telangiectasia. J Am Acad Dermatol 1983; 8: 468–477.

109 Woollons A, Darley CR. Unilateral naevoid telangiectasia syndrome in pregnancy. Clin Exp Dermatol 1996; 21: 459–460.

110 Beacham BE, Kurgansky D. Unilateral naevoid telangiectasia syndrome associated with metastatic carcinoid tumour. Br J Dermatol 1991; 124: 86–88.

111 Hynes LR, Shenefelt PD. Unilateral nevoid telangiectasia: Occurrence in two patients with hepatitis C. J Am Acad Dermatol 1997; 36: 819–822.

112 Uhlin SR, McCarty KS Jr. Unilateral nevoid telangiectatic syndrome. The role of estrogen and progesterone receptors. Arch Dermatol 1983; 119: 226–228.

113 Abrahamian LM, Rothe MJ, Grant-Kels JM. Primary telangiectasia of childhood. Int J Dermatol 1992; 31: 307–313.

114 Smith LL, Conerly SL. Ataxia–telangiectasia or Louis–Bar syndrome. J Am Acad Dermatol 1985; 12: 681–696.

115 Gotz A, Eckert F, Landthaler M. Ataxia–telangiectasia (Louis–Bar syndrome) associated with ulcerating necrobiosis lipoidica. J Am Acad Dermatol 1994; 31: 124–126.

116 Joshi RK, Al Asiri RH, Haleem A et al. Cutaneous granuloma with ataxia telangiectasia – a case report and review of literature. Clin Exp Dermatol 1993; 18: 458–461.

117 Drolet BA, Drolet B, Zvulunov A et al. Cutaneous granulomas as a presenting sign in ataxia–telangiectasia. Dermatology 1997; 194: 273–275.

118 Şentürk N, Hindioğlu U, Şahn S, Gököz A. Granulomatous skin lesions in a patient with ataxia telangiectasia. Br J Dermatol 1998; 139: 543–544.

119 Khumalo NP, Joss DV, Huson SM, Burge S. Pigmentary anomalies in ataxia–telangiectasia: a clue to diagnosis and an example of twin spotting. Br J Dermatol 2001; 144: 369–371.

120 Li A, Swift M. Mutations at the ataxia–telangiectasia locus and clinical phenotypes of A–T patients. Am J Med Genet 2000; 92: 170–177.

121 Bean WB. Vascular spiders and related lesions of the skin. Oxford: Blackwell Scientific Publications, 1958; 3.

122 Wenzl JE, Burgert EO Jr. The spider nevus in infancy and childhood. Pediatrics 1964; 33: 227–232.

123 Bean WB, Walsh JR. Venous lakes. Arch Dermatol 1956; 74: 459–463.

124 Suhonen R, Kuflik EG. Venous lakes treated by liquid nitrogen cryosurgery. Br J Dermatol 1997; 137: 1018–1019.

125 Epstein E, Novy FG Jr, Allington HV. Capillary aneurysms of the skin. Arch Dermatol 1965; 91: 335–341.

126 Imperial R, Helwig EB. Angiokeratoma. A clinicopathological study. Arch Dermatol 1967; 95: 166–175.

127 Haye KR, Rebello DJA. Angiokeratoma of Mibelli. Acta Derm Venereol 1961; 41: 56–60.

128 Imperial R, Helwig EB. Angiokeratoma of the scrotum (Fordyce type). J Urol 1967; 98: 379–387.

129 Bean WB. Vascular spiders and related lesions of the skin. Oxford: Blackwell Scientific Publications, 1958; 262–264.

130 Carrasco L, Izquierdo MJ, Fariña MC et al. Strawberry glans penis: a rare manifestation of angiokeratomas involving the glans penis. Br J Dermatol 2000; 142: 1256–1257.

131 Agger P, Osmundsen PE. Angiokeratoma of the scrotum (Fordyce). A case report on response to surgical treatment of varicocele. Acta Derm Venereol 1970; 50: 221–224.

132 Imperial R, Helwig E. Angiokeratoma of the vulva. Obstet Gynecol 1967; 29: 307–312.

133 Novick NL. Angiokeratoma vulvae. J Am Acad Dermatol 1985; 12: 561–563.

134 Eizaguirre X, Landa N, Raton JA, Diaz-Perez JL. Multiple angiokeratomas with zosteriform distribution in two sisters. Int J Dermatol 1994; 33: 641–642.

135 Shannon PL, Ford MJ. Angiokeratomas in juvenile dermatomyositis. Pediatr Dermatol 1999; 16: 448–451.

136 Lynch PJ, Kosanovich M. Angiokeratoma circumscriptum. Arch Dermatol 1967; 96: 665–668.

137 Holmes RC, Fensom AH, McKee P et al. Angiokeratoma corporis diffusum in a patient with normal enzyme activities. J Am Acad Dermatol 1984; 10: 384–387.

138 Gasparini G, Sarchi G, Cavicchini S, Bertagnolio B. Angiokeratoma corporis diffusum in a patient with normal enzyme activities and Turner's syndrome. Clin Exp Dermatol 1992; 17: 56–59.

139 Fimiani M, Mazzatenta C, Rubegni P, Andreassi L. Idiopathic angiokeratoma corporis diffusum. Clin Exp Dermatol 1997; 22: 205–206.

140 Massi D, Martinelli F, Battini ML et al. Angiokeratoma corporis diffusum (Anderson–Fabry's disease): a case report. J Eur Acad Dermatol Venereol 2000; 14: 127–130.

141 Clarke JTR, Knaack J, Crawhall JC, Wolfe JS. Ceramide trihexosidosis (Fabry's disease) without skin lesions. N Engl J Med 1971; 284: 233–235.

142 Wallace HJ. Anderson–Fabry disease. Br J Dermatol 1973; 88: 1–23.

143 Ostlere L, Hart Y, Misch KJ. Cutaneous and cerebral haemangiomas associated with eruptive angiokeratomas. Br J Dermatol 1996; 135: 98–101.

144 Kanzaki T, Yokota M, Irie F et al. Angiokeratoma corporis diffusum with glycopeptiduria due to deficient lysomal α-N-acetylgalactosaminidase activity. Arch Dermatol 1993; 129: 460–465.

145 Kodama K, Kobayashi H, Abe R et al. A new case of α-N-acetylgalactosaminidase deficiency with angiokeratoma corporis diffusum, with Ménière's syndrome and without mental retardation. Br J Dermatol 2001; 144: 363–368.

146 Rodriguez-Serna M, Botella-Estrada R, Chabás A et al. Angiokeratoma corporis diffusum associated with β-mannosidase deficiency. Arch Dermatol 1996; 132: 1219–1222.

147 Epinette WW, Norins AL, Drew AL et al. Angiokeratoma corporis diffusum with α-L-fucosidase deficiency. Arch Dermatol 1973; 107: 754–757.

148 Ishibashi A, Tsuboi R, Shinmei M. β-galactosidase and neuraminidase deficiency associated with angiokeratoma corporis diffusum. Arch Dermatol 1984; 120: 1344–1346.

149 Kawachi Y, Matsu-ura K, Sakuraba H, Otsuka F. Angiokeratoma corporis diffusum associated with galactosialidosis. Dermatology 1998; 197: 52–54.

150 Calzavara-Pinton PG, Colombi M, Carlino A. Angiokeratoma corporis diffusum and arteriovenous fistulas with dominant transmission in the absence of metabolic disorders. Arch Dermatol 1995; 131: 57–62.

151 Kraus MD, Lind AC, Alder SL, Dehner LP. Angiomatosis with angiokeratoma-like features in children: a light microscopic and immunophenotypic examination of four cases. Am J Dermatopathol 1999; 21: 350–355.

152 Nakamura T, Kaneko H, Nishino I. Angiokeratoma corporis diffusum (Fabry disease): ultrastructural studies of the skin. Acta Derm Venereol 1981; 61: 37–41.

153 Lewis AT, Hsu S, Phillips RM, Lee JA. Computer palms. J Am Acad Dermatol 2000; 42: 1073–1075.

154 Sahn EE, Hussey RH III, Christmann LM. A case of Bloom syndrome with conjunctival telangiectasia. Pediatr Dermatol 1997; 14: 120–124.

155 Salama S, Rosenthal D. Cutaneous collagenous vasculopathy with generalized telangiectasia: an immunohistochemical and ultrastructural study. J Cutan Pathol 2000; 27: 40–48.

156 Basarab T, Yu R, Russell Jones P. Calcium antagonist-induced photo-exposed telangiectasia. Br J Dermatol 1997; 136: 974–975.

157 Borgia F, Vaccaro M, Guarneri F, Cannavò SP. Photodistributed telangiectasia following use of cefotaxime. Br J Dermatol 2000; 143: 674–675.

158 van der Vleuten CJM, Trijbels-Smeulders MAJM, van de Kerkhof PCM. Telangiectasia and gingival hyperplasia as side-effects of amlodipine (Norvasc) in a 3-year-old girl. Acta Derm Venereol 1999; 79: 323–324.

159 Karonen T, Stubb S, Keski-Oja J. Truncal telangiectases coinciding with felodipine. Dermatology 1998; 196: 272–273.

160 Sartori CR, Baker EJ, Hobbs ER. Costal fringe. Arch Dermatol 1991; 127: 1201–1202.

161 Braverman IM. Ultrastructure and organization of the cutaneous microvasculature in normal and pathologic states. J Invest Dermatol 1989; 93: 2S–9S.

162 Buckley DA, Barnes L. Vulvar lymphangiectasia due to recurrent cellulitis. Clin Exp Dermatol 1996; 21: 215–216.

163 Mallett RB, Curley GK, Mortimer PS. Acquired lymphangioma: report of four cases and a discussion of the pathogenesis. Br J Dermatol 1992; 126: 380–382.

164 Moon SE, Youn JI, Lee YS. Acquired cutaneous lymphangiectasia. Br J Dermatol 1993; 129: 193–195.

165 Prioleau PG, Santa Cruz DJ. Lymphangioma circumscriptum following radical mastectomy and radiation therapy. Cancer 1978; 42: 1989–1991.

166 Leshin B, Whitaker DC, Foucar E. Lymphangioma circumscriptum following mastectomy and radiation therapy. J Am Acad Dermatol 1986; 15: 1117–1119.

167 Ziv R, Schewach-Millet M, Trau H. Lymphangiectasia. A complication of thoracotomy for bronchial carcinoid. Int J Dermatol 1988; 27: 123.

168 Weakley DR, Juhlin EA. Lymphangiectases and lymphangiomata. Arch Dermatol 1961; 84: 574–578.

169 Fisher I, Orkin M. Acquired lymphangioma (lymphangiectasis). Report of a case. Arch Dermatol 1970; 101: 230–234.

170 Ambrojo P, Cogolludo EF, Aguilar A et al. Cutaneous lymphangiectases after therapy for carcinoma of the cervix – a case with unusual clinical and histological features. Clin Exp Dermatol 1990; 15: 57–59.

171 LaPolla J, Foucar E, Leshin B et al. Vulvar lymphangioma circumscriptum: a rare complication of therapy for squamous cell carcinoma of the cervix. Gynecol Oncol 1985; 22: 363–366.

172 Harwood CA, Mortimer PS. Acquired vulval lymphangiomata mimicking genital warts. Br J Dermatol 1993; 129: 334–336.

173 Loche F, Schwarze HP, Bazex J. Treatment of acquired cutaneous lymphangiectasis of the thigh and vulva with a carbon dioxide laser. Acta Derm Venereol 1999; 79: 335.

174 Pena JM, Ford MJ. Cutaneous lymphangiectases associated with severe photoaging and topical corticosteroid application. J Cutan Pathol 1996; 23: 175–181.

175 Stone MS. Central-facial papular lymphangiectases: An uncommon manifestation of porphyria. J Am Acad Dermatol 1997; 36: 493–495.

Vascular proliferations (hyperplasias and benign neoplasms)

176 Requena L, Sangueza OP. Cutaneous vascular proliferations. Part II. Hyperplasias and benign neoplasms. J Am Acad Dermatol 1997; 37: 887–920.

177 Metry DW, Hebert AA. Benign cutaneous vascular tumors of infancy. When to worry, what to do. Arch Dermatol 2000; 136: 905–914.

178 Hidano A, Nakajima S. Earliest features of the strawberry mark in the newborn. Br J Dermatol 1972; 87: 138–144.

179 Bowers RE, Graham EA, Tomlinson KM. The natural history of the strawberry nevus. Arch Dermatol 1960; 82: 667–680.

180 Kunkeler ACM, Uitdehaag BMJ, Stoof TJ. Familial cutaneous haemangiomas. Br J Dermatol 1998; 139: 166–167.

181 Walsh TS Jr, Tompkins VN. Some observations on the strawberry nevus of infancy. Cancer 1956; 9: 869–904.

182 Williams HB. Hemangiomas of the parotid gland in children. Plast Reconstr Surg 1975; 56: 29–34.

183 Jacobs AH. Vascular nevi. Pediatr Clin North Am 1983; 30: 465–482.

184 Mancini AJ, Smoller BR. Proliferation and apoptosis within juvenile capillary hemangiomas. Am J Dermatopathol 1996; 18: 505–514.

185 Wallace HJ. Conservative treatment of haemangiomatous naevi. Br J Plast Surg 1953; 6: 78–82.

186 Reischle S, Schuller-Petrovic S. Treatment of capillary hemangiomas of early childhood with a new method of cryosurgery. J Am Acad Dermatol 2000; 42: 809–813.

187 Yap E-Y, Bartley GB, Hohberger GG. Periocular capillary hemangioma: a review for pediatricians and family physicians. Mayo Clin Proc 1998; 73: 753–759.

188 Williams HB. Hemangiomas and lymphangiomas. Adv Surg 1981; 15: 317–349.

189 Patel SD, Cohen BA, Kan JS. Extensive facial hemangioma associated with cardiac and abdominal anomalies. J Am Acad Dermatol 1997; 36: 636–638.

190 Enjolras O, Gelbert F. Superficial hemangiomas: associations and management. Pediatr Dermatol 1997; 14: 173–179.

191 Berg JN, Walter JW, Thisanagayam U et al. Evidence for loss of heterozygosity of 5q in sporadic haemangiomas: are somatic mutations involved in haemangioma formation? J Clin Pathol 2001; 54: 249–252.

192 Blei F, Walter J, Orlow SJ, Marchuk DA. Familial segregation of hemangiomas and vascular malformations as an autosomal dominant trait. Arch Dermatol 1998; 134: 718–722.

193 Bree AF, Siegfried E, Sotelo-Avila C, Nahass G. Infantile hemangiomas. Speculation on placental trophoblastic origin. Arch Dermatol 2001; 137: 573–577.

194 North PE, Waner M, Mizeracki A et al. A unique microvascular phenotype shared by juvenile hemangiomas and human placenta. Arch Dermatol 2001; 137: 559–570.

195 Dosanjh A, Chang J, Bresnick S et al. In vitro characteristics of neonatal hemangioma endothelial cells: similarities and differences between normal neonatal and fetal endothelial cells. J Cutan Pathol 2000; 27: 441–450.

196 North PE, Waner M, Mizeracki A, Mihm MC Jr. GLUT1: a newly discovered immunohistochemical marker for juvenile hemangiomas. Hum Pathol 2000; 31: 11–22.

197 Verkarre V, Patey-Mariaud de Serre N, Vazeux R et al. ICAM-3 and E-selectin endothelial cell expression differentiate two phases of angiogenesis in infantile hemangiomas. J Cutan Pathol 1999; 26: 17–24.

198 Boye E, Yu Y, Paranya G et al. Clonality and altered behavior of endothelial cells from hemangiomas. J Clin Invest 2001; 107: 745–752.

199 Marchuk DA. Pathogenesis of hemangioma. J Clin Invest 2001; 107: 665–666.

200 Gonzalez-Crussi F, Reyes-Mugica M. Cellular hemangiomas ("hemangioendotheliomas") in infants. Am J Surg Pathol 1991; 15: 769–778.

201 Glowacki J, Mulliken JB. Mast cells in hemangiomas and vascular malformations. Pediatrics 1982; 70: 48–51.

202 Calonje E, Mentzel T, Fletcher CDM. Pseudomalignant perineurial invasion in cellular ('infantile') capillary haemangiomas. Histopathology 1995; 26: 159–164.

203 Rositto A, Ranalletta M, Drut R. Congenital hemangioma of eccrine sweat glands. Pediatr Dermatol 1993; 10: 341–343.

204 Smoller BR, Apfelberg DB. Infantile (juvenile) capillary hemangioma: a tumor of heterogeneous cellular elements. J Cutan Pathol 1993; 20: 330–336.

205 Furusato M, Fukunaga M, Kikuchi Y et al. Two- and three-dimensional ultrastructural observations of angiogenesis in juvenile hemangioma. Virchows Arch [B] 1984; 46: 229–237.

206 Pasyk KA, Grabb WC, Cherry GW. Crystalloid inclusions in endothelial cells of cellular and capillary hemangiomas. A possible sign of cellular immaturity. Arch Dermatol 1983; 119: 134–137.

207 Endo H, Kawada A, Aragane Y et al. The successful treatment of diffuse neonatal hemangiomatosis with flashlamp pulsed dye laser. Pediatr Dermatol 2001; 18: 146–148.

208 Holden KR, Alexander F. Diffuse neonatal hemangiomatosis. Pediatrics 1970; 46: 411–421.

209 Burke EC, Winkelmann RK, Strickland MK. Disseminated hemangiomatosis. The newborn with central nervous system involvement. Am J Dis Child 1964; 108: 418–424.

210 Cooper AG, Bolande RP. Multiple hemangiomas in an infant with cardiac hypertrophy. Postmortem angiographic demonstration of the arteriovenous fistulae. Pediatrics 1965; 35: 27–35.

211 Rothe MJ, Rowse D, Grant-Kels JM. Benign neonatal hemangiomatosis with aggressive growth of cutaneous lesions. Pediatr Dermatol 1991; 8: 140–146.

212 Singh G, Rajendran C. Kasabach–Merritt syndrome in two successive pregnancies. Int J Dermatol 1998; 37: 690–693.

213 Geller JD, Topper SF, Hashimoto K. Diffuse neonatal hemangiomatosis: a new constellation of findings. J Am Acad Dermatol 1991; 24: 816–818.

214 Yates R, Syed S, Tsang V, Harper JI. Haemangioma of the head and neck with subglottic involvement and atypical coarctation. Br J Dermatol 2000; 143: 686–688.

215 Stern JK, Wolf JE Jr, Jarratt M. Benign neonatal hemangiomatosis. J Am Acad Dermatol 1981; 4: 442–445.

216 Dyall-Smith D, Cowen P. Benign neonatal hemangiomatosis. Int J Dermatol 1992; 31: 336–338.

217 Keller L, Bluhm JF III. Diffuse neonatal hemangiomatosis. A case with heart failure and thrombocytopenia. Cutis 1979; 23: 295–297.

218 Calonje E, Fletcher CDM. Sinusoidal hemangioma. A distinctive benign vascular neoplasm within the group of cavernous hemangiomas. Am J Surg Pathol 1991; 15: 1130–1135.

219 Nakamura M, Miyachi Y. Calcifying sinusoidal haemangioma on the back. Br J Dermatol 1999; 141: 377–378.

220 Bean WB. Vascular spiders and related lesions of the skin. Oxford: Blackwell Scientific Publications, 1958; 228.

221 Tuder RM, Young R, Karasek M, Bensch K. Adult cutaneous hemangiomas are composed of nonreplicating endothelial cells. J Invest Dermatol 1987; 89: 594–597.

222 Aghassi D, Anderson RR, González S. Time-sequence histologic imaging of laser-treated cherry angiomas with in vivo confocal microscopy. J Am Acad Dermatol 2000; 43: 37–41.

223 Chan JKC, Fletcher CDM, Hicklin GA, Rosai J. Glomeruloid hemangioma. A distinctive cutaneous lesion of multicentric Castleman's disease associated with POEMS syndrome. Am J Surg Pathol 1990; 14: 1036–1046.

224 Kishimoto S, Takenaka H, Shibagaki R et al. Glomeruloid hemangioma in POEMS syndrome shows two different immunophenotypic endothelial cells. J Cutan Pathol 2000; 27: 87–92.

225 Bardwick PA, Zvaifler NJ, Gill GN et al. Plasma cell dyscrasia with polyneuropathy, organomegaly, endocrinopathy, M-protein and skin changes: the POEMS syndrome. Report on 2 cases and a review of the literature. Medicine 1980; 59: 311–322.

226 Shelley WB, Shelley ED. The skin changes in the Crow–Fukase (POEMS) syndrome. A case report. Arch Dermatol 1987; 123: 85–87.

227 Frizzera G. Castleman's disease and related disorders. Semin Diagn Pathol 1988; 5: 346–364.

228 Yang SG, Cho KH, Bang Y-J, Kim CW. A case of glomeruloid hemangioma associated with multicentric Castleman's disease. Am J Dermatopathol 1998; 20: 266–270.

229 Kanitakis J, Roger H, Soubrier M et al. Cutaneous angiomas in POEMS syndrome. An ultrastructural and immunohistochemical study. Arch Dermatol 1988; 124: 695–698.

230 Ardigò N, Brazzelli V, Vassallo C et al. Acquired tufted-glomeruloid hemangioma in a patient with myeloma IgG-κ. Am J Dermatopathol 2000; 22: 358 (abstract).

231 Rongioletti F, Gambini C, Lerza R. Glomeruloid hemangioma. A cutaneous marker of POEMS syndrome. Am J Dermatopathol 1994; 16: 175–178.

232 Puig L, Moreno A, Domingo P et al. Cutaneous angiomas in POEMS syndrome. J Am Acad Dermatol 1985; 12: 961–964.

233 Judge MR, McGibbon DH, Thompson RPH. Angioendotheliomatosis associated with Castleman's lymphoma and POEMS syndrome. Clin Exp Dermatol 1993; 18: 360–362.

234 Girard C, Graham JH, Johnson WC. Arteriovenous hemangioma (arteriovenous shunt). A clinicopathological and histochemical study. J Cutan Pathol 1974; 1: 73–87.

235 Connelly MG, Winkelmann RK. Acral arteriovenous tumor. A clinicopathologic review. Am J Surg Pathol 1985; 9: 15–21.

236 Neumann RA, Knobler RM, Schuller-Petrovic S et al. Giant arteriovenous hemangioma (cirsoid aneurysm) of the nose. J Dermatol Surg Oncol 1989; 15: 739–742.

237 Akiyama M, Inamoto N. Arteriovenous haemangioma in chronic liver disease: clinical and histopathological features of four cases. Br J Dermatol 2001; 144: 604–609.

238 Koutlas IG, Jessurun J. Arteriovenous hemangioma: a clinicopathological and immunohistochemical study. J Cutan Pathol 1994; 21: 343–349.

239 Kadono T, Kishi A, Onishi Y, Ohara K. Acquired digital arteriovenous malformation: a report of six cases. Br J Dermatol 2000; 142: 362–365.

240 Loo WJ, Dawber RPR. Digital arteriovenous malformation. Br J Dermatol 2000; 143: 462.

241 Hunt SJ, Santa Cruz DJ, Barr RJ. Microvenular hemangioma. J Cutan Pathol 1991; 18: 235–240.

242 Aloi F, Tomasini C, Pippione M. Microvenular hemangioma. Am J Dermatopathol 1993; 15: 534–538.

243 Sanz-Trelles A, Ojeda-Martos A, Jimenez-Fernandez A, Vera-Casaño A. Microvenular haemangioma: a new case in a child. Histopathology 1998; 32: 89–90.

244 Black RJ, McCusker GM, Eedy DJ. Microvenular haemangioma. Clin Exp Dermatol 1995; 20: 260–262.

245 Brear SG, Rademaker M, Hasleton P et al. Target-like skin lesions in primary amyloidosis. Br J Dermatol 1985; 112: 209–211.

246 Rapini RP, Golitz LE. Targetoid hemosiderotic hemangioma. J Cutan Pathol 1990; 17: 233–235.

247 Morganroth GS, Tigelaar RE, Longley BJ et al. Targetoid hemangioma associated with pregnancy and the menstrual cycle. J Am Acad Dermatol 1995; 32: 282–284.

248 Vion B, Frenk E. Targetoid hemosiderotic hemangioma. Dermatology 1992; 184: 300–302.

249 Mentzel T, Partanen TA, Kutzner H. Hobnail hemangioma ("targetoid hemosiderotic hemangioma"): clinicopathologic and immunohistochemical analysis of 62 cases. J Cutan Pathol 1999; 26: 279–286.

250 Carlson JA, Daulat S, Goodheart HP. Targetoid hemosiderotic hemangioma – a dynamic vascular tumor: Report of 3 cases with episodic and cyclic changes and comparison with solitary angiokeratomas. J Am Acad Dermatol 1999; 41: 215–224.

251 Santa Cruz DJ, Aronberg J. Targetoid hemosiderotic hemangioma. J Am Acad Dermatol 1988; 19: 550–558.

252 Christenson L, VanBeek M, Davis D. Targetoid hemosiderotic hemangioma occurring in a father and son. Arch Dermatol 2000; 136: 1571–1572.

253 Christenson LJ, Stone MS. Trauma-induced simulator of targetoid hemosiderotic hemangioma. Am J Dermatopathol 2001; 23: 221–223.

254 Rosso R, Brazzelli V, Vassallo C et al. Acral hobnail hemangioma. Am J Dermatopathol 2000; 22: 358 (abstract).

255 Guillou L, Calonje E, Speight P et al. Hobnail hemangioma. A pseudomalignant vascular lesion with a reappraisal of targetoid hemosiderotic hemangioma. Am J Surg Pathol 1999; 23: 97–105.

256 Weiss SW, Enzinger FM. Spindle cell hemangioendothelioma. A low-grade angiosarcoma resembling a cavernous hemangioma and Kaposi's sarcoma. Am J Surg Pathol 1986; 10: 521–530.

257 Fletcher CDM, Beham A, Schmid C. Spindle cell haemangioendothelioma: a clinicopathological and immunohistochemical study indicative of a non-neoplastic lesion. Histopathology 1991; 18: 291–301.

258 Hisaoka M, Kouho H, Aoki T, Hashimoto H. DNA flow cytometric and immunohistochemical analysis of proliferative activity in spindle cell haemangioendothelioma. Histopathology 1995; 27: 451–456.

259 Ding J, Hashimoto H, Imayama S et al. Spindle cell haemangioendothelioma: probably a benign vascular lesion not a low-grade angiosarcoma. Virchows Arch (Pathol Anat) 1992; 420: 77–85.

260 Imayama S, Murakamai Y, Hashimoto H, Hori Y. Spindle cell hemangioendothelioma exhibits the ultrastructural features of reactive vascular proliferation rather than of angiosarcoma. Am J Clin Pathol 1992; 97: 279–287.

261 Perkins P, Weiss SW. Spindle cell hemangioendothelioma. An analysis of 78 cases with reassessment of its pathogenesis and biologic behavior. Am J Surg Pathol 1996; 20: 1196–1204.

262 Setoyama M, Shimada H, Miyazono N et al. Spindle cell hemangioendothelioma: successful treatment with recombinant interleukin-2. Br J Dermatol 2000; 142: 1238–1239.

263 Tomasini C, Aloi F, Soro E, Elia V. Spindle cell hemangioma. Dermatology 1999; 199: 274–276.

264 Requena L, Ackerman AB. Hemangioendothelioma? Dermatopathology: Practical & Conceptual 1999; 5: 110–112.

265 Eltorky M, McChesney T, Sebes J, Hall JC. Spindle cell hemangioendothelioma. Report of three cases and review of the literature. J Dermatol Surg Oncol 1994; 20: 196–202.

266 Fanburg JC, Meis JM, Rosenberg AE. Maffucci's syndrome: Multiple enchondromas and spindle cell haemangioendotheliomas. Mod Pathol 1993; 6: 6a (abstract).

267 Pellegrini AE, Drake RD, Qualman SJ. Spindle cell hemangioendothelioma: a neoplasm associated with Maffucci's syndrome. J Cutan Pathol 1995; 22: 173–176.

268 Scott GA, Rosai J. Spindle cell hemangioendothelioma. Report of seven additional cases of a recently described vascular neoplasm. Am J Dermatopathol 1988; 10: 281–288.

269 Chan JKC. Vascular tumours with a prominent spindle cell component. Curr Diagn Pathol 1997; 4: 76–90.

270 Barker LP, Sachs PM. Angioma serpiginosum. Arch Dermatol 1965; 92: 613–620.

271 Ohnishi T, Nagayama T, Morita T et al. Angioma serpiginosum. A report of 2 cases identified using epiluminescence microscopy. Arch Dermatol 1999; 135: 1366–1368.

272 Marriott PJ, Munro DD, Ryan T. Angioma serpiginosum – familial incidence. Br J Dermatol 1975; 93: 701–706.

273 Kumakiri M, Katoh N, Miura Y. Angioma serpiginosum. J Cutan Pathol 1980; 7: 410–421.

274 Michalowski R, Urban J. Atypical angioma serpiginosum: a case report. Dermatologica 1982; 164: 331–337.

275 Vargas SO, Perez-Atayde AR, González-Crussi F, Kozakewich HP. Giant cell angioblastoma. Three additional occurrences of a distinct pathologic entity. Am J Surg Pathol 2001; 25: 185–196.

276 Wells GC, Whimster IW. Subcutaneous angiolymphoid hyperplasia with eosinophilia. Br J Dermatol 1969; 81: 1–15.

277 Wilson Jones E, Bleehen SS. Inflammatory angiomatous nodules with abnormal blood vessels occurring about the ears and scalp (pseudo or atypical pyogenic granuloma). Br J Dermatol 1969; 81: 804–816.

278 Enzinger FM, Weiss SW. Soft tissue tumors. St Louis: CV Mosby, 1983; 391–397.

279 Rosai J. Angiolymphoid hyperplasia with eosinophilia of the skin. Am J Dermatopathol 1982; 4: 175–184.

280 Rosai J, Akerman LR. Intravenous atypical vascular proliferation. A cutaneous lesion simulating a malignant blood vessel tumor. Arch Dermatol 1974; 109: 714–717.

281 Bendl BJ, Asano K, Lewis RJ. Nodular angioblastic hyperplasia with eosinophilia and lymphofolliculosis. Cutis 1977; 19: 327–329.

282 Kanik AB, Oh CH, Bhawan J. Disseminated cutaneous epithelioid hemangioma. J Am Acad Dermatol 1996; 35: 851–853.

283 Kimura T, Yoshimura S, Ishikawa E. Unusual granulation combined with hyperplastic change of lymphatic tissue. Trans Soc Path Jap 1948; 37: 179–180.

284 Kawada A, Takahashi H, Anzai T. Eosinophilic lymphofolliculosis of the skin (Kimura's disease). Jpn J Dermatol 1966; 76: 61–72.

285 Lenk N, Artüz F, Kulaçoğlu S, Alli N. Kimura's disease. Int J Dermatol 1997; 36: 437–439.

286 Lee JH, Park HJ, Kim YC, Cinn YW. Two cases of Kimura's disease with unusual clinical manifestations. Dermatology 2000; 201: 162–164.

287 Hongcharu W, Baldassano M, Taylor CR. Kimura's disease with oral ulcers: Response to pentoxifylline. J Am Acad Dermatol 2000; 43: 905–907.

288 Kuo T-T, Shih L-Y, Chan H-L. Kimura's disease. Involvement of regional lymph nodes and distinction from angiolymphoid hyperplasia with eosinophilia. Am J Surg Pathol 1988; 12: 843–854.

289 Chan JKC, Hui PK, Ng CS et al. Epithelioid haemangioma (angiolymphoid hyperplasia with eosinophilia) and Kimura's disease in Chinese. Histopathology 1989; 15: 557–574.

290 Helander SD, Peters MS, Kuo T-t, Su WPD. Kimura's disease and angiolymphoid hyperplasia with eosinophilia: new observations from immunohistochemical studies of lymphocyte markers, endothelial antigens, and granulocyte proteins. J Cutan Pathol 1995; 22: 319–326.

291 Zhang J-Z, Zhang C-G, Chen J-M. Thirty-five cases of Kimura's disease (eosinophilic lymphogranuloma). Br J Dermatol 1998; 139: 542–543.

292 Nagore E, Llorca J, Sánchez-Motilla JM et al. Detection of Epstein–Barr virus DNA in a patient with Kimura's disease. Int J Dermatol 2000; 39: 618–620.

293 Arnold M, Geilen CC, Coupland SE et al. Unilateral angiolymphoid hyperplasia with eosinophilia involving the left arm and hand. J Cutan Pathol 1999; 26: 436–440.

294 Blauvelt A, Cobb MW, Turner ML. Widespread cutaneous vascular papules associated with peripheral blood eosinophilia and prominent inguinal lymphadenopathy. J Am Acad Dermatol 2000; 43: 698–700.

295 Burg G. Collision dermatosis: angiolymphoid hyperplasia with eosinophilia developing within a congenital port wine nevus. Dermatology 1993; 187: 293–295.

296 Scurry J, Dennerstein G, Brenan J. Angiolymphoid hyperplasia with eosinophilia of the vulva. Aust NZ J Obstet Gynaecol 1995; 35: 347–348.

297 Lopez JI, Battaglino SB. Angiolymphoid hyperplasia with eosinophilia of the lower lip. Int J Dermatol 1993; 32: 361–362.

298 Misselvish I, Podoshin L, Fradis M, Boss JH. Angiolymphoid hyperplasia with eosinophilia of the oral mucous membrane. Ear Nose Throat J 1995; 74: 122–125.

299 D'Offizi G, Ferrara R, Donati P et al. Angiolymphoid hyperplasia with eosinophils in HIV infection. AIDS 1995; 9: 813–814.

300 Olsen TG, Helwig EB. Angiolymphoid hyperplasia with eosinophilia. A clinicopathologic study of 116 patients. J Am Acad Dermatol 1985; 12: 781–796.

301 Henry PG, Burnett JW. Angiolymphoid hyperplasia with eosinophilia. Arch Dermatol 1978; 114: 1168–1172.

302 Gupta G, Munro CS. Angiolymphoid hyperplasia with eosinophilia: successful treatment with pulsed dye laser using the double pulse technique. Br J Dermatol 2000; 143: 214–215.

303 Shenefelt PD, Rinker M, Caradonna S et al. A case of angiolymphoid hyperplasia with eosinophilia treated with intralesional interferon alfa-2a. Arch Dermatol 2000; 136: 837–839.

304 Oh C-W, Kim K-H. Is angiolymphoid hyperplasia with eosinophilia a benign vascular tumor? A case improved with oral isotretinoin. Dermatology 1998; 197: 189–191.

305 Moy RL, Luftman DB, Nguyen QH, Amenta JS. Estrogen receptors and the response to sex hormones in angiolymphoid hyperplasia with eosinophilia. Arch Dermatol 1992; 128: 825–828.

306 Vadlamudi G, Schinella R. Traumatic pseudoaneurysm: a possible early lesion in the spectrum of epithelioid hemangioma/angiolymphoid hyperplasia with eosinophilia. Am J Dermatopathol 1998; 20: 113–117.

307 Onishi Y, Ohara K. Angiolymphoid hyperplasia with eosinophilia associated with arteriovenous malformation: a clinicopathological correlation with angiography and serial estimation of serum levels of renin, eosinophil cationic protein and interleukin 5. Br J Dermatol 1999; 140: 1153–1156.

303 Kempf W, Haeffner AC, Zepter C et al. Angiolymphoid hyperplasia with eosinophilia: evidence for a T-cell origin. Am J Dermatopathol 2000; 22: 355 (abstract).

309 Sakamoto F, Hashimoto T, Takenouchi T et al. Angiolymphoid hyperplasia with eosinophilia presenting multinucleated cells in histology: an ultrastructural study. J Cutan Pathol 1998; 25: 322–326.

310 Eady RAJ, Wilson Jones E. Pseudopyogenic granuloma: enzyme histochemical and ultrastructural study. Hum Pathol 1977; 8: 653–668.

311 De Kaminsky AR, Otero AC, Kaminsky CA et al. Multiple disseminated pyogenic granuloma. Br J Dermatol 1978; 98: 461–464.

312 Burgdorf WHC, Mukai K, Rosai J. Immunohistochemical identification of factor VIII-related antigen in endothelial cells of cutaneous lesions of alleged vascular nature. Am J Clin Pathol 1981; 75: 167–171.

313 Kung ITM, Gibson JB, Bannatyne PM. Kimura's disease: a clinico-pathological study of 21 cases and its distinction from angiolymphoid hyperplasia with eosinophilia. Pathology 1984; 16: 39–44.

314 Googe PB, Harris NL, Mihm MC Jr. Kimura's disease and angiolymphoid hyperplasia with eosinophilia: two distinct histopathological entities. J Cutan Pathol 1987; 14: 263–271.

315 Wong KT, Shamsoi S. Quantitative study of mast cells in Kimura's disease. J Cutan Pathol 1999; 26: 13–16.

316 Aoki M, Kawana S. The ultrastructural patterns of mast cell degranulation in Kimura's disease. Dermatology 1999; 199: 35–39.

317 Fernández-Figueras M-T, Puig L, Armengol M-P et al. Cutaneous angiolymphoid hyperplasia with high endothelial venules is characterized by endothelial expression of cutaneous lymphocyte antigen. Hum Pathol 2001; 32: 227–229.

318 Padilla RS, Orkin M, Rosai J. Acquired "tufted" angioma (progressive capillary hemangioma). A distinctive clinicopathologic entity related to lobular capillary hemangioma. Am J Dermatopathol 1987; 9: 292–300.

319 LeBoit PE. Lobular capillary proliferation: the underlying process in diverse benign cutaneous vascular neoplasms and reactive conditions. Semin Dermatol 1989; 8: 298–310.

320 Mills SE, Cooper PH, Fechner RE. Lobular capillary hemangioma: the underlying lesion of pyogenic granuloma. A study of 73 cases from the oral and nasal mucous membranes. Am J Surg Pathol 1980; 4: 471–479.

321 Shimizu K, Naito S, Urata Y et al. Inducible nitric oxide synthase is expressed in granuloma pyogenicum. Br J Dermatol 1998; 138: 769–773.

322 Kerr DA. Granuloma pyogenicum. Oral Surgery 1951; 4: 158–176.

323 Patrice SJ, Wiss K, Mulliken JB. Pyogenic granuloma (lobular capillary hemangioma): a clinicopathologic study of 178 cases. Pediatr Dermatol 1991; 8: 267–276.

324 Leyden JL, Master GH. Oral cavity pyogenic granuloma. Arch Dermatol 1973; 108: 226–228.

325 Nappi O, Wick MR. Disseminated lobular capillary hemangioma (pyogenic granuloma). A clinicopathologic study of two cases. Am J Dermatopathol 1986; 8: 379–385.

326 Mussalli NG, Hopps RM, Johnson NW. Oral pyogenic granuloma as a complication of pregnancy and the use of hormonal contraceptives. Int J Gynaecol Obstet 1976; 4: 187–191.

327 Ronchese F. Granuloma pyogenicum. Am J Surg 1965; 109: 430–431.

328 Harris MN, Desai R, Chuang T-Y et al. Lobular capillary hemangiomas: An epidemiologic report, with emphasis on cutaneous lesions. J Am Acad Dermatol 2000; 42: 1012–1016.

329 Juhlin L, Hjertquist S-O, Ponten J, Wallin J. Disseminated granuloma pyogenicum. Acta Derm Venereol 1970; 50: 134–136.

330 Wilson BB, Greer KE, Cooper PH. Eruptive disseminated lobular capillary hemangioma (pyogenic granuloma). J Am Acad Dermatol 1989; 21: 391–394.

331 Shah M, Kingston TP, Cotterill JA. Eruptive pyogenic granulomas: a successfully treated patient and review of the literature. Br J Dermatol 1995; 133: 795–796.

332 Dillman AM, Miller RC, Hansen RC. Multiple pyogenic granulomata in childhood. Pediatr Dermatol 1991; 8: 28–31.

333 Ceyhan M, Erdem G, Kotilo-lu E et al. Pyogenic granuloma with multiple dissemination in a burn lesion. Pediatr Dermatol 1997; 14: 213–215.

334 Warner J, Wilson Jones E. Pyogenic granuloma recurring with multiple satellites. A report of 11 cases. Br J Dermatol 1968; 80: 218–227.

335 Blickenstaff RD, Roenigk RK, Peters MS, Goellner JR. Recurrent pyogenic granuloma with satellitosis. J Am Acad Dermatol 1989; 21: 1241–1244.

336 Taira JW, Hill TL, Everett MA. Lobular capillary hemangioma (pyogenic granuloma) with satellitosis. J Am Acad Dermatol 1992; 27: 297–300.

337 Deroo M, Eeckhout I, Naeyaert J-M. Eruptive satellite vascular malformations after removal of a melanocytic naevus. Br J Dermatol 1997; 137: 292–295.

338 Swerlick RA, Cooper PH. Pyogenic granuloma (lobular capillary hemangioma) within port-wine stains. J Am Acad Dermatol 1983; 8: 627–630.

339 Lee J-B, Kim M, Lee S-C, Won YH. Granuloma pyogenicum arising in an arteriovenous haemangioma associated with a port-wine stain. Br J Dermatol 2000; 143: 669–671.

340 Katta R, Bickle K, Hwang L. Pyogenic granuloma arising in port-wine stain during pregnancy. Br J Dermatol 2001; 144: 644–645.

341 Okada N. Solitary giant spider angioma with an overlying pyogenic granuloma. J Am Acad Dermatol 1987; 16: 1053–1054.

342 MacKenzie-Wood AR, Wood G. Pyogenic granuloma-like lesions in a patient using topical tretinoin. Australas J Dermatol 1998; 39: 248–250.

343 Dawkins MA, Clark AR, Feldman SR. Pyogenic granuloma-like lesion associated with topical tazarotene therapy. J Am Acad Dermatol 2000; 43: 154–155.

344 Momeni A-Z, Enshaieh S, Sodifi M, Aminjawaheri M. Multiple giant disseminated pyogenic granuloma in three patients burned by boiling milk. Int J Dermatol 1995; 34: 707–710.

345 Cecchi R, Giomi A. Pyogenic granuloma as a complication of cryosurgery for venous lake. Br J Dermatol 1999; 140: 373–374.

346 Marsch WCh. The ultrastructure of eruptive hemangioma ('pyogenic granuloma'). J Cutan Pathol 1981; 8: 144–145.

347 Weyers W, Alles JU. Immunocytochemistry of eruptive haemangiomas (pyogenic granulomas). Clin Exp Dermatol 1991; 16: 411–415.

348 Nakamura T. Apoptosis and expression of Bax/Bcl-2 proteins in pyogenic granuloma: a comparative study with granulation tissue and capillary hemangioma. J Cutan Pathol 2000; 27: 400–405.

349 Davies MG, Barton SP, Atai F, Marks R. The abnormal dermis in pyogenic granuloma. Histochemical and ultrastructural observations. J Am Acad Dermatol 1980; 2: 132–142.

350 Fukunaga M. Kaposi's sarcoma-like pyogenic granuloma. Histopathology 2000; 37: 192–193.

351 Rowlands CG, Rapson D, Morell T. Extramedullary hematopoiesis in a pyogenic granuloma. Am J Dermatopathol 2000; 22: 434–438.

352 Cooper PH, McAllister HA, Helwig EB. Intravenous pyogenic granuloma. A study of 18 cases. Am J Surg Pathol 1979; 3: 221–228.

353 Cooper PH, Mills SE. Subcutaneous granuloma pyogenicum. Lobular capillary hemangioma. Arch Dermatol 1982; 118: 30–33.

354 Pesce C, Valente S, Gandolfo AM, Lenti E. Intravascular lobular capillary haemangioma of the lip. Histopathology 1996; 29: 382–384.

355 Song MG, Kim HJ, Lee ES. Intravenous pyogenic granuloma. Int J Dermatol 2001; 40: 57–59.

356 Wilson Jones E. Malignant vascular tumours. Clin Exp Dermatol 1976; 1: 287–312.

357 Wilson Jones E, Orkin M. Tufted angioma (angioblastoma). A benign progressive angioma, not to be confused with Kaposi's sarcoma or low-grade angiosarcoma. J Am Acad Dermatol 1989; 20: 214–225.

358 Macmillan A, Champion RH. Progressive capillary haemangioma. Br J Dermatol 1971; 85: 492–493.

359 Kumakiri M, Muramoto F, Tsukinaga I et al. Crystalline lamellae in the endothelial cells of a type of hemangioma characterized by the proliferation of immature endothelial cells and pericytes – angioblastoma (Nakagawa). J Am Acad Dermatol 1983; 8: 68–75.

360 Cho KH. Tufted angioma: is it the same as angioblastoma (Nakagawa)? Arch Dermatol 1997; 133: 789.

361 Hebeda CL, Scheffer E, Starink ThM. Tufted angioma of late onset. Histopathology 1993; 23: 191–193.

362 Miyamoto T, Mihara M, Mishima E et al. Acquired tufted angioma showing spontaneous regression. Br J Dermatol 1992; 127: 645–648.

363 Vanhooteghem O, André J, Bruderer P et al. Tufted angioma, a particular form of angioma. Dermatology 1997; 194: 402–404.

364 Bernstein EF, Kantor G, Howe N et al. Tufted angioma of the thigh. J Am Acad Dermatol 1994; 31: 307–311.

365 Kleinegger CL, Hammond HL, Vincent SD, Finkelstein MW. Acquired tufted angioma: a unique vascular lesion not previously reported in the oral mucosa. Br J Dermatol 2000; 142: 794–799.

366 Chu P, LeBoit PE. An eruptive vascular proliferation resembling acquired tufted angioma in the recipient of a liver transplant. J Am Acad Dermatol 1992; 26: 322–325.

367 Léauté-Labrèze C, Bioulac-Sage P, Labbé L et al. Tufted angioma associated with platelet trapping syndrome: response to aspirin. Arch Dermatol 1997; 133: 1077–1079.

368 Enjolras O, Mulliken JB, Wassef M et al. Residual lesions after Kasabach–Merritt phenomenon in 41 patients. J Am Acad Dermatol 2000; 42: 225–235.

369 Nakamura E, Ohnishi T, Watanabe S, Takahashi H. Kasabach–Merritt syndrome associated with angioblastoma. Br J Dermatol 1998; 139: 164–166.

370 Seo SK, Suh JC, Na GY et al. Kasabach–Merritt syndrome: identification of platelet trapping in a tufted angioma by immunohistochemistry technique using monoclonal antibody to CD61. Pediatr Dermatol 1999; 16: 392–394.

371 Alvarez-Mendoza A, Lourdes TS, Ridaura-Sanz C, Ruiz-Maldonado R. Histopathology of vascular lesions found in Kasabach–Merritt syndrome: review based on 13 cases. Pediatr Dev Pathol 2000; 3: 556–560.

372 Kim Y-K, Kim H-J, Lee K-G. Acquired tufted angioma associated with pregnancy. Clin Exp Dermatol 1992; 17: 458–459.

373 Alessi E, Bertani E, Sala F. Acquired tufted angioma. Am J Dermatopathol 1986; 8: 426–429.

374 Michel S, Hohenleutner U, Stolz W, Landthaler M. Acquired tufted angioma in association with a complex cutaneous vascular malformation. Br J Dermatol 1999; 141: 1142–1144.

375 Lam WY, Lai FM-M, Look CN et al. Tufted angioma with complete regression. J Cutan Pathol 1994; 21: 461–466.

376 Ohtsuka T, Saegusa M, Yamakage A, Yamazaki S. Angioblastoma (Nakagawa) with hyperhidrosis, and relapse after a 10-year interval. Br J Dermatol 2000; 143: 223–224.

377 Ban M, Kamiya H, Kitajima Y. Tufted angioma of adult onset, revealing abundant eccrine glands and central regression. Dermatology 2000; 201: 68–70.

378 McKenna KE, McCusker G. Spontaneous regression of a tufted angioma. Clin Exp Dermatol 2000; 25: 656–658.

379 Heagerty AHM, Rubin A, Robinson TWE. Familial tufted angioma. Clin Exp Dermatol 1992; 17: 344–345.

380 Munn SE, Jackson JE, Russell Jones R. Tufted haemangioma responding to high-dose systemic steroids: a case report and review of the literature. Clin Exp Dermatol 1994; 19: 511–514.

381 Okada E, Tamura A, Ishikawa O, Miyachi Y. Tufted angioma (angioblastoma): case report and review of 41 cases in the Japanese literature. Clin Exp Dermatol 2000; 25: 627–630.

382 Apfelberg DB, Teasley JL. Unusual locations and manifestations of glomus tumors (glomangiomas). Am J Surg 1968; 116: 62–64.

383 Mackenzie DH. Intraosseous glomus tumours: report of two cases. J Bone Joint Surg (B) 1962; 44: 648–651.

384 Duncan L, Halverson J, DeSchryver-Kecskemeti K. Glomus tumor of the coccyx. Arch Pathol Lab Med 1991; 115: 78–80.

385 Spitzer M, Molho L, Seltzer VL, Lipper S. Vaginal glomus tumor: case presentation and ultrastructural findings. Obstet Gynecol 1985; 66: 86S–88S.

386 García-Prats MD, Sotelo-Rodríguez MT, Ballestín C et al. Glomus tumour of the trachea: report of a case with microscopic, ultrastructural and immunohistochemical examination and review of the literature. Histopathology 1991; 19: 459–464.

387 Mackay B, Legha SS. Coin lesion of the lung in a 19-year-old male. Ultrastruct Pathol 1981; 2: 289–294.

388 Appelman DH, Helwig EB. Glomus tumors of the stomach. Cancer 1969; 23: 203–213.

389 Haque S, Modlin IM, West AB. Multiple glomus tumors of the stomach with intravascular spread. Am J Surg Pathol 1992; 16: 291–299.

390 Ficarra G, Merrell PW, Johnston WH, Hansen LS. Intraoral solitary glomus tumour (glomangioma): a case report and literature review. Oral Surg Oral Med Oral Pathol 1986; 62: 306–311.

391 Potter AJ Jr, Khatib G, Peppard SB. Intranasal glomus tumor. Arch Otolaryngol 1984; 110: 755–756.

392 Hayes MMM, Van der Westhuizen N, Holden GP. Aggressive glomus tumor of the nasal region. Report of a case with multiple local recurrences. Arch Pathol Lab Med 1993; 117: 649–652.

393 Googe PB, Griffin WC. Intravenous glomus tumor of the forearm. J Cutan Pathol 1993; 20: 359–363.

394 Calonje E, Fletcher CDM. Cutaneous intraneural glomus tumor. Am J Dermatopathol 1995; 17: 395–398.

395 Polk P, Biggs PJ. Glomus tumor in neural tissue. Am J Dermatopathol 1996; 18: 444.

396 Acebo E, Val-Bernal JF, Arce F. Giant intravenous glomus tumor. J Cutan Pathol 1997; 24: 384–389.

397 Pepper MC, Laubenheimer R, Cripps DJ. Multiple glomus tumors. J Cutan Pathol 1977; 4: 244–257.

398 Nuovo MA, Grimes A, Knowles DM. Glomus tumors: a clinicopathologic and immunohistochemical analysis of 40 cases. Surg Pathol 1990; 3: 31–45.

399 Landthaler M, Braun-Falco O, Eckert F et al. Congenital multiple plaquelike glomus tumors. Arch Dermatol 1990; 126: 1203–1207.

400 Parsons ME, Russo G, Fucich L et al. Multiple glomus tumors. Int J Dermatol 1997; 36: 894–900.

401 Bhushan M, Kumar S, Griffiths CEM. Multiple glomus tumours, Coats' disease and basic fibroblast growth factor. Br J Dermatol 1997; 137: 454–456.

402 Requena L, Galvan C, Sánchez Yus E et al. Solitary plaque-like telangiectatic glomangioma. Br J Dermatol 1998; 139: 902–905.

403 Yang J-S, Ko J-W, Suh K-S, Kim S-T. Congenital multiple plaque-like glomangiomyoma. Am J Dermatopathol 1999; 21: 454–457.

404 Carvalho VO, Taniguchi K, Giraldi S et al. Congenital plaquelike glomus tumor in a child. Pediatr Dermatol 2001; 18: 223–226.

405 Yoon T-Y, Lee H-T, Chang S-H. Giant congenital multiple patch-like glomus tumors. J Am Acad Dermatol 1999; 40: 826–828.

406 Monteagudo C, Carda C, Llombart-Bosch A et al. Multiple glomangiomyoma versus glomangioma. Conceptual and ultrastructural observations. Am J Dermatopathol 2000; 22: 371–373.

407 Aiba M, Hirayama A, Kuramochi S. Glomangiosarcoma in a glomus tumor. An immunohistochemical and ultrastructural study. Cancer 1988; 61: 1467–1471.

408 Gould EW, Manivel JC, Albores-Saavedra J, Monforte H. Locally infiltrative glomus tumors and glomangiosarcomas. A clinical, ultrastructural, and immunohistochemical study. Cancer 1990; 65: 310–318.

409 Brathwaite CD, Poppiti RJ Jr. Malignant glomus tumor. A case report of widespread metastases in a patient with multiple glomus body hamartomas. Am J Surg Pathol 1996; 20: 233–238.

410 Noer H, Krogdahl A. Glomangiosarcoma of the lower extremity. Histopathology 1991; 18: 365–366.

411 Negri G, Schulte M, Mohr W. Glomus tumor with diffuse infiltration of the quadriceps muscle: a case report. Hum Pathol 1997; 28: 750–752.

412 Graadt van Roggen JF, Joekes EC, Welvaart K, van Krieken JHJM. Unusual presentation of multiple subcutaneous glomus tumours of the lower limb with extensive glomus cell hyperplasia. Histopathology 1999; 34: 474–475.

413 Blume-Peytavi U, Adler YD, Geilen CC et al. Multiple familial cutaneous glomangioma: A pedigree of 4 generations and critical analysis of histologic and genetic differences of glomus tumors. J Am Acad Dermatol 2000; 42: 633–639.

414 Boon LM, Brouillard P, Irrthum A et al. A gene for inherited cutaneous venous anomalies ("glomangiomas") localizes to chromosome 1p21-22. Am J Hum Genet 1999; 65: 125–133.

415 Peretz E, Grunwald MH, Avinoach I, Halevy S. Solitary glomus tumour. Australas J Dermatol 1999; 40: 226–227.

416 Happle R, König A. Type 2 segmental manifestation of multiple glomus tumors: a review and reclassification of 5 case reports. Dermatology 1999; 198: 270–272.

417 Peña-Penabad C, García-Silva J, del Pozo J et al. Two cases of segmental multiple glomangiomas in a family: type 1 or type 2 segmental manifestation? Dermatology 2000; 201: 65–67.

418 Hisa T, Nakagawa K, Wakasa K et al. Solitary glomus tumour with mucinous degeneration. Clin Exp Dermatol 1994; 19: 227–229.

419 Slater DN, Cotton DWK, Azzopardi JG. Oncocytic glomus tumour: a new variant. Histopathology 1987; 11: 523–531.

420 Pulitzer DR, Martin PC, Reed RJ. Epithelioid glomus tumor. Hum Pathol 1995; 26: 1022–1027.

421 Folpe AL, Fanburg-Smith JC, Miettinen M, Weiss SW. Atypical and malignant glomus tumors. Analysis of 52 cases, with a proposal for the reclassification of glomus tumors. Am J Surg Pathol 2001; 25: 1–12.

422 Skelton HG, Smith KJ. Infiltrative glomus tumor arising from a benign glomus tumor. Am J Dermatopathol 1999; 21: 562–566.

423 Dervan PA, Tobbia IN, Casey M et al. Glomus tumours: an immunohistochemical profile of 11 cases. Histopathology 1989; 14: 483–491.

424 Schürch W, Skalli O, Legacé R et al. Intermediate filament proteins and actin isoforms as markers for soft-tissue tumor differentiation and origin. III. Hemangiopericytomas and glomus tumors. Am J Pathol 1990; 136: 771–786.

425 Kishimoto S, Nagatani H, Miyashita A, Kobayashi K. Immunohistochemical demonstration of substance P-containing nerve fibres in glomus tumours. Br J Dermatol 1985; 113: 213–218.

426 Prose NS, Tope W, Miller SE, Kamino H. Eruptive pseudoangiomatosis: a unique childhood exanthem? J Am Acad Dermatol 1993; 29: 857–859.

427 Neri I, Patrizi A, Guerrini V et al. Eruptive pseudoangiomatosis. Br J Dermatol 2000; 143: 435–438.

428 Navarro V, Molina I, Montesinos E et al. Eruptive pseudoangiomatosis in an adult. Int J Dermatol 2000; 39: 237–238.

429 Wilson-Jones E, Marks R. Papular angioplasia. Vascular papules of the face and scalp simulating malignant vascular tumors. Arch Dermatol 1970; 102: 422–427.

430 Smith NP, Wilson Jones E. Multinucleate cell angiohistiocytoma: a new entity. J Cutan Pathol 1986; 13: 77.

431 Wilson Jones E, Cerio R, Smith NP. Multinucleate cell angiohistiocytoma: an acquired vascular anomaly, to be distinguished from Kaposi's sarcoma. Br J Dermatol 1990; 122: 651–663.

432 Smolle J, Auboeck L, Gogg-Retzer I et al. Multinucleate cell angiohistiocytoma: a clinicopathological, immunohistochemical and ultrastructural study. Br J Dermatol 1989; 121: 113–121.

433 Shapiro PE, Nova MP, Rosmarin LA. Multinucleate cell angiohistiocytoma: a distinct entity diagnosable by clinical and histologic features. J Am Acad Dermatol 1994; 30: 417–422.

434 Chang SN, Kim HS, Kim S-C, Yang WI. Generalized multinucleate cell angiohistiocytoma. J Am Acad Dermatol 1996; 35: 320–322.

435 Annessi G, Girolomoni G, Gianetti A. Multinucleate cell angiohistiocytoma. Am J Dermatopathol 1992; 14: 340–344.

436 Kopera D, Smolle J, Kerl H. Multinucleate cell angiohistiocytoma: treatment with argon laser. Br J Dermatol 1995; 133: 308–310.

437 Sass U, Noel J-C, André J, Simonart T. Multinucleate cell angiohistiocytoma: report of two cases with no evidence of human herpesvirus-8 infection. J Cutan Pathol 2000; 27: 258–261.

438 Creamer D, Black MM, Calonje E. Reactive angioendotheliomatosis in association with the antiphospholipid syndrome. J Am Acad Dermatol 2000; 42: 903–906.

439 Bolton-Maggs PHB, Rustin MHA. Diffuse angioma-like changes associated with chronic DIC. Clin Exp Dermatol 1988; 13: 180–182.

440 LeBoit PE, Solomon AR, Santa Cruz DJ, Wick MR. Angiomatosis with luminal cryoprotein deposition. J Am Acad Dermatol 1992; 27: 969–973.

441 Salama SS, Jenkin P. Angiomatosis of skin with local intravascular immunoglobulin deposits, associated with monoclonal gammopathy. A potential cutaneous marker for B-chronic lymphocytic leukemia. J Cutan Pathol 1999; 26: 206–212.

442 Requena L, Fariña MC, Renedo G et al. Intravascular and diffuse dermal reactive angioendotheliomatosis secondary to iatrogenic arteriovenous fistulas. J Cutan Pathol 1999; 26: 159–164.

443 Quinn TR, Alora MBT, Momtaz KT, Taylor CR. Reactive angioendotheliomatosis with underlying hepatopathy and hypertensive portal gastropathy. Int J Dermatol 1998; 37: 382–385.

444 Brazzelli V, Baldini F, Vassallo C et al. Reactive angioendotheliomatosis in an infant. Am J Dermatopathol 1999; 21: 42–45.

445 Snellman E, Niskanen RO, Jeskanen L, Heikkilä H. Cutaneous angiomatosis following implanted osteosynthesis nail: a manifestation of nickel allergy? Br J Dermatol 2000; 142: 1056–1057.

446 Rieger E, Soyer HP, LeBoit PE et al. Reactive angioendotheliomatosis or intravascular histiocytosis? An immunohistochemical and ultrastructural study in two cases of intravascular histiocytic cell proliferation. Br J Dermatol 1999; 140: 497–504.

447 Kimyai-Asadi A, Nousari HC, Ketabchi N et al. Diffuse dermal angiomatosis: A variant of reactive angioendotheliomatosis associated with atherosclerosis. J Am Acad Dermatol 1999; 40: 257–259.

448 Kim S, Elenitsas R, James WD. Diffuse dermal angiomatosis – a case report. J Cutan Pathol 2000; 27: 544 (abstract).

449 Krell JM, Sanchez RL, Solomon AR. Diffuse dermal angiomatosis: a variant of reactive cutaneous angioendotheliomatosis. J Cutan Pathol 1994; 21: 363–370.

450 Masson P. Hemangioendothéliome végétant intravasculaire. Bull Soc Anat (Paris) 1923; 93: 517–532.

451 Kuo T-T, Sayers CP, Rosai J. Masson's "vegetant intravascular hemangioendothelioma": a lesion often mistaken for angiosarcoma. Cancer 1976; 38: 1227–1236.

452 Salyer WR, Salyer DC. Intravascular angiomatosis: development and distinction from angiosarcoma. Cancer 1975; 36: 995–1001.

453 Kumakiri M, Fukaya T, Miura Y. Blue rubber-bleb nevus syndrome with Masson's vegetant intravascular hemangioendothelioma. J Cutan Pathol 1981; 8: 365–373.

454 Clearkin KP, Enzinger FM. Intravascular papillary endothelial hyperplasia. Arch Pathol Lab Med 1976; 100: 441–444.

455 Escasany RT, Millet PU. Masson's pseudoangiosarcoma of the tongue: report of two cases. J Cutan Pathol 1985; 12: 66–71.

456 Albrecht S, Kahn HJ. Immunohistochemistry of intravascular papillary endothelial hyperplasia. J Cutan Pathol 1990; 17: 16–21.

457 İnalöz HS, Patel G, Knight AG. Recurrent intravascular papillary endothelial hyperplasia developing from a pyogenic granuloma. J Eur Acad Dermatol Venereol 2001; 15: 156–158.

458 Kuo T-T, Gomez LG. Papillary endothelial proliferation in cystic lymphangiomas. Arch Pathol Lab Med 1979; 103: 306–308.

459 Pins MR, Rosenthal DI, Springfield DS, Rosenberg AE. Florid extravascular papillary endothelial hyperplasia (Masson's pseudoangiosarcoma) presenting as a soft-tissue sarcoma. Arch Pathol Lab Med 1993; 117: 259–263.

460 Reed CN, Cooper PH, Swerlick RA. Intravascular papillary endothelial hyperplasia. Multiple lesions simulating Kaposi's sarcoma. J Am Acad Dermatol 1984; 10: 110–113.

461 Yamamoto T, Marui T, Mizuno K. Recurrent intravascular papillary endothelial hyperplasia of the toes. Dermatology 2000; 200: 72–74.

462 Renshaw AA, Rosai J. Benign atypical vascular lesions of the lip. A study of 12 cases. Am J Surg Pathol 1993; 17: 557–565.

463 Kreutner A Jr, Smith RM, Trefny FA. Intravascular papillary endothelial hyperplasia. Light and electron microscopic observations of a case. Cancer 1978; 42: 2304–2310.

464 Earhart RN, Aeling JA, Nuss DD, Mellette JR. Pseudo-Kaposi sarcoma. A patient with arteriovenous malformation and skin lesions simulating Kaposi sarcoma. Arch Dermatol 1974; 110: 907–910.

465 Kapdağli H, Gündüz K, Öztürk G, Kandiloğlu G. Pseudo-Kaposi's sarcoma (Mali type). Int J Dermatol 1998; 37: 223–225.

466 Mali JWH, Kuiper JP, Hamers AA. Acro-angiodermatitis of the foot. Arch Dermatol 1965; 92: 515–518.

467 Rikihisa W, Yamamoto O, Kohda F et al. Microvenular haemangioma in a patient with Wiskott–Aldrich syndrome. Br J Dermatol 1999; 141: 752–754.

468 Pires A, Depairon M, Ricci C et al. Effect of compression therapy on a pseudo-Kaposi sarcoma. Dermatology 1999; 198: 439–441.

469 Meynadier J, Malbos S, Guilhou J-J, Barneon G. Pseudo-angiosarcomatose de Kaposi sur membre paralytique. Dermatologica 1980; 160: 190–197.

470 Bluefarb SM, Adams LA. Arteriovenous malformation with angiodermatitis. Stasis dermatitis simulating Kaposi's sarcoma. Arch Dermatol 1967; 96: 176–181.

471 Lee JH, Park CJ, Yi JY. Angiodermatitis associated with congenital arteriovenous malformation on the elbow. Acta Derm Venereol 1999; 79: 238–239.

472 Del-Rio E, Aguilar A, Ambrojo P et al. Pseudo-Kaposi sarcoma induced by minor trauma in a patient with Klippel–Trenaunay–Weber syndrome. Clin Exp Dermatol 1993; 18: 151–153.

473 Landthaler M, Stolz W, Eckert F et al. Pseudo-Kaposi's sarcoma occurring after placement of arteriovenous shunt. A case report with DNA content analysis. J Am Acad Dermatol 1989; 21: 499–505.

474 Goldblum OM, Kraus E, Bronner AK. Pseudo-Kaposi's sarcoma of the hand associated with an acquired, iatrogenic arteriovenous fistula. Arch Dermatol 1985; 121: 1038–1040.

475 Kolde G, Worheide J, Baumgartner R, Brocker E-B. Kaposi-like acroangiodermatitis in an above-knee amputation stump. Br J Dermatol 1989; 120: 575–580.

476 Güçlüer H, Gürbüz O, Kotiloğlu E. Kaposi-like acroangiodermatitis in an amputee. Br J Dermatol 1999; 141: 380–381.

477 Rao B, Unis M, Poulos E. Acroangiodermatitis: a study of ten cases. Int J Dermatol 1994; 33: 179–181.

478 Rüdlinger R. Kaposiforme Akroangiodermatitiden (Pseudokaposi). Hautarzt 1985; 36: 65–68.

479 Gottlieb GJ, Ackerman AB. Kaposi's sarcoma: an extensively disseminated form in young homosexual men. Hum Pathol 1982; 13: 882–892.

480 Strutton G, Weedon D. Acro-angiodermatitis. A simulant of Kaposi's sarcoma. Am J Dermatopathol 1987; 9: 85–89.

481 Martin L, Machet L, Michalak S et al. Acroangiodermatitis in a carrier of the thrombophilic 20210A mutation in the prothrombin gene. Br J Dermatol 1999; 141: 752.

482 Cockerell CJ, LeBoit PE. Bacillary angiomatosis: a newly characterized, pseudoneoplastic, infectious, cutaneous vascular disorder. J Am Acad Dermatol 1990; 22: 501–512.

483 Stoler MH, Bonfiglio TA, Steigbigel RT, Pereira M. An atypical subcutaneous infection associated with acquired immune deficiency syndrome. Am J Clin Pathol 1983; 80: 714–718.

484 Adal KA, Cockerell CJ, Petri WA Jr. Cat scratch disease, bacillary angiomatosis, and other infections due to Rochalimaea. N Engl J Med 1994; 330: 1509–1515.

485 Bruckner DA, Colonna P. Nomenclature for aerobic and facultative bacteria. Clin Infect Dis 1995; 21: 263–272.

486 Bachelez H, Oksenhendler E, Lebbe C et al. Bacillary angiomatosis in HIV-infected patients: report of three cases with different clinical courses and identification of Rochalimaea quintana as the aetiological agent. Br J Dermatol 1995; 133: 983–989.

487 Reed JA, Brigati DJ, Flynn SD et al. Immunocytochemical identification of Rochalimaea henselae in bacillary (epithelioid) angiomatosis, parenchymal bacillary peliosis, and persistent fever with bacteremia. Am J Surg Pathol 1992; 16: 650–657.

488 Santos R, Cardoso O, Rodrigues P et al. Bacillary angiomatosis by Bartonella quintana in an HIV-infected patient. J Am Acad Dermatol 2000; 42: 299–301.

489 LeBoit PE, Berger TG, Egbert BM et al. Bacillary angiomatosis. The histopathology and differential diagnosis of a pseudoneoplastic infection in patients with human immunodeficiency virus disease. Am J Surg Pathol 1989; 13: 909–920.

490 Fagan WA, DeCamp NC, Kraus EW, Pulitzer DR. Widespread cutaneous bacillary angiomatosis and a large fungating mass in an HIV-positive man. J Am Acad Dermatol 1996; 35: 285–287.

491 Plettenberg A, Lorenzen T, Burtsche BT et al. Bacillary angiomatosis in HIV-infected patients – an epidemiological and clinical study. Dermatology 2000; 201: 326–331.

492 Torok L, Viragh SZ, Borka I, Tapai M. Bacillary angiomatosis in a patient with lymphocytic leukaemia. Br J Dermatol 1994; 130: 665–668.

493 Milde P, Brunner M, Borchard F et al. Cutaneous bacillary angiomatosis in a patient with chronic lymphocytic leukemia. Arch Dermatol 1995; 131: 933–936.

494 Schwartz RA, Gallardo MA, Kapila R et al. Bacillary angiomatosis in an HIV seronegative patient on systemic steroid therapy. Br J Dermatol 1996; 135: 982–987.

495 Cockerell CJ, Bergstresser PR, Myrie-Williams C, Tierno PM. Bacillary epithelioid angiomatosis occurring in an immunocompetent individual. Arch Dermatol 1990; 126: 787–790.

496 Paul MA, Fleischer AB Jr, Wieselthier JS, White WL. Bacillary angiomatosis in an immunocompetent child: the first reported case. Pediatr Dermatol 1994; 11: 338–341.

497 Tappero JW, Koehler JE, Berger TG et al. Bacillary angiomatosis and bacillary splenitis in immunocompetent adults. Ann Intern Med 1993; 118: 363–365.

498 Smith KJ, Skelton HG, Tuur S et al. Bacillary angiomatosis in an immunocompetent child. Am J Dermatopathol 1996; 18: 597–600.

499 Karakaş M, Baba M, Aksungur VL et al. Bacillary angiomatosis on a region of burned skin in a immunocompetent patient. Br J Dermatol 2000; 143: 609–611.

500 Tappero JW, Mohle-Boetani J, Koehler JE et al. The epidemiology of bacillary angiomatosis and bacillary peliosis. JAMA 1993; 269: 770–775.

501 Webster GF, Cockerell CJ, Friedman-Kien AE. The clinical spectrum of bacillary angiomatosis. Br J Dermatol 1992; 126: 535–541.

502 Schwartz RA, Nychay SG, Janniger CK, Lambert WC. Bacillary angiomatosis: presentation of six patients, some with unusual features. Br J Dermatol 1997; 136: 60–65.

503 Schlüpen E-M, Schirren CG, Hoegl L et al. Molecular diagnosis of deep nodular bacillary angiomatosis and monitoring of therapeutic success. Br J Dermatol 1997; 136: 747–751.

504 Innocenzi D, Cerio R, Barduagni O et al. Bacillary epithelioid angiomatosis in acquired immunodeficiency syndrome (AIDS) – clinicopathological and ultrastructural study of a case with a review of the literature. Clin Exp Dermatol 1993; 18: 133–137.

505 Berger TG, Tappero JW, Kaymen A, LeBoit PE. Bacillary (epithelioid) angiomatosis and concurrent Kaposi's sarcoma in acquired immunodeficiency syndrome. Arch Dermatol 1989; 125: 1543–1547.

506 Arias-Stella J, Lieberman PH, Erlandson RA, Arias-Stella J Jr. Histology, immunohistochemistry, and ultrastructure of the verruga in Carrion's disease. Am J Surg Pathol 1986; 10: 595–610.

507 Arias-Stella J, Lieberman PH, Garcia-Caceres U et al. Verruga peruana mimicking neoplasms. Am J Dermatopathol 1987; 9: 279–291.

508 Gold SC. Angioendothelioma (lymphatic type). Br J Dermatol 1970; 82: 92–93.

509 Wilson Jones E, Winkelmann RK, Zachary CB, Reda AM. Benign lymphangioendothelioma. J Am Acad Dermatol 1990; 23: 229–235.

510 Zhu W-Y, Penneys NS, Reyes B et al. Acquired progressive lymphangioma. J Am Acad Dermatol 1991; 24: 813–815.

511 Meunier L, Barneon G, Meynadier J. Acquired progressive lymphangioma. Br J Dermatol 1994; 131: 706–708.

512 Renshaw AA, Rosai J. Benign atypical vascular lesions of the lip. A study of 12 cases. Am J Surg Pathol 1993; 17: 557–565.

513 Herron GS, Rouse RV, Kosek JC et al. Benign lymphangioendothelioma. J Am Acad Dermatol 1994; 31: 362–368.

514 Kato H, Kadoya A. Acquired progressive lymphangioma occurring following femoral arteriography. Clin Exp Dermatol 1996; 21: 159–162.

515 Rosso R, Gianelli U, Carnevali L. Acquired progressive lymphangioma of the skin following radiotherapy for breast carcinoma. J Cutan Pathol 1995; 22: 164–167.

516 Wilmer A, Kaatz M, Mentzel T, Wollina U. Lymphangioendothelioma after a tick bite. J Am Acad Dermatol 1998; 39: 126–128.

517 Sevila A, Botella-Estrada R, Sanmartin O et al. Benign lymphangioendothelioma of the thigh simulating a low-grade angiosarcoma. Am J Dermatopathol 2000; 22: 151–154.

518 Mehregan DR, Mehregan AH, Mehregan DA. Benign lymphangioendothelioma: report of 2 cases. J Cutan Pathol 1992; 19: 502–505.

519 Diaz-Cascajo C, Borghi S, Weyers W et al. Benign lymphangiomatous papules of the skin following radiotherapy: a report of five new cases and review of the literature. Histopathology 1999; 35: 319–327.

520 Grunwald MH, Amichai B, Avinoach I. Acquired progressive lymphangioma. J Am Acad Dermatol 1997; 37: 656–657.

521 Guillou L, Fletcher CDM. Benign lymphangioendothelioma (acquired progressive lymphangioma): a lesion not to be confused with well-differentiated angiosarcoma and patch stage Kaposi's sarcoma. Am J Surg Pathol 2000; 24: 1047–1057.

Tumors with variable or uncertain behavior

522 Mentzel T, Kutzner H. Hemangioendotheliomas: heterogeneous vascular neoplasms. Dermatopathology: Practical & Conceptual 1999; 5: 102–109.

523 Kaposi M. Idiopathisches multiple pigmentsarkom der haut. Arch Dermatol Syphilol 1872; 4: 265–273.

524 Centers for Disease Control. Kaposi's sarcoma and *Pneumocystis pneumonia* among homosexual men – New York City and California. MMWR 1981; 30: 305–308.

525 Barete S, Calvez V, Mouquet C et al. Clinical features and contribution of virological findings to the management of Kaposi sarcoma in organ-allograft recipients. Arch Dermatol 2000; 136: 1452–1458.

526 Erdem T, Atasoy M, Akdeniz N et al. A juvenile case of classic Kaposi's sarcoma. Acta Derm Venereol 1999; 79: 492–493.

527 Rothman S. Remarks on sex, age and racial distribution of Kaposi's sarcoma and on possible pathogenetic factors. Acta Un Int Cancer 1962; 18: 326–329.

528 Iscovich J, Boffetta P, Franceschi S et al. Classic Kaposi sarcoma. Epidemiology and risk factors. Cancer 2000; 88: 500–517.

529 Stratigos JD, Potouridou I, Katoulis AC et al. Classic Kaposi's sarcoma in Greece: a clinico-epidemiological profile. Int J Dermatol 1997; 36: 735–740.

530 Cox FH, Helwig EB. Kaposi's sarcoma. Cancer 1959; 12: 289–298.

531 Safai B, Mike V, Giraldo G et al. Association of Kaposi's sarcoma with second primary malignancies. Possible etiopathogenic implications. Cancer 1980; 45: 1472–1479.

532 Piette WW. The incidence of second malignancies in subsets of Kaposi's sarcoma. J Am Acad Dermatol 1987; 16: 855–861.

533 Fossati S, Boneschi V, Ferrucci S, Brambilla L. Human immunodeficiency virus negative Kaposi sarcoma and lymphoproliferative disorders. Cancer 1999; 85: 1611–1615.

534 Cottoni F, Masia IM, Cossu S et al. Classical Kaposi's sarcoma and chronic lymphocytic leukaemia in the same skin biopsy. Report of two cases. Br J Dermatol 1998; 139: 753–754.

535 Abdulla AJJ, Munn SE, Hardwick N et al. Multiple myeloma and Kaposi's sarcoma: what is the association? Br J Dermatol 2000; 142: 818–820.

536 Matsushima AY, Strauchen JA, Lee G et al. Posttransplantation plasmacytic proliferations related to Kaposi's sarcoma-associated herpesvirus. Am J Surg Pathol 1999; 23: 1393–1400.

537 Templeton AC. Kaposi's sarcoma. Pathol Annu 1981; 16 (part 2): 315–336.

538 Taylor JF, Templeton AC, Vogel CL et al. Kaposi's sarcoma in Uganda: a clinico-pathological study. Int J Cancer 1971; 8: 122–135.

539 Slavin G, Cameron HMcD, Forbes C, Smith RM. Kaposi's sarcoma in East African children: a report of 51 cases. J Pathol 1970; 100: 187–199.

540 Taylor JF, Smith PG, Bull D. Kaposi's sarcoma in Uganda. Geographic and ethnic distribution. Br J Cancer 1972; 26: 483–497.

541 Nihal M, Mikkola D, Qian Z et al. The clonality of tumor-infiltrating lymphocytes in African Kaposi's sarcoma. J Cutan Pathol 2001; 28: 200–205.

542 Gange RW, Wilson Jones E. Kaposi's sarcoma and immunosuppressive therapy: an appraisal. Clin Exp Dermatol 1978; 3: 135–146.

543 Harwood AR, Osoba D, Hofstader SL et al. Kaposi's sarcoma in recipients of renal transplants. Am J Med 1979; 67: 759–765.

544 Micali G, Gasparri O, Nasca MR, Sapuppo A. Kaposi's sarcoma occurring de novo in the surgical scar in a heart transplant recipient. J Am Acad Dermatol 1992; 27: 273–274.

545 Trattner A, Hodak E, David M et al. Kaposi sarcoma with visceral involvement after intraarticular and epidural injections of corticosteroids. J Am Acad Dermatol 1993; 29: 890–894.

546 Gaspari AA, Marchese S, Powell D et al. Identification of HHV-8 DNA in the skin lesions of Kaposi's sarcoma in an immunosuppressed patient with bullous pemphigoid. J Am Acad Dermatol 1997; 37: 843–847.

547 Halpern SM, Parslew R, Cerio R et al. Kaposi's sarcoma associated with immunosuppression for bullous pemphigoid. Br J Dermatol 1997; 137: 140–143.

548 Pedagogos E, Nicholls K, Dowling J, Becker G. Kaposi sarcoma post renal transplantation. Aust NZ J Med 1994; 24: 722–723.

549 Montagnino G, Bencini PL, Tarantino A et al. Clinical features and course of Kaposi's sarcoma in kidney transplant patients: report of 13 cases. Am J Nephrol 1994; 14: 121–126.

550 Frances C, Farge D, Desruennes M, Boisnic S. Maladie de Kaposi des transplantés cardiaques. Ann Dermatol Venereol 1991; 118: 864–866.

551 Barre-Sinoussi F, Chermann JC, Rey F et al. Isolation of a T-lymphotropic retrovirus from a patient at risk for acquired immune deficiency syndrome (AIDS). Science 1983; 220: 868–871.

552 Gallo RC, Wong-Staal F. A human T-lymphotropic retrovirus (HTLV-III) as the cause of the acquired immunodeficiency syndrome. Ann Intern Med 1985; 103: 679–689.

553 Coffin J, Haase A, Levy JA et al. Human immunodeficiency viruses. Science 1986; 232: 697.

554 Chavel F, Masinho K, Chamaret S et al. Human immunodeficiency virus type 2 infection associated with AIDS in West Africa. N Engl J Med 1987; 316: 1180–1185.

555 Padilla S, Rivera-Perlman Z, Solomon L. Kaposi's sarcoma in transfusion-associated acquired immunodeficiency syndrome. A case report and review of the literature. Arch Pathol Lab Med 1990; 114: 40–42.

556 Beral V, Peterman TA, Berkelman RL, Jaffe HW. Kaposi's sarcoma among persons with AIDS: a sexually transmitted infection? Lancet 1990; 335: 123–128.

557 Haverkos HW, Drotman DP, Morgan M. Prevalence of Kaposi's sarcoma among patients with AIDS. N Engl J Med 1985; 312: 1518.

558 Orlow SJ, Cooper D, Petrea S et al. AIDS-associated Kaposi's sarcoma in Romanian children. J Am Acad Dermatol 1993; 28: 449–453.

559 Dezube BJ. AIDS-related Kaposi's sarcoma. The role of local therapy for a systemic disease. Arch Dermatol 2000; 136: 1554–1556.

560 Lemich G, Schwan L, Lebwohl M. Kaposi's sarcoma and acquired immunodeficiency syndrome. Postmortem findings in twenty-four cases. J Am Acad Dermatol 1987; 16: 319–325.

561 Gottlieb MS, Groopman JE, Weinstein WM et al. The acquired immunodeficiency syndrome. Ann Intern Med 1983; 99: 208–220.

562 Rothenberg R, Woelfel M, Stoneburner R et al. Survival with the acquired immunodeficiency syndrome. Experience with 5833 cases in New York City. N Engl J Med 1987; 317: 1297–1302.

563 Real FX, Krown SE. Spontaneous regression of Kaposi's sarcoma in patients with AIDS. N Engl J Med 1985; 313: 1659.

564 Schwartz RA, Cohen JB, Watson RA et al. Penile Kaposi's sarcoma preceded by chronic penile lymphoedema. Br J Dermatol 2000; 142: 153–156.

565 De Pasquale R, Nasca MR, Micali G. Postirradiation primary Kaposi's sarcoma of the head and neck. J Am Acad Dermatol 1999; 40: 312–314.

566 Antman K, Chang Y. Kaposi's sarcoma. N Engl J Med 2000; 342: 1027–1038.

567 Li N, Anderson WK, Bhawan J. Further confirmation of the association of human herpesvirus 8 with Kaposi's sarcoma. J Cutan Pathol 1998; 25: 413–419.

568 Herman PS, Shogreen MR, White WL. The evaluation of human herpesvirus 8 (Kaposi's sarcoma-associated herpesvirus) in cutaneous lesions of Kaposi's sarcoma. A study of formalin-fixed paraffin-embedded tissue. Am J Dermatopathol 1998; 20: 7–11.

569 Rady PL, Hodak E, Yen A et al. Detection of human herpesvirus-8 DNA in Kaposi's sarcomas from iatrogenically immunosuppressed patients. J Am Acad Dermatol 1998; 38: 429–437.

570 Warmuth I, Moore PS. Kaposi sarcoma, Kaposi sarcoma-associated herpesvirus, and human T-cell lymphotropic virus type 1. What is the current evidence for causality? Arch Dermatol 1997; 133: 83–85.

571 Lebbé C, Agbalika F, de Crémoux P et al. Detection of human herpesvirus 8 and human T-cell lymphotropic virus type 1 sequences in Kaposi sarcoma. Arch Dermatol 1997; 133: 25–30.

572 du Plessis DG, Schneider JW, Treurnicht FK et al. Absence of human herpesvirus-8 DNA in Kaposi's sarcoma following postmastectomy lymphoedema. Histopathology 2000; 36: 474–475.

573 Soulier J, Grollet L, Oksenhendler E et al. Kaposi's sarcoma-associated herpesvirus-like DNA sequences in multicentric Castleman's disease. Blood 1995; 86: 1276–1280.

574 Cesarman E, Chang Y, Moore PS et al. Kaposi's sarcoma-associated herpesvirus-like DNA sequences in AIDS-related body-cavity-based lymphomas. N Engl J Med 1995; 332: 1186–1191.

575 Cesarman E, Knowles DM. Kaposi's sarcoma-associated herpesvirus: A lymphotropic human herpesvirus associated with Kaposi's sarcoma, primary effusion lymphoma, and multicentric Castleman's disease. Semin Diagn Pathol 1997; 14: 54–66.

576 Kemény L, Gyulai R, Kiss M et al. Kaposi's sarcoma-associated herpesvirus/human herpesvirus-8: A new virus in human pathology. J Am Acad Dermatol 1997; 37: 107–113.

577 Moore PS. The emergence of Kaposi's sarcoma-associated herpesvirus (human herpesvirus 8). N Engl J Med 2000; 343: 1411–1413.

578 Monini P, de-Lellis L, Fabris M et al. Kaposi's sarcoma-associated herpesvirus DNA sequences in prostate tissue and human semen. N Engl J Med 1996; 334: 1168–1172.

579 Brambilla L, Boneschi V, Ferrucci S et al. Human herpesvirus-8 infection among heterosexual partners of patients with classical Kaposi's sarcoma. Br J Dermatol 2000; 143: 1021–1025.

580 Simonart T, Noel J-C, Van Vooren J-P, De Dobbeleer G. Classic Kaposi's sarcoma after multiple-partner heterosexual behavior in Central Africa. J Am Acad Dermatol 1999; 41: 648–649.

581 Cannon MJ, Dollard SC, Smith DK et al. Blood-borne and sexual transmission of human herpesvirus 8 in women with or at risk for human immunodeficiency virus infection. N Engl J Med 2001; 344: 637–643.

582 Henghold WB II, Purvis SF, Schaffer J et al. Kaposi sarcoma-associated herpesvirus/human herpesvirus type 8 and Epstein–Barr virus in iatrogenic Kaposi sarcoma. Arch Dermatol 1997; 133: 109–111.

583 Simonart T, Dargent J-L, Hermans P et al. Penile intraepithelial neoplasia overlying Kaposi's sarcoma lesions. Role of viral synergy? Am J Dermatopathol 1999; 21: 494–497.

584 Kavak A, Akman RY, Alper M, Büyükbabani N. Penile Kaposi's sarcoma in a human immunodeficiency virus-seronegative patient. Br J Dermatol 2001; 144: 207–208.

585 Weissmann A, Linn S, Weltfriend S, Friedman-Birnbaum R. Epidemiological study of classic Kaposi's sarcoma: a retrospective review of 125 cases from Northern Israel. J Eur Acad Dermatol Venereol 2000; 14: 91–95.

586 Kennedy MM, Biddolph S, Lucas SB et al. Cyclin D1 expression and HHV8 in Kaposi sarcoma. J Clin Pathol 1999; 52: 569–573.

587 Li JJ, Huang Y-Q, Cockerell CJ et al. Expression and mutation of the tumor suppressor gene p53 in AIDS-associated Kaposi's sarcoma. Am J Dermatopathol 1997; 19: 373–378.

588 Hodak E, Hammel I, Feinmesser M et al. Differential expression of p53 and Ki-67 proteins in classic and iatrogenic Kaposi's sarcoma. Am J Dermatopathol 1999; 21: 138–145.

589 Bergman R, Ramon M, Kilim S et al. An immunohistochemical study of p53 protein expression in classical Kaposi's sarcoma. Am J Dermatopathol 1996; 18: 367–370.

590 Pollack MS, Safai B, Myskowski PL et al. Frequencies of HLA and Gm immunogenetic markers in Kaposi's sarcoma. Tissue Antigens 1983; 21: 1–8.

591 Prince HE, Schroff RW, Ayoub G et al. HLA studies in acquired immune deficiency syndrome patients with Kaposi's sarcoma. J Clin Immunol 1984; 4: 242–245.

592 Henry M, Uthman A, Geusau A et al. Infection of circulating CD34+ cells by HHV-8 in patients with Kaposi's sarcoma. J Invest Dermatol 1999; 113: 613–616.

593 Dorfman RF. Kaposi's sarcoma with special reference to its manifestations in infants and children and to the concepts of Arthur Purdy Stout. Am J Surg Pathol (Suppl) 1986; 1: 68–77.

594 Requena L, Sangueza OP. Cutaneous vascular proliferations. Part III. Malignant neoplasms, other cutaneous neoplasms with significant vascular component, and disorders erroneously considered as vascular neoplasms. J Am Acad Dermatol 1998; 38: 143–175.

595 Mahmood A, Ackerman AB. Kaposi's sarcoma: the evidence for hyperplasia. Dermatopathology: Practical & Conceptual 2000; 6: 122–127.

596 Delabesse E, Oksenhendler E, Lebbé C et al. Molecular analysis of clonality in Kaposi's sarcoma. J Clin Pathol 1997; 50: 664–668.

597 Puig L, Fernández-Figueras M-T, Penín R-M et al. Differential expression of c-MET in Kaposi's sarcoma according to progression stage and HIV infection status. J Cutan Pathol 1999; 26: 227–231.

598 Smith KJ, Skelton HG III, James WD et al. Angiosarcoma arising in Kaposi's sarcoma (pleomorphic Kaposi's sarcoma) in a patient with human immunodeficiency virus disease. J Am Acad Dermatol 1991; 24: 790–792.

599 Schwartz RA, Kardashian JE, McNutt NS et al. Cutaneous angiosarcoma resembling anaplastic Kaposi's sarcoma in a homosexual man. Cancer 1983; 51: 721–726.

600 Horenstein MG, Cesarman E, Wang X et al. Cyclin D1 and retinoblastoma protein expression in Kaposi's sarcoma. J Cutan Pathol 1997; 24: 585–589.

601 De Thier F, Simonart T, Hermans P et al. Early- and late-stage Kaposi's sarcoma lesions exhibit similar proliferation fraction. Am J Dermatopathol 1999; 21: 25–27.

602 Fernández-Figueras M-T, Armengol P, Puig L et al. Absence of Fas (CD95) and FasL (CD95L) immunohistochemical expression suggests Fas/FasL-mediated apoptotic signal is not relevant in cutaneous Kaposi's sarcoma lesions. J Cutan Pathol 1999; 26: 417–423.

603 MacPhail LA, Dekker NP, Regezi JA. Macrophages and vascular adhesion molecules in oral Kaposi's sarcoma. J Cutan Pathol 1996; 23: 464–472.

604 Dada MA, Chetty R, Biddolph SC et al. The immunoexpression of bcl-2 and p53 in Kaposi's sarcoma. Histopathology 1996; 29: 159–163.

605 Thewes M, Elsner E, Wessner D et al. The urokinase plasminogen activator system in angiosarcoma, Kaposi's sarcoma, granuloma pyogenicum, and angioma: an immunohistochemical study. Int J Dermatol 2000; 39: 188–191.

606 Russell Jones R, Wilson Jones E. The histogenesis of Kaposi's sarcoma. Am J Dermatopathol 1986; 8: 369–370.

607 Nadji M, Morales AR, Ziegles-Weissman J, Penneys NS. Kaposi's sarcoma. Immunohistologic evidence for an endothelial origin. Arch Pathol Lab Med 1981; 105: 274–275.

608 Rutgers JL, Wieczorek R, Bonetti F et al. The expression of endothelial cell surface antigens by AIDS-associated Kaposi's sarcoma. Evidence for a vascular endothelial cell origin. Am J Pathol 1986; 122: 493–499.

609 Holden CA. Histogenesis of Kaposi's sarcoma and angiosarcoma of the face and the scalp. J Invest Dermatol 1989; 93: 119s–124s.

610 Russell Jones R, Spaull J, Spry C, Wilson Jones E. Histogenesis of Kaposi's sarcoma in patients with and without acquired immune deficiency syndrome (AIDS). J Clin Pathol 1986; 39: 742–749.

611 Witte MH, Stuntz M, Witte CL. Kaposi's sarcoma. A lymphologic perspective. Int J Dermatol 1989; 28: 561–570.

612 Beckstead JH, Wood GS, Fletcher V. Evidence for the origin of Kaposi's sarcoma from lymphatic endothelium. Am J Pathol 1985; 119: 294–300.

613 Nickoloff BJ. The human progenitor cell antigen (CD34) is localized on endothelial cells, dermal dendritic cells, and perifollicular cells in formalin-fixed normal skin, and on proliferating endothelial cells and stromal spindle-shaped cells in Kaposi's sarcoma. Arch Dermatol 1991; 127: 523–529.

614 Karasek MA. Origin of spindle-shaped cells in Kaposi sarcoma. Lymphology 1994; 27: 41–44.

615 Sauter B, Böcskör B, Födinger D et al. The histogenesis of Kaposi's sarcoma (KS) cell: immunomorphological comparison with endothelial cells of normal human skin, lymphangioma and hemangioma. Arch Dermatol Res 1994; 286: 212 (abstract).

616 Deichmann M, Thome M, Jäckel A et al. Non-human immunodeficiency virus Kaposi's sarcoma can be effectively treated with low-dose interferon-α despite the persistence of herpesvirus-8. Br J Dermatol 1998; 139: 1052–1054.

617 Pfrommer C, Tebbe B, Tidona CA et al. Progressive HHV-8-positive classic Kaposi's sarcoma: rapid response to interferon α-2a but persistence of HHV-8 DNA sequences in lesional skin. Br J Dermatol 1998; 139: 516–519.

618 Aboulafia DM. Regression of acquired immunodeficiency syndrome-related pulmonary Kaposi's sarcoma after highly active antiretroviral therapy. Mayo Clin Proc 1998; 73: 439–443.

619 Dupin N, Rubin de Cervens V, Gorin I et al. The influence of highly active antiretroviral therapy on AIDS-associated Kaposi's sarcoma. Br J Dermatol 1999; 140: 875–881.

620 Burdick AE, Carmichael C, Rady PL et al. Resolution of Kaposi's sarcoma associated with undetectable level of human herpesvirus 8 DNA in a patient with AIDS after protease inhibitor therapy. J Am Acad Dermatol 1997; 37: 648–649.

621 Eng W, Cockerell CJ. Reconstitution syndrome: a case report of Kaposi's sarcoma in a patient on highly active antiviral therapy. J Cutan Pathol 2000; 27: 555 (abstract).

622 Leu HJ, Odermatt B. Multicentric angiosarcoma (Kaposi's sarcoma). Virchows Arch [A] 1985; 408: 29–41.

623 Chow JWM, Lucas SB. Endemic and atypical Kaposi's sarcoma in Africa – histopathological aspects. Clin Exp Dermatol 1990; 15: 253–259.

624 Cottoni F, Montesu MA. Kaposi's sarcoma classification: a problem not yet defined. Int J Dermatol 1996; 35: 480–483.

625 DeYoung BR, Swanson PE, Argenyi ZB et al. CD31 immunoreactivity in mesenchymal neoplasms of the skin and subcutis: report of 145 cases and review of putative immunohistologic markers of endothelial differentiation. J Cutan Pathol 1995; 22: 215–222.

626 Miettinen M, Lindenmayer AE, Chaubal A. Endothelial cell markers CD31, CD34 and BNH9 antibody to H- and Y-antigens – evaluation of their specificity and sensitivity in the diagnosis of vascular tumors and comparison with von Willebrand factor. Mod Pathol 1994; 7: 82–90.

627 Murray JF, Lothe F. The histopathology of Kaposi's sarcoma. Acta Un Int Cancer 1962; 18: 413–428.

628 Senba M. Autofluorescence of eosinophilic globules in Kaposi's sarcoma. Arch Pathol Lab Med 1985; 109: 703.

629 Kao GF, Johnson FB, Sulica VI. The nature of hyaline (eosinophilic) globules and vascular slits of Kaposi's sarcoma. Am J Dermatopathol 1990; 12: 256–267.

630 Waldo E. Subtle clues to diagnosis by electron microscopy. Kaposi's sarcoma. Am J Dermatopathol 1979; 1: 177–180.

631 Chor PJ, Santa Cruz DJ. Kaposi's sarcoma. A clinicopathologic review and differential diagnosis. J Cutan Pathol 1992; 19: 6–20.

632 Cossu S, Satta R, Cottoni F, Massarelli G. Lymphangioma-like variant of Kaposi's sarcoma: clinicopathologic study of seven cases with review of the literature. Am J Dermatopathol 1997; 19: 16–22.

633 Davis DA, Scott DM. Lymphangioma-like Kaposi's sarcoma: Etiology and literature review. J Am Acad Dermatol 2000; 43: 123–127.

634 Borroni G, Brazzelli V, Vignoli GP, Gaviglio MR. Bullous lesions in Kaposi's sarcoma: case report. Am J Dermatopathol 1997; 19: 379–383.

635 O'Connell KM. Kaposi's sarcoma: histopathological study of 159 cases from Malawi. J Clin Pathol 1977; 30: 687–695.

636 Hengge UR, Stocks K, Goos M. Acquired immune deficiency syndrome-related hyperkeratotic Kaposi's sarcoma with severe lymphoedema: report of five cases. Br J Dermatol 2000; 142: 501–505.

637 Cathomas G, McGandy CE, Terracciano LM et al. PCR on archival skin biopsy specimens of various forms of Kaposi sarcoma. J Clin Pathol 1996; 49: 631–633.

638 Bezold G, Messer G, Peter RU et al. Quantitation of human herpes virus 8 DNA in paraffin-embedded biopsies of HIV-associated and classical Kaposi's sarcoma by PCR. J Cutan Pathol 2001; 28: 127–130.

639 Alkan S, Eltoum IA, Tabbara S et al. Usefulness of molecular detection of human herpesvirus-8 in the diagnosis of Kaposi sarcoma by fine-needle aspiration. Am J Clin Pathol 1999; 111: 91–96.

640 Nuovo M, Nuovo G. Utility of HHV8 RNA detection for differentiating Kaposi's sarcoma from its mimics. J Cutan Pathol 2001; 28: 248–255.

641 Blumenfeld W, Egbert BM, Sagebiel RW. Differential diagnosis of Kaposi's sarcoma. Arch Pathol Lab Med 1985; 109: 123–127.

642 Stout AP, Murray MR. Hemangiopericytoma: a vascular tumor featuring Zimmermann's pericytes. Ann Surg 1942; 116: 26–33.

643 Enzinger FM, Smith BH. Hemangiopericytoma. An analysis of 106 cases. Hum Pathol 1976; 7: 61–82.

644 McMaster MJ, Soule EH, Ivins JC. Hemangiopericytoma. A clinicopathologic study and long-term followup of 60 patients. Cancer 1975; 36: 2232–2244.

645 Angervall L, Kindblom L-G, Nielsen JM et al. Hemangiopericytoma. A clinicopathologic, angiographic and microangiographic study. Cancer 1978; 42: 2412–2427.

646 Kauffman SL, Purdy Stout A. Hemangiopericytoma in children. Cancer 1960; 13: 695–710.

647 Tulenko JF. Congenital hemangiopericytoma: case report. Plast Reconstr Surg 1968; 41: 276–277.

648 Ferreira CMM, Maceira JMP, Coelho JMCO. Congenital hemangiopericytoma of the skin. Int J Dermatol 1997; 36: 521–523.

649 Baker DL, Oda D, Myall RWT. Intraoral infantile hemangiopericytoma: literature review and addition of a case. Oral Surg Oral Med Oral Pathol 1992; 73: 596–602.

650 Hayes MMM, Dietrich BE, Uys CJ. Congenital hemangiopericytomas of skin. Am J Dermatopathol 1986; 8: 148–153.

651 Fletcher CDM. Haemangiopericytoma – a dying breed? Reappraisal of an 'entity' and its variants: a hypothesis. Curr Diagn Pathol 1994; 1: 19–23.

652 Coffin CM, Dehner LP. Vascular tumors in children and adolescents: a clinicopathological study of 228 tumors in 222 patients. Pathol Annu 1993; 28: 97–120.

653 Resnick SD, Lacey S, Jones G. Hemorrhagic complications in a rapidly growing, congenital hemangiopericytoma. Pediatr Dermatol 1993; 10: 267–270.

654 Rodriguez-Galindo C, Ramsey K, Jenkins JJ et al. Hemangiopericytoma in children and infants. Cancer 2000; 88: 198–204.

655 Tsuneyoshi M, Daimaru Y, Enjoji M. Malignant hemangiopericytoma and other sarcomas with hemangiopericytoma-like pattern. Pathol Res Pract 1984; 178: 446–453.

655a Nappi O, Ritter JH, Pettinato G, Wick MR. Hemangiopericytoma: histopathological pattern or clinicopathologic entity? Semin Diagn Pathol 1995; 12: 221–232.

656 Mentzel T, Calonje E, Nascimento AG, Fletcher CDM. Infantile hemangiopericytoma versus infantile myofibromatosis. Study of a series suggesting a continuous spectrum of infantile myofibroblastic lesions. Am J Surg Pathol 1994; 18: 922–930.

657 Folpe AL, Devaney K, Weiss SW. Lipomatous hemangiopericytoma. A rare variant of hemangiopericytoma that may be confused with liposarcoma. Am J Surg Pathol 1999; 23: 1201–1207.

658 Guillou L, Gebhard S, Coindre J-M. Lipomatous hemangiopericytoma: a fat-containing variant of solitary fibrous tumor? clinicopathologic, immunohistochemical, and ultrastructural analysis of a series in favor of a unifying concept. Hum Pathol 2000; 31: 1108–1115.

659 Pollock AM, Sweeney EC. Polypoid dermal hemangiopericytoma. A case report. Am J Dermatopathol 1998; 20: 506–508.

660 Zelger BG, Zelger B. Polypoid dermal hemangiopericytoma? an alternative point of view. Am J Dermatopathol 1999; 21: 588–589.

661 Nemes Z. Differentiation markers in hemangiopericytoma. Cancer 1992; 69: 133–140.

662 Helmbold P, Wohlrab J, Marsch WCh, Nayak RC. Human dermal pericytes express 3G5 ganglioside – A new approach for microvessel histology in the skin. J Cutan Pathol 2001; 28: 206–210.

663 Yu CC-W, Hall PA, Fletcher CDM et al. Haemangiopericytomas: the prognostic value of immunohistochemical staining with a monoclonal antibody to proliferating cell nuclear antigen (PCNA). Histopathology 1991; 19: 29–33.

664 Chung EB, Enzinger FM. Infantile myofibromatosis. Cancer 1981; 48: 1807–1818.

665 Nunnery EW, Kahn LB, Reddick RL, Lipper S. Hemangiopericytoma: a light microscopic and ultrastructural study. Cancer 1981; 47: 906–914.

666 Dardick I, Hammar SP, Scheithauer BW. Ultrastructural spectrum of hemangiopericytoma: a comparative study of fetal, adult and neoplastic pericytes. Ultrastruct Pathol 1989; 13: 111–154.

667 Vin-Christian K, McCalmont TH, Frieden IJ. Kaposiform hemangioendothelioma. An aggressive, locally invasive vascular tumor that can mimic hemangioma of infancy. Arch Dermatol 1997; 133: 1573–1578.

668 Beaubien ER, Ball NJ, Storwick GS. Kaposiform hemangioendothelioma: A locally aggressive vascular tumor. J Am Acad Dermatol 1998; 38: 799–802.

669 Zukerberg LR, Nickoloff BJ, Weiss SW. Kaposiform hemangioendothelioma of infancy and childhood. An aggressive neoplasm associated with Kasabach–Merritt syndrome and lymphangiomatosis. Am J Surg Pathol 1993; 17: 321–328.

670 Tsang WYW, Chan JKC. Kaposi-like infantile haemangioendothelioma: distinctive vascular tumour of the retroperitoneum. Am J Surg Pathol 1991; 15: 982–989.

671 Fukunaga M, Ushigome S, Ishikawa E. Kaposi haemangioendothelioma associated with Kasabach–Merritt syndrome. Histopathology 1996; 28: 281–284.

Malignant tumors

672 Fanburg-Smith JC, Michal M, Partanen TA et al. Papillary intralymphatic angioendothelioma (PILA). A report of twelve cases of a distinctic vascular tumor with phenotypic features of lymphatic vessels. Am J Surg Pathol 1999; 23: 1004–1010.

673 Wilson Jones E. Malignant angioendothelioma of the skin. Br J Dermatol 1964; 76: 21–39.

674 Cooper PH. Angiosarcomas of the skin. Semin Diagn Pathol 1987; 4: 2–17.

675 Rosai J, Sumner HW, Major MC et al. Angiosarcoma of the skin. A clinicopathologic and fine structural study. Hum Pathol 1976; 7: 83–109.

676 Haustein U-F. Angiosarcoma of the face and scalp. Int J Dermatol 1991; 30: 851–856.

677 del Mar Sáez de Ocariz M, de la Barreda F, Angeles LB. Angiosarcoma of the scalp. Int J Dermatol 1999; 38: 697–699.

678 Holden CA, Spittle MF, Wilson Jones E. Angiosarcoma of the face and scalp, prognosis and treatment. Cancer 1987; 59: 1046–1057.

679 Tay YK, Ong BH. Cutaneous angiosarcoma presenting as recurrent angio-oedema of the face. Br J Dermatol 2000; 143: 1346–1348.

680 Diaz-Cascajo C, de la Vega M, Rey-Lopez A. Superinfected cutaneous angiosarcoma: a highly malignant neoplasm simulating an inflammatory process. J Cutan Pathol 1997; 24: 56–60.

681 Mentzel T, Kutzner H, Wollina U. Cutaneous angiosarcoma of the face: Clinicopathologic and immunohistochemical study of a case resembling rosacea clinically. J Am Acad Dermatol 1998; 38: 837–840.

682 Stone NM, Holden CA. Postirradiation angiosarcoma. Clin Exp Dermatol 1997; 22: 46–47.

683 Satoh T, Takahashi Y, Yokozeki H et al. Cutaneous angiosarcoma with thrombocytopenia. J Am Acad Dermatol 1999; 40: 872–876.

684 Tanioka M, Ikoma A, Morita K et al. Angiosarcoma of the scalp: absence of vascular endothelial cadherin in primary and metastatic lesions. Br J Dermatol 2001; 144: 380–383.

685 Cerroni L, Peris K, Legge A, Chimenti S. Angiosarcoma of the face and scalp. A case report with complete spontaneous regression. J Dermatol Surg Oncol 1991; 17: 539–542.

686 Fata F, O'Reilly E, Ilson D et al. Paclitaxel in the treatment of patients with angiosarcoma of the scalp or face. Cancer 1999; 86: 2034–2037.

687 Spieth K, Gille J, Kaufmann R et al. Therapeutic efficacy of interferon alfa-2a and 13-cis-retinoic acid in recurrent angiosarcoma of the head. Arch Dermatol 1999; 135: 1035–1037.

688 Ulrich J, Krause M, Brachmann A et al. Successful treatment of angiosarcoma of the scalp by intralesional cytokine therapy and surface irradiation. J Eur Acad Dermatol Venereol 2000; 14: 412–415.

689 Amato L, Moretti S, Palleschi GM et al. A case of angiosarcoma of the face successfully treated with combined chemotherapy and radiotherapy. Br J Dermatol 2000; 142: 822–824.

690 Stewart FW, Treves N. Lymphangiosarcoma in postmastectomy lymphedema. A report of six cases in elephantiasis chirurgica. Cancer 1948; 1: 64–81.

691 Hallel-Halevy D, Yerushalmi J, Grunwald MH et al. Stewart–Treves syndrome in a patient with elephantiasis. J Am Acad Dermatol 1999; 41: 349–350.

692 Alessi E, Sala F, Berti E. Angiosarcomas in lymphedematous limbs. Am J Dermatopathol 1986; 8: 371–378.

693 Woodward AH, Ivins JC, Soule EH. Lymphangiosarcoma arising in chronic lymphedematous extremities. Cancer 1972; 30: 562–572.

694 Maddox JC, Evans HL. Angiosarcoma of skin and soft tissue: a study of forty-four cases. Cancer 1981; 48: 1907–1921.

695 Offori TW, Platt CC, Stephens M, Hopkinson GB. Angiosarcoma in congenital hereditary lymphoedema (Milroy's disease) – diagnostic beacons and a review of the literature. Clin Exp Dermatol 1993; 18: 174–177.

696 Chan KTK, Bauer V, Flam MS. Angiosarcoma in postsurgical lymphedema. An unusual occurrence in a man. Am J Dermatopathol 1991; 13: 488–492.

697 Simonetti V, Folgaresi M, Motolese A. Angiosarcoma of the lower leg in chronic lymphoedema. Acta Derm Venereol 1999; 79: 251–252.

698 Sinclair SA, Sviland L, Natarajan S. Angiosarcoma arising in a chronically lymph-oedematous leg. Br J Dermatol 1998; 138: 692–694.

699 Muller R, Hajdu SI, Brennan MF. Lymphangiosarcoma associated with chronic filarial lymphedema. Cancer 1987; 59: 179–183.

700 Kirchmann TTT, Smoller BR, McGuire J. Cutaneous angiosarcoma as a second malignancy in a lymphedematous leg in a Hodgkin's disease survivor. J Am Acad Dermatol 1994; 31: 861–866.

701 Azurdia RM, Guerin DM, Verbov JL. Chronic lymphoedema and angiosarcoma. Clin Exp Dermatol 1999; 24: 270–272.

702 Goette DK, Detlefs RL. Postirradiation angiosarcoma. J Am Acad Dermatol 1985; 12: 922–926.

703 Handfield-Jones SE, Kennedy CTC, Bradfield JB. Angiosarcoma arising in an angiomatous naevus following irradiation in childhood. Br J Dermatol 1988; 118: 109–112.

704 Caldwell JB, Ryan MT, Benson PM, James WD. Cutaneous angiosarcoma arising in the radiation site of a congenital hemangioma. J Am Acad Dermatol 1995; 33: 865–870.

705 Cabo H, Cohen ES, Casas GJ et al. Cutaneous angiosarcoma arising on the radiation site of a congenital facial hemangioma. Int J Dermatol 1998; 37: 638–639.

706 Mach K. Zur frage des lymphangioendotheliomas. Klin Exp Dermatol 1966; 226: 318–335.

707 Hodgkinson DJ, Soule EH, Woods JE. Cutaneous angiosarcoma of the head and neck. Cancer 1979; 44: 1106–1113.

708 Fineberg S, Rosen PP. Cutaneous angiosarcoma and atypical vascular lesions of the skin and breast after radiation therapy for breast carcinoma. Am J Clin Pathol 1994; 102: 757–763.

709 Krasagakis K, Hettmannsperger U, Tebbe B, Garbe C. Cutaneous metastatic angiosarcoma with a lethal outcome, following radiotherapy for a cervical carcinoma. Br J Dermatol 1995; 133: 610–614.

710 King DT, Duffy DM, Hirose FM, Gurevitch AW. Lymphangiosarcoma arising from lymphangioma circumscriptum. Arch Dermatol 1979; 115: 969–972.

711 Girard C, Johnson WC, Graham JH. Cutaneous angiosarcoma. Cancer 1970; 26: 868–883.

712 Mentzel T, Katenkamp D. Intraneural angiosarcoma and angiosarcoma arising in benign and malignant peripheral nerve sheath tumours: clinicopathological and immunohistochemical analysis of four cases. Histopathology 1999; 35: 114–120.

713 Al-Najjar AA-W, Harrington CI, Slater DN. Angiosarcoma: a complication of varicose leg ulceration. Acta Derm Venereol 1986; 66: 167–170.

714 Wehrli BM, Janzen DL, Shokeir O et al. Epithelioid angiosarcoma arising in a surgically constructed arteriovenous fistula. A rare complication of chronic immunosuppression in the setting of renal transplantation. Am J Surg Pathol 1998; 22: 1154–1159.

715 Kibe Y, Kishimoto S, Katoh N et al. Angiosarcoma of the scalp associated with renal transplantation. Br J Dermatol 1997; 136: 752–756.

716 Schmutz JL, Kue E, Baylac F et al. Angiosarcoma complicating Hallopeau–Siemens-type hereditary epidermolysis bullosa. Br J Dermatol 1998; 138: 910–912.

717 Ludolph-Hauser D, Thoma-Greber E, Sander C et al. Mast cells in an angiosarcoma complicating xeroderma pigmentosum in a 13-year-old girl. J Am Acad Dermatol 2000; 43: 900–902.

718 Folpe AL, Johnston CA, Weiss SW. Cutaneous angiosarcoma arising in a gouty tophus. Report of a unique case and a review of foreign-material associated angiosarcomas. Am J Dermatopathol 2000; 22: 418–421.

719 Ben-Izhak O, Vlodavsky E, Ofer A et al. Epithelioid angiosarcoma associated with a dacron vascular graft. Am J Surg Pathol 1999; 23: 1418–1422.

720 Gyulai R, Kemény I, Kiss M et al. Human herpesvirus 8 DNA sequences in angiosarcoma of the face. Br J Dermatol 1997; 137: 467.

721 Kárpáti S, Désaknai S, Désaknai M et al. Human herpesvirus type 8-positive facial angiosarcoma developing at the site of botulinum toxin injection for blepharospasm. Br J Dermatol 2000; 143: 660–662.

722 Lin BT-Y, Weiss LM, Battifora H. Intravascularly disseminated angiosarcoma: true neoplastic angioendotheliomatosis? Report of two cases. Am J Surg Pathol 1997; 21: 1138–1143.

723 Yamamoto T, Umeda T, Nishioka K. Immunohistological distribution of stem cell factor and Kit receptor in angiosarcoma. Acta Derm Venereol 2000; 80: 443–445.

724 Arbiser JL, Weiss SW, Arbiser ZK et al. Differential expression of active mitogen-activated protein kinase in cutaneous endothelial neoplasms: Implications for biologic behavior and response to therapy. J Am Acad Dermatol 2001; 44: 193–197.

725 Morgan MB, Stevens GL, Tannenbaum M, Salup R. Expression of the caveolins in dermal vascular tumors. J Cutan Pathol 2001; 28: 24–28.

726 McCluggage WG, Clarke R, Toner PG. Cutaneous epithelioid angiosarcoma exhibiting cytokeratin positivity. Histopathology 1995; 27: 291–294.

727 Hitchcock MG, Hurt MA, Santa Cruz DJ. Cutaneous granular cell angiosarcoma. J Cutan Pathol 1994; 21: 256–262.

728 Miettinen M, Fetsch JF. Distribution of keratins in normal endothelial cells and a spectrum of vascular tumors: implications in tumor diagnosis. Hum Pathol 2000; 31: 1062–1067.

729 Diaz-Cascajo C, Weyers W, Borghi S, Reichel M. Verrucous angiosarcoma of the skin: a distinct variant of cutaneous angiosarcoma. Histopathology 1998; 32: 556–561.

730 Miettinen M, Holthofer H, Lehto V-P. Ulex europaeus I lectin as a marker for tumors derived from endothelial cells. Am J Clin Pathol 1983; 79: 32–36.

731 Burgdorf WHC, Mukai K, Rosai J. Immunohistochemical identification of factor VIII-related antigen in endothelial cells of cutaneous lesions of alleged vascular nature. Am J Clin Pathol 1981; 75: 167–171.

732 Schlingemann RO, Dingjan GM, Emeis JJ. Monoclonal antibody PAL-E specific for endothelium. Lab Invest 1985; 52: 71–76.

733 Battifora HA. Keratin pearls. Hum Pathol 2000; 31: 1009–1010.

734 Ohsawa M, Naka N, Tomita Y et al. Use of histochemical procedures in diagnosing angiosarcoma. Evaluation of 98 cases. Cancer 1995; 75: 2867–2874.

735 Capo V, Ozzello L, Fenoglio CM et al. Angiosarcomas arising in edematous extremities: Immunostaining for factor VIII-related antigen and ultrastructural features. Hum Pathol 1985; 16: 144–150.

736 Svanholm H, Nielsen K, Hauge P. Factor VIII-related antigen and lymphatic collecting vessels. Virchows Arch [A] 1984; 404: 223–228.

737 Kanitakis J, Bendelac A, Marchand C et al. Stewart–Treves syndrome: an histogenetic (ultrastructural and immunohistological) study. J Cutan Pathol 1986; 13: 30–39.

738 McWilliam LJ, Harris M. Histogenesis of post-mastectomy angiosarcoma – an ultrastructural study. Histopathology 1985; 9: 331–343.

739 Schafler K, McKenzie CG, Salm R. Postmastectomy lymphangiosarcoma: a reappraisal of the concept – a critical review and report of an illustrative case. Histopathology 1979; 3: 131–152.

740 Hultberg BM. Angiosarcomas in chronically lymphedematous extremities. Two cases of Stewart–Treves syndrome. Am J Dermatopathol 1987; 9: 406–412.

741 Holden CA, Spaull J, Das AK et al. The histogenesis of angiosarcoma of the face and scalp: an immunohistochemical and ultrastructural study. Histopathology 1987; 11: 37–51.

742 Carstens PHB. The Weibel–Palade body in the diagnosis of endothelial tumors. Ultrastruct Pathol 1981; 2: 315–325.

743 Dabska M. Malignant endovascular papillary angioendothelioma of the skin in childhood. Clinicopathologic study of 6 cases. Cancer 1969; 24: 503–510.

744 Patterson K, Chandra RS. Malignant endovascular papillary angioendothelioma. Cutaneous borderline tumor. Arch Pathol Lab Med 1985; 109: 671–673.

745 Manivel JC, Wick MR, Swanson PE et al. Endovascular papillary angioendothelioma of childhood: a vascular lesion possibly characterized by "high" endothelial cell differentiation. Hum Pathol 1986; 17: 1240–1244.

746 Requena L, Sangueza OP. Cutaneous vascular anomalies. Part I. Hamartomas, malformations, and dilatation of preexisting vessels. J Am Acad Dermatol 1997; 37: 523–549.

747 Schwartz RA, Dąbski C, Dąbska M. The Dąbska tumor: a thirty-year retrospect. Dermatology 2000; 201: 1–5.

748 de Dulanto F, Armijo-Moreno M. Malignant endovascular papillary hemangioendothelioma. Acta Derm Venereol 1973; 53: 403–407.

749 Fukunaga M, Ushigome S, Shishikura Y et al. Endovascular papillary angioendothelioma-like tumour associated with lymphoedema. Histopathology 1995; 27: 243–249.

750 Morgan J, Robinson MJ, Rosen LB et al. Malignant endovascular papillary angioendothelioma (Dabska tumor). A case report and review of the literature. Am J Dermatopathol 1989; 11: 64–68.

751 Monteagudo C, Llombart-Bosch A. Haemangioendothelioma: a current perspective. Curr Diagn Pathol 1995; 2: 65–72.

752 Weiss SW, Enzinger FM. Epithelioid hemangioendothelioma. Cancer 1982; 50: 970–981.

753 Tsunugoshi M, Dorfman HD, Bauer TW. Epithelioid hemangioendothelioma of bone: a clinicopathologic, ultrastructural and immunohistochemical study. Am J Surg Pathol 1986; 10: 754–764.

754 Ishak KG, Sesterhenn IA, Goodman ZD et al. Epithelioid hemangioendothelioma of the liver. Hum Pathol 1984; 15: 839–852.

755 Resnik KS, Kantor GR, Spielvogel RL, Ryan E. Cutaneous epithelioid hemangioendothelioma without systemic involvement. Am J Dermatopathol 1993; 15: 272–276.

756 Malane SL, Sau P, Benson PM. Epithelioid hemangioendothelioma associated with reflux sympathetic dystrophy. J Am Acad Dermatol 1992; 26: 325–328.

757 Mentzel T, Beham A, Calonje E et al. Epithelioid hemangioendothelioma of skin and soft tissues: clinicopathologic and immunohistochemical study of 30 cases. Am J Surg Pathol 1997; 21: 363–374.

758 Polk P, Webb JM. Isolated cutaneous epithelioid hemangioendothelioma. J Am Acad Dermatol 1997; 36: 1026–1028.

759 Zelger BG, Wambacher B, Steiner H, Zelger B. Cutaneous epithelioid hemangioendothelioma, epithelioid cell histiocytoma and Spitz nevus. J Cutan Pathol 1997; 24: 641–647.

760 Roh HS, Kim YS, Suhr KB et al. A case of childhood epithelioid hemangioendothelioma. J Am Acad Dermatol 2000; 42: 897–899.

761 Tyring S, Guest P, Lee P et al. Epithelioid hemangioendothelioma of the skin and femur. J Am Acad Dermatol 1989; 20: 362–366.

762 Mendlick MR, Nelson M, Pickering D et al. Translocation t(1;3)(p36.3;q25) is a nonrandom aberration in epithelioid hemangioendothelioma. Am J Surg Pathol 2001; 25: 684–687.

763 Kanik AB, Hall JD, Bhawan J. Eruptive epithelioid hemangioendothelioma with spindle cells. Am J Dermatopathol 1995; 17: 612–617.

764 Kiryu H, Hashimoto H, Hori Y. Ossifying epithelioid hemangioendothelioma. J Cutan Pathol 1996; 23: 558–561.

765 Gray MH, Rosenberg AE, Dickersin GR, Bhan AK. Cytokeratin expression in epithelioid vascular neoplasms. Hum Pathol 1990; 21: 212–217.

766 Weiss SW, Ishak KG, Dail DH et al. Epithelioid hemangioendothelioma and related lesions. Semin Diagn Pathol 1986; 3: 259–287.

767 Calonje E, Fletcher CDM, Wilson-Jones E, Rosai J. Retiform hemangioendothelioma. A distinctive form of low-grade angiosarcoma delineated in a series of 15 cases. Am J Surg Pathol 1994; 18: 115–125.

768 Schommer M, Herbst RA, Brodersen JP et al. Retiform hemangioendothelioma: Another tumor associated with human herpesvirus type 8? J Am Acad Dermatol 2000; 42: 290–292.

769 Duke D, Dvorak AM, Harris TJ, Cohen LM. Multiple retiform hemangioendotheliomas. A low-grade angiosarcoma. Am J Dermatopathol 1996; 18: 606–610.

770 Sanz-Trelles A, Rodrigo-Fernandez I, Ayala-Carbonero A, Contreras-Rubio F. Retiform hemangioendothelioma. A new case in a child with diffuse endovascular papillary endothelial proliferation. J Cutan Pathol 1997; 24: 440–444.

771 Nayler SJ, Rubin BP, Calonje E et al. Composite hemangioendothelioma. A complex, low-grade vascular lesion mimicking angiosarcoma. Am J Surg Pathol 2000; 24: 352–361.

772 Hegyi L, Cormack GC, Grant JW. Histochemical investigation into the molecular mechanisms of malignant transformation in a benign glomus tumour. J Clin Pathol 1998; 51: 872–874.

773 Hiruta N, Kameda N, Tokudome T et al. Malignant glomus tumor: A case report and review of the literature. Am J Surg Pathol 1997; 21: 1096–1103.

774 Watanabe K, Sugino T, Saito A et al. Glomangiosarcoma of the hip: report of a highly aggressive tumour with widespread distant metastases. Br J Dermatol 1998; 139: 1097–1101.

775 López-Ríos F, Rodriguez-Peralto JL, Castaño E, Ballestín C. Glomangiosarcoma of the lower limb: a case report with a literature review. J Cutan Pathol 1997; 24: 571–574.

776 Enzinger FM, Weiss SW. Soft tissue tumors. St Louis: CV Mosby, 1995; 713.

Cutaneous metastases

39

INTRODUCTION

Metastasis represents the end stage of a complex series of interreactions between the tumor cells and the host tissues.[1,2] There are many factors which influence the localization of metastases other than the natural lymphatic and vascular connections of the primary tumor. In the past, the concept of 'favorable soil' and 'unfavorable soil' was invoked in an attempt to explain why certain organs were only rarely involved by metastases. There are now some scientific explanations available to account for the 'unfavorable soil' of some organs, although none has been advanced that explains satisfactorily why the skin generally is an uncommon site for visceral metastases. The vascularity of the scalp may explain why this is sometimes a favored site. The tumor cells may reach the skin by direct invasion from an underlying tumor, by accidental implantation during a surgical or diagnostic procedure, and by lymphatic and hematogenous spread.

Based on several large autopsy series of patients with visceral cancer, the incidence of cutaneous metastases is about 2% of all cases.[1] The usually quoted range from several different studies is 1.2–4.4%.[3,4] A recent retrospective study of 4020 patients with metastatic disease found that 10% had cutaneous metastases.[5] In one series the skin was the 18th most frequent metastatic site for all tumor types.[6]

There are many generalizations that can be made about cutaneous metastases. These relate to the time interval between their manifestation and the diagnosis of the primary tumor, their clinical appearance, their location, the site of origin of the primary tumor and their prognostic significance.[7] These aspects will be considered below, followed by an account of the cutaneous metastases derived from various viscera.

CLINICAL AND MORPHOLOGICAL FEATURES

Time of development
Cutaneous metastases may be the first indication of a visceral cancer,[8] the incidence in one series being 0.8%.[9] These **precocious metastases** are particularly likely to present at the umbilicus, or less frequently on the scalp. The kidney,[10] lung,[11] thyroid[12] and ovary[8] are organs whose tumors may present in this way.[13]

With most tumors the metastases develop some months or years after the primary malignancy has been diagnosed[8] – so-called **'metachronous metastases'**. In about 7% of cases, this interval exceeds 5 years. Tumors of the breast and kidney and malignant melanomas may give rise to delayed metastases.[14]

The term **'synchronous metastasis'** is used when the cutaneous metastasis and the primary tumor are diagnosed simultaneously.[15] This sometimes occurs with tumors of the breast and oral cavity.

Clinical aspects
Cutaneous metastases are more likely to be found in older individuals.[16] In neonates they are usually derived from a neuroblastoma or, less commonly, from a rhabdomyosarcoma.[17] Metastases from germ cell and trophoblastic tumors, although rare in the skin, develop there particularly in young adults.

Cutaneous metastases usually present as multiple, discrete, painless, freely movable nodules of sudden onset.[5,13,18] Sometimes several small nodules are localized to one area.[19] Solitary metastases occur in about 10% of cases. The nodules are usually 1–3 cm in diameter. Much larger lesions have been recorded.[20] They vary in color from red to bluish-purple to light brown or flesh colored. Occasionally plaques are formed. One variant of this form develops in the scalp as patches of alopecia (alopecia neoplastica), sometimes resembling alopecia areata.[21–24] Cicatricial plaques also form: metastases from the breast,[21,22] lung and kidney may give this pattern on rare occasions.

There are isolated reports of other patterns of cutaneous metastases.[4] For example, they may resemble erythema annulare,[4] a chancre,[25] an epidermal cyst,[26] a condyloma[4] or an ulcer.[4] They may present in a zosteriform pattern.[27–38] In one case, herpes zoster was associated with the metastases.[39] Elephantiasis of the lower limbs due to lymphatic obstruction and facial lymphedema are rare clinical presentations.[40,41] Metastases have also been reported in an area of radiation dermatitis.[42]

There are three clinical patterns of metastasis which are almost exclusively related to carcinomas of the breast: carcinoma erysipelatoides ('inflammatory carcinoma'), carcinoma telangiectaticum, and carcinoma en cuirasse.[16,43–48] The inflammatory pattern presents as a large, tender, warm plaque which may resemble erysipelas.[14,43,49] It is found in less than 2% of all breast carcinomas. Some would regard this as being due to direct extension from the underlying carcinoma, and not a true metastasis.[13] Rarely, this pattern is seen with metastases from melanoma[50] and mesothelioma,[51] and from carcinomas of the esophagus,[52] stomach,[53] pancreas,[54] colon,[47,55] rectum,[56,57] prostate,[44] bladder[58] and lung.[28,59] It follows the obstruction of lymphatics at all levels of the dermis, with resulting edema.[49] There are often some perivascular and perilymphatic inflammatory cells. Carcinoma telangiectaticum presents as a telangiectatic sclerotic plaque, often studded with pink papules and pseudovesicles.[43,60] There is massive subepidermal edema resulting from obstruction by tumor of small blood vessels and lymphatics in the upper dermis. Other vessels are congested. Rarely, metastases from the lung will give this picture. Carcinoma en cuirasse is a diffuse induration of the breast resulting from some dermal fibrosis and a diffuse infiltrate of tumor cells between collagen bundles, sometimes in an Indian-file pattern.[43]

Location of metastases
Metastases tend to occur on the cutaneous surfaces near the site of the primary tumor, although there are many exceptions.[5] Metastases from tumors of the lung often involve the chest wall and proximal parts of the upper extremities, whereas those from the oral cavity and esophagus may metastasize to the head and neck, and those from the gastrointestinal and genitourinary systems to the abdominal wall.[19,61] Approximately 5% of metastases involve the scalp.[5,8,62] This is a common site for metastases from the thyroid.[63]

Metastasis to the umbilicus is also quite common.[64,65] The lesion that results has been called the Sister Mary Joseph nodule, in recognition of a nursing superintendent at the Mayo Clinic, Rochester, Minnesota, who is credited with recognizing the clinical significance of these nodules.[65] The underlying primary tumor is usually an adenocarcinoma of the stomach, large bowel, ovary, pancreas, endometrium or breast (Fig. 39.1).[64,65] Rare primary tumors have included transitional cell carcinoma of the bladder,[66] a peritoneal mesothelioma,[67] a carcinoid, and a leiomyosarcoma of the intestine. Other rare sites are listed in the review of all cases reported between 1960 and 1995.[68] Sister Mary Joseph nodules are usually solitary and firm, sometimes with surface fissuring. In 12 of a series of 85 cases reported in 1984, the umbilical nodule was the initial presentation of the tumor.[65] There are various routes by which tumor cells can reach the umbilicus. These include contiguous extension and spread by lymphatic and venous channels, often associated with embryological vestiges in this region.[65]

The penis may be the site of metastases from the bladder and prostate.[69,70] The deposits are usually multiple and sometimes associated with priapism.[69]

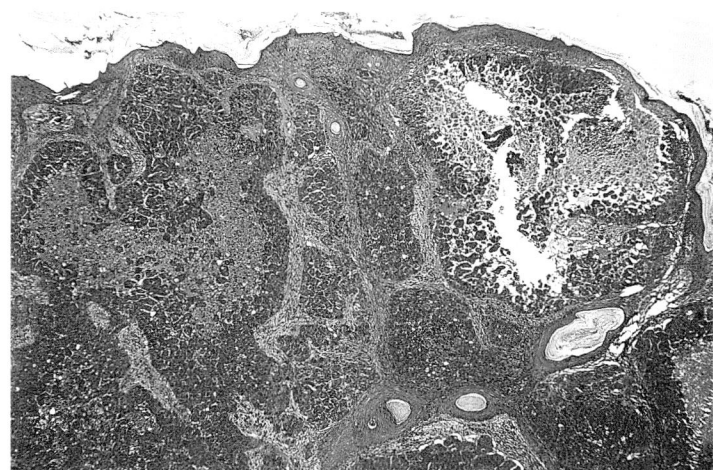

Fig. 39.1 **Umbilicus: Sister Joseph's nodule.** The dermis is replaced by metastatic carcinoma of ovarian origin. (H & E)

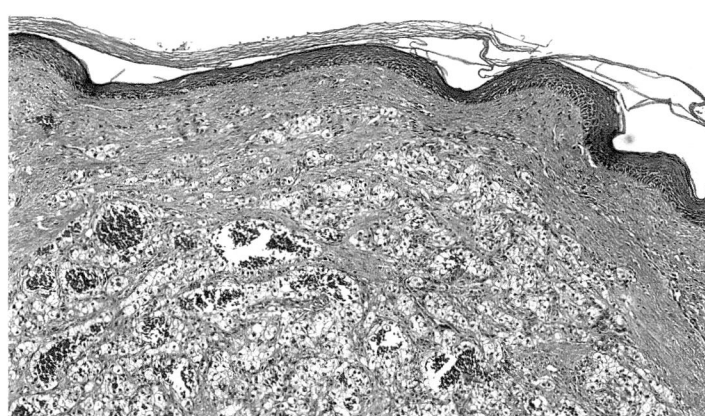

Fig. 39.2 **Metastatic renal cell carcinoma in the skin.** A mistaken diagnosis of eccrine hidradenoma is sometimes made in such a case. (H & E)

The lower extremities, excluding the thighs, are uncommonly involved with metastases.[8] Other rare sites include the nail bed,[71,72] thumb, finger,[73] big toe,[74] scrotum, eyelid, eyebrow, nasal tip and ear.[1,4,75–78]

Cutaneous metastases may develop at the site of a surgical or diagnostic procedure.[1,79–81] Metastases are sometimes seen in abdominal, perineal, mastectomy and nephrectomy scars, around colostomy sites, and along the tract produced by a thoracentesis needle. However, seeding along the needle tract is unexpectedly rare following percutaneous biopsy of prostatic carcinomas.[82]

Metastasis to a nevocellular nevus is a rare event.[83,84]

Sites of the primary tumor

The detailed studies of Brownstein and Helwig (1972) have provided valuable information regarding the most frequent sites of origin of the tumors that give rise to cutaneous metastases.[61] They studied 724 patients in whom there was histopathological confirmation of both the primary tumor and the secondary deposit in the skin. Their studies complement the earlier report by Gates in 1937.[75]

The most frequent primary tumors in men were carcinoma of the lung (24%), carcinoma of the large intestine (19%), melanoma (13%), and squamous cell carcinoma of the oral cavity (12%).[61] In women, they were carcinoma of the breast (69%), carcinoma of the large intestine (9%), melanoma (5%) and carcinoma of the ovary (4%).[61] A more recent study from India (1988) shows the lung and esophagus to be the most common sites of the primary tumor in men and the breast and ovary in women.[85] Breast cancer and melanoma were the most common origins for skin metastases in the recent study of 4020 patients with metastatic carcinoma.[5]

Sometimes, despite exhaustive investigations, no primary lesion can be identified.[86] This may result from an extremely small primary tumor or its regression.

Prognostic aspects

The development of cutaneous metastases is usually a grave prognostic feature, as dissemination to other organs has usually already occurred. The average survival time after the appearance of cutaneous metastases is 3–6 months,[19] although this has improved slightly in recent times.[5] However, there are many reports of patients with carcinoma of the breast, neuroblastoma

and other tumors[12] who survived many years after the appearance of the cutaneous metastases.

Histopathological features

More than 60% of metastases are adenocarcinomas, usually arising in the large intestine, lung or breast.[5,14,19] If the glandular structures are well differentiated, the colon or rectum should be suspected as the primary site. Tumors from the breast usually have a very undifferentiated pattern, with sheets of cells or sometimes columns between the collagen bundles. Signet-ring cells can be found in some metastases of mammary origin, but they are more usual in secondary deposits of gastric origin.[87]

About 15% of metastases are of squamous cell type. They usually arise from the oral cavity, lung or esophagus. The remainder of cutaneous metastases are melanomas, anaplastic tumors, or other rare specific patterns.[88]

Metastases usually resemble the primary tumor, although the features are sometimes more anaplastic.[19] The metastases from a renal clear cell carcinoma can appear disarmingly benign:[89] a mistaken diagnosis of a benign appendage tumor may be made in these circumstances (Fig. 39.2). Clear cell hidradenoma shows a vesicular to finely vacuolated cytoplasm, in contrast to the sometimes granular cytoplasm seen in renal cell carcinoma.[88]

Metastases are centered on the dermis, although there is sometimes extension into the subcutis. The epidermis is usually intact, and there is an underlying narrow zone of compressed collagen separating the tumor from the epidermis (grenz zone). Occasionally a metastatic squamous cell carcinoma will touch the undersurface of the epidermis, making distinction from a primary carcinoma difficult.[90] Epidermotropic metastases are exceedingly rare, except for cutaneous melanomas.[91] Dermal sclerosis is uncommon, but can be seen with some breast carcinomas.

Lymphatic permeation is a prominent feature of the so-called 'inflammatory carcinomas' (see p. 1046). It is sometimes present at the edge of a cutaneous metastasis. Uncommonly, lymphatic channels throughout the dermis are involved (Figs 39.3 and 39.4).

Immunohistochemistry is of increasing value in the interpretation of cutaneous metastases.[88,92] Monoclonal antibodies against thyroglobulin, calcitonin, prostatic antigens, leukocyte common antigen (CD45), epithelial membrane antigen, S100 protein, neuron-specific enolase, various cytokeratins, vimentin and desmin can be used to elucidate or confirm the nature of the primary tumor that gave rise to the cutaneous metastasis. This investigative field is expanding rapidly, with many new markers appearing.

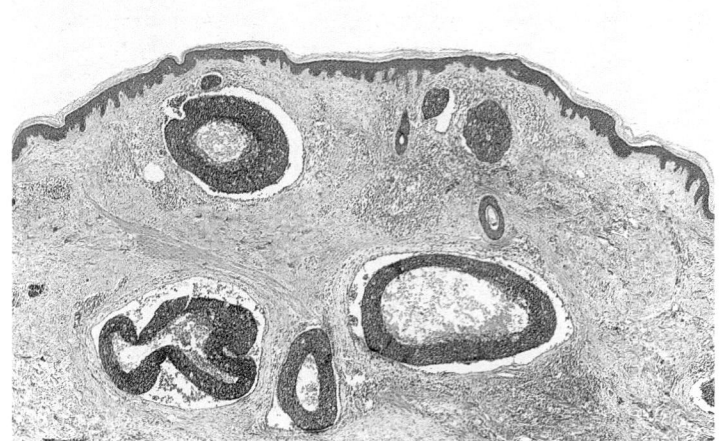

Fig. 39.3 **Metastatic adenocarcinoma with widespread lymphatic permeation.**
(H & E)

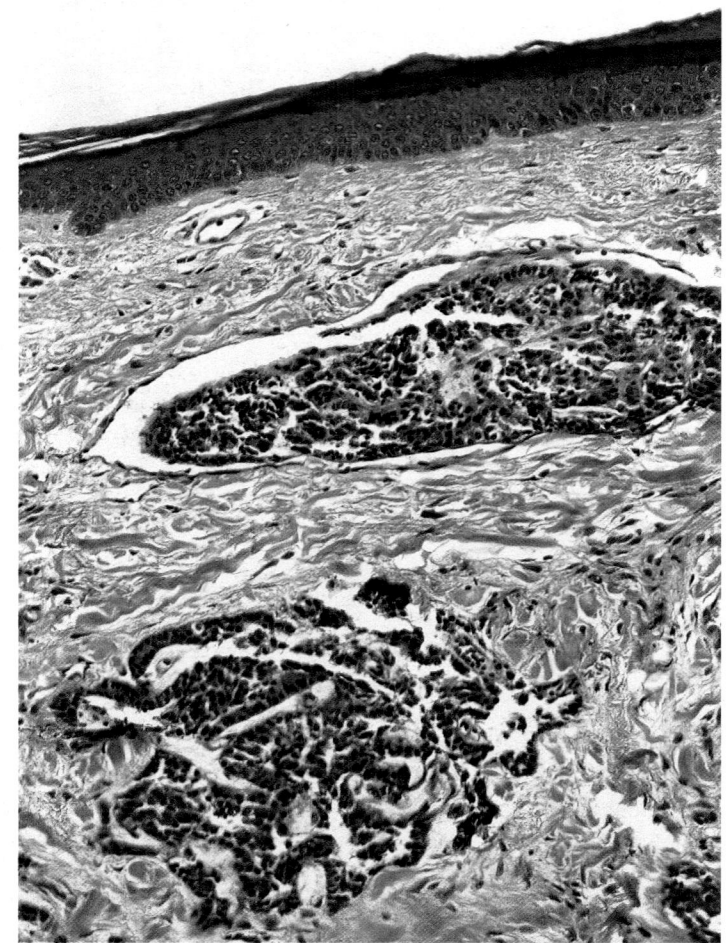

Fig. 39.4 **Lymphatic permeation in another case of metastatic adenocarcinoma.**
(H & E)

SPECIFIC METASTASES

Breast

The anterior chest wall is commonly involved by recurrences of carcinoma of the breast, although distant cutaneous metastases are uncommon.[93,94] In his review of cutaneous metastases, Rosen mentions two autopsy series of carcinoma of the breast where cutaneous metastases were found in 18.6% and 37.7% of cases respectively.[1] Brownstein and Helwig, in their study of 724 patients with cutaneous metastases, recorded 168 cases in women with carcinoma of the breast (69% of the total number of women in the series) and 9 in men.[61] In 20 of these there were single distant metastases; in 3 there were multiple metastases.[61] In the remainder, only the chest wall was involved. Extensive cutaneous metastases are sometimes observed with carcinoma of the breast.[95–97]

The scalp is a favored site of distant metastases.[93] Patches of alopecia resembling alopecia areata (alopecia neoplastica) may result.[21–23,98–101] Other clinical patterns found on the chest wall include the so-called 'inflammatory carcinoma',[44–47] carcinoma telangiectaticum and carcinoma en cuirasse.[43] Prolonged survival has been recorded after the appearance of the cutaneous lesions.[99]

Carcinoma of the inframammary crease is an uncommon but distinctive pattern of presentation which results from early invasion of the skin by a peripherally situated tumor.[102,103] It is exophytic and fissured and may simulate a primary epidermal tumor both clinically and microscopically.[104]

Histopathology

The histopathology is usually that of a poorly differentiated adenocarcinoma (Fig. 39.5). There may be sheets or large clusters of tumor cells in the dermis. Sometimes the cells are in linear array between the collagen bundles, resulting in an 'Indian-file' pattern.[61] Rarely, the cells resemble those seen in a granular cell tumor[105] or have a sarcomatous appearance.[106] Lymphatic permeation may be prominent, particularly in those with an inflammatory or telangiectatic clinical pattern. Prominent epidermotropism has been reported; the pattern mimicked Paget's disease and melanoma.[107] Sclerosis of dermal collagen is sometimes present, particularly in the scalp lesions associated with alopecia neoplastica.[22] Intraepidermal vesicles rarely form, secondary to prolonged lymphatic obstruction. Tumor cells have been seen in these vesicles.[108]

Occasionally only scattered small tumor cells are present in the dermis, and these may be difficult to distinguish from inflammatory cells.[61] Epithelial membrane antigen and some newer mammary specific antigens are detectable on these cells by immunoperoxidase methods. Gross cystic disease fluid protein-15 (GCDFP-15) and estrogen receptor protein are valuable markers for cutaneous metastatic breast carcinoma when used in combination.[109] It should be remembered that an occasional carcinoma of the breast will have S100-positive cells or contain melanin pigment,[110] which could lead to a mistaken diagnosis of malignant melanoma. Breast cancer cells strongly express cathepsin B.[111] Metastasis to a benign intradermal nevus has also been reported.[83]

Lung

Cutaneous metastases are found in 4% or less[112] of patients with carcinoma of the lung. In a small number of cases these are precocious metastases.[11] The chest wall and abdomen are the usual sites, although 'oat-cell' carcinomas appear to have a predilection for metastasizing to the back.[15] Rarely, an inflammatory or zosteriform pattern is produced. Death usually occurs within 3 months of the development of the skin lesions. The histopathological pattern

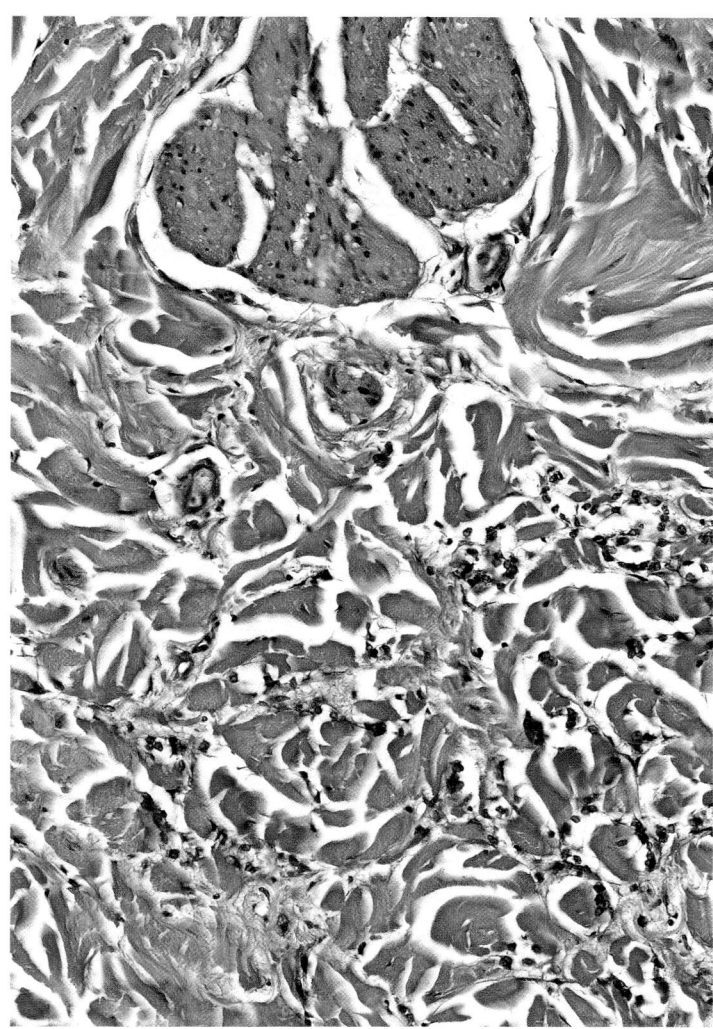

Fig. 39.5 **Metastatic carcinoma of breast origin.** The tumor cells are arranged in an 'Indian-file' pattern. (H & E)

is squamous cell carcinoma in 40%, adenocarcinoma in 20%, and undifferentiated carcinoma in 40%.[15,113,114] One bronchiolar and one mucoepidermoid bronchial carcinoma were among the tumors of lung reported by Brownstein and Helwig in their review on cutaneous metastases.[61] Pleural mesotheliomas rarely metastasize to the skin.[51,115]

Oral cavity and gastrointestinal system

Tumors of the oral cavity usually spread to the face or neck.[61] In some instances this results from direct extension of the tumor rather than true metastasis.[13] The tumors are usually squamous cell carcinomas.

Less than 2% of esophageal carcinomas metastasize to the skin.[15] The primary lesion is usually a squamous cell carcinoma in the lower esophagus;[15] metastatic adenocarcinoma is sometimes seen.[116] The metastases are multiple nodules with a predilection for the upper part of the trunk and the neck. Acral metastases have been recorded.[52]

Brownstein and Helwig reported 29 cases of gastric carcinoma with metastasis to the skin.[61] The trunk, particularly the umbilical area, is a favored site.[65,117,118] The tip of the finger[73,119] and a congenital nevus on the occiput[84] have been involved. The tumors are usually poorly differentiated adenocarcinomas. Signet-ring cells and extracellular mucin pools may be present.

The colon is a common source of cutaneous metastases. Brownstein and Helwig recorded 90 males and 22 females in this category.[61] This makes it the second most common primary site in both males and females. Brady et al reported a 3.5% incidence of cutaneous metastases in patients coming to autopsy with adenocarcinoma of the colon and rectum.[15] The metastases are usually multiple and metachronous, and most often are in the skin of the abdominal wall or perineal region.[15,57,61] The umbilicus may be involved.[65,120,121] The appearance of multiple metastases is a bad prognostic sign. The deposits are usually composed of well-differentiated adenocarcinoma, although mucinous, less well-differentiated variants are found.

A peritoneal mesothelioma, metastatic to the umbilicus, has been reported.[67]

Liver, pancreas and gallbladder

Cutaneous metastases occur in nearly 3% of patients with malignant hepatomas.[122–124] Rarely, it is the presenting manifestation,[125] although death still follows in several weeks.[123] A 12-year-old child with cutaneous metastases on the thorax and epigastrium has been reported.[126] The histopathological pattern may be either a cholangiocarcinoma or a hepatocellular carcinoma.[123,127]

Brownstein and Helwig recorded 15 cases of metastatic pancreatic carcinoma involving the skin.[61] The umbilicus is a favored site for these metastases.[64,128–130] Rarely, an inflammatory pattern is present.[54,131]

There are several reports in which the primary tumor was in the gallbladder.[132–134] Rarely, the metastasis in such cases is to the umbilicus.[65]

Kidney

Metastases have been reported in the skin in from 2.8% to 6.3% of renal carcinomas.[15] They accounted for 6% of the cutaneous metastases in males, and 0.5% in females, in the series of Brownstein and Helwig.[61] As such, they rank after breast, lung, gastrointestinal tract and melanoma in order of frequency.[61] The metastases are solitary in from 15% to 20% of cases.[72,89,135] The head, particularly the scalp, is a common site of involvement.[89,135] They may also be found in nephrectomy scars and the external genitalia.[135] The metastases are sometimes precocious. Metachronous metastases usually appear within 3 years of the nephrectomy,[61] although an interval of 23 years has been recorded.[89] The deposits can be quite vascular, and even resemble a pyogenic granuloma[136] or Kaposi's sarcoma.[137]

Most cases are clear cell carcinomas in which the cells contain considerable glycogen and some fat.[89] Mitoses are sparse. There is usually extravasation of blood, with subsequent deposition of hemosiderin in the stroma. Metastasis to the skin of a transitional cell carcinoma of the renal pelvis[138,139] and of a Wilms' tumor is rarely reported.[89]

Bladder and urethra

Cutaneous metastases from carcinomas of the urinary bladder are rare,[66,140,141] ranging from 0.18%[142] to 1.8%.[15] Brownstein and Helwig reported only 10 cases in their review of 724 patients with cutaneous metastases.[61] The urethra is more rarely the primary site.[140,143]

Metastases from the bladder are usually multiple and at a single site.[15] The upper extremities, trunk, abdomen and penis are the usual sites.[127,140] The tumors are transitional cell carcinomas or anaplastic carcinomas which may show areas of squamous differentiation.[143]

Male genital system

In one study of 321 metastatic lesions in 176 autopsy cases of carcinoma of the prostate, 4 lesions metastatic to the skin were found.[144] Brownstein and Helwig recorded only 5 cases in their large series.[61] The metastases are usually firm violaceous nodules, although unusual clinical patterns[69] such as Sister Mary Joseph nodules (see p. 1046),[65] penile deposits,[69,70,145, 46] metastasis to a gynecomastic breast,[147] a zosteriform pattern[27] and a nodule simulating a sebaceous cyst[26] have been recorded. The primary tumor is usually an adenocarcinoma,[148,149] but one transitional cell carcinoma has been documented.[150] Immunoperoxidase staining for prostate-specific antigen is a useful technique for confirming the prostatic origin of these metastatic adenocarcinomas.[151-153]

There are only several reports of cutaneous metastases from testicular tumors.[154] The histopathological pattern has included seminoma,[154] teratocarcinoma[155] and choriocarcinoma.[19,156,157]

Squamous cell carcinomas of the penis rarely give rise to cutaneous metastases.[14]

Female genital system

Cutaneous metastases are found in approximately 2% of patients with fatal ovarian carcinoma.[15] Brownstein and Helwig recorded 10 cases, which represents 4% of the cutaneous metastatic lesions in females.[61] There are usually multiple nodules at a solitary site on the chest or abdomen. The umbilicus may be involved.[158] The pattern is usually that of a well-differentiated adenocarcinoma, sometimes having a papillary configuration with psammoma bodies.[61] A carcinoma of mucinous pattern and a Brenner tumor[159] have also been reported.

Cutaneous metastases are unusual in carcinoma of the cervix[78,160,161] and uterine body,[162-164] even in the terminal phases.[165,166] They usually involve the lower abdomen, groin, upper thighs[167] or umbilicus.[65,158,163,168,169] Endometrial tumors are adenocarcinomas,[162] whereas those from the cervix may be squamous cell carcinomas,[160,167] adenosquamous carcinomas[18,19] or, rarely, neuroendocrine in type.[170] In a review of the literature of genital carcinomas with metastases to the umbilicus, Galle recorded 18 of ovarian origin, 12 from the uterine body, one squamous cell carcinoma from the cervix, and 2 adenocarcinomas from the fallopian tube.[158] There is one report of cutaneous metastases from an adenocarcinoma of the vulva[171] and another of a deposit of metastatic squamous cell carcinoma from the vagina in the mons pubis.[172]

Skin metastases are an unfavorable prognostic sign in gestational trophoblastic disease. They occur only in association with widespread disease.[173,174] Gluteal metastases[175] and a solitary nodule in the scalp[176] have been reported. There have been several cases of placental choriocarcinoma metastasizing to the skin of a neonate.[177] The histopathology is usually similar to the primary lesion, with large syncytial trophoblastic cells and much hemorrhage.[176] Chorionic gonadotrophin can be demonstrated using immunoperoxidase techniques.

Thyroid

Brownstein and Helwig recorded only 4 cases of metastatic thyroid tumors.[61] In one autopsy study, cutaneous metastases were noted in 2 of 12 medullary carcinomas and 4 of 12 giant-cell carcinomas.[178] Rarely, follicular, papillary and spindle-cell patterns are encountered.[12,179-186] In a review of 43 patients with skin metastases from thyroid carcinoma, a papillary carcinoma was the most common (41%), followed by follicular (28%), anaplastic (15%) and medullary (15%) carcinomas.[63] The scalp was the most common site of metastasis.[63]

A skin nodule may be the presenting sign of the disease.[12] An unusual presentation in one case was the development of multiple pulsatile nodules on the face, suggesting Kaposi's sarcoma.[187] Long survival has been reported after the development of cutaneous metastases,[12] although the average survival in one series was 19 months.[63] Immunoperoxidase methods can be used to demonstrate calcitonin in medullary carcinomas[188] and thyroglobulin in papillary, follicular and some anaplastic tumors.[180,181,189]

Carcinoid tumors

Cutaneous carcinoid tumors may be derived from the bronchus,[190,191] stomach,[192] small bowel, appendix and large bowel.[193-195] The bronchus is the most common primary site. Several cases purporting to be primary cutaneous carcinoids have now been reported.[193,196-198] Metastases are usually multiple, and on the trunk.[190] Solitary[191,194] umbilical metastases[199] and precocious metastases[200] have been recorded. The carcinoid syndrome is sometimes present.[201,202]

Pellagra is a cutaneous manifestation of the carcinoid syndrome, although it is not specifically related to the presence of cutaneous metastases.[203]

Histopathology

Carcinoid tumors are composed of solid islands and nests of uniform cells (Fig. 39.6).[199] Thin collagenous septa extend between the tumor nests. A mucinous stroma was present in one purported case of a primary lesion.[197] The cells may be argentaffin positive if the primary lesion is in the small or large intestine. Cutaneous metastases of bronchial carcinoids are often devoid of both argyrophil and argentaffin granules. The cells in carcinoid tumors are positive for neuron-specific enolase, and often chromogranin as well. Dense-core granules can be seen in the cytoplasm on electron microscopy.[191]

Neuroblastoma

Neuroblastomas are the most common tumors of childhood.[17,204-209] Whereas cutaneous and subcutaneous metastases are found in only 2.6% of cases of neuroblastoma of all ages, they are found in 32% of neonatal tumors.[209] Cutaneous nodules may be the presenting sign of neonatal neuroblastoma.[205,210] They characteristically blanch on pressure.[204,206] The pattern of cutaneous metastases may sometimes resemble that of the 'blueberry muffin baby', which is more usually associated with the congenital rubella syndrome.[207]

Histopathology

The findings are typical of neuroblastoma, with small cells with hyperchromatic nuclei and rosette formation.[208] The cells stain for neuron-specific enolase by immunoperoxidase methods.

Paradoxically, stage IV-s disease in neonates, in whom there is remote spread of tumor to the liver, skin and bone marrow, has a relatively good prognosis.[204] The tumor may remit or transform spontaneously into a benign

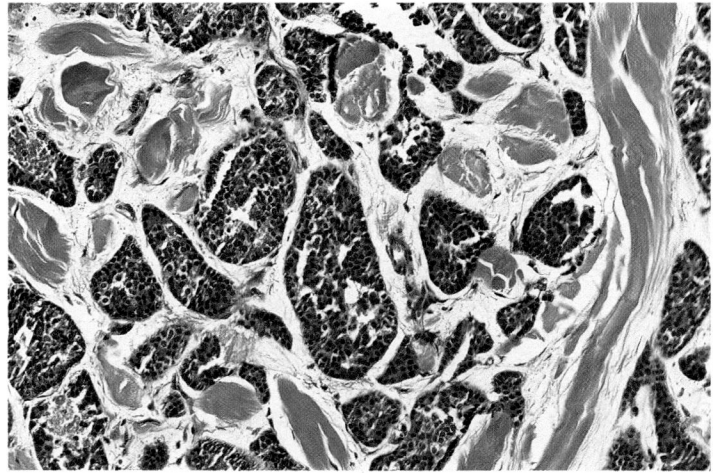

Fig. 39.6 **Metastatic carcinoid of the scalp.** A primary lesion was found in the terminal ileum some months later. (H & E)

ganglioneuroma. With more aggressive treatment protocols, the prognosis is now better than in some of the earlier series of neonatal neuroblastomas.[209]

Melanoma

The skin and subcutaneous tissue are common sites of metastases in melanoma.[5,211] Often they are the first site to become involved.[212] There is great variability in the incidence reported in the literature, which reflects in part the different criteria used for inclusion of cases. Local and in-transit (see below) cutaneous metastases are specifically excluded in some series.[212,213] Metastases to the skin have been present at autopsy in from 10% to 75% of patients with fatal melanoma.[214–216] It has been the site of the first metastasis in from 6% to 22% of cases.[212,213] It has been stated that in nearly 5% of patients a metastasis is the initial presentation of the disease, and no primary lesion can be found.[217] In the author's experience it is less than 0.5%. Usually these individuals present with a lymph node metastasis, but sometimes it is in the skin.[217] Brownstein and Helwig reported 75 cases of metastatic melanoma in the skin, making melanoma the third most common source of cutaneous metastases.[61]

A distinct pattern of cutaneous metastasis which is almost unique to melanoma is the development of multiple small nodular deposits, often on a limb, between the site of the primary lesion and the regional lymph nodes.[218]

These in-transit metastases probably originate from cells trapped in lymphatics.[219] The nodules are bluish, black, or pink in color,[218] and are small and painless. Larger lesions may ulcerate.

Rare clinical presentations have included inflammatory metastases,[50] a zosteriform distribution[31] and diffuse melanosis.[220–222] Vitiligo is an uncommon finding in metastatic melanoma.[223] Although widespread cutaneous metastases are usually a bad prognostic sign, some patients with in-transit metastases localized to a limb can survive for many years.

Histopathology

There is usually no difficulty in diagnosing cutaneous metastatic deposits, although the rare signet-ring cell melanoma may cause problems.[224] They differ in many instances from a primary lesion by the absence of junctional activity and an inflammatory infiltrate.[225] Occasionally lymphatic or vascular permeation is present.[226] Invasion between collagen bundles in the reticular dermis or into fat lobules of the subcutis, accompanied by incorporation of host stroma islands into the tumor bulk, is associated with a bad prognosis.[227,228]

Uncommonly, cutaneous metastases are epidermotropic with nests of tumor cells in the junctional zone and within the epidermis itself.[211,229–232] The criteria originally suggested for an epidermotropic metastasis[229] are no longer regarded as diagnostic (see p. 830).

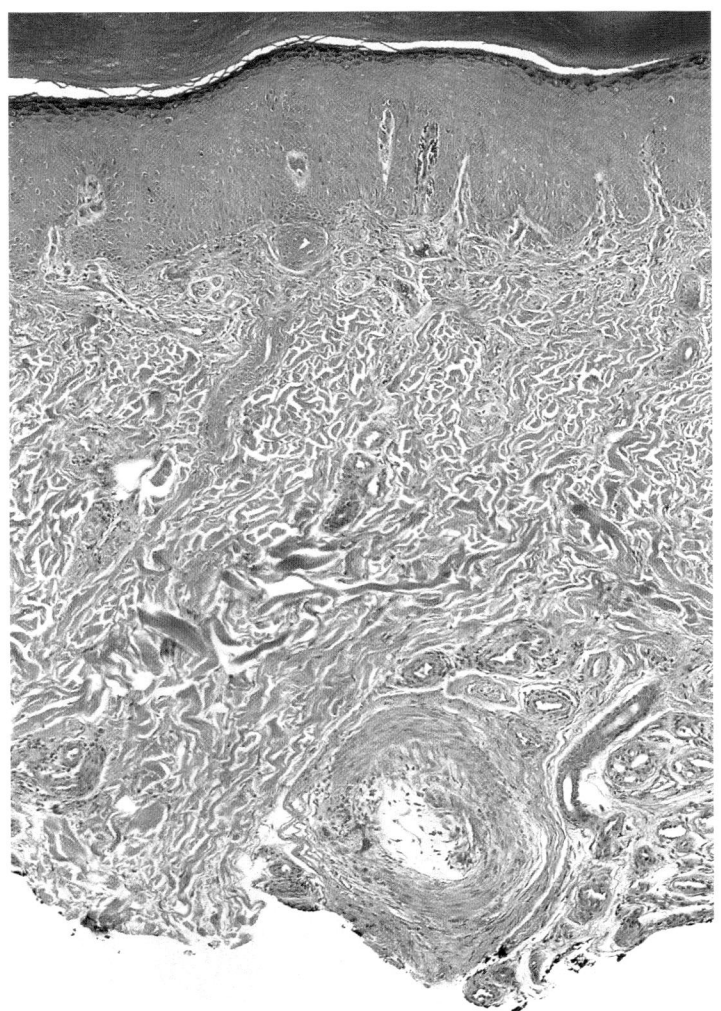
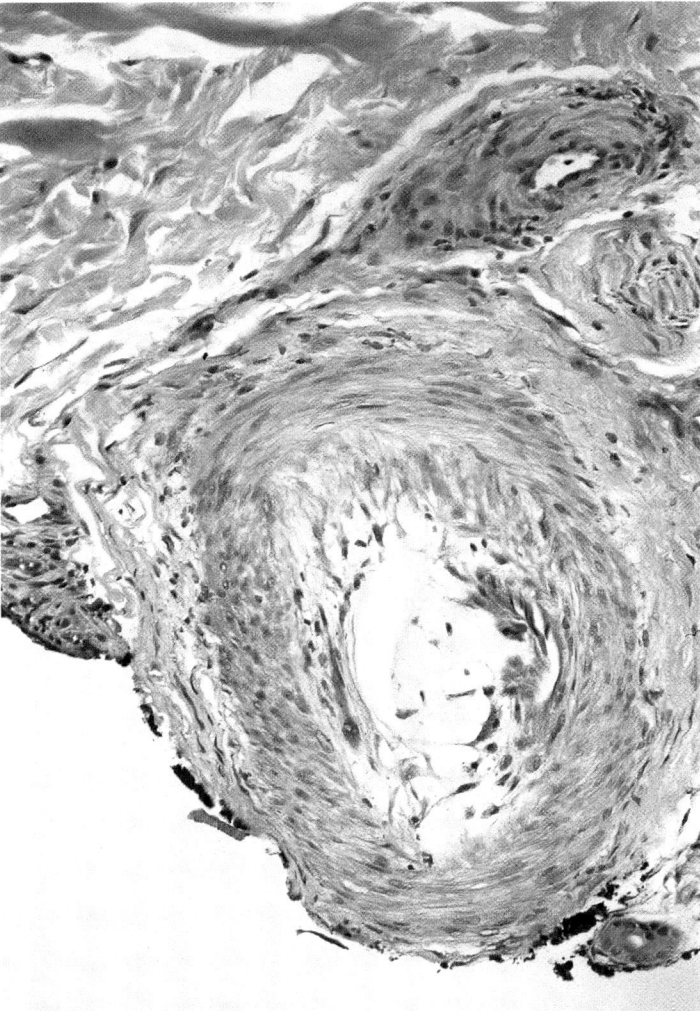

Fig. 39.7 **(A) Atrial myxoma in a deep dermal vessel of the finger. (B)** Loose myxoid tissue is present in the lumen of a small artery. (H & E)

If melanin pigment is absent from the deposit, the diagnosis can be confirmed by immunoperoxidase studies for S100 protein, melan-A or HMB-45. The occasional finding of S100 protein in metastases of mammary carcinoma has already been mentioned.

Miscellaneous tumors

Rare primary lesions that have been known to metastasize to the skin include an adenoid cystic carcinoma and adenocarcinoma of the salivary gland,[233-235] an adenoid cystic carcinoma of the lacrimal gland,[236] an ameloblastoma,[237] a thymoma,[238] an adrenal carcinoma,[239] and carcinomas of the hypopharynx,[240] nasopharynx[25,241] and larynx.[242,243] Medulloblastomas[244] and other intracranial tumors, particularly glioblastomas, rarely metastasize to the skin;[245] when they do so it is usually to the scalp.[246] The author has seen a retinoblastoma metastatic to the skin.

Squamous cell carcinomas of the skin may rarely metastasize to other cutaneous sites.[32,33,36,247]

Brownstein and Helwig reported 19 metastatic sarcomas in their 724 cases of cutaneous metastases.[61] A footnote in the article states that this figure 'includes leiomyosarcoma, rhabdomyosarcoma, fibrosarcoma, chondrosarcoma, Ewing's sarcoma, osteogenic sarcoma, and undifferentiated sarcomas'.[61] Leiomyosarcomas of the uterus,[248] small intestine[249] and colon metastatic to the skin have been recorded, as have rhabdomyosarcomas[17,250] and fibrosarcoma of soft tissues,[18] a giant cell tumor of bone,[251] Ewing's sarcoma,[17] a chondroblastoma,[252] several cases of chondrosarcoma,[253-255] a mesenchymal chondrosarcoma of soft tissue origin,[256] a metaplastic breast carcinoma with chondrosarcomatous features,[106] an osteogenic sarcoma,[257-259] a paraganglionoma[260] and an angiosarcoma of the aorta[261] and heart.[262] Mesotheliomas may rarely metastasize to the skin.[263,264] Two cases of chordoma metastatic to the skin have been reported;[265,266] direct extension to the skin is more common.[267,268]

Finally, atrial myxomas may embolize to the skin, producing a varied clinical appearance.[269,270] The tumor emboli, which have a characteristic myxomatous appearance, do not usually extend beyond the vessel wall (Fig. 39.7).[271]

REFERENCES

Introduction

1 Rosen T. Cutaneous metastases. Med Clin North Am 1980; 64: 885–900.
2 Brodland DG, Zitelli JA. Mechanisms of metastasis. J Am Acad Dermatol 1992; 27: 1–8.
3 Krumerman MS, Garret R. Carcinomas metastatic to skin. NY State J Med 1977; 77: 1900–1903.
4 Su WPD, Powell FC, Goellner JR. In: Wick MR. Pathology of unusual malignant cutaneous tumors. New York: Marcel Dekker, 1985; 357–397.
5 Lookingbill DP, Spangler N, Helm KF. Cutaneous metastases in patients with metastatic carcinoma: a retrospective study of 4020 patients. J Am Acad Dermatol 1993; 29: 228–236.
6 Abrams HL, Spiro R, Goldstein N. Metastases in carcinoma: analysis of 1,000 autopsied cases. Cancer 1950; 3: 74–85.
7 Schwartz RA. Cutaneous metastatic disease. J Am Acad Dermatol 1995; 33: 161–182.

Clinical and morphological features

8 Brownstein MH, Helwig EB. Patterns of cutaneous metastasis. Arch Dermatol 1972; 105: 862–868.
9 Lookingbill DP, Spangler N, Sexton FM. Skin involvement as the presenting sign of internal carcinoma. A retrospective study of 7316 cancer patients. J Am Acad Dermatol 1990; 22: 19–26.
10 Jevtic AP. Skin metastasis from renal carcinoma presenting as an inflammatory lesion. Australas J Dermatol 1987; 28: 18–20.
11 Camiel MR, Aron BS, Alexander LL et al. Metastases to palm, sole, nailbed, nose, face and scalp from unsuspected carcinoma of the lung. Cancer 1969; 23: 214–220.
12 Pitlik S, Kitzes R, Ben-Bassat M, Rosenfeld JB. Thyroid carcinoma presenting as a solitary skin metastasis. Cutis 1983; 31: 532–536.
13 White JW Jr. Evaluating cancer metastatic to the skin. Geriatrics 1985; 40: 67–73.

14 Brownstein MH, Helwig EB. Spread of tumors to the skin. Arch Dermatol 1973; 107: 80–86.
15 Brady LW, O'Neill EA, Farber SH. Unusual sites of metastases. Semin Oncol 1977; 4: 59–64.
16 McKee PH. Cutaneous metastases. J Cutan Pathol 1985; 12: 239–250.
17 Wesche WA, Khare VK, Chesney TM, Jenkins JJ. Non-hematopoietic cutaneous metastases in children and adolescents: thirty years experience at St. Jude Children's Research Hospital. J Cutan Pathol 2000; 27: 485–492.
18 Taboada CF, Fred HL. Cutaneous metastases. Arch Intern Med 1966; 117: 516–519.
19 Reingold IM. Cutaneous metastases from internal carcinoma. Cancer 1966; 19: 162–168.
20 Peris K, Fargnoli MC, Lunghi F, Chimenti S. Unusually large cutaneous metastases of renal cell carcinoma. Acta Derm Venereol 2001; 81: 77–78.
21 Cohen I, Levy E, Schreiber H. Alopecia neoplastica due to breast carcinoma. Arch Dermatol 1961; 84: 490–492.
22 Baum EM, Omura EF, Payne RR, Little WP. Alopecia neoplastica – a rare form of cutaneous metastasis. J Am Acad Dermatol 1981; 4: 688–694.
23 Carson HJ, Pellettiere EV, Lack E. Alopecia neoplastica simulating alopecia areata and antedating the detection of primary breast carcinoma. J Cutan Pathol 1994; 21: 67–70.
24 Kim HJ, Min HG, Lee ES. Alopecia neoplastica in a patient with gastric carcinoma. Br J Dermatol 1999; 141: 1122–1124.
25 Markson LS, Stoops CW, Kanter J. Metastatic transitional cell carcinoma of the penis simulating a chancre. Arch Dermatol 1949; 59: 50–54.
26 Peison B. Metastasis of carcinoma of the prostate to the scalp. Simulation of a large sebaceous cyst. Arch Dermatol 1971; 104: 301–303.
27 Bluefarb SM, Wallk S, Gecht M. Carcinoma of the prostate with zosteriform cutaneous lesions. Arch Dermatol 1957; 76: 402–407.
28 Hodge SJ, Mackel S, Owen LG. Zosteriform inflammatory metastatic carcinoma. Int J Dermatol 1979; 18: 142–145.
29 Matarasso SL, Rosen T. Zosteriform metastasis: case presentation and review of the literature. J Dermatol Surg Oncol 1988; 14: 774–778.
30 Manteaux A, Cohen PR, Rapini RP. Zosteriform and epidermotropic metastasis. Report of two cases. J Dermatol Surg Oncol 1992; 18: 97–100.
31 Itin PH, Lautenschlager S, Buechner SA. Zosteriform metastases in melanoma. J Am Acad Dermatol 1995; 32: 854–857.
32 Shafqat A, Viehman GE, Myers SA. Cutaneous squamous cell carcinoma with zosteriform metastasis in a transplant recipient. J Am Acad Dermatol 1997; 37: 1008–1009.
33 Cuq-Viguier L, Viraben R. Zosteriform cutaneous metastases from squamous cell carcinoma of the stump of an amputated arm. Clin Exp Dermatol 1998; 23: 116–118.
34 Heckmann M, Volkenandt M, Lengyel E-R et al. Cytological diagnosis of zosteriform skin metastases in undiagnosed breast carcinoma. Br J Dermatol 1996; 135: 502–503.
35 Ahmed I, Holley KJ, Charles-Holmes R. Zosteriform metastasis of colonic carcinoma. Br J Dermatol 2000; 142: 182–183.
36 Fearfield LA, Nelson M, Francis N, Bunker CB. Cutaneous squamous cell carcinoma with zosteriform metastases in a human immunodeficiency virus-infected patient. Br J Dermatol 2000; 142: 573–574.
37 Maeda S, Hara H, Morishima T. Zosteriform cutaneous metastases arising from adenocarcinoma of the colon: diagnostic smear cytology from cutaneous lesions. Acta Derm Venereol 1999; 79: 90–91.
38 Bianchi L, Orlandi A, Carboni I et al. Zosteriform metastasis of occult bronchogenic carcinoma. Acta Derm Venereol 2000; 80: 391–392.
39 Cecchi R, Brunetti L, Bartoli L et al. Zosteriform skin metastases from breast carcinoma in association with herpes zoster. Int J Dermatol 1998; 37: 476–477.
40 Lillis PJ, Zuehlke RL. Cutaneous metastatic carcinoma and elephantiasis symptomatica. Arch Dermatol 1979; 115: 83–84.
41 Jang K-A, Choi J-H, Sung K-J et al. Cutaneous metastasis presenting as facial lymphedema. J Am Acad Dermatol 1998; 39: 637–638.
42 Marley NF. Skin metastases in an area of radiation dermatitis. Arch Dermatol 1982; 118: 129–131.
43 Leavell UW Jr, Tillotson FW. Metastatic cutaneous carcinoma from the breast. Arch Dermatol 1951; 64: 774–782.
44 Cox SE, Cruz PD Jr. A spectrum of inflammatory metastasis to skin via lymphatics: three cases of carcinoma erysipeloides. J Am Acad Dermatol 1994; 30: 304–307.
45 Finkel LJ, Griffiths CEM. Inflammatory breast carcinoma (carcinoma erysipeloides): an easily overlooked diagnosis. Br J Dermatol 1993; 129: 324–326.
46 Lever LR, Holt PJA. Carcinoma erysipeloides. Br J Dermatol 1991; 124: 279–282.
47 Ruiz de Erenchun F, Vázquez Doval J, Valérdiz S et al. Inflammatory metastatic carcinoma. A clinical and histopathologic study of three cases. J Dermatol Surg Oncol 1991; 17: 784–787.
48 Hinrichs R, Kirchberg K, Dissemond J et al. Carcinoma erysipeloides of the facial skin in a patient with metastatic breast cancer. Br J Dermatol 1999; 141: 940–941.
49 Siegel JM. Inflammatory carcinoma of the breast. Arch Dermatol 1952; 66: 710–716.

50 Tan BB, Marsden JR, Sanders DSA. Melanoma erysipeloides: inflammatory metastatic melanoma of the skin. Br J Dermatol 1993; 129: 327–329.

51 Prieto VG, Kenet BJ, Varghese M. Malignant mesothelioma metastatic to the skin, presenting as inflammatory carcinoma. Am J Dermatopathol 1997; 19: 261–265.

52 Yasaka N, Ando I, Kukita A. An acral 'inflammatory' cutaneous metastasis of oesophageal carcinoma. Br J Dermatol 1999; 141: 938–939.

53 Şahin S, Hindioğlu U, Benekli M et al. Peculiar inflammatory cutaneous metastasis from stomach adenocarcinoma. Br J Dermatol 1997; 136: 650–652.

54 Edelstein JM. Pancreatic carcinoma with unusual metastasis to the skin and subcutaneous tissue simulating cellulitis. N Engl J Med 1950; 242: 779–781.

55 Webb JM. Carcinoma erysipelatoides from the colon. J Am Acad Dermatol 1996; 34: 1082–1084.

56 Graham BS, Wong SW. Cancer cellulitis. South Med J 1984; 77: 277–278.

57 Kauffman CL, Sina B. Metastatic inflammatory carcinoma of the rectum. Tumor spread by three routes. Am J Dermatopathol 1997; 19: 528–532.

58 Elston DM, Tuthill RJ, Pierson J et al. Carcinoma erysipelatoides resulting from genitourinary cancer. J Am Acad Dermatol 1996; 35: 993–995.

59 Hazelrigg DE, Rudolph AH. Inflammatory metastatic carcinoma. Arch Dermatol 1977; 113: 69–70.

60 Ingram JT. Carcinoma erysipelatoides and carcinoma telangiectaticum. Arch Dermatol 1958; 77: 227–231.

61 Brownstein MH, Helwig EB. Metastatic tumors of the skin. Cancer 1972; 29: 1298–1307.

62 Faust HB, Treadwell PA. Metastatic adenocarcinoma of the scalp mimicking a kerion. J Am Acad Dermatol 1993; 29: 654–655.

63 Dahl PR, Brodland DG, Goellner JR, Hay ID. Thyroid carcinoma metastatic to the skin: A cutaneous manifestation of a widely disseminated malignancy. J Am Acad Dermatol 1997; 36: 531–537.

64 Steck WD, Helwig EB. Tumors of the umbilicus. Cancer 1965; 18: 907–915.

65 Powell FC, Cooper AJ, Massa MC et al. Sister Mary Joseph's nodule: a clinical and histologic study. J Am Acad Dermatol 1984; 10: 610–615.

66 Edoute Y, Ben-Haim SA, Malberger E. Umbilical metastasis from urinary bladder carcinoma. J Am Acad Dermatol 1992; 26: 656–657.

67 Chen KTK. Malignant mesothelioma presenting as Sister Joseph's nodule. Am J Dermatopathol 1991; 13: 300–303.

68 Dubreuil A, Dompmartin A, Barjot P et al. Umbilical metastasis of Sister Mary Joseph's nodule. Int J Dermatol 1998; 37: 7–13.

69 Powell FC, Venencie PY, Winkelmann RK. Metastatic prostate carcinoma manifesting as penile nodules. Arch Dermatol 1984; 120: 1604–1606.

70 Abeshouse BS, Abeshouse GA. Metastatic tumors of the penis: a review of the literature and a report of two cases. J Urol 1961; 86: 99–109.

71 Chang SE, Choi JH, Sung KJ et al. Metastatic squamous cell carcinoma of the nail bed: a presenting sign of lung cancer. Br J Dermatol 1999; 141: 939–940.

72 Vine JE, Cohen PR. Renal cell carcinoma metastatic to the thumb: a case report and review of subungual metastases from all primary sites. Clin Exp Dermatol 1996; 21: 377–380.

73 Okada H, Qing J, Ohnishi T, Watanabe S. Metastasis of gastric carcinoma to a finger. Br J Dermatol 1999; 140: 776–777.

74 Baran R, Tosti A. Metastatic carcinoma to the terminal phalanx of the big toe: report of two cases and review of the literature. J Am Acad Dermatol 1994; 31: 259–263.

75 Gates O. Cutaneous metastases of malignant disease. Am J Cancer 1937; 30: 718–730.

76 Grinspan D, Abulafia J, Abbruzzese M. Metastatic involvement of four eyelids. J Am Acad Dermatol 1997; 37: 362–364.

77 Rubio FA, Pizarro A, Robana G et al. Eyelid metastasis as the presenting sign of recurrent carcinoma of the breast. Br J Dermatol 1997; 137: 1026–1027.

78 Itin PH, Heitzmann F, Stamm B. Metastasis to the nasal tip from a cervical carcinoma. Dermatology 1999; 199: 171–173.

79 Nankhonya JM, Zakhour HD. Malignant seeding of needle aspiration tract: a rare complication. Br J Dermatol 1991; 124: 285–286.

80 Quecedo E, Febrer I, Martínez-Escribano JA et al. Tumoral seeding after pericardiocentesis in a patient with a pulmonary adenocarcinoma. J Am Acad Dermatol 1994; 31: 496–497.

81 Dunn PT, Bigler CF. Metastasis in an electrodesiccation and curettage scar. J Am Acad Dermatol 1997; 36: 117–118.

82 Burkholder GV, Kaufman JJ. Local implantation of carcinoma of the prostate with percutaneous needle biopsy. J Urol 1966; 95: 801–804.

83 Hayes AG, Chesney TMcC. Metastatic adenocarcinoma of the breast located within a benign intradermal naevus. Am J Dermatopathol 1993; 15: 280–282.

84 Betke M, Süss R, Hohenleutner U et al. Gastric carcinoma metastatic to the site of a congenital melanocytic nevus. J Am Acad Dermatol 1993; 28: 866–869.

85 Tharakaram S. Metastases to the skin. Int J Dermatol 1988; 27: 240–242.

86 Alonso-Llamazares J, De Pablo P, Ballestin C et al. Cutaneous metastasis from a presumed signet-ring cell carcinoma in a 10-year-old child. Br J Dermatol 1998; 138: 145–149.

87 Inoue Y, Johno M, Kayashima K et al. Metastatic skin cancer: a case with signet ring cell histology. Br J Dermatol 1996; 135: 634–637.

88 Schwartz RA. Histopathologic aspects of cutaneous metastatic disease. J Am Acad Dermatol 1995; 33: 649–657.

89 Connor DH, Taylor HB, Helwig EB. Cutaneous metastasis of renal cell carcinoma. Arch Pathol 1963; 76: 339–346.

90 Weidner N, Foucar E. Epidermotropic metastatic squamous cell carcinoma. Arch Dermatol 1985; 121: 1041–1043.

91 Aguilar A, Schoendorff C, Lopez Redondo MJ et al. Epidermotropic metastases from internal carcinoma. Am J Dermatopathol 1991; 13: 452–458.

92 Kahn JA, Sinhamohapatra SB, Schneider AF. Hepatoma presenting as a skin metastasis. Arch Dermatol 1971; 104: 299–300.

Specific metastases

93 Peled IJ, Okon E, Weschler Z, Wexler MR. Distant, late metastases to skin of carcinoma of the breast. J Dermatol Surg Oncol 1982; 8: 192–195.

94 Baldari U, Zanelli R, Foschi R, Ridolfi R. Cutaneous metastases from breast carcinoma: a report of 18 cases. Clin Exp Dermatol 1992; 17: 321–323.

95 Gade JN, Kimmick G, Hitchcock MG, McMichael AJ. Generalized cutaneous metastases from breast adenocarcinoma. J Am Acad Dermatol 1997; 37: 129–130.

96 Kim JH, Benson PM, Beard JS, Skelton HG III. Male breast carcinoma with extensive metastases to the skin. J Am Acad Dermatol 1998; 38: 995–996.

97 Peretz E, Hallel-Halevy D, Yanai-Inbar I, Halevy S. Metastatic breast carcinoma: diffuse involvement of the skin. J Eur Acad Dermatol Venereol 2000; 14: 226–227.

98 Schorr WF, Swanson PM, Gomez F, Reyes CN. Alopecia neoplastica. Hair loss resembling alopecia areata caused by metastatic breast cancer. JAMA 1970; 213: 1335–1337.

99 Nelson CT. Alopecia neoplastica (possibly of 28 years' duration). Arch Dermatol 1972; 105: 120.

100 Ronchese F. Alopecia due to metastases from adenocarcinoma of the breast. Arch Dermatol 1949; 59: 329–332.

101 Mallon E, Dawber RPR. Alopecia neoplastica without alopecia: a unique presentation of breast carcinoma scalp metastasis. J Am Acad Dermatol 1994; 31: 319–321.

102 Waisman M. Carcinoma of the inframammary crease. Arch Dermatol 1978; 114: 1520–1521.

103 Watson JR, Watson CG. Carcinoma of the mammary crease. A neglected clinical entity. JAMA 1969; 209: 1718–1719.

104 Dowlati Y, Nedwich A. Carcinoma of mammary crease "simulating basal cell epithelioma". Arch Dermatol 1973; 107: 628–629.

105 Franzblau MJ, Manwaring J, Plumhof C et al. Metastatic breast carcinoma mimicking granular cell tumor. J Cutan Pathol 1989; 16: 218–222.

106 Sexton CW, White WL. Chondrosarcomatous cutaneous metastasis. A unique manifestation of sarcomatoid (metaplastic) breast carcinoma. Am J Dermatopathol 1996; 18: 538–542.

107 Requena L, Sánchez Yus E, Núñez C et al. Epidermotropically metastatic breast carcinomas. Rare histopathologic variants mimicking melanoma and Paget's disease. Am J Dermatopathol 1996; 18: 385–395.

108 Meadows KP, Egan CA. Vesicular carcinoma erysipelatodes. J Am Acad Dermatol 1999; 40: 805–807.

109 Ormsby AH, Snow JL, Su WPD, Goellner JR. Diagnostic immunohistochemistry of cutaneous metastatic breast carcinoma: a statistical analysis of the utility of gross cystic disease fluid protein-15 and estrogen receptor protein. J Am Acad Dermatol 1995; 32: 711–716.

110 Shamai-Lubovitz O, Rothem A, Ben-David E et al. Cutaneous metastatic carcinoma of the breast mimicking malignant melanoma, clinically and histologically. J Am Acad Dermatol 1994; 31: 1058–1060.

111 Inoue H, Kawada A, Takasu H et al. Cathepsin D expression in skin metastasis of breast cancer. J Cutan Pathol 1998; 25: 365–369.

112 Ariel IM, Avery EE, Kanter L et al. Primary carcinoma of the lung. A clinical study of 1205 cases. Cancer 1950; 3: 229–239.

113 Gray LC, Albritton TA, Lesher JL Jr. Adenocarcinoma of the lung with metastasis to the skull presenting as cystic lesions. J Am Acad Dermatol 1997; 36: 644–646.

114 De Argila D, Bureo JC, Márquez FL, Pimentel JJ. Small-cell carcinoma of the lung presenting as a cutaneous metastasis of the lip mimicking a Merkel cell carcinoma. Clin Exp Dermatol 1999; 24: 170–172.

115 Dutt PL, Baxter JW, O'Malley FP et al. Distant cutaneous metastasis of pleural malignant mesothelioma. J Cutan Pathol 1992; 19: 490–495.

116 Toner C, Smith K, Williams J, Skelton H. Metastatic adenocarcinoma of the esophagus to

the skin; new patterns of tumor recurrence and alternate treatments for palliation. J Cutan Pathol 2000; 27: 575 (abstract).

117 Flynn VT, Spurrett BR. Sister Joseph's nodule. Med J Aust 1969; 1: 728–730.

118 Samitz MH. Umbilical metastasis from carcinoma of the stomach. Sister Joseph's nodule. Arch Dermatol 1975; 111: 1478–1479.

119 DiSpaltro FX, Bickley LK, Nissenblatt MJ, Devereux D. Cutaneous acral metastasis in a patient with primary gastric adenocarcinoma. J Am Acad Dermatol 1992; 27: 117–118.

120 Zeligman I, Schwilm A. Umbilical metastasis from carcinoma of the colon. Arch Dermatol 1974; 110: 911–912.

121 Jager RM, Max MH. Umbilical metastasis as the presenting symptom of ceca carcinoma. J Surg Oncol 1979; 12: 41–45.

122 Eppstein S. Primary carcinoma of the liver. Am J Med Sci 1964; 247: 137–144.

123 Reingold IM, Smith BR. Cutaneous metastases from hepatomas. Arch Dermatol 1978; 114: 1045–1046.

124 Kubota Y, Koga T, Nakayama J. Cutaneous metastasis from hepatocellular carcinoma resembling pyogenic granuloma. Clin Exp Dermatol 1999; 24: 78–80.

125 Kahn H, Baumal R, From L. Role of immunohistochemistry in the diagnosis of undifferentiated tumors involving the skin. J Am Acad Dermatol 1986; 14: 1063–1072.

126 Helson L, Garcia EJ. Skin metastases and hepatic cancer in childhood. NY State J Med 1975; 75: 1728–1730.

127 Hollander A, Grots IA. Oculocutaneous metastases from carcinoma of the urinary bladder. Case report and review of the literature. Arch Dermatol 1968; 97: 678–684.

128 Chakraborty AK, Reddy AN, Grosberg SJ, Wapnick S. Pancreatic carcinoma with dissemination to umbilicus and skin. Arch Dermatol 1977; 113: 838–839.

129 Chatterjee SN, Bauer HM. Umbilical metastasis from carcinoma of the pancreas. Arch Dermatol 1980; 116: 954–955.

130 Flórez A, Rosón E, Sánchez-Aguilar D et al. Solitary cutaneous metastasis on the buttock: a disclosing sign of pancreatic adenocarcinoma. Clin Exp Dermatol 2000; 25: 201–203.

131 Taniguchi S, Hisa T, Hamada T. Cutaneous metastases of pancreatic carcinoma with unusual clinical features. J Am Acad Dermatol 1994; 31: 877–880.

132 Padilla RS, Jarmillo M, Dao A, Chapman W. Cutaneous metastatic adenocarcinoma of gallbladder origin. Arch Dermatol 1982; 118: 515–517.

133 Tongco RC. Unusual skin metastases from carcinoma of the gallbladder. Am J Surg 1961; 102: 90–93.

134 Krunic A, Martinovic N, Calonje E, Milinkovic M. Cutaneous metastatic adenocarcinoma of gallbladder origin presenting as carcinoma of unknown primary. Int J Dermatol 1995; 34: 360–362.

135 Rosenthal AL, Lever WF. Involvement of the skin in renal carcinoma. Arch Dermatol 1957; 76: 96–102.

136 Batres E, Knox JM, Wolf JE Jr. Metastatic renal cell carcinoma resembling a pyogenic granuloma. Arch Dermatol 1978; 114: 1082–1083.

137 Rogow L, Rotman M, Roussis K. Renal metastases simulating Kaposi sarcoma. Arch Dermatol 1975; 111: 717–719.

138 Ando K, Goto Y, Kato K et al. Zosteriform inflammatory metastatic carcinoma from transitional cell carcinoma of the renal pelvis. J Am Acad Dermatol 1994; 31: 284–286.

139 Zirwas MJ, Hunt S, Logan TF et al. A painful cutaneous nodule as the presentation of metastatic transitional cell carcinoma of the renal pelvis. J Am Acad Dermatol 2000; 42: 867–868.

140 Scott LS, Head MA, Mack WS. Cutaneous metastases from tumors of the bladder, urethra, and penis. Br J Urol 1954; 26: 387–400.

141 Beautyman EJ, Garcia CJ, Sibulkin D, Snyder PB. Transitional cell bladder carcinoma metastatic to the skin. Arch Dermatol 1983; 119: 705–707.

142 McDonald JH, Heckel NJ, Kretschmer HL. Cutaneous metastases secondary to carcinoma of urinary bladder. Report of two cases and review of the literature. Arch Dermatol 1950; 61: 276–284.

143 Schwartz RA, Fleishman JS. Transitional cell carcinoma of the urinary tract presenting with a cutaneous metastasis. Arch Dermatol 1981; 117: 513–515.

144 Arnheim FK. Carcinoma of the prostate: a study of the postmortem findings in one hundred and seventy-six cases. J Urol 1948; 60: 599–603.

145 Tan HT, Vishniavsky S. Carcinoma of the prostate with metastases to the prepuce. J Urol 1971; 106: 588–589.

146 Oka M, Nakashima K. Carcinoma of the prostate with metastases to the skin and glans penis. Br J Urol 1982; 54: 61.

147 Marcoval J, Moreno A, Jucglà A et al. Prostatic adenocarcinoma with cutaneous metastases overlying oestrogen-induced gynaecomastia. Clin Exp Dermatol 1998; 23: 119–120.

148 Schellhammer PF, Milsten R, Bunts RC. Prostatic carcinoma with cutaneous metastases. Br J Urol 1973; 45: 169–172.

149 Steinkraus V, Lange T, Abeck D et al. Cutaneous metastases from carcinoma of the prostate. J Am Acad Dermatol 1995; 32: 665–666.

150 Razvi M, Firfer R, Berkson B. Occult transitional cell carcinoma of the prostate presenting as skin metastasis. J Urol 1975; 113: 734–735.

151 Scupham R, Beckman E, Fretzin D. Carcinoma of the prostate metastatic to the skin. Am J Dermatopathol 1988; 10: 178–180.

152 Segal R, Penneys NS, Nahass G. Metastatic prostatic carcinoma histologically mimicking malignant melanoma. J Cutan Pathol 1994; 21: 280–282.

153 Rossetti RB, Villaca Neto CM, Paschoal LHC, Burnier M Jr. Cutaneous metastasis originating from prostate adenocarcinoma. Int J Dermatol 1991; 30: 363.

154 Schiff BL. Tumors of testis with cutaneous metastases to scalp. Arch Dermatol 1955; 71: 465–467.

155 Price NM, Kopf AW. Metastases to skin from occult malignant neoplasms. Cutaneous metastases from a teratocarcinoma. Arch Dermatol 1974; 109: 547–550.

156 Chhieng DC, Jennings TA, Slominski A, Mihm MC Jr. Choriocarcinoma presenting as a cutaneous metastasis. J Cutan Pathol 1995; 22: 374–377.

157 Shimizu S, Nagata Y, Han-yaku H. Metastatic testicular choriocarcinoma of the skin. Report and review of the literature. Am J Dermatopathol 1996; 18: 633–636.

158 Galle PC, Jobson VW, Homesley HD. Umbilical metastasis from gynecologic malignancies: a primary carcinoma of the fallopian tube. Obstet Gynecol 1981; 57: 531–533.

159 Beck H, Raahave D, Boiesen P. A malignant Brenner tumor of the ovary with subcutaneous metastases. Acta Pathol Microbiol Scand (A) 1977; 85: 859–863.

160 Freeman CR, Rozenfeld M, Schopflocher P. Cutaneous metastases from carcinoma of the cervix. Arch Dermatol 1982; 118: 40–41.

161 Hayes AG, Berry AD III. Cutaneous metastasis from squamous cell carcinoma of the cervix. J Am Acad Dermatol 1992; 26: 846–850.

162 Debois JM. Endometrial adenocarcinoma metastatic to the scalp. Report of two cases. Arch Dermatol 1982; 118: 42–43.

163 Bukovsky I, Lifshitz Y, Langer R et al. Umbilical mass as a presenting symptom of endometrial adenocarcinoma. Int J Gynaecol Obstet 1979; 17: 229–230.

164 Giardina VN, Morton BF, Potter GK et al. Metastatic endometrial adenocarcinoma to the skin of a toe. Am J Dermatopathol 1996; 18: 94–98.

165 Rasbach D, Hendricks A, Stoltzner G. Endometrial adenocarcinoma metastatic to the scalp. Arch Dermatol 1978; 114: 1708–1709.

166 Damewood MD, Rosenshein NB, Grumbine FC, Parmley TH. Cutaneous metastasis of endometrial carcinoma. Cancer 1980; 46: 1471–1475.

167 Tharakaram S, Rajendran SS, Premalatha S et al. Cutaneous metastasis from carcinoma cervix. Int J Dermatol 1985; 24: 598–599.

168 Daw E, Riley S. Umbilical metastasis from squamous carcinoma of the cervix. Case report. Br J Obstet Gynecol 1982; 89: 1066.

169 Hsu C-T, Sai Y-S. Skin metastases from genital cancer. Report of 2 cases. Obstet Gynecol 1962; 19: 69–75.

170 Fogaca MF, Fedorciw BJ, Tahan SR et al. Cutaneous metastasis of neuroendocrine carcinoma of uterine origin. J Cutan Pathol 1993; 20: 455–458.

171 Prignano F, Vannini P, Wolovsky M et al. Cutaneous metastasis from vulvar adenocarcinoma. Int J Dermatol 1994; 33: 723–724.

172 Kouvaris JR, Plataniotis GA, Sykiotis CA et al. Dermal metastasis from vaginal squamous cell carcinoma. Br J Dermatol 1999; 141: 579–580.

173 Park WW, Lees J. Choriocarcinoma. Arch Pathol 1950; 49: 205–241.

174 Seoud M, Kaspar H, Khalil A et al. Subungual metastatic choriocarcinoma. J Am Acad Dermatol 1996; 34: 511–512.

175 Ertungealp E, Axelrod J, Stanek A et al. Skin metastases from malignant gestational trophoblastic disease: report of two cases. Am J Obstet Gynecol 1982; 143: 843–846.

176 Cosnow I, Fretzin DF. Choriocarcinoma metastatic to skin. Arch Dermatol 1974; 109: 551–553.

177 Avril MF, Mathieu A, Kalifa C, Caillou C. Infantile choriocarcinoma with cutaneous tumors. An additional case and review of the literature. J Am Acad Dermatol 1986; 14: 918–927.

178 Ibanez ML, Russell WO, Albores-Saavedra J et al. Thyroid carcinoma – biologic behavior and mortality. Cancer 1966; 19: 1039–1052.

179 Barr R, Dann F. Anaplastic thyroid carcinoma metastatic to the skin. J Cutan Pathol 1974; 1: 201–206.

180 Rico MJ, Penneys NS. Metastatic follicular carcinoma of the thyroid to the skin: a case confirmed by immunohistochemistry. J Cutan Pathol 1985; 12: 103–105.

181 Horiguchi Y, Takahashi C, Imamura S. Cutaneous metastasis from papillary carcinoma of the thyroid. Report of two cases. J Am Acad Dermatol 1984; 10: 988–992.

182 Hamilton D. Cutaneous metastases from a follicular thyroid carcinoma. J Dermatol Surg Oncol 1980; 6: 116–117.

183 Hoie J, Stenioig AE, Kullmann G, Lindegaard M. Distant metastases in papillary thyroid cancer. A review of 91 patients. Cancer 1988; 61: 1–6.

184 Vives R, Valcayo A, Menendez E, Guarch R. Follicular thyroid carcinoma metastatic to the skin. J Am Acad Dermatol 1992; 27: 276–277.

185 Elgart GW, Patterson JW, Taylor R. Cutaneous metastasis from papillary carcinoma of the thyroid gland. J Am Acad Dermatol 1991; 25: 404–408.

186 Makris A, Goepel JR. Cutaneous metastases from a papillary thyroid carcinoma. Br J Dermatol 1996; 135: 860–861.

187 Auty RM. Dermal metastases from a follicular carcinoma of the thyroid. Arch Dermatol 1977; 113: 675–676.

188 Ordonez NG, Samaan NA. Medullary carcinoma of the thyroid metastatic to the skin: report of two cases. J Cutan Pathol 1987; 14: 251–254.

189 Taniguchi S, Kaneto K, Nishikawa Y et al. Cutaneous metastases from anaplastic thyroid carcinoma. Int J Dermatol 1996; 35: 574–575.

190 Rudner EJ, Lentz C, Brown J. Bronchial carcinoid tumor with skin metastases. Arch Dermatol 1965; 92: 73–75.

191 Keane J, Fretzin DF, Jao W, Shapiro CM. Bronchial carcinoid metastatic to skin. Light and electron microscopic findings. J Cutan Pathol 1980; 7: 43–49.

192 Rodriguez G, Villamizar R. Carcinoid tumor with skin metastasis. Am J Dermatopathol 1992; 14: 263–269.

193 van Dijk C, Ten Seldam REJ. A possible primary cutaneous carcinoid. Cancer 1975; 36: 1016–1020.

194 Norman JL, Cunningham PJ, Cleveland BR. Skin and subcutaneous metastases from gastrointestinal carcinoid tumors. Arch Surg 1971; 103: 767–769.

195 McCracken GA, Washington CV, Templeton SF. Metastatic cutaneous carcinoid. J Am Acad Dermatol 1996; 35: 997–998.

196 Bart RS, Kamino H, Waisman J et al. Carcinoid tumor of skin: report of a possible primary case. J Am Acad Dermatol 1990; 22: 366–370.

197 Sakamoto F, Ito M, Matumura G et al. Ultrastructural study of a mucinous carcinoid of the skin. J Cutan Pathol 1991; 18: 128–133.

198 Courville P, Joly P, Thomine E et al. Primary cutaneous carcinoid tumour. Histopathology 2000; 36: 566–567.

199 Brody HJ, Stallings WP, Fine RM, Someren A. Carcinoid in an umbilical nodule. Arch Dermatol 1978; 114: 570–572.

200 Archer CB, Wells RS, MacDonald DM. Metastatic cutaneous carcinoid. J Am Acad Dermatol 1985; 13: 363–366.

201 Reingold IM, Escovitz WE. Metastatic cutaneous carcinoid. Arch Dermatol 1960; 82: 971–975.

202 Bean SF, Fusaro RM. An unusual manifestation of the carcinoid syndrome. Arch Dermatol 1968; 98: 268–269.

203 Castiello RJ, Lynch PJ. Pellagra and the carcinoid syndrome. Arch Dermatol 1972; 105: 574–577.

204 Lucky AW, McGuire J, Komp DM. Infantile neuroblastoma presenting with cutaneous blanching nodules. J Am Acad Dermatol 1982; 6: 389–391.

205 Nguyen TQ, Fisher GB Jr, Tabbarah SO et al. Stage IV-S metastatic neuroblastoma presenting as skin nodules at birth. Int J Dermatol 1988; 27: 712–713.

206 Hawthorne HC Jr, Nelson JS, Witzleben CL, Giangiacomo J. Blanching subcutaneous nodules in neonatal neuroblastoma. J Pediatr 1970; 77: 297–300.

207 Shown TE, Durfee MF. Blueberry muffin baby: neonatal neuroblastoma with subcutaneous metastases. J Urol 1970; 104: 193–195.

208 Shapiro L. Neuroblastoma with multiple cutaneous metastases. Arch Dermatol 1969; 99: 502–504.

209 Schneider KM, Becker JM, Krasna IH. Neonatal neuroblastoma. Pediatrics 1965; 36: 359–366.

210 Maher-Wiese VL, Wenner NP, Grant-Kels JM. Metastatic cutaneous lesions in children and adolescents with a case report of metastatic neuroblastoma. J Am Acad Dermatol 1992; 26: 620–628.

211 Balch CM, Milton GW. In: Balch CM, Milton GW, Shaw HM, Soong S-J, eds. Cutaneous melanoma. Clinical management and treatment results worldwide. Philadelphia: JB Lippincott, 1985; 221–250.

212 Stehlin JS Jr, Hills WJ, Rufino C. Disseminated melanoma. Biologic behavior and treatment. Arch Surg 1967; 94: 495–501.

213 Karakousis CP, Temple DF, Moore R, Ambrus JL. Prognostic parameters in recurrent malignant melanoma. Cancer 1983; 52: 575–579.

214 Patel JK, Didolkar MS, Pickren JW, Moore RH. Metastatic pattern of malignant melanoma. A study of 216 autopsy cases. Am J Surg 1978; 135: 807–810.

215 Beardmore GL, Davis NC, McLeod R et al. Malignant melanoma in Queensland: a study of 219 deaths. Aust J Dermatol 1969; 10: 158–168.

216 Das Gupta T, Brasfield R. Metastatic melanoma. A clinicopathological study. Cancer 1964; 17: 1323–1339.

217 Baab GH, McBride CM. Malignant melanoma. The patient with an unknown site of primary origin. Arch Surg 1975; 110: 896–900.

218 Balch CM, Urist MM, Maddox WA et al. In: Balch CM, Milton GW, Shaw HM, Soong S-J, eds. Cutaneous melanoma. Clinical management and treatment results worldwide. Philadelphia: JB Lippincott, 1985; 93–130.

219 Marschall S, Welykyj S, Gradini R, Eng A. Unusual presentation of cutaneous metastatic malignant melanoma. J Am Acad Dermatol 1991; 24: 648–650.

220 Steiner A, Rappersberger K, Groh V, Pehamberger H. Diffuse melanosis in metastatic malignant melanoma. J Am Acad Dermatol 1991; 24: 625–628.

221 Péc J, Plank L, Mináriková E et al. Generalized melanosis with malignant melanoma metastasizing to skin – a pathological study with S-100 protein and HMB-45. Clin Exp Dermatol 1993; 18: 454–457.

222 Klaus MV, Shah F. Generalized melanosis caused by melanoma of the rectum J Am Acad Dermatol 1996; 35: 295–297.

223 Cavallari V, Cannavò SP, Ussia AF et al. Vitiligo associated with metastatic malignant melanoma. Int J Dermatol 1996; 35: 738–740.

224 Eckert F, Baricevic B, Landthaler M, Schmid U. Metastatic signet-ring cell melanoma in a patient with an unknown primary tumor. J Am Acad Dermatol 1992; 26: 870–875.

225 Unger SW, Wanebo HJ, Cooper PH. Multiple cutaneous malignant melanomas with features of primary melanoma. Ann Surg 1981; 193: 245–250.

226 Shea CR, Kline MA, Lugo J, McNutt NS. Angiotropic metastatic malignant melanoma. Am J Dermatopathol 1995; 17: 58–62.

227 Smolle J, Hofmann-Wellenhof R, Woltsche-Kahr I et al. Quantitative assessment of fat cells in subcutaneous metastatic melanoma. Am J Dermatopathol 1995; 17: 555–559.

228 Smolle J, Woltsche I, Hofmann-Wellenhof R et al. Pathology of tumor–stroma interaction in melanoma metastatic to the skin. Hum Pathol 1995; 26: 856–861.

229 Kornberg R, Harris M, Ackerman AB. Epidermotropically metastatic malignant melanoma. Arch Dermatol 1978; 114: 67–69.

230 Warner TFCS, Gilbert EF, Ramirez G. Epidermotropism in melanoma. J Cutan Pathol 1980; 7: 50–54.

231 Heenan PJ, Clay CD. Epidermotropic metastatic melanoma simulating multiple primary melanomas. Am J Dermatopathol 1991; 13: 396–402.

232 Abernethy JL, Soyer HP, Kerl H et al. Epidermotropic metastatic malignant melanoma simulating melanoma in situ. Am J Surg Pathol 1994; 18: 1140–1149.

233 Vinod SU, Gay RM. Adenoid cystic carcinoma of the minor salivary glands metastatic to the hand. South Med J 1979; 72: 1483–1485.

234 Tok J, Kao GF, Berberian BJ et al. Cutaneous metastasis from a parotid adenocarcinoma. Am J Dermatopathol 1995; 17: 303–306.

235 Zanca A, Ferracini U, Bertazzoni MG. Telangiectatic metastasis from ductal carcinoma of the parotid gland. J Am Acad Dermatol 1993; 28: 113–114.

236 Nakamura M, Miyachi Y. Cutaneous metastasis from an adenoid cystic carcinoma of the lacrimal gland. Br J Dermatol 1999; 141: 373–374.

237 White RM, Patterson JW. Distant skin metastases in a long-term survivor of malignant ameloblastoma. J Cutan Pathol 1986; 13: 383–389.

238 Bedford GU. A case of carcinoma of the thymus with extensive metastases in a new-born child. Can Med Assoc J 1930; 23: 197–202.

239 Nakada JR. Primary carcinoma of the adrenals with metastases in the skin and myocardium. J Miss State Med Assoc 1930; 27: 367–371.

240 Schultz BM, Schwartz RA. Hypopharyngeal squamous cell carcinoma metastatic to skin. J Am Acad Dermatol 1985; 12: 169–172.

241 Jacyk WK, Dinkel DE, Becker GJ. Cutaneous metastases from carcinoma of the nasopharynx. Br J Dermatol 1998; 139: 344–345.

242 Cawley EP, Hsu YT, Weary PE. The evaluation of neoplastic metastases to the skin. Arch Dermatol 1964; 90: 262–265.

243 Horiuchi N, Tagami H. Skin metastasis in laryngeal carcinoma. Clin Exp Dermatol 1992; 17: 282–283.

244 Kleinman GM, Hochberg FH, Richardson EP Jr. Systemic metastases from medulloblastoma. Report of two cases and review of the literature. Cancer 1981; 48: 2296–2309.

245 Glasauer FE, Yuan RHP. Intracranial tumors with extracranial metastases. Case report and review of the literature. J Neurosurg 1963; 20: 474–493.

246 Campbell AN, Chan HSL, Becker LE et al. Extracranial metastases in childhood primary intracranial tumors. A report of 21 cases and review of the literature. Cancer 1984; 53: 974–981.

247 Youngberg GA, Berro J, Young M, Leicht SS. Metastatic epidermotropic squamous carcinoma histologically simulating primary carcinoma. Am J Dermatopathol 1989; 1: 457–465.

248 Broderick PA, Connors RC. Unusual manifestation of metastatic uterine leiomyosarcoma. Arch Dermatol 1981; 117: 445–446.

249 Powell FC, Cooper AJ, Massa MC et al. Leiomyosarcoma of the small intestine metastatic to the umbilicus. Arch Dermatol 1984; 120: 402–406.

250 Bianchi L, Orlandi A, Iraci S et al. Solid alveolar rhabdomyosarcoma of the hand in adolescence: a clinical, histologic, immunologic, and ultrastructural study. Pediatr Dermatol 1995; 12: 343–347.

251 Cerroni L, Soyer HP, Smolle J, Kerl H. Cutaneous metastases of a giant cell tumor of bone: case report. J Cutan Pathol 1990; 17: 59–63.

252 Seline PC, Jaskierny DJ. Cutaneous metastases from a chondroblastoma initially presenting as unilateral palmar hyperhidrosis. J Am Acad Dermatol 1999; 40: 325–327.

253 King DT, Gurevitch AW, Hirose FM. Multiple cutaneous metastases of a scapular chondrosarcoma. Arch Dermatol 1978; 114: 584–586.

254 Lambert D, Escallier F, Collet E et al. Distal phalangeal metastasis of a chondrosarcoma presenting initially as bilateral onycholysis. Clin Exp Dermatol 1992; 17: 463–465.

255 Leal-Khouri SM, Barnhill RL, Baden HP. An unusual cutaneous metastasis of a chondrosarcoma. J Cutan Pathol 1990; 17: 274–277.

256 Aramburu-González J-A, Rodríguez-Justo M, Jiménez-Reyes J, Santonja C. A case of soft tissue mesenchymal chondrosarcoma metastatic to skin, clinically mimicking keratoacanthoma. Am J Dermatopathol 1999; 21: 392–394.

257 Myhand RC, Hung P-H, Caldwell JB et al. Osteogenic sarcoma with skin metastases. J Am Acad Dermatol 1995; 32: 803–805.

258 Stavrakakis J, Toumbis-Ioannou E, Alexopoulos A, Rigatos GA. Subcutaneous nodules as initial metastatic sites in osteosarcoma. Int J Dermatol 1997; 36: 606–609.

259 Setoyama M, Kanda A, Kanzaki T. Cutaneous metastasis of an osteosarcoma. A case report. Am J Dermatopathol 1996; 18: 629–632.

250 Miller JL, Boyd AS. Metastatic paraganglioma presenting as a scalp nodule. J Am Acad Dermatol 2001; 44: 321–323.

261 Rudd RJ, Fair KP, Patterson JW. Aortic angiosarcoma presenting with cutareous metastasis: Case report and review of the literature. J Am Acad Dermatol 2000; 43: 930–933.

262 Val-Bernal JF, Figols J, Arce FP, Sanz-Ortiz J. Cardiac epithelioid angiosarcoma presenting as cutaneous metastases. J Cutan Pathol 2001; 28: 265–270.

263 Cartwright LE, Steinman HK. Malignant papillary mesothelioma of the tunica vaginalis testes: cutaneous metastases showing pagetoid epidermal invasion. J Am Acad Dermatol 1987; 17: 887–890.

264 Berkowitz RK, Longley J, Buchness MR et al. Malignant mesothelioma: diagnosis by skin biopsy. J Am Acad Dermatol 1989; 21: 1068–1073.

265 Ogi H, Kiryu H, Hori Y, Fukui M. Cutaneous metastasis of CNS chordoma. Am J Dermatopathol 1995; 17: 599–602.

266 Cesinaro AM, Maiorana A, Annessi G, Collina G. Cutaneous metastasis of chordoma. Am J Dermatopathol 1995; 17: 603–605.

267 Gagné EJ, Su WPD. Chordoma involving the skin: an immunohistochemical study of 11 cases. J Cutan Pathol 1992; 19: 469–475.

268 Su WPD, Louback JB, Gagne EJ, Scheithauer BW. Chordoma cutis: a report of nineteen patients with cutaneous involvement of chordoma. J Am Acad Dermatol 1993; 29: 63–66.

269 Feldman AR, Keeling JH III. Cutaneous manifestation of atrial myxoma. J Am Acad Dermatol 1989; 21: 1080–1084.

270 Navarro PH, Bravo FP, Beltran GG. Atrial myxoma with livedoid macules as its sole cutaneous manifestation. J Am Acad Dermatol 1995; 32: 881–883.

271 Reed RJ, Utz MP, Terezakis N. Embolic and metastatic cardiac myxoma. Am J Dermatopathol 1989; 11: 157–165.

Cutaneous infiltrates – non-lymphoid

INTRODUCTION

This chapter includes diseases with an infiltrate in the dermis and/or the subcutaneous tissues of cells, other than lymphocytes, derived from the bone marrow or lymphoid tissues; it specifically covers those conditions in which the cutaneous infiltrate is composed predominantly of one cell type.

The various conditions will be discussed by cell type. For completeness, mention will be made of those conditions fulfilling the definition of 'cutaneous infiltrates' but discussed in other chapters. Special histochemical methods and immunoperoxidase techniques using monoclonal antibodies may be required to characterize fully the particular cell which constitutes the cutaneous infiltrate.

NEUTROPHIL INFILTRATES

Infiltration of the skin by neutrophils is common to numerous diseases of the skin. In most instances the infiltrate is localized to the dermis, although involvement of the epidermis or the subcutaneous fat may occur in various conditions.

Neutrophils

Neutrophils (neutrophil polymorphonuclear leukocytes) measure 10–12 μm in diameter in tissue sections. They have two to five distinct nuclear lobes and their cytoplasm contains two distinct types of granules. The larger ones are azurophilic and constitute approximately 25% of the granules in the cytoplasm. They contain myeloperoxidase, bactericidal substrates, cationic proteins, acid hydrolases and elastase.[1] The smaller granules contain lactoferrin, lysozyme, collagenase and alkaline phosphatase.[1] These enzymes contribute to the neutrophils' vital role in the defense against invading microorganisms.

Neutrophils are produced in the bone marrow; their maturation from myeloblasts through various intermediate stages takes approximately 7–10 days. Their production and maturation is under the influence of a specific glycoprotein known as granulocyte colony-stimulating factor.[2,3] Mature neutrophils are released into the circulation where they spend approximately 7 hours before entering the tissues. Chemotactic substances guide neutrophils to the site of the infective process or another stimulus. They remain functional in the tissues for 1–2 days. Their demise is poorly understood: they can be phagocytosed by macrophages in the tissues or spleen; some appear to be excreted from mucosal surfaces.[1]

The prime function of neutrophils is phagocytosis and the release of the various enzymes stored in the cytoplasmic granules (see above). An unwanted effect is tissue damage caused by some of these enzymes, in particular collagenase and elastase. Although the part played by neutrophils in the phagocytosis and elimination of organisms, immune complexes and damaged tissue is well understood, their role in dermatoses such as psoriasis, dermatitis herpetiformis and the neutrophilic dermatoses is not well understood.

Diseases with neutrophilic infiltrates

All of the conditions characterized by neutrophilic infiltrates in the skin have been discussed in other chapters with the exceptions of Still's disease and congenital and erosive vesicular dermatosis, both of which may have numerous neutrophils in the inflammatory infiltrate.[4,5] They are summarized in Table 40.1.

Table 40.1 **Cutaneous diseases with neutrophilic infiltrates**

Epidermal neutrophilic infiltrates	Erysipelas	Dermatitis herpetiformis
	Erysipeloid	Bullous systemic lupus erythematosus
Impetigo	Cellulitis	Cicatricial pemphigoid
Toxic shock syndrome	Blastomycosis-like pyoderma	Ocular cicatricial pemphigoid
Dermatophytoses	Erosive pustular dermatosis of the scalp	Localized pemphigoid
Chromomycosis	*Mycobacterium ulcerans* infection	Linear IgA bullous dermatosis
Sporotrichosis	Other atypical mycobacterial infections	Epidermolysis bullosa acquisita
Milker's nodule	Erythema nodosum leprosum	Deep lamina lucida pemphigoid
Orf	Chancroid	*Folliculitides*
Yaws	Granuloma inguinale	Bacterial and fungal folliculitis
Subcorneal pustular dermatosis	Kerion	Secondary syphilis
Acute generalized exanthematous pustulosis	Actinomycosis	Perforating folliculitis
Pustular psoriasis	Nocardiosis	*Miscellaneous conditions*
Psoriasis	Mycetoma	Neutrophilic urticaria
Reiter's syndrome	Acute cutaneous leishmaniasis	Polymorphous light eruption
Palmoplantar pustulosis	Secondary syphilis	Cutis laxa (early stage)
Pustular eruption of ulcerative colitis	Bite reactions (fleas, ticks and fire-ants)	Eruptive xanthoma
Infantile acropustulosis	*Neutrophilic dermatoses*	Reticulohistiocytoma
Erythema neonatorum toxicum	Sweet's syndrome	Anaplastic large-cell lymphoma
Transient neonatal pustular melanosis	Pustular vasculitis of the hands	Erythropoietic protoporphyria
Pemphigus foliaceus	Bowel-associated dermatosis–arthritis syndrome	Neutrophilic eccrine hidradenitis
IgA pemphigus	Rheumatoid neutrophilic dermatosis	Familial Mediterranean fever
Miliaria pustulosa	Acute generalized pustulosis	Congenital erosive and vesicular dermatosis
Acute generalized pustulosis	Behçet's syndrome	Still's disease
Glucagonoma syndrome	Pyoderma gangrenosum	
Halogenodermas	*Acute vasculitides*	
Verruciform xanthoma	Hypersensitivity vasculitis and variants	**Subcutaneous neutrophil infiltrates**
Adult T-cell leukemia/lymphoma	Septic vasculitis	
	Erythema elevatum diutinum	Infective panniculitis (causes as for dermal infiltrates – see above); erythema nodosum leprosum
Dermal neutrophilic infiltrates	Granuloma faciale	Factitial panniculitis
	Polyarteritis nodosa	Pustular panniculitis of rheumatoid arthritis
Infections and infestations	*Subepidermal blistering diseases*	α_1-Antitrypsin deficiency
Ecthyma		

EOSINOPHIL INFILTRATES

Eosinophils are readily identified in tissues, but their role in the pathogenesis of the various cutaneous diseases in which they are found has been obscure until comparatively recently.[6] It is now known that they are the effector cells for killing helminths and also for causing tissue damage in hypersensitivity diseases.[6] Eosinophils have also been linked to several inflammatory diseases of the skin associated with edema.[7–9] They appear to have a role in the down-regulation of the inflammation associated with hypersensitivity reactions of immediate type.[6] Eosinophils also possess phagocytic activity, but less than that of neutrophils.[6]

Eosinophils

Eosinophils are polymorphonuclear leukocytes with a bilobed or trilobed nucleus and cytoplasm which contains approximately 20 eosinophilic-staining granules.[10] Ultrastructurally, these granules have an electron-dense core and a relatively radiolucent matrix.[11]

The granular core is the site of production of major basic protein, whereas the other granule proteins (eosinophil cationic protein, eosinophil-derived neurotoxin and eosinophil peroxidase) are found in the matrix.[7] The granule proteins are potent toxins, some of which (major basic protein and eosinophil cationic protein) can directly kill metazoal parasites coated with IgE. Eosinophil cationic protein can also cause local tissue damage when it is released.[12] Major basic protein can cause histamine release from basophils, and most of the granule proteins can induce a wheal-and-flare reaction.[7] Major basic protein can be detected in the tissues in atopic dermatitis[13] and in some cases of urticaria,[11] even in the absence of significant tissue eosinophilia.[7] This has important pathogenetic implications for these two diseases.

Other substances produced by the eosinophil include Charcot–Leyden crystal protein, which has lysophospholipase activity, arylsulfatase, leukotriene C_4 and platelet-activating factor.[7] Thromboembolic disorders are more common in patients with the hypereosinophilic syndrome than in other people, presumably as a consequence of enhanced production of platelet-activating factor.[14]

Eosinophils originate in the bone marrow, where they spend 3–6 days before being released into the circulation.[10] Several factors such as granulocyte–macrophage colony-stimulating factor (GM-CSF), interleukin-3 (IL-3) and interleukin-5 (IL-5) stimulate the production of eosinophils.[15,16] They are in the blood for a short time and then enter the tissues.[10] Only a small proportion of the total number of eosinophils is circulating at any time. Eosinophils appear to go through a late differentiation stage after they have entered the bloodstream.[14,17] Some eosinophils develop low-density cytoplasm ('hypodense eosinophils') which corresponds with activation of the cell.[14,17] Chemotaxis for eosinophils is mediated by GM-CSF, IL-5, leukotriene B_4, platelet activation factor and complement fraction 5.[15] Of particular importance is the role of IL-5, which has selective specificity for eosinophils.[15,16,18] The gene for IL-5 is located on chromosome 5q31.[16] The selectivity of the eosinophil response to a particular stimulus is due to the receptor profile expressed by eosinophils, which is predominantly the CCR3 receptor.[16]

Diseases with conspicuous eosinophils

Eosinophils are a conspicuous component of the inflammatory cell infiltrate in a number of inflammatory and neoplastic disorders. They are listed in Table 40.2.

The distribution of the eosinophils within the skin may be characteristic. This aspect is covered in the discussion of the various entities in other

Table 40.2 **Cutaneous diseases with eosinophilic infiltrates**

Vesiculobullous diseases
Dermatitis herpetiformis (late lesions)
Bullous pemphigoid
Bullous arthropod bite reaction
Pemphigus vegetans
Pemphigoid gestationis
Eosinophilic spongiosis
Erythema neonatorum toxicum

Disorders of blood vessels
Urticaria
Hypersensitivity vasculitis (some cases)
Eosinophilic vasculitis
Allergic granulomatosis (Churg–Strauss)
Juvenile temporal arteritis
Angiolymphoid hyperplasia with eosinophilia
Kimura's disease

Infections/infestations
Parasitic infestations
Dermatophytes (uncommon)

Miscellaneous conditions
Hypereosinophilic syndrome
Wells' syndrome
Pachydermatous eosinophilic dermatitis
Incontinentia pigmenti
Allergic contact dermatitis
Drug reactions
Dermal hypersensitivity
Eosinophilic pustular folliculitis
Eosinophilic pustulosis
Eosinophilic panniculitis
Eosinophilic fasciitis
Eosinophilic, polymorphic and pruritic eruption of radiotherapy

Tumors
Langerhans cell histiocytosis
Tumor-like eosinophilic granuloma
Juvenile xanthogranuloma
Eosinophilic variant, lymphomatoid papulosis
Squamous cell carcinoma
Keratoacanthoma
Malignant melanoma (rare)

sections of the book. One pattern of distribution of eosinophils within the dermis – interstitial eosinophils – is characteristic of certain diseases. The term **'interstitial eosinophils'** refers to the presence of eosinophils between collagen bundles in the intervascular dermis. Eosinophils are invariably present in a perivascular location as well. Interstitial eosinophils are characteristic of various parasitic infestations, particularly arthropod bites (p. 738), but they are also found in certain drug reactions (see Ch. 20), urticaria (p. 227), PUPPP (toxic erythema of pregnancy; p. 244), Wells' syndrome (see below), the urticarial stage of bullous pemphigoid (p. 153), eosinophilic, polymorphic and pruritic eruption of radiotherapy (see p. 100), the hypereosinophilic syndrome (p. 1060) and 'dermal hypersensitivity reaction'.

The term *'dermal hypersensitivity reaction'*, which does not correlate with any defined clinical entity, is used by some dermatopathologists for the morphological finding of a mixed infiltrate of lymphocytes and eosinophils in the upper and mid dermis with perivascular and interstitial eosinophils.[19] It seems to be a 'wastebasket' diagnosis. Clinical follow-up of cases diagnosed as dermal hypersensitivity reaction has shown a diversity of clinical diagnoses including urticaria, drug reaction, eczematous dermatitis and 'idiopathic'.[20] There is a resemblance to the picture seen in arthropod bites, although the infiltrate is not usually as heavy, nor does it extend as deeply in the dermis. This morphological pattern is sometimes seen in patients with an internal cancer who have a non-specific cutaneous eruption. Eosinophils were particularly prominent in one case associated with an islet cell tumor of the pancreas.[21]

A discussion of Wells' syndrome, the hypereosinophilic syndrome, pachydermatous eosinophilic dermatitis and eosinophilic pustulosis follows.

WELLS' SYNDROME (EOSINOPHILIC CELLULITIS)

Wells' syndrome (eosinophilic cellulitis)[22–26] is a disorder of unknown pathogenesis characterized by the tissue reaction pattern known as 'eosinophilic cellulitis with flame figures' (see p. 12).

Clinically, there are edematous infiltrated plaques resembling cellulitis, often with blister formation. This is followed by the development of slate-gray morphea-like induration which resolves, usually without trace, over 4–8 weeks.[23,27] Recurrent lesions may develop over a period of months to years. Milder cases have annular or circinate erythematous plaques. Subcutaneous nodules are extremely rare.[28] There is a predilection for the extremities and trunk; rarely, the face is involved as a major clinical feature.[29] The lesions followed the lines of Blaschko in one case.[30]

Wells' syndrome may occur at any age, although onset in childhood is uncommon.[28,31–36] Several cases occurring in the same family have been documented.[37,38] In one family, the skin lesions were associated with a dysmorphic habitus, mental retardation and elevated plasma IL-5.[38]

Although most cases of Wells' syndrome are idiopathic, some are associated with arthropod bites, parasitic infestation (such as giardiasis and toxocariasis), drug allergy, tetanus vaccine[39] or an atopic history.[23,25,40–44] It has followed varicella infection in a child[34] and been associated with HIV infection[45] and the hypereosinophilic syndrome.[46]

It has been suggested that circulating CD4$^+$ CD7$^-$ T cells play a pivotal role by producing IL-5.[47] Serum and tissue levels of this cytokine appear to correlate with clinical activity.[15]

Histopathology[22,48,49]
In early lesions of Wells' syndrome there is dermal edema and massive infiltration of eosinophils, both interstitial and angiocentric. Subepidermal blisters containing eosinophils may form. After 1 week scattered histiocytes and characteristic 'flame figures' are found. The flame figures are surrounded, in part, by a palisade of histiocytes and a few multinucleate giant cells. Uncommonly, there are numerous multinucleate giant cells present.[50]

The inflammatory process involves the entire thickness of the dermis, and often the subcutis as well. Localization to the subcutis has been reported as eosinophilic panniculitis (see p. 535). Extensive necrotizing granulomas have been reported in the subcutis in this condition.[32] Rarely, the inflammatory infiltrate extends into the fascia and muscle.[51]

The flame figures consist of eosinophil granule major basic protein encrusted on otherwise normal collagen.[27] There is no mucopolysaccharide or lipid, but sometimes basophilic fibrillar material may be seen at the periphery of the eosinophilic material (Fig. 40.1). There is a superficial resemblance to the Splendore–Hoeppli phenomenon, which may develop around metazoal parasites in the tissues.

The tissue reaction pattern of eosinophilic cellulitis with flame figures may be seen in a number of disparate conditions,[22,48,52] including arthropod reactions,[48,53] other parasitic infestations,[54] internal cancers,[55] dermatophyte infections,[22] bullous pemphigoid,[22] herpes gestationis,[22] allergic eczemas[22] and

eosinophilic ulcer of the oral mucosa.[56–58] It is uncommon in all of these conditions, except eosinophilic ulcer of the oral mucosa. This reaction pattern has also been reported in association with eosinophilic folliculitis, as a manifestation of a drug reaction.[59] The clinical setting and other histopathological features allow the conditions listed above to be distinguished from Wells' syndrome.

Electron microscopy
Free eosinophil granules are found coating collagen bundles in the flame figures, but the collagen bundles are not damaged.[49] Numerous intact eosinophils are also present in the adjacent dermis.

HYPEREOSINOPHILIC SYNDROME

The hypereosinophilic syndrome is an idiopathic systemic disorder with involvement of one or more organs and persistent hypereosinophilia ($>1.5 \times 10^9$/l) in the absence of any identifiable cause.[60,61] It encompasses a spectrum of disorders which includes eosinophilic leukemia and Löffler's syndrome. Cardiac involvement, which may be fatal, is quite common; the lungs, skin, liver and central nervous system may also be involved.

Cutaneous lesions, which take the form of pruritic erythematous papules and nodules or urticaria and angioedema, are present in up to one-half of cases. Rarely they are the only manifestation of the syndrome.[62,63] Other mucocutaneous presentations include mucosal ulcerations,[64] erythema annulare centrifugum,[65] purpuric lesions and livedo reticularis.[66] Elevated levels of IgE, IL-2, IL-5, IL-10 and soluble IL-2 receptor may be present.[67]

Cases presenting with episodic or transient angioedema and eosinophilia, but without involvement of other organs, are regarded as a separate entity with a benign clinical course.[9,60,68] Likewise, the syndrome of hyperimmunoglobulinemia-E with recurrent staphylococcal skin infections, defective neutrophil chemotaxis and peripheral eosinophilia is a distinct entity.[69,70] The case that presented with nodular eosinophilic infiltration of the skin and immunoglobulin isotype imbalance is probably a separate condition.[71]

Histopathology[72]
There is a variable superficial and deep, predominantly perivascular, infiltrate of eosinophils, with variable numbers of lymphocytes, plasma cells and mast cells.[73] Dermal edema is present in urticarial lesions. Thrombosis of small vessels in the dermis is a rare finding.[66]

In the syndrome of recurrent angioedema with eosinophilia the infiltrate is primarily mononuclear, with only a few eosinophils.[74] However, with immunofluorescence there is extracellular localization of eosinophil major basic protein.

PACHYDERMATOUS EOSINOPHILIC DERMATITIS

Pachydermatous eosinophilic dermatitis is a recently described entity which is possibly a variant of the hypereosinophilic syndrome. It is associated with a generalized pruritic papular eruption arising on a pachydermatous base, hypertrophic lesions in the genital area, and peripheral blood eosinophilia.[75] The reported cases were in South African black teenage girls. The etiology is unknown.

Histopathology
The lesions showed an eosinophil-rich lymphohistiocytic infiltrate and variable fibrosis of the dermis. The infiltrate varied in amount and distribution. Interstitial

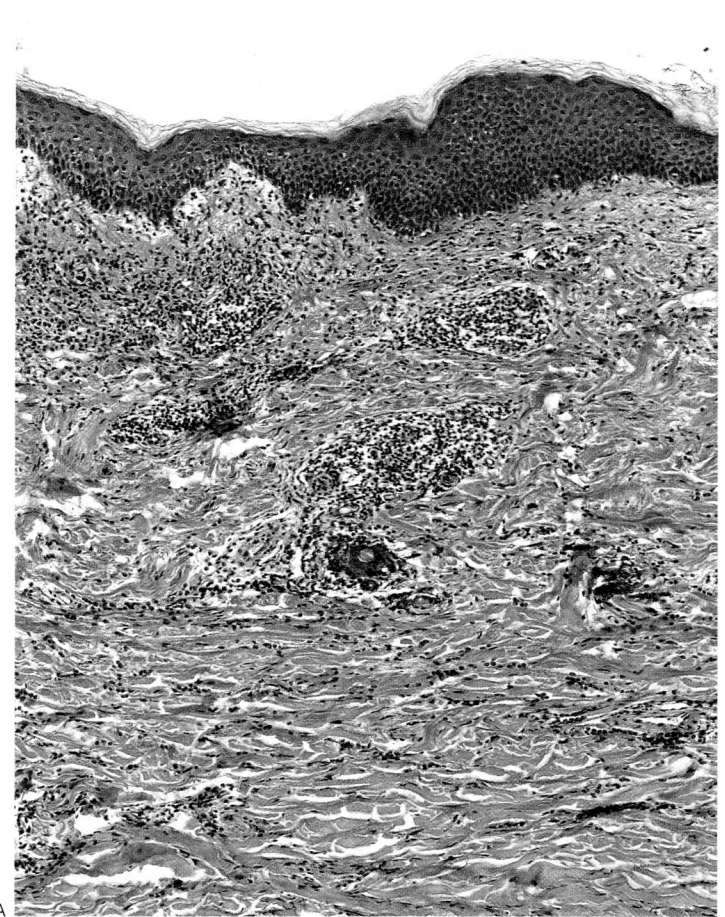
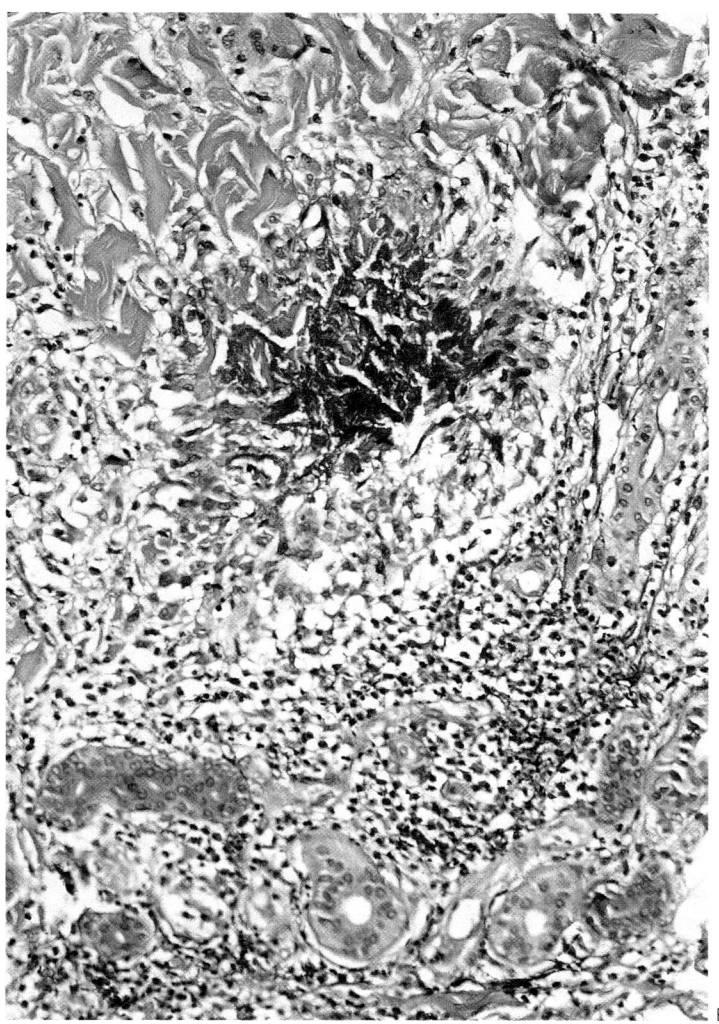

Fig. 40.1 **Wells' syndrome. (A)** A flame figure is shown. **(B)** There are many eosinophils in the surrounding dermis. (H & E)

eosinophils were often present and there was abundant eosinophil granule major basic protein.[75]

EOSINOPHILIC PUSTULOSIS

Eosinophilic pustulosis is an appropriate designation for a spectrum of cases originally reported as eosinophilic pustular folliculitis of infancy (see p. 460). Although it was originally regarded as a dermatosis of the scalp, cases with lesions in other sites have been reported. Furthermore, this condition was originally regarded as a follicular process similar to Ofuji's disease but cases with a predominantly interfollicular infiltrate have since been reported. The papulopustular lesions reported in the genital region appear to belong to this spectrum.[76]

The etiology is unknown. Scabies infection has not been present.

Histopathology

There is a heavy dermal infiltrate of lymphocytes, neutrophils and numerous eosinophils. By definition, there is no primary folliculitis. There is usually no subepidermal edema, and the infiltrate is more polymorphic than in Wells' syndrome.

PLASMA CELL INFILTRATES

Plasma cells are not usually present in the peripheral blood or normal skin, although they may be found in normal mucous membranes. However, they may be a component of the inflammatory infiltrate in a wide range of dermatoses and tumors of the skin.[77] These will be considered after a discussion of the normal plasma cell.

Plasma cells

Plasma cells are terminally differentiated cells which are derived from antigenically stimulated B lymphocytes.[77] During their life span of 2–3 days they continuously synthesize and secrete antibodies that have specificity for the particular antigen that stimulated the plasma cell precursor to proliferate and differentiate.

Plasma cells have abundant basophilic cytoplasm and an eccentrically placed nucleus with coarse chromatin granules, which are often distributed in a cartwheel pattern. Occasionally the cytoplasm contains a round eosinophilic inclusion that may displace the nucleus to the periphery or be liberated into the stroma. These Russell bodies, which may measure up to 20 μm in diameter, result from the accumulation of immunoglobulins and glycoproteins in the cytoplasm.[78] They are PAS positive and diastase resistant. Russell bodies are particularly prominent in the inflammatory infiltrate in rhinoscleroma.

Ultrastructural examination reveals a well-developed rough endoplasmic reticulum with numerous ribosomes. These are involved in the synthesis of a particular immunoglobulin. The endoplasmic reticulum is the site of formation of the Russell bodies. Crystalloid inclusions, iron and even bacteria have been found in the cytoplasm of plasma cells in various circumstances.[77]

Numerous basophilic extracellular bodies, reminiscent of yeast cells, have been found in the dermis in association with plasma cell infiltrates.[79] These structures, known as plasma cell bodies, may measure up to 5 μm in diameter and are derived from the cytoplasm of plasma cells.[79]

In contrast to B lymphocytes, plasma cells have very small amounts of immunoglobulin on their cell membrane, although it may be demonstrated in the cytoplasm by immunoperoxidase methods. This may be useful in distinguishing reactive proliferations of plasma cells, which are polyclonal, from plasmacytomas and myelomatous infiltrates, which are monoclonal. Plasma cells stain for CD79a; CD38 is used as a marker in flow cytometry.

Plasma cell hyperplasias

Plasma cells may be a prominent component of the inflammatory infiltrate in a number of dermatoses and neoplastic disorders.[77] It should be remembered that plasma cells are almost invariably present in any condition involving the lips and other mucous membranes.[80] For some inexplicable reason they may also be prominent in lesions of the forehead and scalp, particularly in keratoses and skin cancers previously subjected to cryotherapy.[81]

Plasma cells are particularly prominent in the inflammatory infiltrate in syphilis (p. 650), granuloma inguinale (p. 633), chancroid (p. 634), yaws (p. 653), rhinoscleroma (p. 635), erythema nodosum leprosum (p. 632, necrobiosis lipoidica (p. 202), the nodular form of primary cutaneous amyloidosis (p. 433), chronic folliculitis (p. 463), Kaposi's sarcoma (p. 1023) and syringocystadenoma papilliferum (p. 878).[77] They may be prominent at the lower edge of the dermal infiltrate in a subgroup of patients with mycosis fungoides (p. 1106),[82] and at the periphery of the rare entity known as inflammatory pseudotumor. This latter has the low-power appearance of a lymph node with variable central fibrosis, but there are no sinuses present.[83–85]

Plasma cells are a less consistent feature in certain deep fungal infections, cutaneous lupus erythematosus, rosacea, scleroderma, pseudolymphoma, persistent light reactions, in drug reactions[86] and the reaction to certain arthropods.[81] A panniculitis rich in plasma cells may be seen in scleroderma, morphea profunda, dermatomyositis and Sjögren's syndrome. Rarely, they are present in lichen planus.[87] Plasma cells are a diagnostic feature of one variant of Castleman's disease (p. 1064). Plasma cells are often present in the stroma of various tumors such as squamous cell carcinomas and basal cell carcinomas, and malignant melanomas, particularly if ulceration has occurred.

PLASMACYTOMAS AND MULTIPLE MYELOMA

Cutaneous plasmacytomas are rare monoclonal proliferations of plasma cells which are usually associated with underlying multiple myeloma, extramedullary (soft tissue) plasmacytomas or, rarely, plasma cell leukemia.[88,89] These secondary cutaneous plasmacytomas are usually multiple. They may arise by direct spread from an underlying tumor deposit in bone or soft tissue, or by metastatic spread via lymphatics or blood vessels.[90] Cutaneous plasmacytomas develop in only a small percentage of cases of multiple myeloma and of extramedullary plasmacytoma.[88,90–92] They are a bad prognostic sign.[90,93] Sometimes cutaneous lesions are the presenting sign of multiple myeloma and, rarely, they may antedate the development of the full-blown disease.[94]

It has been suggested that IgA- and IgD-producing plasmacytomas are disproportionately represented in the skin.[95]

Primary cutaneous plasmacytomas, which by definition arise without concomitant bone marrow or soft tissue disease, are exceedingly rare.[96–99] They usually grow slowly and are solitary; multiple lesions are sometimes present.[100–103] The prognosis is not as good as previously thought: visceral metastases and death occur in over one-third of cases.[104,105]

Plasmacytomas are dusky red or violaceous dome-shaped nodules which measure 1–5 cm in diameter. They have a predilection for the trunk, but they may also develop on the extremities and the face.

Multiple myeloma

Multiple myeloma (myelomatosis) is a malignant proliferation of plasma cells that typically involves the bone marrow but may also involve other tissues.[106] It usually presents with bone pain, anemia, renal insufficiency, hypercalcemia and proteinuria.[106] A monoclonal spike is found in the electrophoretic pattern of the serum, and sometimes of urine, in which Bence Jones protein may also be detected. Amyloidosis may subsequently develop. Cutaneous manifestations of multiple myeloma include the development of xanthomas, amyloid deposits, non-specific erythemas, pyoderma gangrenosum-like lesions, cutaneous infections, including herpes zoster, and hemorrhagic lesions.[106,107]

Histopathology

Cutaneous plasmacytomas are circumscribed non-encapsulated dense infiltrates of plasma cells, situated usually in the reticular dermis but sometimes involving the subcutis as well. The epidermis is often stretched over the deposit, but ulceration is uncommon. The plasma cells show variable maturation (Fig. 40.2). Russell bodies are often present in lesions with many mature plasma cells. In secondary and rapidly growing primary lesions there is more variation in the size and the maturation of the plasma cells, with some binucleate cells and scattered mitoses.[108] Sometimes the cells are immature and resemble immunoblasts or the cells of a malignant lymphoma. These cases with dedifferentiated cells are now classified as lymphoplasmacytoid lymphomas or immunocytomas.[109] Their monoclonal nature can be confirmed by immunohistochemistry. Occasional plasmacytomas are polyclonal.[110] The specific plasma cell antibody PC-1, and CD79a can be used for their confirmation.[77] Plasmacytomas are often negative for CD45 and can be cytokeratin positive, leading to an erroneous interpretation of cancer. The cells do not usually express B-lineage cell surface markers such as L26

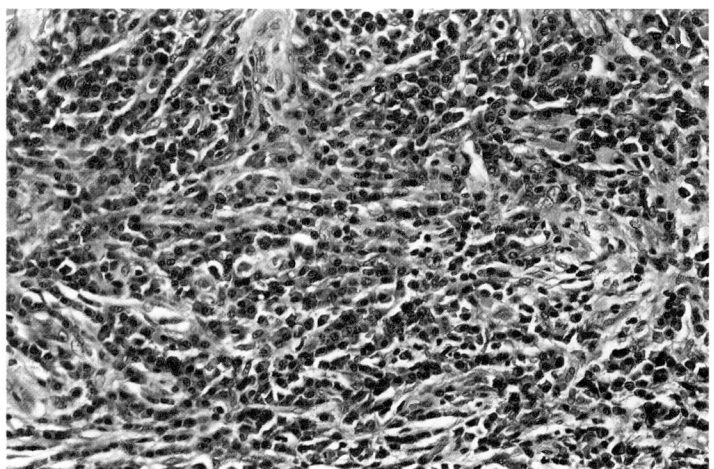

Fig. 40.2 **Plasmacytoma** composed of mature plasma cells. (H & E)

(CD20).[105] The methyl green–pyronin stain, in which the cytoplasm of plasma cells stains red, may be used to confirm the cell type in less well differentiated deposits.[111]

There is one report of needle-like crystalloid inclusions, possibly representing phagocytosed protein, in the cytoplasm of macrophages that were admixed with the plasma cells.[112] A further report documents a patient with myeloma with crystalline deposits in the skin, but without accompanying plasma cells.[113] Amyloid is another uncommon finding in the cutaneous lesions.

Electron microscopy
The immature plasma cells found in some rapidly growing plasmacytomas and cutaneous deposits of multiple myeloma have less abundant rough endoplasmic reticulum than do mature cells.[104]

Cutaneous disorders associated with paraproteinemias
A heterogeneous group of cutaneous diseases have been associated with multiple myeloma or with a monoclonal gammopathy. These include necrobiotic xanthogranuloma, xanthoma disseminatum, generalized plane xanthomas, lichen myxedematosus and scleromyxedema, scleredema, erythema elevatum diutinum, subcorneal pustular dermatosis, pyoderma gangrenosum, dermatitis herpetiformis, a subepidermal bullous dermatosis,[114] acquired angioedema, angioimmunoblastic lymphadenopathy, cutaneous T-cell lymphoma, mycosis fungoides, and the Sézary syndrome.[115]

A monoclonal protein is present in approximately 75% of cases of the POEMS syndrome (*polyneuropathy, organomegaly, endocrinopathy, M-protein and skin lesions*).[116–118] The cutaneous lesions include hyperpigmentation, hypertrichosis and skin thickening. Xanthoma cells have been described in the hyperpigmented patches of one patient.[119]

In Schnitzler's syndrome there is chronic urticaria associated with macroglobulinemia, but criteria for the diagnosis of Waldenström's disease (see below) are lacking.[120]

WALDENSTRÖM'S MACROGLOBULINEMIA

Waldenström's macroglobulinemia is a lymphoproliferative disorder of the elderly in which IgM-producing lymphoplasmacytoid cells proliferate in the bone marrow and/or lymph nodes and spleen.[121,122] Clinical features include weight loss, weakness, anemia and a bleeding diathesis.

Cutaneous manifestations are usually non-specific and result from hyperviscosity of the blood and the bleeding tendency. They include purpura, discoloration of the fingertips and toes, leg ulcers,[123] urticaria and angioedema.[124] Specific skin lesions are quite rare. They take the form of translucent papules composed of deposits of monoclonal IgM (macroglobulinosis cutis),[125,126] and of violaceous plaques, nodules or macular lesions on the face, trunk or proximal parts of the extremities; the plaques, nodules and macules are composed of lymphoplasmacytoid cells.[122,125,127,128] The cutaneous lesions usually develop later in the course of the disease, although they may be the presenting feature.[128]

Histopathology[121]
The rare translucent papules consist of eosinophilic hyaline deposits filling the papillary and upper reticular dermis. Artifactual clefts may be present.[125] Sometimes the material encases the hair follicles; it may undergo transepithelial elimination. The hyaline deposits are strongly PAS positive, but negative with stains for amyloid. They are monoclonal for IgM, using immunofluorescent techniques.

The plaques and tumors are composed of a dense infiltrate of lymphoplasmacytoid cells in the reticular dermis.[121] Occasional binucleate cells and mitotic figures are present. Some of the cells contain intranuclear inclusions which are PAS positive.[127] Hyaline material, which is monoclonal IgM, is sometimes present between the cells. IgM has also been reported along the basement membrane zone of both lesional and non-lesional skin.[129,130]

Electron microscopy
The hyaline deposits are composed of granular material which is electron dense. Fibrils are usually absent,[125,126] although they were present in one case.[131] The lymphoplasmacytoid cells in the infiltrative lesions have abundant ribosomes, and sometimes intranuclear inclusions composed of granular material.

SYSTEMIC AND CUTANEOUS PLASMACYTOSIS

'Systemic plasmacytosis' has been applied in cases with multiple brownish plaques, asymptomatic generalized lymphadenopathy and polyclonal hypergammaglobulinemia.[132–134] There is one report of a patient with systemic plasmacytosis later developing a nodal T-cell lymphoma.[135] The term 'cutaneous plasmacytosis' has been used for the skin lesions when lymphadenopathy is absent.[133,136–140] This distinction is somewhat artificial as rare cases of cutaneous plasmacytosis have subsequently developed systemic disease.[141]

Interleukin-6 (IL-6), thought to be a major plasma cell growth factor, has been increased in the serum in some cases.[142]

Histopathology
Systemic plasmacytosis is characterized by dense perivascular infiltrates in the dermis, composed of mature plasma cells and a small number of lymphocytes.[132] There is some resemblance to the lesions of secondary syphilis.

PLASMACYTOSIS MUCOSAE

An almost endless variety of terms has been used for comparable lesions involving the penis (plasma cell erythroplasia, balanitis circumscripta plasmacellularis, Zoon's balanitis), vulva (vulvitis circumscripta plasmacellularis, Zoon's vulvitis), lips (plasma cell cheilitis), and other mucosal surfaces (plasma cell orificial mucositis,[143,144] atypical gingivostomatitis,[145] plasmocytosis circumorificialis[146]). The term 'plasmacytosis mucosae' has the advantages of relative simplicity, of applying to all mucosal sites, and of indicating that plasma cells are an important component of the inflammatory infiltrate.

Plasmacytosis mucosae is a rare disorder which most frequently involves the glans penis of older men (Zoon's balanitis).[146–151] Vulval lesions (Zoon's vulvitis), which usually involve adults, are exceedingly rare, with fewer than 50 cases reported.[147,152–157] Genital lesions usually take the form of a solitary, asymptomatic, sharply defined red-brown glistening patch measuring 1–3 cm in diameter. Occasionally, several lesions may be present. A tumorous variant has also been described (plasmoacanthoma).[143]

The lesions are usually resistant to treatment, although circumcision has resulted in the disappearance of some lesions of the glans.[150] The etiology is unknown,[152] although herpes simplex antigen has been detected in rare cases[158] and one case has been associated with autoimmune polyglandular endocrine failure, raising the possibility of autoimmunity in the etiology.[159]

Histopathology[147]
There is a dense, often band-like infiltrate of inflammatory cells in the upper dermis, which may extend to the level of the mid-reticular dermis. The

infiltrate is composed predominantly of polyclonal plasma cells,[143,144,151] sometimes containing Russell bodies. There may also be lymphocytes, mast cells, occasional eosinophils and even neutrophils in the infiltrate. The presence of lymphoid follicles is a rare event.

Blood vessels are prominent, with an increase in number and some dilatation. There is often extravasation of erythrocytes. Deposits of hemosiderin may be present, although they have not been a feature of non-genital lesions. With time, there is some fibrosis.

The overlying epidermis is usually attenuated; frank ulceration occurs in only a minority of cases (Fig. 40.3). The epidermis is often mildly edematous and may contain a few inflammatory cells and erythrocytes.

Electron microscopy[146]

The plasma cells in the infiltrate contain considerable rough endoplasmic reticulum. Phagolysosomes may be present. There are also macrophages containing siderosomes.

CASTLEMAN'S DISEASE

Castleman's disease (giant lymph node hyperplasia) is a distinctive lymphoid hyperplasia that occurs predominantly in the mediastinum of young to middle-aged persons.[160] There are two histological variants, a common hyaline vascular type and a less common plasma cell type, which often has systemic manifestations. A mixed variant, the intermediate type, also occurs.

Cutaneous manifestations are usually non-specific. They include plane xanthomas and vasculitis.[161] Cutaneous involvement is exceedingly rare, with only a few cases reported.[160,162] An association with POEMS syndrome (see above) has been recorded.[163]

The pathogenesis is unknown, but elevated levels of interleukin-6, a cytokine necessary for the maturation of B lymphocytes into plasma cells, are often present. Interleukin-6 also stimulates endothelial hyperplasia.[164] Human herpesvirus type 8 (HHV-8) has been implicated in the etiology of multicentric Castleman's disease.[165]

Histopathology

Cutaneous cases are so rare that few histological reports exist. Reported cases have had a circumscribed nodule composed of ill-defined lymphoid follicles with a mantle of small lymphocytes giving an 'onion-skin' appearance. These mantles were traversed by hyalinized capillary-sized vessels. The interfollicular zones were composed of lymphocytes, and plasma cells of polyclonal type.[160]

ANGIOPLASMOCELLULAR HYPERPLASIA

Two cases of the apparently unique condition of angioplasmocellular hyperplasia have been reported. Lesions are composed of a proliferation of small blood vessels, some with vacuolated cytoplasm, and a mixed inflammatory cell infiltrate with a predominance of polyclonal plasma cells.[166] The lesions presented as solitary nodules on the trunk.

MAST CELL INFILTRATES

Although an increase in mast cells is seen in a variety of inflammatory dermatoses and some tumors, the presence of large numbers of these cells is almost confined to mastocytosis. Aspects of the normal mast cell will be considered before describing the pathological conditions.

Mast cells

Mast cells, which measure 8–15 μm in diameter, are round, oval or fusiform in shape and have a central nucleus and cytoplasm which contains lightly basophilic granules.[167] The granules stain metachromatically with the toluidine blue and Giemsa methods. They are orthochromatic (a mixture of blue and red) with an alcian blue–safranin method[168] and orange-red using an enzymatic method (chloroacetate esterase).[169] In formalin-fixed material, toluidine blue may fail to stain up to 20% of mast cells.[170,171] Carnoy's medium appears to be a better fixative than formol saline for their demonstration.[168] Mast cells express tryptase, leukocyte common antigen (CD45), CD43, CD68, MCG-35[172] and CD117, the *c-kit* encoded tyrosine kinase receptor protein.[173,174] Recently, microphthalmia transcription factor has also been detected in mast cells.[175]

The role of genetics in mast cell proliferations has centered on the *c-kit* proto-oncogene which, as mentioned above, encodes a tyrosine kinase transmembrane receptor that is expressed on many cells including mast cells, hemopoietic stem cells and also melanocytes.[176] Its role in piebaldism is mentioned elsewhere (see p. 322). The *c-kit* mutations have been found in sporadic adult mastocytosis and in children at risk for extensive or persistent disease, but not in typical pediatric mastocytosis.[177–180] The *c-kit* gene has been localized to chromosome 4q12.[176]

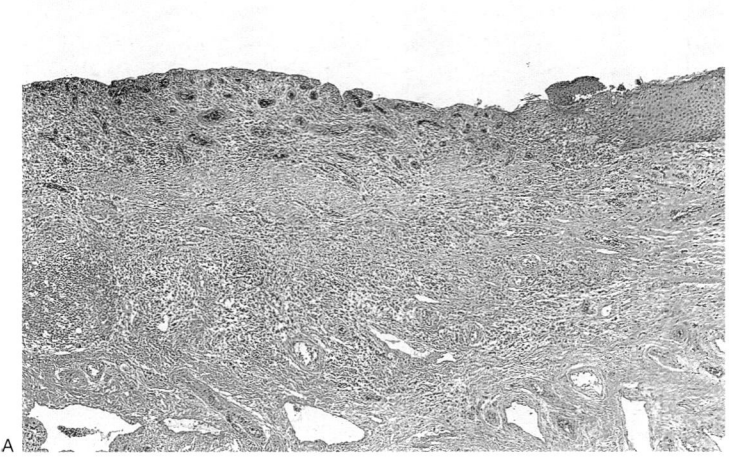
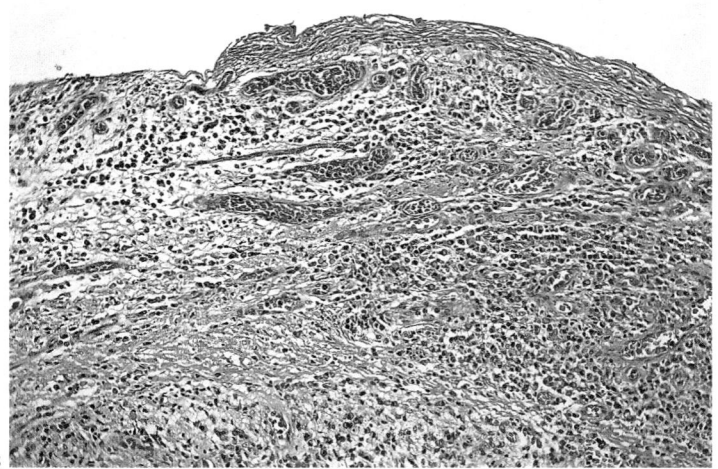

Fig. 40.3 **Zoon's balanitis. (A)** Ulceration is present. **(B)** There is increased vascularity and many plasma cells. (H & E)

In the skin, mast cells are usually found in the dermis with some accentuation around the superficial vascular plexus and appendages.[171,181] They vary in number in the skin of different parts of the body, being most abundant in that of the scrotum.[182] On average, there are approximately 7000 mast cells/mm³ of skin.[183] Mast cells in the mucosa are smaller and contain fewer granules than those in the dermis.[184]

On ultrastructural examination the cytoplasm of mast cells contains 80–300 membrane-bound granules, which are modified lysosomes with a highly structured internal architecture and which appear in sections as whorls or scrolls.[185] Mast cell granules are larger in black skin than in white skin. This larger size appears to result from fusion of granules.[186] Other organelles include mitochondria, lipid droplets, microfilaments and, rarely, melanosomes.[187] There are numerous microvilli projecting from the cell surface, and in mastocytosis these interdigitate with the projections of adjacent cells.[185]

Mast cells, which are derived from a bone marrow stem cell that expresses CD34, produce a variety of pharmacologically active agents which may be preformed or which may form in the cytoplasmic granules in response to various stimuli.[184,188–190] These agents include substances with vasoactive and smooth muscle contracting properties such as histamine, leukotrienes (B_4, C_4, D) and prostaglandin D_2. These substances may be responsible for the pruritus, flushing and syncope that sometimes occur in mast cell disease.[184] Mast cells also manufacture chemotactic factors, enzymes (neutral proteases, acid hydrolases) and heparin. Mast cell degranulation, with release of these substances, is a calcium-dependent process triggered by chemical, physical and immunological stimuli.[188] Mast cells have numerous surface receptors for the Fc part of IgE, and this is responsible for mediating their immunological degranulation.[188,191] One of these receptors (FcεRI), on stimulation, results in the release of an array of cytokines, including various interleukins, interferon-γ, tumor necrosis factor-α and granulocyte–macrophage colony-stimulating factor.[192] Other categories of surface receptors are present, including cytokine receptors and integrins.

The exact role of mast cell growth factor (MGF) in humans remains to be clarified. It is produced by keratinocytes and fibroblasts. It stimulates not only mast cell proliferation but also melanocyte proliferation and melanin pigment production in vitro.[189] This might explain the hyperpigmentation overlying mast cell lesions.

Mast cell hyperplasias

Mast cells appear to participate in nearly all diseases of connective tissue. They are present in wound healing, keloids, chronic inflammation, parasitic infestations, urticarias, atopic eczema, lichen planus, psoriasis, Behçet's syndrome, pretibial myxedema, scleroderma and lichen simplex chronicus, to name just some of the conditions in which mast cells are increased.[183,185,192] They are also increased in the stroma of neurofibromas and other neural tumors, and in mycosis fungoides and basal cell carcinomas.[185] Mast cells are sometimes found in the epidermis in various dermatoses.[193]

Mast cell degranulation has been incriminated in the pathogenesis of the pruritus that occurs in polycythemia rubra vera.[194] This process has also been suggested as a possible cause of the pruritus in chronic renal failure, although in one study there was no correlation between mast cell numbers and the presence or absence of pruritus in patients undergoing hemodialysis for chronic renal failure.[195] Furthermore, antihistamines are unhelpful in controlling the symptoms.[196,197]

MASTOCYTOSIS

Mastocytosis comprises a spectrum of related diseases in which there is an increase in mast cells in one or more organs.[184] It usually occurs as a sporadic disease that is often transient and limited in children and progressive in adults.[179] Monoclonality has been reported.[198] There may be symptoms, such as pruritus, related to the release of various products from these cells. Mastocytosis can be classified as follows:

- *Cutaneous mastocytosis*
  Urticaria pigmentosa
  Solitary mastocytoma
  Diffuse cutaneous mastocytosis
  Telangiectasia macularis eruptiva perstans (TMEP)
- *Systemic mastocytosis*
  With cutaneous lesions
  With extracutaneous lesions only
- *Malignant mast cell disease*
  Malignant mastocytosis
  Mast cell leukemia.

Urticaria pigmentosa

Urticaria pigmentosa is the most common clinical variant of mastocytosis, accounting for approximately 80% of all cases.[199] It usually presents as a generalized eruption of multiple red-brown macules, or rarely papules, predominantly affecting the trunk, but sometimes also the extremities and head. There may be few lesions, which are widely scattered, or hundreds. They are pruritic in less than 50% of cases, although in the majority of cases lesions will develop a wheal and flare when rubbed (Darier's sign).[182] Onset of urticaria pigmentosa is in the first 4 years of life in 75% of cases.[200] Childhood cases have a good prognosis, usually without the occurrence of systemic involvement.[201,202] Most lesions clear by puberty in 80% of affected individuals. Vesiculation is a common transient change in lesions of infancy and childhood.[203,204] Adult-onset disease is marked by persistence of lesions, and the development of systemic disease in approximately 40% of cases.[188,205–207] Bone marrow involvement is common in adults with cutaneous mastocytosis.[208]

Rare clinical presentations of urticaria pigmentosa include a congenital bullous form,[178,209–211] the presence of yellowish lesions resembling xanthoma or pseudoxanthoma elasticum (xanthelasmoid mastocytosis),[212–214] and urticaria, dermatographism,[215] massive peripheral eosinophilia[216] or intractable pruritus without any obvious lesions.[217] Urticaria pigmentosa has been associated with multiple myeloma[218] and juvenile xanthogranuloma.[219] Sporadic familial cases occur.[210,220–223]

Solitary mastocytoma

Solitary lesions account for approximately 10% of childhood mastocytoses.[224] They may occur anywhere on the body, but there is a predilection for the trunk and wrists. The palm is a rare site of involvement.[225] Small solitary lesions are sometimes called 'mast cell nevi', and the term 'mastocytoma' is reserved for larger nodular lesions, which may measure up to 3 cm in diameter.[188] Solitary lesions tend to involute spontaneously, and there is usually no indication for surgical removal.

Diffuse cutaneous mastocytosis

Diffuse cutaneous mastocytosis is a very rare variant that usually begins in early infancy with thickening of the skin, which may be erythematous or yellow-brown in color.[226–229] Pruritus and blistering are common, and the bullae that form are more persistent than in urticaria pigmentosa of childhood. Leathery (pachydermatous) lesions may be present.[179,230] Nodules may develop within the thickened skin, but this does not necessarily indicate a bad prognosis.[231] Systemic involvement is common.[179]

TMEP

TMEP is the universally accepted short designation for telangiectasia macularis eruptiva perstans, a rare adult form of mastocytosis with a high incidence of systemic involvement.[232,233] Childhood cases have been reported.[234] Erythema and telangiectasia are found in faintly pigmented macules on the trunk and proximal parts of the extremities.[167] Facial involvement has been reported.[235,236] Multiple myeloma is a rare association. It has been suggested that aberrations in the *c-kit* pathway may explain the abnormal proliferation of both lineages.[237]

Systemic mastocytosis

In systemic mastocytosis there is a proliferation of mast cells in various tissues apart from or in addition to the skin.[238] Systemic mastocytosis may develop in childhood cases of urticaria pigmentosa that persist beyond puberty, and in approximately 40% of adults with urticaria pigmentosa, usually of long standing.[200,205,239] It may also be associated with TMEP.[240,241] Cutaneous lesions are most common on the trunk, although all skin areas, including mucous membranes, may be involved. Papillomatous and verrucous lesions are rare findings.[242]

The bone marrow is the tissue most frequently involved in systemic mastocytosis, followed by the liver, spleen, gastrointestinal tract lymph nodes and, rarely, other organs.[238,243] Sometimes bone marrow is the only tissue involved besides the skin. Systemic mast cell disease without skin involvement is quite uncommon, and often difficult to diagnose.[232,238] However, the urinary excretion of the histamine metabolite methylimidazoleacetic acid is increased in cases of systemic mastocytosis.[184,244]

Systemic mastocytosis may progress to malignant mastocytosis and/or mast cell leukemia. Various lymphoproliferative and myeloproliferative conditions may sometimes eventuate,[245] particularly myelogenous leukemia.[232,246,247] The hypereosinophilic syndrome is a rare association.[248] It has been claimed that up to one-third of individuals with systemic mastocytosis may progress to malignancy, but this seems unduly pessimistic in the light of other studies, one of which showed that the clinical course of systemic mastocytosis was stable over a period of 10 years in all those followed.[205]

Malignant mast cell disease

There may be a progressive proliferation of atypical mast cells leading to the enlargement of various organs. This usually follows systemic mastocytosis, and has been called malignant mastocytosis and mast cell reticulosis.[249] The extremely rare mast cell sarcoma is a localized mass of malignant mast cells in the soft tissues.[249] Mast cell leukemia may develop in any of these settings or as a progression of systemic mastocytosis.[249] There is extensive bone marrow infiltration and atypical mast cells circulating in the peripheral blood.[250] It has a poor prognosis.[167]

Histopathology[167]

The histological pattern of mastocytosis is similar regardless of the clinical type, although there are major variations in the number of mast cells present.[250] The infiltrate is predominantly in the upper third of the dermis, at times in proximity to the dermoepidermal junction (Fig. 40.4).[250] In the usual macular lesions of *urticaria pigmentosa* the infiltrate may vary from sparse and perivascular to larger aggregates of mast cells. Perivascular mast cells may be cuboidal or fusiform in shape, whereas those in larger aggregates tend to be cuboidal (Fig. 40.5). A scattering of eosinophils is usually present, and there may be superficial edema in lesions that are rubbed prior to removal. Basal hyperpigmentation is a useful clue to the diagnosis of urticaria pigmentosa and some other types of mastocytosis.

In *solitary mastocytoma* there are dense aggregates of mast cells in the dermis, sometimes extending into its deeper levels and even into the subcutis.[167] Eosinophils may be present in small numbers; massive infiltration is a rare occurrence.[251] Localized necrobiosis and stromal fibrosis have been

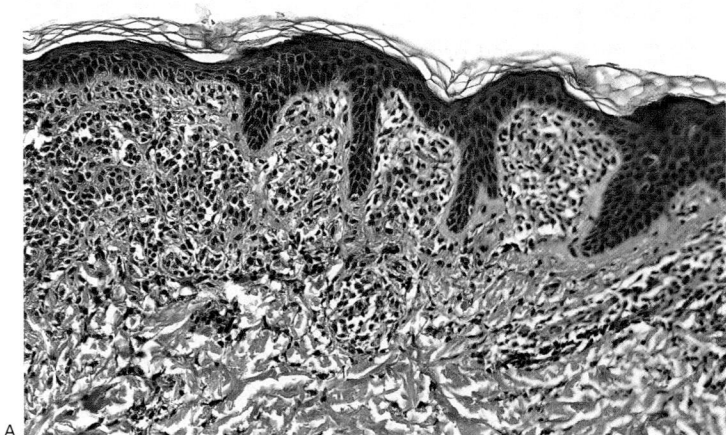
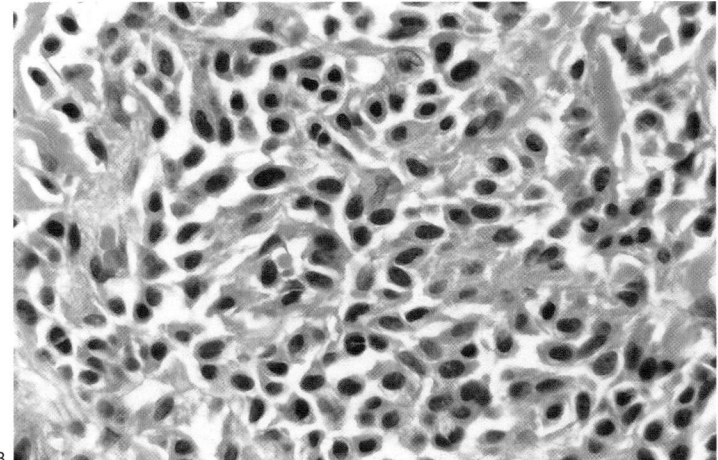

Fig. 40.4 **Urticaria pigmentosa. (A)** Mast cells fill the papillary dermis. **(B)** A higher power view of the mast cells. (H & E)

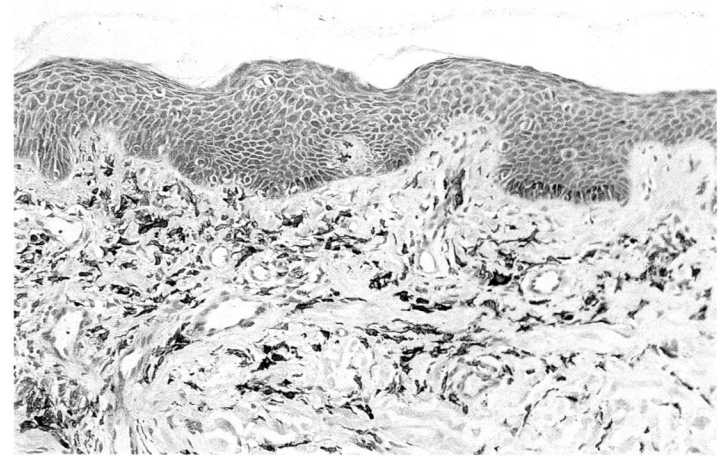

Fig. 40.5 **Urticaria pigmentosa.** Numerous mast cells are present in the upper dermis. There is also mild hyperpigmentation of the basal layer. (Toluidine blue)

reported.[252,253] In *TMEP* there may be only subtle alterations in mast cell numbers; the cells tend to be fusiform and loosely arranged around the dilated vessels of the superficial plexus (Fig. 40.6). Eosinophils are usually absent. In *diffuse cutaneous mastocytosis* there are loosely arranged mast cells throughout the dermis.[231] Fibrosis is sometimes present.[230] The mast cells are deeper in the dermis in the xanthomatous form.

Superficial edema leading to subepidermal vesiculobullous changes is common with mast cell lesions of infancy and childhood.[254] There may be eosinophils, mast cells and occasional neutrophils within the bullae, and a diffuse aggregate of mast cells in the upper dermis below the band of edema or the blister cavity.

Quantitative studies have shown that the number of mast cells in the cutaneous lesions of mastocytosis is from 2 to 160 times that in the adjacent normal skin.[170,255–257] Normal skin may contain up to 15 mast cells per high-power (×40) field. In TMEP, in which the increase may be subtle, it is often useful to have some normal skin at one end of the biopsy for comparison with lesional skin.[167] Qualitatively, the mast cells in mastocytosis resemble normal mast cells, with little atypia and only minor changes detected by morphometry.[258,259] They give the staining reactions described for normal mast cells; the choice of stain (toluidine blue, astra blue, Giemsa or chloroacetate esterase) often depends on individual preference. Immuno-histochemistry for CD117 has also been used.[173,260] In some cases of malignant mastocytosis the cells lack metachromatic granules and fail to stain with routine methods. The antitryptase antibody G3 will stain mast cells in these circumstances.[261]

Electron microscopy

The ultrastructural features of normal mast cells have been described earlier. In mastocytosis the cells have prominent surface projections which inter-digitate with adjacent cells. Other reported findings include giant cytoplasmic granules[262,263] and mast cells with endocytic and autophagic vacuoles.[264] A blue nevus combined with a mastocytoma has been reported, with some cells containing both melanosomes and mast cell granules.[265]

BRACHIORADIAL PRURITUS

Brachioradial pruritus is a rare tropical dermatosis that presents with a chronic intermittent intense pruritus localized to the elbow region in the vicinity of the brachioradialis muscle.[266–269] Sometimes the lateral surface of the upper part of the arm, just below the midpoint, is involved.[270,271] The pruritus, which may be unilateral or bilateral, is often accompanied by a burning sensation.[266] It progressively worsens towards evening.[272] Affected individuals are sometimes referred to a psychiatrist because there is little to see clinically except for mild poikilodermatous mottling suggestive of solar damage.[271]

This condition is seen in Caucasians living in tropical and subtropical climates, suggesting that exposure to the sun is of etiological importance.[266,273] It is therefore regarded as a solar dermopathy and part of the spectrum of solar pruritus.[274–277] However, in some patients clinical improvement has been achieved by cervical spine manipulation, suggesting that in these patients there may be a component of nerve damage from cervical spine disease.[278–280]

Histopathology

Little may be observed on a casual examination of a biopsy. Closer inspection will usually reveal mild, patchy hyperpigmentation of the basal layer with minimal melanin incontinence, mild telangiectasia of superficial blood vessels, and occasional mononuclear cells around dermal vessels and appendages (Fig. 40.7).[271] There is also some solar elastosis.

Stains for mast cells reveal that many of the mononuclear cells are mast cells, and although their increase in number is marginal, they are usually quite plump and contain numerous cytoplasmic granules.[271] This applies particularly to the mast cells in the vicinity of the pilosebaceous follicles and eccrine glands.

HISTIOCYTIC INFILTRATES (NON-LANGERHANS CELL)

The histiocytic infiltrates are a heterogeneous group of disorders which were also known, in the past, as the 'non-X histiocytoses' because the infiltrating cells lack Birbeck granules (Langerhans bodies) and other markers of Langerhans cells, which are the cells found in histiocytosis X.[281–283] Contemporary classifications now regard Langerhans cells as one class of histiocyte, indicating that our concepts have gone 'full circle'. For convenience, the Langerhans cell histiocytes will be considered later in this chapter.

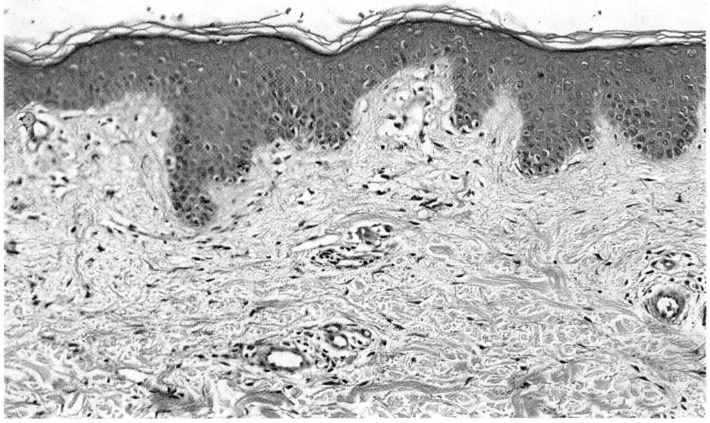

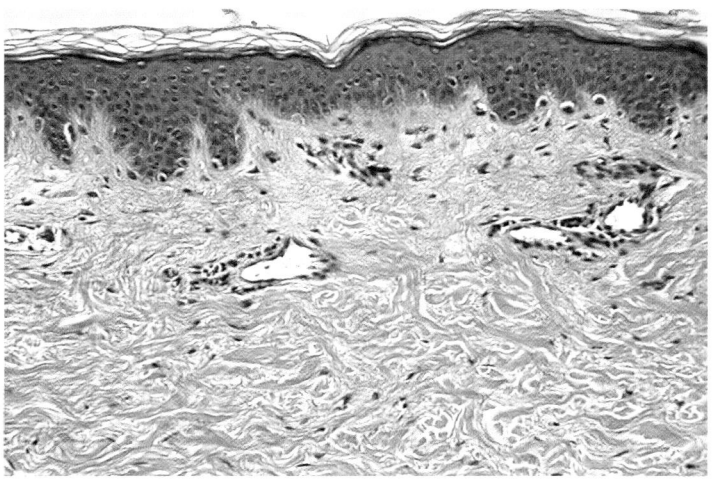

Fig. 40.6 Telangiectasia macularis eruptiva perstans (TMEP). The mast cells are predominantly perivascular in location. The blood vessels are not as telangiectatic as usual. (H & E)

Fig. 40.7 **Brachioradial pruritus.** A few lymphocytes and mast cells surround the telangiectatic vessels in the upper dermis. (H & E)

Histiocytes

The histiocyte is a somewhat controversial cell which still lacks precise definition.[284-287] The term 'histiocyte' has been used in the past for almost any cell with a reniform or indented nucleus, a diameter of 10–25 μm, and a nuclear/cytoplasmic ratio of about 1:1.[284] The advent of immunohistochemistry, with the use of various monoclonal antibodies, has allowed the more precise characterization of cells that resemble each other morphologically. These studies have confirmed that the term 'histiocyte' has been used in the past for a variety of cells, including Langerhans cells and other immune accessory cells and certain subsets of T and B lymphocytes.[284]

In 1997, the Histiocyte Society in conjunction with the WHO Committee on Histiocytic/Reticulum Cell Proliferations published what they called a 'Contemporary Classification of Histiocytic Disorders'.[288] They defined histiocytes as 'a group of immune cells, familiar to morphologists, that includes macrophages and dendritic cells'. They pointed out that macrophages and dendritic cells were polar representatives of one common regulatory system. The origin of the various histiocytes is still controversial but it appears that the macrophage, the indeterminate cell and the Langerhans cell are derived from the CD34+ hemopoietic progenitor, while the dermal dendrocyte is derived from cutaneous mesenchymal (fibroblastic) precursors, although a hemopoietic source has also been proposed.[288] The various types of histiocyte express different antigens that assist in their distinction. They are shown in Table 40.3.

Whereas Langerhans cells and indeterminate cells stain positively for S100 protein and CD1a, cells of the monocyte–macrophage system stain with the CD11B, CD11C, CD14, CD68, HAM-56 and Mac387 antibodies, although Mac387 lacks sensitivity.[288-291] Lysozyme may also be present in these cells. Another marker, MS-1, a high molecular weight extracellular protein specific for sinusoidal endothelial cells and dendritic perivascular macrophages, is expressed by the cells of the various histiocytic tumors but not by Langerhans cells or the palisading histiocytes of granuloma annulare.[292] Although the non-Langerhans histiocytes are usually considered to be S100 negative, scattered cells in some tumors may be positive.[293]

As further immunohistochemical studies come to hand, using expanded panels of monoclonal markers, it may be necessary to recategorize some of these entities.[294] Furthermore, some cases have been reported which defy orderly classification, despite being studied by means of various immunohistochemical markers.[295-300]

As mentioned above, a new classification of histiocytic disorders was published by the Histiocyte Society/WHO group in 1997.[288] As it applies to all body systems, a modified version covering the skin is shown in Table 40.4. It can be seen that many of the diseases to be discussed in this section are dismissed as 'related disorders' of juvenile xanthogranuloma. Unfortunately, it is difficult to classify all of these conditions into one of the various categories of the histiocytoses because of conflicting immunohistochemical results for some of the rarer entities. An attempt will be made to do this below, based on current knowledge. Before doing so, it is worth noting the approach of Zelger and colleagues to this confusing topic.[301] They have attempted a morphological classification of most of the non-Langerhans histiocytoses of presumed dendritic origin. A modified version of their classification is shown in Table 40.5.

The various non-Langerhans histiocytoses will be discussed in the order given below. The categorization is based on the author's interpretation of the current Histiocyte Society/WHO classification and supplemented by published papers,[288,301,302] notwithstanding the problems posed by some apparent discrepancies in published immunohistochemical results. It should be noted that a recent paper has suggested that the plasmacytoid monocyte, rather than the dermal dendrocyte, is the cell of origin of juvenile xanthogranuloma.[303] Other tumors in this same category would presumably have a similar origin.

- *Non-Langerhans histiocytoses of dendritic origin*
  Juvenile xanthogranuloma (including spindle-cell xanthogranuloma)
  Benign cephalic histiocytosis
  Progressive nodular histiocytosis
  Xanthoma disseminatum
  Generalized eruptive histiocytoma
  Progressive mucinous histiocytosis
  Multicentric reticulohistiocytosis
  Reticulohistiocytoma
  Familial histiocytic dermatoarthritis
- *Non-Langerhans histiocytoses of disputed/uncertain origin*
  Necrobiotic xanthogranuloma
  Cutaneous atypical histiocytosis
  Indeterminate cell histiocytosis
- *Histiocytoses of macrophage origin*
  Rosai–Dorfman disease
  Hemophagocytic syndromes
- *Malignant histiocytoses*
  Malignant histiocytosis
- *Miscellaneous*
  Reactive histiocytoses.

Table 40.3 **Distinguishing features of cutaneous histiocytes**

Cell type	Features
Macrophage	CD45, CD14, CD68, lysozyme positive Also, often CD11b, CD11c, HAM-56, Mac387 positive S100, CD1a, factor XIIIa negative
Dermal dendrocyte	Factor XIIIa, CD45, CD68 positive S100, CD1a negative
Indeterminate cell	CD45, S100, CD1a positive Factor XIIIa negative (?) Birbeck granules absent
Langerhans cell	CD45, S100, CD1a, CD101 positive Factor XIIIa negative Birbeck granules present

Table 40.4 **Classification of histiocytic disorders***

Disorders of varied biological behavior

Dendritic cell-related
Langerhans cell histiocytosis
Juvenile xanthogranuloma and related disorders
Solitary histiocytomas with dendritic cell phenotypes

Macrophage-related
Hemophagocytic syndromes (primary and secondary)
Rosai–Dorfman disease
Solitary histiocytoma with macrophage phenotype

Malignant disorders

Monocyte-related (various leukemias)
Dendritic cell-related histiocytic sarcoma
Macrophage-related histiocytic sarcoma

*This classification is based on the Histiocyte Society/WHO classification of 1997, and excludes non-cutaneous diseases.[288]

Table 40.5 Morphological classification of non-Langerhans cell histiocytoses (after Zelger et al)[301]

Cell type	Histiocytoses
Vacuolated	Juvenile xanthogranuloma (mononuclear type)
	Benign cephalic histiocytosis
	Generalized eruptive histiocytosis
	Progressive mucinous histiocytosis
Xanthomatized	Papular xanthoma
	Xanthoma disseminatum (rare)
Spindle-shaped	Spindle-cell xanthogranuloma
	Progressive nodular histiocytosis
	Progressive mucinous histiocytosis
Scalloped	Xanthoma disseminatum
Oncocytic	Multicentric reticulohistiocytosis
Mixed	Juvenile and adult xanthogranuloma
	Reticulohistiocytoma
	Progressive mucinous histiocytosis

Regressing atypical histiocytosis was formerly included with this group, but is now regarded as a T-cell lymphoma on the basis of immunohistochemistry (see p. 1104).

It is becoming increasingly apparent that there is considerable overlap between the clinical and histopathological features of the various cutaneous histiocytoses, suggesting that they possibly represent one disease 'entity' with a wide spectrum of clinical presentations, rather than many discrete disorders.[304] This is particularly so for the non-Langerhans histiocytoses of presumed dendritic origin.

The lesion reported variously as reactive angioendotheliomatosis, intravascular histiocytosis and cutaneous histiocytic lymphangitis (see p. 1018) consists of dilated vascular channels containing histiocytic cells.

JUVENILE XANTHOGRANULOMA

Juvenile xanthogranuloma is a normolipemic histiocytosis composed of cells originally thought to be derived from dermal dendrocytes.[281,288,305–307] However, a recent study has suggested that the plasmacytoid monocyte is a more likely precursor.[303] Solitary or multiple red-brown papulonodules, 1–10 mm in diameter or larger, are found on the head and neck, upper part of the trunk and proximal parts of the limbs.[308,309] The sole of the foot is a rare site.[310] Atypical forms with extensive facial[311] or generalized eruptions[312–314] have been documented. In two-thirds of all cases onset is within the first 6–9 months of life,[315–318] but late onset in adolescence or adult life occurs in a small percentage of cases.[319–323] The term 'xanthogranuloma' or 'adult xanthogranuloma' is used for these cases. Spontaneous involution usually occurs after many months or even years; lesions persist in some individuals who develop their first lesions after the age of 20 years.[324,325]

A small percentage of patients have ocular involvement;[315] visceral, including oral, involvement is exceedingly rare.[305,312,326,327] Rare cases involving a peripheral nerve have been reported.[328] Juvenile xanthogranuloma has been reported in association with neurofibromatosis (sometimes with associated juvenile chronic myelogenous leukemia),[329–332] Niemann–Pick disease (see p. 549),[333] and urticaria pigmentosa.[334]

Although the etiology of juvenile xanthogranuloma is unknown, studies have shown that cholesterol is the principal lipid in the lesions.[335] Furthermore, there are no unusual sterols present.[335]

Histopathology[308,336]

There is a nodular, poorly demarcated dense infiltrate of small histiocytes involving the dermis and sometimes the upper subcutis as well. Rarely, deep extension into skeletal muscle is present.[337,338] The cells are polygonal or spindle-shaped and plump, and have indistinct cytoplasmic borders. Mitoses are rare. Whereas early lesions are fairly monomorphous, with inconspicuous foam cells,[339–344] mature lesions contain foamy histiocytes and varying numbers of Touton cells (Figs 40.8 and 40.9). These cells have a less foamy periphery than those seen in other xanthomatous conditions. Small aggregates of foam cells may be seen in some cases, and fully xanthomatized variants also occur (Fig. 40.10). There are also scattered lymphocytes and neutrophils, rare plasma cells and sometimes eosinophils. Lesions of longer duration will show interstitial fibrosis and proliferating fibroblasts.

The lesion reported as a *spindle-cell xanthogranuloma* is best regarded as a histological variant of the adult form of xanthogranuloma. It is composed of spindle-shaped histiocytes arranged in a storiform pattern. Other mononuclear (xanthomatized, oncocytic, vacuolated and scalloped) and multinucleate (Touton) histiocytes are present.[345]

The *scalloped-cell xanthogranuloma* is another variant in which there is a predominance (>75% of all cells) of scalloped histiocytes. Such cells have an

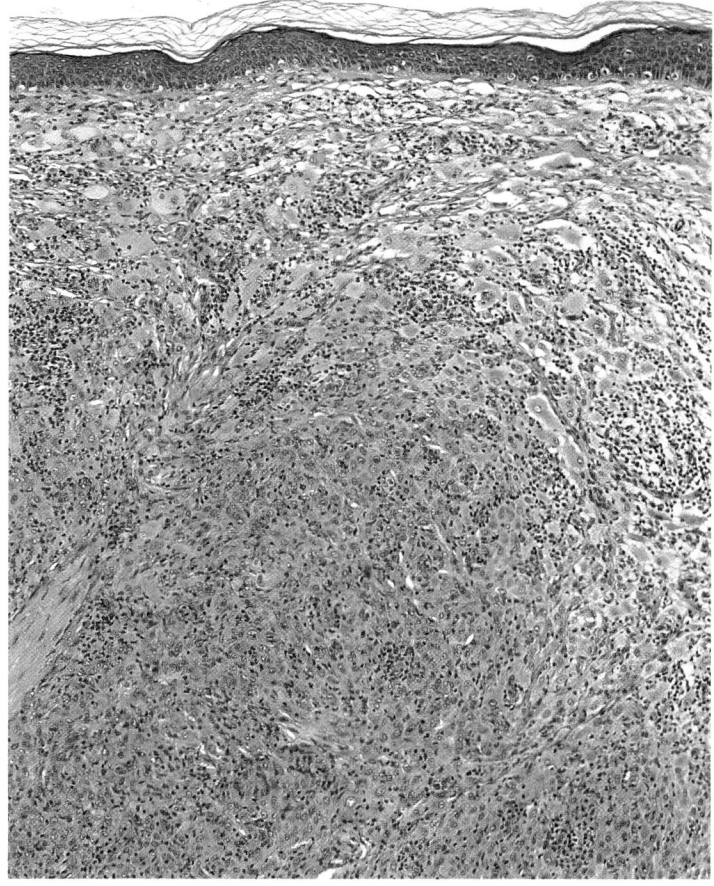

Fig. 40.8 **Juvenile xanthogranuloma.** There is an admixture of several cell types forming a dense infiltrate. (H & E)

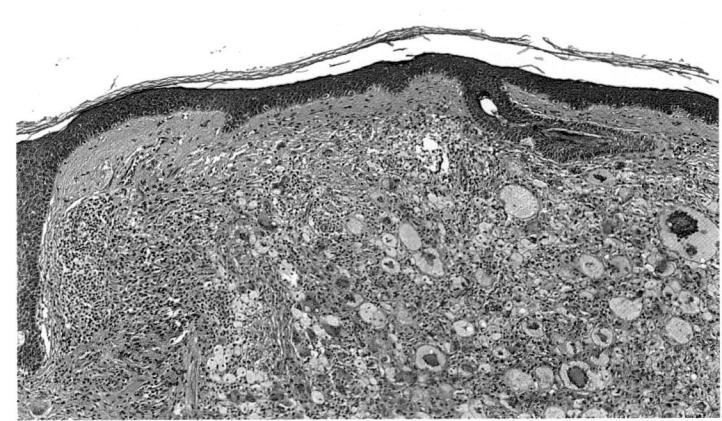

Fig. 40.9 **Juvenile xanthogranuloma.** The Touton giant cells, which are unusually large, are admixed with lymphocytes and histiocytes. (H & E)

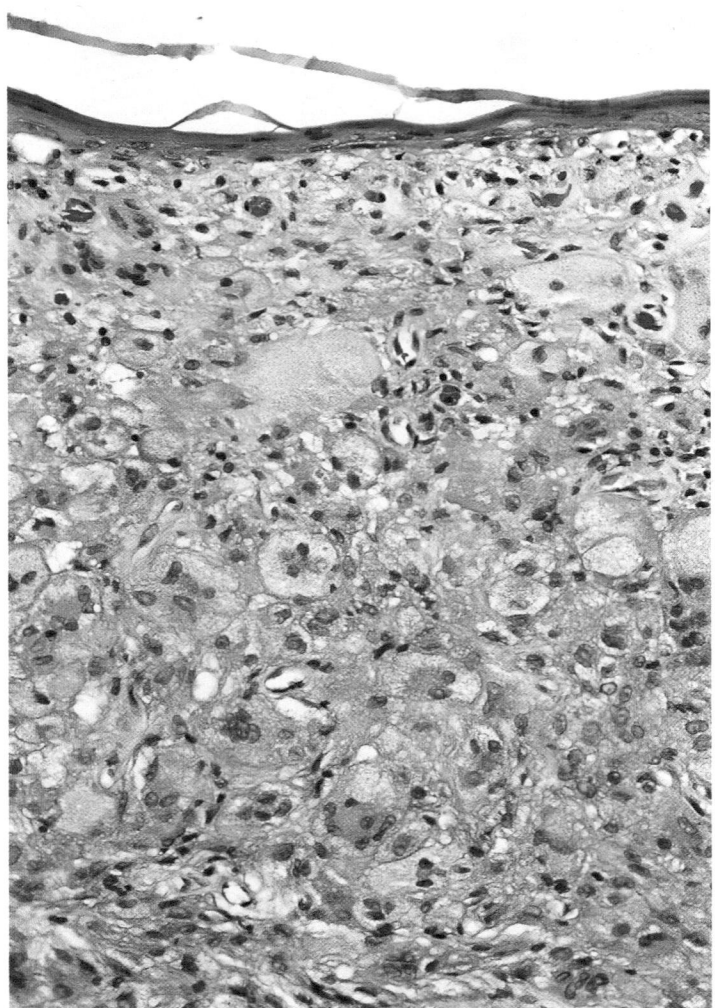

Fig. 40.10 **Juvenile xanthogranuloma.** There is prominent xanthomatization with epidermal atropy. (H & E)

angulated or scalloped border, set apart from one another in a delicate fibrous matrix.[346] The cytoplasm of the cells is homogenous and slightly eosinophilic while the nucleus is round to oval and large.

Fat stains confirm the presence of some lipid. Hemosiderin has been demonstrated in a few cases.[347] The histiocytes are usually positive for CD68, HAM-56, HHF35, cathepsin B, vimentin, factor XIIIa, fascin, CD4, lysozyme and α_1-antichymotrypsin,[308] but negative for Mac387, smooth muscle actin, CD34, CD1a and S100 protein.[312,336] Approximately 1–10% of the other cells in any lesion are S100 positive.[348] Such cells are elongated or dendritic in appearance.[319] Staining for the various markers listed above may be more intense at the periphery of the lesion.

It has been suggested that the deep forms are derived from dermal indeterminate cells (CD1a positive, S100-protein negative), but this is based on only one study.[349] These two markers were not studied in a recent series of three deep cases; the cells were CD68 and factor XIIIa positive.[350]

Electron microscopy[306,351,352]

Ultrastructural examination of mature lesions has shown lipid vacuoles (often without a limiting membrane), lysosomes, cholesterol clefts and myeloid bodies, but no Birbeck granules. Early lesions have only a few lipid-laden cells and there are complex interdigitations of the cell membrane.[353] Fibroblastic cells have also been noted in some lesions.[354]

BENIGN CEPHALIC HISTIOCYTOSIS

Benign cephalic histiocytosis is a clinically distinct non-lipid 'non-X' histiocytic proliferation in children.[355–358] Only 30 cases have been reported. It is characterized by the development of asymptomatic red-brown maculopapules, 2–5 mm or more in diameter, on the face, whence the condition may evolve to affect the neck, upper part of the trunk, arms, and other parts of the body.[359,360] The palmoplantar regions, mucous membranes and viscera are spared;[355] however, a case with diabetes insipidus has recently been reported.[361] Spontaneous regression, complete or partial, occurs during childhood, without scarring.[355,362] Similar lesions have been reported in an adult with T-cell lymphoma. The exact status of this case is uncertain.[363] There is increasing evidence that benign cephalic histiocytosis is a clinico-pathological variant of juvenile xanthogranuloma.[364,365]

Histopathology[355]

There is a diffuse infiltrate of histiocytes, mainly in the upper dermis and in close apposition to the undersurface of the epidermis. The cells have an oval or reniform vesicular nucleus and ill-defined pale cytoplasm.[356] There is usually no cytoplasmic lipid in the early stages of evolution, but xanthomatization can be seen in lesions of long duration.[364] Occasional multinucleate histiocytes are present. There are scattered or grouped lymphocytes within the infiltrate, and occasional eosinophils in some lesions. The histiocytes are negative for S100 protein and CD1a, but positive for CD68, CD11b, CD14, HAM-56 and factor XIIIa.[355,362,364]

Electron microscopy[355]

The most characteristic feature of the histiocytes is the presence of many coated vesicles, 500–1500 nm in diameter, in the cytoplasm. Comma-shaped inclusion bodies are present in 5–30% of the histiocytes.[366] No Birbeck granules or lipid droplets are present. Desmosome-like junctions are present between the histiocytes in densely cellular areas.[355]

PROGRESSIVE NODULAR HISTIOCYTOSIS

The term 'progressive nodular histiocytosis' has been used for a normolipemic histioxanthomatous syndrome in which multiple yellowish-brown papules and nodules develop on the skin and mucous membranes.[367–370] Similar lesions have been noted in a patient with acute myelomonocytic leukemia[371] and in another with chronic myeloid leukemia.[372] It has been suggested that all these cases are variants of, or closely related to, (juvenile) xanthogranuloma. Another confusing feature is the use of the term 'progressive nodular histiocytosis' for cases with morphological features of multicentric reticulohistiocytosis but an absence of the usual systemic symptoms of this disorder (see below).[306] Leonine facies have been present in the latter condition.[306,373,374] In the initial reports of the entity under discussion, the word 'histiocytoma' was used instead of 'histiocytosis' in the title.

Histopathology[282,368,371]

The nodules have a similar appearance to the cellular and fibrous patterns seen in a dermatofibroma. There are histiocytes, foam cells and spindle-shaped cells, sometimes arranged in a storiform pattern.[345] The cells are embedded in a delicate fibrocollagenous matrix. Touton cells may be present. There are usually no other inflammatory cells. Fat and hemosiderin can be demonstrated in the histiocytes with special stains.

Cells express vimentin, CD68, HAM-56 and factor XIIIa, but not CD34, CD1a or S100 protein. Variable staining occurs for Mac387, lysozyme, α_1-antitrypsin and smooth muscle actin.[345]

XANTHOMA DISSEMINATUM

Xanthoma disseminatum is a rare normolipemic histiocytic proliferation of dendrocyte origin. It presents with papules, nodules and plaques that have a predilection for flexural areas, the proximal parts of the extremities, and the trunk. The face is sometimes involved.[375] The lesions are initially reddish-brown in color but become yellow with time.[306] Mucosal lesions and transitory diabetes insipidus are present in approximately 40% of affected individuals.[376–378] Waldenström's macroglobulinemia was present in one case.[379] The condition runs a chronic but usually benign course. Widespread systemic involvement and death have been reported.[380,381]

Xanthoma disseminatum appears to be a clinically distinctive disorder in which there is a primary proliferation of histiocytes with subsequent accumulation of lipid.[382,383] It may represent an evolutionary form of generalized eruptive histiocytoma (see below) and as such be part of the spectrum of dendritic disorders related to (juvenile) xanthogranuloma.

Histopathology[376]

Histiocytes predominate in the early stages, but in established lesions there are histiocytes, foam cells, spindle cells, Touton cells and a moderate number of chronic inflammatory cells.[306] There may be phagocytosis of elastic fibers and sometimes of collagen by macrophages.[382] Siderosis is often observed, and this is quite prominent in the rare variant known as *xanthosiderohistiocytosis*.[384]

Immunohistochemical characterization of the cells has shown HLA-DR positivity but no staining for S100 protein, CD4 or CD1a.[385] The cells express CD68, CD14, CD11b, CD11c and factor XIIIa.[386,387] There is variable staining with Mac387.

Electron microscopy

The cells are similar to those seen in papular xanthoma and juvenile xanthogranuloma, but the plasma membranes of the foamy cells show many microvilli.[306] There are no Birbeck granules.

GENERALIZED ERUPTIVE HISTIOCYTOMA

Generalized eruptive histiocytoma is a rare histiocytosis, characterized clinically by the development of recurrent crops of hundreds of small reddish papules which are distributed symmetrically on the trunk and on the extensor surfaces of the extremities.[388–393] Approximately 30 cases have been reported. It has been documented in children as well as in adults.[388,389,394,395] Lesions usually subside spontaneously, leaving macular hyperpigmentation or no residual features. Evolution into xanthoma disseminatum has been reported, further evidence of the close interrelationship of the various non-Langerhans cell histiocytoses.[396]

Histopathology[391,392]

There is an infiltrate of histiocyte-like cells in the upper and mid dermis. Sometimes the cells are arranged in nests around blood vessels. They have pale cytoplasm and an oval nucleus. No lipid, iron or PAS-positive material is demonstrable in the cytoplasm. A few lymphocytes, and sometimes fibroblasts, are intermingled but there are usually no giant cells or xanthoma cells.[396] The histiocytes are negative for S100 protein and CD1a, but are positive for CD11b, CD14, CD36, factor XIIIa, CD68 and MS-1 protein.[389,396–398] This latter antigen has recently been found in all of the non-Langerhans cell histiocytoses tested. It is specific for sinusoidal endothelial cells and dendritic perivascular macrophages.[292] The cells in generalized eruptive histiocytoma show only patchy positivity for Mac387.[397] A case with some S100-positive cells has been regarded as an indeterminate cell variant.[399]

Benign cephalic histiocytosis and a case reported as 'benign non-X histiocytosis'[400] have features on light microscopy that are similar to those of generalized eruptive histiocytoma, but they differ clinically and ultra-structurally.[389] As mentioned earlier, many of the non-Langerhans histiocytoses of dendritic origin may be different expressions of the same histiocytosis.[390]

Electron microscopy

There are many dense bodies, some with myelin laminations, in the cytoplasm.[391] There are also occasional comma-shaped bodies and lipid droplets, but no Birbeck granules.[389,392]

PROGRESSIVE MUCINOUS HISTIOCYTOSIS

Progressive mucinous histiocytosis, a rare, non-Langerhans cell histiocytosis of childhood, was first described by Bork and Hoede in 1988.[401,402] It is characterized by a progressive eruption of skin-colored to red-brown papules with a predilection for the face and extremities. It appears to have an autosomal dominant mode of inheritance.[403]

Histopathology

There is a dermal infiltrate of epithelioid and spindle-shaped histiocytes, with the latter predominating in older lesions.[404] There are rare giant cells but no foam cells.[405] The cells are set in a collagenous stroma containing abundant mucin (Fig. 40.11). Mast cells can be quite numerous.[406] The cells stain for factor XIIIa, CD68 and vimentin, but not CD1a, S100 protein, CD34 or Mac387.[406]

Electron microscopy

Zebra and myeloid bodies are quite numerous in the cytoplasm of the histiocytes.

MULTICENTRIC RETICULOHISTIOCYTOSIS

Multicentric reticulohistiocytosis is an uncommon normolipemic histiocytosis that is characterized by the presence of an extensive papulonodular cutaneous eruption and a severe, sometimes destructive, arthropathy, the onset of which may precede, follow or accompany the eruption of skin

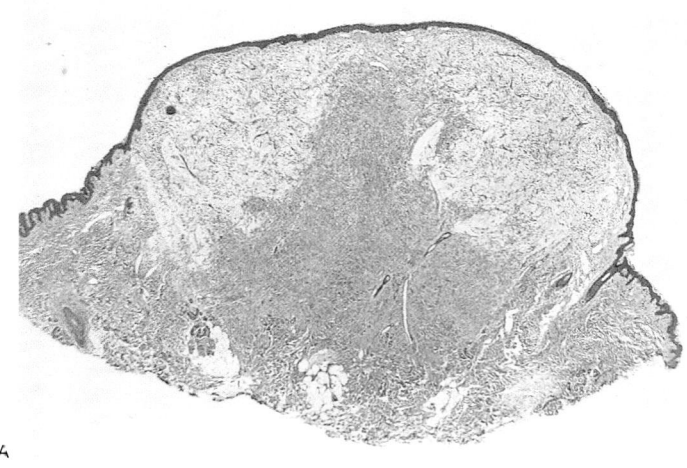

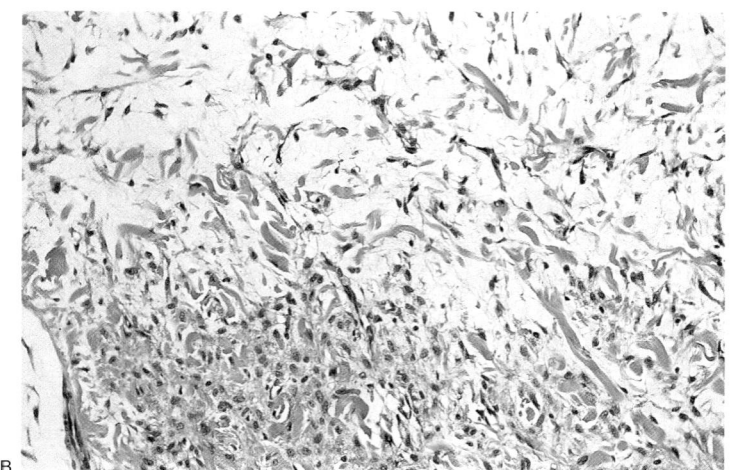

Fig. 40.11 **Mucinous histiocytosis. (A)** There are epithelioid and spindle-cell histiocytes set in a collagenous and mucinous stroma. **(B)** This area is at the interface between the mucinous and more cellular areas seen in (A). (H & E)

lesions.[407–410] The interphalangeal joints of the hands are usually affected. Oral, nasal and pharyngeal mucosae are often involved. There are isolated reports of infiltrates in lymph nodes, lungs, bone marrow, endocardium, stomach, salivary gland[411] and perirenal fat. Xanthelasmas of the eyelids are also common.[408]

The cutaneous lesions, which preferentially involve the face and distal parts of the upper extremities, are multiple brown-yellow papules and nodules measuring 0.3–2 cm in diameter. Rare presentations have included the presence of lesions resembling neurofibromatosis[412] and the localization of lesions to the sites of healed herpes zoster.[413] Onset of the disease is usually in middle life, and there is a predilection for females. Childhood onset is rare.[414] The clinical course is variable, with eventual spontaneous regression of the skin lesions after 5–10 years or more.[415] There may be residual joint impairment. Malignancies of various types may develop in up to 30% of cases.[409,416–418] Systemic vasculitis is rarely associated with multicentric reticulohistiocytosis.

A related entity is **diffuse (multiple) cutaneous reticulohistiocytosis**, in which multiple cutaneous lesions, identical histologically to those seen in multicentric reticulohistiocytosis, develop in the absence of arthritis or systemic lesions.[419–421] The terms 'reticulohistiocytoma' and 'reticulohistiocytic granuloma' have been used for solitary cutaneous lesions of similar histology (see below).

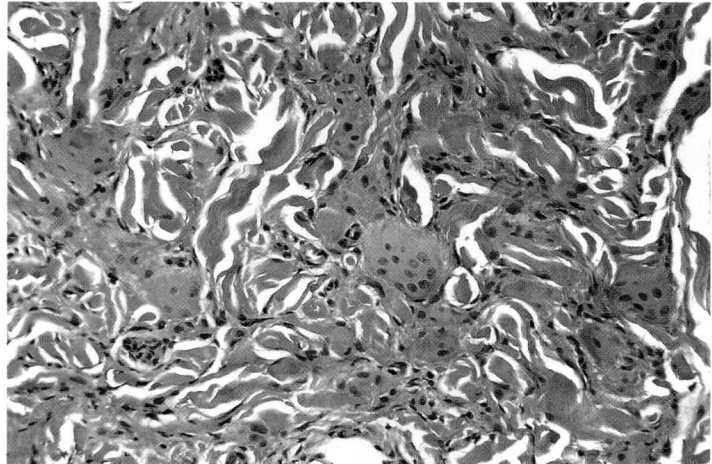

Fig. 40.12 **Multicentric reticulohistiocytosis.** The characteristic multinucleate giant cells are scattered through the collagen of the dermis. (H & E)

Histopathology[407,411,422]

There is a circumscribed non-encapsulated dermal and synovial infiltrate of mononuclear and multinucleate histiocytes with an eosinophilic, finely granular 'ground-glass' cytoplasm. The hallmark of the disease is the presence of the multinucleate cells, which measure 50 μm or more in diameter (Fig. 40.12). They have 3–10 or more nuclei, which may be placed haphazardly, or along the periphery, or clustered in the center of the giant cell. Mitoses are infrequent. Some giant cells may have foamy cytoplasm at the periphery. Phagocytosis of nuclear debris is uncommon. Transition from mononucleate to multinucleate forms can be seen.[423] Giant cells may be sparse in early lesions. The cytoplasm of the histiocytes contains PAS-positive diastase-resistant material, which usually stains with Sudan black as well.[407,424] Reticulin fibers can be demonstrated around individual cells.

Immunohistochemistry shows that the histiocytic cells express CD45, CD68, CD11b and HAM-56, but not S100 protein, Mac387 or CD1a.[419,425,426] There are reports of the cells expressing factor XIIIa, but in one of these cases the cells also stained for S100 protein, suggesting an unusual lineage.[427]

In addition to the histiocytes, small numbers of lymphocytes are scattered through the infiltrate. There may be some perivascular cuffing by lymphocytes in early lesions.[306] The walls of small blood vessels sometimes show 'onion-skin' thickening.[408]

Epidermal changes are variable. There is sometimes thinning of the epidermis overlying the lesion, with loss of rete ridges; ulceration is uncommon. Usually there is a narrow grenz zone of uninvolved collagen which separates the undersurface of the epidermis from the tumor nodule below.

Electron microscopy

The cytoplasm of the histiocytes is rich in organelles. A characteristic feature is the presence of innumerable rounded dense bodies with the morphological structure of lysosomes.[423] Lipid vacuoles are sometimes present, but there are no Birbeck granules.[411] Elastin and collagen in various stages of degeneration may be seen in the cytoplasm of some of the giant cells.[428,429] Intra- and extracytoplasmic long spacing collagen (type VI) has been reported in one case.[430]

RETICULOHISTIOCYTOMA

Reticulohistiocytomas (reticulohistiocytic granulomas) are nodular lesions 0.5–2 cm in diameter, with similar histology to the lesions of multicentric reticulohistiocytosis but without associated arthritis or systemic lesions.[410,431] They are usually solitary, but several may be present.[431–433] There is a predilection for the head and neck, but they may occur anywhere on the skin. Paraproteinemia accompanied several cutaneous nodules in one reported case.[432]

Histopathology[431]

There is a circumscribed dermal nodule, often with overlying epidermal thinning. As with multicentric reticulohistiocytosis, there is an irregular admixture of oncocytic mononuclear histiocytes, multinucleate giant cells with a ground-glass appearance, and inflammatory cells (Fig. 40.13). Phagocytosis of leukocytes is sometimes seen. A few Touton giant cells may be present and these may contain lipid. Reticulin fibers are increased and surround individual cells.

There is usually more of a neutrophilic infiltrate than in multicentric reticulohistiocytosis, and a further point of distinction is the greater propensity for the stroma in reticulohistiocytoma to have many spindle-shaped cells and for there to be xanthomatized cells.[426]

Immunohistochemistry suggests a dendritic cell lineage with staining for factor XIIIa, CD68, HAM-56, lysozyme, α_1-antitrypsin, CD11b and CD14. The cells are negative for CD1a, CD34 and smooth muscle actin.[426,434,435] Positive staining for S100 protein has been reported in several cases, but it is usually negative.[348,436]

FAMILIAL HISTIOCYTIC DERMATOARTHRITIS

Familial histiocytic dermatoarthritis is an exceedingly rare disorder that presents in childhood or adolescence as a papulonodular eruption on the face and limbs associated with a symmetrical destructive arthritis and ocular lesions. A closely related entity is the autosomal recessive dermo-chondro-corneal dystrophy reported in the French literature.[437]

Histopathology

There is a dermal infiltrate of mononuclear histiocytes admixed with some lymphocytes and plasma cells. There is no stored lipid or PAS-positive cytoplasmic material. Fibrosis is conspicuous in older lesions. Recently, two cases were reported in which multinucleate histiocytes were present. PAS-positive material was present in the cytoplasm. The authors suggested that these two

cases had features overlapping with both familial histiocytic dermatoarthritis and multicentric reticulohistiocytosis, which probably form part of a spectrum of dermatoarthritides.[437]

NECROBIOTIC XANTHOGRANULOMA

Necrobiotic xanthogranuloma, a rare chronic disorder, was first delineated by Kossard and Winkelmann in 1980.[438,439] It is characterized by the presence of multiple sharply demarcated nodules and large indurated plaques.[440] A solitary variant has been described.[441] Lesions are violaceous to red, with a partly xanthomatous hue. Central atrophy, ulceration and telangiectasia may develop. There is a predilection for the periorbital area, but other areas of the face, as well as the trunk and limbs, are often involved.[442,443]

Paraproteinemia has been present in nearly all the reported cases.[444–448] Other less frequent findings include leukopenia, bone marrow plasmacytosis, hypocomplementemia[449] and, occasionally, hyperlipidemia. Normolipemic plane xanthoma has been reported in association with necrobiotic xanthogranuloma, suggesting that the two conditions are part of a spectrum.[448,450] Ophthalmic complications are common and include scleritis, episcleritis and keratitis. Cardiac and laryngeal involvement has been recorded.[451,452] The clinical course is chronic and often progressive.[453]

Histopathology[454]

The distinctive changes are found in both the dermis and subcutis, and consist of broad zones of hyaline necrobiosis and granulomatous foci composed of histiocytes, foam cells and multinucleate giant cells (Fig. 40.14). The giant cells are of both Touton and foreign-body type, the latter often having bizarre features with irregular size, shape and distribution of the nuclei. Asteroid bodies and other inclusions are sometimes present.[455] The multinucleate cells may be present in the granulomas and dispersed near the zones of necrobiosis. Sometimes the Touton cells are prominent in the subcutis ('Touton-cell panniculitis'). Giant cells are occasionally quite sparse.[456] Blood vessels may be secondarily involved in the granulomatous process.

The amount of xanthomatization is variable, and sometimes the foam cell population is small.[456] Aggregates of histiocytes may extend into the papillary dermis, and there may be ulceration. Other less constant changes include the presence of cholesterol clefts,[457] rarely with surrounding palisaded granuloma formation, the presence of lymphoid nodules, sometimes with germinal

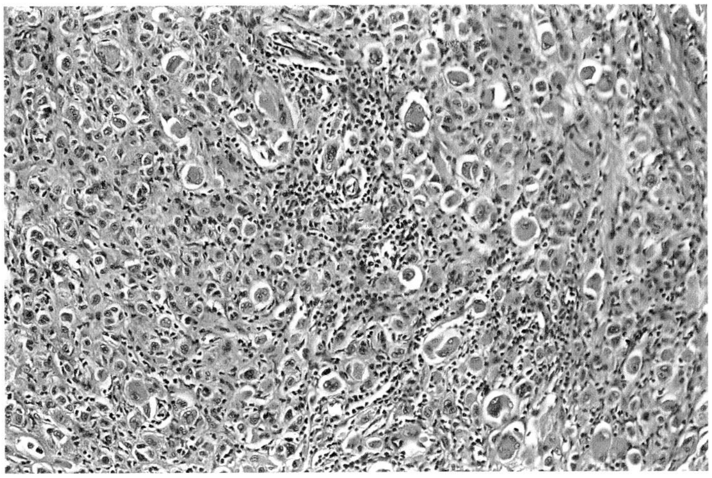

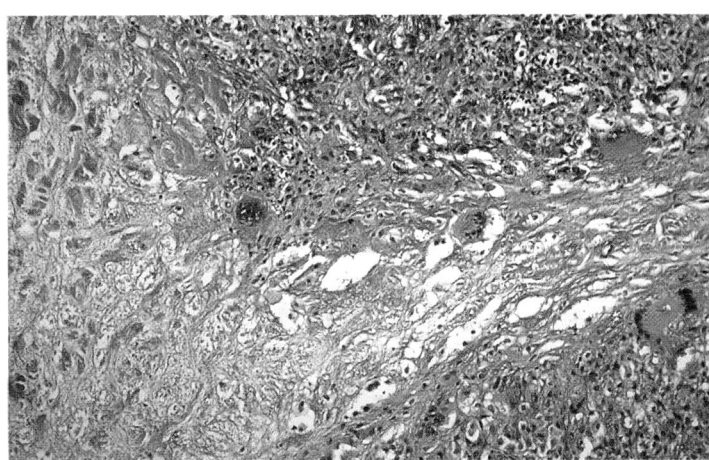

Fig. 40.13 **Solitary reticulohistiocytoma** composed of multinucleate giant cells, histiocytes and lymphocytes. There is some fibrosis of the stroma. (H & E)

Fig. 40.14 **Necrobiotic xanthogranuloma.** A zone of necrobiosis is surrounded by multinucleate giant cells and some histiocytes. (H & E)

centers, and plasma cell collections. Eosinophils are rare. Transepithelial elimination of cholesterol crystals and cellular debris has also been documented.[445] The process is more cellular and has more atypical and prominent giant cells than necrobiosis lipoidica.

Histochemical findings include scant mucin in areas of necrobiosis, sparse or absent elastic fibers, focal lipid droplets in giant cells and histiocytes and in some areas of necrobiosis, and PAS-positive diastase-resistant granules in giant cells. The histiocytes stain with Mac387. Scattered cells are CD68 positive while only isolated cells stain for S100 protein.[456]

Electron microscopy has not contributed any useful further information.

CUTANEOUS ATYPICAL HISTIOCYTOSIS

Only a few cases of cutaneous atypical histiocytosis have been reported.[458,459] It is characterized clinically by the presence of one or more nodular lesions resembling cutaneous lymphoma. There has been a good response to various modes of treatment in the cases reported so far. The status of this entity is doubtful.

Histopathology

There is a monomorphous infiltrate of medium-sized histiocytoid cells with occasional cytoplasmic vacuoles and scattered mitoses.

Electron microscopy

The distinctive feature is the presence in the cells of giant multivesicular bodies and pleomorphic granules.

INDETERMINATE CELL HISTIOCYTOSIS

Indeterminate cells are a class of dendritic cells found in the dermis. They display similar histological and antigenic features to Langerhans cells: both express S100 protein and CD1a surface antigens.[460] They differ by lacking Birbeck granules and by possessing some histiocytic markers.

Only a few cases of indeterminate cell histiocytosis have been reported. They usually present as multiple reddish-brown to yellowish papules.[461,462] A solitary congenital variant has also been reported.[460]

Histopathology

The tumor is composed of a monomorphous infiltrate of mononuclear, and occasionally multinucleate, histiocytes intermingled with clusters of lymphocytes. The cytoplasm is pale and the nucleus is often clefted.[460]

The cells express S100 protein, CD1a, CD68 and HAM-56.[460–462] Although indeterminate cells are said to be factor XIIIa negative,[288] several reports have mentioned positive staining with this marker in this tumor.[462]

ROSAI–DORFMAN DISEASE

The eponymous designation Rosai–Dorfman disease[463] is more appropriate than 'sinus histiocytosis with massive lymphadenopathy', because it is now recognized that in some instances extranodal lesions, including lesions in the skin, may be the sole manifestation of this condition.[464–478] The typical presentation is with painless cervical lymphadenopathy, accompanied by fever, anemia, an elevated erythrocyte sedimentation rate and hypergammaglobulinemia, which has been polyclonal in all but one case.[479,480] Any age may be affected, but 80% of cases develop in the first two decades of life. Extranodal lesions occur in almost one-third of cases, and the skin has been involved in approximately 10% of the 400 or so cases reported.[464,480]

Cutaneous lesions, which are usually multiple, have been varied in their clinical appearance.[464] There may be nodules up to 4 cm or more in diameter,[481] papules which are erythematous or xanthomatous,[464] plaques, pustules, acneiform lesions,[482] pigmented macules,[465] and even a transient panniculitis.[483] The eyelids and the malar regions are the sites of predilection.[465]

The disease usually runs a benign, albeit protracted, clinical course, sometimes with significant morbidity.[480] Death may sometimes result from infiltration of organs or from immunological disturbances.[465,484–486] It is a polyclonal disorder of macrophage origin.[288] Human herpesvirus-6 (HHV-6) has been isolated from a skin lesion in one case.[487]

Histopathology[464]

The pathological changes in the lymph nodes are characteristic, and include expansion of the sinuses by large foamy histiocytes admixed with plasma cells. Cutaneous lesions are not diagnostically specific. There is usually a dense dermal infiltrate of large histiocytes with abundant, lightly eosinophilic cytoplasm and vesicular nuclei.[464] Scattered multinucleate cells and Touton cells and collections of neutrophils may be present.[479] Plasma cells are invariably present, and sometimes contain prominent Russell bodies. Nodular lymphoid aggregates may be conspicuous.

Other features which may be present include phagocytosis of plasma cells and lymphocytes (emperipolesis),[488] xanthoma cells,[489] fibrosis, increased vascularity, and focal necrosis.[464] Histiocytes are often present in dilated lymphatics in the dermis.[471] A mixed septal and lobular panniculitis with some features of cytophagic histiocytic panniculitis (see p. 527) was present in one case.[483]

The large histiocytes of Rosai–Dorfman disease are S100 positive and negative for CD1a.[466,490,491] They also express various macrophage and monocyte markers such as α_1-antitrypsin, lysozyme, CD14, CD68 and Mac387.[470,492] Expression of factor XIIIa, a dendrocyte marker, has also been reported[493] but it has been negative in other cases as might be expected from its presumed cell of origin.[489] There are no Birbeck (Langerhans) inclusions in the histiocytes.[466]

HEMOPHAGOCYTIC SYNDROMES

The hemophagocytic syndromes are macrophage-related histiocytic disorders with significant morbidity and mortality. They present with fever, splenomegaly, liver dysfunction, cytopenia, hypofibrinogenemia and tissue hemophagocytosis. The syndrome may be associated with a variety of infectious agents as well as with drugs, autoimmune diseases and malignancies. The hemophagocytic syndromes are thought to result from a hypercytokinemic state causing poorly controlled activation of macrophages. These changes may turn out to be secondary to lymphocyte dysfunction.[288]

Cutaneous manifestations are a minor component of the illness. There may be hemorrhage from the hypofibrinogenemia. Hemophagocytosis can be seen in cytophagic histiocytic panniculitis (see p. 527). The histiocytes in the skin are S100 negative.

MALIGNANT HISTIOCYTOSIS

Malignant histiocytosis, formerly known as histiocytic medullary reticulosis, is an exceedingly rare and usually fatal systemic proliferation of atypical histiocytes and their precursors.[494,495] Fewer than 10 cases a year are reported in the literature.[288] A review of seven suspected cases seen at the Mayo Clinic over a 20-year period produced only one case that had a true histiocytic origin.[496] Clinical features include fever, generalized lymphadenopathy, hepatosplenomegaly, pancytopenia, and sometimes disseminated intravascular coagulation, night sweats and abdominal pain.[497]

The skin is involved in 10–15% of cases, and in some this is the presenting feature.[498–500] Lesions take the form of papules, nodules or plaques anywhere on the body, but with a predilection for the extremities and buttocks.[501] Sometimes only a solitary nodule is present initially. Spontaneous healing of individual lesions may occur.

Malignant histiocytosis occurs at all ages, but significant numbers of cases have been reported in childhood.[502–504] The prognosis at all ages is poor, although patients presenting with skin lesions form a subgroup with a more favorable outlook.[497,498] At autopsy there is usually involvement of many organs.

The recent classification of histiocytic disorders suggests the use of the term 'histiocytic sarcoma' for this group of tumors, which may be derived from macrophages or dendritic cells.[288] This is likely to prove a controversial term; it has not been used here.

Histopathology

Two patterns of cutaneous involvement may be seen.[499] In one there is a dense, predominantly periadnexal and perivascular infiltrate of atypical histiocytes; in the other there is a diffuse infiltrate of similar cells in the deep dermis and subcutis, with focal necrosis. The papillary dermis is usually spared, but if there are cells in this region there is no associated epidermotropism such as is seen in Langerhans cell histiocytosis.[505]

The cells in the infiltrate show variable pleomorphism, which increases with the passage of time. The cells measure 15–25 μm in diameter and have an oval or reniform nucleus and abundant eosinophilic cytoplasm. Occasional binucleate cells are present. Phagocytosis of erythrocytes and nuclear debris may be seen, but it is not a universal feature.[501] There are also some small lymphocytes and plasma cells in the infiltrate.[505]

The nuclear atypia in malignant histiocytosis allows it to be distinguished from the virus-associated hemophagocytic syndrome, histiocytosis X and cytophagic panniculitis.[498]

Receptors for concanavalin-A, a histochemical marker for macrophages/histiocytes, were present in all cases in one series.[494] Approximately half the cases have some S100-positive cells,[504] a finding that is more likely in children than in adults.[494] The subset of cases which is S100 negative may be positive for NCS (non-specific cross-reacting antigen).[494] Approximately 50% of the cells stain for lysozyme and for α_1-antitrypsin and α_1-antichymotrypsin.[506] Other antigens expressed include CD21, CD35, CD68, Mac387 and epithelial membrane antigen.[288,500]

Electron microscopy

The histiocytes are non-cohesive and sometimes have irregular surface projections[497,507] There are many cytoplasmic organelles, including lysosomes and lipid droplets.[507] There are no Birbeck granules. Phagocytosis is sometimes seen in the more differentiated histiocytes.[508]

REACTIVE HISTIOCYTOSIS

The term 'reactive histiocytosis', also known as secondary histiocytosis, refers to the increased number of histiocytes that may be seen in a variety of cutaneous infections. These include histoplasmosis, toxoplasmosis, brucellosis, tuberculosis, leprosy, rubella and certain infections with the Epstein–Barr virus.[282] Histiocytes are also prominent in actinic reticuloid. In susceptible hosts, particularly those with various immunodeficiency syndromes, infections

may trigger idiopathic histiocytic proliferations indistinguishable from Langerhans cell histiocytosis.[282]

XANTHOMATOUS INFILTRATES

Xanthomas represent the accumulation of lipid-rich macrophages known as foam cells.[509] They present clinically as yellow or yellow-brown papules, nodules or plaques, the color depending on the amount of lipid present and its depth below the surface. They are usually associated with disorders of lipoprotein metabolism, although only a minority of individuals with such disorders develop xanthomas.[509,510]

Xanthomas can be further subdivided on the basis of their clinical morphology, anatomical distribution and mode of development into the following types: eruptive, tuberous, tendinous, planar, verruciform and papular.[509,510] In addition, there are isolated reports in the literature of xanthomas which cannot be fitted into an orderly classification.[511–516] One such example is the occurrence of normolipemic xanthomas in association with HIV infection.[517,518] Another is the solitary xanthoma with prominent epidermotropism simulating balloon cell melanoma.[519] This latter case may have been a fibrous papule with clear cells and not a xanthoma. Specifically excluded, perhaps arbitrarily so, are the xanthogranulomas (which are not related to disorders of lipoprotein metabolism and which usually possess an admixture of cell types) and the histiocytic, dendrocytic and Langerhans cell proliferations in which lipid accumulation (xanthomatization) may be a secondary phenomenon.[510,512,520] Tangier disease and disseminated lipogranulomatosis (Farber's disease), which also possess some xanthoma cells, are not usually included with the xanthomas. The various diseases featuring the presence of xanthoma cells in the skin are summarized in Table 40.6.

Etiology and pathogenesis of xanthomas

Several of the xanthoma types mentioned above are associated with specific abnormalities of lipoprotein metabolism; more than one type of xanthoma may be present in a particular lipoprotein disorder.[510,521] The lipids in xanthomas are primarily free and esterified cholesterol, but occasionally other sterols and even triglycerides accumulate. This is usually the result of a high plasma concentration with subsequent permeation of lipoproteins through the walls of dermal capillaries.[509,522] The lipid is then taken up by dermal macrophages, which evolve into foam cells.[509,522]

There are several possible explanations for the formation of xanthomas in normolipemic states.[522] There may be altered lipoprotein content or structure, or an underlying lymphoproliferative disease with xanthomatization of cells infiltrating the dermis.[522] Finally, local tissue factors may play a role in those cases of xanthoma developing in chronic eczema, photosensitive eruptions, erythroderma and lymphedema, and at sites of injury such as bites, scars and striae and in some regressing tumors. The term 'dystrophic xanthoma' has been used for the accumulation of lipid-rich foam cells within an area of abnormal or damaged skin in both normolipemic and hyperlipoproteinemic states.[523,524] Dystrophic xanthomas may develop in burns scars, lymphedema praecox,[525] laparotomy scars, striae, lichen planus,[526] mycosis fungoides and at the sites of mosquito bites, vaccination, herpes zoster and phlebitis.

The various types of xanthoma will now be considered.

ERUPTIVE XANTHOMA

In the eruptive variant of xanthoma, multiple small red-yellow papules with an erythematous halo develop in crops.[509] There is a predilection for the buttocks

Table 40.6 **Diseases with xanthoma cells in the skin**

Eruptive xanthoma
Tuberous xanthoma
Tendinous xanthoma
Planar xanthoma
Verruciform xanthoma
Papular xanthoma
Facial xanthomatosis
Subcutaneous xanthomatosis
POEMS syndrome
Juvenile xanthogranuloma
Progressive nodular histiocytosis
Necrobiotic xanthogranuloma
Xanthoma disseminatum
Tangier disease
Disseminated lipogranulomatosis
Langerhans cell histiocytosis (histiocytosis X)
Congenital self-healing histiocytosis
Lepromatous leprosy
Rhinoscleroma
Malakoplakia
Scars
Arthropod bites
Lymphedema
Dermatofibroma (histiocytoma)
Hamartoma of dermal dendrocytes
Mycosis fungoides
Erythroderma

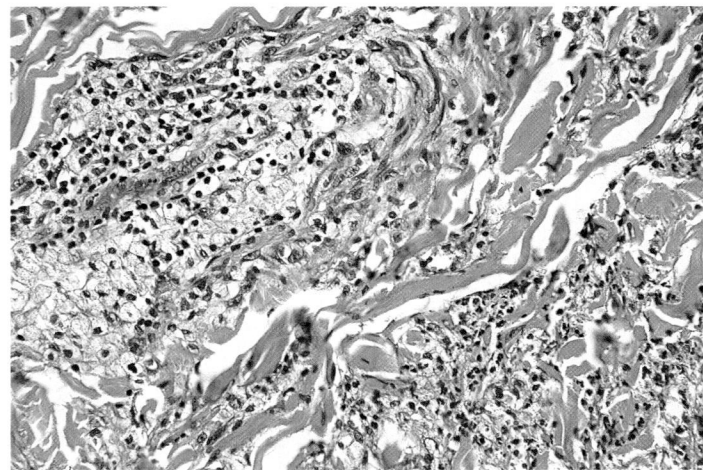

Fig. 40.15 **Eruptive xanthoma.** Small foam cells are admixed with lymphocytes, macrophages and neutrophils. (H & E)

and thighs and the extensor surfaces of the arms and legs.[510] The lesions become progressively more yellow, and eventually resolve spontaneously over several weeks.

Eruptive xanthomas occur in a setting of elevated plasma chylomicrons such as may occur in uncontrolled diabetes mellitus or following the ingestion of alcohol or the use of exogenous estrogens.[510,527] Rare associations include lipoprotein lipase deficiency,[510] types IV and V hyperlipoproteinemia,[528] normolipemia,[529] pregnancy,[530] the nephrotic syndrome,[531] hypothyroidism, the use of intravenous miconazole[532] and the oral ingestion of 13-cis-retinoic acid.[533]

The unique case of normolipemic eruptive xanthomas associated with generalized edema is best regarded as a variant of dystrophic xanthomatosis (see above).[534]

Histopathology[535]

The architecture of the reticular dermis is disturbed by an infiltrate of cells and extravascular lipid deposits in the form of lace-like eosinophilic material between the collagen bundles. The cellular infiltrate cuffs capillaries and extends throughout the dermis.[535] Initially it is composed of neutrophils and lymphocytes, and histiocytes with a finely stippled cytoplasm.[535] Neutrophils may be quite prominent in early lesions, and the absence of foam cells makes the diagnosis difficult on histopathological grounds alone. In established lesions the lipidization of cells is more obvious, although foam cells are never as obvious as in the other variants of xanthoma (Fig. 40.15).[536]

In some stages of their evolution eruptive xanthomas may mimic the changes seen in granuloma annulare, but close inspection for the features mentioned above allows the distinction to be made.[535] Furthermore, doubly-refractile lipid can be seen between foam cells in formalin-fixed material in some cases of eruptive xanthoma, but not in granuloma annulare.[537] In one report, the doubly refractile material was said to resemble urate crystals.[538]

TUBEROUS XANTHOMA

Tuberous xanthomas present a spectrum which ranges from small inflammatory lesions at one end (tuberoeruptive xanthomas) to large nodular lesions at the other. Tuberous xanthomas often form by coalescence of smaller lesions.[509] They are yellowish in color and are found particularly on the elbows, knees and buttocks. With treatment of the underlying hyperlipidemia there is usually slow resolution over many months.

Tuberous xanthomas are most characteristic of familial dysbetalipoproteinemia (type III), but they can be seen rarely in homozygous and heterozygous familial hypercholesterolemia, hepatic cholestasis,[539] cerebrotendinous xanthoma and β-sitosterolemia.[510] This latter condition is autosomal recessive, with the gene localized to 2p21.[540] Tendinous xanthomas are also present in these latter two conditions. Tuberous xanthomas have also been reported in a normolipidemic subject.[541]

Histopathology

There are large aggregates of foam cells throughout the dermis, but usually no Touton giant cells or other inflammatory cells (Fig. 40.16). Fibroblasts are increased in number in older lesions, leading to the progressive deposition of collagen.[541] In one case, concentric layers of xanthoma cells surrounded a cutaneous nerve.[542] In another the cells assumed a plexiform pattern – plexiform xanthoma.[543,544]

The lipid within the foam cells can be stained with oil-red O in frozen sections, or examined polariscopically to confirm its doubly refractile property.

TENDINOUS XANTHOMA

In tendinous xanthoma, lesions of varying size develop in ligaments, fasciae and tendons, especially the extensor tendons of the hands and feet and the Achilles tendon.[510] They are firm to hard, flesh-colored nodules which develop slowly over decades.

Tendinous xanthomas are most commonly associated with heterozygous familial hypercholesterolemia, but they have also been reported in cerebrotendinous xanthoma (caused by a mutation in the sterol 27-hydroxylase gene), β-sitosterolemia, familial dysbetalipoproteinemia (type III) and hepatic cholestasis, and rarely in normolipidemic individuals.[510,541,545]

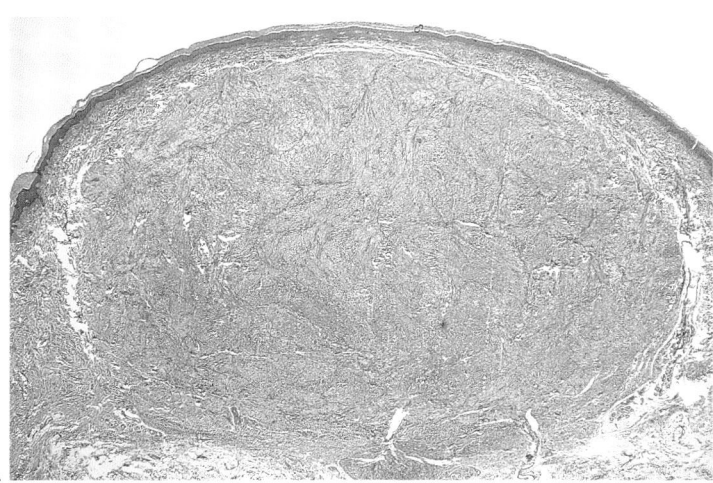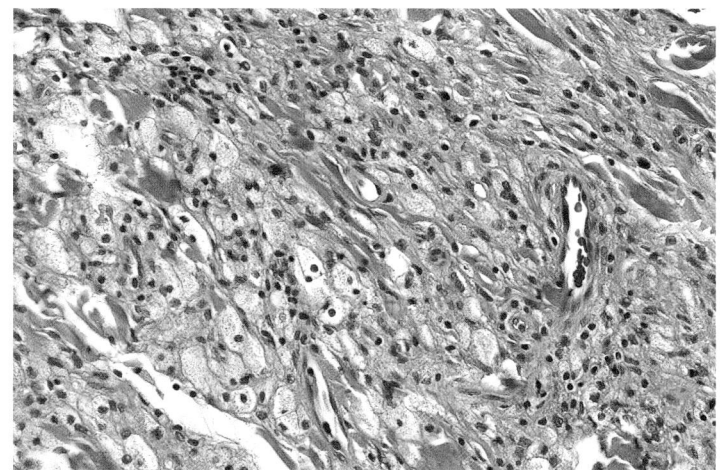

Fig. 40.16 **Xanthoma tuberosum. (A)** Sheets of foam cells involve the dermis. **(B)** Another case. It is early and the xanthoma cells are much smaller than in lesions of long standing. (H & E)

Histopathology

The appearances are similar to those seen in tuberous xanthomas, except for the different tissue substrate.

PLANAR XANTHOMA

Planar xanthomas are yellow, soft macules or slightly elevated plaques which are further subdivided on the basis of their location into xanthelasmas, intertriginous xanthomas,[510] xanthoma striatum palmaris[528,546] and diffuse (generalized) plane xanthomas.[509,510] A further variant, planar xanthoma of cholestasis, is sometimes recognized.[510]

Xanthelasma

Xanthelasma is the best known and most common form of xanthoma and is characterized by one or more yellowish plaques on the eyelids or in periorbital skin.[547] Lipid levels are normal in approximately 50% of affected individuals, although in young affected persons there is a higher incidence of hypercholesterolemia.[509,548] Abnormalities in the apoprotein moiety of lipoproteins have been detected in some of those with normal levels of lipid in the blood.[549] Altered vascular permeability may also play a role.[550]

Intertriginous xanthoma

The variant with localization in intertriginous areas is pathognomonic of homozygous familial hypercholesterolemia.[510]

Xanthoma striatum palmaris

The lesions in xanthoma striatum palmaris, which is characteristic of familial dysbetalipoproteinemia (type III), are present on the palms and volar surfaces of the fingers.[528,546] They are sometimes subtle, requiring proper lighting for their recognition.

Diffuse (generalized) plane xanthomas

The rare condition of diffuse (generalized) plane xanthomas is associated with macular, yellowish discoloration of the skin, involving particularly the trunk and neck, and sometimes the face.[550,551] Yellow-orange plaques are sometimes present.[552] It usually runs a protracted course. The majority of patients are normolipidemic, although several hyperlipoproteinemic states have been associated with this variant.[553] Increased vascular permeability is sometimes

present.[550] There is a significant association with lymphoreticular neoplasms, particularly myeloma, although these disorders may not become manifest until several years after the onset of the xanthomas.[554–559] Sometimes paraproteinemia, without myeloma, is present.[552] Transformation into necrobiotic xanthogranuloma has been reported.[448]

Histopathology

In xanthelasmas there are small aggregates of foam cells in the upper dermis. There is no fibrosis, and no other inflammatory cells are present. Plane xanthomas are composed of small groups and streaks of foam cells in the upper dermis, and sometimes around pilosebaceous follicles. A few perivascular lymphocytes are sometimes present. Fibroblasts may also be increased in number. Uncommonly, there is a more diffuse infiltrate of foamy macrophages and Touton cells, with cholesterol clefts and necrobiosis resembling the pattern seen in necrobiotic xanthogranuloma.[552]

Electron microscopy

Electron microscopy confirms the transition of macrophages into foam cells with lipid inclusions in the cytoplasm.

VERRUCIFORM XANTHOMA

The verruciform variant of xanthoma is composed of asymptomatic, usually solitary, flat plaques or warty lesions up to 2 cm in diameter.[560] They may vary in color from gray to pink or yellow, depending on the thickness of the overlying epithelium. There is a marked predilection for the oral cavity,[561] although lesions have also been reported on the vulva,[562] perianal skin,[563] scrotum,[564,565] penis[566] and occasionally extragenital skin.[567–569] Similar changes have developed in association with epidermal nevi,[570] a fibroepithelial polyp of the vulva,[571] a squamous cell carcinoma,[572,573] an arteriovenous hemangioma,[574] recessive dystrophic epidermolysis bullosa,[568] discoid lupus erythematosus[575] and lymphedema of the leg.[576–578] They have occurred in immunocompromised patients with HIV-1 infection,[579] with graft-versus-host disease[580] and in association with human papillomavirus type 6 (HPV-6).[581] Lesions may persist for long periods. It is assumed that the formation of the xanthoma cells is secondary to degeneration of or damage to cells in the overlying epithelium.[567,579,582,583] The xanthoma cells are thought to be derived from dermal dendrocytes.[584] Lipid metabolism is usually normal, although verruciform xanthoma has been reported in association with an undefined systemic lipid storage disorder.[585]

Histopathology[562]

On low-power magnification the lesions often have a verruca-like configuration. There is hyperkeratosis, focal parakeratosis and verrucous acanthosis (Fig. 40.17). Keratinous columns sometimes extend down into invaginations of the epidermis. There is often prominent exocytosis of neutrophils into the upper layers of the epithelium and the parakeratotic scale.[586] The basal layer usually has reduced amounts of melanin. Cystic invagination of the surface epidermis has been reported.[587]

The papillary dermis is filled with numerous large xanthoma cells. There are variable numbers of lymphocytes, plasma cells, neutrophils and eosinophils beneath and between the xanthoma cells. The cells contain lipid and small amounts of PAS-positive diastase-resistant material between the lipid vacuoles. Perivascular hyalinization of superficial vessels is sometimes present.

The foam cells are positive for CD68 and weakly positive for cytokeratin and factor XIIIa, but negative for S100 protein.[571]

Electron microscopy

Electron microscopy has confirmed the presence of lipid vacuoles within the cytoplasm of the foam cells.[570] One study showed numerous lipid droplets in the cytoplasm of melanocytes in the overlying epidermis. The authors speculated that they were the source of the lipid.[588]

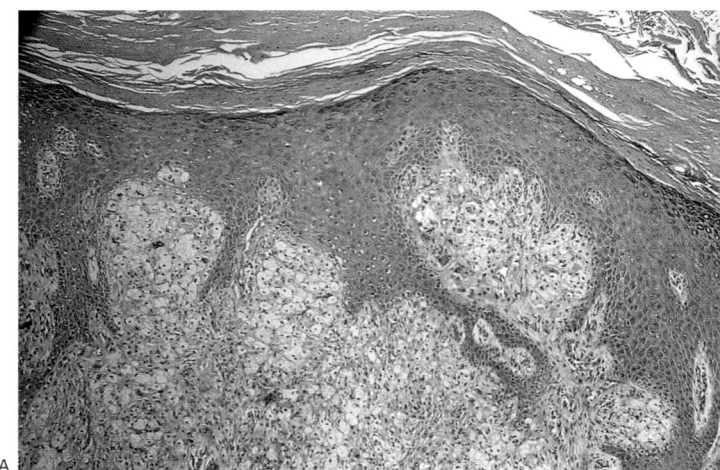

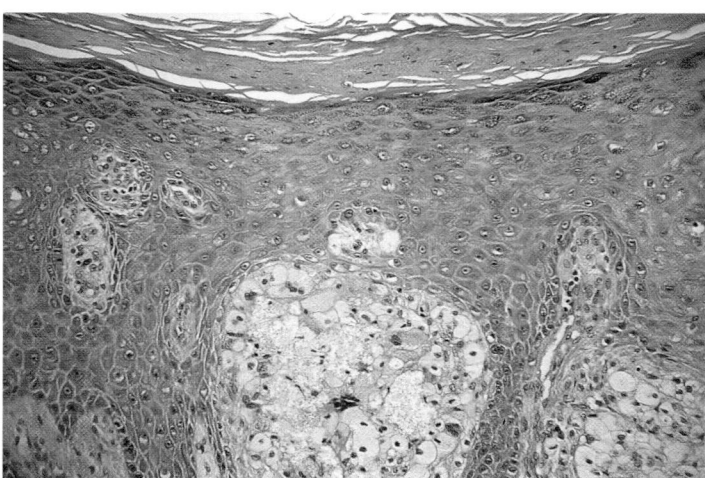

Fig. 40.17 **Verruciform xanthoma. (A)** There is marked hyperkeratosis and verrucous acanthosis, with numerous foam cells in the papillary dermis. **(B)** The foam cells show some nuclear variability. (H & E)

PAPULAR XANTHOMA

Papular xanthoma is a rare condition consisting of multiple discrete yellow-red papules on the face and trunk and occasionally on mucous membranes.[281,306] The condition has been classified with the histiocytic infiltrates because affected individuals are usually normolipidemic,[281] but as there are no primitive histiocytes or other inflammatory cells in the lesions it seems best to classify it as a xanthoma.[589] Furthermore, qualitative abnormalities in the lipoproteins may be present.[590] Papular xanthoma, particularly in children, may be clinically indistinguishable from juvenile xanthogranuloma.[591] Rarely, it is congenital.[592]

Papular xanthomatosis has been reported in a patient with the Sézary syndrome,[593] and in one with erythrodermic atopic dermatitis.[589]

The skin lesions in adults tend to be persistent, although childhood cases are often self-healing within 1 to 5 years.[592]

Histopathology[306,594]

There is an infiltrate of foam cells in the upper and mid dermis, with small numbers of Touton giant cells. There are very few, if any, chronic inflammatory cells within the lesions. Small amounts of hemosiderin are sometimes present within the foam cells and in extracellular locations. The cells are S100 negative. In one reported case the foam cells stained strongly for factor XIIIa, but were negative for Mac387. However, the multinucleate cells expressed this latter marker.[595] In a more recent study, the cells were positive for CD68, but negative for S100 protein, CD1a, CD56 and factor XIIIa. The authors concluded that the cells were of macrophage rather than dendrocyte origin.[596]

The absence of an inflammatory cell component distinguishes papular xanthoma from xanthoma disseminatum, eruptive xanthoma and juvenile xanthogranuloma, and clinical features allow its distinction from the other xanthomas.

Electron microscopy

The foam cells are macrophages with numerous lipid vacuoles and some myelin bodies.[594]

PAPULAR NEUTROPHILIC XANTHOMA

There is one report of three patients with HIV infection who developed a papular facial eruption in association with an IgA gammopathy.[518] Although there is some clinical similarity with the plane or papular xanthomas associated with lymphoproliferative disorders, the histology of these lesions is unique.

Histopathology

The epidermis is intact with a dermal infiltrate of xanthoma cells. Between the xanthoma cells there is hyalinized collagen with neutrophils and nuclear dust. Some of the foamy macrophages contain nuclear debris within their cytoplasm.[518]

LANGERHANS CELL INFILTRATES

The Langerhans cell is one of the dendritic cells, a group of non-phagocytic mononuclear cells which play a role in the trapping and processing of antigens for presentation to lymphocytes.[597,598] Dendritic cells may be of mesenchymal or hemopoietic stem cell origin.[288,599] Other dendritic cells include so-called 'indeterminate cells', 'interdigitating dendritic (reticulum) cells',[600] 'follicular dendritic cells' and 'veiled cells'. Tumors of these other dendritic cells are exceedingly rare, with only a few cases reported.[601–605]

Langerhans cells

The Langerhans cell accounts for approximately 2% of the cells in the epidermis.[597] Like other dendritic cells it specializes in processing and presenting antigens to T lymphocytes.[606] As Langerhans cells move from the skin and travel to draining lymph nodes, they lose their ability to process antigen and acquire the characteristics necessary to present antigen to T lymphocytes.[607] In the lymph nodes, the Langerhans cells may be the cells that have been referred to as veiled cells.[599] Various epidermal cytokines facilitate this functional maturation including granulocyte–macrophage colony-stimulating factor (GM-CSF), tumor necrosis factor (TNF)-α and interleukin-1 (IL-1). This mechanism ensures that antigen presenting at the skin surface is translated into an appropriate immune response.[607]

Langerhans cells are approximately 12–15 μm in diameter with clear cytoplasm and an irregularly shaped nucleus. They are situated in the epidermis above the basal layer, a situation that usually distinguishes them from melanocytes in hematoxylin and eosin-stained sections and in immunoperoxidase preparations for S100 protein. There is considerable regional variation in the number of Langerhans cells in the epidermis.[608,609] Langerhans cells are also found in the pilosebaceous apparatus, where they localize to the infundibular region of the follicle with extension into the germinative sebaceous epithelium.[610]

Ultrastructurally, Langerhans cells possess many organelles, the most characteristic of which is the Birbeck (Langerhans) granule. This is a rod or tennis racquet-shaped organelle of variable length and a constant width of 33 nm.[597] Similar dendritic cells without Birbeck granules are known as indeterminate cells.[597] Of interest is the report of a healthy white male whose epidermal Langerhans cells lacked Birbeck granules. The cells appeared to have normal antigen-presenting capacity, suggesting that Birbeck granules are not a prerequisite for normal function.[611]

Langerhans cells show esterase, acid phosphatase and ATPase activity.[612] They express certain antigens such as CD1a, S100 protein, CD45, CD101 and HLA-DR, and they bind peanut lectin.[612–614] Another marker is Lag, an antigen present in the membranes of the Birbeck granules.[615]

Langerhans cells play an important role in the pathogenesis of allergic contact dermatitis, and a lesser role in various other inflammatory dermatoses, such as lichen planus.[597] They have also been seen in the nodules in scabies, as have indeterminate cells.[616] Langerhans cells are often increased in number in the epidermis overlying various cutaneous tumors.[617] However, significant infiltrates of Langerhans cells are found only in Langerhans cell histiocytosis (formerly known as histiocytosis X) and congenital self-healing histiocytosis, which is now regarded as a self-limited variant of Langerhans cell histiocytosis.[618] The exact nosological position of the exceedingly rare cases reported as 'malignant histiocytic neoplasm of Langerhans cell type' and 'malignant Langerhans cell tumor' is uncertain.[619–621]

LANGERHANS CELL HISTIOCYTOSIS

Langerhans cell histiocytosis, formerly known as histiocytosis X,[622] is the collective designation for a clinical spectrum of diseases which in the past were called Letterer–Siwe disease, Hand–Schüller–Christian disease, and eosinophilic granuloma of bone, as well as intermediate and poorly elucidated forms.[623–626] It is a rare disease with a prevalence of approximately 0.5/100 000 children per year. However, there are many reports of older adults being affected. The traditional classification into three types has largely been abandoned because many cases did not conform to these classic subtypes.[627–630] They are mentioned briefly below because they provide a meaningful insight into the clinical diversity of this condition.

Letterer–Siwe disease

Cutaneous lesions are common and extensive in this acute disseminated form of Langerhans cell histiocytosis. They consist of yellow-brown scaly papules on the scalp, face, trunk and buttocks, which can coalesce to form a weeping erythematous eruption resembling seborrheic dermatitis.[306] Sometimes there is a hemorrhagic component. Cutaneous lesions are accompanied by fever, anemia, lymphadenopathy, osteolytic lesions[631] and often hepatosplenomegaly. This variant has been reported in monozygotic twins.[632]

Hand–Schüller–Christian disease

Hand–Schüller–Christian disease is a chronic multisystem form characterized by the triad of bone lesions, diabetes insipidus and exophthalmos, although it is uncommon for all three to be seen together in the same patient.[306] The skin is involved in one-third or more of cases: the cutaneous manifestations may resemble the lesions of Letterer–Siwe disease, or take the form of papulonodular lesions or granulomatous ulceration in intertriginous areas.[633]

Eosinophilic granuloma

Cutaneous lesions are quite uncommon in eosinophilic granuloma,[634,635] but when they occur they take the form of noduloulcerative lesions in the mouth,[636] or the perineal, perivulval or retroauricular regions.[306,637]

As mentioned above, the categorization of Langerhans cell histiocytosis into three clinical groups is now passé, because many cases do not fit neatly into any category. Rare cutaneous presentations have included cutaneous ulcerations[638,639] resembling pyoderma gangrenosum,[640] child abuse[641] or amebiasis,[642] eruptive xanthoma-like lesions,[643] multiple papules and plaques or nodules,[626,644–647] scattered papular lesions resembling bites,[648] vesicles,[649] pustules,[650] lesions resembling cherry angiomas,[651] verruca plana[652] or Darier's disease,[653] and a solitary lesion on the mons pubis,[654] buttock[655,656] or eyelid.[657] Involvement of the nails,[658] the genitalia of the elderly,[659] and the excision site of a basal cell carcinoma have all been reported.[660] Cutaneous lesions are uncommonly the only manifestation of the disease.[661,662] Many of the cases that were reported as 'familial histiocytosis X' appear to have been immunodeficiency syndromes associated with an idiopathic proliferation of histiocytes.[282,294] Malignant lymphoma has been reported in association with Langerhans cell histiocytosis, either preceding, following or concurrent with it.[663,664]

The prognosis in Langerhans cell histiocytosis depends on the age of the patient, the extent of the disease, and the presence of organ dysfunction.[665] Children under the age of 2 years with multisystem disease and organ dysfunction have a mortality of 50% or more.[666] A study of 314 cases at the Mayo Clinic found that 77 of these patients had skin and/or mucous membrane involvement, but only 14 of this group had isolated skin involvement, the other 63 having multisystem disease. Of the 14 cases with isolated disease, 2 had spontaneous remission and a further 6 were disease free after surgical excision alone.[667] In another study, the prognosis was related to the extent of the disease. If three or more organs/systems were involved, the mortality rate was 26%.[668] Spontaneous healing has been reported in several instances,[669] even with multisystem disease,[670] leading to the suggestion that Langerhans cell histiocytosis is a reactive rather than a malignant neoplastic process.[671,672] However, the cell populations are clonal, although this is not synonymous with a malignant phenotype.[599] An immunohistochemical study of 14 markers showed that the cells in Langerhans cell histiocytosis were 'activated' Langerhans cells,[673] which express various adhesion molecules that are not expressed in normal Langerhans cells.[674] Despite these studies, another used the presence of proliferating cell nuclear antigen (PCNA) in many cases as evidence for a neoplastic rather than a reactive process.[675]

The serum S100-β level is elevated in this disease and may prove to be a useful marker to monitor the progress of the disease.[676]

Human herpesvirus-6 (HHV-6) has been detected by polymerase chain reaction (PCR) techniques in a number of cases. The significance of this observation is currently uncertain.[677]

Histopathology

Langerhans cell histiocytosis is characterized by clusters and sheets of large ovoid cells, 15–25 μm in diameter, with abundant eosinophilic cytoplasm and a nucleus which is indented or reniform and sometimes eccentric – 'coffee-bean' nucleus (Fig. 40.18).[678] The cells are found immediately beneath the epidermis and usually show little tendency to extend into the reticular dermis, except in nodular lesions.[679] The cells often assume a periappendageal distribution in the papules of adult cases.[680,681] Focally, the cells invade the epidermis, sometimes forming small aggregates in the upper epidermis (Fig. 40.19). A few lipidized cells may be present in the papillary dermis, but more marked xanthomatous changes are exceedingly rare,[682] usually being confined to the Hand–Schüller–Christian variant. Occasional binucleate cells are present and there are scattered mitoses.

There is a variable admixture of other inflammatory cells; this will depend on the type of lesion biopsied and, to some extent, the clinical variant of the disease. The cells include neutrophils, eosinophils, lymphocytes and mast cells.[683] In Letterer–Siwe disease the infiltrate is largely of Langerhans cells, with the admixture of relatively few neutrophils, eosinophils and lymphocytes,

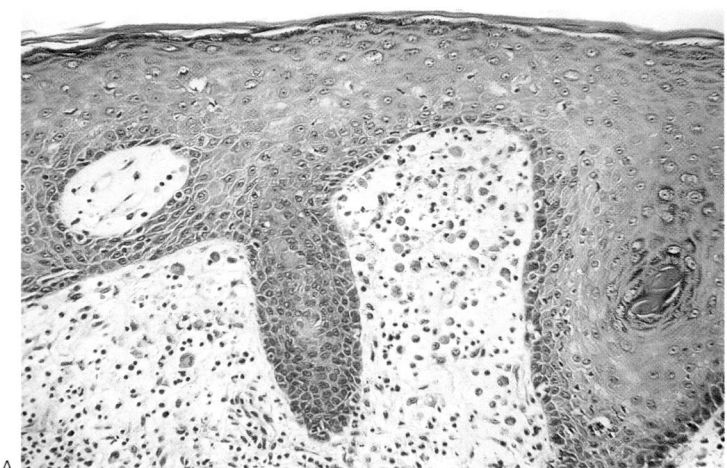

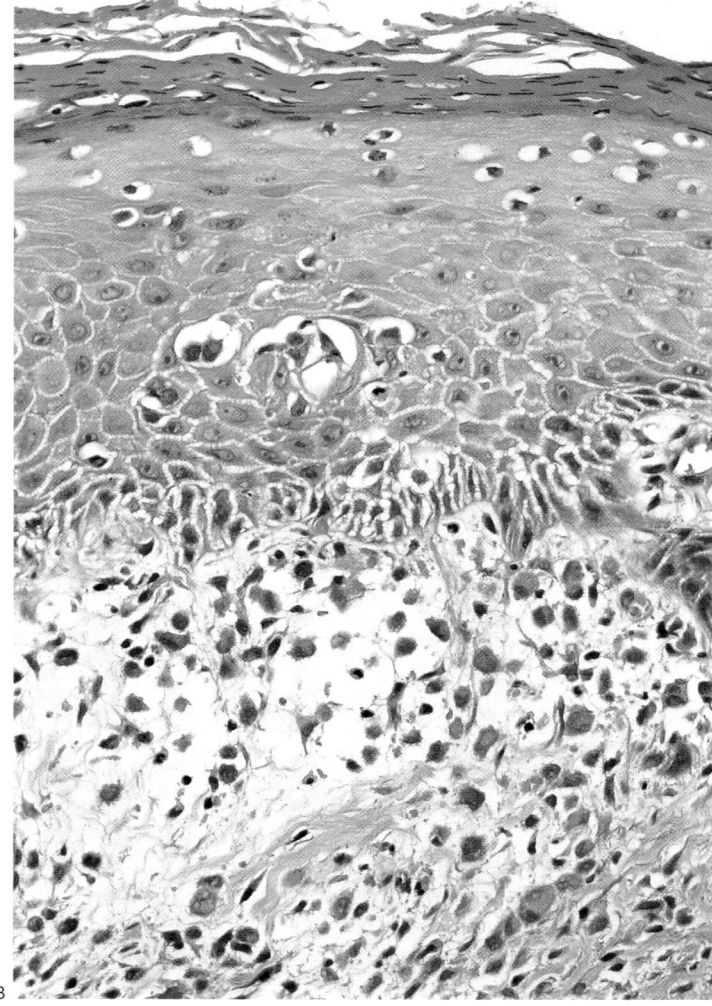

Fig. 40.19 **Langerhans cell histiocytosis. (A)** Langerhans cells and lymphocytes involve the papillary dermis. **(B)** Another case with epidermal involvement as well. (H & E)

Fig. 40.18 **Langerhans cell histiocytosis.** The cells have a characteristic reniform nucleus. (H & E)

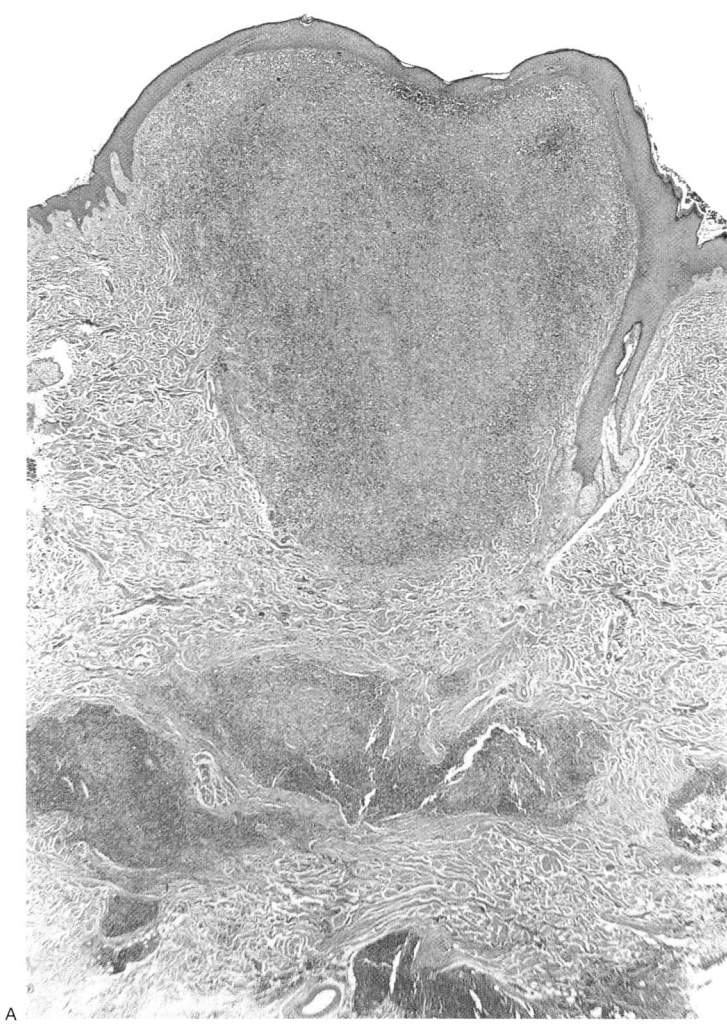

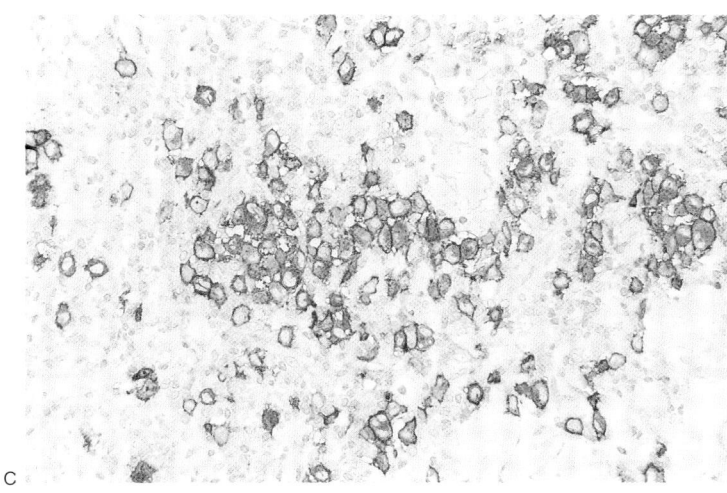

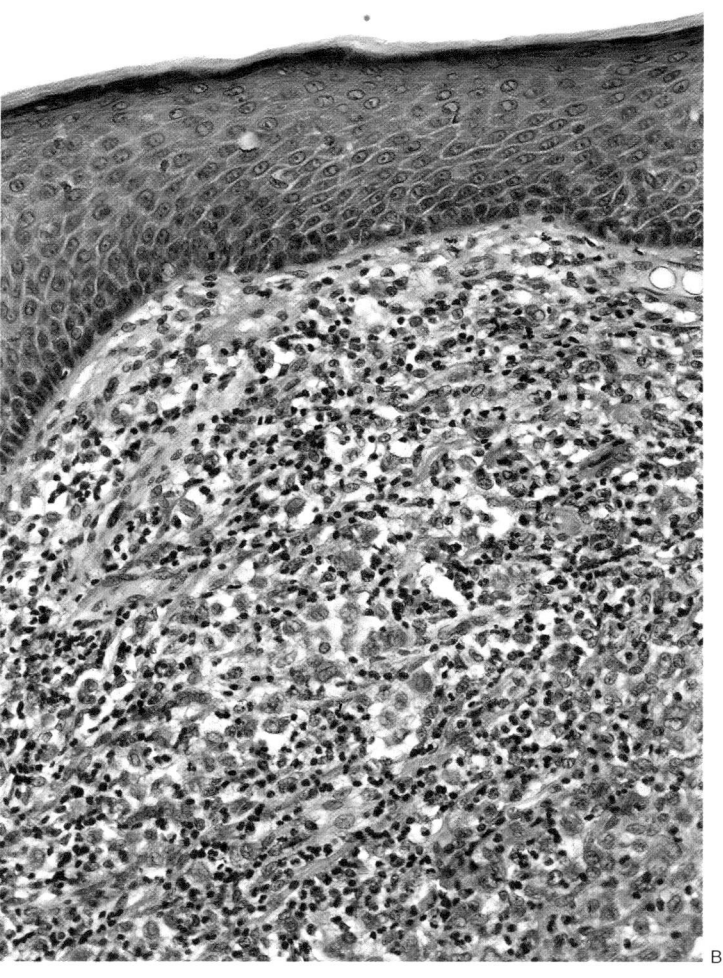

Fig. 40.20 **(A) Langerhans cell histiocytosis. (B)** This is the variant previously known as eosinophilic granuloma, with a mixture of eosinophils and Langerhans cells. (H & E) **(C)** The Langerhans cells stain for S100 protein

whereas in eosinophilic granuloma clusters of eosinophils may form a prominent component of the infiltrate (Fig. 40.20). Multinucleate giant cells may be prominent in both eosinophilic granuloma and Hand–Schüller–Christian disease. Other microscopic changes that are sometimes present include focal necrosis and fibrosis in older lesions.[672] Although the outcome cannot be predicted from the histopathological appearances, strong expression of proliferating cell nuclear antigen (PCNA) by the cells appears to reflect a poor prognosis.[680]

Immunohistochemical markers are those discussed above for the Langerhans cell and include CD1a, HLA-DR and S100 protein.[627,684–686] There appears to be some immunophenotypic heterogeneity, not all cells staining with a particular marker in an individual case.[687] The cells are negative for Mac387, which stains cells of the monocyte–macrophage system but not those of the dendritic cell system.[688] The cells do not express CD34 or MS-1, a marker for sinusoidal endothelial cells and dendritic perivascular macrophages, which is found in the non-Langerhans cell histiocytoses.[292]

Tumor-like eosinophilic granuloma is an extremely rare tumor of the skin composed of eosinophils, neutrophils, and histiocytes that are in part epithelioid and in part foamy.[689] Only sporadic cells stain as Langerhans cells. The lesions may resolve spontaneously. The etiology is unknown.

Electron microscopy

The cells are the same in all three clinical variants, and more or less resemble normal Langerhans cells. Birbeck granules may be absent in a proportion of cells.[665] Interestingly, these granules are relatively resistant to destruction by formalin fixation and paraffin embedding, and accordingly may be seen in material removed from paraffin blocks and reprocessed for electron microscopy.[625]

CONGENITAL SELF-HEALING HISTIOCYTOSIS

Congenital self-healing histiocytosis is a rare infiltrative disorder of the skin described in 1973 by Hashimoto and Pritzker.[690] It is now regarded as a self-limited form of Langerhans cell histiocytosis.[618,691-696]

The usual clinical presentation is with numerous firm red-violaceous or brown papulonodules, 1–10 mm in diameter, scattered over the scalp, face and, to a lesser extent, the trunk and extremities.[691,697,698] Only a solitary lesion was present in several reported cases.[699-702] The tumors are usually present at birth, although early postnatal onset has also been recorded.[703,704] The lesions all regress by 3 months of age, usually leaving residual hyperpigmentation. Relapse and systemic disease are both rare events.[705,706]

Histopathology

The histological picture is often indistinguishable from Langerhans cell histiocytosis.[691] There is usually a dense infiltrate of large histiocytes in the mid and lower dermis. Extension into the subcutis and papillary dermis may occur; there is usually no significant epidermotropism, although this has been described.[704,707] The histiocytes have abundant eosinophilic cytoplasm with a variable number of PAS-positive granules. Some cells have foamy cytoplasm. The nuclei are oval or reniform. Multinucleate giant cells are invariably present. There are also lymphocytes, mast cells and some eosinophils in the infiltrate.[708] Focal necrosis[707] and extravasation of erythrocytes have also been reported.[699] Abundant reticulin fibers are often present around groups of cells, and sometimes between individual cells.[709] It has been suggested that there is a variant with large cells resembling reticulohistiocytoma with intermingled Langerhans cells.[710] The nature of this group of cases is uncertain.

The tumor cells usually express CD1a and S100 protein[691,694] although in one reported case only 30% of the cells were S100 positive.[693,701] In this latter case none of the cells contained Birbeck granules.[693] In congenital self-healing histiocytosis the histiocytes and giant cells are sometimes larger than in Langerhans cell histiocytosis, and some may have foamy cytoplasm.[711] These differences are not regarded as sufficient to justify the continued separation of these two conditions.

Electron microscopy

Contrasting with their immunophenotype, only 5–25% of tumor cells contain Birbeck (Langerhans) granules.[699,709,712] The finding of concentrically laminated dense-core bodies in the same cells that contain Birbeck granules has been proposed as a specific marker for this disease.[713,714] Other cytoplasmic inclusions of unusual shape may also be present, as well as lipid droplets.[713]

REFERENCES

Neutrophil infiltrates

1 Wade BH, Mandell GL. Polymorphonuclear leukocytes: dedicated professional phagocytes. Am J Med 1983; 74: 686–693.

2 Cannistra SA, Griffin JD. Regulation of the production and function of granulocytes and monocytes. Semin Hematol 1988; 25: 173–188.

3 Metcalf D. Peptide regulatory factors. Haemopoietic growth factors 1. Lancet 1989; 1: 825–827.

4 Sadick NS, Shea CR, Schlessel JS. Congenital erosive and vesicular dermatosis with reticulated supple scarring: a neutrophilic dermatosis? J Am Acad Dermatol 1995; 32: 873–877.

5 Lübbe J, Hofer M, Chavaz P et al. Adult-onset Still's disease with persistent plaques. Br J Dermatol 1999; 141: 710–713.

Eosinophil infiltrates

6 Gleich GJ, Adolphson CR. The eosinophilic leukocyte: structure and function. Adv Immunol 1986; 39: 177–253.

7 Leiferman KM, Peters MS, Gleich GJ. The eosinophil and cutaneous edema. J Am Acad Dermatol 1986; 15: 513–517.

8 Wolf C, Pehamberger H, Breyer S et al. Episodic angioedema with eosinophilia. J Am Acad Dermatol 1989; 20: 21–27.

9 Gleich GJ, Schroeter AL, Marcoux JP et al. Episodic angioedema associated with eosinophilia. N Engl J Med 1984; 310: 1621–1626.

10 Berretty PJM, Cormane RH. The eosinophilic granulocyte. Int J Dermatol 1978; 17: 776–784.

11 Peters MS, Winkelmann RK, Greaves MW et al. Extracellular deposition of eosinophil granule major basic protein in pressure urticaria. J Am Acad Dermatol 1987; 16: 513–517.

12 Plötz SG, Abeck D, Seitzer U et al. UVA1 for hypereosinophilic syndrome. Acta Derm Venereol 2000; 80: 221.

13 Leiferman KM, Ackerman SJ, Sampson HA et al. Dermal deposition of eosinophil-granule major basic protein in atopic dermatitis. Comparison with onchocerciasis. N Engl J Med 1985; 313: 282–285.

14 Spry CJF. New properties and roles for eosinophils in disease: discussion paper. J R Soc Med 1985; 78: 844–848.

15 España A, Sanz ML, Sola J, Gil P. Wells' syndrome (eosinophilic cellulitis): correlation between clinical activity, eosinophil levels, eosinophil cation protein and interleukin-5. Br J Dermatol 1999; 140: 127–130.

16 Broide DH, Hoffman H, Sriramarao P. Insights from model systems. Genes that regulate eosinophilic inflammation. Am J Human Genet 1999; 65: 302–307.

17 Fukuda T, Gleich GJ. Heterogeneity of human eosinophils. J Allergy Clin Immunol 1989; 83: 369–373.

18 Kaufman LD, Gleich GJ. The expanding clinical spectrum of multisystem disease associated with eosinophilia. Arch Dermatol 1997; 133: 225–227.

19 Somech R, Arav-Boger R, Assia A et al. Complications of minocycline therapy for acne vulgaris: case reports and review of the literature. Pediatr Dermatol 1999; 16: 469–472.

20 Fung M. The clinical spectrum of dermal hypersensitivity reactions: questions and answers regarding a "wastebasket" diagnosis. J Cutan Pathol 2000; 27: 557 (abstract).

21 Kniffin WD Jr, Spencer SK, Memoli VA, LeMarbre PJ. Metastatic islet cell amphicrine carcinoma of the pancreas. Association with an eosinophilic infiltration of the skin. Cancer 1988; 62: 1999–2004.

22 Wells GC, Smith NP. Eosinophilic cellulitis. Br J Dermatol 1979; 100: 101–109.

23 Dijkstra JWE, Bergfeld WF, Steck WD, Tuthill RJ. Eosinophilic cellulitis associated with urticaria. A report of two cases. J Am Acad Dermatol 1986; 14: 32–38.

24 Fisher GB, Greer KE, Cooper PH. Eosinophilic cellulitis (Wells' syndrome). Int J Dermatol 1985; 24: 101–107.

25 Aberer W, Konrad K, Wolff K. Wells' syndrome is a distinctive disease entity and not a histologic diagnosis. J Am Acad Dermatol 1988; 18: 105–114.

26 Weiss G, Shemer A, Confino Y et al. Wells' syndrome: report of a case and review of the literature. Int J Dermatol 2001; 40: 148–152.

27 Peters MS, Schroeter AL, Gleich GJ. Immunofluorescence identification of eosinophil granule major basic protein in the flame figures of Wells' syndrome. Br J Dermatol 1983; 109: 141–148.

28 Garty B-Z, Feinmesser M, David M et al. Congenital Wells syndrome. Pediatr Dermatol 1997; 14: 312–315.

29 Mitchell AJ, Anderson TF, Headington JT, Rasmussen JE. Recurrent granulomatous dermatitis with eosinophilia. Wells' syndrome. Int J Dermatol 1984; 23: 198–202.

30 Sommer S, Wilkinson SM, Merchant WJ. Eosinophilic cellulitis following the lines of Blaschko. Clin Exp Dermatol 1999; 24: 449–451.

31 Nielsen T, Schmidt H, Søgaard H. Eosinophilic cellulitis (Wells' syndrome) in a child. Arch Dermatol 1981; 117: 427–429.

32 Lindskov R, Illum N, Weismann K, Thomsen OF. Eosinophilic cellulitis: five cases. Acta Derm Venereol 1988; 68: 325–330.

33 Saulsbury FT, Cooper PH, Bracikowski A, Kennaugh JM. Eosinophilic cellulitis in a child. J Pediatr 1983; 102: 266–269.

34 Reichel M, Isseroff RR, Vogt PJ, Gandour-Edwards R. Wells' syndrome in children: varicella infection as a precipitating event. Br J Dermatol 1991; 124: 187–190.

35 Anderson CR, Jenkins D, Tron V, Prendiville JS. Wells' syndrome in childhood: case report and review of the literature. J Am Acad Dermatol 1995; 33: 857–864.

36 Kuwahara RT, Randall MB, Eisner MG. Eosinophilic cellulitis in a newborn. Pediatr Dermatol 2001; 18: 89–90.

37 Kamani N, Lipsitz PJ. Eosinophilic cellulitis in a family. Pediatr Dermatol 1987; 4: 220–224.

38 Davis MDP, Brown AC, Blackston RD et al. Familial eosinophilic cellulitis, dysmorphic habitus, and mental retardation. J Am Acad Dermatol 1998; 38: 919–928.

39 Moreno M, Luelmo J, Monteagudo M et al. Wells' syndrome related to tetanus vaccine. Int J Dermatol 1997; 36: 524–525.

40 Chang DKM, Schloss E, Jimbow K. Wells' syndrome: vesiculobullous presentation and possible role of ectoparasites. Int J Dermatol 1997; 36: 288–291.

41 Friedman IS, Phelps RG, Baral J, Sapadin AN. Wells' syndrome triggered by centipede bite. Int J Dermatol 1998; 37: 602–605.

42 Canonne D, Dubost-Brama A, Segard M et al. Wells' syndrome associated with recurrent giardiasis. Br J Dermatol 2000; 143: 425–427.

43 Hurni MA, Gerbig AW, Braathen LR, Hunziker T. Toxocariasis and Wells' syndrome: a causal relationship? Dermatology 1997; 195: 325–328.

44 Seçkin D, Demirhan B. Drugs and Wells' syndrome: a possible causal relationship? Int J Dermatol 2001; 40: 138–140.

45 Jones-Caballero M, Pérez-Santos S, Bermejo-Martínez G et al. Wells' syndrome and human immunodeficiency virus infection. Br J Dermatol 2000; 143: 672–674.

46 Bogenrieder T, Griese DP, Schiffner R et al. Wells' syndrome associated with idiopathic hypereosinophilic syndrome. Br J Dermatol 1997; 137: 978–982.

47 Yagi H, Tokura Y, Matsushita K et al. Wells' syndrome: a pathogenic role for circulating CD4⁺CD7⁻ T cells expressing interleukin-5 mRNA. Br J Dermatol 1997; 136: 918–923.

48 Wood C, Miller AC, Jacobs A et al. Eosinophilic infiltration with flame figures. A distinctive tissue reaction seen in Wells' syndrome and other diseases. Am J Dermatopathol 1986; 8: 186–193.

49 Stern JB, Sobel HJ, Rotchford JP. Wells' syndrome: is there collagen damage in the flame figures? J Cutan Pathol 1984; 11: 501–505.

50 Newton JA, Greaves MW. Eosinophilic cellulitis (Wells' syndrome) with florid histological changes. Clin Exp Dermatol 1988; 13: 318–320.

51 Trüeb RM, Lübbe J, Torricelli R et al. Eosinophilic myositis with eosinophilic cellulitislike skin lesions. Arch Dermatol 1997; 133: 203–206.

52 Steffen C. Eosinophilic cellulitis. Am J Dermatopathol 1986; 8: 185.

53 Schorr WF, Tauscheck AL, Dickson KB, Melski JW. Eosinophilic cellulitis (Wells' syndrome): histologic and clinical features in arthropod bite reactions. J Am Acad Dermatol 1984; 11: 1043–1049.

54 van den Hoogenband HM. Eosinophilic cellulitis as a result of onchocerciasis. Clin Exp Dermatol 1983; 8: 405–408.

55 Murray D, Eady RAJ. Migratory erythema and eosinophilic cellulitis associated with nasopharyngeal carcinoma. J R Soc Med 1981; 74: 845–847.

56 Mezei MM, Tron VA, Stewart WD, Rivers JK. Eosinophilic ulcer of the oral mucosa. J Am Acad Dermatol 1995; 33: 734–740.

57 Vélez A, Alamillos F-J, Dean A et al. Eosinophilic ulcer of the oral mucosa: report of a recurrent case on the tongue. Clin Exp Dermatol 1997; 22: 154–156.

58 Chung H-S, Kim NS, Kim YB, Kang WH. Eosinophilic ulcer of oral mucosa. Int J Dermatol 1998; 37: 432.

59 Andreano JM, Kantor GR, Bergfeld WF et al. Eosinophilic cellulitis and eosinophilic pustular folliculitis. J Am Acad Dermatol 1989; 20: 934–936.

60 Weller PF, Dvorak AM. The idiopathic hypereosinophilic syndrome. Arch Dermatol 1996; 132: 583–585.

61 May LP, Kelly J, Sanchez M. Hypereosinophilic syndrome with unusual cutaneous manifestations in two men with HIV infection. J Am Acad Dermatol 1990; 23: 202–204.

62 Barna M, Kemény L, Dobozy A. Skin lesions as the only manifestation of the hypereosinophilic syndrome. Br J Dermatol 1997; 136: 646–647.

63 Offidani A, Bernardini ML, Simonetti O et al. Hypereosinophilic dermatosis: skin lesions as the only manifestation of the idiopathic hypereosinophilic syndrome? Br J Dermatol 2000; 143: 675–677.

64 Leiferman KM, O'Duffy JD, Perry HO et al. Recurrent incapacitating mucosal ulcerations. A prodrome of the hypereosinophilic syndrome. JAMA 1982; 247: 1018–1020.

65 Shelley WB, Shelley ED. Erythema annulare centrifugum as the presenting sign of the hypereosinophilic syndrome: observations on therapy. Cutis 1985; 35: 53–55.

66 Fitzpatrick JE, Johnson C, Simon P, Owenby J. Cutaneous microthrombi: a histologic clue to the diagnosis of hypereosinophilic syndrome. Am J Dermatopathol 1987; 9: 419–422.

67 Kanbe N, Kurosawa M, Igarashi N et al. Idiopathic hypereosinophilic syndrome associated with elevated plasma levels of interleukin-10 and soluble interleukin-2 receptor. Br J Dermatol 1998; 139: 916–918.

68 Kühne U, Marsch WC. Episodic angioedema with eosinophilia: precursor lesions and relevance of histology. Acta Derm Venereol 1991; 71: 83–84.

69 Zachary CB, Atherton DJ. Hyper IgE syndrome – case history. Clin Exp Dermatol 1986; 11: 403–408.

70 Blanche P, Bachmeyer C, Buvry C, Sicard D. Hyperimmunoglobulinemia E syndrome in HIV infection. J Am Acad Dermatol 1997; 36: 106–107.

71 Hauser C, Saurat J-H. A syndrome characterized by nodular eosinophilic infiltration of the skin and immunoglobulin isotype imbalance. J Am Acad Dermatol 1991; 24: 352–355.

72 Kazmierowski JA, Chusid MJ, Parrillo JE et al. Dermatologic manifestations of the hypereosinophilic syndrome. Arch Dermatol 1978; 114: 531–535.

73 Lee H-j, Yi J-y, Kim T-y, Kim C-w. Hypereosinophilic syndrome associated with systemic lupus erythematosus. Int J Dermatol 1997; 36: 152–153.

74 Songsiridej V, Peters MS, Dor PJ et al. Facial edema and eosinophilia. Evidence for eosinophil degranulation. Ann Intern Med 1985; 103: 503–506.

75 Jacyk WK, Simson IW, Slater DN, Leiferman KM. Pachydermatous eosinophilic dermatitis. Br J Dermatol 1996; 134: 469–474.

76 Plantin P, Mairesse H, Milochau Ph, Leroy JP. Pyodermatitis of genital areas: an atypical manifestation of eosinophilic pustulosis of childhood. Dermatology 1998; 196: 427–428.

Plasma cell infiltrates

77 Torres SM, Sanchez JL. Cutaneous plasmacytic infiltrates. Am J Dermatopathol 1988; 10: 319–329.

78 Erlach E, Gebhart W, Niebauer G. Ultrastructural investigations on the morphogenesis of Russell bodies. J Cutan Pathol 1976; 3: 145 (abstract).

79 Patterson JW. An extracellular body of plasma cell origin in inflammatory infiltrates within the dermis. Am J Dermatopathol 1986; 8: 117–123.

80 Davies D, Horton PJ, Gow E et al. Ulceration of the urethral meatus after simultaneous pancreas–kidney transplantation. Australas J Dermatol 2000; 41: 95–97.

81 Weedon D. Unpublished observations.

82 Boehncke W-H, Schulte-Rebbelmund H, Sterry W. Plasma cells in the dermal infiltrate of mycosis fungoides are of polyclonal origin. Acta Derm Venereol 1989; 69: 166–169.

83 Hurt MA, Santa Cruz DJ. Cutaneous inflammatory pseudotumor. Am J Surg Pathol 1990; 14: 764–773.

84 Yang M. Cutaneous inflammatory pseudotumor: a case report with immunohistochemical and ultrastructural studies. Pathology 1993; 25: 405–409.

85 Nakajima T, Sano S, Itami S, Yoshikawa K. Cutaneous inflammatory pseudotumour (plasma cell granuloma). Br J Dermatol 2001; 144: 1271–1273.

86 Shelley WB, Rawnsley HM. Plasma cell granulomas in non-lipemic xanthomatosis: apparent induction by indomethacin. Acta Derm Venereol 1975; 55: 489–492.

87 Lupton GP, Goette DK. Lichen planus with plasma cell infiltrate. Arch Dermatol 1981; 117: 124–125.

88 Jorizzo JL, Gammon WR, Briggaman RA. Cutaneous plasmacytomas. A review and presentation of an unusual case. J Am Acad Dermatol 1979; 1: 59–66.

89 Torne R, Su WPD, Winkelmann RK et al. Clinicopathologic study of cutaneous plasmacytoma. Int J Dermatol 1990; 29: 562–566.

90 Patterson JW, Parsons JM, White RM et al. Cutaneous involvement of multiple myeloma and extramedullary plasmacytoma. J Am Acad Dermatol 1988; 19: 879–890.

91 Shpilberg O, Yaniv R, Levy Y et al. Huge cutaneous plasmacytomas complicating multiple myeloma. Clin Exp Dermatol 1994; 19: 324–326.

92 Nandedkar MA, Abbondanzo SL, Miettinen M. Extramedullary manifestation of multiple myeloma (systemic plasmacytoma) that simulates hemangioma. A report of two cases. Arch Pathol Lab Med 2000; 124: 628–631.

93 Schmitz L, Simrell CR, Thorning D. Multiple plasmacytomas in skin. Harbinger of aggressive B-immunocytic malignancy. Arch Pathol Lab Med 1993; 117: 214–216.

94 Hauschild A, Haferlach T, Löffler H, Christophers E. Multiple myeloma first presenting as cutaneous plasmacytoma. J Am Acad Dermatol 1996; 34: 146–148.

95 Swanson NA, Keren DF, Headington JT. Extramedullary IgM plasmacytoma presenting in skin. Am J Dermatopathol 1981; 3: 79–83.

96 Burke WA, Merritt CC, Briggaman RA. Disseminated extramedullary plasmacytomas. J Am Acad Dermatol 1986; 14: 335–339.

97 Llamas-Martin R, Postigo-Llorente C, Vanaclocha-Sebastian F et al. Primary cutaneous extramedullary plasmacytoma secreting λ IgG. Clin Exp Dermatol 1993; 18: 351–355.

98 Chang Y-T, Wong C-K. Primary cutaneous plasmacytomas. Clin Exp Dermatol 1994; 19: 177–180.

99 Tüting T, Bork K. Primary plasmacytoma of the skin. J Am Acad Dermatol 1996; 34: 386–390.

100 Green T, Grant J, Pye R, Marcus R. Multiple primary cutaneous plasmacytomas. Arch Dermatol 1992; 128: 962–965.

101 Tsuboi R, Morioka R, Yaguchi H et al. Primary cutaneous plasmacytoma: treatment with intralesional tumour necrosis factor-α. Br J Dermatol 1992; 126: 395–397.

102 Tamamori T, Nakayama F, Sugimoto H et al. Extramedullary plasmacytoma: cytological and genotypic studies. Br J Dermatol 1993; 129: 468–472.

103 Miyamoto T, Kobayashi T, Hagari Y, Mihara M. The value of genotypic analysis in the assessment of cutaneous plasmacytomas. Br J Dermatol 1997; 137: 418–421.

104 Prost C, Reyes F, Wechsler J et al. High-grade malignant cutaneous plasmacytoma metastatic to the central nervous system. Am J Dermatopathol 1987; 9: 30–36.

105 Wong KF, Chan JKC, Li LPK et al. Primary cutaneous plasmacytoma – report of two cases and review of the literature. Am J Dermatopathol 1994; 16: 392–397.

106 Kyle RA. Multiple myeloma. Review of 869 cases. Mayo Clin Proc 1975; 50: 29–40.

107 Kois JM, Sexton M, Lookingbill DP. Cutaneous manifestations of multiple myeloma. Arch Dermatol 1991; 127: 69–74.

108 Canlas MS, Dillon ML, Loughrin JJ. Primary cutaneous plasmacytoma. Report of a case and review of the literature. Arch Dermatol 1979; 115: 722–724.

109 van der Putte SCJ, Go DMDS, de Kreek EJ, van Unnik JAM. Primary cutaneous lymphoplasmacytoid lymphoma (immunocytoma). Am J Dermatopathol 1984; 6: 15–24.

110 Whittam LR, Coleman R, MacDonald DM. Plasma cell tumour in a renal transplant recipient. Clin Exp Dermatol 1996; 21: 367–369.

111 Wuepper KD, MacKenzie MR. Cutaneous extramedullary plasmacytomas. Arch Dermatol 1969; 100: 155–164.

112 Klein M, Grishman E. Single cutaneous plasmacytoma with crystalloid inclusions. Arch Dermatol 1977; 113: 64–68.

113 Jenkins RE, Calonje E, Fawcett H et al. Cutaneous crystalline deposits in myeloma. Arch Dermatol 1994; 130: 484–488.

114 Vincendeau P, Claudy A, Thivolet J et al. Bullous dermatosis and myeloma. Monoclonal anticytoplasmic antibody activity. Arch Dermatol 1980; 116: 681–682.

115 Daoud MS, Lust JA, Kyle RA, Pittelkow MR. Monoclonal gammopathies and associated skin disorders. J Am Acad Dermatol 1999; 40: 507–535.

116 Ishikawa O, Nihei Y, Ishikawa H. The skin changes of POEMS syndrome. Br J Dermatol 1987; 117: 523–526.

117 Fishel B, Brenner S, Weiss S, Yaron M. POEMS syndrome associated with cryoglobulinemia, lymphoma, multiple seborrheic keratosis, and ichthyosis. J Am Acad Dermatol 1988; 19: 979–982.

118 Feddersen RM, Burgdorf W, Foucar K et al. Plasma cell dyscrasia: a case of POEMS syndrome with a unique dermatologic presentation. J Am Acad Dermatol 1989; 21: 1061–1068.

119 Chang SE, Choi JH, Sung KJ et al. POEMS syndrome with xanthomatous cells. Am J Dermatopathol 1999; 21: 567–570.

120 Janier M, Bonvalet D, Blanc M-F et al. Chronic urticaria and macroglobulinemia (Schnitzler's syndrome): report of two cases. J Am Acad Dermatol 1989; 20: 206–211.

121 Orengo IF, Kettler AH, Bruce S et al. Cutaneous Waldenström's macroglobulinemia. A report of a case successfully treated with radiotherapy. Cancer 1987; 60: 1341–1345.

122 Feiner HD. Pathology of dysproteinemia: light chain amyloidosis, non-amyloid immunoglobulin deposition disease, cryoglobulinemia syndromes, and macroglobulinemia of Waldenström. Hum Pathol 1988; 19: 1255–1272.

123 Nishijima S, Hosokawa H, Yanase K et al. Primary macroglobulinemia presenting as multiple ulcers of the legs. Acta Derm Venereol 1983; 63: 173–175.

124 Jones RR. The cutaneous manifestations of paraproteinaemia. I. Br J Dermatol 1980; 103: 335–345.

125 Mascaro JM, Montserrat E, Estrach T et al. Specific cutaneous manifestations of Waldenström's macroglobulinaemia. A report of two cases. Br J Dermatol 1982; 106: 217–222.

126 Hanke CW, Steck WD, Bergfeld WF et al. Cutaneous macroglobulinosis. Arch Dermatol 1980; 116: 575–577.

127 Swanson NA, Keren DF, Headington JT. Extramedullary IgM plasmacytoma presenting in skin. Am J Dermatopathol 1981; 3: 79–83.

128 Mozzanica N, Finzi AF, Facchetti G, Villa ML. Macular skin lesions and monoclonal lymphoplasmacytoid infiltrates. Arch Dermatol 1984; 120: 778–781.

129 Cobb MW, Domloge-Hultsch N, Frame JN, Yancey KB. Waldenström macroglobulinemia with an IgM-κ antiepidermal basement membrane zone antibody. Arch Dermatol 1992; 128: 372–376.

130 Wuepper KD, Key DJ, Kane PJ. Bullous pemphigoid due to a 19S monoclonal paraprotein in a patient with Waldenström macroglobulinemia. Clin Res 1978; 26: 579A.

131 Lowe L, Fitzpatrick JE, Huff JC et al. Cutaneous macroglobulinosis. Arch Dermatol 1992; 128: 377–380.

132 Watanabe S, Ohara K, Kukita A, Mori S. Systemic plasmacytosis. Arch Dermatol 1986; 122: 1314–1320.

133 Kodama A, Tani M, Hori K et al. Systemic and cutaneous plasmacytosis with multiple skin lesions and polyclonal hypergammaglobulinaemia: significant serum interleukin-6 levels. Br J Dermatol 1992; 127: 49–53.

134 Carey WP, Rico MJ, Nierodzik ML, Sidhu G. Systemic plasmacytosis with cutaneous manifestations in a white man: Successful therapy with cyclophosphamide/prednisone. J Am Acad Dermatol 1998; 38: 629–631.

135 Nitta Y. Case of malignant lymphoma associated with primary systemic plasmacytosis with polyclonal hypergammaglobulinemia. Am J Dermatopathol 1997; 19: 289–293.

136 López-Estebaranz JL, Rodriguez-Peralto JL, Ortiz Romero PL et al. Cutaneous plasmacytosis: report of a case in a white man. J Am Acad Dermatol 1994; 31: 897–900.

137 Uhara H, Saida T, Ikegawa S et al. Primary cutaneous plasmacytosis: report of three cases and review of the literature. Dermatology 1994; 189: 251–255.

138 Shimizu S, Tanaka M, Shimizu H, Han-yaku H. Is cutaneous plasmacytosis a distinct clinical entity? J Am Acad Dermatol 1997; 36: 876–880.

139 Kaneda M, Kuroda K, Fujita M, Shinkai H. Successful treatment with topical PUVA of nodular cutaneous plasmacytosis associated with alopecia of the scalp. Clin Exp Dermatol 1996; 21: 360–364.

140 Cerottini J-P, Guillod J, Vion B, Panizzon RG. Cutaneous plasmacytosis: an unusual presentation sharing features with POEMS syndrome? Dermatology 2001; 202: 49–51.

141 Tada Y, Komine M, Suzuki S et al. Plasmacytosis: systemic or cutaneous, are they distinct? Acta Derm Venereol 2000; 80: 233–235.

142 Yamamoto T, Katayama I, Nishioka K. Increased plasma interleukin-6 in cutaneous plasmacytoma: the effect of intralesional steroid therapy. Br J Dermatol 1997; 137: 631–636.

143 White JW Jr, Olsen KD, Banks PM. Plasma cell orificial mucositis. Report of a case and review of the literature. Arch Dermatol 1986; 122: 1321–1324.

144 Aiba S, Tagami H. Immunoglobulin-producing cells in plasma cell orificial mucositis. J Cutan Pathol 1989; 16: 207–210.

145 Perry HO, Deffner NF, Sheridan PJ. Atypical gingivostomatitis. Nineteen cases. Arch Dermatol 1973; 107: 872–878.

146 Leonforte JF. Balanitis circumscripta plasmacellularis: case report with ultrastructural study. Acta Derm Venereol 1982; 62: 352–356.

147 Souteyrand P, Wong E, MacDonald DM. Zoon's balanitis (balanitis circumscripta plasmacellularis). Br J Dermatol 1981; 105: 195–199.

148 Brodin MB. Balanitis circumscripta plasmacellularis. J Am Acad Dermatol 1980; 2: 33–35.

149 Nishimura M, Matsuda T, Muto M, Hori Y. Balanitis of Zoon. Int J Dermatol 1990; 29: 421–423.

150 Sonnex TS, Dawber RPR, Ryan TJ, Ralfs IG. Zoon's (plasma-cell) balanitis: treatment by circumcision. Br J Dermatol 1982; 106: 585–588.

151 Toonstra J, van Wichen DF. Immunohistochemical characterization of plasma cells in Zoon's balanoposthitis and (pre)malignant skin lesions. Dermatologica 1986; 172: 77–81.

152 Morioka S, Nakajima S, Yaguchi H et al. Vulvitis circumscripta plasmacellularis treated successfully with interferon alpha. J Am Acad Dermatol 1988; 19: 947–950.

153 Davis J, Shapiro L, Baral J. Vulvitis circumscripta plasmacellularis. J Am Acad Dermatol 1983; 8: 413–416.

154 Nedwich JA, Chong KC. Zoon's vulvitis. Australas J Dermatol 1987; 28: 11–13.

155 Kavanagh GM, Burton PA, Kennedy CTC. Vulvitis chronica plasmacellularis (Zoon's vulvitis). Br J Dermatol 1993; 129: 92–93.

156 Hautmann G, Geti V, Difonzo EM. Vulvitis circumscripta plasmacellularis. Int J Dermatol 1994; 33: 496–497.

157 Albers SE, Taylor G, Huyer D et al. Vulvitis circumscripta plasmacellularis mimicking child abuse. J Am Acad Dermatol 2000; 42: 1078–1080.

158 Kuniyuki S, Asada T, Yasumoto R. A case of vulvitis circumscripta plasmacellularis positive for herpes simplex type II antigen. Clin Exp Dermatol 1998; 23: 230–231.

159 Salopek TG, Siminoski K. Vulvitis circumscripta plasmacellularis (Zoon's vulvitis) associated with autoimmune polyglandular endocrine failure. Br J Dermatol 1996; 135: 991–994.

160 Sleater J, Mullins D. Subcutaneous Castleman's disease of the wrist. Am J Dermatopathol 1995; 17: 174–178.

161 Sherman D, Ramsay B, Theodorou NA et al. Reversible plane xanthoma, vasculitis, and peliosis hepatis in giant lymph node hyperplasia (Castleman's disease): a case report and review of the cutaneous manifestations of giant lymph node hyperplasia. J Am Acad Dermatol 1992; 26: 105–109.

162 Kubota Y, Noto S, Takakuwa T et al. Skin involvement in giant lymph node hyperplasia (Castleman's disease). J Am Acad Dermatol 1993; 29: 778–780.

163 Weichenthal M, Stemm AV, Ramsauer J et al. POEMS syndrome: Cicatricial alopecia as an unusual cutaneous manifestation associated with an underlying plasmacytoma. J Am Acad Dermatol 1999; 40: 808–812.

164 Shahidi H, Myers JL, Kuale PA. Castleman's disease. Mayo Clin Proc 1995; 70: 969–977.

165 O'Leary J, Kennedy M, Howells D et al. Cellular localisation of HHV-8 in Castleman's disease: is there a link with lymph node vascularity? J Clin Pathol: Mol Pathol 2000; 53: 69–76.

166 González S, Molgó M. Primary cutaneous angioplasmocellular hyperplasia. Am J Dermatopathol 1995; 17: 307–311.

Mast cell infiltrates

167 Mihm MC, Clark WH, Reed RJ, Caruso MG. Mast cell infiltrates of the skin and the mastocytosis syndrome. Hum Pathol 1973; 4: 231–239.

168 Markey AC, Churchill LJ, MacDonald DM. Human cutaneous mast cells – a study of fixative and staining reactions in normal skin. Br J Dermatol 1989; 120: 625–631.

169 Leder L-D. Subtle clues to diagnosis by histochemistry. Mast cell disease. Am J Dermatopathol 1979; 1: 261–266.

170 Kasper CS, Freeman RG, Tharp MD. Diagnosis of mastocytosis subsets using a morphometric point counting technique. Arch Dermatol 1987; 123: 1017–1021.

171 Olafsson JH, Roupe G, Enerback L. Dermal mast cells in mastocytosis: fixation, distribution and quantitation. Acta Derm Venereol 1986; 66: 16–22.

172 Omerod D, Herriot R, Davidson RJL, Sewell HF. Adult mastocytosis: an immunophenotypic and flow-cytometric investigation. Br J Dermatol 1990; 122: 737–744.

173 Natkunam Y, Rouse RV. Utility of paraffin section immunohistochemistry for C-KIT (CD117) in the differential diagnosis of systemic mast cell disease involving the bone marrow. Am J Surg Pathol 2000; 24: 81–91.

174 Yang F, Tran T-A, Carlson JA et al. Paraffin section immunophenotype of cutaneous and extracutaneous mast cell disease. Comparison to other hematopoietic neoplasms. Am J Surg Pathol 2000; 24: 703–709.

175 King R, Peterson A, Peterson K et al. Microphthalmia transcription factor expression in cutaneous mast cell disease. J Cutan Pathol 2000; 27: 561 (abstract).

176 Rosbotham JL, Malik NM, Syrris P et al. Lack of c-kit mutation in familial urticaria pigmentosa. Br J Dermatol 1999; 140: 849–852.

177 Büttner C, Henz BM, Welker P et al. Identification of activating c-kit mutations in adult-, but not in childhood-onset indolent mastocytosis: a possible explanation for divergent clinical behavior. J Invest Dermatol 1998; 111: 1227–1231.

178 Shah PY, Sharma V, Worobec AS et al. Congenital bullous mastocytosis with myeloproliferative disorder and c-kit mutation. J Am Acad Dermatol 1998; 39: 119–121.

179 Waxtein LM, Vega-Memije ME, Cortés-Franco R, Dominguez-Soto L. Diffuse cutaneous mastocytosis with bone marrow infiltration in a child: a case report. Pediatr Dermatol 2000; 17: 198–201.

180 Hartmann K, Henz BM. Mastocytosis: recent advances in defining the disease. Br J Dermatol 2001; 144: 682–695.

181 Leder LD. Intraepidermal mast cells and their origin. Am J Dermatopathol 1981; 3: 247–250.

182 Fine JD. Mastocytosis. Int J Dermatol 1980; 19: 117–123.

183 Atkins FM, Clark RAF. Mast cells and fibrosis. Arch Dermatol 1987; 123: 191–193.

184 Roupe G. Urticaria pigmentosa and systemic mastocytosis. Semin Dermatol 1987; 6: 334–341.

185 Eady RAJ. The mast cells: distribution and morphology. Clin Exp Dermatol 1976; 1: 313–321.

186 Sueki H, Whitaker-Menezes D, Kligman AM. Structural diversity of mast cell granules in black and white skin. Br J Dermatol 2001; 144: 85–93.

187 Okun MR. Mast cells and melanocytes. Int J Dermatol 1976; 15: 711–722.

188 Stein DH. Mastocytosis: a review. Pediatr Dermatol 1986; 3: 365–375.

189 Longley J, Duffy TP, Kohn S. The mast cell and mast cell disease. J Am Acad Dermatol 1995; 32: 545–561.

190 Hamann K, Haas N, Grabbe J et al. Two novel mast cell phenotypic markers, monoclonal antibodies Ki-MC1 and Ki-M1P, identify distinct mast cell subtypes. Br J Dermatol 1995; 133: 547–552.

191 Melman SA. Mast cells and their mediators. Int J Dermatol 1987; 26: 335–344.

192 Weber S, Krüger-Krasagakes S, Grabbe J et al. Mast cells. Int J Dermatol 1995; 34: 1–10.

193 Tada J, Toi Y, Arata J. Migrating mast cells into the epidermis of wet and inflammatory granuloma. Clin Exp Dermatol 2000; 25: 258–259.

194 Jackson N, Burt D, Crocker J, Boughton B. Skin mast cells in polycythaemia vera: relationship to the pathogenesis and treatment of pruritus. Br J Dermatol 1987; 116: 21–29.

195 Klein LR, Klein JB, Hanno R, Callen JP. Cutaneous mast cell quantity in pruritic and nonpruritic hemodialysis patients. Int J Dermatol 1988; 27: 557–559.

196 Szepietowski JC, Schwartz RA. Uremic pruritus. Int J Dermatol 1998; 37: 247–253.

197 Murphy M, Carmichael AJ. Renal itch. Clin Exp Dermatol 2000; 25: 103–106.

198 Kröber SM, Horny H-P, Ruck P et al. Mastocytosis: reactive or neoplastic? J Clin Pathol 1997; 50: 525–527.

199 Allison MA, Schmidt CP. Urticaria pigmentosa. Int J Dermatol 1997; 36: 321–325.

200 Tharp MD. Southwestern Internal Medical Conference: the spectrum of mastocytosis. Am J Med Sci 1985; 289: 117–132.

201 Kettelhut BV, Parker RI, Travis WD, Metcalfe DD. Hematopathology of the bone marrow in pediatric cutaneous mastocytosis. A study of 17 patients. Am J Clin Pathol 1989; 91: 558–562.

202 Azaña JM, Torrelo A, Mediero IG, Zambrano A. Urticaria pigmentosa: a review of 67 pediatric cases. Pediatr Dermatol 1994; 11: 102–106.

203 Poterack CD, Sheth KJ, Henry DP, Eisenberg C. Shock in an infant with bullous mastocytosis. Pediatr Dermatol 1989; 6: 122–125.

204 Hannaford R, Rogers M. Presentation of cutaneous mastocytosis in 173 children. Australas J Dermatol 2001; 42: 15–21.

205 Czarnetzki BM, Kolde G, Schoemann A et al. Bone marrow findings in adult patients with urticaria pigmentosa. J Am Acad Dermatol 1988; 18: 45–51.

206 Guzzo C, Lavker R, Roberts LJ II et al. Urticaria pigmentosa. Systemic evaluation and successful treatment with topical steroids. Arch Dermatol 1991; 127: 191–196.

207 Tepar G, Staudacher Ch, Geisen F et al. Urticaria pigmentosa – systemic involvement in 31 patients? J Invest Dermatol 1996; 106: 894 (abstract).

208 Fearfield LA, Francis N, Henry K et al. Bone marrow involvement in cutaneous mastocytosis. Br J Dermatol 2001; 144: 561–566.

209 Fenske NA, Lober CW, Pautler SE. Congenital bullous urticaria pigmentosa. Arch Dermatol 1985; 121: 115–118.

210 Oku T, Hashizume H, Yokote R et al. The familial occurrence of bullous mastocytosis (diffuse cutaneous mastocytosis). Arch Dermatol 1990; 126: 1478–1484.

211 Murphy M, Walsh D, Drumm B, Watson R. Bullous mastocytosis: a fatal outcome. Pediatr Dermatol 1999; 16: 452–455.

212 Niemi K-M, Karvonen J. A case of pseudoxanthomatous mastocytosis. Br J Dermatol 1976; 94: 343–344.

213 Revert A, Jordá E, Ramón D et al. Xanthelasmoid mastocytosis. Pediatr Dermatol 1991; 8: 152–154.

214 Husak R, Blume-Peytavi U, Pfrommer C et al. Nodular and bullous cutaneous mastocytosis of the xanthelasmoid type: case report. Br J Dermatol 2001; 144: 355–358.

215 Ruiz-Maldonado R, Tamayo L, Ridaura C. Diffuse dermographic mastocytosis without visible skin lesions. Int J Dermatol 1975; 14: 126–128.

216 Stern RL, Manders SM, Buttress SH, Heymann WR. Urticaria pigmentosa presenting with massive peripheral eosinophilia. Pediatr Dermatol 1997; 14: 284–286.

217 Kendall ME, Fields JP, King LE Jr. Cutaneous mastocytosis without clinically obvious skin lesions. J Am Acad Dermatol 1984; 10: 903–905.

218 Ogg GS, Rosbotham JL, MacDonald DM. Urticaria pigmentosa coexisting with multiple myeloma. Clin Exp Dermatol 1996; 21: 365–366.

219 Tsutsui K, Asai Y, Kawashima Y. Urticaria pigmentosa occurring with juvenile xanthogranuloma. Br J Dermatol 1999; 140: 990–991.

220 Fowler JF Jr, Parsley WM, Cotter PG. Familial urticaria pigmentosa. Arch Dermatol 1986; 122: 80–81.

221 Anstey A, Lowe DG, Kirby JD, Horton MA. Familial mastocytosis: a clinical, immunophenotypic, light and electron microscopic study. Br J Dermatol 1991; 125: 583–587.

222 Offidani A, Cellini A, Simonetti O, Bossi G. Urticaria pigmentosa in monozygotic twins. Arch Dermatol 1994; 130: 935–936.

223 Trevisan G, Pauluzzi P, Gatti A, Semeraro A. Familial mastocytosis associated with neurosensory deafness. J Eur Acad Dermatol Venereol 2000; 14: 119–122.

224 Caplan RM. The natural course of urticaria pigmentosa. Arch Dermatol 1963; 87: 146–157.

225 Lee H-P, Yoon D-H, Kim C-W, Kim T-Y. Solitary mastocytoma on the palm. Pediatr Dermatol 1998; 15: 386–387.

226 Harrison PV, Cook LJ, Lake HJ, Shuster S. Diffuse cutaneous mastocytosis: a report of neonatal onset. Acta Derm Venereol 1979; 59: 541–543.

227 Oranje AP, Soekanto W, Sukardi A et al. Diffuse cutaneous mastocytosis mimicking staphylococcal scalded-skin syndrome: report of three cases. Pediatr Dermatol 1991; 8: 147–151.

228 Enomoto U, Kusakabe H, Matsumura T et al. Diffuse cutaneous mastocytosis responding to cyproheptadine. Clin Exp Dermatol 1999; 24: 16–18.

229 Mackey S, Pride HB, Tyler WB. Diffuse cutaneous mastocytosis. Treatment with oral psoralen plus UV-A. Arch Dermatol 1996; 132: 1429–1430.

230 Meneghini CL, Angelini G. Systemic mastocytosis with diffuse crocodile-like pachydermic skin, pedunculated pseudofibromas and comedones. Br J Dermatol 1980; 103: 329–334.

231 Willemze R, Ruiter DJ, Scheffer E, van Vloten WA. Diffuse cutaneous mastocytosis with multiple cutaneous mastocytomas. Br J Dermatol 1980; 102: 601–607.

232 Bruning RD, McKenna RW, Rosai J et al. Systemic mastocytosis. Extracutaneous manifestations. Am J Surg Pathol 1983; 7: 425–438.

233 Sarkany RPE, Monk BE, Handfield-Jones SE. Telangiectasia macularis eruptiva perstans: a case report and review of the literature. Clin Exp Dermatol 1998; 23: 38–39.

234 Gibbs NF, Friedlander SF, Harpster EF. Telangiectasia macularis eruptiva perstans. Pediatr Dermatol 2000; 17: 194–197.

235 Fried SZ, Lynfield YL. Unilateral facial telangiectasia macularis eruptiva perstans. J Am Acad Dermatol 1987; 16: 250–252.

236 Gonzalez-Castro U, Luelmo-Aguilar J, Castells-Rodellas A. Unilateral facial telangiectasia macularis eruptiva perstans. Int J Dermatol 1993; 32: 123–124.

237 Bachmeyer C, Guillemette J, Blum L et al. Telangiectasia macularis eruptiva perstans and multiple myeloma. J Am Acad Dermatol 2000; 43: 972–974.

238 Webb TA, Li C-Y, Yam LT. Systemic mast cell disease: a clinical and hematopathologic study of 26 cases. Cancer 1982; 49: 927–938.

239 Travis WD, Li C-Y, Su WPD. Adult-onset urticaria pigmentosa and systemic mast cell disease. Am J Clin Pathol 1985; 84: 710–714.

240 Monheit GD, Murad T, Conrad M. Systemic mastocytosis and the mastocytosis syndrome. J Cutan Pathol 1979; 6: 42–52.

241 Tebbe B, Stavropoulos PG, Krasagakis K, Orfanos CE. Cutaneous mastocytosis in adults. Evaluation of 14 patients with respect to systemic disease manifestations. Dermatology 1998; 197: 101–108.

242 Menéndez V, Galán JA, Delgado Y et al. Giant inguinal and suprapubic mastocytomas in an adult with a history of childhood mastocytosis. Br J Dermatol 2001; 144: 208–209.

243 Koeppel MC, Abitan R, Angeli C et al. Cutaneous and gastrointestinal mastocytosis associated with cerebral toxoplasmosis. Br J Dermatol 1998; 139: 881–884.

244 Granerus G, Olafsson JH, Roupe G. Studies on histamine metabolism in mastocytosis. J Invest Dermatol 1983; 80: 410–416.

245 Fromer JL, Jaffe N. Urticaria pigmentosa and acute lymphoblastic leukemia. Arch Dermatol 1973; 107: 283–284.

246 Travis WD, Li C-Y, Bergstralh EJ. Solid and hematologic malignancies in 60 patients with systemic mast cell disease. Arch Pathol Lab Med 1989; 113: 365–368.

247 Petit A, Pulik M, Gaulier A et al. Systemic mastocytosis associated with chronic myelomonocytic leukemia: clinical features and response to interferon alfa therapy. J Am Acad Dermatol 1995; 32: 850–853.

248 McElroy EA Jr, Phyliky RL, Li C-Y. Systemic mast cell disease associated with the hypereosinophilic syndrome. Mayo Clin Proc 1998; 73: 47–50.

249 Lennert K, Parwaresch MR. Mast cells and mast cell neoplasia: a review. Histopathology 1979; 3: 349–365.

250 DiBacco RS, Deleo VA. Mastocytosis and the mast cell. J Am Acad Dermatol 1982; 7: 709–722.

251 Kuramoto Y, Tagami H. Solitary mastocytoma with massive eosinophilic infiltration. Pediatr Dermatol 1994; 11: 256–257.

252 Kamysz JJ, Fretzin DF. Necrobiosis in solitary mastocytoma: coincidence or pathogenesis? J Cutan Pathol 1994; 21: 179–182.

253 Wood C, Sina B, Webster CG et al. Fibrous mastocytoma in a patient with generalized cutaneous mastocytosis. J Cutan Pathol 1992; 19: 128–133.

254 Orkin M, Good RA, Clawson CC et al. Bullous mastocytosis. Arch Dermatol 1970; 101: 547–562.

255 Olafsson JH. Cutaneous and systemic mastocytosis in adults. Acta Derm Venereol (Suppl) 1985; 115: 1–43.

256 Sweet WL, Smoller BR. Perivascular mast cells in urticaria pigmentosa. J Cutan Pathol 1996; 23: 247–253.

257 Wilkinson B, Jones A, Kossard S. Mast cell quantitation by image analysis in adult mastocytosis and inflammatory skin disorders. J Cutan Pathol 1992; 19: 366–370.

258 Tharp MD, Glass MJ, Seelig LL Jr. Ultrastructural morphometric analysis of lesional skin: mast cells from patients with systemic and nonsystemic mastocytosis. J Am Acad Dermatol 1988; 18: 298–306.

259 Tharp MD, Glass MJ, Seelig LL Jr. Ultrastructural morphometric analysis of human mast cells in normal skin and pathological cutaneous lesions. J Cutan Pathol 1988; 15: 78–83.

260 Russell MA, Boyd AS, Patterson JW, Wick MR. Comparison of CD117 (C-Kit) immunostains with histochemical methods in the diagnosis of cutaneous mast cell diseases. J Cutan Pathol 2000; 27: 570 (abstract).

261 Horny H-P, Sillaber C, Menke D et al. Diagnostic value of immunostaining for tryptase in patients with mastocytosis. Am J Surg Pathol 1998; 22: 1132–1140.

262 James MP, Eady RAJ. Familial urticaria pigmentosa with giant mast cell granules Arch Dermatol 1981; 117: 713–718.

263 Kawai S, Okamoto H. Giant mast cell granules in a solitary mastocytoma. Pediatr Dermatol 1993; 10: 12–15.

264 Kruger PG, Nyfors A. Phagocytosis by mast cells in urticaria pigmentosa. Acta Derm Venereol 1984; 64: 373–377.

265 Okun MR, Bhawan J. Combined melanocytoma–mastocytoma in a case of nodular mastocytosis. J Am Acad Dermatol 1979; 1: 338–347.

266 Walcyk PJ, Elpern DJ. Brachioradial pruritus: a tropical dermopathy. Br J Dermatol 1986; 115: 177–180.

267 Goodless DR, Eaglstein WH. Brachioradial pruritus: treatment with topical capsaicin. J Am Acad Dermatol 1993; 29: 783–784.

268 Teixeira F, Miranda-Vega A, Hojyo-Tomoka T et al. Solar (brachioradial) pruritus – response to capsaicin cream. Int J Dermatol 1995; 34: 594–595.

269 Knight TE, Hayashi T. Solar (brachioradial) pruritus – response to capsaicin cream. Int J Dermatol 1994; 33: 206–209.

270 Heyl T. Brachioradial pruritus. Arch Dermatol 1983; 119: 115–116.

271 Weedon D. Unpublished observations.

272 Armstrong DKB, Bingham EA. Brachioradial pruritus – an uncommon photodermatosis presenting in a temperate climate. Dermatology 1997; 195: 414–415.

273 Veien NK, Hattel T, Laurberg G, Spaun E. Brachioradial pruritus. J Am Acad Dermatol 2001; 44: 704–705.

274 Orton DI, Wakelin SH, George SA. Brachioradial photopruritus – a rare chronic photodermatosis in Europe. Br J Dermatol 1996; 135: 486–487.

275 Wallengren J. Brachioradial pruritus: A recurrent solar dermopathy. J Am Acad Dermatol 1998; 39: 803–806.

276 Sassmannshausen J, Lim HW. Action spectrum and response to antihistamine use in solar pruritus. Arch Dermatol 1999; 135: 1122–1123.

277 Hawk JLM. Solar pruritus: a symptom, not a diagnosis. Arch Dermatol 2001; 137: 372.

278 Tait CP, Grigg E, Quirk CJ. Brachioradial pruritus and cervical spine manipulation. Australas J Dermatol 1998; 39: 168–170.

279 Fisher DA. Brachioradial pruritus: A recurrent solar dermopathy. J Am Acad Dermatol 1999; 41: 656–657.

280 Fisher DA. Brachioradial pruritus wanted: a sure cause (and cure) for brachioradial pruritus. Int J Dermatol 1997; 36: 817–818.

Histiocytic infiltrates

281 Winkelmann RK. Cutaneous syndromes of non-X histiocytosis. A review of the macrophage–histiocyte diseases of the skin. Arch Dermatol 1981; 117: 667–672.

282 Roper SS, Spraker MK. Cutaneous histiocytosis syndromes. Pediatr Dermatol 1985; 3: 19–30.

283 Turner RR, Wood GS, Beckstead JH et al. Histiocytic malignancies. Morphologic, immunologic, and enzymatic heterogeneity. Am J Surg Pathol 1984; 8: 485–500.

284 Headington JT. The histiocyte. In memoriam. Arch Dermatol 1986; 122: 532–533.

285 Malone M. The histiocytoses of childhood. Histopathology 1991; 19: 105–119.

286 Foucar K, Foucar E. The mononuclear phagocyte and immunoregulatory effector (M-PIRE) system: evolving concepts. Semin Diagn Pathol 1990; 7: 4–18.

287 Ben-Ezra JM, Koo CH. Langerhans' cell histiocytosis and malignancies of the M-PIRE system. Am J Clin Pathol 1993; 99: 464–471.

288 Favara BE, Feller AC. Contemporary classification of histiocytic disorders. Med Pediatr Oncol 1997; 29: 157–166.

289 Weber-Matthiesen K, Sterry W. Organization of the monocyte/macrophage system of normal human skin. J Invest Dermatol 1990; 95: 83–89.

290 Cerio R, Spaull J, Wilson Jones E. Histiocytoma cutis: a tumour of dermal dendrocytes (dermal dendrocytoma). Br J Dermatol 1989; 120: 197–206.

291 Loftus B, Loh LC, Curran B et al. Mac 387: its non-specificity as a tumour marker or marker of histiocytes. Histopathology 1991; 19: 251–255.

292 Goerdt S, Kolde G, Bonsmann G et al. Immunohistochemical comparison of cutaneous histiocytoses and related skin disorders: diagnostic and histogenetic relevance of MS-1 high molecular weight protein expression. J Pathol 1993; 170: 421–427.

293 Tomaszewski M-M, Lupton GP. Unusual expression of S-100 protein in histiocytic neoplasms. J Cutan Pathol 1998; 25: 129–135.

294 van der Valk P, Meijer CJLM. Cutaneous histiocytic proliferations. Dermatol Clin 1985; 3: 705–717.

295 Horiguchi Y, Tanaka T, Toda K et al. Regressing ulcerative histiocytosis. Am J Dermatopathol 1989; 11: 166–171.

296 Shimizu H, Komatsu T, Harada T et al. An immunohistochemical and ultrastructural study of an unusual case of multiple non-X histiocytoma. Arch Dermatol 1988; 124: 1254–1257.

297 Berti E, Gianotti R, Alessi E. Unusual cutaneous histiocytosis expressing an intermediate immunophenotype between Langerhans' cells and dermal macrophages. Arch Dermatol 1988; 124: 1250–1253.

298 van Haselen CW, Toonstra J, den Hengst CW, van Vloten WA. An unusual form of localized papulonodular cutaneous histiocytosis in a 6-month-old boy. Br J Dermatol 1995; 133: 444–448.

299 Gibbs NF, O'Grady TC. Progressive eruptive histiocytomas. J Am Acad Dermatol 1996; 35: 323–325.

300 Ibbotson SH, Sviland L, Slater DN, Reynolds NJ. Non-Langerhans cell histiocytosis associated with lymphocyte-predominant Hodgkin's disease. Clin Exp Dermatol 1999; 24: 365–367.

301 Zelger BWH, Sidoroff A, Orchard G, Cerio R. Non-Langerhans cell histiocytoses. A new unifying concept. Am J Dermatopathol 1996; 18: 490–504.

302 Chu AC. The confusing state of the histiocytoses. Br J Dermatol 2000; 143: 475–476.

303 Kraus MD, Haley JC, Ruiz R et al. "Juvenile" xanthogranuloma. An immunophenotypic study with a reappraisal of histogenesis. Am J Dermatopathol 2001; 23: 104–111.

304 Mullans EA, Helm TN, Taylor JS et al. Generalized non-Langerhans cell histiocytosis: four cases illustrate a spectrum of disease. Int J Dermatol 1995; 34: 106–112.

305 Helwig EB, Hackney VC. Juvenile xanthogranuloma (nevoxanthoendothelioma). Am J Pathol 1954; 30: 625–626.

306 Gianotti F, Caputo R. Histiocytic syndromes: a review. J Am Acad Dermatol 1985; 13: 383–404.

307 Hernandez-Martin A, Baselga E, Drolet BA, Esterly NB. Juvenile xanthogranuloma. J Am Acad Dermatol 1997; 36: 355–367.

308 Sonoda T, Hashimoto H, Enjoji M. Juvenile xanthogranuloma. Clinicopathologic analysis and immunohistochemical study of 57 patients. Cancer 1985; 56: 2280–2286.

309 Resnick SD, Woosley J, Azizkhan RG. Giant juvenile xanthogranuloma: exophytic and endophytic variants. Pediatr Dermatol 1990; 7: 185–188.

310 Whittam LR, Higgins EH. Juvenile xanthogranuloma on the sole. Pediatr Dermatol 2000; 17: 460–462.

311 Caputo R, Grimalt R, Gelmetti C, Cottoni F. Unusual aspects of juvenile xanthogranuloma. J Am Acad Dermatol 1993; 29: 868–870.

312 Flach DB, Winkelmann RK. Juvenile xanthogranuloma with central nervous system lesions. J Am Acad Dermatol 1986; 14: 405–411.

313 Kolde G, Bonsmann G. Generalized lichenoid juvenile xanthogranuloma. Br J Dermatol 1992; 126: 66–70.

314 Caputo R, Cambiaghi S, Brusasco A, Gelmetti C. Uncommon clinical presentations of juvenile xanthogranuloma. Dermatology 1998; 197: 45–47.

315 Török E, Daróczy J. Juvenile xanthogranuloma: an analysis of 45 cases by clinical follow-up, light- and electron microscopy. Acta Derm Venereol 1985; 65: 167–169.

316 Magaña M, Vázquez R, Fernández-Díez J et al. Giant congenital juvenile xanthogranuloma. Pediatr Dermatol 1994; 11: 227–230.

317 Kobayashi K, Imai T, Adachi S et al. Juvenile xanthogranuloma with hematologic changes in dizygotic twins: report of two newborn infants. Pediatr Dermatol 1998; 15: 203–206.

318 Herbst AM, Laude TA. Juvenile xanthogranuloma: further evidence of a reactive etiology. Pediatr Dermatol 1999; 16: 164.

319 Tahan SR, Pastel-Levy C, Bhan AK, Mihm MC Jr. Juvenile xanthogranuloma. Clinical and pathologic characterization. Arch Pathol Lab Med 1989; 113: 1057–1061.

320 Konohana A, Noda J, Koizumi M. Multiple xanthogranulomas in an adult. Clin Exp Dermatol 1993; 18: 462–463.

321 Whitmore SE. Multiple xanthogranulomas in an adult: case report and literature review. Br J Dermatol 1992; 127: 177–181.

322 Sueki H, Saito T, Iijima M, Fujisawa R. Adult-onset xanthogranuloma appearing symmetrically on the ear lobes. J Am Acad Dermatol 1995; 32: 372–374.

323 Pehr K, Elie J, Watters AK. "Juvenile" xanthogranuloma in a 77-year-old man. Int J Dermatol 1994; 33: 438–441.

324 Cohen BA, Hood A. Xanthogranuloma: report on clinical and histologic findings in 64 patients. Pediatr Dermatol 1989; 6: 262–266.

325 Mancini AJ, Prieto VG, Smoller BR. Role of cellular proliferation and apoptosis in the growth of xanthogranulomas. Am J Dermatopathol 1998; 20: 17–21.

326 Chu AC, Wells RS, MacDonald DM. Juvenile xanthogranuloma with recurrent subdural effusions. Br J Dermatol 1981; 105: 97–101.

327 Satow SJ, Zee S, Dawson KH et al. Juvenile xanthogranuloma of the tongue. J Am Acad Dermatol 1995; 33: 376–379.

328 George DH, Scheithauer BW, Hilton DL et al. Juvenile xanthogranuloma of peripheral nerve. Am J Surg Pathol 2001; 25: 521–526.

329 Zvulunov A, Barak Y, Metzker A. Juvenile xanthogranuloma, neurofibromatosis, and juvenile chronic myelogenous leukemia. Arch Dermatol 1995; 131: 904–908.

330 Ackerman CD, Cohen BA. Juvenile xanthogranuloma and neurofibromatosis. Pediatr Dermatol 1991; 8: 339–340.

331 Gutmann DH, Gurney JG, Shannon KM. Juvenile xanthogranuloma, neurofibromatosis 1, and juvenile chronic myeloid leukemia. Arch Dermatol 1996; 132: 1390.

332 Tan HH, Tay YK. Juvenile xanthogranuloma and neurofibromatosis 1. Dermatology 1998; 197: 43–44.

333 Wood WS, Dimmick JE, Dolman CL. Niemann–Pick disease and juvenile xanthogranuloma. Are they related? Am J Dermatopathol 1987; 9: 433–437.

334 Mann RE, Friedman KJ, Milgraum SS. Urticaria pigmentosa and juvenile xanthogranuloma: case report and review of the literature. Pediatr Dermatol 1996; 13: 122–126.

335 Garvey WT, Grundy SM, Eckel R. Xanthogranulomatosis in an adult: lipid analysis of xanthomas and plasma. J Am Acad Dermatol 1987; 16: 183–187.

336 Sangüeza OP, Salmon JK, White CR Jr, Beckstead JH. Juvenile xanthogranuloma: a clinical, histopathologic and immunohistochemical study. J Cutan Pathol 1995; 22: 327–335.

337 Janney CG, Hurt MA, Santa Cruz DJ. Deep juvenile xanthogranuloma. Subcutaneous and intramuscular forms. Am J Surg Pathol 1991; 15: 150–159.

338 Sánchez Yus E, Requena L, Villegas C, Valle P. Subcutaneous juvenile xanthogranuloma. J Cutan Pathol 1995; 22: 460–465.

339 Tanz WS, Kim YA, Schwartz RA et al. Juvenile xanthogranuloma with inconspicuous foam cells and giant cells. Int J Dermatol 1995; 34: 653–655.

340 Shapiro PE, Silvers DN, Treiber RK et al. Juvenile xanthogranulomas with inconspicuous or absent foam cells and giant cells. J Am Acad Dermatol 1991; 24: 1005–1009.

341 Claudy AL, Misery L, Serre D, Boucheron S. Multiple juvenile xanthogranulomas without foam cells and giant cells. Pediatr Dermatol 1993; 10: 61–63.

342 Busam KJ, Rosai J, Iversen K, Jungbluth AA. Xanthogranulomas with inconspicuous foam cells and giant cells mimicking malignant melanoma. Am J Surg Pathol 2000; 24: 864–869.

343 Newman CC, Raimer SS, Sánchez RL. Nonlipidized juvenile xanthogranuloma: a histologic and immunohistochemical study. Pediatr Dermatol 1997; 14: 98–102.

344 Kubota Y, Kiryu H, Nakayama J, Koga T. Histopathologic maturation of juvenile xanthogranuloma in a short period. Pediatr Dermatol 2001; 18: 127–130.

345 Zelger BWH, Staudacher Ch, Orchard G et al. Solitary and generalized variants of spindle cell xanthogranuloma (progressive nodular histiocytosis). Histopathology 1995; 27: 11–19.

346 Zelger BG, Orchard G, Rudolph P, Zelger B. Scalloped cell xanthogranuloma. Histopathology 1998; 32: 368–374.

347 Gallant CJ, From L. Juvenile xanthogranuloma and xanthoma disseminatum – variations on a single theme. J Am Acad Dermatol 1986; 15: 108–109.

348 Tomaszewski M-M, Lupton GP. Unusual expression of S-100 protein in histiocytic neoplasms. J Cutan Pathol 1996; 23: 63 (abstract).

349 de Graaf JH, Timens W, Tamminga RYJ, Molenaar WM. Deep juvenile xanthogranuloma: a lesion related to dermal indeterminate cells. Hum Pathol 1992; 23: 905–910.

350 Nascimento AG. A clinicopathologic and immunohistochemical comparative study of cutaneous and intramuscular forms of juvenile xanthogranuloma. Am J Surg Pathol 1997; 21: 645–652.

351 Gonzalez-Crussi F, Campbell RJ. Juvenile xanthogranuloma: Ultrastructural study. Arch Pathol 1970; 89: 65–72.

352 Mortensen T, Weismann K, Kobayasi T. Xanthogranuloma juvenile: a case report. Acta Derm Venereol 1983; 63: 79–81.

353 Seifert HW. Membrane activity in juvenile xanthogranuloma. J Cutan Pathol 1981; 8: 25–33.

354 Seo IS, Min KW, Mirkin LD. Juvenile xanthogranuloma. Ultrastructural and immunocytochemical studies. Arch Pathol Lab Med 1986; 110: 911–915.

355 Gianotti F, Caputo R, Ermacora E, Gianni E. Benign cephalic histiocytosis. Arch Dermatol 1986; 122: 1038–1043.

356 Commens C, Jaworski R. Benign cephalic histiocytosis. Australas J Dermatol 1987; 28: 56–61.

357 Godfrey KM, James MP. Benign cephalic histiocytosis: a case report. Br J Dermatol 1990; 123: 245–248.

358 Goday JJ, Raton JA, Landa N et al. Benign cephalic histiocytosis – study of a case. Clin Exp Dermatol 1993; 18: 280–282.

359 Eisenberg EL, Bronson DM, Barsky S. Benign cephalic histiocytosis. A case report and ultrastructural study. J Am Acad Dermatol 1985; 12: 328–331.

360 Peña-Penabad C, Unamuno P, Garcia-Silva J et al. Benign cephalic histiocytosis: case report and literature review. Pediatr Dermatol 1994; 11: 164–167.

361 Weston WL, Travers SH, Mierau GW et al. Benign cephalic histiocytosis with diabetes insipidus. Pediatr Dermatol 2000; 17: 296–298.

362 Larralde de Luna M, Glikin I, Goldberg J et al. Benign cephalic histiocytosis: report of four cases. Pediatr Dermatol 1989; 6: 198–201.

363 Arnold M-L, Anton-Lamprecht I. Multiple eruptive cephalic histiocytomas in a case of T-cell lymphoma. A xanthomatous stage of benign cephalic histiocytosis in an adult patient? Am J Dermatopathol 1993; 15: 581–586.

364 Zelger BG, Zelger B, Steiner H, Mikuz G. Solitary giant xanthogranuloma and benign cephalic histiocytosis – variants of juvenile xanthogranuloma. Br J Dermatol 1995; 133: 598–604.

365 Rodriguez-Jurado R, Duran-McKinster C, Ruiz-Maldonado R. Benign cephalic histiocytosis progressing into juvenile xanthogranuloma. Am J Dermatopathol 2000; 22: 70–74.

366 Ayala F, Balato N, Iandoli R et al. Benign cephalic histiocytosis. Acta Derm Venereol 1988; 63: 264–266.

367 Taunton OD, Yeshurun D, Jarratt M. Progressive nodular histiocytoma. Arch Dermatol 1978; 114: 1505–1508.

368 Burgdorf WHC, Kusch SL, Nix TE Jr, Pitha J. Progressive nodular histiocytoma. Arch Dermatol 1981; 117: 644–649.

369 Vadoud-Seyedi J, Vadoud-Seyedi R, de Dobbeleer G. Progressive nodular histiocytomas. Br J Dermatol 2000; 143: 678–679.

370 Winkelmann RK, Hu C-H, Kossard S. Response of nodular non-X histiocytosis to vinblastine. Arch Dermatol 1982; 118: 913–917.

371 Statham BN, Fairris GM, Cotterill JA. Atypical eruptive histiocytosis – a marker of underlying malignancy? Br J Dermatol 1984; 110: 103–105.

372 Gonzalez Ruíz A, Bernal Ruíz AI, Aragoneses Fraile H et al. Progressive nodular histiocytosis accompanied by systemic disorders. Br J Dermatol 2000; 143: 628–631.

373 Rodríguez HA, Saúl A, Galloso de Bello L et al. Nodular cutaneous reactive histiocytosis caused by an unidentified microorganism: report of a case. Int J Dermatol 1974; 13: 248–260.

374 Torres L, Sánchez JL, Rivera A, González A. Progressive nodular histiocytosis. J Am Acad Dermatol 1993; 29: 278–280.

375 Kuligowski M, Gorkiewicz-Petkow A, Jablonska S. Xanthoma disseminatum. Int J Dermatol 1992; 31: 281–283.

376 Maize JC, Ahmed AR, Provost TT. Xanthoma disseminatum and multiple myeloma. Arch Dermatol 1974; 110: 758–761.

377 Varotti C, Bettoli V, Berti E et al. Xanthoma disseminatum: a case with extensive mucous membrane involvement. J Am Acad Dermatol 1991; 25: 433–436.

378 Woollons A, Darley CR. Xanthoma disseminatum: a case with hepatic involvement, diabetes insipidus and type IIb hyperlipidaemia. Clin Exp Dermatol 1998; 23: 277–280.

379 Goodenberger ME, Piette WW, Macfarlane DE, Argenyi ZB. Xanthoma disseminatum and Waldenström's macroglobulinemia. J Am Acad Dermatol 1990; 23: 1015–1018.

380 Knobler RM, Neumann RA, Gebhart W et al. Xanthoma disseminatum with progressive involvement of the central nervous and hepatobiliary systems. J Am Acad Dermatol 1990; 23: 341–346.

381 Ferrando J, Campo-Voegeli A, Soler-Carrillo J et al. Systemic xanthohistiocytoma: a variant of xanthoma disseminatum? Br J Dermatol 1998; 138: 155–160.

382 Kumakiri M, Sudoh M, Miura Y. Xanthoma disseminatum. Report of a case, with histological and ultrastructural studies of skin lesions. J Am Acad Dermato 1981; 4: 291–299.

333 Mishkel MA, Cockshott WP, Nazir DJ et al. Xanthoma disseminatum. Clinical, metabolic, pathologic, and radiologic aspects. Arch Dermatol 1977; 113: 1094–1100.

384 Battaglini J, Olsen TG. Disseminated xanthosiderohistiocytosis, a variant of xanthoma disseminatum, in a patient with a plasma cell dyscrasia. J Am Acad Dermatol 1984; 11: 750–755.

385 Szekeres E, Tiba A, Korom I. Xanthoma disseminatum: a rare condition with non-X, non-lipid cutaneous histiocytopathy. J Dermatol Surg Oncol 1988; 14: 1021–1024.

386 Zelger B, Cerio R, Orchard G et al. Histologic and immunohistochemical study comparing xanthoma disseminatum and histiocytosis X. Arch Dermatol 1992; 128: 1207–1212.

387 Caputo R, Veraldi S, Grimalt R et al. The various clinical patterns of xanthoma disseminatum. Dermatology 1995; 190: 19–24.

388 Winkelmann RK, Kossard S, Fraga S. Eruptive histiocytoma of childhood. Arch Dermatol 1980; 116: 565–570.

389 Caputo R, Ermacora E, Gelmetti C et al. Generalized eruptive histiocytoma in children. J Am Acad Dermatol 1987; 17: 449–454.

390 Umbert IJ, Winkelmann RK. Eruptive histiocytoma. J Am Acad Dermatol 1989; 20: 958–964.

391 Caputo R, Alessi E, Allegra F. Generalized eruptive histiocytoma. A clinical, histologic, and ultrastructural study. Arch Dermatol 1981; 117: 216–221.

392 Shimizu N, Ito M, Sato Y. Generalized eruptive histiocytoma: an ultrastructural study. J Cutan Pathol 1987; 14: 100–105.

393 Stables GI, MacKie RM. Generalized eruptive histiocytoma. Br J Dermatol 1992; 126: 196–199.

394 Jang KA, Lee HJ, Choi JH et al. Generalized eruptive histiocytoma of childhood. Br J Dermatol 1999; 140: 174–176.

395 Wee SH, Kim HS, Chang S-N et al. Generalized eruptive histiocytoma: a pediatric case. Pediatr Dermatol 2000; 17: 453–455.

396 Repiso T, Roca-Miralles M, Kanitakis J, Castells-Rodellas A. Generalized eruptive histiocytoma evolving into xanthoma disseminatum in a 4-year-old boy. Br J Dermatol 1995; 132: 978–982.

397 Goerdt S, Bonsmann G, Sunderkötter C et al. A unique non-Langerhans cell histiocytosis with some features of generalized eruptive histiocytoma. J Am Acad Dermatol 1994; 31: 322–326.

398 Misery L, Kanitakis J, Hermier C, Cambazard F. Generalized eruptive histiocytoma in an infant with healing in summer: long-term follow-up. Br J Dermatol 2001; 144: 435–437.

399 Saijo S, Hara M, Kuramoto Y, Tagami H. Generalized eruptive histiocytoma: a report of a variant case showing the presence of dermal indeterminate cells. J Cutan Pathol 1991; 18: 134–136.

400 Coldiron BM, Cruz PD Jr, Freeman RG, Sontheimer RD. Benign non-X histiocytosis: a unique case bridging several of the non-X histiocytic syndromes. J Am Acad Dermatol 1988; 18: 1282–1289.

401 Bork K, Hoede N. Hereditary progressive mucinous histiocytosis in women. Report of three members in a family. Arch Dermatol 1988; 124: 1225–1229.

402 Bork K. Hereditary progressive mucinous histiocytosis. Arch Dermatol 1994; 130: 1300–1304.

403 Schröder K, Hettmannsperger U, Schmuth M et al. Hereditary progressive mucinous histiocytosis. J Am Acad Dermatol 1996; 35: 298–303.

404 Wong D, Killingsworth M, Crosland G, Kossard S. Hereditary progressive mucinous histiocytosis. Br J Dermatol 1999; 141: 1101–1105.

405 Mizushima J, Nogita T, Higaki Y, Kawashima M. Hereditary progressive mucinous histiocytosis. Int J Dermatol 1997; 36: 958–960.

406 Sass U, André J, Song M. A sporadic case of progressive mucinous histiocytosis. Br J Dermatol 2000; 142: 133–137.

407 Barrow MV, Holubar K. Multicentric reticulohistiocytosis. A review of 33 patients. Medicine (Baltimore) 1969; 48: 287–305.

408 Lesher JL Jr, Allen BS. Multicentric reticulohistiocytosis. J Am Acad Dermatol 1984; 11: 713–723.

409 Lotti T, Santucci M, Casigliani R et al. Multicentric reticulohistiocytosis. Report of three cases with the evaluation of tissue proteinase activity. Am J Dermatopathol 1988; 10: 497–504.

410 Oliver GF, Umbert I, Winkelmann RK. Reticulohistiocytoma cutis – review of 15 cases and an association with systemic vasculitis in two cases. Clin Exp Dermatol 1990; 15: 1–6.

411 Furey N, Di Mauro J, Eng A, Shaw J. Multicentric reticulohistiocytosis with salivary gland involvement and pericardial effusion. J Am Acad Dermatol 1983; 8: 679–685.

412 Hsu S, Ward SB, Le EH, Lee JB. Multicentric reticulohistiocytosis with neurofibroma-like nodules. J Am Acad Dermatol 2001; 44: 373–375.

413 Verma KK, Mittal R. Cutaneous lesions of multicentric reticulohistiocytosis developing in herpes zoster lesions. Acta Derm Venereol 2000; 80: 150.

414 Havill S, Duffill M, Rademaker M. Multicentric reticulohistiocytosis in a child. Australas J Dermatol 1999; 40: 44–46.

415 Catterall MD. Multicentric reticulohistiocytosis a review of eight cases. Clin Exp Dermatol 1980; 5: 267–279.

416 Coupe MO, Whittaker SJ, Thatcher N. Multicentric reticulohistiocytosis. Br J Dermatol 1987; 116: 245–247.

417 Valencia IC, Colsky A, Berman B. Multicentric reticulohistiocytosis associated with recurrent breast carcinoma. J Am Acad Dermatol 1998; 39: 864–866.

418 Morris-Jones R, Walker M, Hardman C. Multicentric reticulohistiocytosis associated with Sjögren's syndrome. Br J Dermatol 2000; 143: 649–650.

419 Caputo R, Ermacora E, Gelmetti C. Diffuse cutaneous reticulohistiocytosis in a child with tuberous sclerosis. Arch Dermatol 1988; 124: 567–570.

420 Goette DK, Odom RB, Fitzwater JE Jr. Diffuse cutaneous reticulohistiocytosis. Arch Dermatol 1982; 118: 173–176.

421 McKenna DB, Mooney EE, Young MM, Sweeney EC. Multiple cutaneous reticulohistiocytosis. Br J Dermatol 1998; 139: 544–546.

422 Heathcote JG, Guenther LC, Wallace AC. Multicentric reticulohistiocytosis: a report of a case and a review of the pathology. Pathology 1985; 17: 601–608.

423 Coode PE, Ridgway H, Jones DB. Multicentric reticulohistiocytosis: report of two cases with ultrastructure, tissue culture and immunology studies. Clin Exp Dermatol 1980; 5: 281–293.

424 Tani M, Hori K, Nakanishi T et al. Multicentric reticulohistiocytosis. Electron microscopic and ultracytochemical studies. Arch Dermatol 1981; 117: 495–499.

425 Franck N, Amor B, Ayral X et al. Multicentric reticulohistiocytosis and methotrexate. J Am Acad Dermatol 1995; 33: 524–525.

426 Zelger B, Cerio R, Soyer HP et al. Reticulohistiocytoma and multicentric reticulohistiocytosis. Histopathologic and immunophenotypic distinct entities. Am J Dermatopathol 1994; 16: 577–584.

427 Perrin C, Lacour JP, Michiels JF et al. Multicentric reticulohistiocytosis. Immunohistological and ultrastructural study: a pathology of dendritic cell lineage. Am J Dermatopathol 1992; 14: 418–425.

428 Heenan PJ, Quirk CJ, Spagnolo DV. Multicentric reticulohistiocytosis: a light and electron microscopic study. Australas J Dermatol 1983; 24: 122–126.

429 Caputo R, Alessi E, Berti E. Collagen phagocytosis in multicentric reticulohistiocytosis. J Invest Dermatol 1981; 76: 342–346.

430 Fortier-Beaulieu M, Thomine E, Boullie M-C et al. New electron microscopic findings in a case of multicentric reticulohistiocytosis. Long spacing collagen inclusions. Am J Dermatopathol 1993; 15: 587–589.

431 Purvis WE III, Helwig EB. Reticulohistiocytic granuloma ("reticulohistiocytoma") of the skin. Am J Clin Pathol 1954; 24: 1005–1015.

432 Rendall JRS, Vanhegan RI, Robb-Smith AHT et al. Atypical multicentric reticulohistiocytosis with paraproteinemia. Arch Dermatol 1977; 113: 1576–1582.

433 Toporcer MB, Kantor GR, Benedetto AV. Multiple cutaneous reticulohistiocytomas (reticulohistiocytic granulomas). J Am Acad Dermatol 1991; 25: 948–951.

434 Perrin C, Lacour JP, Michiels JF, Ortonne JP. Reticulohistiocytomas versus multicentric reticulohistiocytosis. Am J Dermatopathol 1995; 17: 625.

435 Caputo R, Grimalt R. Solitary reticulohistiocytosis (reticulohistiocytoma) of the skin in children: report of two cases. Arch Dermatol 1992; 128: 698–699.

436 Hunt SJ, Shin SS. Solitary reticulohistiocytoma in pregnancy: immunohistochemical and ultrastructural study of a case with unusual immunophenotype. J Cutan Pathol 1995; 22: 177–181.

437 Valente M, Parenti A, Cipriani R, Peserico A. Familial histiocytic dermatoarthritis. Am J Dermatopathol 1987; 9: 491–496.

438 Kossard S, Winkelmann RK. Necrobiotic xanthogranuloma with paraproteinemia. J Am Acad Dermatol 1980; 3: 257–270.

439 Kossard S, Winkelmann RK. Necrobiotic xanthogranuloma. Australas J Dermatol 1980; 21: 85–88.

440 Holden CA, Winkelmann RK, Wilson Jones E. Necrobiotic xanthogranuloma: a report of four cases. Br J Dermatol 1986; 114: 241–250.

441 Štork J, Kodetová D, Vosmík F, Krejča M. Necrobiotic xanthogranuloma presenting as a solitary tumor. Am J Dermatopathol 2000; 22: 453–456.

442 McGregor JM, Miller J, Smith NP, Hay RJ. Necrobiotic xanthogranuloma without periorbital lesions. J Am Acad Dermatol 1993; 29: 466–469.

443 Chave TA, Chowdhury MMU, Holt PJA. Recalcitrant necrobiotic xanthogranuloma responding to pulsed high-dose oral dexamethasone plus maintenance therapy with oral prednisolone. Br J Dermatol 2001; 144: 158–161.

444 Finan MC, Winkelmann RK. Necrobiotic xanthogranuloma with paraproteinemia. A review of 22 cases. Medicine (Baltimore) 1986; 65: 376–388.

445 Dupre A, Viraben R. Necrobiotic xanthogranuloma: a case without paraproteinemia but with transepithelial elimination. J Cutan Pathol 1988; 15: 116–119.

446 Nishimura M, Takano-Nishimura Y, Yano I et al. Necrobiotic xanthogranuloma in a human T-lymphotropic virus type I carrier. J Am Acad Dermatol 1992; 27: 886–889.

447 Randell PL, Heenan PJ. Necrobiotic xanthogranuloma with paraproteinaemia. Australas J Dermatol 1999; 40: 114–115.

448 Nestle FO, Hofbauer G, Burg G. Necrobiotic xanthogranuloma with monoclonal gammopathy of the IgG lambda type. Dermatology 1999; 198: 434–435.

449 Hauser C, Schifferli J, Saurat J-H. Complement consumption in a patient with necrobiotic xanthogranuloma and paraproteinemia. J Am Acad Dermatol 1991; 24: 908–911.

450 Macfarlane AW, Verbov JL. Necrobiotic xanthogranuloma with paraproteinaemia. Br J Dermatol 1985; 113: 339–343.

451 Umbert I, Winkelmann RK. Necrobiotic xanthogranuloma with cardiac involvement. Br J Dermatol 1995; 133: 438–443.

452 Fortson JS, Schroeter AL. Necrobiotic xanthogranuloma with IgA paraproteinemia and extracutaneous involvement. Am J Dermatopathol 1990; 12: 579–584.

453 Mehregan DA, Winkelmann RK. Necrobiotic xanthogranuloma. Arch Dermatol 1992; 128: 94–100.

454 Finan MC, Winkelmann RK. Histopathology of necrobiotic xanthogranuloma with paraproteinemia. J Cutan Pathol 1987; 14: 92–99.

455 Winkelmann RK, Dahl PM, Perniciaro C. Asteroid bodies and other cytoplasmic inclusions in necrobiotic xanthogranuloma with paraproteinemia. J Am Acad Dermatol 1998; 38: 967–970.

456 Kossard S, Chow E, Wilkinson B, Killingsworth M. Lipid and giant cell poor necrobiotic xanthogranuloma. J Cutan Pathol 2000; 27: 374–378.

457 Gibson LE, Reizner GT, Winkelmann RK. Necrobiosis lipoidica diabeticorum with cholesterol clefts in the differential diagnosis of necrobiotic xanthogranuloma. J Cutan Pathol 1988; 15: 18–21.

458 Furukawa F, Taniguchi S, Oguchi M et al. True histiocytic lymphoma. Arch Dermatol 1980; 116: 915–918.

459 Maier H, Burg G, Schmoeckel C, Braun-Falco O. Primary cutaneous atypical histiocytosis with possible dissemination. Am J Dermatopathol 1985; 7: 373–382.

460 Levisohn D, Seidel D, Phelps A, Burgdorf W. Solitary congenital indeterminate cell histiocytoma. Arch Dermatol 1993; 129: 81–85.

461 Sidoroff A, Zelger B, Steiner H, Smith N. Indeterminate cell histiocytosis – a clinicopathological entity with features of both X- and non-X histiocytosis. Br J Dermatol 1996; 134: 525–532.

462 Manente L, Cotellessa C, Schmitt I et al. Indeterminate cell histiocytosis: a rare histiocytic disorder. Am J Dermatopathol 1997; 19: 276–283.

463 Rosai J, Dorfman RF. Sinus histiocytosis with massive lymphadenopathy. Arch Pathol 1969; 87: 63–70.

464 Thawerani H, Sanchez RL, Rosai J, Dorfman RF. The cutaneous manifestations of sinus histiocytosis with massive lymphadenopathy. Arch Dermatol 1978; 114: 191–197.

465 Wright DH, Richards DB. Sinus histiocytosis with massive lymphadenopathy (Rosai–Dorfman disease): report of a case with widespread nodal and extra nodal

dissemination. Histopathology 1981; 5: 697–709.

466 Lazar AP, Esterly NB, Gonzalez-Crussi F. Sinus histiocytosis clinically limited to the skin. Pediatr Dermatol 1987; 4: 247–253.

467 Viraben R, Dupre A, Gorguet B. Pure cutaneous histiocytosis resembling sinus histiocytosis. Clin Exp Dermatol 1988; 13: 197–199.

468 Nawroz IM, Wilson-Storey D. Sinus histiocytosis with massive lymphadenopathy (Rosai–Dorfman disease). Histopathology 1989; 14: 91–99.

469 Foucar E, Rosai J, Dorfman R. Sinus histiocytosis with massive lymphadenopathy (Rosai–Dorfman disease): review of the entity. Semin Diagn Pathol 1990; 7: 19–73.

470 Annessi G, Giannetti A. Purely cutaneous Rosai–Dorfman disease. Br J Dermatol 1996; 134: 749–753.

471 Chu P, LeBoit PE. Histologic features of cutaneous sinus histiocytosis (Rosai–Dorfman disease): study of cases both with and without systemic involvement. J Cutan Pathol 1992; 19: 201–206.

472 Pérez A, Rodriguez M, Febrer I, Aliaga A. Sinus histiocytosis confined to the skin. Case report and review of the literature. Am J Dermatopathol 1995; 17: 384–388.

473 Child FJ, Fuller LC, Salisbury J, Higgins EM. Cutaneous Rosai–Dorfman disease. Clin Exp Dermatol 1998; 23: 40–42.

474 Innocenzi D, Silipo V, Giombini S et al. Sinus histiocytosis with massive lymphadenopathy (Rosai–Dorfman disease): case report with nodal and diffuse muco-cutaneous involvement. J Cutan Pathol 1998; 25: 563–567.

475 Kang JM, Yang WI, Kim SM, Lee M-G. Sinus histiocytosis (Rosai–Dorfman disease) clinically limited to the skin. Acta Derm Venereol 1999; 79: 363–365.

476 Carrington PR, Reed RJ, Sanusi ID, Fowler M. Extranodal Rosai–Dorfman disease (RDD) of the skin. Int J Dermatol 1998; 37: 271–274.

477 Silvestre JF, Aliaga A. Cutaneous sinus histiocytosis and chronic uveitis. Pediatr Dermatol 2000; 17: 377–380.

478 Braun A, Dugan E. Primary cutaneous Rosai–Dorfman disease in a patient with rheumatoid arthritis. J Cutan Pathol 2000; 27: 550 (abstract).

479 Olsen EA, Crawford JR, Vollmer RT. Sinus histiocytosis with massive lymphadenopathy. Case report and review of a multisystemic disease with cutaneous infiltrates. J Am Acad Dermatol 1988; 18: 1322–1332.

480 Foucar E, Rosai J, Dorfman RF. Sinus histiocytosis with massive lymphadenopathy. Current status and future directions. Arch Dermatol 1988; 124: 1211–1214.

481 Penneys NS, Ahn YS, McKinney EC et al. Sinus histiocytosis with massive lymphadenopathy. Cancer 1982; 49: 1994–1998.

482 Ang P, Tan SH, Ong BH. Cutaneous Rosai–Dorfman disease presenting as pustular and acneiform lesions. J Am Acad Dermatol 1999; 41: 335–337.

483 Suster S, Cartagena N, Cabello-Inchausti B, Robinson MJ. Histiocytic lymphophagocytic panniculitis. An unusual extranodal presentation of sinus histiocytosis with massive lymphadenopathy (Rosai–Dorfman disease). Arch Dermatol 1988; 124: 1246–1249.

484 Buchino JJ, Byrd RP, Kmetz DR. Disseminated sinus histiocytosis with massive lymphadenopathy. Arch Pathol Lab Med 1982; 106: 13–16.

485 Foucar E, Rosai J, Dorfman RF, Eyman JM. Immunologic abnormalities and their significance in sinus histiocytosis with massive lymphadenopathy. Am J Clin Pathol 1984; 82: 515–525.

486 Foucar E, Rosai J, Dorfman RF. Sinus histiocytosis with massive lymphadenopathy. An analysis of 14 deaths occurring in a patient registry. Cancer 1984; 54: 1834–1840.

487 Scheel MM, Rady PL, Tyring SK, Pandya AG. Sinus histiocytosis with massive lymphadenopathy: Presentation as giant granuloma annulare and detection of human herpesvirus 6. J Am Acad Dermatol 1997; 37: 643–646.

488 Veinot JP, Eidus L, Jabi M. Soft tissue Rosai Dorfman disease mimicking inflammatory pseudotumor: a diagnostic pitfall. Pathology 1998; 30: 14–16.

489 Quaglino P, Tomasini C, Novelli M et al. Immunohistologic findings and adhesion molecule pattern in primary pure cutaneous Rosai–Dorfman disease with xanthomatous features. Am J Dermatopathol 1998; 20: 393–398.

490 Bonetti F, Chilosi M, Menestrina F et al. Immunohistological analysis of Rosai–Dorfman histiocytosis. A disease of S-100+ CD1-histiocytes. Virchows Arch [A] 1987; 411: 129–135.

491 Miettinen M, Paljakka P, Haveri P, Saxen E. Sinus histiocytosis with massive lymphadenopathy. A nodal and extranodal proliferation of S-100 protein positive histiocytes? Am J Clin Pathol 1987; 88: 270–277.

492 Paulli M, Rosso R, Kindl S et al. Immunophenotypic characterization of the cell infiltrate in five cases of sinus histiocytosis with massive lymphadenopathy (Rosai–Dorfman disease). Hum Pathol 1992; 23: 647–654.

493 Perrin C, Michiels JF, Lacour JP et al. Sinus histiocytosis (Rosai–Dorfman disease) clinically limited to the skin. J Cutan Pathol 1993; 20: 368–374.

494 Hibi S, Esumi N, Todo S, Imashuku S. Malignant histiocytosis in childhood: clinical, cytochemical, and immunohistochemical studies of seven cases. Hum Pathol 1988; 19: 713–719.

495 Akiyama M, Inamoto N, Kakamura K. Malignant histiocytosis presenting as multiple erythematous plaques and cutaneous depigmentation. Am J Dermatopathol 1997; 19: 299–302.

496 Mongkonsritragoon W, Li C-Y, Phyliky RL. True malignant histiocytosis. Mayo Clin Proc 1998; 73: 520–528.

497 Ducatman BS, Wick MR, Morgan TW et al. Malignant histiocytosis: A clinical, histologic, and immunohistochemical study of 20 cases. Hum Pathol 1984; 15: 368–377.

498 Dodd HJ, Stansfeld AG, Chambers TJ. Cutaneous malignant histiocytosis – a clinicopathological review of five cases. Br J Dermatol 1985; 113: 455–461.

499 Wick MR, Sanchez NP, Crotty CP, Winkelmann RK. Cutaneous malignant histiocytosis: a clinical and histopathologic study of eight cases, with immunohistochemical analysis. J Am Acad Dermatol 1983; 8: 50–62.

500 Nezelov C, Barbey S, Gogusev J, Terrier-Lacombe M-J. Malignant histiocytosis in childhood: a distinctive CD30-positive clinicopathological entity associated with a chromosomal translocation involving 5q35. Semin Diagn Pathol 1992; 9: 75–89.

50 Marshall ME, Farmer ER, Trump DL. Cutaneous involvement in malignant histiocytosis. Case report and review of the literature. Arch Dermatol 1981; 117: 278–281.

502 Zucker JM, Caillaux JM, Vanel D, Gerard-Marchant R. Malignant histiocytosis in childhood. Clinical study and therapeutic results in 22 cases. Cancer 1980; 45: 2821–2829.

503 Jurco S III, Starling K, Hawkins EP. Malignant histiocytosis in childhood: morphologic considerations. Hum Pathol 1983; 14: 1059–1065.

504 Esumi N, Hashida T, Matsumura T et al. Malignant histiocytosis in childhood. Clinical features and therapeutic results by combination chemotherapy. Am J Pediat Hematol Oncol 1986; 8: 300–307.

505 Morgan NE, Fretzin D, Variakojis D, Caro WA. Clinical and pathologic cutaneous manifestations of malignant histiocytosis. Arch Dermatol 1983; 119: 367–372.

506 Nemes Z, Thomazy V. Diagnostic significance of histiocyte-related markers in malignant histiocytosis and true histiocytic lymphoma. Cancer 1988; 62: 1970–1980.

507 Tubbs RR, Sheibani K, Sebek BA, Savage RA. Malignant histiocytosis. Ultrastructural and immunocytochemical characterization. Arch Pathol Lab Med 1980; 104: 26–29.

508 Risdall RJ, Brunning RD, Sibley RK et al. Malignant histiocytosis. A light- and electron-microscopic and histochemical study. Am J Surg Pathol 1980; 4: 439–450.

Xanthomatous infiltrates

509 Parker F. Xanthomas and hyperlipidemias. J Am Acad Dermatol 1985; 13: 1–30.

510 Cruz PD Jr, East C, Bergstresser PR. Dermal, subcutaneous, and tendon xanthomas: diagnostic markers for specific lipoprotein disorders. J Am Acad Dermatol 1988; 19: 95–111.

5 I Smoller BR, McNutt NS, Kline M et al. Xanthomatous infiltrate of the face J Cutan Pathol 1989; 16: 277–280.

512 Vail JT Jr, Adler KR, Rothenberg J. Cutaneous xanthomas associated with chronic myelomonocytic leukemia. Arch Dermatol 1985; 121: 1318–1320.

513 Caputo R, Ermacora E, Gelmetti C, Gianni E. Fatal nodular xanthomatosis in an infant. Pediatr Dermatol 1987; 4: 242–246.

514 Winkelmann RK, Oliver GF. Subcutaneous xanthogranulomatosis: an inflammatory non-X histiocytic syndrome (subcutaneous xanthomatosis). J Am Acad Dermatol 1989; 21: 924–929.

515 Fleischmajer R, Schaefer EJ, Gal AE et al. Normolipemic subcutaneous xanthomatosis. Am J Med 1983; 75: 1065–1070.

516 Archer CB, Sharvill DE, Smith NP. Subcutaneous xanthomatosis. Br J Dermatol 1990; 123: 107–112.

517 Ramsay HM, Garrido MC, Smith AG. Normolipaemic xanthomas in association with human immunodeficiency virus infection. Br J Dermatol 2000; 142: 571–573.

518 Smith KJ, Yeager J, Skelton HG. Histologically distinctive papular neutrophilic xanthomas in HIV-1+ patients. Am J Surg Pathol 1997; 21: 545–549.

519 Northcutt AD. Epidermotropic xanthoma mimicking balloon cell melanoma. Am J Dermatopathol 2000; 22: 176–178.

520 Bork K, Gabbert H, Knop J. Fat-storing hamartoma of dermal dendrocytes. Clinical, histologic, and ultrastructural study. Arch Dermatol 1990; 126: 794–796.

521 Maher-Wiese VL, Marmer EL, Grant-Kels JM. Xanthomas and the inherited hyperlipoproteinemias in children and adolescents. Pediatr Dermatol 1990; 7: 166–173.

522 Parker F. Normocholesterolemic xanthomatosis. Arch Dermatol 1986; 122: 1253–1257.

523 McCradden ME, Glick AD, King LE Jr. Mycosis fungoides associated with cystrophic xanthomatosis. Arch Dermatol 1987; 123: 91–94.

524 Walker EE, Musselman MM. Xanthomas at sites of infection and trauma. Arch Surg 1967; 94: 39–40.

525 Anzilotti MG, Calderon PE. Xanthomatosis associated with lymphedema praecox in a child with congenital pulmonary hypertension. J Am Acad Dermatol 1997; 36: 631–633.

526 Chu C-Y, Yang C-Y, Huang S-F et al. Lichen planus with xanthomatous change in a patient with primary biliary cirrhosis. Br J Dermatol 2000; 142: 377–378.

527 Brunzell JD, Bierman EL. Chylomicronemia syndrome. Med Clin North Am 1982; 66: 455–468.

528 Vermeer BJ, Van Gent CM, Goslings B, Polano MK. Xanthomatosis and other clinical findings in patients with elevated levels of very low density lipoproteins. Br J Dermatol 1979; 100: 657–666.

529 Caputo R, Monti M, Berti E, Gasparini G. Normolipemic eruptive cutaneous xanthomatosis. Arch Dermatol 1986; 122: 1294–1297.

530 Jaber PW, Wilson BB, Johns DW et al. Eruptive xanthomas during pregnancy. J Am Acad Dermatol 1992; 27: 300–302.

531 Teltscher J, Silverman RA, Stock J. Eruptive xanthomas in a child with the nephrotic syndrome. J Am Acad Dermatol 1989; 21: 1147–1149.

532 Barr RJ, Fujita WH, Graham JH. Eruptive xanthomas associated with intravenous miconazole therapy. Arch Dermatol 1978; 114: 1544–1545.

533 Dicken CH, Connolly SM. Eruptive xanthomas associated with isotretinoin (13-cis-retinoic acid). Arch Dermatol 1980; 116: 951–952.

534 Eeckhout I, Vogelaers D, Geerts ML, Naeyaert JM. Xanthomas due to generalized oedema. Br J Dermatol 1997; 136: 601–603.

535 Cooper PH. Eruptive xanthoma: a microscopic simulant of granuloma annulare. J Cutan Pathol 1986; 13: 207–215.

536 Archer CB, MacDonald DM. Eruptive xanthomata in type V hyperlipoproteinaemia associated with diabetes mellitus. Clin Exp Dermatol 1984; 9: 312–316.

537 Poomeechaiwong S, Golitz LE, Brownstein MH. Eruptive xanthomas: evaluation of nineteen cases by polarized light microscopy. J Cutan Pathol 1988; 15: 338 (abstract).

538 Walsh NMG, Murray S, D'Intino Y. Eruptive xanthomata with urate-like crystals. J Cutan Pathol 1994; 21: 350–355.

539 Weston CFM, Burton JL. Xanthomas in the Watson–Alagille syndrome. J Am Acad Dermatol 1987; 16: 1117–1121.

540 Alam M, Garzon MC, Salen G, Starc TJ. Tuberous xanthomas in sitosterolemia. Pediatr Dermatol 2000; 17: 447–449.

541 Fleischmajer R, Tint GS, Bennett HD. Normolipemic tendon and tuberous xanthomas. J Am Acad Dermatol 1981; 5: 290–296.

542 Nakayama H, Mihara M, Shimao S. Perineural xanthoma. Br J Dermatol 1986; 115: 715–720.

543 Behan F, Fletcher CDM. Plexiform xanthoma: an unusual variant. Histopathology 1991; 19: 565–567.

544 El Shabrawi-Caelen L, Kerl H, Soyer HP. Plexiform xanthoma. Dermatopathology: Practical & Conceptual 1999; 5: 124–125.

545 Nakamura S, Tamura T, Takahashi H et al. Cerebrotendinous xanthomatosis: report of a case. Br J Dermatol 2000; 142: 378–380.

546 Friedman SJ, Martin TW. Xanthoma striatum palmare associated with multiple myeloma. J Am Acad Dermatol 1987; 16: 1272–1274.

547 Bergman R. The pathogenesis and clinical significance of xanthelasma palpebrarum. J Am Acad Dermatol 1994; 30: 236–242.

548 Bergman R. Xanthelasma palpebrarum and risk of atherosclerosis. Int J Dermatol 1998; 37: 343–349.

549 Gómez JA, Gónzalez MJ, de Moragas JM et al. Apolipoprotein E phenotypes, lipoprotein composition, and xanthelasmas. Arch Dermatol 1988; 124: 1230–1234.

550 Wilkinson SM, Atkinson A, Neary RH, Smith AG. Normolipaemic plane xanthomas: an association with increased vascular permeability and serum lipoprotein(a) concentration. Clin Exp Dermatol 1992; 17: 211–213.

551 Marcoval J, Moreno A, Bordas X et al. Diffuse plane xanthoma: Clinicopathologic study of 8 cases. J Am Acad Dermatol 1998; 39: 439–442.

552 Williford PM, White WL, Jorizzo JL, Greer K. The spectrum of normolipemic plane xanthoma. Am J Dermatopathol 1993; 15: 572–575.

553 Russell Jones R, Baughan ASJ, Cream JJ et al. Complement abnormalities in diffuse plane xanthomatosis with paraproteinaemia. Br J Dermatol 1979; 101: 711–716.

554 Derrick EK, Price ML. Plane xanthomatosis with chronic lymphatic leukaemia. Clin Exp Dermatol 1993; 18: 259–260.

555 Sharpe PC, Dawson JF, O'Kane MJ et al. Diffuse plane xanthomatosis associated with a monoclonal band displaying anti-smooth muscle antibody activity. Br J Dermatol 1995; 133: 961–966.

556 Winkelmann RK, McEvoy MT. Diffuse-plane normolipaemic xanthoma with aortic-valve xanthoma. Clin Exp Dermatol 1991; 16: 38–40.

557 Loo DS, Kang S. Diffuse normolipidemic plane xanthomas with monoclonal gammopathy presenting as urticarial plaques. J Am Acad Dermatol 1996; 35: 829–832.

558 Ginarte M, Peteiro C, Toribio J. Generalized plane xanthoma and idiopathic Bence-Jones proteinuria. Clin Exp Dermatol 1997; 22: 192–194.

559 Buezo GF, Porras JI, Fraga J et al. Coexistence of diffuse plane normolipaemic xanthoma and amyloidosis in a patient with monoclonal gammopathy. Br J Dermatol 1996; 135: 460–462.

560 Neville B. The verruciform xanthoma. A review and report of eight new cases. Am J Dermatopathol 1986; 8: 247–253.

561 Buchner A, Hansen S, Merrell PW. Verruciform xanthoma of the oral mucosa. Arch Dermatol 1981; 117: 563–565.

562 Santa Cruz DJ, Martin SA. Verruciform xanthoma of the vulva. Report of two cases. Am J Clin Pathol 1979; 71: 224–228.

563 Griffel B, Cordoba M. Verruciform xanthoma in the anal region. Am J Proctol 1980; 32 (4): 24–25.

564 Kimura S. Verruciform xanthoma of the scrotum. Arch Dermatol 1984; 120: 1378–1379.

565 Al-Nafussi AI, Azzopardi JG, Salm R. Verruciform xanthoma of the skin. Histopathology 1985; 9: 245–252.

566 Ronan SG, Bolano J, Manaligod JR. Verruciform xanthoma of penis. Light and electron-microscopic study. Urology 1984; 23: 600–603.

567 Duray PH, Johnston YE. Verruciform xanthoma of the nose in an elderly male. Am J Dermatopathol 1986; 8: 237–240.

568 Cooper TW, Santa Cruz DJ, Bauer EA. Verruciform xanthoma. Occurrence in eroded skin in a patient with recessive dystrophic epidermolysis bullosa. J Am Acad Dermatol 1983; 8: 463–467.

569 Mountcastle EA, Lupton GP. Verruciform xanthomas of the digits. J Am Acad Dermatol 1989; 20: 313–317.

570 Palestine RF, Winkelmann RK. Verruciform xanthoma in an epithelial nevus. Arch Dermatol 1982; 118: 686–691.

571 Kishimoto S, Takenaka H, Shibagaki R et al. Verruciform xanthoma in association with a vulval fibroepithelial polyp. Br J Dermatol 1997; 137: 816–820.

572 Takiwaki H, Yokota M, Ahsan K et al. Squamous cell carcinoma associated with verruciform xanthoma of the penis. Am J Dermatopathol 1996; 18: 551–554.

573 Mannes KD, Dekle CL, Requena L, Sangueza OP. Verruciform xanthoma associated with squamous cell carcinoma. Am J Dermatopathol 1999; 21: 66–69.

574 Kishimoto S, Takenaka H, Shibagaki R et al. Verruciform xanthoma arising in an arteriovenous haemangioma. Br J Dermatol 1998; 139: 546–548.

575 Meyers DC, Woosley JT, Reddick RL. Verruciform xanthoma in association with discoid lupus erythematosus. J Cutan Pathol 1992; 19: 156–158.

576 Chyu J, Medenica M, Whitney DH. Verruciform xanthoma of the lower extremity – report of a case and review of literature. J Am Acad Dermatol 1987; 17: 695–698.

577 Snider RL. Verruciform xanthomas and lymphedema. J Am Acad Dermatol 1992; 27: 1021–1023.

578 Huguet P, Toran N, Tarragona J. Cutaneous verruciform xanthoma arising on a congenital lymphoedematous leg. Histopathology 1995; 26: 277–279.

579 Smith KJ, Skelton HG, Angritt P. Changes of verruciform xanthoma in an HIV-1+ patient with diffuse psoriasiform skin disease. Am J Dermatopathol 1995; 17: 185–188.

580 Helm KF, Höpfl RM, Kreider JW, Lookingbill DP. Verruciform xanthoma in an immunocompromised patient: a case report and immunohistochemical study. J Cutan Pathol 1993; 20: 84–86.

581 Khaskhely NM, Uezata H, Kamiyama T et al. Association of human papillomavirus type 6 with a verruciform xanthoma. Am J Dermatopathol 2000; 22: 447–452.

582 Jensen JL, Liao S-Y, Jeffes EWB III. Verruciform xanthoma of the ear with coexisting epidermal dysplasia. Am J Dermatopathol 1992; 14: 426–430.

583 Connolly SB, Lewis EJ, Lindholm JS et al. Management of cutaneous verruciform xanthoma. J Am Acad Dermatol 2000; 42: 343–347.

584 Mohsin SK, Lee MW, Amin MB et al. Cutaneous verruciform xanthoma. A report of five cases investigating the etiology and nature of xanthomatous cells. Am J Surg Pathol 1998; 22: 479–487.

585 Travis WD, Davis GE, Tsokos M et al. Multifocal verruciform xanthoma of the upper aerodigestive tract in a child with a systemic lipid storage disease. Am J Surg Pathol 1989; 13: 309–316.

586 Lee M, Eyzaguirre E, Ma C et al. Cutaneous verruciform xanthoma: a report of 6 cases with an attempt to explain pathologic features. J Cutan Pathol 1996; 23: 54 (abstract).

587 Poblet E, McCaden ME, Santa Cruz DJ. Cystic verruciform xanthoma. J Am Acad Dermatol 1991; 25: 330–331.

588 Balus S, Breathnach AS, O'Grady AJ. Ultrastructural observations on 'foam cells' and the source of their lipid in verruciform xanthoma. J Am Acad Dermatol 1991; 24: 760–764.

589 Goerdt S, Kretzschmar L, Bonsmann G et al. Normolipemic papular xanthomatosis in erythrodermic atopic dermatitis. J Am Acad Dermatol 1995; 32: 326–335.

590 Meyrick Thomas RH, Miller NE, Rowland Payne CME et al. Papular xanthoma associated with primary dysbetalipoproteinaemia. J R Soc Med 1982; 75: 906–908.

591 Caputo R, Gianni E, Imondi D et al. Papular xanthoma in children. J Am Acad Dermatol 1990; 22: 1052–1056.

592 Kim S-H, Koh K-J, Choi J-H et al. Congenital papular xanthoma. Br J Dermatol 2000; 142: 569–571.

593 Darwin BS, Herzberg AJ, Murray JC, Olsen EA. Generalized papular xanthomatosis in mycosis fungoides. J Am Acad Dermatol 1992; 26: 828–832.

594 Sanchez RL, Raimer SS, Peltier F. Papular xanthoma. A clinical, histologic, and ultrastructural study. Arch Dermatol 1985; 121: 626–631.

595 Fonseca E, Contreras F, Cuevas J. Papular xanthoma in children: report and immunohistochemical study. Pediatr Dermatol 1993; 10: 139–141.

596 Chen C-G, Chen C-L, Liu H-N. Primary papular xanthoma of children. Am J Dermatopathol 1997; 19: 596–601.

Langerhans cell infiltrates

597 Breathnach SM. The Langerhans cell. Br J Dermatol 1988; 119: 463–469.

598 Dezutter-Dambuant C. Role of Langerhans cells in cutaneous immunologic processes. Semin Dermatol 1988; 7: 163–170.

599 Wright-Browne V, McClain KL, Talpaz M et al. Physiology and pathophysiology of dendritic cells. Hum Pathol 1997; 28: 563–579.

600 Hui PK, Feller AC, Kaiserling E et al. Skin tumors of T accessory cells (interdigitating reticulum cells) with high content of T lymphocytes. Am J Dermatopathol 1987; 9: 129–137.

601 Kolde G, Brocker E-B. Multiple skin tumors of indeterminate cells in an adult. J Am Acad Dermatol 1986; 15: 591–597.

602 Wood GS, Hu C-H, Beckstead JH et al. The indeterminate cell proliferative disorder: report of a case manifesting as an unusual cutaneous histiocytosis. J Dermatol Surg Oncol 1985; 11: 1111–1119.

603 Fowler JF, Callen JP, Hodge SJ, Verdi G. Cutaneous non-X histiocytosis: clinical and histologic features and response to dermabrasion. J Am Acad Dermatol 1985; 13: 645–649.

604 Miracco C, Raffaelli M, Margherita de Santi M et al. Solitary cutaneous reticulum cell tumor. Enzyme-immunohistochemical and electron-microscopic analogies with IDRC sarcoma. Am J Dermatopathol 1988; 10: 47–53.

605 Contreras F, Fonseca E, Gamallo C, Burgos E. Multiple self-healing indeterminate cell lesions of the skin in an adult. Am J Dermatopathol 1990; 12: 396–401.

606 Stingl G. New aspects of Langerhans' cell function. Int J Dermatol 1980; 19: 139–213.

607 Cumberbatch M, Dearman RJ, Griffiths CEM, Kimber I. Langerhans cell migration. Clin Exp Dermatol 2000; 25: 413–418.

608 Horton JJ, Allen MH, MacDonald DM. An assessment of Langerhans cell quantification in tissue sections. J Am Acad Dermatol 1984; 11: 591–593.

609 Ashworth J, Turbitt ML, MacKie R. The distribution and quantification of the Langerhans cell in normal human epidermis. Clin Exp Dermatol 1986; 11: 153–158.

610 Moresi JM, Horn TD. Distribution of Langerhans cells in human hair follicle. J Cutan Pathol 1997; 24: 636–640.

611 Mommaas M, Mulder A, Vermeer BJ, Koning F. Functional human epidermal Langerhans cells that lack Birbeck granules. J Invest Dermatol 1994; 103: 807–810.

612 Ishii E, Watanabe S. Biochemistry and biology of the Langerhans cell. Hematol Oncol Clin North Am 1987; 1: 99–118.

613 Writing group of the Histiocyte Society. Histiocytosis syndromes in children. Lancet 1987; 1: 208–209.

614 Bouloc A, Boulland M-L, Geissmann F et al. CD101 expression by Langerhans cell histiocytosis cells. Histopathology 2000; 36: 229–232.

615 Kashihara-Sawami M, Horiguchi Y, Ikai K et al. Letterer–Siwe disease: immunopathologic study with a new monoclonal antibody. J Am Acad Dermatol 1988; 18: 646–654.

616 Talanin NY, Smith SS, Shelley ED, Moores WB. Cutaneous histiocytosis with Langerhans cell features induced by scabies: a case report. Pediatr Dermatol 1994; 11: 327–330.

617 Schreiner TU, Lischka G, Schaumberg-Lever G. Langerhans' cells in skin tumors. Arch Dermatol 1995; 131: 187–190.

618 Lee CW, Park MH, Lee H. Recurrent cutaneous Langerhans cell histiocytosis in infancy. Br J Dermatol 1988; 119: 259–265.

619 Delabie J, de Wolf-Peeters C, de Vos R et al. True histiocytic neoplasm of Langerhans' cell type. J Pathol 1991; 163: 217–223.

620 Tani M, Ishii N, Kumagai M et al. Malignant Langerhans cell tumour. Br J Dermatol 1992; 126: 398–403.

621 Ben-Ezra J, Bailey A, Azumi N et al. Malignant histiocytosis X. A distinct clinicopathologic entity. Cancer 1991; 68: 1050–1060.

622 Lichtenstein L. Histiocytosis X. Arch Pathol 1953; 56: 84–102.

623 Osband ME, Pochedly C. Histiocytosis-X: an overview. Hematol Oncol Clin North Am 1987; 1: 1–7.

624 Osband ME. Histiocytosis X. Langerhans' cell histiocytosis. Hematol Oncol Clin North Am 1987; 1: 737–751.

625 Favara BE, Jaffe R. Pathology of Langerhans cell histiocytosis. Hematol Oncol Clin North Am 1987; 1: 75–97.

626 Munn S, Chu AC. Langerhans cell histiocytosis of the skin. Hematol Oncol Clin North Am 1998; 12: 269–286.

627 Neumann C, Kolde G, Bonsmann G. Histiocytosis X in an elderly patient. Ultrastructure and immunocytochemistry after PUVA photochemotherapy. Br J Dermatol 1983; 119: 385–391.

628 Caputo R, Berti E, Monti M et al. Letterer–Siwe disease in an octogenarian. J Am Acad Dermatol 1984; 10: 226–233.

629 Novice FM, Collison DW, Kleinsmith DM et al. Letterer–Siwe disease in adults. Cancer 1989; 63: 166–174.

630 McLelland J, Chu AC. Multi-system Langerhans-cell histiocytosis in adults. Clin Exp Dermatol 1990; 15: 79–82.

631 Esterly NB, Maurer HS, Gonzalez-Crussi F. Histiocytosis X: a seven-year experience at a children's hospital. J Am Acad Dermatol 1985; 13: 481–496.

632 Katz AM, Rosenthal D, Jakubovic HR et al. Langerhans cell histiocytosis in monozygotic twins. J Am Acad Dermatol 1991; 24: 32–37.

633 Zachary CB, MacDonald DM. Hand–Schüller–Christian disease with secondary cutaneous involvement. Clin Exp Dermatol 1983; 8: 177–183.

634 Winkelmann RK. The skin in histiocytosis X. Mayo Clin Proc 1969; 44: 535–549.

635 Lieberman PH, Jones CR, Steinman RM et al. Langerhans cell (eosinophilic) granulomatosis. A clinicopathologic study encompassing 50 years. Am J Surg Pathol 1996; 20: 519–552.

636 Hashimoto K, Takahashi S, Fligiel A, Savoy LB. Eosinophilic granuloma. Presence of OKT6-positive cells and good response to intralesional steroid. Arch Dermatol 1985; 121: 770–774.

637 Cavender PA, Bennett RG. Perianal eosinophilic granuloma resembling condyloma latum. Pediatr Dermatol 1988; 5: 50–55.

638 Helmbold P, Hegemann B, Holzhausen H-J et al. Low-dose oral etoposide monotherapy in adult Langerhans cell histiocytosis. Arch Dermatol 1998; 134: 1275–1278.

639 Török L, Tiszlavicz L, Somogyi T et al. Perianal ulcer as a leading symptom of pediatric Langerhans' cell histiocytosis. Acta Derm Venereol 2000; 80: 49–51.

640 Norris JFB, Marshall TL, Byrne JPH. Histiocytosis X in an adult mimicking pyoderma gangrenosum. Clin Exp Dermatol 1984; 9: 388–392.

641 Papa CA, Pride HB, Tyler WB, Turkewitz D. Langerhans cell histiocytosis mimicking child abuse. J Am Acad Dermatol 1997; 37: 1002–1004.

642 Modi D, Schulz EJ. Skin ulceration as sole manifestation of Langerhans-cell histiocytosis. Clin Exp Dermatol 1991; 16: 212–215.

643 Chi DH, Sung KJ, Koh JK. Eruptive xanthoma-like cutaneous Langerhans cell histiocytosis in an adult. J Am Acad Dermatol 1996; 34: 688–689.

644 Santhosh-Kumar CR, Al Momen A, Ajarim DSS et al. Unusual skin tumors in Langerhans' cell histiocytosis. Arch Dermatol 1990; 126: 1617–1620.

645 Lichtenwald DJ, Jakubovic HR, Rosenthal D. Primary cutaneous Langerhans cell histiocytosis in an adult. Arch Dermatol 1991; 127: 1545–1548.

646 Kwong YL, Chan ACL, Chan TK. Widespread skin-limited Langerhans cell histiocytosis: Complete remission with interferon alfa. J Am Acad Dermatol 1997; 36: 628–629.

647 Conias S, Strutton G, Stephenson G. Adult cutaneous Langerhans cell histiocytosis. Australas J Dermatol 1998; 39: 106–108.

648 Eng AM. Papular histiocytosis X. Am J Dermatopathol 1981; 3: 203–206.

649 Mejia R, Dano JA, Roberts R et al. Langerhans' cell histiocytosis in adults. J Am Acad Dermatol 1997; 37: 314–317.

650 Gottlöber P, Weber L, Behnisch W et al. Langerhans cell histiocytosis in a child presenting as a pustular eruption. Br J Dermatol 2000; 142: 1234–1235.

651 Messenger GG, Kamei R, Honig PJ. Histiocytosis X resembling cherry angiomas. Pediatr Dermatol 1985; 3: 75–78.

652 Nagy-Vezekényi K, Makai A, Ambró I, Nagy E. Histiocytosis X with unusual skin symptoms. Acta Derm Venereol 1981; 61: 447–451.

653 Vollum DI. Letterer–Siwe disease in the adult. Clin Exp Dermatol 1979; 4: 395–406.

654 Megahed M, Schuppe H-C, Hölzle E et al. Langerhans cell histiocytosis masquerading as lichen aureus. Pediatr Dermatol 1991; 8: 213–216.

655 Taïeb A, de Mascarel A, Surlève-Bazeille JE et al. Solitary Langerhans cell histiocytoma. Arch Dermatol 1986; 122: 1033–1037.

656 Aoki M, Aoki R, Akimoto M, Hara K. Primary cutaneous Langerhans cell histiocytosis in an adult. Am J Dermatopathol 1998; 20: 281–284.

657 Warner TFCS, Hafez GR. Langerhans' cell tumor of the eyelid. J Cutan Pathol 1982; 9: 417–422.

658 Jain S, Sehgal VN, Bajaj P. Nail changes in Langerhans cell histiocytosis. J Eur Acad Dermatol Venereol 2000; 14: 212–215.

659 Meehan SA, Smoller BR. Cutaneous Langerhans cell histiocytosis of the genitalia in the elderly: a report of three cases. J Cutan Pathol 1998; 25: 370–374.

660 Simonart T, Urbain F, Verdebout J-M et al. Langerhans' cell histiocytosis arising at the site of basal cell carcinoma excision. J Cutan Pathol 2000; 27: 476–478.

661 Wolfson SL, Botero F, Hurwitz S, Pearson HA. "Pure" cutaneous histiocytosis-X. Cancer 1981; 48: 2236–2238.

662 Stefanato CM, Andersen WK, Calonje E et al. Langerhans cell histiocytosis in the elderly: A report of three cases. J Am Acad Dermatol 1998; 39: 375–378.

663 Egeler RM, Neglia JP, Puccetti DM et al. Association of Langerhans cell histiocytosis with malignant neoplasms. Cancer 1993; 71: 865–873.

664 Roufosse C, Lespagnard L, Salés F et al. Langerhans' cell histiocytosis associated with simultaneous lymphocyte predominance Hodgkin's disease and malignant melanoma. Hum Pathol 1998; 29: 200–201.

665 Hashimoto K, Kagetsu N, Taniguchi Y et al. Immunohistochemistry and electron microscopy in Langerhans cell histiocytosis confined to the skin. J Am Acad Dermatol 1991; 25: 1044–1053.

666 Greenberger JS, Crocker AC, Vawter G et al. Results of treatment of 127 patients with systemic histiocytosis (Letterer–Siwe syndrome, Schüller–Christian syndrome and multifocal eosinophilic granuloma). Medicine (Baltimore) 1981; 60: 311–338.

667 Howarth DM, Gilchrist GS, Mullan BP et al. Langerhans cell histiocytosis. Diagnosis, natural history, management, and outcome. Cancer 1999; 85: 2278–2290.

668 Yu RC, Chu AC. Langerhans cell histiocytosis – clinicopathological reappraisal and human leucocyte antigen association. Br J Dermatol 1996; 135: 36–41.

669 Corbeel L, Eggermont E, Desmyter J et al. Spontaneous healing of Langerhans cell histiocytosis (histiocytosis X). Eur J Pediatr 1988; 148: 32–33.

670 Broadbent V, Davies EG, Heaf D et al. Spontaneous remission of multi-system histiocytosis X. Lancet 1984; 1: 253–254.

671 Kragballe K, Zachariae H, Herlin T, Jensen J. Histiocytosis X – an immune deficiency disease? Studies on antibody-dependent monocyte-mediated cytotoxicity. Br J Dermatol 1981; 105: 13–18.

672 Risdall RJ, Dehner LP, Duray P et al. Histiocytosis X (Langerhans' cell histiocytosis). Arch Pathol Lab Med 1983; 107: 59–63.

673 Emile J-F, Fraitag S, Leborgne M et al. Langerhans' cell histiocytosis cells are activated Langerhans' cells. J Pathol 1994; 174: 71–76.

674 Ruco LP, Stoppacciaro A, Vitolo D et al. Expression of adhesion molecules in Langerhans' cell histiocytosis. Histopathology 1993; 23: 29–37.

675 Hage C, Willman CL, Favara BE, Isaacson PG. Langerhans' cell histiocytosis (histiocytosis X): immunophenotype and growth fraction. Hum Pathol 1993; 24: 840–845.

676 Ugurel S, Pföhler C, Tilgen W, Reinhold U. S100-β serum protein – a new marker in the diagnosis and monitoring of Langerhans cell histiocytosis? Br J Dermatol 2000; 143: 201–202.

677 Leahy MA, Krejci SM, Friednash M et al. Human herpesvirus 6 is present in lesions of Langerhans cell histiocytosis. J Invest Dermatol 1993; 101: 642–645.

678 Harrist TJ, Bhan AK, Murphy GF et al. Histiocytosis-X. In situ characterization of cutaneous infiltrates with monoclonal antibodies. Am J Clin Pathol 1983; 79: 294–300.

679 Wells GC. The pathology of adult type Letterer–Siwe disease. Clin Exp Dermatol 1979; 4: 407–412.

680 Helm KF, Lookingbill DP, Marks JG Jr. A clinical and pathologic study of histiocytosis X in adults. J Am Acad Dermatol 1993; 29: 166–170.

681 Madden CR, McMichael A, White WL. Folliculocentric Langerhans cell histiocytosis: a distinctive case in an adult confined to the scalp. J Cutan Pathol 2000; 27: 563 (abstract).

682 Altman J, Winkelmann RK. Xanthomatous cutaneous lesions of histiocytosis X. Arch Dermatol 1963; 87: 164–170.

683 Foucar E, Piette WW, Tse DT et al. Urticating histiocytosis: a mast cell-rich variant of histiocytosis X. J Am Acad Dermatol 1986; 14: 867–873.

684 Rowden G, Connelly EM, Winkelmann RK. Cutaneous histiocytosis X. The presence of S-100 protein and its use in diagnosis. Arch Dermatol 1983; 119: 553–559.

685 Rabkin MS, Kjeldsberg CR, Wittwer CT, Marty J. A comparison study of two methods of peanut agglutinin staining with S100 immunostaining in 29 cases of histiocytosis X (Langerhans' cell histiocytosis). Arch Pathol Lab Med 1990; 114: 511–515.

686 Emile J-F, Wechsler J, Brousse N et al. Langerhans' cell histiocytosis. Definitive diagnosis with the use of monoclonal antibody 010 on routinely paraffin-embedded samples. Am J Surg Pathol 1995; 19: 636–641.

687 Groh V, Gadner H, Radaszkiewicz T et al. The phenotypic spectrum of histiocytosis X cells. J Invest Dermatol 1988; 90: 441–447.

688 Fartasch M, Vigneswaran N, Diepgen TL, Hornstein OP. Immunohistochemical and ultrastructural study of histiocytosis X and non-X histiocytoses. J Am Acad Dermatol 1990; 23: 885–892.

689 Gerbig AW, Zala L, Hunziker T. Tumorlike eosinophilic granuloma of the skin. Am J Dermatopathol 2000; 22: 75–78.

690 Hashimoto K, Pritzker MS. Electron microscopic study of reticulohistiocytoma. An unusual case of congenital, self-healing reticulohistiocytosis. Arch Dermatol 1973; 107: 263–270.

691 Kanitakis J, Zambruno G, Schmitt D et al. Congenital self-healing histiocytosis (Hashimoto–Pritzker). An ultrastructural and immunohistochemical study. Cancer 1988; 61: 508–516.

692 Herman LE, Rothman KF, Harawi S, Gonzalez-Serva A. Congenital self-healing reticulohistiocytosis. A new entity in the differential diagnosis of neonatal papulovesicular eruptions. Arch Dermatol 1990; 126: 210–212.

693 Oranje AP, Vuzevski VD, de Groot R, Prins MEF. Congenital self-healing non-Langerhans cell histiocytosis. Eur J Pediatr 1988; 148: 29–31.

694 Whitehead B, Michaels M, Sahni R et al. Congenital self-healing Langerhans cell histiocytosis with persistent cellular immunological abnormalities. Br J Dermatol 1990; 122: 563–568.

695 Larralde M, Rositto A, Giardelli M et al. Congenital self-healing histiocytosis (Hashimoto–Pritzker). Int J Dermatol 1999; 38: 693–696.

696 Jang K-A, Ahn S-J, Choi J-H et al. Histiocytic disorders with spontaneous regression in infancy. Pediatr Dermatol 2000; 17: 364–368.

697 Higgins CR, Tatnall FM, Leigh IM. Vesicular Langerhans cell histiocytosis – an uncommon variant. Clin Exp Dermatol 1994; 19: 350–352.

698 Alexis JB, Poppiti RJ, Turbat-Herrera E, Smith MD. Congenital self-healing reticulohistiocytosis. Report of a case with 7-year follow-up and a review of the literature. Am J Dermatopathol 1991; 13: 189–194.

699 Berger TG, Lane AT, Headington JT et al. A solitary variant of congenital self-healing reticulohistiocytosis: solitary Hashimoto–Pritzker disease. Pediatr Dermatol 1986; 3: 230–236.

700 Ikeda M, Yamamoto Y, Kitagawa N et al. Solitary nodular Langerhans cell histiocytosis. Br J Dermatol 1993; 128: 220–222.

701 Bernstein EF, Resnik KS, Loose JH et al. Solitary congenital self-healing reticulohistiocytosis. Br J Dermatol 1993; 129: 449–454.

702 Divaris DXG, Ling FCK, Prentice RSA. Congenital self-healing histiocytosis. Report of two cases with histochemical and ultrastructural studies. Am J Dermatopathol 1991; 13: 481–487.

703 Hashimoto K, Griffin D, Kohsbaki M. Self-healing reticulohistiocytosis: a clinical, histologic, and ultrastructural study of the fourth case in the literature. Cancer 1982; 49: 331–337.

704 Hashimoto K, Schachner LA, Huneiti A, Tanaka K. Pagetoid self-healing Langerhans cell histiocytosis in an infant. Pediatr Dermatol 1999; 16: 121–127.

705 Longaker MA, Frieden IJ, LeBoit PE, Sherertz EF. Congenital "self-healing" Langerhans cell histiocytosis: the need for long-term follow-up. J Am Acad Dermatol 1994; 31: 910–916.

706 Zaenglein AL, Steele MA, Kamino H, Chang MW. Congenital self-healing reticulohistiocytosis with eye involvement. Pediatr Dermatol 2001; 18: 135–137.

707 Kapila PK, Grant-Kels JM, Alfred C et al. Congenital, spontaneously regressing histiocytosis: case report and review of the literature. Pediatr Dermatol 1985; 2: 312–317.

708 Butler DF, Ranatunge BD, Rapini RP. Urticating Hashimoto–Pritzker Langerhans cell histiocytosis. Pediatr Dermatol 2001; 18: 41–44.

709 Bonifazi E, Caputo R, Ceci A, Meneghini C. Congenital self-healing histiocytosis. Clinical, histologic, and ultrastructural study. Arch Dermatol 1982; 118: 267–272.

710 Dragoš V, Bračko M, Sever-Novosel M. Multiple spontaneously regressing nodules in a newborn. Pediatr Dermatol 2000; 17: 322–324.

711 Hashimoto K, Bale GF, Hawkins HK et al. Congenital self-healing reticulohistiocytosis (Hashimoto–Pritzker type). Int J Dermatol 1986; 25: 516–523.

712 Timpatanapong P, Rochanawutanon M, Siripoonya P, Nitidandhaprabhas P. Congenital self-healing reticulohistiocytosis: report of a patient with a strikingly large tumor mass. Pediatr Dermatol 1989; 6: 28–32.

713 Hashimoto K, Takahashi S, Lee RG, Krull EA. Congenital self-healing reticulohistiocytosis. Report of the seventh case with histochemical and ultrastructural studies. J Am Acad Dermatol 1984; 11: 447–454.

714 Schaumburg-Lever G, Rechowicz E, Fehrenbacher B et al. Congenital self-healing reticulohistiocytosis – a benign Langerhans cell disease. J Cutan Pathol 1994; 21: 59–66.

Cutaneous infiltrates – lymphomatous and leukemic

by Geoffrey Strutton

INTRODUCTION

The diagnosis and classification of cutaneous lymphomas remain one of the most challenging areas in dermatopathology. Most current and widely used classifications of lymphoma and cutaneous lymphoma, such as the Revised European-American Classification of Lymphoid Neoplasms (the REAL classification),[1] the WHO modification of this classification[2] and the classification of the Cutaneous Lymphoma Project Group of the European Organization for Research and Treatment of Cancer (the EORTC classification)[3] are based on a combination of histological, clinical (including site of the process), immunohistochemical and cytogenetic features. It is now clear that simple histological features alone are in many cases insufficient to diagnose these conditions. All the above classifications accept the premise that cell lineage is the starting point for morphological classification, that is, the division into B, T and NK cell types, although the EORTC classification puts more emphasis on clinical features than the other two. These classifications lean heavily for terminology of cell type on the modified Kiel Classification.[4] In previous classifications, apart from mycosis fungoides, cutaneous lymphomas were not included in the general classification of nodal lymphomas.

It is now known that there are a group of lymphomas which appear to arise in the skin – primary cutaneous lymphomas[5] – which, although they have some morphological features in common with nodal lymphomas, have different behavior, prognosis and treatment requirements. This is particularly true for B-cell lymphomas. The EORTC group has importantly drawn attention to the differences between secondary cutaneous lymphomas and those lymphomas which appear to be unique to the skin and which require different therapeutic approaches.

There is still no general agreement as to whether the adoption of a general classification of lymphomas, such as the REAL/WHO classification, or a more skin-specific classification (the EORTC classification) is more applicable to the diagnosis and treatment of cutaneous lymphomas.[6-15] The EORTC classification includes only primary cutaneous lymphomas. The WHO modification of the REAL classification (REAL/WHO) now includes variants of lymphoma peculiar to the skin and has the advantage over the EORTC classification of including other lymphomas and leukemias which not infrequently involve the skin secondarily.[13] The REAL/WHO classification does not classify cutaneous lymphomas separately but includes certain diseases as separate entities if cutaneous involvement is a unique aspect of that disease and considered integral to recognition of that disease. There are also difficulties in defining primary cutaneous lymphomas. The EORTC classification defines primary cutaneous lymphomas as 'lymphomas confined to the skin at presentation and without evidence of extra-cutaneous spread for at least 6 months thereafter'.[3] It does not clearly indicate the extent of staging required to exclude extracutaneous disease.[3] Aggressive primary cutaneous lymphomas (except for Sézary's syndrome) are excluded by this definition. Sézary's syndrome, although included, is a systemic lymphoma at time of diagnosis, whereas adult T-cell leukemia/lymphoma, which involves the skin in the majority of cases, is excluded from the classification.

For the above reasons, the classification of cutaneous lymphomas used here is a modification of the classification suggested by Jaffe et al, based on the REAL/WHO classification (see Table 41.1).[13] The EORTC classification is listed in Table 41.2.

The current diagnosis of lymphomas requires some knowledge of lymphocyte ontogeny and techniques which are used to demonstrate such aspects as cell phenotype, clonality of a proliferation and cytogenetic features, including the presence of viral genetic material. Most laboratories are now able to utilize most of these techniques without difficulty, including immuno-histochemistry and polymerase chain reaction technology (PCR). Flow cytometry is also sometimes used for immunophenotyping but, unlike other organs, the number of neoplastic cells present in skin is sometimes small and cells are technically difficult to extract, particularly those in the epidermis. Enzymatic and mechanical disaggregation methods have been used to extract cells.[16]

The significance of established clonality of either B or T cells in cutaneous lymphoid infiltrates remains a problem of interpretation.[17,18] Although it has often been stated that lymphocyte clonality is not equivalent to malignancy,[19] demonstration of clonality in the appropriate cellular infiltrate and clinical scenario should be regarded as lymphoma.[3,20] Follow-up studies on atypical cutaneous lymphoid infiltrates with demonstrated monoclonal populations of T or B lymphocytes have shown progression to clear-cut lymphoma in some cases.[20,21] Follow-up may need to be over a long period because of the slow evolution and indolent behavior of many cutaneous lymphomas.

Most antibodies used for phenotyping and assessment of proliferation fractions are now available for use on paraffin-embedded tissue. A list of currently used antibodies and their various specificities is included in Table 41.3.[22]

Table 41.1 **Classification of cutaneous lymphomas**

B-cell neoplasms with frequent or constant cutaneous involvement

Precursor B-cell neoplasms
Precursor B-lymphoblastic leukemia/lymphoma
Mature (peripheral) B-cell neoplasms
Follicular lymphoma
- Primary cutaneous follicle center lymphomas
- Secondary
Extranodal marginal zone B-cell lymphoma of MALT type
- Primary
- Secondary
Large B-cell lymphoma
- Immunoblastic, centroblastic, large centrocytic, large cell anaplastic
- Lymphomatoid granulomatosis
- T-cell rich B-cell lymphoma
- Intravascular large B-cell lymphoma
Mantle cell lymphoma
Plasmacytoma

T- and NK-cell neoplasms with frequent or constant cutaneous involvement

Primary cutaneous T-cell lymphomas
Mycosis fungoides (MF)
MF variant
- Pagetoid reticulosis
- MF-associated follicular mucinosis
- Granulomatous slack skin
- Sézary syndrome
Primary cutaneous CD30-positive T-cell lymphoproliferative disorders
- Lymphomatoid papulosis
- Primary cutaneous anaplastic large-cell lymphoma (ALCL)
- Borderline lesions
Subcutaneous panniculitis-like T-cell lymphoma
Other T- or NK-cell neoplasms with frequent cutaneous involvement
Precursor T-lymphoblastic lymphoma/leukemia
T-cell prolymphocytic leukemia
Blastic NK-cell lymphoma
Aggressive NK-cell leukemia
Extranodal NK/T-cell lymphoma, nasal type
Angioimmunoblastic T-cell lymphoma
Adult T-cell leukemia/lymphoma (HTLV-1[+])
Peripheral T-cell lymphoma unspecified
Systemic anaplastic large-cell lymphoma

Table 41.2 EORTC classification of primary cutaneous lymphomas

Primary cutaneous T-cell lymphoma

Indolent
Mycosis fungoides (MF)
MF + follicular mucinosis
Pagetoid reticulosis
Large cell cutaneous T-cell lymphoma, CD30⁺
- Anaplastic
- Immunoblastic
- Pleomorphic
Lymphomatoid papulosis
Aggressive
Sézary syndrome
Large cell cutaneous T-cell lymphoma, CD30⁻
- Immunoblastic
- Pleomorphic
Provisional
Granulomatous slack skin
Cutaneous T-cell lymphoma, pleomorphic small/medium-sized
Subcutaneous panniculitis-like T-cell lymphoma

Primary cutaneous B-cell lymphoma

Indolent
Follicle center cell lymphoma
Immunocytoma (marginal zone B-cell lymphoma)
Intermediate
Large B-cell lymphoma of the leg
Provisional
Intravascular large B-cell lymphoma
Plasmacytoma

Techniques such as laser-based microdissection have also helped to extend our understanding of these disorders.[23,24]

B-CELL LYMPHOMAS WITH FREQUENT OR CONSTANT CUTANEOUS INVOLVEMENT

PRECURSOR B-LYMPHOBLASTIC LEUKEMIA/LYMPHOMA

In the WHO classification, precursor B-lymphoblastic lymphoma (PBLL) and precursor B-cell acute lymphoblastic leukemia (PBALL) are grouped together because they have similar histopathological and immunophenotypic features. Unlike precursor T-lymphoblastic lymphoma (PTLL), which commonly involves lymph nodes and mediastinum, PBLL usually involves extranodal sites, the skin being the most common site of extranodal presentation. Cutaneous presentation of PBLL occurs in children and adults, with the head and neck region being the most commonly involved sites. The lesions are erythematous or violaceous papules or nodules. Although systemic spread is usually demonstrated when staging is undertaken, there are reported cases limited to the skin.[25] Aggressive chemotherapy can prevent progression to leukemia[25] and PBLL appears to have a better prognosis than PBALL.

Histopathology[25,26]
The neoplastic infiltrate involves the dermis and subcutis with sparing of the epidermis. There is commonly a 'starry-sky' pattern. A vague nodular pattern can be produced by collagen compartmentalization. Crush artifact and the 'Azzopardi effect' (basophilic staining of collagen fibers) are common in

biopsies. The cellular infiltrate is monomorphic and consists of medium-sized lymphoid cells with round or convoluted nuclei, inconspicuous nucleoli and little cytoplasm. Numerous mitotic figures, some atypical, can be seen.

Immunohistochemistry and cytogenetics
The neoplastic cells express the B-cell marker CD79a and less commonly CD20 and CD10. TdT (terminal deoxynucleotidyl transferase), CD99 and bcl-2 are positive in all cases.[26] CD99 is particularly useful in distinguishing this lymphoma from other B-cell lymphomas.

FOLLICULAR LYMPHOMA (CUTANEOUS FOLLICLE CENTER LYMPHOMA) AND EXTRANODAL MARGINAL ZONE B-CELL LYMPHOMA OF MALT TYPE

These forms of lymphomas together represent 90% of all forms of cutaneous B-cell lymphoma. They share similar clinical presentations, response to therapy and excellent prognosis.[27] Discussion of this group is confounded by differences in terminology and conceptual problems and for these reasons they are discussed together. The EORTC classification uses the term *'follicle center cell lymphoma'*: the WHO classification uses the term *'cutaneous follicle center lymphoma'* for the cutaneous variant of *follicular lymphoma* (previously *follicle center lymphoma* in the REAL classification). These terms are not necessarily synonymous.

In the EORTC classification, the majority of lymphomas in this group are classified as *follicle center cell lymphomas*. As defined in that classification, neoplastic follicles are rare and cellular infiltrates can be nodular or diffuse. The component cells vary from predominantly small lymphocytes to a monotonous infiltrate of large cells. There are variable numbers of monotypic lymphoplasmacytoid cells and plasma cells.[3]

The REAL/WHO classification requires at least a partial follicular growth pattern for classification as *follicular lymphoma*.[1,2] CD21-positive follicular dendritic cells must be present for a nodule of lymphocytes to be considered a true follicle.[28] In nodal lymphomas, there are only rare cases of diffuse lymphoma which appear to be of follicle center origin. These cases are composed predominantly of centrocytes and rare centroblasts; demonstration of rearrangement of bcl-2 gene and CD10 expression is required for diagnosis.[2]

By these criteria, the majority of lymphomas classified in the EORTC group as follicle center cell lymphomas do not correspond to the follicle center lymphoma of the WHO classification. If carefully defined, primary follicular lymphomas appear to be uncommon, if not rare.[29,30] Even then, there appear to be some differences between cutaneous follicular lymphomas and their presumed nodal equivalent. There are differences in expression of bcl-2 protein and the t(14,18) translocation between cutaneous and nodal lymphomas. Several series report no expression of bcl-2 protein in cutaneous cases or expression in only a small proportion of cases;[23,31,32] nodal follicular lymphomas are positive in approximately 85% of cases.[22] Nodal follicular lymphomas frequently exhibit the t(14,18) translocation involving the bcl-2 oncogene, whereas this is a rare finding in cutaneous follicular lymphomas.[23,31,33–35] Only one study has found a more frequent expression of bcl-2 or the t(14,18) translocation (53%) in cutaneous cases.[32] Unlike nodal cases, the cutaneous follicular lymphomas, whether classified by EORTC or WHO criteria, have an indolent course. Hence the proposal that they represent a different entity, despite similar morphological features.[23]

An alternative viewpoint to that taken by the EORTC group is that the majority of lymphomas in this group represent cutaneous equivalents of MALT (mucosa-associated lymphoid tissue) lymphomas as previously defined.[36]

Table 41.3 **Antibodies used in the diagnosis of cutaneous lymphoma and their specificities**

Antibody	Predominant cells labeled
CD1a	Langerhans cells, Langerhans cell histiocytosis, some T-lymphoblastic lymphomas
CD2	T cells and T-cell lymphomas
CD3	T cells and T-cell lymphomas, NK cells (cytoplasmic staining for CD3e)
CD4	T-helper cells, monocytes, macrophages, Langerhans cells, peripheral T-cell lymphoma, MF, HTLV-1-associated adult T-cell leukemia/lymphoma
CD5	T cells, T-cell lymphoma, B-cell chronic lymphocytic leukemia/small lymphocytic lymphoma, mantle cell lymphoma
CD7	T cells, T-cell lymphomas, myeloid leukemia, NK-cell neoplasms, T-cell lymphoblastic lymphoma/leukemia
CD8	T cytotoxic/suppressor cells, NK cells, T-cell lymphomas, e.g. subcutaneous panniculitis-like T-cell lymphoma
CD10 (CALLA)	Precursor B cells, B-lymphoblastic leukemia/lymphoma, follicular lymphoma
CD15	Neutrophils, monocytes, Reed–Sternberg cells (classical Hodgkin's disease), acute myeloid leukemia
CD20	B cells, B-cell lymphoma
CD21	Follicular dendritic cells, follicular dendritic cell neoplasms, mantle and marginal zone B cells
CD23	Follicular dendritic cells, mantle zone B cells, B-cell small lymphocytic lymphoma/chronic lymphocytic leukemia
CD30	Activated lymphoid cells, anaplastic large cell lymphoma, lymphomatoid papulosis, Reed–Sternberg cells (classical Hodgkin's disease)
CD43	T cells, myeloid cells, mast cells, T-cell lymphomas, some B-cell lymphomas, myeloid leukemia, mast cell neoplasms
CD45 (leukocyte common antigen, LCA)	Hematolymphoid cells, most B- and T-cell lymphomas
CD56	NK cells, subset of activated T cells, T/NK-cell neoplasms, subset of T-cell lymphoma, panniculitis-like T-cell lymphoma (γ/δ type)
CD57	NK cells, T-cell subset, subset of T-cell lymphoma, NK-cell neoplasms
CD68	Histiocytes, myeloid cells, mast cells and their neoplasms
CD79a	Immature and mature B cells, B-cell lymphomas, plasma cells, plasma cell neoplasms
CD99	Lymphoblastic lymphoma/leukemia, small round cell tumors (Ewing's sarcoma/PNET and others)
CD138	Plasma cells, plasmacytoid cells
Cyclin C1 antigen (PRAD 1) – product of Bcl-1 translocation	Mantle cell lymphoma
Bcl-2	Non-germinal center B cells, most T cells, most follicular lymphomas (excluding cutaneous follicle center lymphoma), many other B-cell lymphomas
Bcl-6	Germinal center B cells, follicular lymphoma
Elastase	Myeloid cells, granulocytic tumors, leukemia
Epithelial membrane antigen (EMA)	Plasma cells, plasma cell neoplasms, anaplastic large cell lymphoma, lymphomatoid papulosis, T-cell rich B-cell lymphoma
EBV-latent membrane protein-1 (LMP-1)	AIDS-related non-Hodgkin's lymphomas, post-transplant lymphoproliferations, some NK/T-cell lymphomas
Granzyme B, perforin, TIA-1 (cytotoxic granule associated protein)	NK cells, cytotoxic T cells, subcutaneous panniculitis-like T-cell lymphoma, extranodal NK/T-cell lymphoma, nasal type, aggressive NK-cell leukemia, primary cutaneous CD8+ epidermotropic cytotoxic T-cell lymphoma
Immunoglobulin light chains	Plasma cells, plasma cell and plasmacytoid neoplasms
Myeloperoxidase	Myeloid cells and myeloid leukemia
TdT (terminal (deoxyribonucleotidyl transferase)	Lymphoblastic neoplasms
CD117 (c-kit gene product)	Mast cells and mast cell disorders

Many non-large cell cutaneous B-cell lymphomas have numerous features in common with MALT lymphomas, including excellent survival; involvement of regional nodes and systemic spread are rare events. Although the skin is generally not regarded as a lymphoid organ, T cells and rare B cells can be identified in the epidermis and dermis respectively in normal skin.[37] Chronic antigen stimulation, such as that following infection with *Borrelia burgdorferi* or related to components of tattoos, can be associated with a heavy acquired B-cell rich lymphoid infiltrate.[38–40] The term *'skin associated lymphoid tissue*

(SALT)' has been proposed for this acquired inflammatory infiltrate,[41] and lymphomas arising in this background have been designated *SALT-related B-cell lymphoma*. There have been several studies linking *B. burgdorferi* to the evolution of this group of cutaneous B-cell lymphomas,[42–46] and *B. burgdorferi* DNA has been demonstrated in lesions by PCR techniques. Regression of the lesions following antibiotic therapy has been reported, similar to gastrointestinal MALT lymphomas.[44,47] *B. burgdorferi* DNA was not identified in cutaneous B-cell lymphomas in a study from the United States.[47a]

Currently, the term '*extranodal marginal zone B-cell lymphoma of MALT type*' (MALT-1) is the preferred term in the WHO classification (see below). The term is restricted to lymphomas composed mainly of small cells: areas of large cell lymphoma, if present, are separately diagnosed as *diffuse large cell lymphoma*.[2]

Follicular lymphoma (cutaneous follicle center lymphoma)

There are only a few studies of cutaneous lymphomas of this type defined by REAL/WHO criteria.[23,31,48,49] As discussed above, they may in fact represent a unique entity.[23] Most arise in the head and neck region as single lesions. They are low-grade lymphomas with an indolent clinical course and long-term survival despite relatively frequent recurrences: extracutaneous spread is rare.[23,49]

Histopathology[23,29,48]

The lymphoid infiltrate involves the dermis and sometimes the subcutis without involvement of the epidermis. Infiltrates tend to be bottom heavy. Neoplastic follicles may vary in size and shape and may be widely spaced (Fig. 41.1). They generally have a poorly formed or absent mantle zone (Fig. 41.2). Some cases show fragmentation of the germinal centers with invagination of the mantle zone resembling nodal progressive transformation of germinal centers.[14] Follicles are composed of admixtures of centrocytes (cleaved follicle center cells) and larger centroblasts (large non-cleaved follicle center cells) in various proportions. Follicles can be graded after the system of Mann and Berard (Grade 1: 0–5 centroblasts per high-power field (hpf); Grade 2: 6–15 centroblasts per hpf; Grade 3: >15 per hpf).[50] Tingible bodies are absent or few in number, but they may be more frequent in high-grade tumors.

Interfollicular areas contain small lymphocytes, histiocytes and occasionally eosinophils and plasma cells. Clusters of follicle center cells (highlighted by immunohistochemistry) can be seen outside the follicles sometimes forming a diffuse component.

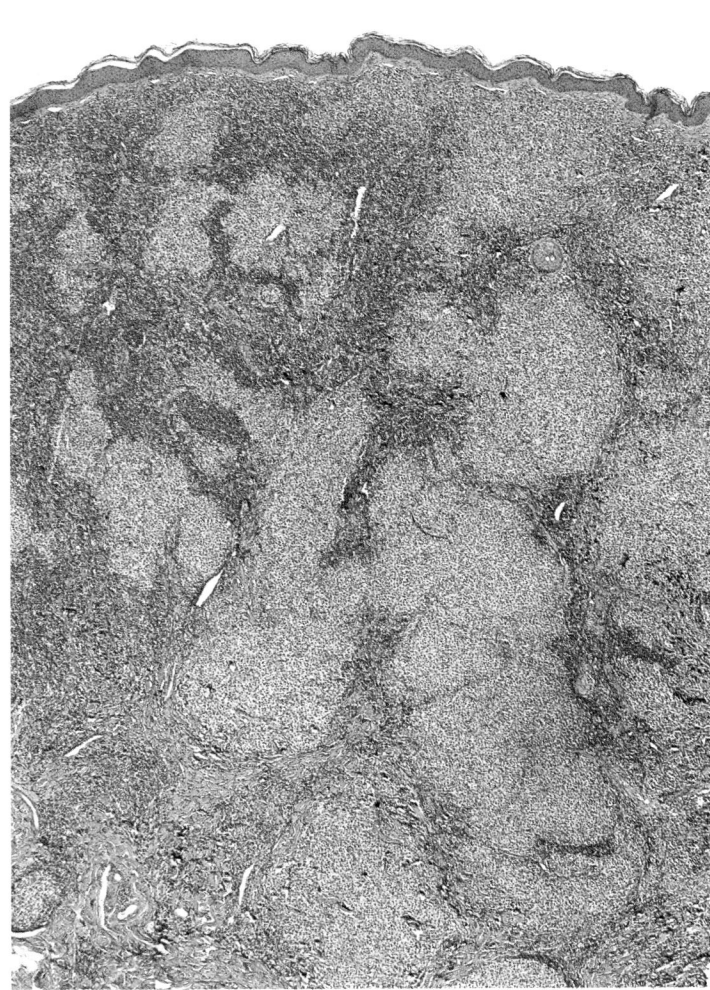

Fig. 41.1 **Follicle center lymphoma.** The follicular structures may be large and irregular. (H & E)

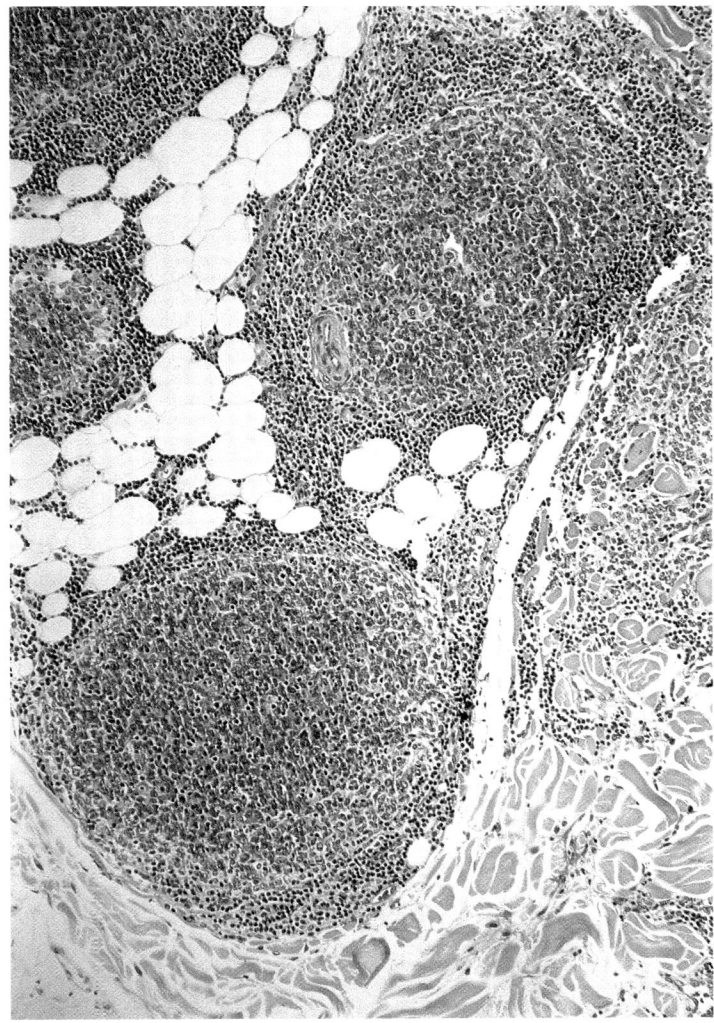

Fig. 41.2 **Follicle center lymphoma.** There is a poorly formed mantle zone and no tingible-body macrophages. (H & E)

Immunohistochemistry and cytogenetics

The follicle center cells express CD20, CD43 and CD10 and/or bcl-6. CD21 outlines the neoplastic follicles. CD10 also demonstrates clusters of follicle center cells outside the follicles. Reactive T cells are present in follicles and interfollicular areas. MIB-1 usually reveals a low proliferation fraction in follicles. Plasma cells are polyclonal. Bcl-2 was found not to be expressed by follicle center cells in some series[23,35] but was present in a proportion of cases in others.[32,48,49] There is similar discrepancy with the t(14;13) translocation; it is found in the majority of nodal follicular lymphomas.[33] Mutations of the bcl-6 gene have been described.[49]

Extranodal marginal zone B-cell lymphoma of MALT type

The majority of low-grade cutaneous B-cell lymphomas appear to be of this type,[30,51] although there is not general agreement on this point.[3] The term 'immunocytoma (marginal B-cell lymphoma)' is used in the EORTC classification. The WHO classification includes previously reported cases of primary cutaneous immunocytoma under the rubric of extranodal marginal zone B-cell lymphoma of MALT type.[52,53] Abandoning the term 'immunocytoma' prevents confusion with nodal lymphoplasmacytoid lymphoma/immunocytoma of the REAL classification and lymphoplasmacytic lymphoma of the WHO classification which is usually accompanied by Waldenström's macroglobulinemia.[7] The nodal form of this lymphoma, however, cannot always be easily distinguished from marginal zone B-cell lymphoma.[54] Cases reported as cutaneous follicular hyperplasia with monotypic plasma cells are also included in this group of cutaneous lymphomas.[55]

Cutaneous lesions are red to purple papules, nodules and plaques. Early studies suggested that lesions occurred most commonly on the arms;[52] however, subsequent studies have shown lesions to have a more common distribution on the head, neck and trunk.[32,48,56–58] Lesions may be multiple and involve more than one site. A dermatomal distribution has been described.[59] Secondary anetoderma has been reported in spontaneously regressing lesions.[60] Although the long-term prognosis is very good, lymphoma may recur at cutaneous sites or in lymph nodes, or rarely appear at other sites, particularly other organs where MALT-type lymphomas occur.[57] Transformation to large cell lymphoma has been reported.[61] Rarely, systemic spread leads to death.[61,62]

Histopathology[23,29,30,56]

Cellular infiltrates involve the dermis and frequently the subcutis. There is usually a nodular pattern about vessels and appendages but occasionally there is a diffuse pattern. A 'bottom heavy' or 'top heavy' arrangement of the cells can be seen and the epidermis is not involved. Follicular structures with reactive germinal centers containing tingible-body macrophages are typically present. These follicles are surrounded by a pale neoplastic infiltrate in a marginal zone pattern: there are interfollicular populations of similar cells. Neoplastic lymphocytes are small to intermediate in size with centrocyte-like (cleaved nuclei) or monocytoid (round nuclei and more prominent pale cytoplasm) features. In the interfollicular areas there are occasional large blasts as well as variable numbers of histiocytes and eosinophils. Where there is a more diffuse pattern, the mantles of follicles may be obliterated by the neoplastic component (follicular colonization). Plasma cells are usually present, often at the periphery of the nodules or beneath the epidermis. Unlike other MALT-type lymphomas, lymphoepithelial lesions involving skin appendages are rare but eccrine ducts or pilosebaceous units may be infiltrated by lymphoid cells.[27,63] In cases previously reported as immunocytoma there are often more diffuse infiltrates with few reactive follicles and more prominent

lymphoplasmacytoid cells (lymphoid nucleus and plasma cell-like cytoplasm) and plasma cells (Fig. 41.3). Dutcher bodies (intranuclear, PAS-positive inclusions) may be present in these cells and are considered to be indicative of a neoplastic process.

Immunohistochemistry and cytogenetics

Neoplastic cells express CD20, CD79a and CD38 (the last two are expressed by plasma cells): they also express bcl-2 but are negative for CD10, CD5, cyclin D1 and bcl-6.[56] Plasma cells and lymphoplasmacytoid cells show cytoplasmic immunoglobulin light-chain restriction.[23,64] Trisomy 3 has been demonstrated in a small number of cases.[65]

Differential diagnosis

The main differential diagnosis for both of these tumors is B-cell cutaneous lymphoid hyperplasia. Separation of these conditions remains one of the most difficult problems in diagnostic dermatopathology. As these forms of lymphoma are indolent low-grade tumors, a favorable clinical course is unreliable in separating lymphoma from lymphoid hyperplasia. Many histological features previously considered to be diagnostic of lymphoma or helpful in separating benign from malignant lymphoid infiltrates are now known to be unreliable, e.g. 'bottom heavy' versus 'top heavy' cellular infiltrates, although malignant infiltrates are more likely to be 'bottom heavy' and deep, often involving the subcutis. Demonstration of B-cell monoclonality by immunohistochemistry, PCR or other techniques is the most reliable tool in separating these conditions[37,51] and should probably be regarded as the gold standard, keeping in mind that PCR on small populations of B lymphocytes may be oversensitive. It has been suggested that pooled repeat PCR reactions helps to avoid this pitfall.[37]

Histopathological criteria helpful in separating hyperplasia from primary follicular lymphoma include follicles with a monotonous appearance, poorly developed or minimal mantle zones, and few or no tingible-body macrophages. The presence or absence of bcl-2 expression is not useful as discussed above. Demonstration of surface light-chain restriction on frozen sections or paraffin sections is unreliable in most laboratories. The presence of clusters of CD10-positive B cells in interfollicular areas is reported to be a useful diagnostic feature.[23]

Collections of pale-staining marginal zone cells in a marginal zone pattern, sheets of plasma cells and Dutcher bodies are helpful in making a diagnosis of marginal zone B-cell lymphoma. Immunohistochemical demonstration of

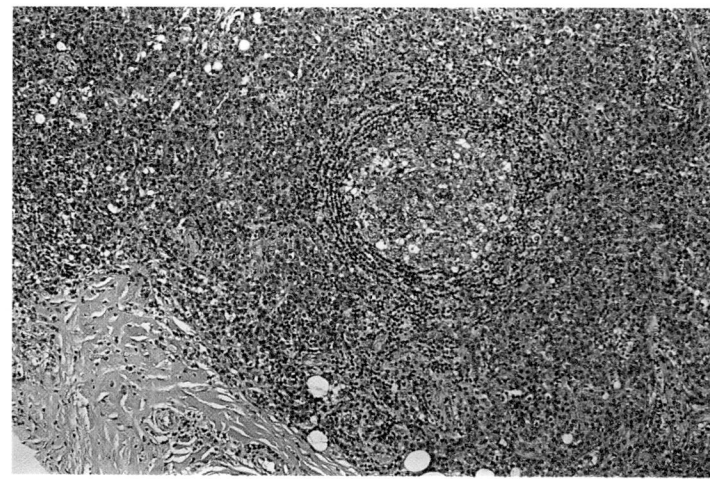

Fig. 41.3 **Marginal zone lymphoma of MALT type.** A reactive follicle is present with sheets of monotypic plasma cells. (H & E)

cytoplasmic light-chain restriction in plasma cells and lymphoplasmacytoid cells in paraffin sections is useful in demonstrating a monoclonal process. Aberrant CD43 expression by neoplastic B cells is considered by some to be a useful discriminator.[29]

Some diffuse, monoclonal, predominantly small cell infiltrates which lack follicular dendritic cells or monotypic plasma cells are not easily categorized as either *follicular lymphoma* or *marginal zone B-cell lymphoma*.[29] Other cases are not clearly neoplastic by either light microscopy or other techniques, and a diagnosis of *atypical cutaneous lymphoid infiltrate* would seem appropriate with clinical follow-up suggested, as even neoplastic infiltrates of this type have an indolent course.

DIFFUSE LARGE B-CELL LYMPHOMA

In the REAL/WHO classifications, diffuse large cell lymphomas are composed of large cells with nuclei at least twice the size of a small lymphocyte and usually larger than a tissue macrophage nucleus. In most cases the cells resemble centroblasts or large non-cleaved cells (cells with scanty basophilic cytoplasm and round nuclei with multiple, medium-sized, usually peripheral nucleoli) or immunoblasts (large cells with more prominent, often amphophilic cytoplasm, oval nuclei and a large, single, central nucleolus).[4] Other cell types include large centrocytes (large cleaved cells), multilobated and anaplastic large cells identical to T-cell and null-cell anaplastic large cell lymphoma.[1] No subclassification is made on histological features although there is some evidence that large cell lymphomas composed predominantly of immunoblasts may have a worse prognosis than the group in general.[2]

Vermeer et al, and subsequently the EORTC classification, distinguish a group of large B-cell lymphomas – *large B-cell lymphoma of the legs* – which they maintain has an intermediate prognosis, but a worse prognosis with a much higher relapse rate than morphologically similar lesions in other sites.[66] As defined by them, this form of cutaneous lymphoma occurs predominantly in the elderly (80% over the age of 70) as red or bluish nodules confined to one or both legs. Females are affected more frequently than males (3–4:1). The 5-year survival rate is 52%, compared with more than 94% for other B-cell lymphomas.[67] It is argued that this group of patients should be identified so that the appropriate therapy can be given, which may include more aggressive therapy than for large cell lymphomas at other sites (which are included in the *follicular center cell lymphoma* in the EORTC classification). This concept of a distinct clinicopathological entity has not been accepted or confirmed by all.[68,69]

Primary cutaneous *diffuse large B-cell lymphoma* is probably a heterogeneous group of large cell lymphomas, some at least representing predominantly diffuse variants of Grade III follicular lymphomas or large cell transformation of a marginal zone lymphoma of MALT type.[30,61,69] Large B-cell lymphoma has been described arising in a leg with lymphedema.[70]

These lymphomas arise on the trunk, head and neck and lower legs, but rarely on the upper extremities.[29] Lesions are usually single or localized papules, nodules or tumors on the upper body but tend to be multiple on the legs.[66] Cases with multiple or disseminated lesions appear to have a worse prognosis independent of site.[71] Sentinel lymph node biopsy has been used to stage apparently localized cutaneous large B-cell lymphoma of the leg.[72] Large B-cell lymphomas of the leg with a round cell morphology (centroblastic and immunoblastic cells) had a worse prognosis than other cell types (large cleaved centrocytic cells) in one series.[67] Most cases of *reticulohistiocytoma of the dorsum (Crosti's lymphoma)*[73,74] and *large cell lymphocytoma*[75,76] represent *large B-cell lymphoma*, although some of the former may represent marginal zone or primary cutaneous follicular lymphoma.[29]

Histopathology

Early lesions may have a perivascular and periappendageal distribution, whereas in most cases there is a diffuse infiltrate involving variable amounts of the dermis and subcutis. There is usually a grenz zone but very rarely there may be some involvement of the epidermis by neoplastic B cells[77] or reactive T cells.[78] The tumor infiltrate may appear polymorphous with an admixture of centroblasts, immunoblasts and commonly large cleaved centrocyte-like cells (Fig. 41.4). Other cell variants include cells with multilobulated nuclei, cells similar to those seen in large cell anaplastic lymphoma, and spindle cells.[79] Areas of necrosis may be present.[71]

Immunohistochemistry and cytogenetics

Tumor cells stain with the pan B-cell markers CD20 and CD79a. A significant number of cases express CD10 and/or bcl-6, including cases from the lower leg.[32,69] *Bcl-2* is expressed in many cases but is not associated with the t(14;18) translocation.[3] Some authors report that bcl-2 is expressed by those tumors classified as *large B-cell lymphoma of the leg* and not large B-cell lymphomas of other sites which are included in the *follicle center cell group*.[3,80] This finding has not been confirmed by others.[61,69,71] The t(14;18) translocation has been reported in cases of secondary large cell B-cell lymphoma and may help to distinguish primary from secondary cases.[80] Cells do not express CD5 or cyclin D1. Occasional cases express CD43 or CD30.[71]

Lymphomatoid granulomatosis

The concept of *lymphomatoid granulomatosis* (LG) has evolved since it was first described by Liebow et al in 1972.[81] It was originally defined as an angiocentric, angiodestructive, lymphohistiocytic disorder which affected the lungs predominantly, but had frequent extrapulmonary manifestations. It was for some time considered to be a T-cell proliferative disorder because of the large number of T cells in lesions, although most studies failed to demonstrate aberrant T-cell phenotypes or a clonal proliferation of T cells.[82] Epstein–Barr virus (EBV) was identified by PCR in most pulmonary cases and some cutaneous lesions, implicating it in the pathogenesis of LG.[83,84] Subsequent studies have localized EBV to a population of large atypical B cells which represent a minor component of the polymorphous infiltrate.[85,86] PCR studies have demonstrated a monoclonal B-cell proliferation.[82,85] Proliferation studies have also shown that B cells are the proliferating population in the lesions and that the accompanying T cells, histiocytes and NK cells are recruited.[87] Consequently, most case of LG are now regarded as an angiocentric T-cell rich B-cell lymphoma.[82] It is classified as a variant of *large B-cell lymphoma* in the WHO classification.[2] Other cases of angiocentric lymphoma involving the lung and skin in which the large atypical cells are T cells and negative for EBV probably represent a different process.[84,85] Chemokines have been implicated in the vascular damage.[88]

Skin lesions are found in 40–60% of cases: these may be the presenting complaint[39–94] and may precede other manifestations by years.[95] They take the form of erythematous or violaceous nodules or plaques which may be widely distributed on the trunk and lower extremities.[90] Rarely, paranasal or ulcerated palatal lesions are present. Any of the lesions may become ulcerated with surface eschar formation: this is more common with nodules on the leg.

The lung is the most commonly affected organ. The kidneys, liver and central and peripheral nervous systems may also be affected, although the skin is the most common extrapulmonary site.[81,96,97] Many patients when investigated are found to have defects in cytotoxic T-cell function and reduced numbers of CD8+ T cells. LG is common in immunodeficiency states such as HIV/AIDS, Wiskott–Aldrich syndrome and following organ transplantation.[88]

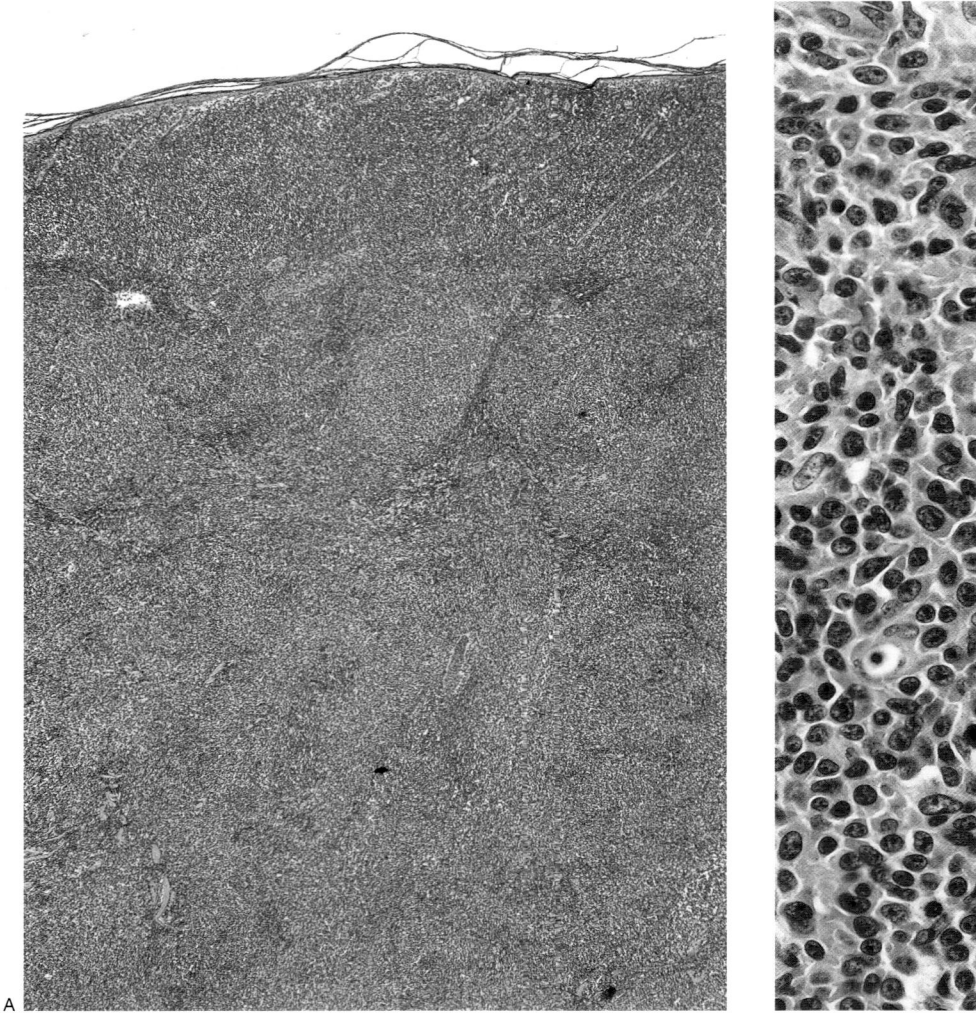
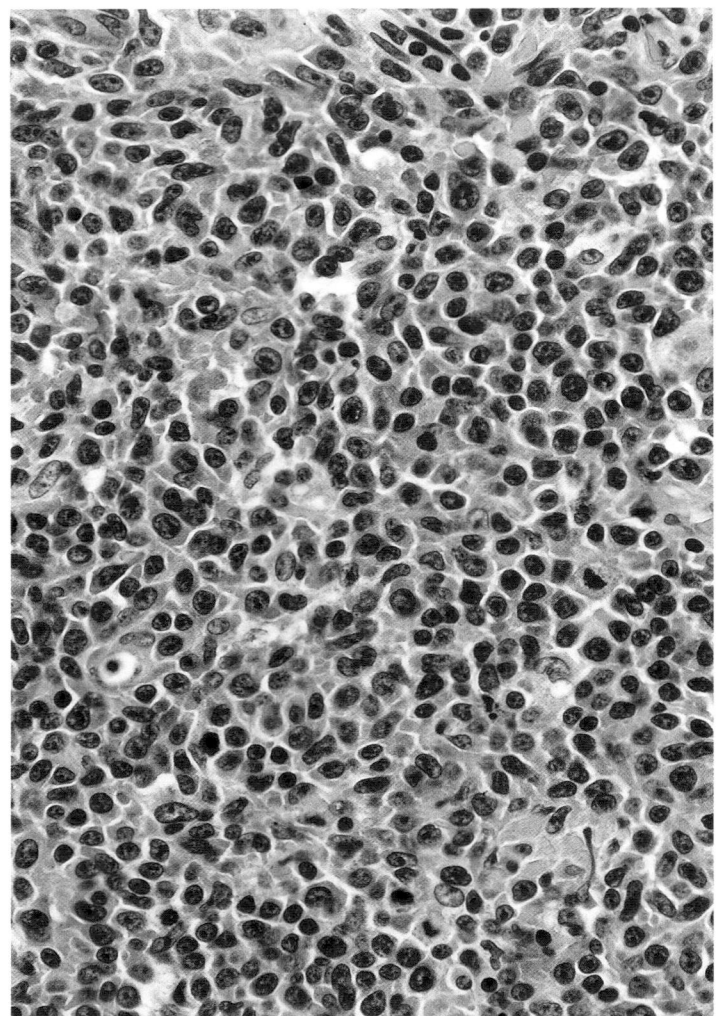

Fig. 41.4 **(A) Diffuse large B-cell lymphoma. (B)** The large B cells are predominantly centroblasts and immunoblasts. (H & E)

Onset is usually in early middle age; it has rarely been reported in children.[98] In older studies there was a rapid downhill clinical course with a median survival of 14 months.[96] Death was usually from respiratory failure. An overt large B-cell lymphoma may develop in the lungs.[87] Currently, longer survivals have been reported with multiagent chemotherapeutic and interferon therapy.[82,85] Spontaneous regression of lesions may occur.[82]

Histopathology

There is a polymorphous infiltrate in the dermis with perivascular, peri-appendageal and perineural accentuation.[89] Sweat glands are particularly involved.[92] The infiltrate is composed of a mixture of small lymphocytes and a variable number of large lymphocytes with vesicular nuclei and prominent nucleoli which may resemble immunoblasts; some multinucleate forms resemble Reed–Sternberg cells.[82,90] Large atypical lymphocytes are more frequent in lung lesions. There are variable numbers of histiocytes, eosinophils and neutrophils only in ulcerated lesions. Multinucleated histiocytes are not usually seen.

As well as being angiocentric, the infiltrate is frequently angioinvasive. Both arteries and veins may be affected. Cells invading vessel walls are predominantly small lymphocytes and histiocytes; large atypical cells are usually rare.[82] Fibrinoid necrosis and infarction are not usually prominent features in the skin. Marked fibroblastic proliferation may be present in some lesions.

Sometimes the histology of the skin lesions is not diagnostic, despite the presence of typical changes in other organs.

The differential diagnosis includes Wegener's granulomatosis (WG), which only displays the classic combination of necrotizing granulomatous inflammation and a necrotizing vasculitis in a minority of cases (see p. 254). Atypical large lymphocytes are not seen in WG but they may be difficult to identify in LG. Neutrophils are not usually seen in LG without ulceration.

The presence of a prominent histiocytic infiltrate and a perineural distribution in biopsies may mimic one of the forms of leprosy.[90]

Immunohistochemistry and cytogenetics

The majority of cells are small CD3[+], CD45RO[+], CD4[+] T cells. Small numbers of CD57[+] cells have also been identified in some cases.[87] The large atypical cells are B cells and are CD20[+], sometimes CD43[+], and CD30[-]. EBV RNA has been demonstrated in the large B cells by in situ hybridization techniques.[82] EBV-positive cells are less frequently identified in skin lesions than lung lesions.[97] Clonal rearrangement of immunoglobulin heavy-chain gene has been demonstrated by PCR in paraffin-embedded material.[82]

T-cell rich B-cell lymphoma

Primary cutaneous *T-cell rich B-cell lymphoma* is a very rare variant of *large B-cell lymphoma* which is characterized by the presence of small numbers of neoplastic large B cells surrounded by large numbers of reactive, small T cells.[99–101] The relative proportions of large B cells and reactive T cells have not been clearly defined.[102] The nodal form of this lymphoma rarely involves the skin secondarily.[103,104] The average age of patients in several series was 42 years. The lesions had no particular anatomical distribution.[105] It may be associated with HIV infection.[102] An angiocentric form has been described which has similarities to *lymphomatoid granulomatosis* (see above).[105] The clinical course is variable in the small number of cases available for study; some cases have progressed to disseminated disease.

Histopathology

Diagnosis is difficult because of the polymorphous nature of the infiltrate and the small numbers of neoplastic cells. There are scattered large B cells which may resemble centroblasts, immunoblasts or Reed–Sternberg-like cells.[100] The majority of cells are small lymphocytes with variable numbers of histiocytes, eosinophils and plasma cells. The differential diagnosis includes Hodgkin's disease, mature (peripheral) T-cell lymphoma, and benign lymphoid hyperplasia. Diagnosis requires demonstration of a monoclonal population of B cells by immunohistochemistry, PCR or other techniques. The neoplastic B cells are positive for CD20, CD79a and other pan-B cell markers. The background population of lymphocytes are predominantly small T cells which are CD3 positive.

Intravascular large B-cell lymphoma

Intravascular large B-cell lymphoma (IVLBL) is a rare form of systemic lymphoma which may first present with skin manifestations.[106] It has also been termed *'intravascular lymphomatosis'* and *'angiotropic large-cell lymphoma'*.[107,108] The term *'malignant angioendotheliomatosis'* is now considered inappropriate for this condition as the intravascular neoplastic cells have been shown to be lymphoid cells by immunohistochemical and molecular techniques.[109] It is characterized by an intravascular proliferation of large atypical lymphoid cells. In the majority of cases there are B cells, but rare cases with a similar histological appearance have a T-cell phenotype.[110–113] It has been suggested in one study that the lack of CD29 (β1 integrin) and CD54 (ICAM-1) adhesion molecules by the lymphoma cells in intravascular lymphomatosis is responsible for its disseminated intravascular pattern, these molecules being important in lymphocyte trafficking and transvascular migration.[114]

Most patients present with multiple neurological defects, including dementia.[115] Skin lesions, seen initially in about one-third of cases, take the form of erythematous to blue plaques and nodules on the extremities, trunk or face[106,116] and may mimic a panniculitis such as erythema nodosum.[117] Unusual presentations reported include generalized telangiectasia[118] and vascular tumors including hemangiomas,[119] angiolipomas[120] and Kaposi's sarcoma in association with HIV/AIDS.[121] It may present as disseminated intravascular coagulation.[115] A form associated with hemophagocytic syndrome has also been described, particularly in Asians. This form rarely presents with neurological complications or skin lesions.[122] There may be an associated extravascular large cell lymphoma, either nodal or extranodal.[123] There are also reports of an association with other types of lymphoma such as follicular lymphoma and MALT lymphoma.[114,124] Some cases have been positive for CD5, suggesting a possible relationship to chronic lymphocytic leukemia/small lymphocytic lymphoma or mantle cell lymphoma.[125] This condition is almost uniformly fatal, although some cases with only skin involvement have had a more prolonged clinical course.[107,126]

Histopathology

Blood vessels in the dermis and subcutis are partially or completely occluded by large atypical lymphoid cells (Fig. 41.5). The cells are several times larger than endothelial cells and have a high nuclear:cytoplasmic ratio. Cell nuclei are round to oval, and nucleoli are often prominent. Mitotic figures are frequent and may be atypical. Fibrin thrombi are often present in vessels, either with or without atypical cells. Extravascular neoplastic cells may also be found in up to 20% of cases.[3] The upper dermis may be spared and a superficial biopsy may not contain the diagnostic changes.[127]

Immunohistochemistry

The majority of cases are large B-cell lymphomas which are positive for CD20 and CD79, and negative for T-cell markers such as CD3. In one series, a subset of cases was also CD5 positive.[125] Monoclonality, with heavy-chain rearrangement, has been demonstrated by PCR on paraffin-embedded tissue.[128] T-cell cases are CD3 positive. T-cell gene rearrangement has been demonstrated by PCR.[112] One rare case was negative for B- and T-cell markers and positive for histiocyte markers Mac387 and CD68.[129]

MANTLE CELL LYMPHOMA

The majority of cases classified as mantle cell lymphoma (MCL) in the skin are secondary to nodal disease.[130] Secondary skin involvement has been reported

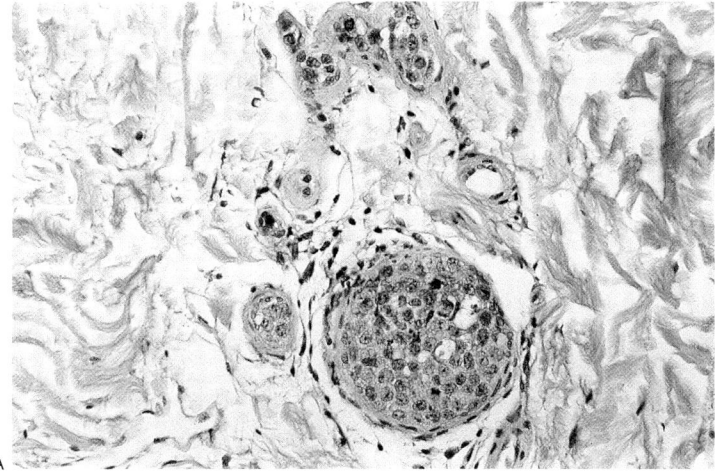
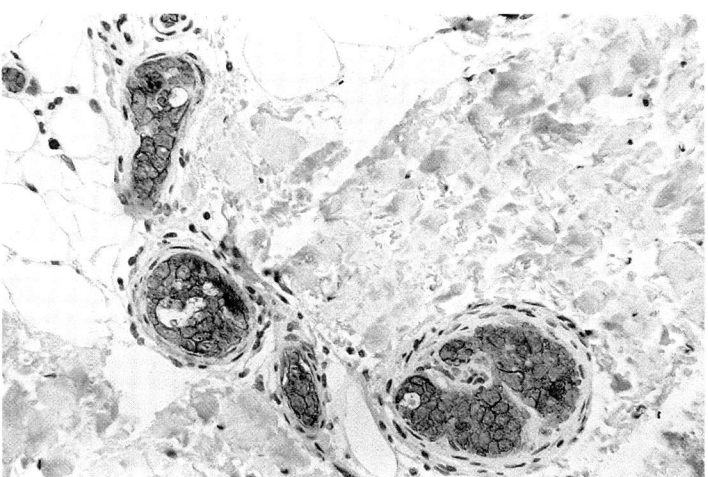

Fig. 41.5 **(A) Intravascular large B-cell lymphoma** (H & E). **(B)** The intravascular cells are positive for CD20. (Immunoperoxidase stain for CD20)

in up to 17% of advanced disease.[131] As defined in the REAL/WHO classification, this is a lymphoma composed of small to medium sized lymphocytes with irregular or cleaved nuclei with dispersed chromatin, inconspicuous nucleoli and scant cytoplasm; large blastic cells are extremely rare or absent.[1] Lymphoblastoid variants have been described with a larger nucleus and more dispersed chromatin,[1] including cases with secondary spread to the skin.[132]

Histopathology

The two possible cases of *primary* MCL were reported to show nodular infiltrates of the characteristic cells surrounding atrophic germinal centers in a mantle zone pattern; the dermis and subcutis were involved with sparing of the epidermis.[133] Plasma cells were present at the periphery of the nodules.

Immunohistochemistry and cytogenetics

The tumor cells were CD20[+], CD5[+] and CD10[-] in these cases. They were reported before the availability of immunohistochemistry for cyclin D1. The detection of this nuclear protein is due to overexpression of the *PRAD1* gene as a result of the translocation t(11:14) involving the immunoglobulin heavy-chain locus and the *bcl-1* locus. The translocation is characteristic of MCL.[134,135] Cases of CD5[+] extranodal marginal cell lymphoma of MALT type have been described.[136] MCL lymphomas are also usually CD23[-] and CD43[+].

PLASMACYTOMA

Plasmacytoma is included in the current classification as a B-cell lymphoma. It has been considered in Chapter 40, page 1062, with the other plasma cell disorders.

T- AND NK-CELL NEOPLASMS WITH FREQUENT OR CONSTANT CUTANEOUS INVOLVEMENT

Classification of this group of lymphomas is generally more complex than for B-cell lymphomas. The REAL/WHO classification has demonstrated the importance of clinical features, including location of the disease, in delineating entities in this group of lymphomas. Cytomorphology alone is insufficient for classification as many distinct T-cell and NK-cell diseases display a range of histological appearances. Immunophenotypic variation exists within disease entities, and different diseases often share similar antigen expression. Most entities do not exhibit characteristic cytogenetic abnormalities. Division into T-cell versus NK lineage and T-cell receptor type is also not a defining feature on its own. Unlike many B-cell lymphomas, demonstration of monoclonality requires more time-consuming techniques than immunohistochemical demonstration of light-chain restriction. An integrated approach including clinical, morphological, immunophenotypic and molecular studies is required for classification in many cases, particularly the uncommon conditions.

Apart from secondary involvement with precursor T-lymphoblastic lymphoma/leukemia, all cutaneous T/NK-cell lymphomas, whether primary or secondary, are mature (peripheral) neoplasms.

The T-cell receptor (TCR) consists of either an $\alpha\beta$ or $\gamma\delta$ heterodimer expressed on the cell surface in association with CD3. Most peripheral T cells express the $\alpha\beta$ TCR and are CD4[+] or CD8[+]. Approximately 5% of T cells express the $\gamma\delta$ TCR. They are almost always CD4[-], CD8[-] but are rarely CD8[+].[137] They are usually found on epithelial surfaces, including the skin.

Normal skin contains small numbers of T cells in the epidermis and dermis, but epidermal cells represent only 2–3% of the total number. The majority express TCR $\alpha\beta$ and are CD4[-]/CD8[+]. Smaller numbers are CD4[+]/CD8[-] or CD4[-]/CD8[-]. Cells also express CD2 and CD5, often lack CD7, and are occasionally CD57[+]. A minor population express TCR $\gamma\delta$; they are usually CD4[-]/CD8[-].[138]

NK cells are large granular cells which represent 10–15% of circulating lymphocytes. They are identified by the expression of antigens such as CD56, CD57 and CD16 and lack B-cell markers and surface CD3 but do express cytoplasmic CD3ϵ. They do not demonstrate rearrangement of immunoglobulin heavy-chain genes or TCR genes.[39] They are usually CD4[-]/CD8[-] but can rarely be CD8[+]. Although CD56, which recognizes the neuronal-cell adhesion molecule (N-CAM), is the most commonly used marker for identification of NK cells, it is not specific, also staining a population of T cells.[140,141] Cytotoxic T cells are closely related cells which express similar surface antigens to NK cells but also express surface CD3 and demonstrate TCR gene rearrangement.[142] The majority express TCR $\alpha\beta$, with only 1–15% expressing TCR $\gamma\delta$.[143] Cytotoxic T cells expressing TCR $\alpha\beta$ are mostly CD4[-]/CD8[+] but can also be CD4[+]/CD8[-] or CD4[-]/CD8[-]. Cells expressing TCR $\gamma\delta$ are usually CD4[-]/CD8[-].[144] Both NK cells and cytotoxic T cells express granzyme B and perforin (when activated) and TIA-1 located in cytoplasmic granules.[22]

MYCOSIS FUNGOIDES

Mycosis fungoides (MF) is a clinically and pathologically distinct form of cutaneous lymphoma characterized by an epidermotropic infiltrate of small to medium sized T lymphocytes. In the WHO classification it is reserved for those cases having classical clinical features in which there is a progression from patches to plaques to tumors.[145]

Although it is overwhelmingly the most common form of primary cutaneous lymphoma,[3,146] it is uncommon, with an annual incidence in the USA of one new case per 1 million population. It usually begins in mid to late adulthood, but earlier onset has been recorded.[147–150] There is a definite male predominance. It has been reported in identical twins.[151] Lesions tend to develop on the lower part of the trunk and thighs, and on the breasts in females.[152] In advanced stages the entire body may be affected, including the face and scalp. The palms and soles have been involved in some cases.[153–155] MF has an indolent course with slow progression over years or decades.[3]

MF is rare in children and young adults but does occur.[156–158] Lesions in children are frequently hypopigmented, particularly in dark-skinned individuals.[157,159–161] A pityriasis lichenoides-like presentation has been reported.[162,163] Some cases with an indolent clinical course are CD8 positive.[164] MF arising in children or young adults is not more aggressive than that appearing in adult life.[157,158] Young patients with limited skin disease may have a slightly better disease-specific survival than older patients.[156]

The etiopathogenesis of MF is unknown. There is no good evidence that is linked to viruses such as HTLV-1, HHV-8 or HTLV-5.[165–175] Classical MF is uncommon in HIV/AIDS.[176] Most cases of cutaneous T-cell lymphoma in HIV/AIDS are erythrodermic, have a CD8[+] phenotype and are rapidly progressive. It has been suggested that MF arises in a background of chronic inflammation as a response to chronic antigen stimulation.[177] There is still considerable controversy as to the existence of a preceding stage (premycotic eruption) and its nature.[178,179] Although it is accepted that MF can evolve from patch through plaque to tumor[180] this is not invariably the case.[156,181]

MF is a monoclonal proliferation of CD4[+] cells. This has been established by PCR for TCR gene rearrangement in from 52% to 90% of cases.[20] Many of the lymphoid cells in the lesions are reactive rather than neoplastic.[182] Micro-manipulation and laser-beam microdissection techniques have demonstrated a monoclonal population of T cells in the epidermis in early (patch stage) lesions of MF.[182,183] Polyclonal (reactive) T lymphocytes are more common in the dermis than clonal T lymphocytes in the early lesions of MF.[182]

Although it is classified as a primary cutaneous lymphoma,[3] circulating clonal T cells have been demonstrated in the peripheral blood even in the early stages of MF by sensitive PCR techniques. Clones are identical to those in the skin.[184]

An MF-like picture has been associated with the therapeutic ingestion of carbamazepine,[185] captopril,[186] quinine,[187] fluoxetine,[188] and phenytoin;[189,190] the eruption cleared in each instance following cessation of the drug.[190]

The patch stage consists of ill-defined patches of varying hue, often with a fine scale. They are irregular in size and shape and have a random distribution, usually on the trunk. This stage may persist for many years before progression occurs.[191] It seems appropriate to regard large plaque parapsoriasis (LPP) as early MF as 10–30% of cases progress to overt MF.[178,192,193] Clonal TCR gene rearrangements have also been identified in a proportion of cases.[194] Poikiloderma atrophicans vasculare is the atrophic form of the patch stage of MF.[195] On the other hand, there is little evidence that small plaque parapsoriasis (digitate dermatosis, chronic superficial scaly dermatitis) is early MF despite views to the contrary (see p. 85).[196–198]

The plaque stage is characterized by well-demarcated lesions which are often annular or arciform in appearance. They are red to violaceous and occasionally scaly.[195] The plaques may develop *de novo* or from patches. In the early stages lesions are often limited to less than 10% of the skin surface, but they may be more widespread, particularly in the late plaque stage.[195] Intractable pruritus is sometimes present, occasionally preceding the appearance of skin lesions by years.[199]

Large plaque parapsoriasis is characterized by irregular erythematous patches and plaques, with minimal scale, on the trunk and major flexures.[192] The lesions are some 10 cm or more in diameter. With time, atrophic (poikilodermatous) change may supervene in a proportion of cases.

Tumors usually develop in pre-existing lesions.[180] The tumors are violaceous to deep red in color, with a tense shiny surface. Ulceration may occur. They measure from 1 cm in diameter to much larger lesions.

The term '*d'emblee* form', used in the past to refer to cases presenting with tumors that were not preceded by patches or plaques, should no longer be used as it has been used for a variety of T- and B-cell lymphomas which presented with tumors.[200,201]

Rare clinical presentations of MF include hypopigmented patches and plaques,[202–208] leukoderma,[209] bullae,[210–214] dyshidrotic lesions,[215] perioral dermatitis-like lesions,[216] pustules, acneiform lesions, hyperkeratotic and verrucous lesions,[217,218] and plaques resembling acanthosis nigricans.[219,220] Acquired epidermal cysts,[221] nail dystrophy,[222] acquired ichthyosis,[223] and second malignancies,[224,225] including skin cancers thought to have resulted from previous topical therapy, have been reported.[226,227] Bullous lesions may develop after interferon therapy.[228] Oral lesions occur rarely.[229] Presentation as keratosis lichenoides chronica has been reported.[230]

MF-associated mucinosis is classified as a variant of mycosis fungoides in the WHO classification.[2] Follicular mucinosis (see p. 414) occurs in approximately 10–15% of cases.

Pilotropic or follicular MF is another variant of MF, possibly related to MF-associated mucinosis.[3] In this form there are alopecia, follicular papules and keratoses, comedo-like lesions and epidermal cysts.[231–235] Lesions are most common on the head and neck region. It may be unilesional.[236] It has presented as dissecting cellulitis of the scalp.[237] In most cases, follicular lesions are found concomitantly with or follow the diagnosis of MF but may also occur without other lesions of MF. Large cell transformation has been reported.[237] This form has been associated with lithium therapy.[238] It has been

suggested that the involvement of hair follicles is related to the overexpression of intercellular adhesion molecule-1 (ICAM-1) by keratinocytes in the hair follicles.[239]

MF may also present as purpuric lesions (see p. 248) which resemble or are indistinguishable from the pigmented purpuric dermatoses (PPD).[240–244] The separation of the two conditions is not always possible by routine histology or even with TCR gene rearrangement studies.[241] Clinical suspicion should be aroused if lesions resembling PPD are extensive, long-standing and have a reticular pattern.[240]

Solitary lesions with the histopathological features of early MF and distinct from pagetoid reticulosis have been reported.[245–248] In one small series of such cases, clonal TCR gene rearrangement was found in 50% of cases. No evidence of progression to classic MF was observed in any of the cases.[246] It is not clear if these lesions represent true lesions of mycosis fungoides or are simulants.[249]

Erythroderma can develop at any stage in the evolution of MF.[180] The distinction between Sézary syndrome and erythrodermic mycosis fungoides has been traditionally based on the absence of circulating 'Sézary cells' in the peripheral blood in the erythrodermic form of MF. Rarely, patients with mycosis fungoides develop a clinical picture indistinguishable from the Sézary syndrome, leading to the view that the latter is a leukemic phase of MF.[191] Circulating T lymphocytes exhibiting the same clonal TCR gene rearrangements as those in skin lesions can be found even in early stages of MF.[184]

Although MF primarily involves the skin, involvement of lymph nodes and other organs may occur in later stages of the disease.[250] Lymphadenopathy in the early stages is due in most cases to dermatopathic lymphadenopathy, a reactive condition that may be seen in lymph nodes draining skin affected by a variety of inflammatory dermatoses as well as MF.[251] However, sensitive PCR techniques have shown involvement of lymph nodes by clonal T lymphocytes even at early stages of MF.[252–254] Molecular biological evaluation of lymph nodes for staging purposes and prognostication may replace older histological techniques.[255,256] One recent study concluded that detection of a monoclonal population of T cells in lymph nodes was predictive of a poor clinical outcome and reduced probability of survival.[257] Detection of a monoclonal population in peripheral blood is also an adverse feature.[258] Visceral involvement is frequently found at autopsy. The lungs, spleen, liver and kidneys are most frequently involved, but every organ can be infiltrated by tumor cells.[259,260] There have been numerous recent studies on prognosis and survival in patients with MF.[261–265]

The clinical course of MF is quite variable; in the majority of cases it is indolent. Spontaneous resolution of individual lesions may occur at any time during the disease. The estimated 5-year survival of patients in the EORTC series was 87%.[3] Patients with only limited plaques (stage IA) have a very favorable outcome; their life expectancy is not altered by the disease.[266] Extensive involvement of the skin, with the development of tumors, lymph node involvement and organomegaly, is a bad prognostic sign.[267–272] Transformation to a CD30+ large cell lymphoma can also occur,[273–275] and is a bad prognostic feature.[275,276]

Histopathology

Mycosis fungoides is characterized by the presence of a variably dense infiltrate of mononuclear cells in the papillary dermis, with extension of these cells into the epidermis (epidermotropism). In establishing the diagnosis in the early stages of the disease these architectural abnormalities are more important than cytological atypia of lymphocytes, which is usually quite mild.[277–279] The histological appearances vary in the different clinical stages of the disease. Appearances may also be altered by corticosteroid or ultraviolet-A radiation therapy, which diminish epidermotropism and the density of the cellular infiltrate.[280] Many studies have shown that interobserver agreement on the histological diagnosis of mycosis is not high.[281]

Patch stage

In the patch stage of MF a relatively sparse infiltrate of lymphocytes is spread along the slightly expanded papillary dermis. The infiltrate shows little tendency to aggregate around the vessels of the superficial plexus. Within the epidermis, lymphocytes are typically confined to the basal layers of the epidermis, either as single cells in a 'string of beads' arrangement or as small groups of cells (Fig. 41.6). These cells are often surrounded by a clear halo but there is usually little or no spongiosis.[277,282] The clear halo around epidermotropic lymphocytes is not caused by mucin accumulation.[283] Pautrier microabscesses (sharply marginated, discrete clusters of lymphocytes in close apposition with one another, within the epidermis) are uncommon in the patch stage (Fig. 41.7).[284] Although they are highly characteristic of MF they are found in only a minority of cases,[285] and cases of MF will be missed if this feature is given undue importance. Occasionally, the histological appearance mimics a melanocytic lesion. Atypia of cells may be minimal in the earlier stages of MF but in some cases the epidermal cells are larger than those in the dermis.[179] Cytological abnormalities may be seen in thin plastic sections that are not apparent in conventional sections.[186] Rare mitotic figures may be seen in the papillary dermis. The presence of mitotic figures may correlate with an unfavorable outcome.[281] There is frequently fibrosis of the papillary dermis in the form of haphazardly arranged wiry bundles of collagen.[179,186] The epidermis may show mild acanthosis; in poikilodermatous and atrophic lesions the epidermis is thin.[277] Basal vacuolar change and pigment incontinence are present in these lesions.[286] In some cases, there is a marked lichenoid tissue reaction with histology resembling lichen planus. Unlike lichen planus there may be plasma cells and eosinophils in the dermal infiltrate as well as atypical lymphocytes.[287] Infiltration of eccrine sweat duct structures may be seen in patch and other stages of MF and may remain after therapy.[288,289]

The diagnostic changes in large plaque parapsoriasis may be subtle with epidermal changes of mild psoriasiform hyperplasia, overlying mild ortho-keratosis and spotty parakeratosis, and a sparse dermal cellular infiltrate. The dermal infiltrate may extend upward into the dermal papillae. Pautrier micro-abscesses are not seen and cellular atypia is often minimal.[290] The atrophic lesions have identical changes to other atrophic lesions of MF.[291]

The pigmented purpuric dermatoses (PPD) and pigmented purpuric dermatitis-like lesions of MF may have a similar histological appearance. In PPD-like MF there may be features typical of MF, but some cases have similar features to PPD. Both PPD and PPD-like MF may have lymphocytes aligned in the basal layer of the epidermis and occasional Civatte bodies. Dermal edema is more common in PPD. Atypia of lymphocytes is seen in MF-like PPD and lymphocytes may be seen in upper levels of the epidermis.[241] PCR studies may show clonal rearrangement of TCR genes in lichenoid forms of PPD, making distinction of some cases from MF difficult.[241]

Plaque stage

Patch and plaque stages are part of a progression. In plaques of mycosis fungoides the infiltrate is more dense and atypical lymphocytes are more common. The lymphocytes measure 10–30 μm in diameter and their nuclei are often indented, cerebriform or prune-like. Prominent convolutions are best appreciated in thin sections. Small collections of cells may aggregate around vessels of the superficial plexus and less often the deep plexus. They also extend around the adnexae, particularly pilosebaceous follicles.[292]

In addition to lymphocytes, the infiltrate usually contains a small number of eosinophils and sometimes plasma cells.[284] Epidermotropism is still a con-spicuous feature. Pautrier microabscesses are seen in more than 50% of biopsies; this proportion increases if step sections are examined. Epidermal changes include parakeratosis, mild to moderate psoriasiform hyperplasia,

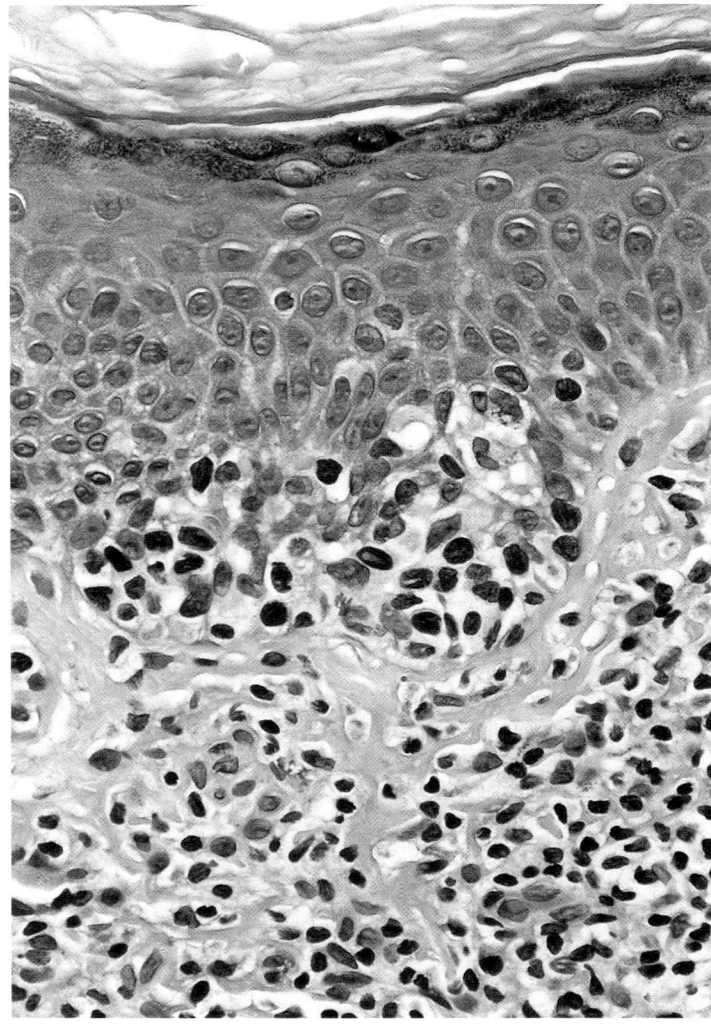

Fig. 41.7 **Mycosis fungoides.** A collection of epidermal atypical lymphocytes forming a Pautrier microabscess. (H & E)

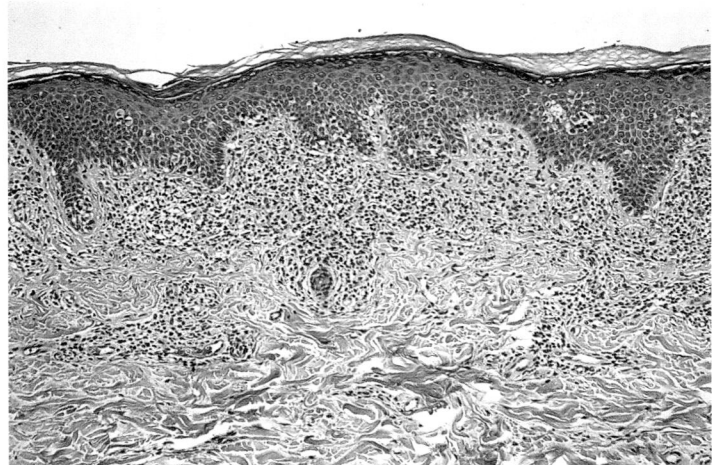

Fig. 41.6 **Mycosis fungoides.** There is a band-like dermal infiltrate with atypical lymphocytes in the basal epidermis. (H & E)

and epidermal mucinosis.[284,293] Mild spongiosis does not exclude the diagnosis of mycosis fungoides as sometimes claimed,[277] but spongiotic microvesiculation is rare.[294] Spongiotic foci resembling Pautrier microabscesses (pseudo-Pautrier microabscesses) sometimes develop in spongiotic diseases such as allergic contact dermatitis and pityriasis rosea.[295] These foci contain monocyte-like cells, Langerhans cells and rare lymphocytes. Cell nuclei are pale and less complex than in true Pautrier microabscesses. These structures are often vase-shaped and appear to open onto the epidermal surface. They may also be seen in MF.[296,297]

Biopsies of apparently normal skin in patients with plaque stage MF sometimes show a mild superficial perivascular infiltrate of lymphocytes, often with epidermotropism.[298]

Tumor stage

In the tumor stage, the infiltrate has a more monomorphic appearance and is dominated by large atypical cells.[299] The proportion of tumor cells relative to reactive cells increases. Mitoses are easily seen. The entire dermis is often involved and extension into the subcutis may occur. Deep dermal and subcutaneous nodules are particularly likely to occur if electron beam therapy has been used on a preceding lesion in the same region.[300] Epidermotropism and Pautrier microabscesses are uncommon in the tumor stage.

The separation of MF from certain inflammatory dermatoses is not as clear cut as has been suggested.[179] There is often disagreement between pathologists in individual cases. Various attempts have been made to provide diagnostic principles and to standardize reporting of cases.[301–305] The important histological features in one study were: Pautrier's microabscesses, lymphocytes with a clear perinuclear halo, lymphocytes aligned along the basal layer, intradermal lymphocytes with hyperconvoluted nuclei, epidermal lymphocytes larger than dermal lymphocytes, and epidermotropism itself.[285]

Histology is not useful in predicting disease course.[306]

Granulomas are a rare finding in mycosis fungoides (granulomatous MF).[294,307–314] They are usually small and tuberculoid in type but they may be palisaded and mimic granuloma annulare.[315] At other times the granulomas are poorly formed and consist of small collections of multinucleate histiocytes. The granulomas are more localized than in granulomatous slack skin. Granulomas in MF should be distinguished from small collections of lipidized macrophages (dystrophic xanthomatosis), which are a rare finding in the dermis in MF.[308,316,317] A variant with interstitial lymphoid infiltrates superficially resembling granuloma annulare or inflammatory morphea has been reported,[318,319] as has generalized granuloma annulare associated with granulomatous MF.[320] Rarely there is extensive fibrosis and mucin in the dermis (fibromucinous variant).[321]

Pilotropic (follicular) MF is characterized by comedo-like dilated follicles plugged with keratin, milia, and larger epidermal (infundibular) cysts which are infiltrated by a heavy lymphoid infiltrate containing atypical forms with convoluted nuclei (pilotropism) (Fig. 41.8).[235,239,322,323] Sebaceous glands may also be involved. There may be destruction of hair follicles in areas of alopecia with only residual follicular epithelial remnants and secondary inflammatory changes.[322,324] Pautrier microabscess equivalents may be seen in the follicular epithelium.[323] Follicular spongiosis and mucinosis are not seen although other lesions may show typical changes of MF-associated follicular mucinosis.[324a] Infiltration of the epidermis (epidermotropism) is sometimes seen. There may also be infiltrates around or infiltrating eccrine sweat duct structures. In some cases there has been a mixed cellular infiltrate including eosinophils, neutrophils and plasma cells.[234]

Other rare histological changes include the presence of a vasculitis,[325] or dermal mucin[294] and the formation of bullae. In the bullous lesions the split

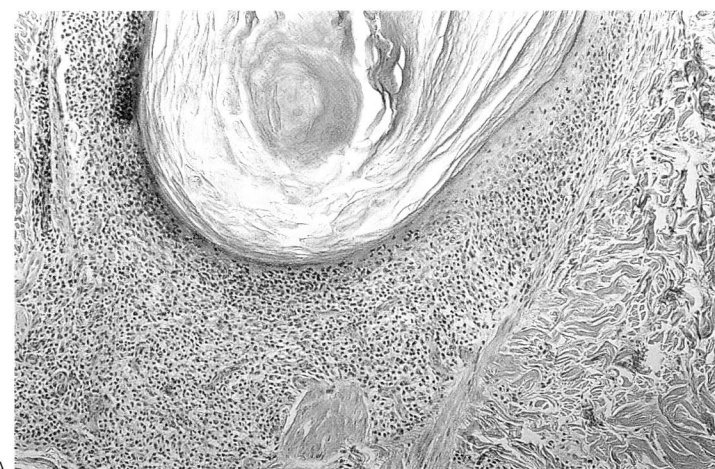

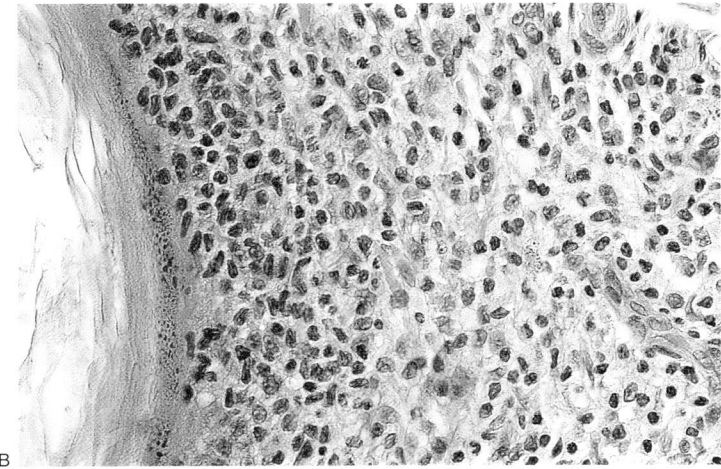

Fig. 41.8 **Pilotropic (follicular) mycosis fungoides. (A)** Dilated follicle with atypical lymphoid infiltrate. **(B)** There is a follicular infiltrate of cerebriform T cells. (H & E)

may occur at any level. The majority of cases have been subepidermal in location with negative immunofluorescence.[210] Signet-ring cells constituted the infiltrate in one case.[326] In hypopigmented lesions of MF, there is a reduction in melanin in the basal layer and, sometimes, melanin incontinence.[327]

Epidermal changes, such as mild epidermal hyperplasia, dyskeratotic cells and atypical keratinocytes with large nuclei, may be seen following topical treatment with nitrogen mustard.[328]

Immunohistochemistry and cytogenetics

The tumor cells are CD2+, CD3+, CD4+, CD45RO+, CD8− and usually CD30−.[329–332] They have the characteristics of mature memory cells of the Th2 subset.[333] Tumor cells frequently lack expression of CD7[334,335] and Leu-8 T-cell antigens.[330,336–339] Although this aberrant feature was thought to be specific for a lymphomatous process and a useful feature in the differential diagnosis of reactive from neoplastic processes, it has also been reported in inflammatory conditions.[340,341] It is, however, unusual to lose both these antigens in a reactive process. Rare cases with a CD3+, CD4−, CD8+ phenotype have been reported. Reactive CD8+ cells can also be found in the lesions of MF. These cells are CD16−, CD56− and CD57−.[342] Their presence may predict a better prognosis.[331,343] In the tumor stage there is commonly an aberrant phenotype with loss of T-cell antigens.[344–347] With progression of the disease, some cases of MF may transform into a CD30+ large cell lymphoma (secondary large cell anaplastic lymphoma).[273–275] Such CD30+ tumors are not associated with the t(2;5) translocation.[348] Rarely, CD30+ cells have been found in appreciable numbers in the patch stage of MF.[349] Expression of certain CD44 splice variants may be linked to systemic spread.[350,351] In addition to lymphocytes, the dermal infiltrate in MF includes numerous dendritic cells that express CD1a or factor XIIIa.[352,353] The T cells within the epidermis usually express proliferating cell nuclear antigen (PCNA). 3 lymphocytes are sometimes present in small numbers.

In most cases, neoplastic lymphocytes of MF express the αβ TCR, but rare cases have been reported in which the γδ receptors are expressed.[354,355] There are many studies in which the detection of clonal TCR gene rearrangements has been used in the diagnosis of MF, particularly in early, histologically equivocal lesions of MF.[20,334,356–361] The significance of demonstrable clonal TCR gene rearrangement in such a setting remains controversial to a certain extent but most authors agree that such a finding warrants clinical monitoring. Many such cases have progressed to frank MF.[20]

Electron microscopy

There is a great diversity in the morphology of the atypical lymphocytes in MF. The characteristic cell has a highly convoluted (cerebriform) nucleus with heterochromatin located predominantly beneath the nuclear membrane (Fig. 41.9). The cytoplasm contains multivesicular bodies and mitochondria, which are sometimes clumped. Some authors use the term 'Sézary cell' for a

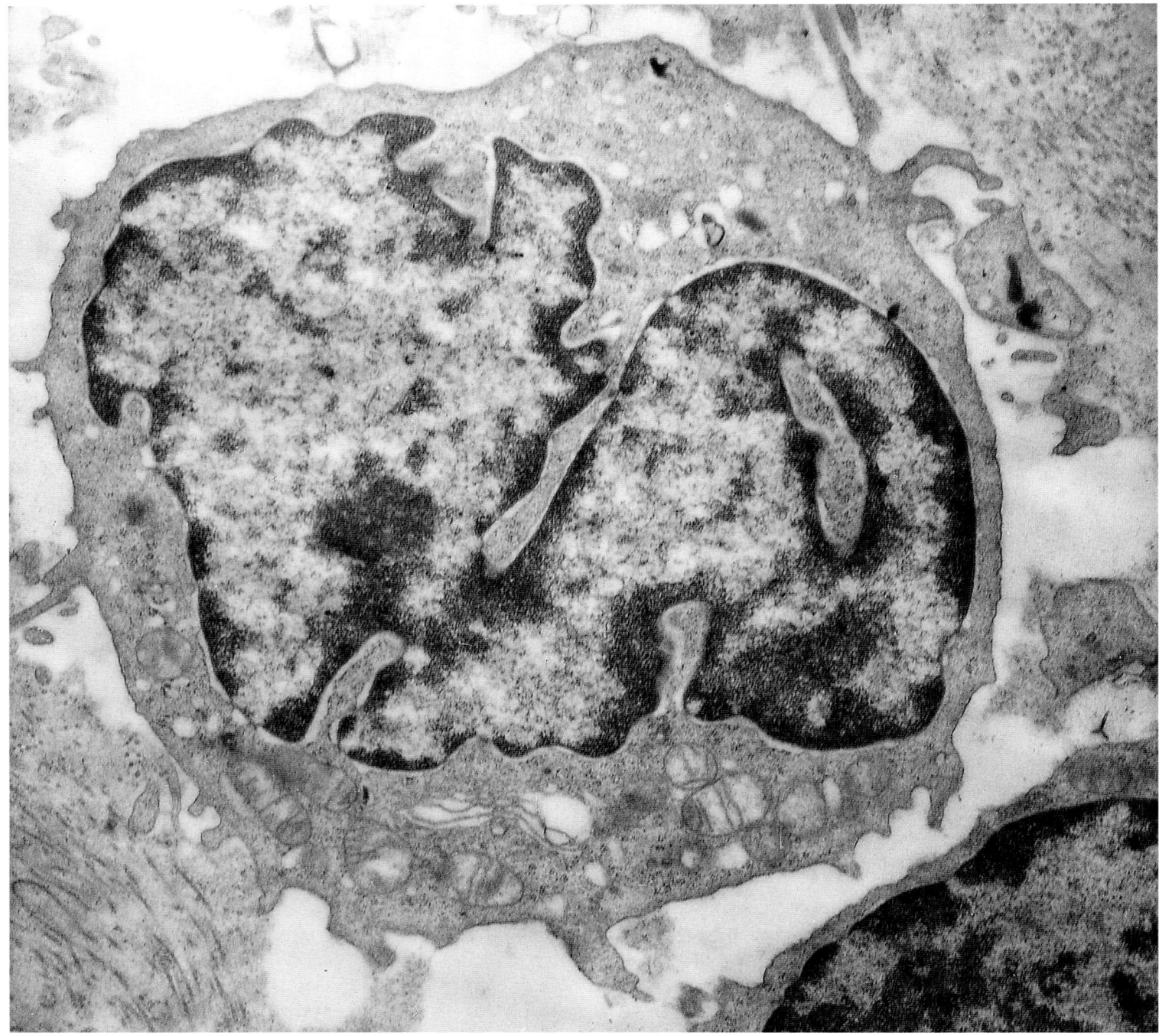

Fig. 41.9 **Mycosis fungoides.** A mycosis cell with its characteristic indented nucleus. (×12 500)

small to medium-sized lymphocyte with a highly convoluted nucleus, and the term 'mycosis cell' for a cell which is slightly larger with fewer nuclear indentations.[278,362] Most authors use the terms 'Sézary cell', 'mycosis cell' and 'Lutzner cell' interchangeably for the various atypical cells, recognizing that intermediate forms also exist.[191,363]

A much larger cell, sometimes called the 'pleomorphic cell', is seen in the tumor stage. It has a vesicular nucleus and a conspicuous nucleolus.[362] The nucleus of the pleomorphic cell may be variably convoluted.

Quantitative electron microscopy has been used to characterize the atypical lymphocytes in MF.[250,364]

Pagetoid reticulosis

Pagetoid reticulosis (Woringer–Kolopp disease) is a rare, distinct variant of mycosis fungoides which presents clinically as large, localized, erythematous, scaly or verrucous patches or plaques.[365,366] Lesions grow slowly and are typically found on the distal part of the limbs. Males are predominantly affected. A disseminated form referred to as Ketron–Goodman disease is now regarded as MF as it has similar clinical behavior. Some cases previously regarded as disseminated pagetoid reticulosis are now classified as primary cutaneous CD8+ epidermotropic cytotoxic T-cell lymphoma.[367,368] A prolonged disease-free survival after simple excision or local irradiation is usual. Extracutaneous dissemination has not been reported.[3]

Histopathology

The epidermis is markedly acanthotic with overlying hyperkeratosis and patchy parakeratosis and is infiltrated by large, atypical mononuclear cells with pale eosinophilic cytoplasm, a large nucleus and a prominent nucleolus (Fig. 41.10).[369,370] Cells are arranged singly or in nests or clusters. This produces a pattern resembling Paget's disease or melanoma. Atypical cells are present at all levels of the epidermis, but are most prominent in the lower third.[365] Cells in the upper layers of the epidermis may show subtle degenerative changes.[369] There are scattered mitotic figures.

Unlike MF, there are no atypical cells in the dermis, which contains a dense, banal infiltrate of non-activated lymphocytes, histiocytes and some plasma cells.[369] There are usually no eosinophils.

Immunohistochemistry and cytogenetics

Tumor cells have a CD3+, CD4+, CD8− or CD3+, CD4−, CD8+ immunophenotype. CD30 is sometimes expressed.[366,371,372] Clonal rearrangement of TCR genes has been demonstrated. This is usually an αβ TCR gene rearrangement.[372,373] A case exhibiting γδ TCR gene rearrangement has been reported.[374] In one case, neoplastic cells expressed cutaneous lymphocyte antigen (HECA 452), a skin homing receptor, which might explain the exquisite epidermotropism of this lesion.[372]

Electron microscopy

Although it is not made clear in most studies, there appear to be two cell populations in the epidermis – histiocytes and stimulated T lymphocytes.[375,376] The latter are the major component.[365]

Mycosis fungoides-associated follicular mucinosis

This variant represents 10–15% of cases of MF and is characterized by folliculotropic lymphomatous infiltrates and mucinous degeneration of the hair follicles. There is sparing of the epidermis. Lesions occur most frequently on the head and neck areas and consist of follicular papules, indurated plaques and tumors. There is often associated alopecia, pruritus and second-

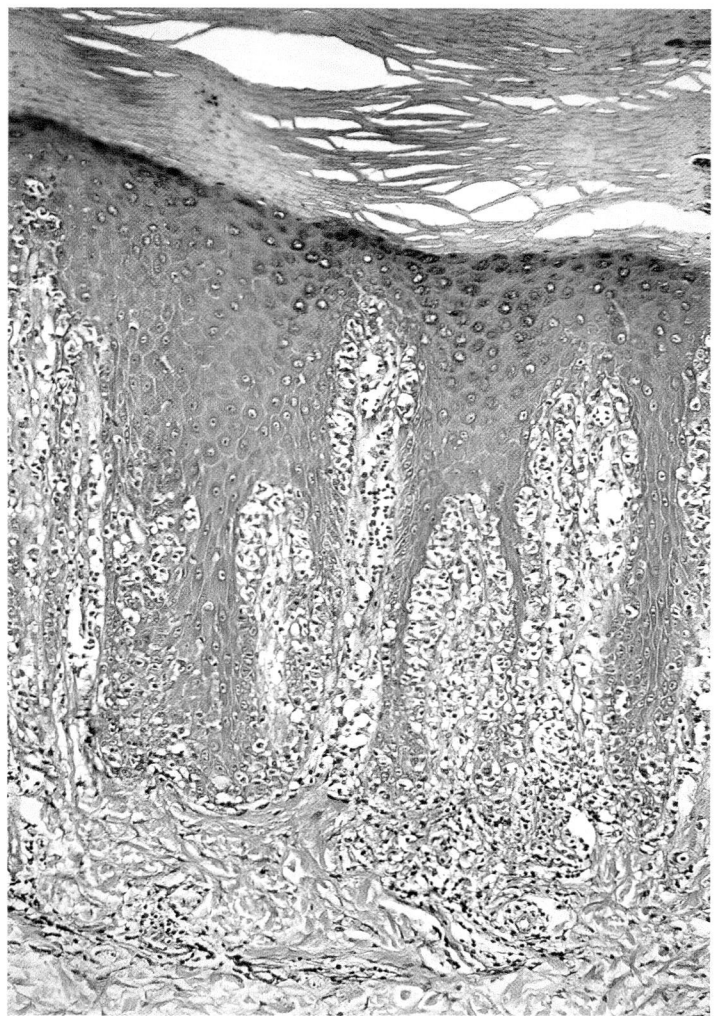

Fig. 41.10 **Pagetoid reticulosis.** There is marked epidermotropism of atypical lymphocytes. (H & E)

ary bacterial infection. An erythrodermic form has been described.[377] The estimated 5-year survival of this form of MF is 70%.[3] Occasionally there may be a rapidly progressive course.[378] The distribution of the lymphomatous infiltrate about follicles means that it is often less responsive to skin-targeted therapies than classic MF.[3]

Histopathology

There is a perivascular and periappendageal infiltrate of atypical lymphocytes of variable size with cerebriform nuclei, admixed in some cases with eosinophils and plasma cells.[379,380] The epidermis is usually spared. The characteristic finding is mucinous degeneration of the hair follicles producing intrafollicular pools of mucin (Fig. 41.11).

Immunohistochemistry and cytogenetics

Neoplastic cells have the same phenotype as classic MF. PCR studies for TCR gene rearrangement are useful in distinguishing MF-associated follicular mucinosis from inflammatory folliculitis.[381,382] Some cases of apparent alopecia mucinosa (see p. 414) have progressed to MF or have been shown to have clonal TCR gene rearrangement of infiltrating lymphocytes, suggesting that long-term follow-up of these patients is necessary.[379,381,383]

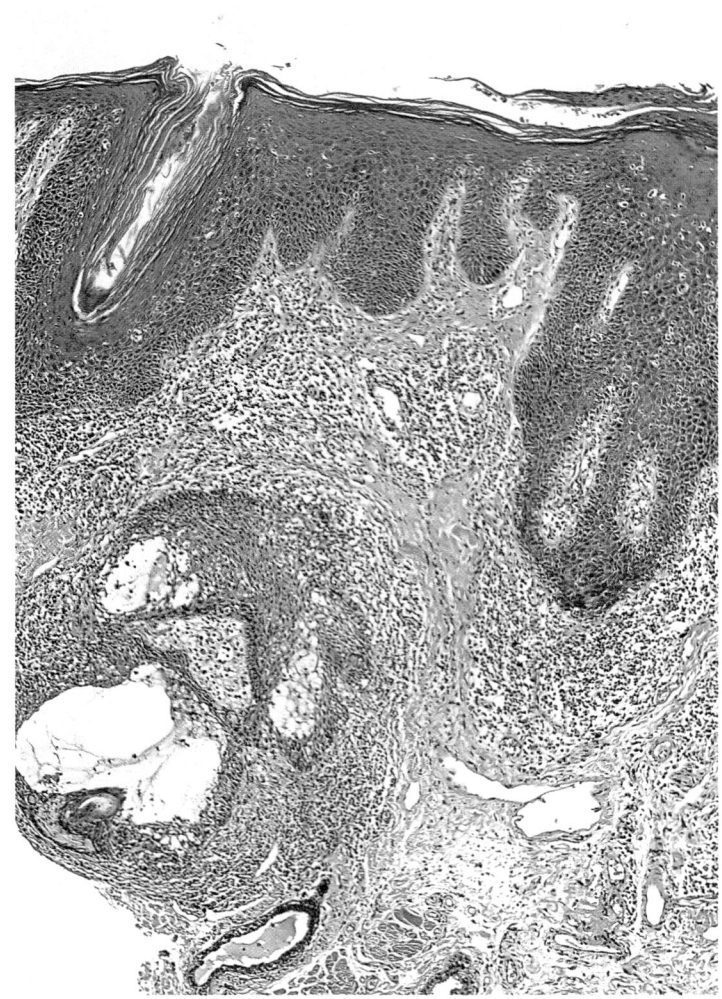

Fig. 41.11 **Mycosis fungoides-associated follicular mucinosis.** (H & E)

Granulomatous slack skin

Granulomatous slack skin is a very rare condition in which pendulous folds of skin develop in large, pre-existing erythematous plaques.[384–387] There is a predilection for flexural areas, particularly the axillae and groin.[388] TCR gene rearrangement studies have demonstrated a clonal infiltrate of CD4+ cells, and it is now regarded as a peculiar T-cell lymphoma, a variant of MF in the WHO classification.[2] Males are predominantly affected.[3] Long survival is the usual outcome, although in a third of patients there is an association with Hodgkin's disease.[308,384,389,390] It may also be associated with classical MF.[391] Most cases have an indolent course. Recurrence of pendulous skin folds after surgical excision has been reported.[384]

Histopathology[384]

Early lesions exhibit a superficial, or superficial and deep perivascular lymphocytic infiltrate, psoriasiform epidermal hyperplasia, slight spongiosis, parakeratosis and occasional lymphocytes in the lower half of the epidermis. Occasional multinucleate histiocytes are seen in the dermal infiltrate. In established lesions, there is permeation of the entire dermis and the subcutis by a dense infiltrate of small, slightly convoluted lymphocytes. Characteristically, there are many multinucleate giant cells scattered uniformly throughout the lymphocytic infiltrate. These giant cells have large numbers of nuclei. Their cytoplasm may contain lymphocytes and elastic fibers. Cellular infiltrates in

the upper dermis may be band like. The dermis between the cellular aggregates is markedly edematous or fibrotic.

Stains for elastic tissue show a complete absence of elastic fibers from the dermis. Occasionally, calcified elastic fibers are seen.[385,392] The epidermis is infiltrated by lymphocytes, either singly or in small clusters in a pattern similar to patch or plaque stage MF.

Immunohistochemistry and cytogenetics

The small lymphoid cells are CD3+, CD4+, CD43+, CD45RO+ T cells. The multinucleate cells express the histiocyte markers CD68 and Mac387.[393,394] Clonal β-chain TCR gene rearrangement of the lymphoid population has been demonstrated.[386,392,395]

Sézary syndrome

The Sézary syndrome (SS) is an uncommon form of cutaneous T-cell lymphoma that is generally considered to represent a leukemic stage of mycosis fungoides.[396] It was defined historically by the triad of erythroderma, lymphadenopathy and circulating atypical mononuclear cells in the peripheral blood.[397] Some authors distinguish between SS and erythrodermic MF by the number of circulating atypical cells (>5% of cells versus <5% of cells).[398] There is characteristically intractable pruritus, and circulating Sézary cell counts usually exceed $1.0 \times 10^9/l$ although there is no consensus on what levels of Sézary cells in the peripheral blood are diagnostic.[3] Some believe that the presence of any number of circulating cells is significant.[396,399] However, Sézary cells can sometimes be found in the peripheral blood of patients with various inflammatory dermatoses.

Less constant clinical features include cutaneous edema, alopecia, nail dystrophy, and palmar and plantar keratoderma.[400] Rarely, bullous lesions,[401] plane xanthomas,[402] vitiligo,[403] or a monoclonal gammopathy[404] may develop. Peripheral blood eosinophilia is present in a small number of cases.[405] Visceral involvement may eventuate, resulting in a shorter survival than the median 2.5 years for all cases.[396] The prognosis is worse in older patients and those in whom the circulating Sézary cells constitute more than 5% of the total lymphocyte count.[406]

The Sézary syndrome usually develops in late adult life. Cases in childhood are extremely rare.[407] It may be preceded by another chronic inflammatory dermatosis such as atopic dermatitis.[408] There is an increased risk of squamous cell carcinoma of the skin, other lymphomas including Hodgkin's disease, and internal malignancies in patients with SS.[409,410] Large cell transformation in skin and peripheral blood has been reported.[411]

Sézary cells can be recognized in blood films stained with the Giemsa or Wright methods. The cells have a high nuclear:cytoplasmic ratio, deep nuclear indentations giving a cerebriform appearance, and condensed chromatin at the nuclear membrane.[412] Sézary cells are the same size as normal lymphocytes or much larger. Cell counts of Sézary cells using smears may underestimate numbers.[413]

Histopathology[402,414,415]

There is great variability in the histological findings. In many cases they are similar to those in MF.[3,416] In the most frequently observed pattern in SS, there is a band-like cellular infiltrate involving the papillary dermis and, sometimes, the upper reticular dermis as well.[415] Epidermotropism is present in some of these cases and Pautrier abscesses may be found, particularly if multiple sections are examined.[415] The infiltrate is of varying density and is composed of small lymphocytes admixed with some larger cells with indented nuclei. The use of ultrathin sections enhances the detection of cells with a convoluted nucleus. These changes occur in a background of irregular acanthosis of the epidermis with orthokeratosis and focal parakeratosis. Spongiosis is sometimes present, although usually mild.[414] The papillary dermis is fibrotic with thickened collagen bundles and scattered melanophages.

In approximately one-third of cases the biopsy appearances are non-specific, with epidermal changes as described above and an infiltrate of lymphocytes in the upper dermis, mostly in a perivascular location.[417] A few larger lymphocytes and macrophages are usually present. Eosinophils and plasma cells may be found in small numbers. Epidermotropism is usually mild. When present, the lymphocytes are not localized to the lower epidermis as in MF. Prominent ectasia of papillary dermal vessels is present in many cases and is more pronounced than in patch/plaque lesions of MF.[398] Rarely, non-caseating granulomas may be seen in the dermal infiltrate.

Multiple biopsies are often needed to make a diagnosis of SS. Topical and other therapy may mask diagnostic histological features. Non-specific histological findings are common in SS even when a circulating T-cell clone is present in the blood.[418]

Immunohistochemistry and cytogenetics

The neoplastic lymphocytes in the skin and in blood are CD3+, CD4+, CD45RO+, CD8− and CD30− and frequently CD7−.[419] Clonal TCR gene rearrangements are present in most cases. Demonstration of clonality in circulating T cells in the peripheral blood aids in the differentiation of SS from other non-neoplastic forms of erythroderma.[420] The small numbers of cells in the dermal infiltrate and problems in extracting cells from skin may make it difficult to demonstrate T-cell clonality in small skin biopsies. Flow cytometric counts of CD4+/CD7− cells in peripheral blood have shown a significant correlation with the number of circulating Sézary cells.[421] In 20% of patients with MF, however, cells are CD4+/CD7+, which obscures the phenotypic distinction between neoplastic cells and normal helper T cells.[422] Diminished expression of CD3 and lack of CD26 expression have also been used to detect and enumerate atypical cells in the blood in SS.[422–424]

Electron microscopy

The Sézary cells have a convoluted nucleus with deep and narrow indentations. The cytoplasm has a number of fibrils. Ultrastructural morphometry has been used to distinguish Sézary cells in the blood from normal and reactive lymphocytes although this technique is rarely used in routine practice.[425]

PRIMARY CUTANEOUS CD8+ EPIDERMOTROPIC CYTOTOXIC T-CELL LYMPHOMA

When carefully defined, primary cutaneous CD8+ epidermotropic cytotoxic T-cell lymphoma appears to be a clinicopathological entity distinct from classical MF and pagetoid reticulosis.[368] It is characterized clinically by generalized patches, plaques, papulonodules and tumors mimicking disseminated pagetoid reticulosis. There is systemic spread to the lungs, testis, central nervous system and oral cavity, but not to lymph nodes. It has an aggressive clinical course (median survival of 32 months).[368]

Histopathology[368]

In early lesions there is an epidermal infiltrate of atypical lymphocytes in a pagetoid pattern. Fully developed lesions are characterized by a band-like dermal infiltrate of atypical cells as well as by diffuse infiltration of the epidermis. Atypical cells vary from small/medium to large pleomorphic cells and immunoblasts. The epidermis is acanthotic and there are frequently secondary changes of spongiosis, vesiculation and necrosis. Unlike MF, a diffuse epidermal infiltrate is present in the tumor stage. Sweat glands and follicular structures are frequently involved, sometimes producing lymphoepithelial lesions. Rare eosinophils and plasma cells are present.

Immunohistochemistry and cytogenetics

The neoplastic lymphocytes have a peripheral T-cell phenotype and are CD3+, CD8+, CD7+, CD45RA+ and express TIA-1. CD2 and CD5 are frequently not expressed. There is a high Ki-67 proliferation index. Unlike pagetoid reticulosis these cases do not express HECA 452. Clonal rearrangement of the TCR γ gene has been demonstrated in all cases.

PRIMARY CUTANEOUS CD30+ T-CELL LYMPHOPROLIFERATIVE DISORDERS

The primary cutaneous CD30+ T-cell lymphoproliferative disorders are linked by the common histological feature of large atypical lymphoid cells expressing CD30.[3] CD30 is a 120 kd transmembrane cytokine receptor of the tumor necrosis factor receptor family and is preferentially expressed by activated lymphoid cells. In normal lymphoid tissue, CD30+ cells are seen in para-follicular areas and in the rim of follicular centers. These are proliferating large T- and B-cell blasts; CD30+ centroblasts are also found within germinal centers.[276,426] Although originally found to strongly label Hodgkin and Reed–Sternberg cells of classical Hodgkin's disease, CD30 is now known to be not specific for that lymphoma.

As well as the group of conditions to be discussed here, it also labels the cells of large B-cell lymphomas and other T-cell lymphomas as well as non-lymphoid neoplasms such as embryonal carcinoma.[426]

The primary cutaneous CD30+ lymphoproliferative disorders include: anaplastic large cell lymphoma-T/null-cell-primary cutaneous type (ALCL), lymphomatoid papulosis (LyP) and borderline cases of the EORTC classification with overlapping features of the other two conditions. Distinction between ALCL and LyP is not always possible on the basis of histological criteria and for this reason the EORTC group uses clinical appearance and course as defining criteria for the definitive diagnosis and treatment of these conditions. The skin may also be secondarily involved by primary systemic ALCL. Patients with primary systemic ALCL that simultaneously or secondarily involves the skin have an unfavorable prognosis.[427]

Anaplastic large cell lymphoma is a group of large cell lymphomas of T/null-cell type defined by the strong expression of CD30.[276] CD30 is expressed on the cell membrane and in the Golgi region of cells. The majority of T/null-cell ALCL are of T-cell type and have clonally rearranged TCR γ and β genes. Cells also express the cytotoxic molecules (perforin, granzyme B, TIA-1) and CD56 in some cases; this immunophenotype, together with the finding that 10% of cases lack detectable TCR gene rearrangements, suggests that a small proportion of cases may be derived from NK cells.[428,429] Large B-cell lymphomas with anaplastic morphology are regarded as morphological variants of diffuse large B-cell lymphoma in the WHO classification. ALCL is rare in HIV-infected individuals; however, cases including apparently primary cutaneous forms have been reported. These have been anaplastic lymphoma kinase fusion protein (ALK) negative.[430–432] It has been suggested that most anaplastic large cell lymphomas in the setting of HIV are anaplastic variants of diffuse large B-cell lymphoma and are associated with EBV infection.[276,433]

The group of ALCLs can be further subdivided into primary systemic, primary cutaneous, and secondary types by clinical and molecular criteria.

Primary systemic ALCL

The primary systemic form can be further subdivided by whether tumor cells express the anaplastic lymphoma kinase fusion protein (ALK) or not. ALK protein is absent in normal tissues except the brain, and expression in other tissues indicates anomalous ALK expression, usually in the form of nucleophosmin (NPM)–ALK fusion protein associated with a t(2:5)(p23;q35) translation. Other translocations such as t(1:2)(q21;p23), t(2:3)(p23;q21) and inversion (2)(p23;q35) have also been reported. Immunohistochemistry, FISH and ALK gene rearrangement studies are equally effective in identifying ALK[+] cases.[434]

Primary cutaneous ALCL is almost invariably ALK negative and does not have the t(2:5) translocation, although rare ALK[+] cases with or without t(2;5) translocation have been reported.[427,435–438]

Systemic ALK[+] and ALK[−] cases have different clinical presentations and response to therapy.[439]

ALK[+] systemic ALCL occurs most commonly in the first three decades of life with a definite male predominance (M:F − 3:1). Extranodal involvement occurs in 60% of cases, with the skin being the most common extranodal site (21% of cases). ALK[−] systemic ALCL is more common in older age groups and there is a much less marked male predominance of cases (M:F − 0.9:1). ALK[+] cases have a better response to therapy and prognosis than ALK[−] cases.[22]

Primary systemic ALCL has been associated with acquired ichthyosis.[440]

Histopathology

The common type of cells in ALCL are large lymphoid cells with chromatin-poor horseshoe-shaped or embryo-shaped nuclei, multiple prominent eosinophilic nucleoli and abundant cytoplasm, often with a pale paranuclear hof. These are sometimes referred to as 'hallmark cells' and are seen in all cytological forms of ALCL. In most cases the cells vary in size but they are sometimes relatively monomorphic.[441] The common type comprises 60–70% of all cases of ALCL. Multinucleate cells resembling Reed–Sternberg cells may also be seen.[276,442] The small cell variant has a mixture of small, medium and large lymphoid cells. Large cells often surround vessels. Small cells are often CD30[−].[443] In the lymphohistiocytic variant there is a heavy histiocytic infiltrate which may mask the smaller neoplastic population of lymphoid cells. Cells are often smaller than those in common ALCL.[444] The small cell type and the lymphohistiocytic type represent approximately 5% and 15% of cases respectively and are predominantly in the pediatric group.[445,446] The giant cell variant is characterized by many multinucleate cells.[276] A sarcomatoid variant resembles a soft tissue sarcoma and contains large atypical, often spindle-shaped cells.[447] Eosinophil-rich and neutrophil-rich variants have also been described.[448–451] A rare signet-ring cell type has also been reported.[452]

Systemic spread to the skin may show the histological appearance of a dermal infiltrate restricted to perivascular and periappendageal sites.[453]

Immunohistochemistry

Tumor cells are by definition predominantly CD30[+] with staining of the cell membrane and Golgi zone. The majority are positive for EMA. CD45 is expressed in 60% of cases. The T-cell antigens CD3 and CD2, CD43 and CD45RO are seen in approximately 50% of cases. A minority are CD4[+] or CD8[+]. CD56, TIA-1, granzyme B and perforin may be expressed. Cells are usually CD15[−]. ALK-1 is positive in 60% of cases.[276,442,454]

Primary cutaneous ALCL

This form of lymphoma represented 9% of primary cutaneous lymphomas in the EORTC series.[3] It occurs predominantly in older adults (median age of 60 years) and is rare in children and adolescents.[455] There is a slight male preponderance of cases (M:F − 3:2).[456] Lesions are solitary or localized grouped nodules or tumors which are red to violaceous in color and may be ulcerated. Partial or complete spontaneous regression occurs in up to 25% of cases.[457] Cases previously reported as regressing atypical histiocytosis represent this form of ALCL.[458,459] The prognosis is favorable (97.5% 5-year survival in one recent series).[427] In most cases only local therapy such as excision or

radiotherapy is required.[3,456,460] Regional lymph nodes may be involved in 25% of cases but this does not necessarily imply an unfavorable prognosis.[456] Five-year survival after systemic spread was 58.3% in one recent series.[427]

Histopathology

There is usually a cohesive diffuse infiltrate in the dermis or subcutis or both. The neoplastic cells are large atypical cells typical of common ALCL or its variants (Fig. 41.12). Reactive lymphocytes may be seen at the periphery of the infiltrate. Eosinophils and neutrophils, sometimes in large numbers, may be seen as a background population.[451] In some cases the number of neoplastic cells is small, producing a LyP-like histology. Epidermal hyperplasia may be present over some lesions.[46] Epidermal hyperplasia, epidermotropism, dermal edema and vascular proliferation are seen in regressing lesions.[462]

Small numbers of CD30[+] large atypical cells can be seen in a variety of cutaneous reactions including drug reactions, viral infections, arthropod bite reactions (scabies) and certain forms of leukemia before or after therapy.[463–465]

Immunohistochemistry and cytogenetics

More than 75% of the neoplastic cells are CD30[+].[456] The majority are CD3[+], CD4[+]/CD8[−].[466] Most but not all are EMA[−] and ALK[−].[276,467] The presence of a positive reaction for ALK generally indicates cutaneous spread of primary systemic ALCL rather than primary cutaneous ALCL.[468] Positive reactions for CD15 in a cytoplasmic and Golgi zone pattern has been reported in a small

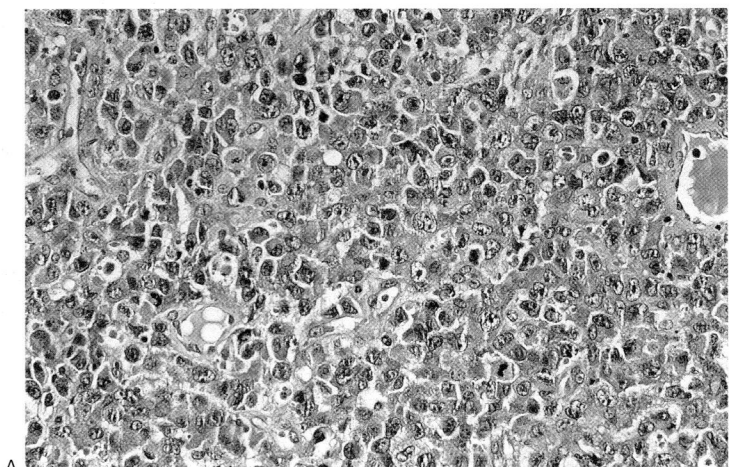

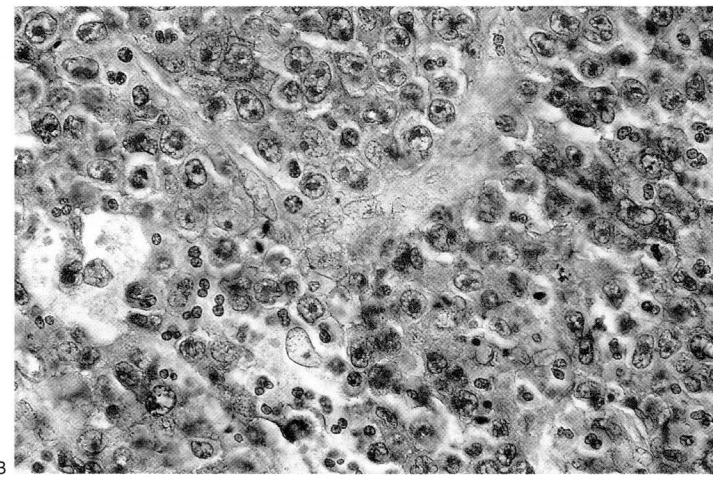

Fig. 41.12 **(A) Primary cutaneous anaplastic large cell lymphoma** (H & E). **(B)** Many cells exhibit a positive Golgi zone. (Immunoperoxidase stain for CD30)

number of cases.[427] Cells may express TIA-1 and granzyme B and rarely CD56.[466,469,470] Neoplastic cells may also express the cutaneous lymphocyte antigen HECA 452 which is not usually expressed in primary systemic ALCL.[460] The translocation t(2;5) is rarely expressed in this form of ALCL.[434,436] Cells are EBV⁻.[467] CD95 (APO-1/Fas) is strongly expressed in ALCL and LyP and may play a role in regression of lesions.[471]

Secondary ALCL

ALCL may arise in the progression of other lymphoproliferative disorders, particularly mycosis fungoides but also peripheral T-cell lymphomas and Hodgkin's disease.[273,274,276,427,472,473] ALCL in this setting is usually ALK⁻ and EMA⁻ and has a poor prognosis. ALCL may also arise in patients with previous LyP and in this setting has a good prognosis.[427]

Lymphomatoid papulosis

Lymphomatoid papulosis (LyP) is a chronic lymphoproliferative disorder characterized by the appearance of recurrent crops of papules, nodules and sometimes large plaques at different stages of development. Lesions spontaneously regress after several weeks or months, sometimes resulting in atrophic scars. The clinical course may extend over decades. Initially the lesions are smooth but later they become necrotic, crusted and ulcerated.[474–480] There may be only a few lesions, or many hundreds present during each exacerbation.[378] They occur mainly on the trunk and proximal parts of the limb, but sometimes also on the face, scalp, palms and soles. Lesions rarely involve mucosal surfaces.[481] There is a predilection for females in the third and fourth decades of life. LyP also occurs in children but transformation to a malignant lymphoma has not been reported.[482] Rare clinical presentations include pustular lesions,[483] a regional distribution of lesions,[484] and a pattern resembling hydroa vacciniforme.[485] It has been associated with the hyper-eosinophilic syndrome.[486,487] Regression of lesions has been reported after cessation of pregnancy.[488]

There is an increased frequency of a prior, coexisting or subsequent lymphoproliferative disorder associated with LyP: this is most commonly mycosis fungoides or Hodgkin's disease.[489–494] It has been claimed that in approximately 5–10% of cases progression to a malignant lymphoma (Hodgkin's disease, mycosis fungoides, ALCL) or a myeloproliferative disorder occurs.[373,378,489,495–507] Subsequent neoplasms may demonstrate identical clonal TCR gene rearrangements to that in LyP.[494,508] In a recent study of 70 patients by the EORTC group no patient died of malignant lymphoma and the 5-year survival was 100%. LyP is not associated with EBV or human herpesvirus type 6, 7 or 8.[467,509,510]

The histological appearance of LyP suggests a lymphomatous process and most would now regard this condition as a low-grade cutaneous T-cell lymphoma, part of a spectrum including ALCL.[511] Some still classify LyP as a 'pseudolymphoma'.[512] Several studies have identified a clonal population of T cells in 60% of the lesions in LyP.[477,513–515] It is, however, not included in the WHO classification of lymphoma because of the benign clinical course.[2] Because the clinical, histopathological and immunophenotypic features of LyP overlap with ALCL, the EORTC group have stressed clinical appearance and course as important features in separating the two conditions and choosing treatment options.[3] Both conditions are proliferations of large atypical CD30⁺ T/null cells.

Lesions of ALCL tend to be few and localized whereas LyP presents as recurring crops of multiple, spontaneously involuting, widely dispersed lesions. Some cases (borderline cases in the EORTC classification) have over-lapping features of both these conditions. Borderline cases have a favorable prognosis.[516] Spontaneous regression occurs in both LyP and ALCL. It has

been suggested that, in LyP, cell-mediated immune reactions involving the small lymphocytes in the infiltrate may play a role in the spontaneous regression of lesions.[517]

Histopathology[3]

The appearance of the lesions varies to a certain extent according to their age. The EORTC group recognizes three histopathological subtypes: LyP types A, B and C.[3]

LyP type A is characterized by a mixed cellular infiltrate which includes a variable number of large atypical cells similar to those seen in ALCL (Fig. 41.13). They may be multinucleate or resemble Reed–Sternberg cells. There is a background population of small lymphocytes, eosinophils, neutrophils and histiocytes. The infiltrate has a wedge-shaped profile in the dermis. Epidermotropism is not seen.

LyP type B has a perivascular or band-like dermal infiltrate with epidermotropism. The predominant cells are small to medium-sized lymphocytes with cerebriform nuclei. This picture resembles plaque stage mycosis fungoides. Some lesions have overlap features of these two types. Different lesions in the same crop may show either of these patterns.

LyP type C lesions resemble ALCL and have a monotonous population of large atypical cells with relatively few admixed inflammatory cells.

Lesions in any of the subtypes may have focal spongiosis in the epidermis, parakeratosis with neutrophils, and ulceration. Epidermal hyperplasia is sometimes present in some cases arising from follicular epithelium.[518] A rare variant in which the infiltrate is centered around hair follicles has been described.[519–521] Mitotic figures are common in all histological subtypes. There is some dermal fibrosis in resolving lesions, particularly in those that have ulcerated. There may be only a few atypical cells in late lesions.

Keratoacanthoma has also been reported in association with LyP.[522,523]

Immunohistochemistry and cytogenetics

The large atypical cells in LyP types A and C are CD30⁺, CD3⁺, CD2⁻/⁺, CD4⁺/⁻, CD8⁻, similar to cells in ALCL. Cells are generally negative for CD15 and EMA but positive reactions have been reported in a few cases, the former being seen in a cytoplasmic and Golgi zone pattern.[427] The atypical cells in type B lesions have a CD3⁺, CD4⁺, CD8⁻ profile. They do not express CD30. Clonal rearrangement of TCR genes has been identified in approximately 60% of lesions.[515,524] As in ALCL, the CD30⁺ cells also express TIA-1, perforin and granzyme B.[466,525] Like primary cutaneous ALCL, CD30⁺ cells are ALK⁻.

SUBCUTANEOUS PANNICULITIS-LIKE T-CELL LYMPHOMA

It is generally considered that most if not all cases of cytophagic histiocytic panniculitis (see p. 527) are in reality not inflammatory in nature but a T-cell lymphoma – subcutaneous panniculitis-like T-cell lymphoma (SPTCL).[526,527]

SPTCL presents as tender, erythematous nodules, predominantly on the legs and less frequently on the trunk, arms and face. The lesions are ulcerated in 20% of cases. The median age at diagnosis is 39 years and there is a slight female preponderance of cases. It is rare in children.[528] Up to 40% of cases have associated fever, weight loss and myalgia. This is generally an aggressive lymphoma although there are reports of cases with a more indolent course.[529,530] Hemophagocytic syndrome occurs in 45% of cases. The mortality rate is 50%, predominantly from hemophagocytic syndrome.[531] Rarely, there is a terminal leukemic phase.[532] The TCR γδ form of SPTCL (see below) is possibly a more aggressive form of the disease.[144,533]

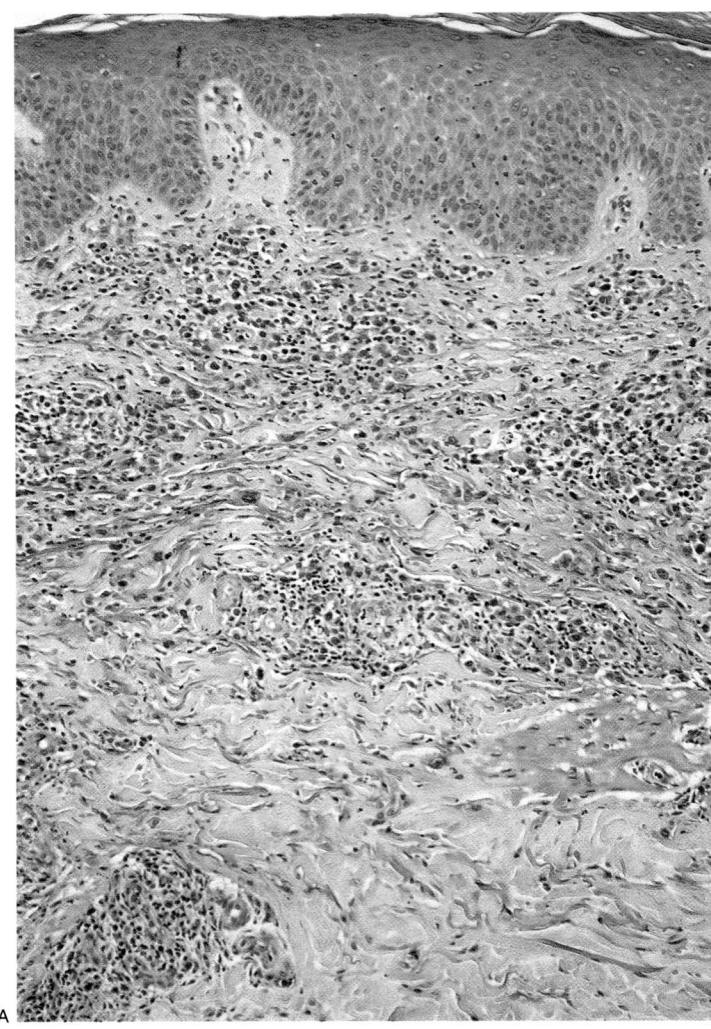

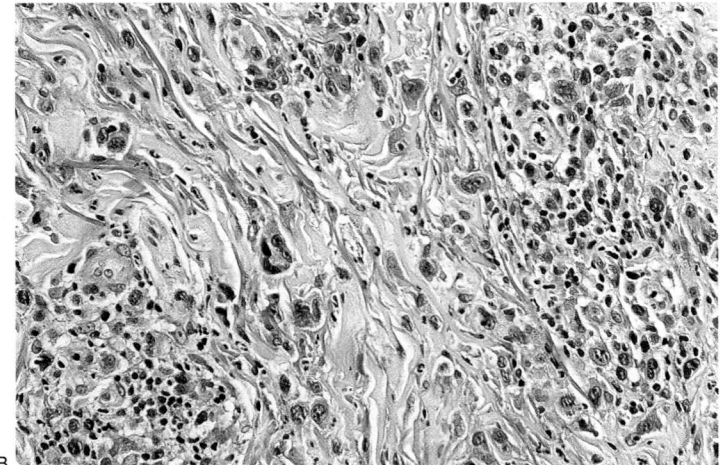

Fig. 41.13 **Lymphomatoid papulosis. (A)** Type A histology. **(B)** There is a mixture of large atypical cells and small lymphocytes. (H & E)

Histopathology[533]

The lymphomatous infiltrate predominantly involves lobules of the subcutis to produce a lobular panniculitis-like pattern (Fig. 41.14). The mid and deep dermis are sometimes involved in a perivascular pattern, particularly in the

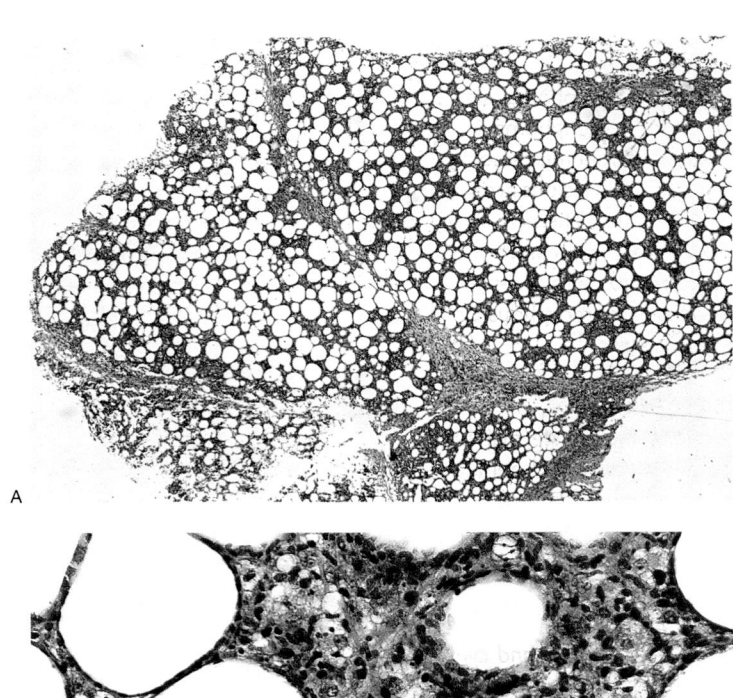

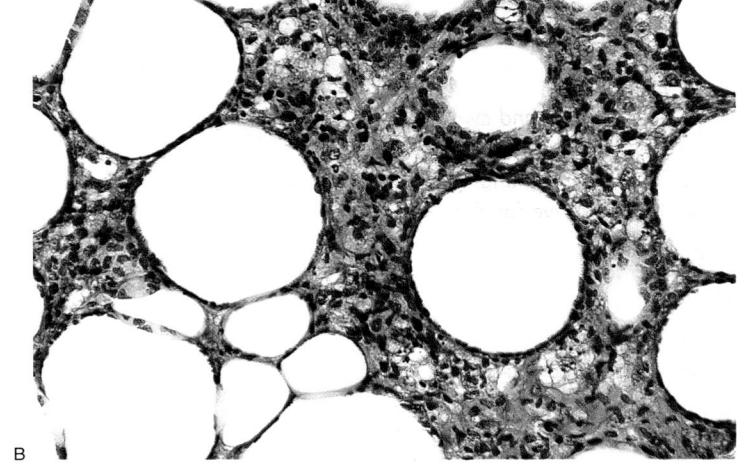

Fig. 41.14 **(A) Subcutaneous panniculitis-like T-cell lymphoma. (B)** There are atypical lymphoid cells ringing adipocytes and histiocytes with cell debris. (H & E)

TCR γδ subset; epidermal involvement is rare. The component cells are small, medium and large lymphocytes with irregular hyperchromatic nuclei. The atypical cells characteristically rim adipocytes to form a lace-like pattern. Apoptotic bodies (karyorrhectic nuclear fragments) are invariably present. A component of large phagocytic histiocytes ('bean-bag histiocytes') containing cell debris or red blood cells (erythrophagocytosis) is sometimes seen. Fat necrosis with foamy histiocytes is present in all cases but epithelioid granulomas are uncommon. Sometimes there is a lipomembranous pattern of fat necrosis.[531] Plasma cells are present in some cases but neutrophils and eosinophils are generally absent. Angiocentricity, angioinvasion and large areas of necrosis, typical of NK/T-cell lymphoma-nasal type, are not typical of SPTCL and if present are only a minor component.

Immunohistochemistry and cytogenetics

The cells of SPTCL are T cells and have the immunophenotype CD3+, CD8+ (or less commonly CD4−/CD8− or CD4+ or CD4+/CD8+). They are TIA+, perforin+ but are usually CD56−, CD16−, CD57− and CD30−. The majority express TCR αβ but up to 25% express TCR γδ.[534] Those cases that express TCR γδ are typically CD56+ and belong to the Vδ2 subset.[534] Cells are negative for EBV in all cases, except for rare cases reported from Asia.[535,536]

BLASTIC NK-CELL LYMPHOMA

Blastic NK-cell lymphoma, also called blastic NK-cell leukemia/lymphoma or blastoid NK-cell lymphoma, is characterized by frequent initial presentation as skin lesions, sometimes associated with lymphadenopathy. Older age groups are affected. Skin lesions are single or multiple plaques and tumors which may be pigmented.[537] There is an aggressive clinical course terminating in bone marrow involvement and overt leukemia.[537–539] The relationship of blastic NK-cell lymphoma to cases showing NK and myeloid features is unclear.[537,540] Cutaneous monomorphous CD4[+], CD56[+] large cell lymphoma appears to be a similar process.[541]

Histopathology

Skin lesions show a dermal and sometimes subcutaneous infiltrate which is either perivascular and periappendageal or diffuse. The tumor cells have a blastic morphology and are intermediate in size with round or slightly indented nuclei and a small amount of cytoplasm. In some cases the cells resemble myeloid blasts. Chromatin is finely particulate and nucleoli are inconspicuous. Mitoses are frequent.[537]

Immunohistochemistry and cytogenetics

The neoplastic cells are CD45[+], CD43[+], CD2[+/−], CD3[−] (surface and cytoplasmic), CD4[+], CD56[+] and CD5[−]. There is no rearrangement of the TCR gene. Cells are negative for EBV.

AGGRESSIVE NK-CELL LEUKEMIA

Aggressive NK-cell leukemia, also known as aggressive NK-cell leukemia/lymphoma, is a very rare disorder in Western countries, most reports coming from Japan.[141,542,543] It occurs in a younger age group than NK/T-cell lymphoma, nasal type (median age of 30 in reported cases).[542] It is characterized by an aggressive disease with fever and hepatosplenomegaly as well as lymph node and bone marrow involvement. There are circulating atypical large lymphoid cells with azurophilic granules. Skin involvement is present in about half the cases.[542]

Immunohistochemistry and cytogenetics

The cells are CD2[+], surface CD3[−] (cytoplasmic CD3ε[+]), CD56[+], CD4[−], CD8[−], CD16[+/−], CD57[−]. There is no TCR gene rearrangement. Cells are positive for EBV (EBER).[141,542,544]

EXTRANODAL NK/T-CELL LYMPHOMA, NASAL TYPE

Extranodal NK/T-cell lymphoma, nasal type, is the best characterized of the NK/T group of lymphomas.[144,545,546] This form of lymphoma is common in Asia, South and Central America and Mexico, but uncommon in the United States and Europe. It is almost always associated with EBV virus when carefully defined, even in Caucasians.[547] The nasal region is the most common site of presentation, often with midline facial destructive disease (lethal midline granuloma) or a nasal mass.[548] The extranasal form of this lymphoma, which appears to be identical to the nasal form, commonly presents in the skin and subcutis and less commonly in the upper respiratory tract to the larynx, gastrointestinal tract, testis and spleen. These are also the sites to which the nasal form commonly disseminates.[549] Nasal metastasis may follow skin presentation.[550] Unlike lymphomatoid granulomatosis, the lung is rarely

involved. Nodal involvement is also very uncommon.[141] Hemophagocytic syndrome is a common complication. This lymphoma has an aggressive behavior with a short median survival and high mortality rate.[547] Some cases with systemic disease have overlap features with aggressive NK/T-cell leukemia/lymphoma.[547] Cutaneous lesions include ulcerated tumors, subcutaneous nodules resembling a panniculitis, erythematous plaques, purpura, bullous lesions and macular papular rashes.[545] Lesions occur on the trunk and extremities.[551]

Histopathology

These lymphomas were previously classified as *angiocentric lymphoma* in the REAL classification.[1] Angiocentricity is a non-specific feature found in other lymphomas, including B-cell neoplasms,[140] and is not seen in all cases of this form of lymphoma.[546]

There is a diffuse or angiocentric and periappendageal cellular infiltrate which involves the dermis and subcutis (Fig. 41.15). The infiltrate consists of variably sized small and intermediate-sized lymphocytes. Cellular pleomorphism may be slight. This feature, together with a background population of other inflammatory cells including eosinophils and plasma cells, may lead to a misdiagnosis of an inflammatory reaction such as a lobular panniculitis.[140,552] Zonal necrosis and karyorrhexis are frequently seen. This may be due to release of cytotoxic granules with the induction of apoptosis[553,554] or production of TNF-α (tumor necrosis factor-α). Angiocentricity is associated with cellular invasion of vessel walls, sometimes with fibrinoid necrosis.[546] Involvement of the subcutis can mimic panniculitis-like T-cell lymphoma, particularly if angiocentricity is absent. Phagocytic macrophages and rimming of adipocytes can be present.[552]

Immunohistochemistry and cytogenetics

The tumor cells are CD56[+], CD2[+], surface CD3[−] and may be TIA-1, perforin and granzyme B positive. They express cytoplasmic CD3ε. There is no TCR or immunoglobulin heavy-chain gene rearrangement. EBV can be detected in most cases by in situ hybridization for EBER (EBV-encoded small RNA) and occasionally by immunohistochemistry (LMP-1). CD7, CD4, CD8 are occasionally positive.[546,555] One case has been reported with TCR γ rearrangement.[556]

ANGIOIMMUNOBLASTIC T-CELL LYMPHOMA

Angioimmunoblastic lymphadenopathy with dysproteinemia (AILD) was originally considered an abnormal immune reaction with B-cell hyperplasia.[557] It is now regarded as a peripheral T-cell lymphoma, as most cases show clonal TCR gene rearrangements.[558] It is characterized by generalized lymphadenopathy, hepatosplenomegaly, constitutional symptoms such as fevers, night sweats and weight loss, polyclonal hypergammaglobulinemia and, in about 50% of cases, a skin rash.[559,560] This often consists of a non-specific, generalized, maculopapular rash resembling a viral exanthem or drug eruption. Lesions may precede or occur concurrently with systemic disease and are commonly on the trunk and limbs. Other cutaneous manifestations include erythematous plaques, nodules, urticarial and purpuric lesions. Lesions may regress spontaneously or after corticosteroid therapy. It occurs most commonly in the elderly. AILD has a moderately aggressive course with a mortality rate of from 50% to 70% and a median survival from 11 to 30 months.[557] Spontaneous remissions or protracted responses to corticosteroids may be seen in the course of the disease. Infections are common complications and there may be progression to a high-grade T-cell or rarely a B-cell lymphoma.[1] Cutaneous B-cell lymphoma has been reported in association with AILD.[561]

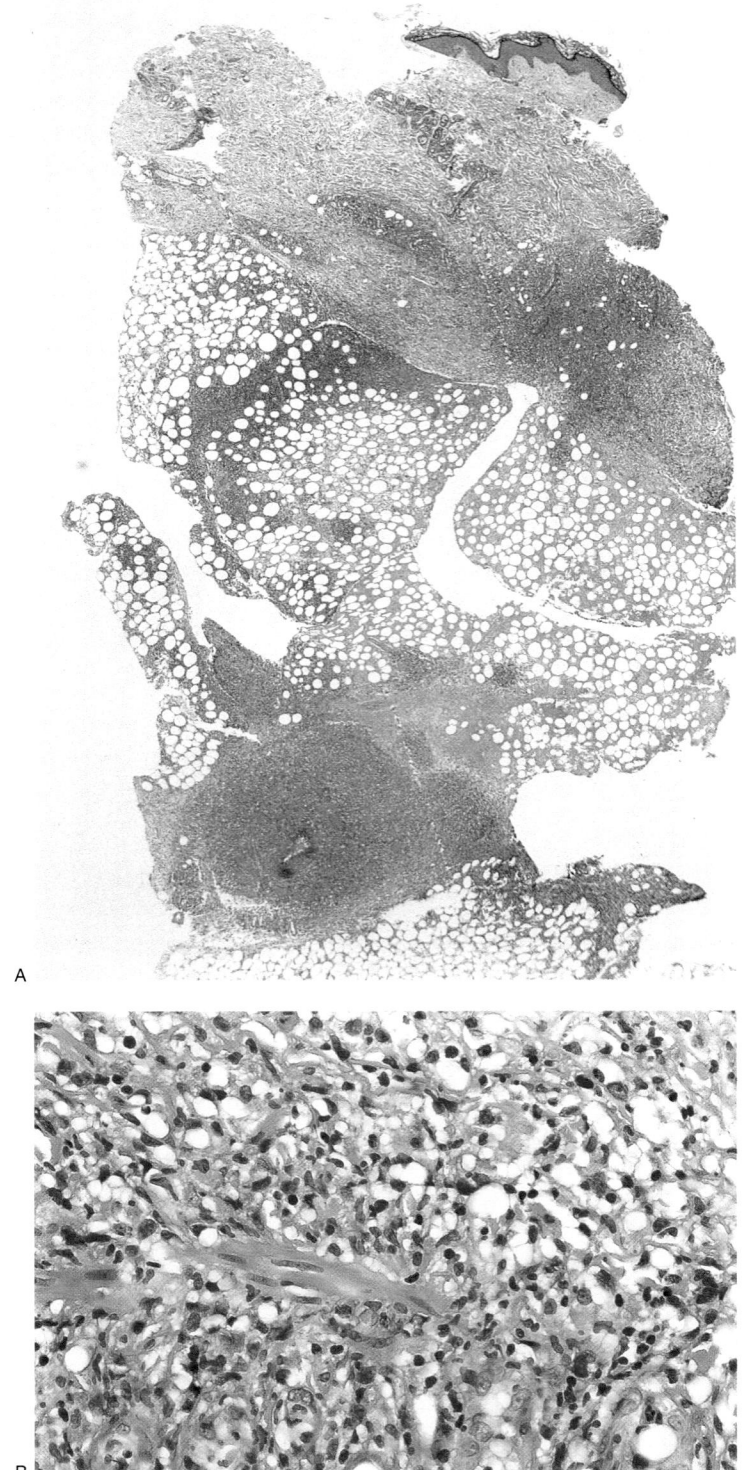

A

B

Fig. 41.15 **Extranodal NK/T-cell lymphoma. (A)** An angiocentric pattern of infiltration is evident. **(B)** A polymorphous lymphoid infiltrate is present in the wall of a vessel. (H & E)

Histopathology[562]

The histological features vary from a mild, non-specific perivascular infiltrate of lymphocytes to variably dense perivascular and periappendageal infiltrates and dense nodular infiltrates which may extend into the subcutis. Cellular infiltrates are polymorphous and include variable numbers of large atypical lymphocytes, medium and small lymphocytes and admixed histiocytes, and occasional plasma cells or eosinophils. Rarely, Reed–Sternberg-like cells are seen.[562] Proliferation of post-capillary venules is also seen in many biopsies, reminiscent of vascular proliferation seen in lymph nodes in AILD. Occasionally there is a leukocytoclastic vasculitis with extravasated red blood cells.

Immunohistochemistry and cytogenetics

Neoplastic lymphocytes express T-cell antigens CD2, CD3, CD45RO, and there is a predominance of CD4+ cells.[562] CD8+ cells may also be expressed in some cells. Clonal TCR genes are rearranged in 75% of lymph nodes and have also been reported in the skin, even in apparently non-specific infiltrates. EBV is detected in lymph nodes in the majority of cases of AILD but only in a few isolated lymphocytes.[562] It has also been reported infrequently in skin lesions.[562–564]

ADULT T-CELL LYMPHOMA/LEUKEMIA (HTLV-1+)

Adult T-cell leukemia (ATLL) is a variant of peripheral T-cell lymphoma resulting from infection with human T-cell lymphotropic virus type 1 (HTLV-1), a type C retrovirus.[565–567]

The virus is endemic in south-western Japan and the Caribbean, but it has also been reported sporadically in parts of Europe, Africa and the south-eastern USA.[568–571] HTLV-1 is transmitted by sexual contact, breast feeding, infected blood products and percutaneously.[568,571] Infection confers a lifetime risk of 2–4% for adult T-cell lymphoma/leukemia.[570] A second related virus, HTLV-2, found particularly in Amerindian groups, parts of Africa and in intravenous drug users, is less clearly linked to lymphoproliferative disorders.[572]

ATLL has variable clinical manifestations which include cutaneous eruptions, bone marrow and peripheral blood involvement, lymphadenopathy, hepatosplenomegaly, pulmonary infiltrates and hypercalcemia. The average age of onset of ATLL in a large series from Japan was 57 years (24 years – 92 years).[573] Immigrant studies suggest there is a long latent period from viral infection to ATLL.[574]

Several clinical forms are recognized including: (1) an aggressive acute form associated with a very high white cell count, hepatosplenomegaly, hypercalcemia and lytic bone lesions; (2) a chronic form associated with lower white cell counts, no hepatosplenomegaly, no hypercalcemia, skin rashes and a slightly longer survival; (3) a smoldering form with a mild clonal lymphocytosis, skin rashes and an indolent course; (4) a rare lymphomatous form with isolated lymphadenopathy or extranodal tumors and without leukemia; and (5) a cutaneous type which resembles mycosis fungoides with the skin alone being involved. Spread to other organs follows.[573,575] The integration pattern of HTLV-1 proviral DNA may be the explanation for the heterogeneity in the behavior of ATTL.[576,577]

Skin lesions are often the initial manifestation of ATTL (50–70% of cases) and are found in all forms of the disease.[578,579] Lesions are often widespread and have many forms including erythematous patches, plaques, papules and nodules. Erythroderma and a pompholyx-like vesicular eruption are less common cutaneous manifestations. Non-specific skin lesions or prurigo may precede the onset of acute ATTL.[580,581]

Atypical lymphocytes are found in 50–80% of patients at presentation; virtually all develop a leukemic phase eventually.[582] The leukemic cells have a distinctive convoluted or clover-shaped appearance.

Histopathology

The cutaneous lesions of ATLL share some features with mycosis fungoides in having an infiltrate of atypical lymphocytes in the upper dermis with variable epidermotropism and occasional Pautrier microabscesses. Unlike mycosis fungoides, these microabscesses may contain prominent apoptotic fragments (Fig. 41.16). The infiltrate in some cases is more massive than in mycosis fungoides, and in others it conforms to a papular outline, an uncommon pattern in mycosis fungoides.[186]

The infiltrating cells may be medium-sized, large or pleomorphic, or a mixture of these types.[568,578] Other elements, such as small lymphocytes, histiocytes, eosinophils and plasma cells, are less common than in mycosis fungoides. Sometimes dermal aggregates of lymphocytes and histiocytes form, resembling granulomas.[583,584]

Atypical lymphocytes are sometimes found in the lumen of blood vessels in the dermis. They occasionally involve the vessel walls, leading to their damage and the extravasation of erythrocytes.[585] Angiocentric and angio-destructive lesions are a rare manifestation of ATLL.[579]

Immunohistochemistry and cytogenetics

The neoplastic lymphocytes are T cells and exhibit clonal rearrangement of the TCR genes. They are CD2[+], CD3[+] and CD4[+]. They also express the IL-2 receptor α chain (CD25), which is a distinguishing feature between ATLL and Sézary syndrome.[585,586] HTLV-1 is clonally integrated in T cells in all cases and can be demonstrated in paraffin-embedded tissue.[587]

Electron microscopy[578]

The tumor cells show slight to marked nuclear irregularity with a convoluted shape and a speckled chromatin pattern. The degree of nuclear indentation is much less than in cells of mycosis fungoides and Sézary syndrome. The cells in ATLL have lysosomal granules and glycogen in their cytoplasm.

PERIPHERAL T-CELL LYMPHOMA (UNSPECIFIED)

The REAL/WHO classification includes under this classification all peripheral T-cell lymphomas not conforming to a known subtype. Although most cases are of nodal origin, cutaneous lesions occur relatively commonly, ranging from 25% to 50% in most series.[7,588–590] The WHO recognizes two variants, lymphoepithelioid type (Lennert's lymphoma) and T-zone type. Stage is regarded as a better prognostic indicator than morphological subtype (cell

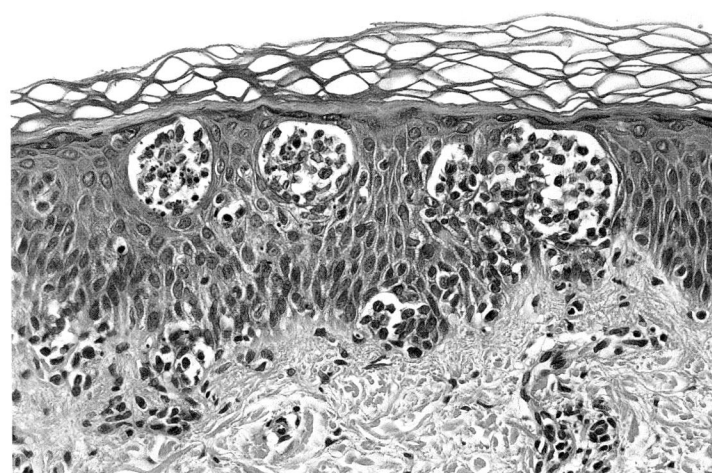

Fig. 41.16 Adult T-cell leukemia/lymphoma. There is extensive epidermotropism with Pautrier microabscess formation. Characteristic apoptotic debris is just visible. (H & E) (Case kindly supplied by Dr Tetsunori Kimura, Section of Dermatology, Sapporo General Hospital, Sapporo, Japan)

size) in primary non-cutaneous lymphomas.[591] The clinical course is usually aggressive.[1]

The EORTC group recognize a primary CD30[-] cutaneous large T-cell lymphoma with an aggressive clinical course. The estimated 5-year survival in their series was 15%.[3] They also include a provisional entity of pleomorphic small/medium-sized cutaneous T-cell lymphoma, distinct from mycosis fungoides.[3,592–594] Cells have a CD4[+] or less commonly a CD8[+] phenotype. The estimated 5-year survival in a small series was 62%.[3] This provisional entity is not accepted by all and may represent a variety of other T-cell lymphomas.[595]

Lennert's lymphoma (lymphoepithelial lymphoma) is an uncommon variant of peripheral T-cell lymphoma. It is generally low grade but sometimes runs a rapid course.[596] There have been comparatively few reports of this entity in recent years.[597] Cutaneous involvement is rare.[597,598] Various skin infections have been reported in patients with this lymphoma.[599] There is one report of this tumor presenting as atypical granuloma annulare.[600]

Histopathology

The cellular infiltrates are polymorphous and contain cells of variable size and shape. In Lennert's lymphoma there is a predominantly dermal infiltrate of neoplastic lymphoid cells without the high content of epithelioid histiocytes that characterize the lymph node changes.[597,598] The abnormal lymphocytes are CD4[+597] or rarely CD8[+].[601]

Immunohistochemistry and cytogenetics

There is variable expression of T-cell associated antigens, CD3, CD2, CD5, CD7. Cells may be CD4[+] or CD8[+] or CD4[-],CD8[-]. TCR genes are usually, but not always, rearranged.[1]

CD4[+], CD56[+] CUTANEOUS NEOPLASMS

There have been recent reports of a neoplastic process presenting with cutaneous papules and nodules in which the neoplastic cells exhibit the phenotype CD4[+], CD56[+], CD45[+], CD43[+]. All other B- and T-cell markers were negative and, except for CD68, the cells were negative for myelomonocytic markers. Other markers for NK cells were also negative (CD16, CD57, TIA-1, granzyme B). No B- or T-cell clonal rearrangements were identified. Some patients had lymph node involvement at presentation or developed bone marrow involvement and leukemia.[602,603] This may be a distinct entity derived from hematological precursor cells.

Histopathology

The dermis and subcutis were infiltrated by a dense infiltrate of small and medium-sized cells with irregular nuclei with finely dispersed chromatin and several small nucleoli. The cells had minimal cytoplasm without demonstrable granularity. Large cells were few in number. Skin appendages were often infiltrated or destroyed by the cellular infiltrate. Angiocentricity was not a feature except in one case.[603]

OTHER LYMPHOMA

HODGKIN'S LYMPHOMA (HODGKIN'S DISEASE)

Infiltration of the skin is usually a late manifestation of Hodgkin's disease, and develops in from 0.5% to 7.5% of patients.[604,605] Lesions often occur in a localized area of the trunk or on the proximal part of the extremities in the vicinity of involved lymph nodes, suggesting retrograde lymphatic spread.[604,606] Hematogenous and in-continuity direct spread are less common routes of dissemination. Direct skin invasion from nodes may mimic scrofuloderma.[607]

Cutaneous lesions may be papules, nodules or plaques, although rare clinical presentations have included multiple ulcers on the scalp,[608] a bullous eruption[609] and widespread lesions. Paradoxically, two of the cases with widespread deposits had a more prolonged survival than is usually seen with cutaneous disease.[610] Spontaneous regression of skin lesions has been reported.[611]

Skin lesions may rarely be the initial manifestation of Hodgkin's disease, with lymph node involvement appearing some months later.[612–616] Primary cutaneous Hodgkin's disease is a controversial entity, although rare cases appear to exist.[617,618] Some cases previously reported may represent lymphomatoid papulosis or anaplastic large cell lymphoma. Cases of lymphomatoid papulosis followed by Hodgkin's disease have been reported.[507,508] Primary cutaneous Hodgkin's disease may pursue a benign course, although up to 50% of patients develop nodal or systemic disease.[617,618]

A variety of non-specific manifestations are commonly found in the skin in Hodgkin's disease. These include pruritus, herpes zoster and acquired ichthyosis. Less common associations have included urticaria, erythema multiforme, drug eruptions, bullous pemphigoid, dermatitis herpetiformis, pemphigus, acquired epidermolysis bullosa, follicular mucinosis, alopecia, lymphedema, dermatomyositis and granuloma annulare. Numerous examples of concurrent Hodgkin's disease and mycosis fungoides have been reported. Rarely, mycosis fungoides and cutaneous Hodgkin's disease have been reported together.[616]

The WHO classification divides Hodgkin's disease into classical Hodgkin's disease (including nodular sclerosis, lymphocyte-rich classical, mixed cellularity and lymphocyte depletion subtypes) and nodular lymphocyte predominance Hodgkin's disease, which is now regarded as a separate clinicopathological entity.[2]

Recent studies have demonstrated that the neoplastic cells of Hodgkin's disease are clonally derived from germinal center B cells that have lost the capacity to produce or express immunoglobulin.[619,620] In addition, many epidemiological and molecular studies suggest that Epstein–Barr virus (EBV) plays a significant etiological role in Hodgkin's disease.[621–623] In situ hybridization for EBV has demonstrated abundant viral transcripts in Reed–Sternberg cells in one case of primary cutaneous Hodgkin's disease.[618]

Histopathology

There is a diffuse infiltrate of cells involving the dermis and upper subcutis. A grenz zone is usually present. Skin appendages and blood vessels are frequently invaded.[613] There is a mixed infiltrate which includes mononuclear variants of Reed–Sternberg cells and variable numbers of classic Reed–Sternberg cells in a background of small lymphocytes, eosinophils, and sometimes neutrophils (Fig. 41.17).[624] Fibrosis is another common feature. The histology may resemble that of nodular sclerosis or mixed cellularity types; lymphocyte depletion may be present in advanced stages.[604] Non-specific changes reported in the skin include small epithelioid granulomas[625] and, in one case, palisading necrobiotic granulomas.[626]

Hodgkin's disease must be distinguished from lymphomatoid papulosis and anaplastic large cell lymphoma with which it has many features in common. Neutrophils and eosinophils have been reported in lesions from all these conditions and are not a discriminating feature. Reed–Sternberg-like cells may be seen in lymphomatoid papulosis and anaplastic large cell lymphoma on occasions. Authentic Reed–Sternberg cells and mononuclear forms are CD30[+], CD15[+] in most cases and also CD45[-], CD45RO[-], CD43[-] and EMA[-].

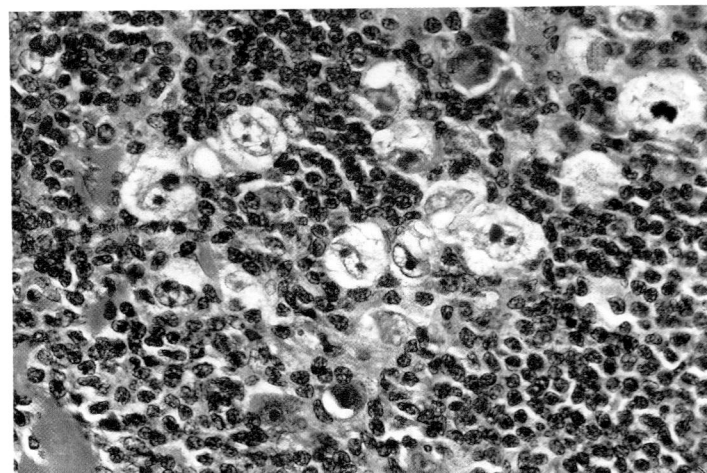

Fig. 41.17 Cutaneous Hodgkin's disease. Several Reed–Sternberg cells are present. (H & E)

Immunoglobulin and TCR genes are germline.[22] Occasionally cells are CD20[+]. EBV-positive cases of classical Hodgkin's disease stain for EBV-LMP. The background population of small lymphocytes are predominantly CD3[+], CD4[+] T cells.

Large cells in primary anaplastic large cell lymphoma and lymphomatoid papulosis are CD30[+], CD15[-], and CD45 may be negative in some cases.[22] They may be EMA[+] more commonly in the primary systemic form than in the primary cutaneous form and lymphomatoid papulosis. ALK-1 is positive in the systemic form and rarely in the cutaneous form but never in Hodgkin's disease.[276] Reed–Sternberg cells are sometimes negative in cutaneous Hodgkin's disease.[605] Stein et al have stated that CD15 and EMA may not help in the distinction between Hodgkin's disease and ALK negative-anaplastic large cell lymphoma.[276]

CUTANEOUS INFILTRATES OF OTHER LEUKEMIAS/LYMPHOMAS

Many of the lymphoma/leukemias associated with frequent cutaneous manifestations have already been described. The following discussion deals predominantly with infiltrates of the myeloproliferative diseases, acute myeloid leukemias and B-chronic lymphocytic leukemia/small lymphocytic lymphoma (B-CLL). The current WHO classification of myeloid neoplasms will be used here.[2]

Cutaneous manifestations of leukemia have been divided into specific (leukemia cutis) and non-specific lesions. Dissemination to the skin is generally associated with a poor prognosis.[627,628] The specific lesions take the form of solitary or multiple, violaceous or reddish-brown and hemorrhagic papules, nodules and plaques of varying sizes.[628] Marked thickening of the gums and oral petechiae are further manifestations of monocytic leukemia.[628] Specific skin lesions usually occur late in the course of the disease, although sometimes they antedate by months the detection of leukemic cells in the blood or bone marrow. The term 'aleukemic leukemia cutis' has been used for this uncommon event, which is seen predominantly with myeloid leukemias.[629–635]

Unusual clinical presentations include eczematous lesions,[636] penile[637] or scrotal ulcers,[638] erythema nodosum-like lesions,[639] acral lividosis,[640] a stasis dermatitis-like presentation,[641] localization at catheter insertion sites,[642] figurate erythema,[643] annular purpuric plaques,[644] hemorrhagic bullae[645,646] and paronychia.[647] Up to 30% of children with congenital leukemia have skin infiltrates[648] and this is one of the causes of the 'blueberry muffin' appearance.[649]

Specific infiltrates occur in 10–50% of forms of acute myeloid leukemia (including myeloid, monocytic and myelomonocytic forms) and myeloproliferative diseases, in 4–20% of B-CLL,[650] and in less than 10% of precursor B- and T-lymphoblastic leukemia/lymphoma and hairy cell leukemia.[651–653]

Non-specific cutaneous manifestations of leukemia are more common than specific leukemic infiltration of the skin, and occur in up to 40% or more of leukemic patients.[654] The most frequent of these are hemorrhagic manifestations, including petechiae, purpura and ecchymoses.[654] *Candida albicans*, *Trichophyton rubrum* and *Cryptococcus neoformans* are the most common causes of cutaneous fungal infections complicating leukemia. Ecthyma gangrenosum (see p. 620) has resulted from severe *Pseudomonas* infection.[655] Herpes zoster is particularly common in patients with B-CLL. Other non-specific cutaneous findings include pyoderma gangrenosum, Sweet's syndrome, erythroderma, intraepidermal blisters, erythema multiforme, urticaria, cutaneous hyperpigmentation, xanthomas[656] and pruritus.

MYELOID LEUKEMIAS, MYELOPROLIFERATIVE DISEASES AND MYELODYSPLASTIC SYNDROMES

Cutaneous infiltrates have been described in all of the forms of acute myeloid leukemia and many forms of myeloproliferative disease, including rare forms.[657–659] In myeloid leukemia lesions may be single or multiple and have no particular distribution. In chronic myelogenous leukemia, lesions are more common on the trunk, head and neck.[660] Rare cases of cutaneous involvement by acute promyelocytic leukemia have been described.[660a]

'Granulocytic sarcoma' was a term originally used for an extramedullary, soft tissue mass composed of neoplastic myeloid cells.[649,661–666] It occurs most often in the orbit, but can arise in any part of the body. 'Chloroma' was another term applied to this tumor mass because of the greenish color that some examples developed on exposure to light due to the presence of myeloperoxidase.[662] It may occur as a manifestation of myeloid leukemia or as the presenting symptom,[667] in the course of chronic myelogenous leukemia or other myeloproliferative syndromes in blast transformation, in myelodysplastic syndromes, and as an isolated form in patients without hematological

abnormalities.[668] Lesions are usually a single, rapidly growing nodular mass. The last form overlaps with lesions that have been called 'aleukemic leukemia cutis', in which there may be widespread papulonodular skin lesions.[669–672] Cutaneous or extracutaneous granulocytic sarcoma can frequently evolve into systemic myeloid leukemia, often within months, but long survivals (usually after chemotherapy) without progression to leukemia have been reported.[649,673,674]

Histopathology[660]

There are nodular and diffuse infiltrates in the dermis and often subcutis; they may be concentrated about vessels or appendages. There is sparing of the upper dermis and characteristically there is prominent percolation of single cells between collagen bundles (Fig. 41.18).

The cellular characteristics depend on the type of leukemia.[660,667,675] In acute myeloid leukemias there are small, medium or large cells representing myeloblasts, atypical myelocytes and monocytoid cells.

In chronic myelogenous leukemia there is either a mixture of mature and immature cells of the granulocytic series (myelocytes, metamyelocytes, eosinophilic metamyelocytes, and neutrophils or eosinophils) or a monomorphous infiltrate of mononuclear cells. Some leukemic infiltrates have a monomorphous appearance resembling a lymphoma and only scattered cells with eosinophilic granules are a clue to a possible leukemic infiltrate (Fig. 41.19). Mitotic figures are quite common. In granulocytic sarcomas there is a dense infiltrate of myeloblasts and myelocytes with some mature cells.[662] Focal necrosis may also be present.

Other histopathological features seen occasionally include the presence of Langhans type giant cells[676] and leukemic vasculitis,[677,678] in which the walls of blood vessels are infiltrated by leukemic cells with variable fibrinoid necrosis. Leukemic infiltrates have also been reported in other skin conditions including basal cell carcinoma[679] and psoriasis.[680]

Histochemistry and immunohistochemistry

Cells stain with napthol AS-D chloroacetate-esterase in up to two-thirds of cases.[660]

CD45, CD74, CD43, lysozyme, elastase or myeloperoxidase are positive in most cases. There is variable positivity for CD68, HAM-56 and Mac387 depending on the degree of monocytic differentiation. CD56 may be positive in up to 30% of cases.[672,681,682] CD30 may be expressed rarely.[683]

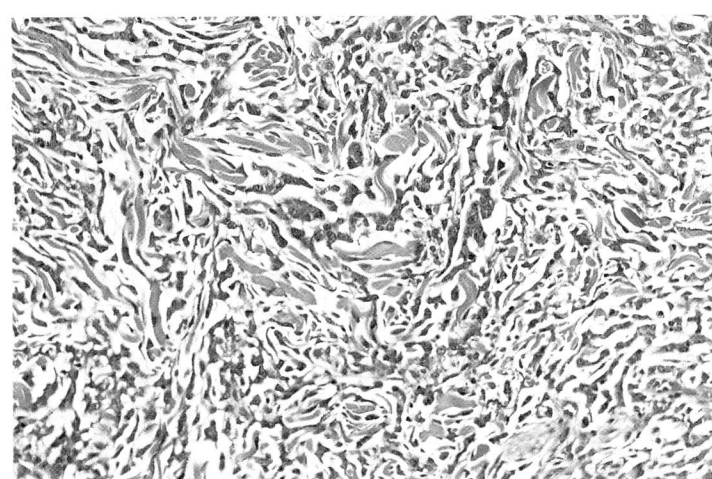

Fig. 41.18 **Cutaneous infiltration by myeloid blasts in a patient with acute myeloid leukemia.** (H & E)

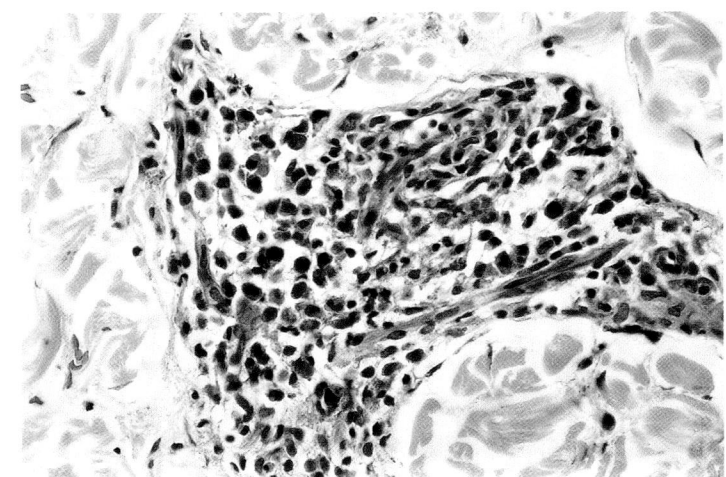

Fig. 41.19 **Myeloid leukemia.** There is only a perivascular infiltrate of myeloid blasts. Some cells contain eosinophilic granules. (H & E)

B-CELL CHRONIC LYMPHOCYTIC LEUKEMIA/SMALL LYMPHOCYTIC LYMPHOMA (B-CLL)

The specific infiltrates of B-CLL include localized or generalized, erythematous papules, plaques, nodules and large tumors. Reflecting the fact that B-CLL occurs predominantly in older adults,[1] the mean age of presentation in one series was 66 years.[684] Uncommonly, skin lesions may represent the first sign of the disease.[684,685] Lesions may present in the scars of herpes zoster or varicella, or herpes simplex lesions.[686–688] Occasionally, B-CLL and mycosis fungoides present together.[689] Cutaneous lesions may also occur frequently in the much rarer T-cell prolymphocytic leukemia (T-cell chronic lymphocytic leukemia).[1,690]

The 5-year survival of B-CLL patients with cutaneous lesions is 66%. Transformation to a large cell lymphoma (Richter's syndrome) is associated with a poor prognosis.[684]

Histopathology

Patterns of dermal infiltration include perivascular and periappendageal, nodular, diffuse and band-like.[684] The cellular infiltrate consists of a monomorphous population of small lymphocytes. Proliferation centers, which are pale areas containing larger prolymphocytes and paraimmunoblasts, are uncommon.[684] Varying numbers of larger cells resembling centroblasts and immunoblasts are present in cases undergoing transformation to a large B-cell lymphoma (Richter's syndrome). There may be epidermal changes of acanthosis and ulceration. Other reactive cells including eosinophils, neutrophils, histiocytes, and plasma cells may be present.[691]

The leukemic infiltrate may surround epithelial neoplasms such as basal cell carcinoma and squamous cell carcinoma (Fig. 41.20).[691a]

Immunohistochemistry and cytogenetics

The small lymphocytes are CD20+, CD5+, CD43+, CD23+ and CD10−.[1,684]

PCR demonstrates clonal immunoglobulin heavy-chain gene rearrangement.

In T-cell prolymphocytic leukemia the cells are CD2+, CD3+, CD5+ and CD7+. Approximately two-thirds of cases are CD4+.[1]

γ HEAVY-CHAIN DISEASE

γ Heavy-chain disease is a biochemical expression of a mutant clone of B cells which produces abnormal incomplete γ heavy chains, devoid of light chains.[692] It is usually associated with a lymphoplasmacytic proliferative disorder, although the associated clinical and histological findings are varied.[693] Cutaneous involvement is rare, being present in less than 5% of the reported cases.[692] The usual skin lesions are erythematous infiltrated plaques and nodules on the trunk and extremities. Livedo reticularis and digital necrosis caused by an associated necrotizing arteritis have been reported.[694]

Histopathology

In the few reported cases of γ heavy-chain disease with cutaneous involvement there has been a dermal infiltrate of lymphoplasmacytic cells, immunoblasts and mature plasma cells.[692] In one case, vascular proliferation and the presence of eosinophils led to an initial diagnosis of angiolymphoid hyperplasia with eosinophilia.[693,695] Sometimes the cells have a conspicuous periadnexal distribution.

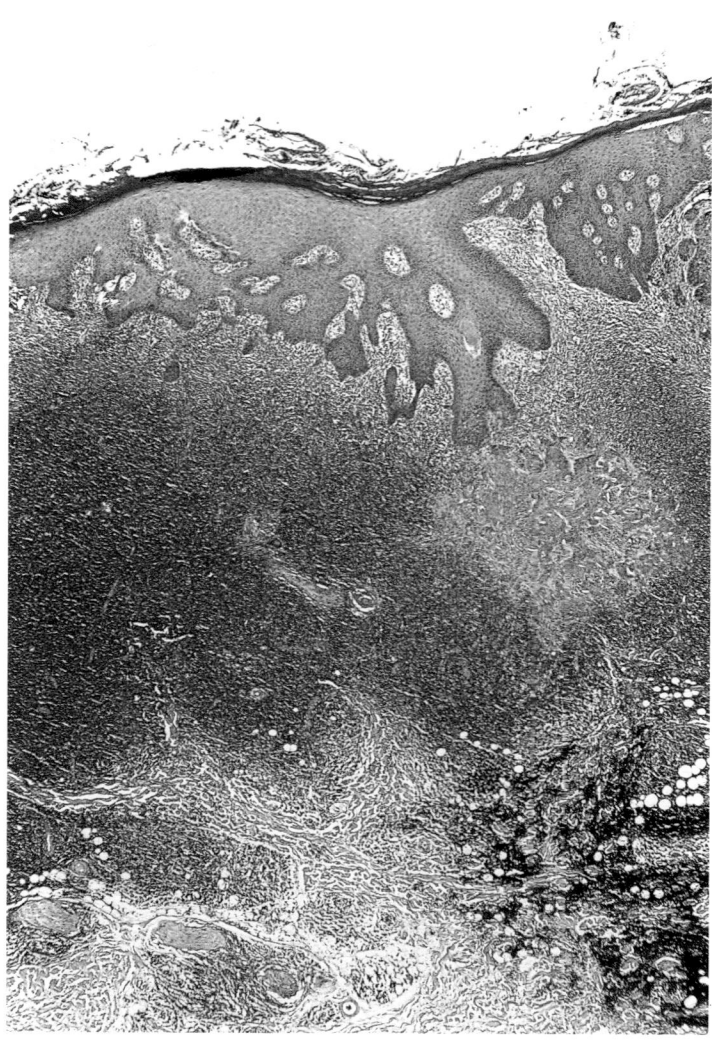

Fig. 41.20 **Basal cell carcinoma associated with an infiltrate of B-cell chronic lymphocytic leukemia.** (H & E)

CUTANEOUS INFILTRATES IN POST-TRANSPLANT LYMPHOPROLIFERATIVE DISORDERS (PT-LPDS)

There is a heterogeneous group of lymphoproliferative disorders, usually of B-cell origin, which occur in the setting of organ transplantation and immunosuppression, particularly with cyclosporin A and monoclonal antibody OKT3. This complication of transplantation varies in incidence from 1% in renal transplant recipients to 10% in heart and combined heart–lung transplant recipients.[696] Approximately 90% of PT-LPDs contain evidence of Epstein–Barr virus (EBV) infection.

Some lesions are hyperplasias that regress after immunosuppression is reduced or stopped. Others are composed of monoclonal B cells,[697] many of which exhibit clonal infection by a single form of EBV.[698]

There have been several classifications of PT-LPDs. The one discussed here is that of Knowles.[699]

Plasmacytic hyperplasia

Plasmacytic hyperplasia is found most commonly in children and young adults and develops shortly after organ transplantation. Most patients have regression of lesions after reduction of immunosuppressive therapy. In lymph nodes or other tissues, there is an infiltrate composed predominantly of small lymphocytes, plasmacytoid lymphocytes, plasma cells and scattered immunoblasts. There is a polyclonal population of cells: there may be a small clonal B-cell population. Many lesions have evidence of EBV infection which may be a polyclonal, oligoclonal or monoclonal infection. There are no structural alterations of oncogenes or tumor suppressor genes.[700]

Polymorphic lymphoproliferative disorder

All ages are affected but the median age is 43. Lymph nodes and extranodal sites are involved shortly after transplantation or after some years. The clinical course is variable and the response to immunotherapy reduction is unpredictable. Histological features vary from infiltrates consisting predominantly of lymphoid cells with plasmacytic differentiation and immunoblasts to atypical lymphoid infiltrates including pleomorphic immunoblasts, some resembling Reed–Sternberg cells. Necrosis and apoptosis are commonly found. Cells may express surface Ig and consistently exhibit clonal Ig heavy-chain and usually light-chain rearrangements. Cells are infected by a single form of EBV. There are no oncogene or tumor suppressor gene alterations.

Malignant lymphoma/multiple myeloma

The malignant lymphoma/multiple myeloma forms of PT-LPD are histologically identical to diffuse large B-cell lymphomas, multiple myeloma or rarely Burkitt's lymphoma. They occur in all ages but patients are generally older and present with disseminated disease. Clinical outcome is poor. Infiltrates involve lymph nodes and other organs including the allograft organ. Large cell lymphomas frequently exhibit immunoblastic or plasmacytoid features. Cells in myeloma are atypical plasma cells. Monoclonal surface or cytoplasmic Ig is expressed and there is clonal Ig heavy-chain and usually light-chain rearrangement. EBV infection by a single form of EBV is usual. There are structural alterations to oncogenes and tumor suppressor genes.

Skin manifestations of PT-LPDs are rare. There may be single or multiple nodules with cellular infiltrates involving dermis and subcutis. The cellular composition is determined by the form of PT-LPD. Loss of elastic tissue associated with elastoclasis by multinucleate giant cells has been observed in regressing lesions after therapy (personal observation).

Post-transplant primary cutaneous T-cell lymphomas have rarely been reported.[701]

CUTANEOUS LYMPHOMAS IN HIV/AIDS

Although mycosis fungoides is the most common primary cutaneous lymphoma in immunocompetent individuals, it is rare during HIV infection.[431] The immunophenotypes of reported cases are heterogeneous[702] and some reported cases may represent non-clonal MF-like CD8[+] cutaneous infiltrates which occur during HIV/AIDS. Granulomatous MF with spontaneous regression has been reported.[703]

The most common type of primary cutaneous lymphomas in the setting of HIV/AIDS are large cell lymphomas, either of T or B phenotype. Large T-cell lymphomas have pleomorphic or anaplastic morphology and are CD30[+].[431,704,705] They may be EMA[+] and EBV[+] (but are usually ALK[−]).[431]

Large B-cell lymphomas have immunoblastic or centroblastic morphology. Some are CD30[+] and EBV[+].

In most cases death is due to the underlying immunodeficiency rather than to spread of cutaneous lymphoma.

LYMPHOID HYPERPLASIA MIMICKING PRIMARY LYMPHOMA

This category includes a variety of benign lymphoid proliferations which simulate cutaneous lymphoma clinically but particularly histopathologically. The term 'pseudolymphoma' has been used for some of these conditions but is best avoided since it suggests a diagnostic category and several conditions included under this umbrella do not pose difficulties in their distinction from lymphoma. Lymphomatoid papulosis, regarded in the past as a pseudomalignancy, is now regarded as a cutaneous lymphoma (see above).[3,706]

Traditionally, this group of conditions has been divided into B-cell and T-cell types based on the pattern of cellular infiltrate. The histological pattern may take the form of a superficial band-like infiltrate in the upper dermis (the so-called 'T-cell pattern'), or a nodular or diffuse infiltrate throughout the dermis (the so-called 'B-cell pattern'). This is an artificial distinction since T-cell 'pseudolymphomas' may have a nodular pattern of dermal infiltration. In cutaneous lymphoid hyperplasia of the B-cell pattern, T cells are in fact more common than B cells.[64]

LYMPHOID HYPERPLASIA SIMULATING B-CELL LYMPHOMA

A plethora of terms have been used for this form of lymphoid hyperplasia: B-cell pseudolymphoma, B-cell cutaneous lymphoid hyperplasia, lymphadenosis benigna cutis, lymphocytoma cutis, cutaneous lymphoplasia.[707,708] These lesions usually present as asymptomatic red-brown or violaceous papules or nodules varying in diameter from 3 mm to 5 cm or more.[709] They may be solitary, grouped or numerous and widespread.[706]

The most common sites of involvement include the face (cheeks, nose and ear lobe), chest and upper extremities.[512] A xanthelasma-like presentation has been reported.[710] Females are affected more often than males. Lesions may resolve spontaneously after months to many years, but there is a tendency for some to recur.[706,709,711] None of the clinical features allow reliable distinction from cutaneous lymphoma.

In most cases, the cause is unknown. Various stimuli are reported to induce this form of lymphoid hyperplasia, including tick and other arthropod bites and stings,[712] *Hirudo medicinalis* (leeches),[713] gold earrings and gold injections,[714] cobalt,[715] tattoos (particularly the red areas),[716–718] a chronic draining sinus,[719] and ingestion of drugs such as phenytoin sodium.[720] Multiple cutaneous lesions have developed following allergen injections given for hyposensitization.[721,722]

In Europe, cutaneous lymphoid hyperplasia has been associated with *Borrelia* infection.[723,724] This is a rare event in North American Lyme disease.[725] In this setting lesions occur particularly on the ears, areolae of the nipples, axillary folds or scrotum. It has been described in association with acrodermatitis chronica atrophicans. The prevalence of borrelial cutaneous lymphoid hyperplasia has been reported to be from 0.6% to 1.3% of cases where there has been a clinical and/or serological diagnosis.[726] It is more common in children than adults.[725]

The use of modern immunohistochemical and molecular techniques and a better understanding of the histopathological subtypes of cutaneous lymphoma has made distinction of cutaneous hyperplasia from low-grade B-cell lymphoma more reproducible. The significance of a clonal proliferation of B cells in a histologically equivocal lesion remains controversial. A monoclonal population of B cells was identified in 14% of cases diagnosed as pseudolymphoma on histological and clinical grounds in one study.[39] It is still not clear in what proportion of cases transformation to cutaneous lymphoma occurs and if 'transformation' may in fact represent undiagnosed early cutaneous lymphoma. Transformation to a malignant lymphoma has been reported to occur in 25% of presumed benign lymphoid hyperplasia where a clonal B-cell population has been identified, compared with 5% of cases without demonstrable clonality.[39]

Histopathology

The histological appearances are varied and there is considerable overlap with cutaneous follicle center lymphoma and extranodal marginal zone B-cell lymphoma of MALT type. There is a variably dense infiltrate which may have a perivascular and periappendageal distribution or be more diffuse. The epidermis is spared. A 'top heavy' infiltrate is more common than a 'bottom heavy' one but is not specific (Fig. 41.21). The infiltrate may extend into the subcutis. Lymphoid follicles with well-developed mantles are seen in a minority of cases (10%),[615] although stains for follicular dendritic cells may demonstrate follicular aggregates without germinal centers. Between these structures, there is an infiltrate rich in small T lymphocytes with admixed scattered T and B immunoblasts. Eosinophils, histiocytes and plasma cells may also be present. In one comparative study of cutaneous lymphoid hyperplasia and cutaneous MALT-type lymphoma, reactive follicles were seen more often in the latter than the former.[64] Although it has been stated that there is B-cell predominance with a variable number of T cells ranging from 5% to 20%,[512] in the same study T cells usually outnumbered B cells. Small blood vessel proliferation may be evident. Features differentiating between hyperplasia and low-grade primary cutaneous lymphomas are discussed elsewhere (see p. 1100).

In a recent study, polyclonality of B cells was demonstrated in all but one of 24 cases of hyperplasia. There was no histological difference between these cases and the one case showing clonality. At the same time, 66% of a group of B-cell lymphomas exhibited clonality of B cells.[727]

LYMPHOMATOID DRUG REACTIONS

The atypical lymphoid infiltrates in some cutaneous drug reactions can resemble mycosis fungoides (the so-called 'T-cell pattern' of pseudo-lymphoma). The lesions associated with ingestion of drugs may present as solitary plaques, nodules or as multiple lesions with a widespread distribution. In addition, erythroderma simulating Sézary syndrome has been reported.[728] Numerous drugs have been implicated including phenytoin sodium (hydantoin), carbamazepine, griseofulvin, atenolol, cyclosporine, allopurinol, ACE inhibitors, antihistamines and mexiletine.[512,729–735]

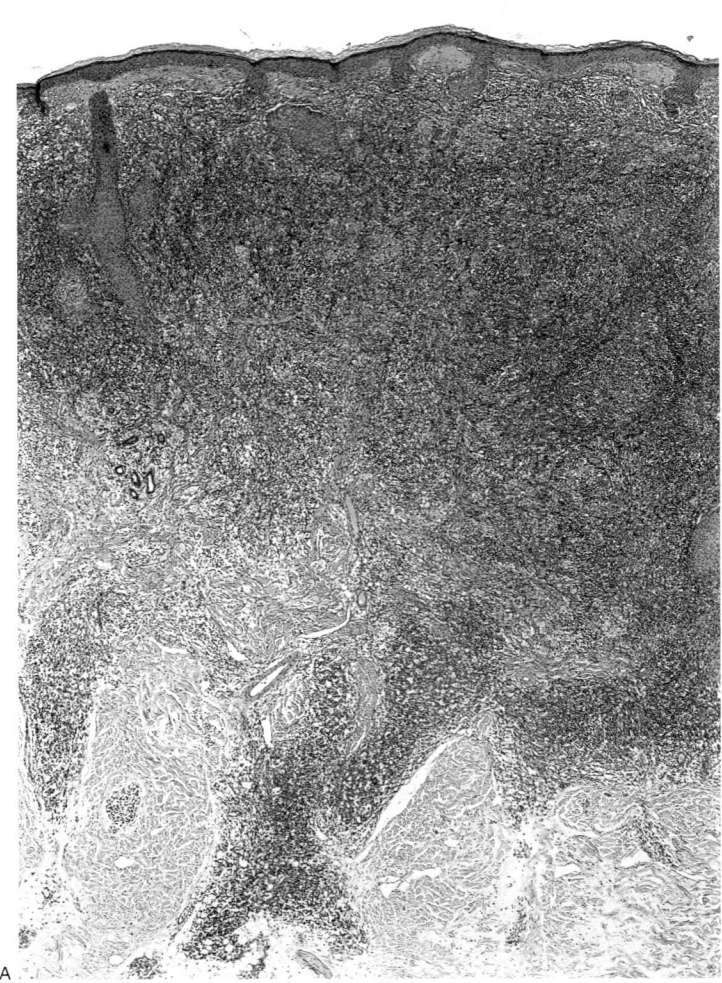

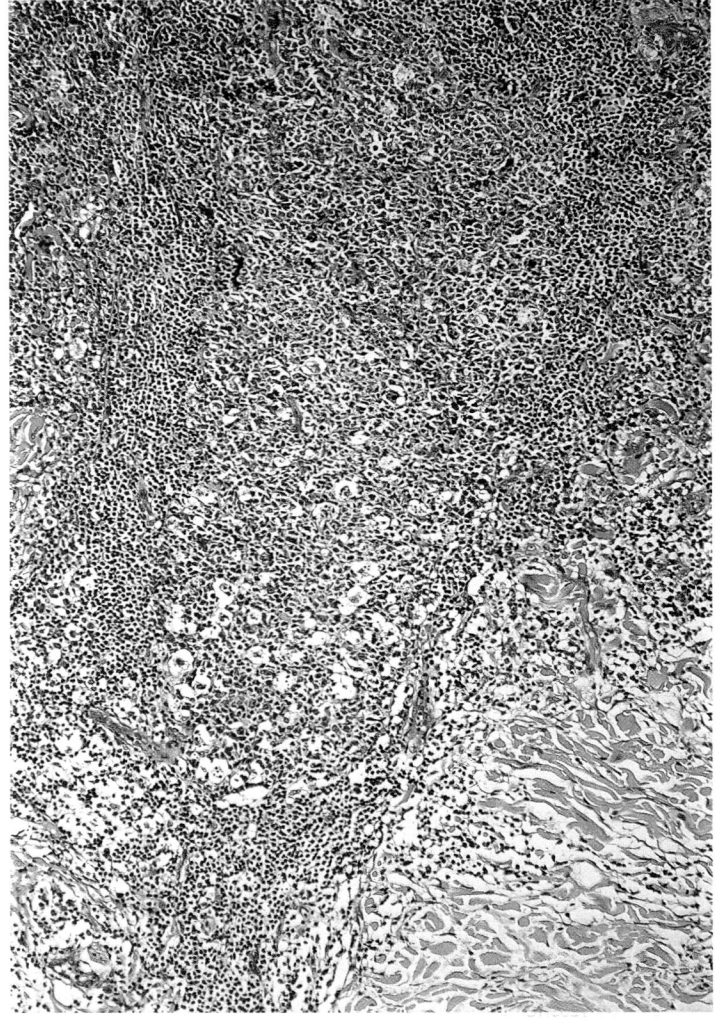

Fig. 41.21 **Cutaneous lymphoid hyperplasia. (A)** The infiltrate is 'top heavy' and contains reactive follicles. **(B)** The germinal centers of reactive follicles contain tingible-body macrophages. (H & E)

The lesions usually regress after withdrawal of the drug, but in the case of the anticonvulsants the lesions may persist for 12 months or more.[736,737]

Histopathology

There is an infiltrate of lymphocytes in the dermis which may be band-like, resembling mycosis fungoides, or nodular.[729]

The infiltrate often contains atypical nuclei which have a cerebriform outline. There is usually a substantial histiocytic component, particularly in the nodular lesions. Eosinophils and plasma cells are usually sparse or absent, although they may be more obvious in the nodular infiltrates.[735]

Epidermotropism may be observed.[738] Large CD30⁺ T cells, together with Pautrier microabscess-like collections, have been reported in a reaction to carbamazepine.[463]

Immunohistochemistry and cytogenetics

Infiltrates usually consist predominantly of T cells, but rarely B cells predominate. This occurs with some antihistamines[735] and thioridazine.[739]

Most T cells are CD4⁺ and there is usually no shedding of pan-T cell markers (CD2, CD3, CD5).[740]

PCR analysis of TCR and immunoglobulin heavy-chain (IgH) genes shows polyclonal infiltrates in most cases.[738,741]

REACTIONS RESEMBLING CD30⁺ LYMPHOPROLIFERATIVE DISORDERS

Atypical histological infiltrates with large CD30⁺ cells can occur in a variety of situations,[464] including carbamazepine-induced drug eruptions,[463] granulocytic sarcoma,[633] atypical eruption of lymphocyte recovery[742] and viral infections including molluscum contagiosum (Fig. 41.22), herpes simplex[593] and lymphoproliferative lesions associated with EBV,[743] and arthropod bites (scabies).[465]

PSEUDOLYMPHOMATOUS FOLLICULITIS

Pseudolymphomatous folliculitis is a recently described condition which may mimic a cutaneous lymphoma clinically and folliculotropic mycosis fungoides histologically. Solitary, flat or dome-shaped lesions up to 1.5 cm in diameter are situated on the face. Regression occurs in some cases after biopsy.

Histopathology

There is a diffuse, predominantly perifollicular infiltrate of lymphocytes with infiltration of follicular structures together with enlargement and distortion of these structures. Aggregates of histiocytes, or granulomas related to disrupted follicles, may be seen. Lymphoid follicles are rarely seen. The epidermis is not involved. Occasional large atypical cells may be identified (see p. 466).

Immunohistochemistry and cytogenetics

There is a mixture of B and T cells identifiable by conventional markers (CD20, CD79a, CD3, CD45RO). Either B or T cells may predominate. Aggregates of perifollicular dendritic cells which are CD1a⁺ and S100⁺ are seen. Cells are negative for EBER-1, and neither B- nor T-cell clonality has been identified by PCR.

JESSNER'S LYMPHOCYTIC INFILTRATE

Jessner's lymphocytic infiltrate is a relatively uncommon condition that was first delineated by Jessner and Kanof in 1953.[744] In this condition there are asymptomatic, erythematous plaques, usually on the face or neck.[745] The

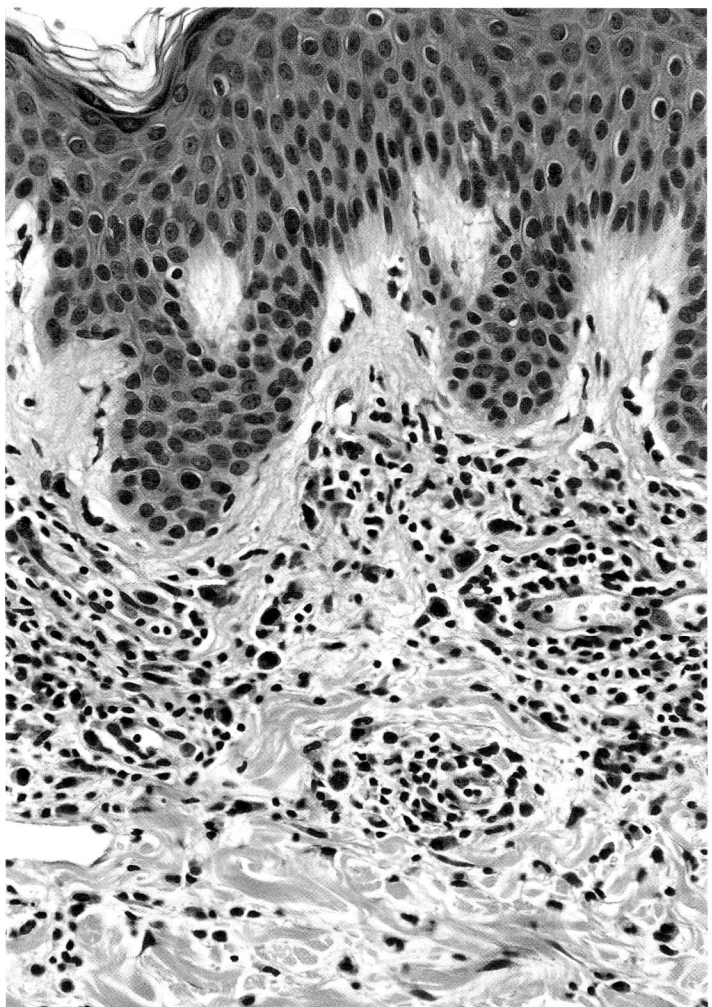

Fig. 41.22 Atypical inflammatory cell infiltrate adjacent to molluscum contagiosum. The large cells are CD30-positive T cells. (H & E)

upper part of the trunk and other sites are occasionally involved.[709] It occurs predominantly in men, but has been reported in children,[746,747] and also in a familial setting.[748]

This condition is not regarded by all as a distinct entity.[749] Others believe that it is part of the spectrum of lupus erythematosus or polymorphous light eruption.[750,751] It is classified by some as a pseudolymphoma[729] although the histology is often not atypical and does not suggest a malignant process.

Jessner's lymphocytic infiltrate has a benign, but somewhat unpredictable course. Individual lesions may show central clearing and even regression, but there may be recurrences in the same or other areas. The average duration of the disease is 5 years. Its etiology is unknown. Only time will tell if it will continue to be recognized as an authentic disease (see p. 48).

Histopathology

There is usually a moderately dense, perivascular infiltrate of small lymphocytes (predominantly T lymphocytes),[752–754] involving the superficial and deep vascular plexuses of the dermis.[755] The infiltrate may extend around the pilosebaceous follicles and occasionally even into the subcutis.[754–756] Occasional larger lymphocytes, plasma cells and plasmacytoid monocytes may be present.[757,758]

A small amount of mucin may be seen between the collagen bundles.

The epidermis is usually normal, with no evidence of atrophy, basal vacuolar change or follicular plugging. These features, together with negative immunofluorescence, are said to distinguish this condition from lupus erythematosus. In 10–20% of cases of lupus, however, immunofluorescence is negative.[750]

Immunohistochemistry

Investigations have shown a predominantly T-cell population admixed with some B cells. Clear distinction between cutaneous lupus and Jessner's lymphocytic infiltrate cannot be made based on the relative proportions of B and T cells in lesions.[759] Past studies have reported a higher number of Leu-8 positive lymphocytes in Jessner's lymphocytic infiltrate than in cutaneous lupus,[760,761] although this has been disputed.[762]

CUTANEOUS CD8+ T-CELL INFILTRATES IN HIV/AIDS

Cutaneous CD8+ T-cell infiltrates in HIV/AIDS present as plaques and nodules, primarily on the face and extremities, or with generalized erythroderma.[763,764]

Histopathology[763]

Histopathology in these cases has shown a papillary and mid-dermal infiltrate of small cerebriform lymphocytes or a mixed population of lymphocytes including larger cells. Eosinophils are common in the infiltrate. There is mild epidermotropism and occasionally Pautrier microabscesses. Epidermal alterations such as acanthosis and hyperkeratosis may also be present as well as a lichenoid reaction with vacuolar change and apoptotic bodies at the dermoepidermal junction. Papillary dermal fibrosis and granulomas are other changes.

Immunohistochemistry and cytogenetics

The cellular infiltrate consists predominantly of T cells which are CD2+, CD3+, CD5+ and CD8+. CD7 and CD4 are expressed by some cells. Clonal TCR gene rearrangements are not present.

PSEUDOLYMPHOMATOUS ANGIOKERATOMA

Pseudolymphomatous angiokeratoma (originally reported as 'acral pseudo-lymphomatous angiokeratoma of children' – APACHE) is a rare entity in which angiomatous papules develop on the extremities.[765] Rarely, a solitary lesion may be present.[765a]

Histopathology

There is a dense infiltrate of lymphocytes and some plasma cells in the upper dermis. Small vessels are sometimes prominent, leading to the initial suggestion that this entity was a vascular proliferation rather than a reactive lymphoid hyperplasia. The endothelial cells show hyperplasia. There are no vacuolated endothelial cells as seen in angioplasmocellular hyperplasia (see p. 1064).

The majority of the lymphocytes in this condition are of T-cell lineage.

MISCELLANEOUS

EXTRAMEDULLARY HEMATOPOIESIS

Hematopoiesis takes place in the skin in early embryonic life. This process has also been reported in neonates as a consequence of intrauterine viral infection (rubella, cytomegalovirus and coxsackievirus)[766] and of congenital hematological dyscrasias (hemolytic disease of the newborn and the 'twin transfusion' syndrome).[767,768] In adults it is an extremely rare complication of myelofibrosis, particularly following splenectomy.[769–773] It has also been reported in pilomatrixomas of the skin (see p. 870).

The clinical features of extramedullary hematopoiesis are quite variable and include solitary lesions, plaque-like lesions, leg ulcers,[774] and bullae and erythema in the margins of a surgical wound.[769] In neonates there are often multiple violaceous papulonodular lesions (the so-called 'blueberry muffin' eruption).[767,775,776]

Histopathology

Extramedullary hematopoiesis presents as a polymorphic dermal infiltrate consisting predominantly of myeloid and erythroid elements; sometimes megakaryocytes are a conspicuous component of the infiltrate.[772,775,777,778] Cells in all stages of maturation can usually be found. The infiltrate is present in the superficial and deep dermis, particularly in a perivascular position.[770]

The Leder stain can be used to confirm the presence of the myeloid elements in the infiltrate. They also stain with Mac387, whereas the megakaryocytes stain for factor XIIIa and factor VIII-related antigen.[773]

REFERENCES

Introduction

1 Harris NL, Jaffe ES, Stein H et al. A revised European-American Classification of Lymphoid Neoplasms: A proposal from the International Lymphoma Study Group. Blood 1994; 84: 1361–1392.

2 Harris NL, Jaffe ES, Diebold J et al. The World Health Organization classification of neoplastic diseases of the haematopoietic and lymphoid tissues: report of the Clinical Advisory Committee meeting, Airlie House, Virginia, November 1997. Histopathology 2000; 36: 69–87.

3 Willemze R, Kerl H, Sterry W et al. EORTC classification for primary cutaneous lymphomas: a proposal from the Cutaneous Lymphoma Study Group of the European Organization for Research and Treatment of Cancer. Blood 1997; 90: 354–371.

4 Lennert K, Feller AC. Histopathology of non-Hodgkin's lymphomas (based on the updated Kiel Classification). Berlin: Springer-Verlag, 1992.

5 Cerroni L. Primary cutaneous lymphomas? Am J Dermatopathol 1999; 21: 578–579.

6 Willemze R, Meijer CJLM. Classification of cutaneous lymphomas: crosstalk between pathologist and clinician. Curr Diagn Pathol 1998; 5: 23–33.

7 Sander CA, Kind P, Kaudewitz P et al. The Revised European-American Classification of Lymphoid Neoplasms (REAL): a new perspective for the classification of cutaneous lymphomas. J Cutan Pathol 1997; 24: 329–341.

8 Russell-Jones R. Primary cutaneous B-cell lymphoma: how useful is the new European Organization for Research and Treatment of Cancer (EORTC) classification? Br J Dermatol 1998; 139: 945–949.

9 Slater DN. Is the WHO classification suitable for skin lymphoma? Histopathology 2000; 37: 282–283.

10 Slater D. Classification of cutaneous lymphomas. Arch Dermatol 1996; 132: 972–973.

11 Willemze R, Meijer CJLM. Classification of primary cutaneous B-cell lymphomas: EORTC classification or REAL classification? Br J Dermatol 1999; 141: 350–352.

12 Slater DN. Primary cutaneous B-cell lymphoma: how useful is the new European Organisation for Research and Treatment of Cancer classification? Br J Dermatol 1999; 141: 352–353.

13 Jaffe ES, Sander CA, Flaig MJ. Cutaneous lymphomas: a proposal for a unified approach to classification using the R.E.A.L./WHO classification. Ann Oncol 2000; 11 (Suppl 1): S17–S21.

14 Norton AJ. Classification of cutaneous lymphoma. A critical appraisal of recent proposals. Am J Dermatopathol 1999; 21: 279–287.

15 Willemze R, Meijer CJLM. EORTC classification for primary cutaneous lymphomas: the best guide to good clinical management. Am J Dermatopathol 1999; 21: 265–273.

16 Novelli M, Savoia P, Cambieri I et al. Collagenase digestion and mechanical disaggregation as a method to extract and immunophenotype tumour lymphocytes in cutaneous T-cell lymphomas. Clin Exp Dermatol 2000; 25: 423–431.

17 Slater D. Clonal dermatoses: a conceptual and diagnostic dilemma. J Pathol 1990; 162: 1–3.

18 Bachelez H. The clinical use of molecular analysis of clonality in cutaneous lymphocytic infiltrates. Arch Dermatol 1999; 135: 200–202.

19 Collins RD. Is clonality equivalent to malignancy: specifically, is immunoglobulin gene rearrangement diagnostic of malignant lymphoma? Hum Pathol 1997; 28: 757–759.

20 Ashton-Key M, Diss TC, Du MQ et al. The value of the polymerase chain reaction in the diagnosis of cutaneous T-cell infiltrates. Am J Surg Pathol 1997; 21: 743–747.

21 Wood GS, Ngan B-Y, Tung R et al. Clonal rearrangements of immunoglobulin genes and progression to B cell lymphoma in cutaneous lymphoid hyperplasia. Am J Pathol 1989; 135: 13–19.

22 Chu PG, Chang KL, Arber DA, Weiss LM. Immunophenotyping of hematopoietic neoplasms. Semin Diagn Pathol 2000; 17: 236–256.

23 Cerroni L, Arzberger E, Pütz B et al. Primary cutaneous follicle center lymphoma with follicular growth pattern. Blood 2000; 95: 3922–3928.

24 Cerroni L, Arzberger E, Ardigò M et al. Monoclonality of intraepidermal T lymphocytes in early mycosis fungoides detected by molecular analysis after laser-beam-based microdissection. J Invest Dermatol 2000; 114: 1154–1157.

B-cell lymphomas with frequent or constant cutaneous involvement

25 Lin P, Jones D, Dorfman DM, Medeiros LJ. Precursor B-cell lymphoblastic lymphoma. A predominantly extranodal tumor with low propensity for leukemic involvement. Am J Surg Pathol 2000; 24: 1480–1490.

26 Chimenti S, Fink-Puches R, Peris K et al. Cutaneous involvement in lymphoblastic lymphoma. J Cutan Pathol 1999; 26: 379–385.

27 Santucci M, Pimpinelli N, Arganini L. Primary cutaneous B-cell lymphoma: a unique type of low-grade lymphoma. Clinicopathologic and immunologic study of 83 cases. Cancer 1991; 67: 2311–2326.

28 Isaacson PG. Malignant lymphomas with a follicular growth pattern. Histopathology 1996; 28: 487–495.

29 Goodlad JR, Hollowood K. Primary cutaneous B-cell lymphoma. Curr Diagn Pathol 2001; 7: 33–44.

30 Isaacson PG, Norton AJ. Cutaneous lymphoma. In: Extranodal lymphomas. Edinburgh: Churchill Livingstone, 1994; 131–191.

31 Bergman R, Kurtin PJ, Gibson LE et al. Clinicopathologic, immunophenotypic, and molecular characterization of primary cutaneous follicular B-cell lymphoma. Arch Dermatol 2001; 137: 432–439.

32 Yang B, Tubbs RR, Finn W et al. Clinicopathologic reassessment of primary cutaneous B-cell lymphomas with immunophenotypic and molecular genetic characterization. Am J Surg Pathol 2000; 24: 694–702.

33 Weiss LM, Warnke RA, Sklar J, Cleary ML. Molecular analysis of the t(14;18) chromosomal translocation in malignant lymphomas. N Engl J Med 1987; 317: 1185–1189.

34 Cerroni L, Volkenandt M, Rieger E et al. bcl-2 protein expression and correlation with the interchromosomal 14;18 translocation in cutaneous lymphomas and pseudolymphomas. J Invest Dermatol 1994; 102: 231–235.

35 Child FJ, Russell-Jones R, Woolford AJ et al. Absence of the t(14;18) chromosomal translocation in primary cutaneous B-cell lymphoma. Br J Dermatol 2001; 144: 735–744.

36 Isaacson P, Wright DH. Malignant lymphoma of mucosa-associated lymphoid tissue: a distinctive type of B-cell lymphoma. Cancer 1983; 52: 1410–1416.

37 Nihal M, Mikkola D, Wood GS. Detection of clonally restricted immunoglobulin heavy chain gene rearrangements in normal and lesional skin. J Mol Diagn 2000; 2: 5–10.

38 Slater DN. MALT and SALT: the clue to cutaneous B-cell lymphoproliferative disease. Br J Dermatol 1994; 131: 557–561.

39 Slater D. Cutaneous B-cell lymphoproliferative diseases: a centenary celebration classification. J Pathol 1994; 172: 301–305.

40 Willemze R, Rijlaarsdam JU, Meijer CJLM. Are most primary cutaneous B-cell lymphomas 'marginal cell lymphomas'? Br J Dermatol 1995; 133: 950–954.

41 Giannotti B, Santucci M. Skin-associated lymphoid tissue (SALT)-related B-cell lymphoma (primary cutaneous B-cell lymphoma). Arch Dermatol 1993; 129: 353–355.

42 Goodlad JR, Davidson MM, Hollowood K et al. Borrelia burgdorferi-associated cutaneous marginal zone lymphoma: a clinicopathological study of two cases illustrating the temporal progression of B. burgdorferi-associated B-cell proliferation in the skin. Histopathology 2000; 37: 501–508.

43 Slater DN. Borrelia burgdorferi-associated primary cutaneous B-cell lymphoma. Histopathology 2001; 38: 73–77.

44 Kütting B, Bonsmann G, Metze D et al. Borrelia burgdorferi-associated primary cutaneous B cell lymphoma: complete clearing of skin lesions after antibiotic pulse therapy or intralesional injection of interferon alfa-2a. J Am Acad Dermatol 1997; 36: 311–314.

45 Cerroni L, Zöchling N, Pütz B, Kerl H. Infection by Borrelia burgdorferi and cutaneous B-cell lymphoma. J Cutan Pathol 1997; 24: 457–461.

46 Goodlad JR, Davidson MM, Hollowood K et al. Primary cutaneous B-cell lymphoma and Borrelia burgdorferi infection in patients from the highlands of Scotland. Am J Surg Pathol 2000; 24: 1279–1285.

47 Roggero E, Zucca E, Mainetti C et al. Eradication of Borrelia burgdorferi infection in primary marginal zone B-cell lymphoma of the skin. Hum Pathol 2000; 31: 263–268.

47a. Wood GS, Kamath NV, Guitart J et al. Absence of Borrelia burgdorferi DNA in cutaneous B-cell lymphomas from the United States. J Cutan Pathol 2001; 28: 502–507.

48 ce Leval L, Harris NL, Longtine J et al. Cutaneous B-cell lymphomas of follicular and marginal zone types. Use of Bcl-6, CD10, Bcl-2 and CD21 in differential diagnosis and classification. Am J Surg Pathol 2001; 25: 732–741.

49 Franco R, Fernandez-Vazquez A, Rodriguez-Peralco JL et al. Cutaneous follicular B-cell lymphoma. Description of a series of 18 cases. Am J Surg Pathol 2001; 25: 875–883.

50 Mann R, Berard C. Criteria for the cytologic subclassification of follicular lymphomas: a proposed alternative method. Hematol Oncol 1982; 1: 187–192.

51 Pimpinelli N, Santucci M, Mori M et al. Primary cutaneous B-cell lymphoma: A clinically homogeneous entity? J Am Acad Dermatol 1997; 37: 1012–1016.

52 Rijlaarsdam JU, van der Putte SCJ, Berti E et al. Cutaneous immunocytomas: a clinicopathologic study of 26 cases. Histopathology 1993; 23: 117–125.

53 LeBoit PE, McNutt NS, Reed JA et al. Primary cutaneous immunocytoma. A B-cell lymphoma that can easily be mistaken for cutaneous lymphoid hyperplasia. Am J Surg Pathol 1994; 18: 969–978.

54 Andriko J-AW, Swerdlow SH, Aguilera NI, Abbondanzo SL. Is lymphoplasmacytic lymphoma/immunocytoma a distinct entity? A clinicopathologic study of 20 cases. Am J Surg Pathol 2001; 25: 742–751.

55 Schmid U, Eckert F, Griesser H et al. Cutaneous follicular lymphoid hyperplasia with monotypic plasma cells. A clinicopathologic study of 18 patients. Am J Surg Pathol 1995; 19: 12–20.

56 Cerroni L, Signoretti S, Höfler G et al. Primary cutaneous marginal zone B-cell lymphoma: a recently described entity of low-grade malignant cutaneous B-cell lymphoma. Am J Surg Pathol 1997; 21: 1307–1315.

57 de la Fouchardière A, Balme B, Chouvet B et al. Primary cutaneous marginal zone B-cell lymphoma: A report of 9 cases. J Am Acad Dermatol 1999; 41: 181–188.

58 Tomaszewski M-M, Abbondanzo SL, Lupton GP. Extranodal marginal zone B-cell lymphoma of the skin: a morphologic and immunophenotypic study of 11 cases. Am J Dermatopathol 2000; 22: 205–211.

59 Marzano AV, Berti E, Alessi E. Primary cutaneous B-cell lymphoma with a dermatomal distribution. J Am Acad Dermatol 1999; 41: 884–886.

60 Child FJ, Woollons A, Price ML et al. Multiple cutaneous immunocytoma with secondary anetoderma: a report of two cases. Br J Dermatol 2000; 143: 165–170.

61 Grønbæk K, Møller PH, Nedergaard T et al. Primary cutaneous B-cell lymphoma: a clinical, histological, phenotypic and genotypic study of 21 cases. Br J Dermatol 2000; 142: 913–923.

62 Goodlad JR, Dunn-Walters D, Davidson MM et al. Primary cutaneous marginal zone lymphoma of the skin and its relationship to Borrelia burgdorferi infection. J Pathol 1999; 189 (Suppl): 20A.

63 Pelstring RJ, Essell JH, Kurtin PJ et al. Diversity of organ site involvement among malignant lymphomas of mucosa-associated tissues. Am J Clin Pathol 1991; 96: 738–745.

64 Baldassano MF, Bailey EM, Ferry JA et al. Cutaneous lymphoid hyperplasia and cutaneous marginal zone lymphoma. Comparison of morphologic and immunophenotypic features. Am J Surg Pathol 1999; 23: 88–96.

65 Baldassano MF, Harris NL, Duncan LM. Trisomy 3 in cutaneous marginal zone B-cell lymphoma. J Cutan Pathol 1999; 26: 459 (abstract).

66 Vermeer MH, Geelen FAMJ, van Haselen CW et al. Primary cutaneous large B-cell lymphomas of the legs. A distinct type of cutaneous B-cell lymphoma with an intermediate prognosis. Arch Dermatol 1996; 132: 1304–1308.

67 Grange F, Bekkenk MW, Wechsler J et al. Prognostic factors in primary cutaneous large B-cell lymphomas: a European multicenter study. J Clin Oncol 2001; 19: 3602–3610.

68 Russell-Jones R. Primary cutaneous B-cell lymphoma: how useful is the new European Organization for Research and Treatment of Cancer (EORTC) classification? Br J Dermatol 1998; 139: 945–949.

69 Fernández-Vázquez A, Rodriguez-Peralto JL, Martínez MA et al. Primary cutaneous large B-cell lymphoma. The relation between morphology, clinical presentation, immunohistochemical markers, and survival. Am J Surg Pathol 2001; 25: 307–315.

70 Torres-Paoli D, Sánchez JL. Primary cutaneous B-cell lymphoma of the leg in a chronic lymphedematous extremity. Am J Dermatopathol 2000; 22: 257–260.

71 Kurtin PJ, DiCaudo DJ, Habermann TM et al. Primary cutaneous large-cell lymphomas. Morphologic, immunophenotypic, and clinical features of 20 cases. Am J Surg Pathol 1994; 18: 1183–1191.

72 Starz H, Balda B-R, Bachter D et al. Secondary lymph node involvement from primary cutaneous large B-cell lymphoma of the leg. Cancer 1999; 85: 199–207.

73 Berti E, Alessi E, Caputo R et al. Reticulohistiocytoma of the dorsum. J Am Acad Dermatol 1988; 19: 259–272.

74 Berti E, Alessi E, Caputo R. Reticulohistiocytoma of the dorsum (Crosti's disease) and other B-cell lymphomas. Semin Diagn Pathol 1991; 8: 82–90.

75 Duncan SC, Evans HL, Winkelmann RK. Large cell lymphocytoma. Arch Dermatol 1980; 116: 1142–1146.

76 Winkelmann RK, Dabski K. Large cell lymphocytoma: follow up, immunopathology studies, and comparison to cutaneous follicular and Crosti lymphoma. Arch Dermatol Res 1987; 279: s81–s87.

77 Chui CT, Hoppe RT, Kohler S, Kim YH. Epidermotropic cutaneous B-cell lymphoma mimicking mycosis fungoides. J Am Acad Dermatol 1999; 41: 271–274.

78 Landa NG, Zelickson BD, Kurtin PJ, Winkelmann RK. Primary B-cell lymphoma with histologic features of a T-cell neoplasm. J Am Acad Dermatol 1992; 26: 288–291.

79 Cerroni L, El-Shabrawi-Caelen L, Fink-Puches R et al. Cutaneous spindle-cell B-cell lymphoma. A morphologic variant of cutaneous large B-cell lymphoma Am J Dermatopathol 2000; 22: 299–304.

80 Geelen FAMJ, Vermeer MH, Meijer CJLM et al. bcl-2 protein expression in primary cutaneous large B-cell lymphoma is site-related. J Clin Oncol 1998; 16: 2080–2085.

81 Liebow AA, Carrington CRB, Friedman PJ. Lymphomatoid granulomatosis. Hum Pathol 1972; 3: 457–533.

82 McNiff JM, Cooper D, Howe G et al. Lymphomatoid granulomatosis of the skin and lung. An angiocentric T-cell-rich B-cell lymphoproliferative disorder. Arch Dermatol 1996; 132: 1464–1470.

83 Katzenstein AL, Peiper SC. Detection of Epstein–Barr virus genomes in lymphomatoid granulomatosis: analysis of 29 cases by the polymerase chain reaction technique. Mod Pathol 1990; 3: 435–441.

84 Angel CA, Slater DN, Royds JA et al. Epstein–Barr virus in cutaneous lymphomatoid granulomatosis. Histopathology 1994; 25: 545–548.

85 Myers JL, Kurtin PJ, Katzenstein A-LA et al. Lymphomatoid granulomatosis. Evidence of immunophenotypic diversity and relationship to Epstein–Barr virus infection. Am J Surg Pathol 1995; 19: 1300–1312.

86 Guinee D Jr, Jaffe E, Kingma D et al. Pulmonary lymphomatoid granulomatosis. Evidence for a proliferation of Epstein–Barr virus infected B-lymphocytes with a prominent T-cell component and vasculitis. Am J Surg Pathol 1994; 18: 753–764.

87 Guinee DG, Perkins SL, Travis WD et al. Proliferation and cellular phenotype in lymphomatoid granulomatosis. Implications of a higher proliferation index in B cells. Am J Surg Pathol 1998; 22: 1093–1100.

88 Jaffe ES, Wilson WH. Lymphomatoid granulomatosis: pathogenesis, pathology and clinical implications. Cancer Surv 1997; 30: 233–248.

89 Jambrosic J, From L, Assaad DA et al. Lymphomatoid granulomatosis. J Am Acad Dermatol 1987; 17: 621–631.

90 James WD, Odom RB, Katzenstein A-LA. Cutaneous manifestations of lymphomatoid granulomatosis. Report of 44 cases and a review of the literature. Arch Dermatol 1981; 117: 196–202.

91 Camisa C. Lymphomatoid granulomatosis: Two cases with skin involvement. J Am Acad Dermatol 1989; 20: 571–578.

92 Wood ML, Harrington CI, Slater DN et al. Cutaneous lymphomatoic granulomatosis: a rare cause of recurrent skin ulceration. Br J Dermatol 1984; 110: 619–625.

93 Tawfik NH, Magro CMJ, Crowson AN, Maxwell I. Lymphomatoid granulomatosis presenting as a solitary cutaneous lesion. Int J Dermatol 1994; 33: 188–189.

94 Tong MM, Cooke B, Barnetson RStC. Lymphomatoid granulomatosis. J Am Acad Dermatol 1992; 27: 872–876.

95 Wood ML, Harrington CI, Slater DN et al. Cutaneous lymphomatoid granulomatosis: a rare cause of recurrent skin ulceration. Br J Dermatol 1984; 110: 619–625.

96 Katzenstein A-LA, Carrington CB, Liebow AA. Lymphomatoid granulomatosis. A clinicopathologic study of 152 cases. Cancer 1979; 43: 360–373.

97 Beaty MW, Toro J, Sorbara L et al. Cutaneous lymphomatoid granulomatosis. Correlation of clinical and biologic features. Am J Surg Pathol 2001; 25: 1111–1120.

98 LeSueur BW, Ellsworth L, Bangert JL, Hansen RC. Lymphomatoid granulomatosis in a 4-year-old boy. Pediatr Dermatol 2000; 17: 369–372.

99 Arai E, Sakurai M, Nakayama H et al. Primary cutaneous T-cell-rich B-cell lymphoma. Br J Dermatol 1993; 129: 196–200.

100 Dommann SNW, Dommann-Scherrer CC, Zimmerman D et al. Primary cutaneous T-cell-rich B-cell lymphoma. A case report with a 13-year follow-up. Am J Dermatopathol 1995; 17: 618–624.

101 Sander CA, Kaudewitz P, Kutzner H et al. T-cell-rich B-cell lymphoma presenting in skin. J Cutan Pathol 1996; 23: 101–108.

102 Krishnan J, Wallberg K, Frizzera G. T-cell-rich large B-cell lymphoma. A study of 30 cases, supporting its histologic heterogeneity and lack of clinical distinctiveness. Am J Surg Pathol 1994; 18: 455–465.

103 Ramsay AD, Smith WJ, Isaacson PG. T-cell rich B-cell lymphoma. Am J Surg Pathol 1988; 12: 433–443.

104 Macon WR, Williams ME, Greer JP et al. T-cell-rich B-cell lymphomas. A clinicopathologic study of 19 cases. Am J Surg Pathol 1992; 16: 351–363.

105 Gogstetter D, Brown M, Seab J, Scott G. Angiocentric primary cutaneous T-cell-rich B-cell lymphoma: a case report and review of the literature. J Cutan Pathol 2000; 27: 516–525.

106 Wick MR, Mills SE. Intravascular lymphomatosis: clinicopathologic features and differential diagnosis. Semin Diagn Pathol 1991; 8: 91–101.

107 Willemze R, Kruyswijk MRJ, de Bruin CD et al. Angiotropic (intravascular) large-cell lymphoma of the skin previously classified as malignant angioendotheliomatosis. Br J Dermatol 1987; 116: 393–399.

108 Petroff N, Koger O'NW, Fleming MG et al. Malignant angioendotheliomatosis: an angiotropic lymphoma. J Am Acad Dermatol 1989; 21: 727–733.

109 Wick MR, Mills SE, Scheithauer BW et al. Reassessment of malignant "angioendotheliomatosis". Evidence in favor of its reclassification as "intravascular lymphomatosis". Am J Surg Pathol 1986; 10: 112–123.

110 Sepp N, Schuler G, Romani N et al. "Intravascular lymphomatosis" (angioendotheliomatosis): evidence for a T-cell origin in two cases. Hum Pathol 1990; 21: 1051–1058.

111 Sangueza O, Hyder DM, Sangueza P. Intravascular lymphomatosis: report of an unusual case with T cell phenotype occurring in an adolescent male. J Cutan Pathol 1992; 19: 226–231.

112 Lakhani SR, Hulman G, Hall JM et al. Intravascular malignant lymphomatosis (angiotropic large-cell lymphoma). A case report with evidence of T-cell lineage with polymerase chain reaction analysis. Histopathology 1994; 25: 283–286.

113 Au WY, Shek WH, Nicholls J et al. T-cell intravascular lymphomatosis (angiotropic large cell lymphoma): association with Epstein–Barr viral infection. Histopathology 1997; 31: 563–567.

114 Ponzoni M, Arrigoni G, Gould VE et al. Lack of CD29 (β1 integrin) and CD54 (ICAM-1) adhesion molecules in intravascular lymphomatosis. Hum Pathol 2000; 31: 220–226.

115 Stahl RL, Chan W, Duncan A, Corley CC Jr. Malignant angioendotheliomatosis presenting as disseminated intravascular coagulopathy. Cancer 1991; 68: 2319–2323.

116 Berger TG, Dawson N A. Angioendotheliomatosis. J Am Acad Dermatol 1988; 18: 407–412.

117 Kiyohara T, Kumakiri M, Kobayashi H et al. A case of intravascular large B-cell lymphoma mimicking erythema nodosum: the importance of multiple skin biopsies. J Cutan Pathol 2000; 27: 413–418.

118 Özgüroğlu E, Büyülbabani N, Özgüroğlu M, Baykal C. Generalized telangiectasia as the major manifestation of angiotropic (intravascular) lymphoma. Br J Dermatol 1997; 137: 422–425.

119 Rubin MA, Cossman J, Freter CE, Azumi N. Intravascular large cell lymphoma coexisting with hemangiomas of the skin. Am J Surg Pathol 1997; 21: 860–864.

120 Smith ME, Stamatakos MD, Neuhauser TS. Intravascular lymphomatosis presenting within angiolipomas. Ann Diagn Pathol 2001; 5: 103–106.

121 Au WY, Shek TW, Kwong YL. Epstein–Barr virus-related intravascular lymphomatosis. Am J Surg Pathol 2000; 24: 309–310.

122 Murase T, Nakamura S, Kawauchi K et al. An Asian variant of intravascular large B-cell lymphoma: clinical, pathological and cytogenetic approaches to diffuse large B-cell lymphoma associated with haemophagocytic syndrome. Br J Haematol 2000; 111: 826–834.

123 López-Gil F, Roura M, Umbert I, Umbert P. Malignant proliferative angioendotheliomatosis or angiotropic lymphoma associated with a soft-tissue lymphoma. J Am Acad Dermatol 1992; 26: 101–104.

124 Carter DK, Batts KP, de Groen PC, Kurtin PJ. Angiotropic large cell lymphoma (intravascular lymphomatosis) occurring after follicular small cleaved cell lymphoma. Mayo Clin Proc 1996; 71: 869–873.

125 Khalidi HS, Brynes RK, Browne P et al. Intravascular large B-cell lymphoma: the CD5 antigen is expressed by a subset of cases. Mod Pathol 1998; 11: 983–988.

126 Chang A, Zic JA, Boyd AS. Intravascular large cell lymphoma: A patient with asymptomatic purpuric patches and a chronic clinical course. J Am Acad Dermatol 1998; 39: 318–321.

127 Perniciaro C, Winkelmann RK, Daoud MS, Su WPD. Malignant angioendotheliomatosis is an angiotropic intravascular lymphoma. Am J Dermatopathol 1995; 17: 242–248.

128 Sleater JP, Segal GH, Scott MD, Masih AS. Intravascular (angiotropic) large cell lymphoma: determination of monoclonality by polymerase chain reaction on paraffin-embedded tissues. Mod Pathol 1994; 7: 593–598.

129 Snowden JA, Angel CA, Winfield DA et al. Angiotropic lymphoma: report of a case with histiocytic features. J Clin Pathol 1997; 50: 67–70.

130 Samaha H, Dumontet C, Ketterer N et al. Mantle cell lymphoma: a retrospective study of 121 cases. Leukemia 1998; 12: 1281–1287.

131 Ellison DJ, Turner RR, Van Antwerp R et al. High-grade mantle zone lymphoma. Cancer 1987; 60: 2717–2720.

132 Marti RM, Campo E, Bosch F et al. Cutaneous lymphocyte-associated antigen (CLA) expression in a lymphoblastoid mantle cell lymphoma presenting with skin lesions. Comparison with other clinicopathologic presentations of mantle cell lymphoma. J Cutan Pathol 2001; 28: 256–264.

133 Bertero M, Novelli M, Fierro MT, Bernengo MG. Mantle zone lymphoma: an immunohistologic study of skin lesions. J Am Acad Dermatol 1994; 30: 23–30.

134 Raffeld M, Jaffe ES. bcl-1, t(11;14), and mantle cell-derived neoplasms. Blood 1991; 78: 259–263.

135 Moody BR, Bartlett NL, George DW et al. Cyclin D1 as an aid in the diagnosis of mantle cell lymphoma in skin biopsies. A case report. Am J Dermatopathol 2001; 23: 470–476.

136 Ferry JA, Yang W-I, Zukerberg LR et al. CD5+ extranodal marginal zone B-cell (MALT) lymphoma. A low grade neoplasm with a propensity for bone marrow involvement and relapse. Am J Clin Pathol 1996; 105: 31–37.

T- and NK-cell neoplasms with frequent or constant cutaneous involvement

137 Toro JR, Beaty M, Sorbara L et al. γδ T-cell lymphoma of the skin. A clinical, microscopic, and molecular study. Arch Dermatol 2000; 136: 1024–1032.

138 Friedberg IM, Eisen AZ, Wolf K et al, eds. Fitzpatrick's Dermatology in general medicine, 5th ed. Vol 1. New York: McGraw Hill, 1999; 360–363.

139 Robertson MJ, Ritz J. Biology and clinical relevance of human natural killer cells. Blood 1990; 76: 2421–2438.

140 Tsang WYW, Chan JKC, Ng CS, Pau MY. Utility of a paraffin section-reactive CD56 antibody (123C3) for characterization and diagnosis of lymphomas. Am J Surg Pathol 1996; 20: 202–210.

141 Kluin PM, Feller A, Gaulard P et al. Peripheral T/NK-cell lymphoma: a report of the IXth Workshop of the European Association for Haematopathology. Histopathology 2001; 38: 250–270.

142 Spits H, Lanier LL, Phillips JH. Development of human T and natural killer cells. Blood 1995; 85: 2654–2670.

143 Arnulf B, Copie-Bergman C, Delfau-Larue M-H et al. Nonhepatosplenic γδ T-cell lymphoma: a subset of cytotoxic lymphomas with mucosal or skin localization. Blood 1998; 91: 1723–1731.

144 de Wolf-Peeters C, Achten R. γδ T-cell lymphomas: a homogeneous entity? Histopathology 2000; 36: 294–305.

145 Harris NL. Question: How do you define, succinctly, mycosis fungoides? Dermatopathology: Practical & Conceptual 2000; 6: 402–405.

146 Zackheim HS, Vonderheid EC, Ramsay DL et al. Relative frequency of various forms of primary cutaneous lymphomas. J Am Acad Dermatol 2000; 43: 793–796.

147 Koch SE, Zackheim HS, Williams ML et al. Mycosis fungoides beginning in childhood and adolescence. J Am Acad Dermatol 1987; 17: 563–570.

148 Peters MS, Thibodeau SN, White JW Jr, Winkelmann RK. Mycosis fungoides of childhood and adolescents. J Am Acad Dermatol 1990; 22: 1011–1018.

149 Wilson AGMcT, Cotter FE, Lowe DG et al. Mycosis fungoides in childhood: an unusual presentation. J Am Acad Dermatol 1991; 25: 370–372.

150 Burns MK, Ellis CN, Cooper KD. Mycosis-fungoides-type cutaneous T-cell lymphoma arising before 30 years of age. J Am Acad Dermatol 1992; 27: 974–978.

151 Naji AA, Waiz MM, Sharquie KE. Mycosis fungoides in identical twins. J Am Acad Dermatol 2001; 44: 532–533.

152 Schwartz JG, Clark EGI. Fine-needle aspiration biopsy of mycosis fungoides presenting as an ulcerating breast mass. Arch Dermatol 1988; 124: 409–413.

153 Agnarsson BA, Vonderheid EC, Kadin ME. Cutaneous T cell lymphoma with suppressor/cytotoxic (CD8) phenotype: Identification of rapidly progressive and chronic subtypes. J Am Acad Dermatol 1990; 22: 569–577.

154 Resnik KS, Kantor GR, Lessin SR et al. Mycosis fungoides palmaris et plantaris. Arch Dermatol 1995; 131: 1052–1056.

155 Sandwich JT, Davis LS. Mycosis fungoides palmaris et plantaris. Arch Dermatol 1996; 132: 971.

156 Crowley JJ, Nikko A, Varghese A et al. Mycosis fungoides in young patients: Clinical characteristics and outcome. J Am Acad Dermatol 1998; 38: 696–701.

157 Zackheim HS, McCalmont TH, Deanovic FW, Odom RB. Mycosis fungoides with onset before 20 years of age. Review of 24 patients and report of a case diagnosed at age 22 months. J Am Acad Dermatol 1997; 36: 557–562.

158 Quaglino P, Zaccagna A, Verrone A et al. Mycosis fungoides in patients under 20 years of age: report of 7 cases, review of the literature and study of the clinical course. Dermatology 1999; 199: 8–14.

159 Neuhaus IM, Ramos-Caro FA, Hassanein AM. Hypopigmented mycosis fungoides in childhood and adolescence. Pediatr Dermatol 2000; 17: 403–406.

160 Tan E, Tay Y-K, Giam Y-C. Profile and outcome of childhood mycosis fungoides in Singapore. Pediatr Dermatol 2000; 17: 352–356.

161 Di Landro A, Marchesi L, Naldi L et al. A case of hypopigmented mycosis fungoides in a young Caucasian boy. Pediatr Dermatol 1997; 14: 449–452.

162 Ko J-W, Seong J-Y, Suh K-S, Kim S-T. Pityriasis lichenoides-like mycosis fungoides in children. Br J Dermatol 2000; 142: 347–352.

163 Thomson KF, Whittaker SJ, Russell-Jones R, Charles-Holmes R. Childhood cutaneous T-cell lymphoma in association with pityriasis lichenoides chronica. Br J Dermatol 1999; 141: 1146–1148.

164 Whittam LR, Calonje E, Orchard G et al. CD8-positive juvenile onset mycosis fungoides: an immunohistochemical and genotypic analysis of six cases. Br J Dermatol 2000; 143: 1199–1204.

165 Lange Wantzin G, Thomsen K, Nissen NI et al. Occurrence of human T cell lymphotropic virus (type 1) antibodies in cutaneous T cell lymphoma. J Am Acad Dermatol 1986; 15: 598–602.

166 Peterman A, Jerdan M, Staal S et al. Evidence for HTLV-1 associated with mycosis fungoides and B-cell chronic lymphocytic leukemia. Arch Dermatol 1986; 122: 568–571.

167 Khan ZM, Sebenik M, Zucker-Franklin D. Localization of human T-cell lymphotropic virus-1 tax proviral sequences in skin biopsies of patients with mycosis fungoides by in situ polymerase chain reaction. J Invest Dermatol 1996; 106: 667–672.

168 Detmar M, Pauli G, Anagnostopoulos I et al. A case of classical mycosis fungoides associated with human T-cell lymphotropic virus type 1. Br J Dermatol 1991; 124: 198–202.

169 D'Incan M, Antoniotto O, Gasmi M et al. HTLV-1-associated lymphoma presenting as mycosis fungoides in an HTLV-1 non-endemic area: a viro-molecular study. Br J Dermatol 1995; 132: 983–988.

170 Longacre TA, Foucar K, Koster F, Burgdorf W. Atypical cutaneous lymphoproliferative disorder resembling mycosis fungoides in AIDS. Am J Dermatopathol 1989; 11: 451–456.

171 Kerschmann RL, Berger TG, Weiss LM. Cutaneous presentations of lymphoma in human immunodeficiency virus disease. Predominance of T-cell lineage. Arch Dermatol 1995; 131: 1281–1288.

172 Burns MK, Cooper KD. Cutaneous T-cell lymphoma associated with HIV infection. J Am Acad Dermatol 1993; 29: 394–399.

173 Zhang P, Chiriboga L, Jacobson M et al. Mycosis fungoideslike T-cell cutaneous lymphoid infiltrates in patients with HIV infection. Am J Dermatopathol 1995; 17: 29–35.

174 Morales Suárez-Varela MM, Llopis González A, Marquina Vila A, Bell J. Mycosis fungoides: review of epidemiological observations. Dermatology 2000; 201: 21–28.

175 Manzari V, Gismondi A, Barillari G et al. HTLV-V: a new human retrovirus isolated in a Tac-negative T cell lymphoma/leukemia. Science 1987; 238: 1581–1583.

176 Burns MK, Cooper KD. Cutaneous T-cell lymphoma associated with HIV infection. J Am Acad Dermatol 1993; 29: 394–399.

177 Burg G, Dummer R, Haeffner A et al. From inflammation to neoplasia. Mycosis fungoides evolves from reactive inflammatory conditions (lymphoid infiltrates) transforming into neoplastic plaques and tumors. Arch Dermatol 2001; 137: 949–952.

178 Lambert WC. Premycotic eruptions. Dermatol Clin 1985; 3: 629–645.

179 Hilbrich D, Ackerman AB. Mycosis fungoides is common, rarely fatal, and diagnosable when lesions are flat. Dermatopathology: Practical & Conceptual 1997; 3: 24–37.

180 Grekin DA, Zackheim HS. Mycosis fungoides. Med Clin North Am 1980; 64: 1005–1016.

181 Kim YH, Jensen RA, Watanabe GL et al. Clinical stage IA (limited patch and plaque) mycosis fungoides. A long-term outcome analysis. Arch Dermatol 1996; 132: 1309–1313.

182 Gelbrich S, Lukowsky A, Schilling T et al. Microanatomical compartments of clonal and reactive T cells in mycosis fungoides: molecular demonstration by single cell polymerase chain reaction of T cell receptor gene rearrangements. J Invest Dermatol 2000; 115: 620–624.

183 Cerroni L, Arzberger E, Ardigò M et al. Monoclonality of intraepidermal T lymphocytes in early mycosis fungoides detected by molecular analysis after laser-beam-based microdissection. J Invest Dermatol 2000; 114: 1154–1157.

184 Muche JM, Lukowsky A, Asadullah K et al. Demonstration of frequent occurrence of clonal T cells in the peripheral blood of patients with primary cutaneous T-cell lymphoma. Blood 1997; 90: 1636–1642.

185 Rijlaarsdam U, Scheffer E, Meijer CJLM et al. Mycosis fungoides-like lesions associated with phenytoin and carbamazepine therapy. J Am Acad Dermatol 1991; 24: 216–220.

186 LeBoit PE. Cutaneous lymphomas and their histopathologic imitators. Semin Dermatol 1986; 5: 322–333.

187 Okun MM, Henner M, Paulson C. A quinine-induced drug reaction of photosensitive distribution with histological features mimicking mycosis fungoides. Clin Exp Dermatol 1994; 19: 246–248.

188 Gordon KB, Guitart J, Kuzel T et al. Pseudo-mycosis fungoides in a patient taking clonazepam and fluoxetine. J Am Acad Dermatol 1996; 34: 304–306.

189 Wolf R, Kahane E, Sandbank M. Mycosis fungoides-like lesions associated with phenytoin therapy. Arch Dermatol 1985; 121: 1181–1182.

190 Rosenthal CJ, Noguera CA, Coppola A, Kapelner SN. Pseudolymphoma with mycosis fungoides manifestations, hyperresponsiveness to diphenylhydantoin, and lymphocyte disregulation. Cancer 1982; 49: 2305–2314.

191 Thiers BH. Controversies in mycosis fungoides. J Am Acad Dermatol 1982; 7: 1–16.

192 Lambert WC, Everett MA. The nosology of parapsoriasis. J Am Acad Dermatol 1981; 5: 373–395.

193 Kikuchi A, Naka W, Harada T et al. Parapsoriasis en plaques: its potential for progression to malignant lymphoma. J Am Acad Dermatol 1993; 29: 419–422.

194 Simon M, Flaig MJ, Kind P et al. Large plaque parapsoriasis: clinical and genotypic correlations. J Cutan Pathol 2000; 27: 57–60.

195 Abel EA. Clinical features of cutaneous T-cell lymphoma. Dermatol Clin 1985; 3: 647–664.

196 Smith NP. Histologic criteria for early diagnosis of cutaneous T-cell lymphoma. Dermatol Clin 1994; 12: 315–322.

197 Ackerman AB, Schiff TA. If small plaque (digitate) parapsoriasis is a cutaneous T-cell lymphoma, even an 'abortive' one, it must be mycosis fungoides! Arch Dermatol 1996; 132: 562–566.

198 King-Ismael D, Ackerman AB. Guttate parapsoriasis/digitate dermatosis (small plaque parapsoriasis) is mycosis fungoides. Am J Dermatopathol 1992; 14: 518–530.

199 Pujol RM, Gallardo F, Llistosella E et al. Invisible mycosis fungoides: A diagnostic challenge. J Am Acad Dermatol 2000; 42: 324–328.

200 O'Quinn RP, Zic JA, Boyd AS. Mycosis fungoides d'emblee: CD30-negative cutaneous large T-cell lymphoma. J Am Acad Dermatol 2000; 43: 861–863.

201 Beljaards RC, Meijer CJLM, Sebastiaan CJ et al. Primary cutaneous T-cell lymphoma: clinicopathological features and prognostic parameters of 35 cases other than mycosis fungoides and CD30-positive large cell lymphoma. J Pathol 1994; 172: 63–60.

202 Rustin MHA, Griffiths M, Ridley CM. The immunopathology of hypopigmented mycosis fungoides. Clin Exp Dermatol 1986; 11: 332–339.

203 Misch KJ, Maclennan KA, Marsden RA. Hypopigmented mycosis fungoides. Clin Exp Dermatol 1987; 12: 53–55.

204 Sigal M, Grossin M, Laroche L et al. Hypopigmented mycosis fungoides. Clin Exp Dermatol 1987; 12: 453–454.

205 Goldberg DJ, Schinella RS, Kechijian P. Hypopigmented mycosis fungoides. Speculations about the mechanism of hypopigmentation. Am J Dermatopathol 1986; 8: 326–330.

206 Whitmore SE, Simmons-O'Brien E, Rotter FS. Hypopigmented mycosis fungoides. Arch Dermatol 1994; 130: 476–480.

207 Lambroza E, Cohen SR, Phelps R et al. Hypopigmented variant of mycosis fungoides: demography, histopathology, and treatment of seven cases. J Am Acad Dermatol 1995; 32: 987–993.

208 Handfield-Jones SE, Smith NP, Breathnach SM. Hypopigmented mycosis fungoides. Clin Exp Dermatol 1992; 17: 374–375.

209 Bouloc A, Grange F, Delfau-Larue MH et al. Leucoderma associated with flares of erythrodermic cutaneous T-cell lymphomas: four cases. Br J Dermatol 2000; 143: 832–836.

210 Kartsonis J, Brettschneider F, Weissmann A, Rosen L. Mycosis fungoides bullosa. Am J Dermatopathol 1990; 12: 76–80.

211 Okano M, Nakajima C, Uehara H, Tsujimoto T. Bullous lymphoma of the skin. Br J Dermatol 1994; 131: 709–712.

212 McBride SR, Dahl MGC, Slater DN, Sviland L. Vesicular mycosis fungoides. Br J Dermatol 1998; 138: 141–144.

213 Ho KK-L, Browne A, Fitzgibbons J et al. Mycosis fungoides bullosa simulating pyoderma gangrenosum. Br J Dermatol 2000; 142: 124–127.

214 Córdoba S, Fernández-Herrera J, Sánchez-Pérez J et al. Vesiculobullous mycosis fungoides. Br J Dermatol 1999; 141: 164–166.

215 Jakob T, Tiemann M, Kuwert C et al. Dyshidrotic cutaneous T-cell lymphoma. J Am Acad Dermatol 1996; 34: 295–297.

216 Wolf P, Cerroni L, Kerl H. Mycosis fungoides mimicking perioral dermatitis. Clin Exp Dermatol 1992; 17: 132–134.

217 Price NM, Fuks ZY, Hoffman TE. Hyperkeratotic and verrucous features of mycosis fungoides. Arch Dermatol 1977; 113: 57–60.

218 Wakelin SH, Stewart EJC, Emmerson RW. Poikilodermatous and verrucous mycosis fungoides. Clin Exp Dermatol 1996; 21: 205–208.

219 Willemze R, Scheffer E, van Vloten WA. Mycosis fungoides simulating acanthosis nigricans. Am J Dermatopathol 1985; 7: 365–371.

220 Puig L, Musulén E, Fernández-Figueras M-T et al. Mycosis fungoides associated with unusual epidermal hyperplasia. Clin Exp Dermatol 1996; 21: 61–64.

221 Radeff B, Merot Y, Saurat J-H. Acquired epidermal cysts and mycosis fungoides. A possible pitfall in clinical staging. Am J Dermatopathol 1988; 10: 424–429.

222 Dalziel KL, Telfer NR, Dawber RPR. Nail dystrophy in cutaneous T-cell lymphoma. Br J Dermatol 1989; 120: 571–574.

223 Kütting B, Metze D, Luger TA, Bonsmann G. Mycosis fungoides presenting as an acquired ichthyosis. J Am Acad Dermatol 1996; 34: 887–889.

224 Caya JG, Choi H, Tieu TM et al. Hodgkin's disease followed by mycosis fungoides in the same patient. Case report and literature review. Cancer 1984; 53: 463–467.

225 Olsen EA, Delzell E, Jegasothy BV. Second malignancies in cutaneous T cell lymphoma. J Am Acad Dermatol 1984; 10: 197–204.

226 Abel EA, Sendagorta E, Hoppe RT. Cutaneous malignancies and metastatic squamous cell carcinoma following topical therapies for mycosis fungoides. J Am Acad Dermatol 1986; 14: 1029–1038.

227 Smoller BR, Marcus R. Risk of secondary cutaneous malignancies in patients with long-standing mycosis fungoides. J Am Acad Dermatol 1994; 30: 201–204.

228 Pföhler C, Ugurel S, Seiter S et al. Interferon-alpha-associated development of bullous lesions in mycosis fungoides. Dermatology 2000; 200: 51–53.

229 Gomez-de la Fuente E, Rodriguez-Peralto JL, Ortiz PL et al. Oral involvement in mycosis fungoides: report of two cases and a literature review. Acta Derm Venereol 2000; 80: 299–301.

230 Bahadoran P, Wechsler J, Delfau-Larue M-H et al. Mycosis fungoides presenting as keratosis lichenoides chronica. Br J Dermatol 1998; 138: 1067–1069.

231 Goldenhersh MA, Zlotogorski A, Rosenmann E. Follicular mycosis fungoides. Am J Dermatopathol 1994; 16: 52–55.

232 Lacour J-P, Castanet J, Perrin C, Ortonne J-P. Follicular mycosis fungoides. J Am Acad Dermatol 1993; 29: 330–334.

233 Vergier B, Beylot-Barry M, Beylot C et al. Pilotropic cutaneous T-cell lymphoma without mucinosis. A variant of mycosis fungoides? Arch Dermatol 1996; 132: 683–687.

234 Peris K, Chimenti S, Sacerdoti G et al. Pilotropic mycosis fungoides. Dermatology 1999; 199: 192–194.

235 Kossard S, White A, Killingsworth M. Basaloid folliculolymphoid hyperplasia with alopecia as an expression of mycosis fungoides (CTCL). J Cutan Pathol 1995; 22: 466–471.

236 Marzano AV, Berti E, Lupica L, Alessi E. Unilesional follicular mycosis fungoides. Dermatology 1999; 199: 174–176.

237 Gilliam AC, Lessin SR, Wilson DM, Salhany KE. Folliculotropic mycosis fungoides with large-cell transformation presenting as dissecting cellulitis of the scalp. J Cutan Pathol 1997; 24: 169–175.

238 Francis GJ, Silverman AR, Saleh O, Lee GJ. Follicular mycosis fungoides associated with lithium. J Am Acad Dermatol 2001; 44: 308–309.

239 Beylot-Barry M, Vergier B. Pilotropic mycosis fungoides. J Am Acad Dermatol 1998; 38: 501.

240 Lipsker D, Cribier B, Hud E, Grosshans E. [Cutaneous lymphoma manifesting as pigmented, purpuric capillaries.] Ann Dermatol Venereol 1999; 126: 321–326.

241 Toro JR, Sander CA, LeBoit PE. Persistent pigmented purpuric dermatitis and mycosis fungoides: simulant, precursor, or both? A study by light microscopy and molecular methods. Am J Dermatopathol 1997; 19: 108–118.

242 Barnhill RL, Braverman IM. Progression of pigmented purpura-like eruptions to mycosis fungoides: Report of three cases. J Am Acad Dermatol 1988; 19: 25–31.

243 Cather JC, Farmer A, Jackow C et al. Unusual presentation of mycosis fungoides as pigmented purpura with malignant thymoma. J Am Acad Dermatol 1998; 39: 858–863.

244 Ameen M, Darva A, Black MM et al. CD8-positive mycosis fungoides presenting as capillaritis. Br J Dermatol 2000; 142: 564–567.

245 Oliver GF, Winkelmann RK. Unilesional mycosis fungoides: a distinct entity. J Am Acad Dermatol 1989; 20: 63–70.

246 Cerroni L, Fink-Puches R, El-Shabrawi-Caelen L et al. Solitary skin lesions with histopathologic features of early mycosis fungoides. Am J Dermatopathol 1999; 21: 518–524.

247 Heald PW, Glusac EJ. Unilesional cutaneous T-cell lymphoma: Clinical features, therapy, and follow-up of 10 patients with a treatment-responsive mycosis fungoides variant. J Am Acad Dermatol 2000; 42: 283–285.

248 Hodak E, Phenig E, Amichai B et al. Unilesional mycosis fungoides. A study of seven cases. Dermatology 2000; 201: 300–306.

249 Kossard S. Unilesional mycosis fungoides or lymphomatoid keratosis? Arch Dermatol 1997; 133: 1312–1313.

250 Slater DN, Rooney N, Bleehen S, Hamed A. The lymph node in mycosis fungoides: a light and electron microscopy and immunohistological study supporting the Langerhans' cell-retrovirus hypothesis. Histopathology 1985; 9: 587–621.

251 Scheffer E, Meijer CJLM, van Vloten WA. Dermatopathic lymphadenopathy and lymph node involvement in mycosis fungoides. Cancer 1980; 45: 137–148.

252 Veelken H, Wood GS, Sklar J. Molecular staging of cutaneous T-cell lymphoma: evidence for systemic involvement in early disease. J Invest Dermatol 1995; 104: 889–894.

253 Kern DE, Kidd PG, Moe R et al. Analysis of T-cell receptor gene rearrangement in lymph nodes of patients with mycosis fungoides. Prognostic implications. Arch Dermatol 1998; 134: 158–164.

254 Wood GS. Using molecular biologic analysis of T-cell receptor gene rearrangements to stage cutaneous T-cell lymphoma. Arch Dermatol 1998; 134: 221–223.

255 Sausville EA, Worsham GF, Matthews MJ et al. Histologic assessment of lymph nodes in mycosis fungoides/Sézary syndrome (cutaneous T-cell lymphoma): clinical correlations and prognostic import of a new classification system. Hum Pathol 1985; 16: 1098–1109.

256 Sausville EA, Eddy JL, Makuch RW et al. Histopathologic staging at initial diagnosis of mycosis fungoides and the Sézary syndrome. Definition of three distinctive prognostic groups. Ann Intern Med 1988; 109: 372–382.

257 Kern DE, Kidd PG, Moe R et al. Analysis of T-cell receptor gene rearrangement in lymph nodes of patients with mycosis fungoides. Prognostic implications. Arch Dermatol 1998; 134: 158–164.

258 Fraser-Andrews EA, Woolford AJ, Russell-Jones R et al. Detection of a peripheral blood T cell clone is an independent prognostic marker in mycosis fungoides. J Invest Dermatol 2000; 114: 117–121.

259 Camisa C, Goldstein A. Mycosis fungoides. Small-bowel involvement complicated by perforation and peritonitis. Arch Dermatol 1981; 117: 234–237.

260 Zackheim HS, Lebo CF, Wasserstein P et al. Mycosis fungoides of the mastoid, middle ear, and CNS. Literature review of mycosis fungoides of the CNS. Arch Dermatol 1983; 119: 311–318.

261 Weinstock MA, Reynes JF. The changing survival of patients with mycosis fungoides. Cancer 1999; 85: 208–212.

262 Jones GW, Wilson LD. The changing survival of patients with mycosis fungoides. A population-based assessment of trends in the United States. Cancer 1999; 86: 191–193.

263 Kim YH, Chow S, Varghese A, Hoppe RT. Clinical characteristics and long-term outcome of patients with generalized patch and/or plaque (T2) mycosis fungoides. Arch Dermatol 1999; 135: 26–32.

264 Yen A, McMichael A, Kilkenny M, Rotstein H. Mycosis fungoides: an Australian experience. Australas J Dermatol 1997; 38 (Suppl): S86–S90.

265 Toro JR, Stoll HL Jr, Stomper PC, Oseroff AR. Prognostic factors and evaluation of mycosis fungoides and Sézary syndrome. J Am Acad Dermatol 1997; 37: 58–67.

266 Kim YH, Jensen RA, Watanabe GL et al. Clinical stage IA (limited plaque) mycosis fungoides: a long-term outcome analysis. J Invest Dermatol 1996; 106: 844 (abstract).

267 Hamminga L, Hermans J, Noordijk EM et al. Cutaneous T-cell lymphoma: clinicopathological relationships, therapy and survival in ninety-two patients. Br J Dermatol 1982; 107: 145–156.

268 Green SB, Byar DP, Lamberg SI. Prognostic variables in mycosis fungoides. Cancer 1981; 47: 2671–2677.

269 Cohen SR, Stenn KS, Braverman IM, Beck GJ. Mycosis fungoides. Clinicopathologic relationships, survival, and therapy in 59 patients with observations on occupation as a new prognostic factor. Cancer 1980; 46: 2654–2666.

270 Sausville EA, Worsham GF, Matthews MJ et al. Histologic assessment of lymph nodes in mycosis fungoides/Sézary syndrome (cutaneous T-cell lymphoma): clinical correlations and prognostic import of a new classification system. Hum Pathol 1985; 16: 1098–1109.

271 Sausville EA, Eddy JL, Makuch RW et al. Histopathologic staging at initial diagnosis of mycosis fungoides and the Sézary syndrome. Definition of three distinctive prognostic groups. Ann Intern Med 1988; 109: 372–382.

272 Yamamura T, Aozasa K, Sano S. The cutaneous lymphomas with convoluted nucleus. Analysis of thirty-nine cases. J Am Acad Dermatol 1984; 10: 796–803.

273 Cerroni L, Rieger E, Hödl S, Kerl H. Clinicopathologic and immunologic features associated with transformation of mycosis fungoides to large-cell lymphoma. Am J Surg Pathol 1992; 16: 543–552.

274 Wood GS, Bahler DW, Hoppe RT et al. Transformation of mycosis fungoides: T-cell receptor β gene analysis demonstrates a common clonal origin for plaque-type mycosis fungoides and CD30⁺ large-cell lymphoma. J Invest Dermatol 1993; 101: 296–300.

275 Kaudewitz P, Stein H, Dallenbach F et al. Primary and secondary cutaneous Ki-1⁺ (CD30⁺) anaplastic large cell lymphomas. Morphologic, immunohistologic, and clinical characteristics. Am J Pathol 1989; 135: 359–367.

276 Stein H, Foss H-D, Dürkop H et al. CD30+ anaplastic large cell lymphoma: a review of its histopathologic, genetic, and clinical features. Blood 2000; 96: 3681–3695.

277 Sanchez JL, Ackerman AB. The patch stage of mycosis fungoides. Criteria for histologic diagnosis. Am J Dermatopathol 1979; 1: 5–26.

278 Eng AM, Blekys I, Worobec SM. Clinicopathologic correlations in Alibert-type mycosis fungoides. Arch Dermatol 1981; 117: 332–337.

279 Lefeber WP, Robinson JK, Clendenning WE et al. Attempts to enhance light microscopic diagnosis of cutaneous T-cell lymphoma (mycosis fungoides). Arch Dermatol 1981; 117: 408–411.

280 MacKie RM, Foulds IS, McMillan EM, Nelson HM. Histological changes observed in the skin of patients with mycosis fungoides receiving photochemotherapy. Clin Exp Dermatol 1980; 5: 405–413.

281 Olerud JE, Kulin PA, Chew DE et al. Cutaneous T-cell lymphoma. Arch Dermatol 1992; 128: 501–507.

282 Shapiro PE, Pinto FJ. The histologic spectrum of mycosis fungoides/Sézary syndrome (cutaneous T-cell lymphoma). Am J Surg Pathol 1994; 18: 645–667.

283 El Darouti M, Marzouk SA, Horn TD. Failure of detection of mucin in the clear halos around the epidermotropic lymphocytes in mycosis fungoides. J Cutan Pathol 2000; 27: 183–185.

284 Nickoloff BJ. Light-microscopic assessment of 100 patients with patch/plaque-stage mycosis fungoides. Am J Dermatopathol 1988; 10: 469–477.

285 Smoller BR, Bishop K, Glusac E et al. Reassessment of histologic parameters in the diagnosis of mycosis fungoides. Am J Surg Pathol 1995; 19: 1423–1430.

286 Everett MA. Early diagnosis of mycosis fungoides: vacuolar interface dermatitis. J Cutan Pathol 1985; 12: 271–278.

287 Guitart J, Peduto M, Caro WA, Roenigk HH. Lichenoid changes in mycosis fungoides. J Am Acad Dermatol 1997; 36: 417–422.

288 Hitchcock MG, Burchette JL Jr, Olsen EA et al. Eccrine gland infiltration by mycosis fungoides. Am J Dermatopathol 1996; 18: 447–453.

289 Rongioletti F, Smoller B. The histologic value of adnexal (eccrine gland and follicle) infiltration in mycosis fungoides. J Cutan Pathol 2000; 27: 406–409.

290 Altman J. Parapsoriasis: a histopathologic review and classification. Semin Dermatol 1984; 3: 14–21.

291 McMillan EM, Wasik R, Martin D et al. Immuno-electron microscopy of "T" cells in large plaque parapsoriasis. J Cutan Pathol 1981; 8: 385–392.

292 Kim SY. Follicular mycosis fungoides. Am J Dermatopathol 1985; 7: 300.

293 Nickoloff BJ. Epidermal mucinosis in mycosis fungoides. J Am Acad Dermatol 1986; 15: 83–86.

294 LeBoit PE. Variants of mycosis fungoides and related cutaneous T-cell lymphomas. Semin Diagn Pathol 1991; 8: 73–81.

295 Ackerman AB, Breza TS, Capland L. Spongiotic simulants of mycosis fungoides. Arch Dermatol 1974; 109: 218–220.

296 Candiago E, Marocolo D, Manganoni MA et al. Nonlymphoid intraepidermal mononuclear collections (pseudo-Pautrier abscesses). A morphologic and immunophenotypical characterization. Am J Dermatopathol 2000; 22: 1–6.

297 LeBoit PE, Epstein BA. A vase-like shape characterizes the epidermal-mononuclear cell collections seen in spongiotic dermatitis. Am J Dermatopathol 1990; 12: 612–616.

298 Bergman R, Cohen A, Harth Y et al. Histopathologic findings in the clinically uninvolved skin of patients with mycosis fungoides. Am J Dermatopathol 1995; 17: 452–456.

299 Horiuchi Y, Tone T, Umezawa A, Takezaki S. Large cell mycosis fungoides at the tumor stage. Unusual T8, T4, T6 phenotypic expression. Am J Dermatopathol 1988; 10: 54–58.

300 Proctor MS, Price NM, Cox AJ, Hoppe RT. Subcutaneous mycosis fungoides. Arch Dermatol 1978; 114: 1326–1328.

301 Santucci M, Biggeri A, Feller AC, Burg G. Accuracy, concordance, and reproducibility of histologic diagnosis in cutaneous T-cell lymphoma. Arch Dermatol 2000; 136: 497–502.

302 Santucci M, Biggeri A, Feller AC et al. Efficacy of histologic criteria for diagnosing early mycosis fungoides. An EORTC Cutaneous Lymphoma Study Group Investigation. Am J Surg Pathol 2000; 24: 40–50.

303 Ming M, LeBoit PE. Can dermatopathologists reliably make the diagnosis of mycosis fungoides? If not, who can? Arch Dermatol 2000; 136: 543–546.

304 Glusac EJ. Of cells and architecture: new approaches to old criteria in mycosis fungoides. J Cutan Pathol 2001; 28: 169–173.

305 Guitart J, Kennedy J, Ronan S et al. Histologic criteria for the diagnosis of mycosis fungoides: proposal for a grading system to standardize pathology reporting. J Cutan Pathol 2001; 28: 174–183.

306 Smoller BR, Detwiler SP, Kohler S et al. Role of histology in providing prognostic information in mycosis fungoides. J Cutan Pathol 1998; 25: 311–315.

307 Flaxman BA, Koumans JAD, Ackerman AB. Granulomatous mycosis fungoides. A 14-year follow-up of a case. Am J Dermatopathol 1983; 5: 145–151.

308 LeBoit PE, Zackheim HS, White CR Jr. Granulomatous variants of cutaneous T-cell lymphoma. The histopathology of granulomatous mycosis fungoides and granulomatous slack skin. Am J Surg Pathol 1988; 12: 83–95.

309 Papadavid E, Yu RC, Bunker C et al. Tumour progression in a patient with granulomatous mycosis fungoides. Br J Dermatol 1996; 134: 740–743.

310 Argenyi ZB, Goeken JA, Piette WW, Madison KC. Granulomatous mycosis fungoides. Clinicopathologic study of two cases. Am J Dermatopathol 1992; 14: 200–210.

311 Chen K-R, Tanaka M, Miyakawa S. Granulomatous mycosis fungoides with small intestinal involvement and a fatal outcome. Br J Dermatol 1998; 138: 522–525.

312 Metzler G, Schlagenhauff B, Kröber S-M et al. Granulomatous mycosis fungoides. Report of a case with some histopathologic features of granulomatous slack skin. Am J Dermatopathol 1999; 21: 156–160.

313 Gómez-de la Fuente E, Ortiz PL, Vanaclocha F et al. Aggressive granulomatous mycosis fungoides with clinical pulmonary and thyroid involvement. Br J Dermatol 2000; 142: 1026–1029.

314 Fischer M, Wohlrab J, Audring H et al. Granulomatous mycosis fungoides. Report of two cases and review of the literature. J Eur Acad Dermatol Venereol 2000; 14: 196–202.

315 Woollons A, Darvay A, Khorshid SM et al. Necrobiotic cutaneous T-cell lymphoma. J Am Acad Dermatol 1999; 41: 815–819.

316 Darwin BS, Herzberg AJ, Murray JC, Olsen EA. Generalized papular xanthomatosis in mycosis fungoides. J Am Acad Dermatol 1992; 26: 828–832.

317 Ross EV, Roman L, Rushin JM et al. Xanthomatized atypical T cells in a patient with mycosis fungoides and hyperlipidemia. Arch Dermatol 1992; 128: 1499–1502.

318 Su LD, Kim YH, LeBoit PE et al. Interstitial mycosis fungoides, a variant of mycosis fungoides resembling granuloma annulare and inflammatory morphea. J Cutan Pathol 2000; 27: 574 (abstract).

319 Freedman AM, Ackerman AB. What is the clue and what is the diagnosis? Dermatopathology: Practical & Conceptual 1997; 3: 171–174.

320 Wong W-R, Yang L-J, Kuo T-t, Chan H-L. Generalized granuloma annulare associated with granulomatous mycosis fungoides. Dermatology 2000; 200: 54–56.

321 Fairbee SI, Morgan MB, Tannenbaum MT, Glass LF. Fibromucinous T-cell lymphoma. A new clinicopathologic variant of mycosis fungoides? Am J Dermatopathol 2000; 22: 515–518.

322 Hodak E, Feinmesser M, Segal T et al. Follicular cutaneous T-cell lymphoma: a clinicopathological study of nine cases. Br J Dermatol 1999; 141: 315–322.

323 Pereyo NG, Requena L, Galloway J, Sangüeza OP. Follicular mycosis fungoides: A clinicohistopathologic study. J Am Acad Dermatol 1997; 36: 563–568.

324 Fraser-Andrews E, Ashton R, Russell-Jones R. Pilotropic mycosis fungoides presenting with multiple cysts, comedones and alopecia. Br J Dermatol 1999; 140: 141–144.

324a Flaig MJ, Cerroni L, Schuhmann K et al. Follicular mycosis fungoides. A histopathologic analysis of nine cases. J Cutan Pathol 2001; 28: 525–530.

325 Granstein RD, Soter NA, Haynes HA. Necrotizing vasculitis within cutaneous lesions of mycosis fungoides. J Am Acad Dermatol 1983; 9: 128–133.

326 De Misa RF, Azaña JM, Bellas C et al. Mycosis fungoides with signet-ring cells and monoclonal gammopathy. Int J Dermatol 1994; 33: 652–653.

327 Goldberg DJ, Schinella RS, Kechijian P. Hypopigmented mycosis fungoides. Speculations about the mechanism of hypopigmentation. Am J Dermatopathol 1986; 8: 326–330.

328 Reddy VB, Ramsay D, Garcia JA, Kamino H. Atypical cutaneous changes after topical treatment with nitrogen mustard in patients with mycosis fungoides. Am J Dermatopathol 1996; 18: 19–23.

329 Michie SA, Abel EA, Hoppe RT et al. Expression of T-cell receptor antigens in mycosis fungoides and inflammatory skin lesions. J Invest Dermatol 1989; 93: 116–120.

330 Wood NL, Kitces EN, Blaylock WK. Depressed lymphokine activated killer cell activity in mycosis fungoides. A possible marker for aggressive disease. Arch Dermatol 1990; 126: 907–913.

331 Wood GS. Lymphocyte activation in cutaneous T-cell lymphoma. J Invest Dermatol 1995; 105: 105S–109S.

332 Ralfkiaer E. Immunohistochemical markers for the diagnosis of cutaneous lymphomas. Semin Diagn Pathol 1991; 8: 62–72.

333 Vonderheid EC, Tan E, Sobel EL et al. Clinical implications of immunologic phenotyping in cutaneous T cell lymphoma. J Am Acad Dermatol 1987; 17: 40–52.

334 Ormsby A, Bergfeld WF, Tubbs RR, Hsi ED. Evaluation of a new paraffin-reactive CD7 T-cell deletion marker and a polymerase chain reaction-based T-cell receptor gene rearrangement assay: implications for diagnosis of mycosis fungoides in community clinical practice. J Am Acad Dermatol 2001; 45: 405–413.

335 Ormsby AH, Tubbs RR, Bergfeld WF, Hsi ED. A new CD7 paraffin reactive antibody and T-γ PCR monoclonality are sensitive and specific for a diagnosis of mycosis fungoides (MF). J Cutan Pathol 2000; 27: 567 (abstract).

336 Lindae ML, Abel EA, Hoppe RT, Wood GS. Poikilodermatous mycosis fungoides and atrophic large-plaque parapsoriasis exhibit similar abnormalities of T-cell antigen expression. Arch Dermatol 1988; 124: 366–372.

337 Wood GS, Abel EA, Hoppe RT, Warnke RA. Leu-8 and Leu-9 antigen phenotypes: immunologic criteria for the distinction of mycosis fungoides from cutaneous inflammation. J Am Acad Dermatol 1986; 14: 1006–1013.

338 Wood GS, Hong SR, Sasaki DT et al. Leu-8/CD7 antigen expression by CD3+ T cells: comparative analysis of skin and blood in mycosis fungoides/Sézary syndrome relative to normal blood values. J Am Acad Dermatol 1990; 22: 602–607.

339 Turbitt ML, MacKie RM. An assessment of the diagnostic value of the monoclonal antibodies Leu 8, OKT9, OKT10 and Ki67 in cutaneous lymphocytic infiltrates. Br J Dermatol 1986; 115: 151–158.

340 Harmon CB, Witzig TE, Katzmann JA, Pittelkow MR. Detection of circulating T cells with CD4+CD7– immunophenotype in patients with benign and malignant lymphoproliferative dermatoses. J Am Acad Dermatol 1996; 35: 404–410.

341 Murphy M, Fullen D, Carlson JA. CD7 paraffin reactive antibody: loss of expression in benign and malignant cutaneous lymphocytic infiltrates. J Cutan Pathol 2000; 27: 566 (abstract).

342 Wood GS, Dubiel C, Mueller C et al. Most CD8+ cells in skin lesions of CD3+ CD4+ mycosis fungoides are CD3+ T cells that lack CD11b, CD16, CD56, CD57, and human Hanukah factor mRNA. Am J Pathol 1991; 138: 1545–1552.

343 Hoppe RT, Medeiros LJ, Warnke RA, Wood GS. CD8-positive tumor-infiltrating lymphocytes influence the long-term survival of patients with mycosis fungoides. J Am Acad Dermatol 1995; 32: 448–453.

344 Willemze R, de Graaff-Reitsma CB, Cnossen J et al. Characterization of T-cell subpopulations in skin and peripheral blood of patients with cutaneous T-cell lymphomas and benign inflammatory dermatoses. J Invest Dermatol 1983; 80: 60–66.

345 van der Putte SCJ, Toonstra J, van Wichen DF et al. Aberrant immunophenotypes in mycosis fungoides. Arch Dermatol 1988; 124: 373–380.

346 McMillan EM, Wasik R, Beeman K, Everett MA. In situ immunologic phenotyping of mycosis fungoides. J Am Acad Dermatol 1982; 6: 888–897.

347 Preesman AH, Toonstra J, van der Putte SCJ, van Vloten WA. Immunophenotyping on simultaneously occurring plaques and tumors in mycosis fungoides and Sézary syndrome. Br J Dermatol 1993; 129: 660–666.

348 Li G, Salhany KE, Rook AH, Lessin SR. The pathogenesis of large cell transformation in cutaneous T-cell lymphoma is not associated with t(2;5)(p23;q35) chromosomal translocation. J Cutan Pathol 1997; 24: 403–408.

349 Wu H, Telang GH, Lessin SR, Vonderheid EC. Mycosis fungoides with CD30-positive cells in the epidermis. Am J Dermatopathol 2000; 22: 212–216.

350 Dommann SNW, Ziegler T, Dommann-Scherrer CC et al. CD44v6 is a marker for systemic spread in cutaneous T-cell lymphoma. J Cutan Pathol 1995; 22: 407–412.

351 Wagner SN, Wagner C, Reinhold U et al. Predominant expression of CD44 splice variant v10 in malignant and reactive human skin lymphocytes. J Invest Dermatol 1998; 111: 464–471.

352 Hansen ER. Immunoregulatory events in the skin of patients with cutaneous T-cell lymphoma. Arch Dermatol 1996; 132: 554–561.

353 Fivenson DP, Nickoloff BJ. Distinctive dendritic cell subsets expressing factor XIIIa, CD1a, CD1b and CD1c in mycosis fungoides and psoriasis. J Cutan Pathol 1995; 22: 223–228.

354 Barzilai A, Goldberg I, Shibi R et al. Mycosis fungoides expressing γ/δ T-cell receptors. J Am Acad Dermatol 1996; 34: 301–302.

355 Munn SE, McGregor JM, Jones A et al. Clinical and pathological heterogeneity in cutaneous gamma-delta T-cell lymphoma: a report of three cases and a review of the literature. Br J Dermatol 1996; 135: 976–981.

356 Fucich LF, Freeman SF, Boh EE et al. Atypical cutaneous lymphocytic infiltrate and a role for quantitative immunohistochemistry and gene rearrangement studies. Int J Dermatol 1999; 38: 749–756.

357 Curcó N, Servitje O, Llucià M et al. Genotypic analysis of cutaneous T-cell lymphoma: a comparative study of Southern blot analysis with polymerase chain reaction amplification of the T-cell receptor-γ gene. Br J Dermatol 1997; 137: 673–679.

358 Bergman R. How useful are T-cell receptor gene rearrangement studies as an adjunct to the histopathologic diagnosis of mycosis fungoides? Am J Dermatopathol 1999; 21: 498–502.

359 Tok J, Szabolcs MJ, Silvers DN et al. Detection of clonal T-cell receptor γ chain gene rearrangements by polymerase chain reaction and denaturing gradient gel electrophoresis (PCR/DGGE) in archival specimens from patients with early cutaneous T-cell lymphoma: Correlation of histologic findings with PCR/DGGE. J Am Acad Dermatol 1998; 38: 453–460.

360 Murphy M, Signoretti S, Kadin ME, Loda M. Detection of TCR-γ gene rearrangements in early mycosis fungoides by non-radioactive PCR-SSCP. J Cutan Pathol 2000; 27: 228–234.

361 Bergman R, Faclieru D, Sahar D et al. Immunophenotyping and T-cell receptor γ gene rearrangement analysis as an adjunct to the histopathologic diagnosis of mycosis fungoides. J Am Acad Dermatol 1998; 39: 554–559.

362 Tykocinski M, Schinella R, Greco A. The pleomorphic cells of advanced mycosis fungoides. An ultrastructural study. Arch Pathol Lab Med 1984; 108: 387–391.

363 van der Putte SCJ, van der Meer JB. Mycosis fungoides: a morphological study. Clin Exp Dermatol 1981; 6: 57–76.

364 McMillan EM, Beeman K, Wasik R, Everett MA. Demonstration of OKT6-reactive cells in mycosis fungoides. J Am Acad Dermatol 1982; 6: 880–887.

365 Mandojana RM, Helwig EB. Localized epidermotropic reticulosis (Woringer–Kolopp disease). A clinicopathologic study of 15 new cases. J Am Acad Dermatol 1983; 8: 813–829.

366 Burns MK, Chan LS, Cooper KD. Woringer–Kolopp disease (localized pagetoid reticulosis) or unilesional mycosis fungoides? An analysis of eight cases with benign disease. Arch Dermatol 1995; 131: 325–329.

367 Berti E, Cerri A, Cavicchini S et al. Primary cutaneous γ/δ T-cell lymphoma presenting as disseminated pagetoid reticulosis. J Invest Dermatol 1991; 96: 718–723.

368 Berti E, Tomasini D, Vermeer MH et al. Primary cutaneous CD8-positive epidermotropic cytotoxic T cell lymphomas. A distinct clinicopathological entity with an aggressive clinical behavior. Am J Pathol 1999; 155: 483–492.

369 Wood WS, Killby VAA, Stewart WD. Pagetoid reticulosis (Woringer–Kolopp disease). J Cutan Pathol 1979; 6: 113–123.

370 Lever WF. Localized mycosis fungoides with prominent epidermotropism. Woringer–Kolopp disease. Arch Dermatol 1977; 113: 1254–1256.

371 Mielke V, Wolff HH, Winzer M, Sterry W. Localized and disseminated pagetoid reticulosis. Diagnostic immunophenotypical findings. Arch Dermatol 1989; 125: 402–406.

372 Drillenburg P, Bronkhorst CM, van der Wal AC et al. Expression of adhesion molecules in pagetoid reticulosis (Woringer–Kolopp disease). Br J Dermatol 1997; 136: 613–616.

373 Wood GS, Weiss LM, Hu C-H et al. T-cell antigen deficiencies and clonal rearrangements of T-cell receptor genes in pagetoid reticulosis (Woringer–Kolopp disease). N Engl J Med 1988; 318: 164–167.

374 Alaibac M, Chu AC. Woringer–Kolopp disease. Am J Surg Pathol 1996; 20: 1153–1154.

375 MacKie RM, Turbitt ML. A case of Pagetoid reticulosis bearing the T cytotoxic suppressor surface marker on the lymphoid infiltrate: further evidence that Pagetoid reticulosis is not a variant of mycosis fungoides. Br J Dermatol 1984; 110: 89–94.

376 Russell Jones R, Chu A. Pagetoid reticulosis and solitary mycosis fungoides. Distinct clinicopathological entities. J Cutan Pathol 1981; 8: 40–51.

377 LeBoit PE, Abel EA, Cleary ML et al. Clonal rearrangement of the T-cell receptor β gene in the circulating lymphocytes of erythrodermic follicular mucinosis. Blood 1988; 71: 1329–1333.

378 Bonta MD, Tannous ZS, Demierre M-F et al. Rapidly progressing mycosis fungoides presenting as follicular mucinosis. J Am Acad Dermatol 2000; 43: 635–640.

379 Sentis HJ, Willemze R, Scheffer E. Alopecia mucinosa progressing into mycosis fungoides. A long-term follow-up of two patients. Am J Dermatopathol 1988; 10: 478–486.

380 Nickoloff BJ, Wood C. Benign idiopathic versus mycosis fungoides-associated follicular mucinosis. Pediatr Dermatol 1985; 2: 201–206.

381 Pujol RM, Alonso J, Gibson LE et al. Follicular mucinosis: clinicopathologic evaluation and genotypic analysis of 25 cases, with clonality evaluation by TCR gamma chain PCR amplification. J Cutan Pathol 1996; 23: 58 (abstract).

382 Zelickson BD, Peters MS, Muller SA et al. T-cell receptor gene rearrangement analysis: cutaneous T-cell lymphoma, peripheral T-cell lymphoma, and premalignant and benign cutaneous lymphoproliferative disorders. J Am Acad Dermatol 1991; 25: 787–796.

383 Gibson LE, Muller SA, Leiferman KM, Peters MS. Follicular mucinosis: clinical and histopathologic study. J Am Acad Dermatol 1989; 20: 441–446.

384 LeBoit PE. Granulomatous slack skin. Dermatol Clin 1994; 12: 375–389.

385 Ackerman AB. Histologic diagnosis of inflammatory skin diseases. Philadelphia: Lea & Febiger, 1978; 483–485.

386 Helm KF, Cerio R, Winkelmann RK. Granulomatous slack skin: a clinicopathological and immunohistochemical study of three cases. Br J Dermatol 1992; 126: 142–147.

387 Mouly F, Baccard M, Cayuela J-M et al. Cutaneous T-cell lymphoma associated with granulomatous slack skin. Dermatology 1996; 192: 288–290.

388 Alessi E, Crosti C, Sala F. Unusual case of granulomatous dermohypodermitis with giant cells and elastophagocytosis. Dermatologica 1986; 172: 218–221.

389 DeGregorio R, Fenske NA, Glass LF. Granulomatous slack skin: a possible precursor of Hodgkin's disease. J Am Acad Dermatol 1995; 33: 1044–1047.

390 Noto G, Pravatá G, Miceli S, Aricò M. Granulomatous slack skin: report of a case associated with Hodgkin's disease and a review of the literature. Br J Dermatol 1994; 131: 275–279.

391 Mouly F, Baccard M, Cayuela J-M et al. Cutaneous T-cell lymphoma associated with granulomatous slack skin. Dermatology 1996; 192: 288–290.

392 Puig S, Iranzo P, Palou J et al. Lymphoproliferative nature of granulomatous slack skin. Clonal rearrangement of the T-cell receptor β-gene. Arch Dermatol 1992; 128: 562–563.

393 Tsang WYW, Chan JKC, Loo KT et al. Granulomatous slack skin. Histopathology 1994; 25: 49–55.

394 Balus L, Manente L, Remotti D et al. Granulomatous slack skin. Report of a case and review of the literature. Am J Dermatopathol 1996; 18: 199–206.

395 LeBoit PE, Beckstead JH, Bond B et al. Granulomatous slack skin: clonal rearrangement of the T-cell receptor β gene is evidence for the lymphoproliferative nature of a cutaneous elastolytic disorder. J Invest Dermatol 1987; 89: 183–186.

396 Wieselthier JS, Koh HK. Sézary syndrome: diagnosis, prognosis, and critical review of treatment options. J Am Acad Dermatol 1990; 22: 381–401.

397 Sézary A, Bouvrain Y. Erythrodermie avec présence de cellules monstreuses dans le derme et le sang circulant. Bull Soc Fr Dermatol Syph 1938; 45: 254–260.

398 Kohler S, Kim YH, Smoller BR. Histologic criteria for the diagnosis of erythrodermic mycosis fungoides and Sézary syndrome: a critical reappraisal. J Cutan Pathol 1997; 24: 292–297.

399 Winkelmann RK, Buechner SA, Diaz-Perez JL. Pre-Sézary syndrome. J Am Acad Dermatol 1984; 10: 992–999.

400 Buzzanga J, Banks PM, Winkelmann RK. Lymph node histopathology in Sézary syndrome. J Am Acad Dermatol 1984; 11: 880–888.

401 Zina G, Bernengo MG, Zina AM. Bullous Sézary syndrome. Dermatologica 1981; 163: 25–33.

402 Holdaway DR, Winkelmann RK. Histopathology of Sézary syndrome. Mayo Clin Proc 1974; 49: 541–547.

403 Alcalay J, David M, Shohat B, Sandbank M. Generalized vitiligo following Sézary syndrome. Br J Dermatol 1987; 116: 851–855.

404 Venencie PY, Winkelmann RK, Puissant A, Kyle RA. Monoclonal gammopathy in Sézary syndrome. Report of three cases and review of the literature. Arch Dermatol 1984; 120: 605–608.

405 Suchin KR, Cassin M, Gottlieb SL et al. Increased interleukin 5 production in eosinophilic Sézary syndrome: Regulation by interferon alfa and interleukin 12. J Am Acad Dermatol 2001; 44: 28–32.

406 Kim YH, Bishop K, Varghese A, Hoppe RT. Prognostic factors in erythrodermic mycosis fungcides and the Sézary syndrome. Arch Dermatol 1995; 131: 1003–1008.

407 Meister L, Duarte AM, Davis J et al. Sézary syndrome in an 11-year-old girl. J Am Acad Dermatol 1993; 28: 93–95.

408 van Haselen CW, Toonstra J, Preesman AH et al. Sézary syndrome in a young man with severe atopic dermatitis. Br J Dermatol 1999; 140: 704–707.

409 Scarisbrick JJ, Child FJ, Evans AV et al. Secondary malignant neoplasms in 71 patients with Sézary syndrome. Arch Dermatol 1999; 135: 1381–1385.

410 Scarisbrick JJ, Child F, Spittle M et al. Systemic Hodgkin's lymphoma in a patient with Sézary syndrome. Br J Dermatol 2000; 142: 771–775.

411 So C-c, Wong K-f, Siu LLP, Kwong Y-l. Large cell transformation of Sézary syndrome. A conventional and molecular cytogenetic study. Am J Clin Pathol 2000; 113: 792–797.

412 Hamminga L, Hartgrink-Groeneveld CA, van Vloten WA. Sézary's syndrome: a clinical evaluation of eight patients. Br J Dermatol 1979; 100: 291–296.

413 Heald P, Yan S-L, Edelson R. Profound deficiency in normal circulating T cells in erythrodermic cutaneous T-cell lymphoma. Arch Dermatol 1994; 130: 198–203.

414 Buechner SA, Winkelmann RK. Sézary syndrome. A clinicopathologic study of 39 cases. Arch Dermatol 1983; 119: 979–986.

415 Sentis HJ, Willemze R, Scheffer E. Histopathologic studies in Sézary syndrome and erythrodermic mycosis fungoides: a comparison with benign forms of erythroderma. J Am Acad Dermatol 1986; 15: 1217–1226.

416 Kamarashev J, Burg G, Kempf W et al. Comparative analysis of histological and immunohistological features in mycosis fungoides and Sézary syndrome. J Cutan Pathol 1998; 25: 407–412.

417 Kuzel TM, Roenigk HH, Rosen ST. Mycosis fungoides and the Sézary syndrome: a review of pathogenesis, diagnosis, and therapy. J Clin Oncol 1991; 9: 1298–1308.

418 Trotter MJ, Whittaker SJ, Orchard GE, Smith NP. Cutaneous histopathology of Sézary syndrome: a study of 41 cases with a proven circulating T-cell clone. J Cutan Pathol 1997; 24: 286–291.

419 Rappl G, Muche JM, Abken H et al. CD4+CD7− T cells compose the dominant T-cell clone in the peripheral blood of patients with Sézary syndrome. J Am Acad Dermatol 2001; 44: 456–461.

420 Bakels V, van Oostveen JW, Gordijn RLJ et al. Diagnostic value of T-cell receptor beta gene rearrangement analysis on peripheral blood lymphocytes of patients with erythroderma. J Invest Dermatol 1991; 97: 782–786.

421 Laetsch B, Häffner AC, Döbbeling U et al. CD4+/CD7− T cell frequency and polymerase chain reaction-based clonality assay correlate with stage in cutaneous T cell lymphomas. J Invest Dermatol 2000; 114: 107–111.

422 Edelman J, Meyerson HJ. Diminished CD3 expression is useful for detecting and enumerating Sézary cells. Am J Clin Pathol 2000; 114: 467–477.

423 Bernengo MG, Novelli M, Quaglino P et al. The relevance of the CD4+ CD26− subset in the identification of circulating Sézary cells. Br J Dermatol 2001; 144: 125–135.

424 Russell-Jones R. Immunophenotyping of Sézary cells. Br J Dermatol 2001; 144: 2–3.

425 Payne CM, Glasser L. Ultrastructural morphometry in the diagnosis of Sézary syndrome. Arch Pathol Lab Med 1990; 114: 661–671.

426 Chiarle R, Podda A, Prolla G et al. CD30 in normal and neoplastic cells. Clin Immunol 1999; 90: 157–164.

427 Vergier B, Beylot-Barry M, Pulford K et al. Statistical evaluaton of diagnostic and prognostic features of CD30+ cutaneous lymphoproliferative disorders. A clinicopathologic study of 65 cases. Am J Surg Pathol 1998; 22: 1192– 202.

428 Felgar RE, Salhany KE, Macon WR et al. The expression of TIA-1+ cytolytic-type granules and other cytolytic lymphocyte-associated markers in CD30+ anaplastic large cell lymphomas (ALCL): correlation with morphology, immunophenotype, ultrastructure, and clinical features. Hum Pathol 1999; 30: 228–236.

429 Foss H-D, Anagnostopoulos I, Araujo I et al. Anaplastic large-cell lymphomas of T-cell and null-cell phenotype express cytotoxic molecules. Blood 1996; 88: 4005–4011.

430 Viraben R, Brousset P, Aquilina C, Lamant L. Cutaneous non-epidermotropic lymphoma associated with human immunodeficiency virus infection. Clin Exp Dermatol 1997; 22: 262–264.

431 Beylot-Barry M, Vergier B, Masquelier B et al. The spectrum of cutaneous lymphomas in HIV infection. A study of 21 cases. Am J Surg Pathol 1999; 23: 1208–1216.

432 Jhala DN, Medeiros LJ, Lopez-Terrada D et al. Neutrophil-rich anap astic large cell lymphoma of T-cell lineage. A report of two cases arising in HIV-positive patients. Am J Clin Pathol 2000; 114: 478–482.

433 Nakamura K, Katano H, Hoshino Y et al. Human herpesvirus type 8 and Epstein–Barr virus-associated cutaneous lymphoma taking anaplastic large cell morphology in a man with HIV infection. Br J Dermatol 1999; 141: 141–145.

434 Cataldo KA, Jalal SM, Law ME et al. Detection of t(2;5) in anaplastic large cell lymphoma. Comparison of immunohistochemical studies, FISH, and RT-PCR in paraffin-embedded tissue. Am J Surg Pathol 1999; 23: 1386–1392.

435 DeCoteau JF, Butmarc JR, Kinney MC, Kadin ME. The t(2;5) chromosomal translocation is not a common feature of primary cutaneous CD30⁺ lymphoproliferative disorders: comparison with anaplastic large-cell lymphoma of nodal origin. Blood 1996; 87: 3437–3441.

436 Su LD, Schnitzer B, Ross CW et al. The t(2;5)-associated p80 NPM/ALK fusion protein in nodal and cutaneous CD30+ lymphoproliferative disorders. J Cutan Pathol 1997; 24: 597–603.

437 Gould JW, Eppes RB, Gilliam AC et al. Solitary primary cutaneous CD30+ large cell lymphoma of natural killer cell phenotype bearing the t(2;5)(p23;q35) translocation and presenting in a child. Am J Dermatopathol 2000; 22: 422–428.

438 Wood GS. Analysis of the t(2;5)(p23;q35) translocation in CD30+ primary cutaneous lymphoproliferative disorders and Hodgkin's disease. Leuk Lymphoma 1998; 29: 93–101.

439 Falini B, Pileri S, Zinzani I et al. ALK+ lymphoma: clinico-pathological findings and outcome. Blood 1999; 95: 2697–2706.

440 Kato N, Yasukawa K, Kimura K, Yoshida K. Anaplastic large-cell lymphoma associated with acquired ichthyosis. J Am Acad Dermatol 2000; 42: 914–920.

441 Chott A, Kaserer K, Augustin I et al. Ki-1-positive large-cell lymphoma. A clinicopathologic study of 41 cases. Am J Surg Pathol 1990; 14: 439–448.

442 MacLennan KA, Diebold J. Anaplastic large cell lymphoma. Curr Diagn Pathol 1998; 5: 165–173.

443 Kinney MC, Collins RD, Greer JP et al. A small-cell-predominant variant of primary Ki-1 (CD30)+ T-cell lymphoma. Am J Surg Pathol 1993; 17: 859–868.

444 Pileri S, Falini B, Delsol G et al. Lymphohistiocytic T-cell lymphoma (araplastic large cell lymphoma CD30+/Ki-1+ with a high content of reactive histiocytes). Histopathology 1990; 16: 383–391.

445 Benharroch D, Meguerian-Bedoyan Z, Lamat L et al. ALK-positive lymphoma: a single disease with a broad spectrum of morphology. Blood 1998; 91: 2076–2084.

446 Brugières L, Le Deley MC, Pacquement H et al. CD30+ anaplastic large-cell lymphoma in children: analysis of 82 patients enrolled in two consecutive studies of the French Society of Pediatric Oncology. Blood 1998; 92: 3591–3598.

447 Chan JKC, Buchanan R, Fletcher CDM. Sarcomatoid variant of anaplastic large-cell Ki-1 lymphoma. Am J Surg Pathol 1990; 14: 983–988.

448 Mann KP, Hall B, Kamino H et al. Neutrophil-rich, Ki-1-positive anaplastic large-cell malignant lymphoma. Am J Surg Pathol 1995; 19: 407–416.

449 McCluggage WG, Walsh MY, Bharucha H. Anaplastic large cell malignant lymphoma with extensive eosinophilic or neutrophilic infiltration. Histopathology 1998; 32: 110–115.

450 Camisa C, Helm TN, Sexton C, Tuthill R. Ki-1-positive anaplastic large-cell lymphoma can mimic benign dermatoses. J Am Acad Dermatol 1993; 29: 696–700.

451 Simonart T, Kentos A, Renoirte C et al. Cutaneous involvement by neutrophil rich, CD30-positive anaplastic large cell lymphoma mimicking deep pustules. Am J Surg Pathol 1999; 23: 244–246.

452 Bellas C, Molina A, Montalban C, Mampaso F. Signet ring cell lymphoma of T-cell type with CD30 expression. Histopathology 1993; 22: 188–189.

453 Derringer GA, Cotton JP, Melemed AS et al. Extranodal spread of anaplastic large cell

454 Krenacs L, Wellman A, Sorbara L et al. Cytotoxic cell antigen expression in anaplastic large cell lymphomas of T- and null-cell type and Hodgkin's disease: evidence for distinct cellular origin. Blood 1997; 89: 980–989.

455 Tomaszewski M-M, Moad JC, Lupton GP. Primary cutaneous Ki-1 (CD30) positive anaplastic large cell lymphoma in childhood. J Am Acad Dermatol 1999; 40: 857–861.

456 Beljaards RC, Kaudewitz P, Berti E et al. Primary cutaneous CD30-positive large-cell lymphoma: definition of a new type of cutaneous lymphoma with a favorable prognosis. Cancer 1993; 71: 2097–2104.

457 Artemi P, Wong DA, Mann S, Regan W. CD30 (Ki-1)-positive primary cutaneous T-cell lymphoma: report of spontaneous resolution. Australas J Dermatol 1997; 38: 206–208.

458 Headington JT, Roth MS, Schnitzer B. Regressing atypical histiocytosis: a review and critical appraisal. Semin Diagn Pathol 1987; 4: 28–37.

459 Motley RJ, Jasani B, Ford AM et al. Regressing atypical histiocytosis, a regressing cutaneous phase of Ki-1-positive anaplastic large-cell lymphoma. Cancer 1992; 70: 476–483.

460 de Bruin PC, Beljaards RC, van Heerde P et al. Differences in clinical behaviour and immunophenotype between primary cutaneous and primary nodal anaplastic large-cell lymphoma of T-cell or null cell phenotype. Histopathology 1993; 23: 127–135.

461 Scarisbrick JJ, Calonje E, Orchard G et al. Pseudocarcinomatous change in lymphomatoid papulosis and primary cutaneous CD30⁺ lymphoma: A clinicopathologic and immunohistochemical study of 6 patients. J Am Acad Dermatol 2001; 44: 239–247.

462 Bernier M, Bagot M, Broyer M et al. Distinctive clinicopathologic features associated with regressive primary CD30 positive cutaneous lymphomas: analysis of 6 cases. J Cutan Pathol 1997; 24: 157–163.

463 Nathan DL, Belsito DV. Carbamazepine-induced pseudolymphoma with CD-30 positive cells. J Am Acad Dermatol 1998; 38: 806–809.

464 Su LD, Duncan LM. Lymphoma- and leukemia-associated cutaneous atypical CD30+ T-cell reactions. J Cutan Pathol 2000; 27: 249–254.

465 McCalmont TH, LeBoit PE. A lymphomatoid papule, but not lymphomatoid papulosis! Am J Dermatopathol 2000; 22: 188–190.

466 Kummer JA, Vermeer MH, Dukers D et al. Most primary cutaneous CD30-positive lymphoproliferative disorders have a CD4-positive cytotoxic T-cell phenotype. J Invest Dermatol 1997; 109: 636–640.

467 Herbst H, Sander C, Tronnier M et al. Absence of anaplastic lymphoma kinase (ALK) and Epstein–Barr virus gene products in primary cutaneous anaplastic large cell lymphoma and lymphomatoid papulosis. Br J Dermatol 1997; 137: 680–686.

468 Simonart T, Kentos A, Renoirte C et al. Cutaneous involvement by neutrophil-rich, CD30-positive anaplastic large cell lymphoma mimicking deep pustules. Am J Surg Pathol 1999; 23: 244–246.

469 Natkunam Y, Warnke RA, Haghighi B et al. Co-expression of CD56 and CD30 in lymphomas with primary presentation in the skin: clinicopathologic, immunohistochemical and molecular analyses of seven cases. J Cutan Pathol 2000; 27: 392–399.

470 Chang S-E, Park I-J, Hugh J et al. CD56 expression in a case of primary cutaneous CD30+ anaplastic large cell lymphoma. Br J Dermatol 2000; 142: 766–770.

471 Paulli M, Berti E, Boveri E et al. Cutaneous CD30+ lymphoproliferative disorders: expression of bcl-2 and proteins of the tumor necrosis factor receptor superfamily. Hum Pathol 1998; 29: 1223–1230.

472 Kudo Y, Katagiri K, Ise T et al. A case of Ki-1 positive anaplastic large cell lymphoma transformed from mycosis fungoides. J Dermatol 1996; 23: 606–613.

473 Terao H, Kiryu H, Ohshima K et al. Cutaneous CD30 (Ki-1)-positive anaplastic large cell lymphoma preceded by Hodgkin's disease. J Dermatol 2000; 27: 170–173.

474 Macaulay WL. Lymphomatoid papulosis update. A historical perspective. Arch Dermatol 1989; 125: 1387–1389.

475 Willemze R. Lymphomatoid papulosis. Dermatol Clin 1985; 3: 735–757.

476 Wood GS, Strickler JG, Deneau DG et al. Lymphomatoid papulosis expresses immunophenotypes associated with T cell lymphoma but not inflammation. J Am Acad Dermatol 1986; 15: 444–458.

477 Karp DL, Horn TD. Lymphomatoid papulosis. J Am Acad Dermatol 1994; 30: 379–395.

478 Vonderheid EC, Sajjadian A, Kadin ME. Methotrexate is effective therapy for lymphomatoid papulosis and other primary cutaneous CD30-positive lymphoproliferative disorders. J Am Acad Dermatol 1996; 34: 470–481.

479 Tomaszewski M-M, Lupton GP, Krishnan J, May DL. A comparison of clinical, morphological and immunohistochemical features of lymphomatoid papulosis and primary cutaneous CD30 (Ki-1)-positive anaplastic large-cell lymphoma. J Cutan Pathol 1995; 22: 310–318.

480 Jones RE Jr. Questions to the Editorial Board and other authorities. Lymphomatoid papulosis. Am J Dermatopathol 1995; 17: 197–208.

(CD30+) lymphoma presenting as a cutaneous perivascular infiltrate. J Cutan Pathol 1996; 23: 323–327.

481 Chimenti S, Fargnoli MC, Pacifico A, Peris K. Mucosal involvement in a patient with lymphomatoid papulosis. J Am Acad Dermatol 2001; 44: 339–341.

482 van Neer FJMA, Toonstra J, van Voorst Vader PC et al. Lymphomatoid papulosis in children: a study of 10 children registered by the Dutch Cutaneous Lymphoma Working Group. Br J Dermatol 2001; 144: 351–354.

483 Barnadas MA, López D, Pujol RM et al. Pustular lymphomatoid papulosis in childhood. J Am Acad Dermatol 1992; 27: 627–628.

484 Scarisbrick JJ, Evans AV, Woolford AJ et al. Regional lymphomatoid papulosis: a report of four cases. Br J Dermatol 1999; 141: 1125–1128.

485 Tabata N, Aiba S, Ichinohazama R et al. Hydroa vacciniforme-like lymphomatoid papulosis in a Japanese child: a new subset. J Am Acad Dermatol 1995; 32: 378–381.

486 Whittaker SJ, Russel Jones R, Spry CJF. Lymphomatoid paulosis and its relationship to "idiopathic" hypereosinophilic syndrome. J Am Acad Dermatol 1988; 18: 339–344.

487 Granel B, Serratrice J, Swiader L et al. Lymphomatoid papulosis associated with both severe hypereosinophilic syndrome and CD30 positive large T-cell lymphoma. Cancer 2000; 89: 2138–2143.

488 Yamamoto O, Tajiri M, Asahi M. Lymphomatoid papulosis associated with pregnancy. Clin Exp Dermatol 1997; 22: 141–143.

489 LeBoit PE. Epstein–Barr virus and lymphomatoid papulosis. A suspect exonerated (at least for now). Arch Dermatol 1996; 132: 335–337.

490 Kardashian JL, Zackheim HS, Egbert BM. Lymphomatoid papulosis associated with plaque-stage and granulomatous mycosis fungoides. Arch Dermatol 1985; 121: 1175–1180.

491 Thomsen K, Wantzin GL. Lymphomatoid papulosis. A follow-up study of 30 patients. J Am Acad Dermatol 1987; 17: 632–636.

492 Wang HH, Lach L, Kadin ME. Epidemiology of lymphomatoid papulosis. Cancer 1992; 70: 2951–2957.

493 Wolf P, Cerroni L, Smolle J, Kerl H. PUVA-induced lymphomatoid papulosis in a patient with mycosis fungoides. J Am Acad Dermatol 1991; 25: 422–426.

494 Basarab T, Fraser-Andrews EA, Orchard G et al. Lymphomatoid papulosis in association with mycosis fungoides: a study of 15 cases. Br J Dermatol 1998; 139: 630–638.

495 Madison JF, O'Keefe TE, Meier FA, Clendenning WE. Lymphomatoid papulosis terminating as cutaneous T cell lymphoma (mycosis fungoides). J Am Acad Dermatol 1983; 9: 743–747.

496 Scheen SR III, Doyle JA, Winkelmann RK. Lymphoma-associated papulosis: lymphomatoid papulosis associated with lymphoma. J Am Acad Dermatol 1981; 4: 451–457.

497 Tucker WFG, Leonard JN, Smith N et al. Lymphomatoid papulosis progressing to immunoblastic lymphoma. Clin Exp Dermatol 1984; 9: 190–195.

498 Lange Wantzin G, Thomsen K, Brandrup F, Larsen JK. Lymphomatoid papulosis. Development into cutaneous T-cell lymphoma. Arch Dermatol 1985; 121: 792–794.

499 Espinoza CG, Erkman-Balis B, Fenske NA. Lymphomatoid papulosis: a premalignant T cell disorder. J Am Acad Dermatol 1985; 13: 736–743.

500 Harrington DS, Braddock SW, Blocher KS et al. Lymphomatoid papulosis and progression to T cell lymphoma: an immunophenotypic and genotypic analysis. J Am Acad Dermatol 1989; 21: 951–957.

501 Marques Pinto G, Gonçalves L, Gonçalves H et al. A case of lymphomatoid papulosis and Hodgkin's disease. J Am Acad Dermatol 1989; 21: 1051–1056.

502 Kadin ME. Lymphomatoid papulosis and associated lymphomas. How are they related? Arch Dermatol 1993; 129: 351–353.

503 Zackheim HS, LeBoit PE, Gordon BI, Glassberg AB. Lymphomatoid papulosis followed by Hodgkin's lymphoma. Differential response to therapy. Arch Dermatol 1993; 129: 86–91.

504 Kaudewitz P, Herbst H, Anagnostopoulos I et al. Lymphomatoid papulosis followed by large-cell lymphoma: immunophenotypical and genotypical analysis. Br J Dermatol 1991; 124: 465–469.

505 Lish KM, Ramsay DL, Raphael BG et al. Lymphomatoid papulosis followed by acute myeloblastic leukemia. J Am Acad Dermatol 1993; 29: 112–115.

506 Harabuchi Y, Kataura A, Kobayashi K et al. Lethal midline granuloma (peripheral T-cell lymphoma) after lymphomatoid papulosis. Cancer 1992; 70: 835–839.

507 Silva MM, Morais JC, Spector N et al. Lymphomatoid papulosis followed by Hodgkin's disease. Int J Dermatol 1998; 37: 541–543.

508 Davis TH, Morton CC, Miller-Cassman R et al. Hodgkin's disease, lymphomatoid papulosis, and cutaneous T-cell lymphoma derived from a common T-cell clone. N Engl J Med 1992; 326: 1115–1122.

509 Sangüeza OP, Galloway J, Eagan PA et al. Absence of Epstein–Barr virus in lymphomatoid papulosis. Arch Dermatol 1996; 132: 279–282.

510 Kempf W, Kadin ME, Kutzner H et al. Lymphomatoid papulosis and human herpesviruses – a PCR-based evaluation for the presence of human herpesvirus 6, 7 and 8 and related herpesviruses. J Cutan Pathol 2001; 28: 29–33.

511 Cerroni L. Lymphomatoid papulosis, pityriasis lichenoides et varioliformis acuta, and anaplastic large-cell (Ki-1+) lymphoma. J Am Acad Dermatol 1997; 37: 287.

512 Ploysangam T, Breneman DL, Mutasim DF. Cutaneous pseudolymphomas. J Am Acad Dermatol 1998; 38: 877–905.

513 Orchard GE, Ng Y, Smith NP et al. Lymphomatoid papulosis: analysis of TCR genes using Southern blot and PCR-SSCP. J Pathol (Suppl) 1996; 178: 54A (abstract).

514 Chott A, Vonderheid EC, Olbricht S et al. The same dominant T cell clone is present in multiple regressing skin lesions and associated T cell lymphomas of patients with lymphomatoid papulosis. J Invest Dermatol 1996; 106; 696–700.

515 Whittaker S, Smith N, Russell Jones R, Luzzatto L. Analysis of β, γ and δ T-cell receptor genes in lymphomatoid papulosis: cellular basis of two distinct histologic subsets. J Invest Dermatol 1991; 96: 786–791.

516 Paulli M, Berti E, Rosso R et al. CD30/Ki-1-positive lymphoproliferative disorders of the skin – clinicopathologic correlation and statistical analysis of 86 cases: a multicentric study from the European Organization for Research and Treatment of Cancer Cutaneous Lymphoma Project Group. J Clin Oncol 1995; 13: 1343–1354.

517 Agnarsson BA, Kadin ME. Host response in lymphomatoid papulosis. Hum Pathol 1989; 20: 747–752.

518 Kato N, Matsue K. Follicular lymphomatoid papulosis. Am J Dermatopathol 1997; 19: 189–196.

519 Pierard GE, Ackerman AB, Lapiere CM. Follicular lymphomatoid papulosis. Am J Dermatopathol 1980; 2: 173–180.

520 Sexton FM, Maize JC. Follicular lymphomatoid papulosis. Am J Dermatopathol 1986; 8: 496–500.

521 Requena L, Sanchez M, Coca S, Sanchez Yus E. Follicular lymphomatoid papulosis. Am J Dermatopathol 1990; 12: 67–75.

522 Cespedes YP, Rockley PF, Flores F et al. Is there a special relationship between CD30-positive lymphoproliferative disorders and epidermal proliferation? J Cutan Pathol 2000; 27: 271–275.

523 Guitart J, Gordon K. Keratoacanthomas and lymphomatoid papulosis. Am J Dermatopathol 1998; 20: 430–432.

524 Kadin ME. The spectrum of Ki-1+ cutaneous lymphomas. Curr Probl Dermatol 1990; 19: 132–143.

525 Boulland M-L, Wechsler J, Bagot M et al. Primary CD30-positive cutaneous T-cell lymphomas and lymphomatoid papulosis frequently express cytotoxic proteins. Histopathology 2000; 36: 136–144.

526 Gonzalez CL, Medeiros LJ, Braziel RM, Jaffe ES. T-cell lymphoma involving subcutaneous tissue A clinicopathologic entity commonly associated with hemophagocytic syndrome. Am J Surg Pathol 1991; 15: 17–27.

527 Wick MR, Patterson JW. Cytophagic histiocytic panniculitis – a critical reappraisal. Arch Dermatol 2000; 136: 922–924.

528 Taniguchi S, Kono T. Subcutaneous T-cell lymphoma in a child with eosinophilia. Br J Dermatol 2000; 142: 183–184.

529 Perniciaro C, Zalla MJ, White JW Jr, Menke DM. Subcutaneous T-cell lymphoma. Arch Dermatol 1993; 129: 1171–1176.

530 Marzano AV, Berti E, Paulli M, Caputo R. Cytophagic histiocytic panniculitis and subcutaneous panniculitis-like T-cell lymphoma. Report of 7 cases. Arch Dermatol 2000; 136: 889–896.

531 Weenig RH, Ng CS, Perniciaro C. Subcutaneous panniculitis-like T-cell lymphoma. An elusive case presenting as lipomembranous panniculitis and a review of 72 cases in the literature. Am J Dermatopathol 2001; 23: 206–215.

532 Romero LS, Goltz RW, Nagi C et al. Subcutaneous T-cell lymphoma with associated hemophagocytic syndrome and terminal leukemic transformation. J Am Acad Dermatol 1996; 34: 904–910.

533 Salhany KE, Macon WR, Choi JK et al. Subcutaneous panniculitis-like T-cell lymphoma. Clinicopathologic, immunophenotypic, and genotypic analysis of alpha/beta and gamma/delta subtypes. Am J Surg Pathol 1998; 22: 881–893.

534 Przybylski GK, Wu H, Macon WR et al. Hepatosplenic and subcutaneous panniculitis-like γ/δ T cell lymphomas are derived from different Vδ subsets of γ/δ T lymphocytes. J Mol Diagn 2000; 2: 11–19.

535 Iwatsuki K, Harada H, Ohtsuka M et al. Latent Epstein–Barr virus infection is frequently detected in subcutaneous lymphoma associated with hemophagocytosis but not in nonfatal cytophagic histiocytic panniculitis. Arch Dermatol 1997; 133: 787–788.

536 Chan JKC, Tsang WYW, Lo ESF. Cutaneous angiocentric 'T' cell lymphoma and subcutaneous panniculitic T cell lymphomas are distinct entities. Mod Pathol 1996; 9: 109 (abstract).

537 DiGuiseppe JA, Louie DC, Williams JE et al. Blastic natural killer leukemia/lymphoma: a clinicopathologic study. Am J Surg Pathol 1997; 21: 1223–1230.

538 Bower CPR, Standen GR, Pawade J et al. Cutaneous presentation of steroid responsive blastoid natural killer cell lymphoma. Br J Dermatol 2000; 142: 1017–1020.

539 Ginarte M, Abalde MT, Peteiro C et al. Blastoid NK cell leukemia/lymphoma with cutaneous involvement. Dermatology 2000; 201: 268–271.

540 Scott AA, Head DR, Kopecky KJ et al. HLA-DR⁻, CD33⁺, CD56⁺, CD16⁻ myeloid/natural killer cell acute leukemia: A previously unrecognized form of acute leukemia potentially misdiagnosed as French-American-British acute myeloid leukemia-M3. Blood 1994; 84: 244–255.

541 Nagatani T, Okazawa H, Kambara T et al. Cutaneous monomorphous CD4- and CD56-positive large-cell lymphoma. Dermatology 2000; 200: 202–208.

542 Sun T, Brody J, Susin M et al. Aggressive natural killer cell lymphoma/leukemia. Am J Surg Pathol 1993; 17: 1289–1299.

543 Imamura N, Kusunoki Y, Kawa-Ha K et al. Aggressive natural killer cell leukemia/lymphoma: report of four cases and review of the literature. Possible existence of a new clinical entity originating from the third lineage of lymphoid cells. Br J Haematol 1990; 75: 49–59.

544 Chan JKC, Sin VC, Wong KF et al. Nonnasal lymphoma expressing the natural killer cell marker CD56: a clinicopathologic study of 49 cases of an uncommon aggressive neoplasm. Blood 1997; 89: 4501–4513.

545 El Shabrawi-Caelen L, Cerroni L, Kerl H. The clinicopathologic spectrum of cytotoxic lymphomas of the skin. Semin Cutan Med Surg 2000; 19: 118–123.

546 Jaffe ES, Chan JKC, Su I-J et al. Report of the Workshop on Nasal and Related Extranodal Angiocentric T/Natural Killer Cell Lymphomas. Definitions, differential diagnosis, and epidemiology. Am J Surg Pathol 1996; 20: 103–111.

547 Chan JKC, Sin VC, Wong KF et al. Nonnasal lymphoma expressing the natural killer cell marker CD56: a clinicopathologic study of 49 cases of an uncommon aggressive neoplasm. Blood 1997; 89: 4501–4513.

548 Yamazaki M, Kakuta M, Takimoto R et al. Nasal natural killer cell lymphoma presenting as lethal midline granuloma. Int J Dermatol 2000; 39: 931–934.

549 Hirakawa S, Kuyama M, Takahashi S et al. Nasal and nasal-type natural killer/T-cell lymphoma. J Am Acad Dermatol 1999; 40: 268–272.

550 Miyamoto T, Yoshino T, Takehisa T et al. Cutaneous presentation of nasal/nasal type T/NK cell lymphoma: clinicopathological findings of four cases. Br J Dermatol 1998; 139: 481–487.

551 Natkunam Y, Smoller BR, Zehnder JL et al. Aggressive cutaneous NK and NK-like T-cell lymphomas. Clinicopathologic, immunohistochemical, and molecular analyses of 12 cases. Am J Surg Pathol 1999; 23: 571–581.

552 Chang S-E, Huh J, Choi J-H et al. Clinicopathological features of CD56+ nasal-type T/natural killer cell lymphomas with lobular panniculitis. Br J Dermato 2000; 142: 924–930.

553 Takeshita M, Yamamoto M, Kikuchi M et al. Angiodestruction and tissue necrosis of skin-involving CD56+ NK/T-cell lymphoma are influenced by expression of cell adhesion molecules and cytotoxic granule and apoptosis-related proteins. Am J Clin Pathol 2000; 113: 201–211.

554 Ng C-S, Lo STH, Chan JKC, Chan WC. CD56⁺ putative natural killer cell lymphomas: production of cytolytic effectors and related proteins mediating tumor cell apoptosis? Hum Pathol 1997; 28: 1276–1282.

555 Savoia P, Fierro MT, Novelli M et al. CD56-positive cutaneous lymphoma: a poorly recognized entity in the spectrum of primary cutaneous disease. Br J Dermatol 1997; 137: 966–971.

556 Yoon T-Y, Lee H-T, Chang S-H. Nasal-type T/natural killer cell angiocentric lymphoma, Epstein–Barr virus-associated, and showing clonal T-cell receptor γ gene rearrangement. Br J Dermatol 1999; 140: 505–508.

557 Frizzera G, Moran EM, Rappaport H. Angio-immunoblastic lymphadenopathy with dysproteinaemia. Lancet 1974; 1: 1070–1073.

558 Feller AC, Griesser H, Schilling CV et al. Clonal gene rearrangement patterns correlate with immunophenotype and clinical parameters in patients with angioimmunoblastic lymphadenopathy. Am J Pathol 1988; 133: 549–556.

559 Siegert W, Nerl C, Agthe A et al. Angioimmunoblastic lymphadenopathy (AILD)-type T-cell lymphoma: prognostic impact of clinical observations and laboratory findings at presentation. The Kiel Lymphoma Study Group. Ann Oncol 1995; 6: 659–664.

560 Freter CE, Cossman J. Angioimmunoblastic lymphadenopathy with dysproteinemia. Semin Oncol 1993; 20: 627–635.

561 Viraben R, Brousset P, Lamant L. Cutaneous B-cell lymphoma associated with angioimmunoblastic lymphadenopathy. J Am Acad Dermatol 1998; 38: 992–994.

562 Brown HA, Macon WR, Kurtin PJ, Gibson LE. Cutaneous involvement by angioimmunoblastic T-cell lymphoma with remarkable heterogeneous Epstein–Barr virus expression. J Cutan Pathol 2001; 28: 432–438.

563 Martel P, Laroche L, Courville P et al. Cutaneous involvement in patients with angioimmunoblastic lymphadenopathy with dysproteinemia. Arch Dermatol 2000; 136: 881–886.

564 Salama S. Epstein–Barr virus (EBV) associated cutaneous lympho-proliferative disorders (LPDs). J Cutan Pathol 2000; 27: 571 (abstract).

565 Yamada M, Takigawa M, Iwatsuki K, Inoue F. Adult T-cell leukemia/lymphoma and cutaneous T-cell lymphoma. Are they related? Int J Dermatol 1989; 28: 107–113.

566 Wood GS, Weiss LM, Warnke RA, Sklar J. The immunopathology of cutaneous lymphomas: immunophenotypic and immunogenotypic characteristics. Semin Dermatol 1986; 5: 334–345.

567 Wright SA, Rothe MJ, Sporn J et al. Acute adult T-cell leukemia/lymphoma presenting with florid cutaneous disease. Int J Dermatol 1992; 31: 582–587.

568 Gross DJ, Kavanaugh A. HTLV-I. Int J Dermatol 1990; 29: 161–165.

569 Knobler RM, Rehle T, Grossman M et al. Clinical evolution of cutaneous T cell lymphoma in a patient with antibodies to human T-lymphotropic virus type I. J Am Acad Dermatol 1987; 17: 903–909.

570 Donati M, Seyedzadeh H, Leung T et al. Prevalence of antibody to human T cell leukaemia/lymphoma virus in women attending antenatal clinic in southeast London: retrospective study. BMJ 2000; 320: 92–93.

571 Ades AE, Parker S, Walker J et al. Human T cell leukaemia/lymphoma virus infection in pregnant women in the United Kingdom: population study. BMJ 2000; 320: 1497–1501.

572 Hall WW, Ishak R, Zhu SW et al. Human T lymphotropic virus II (HTLV-II): epidemiology, molecular properties and clinical features of infection. J Acquir Immune Defic Syndr Hum Retrovirol 1996; 13 (Suppl 1): S204–S214.

573 Shimoyama M, and members of the Lymphoma Study Group (1984–87). Diagnostic criteria and classification of clinical subtypes of adult T-cell leukaemia-lymphoma. A report from the Lymphoma Study Group (1984–87). Br J Haematol 1991; 79: 428–437.

574 Greaves MF, Verbi W, Tilley R et al. Human T-cell leukaemia virus (HTLV) in the United Kingdom. Int J Cancer 1984; 33: 795–806.

575 Dosaka N, Tanaka T, Miyachi Y et al. Examination of HTLV-I integration in the skin lesions of various types of adult T-cell leukemia (ATL): independence of cutaneous-type ATL confirmed by Southern blot analysis. J Invest Dermatol 1991; 96: 196–200.

576 Shimamoto Y, Suga K, Shibata K et al. Clinical importance of extraordinary integration patterns of human T-cell lymphotrophic virus type I proviral DNA in adult T-cell leukemia/lymphoma. Blood 1994; 84: 853–858.

577 Kato N, Sugawara H, Aoyagi S, Mayuzumi M. Lymphoma-type adult T-cell leukaemia-lymphoma with a bulky cutaneous tumour showing multiple human T-lymphotropic virus-I DNA integration. Br J Dermatol 2001; 144: 1244–1248.

578 Zimbow K, Takami T. Cutaneous T-cell lymphoma and related disorders. Int J Dermatol 1986; 25: 485–497.

579 Manabe T, Hirokawa M, Sugihara K et al. Angiocentric and angiodestructive infiltration of adult T-cell leukemia/lymphoma (ATLL) in the skin. Report of two cases. Am J Dermatopathol 1988; 10: 487–496.

580 Bunker CB, Whitaker S, Luzzatto L et al. Indolent cutaneous prodrome of fatal HTLV-I infection. Lancet 1990; 335: 426.

581 Setoyama M, Mizoguchi S, Kanzaki T. Prurigo as a clinical prodrome to adult T-cell leukaemia/lymphoma. Br J Dermatol 1998; 138: 137–140.

582 Jaffe ES. The morphologic spectrum of T-cell lymphoma. Am J Surg Pathol 1988; 12: 158–159.

583 DiCaudo DJ, Perniciaro C, Worrell JT et al. Clinical and histologic spectrum of human T-cell lymphotropic virus type I-associated lymphoma involving the skin. J Am Acad Dermatol 1996; 34: 69–76.

584 Setoyama M, Katahira Y, Kanzaki T et al. Adult T-cell leukemia/lymphoma associated with noninfectious epithelioid granuloma in the skin: a clinicopathologic study. Am J Dermatopathol 1997; 19: 591–595.

585 Maeda K, Takahashi M. Characterization of skin infiltrating cells in adult T-cell leukemia/lymphoma (ATLL): clinical, histological and immunohistochemical studies on eight cases. Br J Dermatol 1989; 121: 603–612.

586 Lando Z, Sarin P, Megson M et al. Association of human T-cell leukemia/lymphoma virus with the Tac antigen marker for the human T-cell growth factor receptor. Nature 1983; 305: 733–736.

587 Wood GS, Ruffo A, Salvekar A et al. Detection of human T-cell lymphotrophic virus type I in archival tissue specimens. Arch Dermatol 1996; 132: 1339–1343.

588 Armitage JO, Greer JP, Levine AM et al. Peripheral T-cell lymphoma. Cancer 1989; 63: 158–163.

589 Coiffier B, Berger F, Bryon PA, Magaud JP. T-cell lymphomas: immunologic, histologic, clinical, and therapeutic analysis of 63 cases. J Clin Oncol 1988; 6: 1584–1589.

590 Horning SJ, Weiss LM, Crabtree GS, Warnke RA. Clinical and phenotypic diversity of T cell lymphomas. Blood 1986; 67: 1578–1582.

591 Noorduyn LA, Van der Valk P, Van Heerde P et al. Stage is a better prognostic indicator than morphologic subtype in primary noncutaneous T-cell lymphoma. Am J Clin Pathol 1990; 93: 49–57.

592 Kim Y-C, Vandersteen DP. Primary cutaneous pleomorphic small/medium-sized T-cell lymphoma in a young man. Br J Dermatol 2001; 144: 903–905.

593 Crawford RI, McCalmont TH. The specificity of CD30 immunohistochemical staining in the diagnosis of cutaneous CD30-positive lymphoproliferative disease. J Cutan Pathol 1997; 24: 92 (abstract).

594 Beljaards RC, Meijer CJLM, van der Putte SCJ et al. Primary cutaneous T-cell lymphoma: clinicopathological features and prognostic parameters of 35 cases other than mycosis fungoides and CD38-positive large cell lymphoma. J Pathol 1994; 172: 53–60.

595 Kerl H, Cerroni L. Is small/medium-sized pleomorphic T-cell lymphoma a distinct cutaneous lymphoma? Dermatopathology: Practical & Conceptual 2000; 6: 298–300.

596 Weis JW, Winter MW, Phyliky RL, Banks PM. Peripheral T-cell lymphomas: histologic, immunohistologic and clinical characterization. Mayo Clin Proc 1986; 61: 411–426.

597 Kiesewetter F, Haneke E, Lennert K et al. Cutaneous lymphoepithelioid lymphoma (Lennert's lymphoma). Combined immunohistological, ultrastructural, and DNA-flow-cytometric analysis. Am J Dermatopathol 1989; 11: 549–554.

598 Roundtree JM, Burgdorf W, Harkey MR. Cutaneous involvement in Lennert's lymphoma. Arch Dermatol 1980; 116: 1291–1294.

599 Zamora I, Nunez C, Hu C-H. Lennert's lymphoma presenting with clusters of cutaneous infection. J Am Acad Dermatol 1981; 5: 450–454.

600 Bhushan M, Craven NM, Armstrong GR, Chalmers RJG. Lymphoepithelioid cell lymphoma (Lennert's lymphoma) presenting as atypical granuloma annulare. Br J Dermatol 2000; 142: 776–780.

601 Kikuchi A, Naka W, Harada T, Nishikawa T. Primary CD8+ lymphoepithelioid lymphoma of the skin. J Am Acad Dermatol 1993; 29: 871–875.

602 Uchiyama N, Ito K, Kawai K et al. CD2–, CD4+, CD56+ agranular natural killer cell lymphoma of the skin. Am J Dermatopathol 1998; 20: 513–517.

603 Petrella T, Dalac S, Maynadié M et al. CD4+ CD56+ cutaneous neoplasms: a distinct hematological entity? Am J Surg Pathol 1999; 23: 137–146.

Other lymphoma

604 Smith JL Jr, Butler JJ. Skin involvement in Hodgkin's disease. Cancer 1980; 45: 354–361.

605 Cerroni L, Beham-Schmid C, Kerl H. Cutaneous Hodgkin's disease: an immunohistochemical analysis. J Cutan Pathol 1995; 22: 229–235.

606 Heyd J, Weissberg N, Gottschalk S. Hodgkin's disease of the skin. A case report. Cancer 1989; 63: 924–929.

607 Takagawa S, Maruyama R, Yokozeki H et al. Skin invasion of Hodgkin's disease mimicking scrofuloderma. Dermatology 1999; 199: 268–270.

608 Misra RS, Mukherjee A, Ramesh V et al. Specific skin ulcers in Hodgkin's disease. Cutis 1987; 39: 247–248.

609 Hanno R, Bean SF. Hodgkin's disease with specific bullous lesions. Am J Dermatopathol 1980; 2: 363–366.

610 Gordon RA, Lookingbill DP, Abt AB. Skin infiltration in Hodgkin's disease. Arch Dermatol 1980; 116: 1038–1040.

611 Williams MV. Spontaneous regression of cutaneous Hodgkin's disease. BMJ 1980; 280: 903.

612 O'Bryan-Tear CG, Burke M, Coulson IH, Marsden RA. Hodgkin's disease presenting in the skin. Clin Exp Dermatol 1987; 12: 69–71.

613 Silverman CL, Strayer DS, Wasserman TH. Cutaneous Hodgkin's disease. Arch Dermatol 1982; 118: 918–921.

614 Hayes TG, Rabin VR, Rosen T, Zubler MA. Hodgkin's disease presenting in the skin: case report and review of the literature. J Am Acad Dermatol 1990; 22: 944–947.

615 Guitart J, Fretzin D. Skin as the primary site of Hodgkin's disease: a case report of primary cutaneous Hodgkin's disease and review of its relationship with non-Hodgkin's lymphoma. Am J Dermatopathol 1998; 20: 218–222.

616 Geldenhuys L, Radhi J, Hull PR. Mycosis fungoides and cutaneous Hodgkin's disease in the same patient: a case report. J Cutan Pathol 1999; 26: 311–314.

617 Sioutos N, Kerl H, Murphy SB, Kadin ME. Primary cutaneous Hodgkin's disease. Unique clinical, morphologic, and immunophenotypic findings. Am J Dermatopathol 1994; 16: 2–8.

618 Kumar S, Kingma DW, Weiss WB et al. Primary cutaneous Hodgkin's disease with evolution to systemic disease. Association with the Epstein–Barr virus. Am J Surg Pathol 1996; 20: 754–759.

619 Stein H, Hummel M. Cellular origin and clonality of classic Hodgkin's lymphoma: immunophenotypic and molecular studies. Semin Hematol 1999; 36: 233–241.

620 Cossman J, Annunziata CM, Barash S et al. Reed–Sternberg cell genome expression supports a B-cell lineage. Blood 1999; 94: 411–416.

621 Gutensohn N, Cole P. Epidemiology of Hodgkin's disease in the young. Int J Cancer 1977; 19: 595–604.

622 Weiss LM, Movahed LA, Warnke RA et al. Detection of Epstein–Barr viral genomes in Reed–Sternberg cells of Hodgkin's disease. N Engl J Med 1989; 320: 502–506.

623 Wu T-C, Mann RB, Charache P et al. Detection of EBV gene expression in Reed–Sternberg cells of Hodgkin's disease. Int J Cancer 1990; 46: 801–804.

624 Torne R, Umbert P. Hodgkin's disease presenting with superficial lymph nodes and tumors of the scalp. Dermatologica 1986; 172: 225–228.

625 Randle HW, Banks PM, Winkelmann RK. Cutaneous granulomas in malignant lymphoma. Arch Dermatol 1980; 116: 441–443.

626 Peltier FA, Pursley TV, Apisarnthanarax P, Raimer SS. Necrobiotic granulomas of the skin associated with Hodgkin's disease. Arch Dermatol 1981; 117: 123–124.

Cutaneous infiltrates of other leukemias/lymphomas

627 Shaikh BS, Frantz E, Lookingbill DP. Histologically proven leukemia cutis carries a poor prognosis in acute nonlymphocytic leukemia. Cutis 1987; 39: 57–60.

628 Su WPD, Buechner SA, Li C-Y. Clinicopathologic correlations in leukemia cutis. J Am Acad Dermatol 1984; 11: 121–128.

629 Ohno S, Yokoo T, Ohta M et al. Aleukemic leukemia cutis. J Am Acad Dermatol 1990; 22: 374–377.

630 Hansen RM, Barnett J, Hanson G et al. Aleukemic leukemia cutis. Arch Dermatol 1986; 122: 812–814.

631 Heskel NS, White CR, Fryberger S et al. Aleukemic leukemia cutis: juvenile chronic granulocytic leukemia presenting with figurate cutaneous lesions. J Am Acad Dermatol 1983; 9: 423–427.

632 Horlick HP, Silvers DN, Knobler EH, Cole JT. Acute myelomonocytic leukemia presenting as a benign-appearing cutaneous eruption. Arch Dermatol 1990; 126: 653–656.

633 Aractingi S, Bachmeyer C, Miclea J-M et al. Unusual specific cutaneous lesions in myelodysplastic syndromes. J Am Acad Dermatol 1995; 33: 187–191.

634 Daoud MS, Snow JL, Gibson LE, Daoud S. Aleukemic monocytic leukemia cutis. Mayo Clin Proc 1996; 71: 166–168.

635 Canioni D, Fraitag S, Thomas C et al. Skin lesions revealing neonatal acute leukemias with monocytic differentiation. A report of 3 cases. J Cutan Pathol 1996; 23: 254–258.

636 O'Connell DM, Fagan WA, Skinner SM et al. Cutaneous involvement in chronic myelomonocytic leukemia. Int J Dermatol 1994; 33: 628–631.

637 Czarnecki DB, O'Brien TJ, Rotstein H, Brenan J. Leukaemia cutis mimicking primary syphilis. Acta Derm Venereol 1981; 61: 368–369.

638 Zax RH. Kulp-Shorten CL, Callen JP. Leukemia cutis presenting as a scrotal ulcer. J Am Acad Dermatol 1989; 21: 410–413.

639 Sumaya CV, Babu S, Reed RJ. Erythema nodosum-like lesions of leukemia. Arch Dermatol 1974; 110: 415–418.

640 Frankel DH, Larson RA, Lorincz AL. Acral lividosis – a sign of myeloproliferative diseases. Hyperleukocytosis syndrome in chronic myelogenous leukemia. Arch Dermatol 1987; 123: 921–924.

641 Butler DF, Berger TG, Rodman OG. Leukemia cutis mimicking stasis dermatitis. Cutis 1985; 35: 47–48.

642 Baden TJ, Gammon WR. Leukemia cutis in acute myelomonocytic leukemia. Preferential localization in a recent Hickman catheter scar. Arch Dermatol 1987; 123: 88–90.

643 Anzai H, Kikuchi A, Kinoshita A, Nishikawa T. Recurrent annular erythema in juvenile chronic myelogenous leukaemia. Br J Dermatol 1998; 138: 1058–1060.

644 Logan RA, Smith NP. Cutaneous presentation of prolymphocytic leukemia. Br J Dermatol 1988; 118: 553–558.

645 Côté J, Trudel M, Gratton D. T cell chronic lymphocytic leukemia with bullous manifestations. J Am Acad Dermatol 1983; 8: 874–878.

646 Eubanks SW, Patterson JW. Subacute myelomonocytic leukemia – an unusual skin manifestation. J Am Acad Dermatol 1983; 9: 581–584.

647 High DA, Luscombe HA, Kauh YC. Leukemia cutis masquerading as chronic paronychia. Int J Dermatol 1985; 24: 595–597.

648 Resnik KS, Brod BB. Leukemia cutis in congenital leukemia. Arch Dermatol 1993; 129: 1301–1306.

649 Meis JM, Butler JJ, Osborne BM, Manning JT. Granulocytic sarcoma in nonleukemic patients. Cancer 1986; 58: 2697–2709.

650 Yen A, Sanchez R, Oblender M, Raimer S. Leukemia cutis: Darier's sign in a neonate with acute lymphoblastic leukemia. J Am Acad Dermatol 1996; 34: 375–378.

651 Lawrence DM, Sun NCJ, Mena R, Moss R. Cutaneous lesions in hairy-cell leukemia. Case report and review of the literature. Arch Dermatol 1983; 119: 322–325.

652 Finan MC, Su WPD, Li C-Y. Cutaneous findings in hairy cell leukemia. J Am Acad Dermatol 1984; 11: 788–797.

653 Aboud H, Treleaven J, Carter R et al. An adult with common acute lymphoblastic leukemia (C-ALL) presenting with skin infiltration. Br J Dermatol 1991; 124: 84–85.

654 Stawiski MA. Skin manifestations of leukemias and lymphomas. Cutis 1978; 21: 814–818.

655 Koriech OM, Al-Dash FZ. Skin and bone necrosis following ecthyma gangrenosum in acute leukemia – report of three cases. Clin Exp Dermatol 1988; 13: 78–81.

656 Miralles ES, Escribano L, Bellas C et al. Cutaneous xanthomatous tumors as an expression of chronic myelomonocytic leukemia? Clin Exp Dermatol 1996; 21: 145–147.

657 Macfarlane AW, Parry DH, Caslin AW, Hughes M. Cutaneous lesions in a case of acute megakaryoblastic leukaemia. Clin Exp Dermatol 1996; 21: 201–204.

658 Janier M, Raynaud E, Blanche P et al. Leukaemia cutis and erythroleukaemia. Br J Dermatol 1999; 141: 372–373.

659 Willard RJ, Turiansky GW, Genest GP et al. Leukemia cutis in a patient with chronic neutrophilic leukemia. J Am Acad Dermatol 2001; 44: 365–369.

660 Kaddu S, Zenahlik P, Beham-Schmid C et al. Specific cutaneous infiltrates in patients with myelogenous leukemia: A clinicopathologic study of 26 patients with assessment of diagnostic criteria. J Am Acad Dermatol 1999; 40: 966–978.

660a Ueda K, Kume A, Furukawa Y, Higashi N. Cutaneous infiltration in acute promyelocytic leukemia. J Am Acad Dermatol 1997; 36: 104–106.

661 Sadick N, Edlin D, Myskowski PL et al. Granulocytic sarcoma. A new finding in the setting of preleukemia. Arch Dermatol 1984; 120: 1341–1343.

662 Choi H-SH, Orentreich D, Kornblee L, Muhlfelder TW. Granulocytic sarcoma presenting as a solitary nodule of skin in a patient with Waldenström's macroglobulinemia. An immunohistochemical and electron-microscopic study. Am J Dermatopathol 1989; 11: 51–57.

663 Raman BKS, Janakiraman N, Raju UR et al. Osteomyelosclerosis with granulocytic sarcoma of chest wall. Morphological, ultrastructural, immunologic, and cytogenetic study. Arch Pathol Lab Med 1990; 114: 426–429.

664 Harris DWS, Ostlere LS, Rustin MHA. Cutaneous granulocytic sarcoma (chloroma) presenting as the first sign of relapse following autologous bone marrow transplantation for acute myeloid leukemia. Br J Dermatol 1992; 127: 182–184.

665 Ritter JH, Goldstein NS, Argenyi Z, Wick MR. Granulocytic sarcoma: an immunohistologic comparison with peripheral T-cell lymphoma in paraffin sections. J Cutan Pathol 1994; 21: 207–216.

666 Ostlere L, Harris D, Scott F et al. Granulocytic sarcoma (chloroma) of chest wall at site of Hickman line. Int J Dermatol 1993; 32: 299–300.

667 Benucci R, Annessi G, Signoretti S, Simoni R. Minimally differentiated acute myeloid leukemia revealed by specific cutaneous lesions. Br J Dermatol 1996; 135: 119–123.

668 Pulsoni A, Falcucci P, Anghel G et al. Isolated granulocytic sarcoma of the skin in an elderly patient: good response to treatment with local radiotherapy and low-dose methotrexate. J Eur Acad Dermatol Venereol 2000; 14: 216–218.

669 Tomasini C, Quaglino P, Novelli M, Fierro MT. "Aleukemic" granulomatous leukemia cutis. Am J Dermatopathol 1998; 20: 417–421.

670 Sisack MJ, Dunsmore K, Sidhu-Malik N. Granulocytic sarcoma in the absence of myeloid leukemia. J Am Acad Dermatol 1997; 37: 308–311.

671 Gil-Mateo MP, Miquel FJ, Piris MA et al. Aleukemic "leukemia cutis" of monocytic lineage. J Am Acad Dermatol 1997; 36: 837–840.

672 Murakami Y, Nagae S, Matsuishi E et al. A case of CD56+ cutaneous aeukaemic granulocytic sarcoma with myelodysplastic syndrome. Br J Dermatol 2000; 143: 587–590.

673 Eshghabadi M, Shojania AM, Carr I. Isolated granulocytic sarcoma: report of a case and review of the literature. J Clin Oncol 1986; 4: 912–917.

674 Byrd JC, Edenfield WJ, Dow NS et al. Extramedullary myeloid cell tumors in myelodysplastic-syndromes: not a true indication of impending acute myeloid leukemia. Leuk Lymphoma 1996; 21: 153–159.

675 Buechner SA, Li C-Y, Su WPD. Leukemia cutis. A histopathologic study of 42 cases. Am J Dermatopathol 1985; 7: 109–119.

676 Baksh FK, Nathan D, Richardson W et al. Leukemia cutis with prominent giant cell reaction. Am J Dermatopathol 1998; 20: 48–52.

677 Jones D, Dorfman DM, Barnhill RL, Granter SR. Leukemic vasculitis: a feature of leukemia cutis in some patients. Am J Clin Pathol 1997; 107: 637–642.

678 Smoller BR. Leukemic vasculitis: a newly described pattern of cutaneous involvement. Am J Clin Pathol 1997; 107: 627–629.

679 Diaz-Cascajo C, Bloedern-Schlicht N. Cutaneous infiltrates of myelogenous leukemia in association with pre-existing skin diseases. J Cutan Pathol 1998; 25: 185–186.

680 Metzler G, Cerroni L, Schmidt H et al. Leukemic cells within skin lesions of psoriasis in a patient with acute myelogenous leukemia. J Cutan Pathol 1997; 24: 445–448.

681 Kuwabara H, Nagai M, Yamaoka G et al. Specific skin manifestations in CD56 positive acute myeloid leukemia. J Cutan Pathol 1999; 26: 1–5.

682 Kaddu S, Beham-Schmid C, Zenahlik P et al. CD56+ blastic transformation of chronic myeloid leukemia involving the skin. J Cutan Pathol 1999; 26: 497–503.

683 Fickers M, Theunissen P. Granulocytic sarcoma with expression of CD30. J Clin Pathol 1996; 49: 762–763.

684 Cerroni L, Zenahlik P, Höfler G et al. Specific cutaneous infiltrates of B-cell chronic lymphocytic leukemia. A clinicopathologic and prognostic study of 42 patients. Am J Surg Pathol 1996; 20: 1000–1010.

685 Stefanidou MP, Kanavaros PE, Tosca AD. Chronic lymphocytic leukemia presenting as cutaneous and bone involvement. Int J Dermatol 2001; 40: 50–52.

686 Wakelin SH, Young E, Kelly S, Turner M. Transient leukaemia cutis in chronic lymphocytic leukaemia. Clin Exp Dermatol 1997; 22: 37–40.

687 Doutre M-S, Beylot-Barry M, Beylot C et al. Cutaneous localization of chronic lymphocytic leukemia at the site of chickenpox. J Am Acad Dermatol 1997; 36: 98–99.

688 Wakelin SH, Young E, Kelly S, Turner M. Transient leukaemia cutis in chronic lymphocytic leukaemia. Clin Exp Dermatol 1997; 22: 148–151.

689 Hull PR, Saxena A. Mycosis fungoides and chronic lymphocytic leukaemia – composite T-cell and B-cell lymphomas presenting in the skin. Br J Dermatol 2000; 143: 439–444.

690 Nousari HC, Kimyai-Asadi A, Huang C-HV, Tausk FA. T-cell chronic lymphocytic leukemia mimicking dermatomyositis. Int J Dermatol 2000; 39: 144–146.

691 Kaddu S, Smolle J, Cerroni L, Kerl H. Prognostic evaluation of specific cutaneous infiltrates in B-chronic lymphocytic leukemia. J Cutan Pathol 1996; 23: 487–494.

691a Smoller BR, Warnke RA. Cutaneous infiltrate of chronic lymphocytic leukemia and relationship to primary cutaneous epithelial neoplasms. J Cutan Pathol 1998; 25: 160–164.

692 Kanoh T, Takigawa M, Niwa Y. Cutaneous lesions in γ heavy-chain disease. Arch Dermatol 1988; 124: 1538–1540.

693 Wester SM, Banks PM, Li C-Y. The histopathology of γ heavy-chain disease. Am J Clin Pathol 1982; 78: 427–436.

694 Lassoued K, Picard C, Danon F et al. Cutaneous manifestations associated with gamma heavy chain disease. J Am Acad Dermatol 1990; 23: 988–991.

695 Kyle RA, Greipp PR, Banks PM. The diverse picture of gamma heavy-chain disease. Report of seven cases and review of the literature. Mayo Clin Proc 1981; 56: 439–451.

Cutaneous infiltrates in post-transplant lymphoproliferative disorders (PT-LPDS)

696 Chadburn A, Cesarman E, Knowles DM. Molecular pathology of the posttransplantation lymphoproliferative disorders. Semin Diagn Pathol 1997; 14: 15–26.

697 Frizzera G, Hanto DW, Gajl-Peczalska KJ et al. Polymorphic diffuse B-cell hyperplasias and lymphomas in renal transplant recipients. Cancer Res 1981; 41: 4262–4279.

698 Cleary ML, Sklar J. Lymphoproliferative disorders in cardiac transplant recipients are multiclonal lymphomas. Lancet 1984; ii: 489–493.

699 Knowles DM. Immunodeficiency-associated lymphoproliferative disorders. Mod Pathol 1999; 12: 200–217.

700 Knowles DM, Cesarman E, Chadburn A et al. Correlative morphologic and molecular genetic analysis demonstrates three distinct categories of posttransplantation lymphoproliferative disorders. Blood 1995; 85: 552–565.

701 Raftery MJ, Tidman MJ, Koffman G et al. Posttransplantation T-cell lymphoma of the skin. Transplantation 1988; 46: 475–477.

Cutaneous lymphomas in HIV/AIDS

702 Myskowski PL. Cutaneous T-cell lymphoma and human immunodeficiency. The spectrum broadens. Arch Dermatol 1991; 127: 1045–1047.

703 Sorrells T, Pratt L, Newton J et al. Spontaneous regression of granulomatous mycosis fungoides in an HIV positive patient. J Am Acad Dermatol 1997; 37: 876–880.

704 Dreno B, Milpied-Homsi B, Moreau P et al. Cutaneous anaplastic T-cell lymphoma in a patient with human immunodeficiency virus infection: detection of Epstein–Barr virus DNA. Br J Dermatol 1993; 129: 77–81.

705 Chadburn A, Cesarman E, Jagirdar J et al. CD30 (Ki-1) positive anaplastic large cell lymphomas in individuals infected with the human immunodeficiency virus. Cancer 1993; 72: 3078–3090.

Lymphoid hyperplasia mimicking primary lymphoma

706 Zackheim HS, LeBoit PE, Stein KM. Disseminated recurrent papular B-cell pseudolymphoma. Int J Dermatol 1997; 36: 614–618.

707 Wirt DP, Grogan TM, Jolley CS et al. The immunoarchitecture of cutaneous pseudolymphoma. Hum Pathol 1985; 6: 492–510.

708 Brodell RT, Santa Cruz DJ. Cutaneous pseudolymphomas. Dermatol Clin 1985; 3: 719–734.

709 Lange Wantzin G, Hou-Jensen K, Nielsen M et al. Cutaneous lymphocytomas: clinical and histological aspects. Acta Derm Venereol 1982; 62: 119–124.

710 Egan CA, Patel BCK, Morschbacher R et al. Atypical lymphoid hyperplasia of the eyelids manifesting as xanthelasma-like lesions. J Am Acad Dermatol 1997; 37: 839–842.

711 Sangueza OP, Yadav S, White CR Jr, Braziel RM. Evolution of B-cell lymphoma from pseudolymphoma. Am J Dermatopathol 1992; 14: 408–413.

712 Peretz E, Grunwald MH, Cagnano E, Halevy S. Follicular B-cell pseudolymphoma. Australas J Dermatol 2000; 41: 48–49.

713 Smolle J, Cerroni L, Kerl H. Multiple pseudolymphomas caused by *Hirudo medicinalis* therapy. J Am Acad Dermatol 2000; 43: 867–869.

714 Kalimo K, Räsänen L, Aho H et al. Persistent cutaneous pseudolymphoma after intradermal gold injection. J Cutan Pathol 1996; 23: 328–334.

715 Miyamoto T, Iwasaki K, Mihara Y et al. Lymphocytoma cutis induced by cobalt. Br J Dermatol 1997; 137: 469–471.

716 Blumental G, Okun MR, Ponitch JA. Pseudolymphomatous reaction to tattoos. Report of three cases. J Am Acad Dermatol 1982; 6: 485–488.

717 Zinberg M, Heilman E, Glickman F. Cutaneous pseudolymphoma resulting from a tattoo. J Dermatol Surg Oncol 1982; 8: 955–958.

718 Rijlaarsdam JU, Bruynzeel DP, Vos W et al. Immunohistochemical studies of lymphadenosis benigna cutis occurring in a tattoo. Am J Dermatopathol 1988; 10: 518–523.

719 Sidwell RU. Doe PT, Sinett D et al. Lymphocytoma cutis and chronic infection. Br J Dermatol 2000; 143: 909–910.

720 Adams JD. Localized cutaneous pseudolymphoma associated with phenytoin therapy: a case report. Australas J Dermatol 1981; 22: 28–29.

721 Goerdt S, Spieker T, Wölffer L-U et al. Multiple cutaneous B-cell pseudolymphomas after allergen injections. J Am Acad Dermatol 1996; 34: 1072–1074.

722 Bernstein H, Shupack J, Ackerman AB. Cutaneous pseudolymphoma resulting from antigen injections. Arch Dermatol 1974; 110: 756–757.

723 Albrecht S, Hofstadter S, Artsob H et al. Lymphadenosis benigna cutis resulting from *Borrelia* infection (*Borrelia* lymphocytoma). J Am Acad Dermatol 1991; 24: 621–625.

724 Rabb DC, Lesher JL Jr, Chandler FW. Polymerase chain reaction confirmation of *Borrelia burgdorferi* in benign lymphocytic infiltrate of dermis. J Am Acad Dermatol 1992; 26: 267–268.

725 Hovmark A, Åsbrink E, Olsson I. The spirochetal etiology of lymphadenosis benigna cutis solitaria. Acta Derm Venereol 1986; 66: 479–484.

726 Stanek G, Wewalka G, Groh V et al. Differences between lyme disease and European arthropod-borne borrelia infections. (letter) Lancet 1985; 1: 401.

727 Bouloc A, Delfau-Larue M-H, Lenormand B et al. Polymerase chain reaction analysis of immunoglobulin gene rearrangement in cutaneous lymphoid hyperplasias. Arch Dermatol 1999; 135: 168–172.

728 D'Incan M, Souteyrand P, Bignon YJ et al. Hydantoin-induced cutaneous pseudolymphoma with clinical, pathologic, and immunologic aspects of Sézary syndrome. Arch Dermatol 1992; 128: 1371–1374.

729 Rijlaarsdam U, Willemze R. Cutaneous pseudo-T-cell lymphomas. Semin Diagn Pathol 1991; 8: 102–108.

730 Kardaun SH, Scheffer E, Vermeer BJ. Drug-induced pseudolymphomatous skin reactions. Br J Dermatol 1988; 118: 545–552.

731 Schreiber MM, McGregor JG. Pseudolymphoma syndrome. A sensitivity to anticonvulsant drugs. Arch Dermatol 1968; 97: 297–300.

732 Henderson CA, Shamy HK. Atenolol-induced pseudolymphoma. Clin Exp Dermatol 1990; 15: 119–120.

733 Gupta AK, Cooper KD, Ellis CN et al. Lymphocytic infiltrates of the skin in association with cyclosporine therapy. J Am Acad Dermatol 1990; 23: 1137–1141.

734 D'Incan M, Souteyrand P, Bignon YJ et al. Hydantoin-induced cutaneous pseudolymphoma with clinical, pathologic, and immunologic aspects of Sézary syndrome. Arch Dermatol 1992; 128: 1371–1374.

735 Magro CM, Crowson AN. Drugs with antihistaminic properties as a cause of atypical cutaneous lymphoid hyperplasia. J Am Acad Dermatol 1995; 32: 419–428.

736 Harris DWS, Ostlere L, Buckley C et al. Phenytoin-induced pseudolymphoma. A report of a case and review of the literature. Br J Dermatol 1992; 127: 403–406.

737 Braddock SW, Harrington D, Vose J. Generalized nodular cutaneous pseudolymphoma associated with phenytoin therapy. J Am Acad Dermatol 1992; 27: 337–340.

738 Callot V, Roujeau J-C, Bagot M et al. Drug-induced pseudolymphoma and hypersensitivity syndrome. Two different clinical entities. Arch Dermatol 1996; 132: 1315–1321.

739 Aguilar JL, Barceló CM, Martín-Urda MT et al. Generalized cutaneous B-cell pseudolymphoma induced by neuroleptics. Arch Dermatol 1992; 128: 121–123.

740 Rijlaarsdam JU, Scheffer E, Meijer CJLM, Willemze R. Cutaneous pseudo-T-cell lymphomas. A clinicopathologic study of 20 patients. Cancer 1992; 69: 717–724.

741 Brady SP, Magro CM, Diaz-Cano SJ, Wolfe HJ. Analysis of clonality of atypical cutaneous lymphoid infiltrates associated with drug therapy by PCR/DGGE. Hum Pathol 1999; 30: 130–136.

742 Horn T, Lehmkuhle MA, Gore S et al. Systemic cytokine administration alters the histology of the eruption of lymphocyte recovery. J Cutan Pathol 1996; 23: 242–246.

743 Chai C, White WL, Shea CR, Prieto VG. Epstein–Barr virus-associated lymphoproliferative-disorder primarily involving the skin. J Cutan Pathol 1999; 26: 242–247.

744 Jessner M, Kanof NB. Lymphocytic infiltration of the skin. Arch Dermatol 1953; 68: 447–449.

745 Toonstra J, Wildschut A, Boer J et al. Jessner's lymphocytic infiltration of the skin. A clinical study of 100 patients. Arch Dermatol 1989; 125: 1525–1530.

746 Mullen RH, Jacobs AH. Jessner's lymphocytic infiltrate in two girls. Arch Dermatol 1988; 124: 1091–1093.

747 Higgins CR, Wakeel RAP, Cerio R. Childhood Jessner's lymphocytic infiltrate of the skin. Br J Dermatol 1994; 131: 99–101.

748 Toonstra J, van der Putte SCJ, Baart de la Faille H, van Vloten WA. Familial Jessner's lymphocytic infiltration of the skin, occurring in a father and daughter. Clin Exp Dermatol 1993; 18: 142–145.

749 Ackerman AB, Chongchitnant N, Sanchez J et al. Histologic diagnosis of inflammatory skin diseases. An algorithmic method based on pattern analysis. 2nd ed. Baltimore: Williams and Wilkins, 1997: 943.

750 Gately LE, Nesbitt LT. Update on immunofluorescent testing in bullous diseases and lupus erythematosus. Dermatol Clin 1994; 12: 133–142.

751 O'Toole EA, Powell F, Barnes L. Jessner's lymphocytic infiltrate and probable discoid lupus erythematosus occurring separately in two sisters. Clin Exp Dermatol 1999; 24: 90–93.

752 Willemze R, Dijkstra A, Meijer CJLM. Lymphocytic infiltration of the skin (Jessner): a T-cell lymphoproliferative disease. Br J Dermatol 1984; 110: 523–529.

753 Konttinen YT, Bergroth V, Johansson E et al. A long-term clinicopathologic survey of patients with Jessner's lymphocytic infiltration of the skin. J Invest Dermatol 1987; 89: 205–208.

754 Cerio R, Oliver GF, Wilson Jones E, Winkelmann RK. The heterogeneity of Jessner's lymphocytic infiltration of the skin. J Am Acad Dermatol 1990; 23: 63–67.

755 Kuo T-t, Lo S-K, Chan H-L. Immunohistochemical analysis of dermal mononuclear cell infiltrates in cutaneous lupus erythematosus, polymorphous light eruption, lymphocytic infiltration of Jessner, and cutaneous lymphoid hyperplasia: a comparative differential study. J Cutan Pathol 1994; 21: 430–436.

756 Helm KF, Muller SA. Benign lymphocytic infiltrate of the skin: correlation of clinical and pathologic findings. Mayo Clin Proc 1992; 67: 748–754.

757 Facchetti F, Boden G, de Wolf-Peeters C et al. Plasmacytoid monocytes in Jessner's lymphocytic infiltration of the skin. Am J Dermatopathol 1990; 12: 363–369.

758 Toonstra J, van der Putte SCJ. Plasmacytoid monocytes in Jessner's lymphocytic infiltration of the skin. A valuable clue for the diagnosis. Am J Dermatopathol 1991; 13: 321–328.

759 Akasu R, Kahn HJ, From L. Lymphocyte markers on formalin-fixed tissue in Jessner's lymphocytic infiltrate and lupus erythematosus. J Cutan Pathol 1992; 19: 59–65.

760 Ashworth J, Turbitt M, Mackie R. A comparison of the dermal lymphoid infiltrates in discoid lupus erythematosus and Jessner's lymphocytic infiltrate of the skin using the monoclonal antibody Leu 8. J Cutan Pathol 1987; 14: 198–201.

761 Rijlaarsdam JU, Nieboer C, de Vries E, Willemze R. Characterization of the dermal infiltrates in Jessner's lymphocytic infiltrate of the skin, polymorphous light eruption and cutaneous lupus erythematosus: differential diagnostic and pathogenetic aspects. J Cutan Pathol 1990; 17: 2–8.

762 Merot Y, French L, Saurat J-H. Leu 8-positive cells in discoid lupus erythematosus and Jessner–Kanof's lymphocytic infiltrate of the skin. J Cutan Pathol 1988; 15: 412–413.

763 Guitart J, Variakojis D, Kuzel T, Rosen S. Cutaneous CD8+ T cell infiltrates in advanced HIV infection. J Am Acad Dermatol 1999; 41: 722–727.

764 Zhang P, Chiriboga L, Jacobson M et al. Mycosis fungoideslike T-cell cutaneous lymphoid infiltrates in patients with HIV infection. Am J Dermatopathol 1995; 17: 29–35.

765 Hara M, Matsunaga J, Tagami H. Acral pseudolymphomatous angiokeratoma of children (APACHE): a case report and immunohistological study. Br J Dermatol 1991; 124: 387–388.

765a Fernández-Figueres M-T, Puig L. Of APACHEs and PALEFACEs. Am J Dermatopathol 1995; 17: 209–211.

Miscellaneous

766 Brough AJ, Jones D, Page RH, Mizukami I. Dermal erythropoiesis in neonatal infants. A manifestation of intra-uterine viral disease. Pediatrics 1967; 40: 627–635.

767 Bowden JB, Hebert AA, Rapini RP. Dermal hematopoiesis in neonates: report of five cases. J Am Acad Dermatol 1989; 20: 1104–1110.

768 Pagerols X, Curcó N, Martí JM, Vives P. Cutaneous extramedullary haematopoiesis associated with blast crisis in myelofibrosis. Clin Exp Dermatol 1998; 23: 296–297.

769 Hocking WG, Lazar GS, Lipsett JA, Busuttil RW. Cutaneous extramedullary hematopoiesis following splenectomy for idiopathic myelofibrosis. Am J Med 1984; 76: 955–958.

770 Sarma DP. Extramedullary hemopoiesis of the skin. Arch Dermatol 1981; 117: 58–59.

771 Mizoguchi M, Kawa Y, Minami T et al. Cutaneous extramedullary hematopoiesis in myelofibrosis. J Am Acad Dermatol 1990; 22: 351–355.

772 Schofield JK, Shun JLK, Cerio R, Grice K. Cutaneous extramedullary hematopoiesis with a preponderance of atypical megakaryocytes in myelofibrosis. J Am Acad Dermatol 1990; 22: 334–337.

773 Hoss DM, McNutt NS. Cutaneous myelofibrosis. J Cutan Pathol 1992; 19: 221–225.

774 Kuo T. Cutaneous extramedullary hematopoiesis presenting as leg ulcers. J Am Acad Dermatol 1981; 4: 592–596.

775 Tagami H, Tashima M, Uehara N. Myelofibrosis with skin lesions. Br J Dermatol 1980; 102: 109–112.

776 Pizarro A, Elorza D, Gamallo C et al. Neonatal dermal erythropoiesis associated with severe rhesus immunization: amelioration by high-dose intravenous immunoglobulin. Br J Dermatol 1995; 133: 334–336.

777 Pedro-Botet J, Feliu E, Rozman C et al. Cutaneous myeloid metaplasia with dysplastic features in idiopathic myelofibrosis. Int J Dermatol 1988; 27: 179–180.

778 Patel BM, Su WPD, Perniciaro C, Gertz MA. Cutaneous extramedullary hematopoiesis. J Am Acad Dermatol 1995; 32: 805–807.

Index

U